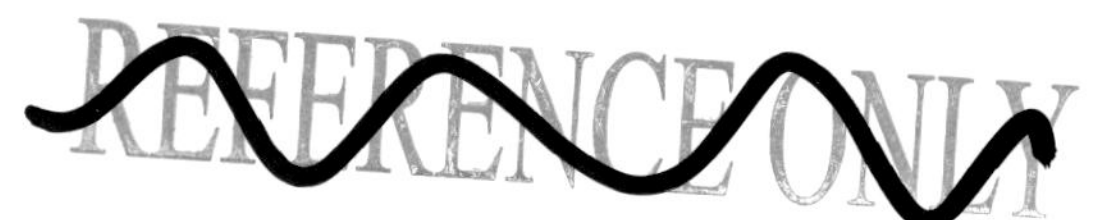

Pediatric Neurology

Pediatric Neurology

Principles & Practice

Volume 2
Fourth Edition

Kenneth F. Swaiman, MD
Director Emeritus, Division of Pediatric Neurology
Professor Emeritus of Neurology and Pediatrics
University of Minnesota Medical School
Minneapolis, Minnesota

Stephen Ashwal, MD
Distinguished Professor of Pediatrics
Chief of the Division of Child Neurology
Loma Linda University School of Medicine
Loma Linda, California

Donna M. Ferriero, MD
Professor, Departments of Neurology and Pediatrics
Division Chief, Child Neurology
Director of the Neonatal Brain Disorders Center
University of California, San Francisco, School of Medicine
San Francisco, California

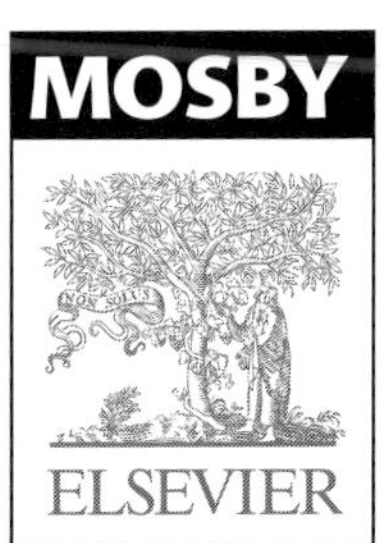

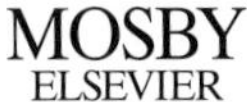

1600 John F. Kennedy Blvd.
Ste 1800
Philadelphia, PA 19103-2899

PEDIATRIC NEUROLOGY: PRINCIPLES & PRACTICE

ISBN-13: 9780323033657
Volume 1: Part no. 9996004716
Volume 2: Part no. 9996004775
ISBN-10: 0-323-03365-2

Library of Congress Cataloging-in-Publication Data

Pediatric neurology : principles & practice / [edited by] Kenneth F. Swaiman, Stephen Ashwal, Donna M. Ferriero.—4th ed.
p. ; cm.
Includes bibliographical references and index.
ISBN 0-323-03365-2
1. Pediatric neurology. I. Swaiman, Kenneth F., 1931– II. Ashwal, Stephen, 1945– III. Ferriero, Donna M.
[DNLM: 1. Nervous System Diseases—Child. 2. Nervous System Diseases—Infant. WS 340 P3713 2006]
RJ486.P336.2006
618.92'8—dc22

2005043798

Acquisitions Editor: Susan Pioli
Developmental Editor: Jennifer Shreiner
Publishing Services Manager: Frank Polizzano
Project Manager: Lee Ann Draud
Design Direction: Steve Stave

Printed in the United States of America

Last digit is the print number: 9 8 7 6 5 4 3 2 1

DEDICATION

It is our pleasure to dedicate this book to our spouses, Phyllis Sher, Eileen Ashwal, and Thomas Rando, who made it possible for us to spend the enormous amount of time planning, reading, and editing that was necessary to bring this text to fruition. It is impossible to adequately describe the value of their encouragement and support.

No dedication of a book embracing this field would be meaningful without a tribute to the courage and perserverance of neurologically impaired children and their caretakers.

CONTRIBUTORS

Anthony A. Amato, MD
Associate Professor of Neurology, Harvard Medical School; Vice-Chairman, Department of Neurology, Brigham and Women's Hospital, Boston, Massachusetts
Inflammatory Myopathies

Stephen Ashwal, MD
Distinguished Professor of Pediatrics and Chief of the Division of Child Neurology, Loma Linda University School of Medicine, Loma Linda, California
Pediatric Neuroimaging; Congenital Structural Defects; Impairment of Consciousness and Coma; Hypoxic-Ischemic Encephalopathy in Infants and Older Children; Determination of Brain Death in Infants and Children; Neurologic Manifestations of Rheumatic Disorders of Childhood; Inflammatory Neuropathies; Neurologic Disorders Associated with Gastrointestinal Diseases, Nutritional Deficiencies, and Fluid-Electrolyte Disorders

James F. Bale, Jr., MD
Associate Chair and Professor, Department of Pediatrics, University of Utah School of Medicine; Attending Physician, Department of Pediatrics, Primary Children's Medical Group, Salt Lake City, Utah
Viral Infections of the Nervous System

Tallie Z. Baram, MD, PhD
Professor of Pediatrics, Anatomy/Neurobiology, and Neurology, University of California, Irvine, School of Medicine, Irvine, California
Myoclonus, Myoclonic Seizures, and Infantile Spasms

Richard J. Barohn, MD
Professor and Chair, Department of Neurology, University of Kansas Medical Center and University of Kansas Hospital, Kansas City, Kansas
Diseases of the Neuromuscular Junction

Mark L. Batshaw, MD
Associate Dean for Academic Affairs and Professor and Chair, Department of Pediatrics, George Washington University School of Medicine and Health Sciences; Chief Academic Officer, Children's National Medical Center, Washington, DC
Inborn Errors of Urea Synthesis

Samuel F. Berkovic, MD
Epilepsy Research Centre and Department of Medicine, University of Melbourne, Melbourne; Director, Comprehensive Epilepsy Program, Austin Health, Heidelberg, Victoria, Australia
Genetics of Epilepsy

Angela K. Birnbaum, PhD
Associate Professor of Experimental and Clinical Pharmacology, College of Pharmacy, University of Minnesota, Minneapolis Minnesota
Antiepileptic Drug Therapy in Children

Rose-Mary N. Boustany, MD
Professor of Pediatrics and Neurobiology, Duke University Medical Center, Durham, North Carolina; Professor of Pediatrics and Biochemistry and Head, Clinical and Basic Neuroscience, American University of Beirut, Beirut, Lebanon
Degenerative Diseases Primarily of Gray Matter

Carol S. Camfield, MD
Professor, Department of Pediatrics, Dalhousie University Faculty of Medicine; Pediatrician, IWK Health Centre, Halifax, Nova Scotia, Canada
Pediatric Epilepsy: An Overview

Peter R. Camfield, MD
Professor, Department of Pediatrics, Dalhousie University Faculty of Medicine; Pediatric Neurologist, IWK Health Centre, Halifax, Nova Scotia, Canada
Pediatric Epilepsy: An Overview

Enrique Chaves-Carballo, MD
Clinical Professor, Departments of Pediatrics and History of Medicine, Kansas University Medical Center, Kansas City, Kansas
Syncope and Paroxysmal Disorders Other than Epilepsy

Claudia A. Chiriboga, MD, MPH
Associate Professor of Clinical Neurology and Pediatrics, Columbia University College of Physicians and Surgeons; Associate Attending Physician, Department of Neurology, Columbia University Medical Center, New York, New York
Neurologic Complications of Immunization

Raymond W. M. Chun, MD
Professor Emeritus of Neurology and Pediatrics, University of Wisconsin Medical School, Madison, Wisconsin
Interrelationships between Renal and Neurologic Diseases and Therapies

Michael E. Cohen, MD
Professor of Neurology and Pediatrics, State University of New York at Buffalo School of Medicine and Biomedical Sciences; Attending Physician, Women and Children's Hospital, Buffalo, New York
Tumors of the Brain and Spinal Cord, Including Leukemic Involvement

Anne M. Connolly, MD
Associate Professor of Neurology and Pediatrics, Washington University School of Medicine; Attending Physician, St. Louis Children's Hospital and Barnes Jewish Hospital, St. Louis, Missouri
Anterior Horn Cell and Cranial Motor Neuron Disease

Jeannine M. Conway, PharmD, BCPS
Assistant Professor, Experimental and Clinical Pharmacology, College of Pharmacy, University of Minnesota, Minneapolis, Minnesota
Antiepileptic Drug Therapy in Children

David L. Coulter, MD
Associate Professor of Neurology, Harvard Medical School; Attending Neurologist, Children's Hospital Boston, Boston, Massachusetts
Ethical Issues in Child Neurology

Tina M. Cowan, PhD
Associate Professor, Department of Pathology, Stanford University School of Medicine; Director, Biochemical Genetics Laboratory, Stanford University Medical Center, Stanford, California
Aminoacidemias and Organic Acidemias

Natalie Z. Cvijanovich, MD
Clinical Assistant Professor, University of California, San Francisco, School of Medicine, San Francisco; Associate Physician, Critical Care, Children's Hospital and Research Center at Oakland, Oakland, California
Neonatal Brain Injury

Soma Das, PhD
Assistant Professor and Director, Clinical Molecular Genetics Laboratory, Department of Human Genetics, Pritzker School of Medicine at the University of Chicago, Chicago, Illinois
Introduction to Genetics

Maria Descartes, MD
Associate Professor, Department of Genetics and Department of Pediatrics, University of Alabama School of Medicine; Attending Physician, Children's Hospital, Birmingham, Alabama
Chromosomes and Chromosomal Abnormalities

Gabrielle Aline deVeber, MD, MHSc
Associate Professor of Pediatrics, University of Toronto Faculty of Medicine; Staff Neurologist and Director, Children's Stroke Program, The Hospital for Sick Children; Scientist, Population Health Sciences and Brain and Behavior Programs, The Hospital for Sick Children Research Institute, Toronto, Ontario, Canada
Cerebrovascular Disease

Darryl C. De Vivo, MD
Sidney Carter Professor of Neurology, Professor of Pediatrics, and Director Emeritus, Pediatric Neurology Division, Columbia University College of Physicians and Surgeons; Attending Neurologist and Attending Pediatrician, Columbia University Medical Center and New York–Presbyterian Hospital, New York, New York
Mitochondrial Diseases

Salvatore DiMauro, MD
Lucy G. Moses Professor of Neurology, Columbia University College of Physicians and Surgeons, New York, New York
Mitochondrial Diseases

William B. Dobyns, MD
Professor of Human Genetics, Neurology, and Pediatrics, Pritzker School of Medicine at the University of Chicago, Chicago, Illinois
Congenital Structural Defects; Introduction to Genetics

Qing Dong, MD, PhD
Adjunct Instructor, Department of Pediatrics, University of California, San Francisco, School of Medicine; Attending Physician, UCSF Children's Hospital, San Francisco, California
Endocrine Disorders of the Hypothalamus and Pituitary

Patricia K. Duffner, MD
Professor of Neurology and Pediatrics, State University of New York at Buffalo School of Medicine and Biomedical Sciences; Women and Children's Hospital of Buffalo, Buffalo, New York
Tumors of the Brain and Spinal Cord, Including Leukemic Involvement

Ann-Christine Duhaime, MD
Professor of Neurosurgery, Dartmouth Medical School, Hanover; Director, Pediatric Neurosurgery, Children's Hospital at Dartmouth, Dartmouth-Hitchcock Medical Center, Lebanon, New Hampshire
Inflicted Childhood Neurotrauma

Adré J. du Plessis, MBChB, MPH
Associate Professor of Neurology, Harvard Medical School; Senior Associate, Neurology, and Director, Fetal-Neonatal Neurology, Children's Hospital Boston, Boston, Massachusetts
Neurologic Disorders Associated with Cardiac Disease

Gregory M. Enns, MB, ChB
Assistant Professor of Pediatrics and Director, Biochemical Genetics Program, Stanford University School of Medicine; Attending Physician, Lucile Packard Children's Hospital, Stanford, California
Aminoacidemias and Organic Acidemias

Diana M. Escolar, MD
Associate Professor of Neurology and Pediatrics, Department of Neurology, George Washington University School of Medicine and Health Sciences; Investigator, Research Center for Genetic Medicine, and Director, Neuromuscular Program, Children's National Medical Center and Children's Research Institute, Washington, DC
Muscular Dystrophies

Owen B. Evans, Jr., MD
Professor and Chairman, Department of Pediatrics, University of Mississippi Medical Center, Jackson, Mississippi
Normal Muscle

Lydia Eviatar, MD
Professor of Neurology and Pediatrics, Albert Einstein College of Medicine, Bronx; Chief Emeritus, Pediatric Neurology, Schneider Children's Hospital of Long Island Jewish Medical Center Health System, New Hyde Park, New York
Vertigo

Donna M. Ferriero, MD
Professor, Departments of Neurology and Pediatrics; Division Chief, Child Neurology; and Director, Neonatal Brain Disorders Center, University of California, San Francisco, School of Medicine, San Francisco, California
Pathophysiology of Neonatal Hypoxic-Ischemic Brain Injury; Neonatal Brain Injury

Pauline A. Filipek, MD
Associate Professor of Clinical Pediatrics and Neurology, University of California, Irvine, School of Medicine, Irvine; Director, For OC Kids, University Children's Hospital at UCI Medical Center, Orange, California
Autistic Spectrum Disorders

Yitzchak Frank, MD
Professor of Clinical Neurology and Pediatrics, Mount Sinai School of Medicine; Adjunct Professor of Neurology, New York University School of Medicine; Pediatric Neurologist, Mount Sinai Medical Center, New York, New York
Neurologic Disorders Associated with Gastrointestinal Diseases, Nutritional Deficiencies, and Fluid-Electrolyte Disorders

Douglas Fredrick, MD
Associate Professor of Clinical Ophthalmology and Pediatrics, University of California, San Francisco, School of Medicine; Director of Pediatric Ophthalmology, University of California, San Francisco, Medical Center, San Francisco, California
Vision Loss

Hudson H. Freeze, PhD
Adjunct Professor of Medicine, University of California, San Diego, School of Medicine; Professor and Director, Glycobiology and Carbohydrate Chemistry Program, The Burnham Institute, La Jolla, California
Disorders of Glycosylation

Bhuwan P. Garg, MB, BS
Professor of Neurology, Indiana University School of Medicine; Department of Child Neurology, James Whitcomb Riley Hospital for Children, Indianapolis, Indiana
Disorders of Micturition and Defecation; Poisoning and Drug-Induced Neurologic Diseases

Elizabeth E. Gilles, MD
Assistant Professor of Pediatrics and Neurology, University of Minnesota Medical School, Minneapolis; Staff Child Neurologist, Gillette Children's Specialty Healthcare, St. Paul, Minnesota
Inflicted Childhood Neurotrauma

Christopher C. Giza, MD
Assistant Professor, Divisions of Neurosurgery and Pediatric Neurology, David Geffen School of Medicine at UCLA, Los Angeles, California
Traumatic Brain Injury in Children

Carol A. Glaser, DVM, MD
Associate Clinical Professor of Pediatrics, University of California, San Francisco, School of Medicine, San Francisco; Chief, Viral and Rickettsial Disease Laboratory, California Department of Health Services, Richmond, California
Fungal, Rickettsial, and Parasitic Diseases of the Nervous System

Joseph G. Gleeson, MD
Associate Professor of Neurosciences, University of California, San Diego, School of Medicine, La Jolla; Attending Physician, Children's Hospital and Health Center, San Diego, California
Congenital Structural Defects

Meredith Rose Golomb, MD, MSc
Assistant Professor, Indiana University School of Medicine; Attending Physician, Riley Hospital for Children, Indianapolis, Indiana
Neonatal Brain Injury

Cecil D. Hahn, MD, MPH
Instructor, Department of Neurology, Harvard Medical School; Staff Physician, Department of Neurology, Children's Hospital Boston, Boston, Massachusetts
Neurologic Disorders Associated with Cardiac Disease

Chellamani Harini, MD
Fellow in Epilepsy and Clinical Neurophysiology, Children's Hospital Boston, Boston, Massachusetts
Spinal Cord Injury

Alan Hill, MD, PhD
Professor, Department of Pediatrics, Division of Neurology, University of British Columbia Faculty of Medicine; Division of Neurology, British Columbia Children's Hospital, Vancouver, British Columbia, Canada
Hypoxic-Ischemic Cerebral Injury in the Newborn

Deborah G. Hirtz, MD
Program Director, Clinical Trials, National Institute of Neurological Disorders and Stroke, National Institutes of Health, Bethesda, Maryland
Autistic Spectrum Disorders

Gregory L. Holmes, MD
Professor of Medicine (Neurology) and Pediatrics, Dartmouth Medical School, Hanover; Chief, Section of Neurology, Dartmouth-Hitchcock Medical Center, Lebanon, New Hampshire
Generalized Seizures

Barbara A. Holshouser, PhD
Associate Professor of Radiology, Loma Linda University School of Medicine; Medical Physicist, Department of Radiology, Loma Linda University Medical Center, Loma Linda, California
Pediatric Neuroimaging

Susan T. Iannaccone, MD
Jimmy and Elizabeth Wescott Distinguished Chair in Pediatric Neurology and Professor of Neurology and Pediatrics, University of Texas Southwestern Medical Center at Dallas; Director of Child Neurology, Children's Medical Center; Director of Neuromuscular Disease and Neurorehabilitation, Texas Scottish Rite Hospital for Children, Dallas, Texas
Anterior Horn Cell and Cranial Motor Neuron Disease

Rebecca N. Ichord, MD
Assistant Professor, Departments of Neurology and Pediatrics, University of Pennsylvania School of Medicine; Attending Physician, Department of Neurology, Children's Hospital of Philadelphia, Philadelphia, Pennsylvania
Perinatal Metabolic Encephalopathies

Edward M. Kaye, MD
Consulting Neurologist, Children's Hospital Boston, Boston; Vice President for Clinical Research, Genzyme Corporation, Cambridge, Massachusetts
Disorders Primarily of White Matter

John T. Kissel, MD
Professor and Interim Chair, Department of Neurology, The Ohio State University, Columbus, Ohio
Inflammatory Myopathies

Ophir Klein, MD, PhD
Clinical Fellow, Division of Genetics, Department of Pediatrics, University of California, San Francisco, School of Medicine, San Francisco, California
Aminoacidemias and Organic Acidemias

Edwin H. Kolodny, MD
Bernard A. and Charlotte Marden Professor and Chairman, Department of Neurology, New York University School of Medicine; Director, Department of Neurology, New York Medical Center, New York, New York
Lysosomal Storage Diseases

Bruce R. Korf, MD, PhD
Wayne H. and Sara Crews Finley Professor of Medical Genetics and Chair, Department of Genetics, University of Alabama at Birmingham School of Medicine, Birmingham, Alabama
Chromosomes and Chromosomal Abnormalities; Phakomatoses and Allied Conditions

Suresh Kotagal, MD
Professor, Department of Neurology, Mayo Clinic College of Medicine; Chair, Division of Child Neurology, and Consultant, Department of Child Neurology, Mayo Clinic, Rochester, Minnesota
Sleep-Wake Disorders; Increased Intracranial Pressure

Robert L. Kriel, MD
Professor, Departments of Neurology, Pediatrics, and College of Pharmacy, University of Minnesota Medical School; Pediatric Neurologist, Hennepin County Medical Center, Minneapolis, Minnesota
Antiepileptic Drug Therapy in Children

Steven M. Leber, MD, PhD
Professor of Pediatrics and Neurology, University of Michigan Medical School and C. S. Mott Children's Hospital, Ann Arbor, Michigan
The Internet and Its Resources for the Child Neurologist

Melissa Lee, MD
Assistant Professor, Department of Psychiatry and Behavioral Sciences, Johns Hopkins University School of Medicine, Baltimore, Maryland
Neuropsychopharmacology

Robert T. Leshner, MD
Professor of Neurology and Pediatrics, George Washington University School of Medicine and Health Sciences; Attending Neurologist, Center for Genetic Medicine, Department of Neurology, Children's National Medical Center, Washington, DC
Muscular Dystrophies

Donald W. Lewis, MD
Professor of Pediatrics and Neurology, Eastern Virginia Medical School; Pediatric Neurologist, Children's Hospital of the King's Daughters, Norfolk, Virginia
Headaches in Infants and Children

Paul F. Lewis, MD
Associate Professor of Pediatrics, Oregon Health and Science University; Public Health Physician, Acute and Communicable Disease Program, Oregon Department of Human Services, Portland, Oregon
Fungal, Rickettsial, and Parasitic Diseases of the Nervous System

Uta Lichter-Konecki, MD, PhD
Assistant Professor of Pediatrics, George Washington University School of Medicine and Health Sciences; Assistant Professor of Pediatrics, Children's Research Institute, Children's National Medical Center, Washington, DC
Inborn Errors of Urea Synthesis

Kenneth J. Mack, MD, PhD
Associate Professor of Neurology, Mayo Clinic, Rochester, Minnesota
The Internet and Its Resources for the Child Neurologist

David E. Mandelbaum, MD, PhD
Professor of Clinical Neurosciences and Pediatrics, Brown Medical School; Director, Division of Child Neurology, Rhode Island and Hasbro Children's Hospitals, Providence, Rhode Island
Attention-Deficit–Hyperactivity Disorder

Stephen M. Maricich, PhD, MD
Fellow, Baylor College of Medicine; Fellow, Texas Children's Hospital, Houston, Texas
The Cerebellum and the Hereditary Ataxias

Christopher J. Mathias, DPhil, DSc
Professor of Neurovascular Medicine, National Hospital for Neurology and Neurosurgery, University College London; Professor of Neurovascular Medicine, Imperial College London at St. Mary's Hospital, London, United Kingdom
Disorders of the Autonomic Nervous System: Autonomic Dysfunction in Pediatric Practice

Claire McLean, MD
Assistant Professor of Pediatrics, Keck School of Medicine of University of Southern California; Attending Physician, Children's Hospital of Los Angeles, Los Angeles, California
Pathophysiology of Neonatal Hypoxic-Ischemic Brain Injury

Julie A. Mennella, PhD
Member and Director of Education Outreach, Monell Chemical Senses Center, Philadelphia, Pennsylvania
Taste and Smell

Laura R. Ment, MD
Professor, Departments of Pediatrics and Neurology, Yale University School of Medicine; Attending Physician, Yale–New Haven Hospital, New Haven, Connecticut
Intraventricular Hemorrhage of the Preterm Neonate

David J. Michelson, MD
Assistant Professor of Child Neurology, Loma Linda University School of Medicine, Loma Linda, California
Spinal Fluid Examination; Cognitive and Motor Regression

Jonathan W. Mink, MD, PhD
Associate Professor of Neurology, Neurobiology and Anatomy, and Pediatrics, University of Rochester Medical Center School of Medicine and Dentistry; Chief, Child Neurology, Golisano Children's Hospital at Strong Memorial Hospital, Rochester, New York
Movement Disorders

Wendy G. Mitchell, MD
Professor of Neurology and Pediatrics, Keck School of Medicine of the University of Southern California; Director, Child Neurology Training Program, Children's Hospital of Los Angeles, Los Angeles, California
Behavioral, Cognitive, and Social Aspects of Childhood Epilepsy

Eli M. Mizrahi, MD
Head, Peter Kellaway Section of Neurophysiology; Vice-Chairman, Department of Neurology; and Professor of Neurology and Pediatrics, Baylor College of Medicine; Chief, Neurophysiology Service, Methodist Hospital and St. Luke's Episcopal Hospital; Chief, Clinical Neurophysiology Laboratory Services, Texas Children's Hospital, Houston, Texas
Neonatal Seizures

Lawrence D. Morton, MD
Associate Professor of Neurology and Pediatrics, Medical College of Virginia Campus of Virginia Commonwealth University School of Medicine; Director, Clinical Neurophysiology, Virginia Commonwealth University Health Systems, Richmond, Virginia
Status Epilepticus

Hugo W. Moser, MD
Professor, Departments of Neurology and Pediatrics, Johns Hopkins University School of Medicine; Director, Neurogenetics Research Center, Kennedy Krieger Institute, Baltimore, Maryland
Peroxisomal Disorders

Richard T. Moxley III, MD
Professor of Neurology and Pediatrics, University of Rochester Medical Center School of Medicine and Dentistry; Director, Neuromuscular Disease Center, University of Rochester Medical Center, Rochester, New York
Chanellopathies: Myotonic Disorders and Periodic Paralysis

SakkuBai Naidu, MD
Professor, Department of Neurology, Johns Hopkins University School of Medicine; Director, Neurogenetics Unit, Kennedy Krieger Institute, Baltimore, Maryland
Peroxisomal Disorders

Ruth Nass, MD
Professor of Clinical Neurology, New York University School of Medicine, New York, New York
Developmental Language Disorders

Douglas R. Nordli, Jr., MD
Associate Professor of Pediatrics and Neurology, Feinberg School of Medicine, Northwestern University; Lorna S. and James P. Langdon Chair of Pediatric Epilepsy, Children's Memorial Hospital, Chicago, Illinois
Focal and Multifocal Seizures

Robert Ouvrier, MD
Petre Foundation Professor of Paediatric Neurology, Department of Paediatrics, University of Sydney, Sydney; Attending Physician, Children's Hospital at Westmead, Westmead, New South Wales, Australia
Peripheral Neuropathies

Seymour Packman, MD
Professor, Department of Pediatrics, and Director, Biochemical Genetics Service and Neurometabolic Program and Clinics, University of California, San Francisco, School of Medicine, San Francisco, California
Aminoacidemias and Organic Acidemias

John Colin Partridge, MD, MPH
Clinical Professor, Department of Pediatrics, University of California, San Francisco, School of Medicine; Attending Neonatologist, University of California, San Francisco, Medical Center and San Francisco General Hospital, San Francisco, California
Pain Management and Palliative Care

Gregory M. Pastores, MD
Associate Professor of Neurology and Pediatrics, New York University School of Medicine; Director, Neurogenetics Laboratory, New York University Medical Center, New York, New York
Lysosomal Storage Diseases

Marc C. Patterson, MD
Professor and Head, Division of Pediatric Neurology, Departments of Neurology and Pediatrics, Columbia University College of Physicians and Surgeons; Director of Pediatric Neurology, Morgan Stanley Children's Hospital of New York–Presbyterian, New York, New York
Diseases Associated with Primary Abnormalities in Carbohydrate Metabolism; Disorders of Glycosylation

John M. Pellock, MD
Professor and Chairman, Division of Child Neurology, and Vice Chairman, Department of Neurology, Medical College of Virginia Campus of Virginia Commonwealth University School of Medicine, Richmond, Virginia
Status Epilepticus

Ronald M. Perkin, MD, MA
Professor and Chairman, Department of Pediatrics, Brody School of Medicine at East Carolina University; Medical Director, Children's Hospital of Eastern North Carolina; Chief of Pediatrics, Pitt County Memorial Hospital, Greenville, North Carolina
Hypoxic-Ischemic Encephalopathy in Infants and Older Children

Lauren Plawner, MD
Assistant Clinical Professor, Departments of Pediatrics and Neurology, University of California, San Francisco, School of Medicine; Pediatric Neurologist, Department of Pediatrics, Kaiser Permanente Medical Center, San Francisco, California
Congenital Structural Defects

Isabelle Rapin, MD
Professor of Neurology and Pediatrics, Albert Einstein College of Medicine; Attending Neurologist and Child Neurologist, Jacobi Medical Center and Montefiore Medical Center, Bronx, New York
Hearing Impairment

Gerald V. Raymond, MD
Associate Professor, Department of Neurology, Johns Hopkins University School of Medicine; Neurologist, Neurogenetics Research Center, Kennedy Krieger Institute, Baltimore, Maryland
Peroxisomal Disorders

Jong M. Rho, MD
Associate Professor of Clinical Neurology, University of Arizona College of Medicine, Tucson; Associate Director of Child Neurology, Children's Health Center, St. Joseph's Hospital and Medical Center, Phoenix; Director of Pediatric Epilepsy Research, Barrow Neurological Institute, Phoenix, Arizona
Neurophysiology of Epilepsy

Sarah M. Roddy, MD
Associate Professor of Pediatrics and Neurology, Loma Linda University School of Medicine; Attending Physician, Loma Linda University Children's Hospital, Loma Linda, California
Breath-Holding Spells and Reflex Anoxic Seizures

Stephen M. Rosenthal, MD
Professor of Pediatrics, University of California, San Francisco, School of Medicine, San Francisco, California
Endocrine Disorders of the Hypothalamus and Pituitary

N. Paul Rosman, MD
Professor of Pediatrics and Neurology, Boston University School of Medicine; Pediatric Neurologist, Boston Medical Center, Boston, Massachusetts
Spinal Cord Injury

Robert S. Rust, MD, MA
Worrell Professor of Epileptology and Neurology and Professor of Pediatrics, University of Virginia School of Medicine, Charlottesville, Virginia
Interrelationships between Renal and Neurologic Diseases and Therapies

Terence D. Sanger, MD, PhD
Assistant Professor, Stanford University School of Medicine; Division of Child Neurology, Lucile Packard Children's Hospital, Stanford, California
Movement Disorders

Urs B. Schaad, MD
Professor of Pediatrics, University of Basel; Medical Director and Chairman, Department of Pediatrics, University Children's Hospital, Basel, Switzerland
Bacterial Infections of the Nervous System

Ingrid E. Scheffer, MBBS, PhD
Professor, Department of Medicine and Paediatrics, University of Melbourne, Melbourne; Paediatric Neurologist, Austin Health, Heidelberg; Paediatric Neurologist, Monash Medical Centre, Clayton, Victoria, Australia
Genetics of Epilepsy

Mark S. Scher, MD
Professor of Pediatrics, Case Western Reserve University School of Medicine; Division Chief, Pediatric Neurology, and Director of Pediatric Sleep/Epilepsy and Fetal Neonatal Neurology Programs, Rainbow Babies and Children's Hospital and University Hospitals of Cleveland, Cleveland, Ohio
Pediatric Neurophysiologic Evaluation

Nina Felice Schor, MD, PhD
Professor of Pediatrics, Neurology, and Pharmacology; Chief, Division of Child Neurology; Associate Dean for Medical Student Research, University of Pittsburgh School of Medicine; Carol Ann Craumer Chair of Pediatric Research and Director, Pediatric Center for Neuroscience, Children's Hospital of Pittsburgh, Pittsburgh, Pennsylvania
Neurologic Manifestations of Rheumatic Disorders of Childhood

Frederick L. Schuster, PhD
Viral and Rickettsial Disease Laboratory, California Department of Health Services, Richmond, California
Fungal, Rickettsial, and Parasitic Diseases of the Nervous System

Bennett A. Shaywitz, MD
Professor of Pediatrics and Neurology, Yale University School of Medicine, New Haven, Connecticut
Dyslexia

Sally E. Shaywitz, MD
Professor of Pediatrics, Yale University School of Medicine, New Haven, Connecticut
Dyslexia

Robert Sheets, MD
Assistant Clinical Professor of Pediatrics, University of California, San Diego, School of Medicine, La Jolla; Pediatric Rheumatologist, Children's Hospital of San Diego, San Diego, California
Neurologic Manifestations of Rheumatic Disorders of Childhood

Elliott H. Sherr, MD, PhD
Assistant Professor of Neurology, University of California, San Francisco, School of Medicine; Attending Physician, UCSF Children's Hospital, San Francisco, California
Mental Retardation and Global Developmental Delay

Michael I. Shevell, MD
Professor, Departments of Neurology/Neurosurgery and Pediatrics, McGill University Faculty of Medicine; Division of Pediatric Neurology, Montreal Children's Hospital–McGill University Health Centre, Montreal, Quebec, Canada
Mental Retardation and Global Developmental Delay

Shlomo Shinnar, MD, PhD
Professor of Neurology and Pediatrics and Hyman Climenko Professor of Neuroscience Research, Albert Einstein College of Medicine; Director, Comprehensive Epilepsy Management Center, Montefiore Medical Center, Bronx, New York
Febrile Seizures

Stanford K. Shu, MD
Assistant Professor of Child Neurology, Loma Linda University School of Medicine, Loma Linda, California
Cognitive and Motor Regression

Faye S. Silverstein, MD
Professor of Pediatrics and Neurology, University of Michigan Medical School, Ann Arbor, Michigan
Pathophysiology of Neonatal Hypoxic-Ischemic Brain Injury

Harvey S. Singer, MD
Haller Professor of Pediatric Neurology, Johns Hopkins University School of Medicine; Director, Child Neurology, Johns Hopkins Hospital, Baltimore, Maryland
Tourette Syndrome and Its Associated Neurobehavioral Problems

John T. Sladky, MD
Professor of Pediatrics and Neurology, Emory University School of Medicine; Division Chief, Child Neurology, Children's Healthcare of Atlanta; Division Chief, Child Neurology, Grady Health System, Atlanta, Georgia
Inflammatory Neuropathies

Stephen A. Smith, MD
Director, Neuromuscular Laboratory, Department of Pathology, Hennepin County Medical Center, Minneapolis, Minnesota; Director, Neuromuscular Program, Department of Neurology, Gillette Children's Specialty Healthcare, St. Paul, Minnesota; Director, Neuromuscular Laboratory, Department of Pathology, Parkview Hospital, Pueblo, Colorado
Peripheral Neuropathies

Carl E. Stafstrom, MD, PhD
Professor of Neurology and Pediatrics, University of Wisconsin Medical School; Chief, Section of Pediatric Neurology, University of Wisconsin Hospital, Madison, Wisconsin
Neurophysiology of Epilepsy

Jonathan B. Strober, MD
Assistant Clinical Professor of Neurology and Pediatrics, University of California, San Francisco, School of Medicine, San Francisco, California
Congenital Myopathies

Kenneth F. Swaiman, MD
Director Emeritus, Division of Pediatric Neurology, and Professor Emeritus of Neurology and Pediatrics, University of Minnesota Medical School, Minneapolis, Minnesota
General Aspects of the Patient's Neurologic History; Neurologic Examination of the Older Child; Neurologic Examination after the Newborn Period until 2 Years of Age; Neurologic Examination of the Term and Preterm Infant; Muscular Tone and Gait Disturbances; Cerebral Palsy; Diseases Associated with Primary Abnormalities in Carbohydrate Metabolism

Kathryn J. Swoboda, MD
Associate Professor of Neurology and Adjunct Associate Professor of Pediatrics, University of Utah School of Medicine, Salt Lake City, Utah
Diagnosis and Treatment of Neurotransmitter-Related Disorders

Ilona S. Szer, MD
Professor of Clinical Pediatrics, University of California, San Diego, School of Medicine, La Jolla; Director, Pediatric Rheumatology, Children's Hospital of San Diego, San Diego, California
Neurologic Manifestations of Rheumatic Disorders of Childhood

Martin G. Täuber, MD
Professor and Co-Director, Institute for Infectious Diseases, University of Bern; Director, Clinic and Policlinic for Infectious Diseases, University Hospital Insel, Bern, Switzerland
Bacterial Infections of the Nervous System

Rabi Tawil, MD
Associate Professor of Neurology, Pathology, and Laboratory Medicine, University of Rochester Medical Center School of Medicine and Dentistry; Co-Director; Neuromuscular Disease Clinic, University of Rochester Medical Center, Rochester, New York
Chanellopathies: Myotonic Disorders and Periodic Paralysis

Donald A. Taylor, MD
Director of Pediatric Clinical Neurophysiology, St. Mary's Hospital, Richmond, Virginia
Impairment of Consciousness and Coma

Ingrid Tein, MD, BSc
Associate Professor of Pediatrics, Laboratory Medicine, and Pathobiology, University of Toronto Faculty of Medicine; Director, Neurometabolic Clinic and Research Laboratory, and Senior Scientist, The Research Institute, The Hospital for Sick Children, Toronto, Ontario, Canada
Metabolic Myopathies

Elizabeth A. Thiele, MD, PhD
Associate Professor of Neurology, Harvard Medical School; Director, Carol and James Herscot Center for Tuberous Sclerosis Complex, Massachusetts General Hospital, Boston, Massachusetts
Phakomatoses and Allied Conditions

Joseph R. Thompson, MD
Professor of Radiology, Loma Linda University School of Medicine; Pediatric Neuroradiologist, Department of Radiology, Loma Linda University Medical Center, Loma Linda, California
Pediatric Neuroimaging

Ann H. Tilton, MD
Professor and Section Chair of Child Neurology, Louisiana State University Health Sciences Center; Co-Director of Rehabilitation, Child Neurology, Children's Hospital of New Orleans, New Orleans, Louisiana
Pediatric Neurorehabilitation Medicine

Doris A. Trauner, MD
Professor and Chief of Pediatric Neurology, University of California, San Diego, School of Medicine, La Jolla, California
Developmental Language Disorders

Mendel Tuchman, MD
Professor of Pediatrics, Biochemistry, and Molecular Biology, George Washington University School of Medicine and Health Sciences; Vice Chair for Research and Scientific Director, Children's Research Institute, Children's National Medical Center, Washington, DC
Inborn Errors of Urea Synthesis

Roberto Tuchman, MD
Associate Professor of Neurology, University of Miami Miller School of Medicine, Miami; Director, Developmental and Behavioral Neurology, Miami Children's Hospital Dan Marino Center, Weston, Florida
Epileptiform Disorders with Cognitive Systems

Marjo S. van der Knaap, MD, PhD
Professor of Child Neurology, University Medical Center, Amsterdam, The Netherlands
Disorders Primarily of White Matter

Michèle Van Hirtum-Das, MD
Resident, Child Neurology, Children's Hospital of Los Angeles, Los Angeles, California
Behavioral, Cognitive, and Social Aspects of Childhood Epilepsy

V. Venkataraman Vedanarayanan, MD
Professor of Neurology and Professor of Pediatrics, University of Mississippi School of Medicine; Attending Physician, University of Mississippi Medical Center, Jackson, Mississippi
Normal Muscle

Ann Wagner, PhD
Chief, Neurodevelopmental Disorders Branch, Division of Pediatric Translational Research and Treatment Development, National Institute of Mental Health, National Institutes of Health, Bethesda, Maryland
Autistic Spectrum Disorders

John T. Walkup, MD
Associate Professor, Department of Psychiatry and Behavioral Sciences, Johns Hopkins University School of Medicine; Deputy Director, Division of Child and Adolescent Psychiatry, Johns Hopkins Hospital, Baltimore, Maryland
Neuropsychopharmacology

Laurence E. Walsh, MD
Assistant Professor of Clinical Neurology and Medical and Molecular Genetics, Indiana University School of Medicine; Director, Section of Child Neurology, James Whitcomb Riley Hospital for Children, Indianapolis, Indiana
Poisoning and Drug-Induced Neurologic Diseases

Maria B. Weimer, MD
Assistant Professor of Clinical Neurology, Louisiana State University Health Sciences Center; Staff Child Neurologist, Children's Hospital, New Orleans, Louisiana
Pediatric Neurorehabilitation Medicine

James W. Wheless, MD
Professor of Neurology and Pediatrics and Director, Texas Comprehensive Epilepsy Program, University of Texas Health Science Center at Houston–Medical School; Director, Epilepsy Monitoring Unit, and Director, EEG and Clinical Neurophysiology, Memorial Hermann and Memorial Hermann Children's Hospitals, Houston, Texas
The Ketogenic Diet

Gil I. Wolfe, MD
Dr. Bob and Jean Smith Foundation Distinguished Chair in Neuromuscular Disease Research and Associate Professor, Department of Neurology, University of Texas Southwestern Medical Center, Dallas, Texas
Diseases of the Neuromuscular Junction

Yvonne Wu, MD, MPH
Assistant Professor, Departments of Neurology and Pediatrics, University of California, San Francisco, School of Medicine, San Francisco, California
Cerebral Palsy

Nathaniel D. Wycliffe, MD
Assistant Professor of Radiology, Loma Linda University School of Medicine; Neuroradiologist and Director of Head and Neck Radiology, Department of Radiology, Loma Linda University Medical Center, Loma Linda, California
Pediatric Neuroimaging

Huda Y. Zoghbi, MD
Professor of Pediatrics, Molecular and Human Genetics, Neurology, and Neuroscience, Baylor College of Medicine; Investigator, Howard Hughes Medical Institute, Houston, Texas
The Cerebellum and the Hereditary Ataxias

Adam Zucker, MD
Duke University Medical Center, Durham, North Carolina
Degenerative Diseases Primarily of Gray Matter

Mary L. Zupanc, MD
Professor, Departments of Neurology and Pediatrics, Medical College of Wisconsin; Director Comprehensive Epilepsy Center, Children's Hospital of Wisconsin, Milwaukee, Wisconsin
Epilepsy Surgery in the Pediatric Population

PREFACE TO THE FOURTH EDITION

Since publication in 1999 of the third edition of *Pediatric Neurology: Principles & Practice*, the discipline of child neurology has progressed and reached new levels of complexity. Advances in molecular biology and neuroimaging have fueled an explosion of knowledge that has translated into a richer understanding of nervous system development and function. Researchers and clinicians alike believe that, during the next decade, novel and targeted treatments will be the product of such fundamental advances in knowledge. Successful treatment of children with both common and rare neurologic disorders will be a reality.

This fourth edition reflects the enormous growth and intricacy of the basic and clinical neurosciences. The entire text has been revised and reorganized. There are many new chapters that reflect areas of child neurology that are becoming increasingly relevant clinically (e.g., neurogenetics, neuropsychopharmacology, neurorehabilitation, ethics), as well as new chapters on diseases that were previously unrecognized (e.g., PNTD, CDG). Many chapters have new authors who bring to these discussions new insights into disease mechanisms. Also, the two senior editors are extremely fortunate to have Donna M. Ferriero join us to provide her expertise to ensure maintenance of the quality of this publication.

The two volumes are divided into 16 parts, encompassing 95 chapters as outlined in the table of contents. Parts I and II contain information regarding selected aspects of the pediatric neurologic examination in a general sense, as well as the different motor and sensory systems, and these discussions are followed by a comprehensive review of the pertinent neurodiagnostic testing procedures and their clinical application. Part III covers important aspects of neonatal neurology and the long-term sequelae of acquired and developmental abnormalities that can result in chronic disorders, such as cerebral palsy, developmental delay, and epilepsy. Part IV documents the vast array of genetic and neurometabolic disorders that occur in infants and children; this section also provides many of the fundamental concepts of molecular biology and neurochemistry that constitute the scientific basis of these diseases. Part V describes the major neurobehavioral disorders of childhood and includes chapters on autism and the neuropsychiatric problems that accompany Tourette syndrome and a new chapter on neuropsychopharmacology. Part VI focuses on pediatric epilepsy and contains new chapters on the neurophysiology and neurogenetics of pediatric epilepsy. Also included are chapters on the various types of pediatric epilepsy, epileptiform disorders with cognitive symptomatology, the ketogenic diet, surgical treatment, and the learning and behavioral problems associated with epilepsy.

The second volume encompasses many of the serious and complex central and peripheral nervous system diseases that confront child neurologists and allied health professionals. Part VII reviews the nonepileptiform paroxysmal disorders, including headache, syncope, and sleep disorders. Parts VIII and IX deal with conditions that are degenerative in nature and cause severe loss of motor and mental function. These conditions include gray and white matter diseases that can cause ataxia, movement disorders, progressive spasticity, and dementia. Part X contains chapters on traumatic and nontraumatic brain injury in infants and older children. Because neurologists are frequently asked to provide consultation for many of these conditions, chapters on disorders of consciousness, nonaccidental trauma, anoxic brain injury, and traumatic brain and spinal cord injury are included, as well as a current review of the issues related to brain death determination. Parts XI (infection) and XII (tumors and cerebrovascular and vasculitic diseases) extensively cover the major diseases that directly or indirectly cause serious neurologic symptoms and are presented primarily from a clinical perspective. The neuromuscular diseases are reviewed in Part XIII, which contains chapters on the classic neuromuscular disorders including the anterior horn cell diseases, disorders of the peripheral nervous system, neuromuscular junction, inflammatory neuropathies, metabolic myopathies, and channelopathies. Parts XIV and XV include important chapters that review many pediatric systemic (e.g., endocrine, renal, cardiac, gastrointestinal) conditions that are known to cause neurologic symptoms, as well as chapters on poisonings, complications of immunizations, and autonomic nervous system disorders. This volume concludes with Part XVI, which has been revised extensively and includes new and revised chapters on pediatric neurorehabilitation, pain and palliative care management, ethical issues in child neurology, and an update on the Internet as it relates to child neurology.

We hope that the reader will find this book a useful resource and that the information will benefit the many children who suffer from these conditions. It is our wish that the greater world community will increase support for the care of neurologically impaired children and the research necessary to provide further understanding of neurologic diseases. This support is necessary to facilitate discovery of new therapies that will improve the survival and quality of life of these unfortunate and brave children.

Kenneth F. Swaiman
Stephen Ashwal
Donna M. Ferriero

PREFACE TO THE FIRST EDITION

It is concurrently tiring, humiliating, and intellectually revitalizing to compile a book containing the essence of the information that embraces one's life work and professional preoccupation. For me, there is a certain moth-to-the-flame phenomenon that cannot be resisted; therefore this new book has been produced.

Pediatric neurology has come of age since my initial interest and subsequent immersion in the field. Concentrated attention to the details of brain development and function has brought much progress and understanding. Studies of disease processes by dedicated and intelligent individuals accompanied by a cascade of new technology (e.g., neuroimaging techniques, positron emission tomography, DNA probes, synthesis of gene products, sophisticated lipid chemistry) have propelled the field forward. The simultaneous increase of knowledge and capability of pediatric neurologists and others who diagnose and treat children with nervous system dysfunction has been extremely gratifying.

Although once within the realm of honest delusion of a seemingly sane (but unrealistic) devotee of the field, it is no longer possible to believe that a single individual can fathom, much less explore, the innumerable rivulets that coalesce to form the river of knowledge that currently is pediatric neurology. Streams of information in certain areas sometimes peacefully meander for years; suddenly, when knowledge of previously obscure areas is advanced and the newly gained information becomes central to understanding basic pathophysiologic entities, a once small stream gains momentum and abruptly flows with torrential force.

This text is an attempt to gather the most important aspects of current pediatric neurology and display them in a comprehensible manner. The task, although consuming great energies and concentration, cannot be accomplished completely because new conditions are described daily.

The advancement of the field necessitated that preparation of this text keep pace with current knowledge and present new and valuable techniques. My colleagues and I have made every effort to discharge this responsibility. Because of continuous scientific progress, controversies are extant in some areas for varying periods; wherever possible, these areas of conflict are indicated.

This book is divided into four unequal parts. Part I contains a discussion of the historic and clinical examination. Part II contains information concerning laboratory examination. Chapters relating to the symptom complexes that often reflect the chief complaints of neurologically impaired children compose Part III. Part IV provides detailed discussion of various neurologic diseases that afflict children.

Although every precaution has been taken to avoid error, bias, and prejudice, inevitably some of these demons have become embedded in the text. The editor assumes full responsibility for these indiscretions.

It is my fervent hope that the reader will find this book informative and stimulating and that the contents will provide an introduction to the understanding of many of the conditions that remain mysterious and poorly explained.

Kenneth F. Swaiman, MD
Autumn 1988

ACKNOWLEDGMENTS

We wish to thank Arlene Carpenter, Diana Laulainen-Schein, Ann Elliott, and Kei Kaneshiro for their time and effort, which so efficiently affected manuscript flow, editing, and preparation, as well as the innumerable other tasks necessary to complete this book. We also wish to thank the librarians at the University of Minnesota Medical School and at the Coleman and Del Webb Libraries at Loma Linda University School of Medicine for their help, advice, and willingness at any time to obtain information that we required.

In addition, we wish to thank the editorial and publishing staff at Elsevier, especially Susan Pioli, Jennifer Shreiner, and Lee Ann Draud. Without their diligence, persistence, insight, and flexibility, we would have never been able to complete this project.

CONTENTS

Volume I

Volume II

PART VII

Nonepileptiform Paroxysmal Disorders and Disorders of Sleep

CHAPTER 53

Headaches in Infants and Children

Donald W. Lewis

Headache is a universal affliction of humankind from which children are not spared. Headache is the most common reason that children are referred to child neurology practices. It is therefore essential for clinicians to have a thorough, systematic approach to the evaluation and management of the child or adolescent with the complaint of headache.

Headaches are classified into two categories, *primary* and *secondary* (Box 53-1). Migraine and tension-type are examples of primary headache in which there is no underlying pathology and the pain arises from intrinsic processes. Alternatively, the headache pain may result from secondary causes such as brain tumors, increased intracranial pressure, drug intoxications, paranasal sinus disease, or acute febrile illnesses such as influenza. The evaluation of a child presenting with headache follows the traditional medical model with extraction of necessary history and performance of a thorough physical and neurologic examination. In most instances, this initial process will yield a diagnosis or indicate the need for further ancillary testing. Once the diagnosis is established, a comprehensive treatment program can be put into place, blending pharmacologic and biobehavioral measures and being mindful of both physical and emotional factors.

The purpose of this chapter is to explore the symptom of headache, reviewing the epidemiology, current classification system, appropriate evaluation, and differential diagnosis.

EPIDEMIOLOGY

Headaches are common during childhood and become increasingly more frequent during adolescence. The prevalence of headache ranges from 37% to 51% in 7 year olds, gradually rising to 57% to 82% by age 15. Recurring or frequent headaches occurred in 2.5% of 7 year olds and 15% of 15 year olds [Bille, 1962]. Before puberty, boys are affected more frequently than girls, but after puberty, headaches occur more frequently in girls [Dalsgaard-Nielsen, 1970; Deubner, 1977; Laurell et al., 2004; Sillanpaa, 1983].

The prevalence of migraine headache steadily increases throughout childhood, and the male-to-female ratio shifts during adolescence. The prevalence rises from 3% at ages 3 to 7 years, to 4% to 11% by ages 7 through 11, and up to 8% to 23% during adolescence (Table 53-1). The mean age of onset of migraine is 7.2 years for boys and 10.9 years for girls [Dalsgaard-Nielsen, 1970; Lipton et al., 1994; Mortimer et al., 1992; Sillanpaa, 1976; Small and Waters, 1974; Stewart et al., 1991; Stewart et al., 1992; Valquist, 1955].

Data regarding tension-type headache are limited. Two recent studies including school children, ages 7 to 19 years, using the International Headache Society criteria found a 1-year prevalence of tension-type headache to be 10% to 23%. The prevalence of tension-type headache increased with age in both boys and girls, up to age 11 years, and thereafter increased only in girls [Laurell et al., 2004; Zwart et al., 2004].

CLASSIFICATION

The International Headache Society has recently published an updated classification system for headache disorders (see Box 53-1) that is available online at www.ihs.org.

Each headache category is further subclassified. The classification for the most common primary headache disorder, migraine, has been modified based on current views of the pathophysiology of migraine, in that the focal, com-

TABLE 53-1

The Prevalence of Migraine Headache through Childhood

By age	3–7 years	7–11 years	15 years
Prevalence	1.2%–3.2%	4%–11%	8%–23%
Gender ratio	boys > girls	boys = girls	girls > boys

Box 53-1 THE INTERNATIONAL CLASSIFICATION OF HEADACHE DISORDERS

Primary Headache Disorders

1. Migraine
2. Tension-type
3. Cluster headache
4. Other primary headache disorders

Secondary Headaches

5. Headache attributed to head or neck trauma
6. Headache attributed to cranial or cervical vascular disorder
7. Headache attributed to nonvascular intracranial disorder
8. Headache attributed to substance or withdrawal from substances
9. Headache attributed to infection
10. Headache attributed to disorders of homeostasis
11. Headache attributed to disorders of the cranium, neck, eyes, ears, nose, sinuses, teeth, or other facial or cranial structures
12. Headache attributed to psychiatric disorders
13. Cranial neuralgia and central causes of facial pain
14. Other headache, cranial neuralgia, central or primary facial pain

BOX 53-2 2003 INTERNATIONAL CLASSIFICATION OF HEADACHE DISORDERS CRITERIA FOR MIGRAINE

Migraine
- Migraine without aura
- Migraine with aura
  - Typical aura with migraine headache
  - Typical aura with nonmigraine headache
  - Typical aura without headache
  - Familial hemiplegic migraine
  - Sporadic hemiplegic migraine
  - Basilar-type migraine
- Childhood periodic syndromes that are commonly precursors of migraine
  - Cyclical vomiting
  - Abdominal migraine
  - Benign paroxysmal vertigo of childhood
- Retinal migraine
- Complications of migraine
  - Chronic migraine
  - Status migraine
  - Persistent aura without infarction
  - Migrainous infarction
- Probable migraine

plicated, or variants of migraine are all included under migraine with aura (Box 53-2). For example, a migraine with hemiparesis (e.g., familial or sporadic hemiplegic migraine) falls in the category of migraine with aura. Another change in the new classification system is the inclusion of cyclic vomiting and abdominal migraine within the category of "Childhood periodic syndromes that are commonly precursors of migraine." The new classification system also recognizes that many patients experience frequent or near daily migraine (more than 15 headaches per month) in a category of "chronic migraine" (see "Chronic Daily Headache").

Omitted from the 2004 classification are "Alternating hemiparesis of childhood" and the "Alice in Wonderland" syndrome. The rare and bizarre entity of alternating hemiparesis of childhood, once thought to be a migrainous phenomenon, is viewed as a metabolic disorder, probably because of a mitochondrial disorder or a channelopathy. Recently, however, a novel ATP1A2 mutation in a kindred with features that bridge the phenotypic spectrum between alternating hemiparesis of childhood and familial hemiplegic migraine has been reported, which may draw alternating hemiparesis of childhood back into the migraine spectrum [Swoboda et al., 2004]. The Alice in Wonderland syndrome represents transient visual or perceptual disturbances with micropsia or macropsia and, when heralding an otherwise typical migraine headache, is appropriately viewed as migraine with aura. Anatomically, the aura is arising from the occipital, parietal, or posterior temporal lobes to produce these distorted visual symptoms.

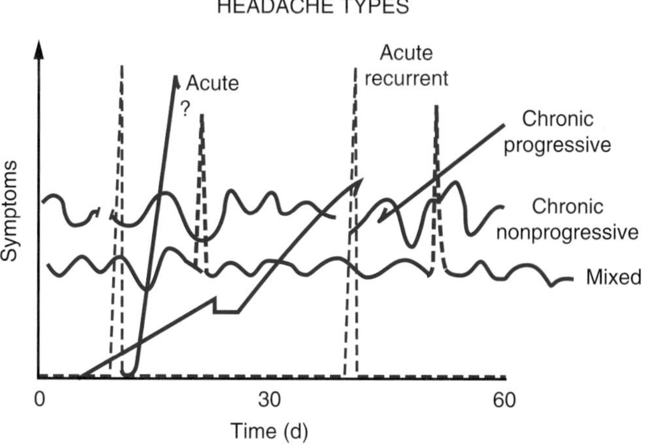

FIGURE 53-1. Five temporal patterns of pediatric headache.

Another modification in the new classification is to remove "Ophthalmoplegic migraine" from the category of migraine to the group of cranial neuralgias. Although paradoxically still labeled as "migraine," this clinical entity is characterized by transient disturbances of cranial nerves III, IV, or VI coupled with intense peri- or retro-orbital pain.

A separate, clinically useful classification system was proposed by Rothner that divides headache into five temporal patterns (Fig. 53-1): acute, acute-recurrent, chronic-progressive, chronic-nonprogressive, and mixed. Each of these temporal patterns suggests differing pathophysiologic processes and has distinctive differential diagnoses (Table 53-2).

TABLE 53-2

Examples of Syndromes That Cause Headaches

ACUTE GENERALIZED	ACUTE LOCALIZED	ACUTE RECURRENT	CHRONIC PROGRESSIVE	CHRONIC NONPROGRESSIVE
Fever	Sinusitis	Migraine	Tumor	Muscle contraction
Systemic infection	Otitis	Complex migraine	Pseudotumor	Conversion
Central nervous system infection	Ocular abnormality	Migraine variants	Brain abscess	Malingering
Toxins: lead CO_2	Dental disease	Cluster	Subdural hematoma	After concussion
After seizure	Trauma	Paroxysmal hemicrania	Hydrocephalus	Depression
Electrolyte imbalance	Occipital neuralgia	After seizure	Hemorrhage	Anxiety
Hypertension	Temporomandibular joint dysfunction	Tic douloureux	Hypertension	Adjustment reaction
Hypoglycemia		Exertional	Vasculitis	Hemicrania continua
After lumbar puncture				
Trauma				
Embolic				
Vascular thrombosis				
Hemorrhage				
Collagen disease				
Exertional				

The *acute*, sudden onset of headache in an otherwise healthy child is usually due to intercurrent viral infection (e.g., upper respiratory infection or pharyngitis). The acute headache with focal neurologic signs must raise concerns for intracranial hemorrhage from aneurysm, vascular malformation, or coagulopathy. Sudden headache with fever warrants consideration of cerebrospinal fluid analysis for the possibility of meningitis.

Acute-recurrent pattern implies attacks of headache, separated by symptom-free intervals. The primary headache disorders—migraine and tension-type—are the most common causes of this pattern, although, infrequently, complex partial seizures, substance abuse, cluster headache, and recurrent trauma can produce recurring headache syndromes.

Chronic-progressive headaches implies a gradually increasing frequency and severity of headache and is the most ominous of the five temporal patterns. The pathologic correlate is increasing intracranial pressure. Causes of this pattern include brain tumor, hydrocephalus, pseudotumor cerebri, chronic meningitis, brain abscess, or subdural collections.

Chronic-nonprogressive or chronic daily headache represents a pattern of frequent or near-constant headache. The definition of CDH requires a period longer than 4 months during which the patient experiences more than 15 headaches per month and the headaches last more than 4 hours per day. Many adolescents will have continual, unremitting, disabling daily headache. Affected patients generally have normal neurologic examinations, and there are usually interwoven psychologic factors and heightened anxiety about unrecognized, underlying organic causes.

"Mixed" headache pattern represents the superimposition of acute-recurrent headache (usually migraine) upon a chronic daily background pattern; therefore, it represents a variant of chronic-nonprogressive headache (see later sections).

DIAGNOSTIC CRITERIA

The 2004 International Classification of Headache Disorders also establishes the diagnostic criteria for the primary headache disorders (Box 53-3). Beginning in the 1950s, efforts were made to define migraine in children. Valquist, Bille, and later, Prensky and Sommer all proposed the criteria for pediatric migraine, which included the following features:

1. Paroxysmal headache separated by pain-free intervals
2. Accompanied by a variable number of associated features including:
   Visual aura
   Nausea
   Abdominal pain
   Throbbing quality
   Unilateral pain
   Family history of migraine [Bille, 1962; Prensky and Sommer, 1979; Valquist, 1955]

In 1988, the International Headache Society established the gold standard for the definition of migraine [Olesen, 1988]. Although these criteria provided a solid framework for adult migraine, their sensitivity for the pediatric population was less than satisfactory. Therefore, in 2003, the International Headache Society revised the diagnostic criteria, incorporating many developmentally sensitive changes that permit a broader applicability for children and adolescents, maintaining specificity and improving sensitivity [Olesen, 2004]. These new criteria accept the clinical observations that pediatric migraine may be brief (≈1 hour) and bifrontal, and that the associated symptoms of photophobia and phonophobia may be inferred by the child's behavior, such as withdrawing to a dark, quiet room to rest during the headache attack. The diagnostic criteria also include cyclic vomiting and abdominal migraine (Boxes 53-4 and 53-5).

Box 53-3 2003 International Headache Society Diagnostic Criteria for the Primary Headache Disorders: Migraine and Tension-Type

Pediatric Migraine without Aura

A. At least five attacks fulfilling criteria B through D
B. Headache attacks lasting 1 to 72 hours
C. Headache has at least two of the following characteristics:
 1. Unilateral location, may be bilateral, frontotemporal (not occipital)
 2. Pulsing quality
 3. Moderate or severe pain intensity
 4. Aggravation by or causing avoidance of routine physical activity (e.g., walking or climbing stairs)
D. During the headache, at least one of the following:
 1. Nausea and/or vomiting
 2. Photophobia and phonophobia, which may be *inferred* from behavior
E. Not attributed to another disorder

Episodic Tension-Type Headache

A. At least 10 episodes occurring on more than 1, but fewer than 15 days per month for at least 3 months and fulfilling criteria B through D.
B. Headache lasting 30 minutes to 7 days.
C. Headache has at least two of the following characteristics:
 1. Bilateral location
 2. Pressing or tightening (nonpulsing) quality
 3. Mild or moderate intensity
 4. Not aggravated by routine physical activity such as walking or climbing stairs.
D. Both of the following:
 5. No nausea or vomiting (anorexia may occur)
 6. Photophobia or phonophobia (but not both)
F. Not attributed to another structural or metabolic disorder

EVALUATION OF THE CHILD WITH HEADACHE

The evaluation of a child with headaches follows the traditional medical model and begins with a thorough medical history and complete physical and neurologic examination. A brief series of questions shown in Box 53-6 provides a logical framework for evaluating headaches and generally yields sufficient information to diagnose most primary headaches and reveal clues to the presence of secondary headache disorders.

Box 53-4 International Classification of Headache Disorders Criteria for Cyclic Vomiting

Description
Recurrent episodic attacks, usually stereotypical in the individual patient, of vomiting and intense nausea. Attacks are associated with pallor and lethargy. There is complete resolution of symptoms between attacks.

Diagnostic Criteria

A. At least five attacks fulfilling criteria B and C

B. Episodic attacks, stereotypical in the individual patient, of intense nausea and vomiting lasting 1 to 5 days

C. Vomiting during attacks occurs at least 5 times/hour for at least 1 hour

D. Symptom-free between attacks

E. Not attributed to another disorder. History and physical examination do not reveal signs of gastrointestinal disease.

Box 53-5 International Classification of Headache Disorders Criteria for Abdominal Migraine

Description
An idiopathic recurrent disorder seen mainly in children and characterized by episodic midline abdominal pain manifesting in attacks lasting 1 to 72 hours with normality between episodes. The pain is of moderate-to-severe intensity and associated with vasomotor symptoms, nausea, and vomiting.

Diagnostic Criteria

A. At least five attacks fulfilling criteria B through D

B. Attacks of abdominal pain lasting 1 to 72 hours

C. Abdominal pain has all of the following characteristics:

1. Midline location, periumbilical or poorly localized
2. Dull or "just sore" quality
3. Moderate or severe intensity

D. During abdominal pain, at least two of the following:

1. Anorexia
2. Nausea
3. Vomiting
4. Pallor

Not attributed to another disorder. History and physical examination do not indicate signs of gastrointestinal or renal disease, or such disease has been ruled out by appropriate investigations.

The role of further ancillary diagnostic studies such as laboratory testing, electroencephalography (EEG), and neuroimaging has been extensively reviewed in a practice parameter of the American Academy of Neurology [Lewis et al., 2002]. The practice parameter determined that there is inadequate documentation in the literature to support any recommendation as to the appropriateness of routine laboratory studies (e.g., hematology or chemistry panels) or performance of lumbar puncture. Routine EEG is not recommended as part of the headache evaluation. Data compiled from eight studies demonstrated that the EEG was not necessary for differentiation of primary headache (e.g., migraine, tension-type) from secondary headache due to structural disease involving the head and neck or from headaches due to a psychogenic etiology. EEG is unlikely to define or determine an etiology of the headache or distinguish migraine from other types of headaches. Furthermore, in those children undergoing evaluation for recurrent headache who were found to have paroxysmal EEGs, the risk of future seizures is negligible.

The role of neuroimaging is better defined. Data compiled from six pediatric studies permitted the following recommendations:

1. Obtaining a neuroimaging study on a routine basis is not indicated in children with recurrent headaches and a normal neurologic examination.
2. Neuroimaging should be considered in children in whom there are historical features to suggest the following:
   a. Recent onset of severe headache
   b. Change in the type of headache
   c. Neurologic dysfunction

Box 53-6 Key Questions to Ask in the Evaluation of Children with Headaches

Headache Database

1. How and when did your headache(s) begin?
2. What is the time pattern of your headache: sudden first headache, episodes of headache, an everyday headache, gradually worsening, or a mixture?
3. Do you have one type of headache or more than one type?
4. How often does the headache occur and how long does it last?
5. Can you tell that a headache is coming?
6. Where is the pain located and what is the quality of the pain: pounding, squeezing, stabbing, or other?
7. Are there any other symptoms that accompany your headache: nausea, vomiting, dizziness, numbness, weakness, or other?
8. What makes the headache better or worse? Do any activities, medications, or foods tend to cause or aggravate your headaches?
9. Do you have to stop your activities when you get a headache?
10. Do the headaches occur under any special circumstances or at any particular time?
11. Do you have other symptoms between headaches?
12. Are you taking or are you being treated with any medications (for the headache or other purposes)?
13. Do you have any other medical problems?
14. Does anyone in your family suffer from headaches?
15. What do you think might be causing your headache?

Adapted from Rothner, 1995.

3. Neuroimaging should be considered in children with an abnormal neurologic examination (e.g., focal findings, signs of increased intracranial pressure, significant alteration of consciousness) and the coexistence of seizures.

Care must be taken not to over- or underinterpret these recommendations. Neuroimaging may be considered in children with recurrent headache based on clues extracted from the medical history or on the findings of neurologic examination. Since publication of this parameter, feedback from clinicians and personal experience has demonstrated that many in the "managed care industry" have focused only on recommendation number one and not recognized numbers two and three, which clearly places the responsibility in the hands of the clinician to make the decision to perform ancillary testing, including neuroimaging, based on good clinical judgment. The findings of the American Academy of Neurology support the medical decision to perform scans or to withhold scans, based on clinical determinants for the individual patient.

PRIMARY HEADACHE SYNDROMES

Migraine

Migraine is the most common acute-recurrent headache syndrome. The classifications of migraine are shown in Box 53-2 and the cardinal diagnostic features are shown in Box 53-3.

Pathophysiology

Migraine is considered to be a primary neuronal process (Fig. 53-2) [Pietrobon and Striessnig, 2003; Silberstein, 2004]. The principal underlying phenomenon of migraine is a hyperexcitable cerebral cortex. Polygenic influences produce disturbances of neuronal ion channels (e.g., calcium channels), leading to a lowered threshold for external and/or internal factors that trigger episodes of cortical spreading depression. Cortical spreading depression represents a slowly propagating wave (≈2 to 6 mm/minute) of neuronal depolarization and is now viewed as the key initial phase that is responsible for (1) migraine aura and (2) activation of the "trigeminovascular system."

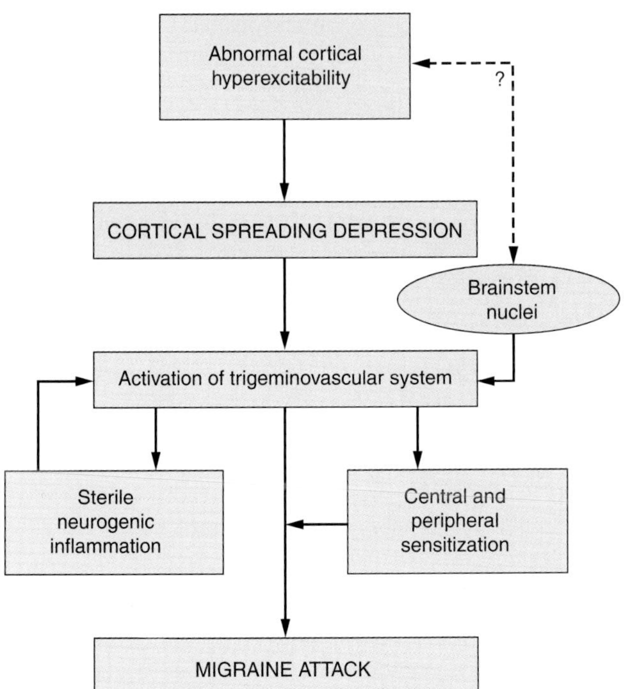

FIGURE 53-2. Migraine pathophysiology. (Adapted from Pietrobon D, Striessnig J. Neurobiology of migraine. Nat Rev 2003;4:386.)

The aura of migraine represents transient, focal somatosensory phenomena such as visual scotomata or distortions, dysesthesias, hemiparesis, or aphasia. The aura is viewed to be caused by the regional neuronal depolarization and/or the accompanying regional oligemia observed with cortical spreading depression.

In addition to sustained cortical oligemia, cortical spreading depression is accompanied by extravasation of plasma proteins from dural vessels and activation of meningeal afferents. The sum of these effects is to increase *FOS* expression in the trigeminal nucleus within the brainstem [Prensky and Sommer, 1979]. Cortical spreading depression, then, is the key event for episodic activation of the trigeminal vascular system that culminates in the migraine attack.

The role played by the brainstem nuclei is controversial. Some investigators believe the locus ceruleus and dorsal raphe nuclei act as the "migraine generator," initiating noradrenergic and serotonergic signals to the cortex and dural vessels in a parallel fashion. Other investigators favor the view that cortical spreading depression is the initiating phenomenon and believe that the brainstem nuclei provide a "permissive" role, favoring "central trigeminal hyperexcitability."

Although cortical spreading depression nicely explains the somatosensory aura, only about 30% of children and adolescents experience aura. Clearly, the processes leading to pain may occur in the absence of a perceived aura. Two mechanisms are thought to be responsible for the generation of the pain of migraine: (1) neurogenic inflammation of the meningeal vessels and (2) "sensitization" of peripheral and central trigeminal afferents.

Cortical spreading depression initiates vascular dilation with extravasation of plasma proteins from dural vessels and activates trigeminal meningeal afferents. These processes set the stage for "neurogenic" inflammation of the dural and pial vessels, mediated principally by neuropeptides and calcitonin gene-related protein. The inflammatory cascade stimulates nociceptive afferents, leading to pain. Many authors question whether neurogenic inflammation alone is sufficient to produce the pain of migraine.

One of the striking features noted during an attack of migraine is that seemingly innocuous activities, such as coughing, walking up stairs, or bending over greatly intensify the pain. In fact, the International Classification of Headache Disorders criteria include "aggravation" by activities as one of the diagnostic features of migraine. This observation coupled with elegant research has led to the concepts of "sensitization" of trigeminal vascular afferents, whereby both peripheral and central afferent circuits become exceptionally sensitive to mechanical, thermal, and chemical stimuli. These circuits become so sensitive that virtually any stimulation is perceived as painful, the concept of allodynia [Burstein et al., 2000; Burstein et al., 2004; Burstein and Jakubowski, 2004].

Therefore, the current view of the pathophysiology of migraine begins with an inherited vulnerability with a hyperexcitable cerebral cortex. A variety of stimuli may trigger episodes of cortical spreading depression, which, in turn, initiates the processes of localized, neurogenic inflammation and of sensitization of both peripheral and central afferent circuitry.

Clinical Manifestations

MIGRAINE WITHOUT AURA

The diagnostic criteria for migraine without aura are shown in Box 53-3. Migraine without aura is the most frequent form, accounting for 60% to 85% of all migraine in children and adolescents. Patients often recognize prodromal features: mood changes (euphoria to depression), irritability, lethargy, yawning, food cravings, or increased thirst. Perhaps the most frequent heralding feature is a change in behavioral patterns or withdrawal from activities.

A migraine headache begins gradually and is usually localized to the frontal or temporal region. The pain may be unilateral. The quality is generally described as pounding, pulsing, or throbbing, but the key feature is its intensity. Routine activities will be interrupted. Photophobia and phonophobia are common and may be inferred by the child's desire to seek a quiet, dark place to rest or even to sleep because sleep often produces significant relief.

Nausea, vomiting, and abdominal pain may be the most disabling feature because a student with headache may be able to stay in the classroom with pain, but the onset of nausea or vomiting necessitates a visit to the school nurse.

A migraine headache typically last for hours, even days (1 to 72 hours) but does not generally occur more frequently than 6 to 8 times per month. More than 8 to 10 attacks per month must warrant consideration of alternative diagnoses such as organic conditions (i.e., pseudotumor cerebri) or the chronic daily headache syndromes [American College of Emergency Physicians, 1996; Gladstein et al., 1997].

The time of day when the headache occurs tends to shift through childhood. Younger children often complain in the afternoon, after school. Younger teenagers frequently begin to report their headaches about lunchtime, often precipitated by the chaos of the school cafeteria with its combination of bright lights, loud noise, and peer pressure. Older teens acquire the more adult patterns of morning headache, often a concern because morning occurrence frequently raises suspicion of space-occupying lesions.

Although most verbal children can readily relate to these symptoms, the developmentally challenged child may be unable to express these complaints. Caregivers report repeated cycling events of quiet, withdrawn behavior with pallor, regurgitation, vomiting, and desire to rest. These stereotyped episodes may prompt investigation for epilepsy, gastroesophageal reflux, or hydrocephalus, when in fact they may represent migraine.

TABLE 53-3

Migraine Aura

Visual:	Negative scotoma
	"Fortification" scotoma
	Field deficits:
	  Hemianopsia
	  Quadrantanopsia
	Photopsia
	Visual distortions:
	  Teichopsia
	  Metamorphopsia
	  Prosopagnosia
	  "Alice in Wonderland"

Sensory:	Parasthesias Dysesthesias Perioral and/or hand numbness (chiro-oral)
Motor:	Hemiparesis Monoparesis
Aphasia	
Psychic:	Confusion Dysphasia Amnesia Disequilibrium

MIGRAINE WITH AURA

Approximately 14% to 30% of children report visual disturbances, distortions, or obscuration before or as the headache begins (Table 53-3) [Lewis, 1995]. The aura ("cool breeze") is, however, an inconsistent feature in childhood and adolescents. The presence of an aura must be elicited with very specific questions: "Do you have spots, colors, lights, or dots in your eyes before or as you are getting a headache?"

Typically, the aura is a visual phenomenon, but, as discussed in the pathophysiology section previously, the cortical spreading depression responsible for the aura may disturb virtually any cortical region including language, motor, or sensory areas. The classic visual symptomatology during migraine include three dominant visual phenomena:

1. Binocular visual impairment with scotoma (77%)
2. Distortion or hallucinations (16%)
3. Monocular visual impairment or scotoma (7%) [Hachinshi et al., 1973]

The onset of the visual aura is gradual and lasts minutes. Sudden images and complicated visual perceptions should prompt consideration of complex partial seizures, even if followed by headache. Young adolescents may experience strange visual effects (distortions, illusions, micropsia, and macropsia) within the spectrum of the Alice in Wonderland syndrome. Transient visual obscurations, brief episodes of near-complete blindness, are also features of pseudotumor cerebri.

The aura has long been thought to be an extremely useful feature therapeutically, with early warning of an impending headache permitting the institution of abortive measures such as ergotamine or the "triptan" agents. Unfortunately, the therapeutic utility of treating the headache at the onset of the aura in adolescent migraine is not reliable or effective.

Alice in Wonderland Syndrome

Bizarre visual illusions and spatial distortions occasionally precede migraine headaches. Similar to Alice's visual distortions after eating mushrooms in *Through the Looking Glass,* affected children describe visual distortions before or as the headache is beginning. The children may describe bizarre or vivid visual illusions, such as the following:

Macropsia: objects appear larger
Micropsia: objects appear smaller
Metamorphopsia: objects (such as faces) appear distorted
Teleopsia: objects appear far away

These patients are often not confused or frightened by these illusions and are able to relate the experience in enthusiastic detail. This unusual visual symptomatology is best considered as migraine with aura, though historically, Alice-in-Wonderland syndrome is included as a distinct variant. This type of visuoperceptual abnormality has been reported with infectious mononucleosis, complex partial seizures, and hallucinogenic drug ingestion.

Retinal Migraine

Also referred to as *ocular, ophthalmic*, or *anterior visual pathway* migraine, retinal migraine is uncommon in young children but occurs during adolescence. Affected patients will report brief (seconds to <60 minutes), sudden, monocular blackouts or gray-outs, or bright, blinding episodes (e.g., photopsia) of visual disturbance, before, after, or during the headache. A 60-minute interval between visual symptom and headache may occur. As with ophthalmoplegic migraine, the pain is often described as retro-orbital and ipsilateral to the visual disturbance.

Examination of the optic fundus during an attack may disclose constriction of retinal veins and arteries with marked retinal pallor. An occasional patient may suffer significant visual sequelae (e.g., scotoma, altitudinal defects, or monocular blindness) in retinal migraine presumably due to vasoconstriction with retinal infarction. Although the patient population with retinal migraine is generally much younger than those who experience amaurosis fugax from atheromatous carotid disease, evaluation for hypercoagulable states, embolic sources, and carotid dissection must be considered.

Basilar-Type Migraine

Also known as *basilar artery* or *vertebrobasilar migraine*, basilar-type migraine is the most frequent of complicated migraine variants and is estimated to represent 3% to 19% of all migraine [Bickerstaff, 1961; Golden and French, 1975; Lapkin and Golden, 1978]. This wide range of frequency relates to the rigorousness of the definition. Some authors included any headache with dizziness to be within the spectrum of basilar migraine, whereas others require the presence of clear signs and symptoms of posterior fossa involvement before establishing this diagnosis. The International Classification of Headache Disorders criteria require two or more symptoms (Table 53-4) and emphasize bulbar and bilateral sensorimotor features.

Onset of basilar migraine tends to occur in younger children, with a mean age of 7 years, although the clinical entity probably appears as early as 12 to 18 months in the form of "benign paroxysmal vertigo" with episodes of ataxia, vertigo, clumsiness, pallor, and vomiting.

TABLE 53-4

Signs and Symptoms of Basilar-Type Migraine

Vertigo	73%
Nausea or vomiting	30%-50%
Ataxia	43%-50%
Visual field deficits	43%
Diplopia	30%
Tinnitus	13%
Vertigo	73%
Hearing loss	*
Confusion	20%
Dysarthria	*
Weakness (hemiplegia, quadriplegia, diplegia)	20%
Syncope	*

*No figures available.

Affected children have attacks of intense dizziness, vertigo, visual disturbances, ataxia, and diplopia. These early, transient features last from minutes up to an hour and are followed by the headache phase. The headache may be occipital. The quality of the pain may be ill defined and the terms such as *pulsing* or *throbbing* may not be used. A small subset of patients with basilar migraine will have their posterior fossa symptoms after the headache phase is well established.

The pathogenesis of basilar migraine is not well understood. Although focal cortical processes, oligemia or depolarization, can explain the deficits in hemiplegic migraine, the posterior fossa signs of basilar migraine are more problematic. A single case report of a 25-year-old woman with basilar migraine exists wherein transcranial Doppler and single photon emission tomography were performed through the course of a basilar migraine attack. These data suggest decreased posterior cerebral artery perfusion through the aura phase at a time when the described patient was experiencing transient bilateral blindness and ataxia [LaSpina et al., 1997].

The sudden appearance of diplopia, vertigo, and vomiting must prompt consideration of disorders within the posterior fossa such as arteriovenous malformations, cavernous angiomas, tumors (medulloblastoma, ependymoma, brainstem glioma), congenital malformations (e.g. Chiari, Dandy-Walker), or vertebrobasilar insufficiency (e.g., vertebral dissection or thrombosis). Acute labyrinthitis or positional vertigo can mimic basilar migraine. Complex partial seizures and drug ingestions must be considered at any age. Rarely, metabolic diseases such as Hartnup's disease, hyperammonemias (urea cycle or organic acidemias), or disorders of pyruvate or lactate metabolism may present with episodic vertigo, but these inborn errors of metabolism usually have some degree of altered consciousness, even coma.

Hemiplegic Migraine

Familial Hemiplegic Migraine

Familial hemiplegic migraine is an uncommon autosomal-dominant form of migraine headache in which the aura has a "strokelike" quality, producing some degree of hemiparesis. The nosology is somewhat misleading because there is actually a wide diversity of focal symptoms and signs that can accompany this migraine variant beyond motor deficits. Barlow proposed the more appropriate term *hemi-syndrome migraine* to emphasize the diversity of associated symptoms, but this term has not received broad acceptance [Barlow, 1984]. The International Headache Society criteria clearly require that "some degree of hemiparesis" must be present, so the term will likely persist.

A series of recent exciting discoveries into the molecular genetics of familial hemiplegic migraine have broadened the understanding of the fundamental mechanisms of migraine and demonstrated the overlap with other paroxysmal disorders such as acetazolamide-responsive episodic ataxia [Joutel et al., 1993]. Genetic linkage to chromosome 19p13 has been identified in half of the known familial hemiplegic migraine pedigrees and, more recently, a separate pedigree with linkage to chromosome 1q31 has been reported [Gardner et al., 1997; Ophoff et al., 1997]. The chromosomal 19 defect produces a missense mutation in a neuronal calcium channel gene providing compelling evidence that familial hemiplegic migraine represents a channelopathy. These discoveries have revolutionized the understanding of migraine and may open new territory for pharmacologic interventions.

From the clinical perspective, hemiplegic migraine is characterized by transient (hours to days) episodes of focal neurologic deficits, hemiparesis, hemisensory changes, aphasia, and visual field defects that precede the headache phase by 30 to 60 minutes but occasionally extend well beyond the headache itself. The headache is often, but not invariably, contralateral to the focal deficit.

The appearance of acute, focal neurologic deficits in the setting of headache in an adolescent necessitates vigorous investigation for disorders such as intracranial hemorrhage, stroke, tumor, vascular malformations, acute disseminated encephalomyelitis, or focal infection. Complex partial seizure or drug intoxication with a sympathomimetic must also be considered. Neuroimaging (magnetic resonance imaging [MRI] and magnetic resonance angiography) and EEG may be indicated. Investigations for embolic sources or hypercoagulable states and for mitochondrial disorders (MELAS—mitochondrial myopathy, encephalography, lactic acidosis and stroke-like attacks) are likewise appropriate.

Sporadic hemiplegic migraine represents an identical clinical phenomenon but lacks the identifiable family history.

Alternating Hemiplegia of Childhood

Traditionally, alternating hemiplegia of childhood has been considered a variant of hemiplegic migraine, but more recent perspectives suggest other mechanisms, and the 2003 International Classification of Headache Disorders has omitted it from the migraine spectrum. Affected patients have their initial symptoms before 18 months of life. These unfortunate children have attacks of paralysis (hemiparesis, monoparesis, diparesis, ophthalmoparesis, and bulbar paralysis) that may be accompanied by variable tone changes (flaccid, spastic, or rigid). A variety of paroxysmal involuntary movements, including chorea, athetosis, dystonia, nystagmus, and respiratory irregularities (hyperpnea), can be seen. The attacks of paralysis can be brief (minutes) or prolonged (days) and potentially life threatening during periods of bulbar paralysis. Curiously, the attacks generally subside after sleep. Affected children are frequently developmentally challenged [Aicardi et al., 1995; Verret and Steele, 1971].

The link to migraine was tenuous but was based on the presence of a high prevalence of migraine in the families of affected children and on cerebral blood flow data that suggest a "migrainous" mechanism. In 1997, an international workshop was conducted to address the various hypotheses surrounding alternating hemiparesis of childhood and the proceedings have been reviewed by Rho and Chugani, [1998]. Proposed mechanisms include channelopathy, mitochondrial cytopathy, and cerebrovascular dysfunction, though the former seems to be the most likely hypothesis. Recently however, a novel ATP1A2 mutation in a kindred with features that bridge the phenotypic spectrum between alternating hemiparesis of childhood and familial hemiplegic migraine has been reported that may draw alternating hemiplegia of childhood back into the migraine spectrum [Swoboda et al., 2004].

Investigations into the etiology of this entity warrant aggressive evaluation for vascular disorders, inborn errors of metabolism, mitochondrial encephalomyopathies, or epileptic variants.

Management is difficult. The calcium channel blocker flunarezine not available through U.S. pharmacies, can be remarkably effective in reducing attack frequency and severity.

Confusional Migraine

Omitted from the International Classification of Headache Disorders classification system is the entity "Confusional migraine," which most likely represents a hybrid or overlap between hemiplegic and basilar-type migraine. The term *confusional migraine* was omitted with the expectation that those patients who have attacks associated with language disturbances, hemiparesis, and confusion represent the spectrum of hemiplegic migraine and those with bilateral blindness, ataxia, vertigo, and confusion represent the spectrum of basilar-type migraine.

The clinical entity was first described in 1970 by Garcon and Barlow, who reported a series of children, ages 8 to 16 years, with acute confusional states lasting 4 to 24 hours, associated with agitation and aphasia. The authors suggested the confusional state was a manifestation of juvenile migraine [Garcon and Barlow, 1970]. Ehyai and Fenichel [1978] later introduced the term *acute confusional migraine*. Subsequent reports have broadened the clinical phenomenology to include blindness, paresthesias, hemiparesis and amnesia. Amnesia can be such a prominent feature that Jensen [1980] proposed the term *transient global amnesia of childhood*, but amnesia is only part of the clinical spectrum.

Affected children, more commonly males, become agitated, restless, disoriented, and, occasionally, combative for minutes to hours. Once consciousness has returned to baseline, the patients may describe an inability to communicate, frustration, confusion, loss of orientation to time, and may not recall a headache phase at all. A strong family history of migraine is elicited in 75% of patients.

There is a clear link to head trauma in many cases [Ferrera and Reicho, 1996]. The term *footballer's migraine* is applied in Europe when a soccer player, after "heading" the ball, develops an acute confusional state with headache. Similar symptoms may follow other causes of minor head injury. This variant should be viewed within the spectrum of trauma-triggered migraine.

Acute confusional states in children and adolescents warrant aggressive investigation for encephalitis, brain abscess, drug intoxication, cerebrovascular disease, vasculitis, or metabolic encephalopathies [Amit, 1988]. Particular attention must be focused on the possibility of complex partial seizures or postictal states.

CHILDHOOD "PERIODIC SYNDROMES"

The following curious and pediatric-specific clinical entities represent episodic conditions with stereotyped features that are considered precursors of migraine.

Cyclic vomiting syndrome is a disorder characterized by recurrent self-episodes of intense vomiting (more than four emeses/hour), recognizable by their stereotypical time of onset, duration, and symptomatology in the individual (see Box 53-4). The vomiting is uniquely intense, the subjective nausea disabling, and the resultant dehydration often necessitates hospital-based treatment. The attacks are accompanied by pallor, listlessness, anorexia, abdominal pain, retching, headache, and photophobia. The interval between attacks is 2 to 4 weeks and a typical attack lasts 24 to 48 hours. The children are, by definition, healthy between attacks.

Boys and girls are equally affected by cyclic vomiting syndrome. The usual age of onset is 5 years, but the diagnosis is often delayed until age 8 and many, if not most, children "outgrow" these attacks by age 10.

A thorough diagnostic evaluation must be performed to rule out intermittent bowel obstruction, elevated intracranial pressure, epilepsy, and metabolic disorders such as urea cycle defects and organic acidurias. The pediatric gastroenterology community is currently developing practice guidelines.

The link to migraine is based on natural history data that suggest the evolution toward more typical migraine, parallels based on autonomic data (i.e., "neurocardiac"), and presence of family history of migraine in children with cyclic vomiting syndrome.

The management of cyclic vomiting syndrome involves both acute strategies and preventive measures. As soon as an attack begins, these patients must be volume replenished with glucose-containing solutions. Pharmacologic options have not been systematically investigated, but anecdotal information suggests a role for antiemetics (e.g., ondansetron, promethazine, or prochlorperazine) and sedation (e.g., diphenhydramine, benzodiazepine). Subcutaneous sumatriptan (2 to 3 mg) has been used widely but no controlled trials have been conducted. Preventive agents such as cyproheptadine, amitriptyline or nortriptyline, valproate, topiramate, propranolol, or verapamil have all been used, but again no clinical trials have been reported.

Abdominal migraine is a new addition to the International Headache Society classification. The diagnostic criteria for abdominal migraine are shown in Box 53-5. This clinical entity is characterized by recurrent episodes of midline epigastric abdominal pain lasting 1 to 72 hours. The pain is of moderate-to-severe intensity and associated with vasomotor symptoms (e.g., flushing, pallor), as well as nausea and vomiting. The patients are well between attacks. Clearly, thorough gastrointestinal and renal investigation must be conducted before this diagnosis is entertained.

Benign paroxysmal vertigo of childhood is common and occurs in young children as abrupt, brief episodes of unexplained unsteadiness, with the child appearing to be "off balance" or falling. Careful observation may disclose nystagmus. Older children may be able to report symptoms of dizziness, clumsiness, headache, and nausea. The attacks may occur in clusters and typically resolve with sleep. In a small series of patients with long-term follow-up, most of the children had resolution of the episodes of vertigo but later developed migraine.

The diagnosis of benign paroxysmal vertigo is one of exclusion. Epilepsy, otologic pathology, and central nervous system pathology should be considered.

Treatment for benign paroxysmal vertigo can include symptomatic treatment such as antiemetics, although sleep aborts the attack in most patients. For a child in whom frequent events occur, a trial of cyproheptadine prophylaxis may be helpful in aborting attacks. A dosage of 2 to 4 mg nightly may be all that is required, and medication should be discontinued after the attacks have stopped. The majority of patients do not require any treatment. Reassurance regarding the benign nature of the condition may be all that is required.

Benign paroxysmal torticollis is a rare paroxysmal dyskinesia characterized by attacks of head tilt alone or tilt accompanied by vomiting and ataxia that may last hours to days [Chaves-Carballo, 1996]. Other tortional or dystonic features, including truncal or pelvic posturing, are described by Chutorian [1974]. Attacks first manifest during infancy between 2 and 8 months of age. The original descriptions of benign paroxysmal torticollis by Snyder [1969] suggested a form of labyrinthitis and demonstrated abnormal vestibular reflexes.

The link to migraine is strengthening. Paroxysmal torticollis is likely an early onset variant of basilar migraine, which itself is a variant of benign paroxysmal vertigo. Additionally, there is often a family history of migraine. More intriguing information has recently been reported wherein four children with this clinical entity have been found to have the mutation in the *CACNA1A* gene [Giffin et al., 2002].

The differential diagnosis must include gastroesophageal reflux (e.g., Sandifer's syndrome), idiopathic torsional dystonia, and complex partial seizure, but particular attention must be paid to the posterior fossa and craniocervical junction, where congenital or acquired lesions may produce torticollis. Rarely, trochlear nerve dysfunction produces compensatory head tilt.

If the episodes continue to recur, the management is unclear. There are no clinical trials reported. There is clearly the question of whether these events, once determined to be benign, require any treatment beyond reassurance. The author suggests a trial of cyproheptadine as a safe measure that may provide some benefit if the episodes are judged to be painful in an individual patient.

MANAGEMENT OF PEDIATRIC MIGRAINE

Once the diagnosis of migraine is established and appropriate reassurances provided, a balanced and individually tailored treatment plan can be instituted. The first step is to appreciate the degree of disability imposed by the patient's headache. Understanding of the impact of the headache on the quality of life should guide the decisions regarding the most appropriate therapeutic course [Powers et al., 2003; 2004].

An American Academy of Neurology Practice Parameter has established the general principles for the management of migraine headache. The fundamental goals of long-term migraine treatment include the following:

1. Reduction of headache frequency, severity, duration, and disability
2. Reduction of reliance on poorly tolerated, ineffective, or unwanted acute pharmacotherapy
3. Improvement in the quality of life
4. Avoidance of acute headache medication escalation
5. Education and enablement of patients to manage their disease
6. Reduction of headache-related distress and psychologic symptoms [Silberstein, 2000]

To achieve these goals, it is becoming increasingly clear that a balanced treatment must include biobehavioral strategies and nonpharmacologic methods, as well as pharmacologic measures. Biobehavioral treatments include biofeedback, stress management, sleep hygiene, exercise, and dietary modifications (Box 53-7) [Holroyd and Mauskop, 2003].

Box 53-7 Complementary and Alternative Treatments

- Identification of migraine triggers
- Biobehavioral
- Biofeedback
  - Electromyographic biofeedback
  - Electroencephalography
  - Thermal hand warming
  - Galvanic skin resistance feedback
- Relaxation therapy
  - Progressive muscle relaxation
  - Autogenic training
  - Meditation
  - Passive relaxation
  - Self-hypnosis
- Cognitive therapy/stress management
  - Cognitive control
  - Guided imagery
- Dietary measures
  - "Avoidance diets"
  - Caffeine moderation
  - Herbs
    - Feverfew *(Tanacetum parthenium)*
    - Ginkgo
    - Valerian root
  - Minerals
    - Magnesium
  - Vitamins
    - Riboflavin (B_2)
- Acupuncture
- Massage therapy
- Aroma therapy

Biofeedback has demonstrated effectiveness in the treatment of both adults and children with migraine in controlled trials. Although the physiologic basis for its effectiveness is unclear, data suggest that levels of plasma beta-endorphin can be altered by biofeedback therapies [Baumann, 2002]. Biofeedback therapies commonly use electrical devices that provide audio or visual displays to demonstrate a physiologic effect. Thermal biofeedback is the most commonly used technique in pediatrics wherein children are taught to raise the temperature of one of their fingers. These techniques can easily be taught to children, and their use is associated with fewer and briefer migraine headaches. Once taught these methods, children can manage headaches, allowing them to have greater control of their health.

Stress management and relaxation therapies use techniques such as progressive relaxation, self-hypnosis, and guided imagery. Controlled trials have found relaxation therapies to be as effective in reducing the frequency of migraine attacks as the beta-blocker propranolol [Olness et al., 1987].

Sleep disturbances occur in 25% to 40% of children with migraine. One recent study found too little sleep (42%), bruxism (29%), co-sleeping (25%), and snoring (23%) in a population of 118 children. When children with migraine were compared with matched controls, statistically significant differences were found in sleep duration, daytime sleepiness, night awakenings, sleep anxiety, parasomnias, sleep-onset delay, bedtime resistance, and sleep-disordered breathing [Miller et al., 2003]. It remains unclear, however, whether sleep disturbances increase the occurrence of migraine, whether frequent and intense migraine leads to sleep disturbances, or whether the two are unrelated. Current practice is to recommend good sleep hygiene.

Exercise is recommended for patients with frequent migraines, and a review of Internet web sites serving headache sufferers reveals the common endorsement of regular physical activity. A recent study to evaluate the effects of exercise on plasma beta-endorphin levels in 40 migraine patients found beneficial effects on all migraine parameters [Koseoglu et al., 2003].

The role of dietary measures has recently been reviewed, yet the subject remains controversial [Millichap and Yee, 2003]. Seven to 44% of children and adults with migraine report that a particular food or drink can precipitate a migraine attack [Stang et al., 1992; Van den Bergh et al., 1987]. In children, the principal dietary triggers were cheese, chocolates, and citrus fruits. Other purported dietary precipitants include processed meats, yogurt, fried foods, monosodium glutamate, aspartame, and alcoholic beverages. For chocolate, the median time interval to the onset of headache after ingestion was 22 hours (3.5 to 27 hours) [Gibb et al., 1991].

Nonetheless, wholesale dietary elimination of a laundry list of foods is not recommended. Once popular, elimination diets are now judged to be excessive and generally set the stage for a battleground at home when parents attempt to enforce a restrictive diet on an unwilling adolescent, ultimately producing heightened tensions. A more reasonable approach is to review the list of foods thought to be linked to migraine and invite the patient to keep a headache diary to see if a temporal relationship exists between ingestion of one or more of those foods and the development of headache. If a link is found, prudence dictates avoidance of the offending food substance.

In addition to paying attention to what is eaten, it is important to encourage regular meals and drinking plenty of fluids. Many teenagers routinely skip breakfast. Missing meals is a common precipitant of migraine and identified by adolescents as one of the leading triggers [Lewis et al., 2004a]. A simple lifestyle modification for adolescents with frequent migraine includes eating three meals a day, including breakfast, and consuming plenty of water.

Overuse of over-the-counter analgesics has been a particular focus recently. Recognized in adults some years ago, overuse (more than five times per week) of acetaminophen, ibuprofen, and, to a lesser extent, aspirin-containing compounds can be a contributing factor to frequent, even daily, headache patterns. When recognized, patients who are overusing analgesics must be educated to discontinue the practice. Retrospective studies have suggested that this recommendation alone can decrease headache frequency [Reimschisel, 2003; Rothner and Guo, 2004].

Caffeine in coffee and sodas warrants special mention. A link between caffeine and migraine has been established [James, 1998; Mannix et al., 1997]. Not only does caffeine seem to have an influence on headache, it also may disrupt sleep or aggravate mood, both of which can exacerbate headache. Furthermore, caffeine withdrawal headache, which begins 1 to 2 days after cessation of regular caffeine use, can last up to a week [Dusseldorp and Katan, 1990]. Every effort must be made to moderate caffeine use.

The pharmacologic management of pediatric migraine has been subjected to thorough review, and controlled data are, unfortunately, limited (Table 53-5) [Lewis et al., 2004a; Victor and Ryan, 2003].

For the acute treatment of migraine, the most rigorously studied agents are ibuprofen, acetaminophen, and sumatriptan nasal spray, all of which have been found to be safe and efficacious in controlled trials. Although none of the triptan agents has yet been approved by the U.S. Food and Drug Administration for use in children and adolescents, multiple studies have demonstrated the safety of their use in children [Major et al., 2003]. Thus far, only sumatriptan in the nasal spray form (5 and 20 mg) has demonstrated efficacy in adolescents [Ahonen et al., 2004; Ueberall, 2001; Winner et al., 2000]. For young children, younger than 12 years of age, ibuprofen (7.5 to 10 mg/kg) and acetaminophen (15 mg/kg) have demonstrated efficacy and safety for the acute treatment of migraine [Hamalainen et al., 1997; Lewis et al., 2002b]. Butalbital preparations are no longer recommended.

For preventive or prophylactic treatment in the population of children and adolescents with frequent, disabling migraine, flunarizine (not available in the United States) is the most efficacious agent, but encouraging data are emerging regarding several antiepileptic agents such as topiramate, sodium valproate, and levetiracetam, as well as the antihistamine cyproheptadine and the antidepressant amitriptyline [Ferrera and Reicho, 1996; Hershey et al., 2002; Lewis et al., 2004b; Miller, 2004; Serdaroglu et al., 2002].

OTHER PRIMARY HEADACHE SYNDROMES

Chronic Daily Headache

Many adolescents report the experience of headache virtually every day, sometimes, during every waking hour. This chronic, nonprogressive, unremitting, daily, or near daily, pattern of headache represents one of the most difficult subsets of headache known as *chronic daily headache*. Chronic daily headache may be formally defined as longer than 4 months during which the patient has more than 15 headaches per month, with the headaches lasting more than 4 hours per day. The estimated prevalence of chronic daily headache in adolescents is about 1% and may be as high as 4% of the adult population [Abu-Arefeh and Russell, 1994; Castillo et al., 1999; Lipton and Stewart, 1997]. Chronic daily headache is very common in referral headache clinics, where up to 15% to 20% of patients present with daily or near-daily head pain [Viswanathan et al., 1998].

Understandably, the quality of life of patients with chronic daily headache is significantly influenced. The negative effect extends beyond the affected patient to family, friends, and society as a whole. The extensive disability that results from chronic daily headache can be measured in school absence, abstinence from after-school activities, and family discord that invariably results. Therefore early diagnosis and management of frequent or chronic daily headaches are essential.

Four primary chronic headache categories have been identified:

Chronic migraine ("transformed" migraine)
Chronic tension-type
New daily persistent headache
Hemicranium continuum

Chronic ("transformed") migraine represents chronic daily migraines that have slowly evolved from episodic migraine headache, whereas the chronic tension-type headaches evolved from episodic tension-type headaches. The new daily persistent headaches appeared to represent a unique entity in that the chronic daily headaches started quite abruptly, de nouveau, without any history of previous headache syndrome. Uncommon in children, hemicrania continua represented a cluster variant with daily or continuous unilateral pain with conjunctival injection, lacrimation, rhinorrhea and, occasionally, ptosis. One of the key features of hemicrania continua is responsiveness to indomethacin.

Each of these four types of chronic daily headache is further separated into those with or without superimposed analgesic overuse. The medications implicated in this analgesic overuse syndrome include most over-the-counter analgesics (e.g., acetaminophen, aspirin, ibuprofen), opioids, butalbital, isometheptene, benzodiazepines, ergotamine, and the triptans [Mathew et al., 1990].

Secondary causes of the chronic daily headache pattern in children and adolescents include neoplasm, idiopathic intracranial hypertension (pseudotumor cerebri), hydrocephalus, chronic subdural hematomas, chronic sinusitis, glaucoma, malocclusion, temporomandibular dysfunction, and psychologic conditions. The "medicolegal headache" falls into this category as pending litigation tends to exacerbate stress

TABLE 53-5

Acute and Preventive Agents for Childhood Migraine

Acute Therapies					
AGENTS	**CLASSIFICATION OF EVIDENCE***	**"N"**	**EFFICACY**	**CLINICAL IMPRESSION OF EFFECT†**	**ADVERSE EFFECTS**
NSAIDs and Nonopiate Analgesics					
Ibuprofen	I	88	$P<0.05$*	+++	Infrequent
	I	84	$P<0.006$		
Acetaminophen	I	88	$P<0.05$*	++	Infrequent
Triptan agents					
Sumatriptan					
Nasal	I	14	$P<0.03$	+++	Occasional to frequent
	I	510	$P<0.05$		
	IV	58	78%		
	I	83	$P<0.003$		
Oral	IV	23	NS	++	Occasional to frequent
Subcutaneous	IV	17	64%	++	Occasional to frequent
	IV	50	78%		
Other oral triptans					Occasional to frequent
Rizatriptan	I	296	NS 66% active, 56% placebo	++	Occasional to frequent
Zolmitriptan	IV	38	85% 2.5 mg 70% 5.0 mg	++	Occasional to frequent

Commonly Used Agents for the Acute Treatment of Migraine

AGENTS	**DOSE**
Ibuprofen	7.5-10 mg/kg
Acetaminophen	15 mg/kg
Naproxen sodium	2.5-5 mg/kg
Triptans	
Sumatriptan	
Subcutaneous	6 mg
Tablets	25, 50, 100 mg
Nasal spray	5, 20 mg
Rizatriptan	5, 10 mg tablets 5, 10 mg oral disintegrating tablets
Zolmitriptan	2.5, 5 mg tablet 2.5, 5, mg oral disintegrating tablets 2.5 mg nasal spray
Frovatriptan	2.5 mg tablets
Almotriptan	6, 12.5 mg tablets
Eletriptan	20, 40 mg tablets
Naratriptan	1.0, 2.5 mg tablets

Preventive Therapies					
AGENTS	**CLASSIFICATION OF EVIDENCE***	**"N"**	**EFFICACY**	**CLINICAL IMPRESSION OF EFFECT†**	**ADVERSE EFFECTS**
Antiepileptic Medications					
Divalproex sodium/ sodium valproate	IV IV	42 10	76% had >50% reduction in headache frequency $P=0$	++ +++	Occasional to frequent
Topiramate	IV	75	$P<0.001$	+++	Occasional to frequent
Levetiracetam	IV	19	$P<0.0001$	+++	Occasional to frequent
Gabapentin	IV	18	80% ≥ 50% reduction in headache frequency and severity	++	Occasional

TABLE 53-5, *cont'd*

Acute and Preventive Agents for Childhood Migraine

AGENTS	CLASSIFICATION OF EVIDENCE*	"N"	EFFICACY	CLINICAL IMPRESSION OF EFFECT†	ADVERSE EFFECTS
Antidepressant Medications					
Trazodone	II	35	NS	0	Occasional to frequent
Pizotifen	I	47	NS	0	Occasional to frequent
Amitriptyline	IV	192			
	IV	73	80%		
			89%	+++	Occasional to frequent
Antihistamines					
Cyproheptadine	IV	30	83%	+++	Occasional to frequent
Calcium Channel Blockers					
Flunarizine	I	42	$P < 0.001$	+++	Occasional
	I	63	$P < 0.001$		
	IV	12	75% had 75%-100% reduction in headache frequency		
Nimodipine	I	37	NS	0	Occasional
Antihypertensive Agents					
Propranolol	II	39	81% had >66% reduction in headache frequency	++	Occasional to frequent
	II	28	NS	0	
	II	28	NS	0	
Timolol	II	19	NS	0	Occasional
Clonidine	II	43	NS	0	Occasional to frequent
	II	57	NS		
NSAID					
Naproxen sodium	IV	10	60% had >60% reduction in headache frequency	++	Occasional

Commonly Used Preventive Agents for Migraine Management

AGENTS	DOSE
Calcium Channel Blocker	
Flunarizine	5-10 mg daily
Antidepressant	
Amitriptyline	5-25 mg orally at bedtime
Antiepileptic Agents	
Topiramate	1-10 mg/kg divided bid
Sodium valproate	10-40 mg/kg Usual (250-500 mg extended release at bedtime)
Antihistamine	
Cyproheptadine	2-8 mg/day (at bedtime or divided bid)
Beta-Blockers	
Propranolol	2-4 mg/kg/day
Metoprolol	2-6 mg/kg/day
Atenolol	2-6 mg/kg/day
NSAID	
Naproxen sodium	250-500 mg bid

***American Academy of Neurology classification of evidence:**

Class I: Prospective, randomized, controlled clinical trial with masked outcome assessment, in a representative population.

The following are required:

A. Primary outcome(s) is/are clearly defined.

B. Exclusion/inclusion criteria are clearly defined.

C. Adequate accounting for dropouts and crossovers with numbers sufficiently low to have minimal potential for bias.

D. Relevant baseline characteristics are presented and are substantially equivalent among treatment groups, or there is appropriate statistical adjustment for differences.

Class II: Prospective matched group cohort study in a representative population with masked outcome assessment that meets A-D above *or* a randomized controlled trial in a representative population that lacks one criterion in A-D.

Class III: All other controlled trials (including well-defined natural history controls or patients serving as own controls) in a representative population in which outcome is independently assessed or independently derived by objective outcome measurement.

Class IV: Evidence from uncontrolled studies, case series, case reports, or expert opinion.

†**Classification of effect:** 0, ineffective: most patients get no improvement; +, somewhat effective: few patients get clinically significant improvement; ++, effective: some patients get clinically significant improvement; +++, very effective: most patients get clinically significant improvement.

NS, not significant; NSAID, nonsteroidal anti-inflammatory drug.

levels and contribute to prolongation of the headache syndrome. Because the patient and family who present with the complaint of chronic daily headache are understandably concerned about the possibility of organic causes, it is critical to consider and exclude possible secondary causes for the headache. No treatment regimen will be successful until clear and confident reassurances as to the absence of serious underlying disease are provided.

Breaking the cycle of chronic daily headache is the principal goal of management. Pharmacologic efforts, however, used in isolation, will be uniformly unsuccessful. Therefore, initiation of a multidisciplined approach with emphasis on preventive strategies takes precedence over the use of intermittent analgesics. This population of patients has already likely been overusing over-the-counter analgesic agents, so a fundamental change in treatment philosophy must be taught to the patient and family.

An integral part of the educational process will be the incorporation of wholesale lifestyle changes, such as regulation of sleep and eating habits, regular exercise, identification of triggering factors, stress management, biofeedback-assisted relaxation therapy, and biobehavioral programs (see Box 53-7) [Rothrock, 1999].

The genesis of the chronic daily headache pattern may have its roots in psychosocial factors. Therefore, thorough social and educational history must be explored. Issues relating to life at school (e.g., bullying, learning disabilities), family conflict (e.g., parental discord, impending divorce), grief and loss (e.g., grandparent's illness, break-up of personal relationship), drug and alcohol use, and other factors shed light on a teenager's world that help the practitioner and patient understand some of the issues that may complicate management.

For the chronic daily headache population, a group of lifestyle changes must be incorporated into the treatment plan. This maintenance of a healthy lifestyle includes the following five major components:

1. Return to the routine of adolescent "life"
2. Adequate and regular sleep
3. Regular exercise (20 to 30 minutes per day of aerobic exercise)
4. Balanced nutrition, including avoidance of skipping meals
5. Adequate fluid intake with avoidance of caffeine

The pharmacologic treatment of chronic daily headaches requires an individually tailored regimen with the judicious use of appropriate prophylactic and analgesic agents. Recognizing the degree of disability helps guide the aggressiveness of the management. Unfortunately, no controlled studies have explored the pharmacologic management of chronic daily headache in children.

Preventive Therapy for Chronic Daily Headache

For the population of children and adolescents with chronic daily headache, preventive therapy takes center stage and represents the mainstay of drug treatment (Table 53-6). Because the majority of children with chronic daily headache have chronic migraine or have prominent migrainous features, a modification of standard migraine therapy is appropriate, but emphasis must be placed on prevention measures rather than analgesic or abortive strategies. The one exception may be patients with a recent onset of chronic daily headache attributed almost exclusively to analgesic rebound. In this infrequent group, a trial of an analgesic-free period as noted earlier may be the sole successful treatment.

Preventive therapies used for chronic daily headache include tricyclic antidepressants, antiepileptic agents, beta-blockers, serotonergic agents, and calcium channel blockers; however, none of these medications have been subjected to control trials and none are currently approved for the prevention of headaches in children [Redillas and Solomons, 2000].

When making the clinical decision regarding choice of pharmacologic agents, it is important to consider comorbid conditions. For the patient with difficulty falling asleep, amitriptyline at bedtime may provide dual benefits. Similarly, if there are mild-to-moderate affective issues, amitriptyline, valproic acid, or one of the selective serotonin reuptake inhibitors may be beneficial. If there is comorbid obesity, topiramate may decrease the appetite. Alternatively, if the patient's appetite is low, valproate often stimulates the appetite.

TABLE 53-6

Preventive Agents for the Treatment of Chronic Daily Headache in Adolescents

Antidepressant Agents	
Amitriptyline	5-25 mg orally at bedtime
Antiepileptic Agents	
Topiramate	50-100 mg orally bid
Sodium valproate	250-500 mg orally bid
	500 mg extended-release preparation
Nonsteroidal Anti-inflammatory Agents	
Naproxen	250-500 mg orally bid
Antihypertensive Agents	
Propranolol	60-120 mg orally once a day
Antihistamines	
Cyproheptadine	2–8 mg orally divided tid, bid, or at bedtime

ANTIDEPRESSANTS

The tricyclic antidepressant amitriptyline has been widely used for the prevention of migraine headaches. The mechanism of action is unclear but thought to be due to a multiple reuptake inhibitor action. The agent is well tolerated in children and adolescents; its side effects are attributable to their anticholinergic effects with additional concerns of cardiac dysrhythmias. The most frequently cited side effect is sedation. To minimize the side effects, a slow taper starting at 0.25 mg/kg (5 to 10 mg) and increasing by 0.25 mg every 2 to 3 weeks until dose of 1 mg/kg (10 to 25 mg) results in a well-tolerated, effective management [Hershey et al., 2000]. Selective serotonin reuptake inhibitors have not been studied for chronic daily headache, but may have a role in those patients with comorbid depression.

ANTIEPILEPTICS

Several antiepileptic drugs have been effective in preventing adult migraine; however, very limited evidence is available for children.

Topiramate, one of the newer antiepileptic drugs, has demonstrated efficacy in preventing adult and adolescent migraine [Brandes et al., 2004]. A multicenter, double-blind, placebo-controlled multidose trial included patients between the ages of 12 and 65 years with a 6-month history of International Headache Society migraine and 3 to 12 migraines per month but excluded patients with more than 15 headache days per month. A significant reduction in headache frequency was demonstrated at doses of 50 to 100 mg twice a day. Adverse events resulting in discontinuation in the topiramate groups included paresthesias, fatigue, and nausea.

One retrospective study assessing the efficacy of topiramate for pediatric headache included 41 evaluable patients. Topiramate at daily doses of 1.4 (± 0.74) mg/kg/day were reached and headache frequency was reduced from 16.5 (± 10) headaches per month to 11.6 (± 10) headaches per month ($P < 0.001$). Mean headache severity, duration, and accompanying disability were also reduced. Side effects included cognitive changes (12.5%), weight loss (5.6%), and sensory symptoms (2.8%) [Hershey et al., 2002]. This study population was predominantly children with very frequent migraine headaches approaching the spectrum of chronic daily headache as defined by more than 15 headaches per month.

The most common side effects observed included paresthesias, weight loss, and cognitive problems. The cognitive problems appear to decline with use, and can be minimized by slow taper, starting at a very low dose. This starting dose may be as low as 12.5 mg. per day, and slowly increased by 12.5 to 25 mg every 2 weeks to a dose of 50 mg twice a day [Hershey et al., 2002]. The weight loss needs to be monitored, although for the majority it does not appear to be significant.

Sodium valproate is effective and approved for the prevention of migraines in adults [Mathew et al., 1995]. It is also effective for chronic daily headache and in an extended-release formulation [Freitag et al., 2001; 2002]. A small study of 42 patients, demonstrated that it was effective and well tolerated in 7- to 16-year-olds [Caruso et al., 2000]. Two of the side effects that may limit its use in adolescents include weight gain and the development of ovarian cysts.

Gabapentin has also been used for prevention of adult headaches. It appears to be well tolerated; however, its effectiveness in children and adolescents is unknown [Mathew et al., 2001].

ANTIHISTAMINES

The antihistamine cyproheptadine has been widely used for the prevention of migraine headaches in young children, but it has not been studied in chronic daily headache [Bille et al., 1977]. It tends to be very well tolerated, with its most significant side effects being sedation and weight gain, specifically limiting its tolerability in adolescents.

BETA-BLOCKERS

Both propranolol and atenolol have been approved for the prevention of migraines in adults. There are conflicting data regarding the efficacy of propranolol for migraine in children and there are no data regarding its use in chronic daily headache. The exact dosing parameters have also not been identified. Two of its more common side effects of concern for children include exacerbation of reactive airway disease and depression. This reactive airway disease may be of special concern for the athletic adolescent who is unaware of the conditon until the combination of exercise and a beta-blocker results in shortness of breath.

NONSTEROIDAL ANTI-INFLAMMATORY AGENTS

Naproxen sodium was shown to be effective in adolescent migraine in one small (n = 10) trial using a double-blind, placebo-controlled crossover design [Lewis et al., 1994]. Sixty percent of the patients experienced a more than 60% reduction in headache frequency and severity with naproxen 250 mg twice a day, whereas only 40% responded favorably to placebo. No adverse effects were noted in this study. Naproxen should not be used for longer than 8 weeks because of potential gastrointestinal toxicity.

Naproxen is often used in conjunction with amitriptyline or topiramate. Patients are begun on a schedule of 250 to 500 mg twice a day and at the same time an evening dose of 5 to 25 mg of amitriptyline is started. After about 4 to 6 weeks, the naproxen is discontinued and the amitriptyline continued. Alternatively, naproxen is begun and topiramate titrated upward by 25 mg per week to a target dose of 50 to 100 mg twice a day. Naproxen is then discontinued after 6 to 8 weeks and topiramate continued.

Analgesic Agents for Chronic Daily Headache

The use of analgesic agents for children and adolescents with chronic daily headache is controversial, particularly in view of a growing body of literature regarding analgesic overuse in children. Because the children describe continuous or near-continuous pain, it is often difficult to decide when and how to use analgesics to avoid the "slippery slope" of analgesic overuse. One approach is to map or graph the pattern of headaches to identify the epochs of intense migraine pain when it arises from the background daily pain, at which time analgesics, including the triptan agents, may be most useful. Patients with chronic daily headache are often able to report that they may have headache every waking hour, but twice a week they have an intense headache that likely represents the migraine component. Once this is teased out of the history, analgesics can be more rationally used. Analgesic overuse may be one of the leading precipitants of the phenomenon of chronic daily headache, so care must be taken not to fan the flames further with overuse. The keys for effective use include catching the migraine component of the headache as soon as it starts, using an adequate dose, and avoiding overuse.

Nonpharmacologic Measures for Chronic Daily Headache

A variety of vitamins (e.g., riboflavin), minerals (e.g., magnesium), and herbal remedies (e.g., feverfew) have been attempted for prevention of headaches. Unfortunately, none of these remedies has been thoroughly evaluated in children with chronic daily headache but may play a role, particularly in families in which traditional pharmacologic approaches are considered unacceptable (see Box 53-7).

Biofeedback-assisted relaxation training has been shown to be an effective treatment for aborting and preventing recurrent headaches in a large number of studies in children. This technique is typically taught over a multisession analysis. It is also effective in a single session with tape recordings provided for home practie [Powers et al., 2001]. It does require a degree of motivation in the child and is difficult to assess effectiveness in isolation. However, it has low side effect potential, and may provide a benefit, including moderation of stress as well as sleep-onset difficulties.

Psychologic or psychiatric intervention is quite valuable if emotional comorbidity has been demonstrated [Juant et al., 2000]. In addition, if stress has been implicated as a possible migraine trigger, psychologic or psychiatric intervention, stress management, or self-hypnosis may be beneficial for chronic daily headache treatment and management.

The outcome of adolescents with chronic daily headache is poorly understood. No long-term follow-up data exist. One abstracted report provides short-term follow-up of 24 adolescents with a peak age 13 years and chronic daily headache of whom greater than half experienced a more than 75% reduction in headache frequency and one third experienced a greater than 90% improvement in a 6-month follow-up. A wide variety of preventive agents were used, but amitriptyline and topiramate provided the largest proportion of successful outcomes.

Tension-Type Headache

Tension-type headache may be episodic or chronic, the differentiation being a lower frequency (fewer than 15 days per month) with episodic and greater frequency (more than 15 days per month) for chronic tension-type headache. Episodic tension-type headache may be the most prevalent type of all primary headaches, but infrequently prompts referral to subspecialty clinics. Pathophysiologically, tension-type and migraine headaches may be similar, and there is a growing appreciation that the two may lie within the same spectrum, with milder, less disabling headache being tension-type and the more severe patterns being migraine. The diagnostic criteria for tension-type headache (see Box 53-3) emphasize the distinction from migraine. Generally, nausea and vomiting are not present in tension-type headache, and either photophobia or phonophobia may be present, but not both. On occasion, associated symptoms such as tiredness, sleep disturbances, and light-headedness may occur with episodic tension-type headache.

The management of tension-type headache has not been rigorously studied, but simple over-the-counter analgesics are commonly used. Various agents such as acetaminophen (1000 mg), ibuprofen (400 to 600 mg), or naproxen (220-500 mg) may be very helpful. A major concern is with overuse of these types of medications. Chronic tension-type headache is often associated with a significant degree of stress and anxiety for the child and family because of the frequent, unrelenting nature of this type of headache (see "Chronic Daily Headache").

Cranial Neuralgias

Ophthalmoplegic Migraine

Once classified as migraine, ophthalmoplegic migraine is now viewed as a cranial neuralgia but oddly is still called migraine. Migraine is one of the most dramatic and clinically challenging headache syndromes and, fortunately, one of the least common. Available epidemiologic data suggest an annual incidence of 0.7 per million [Hansen et al., 1990]. The two key features are ophthalmoparesis and headache, although the headache may be mild or a nondescript retro-orbital discomfort. Ptosis, adduction defects, and skew deviations are the common objective findings.

The clinical course of ophthalmoplegic migraine is quite different from that of the more commonly encountered migraine with a heralding "aura." Symptoms and signs of oculomotor dysfunction may appear well into the headache phase rather than precede the headache. The signs may persist for days or even weeks after the headache has resolved.

The oculomotor nerve, or its divisions, is most frequently involved, but pupillary involvement is inconsistent and controversial. Some authors report pupillary involvement in only one third of patients [Vijayan, 1980]. The third nerve involvement may be incomplete, with partial deficits in both inferior and superior division of the third nerve. Abduction defects, due to abducens involvement, are the second most frequent reported variants of ophthalmoplegic migraine, and trochlear nerve involvement is the least common.

The mechanism of ophthalmoplegic migraine is controversial. The primary theories suggest ischemic, compressive, or inflammatory processes [Stommel et al., 1994]. Lack of pupillary involvement argues for an ischemic mechanism, whereas a higher incidence of pupillary involvement weighs toward a compressive mechanism. Alternatively, recent reports have questioned whether ophthalmoplegic migraine may be an inflammatory process within the spectrum of Tolosa-Hunt syndrome, particularly given the steroid responsiveness of many patients. Furthermore, high-resolution neuroimaging has demonstrated a reversible enhancement and even thickening of the oculomotor nerve during attacks, which lends further credence to an inflammatory mechanism [Mark et al., 1998]. The most recent International Headache Society classification comments that ophthalmoplegic migraine may be a recurrent demyelinating neuropathy.

The differential diagnosis for ophthalmoplegic migraine includes aneurysm or mass lesion in or around the orbital apex and parasellar region. Imaging study with MRI or magnetic resonance angiography is usually indicated.

Repeated attacks of ophthalmoplegic migraine can lead to permanent deficits; therefore, acute treatment with steroids and prophylactic treatment must be considered.

Occipital neuralgia is characterized by a stabbing pain in the upper neck or occipital region, often precipitated by neck flexion or head rotation. It may occur post-traumatically. Examination of the craniocervical region may disclose point tenderness, C-2 distribution sensory changes, or limitation of motion. MRI of the craniocervical junction is warranted to exclude congenital or pathologic processes.

Treatment includes soft collars, nonsteroidal anti-inflammatory drugs (naproxen), muscle relaxants, local injections, and physical therapy. The prognosis is good.

A similar entity is neck-tongue syndrome, wherein head movements trigger occipital pain accompanied by ipsilateral tongue numbness. Again, craniocervical anomalies must be sought, though the majority of children and adolescents have not demonstrated abnormalities, and it occasionally occurs in families.

Cluster Headache

Cluster headache is uncommon in children and adolescents. The prevalence of childhood onset of cluster is approximately 0.1% [Lampl, 2002].

The diagnostic criteria require at least five attacks of severe unilateral orbital pain lasting 15 to 180 minutes with a sense of restless agitation accompanied by ipsilateral conjunctival injection, lacrimation, nasal congestion, rhinorrhea, eyelid edema, forehead sweating, miosis, or ptosis. Cluster headaches may be episodic or chronic, and attacks occur in series that last for weeks or even months. A cluster headache may be precipitated by alcohol, histamine, or nitroglycerin. Males are three times more likely to be affected than females.

Management is difficult. Acute treatments include inhalation of 100% oxygen at 8 to 10 L/minute for 10 to 15 minutes through a nonrebreathing facemask; sumatriptan 6 mg subcutaneous injections or 20 mg intranasally; and intravenous, intramuscular, or subcutaneous injections of dihydroergotamine, 0.5 to 1 mg, at headache onset. Prophylactic medications useful in preventing attacks during cluster cycles include verapamil, sodium valproate, lithium carbonate, methysergide, and ergotamine tartrate [Newman et al., 2001].

Paroxysmal Hemicrania

Paroxysmal hemicrania is a cluster-like syndrome characterized by intense attacks of periorbital pain lasting only 5 to 30 minutes but occurring up to dozens of times per day. In distinction to cluster headache, there are no accompanying autonomic symptoms of lacrimation or rhinorrhea. One of the most striking features is the exquisite responsiveness to indomethacin (25 to 50 mg/day), which has prompted the alternative nosology, "indomethacin-sensitive" headache.

Temporomandibular Joint Dysfunction

Temporomandibular joint dysfunction manifests with unilateral pain just anterior or inferior to the ear. The pain is aggravated by chewing, teeth clenching, or yawning. Patients may describe a clicking or locking of their jaw. Family members may describe bruxism, and there may be antecedent trauma. Examination reveals tenderness over the temporomandibular joint and limitation of mouth opening. Treatment includes nonsteroidal anti-inflammatory drugs, muscle relaxation, and avoidance of provocative processes like chewing gum or hard candy. Major oral surgery is rarely necessary.

SPECIFIC SECONDARY HEADACHE SYNDROMES

Post-traumatic Headache

Headache following closed-head injury or neck trauma in children is one of the most common secondary headache syndromes but has not been systematically studied. No epidemiologic data are available. Post-traumatic headache is divided into acute and chronic patterns based on duration of symptoms, less than 3 months being acute, and greater than 3 months being chronic.

Acute post-traumatic headache must immediately raise concerns for traumatic brain injury such as cerebral hematoma (subdural or epidural), subarachnoid hemorrhage, cerebral contusion, or skull fracture and warrant urgent neuroimaging, particularly if associated with alteration of consciousness, seizures or Glasgow Coma Scale less than 13. Cerebrospinal fluid leaks following meningeal tears can lead to positional, or "low pressure" headaches.

Post-traumatic headache may arise within hours or up to a week after head injury, and the clinical manifestations are quite variable. "Footballer's migraine" may occur immediately after relatively minor head trauma that occurs playing sports such as soccer or football, and may happen after accidental head injury. The clinical features of confusion, language disorders, and agitation are discussed in earlier sections of this chapter (see "Confusional Migraine").

Chronic post-traumatic headache may be part of a global postconcussive syndrome with behavioral changes (e.g., hyperactivity, hypoactivity), dizziness, tinnitus, vertigo, blurred vision, memory changes, sleep disorder, irritability, and attentional disorders. The duration of symptoms is variable, with some patients having brief, self-limited syndromes, others suffering from headaches for greater than 6 months. One retrospective study of 23 children with chronic post-traumatic headache found a mean duration of 13.3 months (range 2 to 60 months, median 7 months) [Callaghan, 2001]. The headache forms span the spectrum from tension-type, migraine, chronic daily headache, neuralgias (e.g., occipital neuralgia), temporomandibular joint, and on rare occasions, cluster headache.

Many athletes competing in contact sports experience post-traumatic headache as part of a postconcussion syndrome. A common question is when it is safe to return to a full-contact sport. Two organizations, the American Academy of Neurology and the American College of Sports Medicine, have provided guidelines regarding return to activities, which range from 1 to 4 weeks [American College of Sports Medicine, 1991; Quality Standards Subcommittee, American Academy of Neurology, 1997]. Both guidelines are available online.

The management of post-traumatic headache requires an appreciation of the degree of disability produced by the headache. Post-traumatic tension-type headaches can generally be managed with nonsteroidal anti-inflammatory agents such as ibuprofen or naproxen sodium. Post-traumatic migraine is treated as discussed earlier with a balance of analgesic or triptan agents and, if warranted, daily preventive therapies. For patients with frequent or daily headaches, the management strategies in the chronic daily headache discussion apply with daily preventive programs, both pharmacologic and nonpharmacologic, as well as analgesics, for episodes of intense pain.

There are no outcome data on post-traumatic headache in children and adolescents, but typically, 3 to 6 months is the anticipated course of recovery. If the post-traumatic headache syndrome is associated with pending "personal injury" litigation, stress levels and compensation issues may contribute to prolongation of the headache syndrome.

Idiopathic Intracranial Hypertension

Also known as *pseudotumor cerebri*, idiopathic intracranial hypertension produces a global, daily, pounding headache and is an important consideration in the differential diagnosis of chronic daily headache. The incidence of idiopathic intracranial hypertension is 3.5 to 19 per 100,000 population; the majority of sufferers are female. Neck stiffness (30% to 59%) and transient visual disturbances may be present. The key finding on physical examination is papilledema. Neuroimaging will likely be normal. The pathogenesis of idiopathic intracranial hypertension is unclear but somehow involves impairment of cerebrospinal reabsorption. Idiopathic intracranial hypertension can be caused by multiple disorders including endocrinopathies (e.g., hypothyroidism, Addison's disease, oral steroids), pregnancy, drugs (e.g., tetracycline, oral contraceptive agents), vitamin A intoxication, anemia, systemic lupus erythematosus, chronic sinopulmonary infection, and obesity, or it may be idiopathic.

Other secondary headaches that present with chronic daily headache include intoxications of lead or other heavy metals, chronic carbon monoxide poisoning, chronic meningitis with such pathogens as tuberculosis, fungi, or spirochetal syphilis and Lyme disease. A chronic daily pattern can also be seen with central nervous system leukemia or lymphoma or leptomeningeal metastasis. Rarely, diffuse "butterfly" gliomatosis of the brain can produce this picture, but cognitive decline and pyramidal tract signs would be expected. Uncontrolled hypertension can lead to optic disc changes with headache, but this would be uncommon during adolescence. Chronic sinusitis or venous sinus thrombosis can also produce a pattern of slowly increasing intracranial pressure with normal computed tomography scan.

The diagnostic test of choice for idiopathic intracranial hypertension is lumbar puncture with measurement of opening pressure. Given a normal computed tomography scan, the test can be accomplished safely even though the examination shows a fifth nerve palsy because this can be a "false localizing" sign, indicative of diffuse increase in intracranial pressure. The mechanism is likely compressive, though some degree of ischemia to the fifth nerve can occur in this setting.

The normal cerebrospinal fluid opening pressure is less than 180 mm of water; in idiopathic intracranial hypertension, the opening pressure will exceed 200 mm of water, often exceeding 400 mm of water. Cerebrospinal fluid must be collected for glucose, protein, cell counts, and bacterial cultures. Neuroborreliosis can mimic idiopathic intracranial hypertension, so polymerase chain reaction studies for Lyme disease may be indicated. If cerebrospinal fluid pleocytosis is found, cultures (fungal and tuberculosis) and special studies for detection of fungi (cryptococcal antigen), syphilis, and cytopathology may be considered.

Not only does the lumbar puncture yield critical diagnostic information, but the relief of pressure also usually provides significant decrease in headache symptoms. The volume of cerebrospinal fluid to be removed is controversial. Generally, removal of sufficient volume to lower the pressure down to about 200 mm of water is valid and safe. Care must be taken to limit the risk of post–lumbar puncture headache by keeping the patient recumbent for several hours after the lumbar puncture.

Once the diagnosis is established, the carbonic anhydrase inhibitor acetazolamide can be used to lower cerebrospinal fluid pressures, probably by a diuretic mechanism. The side effects are few and include paresthesias, polyuria, and sedation. The dose is typically 250 mg twice a day up to 1000 mg per day. There is a once daily preparation available. The recovery is slow, taking weeks or months. If obesity is a contributing factor, a weight loss program is recommended. If the visual symptoms are severe, progressive, or if there is visual compromise, ophthalmologic intervention may be necessary with performance of an optic nerve sheath fenestration.

Brain Tumor Headache

About two thirds of children with brain tumors have headache as a presenting symptom. There is, however, no invariable "brain tumor headache" profile. A steady, gradual rise in intracranial pressure typically produces the chronic progressive pattern, but on occasion an anaplastic tumor or hemorrhage into tumor may cause an acute pattern (see Fig. 53-1). Several historical clues suggest space-occupying lesions such as brain tumors, but these clues may also be present in other expanding masses such as brain abscess, hematoma, or vascular anomaly. Morning headache or headaches that awaken the child from sleep are classic symptoms of the dependent edema of intracranial lesions. Likewise, nocturnal or morning emesis, with or without headache, suggests increased intracranial pressure and is a particularly common symptom of tumors arising near the floor of the fourth ventricle. Head pain aggravated by exertion or Valsalva's maneuver suggests a mass lesion. In addition to headache, parents may note behavioral or mood changes, cognitive changes, or declining school performance.

Accompanying symptoms may suggest localized disturbances of neurologic function. Ocular symptoms are common: loss of vision (e.g., craniopharyngioma, optic pathway tumors) or diplopia (e.g., brainstem glioma, medulloblastoma). Disorders of coordination such as truncal ataxia (e.g., medulloblastoma, ependymoma) or dysmetria (e.g., cerebellar astrocytoma) suggest posterior fossa tumors. The presence of seizures indicates cortical disturbances often localized to the temporal lobes.

The key physical examination signs that indicate brain tumor include the following:

Papilledema
Abnormal eye movements
Hemiparesis
Ataxia (truncal or appendicular)
Abnormal tendon reflexes [The Childhood Brain Tumor Consortium, 1991]

As stated in the American Academy of Neurology practice parameter, neuroimaging (MRI or CT) is appropriate for children with headache in whom there are historical features or recent onset of severe headache, a change in the type of headache, or focal neurologic dysfunction. Neuroimaging should also be considered in children with an abnormal neurologic examination (e.g., focal findings, signs of increased intracranial pressure, significant alteration of consciousness) or coexisting seizures.

REFERENCES

Abu-Arefeh I, Russell G. Prevalence of headache and migraine in schoolchildren. BMJ 1994;309:765.

Ahonen K, Hamalainen ML, Rantala H, et al. Nasal sumatriptan is effective in the treatment of migraine attacks in children. Neurology 2004;62:883.

Aicardi J, Bourgeois M, Goutieres F. Alternating hemiplegia of childhood: Clinical findings and diagnostic criteria. In: Andermann F, Aicardi J, Vigevano F, eds. Alternating hemiplegia of childhood. New York: Raven Press, 1995;3.

American College of Emergency Physicians: Clinical policy for the initial approach to adolescents and adults presenting to the emergency department with a chief complaint of headache. Ann Emerg Med 1996;27:821.

American College of Sports Medicine. Guidelines for the management of concussion in sports, Rev. ed. Denver: Colorado Medical Society; 1991.

Amit R. Acute confusional state in childhood. Child Nerv Syst 1988;4:255.

Barlow CF. Headaches and migraine in childhood. Clin Devel Med 1984;91:93.

Baumann RJ. Behavioral treatment of migraine in children and adolescents. Paediatr Drugs 2002;4(9):555.

Bickerstaff ER. Basilar artery migraine. Lancet 1961;1:15.

Bille B. Migraine in school children. Acta Paediatr 1962;51 (Suppl 136): 1.

Bille B, Ludvigsson J, Sanner G. Prophylaxis of migraine in children. Headache 1977;17:61.

Brandes JL, Saper JR, Diamond M, et al. Topiramate for migraine prevention: A randomized controlled trial. JAMA. 2004;291:965.

Burstein R, Jakubowski M. Analgesic triptan action in an animal model of intracranial pain: A race against the development of control sensitization. Ann Neurol 2004;55:27.

Burstein R, Collins B, Jakubowski M. Defeating migraine pain with triptans: A race against the development of cutaneous allodynia. Ann Neurol 2004;55:19.

Burstein R, Yarnitsky D, Goor-Aryeh I, et al. An association between migraine and cutaneous allodynia. Ann Neurol 2000;47:614.

Callaghan M. Chronic posttraumatic headache in children and adolescents. Dev Med Child Neurol 2001;43:819.

Caruso J, Brown W, Exil G, et al. The efficacy of divalproex sodium in the prophylactic treatment of children with migraine. Headache 2000;40:672.

Castillo J, Munoz P, Guitera V, et al. Epidemiology of chronic daily headache in the general population. Headache 1999;39:190.

Chaves-Carballo E. Paroxysmal torticollis. Semin Pediatr Neurol 1996;3:255.

The Childhood Brain Tumor Consortium.The epidemiology of headache among children with brain tumor. Headache in children with brain tumors. J Neurooncol 1991;10:31.

Chutorian AM. Benign paroxysmal torticollis, tortipelvis and retrocollis of infancy. Neurology 1974;24:366.

Dalsgaard-Nielsen T. Some aspects of the epidemiology of migraine in Denmark. Headache 1970;10:14.

Deubner DC. An epidemiologic study of migraine and headache in 10–20 year olds. Headache 1977;17:173.

Dusseldorp M, Katan M. Headache caused by caffeine withdrawal among moderate coffee drinkers switched from ordinary to decaffeinated coffee: A 12 week double-blind trial. BMJ 1990; 300: 1558.

Ehyai A, Fenichel G. The natural history of acute confusional migraine. Arch Neurol 1978;35:368.

Ferrera PC, Reicho PR. Acute confusional migraine and trauma-triggered migraine. Am J Emerg Med 1996;14:276.

Freitag F, Collins S, Carlson H, et al. A randomized trial of divalproex sodium extended-release tablets in migraine prophylaxis. Neurology 2002;58:1652.

Freitag F, Diamond S, Diamond M, et al. Divalproex in the long-term treatment of chronic daily headache. Headache 2001;41:271.

Garcon G, Barlow CF. Juvenile migraine presenting as acute confusional states. Pediatrics 1970;45:628.

Gardner K, Barmada MM, Ptacek LJ, et al. A new locus for hemiplegic migraine maps to chromosome 1q31. Neurology 1997;49:1231.

Gibb C, Davies P, Glover V, et al. Chocolate is a migraine-provoking agent. Cephalalgia 1991;11:93.

Giffin NJ, Benton S, Goadsby PJ. Benign paroxysmal torticollis of infancy: Four new cases and linkage to CACNA1A mutation. Dev Med Child Neurol 2002;44:490.

Gladstein J, Holden E, Winner P, et al. Chronic daily headache in children and adolescents: Current status and recommendations for the future. Headache 1997;37:626.

Golden GS, French JH. Basilar artery migraine in young children. Pediatrics 1975;56:722.

Hachinshi VC, Porchawka J, Steele JC. Visual symptoms in the migraine syndrome. Neurology 1973;23:570.

Hamalainen ML, Hoppu K, Valkeila E, et al. Ibuprofen or acetaminophen for the acute treatment of migraine in children: A double-blind, randomized, placebo-controlled, crossover study. Neurology 1997;48:102.

Hansen SL, Borelli-Moller L, Strange P, et al. Ophthalmoplegic migraine: Diagnostic criteria, incidence of hospitalization, and possible etiology. Acta Neurol Scand 1990;81:54.

Hershey A, Powers S, Bentti A, et al. Effectiveness of amitriptyline in the prophylactic management of childhood headaches. Headache 2000;40:539.

Hershey AD, Powers SW, Vockell AL, et al. Effectiveness of topiramate in the prevention of childhood headache. Headache 2002;42:810.

Holroyd K, Mauskop A. Complementary and alternative treatments. Neurology 2003;60(Suppl 2):58.

James JE. Acute and chronic effects of caffeine on performance, mood, headache, and sleep. Neuropsychobiology 1998;38:32.

Jensen TS. Transient global amnesia in childhood. Dev Med Child Neurol 1980;5:654.

Joutel A, Bousser M-G, Biousse V, et al. A gene for familial hemiplegic migraine maps to chromosome 19. Nat Genet 1993;5:40.

Juant K, Wang S, Fuh J, et al. Comorbidity of depressive and anxiety disorders in chronic daily headache and its subtypes. Headache 2000;40:818.

Koseoglu E, Akboyraz A, Soyuer A, Ersoy AO. Aerobic exercise and plasma beta endorphin levels in patients with migrainous headache without aura. Cephalalgia 2003;10:972.

Lampl C. Childhood-onset cluster headache. Pediatr Neurol 2002;27:138.

Lapkin ML, Golden GS. Basilar artery migraine, a review of 30 cases. Am J Dis Child 1978;132:278.

La Spina I, Vignati A, Porazzi D, et al. Basilar artery migraine: Transcranial Doppler EEG and SPECT from the aura phase to the end. Headache 1997;37:43.

Laurell K, Larsson B, Eeg-Olofsson O. Prevalence of headache in Swedish schoolchildren, with a focus on tension-type headache. Cephalalgia 2004;24:380.

Lewis DW. Migraine and migraine variant in childhood and adolescence. Semin Pediatr Neurol 1995;2:127

Lewis DW, Ashwal S, Dahl G, et al. Practice parameter: Evaluation of children and adolescents with recurrent headache. Neurology 2002;59:490.

Lewis D, Ashwal S, Hershey A, Hirtz D, et al. Practice parameter: Pharmacological treatment of migraine headache in children and adolescents. Neurology 2004;63:2215.

Lewis D, Diamond S, Scott D, et al. Prophylactic treatment of pediatric migraine. Headache 2004;44:230.

Lewis DW, Kellstein D, Burke B, et al. Children's ibuprofen suspension for the acute treatment of pediatric migraine headache. Headache 2002;42:780.

Lewis DW, Middlebrook MT, Deline C. Naproxen sodium for chemoprophylaxis of adolescent migraine. Ann Neurol 1994;36:542.

Lewis DW, Middlebrook MT, Mehallick L, Rouch TM. Pediatric headaches: What do the children want? Headache 1996;36:224.

Lipton RB, Silberstein SD, Stewart WF. An update on the epidemiology of migraine. Headache 1994;34:319.

Lipton R, Stewart W. Prevalence and impact of migraine. Neurol Clin1997;15:1.

Major P, Grubisa H, Thie N. Triptans for the treatment of acute pediatric migraine: A systematic literature review. Pediatr Neurol 2003;29:425.

Mannix LK, Frame JR, Soloman GD. Alcohol, smoking and caffeine use among headache patients. Headache 1997;37:572.

Mark AS, Casselman J, Brown D, et al. Ophthalmoplegic migraine: Reversible enhancement and thickening of the cisternal segment of the oculomotor nerve on contrast-enhanced MR images. Am J Neuroradiol 1998;9:1887.

Mathew NT, Kurman R, Perez F. Drug-induced refractory headache—Clinical features and management. Headache 1990;30:634.

Mathew N, Rapoport A, Saper J, et al. Efficacy of gabapentin in migraine prophylaxis. Headache 2001; 41:119.

Mathew N, Saper J, Siberstein S, et al. Migraine prophylaxis with divalproex. Arch Neurol 1995;52:281.

Miller GS. Efficacy and safety of levetiracetam in pediatric migraine. Headache 2004;44:238.

Miller V, Palermao T, Powers S, et al. Migraine headaches and sleep disturbances in children. Headache 2003;43:362.

Millichap J, Yee M. The diet factor in pediatric and adolescent migraine. Pediatr Neurol 2003;28:9.

Mortimer MJ, Kay J, Jaron A. Epidemiology of headache and childhood migraine in an urban general practice using ad hoc, Vahlquist and IHS criteria. Dev Med Child Neurol 1992;34:1095.

Newman L, Goadsby P, Lipton R. Cluster and related headaches. Med Clin North Am 2001;85:997.

Olesen J. Headache Classification Committee of the International Headache Society. Classification and diagnostic criteria for headache disorders, cranial neuralgia, and facial pain. Cephalgia 1988;8(Suppl 7): 1.

Oleson J. The international classification of headache disorders. Cephalalgia 2004;24(Suppl 1): 1.

Olness K, MacDonald JT, Uden DL. Comparison of self-hypnosis and propranolol in the treatment of juvenile classic migraine. Pediatrics 1987;79:593.

Ophoff RA, Terwindt GM, Vergouwe MN, et al. Involvement of a Ca^{2+} channel gene in familial hemiplegic migraine and migraine with and without aura. Headache 1997;37:479.

Pietrobon D, Striessnig J. Neurobiology of migraine. Nature Revs 2003;4:386.

Powers S, Mitchell M, Byars K, et al. Effectiveness of one-session biofeedback training in a pediatric headache center: A pilot study. Neurology 2001;56:133.

Powers S, Patton S, Hommel K, Hershey A. Quality of life in childhood migraine: Clinical aspects and comparison to other chronic illness. Pediatrics 2003;112:e1.

Powers S, Patton S, Hommell K, Hershey A. Quality of life in paediatric migraine: Characterization of age-related effects using PedsQL 4.0. Cephalalgia 2004;24:120.

Prensky AL, Sommer D. Diagnosis and treatment of migraine in children. Neurology 1979;29:506.

Quality Standards Subcommittee, American Academy of Neurology. Practice parameter. The management of concussions in sports. Neurology 1997;48:581.

Redillas C, Solomons S. Prophylactic pharmacological treatment of chronic daily headache. Headache 2000;40:83.

Reimschisel T. Breaking the cycle of medication overuse headache. Contemp Pediatr 2003;20:101.

Rho JM, Chugani HT. Alternating hemiplegia of childhood: Insights into its pathogenesis. J Child Neurol 1998;13:39.

Rothner A, Guo Y. An analysis of headache types, over-the-counter (OTC) medication overuse and school absences in a pediatric/adolescent headache clinic. Headache 2004;44:490.

Rothner AD. Miscellaneous headache syndromes in children and adolescents. Semin Pediatr Neurol 1995;2:159.

Rothrock J. Management of chronic daily headache utilizing a uniform treatment pathway. Headache 1999;39:650.

Serdaroglu G, Erhan E, Tekgul, et al. Sodium valproate prophylaxis in childhood migraine. Headache 2002;42:819.

Silberstein S. Migraine. Lancet 2004;31:381.

Silberstein SD. Practice parameter: Evidence-based guidelines for migraine headache (an evidence-based review). Neurology 2000;55:754.

Sillanpaa M. Prevalence of migraine and other headache in Finnish children starting school. Headache 1976;15:288.

Sillanpaa M. Changes in the prevalence of migraine and other headache during the first seven school years. Headache 1983;23:15.

Small P, Waters WE. Headache and migraine in a comprehensive school. In: Waters, ed. The epidemiology of migraine. Bracknell-Berkshire, England: Boehringer Ingel-helm, Ltd., 1974;56.

Snyder CH. Paroxysmal torticollis in infancy. A possible form of labyrinthitis. Am J Dis Child 1969;117:458.

Stang P, Yanagihar P, Swanson J, et al. Incidnece of migraine headache: A population based study in Olmsted County, Minn. Neurology 1992;42: 1657.

Stewart WF, Linet MS, Celentano DD, et al. Age and sex-specific incidence rates of migraine with and without visual aura. Am J Epidemiol 1991;34:1111.

Stewart WF, Lipton RB, Celentano DD, Reed ML. Prevalence of migraine headache in the United States. JAMA 1992;267:64.

Stommel EW, Ward D, Harris R, et al. Ophthalmoplegic migraine or Tolosa-Hunt syndrome? Headache 1994;34:177.

Swoboda KJ, Kanavakis E, Xaidara A, et al. Alternating hemiplegia of childhood or familial hemiplegic migraine? A novel ATP1A2 mutation. Ann Neurol 2004;55:884.

Ueberall M. Sumatriptan in paediatric and adolescent migraine. Cephalalgia 2001;21(Suppl 1):21.

Valquist B. Migraine in children. Int Arch Allergy 1955; 7:348.

Van den Bergh V, Amery W, Waelkens J. Trigger factors in migraine: A study conducted by the Belgian Migraine Society. Headache 1987;27:191.

Verret S, Steele JC. Alternating hemiplegia in childhood: A report of eight patients with complicated migraine beginning in infancy. Pediatrics 1971;47:675.

Victor S, Ryan S. Drugs for preventing migraine headaches in children. Cochrane Database System Reviews 2003;4:CD 002761.

Vijayan N. Ophthalmoplegic migraine: Ischemic or compressive neuropathy? Headache 1980;20:300.

Viswanathan V, Bridges SJ, Whitehouse W, et al. Childhood headaches: Discrete entities or continuum? Dev Med Child Neurol 1998;40:544.

Winner P, Rothner AD, Saper J, et al. A randomized, double-blind, placebo-controlled study of sumatriptan nasal spray in the treatment of acute migraine in adolescents. Pediatrics 2000;106:989.

Zwart JA, Dyb G, Holmen TL, et al. The prevalence of migraine and tension-type headaches among adolescents in Norway. The Nord-Trondelag Health Study (Head-HUNT-Youth), a large population-based epidemiological study. Cephalalgia. 2004;24:373.

CHAPTER 54

Breath-Holding Spells and Reflex Anoxic Seizures

Sarah M. Roddy

Breath-holding spells and reflex anoxic seizures are nonepileptic paroxysmal events. The events are benign but can be frightening to parents and others observing an episode. It is important to differentiate these episodes from epileptic seizures so that the child is not inappropriately treated with antiepileptic medication.

Possibly the earliest report of breath-holding spells was published in 1737 by Nicholas Culpepper, who gave the following description:

> There is a disease … in children from anger or grief, when the spirits are much stirred and run from the heart to the diaphragms forceably, and hinder or stop the breath … but when the passion ceaseth, this symptom ceaseth.

The clinical characteristics were well recognized and described in the pediatric literature in the 19th and early 20th centuries. More recent reports have provided a better understanding of the pathophysiology of these events.

BREATH-HOLDING SPELLS

Clinical Features

The term *breath holding* is a misnomer and implies that the child is voluntarily holding his or her breath in a prolonged inspiration. Breath-holding episodes actually occur during expiration and are involuntary. Breath-holding spells are not uncommon, with an incidence of 4.6% to 4.7% [Linder, 1968; Lombroso and Lerman, 1967]. The typical age of onset is between 6 and 18 months, although occasionally the onset may occur in the first few weeks of life [Breukels et al., 2002]. Less than 10% have onset after 2 years of age [DiMario, 1992]. The frequency of episodes ranges from several times daily to once yearly. The spells are often spaced weeks to months apart at onset and increase in frequency to as many as several per day during the second year of life [Laxdal et al., 1969; DiMario, 2001]. Breath-holding spells are classified by the color change manifested in the child during an event. Cyanotic episodes are more common than pallid episodes. In some instances, there are features of both cyanosis and pallor, and these are termed *mixed episodes.*

Cyanotic breath-holding spells are often precipitated by emotional stimuli, such as anger or frustration. The child typically cries vigorously but usually for less than 15 seconds, then becomes silent, and holds the breath in expiration. The apnea is associated with the rapid onset of cyanosis. Some episodes may resolve at this point, but there may be loss of consciousness and a brief period of limpness followed by opisthotonic posturing. Recovery is usually within 1 minute, with the child having a few gasping respirations and then a return to regular breathing and consciousness.

Pallid breath-holding spells are usually provoked by sudden fright or pain. A fall with a minor injury to the head is frequently the precipitating event. An unexpected event or a surprise seems to play a role in triggering the spell. Sometimes the provoking event is not witnessed, and the child is found already in an episode. The child may gasp and cry, although it is usually for only a brief period of time. The child then becomes quiet, loses consciousness, and becomes pale. Limpness and diaphoresis are common. Clonic movements of the extremities and incontinence may occur with more severe episodes. Cyanosis may occur during the episode but is much milder than with cyanotic breath-holding spells. The child typically regains consciousness in less than 1 minute but may sleep for several hours after the episode.

An association between behavior problems, emotional factors, and breath-holding spells has been discussed by many investigators. Breath-holding spells were described by Abt [1918] as occurring in "neuropathic children of neuropathic parents." Bridge and colleagues [1943] stated that children susceptible to breath holding are usually of the active energetic type who react vigorously to situations and that episodes were precipitated by "spoiled child reactions." Breath-holding spells were felt to be a sign of a disturbed parent-child relationship by Kanner [1935]. Laxdal and associates [1969] reported that 30% of the children with breath-holding spells had abnormal behavior, including temper tantrums, hyperactivity, and stubbornness. To further investigate the role of behavior and breath holding, DiMario and Burleson [1993b] studied behavior in children with breath-holding spells compared with controls and found no differences in the behavioral profiles, suggesting that breath-holding spells are nonvolitional and cannot be equated with a temperamentally difficult child.

Breath-holding spells generally decrease in frequency during the second year of life. By 4 years of age, 50% of children will no longer have episodes. Almost all will have stopped having episodes by age 7 to 8 years [DiMario, 1992: Goraya and Virdi, 2001]. Syncopal episodes occur in late childhood or adolescence in as many as 17% of patients with breath-holding spells [Lombroso and Lerman, 1967].

Serious complications with breath-holding spells are rare. Taiwo and Hamilton [1993] reported a prolonged cardiac arrest in a patient with breath-holding spells. The few reported deaths may have been precipitated by aspiration or occurred in children who were at the severe end of the spectrum of breath holders, often with structural abnormalities of the respiratory tract or complicated medical histories [Paulson, 1963; Southall et al., 1987; 1990].

Clinical Laboratory Tests

A detailed history of the event, including the precipitating circumstances, is essential in making the diagnosis of breath-holding spells. If the event was not witnessed from onset, important details may not be available. A video recording by the parents may be helpful in confirming the diagnosis. Usually no laboratory tests are needed to make the diagnosis. An electroencephalogram (EEG) is usually not indicated unless the convulsive activity is prolonged or the clinical description is incomplete and epileptic seizures cannot be ruled out. If ocular compression is performed in patients with pallid breath-holding spells, there may be asystole on cardiac monitoring and slowing or suppression of voltage on EEG [Lombroso and Lerman, 1967; Stephenson, 1978]. Long-QT syndrome is rare but should be considered as part of the differential diagnosis in a child with breath-holding spells. Patients with long-QT syndrome have episodes of loss of consciousness that may be induced by injury, fright, or excitement. An electrocardiogram should be considered in any patient with breath-holding spells [Breningstall, 1996; Franklin and Hickey, 1995].

Pathophysiology

Cyanotic Spells

The pathophysiology of cyanotic breath-holding spells is complex and not completely understood. Cyanosis occurs early in the episode, which is unusual during voluntary breath holding. In breath-holding spells, the breath is held in full expiration, which also is not typical with voluntary breath holding [Livingston, 1970]. Gauk and colleagues [1963] studied a child during a cyanotic breath-holding episode with cinefluorography and noted the diaphragm to be high, as would be seen in full expiration, and motionless during the period of apnea. Peiper [1939] studied a child during intentionally precipitated breath-holding spells and noted small periodic movements of the diaphragm during the expiratory apnea without corresponding effects on pulmonary ventilation or the degree of cyanosis, indicating that spasm of the glottis occurred as part of the generalized rigidity. Spasm of the glottis and respiratory muscles with increased intrathoracic pressure occurs during expiration. Increased intrathoracic pressure reduces cardiac output, causing a decrease in cerebral perfusion. Lombroso and Lerman [1967] suggested that violent crying could lead to hypocapnia, which would also impair cerebral circulation.

Southall and associates [1985] further evaluated the prolonged expiratory mechanism in nine infants with cyanotic episodes that were usually triggered by noxious stimuli. Arterial oxygen saturation fell below 20 mm Hg within 20 seconds. Loss of consciousness occurred after 30 seconds. Measurements of respiratory movements, airflow, and esophageal pressure and, in some patients, microlaryngoscopy and chest fluoroscopy were obtained. They documented no inspiratory flow during the period of apnea but continued expiratory muscle activity at low lung volumes with partial or complete glottic closure. No intracardiac shunt could be demonstrated. The rapid fall in arterial oxygen saturation was attributed to lack of ventilation at a maximum expiratory position in the presence of a rapid circulation time. They hypothesized that central and peripheral neural respiratory control was functioning normally but was interfered with by a mechanical defect involving lung-volume maintenance. This defect could occur because of an excessively compliant rib cage, allowing alveolar collapse. This collapse in turn could lead to stretching of the airways and their stretch receptors, inappropriately simulating maximum lung volumes and thereby inhibiting inspiration. Southall and colleagues [1990] did further evaluations of prolonged expiratory apnea with krypton infusion scans and demonstrated krypton outside the lung fields, without evidence of an intracardiac shunt. They felt there was intrapulmonary shunting that contributed to the rapid onset and severity of the hypoxemia.

The relation between breath holding and chemosensitivity has also been investigated. Anas and associates [1985] hypothesized that persons with cyanotic breath-holding episodes have blunted ventilatory chemosensitivity. Because of the difficulty of measuring chemosensitivity in toddlers, they measured ventilatory responses to progressive hypercapnia and to progressive hypoxia in subjects ages 11 to 50 who had a history of cyanotic breath-holding spells and compared the results with a control group. Contrary to their hypothesis, the majority of persons with a history of cyanotic breath-holding spells had normal ventilatory responses. However, no one with a history of breath-holding spells had high normal responses to hypercapnia or hypoxia, as did some individuals in the control group. They postulated that the difference between the groups might represent the vestige of a disorder of ventilatory chemosensitivity that resolved with maturation.

Kahn and colleagues [1990] also investigated the relation between breath holding and cardiorespiratory control. The study included 71 infants with a history of breath-holding spells and age- and gender-matched controls. The median age of infants in the study was 14 weeks, which is younger than the typical age for onset of breath-holding episodes. The infants with breath-holding spells were significantly more often covered with sweat during sleep and wakefulness compared with control infants. One-night sleep studies were obtained in each infant. The infants with breath-holding spells had significantly less non–rapid eye movement stage III sleep, more indeterminate sleep, more arousals, and more sleep-stage changes than the control infants. Airway obstructions during sleep occurred in 41 infants with a history of breath holding compared with 6 in the control group. The obstructions were generally short and not accompanied by significant bradycardia or oxygen desaturation. They concluded that there was a common underlying mechanism resulting in airway obstruction during breath-holding spells and sleep, which possibly involved the autonomic nervous system because the autonomic nervous system controls the patency of the upper airways.

Kohyama and associates [2000] did polysomnography to evaluate rapid eye movement sleep in seven children with breath-holding spells and nine normal age-matched controls. The children with breath-holding spells had a significant decrease in ocular activity during rapid eye movement sleep, especially during the last third of the night, compared with the controls. Relative elevation of cholinergic tone compared with monoaminergic tone is considered to be involved in the physiologic increase of rapid eye movement sleep in the later cycles of the night. The vestibular nucleus and the medioventral caudal pons are believed to be involved in bursts of eye movements during rapid eye movement sleep. They hypothesized that there was a functional disturbance in the pons of children with breath-holding spells. The study also suggests that the autonomic nervous system is involved because of the more pronounced decrease in eye movement in the later cycles of the night, which are regulated by the autonomic nervous system.

DiMario and Burleson [1993a] used noninvasive methods to evaluate autonomic nervous system function in children with severe cyanotic breath-holding spells. Compared with controls, the breath holders had a significantly greater increase in pulse rate at 15 seconds of standing after rising from the supine position. Breath holders also had a greater decrease in diastolic blood pressure without an increase in systolic blood pressure after standing from the supine position. These results suggest that there is autonomic dysregulation in children with cyanotic breath-holding spells. Based on the results of this study and prior studies, DiMario and Burleson postulated that in addition to evidence of parasympathetic excess, children with cyanotic breath holding exhibit subtle sympathetic excess, which mediates vascular resistance, arterial distensibility, and blood flow through the lungs. This sympathetic overactivity could cause the intrapulmonary shunting and subsequent hypoxemia [Southall et al., 1990].

Pallid Spells

Excessive vagal tone leading to cerebral hypoperfusion is the underlying cause of pallid breath-holding spells. Observation of children during a typical episode reveals marked bradycardia or asystole [Bridge et al., 1943]. Ocular compression that triggers the oculocardiac reflex has been used to evaluate vagal tone in children with breath holding [Lombroso and Lerman, 1967; Stephenson, 1978]. This maneuver results in transmission of afferent signals to the brainstem via the ophthalmic division of the trigeminal nerve and efferent parasympathetic signals via the vagus nerve. In 61% to 78% of children with pallid breath-holding spells, ocular compression resulted in asystole of 2 seconds or longer compared with 23% to 26% of children with cyanotic breath-holding spells [Lombroso and Lerman, 1967; Stephenson, 1978]. Episodes that occurred spontaneously during cardiac monitoring were also associated with asystole [Lombroso and Lerman, 1967; Maulsby and Kellaway, 1964]. The asystole during spontaneous episodes is believed to be vagally mediated. When asystole is prolonged, a reflex anoxic seizure may occur.

The role of underlying autonomic dysfunction in children with pallid breath-holding spells has been investigated in a small number of patients. Measurements of mean arterial pressures, pulse rates, electrocardiograms, and plasma norepinephrine levels were obtained in patients and controls during changes in position. The breath holders had a statistically significant decrease in mean arterial pressure and an unsustained increase in pulse rate during the prone to standing maneuver. One child with pallid breath-holding spells had a plasma norepinephrine level that was 60% below the mean for both groups [DiMario et al., 1990]. Further evaluation of autonomic function was performed in children with either pallid or cyanotic breath-holding spells. Respiratory sinus arrhythmia, which is an established measure of vagal tone, was measured. There were no significant differences between controls and children with cyanotic breath-holding spells. The children with pallid spells, however, had a marked difference in respiratory sinus dysrhythmia with less variability compared with controls and those with cyanotic episodes [DiMario et al., 1998]. These studies suggest that there may be an underlying parasympathetic dysregulation in children with pallid breath-holding spells.

The role of anemia in the pathophysiology of breath-holding spells was suggested by Holowach and Thurston [1963]. They found that 23.5% of 102 children with breath holding had a hemoglobin level less than 8 grams/100 mL compared with 7% and 2.6% in two control groups. Subsequent studies did not find any significant difference in hemoglobin levels in the breath-holding group compared with the control group [Laxdal et al., 1969; Maulsby and Kellaway, 1964]. There are reports of children with breath-holding spells and concomitant anemia who had resolution of their spells with correction of the anemia [Bhatia et al., 1990; Colina and Abelson, 1995; DiMario, 1992; Mocan et al., 1999; Orii et al., 2002]. Tam and Rash [1997] described a child with pallid breath-holding spells associated with transient erythroblastopenia of childhood. The spells resolved after treatment with iron but before the anemia resolved. Daoud and colleagues [1997] studied 67 children with breath-holding spells to investigate the effect of iron therapy. Treatment and placebo groups were similar in respect to gender, age at onset, and frequency and type of spells and had similar blood indices, including packed cell volume, mean corpuscular volume, saturation index, total iron binding capacity, and serum iron. At the end of the treatment period, 51.5% of the children treated with ferrous sulfate had complete remission of spells and an additional 36.4% experienced a greater than 50% reduction. No children in the placebo group had total remission of spells, and only 5.9% had a greater than 50% reduction. As expected, the treatment group experienced significant improvement in the hemoglobin level and total iron-binding capacity. However, some children who were not iron deficient had a favorable response to iron therapy and some who were iron deficient did not respond. Iron deficiency may play a role in the pathophysiology of breath-holding spells because iron is important for catecholamine metabolism and neurotransmitter function [Daoud et al., 1997].

Genetics

In children with breath-holding spells, there is a positive family history of similar episodes in 23% to 38%, suggesting a genetic influence [Laxdal et al., 1969; Lombroso and Lerman, 1967]. An evaluation of family pedigrees found that 27% of 114 proband parents and 21% of proband siblings had a history of breath holding. Several families had some members with pallid spells and other members with cyanotic spells. The male-to-female ratio was 1:1.2 and the risk of transmission from parent to child was 50:50. There were seven instances of father-to-son transmission, ruling out an X-linked inheritance. Using a regression model for pedigree analysis, the inheritance pattern was consistent with an autosomal-dominant pattern with reduced penetrance [DiMario and Sarfarazi, 1997].

Treatment

The most important aspect of treatment of breath-holding spells is to reassure the family of the benign nature of the spells. It is important to emphasize that the episodes do not lead to mental retardation or epilepsy. Although parents are inclined to pick up a child who is having a breath-holding spell, they should be instructed to place the child in a lateral recumbent position so as not to prolong the period of cerebral anoxia. Initiation of cardiopulmonary resuscitation should be avoided. Although anger and frustration are often precipitants for breath-holding spells, parents should be encouraged not to alter customary discipline for fear of triggering an episode [DiMario, 1992]. Parenting a child with breath-holding spells has been associated with more maternal stress than parenting a child with a convulsive seizure disorder, and parents of children with breath-holding spells are at risk for developing dysfunctional parenting behaviors [Mattie-Luksic et al., 2000]. Referral of parents to professionals to help with stress and parenting skills should be considered.

Treatment with iron therapy should be initiated in any child who has iron deficiency anemia and should be considered in any child with breath-holding spells because children without anemia may have improvement in their breath-holding spells. The convulsive movements seen during breath-holding spells are reflex anoxic seizures, which are not epileptic and do not require antiepileptic treatment. There have been a few patients who have been reported to have prolonged seizures and even status epilepticus from breath-holding spells [Emery, 1990; Kuhle et al., 2000; Moorjani et al., 1995; Nirale and Bharucha, 1991]. It is presumed that these patients have a lowered seizure threshold and that hypoxia-ischemia triggered the seizures [Emery, 1990]. Stephenson [1990] has termed these events *anoxic-epileptic seizures.* Treatment with antiepileptic medication may stop the seizure activity but not the breath-holding spells. Atropine (0.01 mg/kg two or three times daily) is effective for pallid breath-holding spells, but its use is rarely warranted [McWilliam and Stephenson, 1984; Stephenson, 1980]. Piracetam, which has a chemical structure similar to γ-aminobutyric acid, has been used to treat children with breath-holding spells. In a study of 76 children with breath-holding spells, treatment with piracetam for 2 months resulted in 92% having no recurrence of episodes for 6 months after treatment compared with 30% who received placebo [Donma, 1998]. Piracetam has not received approval from the U.S. Food and Drug Administration and is designated only as an orphan drug for use in myoclonus.

REFLEX ANOXIC SEIZURES

Reflex anoxic seizures are nonepileptic events resulting from cardiac asystole of vagal origin [Stephenson, 1990, 2001]. Pain and surprise are common provoking factors for the events [Stephenson, 1980]. Reflex anoxic seizures may occur with pallid breath-holding spells but also have been reported with minor blows to the occiput, expelling hard stools past an anal fissure, venipuncture, intramuscular injections, and seeing an intravenous scalp drip [Braham et al., 1981; Gordon, 1982; Lombroso and Lerman, 1967; Roddy et al., 1983; Stephenson, 1980]. Nonepileptic anoxic seizures may also occur after syncope, cyanotic breath-holding spells, or any event that results in a sudden reduction in cerebral perfusion or hypoxia.

Clinical Features

Reflex anoxic seizures occur a few seconds after the provocation and are characterized by loss of muscle tone initially and later by tonic posturing. There may be opisthotonic posturing in some patients. A few jerks at the onset and end of an anoxic seizure may occur and probably represent myoclonic phenomena. A snoring type of inspiration or snort occurring close to the restoration of the cardiac rhythm is often noted. Urinary incontinence happens in approximately 10% of children with anoxic seizures, with bowel incontinence occurring less commonly [Stephenson, 1990]. Other less common features include adversive head movements, limb quivering or twitching, agitation or fear, vomiting, and tongue biting. The color change seen with an anoxic seizure may be cyanosis or pallor, depending on the mechanism producing loss of consciousness. The duration of unconsciousness is almost always less than 1 minute. Most patients experience a rapid recovery of consciousness, but some will be dazed or disoriented for a short period. Some will be drowsy after an episode and may sleep [Stephenson, 1990]. Occasionally patients will have prolonged seizure activity after syncopal spells. These events, termed *anoxic-epileptic seizures,* are epileptic seizures triggered by hypoxia in patients with a lowered seizure threshold [Stephenson, 1990].

Pathophysiology

The mechanism of reflex anoxic seizures has been studied by using ocular compression with EEG and cardiac monitoring [Gastaut and Fischer-Williams, 1957; Gastaut and Gastaut, 1958; Lombroso and Lerman, 1967; Stephenson, 1978;]. Ocular compression induced asystole in susceptible patients. If asystole lasted 3 to 6 seconds, there were no clinical symptoms and the EEG demonstrated only desynchronization. When asystole lasted 7 to 13 seconds, slow waves appeared, usually associated with altered consciousness. If asystole was prolonged for 14 seconds or more, there were often myoclonic jerks or tonic posturing. The EEG during this time reveals no electrocerebral activity. With return of cardiac activity, there was again high-voltage slow-wave activity on the EEG with return of normal activity over 20 to 30 seconds [Gastaut and Fischer-Williams, 1957]. At no time during EEG monitoring were epileptiform discharges present. Some patients have had spontaneous episodes or episodes triggered by other stimuli, such as venipuncture during EEG and cardiac monitoring, and have demonstrated similar changes to those seen with ocular compression [Braham et al., 1981; Gordon, 1982; Lombroso and Lerman, 1967; Roddy et al., 1983]. Ocular compression increases vagal tone with the afferent pathway involving fibers from the trigeminal nerve originating from the cornea, iris, and eyelids. In contrast, episodes induced by exteroceptive stimulation, such as pain and emotion, have afferent fibers in various sensory pathways. In both situations the vagal reflex centers are located in the brainstem in the nucleus ambiguus [Chen and Chai, 1976]. The efferent pathway involves the cardioinhibitory fibers of the vagus nerve.

Laboratory Tests

Diagnosis of reflex anoxic seizures is usually made by obtaining a history of the episode. Details about the precipitating circumstances and onset are essential. Parents may state that their child had a seizure, and a careful description of the movements and posture, length of the episode, and recovery period will be helpful. Usually no laboratory tests are needed, although consideration should be given to obtaining an electrocardiogram to evaluate for a cardiac cause if the episodes are not typical. Rarely is it necessary to obtain an EEG. If an EEG is obtained, ocular compression may be helpful in confirming the diagnosis.

Treatment

Treatment of reflex anoxic seizures focuses on explaining the nature of the event to the parents and reassuring them that the episodes are not epileptic seizures and do not need treatment with antiepileptic medication. In more severe cases atropine, theophylline, and transdermal scopolamine have been helpful [Benditt et al., 1983; McWilliam and Stephenson, 1984; Palm and Blennow, 1985; Stephenson, 1979]. Pacemaker implantation has also been useful in the rare patient with severe episodes [Kelly et al., 2001; McLeod et al., 1999; Porter et al., 1994; Sapire et al., 1983]. Children with reflex anoxic seizures are at risk of bradycardia during surgical procedures, and modifications in the anesthesia protocol may be warranted [Onslow and Burden, 2003; Pollard, 1999].

REFERENCES

Abt IA. Breath holding in infants. Am J Dis Child 1918;16:118.

Anas NG, McBride JT, Boettrich C, et al. Ventilatory chemosensitivity in subjects with a history of childhood cyanotic breath-holding spells. Pediatrics 1985;75:76.

Benditt DG, Benson DW, Kreitt J, et al. Electrophysiologic effects of theophylline in young patients with recurrent symptomatic bradyarrhythmias. Am J Cardiol 1983;52:1223.

Bhatia MS, Singhal PK, Dhar NK, et al. Breath holding spell: An analysis of 50 cases. Indian Pediatr 1990;27:1073.

Braham J, Hertzeanu H, Yahini JH, et al. Reflex cardiac arrest presenting as epilepsy. Ann Neurol 1981;10:277.

Breningstall GN. Breath-holding spells. Pediatr Neurol 1996;14:91.

Bridge EM, Livingston S, Tietze C. Breath-holding spells: Their relationship to syncope, convulsions, and other phenomena. J Pediatr 1943;23:539.

Breukels MA, Plotz FB, van Nieuwenhulzen O, et al. Breath holding spells in a 3-day-old neonate: An unusual early presentation in a family with a history of breath holding spells. Neuropediatrics 2002;33:41.

Chen HI, Chai CY. Integration of the cardiovagal mechanism in the medulla oblongata of the cat. Am J Physiol 1976;231:454.

Colina KF, Abelson HT. Resolution of breath-holding spells with treatment of concomitant anemia. J Pediatr 1995;126:395.

Culpepper N. A directory for midwives: Or a guide for women in their conception, rearing, and suckling their children. London: A. Bettesworth and C. Hitch, 1737.

Daoud AS, Batieha A, Al-Sheyyab M, et al. Effectiveness of iron therapy on breath-holding spells. J Pediatr 1997;130:547.

DiMario FJ Jr. Breath-holding spells in childhood. Am J Dis Child 1992;146:125.

DiMario FJ Jr. Prospective study of children with cyanotic and pallid breath-holding spells. Pediatrics 2001;107:265.

DiMario FJ Jr, Bauer L, Baxter D. Respiratory sinus arrhythmia in children with severe cyanotic and pallid breath-holding spells. J Child Neurol 1998;13:440.

DiMario FJ Jr, Burleson JA. Autonomic nervous system function in severe breath-holding spells. Pediatr Neurol 1993a;9:268.

DiMario FJ Jr, Burleson JA. Behavior profile of children with severe breath-holding spells. J Pediatr 1993b;122:488.

DiMario FJ Jr, Chee CM, Berman P. Pallid breath-holding spells. Evaluation of the autonomic nervous system. Clin Pediatr 1990;29:17.

DiMario FJ Jr, Sarfarazi M. Family pedigree analysis of children with severe breath-holding spells. J Pediatr 1997;130:647.

Donma MM. Clinical efficacy of piracetam in the treatment of breath-holding spells. Pediatr Neurol 1998;18:41.

Emery ES. Status epilepticus secondary to breath-holding and pallid syncopal spells. Neurology 1990;40:859.

Franklin WH, Hickey RW. Long-QT syndrome. N Engl J Med 1995;333:335.

Gastaut H, Fischer-Williams M. Electroencephalographic study of syncope: Its differentiation from epilepsy. Lancet 1957;2:1018.

Gastaut H, Gastaut Y. Electroencephalographic and clinical study of anoxic convulsions in children. Electroencephalogr Clin Neurophysiol 1958;10:607.

Gauk EW, Kidd L, Prichard JS. Mechanism of seizures associated with breath-holding spells. N Engl J Med 1963;268:1436.

Goraya JS, Virdi VS. Persistence of breath-holding spells into late childhood. J Child Neurol 2001;16:697.

Gordon N. The differential diagnosis of epilepsy and the use of the ambulatory electroencephalogram. J Electrophysiol Tech 1982;8:15.

Holowach J, Thurston DL. Breath-holding spells and anemia. N Engl J Med 1963;268:21.

Kahn A, Rebuffat E, Sottiaux M, et al. Brief airway obstructions during sleep in infants with breath-holding spells. J Pediatr 1990;117:188.

Kanner L. Child psychiatry. Springfield, IL: Charles C Thomas, 1935.

Kelly AM, Porter CJ, McGoon MD, et al. Breath-holding spells associated with significant bradycardia: Successful treatment with permanent pacemaker implantation. Pediatrics 2001;108:698.

Kohyama J, Hasegawa T, Shimohira M, et al. Rapid eye movement sleep in breath holders. J Child Neurol 2000;15:449.

Kuhle S, Tiefenthaler M, Seidl, R, et al. Prolonged generalized epileptic seizures triggered by breath-holding spells. Pediatr Neurol 2000;23:271.

Laxdal T, Gomez MR, Reiher J. Cyanotic and pallid syncopal attacks in children (breath-holding spells). Dev Med Child Neurol 1969;11:755.

Linder CW. Breath-holding spells in children. Clin Pediatr 1968;7:88.

Livingston S. Breathholding spells in children: Differentiation from epileptic attacks. JAMA 1970;212:2231.

Lombroso CT, Lerman P. Breathholding spells (cyanotic and pallid infantile syncope). Pediatrics 1967;39:563.

Mattie-Luksic M, Javornisky G, DiMario FJ Jr. Assessment of stress in mothers of children with severe breath-holding spells. Pediatrics 2000;106:1.

Maulsby R, Kellaway P. Transient hypoxic crises in children. In: Kellaway P, Petersen I, eds. Neurological and electroencephalographic correlative studies in infancy. New York: Grune and Stratton, 1964.

McLeod KA, Wilson N, Hewitt J, et al. Cardiac pacing for severe childhood neurally mediated syncope with reflex anoxic seizures. Heart 1999;82:721.

McWilliam RC, Stephenson JBP. Atropine treatment of reflex anoxic seizures. Arch Dis Child 1984;59:473.

Mocan H, Yildiran A, Orhan F, et al. Breath holding spells in 91 children and response to treatment with iron. Arch Dis Child 1999;81:261.

Moorjani BI, Rothner D, Kotagal P. Breath-holding spells and prolonged seizures. Ann Neurol 1995;38:512.

Nirale S, Bharucha NE. Breath-holding spells and status epilepticus. Neurology 1991;41:159.

Onslow JM, Burden J. Anaesthetic considerations for a child with reflex anoxic seizures. Paediatr Anaesth 2003;13:550.

Orii KE, Kato Z, Osamu F, et al. Changes of autonomic nervous system function in patients with breath-holding spells treated with iron. J Child Neurol 2002;17:337.

Palm L, Blennow G. Transdermal anticholinergic treatment of reflex anoxic seizures. Acta Paediatr Scand 1985;74:803.
Paulson G. Breath holding spells: A fatal case. Dev Med Child Neurol 1963;5:246.
Peiper A. Das "Wegbleiben." Monatschr Kinderh 1939;79:236.
Pollard RC. Reflex anoxic seizures and anaesthesia. Paediatr Anaesth 1999;9:467.
Porter CJ, McGoon MD, Espinosa RE, et al. Apparent breath-holding spells associated with life-threatening bradycardia treated by permanent pacing. Pediatr Cardiol 1994;15:260.
Roddy SM, Ashwal S, Schneider S. Venipuncture fits: A form of reflex anoxic seizures. Pediatrics 1983;72:715.
Sapire DW, Casta A, Safley W, et al. Vasovagal syncope in children requiring pacemaker implantation. Am Heart J 1983;106:1406.
Southall DP, Samuels MP, Talbert DG. Recurrent cyanotic episodes with severe arterial hypoxaemia and intrapulmonary shunting: A mechanism for sudden death. Arch Dis Child 1990;65:953.
Southall DP, Stebbens V, Shinebourne EA. Sudden and unexpected death between 1 and 5 years. Arch Dis Child 1987;62:700.
Southall DP, Talbert DG, Johnson P, et al. Prolonged expiratory apnoea: A disorder resulting in episodes of severe arterial hypoxaemia in infants and young children. Lancet 1985;2:8455.
Stephenson JBP. Reflex anoxic seizures ("white breath-holding"): Nonepileptic vagal attacks. Arch Dis Child 1978;53:193.
Stephenson JBP. Atropine methonitrate in management of near-fatal reflex anoxic seizures. Lancet 1979;2:955.
Stephenson JBP. Reflex anoxic seizures and ocular compression. Dev Med Child Neurol 1980;22:380.
Stephenson JBP. Fits and faints. Philadelphia: JB Lippincott, 1990.
Stephenson JPB. Anoxic seizures: Self-terminating syncopes. Epileptic Disord 2001;3:3.
Taiwo B, Hamilton AH. Cardiac arrest: A rare complication of pallid syncope? Postgrad Med J 1993;69:738.
Tam DA, Rash FC. Breath-holding spells in a patient with transient erythroblastopenia of childhood. J Pediatr 1997;130:651.

CHAPTER 55

Syncope and Paroxysmal Disorders Other than Epilepsy

Enrique Chaves-Carballo

Epilepsy is the most common paroxysmal disorder seen in the practice of pediatric neurology. However, other paroxysmal events are confused with epilepsy or have unusual clinical features [Bleasel and Kotagal, 1995; Bye et al., 2000; Donat and Wright, 1990; Kotagal et al., 2002; Sotero, 2002; Stephenson, 1990a]. Paroxysmal disorders other than epilepsy are described in this chapter (Box 55-1). Breath-holding spells, migraine, pseudoseizures, and sleep-related paroxysmal disorders are reviewed elsewhere in this book.

SYNCOPE

Syncope (derived from the Greek *synkoptein,* "to cut or break") is defined as a sudden loss of consciousness and postural tone, because of transient cerebral hypoperfusion, followed by spontaneous recovery [Feit, 1996; Gastaut, 1974; Grubb and Kosinski, 1996; Kapoor, 2000]. Transient interruption of cerebral blood flow is followed by loss of consciousness within 8 to 10 seconds [Manolis et al., 1990]. More relevant to syncope is the rate of cerebral perfusion; less than 30 mL per 100 grams of brain tissue per minute results in syncope [Schraeder et al., 1994]. The critical threshold of cerebral hypoperfusion at which syncope ensues is 50% below baseline (horizontal) mean cerebral flow velocity [Njemanze, 1992].

Although syncope in children is usually benign and self-limiting, physical injury may result from unprotected falls. Older children and adolescents may suffer emotional trauma from embarrassment or fear of having epilepsy, cardiac disease, or sudden death.

Incidence

Syncope is seldom brought to medical attention and, therefore, its incidence is unknown. An estimated 30% to 50% of children have at least one episode by adolescence, yet syncope accounts for only about 1% of pediatric emergency room visits [Kudenchuk and McAnulty, 1985; Pratt and Fleischer, 1989]. Among 5207 adults in the Framingham study cohort, 3% of the men and 3.5% of the women had a syncopal episode [Savage et al., 1985]. Of 7814 adult participants in the Framingham study followed for an average of 17 years, 822 (10.5%) reported syncope, and the incidence of a first report of syncope was 6.2 per 1000 person-years [Soteriades et al., 2002]. In the Rochester Epidemiological Project, the incidence of syncope brought to medical attention was 125.8 per 100,000 for the 5-year period between 1987 and 1991, with this incidence peaking among adolescents 15 to 19 years of age [Driscoll et al., 1997]. The recurrence rate of syncope ranges from 33% to 51% when patients are followed up to 5 years [Kapoor, 1990].

Syncope may result from cardiovascular or neurologic causes (cardiovascular-mediated or neurally mediated syncope). Each of these categories accounts for about 50% of

Box 55-1 Syncope and Other Nonepileptic Paroxysmal Disorders

Syncope
- Cardiovascular-mediated syncope
- Neurocardiogenic syncope
- Convulsive syncope
- Reflex syncope
- Situational syncope
- Cough syncope
- Defecation syncope
- Deglutition syncope
- Diving syncope
- Hair-grooming syncope
- Micturition syncope
- Sneeze syncope
- Trumpet-playing syncope
- Weight-lifting syncope
- Hyperventilation syncope
- Suffocation syncope
- Drug-induced syncope
- Psychogenic syncope

Other Nonepileptic Paroxysmal Disorders
- Benign paroxysmal vertigo
- Paroxysmal dystonic choreoathetosis
- Paroxysmal kinesigenic choreoathetosis
- Dopa-responsive dystonia with diurnal variation
- Acetazolamide-responsive paroxysmal ataxia
- Benign paroxysmal tonic upgaze
- Benign paroxysmal torticollis
- Sandifer's syndrome
- Cyclic vomiting
- Benign myoclonus of early infancy
- Hyperekplexia
- Spasmus nutans
- Shuddering attacks
- Hyperventilation syndrome
- Rhythmic movements
- Stereotypes
- Gratification phenomena
- Masturbation

adult syncope [Kapoor et al., 1983]. Cardiovascular-mediated syncope is less frequent in children than it is in adults.

Cardiovascular-Mediated Syncope

Cardiovascular-mediated syncope has a higher mortality and a higher incidence of sudden death than neurally mediated syncope [Kapoor et al., 1983; Kapoor, 2000]. Pediatric neurologists should become familiar with risk factors that suggest structural or conduction heart defects [Aicardi, 1992]. A previous history of heart murmur or congenital heart disease, acute attacks associated with hyperpnea or cyanosis, abrupt loss of consciousness during exercise, and absence of the usual premonitory symptoms or precipitating factors associated with neurally mediated syncope are suggestive of cardiovascular-mediated syncope. If any of these risk factors are present, an appropriate referral should be made for cardiac evaluation. Cardiovascular causes of syncope in children include aortic stenosis, hypertrophic obstructive cardiomyopathy, primary pulmonary hypertension, sick-sinus syndrome, long Q-T syndrome, supraventricular tachycardia, ventricular tachycardia, and heart block [Feit, 1996]. Further discussion of cardiovascular-mediated syncope is outside the scope of this chapter and the interested reader is referred elsewhere [e.g., Fogoros, 1993; Kapoor, 2000; Linzer et al., 1997a; 1997b; Manolis et al., 1990; Shen and Gersh, 1993].

An acceptable classification of syncope is hampered by a lack of uniform terminology. Some refer to syncope as *generalized anoxic seizures*, whereas others object to the implication of epilepsy in syncope [Aicardi, 1992; Gastaut, 1974; Stephenson, 1990b]. Thomas Lewis reintroduced the term *vasovagal syncope* more than 50 years after Gowers identified the term in 1882 [Lewis, 1932]. However, this designation is under scrutiny as inconsistent with current understanding of the pathophysiology of syncope [Kosinski et al., 1995]. *Neurocardiogenic syncope* has been proposed as a more meaningful and descriptive term [Abboud, 1993; Sra et al., 1991]. Despite objections, the recent literature evidences acceptance of the new terminology [Landau and Nelson, 1996].

Neurocardiogenic Syncope

Neurocardiogenic syncope, previously known as *vasodepressor, vasovagal,* or *neurally mediated syncope,* is commonly confused with epilepsy [Stephenson, 1990c].

CLINICAL FEATURES

A diagnosis of syncope rests mainly on clinical grounds [Kapoor, 2000; Lerman-Sagie et al., 1994]. A prodromal phase or presyncope consists of light-headedness, blurred vision, epigastric discomfort, nausea, pallor, or diaphoresis [Manolis et al., 1990; Feit, 1996]. When present, these clinical features help to differentiate syncope from epilepsy. A detailed history usually reveals contributory environmental factors before the loss of consciousness and postural tone. These environmental factors include upright posture, prolonged standing, change in posture (orthostasis), crowding, heat, fatigue, hunger, or a concurrent illness [Sutton, 1996]. Emotional or stress factors, such as venipuncture, public speaking, "fight-or-flight" situations, pain, and fear, are also commonly identified [Driscoll et al., 1997]. The loss of consciousness is usually brief, lasting from a few seconds to 1 or 2 minutes, followed by rapid spontaneous recovery without persistent neurologic deficits. During the ictus the patient may have tonic posturing or a brief clonic seizure, rarely associated with incontinence. The postictal period may be accompanied by nausea, pallor, diaphoresis, and a generally "washed-out" appearance. Complete recovery usually evolves in less than an hour [Feit, 1996].

Differentiation of neurocardiogenic syncope from an epileptic seizure is mainly based on the clinical features. However, interobserver agreement is poor when a retrospective diagnosis is made on information obtained after a single syncopal episode [Hoefnagels et al., 1992]. The evaluation of syncope may result in unnecessary and costly tests [Landau and Nelson, 1996]. A complete investigation includes neuroimaging studies, Holter monitoring, electroencephalography, glucose tolerance test, and, in selected cases, intracardiac electrophysiologic studies [Grubb et al., 1992] or implantable continuous loop-recordings [Krahn et al., 1999]. More than 40% of patients with recurrent syncope do not have a specific diagnosis after extensive investigation [Kapoor, 1991]. Introduction of the tilt-table test may help to resolve some of these problems.

PATHOPHYSIOLOGY

Explanation of the pathophysiology of neurocardiogenic syncope has been revised [Abboud, 1993; Benditt et al., 1996b; Grubb and Kosinski, 1996; Kosinski et al., 1995; Mosqueda-García et al., 2000]. Among predisposed individuals who experience recurrent syncope, excess peripheral venous pooling on prolonged standing results in diminished venous return. Decreased cardiac ventricular filling activates mechanoreceptors located mainly in the inferoposterior wall of the left ventricle that send afferent impulses via C-fibers to the dorsal nucleus of the vagus [Lieshout et al., 1991]. Arterial baroreceptors and carotid sinus afferent activation may also contribute to the complex pathophysiology of syncope [Kinsella and Tuckey, 2001]. These inhibitory cardiac and arterial receptors mediate increased parasympathetic activity and inhibit sympathetic activity that result in bradycardia, vasodilation, and hypotension (Bezold-Jarisch reflex) [Kinsella and Tuckey, 2001; Shen and Gersh, 1993]. The normal response during upright posture is an increased heart rate and diastolic pressure and an unchanged or slightly decreased systolic pressure [Rea and Thames, 1993]. In individuals susceptible to recurrent syncope, a "paradoxical" reflex bradycardia and peripheral vascular dilation occur [Grubb and Kosinski, 1996]. The previous emphasis on parasympathetic (vagal) output is shifting to sympathetic withdrawal as the main mechanism responsible for the bradycardia or asystole (cardioinhibitory response) and hypotension (vasodepressor response) that accompany neurocardiogenic syncope [Hannon and Knilans, 1993]. Although parasympathetic-mediated bradycardia remains a contributory factor in syncope, the responsible phenomena are vasodilation and hypotension [Kosinski et al., 1995]. Current hypotheses propose that the primary efferent event is systemic vasodilation and that this vasodepressor element is mediated by a profound centrally mediated sympathetic withdrawal [Kosinski et al., 1995]. The persistence of neurocardiogenic syncope in subjects who had cardiac transplants and, therefore, technically denervated hearts, as well as the finding of increased epinephrine levels during upright position and syncope, are strong evidence supporting a sympathetic withdrawal mechanism in syncope [Fitzpatrick et al., 1993; Njemanze, 1993; Sra et al., 1994]. Altered cerebral autoregulation may also be contributory in neurocardiogenic syncope [Rodríguez-Nuñez et al., 1997]. Transcranial Doppler studies have demonstrated cerebral vasoconstriction during tilt-table–induced syncope [Grubb et al., 1991]. These observations may stimulate future research and modify current insight about neurocardiogenic syncope.

Tilt-Table Testing

The tilt-table test was developed during World War II to study the effect of centrifugal forces on pilots during aircraft operation [Graybiel and McFarland, 1941]. Almost half a century later, the head-upright tilt-table test was introduced for clinical use to induce hypotension and bradycardia and confirm the diagnosis of neurocardiogenic syncope among individuals susceptible to recurrent syncope [Kapoor, 1996; Kenny et al., 1986; Sra et al., 1991].

Despite criticism that this provocative test suffers from "naive rationale," lacks patient selection standards, and needs controlled treatment and outcome studies [Landau and Nelson, 1996], the tilt-table test continues to enjoy popularity as a noninvasive and physiologically appropriate neurophysiologic test for the diagnosis of neurocardiogenic syncope [Dijane et al., 1996; Kapoor, 1999].

The test is done by positioning the patient head-upright at an angle of 60 to 80 degrees for 15 to 60 minutes on a tilt table with a supporting footboard. A tilt-table test result is positive when the symptoms of syncope or presyncope are reproduced [Sra et al., 1991]. If the result is negative, isoproterenol is administered intravenously and the dose increased until the heart rate increases by at least 20%. To standardize the test, the duration of head-up tilting has been increased to 45 minutes or two standard deviations of the mean time required to reproduce syncope [Sneddon and Camm, 1993]. A comprehensive analysis of available tilt-table data suggests that administration of isoproterenol has no added benefit, and 60 degrees for 45 to 60 minutes is recommended [Kapoor et al., 1994].

Experience with tilt-table test among pediatric populations is limited. Of 35 adolescents who had recurrent presyncope or syncope, 26 had positive tilt-table test results at 60 degrees for 30 to 60 minutes and isoproterenol infusion from 1 to 5 μg/minute [Thilenius et al., 1991]. Among 54 pediatric patients who had recurrent syncope, tilt-table testing at 80 degrees for 30 minutes was superior to studies, such as chest radiograph, electrocardiogram, echocardiogram, EEG, or neuroimaging, in arriving at a diagnosis of neurocardiogenic syncope [Strieper et al., 1994]. Tilt-table studies in 20 children with unexplained syncope and 10 controls using 60 degrees for 25 minutes and isoproterenol infusion from 0.02 to 0.08 μg/kg/minute were positive in 75% of patients and in 10% of controls for a sensitivity of 75% and a specificity of 90% [Alehan et al., 1996]. The tilt-table test has been used in children as young as 3 years of age [Grubb et al., 1992].

In addition to heart rate and blood pressure monitoring during tilt-table testing, electroencephalographic recording may be used to differentiate anoxic from epileptic seizures [Grubb et al., 1992]. More controlled studies and standardization of degree and duration of tilting are necessary to validate the tilt-table test as a safe, practical, and useful diagnostic tool for neurocardiogenic syncope in children [Benditt and Lurie, 1996a; Mansourati and Blanc, 1996; Moya et al., 1996a; 1996b; Victor, 1996].

TREATMENT

Once a diagnosis of neurocardiogenic syncope is confirmed, treatment requires counseling of the patient (when appropriate) and his or her parents. The benign nature of these events should be explained to allay concerns about epilepsy or sudden death. Avoidance of identified environmental factors may remediate or prevent most attacks. If a prodromal phase is consistently present, the patient may be taught to recline or sit to avoid injury from a fall. Supplemental fluids and electrolytes may be beneficial when excess environmental heat or diaphoresis is contributory. If these conservative measures fail to prevent recurrent syncope, several medications may be tried [Grubb and Kosinski, 1996]. Favorable response to treatment has been reported with beta-blockers, anticholinergics, serotonin reuptake inhibitors, methylxanthines, mineralocorticosteroids, and estrogens (Box 55-2) [Boehm et al., 1997; Milstein et al., 1990; O'Marcaigh et al., 1994; Raviale et al., 1996; Scott et al., 1995; Sra et al., 1991]. Subjects who require isoproterenol

Box 55-2 Medications for Treatment of Neurocardiogenic Syncope*

Beta-Adrenergic Blockers	
Atenolol	1 to 2 mg/kg/day
Esmolol	
Metoprolol	1 to 2 mg/kg/day
Nadolol	
Propranolol	0.5 to 4 mg/kg/day
Anticholinergics	
Disopyramide	10 to 15 mg/kg/day
Hyoscine	
Propantheline	
Scopolamine	
Alpha-Adrenergic Agonists	
Ephedrine	
Methylphenidate	5 to 10 mg tid
Midodrine	
Pseudoephedrine	60 mg bid
Serotonin Receptor Uptake Inhibitors	
Fluoxetine	
Sertraline	
Mineralocorticoids	
Fludrocortisone	0.1 to 0.3 mg/day

*Pediatric doses are given for those medications used in children in which dosages have been recommended.

Data from Grubb and Kosinski, 1996; Lazarus and Mauro, 1996; Raviele et al., 1996; Sra et al., 1997.

to induce syncope during tilt-table testing or who experience tachycardia before syncope may respond better to beta-blocker therapy [Leor et al., 1994; Sra et al., 1992].

Convulsive Syncope

A brief tonic or, rarely, a clonic seizure may accompany syncope. In a study of blood donors, 0.05% suffered a convulsion associated with syncope (convulsive syncope) [Lin et al., 1982]. Among 216 children who had a positive tilt-table test, 25 (11.6%) had seizures during the test [Fernández Sanmartín et al., 2003]. Most convulsions consisted of tonic spasms (65%) characterized by eye rolling, nuchal rigidity, arms flexed at the elbow, and fists clenched, followed usually by prompt recovery [Lin et al., 1982]. Other types of convulsions were myoclonic (23%), clonic (6%), and tonic-clonic (6%). No difference was found in severity of bradycardia or hypotension among those who had syncope associated with convulsion and those who did not [Lin et al., 1982]. In subjects who had cardiac asystole induced by ocular compression, only those who remained asystolic for more than 14 seconds experienced convulsive phenomena [Lin et al., 1982]. Convulsive syncope results from cerebral ischemia and is not indicative of an epileptic predisposition. The electroencephalogram (EEG) reveals diffuse slowing followed by loss of electrocerebral activity; epileptiform activity is absent [Fernández Sanmartín et al, 2003; Stephenson, 1990d]. Rarely, an epileptic seizure is triggered by syncope. In such cases the EEG, in contrast to what is seen in convulsive syncope, reveals epileptiform activity [Stephenson, 1990g].

Reflex Syncope

Syncope that is triggered by specific factors or events is known as *reflex* or *situational syncope.* The most common of these among infants and children is breath-holding spells. These are discussed in greater detail in Chapter 54. A related but distinctive type of syncope (known by various names in the past, including *pallid breath-holding spells* or *pallid infantile syncope*) is frequently confused with breath-holding spells. A simple and more appropriate designation for this type of paroxysm is *reflex syncope.*

In reflex syncope the antecedent event is minor trauma (usually to the head) before loss of postural tone and consciousness, without any audible inspiratory stridor or expiratory cry. Reflex syncopal episodes are easily confused with typical breath-holding spells, but evidence is lacking that these result from transient cerebral hypoxia because of breath holding. The rapid or immediate onset of syncope after minor trauma or other unexpected painful stimuli differentiates reflex syncope from breath-holding spells. In breath-holding spells, several seconds may elapse before loss of consciousness. There is general agreement that reflex syncopal attacks do not represent epileptic seizures, but the mechanism responsible is less clear. Some refer to these events as *reflex anoxic seizures* [Stephenson, 1978]. According to Stephenson, cardiac arrest is inducible in individuals susceptible to reflex syncope by the ocular compression test. This test is performed by applying pressure over the closed eyelids for 10 seconds during cardiac and electroencephalographic monitoring [Stephenson, 1980a]. After 7 to 15 seconds of asystole, a typical paroxysm is reproduced, thus confirming the diagnosis of reflex syncope. Reproduction of reflex syncope by ocular compression suggests that these children have an exaggerated oculocardiac reflex [Stephenson, 1990f]. Despite assurances about the safety and diagnostic usefulness of the ocular compression test to reproduce this type of syncope [Gastaut, 1974; Stephenson, 1980a; 1990f], its acceptance as a provocative test has been limited.

Situational Syncope

Other triggering factors associated with syncope include cough, deglutition (cold liquids), defecation, diving, micturition, sneezing, trumpet-playing, and weight lifting [Hannon and Knilans, 1993]. These events are more common in adults than in children and are referred to as *situational syncope.* A common denominator in situational syncope is that most of the triggering factors are accompanied by a Valsalva-like maneuver. Hair-grooming syncope is an uncommon type of situational syncope among adolescent females; it is often followed by brief seizure activity [Igarashi et al., 1988; Lewis and Frank, 1993].

Hyperventilation Syncope

Loss of postural tone and consciousness during hyperventilation is thought to result from cerebral vasoconstriction induced by hypocapnia. This type of syncope is discussed in more detail in a later section (see the section on hyperventilation syndrome).

Suffocation or Strangulation Syncope

Meadow's syndrome (Munchausen by proxy) is a rarely suspected cause of syncope. A caretaker induces loss of consciousness by obstructing the infant's airway using a pillow or by pressing the infant's face against the caretaker's trunk [Stephenson, 1990e]. In other cases, compression of the neck by strangulation results in cerebral hypoxia and, after repeated attempts, brain damage. A solicitous and omnipresent caretaker should raise suspicion of foul play [Folks, 1995]. The morbid events have been documented in some cases during video/EEG monitoring, but the incriminating evidence may not be admissible in court.

Drug-Induced Syncope

Among the medications that can cause syncope are those that induce ventricular tachycardia or cause hypotension. Cardiovascular medications (vasodilators and antiarrhythmics), psychotropics, diuretics, and glucose-controlling medications are the most common drugs associated with syncope [Lazarus and Mauro, 1996]. Illicit drugs may also cause syncope (particularly alcohol but also cocaine and marijuana). Drug-induced syncope is common among the elderly but rare among children.

Psychogenic Syncope

Failure to rapidly regain consciousness after a syncopal episode should raise suspicion of psychogenic syncope.

Psychogenic syncope is seen mainly among adolescents who demonstrate no cardiovascular or neurologic abnormalities and, in addition, lack any of the usual precipitating or triggering factors. A detailed psychosocial history may provide clues about the possible mechanisms involved. The general (including pulses, heart rate, and blood pressure) and neurologic examinations are unremarkable. A useful clinical maneuver in the unresponsive patient whose eyes are closed is to gently touch the eyelashes. This touch elicits a blink reflex in the conscious patient and alerts the examiner about the underlying psychopathology. Appropriate referral to a behavioral specialist should be made for further evaluation and management.

Other Nonepileptic Paroxysmal Disorders

Benign Paroxysmal Vertigo

Since Basser [1964] described benign paroxysmal vertigo, few studies have contributed additional information to clarify its etiology, pathophysiology, and presumed relationship to migraine. The paroxysms are stereotyped and easily recognized in the typical case. The child suddenly appears frightened and falls unless supported or, alternatively, holds on to the nearest person or object to maintain balance and upright posture [Finkelhor and Harker, 1987]. The duration of the episode is usually less than 1 minute. There is no associated impairment of consciousness and rarely is there vomiting. Recovery is rapid and complete. Nystagmus during the ictus is seldom described and its presence is usually unknown in most cases unless witnessed by a physician or other reliable observer. The majority of cases are observed in early childhood. The frequency of the attacks ranges from several daily to only one or two per month until these disappear spontaneously several months or years later. Older children may report vertigo as a spinning sensation and may experience nausea. The disorder is benign and resolves spontaneously without any specific treatment [Finkelhor and Harker, 1987].

Results of oculovestibular testing with ice-water calorics vary, probably because of different techniques used, as well as the difficulties in performing this test in younger children. Because ocular fixation suppresses nystagmus, the test must be carried out in a dark room [Finkelhor and Harker, 1987]. When properly done, no abnormalities in vestibular function have been detected [Eeg-Olofsson et al., 1982; Finkelhor and Harker, 1987]. The pathophysiology of benign paroxysmal vertigo is not understood. Evidence to support vestibular or labyrinthine dysfunction in children is incomplete. The rapidity of the onset of the vertiginous attacks and their abrupt cessation favor a vascular etiology. Some consider these as transient ischemic attacks of the posterior circulation, but supportive evidence is lacking.

The relationship between benign paroxysmal vertigo and childhood migraine remains conjectural [Fenichel, 1967]. It is not unusual to find a positive family history of migraine among immediate relatives. The possibility that benign paroxysmal vertigo represents a "migraine equivalent" is strengthened when a child with the typical syndrome reports associated headache and subsequently develops classic or vertebrobasilar migraine.

In the typical case of benign paroxysmal vertigo, neurophysiologic studies are unnecessary [Drigo et al., 2001].

TABLE 55-1

Medications for Treatment of Nonepileptic Paroxysmal Disorders

DISORDER	MEDICATION
Acetazolamide-responsive paroxysmal ataxia	Acetazolamide*
Benign paroxysmal tonic upgaze	Levodopa
Benign paroxysmal vertigo	Diphenhydramine, meclizine
Cyclic vomiting	Lorazepam, propranolol, amitriptyline, erythromycin succinate
Dopa-responsive dystonia with diurnal variation	Levodopa*
Hyperekplexia	Clonazepam,* valproic acid
Paroxysmal dystonic choreoathetosis	Clonazepam,* haloperidol, acetazolamide, valproic acid
Paroxysmal kinesigenic choreoathetosis	Carbamazepine,* phenytoin,* barbiturates, scopolamine, levodopa, belladona, chlordiazepoxide, diphenhydramine, oxcarbazepine
Sandifer's syndrome	Antigastroesophageal reflux medications (ranitidine, cimetidine, omeprazole)
Shuddering attacks	Propranolol

*Treatment medication of choice.

Brainstem auditory-evoked potentials are seldom abnormal. Treatment is also of limited value unless the episodes are unusually frequent or severe. Diphenhydramine or meclizine may be helpful in such children (Table 55-1). The most important aspect of management is reassurance that the attacks are not epileptic seizures or life threatening [Dunn and Snyder, 1976].

Paroxysmal Dystonic Choreoathetosis

Paroxysmal choreoathetosis is the essential symptomatology in the following four syndromes: paroxysmal dystonic (nonkinesigenic) choreoathetosis of Mount and Reback, paroxysmal kinesigenic choreoathetosis, supplementary sensorimotor seizures, and paroxysmal nocturnal dystonia [Luders, 1996]. The last disorder has been reported in children [Oguni et al., 1992; de Saint-Martin et al., 1997; Veggiotti et al., 1993] and is characterized by paroxysmal dystonic posturing in which the EEG shows interictal epileptiform discharges; such discharges are not usually observed during the periods of posturing. Tonic limb and body movements, automatisms, behavioral changes, and vocalizations may also be seen [Hirsch et al., 1996].

The description of paroxysmal choreoathetosis by Mount and Reback in 1940 established as a nosologic entity a familial paroxysmal movement disorder manifested by involuntary writhing and posturing of the trunk and extremities, more correctly labeled as *paroxysmal dystonic choreoathetosis* [Mount and Reback, 1940]. Kertesz introduced the term *paroxysmal kinesigenic choreoathetosis* to differentiate cases in which the episodes were brief and precipitated by movement instead of by prolonged immobility or intake of specific beverages (coffee, tea, cola drinks, alcohol), as in the cases of Mount and Reback [Kertesz, 1967]. Both paroxysmal dystonic (nonkinesigenic) choreoathetosis and paroxysmal kinesigenic choreoathetosis are included under the *paroxysmal dyskinesias* [Demirkiran and Jankovic, 1995; Shulman and Weiner, 1995]. A revised classification of the paroxysmal dyskinesias based on phenomenology, duration of the attacks (5 minutes or less and longer than 5 minutes), and etiology (idiopathic or secondary) was introduced by Demirkiran and Jankovic and has gained acceptance [Demirkiran and Jankovic, 1995; Jankovic and Demirkiran, 2002; Temudo, 2004]. Furthermore, these authors prefer the designations *paroxysmal kinesigenic dyskinesia* and *paroxysmal nonkinesigenic dyskinesia* because the paroxysmal attacks may include any combination of dystonia, chorea, athetosis, and ballism [Jankovic and Demirkiran, 2002].

Paroxysmal dystonic (nonkinesigenic) choreoathetosis is characterized by episodes of dystonia and choreoathetosis involving the face, trunk, and extremities, often associated with dysarthria and dysphagia lasting from minutes to several hours and occurring up to several times a week [Bressman et al., 1988; Demirkiran and Jankovic, 1995; Kinast et al., 1980; Lance, 1977; Pryles et al., 1952; Tibbles and Barnes, 1980]. The attacks begin spontaneously at rest or after intake of caffeine or alcohol. Other precipitating factors are fatigue, stress, hunger, and excitement. An aura consisting of twitching, feeling funny, or light-headedness has been noted [Williams and Stevens, 1963]. The disorder begins in early childhood and is inherited in most cases by autosomal dominant transmission. Linkage analysis has established a locus for paroxysmal dystonic choreoathetosis on distal chromosome 2q in an affected kindred [Fink et al., 1996]. Response to treatment with antiepileptic drugs is poor. Clonazepam is the treatment of choice for the majority of patients. Others respond to haloperidol, acetazolamide, or valproic acid [Przuntec and Monninger, 1983].

Paroxysmal Kinesigenic Choreoathetosis

The attacks are brief (usually lasting less than 2 minutes) and characterized by dystonic posturing, choreoathetosis, or ballistic movements, either singly or in combination, and affecting one or both sides concomitantly [Lance, 1977]. The patient remains conscious throughout the episodes, which may be as many as 100 daily, and without any postictal impairment. In a review of 100 cases of paroxysmal kinesigenic choreoathetosis, 79 were male and 21 female [Lance, 1977]. Seventy-two were familial, and the majority of these were consistent with autosomal-dominant inheritance. The age at onset in the familial cases was between 5 and 15 years. An aura consisting of tightness, numbness, tingling, or paresthesias in the extremities was not uncommon. The ictus consisted of dystonic posturing, choreoathetosis, or ballistic movements alone or in combination. In these cases the most common precipitating factor was sudden movement after rest. In some, however, startle, excitement, stress, and hyperventilation could induce the paroxysmal movements [Lance, 1977]. In a series of 23 men and 3 women with paroxysmal kinesigenic choreoathetosis, two thirds had attacks lasting between 30 and 60 seconds, more than one half experienced 1 to 10 attacks daily, and most consisted of pure dystonia [Houser et al., 1999].

Neurophysiologic and neuroimaging studies are normal, except for occasional slowing noted in the EEG [Buruma and Roos, 1986]. No epileptiform activity is usually seen, even when recordings are made during an episode. Nevertheless, reports of epilepsy among members of the same family raise the question about the possible association between these disorders [Demirkiran and Jankovic, 1995]. Lombroso has demonstrated ictal discharges emanating from the supplementary sensorimotor cortex and ipsilateral caudate nucleus in a female with paroxysmal kinesigenic choreoathetosis by invasive long-term monitoring [Lombroso, 1995].

Treatment of paroxysmal kinesigenic choreoathetosis is facilitated by an exquisite sensitivity to antiepileptic medications [Wein et al., 1996]. Paroxysmal control may be achieved even with subtherapeutic levels of phenytoin or carbamazepine. Other medications found to be effective, but to a lesser degree, are barbiturates, scopolamine, levodopa, belladonna, chlordiazepoxide, and diphenhydramine [Kinast et al., 1980]. This marked sensitivity to antiepileptic medications has been used to differentiate paroxysmal dystonic choreoathetosis of Mount and Reback from paroxysmal kinesigenic choreoathetosis.

The etiology of these disorders is unknown. The obvious localization to the basal ganglia lacks supporting evidence from available neuropathologic and neuroimaging studies [Demirkiran and Jankovic, 1995]. The proximity of the paroxysmal dystonic choreoathetosis gene locus to a cluster of ion-channel genes on distal chromosome 2q raises the possibility that, as in several other paroxysmal neurologic disorders (periodic ataxia with myokymia and potassium-related periodic paralyses), the underlying cause may be

TABLE 55-2

Genetics of Nonepileptic Paroxysmal Disorders

DISORDER	INHERITANCE	CHROMOSOME	GENE	CHANNELOPATHY
Acetazolamide-responsive paroxysmal ataxia	AD	19p	*CACNA1A*	Calcium
Dopa-responsive dystonia	AD	14q	*GCH-I*	
Hyperekplexia	AD	5q	*GLRA1*	Glycine (α_1 subunit)
	AR	4q		Glycine (β subunit)
Paroxysmal dystonic choreoathetosis	AD	21		
Paroxysmal kinesigenic choreoathetosis	AD	16p		

AD, autosomal dominant; AR, autosomal recessive.

Data from Ducros et al., 2001; Hejazi et al., 2001; Jankovic and Demirkiran, 2002.

related to ion-channel gene mutations (Table 55-2) [Fink et al., 1996].

Dopa-Responsive Dystonia with Diurnal Variation

Few disorders in the practice of pediatric neurology provide the opportunity to reverse a disabling condition in the dramatic manner afforded by dopa-responsive dystonia with diurnal variation. The condition was not recognized until 1971, when Segawa reported two children with the typical clinical features [Segawa et al., 1986]. The mode of inheritance is thought to be autosomal dominant, and more than 200 cases have been reported [Nygaard, 1993]. The estimated prevalence in England and Japan is 0.5 per million [Nygaard, 1993]. The onset presents between 1 and 9 years of age (average is 5 years) with fatigability and foot dystonia. These symptoms are aggravated by standing, by assuming a certain posture, or by voluntary movements. The most characteristic feature is the diurnal variation of the dystonia, which worsens in the evening and improves in the morning. According to Segawa, the dystonia progresses to involve all extremities within 5 or 6 years from onset and usually follows a letter N pattern, affecting the ipsilateral upper extremity, followed by the contralateral lower extremity and, finally, the contralateral upper extremity [Segawa et al., 1986]. The foot dystonia is mainly flexion inversion (pes equinovarus), whereas the arm is that of flexion pronation at the elbow and palmar flexion at the wrist with thumb adduction. When assuming the standing posture, the knee joint ipsilateral to the affected foot is hyperextended and the lumbar lordosis is exaggerated [Segawa et al., 1986]. Dystonic posturing of the big toe (striatal toe) may mimic a positive plantar (Babinski) response [Iivanainen and Kaakola, 1993]. Features of parkinsonism, such as rigidity, bradykinesia, postural instability, action, postural tremor of the arms, and, rarely, a resting tremor, may also be present and eventually develop in most cases [Nygaard et al., 1994]. The unusual presentation may be confused with cerebral palsy, spastic paraparesis, or hysteria [Nygaard et al., 1994].

Response to treatment is dramatic. Fatigability is usually alleviated within a week and dystonia within 6 weeks. A 20 mg/kg/day dose of levodopa without inhibitor is effective in most cases. A few patients benefit from increased doses of levodopa to 30 mg/kg/day. The therapeutic response is sustained and cumulative side effects are few [Segawa et al., 1986].

The neurophysiologic mechanisms involved in this disorder implicate the nigrostriatal dopaminergic system. Cerebrospinal fluid homovanillic acid levels are reduced, and biopterin concentrations are markedly reduced in all patients studied [Nygaard, 1995]. Positron emission tomography studies have been normal in most cases [Snow et al., 1993]. Neuropathologic data in one case demonstrated marked reduction of dopamine levels in the substantia nigra and in the striatum [Rajput et al., 1994]. The gene responsible for autosomal dominant hereditary progressive dystonia with marked diurnal fluctuation has been identified as guanosine triphosphate cyclohydrolase I located on 14q22.1-q22.2 [Furukawa et al., 1995; Segawa, 2000; Segawa et al., 2003; Tanaka et al., 1995].

Acetazolamide-Responsive Paroxysmal Ataxia

Recurrent episodes of vertigo, dysarthria, nystagmus, and gait ataxia starting in childhood and lasting for minutes or hours have been reported in several kindreds. The mode of inheritance of paroxysmal ataxia is autosomal dominant. Although asymptomatic between attacks, neurologic examination may reveal ocular abnormalities, including gaze-evoked nystagmus, abnormal optokinetic nystagmus, and hypermetric saccades [Van Bogaert et al., 1993]. Acetazolamide-responsive paroxysmal ataxia is also known as *episodic ataxia associated with nystagmus (EA-2)* [Jankovic and Demirkiran, 2002]. MRI and positron emission tomography studies may demonstrate atrophy of the anterosuperior aspect of the cerebellar vermis [Vighetto et al., 1988]. Intermittent rhythmic delta activity, sometimes associated with low-amplitude spikes and resulting in irregular spike-and-wave patterns, has been reported in EEG studies [Van Bogaert and Szliwowski, 1996]. Paroxysmal ataxia is almost always responsive to treatment with acetazolamide and the favorable response has been sustained for up to 5 years [Griggs et al., 1978]. The responsible gene has been mapped to the short arm of chromosome 19p [von Brederlow et al., 1995]. Localization of the gene responsible for familial hemiplegic migraine also to chromosome 19 suggested that these paroxysmal disorders were allelic [Joutel et al., 1993]. Acetazolamide-responsive paroxysmal ataxia and familial hemiplegic migraine are both associated with mutations in the gene *CACNA1A*, which encodes the α_{1A} subunit of voltage-gated neuronal calcium channels [Ducros et al., 2001; Ophoff et al., 1996]. Other closely related autosomal-dominant paroxysmal ataxias associated with myokymia (also known as *episodic ataxia type 1, or EA-1)* have been mapped to the short arm of chromosome 12p [Lubbers et al., 1995].

Benign Paroxysmal Tonic Upgaze

Sudden onset of constant or variably sustained upward deviation of the eyes with or without ataxia was described only recently [Deonna et al., 1990; Ouvrier and Billson, 1988]. More than 30 cases have been reported to date [Merino-Andreu et al., 2004]. The episodes are usually brief (lasting about 2 minutes each) recurring over a period of several hours or days, and may be exacerbated by infections, fatigue, or stress [Merino-Andeu et al., 2004; Temudo, 2004]. The paroxysmal upward gaze is accompanied by compensatory flexion of the neck and downward deviation of the chin [Merino-Andreu et al., 2004]. On attempted downward gaze below horizontal, nystagmus or down-beating saccades are elicited. The onset is usually in early life (within the first 12 months) and the abnormal eye movements improve or resolve spontaneously within a few years [Verrotti et al., 2001]. Associated findings, in addition to ataxia, may include developmental delay, intellectual disability, and language delay [Hayman et al., 1998]. Familial cases suggest an autosomal-dominant mode of inheritance [Guerrini et al., 1998]. Response to treatment with levodopa has been, with few exceptions, poor.

Neuroradiologic and neurophysiologic studies usually have normal results. However, focal or generalized epileptiform discharges recorded by polysomnography in four cases require further studies for confirmation [Merino-Andreu et al., 2004].

Benign Paroxysmal Torticollis

Intermittent twisting of the neck (wryneck or torticollis), without persistent or obligatory abnormal head positioning, followed by subsequent spontaneous resolution is characteristic of benign paroxysmal torticollis. The onset is seen more often between 2 and 8 months of age. Truncal posturing (retrocollis and tortipelvis) is an added feature in some cases [Chutorian, 1974]. The episodes may last from 10 minutes to 14 days, recur two or three times a month, and involve either side [Snyder, 1969]. An attack may be anticipated by the onset of irritability, distress, or vomiting [Chaves-Carballo, 1996]. Most affected individuals recover by 2 to 3 years of age without treatment. A few cases have been familial [Gilbert, 1977; Lipson and Robertson, 1978]. Most cases described since the initial report by Snyder conform to this clinical description [Bratt and Menelaus, 1992; Cataltepe and Barron, 1993; Cohen et al., 1993; Hanukoglu et al., 1984; Sanner and Bergstrom, 1979; Snyder, 1969].

The pathophysiology of benign paroxysmal torticollis is subject to speculation. The observation of eye rolling or deviation in some cases suggests labyrinthine involvement. Abnormal oculovestibular function was found in 9 of 12 cases [Snyder, 1969]. Others believe that benign paroxysmal torticollis is related to benign paroxysmal vertigo or migraine [Deonna and Martin, 1981; Dunn and Snyder, 1976; Eviatar, 1994; Giffin et al., 2002].

The differential diagnosis includes seizures, vertigo, gastroesophageal reflux, diaphragmatic hernia (Sandifer's syndrome), dystonia, posterior fossa, and craniocervical junction abnormalities (basilar impression, platybasia, atlantoaxial instability, Chiari malformation, and Klippel-Feil syndrome). Vestibular testing may be difficult to perform and interpret in young children. Brainstem auditory-evoked potentials are of interest because hearing impairment may be an associated finding. Neuroimaging studies are necessary to exclude congenital and acquired lesions involving the craniocervical region.

Treatment with diphenhydramine, meclizine, and chlorpromazine has not been successful [Snyder, 1969]. The prognosis, however, is favorable and follow-up studies suggest spontaneous resolution in most cases [Dunn and Snyder, 1976].

Sandifer's Syndrome

Sandifer's syndrome or complex consists of torsion spasms and abnormal posturing with or without gastroesophageal reflux or hiatal hernia [Gellis and Feingold, 1971; Kinsbourne and Oxon, 1964; Werlin et al., 1980]. The paucity of reports suggests that the disorder may not be well recognized [Kotagal et al., 2002]. It is not uncommon for a diagnosis of neurologic disease, such as dystonia or epilepsy, to be entertained before the true nature of the problem is identified [Mandel et al., 1989]. Among 126 infants and children with gastroesophageal reflux studied at a children's hospital, 7.6% had Sandifer's syndrome [Shepherd et al., 1987].

Abnormal posturing of the neck, trunk, and limbs results in bizarre positions. The torticollis is not associated with spasm of the neck muscles. At times, head nodding and gurgling sounds are noted. However, it is not necessary to demonstrate gastroesophageal reflux or hiatal hernia to make a diagnosis of Sandifer's syndrome [Werlin et al., 1980]. The initial explanations given for the contortions focused on the relief these positions afforded from the discomfort of acid regurgitation. However, there has been no correlation between the frequency or severity of gastroesophageal reflux and contortions. More sophisticated techniques and criteria for diagnosis of gastroesophageal reflux cast doubts on the validity of the association between Sandifer's syndrome and gastroesophageal reflux. In a study of eight patients with Sandifer's syndrome who had a barium swallow, pH monitoring, esophageal manometry, endoscopy, and biopsy for esophagitis, the most frequent finding was esophageal dysmotility [Gorrotxategi et al., 1995].

Because medical or surgical treatment of gastroesophageal reflux is effective, recognition of Sandifer's syndrome may carry a good prognosis for amelioration of the contortions. Children who have a diagnosis of paroxysmal torticollis, paroxysmal dystonia of the neck without palpable increased tone of the corresponding muscle groups, or adversive seizures without alteration of the level of consciousness should have Sandifer's syndrome included in their differential diagnosis.

Cyclic Vomiting

The syndrome of cyclic vomiting is characterized by repeated, unpredictable, explosive episodes of nausea and vomiting lasting for hours or days and separated by asymptomatic intervals [Li, 1995]. Although there are no diagnostic laboratory or neurophysiologic markers, the clinical features are sufficiently distinctive to allow a clinical diagnosis to be made confidently in most cases. The etiology and pathogenesis of cyclic vomiting remain elusive more than a century since the initial description as "fitful or recurrent vomiting" [Walker-Smith, 1995].

Among school-aged children, the prevalence of cyclic vomiting is 1.9% [Abu-Arafeh and Russell, 1995]. This figure agrees with a prevalence rate of 2.3% in a population-based study among 4- to 15-year-old children in western Australia [Cullen and MacDonald, 1963]. It is suspected, based on these reports, that cyclic vomiting remains underreported.

The age at onset is variable. Of the 44 patients reported from the Mayo Clinic, 82% had the onset of recurrent vomiting before the age of 6 years [Hoyt and Stickler, 1960]. Among 141 patients from three combined series, the peak age at onset was 3 years [Fleisher, 1995]. Although cyclic vomiting usually begins in early childhood, cases among preadolescents are not uncommon [Fleisher and Matar, 1993].

A typical episode is characterized by persistent nausea accompanied by intense vomiting, gagging, or retching [Fleisher, 1995]. The onset may be abrupt or be preceded by malaise, anxiety, or mild nausea lasting for minutes to hours [Fleisher, 1995]. Abdominal pain, diarrhea, headache, low-grade fever, tachycardia, and hypertension may be additional features. The attack is more common at night or in the early morning. The duration of the episodes is more often between 6 and 48 hours. The episodes are regular or cyclic in only about half of the patients. Precipitating or triggering factors are identified in about 80% of patients [Fleisher and Matar, 1993]. These are most often emotional stress, excitement, or concomitant infections. The peak intensity (number of emeses per hour) and frequency (number of attacks per month) may help to differentiate cyclic vomiting from chronic vomiting caused by other gastrointestinal disorders. Children who have cyclic vomiting experience more intense emesis (12.6 times per hour versus 1.9 times per hour) and fewer episodes (1.9 attacks per month versus 36.6 attacks per month) than children who have chronic vomiting from identifiable causes [Pfau et al., 1996]. About one third of affected children continue to have episodes of cyclic vomiting well into their teens [Dignan et al., 2001].

A diagnosis of cyclic vomiting requires exclusion of other causes. The differential diagnosis is extensive and should consider gastrointestinal, neurologic, renal, endocrine, and metabolic etiologies. Recommended studies include blood, urine, and stool examinations; gastrointestinal ultrasonography, endoscopy, and motility studies; and electroencephalographic and neuroimaging tests [Fleisher and Matar, 1993]. However, each case needs to be investigated individually, taking into consideration the circumstances associated with the recurrent bouts of vomiting. Olson and Li found upper gastrointestinal studies with small bowel follow-through (combined with empiric antimigraine therapy) to be more cost effective than extensive diagnostic evaluation in children with cyclic vomiting [Olson and Li, 2002].

There is no uniform recommended management for children with cyclic vomiting. Supportive measures may require administration of parenteral fluids and electrolytes. The use of antiemetics is elective. These are more effective when given during the first hour of emesis. Some prefer to induce sleep and use lorazepam, which has antiemetic, anxiolytic, and sedative properties, at a dose of 0.05 to 0.2 mg/kg intravenously. Long-term therapy using propranolol or amitriptyline has been successful in many cases [Fleisher and Matar, 1993]. Treatment with erythromycin ethylsuccinate, an agonist of the neuroenteric peptide, at a dose of approximately 20 mg/kg/day in two to four divided doses daily for 7 days ameliorated the symptoms in 18 of 24 children with cyclic vomiting [Vanderhoof et al., 1995].

Cyclic vomiting has been known in the past by different names, including periodic syndrome, acetonemic vomiting, autonomic epilepsy, abdominal epilepsy, migraine or convulsive equivalent, and abdominal migraine [Pfau et al., 1996]. Although the etiology of cyclic vomiting is unknown, suspicions abound that it is related to migraine. Headaches are present in about half of the children with cyclic vomiting [Fleisher and Matar, 1993]. Migraine headaches were found in 38% of children with cyclic vomiting in the Aberdeen-Hartlepool Childhood Migraine database [Symon and Russell, 1995]. Family history is positive for migraine in 40% of first- and second-degree relatives [Fleisher and Matar, 1993]. The prevalence rate of migraine in children with cyclic vomiting is twice that of the general childhood population (21% versus 10.6%) [Abu-Arafen and Russell, 1995]. Many of the following clinical features are common to both disorders: mode of presentation, triggering and relieving factors, associated gastrointestinal and sensory symptoms, vasomotor changes, electroencephalographic findings, and associated personality and psychosocial dysfunction [Fleisher and Matar, 1993]. For these reasons, cyclic vomiting has been grouped among the "migraine equivalents." The importance of stress stemming from psychologic conflicts in children with cyclic vomiting has been emphasized [Hammond, 1974; Reinhart et al., 1977]. However, cyclic vomiting as a major symptom of epilepsy is rare [Mitchell et al., 1983].

Benign Myoclonus of Early Infancy

Benign myoclonus of early infancy describes a group of infants between 3 and 8 months of age who develop myoclonic activity, usually in flurries and predominantly involving flexion or extension of the neck and rarely demonstrating adversive clonic activity of the head (cephalic myoclonus) [Lombroso and Fejerman, 1977]. Additional abnormal movements may include spasms of the head, trunk, or extremities; eye blinking; and brief jerking of the upper extremities or trunk [Maydell et al., 2001]. The paroxysmal activity resembles infantile spasms but lacks the electroencephalographic correlate of hypsarrhythmia and the associated neurologic abnormalities seen in West's syndrome. The myoclonic activity increases for a few weeks or months after onset but within an average of 3 months decreases considerably in most infants and disappears spontaneously by 2 years of age [Lombroso and Fejerman, 1977]. The condition is differentiated from stimulus-sensitive or action myoclonus as seen in posthypoxic encephalopathies; periodic myoclonus noted in subacute sclerosing panencephalitis and herpes simplex encephalitis; burst myoclonus encountered in Lennox-Gastaut syndrome; and from degenerative disorders of gray or white matter including gangliosidoses, leukodystrophies, and Unverricht-Lundborg and Lafora body diseases [Lombroso and Fejerman, 1977]. Other protracted but eventually self-limiting disorders, such as myoclonic infantile encephalopathy, hereditary essential myoclonus, benign essential myoclonus, and shuddering attacks, are also excluded. The condition is also differentiated from benign neonatal sleep myoclonus, which represents an exaggeration of normal physiologic phenomena during sleep [Noone et al., 1995]. Although initially some thought this could represent "stomach fits" instead of "brain fits" as manifestations of gastroesophageal reflux mimicking neurologic syndromes [Bray, 1977], benign myoclonus of early infancy is recognized as a distinct syndrome [Dravet et al., 1986]. Electroencephalographic studies fail to reveal any epileptiform activity during the paroxysmal episodes of myoclonus; however, more prolonged video/EEG monitoring may be required to establish the nonepileptic nature of the myoclonus [Bleasel and Kotagal, 1995; Pachatz et al., 1999].

Hyperekplexia

An exaggerated startle response may be a component of epilepsy (startle epilepsy) or of nonepileptiform paroxysmal disorders (jumping and hyperekplexia) [Andermann and Andermann, 1988]. The term *hyperekplexia* is derived from Greek and means excessive jerking or jumping. It refers to a strikingly excessive response to startle elicited by visual, auditory, or proprioceptive stimuli that fail to produce a startle response in most normal individuals [Aicardi, 1992]. In the normal individual the startle response is a basic alerting reaction with stereotyped features consisting of eye blinking, facial grimacing, flexion of the head, elevation of the shoulders, and flexion of the elbows, trunk, and knees [Andermann et al., 1980]. This involuntary reflex is enhanced by tension, fatigue, and heightened expectation and decreased with repeated stimulation. The reflex is said to appear during infancy at the same time as the Moro reflex [Andermann and Andermann, 1988]. The abnormal or pathologic response consists of an exaggerated startle response associated with generalized muscle stiffness and loss of postural control, causing the subject to fall en statue without loss of consciousness [Aicardi, 1992]. This propensity to fall may result in injuries, including head trauma.

Hyperekplexia presents in its major form during the neonatal period as stiff-baby syndrome (stiff-man syndrome in the newborn) [Klein et al., 1972; Lingam et al., 1981; Stephenson, 1980b]. The onset of stiffness becomes evident a few hours after birth and the shoulder-girdle muscles are hypertonic. There may be difficulty in swallowing and frequent choking. Apnea may result from hyperekplexia and cause death [Kurczynski, 1983; Nigro and Lim, 1992]. The hypertonia usually disappears during sleep, although repetitive and violent movements of the extremities may be seen during the hypnagogic stage, which lifts the child off the bed [Aicardi, 1992; Andermann and Andermann, 1988]. The neonatal form improves spontaneously during the first year of life, although later on there may be absence of crawling and delay in walking. Hip dislocation, as well as umbilical, inguinal, and diaphragmatic hernias, result from increased intra-abdominal pressure and muscle stiffness [Aicardi, 1992; Gordon, 1993]. A clinically useful maneuver is to tap the tip of the nose or the glabella (glabellar tap). This maneuver will elicit an exaggerated nonhabituating startle response in affected individuals [Shahar et al., 1991]. Similar results may be obtained by blowing air directly on the face of neonates and infants with hyperekplexia [Shahar and Raviv, 2004].

Neurophysiologic studies demonstrate that hyperekplexia is not an exaggerated normal startle response [Hallet et al., 1986]. Electromyogram latencies are shorter than normal. EEG studies may reveal an initial spike maximally in the frontocentral region followed by slow waves and desynchronization of background activity [Andermann and Andermann, 1988]. Auditory- and somatosensory-evoked potentials are reported as increased or normal [Andermann and Andermann, 1988; Hallet et al., 1986]. Caudorostral recruitment of cranial nerve innervated muscles supports a brainstem origin for the abnormal startle response in hyperekplexia [Brown, 2002].

The condition is familial and transmitted as an autosomal-dominant trait. Linkage analyses demonstrate genetic homogeneity in typical cases linked to DNA markers in the long arm of chromosome 5q [Ryan et al., 1992; Shiang et al., 1993]. Familial cases demonstrate point mutations in the α_1 subunit of the inhibitory glycine receptor (*GLRA1*) [Shiang et al., 1995]. Sporadic and autosomal-recessive hyperekplexia cases may show abnormalities in the β subunit of the glycine receptor (*GLRB*) [Hejazi et al., 2001; Rees et al., 2002]. Glycine receptors are found primarily in the brainstem and spinal cord [Rajendra et al., 1997]. The main inhibitory neurotransmitter receptor is the γ-aminobutyric acid type A receptor. Affected individuals usually reveal a favorable response to treatment with clonazepam, an agonist of γ-aminobutyric acid type A receptors [Shiang et al., 1995].

The relationship of hyperekplexia to other nonepileptic startle disorders, such as jumping (jumping Frenchmen of Maine), latah (ticklishness associated with echopraxia and coprolalia in Malaysia), and myriachit (to act foolishly as reported from Siberia, Asia, and Africa), although discussed a century ago by Gilles de la Tourette [1884; 1899] in the context of tic convulsif, remains conjectural [Andermann and Andermann, 1988].

Treatment is most effective with clonazepam (0.1 to 0.2 mg/kg/day), but in some cases symptoms may not be totally suppressed [Aicardi, 1992]. Valproic acid is recommended in cases of late onset [Dooley and Andermann, 1989]. Vigabatrin did not reduce startle activity among four patients with hyperekplexia [Tijssen et al., 1997].

The prognosis is variable. Neonatal hyperekplexia may result in apnea, neonatal encephalopathy, cerebral palsy, and unexpected death [Chaves-Carballo et al., 1999]. Early identification and treatment improve the outcome in most children. Although hyperekplexia may persist into adult life, in some families the exaggerated startle response ameliorates or disappears spontaneously by 2 years of age [Shahar et al., 1991].

In the minor form of hyperekplexia, there is only an abnormal startle response without generalized stiffness or tonic spasms. The minor form is not associated with neurologic or catastrophic sequelae and no mutations have been detected in the genes encoding the glycine receptor [Tijssen et al., 1997].

Spasmus Nutans

Spasmus nutans is a benign, self-limiting condition manifested by the clinical triad of asymmetric ocular oscillations, head nodding, and anomalous head positions in infants. Differentiation of spasmus nutans from other similar but more serious disorders has been hampered by the fact that patients often do not demonstrate all of the typical diagnostic features [Gottlob et al., 1990]. Furthermore, clinical detection of asymmetric nystagmus and head nodding may be difficult. Monocular or dissociated nystagmus occurs also in spasmus nutans [Farmer and Hoyt, 1984]. The head nodding corresponds to a normal compensatory oculovestibular reflex [Gottlob et al., 1992]. The pathophysiologic mechanisms involved in spasmus nutans are undetermined. The initial speculation that spasmus nutans results from environmental deprivation of sunlight has not been substantiated. Certain demographic and low socioeceonomic conditions may, however, represent risk factors for the development of spasmus nutans [Wizov et al., 2002].

Numerous cases of spasmus nutans have been associated with chiasmatic lesions [Albright et al., 1984; Anthony et al., 1980; Farmer and Hoyt, 1984; Kelly, 1970], diencephalic syndrome, porencephalic cysts [Gottlob et al., 1990], opsoclonus-myoclonus [Allarakhia and Trobe, 1995], empty sella [Gottlob et al., 1990], ependymoma [Gottlob et al., 1990], and retinal disorders [Gottlob et al., 1995a; Lambert and Newman, 1993]. Spasmus nutans is no longer regarded as a benign entity [Hoefnagel and Biery, 1968; Norton and Cogan, 1954].

To differentiate congenital nystagmus from spasmus nutans, eye and head movements were recorded in 23 patients with spasmus nutans, 10 patients with spasmus nutans-like disease (associated with central nervous sytem [CNS] lesions), and 25 patients with congenital nystagmus [Gottlob et al., 1990]. The mean onset of nystagmus and head nodding was 8 months, and the mean onset of head tilt was 15 months in the spasmus nutans group. These findings permitted differentiation of spasmus nutans from infantile nystagmus: ocular oscillations were of later onset; head nodding was more frequent, of larger amplitude, and clinically easier to detect; and nystagmus was asymmetric and intermittent in spasmus nutans compared with infantile nystagmus. Optokinetic nystagmus was usually present in spasmus nutans and absent in most patients with infantile nystagmus. Head tilt was not found to be a useful differentiating criterion. The recordings were unable to differentiate spasmus nutans from spasmus nutans associated with neurologic abnormalities. The authors concluded that patients with signs suggestive of spasmus nutans should have neuroimaging studies [Gottlob et al., 1990]. A normal electroretinogram may help to substantiate a diagnosis of spasmus nutans [Smith et al., 2000]. Long-term follow-up studies are important to substantiate a diagnosis of spasmus nutans. Most patients eventually attain good visual acuity. However, subclinical nystagmus persists until at least 5 to 12 years of age [Gottlob et al., 1995b].

Shuddering Attacks

Shuddering or shivering attacks are uncommon paroxysmal events rarely reported and poorly understood. These may start as early as 4 to 6 months of age or after 3 years of age and are precipitated or aggravated by fear, anger, frustration, or embarrassment [Vanesse et al., 1976]. The episodes last usually for a few seconds and are characterized by stiffening; adduction of the knees and arms; flexion of the head, elbows, trunk and knees; and flexion or extension of the neck. There is no change in the level of consciousness associated with the abnormal movements. In five of six cases reported, one of the parents had an essential tremor [Vanesse et al., 1976]. These characteristics suggested that shuddering attacks represent "the expression of an essential tremor in the immature brain." Head tremor may evolve from shuddering attacks [DiMario, 2000]. Electroencephalographic recording of shuddering attacks in seven children failed to reveal any epileptiform activity [Holmes and Russman, 1986; Kanazawa, 2000]. Treatment with antiepileptic medications has not been effective. Propranolol, however, has eliminated shuddering attacks [Barron and Younkin, 1992]. Monosodium glutamate has been implicated in other cases, and avoidance or elimination from the diet has been effective [Reif-Lehrer and Stemmermann, 1975]. The prognosis is favorable; most children improve spontaneously before 10 years of age [Kanazawa, 2000; Vanesse et al., 1976].

Hyperventilation Syndrome

Although hyperventilation syndrome has been known in the medical literature for more than 50 years, it frequently remains unrecognized by both patients and physicians [Evans, 1995]. The syndrome is defined by its symptoms, which are commonly related to anxiety, and by their reproducibility during voluntary hyperventilation [Evans, 1995]. Common chronic symptoms manifested in children with hyperventilation syndrome include anxiety, headaches, depression, and irritable bowel [Herman et al., 1981]. During attacks of hyperventilation, tachypnea, anxiety, breathlessness, light-headedness, and paresthesias are predominant. Among pediatric patients, the syndrome is more frequent among adolescents, although it has been recorded as early as 6 years of age. Many of the affected children have psychiatric problems before the onset of hyperventilation attacks. Unfortunately, 40% of surveyed patients are still having hyperventilation episodes when they reach adulthood [Herman et al., 1981].

Diagnosis requires a high index of suspicion and reproduction of the symptoms during voluntary hyperventilation. Inability to reproduce these symptoms does not necessarily negate the diagnosis. In such cases, empiric treatment consisting of breath holding, slow breathing, or breathing into a paper bag may be worthwhile. Treatment in the majority, however, requires more than reassurance and physiologic remediation of hypocapnia and alkalosis. The underlying psychopathology may be recalcitrant to such simple measures and will require careful follow-up and psychiatric intervention. Recent studies question the pathophysiology and validity of the hyperventilation syndrome [Bass, 1997].

Rhythmic Movements, Stereotypes, Gratification Phenomena, and Masturbation

Repetitive stereotyped movements are not uncommon among both normal and neurologically impaired children. Examples of such self-stimulating or gratification phenomena are body rocking, head banging (jactatio capitis), and head rolling [Sallustro and Atwell, 1978]. Rocking motions of the trunk observed among mentally and visually impaired children may represent a form of vestibular stimulation akin to the maternal rocking that effectively comforts a crying, tired, or sleepy infant. The peculiar purposeless hand-wringing, repetitive hand movements seen among autistic children and in Rett's syndrome may also be grouped into the category of self-stimulating behavior. Children who have a photoconvulsive response may learn to induce a seizure by repetitive hand movements in front of their eyes as a form of photic stimulation.

More difficult to recognize is masturbatory behavior, particularly when this occurs in young children and infants [Fleisher and Morrison, 1990; Nechay et al., 2004]. The repetitive movements usually involve the lower trunk and may be accompanied by pelvic thrusting or contractions of the gluteal muscles. The physical effort may be prolonged and lead to diaphoresis, hyperpnea, flushing, and grunting [Fleisher and Morrison, 1990]. The paroxysms may terminate in fatigue, exhaustion, or sleep. The pediatric neurologist is usually asked to evaluate the child because of concern that these events may represent a form of epilepsy. Detailed observation of an episode or review of a videotaped event may be necessary to clarify the diagnosis, particularly in infants younger than 1 year of age [Casteels et al., 2004]. Any explanation of the benign nature of the paroxysms should take into account unusually sensitive or incredulous parents [Leung and Robson, 1993]. Reassurance that the episodes are benign and self-limiting should help to avoid unjustified concerns and unnecessary investigations [Mink and Neil, 1995].

Paroxysmal Disorders and Channelopathies

Mutations in the genes encoding ion channels may disrupt excitability of cellular membranes and result in paroxysmal disorders such as epilepsy, periodic paralysis, myotonic dystrophy, and malignant hyperthermia. Among the nonepileptic paroxysmal disorders discussed in this chapter, acetazolamide-responsive paroxysmal ataxia and hyperekplexia are identified as channelopathies. Proximity of the gene locus for paroxysmal dystonic choreoathetosis to a cluster of ion-channel genes on chromosome 2q raises the possibility that this also is a channelopathy. Distinct types of *CACNA1A* gene mutations located in chromosome 19 are found in acetazolamide-responsive paroxysmal ataxia, familial hemiplegic migraine, and spinocerebellar ataxia type 6 [Ducros et al., 2001]. Such broad clinical manifestations, derived from mutations of a gene that encodes the α_{1A} subunit of voltage-gated neuronal calcium channels, may help to understand the common association of migraine, epilepsy, ataxia and other paroxysmal disorders [Jancovic and Demirkiran, 2002].

REFERENCES

Abboud FM. Neurocardiogenic syncope. New Engl J Med 1993;328:1118.

Abu-Arafeh I, Russell G. Cyclical vomiting syndrome in children: A population-based study. J Pediatr Gastroenterol Nutr 1995;21:454.

Aicardi J. Paroxysmal disorders other than epilepsy. In: Aicardi J, ed. Diseases of the nervous system in childhood. Oxford: Blackwell, 1992.

Albright AL, Sclabassi RJ, Slamovits TL, et al. Spasmus nutans associated with optic gliomas in infants. J Pediatr 1984;105:778.

Alehan D, Celiker A, Ozme S. Head-up tilt test: A highly sensitive, specific test for children with unexplained syncope. Pediatr Cardiol 1996;17:86.

Allarakhia IN, Trobe DJ. Opsoclonus-myoclonus presenting with features of spasmus nutans. J Child Neurol 1995;10:67.

Andermann F, Andermann E. Startle disorders in man: Hyperekplexia, jumping and startle epilepsy. Brain Dev 1988;10:213.

Andermann F, Keene DL, Andermann E, et al. Startle disease or hyperekplexia. Further delineation of the syndrome. Brain 1980;103:985.

Anthony JH, Ouvrier RA, Wise G. Spasmus nutans: a mistaken identity. Arch Neurol 1980;37:373.

Barron TF, Younkin DP. Propranolol therapy for shuddering attacks. Neurology 1992;42:258.

Bass C. Hyperventilation syndrome: A chimera? J Psychosom Res 1997;42:421.

Basser LS. Benign paroxysmal vertigo of childhood (a variety of vestibular neuronitis). Brain 1964;87:141.

Benditt DG, Lurie KG, Adler SW, et al. Pathophysiology of vasovagal syncope. In: Blanc JJ, Benditt D, Sutton R, eds. Neurally mediated syncope: Pathophysiology, investigations, and treatment. Armonk, NY: Futura, 1996a.

Benditt DG, Lurie KG. Tilt-table testing: toward a "universal" protocol. In: Blanc JJ, Benditt D, Sutton R, eds. Neurally mediated syncope: Pathophysiology, investigations, and treatment. Armonk, NY: Futura, 1996b.

Bleasel A, Kotagal P. Paroxysmal nonepileptic disorders in children and adolescents. Sem Neurol 1995;15:203.

Boehm KE, Kip KT, Grubb BP, et al. Neurocardiogenic syncope: Response to hormonal therapy. Pediatrics 1997;99:623.

Bratt HD, Menelaus MB. Benign paroxysmal torticollis of infancy. J Bone Joint Surg [Br] 1992;74B:449.

Bray PF. "Brain fits" or "stomach fits"? Ann Neurol 1977;2:176.

Bressman SB, Fahn S, Burke RE. Paroxysmal non-kinesigenic dystonia. Adv Neurol 1988;50:403.

Brown P. Neurophysiology of the startle syndrome and hyperekplexia. Adv Neurol 2002;89:153.

Buruma OJS, Roos RAC. Paroxysmal choreoathetosis. In: Vinken PJ, Bruyn GW, Klawans HL, eds. Handbook of clinical neurology, Vol. 49 (Revised Series 5), Extrapyramidal disorders. Amsterdam: Elsevier, 1986.

Bye AM, Kok DJ, Ferenschild FT, et al. Paroxysmal non-epileptic events in children: A retrospective study over a period of 10 years. J Paediatr Child Health 2000;36:244.

Casteels K, Wouters C, Van Geet C, et al. Video reveals self-stimulation in infancy. Acta Paediatr 2004;93:844.

Cataltepe SE, Barron TF. Benign paroxysmal torticollis presenting as "seizures" in infancy. Clin Pediatr 1993;32:564.

Chaves-Carballo E. Paroxysmal torticollis. Sem Pediatr Neurol 1996;3:255.

Chaves-Carballo E, Dabbagh O, Essa M, et al. Neurological complications of hyperekplexia in infancy. Ann Neurol 1999;46:466.

Chutorian AM. Benign paroxysmal torticollis, tortipelvis and retrocollis in infancy. Neurology 1974;24:366.

Cohen HA, Nussinovitch M, Ashkenasi A, et al. Benign paroxysmal torticollis in infancy. Pediatr Neurol 1993;9:488.

Cullen KJ, MacDonald WB. The periodic syndrome: Its nature and prevalence. Med J Austral 1963;2:167.

Demirkiran M, Jankovic J. Paroxysmal dyskinesias: Clinical features and a new classification. Ann Neurol 1995;38:571.

Deonna T, Martin D. Benign paroxysmal torticollis in infancy. Arch Dis Child 1981;56:956.

Deonna T, Roulet E, Meyer HU. Benign paroxysmal tonic upgaze of childhood—A new syndrome. Neuropediatrics 1990;21:213.

de Saint-Martin A, Badinand N, Picard F, et al. Diurnal and nocturnal dyskinesia in young children: A new entity? Rev Neurol (Paris) 1997;153:262.

Dignan F, Symon DNK, AbuArafeh I, et al. The prognosis of cyclical vomiting syndrome. Arch Dis Child 2001;84:55.

Dijane P, Deharo J-P, Macaluso G. Use of tilt table testing in clinical practice: Its role in the evaluation of syncope and dizziness. In: Blanc JJ, Benditt D, Sutton R, eds. Neurally mediated syncope: Pathophysiology, investigations, and treatment. Armonk, NY: Futura, 1996.

DiMario FJ Jr. Childhood head tremor. J Child Neurol 2000;15:22.

Donat JF, Wright FS. Episodic symptoms mistaken for seizures in the neurologically impaired child. Neurology 1990;40:156.

Dooley JM, Andermann F. Startle disease or hyperekplexia: Adolescent onset and response to valproate. Pediatr Neurol 1989;5:126.

Dravet C, Giraud N, Bureau M, et al. Benign myoclonus of early infancy or benign non-epileptic infantile spasms. Neuropediatr 1986;17:33.

Drigo P, Carli G, Laverda AM. Benign paroxysmal vertigo of childhood. Brain Dev 2001;23:38.

Driscoll DJ, Jacobsen SJ, Porter CJ, et al. Syncope in children and adolescents. J Am Coll Cardiol 1997;29:1030.

Ducros A, Denier C, Joutel A, et al. The clinical spectrum of familial hemiplegic migraine associated with mutations in a neuronal calcium channel. N Engl J Med 2001;345:17.

Dunn DW, Snyder CH. Benign paroxysmal vertigo of childhood. Am J Dis Child 1976;130:1099.

Eeg-Olofsson O, Odkvist L, Lindskog U, et al. Benign paroxysmal vertigo in childhood. Acta Otolaryngol 1982;93:283.

Evans RW. Neurologic aspects of hyperventilation syndrome. Sem Neurol 1995;15:115.

Eviatar L. Benign paroxysmal torticollis. Pediatr Neurol 1994;11:72.

Farmer J, Hoyt CS. Monocular nystagmus in infancy and early childhood. Am J Ophthalmol 1984;98:504.

Feit LR. Syncope in the pediatric patient: Diagnosis, pathophysiology, and treatment. Adv Pediatr 1996;43:469.

Fenichel GM. Migraine as a cause of benign paroxysmal vertigo in childhood. J Pediatr 1967;71:114.

Fernández Sanmartín M, Rodríguez Núñez A, Martinón-Torres F, et al. Síncope convulsivo: Características y reproducibilidad mediante la prueba de la cama basculante [Convulsive syncope: Characteristics and reproducibility using the tilt test]. Ann Pediatr (Barc) 2003;59:441.

Fink JK, Rainer S, Wilkowski J, et al. Paroxysmal dystonic choreoathetosis: Tight linkage to chromosome 2q. Am J Hum Genet 1996;59:140.

Finkhelhor BK, Harker LA. Benign paroxysmal vertigo of childhood. Laryngoscope 1987;97:1161.

Fitzpatrick A, Banner N, Cheng A, et al. Vasovagal reactions may occur after orthoptic heart transplantation. J Am Coll Cardiol 1993;21:1132.

Fleisher DR. The cyclic vomiting syndrome described. J Pediatr Gastroenterol Nutr 1995;21(Suppl 1):S1.

Fleisher DR, Matar M. The cyclic vomiting syndrome: A report of 71 cases and literature review. J Pediatr Gastroenterol Nutr 1993;17:361.

Fleisher DR, Morrison A. Masturbation mimicking abdominal pain or seizures in young girls. J Pediatr 1990;116:810.

Fogoros RN. Cardiac arrhythmias, syncope and stroke. Neurol Clin 1993;11:375.

Folks DG. Munchausen's syndrome and other factitious disorders. Neurol Clin 1995;13:267.

Furukawa Y, Mizuno Y, Nishi K, et al. A clue to the pathogenesis of dopa-responsive dystonia. Ann Neurol 1995;37:139.

Gastaut H. Syncope: Generalized anoxic cerebral seizures. In: Vinken PJ, Bruyn GW, eds. Handbook of clinical neurology, Vol. 15. The epilepsies. Amsterdam: North-Holland, 1974.

Gellis SS, Feingold M. Syndrome of hiatus hernia with torsion spasms and abnormal posturing (Sandifer's syndrome). Am J Dis Child 1971;121:53.

Gilbert GJ. Familial spasmodic torticollis. Neurology 1977;27:11.

Giffin NJ, Benton S, Goadsby PJ. Benign paroxysmal torticollis of infancy: Four new cases and linkage to CACNA1A mutation. Dev Med Child Neurol 2002;44:490.

Gilles de la Tourette G. Jumping, latah, myriachit. Arch Neurol 1884;8:68.

Gilles de la Tourette G. La maladie des tics convulsifs. La Semaine Medicale 1899;19:153.

Gordon N. Startle disease or hyperekplexia. Dev Med Child Neurol 1993;35:1015.

Gorrotxategi P, Reguikon MJ, Arana J, et al. Gastroesphageal reflux in association with the Sandifer syndrome. Eur J Pediatr Surg 1995;5:203.

Gottlob I, Zubcov A, Catalano RA, et al. Signs distinguishing spasmus nutans (with and without central nervous system lesions) from infantile nystagmus. Ophthalmology 1990;97:1166.

Gottlob I, Zubcov AA, Wizov SS, et al. Head nodding is compensatory in spasmus nutans. Ophthalmology 1992; 99:1024.

Gottlob I, Wizov SS, Reinecke RD. Quantitative eye and head movement recordings of retinal disease mimicking spasmus nutans. Am J Ophthalmol 1995a;119:374.

Gottlob I, Wizov SS, Reinecke RD. Spasmus nutans. A long-term follow-up. Invest Ophthalmol Vis Sci 1995b;36:2768.

Graybiel A, McFarland R. Use of tilt-table test in aviation medicine. J Aviation Med 1941;12:194.

Griggs RC, Moxley RT, Lafrance RA, et al. Hereditary paroxysmal ataxia: Response to acetazolamide. Neurology 1978;28:1259.

Grubb BP, Gerard G, Roush K, et al. Cerebral vasoconstriction during head-upright tilt-induced vasovagal syncope. A paradoxic and unexpected response. Circulation 1991;84:1157.

Grubb BP, Kosinski D. Current trends in etiology, diagnosis and management of neurocardiogenic syncope. Curr Opin Cardiol 1996;11:32.

Grubb BP, Orecchio E, Kurczynski TW. Head-upright tilt table testing in evaluation of recurrent, unexplained syncope. Pediatr Neurol 1992;8:423.

Guerrini R, Belmonte A, Carrozzo R. Paroxysmal tonic upgaze of childhood with ataxia: A benign transient dystonia with autosomal dominant inheritance. Brain Dev 1998;20:116.

Hallett M, Marsden CD, Fahn S. Myoclonus. In: Vinken PJ, Bruyn GW, Klawans HL, eds. Handbook of clinical neurology, Vol. 49 (revised series 5). Extrapyramidal disorders. Amsterdam: Elsevier, 1986.

Hammond J. The late sequelae of recurrent vomiting of childhood. Dev Med Child Neurol 1974;16:15.

Hannon DW, Knilans TK. Syncope in children and adolescents. Current Probl Pediatr 1993;23:358.

Hanukoglu A, Somekh E, Fried D. Benign paroxysmal torticollis in infancy. Clin Pediatr 1984;23:272.

Hayman M, Harvey AS, Hopkins IJ, et al. Paroxysmal tonic upgaze: A reappraisal of outcome. Ann Neurol 1998;43:514.

Hejazi NS, Chaves EC, Boumah C, et al. Linkage of hyperekplexia (HEK) in three Saudi families to chromosome 4q31.3 associated with the glycine receptor beta subunit (GLRβ). Neurology 2001;56(Suppl 3):A132.

Herman SP, Stickler GB, Lucas AR. Hyperventilation syndrome in children and adolescents: long-term follow-up. Pediatrics 1981;67:183.

Hirsch E, Sellal F, Maton B, et al. Nocturnal paroxysmal dystonia: A clinical form of focal epilepsy. Neurophysiol Clin 1994;24:207.

Hoefnagel D, Biery B. Spasmus nutans. Dev Med Child Neurol 1968;10:32.

Hoefnagels WAJ, Padberg GW, Overweg J, et al: Syncope or seizures? A matter of opinion. Clin Neurol Neurosurg 1992;94:153.

Holmes GL, Russman BS. Shuddering attacks. Evaluation using electroencephalographic frequency modulation radiotelemetry and videotape monitoring. Am J Dis Child 1986;140:72.

Houser MK, Soland VL, Bhatia KP, et al. Paroxysmal kinesigenic choreoathetosis: A report of 26 patients. J Neurol 1999;246:120.

Hoyt SC, Stickler GB. A study of 44 children with the syndrome of recurrent (cyclic) vomiting. Pediatrics 1960;25:775.

Igarashi M, Boehm RM Jr, May WN, et al. Syncope associated with hair-grooming. Brain Dev 1988;10:249.

Iivanainen M, Kaakola S. Dopa-responsive dystonia of childhood. Dev Med Child Neurol 1993;35:362.

Jankovic J, Demirkiran M. Classification of paroxysmal dyskinesias and ataxias. Adv Neurol 2002;89:387.

Joutel A, Bousser MG, Biousse V, et al. A gene for familial hemiplegic migraine maps to chromosome 19. Nat Gen 1993;5:40.

Kanazawa O. Shuddering attacks-report of four children. Pediatr Neurol 2000;23:421.

Kapoor WN. Evaluation and outcome of patients with syncope. Medicine 1990;69:160.

Kapoor WN. Diagnostic evaluation of syncope. Am J Med 1991;90:91.

Kapoor WN. Importance of neurocardiogenic causes in etiology of syncope. In: Blanc JJ, Benditt D, Sutton R, eds. Neurally mediated syncope: Pathophysiology, investigations, and treatment. Armonk, NY: Futura, 1996.

Kapoor WN, Karpf M, Wieand S, et al. A prospective evaluation and follow-up of patients with syncope. New Engl J Med 1983;309:197.

Kapoor WN, Smith MA, Miller NL, et al. Upright tilt testing in evaluating syncope: A comprehensive literature review. Am J Med 1994;97:78.

Kapoor WN. Using a tilt table to evaluate syncope. Am J Med Sci 1999;317:110.

Kapoor WN. Syncope. New Engl J Med 2000;343:1856.

Kelly TW. Optic glioma presenting as spasmus nutans. Pediatrics 1970;45:295.

Kenny RA, Ingram A, Bayliss J, et al. Head-up tilt: A useful test for investigating unexplained syncope. Lancet 1986;1:1352.

Kertesz A. Paroxysmal kinesigenic choreoathetosis. An entity within paroxysmal choreoathetosis syndrome. Description of 10 cases, including 1 autopsied. Neurology 1967;17:680.

Kinast M, Erenberg G, Rothner DA. Paroxysmal choreoathetosis: Report of five cases and review of the literature. Pediatrics 1980;65:74.

Kinsbourne M, Oxon DM. Hiatus hernia with contortions of the neck. Lancet 1964;1:1048.

Kinsella SM, Tuckey JP. Perioperative bradycardia and asystole: Relationship to vasovagal syncope and the Bezold-Jarisch reflex. Brit J Anesth 2001;86:859.

Klein R, Haddow JE, DeLuca C. Familial congenital disorder resembling stiff-man syndrome. Am J Dis Child 1972;124:730.

Kosinski D, Grubb BP, Temesy-Armos P. Pathophysiological aspects of neurocardiogenic syncope: Current concepts and new perspectives. PACE Pacing Clin Electrophysiol 1995;18:716.

Kotagal P, Costa M, Wyllie E, et al. Paroxysmal nonepileptic events in children and adolescents. Pediatrics 2002;110:e46.

Krahn AD, Klein GJ, Yee R, et al. Use of an extended monitoring strategy in patients with problematic syncope. Circulation 1999;99:406.

Kudenchuk PJ, McAnulty JH. Syncope: Evaluation and treatment. Modern Concepts Cardiovasc Dis 1985;54:25.

Kurczynski TW. Hyperekplexia. Arch Neurol 1983;40:246.

Lambert SR, Newman NJ. Retinal disease masquerading as spasmus nutans. Neurology 1993;43:1607.

Lance JW. Familial paroxysmal dystonic choreoathetosis and its differentiation from related syndromes. Ann Neurol 1977;2:285.

Landau WM, Nelson DA. Clinical neuromythology XV. Feinting science: Neurocardiogenic syncope and collateral vasovagal confusion. Neurology 1996;46:609.

Lazarus JC, Mauro VF. Syncope: Pathophysiology, diagnosis, and pharmacotherapy. Ann Pharmacother 1996;30:994.

Leor J, Rotstein Z, Vered Z, et al. Absence of tachycardia during tilt test predicts failure of beta-blocker therapy in patients with neurocardiogenic syncope. Am Heart J 1994;127:1539.

Lerman-Sagie T, Lerman P, Mukamel M, et al. A prospective evaluation of pediatric patients with syncope. Clin Pediatr 1994;33:67.
Leung AKC, Robson WLM. Childhood masturbation. Clin Pediatr 1993;32:238.
Lewis T. A lecture on vasovagal syncope and the carotid sinus mechanism with comments on Gowers' and Nothnagel's syndrome. BMJ 1932;1:873.
Lewis DW, Frank LM. Hair-grooming syncope seizures. Pediatrics 1993;91:836.
Li BUK. Cyclic vomiting: The pattern and syndrome paradigm. J Pediatr Gastroenterol Nutr 1995;21(Suppl 1):S6.
Lieshout JJV, Wieling W, Karemaker JM, et al. The vasovagal response. Clin Sci 1991;81:575.
Lin JT-W, Ziegler DK, Lai C-W, et al. Convulsive syncope in blood donors. Ann Neurol 1982;11:525.
Lingam S, Wilson J, Hart EW. Hereditary stiff-baby syndrome. Am J Dis Child 1981;135:909.
Linzer M, Yang EH, Mark Estes NA, et al. Diagnosing syncope. Part 1: Value of history, physical examination, and electrocardiography. Ann Int Med 1997a;126:989.
Linzer M, Yang EH, Mark Estes NA, et al. Diagnosing syncope. Part 2: Unexplained syncope. Ann Int Med 1997b;127:76.
Lipson EH, Robertson WC. Paroxysmal torticollis of infancy: Familial occurrence. Am J Dis Child 1978;132:422.
Lombroso CT. Paroxysmal choreoathetosis. An epileptic or non-epileptic disorder? Italian J Neurol Sci 1995;16:271.
Lombroso CT, Fejerman N. Benign myoclonus of early infancy. Ann Neurol 1977;1:138.
Lubbers WJ, Brunt ER, Scheffer H, et al. Hereditary myokymia and paroxysmal ataxia linked to chromosome 12 is responsive to acetazolamide. J Neurol Neurosurg Psych 1995;59:400.
Luders HO. Paroxysmal choreoathetosis. Europ Neurol 1996;36(Suppl 1):20.
Mandel H, Tirosh E, Berant M. Sandifer syndrome reconsidered. Acta Paediatr Scand 1989;78:797.
Manolis AS, Linzer M, Salem D, et al. Syncope: Current diagnostic evaluation and management. Ann Int Med 1990;112:850.
Mansourati J, Blanc JJ. Tilt test procedure: Angle, duration, positive criteria. In: Blanc JJ, Benditt D, Sutton R, eds. Neurally mediated syncope: Pathophysiology, investigations, and treatment. Armonk, NY: Futura, 1996.
Maydell BV, Berenson F, Rothner AD, et al. Benign myoclonus of early infancy: An imitator of West's syndrome. J Child Neurol 2001;16:109.
Merino-Andreu M, Arcas J, Izal-Linares E, et al. Desviación ocular paroxística benigna infantil: Un trastorno no epiléptico? Rev Neurol 2004;39:129.
Milstein S, Buetikofer J, Dunnigan A, et al: Usefulness of disopyramide for prevention of upright tilt-induced hypotension-bradycardia. Am J Cardiol 1990;54:1339.
Mink JW, Neil JJ. Masturbation mimicking paroxysmal dystonia or dyskinesia in a young girl. Movement Disorders 1995;10:518.
Mitchell WG, Greenwood RS, Messenheimer JA. Abdominal epilepsy. Cyclic vomiting as the major symptom of simple partial seizures. Arch Neurol 1983;40:251.
Mosqueda-García R, Furlan R, Tank J, et al. The elusive pathophysiology of neurally mediated syncope. Circulation 2000;102:2898.
Mount LA, Reback S. Familial paroxysmal choreoathetosis: Preliminary report on a hitherto undescribed clinical syndrome. Arch Neurol 1940;44:841.
Moya A, Permanyer-Miralda G, Sagrista J, et al. Is there a role for tilt testing in the evaluation of treatment of vasovagal syncope? In: Blanc JJ, Benditt D, Sutton R, eds. Neurally mediated syncope: Pathophysiology, investigations, and treatment. Armonk, NY: Futura, 1996a.
Moya A, Sgrista J, Permanyer-Miralda G, et al. Isoproterenol and tilt test: Protocol, importance, contraindications. In: Blanc JJ, Benditt D, Sutton R, eds. Neurally mediated syncope: Pathophysiology, investigations, and treatment. Armonk, NY: Futura, 1996b.
Nechay A, Ross LM, Stephenson JB, et al. Gratification disorder ("infantile masturbation"): A review. Arch Dis child 2004;89:225.
Nigro M, Lim HC. Hyperekplexia and sudden neonatal death. Pediatr Neurol 1992;8:221.
Njemanze PC. Critical limits of pressure-flow relation in the human brain. Stroke 1992;23:1743.
Njemanze PC. Isoproterenol induced cerebral hypoperfusion in a heart transplant recipient. PACE Pacing Clin Electrophysiol 1993;16:491.
Noone PG, King M, Loftus BG. Benign neonatal sleep myoclonus. Irish Med J 1995;88:172.
Norton EWD, Cogan DG. Spasmus nutans: A clinical study of twenty cases followed two years or more since onset. Arch Ophthalmol 1954;52:442.
Nygaard TG. Dopa-responsive dystonia. Delineation of the clinical syndrome and clues to the pathogenesis. Adv Neurol 1993;60:577.
Nygaard TG. Dopa-responsive dystonia. Curr Opinion Neurol 1995;8:310.
Nygaard TG, Waran SP, Levine RA, et al. Dopa-responsive dystonia simulating cerebral palsy. Pediatr Neurol 1994;11:236.
Oguni M, Oguni H, Kozasa M, et al. A case of nocturnal paroxysmal unilateral dystonia and interictal right frontal epileptic EEG focus: A lateralized variant of nocturnal paroxysmal dystonia. Brain Dev 1992;14:412.
Olson AD, Li BU. The diagnostic evaluation of children with cyclic vomiting: A cost-effectiveness assessment. J Pediatr 2002;141:724.
O'Marcaigh AS, MacLellan-Tobert S, Coburn JP. Tilt-table testing and oral metoprolol in young patients with unexplained syncope. Pediatrics 1994;93:278.
Ophoff RA, Terwindt GM, Vergouwe MN, et al. Familial hemiplegic migraine and episodic ataxia type 2 are caused by mutations in the Ca2+ channel gene CACNL1A4. Cell 1996;87:543.
Ouvrier RA, Billson F. Benign paroxysmal tonic upgaze of childhood. J Child Neurol 1988;3:177.
Pachatz C, Fusco L, Vigevano F. Benign myoclonus of early infancy. Epileptic Disord 1999;1:57.
Pfau BT, Li BUK, Murray RD, et al. Differentiating cyclic from chronic vomiting patterns in children: Quantitative criteria and diagnostic implications. Pediatrics 1996;97:364.
Pratt JL, Fleisher GR. Syncope in children and adolescents. Pediatr Emerg Care 1989;5:80.
Pryles CV, Livingston S, Ford FR. Familial paroxysmal choreoathetosis of Mount and Reback. Pediatrics 1952;9:44.
Przuntek H, Monninger P. Therapeutic aspects of kinesiogenic paroxysmal choreoathetosis and familial paroxysmal choreoathetosis of the mount and reback type. J Neurol 1983;230:163.
Rajendra S, Lynch JW, Schofield PR. The glycine receptor. Pharmacol Therap 1997;73:121.
Rajput AH, Gibb WRG, Zhong XH, et al. Dopa-responsive dystonia: Pathological and biochemical observations in a case. Ann Neurol 1994;35:396.
Raviele A, Themistoclakis S, Gasparini G. Drug treatment of vasovagal syncope. In: Blanc JJ, Benditt D, Sutton R, eds. Neurally mediated syncope: Pathophysiology, investigations, and treatment. Armonk, NY: Futura, 1996.
Rea R, Thames MD. Neural control mechanisms and vasovagal syncope. J Cardiovasc Electrophysiol 1993;4:587.
Rees MI, Lewis TM, Kwok JBJ, et al. Hyperekplexia associated with compound heterozygote mutations in the β-subunit of the human inhibitory glycine receptor (*GLRB*). Hum Mol Genet 2002;11:853.
Reif-Lehrer L, Stemmermann MG. Monosodium glutamate intolerance in children. New Engl J Med 1975;293:1204.
Reinhart JB, Evans SI, McFadden DL. Cyclic vomiting in children: Seen through the psychiatrist's eye. Pediatrics 1977;59:371.
Rodríguez-Nuñez A, Couceiro J, Alonso C, et al. Cerebral oxygenation in children with syncope during head-upright tilt test. Pediatr Cardiol 1997;18:406.
Ryan SG, Sherman SL, Terry JC, et al. Startle disease, or hyperekplexia: Response to clonazepam and assignment of the gene (STHE) to chromosome 5q by linkage analysis. Ann Neurol 1992;31:663.
Sallustro F, Atwell CW. Body rocking, head banging, and head rolling in normal children. J Pediatr 1978;93:704.
Sanner G, Bergstrom B. Benign paroxysmal torticollis in infancy. Acta Paediatr Scand 1979;68:219.
Savage DD, Corwin L, McGee DL, et al. Epidemiological features of isolated syncope: The Framingham study. Stroke 1985;16:626.
Schraeder PL, Lathers CM, Charles JB. The spectrum of syncope. J Clin Pharmacol 1994;34:454.
Scott WA, Pongiglione G, Bromberg BI, et al. Randomized comparison of atenolol and fludrocortisone acetate in the treatment of pediatric neurally mediated syncope. Am J Cardiol 1995;76:400.
Segawa M, Nomura Y, Kase M. Diurnally fluctuating hereditary progressive dystonia. In: Vinken PJ, Bruyn GW, Klawans HL, eds. Handbook of clinical neurology, Vol. 5 (Revised Series) (49). Amsterdam: Elsevier, 1986.

Segawa M. Hereditary progressive dystonia with marked diurnal fluctuation. Brain Dev 2000;22 (Suppl 1):S65.

Segawa M, Nomura Y, Nishiyama N. Autosomal dominant guanosine triphosphate cyclohydrolase I deficiency (Segawa disease). Ann Neurol 2003;54(Suppl 6):S32.

Shahar E, Brand N, Uziel Y, et al. Nose tapping test inducing a generalized flexor spasm: A hallmark of hyperekplexia. Acta Paediatr Scand 1991;80:1073.

Shahar E, Raviv R. Sporadic major hyperekplexia in neonates and infants: Clinical manifestations and outcome. Pediatr Neurol 2004;31:30.

Shen W-K, Gersh BJ. Syncope: mechanisms, approach, and management. In: Low PA, ed. Clinical autonomic disorders. Boston: Little, Brown & Co, 1993.

Shepherd RW, Wren J, Evans S, et al. Gastroesophageal reflux in children. Clinical profile, course and outcome with active therapy in 126 cases. Clin Pediatr 1987;26:55.

Shiang R, Ryan SG, Zhu Y-Z, et al. Mutations in alpha-1 subunit of the inhibitory glycine receptor cause the dominant neurologic disorders, hyperekplexia. Nature (Genetics) 1993;5:351.

Shiang R, Ryan SG, Zhu Y-Z, et al. Mutational analysis of familial and sporadic hyperekplexia. Ann Neurol 1995;38:85.

Shulman LM, Weiner WJ. Paroxysmal movement disorders. Sem Neurol 1995;15:188.

Smith DE, Fitzgerald K, Stass-Isern M, et al. Electroretinography is necessary for spasmus nutans diagnosis. Pediatr Neurol 2000;23:33.

Sneddon JF, Camm AJ. Vasovagal syncope: Classification, investigation and treatment. Br J Hosp Med 1993;49:329.

Snow BJ, Nygaard TG, Takahashi H, et al. Positron emission tomographic studies of dopa-responsive dystonia and early-onset parkinsonism. Ann Neurol 1993;34:733.

Snyder CH. Paroxysmal torticollis in infancy. A possible form of labyrinthitis. Am J Dis Child 1969;117:458.

Soteriades ES, Evans JC, Larson MG, et al. Incidence and prognosis of syncope. New Engl J Med 2002;347:878.

Sotero de Menezes MA. Paroxysmal non-epileptic events. J Pediatr (Rio J) 2002;78(Suppl 1):73.

Sra J, Maglio C, Biehl M, et al. Efficacy of midodrine hydrochloride in neurocardiogenic syncope refractory to standard therapy. J Cardiovasc Electrophysiol 1997;8:42.

Sra JS, Anderson AJ, Sheikh SH, et al. Unexplained syncope evaluated by electrophysiologic studies and head-up tilt testing. Ann Int Med 1991;114:1013.

Sra JS, Murthy VS, Jazayeri MR, et al. Use of intravenous esmolol to predict efficacy of oral beta-adrenergic blocker therapy in patients with neurocardiogenic syncope. J Am Coll Cardiol 1992;19:402.

Sra JS, Murthy V, Natale A, et al. Circulatory and catecholamine changes during head-up tilt testing in neurocardiogenic (vasovagal) syncope. Am J Cardiol 1994;73:33.

Stephenson JBP. Reflex anoxic seizures ("white breath-holding"): Non-epileptic vagal attacks. Arch Dis Child 1978;53:193.

Stephenson JBP. Reflex anoxic seizures and ocular compression. Dev Med Child Neurol 1980a;22:380.

Stephenson JBP. Benign familial stiff baby syndrome. Arch Dis Child 1980b;55:907.

Stephenson JBP. Fits and faints. Oxford: Blackwell, 1990a.

Stephenson JBP. Epileptic and non-epileptic seizures: Words and meanings. In: Stephenson JBP. Fits and faints. Oxford: Blackwell, 1990b.

Stephenson JBP. Size of the problem. In: Stephenson JBP. Fits and faints. Oxford: Blackwell, 1990c.

Stephenson JBP. Anoxic seizures or syncopes. In: Stephenson JBP. Fits and faints. Oxford: Blackwell, 1990d.

Stephenson JBP. Specific syncopes and anoxic seizure types. In: Stephenson JBP. Fits and faints. Oxford: Blackwell, 1990e.

Stephenson JBP. Vagocardiac syncope and reflex anoxic seizures. In: Stephenson JBP. Fits and faints. Oxford: Blackwell, 1990f.

Stephenson JBP. Anoxic-epileptic seizures. In: Stephenson JBP. Fits and faints. Oxford: Blackwell, 1990g.

Strieper MJ, Auld DO, Hulse JE, et al. Evaluation of recurrent pediatric syncope: Role of tilt table testing. Pediatrics 1994;93:660.

Sutton R. Vasovagal syncope: Clinical features, epidemiology, and natural history. In: Blanc JJ, Benditt D, Sutton R, eds. Neurally mediated syncope: Pathophysiology, investigations, and treatment. Armonk, NY: Futura, 1996.

Symon DNK, Russell G. The relationship between cyclic vomiting syndrome and abdominal migraine. J Pediatr Gastroenterol Nutr 1995;21(Suppl 1):S42.

Tanaka H, Endo K, Tsuji S, et al. The gene for hereditary progressive dystonia with marked diurnal fluctuation maps to chromosome 14q. Ann Neurol 1995;37:405.

Temudo T. Discinesia paroxística en la infancia. Rev Neurol 2004;38:53.

Thilenius OG, Quinones JA, Husayni TS, et al. Tilt test for diagnosis of unexplained syncope in pediatric patients. Pediatrics 1991;87:334.

Tibbles JAR, Barnes SE. Paroxysmal dystonic choreoathetosis of Mount and Reback. Pediatrics 1980;65:149.

Tijssen MA, Schoemaker HC, Edelbroek PJ, et al. The effects of clonazepam and vigabatrin in hyperekplexia. J Neurol Sci 1997;149:63.

Tijssen MA, Vergouwe MN, van Dijk JG, et al. Major and minor form of hereditary hyperekplexia. Mov Disord 2002;17:826.

Van Bogaert P, Van Nechel C, Goldman S, et al. Acetazolamide-responsive hereditary paroxysmal ataxia: Report of a new family. Acta Neurol Belg 1993;93:268.

Van Bogaert P, Szliwowski HB. EEG findings in acetazolamide-responsive hereditary paroxysmal ataxia. Neurophysiol Clin 1996;26:335.

Vanderhoof JA, Young R, Kaufman SS, et al. Treatment of cyclic vomiting in childhood with erythromycin. J Pediatr Gastroenterol Nutr 1995;21(Suppl 1):S60.

Vanesse M, Bedard P, Andermann F. Shuddering attacks in children: An early clinical manifestation of early tremor. Neurology 1976;26:1027.

Veggiotti P, Zambrino CA, Balottin U, et al. Concurrent nocturnal and diurnal paroxysmal dystonia. Childs Nerv Syst 1993;9:458.

Verrotti A, Trotta D, Blasetti A, et al. Paroxysmal tonic upgaze of childhood: Effect of age-of-onset on prognosis. Acta Paediatr 2001;90:1343.

Victor J. Tilt test. Environment, material, patient preparation. In: Blanc JJ, Benditt D, Sutton R, eds. Neurally mediated syncope: Pathophysiology, investigations, and treatment. Armonk, NY: Futura, 1996.

Vighetto A, Forment JC, Trillet M, et al. Magnetic resonance imaging in familial paroxysmal ataxia. Arch Neurol 1988;45:547.

Von Brederlow B, Hahn AF, Koopman WJ, et al. Mapping the gene for acetazolamide responsive hereditary paroxysmal cerebellar ataxia to chromosome 19p. Hum Mol Genet 1995;4:279.

Walker-Smith J. Historical perspectives of cyclic vomiting. J Pediatr Gastroenterol Nutr 1995;21(Suppl 1):ix.

Wein T, Andermann F, Silver K, et al. Exquisite sensitivity of paroxysmal kinesigenic choreoathetosis to carbamazepine. Neurology 1996;47:1104.

Werlin SL, D'Souza BJ, Hogan WJ, et al. Sandifer syndrome: An unappreciated clinical entity. Dev Med Child Neurol 1980;22:374.

Williams J, Stevens H. Familial paroxysmal chorea-athetosis. Pediatrics 1963;31:656.

Wizov S, Reinecke RD, Bocarnea M, et al. A comparative demographic and socioeceonomic study of spasmus nutans and infantile nystagmus. Am J Ophthalmol 2002;133:256.

CHAPTER 56

Sleep-Wake Disorders

Suresh Kotagal

Complaints about insufficient or nonrestorative sleep are quite common during childhood and adolescence. In a questionnaire survey of 332 children of 11 through 15 years of age, Ipsiroglu and associates [2001] observed that 28% of the subjects complained of snoring, insomnia, or a parasomnia. In another study of 472, 4- to 12-year-old urban and rural children receiving routine pediatric care, Stein and co-workers [2001] noted a 10% prevalence of sleep disorders on a questionnaire survey, but that less than one half of the parents had discussed the sleep problems with the child's pediatrician. Childhood sleep disorders can have a significant effect on the quality of life. Many are also easily treatable, thus underscoring the importance of their prompt recognition and management. This chapter covers salient aspects of childhood sleep-wake function and common pediatric sleep disorders.

SLEEP PHYSIOLOGY AND ONTOGENY

Sleep onset is facilitated by melatonin, which is a hormone released by the pineal gland. Bright light suppresses melatonin release, whereas dim light facilitates its release. The ultimate command center for the once-a-day (circadian) rhythm of sleep and wakefulness is the *suprachiasmatic nucleus* of the hypothalamus [Miller et al., 1996; Steriade et al., 1993], which has cells with receptors for melatonin. The suprachiasmatic nucleus is also strongly infiuenced by light-mediated impulses received through the retino-hypothalamic tract. Clock and period genes, remarkably preserved across various phyla, were studied initially in *Drosophila melanogaster;* they also influence the timing of activity of the suprachiasmatic nucleus cells [Challet et al., 2003; Hamada et al., 2001]. The body temperature rhythm is also regulated by the hypothalamus [van Someren, 2000]—a rise in body temperature leads to postponement of sleep. Conversely, individuals are most sleepy around the nadir of body temperature, that is, around 0400 hours. An artificial increase in body temperature in the 1 to 2 hours before bedtime, such as through vigorous exercise, may provoke sleep-onset insomnia.

Wakefulness can be differentiated from sleep by 27 to 28 weeks' postconceptional age in the preterm infant. At this age, sleep is primarily of the active or rapid eye movement type, which is associated with irregular breathing, phasic or intermittent electromyographic activity, and low-voltage electroencephalographic activity. Cerebral blood fiow and cerebral metabolism are higher in rapid eye movement relative to non–rapid eye movement sleep (also termed *quiet sleep* in newborns). By 40 weeks' postconceptional age, active (rapid eye movement) sleep decreases to about 50% of the total sleep time, with a corresponding rise in the proportion of quiet (non–rapid eye movement) sleep. By 46 to 48 weeks postconceptional age, sleep spindles appear during stages II and III of non–rapid eye movement sleep. By 4 to 6 months of age, non–rapid eye movement has fully differentiated into four stages. Stages III and IV non–rapid eye movement sleep together are also termed *slow wave sleep*, and are characterized by the presence of slow electroencephalogram (EEG) activity of predominantly the delta frequency, that is, less than 4 hertz (Fig. 56-1). The bulk of slow wave sleep occurs during the first third of the night. Growth hormone release is closely linked to slow wave sleep [Van Cauter and Plat, 1996], with suppression of the last leading to impaired growth hormone release. Rapid eye movement sleep decreases to about 20 to 25 percent of total sleep time by the age of 3 years. Until the age of 3 months, the initial transition from wakefulness is into rapid eye movement sleep. Subsequently, however, the physiologic transition from wakefulness is first into non–rapid eye movement sleep, with rapid eye movement sleep occurring 90 to 140 minutes later.

Physiologic sleep-onset time in elementary school-age children is usually around 8:00 PM to 8:30 PM. Around adolescence, there is a physiologic delay in sleep-onset time, which shifts to around 10:30 PM TO 11:00 PM [Carskadon et al., 1998]. Teenage girls generally have their final morning awakening about one half hour earlier than boys. When juxtaposed with early high school start times of around 7:30 AM, it is easy to understand why most teenagers are chronically sleep deprived.

THE INTERNATIONAL CLASSIFICATION OF SLEEP DISORDERS

The International Classification of Sleep Disorders [American Sleep Disorders Association, 1997] was introduced in 1990. It was developed through collaborative efforts of the American Sleep Disorders Association, the European Sleep Research Society, the Japanese Society of Sleep Research, and the Latin American Sleep Society. Primary sleep disorders are separated from those due to medical or psychiatric conditions (Table 56-1). Primary sleep disorders are further subdivided into (1) *dyssomnias*, or disorders that are accompanied by excessive sleepiness or insomnia, and (2) *parasomnias,* or disorders that intrude onto sleep, but are not associated with complaints of insomnia or sleepiness. Dyssomnias are further subdivided into intrinsic, extrinsic, and circadian rhythm sleep disorders. The classification

*Portions of this chapter have appeared in Kotagal S. Sleep disorders in childhood. Neurol Clin 21:961;81, 2003.

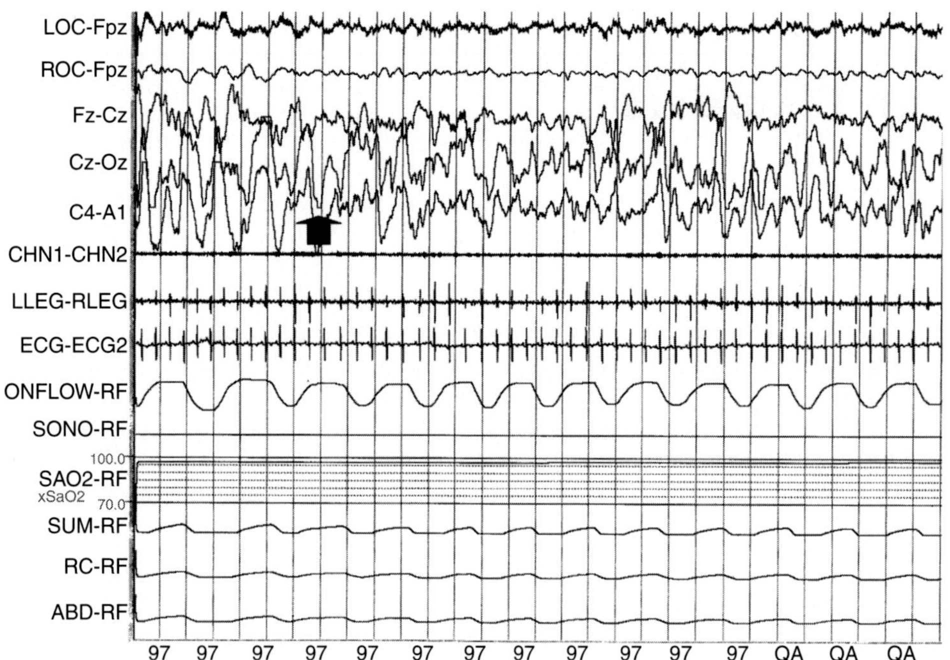

FIGURE 56-1. Normal nocturnal polysomnogram during stage III of non–rapid eye movement sleep, showing continuous delta (<4 hertz) activity on the EEG *(arrow)*, regular respiration, and tonic chin electromyographic activity. Stage III and stage IV non–rapid eye movement sleep are together also termed "slow wave" sleep, which is most abundant in the first third of the night's sleep. Nocturnal growth hormone release is closely linked to slow wave sleep. Parasomnias such as sleepwalking and confusional arousals generally occur during the transition from slow wave sleep to the lighter stages of non–rapid eye movement sleep. (Paper speed 10 mm/second.)

provides a unique code number for each sleep disorder so that disorders can be efficiently tabulated for diagnostic, statistical, and research purposes. Diagnostic severity, duration, and duration criteria are presented in an axial system so that clinicians can standardize the relevant information about their patients. Axis A contains the primary sleep diagnosis. Axis B lists the procedures that are performed in the practice of sleep medicine, and axis C comprises the medical and psychiatric disorders that are not primarily sleep disorders in and of themselves. Numbers in parentheses after each diagnosis or procedure indicate its specific International Classification of Disease code number. As an example, narcolepsy is recorded as:

Axis A: Narcolepsy, moderate, chronic, with excessive daytime sleepiness and cataplexy (347)

Axis B: Nocturnal polysomnogram (89.17)
Multiple sleep latency test (89.18)

The International Classification of Sleep Disorders is undergoing revision, and a new version (International Classification of Sleep Disorders-2) that reflects recent advances in the field of sleep medicine will be released shortly. An abbreviated classification is presented in Table 56-1.

ASSESSMENT OF SLEEP-WAKE COMPLAINTS

Sleep History

The sleep history is provided by the patient, parent, or guardian. It is crucial to the planning of appropriate

TABLE 56-1

The International Classification of Sleep Disorders

Dyssomnias	*Intrinsic sleep disorders (examples):* idiopathic insomnia, narcolepsy, idiopathic hypersomnia, post-traumatic hypersomnia, obstructive sleep apnea, central alveolar hypoventilation syndrome, restless legs syndrome, periodic limb movement disorder
	Extrinsic sleep disorders (examples): inadequate sleep hygiene, environmental sleep disorder, limit-setting sleep disorder, sleep-onset association disorder, hypnotic-dependent sleep disorder, stimulant-dependent sleep disorder, nocturnal eating-drinking syndrome
	Circadian rhythm sleep disorders (examples): irregular sleep-wake patterns, jet lag, non–24-hour sleep disorder, advanced sleep phase syndrome, delayed sleep phase syndrome
Parasomnias	*Arousal disorders:* confusional arousals, sleepwalking, sleep terrors
	Sleep-wake transition disorders: rhythmic movement disorder, sleep starts, sleeptalking, nocturnal leg cramps
	Parasomnias usually associated with REM sleep (examples): nightmares, sleep paralysis, REM-sleep-related sinus arrest, REM-sleep behavior disorder
	Other parasomnias (examples): bruxism (teeth grinding), sleep enuresis, benign neonatal sleep myoclonus
Disorders associated with psychiatric, neurologic, or medical disorders	*With mental disorders (examples):* psychoses, mood disorders, anxiety disorders, panic disorders
	With neurologic disorders (examples): cerebral degenerative disorders, parkinsonism, fatal familial insomnia, sleep-related epilepsy, electrical status epilepticus of sleep, sleep-related headaches
	With other medical disorders (examples): sleep-related asthma, sleep-related gastroesophageal reflux, fibromyalgia, nocturnal cardiac ischemia
Proposed sleep disorders	*Examples*: Terrifying hypnagogic hallucinations, sleep hyperhidrosis

Source: American Sleep Disorders Association, 1997.

diagnostic procedures and arriving at a specific diagnosis. Questions relevant to infants and preschool-age children include the following:

- The sleeping environment (e.g., crib, bassinet, parent's room)
- The sleeping position (e.g., prone or supine, semiupright)
- Habitual need for sleep aids (e.g., pacifier, rocking, patting)
- The time of going to bed, sleep onset, and the final morning awakening
- Sensation of restlessness in the legs before sleep onset, intrusive thoughts or worries that interfere with sleep onset
- Presence of habitual snoring, mouth breathing, observed apnea, restless sleep, sweating, gastroesophageal refiux, and abnormal behavior at night suggestive of seizures or parasomnias
- Behavior during the daytime (irritability, inattentiveness, hyperactivity, sleepiness)
- Number of daytime naps and their duration
- Medications that may affect sleep-wake function (e.g., sedatives, stimulants)
- Interventions that the parents have used to improve sleep

In adolescents, one should also inquire about events in the 3 to 4 hours before bedtime like after-school employment, vigorous exercise, heavy meals, caffeine use, nicotine or substance abuse that may interfere with sleep onset, as well as about hypnagogic hallucinations, or sleep paralysis. Daytime sleepiness assessment should include questions about taking involuntary naps in the classroom, automatic behavior, and the impact of sleepiness on driving, cataplexy, hypnagogic hallucinations, medications used to promote alertness, academic function and behavioral and mood problems, and the number of school days missed because of sleepiness.

Sleep-Related Examination

Height, weight, and body mass index should be recorded because obstructive sleep apnea may be associated with poor weight gain during infancy, and with obesity in adolescents. The blood pressure should be recorded because patients with long-standing and severe obstructive sleep apnea may develop hypertension. The patient should also be evaluated for craniofacial abnormalities like micrognathia, dental malocclusion, macroglossia, myopathic face and midface hypoplasia [Brooks, 2002; Colmenero et al., 1991]. Deviated nasal septum, swollen inferior turbinates, tonsillar hypertrophy and mouth breathing may accompany obstructive sleep apnea. Consultation with an otolaryngologist may be required to exclude adenoidal hypertrophy. Inattentiveness, irritability, and mood swings may suggest daytime sleepiness. Obstructive sleep apnea related to brainstem abnormalities like the Chiari type I or II malformations [Doherty et al., 1995] can lead to hoarseness of voice, decreased gag reflex, and changes in the amplitude of the jaw jerk relative to that of other tendon reflexes. Neuromuscular disorders like myotonic dystrophy may be associated with chronic obstructive hypoventilation from a combination of upper airway collapse and diminished chest wall–abdominal excursion [Givan, 2002; Labanowski et al., 1996; Misuri et al., 2001]. The parent-child interaction should be observed not only for clues toward parental anxiety and reluctance to set limits on inappropriate behaviors that sometimes perpetuate insomnia in toddlers, but also for subtle clues to a child maltreatment syndrome. Home videos, if available, may also provide valuable clues to etiology for disorders such as restless legs syndrome, confusional arousals, and nocturnal seizures.

Nocturnal Polysomnography

The technique of nocturnal polysomnography is useful for monitoring multiple physiologic parameters during sleep in the evaluation of intrinsic sleep disorders like narcolepsy, obstructive sleep apnea, the upper airway resistance syndrome, and the periodic limb movement disorder. It is not indicated for diagnosing obstructive sleep apnea secondary to *severe* adenotonsillar enlargement, which can be easily recognized on the basis of clinical findings combined with severe oxygen desaturation on overnight oximetry. The nocturnal polysomnogram usually consists of simultaneous monitoring of two to four channels of the EEG, eye movements, chin and leg electromyogram, nasal pressure, thoracic and abdominal respiratory effort, electrocardiogram, and oxygen saturation [Kotagal and Goulding, 1996; Kotagal and Herold, 2002]. Patients with Down syndrome, neuromuscular disorders, and obesity have hypoventilation, characterized by shallow chest and abdominal wall movement with resultant CO_2 retention. It is therefore important to also measure end-tidal CO_2 levels in these patients. Esophageal pH can be monitored simultaneously when there is a suspicion of gastroesophageal reflux.

In patients with obvious upper airway obstruction secondary to obesity or neuromuscular disorders like myotonic dystrophy, a therapeutic trial of continuous positive pressure airway breathing can be attempted midway during the course of the sleep recording. Synchronized video monitoring and a full 16- to 20-channel EEG montage are recommended when nonepileptic parasomnias need to be distinguished from nocturnal seizures. Normative data for commonly used polysomnographic variables are listed in Table 56-2 [Marcus and Loughlin, 1996]. There is insufficient evidence to determine the utility of ambulatory, in-home polygraphic monitoring, especially in the preschool age group; thus, traditional sleep laboratory monitoring is the gold standard.

Multiple Sleep Latency Test

The multiple sleep latency test measures the speed with which one falls asleep, as well as the nature of the transition from wakefulness into sleep, that is, into non–rapid eye movement or rapid eye movement sleep. It can reliably detect sleepiness under clinical and experimental conditions [Carskadon et al., 1986]. The lower age limit at which one can use the multiple sleep latency test is about 6 to 7 years. Application in children younger than 6 years is unhelpful because younger children experience physiologic napping during the daytime. In order to derive valid conclusions, the multiple sleep latency test must be preceded the night before by a polysomnogram in which the total sleep time should approximate that observed at home.

TABLE 56-2

Normal Polysomnographic Values in Children

PARAMETER	VALUE	COMMENTS
Total sleep time (hours)	6-7 hours	"Acceptable" value during laboratory conditions
Sleep efficiency (%)	>90	"Acceptable" value during laboratory conditions
REM sleep (% of TST)	15-30	Higher values of REM sleep are seen during infancy
Slow wave sleep (stage III–stage IV of NREM sleep; % of TST)	10-40	
Apnea index (events per hour of sleep)	<1	Normal peak CO_2 may be lower during infancy
Peak end-tidal CO_2	<53 mm Hg	
Duration of hypoventilation ($P_{ET}CO_2$ > 50 mm Hg as % of TST)	<8 %	
Oxygen saturation nadir	92%	
Oxygen desaturations > 4% (number/hour of TST)	1.4	

NREM, non–rapid eye movement; REM, rapid eye movement; TST, total sleep time.
From: Marcus and Loughlin, 1996.

The multiple sleep latency test consists of the provision of four or five daytime nap opportunities at 2-hour intervals, for example, 1000, 1200, 1400, and 1600 hours while the EEG, chin electromyogram, and eye movements are being monitored. The patient should be dressed in street clothes. The attending parent or guardian should prevent the child from dozing off involuntarily in between the scheduled naptimes. At each planned nap opportunity, the lights are turned off and the patient is invited to try to sleep. The time from "lights out" to sleep onset is measured, and constitutes the *sleep latency*. The nap opportunity is terminated either 15 minutes after sleep onset, or if the patient does not fall asleep, at 20 minutes after "lights out." A *mean sleep latency* is also derived for the four naps. Normative values have been established for the mean sleep latency. Mean sleep latency decreases inversely with an increase in the Tanner stage of sexual development, and ranges between 12 to 18 minutes [Carskadon, 1982]. A mean sleep latency of less than 5 minutes indicates severe daytime sleepiness; a value between 5-10 minutes indicates moderate daytime sleepiness. A urine drug screen is obtained in between the naps if stimulant or hypnotic abuse is suspected. The occurrence of rapid eye movement sleep within 15 minutes of sleep onset constitutes a *sleep-onset rapid eye movement period (SOREMP)*. The presence of SOREMPs on two to four or more multiple sleep latency test nap opportunities in association with shortened mean sleep latency of less than 5 minutes is highly suggestive of narcolepsy.

In adults, a mean sleep latency of less than 5 minutes in association with two or more SOREMPs is 70% sensitive and 97% specific for the diagnosis of narcolepsy [Aldrich et al., 1997]. Comparable data on the sensitivity and specificity are not available for children and adolescents. The recent work of Gozal and associates [2001] suggests that in prepubertal children, the normal mean sleep latency is 23.7 minutes, plus or minus 3.1 minutes. Palm and co-workers [1989] also found a mean sleep latency of 26.4 minutes plus or minus 2.8 minutes in 18 prepubertal children. These data suggest that the normal mean sleep latency in children may be actually higher than previously reported and that normative data for the multiple sleep latency test in childhood might perhaps need revision. One of the merits of the multiple sleep latency test is that it provides reliable and quantitative information about the propensity for sleepiness. It has been validated as a measure of daytime sleepiness following episodes of sleep loss [Rosenthal et al., 1993], sleep disruption [Stepanski et al., 1987], and hypnotic drug and alcohol abuse [Billiard et al., 1987; Papineau et al., 1998]. The effects of treatment of daytime sleepiness with stimulants cannot be reliably measured, however. In addition, although one can control ambient noise and light that might affect sleep during the testing process, one cannot control for internal factors like anxiety and apprehension that also affect sleep propensity.

Maintenance of Wakefulness Test

The maintenance of wakefulness test is the mirror image of the multiple sleep latency test in that it measures the ability to stay awake in a darkened, quiet environment during the daytime while the patient is seated in a semireclining position [Mitler et al., 1982, 2000]. EEG, eye movements, and chin electromyography are monitored in a manner identical to that in the multiple sleep latency test. The patient is provided four or five nap opportunities. The duration of each session is set at 20 or 40 minutes. The average mean sleep latency for normal adults is 35.2 minutes. Normative values have not been established for children. The test is useful in documenting the effect of therapeutic interventions on daytime sleepiness, for example, stimulant medications [Mitler, 1994].

Actigraphy

The technique involves the recording and storing of skeletal muscle activity continuously for 1 to 2 weeks, generally from the nondominant forearm, using a wristwatch-shaped microcomputer device that records linear acceleration and translates it into a numeric and graphic representation. This numeric representation is sampled frequently, that is, every 0.1 second, and aggregated at a constant interval or epoch length [Sadeh et al., 1995]. The device captures signals during periods of muscle activity (generally correlating with

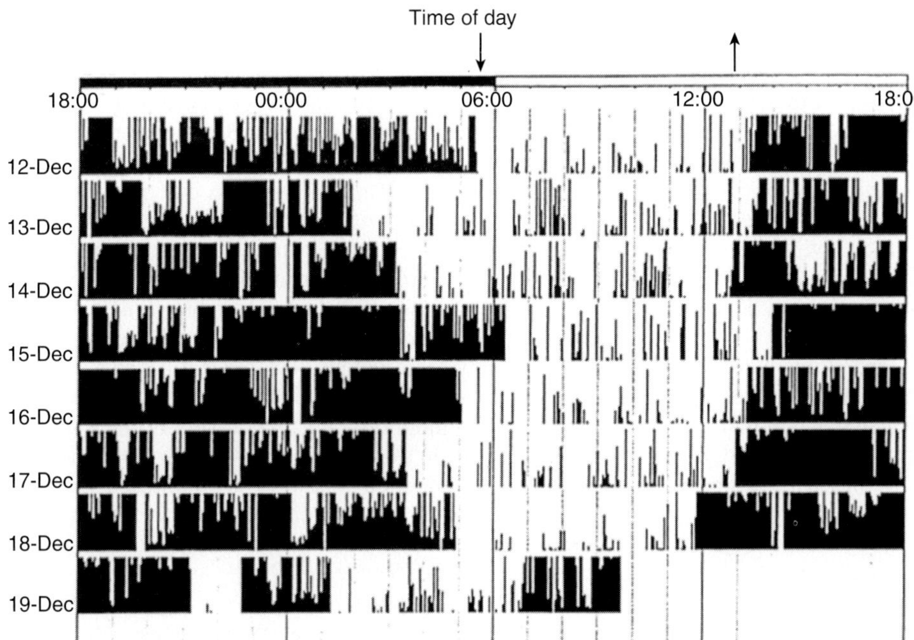

FIGURE 56-2. Wrist actigraph showing 2 weeks of sleep-wake recording in a teenager with delayed sleep phase syndrome, who presented with difficulty falling asleep. The dark bars indicate presence of muscle activity, which correlates closely with wakefulness, and the clear areas indicate lack of muscle activity, which generally correlates with sleep. Notice sleep onset late in the early morning hours *(down arrow)* and awakening in the afternoon *(up arrow).*

wakefulness) and periods of no muscle activity (generally correlating with sleep; Fig. 56-2). There is a close correlation with polysomnographically defined total sleep time, sleep latency, and sleep efficiency (total sleep time or total time in bed × 100; [Sadeh et al., 1995]). Wrist actigraphy should be combined with 1 to 2 weeks of "sleep logs" that detail specific wake-up and sleep-onset times, daytime naps, and so on. Wrist actigraphy is useful in the study of insomnia and circadian rhythm disorders like the delayed sleep phase syndrome. In the latter instance, it will show sleep onset late at night or in the early morning hours, uninterrupted sleep thereafter, with a final awakening late in the morning or early afternoon (see Fig. 56-1). In patients being evaluated for suspected narcolepsy, two weeks of actigraphy before nocturnal polysomnography and the multiple sleep latency test helps exclude the possibility of sleepiness resulting from a circadian rhythm disorder or insufficient night sleep.

COMMON CHILDHOOD SLEEP DISORDERS

Sleep-Related Breathing Disturbances

Between 10% and 12% of children snore on a habitual basis [Corbo et al., 2001; O'brien et al., 2003]. The snoring sound

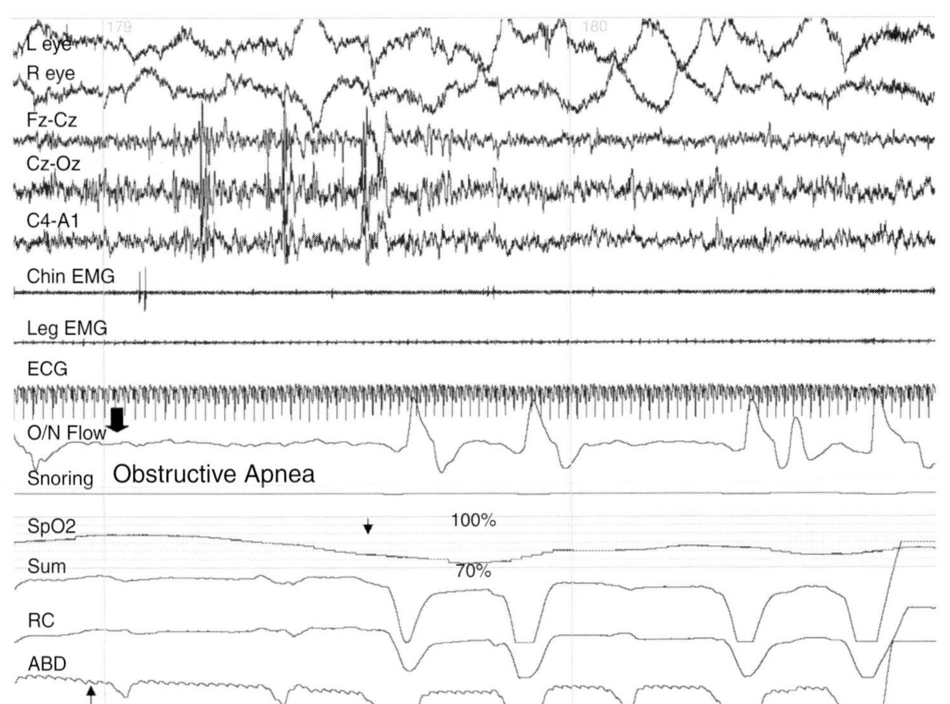

FIGURE 56-3. Nocturnal polysomnogram showing obstructive sleep apnea. Notice lack of signal in the nasal pressure channel *(bold down arrow)* despite persistence of abdominal respiratory effort *(upward arrow).* The oxygen desaturation resulting from the obstructive apnea event triggers an EEG arousal *(small downward arrow).* (Paper speed 10 mm/second.)

is largely caused by vibration of the soft palate as a result of narrowing of the oropharynx. Children who snore but do not fulfill the polysomnographic criteria for obstructive sleep apnea are defined as having primary snoring. Although some guidelines [American Academy of Pediatrics, 2002] suggest that primary snoring may be a "benign condition that does not warrant any specific therapy," a recent study of 87 5- to 7-year-olds [O'brien et al., 2004] found that compared with age-matched nonsnoring children, those with primary snoring performed worse on neuropsychologic measures of attention and had more social problems and anxious or depressive symptoms.

Obstructive sleep apnea is characterized by partial or complete upper airway occlusion with impaired oronasal air exchange despite persistence of thoracic and abdominal respiratory effort, in association with transient oxygen desaturation of 4% (Fig. 56-3). Community-based studies have determined the prevalence of childhood obstructive sleep apnea at 1.1% to 2.9% [Ali et al., 1993; Brunetti et al., 2001]. The most common etiologic factors are adenotonsillar hypertrophy, craniofacial anomalies like micrognathia or maxillary hypoplasia, neuromuscular disorders such as myotonic dystrophy or congenital nonprogressive myopathies, and obesity [Marcus and Loughlin, 1996]. Repetitive occlusion of the upper airway during sleep with resultant oxygen desaturation provokes cortical arousals, and suppression in the proportion of rapid eye movement sleep and slow wave sleep. Nocturnal symptoms of childhood obstructive sleep apnea include habitual snoring, restless sleep with snort arousals, increased frequency of parasomnias such as confusional arousals, excessive sweating, mouth breathing, choking sounds, and parental reports of having observed apnea. Daytime symptoms consist of inattentiveness, impaired academic performance [Chervin et al., 2002], hyperactivity (in preschool children), and sleepiness. Nocturnal polysomnography is not needed to confirm the diagnosis in patients with severe symptoms of obstructive sleep apnea who have severe tonsillar hypertrophy—one night of oximetry in the home environment that documents recurrent oxygen desaturation is sufficient for establishing the diagnosis [Brouilette et al., 2000]. Nocturnal polysomnography in the sleep laboratory is, however, indicated for patients with less obvious symptoms and etiology; in those with multiple neurologic handicaps, for example, Down syndrome patients; and when the patient needs to be considered for nonsurgical therapeutic options like continuous positive airway pressure breathing. Obstructive sleep apnea secondary to adenotonsillar hypertrophy responds favorably to adenotonsillectomy, but patients younger than 3 years old and those with severe obstructive sleep apnea should be monitored postoperatively in the intensive care unit for respiratory compromise from upper airway edema. Weight-reduction measures are indicated in obese patients. Orthodontic consultation and the use of oral appliances during sleep is indicated in those with retrognathia and tongue prolapse [Rondeau, 1998].

The *upper airway resistance syndrome* is a form of upper airway obstruction in which no frank apneas or oxygen desaturation are observed during sleep, but the airway narrowing leads to recurrent arousals, fragmented sleep, and daytime sleepiness [Guilleminault et al., 1996]. Some patients exhibit subtle posterior displacement of the tongue, narrow nostrils, or a high-arched palate, but others might not show any craniofacial anomalies. The nocturnal polysomnogram may appear superficially normal, with the exception of snoring and increased EEG arousals of 3 or more seconds (normally less than 10 to 12 per hour of sleep). Simultaneously obtained intraluminal pressures from an esophageal balloon demonstrate a marked increase in the intrathoracic negative pressure during the upper airway resistance syndrome episodes. The management is the same as for obstructive sleep apnea.

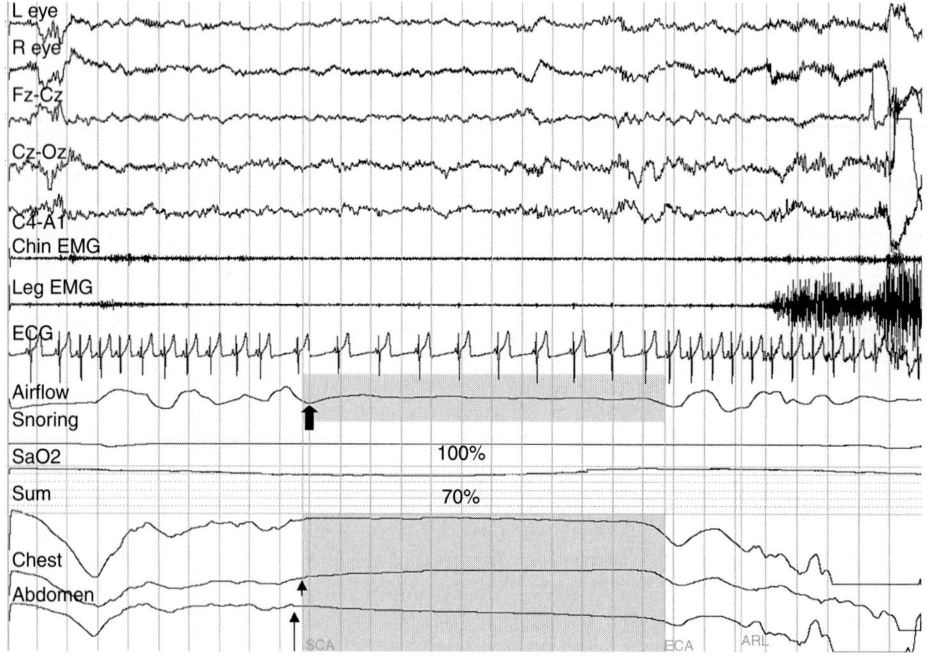

FIGURE 56-4. Central sleep apnea in a child with a primary brainstem tumor involving the medulla. Notice the simultaneous cessation of signal in the airflow channel *(wide arrow)* as well as in the thoracic and abdominal effort channels *(thin arrows).*

Central Hypoventilation Syndrome

Defective automatic regulation of breathing during sleep due to brainstem dysfunction is characteristic of this syndrome. The disorder may present in infancy or childhood. Developmental malformations of the brainstem are common, but may be visible only on microscopic examination. Head injury, bulbar poliomyelitis, syringobulbia, hyperendorphinism, Chiari type II malformation [Zolty et al., 2000], and inborn errors of metabolism (e.g., Leigh's syndrome) are other predisposing factors. Polysomnography may reveal central sleep apnea (Fig. 56-4). Except for surgical decompression in Chiari malformation and syringobulbia-associated hypoventilation, the management in these secondary central hypoventilation syndromes is similar to that for idiopathic *congenital central alveolar hypoventilation,* discussed below.

Congenital central alveolar hypoventilation is a disorder in which no obvious structural or metabolic etiology is found for the defective control of breathing during sleep [Gozal, 2004; Gozal and Harper, 1999]. Onset of symptoms may be in infancy or early childhood. From a clinical standpoint, the respiratory rate and depth are initially normal during wakefulness, but shallow breathing (hypoventilation), hypercarbia, and oxygen desaturation appear during sleep. Ventilatory challenge with inhalation of a mixture of 5% CO_2 and 95% O_2 fails to evoke the physiologic, three- to fivefold increase in minute volume. Common sites of neuronal loss and gliosis include the arcuate nucleus in the medulla, the ventrolateral nucleus of the tractus solitarius, nucleus ambiguus, nucleus retroambigualis, the chemosensitive ventral medullary surface, and the nucleus parabrachialis in the dorsolateral pons. Between 15% and 20% of congenital central alveolar hypoventilation patients have coexisting Hirschprung's disease or neural crest tumors such as neuroblastoma or ganglioneuroma [Roshkow et al., 1988; Swaminathan et al., 1989]. It has been hypothesized that congenital central alveolar hypoventilation is a neural crest disorder, because brainstem neurons that regulate chemosensitivity are derived from the neural crest during fetal development. The proto-oncogene, receptor tyrosine kinase, is involved in this process [Bolk et al., 1996]. Recently mutations in the *PHOX2B* gene have been identified in more than 90 percent of patients with central hypoventilation syndrome [Traochet et al., 2005]. There is no definitive and satisfactory treatment for congenital central alveolar hypoventilation, though acetazolamide and theophylline enhance chemoreceptivity of the brainstem respiratory neurons to a modest degree. Home ventilation via tracheostomy and diaphragmatic pacing are other therapeutic modalities. Patients may die in infancy or early childhood.

Narcolepsy

Chronic daytime sleepiness, hypnagogic hallucinations (vivid dreams at sleep onset), sleep paralysis, cataplexy (sudden loss of skeletal muscle tone in response to emotional triggers like laughter, fright, or surprise), and fragmented night sleep are the characteristic clinical features of narcolepsy. The incidence of narcolepsy in the United States is 1.37 per 100,000 persons per year (1.72 for men and 1.05 for women; 35). It is highest in the second decade, followed by a gradual decline. The prevalence is approximately 56 per 100,000 persons [Silber et al., 2002]. A meta-analysis of 235 pediatric cases derived from three studies [Challamel et al., 1994] found that 34% of all narcolepsy subjects had onset of symptoms before the age of 15 years, 16% before the age 10 years, and 4.5 % before age 5 years (Fig. 56-5). Although the age of onset is generally in the latter half of the first decade or the second decade, rare cases with onset of extreme sleepiness and cataplexy during infancy have also been reported [Nevsimalova et al., 1986; Sharp and D'Cruz, 2001]. Childhood daytime sleepiness may be overlooked by parents, schoolteachers, and physicians alike. Sleepy children are frequently mistaken for being "lazy." They may exhibit mood swings and inattentiveness. Cataplexy, present in about two thirds of patients, is due to abrupt hyperpolarization of the spinal alpha motor neurons. The cataplectic muscle weakness generally lasts for a few minutes, and is associated with muscle atonia, absence of muscle stretch reflexes, and full preservation of consciousness. Because it can be very subtle, the examiner might need to ask leading questions about sudden muscle weakness in the lower extremities, neck, or trunk in response to laughter, fright, excitement, or anger. Children younger than 7 or 8 years do not provide a reliable history of hypnagogic hallucinations or sleep paralysis. Fragmentation of night sleep is also common in narcolepsy. This fragmentation may or may not be accompanied by periodic limb movement activity [Wittig et al., 1983]. Patients exhibit less circadian clock–dependent alertness during the daytime and also less circadian clock– dependent sleepiness at night [Broughton et al., 1998]. In rare instances secondary narcolepsy may develop in patients after closed head injuries, primary brain tumors, lymphomas, and encephalitis [Autret et al., 1994].

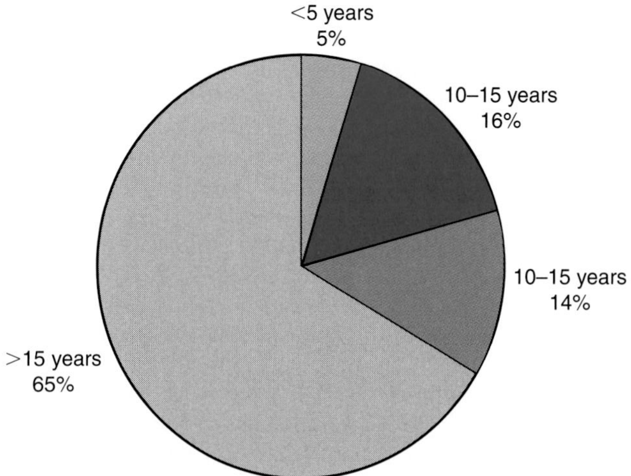

FIGURE 56-5. Graph depicting the age of onset of narcolepsy. Data derived from: Challamel, et al., 1994.

The presence of the histocompatibility antigen DQB1*0602 in close to 100% of persons with narcolepsy, as compared with a 12% to 32% prevalence in the general population indicates a genetic susceptibility, which is insufficient to precipitate the clinical syndrome. Monozygotic twins have been reported to be discordant for narcolepsy [Langdon et al., 1986; Mignot et al., 1999, 2001]. In genetically susceptible individuals, acquired life stresses like minor head injury, systemic illnesses such as infectious mononucleosis, and bereavement may play a role in triggering the disorder, and have been reported in close to two thirds of subjects—"the two-hit hypothesis" [Billiard et al., 1986].

The defining pathophysiologic event in narcolepsy-cataplexy is hypocretin deficiency [Nishino et al., 2000, 2001]. Hypocretin (orexin) is a peptide that is produced by neurons of the dorsolateral hypothalamus. Hypocretins 1 and 2 (synonymous with orexins A and B) are peptides that are synthesized from preprohypocretin. They have corresponding receptors. Whereas the hypocretin type 1 receptor binds only to hypocretin-1, the hypocretin type 2 receptor binds to both type 1 and 2 ligands [Hungs et al., 2001]. Hypocretin neurons have widespread projections to the forebrain and brainstem. Hypocretin promotes alertness and increases motor activity and basal metabolic rate [John et al., 2000]. Of significance is the postmortem examination finding in humans with narcolepsy of Thannickal and colleagues [2000], documenting an 85% to 95% reduction in the number of hypocretin neurons in the hypothalamus, whereas melanin-concentrating hormone neurons that are intermingled with hypocretin neurons remained unaffected, thus suggesting a targeted neurodegenerative process. It is hypothesized that degeneration of the hypocretin-producing cells of the hypothalamus (perhaps linked to HLA DQB1*0602 by mechanisms yet unknown) provokes a decrease in forebrain noradrenergic activation, which in turn decreases alertness. A corresponding decrease of noradrenergic activity in the brainstem leads to disinhibition of brainstem cholinergic systems, thus triggering cataplexy and other phenomena of rapid eye movement sleep such as hypnagogic hallucinations and sleep paralysis.

The decrease in secretion of hypocretin-1 that is characteristic of human narcolepsy-cataplexy is also reflected in the cerebrospinal fluid. Using a radioimmunoassay, Nishino and associates [2000, 2001] found that the mean level of hypocretin-1 in healthy controls was 280.3 plus or minus 33.0 pg/mL; in neurologic controls it was 260.5 plus or minus 37.1 pg/mL; and in those with narcolepsy, hypocretin-1 was either undetectable or less than 100 pg/mL. Low-to-absent levels were found in 32 of 38 narcolepsy patients, who were all also HLA DQB1*0602 positive. Narcolepsy patients who were HLA DQB1*0602 antigen negative tended to have normal to high cerebrospinal fluid hypocretin-1 levels. In another study of narcolepsy with cataplexy, narcolepsy without cataplexy, and idiopathic hypersomnia, Kanbayashi and associates [2002] found that their nine cerebrospinal fluid hypocretin–deficient patients were all HLA DQB1*0602 positive, including three preadolescents. In contrast, narcolepsy without cataplexy and idiopathic hypersomnia patients exhibited normal cerebrospinal fluid hypocretin levels (Fig. 56-6). The assay may be most useful when an HLA DQB1*0602–positive patient with suspected narcolepsy-cataplexy is already receiving central nervous system stimulants on initial presentation, and when discontinuation of these medications for the purpose of obtaining polysomnography and a multiple sleep latency test is inconvenient or impractical.

A combined battery of nocturnal polysomnogram and multiple sleep latency test remains the most widely used method to diagnose narcolepsy. The nocturnal polysomnogram demonstrates increased arousals, decreased initial rapid eye movement latency of less than 70 minutes (time from sleep onset to onset of the first rapid eye movement sleep epoch; normal value in teenagers is around 140 minutes), and absence of any other significant sleep pathology such as obstructive sleep apnea. The multiple sleep latency test, which is obtained on the day after the nocturnal polysomnogram, records sleep onset on each of the four nap opportunities within 5 minutes of "lights out," whereas the reference value is approximately 16 to 18 minutes. Sleep-onset rapid eye movement periods are also seen during at least two out of four nap opportunities. Because narcolepsy is a lifelong condition, the diagnostic test results need to be clear and unambiguous.

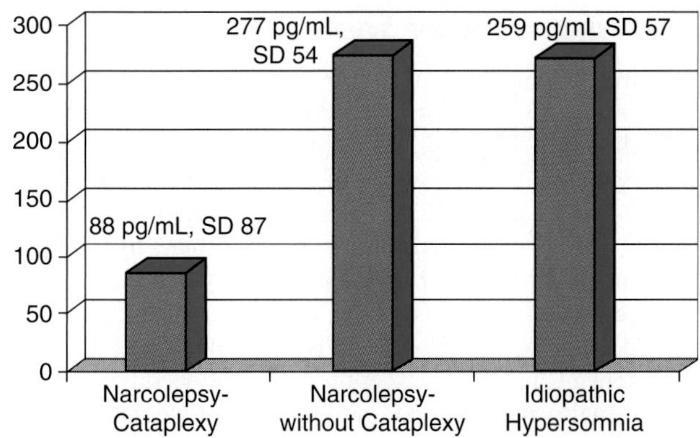

FIGURE 56-6. Cerebrospinal fluid levels of hypocretin-1 in patients with narcolepsy-cataplexy, narcolepsy without cataplexy, and idiopathic hypersomnia. Data derived from Kanbayashi, et al., 2002.

Management of narcolepsy requires a combination of lifestyle changes and pharmacotherapy. A planned daytime nap of 20 to 30 minutes at school and another one in the afternoon upon return home may enhance alertness. The patient should observe regular sleep onset and morning wake-up times, avoid alcohol, and exercise regularly. To minimize the risk of accidents, the patient should avoid sharp, moving objects. Daytime sleepiness is treated pharmacologically with modafinil (100 to 400 mg/day in two divided doses) or regular or extended-release preparations of methylphenidate (20 to 60 mg/day in two divided doses) and dextroamphetamine (10 to 30 mg/day in two divided doses) [Littner et al., 2001]. Cataplexy is treated using clomipramine (25 mg at bedtime) or protryptiline (2.5 to 5 mg/day in two divided doses) or sodium oxybate (gamma hydroxybutyrate). Sodium oxybate is administered in two divided doses or at night, and seems to work by improving noc-turnal sleep architecture. There are insufficient data on its use in childhood. Emotional and behavioral problems that commonly accompany childhood narcolepsy may require the addition of fluoxetine (10 to 30 mg every morning) or sertraline (25 to 50 mg twice daily) and supportive psychotherapy. Teenagers should be counseled against driving if they have uncontrolled sleepiness. They should also avoid work and social situations in which they could endanger themselves or others.

Idiopathic Hypersomnia

Idiopathic hypersomnia is defined by the International Classification of Sleep Disorders as "a disorder of presumed central nervous system cause that is associated with a normal or prolonged major sleep episode and excessive sleepiness consisting of prolonged (1 to 2 hour) sleep episodes of non-rapid eye movement sleep" [Roth, 1976]. In contrast with the mean sleep latency on the multiple sleep latency test of less than 5 minutes that is typically observed in narcolepsy, the mean sleep latency in idiopathic hypersomnia is generally in the 5- to 10-minute range. Patients do not exhibit cataplexy, hypnagogic hallucinations, or sleep paralysis. Two or more SOREMPs that are typically seen on the multiple sleep latency test in patients with narcolepsy are also not present. In a review of 42 patients evaluated at the University of Michigan over a 10-year period, Basetti and Aldrich [1997] observed that hypersomnia began at a mean age of 19 plus or minus 8 years (range 6 to 43). Almost half of the subjects described restless sleep with frequent arousals. Habitual dreaming was present in about 40% of the subjects. They described three subtypes of idiopathic hypersomnia:

1. The classic form, in which sleepiness was not overwhelming, and there was a tendency to take long, unrefreshing naps, prolonged nighttime sleep, and difficulty awakening
2. The narcolepsy-like idiopathic hypersomnia, with overwhelming daytime sleepiness, a tendency to take short, refreshing naps, and awakening without difficulty; sleep attacks tended to occur even while standing
3. The "mixed" form, in which the naps were brief, but unrefreshing

They mention that there is substantial clinical overlap between narcolepsy and idiopathic hypersomnia. In a subset of children, idiopathic hypersomnia may represent a transitional phase en route to the development of classic narcolepsy [Kotagal and Swink, 1996].

Restless Legs Syndrome

Restless legs syndrome is an autosomal-dominant, sensorimotor disorder in which the subject complains of a peculiar "creepy or crawling" feeling in the extremities. There is an urge to move the limbs. The discomfort appears in the evening and nighttime hours, is exacerbated by immobility, and is momentarily relieved by movement of the limb [Allen et al., 2003]. This discomfort interferes with sleep initiation and maintenance, and may be accompanied by daytime fatigue, inattentiveness, or sleepiness. Childhood restless legs syndrome may be synonymous with "growing pains" in some children [Walters, 2002]. On nocturnal polysomnography, the patient may or may not demonstrate periodic limb movements, which are defined as a series of three or more rhythmic, electromyographically recorded movements of the legs lasting 0.5 to 5 seconds and occurring 5 to 90 seconds apart, generally during stages I or II of non–rapid eye movement sleep. The favorable response to dopamine receptor agonists like pramipexole and carbidopa-levodopa suggests that central nervous system dopamine deficiency is a pathophysiologic feature. There may be an associated systemic iron deficiency in the form of low levels of serum ferritin [Kotagal and Silber, 2004] because iron is a cofactor in the synthesis of dopamine. There also appears to be an association between restless legs syndrome and attention-deficit disorder [Chervin et al., 2002; Picchietti et al., 1999]—in a community-based questionnaire survey of 866 children ages 2 to 13.9 years, Chervin and co-workers [2002] found an odds ratio for significant hyperactivity and restless legs of 1: 9. Besides dopamine agonists, oral iron, clonazepam, and gabapentin have also been used to treat restless legs syndrome, but there have been no randomized controlled trials to determine which drug is the most effective.

Periodic Hypersomnia (Kleine-Levin Syndrome)

Periodic hypersomnia is generally seen in adolescents with a male predominance. Patients develop 1- to 2-week periods of hypersomnolence, characterized by sleeping 18 to 20 hours per day, cognitive and mood disturbances in association with compulsive hyperphagia, and hypersexual behavior, with intervening 2 to 4 months of normal alertness and behavior [Brown and Billiard, 1995]. Incomplete forms of the syndrome have also been recognized. The hyperphagia may be in the form of binge eating, and can actually be associated with a 2- to 5-kg increase in body weight. Nocturnal polysomnography during the sleepy periods exhibits decreased sleep efficiency, shortened rapid eye movement latency, and decreased percentage of time spent in stages III and IV of non–rapid eye movement sleep and rapid eye movement sleep. The multiple sleep latency test reveals moderately shortened mean sleep latency in the 5- to 10-minute range, but lacks the two or more SOREMPs typically seen in narcolepsy. The episodic hypersomnia gradually diminishes, ultimately resolving completely over 2 to 3 years or evolving into classic depression, thus bringing up the issue of whether the disorder is a variant of depression. A disturbance of hypothalamic-thalamic function has been hypothesized but not established. The association of Kleine-Levin syndrome with histocompatibility antigen DQB1*0201, the occasional precipitation after systemic infections, as well as the relapsing and remitting nature, are suspicious for an autoimmune etiology [Dauvilliers et al., 2002]. There is no satisfactory treatment, although lithium has been reported to be effective in case reports [Poppe et al., 2003].

Delayed Sleep Phase Syndrome

Delayed sleep phase syndrome is a circadian rhythm disorder initially described in a medical student who was unable to wake up in time to attend his morning classes [Weitzman et al., 1981]. Despite hypnotic use, the patient was unable to fall asleep before the early morning hours and was mistaken initially to have insomnia. Sleep in the laboratory was, however, quantitatively and qualitatively normal. The delay in the timing of occurrence of the sleeping phase of the 24-hour sleep-wake cycle was due to a constitutional inability to prepone sleep, which in turn is secondary to altered function of the circadian timekeeper, that is, the suprachiasmatic nucleus. The disorder typically has onset in adolescence, with a male predominance. The increased frequency of HLA DR1 and the occasional familial clustering of delayed sleep phase syndrome suggest a genetic predisposition [Garcia et al., 2001]. The condition must, however, be differentiated from school avoidance seen in adolescents with delinquent and antisocial behavior, because these individuals can fall asleep at an earlier hour at night in the controlled sleep laboratory setting. Maintenance of sleep logs and wrist actigraphy for 1 to 2 weeks is helpful in establishing the diagnosis of delayed sleep phase syndrome (see Fig. 56-2). "Bright light" therapy is helpful in advancing the sleep-onset time [Cole et al., 2002]. It consists of the provision of 2700 to 10,000 lux of bright light via a "light box" for 20 to 30 minutes immediately upon awakening in the morning. The light box is kept at a distance of 18 to 24 inches from the face. The phototherapy leads to a gradual advancement (shifting back) of the sleep-onset time at night. Bright light therapy may be combined with administration of melatonin about 5 to 5.5 hours before the required bedtime in a dose of 0.5 to 1 mg. The other therapeutic option is one of gradually delaying bedtimes by 3 to 4 hours per day until it becomes synchronized with socially acceptable sleep-wake times, and then adhering to this schedule (chronotherapy). Over time, however, all delayed sleep phase syndrome patients are at risk for drifting back to progressively later and later bedtimes. Daytime stimulants like modafinil (100 to 400 mg/day in two divided doses) may also improve the level of daytime alertness. The physician may also need to write a letter to the school, requesting a late midmorning school starting time on medical grounds.

The Relationship between Sleep and Epilepsy

The onset of sleep may be associated with increased interictal spiking, as well as with an increased propensity for clinical seizures. Frontal and temporal lobe seizures are especially prone to occur during sleep, and to secondarily generalize during sleep [Bourgeois, 1996; Kotagal P, 2001]. Interictal epileptiform discharges may at times be observed only during sleep [Shinnar et al., 1994]. Nocturnal seizures are most likely to occur during stage II, followed by stage I, stage III, stage IV of non–rapid eye movement, and rapid eye movement sleep, in that order.

The syndrome of *electrical status epilepticus during slow wave sleep* is characterized by continuous spike and wave discharges during 85% or more of nocturnal non–rapid eye movement sleep, along with cognitive and behavioral regression. Landau-Kleffner syndrome is characterized by regression in language function, typically in the form of auditory verbal agnosia, in association with continuous epileptiform activity during both rapid eye movement and non–rapid eye movement sleep [Landau and Kleffner, 1957]. Prolonged daytime and nighttime EEG may be needed to establish the diagnosis of either entity. Intravenous lorazepam or diazepam may transiently suppress the epileptiform discharges. Long-term maintenance with valproic acid is modestly effective.

Sleep deprivation leads to activation of seizures. Ellingson and colleagues [1984] observed that clinical seizures occurred after sleep deprivation in 19 of 788 (2.4%) otherwise healthy subjects. Patterns of epileptiform abnormality are also considerably infiuenced by sleep. [Kotagal P, 2001]. For example, the three-per-second spike and wave complexes of absence seizures are replaced by single spike and waves or by polyspike and wave complexes. The hypsarrythmia of infantile spasms is replaced during sleep by brief periods of generalized voltage attenuation. Patients with Lennox-Gastaut syndrome may manifest long runs of generalized spike and wave discharges.

Conversely, seizures also influence sleep by suppressing rapid eye movement sleep, with a corresponding increase in slow wave sleep. This effect of slowing of the background EEG frequency may persist for days after a seizure. Frequent nocturnal seizures also tend to disrupt sleep continuity, with an increased number of arousals. Patients with Lennox-Gastaut syndrome frequently exhibit tonic seizures during sleep.

Sleep disorders can also adversely affect seizure control. Patients with obstructive sleep apnea may manifest poor seizure control, which improves after correction of obstructive sleep apnea with CPAP, positional therapy, or tracheostomy [Britton et al., 1997]. In some instances, the daytime somnolence sleep apnea may be mistaken as a side effect of antiepileptic therapy when in fact it is a consequence of an associated sleep disorder.

Antiepileptic drugs in general lead to stabilization of sleep, with a decrease in the amount of sleep fragmentation. Phenobarbital therapy is associated with suppression in the proportion of time spent in rapid eye movement sleep and increased stage III and IV non–rapid eye movement sleep (slow wave sleep). Both phenytoin and carbamazepine also increase stage III and IV non–rapid eye movement sleep at the expense of stages I and II non–rapid eye movement sleep. Benzodiazepines increase stages III and IV non–rapid eye movement sleep at the expense of stages I and II rapid eye movement sleep. Lamotrigine therapy is associated with an increase in the proportion of time spent in rapid eye movement sleep, with fewer sleep stage shifts [Kotagal P, 2001]. Felbamate is associated with insomnia in about 11 % of subjects [Cilio et al., 2001].

Sleep in Neurologically Compromised Children

Children with spastic quadriparetic cerebral palsy may exhibit daytime irritability, fragmented sleep with frequent nighttime awakenings, and oxygen desaturation from obstructive sleep apnea due to upper airway collapse or adenotonsillar hypertrophy [Kotagal et al., 1994]. They are unable to compensate for the disordered breathing by changes in body position, which makes obstructive sleep apnea especially severe for them. Jouvet and Petre-Quadens [1966] described prolonged initial rapid eye movement latency and suppression in the proportion of time spent in rapid eye movement sleep in patients with severe mental retardation. Decreased rapid eye movements and spindle density, as well as the presence of "undifferentiated" sleep correlate with low levels of intelligence [Zucconi, 2000].

Patients with Leigh's syndrome manifest recurrent central apneas or hypoventilation as a consequence of brainstem involvement [Cummiskey et al., 1987]. Joubert's syndrome is associated with periods of hyperpnea and panting respiration. Rett's syndrome is characterized by deep, sighing respiration during wakefulness and normal breathing patterns during sleep, consistent with impairment of the voluntary, cortical control of breathing, and a normal automatic or brainstem control of respiration [Zucconi, 2000]. Patients with Down syndrome have a complicated set of sleep problems. First, they develop obstructive sleep apnea from the combination of macroglossia, midface hypoplasia, and hypotonic upper airway musculature [Levanon et al., 1999]. Superimposed on this is an element of hypoventilation and CO_2 retention due to the hypotonic intercostal and diaphragmatic musculature. Sleep architecture is frequently disrupted, with decreased sleep efficiency, increased arousals, suppression of slow wave sleep, and rapid eye movement sleep. Patients with achondroplasia may develop obstructive and central apnea in infancy as a result of macroglossia. Zucconi and colleagues [1996] found sleep-related breathing disorders in close to 75% of achondroplasia patients. There is no correlation between the diameter of the foramen magnum and severity of the sleep apnea, but patients need close follow-up of their neurologic and respiratory function. Certain lysosomal storage disorders like the mucopolysaccharidoses, especially Hurler syndrome, have been associated with severe obstructive sleep apnea that resolves with reduction in macroglossia and augmentation of upper airway diameter after bone marrow transplantation. Patients with Niemann-Pick type C disease frequently manifest cataplexy from brainstem involvement, but lack other features characteristic of narcolepsy [Kandt et al., 1982].

Circadian rhythm disorders like irregular sleep-wake rhythms are also common in patients with severe mental retardation and cerebral palsy, especially if there is associated blindness with impaired light perception, which interferes with light-dark entrainment, melatonin secretion, and the development of circadian rhythms. Many blind patients with complete lack of light perception fall asleep relatively early in the evening and are wide awake in early morning hours (3 or 4 AM) or exhibit multiple periods of daytime sleepiness. Melatonin administration and bright light (if light perception is intact) may be used to manipulate the sleep schedule in these patients.

Parasomnias

Parasomnias are unpleasant or undesirable events that intrude onto sleep, without altering sleep quality or quantity. These events may occur during the transition to sleep, during rapid eye movement sleep, or in the transition from the deeper stages to the lighter stages of non–rapid eye movement sleep. The incidence of parasomnias is variable, though 30% of children have at least one episode of sleepwalking, and sleeptalking is noted in about half the population [D'Cruz and Vaughn, 2001]. Frequently, the patient remains unaware of the events but medical attention is sought owing to disruption of the sleep of other family members or serious injury to the patient.

Non–rapid eye movement parasomnias such as confusional arousals, sleepwalking, and sleep terrors are most commonly seen during stages III and IV of non–rapid eye movement sleep, and thus in the first third of night sleep. They are linked to attempted transition from stages III and IV non–rapid eye movement sleep into stage I or II of non–rapid eye movement sleep. Confusional arousals are seen in toddlers, whereas sleepwalking and sleep terrors may occur throughout the first decade. Because non–rapid eye movement sleep is most abundant during the first third of night sleep, a useful historical clue for non–rapid eye movement parasomnias is the occurrence of the events during the 2 to 3 hours after initial sleep onset. Children with confusional arousals may sit up in bed, moan or whimper inconsolably, and utter words like "no" or "go away." Autonomic activity is minimal. The events may last 5 to 30 minutes, after which the patient goes right back to sleep and has no recollection of the events whatsoever on the following morning. A simultaneously obtained EEG recording reveals rhythmic delta activity consistent with slow wave sleep in all of these three non–rapid eye movement parasomnias. Patients with night terrors and sleepwalking may exhibit flushing of the face, increased sweating, inconsolability, and agitation, with complete amnesia for the events the following morning. The events may last 2 to 20 minutes during which the EEG might show continuous slow activity in the delta range. A low dose of clonazepam (0.25 to 0.5 mg at bedtime) is helpful in preventing most non-rapid eye movement parasomnias. Attention to environmental safety, like installing a deadbolt lock on the door may also be necessary in patients with habitual sleep walking. Most non–rapid eye movement parasomnias subside after 10-12 years of age.

Common rapid eye movement parasomnias include nightmares (scary dreams), terrifying hypnagogic hallucinations, and the rapid eye movement sleep behavior disorder. Because rapid eye movement sleep is most abundant during the final third of night sleep, nightmares and rapid eye movement sleep behavior disorder tend to occur during the early morning hours. The rapid eye movement sleep behavior disorder is characterized by actual motoric dream enactment during which the patient might kick, jump, or struggle against an imaginary assailant as a result of failure of the customary inhibition of skeletal muscle activity in rapid eye movement sleep by the medullary nucleus gigantocellularis. The nocturnal polysomnogram reveals increased phasic electromyographic activity during rapid eye movement sleep. Although rapid eye movement sleep behavior disorder is infrequent during childhood, sporadic cases do occur. Treatment with clonazepam (0.25 to 0.5 mg at bedtime) is effective in preventing most rapid eye movement parasomnias.

Nocturnal paroxysmal dystonia was initially described as a sleep-related movement disorder and a parasomnia of non–rapid eye movement sleep that responded favorably to treatment with carbamazepine. Detailed video-EEG studies have now confirmed, however, that the disorder is a form of nocturnal frontal lobe epilepsy [Zucconi et al., 1998]. It often becomes difficult to distinguish nocturnal seizures from parasomnias. Non–rapid eye movement parasomnias can be distinguished by history from nocturnal seizures because the former are generally time-locked to occur within 2 to 3 hours of initial sleep onset, whereas nocturnal seizures tend to occur randomly through night sleep, sometimes on more than one occasion on a given night. Video-EEG polysomnography plays a crucial role in accurately characterizing the nature of nocturnal spells.

FUTURE TRENDS

Future revisions in the International Classification of Sleep Disorders might need to consider the inclusion of some of the newer sleep disorders such as the upper airway resistance syndrome. Normative values for polysomnographic variables in infants and children will become better defined. Improvements in technology and pressures from third party payers are leading to a re-assessment of the role of ambulatory (in-home) polysomnography as an alternative to the relatively more expensive sleep laboratory testing. The recent discovery of hypocretin deficiency as the pathophysiologic basis for narcolepsy-cataplexy is likely to spur the development of hypocretin analogs for definitive treatment [John et al., 2000; Mignot et al., 2002]. The link between disrupted sleep, inattentiveness, and impaired learning remains a challenging area of behavioral child neurology, wherein progress is likely once methodologic issues pertaining to the correlation of sleepiness with neuropsychologic disturbance has been firmly established. There may be a greater application of functional neuroimaging to the study of sleep-wake disorders. The discovery of the clock and period genes in *Drosophila* has also stimulated the study of human chronobiology. In many ways, therefore, sleep medicine is benefiting from recent advances in the neurosciences, genetics, bioinformatics, and biotechnology.

REFERENCES

Aldrich MS, Chervin RD, Malow BA. Value of the multiple sleep latency test (MSLT) for the diagnosis of narcolepsy. Sleep 1997;20(8):620.

Ali NJ, Pitson DJ, Stradling JR. Snoring, sleep disturbance and behavior in 4-5 year olds. Arch Dis Child 1993;68:360.

Allen RP, Picchietti D, Hening WA, et al. Restless legs syndrome: Diagnostic criteria, special considerations, and epidemiology. A report from the restless legs syndrome diagnosis and epidemiology workshop at the National Institutes of Health. Sleep Med 2003;4:101.

American Academy of Pediatrics Policy Statement. Clinical practice guideline: Diagnosis and management of childhood obstructive sleep apnea syndrome. Pediatrics 2002;109:704.

American Sleep Disorders Association: The International Classification of Sleep Disorders: Diagnostic and coding manual. Rochester, MN: American Sleep Disorders Association, 1997.

Autret A, Lucas F, Henry-Lebras F, de Toffol B. Symptomatic narcolepsies. Sleep 1994;17(Suppl 1):21.

Basetti C, Aldrich MS. Idiopathic hypersomnia: A series of 42 patients. Brain 1997;120:1423.

Billiard M, Besset A, de Lustrac C, Brissaud L. Dose response effects of zopiclone on night sleep and on night time and day time functioning. Sleep 1987;10(Suppl 1):27.

Billiard M, Seignalet J, Besset A, Cadilhac J. HLA DR2 and narcolepsy. Sleep 1986;9:149.

Bolk S, Augrist M, Schwartz S, et al. Congenital central hypoventilation syndrome: Mutation analysis of the receptor tyrosine kinase (RET). Am J Med Genet 1996;63:603.

Bourgeois B. The relationship between sleep and epilepsy in children. Semin Pediatr Neurol 1996;3(1):29.

Britton TC, O'Donoghue M, Duncan JS. Exacerbation of epilepsy by sleep apnea. J Neurol Neurosurg Psychiatry 1997;63:808.

Brooks LJ. Genetic syndromes affecting breathing during sleep. In: Lee-Chiong TL, Sateia M, Carskadon MA, eds. Sleep medicine. Philadelphia: Hanley and Belfus, 2002;305.

Broughton R, Krupa S, Boucher B, et al. Impaired circadian waking arousal in narcolepsy-cataplexy. Sleep Res Online 1998;1(4):159.

Brouillette RT, Morielli A, Leimanis A, et al. Nocturnal pulse oximetry as an abbreviated testing modality for pediatric obstructive sleep apnea. Pediatrics 2000;105:405.

Brown LW, Billiard M. Narcolepsy, Kleine-Levin syndrome, and other causes of sleepiness in children. In: Ferber R, Kryger M, eds. Principles and practice of sleep medicine in the child. Philadelphia: WB Saunders, 1995;125.

Brunetti L, Rana S, Losppalluti ML, et al. Prevalence of obstructive sleep apnea syndrome in a cohort of 1207 children of Southern Italy. Chest 2001;120:1930.

Carskadon MA. The second decade. In: Guillleminault C, ed. Sleeping and waking disorders. Indications and techniques. Menlo Park, CA: Addison Wesley, 1982;99.

Carskadon MA, Dement WC, Mitler MM, et al. Guidelines for the multiple sleep latency test (MSLT): A standard measure of sleepiness. Sleep 1986;9:519.

Carskadon MA, Wolfson AR, Acebo C, et al. Adolescent sleep patterns, circadian timing, and sleepiness at a transition to early school days. Sleep 1998;21:871.

Challamel MJ, Mazzola ME, Nevsimalova S, et al. Narcolepsy in children. Sleep 1994;17S:17.

Challet E, Caldelas I, Graff C, Pevet P. Synchronization of the molecular clockwork by light- and food-related cues in mammals. Biol Chem 2003;384:711.

Chervin RD, Archbold KH, Dillon JE, et al. Associations between symptoms of inattention, hyperactivity, restless legs, and periodic leg movements. Sleep 2002;25:213.

Cilio MR, Kartashov AI, Vigevano F. The long-term use of felbamate in children with severe refractory epilepsy. Epilepsy Res 2001;47:1.

Cole RJ, Smith JS, Alcala YC, et al. Bright-light mask treatment of delayed sleep phase syndrome. J Biol Rhythms 2002;17:89.

Colmenero C, Esteban R, Albarino AR, et al. Sleep apnea syndrome associated with maxillofacial abnormalities. J Laryngol Otol 1991;105:94.

Corbo GM, Forastiere F, Abigail N, et al. Snoring in 9 to 15 year old children: Risk factors and clinical relevance. Pediatrics 2001;180:1149.

Cummiskey J, Guilleminault C, Davis R, et al. Automatic respiratory failure: Sleep studies and Leigh's disease. Neurology 1987;37:1876.

Dauvilliers Y, Mayer G, Lecendreux M, et al. Kleine Levin syndrome. An autoimmune hypothesis based on clinical and genetic analyses. Neurology 2002;59:1739.

D'Cruz FO, Vaughn BV. Parasomnias—An update. Semin Pediatr Neurol 2001;8:251.

Doherty MJ, Spence DPS, Young C, et al. Obstructive sleep apnea with Chiari malformation. Thorax 1995;50:690.

Ellingson RJ, Wilken K, Bennet DR. Efficacy of sleep deprivation as an activating procedure in epilepsy patients. J Clin Neurophysiol 1984;1:83.

Garcia J, Rosen G, Mahowald M. Circadian rhythms and circadian rhythm disorders in children and adolescents. Semin Pediatr Neurol 2001;8:229.

Givan DC. Sleep in children with neuromuscular disorders. In Lee-Chiong TL, Sateia M, Carskadon MA, eds. Sleep medicine. Philadelphia: Hanley and Belfus, 2002;297.

Gozal D. New concepts in abnormalities of respiratory control in children. Curr Opin Pediatr 2004;16:305.

Gozal D, Harper RM. Novel insights into congenital hypoventilation syndrome. Curr Opin Pulm Med 1999;5:335.

Gozal D, Wang M, Pope DW. Objective sleepiness measures in pediatric obstructive sleep apnea. Pediatrics 2001;108:693.

Guilleminault C, Pelayo R, Leger D, et al. Recognition of sleep-disordered breathing in children. Pediatrics 1996;98:871.

Hamada T, LeSauter J, Venuti JM, Silver R. Expression of *Period* genes: Rhythmic and nonrhythmic compartments of the suprachiasmatic nucleus pacemaker. J Neurosci 2001;21:7742.

Hungs Fan J, Lin X, Maki RA, Mignot E. Identification and functional analysis of mutations in the hypocretin (orexin) genes of narcoleptic canines. Genome Res 2001;11:531.

Ipsiroglu OS, Fatemi A, Werner I, et al. Prevalence of sleep disorders in school children between 11 and 15 years of age (German). Wiener Klinische Wochenschrift 2001;113:235.

John J, Wu M-F, Siegel JM. Systemic administration of hypocretin-1 reduces cataplexy and normalizes sleep and waking durations in narcoleptic dogs. Sleep Res Online 2000;3:23.

Jouvet M, Petre-Quadens O. Paradoxical sleep and dreaming in the mentally deficient. Acta Neurol Psychiatr Belg 1966;66:116.

Kanbayashi T, Inoue Y, Chiba S, et al. CSF hypocretin-1 (orexin-A) concentrations in narcolepsy with and without cataplexy and idiopathic hypersomnia. J Sleep Res 2002;11:91.

Kandt RS, Emerson RG, Singer HS, et al. Cataplexy in variant forms of Niemann-Pick disease. Ann Neurol 1982;12:284.

Kotagal P. The relationship between sleep and epilepsy. Semin Pediatr Neurol 2001;8:241.

Kotagal S. A developmental perspective on narcolepsy. In: Loughlin GM, Carroll JL, Marcus CL, eds. Sleep and breathing. A developmental approach. New York: Marcel Dekker, 2000;347.

Kotagal S, Gibbons VP, Stith J. Sleep abnormalities in patients with severe cerebral palsy. Dev Med Child Neurol 1994;36:304.

Kotagal S, Goulding PM. The laboratory assessment of daytime sleepiness in childhood. J Clin Neurophysiol 1996;13:208.

Kotagal S, Herold DL. The laboratory assessment of childhood sleep-wake disorders. Am J End Technol 2002;42:73.

Kotagal S, Silber MH. Childhood-onset restless legs syndrome. Ann Neurol 2004;56:803.

Kotagal S, Swink TD. Excessive daytime sleepiness in a 13-year old. Semin Pediatr Neurol 1996;3:170.

Labanowski M, Schmidt-Nowara W, Guilleminault C. Sleep and neuromuscular disease: Frequency of sleep-disordered breathing in a neuromuscular disease clinic population. Neurology 1996;47:1173.

Landau WM, Kleffner FR. Syndrome of acquired aphasia with convulsive disorder in children. Neurology 1957;7:523.

Langdon N, Lock C, Welsh K, et al. Immune factors in narcolepsy. Sleep 1986;9:143.

Levanon A, Tarasiuk A, Tal A. Sleep characteristics in children with Down syndrome. J Pediatr 1999;134:755.

Littner M, Johnson SF, McCall WV, et al. Practice parameters for treatment of narcolepsy: An update for 2000. Sleep 2001;24:451.

Marcus CL, Loughlin GM. Obstructive sleep apnea in children. Semin Pediatr Neurol 1996;3:23.

Mignot E, Lin L, Rogers W, et al. Complex HLA-DR and -DQ interactions confer risk of narcolepsy-cataplexy in three ethnic groups. Am J Hum Genet 2001;68:686.

Mignot E, Taheri S, Nishino S. Sleeping with the hypothalamus: Emerging therapeutic targets for sleep disorders. Nat Neurosci Suppl 2002;5:1071.

Mignot E, Young T, Lin L, Fin L. Nocturnal sleep and daytime sleepiness in normal subjects with HLA-DQB1*0602. Sleep 1999;22:347.

Miller JD, MorinLP, Schwartz WJ, Moore RY. New insights into the mammalian circadian clock. Sleep 1996;19:641.

Misuri G, Lanini B, Gigliotti F, et al. Mechanisms of CO_2 retention in patients with neuromuscular disease. Chest 2000;117:447.

Mitler MM. Evaluation of treatment with stimulants in narcolepsy. Sleep 1994;17(Suppl 8):103.

Mitler MM, Doghramji K, Shapiro C. The maintenance of wakefulness test. Normative data by age. J Psychosom Res 2000;9:63.

Mitler MM, Gujavarty KS, Brownman CP. Maintenance of wakefulness test: A polysomnographic technique for evaluation of treatment efficacy in patients with excessive somnolence. Electroencephalogr Clin Neurophysiol 1982;53:658.

Nevsimalova S, Roth B, Zouhar A, Zemanova H. Narkolepsie-kataplexie a periodicka hypersomnie se zacatkem v kojeneckem veku. Cs Pediatr 1986;41:324.

Nishino S, Ripley B, Overeem S, et al. Hypocretin (orexin) deficiency in human narcolepsy. Lancet 2000;355:39.

Nishino S, Ripley B, Overeem S, et al. Low cerebrospinal fiuid hypocretin (orexin) and altered energy homeostasis in human narcolepsy. Ann Neurol 2001;50:381.

O'brien LM, Holbrook CR, Mervis CB, et al. Sleep and neurobehavioral characteristics in 5–7 year old hyperactive children. Pediatrics 2003;111:554.

O'brien LM, Mervis CB, Holbrook CR, et al. Neurobehavioral implications of habitual snoring in children. Pediatrics 2004;114:44.

Palm L, Persson E, Elmquist D, Blennow G. Sleep and wakefulness in normal pre-adolescents. Sleep 1989;12: 299.

Papineau KL, Roehts TA, Petrucelli N, et al. Elecrophysiological Assessment (the multiple sleep latency test) of the biphasic effects of ethanol in humans. Alcohol Clin Exp Res 1998; 2:231.

Picchietti DL, Underwood DJ, Farris WA, et al. Further studies on periodic limb movement disorder and restless legs syndrome in children with attention deficit-hyperactivity disorder. Movement Disorders. 1999;14:1000.

Poppe M, Friebel D, Reuner U, et al. The Kleine-Levin syndrome—Effects of treatment with lithium. Neuropediatrics 2003;34:113.

Rondeau BH. Dentist's role in the treatment of snoring and sleep apnea. Funct Orthodont 1998;15:4.

Rosenthal L, Roehrs TA, Rosen A, Roth T. Level of sleepiness and total sleep time following various time in bed conditions. Sleep 1993;16:226.

Roshkow JE, Haller JO, Berdon WE, Sane SM. Hirschprung's disease, Ondine's curse, and neuroblastoma—Manifestations of neurocristopathy. Pediatr Radiol 1988;19:45.

Roth B. Narcolepsy and hypersomnia: Review and classification of 642 personally observed cases. Schweiz Arch Neurol Neurochir Psychiatr 1976;119:31.

Sadeh A, Hauri PJ, Kripke DF, Lavie P. The role of actigraphy in the evaluation of sleep disorders. Sleep 1995;18:288.

Sharp SJ, D'Cruz OF. Narcolepsy in a 12 month old boy. J Child Neurol 2001;16:145.

Shinnar S, Kang H, Berg AT, et al. EEG abnormalities in children with a first unprovoked seizure. Epilepsia 1994;35:471.

Silber MH, Krahn LE, Olson EJ, Pankrantz S. Epidemiology of narcolepsy in Olmstead County, Minnesota. Sleep 2002;25:197.

Stein MA, Mendelsohn J, Obermeyer WH, et al. Sleep and behavior problems in school-aged children. Pediatrics 2001;107:E60.

Stepanski E, Lamphere J, Roehrs T, et al. Experimental sleep fragmentation in normal subjects. Int J Neurosci 1987;33:207.

Steriade M, Contreras D, Curro Dossi R, Nunez A. The slow (< 1 Hz) oscillation in reticular thalamic and thalamocortical neurons: Scenario of sleep rhythm generation in interacting thalamic and neocortical networks. J Neurosci 1993;13:3284.

Swaminathan S, Gilsanz V, Atkinson J, Keens TG. Congenital central hypoventilation syndrome associated with multiple ganglioneuromas. Chest 1989;96:423.

Thannickal TC, Moore RY, Nienhuis R, et al. Reduced number of hypocretin neurons in human narcolepsy. Neuron 2000;27:469.

Trochet D, O'brien LM, Gozal D, et al. PHOX2B genotype allows for prediction of tumor risk in congenital central hypoventilation syndrome. Am J Hum Genet 2005;76:421.

Van Cauter E, Plat L. Physiology of growth hormone secretion during sleep. J Pediatr 1996;128(Part 2):S32.

Van Someren EJ. More than a marker: Interaction between the circadian regulation of temperature and sleep, age-related changes, and treatment possibilities. Chronobiol Int 2000;17:313.

Walters AS. Is there a subpopulation of children with growing pains who really have restless legs syndrome? A review of the literature. Sleep Med 2002;3:93.

Weitzman ED, Czeisler CA, Coleman RM, et al. Delayed sleep phase syndrome. A chronobiological disorder with sleep-onset insomnia. Arch Gen Psychiatry 1981;38:737.

Wittig R, Zorick F, Roehrs T, et al. Narcolepsy in a 7 year old. J Pediatr 1983;102:725.

Zolty P, Sanders MH, Pollack IF. Chiari malformation and sleep-disordered breathing: A review of diagnostic and management issues. Sleep 2000;23:637.

Zucconi M. Sleep disorders in children with neurological disease. In: Loughlin GM, Carroll JL, Marcus CL, eds. Sleep and breathing in children. A developmental approach. New York: Marcel Dekker, 2000;363.

Zucconi M, Ferini-Strambi L, Oldani A, et al. Nocturnal motor behaviors in children: A video- polysomnographic study. Sleep 1998;21(Suppl):148.

Zucconi M, Weber G, Castronovo V, et al. Sleep and upper airway obstruction in children with achondroplasia. J Pediatr 1996;129:743.

PART VIII

Disorders of Balance and Movement

CHAPTER 57

The Cerebellum and the Hereditary Ataxias

Stephen M. Maricich and Huda Y. Zoghbi

The cerebellum functions mainly to monitor and coordinate complex motor movements. Disruptions of its input or basic structure secondary to developmental anomalies, degenerative diseases, vascular insults, or trauma result in a characteristic spectrum of motor symptoms and signs. Advances in understanding the cellular, molecular, and physiologic composition of the cerebellum have provided new insights into both its normal functions and disruptions in specific disease processes. This chapter begins by describing the basic structure, connectivity, and functions of the cerebellum because this provides a starting point for understanding how the organ functions within the rest of the central nervous system (CNS). Next, derangements of cerebellar function are considered, with a primary emphasis on the hereditary ataxias. Other conditions associated with cerebellar dysfunction also are discussed in this text.

BASIC CEREBELLAR STRUCTURE, FUNCTION AND DYSFUNCTION

Cerebellar Structure

Anatomically, the cerebellum can be divided in the anteroposterior and mediolateral dimensions (Fig. 57-1A and B). Fissures divide the rostrocaudal length of the cerebellum into 10 lobules, which are analogous to the gyri of the cerebral cortex. These lobules can be grouped into three lobes: the *anterior lobe* (lobules I through V), the *posterior lobe* (lobules VI through IX), and the *flocculonodular lobe* (lobule X) (see Fig. 57-1C). The mediolateral divisions are the *vermis,* which lies medially, and the *hemispheres,* which lie laterally and are separated from the vermis by shallow grooves.

Functional regions of the cerebral cortex, which roughly correspond to Brodmann's areas, differ in their cellular histology. The same is not true of the cerebellar cortex. Rather, the same five cell types, arranged in the same relative orientation, are present regardless of anatomic or functional location (Fig. 57-2A). *Purkinje cells* are among the largest neurons in the CNS, and represent the sole output of the cerebellar cortex. Cerebellar *granule cells,* which reside in the *internal granular layer,* form the most numerous neuronal population in the central nervous system (their numbers are nearly equal to all other CNS neurons combined). Granule cells extend long, bifurcated axons *(parallel fibers)* into the molecular layer, where they travel for several millimeters and synapse with 1000 to 2000 Purkinje cells on their dendritic arbors; in turn, each Purkinje cell forms synapses with as many as 1 million parallel fibers. Granule cells are the only excitatory cell type in the cerebellar cortex. Three local inhibitory interneurons also reside in the cortex. *Golgi type II* cells are large neurons found in the internal granular layer that receive mossy fiber inputs and inhibit granule cells. *Basket* and *stellate cells* are found in the *molecular layer,* where they receive excitatory inputs from parallel fibers and are inhibitory to Purkinje cells.

The neurons of the *deep cerebellar nuclei* form four separate clusters in the cerebellar white matter (see Fig. 57-1A). These cells receive inhibitory cortical input from the Purkinje cells and excitatory extracerebellar afferents from climbing and mossy fibers. The *fastigial nuclei* lie most medially, and receive input from vermal Purkinje cells. The *interposed nuclei (nucleus globose* and *nucleus emboliform)* receive input from paravermal Purkinje cells. The *dentate nuclei,* which are the largest deep cerebellar nuclei in primates, receive input from the cerebellar hemispheres. Along with some Purkinje cells found in the flocculonodular lobe, the deep cerebellar nuclei represent the sole efferent output of the cerebellum, projecting to multiple brainstem nuclei in the medulla and pons, as well as the red nucleus and thalamus.

Cerebellar input consists of three classes of afferents. *Climbing fibers* originate in the inferior olives, which project to the contralateral cerebellar hemisphere. They provide strong excitatory input to Purkinje cells and neurons of the deep cerebellar nuclei. Each climbing fiber synapses on no more than 10 Purkinje cells, whereas each Purkinje cell receives input from only one climbing fiber. *Mossy fibers* originate in multiple locations in the thalamus, brainstem, and spinal cord and form excitatory synapses on granule cells and Golgi type II neurons in the internal granular layer, as well as on neurons of the deep cerebellar nuclei. Climbing fibers, and to a lesser extent mossy fibers, are arranged in a series of parasagittal bands that "stack" next to one another in the mediolateral dimension (see Fig. 57-2B); the functional significance of this arrangement is discussed later in the chapter. Finally, *multilayer fibers* originate in the hypothalamus, locus ceruleus, and raphe nuclei and form a diffuse fiber network in the cortex and deep cerebellar nuclei.

Like the cerebral cortex, cerebellar cortical afferents and efferents are arranged in a somatotopic manner [Manni and Petrosini, 2004]. This organization is more complex than that of the cerebral cortex in two ways. First, at least three separate homunculi (one in the anterior lobe and one in each of the paravermian lobules) can be identified (Fig. 57-3A). These are believed to converge on separate, continuous somatotopic maps in the four cerebellar nuclei. This arrangement, which was initially described in other species, has recently been directly demonstrated in humans using functional neuroimaging [Bushara et al., 2001; Manni and

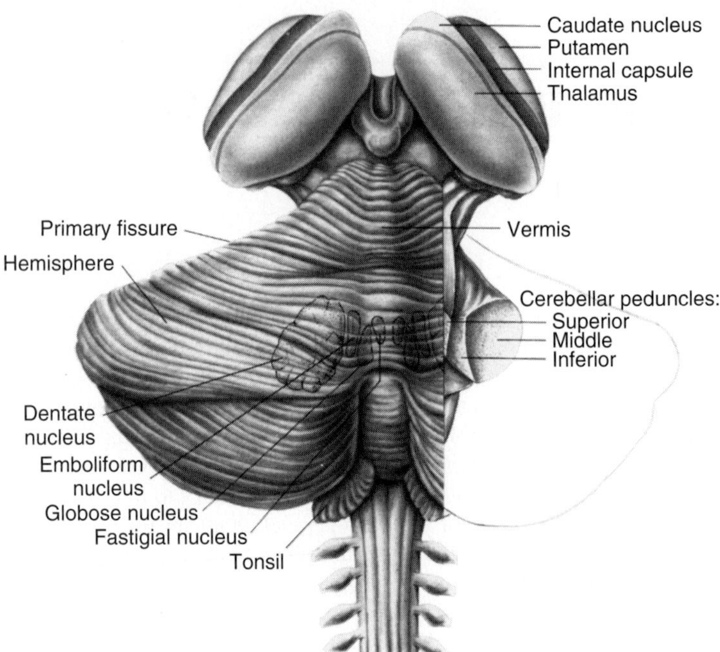

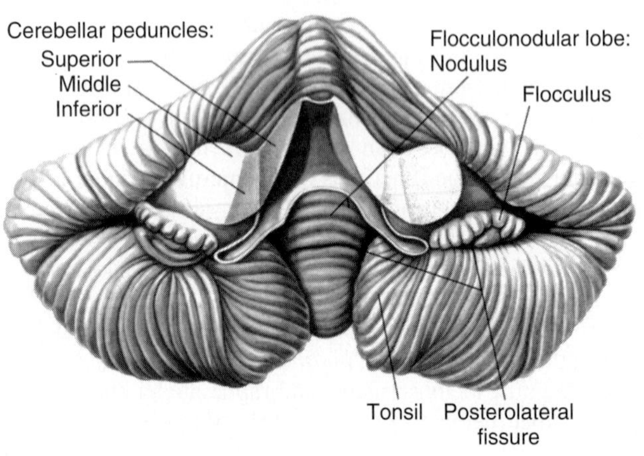

C

FIGURE 57-1. **A,** Dorsal view of the human cerebellum. The deep cerebellar nuclei are shown in their approximate positions. **B,** Ventral view of the human cerebellum. The brainstem is cut away, and the cerebellar peduncles are labeled. **C,** Sagittal midline section of human cerebellum. The lobules are labeled, and the anterior, posterior and flocculonodular lobes are shaded with different tones for easier distinction. Dorsal is at the top of the photograph, and anterior is to the right. (**A** and **B**, From Kandel ER and Schwartz, JH, eds. Principles of neural science, 2nd ed. New York: Elsevier, 1985;504; **C**, Photograph courtesy of Dr. Dawna Armstrong.)

Petrosini, 2004; Rijntjes et al., 1999]. Second, the sensory map within a cerebellar folium is not continuous. Instead, a *fractured somatotopy* exists, in which each region of the face or limb has multiple representations within the folium that may not be directly adjacent to one another (see Fig. 57-3B). The reason for this arrangement is unknown but may be necessary to bring climbing fiber and mossy fiber inputs into register with one another.

Three major fiber tracts connect the cerebellum with the rest of the neuraxis. The *inferior cerebellar peduncle,* or *restiform body,* contains mossy fiber projections from the spinal cord (dorsal spinocerebellar tract) and medulla (cuneocerebellar, vestibulocerebellar, reticulocerebellar, arcuatocerebellar, and trigeminocerebellar tracts) and climbing fibers from the inferior olives. Cerebellovestibular and cerebelloreticular efferents also course through this

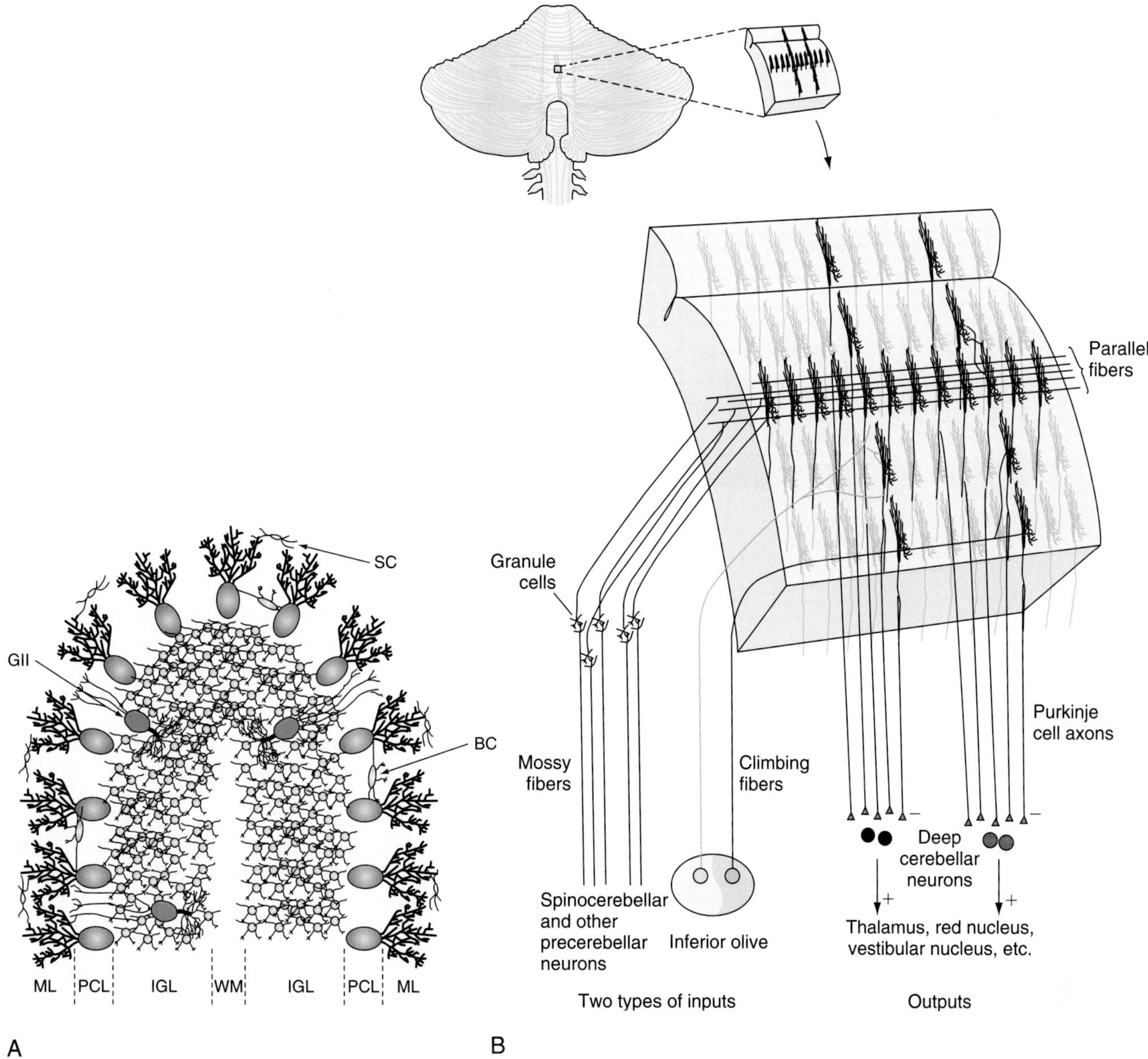

FIGURE 57-2. **A,** Major cell types of the cerebellar cortex. This is a representation of a sagittal section through a cerebellar folium. Granule cell parallel fibers are omitted for clarity. **B,** Climbing fiber input delineates parasagittal Purkinje cell bands that run perpendicular to parallel fiber input. Purkinje cells in the same band tend to project to the same cells in the deep cerebellar nuclei. (**B,** From Kandel ER, Schwartz JH, and Jessel TM, eds. Principles of neural science, 4th ed. New York: McGraw-Hill, 2003;838.)

tract. The *middle cerebellar peduncle,* or *brachium pontis,* is the largest peduncle and contains primarily cerebellar afferents from the pons. The *superior cerebellar peduncle,* or *brachium conjunctivum,* connects the cerebellum to the midbrain. It is mainly an efferent pathway, connecting the cerebellum to the red nucleus and thalamus via the dentatorubral and dentatothalamic tracts, and contains outputs to the vestibular nuclei and reticular formation as well. Afferents from the ventral spinocerebellar, tectocerebellar, trigeminocerebellar, and cerulocerebellar tracts also travel within it.

Cerebellar Function

As a whole, the cerebellum functions to integrate multiple sources of sensory information, then uses this information to coordinate motor movements and direct motor learning. Three main anatomic regions divide up these tasks. The *archicerebellum,* also called the *vestibulocerebellum,* roughly corresponds to the flocculonodular lobe. This division makes connections with the vestibular nuclei and is integrally involved in the maintenance of balance and the control of reflexive head and eye movements. The *paleocerebellum,* or *spinocerebellum,* consists of the vermis and paravermal (intermediate) regions of the cerebellar hemispheres, and the fastigial and interposed nuclei. The spinocerebellum functions in the regulation of limb movement and posture. The *neocerebellum,* or *cerebrocerebellum,* is made up of the lateral hemispheres and dentate nuclei. In primates, the cerebrocerebellum is the largest division and is involved not only in the planning of movements but also in motor learning.

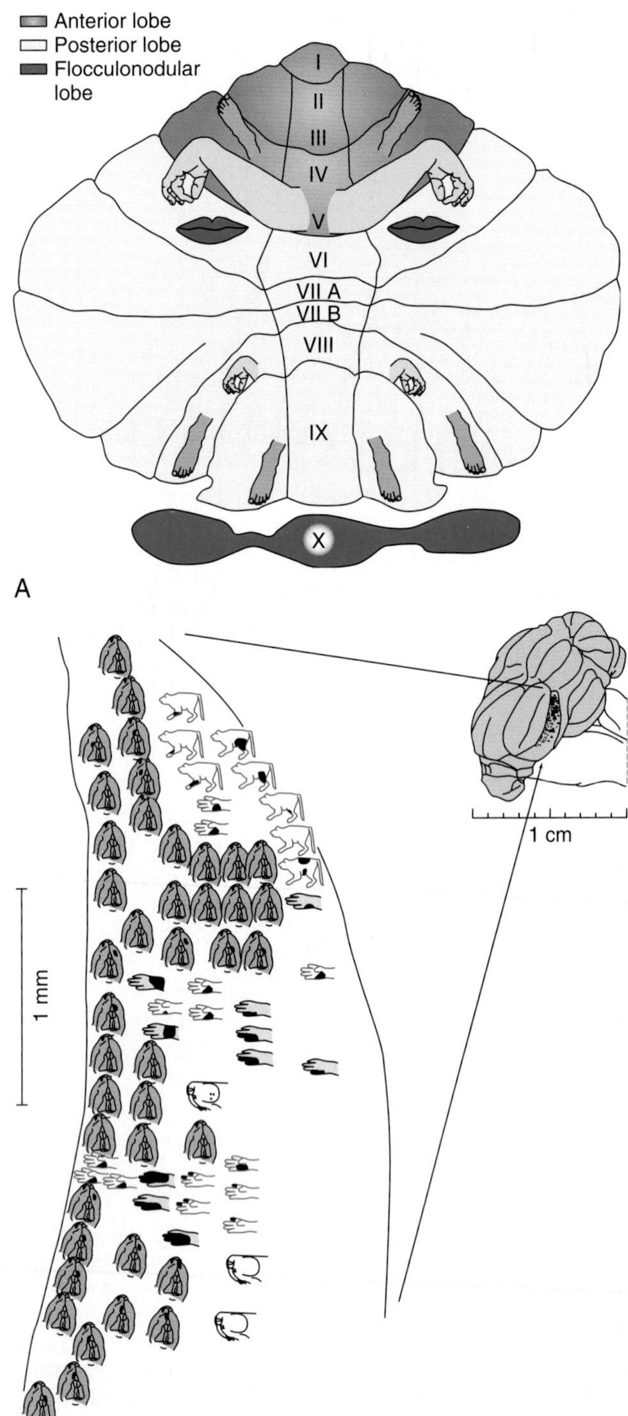

FIGURE 57-3. A, Sensorimotor representation in the human cerebellar cortex based on functional MRI data. The face representation is not shown. **B,** Fractured somatotopy of the cerebellum. Patches of tactile projections to left paramedian lobe. Black patches on body figurines depict receptive fields, which optimally activate multiple units in granular cell layer at sites marked by black dots in inset. MRI, magnetic resonance imaging. (**A**, From Manni E and Petrosini L. A century of cerebellar somatotopy: A debated representation. Nat Rev Neurosci 2004:5;241; **B,** From King JS, ed. Neurology and neurobiology, vol. 22. New York: AR Liss, 1987. Reprinted with permission of Wiley-Liss Inc., a subsidiary of John Wiley & Sons, Inc.)

As previously described, cerebellar afferent input is predominantly segregated into a series of parasagittal bands. This parasagittal arrangement is thought to be essential to the underlying function of the cerebellum. Comparison of climbing fiber to mossy fiber excitatory inputs within these bands may be important for refining movements and motor learning [Ito, 2002]. It has also been proposed that mossy fiber input, which is translated through granule cells and their parallel fibers, could transform spatial relationships into temporal ones as the signal beam passes from Purkinje cells closest to the granule cells to those farther down the parallel fiber path. The receptive Purkinje cells could then detect timing differences between the incoming granule cell and climbing fiber signals. Thus, the cerebellum could act as an alarm clock, stopwatch, or coincidence/time shift detector [Braitenberg, 1961, 1967].

Recent studies using advanced imaging techniques such as functional magnetic resonance imaging and positron-emission tomography scanning suggest that the cerebellum is also involved in several nonmotor functions. These include sensory discrimination, attention, working memory, semantic association, verbal learning, memory, and complex problem solving [Allen et al., 1997]. In addition, a number of studies have linked the cerebellum to various higher-order cognitive processes [Daum and Ackermann, 1995; Leiner and Leiner, 1991; Middleton and Strick, 1994]. Most of these functions are subserved by the cerebellar hemispheres and the dentate nuclei.

Cerebellar Dysfunction

Cerebellar lesions or dysfunction disturb regulation of muscle tone, motor control, and coordination of movement. The constellation of symptoms is sometimes useful for localizing the cerebellar lesion, but often there is considerable overlap.

Hypotonia is a decrease in muscle tone in response to stretch. It is typically seen with acute cerebellar hemispheral lesions and is often accompanied by hyporeflexia. Hypotonia likely results from decreased fusimotor activity resulting in decreased muscle spindle afferent response. It is usually a transient phenomenon after an acute lesion but can be seen in chronic lesions as well.

Ataxia is a broad term that refers to a disturbance in the smooth performance of voluntary motor acts. It includes *abasia* (unsteadiness of stance), *asynergia* (decomposition of complex movements into isolated, successive parts), *dysmetria* (abnormal excursions in movement), *dysdiadochokinesis* (impaired performance of rapid alternating movements), and impaired check/excessive rebound responses. Vermal lesions result in truncal ataxia and *titubation* (a bobbing of the head predominantly in the anteroposterior dimension), whereas hemispheric lesions cause limb ataxia.

Cerebellar dysarthria is characterized by abnormalities in articulation and prosody of speech. Slow, staccato, or scanning speech with uneven articulation or phonation can result from hemispheric damage and may be a manifestation of dysdiadochokinesis or hypotonia, or both. There is also evidence that left cerebellar lesions interfere with speech prosody because of disruptions of interconnections with the right cerebral hemisphere, which mediates this process [Brazis et al., 2001]. *Cerebellar mutism* is sometimes seen after removal of vermian tumors and may result from bilateral involvement of the dentatorubrothalamic tracts.

Intention tremor can occur after lesions of the dentate nuclei and is manifest only when the individual attempts to make a directed movement. Postural tremor is a rare manifestation of cerebellar damage.

Eye movement abnormalities, predominantly in the form of nystagmus, are also a manifestation of cerebellar disease. They usually occur when the vermis or flocculonodular lobe is affected. *Ocular dysmetria* (conjugate overshoot or undershoot of a visual target accompanied by voluntary saccades) can result from midline or hemispheric lesions.

Nonmotor manifestations of cerebellar disease can also occur. A cerebellar cognitive affective syndrome has been described in patients with isolated cerebellar lesions resulting from a number of different etiologies [Schmahmann and Sherman, 1998]. In this syndrome, executive functions, spatial cognition, personality changes, and language deficits are present. The postulated neural substrate involves circuits that link prefrontal, posterior parietal, superior temporal, and limbic cortices to the cerebellum.

Disorders that specifically affect different cerebellar subdivisions lead to a characteristic spectrum of motor abnormalities. Midline cerebellar disease causes disorders of stance and gait, truncal titubation, rotated postures of the head, and disturbances in eye movements. These can be subdivided into rostral vermal lesions that result in abasia and gait ataxia, and caudal vermal lesions that add nystagmus as well. Likewise, lesions of the fastigial nuclei, which receive their input from the vermis, also result in abasia. Intermediate hemisphere disease or lesions of the interposed nuclei cause delayed check (rebound) responses, truncal titubation, abnormal rapid alternating movements, action tremor, oscillation of outstretched extremities, and ataxia on finger-nose-finger and heel-knee-shin maneuvers. Disruption of the cerebellar hemispheres and dentate nuclei result in dysarthria, limb ataxia, hypotonia, terminal and intention tremor, and abnormal eye movements.

DIFFERENTIAL DIAGNOSIS OF ATAXIA

The underlying cause of ataxia is virtually always primary or secondary dysfunction of the cerebellum. Cerebellar disease is a result of a number of underlying conditions, many of which are listed in Box 57-1. The most prevalent causes of acute cerebellar ataxia are viral infections (e.g., coxsackievirus, rubeola, varicella), toxins (e.g., alcohol, barbiturates, antiepileptic drugs), and trauma. Tumors of the cerebellum (vermal and hemispheric) and tumors of the brainstem, particularly pontine gliomas, are also relatively common. Numerous metabolic conditions affecting the central and peripheral nervous systems lead to ataxia. Congenital abnormalities of the nervous system, particularly those related to Chiari malformation, Dandy-Walker malformation, and basilar impression, are associated with ataxia. Endocrinologic abnormalities, particularly hypothyroidism, may also present with ataxia as the predominant manifestation. Vascular abnormalities are unusual, but cerebellar hemorrhage, infarction, and embolism do occur. Angioblastomas of the cerebellum are rare; von Hippel-Lindau disease, a neurocutaneous condition, is associated with vascular lesions of the cerebellum, as is the PHACE (*P*osterior fossa malformations, *H*emangiomas, *A*rterial anomalies, *C*oarctation of aorta and *C*ardiac defects, and *E*ye abnormalities) syndrome [Frieden et al., 1996]. Although psychogenic presentation in the form of conversion reaction can suggest the presence of ataxia, careful examination often discloses incongruencies in the findings, distinguishing the motor difficulties from true ataxia.

MANAGEMENT OF CEREBELLAR DYSFUNCTION AND ATAXIA

When ataxia is the result of specific metabolic disorders, specific therapies are sometimes possible (Table 57-1). The presence of toxins, trauma, and neoplasms requires specific therapy for the underlying condition. Patients may require various aids for ambulation. Most often, physical therapy and occupational therapy are not significantly helpful in moderate-to-severe ataxia.

THE HEREDITARY ATAXIAS

Classification of the hereditary ataxias has long posed a significant challenge. Before the advent of gene cloning technology, these conditions were classified based on their mode of inheritance, clinical features, and pathologic findings. These approaches ultimately proved to be unsatisfactory and often led to more confusion than clarity. Patients with known hereditary ataxia have a range of cerebellar dysfunction that may be exclusively cerebellar in origin or combined with other features including brainstem dysfunction, spinal cord abnormalities, extrapyramidal findings, neuropathy, retinopathy, deafness, cataracts, seizures, and dementia [Berciano, 1982; Greenfield, 1954; Harding et al., 1985; Koeppen and Barron, 1984; Zoghbi, 1993]. The age of onset and clinical manifestations of any given disorder may differ significantly from family to family and even in the same kindred, making specific assignment beyond mode of inheritance difficult [Currier et al., 1972; Zoghbi and Caskey, 1998]. Likewise, attempts to classify ataxia according to the anatomic site of the most dominant pathology (e.g., spinal cord, cerebellum) are also flawed. Descriptors such as "olivopontocerebellar atrophy," a pathologic finding seen most predominantly in the dominantly inherited ataxias, do not adequately serve to distinguish between them.

The application of genetic and molecular biologic techniques to the hereditary ataxias has resulted in the most precise classification scheme to date and will ultimately provide insight into pathologic mechanisms and possible therapeutic interventions. There has been an explosion of knowledge in this area over the past 20 years, with a concomitant expansion in the number of new hereditary ataxias identified as old classifications are found to be groupings of genetically unrelated disorders.

The following sections subdivide the hereditary ataxias by their predominant mode of inheritance. Chromosomal loci, genes and gene products, and molecular mechanisms are presented where they are known.

Autosomal-Recessive Inherited Syndromes

The autosomal-recessive inherited ataxias (summarized in Table 57-2) are a varied group of disorders that tend to have

Box 57-1 Selected Causes of Ataxia in Childhood

Congenital
Agenesis of vermis of the cerebellum
Aplasia or dysplasia of the cerebellum
Basilar impression
Chiari malformation
Cerebellar dysplasia with microgyria, macrogyria, or agyria
Cervical spinal bifida with herniation of the cerebellum (Chiari malformation, type 3)
Dandy-Walker syndrome
Encephalocele
Hydrocephalus (progressive)
Hypoplasia of the cerebellum

Degenerative and/or Genetic
Acute intermittent cerebellar ataxia [Hill and Sherman*]
Ataxia, retinitis pigmentosa, deafness, vestibular abnormality, and intellectual deterioration [Francois and Descampas*]
Ataxia-telangiectasia
Biemond's posterior column ataxia
Cerebellar ataxia with deafness, anosmia, absent caloric responses, nonreactive pupils, and hyporeflexia [Brown, 1959]
Cockayne's syndrome
Dentate cerebellar ataxia (dyssynergia cerebellaris progressiva)
Familial ataxia with macular degeneration [Foster and Ingram*]
Friedreich's ataxia
Hereditary cerebellar ataxia, intellectual retardation, choreoathetosis, and eunuchoidism [Altchule and Kotowski*]
Hereditary cerebellar ataxia with myotonia and cataracts [Brown, 1959]
Hypertrophic interstitial neuritis
Marie's ataxia
Marinesco-Sjögren syndrome
Pelizaeus-Merzbacher disease
Periodic attacks of vertigo, diplopia, and ataxia—autosomal-dominant inheritance [Farmer and Mustian*]
Posterior and lateral column difficulties, nystagmus, and muscle atrophy [Burge and Wuthrich*]
Progressive cerebellar ataxia and epilepsy [von Bogaert and Colle*]
Ramsay Hunt disease (myoclonic seizures and ataxia)
Roussy-Lévy disease
Spinocerebellar ataxia (SCA); olivopontocerebellar ataxias

Endocrinologic
Acquired hypothyroidism
Cretinism

Infectious or Postinfectious
Acute cerebellar ataxia
Acute disseminated encephalomyelitis
Cerebellar abscess
Coxsackievirus
Diphtheria
Echovirus
Fisher's syndrome
Infectious mononucleosis (Epstein-Barr virus infection)
Infectious polyneuropathy
Japanese B encephalitis
Mumps encephalitis
Mycoplasma pneumoniae
Pertussis
Polio
Postbacterial meningitis
Rubeola
Tuberculosis
Typhoid
Varicella

Metabolic
Abetalipoproteinemia
Argininosuccinic aciduria
Ataxia with vitamin E deficiency (AVED)
GM2 gangliosidosis (late)
Hartnup's disease
Hyperalaninemia
Hyperammonemia I and II
Hypoglycemia
Kearns-Sayre syndrome
Leigh's disease
Maple syrup urine disease (intermittent)
Myoclonic epilepsy with ragged red fibers
Metachromatic leukodystrophy
Mitochondrial complex defects (I, III, IV)
Multiple carboxylase deficiency (biotinidase deficiency)
Neuronal ceroid-lipofuscinosis
Neuropathy, ataxia, retinitis pigmentosa (NARP)
Niemann-Pick disease (late infantile)
5-Oxoprolinuria
Pyruvate decarboxylase deficiency
Refsum's disease
Sialidosis
Triose-phosphate isomerase deficiency
Tryptophanuria
Wernicke's encephalopathy

Neoplastic
Frontal lobe tumors
Hemispheric cerebellar tumors
Midline cerebellar tumors
Neuroblastoma
Pontine tumors (primarily gliomas)
Spinal cord tumors

Primary Psychogenic
Conversion reaction

Toxic
Alcohol
Benzodiazepines
Carbamazepine
Clonazepam
Lead encephalopathy
Neuroblastoma
Phenobarbital
Phenytoin
Primidone
Tic paralysis poisoning

Traumatic
Acute cerebellar edema
Acute frontal lobe edema

Vascular
Angioblastoma of cerebellum
Basilar migraine
Cerebellar embolism
Cerebellar hemorrhage
Cerebellar thrombosis
Posterior cerebellar artery disease
Vasculitis
von Hippel-Lindau disease

*Cited in Brown, 1962.

TABLE 57-1

Treatable Causes of Inherited Ataxia

DISORDER	METABOLIC ABNORMALITY	DISTINGUISHING CLINICAL FEATURES	TREATMENT
Ataxia with vitamin E deficiency	Mutation in α-tocopherol transfer protein	Ataxia, areflexia, retinopathy	Vitamin E
Bassen-Kornzweig syndrome	Abetalipoproteinemia	Acanthocytosis, retinitis pigmentosa, fat malabsorption	Vitamin E
Hartnup's disease	Tryptophan malabsorption	Pellagra rash, intermittent ataxia	Niacin
Familial episodic ataxia type 1 and type 2	Mutations in potassium channel (KCNA1) and α_{1A} voltage-gated calcium channel, respectively	Episodic attacks, worse with pregnancy or birth control pills	Acetazolamide
Mitochondrial complex defects	Complexes I, III, IV	Encephalomyelopathy	Possibly riboflavin, CoQ_{10}, dichloroacetate
Multiple carboxylase deficiency	Biotinidase deficiency	Alopecia, recurrent infections, variable organic aciduria	Biotin
Pyruvate dehydrogenase deficiency	Block in E-M and Krebs cycle interface	Lactic acidosis, ataxia	Ketogenic diet, possibly dichloroacetate
Refsum's disease	Phytanic acid, α-hydroxylase	Retinitis pigmentosa, cardiomyopathy, hypertrophic neuropathy, ichthyosis	Dietary restriction of phytanic acid
Urea cycle defects	Urea cycle enzymes	Hyperammonemia	Protein restriction, arginine, benzoate, α-ketoacids

Modified from Stumpf DA. The inherited ataxias. Pediatr Neurol 1985;1:129.

an early age of onset in infancy or childhood. They can involve multiple regions of the central and peripheral nervous systems. In general, earlier age of onset usually heralds a more aggressive disease course. Several causative mutations have been identified, leading to a clear genetic classification scheme.

Friedreich's Ataxia (Spinocerebellar Ataxia; MIM 229300)

Friedreich's ataxia is one of the most common hereditary ataxias, with a prevalence of approximately 1 to 2 per 100,000 in the general population [Harding, 1984]. Whites are affected more often than other racial groups, with a prevalence closer to 1 per 50,000 [Cossée et al., 1997]. Clinically, the disease is signaled by the presence of ataxia and corticospinal tract impairment. Other associated features include nystagmus, kyphoscoliosis, and an unusual cardiomyopathy. Originally reported by Friedreich [1863], who believed the disease was associated only with spinal cord abnormalities, subsequent findings demonstrated involvement of the medulla, peripheral nerves, and cerebral cortex in some cases.

CLINICAL MANIFESTATIONS

Symptoms typically begin in the last half of the first decade, although onset may be detected at age 2 years or may be delayed until the second decade [Harding, 1981]. The initial

TABLE 57-2

Autosomal Recessive Cerebellar Ataxias

ATAXIA	CHROMOSOME	GENE	GENE PRODUCT	MECHANISM	AGE OF ONSET (YEARS)
Friedreich's ataxia	9q13	*X25*	Frataxin	GAA repeat	2-51
Friedreich's ataxia 2	9p23-p11	Unknown	Unknown	Unknown	5-20
AVED	8q13	*TTP1*	TTPA	Missense mutation, deletion, insertion	2-52
Ataxia-telangiectasia	11q22.3	*ATM*	ATM	Missense and deletion mutations	Infancy
Ataxia-telangiectasia–like disorder	11q21	*hMRE11*	MRE11A	Missense and deletion mutations	9-48 months
Ataxia-ocular apraxia 1	9p13.3	*APTX*	Aprataxin	Frameshift, missense, nonsense mutations	2-18
Ataxia-ocular apraxia 2	9q34	*SETX*	Senataxin	Frameshift, missense, nonsense mutations	9-22
Ataxia, Cayman type	19q13.3	*ATCAY*	Caytaxin	Missense mutation	Birth
IOSCA	10q24	Unknown	Unknown	Unknown	9-24 months
Progressive Myoclonic Epilepsy	21q22.3	*CST6*	Cystatin B	5′ Dodecamer repeat	6-13
ARSACS	13q12	*SACS*	Sacsin	Frameshift and nonsense mutations	1-20

APTX, apraxatin gene; ARSACS, autosomal recessive spastic ataxia of Charlevoix-Saguenay; *ATCAY*, Cayman-type cerebellar ataxia gene; *ATM*, ataxia-telangiectasia mutated gene; AVED, ataxia with vitamin E deficiency; *CST6*, cystatin 6 gene, *hMRE11*, meiotic recombination 11 gene; IOSCA, infantile-onset spinocerebellar ataxia; *SACS*, sacsin gene; *SETX*, senataxin gene; *TTP1*, tocopherol transfer protein 1 gene.

presentation is usually progressive gait ataxia and slowing. The pattern of gait may be extremely wide, and may have a reeling or lurching quality. Asymmetries are sometimes present but more commonly both legs are equally involved. Bladder dysfunction may manifest at any time during the disease course; symptoms of spastic bladder are common. Difficulties with the upper extremities and distal muscle wasting become apparent as the disease progresses. Incoordination of the arms becomes evident, limb and head tremor begins, and choreiform movements of the arms and face are often seen. Lateral or horizontal nystagmus may be prominent, and visual pursuit is punctuated with small jerks. Muscles of speech become involved, and cerebellar dysarthria is seen. The dysarthria rapidly worsens, and the patient's speech is rendered ineffective early in the disease course. Difficulties in swallowing, if present, are delayed until the terminal phases.

Cranial nerve involvement is not limited to nerves VII, XI, and XII. Impairment of pupillary responsivity and limited extraocular movements are also common. Additional ophthalmologic abnormalities include cataracts, retinitis pigmentosa, and optic atrophy. Auditory dysfunction is common [Cassandro et al., 1986] and is documented by abnormal brainstem auditory-evoked potentials that are likely the result of impairment of both central and peripheral acoustic pathways [De Pablos et al., 1991; Knezevic and Stewart-Wynne, 1985]. The degree of hearing compromise is variable. Vertigo has been reported to accompany this condition. Although higher cortical function appears intact when evaluated clinically, some studies suggest a decrease in speed of information processing [Hart et al., 1985; 1986].

Examination reveals that deep tendon reflexes are absent after the illness has been present for a short time; the patellar reflexes are often lost first. The deep tendon reflexes may be preserved for a longer period in young children [Salih et al., 1990]. Bilateral extensor toe signs are easily elicitable. Cremasteric and abdominal reflexes may be lost. The masseter reflex remains intact [Auger, 1992]. Occasionally weakness, muscle atrophy, and profound hypotonia may be evident, usually associated with spinal nerve disintegration. As mentioned, virtually all facets of cerebellar function are involved, and both gross and fine coordination are affected. Position sense, vibration sense, and other skills requiring normal posterior column function are grossly impaired. Autonomic innervation of superficial layers of skin may be involved. Pain and temperature sensation are usually intact, although some impairment may be present late in the course of the illness. Evidence of axonal sensory neuropathy indicated by electrodiagnostic studies is invariably present. Somatosensory-evoked potentials are abnormal, as is central motor function as determined by magnetic stimulation [Claus et al., 1988].

Patients with Friedreich's ataxia virtually always have talipes equinovarus and pes cavus. Grotesque deformities of the hand, including the claw deformity, can occur. Flexor spasms with attendant pain may be a great source of discomfort. Many patients suffer from kyphoscoliosis [Daher et al., 1985; Labelle et al., 1986] and may be unable to walk secondary to poor balance and an abnormally shifted center of gravity (Fig. 57-4). Surgical intervention may correct the abnormal spinal curve, but an absence of compensation by the impaired motor system may still render the patient unable to ambulate.

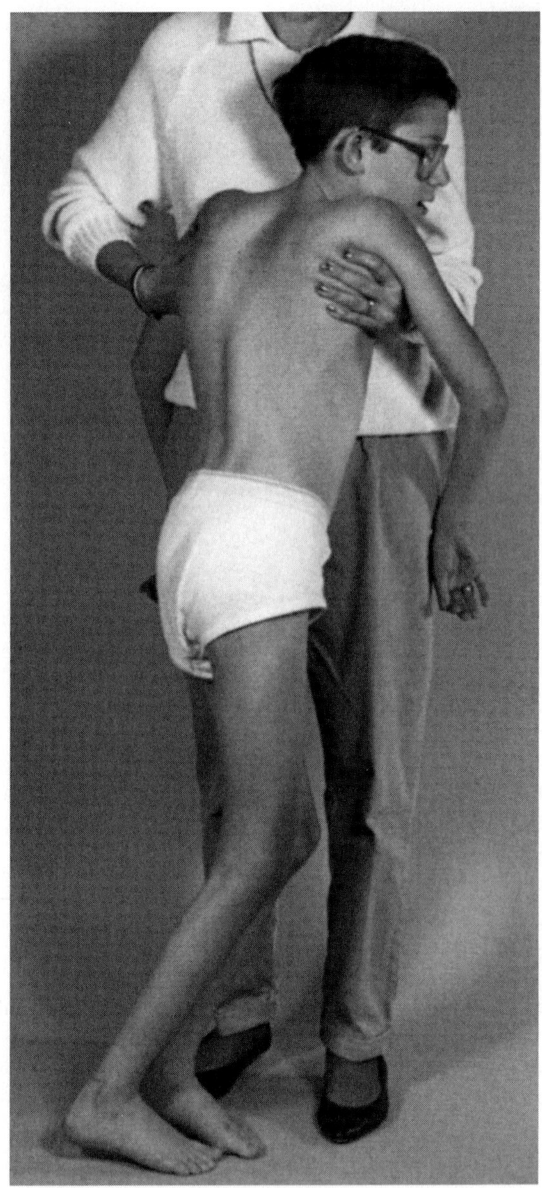

FIGURE 57-4. Friedreich's ataxia and moderate scoliosis in a 13-year-old boy who is unable to walk independently.

Cardiomyopathies are the most common accompanying cardiac abnormalities, although congenital heart disease has been described. The cardiomyopathy is often progressive and is documented even before clinical manifestations by the presence of electrocardiogram abnormalities (e.g., deep Q waves, low wave QRS complexes, S-T segment changes, T-wave inversion) [Child et al., 1986; Harding and Hewer, 1983; Heck, 1963]. Dysrhythmias may be particularly worrisome and life threatening [Baldwin and Lane, 1987]. Electrocardiogram and vectorcardiographic changes are demonstrable in more than 90% of patients [Child et al., 1986]. Left ventricular hypertrophy or symmetric ventricular hypertrophy is frequently evident on echocardiography [Pentland and Fox, 1983]. Hypertrophic cardiomyopathy is the leading cause of death in Friedreich's ataxia patients.

Diabetes mellitus is associated with Friedreich's ataxia; even in its absence, the glucose tolerance curve may be abnormal. Insulin resistance appears to be the explanation

[Fantus et al., 1991; Khan et al., 1986]. Unaffected relatives may also manifest insulin resistance. Episodic hypothermia, intermittent vomiting, and ventilatory dysfunction have also been reported [Heck, 1963; Thoren, 1959, 1962].

Imaging studies reveal both structural and functional changes that correlate with pathologic changes. MRI studies document atrophy of the upper cervical spinal cord and cerebellum [Wessel et al., 1989]. Positron emission tomography demonstrates a widespread increase in cerebral metabolic rate for glucose in the brain of ambulatory patients with Friedreich's ataxia. As the disease progresses, glucose metabolism decreases in a regionally specific manner; only the caudate and lenticular nuclei have increased metabolic rate in nonambulatory patients [Gilman et al., 1990].

Diagnosis is suggested by the presence of the expected clinical manifestations and sometimes by family history. Distinct diagnostic criteria for diagnosing Friedreich's ataxia were advanced by Geoffroy and colleagues [1976]. These criteria included autosomal-recessive inheritance, onset before 10 years of age, gait ataxia, dysarthria, absent deep tendon reflexes, dorsal column signs, and weakness. The presence of an abnormal 5-hour glucose tolerance curve may be corroborative. Spinal fluid findings may include elevated protein content and mild pleocytosis.

PATHOLOGY

The primary site of involvement on pathologic examination is the spinal cord. Gross examination reveals a shrunken cord with the posterior columns, spinocerebellar tracts, corticospinal tracts, and posterior rootlets strikingly involved by varying degrees of fiber loss, demyelination, and gliosis. Axons and myelin alike are involved, although the medullary nuclei (Burdach's nuclei) are usually spared [Greenfield, 1954]. Structures in the medial root zone, including ganglion cells and the posterior roots that terminate within them, manifest varying degrees of involvement but are typically decreased in number. The lumbar and sacral roots are most severely affected, and the large, myelinated lumbar spinal nerves lose many axons. In contrast, anterior horn cells and their rootlets are usually uninvolved; however, minor pathologic alterations may be evident. Although reported, myopathic changes are rare.

At the gross level the cerebellum, brainstem, and cerebral hemispheres are relatively normal. However, microscopic study of the cerebellum often reveals varying degrees of cerebellar cortical degeneration with minimal involvement of the deep nuclei. The inferior olives, vestibular nuclei, and pontine nuclei may be involved to varying degrees. In the cerebrum, subtle neuronal changes affecting Betz cells in the motor strip have been reported.

Reduction in the density of large myelinated fibers in sural nerve biopsies can be present even in young children, and often worsens with age [Said et al., 1986].

Pathologic changes in the heart include evidence of cardiomyopathy and involvement of blood vessels, nerves, and ganglia [James et al., 1987].

GENETICS

Friedreich's ataxia is transmitted as an autosomal-recessive disorder; the finding of consanguinity among several families clearly supported the autosomal-recessive inheritance pattern. The disease affects males and females equally. The establishment of the criteria proposed by Geoffroy and co-workers [1976] provides a basis for research studies and allows clinical identification of families for linkage studies. Genetic linkage studies mapped the Friedreich's ataxia gene to chromosome 9 and confirmed that the "Acadian" form of ataxia characterized by a slower course of degeneration [Barbeau et al., 1984; Keats et al., 1989] also maps to chromosome 9 [Chamberlain et al., 1988; Fujita et al., 1989; Keats et al., 1989]. Friedreich's ataxia is caused by the decreased expression of a mitochondrial protein, frataxin, encoded by the *X25* gene located at 9q13 [Bidichandani et al., 1998; Koeppen, 1998; Montermini et al., 1995].

Campuzano and co-workers [1996] were the first to identify an unstable GAA trinucleotide repeat in the first intron of *X25* [Campuzano et al., 1996]. They also identified three different point mutations. In the group of 74 patients without a point mutation, 71 were homozygous for expanded alleles, and 3 were heterozygous for the expanded repeat. Five patients with point mutations were heterozygous for the expansion. The size of the repeat ranged from 7 to 22 on normal alleles and from 200 to 900 on Friedreich's ataxia chromosomes. Further studies revealed that the triplet repeat could get as large as 1700 units, and that the lengths of both the larger and smaller expanded alleles correlated inversely with the age of onset and severity of disease [Durr et al., 1996; Filla et al., 1996]. The mean allele length is significantly higher in Friedreich's ataxia patients with diabetes, cardiomyopathy, and loss of reflexes in the upper extremities. Of 187 patients with autosomal-recessive ataxia, 140 were homozygous for a GAA expansion [Durr et al., 1996]. Approximately one fourth of the patients had atypical Friedreich's ataxia with retained deep tendon reflexes and/or later onset of disease, suggesting that the clinical spectrum of Friedreich's ataxia is wider than expected, and that deoxyribonucleic acid (DNA)–based testing is the most accurate means for diagnosis and subsequent genetic counseling.

Frataxin is localized to the inner mitochondrial membrane and is thought to play a role in mitochondrial respiration and iron accumulation. Deletion of the frataxin homolog in yeast leads to mitochondrial iron accumulation and increased susceptibility to oxidative stress, with an increased production of free radicals [reviewed in Voncken et al., 2004]. These observations, coupled with the fact that expanded trinucleotide repeats interfere with transcription elongation of the *X25* gene and cause a frataxin deficiency state, might explain the human phenotype [Bidichandani et al., 1998]. The production of a viable animal model has been complicated by early embryonic lethality in *X25*-null mice and absence of a phenotype in mice that have had a human FRDA allele "knocked-in" to the murine locus. Data from yeast, a mouse model, and human fibroblast experiments have led to the hypothesis that frataxin plays a role in the biosynthesis of iron/sulfur complex–containing proteins, which are critical elements in the mitochondrial respiratory chain [Voncken et al., 2004]. Frataxin has also been found to function as an iron chaperone protein that aids in the regeneration of aconitase, an enzyme essential in the citric acid cycle [Bulteau et al., 2004]. Why only selective neuronal systems are vulnerable to the loss of frataxin function remains unknown.

TREATMENT

Given the proposed function of frataxin protein in iron or sulfur cluster biosynthesis and the increased oxidative stress found with decreased protein levels, several groups have initiated treatment with idebenone, a short-chain analog of coenzyme Q_{10} [Buyse et al., 2003; Hausse et al., 2002; Mariotti et al., 2003; Rustin et al., 1999; Schols et al., 2001]. All but one of these trials (the shortest trial) have demonstrated improved cardiac function and decreased ventricular mass, which are important findings because cardiac dysfunction is the leading cause of death in Friedreich's ataxia patients. Unfortunately, idebenone treatment has no effect on the progression of ataxia. Therapy with other antioxidants, iron chelators, or glutathione peroxidase mimetics has been suggested (and in some cases tried), but no clear beneficial effect has been established.

Symptomatic treatment in the form of antispasticity agents can be helpful to relieve painful muscle spasms, and surgical correction of scoliosis can sometimes be palliative, at least for a time.

Friedreich's Ataxia 2 (MIM 601992)

Other families with a Friedreich's ataxia disease phenotype but without point mutations or GAA expansions in the *X25* gene have been described [Christodoulou et al., 2001; Kostrzewa et al., 1997]. In one family, linkage to a locus on chromosome 9p23-p11 has been found [Christodoulou et al., 2001]. The biologic basis for the genocopy is not known, but it has been proposed that mutations in genes in the iron metabolism pathway may be responsible.

Vitamin E Deficiency and Related Syndromes

Ataxia with isolated vitamin E deficiency (MIM 277460) is a rare but important cause of early onset ataxia. The clinical presentation closely resembles that of Friedreich's ataxia with the exceptions that cardiac involvement is rarely seen, diabetes is not part of the clinical constellation, and occasionally head titubation and/or dystonia is present. Symptoms typically begin in childhood or adolescence. Similar features can be seen in individuals with malabsorption syndromes, chronic steatorrhea, abetalipoproteinemia (Bassen-Kornzweig disease), or primary vitamin E deficiency; these individuals should be identified by their risk factors.

Numerous mutations have been identified in the tocopherol transfer protein gene (*TTP1*), which encodes the α-tocopherol transfer protein (TTPA) [Cavalier et al., 1998; Ouahchi et al., 1995]. TTPA is expressed in the liver and is responsible for the incorporation of tocopherol (vitamin E) into very-low-density lipoprotein [Traber et al., 1990]. Mutations in the gene disrupt vitamin E recycling, leading to its rapid elimination from the body and a profound deficiency state.

Because this disease is treatable, all patients with a Friedreich's ataxia phenotype should be evaluated for vitamin E deficiency. Supplementation rapidly normalizes plasma vitamin E levels and halts disease progression. Unfortunately, once symptoms occur, recovery of neurologic deficits may be incomplete.

Ataxia-Telangiectasia (Louis-Bar Syndrome; MIM 208900)

Ataxia-telangiectasia is one of the most common inherited causes of early childhood–onset ataxia in most countries, with a prevalence of one in 40,000 to 100,000 live births in the United States. The disease is characterized by progressive cerebellar ataxia, ocular apraxia, oculocutaneous telangiectasias, choreoathetosis, proclivity to sinopulmonary infections, and lymphoreticular neoplasia. Death often occurs by the fourth or fifth decade of life, typically resulting from sinopulmonary disease, neoplasms, or neurologic deterioration.

The initial clinical description of this disease was reported by Syllaba and Henner [1926], who called it *congenital double athetosis-aconjunctival vascular plexus syndrome* [Syllaba and Henner, 1926]. Louis-Bar [1941] reported a 9-year-old male with associated ataxia and cutaneous telangiectasias, classifying the case as a previously unrecognized phakomatosis [Louis-Bar, 1941]. Three additional independent reports subsequently appeared in the literature [Biemond, 1957; Boder and Sedgwick, 1957, 1958], and Boder and Sedgwick named the condition *ataxia-telangiectasia.*

CLINICAL MANIFESTATIONS

Early motor development appears to be normal until the onset of ataxia, which often begins during infancy but is not noted until around the time that the child starts walking. The ataxia is progressive and ultimately leads to an inability to ambulate by the beginning of the second decade. Choreoathetosis and dystonia occur in up to 90% of patients, and these motor findings become more prominent with increasing age. A characteristic impassive facies, as well as drooling and dysarthria, are common features as well. Although strength is initially normal, many patients in their 20s and 30s develop progressive spinal muscular atrophy, predominantly affecting the hands and feet [Gatti et al., 1991]. Peripheral neuropathy in the form of diminished deep tendon reflexes and loss of large fiber sensation is also seen. Mental function is well preserved, although deficits in short-term memory can occur in the third and fourth decades [Gatti et al., 1991].

Oculomotor apraxia is a distinguishing feature of the disease. The apraxia commonly presents before the appearance of conjunctival telangiectasias and is characterized by defects of initiating voluntary saccades, hypometric voluntary saccades accompanied by compensatory eye blinking and/or head thrusting movements, and disrupted smooth pursuit movements [Baloh et al., 1978; Sedgwick and Boder, 1972; Smith and Cogan, 1959]. Involuntary saccade initiation and optokinetic nystagmus can be impaired as well, and vestibulo-ocular reflexes can be increased.

Telangiectasias are usually first observed in patients between the ages of 2 and 4 years, although they can occur as early as birth and as late as 14 years of age [Centerwall and Miller, 1958; McFarlin et al., 1972] (Fig. 57-5). In addition to the conjunctivae, they appear on exposed areas of the skin, particularly areas of friction and trauma such as the auricle, nasal bridge, and antecubital and popliteal spaces. Exposure to sun enhances their appearance. Pre-

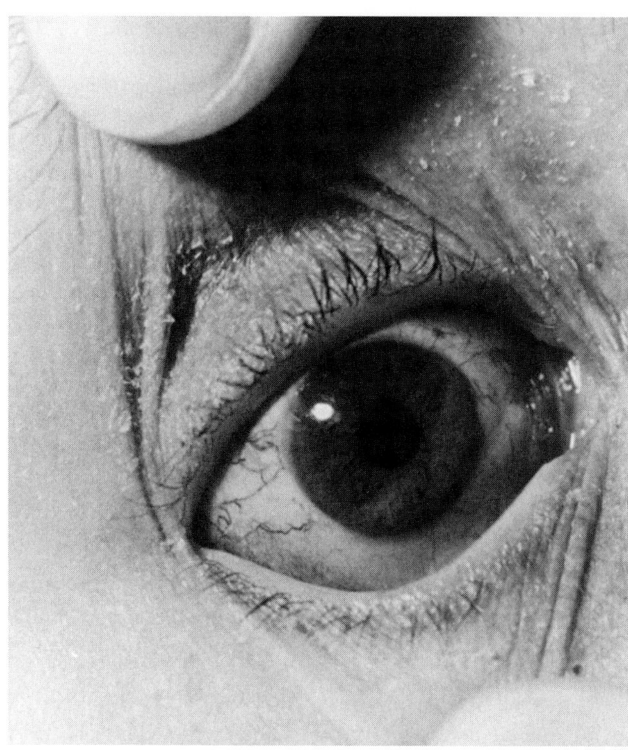

FIGURE 57-5. Characteristic conjunctival telangiectasias observed in a 12 year old with ataxia-telangiectasia.

mature aging of hair and skin is frequent, as are skin infections, including chronic blepharitis. Other skin changes consisting of vitiligo and café au lait spots can be seen. Rarely, scleroderma-like lesions occur.

Recurrent sinopulmonary infections are common, affecting 90% of patients, and usually result in chronic bronchitis, bronchiectasis, or both. The impairment of cellular immunity is also manifest by abnormally developed or absent adenoids, tonsils, lymphoid tissue, and thymus gland. Patients have an impaired delayed hypersensitivity response to skin-sensitizing antigens and a delayed homograft-rejection response [McFarlin and Oppenheim, 1969].

Patients with ataxia-telangiectasia are prone to develop tumors and are more likely than the general population to have Hodgkin's disease, leukemia, lymphoma, and lymphosarcoma. Other associated neoplasms include brain tumors, gastric adenocarcinomas, ovarian dysgerminomas, gonadoblastomas, cystic adenofibromas, uterine leiomyomas, and thyroid adenomas [Gatti and Good, 1971; Miller and Chatten, 1967; Spector et al., 1982].

Hypogonadism is frequent in both genders, and growth retardation is notable despite normal levels of growth hormone. Insulin-resistant diabetes is also occasionally seen as part of the clinical constellation.

Patients with less severe variant forms of ataxia-telangiectasia have been described [Gilad et al., 1998; Saviozzi et al., 2002]. Immunodeficiency, telangiectasias, cancer, and sinopulmonary infections may be absent or reduced, but the neurologic manifestations still occur. These individuals have a later onset and slower progression of neurologic signs, longer life spans, and decreased chromosomal instability and cellular radiosensitivity.

LABORATORY FINDINGS

Serum α-fetoprotein and carcinoembryonic antigen levels are often elevated in affected individuals. Most patients have decreased concentrations or absence of immunoglobulins A and E secondary to reduced synthesis, even though a high catabolic rate has been reported. Immunoglobulin M, G1, and G3 concentrations are normal or elevated, and immunoglobulin G2 and G4 concentrations are generally decreased. These humoral defects result in impaired antibody response to various bacterial and viral antigens.

Fibroblast and lymphoid cell lines from ataxia-telangiectasia patients exhibit increased radiosensitivity, leading to spontaneous and radiation-induced chromosomal breakage and rearrangement that can be assessed in culture [Shiloh et al., 1985]. In lymphoid cell lines, the chromosomal breaks occur at the loci of T-cell antigen receptors and immunoglobulin genes, where DNA rearrangements and deletions naturally occur [Arlett and Priestley, 1985; Davis et al., 1985; Hecht and Hecht, 1985].

Whereas these tests can be useful for screening, genetic analysis has become the gold standard for diagnosis (see later discussion).

PATHOLOGY

Cerebellar atrophy primarily affects the Purkinje and granular cells, although basket cells can also be involved. Neuronal degeneration of the dentate and olivary nuclei and the substantia nigra has been demonstrated, and nuclear changes occur in the cells of the oculomotor complex, pretectal nuclei, and hypothalamus. Pituitary cells often have enlarged or dysplastic nuclei. Older patients have denervation of the posterior columns of the spinal cord. Degeneration of the anterior horn cells, decreased numbers of satellite cells in the dorsal root ganglia, and nucleomegaly of Schwann cells have been described [Boder, 1987; De Leon et al., 1976; Sourander et al., 1966].

GENETICS

The worldwide incidence of ataxia-telangiectasia is approximately 1 in 40,000 to 100,000 live births; the carrier frequency ranges from 0.5% to 1%. The gene locus maps to chromosome 11q22-23 [Gatti et al., 1988]. The *ATM* (ataxia-telangiectasia mutated) gene is very large, with 66 exons spanning 150kb of genomic DNA [Uziel et al., 1996]; this fact makes mutation detection a challenge. In addition, because of the large number of different mutations the majority of patients are compound heterozygotes. Still, using a combination of techniques the estimated mutation detection rate is greater than 95% in affected individuals. It is estimated that truncating mutations account for about 85% of mutations, whereas point mutations are responsible for the rest [Buzin et al., 2002].

The ATM protein is a nuclear phosphoprotein homologous to a family of phosphatidylinositol kinase-related proteins that functions in the DNA damage response and in cell cycle regulation [Savitsky et al., 1995a; 1995b]. Individuals with classic ataxia-telangiectasia have little or no active ATM protein, whereas most individuals with variant ataxia-telangiectasia have one severe mutation coupled with a mild mutation. In this latter condition some ATM activity is preserved, which probably explains the milder phenotype [Saviozzi et al., 2002].

Loss of ATM activity could lead to neuronal degeneration in at least two ways. As a monitor of DNA strand breaks important for initiating repair, it has been suggested that the ATM protein is necessary for the elimination of neural cells with genomic damage and that the preservation of those cells may contribute to neuronal dysfunction [Herzog et al., 1998]. Several other diseases that affect DNA repair (ataxia-telangiectasia–like disorder, ataxia-ocular apraxia 1, xeroderma pigmentosum, Cockayne's syndrome, Nijmegen's breakage syndrome and de Sanctis-Cacchione syndrome) have a cerebellar phenotype, suggesting that cerebellar neurons may be sensitive to DNA damage. This hypothesis highlights a nuclear role for the ATM protein. In neurons, however, a large percentage of the protein is found in the cytoplasm and axons. Increased numbers of lysosomes are found in Purkinje cell bodies and axons in ATM-deficient mice [Barlow et al., 2000]. This increase, coupled with an observed interaction with β-adaptin, a protein important for clathrin-mediated endocytosis, suggests that vesicle/protein transport may also be disrupted in ATM-defective cells [Lim et al., 1998].

TREATMENT

Patients should receive vigorous supportive therapy, with particular attention directed to recurrent sinopulmonary infection. Attempts to improve immunologic status by plasma transfusion of thymosin and provision of fetal thymus transplants have not altered the course of the neurologic signs and symptoms [Wara and Ammann, 1978]. Treatment of neoplasms must proceed with caution because patients are extremely sensitive to radiation and chemotherapy, and demonstrate resultant ulcerative dermatitis, severe esophagitis, dysphagia, and deep-tissue necrosis [Gotoff et al., 1967; Morgan et al., 1968].

Ataxia-Telangiectasia–like Disorder (MIM 604391)

Four patients have been described with clinical presentations that are essentially identical to that of ataxia-telangiectasia except that ocular telangiectasias are absent [Hernandez et al., 1993; Klein et al., 1996]. Two of the patients, who are brothers, presented first with chorea that later progressed to ataxia. Increased susceptibility to DNA damage was noted in all four patients. Stewart and colleagues [1999] found that the disorder maps to chromosome 11q21 in all four patients. Loss-of-function mutations in the *hMRE11A* gene are causative. Like ATM, MRE11A is important for DNA repair and may act as a sensor of DNA damage. Stewart and associates [1999] estimate that approximately 6% of ataxia-telangiectasia patients may in fact have ataxia-telangiectasia–like disorder.

Ataxia-Oculomotor Apraxia 1 (Early Onset Ataxia with Oculomotor Apraxia and Hypoalbuminemia; MIM 208920)

Ataxia-oculomotor apraxia is an autosomal-recessive ataxia that was initially described in Japanese families but has subsequently been described in other areas of the world as well [Tranchant et al., 2003]. It is the most frequent cause of autosomal-recessive cerebellar ataxia in Japan and the second most common cause in Portugal. The presentation is nearly identical to that of ataxia-telangiectasia without the non-neurologic features [Aicardi et al., 1988], and accounts for up to 10% of autosomal-recessive cerebellar ataxias [Le Ber et al., 2003]. Gait imbalance and dysarthria are the typical presenting features, although chorea can sometimes be the presenting symptom. Ocular apraxia typically occurs a few years after symptom onset; with time, progressive ophthalmoplegia occurs as well. Areflexia, dystonia, choreoathetosis, sensory and motor neuropathy, mental retardation, and retinal/macular lesions seen on funduscopy can also be part of the presentation. Life span is not affected. Laboratory studies reveal hypoalbuminemia and hypercholesterolemia in the majority of cases as a later manifestation of the disease. Neuroimaging demonstrates cerebellar and sometimes brainstem atrophy. Pathology studies report loss of Purkinje cells in the cerebellum, degeneration of the posterior columns, spinocerebellar tracts, and anterior horn cells of the spinal cord [Sekijima et al., 1998].

The gene *APTX* maps to chromosome 9p13.3 and is expressed in all body tissues [Date et al., 2001; Moreira et al., 2001]. Several mutations have been described, as have compound heterozygotes; frameshift and nonsense mutations result in more severe phenotypes than missense mutations. The *APTX* gene product, aprataxin, has domains that suggest a potential role in single-strand DNA repair and has been found to interact with another protein implicated in this process [Sano et al., 2004].

Ataxia-Oculomotor Apraxia 2 (Spinocerebellar Ataxia, Recessive, Non-Friedreich's Type 1; MIM 606002)

A second ataxia-telangiectasia–like spinocerebellar ataxia with slightly different features than ataxia-oculomotor apraxia type 1 has been described in families of several different ethnic backgrounds. The clinical features of ataxia-oculomotor apraxia type 2 include gait ataxia, sensorimotor neuropathy, and ocular apraxia, with the latter occurring about 50% of the time. Although overall cognitive function is normal, subtle changes in executive function can be seen on neuropsychologic testing [Le Ber et al., 2004]. Neuroimaging demonstrates cerebellar atrophy. Ataxia-oculomotor apraxia type 2 is distinguished from ataxia-oculomotor apraxia type 1 by the later age of onset, less common ocular apraxia, high levels of serum α-fetoprotein, and normal serum albumin. The functional prognosis is also better in ataxia-oculomotor apraxia type 2. The gene *SETX* maps to chromosome 9q34 [Nemeth et al., 2000]. Mutations cause premature termination of the senataxin protein, which is a member of the helicase family and is involved in ribonucleic acid maturation and termination [Moreira et al., 2004]. Interestingly, other mutations in senataxin are transmitted in an autosomal-dominant manner and cause juvenile amyotrophic lateral sclerosis [Chen et al., 2004a]; the basis for the dramatic phenotypic difference between the two diseases is unknown.

Cerebellar Ataxia, Cayman Type (MIM 601238)

Cerebellar ataxia, Cayman type, is a recessive disorder described in an isolated population from Grand Cayman Island, mapping to chromosome 19q13.3 [Brown et al., 1984; Johnson et al., 1978; Nystuen et al., 1996]. The disorder consists of hypotonia from birth, followed by psychomotor retardation, nystagmus, intention tremor, dysarthria, and ataxic gait. The cerebellar findings are typically nonprogressive. Brain imaging demonstrates isolated cerebellar atrophy. The *ATCAY* gene is expressed only in neurons in the brain and in components of the spinal cord and peripheral nervous system. Two nucleotide substitutions, one in exon 9 resulting in a serine to arginine substitution, and one in intron 9 that interferes with splicing, have been identified as causative [Bomar et al., 2003]. *ATCAY* codes for the caytaxin protein, a protein that shares a conserved domain with TTPA (see earlier section on vitamin E deficiency syndromes). However, it does not appear that caytaxin binds vitamin E, and its function is currently unknown.

Infantile-Onset Spinocerebellar Ataxia (MIM 271245)

Infantile-onset spinocerebellar ataxia has been described in 19 patients from 13 Finnish families, and maps to chromosome 10q24 [Koskinen et al., 1994; Nikali et al., 1995; 1997]. It is thought that a single founder mutation occurred 30 to 40 generations ago in an ancestral Finnish kindred, with subsequent spread of the mutation throughout Finland. Affected children are healthy and develop normally until the onset of symptoms, usually between the ages of 1 and 2 years. Clumsiness, head tilt, athetosis of the arms and face, and loss of the ability to walk are the typical presenting symptoms, and they can begin in the setting of an acute infection. Ataxia, hypotonia, muscle atrophy, loss of deep tendon reflexes, and loss of proprioceptive sense are found on initial examination. Abnormal eye movements culminate in ophthalmoplegia by age 5. Mild-to-moderate sensorineural hearing loss starts at 2 to 5 years of age and progresses to a severe hearing deficit. Sensory axonal neuropathy, optic atrophy, decreased cognitive performance, and epilepsy occur by adolescence. Patients can present in status epilepticus that is refractory to medical management and can result in death. Female patients have primary hypogonadism, with amenorrhea and poor development of secondary sexual characteristics; sexual maturation appears to be normal in males [Koskinen et al., 1994; Koskinen et al., 1995a]. Although the early onset, progressive nature of the disease, and exacerbation with illness suggest a mitochondrial disorder, metabolic analyses, mtDNA testing, and muscle biopsy are normal in these patients. On neuroimaging, cerebellar atrophy is absent until about 5 years of age, and then progresses to olivopontocerebellar and spinocerebellar atrophy with time [Koskinen et al., 1995b]. Pathology studies reveal atrophy that is most pronounced in the posterior columns of the spinal cord and dorsal roots, with loss of myelinated fibers in the sural nerve; the cerebellar cortex and dentate nuclei, inferior olives, oculomotor nuclei, trochlear nuclei, abducens nuclei, and cochlear nerve and nuclei are all affected [Lonnqvist et al., 1998]. Based on these findings it is postulated that, as in Friedreich's ataxia, the sensory degeneration may be the primary process with secondary degeneration of the cerebellar system. The genetic defect is not known.

Ramsay Hunt Syndrome: Progressive Myoclonic Ataxia and Progressive Myoclonic Epilepsy (Baltic Myoclonus, Mediterranean Myoclonus, Unverricht-Lundborg Syndrome)

The Ramsay Hunt syndrome is a heterogeneous group of disorders whose clinical hallmarks are cerebellar ataxia and myoclonus [Hunt, 1922]. The presentation and severity can be quite variable, and the differential diagnosis includes myoclonic epilepsy with ragged red fibers, sialidosis, and progressive myoclonic epilepsy. These disorders are described in other chapters in this text.

Progressive myoclonic epilepsy (MIM 254800) was first described in families from Estonia and eastern Sweden, but is most common in Finland. The disease typically presents with generalized tonic-clonic seizures and myoclonus, with ataxia seen later in the course. Dodecamer repeats in the promoter region of the *cystatin B* gene are the most frequent cause [Lafreniere et al., 1997; Virtaneva et al., 1997].

Other Childhood-Onset Ataxias

Other early onset ataxias with associated deafness and varying degrees of mental retardation have been reported. In Behr's syndrome, mental retardation, ataxia, sensory neuropathy, spasticity, and optic atrophy are the predominant findings [Thomas et al., 1984]. Mental retardation, ataxia, cataracts, short stature, and limited sexual maturation characterize Marinesco-Sjögren syndrome.

Yet other conditions have been reported associated with atypical findings of dementia, muscular atrophy, ichthyosis, and familial spastic paralysis. Both autosomal-dominant and X-linked transmission have been described in these patients [Bell and Carmichael, 1939; Farlow et al., 1987; Spira et al., 1979].

Autosomal-Dominant Inherited Ataxias (Spinocerebellar Ataxias)

The dominantly inherited spinocerebellar ataxias (Table 57-3) are a group of conditions characterized by premature cerebellar neuronal loss, with some types involving other structures such as the optic nerve, basal ganglia, brainstem, and spinal cord. These heterogeneous disorders were often referred to in the past as the *olivopontocerebellar atrophies,* a descriptive pathology term used because of the frequent presence of atrophy involving the cerebellum, and pontine and olivary nuclei [Koeppen and Barron, 1984]. Parallel with the pathologic abnormalities, patients with spinocerebellar ataxia display various clinical features of progressive ataxia, motor impairment, extrapyramidal symptoms, retinal degeneration, deafness, ophthalmoplegia, dorsal column dysfunction, and peripheral neuropathy. The overall incidence of spinocerebellar ataxia is 1 to 5 per 100,000, with an average age of onset in the third decade of life.

Harding proposed a classification system for the autosomal-dominant cerebellar ataxias that uses the constellation of

TABLE 57-3

Autosomal Dominant Cerebellar Ataxias

ATAXIA	CHROMOSOME	GENE	GENE PRODUCT	MECHANISM	AGE OF ONSET (YEARS)	NORMAL REPEAT	EXPANDED REPEAT
Polyglutamine Expansion							
SCA1	6p23	*SCA1*	Ataxin-1	CAG repeat	6-60	6-44*	39-82*
SCA2	12q24	*SCA2*	Ataxin-2	CAG repeat	2-65	15-24	35-59
SCA3/MJD	14q24.3-q31	*MJD1*	Ataxin-3	CAG repeat	11-70	13-36	61-84
SCA6	19q13	*CACNA1A*	CACNA1A	CAG repeat	16-73	4-20	21-33
SCA7	3p21.1-p12	*SCA7*	Ataxin-7	CAG repeat	Birth-53	4-35	37-460
SCA17	6q27	*SCA17*	TBP	CAG repeat	3-48	25-42	45-66
DRPLA	12p13.31	*DRPLA*	Atrophin-1	CAG repeat	4 months-55	7-34	53-93
Noncoding Expansion							
SCA8	13q21	*SCA8*	SCA8 RNA	CTG repeat in 3′ UTR	18-72	2-91*	110-155*
SCA10	22q13	*SCA10*	Ataxin-10	ATTCT repeat in intron 9	14-45	10-22	750-4500
SCA12	5q31-q33	*SCA12*	PPP2R2B	CAG repeat in 5′ UTR	8-55	7-32	55-78
Missense Mutation							
SCA14	19q13.4	*PKC-γ*	PKC-γ	Missense mutation	10-69		
FGF14-SCA	13q34	*FGF14*	FGF14	Fibroblast growth factor deficiency	15-20		
Channelopathy							
EA1	12p13	*EA1*	KCNA1	Channelopathy	Early Childhood		
EA2/FHM	19p13	*CACNA1A*	CACNA1A	Channelopathy: missense and nonsense mutations	4-30		
Mutation Unknown							
SCA4	16q22	Unknown	Unknown	Unknown	19-59		
SCA5	11p11-q11	Unknown	Unknown	Unknown	10-68		
SCA11	15q14-q21.3	Unknown	Unknown	Unknown	15-43		
SCA13	19q13.3-q13.4	Unknown	Unknown	Unknown	<1-45		
SCA15	3p24.2-3pter	Unknown	Unknown	Unknown	Child–Adult		
SCA16	8q22.1-q24.1	Unknown	Unknown	Unknown	20-66		
SCA18/SMNA	7q31-q32	Unknown	Unknown	Unknown	12-25		
SCA19	1p21-q21	Unknown	Unknown	Unknown	10-45		
SCA20	11	Unknown	Unknown	Unknown	19-64		
SCA21	7p21.3-p15.1	Unknown	Unknown	Unknown	6-30		
SCA22	1p21-q23	Unknown	Unknown	Unknown	10-46		
SCA23	20p13-p12.2	Unknown	Unknown	Unknown	43-56		
SCA25	2p	Unknown	Unknown	Unknown	1.5-39		
EA3	Unknown	Unknown	Unknown	Unknown	23-42		
EA4	Unknown	Unknown	Unknown	Unknown	1-42		
SAX1	12p13	Unknown	Unknown	Unknown	Early childhood-early 20s		
SPAR	Unknown	Unknown	Unknown	Unknown	15-35		

*There is some ovelap of pathogenic and nonpathogenic repeat length. See text for details.

DRPLA, dentatorubral-pallidoluysian atrophy; EA, episodic ataxia; FHM, familial hemiplegic migraine; SAX, spastic ataxia; SCA, spinocerebellar ataxia; SMNA, sensorimotor neuropathy with ataxia; SPAR, spastic paraplegia, ataxia, and mental retardation; TBP, TATA-binding protein; UTR, untranslated region.

clinical symptoms for categorization [Harding, 1993]. Type I autosomal-dominant cerebellar ataxias have a cerebellar syndrome plus pyramidal signs, supranuclear ophthalmoplegia, extrapyramidal signs, and dementia. Type II autosomal-dominant cerebellar ataxias demonstrate a cerebellar syndrome plus pigmentary maculopathy. Type III autosomal-dominant cerebellar ataxias are "pure" cerebellar syndromes that have mild, if any, pyramidal symptoms. Some authors have attempted to keep these clinical categories and assign genetically defined spinocerebellar ataxias to them. Practically speaking, however, the age of onset and the clinical findings vary not only from family to family but within the same kindred as well [Berciano, 1982; Currier et al., 1972; Nino et al., 1980; Schut, 1954; Zoghbi et al., 1988].

Genetic studies over the past 20 years have been directed at mapping the gene loci for many of these disorders. These studies confirmed genetic heterogeneity in addition to the clinical heterogeneity, identifying 28 separate genetic loci. The next section describes the clinical features and molecular genetic profiles of the various spinocerebellar ataxias, including the periodic ataxias and dentatorubral-pallidoluysian atrophy.

Spinocerebellar Ataxia Type 1 (MIM 164400)

Spinocerebellar ataxia type 1 is characterized by progressive loss of balance and coordination, mild cognitive impairments, oculomotor deficits including gaze palsy and slowing of saccades, speaking and swallowing difficulties, and eventually respiratory failure. The primary sites of neurodegeneration in spinocerebellar ataxia type 1 include cerebellar Purkinje cells, brainstem cranial nerve nuclei, and the inferior olive and spinocerebellar tracts [Zoghbi and Orr, 2000]. The onset is typically in the third or fourth decade of life, but patients with onset as early as 4 years of age and as late as 60 years of age have been reported [Zoghbi and Orr, 2000]. The disorder has been described in many ethnic groups including whites, blacks, Asians, and Iakuts [Ranum et al., 1994a].

The spinocerebellar ataxia type 1 gene was mapped to chromosome 6p22-23 and the mutation identified using a positional cloning approach [Banfi et al., 1994; Orr et al., 1993]. A highly polymorphic CAG repeat was found to be unstable and expanded in all individuals with spinocerebellar ataxia type 1 [Orr et al., 1993]. The number of CAG repeats ranges from 6 to 44 on normal chromosomes and from 39 to 82 on spinocerebellar ataxia type 1 chromosomes [Servadio et al., 1995]. The repeat configuration on normal chromosomes is interrupted by 1 to 4 CAT trinucleotides in alleles with 20 or more repeats, whereas a perfect CAG repeat configuration is found on spinocerebellar ataxia type 1 chromosomes [Chung et al., 1993]. This finding led to the hypothesis that loss of the CAT interruption rendered the spinocerebellar ataxia type 1 CAG repeat unstable [Chong et al., 1995; Chung et al., 1993]. The presence of CAT interruptions in normal alleles containing 39 to 44 repeats is useful for distinguishing them from disease-associated alleles. There is a strong inverse correlation between repeat size and age of onset; individuals with 70 or more CAG repeats have childhood onset, a rapidly deteriorating course, and death within 4 to 5 years, whereas adult-onset cases have fewer than 70 repeats and typically live 10 to 20 years after symptoms appear [Zoghbi and Orr, 2000]. Genetic anticipation, or the tendency of affected individuals in successive generations of a kindred to have decreasing ages of disease onset, is a prominent feature of this and other polyglutamine repeat diseases. The mechanism involves progressive expansion of the polyglutamine repeats in disease alleles, particularly those that are paternally transmitted [Orr et al., 1993]

The spinocerebellar ataxia type 1 CAG repeat falls within the open reading frame of a transcript that is widely expressed and whose size is approximately 11.5 kb [Orr et al., 1993]. The CAG repeat codes for polyglutamine within ataxin-1, a protein predicted to contain 792 to 830 amino acids according to the size of the repeat [Banfi et al., 1994]. Ataxin-1 is predominantly nuclear in neurons and cytoplasmic in peripheral cells; shuttling between the two compartments may occur in neurons [Servadio et al., 1995]. A 120-residue region of the protein (573-694 in alleles containing 30 glutamines) shares significant sequence similarity with the HMG-box transcription factor HBP1 and has been implicated in protein-protein interactions and possibly in protein–ribonucleic acid interactions [Chen et al., 2004b].

The exact cellular functions of ataxin-1 are currently unknown, but data from animal models are providing some useful clues. Mice lacking ataxin-1 have spatial and motor learning deficiencies, as well as impairment of short-term plasticity [Matilla et al., 1998], but do not display ataxia or neuronal degeneration. These findings argue that spinocerebellar ataxia type 1 is not caused by loss of function of ataxin-1. Support for a gain-of-function pathogenic mechanism first came from mice overexpressing a mutant *SCA1* cDNA with 82 glutamines (82Q) specifically in Purkinje cells. These mice developed progressive ataxia and Purkinje cell degeneration [Burright et al., 1995]. The mutant ataxin-1 accumulates in nuclear inclusions [Skinner et al., 1997] along with components of the proteasome, suggesting that mutant ataxin-1 might misfold and resist degradation [Cummings et al., 1998]. Similarly, fruitflies that overexpress human ataxin-1 (82Q) also developed progressive neuronal degeneration and ataxin-1-containing nuclear inclusions that co-localized with chaperones and ubiquitin. To characterize the effects of the spinocerebellar ataxia type 1 mutation on all ataxin-1-expressing neurons, an expanded CAG tract of 154 repeats was targeted in place of the typical 2 CAGs present in the endogenous mouse locus. $Sca1^{154Q/+}$ mice reproduced all features of human spinocerebellar ataxia type 1 including ataxia, brainstem dysfunction, Purkinje cell degeneration, and premature death [Watase et al., 2002]. Consistent with the in vivo data, cellular and in vitro studies demonstrated that ataxin-1 is ubiquitinated, the expanded polyglutamine tract retards its degradation, and inhibition of the proteasome enhances its accumulation [Cummings et al., 1998; 1999]. Chaperone overexpression, which presumably aids in the folding or elimination of the expanded protein, resulted in improved motor coordination and suppressed Purkinje cell degeneration in *SCA1* (82Q) transgenic mice [Cummings et al., 2001]. The important roles of protein misfolding and degradation have also been demonstrated in several other polyglutamine diseases [Opal and Zoghbi, 2002; Paulson, 1999].

Ataxin-1 is phosphorylated at serine 776 (S776); when this serine is mutated to alanine (S776A), mutant ataxin-1 does not accumulate when overexpressed in cultured cells. Moreover, mice that express ataxin-1 (82Q) with an alanine at position 776 do not develop ataxia or pathology in spite of the long glutamine tract. These data show that (1) toxicity is mediated by the protein and not ribonucleic acid; (2) that the protein context is important given that a single amino acid change abrogated accumulation and toxicity; and (3) that a long polyglutamine tract can be efficiently handled by the cell's degradation machinery [Emamian et al., 2003]. Akt is the kinase that phosphorylates ataxin-1 at S776, allowing interactions between ataxin-1 and the 14-3-3 proteins. The binding of 14-3-3 to ataxin-1 enhances its levels both in cells and in vivo (*Drosophila* model) and hence provides an explanation for the importance of S776 in ataxin-1's pathogenicity. Genetic interaction studies in *Drosophila* indicated that overexpression of 14-3-3, phosphatidylinositol 3-kinase (PI3K, which activates Akt), and Akt enhanced neurodegeneration, whereas decreasing Akt levels by half suppressed ataxin-1–induced degeneration and decreased ataxin-1 levels [Chen et al., 2003b]. These studies identified a pathway that can be targeted pharmacologically (the PI3kinase/Akt pathway) to decrease mutant ataxin-1's toxicity. Preclinical studies using PI3K/Akt inhibitors are being conducted in spinocerebellar ataxia type 1 mouse models to evaluate their potential benefit for this disease.

Spinocerebellar Ataxia Type 2 (MIM 183090)

In 1989, Orozco and associates [1989] described a form of dominantly inherited spinocerebellar ataxia that occurs at an estimated frequency of 41 per 100,000 in the province of Holguine, Cuba. Age of onset varies from 2 to 65 years, with 40% of the patients presenting with symptoms before 25 years of age. Onset before the age of 20 years correlates with a more aggressive disease course. The clinical features include ataxia, dysarthria, tremor, and extremely slow saccades. Hyporeflexia of the upper limbs and ophthalmoparesis are seen in over half the patients. Dementia occurs in a significant minority of patients. The locus was termed *spinocerebellar ataxia type 2* and mapped to chromosome 12q24 [Gispert et al., 1993]. Families with this disorder have been described from other regions of the world outside of Cuba as well [Lopes-Cendes et al., 1994].

Pathology specimens demonstrate severe loss of Purkinje cells and of neurons in the substantia nigra and basis pontis. Mild-to-moderate neuronal loss is seen in the inferior and accessory olives; dentate, arcuate, gracile, and accessory cuneate nuclei; internal granule cell layer of the cerebellum; and in the anterior horns of the spinal cord. Axonal loss from the dorsal roots and posterior columns, the dorsal spinocerebellar tract, and often from the anterior spinal roots is also found. Reactive gliosis can be seen in the globus pallidus, thalamus, subthalamus, and periaqueductal regions [Durr et al., 1995; Hunyh et al., 1999; Koeppen, 1998].

By using three different approaches the spinocerebellar ataxia type 2 gene was identified, and the mutation was determined to involve an expansion of a CAG trinucleotide repeat that lies within the coding region of a novel protein termed ataxin-2 [Imbert et al., 1996; Pulst et al., 1996; Sanpei et al., 1996]. Normal *ataxin-2* alleles contain 15-24 CAG repeats (with 22 repeats found 94% of the time), whereas disease alleles have 35 to 59 repeats. The range of pathogenic alleles in spinocerebellar ataxia type 1 is shifted toward shorter repeats compared with other spinocerebellar ataxias, suggesting that the expanded repeat within ataxin-2 is more deleterious to neurons. The CAG repeat in the spinocerebellar ataxia type 2 gene is interrupted by one to three CAA units only on normal alleles, suggesting that, as in spinocerebellar ataxia type 1, interruption of CAG repeats may confer stability. Finally, there is a strong inverse correlation between the size of the repeat and the age of onset of symptoms.

The spinocerebellar ataxia type 2 gene, *ataxin-2*, contains 25 exons and spans approximately 130 kb of genomic DNA. Two alternately spliced forms of messenger ribonucleic acids are generated, one of which results in a protein that is truncated by 70 amino acids [Sahba et al., 1998]. *Ataxin-2* messenger ribonucleic acid is found in multiple tissues and in all regions of the CNS [Imbert et al., 1996; Pulst et al., 1996; Sanpei et al., 1996], where it is present predominantly in neurons and is highly expressed in Purkinje cells [Hunyh et al., 1999]. Ataxin-2 is a cytoplasmic protein and is subcellularly localized to the Golgi apparatus [Shibata et al., 2000]. Although a definitive function of ataxin-2 has not been established, several lines of evidence suggest that the protein may function in messenger ribonucleic acid processing, stability, and transport. First, ataxin-2 contains two domains that have been implicated in ribonucleic acid splicing. Second, a ribonucleic acid–binding protein (ataxin-2 binding protein 1) with a similar expression pattern has been found to interact with ataxin-2 [Shibata et al., 2000]. Third, related proteins from other species are involved in ribonucleic aicd processing. The morphologic changes seen in diseased Purkinje cells may result from abnormal cytoskeletal architecture, as suggested by two further studies. Purkinje cells in transgenic mice that express mutant ataxin-2 lose their dendritic arbors before cell body degeneration [Huynh et al., 2000], and a *Drosophila* homolog of ataxin-2 (Datx2) is involved in microtubule assembly through an indirect mechanism [Satterfield et al., 2002]. Whether these effects are mediated through ribonucleic acid interactions is unknown.

Machado-Joseph Disease and Spinocerebellar Ataxia Type 3 (MIM 109150)

More than 100 families with Machado-Joseph disease have been evaluated [Coutinho and Andrade, 1978; Fowler, 1984; Rosenberg et al., 1976]. First described in families of Azorean-Portuguese origin, Machado-Joseph disease or spinocerebellar ataxia type 3 has subsequently been described in families from around the world [Bharucha et al., 1986; Sasaki et al., 1992a; 1992b]. The vast majority of cases are linked to a single haplotype that probably originated in mainland Portugal, with subsequent spread to the Azores and beyond [Gaspar et al., 2001].

The clinical features of Machado-Joseph disease include progressive ataxia, areflexia, peripheral amyotrophy, external ophthalmoplegia, bulging eyes, facial and lingual fasciculations, muscle atrophy, parkinsonian features, dystonia, and spasticity. Based on the constellation of clinical findings and the age of onset of symptoms, attempts have been made to categorize this disorder into different clinical subtypes [Barbeau et al., 1984; Coutinho and Andrade, 1978; Rosenberg et al., 1976]. However, this approach has not proven diagnostically useful because different subtypes occur in the same kindred, and affected individuals often evolve from one subtype to another.

The Machado-Joseph disease gene was mapped to the long arm of chromosome 14 (14q24.3-q32) [Takiyama et al., 1993]. Subsequently, Stevanin and colleagues [1994] mapped the gene in a family with a dominantly inherited spinocerebellar ataxia to chromosome 14q24.3-qter. They designated the new locus as spinocerebellar ataxia type 3 because the familial phenotype was clinically distinct from Machado-Joseph disease and more closely resembled that of spinocerebellar ataxia type 1. Further studies have demonstrated that both spinocerebellar ataxia type 3 and Machado-Joseph disease result from a CAG repeat expansion in the *MJD1* gene and emphasize the marked clinical heterogeneity associated with this mutation [Cancel et al., 1995; Kawaguchi et al., 1994; Maciel et al., 1995; Maruyama et al., 1995; Matilla et al., 1995; Ranum et al., 1995]. Normal *MJD1* alleles contain 13-36 CAG repeats, and expanded alleles contain 61 to 84 repeats.

Ataxin-3 is the smallest of the polyglutamine proteins. Its normal function is unknown, and the pathogenesis of Machado-Joseph disease or spinocerebellar ataxia type 3 is poorly understood. The introduction of ataxin-3 with an expanded polyglutamine tract into cultured cells induces apoptosis, suggesting that the mutant protein is either directly or indirectly involved with a cellular suicide pathway [Ikeda et al., 1996]. Other studies suggest that protein misfolding, presumably initiated by the expanded polyglutamine tract, leads to ubiquitination and subsequent formation of intranuclear inclusions [Chai et al., 1999]. This is a common pathway in polyglutamine expansion diseases. How this leads to cell dysfunction and death and why the clinical time course takes so long to evolve remain unknown.

Spinocerebellar Ataxia Type 4 (MIM 600223)

Seven kindreds (one from Utah and six from Japan) have been described thus far [Gardner et al., 1994; Nagaoka et al., 2000]. Clinically, affected individuals in the Japanese families have a pure cerebellar ataxia, whereas those in the Utah kindred also have dysarthria and sensory axonal neuropathy [Flanigan et al., 1996]. Detailed genetic mapping studies show that the gene involved in spinocerebellar ataxia type 4 maps to the long arm of human chromosome 16. Anticipation does not occur.

Spinocerebellar Ataxia Type 5 (MIM 600224)

The locus for spinocerebellar ataxia type 5 was localized to the centromeric region of human chromosome 11 based on detailed mapping studies on two major branches of a family descended from the paternal grandparents of President Abraham Lincoln [Ranum et al., 1994b]. The phenotype is that of pure cerebellar ataxia and dysarthria. The disease is milder than that observed in other spinocerebellar ataxias, without substantial effects on life span.

Spinocerebellar Ataxia Type 6 (MIM 183086)

Spinocerebellar ataxia type 6 accounts for 1% to 13% of families with autosomal-dominant cerebellar ataxia from European centers, 6% to 31% from Japanese centers, and zero to 11% in Chinese series [Mantuano et al., 2003; Schöls et al., 1998;]. The mutation is occasionally found in sporadic cases as well.

The clinical features consist predominantly of mild but slowly progressive cerebellar ataxia of the limbs, gait ataxia, dysarthria, nystagmus, and mild vibratory and proprioceptive sensory loss. Cognitive function is not affected. Patients often have acute episodes of ataxia or vertigo that are responsive to acetazolamide. Onset is later than the other dominantly inherited spinocerebellar ataxias, typically occurring in the third decade at the earliest. Brain imaging reveals atrophy of the cerebellum.

Pathology specimens demonstrate loss of Purkinje and granule cells, with proliferation of Bergmann glia, which is more prominent in the vermis than in the hemispheres [Gomez et al., 1997; Takahashi et al., 2004; Tsuchiya et al., 1998]. Loss of inferior olive neurons also occurs, but may be secondary to the cerebellar changes.

The genetic locus was mapped to chromosome 19q13, where a CAG repeat expansion in exon 47 at the 3′ region of the *CACNA1A* gene was identified as the causative mutation [Zhuchenko et al., 1997]. *CACNA1A* codes for the brain-specific, voltage-sensitive α_{1A} ($Ca_v2.1$) subunit of the P/Q-type calcium channel, which is highly expressed in Purkinje cells [Ishikawa et al., 1999]. Alternative splicing leads to six isoforms, three of which contain the polyglutamine sequence. Repeat expansions are the smallest of the triplet repeat diseases, with 21 or more repeats being pathogenic. Individuals who are homozygous for expanded repeats have no phenotypic or age of onset differences [Takiyama et al., 1998]. Phenotypic severity is inversely correlated with the number of CAG repeats, as is the age of onset [Takahashi et al., 2004]. Clinical anticipation has been observed, but does not always appear to stem from CAG repeat instability. No CAA interruptions are present in the repeats.

Proteins with the expanded repeat aggregate specifically in the cytoplasm of Purkinje cells [Ishikawa et al., 1999]. These inclusions are not ubiquitinated and lack several other components found in the inclusions of other CAG repeat disorders. It is not clear whether spinocerebellar ataxia type 6 is caused by a "gain-of-function" mechanism similar to that in other polyglutamine diseases or a channelopathy that alters calcium homeostasis. As will be discussed later (see "Episodic Ataxias"), point mutations and deletions in the *CACNA1A* coding sequence cause episodic ataxia type 2 and familial hemiplegic migraine type 1. Families with significant phenotypic overlap have been identified, leading some to postulate that the three disorders represent a spectrum of disease rather than truly separate entities. The identification of small triplet expansions (20 and 23 repeats) in two kindreds whose members presented with EA2, and the identification of a point mutation leading to early hemiplegic migraine and later progressive ataxia, is supportive of this interpretation [Alonso et al., 2003; Jodice et al., 1997].

Spinocerebellar Ataxia Type 7 (MIM 164500)

Spinocerebellar ataxia type 7 is distinguished clinically from the other spinocerebellar ataxias by the presence of macular dystrophy leading to pigmentary retinal degeneration [Bjork et al., 1956; Colan et al., 1981; Enevoldson et al., 1994; Gouw et al., 1994; Havener, 1951; Jampel et al., 1961]. The retinal changes in spinocerebellar ataxia type 7 start in a central location and move peripherally as the disease progresses, thus distinguishing the eye findings from those in retinitis pigmentosa. Progressive ataxia or dysmetria, pyramidal tract signs, supranuclear ophthalmoplegia, and dysarthria or dysphagia are also present, and occasionally dementia and deafness are seen as well [Benton et al., 1998]. Either ataxia or visual changes can be the presenting symptom, depending on the number of CAG repeats in the expanded allele (see later). Brain imaging in all cases typically demonstrates cerebellar atrophy; ventricular dilation and delayed myelination can be found in infantile cases. Brain pathologic specimens reveal atrophy of the cerebellum with loss of dentate neurons and Purkinje cells and loss of inferior olivary neurons in the brainstem; posterior column, dorsal and ventral spinocerebellar tract loss in the spinal cord; and macular degeneration with loss of photoreceptive cells in the retina.

An extremely aggressive infantile-onset form of spinocerebellar ataxia type 7 that occurs only on paternal transmission has been described [Benton et al., 1998; Enevoldson et al., 1994]. It presents with hypotonia, dysphagia, myoclonic seizures, and visual disturbances that typically lead to rapid mental deterioration and severe physical disability culminating in death by age 3 or earlier. The infantile-onset form is also associated with cardiac abnormalities, particularly patent ductus arteriosus [Benton et al., 1998; Johansson et al., 1998; van de Warrenburg et al., 2001]. Childhood-onset spinocerebellar ataxia type 7 is less aggressive than the infantile-onset form but more progressive than the adult-onset form.

Spinocerebellar ataxia type 7 maps to the short arm of chromosome 3 [Benomar et al., 1995; Gouw et al., 1995; Holmberg et al., 1998]. By using an antibody that selectively detects proteins containing an expanded polyglutamine tract, it was demonstrated that the mutational mechanism in spinocerebellar ataxia type 7 is expansion of a CAG repeat [Trottier et al., 1995]. *SCA7* encodes a novel protein, ataxin-7, with a polyglutamine tract at the amino terminus [David et al., 1997]. The *SCA7* CAG repeat ranges in size from 4 to 35 repeats in normal alleles, and from 37 to 306 repeats in expanded alleles. Typically, larger expansions are paternally inherited and result from significant intergenerational repeat instability. An inverse correlation exists between repeat length and age of onset, and repeat expansions larger than 59 repeats tend to develop visual impairment prior to ataxia [Johansson et al., 1998]. Alleles ranging in size from 34 to 36 repeats have been observed in individuals who are at risk but asymptomatic at the time of evaluation [Benton et al., 1998; David et al., 1997, 1998; Del-Favero et al., 1998; Gouw et al., 1998; Holmberg et al., 1998; Johansson et al., 1998; Moseley et al., 1998].

Mouse models of spinocerebellar ataxia type 7 have provided some insight into the pathogenesis of the disease. Expression of the expanded ataxin-7 protein in transgenic mice leads to the development of intranuclear inclusions and the degeneration of rod photoreceptors and Purkinje cells, findings consistent with the human phenotype [Yvert et al., 2000]. In retinal photoreceptor cells, the expression of expanded ataxin-7 is associated with alterations in gene expression that predate photoreceptor degeneration [La Spada et al., 2001; Yoo et al., 2003]. Another interesting finding is that the speed of ataxin-7 accumulation varies in different neuronal populations, suggesting that intrinsic differences in the ability to clear mutant protein may explain the variable susceptibility of different cell types in this and other polyglutamine diseases. Finally, cellular dysfunction predates the appearance of neuronal inclusions, suggesting that although they are part of the pathogenesis, inclusions in and of themselves are not the primary cause of dysfunction [Yoo et al., 2003].

Spinocerebellar Ataxia Type 8 (MIM 608768)

Described predominantly in white families from the United States and Canada, the clinical presentation of spinocerebellar ataxia type 8 is similar to that of the other slowly progressive spinocerebellar ataxias. Ataxic dysarthria, nystagmus, limb and gait ataxia, limb spasticity, and diminished vibratory sense are present [Koob et al., 1999]. MRI of the brain demonstrates cerebellar atrophy. Spinocerebellar ataxia type 8 was mapped to chromosome 13q21, and the vast majority of disease alleles in individuals of European descent share a common haplotype [Ikeda et al., 2004].

Unlike other repeat disorders (with the exception of myotonic dystrophy) that are caused by polyglutamine expansions, spinocerebellar ataxia type 8 is caused by a CTG repeat in a noncoding gene; that is, no open reading frame is present in the gene, suggesting that it is transcribed into messenger ribonucleic acid but not translated into protein [Koob et al., 1999]. This is only one of several unusual characteristics of spinocerebellar ataxia type 8. There is high variability in the repeat length of the wild-type allele, with some unaffected individuals having repeat lengths as high as 174, by far the largest number of wild-type repeats of any spinocerebellar ataxia. The substantial overlap of repeat size in pathogenic and nonpathogenic alleles is also unique among the spinocerebellar ataxias. Furthermore, homozygosity for an expanded allele does not appear to exacerbate the disease phenotype as it does in spinocerebellar ataxia type 1 and dentatorubral-pallidoluysian atrophy. Repeat lengths contract with paternal transmission and expand with maternal transmission, another unusual finding of this disease. Although a relationship between repeat size and clinical effects was demonstrated in the initial report, other families with this disorder have greater variability in penetrance [Ikeda et al., 2004]. Further confusing the picture is the coexistence of spinocerebellar ataxia type 8 expansions with those of spinocerebellar ataxia type 1 or spinocerebellar ataxia type 6 in some kindreds [Izumi et al., 2003; Sulek et al., 2003]. Spinocerebellar ataxia type 8 expansions have also been found in patients with Alzheimer's disease, Parkinson's disease, and an individual with vitamin E deficiency heterozygous for the TTPA mutation [Cellini et al., 2002; Izumi et al., 2003; Sobrido et al., 2001]. How these factors influence the pathogenesis of the disease is unknown and has led some authors to question the pathogenesis of the expansion itself [Schols et al., 2003; Stevanin et al., 2000; Worth et al., 2000].

The genomic arrangement of the spinocerebellar ataxia type 8 locus suggests a potential function of the gene. The *SCA8* gene lies in a reverse orientation to and partially overlaps the locus of another gene (*KLHL1*). It has been suggested that the *SCA8* messenger ribonucleic acid functions as an endogenous inhibitory RNA for *KLHL1*, or as a regulator of ribonucleic acid–binding proteins [Mutsuddi et al., 2004], although further evidence of these functions is needed.

Spinocerebellar Ataxia Type 10 (MIM 603516)

Grewal and associates [1998] described a dominantly inherited spinocerebellar ataxia in a single four-generation Mexican kindred. The locus was independently mapped to chromosome 22q13 by two different groups [Matsuura et al., 1999; Zu et al., 1999]. Spinocerebellar ataxia type 10 is the second most common form of dominantly inherited ataxia (spinocerebellar ataxia type 2 is the most common) in people of Mexican descent; this fact, coupled with the rarity of expanded alleles in other populations, has led to the hypothesis that the mutation arose in the New World [Matsuura et al., 2002]. The phenotype consists of ataxia, dysarthria, nystagmus, and epilepsy. Mood disorders and polyneuropathy diagnosed by nerve conduction studies can also be seen. A pentanucleotide (ATTCT) repeat in intron 9 of the *ataxin-10* gene is responsible for the phenotype; instability of the repeat region can lead to as many as 4500 repeats [Matsuura et al., 2000]. There is an inverse correlation between expansion size and the age of onset, and genetic anticipation is present. The repeats are highly unstable when transmitted paternally, whereas maternal transmission results in more stable repeats. Brain imaging reveals cerebellar atrophy.

Ataxin-10 is a protein that is widely expressed throughout the brain and in several other tissues [Marz et al., 2004]. It is localized to the cytosol and perinuclear region in neurons. Whether the disease phenotype stems from genomic disruption, ribonucleic acid gain-of-function, or ataxin-10 loss of function is unknown, although decreased ataxin-10 ribonucleic acid levels in primary cerebellar and cortical neuronal culture result in increased apoptosis, suggesting that loss of function may be the pathogenetic mechanism [Marz et al., 2004].

Spinocerebellar Ataxia Type 11 (MIM 604432)

Worth and colleagues [1999] described a single family with a benign, slowly progressive, pure cerebellar syndrome linked to chromosome 15. Mean age of onset was about 25 years; genetic anticipation did not appear to be present. The gene has yet to be identified.

Spinocerebellar Ataxia Type 12 (MIM 604326)

Identified in a family of German descent [Holmes et al., 1999], spinocerebellar ataxia type 12 is unique in that action tremor is the most distinguishing clinical feature and is typically the initial symptom. Slow progression over several decades leads to head tremor, gait ataxia, dysmetria, dysarthria, hyperreflexia, parkinsonian signs, abnormal eye movements, and occasionally dementia. Two patients in the initial kindred were reported with childhood-onset symptoms: one had nystagmus from birth; the other had lower extremity dystonia that developed in childhood [O'Hearn et al., 2001]. Brain imaging reveals both cortical and cerebellar atrophy. Pathology is available only on a single brain, and revealed diffuse atrophy of cerebral and cerebellar cortices and specifically loss of Purkinje cells. Spinocerebellar ataxia type 12 is rare except in India, where it is the third most common spinocerebellar ataxia [Holmes et al., 2003; Srivastava et al., 2001].

Genetic analysis revealed a triplet CAG expansion on chromosome 5q31-q33. No apparent relationship exists between repeat size and age of onset. Unlike other spinocerebellar ataxias with CAG expansions, the expanded allele does not lead to a polyglutamine tract. Rather, the CAG expansion is found 133 nucleotides upstream of the transcription start site for PPP2R2B, a brain-specific regulatory subunit of protein phosphatase 2A. The B subunits are thought to modulate PP2A function by regulating substrate specificity and intracellular targeting [Holmes et al., 2003]. How this expansion affects PPP2R2B function is unknown.

Spinocerebellar Ataxia Type 13 (MIM 605259)

A dominantly inherited disorder of slowly progressive childhood-onset cerebellar gait ataxia associated with cerebellar dysarthria, moderate mental retardation (IQ = 62 to 76), and mild developmental delays in motor skills acquisition has been described in a single French kindred [Herman-Bert et al., 2000]. Nystagmus and pyramidal signs were also observed in some affected individuals. Cerebral magnetic resonance imaging in two patients revealed moderate cerebellar and pontine atrophy. No evidence of genetic anticipation was found.

Spinocerebellar Ataxia Type 14 (MIM 605361)

Three families (one Japanese, one Dutch, and one English/Dutch) have been described, all with a locus mapping to 19q13.4 telomeric to the locus for spinocerebellar ataxia type 13 [Brkanac et al., 2002a; van de Warrenburg et al., 2003; Yamashita et al., 2000]. The phenotype varies from family to family and within families as well. In the Japanese kindred, subjects with onset of symptoms before 27 years of age presented with axial myoclonus before development of ataxia, whereas those with onset after age 39 presented with a pure cerebellar ataxia. Gait ataxia, dysarthria, horizontal gaze nystagmus, abnormal smooth pursuit movements, hyper- and hyporeflexia, and peripheral neuropathy were described in all of the families [Brkanac et al., 2002a; van de Warrenburg et al., 2003; Yamashita et al., 2000]. Imaging reveals atrophy of the cerebellar vermis and hemispheres. Life span does not appear to be affected in any of the kindreds, and ataxia displays a slowly progressive course. Genetic anticipation occurs. Limited pathologic specimens suggest a primary Purkinje cell defect [Brkanac et al., 2002a]. Molecular studies reveal that missense point mutations in exon 4 of the protein kinase C gamma gene are responsible, although the mechanism of pathogenesis remains unknown [Chen et al., 2003a; van de Warrenburg et al., 2003; Yabe et al., 2003].

Spinocerebellar Ataxia Type 15 (MIM 606658)

Spinocerebellar ataxia type 15 was described in a single Australian family with Anglo-Celtic ancestry, whose affected members had a slowly progressive ataxia with associated nystagmus and dysarthria [Storey et al., 2001]. Age of onset was not reported, although it was commented that childhood and adolescence fell in the spectrum. Neuroimaging demonstrated cerebellar vermal atrophy. A candidate gene approach has thus far failed to identify the target gene.

Spinocerebellar Ataxia Type 16 (MIM 606364)

Miyoshi and co-workers [2001] reported a single Japanese family with adult-onset gait ataxia, dysarthria, nystagmus, impaired smooth pursuit movements, and head tremor. Linkage to chromosome 8q22.1-q24.1 was established. Imaging demonstrated cerebellar vermal atrophy. Anticipation was not present.

Spinocerebellar Ataxia Type 17 (MIM 607136)

This spinocerebellar ataxia may variably present with predominant symptoms of cerebellar ataxia associated with dysarthria and extrapyramidal symptoms (e.g., parkinsonism and dystonia), with mental deterioration or dementia and psychiatric symptoms such as depression and hallucinations, or as a Huntington's disease phenocopy with chorea as a major manifestation [Bauer et al., 2004; Koide et al., 1999; Maltecca et al., 2003; Nakamura et al., 2001; Rolfs et al., 2003; Stevanin et al., 2003; Toyoshima et al., 2004]. Different individuals in the same family may have dramatically different presenting phenotypes and, as the disease progresses, symptoms from each of the subtypes can occur in the same individual. Neuroimaging demonstrates diffuse cortical and cerebellar atrophy that is most pronounced in the vermis. Pathologic specimens reveal neuronal loss in many brain areas, including loss of Purkinje cells [Nakamura et al., 2001; Rolfs et al., 2003].

Spinocerebellar ataxia type 17 is caused by CAG repeat expansions in the TATA-binding protein *(TBP)* gene on chromosome 6q27 [Nakamura et al., 2001]. Like other spinocerebellar ataxias, short CAA tracts interrupt the CAG repeats; however, both the CAG and CAA tracts are replicated in the expansions, distinguishing this spinocerebellar ataxia from the others. Marked anticipation was observed in an Italian kindred, with the youngest family member in the fourth generation presenting with dysarthria and ataxia at age 3 [Maltecca et al., 2003]. Repeat sizes of 42 to 48 repeats have variable penetrance. Like other expansion diseases, an inverse correlation exists between repeat size and age of onset.

TBP is the DNA-binding subunit of ribonucleic acid polymerase II transcription factor D complex, which is important in general gene transcription [Tsuji, 2004]. Immunostaining for ubiquitin, TBP, and polyglutamine tracts demonstrates their presence in intranuclear inclusions in several neuronal cell types, including Purkinje cells [Nakamura et al., 2001; Rolfs et al., 2003].

Spinocerebellar Ataxia Type 18 (Sensorimotor Neuropathy with Ataxia; MIM 607458)

Spinocerebellar ataxia type 18, or sensorimotor neuropathy with ataxia, was described in a five-generation American family of Irish descent [Brkanac et al., 2002b]. Clinically, affected individuals present first with gait instability in the dark, followed by limb ataxia, nystagmus, decreased vibratory and position sense, decreased deep tendon reflexes, and proximal or distal muscle weakness and atrophy. Upgoing plantar responses and pes cavus are occasionally seen. Neuroimaging is either normal or demonstrates mild cerebellar atrophy. Electromyography/nerve conduction velocities show evidence of denervation and axonal sensory neuropathy. Thus, the overall picture is one of a mixed cerebellar degeneration and peripheral neuropathy. The disorder was mapped to chromosome 7q31-32; the causative gene has yet to be identified.

Spinocerebellar Ataxia Type 19 (MIM 607346)

A single Dutch family with ataxia, cognitive impairment, irregular postural tremor, myoclonus, and poor performance on the Wisconsin Card Sorting Test has been described [Schelhaas et al., 2001; Verbeek et al., 2002]. Imaging reveals atrophy of the cerebellar hemispheres or vermis. The genetic locus maps to chromosome 1p21-q21, where it overlaps with the locus for spinocerebellar ataxia type 22 (see later).

Spinocerebellar Ataxia Type 20 (MIM 608687)

A dominantly inherited cerebellar ataxia associated with palatal tremor and a characteristic dysphonia has been described in a single Anglo-Celtic kindred [Knight et al., 2004]. Imaging demonstrates mild-to-moderate cerebellar atrophy and the unique finding of dentate calcification in the absence of basal ganglia calcification. The genetic locus overlaps that of spinocerebellar ataxia type 5, so the separate identity of this spinocerebellar ataxia remains to be established.

Spinocerebellar Ataxia Type 21 (MIM 607454)

Spinocerebellar ataxia type 21 was described in a single French kindred with gait ataxia; extrapyramidal signs such as tremor, akinesia, and cogwheeling; and mental impairment mapping to chromosome 7p21.3-p15.1 [Devos et al., 2001; Vuillaume et al., 2002]. Eye movements are normal, and disease progression is slow. Anticipation is suggested. Brain imaging reveals marked atrophy of the cerebellum. The responsible gene has not yet been identified.

Spinocerebellar Ataxia Type 22

Chung and associates [2003] reported a pure cerebellar ataxia syndrome consisting of gait and limb ataxia, dysarthria, and nystagmus in a single Chinese kindred mapping to chromosome 1p21-q23 [Chung et al., 2003]. Neuroimaging found diffuse involvement of the cerebellum. Anticipation is suggested. Based on their chromosomal loci, it has been suggested that spinocerebellar ataxia type 19 and spinocerebellar ataxia type 22 might be the same disorder [Schelhaas et al., 2004]; identification of the responsible gene(s) should answer this question.

Spinocerebellar Ataxia Type 23

A single, three-generation Dutch family with a late onset (>40 years), slowly progressive spinocerebellar ataxia was identified with locus linkage at 20p13-p12.2 [Verbeek et al., 2004]. The clinical presentation includes gait and limb ataxia, disturbance of oculomotor control, dysarthria, and hyperreflexia. Neuroimaging demonstrates severe cerebellar atrophy. Pathology in a single individual who died at 80 years of age exhibited loss of Purkinje cells and of neurons in the dentate nuclei and inferior olives; thinning of the cerebellopontine tracts; demyelination of the posterior and lateral columns in the spinal cord; and ubiquitin-positive, polyglutamine-negative intranuclear inclusions in nigral neurons that resembled Marinesco bodies. The pathogenic significance of this last finding is uncertain. A candidate gene approach has thus far failed to identify the responsible gene.

Spinocerebellar Ataxia Type 25 (MIM 608703)

Stevanin and colleagues [2004] reported a single French kindred with cerebellar ataxia and peripheral sensory neuropathy manifest as loss of vibratory, light, touch, and pain sensation. Initial symptoms often include vomiting and gastrointestinal features. No evidence of anticipation was found. Brain imaging demonstrates global cerebellar atrophy. A candidate gene search failed to identify the affected gene.

Fibroblast Growth Factor 14—Spinocerebellar Ataxia (MIM 601515)

A single Dutch kindred was described with a spinocerebellar ataxia that begins with trembling of the hands during childhood [van Swieten et al., 2003]. Limb ataxia develops between the ages of 15 and 20 years. Ataxia, dysmetric saccades and smooth pursuit movements, nystagmus, small-amplitude hand tremor, psychiatric symptoms, and decreased cognitive performance are part of this slowly progressive disease. Brain imaging is normal or reveals cerebellar atrophy.

The same investigators demonstrated that a single nucleotide change in exon 4 of the FGF14 gene, resulting in a phenylalanine to serine substitution and a predicted destabilization of the protein structure, is the responsible mutation. Although the effects of this mutation have not been examined in an animal model, mice lacking FGF14 are ataxic and have a paroxysmal dystonia [Wang et al., 2002]. The authors also demonstrated that FGF14 is transported into neuronal processes, suggesting that disruption of this process may lead to the clinical phenotype.

Episodic Ataxia

There are four episodic ataxias, all of which are rare dominant disorders characterized by intermittent ataxia. Episodic ataxias type 1 and type 2 are caused by channelopathies; the pathogenesis of episodic ataxia type 3 and episodic ataxia type 4 is unknown, but channelopathies are also suspected in the latter two diseases. Acetazolamide is useful for treating three of the four disorders [Griggs et al., 1978].

Episodic ataxia type 1 (MIM 160120), also known as *episodic ataxia with myokymia*, is characterized by intermittent episodes of ataxia that may occur spontaneously but are often precipitated by exercise, fever, stress, or even sudden movement. The attacks may last seconds to minutes and may occur several times per day. *Myokymia*, a rippling movement of muscle, is usually observed in the periorbital and small hand muscles and persists between ataxic attacks. Episodic ataxia type 1 maps to human chromosome 12p13, and the disease is caused by point mutations in the potassium channel gene *KCNA1* (Kv1.1) [Browne et al., 1994; 1995; Comu et al., 1996]. All affected individuals are heterozygous.

Episodic ataxia type 2 (MIM 108500), also known as *hereditary paroxysmal cerebellar ataxia*, is characterized by intermittent attacks of ataxia and dysarthria lasting from a few minutes to a few days. Nausea, migraine, weakness, vertigo, diplopia, oscillopsia, or dystonia may accompany an attack. Attacks are often followed by a period of fatigue. Interictal neurologic findings include nystagmus (either gaze evoked or downbeat), mild cerebellar ataxia, and occasionally epilepsy. A progressive cerebellar ataxia is seen in some kindreds. The ataxia and number of attacks typically decrease with acetazolamide treatment; 4-aminopyridine may be a useful alternative if acetazolamide fails or loses effectiveness [Strupp et al., 2004]. The gene locus for this disease was mapped to the short arm of chromosome 19 in a position that overlaps the locus for familial hemiplegic migraine [Joutel et al, 1993; Vahedi et al., 1995; von Brederlow et al., 1995]. Ophoff and associates [1996] subsequently demonstrated that both episodic ataxia type 2 and FHM are caused by mutations in the *CACNA1A* gene. Thus, episodic ataxia type 2, familial hemiplegic migraine, and spinocerebellar ataxia type 6 are allelic disorders. *CACNA1A* codes for the brain-specific, voltage-sensitive α_{1A} ($Ca_v2.1$) subunit of the P/Q-type calcium channel, which is highly expressed in Purkinje cells [Ishikawa et al., 1999]. Several different missense and nonsense mutations in the gene are associated with episodic ataxia type 2 [Jen et al., 2004]. Although there initially appeared to be a clear genotype-phenotype relationship, further studies have demonstrated that the nature of the mutation in the gene is not predictive of whether an individual will clinically present with episodic ataxia type 2 or familial hemiplegic migraine.

Episodic ataxia type 3, or periodic vestibulocerebellar ataxia (MIM 606552), has been described in two white families from North Carolina [Farmer and Mustian, 1963; Vance et al., 1984]. Clinically, the disorder consists of episodic attacks of vertigo, nausea, tinnitus, horizontal nystagmus, oscillopsia, and ataxia that begin in the third decade and may evolve into a constant condition. The visual sensation of objects moving past the patient, such as occurs while riding in a car, can exacerbate attacks, but lying quietly for 15 to 30 minutes can alleviate an attack. Acetazolamide is not therapeutic, although antihistamines have been anecdotally reported to decrease the frequency and severity of attacks in at least some individuals [Farmer and Mustian, 1963]. Neuroimaging and pathology studies have not been done. Several spinocerebellar ataxias, as well as episodic ataxias type 1 and type 2, have been eliminated as causative [Damji et al., 1996]. The gene locus is not known.

Episodic ataxia type 4 (MIM 606554) was described in a large Canadian kindred [Steckley et al., 2001]. Clinical attacks consist of vertigo, incoordination, imbalance, tinnitus, diplopia, or visual blurring lasting for 1 minute to 6 hours. Interictal myokymia or ataxia is also present. Attacks often occur once or twice per day, followed by a refractory period. Generalized seizures occur in some members of the kindred, suggesting that a channelopathy might be reponsible. Acetazolamide was useful for reducing the frequency of attacks in one patient. Episodic ataxias type 1 and type 2 loci were excluded by mapping studies.

Dentatorubral-Pallidoluysian Atrophy (MIM 125370)

Dentatorubral-pallidoluysian atrophy is a rare autosomal-dominant, neurodegenerative disorder characterized by progressive ataxia, myoclonus, epilepsy, chorea, athetosis, and dementia [Smith, 1975; Smith et al., 1958]. The hereditary nature of the disease was confirmed through detailed clinical, genetic, and neuropathologic studies of five Japanese families with familial myoclonic epilepsy and choreoathetosis [Naito and Oyanagi, 1982]. Clinically, age of onset is linked to disease phenotype. Early onset cases (<20 years of age) tend to present with a progressive myoclonic epilepsy syndrome consisting of epilepsy, myoclonus, cerebellar ataxia, and mental retardation, whereas adult onset cases (>20 years of age) tend to present with cerebellar ataxia, choreoathetosis, or dementia. The phenotypic diversity within and among families is striking, as is the overlap with the clinical presentation of Huntington's chorea. Imaging studies demonstrate cerebellar, tegmental, and cerebral atrophy, as well as signal changes in the white matter. In late onset cases, signal change can also be found in the pons, midbrain, thalamus, and globus pallidus [Kanazawa, 1998]. Pathologic findings in dentatorubral-pallidoluysian atrophy include neuronal loss in the dentate nucleus, red nucleus, globus pallidus, and subthalamic nucleus. There is also diffuse loss of myelin staining in the cerebral white matter [Kanazawa, 1998; Munoz et al., 2004]. The disorder is very rare except in Japan, where it accounts for a significant proportion of autosomal-dominant spinocerebellar ataxias [Watanabe et al., 1998].

By using a candidate gene approach, the mutation causing dentatorubral-pallidoluysian atrophy was identified by two research groups [Koide et al., 1994; Nagafuchi et al., 1994]. They both found linkage to chromosome 12 and identified a CAG repeat as responsible for the disorder. An inverse correlation exists between the number of repeat units and the age of onset. Anticipation has been demonstrated in both paternal and maternal transmission of the disease allele, and extreme expansions (>90 repeats) can lead to infantile disease [Shimojo et al., 2001]. Gene dosage also plays a role in severity of phenotype, with homozygosity for a pathogenic allele causing more severe clinical manifestations than would otherwise be predicted based on repeat length [Sato et al., 1995].

The clinical heterogeneity of dentatorubral-pallidoluysian atrophy belies its genetic cause. Haw River syndrome shares many clinical and neuropathologic features with dentatorubral-pallidoluysian atrophy, Huntington's disease, and the spinocerebellar ataxias. However, this clinical entity differs from dentatorubral-pallidoluysian atrophy in the absence of myoclonic epilepsy, as well as the presence of basal ganglia calcifications and neuroaxonal dystrophy. Despite these phenotypic differences, the dentatorubral-pallidoluysian atrophy expansion was detected in a black family with Haw River syndrome [Burke et al., 1994]. Similarly, Warner and co-workers [1994] reported the CAG repeat expansion in a family of Maltese origin with variable clinical features that included dementia and seizures in younger patients, and dementia, psychosis, ataxia, and chorea in older patients. The neuropathologic findings in this family were not consistent with dentatorubral-pallidoluysian atrophy. These examples illustrate the wide phenotypic diversity encountered in dentatorubral-pallidoluysian atrophy. Genetic testing for the disorder is therefore indicated in patients with an autosomal dominant disorder causing dementia, ataxia, seizures, psychiatric symptoms, dystonia, chorea, or myoclonus. Also, patients with features of Huntington's disease but no evidence of expansion of the Huntington's disease CAG repeat should be evaluated for the CAG repeat at the dentatorubral-pallidoluysian atrophy locus.

The pathogenesis of dentatorubral-pallidoluysian atrophy remains a mystery. The number of CAG repeats varies in different tissues and tends to be larger in brain, suggesting somatic instability of the repeat [Ueno et al., 1995]. However, the degree of expansion does not seem to parallel neuropathologic involvement. Intranuclear inclusions are found in both neurons and glia; their presence in oligodendrocytes may cause the white matter lesions that are sometimes seen [Hayashi et al., 1998]. Atrophin-1, the *DRPLA* gene product, is expressed ubiquitously in human tissue. Several proteins proposed to interact with atrophin-1 have been identified using a yeast two-hybrid screen [Wood et al., 1998]. Recent evidence suggests that the wild-type atrophin-1 protein is involved in regulation of transcription, both positively and negatively [Shimohata, 2000; Zhang, 2002]. The target genes and the effect of polyglutamine expansion on this function remain unknown.

Hereditary Spastic Ataxia

The hereditary spastic ataxias are a heterogeneous group of disorders that combine the features of hereditary spastic paralysis and spinocerebellar ataxia. They typically present first with lower limb spasticity followed by ataxia, dysarthria, and gait disturbance. Autosomal-dominant, recessive, and X-linked forms have been described.

Autosomal-dominant hereditary spastic ataxia (SAX1-MIM 108600): Described in three kindreds from Newfoundland, these patients typically present first with progressive leg spasticity, followed by dysarthria and ocular movement abnormalities [Meijer et al., 2002]. The dentatorubral-pallidoluysian atrophy locus has not been excluded, although genetic anticipation is not observed.

Autosomal-recessive spastic ataxia of Charlevoix-Saguenay (ARSACS-MIM 270550): Originally described in French-Canadians from the Charlevoix-Saguenay region of Quebec, this autosomal-recessive disorder has also been found in a large Tunisian family [Bouchard, 1978; Mrissa et al., 2000]. Early onset is a rule, with the condition first being noticed when a child begins to walk; however, age of onset can be as late as 20 years. In addition to spasticity and ataxia, affected individuals also have sensory disturbances in the lower limbs (electromyography shows absent sensory-nerve conduction and reduced motor-nerve velocity), as well as hypermyelination of retinal-nerve fibers. Physical examination often reveals absent or reduced tendon reflexes in the lower limbs with a present Babinski sign; claw hand deformity and pes cavus can also be seen. Eye movements are not affected. Nonverbal intelligence quotient scores are often at the low end of normal. The *SACS* gene was mapped to chromosome 13q12. Frameshift and nonsense mutations lead to truncations in the gene product, sacsin, which is expressed throughout the CNS and may be involved in chaperone-mediated protein folding [Engert et al., 2000].

Spastic Paraplegia, Ataxia, and Mental Retardation (MIM 607565)

Hedera and colleagues [2002] identified a single kindred whose older members presented with uncomplicated spastic paraplegia, whereas later generations had either spastic paraplegia and ataxia or spastic paraplegia, ataxia, and mental retardation. Multiple spinocerebellar ataxias and hereditary spastic paraplegias were excluded by gene tests and linkage analysis, demonstrating that spastic paraplegia, ataxia, and mental retardation is a distinct disorder. Neuroimaging demonstrates dorsal column atrophy in all three types, although only the latter two had cerebellar atrophy. Pathologic studies are not available. Genetic anticipation, both in age of onset and disease severity, was suggested. The causative gene is unknown.

X-Linked Spinocerebellar Ataxia

A group of hereditary ataxias can be classified as X-linked based on the pattern of inheritance in specific kindreds. Shokeir [1970] described three families with an X-linked recessive pattern of inheritance and onset of ataxia in the late teens or early 20s. No extrapyramidal or posterior column deficits were noted. Another syndrome of X-linked cerebellar ataxia with hypotonia, optic atrophy, and sensorineural deafness has been described [Schmidley et al., 1987]. The disease occurs in infancy, is progressive, and causes death in childhood. Remarkable degeneration occurs in the red nucleus, dorsal motor nucleus of the vagus nerve, and auditory pathway, with some neuronal loss and gliosis in the dentate nucleus and inferior olive. Apak and associates [1989] described a progressive ataxia combined with paraplegia in a family in which seven males were affected; death typically occurred in the third or fourth decade. A pure X-linked cerebellar ataxia with slow progression has also been seen [Lutz et al., 1989]. An X-linked recessive disease characterized by ataxia, early onset floppiness, liability to infections (especially of the upper respiratory tract), deafness, and eventually flaccid quadriplegia and areflexia was reported [Arts et al., 1993]. This disease is rapidly progressive and results in death in early childhood. No precise genetic localization of the X-linked ataxias has been established.

PROPOSED DIAGNOSTIC APPROACH TO THE HEREDITARY ATAXIAS

Although the constellation of symptoms and signs may be suggestive of a hereditary ataxia, the clinical overlap of these disorders often precludes precise classification on clinical grounds alone. Still, important clues can be gleaned from the history and physical examination. Involvement of non-neural systems (e.g., frequent infections; ataxia-telangiectasia; absence of female sexual maturation; ataxia-telangiectasia, ataxia-oculomotor apraxia type 1; diabetes mellitus; Friedreich's ataxia) or intermittent symptoms (episodic ataxias) can suggest a diagnosis. A careful family history (including possible consanguinity) is needed to separate dominant from recessive conditions, although the sporadic appearance of a dominant disorder can sometimes create confusion. Physical examination findings such as the presence of pes cavus (Friedreich's ataxia, ataxia-telangiectasia), telangiectasias (ataxia-telangiectasia), or bulging eyes (Machado-Joseph disease or spinocerebellar ataxia) may also suggest a particular disorder.

Laboratory testing, such as measuring serum vitamin E (low in AVED) or albumin levels (low in ataxia-oculomotor apraxia type 1) can be useful. Ancillary tests such as EEG to further evaluate seizures and nerve conduction studies/electromyography to characterize peripheral nerve involvement can be helpful as well. MRI of the brain and spinal cord can help to distinguish "pure" cerebellar ataxias (such as spinocerebellar ataxia type 5) from those that involve multiple CNS regions (such as dentatorubral-pallidoluysian atrophy and Friedreich's ataxia). However, all of these tests have their limitations and may not provide the correct diagnosis.

In the current age of molecular diagnostics, the gold standard is genetic testing. Genetic testing has the added benefit of providing information that can be used for genetic counseling. Mutation testing is available for all of the disorders presented in this chapter whose causative gene has been identified. Although the majority of mutations will be detected by this analysis, these tests occasionally miss certain abnormalities such as single nucleotide substitutions (e.g., FRDA) or massive repeat expansions. When the constellation of clinical features suggests a particular disorder, directed testing for that disorder is appropriate. However, in new-onset cases lacking a specific presentation, a more comprehensive approach may be needed to identify the correct diagnosis.

ACKNOWLEDGMENT

The section on ataxia-telangiectasia was modified from Chapter 29 by Bruce O. Berg from the 3rd edition (1999) of this book.

REFERENCES

Aicardi J, Barbosa C, Andermann E, et al. Ataxia-ocular motor apraxia: A syndrome mimicking ataxia-telangiectasia. Ann Neurol 1988;24:497.

Allen G, Buxton RB, Wong EC, et al. Attentional activation of the cerebellum independent of motor involvement. Science 1997;275:1940.

Alonso I, Barros J, Tuna A, et al. Phenotypes of spinocerebellar ataxia type 6 and familial hemiplegic migraine caused by a unique CACNA1A missense mutation in patients from a large family. Arch Neurol 2003;60:610.

Apak S, Yuksel M, Ozmen M, et al. Heterogeneity of X-linked recessive (spino)cerebellar ataxia with or without spastic diplegia. Am J Hum Genet 1989;34:155.

Arlett CF, Priestley A. An assessment of the radiosensitivity in ataxia-telangiectasia heterozygotes. Kroc Found Ser 1985;19:101.

Arts WFM, Loonen MCB, Sengers RCA, et al. X-linked ataxia, weakness, deafness, and loss of vision in early childhood with a fatal course. Ann Neurol 1993;33:535.

Auger RG. Preservation of the masseter reflex in Friedreich's ataxia. Neurology 1992;42:875.

Baldwin RN, Lane RJ. Development of Wolff-Parkinson-White syndrome in a patient with Friedreich's ataxia. J Neurol Neurosurg Psychiatry 1987;50:235.

Baloh R, Yee RD, Boder E. Eye movements in ataxia-telangiectasia. Neurology 1978;28:1099.

Banfi S, Servadio A, Chung M, et al. Identification and characterization of the gene causing type 1 spinocerebellar ataxia. Nat Genet 1994;7:513.

Barbeau A, Roy M, Sadibelouiz M, et al. Recessive ataxia in Acadians and "Cajuns." Can J Neurol Sci 1984;11:526.

Barlow C, Ribaut-Barassin C, Zwingman TA, et al. ATM is a cytoplasmic protein in mouse brain required to prevent lysosomal accumulation. Proc Natl Acad Sci U S A 2000;97:871.

Bauer P, Laccone F, Rolfs A, et al. Trinucleotide repeat expansion in SCA17/TBP in white patients with Huntington's disease-like phenotype. J Med Genet 2004;41:230.

Bell J, Carmichael EA. On hereditary ataxia and spastic paraplegia. Treas Hum Inherit 1939;5:141.

Benomar A, Krols L, Stevanin G, et al. The gene for autosomal dominant cerebellar ataxia with pigmentary macular dystrophy maps to chromosome 3p12-p21.1. Nat Genet 1995;10:84.

Benton CS, de Silva R, Rutledge SL, et al. Molecular and clinical studies in SCA-7 define a broad clinical spectrum and the infantile phenotype. Neurology 1998;51:1081.

Berciano J. Olivopontocerebellar atrophy: A review of 117 cases. J Neurol Sci 1982;53:253.

Bharucha NE, Bharucha EP, Bhabha SK. Machado-Joseph-Azorean disease in India. Arch Neurol 1986;43:142.

Bidichandani SI, Ashizawa T, Patel PI. The GAA triplet-repeat expansion in Friedreich ataxia interferes with transcription and may be associated with an unusual DNA structure. Am J Hum Genet 1998;62:111.

Biemond A. Paleocerebellar atrophy with extrapyramidal manifestations in association with bronchiectasis and telangiectasis of the conjunctiva bulb as a familial syndrome. Proceedings: First International Congress of Neurological Sciences. London: Pergamon Press, 1957.

Bjork A, Lindblom U, Wadensten L. Retinal degeneration in hereditary ataxia. J Neurol Neurosurg Psychiatry 1956;19:186.

Boder E. Ataxia telangiectasia. In: Gomez MR, ed. Neurocutaneous disorders: A practical approach. Boston: Butterworth, 1987.

Boder E, Sedgwick RP. Ataxia-telangiectasia and frequent pulmonary infection: A preliminary report on 7 children, an autopsy and a case history. USC Med Bull 1957;9:15.

Boder E, Sedgwick RP. Ataxia-telangiectasia: A familial syndrome of progressive cerebellar ataxia, oculocutaneous telangiectasia and frequent pulmonary infections. Pediatrics 1958;21:526.

Bomar JM, Benke PJ, Slattery EL, et al. Mutations in a novel gene encoding a CRAL-TRIO domain cause human Cayman ataxia and ataxia/dystonia in the jittery mouse. Nat Genet 2003;35:264.

Bouchard JP, Barbeaw A, Bouchard R, Bouchard RW. Autosomal recessive spastic ataxia of Charlevoix-Saguenay. Can J Neurol Sci 1978;5:61.

Braitenberg V. Functional interpretation of cerebellar histology. Nature 1961;190:539.

Braitenberg V. Is the cerebellar cortex a biological clock in the millisecond range? Prog Brain Res 1967;25:334.

Brazis PW, Masdeu JC, Biller J. Localization in clinical neurology, 4th ed. Philadelphia: Lippincott Williams & Wilkins, 2001.

Brkanac Z, Bylenok L, Fernandez M, et al. A new dominant spinocerebellar ataxia linked to chromosome 19q13.4-qter. Arch Neurol 2002a;59:1291.

Brkanac Z, Fernandez M, Matsushita M, et al. Autosomal dominant sensory/motor neuropathy with Ataxia (SMNA): Linkage to chromosome 7q22-q32. Am J Med Genet 2002b;114:450.

Brown JR. Disorders of the cerebellum. In: Baker AB, Baker LH, eds. Clinical neurology. New York: Harper & Row, 1962.

Brown L, Mueller M, Benke PJ. A non-progressive cerebellar ataxia on Grand Cayman Island. Neurology 1984;34:273.

Browne DL, Brunt ERP, Griggs RC, et al. Identification of two new KCNA1 mutations in episodic ataxia/myokymia families. Hum Mol Genet 1995;4:1671.

Browne DL, Gancher ST, Nutt JG, et al. Episodic ataxia/myokymia syndrome is associated with point mutations in the human potassium channel gene, *KCNA1*. Nat Genet 1994;8:136.

Bulteau A-L, O'Neill HA, Kennedy MC, et al. Frataxin acts as an iron chaperone protein to modulate mitochondrial aconitase activity. Science 2004;305:242.

Burke JR, Wingfield MS, Lewis KE, et al. The Haw River syndrome: Dentatorubropallidoluysian atrophy (DRPLA) in an African-American family. Nat Genet 1994;7:521.

Burright EN, Clark HB, Servadio A, et al. SCA1 transgenic mice: A model for neurodegeneration caused by an expanded CAG trinucleotide repeat. Cell 1995;82:937.

Bushara KO, Wheat JM, Khan A, et al. Multiple tactile maps in the human cerebellum. Neuroreport 2001;12:2483.

Buyse G, Mertens L, Di Salvo G, et al. Idebenone treatment in Friedreich's ataxia: Neurological, cardiac, and biochemical monitoring. Neurology 2003;60:1679.

Buzin CH, Gatti RA, Nguyen VQ, et al. Comprehensive scanning of the *ATM* gene with DOVAM-S. Hum Mutat 2002;21:123.

Campuzano V, Montermini L, Molto MD, et al. Friedreich's ataxia: Autosomal recessive disease caused by an intronic GAA triplet repeat expansion. Science 1996;271:1423.

Cancel G, Abbas N, Stevanin G, et al. Marked phenotypic heterogeneity associated with expansion of a CAG repeat sequence at the spinocerebellar ataxia 3/Machado-Joseph disease locus. Am J Hum Genet 1995;57:809.

Cassandro E, Mosca F, Sequino L, et al. Otoneurological findings in Friedreich's ataxia and other inherited neuropathies. Audiology 1986;25:84.

Cavalier L, Ouahchi K, Kayden HJ, et al. Ataxia with isolated vitamin E deficiency: Heterogeneity of mutations and phenotypic variability in a large number of families. Am J Hum Genet 1998;62:301.

Cellini E, Piacentini S, Nacmias B, et al. A family with spinocerebellar ataxia type 8 expansion and vitamin E deficiency ataxia. Arch Neurol 2002;59:1952.

Centerwall WR, Miller MM. Ataxia, telangiectasia and sinopulmonary infections: A syndrome of slowly progressive deterioration in childhood. Am J Dis Child 1958;95:385.

Chai Y, Koppenhafer SL, Shoesmith SJ, et al. Evidence for proteasome involvement in polyglutamine disease: Localization to nuclear inclusions in SCA3/MJD and suppression of polyglutamine aggregation in vitro. Hum Mol Genet 1999;8:673.

Chamberlain S, Shaw J, Rowland A, et al. Mapping of mutation causing Friedreich's ataxia to human chromosome 9. Nature 1988;334:248.

Chen D-H, Brkanac Z, Verlinde CLMJ, et al. Missense mutations in the regulatory domain of PKC-gamma: A new mechanism for dominant nonepisodic cerebellar ataxia. Am J Hum Genet 2003a;72:839.

Chen HK, Fernandez-Funez P, Acevedo SF, et al. Interaction of Akt-phosphorylated ataxin-1 with 14-3-3 mediates neurodegeneration in spinocerebellar ataxia type 1. Cell 2003b;113:457.

Chen YW, Allen MD, Veprintsev DB, et al. The structure of the AXH domain of spinocerebellar ataxin-1. J Biol Chem 2004a;279:3758.

Chen Y-Z, Bennett CL, Huynh HM, et al. DNA/RNA helicase gene mutations in a form of juvenile amyotrophic lateral sclerosis (ALS4). Am J Hum Genet 2004b;74:1178.

Child JS, Perloff JK, Bach PB, et al. Cardiac involvement in Friedreich's ataxia: A clinical study of 75 patients. J Am Coll Cardiol 1986;7:1370.

Chong SS, McCall AE, Cota J, et al. Gametic and somatic tissue-specific heterogeneity of the expanded SCA1 CAG repeat in spinocerebellar ataxia type 1. Nat Genet 1995;10:344.

Christodoulou K, Deymeer F, Serdaroglu P, et al. Mapping of the second Friedreich's ataxia (FRDA2) locus to chromosome 9p23-p11: Evidence for further locus heterogeneity. Neurogenetics 2001;3:127.

Chung M, Ranum LPW, Duvick LA, et al. Evidence for a mechanism predisposing to intergenerational CAG repeat instability in spinocerebellar ataxia type 1. Nat Genet 1993;5:254.

Chung M-Y, Lu Y-C, Cheng N-C, et al. A novel autosomal dominant spinocerebellar ataxia (SCA22) linked to chromosome 1p21-q23. Brain 2003;126:1293.

Claus D, Harding AE, Hess CW, et al. Central motor conduction in degenerative ataxic disorders: A magnetic stimulation study. J Neurol Neurosurg Psychiatry 1988;51:790.

Colan RV, Snead OC, Ceballos R. Olivopontocerebellar atrophy in children: A report of seven cases in two families. Ann Neurol 1981;10:355.

Comu S, Giuliani M, Narayanan V. Episodic ataxia and myokymia syndrome: A new mutation of potassium channel gene Kv1.1. Ann Neurol 1996;40:684.

Cossée M, Schmitt M, Campuzano V, et al. Evolution of the Friedreich's ataxia trinucleotide repeat expansion: Founder effect and premutations. Proc Natl Acad Sci U S A 1997;94:7452.

Coutinho P, Andrade C. Autosomal dominant system degeneration in Portuguese families of the Azore Islands. A new genetic disorder involving cerebellar, pyramidal, extrapyramidal and spinal cord motor functions. Neurology 1978;28:703.

Cummings CJ, Mancini MA, Antalffy B, et al. Chaperone suppression of aggregation and altered subcellular proteasome localization imply protein misfolding in SCA1. Nat Genet 1998;19:148.

Cummings CJ, Reinstein E, Sun Y, et al. Mutation of the E6-AP ubiquitin ligase reduces nuclear inclusion frequency while accelerating polyglutamine-induced pathology in SCA1 mice. Neuron 1999;24:879.

Cummings CJ, Sun Y, Opal P, et al. Over-expression of inducible HSP70 chaperone suppresses neuropathology and improves motor function in SCA1 mice. Hum Mol Genet 2001;10:1511.

Currier RD, Glover G, Jackson JF, et al. Spinocerebellar ataxia: Study of a large kindred. Neurology 1972;22:1040.

Daher YH, Lonstein JE, Winter RB, et al. Spinal deformities in patients with Friedreich ataxia: A review of 19 patients. J Pediatr Orthop 1985;5:553.

Damji KF, Allingham RR, Pollock SC, et al. Periodic vestibulocerebellar ataxia, an autosomal dominant ataxia with defective smooth pursuit, is genetically distinct from other autosomal dominant ataxias. Arch Neurol 1996;53:338.

Date H, Onodera O, Tanaka H, et al. Early-onset ataxia with ocular motor apraxia and hypoalbuminemia is caused by mutations in a new HIT superfamily gene. Nat Genet 2001;29:184.
Daum I, Ackermann H. Cerebellar contributions to cognition. Behav Brain Res 1995;67:201.
David G, Abbas N, Stevanin G, et al. Cloning of the SCA7 gene reveals a highly unstable CAG repeat expansion. Nat Genet 1997;17:65.
David G, Durr A, Stevanin G, et al. Molecular and clinical correlations in autosomal dominant cerebellar ataxia with progressive macular dystrophy (SCA7). Hum Mol Genet 1998;2:165.
Davis MM, Gatti RA, Sparkes RS. Neoplasia and chromosomal breakage in ataxia-telangiectasia: A 2:14 translocation. Kroc Found Ser 1985;19:197.
De Leon GA, Grover WD, Huff DS. Neuropathologic changes in ataxia-telangiectasia. Neurology 1976;26:947.
De Pablos C, Berciano JCalleja J. Brain-stem auditory evoked potentials and blink reflex in Friedreich's ataxia. J Neurol 1991;238:212.
Del-Favero J, Krols L, Michalik A, et al. Molecular genetic analysis of autosomal dominant cerebellar ataxia with retinal degeneration (ADCA type II) caused by CAG triplet repeat expansion. Hum Mol Genet 1998;7:177.
Devos D, Schraen-Maschke S, Vuillaume I, et al. Clinical features and genetic analysis of a new form of spinocerebellar ataxia. Neurology 2001;56:234.
Durr A, Smadja D, Cancel G, et al. Autosomal dominant cerebellar ataxia type I in Martinique (French West Indies). Clinical and neuropathological analysis of 53 patients from three unrelated SCA2 families. Brain 1995;118:1573.
Durr A, Cossee M, Agid Y, et al. Clinical and genetic abnormalities in patients with Friedreich's ataxia. N Engl J Med 1996;335:1169.
Emamian ES, Kaytor MD, Duvick LA, et al. Serine 776 of ataxin-1 is critical for polyglutamine-induced disease in SCA1 transgenic mice. Neuron 2003;38:375.
Enevoldson TP, Sanders MD, Harding AE. Autosomal dominant cerebellar ataxia with pigmentary macular dystrophy: A clinical and genetic study of eight families. Brain 1994;117:445.
Engert JC, Berube P, Mercier J, et al. ARSACS, a spastic ataxia common in northeastern Quebec, is caused by mutations in a new gene encoding an 11.5-kb ORF. Nat Genet 2000;24:120.
Fantus IG, Janjua N, Senni H, et al. Glucose intolerance in first-degree relatives of patients with Friedreich's ataxia is associated with insulin resistance: Evidence for a closely linked inherited trait. Metabolism 1991;40:788.
Farlow MR, DeMyer W, Dlouhy SR, et al. X-linked recessive inheritance of ataxia and adult-onset dementia: Clinical features and preliminary linkage analysis. Neurology 1987;37:602.
Farmer TW, Mustian VM. Vestibulo-cerebellar ataxia: A newly defined hereditary syndrome with periodic manifestations. Arch Neurol 1963;8:471.
Filla A, De Michele G, Cavalcanti F, et al. The relationship between trinucleotide (GAA) repeat length and clinical features in Friedreich ataxia. Am J Hum Genet 1996;59:554.
Flanigan K, Gardner K, Alderson K, et al. Autosomal dominant spinocerebellar ataxia with sensory axonal neuropathy (SCA4): Clinical description and genetic localization to chromosome. Am J Hum Genet 1996;59:392.
Fowler HL. Machado-Joseph-Azorean disease: A ten year study. Arch Neurol 1984;41:921.
Frieden IJ, Reese V, Cohen D. PHACE syndrome. The association of posterior fossa brain malformations, hemangiomas, arterial anomalies, coarctation of the aorta and cardiac defects, and eye abnormalities. Arch Dermatol 1996;132:307.
Friedreich N. Über degenerative Atrophie der spinalen Hinterstrange. Virchows Arch Pathol Anat 1863;26:433.
Fujita R, Agid Y, Trouillas P, et al. Confirmation of linkage of Friedreich ataxia to chromosome 9 and identification of a new closely linked marker. Genomics 1989;4:110.
Gardner K, Alderson K, Galster B, et al. Autosomal dominant spinocerebellar ataxia: Clinical description of a distinct hereditary ataxia and genetic localization to chromosome 16 (SCA4) in a Utah kindred. Neurology 1994;A361.
Gaspar C, Lopes-Cendes I, Hayes S, et al. Ancestral origins of the Machado-Joseph disease mutation: A worldwide haplotype study. Am J Hum Genet 2001;68:523.
Gatti RA, Berkel I, Boder E, et al. Localization of an ataxia-telangiectasia gene to chromosome 11q22-23. Nature 1988; 336:577.
Gatti RA, Boder E, Vinters HV, et al. Ataxia-telangiectasia: An interdisciplinary approach to pathogenesis. Medicine (Baltimore) 1991;70:99.
Gatti RA, Good RA. Occurrence of malignancy in immunodeficiency diseases. Cancer 1971;28:89.
Geoffroy G, Barbeau AS, Brehon G, et al. Clinical and roentgenologic evaluation of patients with Friedreich's ataxia. Can J Neurol Sci 1976;3:279.
Gilad S, Chessa L, Khosravi R, et al. Genotype-phenotype relationships in ataxia-telangiectasia and variants. Am J Hum Genet 1998;62:551.
Gilman S, Junck L, Markel DS, et al. Cerebral glucose hypermetabolism in Friedreich's ataxia detected with positron emission tomography. Ann Neurol 1990;28:750.
Gispert S, Twells R, Orozco G, et al. Chromosomal assignment of the second locus for autosomal dominant cerebellar ataxia (SCA2) to chromosome 12q23-24.1. Nat Genet 1993;4:295.
Gomez CM, Thompson RM, Gammack JT, et al. Spinocerebellar ataxia type 6: Gaze-evoked and vertical nystagmus, Purkinje cell degeneration, and variable age of onset. Ann Neurol 1997;42:933.
Gotoff SP, Amirmokri E, Liebner EJ. Ataxia-telangiectasia, neoplasia, untoward response to x-irradiation and tuberous sclerosis. Am J Dis Child 1967;114:617.
Gouw LG, Castaneda MA, McKenna CK, et al. Analysis of the dynamic mutation in the SCA7 gene shows marked parental effects on CAG repeat transmission. Hum Mol Genet 1998;7:525.
Gouw LG, Digre KB, Harris CP, et al. Autosomal dominant cerebellar ataxia with retinal degeneration: Clinical, neuropathologic, and genetic analysis of a large kindred. Neurology 1994;44:1441.
Gouw LG, Kaplan CD, Haines JH, et al. Retinal degeneration characterizes a spinocerebellar ataxia mapping to chromosome 3p. Nat Genet 1995;10:89.
Greenfield JG. The spino-cerebellar degenerations. Springfield, IL: Charles C Thomas, 1954.
Grewal RP, Tayag E, Figueroa KP, et al. Clinical and genetic analysis of a distinct autosomal dominant spinocerebellar ataxia. Neurology 1998;51:1423.
Griggs RC, Moxley RT, Lafrance RA, et al. Hereditary paroxysmal ataxia: Response to acetazolamide. Neurology 1978;28:1259.
Harding A. Friedreich's ataxia: A clinical and genetic study of 90 families with an analysis of early diagnostic criteria and intrafamilial clustering of clinical features. Brain 1981;104:589.
Harding AE. The hereditary ataxias and related disorders. Edinburgh: Churchill Livingstone, 1984.
Harding AE. Clinical features and classification of inherited ataxias. Adv Neurol 1993;61:1.
Harding A, Hewer RL. The heart disease in Friedreich's ataxia; a clinical and electrocardiographic study of 115 patients with an analysis of serial electrocardiographic changes in 30 cases. Quart J Med 1983;28:489.
Harding AE, Matthews S, Jones S, et al. Spinocerebellar degeneration associated with a selective defect of vitamin E absorption. N Engl J Med 1985;313:32.
Hart RP, Henry GK, Kwentus JA, et al. Information processing speed of children with Friedreich's ataxia. Dev Med Child Neurol 1986;28:310.
Hart RP, Kwentus JA, Leshner RT, et al. Information processing speed in Friedreich's ataxia. Ann Neurol 1985;17:612.
Hausse AO, Aggoun Y, Bonnet D, et al. Idebenone and reduced cardiac hypertrophy in Friedreich's ataxia. Heart 2002;87:346.
Havener WH. Cerebellar-macular abiotrophy. Arch Ophthalmol 1951;45:40.
Hayashi Y, Kakita A, Yamada M, et al. Hereditary dentatorubral-pallidoluysian atrophy: Detection of widespread ubiquitinated neuronal and glial intranuclear inclusions in the brain. Acta Neuropathol (Berl) 1998;96:547.
Hecht F, Hecht BK. Ataxia-telangiectasia breakpoints in chromosome rearrangements reflects gene important to T and B lymphocytes. Kroc Found Ser 1985;19:189.
Heck AF. Heart disease in Friedreich's ataxia: Clinical studies and review of the literature. Neurology 1963;13:587.
Hedera P, Rainier S, Zhao XP, et al. Spastic paraplegia, ataxia, mental retardation (SPAR): A novel genetic disorder. Neurology 2002;58:411.
Herman-Bert A, Stevanin G, Netter J-C, et al. Mapping of spinocerebellar ataxia 13 to chromosome 19q13.3-q13.4 in a family with autosomal dominant cerebellar ataxia and mental retardation. Am J Hum Genet 2000;67:229.

Hernandez D, McConville CM, Stacey M, et al. A family showing no evidence of linkage between the ataxia telangiectasia gene and chromosome 1q22-23. J Med Genet 1993;30:135.

Herzog K-H, Chong MJ, Kapsetaki M, et al. Requirement for Atm in ionizing radiation-induced cell death in the developing central nervous system. Science 1998; 80:1089.

Holmberg M, Duyckaerts C, Durr, A., et al. Spinocerebellar ataxia type 7 (SCA7): A neurodegenerative disorder with neuronal intranuclear inclusions. Hum Mol Genet 1998;7:913.

Holmes SE, O'Hearn EE, Margolis RL. Why is SCA12 different from other SCAs? Cytogenet Gen Res 2003;100:189.

Holmes SE, O'Hearn EE, McInnis MG, et al. Expansion of a novel CAG trinucleotide repeat in the 5-prime region of PPP2R2B is associated with SCA12. Nat Genet 1999;23:391.

Hunt JR. Dyssynergia cerebellaris myoclonica—primary atrophy of the dentate system: Contribution to the pathology and symptomatology of the cerebellum. Brain 1922;44:490.

Hunyh DP, Del Bigio MR, Ho DH, et al. Expression of ataxin-2 in brains from normal individuals and patients with Alzheimer's disase and spinocerebellar ataxia 2. Ann Neurol 1999;45:232.

Huynh DP, Figueroa K, Hoang N, et al. Nuclear localization or inclusion body formation of ataxin-2 are not necessary for SCA2 pathogenesis in mouse or human. Nat Genet 2000;26:44.

Ikeda H, Yamaguchi M, Sugai S, et al. Expanded polyglutamine in the Machado-Joseph disease protein induces cell death in vitro and in vivo. Nat Genet 1996;13:196.

Ikeda Y, Dalton JC, Moseley ML, et al. Spinocerebellar ataxia type 8: Molecular genetic comparisons and haplotype analysis of 37 families with ataxia. Am J Hum Genet 2004;75:3.

Imbert G, Saudou F, Yvert G, et al. Cloning of the gene for spinocerebellar ataxia 2 reveals a locus with high sensitivity to expanded CAG/glutamine repeats. Nat Genet 1996;14:285.

Ishikawa K, Fujigasaki H, Saegusa H, et al. Abundant expression and cytoplasmic aggregations of alpha-1A voltage-dependent calcium channel protein associated with neurodegeneration in spinocerebellar ataxia type 6. Hum Mol Genet 1999;8:1185.

Ito M. Historical review of the significance of the cerebellum and the role of purkinje cells in motor learning. Ann N Y Acad Sci 2002;978:273.

Izumi Y, Maruyama H, Oda M, et al. SCA8 repeat expansion: Large CTA/CTG repeat alleles are more common in ataxic patients, including those with SCA6. Am J Hum Genet 2003;72:704.

James TN, Cobbs BW, Coghlan HC, et al. Coronary disease, cardioneuropathy, and conduction system abnormalities in the cardiomyopathy of Friedreich's ataxia. Br Heart J 1987;57:446.

Jampel RS, Okazaki H, Berstein H. Ophthalmoplegia and retinal degeneration associated with spinocerebellar ataxia. Arch Ophthalmol 1961;66:247.

Jen J, Kim GW, Baloh RW. Clinical spectrum of episodic ataxia type 2. Neurology 2004;62:17.

Jodice C, Mantuano E, Veneziano L, et al. Episodic ataxia type 2 (EA2) and spinocerebellar ataxia type 6 (SCA6) due to CAG repeat expansion in the CACNA1A gene on chromosome 19p. Mol Genet 1997;6:1973.

Johansson J, Forsgren L, Sandgren O, et al. Expanded CAG repeats in Swedish spinocerebellar ataxia type 7 (SCA7) patients: Effect of CAG repeat length on the clinical manifestation. Hum Mol Genet 1998;7:171.

Johnson WG, Murphy M, Murphy WI, et al. Recessive congenital cerebellar disorder in a genetic isolate: CPD type VII? Neurology 1978;28:352.

Joutel A, Bousser MG, Biousse V, et al. A gene for familial hemiplegic migraine maps to chromosome 19. Nat Genet 1993;5:40.

Kanazawa I. Dentatorubral-pallidoluysian atrophy or Naito-Oyanagi disease. Neurogenetics 1998;2:1.

Kawaguchi Y, Okamoto T, Taniwaki M, et al. CAG expansions in a novel gene for Machado-Joseph disease at chromosome 14q32.1. Nat Genet 1994;8:221.

Keats BJ, Ward LJ, Shaw J, et al. "Acadian" and "classical" forms of Friedreich ataxia are most probably caused by mutations at the same locus. Am J Med Genet 1989;1989:2.

Khan RJ, Andermann E, Fantus IG. Glucose intolerance in Friedreich's ataxia: Association with insulin resistance and decreased insulin binding. Metabolism 1986;35:1017.

Klein C, Wenning GK, Quinn NP, et al. Ataxia without telangiectasia masquerading as benign hereditary chorea. Mov Disord 1996;11:217.

Knezevic W, Stewart-Wynne EG. Brainstem auditory evoked responses in hereditary spinocerebellar ataxias. Clin Exp Neurol 1985;21:149.

Knight MA, McKinlay Gardner RJ, Bahlo M, et al. Dominantly inherited ataxia and dysphonia with dentate calcification: Spinocerebellar ataxia type 20. Brain 2004;127:1172.

Koeppen AH. The hereditary ataxias. J Neuropathol Exp Neurol 1998;57:531.

Koeppen AH, Barron KD. The neuropathology of olivopontocerebellar atrophy. In: Duvoisin RC, Plaitakis A, eds. The olivopontocerebellar atrophies, New York: Raven Press, 1984;13–38.

Koide R, Ikeuchi T, Onodera O, et al. Unstable expansion of CAG repeat in hereditary dentatorubral-pallidoluysian atrophy (DRPLA). Nat Genet 1994;6:9.

Koide R, Kobayashi S, Shimohata T, et al. A neurological disease caused by an expanded CAG trinucleotide repeat in the TATA-binding protein gene: A new polyglutamine disease? Hum Mol Genet 1999;8:2047.

Koob MD, Moseley ML, Schut LJ, et al. An untranslated CTG expansion causes a novel form of spinocerebellar ataxia (SCA8). Nat Genet 1999;21:379.

Koskinen T, Santavuori P, Sainio K, et al. Infantile onset spinocerebellar ataxia with sensory neuropathy: A new inherited disease. J Neurol Sci 1994;121:50.

Koskinen T, Pihko H, Voutilainen R. Primary hypogonadism in females with infantile onset spinocerebellar ataxia. Neuropediatrics 1995a;26:263.

Koskinen T, Valanne L, Ketonen LM, et al. Infantile-onset spinocerebellar ataxia: MR and CT findings. Am J Neurorad 1995b;16:1427.

Kostrzewa M, Klockgether T, Damian MS, et al. Locus heterogeneity in Friedreich ataxia. Neurogenetics 1997;1:43.

La Spada AR, Fu Y-H, Sopher BL, et al. Polyglutamine-expanded ataxin-7 antagonizes CRX function and induces cone-rod dystrophy in a mouse model of SCA7. Neuron 2001;31:913.

Labelle H, Tohme S, Duhaime M, et al. Natural history of scoliosis in Friedreich's ataxia. Bone Joint Surg 1986;68:564.

Lafreniere RG, Rochefort DL, Chretien N, et al. Unstable insertion of the 5-prime flanking region of the cystatin B gene is the most common mutation in progressive myoclonus epilepsy type 1, EPM1. Nat Genet 1997;15:298.

Le Ber I, Bouslam N, Rivaud-Pechoux S, et al. Frequency and phenotypic spectrum of ataxia with oculomotor apraxia 2: A clinical and genetic study in 18 patients. Brain 2004;127:759.

Le Ber I, Moreira M-C, Rivaud-Pechoux R, et al. Cerebellar ataxia with oculomotor apraxia type 1: Clinical and genetic studies. Brain 2003;126:2761.

Leiner HC, Leiner AL. The human cerebro-cerebellar system: Its computing, cognitive and language skills. Behav Brain Res 1991;44:113.

Lim DS, Kirsch DG, Canman CE, et al. ATM binds to beta-adaptin in cytoplasmic vesicles. Proc Natl Acad Sci U S A 1998;95:10146.

Lonnqvist T, Paetau A, Nikali K, et al. Infantile onset spinocerebellar ataxia with sensory neuropathy (IOSCA): Neuropathological features. J Neurol Sci 1998;161:57.

Lopes-Cendes I, Andermann E, Attig E, et al. Confirmation of the SCA-2 locus as an alternative locus for dominantly inherited spinocerebellar ataxias and refinement of the candidate region. Am J Hum Genet 1994;54:774.

Louis-Bar D. Sur un syndrome professif comprenant des telangiectasis capillaries cutanees et conjunctivales symetriques a disposition naevoide et des troubles cerebelleux. Confin Neurol 1941;4:32.

Lutz R, Bodensteiner J, Schaeffer B, et al. X-linked olivopontocerebellar atrophy. Clin Genet 1989;35:417.

Maciel P, Gaspar C, DeStefano AL, et al. Correlation between CAG repeat length and clinical features in Machado-Joseph disease. Am J Hum Genet 1995;57:54.

Maltecca F, Filla A, Castaldo I, et al. Intergenerational instability and marked anticipation in SCA-17. 2003;61:1441.

Manni E, Petrosini L. A century of cerebellar somatotopy: A debated representation. Nat Neurosci Rev 2004;5:241.

Mantuano E, Veneziano L, Jodice C, et al. Spinocerebellar ataxia type 6 and episodic ataxia type 2: Differences and similarities between two allelic disorders. Cytogenet Gen Res 2003;100:147.

Mariotti C, Solari A, Torta D, et al. Idebenone treatment in Friedreich patients: One-year-long randomized placebo-controlled trial. Neurology 2003;60:1676.

Maruyama H, Nakamura S, Matsuyama Z, et al. Molecular features of the CAG repeats and clinical manifestation of Machado-Joseph disease. Hum Mol Genet 1995;4:807.

Marz P, Probst A, Lang S, et al. Ataxin-10, the SCA10 neurodegenerative disorder protein, is essential for survival of cerebellar neurons. J Biol Chem 2004;279:35542.

Matilla T, McCall A, Subramony SH, et al. Molecular and clinical correlations in spinocerebellar ataxia type 3 and Machado-Joseph disease. Ann Neurol 1995;38:68.

Matilla A, Roberson ED, Banfi S, et al. Mice lacking ataxin-1 display learning deficits and decreased hippocampal paired-pulse facilitation. J Neurosci 1998;18:5508.

Matsuura T, Achari M, Khajavi M, et al. Mapping of the gene for a novel spinocerebellar ataxia with pure cerebellar signs and epilepsy. Ann Neurol 1999;45:407.

Matsuura T, Ranum LPW, Volpini V, et al. Spinocerebellar ataxia type 10 is rare in populations other than Mexicans. Neurology 2002;58:983.

Matsuura T, Yamagata T, Burgess DL, et al. Large expansion of the ATTCT pentanucleotide repeat in spinocerebellar ataxia type 10. Nat Genet 2000;26:191.

McFarlin DE, Oppenheim JJ. Impaired lymphocyte transformation in ataxia-telangiectasia in part due to a plasma inhibitory factor. J Immunol 1969;103:1212.

McFarlin DE, Strober W, Waldman TA. Ataxia-telangiectasia. Medicine (Baltimore) 1972;51:281.

Meijer IA, Hand CK, Grewal KK, et al. A locus for autosomal dominant hereditary spastic ataxia, SAX1, maps to chromosome 12p13. Am J Hum Genet 2002;70:763.

Middleton FA, Strick PL. Anatomical evidence for cerebellar and basal ganglia involvement in higher cognitive function. Science 1994;266:458.

Miller ME, Chatten J. Ovarian changes in ataxia telangiectasia. Acta Paediatr Scand 1967;56:559.

Miyoshi Y, Yamada T, Tanimura M, et al. A novel autosomal dominant spinocerebellar ataxia (SCA16) linked to chromosome 8q22.1-24.1. Neurology 2001;57:96.

Montermini L, Rodius F, Pianese L, et al. The Friedreich ataxia critical region spans a 150-kb interval on chromosome 9q13. Am J Hum Genet 1995;57:1061.

Moreira M-C, Barbot C, Tachi N, et al. The gene mutated in ataxia-oculomotor apraxia 1 encodes the new HIT/Zn-finger protein aprataxin. Nat Genet 2001;29:189.

Moreira M-C, Klur S, Watanabe M, et al. Senataxin, the ortholog of a yeast RNA helicase, is mutant in ataxia-ocular apraxia 2. Nat Genet 2004;36:225.

Morgan JL, Holcomb TM, Morrissey RW. Radiation reaction in ataxia-telangiectasia. Am J Dis Child 1968;116:557.

Moseley ML, Benzow KA, Schut LJ, et al. Incidence of dominant spinocerebellar and Friedreich triplet repeats among 361 ataxia families. Neurology 1998;51:1666.

Mrissa N, Belal S, Ben Hamida C, et al. Linkage to chromosome 13q11-12 of an autosomal recessive cerebellar ataxia in a Tunisian family. Neurology 2000;54:1408.

Munoz E, Campdelacreu J, Ferrer I, et al. Severe cerebral white matter involvement in a case of dentatorubropallidoluysian atrophy studied at autopsy. Arch Neurol 2004;61:946.

Mutsuddi M, Marshall CM, Benzow KA, et al. The spinocerebellar ataxia 8 noncoding RNA causes neurodegeneration and associates with stafuen in *Drosophila*. Curr Biol 2004;14:302.

Nagafuchi S, Yanagisawa H, Sato K, et al. Dentatorubral and pallidoluysian atrophy expansion of an unstable CAG trinucleotide on chromosome 12p. Nat Genet 1994;6:14.

Nagaoka U, Takashima M, Ishikawa K, et al. A gene on SCA4 locus causes dominantly inherited pure cerebellar ataxia. Neurology 2000;54:1971.

Naito H, Oyanagi S. Familial myoclonus epilepsy and choreoathetosis: Hereditary dentatorubral-pallidoluysian atrophy. Neurology 1982;32:798.

Nakamura K, Jeong S-Y, Uchihara T, et al. SCA17, a novel autosomal dominant cerebellar ataxia caused by an expanded polyglutamine in TATA-binding protein. Hum Mol Genet 2001;10:1441.

Nemeth AH, Bochukova E, Dunne E, et al. Autosomal recessive cerebellar ataxia with oculomotor apraxia (ataxia-telangiectasia–like syndrome) is linked to chromosome 9q34. Am J Hum Genet 2000;67:1320.

Nikali K, Suomalainen A, Terwilliger J, et al. Random search for shared chromosomal regions in four affected individuals: The assignment of a new hereditary ataxia locus. Am J Hum Genet 1995;56:1088.

Nikali K, Isosomppi J, Lonnqvist T, et al. Toward cloning of a novel ataxia gene: Refined assignment and physical map of the IOSCA locus (SCA8) on 10q24. Genomics 1997;39:185.

Nino HE, Noreen HJDubey DP. A family with hereditary ataxia: HLA typing. Neurology 1980;30:12.

Nystuen A, Benke PJ, Merren J, et al. A cerebellar ataxia locus identified by DNA pooling to search for linkage disequilibrium in an isolated population from the Cayman Islands. Hum Mol Genet 1996;5:525.

O'Hearn E, Holmes SE, Calvert PC, et al. SCA-12: Tremor with cerebellar and cortical atrophy is associated with a CAG repeat expansion. Neurology 2001;56:299.

Opal P, Zoghbi HY. The role of chaperones in polyglutamine disease. Trends Mol Med 2002;8:232.

Ophoff RA, Terwindt GM, Vergouwe MN, et al. Familial hemiplegic migraine and episodic ataxia type-2 are caused by mutations in the Ca(2+) channel gene CACNL1A4. Cell 1996;87:543.

Orozco G, Estrada R, Perry TL, et al. Dominantly inherited olivopontocerebellar atrophy from eastern Cuba: Clinical, neuropathological, and biochemical findings. J Neurol Sci 1989;93:37.

Orr HT, Chung M, Banfi S, et al. Expansion of an unstable trinucleotide CAG repeat in spinocerebellar ataxia type 1. Nat Genet 1993;4:221.

Ouahchi K, Arita M, Kayden H, et al. Ataxia with isolated vitamin E deficiency is caused by mutations in the alpha-tocopherol transfer protein. Nat Genet 1995;9:141.

Paulson HL. Protein fate in neurodegenerative proteinopathies: Polyglutamine diseases join the (mis)fold. Am J Hum Genet 1999;64:339.

Pentland B, Fox KA. The heart in Friedreich's ataxia. J Neurol Neurosurg Psychiatry 1983;46:1138.

Pulst S-M, Nechiporuk A, Nechiporuk T, et al. Moderate expansion of a normally biallelic trinucleotide repeat in spinocerebellar ataxia type 2. Nat Genet 1996;14:269.

Ranum LPW, Chung M, Banfi S, et al. Molecular and clinical correlations in spinocerebellar ataxia type I: Evidence for familial effects on the age at onset. Am J Hum Genet 1994a;55:244.

Ranum LPW, Schut LJ, Lundgren JK, et al. Spinocerebellar ataxia type 5 in a family descended from the grandparents of President Lincoln maps to chromosome 11. Nat Genet 1994b;8:280.

Ranum LPW, Lundgren JK, Schut LJ, et al. Spinocerebellar ataxia type 1 and Machado-Joseph disease: Incidence of CAG expansions among adult-onset ataxia patients from 311 families with dominant, recessive, or sporadic ataxia. Am J Hum Genet 1995;57:603.

Rijntjes M, Buechel C, Kiebel S, et al. Multiple somatotopic representations in the human cerebellum. Neuroreport 1999;10:3653.

Rolfs A, Koeppen AH, Bauer I, et al. Clinical features and neuropathology of autosomal dominant spinocerebellar ataxia (SCA17). Ann Neurol 2003;54:367.

Rosenberg RN, Nyhan WL, Bay C, et al. Autosomal dominant striatonigral degeneration: A clinical, pathologic and biochemical study of a new genetic disorder. Neurology 1976;26:703.

Rustin P, von Kleist-Retzow J-C, Chantrel-Groussard K, et al. Effect of idebenone on cardiomyopathy in Friedreich's ataxia: A preliminary study. Lancet 1999;354:477.

Sahba S, Nechiporuk A, Figueroa KP, et al. Genomic structure of the human gene for spinocerebellar ataxia type 2 (*SCA2*) on chromosome 12q24.1. Genomics 1998;47:359.

Said G, Marion MH, Selva J, et al. Hypotrophic and dying-back nerve fibers in Friedreich's ataxia. Neurology 1986;36:1292.

Salih MA, Ahlsten G, Stalberg E, et al. Friedreich's ataxia in 13 children: Presentation and evolution with neurophysiologic, electrocardiographic, and echocardiographic features. J Child Neurol 1990;5:321.

Sano Y, Date H, Igarashi S, et al. Aprataxin, the causative protein for EAOH is a nuclear protein with a potential role as a DNA repair protein. Ann Neurol 2004;55:241.

Sanpei K, Takano H, Igarashi S, et al. Identification of the spinocerebellar ataxia type 2 gene using a direct identification of repeat expansion and cloning technique, DIRECT. Nat Genet 1996;14:277.

Sasaki H, Wakisaka A, Hamada K, et al. Clinicopathological study of Joseph disease: Report of 4 pedigrees and its nosological consideration. Hokkaido Igaku Zasshi 1992a;67:174.

Sasaki H, Wakisaka A, Tashiro K, et al. Linkage study of Machado-Joseph disease: Genetic evidence for the locus different from SCA1. Rinsho Shinkeigaku 1992b;32:13.

Sato K, Kashihara K, Okada S, et al. Does homozygosity advance the onset of dentatorubral-pallidoluysian atrophy? Neurology 1995;45:1934.

Satterfield TF, Jackson SM, Pallanck LJ. A *Drosophila* homolog of the polyglutamine disease gene *SCA2* is a dosage-sensitive regulator of actin filament formation. Genetics 2002;162:1687.

Saviozzi S, Saluto A, Taylor AMR, et al. A late onset variant of ataxia-telangectasia with a compound heterozygous genotype, A8030G/7481 insA. J Med Genet 2002;39:57.

Savitsky K, Bar-Shira A, Gilad S, et al. A single ataxia telangiectasia gene with a product similar to PI-3 kinase. Science 1995a;268:1749.

Savitsky K, Sfez S, Tagle DA, et al. The complete sequence of the coding region of the ATM gene reveals similarity to cell cycle regulators in different species. Hum Mol Genet 1995b;4:2025.

Schelhaas HJ, Ippel PF, Hageman G, et al. Clinical and genetic analysis of a four-generation family with a distinct autosomal dominant cerebellar ataxia. J Neurol 2001; 248:113.

Schelhaas HJ, Verbeek DS, Van de Warrenburg BPC, et al. SCA19 and SCA22: Evidence for one locus with a worldwide distribution. Brain 2004;127:e6.

Schmahmann JD, Sherman JC. The cerebellar cognitive affective syndrome. Brain 1998;121:561.

Schmidley JW, Levinsohn MW, Manetto V. Infantile X-linked ataxia and deafness: A new clinicopathologic entity. Neurology 1987;37:1344.

Schols L, Vorgerd M, Schillings M, et al. Idebenone in patients with Friedreich ataxia. Neurosci Lett 2001;306:169.

Schols L, Bauer I, Zuhlke C, et al. Do CTG expansions at the SCA8 locus cause ataxia? Ann Neurol 2003;54:110.

Schöls L, Krüger R, Amoiridis G, et al. Spinocerebellar ataxia type 6: Genotype and phenotype in German kindreds. J Neurol Neurosurg Psychiatry 1998;64:67.

Schut JW. Hereditary ataxia: Clinical study through six generations. Arch Neurol Psychiat 1954;63:535.

Sedgwick RP, Boder E. Ataxia-telangiectasia. In: Vinken PJ, Bruyn GW, eds. Handbook of clinical neurology. Amsterdam: North-Holland, 1972.

Sekijima Y, Ohara S, Nakagawa S, et al. Hereditary motor and sensory neuropathy associated with cerebellar atrophy (HMSNCA): Clinical and neuropathological features of a Japanese family. J Neurol Sci 1998;158:30.

Servadio A, McCall A, Zoghbi HY, et al. Expression analysis of the ataxin-1 protein in tissues from normal and spinocerebellar ataxia type 1 individuals. Nat Genet 1995;10:94.

Shibata H, Huynh DO, Pulst S-M. A novel protein with RNA-binding motifs interacts with ataxin-2. Hum Mol Genet 2000;9:1303.

Shiloh Y, Tabor EBecker Y. In vitro phenotype of ataxia-telangiectasia (AT) fibroblast strains: Clues to the nature of the AT DNA lesion and the molecular defect in AT. Kroc Found Ser 1985;19:111.

Shimohata T, Nakajima T, Yamada M, et al. Expanded polyglutamine stretches interact with TAFII130, interfering with CREB-dependent transcription. Nat Genet 2000;26:29.

Shimojo Y, Osawa Y, Fukumizu M, et al. Severe infantile dentatorubral pallidoluysian atrophy with extreme expansion of CAG repeats. Neurology 2001;56:277.

Shokeir MHK. X-linked cerebellar ataxia. Clin Genet 1970;1:225.

Skinner PJ, Koshy B, Cummings C, et al. Ataxin-1 with extra glutamines induces alterations in nuclear matrix-associated structures. Nature 1997;389:971.

Smith JK. Dentatorubropallidoluysian atrophy. In: Vinken PJ, Bruyn GW, eds. Handbook of clinical neurology. Amsterdam: North-Holland, 1975.

Smith JK, Gonda VE, Malamud N. Unusual form of cerebellar ataxia; combined dentato-rubral and pallido-Luysian degeneration. Neurology 1958;8:205.

Smith JL, Cogan DD. Ataxia-telangiectasia. Arch Ophthalmol 1959;62:364.

Sobrido M-J, Cholfin JA, Perlman S, et al. SCA8 repeat expansions in ataxia: A controversial association. Neurology 2001;57:1310.

Sourander P, Bonnevier JO, Olsson Y. A case of ataxia-telangiectasia. J Neurol Neurosurg Psychiatry 1966;42:354.

Spector BD, Filipovich AHG, Perry GS, et al. Epidemiology of cancer in ataxia-telangiectasia. In: Bridges BA, Harnden D, eds. Ataxia-telangiectasia. New York: John Wiley & Sons, 1982.

Spira PJ, McLeod JG, Evans WA. A spinocerebellar degeneration with X-linked inheritance. Brain 1979;102:27.

Srivastava AK, Choudhry S, Gopinath MS, et al. Molecular and clinical correlation in five Indian families with spinocerebellar ataxia 12. Ann Neurol 2001;50:796.

Steckley JL, Ebers GC, Cader MZ, et al. An autosomal dominant disorder with episodic ataxia, vertigo, and tinnitus. Neurology 2001;57:1499.

Stevanin G, Le Guern E, Ravise N, et al. A third locus for autosomal dominant cerebellar ataxia type 1 maps to chromosome 14q24.3-qter: Evidence for the existence of a fourth locus. Am J Hum Genet 1994;54:11.

Stevanin G, Herman A, Durr A, et al. Are (CTG)n expansions at the SCA8 locus rare polymorphisms? Nat Genet 2000;24:213.

Stevanin G, Fujigasaki H, Lebre A-S, et al. Huntington's disease–like phenotype due to trinucleotide repeat expansions in the TBP and JPH3 genes. Brain 2003;126:1599.

Stevanin G, Bouslam N, Thobois S, et al. Spinocerebellar ataxia with sensory neuropathy (SCA25) maps to chromosome 2p. Ann Neurol 2004;55:97.

Stewart GS, Maser RS, Stankovic T, et al. The DNA double-strand break repair gene hMRE11 is mutated in individuals with an ataxia-telangiectasia-like disorder. Cell 1999;99:577.

Storey E, Gardner RJM, Knight MA, et al. A new autosomal dominant pure cerebellar ataxia. Neurology 2001;57:1913.

Strupp M, Kalla R, Dichgans M, et al. Treatment of episodic ataxia type 2 with the potassium channel blocker 4-aminopyridine. Neurology 2004;62:1623.

Sulek A, Hoffman-Zacharska D, Zdzienicka E, et al. SCA8 repeat expansion coexists with SCA1—not only with SCA6. Am J Hum Genet 2003;73:972.

Syllaba L, Henner K. Contribution a l'independence de l'athetose double idiopathique et congenitale: Atteinte familiale, syndrome dystrophique, signe du reseau vasculaire conjunctival, integrite psychique. Rev Neurol 1926;1:541.

Takahashi H, Ishikawa K, Tsutsumi T, et al. A clinical and genetic study in a large cohort of patients with spinocerebellar ataxia type 6. J Hum Genet 2004;49:256.

Takiyama Y, Nishizawa M, Tanaka H, et al. The gene for Machado-Joseph disease maps to human chromosome 14q. Nat Genet 1993;4:300.

Takiyama Y, Sakoe K, Namekawa M, et al. A Japanese family with spinocerebellar ataxia type 6 which includes three individuals homozygous for an expanded CAG repeat in the *SCA6/CACNL1A4* gene. J Neurol Sci 1998;158:141.

Thomas PK, Workman JM, Thage O. Behr's syndrome: A family exhibiting pseudodominant inheritance. J Neurol Sci 1984;64:137.

Thoren C. Cardiomyopathy in Friedreich's ataxia. Acta Paediatr 1959;48:100.

Thoren C. Diabetes mellitus in Friedreich's ataxia. Acta Paediatr 1962;51:239.

Toyoshima Y, Yamada M, Onodera O, et al. SCA17 homozygote showing Huntington's disease–like phenotype. Ann Neurol 2004;55:281.

Traber MG, Sokol RJ, Burton GW, et al. Impaired ability of patients with familial isolated vitamin E deficiency to incorporate α-tocopherol into lipoproteins secreted by the liver. J Clin Invest 1990;85:397.

Tranchant C, Fleury M, Moreira M-C, et al. Phenotypic variability of *aprataxin* gene mutations. Neurology 2003;60:868.

Trottier Y, Lutz Y, Stevanin G, et al. Polyglutamine expansion as a pathological epitope in Huntington's disease and four dominant cerebellar ataxias. Nature 1995;378:403.

Tsuchiya K, Ishikawa K, Watabiki S, et al. A clinical, genetic, neuropathological study in a Japanese family with SCA 6 and a review of Japanese autopsy cases of autosomal dominant cortical cerebellar atrophy. J Neurol Sci 1998;160:54.

Tsuji S. Spinocerebellar ataxia type 17. Arch Neurol 2004;61:183.

Ueno S, Kondoh K, Kotani Y, et al. Somatic mosaicism of CAG repeat in dentatorubral-pallidoluysian atrophy (DRPLA). Hum Mol Genet 1995;4:663.

Uziel T, Savitsky K, Platzer M, et al. Genomic organization of the ATM gene. Genomics 1996;33:317.

Vahedi K, Joutel A, Von Bogaert P, et al. A gene for hereditary paroxysmal cerebellar ataxia maps to chromosome 19p. Ann Neurol 1995;37:289.

van de Warrenburg BP, Frenken CW, Ausems MG, et al. Striking anticipation in spinocerebellar ataxia type 7: The infantile phenotype. J Neurol 2001;248:911.

van de Warrenburg BPC, Verbeek DS, Piersma SJ, et al. Identification of a novel SCA14 mutation in a Dutch autosomal dominant cerebellar ataxia family. Neurology 2003;61:1760.

van Swieten JC, Brusse E, de Graaf BM, et al. A mutation in the fibroblast growth factor 14 gene is associated with autosomal dominant cerebral ataxia. Am J Hum Genet 2003;72:191.

Vance JM, Pericak-Vance MA, Payne CS, et al. Linkage and genetic analysis in adult onset periodic vestibulo-cerebellar ataxia: Report of a new family. Am J Hum Genet 1984;36:78S.

Verbeek DS, Schelhaas JH, Ippel EF, et al. Identification of a novel SCA locus (SCA19) in a Dutch autosomal dominant cerebellar ataxia family on chromosome region 1p21-q21. Hum Genet 2002;111:388.

Verbeek DS, Van de Warrenburg BPC, Wesseling P, et al. Mapping of the SCA23 locus involved in autosomal dominant cerebellar ataxia to chromosome region 20p13-12.3. Brain 2004;127:2551.

Virtaneva K, D'Amato E, Miao J, et al. Unstable minisatellite expansion causing recessively inherited myoclonus epilepsy, EPM1. Nat Genet 1997;15:393.

von Brederlow B, Hahn AF, Koopman WJ, et al. Mapping the gene for acetazolamide responsive hereditary paroxysmal cerebellar ataxia to chromosome 19p. Hum Mol Genet 1995:4:279.

Voncken M, Ioannou P, Delatycki MB. Friedreich ataxia—Update on pathogenesis and possible therapies. Neurogenetics 2004;5:1.

Vuillaume I, Devos D, Schraen-Maschke S, et al. A new locus for spinocerebellar ataxia (SCA21) maps to chromosome 7p21.3-p15.1. Ann Neurol 2002;52:666.

Wang Q, Bardgett ME, Wong M, et al. Ataxia and paroxysmal dyskinesia in mice lacking axonally transported FGF14. Neuron 2002;35:25.

Wara DW, Ammann AJ. Thymosin treatment of children with primary immunodeficiency disease. Transplant Proc 1978;10:203.

Warner TT, Williams L, Harding AE. DRPLA in Europe. Nat Genet 1994;6:225.

Watanabe H, Tanaka F, Matsumoto M, et al. Frequency analysis of autosomal dominant cerebellar ataxias in Japanese patients and clinical characterization of spinocerebellar ataxia type 6. Clin Genet 1998;53:13.

Watase K, Weeber EJ, Xu B, et al. A long CAG repeat in the mouse Sca1 locus replicates SCA1 features and reveals the impact of protein solubility on selective neurodegeneration. Neuron 2002;34:905.

Wessel K, Schroth G, Diener HC, et al. Significance of MRI-confirmed atrophy of the cranial spinal cord in Friedreich's ataxia. Eur Arch Psychiatry Neurol Sci 1989;238:225.

Wood JD, Yuan J, Margolis RL, et al. Atrophin-1, the DRPLA gene product, interacts with two families of WW domain-containing proteins. Mol Cell Neurosci 1998;11:149.

Worth PF, Giunti P, Gardner-Thorpe C, et al. Autosomal dominant cerebellar ataxia type III: Linkage in a large British family to a 7.6-cM region on chromosome 15q14-21.3. Am J Hum Genet 1999;65:420.

Worth PF, Houlden H, Giunti P, et al. Large, expanded repeats in SCA8 are not confined to patients with cerebellar ataxia. Nat Genet 2000;24:214.

Yabe I, Sasaki H, Chen D-H, et al. Spinocerebellar ataxia type 14 caused by a mutation in protein kinase C gamma. Arch Neurol 2003;60:1749.

Yamashita I, Sasaki H, Yabe I, et al. A novel locus for dominant cerebellar ataxia (SCA14) maps to a 10.2-cM interval flanked by D19S206 and D19S605 on chromosome 19q13.4-qter. Ann Neurol 2000;48:156.

Yoo S-Y, Pennesi ME, Weeber EJ, et al. SCA7 knockin mice model human SCA7 and reveal gradual accumulation of mutant ataxin-7 in neurons and abnormalities in short-term plasticity. Neuron 2003;37:383.

Yvert G, Lindenberg KS, Picaud S, et al. Expanded polyglutamines induce neurodegeneration and trans-neuronal alterations in cerebellum and retina of SCA7 transgenic mice. Hum Mol Genet 2000;9:2491.

Zhang S, Xu L, Lee J, et al. *Drosophila atrophin* homolog functions as a transcriptional corepressor in multiple developmental processes. Cell 2002;108:45.

Zhuchenko O, Bailey J, Bonnen P, et al. Autosomal dominant cerebellar ataxia (SCA6) associated with small polyglutamine expansions in the alpha 1A-voltage-dependent calcium channel. Nat Genet 1997;15:62.

Zoghbi HY, Caskey CT. Inherited disorders caused by trinucleotide repeat expansions. In: Harris H, Hirschorn KH, eds. Advances in human genetics. New York; Plenum, 1998.

Zoghbi HY, Pollack MS, Lyons LA, et al. Spinocerebellar ataxia: Variable age of onset and linkage to human leukocyte antigen in a large kindred. Ann Neurol 1988;23:580.

Zoghbi HY, Orr HT. Glutamine repeats and neurodegeneration. Ann Rev Neurosci 2000;23:217.

Zu L, Figueroa KP, Grewal R, et al. Mapping of a new autosomal dominant spinocerebellar ataxia to chromosome 22. Am J Hum Genet 1999;64:594.

CHAPTER 58

Movement Disorders

Terence D. Sanger and Jonathan W. Mink

APPROACH TO CHILDHOOD MOVEMENT DISORDERS

Movement disorders are syndromes characterized by impaired voluntary movement, presence of involuntary movements, or both. There may be impaired targeting and velocity of intended movements, abnormal involuntary movements, abnormal postures, or excessive normal-appearing movements at inappropriate or unintended times. Movement disorders in children include athetosis, chorea, dystonia, myoclonus, parkinsonism, stereotypies, tics, and tremor [Sanger, 2003b]. Movement disorders may be accompanied by weakness, spasticity, hypotonia, ataxia, apraxia [Koski et al., 2002], and other motor deficits, although many authors do not include these accompanying deficits among the movement disorders.

Movement disorders have been divided into *hyperkinetic* disorders in which there is excessive movement, and *hypokinetic* disorders in which there is a paucity of movement. Hyperkinetic disorders consist of abnormal, repetitive involuntary movements and include most of the childhood movement disorders such as chorea, dystonia, athetosis, myoclonus, stereotypies, tics, and tremor. Hypokinetic movement disorders are primarily akinetic or rigid. The primary syndrome in this category is parkinsonism, occurring most commonly in adulthood as Parkinson's disease or one of the many forms of secondary parkinsonism. In children, hypokinetic disorders are much less common than hyperkinetic disorders.

Abnormalities of movement that are presumed to be due to central nervous system disorders are typically divided into two primary categories: pyramidal and extrapyramidal. Many authors consider only the extrapyramidal symptoms to be movement disorders. Pyramidal symptoms typically involve weakness, specific patterns of weakness, or spasticity. Pyramidal symptoms are thought to be due to injury to the pyramidal tract, including the corticospinal tract, and therefore to represent, to some extent, the effect of a denervated spinal cord. Extrapyramidal disorders are often described as everything that is not a pyramidal disorder. In particular, the term usually includes disorders of movement that are not due to weakness.

Movement disorder terminology has been well defined for adults but less so for children. Therefore, it is likely that movement disorders are underreported in children and that there is inconsistent terminology. Recently, there have been attempts to provide specific definitions of childhood hypertonic disorders, including dystonia and rigidity [Sanger et al., 2003]. The prevalence in children of different types of hypertonic disorders, as well as other movement disorders, is not well known, although there have been studies investigating this in certain populations. Consistent definitions of nonhypertonic disorders in childhood are not yet available. In this chapter, use of terminology for nonhypertonic disorders is based on current adult definitions.

In adult movement disorders, it is frequently helpful to divide disorders into primary and secondary disorders, although there is no consistent definition of these terms. Many authors refer to disorders as primary if there is only a single dominant symptom and the underlying cause is presumably genetic or is due to an identified gene. However, the existence of a single symptom in childhood movement disorders is probably the exception rather than the rule.

Characteristic Features of Pediatric Movement Disorders

Movement disorders in children differ from those in adults in several important aspects. Perhaps the most important is that movement disorders in childhood are primarily symptoms of other diseases, rather than diseases in and of themselves [Sanger, 2003b; Sanger et al., 2003). In adults, dystonia and parkinsonism are usually due to primary dystonia or idiopathic Parkinson's disease, respectively. However, dystonia or parkinsonism in children are more likely to be features of an underlying static or progressive neurologic disorder. Diagnosis in children is complicated by the fact that many symptoms have more than one cause, and any particular underlying pathophysiology may lead to a complex combination of symptoms. The diagnostic evaluation in children is guided by symptoms, but the existence of a large class of diseases that can lead to the same set of symptoms often necessitates a broad etiologic evaluation. There may be specific etiologic treatments and symptomatic treatments, both of which may be beneficial in an individual child. In particular, many of the causes of childhood movement disorders do not yet have any specific treatment, yet symptomatic treatment for the resulting movement disorder can be extremely helpful and lead to improvement in quality of life.

Another distinction between movement disorders in adults and children is that many adult neurologic disorders can be attributed to anatomically localized injury, but childhood disorders frequently result from a global or multifocal injury that may affect particular cell types, receptor types, or metabolic pathways. Therefore in children, the injury is often sparse but global, with manifestations across multiple areas of function, including sensorimotor and cognitive functions.

The clinical manifestations of a movement disorder will depend on the child's developmental stage. The same illness may present differently depending on the age at onset of symptoms. Detection of a progressive disorder may be complicated by superposition of a progressive disorder on the natural improvement of function that is expected throughout childhood. Therefore, a child with a progressive movement disorder may continue to develop new skills despite falling further and further behind in age-appropriate behavior. The presence of a movement disorder may affect the current and continuing development of the child's normal motor and cognitive abilities. Therefore, an acute illness may have developmental consequences that outlast the duration of the injury itself.

Diagnosis of Movement Disorders

Classification of the movement disorder based on the spatial and temporal pattern is essential for diagnosis. It is also important to define the context in which the movements occur. Although it is often helpful to list the characteristics of the movements (Table 58-1), the diagnosis relies on pattern recognition, and the clinician must see the movements. If the movements are not apparent during the neurologic examination, repeating the examination at another time or obtaining video recordings of the movements is essential. The widespread availability of video cameras has substantially improved diagnosis of movement disorders.

When approaching a patient with a movement disorder, it is helpful to determine the answers to some key questions: (1) Is the number of movements excessive (hyperkinetic) or diminished (hypokinetic)? (2) If hyperkinetic, do the individual movements appear normal or abnormal? (3) Is the movement paroxysmal (sudden onset and offset), continual (repeated again and again), or continuous (without stop)? (4) What is the developmental stage of the child, and has the development been normal? (5) How does voluntary movement affect the movement disorder? Are the symptoms and signs present at rest (body part supported against gravity), with maintained posture, with action, with approach to a target (intention), or a combination? (6) Has the movement disorder changed over time? (7) Do environmental stimuli or emotional states precipitate, exacerbate, or alleviate the movement disorder? (8) Is the patient aware of the movements? (9) Can the movements be suppressed voluntarily? (10) Are the movements heralded by a premonitory sensation or urge? (It may be helpful to ask the patient, "Why do you do that?") (11) Does the movement disorder abate with sleep? (12) Are there other findings on the examination suggestive of focal neurologic deficit or systemic disease? (13) Is there a family history of a similar or related condition?

TABLE 58-1

Phenomenologic Classification of Movement Disorders

MOVEMENT DISORDER	BRIEF DESCRIPTION
Athetosis	Slow, continuous writhing movements of distal body parts, especially the fingers and hands
Chorea, ballism	Chaotic, random, repetitive, brief, purposeless movements. Rapid, but not as rapid as myoclonus. When very large amplitude affecting proximal joints, choreic limb movements are often called *ballism*.
Dystonia	Repetitive, sustained, abnormal postures or movements. Abnormal postures typically have a twisting quality.
Myoclonus	Sudden, brief, shocklike movements that may be repetitive or rhythmic
Parkinsonism	Hypokinetic syndrome characterized by a combination of rest tremor, slow movement (bradykinesia), rigidity, and postural instability
Stereotypy	Patterned, episodic, repetitive, purposeless, rhythmic movements
Tics	Stereotyped intermittent, sudden, discrete, repetitive, nonrhythmic movements, most frequently involving head and upper body
Tremor	Rhythmic oscillation around a central point or position involving any one body part or more than one

Laboratory tests, imaging, and other diagnostic testing should be based on the specific movement disorder. There is no universal "movement disorder workup" because the causes are varied and some movement disorders (e.g., tics) are rarely symptomatic of an underlying disease.

Movement disorders may be difficult to characterize unless other symptoms and behavioral context are taken into account. Chorea can resemble myoclonus. Dystonia can resemble spasticity. Paroxysmal movement disorders such as dystonia and tics may resemble seizures. Movements in some contexts may be normal and in others may indicate underlying pathology. For example, frequent eye blinking can be perfectly normal and appropriate in one setting (a windy day on the beach) but excessive in another (tics). Movements that raise concern about a degenerative disorder in older children (progressive myoclonus) may be completely normal in an infant (benign neonatal myoclonus). Thus, it is important to view the movement disorder in the context of a complete history and neurologic examination.

Role of the Basal Ganglia in Movement Disorders

Most movement disorders can be attributed to dysfunction of the basal ganglia. However, *basal ganglia disorder* and *movement disorder* are not synonymous. Some movement disorders (e.g., tremor and myoclonus) may have little to do with the basal ganglia. Conversely, basal ganglia lesions may cause cognitive or affective symptoms and minimal or no motor impairment. Nonetheless, because most movement disorders involve the basal ganglia, it is useful to have some understanding how this system is organized.

The basal ganglia are subcortical structures comprising several interconnected nuclei in the forebrain, midbrain, and diencephalon (Fig. 58-1). They include the striatum (caudate, putamen, nucleus accumbens); the subthalamic nucleus; the globus pallidus (internal segment [GPi], external segment [GPe], and ventral pallidum); and the substantia nigra (pars compacta [SNpc] and pars reticulata [SNpr]). The striatum and subthalamic nucleus are the primary input structures of the basal ganglia, receiving excitatory input from cerebral cortex. The GPi and SNpr are the primary output nuclei, sending inhibitory output to thalamus and brainstem targets. Acting through the thalamus, the basal ganglia output influences frontal lobe cortical neurons. By virtue of the inhibitory output from the basal ganglia, conditions associated with destruction of the output nuclei are associated with unwanted and nonspecific overactivity of thalamocortical and brainstem targets.

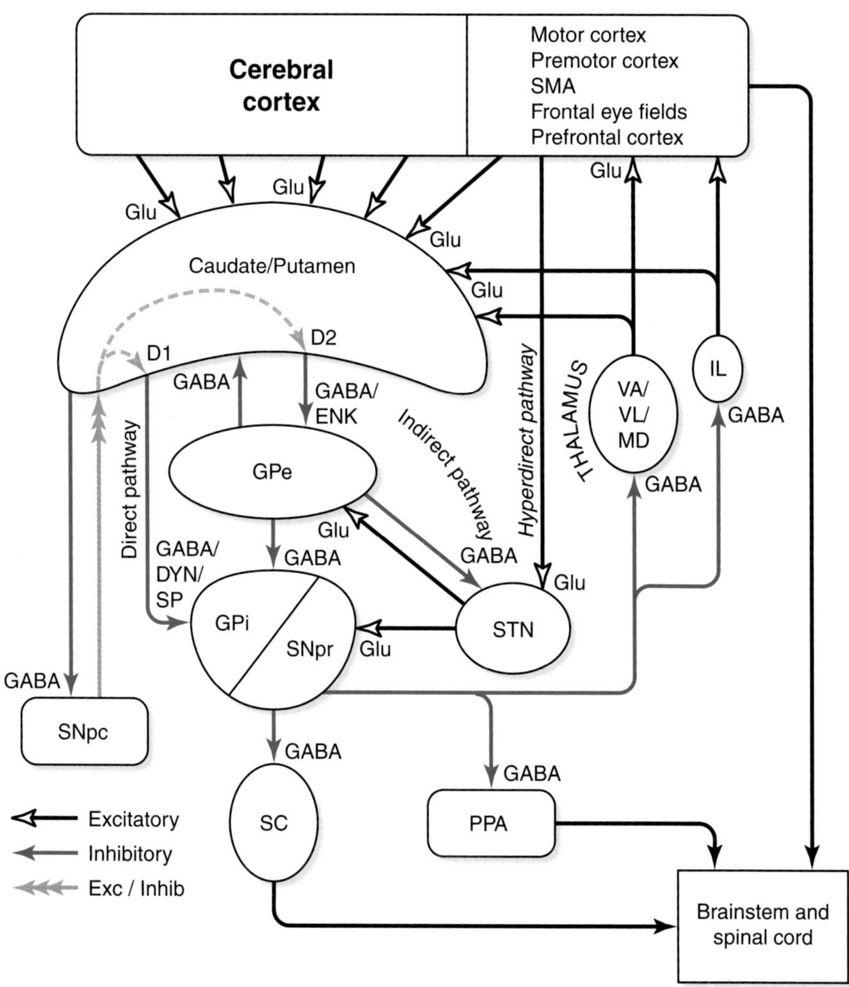

FIGURE 58-1. Simplified schematic diagram of basal ganglia circuitry. Excitatory connections are indicated by *open arrows*, inhibitory connections by *filled arrows*, and the modulatory dopamine projection is indicated by a *three-headed arrow*. DYN, dynorphin; ENK, enkephalin; glu, glutamate; GPe, globus pallidus external segment; GPi, globus pallidus internal segment; IL, intralaminar thalamic nuclei; MD, mediodorsal nucleus; PPA, pedunculopontine area; SC, superior colliculus; SMA, supplementary motor area; SNpc, substantia nigra pars compacta; SNpr, substantia nigra pars reticulata; SP, substance P; STN, subthalamic nucleus; VA ventral anterior nucleus; VL, ventral lateral nucleus.

The striatum receives excitatory input from virtually all of cerebral cortex. In addition to the cortical input, the striatum receives a dense input from dopamine-containing neurons in the SNpc. The action of dopamine on striatal neurons depends on the type of dopamine receptor involved. Five types of G protein–coupled dopamine receptors have been described (D1 to D5) and have been grouped into two families. The D1 family includes D1 and D5 receptors and the D2 family includes D2, D3, and D4 receptors. D1 receptors potentiate the effect of cortical input to striatal neurons, whereas D2 receptors decrease the effect of cortical input to striatal neurons. The main neuron type is the medium spiny neuron, accounting for 95% of striatal neurons. In addition to cortical and nigral inputs, medium spiny striatal neurons receive a number of other inputs, including (1) excitatory glutamatergic inputs from thalamus; (2) cholinergic input from striatal interneurons; (3) γ-aminobutyric acid (GABA), substance P, and enkephalin input from adjacent medium spiny striatal neurons; and (4) GABA input from local inhibitory interneurons. The neurochemistry of the striatum is complicated but provides many options for pharmacologic therapeutics. Both dopamine and acetylcholine modulate the activity of striatal output neurons and are the targets for the most commonly used medications for treating movement disorders. GABA is ubiquitous in the basal ganglia and is another target for pharmacologic therapeutics, but because it is ubiquitous, the effects of medications such as benzodiazepines and baclofen may be rather nonspecific.

Medium spiny striatal neurons contain the inhibitory neurotransmitter GABA and are inhibitory to their targets. In addition, they have peptide neurotransmitters that are colocalized with GABA. Based on the type of neurotransmitters and the predominant type of dopamine receptor they contain, the medium spiny neurons can be divided into two populations. One population contains GABA, dynorphin, and substance P and primarily expresses D1 dopamine receptors. These neurons project to the basal ganglia output nuclei, GPi and SNpr, and form the "direct pathway" [Albin et al., 1989; Alexander and Crutcher, 1990; DeLong, 1990]. The second population contains GABA and enkephalin and primarily expresses D2 dopamine receptors. These neurons project to GPe and form the first limb of the "indirect pathway" [Albin et al., 1989; Alexander and Crutcher, 1990; DeLong, 1990].

The subthalamic nucleus receives an excitatory, glutamatergic input from many areas of frontal lobes with especially large inputs from motor areas of cortex. The subthalamic nucleus also receives an inhibitory GABA input from GPe. The output from the subthalamic nucleus is glutamatergic and excitatory to the basal ganglia output nuclei, GPi and SNpr. This projection forms the second limb of the indirect pathway [Albin et al., 1989; Alexander and Crutcher, 1990; DeLong, 1990].

There are several routes through which information flows from the cerebral cortex to the basal ganglia output nuclei. The two most direct are the disynaptic, inhibitory, direct pathway from cortex to striatum to GPi and SNpr and the disynaptic, excitatory, "hyperdirect pathway" [Nambu et al., 2000] from cortex to subthalamic nucleus to GPi and SNpr. The direct pathway is inhibitory to GPi and SNpr; the hyperdirect pathway is excitatory to GPi and SNpr. The hyperdirect pathway is the fastest route through the basal ganglia. There are several indirect routes, but the most important is the indirect pathway from cortex to striatum to GPe to subthalamic nucleus to GPi and SNpr. Organization of these pathways confers a pattern of fast, powerful, and relatively broad excitation through the hyperdirect pathway and more focused inhibition through the direct pathway (Fig. 58-2) [Mink, 1996; Nambu et al., 2000; Parent and Hazrati, 1993]. The indirect pathway confers additional focus.

The primary basal ganglia output arises from GPi and SNpr, uses GABA, and is entirely inhibitory. The outputs from GPi and SNpr project to parts of the ventral anterior, ventral lateral, and mediodorsal thalamic nuclei. GPi and SNpr also project to the brainstem in the area of the pedunculopontine nucleus and to the intralaminar centromedian-parafascicular complex of the thalamus. A portion of the SNpr projects to the superior colliculus, where it contributes to eye movement control.

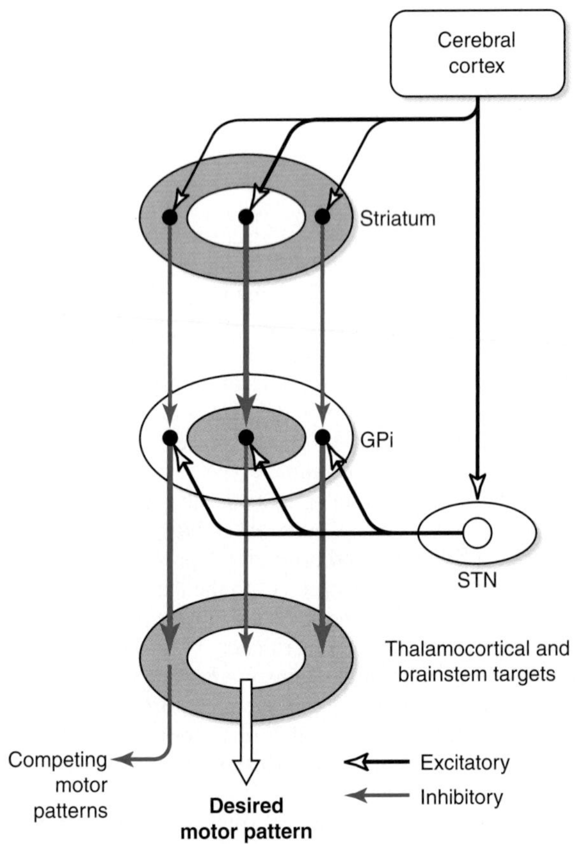

FIGURE 58-2. Model of the functional organization of basal ganglia output for selective facilitation and surround inhibition of competing motor patterns. Excitatory projections are indicated with *open arrows*; inhibitory projections are indicated with *filled arrows*. Relative magnitude of activity is represented by line thickness. GPi, globus pallidus internal segment; STN, subthalamic nucleus.

The output from basal ganglia to thalamocortical circuits appears to be segregated anatomically and possibly functionally. The thalamic targets of GPi and SNpr project, in turn, to frontal lobe, with the strongest output going to motor areas. The basal ganglia motor circuit has a somatotopic organization, with separate representation of different body parts maintained throughout the basal ganglia. There also appears to be relative segregation of motor from nonmotor basal ganglia circuits [Hoover and Strick, 1993].

A popular model of basal ganglia dysfunction in movement disorders was developed in the late 1980s (Fig. 58-3) [Albin et al., 1989, 1995; DeLong, 1990]. In simple terms, the model proposes that hypokinetic movement disorders (e.g., parkinsonism) can be distinguished from hyperkinetic movement disorders (e.g., chorea, dystonia, tics) based on the magnitude and pattern of the basal ganglia output neurons in GPi and SNpr [Wichmann and DeLong, 1996]. Because basal ganglia output neurons are inhibitory to thalamus and the pedunculopontine nucleus, their function is analogous to a braking mechanism such that increased activity inhibits and decreased activity facilitates motor pattern generators in cerebral cortex and brainstem [Mink, 1996]. As described earlier, the anatomic organization of the basal ganglia confers a pattern of focused facilitation and surround inhibition of motor mechanisms in thalamocortical and brainstem circuits (see Fig. 58-2). The normal function of this organization is to selectively facilitate desired movements and to inhibit potentially competing movements [Mink, 1996; Mink, 2003].

Basal Ganglia Pathophysiology in Movement Disorders

Basal ganglia dysfunction can occur on many levels. There can be destructive lesions of specific nuclei (e.g., infarction, hemorrhage, metabolic disorders) that may result in specific movement disorders. There can also be injury to multiple nuclei than may result in single or multiple movement disorders (e.g., hypoxia, carbon monoxide poisoning, metabolic disorders). Movement disorders can also be caused by loss of specific neuron types (e.g., Huntington's disease, Parkinson's disease) or by cellular dysfunction without neuronal death (e.g., DYT1 dystonia). As in other areas of neurology, lesion localization is important in movement disorders and may often provide important clues to guide an efficient evaluation and treatment plan.

Lesions in the striatum produce variable results that depend in part on the location of the lesion, in part on the lesion method, and in part on what is measured. Lesions in the caudate nucleus most commonly cause behavioral disturbance such as abulia but may also cause chorea or dystonia. Lesions in the putamen are likely to produce movement deficits and typically cause dystonia (most common) or parkinsonism [Bhatia and Marsden, 1994].

A unilateral subthalamic nucleus lesion is the classic cause of hemiballism; smaller amplitude chorea can also result from subthalamic nucleus lesions [Carpenter and Carpenter, 1951]. When bilateral, subthalamic nucleus lesions cause bilateral chorea or ballism. Most commonly, the

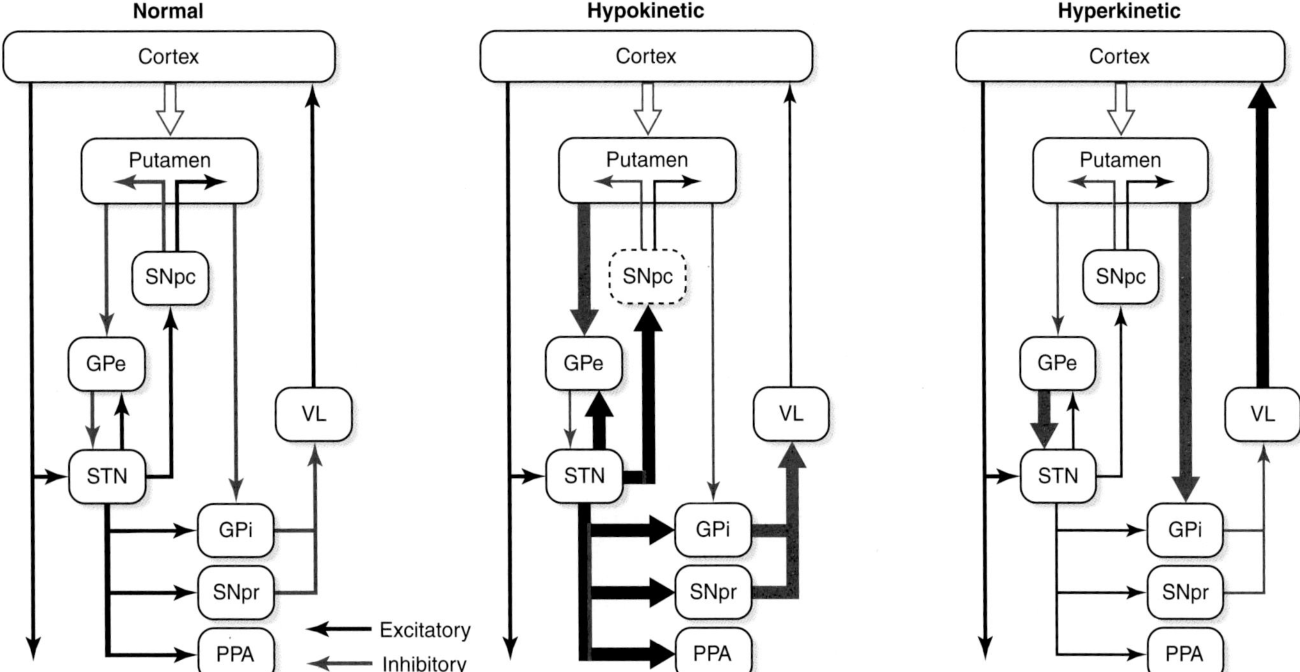

FIGURE 58-3. Summary of the main connections of the "motor circuit" of the basal ganglia and a model for the role of dopamine in hyperkinetic and hypokinetic disorders. In the normal state, the putamen receives afferents from the motor and somatosensory cortical areas and communicates with the globus pallidus internal segment (GPi)/substantia nigra reticulata (SNpr) through a direct inhibitory pathway and though a multisynaptic (globus pallidus external segment [GPe], subthalamic nucleus [STN]) indirect pathway. Dopamine is believed to modulate striatal activity, mainly by inhibiting the indirect and facilitating the direct pathways. In hypokinetic movement disorders, dopamine deficiency may lead to increased inhibitory activity from the putamen onto the GPe and disinhibition of the STN. STN hyperactivity produces excessive excitation of the GPi/SNr neurons, which overinhibit the thalamocortical and brainstem motor centers. In some hyperkinetic movement disorders, decreased activity of the STN may lead to disinhibition of the GPi output to the thalamocortical projection. PPA, pedunculopontine area; SNpc, substantia nigra compacta; VL, ventral lateral nucleus.(From Obeso JA, Rodriguez-Oroz MC, Rodriguez M, et al. The basal ganglia and disorders of movement: Pathophysiological mechanisms. News Physiol Sci 2002;17:51.)

chorea or hemiballism resulting from subthalamic nucleus lesions involves the lower extremities more than the upper extremities and can persist for days to months. The intensity of hemiballism usually diminishes over time. Lesions of globus pallidus usually involve GPe and GPi, GPe and putamen, or GPi and SNpr. Lesions involving globus pallidus can cause dystonia, parkinsonism, or both [Bhatia and Marsden, 1994; Heidenreich et al., 1988; Mink, 1996]. Chorea rarely accompanies globus pallidus lesions. Focal lesions of SNpr can cause involuntary eye movements [Hikosaka and Wurtz, 1985]. Lesion of SNpc dopamine neurons cause depletion of dopamine in the striatum, resulting in parkinsonism, dystonia, or both [Calne et al., 1997].

Focal basal ganglia lesions are uncommon in children. Movement disorders in children most likely result from global dysfunction of basal ganglia circuits. The model shown in Figure 58-3 has been used to explain the basis for hypokinetic and hyperkinetic movement disorders but does not distinguish among the different hyperkinetic movement disorders. However, based on what is known about these disorders and the underlying neural circuitry, specific models have been proposed [Mink, 2003]. Diseases affecting the basal ganglia cause movement disorders that can be understood as failure to facilitate desired movements (e.g., Parkinson's disease), failure to inhibit unwanted movements (e.g., chorea, dystonia, tics), or both [Albin et al., 1989; DeLong, 1990; Mink, 1996; Mink, 2003]. The involuntary movements of chorea, dystonia, and tics differ in important spatial and temporal characteristics that reflect important pathophysiologic differences. More extensive discussion of the neural basis of these disorders has been undertaken [Mink, 2003].

Etiology of Movement Disorders in Children

The etiology of movement disorders in children is extensive and is discussed further below. The most common cause of secondary disorders is likely to be cerebral palsy, with a prevalence of 2 per 1000. However, cerebral palsy itself represents a constellation of both injuries and symptoms, and there is a wide range of types of injury, localization, and combinations of symptoms [Surveillance of Cerebral Palsy in Europe, 2002]. Cerebral palsy can be associated with almost all forms of childhood movement disorders, and despite the lack of an ongoing destructive process, the clinical picture may change during development. The diagnosis and management of cerebral palsy are complex and are discussed in Chapter 20.

Specific types of movement disorders may represent injury to particular localized regions of the central nervous system [Sanger, 2003a]. Ataxia most likely results from injury to the cerebellum or its inflow and outflow [Taroni and DiDonato, 2004]. Bradykinesia most likely occurs with injury to the substantia nigra or striatum of the basal ganglia leading to either presynaptic or postsynaptic failure of dopaminergic transmission [Albin et al., 1989]. Chorea occurs in severe cortical injury or basal ganglia injury, particularly if the subthalamic nucleus is involved. Dystonia most likely involves injury to basal ganglia, but the possibility of cortical or cerebellar abnormalities cannot be excluded as contributors [Hallett, 1998; Sanger, 2003a]. Myoclonus most likely involves cortical, brainstem, or spinal injury to gray matter [Caviness and Brown, 2004]. The localization of tremor depends on the type, but some forms of tremor involve cerebellum or brainstem circuits [Jankovic et al., 2004; Uddin and Rodnitzky, 2003]. Tic disorders probably involve an abnormality of the basal ganglia, but cortical mechanisms may also contribute [Mink, 2001a].

Approach to Treatment

Treatment of childhood movement disorders is based primarily on symptomatology independent of the underlying cause. When a specific treatment for the underlying cause is available, certainly this should be applied, but in many cases such treatment is only partly effective. The goal of symptomatic treatment is to break the connection between the pathophysiology and the expression of clinical impairment.

It is essential to ask both the child and the parents for the most significant cause of disability. In some children, the impairment that is most evident to the clinician is not the primary cause of disability. Sometimes treatment of the functional limitation or direct treatment of a disability is more effective, less time-consuming, and less risky than attempts to treat the underlying pathophysiology, and therefore it is essential to be certain that any treatment addresses the needs and goals of the child and family. In particular, it is usually neither necessary nor possible to treat all symptoms. It is most helpful to pick specific goals and to monitor progress toward those goals. In many cases, a team approach has been found to be helpful, particularly when there are multiple impairments leading to disability, and the team approach allows appropriate focusing and selection of interventions. In some individuals, a supportive environment and adaptive equipment are more effective than any medical intervention.

CLASSIFICATION OF CHILDHOOD MOVEMENT DISORDERS

The first step to diagnosing and treating a movement disorder is to define the disorder (see Table 58-1). Individual names of movement disorders can refer to neurologic signs or to neurologic syndromes or diseases, which can cause some confusion. In this section, the definitions are limited to the neurologic signs to which they refer. Subsequent sections present a more complete discussion of the syndromes and diseases in which the different signs are seen either alone or in combination with other signs.

The most common movement disorder in the pediatric population is the group of tic disorders. The prevalence of tic disorders in schoolchildren may be as high as 25% [Snider et al., 2002]. Most tic disorders are not severe, and the level of morbidity is low. Nevertheless, because of the lack of association with other neurologic symptoms, it is not unreasonable to consider a tic disorder as a primary disorder in idiopathic cases. There are rare exceptions in which tics are due to secondary disorders, such as brain injury or neuroacanthocytosis.

Dystonia is a relatively prevalent disorder in children, most likely because of its incidence in cerebral palsy. Dystonia as the primary symptom in cerebral palsy is less common, but dystonia as a complicating factor, particularly in the upper extremities of children with cerebral palsy otherwise characterized by weakness or spasticity, is probably more common. The incidence and classification of cerebral palsy are discussed in Chapter 20.

In contrast to adults, task-specific dystonia, or occupational cramps, is not seen in younger children. Certainly focal dystonias do occur, but the task specificity seems to be a consequence of practiced skill, which would not be expected to present in the early childhood years. The incidence of parkinsonism, including bradykinesia and rigidity, is unknown in children and probably underreported. However, it is likely that parkinsonism is less common in children, given that its primary cause in adults is dopaminergic failure, whereas disorders known to cause failure of dopamine transmission in children more commonly present as dystonia.

Choreoathetosis is a term that has been applied to a specific subset of children with a dyskinetic form of cerebral palsy. This term is not generally used in adults. It is not known whether choreoathetosis represents a form of dystonia, chorea, or an entirely different disorder [Turny et al., 2004]. Choreoathetotic cerebral palsy is an easily recognized syndrome, and because many of these children also possess some degree of dystonia, as well as chorea, choreoathetosis may simply be the expression of a combination of other movement disorders [Morris et al., 2002b]. Spasticity and weakness are very common in childhood motor disorders, again owing to the higher prevalence of cerebral palsy. However, these are not discussed further in this chapter.

Hypotonia, or decreased muscle tone, is a disorder that appears to be unique to children and is not traditionally classified as a movement disorder, although it may be associated with movement disorders. Certainly flaccid paralysis is described in adults, but the particular picture of a generalized hypotonia without significant weakness, or disproportionate to the degree of weakness, seems to occur only in young children, generally younger than 2 years. In many cases, hypotonia is associated with abnormalities of cerebellar development or cerebellar injury, and many of these children subsequently develop ataxia. Therefore, it is possible to hypothesize that hypotonia may be the early childhood or infantile expression of cerebellar disease, whereas ataxia is the later childhood, juvenile, or adult expression of cerebellar disease.

Chorea

Chorea describes an apparently random, nonrhythmic, purposeless set of movements of either distal or proximal muscles that appears to flow from one muscle or muscle group to another without any evident pattern. Chorea occurs at rest and with action and gives the child a "fidgety" appearance and the inability to hold still. It is associated with motor impersistence (e.g., the inability to maintain the tongue extended). Chorea may worsen or improve with voluntary movement, but even very severe chorea may not prevent accurate voluntary movement for some children, suggesting that compensatory mechanisms exist. Many individuals with chorea incorporate the involuntary movements into a voluntary movement to mask the impairment. However, the involuntary movements can lead to significant disability, and some children will injure themselves or others as a result of rapid ballistic flinging movements of the arms or legs. Tone is normal or reduced in pure chorea, but in children chorea may occur in the presence of hypertonic disorders including dystonia. As with most movement disorders, chorea disappears in sleep, but it may be at its worst when the child is drowsy. The term *choreiform* is often used to describe the minimal twitching or "piano playing" movements seen in many normal young children when arms are extended during the neurologic examination. The movements of chorea are briefer than the sustained muscle contractions seen in dystonia and are longer in duration than the shocklike movements of myoclonus [Marsden et al., 1983].

Primary Chorea

HUNTINGTON'S DISEASE

Huntington's disease is autosomal dominant, caused by a trinucleotide repeat expansion within the *IT-15* gene on chromosome 4 [Li et al., 1993]. This disorder is characterized by a combination of dystonia, chorea, myoclonus, behavioral abnormalities, ataxia, and ultimately dementia. When Huntington's disease begins in childhood, the typical presentation is dystonia and rigidity, and not chorea. This has been referred to as the *Westphal variant of Huntington's disease* [Quinn and Schrag, 1998; Topper et al., 1998]. The age of onset is earlier for children with a higher number of repeats [Langbehn et al., 2004]. There tends to be amplification of the number of repeats, particularly when it is transmitted from father to child, and therefore most cases of juvenile Huntington's disease are inherited from the father and involve repeat lengths that are significantly higher than those seen in adults.

Diagnosis is based on identification of the trinucleotide repeat sequence. Although at least 38 repeats are usually required for the occurrence of symptoms in adults, a larger number of repeats would be expected when symptoms present in childhood [Langbehn et al., 2004; Quinn and Schrag, 1998]. Magnetic resonance imaging (MRI) reveals atrophy of the caudate heads and, in later stages, generalized cerebral and cerebellar atrophy.

In teenagers, the initial presentation of Huntington's disease may be with psychiatric illness, and in particular, major depression may be the presenting symptom [Tost et al., 2004]. Dystonia or chorea supervenes later. The pathology includes basal ganglia, cerebellar, and cortical degeneration [de la Monte et al., 1988; Myers et al., 1988; Vonsattel et al., 1985]. The origin of the chorea has been hypothesized to be a primary loss of medium spiny cells in the striatum that bear D2-like receptors [Deng et al., 2004]. In children, there may be a relatively symmetric loss of D1-bearing and D2-bearing medium spiny neurons, which could account for the primarily dystonic rather than choreatic presentation [Albin et al., 1990; Augood et al., 1997].

Treatment of Huntington's chorea in adults is typically based on modification of the chorea or myoclonus. Because the chorea has been presumed to be due to loss of medium spiny neurons in the indirect pathway, neuroleptic medications have been most frequently used in the adult population [Bonelli and Hofmann, 2004; Bonelli et al., 2004]. Neuroleptic agents would be expected to partially compensate for early loss of indirect pathway neurons by blocking the inhibitory effects of dopamine and thereby disinhibiting the remaining neurons. There is much less experience in children, in whom dystonia and rigidity may be greater contributors to disability. Other medications that have been used successfully in Huntington's disease include tetrabenazine [Asher and Aminoff, 1981; Ondo et al., 2002], clonazepam [Thompson et al., 1994], and valproic acid [Grove et al., 2000]. There is currently no treatment that modifies the progression of the disease.

Prognosis is poor for childhood-onset Huntington's disease, and the movement disorder is expected to worsen progressively over the years after diagnosis. Life expectancy depends on the severity of symptoms and the number of repeats, but typically children will survive 10 to 15 years from the time of diagnosis.

ATAXIA-TELANGIECTASIA

Despite the name of this disorder, ataxia is not always the presenting finding, and ataxia may be a much less prominent early symptom than upper extremity chorea (see Chapter 57). However, the chorea is usually less disabling than the ataxia. Other symptoms associated with ataxia-telangiectasia include dystonia, which is often proximal [Bodensteiner et al., 1980]. Ataxia-telangiectasia (Louis-Bar syndrome) is most commonly due to mutations in the *ATM* (ataxia-telangiectasia mutated) gene on chromosome 11q22-23 [Chun and Gatti, 2004; Coutinho et al., 2004; Gatti et al., 1998]. Mutation in this gene leads to decreased inhibition of cell cycling in the context of injury to nuclear DNA, and this leads to an accumulation of mutations at known "hot spots," including translocations between regions on chromosome 7 and 14 known to be involved with immune function [Farina et al., 1994]. Therefore, one of the cardinal features of this disorder is a history of frequent sinopulmonary infections [Centerwall and Miller, 1958], which requires very close attention to pulmonary function and aggressive treatment of pulmonary infections at all ages. In later stages of the disorder, hematologic malignancy may occur [Stankovic et al., 1998]. Children with ataxia-telangiectasia may be particularly vulnerable to injury from ionizing radiation and certain chemotherapy agents, and this must be taken into consideration in planning any treatment for malignancy.

The cause of the cerebellar degeneration is discussed further in Chapter 57. The pathology suggests a characteristic loss of Purkinje cells, such that by late stages in the disease, Purkinje cells are often completely absent. The cause of the chorea is not known, and basal ganglia pathology is minimal. Eye movement disorders are well described and include an inability to suppress and an inability to initiate saccades [Bundey, 1994; Lewis et al., 1999]. The inability to initiate saccades leads to a characteristic finding of oculomotor apraxia, in which a child will use thrusts of the head to position the eyes on the target. Diagnosis is based on laboratory testing, including decreased immunoglobulin G2 and immunoglobulin A, abnormalities in T-cell subsets, elevated α-fetoprotein, increased lymphocyte radiosensitivity, and decreased radiation-induced mitotic suppression [Stray-Pedersen et al., 2004]. Treatment of this disorder is primarily supportive, although there are isolated reports of dystonic symptoms responding to either trihexyphenidyl or levodopa. The chorea generally is mild and does not require specific treatment. There is no known treatment for the ataxia.

Ataxia–oculomotor apraxia is an autosomal-recessive disorder with similar motor symptoms caused in some cases by mutations in the aprataxin gene *AOA-1* [Moreira et al., 2001; Shimazaki et al., 2002; Tranchant et al., 2003]. This disorder commonly presents with chorea, ataxia, and oculomotor apraxia [Sano et al., 2004]. It is most prevalent in Japan and Europe. *AOA-1* does not seem to be involved with cell cycle regulation, and therefore the DNA breakage, immune abnormalities, and malignancies seen in ataxia-telangiectasia do not occur. These patients have hypoalbuminemia [Shimazaki et al., 2002]. The long-term prognosis is considerably better than for ataxia-telangiectasia.

OTHER PRIMARY CHOREAS

Other primary causes of chorea include familial benign hereditary chorea [Breedveld et al., 2002a; Kleiner-Fisman et al., 2003], which is an autosomal-dominant disorder that in some cases is due to mutations in the *TITF-1* gene on chromosome 14 [Breedveld et al., 2002b]. Affected family members have normal or near-normal intelligence, and chorea is often the only complaint, although mild truncal dystonia and gait ataxia have been reported [Fernandez et al., 2001]. The severity of chorea can vary among different affected family members. Symptomatic treatment may yield some mild benefit.

Neuroacanthocytosis is also a potential cause of chorea [Marson et al., 2003], although classification as a primary or secondary chorea is not universally agreed on.

Secondary Chorea

There is a very long list of secondary causes of chorea in children, and these can be divided into several categories. The categories and disorders are summarized in Table 58-2.

SYDENHAM'S CHOREA

Of the secondary causes of chorea in children, Sydenham's chorea is the most common [Garvey and Swedo, 1997; Jordan and Singer, 2003; Jummani and Okun, 2001]. It has onset weeks or months after an acute infection with group A β-hemolytic streptococcus and is one of the cardinal symptoms of rheumatic fever (see Chapter 73). Symptoms may persist for weeks or months, but chorea almost always resolves spontaneously within 6 months [Jordan and Singer, 2003], although there have been a few reported cases of continued or recurring symptoms [Faustino et al., 2003]. The chorea is typically described involving distal musculature of the hands with a "piano playing" pattern, but other forms of chorea, including ballism, have been observed. Large generalized body movements in some patients previously inspired the term *St. Vitus's dance.*

Anti–basal ganglia antibodies are found in some children [Church et al., 2002], and it has been hypothesized that production of these antibodies is triggered because of molecular mimicry by streptococcal antigens [Goldenberg et al., 1992; Kirvan et al., 2003; Loiselle and Singer, 2001; Singer et al., 2003]. Anti–basal ganglia antibodies can be detected

TABLE 58-2

Causes of Chorea

Static Injury, Structural
Cerebral palsy, stroke, trauma, moyamoya disease, vasculitis, tumors, congenital malformations, Joubert's syndrome
Hereditary, Degenerative
Ataxia-telangiectasia, ataxia ocular motor apraxia (includes AOA-1 and early-onset cerebellar ataxia and hypoalbuminemia, EOCA-HA), Fahr's disease, pantothenate kinase–associated neurodegeneration (PKAN associated with mutations in *PANK-2*, the pantothenate kinase-2 gene), Huntington-disease–like disorder type 2 (associated with mutation in junctophilin), Rett's syndrome, HARP syndrome (hypoprebetalipoproteinemia, acanthocytosis, retinitis pigmentosa, and pallidal degeneration)
Metabolic Disease
Acyl–coenzyme-A dehydrogenase deficiency, mitochondrial disorders, including Leigh's syndrome, Wilson's disease, GM1 gangliosidosis, metachromatic leukodystrophy, Lesch-Nyhan disease, Niemann-Pick type C, methylmalonic aciduria, nonketotic hyperglycinemia, Pelizaeus-Merzbacher disease (now classified as a form of hereditary spastic paraparesis), kernicterus, hypoparathyroidism, hyperthyroidism, propionic acidemia, hypernatremia, hypomagnesemia, hypocalcemia, hypoglycemia or hyperglycemia, vitamin E deficiency or malabsorption, Bassen-Kornzweig disease, and complications of cardiac bypass
Infectious, Parainfectious
Encephalitis and postencephalitis
Immune Mediated
Sydenham's chorea, lupus erythematosus, Henoch-Schönlein purpura, anticardiolipin or antiphospholipid antibody syndrome, chorea gravidarum
Drugs, Toxins
Neuroleptic medications, including antiemetics (haloperidol, chlorpromazine [Thorazine], pimozide, prochlorperazine [Compazine], metoclopramide), calcium channel blockers (flunarizine, cinnarizine), antiseizure medications (phenytoin, carbamazepine, valproate, phenobarbital), anticholinergic medications (trihexyphenidyl, benztropine), antihistamines, tricyclic antidepressants, clomipramine, benzodiazepines, stimulants (including methylphenidate, dextroamphetamine, pemoline, and bronchodilators), clonidine, levodopa, cocaine, bismuth, lithium, manganese, ethanol, carbon monoxide, oral contraceptives, general anesthesia (including propofol)
Paroxysmal Disorders
Complex migraine, alternating hemiplegia, paroxysmal kinesigenic choreoathetosis (PKC), paroxysmal nonkinesigenic choreoathetosis (PNKC, or paroxysmal dystonic choreoathetosis [PDC], or Mount and Reback disease), paroxysmal choreoathetosis and spasticity, paroxysmal exercise-induced choreoathetosis (PEC)
Physiologic Chorea
This is seen in normal development before 1 year of age.
Disorders That Mimic Chorea
Spasmus nutans, tics, shaking and shuddering spells, proprioceptive loss, masturbation, psychogenic disorders

in cerebrospinal fluid [Singer et al., 2003], and antistreptolysin antibodies can be detected in serum. However, the high prevalence of positive antistreptolysin antibody titers in the general population means that both acute and convalescent titers must be measured to confirm an acute infection. The clinical situation often provides a strong indication for the diagnosis, but if other neurologic symptoms are present or there is doubt about etiology, a more complete evaluation may be needed, including tests for thyroid function, toxins, metabolic disorders, or encephalitis.

Sydenham's chorea usually does not require treatment, although the acute streptococcal infection should be treated to reduce the incidence of rheumatic fever. Valproic acid, carbamazepine, or neuroleptics may have some benefit [Genel et al., 2002; Kulkarni and Anees, 1996; Pena et al., 2002]. Treatment with immune suppressant medication, including corticosteroids or intravenous immunoglobulin preparations, has been studied, but the natural history with spontaneous resolution of symptoms makes interpretation of efficacy in open-label clinical trials difficult [Cardoso et al., 2003; Garvey and Swedo, 1997; Green, 1978]. Long-term treatment with antibiotics may reduce the low risk for recurrence [Gebremariam, 1999]. There are sometimes associated obsessive-compulsive or behavioral symptoms [Moore, 1996; Wilcox and Nasrallah, 1988], and these symptoms are often managed with selective serotonin reuptake inhibitors. Acute streptococcal illness needs to be treated, and prolonged antibiotic prophylaxis is usually needed in cases of rheumatic fever. The prognosis for the movement disorder is excellent, and complete resolution occurs in most cases. Recurrence is rare and is sometimes associated with recurrence of other symptoms of rheumatic fever [Korn-Lubetzki et al., 2004]. There appears to be a higher risk for chorea gravidarum in women with a previous history of Sydenham's chorea [Korn-Lubetzki et al., 2004].

The rapid onset of Sydenham's chorea has raised the question of whether an autoimmune mechanism could be responsible for other acute-onset movement disorders. This has led to the hypothesis of pediatric autoimmune neuropsychiatric disorders associated with streptococcus (PANDAS) [March, 2004; Trifiletti and Packard, 1999]. PANDAS are characterized by an abrupt or explosive onset of tics, obsessive-compulsive behavior, and a movement disorder (usually chorea) that is temporally associated with streptococcal infection [Chmelik et al., 2004; Pavone et al., 2004; Snider and Swedo, 2004; Swedo, 2002]. Symptoms may persist with a relapsing and remitting course. The existence of this disorder has been debated [Kurlan, 2004; Kurlan and Kaplan, 2004; Singer and Loiselle, 2003; Swedo et al., 2004], and anti–basal ganglia antibodies have not been found to be elevated [Singer et al., 2004]. It has not been possible to transmit the disorder passively to animals by inoculation with antibodies from affected humans [Loiselle et al., 2004]. Nevertheless, there have been an increasing number of case reports of explosive onset of neurobehavioral disorders, including tic disorders, chorea, and obsessive-compulsive disorder, after streptococcal infections, and therefore the hypothesis merits further investigation. It is not clear that there is any specific treatment, although some authors advocate immune modulation, long-term antibiotics, or tonsillectomy [Araujo et al., 2002; Gebremariam, 1999; Green, 1978; Heubi and Shott, 2003; Leonard and Swedo, 2001; van Toorn et al., 2004].

MEDICATION-INDUCED CHOREA

Chorea is frequently associated with administration of medications, and any child with chorea needs to be carefully examined for the possibility of iatrogenic causes. In particular, treatment of other movement disorders with anticholinergic medication such as trihexyphenidyl can precipitate chorea, even at relatively low doses [Nomoto et al., 1987]. Antiepileptic medications, including carbamazepine and phenytoin, have been associated with precipitation of chorea, and in children with diffuse brain injury, sedating medications can sometimes precipitate chorea.

Chorea can appear as a tardive symptom many months after being on a medication, or after discontinuing a medication. Tardive chorea is probably less common than tardive dystonia or dyskinesia, but it nevertheless does occur, and the onset of chorea, even many months or years after being treated with neuroleptic or anticholinergic medications, should raise suspicion of a tardive medication effect. There is a more complete description of tardive syndromes later in this chapter.

CHOREA ASSOCIATED WITH BRAIN INJURY

Chorea is frequently seen in children with cerebral palsy on awakening or when drowsy. A common form of more persistent chorea that can last several months often follows encephalitis. In particular, children with encephalitis, in many cases, develop a severe and persistent chorea within several weeks of recovery from the acute phase of the illness. This chorea often lasts 6 to 12 months. It may respond to treatment with benzodiazepines, including clonazepam, or valproic acid. It does not appear to respond to other antichorea treatments, such as neuroleptic medication or tetrabenazine. Whether treatment of the chorea hastens its improvement or in any way alters the natural course is not known, but treatment may help with feeding and rehabilitation.

A severe form of chorea or ballism can occur in children with cerebral palsy or other static brain injury after the onset of an otherwise unremarkable febrile illness. Often there is a combination of chorea and dystonia, and this syndrome is described below in the section on dystonic storm.

CHOREA ASSOCIATED WITH SYSTEMIC ILLNESS

Hyperthyroidism can be a cause of chorea, and any child with unexplained acute or persistent chorea should have serum testing for thyroid function. The mechanism is unknown. It should be noted that the *TITF-1* gene responsible for benign hereditary chorea is a transcription factor involved with both thyroid and basal ganglia development, although in this disorder thyroid function is reduced.

Autoimmune diseases including lupus erythematosus and antiphospholipid antibody syndromes can be a cause of chorea, possibly through an autoimmune mechanism. In such cases, treatment should be directed at the underlying autoimmune disorder. This class of disorders may be a relatively common cause of chorea in children, and it is particularly important because of the potential for response to treatment.

Ballism

Ballism is a high-amplitude, flinging movement, usually due to involuntary movements of proximal joints. Ballism is part of the spectrum of chorea and involves similar pathophysiologic mechanisms [Albin et al., 1989; DeLong, 1990]. When ballism involves one side of the body, it is called *hemiballism*. Hemiballism is the classic manifestation of vascular events affecting the subthalamic nucleus but can be associated with lesions in other parts of the basal ganglia.

Treatment of Chorea

Chorea is often difficult to treat. Secondary chorea may respond to a combination of clonazepam and valproic acid. Sedation may be helpful for short-term management. In some cases, tetrabenazine [Asher and Aminoff, 1981; Chatterjee and Frucht, 2003; Jankovic and Orman, 1988], reserpine, or neuroleptics may be helpful, but the use of neuroleptics requires caution because chorea may mask the onset of tardive dyskinesia or tardive dystonia. If dystonia is present with chorea, then neuroleptics should be used only with great caution because of their ability to precipitate acute or tardive dystonia and the potential for worsening dystonia owing to dopaminergic failure. Trihexyphenidyl, levodopa, carbamazepine, and phenytoin can worsen chorea and should be avoided in most cases. Chorea that is due to global cerebral injury, such as that following encephalitis, may worsen when the child is sleepy, and therefore sedating medications should be avoided if possible, although clonazepam is sometimes helpful. Some forms of chorea are time limited and may only require brief treatment. It is possible that there may be a role for deep brain stimulation in some forms [Thompson et al., 2000]. Before any treatment for chorea, it is important to evaluate the child's current medications to rule out an iatrogenic cause.

Dystonia

Dystonia is probably the next most common movement disorder in children after tics. This prevalence is because dystonia can occur as an associated feature in many static and degenerative childhood disorders. In children, dystonia is defined as "a movement disorder in which involuntary sustained or intermittent muscle contractions cause twisting and repetitive movements, abnormal postures, or both" [Fahn and Williams, 1988; Sanger et al., 2003]. Although the term seems to imply an abnormality of tone, dystonia is not primarily a disorder of tone, but rather a disorder of movement. When individuals with dystonia are at rest, tone is often diminished, although in severe dystonia, involuntary contractions persist during attempted rest, and tone may be increased. Dystonia can manifest as hypertonic dystonia with increased stiffness, hyperkinetic dystonia with increased movements, or a combination of the two. Dystonia can also be reflected in very slow twisting or writhing movements or very quick ballistic movements, and it can have rhythmicity, appearing like tremor, in which case it would be referred to as *dystonic tremor*.

Dystonia is commonly triggered or exacerbated by voluntary movement, and it may fluctuate in presence and severity over minutes, weeks, or months. Dystonia can be task or movement specific, so that a muscle may exhibit involuntary contraction only during certain voluntary movements and not others. For example, walking forward may elicit severe lower extremity and truncal twisting, yet walking backward, running, or swimming may be completely unaffected. Stress or excitement exacerbates most forms of dystonia. Dystonic contractions resolve during sleep. Individuals with dystonia sometimes discover that touching one part of the body may relieve the dystonic spasms; this phenomenon is called a *sensory trick* or *geste antagoniste*. Dystonia may be generalized or focal, involving just a single body part. Childhood-onset dystonia is more likely to be generalized than adult dystonia [Bressman et al., 1994]. Task-specific dystonia in which symptoms occur only during performance of a specific skilled action does not occur commonly in children, although focal dystonia that affects one part of the body during many actions certainly is seen.

Classification

Dystonia is classified by etiology as either primary or secondary, and by location as focal, segmental, hemidystonia, multifocal, or generalized dystonia [Fahn et al., 1998]. Focal dystonia involves a single part of the body such as a limb, the neck, or the face. Examples include blepharospasm (forceful eye closure), oromandibular dystonia (involving the jaw or mouth musculature, or both), spasmodic dysphonia (vocal cord involvement), torticollis (twisting or tilting of the neck), or focal hand or foot dystonia. Segmental dystonia involves the muscles of two contiguous body parts, for example, cranial segmental dystonia involving multiple muscles of the face and neck, axial dystonia involving the neck and trunk, brachial dystonia involving the arm and trunk, and crural dystonia involving one or both legs and the trunk. Hemidystonia involves all or most muscles on one side of the body. Multifocal dystonia involves two or more noncontiguous body regions. Generalized dystonia involves multiple limbs on both sides of the body including at least one leg.

In children, dystonia often starts distally, and it may initially involve only a hand or foot. Typical patterns include spooning deformity of the fingers, with forceful extension at the metacarpal-phalangeal and interphalangeal joints of the hand, or a combination of inversion (supination) and extension of the ankle. An upgoing "striatal toe" is a common finding that is often confused with the Babinski sign but that seems to be due to extrapyramidal dysfunction. Proximal forms of dystonia include opisthotonus (arching), truncal sway, side bending, twisting of the neck, and proximal fixed postures or random movements of the large muscles of the legs or arms. Orofacial movements include dysarthria, involuntary tongue protrusion, involuntary jaw opening or closing, blinking, and facial contortions.

Dystonia is considered primary when it is the predominant or only clinical feature (Table 58-3). At least 17 different inherited phenotypes designated with the "DYT" genetic locus specification have been defined so far [Bressman, 2004; Misbahuddin and Warner, 2001; Nishiyama et al., 2000]. Most of these are quite rare. Only seven

TABLE 58-3

Causes of Dystonia

Static Injury, Structural
Cerebral palsy, hypoxic-ischemic injury, kernicterus, head trauma, encephalitis, tumors, stroke in the basal ganglia (which may be due to vascular abnormalities or varicella), congenital malformations
Hereditary, Degenerative
DYT1 (9q34, encodes torsin-A), DYT2 (autosomal recessive), DYT3 (X-linked dystonia-parkinsonism syndrome of Lubag-Xq13), DYT4, DYT5 (14q22.1-2, encodes GTP cyclohydrolase I, leading to dopa-responsive dystonia or Segawa's disease), DYT6 (8p21-q22), DYT7 (18p), DYT8 (2q33-q35, causing paroxysmal nonkinesigenic choreoathetosis [PNKC]), DYT9 (1p, causing PNKD and spasticity), DYT10 (16p11.2-q12.1, causing paroxysmal kinesigenic choreoathetosis [PKC]), DYT11 (heterogeneous, causing familial myoclonus-dystonia). Rapid-onset dystonia-parkinsonism (linked to chromosome 19), Fahr's disease (often due to hypoparathyroid disease), pantothenate kinase–associated neurodegeneration (PKAN, neuronal brain iron accumulation type 1, formerly Hallervorden-Spatz disease, sometimes due to mutations in pantothenate-kinase-2 [*PANK-2*]), Huntington's disease (particularly the Westphal variant, IT15-4p16.3), spinocerebellar ataxias (SCAs), including SCA3/Machado-Joseph disease, neuronal ceroid lipofuscinoses (NCL), Rett's syndrome, striatal necrosis, Leigh's disease, neuroacanthocytosis, HARP syndrome (hypoprebetalipoproteinemia, acanthocytosis, retinitis pigmentosa, and pallidal degeneration), ataxia-telangiectasia, Tay-Sachs disease, Sandhoff's disease, Niemann-Pick type C, GM1 gangliosidosis, metachromatic leukodystrophy (MLD), Lesch-Nyhan disease
Metabolic Disease
Glutaric aciduria types 1 and 2, acyl coenzyme A dehydrogenase deficiency, dopa-responsive dystonia (tyrosine hydroxylase deficiency, GTP cyclohydrolase 1 deficiency, DYT5), dopamine agonist–responsive dystonia (aromatic L-amino acid decarboxylase deficiency [ALAD]), mitochondrial disorders, Wilson's disease, vitamin E deficiency, homocystinuria, methylmalonic aciduria, tyrosinemia
Drugs, Toxins
Neuroleptic and antiemetic medications (haloperidol, chlorpromazine [Thorazine], olanzapine, risperidone, prochlorperazine [Compazine]), calcium channel blockers, stimulants (amphetamine, cocaine, ergot alkaloids), anticonvulsants (carbamazepine, phenytoin), thallium, manganese, carbon monoxide, ethylene glycol, cyanide, methanol, wasp sting
Paroxysmal
PKC, PNKC, exercise-induced dystonia, complex migraine, alternating hemiplegia of childhood (AHC), paroxysmal torticollis of infancy
Disorders That Mimic Dystonia
Tonic seizures (including paroxysmal nocturnal dystonia caused by nocturnal frontal lobe seizures), Arnold-Chiari malformation type II, atlantoaxial subluxation, syringomyelia, posterior fossa mass, cervical spine malformation (including Klippel-Feil syndrome), skew deviation with vertical diplopia causing neck twisting, juvenile rheumatoid arthritis, Sandifer's syndrome (associated with hiatus hernia in infants), spasmus nutans, tics, masturbation, spasticity, myotonia, rigidity, stiff-person syndrome, Isaac's syndrome (neuromyotonia), startle disease (hyperekplexia), neuroleptic malignant syndrome, central herniation with posturing, psychogenic dystonia

of the genes have been identified. Many of these disorders do not present in childhood. Many of these disorders represent "dystonia-plus" syndromes that include dystonia as a primary feature but also have other associated movement disorders. Examples of dystonia-plus syndromes include dopa-responsive dystonia, myoclonus dystonia, and rapid-onset dystonia-parkinsonism.

Diagnosis

Dystonia must be distinguished from other disorders, including spasticity, rigidity, tics, tremor, and ataxia, although in some cases this is difficult. Spasticity is associated with increased reflexes and frequently has a spastic catch whose position depends on the velocity of movement [Sanger et al., 2003]. Rigidity does not tend to have a particular fixed posture; it has a "lead pipe" quality and resists attempts at passive movement of the arm or leg, although the limb can be placed into an arbitrary posture by the examiner [Sanger et al., 2003]. Tics can be differentiated by their episodic and repeatable nature and normal posture and function between tics. In addition, tics rarely have the same degree of motor disability as is seen in dystonia. Dystonic tremor tends to be less rhythmic than regular tremor, and often exhibits a "null point," in which there exists a particular joint angle at which the tremor decreases or is absent [Deuschl, 2003]. To one side of that joint angle, movement in one direction will cause the tremor to worsen, but often beating in a particular direction that is different from the direction in which the tremor will beat if the joint is moved in the opposite direction. Ataxia does not have characteristic postures, it does not have overflow of muscle activity, and quality of movement may improve at slow speeds [Paulson and Ammache, 2001].

Dystonic Storm

A particularly dramatic presentation of dystonia that is seen primarily in children with preexisting motor abnormalities is dystonic storm [Dalvi et al., 1998; Opal et al., 2002]. Usually this is seen in the context of an acute illness in a child with a previous history of dystonia, cerebral palsy, or other movement disorder. The child will become ill with an otherwise unremarkable disease such as a respiratory illness but then will rapidly develop severe and intractable hyperkinetic dystonia with ballistic or flinging movements of the arms, legs, or head. This dystonia can also be associated with severe limb extension or opisthotonic posturing with dorsiflexion at the neck or trunk. In many cases, these symptoms will not have been seen previously. In some cases, this clinical picture is associated with encephalitis or other causes of acute striatal injury. Treatment is extremely difficult and may require general anesthesia to abate the movement. Multiple medications have been tried, including benzodiazepines, levodopa, anticholinergic medications, tetrabenazine, reserpine, dantrolene, and baclofen. It is possible that intrathecal baclofen [Dalvi et al., 1998] or deep brain stimulation [Angelini et al., 2000] could be helpful in severe cases when medications are ineffective [Kyriagis et al., 2004]. Dystonic storm can continue for months and can be life-threatening, usually requiring intensive care monitoring. It can recur in the context of a subsequent illness.

Associated Movement Disorders

Athetosis literally means "not fixed," which refers to the continuous writhing movements that characterize this disorder [Morris et al., 2002b]. Athetotic movements are often caused or worsened by attempts at voluntary movement. In this respect, athetosis is very similar to dystonia, and particular dystonic postures of the arms or hands can occur simultaneously. The use of the term *athetosis* has diminished substantially in recent years. It has been argued that in most cases, athetosis is actually a form of dystonia [Turny et al., 2004]. Currently, the term is used most commonly to describe a form of cerebral palsy (athetoid) but is also used in conjunction with the term *chorea* (choreoathetosis) to describe the apparent random and hyperkinetic quality of the movements [Morris et al., 2002a].

Dystonia in children is frequently associated with bradykinesia [Nygaard and Duvoisin, 1986], possibly because both dystonia and bradykinesia can be caused by failure of dopamine transmission [Riederer and Foley, 2002; Segawa et al., 1999]. Bradykinesia may be a relatively common finding in children with hypertonic disorders, but it is likely to be underreported because the slow movement may be attributed to the hypertonia rather than to the underlying bradykinesia.

Primary Dystonias

DYT1 DYSTONIA

DYT1 dystonia is known as *Oppenheim's dystonia* after Hermann Oppenheim, who first described it in 1911. It has also been referred to as *dystonia musculorum deformans*, which was Oppenheim's original term. This is probably the most common genetically determined cause of dystonia in children. In some populations, this is the most common explanation for dystonia with onset in the foot before the age of 20 years [Klein et al., 1999; O'Riordan et al., 2004]. The median age at onset is 10 years, with a range of 4 years to adulthood. Usually onset is in a lower extremity, but upper extremity onset has been described. The general features include a gradually progressive dystonia that eventually involves multiple limbs and progresses to generalized dystonia, often involving both distal and proximal musculature [Bressman et al., 2002]. However, there is great variation in the progression and severity. When DYT1 dystonia presents in adulthood, it is usually mild.

DYT1 dystonia is autosomal dominant, but it has about 30% penetrance [Saunders-Pullman et al., 2004b]. Recent evidence suggests that nonmanifesting carriers do have abnormalities of brain networks on fluorodeoxyglucose positron-emission tomography, but the reason that they do not express symptoms of the disease is currently not known [Eidelberg et al., 1998]. The gene is on chromosome 9Q34, and its product is torsin-A [Bressman et al., 1994; Ozelius et al., 1999]. Torsin-A is an adenosine triphosphate–binding protein with homology to heat shock and chaperone proteins [Ozelius et al., 1997]. The homology to heat shock proteins has been proposed as a possible explanation for the onset of symptoms after injury, surgery, or other situations in which such proteins would be expected to be expressed. The common deletion is a three-base-pair GAG deletion, resulting in loss of a single glutamate from a highly conserved region of the protein [Ozelius et al., 1999]. This mutation seems to have arisen independently from founders in different populations. The prevalence of manifesting DYT1 dystonia is higher in Ashkenazi Jews, for whom it is about 1 in 5000. The general population has a rate of 1 in 15,000 worldwide, but there may be other groups for whom higher prevalence occurs.

There are very little data on pathology, and many of the early pathologic reports did not detect abnormalities. More recent reports suggest that there may be some abnormalities in brainstem nuclei, but no specific abnormalities of the dopaminergic or basal ganglia systems have been found. Gene testing is currently available for the common GAG deletion.

DYT1 dystonia does not respond to dopaminergic medication. The mainstay of treatment is anticholinergic medication, but often very high doses are required [Bressman, 2000; Bressman and Greene, 2000]. Other medications such as benzodiazepines, baclofen, carbamazepine, neuroleptics, and tetrabenazine have been tried with varied success, and these are summarized below. In multiple case reports, pallidotomy or deep brain stimulation seems to be particularly helpful in DYT1-positive patients with dystonia [Cif et al., 2003; Coubes et al., 2004; Coubes et al., 2000; Eltahawy et al., 2004]. Untreated, DYT1 dystonia will progress gradually over many years, although it may reach a plateau in adulthood. The prognosis and life span depend on the severity of the disorder. There do not appear to be associated abnormalities in other organ systems, and mortality is usually due to pulmonary complications of the motor dysfunction.

DOPA-RESPONSIVE DYSTONIA

Dopa-responsive dystonia is labeled DYT5 dystonia [Bandmann et al., 1998b] and is also known as *Segawa's disease* after Segawa first described it in 1976 [Bandmann and Wood, 2002; Segawa et al., 1999; Segawa et al., 2003]. The presentation is very similar to DYT1 dystonia in many cases, although it can have onset at an earlier age. The average age of onset is 6 years, with a range of onset from 1 to 12 years. It frequently starts in a limb in children. In adults, it has been reported as a cause of parkinsonism, with a bradykinetic rigid onset rather than limb dystonia onset [Uncini et al., 2004]. In children, the dystonia is often combined with parkinsonism, although without tremor [Nygaard et al., 1990; Uncini et al., 2004]. The combination of dystonia and parkinsonism is due to decreased but not absent dopamine production. Diurnal variation is present in 77% of children [Nygaard et al., 1988]. Such children appear to be significantly improved upon awakening in the morning or after a nap, with a gradual worsening of symptoms the longer they remain awake and active. Dopa-responsive dystonia can mimic many of the features of cerebral palsy [Jan, 2004], and there have been reported cases of associated hyperreflexia [Bandmann et al., 1998a]. Untreated, dopa-responsive dystonia is a progressive disorder, and this helps to distinguish it from static disorders such as cerebral palsy.

Dopa-responsive dystonia is due to mutations in either the guanosine triphosphate cyclohydrolase 1 gene [Bandmann et al., 1996; Bandmann et al., 1998b; Furukawa et al., 2000] or the tyrosine hydroxylase gene [Grattan-Smith et al., 2002; Ichinose et al., 1999]. Guanosine triphosphate cyclohydrolase 1 is on chromosome 14Q22.1-2, and expression is autosomal dominant with variable penetrance [Uncini et al., 2004], which may be greater in girls than in boys [Furukawa et al., 1998]. Guanosine triphosphate cyclohydrolase is an enzyme that is important for the synthesis of biopterins and neopterins, which are cofactors for the enzyme tyrosine hydroxylase (see Chapter 30). The pterins are also cofactors for tryptophan hydroxylase and phenylalanine hydroxylase, although reduced function of these enzymes does not seem to be a cause of symptoms. Rare cases of homozygosity for guanosine triphosphate cyclohydrolase mutations have been reported, with a more severe phenotype [Thony and Blau, 1997].

Significant improvement during a trial with levodopa strongly suggests the diagnosis, although a similar response can be seen in juvenile Parkinson's disease and even in some cases of secondary dystonia. The diagnosis can be confirmed by quantitative evaluation of cerebrospinal fluid neurotransmitters and pterins. In particular, biopterin, neopterin, and homovanillic acid (a dopamine metabolite) are low in cerebrospinal fluid. Another test that has been used is the phenylalanine loading test [Bandmann et al., 2003; Hyland et al., 1997; Ponzone et al., 1994; Saunders-Pullman et al., 2004a]. This test reflects a defect in phenylalanine hydroxylase that is present in liver and depends on biopterin as a cofactor. To perform the test, 100 mg/kg of phenylalanine is given orally, and the serum phenylalanine to tyrosine ratio is measured at intervals over 6 hours. However, this test may not be as sensitive and specific as cerebrospinal fluid neurotransmitter metabolite measurement. There is no common mutation in guanosine triphosphate cyclohydrolase 1 [Ichinose et al., 1999; Nishiyama et al., 2000], so full sequencing of the gene is usually required for genetic diagnosis; sequencing detects about 60% of cases.

Tyrosine hydroxylase deficiency is due to mutations in the tyrosine hydroxylase gene on chromosome 11P15.5 [Nagatsu and Ichinose, 1996; Royo et al., 2005]. Expression is autosomal recessive with full penetrance. The onset of the dystonia tends to be earlier, usually in infancy, with more severe symptoms [Brautigam et al., 1999; Furukawa et al., 2001], but mild forms have been reported [Furukawa et al., 2004b]. Examination of the cerebrospinal fluid reveals normal biopterins and neopterins but low homovanillic acid [Wevers et al., 1999]. Confirmation of the diagnosis requires demonstration of low tyrosine hydroxylase function in fibroblasts or lymphocytes, or sequencing of the tyrosine hydroxylase gene.

In both autosomal-recessive and autosomal-dominant dopa-responsive dystonia, treatment involves replacement of dopamine using oral levodopa [Nutt and Nygaard, 2001]. In particular, the combination of levodopa and a peripheral dopa decarboxylase inhibitor such as carbidopa usually results in a dramatic improvement in symptoms with minimal side effects [Hwang et al., 2001; Nutt and Nygaard, 2001]. Often very low doses are required, and treatment can be continued throughout life with no adverse events. In particular, the escalation of dose frequently seen in Parkinson's disease and the development of motor dyskinesias over time does not seem to occur or occurs only rarely. There are reports that a gradual escalation of dose may be needed after several years. Although many children and adults will achieve complete resolution with doses of 100 mg/day or less of levodopa, some children have required up to 10 mg/kg/day. Medication is usually given three times per day. Other medications for Parkinson's disease will also work, including anticholinergic medication, dopamine agonists, and amantadine, although these are usually not needed. Peripherally induced side effects of levodopa include nausea and hypotension, and these can often be ameliorated by giving an extra dose of carbidopa 30 minutes before administration of the levodopa-carbidopa combination. Intestinal absorption of levodopa is increased by simultaneous carbohydrate intake and decreased by simultaneous protein intake. The prognosis is excellent with treatment [Nygaard et al., 1991], but untreated children are at risk for severe dystonia with progressive orthopedic deformities.

MYOCLONUS DYSTONIA

Myoclonus dystonia is a disorder with a combination of both symptoms [Asmus and Gasser, 2004; Lang, 1997]. In some but not all families with these symptoms, the disorder is due to a mutation in the epsilon-sarcoglycan gene on chromosome 7Q21 [Nygaard et al., 1999], and this has been designated *DYT11* [Furukawa and Rajput, 2002; Schule et al., 2004; Valente et al., 2003]. The details of the myoclonus are discussed further in the section on myoclonus. Myoclonus involves the neck, trunk, and arms and is often alcohol responsive. Dystonia occurs in about half of patients and can be the only manifestation. Dystonia usually expresses as either torticollis or arm dystonia. In addition, behavioral symptoms and obsessive-compulsive disorder have been associated with gene mutations. Onset is in late childhood or adolescence.

This disorder is autosomal dominant, although de novo mutations are frequent [Hedrich et al., 2004]. When the epsilon-sarcoglycan gene is inherited from the father, there is about 100% symptomatic expression, but when inherited from the mother, there is only 10% symptomatic expression, suggesting an important role of maternal imprinting [Grabowski et al., 2003; Muller et al., 2002]. It can be diagnosed by sequencing of the epsilon-sarcoglycan gene, and this detects 95% of patients in affected families. Treatment is with benzodiazepines, valproate, and alcohol, although chronic use of alcohol frequently leads to dependence, and this has not been proposed as an appropriate long-term therapy. Some reports have suggested the use of γ-hydroxybutyrate, which has alcohol-like effects and seems to be helpful in small case series [Priori et al., 2000]. There have also been reports of the use of deep brain stimulation in both the globus pallidus and the ventral intermediate nucleus of the thalamus with symptomatic relief [Cif et al., 2004]. The prognosis is excellent, and children would be expected to have a normal life span, although symptoms do not spontaneously resolve.

OTHER IDENTIFIED PRIMARY DYSTONIAS

DYT8 is the designation for paroxysmal nonkinesigenic dyskinesia, and DYT10 is the designation for paroxysmal kinesigenic choreoathetosis, and both of these are discussed in the section on paroxysmal disorders.

DYT12 is the designation for rapid-onset dystonia parkinsonism, which has been associated with the *ATP-1A3* gene [de Carvalho Aguiar et al., 2004]. In this disorder, a combination of dystonia and bradykinesia can develop over hours to days. It is autosomal dominant with variable penetrance [Brashear et al., 1998]. Once the dystonia has developed, it does not resolve [Dobyns et al., 1993]. Treatment is entirely symptomatic. The disorder does not appear to be progressive, and once the initial symptoms have developed, they remain at about the same level of severity or progress only gradually [Dobyns et al., 1993].

PSYCHOGENIC DYSTONIA

Dystonia as a manifestation of psychiatric disorders is not uncommon. It is most often a form of conversion reaction. Common features of psychogenic disorders include maximal severity at onset, entraining to rhythmic stimuli, distractibility, suggestibility, and a posture or presentation that is otherwise atypical for the disease [Fahn and Williams, 1988; Kirsch and Mink, 2004; Ozekmekci et al., 2003; Pringsheim and Lang, 2003; Thomas and Jankovic, 2004]. Children may not be aware of the psychogenic origin, and there may be no history of other psychopathology. There may be no secondary gain. In some cases, psychogenic dystonia occurs in the presence of true dystonia, worsening its apparent severity [Bentivoglio et al., 2002]. It can also appear in families in which other family members have dystonia or other movement disorders. It is essential to exclude organic causes in testing. Surface or needle electromyography can be helpful because certain patterns of rhythmic contraction sometimes seen in dystonia cannot be mimicked voluntarily [Hallett, 1983], and if these patterns occur, that would be a clue to an organic cause. The primary treatment is psychiatric, but this is considered a very primitive psychiatric defense mechanism, and the prognosis for spontaneous resolution is poor [Feinstein et al., 2001; Miyasaki et al., 2003].

Secondary Dystonia

There is a long list of possible secondary causes for dystonia, as shown in the Table 58-3. This section reviews several of the most important causes. Many of these disorders are discussed elsewhere or in other chapters.

CEREBRAL PALSY

Cerebral palsy is probably the most common cause of dystonia in childhood. This is because of its relatively high prevalence. Further details about this disorder, including the etiology and details of the symptomatology, can be found in Chapter 20. Only the elements contributing to dystonia are summarized here. Dyskinetic cerebral palsy represents between 6% and 15% of all cases of cerebral palsy [Surveillance of Cerebral Palsy in Europe (SCPE), 2002], and in dyskinetic cerebral palsy, dystonia is usually the primary feature. Dystonia occurs frequently as an associated feature in other forms of cerebral palsy, including tetraplegic and hemiplegic cerebral palsy. Dystonia is usually associated with lesions of the basal ganglia or thalamus [Krageloh-Mann et al., 2002], and these lesions are commonly caused by hypoxic-ischemic injury in the full-term neonate [Volpe, 2000]. A similar syndrome can occur in victims of near drowning or other forms of asphyxia, as well as in stroke and sometimes head trauma. Symptoms most often affect the arms, with the legs often being affected either by spasticity or a combination of spasticity and dystonia. There may be associated bradykinesia or choreoathetosis.

Although the dystonia in cerebral palsy presumably is due to a static injury, the symptom can worsen over time. In fact, the onset of dystonia may be many years after the initial injury leading to cerebral palsy [Saint Hilaire et al., 1991].

KERNICTERUS

Kernicterus occurs because of high bilirubin levels in the perinatal period, but the effects are variable and unpredictable (see Chapter 90) [Shapiro, 2005]. There is probably an increased susceptibility to hyperbilirubinemia with prematurity, hypoxia, or infection [Volpe, 2000]. It has been hypothesized that in such cases there is a reduction of the efficacy of the blood-brain barrier, which allows unconjugated bilirubin to penetrate and affect multiple brain regions including the globus pallidus. Injury to the globus pallidus is thought to be the etiology of the movement disorder [Govaert et al., 2003; Johnston and Hoon, 2000]. The overall severity later in life is quite variable, and symptoms include choreoathetosis, dystonia (which can be progressive), sensorineural hearing loss, and supranuclear gaze palsy [Shapiro, 2005]. In the absence of other associated injury, the intellect is usually normal, and the motor disorder is often the single greatest cause of disability.

The acute toxicity of bilirubin is described by three distinct clinical phases. In phase one, there is hypotonia and lethargy for the first few days, which is often misinterpreted as perinatal depression from hypoxic injury. In phase two, starting after the first few days, there is a sudden rise in tone, with hypertonia manifesting primarily as extension of the neck and back with opisthotonus. This may be associated with an otherwise unexplained fever. The presence of early extensor posturing is probably a poor prognostic sign for later development, but this early symptom will resolve after 1 to 2 weeks. Subsequently, in phase three, the child is normal or hypotonic. The child will remain hypotonic during much of the first year, although with delayed motor milestones. The hypertonia will subsequently return after months, or in some cases years, with development of dystonia and choreoathetosis. Children may have seizures and oculogyric crises. Diagnosis is based on the characteristic history, although it is often difficult to verify.

The most effective treatment is prevention of neonatal hyperbilirubinemia [Bhutani et al., 2004; Blackmon et al., 2004; Rubaltelli, 1998; Stevenson et al., 2004]. Treatment of symptomatic cases is often quite difficult. Many children receive cochlear implants for the hearing loss. There is only a slight benefit of anticholinergic medications, valproic acid [Kulkarni, 1992], benzodiazepines, or botulinum toxin. Some children have benefited from intrathecal baclofen. In general, treatment of this disorder is frustrating. Life span is shortened in severely affected children because of pulmonary complications.

PANTOTHENATE KINASE–ASSOCIATED NEURODEGENERATION

Pantothenate kinase–associated neurodegeneration is a member of the group of diseases now referred to as *neuronal brain iron accumulation* [Bertrand, 2002a, 2002b]. Pantothenate kinase–associated neurodegeneration was previously referred to as *Hallervorden-Spatz disease*, although this eponym is no longer favored because of unethical behavior of the physicians who initially described the disorder. Symptoms of pantothenate kinase–associated neurodegeneration include progressive dystonia, dysarthria, rigidity, ballism, choreoathetosis, spasticity, dementia, and pigmentary retinal degeneration [Swaiman, 1991]. In its later stages, this disorder has characteristic ballistic flinging movements of arms and legs, as well as involuntary and repetitive tongue protrusion. The limb and tongue movements may lead to injury, requiring restraint of the arms and legs and dental extraction [Sheehy et al., 1999]. There is a gradual progression over years, with loss of ambulation within 5 to 15 years of onset. The initial symptoms usually occur either in the childhood or juvenile years.

Pantothenate kinase–associated neurodegeneration has been divided into the characteristic type with presentation in the first decade (average onset at 3 years), and an atypical form with onset in the second decade, which seems to have slower progression and lesser severity [Thomas et al., 2004]. Dystonia in pantothenate kinase–associated neurodegeneration usually starts in the leg, but sometimes the earliest presenting sign is visual loss. There is often associated bradykinesia. The rate of progression is more rapid with younger onset. The overall incidence is estimated to be about 3 cases per 1 million population. The amount of dementia is variable and unknown because the severity of the movement disorder makes assessment of cognitive function in later stages difficult.

The atypical form generally starts later, between 10 and 30 years of age at onset, with a mean of 13 years. It has slower progression, and retinopathy is quite rare. The atypical form presents with dysarthria and psychiatric disturbances, which include emotional lability, depression, and sometimes aggressive or violent behavior. There are also freezing episodes similar to those seen in Parkinson's disease.

The gene responsible for pantothenate kinase–associated neurodegeneration is pantothenate-kinase-2 (*PANK-2*) on chromosome 20p13-p12.3 [Hayflick, 2003b; Zhou et al., 2001]. Inheritance is autosomal recessive. Pantothenate kinase is responsible for synthesis of coenzyme A, and the neurologic abnormalities may be due to a combination of factors, including accumulation of upstream metabolites causing iron chelation and decreased availability of coenzyme A for fatty acid metabolism [Gordon, 2002; Hayflick, 2003a]. The pathophysiology is characterized by rust-colored iron pigmentation of the globus pallidus and SNpr. Injury to the globus pallidus with consequent abnormalities of outflow patterns may be responsible for the movement disorder [Mink, 2001b]. In addition, there are axonal spheroids similar to those seen in neuroaxonal dystrophy [Gordon, 2002].

MRI reveals a characteristic "eye of the tiger" sign. This sign consists of a dark globus pallidus internus on T2-weighted imaging, with a bright region in the center of the globus pallidus that is thought to be due to central necrosis (Fig. 58-4). The dark signal is due to iron accumulation [Hayflick et al., 2001], although deposition of iron may be secondary to other metabolic deficits rather than the primary cause of symptoms [Koeppen and Dickson, 2001]. When the full eye of the tiger sign is present in childhood, 100% of such cases have the *PANK-2* mutation [Hayflick et al., 2003]. Similarly, 100% of children with *PANK-2* mutations exhibit the eye of the tiger sign at some point during the illness [Trimble, 2003]. Children with clinical features of pantothenate kinase–associated neurodegeneration but without the eye of the tiger sign only have a 50% chance of being positive for the *PANK-2* mutation. Ophthalmologic examination and electroretinogram may detect presymptomatic retinopathic changes and early visual loss [Swaiman, 1991]. Acanthocytes are sometimes, but not always, present, and there may be a low level of prebetalipoprotein. These findings are similar to those seen in the HARP syndrome (hypoprebetalipoproteinemia, acanthocytosis, retinitis pigmentosa, and pallidal degeneration). Some families with HARP syndrome have the *PANK-2* mutation, and therefore it is not known whether this is a separate disorder or a variant of pantothenate kinase–associated neurodegeneration [Houlden et al., 2003]. It is important to test for other disorders that can present with similar generalized dystonia in childhood, including Huntington's disease, neuronal ceroid lipofuscinosis, and hexosaminidase A deficiency (Tay-Sachs disease).

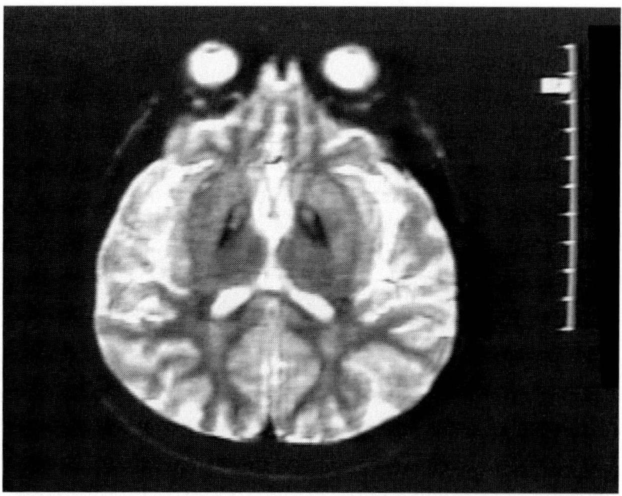

FIGURE 58-4. T2-weighted magnetic resonance imaging (MRI) view of an 11-year old patient with pantothenate kinase–associated neurodegeneration, showing the characteristic "eye of the tiger" sign within the internal globus pallidus.

Treatment is symptomatic. Some children benefit from benzodiazepines, anticholinergic medications, botulinum toxin, baclofen, or intrathecal baclofen. It is unlikely that any of these treatments slow the progression of the underlying disease, but several case reports of treatment with pallidotomy or deep brain stimulation of the globus pallidus internus suggest the possibility of symptomatic improvement [Justesen et al., 1999; Umemura et al., 2004]. The prognosis is universally poor, with death from medical complications usually within 10 to 20 years of onset in the typical form; in the atypical form, survival may be longer.

LESCH-NYHAN DISEASE

Lesch-Nyhan disease is a progressive neurodegenerative disorder that initially presents with hypotonia and developmental delay in the first year of life. It progresses over several years and can mimic athetotic cerebral palsy, with ballism, choreoathetosis, axial dystonia, and spasticity [Nyhan, 1968a, 1968b, 1972]. There is a striking prevalence of self-mutilation behavior, including tongue biting, head banging, biting the fingers and lips, and thrusting arms or legs against objects [Lee et al., 2002; Robey et al., 2003]. There are also compulsive behaviors, and slowly progressive dementia is characteristic [Matthews et al., 1999]. There is increase in uric acid in both the blood and the urine, and this leads to symptoms of gout in advanced cases, as well as in some late onset cases, although this is less common in children. Both arthritis and renal stones have been reported but usually at older ages.

The responsible gene is *HPRT-1* (hypoxanthine-guanine phosphoribosyltransferase) [Mak et al., 2000]. Deficiency of *HPRT-1* can be detected in fibroblasts and leukocytes. The disorder is X-linked recessive, and the incidence of symptomatic cases is about 1 in 400,000 boys. MRI shows only nonspecific atrophy.

Treatment is symptomatic. Allopurinol may alleviate signs of gout and prevent renal calculi [Brock et al., 1983; Hiraishi et al., 1987]. Behavioral programs can be used to reduce self-mutilation [Olson and Houlihan, 2000]. Benzodiazepines, carbamazepine, and possibly selective serotonin reuptake inhibitors can be helpful for the behavior disorder [Cusumano et al., 2001; Roach et al., 1996; Saito and Takashima, 2000]. Tetrabenazine or levodopa may be helpful to treat the dystonia [Jankovic et al., 1988]. Naltrexone has been attempted to reduce self-mutilation with only limited success. In some cases, restraint and removal of dentition are required to prevent self-mutilation, and patients who can communicate often request to be placed in restraint to reduce self-injury. The injury behavior seems to become worse in times of stress, and avoidance of stressful situations may be helpful. A single case report suggests the possibility of treatment with deep brain stimulation [Taira et al., 2003]. The prognosis is poor. Most children never walk, and there is progression of symptoms and dementia over several years. Survival is possible into the second or third decade.

SPINOCEREBELLAR ATAXIA

The spinocerebellar ataxias are reviewed in Chapter 57. However, it is worth mentioning that spinocerebellar ataxia type 3 (Machado-Joseph disease) has a characteristic presentation with a dystonic-rigid or parkinsonian syndrome. This is referred to as *type 1 Machado-Joseph disease*, with type 2 presenting more typically with ataxia and spasticity. The type 1 dystonic-rigid form tends to present more commonly in children and can resemble juvenile Huntington's disease [Jardim et al., 2001a, 2001b]. There is often progressive external ophthalmoplegia and bulging eyes, superimposed on a nuclear or supranuclear gaze palsy. Presentation can be as early as 5 years of age, although it is more common to present in the second decade or later. Machado-Joseph disease is due to a CAG triplet repeat on chromosome 14Q24.3-Q31, and children with 53 to 86 repeats are symptomatic. Higher numbers of repeats are associated with earlier onset and greater severity. Inheritance is autosomal dominant. Treatment is primarily symptomatic, although some cases have responded to treatment with levodopa early in the course.

ORGANIC ACIDEMIAS

Organic acidemias, including methylmalonic aciduria, glutaric aciduria types 1 and 2, biotinidase deficiency, disorders of fatty acid oxidation, and mitochondrial respiratory chain disorders can lead to dystonia. Many of these disorders do not present until a time of metabolic stress, at which time a rapid decompensation with onset of severe generalized dystonia over a period of hours to days is possible. Once dystonia has occurred, symptoms are often irreversible. Specific treatment is usually urgently needed, and, in some cases, this requires limitation of intake of specific amino acids, whereas in other cases, specific medications or enzyme replacement is needed.

Many of these disorders can be detected with newborn screening. For children with new onset of symptoms or rapid progression of symptoms, there needs to be high index of suspicion to detect these disorders because any delay in treatment usually leads to significantly worse prognosis. Most of these diseases are autosomal recessive.

A particularly striking presentation that often occurs in infancy, but that can occur later in childhood, has been referred to as *infantile bilateral striatal necrosis* [Basel-Vanagaite et al., 2004; Straussberg et al., 2002]. This presentation can occur with any of these metabolic disorders, but it also seems to be able to occur in the context of acute infections, particularly with mycoplasma, and it has been reported in children with *PANK-2* mutations. Most often the cause is unknown. There have been some rare familial cases. This disorder is characterized by a rapid onset of dystonia and dyskinesia, sometimes associated with chorea [Mito et al., 1986; Roytta et al., 1981], and MRI often exhibits evidence of irreversible striatal and sometimes pallidal injury on diffusion T2-weighted or enhanced images [Mito et al., 1986; Roytta et al., 1981].

Early diagnosis of a possible metabolic defect is essential, and treatment of any precipitating infectious process should be initiated rapidly. Once the injury has occurred, usually only symptomatic treatment is available. There have been a few reported cases of a biotin-responsive type of striatal necrosis that has been thought to be due to an abnormality of biotin transport, and such cases may have rapid and effective resolution when treated with biotin [Straussberg et al., 2002]. There have been reported cases of trauma being the inciting event, but whether trauma by itself is able to cause this, or whether another associated metabolic abnormality is required, is not known.

FAHR'S DISEASE

Fahr's disease is characterized by basal ganglia calcification, as well as calcification of other gray matter structures, including cerebellar nuclei and punctate calcifications in thalamus and sometimes cortex [Oliveira et al., 2004]. This is usually an adult-onset disease, but in rare cases can occur in the second decade of life. When it does, it is characterized by microcephaly, hypertonia, and choreoathetosis. The etiology is often unknown, but in some cases it is due to hypoparathyroidism, and therefore parathyroid function should be checked. It is autosomal dominant, with reduced penetrance in most families, and appears to be slowly progressive. Diagnosis is based on evidence of calcification detected

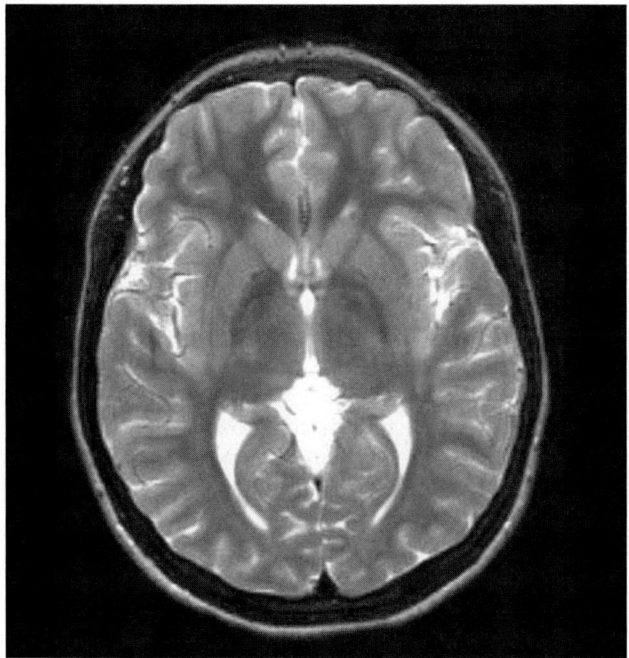

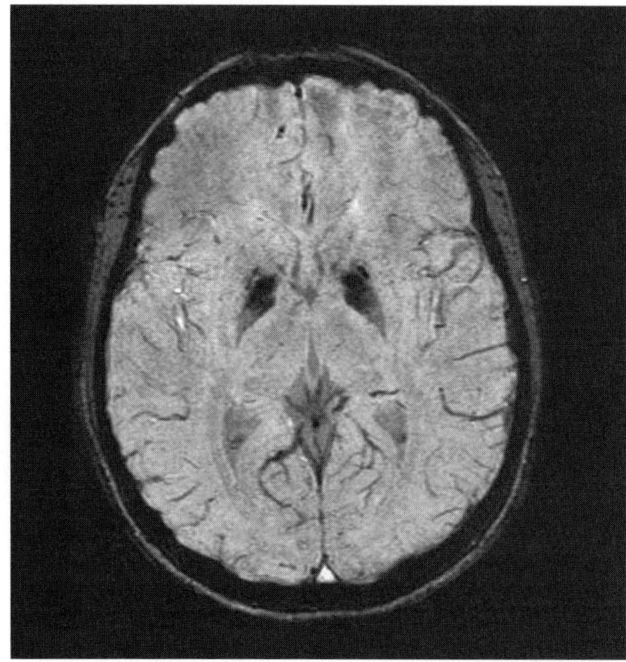

FIGURE 58-5. Magnetic resonance imaging view of an adolescent with Fahr's disease. **A**, T2-weighted axial image shows low signal in the basal ganglia secondary to calcification. Calcification was noted in the corresponding area in a previous computed tomography scan. **B**, Same patient with susceptibility weighted axial (SWI) image showing low signal in the basal ganglia secondary to calcification. Accentuated susceptibility effect in this imaging technique has resulted in more intense signal change due to the calcification. (Courtesy of Dr. Daniel Wycliffe, Department of Radiology, Loma Linda University Medical Center, Loma Linda, CA.)

by head computed tomography scanning [Koller et al., 1979; Koller and Klawans, 1980; Oliveira et al., 2004] or MRI (Fig. 58-5). Treatment is supportive, unless a specific disorder of parathyroid hormone can be found, in which case specific treatment will be available.

NEUROACANTHOCYTOSIS

Neuroacanthocytosis has also been referred to as *chorea acanthocytosis* or *Levine-Critchley syndrome*. It is characterized by spiky projections on erythrocytes (Fig. 58-6), although such projections are often seen in non-neurologic disease, including hepatic disease. Acanthocytes are also seen in abetalipoproteinemia (Bassen-Kornzweig disease) [Bohlega et al., 1998], vitamin E deficiency, hypoprebetalipoproteinemia, HARP syndrome, and with abnormal Kell blood group antigens (McLeod syndrome) [Danek et al., 2001; Dotti et al., 2000; Mehndiratta et al., 2000; Rampoldi et al., 2002]. Onset is usually in the adult years, but onset as early as 8 years of age has been reported. Symptoms in childhood resemble juvenile Huntington's disease, with dystonia and an akinetic-rigid syndrome, as well as a severe and progressive tic disorder [Kutcher et al., 1999; Yamamoto et al., 1982]. Presentation in adults is more typically with chorea or psychiatric illness [Bruneau et al., 2003; Dixit et al., 1993; Robinson et al., 2004]. There is frequent tongue protrusion and difficulty eating, and severe dysarthria is often a presenting feature. Some children and adults show areflexia or impulsive behavior, and there is occasionally mild dementia.

Testing for this disease requires examination of a fixed smear of blood under the microscope, stressed by mixing 1:1 with normal saline, and this requires an experienced and knowledgeable technician. Greater than 3% acanthocytes is diagnostic. MRI shows caudate atrophy [Kutcher et al., 1999; Okamoto et al., 1997]. Positron-emission tomography scanning shows decreased fluoro-dopa uptake and decreased raclopride binding, suggesting both presynaptic and postsynaptic disorders of striatal function [Brooks et al., 1991; Peppard et al., 1990]. Treatment is symptomatic. Benzo-

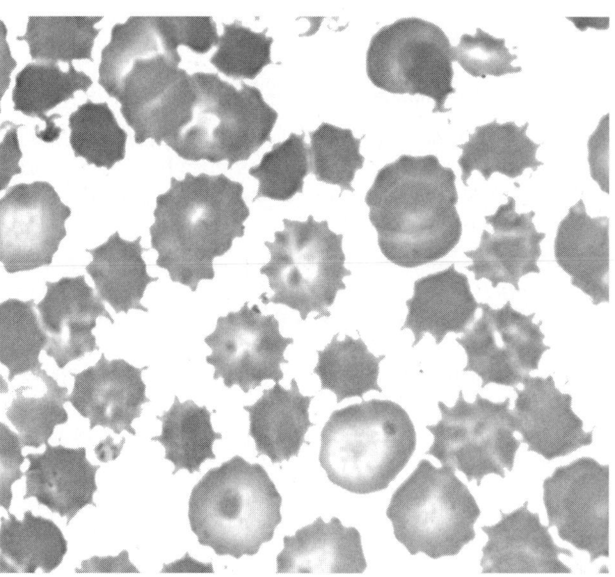

FIGURE 58-6. Stressed blood smear showing acanthocytes. (Courtesy of Tracy George, MD.)

diazepines are often helpful. When chorea is present, neuroleptics are helpful, but this is probably less useful in childhood. There has been an isolated report of improvement with calcium channel blockers.

Although the use of the term *neuroacanthocytosis* is intended for the lack of other known causes of acanthocytes, many of these other known causes do present with dystonia, and some with peripheral neuropathy and retinal degeneration. In particular, vitamin E deficiency, Bassen-Kornzweig disease, and HARP syndrome can have a similar neurologic presentation.

MEDICATION-INDUCED DYSTONIA

Medications are able to cause dystonia, and this is most commonly seen with neuroleptic medications. In particular, there is a higher rate of acute dystonic reactions in children than in adults, and this has been reported to be as high as 10% to 20% in some series [Ayers and Dawson, 1980; Olsen et al., 2000; Spina et al., 1993]. Acute dystonic reactions are easily treated with diphenhydramine (1 mg/kg usually given intravenously) or other anticholinergics [Dahiya and Noronha, 1984]. Other types of acute reactions to neuroleptics such as akathisia can be more difficult to treat, but in some cases respond to benzodiazepines. Acute dystonic reactions often present with uncontrollable tongue movements, opisthotonus, and neck hyperextension or torticollis. Medications not normally classed with the neuroleptics, including antiemetic medications such as metoclopramide [Cowan, 1982; Lu and Chu, 1988; Renwick, 1990], domperidone [Madej, 1985], and prochlorperazine [Leeman, 1965], are able to produce the full range of neuroleptic side effects. It is likely that any medication that either blocks or depletes central catecholamines has the potential to cause an acute dystonic reaction [Burke et al., 1985; McCann et al., 1990].

Tardive dystonia and tardive dyskinesia are particularly worrisome consequences of neuroleptic use because symptoms may not resolve following discontinuation of the causative medication [Burke et al., 1982]. Tardive syndromes and their treatment are described in a separate section.

OTHER DISORDERS CAUSING SECONDARY DYSTONIA

Aromatic L-amino acid decarboxylase deficiency leads to dopamine agonist–responsive dystonia. In this disorder, conversion of levodopa to dopamine is impaired, and therefore administration of levodopa is not helpful [Swoboda et al., 1999; Swoboda et al., 2003]. This disorder does respond to dopamine agonists, but because of the combination of severe autonomic and sleep disturbances, treatment with serotonergic medication is often required as well [Swoboda et al., 1999]. Very few cases have been reported. This disorder is detectable by a characteristic pattern of cerebrospinal fluid neurotransmitter metabolites. Symptoms include dysautonomia, sleep disturbances, eye movement disturbances, and severe generalized dystonia, usually with onset in the first year of life. It appears to be autosomal recessive.

Juvenile Parkinson's disease can present with a picture very similar to dopa-responsive dystonia, with a combination of progressive dystonia and bradykinesia, and this is described further in the next section. Huntington's disease in children often presents with a rigid-akinetic syndrome and severe dystonia, as described earlier in this chapter. Pontocerebellar hypoplasia type 2 is characterized by infantile onset of a combination of extrapyramidal symptoms, dyskinesia, and dystonia [Coppola et al., 2000; Grellner et al., 2000; Grosso et al., 2002].

Alternating hemiplegia is characterized by episodes of hemiplegia or dystonia that can last for hours to days and then resolve [Bassi et al., 2004; Saltik et al., 2004]. Transmission appears to be recessive, although in some cases, there is autosomal dominant transmission [Kanavakis et al., 2003]. Cases with dominant transmission must be distinguished from familial hemiplegic migraine. There is usually a slowly progressive generalized dystonia between episodes [Swoboda et al., 2004]. Treatment for alternating hemiplegia with calcium channel blockers, in particular flunarizine (5 to 15 mg/day), may reduce the frequency and severity of attacks. Symptomatic treatment, including anticholinergic medication, amantadine, and levodopa, may help in some cases [Sasaki et al., 2001; Sone et al., 2000].

Treatments for Dystonia

Because dopa-responsive dystonia can mimic cerebral palsy, it has been recommended that all children with unexplained dystonia or cerebral palsy be given a trial of levodopa [Jan, 2004; Nygaard et al., 1988]. Levodopa may be helpful in some children even with secondary dystonia [Brunstrom et al., 2000]. The required dose of levodopa is very low in dopa-responsive dystonia (typically 50 to 100 mg/day) but may be much higher in juvenile Parkinson's disease and secondary causes of dystonia, including cerebral palsy. Dosages as high as 10 mg/kg/day divided three times per day are sometimes needed. Common side effects of levodopa include nausea, vomiting, and diarrhea. Orthostatic hypotension occurs rarely in children. Levodopa must be combined with a peripheral decarboxylase inhibitor, such as carbidopa, to increase central uptake and decrease peripheral side effects. Commercial preparations with a ratio of levodopa to carbidopa of 4:1 are typically used. Peripheral side effects can often be reduced by an additional dose of the peripheral decarboxylase inhibitor given one half hour before the levodopa dose. Levodopa competes for absorption with neutral amino acids, and therefore absorption is slowed and the peak effect is less when it is taken with a protein meal. Conversely, absorption rate is increased, the peak effect is greatest, and the side effects may be greatest when it is taken with carbohydrates. Levodopa and anticholinergic medications are frequently used together. The appropriate dose of levodopa is difficult to determine, and it needs to be titrated gradually over a period of 2 weeks to 2 months. Rapid titration is possible, but the purpose of gradual titration is to find the optimal dose. Excessive doses of levodopa usually cause dyskinesias or worsen dystonia, and often an intermediate dose is most effective. Rapid withdrawal can lead to worsening of dystonia, and there are rare reports of symptoms similar to neuroleptic malignant syndrome after rapid withdrawal in adults.

Anticholinergic medication is very effective in acute dystonic reactions, as described earlier. It is partly effective in a subset of children with chronic dystonia [Hoon et al., 2001], and trihexyphenidyl remains the best studied centrally active antidystonia medication [Burke and Fahn, 1983; Burke et al., 1986; Greene et al., 1988]. Its mechanism of action for dystonia is not known, although it is presumed to have an effect on the large cholinergic interneurons of the striatum. Its anticholinergic effects would be expected to be widespread throughout the basal ganglia and cortex [Fahn, 1987]. It is often necessary to proceed to very high doses: 1 mg/kg, and in some cases higher [Fahn, 1983a, 1983b]. In younger children, lower doses may be sufficient, but children will tolerate the high doses better than adults. In particular, adults and older children are more likely to develop confusion or behavior changes on high doses. The effectiveness may be greater in young children, and speech and hand function seem to improve the most [Hoon et al., 2001]. The dose must be increased gradually, and it may often take 3 to 4 months to achieve an appropriate dosage. Appropriate initial dosage is 0.1 mg/kg/day or less. The medication is usually divided three times per day and given during the day. Side effects are similar to those of other anticholinergic medications. Behavior changes are not uncommon, and deficits in attention have been reported in adult trials. Anticholinergic medications can worsen chorea and possibly choreoathetosis. The benefit on dystonia is often delayed, and there may be no apparent benefit for several months after starting the medication. At high doses, abrupt withdrawal could be dangerous, and there are rare reports of neuroleptic malignant syndrome following abrupt withdrawal of high doses of trihexyphenidyl in adults. Other anticholinergic medications may work as well, but others have not been extensively tested.

Diazepam and other benzodiazepines or sedative medications can occasionally be helpful. Orthopedic procedures may not have expected outcomes in children with dystonia because there is a tendency for dystonia to transfer to other muscles following an orthopedic procedure. Restraint of a dystonic limb, casting, or braces may make the dystonia worse, and there is a tendency for the dystonia to "fight against" any restraining force. This problem needs to be considered very carefully when planning prolonged casting of the lower extremities, such as after hip surgery, because the dystonia may worsen significantly after removal of the cast. Selective dorsal rhizotomy has been reported to have a very poor outcome in dystonia, and it is therefore essential to exclude dystonia when selecting cases for this intervention.

When dystonia is associated with increased tone, botulinum toxin has been found to be very effective [Boyd et al., 2001; Graham et al., 2003]. It may be effective in directly reducing the tone in the hypertonic muscles, but may also be effective in changing the overall pattern of dystonia. In particular, it is sometimes observed that botulinum toxin injection into one muscle will relax other muscles of the same limb. Injection is often performed with electromyographic guidance, and although some practitioners perform this procedure using general anesthesia, many have now chosen to use only local anesthesia. The procedure should not be performed more frequently than every 3 months because of the risk for buildup of neutralizing antibodies. In some individuals, repeated doses of botulinum toxin every 3 months are needed, but in others, short-term treatment can be effective. Neurolysis and dantrolene have not been commonly used in dystonia.

Baclofen has been used and may be effective in some cases, although its mechanism of effectiveness in dystonia remains unknown. Intrathecal baclofen can reduce tone in generalized dystonia if the catheter is placed at cervical levels [Albright et al., 1996; Albright et al., 1998; Albright et al., 2001; Butler and Campbell, 2000; Ford et al., 1998]. There is a high rate of complications, up to 35% in some series [Campbell et al., 2002]. Complications can be serious and can include meningitis. Overdoses are rare, but pump failure or catheter disconnection with acute and possibly life-threatening baclofen withdrawal can occur. Withdrawal needs to be treated with a combination of oral baclofen and intravenous diazepam, as well as surgical reimplantation of the catheter as soon as possible. For this reason, many clinicians recommend that children with intrathecal baclofen pumps remain within 30 minutes of an appropriately trained emergency room at all times.

Neurosurgical intervention is reserved for the most severe cases, but the possibility that earlier surgical intervention may slow progression of the disease or lead to a longer disease-free interval has been raised. Pallidotomy and thalamotomy have been in use for many years with some success [Gros et al., 1976a; Gros et al., 1976b; Vercueil, 2003]. More recently, deep brain stimulation has become available, and multiple targets have been attempted, including the ventrolateral thalamus [Ghika et al., 2002; Thompson et al., 2000], internal globus pallidus [Coubes et al., 2000; Tronnier and Fogel, 2000; Vercueil et al., 2001], and most recently subthalamic nucleus [Benabid et al., 2001]. The advantage of deep brain stimulation is the ability to control the current delivery and the ability to select one or a combination of up to four electrodes through an external programmer. The stimulation wire is implanted using a combination of stereotactic neurosurgical techniques and usually microelectrode recording for precise localization. There is emerging evidence that the precision of implantation affects the outcome. The lead is connected to a pacemaker implanted in the chest. For generalized dystonia, usually both sides need to be implanted. The full effect of ablative surgery or stimulation implantation is often not seen for many months, and there are reports of continued improvement up to 1 year after pallidotomy [Lin et al., 2001]. Surgical procedures in the globus pallidus internus seem to be particularly effective in DYT1 and other primary dystonias [Coubes et al., 2004; Eltahawy et al., 2004; Ford, 2004; Lozano et al., 1997; Vercueil et al., 2002; Vitek et al., 1998], and these are cases in which earlier intervention may be most effective [Coubes et al., 2000]. The secondary causes of dystonia may also respond [Ghika et al., 2002; Rakocevic et al., 2004], but surgery seems to be less effective for secondary dystonia [Cif et al., 2003; Coubes et al., 2002; Krack and Vercueil, 2001; Teive et al., 2001]. The largest case series suggests up to 50% effectiveness in children with secondary dystonia but up to 80% effectiveness in children with primary dystonia. Complications are essentially those of the implantation procedure. Infections do occur, but these are rare outside of the immediate perioperative period. Batteries need to be replaced every 3 to 5 years, and this requires a brief surgical procedure. The long-term efficacy of deep brain stimulation is not known. Whether there is a difference in programming parameters between children and adults is likewise not known.

Treatment of Dyskinesia and Hyperkinetic Dystonia

Hyperkinetic disorders are more difficult to treat, and although they represent a positive symptom, it is often difficult to remove the effects of dyskinetic movements through botulinum toxin owing to the likely need to completely paralyze the affected muscle. Trihexyphenidyl can often make dyskinesia worse, as can levodopa. There is some effectiveness of clonazepam and valproate. Tetrabenazine [Jankovic and Beach, 1997; Jankovic and Orman, 1988], reserpine, and amantadine have been tried, but there are no consistent reports of benefit. Whether hyperkinetic dystonia and dyskinesia respond to pallidotomy or deep brain stimulation is not currently known. In Parkinson's disease, pallidotomy does seem to improve dyskinesias, but the mechanism of dyskinesia in this case may be very different from the hyperkinetic symptoms seen in children, and there is not yet adequate data to guide therapy.

Tremor

Classification of Tremor

Tremor has been described as "a rhythmical, involuntary, oscillatory movement of a body part" [Deuschl et al., 1998]. It can be classified based on the time of greatest severity at rest, postural, action, or intention tremor. Rest tremor is defined as tremor involving a body part that is inactive and supported against gravity. It may improve during movement. Rest tremor is most commonly associated with other signs of parkinsonism but may occur in isolation. Postural tremor is worse when a child attempts to sustain a posture against gravity, such as with the arms outstretched in front or with the hands near the nose. It may improve with movement or with rest supported against gravity. Action tremor is worse during active movement, but postural or rest components may be present as well. Intention tremor is a specific form of tremor associated with cerebellar disorders, in which the tremor becomes worse as the arm approaches an end point or target, and there is great difficulty achieving target accuracy. Tremor can affect the head [DiMario, 2000], extremities, trunk, or voice.

Tremor can be described in terms of its frequency. Tremor associated with Parkinson's disease or parkinsonism is between 4 and 6 Hz [Findley et al., 1981], whereas essential tremor is more likely at 5 to 8 Hz [Elble, 2000], and physiologic tremor has two components at 8 to 12 Hz and at 20 to 25 Hz [Makabe and Sakamoto, 2002; Takanokura et al., 2002]. In diagnosing tremor, it is important to distinguish it from dystonic tremor and myoclonus. Dystonic tremor, as described earlier, tends to be less regular and often exhibits a null point. Myoclonus can be rhythmic and can be a form of tremor, but the rapid shocklike quality distinguishes it. Electromyography may be helpful in distinguishing myoclonic-type tremor from other forms of tremor, because of the short bursts of less than 50 milliseconds and correlation with scalp potentials that are often seen with myoclonus [Shibasaki, 2000; Shibasaki et al., 1986].

Primary Tremor

The various etiologies of tremor are listed in Table 58-4. Familial essential tremor is an autosomal-dominant disorder with variable penetrance and severity. It can present in childhood and often is slowly progressive over many years [Jankovic et al., 2004; Louis et al., 2001; Paulson, 1976]. It is rarely disabling in childhood, except in extreme cases. Tremor is primarily postural but can also be worsened with action. Tremors when holding a cup or with handwriting are often some of the earliest complaints, but head, trunk, and voice can be affected [Jankovic, 2000]. There is no specific treatment. In adults, there may be a statistical association between essential tremor and Parkinson's disease [Yahr et al., 2003].

Task-specific tremor is rare in children, and when it occurs, it most often seems to involve handwriting. Whether task-specific tremors are a variant of dystonic tremor with task specificity or whether this is a form of essential tremor is not known [Rosenbaum and Jankovic, 1988]. It is important to examine the child for other evidence of dystonia either in the affected limb or elsewhere. Medical treatment is usually ineffective, but occupational therapy may be helpful to develop compensatory strategies.

Physiologic tremor is a normal response that becomes particularly noticeable when a muscle is exerting high levels of force [Makabe and Sakamoto, 2002; Takanokura et al., 2002]. The characteristic of physiologic tremor is that it occurs only with or worsens only when the child is carrying a heavy object or otherwise needs to contract the muscle against high resistance. Some children have an enhanced physiologic tremor that can become noticeable but is only rarely bothersome. There is no effective treatment for enhanced physiologic tremor, but progression is probably rare.

Tremor is a frequent manifestation seen in psychogenic movement disorders. As noted in the section on Psychogenic Dystonia, psychogenic tremor likely represents a conversion reaction and may reflect relatively serious psychopathology

TABLE 58-4

Causes of Tremor

Benign
Enhanced physiologic tremor, shaking and shuddering episodes, spasmus nutans
Static Injury, Structural
Stroke (particularly in the midbrain or cerebellum), multiple sclerosis
Hereditary, Degenerative
Familial essential tremor, juvenile parkinsonism (tremor is rare), pallidonigral degeneration, Wilson's disease, Huntington's disease
Metabolic
Hyperthyroidism, hyperadrenergic state (including pheochromocytoma and neuroblastoma), hypomagnesemia, hypocalcemia, hypoglycemia, hepatic encephalopathy, vitamin B_{12} deficiency
Drugs, Toxins
Valproate, lithium, tricyclic antidepressants, stimulants (cocaine, amphetamine, caffeine, thyroxine, bronchodilators), neuroleptics, cyclosporine, toluene, mercury, thallium, amiodarone, nicotine, lead, manganese, arsenic, cyanide, naphthalene, ethanol, lindane, serotonin reuptake inhibitors
Other Causes of Tremor
Peripheral neuropathy, cerebellar disease or malformation, anxiety, psychogenic tremor

with consequent poor prognosis [Kim et al., 1999; Miyasaki et al., 2003]. Psychogenic tremor can often be distinguished from organic bases of tremor by entrainment to the examiner. In particular, when a child is asked to make a rhythmic movement with a hand or foot at a rhythm different from the tremor, often the tremor will entrain to the rhythmic movement, or the rhythmic movement will entrain to the tremor, such that either the tremor becomes irregular during accurate performance of the rhythmic movement or performance of the rhythmic movement is impossible [Zeuner et al., 2003]. Similarly, distraction using mathematical tasks or other difficult cognitive tasks can often change the nature or frequency of a physiologic tremor, but this would not be expected to occur for an organic tremor. However, the severity (but usually not the frequency) of an organic tremor could worsen in the context of a cognitive performance task if it were worsened by stress.

Other causes of tremor include Parkinson's disease, although the tremor-dominant form is much more common in adults than children. Huntington's disease can cause tremor, although other symptoms usually dominate. Spasmus nutans is an unusual tremor-like disorder seen in young children, usually starting as early as 4 months of age and lasting several years. It is described in a separate section. Shaking and shuddering spells are rarely observed in the clinic, and diagnosis rests on parental description of the typical episodes. These are a benign phenomenon described in a separate section.

Secondary Tremor

There are a large number of secondary causes of tremor, and most of these are listed in the table. It is important to exclude Wilson's disease. This disorder is characterized by a wing-beating tremor that often involves the adductors of the arm, and is seen when the child is asked to abduct the arms with elbows bent [Saito, 1987; Stremmel et al., 1991]. The tremor is primarily postural but may occur at rest. Other forms of tremor are possible in Wilson's disease. Other symptoms include dystonia, rigidity, dysarthria, and psychiatric disorders. The defect is due a mutation in the *ATP7B* copper-transport *atp-ase* gene on 13q14.3, which leads to reduced biliary excretion of copper and consequent accumulation of copper in multiple tissues. Symptom onset is between 6 and 45 years of age. Diagnosis of Wilson's disease is made by noting a low serum ceruloplasmin and elevated excretion of copper in the urine, as measured by a 24-hour urine collection with measurement of the copper-to-creatinine ratio. In patients with neurologic symptoms, slit-lamp examination almost always reveals Kayser-Fleischer rings. Overt or occult liver disease is usually present. Because Wilson's disease is treatable, it is extremely important to exclude this disorder. Common treatments include zinc acetate, trientine, or penicillamine, although if not detected early, liver transplantation may be needed [Roberts and Schilsky, 2003].

Rubral tremor describes a large-amplitude rhythmic but partly ballistic movement that often affects the arms and can be unilateral. It is associated with attempts at movement and is therefore an action tremor. In some cases it can be difficult to distinguish chorea from rubral tremor, although rubral tremor is much less common. It is associated with lesions in the thalamus [Tan et al., 2001], midbrain [Leung et al., 1999], pons, or cerebellar peduncles, although not necessarily the red nucleus. Rubral tremor is usually nonprogressive, but it can be severely disabling.

It is important in the evaluation of a tremor to exclude hyperthyroid states, and this can either be a primary cause of tremor or can worsen a preexisting tremor. Hyperadrenergic states can cause tremor, and this may occur in the presence of tumors that secrete epinephrine, such as pheochromocytoma or neuroblastoma, but it can also occur in the context of severe anxiety disorders. Tremor can occur with electrolyte or glucose abnormalities, vitamin B_{12} deficiency, and in response to medication, including valproate, lithium, tricyclic antidepressants, and stimulant medication such as methylphenidate.

Treatment of Tremor

The first goal in treatment of tremor is to exclude other possible causes of rhythmic movement, including myoclonus, dystonia, seizures, or cerebellar dysfunction. Any underlying metabolic or hormonal cause must be corrected. Essential tremor is treated with propranolol, primidone, benzodiazepines (clonazepam may be particularly effective), or gabapentin [Gironell et al., 1999; Jankovic et al., 2004; Paulson, 1976; Rajput et al., 2004]. If tremor is caused or worsened by anxiety, benzodiazepines may be particularly helpful. Tremor due to stage fright, social phobia, or panic disorder often responds to propranolol.

These same medications can be tried in other forms of tremor, but usually there is minimal responsiveness. Rubral tremor is notoriously refractory to all attempts at intervention, although some cases respond to levodopa [Findley and Gresty, 1980; Yuill, 1980], clonazepam [Jacob and Pratap Chand, 1998], or thalamic deep brain stimulation [Nikkhah et al., 2004].

Parkinsonism

Parkinsonism is defined by presence of two or more of the cardinal signs of Parkinson's disease. These signs are tremor at rest, bradykinesia, rigidity, and postural instability. Tremor is rare in childhood parkinsonism. *Bradykinesia* is slowness of movement in the absence of weakness or ataxia. There may also be *hypokinesia* with paucity of movement, few spontaneous movements, and decreased amplitude of movement. Hypokinesia is often seen as diminished spontaneous facial expression, soft speech (hypophonia), small handwriting (micrographia), and general slowness. *Rigidity* is increased muscle tone that is equal in all directions of movement, does not increase with increased velocity of passive movement, and does not have a particular preferred posture. Rigidity may have a "lead pipe" quality, in which the limb can be moved with difficulty into arbitrary postures, but once placed in a posture, will remain there against gravity. If there is superimposed tremor, the rigidity can feel ratchety, like a cogwheel. *Postural instability* manifests as increased likelihood of falling and is due to dysregulation of postural reflexes. Clinically, it is evaluated with the "pull test," in which the patient stands, facing away from the examiner with feet apart at shoulder width. The examiner gives a gentle pull backward at the shoulders bilaterally. A normal individual may take a step backward, but an individual with parkinsonian postural instability will take many steps backward (retropulsion) or may fall backward with no attempt to compensate.

Bradykinesia can be difficult to detect when hypertonia is present because hypertonia may be interpreted as the reason for slow movement. In parkinsonian syndromes in children, bradykinesia is likely to be a more disabling symptom than rigidity. Rigidity can be difficult to distinguish from other causes of hypertonia, including dystonia or spasticity. The absence of a spastic catch or fixed posture distinguishes rigidity from spasticity. The absence of overflow movements or a fixed abnormal posture helps to distinguish rigidity from dystonia, although both may exhibit co-contraction [Sanger et al., 2003]. Arm rigidity is often suspected by observing decreased arm swing when examining the patient's gait and is most easily seen when it is asymmetric. Rigidity can be brought out by facilitation maneuvers, such as having the child open and close one fist while the resistance to movement at the opposite elbow is tested.

In adults, the most common cause of parkinsonism is Parkinson's disease. In children, parkinsonism is uncommon but can be a manifestation of several different disorders, as discussed later [Riederer and Foley, 2002]. It is often associated with a dopaminergic deficit, and because dopaminergic deficits can produce dystonia in children, dystonia may be present as well [Yokochi, 2000].

Parkinson's Disease

Primary causes of parkinsonism in children are rare [Pranzatelli et al., 1994]. Dopa-responsive dystonia may be a relatively common cause compared with others, and has been described previously. Juvenile Parkinson's disease presents with leg dystonia in younger children and bradykinesia and rigidity in older children. It rarely demonstrates tremor. It most commonly presents in young adults, and childhood or juvenile onset is rare. Many cases are due to mutations in the parkin gene, labeled *PARK-2*, on chromosome 6q25.2-27 [Huynh et al., 2003; Ruiz-Linares, 2004]. This is autosomal-recessive and can be contrasted with the autosomal-dominant inheritance of some forms of adult parkinsonism associated with mutations in the α-synuclein gene. The autosomal-dominant form does not appear to occur in childhood. Other genes have been identified in specific families [Bentivoglio et al., 2001; DeStefano et al., 2002; Valente et al., 2002; West et al., 2002a; West et al., 2002b; West et al., 2003]. The pathology of parkin-associated Parkinson's disease does not show Lewy bodies, although there is neuronal loss and neurofibrillary tangles. Fluoro-dopa positron-emission tomography scanning can reveal decreased uptake, suggesting a presynaptic abnormality consistent with degeneration of the nigro-striatal pathways, rather than a metabolic defect in the synthesis of dopamine, as seen in dopa-responsive dystonia [Khan et al., 2002; Pal et al., 2002].

Juvenile Parkinson's disease is levodopa responsive in the early years. It will also respond to anticholinergic medication, dopamine agonists, and inhibitors of dopamine breakdown. However, escalating doses are required, and children eventually develop dyskinesias similar to those seen in adults on chronic dopaminergic therapy. It is important to differentiate this disorder from dopamine-responsive dystonia, as well as from other disorders that may respond to dopaminergic medication, because the prognosis is different and it may be helpful to consider treatment with dopamine-sparing medications, including dopamine agonists or inhibitors of dopamine breakdown, to prolong the efficacy and delay the onset of dyskinesias.

Secondary Parkinsonism

Causes of secondary parkinsonism are listed in Table 58-5. These include infarcts, particularly in the striatum or pallidum, as well as the ceroid lipofuscinoses, in which a combination of bradykinesia and visual loss leads to a very striking hesitancy of gait [Nijssen et al., 2002]. Pantothenate kinase–associated neurodegeneration can be a cause of bradykinesia. Similarly, spinocerebellar ataxia, Rett's syndrome, Huntington's disease, and Wilson's disease can be a cause of bradykinesia. Parkinsonism can be associated with acute encephalitis or postencephalitic parkinsonism. The widespread epidemic of encephalitic parkinsonism (von Economo's disease) that occurred between 1916 and 1930 has not recurred, and the term *encephalitis lethargica* should probably be reserved for patients who were victims of that epidemic. There are reported cases of a similar syndrome after streptococcal illness [Dale et al., 2004; Kiley and Esiri, 2001; Vincent, 2004]. Whether the original epidemic of encephalitis lethargica was due to influenza virus has been called into doubt recently [Jellinger, 2001; Lo et al., 2003].

Several medications and toxins are known to be able to cause parkinsonism [Pranzatelli et al., 1994]. Parkinsonism is a common side effect of tetrabenazine and reserpine and can be seen with neuroleptic treatment as well. The chemical MPTP, which is a synthetic methamphetamine derivative used for illicit recreational purposes, led to several cases of very rapid onset of irreversible parkinsonism; its use also has

TABLE 58-5

Causes of Parkinsonism

Static Injury, Structural
Basal ganglia infarcts, brain tumor, hydrocephalus
Hereditary, Degenerative
Juvenile Parkinson's disease, spinocerebellar ataxia, Huntington's disease (Westphal variant), PKAN, Rett's syndrome, Pelizaeus-Merzbacher disease, Machado-Joseph disease (SCA3)
Metabolic
Dopa-responsive dystonia, tyrosine hydroxylase deficiency and other abnormalities of bioamine metabolism, abnormalities of folate metabolism, Wilson's disease, basal ganglia calcification (Fahr's disease, hypoparathyroidism)
Infectious, Parainfectious
Encephalitis lethargica (Von Economo's disease), viral encephalitis, acute demyelinating encephalomyelitis
Drugs, Toxins
MPTP poisoning, rotenone, tetrabenazine, reserpine, methyldopa, sedatives, neuroleptics, antiemetics, calcium channel blockers, isoniazid, serotonin reuptake inhibitors (sertraline, fluoxetine), meperidine
Disorders That Mimic Parkinsonism
Catatonia, spasticity, hypothyroidism, depression

PKAN, pantothenate kinase–associated neurodegeneration; SCA, spinocerebellar ataxia.

become very important in research into the pathogenesis and treatment of parkinsonian syndromes [Burns et al., 1985; Eldridge and Rocca, 1985].

Treatment of Parkinsonism

Bradykinesia is the primary symptom that is responsive to treatment in childhood parkinsonism. It is usually assumed to be due to dopamine deficiency and therefore is treated with levodopa or dopamine agonists. Levodopa is combined with a peripheral decarboxylase inhibitor such as carbidopa to reduce side effects and increase delivery to the brain. Treatment is often initiated with a single dose of levodopa, 1 mg/kg (or 50 to 100 mg total) given in the morning, to evaluate for potential side effects including nausea or postural hypotension. If this dose is tolerated for 3 or 4 days, then therapeutic treatment can be initiated three times per day. Unless symptoms are present at night, the doses are usually given during the daytime to maximize effect. Dosage can be increased to a maximum of 10 to 15 mg/kg/day depending on effectiveness. In addition to nausea and hypotension, common side effects can include dystonia, agitation, sleeplessness, and behavior changes. The dosage must be adjusted gradually to find the optimal dose, and the optimal dose may change as the child grows. Additional carbidopa may be given to decrease nausea.

In adults and children with Parkinson's disease, long-term treatment with dopamine or dopamine agonists will eventually lead to dyskinesias and freezing episodes that can limit its use. Some authors have advocated "dopamine-sparing" strategies that involve the early use of dopamine agonists such as pergolide, pramipexole, or ropinirole, or dopamine breakdown inhibitors such as entacapone or selegiline [Jenner, 2003]. This approach remains controversial and has not been studied in children.

Amantadine may be used to treat dyskinesias associated with acute or chronic use of levodopa [Furukawa et al., 2004a], and it has some antiparkinsonian effects as well [Crosby et al., 2003; Paci et al., 2001]. Anticholinergic medication will improve parkinsonism, but it is more commonly used to treat associated dystonia. Deep brain stimulation in the internal globus pallidus or subthalamic nucleus has met with tremendous success in ameliorating symptoms of adult Parkinson's disease [Germano et al., 2004; Peppe et al., 2004]. Whether similar neurosurgical procedures would be effective in children is not known.

Failure of dopaminergic transmission can be divided into presynaptic and postsynaptic forms. In presynaptic failure, there is reduced production or release of dopamine at nigro-striatal nerve terminals. These reductions are typical in juvenile Parkinson's disease and dopa-responsive dystonia. In postsynaptic failure, there is injury to the striatal targets. This is typical following encephalitis or hypoxic injury. Treatment with dopaminergic medication is most successful when there is presynaptic failure. If injury is primarily postsynaptic, there may be some mild benefit from dopaminergic medication, but the effect is limited.

Myoclonus

Myoclonus is very brief, abrupt, involuntary, nonsuppressible, jerky contractions (or interruption of contraction) involving a single muscle or muscle group. The rapidity of these movements warrants the descriptor "shocklike," as if an electric shock had just been applied to the peripheral nerve innervating the muscle [Marsden et al., 1983]. Myoclonus can be rhythmic, in which case it often appears tremor-like. However, in true tremor, the movement oscillates with near equal amplitude around a midpoint, whereas in myoclonus, the movement has a more sawtooth character. In some cases, myoclonus can be elicited by a sensory stimulus (reflex myoclonus; the most famous example is the acoustic startle response in infancy) or volitional movement (action myoclonus). Myoclonus is perhaps the most protean of abnormal movements. It is present in normal (associated with sleep, exercise, anxiety) and pathologic situations, both epileptic and nonepileptic. Epileptic myoclonus is discussed in Chapter 46. This chapter limits its focus to nonepileptic myoclonus.

Classification of Myoclonus

Several different schemes have been used to classify myoclonus, using clinical, anatomic, or etiologic criteria. Perhaps the simplest classification is based on when the myoclonus occurs. Thus, myoclonus may occur at rest, with action, or in response to a sensory stimulus (reflex myoclonus). In adults it is helpful to classify myoclonus based on presumed neuroanatomic location (e.g., cerebral cortex, thalamus, brainstem, or spinal cord). The neurophysiology of myoclonus has been reviewed elsewhere [Caviness and Brown, 2004; Shibasaki and Hallett, 2004]. In children, etiologic classification is the most useful. This classification is summarized in Table 58-6.

Physiologic and Developmental Myoclonus

Physiologic myoclonus is that which occurs in normal individuals in specific settings. It includes such entities as hiccups, sleep starts, and sleep myoclonus. Sleep starts, also known as *hypnic myoclonus*, occur with sleep initiation [Montagna, 2004]. They are often accompanied by a sense of falling. Sleep starts are normal physiologic phenomena, and no treatment is required. Sleep myoclonus (nocturnal myoclonus) is also a part of normal sleep physiology. It is thought to result from paradoxical excitation during rapid-eye-movement sleep due to transient failure of brainstem inhibition [Montagna, 2004]. Sleep myoclonus in older children is more fragmentary than neonatal sleep myoclonus and tends to persist throughout life. No treatment is required.

Benign myoclonus may occur in association with specific developmental stages. Benign neonatal sleep myoclonus and benign myoclonus of early infancy are discussed in other sections of this chapter. Myoclonus can also occur with fever in otherwise normal children [Dooley and Hayden, 2004]. The myoclonic jerks may be quite frequent, but they are self-limited, ceasing when the fever resolves. Febrile myoclonus may be more common in younger children. No treatment is required.

Essential Myoclonus

Essential myoclonus is a relatively mild condition starting in the first or second decade. It is inherited as an autosomal-

TABLE 58-6

Causes of Myoclonus

Physiologic
Hiccups, hypnic jerks (sleep starts), nocturnal (sleep) myoclonus
Developmental
Benign neonatal sleep myoclonus, benign myoclonus of early infancy, myoclonus with fever
Essential (familial myoclonus dystonia syndrome)
Psychogenic
Storage diseases
Juvenile Gaucher's disease (type III), sialidosis type 1 (cherry red spot myoclonus), GM-1 gangliosidosis, neuronal ceroid lipofuscinosis (late infantile to juvenile)
Degenerative Conditions
Dentatorubro-pallidoluysian atrophy (DRPLA), Huntington's disease, progressive myoclonus, ataxia, Ramsay Hunt syndrome, dementias, bovine spongiform encephalopathy, Creutzfeldt-Jacob disease
Infectious and Postinfectious
Meningitis (viral or bacterial), encephalitis, Epstein-Barr virus, coxsackievirus, influenza, human immunodeficiency syndrome, acute disseminated encephalomyelitis
Metabolic
Uremia, hepatic failure, electrolyte disturbances, hypoglycemia or hyperglycemia, aminoacidurias, organic acidurias, urea cycle disorders, myoclonus epilepsy with ragged red fibers (MERRF), mitochondrial encephalomyopathy–lactic acidosis–and strokelike symptoms (MELAS), biotinidase deficiency (usually epileptic), cobalamin deficiency (infantile), opsoclonus-myoclonus syndrome (myoclonic encephalopathy of infancy)
Toxic
Psychotropic medications (tricyclic antidepressants, lithium, selective serotonin reuptake inhibitors, monoamine oxidase inhibitors, neuroleptics)
Antibiotics (penicillin, cephalosporins, quinolones)
Antiepileptics (phenytoin, carbamazepine, lamotrigine, gabapentin, benzodiazepines [in infants], vigabatrin)
Opioids
General anesthetics
Antineoplastic drugs
Strychnine, toluene, lead, CO, mercury
Hypoxia (Lance-Adams syndrome)
Focal lesions

dominant trait with incomplete penetrance [Fahn and Sjaastad, 1991; Quinn, 1996]. It is usually slowly progressive for a few years after onset and then stabilizes. The myoclonus may fluctuate slightly over the years, or may demonstrate mild spontaneous improvement. The myoclonus usually responds to ethanol, but the magnitude of benefit varies across individuals. The most common mutation identified is in the epsilon-sarcoglycan gene (7q21-q31). Mutations in this gene have also been associated with myoclonus-dystonia syndrome (see section on Myoclonus Dystonia). Many patients with essential myoclonus also have dystonia, and it appears that the two clinical syndromes may have the same underlying genetic basis [Nygaard et al., 1999; Quinn, 1996]. Some family members may have only myoclonus, others may have only dystonia, and others may have both myoclonus and dystonia. Essential myoclonus may respond to benzodiazepines, primidone, or propranolol.

Symptomatic Myoclonus

Myoclonus can be symptomatic of many disorders, as listed in Table 58-6. Many of these conditions are discussed elsewhere in this text. This section covers specific conditions in which myoclonus can be the primary feature.

MYOCLONIC ENCEPHALOPATHY OF INFANCY (OPSOCLONUS-MYOCLONUS SYNDROME)

Myoclonic encephalopathy is an uncommon acquired disorder of late infancy. It was first described by Kinsbourne and often is referred to as *Kinsbourne's syndrome* [Kinsbourne, 1962]. It has also been called *infantile polymyoclonia* [Dyken and Kolar, 1968] and *opsoclonus-myoclonus syndrome.* The clinical features of the syndrome include acute or subacute onset of rapid, dancing eye movements and myoclonic jerking of the limbs and trunk. The eye movements (opsoclonus) are usually conjugate but can be dysconjugate. As the disorder progresses, there is increased severity of the truncal myoclonus, which often prevents children from standing or walking. The myoclonus usually ceases during sleep but may persist. The opsoclonus may also persist during sleep. In some children, the myoclonus is stimulus sensitive, and it usually increases with action. The marked increase of myoclonus with action may make it difficult to distinguish this from ataxia. Many children with this condition have prominent irritability.

Myoclonic encephalopathy has several potential causes. An important association has been made between myoclonic encephalopathy and neuroblastoma [Warrier et al., 1985]. The opsoclonus and myoclonus typically occur before the tumor is diagnosed [Dyken and Kolar, 1968]. The pathophysiology of myoclonic encephalopathy associated with neuroblastoma is unknown but is presumed to be immune mediated [Pranzatelli et al., 2004]. Removal of the tumor does not prevent relapse or permanent sequelae. Immunomodulatory therapy can be effective in some patients, but even with treatment, most patients have at least mild neurologic sequelae [Hayward et al., 2001].

About half the patients with myoclonic encephalopathy do not have an identifiable neuroblastoma [Tate et al., 2005]. In some instances the cause is most likely infectious or postinfectious. It has been associated with aseptic meningitis but more commonly follows a viral infection [Kinsbourne, 1962; Sheth et al., 1995]. There can be elevation of cerebrospinal fluid protein and mild lymphocytic pleocytosis, but the presence of cerebrospinal fluid pleocytosis does not distinguish paraneoplastic from infectious opsoclonus-myoclonus syndrome [Mitchell and Snodgrass, 1990; Tate et al., 2005]. Similar serum antineuronal antibodies have been detected in patients with postinfectious or neuroblastoma-associated opsoclonus-myoclonus syndrome [Connolly et al., 1997].

It is necessary to undertake a careful investigation for occult neuroblastoma in all infants and children with myoclonic encephalopathy unless the cause is obvious. The symptoms of children with and without neuroblastoma respond to adrenocorticotropic hormone therapy [Tate et al., 2005] (40 units/m^2/day), which has proved highly effective in many instances. Removal of the tumor may lead to symptom resolution, but it may be followed by recurrence.

DYSSYNERGIA CEREBELLARIS MYOCLONICA (RAMSAY HUNT SYNDROME)

Hunt reported six patients with seizures, action myoclonus, and intention tremor and termed their condition *dyssynergia cerebellaris myoclonica* [Hunt, 1921]. One twin whose progressive neurologic symptoms began in the third decade of life came to postmortem examination; the other twin experienced myoclonus 2 years before seizures began. Atrophy of the dentate nucleus and hypodense myelin in the superior cerebellar peduncle were evident, as was disruption of the spinocerebellar tracts. Hunt ascribed the clinical findings to the dentate nucleus pathology. A familial pattern was suggested. A number of patients have been reported since the first description. There is not a single underlying cause for this syndrome, and it has been debated whether this is even a unique syndrome.

DENTATORUBRO-PALLIDOLUYSIAN ATROPHY

Dentato-rubropallidoluysian atrophy (DRPLA) is an autosomal-dominant, degenerative disorder of the dentate nucleus, red nucleus, globus pallidus, and subthalamic nucleus [Becher et al., 1997]. Clinical features include myoclonus (see Chapter 57), cerebellar ataxia, epilepsy, choreoathetosis, and dementia. The disease is caused by a CAG repeat expansion in the *DRPLA* gene, on chromosome 12p13. It is most common in people of Japanese or Portuguese origin, but it has been reported in other groups.

POSTANOXIC MYOCLONUS

Lance and Adams described myoclonus as a consequence of severe hypoxia during surgery in adults [Lance and Adams, 1963]. Postanoxic myoclonus is primarily an action or intention myoclonus. It can be disabling and can include negative myoclonus that may lead to falls. Some infants who undergo hypoxic-ischemic brain injury at birth develop continuous myoclonic activity of the face and limbs. This condition has been called *polymyoclonus* but may be a variant of Lance-Adams syndrome.

Treatment of Myoclonus

Myoclonus is often refractory to medical treatment. Cortical myoclonus may respond to benzodiazepines and is commonly treated with clonazepam (although sleep myoclonus may worsen [Reggin and Johnson, 1989]). Valproic acid is sometimes helpful, but it must be used with caution because of the ability to cause tremor as a side effect with consequent confusion of symptoms. Piracetam has been used for many years to treat myoclonus with good efficacy. Levetiracetam is a piracetam analogue but does not seem to have equivalent efficacy to piracetam. There are recent reports of efficacy with zonisamide, but this is still under evaluation. Posthypoxic myoclonus seems to be particularly responsive to serotonergic medications, including selective serotonin reuptake inhibitors and oral administration of 5-hydroxytryptophan or 5-hydroxytryptamine. Baclofen has been occasionally used, but the mechanism of action is not clear. Carbamazepine can make myoclonus worse.

Ataxia

Ataxia is discussed in detail in Chapter 57 and in several other chapters of this textbook. For a detailed list of the causes of ataxia in children, see Table 58-7. Ataxia can be defined by a combination of features that lead to poor coordination. Children with ataxia exhibit intention tremor with worsening amplitude and frequency of tremor on approach to a target, particularly with finger-to-nose testing. They also display dysmetria with inaccuracy pointing to a target with either the hand or the foot, and poor coordination. Gait often is wide based and unsteady, and when ataxia affects the mouth, it leads to dysarthria, without the abnormal muscle contractions seen in spasmodic dysphonia

TABLE 58-7

Causes of Ataxia

Causes
Static Injury, Structural
Cerebral palsy, stroke, trauma, hypoxic injury, Joubert's syndrome, Dandy-Walker malformation, basilar impression, vermian agenesis, cerebellar dysgenesis, rhombencephalosynapsis, Chiari malformation types 2 and 3, pontocerebellar hypoplasia
Hereditary, Degenerative
Ataxia-telangiectasia, ataxia oculomotor apraxia, Friedreich's ataxia, spinocerebellar ataxia (including Machado-Joseph disease), dentatorubro-pallidoluysian atrophy (DRPLA), olivopontocerebellar atrophy (OPCA), Marinesco-Sjögren syndrome, Pelizaeus-Merzbacher disease, childhood ataxia with central hypomyelination (CACH) syndrome
Metabolic
Hartnup's disease, lipidoses, mitochondrial disorders (including Leigh's disease, myoclonus epilepsy with ragged red fibers [MERRF], NARP, and pyruvate dehydrogenase complex deficiency), glutaric aciduria, Refsum's disease, vitamin deficiency (B_{12}, E, thiamine), abetalipoproteinemia (Bassen-Kornzweig disease), lysosomal storage disorders (including Krabbe's disease, metachromatic leukodystrophy, carnitine acetyltransferase deficiencies, juvenile Gaucher's disease, Tay-Sachs disease), ceroid lipofuscinosis, congenital disorders of glycosylation (CDG), biotinidase deficiency, holocarboxylase deficiency, Niemann-Pick type C, hypothyroidism, propionic acidemia, maple syrup urine disease and its thiamine-responsive variant, urea cycle disorders, porphyria, and electrolyte or glucose abnormalities
Neoplastic, Paraneoplastic
Tumors of the cerebellum or brainstem, neuroblastoma in the chest or abdomen (associated with the opsoclonus-myoclonus-ataxia syndrome)
Immune Mediated, Demyelinating
Acute postinfectious cerebellar ataxia, antigliadin antibody (gluten enteropathy), Miller-Fisher variant of Guillain-Barré syndrome, multiple sclerosis
Drugs, Toxins
Antiepileptic medication (particularly phenytoin and carbamazepine), antihistamines, barbiturates, lithium, alcohol, chemotherapy, heavy metal poisoning (lead, mercury, thallium), bromide intoxication
Paroxysmal
Dominant familial episodic ataxias (EA1, EA2), calcium channel disorders, basilar migraine
Disorders that Mimic Ataxia
Weakness, low blood pressure, any peripheral neuropathy or central cause of proprioceptive loss (with lack of sensation in the feet), astasia-abasia (usually psychogenic), seizures (pseudo ataxia), paroxysmal vertigo (may be a migraine variant)

or dystonic dysarthria. Movements in ataxia appear to be disjointed, with a lack of coordination between the movements of different joints, and in some cases movement of one joint will lead to a loss of balance owing to inappropriate compensation for the resulting forces. Children appear very unsteady in all their movements, with reduced accuracy. Slow movements tend to be performed much more accurately than fast movements, and this has led to the hypothesis that in ataxia there is difficulty compensating for the dynamics of movement and difficulty with accurate estimation of the forces required to both accelerate and decelerate objects of known mass. Rapid repetitive or small cyclic movements may be particularly difficult, a symptom referred to as *dysdiadochokinesia*. It is important to distinguish ataxia from weakness, dystonia, chorea, athetosis, and tremor, all of which can lead to inaccurate or apparently uncoordinated movements. Weakness exacerbates or mimics ataxia, and therefore adequate strength needs to be tested. Ataxia is worsened if there is poor support of proximal joints. For example, a child with ataxia affecting reaching appears much worse if he or she must reach with the trunk unsupported.

The primary causes of ataxia include the spinocerebellar ataxias, ataxia-telangiectasia, ataxia-oculomotor apraxia, Friedreich's ataxia, DRPLA, and other genetic causes known to lead to ataxia. In addition, certain congenital malformations, including Joubert's syndrome, pontocerebellar hypoplasia, Dandy-Walker syndrome and its variants, and vermian agenesis, can cause of ataxia.

Secondary causes of ataxia include cerebral palsy, of which the ataxic form is rare, but this term is often used to encompass some of the malformations described earlier. Metabolic disease can lead to intermittent ataxia [Parker and Evans, 2003] or secondary cerebellar degenerative diseases. Such metabolic diseases include congenital disorders of glycosylation, mitochondrial disorders, vitamin E deficiency, and Refsum's disease, with abnormalities of processing of phytanic acid. It is important to exclude opsoclonus-myoclonus ataxia, even when neither opsoclonus nor myoclonus is present [Mitchell et al., 2002]. This disorder presents in early childhood but can present later in the juvenile years, and is thought to be due to cross-reactivity of antibodies against neuroblastoma. Even after removal of the tumor the antibodies may persist, and long-term immunosuppressive treatment with corticosteroids, adrenocorticotropic hormone, intravenous immunoglobulins, or chemotherapeutic agents may be required. If left untreated, the ataxia will worsen, and there may be progressive cognitive decline.

Acute Cerebellar Ataxia

Acute cerebellar ataxia is a clinical syndrome defined by the rapid onset of cerebellar dysfunction, which manifests primarily as gait disturbance and incoordination [Davis et al., 2003; Connolly et al., 1994; Gieron-Korthals et al., 1994]. Acute cerebellar ataxia is relatively rare and the annual incidence has been estimated to be approximately 1 case in 100,000 to 500,000 children [Davis and Marino, 2003]. A recent study of 39 children with acute cerebellar ataxia found the mean age of children presenting with this disorder to be 4.8 years [Nussinovitch et al., 2003]. A prodromal febrile illness was noted in about 75%, and the latency from the prodromal illness to the onset of ataxia was approximately 9 days. The most common infections included varicella (31%), mumps (20%), nonspecific viral infection (15.4%), mycoplasma (5%), and Epstein-Barr virus (3%). Other studies have found that enterovirus [Huang et al., 1999] and parvovirus [Shimizu et al., 1999] infections also can cause acute cerebellar ataxia. Acute cerebellar ataxia may also occur after immunizations for varicella, hepatitis B, and rabies. Symptoms typically include ataxia and difficulties with fine motor coordination; some patients develop headache. The occur-rence of fever, altered mental status, or nuchal rigidity should prompt evaluation for a central nervous system (CNS) infection (Chapter 68). In a study of 39 children, recovery occurred within a mean of 2 weeks but took up to 24 days in some patients, a time frame shorter than that previously reported [Nussinovitch et al., 2003]. About 90% of patients with acute cerebellar ataxia will make a complete recovery [Connolly et al., 1994]. The risk of chronic cerebellar symptoms is associated with an older age or if Epstein-Barr virus infection is present [Davis and Marino, 2003]. About 20% of children have transient behavioral or intellectual difficulties and only rarely will long-term learning problems persist [Connolly et al., 1994].

The etiology of acute cerebellar ataxia is uncertain, but it is considered, in part, to be a postviral inflammatory disease. Viral nucleic acids and antiviral antibodies have been isolated from the cerebrospinal fluid of affected patients [Abdul Hafiz et al., 1996; Adams et al., 2000; Davis and Marino, 2003].

The evaluation of the child with acute cerebellar ataxia initially should focus on whether there may be a mass lesion or infection in the CNS, to determine whether neuroimaging and lumbar puncture are indicated. Neuroimaging, including computed tomography (CT) and magnetic resonance imaging (MRI), is normal in the majority of patients with acute cerebellar ataxia, but in some patients evidence of cerebellar inflammation is present [Connolly et al., 1994; Soussan et al., 2003]. It has been suggested that the presence of lesions on MRI is associated with a poorer prognosis but this observation is inconsistent. Likewise children with normal neuroimaging may have sequelae of chronic ataxia. An increase in the number of white cells may be seen on cerebrospinal fluid examination, and on occasion the cerebrospinal fluid protein is elevated [Gieron-Korthals et al., 1994]. Early in the course, it may be difficult to distinguish a para-infectious acute cerebellar ataxia syndrome from an acute viral or bacterial CNS infection, and in such cases, antiviral agents or antibiotics should be administered until cultures and serologic test results become available. Currently, routine assays for cerebrospinal fluid autoantibodies or for myelin basic protein do not appear to be clinically indicated, because the yield from such testing is unknown.

There is no specific therapy for acute cerebellar ataxia. Steroids and intravenous immune globulin have been anecdotally used for treatment but no class I studies have been conducted to ascertain whether either is of clinical benefit. Because of the association with varicella, antiviral therapy with acyclovir has been used in patients with immune deficiency syndromes, but this treatment also has not been prospectively evaluated. Pleconaril, which is believed to be of benefit in treating enteroviral meningitis, is another potential treatment option, but recent small studies have shown that it is not effective in enteroviral meningitis in children [Tunkel, 2004].

In addition to infectious causes, the differential diagnosis of acute onset of ataxia includes several metabolic diseases. In particular the urea cycle disorders need to be excluded because these can present with episodic ataxia. Other disorders, including mitochondrial disease and congenital disorders of glycosylation, can present with acute onset or episodic ataxia.

Developmental disorders that lead to ataxia and that present in the first year of life often exhibit hypotonia, which only later evolves to ataxia. Because it is known that the cerebellum is involved with the control of tone, it is not surprising that early cerebellar abnormalities might lead to hypotonia, but whether this is an obligate feature of later ataxia is not known.

Ataxia is very difficult to treat and constitutes a negative symptom, meaning that it is lack of a particular skill rather than an excess of muscle activity. The mainstay of treatment is physical and occupational therapy, and in some cases adaptation of the environment may be successful. Nevertheless, treatment is often not successful, and children with even static forms of ataxia generally fail to improve despite intervention.

Paroxysmal Dyskinesia

Paroxysmal dyskinesias are a relatively rare subset of hyperkinetic movement disorders that are defined by their episodic nature. Mount and Reback reported an apparent familial form in which the proband had infantile onset of episodes that began with a tight sensation in the neck and abdomen and a sense of fatigue followed by involuntary flexion of the arms and extension of the legs (dystonia) [Mount and Reback, 1940]. The spells progressed to involuntary choreoathetosis and dysarthria despite normal consciousness; Mount and Reback called the condition *familial paroxysmal choreoathetosis*. Kertesz described a group of patients who primarily had a childhood onset of movement-induced paroxysmal choreoathetosis. He highlighted the kinesigenic component and coined the term *paroxysmal kinesigenic choreoathetosis* [Kertesz, 1967]. The kinesigenic form was defined by a brief (seconds to minutes) duration of the episode, whereas the nonkinesigenic form was defined to be longer lasting (minutes to hours). Subsequently, the term *paroxysmal dystonic choreoathetosis of Mount and Reback* was used to delineate this form from the more common paroxysmal kinesigenic choreoathetosis [Richards and Barnett, 1968]. Another form with intermediate-duration attacks precipitated by prolonged exercise has been described [Lance, 1977].

The traditional terminology has been a cause for confusion about the types of movements and the relationship between precipitating factors and the duration of episodes. The paroxysmal dyskinesias can manifest as chorea, dystonia, or both. Specifically, paroxysmal dystonic choreoathetosis is not always dystonic, and paroxysmal kinesigenic choreoathetosis may be purely dystonic. The kinesigenic form is not always brief, and the Mount and Reback form is not always of long duration. Therefore, Demirkiran and Jankovic [1995] developed a classification scheme that was based primarily on the precipitating events, arguing that the precipitant is the best predictor of clinical course and response to specific medications. They proposed the following classification of paroxysmal dyskinesias: kinesigenic, nonkinesigenic, exertion induced, and hypnogenic (also called *paroxysmal nocturnal dystonia of sleep*). Secondary categorization is based on duration; short is less than or equal to 5 minutes, and long is greater than 5 minutes. The tertiary classification is based on etiology: idiopathic (familial versus sporadic) and secondary.

Paroxysmal Kinesigenic Dyskinesia

Paroxysmal kinesigenic dyskinesia is often inherited in an autosomal dominant fashion, but one fourth of the cases are sporadic. Males are affected more often than females by a ratio of 4:1 [Goodenough et al., 1978; Lotze and Jankovic, 2003]. The age of onset is 5 to 15 years in familial cases but may be variable in sporadic cases. The attacks are typically precipitated by startle or making a sudden movement after a period of rest. There is often a refractory period after an episode during which a sudden movement will not provoke an attack. The attacks may occur up to 100 times per day. The duration is typically a few seconds to a few minutes, but longer-lasting attacks may occur [Demirkiran and Jankovic, 1995]. The movements may be preceded by an abnormal sensation in the affected limbs, and some patients may only have an abnormal sensation without developing involuntary movements. Most patients have dystonia, but some have a combination of chorea and dystonia and rarely ballism. The attacks may be limited to one side of the body or even one limb. The attacks decrease in frequency during adulthood [Kertesz, 1967; Lotze and Jankovic, 2003].

Three types of paroxysmal kinesigenic dyskinesia have been linked to chromosome 16. The first is the syndrome of familial infantile convulsions and paroxysmal choreoathetosis, which has been linked to the pericentromeric region of chromosome 16 [Swoboda et al., 2000; Szepetowski et al., 1997]. Individuals homozygous for the disease haplotype in the pericentromeric region of chromosome 16 have earlier age of onset and higher frequency of attacks than heterozygous family members [Demir et al., 2004].

A syndrome of paroxysmal kinesigenic dyskinesia without infantile convulsions has also been linked to the pericentromeric region of chromosome 16 that overlaps with the region for infantile convulsions and paroxysmal choreoathetosis [Bennett et al., 2000]. A family with paroxysmal kinesigenic dyskinesia has been described with linkage to 16q and with no overlap with the pericentromeric region reported for the other families [Spacey et al., 2002].

In addition to idiopathic or genetic causes, there are many other causes of paroxysmal kinesigenic dyskinesia. These include multiple sclerosis, cerebral palsy, head trauma, strokes, hypoparathyroidism, maple syrup urine disease, infection, and methylphenidate therapy [Blakeley and Jankovic, 2002; Gay and Ryan, 1994; Kato et al., 1987; Temudo et al., 2004].

Paroxysmal kinesigenic dyskinesia responds well to antiepileptic drugs, including phenytoin, carbamazepine, phenobarbital, and levetiracetam [Chatterjee et al., 2002; Goodenough et al., 1978]. The dose required is usually less than the standard antiepileptic dosage, and familial paroxysmal kinesigenic dyskinesia is exquisitely responsive to carbamazepine [Wein et al., 1996]. With or without treatment, the attacks tend to diminish during adulthood, and individuals do not have progressive neurologic deficits.

Paroxysmal Nonkinesigenic Dyskinesia

Paroxysmal nonkinesigenic dyskinesia is usually inherited as an autosomal-dominant trait. Males are affected more often than females (2:1 ratio). The age of onset is usually in early childhood, but attacks may not start until the early 20s. The frequency varies from three per day to two or fewer per year. Typical precipitating factors are fatigue, alcohol, caffeine, and emotional excitement. An episode may start with involuntary movements of a single limb, but may spread to involve all extremities and the face. The usual duration is minutes to 3 to 4 hours, but shorter and longer episodes have been reported [Demirkiran and Jankovic, 1995]. During the attack, the patient may be unable to communicate, but remains conscious and continues to breathe normally. Some individuals have mostly dystonia [Forssman, 1961], whereas others have predominant chorea [Mount and Reback, 1940]. Attacks may be relieved by sleep.

Paroxysmal nonkinesigenic dyskinesia has been linked to chromosome 2q in the region of a putative ion channel gene [Fink et al., 1997; Hofele et al., 1997]. Nongenetic causes include multiple sclerosis, infection, hypoglycemia, thyrotoxicosis, hypoparathyroidism, moyamoya disease, pseudohypoparathyroidism, and biopterin synthesis defects [Blakeley and Jankovic, 2002; Dure and Mussell, 1998; Factor et al., 1991; Gonzalez-Alegre et al., 2003].

Management of paroxysmal nonkinesigenic dyskinesia relies on avoidance of precipitating factors such as alcohol, caffeine, and stress. Several medications have been used, including clonazepam, haloperidol, oxazepam, acetazolamide, and anticholinergics [Micheli et al., 1987]. Antiepileptic drugs are ineffective in most cases. Prognosis is variable and depends on the underlying cause. In familial cases, neurologic function between the attacks is normal, even after repeated attacks.

Paroxysmal Exertion-Induced Dyskinesia

Paroxysmal exertion-induced dyskinesia is usually inherited in an autosomal-dominant fashion, although sporadic cases have been described [Bhatia et al., 1997]. The attacks are triggered by prolonged exercise [Lance, 1977]. The frequency varies from one per day to two per month. The usual duration is 5 to 30 minutes.

Autosomal-dominant paroxysmal choreoathetosis-spasticity, an exercise-induced dyskinesia frequently with spastic paraplegia during the episode, has been mapped to a 12 cM region on chromosome 1p in the vicinity of a potassium channel gene cluster [Auburger et al., 1996]. Another family has been described with paroxysmal exercise-induced dystonia and migraine that was not linked to the paroxysmal nonkinesigenic dyskinesia locus on chromosome 2, the infantile convulsions and paroxysmal kinesigenic dyskinesia locus on chromosome 16, or the familial hemiplegic migraine locus on chromosome 19, suggesting that other loci exist for paroxysmal exertion-induced dyskinesia [Munchau et al., 2000]. In addition to genetic causes, paroxysmal exertion-induced dyskinesia has been reported after head trauma [Demirkiran and Jankovic, 1995].

Avoidance of prolonged exercise may help diminish the frequency of attacks. Drug therapy is often ineffective, but there are isolated reports of improvement with levodopa and acetazolamide [Bhatia et al., 1997; Demirkiran and Jankovic, 1995]. Prognosis is variable; neurologic function remains normal between attacks in familial and idiopathic forms.

Paroxysmal Hypnogenic Dyskinesia

Paroxysmal hypnogenic dyskinesia is sometimes known as *paroxysmal nocturnal dystonia*. It is characterized by attacks of dystonia, chorea, or ballism during non–rapid-eye-movement sleep [Lugaresi and Cirignotta, 1981; Lugaresi et al., 1986]. The frequency may be from five times per year to five times per night. These attacks may be associated with electroencephalographic signs of arousal, and the patient usually falls asleep after the attack. The usual duration of the attacks is 30 to 45 seconds but may be longer. Sometimes the patients may have daytime attacks of dyskinesia. Paroxysmal hypnogenic dyskinesia is probably a heterogeneous condition comprising attacks of different durations and clinical features, but it appears that many cases result from frontal lobe seizures, and it has been reported in association with orbitofrontal cortical dysplasia [Lombroso, 2000; Provini et al., 2000].

Short-duration paroxysmal hypnogenic dyskinesia may respond to antiepileptic drugs, including carbamazepine and phenytoin. The longer-lasting attacks respond less well but may improve with haloperidol or acetazolamide. It is essential to rule out frontal lobe epilepsy as the underlying cause. Prognosis depends on the etiology.

Tic Disorders

Tics are the most common movement disorder in children. Tics are repeated sudden, stereotyped, discrete, intermittent movements. When movements involve skeletal muscle, they are called *motor tics*. When the movements involve the diaphragm or laryngeal-pharyngeal muscles, and a sound is produced, they are called *phonic* or *vocal tics*. There is a great range of severity, and mild tics are not uncommon in healthy children [Kurlan et al., 1988]. Tics occur many times a day, nearly every day. They typically change anatomic location, frequency, type, complexity, and severity over time. Tics can be classified by mode of manifestation (motor or vocal) and complexity (simple or complex). Motor tics can be further classified by speed and quality as clonic (abrupt and fast) or dystonic-tonic (slow and sustained). Simple motor tics include blinking, nose twitching, grimacing, neck jerking, shoulder elevation, sustained eye closure, gaze shifts, bruxism, and abdominal tensing. Simple vocal tics include sniffing, throat clearing, grunting, squeaking, humming, coughing, blowing, and sucking sounds. Complex tics appear more "purposeful" than simple tics and may include combinations of movements of multiple body parts. Complex motor tics include head shaking, trunk flexion, scratching, touching, finger tapping, hitting, jumping, kicking, and gestures (obscene gestures are termed *copropraxia*). Complex vocal tics include spoken syllables words or phrases, shouting of obscenities or profanities (coprolalia), repetition of the words of others (echolalia), and repetition of final syllable, word, or phrase of one's own words (palilalia) [Robertson, 2003]. Tics and Tourette's syndrome are described in greater detail in Chapter 37.

Treatment of Tic Disorders

Mild or moderate tic disorders often do not require treatment, and appropriate modification of the environment and reassurance of parents may be all that is needed [Bower, 1981]. For example, a child who is having social difficulty because of a tic may be able to do a class presentation or otherwise explain to their friends the nature of the disease, and the demystification of the disease may resolve the social complications. Anxiety, depression, or stress can often be triggers, and treatment of the triggers may be more helpful than treatment of the resulting tics. Treatment should be directed at improvement of specific abilities of the child, usually involving school participation or the ability to work. Discomfort or embarrassment of the parents should not be the sole indication for treatment.

Medications that are effective include clonidine, guanfacine, benzodiazepines, and neuroleptics. Neuroleptics must be used with caution but these are often the most effective medicines. The goal of medication is not to completely eliminate the tics, but rather to reduce them to an adequate level that allows the child to achieve his or her functional goals. Complete elimination of tics is generally not possible. Because tic disorders wax and wane over time, it is essential to make frequent attempts to discontinue medications because apparent success of the medication may instead be the result of waning of the underlying disorder rather than any direct effect of the intervention. Similarly, apparent lack of effect could be due to a worsening of the disorder, and therefore it is essential to continually reevaluate the use of all medications, particularly when children are taking multiple medications. The use of multiple neuroleptics simultaneously is strongly discouraged because this seems to increase the risk for tardive symptoms.

Tic disorders are frequently associated with obsessive-compulsive disorder or attention-deficit disorder, and these disorders may be much more disabling and lead to much more significant effects on school performance than the tic disorder itself. Therefore, it is important to screen for these disorders and treat them appropriately.

Stereotypy

Motor stereotypies are rhythmic, patterned, repetitive, involuntary movements that can occur in association with specific diseases or in otherwise normal children [Bodfish et al., 2000; Mahone et al., 2004]. In the minds of many physicians, stereotypies are associated with autism, sensory deficits, or mental retardation. However, they are not uncommon in normal children. The term *physiologic stereotypies* has been suggested for when these movements occur in normal children [Mahone et al., 2004]. Typical movements include repeated recurrent raising and lowering of the arms, flapping, waving, wrist rotation, and finger wiggling. They are often accompanied by facial movements or grimacing. Other terms have been used to describe stereotypies, including *rhythmic habit patterns, gratification phenomena, self-stimulation,* and *motor rhythmias*. Physiologic stereotypies may be present in any setting but are most common when the child is excited, mentally engaged, stressed, or bored. They may increase with fatigue. A hallmark of stereotypies is that they usually cease when the child is distracted or engaged in a new activity. Most children appear to be unaware of the stereotypies. When a child is asked during the movement, "Why are you doing that?" the most common response is "Doing what?"

The clinical characteristics of physiologic stereotypes have been described in a small number of studies [Mahone et al., 2004; Tan et al., 1997]. The typical age of onset for childhood stereotypies is less than 2 years. They are more common in boys (almost a 2:1 ratio). Unlike tics, stereotypies tend not to change in anatomic location or complexity over time. Stereotypies are not preceded by an urge or thought as is common with tics or compulsions. Physiologic stereotypies last for multiple years in most children. In some children, they disappear over time, but in other cases, they persist into adulthood. Although commonly seen in otherwise normal children, there appears to be an increased incidence of attention-deficit–hyperactivity disorder or learning disabilities in children with stereotypies.

There is no consistently effective pharmacologic treatment for physiologic stereotypies. Stereotypies typically do not bother the patient but can be distressing to the parents. They rarely interfere with task performance by the individual with stereotypies but may cause embarrassment or have other social impact. Behavioral therapy may be effective [Miller, 2004]. Repeated instruction to the child to "stop that" is usually not effective.

Transient Developmental Movement Disorders

The presence of a movement disorder in a child usually raises concerns about an underlying serious, progressive, degenerative, or metabolic disease. However, many movement disorders are benign and related to normal stages of development. In fact, it may be difficult to justify the term *disorder* in describing many of these movements. The developing nervous system may produce a variety of motor patterns that would be pathologic in older children and adults but are simply a manifestation of central nervous system immaturity. Like many of the neonatal reflexes (e.g., grasping, rooting, placing, tonic neck reflexes), these motor patterns disappear as neuron connectivity and myelination matures. Examples include the minimal chorea of infants, the mild action dystonia commonly seen in toddlers, and the overflow movements that are commonly seen in young children. Other transient or developmental movement disorders may be manifestations of abnormal neural function but do not correlate with serious underlying pathology. These are typically associated with complete resolution of the abnormal movements and ultimately normal development and neurologic function. Most of these conditions occur during infancy or early childhood. It is important to recognize these transient developmental movement disorders, distinguish them from more serious disorders, and be able to provide reassurance when possible.

Benign Neonatal Sleep Myoclonus

Benign neonatal sleep myoclonus is characterized by repetitive myoclonic jerks occurring during sleep [Coulter and

Allen, 1982]. The myoclonic jerks are typically in the distal more than proximal limbs and are more prominent in the upper than lower extremities. In some cases, jerks of axial or facial muscles can be seen. The myoclonus can be focal, multifocal, unilateral, or bilateral. The movements can be rhythmic or nonrhythmic. Typically, the movements occur in clusters of jerks at 1 to 5 Hz over a period of several seconds. Benign neonatal sleep myoclonus begins during the first week of life, diminishes in the second month, and is usually gone before 6 months of age but has been reported to persist as long as 3 years in one patient [Egger et al., 2003]. Ictal and interictal electroencephalograms are typically normal [DiCapua et al., 1993]. The movements are most likely to occur during quiet (non–rapid-eye-movement) sleep [Resnick et al., 1986]. Waking the infant causes the movements to cease. Episodes of myoclonus can be exacerbated by treatment with benzodiazepines [Reggin and Johnson, 1989]. Treatment is not required, and neurologic outcome is normal.

Benign Myoclonus of Early Infancy

Benign myoclonus of early infancy is characterized by episodes of myoclonic spasms involving flexion of the trunk, neck, and extremities in a manner resembling the infantile spasms of West's syndrome [Lombroso, 1990; Lombroso and Fejerman, 1977]. The myoclonic spasms typically occur in clusters. In some cases they involve a shuddering movement of the head and shoulders, and in others the movements of the trunk and limbs are extensor. There is no change in consciousness during the spells. Unlike benign neonatal sleep myoclonus, the movements in benign myoclonus of early infancy occur only in the waking state. The onset of these spells is usually between ages 3 and 9 months, but they may begin in the first month of life. The spells usually cease within 2 weeks to 8 months of onset [Maydell et al., 2001] but may persist for 1 to 2 years [Lombroso, 1990]. Both ictal and interictal electroencephalograms are normal, distinguishing this entity from infantile spasms. Treatment is not required, but an electroencephalogram is usually needed to exclude infantile spasms or infantile myoclonic epilepsy syndromes. Development and neurologic outcome are normal.

Jitteriness

Jitteriness is a movement disorder that is commonly observed in the neonatal period. Jitteriness manifests as generalized, symmetric, rhythmic oscillatory movements that resemble tremor or clonus. Up to 50% of term infants exhibit jitteriness during the first few days of life, especially when stimulated or crying. Jitteriness usually disappears shortly after birth but can persist for months or recur after being gone for several weeks [Kramer et al., 1994; Shuper et al., 1991]. Persistent jitteriness has been associated with hypoxic-ischemic injury, hypocalcemia, hypoglycemia, drug withdrawal, and other causes of metabolic encephalopathies. Jitteriness is highly stimulus sensitive. It can be precipitated by startle and suppressed by gentle passive flexion of the limb. Unlike seizures, there are no associated abnormal eye movements or autonomic changes [Volpe, 2000]. Idiopathic jitteriness is usually associated with normal development and neurologic outcome. The outcome of infants with symptomatic jitteriness depends on the underlying cause.

Shuddering

Shuddering episodes are characterized by periods of rapid tremor of the head, shoulders, and arms that resemble shivering [Holmes and Russman, 1986; Kanazawa, 2000]. Onset is in infancy or early childhood but can occur as late as 10 years of age. The episodes last several seconds and can occur up to 100 times per day, often triggered by excitement or surprise. During a spell, there is no change in consciousness. Ictal and interictal electroencephalograms are normal. Preservation of consciousness, predictable triggers, ability to abort an episode when distracted by a parent, and normal electroencephalogram distinguish this entity from seizures. Similarity to benign myoclonus of early infancy has been suggested [Kanazawa, 2000], but shuddering is better classified as tremor than myoclonus. Shuddering episodes typically abate as the child grows older. The prognosis for development and neurologic function is uniformly good.

Paroxysmal Tonic Upgaze of Infancy

Paroxysmal tonic upgaze of infancy is a disorder characterized by repeated episodes of upward gaze deviation [Ouvrier and Billson, 1988]. The gaze deviation can be sustained or intermittent during an episode. The typical episode lasts for a few hours but can persist for days. Attempts to look downward are accompanied by down-beating nystagmus. Horizontal eye movements are normal during an episode. Spells may resolve with sleep and be aggravated by fatigue or infection. This condition remits spontaneously and completely within 1 to 4 years [Verrotti et al., 2001]. Some infants may have ataxia during episodes. There can be a positive family history in some cases. Laboratory investigations and imaging are usually unrevealing, although there is one report of a child with this condition with psychomotor retardation and MRI findings of periventricular leukomalacia [Campistol et al., 1993; Ouvrier and Billson, 1988]. There is no specific treatment, but there have been a few reports of improvement with levodopa treatment [Campistol et al., 1993; Ouvrier and Billson, 1988].

Spasmus Nutans

Spasmus nutans is a condition beginning in late infancy (3 to 8 months) that is characterized by a slow head tremor (about 2 Hz) that can be horizontal ("no-no") or vertical ("yes-yes"). The head movements are accompanied by a small-amplitude nystagmus that can be dysconjugate, conjugate, or uniocular [Anthony et al., 1980]. When the child is looking at an object, the nodding or nystagmus may increase, and if the head is held, the nystagmus typically increases. These observations have led to the suggestion that the head nodding is compensatory for the nystagmus [Gottlob et al., 1992]. Spasmus nutans generally resolves within several months, but most patients continue to have a fine subclinical nystagmus until at least 5 to 12 years of age [Gottlob et al., 1995]. Long-term outcome for visual acuity is good.

Spasmus nutans must be distinguished from congenital nystagmus [Gottlob et al., 1990]. Congenital nystagmus usually begins in the newborn period before 6 months of age. Congenital nystagmus is usually bilaterally symmetric, whereas spasmus nutans is often asymmetric. Congenital nystagmus persists beyond a few months. Visual acuity is abnormal in about 90% of children with congenital nystagmus. Although these features are useful in distinguishing congenital nystagmus from spasmus nutans, some children who clinically appear to have spasmus nutans at the time of presentation have been found to have retinal abnormalities by electroretinography [Smith et al., 2000]. Neuroimaging abnormalities, including tumor and aplasia of the cerebellar vermis, have been described in patients with spasmus nutans, but this is a rare association [Kim et al., 2003; Unsold and Ostertag, 2002]. Routine neuroimaging in the absence of other evidence for intracranial pathology has limited yield [Arnoldi and Tychsen, 1995], but the possibility of a mass lesion or destructive process in the posterior fossa must be considered.

Head Nodding

Head nodding without accompanying nystagmus can occur as paroxysmal events in older infants and toddlers [Nellhaus, 1983]. These head movements can be lateral ("no-no"), vertical ("yes-yes"), or oblique. The episodes may occur several times per day. The frequency (1 to 2 Hz) is slower than that of shuddering. The movements do not occur when the child is lying down but can occur in the sitting or standing position. The movements typically resolve within months but can persist longer. Some children with head nodding have a prior history of shuddering spells; others may have a family history of essential tremor [DiMario, 2000]. Development and neurologic outcome are unaffected by this condition.

Benign Paroxysmal Torticollis

Benign paroxysmal torticollis is an episodic disorder starting in the first year of life. It typically manifests as a head tilt to one side for a few hours or days. Spells can last as little as 10 minutes or as long as 2 months, but this is uncommon [Giffin et al., 2002]. The torticollis may occur without any associated symptoms or may be accompanied by pallor, vomiting, irritability, or ataxia. Episodes typically recur with some regularity, up to twice a month initially and becoming less frequent as the child grows older. The spells abate spontaneously, usually by 2 to 3 years of age but always by age 5. The child is normal between spells. Interictal and ictal electroencephalograms are normal.

It has been suggested that benign paroxysmal torticollis is a migraine variant [Al-Twaijri and Shevell, 2002]. There is often a family history of migraine. Some older children complain of headache during a spell, and many children go on to develop typical migraine after they have "outgrown" the paroxysmal torticollis [Deonna and Martin, 1981; Roulet and Deonna, 1988]. Two patients with benign paroxysmal torticollis have been reported from a kindred with familial hemiplegic migraine linked to a *CACNA1A* mutation [Giffin et al., 2002].

The differential diagnosis is broad, and diagnosis of benign paroxysmal torticollis is one of exclusion. Torticollis can be seen as an acute dystonic reaction to medication, as a symptom of a posterior fossa or cervical cord lesion, or as a cervical vertebral abnormality, such as Klippel-Feil syndrome. It is important to exclude posterior fossa abnormalities, such as Chiari syndrome or a mass. In the case of structural lesions, the torticollis tends to be persistent and not paroxysmal. Torticollis can also be a sign of cranial nerve palsy. Congenital muscular torticollis is another possibility; it is present from birth, is nonparoxysmal, and is associated with palpable tightness or fibrosis of the sternocleidomastoid muscle unilaterally.

Benign Idiopathic Dystonia of Infancy

Benign idiopathic dystonia of infancy is a rare disorder characterized by a segmental dystonia, usually of one upper extremity, that can be intermittent or persistent [Deonna et al., 1991; Willemse, 1986]. The syndrome usually appears before 5 months of age and disappears by 1 year of age. The characteristic posture is of shoulder abduction, pronation of the forearm, and flexion of the wrist. The posture occurs when the infant is at rest and disappears completely with volitional movement. Occasionally, both arms, an arm and leg on one side of the body, or the trunk can be involved. In some infants the posture is only apparent with relaxation or in certain positions. In others it may be present during all waking hours. The rest of the neurologic examination is normal, and the developmental and neurologic outcome is normal. Exclusion of progressive dystonia, brachial plexus injury, infantile hemiplegia, and orthopedic abnormalities is important.

Posturing during Masturbation

Masturbation is a normal behavior that occurs in both boys and girls. Although masturbation occurs at all ages and has even been observed in utero, it is most common at about 4 years of age and during adolescence [Leung and Robson, 1993]. Masturbation in young children may involve unusual postures or movements [Bower, 1981], which may be mistaken for abdominal pain or seizures [Fleisher and Morrison, 1990]. Masturbatory movements in boys are usually obvious to the observer because of direct genital manipulation. In girls, they are more subtle and often involve adduction of the thighs, or sitting on a hand or foot and rocking. When the movements are accompanied by posturing of the limbs they are often mistaken for paroxysmal dystonia. Several characteristic features of masturbating girls who present for diagnosis have been identified [Fleisher and Morrison, 1990; Mink and Neil, 1995]: (1) onset after 2 months of age and before 3 years of age; (2) stereotyped posturing with pressure applied to the pubic area; (3) quiet grunting, diaphoresis, or facial flushing; (4) episode duration of less than a minute to several hours; (5) no alteration of consciousness; (6) normal findings on examination; and (7) cessation with distraction or engagement of the child in another activity. Multiple diagnostic tests are often performed before the true nature of the behavior is recognized. No imaging or laboratory evaluation is required if the movements abate when the child is distracted, the movements involve irregular rocking, the child remains interactive, there is some degree of volitional control, direct genital stimulation is involved, and the neurologic and physical examinations are normal. There appears to be no association with sexual thoughts in the child. Instead, it is probably better to view these movements on the spectrum of other self-comforting behaviors such as thumb sucking or rocking, which have no concerning connotations for the parents [Mink and Neil, 1995]. Masturbation is a normal human behavior, so there is no expectation that this behavior will cease as the child grows older. However, the frequency of the behavior usually decreases as the child gets older, and the behavior is less likely to occur under the observation of the parents. Neurologic and developmental outcome is normal.

Transient Tic Disorder

Transient tic disorder is a disorder of childhood with one or several tics that are indistinguishable from the tics of chronic tic disorder but that last only several months. The diagnosis is made in retrospect because only with complete resolution can this be distinguished from a chronic tic disorder or Tourette syndrome. Transient tics can occur at any time during childhood but are most commonly seen in children of preschool and primary school age. About 10% of children may have a transient tic or tics [Robertson, 2003]. In most cases, transient tics do not require treatment. The cause is unknown, but transient tic disorder has been reported in members of a large kindred with Tourette syndrome, suggesting that transient tic disorder is a possible expression of the Tourette syndrome gene or genes [Kurlan et al., 1988]. Once the tics have resolved, they usually do not recur, and long-term prognosis is excellent.

Tardive Movement Disorders

Many medicines and environmental toxins are able to cause movement disorders, and examples were listed earlier under the specific relevant disorders. A particularly frustrating class of chemical-induced movement disorders is the tardive syndromes, including tardive dyskinesia, tardive dystonia, and tardive chorea. Tardive syndromes are most often caused by high-potency neuroleptic medications, including haloperidol, pimozide, or fluphenazine but can also be caused by atypical neuroleptics such as risperidone, olanzapine, and quetiapine and by medium- or low-potency neuroleptics used as antiemetics such as metoclopramide, chlorpromazine, and droperidol. All neuroleptics, with the exception of clozapine, are able to cause tardive reactions. Whether some neuroleptics have a lower rate of tardive movement disorders than others is not yet known. Children with preexisting mild brain injury may be at particularly high risk [Pourcher et al., 1995].

Symptoms of Tardive Movement Disorders

Onset of symptoms can occur shortly after starting the medication, or months or years later. In some cases, symptom onset can occur after termination of the medication, although this is rare. When symptoms start at the time of withdrawal of medication they are called *withdrawal emergent.* Tardive symptoms, when recognized rapidly, often resolve after discontinuation of the causative agent. However, in some cases tardive symptoms persist and may present a greater cause of disability than the original disorder for which the causative medication was prescribed.

Tardive dyskinesia involves rabbit-like mouth movements with pursing of the lips, rotational jaw and tongue movements, and other uncontrolled continuous but usually nonrhythmic facial movements. Limbs and trunk may be involved as well, but this is more common with tardive dystonia. Tardive dystonia can present as any of the forms of dystonia, involving a single limb or multiple body segments. Tardive chorea appears similar to other forms of chorea but can be severe with large proximal movements or ballism.

Treatment of Tardive Movement Disorders

Treatment of tardive symptoms relies on rapid withdrawal of the offending medication; therefore, patients must be warned of the possibility of these symptoms, so that they can alert their physicians and be taken off the medications as soon as possible after symptoms occur. Often the symptoms resolve spontaneously, in which case a rechallenge with neuroleptics should be avoided [Simpson, 2000]. If symptoms do not resolve, treatment with tetrabenazine may be helpful [Swash et al., 1972]. Tetrabenazine is a presynaptic dopamine depleter. It may be effective in dystonia but seems to be particularly effective in tardive dystonia and tardive dyskinesia [Asher and Aminoff, 1981]. Reserpine has a similar mechanism of action and may also be effective [Kang et al., 1986]. Treatment with a combination of large neutral amino acids (Tarvil), including phenylalanine and tyrosine, decreases the uptake of dopamine precursors and therefore is expected to have a similar effect to tetrabenazine. Pilot trials in tardive dyskinesia have shown promise [Richardson et al., 2003; Richardson et al., 1999; Richardson et al., 2004]. Neuroleptic medications themselves reduce tardive symptoms that persist after withdrawal from neuroleptics [Lucetti et al., 2002; Sasaki et al., 2004]; however, such treatment may perpetuate the disorder.

Other Movement Disorders

Restless Leg Syndrome and Periodic Leg Movements of Sleep

Restless leg syndrome manifests as an uncomfortable sensation in the legs that is typically relieved by movement. The sensation is poorly described by most children, but adults often use the descriptors "crawling," "pulling," or a "creeping" sensation under the skin. The sensation and movements occur most often at night and usually peak within the first 20 minutes of lying down. Relief is obtained by moving the legs while lying down or by walking. Restless leg syndrome responds to treatment with dopaminergic medication, and dopamine agonists are most often used for adults with this condition [Allen et al., 2004; Earley and Allen, 1996]. Treatment may not be needed in most children. It is frequently associated with periodic leg movements of sleep, which most often consist of brief flexion movements at the hip, knee, and ankle, occurring every few seconds while the child is asleep [Mahowald, 2003]. Periodic leg movements of sleep do not require treatment but can be helpful in the diagnosis of restless leg syndrome symptoms appearing while awake. There appears to be increased risk for both syndromes in children with symptoms of attention-deficit–hyperactivity disorder [Chervin et al., 2002; Picchietti et al., 1998].

Hyperekplexia

Hyperekplexia, otherwise known as *familial startle disease*, is an autosomal-dominant disorder characterized by an exaggerated startle reaction in response to sudden, unexpected auditory or tactile stimuli [Ryan et al., 1992]. Symptoms may begin in the neonatal period with profound and potentially fatal paroxysmal hypertonia and opisthotonic extensor posturing. Such episodes often resolve if the examiner flexes the neck, back, and knees of the child. Older children and adults may display nonadapting head retraction in response to nose tapping. The disorder is associated with mutations in the α_1 subunit of the glycine receptor [Shiang et al., 1993]. Symptoms respond well to treatment with clonazepam.

Bobble-Head Doll Syndrome

The bobble-head doll syndrome is a condition in which an infant or child has jerky head movements similar to certain types of toy dolls [Benton et al., 1966]. The movement is a continuous or episodic involuntary forward and backward or side to side movement of the head at the frequency of 2 to 3 Hz. The condition is usually associated with structural abnormalities leading to third ventricular dilation, including third ventricular cyst, aqueductal stenosis, or tumor [Mussell et al., 1997; Wiese et al., 1985]. It has been suggested that the tremor results from pressure on the red nucleus and that the bobbing behavior lessens the symptoms of hydrocephalus [Wiese et al., 1985]. However, most authors view the movement as involuntary and not compensatory [Mussell et al., 1997].

Volitional restraint momentarily controls the movements, but the movements recur when the patient ceases to concentrate on restraining them. Brain imaging virtually always confirms the presence of a structural abnormality. Surgical treatment is usually beneficial [Goikhman et al., 1998].

Spasticity

Spasticity is described in Chapter 20 on cerebral palsy. However, it is frequently associated with other movement disorders and is thus briefly addressed here. Along with dystonia and rigidity, spasticity is an important cause of hypertonia in childhood. Children with hypoxic-ischemic injury or other causes of cerebral palsy often have a combination of spasticity and dystonia [Sanger et al., 2003]. In some cases, treatment can be directed at both symptoms simultaneously.

Although spasticity is a reflection of increased sensitivity of the spinal motor neuron pools, prolonged spasticity leads to changes in the muscle and tendon and potential changes in the joint that may require mechanical treatment [Gracies, 2001]. In particular, long-standing spasticity and weakness are known to lead to shortening of the muscle-tendon unit, and therefore stretching, serial casting, and orthopedic procedures including tenotomy or tendon-lengthening procedures may be needed. Mechanical shortening of the muscle will not respond to centrally acting medications, neurolysis, or neuromuscular blockade.

Treatment planning requires careful attention to the relation between different movement disorders because in some cases successful treatment of one disorder may worsen symptoms associated with another. In some children, spasticity may partly compensate for weakness in antigravity muscles [Burne et al., 2005; Damiano et al., 2001]. Therefore, reduction of spasticity may lead to worsened standing or seated posture. For example, reduction of spasticity with oral baclofen is frequently accompanied by decreased trunk and neck tone. Thus, it is important to distinguish spastic and dystonic contributions to hypertonia so that dystonia can be treated aggressively while helpful components of spasticity can be preserved. It is also important to determine whether dystonia or other movement disorders are the primary cause of disability. For many children, the "negative symptoms," such as weakness or ataxia, may be greater contributors to disability, and treatment of the movement disorder or spasticity may not lead to improved function.

REFERENCES

Abdul Hafiz KM, Abdul Moneim AA, Betar B, et al. The immunological aspects of acute C.N.S. complications of the exanthematous viral diseases. J Egypt Soc Parasitol 1996;26:169.

Adams C, Diadori P, Schoenroth L, et al. Autoantibodies in childhood post-varicella acute cerebellar ataxia. Can J Neuol Sci 2000;27:316.

Albin RL, Reiner A, Anderson KD, et al. Striatal and nigral neuron subpopulations in rigid Huntington's disease: Implications for the functional anatomy of chorea and rigidity-akinesia. Ann Neurol 1990;27:357.

Albin RL, Young AB, Penney JB. The functional anatomy of basal ganglia disorders. Trends Neurosci 1989;12:366.

Albin RL, Young AB, Penney JB. The functional anatomy of disorders of the basal ganglia. Trends Neurosci 1995;18:63.

Albright AL, Barry MJ, Fasick P, et al. Continuous intrathecal baclofen infusion for symptomatic generalized dystonia. Neurosurgery 1996;38:934; discussion, 938.

Albright AL, Barry MJ, Painter MJ, et al. Infusion of intrathecal baclofen for generalized dystonia in cerebral palsy. J Neurosurg 1998;88:73.

Albright AL, Barry MJ, Shafton DH, et al. Intrathecal baclofen for generalized dystonia. Dev Med Child Neurol 2001;43:652.

Alexander GE, Crutcher MD. Functional architecture of basal ganglia circuits: Neural substrates of parallel processing. Trends Neurosci 1990;13:266.

Allen R, Becker PM, Bogan R, et al. Ropinirole decreases periodic leg movements and improves sleep parameters in patients with restless legs syndrome. Sleep 2004;27:907.

Al-Twaijri W, Shevell M. Pediatric migraine equivalents: Occurrence and clinical features in practice. Pediatr Neurol 2002;26:365.

Angelini L, Nardocci N, Estienne M, et al. Life-threatening dystonia-dyskinesias in a child: Successful treatment with bilateral pallidal stimulation. Mov Disord 2000;15:1010.

Anthony J, Ouvrier R, Wise G. Spasmus nutans, a mistaken entity. Arch Neurol 1980;37:373.

Araujo AP, Padua PA, Maia Filho HS. Management of rheumatic chorea: An observational study. Arq Neuropsiquiatr 2002;60:231.

Arnoldi K, Tychsen L. Prevalence of intracranial lesions in children initially diagnosed with disconjugate nystagmus (spasmus nutans). J Pediatr Ophthalm Strabismus 1995;32:296.

Asher SW, Aminoff MJ. Tetrabenazine and movement disorders. Neurology 1981;31:1051.

Asmus F, Gasser T. Inherited myoclonus-dystonia. Adv Neurol 2004;94:113.

Auburger G, Ratzlaff T, Lunkes A, et al. A gene for autosomal dominant paroxysmal choreoathetosis/spasticity (CSE) maps to the vicinity of a potassium channel gene cluster on chromosome 1p, probably within 2 cM between D1S443 and D1S197. Genomics 1996;31:90.

Augood SJ, Faull RL, Emson PC. Dopamine D1 and D2 receptor gene expression in the striatum in Huntington's disease. Ann Neurol 1997;42:215.

Ayers JL, Dawson KP. Acute dystonic reactions in childhood to drugs. N Z Med J 1980;92:464.
Bandmann O, Goertz M, Zschocke J, et al. The phenylalanine loading test in the differential diagnosis of dystonia. Neurology 2003;60:700.
Bandmann O, Marsden CD, Wood NW. Atypical presentations of dopa-responsive dystonia. Adv Neurol 1998a;78:283.
Bandmann O, Nygaard TG, Surtees R, et al. Dopa-responsive dystonia in British patients: New mutations of the GTP-cyclohydrolase I gene and evidence for genetic heterogeneity. Hum Mol Genet 1996;5:403.
Bandmann O, Valente EM, Holmans P, et al. Dopa-responsive dystonia: A clinical and molecular genetic study. Ann Neurol 1998b;44:649.
Bandmann O, Wood NW. Dopa-responsive dystonia—the story so far. Neuropediatrics 2002;33:1.
Basel-Vanagaite L, Straussberg R, Ovadia H, et al. Infantile bilateral striatal necrosis maps to chromosome 19q. Neurology 2004;62:87.
Bassi MT, Bresolin N, Tonelli A, et al. A novel mutation in the ATP1A2 gene causes alternating hemiplegia of childhood. J Med Genet 2004;41:621.
Becher MW, Rubinsztein DC, Leggo J, et al. Dentatorubral and pallidoluysian atrophy (DRPLA). Clinical and neuropathological findings in genetically confirmed North American and European pedigrees. Mov Disord 1997;12:519.
Benabid AL, Koudsie A, Benazzouz A, et al. Deep brain stimulation of the corpus luysi (subthalamic nucleus) and other targets in Parkinson's disease. Extension to new indications such as dystonia and epilepsy. J Neurol 2001;248(Suppl 3):III37.
Bennett LB, Roach ES, Bowcock AM. A locus for paroxysmal kinesigenic dyskinesia maps to human chromosome 16. Neurology 2000;54:125.
Bentivoglio AR, Cortelli P, Valente EM, et al. Phenotypic characterisation of autosomal recessive PARK6-linked Parkinsonism in three unrelated Italian families. Mov Disord 2001;16:999.
Bentivoglio AR, Loi M, Valente EM, et al. Phenotypic variability of DYT1-PTD: Does the clinical spectrum include psychogenic dystonia? Mov Disord 2002;17:1058.
Benton JW, Nellhaus G, Huttenlocher PR, et al. The bobble-head doll syndrome. Report of a unique truncal tremor associated with third ventricular cyst and hydrocephalus in children. Neurology 1966;16:725.
Bertrand E. Neurodegeneration with brain iron accumulation, type-I (NBIA-I) (formerly Hallervorden-Spatz, disease). I. Clinical manifestation and treatment. Neurol Neurochir Pol 2002a;36:947.
Bertrand E. Type I neurodegeneration with brain iron accumulation (NBIA-I, formerly Hallervorden-Spatz disease). II. Neuropathologic manifestation, novel genetic aspects and pathogenesis. Neurol Neurochir Pol 2002b;36:1163.
Bhatia KP, Marsden CD. The behavioural and motor consequences of focal lesions of the basal ganglia in man. Brain 1994;117:859.
Bhatia KP, Soland VL, Bhatt MH, et al. Paroxysmal exercise-induced dystonia: Eight new sporadic cases and a review of the literature. Mov Disord 1997;12:1007.
Bhutani VK, Johnson LH, Jeffrey Maisels M, et al. Kernicterus: Epidemiological strategies for its prevention through systems-based approaches. J Perinatol 2004;24:650.
Blackmon LR, Fanaroff AA, Raju TN. Research on prevention of bilirubin-induced brain injury and kernicterus: National Institute of Child Health and Human Development conference executive summary 2003. Pediatrics 2004;114:229.
Blakeley J, Jankovic J. Secondary paroxysmal dyskinesias. Mov Disord 2002;17:726.
Bodensteiner JB, Goldblum RM, Goldman AS. Progressive dystonia masking ataxia in ataxia-telangiectasia. Arch Neurol 1980;37:464.
Bodfish JW, Symons FJ, Parker DE, et al. Varieties of repetitive behavior in autism: Comparisons to mental retardation. J Autism Dev Dis 2000;30:237.
Bohlega S, Riley W, Powe J, et al. Neuroacanthocytosis and aprebetalipoproteinemia. Neurology 1998;50:1912.
Bonelli RM, Hofmann P. A review of the treatment options for Huntington's disease. Expert Opin Pharmacother 2004;5:767.
Bonelli RM, Wenning GK, Kapfhammer HP. Huntington's disease: Present treatments and future therapeutic modalities. Int Clin Psychopharmacol 2004;19:51.
Bower B. Fits and other frightening or funny turns in young people. Practitioner 1981;225:297.
Boyd RN, Morris ME, Graham HK. Management of upper limb dysfunction in children with cerebral palsy: A systematic review. Eur J Neurol 2001;8(Suppl 5):150.
Brashear A, Butler IJ, Ozelius LJ, et al. Rapid-onset dystonia-parkinsonism: A report of clinical, biochemical, and genetic studies in two families. Adv Neurol 1998;78:335.
Brautigam C, Steenbergen-Spanjers GC, Hoffmann GF, et al. Biochemical and molecular genetic characteristics of the severe form of tyrosine hydroxylase deficiency. Clin Chem 1999;45:2073.
Breedveld GJ, Percy AK, MacDonald ME, et al. Clinical and genetic heterogeneity in benign hereditary chorea. Neurology 2002a;59:579.
Breedveld GJ, van Dongen JW, Danesino C, et al. Mutations in TITF-1 are associated with benign hereditary chorea. Hum Mol Genet 2002b;11:971.
Bressman SB. Dystonia update. Clin Neuropharmacol 2000;23:239.
Bressman SB. Dystonia genotypes, phenotypes, and classification. Adv Neurol 2004;94:101.
Bressman SB, de Leon D, Kramer PL, et al. Dystonia in Ashkenazi Jews: Clinical characterization of a founder mutation. Ann Neurol 1994;36:771.
Bressman SB, Greene PE. Dystonia. Curr Treat Options Neurol 2000;2:275.
Bressman SB, Raymond D, Wendt K, et al. Diagnostic criteria for dystonia in DYT1 families. Neurology 2002;59:1780.
Brock WA, Golden J, Kaplan GW. Xanthine calculi in the Lesch-Nyhan syndrome. J Urol 1983;130:157.
Brooks DJ, Ibanez V, Playford ED, et al. Presynaptic and postsynaptic striatal dopaminergic function in neuroacanthocytosis: A positron emission tomographic study. Ann Neurol 1991;30:166.
Bruneau MA, Lesperance P, Chouinard S. Schizophrenia-like presentation of neuroacanthocytosis. J Neuropsychiatry Clin Neurosci 2003;15:378.
Brunstrom JE, Bastian AJ, Wong M, et al. Motor benefit from levodopa in spastic quadriplegic cerebral palsy. Ann Neurol 2000;47:662.
Bundey S. Clinical and genetic features of ataxia-telangiectasia. Int J Radiat Biol 1994;66(Suppl 6):S23.
Burke RE, Fahn S. Double-blind evaluation of trihexyphenidyl in dystonia. Adv Neurol 1983;37:189.
Burke RE, Fahn S, Jankovic J, et al. Tardive dystonia and inappropriate use of neuroleptic drugs. Lancet 1982;1:1299.
Burke RE, Fahn S, Marsden CD. Torsion dystonia: A double-blind, prospective trial of high-dosage trihexyphenidyl. Neurology 1986;36:160.
Burke RE, Reches A, Traub MM, et al. Tetrabenazine induces acute dystonic reactions. Ann Neurol 1985;17:200.
Burne JA, Carleton VL, O'Dwyer NJ. The spasticity paradox: Movement disorder or disorder of resting limbs? J Neurol Neurosurg Psychiatry 2005;76:47.
Burns RS, LeWitt PA, Ebert MH, et al. The clinical syndrome of striatal dopamine deficiency. Parkinsonism induced by 1-methyl-4-phenyl-1,2,3,6-tetrahydropyridine (MPTP). N Engl J Med 1985;312:1418.
Butler C, Campbell S. Evidence of the effects of intrathecal baclofen for spastic and dystonic cerebral palsy. AACPDM Treatment Outcomes Committee Review Panel. Dev Med Child Neurol 2000;42:634.
Calne DB, de la Fuente-Fernandez R, Kishore A. Contributions of positron emission tomography to elucidating the pathogenesis of idiopathic parkinsonism and dopa responsive dystonia. J Neural Transm Suppl 1997;50:47.
Campbell WM, Ferrel A, McLaughlin JF, et al. Long-term safety and efficacy of continuous intrathecal baclofen. Dev Med Child Neurol 2002;44:660.
Campistol J, Prats J, Garaizar C. Benign paroxysmal tonic upgaze of childhood with ataxia. A neurophthalmological syndrome of familial origin? Dev Med Child Neurol 1993;35:436.
Cardoso F, Maia D, Cunningham MC, et al. Treatment of Sydenham chorea with corticosteroids. Mov Disord 2003;18:1374.
Carpenter MB, Carpenter CS. Analysis of somatotopic relations of the corpus Luysi in man and monkey. J Comp Neurol 1951;95:349.
Caviness JN, Brown P. Myoclonus: Current concepts and recent advances. Lancet Neurol 2004;3:598.
Centerwall WR, Miller MM. Ataxia, telangiectasia, and sinopulmonary infections: A syndrome of slowly progressive deterioration in childhood. AMA J Dis Child 1958;95:385.
Chatterjee A, Frucht SJ. Tetrabenazine in the treatment of severe pediatric chorea. Mov Disord 2003;18:703.
Chatterjee A, Louis ED, Frucht S. Levetiracetam in the treatment of paroxysmal kinesigenic choreoathetosis. Mov Disord 2002;17:614.
Chervin RD, Archbold KH, Dillon JE, et al. Associations between symptoms of inattention, hyperactivity, restless legs, and periodic leg movements. Sleep 2002;25:213.

Chmelik E, Awadallah N, Hadi FS, et al. Varied presentation of PANDAS: A case series. Clin Pediatr (Phila) 2004;43:379.

Chun HH, Gatti RA. Ataxia-telangiectasia, an evolving phenotype. DNA Repair (Amst) 2004;3:1187.

Church AJ, Cardoso F, Dale RC, et al. Anti-basal ganglia antibodies in acute and persistent Sydenham's chorea. Neurology 2002;59:227.

Cif L, El Fertit H, Vayssiere N, et al. Treatment of dystonic syndromes by chronic electrical stimulation of the internal globus pallidus. J Neurosurg Sci 2003;47:52.

Cif L, Valente EM, Hemm S, et al. Deep brain stimulation in myoclonus-dystonia syndrome. Mov Disord 2004;19:724.

Connolly AM, Dodson WE, Prensky AL, Rust RS. Course and outcome of acute cerebellar ataxia. Ann Neurol 994;35673.

Connolly AM, Pestronk A, Mehta S, et al. Serum autoantibodies in childhood opsoclonus-myoclonus syndrome: An analysis of antigenic targets in neural tissues. J Pediatr 1997;130:878.

Coppola G, Muras I, Pascotto A. Pontocerebellar hypoplasia type 2 (PCH2): Report of two siblings. Brain Dev 2000;22:188.

Coubes P, Cif L, Azais M, et al. Treatment of dystonia syndrome by chronic electric stimulation of the internal globus pallidus. Arch Pediatr 2002;9(Suppl 2):84s.

Coubes P, Cif L, El Fertit H, et al. Electrical stimulation of the globus pallidus internus in patients with primary generalized dystonia: long-term results. J Neurosurg 2004;101:189.

Coubes P, Roubertie A, Vayssiere N, et al. Treatment of DYT1-generalised dystonia by stimulation of the internal globus pallidus. Lancet 2000;355:2220.

Coulter D, Allen R. Benign neonatal myoclonus. Arch Neurol 1982;39:191.

Coutinho G, Mitui M, Campbell C, et al. Five haplotypes account for fifty-five percent of ATM mutations in Brazilian patients with ataxia telangiectasia: Seven new mutations. Am J Med Genet 2004;126:33.

Cowan AN. Acute dystonic reaction to Maxolon (metoclopramide). Med J Aust 1982;2:215.

Crosby NJ, Deane KH, Clarke CE. Amantadine for dyskinesia in Parkinson's disease. Cochrane Database Syst 2003;(Rev 2): CD003467.

Cusumano FJ, Penna KJ, Panossian G. Prevention of self-mutilation in patients with Lesch-Nyhan syndrome: Review of literature. ASDC J Dent Child 2001;68:175.

Dahiya U, Noronha P. Drug-induced acute dystonic reactions in children. Alternatives to diphenhydramine therapy. Postgrad Med 1984;75:286, 290.

Dale RC, Church AJ, Surtees RA, et al. Encephalitis lethargica syndrome: 20 New cases and evidence of basal ganglia autoimmunity. Brain 2004;127:21.

Dalvi A, Fahn S, Ford B. Intrathecal baclofen in the treatment of dystonic storm. Mov Disord 1998;13:611.

Damiano DL, Quinlivan J, Owen BF, et al. Spasticity versus strength in cerebral palsy: Relationships among involuntary resistance, voluntary torque, and motor function. Eur J Neurol 2001;5(Suppl 8):40.

Danek A, Rubio JP, Rampoldi L, et al. McLeod neuroacanthocytosis: Genotype and phenotype. Ann Neurol 2001;50:755.

Davis DP, Marino A. Acute cerebellar ataxia in a toddler: Case report and literature review. J Emerg Med 2003;24:281.

de Carvalho Aguiar P, Sweadner KJ, Penniston JT, et al. Mutations in the Na+/K+-ATPase alpha3 gene ATP1A3 are associated with rapid-onset dystonia parkinsonism. Neuron 2004;43:169.

Deep-Brain Stimulation for Parkinson's Disease Study Group. Deep-brain stimulation of the subthalamic nucleus or the pars interna of the globus pallidus in Parkinson's disease. N Engl J Med 2001;345:956.

de la Monte SM, Vonsattel JP, Richardson EP Jr. Morphometric demonstration of atrophic changes in the cerebral cortex, white matter, and neostriatum in Huntington's disease. J Neuropathol Exp Neurol 1998;47:516.

DeLong MR. Primate models of movement disorders of basal ganglia origin. Trends Neurosci 1990;13:281.

Demir E, Prud'homme JF, Topcu M. Infantile convulsions and paroxysmal choreoathetosis in a consanguineous family. Pediatr Neurol 2004;30:349.

Demirkiran M, Jankovic J. Paroxysmal dyskinesias: Clinical features and classification. Ann Neurol 1995;38:571.

Deng YP, Albin RL, Penney JB, et al. Differential loss of striatal projection systems in Huntington's disease: A quantitative immunohistochemical study. J Chem Neuroanat 2004;27:143.

Deonna T, Martin D. Benign paroxysmal torticollis in infancy. Arch Dis Child 1981;56:956.

Deonna T, Ziegler A, Nielsen J. Transient idiopathic dystonia in infancy. Neuropediatrics 1991;22:220.

DeStefano AL, Lew MF, Golbe LI, et al. PARK3 influences age at onset in Parkinson disease: A genome scan in the GenePD study. Am J Hum Genet 2002;70:1089.

Deuschl G. Dystonic tremor. Rev Neurol (Paris) 2003;159:900.

Deuschl G, Bain P, Brin M. Consensus statement of the Movement Disorder Society on Tremor. Ad Hoc Scientific Committee. Mov Disord 1998;13(Suppl 3):2.

DiCapua M, Fusco L, Ricci S, et al. Benign neonatal sleep myoclonus: Clinical features and videopolygraphic recordings. Mov Disord 1993;8:191.

DiMario FJ. Childhood head tremor. J Child Neurol 2000;15:22.

Dixit SN, Sharma S, Behari M, et al. Neuroacanthocytosis with pure chorea. J Assoc Physicians India 1993;41:613.

Dobyns WB, Ozelius LJ, Kramer PL, et al. Rapid-onset dystonia-parkinsonism. Neurology 1993;43:2596.

Dogulu F, Onk A, Kaymaz M, et al. Acute cerebellitis with hydrocephalus. Neurology 2003;60:1717.

Dooley JM, Hayden JD. Benign febrile myoclonus in childhood. Can J Neurol Sci 2004;31:504.

Dotti MT, Battisti C, Malandrini A, et al. McLeod syndrome and neuroacanthocytosis with a novel mutation in the XK gene. Mov Disord 2000;15:1282.

Dure LS, Mussell HG. Paroxysmal dyskinesia in a patient with pseudohypoparathyroidism. Mov Disord 1998;13:746.

Dyken P, Kolar O. Dancing eyes, dancing feet: Infantile polymyoclonia. Brain 1968;91:305.

Earley CJ, Allen RP. Pergolide and carbidopa/levodopa treatment of the restless legs syndrome and periodic leg movements in sleep in a consecutive series of patients. Sleep 1996;19:801.

Egger J, Grossmann G, Auchterlonie IA. Lesson of the week: Benign sleep myoclonus in infancy mistaken for epilepsy. BMJ 2003;326:975.

Eidelberg D, Moeller JR, Antonini A, et al. Functional brain networks in DYT1 dystonia. Ann Neurol 1998;44:303.

Elble RJ. Essential tremor frequency decreases with time. Neurology 2000;55:1547.

Eldridge R, Rocca WA. The clinical syndrome of striatal dopamine deficiency: Parkinsonism induced by MPTP. N Engl J Med 1985;313:1159.

Eltahawy HA, Saint-Cyr J, Giladi N, et al. Primary dystonia is more responsive than secondary dystonia to pallidal interventions: Outcome after pallidotomy or pallidal deep brain stimulation. Neurosurgery 2004;54:613; discussion, 619.

Factor SA, Coni RJ, Cowger M, et al. Paroxysmal tremor and orofacial dyskinesia secondary to a biopterin synthesis defect. Neurology 1991;41:930.

Fahn S. High dosage anticholinergic therapy in dystonia. Neurology 1983a;33:1255.

Fahn S. High-dosage anticholinergic therapy in dystonia. Adv Neurol 1983b;37:177.

Fahn S. Systemic therapy of dystonia. Can J Neurol Sci 1987;14(Suppl 3): 528.

Fahn S, Bressman SB, Marsden CD. Classification of dystonia. Adv Neurol 1998;78:1.

Fahn S, Sjaastad O. Hereditary essential myoclonus in a large Norwegian family. Mov Disord 1991;6:237.

Fahn S, Williams DT. Psychogenic dystonia. Adv Neurol 1988;50:431.

Farina L, Uggetti C, Ottolini A, et al. Ataxia-telangiectasia: MR and CT findings. J Comput Assist Tomogr 1994;18:724.

Faustino PC, Terreri MT, da Rocha AJ, et al. Clinical, laboratory, psychiatric and magnetic resonance findings in patients with Sydenham chorea. Neuroradiology 2003;45:456.

Feinstein A, Stergiopoulos V, Fine J, et al. Psychiatric outcome in patients with a psychogenic movement disorder: A prospective study. Neuropsychiatry Neuropsychol Behav Neurol 2001;14:169.

Fernandez M, Raskind W, Matsushita M, et al. Hereditary benign chorea: Clinical and genetic features of a distinct disease. Neurology 2001;57:106.

Findley LJ, Gresty MA. Suppression of rubral tremor with levodopa. BMJ 1980;281:1043.

Findley LJ, Gresty MA, Halmagyi GM. Tremor, the cogwheel phenomenon and clonus in Parkinson's disease. J Neurol Neurosurg Psychiatry 1981;44:534.

Fink JK, Hedera P, Mathay JG, et al. Paroxysmal dystonic choreoathetosis linked to chromosome 2q: Clinical analysis and proposed pathophysiology. Neurology 1997;49:177.
Fleisher DR, Morrison A. Masturbation mimicking abdominal pain or seizures in young girls. J Pediatr 1990;116:810.
Ford B. Pallidotomy for generalized dystonia. Adv Neurol 2004;94:287.
Ford B, Greene PE, Louis ED, et al. Intrathecal baclofen in the treatment of dystonia. Adv Neurol 1998;78:199.
Forssman H. Hereditary disorder characterized by attacks of muscular contraction, induced by alcohol amongst other factors. Acta Med Scand 1961;170:517.
Furukawa Y, Filiano JJ, Kish SJ. Amantadine for levodopa-induced choreic dyskinesia in compound heterozygotes for GCH1 mutations. Mov Disord 2004a;19:1256.
Furukawa Y, Graf WD, Wong H, et al. Dopa-responsive dystonia simulating spastic paraplegia due to tyrosine hydroxylase (TH) gene mutations. Neurology 2001;56:260.
Furukawa Y, Guttman M, Sparagana SP, et al. Dopa-responsive dystonia due to a large deletion in the GTP cyclohydrolase I gene. Ann Neurol 2000;47:517.
Furukawa Y, Kish SJ, Fahn S. Dopa-responsive dystonia due to mild tyrosine hydroxylase deficiency. Ann Neurol 2004b;55:147.
Furukawa Y, Lang AE, Trugman JM, et al. Gender-related penetrance and de novo GTP-cyclohydrolase I gene mutations in dopa-responsive dystonia. Neurology 1998;50:1015.
Furukawa Y, Rajput AH. Inherited myoclonus-dystonia: How many causative genes and clinical phenotypes? Neurology 2002;59:1130.
Garvey MA, Swedo SE. Sydenham's chorea. Clinical and therapeutic update. Adv Exp Med Biol 1997;418:115.
Gatti RA, Berkel I, Boder E, et al. Localization of an ataxia-telangiectasia gene to chromosome 11q22-23. Nature 1988;336:577.
Gay CT, Ryan SG. Paroxysmal kinesigenic dystonia after methylphenidate administration. J Child Neurol 1994;9:45.
Gebremariam A. Sydenham's chorea: Risk factors and the role of prophylactic benzathine penicillin G in preventing recurrence. Ann Trop Paediatr 1999;19:161.
Genel F, Arslanoglu S, Uran N, et al. Sydenham's chorea: Clinical findings and comparison of the efficacies of sodium valproate and carbamazepine regimens. Brain Dev 2002;24:73.
Germano IM, Gracies JM, Weisz DJ, et al. Unilateral stimulation of the subthalamic nucleus in Parkinson disease: A double-blind 12-month evaluation study. J Neurosurg 2004;101:36.
Ghika J, Villemure JG, Miklossy J, et al. Postanoxic generalized dystonia improved by bilateral Voa thalamic deep brain stimulation. Neurology 2002;58:311.
Gieron-Korthals MA, Westberry KR, Emmanuel PJ. Acute childhood ataxia: 10-year experience. J Child Neurol 1994;9:381.
Giffin NJ, Benton S, Goadsby PJ. Benign paroxysmal torticollis of infancy: Four new cases and linkage to CACNA1A mutation. Dev Med Child Neurol 2002;44:490.
Gironell A, Kulisevsky J, Barbanoj M, et al. A randomized placebo-controlled comparative trial of gabapentin and propranolol in essential tremor. Arch Neurol 1999;56:475.
Goikhman I, Zelnik N, Peled N, et al. Bobble-head doll syndrome: A surgically treatable condition manifested as a rare movement disorder. Mov Disord 1998;13:192.
Goldenberg J, Ferraz MB, Fonseca AS, et al. Sydenham chorea: Clinical and laboratory findings. Analysis of 187 cases. Rev Paul Med 1992;110:152.
Gonzalez-Alegre P, Ammache Z, Davis PH, et al. Moyamoya-induced paroxysmal dyskinesia. Mov Disord 2003;18:1051.
Goodenough DJ, Fariello RG, Annis BL, et al. Familial and acquired paroxysmal dyskinesias. A proposed classification with delineation of clinical features. Arch Neurol 1978;35:827.
Gordon N. Pantothenate kinase-associated neurodegeneration (Hallervorden-Spatz syndrome). Eur J Paediatr Neurol 2002;6:243.
Gosalakkal JA. Epstein-Barr virus cerebellitis presenting as obstructive hydrocephalus. Clin Pediatr (Phila) 2001;40:229.
Gottlob I, Wizov S, Reinecke R. Spasmus nutans. A long-term follow-up. Invest Ophthalmol Vis Sci 1995;36:2768.
Gottlob I, Zubcov A, Catalano R, et al. Signs distinguishing spasmus nutans (with and without central nervous system lesions) from infantile nystagmus. Ophthalmology 1990;97:1166.
Gottlob I, Zubcov A, Wizov S, et al. Head nodding is compensatory in spasmus nutans. Ophthalmology 1992;99:1024.
Govaert P, Lequin M, Swarte R, et al. Changes in globus pallidus with (pre)term kernicterus. Pediatrics 2003;112:1256.
Grabowski M, Zimprich A, Lorenz-Depiereux B, et al. The epsilon-sarcoglycan gene (SGCE), mutated in myoclonus-dystonia syndrome, is maternally imprinted. Eur J Hum Genet 2003;11:138.
Gracies JM. Pathophysiology of impairment in patients with spasticity and use of stretch as a treatment of spastic hypertonia. Phys Med Rehabil Clin N Am 2001;2:747.
Graham HK, Boyd RN, Fehlings D. Does intramuscular botulinum toxin A injection improve upper-limb function in children with hemiplegic cerebral palsy? Med J Aust 2003;178:95.
Grattan-Smith PJ, Wevers RA, Steenbergen-Spanjers GC, et al. Tyrosine hydroxylase deficiency: Clinical manifestations of catecholamine insufficiency in infancy. Mov Disord 2002;17:354.
Green LN. Corticosteroids in the treatment of Sydenham's chorea. Arch Neurol 1978;35:53.
Greene P, Shale H, Fahn S. Analysis of open-label trials in torsion dystonia using high dosages of anticholinergics and other drugs. Mov Disord 1988;3:46.
Grellner W, Rohde K, Wilske J. Fatal outcome in a case of pontocerebellar hypoplasia type 2. Forensic Sci Int 2000;113:165.
Gros C, Frerebeau P, Perez-Dominguez E, et al. Long term results of stereotaxic surgery for infantile dystonia and dyskinesia. Neurochirurgia (Stuttg) 1976a;19:171.
Gros C, Frerebeau P, Privat JM, et al. Stereotaxic surgery of non-Parkinsonian dystonias and dyskinesias. Neurochirurgie 1976b;22:539.
Grosso S, Mostadini R, Cioni M, et al. Pontocerebellar hypoplasia type 2: Further clinical characterization and evidence of positive response of dyskinesia to levodopa. J Neurol 2002;249:596.
Grove VE Jr, Quintanilla J, DeVaney GT. Improvement of Huntington's disease with olanzapine and valproate. N Engl J Med 2000;343:973.
Hallett M. Analysis of abnormal voluntary and involuntary movements with surface electromyography. Adv Neurol 1983;39:907.
Hallett M. The neurophysiology of dystonia. Arch Neurol 1998;55:601.
Hamada H, Kurimoto M, Masuoka T, et al. A case of surgically treated acute cerebellitis with hydrocephalus. Childs Nerv Syst 2001;17:500.
Hayflick SJ. Pantothenate kinase-associated neurodegeneration (formerly Hallervorden-Spatz syndrome). J Neurol Sci 2003a;207:106.
Hayflick SJ. Unraveling the Hallervorden-Spatz syndrome: Pantothenate kinase-associated neurodegeneration is the name. Curr Opin Pediatr 2003b;15:572.
Hayflick SJ, Penzien JM, Michl W, et al. Cranial MRI changes may precede symptoms in Hallervorden-Spatz syndrome. Pediatr Neurol 2001;25:166.
Hayflick SJ, Westaway SK, Levinson B, et al. Genetic, clinical, and radiographic delineation of Hallervorden-Spatz syndrome. N Engl J Med 2003;348:33.
Hayward K, Jeremy RJ, Jenkins S, et al. Long-term neurobehavioral outcomes in children with neuroblastoma and opsoclonus-myoclonus-ataxia syndrome: Relationship to MRI findings and anti-neuronal antibodies. J Pediatr 2001;139:552.
Hedrich K, Meyer EM, Schule B, et al. Myoclonus-dystonia: Detection of novel, recurrent, and de novo SGCE mutations. Neurology 2004;62:1229.
Heidenreich R, Natowicz M, Hainline BE, et al. Acute extrapyramidal syndrome in methylmalonic acidemia: Metabolic stroke involving the globus pallidus. J Pediatr 1988;113:1022.
Heubi C, Shott SR. PANDAS: Pediatric autoimmune neuropsychiatric disorders associated with streptococcal infections—an uncommon, but important indication for tonsillectomy. Int J Pediatr Otorhinolaryngol 2003;67:837.
Hikosaka O, Wurtz RH. Modification of saccadic eye movements by GABA-related substances. II. Effects of muscimol in monkey substantia nigra pars reticulata. J Neurophysiol 1985;53:292.
Hiraishi K, Nakamura S, Yamamoto S, Kurokawa K. Prevention of xanthine stone formation by augmented dose of allopurinol in the Lesch-Nyhan syndrome. Br J Urol 1987;59:362.
Hofele K, Benecke R, Auburger G. Gene locus FPD1 of the dystonic Mount-Reback type of autosomal dominant paroxysmal choreoathetosis. Neurology 1997;49:1252.
Holmes G, Russman B. Shuddering attacks. Evaluation using electroencephalographic frequency modulation radiotelemetry and videotape monitoring. Am J Dis Child 1986;140:72.
Hoon AH Jr, Freese PO, Reinhardt EM, et al. Age-dependent effects of trihexyphenidyl in extrapyramidal cerebral palsy. Pediatr Neurol 2001;25:55.
Hoover JE, Strick PL. Multiple output channels in the basal ganglia. Science 1993;259:819.

Houlden H, Lincoln S, Farrer M, et al. Compound heterozygous PANK2 mutations confirm HARP and Hallervorden-Spatz syndromes are allelic. Neurology 2003;61:1423.

Huang CC, Liu CC, Chang YC, et al. Neurologic complications in children with enterovirus 71 infection. N Engl J Med 1999;341:936.

Hunt J. Dyssynergi cerebellaris myoclonica: Primary atrophy of the dentate system. A contribution to the pathology and symptomatology of the cerebellum. Brain 1921;44:490.

Huynh DP, Scoles DR, Nguyen D, et al. The autosomal recessive juvenile Parkinson disease gene product, parkin, interacts with and ubiquitinates synaptotagmin XI. Hum Mol Genet 2003;12:2587.

Hwang WJ, Calne DB, Tsui JK, et al. The long-term response to levodopa in dopa-responsive dystonia. Parkinsonism Relat Disord 2001;8:1.

Hyland K, Fryburg JS, Wilson WG, et al. Oral phenylalanine loading in dopa-responsive dystonia: A possible diagnostic test. Neurology 1997;48:1290.

Ichinose H, Suzuki T, Inagaki H, et al. Molecular genetics of dopa-responsive dystonia. Biol Chem 1999;380:1355.

Jacob PC, Pratap Chand R. Posttraumatic rubral tremor responsive to clonazepam. Mov Disord 1998;13:977.

Jan MM. Misdiagnoses in children with dopa-responsive dystonia. Pediatr Neurol 2004;31:298.

Jankovic J. Essential tremor: Clinical characteristics. Neurology 2000;54(Suppl 4):S21.

Jankovic J, Beach J. Long-term effects of tetrabenazine in hyperkinetic movement disorders. Neurology 1997;48:358.

Jankovic J, Caskey TC, Stout JT, et al. Lesch-Nyhan syndrome: A study of motor behavior and cerebrospinal fluid neurotransmitters. Ann Neurol 1988;23:466.

Jankovic J, Madisetty J, Vuong KD. Essential tremor among children. Pediatrics 2004;114:1203.

Jankovic J, Orman J. Tetrabenazine therapy of dystonia, chorea, tics, and other dyskinesias. Neurology 1988;38:391.

Jardim LB, Pereira ML, Silveira I, et al. Machado-Joseph disease in South Brazil: Clinical and molecular characterization of kindreds. Acta Neurol Scand 2001a;104:224.

Jardim LB, Pereira ML, Silveira I, et al. Neurologic findings in Machado-Joseph disease: Relation with disease duration, subtypes, and (CAG)n. Arch Neurol 2001b;58:899.

Jellinger KA. Influenza RNA not detected in archival brain tissues from acute encephalitis lethargica cases or in postencephalitic Parkinson cases. J Neuropathol Exp Neurol 2001;60:1121.

Jenner P. Dopamine agonists, receptor selectivity and dyskinesia induction in Parkinson's disease. Curr Opin Neurol 2003;16(Suppl 1):S3.

Johnston MV, Hoon AH Jr. Possible mechanisms in infants for selective basal ganglia damage from asphyxia, kernicterus, or mitochondrial encephalopathies. J Child Neurol 2000;15:588.

Jordan LC, Singer HS. Sydenham chorea in children. Curr Treat Options Neurol 2003;5:283.

Jummani R, Okun M. Sydenham chorea. Arch Neurol 2001;58:311.

Justesen CR, Penn RD, Kroin JS, et al. Stereotactic pallidotomy in a child with Hallervorden-Spatz disease. Case report. J Neurosurg 1999;90:551.

Kanavakis E, Xaidara A, Papathanasiou-Klontza D, et al. Alternating hemiplegia of childhood: A syndrome inherited with an autosomal dominant trait. Dev Med Child Neurol 2003;45:833.

Kanazawa O. Shuddering attacks-report of four children. Pediatr Neurol 2000;23:421.

Kang UJ, Burke RE, Fahn S. Natural history and treatment of tardive dystonia. Mov Disorder 1986;1:193.

Kato H, Kobayashi K, Kohari S, et al. Paroxysmal kinesigenic choreoathetosis and paroxysmal dystonic choreoathetosis in a patient with familial idiopathic hypoparathyroidism. Tohoku J Exp Med 1987;151:233.

Kertesz A. Paroxysmal kinesigenic choreoathetosis. Neurology 1967;17:680.

Khan NL, Valente EM, Bentivoglio AR, et al. Clinical and subclinical dopaminergic dysfunction in PARK6-linked parkinsonism: An 18F-dopa PET study. Ann Neurol 2002;52:849.

Kiley M, Esiri MM. A contemporary case of encephalitis lethargica. Clin Neuropathol 2001;20:2.

Kim JS, Park SH, Lee KW. Spasmus nutans and congenital ocular motor apraxia with cerebellar vermian hypoplasia. Arch Neurol 2003;60:1621.

Kim YJ, Pakiam AS, Lang AE. Historical and clinical features of psychogenic tremor: A review of 70 cases. Can J Neurol Sci 1999;26:190.

Kinsbourne M. Myoclonic encephalopathy of infants. J Neurol 1962;25:271.

Kirsch DB, Mink JW. Psychogenic movement disorders in children. Pediatr Neurol 2004;30:1.

Kirvan CA, Swedo SE, Heuser JS, et al. Mimicry and autoantibody-mediated neuronal cell signaling in Sydenham chorea. Nat Med 2003;9:914.

Klein C, Friedman J, Bressman S, et al. Genetic testing for early-onset torsion dystonia (DYT1): Introduction of a simple screening method, experiences from testing of a large patient cohort, and ethical aspects. Genet Test 1999;3:323.

Kleiner-Fisman G, Rogaeva E, Halliday W, et al. Benign hereditary chorea: Clinical, genetic, and pathological findings. Ann Neurol 2003;54:244.

Koeppen AH, Dickson AC. Iron in the Hallervorden-Spatz syndrome. Pediatr Neurol 2001;25:148.

Koller WC, Cochran JW, Klawans HL. Calcification of the basal ganglia: Computerized tomography and clinical correlation. Neurology 1979;29:328.

Koller WC, Klawans HL. Cerebellar calcification on computerized tomography. Ann Neurol 1980;7:193.

Korn-Lubetzki I, Brand A, Steiner I. Recurrence of Sydenham chorea: Implications for pathogenesis. Arch Neurol 2004;61:1261.

Koski L, Iacoboni M, Mazziotta JC. Deconstructing apraxia: Understanding disorders of intentional movement after stroke. Curr Opin Neurol 2002;15:71.

Krack P, Vercueil L. Review of the functional surgical treatment of dystonia. Eur J Neurol 2001;8:389.

Krageloh-Mann I, Helber A, Mader I, et al. Bilateral lesions of thalamus and basal ganglia: Origin and outcome. Dev Med Child Neurol 2002;44:477.

Kramer U, Nevo Y, Harel S. Jittery babies: A short term follow-up. Brain Dev 1994;16:112.

Kulkarni ML. Sodium valproate controls choreoathetoid movements of kernicterus. Indian Pediatr 1992;29:1029.

Kulkarni ML, Anees S. Sydenham's chorea. Indian Pediatr 1996;33:112.

Kurlan R. The PANDAS hypothesis: Losing its bite? Mov Disord 2004;19:371.

Kurlan R, Behr J, Medved L, et al. Transient tic disorder and the spectrum of Tourette's syndrome. Arch Neurol 1988;45:1200.

Kurlan R, Kaplan EL. The pediatric autoimmune neuropsychiatric disorders associated with streptococcal infection (PANDAS) etiology for tics and obsessive-compulsive symptoms: Hypothesis or entity? Practical considerations for the clinician. Pediatrics 2004;113:883.

Kutcher JS, Kahn MJ, Andersson HC, et al. Neuroacanthocytosis masquerading as Huntington's disease: CT/MRI findings. J Neuroimaging 1999;9:187.

Kyriagis M, Grattan-Smith P, Scheinberg A, et al. Status dystonicus and Hallervorden-Spatz disease: Treatment with intrathecal baclofen and pallidotomy. J Paediatr Child Health 2004;40:322.

Lance J, Adams R. The syndrome of intention or action myoclonus as a sequel to hypoxic encephalopathy. Brain 1963;86:111.

Lance JW. Familial paroxysmal dystonic choreoathetosis and its differentiation from related syndromes. Ann Neurol 1977;2:285.

Lang AE. Essential myoclonus and myoclonic dystonia. Mov Disord 1997;12:127.

Langbehn DR, Brinkman RR, Falush D, et al. A new model for prediction of the age of onset and penetrance for Huntington's disease based on CAG length. Clin Genet 2004;65:267.

Lee JH, Berkowitz RJ, Choi BJ. Oral self-mutilation in the Lesch-Nyhan syndrome. ASDC J Dent Child 2002;69:66, 12.

Leeman CP. Acute dystonic reactions to small doses of prochlorperazine: Report of three cases misdiagnosed as hysteria. JAMA 1965;193:839.

Leonard HL, Swedo SE. Paediatric autoimmune neuropsychiatric disorders associated with streptococcal infection (PANDAS). Int J Neuropsychopharmacol 2001;4:191.

Leung AKC, Robson WLM. Childhood masturbation. Clin Pediatr 1993;32:238.

Leung GK, Fan YW, Ho SL. Rubral tremor associated with cavernous angioma of the midbrain. Mov Disord 1999;14:191.

Levy EI, Harris AE, Omalu BI, et al. Sudden death from fulminant acute cerebellitis. Pediatr Neurosurg 2001;35:24.

Lewis RF, Lederman HM, Crawford TO. Ocular motor abnormalities in ataxia telangiectasia. Ann Neurol 1999;46:287.

Li SH, Schilling G, Young WS 3rd, et al. Huntington's disease gene (IT15) is widely expressed in human and rat tissues. Neuron 1993;11:985.

Lin JJ, Lin SZ, Lin GY, et al. Treatment of intractable generalized dystonia by bilateral posteroventral pallidotomy: One-year results. Zhonghua Yi Xue Za Zhi (Taipei) 2001;64:231.

Lo KC, Geddes JF, Daniels RS, et al. Lack of detection of influenza genes in archived formalin-fixed, paraffin wax-embedded brain samples of encephalitis lethargica patients from 1916 to 1920. Virchows Arch 2003;442:591.

Loiselle CR, Lee O, Moran TH, et al. Striatal microinfusion of Tourette syndrome and PANDAS sera: Failure to induce behavioral changes. Mov Disord 2004;19:390.

Loiselle CR, Singer HS. Genetics of childhood disorders. XXXI. Autoimmune disorders, part 4: Is Sydenham chorea an autoimmune disorder? J Am Acad Child Adolesc Psychiatry 2001;40:1234.

Lombroso C. Early myoclonic encephalopathy, early infantile epileptic encephalopathy, and benign and severe infantile myoclonic epilepsies: A critical review and personal contributions. J Clin Neurophysiol 1990;7:80.

Lombroso CT. Nocturnal paroxysmal dystonia due to a subfrontal cortical dysplasia. Epileptic Disord 2000;2:15.

Lombroso C, Fejerman N. Benign myoclonus of early infancy. Ann Neurol 1977;1:138.

Lotze T, Jankovic J. Paroxysmal kinesigenic dyskinesias. Semin Pediatr Neurol 2003;10:68.

Louis ED, Dure LS 4th, Pullman S. Essential tremor in childhood: A series of nineteen cases. Mov Disord 2001;16:921.

Lozano AM, Kumar R, Gross RE, et al. Globus pallidus internus pallidotomy for generalized dystonia. Mov Disord 1997;12:865.

Lu CS, Chu NS. Acute dystonic reaction with asterixis and myoclonus following metoclopramide therapy. J Neurol Neurosurg Psychiatry 1988;51:1002.

Lucetti C, Bellini G, Nuti A, et al. Treatment of patients with tardive dystonia with olanzapine. Clin Neuropharmacol 2002;25:71.

Lugaresi E, Cirignotta F. Hypnogenic paroxysmal dystonia: Epileptic seizure or a new syndrome? Sleep 1981;4:129.

Lugaresi E, Cirignotta F, Montagna P. Nocturnal paroxysmal dystonia. J Neurol Neurosurg Psychiatry 1986;49:375.

Madej TH. Domperidone: An acute dystonic reaction. Anaesthesia 1985;40:202.

Mahone EM, Bridges D, Prahme C, et al. Repetitive arm and hand movements (complex motor stereotypies) in children. J Pediatr 2004;145:391.

Mahowald MW. Restless leg syndrome and periodic limb movements of sleep. Curr Treat Options Neurol 2003;5:251.

Mak BS, Chi CS, Tsai CR, et al. New mutations of the HPRT gene in Lesch-Nyhan syndrome. Pediatr Neurol 2000;23:332.

Makabe H, Sakamoto K. Evaluation of postural tremor of finger for neuromuscular diseases and its application to the classification. Electromyogr Clin Neurophysiol 2002;42:205.

March JS. Pediatric autoimmune neuropsychiatric disorders associated with streptococcal infection (PANDAS): Implications for clinical practice. Arch Pediatr Adolesc Med 2004;158:927.

Marsden CD, Obeso JA, Rothwell JC. Clinical neurophysiology of muscle jerks: Myoclonus, chorea, and tics. Adv Neurol 1983;39:865.

Marson AM, Bucciantini E, Gentile E, et al. Neuroacanthocytosis: Clinical, radiological, and neurophysiological findings in an Italian family. Neurol Sci 2003;24:188.

Matthews WS, Solan A, Barabas G, et al. Cognitive functioning in Lesch-Nyhan syndrome: A 4-year follow-up study. Dev Med Child Neurol 1999;41:260.

Maydell BV, Berenson F, Rothner AD, et al. Benign myoclonus of early infancy: An imitator of West's syndrome. J Child Neurol 2001;16:109.

McCann UD, Penetar DM, Belenky G. Acute dystonic reaction in normal humans caused by catecholamine depletion. Clin Neuropharmacol 1990;13:565.

Mehndiratta MM, Malik S, Kumar S, et al. McLeod syndrome (a variant of neuroacanthocytosis). J Assoc Physicians India 2000;48:356.

Micheli F, Fernandez Pardal M, de Arbelaiz R, et al. Paroxysmal dystonia responsive to anticholinergic drugs. Clin Neuropharmacol 1987;10:365.

Miller J, Singer HS, Waranch HR. Behavior therapy for the treatment of stereotypic movements in non-autistic children. Ann Neurol 2004;56(Suppl 8):S109.

Mink JW. The basal ganglia: Focused selection and inhibition of competing motor programs. Prog Neurobiol 1996;50:381.

Mink JW. Basal ganglia dysfunction in Tourette's syndrome: A new hypothesis. Pediatr Neurol 2001a;25:190.

Mink JW. Basal ganglia motor function in relation to Hallervorden-Spatz syndrome. Pediatr Neurol 2001b;25:112.

Mink J. The basal ganglia and involuntary movements: Impaired inhibition of competing motor patterns. Arch Neurol 2003;60:1365.

Mink J, Neil J. Masturbation mimicking paroxysmal dystonia or dyskinesia in a young girl. Mov Disord 1995;10:518.

Misbahuddin A, Warner TT. Dystonia: An update on genetics and treatment. Curr Opin Neurol 2001;14:471.

Mitchell WG, Davalos-Gonzalez Y, Brumm VL, et al. Opsoclonus-ataxia caused by childhood neuroblastoma: Developmental and neurologic sequelae. Pediatrics 2002;109:86.

Mitchell WG, Snodgrass SR. Opsoclonus-ataxia due to childhood neural crest tumors: A chronic neurologic syndrome. J Child Neurol 1990;5:153.

Mito T, Tanaka T, Becker LE, et al. Infantile bilateral striatal necrosis. Clinicopathological classification. Arch Neurol 1986;43:677.

Miyasaki JM, Sa DS, Galvez-Jimenez N, et al. Psychogenic movement disorders. Can J Neurol Sci 2003;30(Suppl 1):S94.

Montagna P. Sleep-related non-epileptic motor disorders. J Neurol 2004;251:781.

Moore DP. Neuropsychiatric aspects of Sydenham's chorea: A comprehensive review. J Clin Psychiatry 1996;57:407.

Moreira MC, Barbot C, Tachi N, e al. The gene mutated in ataxia-ocular apraxia 1 encodes the new HIT/Zn-finger protein aprataxin. Nat Genet 2001;29:189.

Morris JG, Grattan-Smith P, Jankelowitz SK, et al. Athetosis. II. The syndrome of mild athetoid cerebral palsy. Mov Disord 2002a;17:1281.

Morris JG, Jankelowitz SK, Fung VS, et al. Athetosis. I. Historical considerations. Mov Disord 2002b;17:1278.

Mount LA, Reback S. Familial paroxysmal choreoathetosis. Arch Neurol Psychiatry 1940;44:841.

Muller B, Hedrich K, Kock N, et al. Evidence that paternal expression of the epsilon-sarcoglycan gene accounts for reduced penetrance in myoclonus-dystonia. Am J Hum Genet 2002;71:1303.

Munchau A, Valente EM, Shahidi GA, et al. A new family with paroxysmal exercise induced dystonia and migraine: A clinical and genetic study. J Neurol Neurosurg Psychiatry 2000;68:609.

Mussell HG, Dure LS, Percy AK, et al. Bobble-head doll syndrome: Report of a case and review of the literature. Mov Disord 1997;12:810.

Myers RH, Vonsattel JP, Stevens TJ, et al. Clinical and neuropathologic assessment of severity in Huntington's disease. Neurology 1988;38:341.

Nagatsu T, Ichinose H. GTP cyclohydrolase I gene, tetrahydrobiopterin, and tyrosine hydroxylase gene: Their relations to dystonia and Parkinsonism. Neurochem Res 1996;21:245.

Nambu A, Tokuno H, Hamada I, et al. Excitatory cortical inputs to pallidal neurons via the subthalamic nucleus in the monkey. J Neurophysiol 2000;84:289.

Nellhaus G. Abnormal head movements of young children. Dev Med Child Neurol 1983;25:384.

Nijssen PC, Brusse E, Leyten AC, et al. Autosomal dominant adult neuronal ceroid lipofuscinosis: Parkinsonism due to both striatal and nigral dysfunction. Mov Disord 2002;17:482.

Nikkhah G, Prokop T, Hellwig B, et al. Deep brain stimulation of the nucleus ventralis intermedius for Holmes (rubral) tremor and associated dystonia caused by upper brainstem lesions. Report of two cases. J Neurosurg 2004;100:1079.

Nishiyama N, Yukishita S, Hagiwara H, et al. Gene mutation in hereditary progressive dystonia with marked diurnal fluctuation (HPD), strictly defined dopa-responsive dystonia. Brain Dev 2000;22(Suppl 1):S102.

Nomoto M, Thompson PD, Sheehy MP, et al. Anticholinergic-induced chorea in the treatment of focal dystonia. Mov Disord 1987;2:53.

Nussinovitch M, Prais D, Volovitz B, et al. Post-infectious acute cerebellar ataxia in children. Clin Pediatr 2003;42:581.

Nutt JG, Nygaard TG. Response to levodopa treatment in dopa-responsive dystonia. Arch Neurol 2001;58:905.

Nygaard TG, Duvoisin RC. Hereditary dystonia-parkinsonism syndrome of juvenile onset. Neurology 1986;36:1424.

Nygaard TG, Marsden CD, Duvoisin RC. Dopa-responsive dystonia. Adv Neurol 1988;50:377.

Nygaard TG, Marsden CD, Fahn S. Dopa-responsive dystonia: Long-term treatment response and prognosis. Neurology 1991;41:174.

Nygaard TG, Raymond D, Chen C, et al. Localization of a gene for myoclonus-dystonia to chromosome 7q21-q31. Ann Neurol 1999;46:794.

Nygaard TG, Trugman JM, de Yebenes JG, et al. Dopa-responsive dystonia: The spectrum of clinical manifestations in a large North American family. Neurology 1990;40:66.

Nyhan WL. Clinical features of the Lesch-Nyhan syndrome. Introduction: Clinical and genetic features. Fed Proc 1968a;27:1027.

Nyhan WL. Lesch-Nyhan syndrome. Summary of clinical features. Fed Proc 1968b;27:1034.

Nyhan WL. Clinical features of the Lesch-Nyhan syndrome. Arch Intern Med 1972;130:186.

Obeso JA, Rodriguez-Oroz MC, Rodriguez M, et al. The basal ganglia and disorders of movement: Pathophysiological mechanisms. News Physiol Sci 2002;17:51.

Okamoto K, Ito J, Furusawa T, et al. CT and MR findings of neuroacanthocytosis. J Comput Assist Tomogr 1997;21:221.

Oliveira JR, Spiteri E, Sobrido MJ, et al. Genetic heterogeneity in familial idiopathic basal ganglia calcification (Fahr disease). Neurology 2004;63:2165.

Olsen JC, Keng JA, Clark JA. Frequency of adverse reactions to prochlorperazine in the ED. Am J Emerg Med 2000;18:609.

Olson L, Houlihan D. A review of behavioral treatments used for Lesch-Nyhan syndrome. Behav Modif 2000;24:202.

Ondo WG, Tintner R, Thomas M, et al. Tetrabenazine treatment for Huntington's disease-associated chorea. Clin Neuropharmacol 2002;25:300.

Opal P, Tintner R, Jankovic J, et al. Intrafamilial phenotypic variability of the DYT1 dystonia: From asymptomatic TOR1A gene carrier status to dystonic storm. Mov Disord 2002;17:339.

O'Riordan S, Raymond D, Lynch T, et al. Age at onset as a factor in determining the phenotype of primary torsion dystonia. Neurology 2004;63:1423.

Ouvrier R, Billson F. Benign paroxysmal upgaze of childhood. J Child Neurol 1988;3:177.

Ozekmekci S, Apaydin H, Ekinci B, et al. Psychogenic movement disorders in two children. Mov Disord 2003;18:1395.

Ozelius LJ, Hewett JW, Page CE, et al. The early-onset torsion dystonia gene (DYT1) encodes an ATP-binding protein. Nat Genet 1997;17:40.

Ozelius LJ, Page CE, Klein C, et al. The TOR1A (DYT1) gene family and its role in early onset torsion dystonia. Genomics 1999;62:377.

Paci C, Thomas A, Onofrj M. Amantadine for dyskinesia in patients affected by severe Parkinson's disease. Neurol Sci 2001;22:75.

Pal PK, Leung J, Hedrich K, et al. [18F]-Dopa positron emission tomography imaging in early-stage, non-parkin juvenile parkinsonism. Mov Disord 2002;17:789.

Parent A, Hazrati LN. Anatomical aspects of information processing in primate basal ganglia. Trends Neurosci 1993;16:111.

Parker CC, Evans OB. Metabolic disorders causing childhood ataxia. Semin Pediatr Neurol 2003;10:193.

Paulson GW. Benign essential tremor in childhood: Symptoms, pathogenesis, treatment. Clin Pediatr 1976;15:67.

Paulson H, Ammache Z. Ataxia and hereditary disorders. Neurol Clin 2001;19:759, viii.

Pavone P, Bianchini R, Parano E, et al. Anti-brain antibodies in PANDAS versus uncomplicated streptococcal infection. Pediatr Neurol 2004;30:107.

Pena J, Mora E, Cardozo J, et al. Comparison of the efficacy of carbamazepine, haloperidol and valproic acid in the treatment of children with Sydenham's chorea: Clinical follow-up of 18 patients. Arq Neuropsiquiatr 2002;60(2-B):374.

Peppard RF, Lu CS, Chu NS, et al. Parkinsonism with neuroacanthocytosis. Can J Neurol Sci 1990;17:298.

Peppe A, Pierantozzi M, Bassi A, et al. Stimulation of the subthalamic nucleus compared with the globus pallidus internus in patients with Parkinson disease. J Neurosurg 2004;101:195.

Picchietti DL, England SJ, Walters AS, et al. Periodic limb movement disorder and restless legs syndrome in children with attention-deficit hyperactivity disorder. J Child Neurol 1998;13:588.

Ponzone A, Ferraris S, Spada M, et al. Combined phenylalanine-tetrahydrobiopterin loading test in GTP cyclohydrolase 1 deficiency. Eur J Pediatr 1994;153:616.

Pourcher E, Baruch P, Bouchard RH, et al. Neuroleptic associated tardive dyskinesias in young people with psychoses. Br J Psychiatry 1995;166:768.

Pranzatelli MR, Mott SH, Pavlakis SG, et al. Clinical spectrum of secondary parkinsonism in childhood: A reversible disorder. Pediatr Neurol 1994;10:131.

Pranzatelli MR, Travelstead AL, Tate ED, et al. B- and T-cell markers in opsoclonus-myoclonus syndrome: Immunophenotyping of CSF lymphocytes. Neurology 2004;62:1526.

Pringsheim T, Lang AE. Psychogenic dystonia. Rev Neurol 2003;159:885.

Priori A, Bertolasi L, Pesenti A, et al. Gamma-hydroxybutyric acid for alcohol-sensitive myoclonus with dystonia. Neurology 2000;54:1706.

Provini F, Plazzi G, Lugaresi E. From nocturnal paroxysmal dystonia to nocturnal frontal lobe epilepsy. Clin Neurophysiol 2000;111(Suppl 2):S2.

Quinn NP. Essential myoclonus and myoclonic dystonia. Mov Disord 1996;11:119.

Quinn N, Schrag A. Huntington's disease and other choreas. J Neurol 1998;245:709.

Rajput A, Robinson CA, Rajput AH. Essential tremor course and disability: A clinicopathologic study of 20 cases. Neurology 2004;62:932.

Rakocevic G, Lyons KE, Wilkinson SB, et al. Bilateral pallidotomy for severe dystonia in an 18-month-old child with glutaric aciduria. Stereotact Funct Neurosurg 2004;82:80.

Rampoldi L, Danek A, Monaco AP. Clinical features and molecular bases of neuroacanthocytosis. J Mol Med 2002;80:475.

Reggin J, Johnson M. Exacerbation of benign sleep myoclonus by benzodiazepine treatment. Ann Neurol 1989;26:455.

Renwick J. Metoclopramide: Acute dystonic reactions. Aust Nurses J 1990;20:28.

Resnick TJ, Moshe SL, Perotta L, et al. Benign neonatal sleep myoclonus. Relationship to sleep states. Arch Neurol 1986;43:266.

Richards RN, Barnett HJM. Paroxysmal dystonic choreoathetosis: A family study and review of the literature. Neurology 1968;18:461.

Richardson MA, Bevans ML, Read LL, et al. Efficacy of the branched-chain amino acids in the treatment of tardive dyskinesia in men. Am J Psychiatry 2003;160:1117.

Richardson MA, Bevans ML, Weber JB, et al. Branched chain amino acids decrease tardive dyskinesia symptoms. Psychopharmacology 1999;143:358.

Richardson MA, Small AM, Read LL, et al. Branched chain amino acid treatment of tardive dyskinesia in children and adolescents. J Clin Psychiatry 2004;65:92.

Riederer P, Foley P. Mini-review: Multiple developmental forms of parkinsonism. The basis for further research as to the pathogenesis of parkinsonism. J Neural Transm 2002;109:1469.

Roach ES, Delgado M, Anderson L, et al. Carbamazepine trial for Lesch-Nyhan self-mutilation. J Child Neurol 1996;11:476.

Roberts EA, Schilsky ML. A practice guideline on Wilson disease. Hepatology 2003;37:1475.

Robertson MM. Diagnosing Tourette syndrome: Is it a common disorder? J Psychosom Res 2003;55:3.

Robey KL, Reck JF, Giacomini KD, et al. Modes and patterns of self-mutilation in persons with Lesch-Nyhan disease. Dev Med Child Neurol 2003;45:167.

Robinson D, Smith M, Reddy R. Neuroacanthocytosis. Am J Psychiatry 2004;161:1716.

Rosenbaum F, Jankovic J. Focal task-specific tremor and dystonia: Categorization of occupational movement disorders. Neurology 1988;38:522.

Roulet E, Deonna T. Benign paroxysmal torticollis in infancy. Dev Med Child Neurol 1988;30:409.

Royo M, Daubner SC, Fitzpatrick PF. Effects of mutations in tyrosine hydroxylase associated with progressive dystonia on the activity and stability of the protein. Proteins 2005;58:14.

Roytta M, Olsson I, Sourander P, et al. Infantile bilateral striatal necrosis. Clinical and morphological report of a case and a review of the literature. Acta Neuropathol 1981;55:97.

Rubaltelli FF. Current drug treatment options in neonatal hyperbilirubinaemia and the prevention of kernicterus. Drugs 1998;56:23.

Ruiz-Linares A. Juvenile Parkinson disease and the C212Y mutation of parkin. Arch Neurol 2004;61:444..

Ryan MM, Engle EC. Acute ataxia in childhood. J Child Neurol 2003;18:309.

Ryan SG, Sherman SL, Terry JC, et al. Startle disease, or hyperekplexia: Response to clonazepam and assignment of the gene (STHE) to chromosome 5q by linkage analysis. Ann Neurol 1992;31:663.

Saint Hilaire MH, Burke RE, Bressman SB, et al. Delayed-onset dystonia due to perinatal or early childhood asphyxia. Neurology 1991;41:216.

Saito T. Presenting symptoms and natural history of Wilson disease. Eur J Pediatr 1987;146:261.

Saito Y, Takashima S. Neurotransmitter changes in the pathophysiology of Lesch-Nyhan syndrome. Brain Dev 2000;22(Suppl 1):S122.

Saltik S, Cokar O, Uslu T, et al. Alternating hemiplegia of childhood: Presentation of two cases regarding the extent of variability. Epileptic Disord 2004;6:45.

Sanger TD. Pathophysiology of pediatric movement disorders. J Child Neurol 2003a;18(Suppl 1):S9.

Sanger TD. Pediatric movement disorders. Curr Opin Neurol 2003b;16:529.

Sanger TD, Delgado MR, Gaebler-Spira D, et al. Classification and definition of disorders causing hypertonia in childhood. Pediatrics 2003;111:e89.

Sano Y, Date H, Igarashi S, et al. Aprataxin, the causative protein for EAOH is a nuclear protein with a potential role as a DNA repair protein. Ann Neurol 2004;55:241.

Sasaki M, Sakuragawa N, Osawa M. Long-term effect of flunarizine on patients with alternating hemiplegia of childhood in Japan. Brain Dev 2001;23:303.

Sasaki Y, Kusumi I, Koyama T. A case of tardive dystonia successfully managed with quetiapine. J Clin Psychiatry 2004;65:583.

Saunders-Pullman R, Blau N, Hyland K, et al. Phenylalanine loading as a diagnostic test for DRD: Interpreting the utility of the test. Mol Genet Metab 2004a;83:207.

Saunders-Pullman R, Shriberg J, Shanker V, et al. Penetrance and expression of dystonia genes. Adv Neurol 2004b;94:121.

Schule B, Kock N, Svetel M, et al. Genetic heterogeneity in ten families with myoclonus-dystonia. J Neurol Neurosurg Psychiatry 2004;75:1181.

Segawa M, Nishiyama N, Nomura Y. DOPA-responsive dystonic parkinsonism: Pathophysiologic considerations. Adv Neurol 1999;80:389.

Segawa M, Nomura Y, Nishiyama N. Autosomal dominant guanosine triphosphate cyclohydrolase I deficiency (Segawa disease). Ann Neurol 2003;54(Suppl 6):S32.

Shapiro SM. Definition of the clinical spectrum of kernicterus and bilirubin-induced neurologic dysfunction (BIND). J Perinatol 2005;25:54.

Sheehy EC, Longhurst P, Pool D, et al. Self-inflicted injury in a case of Hallervorden-Spatz disease. Int J Paediatr Dent 1999;9:299.

Sheth RD, Horwitz SJ, Aronoff S, et al. Opsoclonus myoclonus syndrome secondary to Epstein-Barr virus infection. J Child Neurol 1995;10:297.

Shiang R, Ryan SG, Zhu YZ, et al. Mutations in the alpha 1 subunit of the inhibitory glycine receptor cause the dominant neurologic disorder, hyperekplexia. Nat Genet 1993;5:351.

Shibasaki H. Electrophysiological studies of myoclonus. Muscle Nerve 2000;23:321.

Shibasaki H, Hallett M. Electrophysiological studies of myoclonus. Muscle Nerve 2004;31:157.

Shibasaki H, Yamashita Y, Tobimatsu S, et al. Electroencephalographic correlates of myoclonus. Adv Neurol 1986;43:357.

Shimazaki H, Takiyama Y, Sakoe K, et al. Early-onset ataxia with ocular motor apraxia and hypoalbuminemia: The aprataxin gene mutations. Neurology 2002;59:590.

Shimizu Y, Ueno T, Komatsu H, et al. Acute cerebellar ataxia with human parvovirus B19 infection. Arch Dis Child 1999;80:72.

Shuper A, Zalzberg J, Weitz R, et al. Jitteriness beyond the neonatal period: A benign pattern of movement in infancy. J Child Neurol 1991;6:243.

Simpson GM. The treatment of tardive dyskinesia and tardive dystonia. J Clin Psychiatry 2000;61(Suppl 4):39.

Singer HS, Loiselle C. PANDAS: A commentary. J Psychosom Res 2003;55:31.

Singer HS, Loiselle CR, Lee O, et al. Anti-basal ganglia antibody abnormalities in Sydenham chorea. J Neuroimmunol 2003;136:154.

Singer HS, Loiselle CR, Lee O, et al. Anti-basal ganglia antibodies in PANDAS. Mov Disord 2004;19:406.

Smith D, Fitzgerald K, Stass-Isern M, et al. Electroretinography is necessary for spasmus nutans diagnosis. Pediatr Neurol 2000;23:33.

Snider LA, Seligman LD, Ketchen BR, et al. Tics and problem behaviors in schoolchildren: Prevalence, characterization, and associations. Pediatrics 2002;110:331.

Snider LA, Swedo SE. PANDAS: Current status and directions for research. Mol Psychiatry 2004;9:900.

Sone K, Oguni H, Katsumori H, et al. Successful trial of amantadine hydrochloride for two patients with alternating hemiplegia of childhood. Neuropediatrics 2000;31:307.

Soussan V, Husson B, Tardieu M. [Description and prognostic value of cerebellar MRI lesions in children with severe acute ataxia.] Arch Pediatr 2003;10:604.

Spacey SD, Valente EM, Wali GM, et al. Genetic and clinical heterogeneity in paroxysmal kinesigenic dyskinesia: Evidence for a third EKD gene. Mov Disord 2002;17:717.

Spina E, Sturiale V, Valvo S, et al. Prevalence of acute dystonic reactions associated with neuroleptic treatment with and without anticholinergic prophylaxis. Int Clin Psychopharmacol 1993;8:21.

Stankovic T, Kidd AM, Sutcliffe A, et al. ATM mutations and phenotypes in ataxia-telangiectasia families in the British Isles: Expression of mutant ATM and the risk of leukemia, lymphoma, and breast cancer. Am J Hum Genet 1998;62:334.

Stevenson DK, Wong RJ, Vreman HJ, et al. NICHD conference on kernicterus. Research on prevention of bilirubin-induced brain injury and kernicterus: Bench-to-bedside—diagnostic methods and prevention and treatment strategies. J Perinatol 2004;24:521.

Straussberg R, Shorer Z, Weitz R, et al. Familial infantile bilateral striatal necrosis: Clinical features and response to biotin treatment. Neurology 2002;59:983.

Stray-Pedersen A, Jonsson T, Heiberg A, et al. The impact of an early truncating founder ATM mutation on immunoglobulins, specific antibodies and lymphocyte populations in ataxia-telangiectasia patients and their parents. Clin Exp Immunol 2004;137:179.

Stremmel W, Meyerrose KW, Niederau C, et al. Wilson disease: Clinical presentation, treatment, and survival. Ann Intern Med 1991;115:720.

Surveillance of Cerebral Palsy in Europe (SCPE). A collaboration of cerebral palsy surveys and registers. Dev Med Child Neurol 2000;42:816.

Surveillance of Cerebral Palsy in Europe (SCPE). Prevalence and characteristics of children with cerebral palsy in Europe. Dev Med Child Neurol 2002;44:633.

Swaiman KF. Hallervorden-Spatz syndrome and brain iron metabolism. Arch Neurol 1991;48:1285.

Swash M, Roberts AH, Zakko H, et al. Treatment of involuntary movement disorders with tetrabenazine. J Neurol Neurosurg Psychiatry 1972;35:186.

Swedo SE. Pediatric autoimmune neuropsychiatric disorders associated with streptococcal infections (PANDAS). Mol Psychiatry 2002;7(Suppl 2):S24.

Swedo SE, Leonard HL, Rapoport JL. The pediatric autoimmune neuropsychiatric disorders associated with streptococcal infection (PANDAS) subgroup: Separating fact from fiction. Pediatrics 2004;113:907.

Swoboda KJ, Hyland K, Goldstein DS, et al. Clinical and therapeutic observations in aromatic L-amino acid decarboxylase deficiency. Neurology 1999;53:1205.

Swoboda KJ, Kanavakis E, Xaidara A, et al. Alternating hemiplegia of childhood or familial hemiplegic migraine? A novel ATP1A2 mutation. Ann Neurol 2004;55:884.

Swoboda KJ, Saul JP, McKenna CE, et al. Aromatic L-amino acid decarboxylase deficiency: Overview of clinical features and outcomes. Ann Neurol 2003;54(Suppl 6):S49.

Swoboda KJ, Soong BW, McKenna C, et al. Paroxysmal kinesigenic dyskinesia and infantile convulsions: Clinical and linkage studies. Neurology 2000;55:224.

Szepetowski P, Rochette J, Berquin P, et al. Familial infantile convulsions and paroxysmal choreoathetosis: A new neurological syndrome linked to the pericentromeric region of human chromosome 16. Am J Human Genet 1997;61:889.

Taira T, Kobayashi T, Hori T. Disappearance of self-mutilating behavior in a patient with Lesch-Nyhan syndrome after bilateral chronic stimulation of the globus pallidus internus. Case report. J Neurosurg 2003;98:414.

Takanokura M, Kokuzawa N, Sakamoto K. The origins of physiological tremor as deduced from immersions of the finger in various liquids. Eur J Appl Physiol 2002;88:29.

Tan A, Salgado M, Fahn S. The characterization and outcome of stereotypical movements in nonautistic children. Mov Disord 1997;12:47.

Tan H, Turanli G, Ay H, et al. Rubral tremor after thalamic infarction in childhood. Pediatr Neurol 2001;25:409.

Taroni F, DiDonato S. Pathways to motor incoordination: The inherited ataxias. Nat Rev Neurosci 2004;5:641.

Tate ED, Allison TJ, Pranzatelli MR, et al. Neuroepidemiologic trends in 105 US cases of pediatric opsoclonus-myoclonus syndrome. J Pediatr Oncol Nurs 2005;22:8.

Teive HA, Sa DS, Grande CV, et al. Bilateral pallidotomy for generalized dystonia. Arq Neuropsiquiatr 2001;59:353.

Temudo T, Martins E, Pocas F, et al. Maple syrup disease presenting as paroxysmal dystonia. Ann Neurol 2004;56:749.

Thomas M, Hayflick SJ, Jankovic J. Clinical heterogeneity of neurodegeneration with brain iron accumulation (Hallervorden-Spatz syndrome) and pantothenate kinase-associated neurodegeneration. Mov Disord 2004;19:36.

Thomas M, Jankovic J. Psychogenic movement disorders: Diagnosis and management. CNS Drugs 2004;18:437.

Thompson PD, Bhatia KP, Brown P, et al. Cortical myoclonus in Huntington's disease. Mov Disord 1994;9:633.

Thompson TP, Kondziolka D, Albright AL. Thalamic stimulation for choreiform movement disorders in children. Report of two cases. J Neurosurg 2000;92:718.

Thony B, Blau N. Mutations in the GTP cyclohydrolase I and 6-pyruvoyl-tetrahydropterin synthase genes. Hum Mutat 1997;10:11.

Topper R, Schwarz M, Lange HW, et al. Neurophysiological abnormalities in the Westphal variant of Huntington's disease. Mov Disord 1998;13:920.

Tost H, Wendt CS, Schmitt A, et al. Huntington's disease: Phenomenological diversity of a neuropsychiatric condition that challenges traditional concepts in neurology and psychiatry. Am J Psychiatry 2004;161:28.

Tranchant C, Fleury M, Moreira MC, et al. Phenotypic variability of aprataxin gene mutations. Neurology 2003;60:868.

Trifiletti RR, Packard AM. Immune mechanisms in pediatric neuropsychiatric disorders. Tourette's syndrome, OCD, and PANDAS. Child Adolesc Psychiatr Clin N Am 1999;8:767.

Trimble M. Magnetic resonance imaging and Hallervorden-Spatz syndrome. CNS Spectr 2003;8:420.

Tronnier VM, Fogel W. Pallidal stimulation for generalized dystonia. Report of three cases. J Neurosurg 2000;92:453.

Tunkel AR. Double-blind placebo-controlled trial of pleconaril in infants with enteroviral meningitis. Curr Infect Dis Rep 2004;6:295.

Turny F, Jedynak P, Agid Y. Athetosis or dystonia? Rev Neurol 2004;160:759.

Uddin MK, Rodnitzky RL. Tremor in children. Semin Pediatr Neurol 2003;10:26.

Umemura A, Jaggi JL, Dolinskas CA, et al. Pallidal deep brain stimulation for longstanding severe generalized dystonia in Hallervorden-Spatz syndrome. Case report. J Neurosurg 2004;100:706.

Uncini A, De Angelis MV, Di Fulvio P, et al. Wide expressivity variation and high but no gender-related penetrance in two dopa-responsive dystonia families with a novel GCH-I mutation. Mov Disord 2004;19:1139.

Unsold R, Ostertag C. Nystagmus in suprasellar tumors: Recent advances in diagnosis and therapy. Strabismus 2002;10:173.

Valente EM, Brancati F, Ferraris A, et al. PARK6-linked parkinsonism occurs in several European families. Ann Neurol 2002;51:14.

Valente EM, Misbahuddin A, Brancati F, et al. Analysis of the epsilon-sarcoglycan gene in familial and sporadic myoclonus-dystonia: Evidence for genetic heterogeneity. Mov Disord 2003;18:1047.

Van Lierde A, Righini A, Tremolati E. Acute cerebellitis with tonsillar herniation and hydrocephalus in Epstein-Barr virus infection. Eur J Pediatr 2004;163:689.

van Toorn R, Weyers HH, Schoeman JF. Distinguishing PANDAS from Sydenham's chorea: Case report and review of the literature. Eur J Paediatr Neurol 2004;8:211.

Vercueil L. Fifty years of brain surgery for dystonia: Revisiting the Irving S. Cooper's legacy, and looking forward. Acta Neurol Belg 2003;103:125.

Vercueil L, Krack P, Pollak P. Results of deep brain stimulation for dystonia: A critical reappraisal. Mov Disord 2002;17(Suppl 3):S89.

Vercueil L, Pollak P, Fraix V, et al. Deep brain stimulation in the treatment of severe dystonia. J Neurol 2001;248:695.

Verrotti A, Trotta D, Blasetti A, et al. Paroxysmal tonic upgaze of childhood: Effect of age-of-onset on prognosis. Acta Paediatr 2001;90:1343.

Vincent A. Encephalitis lethargica: Part of a spectrum of post-streptococcal autoimmune diseases? Brain 2004;127:2.

Vitek JL, Zhang J, Evatt M, et al. GPi pallidotomy for dystonia: Clinical outcome and neuronal activity. Adv Neurol 1998;78:211

Volpe JJ. Neurology of the newborn. Philadelphia: WB Saunders, 2000.

Vonsattel JP, Myers RH, Stevens TJ, et al. Neuropathological classification of Huntington's disease. J Neuropathol Exp Neurol 1985;44:559.

Warrier RP, Kini R, Besser A, et al. Opsomyoclonus and neuroblastoma. Clin Pediatr 1985;24:32.

Wein T, Andermann F, Silver K, et al. Exquisite sensitivity of paroxysmal kinesigenic choreoathetosis to carbamazepine. Neurology 1996;47:1104.

West A, Periquet M, Lincoln S, et al. Complex relationship between Parkin mutations and Parkinson disease. Am J Med Genet 2002a;114:584.

West AB, Lockhart PJ, O'Farell C, et al. Identification of a novel gene linked to parkin via a bi-directional promoter. J Mol Biol 2003;326:11.

West AB, Maraganore D, Crook J, et al. Functional association of the parkin gene promoter with idiopathic Parkinson's disease. Hum Mol Genet 2002b;11:2787.

Wevers RA, de Rijk-van Andel JF, Brautigam C, et al. A review of biochemical and molecular genetic aspects of tyrosine hydroxylase deficiency including a novel mutation (291delC). J Inherit Metab Dis 1999;22:364.

Wichmann T, DeLong MR. Functional and pathophysiological models of the basal ganglia. Curr Opin Neurobiol 1996;6:751.

Wiese JA, Gentry LR, Menezes AH. Bobble-head doll syndrome: Review of the pathophysiology and CSF dynamics. Pediatr Neurol 1996;1:361.

Wilcox JA, Nasrallah H. Sydenham's chorea and psychopathology. Neuropsychobiology 1988;19:6.

Willemse J. Benign idiopathic dystonia in the first year of life. Dev Med Child Neurol 1986;28:355.

Yahr MD, Orosz D, Purohit DP. Co-occurrence of essential tremor and Parkinson's disease: Clinical study of a large kindred with autopsy findings. Parkinsonism Relat Disord 2003;9:225.

Yamamoto T, Hirose G, Shimazaki K, et al. Movement disorders of familial neuroacanthocytosis syndrome. Arch Neurol 1982;39:298.

Yokochi M. Development of the nosological analysis of juvenile parkinsonism. Brain Dev 2000;22(Suppl 1):S81.

Yuill GM. Suppression of rubral tremor with levodopa. BMJ 1980;281:1428.

Zeuner KE, Shoge RO, Goldstein SR, et al. Accelerometry to distinguish psychogenic from essential or parkinsonian tremor. Neurology 2003;61:548.

Zhou B, Westaway SK, Levinson B, et al. A novel pantothenate kinase gene (PANK2) is defective in Hallervorden-Spatz syndrome. Nat Genet 2001;28:345.

PART IX

Gray and White Matter Degenerative Disorders

CHAPTER 59

Degenerative Diseases Primarily of Gray Matter

Rose-Mary N. Boustany and Adam Zucker

This chapter groups together the seemingly disparate entities of Rett's syndrome, Menkes' disease, Alpers' disease, and various forms of Batten's disease. The first assumption is that they are neurodegenerative diseases that progress after a relatively normal period of early development. That is true for most, with the exception of Menkes' disease, for which affected children are abnormal from birth. The second assumption is that cerebral and cerebellar cortex and deep gray structures are affected, with neuronal loss occurring in most and defective cellular function occurring in all. The third and most tenuous assumption is that the white matter or myelin is spared or only secondarily affected because of wallerian degeneration. As more is learned about the cellular pathobiology of these disorders, it has become apparent that myelin and white matter are affected in a primary way and as a result of neuronal loss or malfunction. Great strides have been made in defining the underlying genetics and molecular defects of these diseases. The next frontier is to understand function of the identified proteins and to devise intelligent, effective, and targeted therapies for these devastating disorders.

RETT'S SYNDROME

Rett's syndrome is an X-linked disease that primarily affects females. It is the second leading cause of mental retardation in females, with an incidence of 1 case per 10,000 to 22,000 females [Hagberg et al., 1985; Kozinetz et al., 1993]. All ethnicities are equally affected. The hallmarks of this syndrome are a period of normal development followed by regression of speech and development of stereotypical hand gestures. The gene that causes this syndrome is *MECP2*, which maps to the Xq28 locus. The MECP2 protein is thought to be necessary for the maintenance of neurons during the later stages of development and after neuronal maturation is complete. The structure and function of the MECP2 protein continue to be the focus of intense scrutiny. Although this syndrome has many severe manifestations, approximately 50% of affected individuals live into the third decade of life. Despite the advances in knowledge about the cause and defects of Rett's syndrome during the past decade, treatment remains primarily supportive.

History

Rett's syndrome was first reported in 1966 by Dr. Andreas Rett [Rett, 1966]. This initial case report was followed in 1978 with a report of Japanese female patients with a particular pattern of symptoms, including mental retardation and stereotypical hand-wringing [Ishikawa et al., 1978]. It was not until 1983, when Hagberg and colleagues [1983] published a case report of 35 female patients, that Rett's syndrome gained international attention. Intense investigation of Rett's syndrome over the past 20 years led to identification of the genetic defect in 1999 [Amir et al., 1999].

Clinical Description

The diagnosis of Rett's syndrome is based on a set of clinical observations accompanied by changes in various laboratory test results. The clinical criteria for classic Rett's syndrome were established in the 1980s [Hagberg et al., 1985; Trevathan and Moser, 1988] and include loss of speech, seizures, mental retardation, and classic motor (specifically hand) movements. Criteria for atypical Rett's syndrome were reported in 1993 [Hagberg and Gillberg, 1993]. More than 75% of patients have classic Rett's syndrome, whereas 25% have atypical Rett's syndrome variants [Hagberg, 2002].

In classic Rett's syndrome (Table 59-1), the newborn initially appears developmentally normal. This period is followed by deceleration of head growth, loss of purposeful hand movements, development of stereotypic hand movements, and gait dyspraxia. These five criteria must be met for the diagnosis of classic Rett's syndrome [Hagberg, 1995]. The chronology of these symptoms is critical for the diagnosis. Normal development is typical for the first 3 to 6 months of life. Deceleration in the rate of head growth occurs between 3 months and 4 years. Patients lose the ability to use their hands in a purposeful manner between 9 months and 2.5 years. Stereotypic hand movements appear between 1 and 3 years of age, and a dyspraxic gait manifests between 2 and 4 years of age if the patient is ambulatory.

Clinical manifestations of classic Rett's syndrome are grouped into four stages: early onset (3 to 6 months of age), regression (1 to 4 years of age), stabilization, and late motor impairment (after the age of 3 years) [Jellinger, 2003]. The early-onset stage is characterized by developmental delay, deceleration of head growth [Neul and Zoghbi, 2004; Schultz et al., 1993], onset of autistic-like behavior, and classic hand-wringing [Jellinger, 2003]. Weight and height percentiles for age also decrease; the median values fall below the fifth percentile by age 7 years [Percy, 2002]. Although Rett's syndrome can manifest earlier, clear signs of a central nervous system abnormality are usually not evident until 6 months of age [Akbarian, 2003]. The second stage of the syndrome is characterized by cognitive decline and regression [Hagberg, 2002]. Loss of speech and purposeful hand movements, emergence of stereotypic movements, seizures, breathing irregularities, other signs of autonomic instability, inattentive behavior, and hypotonia appear [Hagberg, 2002;

TABLE 59-1

Obligatory Criteria for the Diagnosis of Rett's Syndrome

MANIFESTATION	AGE	COMMENTS
Period of normal neonatal development	0–6 mo	Prenatal or perinatal period into the first 6 months of life, sometimes longer
Stagnation of rate of head circumference growth	3 mo–4 yr	Normal at birth, then decelerates
Loss of purposeful hand skills	9 mo–2.5 yr	Communicative dysfunction, social withdrawal, mental deficiency, loss of speech or babbling
Classic stereotypic hand movements	1–3 yr	Hand-washing or hand-wringing and variants, including clapping and tapping, are common.
Gait or posture dyspraxia	2–4 yr	Truncal "ataxia"
Absence of organomegaly, optic atrophy, retinal changes, or delayed intrauterine growth		

Data from Hagberg B. Clinical manifestations and stages of Rett syndrome. Ment Retard Dev Disabil 2002;8:61–65, and from Percy AK. Clinical trials and treatment prospects. Ment Retard Dev Disabil 2002;8:106–111.

Jellinger, 2003; Kerr et al., 2001]. The third stage consists of stabilization of symptoms; this stage differentiates Rett's syndrome clinically from other pediatric neurodegenerative disorders. Sometimes there is a return of communication skills, with preservation of remaining ambulatory skills. This stage is also known as the *pseudostationary stage* because slow neuromotor regression continues [Hagberg, 1995]. In patients older than 3 years, bradykinesia and rigidity set in [Fitzgerald et al., 1990]. Stabilization can last years to decades. Late motor impairment begins when ambulation ceases; this signals the end of the stabilization or pseudostationary stage. This final stage of Rett's syndrome is characterized by nonambulation and severe disability. The length of late motor impairment is variable and can last decades.

Common clinical manifestations of classic Rett's syndrome include stereotypical hand movements, intense staring, breathing irregularities, bruxism, sleep disturbances and night laughter, scoliosis, lower limb spasticity and dystonia, seizures, swallowing dysfunction, constipation, gastroesophageal reflux, and small, bluish or red feet. The stereotypic hand movements occur while the individual is awake. These gestures are individualized, but they typically include continuous and repetitive twisting, wringing, knitting, and clapping motions. The intense eye communication may be compensatory for the loss of speech. This eye pointing has been observed in many individuals with Rett's syndrome. The breathing irregularities are of two types: hyperventilation and breath-holding. Typically, they occur only while the individual is awake.

Periods of apnea can last 30 to 40 seconds, and they disrupt stretches of hyperventilation. Most individuals with Rett's syndrome experience sleep disturbances. It has also been reported that up to 90% of young children interrupt sleep with night laughter.

Although not pathognomonic, many individuals with Rett's syndrome have early growth retardation of their feet. The nails and skin demonstrate trophic changes, and the skin is cool to touch and discolored with a blue-red color. Autonomic dysregulation may produce some of these changes. The scoliosis in Rett's syndrome is a double-curve deformation that develops during the first decade of life. Most commonly, the double curve has a longer upper curve and a shorter lower curve. The incidence of scoliosis increases with age, occurring in 8% of preschool patients and 80% of patients older than 16 years. Abnormalities of the lower extremities in Rett's syndrome include asymmetric distal dystonia, mild spasticity, and feet that tend to orient in a flexed and supinated position.

Seizures are reported in 30% to 80% of individuals with Rett's syndrome. The electroencephalogram (EEG) is always abnormal after the age of 2 years. Infrequent clinical manifestations of classic Rett's syndrome include bloating, violent screaming, and abnormal nociception. Bloating or air swallowing is generally mild, but 5% to 10% of individuals with Rett's syndrome demonstrate severe bloating. The gastrointestinal disturbances are attributed to changes within the autonomic nervous system. Screaming typically is encountered in teenage patients. The screaming may be associated with ill-defined pain, but no known pathology can be found. Occasionally, patients have abnormally prolonged responses to pain. Although a decreased life span is characteristic for this syndrome, many patients to survive into adulthood [Sekul and Percy, 1992], with 50% still alive in their 30s [Akbarian, 2003].

The three most common atypical Rett's syndrome variants include a forme fruste variant, a preserved speech variant, and congenital Rett's syndrome. Diagnosis of atypical Rett's syndrome is complex. The criteria for variants of classic Rett's syndrome as outlined by Hagberg and Skjeldal [1994] are especially helpful (Box 59-1). Forme fruste is the most common atypical variant, accounting for about 80% of nonclassic Rett's syndrome. There is a wide variability of function in forme fruste; it is a milder variant. It is seldom diagnosed before 8 to 10 years of age, and it is usually suspected in older individuals who are just beginning to develop symptoms of Rett's syndrome. The preserved speech variant was first described in 1992 [Zappella, 1992]. It is characterized by the preservation of speech, but preserved head size and obesity are also common features [Zappella, 1992; Zappella et al., 2001]. There is some debate about whether the preserved speech variant is part of the autistic spectrum disorders, as well as the Rett's syndrome spectrum [Percy et al., 1990]. Congenital Rett's syndrome is rare. It differs from classic Rett's syndrome because of the absence of the 3- to 6-month period of normal development [Hagberg and Skjeldal, 1994].

Clinical Diagnostic Tests

Routine Laboratory Tests

Levels of lactate, pyruvate, and glutamate are increased in cerebrospinal fluid [Budden et al., 1990; Lappalainen et al., 1997]. Cerebrospinal fluid testing yields decreased levels of β-phenylalanine, substance P, and gangliosides [Lekman

Box 59-1 Defining Variants of Rett's Syndrome

Inclusion Criteria

1. A girl of at least 10 years of age with mental retardation of unexplained origin
2. *And* three of the six primary criteria defined below
3. *And* six of the eleven supportive manifestations defined below

Primary Criteria

1. Partial or subtotal loss of acquired fine finger skill in late infancy or early childhood
2. Loss of acquired single words, phrases, or nuanced babble
3. Stereotypic Rett's syndrome hand movements, with hands together or apart
4. Early deviant communicative ability
5. Deceleration in head growth of two standard deviations below the mean (even if head growth or circumference is still within normal limits)
6. Rett's syndrome profile
   - Stage I—early-onset stagnation
   - Stage II—period of regression
   - Stage III—recovery of some contact and communicative abilities after stage II. Slow neuromotor regression that lasts through school age and adolescence
   - Stage IV—late motor deterioration. Slow neuromotor regression that lasts through school age and adolescence

Supportive Manifestations

1. Breathing irregularities (e.g., hyperventilation, breath-holding)
2. Bloating or air swallowing
3. Teeth grinding
4. Gait dyspraxia
5. Neurogenic scoliosis or high kyphosis (in ambulant girls)
6. Development of abnormal lower limb neurology
7. Small, blue or cold, impaired feet; autonomic or trophic dysfunction
8. Abnormal electroencephalogram, consistent with Rett's syndrome
9. Unprompted laughing or screaming spells
10. Impaired or delayed nociception
11. Intensive eye communication (i.e., eye pointing)

et al., 1991; Matsuishi et al., 1997; Satoi et al., 2000]. There are increased levels of biogenic amines and creatine in the urine [Lekman et al., 1990]. Plasma levels of levels of β-endorphin and prolactin are decreased [Fanchetti et al., 1986]. The increased levels of lactate and pyruvate in the cerebrospinal fluid may result from hyperventilation [Budden et al., 1990], whereas the decreased levels of cerebrospinal fluid β-phenylalanine are caused by dysregulation of the dopaminergic pathways in patients with Rett's syndrome [Satoi et al., 2000].

Neurophysiologic Tests

The EEG is abnormal in Rett's syndrome. Initial abnormalities are noticed in the rapid eye movement stage of sleep [Kudo et al., 2003]. During the stabilization stage of Rett's syndrome, a slow spike-wave pattern resembling that in Lennox-Gastaut syndrome is observed [Glaze, 1987]. After 3 years of age, there is a decrease in alpha activity with a subsequent increase in theta activity [Bashina et al., 1994]. There is a prolongation of somatosensory-evoked responses in older patients, suggesting involvement of the upper spinal cord and spinothalamic tracts [Bader et al., 1989]. Results of nerve conduction studies are consistent with an axonopathy and denervation indicative of lower motor dysfunction [Jellinger et al., 1990].

Neuroimaging Studies

Initial cranial computed tomographic (CT) scans and magnetic resonance imaging (MRI) are normal. As the patient ages and neurologic symptoms develop, generalized atrophy of the cerebral hemispheres and decreased volume of the caudate nucleus become apparent [Reiss et al., 1993]. Imaging of the basal ganglia reveals decreased volume of the caudate head [Dunn et al., 2002]. Commonly, there is a decrease in gray and white matter volumes, specifically within the frontal and temporal regions of the midbrain and cerebellum [Subramaniam et al., 1997]. Hypoperfusion of the prefrontal and temporoparietal regions is also reported [Lappalainen et al., 1997]. Although imaging studies can help in making the diagnosis, there is no correlation between spectroscopic changes and clinical status [Gokcay et al., 2002]. One study reported an association between the level of hypoperfusion and early-onset Rett's syndrome [Lappalainen et al., 1997].

Pathology

Brain

Gross findings include generalized atrophy of the frontal and temporal regions, the cerebellum, and especially the vermis. The corpus callosum decreases in size by as much as 30% [Oldfors et al., 1990; Reiss et al., 1993]. The brain is the only organ that is decreased in size compared with height [Armstrong et al., 1999]. Cerebellar volume is reported to remain relatively normal. The average weight of a brain from a patient with Rett's syndrome is about 950 grams, equivalent to the weight of a brain from a developmentally normal 1-year-old child [Armstrong, 2000]. More importantly, the brain weight does not continue to decrease with age, because Rett's syndrome is not a progressive neurodevelopmental disorder in the classic sense.

There are many microscopic findings in the brain tissue from Rett's syndrome patients. Neuronal size is decreased, but cell density in the cerebral cortex, thalamus, basal ganglia, amygdala, and hippocampus is increased [Bauman et al., 1995]. The previous findings contrast with a report of an overall decrease in the number of neurons in the frontal cortex, the temporal cortex, and the cholinergic nucleus basalis of Meynert [Belichenko et al., 1994; Kitt and Wilcox, 1995]. Decreases in dendritic branching and dendritic number are found in the frontal, motor, and subicular areas [Armstrong, 1997; Armstrong et al., 1995; Cornford, 1994]. In addition to decreases in dendritic number and branches, shortening of the apical and basilar dendritic branches within these same regions of the brain has been reported [Armstrong et al., 1998]. Afferent neurons have decreased synaptic contacts. The striatum and internal pallidum exhibit hypochromia, whereas hypomyelination is observed in the substantia nigra pars compacta [Jellinger et al., 1988]. The neocortex has decreased expression of microtubule-associated protein 2, and disruption of the cytoskeleton within the neocortex is apparent [Kaufmann et al., 1995]. The caudate nucleus and putamen exhibit reduced levels of dopamine transporter protein [Wong et al., 1998].

There are conflicting results regarding the expression of nerve growth factor in Rett's syndrome patients. One study documented no reduction in the cortical levels of nerve growth factor [Wenk and Hauss-Wgrzyniak, 1999], and others demonstrated large decreases in the expression of nerve growth factor and the neurotrophic tyrosine kinase type receptor, which binds to nerve growth factor with high affinity [Lipani et al., 2000]. Adults with Rett's syndrome also have axonal degeneration, loss of motor neurons, loss of spinal ganglion cells, and decreased glutamate and γ-aminobutyric acid type B ($GABA_B$) receptor density [Oldfors et al., 1988; Blue et al., 1999]. Blue and colleagues [1999] reported age-specific alterations in amino acid neurotransmitter receptors within the basal ganglia of adults.

Electron microscopy of neurons depicts distinct abnormalities [Papadimitriou et al., 1988]. These changes include abnormal neurites that are filled with lysosomes and laminate bodies. Axonal swellings, large mitochondria, and membranous multilamellar bodies are seen. Although electron microscopy reveals intraneuronal inclusion bodies that contain lipofuscin-like material, there are no other characteristics of a lipid storage disorder.

Muscle

Type I and type II fiber atrophy are sometimes seen on muscle biopsy [Wakia et al., 1990]. Decreased cytochrome *c* oxidase and succinate cytochrome *c* reductase activities in muscle biopsies have also been reported [Coker and Melnyk, 1991]. The myocardium has no gross abnormalities. The atrioventricular node has an abnormal or immature rearrangement of muscle fibers within the conduction system [Armstrong, 1997]. Electron microscopy of muscle biopsy specimens reveals dumbbell-shaped mitochondria with foamy vacuoles [Ruch et al., 1989].

Genetics

Rett's syndrome is an X-linked dominant disorder that has been mapped to the Xq28 locus [Ellison et al., 1992; Sirianni et al., 1998]. Although most cases of Rett's syndrome are sporadic, genetic mapping was possible because familial inheritance does occur, and there is concordance in monozygotic twins [Jellinger, 2003]. Mutations within the methyl-CpG-binding protein 2 gene *(MECP2)* cause 70% to 80% of reported cases of Rett's syndrome in females [Auranen et al., 2001; Van den Veyver and Zoghbi, 2002]. This gene was identified in 1999 [Amir et al., 1999]. Most mutations in males lead to fetal demise. Although DNA mitochondrial mutations are found in some cases of Rett's syndrome, there is no indication that mitochondrial DNA plays a part in the development of this syndrome [Nielson et al., 1993; Colantuoni et al., 2001]. Mutations within *MECP2* have also been linked to childhood-onset schizophrenia, Angelman's syndrome, and mild mental retardation [Watson et al., 2001].

The MECP2 protein has three known functional domains: an amino-terminal methyl-CpG-binding domain [Lewis et al., 1992], a transcriptional repressor domain, and a carboxyl-terminal domain [Chandler et al., 1999]. The MECP2 protein binds to methylated CpG dinucleotides by the methyl-CpG-binding domain [Nan et al., 1993]. The transcriptional repressor domain interacts with various co-repressor complexes and disrupts transcription [Nan et al., 1996, 1997]. The nuclear localization signal (NLS), consisting of amino acid residues 265-271, is contained within the transcriptional repressor domain. The biochemical function of the carboxyl-terminal region is unknown [Kriaucionis and Bird, 2003]. Seventy percent of the mutations within *MECP2* are in eight hotspots affecting translation of the following amino acids: R106, R133, T158, R168, R255, R270, R294, and R306. Seven of these eight mutation hotspots affect arginine, which contains a CpG in its codon. These mutations may result from unrepaired deamination of 5-methylcytosine. This mechanism is thought to cause one third of all point mutations that lead to human genetic disease [Cooper and Youssoufian, 1988]. Eighty percent of females with classic Rett's syndrome have nonsense or frameshift mutations within the *MECP2* gene [Van den Veyver and Zoghbi, 2002].

Genotype-Phenotype Correlation

Genotype-phenotype correlation has been attempted, but it is complicated by *MECP2* gene X-chromosome inactivation. This inactivity allows a mother with a mutation of *MECP2* to have a normal phenotype because of skewing of X-chromosome inactivation. If this mother has a daughter with the mutation of *MECP2* but balanced X-chromosome inactivation, the daughter will have Rett's syndrome [Amir et al., 2000]. Despite the problems with X-chromosome inactivation, many studies of genotype-phenotype correlations exist. It is reported that truncated mutations of *MECP2* are more severe than missense mutations [Chae et al., 2002; Cheadle et al., 2000; Monros et al., 2001]. The location of the truncation generally does not affect the phenotype [Bienvenu et al., 2000; Giunti et al., 2001; Huppke et al., 2000; Satoi et al., 2000]. Amir and coworkers [2002] reported that truncation mutations led to increased levels of homovanillic acid in cerebrospinal fluid and to increased respiratory problems. The same study reported an increased incidence of scoliosis in cases of missense mutations. Huppke and colleagues [2002] examined mutations from 123 patients with Rett's syndrome. They determined that mutations affecting the NLS caused the most severe phenotype. They also reported that deletions within the carboxyl terminus caused the least severe clinical presentation. Truncations result in more severe disease than missense mutations, except when the truncation affects the carboxyl terminus. Single–amino acid mutations cause less severe phenotypes, presumably because they lead to mild impairment of protein function [Laccone et al., 2002].

Rett's Syndrome Variants

Most of the mutations within *MECP2* cause classic Rett's syndrome. Twenty-nine cases of the preserved speech variant of Rett's syndrome have mutations within the *MECP2* gene [Conforti et al., 2003; Hoffbuhr et al., 2001; Huppke et al., 2000; Neul and Zoghbi, 2004; Nielsen et al., 2001; Obata et al., 2000; Weaving et al., 2003; Yamashita et al., 2001; Zappella et al., 2001]. These mutations were evenly distributed among the three known functional domains of the *MECP2* gene—the methyl-CpG-binding domain, the transcriptional repressor domain, and the carboxyl-terminal domain. Mutations resulting in less severe phenotypes (i.e., mutations within the carboxyl terminus or a truncation after the NLS motif) were common in patients with the preserved speech variant of Rett's syndrome. Patients with the preserved speech variant who had mutations normally associated with severe disease had skewed X-chromosome inactivation (92:8 in one case), explaining the less severe phenotypes [Hoffbuhr et al., 2001; Zappella et al., 2001].

MECP2 Mutations in Males

Three outcomes occur in males: Rett's syndrome, severe encephalopathy with neonatal fatality, and mild neuropsychiatric phenotypes [Geerdink et al., 2002; Villard et al., 2000; Wan et al., 1999; Zeev et al., 2002]. The classic form of Rett's syndrome can occur in males [Jan et al., 1999]. Although similar mutations are seen in males and females with this disease, there is a report of a unique mutation within *MECP2* that causes Rett's syndrome in males [Ravn et al., 2003]. Male siblings of female Rett's syndrome patients with identical *MECP2* mutations develop a severe encephalopathy and die by 1 to 2 years of age. These mutations typically affect the methyl-CpG-binding domain or the NLS portion of the MECP2 protein.

Rett's syndrome is produced as a result of somatic mosaicism, meaning there is a mixed population of cells with the wild type of *MECP2* and mutated *MECP2* [Armstrong et al., 2001; Clayton-Smith et al., 2000; Topcu et al., 2002a]. Males with Rett's syndrome have a unique genetic composition. Klinefelter's syndrome (46,XXY) allows phenotypic males to replicate the somatic mosaicism achieved by females and avoid neonatal fatality [Leonard et al., 2003; Schwartzman et al., 2001]. There are case reports of Rett's syndrome occurring in a phenotypic male, in whom the *SRY* region of the Y chromosome that produces "maleness" is translocated onto an X chromosome, so that a phenotypic male is genotypically a female (46,XX) [Maiwald et al., 2002]. Mutations in the *MECP2* gene also occur in males with mental retardation and no other symptoms of Rett's syndrome. These mutations generally affect the carboxyl terminus of the methyl-CpG-binding domain region of the MECP2 protein [Couvert et al., 2001; Kleefstra et al., 2002; Yntema et al., 2002a]. Whether these mutations contribute to the phenotypes observed, or are normal polymorphisms is being explored [Laccone et al., 2002; Yntema et al., 2002b].

Cell Biology

Because Rett's syndrome is caused primarily by mutations within the *MECP2* gene, it is necessary to understand the function and interactions of the MECP2 protein. The *MECP2* gene encodes a protein with three known functional domains: the methyl-CpG-binding domain, the transcriptional repressor domain, and the carboxyl terminus. Human MECP2 has 48 amino acids (about 80 kDa) [Akbarian, 2003]. The methyl-CpG-binding domain contains 85 amino acids [Nan et al., 1993] and binds to single- and double-methylated CpG dinucleotides [Bird and Wolfe, 1999; Lewis et al., 1992]. There is a correlation between the capability of the methyl-CpG-binding domain to bind to pericentromeric heterochromatic regions of DNA and the ability of the protein to repress methylated promoters [Kudo et al., 2003]. Residues R111, R133C, and R134C within the methyl-CpG-binding domain are thought to come into contact with methylated cystines. Mutations affecting R111 cause the MECP2 protein to lose its binding ability to heterochromatic DNA and its capability to repress transcription. Mutations resulting in R133C or R134C affect neither of the aforementioned protein properties. The MECP2 protein associates with chromatin remodeling complexes and aids in the regulation of the structure and function of chromatin.

The transcriptional repressor domain is 100 base pairs (bp) long, and it interacts with various corepressor complexes [Nan et al., 1997]. One of these complexes is the Sin3A corepressor complex. This complex contains histone deacetylases 1 and 2, which remove acetyl groups from histones and create a compressed form of chromatin that then inhibits or represses gene expression [Nan et al., 1998]. The action of the transcriptional repressor domain is partially reversed by trichostatin A, a histone deacetylase inhibitor. This finding suggests that repression by means of the transcriptional repressor domain is caused by histone deacetylation. *MECP2* recruits these histone deacetylases and other chromatin remodeling complexes to methylated CpG dinucleotides. This leads to chromatin condensation that interferes with the binding of transcription complexes [Akbarian, 2003]. The transcriptional repressor domain has also been seen to bind to *TFIIB* (also designated *GTF2B*), *SKI* (a proto-oncogene), DNMT1 (which codes for a DNA methyltransferase), and *SUV39H1* (which codes for a histone methyltransferase), although the importance of these interactions is unknown [Fuks et al., 2003; Kaludov and Wolffe, 2000; Kimura and Shiota, 2003]. Repression can be mediated in other ways, because the MECP2 protein binds to general transcription factors and interferes with the binding of transcription complexes. The transcriptional repressor domain is able to repress transcription when bound as far as 2000 bp from the transcription initiation site. The carboxyl terminus is thought to be involved in the binding of MECP2 to naked and nucleosomal DNA. Specifically, the carboxyl-terminal region of the MECP2 protein binds to DNA that is coiled around histone octamers [Chandler et al., 1999].

The MECP2 protein is mostly located within the nucleus of cells, and a small portion is seen within the perikarya [Kaufmann et al., 1995]. Although MECP2 binds throughout chromosomes, binding is most dense around pericentromeric heterochromatic regions of DNA. Forty percent of methyl-CpGs (i.e., binding sites for the methyl-CpG-binding domain) are found within pericentromeric heterochromatic DNA. The immunoreactivity of MECP2 is increased around centromeric and perinucleolar heterochromatin. MECP2 does not associate with ribosomal DNA, despite its many methylations. MECP2 distribution is regulated by unknown factors and does not simply distribute to where methylated CpGs are found. The MECP2 protein is thought to play a role in the maintenance of neuronal nuclei in the later stages of development and within the mature brain [Akbarian, 2003]. It is hypothesized that MECP2 makes chromatin more stable and less accessible to transcription factors by anchoring chromatin fibers into the nuclear matrix.

There are reduced levels of dopamine, serotonin, and their metabolites homovanillic acid and 5-hydroxy-indole acetic acid in Rett's syndrome [Lekman et al., 1990]. Some researchers have noticed a decreased density of postsynaptic D_2 receptors in older patients with Rett's syndrome [Dunn, 2001], whereas others describe increased specific binding at D_2 receptors. The latter finding implies that the decreased levels of dopamine are causing increased levels or density of postsynaptic receptors [Chiron et al., 1993; Dunn et al., 2002]. The D_1 receptor density is unchanged [Wenk, 1995]. Jellinger and associates [1990] proposed that the different densities of postsynaptic receptors within the dopaminergic pathways might be age specific. Increased choline concentrations and decreased choline acetyltransferase levels are thought to result from problems within the cholinergic system in the forebrain [Gokcay et al., 2002]. The frontal cortex and striatum have decreased levels of ferritin [Sofic et al., 1987]. Decreased levels of binding protein for the benzodiazepine receptor in the frontotemporal, parietal, and occipital regions of the brain also have been reported [Yamashita et al., 1998].

Animal Models

In a model of MECP2-null mice, males and females were affected. Homozygous female mice and heterozygous male mice were developmentally normal for the first several weeks of life, but they died soon after neurologic symptoms appeared [Chen et al., 2001; Guy et al., 2001]. This model replicates the genetic component of Rett's syndrome, but it was difficult to study because of the rapid deterioration and early death of the animals after symptoms appeared. Shahbazian and co-workers [2002b] developed a mouse model that has a truncation mutation within the *MECP2* gene with a less severe phenotype than the MECP2-null mice. The truncated protein mimics a commonly observed human mutation, and it is partially functional, containing the methyl-CpG-binding domain and transcriptional repressor domain. This group observed that the mice appeared developmentally normal up to 6 weeks after birth. After this period of normal development, the mice developed neurologic symptoms, including tremors, motor impairment, hypoactivity, seizures, kyphosis, and the classic forearm movements associated with human Rett's syndrome [Shahbazian et al., 2002b]. Random X inactivation causes a variety of phenotypes due to a single genotype in females, which makes analysis of the mouse model difficult [Young and Zoghbi, 2004]. One solution is to use male mice, because they are not subject to random X inactivation.

Luikenhuis and colleagues [2004] overexpressed MECP2 in postmitotic neurons of homozygous MECP2-null mice. These mice did not display any neurologic symptoms, and they were developmentally equivalent to the control population. In normal mice, *MECP2*-encoded RNA is not expressed until about 10 days after conception, and it reaches adult levels by 16 days after conception. It has been postulated that the defect in Rett's syndrome involves neuronal maintenance and maturation and therefore affects developmental stability.

Pathogenesis

The timeline of MECP2 expression suggests that it is needed in the later phase of cortical development in neonates and after maturation in adults. MECP2 is expressed in normal fetal brains until 20 weeks' gestation, after which it disappears from the cerebellum. It disappears from the brainstem after the perinatal period. MECP2 does not reappear in the brain until after adolescence. Lack of MECP2 during any of these developmental periods may lead to synaptic and neuronal dysfunction of the catecholaminergic neurons in patients with Rett's syndrome [Itoh and Takashima, 2002]. Mice with MECP2 overexpressed in postmitotic neurons are rescued from the Rett's syndrome phenotype. A decrease in MECP2 in postmitotic neurons during the later stages of development is sufficient to cause Rett's syndrome [Chen et al., 2001], but MECP2 deficiency in neuronal precursors is probably not a major contributor to the pathogenesis in Rett's syndrome.

MECP2 causes transcriptional repression, and loss of function of this protein may cause an imbalance between transcription and gene silencing, leading to dysregulated gene expression and pathologic changes. Some groups have found no evidence for MECP2 transcriptional repression in neurons or glia. Gene expression studies found an increase in glial transcription, in contrast to the predicted decrease. Levels of presynaptic proteins, however, were decreased. MECP2 may be causing perturbations within the presynaptic signal transduction pathway [Colantuoni et al., 2001]. The critics of this theory point out that these studies were performed on postmortem brains, suggesting that relevant time points in gene expression may have been missed. Additional evidence argues against MECP2 deficiency unsilencing transcription and causing Rett's syndrome. Affymetrix GeneChip analysis of MECP2-deficient human fibroblasts did not demonstrate any large-scale dysregulation of gene expression. There were only small differences in gene expression in presymptomatic, early symptomatic, and late symptomatic MECP2-deficient mouse brains [Tudor et al., 2002].

If MECP2 does not act as a transcriptional repressor, it may play a maintenance role during development. *MECP2*-encoded mRNA is undetectable in the mouse forebrain during mid-gestation [Coy et al., 1999]. Immunohistochemical studies in nonhuman primates and mice demonstrate MECP2 expression in neuronal nuclei correlates with neuronal maturity, and levels of expression are highest in the adult cerebral cortex [Akbarian et al., 2001]. In human cerebral cortex, MECP2 is seen only in Cajal-Retzius cells, the earliest maturing neurons [Marin-Padilla, 1998], at 14 weeks' gestation. At 26 weeks' gestation, MECP2-immunoreactive neurons are seen in the deeper, more differentiated cortical layers. MECP2 neuronal immunoreactivity increases with age. Only about 10% of cells are immunoreactive during the third trimester of pregnancy, but approximately

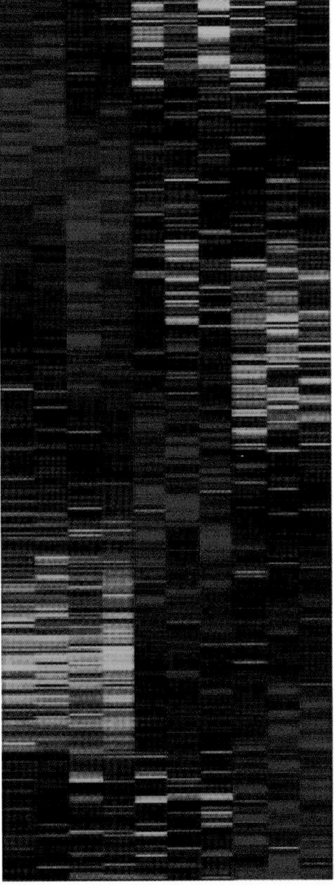

FIGURE 59-1. Partial dendrogram depicting gene expression pattern for *CLN1-, CLN2-, CLN3-, CLN6-, CLN9*-deficient and normal fibroblast RNA. Upregulated genes are *red*, downregulated genes are *green*, and no change from control is *black*. Notice the similarity of gene expression in the CLN9(1) and CLN9(2) patients. CLN, ceroid-lipofuscinosis, neuronal.

80% of neurons demonstrate immunoreactivity for MECP2 at 10 years of age [Shahbazian et al., 2002a]. These findings are also seen in rodents and nonhuman primates. The observation that MECP2 expression is decreased in immature neurons and elevated in mature neurons suggests a role for MECP2 in neuronal maintenance. MECP2 expression studies show high levels of the protein in mature neurons but not in glia or astrocytes.

MECP2 may also play a role in cell division. Removing pericentromeric heterochromatin or disrupting heterochromatin silencing by inhibition of histone deacetylases in *Drosophila* and yeast reduced chromosome transmission during cell division [Henikoff, 2001]. Because MECP2 associates with pericentromeric heterochromatin, it may influence cell division.

Treatment

Rett's syndrome has no cure. The treatments available have been empirically derived and are designed to combat specific symptoms. Antiepileptic agents include carbamazepine, valproic acid, and lamotrigine. The use of L-dopa and dopamine agonists to increase motor ability in Rett's syndrome patients is controversial. [Zappella, 1990]. The breathing irregularities associated with Rett's syndrome can be treated with naltrexone, an opiate antagonist. Naltrexone (1 to 3 mg/kg/day) can reduce disorganized breathing and increases oxygen saturation levels [Percy, 2002]. Use of high-fat, high-calorie diets is recommended in the late stages of the disease, and it has been suggested that individuals with Rett's syndrome require a higher protein intake [Motil et al., 1999]. Feeding by means of a gastrostomy tube is sometimes indicated [Jellinger, 2003]. Constipation in Rett's syndrome has been managed with high-fiber foods, enemas, mineral oils, milk of magnesia, and polyethylene glycol or MiraLax, with various degrees of success. Orthopedists and physical therapists routinely see individuals with Rett's syndrome. The goals are to improve balance, enhance flexibility, and strengthen atrophying muscles. Bracing for scoliosis is necessary when a 25-degree curvature exists, and surgery is advised when the curvature exceeds 40 degrees. Speech and occupational therapy are occasionally used to improve communication.

Small-scale clinical trials using L-carnitine and the ketogenic diet have been completed. L-Carnitine has been reported to improve the respiratory features of Rett's syndrome [Ellaway et al., 2001], and the ketogenic diet may reduce seizure frequency during the first 3 months, but no long-term clinical trials have been reported.

MENKES' DISEASE

Menkes' disease is an X-linked disorder caused by mutations in the *ATP7A* gene. The protein it encodes is necessary for absorption of copper from the intestinal epithelium and for transport of copper across the blood-brain barrier. The reported incidence is 1 case per 100,000 to 300,000 persons. Menkes' disease has three variants: classic disease, mild disease, and occipital horn syndrome. In classic disease, a 2- to 3-month period of normal development is followed by severe neurologic regression characterized by seizures, hypotonia, visual impairment, and failure to thrive. Death ensues by 4 years of age. Kinky, coarse, and lightly pigmented hair is pathognomonic for this disease, although many other phenotypic features may be observed. Connective tissue disorders are common in all three variants because of dysfunction of the cupric enzyme lysyl oxidase. Two biochemical markers, decreased serum copper and ceruplasmin, in conjunction with clinical manifestations aid in the diagnosis. The only available treatment is replacement therapy using copper histidine. Early intervention is essential for the therapy to be neuroprotective.

History

The story of the discovery of Menkes' disease begins in 1930s, when veterinary physicians in Australia noticed the importance of copper for the normal development of sheep [Bennetts and Chapman, 1937]. They observed that mothers that grazed in copper-deficient pastures had offspring with cerebral demyelination, ataxia, and porencephaly. They concluded that copper deficiency in sheep was associated with ataxia and a demyelinating disease. The disease was described in 1962 by John Menkes [Menkes et al., 1962]. He described five males of English-Irish heritage who had peculiar hair, failure to thrive, and a neurodegenerative disorder. The syndrome was initially called Menkes' kinky hair syndrome in reference to the peculiar hair that was unique to these patients. The basis for Menkes' disease was not known until the association was made with the illness in sheep [Danks et al., 1972, 1973]. The distinctive hair found in the copper-deficient sheep and in patients provided the necessary link. Serum testing revealed that patients who had this distinctive hair also had decreased serum copper and ceruplasmin levels. Danks and colleagues [1972, 1973] then concluded that Menkes' disease was a human example of a neurodevelopmental disorder caused by copper deficiency. In 1993, three groups used positional cloning to discover the *ATP7A* gene [Chelly et al., 1993; Mercer et al., 1993].

Clinical Description

Menkes' disease typically occurs in males and has an incidence of 1 case per 100,000 to 300,000 people [Kaler, 1994]. Menkes' disease has three clinical variants: classic Menkes' disease, mild Menkes' disease, and occipital horn syndrome, also known as *X-linked cutis laxa* [Danks, 1995]. In classic Menkes' disease, there is a period of normal development that typically lasts for 2 to 3 months [Kaler, 1994]. Developmental regression follows with seizures, hypotonia, and failure to thrive [Kaler, 1998]. Patients exhibit severe mental retardation with symptoms of neurodegeneration [Mercer, 1998]. Most individuals with classic Menkes' disease die between the ages of 7 months and 4 years [Bankier, 1995]. Occipital horn syndrome is characterized by a less severe genetic mutation that results in a connective tissue disorder.

The characteristic findings in classic Menkes' disease are related to the patient's hair. Commonly described as steel-woolish, the hair on the scalp and eyebrows is short, sparse, coarse, and twisted. The amount of hair is decreased, and it is generally shorter on the sides of the head. Color is often light, with white, silver, and gray being common. Light microscopy of hair reveals three characteristic findings [Kaler, 1998; Moore and Howell, 1985]:

1. *Pili torti* is a 180-degree twisting of the hair shaft that is pathognomonic for Menkes' disease.
2. *Trichoclasis* is a transverse fracture of the hair shaft.
3. *Trichoptilosis* is longitudinal splitting of the hair shaft.

Hypopigmentation is common but not the rule, and it is caused by a deficiency of catechol oxidase. Patients typically have large jowls, sagging cheeks, large ears, and a high-arched palate. The skin appears loose at the nape of the neck, in the axillae, and on the trunk. Delayed tooth eruption and pectus excavatum are common, and the incidence of umbilical hernias is increased.

Classic Menkes' disease has several distinctive neurologic findings. These patients exhibit truncal hypotonia with poor head control, hyperactive deep tendon reflexes, impaired visual fixation or tracking, and cortical adducted thumbs. There is increased appendicular tone, and asymmetric growth failure that appears shortly after neurodegeneration begins. EEGs are moderately or severely abnormal, and hypsarrhythmia occurs frequently [Venta-Sobero et al., 2004]. Ophthalmologic findings common in Menkes' disease include myopia, strabismus, and problems with visual fixation and tracking.

Connective tissue disorders are common in the three variants. Pelvic ultrasound and cystograms reveal diverticula of the urinary bladder [Daly and Rabinovitch, 1981; Harke et al., 1977]. Skull and skeletal radiographs are notable for wormian bones in the skull, metaphyseal spurring of the long bones, and anterior flaring or multiple fractures of the ribs [Adams et al., 1974; Capesius et al., 1977; Koslowski and McCrossin, 1979; Stanley et al., 1976]. MRI demonstrates white matter changes and impaired myelination, cerebral blood vessel tortuosity, ventriculomegaly, and diffuse cerebral atrophy [Faerber et al., 1989; Johnsen et al., 1991].

Patients with occipital horn syndrome have hyperelastic skin and may develop other connective tissue disorders, including aortic aneurysms, hernias, bladder diverticula, and skeletal abnormalities, which most likely result from lysyl oxidase deficiency. These individuals also have mild mental retardation and autonomic dysfunction that manifests as syncope, hypothermia, and diarrhea [Byers et al., 1980]. The severity of mild Menkes' disease falls between that in the classic form and the much milder occipital horn syndrome [Procopis et al., 1981]. It is important for patients with milder variations of Menkes' disease to have frequent vision examinations because ophthalmologic problems can greatly impair functioning of affected individuals.

Clinical and Biochemical Diagnoses

The clinical diagnosis of Menkes' disease is supported by specific laboratory findings [Poulsen et al., 2002]. Early diagnosis of affected newborns is necessary for the institution of appropriate therapy and survival. A high index of suspicion based on clinical grounds is essential because supportive laboratory findings may be problematic in the first few months of life.

Initially, few or no neurologic manifestations occur [Gunn et al., 1984]. Kinky hair with light hair pigmentation is most suggestive of Menkes' disease. The pili torti pathognomonic for Menkes' disease are usually seen only in older patients. The diagnosis should be considered for a neonate born after premature labor and delivery with large cephalohematomas, unexplained hypothermia or hypoglycemia, jaundice requiring phototherapy, pectus excavatum, and inguinal or umbilical hernias [Kaler, 1998].

The classic biochemical markers of Menkes' disease are low serum levels of copper and ceruplasmin. Decreased intestinal copper absorption leads to low levels of copper in the plasma, liver, and brain. In contrast, copper stores are increased in the duodenum, kidney, spleen, pancreas, and skeletal muscle [Heydorn et al., 1975; Horn, 1984; Williams and Atkins, 1981].

Early laboratory diagnosis of neonates is complicated by the fact that copper and ceruloplasmin concentrations are normally low in healthy newborns, and these values can overlap with those typically found for older patients with Menkes' disease [Lockitch et al., 1986, 1988]. Copper egress assay in cultured fibroblasts is the definitive diagnostic study at this age, but the test is lengthy and requires several weeks of cell culture. Rapid diagnosis of Menkes' disease can be achieved by measurement of plasma catecholamines or polymerase chain reaction (PCR) detection of known deletions or point mutations in the *ATP7A* gene. The copper deficiency in Menkes' disease affects the function of many enzymes requiring copper. Dopamine monooxygenase is one of the cuproenzymes that is dysfunctional in Menkes' disease, resulting in abnormal plasma catechol concentrations in newborns and fetuses [Kaler et al., 1993a, 1993b, 1993c]. The plasma catecholamine profile is considered to be the most rapid and reliable way to diagnose Menkes' disease during the neonatal period. PCR methods are helpful in the diagnosis of partial deletions and point mutations when they are already identified for a specific family. The DNA-based technologies used for screening *ATP7A* for point mutations are chemical cleavage mismatch detection [Das et al., 1994], single-strand conformational polymorphism analysis [Tumer et al., 1997], and dideoxy fingerprinting [Moller et al., 2000]. PCR-based methods for screening *ATP7A* for large partial deletions include multiplex PCR, genomic PCR, and reverse transcriptase PCR [Poulsen et al., 2002]. These PCR methods are useful in neonatal and prenatal diagnosis, and they are helpful for carrier screening.

Prenatal diagnosis and identification of carrier status are important for families that are at risk for Menkes' disease. Assays looking for increased levels of copper in cultured fibroblasts also can be used for prenatal diagnosis and for testing of potential carriers [Goka et al., 1976; Poulsen et al., 2002; Tumer et al., 2003], but random X inactivation renders carrier testing using this technique uninformative when negative. The only definitive tests that can exclude this disease are DNA-based assays.

An important component of all variants of Menkes' disease is connective tissue involvement. Deoxypyridinoline is a cross-linking residue of type I collagen and is a good marker for lysyl oxidase activity, the cuproenzyme deficiency that is responsible for the connective tissue disorders observed in these patients. Deoxypyridinoline has been proposed as a marker for the presence of connective tissue disorders associated with Menkes' disease [Kodama et al., 2003].

Genetics

Menkes' disease is an X-linked disease, and one third of cases are thought to represent new mutations [Haldane, 1935]. The gene responsible for Menkes' disease, *ATP7A*, was discovered in 1993 [Chelly et al., 1993; Mercer et al., 1993; Vulpe et al., 1993]. The gene encodes the copper transporting ATPase known as ATP7A [Mercer, 1998]. ATP7A is part of a highly conserved family of cation transporting ATPase proteins [Odermatt et al., 1993; Pederson and Carafoli, 1987]. This protein family includes the protein WD that is defective in Wilson's disease. The *ATP7A* gene (formerly known as *MNK*) is located at Xq13.2-q13.3 [Tumer et al., 2003]. It has 23 exons and is about 140 kb long [Dierick et al., 1995]. *ATP7A* is 8.5 kDa.

Occipital horn syndrome results from point mutations (75%), chromosomal rearrangements (about 1%), and large or partial deletions (about 15%) in the *ATP7A* gene [Liu et al., 1999; Tumer et al., 1999]. Severe classic Menkes' disease RNA contains low levels of active ATP7A mRNA, whereas mild variants of Menkes' disease have higher levels of active ATP7A mRNA. Occipital horn syndrome has 20% to 35% residual ATP7A mRNA in cultured cells, whereas classic Menkes' disease has lower levels of mRNA in the cells [Kaler, 1994, 1998]. Decreased mRNA levels result from premature stop codons, missense mutations, frame shifts, and other deletions or mutations that affect RNA splicing [Das et al., 1995]. Patients with the identical deletion or mutation may have different clinical outcomes [Tumer et al., 2003]. This finding suggests that other modifying genes or proteins must play a role in the pathogenesis of this disease. Alternatively, other pathways for copper transport may exist at the cellular level.

Alternate splice products of *ATP7A* exist. One of the splice variants lacks exon 10, but the product is in-frame. This exon encodes transmembrane domains 3 and 4. This protein may act as a copper transporter, but it may not be able to function as a copper-transporting ATPase. It is also possible that alternate exons exist within intronic sequences.

Biochemistry

The genetic mutation of the *ATP7A* gene leads to problems with copper transport within the body. Normally, ATP7A allows efflux of copper from gut epithelium into the portal circulation, transport of copper across the blood-brain barrier, and transfer of copper that is reabsorbed by the kidney back into circulation. ATP7A protein deficiency results in an inability of the body to absorb copper from the gastrointestinal tract in amounts required to satisfy nutritional needs, as well as in impaired use and handling of the copper that is absorbed from the intestine. Copper is mobilized from the cytoplasm of cells so that it can be incorporated into secretory pathways [Tumer et al., 2003]. The mutation of a copper-transporting ATPase causes impaired cellular copper efflux, leading to increased intracellular copper concentrations. Patients with Menkes' disease have high concentrations of copper in gut epithelial cells, and they absorb little copper from their diet. Copper accumulates in kidney tubules. At high levels, copper causes lipid peroxidation, protein cleavage, enzyme inhibition, and DNA damage. Normally, basal intracellular stores are maintained at low levels [Rae et al., 1999; Voskoboinik and Camakaris 2002]. The disease is caused by a decreased amount of the ATP7A protein, or it can result from alterations to the protein that impair its ability to transport copper.

ATP7A has six to eight transmembrane domains, and it transports Cu^{2+} ions using energy from ATP hydrolysis [Vulpe et al., 1993]. The protein has several known motifs or domains within it, such as the ATP binding domain. The phosphorylation motif (DKTG) contains an aspartic acid that becomes phosphorylated during the protein's cycle (present in all P-type ATPases). The cation transduction motif (CPC) features a conserved proline, which plays a role in the conformation changes that occur with cation transport [Silver et al., 1989]. There are six metal binding sites (MBSs) in the amino-terminal region of ATP7A. The consensus sequence of the MBS is GMxCxxC. Although human ATP7A has six different forms of MBSs, microbial cells show that only one or two are necessary for a functional protein [Odermatt et al., 1993; Solioz et al., 1994]. Human ATP7A does not need a MBSs, demonstrated by the fact that mutations in all six MBSs do not stop ATP7A from functioning [Forbes et al., 1999; Payne and Gitlin, 1998; Tsivkovskii et al., 2002]. The MBS may act as a sensor for intracellular copper levels, and it may play a regulatory role when concentrations are low [Goodyer et al., 1999; Strausak et al., 1999; Voskoboinik and Camakaris 2002]. ATP7A also features a magnesium binding motif (TGE), the "hinge" domain of the protein, and a phosphatase motif (DKTG).

ATP7A-encoded mRNA is found is most cell types, but it is missing in liver. ATP7B, the protein mutated in Wilson's disease (Table 59-2), transports copper in the liver [Vulpe et al., 1993; Paynter et al., 1994]. ATP7A and ATP7B are members of the P-type ATPases group IB family, as are bacterial heavy metal transporters [Tsivkovskii et al., 2002; Voskoboinik et al., 2001]. ATP7A has been localized to the *trans*-Golgi compartment under basal conditions [Petris et al., 1996]. This is consistent with the ability of ATP7A to supply cuproenzymes (i.e., lysyl oxidase) that are in secretory pathways. There is continuous recycling of ATP7A between the plasma membrane and the *trans*-Golgi compartment [Petris and Mercer, 1999]. ATP7A traffics to the plasma membrane with increased extracellular copper concentrations and is endocytosed back to the *trans*-Golgi compartment after extracellular levels decrease to normal. Copper-dependent vesicular trafficking moves ATP7A from the plasma membrane to the *trans*-Golgi network and back. Lower organisms have two copper ATPases, but this is unnecessary in humans because ATP7A traffics between the two areas where such ATPases are needed [Yuan et al., 1997]. Cu(I) may be the type of copper used by ATP7A as its substrate. It is unknown whether Cu(I) becomes Cu(II) before or after it is released in the Golgi lumen.

Menkes' disease is caused by mutations that result in a substitution of highly conserved amino acids or those in highly conserved motifs. Any mutation that affects the structure and function of the *ATP7A* gene will lead to disease [Guy et al., 2001]. Mutations that induce Menkes' disease include those that abolish the Mg^{2+} binding domain [Seidel et al., 2001] and those that change the cation transduction motif. Classic Menkes' disease is usually caused by a premature truncation, typically occurring before the first

TABLE 59-2

Comparison of Menkes' Disease and Wilson's Disease

CHARACTERISTIC	MENKES' DISEASE	WILSON'S DISEASE
Inheritance pattern	X-linked recessive	Autosomal recessive
Location	Xq13.3	13q14.3
Incidence	1:300,000	1:100,000
Clinical manifestations	Onset at birth Cerebral degeneration Global delay Kinky hair Pili torti Abnormal facies Hypopigmentation Arterial rupture or thrombosis Bone changes or cutis laxa	Dysarthria Kayser-Fleisher rings
Laboratory test findings	↓ Serum Cu ↓ Serum ceruloplasmin ↑ Intestinal or kidney Cu ↓ Liver Cu	↓ Serum Cu ↓ Serum ceruloplasmin ↑ Urinary Cu ↑ Liver Cu
Prognosis	Lethal in classic cases Death < 3 yr	Can be treated effectively with chelating agents
Gene product	1500–amino acid copper-binding ATPase	1411–amino acid copper-binding ATPase
Location, expression	All tissues except liver	Liver, kidney, and placenta
Mutation	Partial deletions in 15%; most others are point mutations	Point mutations and small rearrangements

transmembrane domain and resulting in loss of all catalytic activity. Occipital horn syndrome and mild Menkes' disease usually result from missense or splice mutations. It is unknown how much catalytic activity is needed to result in a milder phenotype (i.e., ATP7A still able to absorb sufficient amounts of intestinal copper and enable its delivery to the requisite enzymes) [Tumer et al., 1997]. A case study of a patient with occipital horn syndrome showed that the splice mutation allowed 2% to 5% of ATP7A transcripts to be produced. This amount of protein was sufficient to allow partial absorption of copper from the gut epithelium and partial transport across the blood-brain barrier [Moller et al., 2000]. There was, however, too little protein for lysyl oxidase to function correctly. Between 2% and 5% of ATP7A activity is the proposed amount of protein necessary to decrease the severity of the Menkes' disease phenotype.

Most of the clinical manifestations of Menkes' disease can be explained by understanding which cuproenzymes are affected. Intracellular copper is necessary for oxidative reactions. Most clinical symptoms are caused by dysfuntion of dopamine monooxygenase, peptidylglycine monooxygenase, cytochrome *c* oxidase, lysyl oxidase, and Cu/Zn superoxide dismutase (SOD).

Dopamine monooxygenase, also known as dopamine β-hydroxylase, is part of the catecholamine biosynthetic pathway. In Menkes' disease, there is complete or partial deficiency of dopamine β-hydroxylase. This deficiency causes abnormal plasma and cerebrospinal fluid patterns. The degree of deficiency can be evaluated by looking at norepinephrine concentrations or looking at the ratio of dihydroxyphenylalanine to dihydroxyphenylglycol. Cases of Menkes' disease with deficient dopamine β-hydroxylase exist that have normal plasma and cerebrospinal fluid concentrations of norepinephrine. It is unknown why compensatory mechanisms are active in some patients but not in others. In the mouse model of Menkes' disease, normal concentrations of norepinephrine are observed in certain areas of the brain [Prohaska and Bailey, 1994]. The dopamine β-hydroxylase deficiency causes temperature instability, hypoglycemia, eyelid ptosis, and loss of sympathetic adrenergic function [Biaggioni et al., 1990; Robertson et al., 1986].

Peptidylglycine monooxygenase is a cuproenzyme necessary for the removal of the carboxyl-terminal glycine residue from neuroendocrine precursors, including gastrin, cholecystokinin, vasoactive intestinal peptide, corticotropin releasing factor, calcitonin, vasopressin, and thyrotropin-releasing hormone [Eipper et al., 1983, 1992]. When this enzyme is deficient, these neuroendocrine factors have 100- to 1000-fold decreased bioactivity. Affected animal models of Menkes' disease have decreased peptidylglycine monooxygenase activity within their brains [Prohaska and Bailey, 1995]. The decreased activity of these neuroendocrine factors contributes to the phenotype of Menkes' disease.

Cytochrome *c* oxidase is a copper-dependent enzyme that is deficient in Menkes' disease. The decreased cytochrome *c* oxidase activity causes a subacute necrotizing encephalomyelitis without the severe lactic acidemia that is generally associated with complex IV defects [DiMauro et al., 1990; Robinson, 1989; Robinson et al., 1987]. Peripheral hypotonia and muscle weakness in patients with Menkes' disease is partially caused by decreased activity of this enzyme.

The normal function of lysyl oxidase (protein lysine 6-oxidase) is to deaminate lysine and hydroxylysine during the first step of collagen cross-link formation [Siegel, 1979]. ATP7A may be needed to transport copper into the *trans*-Golgi for use by lysyl oxidase. Deficiency of lysyl oxidase decreases the strength of connective tissue in certain tissues or organs and leads to a host of connective tissue disorders that usually are associated with Menkes' disease, including vascular tortuosity [Royce and Steinmann, 1990], bladder diverticula [Daly and Rabinovitch, 1981; Harke et al., 1977], and gastric polyps. ATP7A deficiency affects lysyl oxidase more profoundly than any of the other cuproenzymes [Gacheru et al., 1993]. It is possible that other cuproenzymes can acquire copper from cytoplasmic carriers without using ATP7A (an intermediate carrier), and this may explain why some mutations of ATP7A lead to the less severe occipital horn syndrome.

Cu/Zn SOD is also deficient in this disease [Rohmer et al., 1977]. Lowered levels of Cu/Zn SOD can increase susceptibility to damage by oxygen free radicals. It is not known whether decreased Cu/Zn SOD causes any developmental regression, because animal models without Cu/Zn SOD have normal development [Reaume et al., 1996]. Postmortem studies of patient with Menkes' disease have found increased levels of manganese SOD, which may be a compensatory change for the decreased levels of Cu/Zn SOD [Shibata et al., 1995]. It is unknown whether the decrease in this enzyme contributes to the phenotype observed in Menkes' disease.

Pathology

Kidney

Copper accumulation within the kidneys leads to problems with renal reabsorption. Animal models of Menkes' disease demonstrate an accumulation of copper within the proximal tubules of the kidney [Kodama and Murata, 1999]. β_2-Microglobulin is absorbed by the renal proximal tubules. Urinary β_2-microglobulin levels increase with increasing age of Menkes' disease patients, regardless of whether they undergo treatment [Ozawa et al., 2003].

Brain

Microscopy of tissues from animal models of Menkes' disease reveal an increased number of apoptotic cells within the neocortex and the hippocampus [Rossi et al., 2001]. Brain CT scans demonstrate atrophy that is generalized or diffuse. Brain MRI reveals infarcts that result from tortuous arteries [Venta-Sobero et al., 2004]. MRI also demonstrates white matter disturbances, ventriculomegaly, and diffuse atrophy [Faerber et al., 1989].

Connective Tissue

Urinary diverticula can be seen on pelvic ultrasound and cystography. Bone abnormalities are common and include wormian bones in the skull, metaphyseal spurring of the long bones, and anterior flaring and multiple fractures of the ribs [Adams et al., 1974; Stanley et al., 1976].

Pathogenesis

Defective copper trafficking explains most changes seen in Menkes' disease. Nutritional needs of the body for copper are crucial the first 12 months of life. Brain growth and motor development are most rapid during this phase. Neurodevelopment and motor development are processes that require copper [Berg, 1994]. Expression of BCL2, an antiapoptotic protein, is decreased in children with Menkes' disease. Decreased levels of copper lead to mitochondrial damage that causes decreased levels of BCL2 [Rossi et al., 2001]. These decreased levels of BCL2 may explain the increased number of apoptotic cells seen in the brain of the animal model, as well as the mechanism behind neurodegeneration in Menkes' disease.

Phenotypic differences in animal models and in humans appear to depend on the amount of functional *ATP7A*-encoded mRNA. During different stages of development, the various organs and tissues have different copper requirements. If the requirement is not met, the organ or tissue undergoes developmental failure.

Animal Models

Complete deficiency of the Menkes' protein in mice causes lethality before birth, whereas humans can survive for a limited time without ATP7A [Mercer, 1998]. The murine homolog of ATP7A is Atp7a [Levinson et al., 1994; Mercer et al., 1994]. Just as in humans, there are a variety of observed phenotypes, with most of them reflecting their human counterparts. The severity of the murine phenotypes depends on the amount of *ATP7A*-encoded mRNA. Four murine genotypes are used to study Menkes' disease:

1. Jax brindled, akin to classic Menkes' disease, does not respond to copper treatment.
2. Macular brindled corresponds to classic Menkes' disease. Mice are hypopigmented because of catechol oxidase deficiency. They have severe neurologic deficits and die about 15 days after birth if untreated. However, if copper is given before the seventh day of life, the mice are able to survive [Fujii et al., 1990; Mercer, 1998].
3. Viable brindled corresponds to mild Menkes' disease. These mice are similar to the other brindled mutants, but they have increased viability.
4. Blotchy corresponds to occipital horn syndrome. These mice display less severe phenotypes than the other mutants. Their defects are mostly limited to connective tissue abnormalities. Assays reveal that full-length Atp7a-encoded mRNA is present [Levinson et al., 1994; Mercer et al., 1994].

Treatment

Treatment of Menkes' disease is limited to supportive therapy and supplementation with copper histidine. Unlike nutritional copper deficiency, Menkes' disease cannot be cured by copper replacement. Copper histidine is more effective in patients with milder phenotypes. A small subset of patients can achieve normal neurodevelopment. Early detection and intervention are critical for the copper histidine treatment to have an effect. Many individuals with Menkes' disease fare poorly, with little or no developmental improvement despite early intervention. Older patients with neurologic signs of Menkes' disease demonstrate little improvement with copper histidine replacement. Therapy may, however, reduce irritability and allow for calmer sleeping patterns and minor improvements in personal and social development [Kaler, 1998]. These minor responses to therapy may help lessen the burden placed on caretakers. Copper histidine therapy helps the neurologic signs and symptoms of Menkes' disease, but it has no effect on connective tissue disorders associated with this disease.

Early copper histidine replacement therapy is most effective in patients with milder phenotypes who have some residual copper transport activity. These milder variants result from mutations that do not affect the regions of ATP7A necessary for catalytic activity and allow for residual levels of copper transport. The beneficial response to copper histidine therapy can be predicted by PCR-based analysis of mutations.

Future Directions

Improved therapeutic strategies are critical for better outcomes. Biochemical approaches to bypass the block in copper absorption from the intestine and allow requisite copper absorption are needed. Affected individuals must be identified early to initiate treatment before manifestations of neurologic signs and symptoms occur. This is the period when treatment has the most potential. ATP7A is necessary for the transport of copper through the blood-brain barrier. To prevent neurologic developmental regression, other ways of delivering copper stores to the brain must be identified. The symptoms of Menkes' disease result from the dysfunction of multiple cuproenzymes, and copper must be made available to these enzymes to reduce the non-neurologic symptoms experienced by these patients [Kaler, 1998]. Although advances have been made in early detection of affected individuals, there has been little progress in finding ways to deliver copper to the necessary cuproenzymes or through the blood-brain barrier. Because classic Menkes' disease is the result of the partial or complete absence of the traditional copper transport pathway, identification of alternate routes may allow the delivery essential for normal development.

ALPERS' DISEASE

Alpers' disease is a fatal, progressive disease that affects the gray matter of the brain [Simonati et al., 2003]. This disease was initially described formally in 1931 [Alpers, 1931]. Alpers' disease is known by other names: diffuse progressive degeneration of the gray matter, poliodystrophia cerebri progressiva, degeneration of the cerebral gray matter of Alpers [Ford et al., 1951], diffuse cerebral degeneration of infancy [Blackwood et al., 1963], progressive poliodystrophy [Dreifuss and Netsky, 1964], spongy glioneuronal dystrophy [Klein and Dichgans, 1969], spongy degeneration of the gray matter [Janota, 1974], and progressive neuronal degeneration of childhood with liver disease [Harding et al., 1986]. Characteristic manifestations include neurologic deterioration, intractable seizures, and liver failure [Harding, 1990]. There is no known treatment. The clinical manifestations of Alpers' disease are caused by myriad genetic defects with various forms of inheritance. Most of the genetic mutations that lead to Alpers' disease are still unknown.

History

While visiting a colleague's laboratory in Hamburg, American neuropathologist Bernard Alpers conducted a detailed study of a 4-month-old girl who died after a month of intractable seizures. The patient had a normal birth and normal development until age 4 months. There was necrosis of the deep gray matter nuclei and diffuse loss of ganglion cells in the third layer of the cortex. Alpers believed that the degeneration had a toxic cause. Many similar case reports have been made since then. Huttenlocher and co-workers [1976] were first to report that the neuronal degeneration was associated with liver failure. Alpers' disease is also referred to as *Alpers-Huttenlocher syndrome*. The pattern of inheritance has been postulated to be autosomal recessive [Sandbank and Lerman, 1972]. A mitochondrial defect leading to Alpers' disease has also been hypothesized [Naviaux et al., 1999]. The disease most likely has several causes, accounting for subtypes such as hepatocerebral or myopathic Alpers' disease.

Clinical Features

Alpers' disease is a clinical diagnosis that is documented on MRI but confirmed on postmortem examination. The disease is a diagnosis of exclusion, but specific clinical findings suggest its presence. Characteristic manifestations are liver failure, refractory seizures, and psychomotor retardation [Wefring and Lamvik, 1967]. Patients with Alpers' disease are initially developmentally normal. Onset can occur between 1 month and 25 years of age [Harding et al., 1995]. Onset is more common during a patient's infancy and adolescence, with most cases showing initial symptoms in infancy, usually before the age of 5.

Death occurs between 3 months and 12 years of age, with most patients dying before the age of 3 years. The course of Alpers' disease is variable, alternating among periods of development, degeneration, and mild recovery or stasis. Rare cases of Alpers' disease have been reported in individuals as old as 25 years. Because of the variable age of onset, Alpers' disease has been categorized as juvenile, infantile, and prenatal forms [Frydman et al., 1993; Harding et al., 1995; Montine et al., 1995; Simonati et al., 2003; Worle et al., 1998]. Prenatal Alpers' disease has been described in one family, and it is characterized by microcephaly, intrauterine growth retardation, retrognathia, joint limitations, and chest deformity. The infantile form manifests with early onset, a slowly progressive course, and late-occurring severe signs and symptoms. The juvenile form of Alpers' disease is identical to the infantile form, but it is notable for a peripheral ataxia resulting from central and peripheral sensory axonopathy.

In addition to the classic triad of symptoms (i.e., psychomotor retardation, intractable seizures, and liver failure), patients with Alpers' disease may have other manifestations. Hypotonia may occur initially [Egger et al., 1987]. Ataxia, febrile illness, and cortical blindness are less common [Naviaux and Nguyen, 2004]. A progressive ataxia that involves the sensory pathways has been described. This occurrence is similar to other sensory neuropathies caused by mitochondrial disorders [Fadic et al., 1997].

Liver failure is a complication that manifests late in the course of the disease [Smith et al., 1996], and it is usually the cause of death. Most cases of liver failure in these patients were attributed to hepatotoxicity caused by antiepileptic drugs, specifically valproic acid. However, some cases of liver failure and identical hepatic histology have occurred in patients who did not receive antiepileptic drugs. Valproic acid may cause hepatotoxicity in some cases of Alpers' disease, but it cannot explain all cases. Orthotopic liver transplantation has not been helpful in cases with liver failure. Liver transplantation in patients with Alpers' disease has been associated with neurologic deterioration [Delarue et al., 2000; Kayihan et al., 2000]. Complications of neuronal degeneration can lead to death from respiratory failure or primary hypoventilation.

Clinical Laboratory Tests

Initial laboratory test results can be normal. Liver function test results can be elevated initially, although this finding is rare [Egger et al., 1987]. Values are elevated in the later stages of the disease because of liver cirrhosis. There are no specific in vivo serum or cerebrospinal fluid markers for Alpers' disease, and the diagnosis must rely on neuropathologic evaluation.

Cranial CT scans demonstrate progressive atrophy and low densities in the occipital and temporal lobes. There is involvement of the cortex and the white matter [Kendall et al., 1987; Flemming et al., 2002]. Generalized atrophy is common throughout the brain in the later stages of the disease. Multiple findings are apparent on conventional MRI scans. These include diminished white matter and cortical thinning of the frontal, posterotemporal, and occipital lobes [Barkovich et al., 1993]. Lesions of the thalamus also have been reported. Occipital lobe atrophy is widespread. Proton MR spectroscopy reveals increased cerebrospinal fluid levels of lactate [Charles et al., 1994] and a reduced *N*-acetylaspartate-to-creatine ratio. The increase in lactate marks the switch from oxidative to anaerobic metabolism. *N*-acetylaspartate is an indicator of neuronal viability [Neumann-Haefelin et al., 2000].

Electroencephalographic findings correlate with the lesions seen on MRI most apparent in the occipital lobes. The EEG of Alpers' disease is described as slow (<1 Hz) with high-amplitude activity (0.2 to 1.0 mV). Lower-amplitude polyspikes are also recognized on the EEG. This pattern is seen in 75% of patients, but it may be present only transiently in periodic bursts [Martinez-Mena et al., 1998]. These bursts increase in number and duration as the disease progresses. The triad of requisite clinical symptoms and MRI and electroencephalographic findings suggest the diagnosis of Alpers' disease.

Pathology

Alpers originally described the neuronal pathology as cortical lesions with reactive gliosis, demyelination, nerve cell loss, spongy degeneration, and accumulation of neutral lipids. The occipital cortices are usually involved, and involvement can be symmetric or asymmetric. Patchy cerebral cortical destruction usually is worst within the striate cortex. Striate cortex involvement is a hallmark of Alpers' disease [Harding, 1990; Harding et al., 1986]. Because of the destruction of the visual cortices, patient often have cortical blindness [Charles et al., 1994; Dietrich et al., 2001; Parsons et al., 2000]. Multiple case studies have described the cortical destruction as neuronal loss, spongiosis, astrocytosis, and gliosis. Milder changes are seen in the parietal cortices [Montine et al., 1995]. Necroses in the hippocampi, lateral geniculate nuclei, amygdala, substantia nigra, and dorsal columns may be evident. In patients with severe liver failure in the late stages of Alpers' disease, Alzheimer's disease type II astrocytes are seen. The white matter is only minimally affected.

Premortem liver biopsies reveal lobular disarray, microvesicular steatosis, and inflammation with acute and chronic hepatocyte necrosis [Narkewicz et al., 1991]. Common hepatic findings at autopsy are fibrosis, regenerative nodules, hepatocyte dropout, bile duct proliferation, fatty changes, and bile stasis. Pancreatitis is infrequently observed in these patients. Muscle biopsies may contain ragged red fibers and cytochrome *c* oxidase–negative fibers when Alpers' disease is caused by a mitochondrial defect. A subset of patients with Alpers' disease lack any detectable energy metabolism defect and have normal hepatic histology [Frydman et al., 1993].

Biochemistry

The clinical manifestations of Alpers' disease have several causes. Abnormalities within the citric acid cycle of leukocytes, cultured fibroblasts, and hepatocytes due to a defect in pyruvate metabolism or mitochondria have been suggested [Gabreels et al., 1984; Prick et al., 1981]. These defects result in deficiencies of cytochrome *c* oxidase, pyruvate cocarboxylase, and mitochondrial electron transport chain complex I. Mitochondrial DNA (mtDNA) polymerase gamma activity is less than 5% of normal in muscle and liver cells [Naviaux and Nguyen, 2004]. Immunoreactive subunits of the mtDNA polymerase are still present in patients. The deletion that causes the reduced amount of mtDNA polymerase is small because detectable levels of protein are still present. Southern blot analysis of two infants with Alpers' disease revealed decreased mtDNA in muscle, liver, brain, and fibroblasts. The loss of mtDNA may be tissue specific [Tesarova et al., 2004].

Genetics

The mode of transmission of Alpers' disease is understood, and it is consistent between families. Case studies and biochemical evidence support autosomal recessive inheritance and maternal or mitochondrial inheritance patterns. Cases with autosomal-recessive inheritance patterns have no mitochondrial deficiencies [Harding, 1990]. Simonati and associates [2003] observed that although the disease affects both genders, there appears to be a mild male predominance. The same group also observed that children with juvenile Alpers' disease do not have depletion or significant mutations in mtDNA.

Two mutations within the polymerase gamma gene *(POLG)* are associated with Alpers' disease: G2899T and G1681A. G2899T causes a premature stop codon (Glu873Stop). Some Alpers' disease patients are heterozygous for the *POLG* mutation Glu873Stop. It has been theorized that this stop codon is incomplete and allows a small number of ribosomes to be read. The number of ribosomes that are able to bypass the premature stop codon may be regulated in an age- and tissue-dependent manner, allowing Alpers' disease to manifest at different ages and in different tissue types. In *Drosophila melanogaster*, proteins are regulated in a tissue-specific manner by changing the ratio of short to long forms of the protein [Robinson and Cooley, 1997]. The premature stop codon in *POLG* may change the ratio and cause tissue-dependent regulation.

The G1681A causes an Ala167Thr substitution. This corresponds to the linker region of the POLG protein. *POLG* is located on chromosome 15q24-26 [Zullo et al., 1977]. No other polymerase can substituted for decreased POLG activity. POLG is the only polymerase of the 15 known DNA polymerases that has a mitochondrial import signal. Mutations within POLG are found in other mitochondrial diseases: progressive external ophthalmoplegia (autosomal recessive and dominant forms) [Van Goethem et al., 2002, 2003], ophthalmoparesis, sensory ataxia, neuropathy, dysarthria, and male infertility. Children homozygous for the G2899T mutation are affected with Alpers' disease, whereas control groups consisting of patients with neuromuscular diseases or patients with other mitochondrial diseases do not have this mutation. Many patients with Alpers' disease are heterozygous for G1681A, but the mutation is not specific. Heterozygous G1681A mutations are also seen in ophthalmoparesis, both types of progressive external ophthalmoplegia, and in the asymptomatic parents of children with Alpers' disease.

Pathogenesis

Alpers' disease was originally believed to be a complication of concomitant hypoxia and epilepsy. Comparisons with status epilepticus cases are not valid because the cortical lesions in the two diseases differ significantly. Others have proposed that the underlying defect is metabolic. Alpers' disease most likely can be caused by multiple metabolic defects. The cerebral destruction of the striate cortex in Alpers' disease may result from a novel form of hepatocerebral toxicity, which is different from that seen in wilsonian hepatocerebral degeneration.

Management

There is no known treatment for Alpers' disease. It is important to recognize this disease early and avoid the use of valproic acid, because it increases the incidence of hepatotoxicity in these patients. Although some patients may respond to antiepileptic medications early in their disease course, the seizures become refractory to treatment.

NEURONAL CEROID-LIPOFUSCINOSIS: BATTEN'S DISEASE

The neuronal ceroid-lipofuscinoses, or Batten's disease, comprise a group of inherited neurodegenerative diseases of childhood caused by defects in different genes and proteins. Their unifying clinical hallmarks are seizures, blindness, cognitive and motor decline, and early death. Six genes and their protein products have been identified to account for 8 of the 10 or more described clinical entities: CLN1/protein palmitoyl thioesterase (PPT1), CLN2/tripeptidyl peptidase (TTP1), CLN3/battenin, CLN5, CLN6, and CLN8/EPMR. The clinical types are classic infantile (INCL/CLN1); classic late infantile (LINCL/CLN2); variant late infantile Finnish (CLN5); variant late infantile, also known as Costa Rican or Portuguese but not limited to these populations (CLN6); classic juvenile (JNCL/CLN3); Scottish juvenile (CLN1); epilepsy with mental retardation (EPMR/CLN8); Turkish variant infantile, previously classified as CLN7 (with defects in the *CLN8* gene); CLN9 variant (CLN9; gene location yet to be identified); and a number of adult-onset variants that are dominantly or recessively inherited (CLN4, gene location yet to be identified) [Boustany, 1996; Goebel et al., 1999; Mole 2004] (Table 59-3).

Most of the variants manifest neuronal and photoreceptor programmed cell death. Massive neuronal loss is documented as cerebral and cerebellar cortical atrophy on CT scans and by MRI, and photoreceptor loss as attenuated a and b waves is demonstrated on electroretinograms (ERGs). Autofluorescent material accumulates in these cells. Ultrastructural features characteristic for the clinical types consist of granular osmiophilic deposits (GRODs) in INCL, curvilinear bodies in LINCL, curvilinear and fingerprint-like inclusions in JNCL, and combinations of these features in the others. These inclusions have been observed in neurons, liver, muscle, conjunctival, and other cell types from affected patients.

A plethora of novel information has emerged over the past decade regarding the genetics, molecular and cell biology, and biochemistry of this group of disorders. [Gao et al., 2002; Persaud-Sawin, 2004; Puranam et al., 1997; Ranta et al., 1999; Schulz et al., 2004; Sleat et al., 1997]. Two of the proteins identified, protein palmitoyl thioesterase and tripeptidyl peptidase, are soluble lysosomal proteins, although INCL and LINCL are not typical lysosomal storage diseases. Two other proteins, CLN6 and CLN8, are resident proteins in the endoplasmic reticulum, and CLN3 is a protein that traffics among the Golgi, early recycling endosomes, and lipid rafts in the plasma membrane. CLN3, CLN6, and CLN8 are hydrophobic membrane proteins. CLN5 is characterized as a lysosomal membrane glycoprotein. There are many naturally occurring animal models. Two of these, the nclf mouse and the New Zealand Southhampshire sheep, are models for CLN6. Transgenic models for INCL, LINCL, and CLN6-deficient variant LINCL also are available.

Diagnosis is primarily made on clinical grounds, documented by appropriate neuroradiologic and electrophysiologic studies, and confirmed by the appropriate enzymatic (PPT1 or TTP1 activity in CLN1 and CLN2 deficiencies, respectively) or DNA-based laboratory tests. Ultrastructural examination of skin fibroblasts continues to be a valuable diagnostic tool, particularly for identification of novel clinical variants not accounted for by the known genetic defects. Abnormal ultrastructural findings in the setting of a convincing clinical picture is what led to pursuit of the cause, genetics, and biochemistry of the CLN8-, CLN6- and CLN9-deficient variants.

Treatment options are beginning to expand beyond anticonvulsants and supportive nutritional and physical measures. Targeted therapies have been used in patients with known biochemical and cell biologic processes, such as cysteamine in INCL and flupirtine in INCL, LINCL, variant forms of LINCL, JNCL, and CLN6- and CLN9-deficient variants [Batten and Mayou, 1915; Dhar et al., 2002; Mayou, 1904]. Gene- and protein-based delivery systems are being developed for the classic late infantile and infantile types with defects in soluble proteins, and they are being tested in transgenic mouse models. Stem cell replacement is being explored in animal models as potential therapy for these terminal diseases.

History and Terminology

The first clinical description of neuronal ceroid-lipofuscinosis was that of the juvenile form Stengel [1826]. This description was soon followed by clinical and pathologic descriptions by Batten, Mayou, Spielmeyer, Vogt, and Sjögren [Batten and Mayou, 1915; Mayou, 1904; Spielmeyer, 1923; Vogt, 1909]. The *CLN3* gene responsible for the juvenile form (JNCL) was discovered in 1995 [Lerner et al., 1995]. The late infantile form (LINCL) was described by Jansky and Bielchowski in 1908 and 1913 [Jansky, 1908]. These two variants were previously referred to as *Batten's disease*, a term that now refers to all variants. The adult form or Kufs disease, an early-onset dementia with seizures and absence of visual findings was described in 1925 [Dom et al., 1979]. The adult form (ANCL) has been described in sporadic cases and familial cases, with some families suggesting a dominant pattern of inheritance. Chromosomal location of the *CLN4* gene or genes responsible for the adult disease remains unknown.

The term *neuronal ceroid-lipofuscinosis* was introduced by Zeman and Dyken in 1969 as a descriptive term referring to the autofluorescent, waxy, dusky lipid accumulating in

TABLE 59-3

Batten's Disease Variants

GENE	EPONYM FOR MAJOR CLINICAL PRESENTATION	AGE OF ONSET	AFFECTED ETHNICITIES	MAIN CLINICAL FEATURES	EM-DETECTED PROTEIN	DIAGNOSTIC TESTS	MRI And CT FINDINGS	PROTEIN TYPE, LOCATION
*CLN1**	INCL, Haltia-Santavuori	9–18 mo	Primarily Finnish, described in others	Seizures, cognitive and motor decline, blindness, microcephaly	GRODs, saposins A and D	PPT1 enzymatic assay, gene-based test, skin biopsy, isoelectric EEG by age 3 yr	Signal loss in the thalami, T2-weighted high signal intensity for periventricular rims, cerebral atrophy	Soluble lysosomal protein, lysosome
CLN2†	LINCL, Jansky-Bielchowski	2.5–3.5 yr	Pan-ethnic	Seizures, ataxia, cognitive and motor decline, retinitis pigmentosa	Curvilinear inclusions, subunit C or 9 of ATP synthase	TTP1 enzymatic assay, gene-based test, giant occipital EEG spike, ERG	Increased T2 periventricular signal; signal loss in thalami; caudate, cerebral, and cerebellar atrophy	Soluble lysosomal protein, lysosome and PM
CLN3	JNCL, Spielmeier-Vogt	4–8 yr	Northern European, described in many others	Retinitis pigmentosa, seizures, echolalia, psychosis, dystonia, tremor, bradycardia	Fingerprint or curvilinear inclusions, subunit C or 9 of ATP synthase	Gene-based test, ERG	Cerebellar and cerebral atrophy, caudate and putamen atrophy, decreased thalamic density	Membrane protein, PM, Golgi, early endosomes, lipid rafts
CLN4‡	ANCL, Kufs' disease, dominant forms known as Parry's disease	30 yr		Early dementia, psychosis; type A myoclonic seizures; type B extrapyramidal signs and facial dyskinesias	Fingerprint inclusions, pigmentation, subunit C of ATP synthase	Clinical, pathologic examinations; exclude other dementias	Normal or mild cerebral cortical atrophy	Unknown
CLN5	vLINCL, Finnish late infantile	5–7 yr	Finnish	Clumsiness, visual failure, cognitive and motor decline, seizures	Curvilinear or fingerprint inclusions, subunit C of ATP synthase, saposins A and D	Gene-based test	Severe early cerebellar atrophy, cerebral atrophy	Soluble lysosomal glyco-protein, lysosome, ER
CLN6	vLINCL, Costa Rican, Portuguese, Indian	4–6 yr	Costa Rican, Portuguese, Indian, Pakistani	Loss of speech, seizures, retinitis, cognitive and motor decline	Fingerprint, curvilinear, or rectilinear inclusions; lipid drops; subunit C of ATP synthase	Gene-based test	Increased T2 periventricular signal, cerebellar and cerebral atrophy, decreased T2 signal for the thalamus and putamen	Membrane protein, ER, PM
CLN7‡	vLINCL, Turkish	5–7 yr	Turkish		Fingerprint or curvilinear inclusions		Similar to findings for CLN2, CLN6	Unknown
CLN8	EPMR or northern epilepsy with mental retardation	5–8 yr	Finnish	Seizures increased with puberty and decreased with age; clumsiness, dysarthria, decreased cognition, agitation, decreased visual acuity	Curvilinear inclusions, fine GRODs, lipid drops, subunit C of ATP synthase, saposin D	Gene-based test, EEG	Cerebral cortical atrophy	Membrane protein, ER, ER-Golgi inter-mediate compart-ment

Continued

TABLE 59-3, cont'd

Batten's Disease Variants

GENE	EPONYM FOR MAJOR CLINICAL PRESENTATION	AGE OF ONSET	AFFECTED ETHNICITIES	MAIN CLINICAL FEATURES	DIAGNOSTIC PROTEIN	EM-DETECTED TESTS	MRI And CT FINDINGS	PROTEIN TYPE, LOCATION
CLN8	vLINCL Turkish (previously classified as CLN7)	5–7 yr	Turkish	Loss of speech, seizures, retinitis, cognitive and motor decline	Curvilinear or fingerprint inclusions, subunit C of ATP synthase	Clinical, exclude CLN2, CLN5, CLN6 forms	Cerebral cortical atrophy	Membrane protein, ER, ER-Golgi intermediate compartment
CLN9‡	vJNCL	4–8 yr	Serbian, German	Myoclonus, seizures, cognitive and motor decline	Fingerprint or curvilinear inclusions, GRODs, subunit C of ATP synthase	EM, increased cell growth, decreased cell adhesion, GeneChip analysis	Cerebellar and cerebral cortical atrophy	Unknown

*Rare cases of adolescent and adult forms of CLN1 deficiency have been described. The *CLN1* gene is also designated *PPT1*.
†Patients with CLN2 deficiency of later onset survive into the fourth and fifth decades.
‡*CLN4*, *CLN7*, and *CLN9* genes are unidentified.
ANCL, adult neuronal ceroid-lipofuscinosis; CLN, ceroid-lipofuscinosis, neuronal; CT, computed tomography; EEG, electroencephalogram; EM, electron microscopy; EPMR, epilepsy with mental retardation; ER, endoplasmic reticulum; ERG, electroretinography; GRODs, granular osmiophilic deposits; INCL, infantile neuronal ceroid-lipofuscinosis; JNCL, juvenile neuronal ceroid-lipofuscinosis; LINCL, late infantile neuronal ceroid-lipofuscinosis; MRI, magnetic resonance imaging; PM, plasma membrane; PPT1, palmitoyl protein thioesterase-1; TTP1, tripeptidyl peptidase-1; v, variant.

neuronal endosomes, reminiscent of lipofuscin, the aging pigment [Zeman et al., 1970]. The infantile form (INCL) was described by Hagberg and then by Haltia and Santavuori in 1973 [Hagberg et al., 1968; Haltia et al., 1973a, 1973b; Santavuori et al., 1973]. The *CLN1* gene was identified in 1995, followed by the *CLN2* gene responsible for LINCL [Sleat et al., 1997]. Other types have been described since then, including variant late infantile forms and early juvenile forms due to defects in the *CLN5*, *CLN6*, and *CLN8* genes [Gao et al., 2002; Klockars et al., 1998; Ranta et al., 2001; Savukoski et al., 1998; Wheeler et al., 2002]. A CLN9 form is also described that is clinically similar to the juvenile form [Lin et al., 2001; Schulz, Dhar et al., 2004]. The *CLN9* gene remains to be characterized.

The terminology is confusing because it was established before many variants or clinical forms were defined and before any of the genes were identified. The terms INCL, LINCL, JNCL, and ANCL were initially chosen to separate the forms according to age of onset. This holds true for the main classic variants described. Since discovery of the various genes, many atypical cases have been described with variable ages of onset. Different defects in one gene can manifest with dissimilar ages of onset and a variety of clinical phenotypes. The best approach may be to refer to CLN1-, CLN2-, CLN3-, CLN5-, CLN6- and CLN8-deficient types (see Table 59-3).

The decision to name the genes CLN as opposed to neuronal ceroid-lipofuscinosis genes is most unfortunate, because it causes confusion with yeast cyclin genes, especially in scientific and medical literature searches. The decision to refer to all forms as Batten's disease, although historically incorrect, is a simple and practical one, because of the length and wordiness of *neuronal ceroid-lipofuscinoses*. The term *Batten's disease* has been universally adopted and accepted by family groups, private foundations, and U.S. government agencies.

Major Neuronal Ceroid-Lipofuscinosis Clinical Types or Syndromes

The clinical features, laboratory tests, pathology, biochemistry, and genetics are summarized for each of the major types (see Table 59-3).

Infantile Neuronal Ceroid-Lipofuscinosis

INCL (i.e., Haltia-Santavuori variant, CLN1-defective, PPT1-deficient form) is caused by a deficiency in palmitoyl protein thioesterase. The function of this lysosomal thioesterase is to remove fatty acids attached in thioester linkages to cysteine residues in proteins [Schriner et al., 1996]. The first description of this disease was in 1968 by Hagberg and colleagues [1968]. A comprehensive clinical and pathologic characterization of this autosomal-recessive disorder was provided later from Finland [Haltia et al., 1973b; Santavuori et al., 1973].

CLINICAL DESCRIPTION

The Finnish cases represent the most severe form of the disease. Development is normal until 10 to 18 months of age. Deceleration of head growth can start as early as 5 months of age. Developmental arrest, hypotonia, and ataxia ensue. All children become microcephalic. Visual impairment is apparent at 1 year of age, and children are blind by the age of 2 years. Optic atrophy, thinned retinal vessels, and a discolored, brownish macula are seen funduscopically. Frequent myoclonic jerks begin after year 1, and many affected children develop generalized seizures. Hand-knitting movements reminiscent of Rett's syndrome are observed early but disappear by age 2 years. By the third year of life, patients are bedridden, hypotonic, irritable, and spastic. At age

5 years, severe flexion contractures, acne, hirsutism, and rarely, precocious puberty are observed. Most children die between the ages of 7 and 13 years. There are rare cases in which the age of onset may be as late as 4 years. A distinct adolescent phenotype reminiscent of the classic juvenile variant has been described in some patients of Scottish descent [Mitchison et al., 1998].

CLINICAL DIAGNOSTIC TESTS

The single best diagnostic test is measurement of PPT1 enzyme activity in leukocytes [Das et al., 1998]. Enzyme activity can be measured from a dried blood spot on filter paper or from cultured fibroblasts. In the proper clinical setting, an enzyme activity less than 5% of normal is diagnostic for INCL. DNA diagnostics are also widely available. Before the availability of the enzyme assay or DNA diagnostics for this disease, the diagnosis was based on the clinical presentation and electron microscopic examination of skin or other available tissue. The characteristic finding is membrane-bound GRODs, which typically are seen in endothelial, periepithelial, and autonomic nerve cells of the submucosal myenteric nerve plexus, but they also have been reported in other cell types. The EEG may initially be normal but then reveals lack of sleep spindles and absence of the attenuation in amplitude seen with eye opening by the ages of 16 to 24 months. There is gradual loss of amplitude, and the EEG becomes isoelectric by age 3 years. The ERGs, visual-evoked responses, and somatosensory-evoked responses are also abnormal but tedious to demonstrate in young children, and they are they not needed for the diagnosis. The ERG is abnormal, with cone function affected before rod function. CT and MRI findings are present early and include signal loss in the thalami and cerebral atrophy with high-signal-intensity, thinned periventricular rims. Postmortem T2-weighted MRI scans reveal a remarkable hypointensity of the gray matter with respect to the white matter. Prenatal diagnosis has been performed on chorionic villus samples as early as 11 weeks, and it can be achieved by examining amniocytes at a later stage (16 to 18 weeks). Initially, electron microscopic or ultrastructural studies were performed to look for GRODs, but the PPT1 enzyme assay and a DNA analysis can be performed instead. There remains a role for electron microscopy when enzymatic diagnosis is not available, when enzyme activities and DNA analysis are not clear-cut or when identification of the existing mutation is absent. Ideally, all three diagnostic methods should be used because of the importance of the decision based on these results to be taken by the family, treating obstetrician, and geneticist. The diagnosis of a normal or carrier fetus should be confirmed at birth by analysis of cord blood.

PATHOLOGY

At the time of death, brain weight is drastically reduced to 250 to 400 grams. Serial pathologic studies in Finland revealed progressive cortical neuronal beginning at 1 year of age, with a subtotal loss of neurons by 4 years. Giant Betz cells and neurons of the hippocampal CA1 and CA4 sectors are relatively preserved. Reactive astrocytes become more prominent with time. GRODs are apparent in neurons and macrophages as early as 8 weeks' gestation. Ultimately, cerebellar Purkinje cells and granule cells are destroyed and are replaced by a rim of Bergman glia. The white matter appears gliotic. The brainstem and basal ganglia are also involved. The spinal cord is relatively preserved with anterior horn cells that demonstrate storage only. Storage granules can be seen in many different tissues of the body, but tissue destruction is reserved for the brain and retina [Goebel and Wisniewski 2004; Wisniewski et al., 2004b].

BIOCHEMISTRY, CELL BIOLOGY, AND PATHOPHYSIOLOGY

There is loss of function of PPT1, which removes long-chain fatty acids attached in thioester linkage to the cysteine residues of proteins. Proteins containing the fatty acylated cysteine residues are usually found at the inner plasma membrane leaflet. Normally, reversible acylation and deacylation of these may have impact on protein-protein and protein-lipid membrane interactions. *S*-acylated proteins are degraded in lysosomes, and this function also may be impaired in INCL. INCL, like other neuronal ceroid-lipofuscinosis disorders, differs from other storage diseases in that the material that accumulates in the cell has no demonstrable link to the actual defect and may be a secondary occurrence. PPT1 is located in the lysosome and taken up in a mannose-6 phosphate– dependent manner, but it is also activated at neutral and basic pH and likely functions in the lysosome and elsewhere in the cell. PPT1 colocalizes with synaptophysin to presynaptic vesicles in neurons. Sphingolipid activator proteins A and D accumulate in storage cytosomes, probably as a secondary phenomenon [Tyynela et al., 1993]. There are reported abnormalities in brain sphingomyelin and other phospholipids, levels of which are decreased in the INCL brain. There are reports of increased rates of apoptosis in lymphocytes, cultured lymphoblasts, and fibroblasts from patients, as well as neurons rendered deficient in PPT1 [Cho et al., 2001].

Increased apoptosis is a common finding in a number of neurodegenerative disorders such as Alzheimer's disease, Parkinson's disease, amyotrophic lateral sclerosis, and other forms of Batten's disease. Recognizing the defect in deacylation of *S*-acylated proteins and the increased apoptosis rate of PPT1-deficient cells and neurons has led to some targeted therapies (see "Management and Treatment").

GENETICS

All cases of INCL in Finland are caused by an identical common missense mutation (R122W, arginine to tryptophan) that leads to an unstable protein that is degraded in the endoplasmic reticulum [Mole et al., 1999]. At 1 in 70, the carrier frequency is high in Finland, and the incidence of the disease is 1 case per 20,000 individuals. The incidence in the United States has never been accurately computed, but it probably accounts for about 20% of all diagnosed cases of Batten's disease. A juvenile-onset variant of this disorder was first described in a person from Scotland; it has a threonine to proline substitution at position 75 [Mitchison et al., 1998]. This mutation and another with a premature stop codon at arginine 151 account for most alleles from patients in the United States, all of whom have Irish or Scottish ancestry. The former is found in juvenile cases and the latter in infantile cases. At least 40 mutations in the *CLN1* gene have been described.

MANAGEMENT AND TREATMENT

Supportive therapies are still the mainstay. Muscle relaxants, including baclofen and benzodiazepine derivatives, are given to combat irritability, sleep problems, athetosis, spasticity, and rigidity. Lamotrigine, valproic acid, and many of the benzodiazepine derivatives are used to manage the seizures and the previously described symptoms. Pain is a common feature that is helped by these medications. Physical therapy plays a role early in the course and delays the onset of painful contractures.

In a mouse model for PPT1 deficiency, virally mediated *CLN1* gene delivery has cleared storage and improved the clinical condition of these neurologically impaired mice. This therapy is being developed for use in humans. Enzyme replacement is a theoretical possibility, although protein delivery to the central nervous system is not trivial. Under development are methods to chemically open the blood-brain barrier or chemically camouflage proteins to enable them to selectively cross it. Bone marrow replacement has failed, but stem cell therapies are being explored. An ongoing clinical trial is using phosphocysteamine, an oral and safe drug that deacylates proteins and is anti-apoptotic. Clinical efficacy is unknown, but the drug clears storage material and decreases apoptosis in vitro [Zhang et al., 2001]. Flupirtine is an oral anti-apoptotic drug with analgesic, antispasmodic, and weak antiepileptic properties that protects PPT1-deficient cells from apoptosis. It is approved for use as an analgesic and antispasmodic in Europe, but it has not been approved by the U.S. Food and Drug Administration. Its clinical efficacy in INCL remains unknown.

Classic Late Infantile Neuronal Ceroid-Lipofuscinosis or Late Infantile Batten's Disease

LINCL (i.e., Jansky-Bielchowski, CLN2-defective, TPP1-deficient form) results from a deficiency of lysosomal tripeptidyl peptidase. The defect was discovered by comparing mannose-6-phosphate–modified lysosomal proteins from a normal and an LINCL-affected brain [Sleat et al., 1997]. It was first described by Jansky in 1908 and then by Bielchowski in 1913. It is the most pan-ethnic of neuronal ceroid-lipofuscinosis disorders, having been described in European, Middle-Eastern, Chinese, Pakistani, and Indian patients. It is the second most common form of Batten's disease in the United States, although the total number of cases at any time is less than 500, making it an orphan disease according to the Food and Drug Administration. It is thought that a large number of cases originate from Europe.

CLINICAL DESCRIPTION

LINCL manifests with a generalized seizure disorder and ataxia due to unrecognized, frequent absence seizures occurring between the ages of 2.5 and 3.5 years. Within 6 months, vision, motor, and cognitive skills deteriorate rapidly. Affected children are blind by age 4 years because of tapetoretinal degeneration. Most children are nonambulatory and mute by age 5 years, and they require gavage feeding. In addition to prolonged, generalized tonic-clonic seizures, all have frequent myoclonic jerks, which are most prominent in the face but are also observed in the trunk and extremities. An early hypotonia gives way to severe spasticity with flexion contractures. Autoregulation of vascular tone is lost, resulting in mottled, cold hands and feet. Hypothalamic involvement leads to temperature instability vacillating between hyperthermia and hypothermia. Hyperthermia often leads to unnecessary fever evaluations. Copious secretions and shallow breathing resulting from poor chest wall excursions often cause pneumonias. Sepsis and uncontrollable seizures are frequently the cause of death at the end of the first decade or in the early teens [Boustany, 1996; Zhong et al., 2000]. Some atypical cases have a later onset and protracted course [Wisniewski et al., 2004c].

CLINICAL DIAGNOSTIC TESTS

The most definitive test for is measurement of TPP1 enzyme activity when the clinical history and course fit the description. Typically, enzyme activity less than 5% of normal is diagnostic for LINCL. This test can be performed on leukocytes, cultured fibroblasts, or amniocytes and on dried blood from a filter paper. DNA-based diagnosis is also available, but it is more tedious, particularly if the specific family mutation or mutations are not known. In this instance, the diagnostic laboratory excludes the most commonly reported mutations first. Before availability of enzyme or DNA diagnosis, ultrastructural study of a skin biopsy provided objective proof for the disease. The appearance of curvilinear bodies enclosed within unilamellar endosomes in multiple cell types (i.e., endothelial cell, pericyte, Schwann cell, and others) is the most characteristic feature. Rarely, few fingerprint profiles may be seen. Electron microscopy continues to be a valuable diagnostic tool when other forms of diagnosis are not available and in evaluating atypical cases. It has sometimes led to identification of novel neuronal ceroid-lipofuscinosis variant. The ERG reveals reduced amplitudes early in the course of this illness, even before changes of thinned vessels and pale discs become apparent. The process is extinguished within a few months of presentation. Characteristic giant occipital polyspike-spike discharges are seen on the EEG in response to a single flash of light or to low-frequency, repetitive stimulation. These discharges represent the early phase of an exaggerated visual-evoked response. Wave amplitudes of visual-evoked and somatosensory-evoked responses are also high. These tests are seldom used diagnostically. Neuroimaging studies often help to confirm the diagnosis. An initial CT or MRI scan may be normal, but usually within 6 months of onset and before the age of 4 years, cerebral and cerebellar atrophy is prominent. Within 2 years of onset, there is a 40% loss of volume of the cerebellum and a fivefold increase in lateral ventricle-to-hemisphere volume ratio. Caudate and thalamic volumes are markedly reduced compared with age-matched controls, and there is relative preservation of brainstem volume early in the course [Boustany and Filipek, 1993].

PATHOLOGY

Brain weight at the time of death is markedly diminished to between 250 and 700 grams. The calvarium is thickened, and the sulci are prominent, particularly in the occipital regions. Cerebellar folia are prominent, the ventricles are widened, and laminar necrosis is observed. There is massive neuronal loss, with some neurons preserved in layer III. Those cells demonstrate meganeurites. Purkinje and granule cells are almost completely absent from the cerebellum. The putamen and subthalamic nuclei, as well as nuclei in the brainstem, manifest neuronal loss. There is pallor of the white matter. A reactive astrocytosis is seen with activation of microglia, but monocyte-derived macrophages seen in chronic and acute inflammation are conspicuously absent. This absence suggests that the initial event in LINCL is neuronal destruction and loss with a secondary, reactive gliosis.

The small number of remaining neurons has distended cell bodies and granular cytoplasm. This material is periodic acid–Schiff (PAS), Luxol fast blue, and Sudan black B positive in light microscopy sections. White matter appears relatively intact, strongly speaking against a primary inflammatory component in LINCL. Condensed chromatin identified by electron microscopy, upregulation of BCL2 protein, and positive TUNEL stains all provide evidence for the occurrence of apoptosis, a feature common to multiple neurodegenerative diseases [Puranam et al., 1995, 1997]. There is strong reactivity with an antibody to subunit C of mitochondrial ATP synthase [Johnson et al., 1995]. The reason for this is still unknown, but it may represent a form of apoptosis observed in neurodegenerative illnesses called *mitopsis*.

Ultrastructurally, neurons and many other cells contain curvilinear inclusions enclosed within a single membrane. Frequently, these inclusions are admixed with fingerprint profiles. This is more commonly observed in cells outside the central nervous system, such as smooth muscle cells, eccrine sweat glands, endothelial cells, and pericytes. Before the availability of enzymatic diagnosis, prenatal diagnosis was determined by analyzing the ultrastructure of amniocytes obtained at 16 to 17 weeks' gestation [Wisniewski et al., 2004a].

BIOCHEMISTRY

LINCL is caused by defects in a pepstatin-insensitive lysosomal tripeptidyl peptidase that normally removes tripeptides from the amino terminus of proteins. The defect was discovered by comparing mannose-6-phosphorylated glycoproteins from a normal and an LINCL-affected brain. TPP1 is a 46-kDa protein with strong similarity to bacterial proteases. Subunit C or 9 of mitochondrial ATP synthase accumulates. It is unknown how or whether this relates to the TPP1 deficiency. Other neuronal ceroid-lipofuscinosis disorders with normal TPP1 activity (i.e., CLN3, CLN4, CLN6, and CLN8 forms) also accumulate subunit C. It is most likely a secondary process and may be related to the increase in apoptotic activity observed in CLN2, CLN3-, CLN6- and CLN8-deficient cells. TPP1 deficiency and measurement of its activity constitute the cornerstone of diagnostic tools available to the clinician for objective diagnosis of LINCL. This test can also be performed on dried blood filter paper spots.

GENETICS

LINCL is an autosomal-recessive disorder that appears to be pan-ethnic, with cases diagnosed from many countries from all continents except Africa. There is a notable lack of African and Jewish cases. It is the second most common form of Batten's disease in the United States, accounting for one third of diagnosed cases. More than 53 mutations have been described. In the United States, two common mutations account for 65% of diagnosed cases. One is a nonsense mutation, Arg208X, and the other affects a splice junction site, IVS5-1G>C. The few cases with a milder course and later onset carry one of these two mutations on one allele and an Arg447His on the other. A mouse model for this disease has been developed [Sleat et al., 2004].

MANAGEMENT AND TREATMENT

Treatment is primarily supportive. Areas requiring attention include seizures that become uncontrollable with antiepileptic drug monotherapy. Single or combined use of valproic acid, clonazepam, and clorazepate is helpful, particularly in the early stages. There is also a role for phenobarbital, zonisamide, and levetiracetam. Gavage feeding becomes a necessity by age 5 to7 years, when frequent pneumonias imply difficulty swallowing and aspiration. Attention should be given to development of contractures. Bone marrow transplantation has been tried and has failed [Lake et al., 1997]. Gene and enzyme replacement strategies are being developed and soon may be tried in a developed mouse model. Gene replacement achieved by a number of strategically placed burr holes in three patients with advanced disease is being evaluated. Stem cell therapy also is being developed as a treatment option. It has been proposed that oral use of an anti-apoptotic drug such as flupirtine may slow the progression of this disease. The safety of this drug and its analgesic, antispasmodic, and weak antiepileptic effects make it particularly attractive [Dhar et al., 2002]. The efficacy of this drug in LINCL remains unproven.

Variant Late Infantile Forms

Several variant late infantile types (i.e., vLINCL; Finnish type: CLN5-deficient form; Costa Rican/Portuguese/Lake Cavanaugh variant: CLN6-deficient form; northern epilepsy or epilepsy with mental retardation [EPMR] and Turkish vLINCL or tLINCL: CLN8-deficient form) have been described with an age of onset between 5 and 8 years and a clinical profile reminiscent of the late infantile type but with a more protracted course.

Three genes have been described. The gene for the variant Finnish type, *CLN5*, was the first to be identified. This rare variant is mostly restricted to a region in Finland and has been found in 16 families, with one Swedish and one Dutch case also reported. Northern epilepsy and its gene, *CLN8*, were identified in cases from the northeast part of Finland. A subset of Turkish cases with variant LINCL are also caused by mutations in the *CLN8* gene. The variant LINCL type referred to as Costa Rican/Portuguese or CLN6 deficient has been identified in patients of Venezuelan, Pakistani, and Indian descent, as well as in a case from the United States. It had been previously described as an early juvenile form, and it is also referred to as the Lake Cavanaugh variant [Gao et al., 2002; Savukoski et al., 1998; Wheeler et al., 2002].

CLINICAL DESCRIPTION

For the Finnish variant LINCL (i.e., CLN5-deficient form), the initial symptoms are motor clumsiness at age 4.5 years, followed by cognitive decline at age 6 years and by generalized and myoclonic epilepsy at age 8 years. Blindness due to macular degeneration is evident by age 8 years. Children lose the ability to ambulate by age 10 years, and most die between the ages of 14 and 34 years.

For northern epilepsy or EPMR (i.e., CLN8-deficient form) [Ranta et al., 1999], the first stage of disease occurs from age 5 to puberty and is characterized by frequent but short generalized tonic-clonic convulsions and complex partial seizures, as well as by cognitive decline to a low average level. After puberty, the second stage is notable for slowness of movement and a slowing of the rate of cognitive decline. In the final stage of the illness, seizures diminish in frequency, but mental dullness and cognitive decline lead to moderate mental retardation by the end of the third decade. This stage is also notable for clumsiness, ataxia, and impaired vision. Age at death varies from 17 years to late middle age.

For Turkish vLINCL (i.e., tLINCL or CLN8-deficient form), the clinical phenotype is substantially more severe than that of EPMR. Patients present between the ages of 2 and 5 with severe seizures. Intellectual decline, blindness, and behavioral problems follow and are prominent by age 8 or 9 years. By 10 years of age, most of the children are wheelchair bound.

For the Costa Rican/Portuguese vLINCL/Lake Cavanaugh variant (i.e., CLN6-deficient form) [Teixeira et al., 2003], the initial presenting symptoms at the age of 4 years are ataxia and speech difficulties after a period of normal development. Visual failure due to retinitis pigmentosa, myoclonic jerks, and seizures are accompanied by ataxia and intellectual decline. Death occurs in the early to middle teens.

CLINICAL DIAGNOSTIC TESTS

Presenting symptoms suggesting classic LINCL or JNCL with atypical features, normal TPP1 enzyme activities, absence of vacuolated lymphocytes, and a normal *CLN3* gene screen strongly suggest one of the variant LINCL types. Electron microscopic results of a skin biopsy, the patient's ethnic background, and subtle characteristic clinical features for one of these subtypes may tip the scale in favor of one of the LINCL variants over the others. Fingerprint and rectilinear structures favor the Finnish variant. A combination of curvilinear and fingerprint bodies favors the Costa Rican/Portuguese variant. Electron microscopic findings for the Finnish CLN8 variant include loose curvilinear-like structures, and electron microscopic assessment of the Turkish variant demonstrates dense fingerprint profiles in addition to dark amorphous material. The definitive confirmatory test is DNA-based proof of defects in one of the relevant genes: *CLN5*, *CLN6*, or *CLN8*. MRI scans of Costa Rican/Portuguese/Venezuelan CLN6-deficient patients and those with Finnish vLINCL demonstrate severe cerebral and cerebellar cortical atrophy, low densities in the thalami and basal ganglia, and hyperintensities of the white matter. MRI scans of patients with tLINCL demonstrate cerebellar and cerebral atrophy and tissue loss in the brainstem. The EEGs for all of these variants record large-amplitude occipital spikes in response to low-frequency photic stimulation.

PATHOLOGY

In cases of Finnish variant LINCL (i.e., CLN5-deficient form), the brain weighs about 500 grams at postmortem examination. Most notable is the severe cerebellar atrophy. Findings are otherwise quite similar to those for classic LINCL. There is strong immunoreactivity to subunit C or 9 of mitochondrial ATP synthase and weak immunoreactivity to the saposins. Electron microscopic findings are notable for the presence of rectilinear profiles and curvilinear and fingerprint bodies [Goebel and Wisniewski, 2004; Goebel et al., 1999; Topcu et al., 2004b; Wisniewski et al., 2004b].

For the Costa Rican/Portuguese vLINCL/Lake Cavanaugh variant (i.e., CLN6-deficient form), the brain weighs between 600 and 900 grams at postmortem examination. Neuronal loss is pervasive and particularly prominent in neocortex layer V. Although granule cells in the cerebellum are completely eliminated, some Purkinje cells remain. There is strong immunoreactivity with subunit C of mitochondrial ATP synthase in neuronal tissues. It is, however, absent from peripheral organs. At the electron microscopic level, there are primarily fingerprint bodies and, to a lesser extent, rectilinear profiles in the brain. Rectilinear, fingerprint, and curvilinear components are found in organs.

For northern epilepsy or EPMR (i.e., CLN8-deficient form), the brain weight at postmortem examination has been in excess of 100 grams but less than 1600 grams. The brain may appear entirely normal, or mild atrophy can be observed. Most storage material is seen in layer III of the cortex. Neuronal loss is most prominent in cortex layer V. Deep gray structures and cerebellar Purkinje cells demonstrate little storage. There is strong reactivity with antibodies to β-amyloid, subunit C, and saposin D. Ultrastructure of the storage bodies demonstrates curvilinear bodies and granular material.

For Turkish vLINCL or tLINCL (i.e., CLN8-deficient form), no pathology reports of are available in the literature. The ultrastructure of skin fibroblasts reveals the presence of curvilinear, rectilinear, and fingerprint profiles [Topcu et al., 2004b].

GENETICS

For the Finnish vLINCL (i.e., CLN5-deficient form), the major mutation accounting for 94% of Finnish cases is a 2-bp deletion in exon 4 (c.1175delAT). There is a minor Finnish mutation, D279N, and two other mutations, W75X and c669insC, reported in rare Dutch and Swedish cases.

For the Costa Rican/Portuguese vLINCL/Lake Cavanaugh variant (i.e., CLN6-deficient form), more than 19 mutations are recognized. The most prevalent are the nonsense mutation (c.214G>T) reported in 20 Costa Rican families and the 3-bp deletion (I154del) in 6 Portuguese families [Teixeira et al., 2003]. Other mutations have been described in those of Venezuelan, Indian, Pakistani, Greek, U.S., Trinidadian, or East Indian ancestry. The nclf mouse is a naturally occurring model for CLN6-deficient vLINCL [Mole, 2004].

For northern epilepsy or EPMR (i.e., CLN8-deficient form) and variant Turkish tLINCL, one mutation, R24G, accounts for all patients with northern epilepsy. The four other mutations result in the more severe phenotype of tLINCL. Two missense mutations (R204C and W263C) occur in exon 3, and two others, L16M and T170M, occur in exon 2 and are also missense mutations. R204C occurs in the conserved TLC lipid-sensing domain and predicts a potential role for CLN8 in the sphingolipid synthetic pathways. The mnd mouse is a naturally occurring mouse model for

CLN8-deficient forms of neuronal ceroid-lipofuscinosis [Ranta et al., 2004].

BIOCHEMISTRY AND CELL BIOLOGY

CLN6 and CLN8 are transmembrane proteins that reside in the endoplasmic reticulum. The CLN5 protein has been reported as being a transmembrane protein in some papers and a secreted lysosomal glycoprotein in others [Holmberg et al., 2004; Savukoski et al., 1998]. CLN5 has been reported to co-immunoprecipitate with CLN2 protein and with CLN3 protein [Vesa et al., 2002]. This interaction implies that these are dynamic proteins that most likely exist in many subcellular locations and that they may functionally interact forming a complex whereby one protein may substitute for the other. This finding can have great implications for therapy, because some of these proteins, such as CLN2, are soluble and amenable to protein or gene replacement therapy, whereas transmembrane proteins such as CLN3 are not.

MANAGEMENT AND THERAPY

Treatment for these variants is almost identical to that outlined for the classic LINCL and JNCL types. The relatively mild northern epilepsy variant responds very well to monotherapy with clonazepam. Patients have been reported to remain seizure free for a number of years on this drug. Seizure frequency in this variant tends to wane with age.

Juvenile Neuronal Ceroid-Lipofuscinosis or Juvenile Batten's Disease

Although cases of JNCL (i.e., JNCL, Spielmeier-Vogt-Batten-Mayou, CLN3-defective or -deficient form) from all over the world have been described, there is a preponderance of cases with Northern European ancestry (i.e., Finland, Iceland, Norway, Sweden, Denmark, Germany, and Holland). There is a notable absence of African or Jewish cases. Japanese, Portuguese, Polish British, Turkish, Moroccan, and Lebanese cases and cases from other countries have been described. It is the most prevalent type of neuronal ceroid-lipofuscinosis in the United States [Boustany, 1996]. JNCL was the first Batten variant to be recognized, and the gene responsible for it, *CLN3*, was the first to be cloned [Lerner et al., 1995]. Description of the first juvenile cases is credited to a Danish physician, Otto Christian Stengel [Stengel, 1826]. The genetic nature of the illness was established in the Norwegian family he described who had four affected siblings. Because they were raised in different geographic areas by different family members, an environmental cause for the illness was eliminated.

CLINICAL DESCRIPTION

Early development is normal. The first sign of trouble is decreased central vision caused by retinitis pigmentosa. This sets in between 4 and 6 years of age. These children are followed by ophthalmologists as normal children with retinitis pigmentosa. They ultimately are enrolled in schools for the visually impaired. Patients become completely blind between the ages of 10 and 14 years, but sometimes even later. Complete blindness is accompanied by a disturbed sleep-wake cycle and insomnia. Retrospectively, a subset of affected children may manifest difficult behavior between the ages of 7 and 9 years. By age 10 years, cognitive decline sets in. The diagnosis is first suspected by teachers, who may be familiar with this condition in the pediatric visually impaired population. Seizures make their appearance as early as age 12 years, but they often do not occur until 14 years of age. Early-onset seizures that are difficult to control often foretell a more rapidly declining course. Speech becomes echolalic. Perseveration of speech and actions becomes routine. A cogwheel rigidity of the limbs sets in. Patients walk with a stooped, shuffling gait reminiscent of patients with Parkinson's disease. An intention tremor of variable severity is often observed.

Patients generally plateau in their middle teens. A large number of patients become depressed and agitated, and a small number become aggressive and psychotic. These adolescents often have a positive family history for unipolar or bipolar illness. Treatment is often necessary. It can aggravate extrapyramidal signs and symptoms. Hallucinations are common. They can, however, be of a pleasant and repetitive nature. A number of patients have imaginary friends with names and include them in their daily routine. Growth and physical maturity are not affected, which can make sexual development a problem, particularly for teenage girls. Contraception is often sought by parents for affected teenage daughters. Late-stage symptoms include drooling, difficulty swallowing, and weight loss. These problems are obviated by the use of feeding tubes. Temperature instability with episodes of extreme hypothermia down to 92° F alternating with hyperthermia points to hypothalamic involvement. Seizures increase in number and are difficult to control. Some patients develop a cardiomyopathy or sick sinus syndrome with bradycardia. Most patients succumb in their early to mid-20s to seizures and cardiopulmonary arrest. A small number can survive into the fourth decade of life.

CLINICAL DIAGNOSTIC TESTS

When clinical suspicion is strong, DNA-based *CLN3* gene tests can confirm the diagnosis (see "Genetics"). The EEG is abnormal from age 9 years onward. Large-amplitude spike and slow-wave complexes are observed. CT and MRI scans may initially be normal and can remain so until age 12 years. Ultimately, cerebral atrophy with gaping sulci and large ventricles is the norm. Cerebellar atrophy is often present. Morphometric MRI measurements indicate loss of hemispheric, caudate, thalamic, and lenticular volumes [Boustany and Filipek, 1993]. There is a low signal in the white matter seen in T2-weighted images. Positron emission tomography has demonstrated decreased glucose use that starts in the calcarine area and progresses to involve all gray matter structures. The latter two techniques are not done routinely on patients, but when carried out, they can help to better understand disease progression. The ERG is often abnormal, even before the patients complain of decreased vision. Visual-evoked potentials reveal reduced-amplitude potentials, and somatosensory-evoked potentials are enhanced, but these are not particularly useful tests. The ultrastructure of the skin biopsy sample is often helpful, particularly if the common 1-kb deletion is absent from one or both alleles. Schwann cells, endothelial cells, pericytes, neurons, macrophages, and eccrine sweat glands all show inclusions. Fingerprint-like inclusions enclosed by a unit membrane are typical. Curvilinear inclusions are frequently seen, sometimes within the same cell. Vacuolated lymphocytes are a hallmark of JNCL, but these have to be processed swiftly and correctly, otherwise the number of false-positive results becomes high. Unfortunately, very few diagnostic laboratories can accurately evaluate vacuolated lymphocytes. Skin fibroblast electron microscopy is a more robust test that has proved extremely helpful over the years.

PATHOLOGY

Brain weight at the time of death is 450 to 1100 grams. There is thinning of the cortical mantle. There is moderate neuronal loss with gliosis and accumulation of autofluorescent material. This material is Sudan black B and PAS positive. Meganeurites are seen in the basolateral amygdaloid complex and in cortical layer V. Purkinje cell and granule cell dropout is observed in the cerebellum. Electron microscopy reveals apoptotic neurons with dark, shrunken, and fragmented chromatin in the cerebral cortex. A number of neurons are TUNEL stain–positive, confirming the existence of apoptotic neurons. Surviving neurons demonstrate immunoreactivity with antibodies to BCL2, a neuroprotective protein, and to subunit C or 9 of mitochondrial ATP synthase. Lipopigment accumulates in anterior horn cells of the spinal cord and the receptor cells of the organ of Corti. In neuronal cells, fingerprint profiles predominate, whereas in non-neuronal cells, curvilinear inclusions are common.

BIOCHEMISTRY, CELL BIOLOGY, AND PATHOPHYSIOLOGY

An initial observation was that ceramide, the pro-apoptotic lipid second messenger was elevated in JNCL brains [Puranam et al., 1999]. This elevation correlated with the identification of apoptosis in JNCL brains and anti-apoptotic amino acid stretches within the CLN3 protein [Persaud-Sawin et al., 2002]. In addition to ceramide, galactosyl-ceramide, glucosylceramide, ceramide trihexoside, and sphingomyelin levels are elevated, pointing to sphingolipid overproduction [Persaud-Sawin et al., 2004]. The CLN3 protein is upregulated in a number of human and mouse cancer cell lines and in solid colon cancer specimens [Rylova et al., 2002]. The CLN3 protein localizes to the Golgi, early recycling endosomes, and lipid rafts in plasma membranes. The VYFAE motif within the CLN3 protein is embedded in a larger galactosylceramide lipid raft binding domain. In CLN3-deficient cells, mutant CLN3 incorrectly localizes to late endosomes and lysosomes, and mutant CLN3 protein and galactosylceramide, an important component of lipid rafts, remain stuck in the Golgi, never reaching the plasma membrane and lipid rafts. Reversal of this after restoring CLN3 to the deficient cells suggests that CLN3 normally functions as a galactosylceramide transporter from the Golgi to lipid rafts by recycling endosomes. This may explain the increase in apoptosis that is often initiated from lipid rafts and the increased production of sphingolipids in an attempt to rectify the galactosylceramide deficiency in lipid rafts.

GENETICS

JNCL is the most common form of Batten's diseases in the United States. This autosomal-recessive disease has a prevalence of 7 per 100,000 live births in Iceland and 0.71 per 100,000 live births in Germany. The prevalence decreases as the distance increases from Scandinavian countries, and the prevalence in the United States therefore is much less. JNCL is classified as an orphan disease according to Food and Drug Administration guidelines.

The gene has 15 exons, which translates into a protein that is 438 amino acids long. The hydrophobic protein has five to seven potential transmembrane domains. This protein is highly conserved among species, indicating a significant role for cell maintenance. Thirty-six mutations have been described. The same 1.02-kb deletion accounts for 85% of cases in the United States. DNA-based carrier testing is available, provided the family mutation is known. Prenatal diagnosis has been performed using ultrastructure and DNA-based tests as early as 11 weeks' gestation. It is best to confirm diagnosis again at birth using cord blood.

MANAGEMENT AND TREATMENT

JNCL is the most challenging of the clinical types to manage. Although initially seizure control is easily achieved with one drug, as the disease advances, some patients progress to having over 100 seizures per day despite use of a multitude of antiepileptic medications. The seizures are of mixed type, including generalized, myoclonic, and partial complex seizures. The emotional and psychiatric aspects of this disorder present a therapeutic dilemma. Many patients require antipsychotic drugs and mood stabilizers, which lower seizure threshold and aggravate parkinsonian symptoms. Insomnia is a problem that should be addressed with the use of benzodiazepines and other drugs. Weight loss becomes an issue in the final few years. It requires gastrostomy tubes for adequate provision of calories, liquids, and anticonvulsants. Anecdotal reports of the use of the anti-apoptotic medication flupirtine suggests improved seizure control and sleep patterns. Of those patients that develop bradycardia, only a handful have needed pacemakers placed.

Death invariably ensues in the early to middle 20s, with some patients dying as young as age 13 and others surviving to age 40 years. The average survival has increased with the advent of vigorous treatment of infections, use of feeding tubes, and better antiepileptic drugs. Unfortunately, because CLN3 is a membrane protein, there is little enthusiasm for protein or gene replacement strategies. Stem cell approaches have not been explored but may some day have a role in therapy. There are multiple mouse models for this disease. The hope for lessening the burden of JNCL continues to rely on achievement of a better understanding of the pathobiology and biochemistry of this disorder.

CLN9-Deficient Juvenile-like Variant

Two German brothers and two American sisters of Serbian descent had been clinically diagnosed with the JNCL variant before identification of the *CLN3* gene [Lin et al., 2001; Schulz, Dhar et al., 2004]. When DNA from these cases was examined, it was determined that they had no defects in the

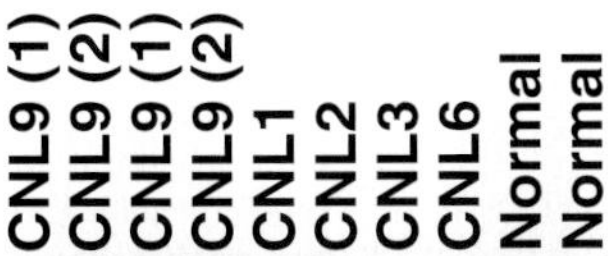

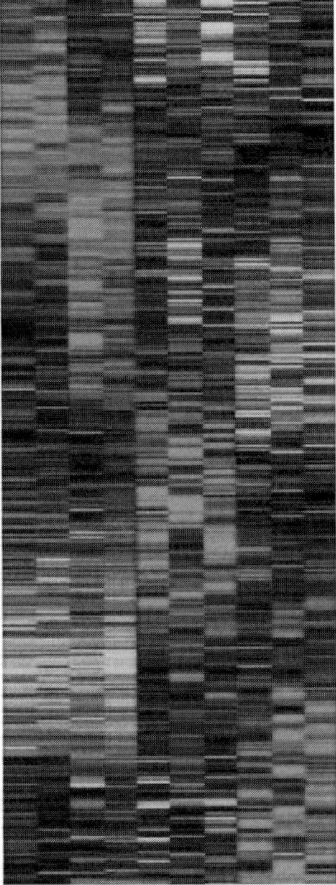

FIGURE 59-1. Partial dendrogram depicting gene expression pattern for *CLN1-, CLN2-, CLN3-, CLN6-, CLN9*-deficient and normal fibroblast RNA. Upregulated genes are *red*, downregulated genes are *green*, and no change from control is *black*. Notice the similarity of gene expression in the CLN9(1) and CLN9(2) patients. CLN, ceroid-lipofuscinosis, neuronal. See also Color Plate.

CLN3 gene, and they had normal levels of CLN3 mRNA. Analysis of cDNA from CLN3-, CLN1-, CLN2-, and CLN6-deficient variants, together with cDNA from these unknown cases, using Affymetrix GeneChips revealed a distinctive gene profile that grouped them together as a separate variant (Fig. 59-1). Results of enzyme assays and molecular tests for all other known neuronal ceroid-lipofuscinosis variants were normal.

CLINICAL DESCRIPTION

The clinical course for CLN9-deficient juvenile-like variant is almost identical to that of JNCL, with decreased vision occurring at age 4 years, cognitive decline at age 6 years, and ataxia and rigidity by age 9 years. These patients develop dysarthria and scanning speech, and they are mute by age 12 years. One of the German brothers developed hallucinations and behavior problems. All four patients developed intractable seizures in their early to middle teens that eventually diminished. Retinitis with pigmentary changes was documented in one of the two brothers. One of the brothers died of pneumonia at age 15 years, and the other died at age 19 years after suffering from swallowing difficulties and many seizures. The two sisters remain alive. One is in her early 20s and has been bedridden since she was 14 years old. She has well-controlled seizures and requires a feeding tube. The younger sister is now 12 years old and is following a similar course.

CLINICAL DIAGNOSTIC TEST

The ERG showed diminished wave amplitudes in one of the brothers with JNCL variant. The EEGs in all four patients demonstrated slowing and frequent polyspike discharges.

Electron micrographs of lymphocytes show numerous membrane-bound inclusions containing a mixture of electron-dense storage material and fingerprint patterns. CT and MRI scans showed progressive cerebral and cerebellar cortical atrophy. Abnormal signal intensity was observed in the periventricular white matter. A diagnostic brain biopsy from one of the sisters showed neurons that contained granular osmiophilic inclusions and curvilinear bodies.

PATHOLOGY

The brain weight of the older brother at the time of death was 1140 grams. Neurons were ballooned with fine, granular material. Large neurons remaining in the cerebral cortex and the deep gray structures were ballooned. The substantia nigra and nuclear thalami showed moderate-to-severe astrogliosis, as did the spinal cord. The storage material was stained gray with Sudan black, and it had a yellow autofluorescence. The ultrastructure of neurons reveals GRODs and curvilinear bodies (Fig. 59-2). Neurons also demonstrated immunoreactivity to subunit C or 9 of mitochondrial ATP synthase.

GENETICS

Chromosomal location of the underlying *CLN9* gene remains unknown, but candidate genes include those encoding for proteins that impact the ceramide synthetic and catabolic pathways. The small number of affected cases has precluded traditional linkage analysis studies.

BIOCHEMISTRY AND CELL BIOLOGY

Although the gene remains unidentified, the biochemistry and cell biology of this variant is well understood. CLN9-deficient cells have a distinctive morphology and phenotype. Cells are small and rounded rather than elongated, and they have prominent nucleoli as seen by filipin staining. They have rapid growth rates because of increased DNA synthesis, but they have an increased sensitivity to apoptosis. They have an adhesion defect, and a number of the genes involved in cell adhesion and apoptosis are dysregulated, as determined by gene profiling and as listed in a table posted at www.dbsr.duke.edu/pub/cln9/. Gene expression of cyclins A_2, B_1, C, E_2, G_1, and T_2 were increased. Cyclin D_1, encoded by a proto-oncogene involved in malignant transformation of breast tissue, was significantly downregulated, as was member 1A of the tumor necrosis factor superfamily. Expression of subunits of cytochrome *c* oxidases and glutathione *S*-transferase was also increased. Ceramide,

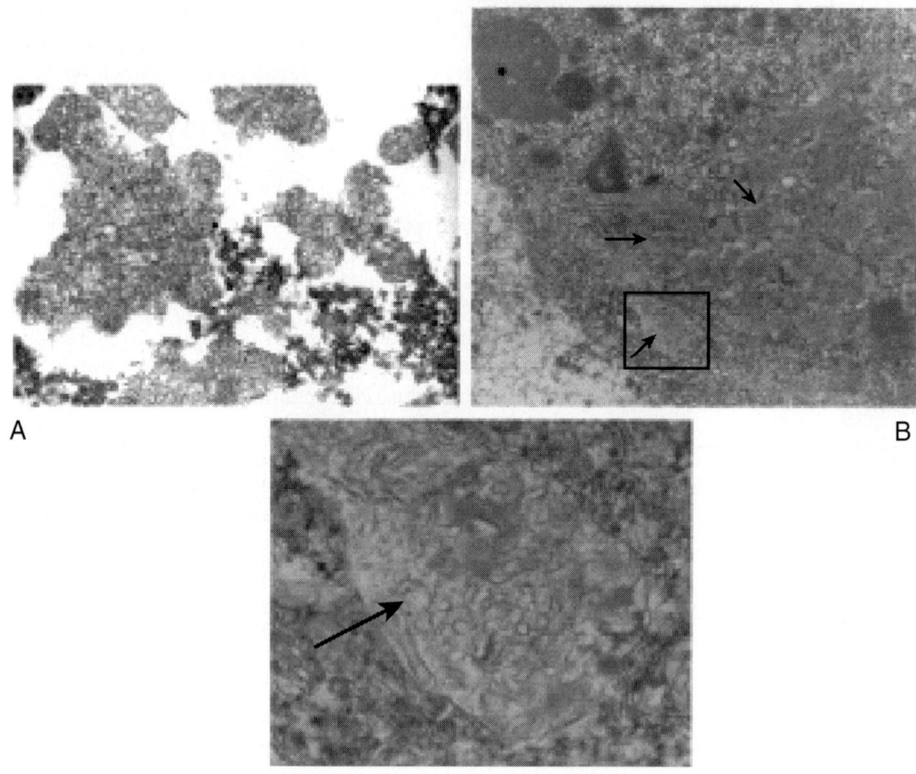

FIGURE 59-2. Electron micrographs of *CLN9*-deficient frontal cortex. **A,** Notice the secondary lysosomes with curvilinear bodies (magnification ×20,000). **B,** Granular osmiophilic deposits (GRODs) are denoted by *arrows*, and curvilinear bodies are denoted by a *framed arrow* (magnification ×54,000). **C,** Enlarged inset from **B** (magnification ×100,000).

sphingomyelin, lactosylceramide, ceramide trihexoside, and globoside levels were decreased by 60% to 100%. The key regulating enzyme in the ceramide de novo synthetic pathway, serine palmitoyl transferase, was threefold to fourfold upregulated, suggesting a block further downstream. The low levels of glycosphingolipids can explain the defect in cell adhesion observed in CLN9-deficient fibroblasts.

MANAGEMENT AND TREATMENT

Treatment is similar to that outlined for the JNCL variant. Flupirtine used empirically in the two sisters has led to stabilization of the course and better control of seizures. After the entire sphingolipid pathway and its perturbations are better defined for this variant, it will become possible to use drugs to correct defects in the pathway.

REFERENCES

Adams P, Strand R, Bresnan MJ, et al. Kinky hair syndrome: Serial study of radiological findings with emphasis on the similarity to the battered child syndrome. Radiology 1974;112:401–407.

Akbarian S. The neurobiology of Rett syndrome. Neuroscientist 2003;9:57–63.

Akbarian S, Chen RZ, Gribnau J, et al. Expression pattern of the Rett syndrome gene MeCP2 in primate prefrontal cortex. Neurobiol Dis 2001;87:84–91.

Alpers B. Diffuse progressive degeneration of the gray matter of the cerebrum. Arch Neurol Psychiatry 1931;25:469–505.

Amir RE, Van den Veyver IB, et al. Influence of mutation type and X chromosome inactivation on Rett syndrome phenotypes. Ann Neurol 2000;47:670–679.

Amir RE, Van den Veyver IB, et al. Rett syndrome is caused by mutations in X-linked MeCP2, encoding methyl-CpG-binding protein 2. Nat Genet 1999;23:185–188.

Armstrong DD. Review of Rett syndrome. J Neuropathol Exp Neurol 1997;56:843–749.

Armstrong DD. Rett syndrome: Neuropathology review. Brain Dev 2000;23 (Suppl 1):S72–S76.

Armstrong D, Dunn K, et al. Decreased dendritic branching in frontal, motor and limbic cortex in Rett syndrome compared with trisomy 21. J Neuropathol Exp Neurol 1998;57:1013–1017.

Armstrong DD, Dunn JK, et al. Selective dendritic alterations in the cortex of Rett syndrome. J. Neuropathol Exp Neurol 1995;54:195–201.

Armstrong DD, Dunn JK, et al. Organ growth in Rett syndrome, a post mortem examination analysis. Pediatr Neurol 1999;20:125–129.

Armstrong J, Pineda M, et al. Classic Rett syndrome in a boy as a result of a somatic mosaicism for a MECP2 mutation. Ann Neurol 2001;50:692.

Auranen M, Vanhala R, et al. MeCP2 gene analysis in classical Rett syndrome and in patients with Rett-like features. Neurology 2001;56:611–617.

Bader GG, Witt-Engerstrom I, et al. Neurophysiological findings in the Rett syndrome. II. Visual and auditory brainstem, middle and late evoked responses. Brain Dev 1989;11:110–114.

Bankier A. Menkes disease. J Med Genet 1995;32:213–215.

Barkovich A, Good W, et al. Mitochondrial disorders: Analysis of their clinical and imaging characteristics. AJNR Am J Neuroradiol 1993;14:1119–1137.

Bashina VM, Gorbachevskaya NL, et al. Clinical, neurophysiological and differential diagnostic aspects of severe early childhood autism. J. Neuropathol 1994;4:68–71.

Batten FE, Mayou MS. Family cerebral degeneration with macular changes. Proc R Soc Med 1915;8:70–90.

Bauman JL, Kemper TL, et al. Pervasive neuroanatomic abnormalities of the brain in three cases of Rett's syndrome. Neurology 1995;45:1581–1586.

Belichenko PV, Oldfors A, et al. Rett syndrome: 3-D confocal microscopy of cortical pyramidal dendrites and afferents. Neuroreport 1994;5:1509–1513.

Bennetts H, Chapman F. Copper deficiency in sheep in western Australia: A preliminary account of the aetiology of enzootic ataxia of lambs and anaemia of ewes. Aust Vet J 1937;13:138–149.

Berg B. The neurologic examination. In: Berg B, ed. Child neurology: A clinical manual. Philadelphia: JB Lippincott, 1994:1–26.

Biaggioni I, Goldstein D, et al. Dopamine-beta-hydroxylase deficiency in humans. Neurology 1990;40:370–373.

Bienvenu T, Carrie A, et al. MECP2 mutations account for most cases of typical forms of Rett syndrome. Hum Mol Genet 2000;9:1377–1384.

Bird AP, Wolfe AP. Methylation-induced repression-belts, braces, and chromatin. Cell 1999;99:451–454.

Blackwood W, Buxton P, et al. Diffuse cerebral degeneration in infancy (Alpers' disease). Arch Dis Child 1963;38:193–204.

Blue ME, Naidu S, et al. Altered development of glutamate and GABA receptors in the basal ganglia of girls with Rett syndrome. Exp Neurol 1999;156:345–352.

Boustany RM. Batten disease or neuronal ceroid lipofuscinosis. In: Handbook of clinical neurology: Neurodystrophies and neurolipidoses. New York: Elsevier, 1996:671–900.

Boustany RM, Filipek P. Seizures, depression and dementia in teenagers with Batten disease. J Inherit Metab Dis 1993;16:252–255.

Budden SS, Myer EC, et al. Cerebrospinal fluid studies in the Rett syndrome: Biogenic amines and P-endorphins. Brain Dev 1990;12:81–84.

Byers P, Siegel R, et al. X-linked cutis laxa: Defective cross-link formation in collagen due to decreased lysyl oxidase activity. N Engl J Med 1980;303:61–65.

Capesius P, Van Damme W, et al. The metaphyseal lesions of the Menkes' syndrome—a case report. J Belge Radiol 1977;60:345–350.

Chae JH, Hwang YS, et al. Mutation analysis of MECP2 and clinical characterization in Korean patients with Rett syndrome. J Child Neurol 2002;17:33–36.

Chandler SP, Guschin D, Landsberger N, et al. The methyl-CpG binding transcriptional repressor MeCP2 stably associates with nucleosomal DNA. Biochemistry 1999;38:7008–7018.

Charles H, Lazeyras F, et al. Proton spectroscopy of human brain: Effects of age and sex. Prog Neuropsychopharmacol Biol Psychiatry 1994;18:995–1004.

Cheadle J, Gill H, Fleming N, et al. Long-read sequence analysis of the MECP2 gene in Rett syndrome patients: Correlation of disease severity with mutation type and location. Hum Mol Genet 2000;9:1119–1129.

Chelly J, Tumer Z, et al. Isolation of a candidate gene for Menkes disease that encodes a potential heavy mental binding protein. Nat Genet 1993;3:14–19.

Chen RZ, Akbaraian S, et al. Deficiency of methyl-CpG binding protein-2 in CNS neurons results in a Rett-like phenotype in mice. Nat Genet 2001;27:327–331.

Chiron C, Bulteau C, et al. Dopaminergic D2 receptor SPECT imaging in Rett syndrome: Increase of specific binding in striatum. J Nucl Med 1993;34:1717–1721.

Cho S, Dawson PE, et al. Role of palmitoyl-protein thioesterase in cell death: Implications for infantile neuronal ceroid lipofuscinosis. Eur J Paediatr Neurol 2001;5 (Suppl A):53–55.

Clayton-Smith J, Watson P, et al. Somatic mutation in MECP2 as a non-fatal neurodevelopment disorder in males. Lancet 2000;356:830–832.

Coker SB, Melnyk AR. Rett syndrome and mitochondrial enzyme deficiencies. J Child Neurol 1991;6:164–166.

Colantuoni C, Jeon OH, Hyder K, et al. Gene expression profiling in postmortem Rett syndrome brain: Differential gene expression and patient classification. Neurobiol Dis 2001;8:847–865.

Conforti FL, Mazzei R, Magariello A, et al. Mutation analysis of the MECP2 gene in patients with Rett syndrome. Am J Med Genet A 2003;117:184–187.

Cooper DN, Youssoufian H. The CpG dinucleotide and human genetic disease. Hum Genet 1988;78:151–155.

Cornford ME. Neuropatholgoy of Rett syndrome: Case report with neuronal and mitochondrial abnormalities in the brain. J Child Neurol 1994;9:424–431.

Couvert P, Bienvenu T, et al. MECP2 is highly mutated in X-liked mental retardation. Hum Mol Genet 2001;10:941–946.

Coy J, Sedlacek Z, et al. A complex pattern of evolutionary conservation and alternative polyadenylation within the long 3-untranslated region of the methyl-CpG-binding protein 2 gene (MeCP2) suggests a regulatory role in gene expression. Hum Mol Genet 1999;8:1253–1262.

Daly W, Rabinovitch H. Urologic abnormalities in Menkes' syndrome. J Utol 1981;126:262–264.

Danks D. Disorders of copper transport. In: Scriver C, Beaudet A, Sly W, Valle D, eds. The metabolic and molecular basis of inherited disease. New York: McGraw-Hill, 1995:2211–2235.

Danks D, Cartwright E, et al. Menkes' kinky hair disease: Further definition of the defect in copper transport. Science 1973;179:1140–1142.

Danks D, Stevens, et al. Menkes' kinky hair syndrome. Lancet 1972;1:1100–1102.

Das AK, Becerra CHR, et al. Molecular genetics of palmitoyl-protein thioesterase deficiency in the U.S. J Clin Invest 1998;102:361.

Das S, Levinson B, et al. Similar splicing mutations of the Menkes/mottled copper-transporting ATPase gene in occipital horn syndrome and the blotchy mouse. Am J Hum Gen 1995;56:570–576.

Das S, Levinson B, et al. Diverse mutations in patients with Menkes disease often leads to exon skipping. Am J Hum Genet 1994;55:883–889.

Delarue A, Paut O, Guys JM, et al. Inappropriate liver transplantation in a child with Alpers-Huttenlocher syndrome misdiagnosed as valproate-induced acute liver failure. Pediatr Transplant 2000;4:67–71.

Dhar S, Bitting RL, et al. Flupirtine blocks apoptosis in Batten patient lymphoblasts and in human postmitotic CLN3- and CLN2-deficient neurons. Ann Neurol 2002;51:448–466.

Dierick H, Ambrosini L, et al. Molecular structure of the Menkes disease gene (ATP7A). Genomics 1995;28:462–469.

Dietrich O, Heiland S, et al. Noise correction for exact determination of apparent diffusion coefficients at low SNR. Magn Reson Med 2001;45:448–453.

DiMauro S, Lombes, et al. Cytochrome *c* oxidase deficiency. Pediatr Res 1990;28:536–541.

Dom R, Brucher JM, et al. Adult ceroid-lipofuscinosis (Kufs disease) in two brothers: Retinal and visceral storage in one; diagnostic muscle biopsy in the other. Acta Neuropathol 1979;45:67–72.

Dreifuss F, Netsky M. Progressive poliodystrophy. Am J Dis Child 1964;107:649–656.

Dunn HG. Rett syndrome: Review of biological abnormalities. Can J Neurol Sci 2001;28:16–29.

Dunn HG, Stoessl AJ, et al. Rett syndrome: Investigation of nine patients, including PET scan. Can J Neurol Sci 2002;29:345–357.

Egger J, Harding B, et al. Progressive neuronal degeneration of childhood (PNDC) with liver disease. Clin Pediatr 1987;26:167–73.

Eipper B, Mains R, Glembotski CC. Identification in pituitary tissue of a peptide alpha-amidation activity that acts on glycine extended peptides and requires molecular oxygen, copper, and ascorbic acid. Proc Natl Acad Sci U S A 1983;80:5144–8514.

Eipper B, Stoffers D, et al. The biosynthesis of neuropeptides. Peptide alpha-amidation. Annu Rev Neurosci 1992;15:57–85.

Ellaway C, Peat J, et al. Medium-term open label trial of L-carnitine in Rett syndrome. Brain Dev 2001;23 (Suppl):S85–S89.

Ellison KA, Fill CP, et al. Examination of X chromosome markers in Rett syndrome: Exclusion mapping with a novel variation on multilocus linkage analysis. Am J Hum Genet 1992;50:278–287.

Fadic R, Russell J, et al. Sensory ataxic neuropathy as the presenting feature of a novel mitochondrial disease. Neurology 1997;49:239–245.

Faerber E, Grover W, et al. Cerebral MR of Menkes' kinky hair disease. AJNR Am J Neuroradiol 1989;10:190–192.

Fanchetti E, Zappela M, et al. Plasma endorphins in Rett syndrome. Preliminary data. Am J Med Genet 1986;24:331–338.

Fitzgerald PM, Jankovic J, et al. Rett syndrome and associated movement disorders. Mov Disord 1990;5:195–202.

Flemming K, Ulmer S, et al. MR spectroscopic findings in a case of Alpers-Huttenlocher syndrome. AJNR Am J Neuroradiol 2002;23:1421–1423.

Forbes J, His G, et al. Role of the copper-binding domain in the copper transport function of ATP7B, the P-type ATPase defective in Wilson disease. J Biol Chem 1999;274:12408–12413.

Ford F, Livingston S, et al. Familial degeneration of the cerebral gray matter in childhood, with convulsions, myoclonus, spasticity, cerebellar ataxia, choreoathetosis, dementia, and death in status epilepticus: Differentiation of infantile and juvenile types. J Pediatr 1951;39:33–43.

Frydman M, Jager-Roman E, et al. Alpers progressive infantile neuronal poliodystrophy: An acute neonatal form with findings of the fetal akinesia syndrome. Am J Med Genet 1993;47:31–36.

Fujii T, Ito M, et al. Biochemical study on the critical period for treatment of the mottled brindled mouse. J Neurol 1990;55:885–889.

Fuks F, Hurd P, et al. The methyl-CpG-binding protein MeCP2 links DNA methylation to histone methylation. J Biol Chem 2003;278:4035–4040.

Gabreels F, Prick M, et al. Defects in citric acid cycle and the electron transport chain in progressive poliodystrophy. Acta Neurol Scand 1984;70:145–154.

Gacheru S, McGee C, et al. Expression and accumulation of lysyl oxidase, elastin, and type 1 procollagen in human Menkes and mottle mouse fibroblasts. Arch Biochem Biophys 1993;301:325–329.

Gao H, Boustany RM, et al. Mutations in a novel CLN6 encoded transmembrane protein cause variant neuronal ceroid lipofuscinosis in mouse and man. Am J Hum Genet 2002;70:324–335.

Geerdink N, Rotteveel JJ, et al. MECP2 mutation in a boy with severe neonatal encephalopathy: Clinical, neuropathological and molecular findings. Neuropediatrics 2002;33:33–36.

Giunti L, Pelagatti S, et al. Spectrum and distribution of MECP2 mutations in 64 Italian Rett syndrome girls: Tentative genotype/ phenotype correlation. Brain Dev 2001;23 (Suppl 1): S242–S245.

Glaze DG. Rett's syndrome: Characterization of respiratory patterns and sleep. Ann Neurol 1987;21:377–382.

Goebel HH, Mole SE, et al., eds. The neuronal ceroid lipofuscinoses (Batten disease). Burke, VA: IOS Press, 1999.

Goebel HH, Wisniewski KE. Current state of clinical and morphological features in human NCL. Brain Pathol 2004;14:61–69.

Goka T, Stevenson R, et al. Menkes disease: A biochemical abnormality in cultured human fibroblasts. Proc Natl Acad Sci U S A 1976;73:604–606.

Gokcay A, Kitis O, et al. Proton MR spectroscopy in Rett syndrome. Comput Med Imaging Graph 2002;26:271–275.

Goodyer I, Jones E, et al. Characterization of the Menkes protein copper-binding domains and their role in copper-induced protein relocalization. Hum Mol Genet 1999;8:1473–1478.

Gunn T, McFarlane S, et al. Difficulties in the neonatal diagnosis of Menkes' kinky hair syndrome-trichopoliodystrophy. Clin Pediatr 1984;23:514–516.

Guy J, Hendrich B, et al. A mouse Mecp2-null mutation causes neurological symptoms that mimic Rett syndrome. Nat Genet 2001;27:322–326.

Hagberg B. Rett syndrome: Clinical peculiarities and biologic mysteries. Acta Paediatr 1995;84:971–976.

Hagberg B. Clinical manifestations and stages of Rett syndrome. Ment Retard Dev Disabil 2002;8:61–65.

Hagberg B, Aicardi J, et al. A progressive syndrome of autism, dementia, ataxia and loss of purposeful hand use in girls: Rett syndrome. Report of 35 cases. Ann Neurol 1983;14:471–479.

Hagberg B, Gillberg C. Rett variants—retoid phenotypes. Clin Dev Med 1993;127:40–60.

Hagberg B, Goutieres F, et al. Rett syndrome: Criteria for inclusion and exclusion. Brain Dev 1985;7:372–373.

Hagberg B, Skjeldal OH. Rett variants: A suggested model for inclusion criteria. Pediatr Neurol 1994;11:5–11.

Hagberg B, Sourander P, et al. Late Infantile progressive encephalopathy with disturbed polyunsaturated fat metabolism. Acta Paediatr Scand 1968;57:495–499.

Haldane J. The rate of spontaneous mutation of a human gene. J Genet 1935;31:317–326.

Haltia M, Rapola J, et al. Infantile type of so-called neuronal ceroid lipofuscinosis. Part II. Histological and electron microscopic studies. Acta Neuropathol 1973a;26:157.

Haltia M, Rapola J, et al. Infantile type of so-called neuronal ceroid-lipofuscinosis. Part 2. Morphological and biochemical studies. J Neurol Sci 1973b;18:269.

Harding B. Progressive neuronal degeneration of childhood with liver disease (Alpers-Huttenlocher syndrome): A personal review. J Child Neurol 1990;5:273–287.

Harding B, Alsanjari N, et al. Progressive neuronal degeneration of childhood with liver disease (Alpers' disease) presenting in young adults. J Neurol Neurosurg Psychiatry 1995;58:320–325.

Harding B, Egger J, et al. Progressive neuronal degeneration of childhood with liver disease. Brain 1986;109:181–206.

Harke HJ, Capitanio M, et al. Bladder diverticula and Menkes' syndrome. Radiology 1977;124:459–461.

Henikoff S. Chromosomes on the move. Trends Genet 2001;17:689–690.

Heydorn K, Damsgaard E, et al. Extrahepatic storage of copper. A male foetus suspected of Menkes' disease. Hum Genet 1975;29:171–175.

Hoffbuhr K, Devaney JM, et al. MeCP2 mutations in children with and without the phenotype of Rett syndrome. Neurology 2001;56:1486–1495.

Holmberg V, Jalanko A, Isosomppi J et al. The mouse ortholog of the neuronal ceroid lipofuscinosis CLN5 gene encodes a soluble lysosomal glycoprotein expressed in the developing brain. Neurobiol Dis 2004;16:29–40.

Horn N. Copper metabolism in Menkes' disease. In: Rennert O, Chan WY, eds. Metabolism of trace elements in man, Vol. II. Genetic implications. Boca Raton, FL: CRC Press, 1984:25–51.

Huppke P, Held M, Hanefield F, et al. Influence of mutation type and location on phenotype in 123 patients with Rett syndrome. Neuropediatrics 2002;33:63–68.

Huppke P, Laccone F, et al. Rett syndrome: Analysis of MECP2 and clinical characterization of 31 patients. Hum Mol Genet 2000;9:1369–1375.

Huttenlocher P, Solitare G, et al. Infantile diffuse cerebral degeneration with hepatic cirrhosis. Arch Neurol 1976;33:186–192.

Ishikawa A, Goto T, et al. A new syndrome (?) of progressive psychomotor deterioration with peculiar stereotype movement and autistic tendency: A report of three cases. Brain Dev 1978;3:258.

Itoh M, Takashima S. Neuropathology and immunohistochemistry of brains with Rett syndrome. No To Hattatsu 2002;34:211–216.

Jan MM, Dooley JM, et al. Male Rett syndrome variant: Application of diagnostic criteria. Pediatr Neurol 1999;20:238–240.

Janota I. Spongy degeneration of grey matter in three children: Neuropathological report. Arch Dis Child 1974;49:571–575.

Jansky J. Dosud nepopsany pripad familiarni amazuroticke idiotie komplikovanem a hypoplasii mozeckovou. Sborn Lek 1908;13:165–196.

Jellinger K, Armstrong D, et al. Neuropathology of Rett syndrome. Acta Neuropathol 1988;76:142–158.

Jellinger K, Grisold W, et al. Peripheral nerve involvement in the Rett syndrome. Brain Dev 1990;12:109–114.

Jellinger KA. Rett syndrome—an update. J Neural Transm 2003;110:681–701.

Johnsen D, Coleman L, et al. MR of progressive neurodegenerative change in treated Menkes' kinky hair disease. Neuroradiology 1991;33:181–2.

Johnson DW, Speier S, et al. Role of subunit-9 of mitochondrial ATP synthase in Batten disease. Am J Med Genet 1995;57:350–360.

Kaler S. Menkes disease. Adv Pediatr 1994;41:262–303.

Kaler S. Diagnosis and therapy of Menkes syndrome, a genetic form of copper deficiency. Am J Clin Nutr 1998;67 (Suppl):1029S–1034S.

Kaler S, Goldstein D, et al. Plasma and cerebrospinal fluid neurochemical pattern in Menkes disease. Ann Neurol 1993a;33:171–175.

Kaler S, Miller R, et al. In utero treatment of Menkes disease [Abstract]. Pediatr Res 1993b;33:192A.

Kaler S, Westman J, et al. Gastrointestinal hemorrhage associated with gastric polyps in Menkes disease. J Pediatr 1993c;122:93–95.

Kaludov N, Wolffe A. MeCP2 driven transcriptional repression in vitro: Selectivity for methylated DNA, action at a distance and contacts with the basal transcription machinery. Nucleic Acids Res 2000;28:1921–1928.

Kaufmann WE, Naidu S, et al. Abnormal expression of microtubule-associated protein 2 (MAP-2) in neocortex in Rett syndrome. Neuropediatrics 1995;26:109–113.

Kayihan N, Nennesomo I, et al. Fatal deterioration of neurological disease after orthotopic liver transplantation for valproic acid-induced liver damage. Pediatr Transplant 2000;4:211–214.

Kendall B, Boyd S, et al. Progressive neuronal degeneration of childhood with liver disease. Computed tomographic features. Neuroradiology 1987;29:174–180.

Kerr AM, Nomura Y, et al. Guidelines for reporting clinical features in cases with MECP2 mutations. Brain Development 2001;23:208–211.

Kimura H, Shiota K. Methyl-CpG-binding protein, MeCP2, is a target molecule for maintenance DNA methyltransferase, Dnmt1. J Biol Chem 2003;278:4806–4812.

Kitt CA, Wilcox BJ. Preliminary evidence for neurodegenerative changes in the substantia nigra of Rett syndrome. Neuropediatrics 1995;26:114–118.

Kleefstra T, Yntema HG, et al. De novo MECP2 frameshift mutation in a boy with moderate retardation, obesity and gynaecomastia. Clin Genet 2002;61:359–362.

Klein H, Dichgans J. Familiare juvenile glio-neurale Dystrophie: Akut beginnende progressive Encephalopathie mit rechtsseitigen occipito-parietalen Herdsymptomen und Status epilepticus. Arch Psychiatr Nervenkr 1969;212:400–22.

Kodama H, Murata Y. Molecular genetics and pathophysiology of Menkes disease. Pediatr Int 1999;41:430–435.

Kodama H, Sato E, et al. Biochemical indicator for evaluation of connective tissue abnormalities in Menkes' disease. J Pediatr 2003;142:726–728.

Koslowski K, McCrossin R. Early osseous abnormalities in Menkes kinky hair syndrome. Pediatr Radiol 1979;8:191–194.

Kozinetz CA, Skender ML, et al. Epidemiology of Rett syndrome: A population-based registry. Pediatrics 1993;91:445–450.

Kriaucionis S, Bird A. DNA methylation and Rett syndrome. Hum Mol Genet 2003;12:R221–R227.

Kudo S, Nomura Y, et al. Heterogeneity in residual function of MeCP2 carrying missense mutations in the methyl CpG binding domain. J Med Genet 40 2003;7:487–493.

Laccone F, Zoll B, et al. MECP2 gene nucleotide changes and their pathogenicity in males: Proceed with caution. J Med Genet 2002;39:586–588.

Lake BD, Steward CG, Oakhill A, et al. Bone marrow transplantation in late infantile Batten disease and juvenile Batten disease. Neuropediatrics 1997;28:80–81.

Lappalainen R, Liewendahl K, et al. Brain perfusion SPECT and EEG findings in Rett syndrome. Acta Neurol Scand 1997;95:44–50.

Lappalainen R, Lindholm D, et al. Low levels of nerve growth factor in cerebrospinal fluid of children with Rett syndrome. J Child Neurol 1997;11:296–300.

Lekman A, Hagberg B, et al. Membrane cerebral lipids in Rett syndrome. Pediatr Neurol 1991;7:186–190.

Lekman A, Witt-Engerstrom I, et al. CSF and urine biogenic amine metabolites in Rett syndrome. Clin Genet 1990;37:173–178.

Leonard H, Colvin L, Christodoulou J, et al. Patients with the R133C mutation: Is their phenotype different from patients with Rett syndrome with other mutations? J Med Genet 2003;40:E52.

Lerner TJ, Boustant RM, et al. Isolation of a novel gene underlying Batten disease, CLN3. Cell 1995;82:949–957.

Levinson B, Vulpe C, et al. The mottled gene is the mouse homologue of the Menkes disease gene. Nat Genet 1994;6:369–373.

Lewis JD, Meehan RR, et al. Purification, sequence, and cellular localization of a novel chromosomal protein that binds to methylated DNA. Cell 1992;69:905–814.

Lin SM, Dhar S, et al. Extracting knowledge from gene expression data: A case study of Batten Disease. Proceedings of Data Mining in Bioinformatics. San Francisco, CA: Association for Computing Machinery–Knowledge Discovery and Data Mining (ACM-KDD), 2001

Lipani JD, Bhattacharjee MB, et al. Reduced nerve growth factor in Rett syndrome postmortem brain tissue. J Neuropathol Exp Neurol 2000;59:889–895.

Liu Y, Wada R, et al. A genetic model of substrate deprivation therapy for a glycosphingolipid storage disorder. J Clin Invest 1999;103:439–440.

Lockitch G, Halstead A, et al. Age- and sex-specific pediatric reference intervals and correlations for zinc, copper, selenium, iron, vitamins A and E and related proteins. Clin Chem 1988;34:1625–1628.

Lockitch G, McCallum C, et al. Reference intervals for eight plasma proteins in preterm and term newborns by laser nephelometry [Letter]. Clin Chem 1986;32:2106.

Luikenhuis S, Giacometti E, et al. Expression of MeCP2 in postmitotic neurons rescues Rett syndrome in mice. Proc Natl Acad Sci U S A 2004;101:6033–6038.

Maiwald R, Bonte A, et al. De novo MECP2 mutation in a 46, XX male patient with Rett syndrome. Neurogenetics 2002;4:107–108.

Marin-Padilla M. Cajal-Retzius cells and the development of the neocortex. Trends Neurosci 1998;21:64–71.

Martinez-Mena J, Manquillo A, et al. Neurophysiological study in Alpers syndrome [in Spanish]. Rev Neurol 1998;26:70–77.

Matsuishi T, Nagamitsu S, et al. Decreased cerebrospinal fluid levels of substance P in patients with Rett syndrome. Ann Neurol 1997;42:978–981.

Mayou MS. Cerebral degeneration with symmetrical changes in the maculae in three members of a family. Trans Ophthalmol Soc U K 1904;24:142–145.

Menkes J, Alter M, et al. A sex-linked recessive disorder with retardation of growth, peculiar hair and focal cerebellar degeneration. Pediatrics 1962;29:764–769.

Mercer J. Menkes syndrome and animal models. Am J Clin Nutr 1998;67 (Suppl):1022S–1028S.

Mercer J, Grimers A, et al. Mutations in the murine homologue of the Menkes disease gene in dappled and blotchy mice. Nat Genet 1994;6:374–378.

Mercer J, Livingston J, et al. Isolation of a partial candidate gene for Menkes disease by positional cloning. Nat Genet 1993;3:20–25.

Mitchison HM, Hofmann SL, Becerra CH, et al. Mutations in the palmitoyl-protein thioesterase gene (PPT; CLN1) causing juvenile neuronal ceroid lipofuscinosis with granular osmiophilic deposits. Hum Mol Genet 1998;7:291–297.

Mole SE. The genetic spectrum of human neuronal ceroid-lipofuscinoses. Brain Pathol 2004;14:70–76.

Mole SE, Mitchison HM, et al. Molecular basis of the neuronal ceroid lipofuscinoses: Mutations in CLN1, CLN2, CLN3, and CLN5. Hum Mutat 1999;14:199–215.

Moller L, Tumer Z, et al. Similar splice-site mutations of the ATP7A gene lead to different phenotypes: Classical Menkes disease or occipital horn syndrome. Am J Hum Genet 2000;66:1211–1220.

Monros E, Armstrong J, et al. Rett syndrome in Spain: Mutation analysis and clinical correlations. Brain Dev 2001;23 (Suppl 1):S251–S253.

Montine T, Powers J, et al. Alpers' syndrome presenting with seizures and multiple stroke-like episodes in a 17-year-old male. Clin Neuropathol 1995;14:322–326.

Moore C, Howell R. Ectodermal manifestation in Menkes' disease. Clin Genet 1985;28:532–537.

Motil K, Schultz R, et al. Oropharyngeal dysfunction and gastroesophageal dysmotility are present in girls and women with Rett syndrome. J Pediatr Gastroenterol Nutr 1999;29:31–37.

Nan X, Campoy FJ, et al. McCP2 is a transcriptional repressor with abundant binding sites in genomic chromatin. Cell 1997;88:471–481.

Nan X, Meehan RR, et al. Dissection of the methyl-CpG binding domain from the chromosomal protein McCP2. Nucleic Acids Res 1993;21:4886–4892.

Nan X, Ng H, et al. Transcriptional repression by the methyl-CpG-binding protein MeCP2 involves a histone deacetylase complex. Nature 1998;393:386–389.

Nan X, Tate P, et al. DNA methylation specifies chromosomal localization of MeCP2. Mol Cell Biol 1996;16:414–421.

Narkewicz M, Sokol R, et al. Liver involvement in Alpers disease. J Pediatr 1991;119:260–267.

Naviaux R, Nguyen K. POLG mutations associated with Alpers' syndrome and mitochondrial DNA depletion. Ann Neurol 2004;55:706–712.

Naviaux R, Nyhan W, et al. Mitochondrial DNA polymerase gamma deficiency and mtDNA depletion in a child with Alpers' syndrome. Ann Neurol 1999;45:54–58.

Neul JL, Zoghbi Y. Rett syndrome: A prototypical neurodevelopmental disorder. Neuroscientist 2004;10:118–128.

Neumann-Haefelin T, Wittask H, et al. Diffusion- and perfusion-weighted MRI: Influence of severe carotid artery stenosis on the DWI/ PWI mismatch in acute stroke. Stroke 2000;31:1311–1317.

Nielsen JB, Henriksen KF, et al. MECP2 mutations in Danish patients with Rett syndrome: High frequency of mutations but no consistent correlations with clinical severity or with the X chromosome inactivation pattern. Eur J Hum Genet 2001;9:178–184.

Nielson JB, Toft PB, et al. Cerebral magnetic resonance spectroscopy in Rett syndrome. Failure to detect mitochondrial disorder. Brain Dev 1993;15:107–112.

Obata K, Matsuishi T, et al. Mutation analysis of the methyl-CpG biding protein 2 gene (MECP2) in patients with Rett syndrome. J Med Genet 2000;37:608–610.

Odermatt A, Suter H, Krapf R, et al. Primary structure of two P-type ATPases involved in copper homeostasis in *Enterococcus hirae*. J Biol Chem 1993;268:12775–12779.

Oldfors A, Hagberg B, et al. Rett syndrome: Spinal cord pathology. Pediatr Neurol 1988;4:172–174.

Oldfors A, Sourander P, et al. Rett syndrome: Cerebellar pathology. Pediatr Neurol 1990;6:310–331.

Ozawa H, Kodama H, Kawaguchi H, et al. Renal function in patients with Menkes disease. Eur J Pediatr 2003;162:51–52.

Papadimitriou JM, Hockey A, Tan N, et al. Rett syndrome: Abnormal membrane-bound lamellated inclusions in neurons and oligodendroglia. Am J Med Genet 1988;29:365–368.

Parsons M, Li T, et al. Combined (1)H MR spectroscopy and diffusion-weighted MRI improves the prediction of stroke outcome. Neurology 2000;55:498–505.

Payne A, Gitlin J. Functional expression of the Menkes disease protein reveals common biochemical mechanisms among the copper-transporting P-type ATPases. J Biol Chem 1998;273:3765–3770.

Paynter J, Grimers A, et al. Expression of the Menkes gene homologue in mouse tissue: Lack of effect of copper on the mRNA levels. FEBS Lett 1994;351:186–190.

Pederson P, Carafoli E. Ion motive ATPases. I. Ubiquity, properties, and significance to the cell function. Trends Biochem Sci 1987;12:146–50.

Percy AK. Clinical trials and treatment prospects. Ment Retard Dev Disabil 2002;8:106–111.

Percy AK, Gillberg C, et al. Rett syndrome and the autistic disorders. Neurol Clin 1990;8:659–676.

Persaud-Sawin DA, McNamara J 2nd, Rylova S, et al. A galactosylceramide binding motif is involved in trafficking of CLN3 from Golgi to rafts via recycling endosomes. Pediatr Res 2004;56:449–463.

Persaud-Sawin DA, VanDongen A, et al. Motifs within the CLN3 protein: Modulation of cell growth rates and apoptosis. Hum Mol Genet 2002;11:2129–2142.

Petris M, Mercer J. The Menkes protein (ATP7A; MNK) cycles via the plasma membrane both in basal and elevated extracellular copper using a C-terminal di-leucine endocytic signal. Hum Mol Genet 1999;8:2107–2115.

Petris M, Mercer J, et al. Ligand-regulated transport of the Menkes copper P-type ATPase efflux pump from the Golgi apparatus to the plasma membrane: A novel mechanism of regulated trafficking. EMBO J 1997;15:6084–6095.

Poulsen L, Horn N, et al. X-linked recessive Menkes disease: Identification of a partial gene deletions in affected males. Clin Genet 2002;62:449–457.

Prick M, Gabreels F, et al. Pyruvate dehydrogenase deficiency restricted to the brain. Neurology 1981;31:398–404.

Procopis P, Camakaris J, et al. A mild form of Menkes syndrome. J Pediatr 1981;98:97–100.

Prohaska J, Bailey W. Regional specificity in alterations of rat brain copper and catecholamines following perinatal copper deficiency. J Neurochem 1994;63:1551–1557.

Prohaska J, Bailey W. Alterations of peptidylglycine alpha-amidating monooxygenase and other cuproenzyme activities following perinatal copper deficiency. Proc Soc Exp Biol Med 1995;210:107–116.

Puranam K, Lane SC, et al. Overexpression of Bcl–2 is associated with apoptosis in neuronal death. J Cell Biochem 1995;19 (Suppl B):318.

Puranam K, Qian WH, et al. Upregulation of Bcl-2 and elevation of ceramide in Batten disease. Neuropediatrics 1997;28:37–41.

Puranam KL, Guo WX, et al. CLN3 defines a novel antiapoptotic pathway operative in neurodegeneration and mediated by ceramide. Mol Genet Metab 1999;66:294–308.

Rae T, Schmidt P, et al. Undetectable intracellular free copper: The requirement of a copper chaperone for superoxide dismutase. Science 1999;184:805–808.

Ranta S, Savukoski M, et al. Studies of homogenous populations: CLN5 and CLN8. Adv Genet 2001;45:123–140.

Ranta S, Topcu M, et al. Variant late infantile neuronal ceroid lipofuscinosis in a subset of Turkish patients is allelic to Northern epilepsy. Hum Mutat 2004;23:300–3005.

Ranta S, Zhang Y, et al. The neuronal ceroid lipofuscinoses in human EPMR and mnd mutant mice are associated with mutations in CLN8. Nat Genet 1999;23:233–236.

Ravn K, Nielsen JB, Uldall P, et al. No correlation between phenotype and genotype in boys with a truncating MECP2 mutation. J Med Genet 2003;40:E5.

Reaume A, Elliott J, Hoffman EK, et al. Motor neurons in Cu/Zn superoxide dismutase-deficient mice develop normally but exhibit enhanced cell death after axonal injury. Nat Genet 1996;13:43–47.

Reiss AL, Farugue F, et al. Neuroanatomy of Rett syndrome: A volumetric imaging study. Ann Neurol 1993;34:227–234.

Rett A. Uber ein eigenartiges hirnatrophisches Syndrom bei Hyperammonamie im Kindesalter. Wien Klin Wochenschr 1966;116:723–725.

Robertson D, Goldberg M, et al. Isolated failure of autonomic noradrenergic neurotransmission. N Engl J Med 1986;314:1494–1487.

Robinson B. Lactic acidemia. In: Scriver C, Beaudet A, Sly W, Valle D, eds. The metabolic and molecular basis of inherited disease. New York: McGraw-Hill, 1989:879–882.

Robinson B, De Meirleir L, et al. Clinical presentation of patients with mitochondrial respiratory chain defects in NADH-coenzyme Q reductase and cytochrome oxidase: Clues to the pathogenesis of Leigh disease. J Pediatr 1987;110:216–222.

Robinson D, Cooley L. Genetic analysis of the actin cytoskeleton in the *Drosophila* ovary. Annu Rev Cell Biol 1997;13:147–170.

Rohmer A, Krug J, et al. Maladie de Menkes: Etude de deux enzymes cupro-dependants. Pediatrie 1977;32:447–456.

Rossi L, DeMartino A, et al. Neurodegeneration in the animal model of Menkes' disease involves Bcl-2-linked apoptosis. Neuroscience 2001;103:181–188.

Royce P, Steinmann B. Markedly reduced activity of lysyl oxidase in skin and aorta from a patient with Menkes disease showing unusually severe connective tissue manifestations. Pediatr Res 1990;28:137–141.

Ruch A, Kurczynski TW, et al. Mitochondrial alterations in Rett syndrome. Pediatr Neurol 1989;5:320–323.

Rylova SN, Amalfitano A, et al. The CLN3 gene is a novel molecular target for cancer drug discovery. Cancer Res 2002;62:801–808.

Sandbank U, Lerman P. Progressive cerebral poliodystrophy—Alpers' disease. Disorganized giant neuronal mitochondria on electron microscopy. J Neurol Neurosurg Psychiatry 1972;35:749–755.

Santavuori P, Haltia M, et al. Infantile type of so-called neuronal ceroid-lipofuscinosis: Part 1, a clinical study of 15 patients. J Neurol Sci 1973;18:257–267.

Satoi M, Matsuishi T, et al. Decreased cerebrospinal fluid levels of beta-phenylethylamine in patients with Rett syndrome. Ann Neurol 2000;47:801–803.

Savukoski M, Klockars T, et al. CLN5, a novel gene encoding a putative transmembrane protein mutated in Finnish variant late infantile neuronal ceroid lipofuscinosis. Nat Genet 1998;19:286–288.

Schriner JE, Yi W, et al. cDNA and genomic cloning of human palmitoyl-protein thioesterase (PPT), the enzyme defective in infantile neuronal ceroid lipofuscinosis [published erratum appears in Genomics 1996;38:458]. Genomics 1996;34:317.

Schultz RJ, Glaze DG, et al. The pattern of growth failure in Rett syndrome. Am J Dis Child 1993;147:663-667.

Schulz A, Dhar S, et al. Impaired cell adhesion and apoptosis in the novel CLN9 Batten Disease variant. Ann Neurol 2004;56:342–350.

Schwartzman JS, Bernardino A, et al. Rett syndrome in a boy with a 47,XXY karyotype confirmed by a rare mutation in the MECP2 gene. Neuropediatrics 2001;32:164–164.

Seidel J, Moller L, et al. Disturbed copper transport in humans. Part 1. Mutations of the ATP7A gene lead to Menkes disease and occipital horn syndrome. Cell Mol Biol 2001;47:141–148.

Sekul EA, Percy AK. Rett syndrome: Clinical features, genetic considerations, and the search for a biological marker. Curr Neurol 1992;12:173–200.

Shahbazian M, Sun Y, et al. Balanced X chromosome inactivation patterns in the Rett syndrome brain. Am J Med Genet 2002a;111:164–168.

Shahbazian M, Young J, Yuva-Paylor L, et al. Mice with truncated MeCP2 recapitulate many Rett syndrome features and display hyperacetylation of histone H3. Neuron 2002b;35:243–254.

Shibata N, Hirano A, et al. Cerebellar superoxide dismutase expression in Menkes kinky hair disease: An immunohistochemical investigation. Acta Neuropathol 1995;90:198–202.

Silver S, Nucifora G, et al. Bacterial resistance ATPases: Primary pumps for exporting toxic cations and anions. Trends Biochem Sci 1989;14:76–80.

Simonati A, Filosto M, et al. Central-peripheral sensory axonopathy in a juvenile case of Alpers-Huttenlocher disease. J Neurol 2003;250:702–706.

Sirianni N, Naidu S, et al. Rett syndrome: Confirmation of X-linked dominant inheritance, and localization of the gene to Xq28. Am J Hum Gen 1998;63:1552–1558.

Sleat D, Wiseman J, et al. A mouse model of classical late-infantile neuronal ceroid lipofuscinosis based on targeted disruption of the CLN2 gene results in a loss of tripeptidyl-peptidase I activity and progressive neurodegeneration. J Neurosci 2004;24:9117–9126.

Sleat DE, Donnelly RJ, et al. Associations of mutations in a lysosomal protein with classical late-infantile neuronal ceroid lipofuscinosis. Science 1997;277:1802–1805.

Smith J, Mah J, et al. Brain MR imaging findings in two patients with Alpers' syndrome. Clin Imaging 1996;20:235–237.

Sofic E, Riederer P, Killian W, et al. Reduced concentration of ascorbic acid and glutathione in a single case of Rett syndrome: A postmortem brain study. Brain Dev 1987;9:529–532.

Solioz M, Odermatt A, et al. Copper pumping ATPases: Common concepts in bacteria and man. FEBS Lett 1994;346:44–47.

Spielmeyer W. Familiare amaurotische Idiotie. Zentralbl Gesamte Ophthalmol 1923;10:161–208.

Stanley P, Gwinn J, et al. The osseous abnormalities in Menkes syndrome. Ann Radiol 1976;19:167–172.

Stengel E. Beretning om et maerkeligt Sygdomstilfoelde hos fire Sodskende i Naerheden af Roraas. Eyr Med Tidskr 1826;1:347–352.

Strausak D, La Fontaine S, Hill J, et al. The role of GMXCXXC metal binding sites in the copper-induced redistribution of the Menkes protein. J Biol Chem 1999;274:11170–11177.

Subramaniam B, Naidu S, et al. Neuroanatomy in Rett syndrome: Cerebral cortex and posterior fossa. Neurology 1997;48:399–407.

Teixeira CA, Espinola J, et al. Novel mutations in the CLN6 gene causing a variant late infantile neuronal ceroid lipofuscinosis. Hum Mutat 2003;21:502–508.

Tesarova M, Mayr J, et al. Mitochondrial DNA depletion in Alpers syndrome. Neuropediatrics 2004;35:217–223.

Topcu M, Akyerli C, et al. Somatic mosaicism for a MECP2 mutation associated with classic Rett syndrome in a boy. Eur J Hum Genet 2002;10:77–81.

Topcu M, Tan H, et al. Evaluation of 36 patients from Turkey with neuronal ceroid lipofuscinosis: Clinical, neurophysiological, neuroradiological and histopathologic studies. Turk J Pediatr 2004;46:1–10.

Trevathan E, Moser HW. Diagnostic criteria for Rett syndrome. The Rett Syndrome Diagnostic Criteria Work Group. Ann Neurol 1988;23:425–428.

Tsivkovskii R, Eisses J, et al. Functional properties of the copper-transporting ATPase ATP7B (the Wilson's disease protein) expressed in insect cells. J Biol Chem 2002;277:976–983.

Tudor M, Akbarian S, et al. Transcriptional profiling of a mouse model for Rett syndrome reveals subtle transcriptional changes in the brain. Proc Natl Acad Sci U S A 2002;99:15536–15541.

Tumer Z, Lund C, et al. Identification of point mutations in 41 unrelated patients affected with Menkes disease. Am J Hum Genet 1997;60:63–71.

Tumer Z, Moller L, et al. Mutation spectrum of ATP7A, the gene defective in Menkes disease. Adv Exp Med Biol 1999;448:83–95.

Tumer Z, Moller L, et al. Screening of 383 unrelated patients affected with Menkes disease and findings of 57 gross deletions in ATP7A. Hum Mutat 2003;22:457–464.

Tyynela J, Palmer DN, et al. Storage of saposins A and D in infantile neuronal ceroid-lipofuscinosis. Fed Eur Biochem Soc 1993;330:1:8–12.

Van den Veyver IB, Zoghbi HY. Genetic basis of Rett syndrome. Ment Retard Dev Disabil Res Rev 2002;8:82–86.

Van Goethem G, Martin J, et al. Progressive external ophthalmoplegia and multiple mitochondrial DNA deletions. Acta Neurol Belg 2002;102:39–42.

Van Goethem G, Martin J, Van Broeckhoven C. Progressive external ophthalmoplegia characterized by multiple deletions of mitochondrial DNA: Unraveling the pathogenesis of human mitochondrial DNA instability and the initiation of a genetic classification. Neuromol Med 2003;3:129–146.

Venta-Sobero JA, Porras-Kattz E, et al. West syndrome as an epileptic presentation in Menkes' disease. Rev Neurol 2004;39:133–136.

Vesa J, Chin MH, et al. Neuronal ceroid lipofuscinoses are connected at molecular level: Interaction of CLN5 protein with CLN2 and CLN3. Mol Biol Cell 2002;13:2410–2420.

Villard L, Kpebe A, et al. Two affected boys in a Rett syndrome family: Clinical and molecular findings. Neurology 2000;55:1188–1193.

Vogt H. Familiare amaurotische Idiotie, histologische und histopathologische Studien. Arch Kinderheilkd 1909;51:1–35.

Voskoboinik I, Camakaris J. Menkes copper-translocating P-type ATPases (ATP7A): Biochemical and cell biology properties, and role in Menkes disease. J Bioenerg Biomembr 2002;34:363–371.

Voskoboinik I, Greenough M, et al. Functional studies on the Wilson copper P-type ATPase and toxic milk mouse mutant. Biochem Biophys Res Commun 2001;281:966–970.

Vulpe C, Levinson B, et al. Isolation of a candidate gene for Menkes disease and evidence that it encodes a copper-transporting ATPase. Nat Genet 1993;3:7–13.

Wakia S, Kameda I, et al. Rett syndrome: Findings suggesting axonopathy and mitochondrial abnormalities. Pediatr Neurol 1990;6:339–343.

Wan M, Lee SS, et al. Rett syndrome and beyond: Recurrent spontaneous and familial MECP2 mutations at CpG hotspots. Am J Hum Genet 1999;65:1520–1529.

Watson P, Black G, et al. Angelman syndrome phenotype associated with mutations in MECP2, a gene encoding a methyl CpG binding protein. J Med Genet 2001;38:224–228.

Weaving LS, Williamson SL, Bennetts B, et al. Effects of MECP2 mutation type, location and X-inactivation in modulating Rett syndrome phenotype. Am J Med Genet A 2003;118:103–114.

Wefring K, Lamvik J. Familial progressive poliodystrophy with cirrhosis of the liver. Acta Paediatr Scand 1967;56:295–300.

Wenk GL. Alterations in dopaminergic function in Rett syndrome. Neuropediatrics 1995;26:123–125.

Wenk GL, Hauss-Wgrzyniak B. Altered cholinergic function in the basal forebrain of girls with Rett syndrome. Neuropediatrics 1999;30:125–129.

Wheeler RB, Sharp JD, Schultz RA, et al. The gene mutated in variant late-infantile neuronal ceroid lipofuscinosis (CLN6) and in nclf mutant mice encodes a novel predicted transmembrane protein. Am J Hum Genet 2002;70:537–542.

Williams D, Atkins C. Tissue copper concentrations of patients with Menkes' kinky hair disease. Am J Dis Child 1981;135:375–376.

Wisniewski K, Golabek A, et al. Classic late-infantile NCL with tripeptidyl-peptidase I deficiency (CLN2). Pathology and genetics. In: Golden J, Harding B, eds. Developmental neuropathology. Basel, ISN Neuropath Press, 2004a:274–276.

Wisniewski K, Golabek A, et al. Palmitoyl-protein thioesterase 1 deficiency with granular osmiophilic deposits (CLN1). Pathology and genetics. In: Golden J, Harding B, eds. Developmental neuropathology. Basel, ISN Neuropath Press, 2004b:271–273.

Wisniewski K, Golabek A, et al. Rare forms of neuronal ceroid lipofuscinoses. Pathology and genetics. In: Golden J, Harding B, eds. Developmental neuropathology. Basel, ISN Neuropath Press, 2004c:280–282.

Wong DF, Ricaurte G, et al. Dopamine transporter changes in neuropsychiatric disorders. Adv Pharmacol 1998;42:219–223.

Worle H, Kohler B, et al. Progressive cerebral degeneration of childhood with liver disease (Alpers-Huttenlocher disease) with cytochrome oxidase deficiency presenting with epilepsia partialis continua as the first clinical manifestation. Clin Neuropathol 1998;17:63–68.

Yamashita Y, Kondo I, et al. Mutation analysis of the methyl-CpG–binding protein 2 gene (MECP2) in Rett patients with preserved speech. Brain Dev 2001;23 (Suppl 1): S157–S1560.

Yamashita Y, Matsuishi T, et al. Decrease in benzodiazepine receptor binding in the brains of adult patients with Rett syndrome. J Neurol Sci 1998;154:146–150.

Yntema HG, Kleefstra T, et al. Low frequency of MECP2 mutations in mentally retarded males. Eur J Hum Genet 2002a;10:487–490.

Yntema HG, Oudakker AR, et al. In-frame deletion in MECP2 causes mild nonspecific mental retardation. Am J Med Genet 2002b;107:81–83.

Young JI, Zoghbi HY. X-chromosome inactivation patterns are unbalanced and affect the phenotypic outcome in a mouse model of Rett syndrome. Am J Hum Genet 2004;74:511–520.

Yuan D, Dancis A, et al. Restriction of copper export in *Saccharomyces cerevisiae* to a late Golgi or post-Golgi compartment in the secretory pathway. J Biol Chem 1997;272:25787–25793.

Zappella M. A double blind trial of bromocriptine in the Rett syndrome. Brain Dev 1990;12:148–150.

Zappella M. The Rett girls with preserved speech. Brain Dev 1992;14:98–101.

Zappella M, Meloni I, et al. Preserved speech variants of the Rett syndrome: Molecular and clinical analysis. Am J Med Genet 2001;104:14–22.

Zeev BB, Yaron Y, et al. Rett syndrome: Clinical manifestations in males with MECP2 mutations. J Child Neurol 2002;17:20–24.

Zeman W, Donahue P, et al. The neuronal ceroid-lipofuscinoses (Batten-Vogt syndrome). In: Vinken PJ, Bruyn GW, eds. Handbook of clinical neurology: Leukodystrophies and poliodystrophies. Amsterdam: North-Holland Publishing, 1970:588–687.

Zhong N, Moroziewicz DN, et al. Heterogeneity of late-infantile neuronal ceroid lipofuscinosis. Genet Med 2000;2:312–318.

Zullo SJ, Butler L, Zahorchak RJ, et al. Localization by fluorescence in situ hybridization (FISH) of human mitochondrial polymerase gamma (POLG) to human chromosome band 15q24→q26, and of mouse mitochondrial polymerase gamma (Polg) to mouse chromosome band 7E, with confirmation by direct sequence analysis of bacterial artificial chromosomes (BACs). Cytogenet Cell Genet 1997;78:281–284.

CHAPTER 60

Disorders Primarily of White Matter

Edward M. Kaye and Marjo S. van der Knaap

The concept of a leukodystrophy has changed considerably from its original pathologic definition, which was first introduced by Bielschowski and Henneberg in 1928 [Bielschowsky and Henneberg, 1928]. The sensitivity of magnetic resonance imaging (MRI) to demonstrate abnormalities in myelin development and maintenance has also expanded our concept of the disorders affecting myelin. The understanding of the pathophysiology of leukodystrophies is evolving, and the classification of the leukodystrophies must continue to be arbitrary. The term *leukodystrophy* should be restricted to inherited diseases that affect myelin development and maintenance and should exclude acquired disorders affecting myelin, such as multiple sclerosis and other disorders that are associated with inflammatory lesions affecting myelin, and toxic disorders, such as organic solvent exposure. The term *leukodystrophy* is controversial because many genetic diseases that affect the white matter, even those disorders that are considered primary leukodystrophies, may involve non–white matter regions of the nervous system but not primarily or not only the myelin, and even the primary leukodystrophies may involve non–white matter regions of the nervous system. The term *leukoencephalopathy* is more neutral and may also be more accurate.

Leukoencephalopathies comprise all inherited and acquired disorders that selectively or predominantly involve the white matter of the central nervous system (CNS), irrespective of the underlying pathophysiologic mechanism and histopathologic basis. In the *pathologic classification*, leukoencephalopathies can be grossly divided into (1) dysmyelinating (abnormal formation of myelin with disturbed myelination); (2) hypomyelinating (decreased myelin production); (3) demyelinating (loss of previously normal myelin both morphologically and functionally normal myelin), (4) spongiform (splitting of myelin and intramyelinic vacuole formation), and (5) cystic (white matter rarefaction and cystic degeneration) (Table 60-1). An etiologic classification can also be used to classify leukoencephalopathies into the following categories: (1) immune mediated, (2) lipid disorders, (3) protein disorders, (4) amino or organic acid disorders, (5) defects of energy metabolism, and (6) other causes (Table 60-2). As might be expected, some diseases, such as X-linked adrenoleukodystrophy, resist being placed into a distinct category because, although it is usually considered a lipid disorder, there is an inflammatory response similar to the immune-mediated disorders. These classifications will certainly change as the molecular mechanisms for more of the leukoencephalopathies become elucidated.

It is important to realize that the classification of diseases into disorders primarily affecting gray matter and disorders primarily affecting white matter is quite artificial. Although conceptually easier to consider, neurologic diseases often cannot be easily separated into highly compartmentalized disorders. For example, hypomyelinating and dysmyelinating disorders are frequently noted as a consequence of generalized metabolic diseases that secondarily affect the nervous system, such as galactosemia, phenylketonuria, glutaricaciduria type I, pyridoxine-dependent seizures, and Pompe's disease, among others [Kolodny, 1993].

IMMUNE-MEDIATED DEMYELINATING DISORDERS

The lack in understanding the basic pathophysiology of many of the diseases that affect white matter has led to a somewhat arbitrary categorization, which will evolve as the molecular and genetic causes of myelin diseases become elucidated. Childhood demyelinating disorders, which appear to be immunologically mediated, are characteristically the most difficult to separate because of the overlap and clinical similarities. These diseases consist of multiple sclerosis, acute disseminated encephalomyelitis, acute hemorrhagic leukoencephalitis, and myelinoclastic diffuse cerebral scler-

TABLE 60-1

Pathologic Classification of the Leukoencephalopathies

DEMYELINATING OR DYSMYELINATING	HYPOMYELINATING	SPONGIFORM	CYSTIC
X-linked adrenoleukodystrophy	Pelizaeus-Merzbacher disease	Canavan's disease	Vanishing white matter disease/childhood ataxia with cerebral hypomyelination
Globoid cell leukodystrophy	Alexander's disease	Megaloencephalic leukoencephalopathy	Alexander's disease
Metachromatic leukodystrophy Glutaric aciduria type I Phenylketonuria	Myelin basic protein deficiency Aicardi-Goutières syndrome	Maple syrup urine disease	Mitochondrial disorders

TABLE 60-2

Etiologic Classification of the Leukoencephalopathies

IMMUNE MEDIATED	LIPID ABNORMALITIES	PROTEIN ABNORMALITIES	AMINO/ORGANIC ACID DISORDERS	ENERGY DEFECTS	OTHER CAUSES
Multiple sclerosis	Adrenoleukodystrophy	Pelizaeus-Merzbacher disease	Canavan's disease	MELAS syndrome (mitochondrial encephalomyopathy, lactic acidosis, and stroke)	Vanishing white matter disease/childhood ataxia with cerebral hypomyelination
Schilder's disease	Globoid cell leukodystrophy	Myelin basic protein deficiency	Methylmalonic aciduria	Leber's disease	
Acute disseminated encephalomyelitis	Metachromatic leukodystrophy	Alexander's disease	Propionic aciduria	Complex I deficiency	
Acute hemorrhagic leukoencephalitis	Sjögren-Larsson syndrome	Merosin deficiency	Maple syrup urine disease	Complex II deficiency	
Aicardi-Goutières syndrome	Cerebrotendinous xanthomatoses	Megaloencephalic leukoencephalopathy	Phenylketonuria	Cytochrome oxidase deficiency	

osis of Schilder. An interesting hypothesis that tries to explain some of the similarities of these disorders is based on the age of exposure to certain viral antigens that share homologous regions with potentially encephalitogenic peptides, such as myelin basic protein and proteolipid protein [Alvord et al., 1987]. According to this theory, very young children develop complete immunity to certain pathogens, but intermediate-aged children may develop a fulminant hypersensitivity to these epitopes, resulting in acute immune-mediated demyelination or an intermediate response with perhaps relapsing-remitting symptoms. Until the basic mechanisms of immune-mediated demyelination are better understood, the classification of these diseases will remain difficult.

Multiple Sclerosis

Multiple sclerosis is a demyelinating disorder that affects discrete areas of the CNS, including the optic nerves, in a quite variable relapsing-remitting fashion over a prolonged period of time. The disorder occurs worldwide and has a twofold more common incidence in females than males. Although usually considered to be a disease that affects people in early to middle adulthood, children develop multiple sclerosis and may account for up to 4% to 5% of all reported cases [Ghezzi et al., 1997; Ruggieri et al., 1999; Sindern et al., 1992]. The disease may be divided into a true childhood onset when it begins before age 10 and juvenile onset when it begins between the ages of 10 and 15 years [Hanefeld et al., 1991]. Multiple sclerosis in children younger than 10 years is considered unusual, but children younger than 6 years have been diagnosed using the standard diagnostic criteria used in adults [Ruggieri et al., 1999]. The juvenile onset, which appears to follow a course very similar to the adult-onset disorder, is the most common age for presentation, accounting for 80% of the childhood cases.

The etiology for multiple sclerosis continues to be elusive. Many theories have been proposed and have included environmental, infectious, toxic, immunologic, and genetic causes for multiple sclerosis. The environmental or ecologic causes for multiple sclerosis have been difficult to study because of variability of disease and exposure rates. Climactic features such as low temperature, high humidity, and precipitation in the winter, for which respiratory tract infections were considered an intermediary, have been associated with a higher risk for the development of multiple sclerosis, especially if these environmental factors are present in the first 15 years of life. Infections, especially viral, have been proposed as etiologic factors for the development of multiple sclerosis [Delasnerie-Laupretre and Alperovitch, 1990]. Antibodies to measles, in addition to other viruses such as herpes simplex, varicella, rubella, Epstein-Barr, influenza C, and some parainfluenza viruses, have been detected in the serum and cerebrospinal fluid of multiple sclerosis cases [Kurtzke, 1995]. To date, no specific virus has been consistently isolated from people with multiple sclerosis. Nonviral organisms have been implicated in demyelination, including *Acanthamoeba, Borrelia, Brucella, Campylobacter,* and *Hartmannella* species; *Chlamydia pneumonia;* and mycobacterium, trypanosomes, diphtheria toxin, human herpes virus type 6, and tetanus toxoid. Dietary features, such as higher consumption of animal fat, protein, and meat, appear to correlate with an increased risk for development of multiple sclerosis. Toxic exposure to such items as organic solvents has been suggested but not proved as an etiologic factor in the development of multiple sclerosis.

An immunopathogenic hypothesis has been proposed for the etiology of multiple sclerosis, which suggests that potentially autoaggressive T lymphocytes specific for myelin basic protein preexist in the normal immune system. One proposal suggests that the activation of autoreactive T cells occurs through molecular mimicry during bacterial or viral infection, which is likely to occur outside the CNS. The activated T cells then are likely to enter the CNS irrespective of their antigen specificity. Once inside the CNS, the recognition of an autoantigen within the CNS initiates a cascade of immunopathologic reactions, which include a pronounced inflammatory response and a breakdown of the blood-brain barrier. It is also probable that B cells are equally important in multiple sclerosis, especially for the development of demyelination. It appears that autoantibodies against surface antigens of myelin or oligodendrocytes are necessary to produce severe demyelination. Once these demyelinating antibodies have adhered to the myelin surface, complement is activated and macrophages and microglia enter the region. The macrophages not only physically strip the myelin but also release complement, inflammatory mediators, and tumor necrosis factor-α, and they produce inducible nitric oxide synthase, which all participate in the injury to myelin. Studies in experimental autoimmune encephalomyelitis have documented the role of tumor necrosis factor-α in demyelination because administration of tumor necrosis factor-α augments experimental autoimmune encephalomyelitis, whereas inhibitors of tumor necrosis factor-α or its receptor will ameliorate the disorder [Kuroda and Shimamoto, 1991; Ruddle et al., 1990]. Adhesion molecules, such as the integrins leukocyte function-associated antigen 1 and very late appearing antigen 4, are cell surface proteins that participate in leukocyte circulation and in transendothelial migration [Hohlfeld, 1997]. These adhesion molecules can be found on activated leukocytes and likely participate in the migration of leukocytes across the vascular endothelium into the brain.

Clinical Characteristics and Subclassification

Because of the slow, intermittent course and variety of symptoms in multiple sclerosis, the diagnosis may be difficult, especially in children. Various algorithms and classification schemes have been proposed over the years to address this issue [Poser and Brinar, 2001]. The Poser Criteria [Poser et al., 1983], widely adopted during the past two decades, advanced the diagnostic schema by integrating the results of laboratory, neuroimaging, and neurophysiologic tests with the clinical criteria. More recently, the International Panel on Multiple Sclerosis Diagnosis presented revised diagnostic criteria for multiple sclerosis, commonly known as the *McDonald criteria* [McDonald et al., 2001]. The McDonald criteria integrate MRI into the overall diagnostic scheme that establishes the dissemination of lesions in time and space. Unfortunately, the MRI criterion used in the McDonald criteria may not always be applicable to the pediatric population because the MRI lesions in childhood multiple sclerosis may be fewer and less dramatic than those seen in adult multiple sclerosis patients [Hahn et al., 2004]. Additionally, the new criteria simplified the diagnostic classification. In particular, previously used terms such as "clinically definite" and "probable multiple sclerosis" are no longer recommended. The outcome of a diagnostic evaluation is either "multiple sclerosis," "possible multiple sclerosis," or "not multiple sclerosis." A summary of the McDonald criteria is available from the web site of the National Multiple Sclerosis Society at http://www.nationalmssociety.org/pdf/forpros/dx_tipsheet.pdf.

The category of possible multiple sclerosis describes patients who have a clinical condition consistent with multiple sclerosis but who do not at present fully meet the diagnostic criteria. One of the diagnostic requisites is that there must be no better explanation for the clinical and paraclinical abnormalities. This category is particularly useful in children because other diseases, which include other leukodystrophies such as X-linked adrenoleukodystophy, Leber's hereditary optic neuropathy, and acute disseminated encephalomyelitis, can appear clinically as multiple sclerosis.

Subtypes of multiple sclerosis can be defined by the clinical course. An international consensus definition proposed these four categories for subgroups of multiple sclerosis [Lublin and Reingold, 1996]:

1. Relapsing-remitting multiple sclerosis. Clearly defined disease relapses with full recovery or with sequelae and residual deficit upon recovery.
2. Secondary progressive multiple sclerosis. Initial relapsing-remitting course is followed by progression.
3. Primary progressive multiple sclerosis. Disease is progressive from onset with only temporary plateaus and minor improvements allowed.
4. Progressive-relapsing multiple sclerosis. Progressive disease from onset with clear acute relapses.

The same categories may apply in pediatric multiple sclerosis. In children, multiple sclerosis presents most often as a relapsing-remitting disease, but it may appear as a primary progressive form. In one study, 56% of children with multiple sclerosis had a relapsing-remitting course, 22% had an initially progressive course, and 22% had a mixed course [Duquette et al., 1987].

The clinical symptoms in children are much like those in adults. Common symptoms are visual changes, paresthesias, focal weakness, ataxia or unstable gait, vertigo, sphincteric problems, and cognitive changes. In a large study of 149 children with multiple sclerosis diagnosed before age 16, brainstem dysfunction was noted in 25%, motor and sensory disturbance in 17.5%, optic neuritis in 16.5%, and cerebellar disturbance in 9.1% [Ghezzi et al., 1997]. Visual disturbances are particularly common in pediatric multiple sclerosis, with optic neuritis occurring in as many as 25% to 70% of children [Ghezzi et al., 1997]. Other visual findings include nystagmus, dysmetria, diplopia, internuclear ophthalmoplegia, abducens nerve palsy, and saccadic pursuits. The long-term prognosis for childhood multiple sclerosis does not appear to be more severe than for adults, and in some cases, a more favorable outcome was noted in children when compared with adults, although the difference did not reach statistical significance because of the small number of children studied [Cole et al., 1995]. Very young children presenting with multiple sclerosis symptoms before 24 months of age may have a more unfavorable outcome [Ruggieri et al., 1999].

Clinical Studies

Laboratory studies have proved extremely useful to augment the clinical diagnosis of multiple sclerosis. MRI and cerebrospinal fluid examination appear to be the most reliable tests in children with multiple sclerosis. MRI may be positive in as many as 80% of cases and demonstrates lesions on T2-weighted images in the cerebellum, brainstem, and central white matter, especially in the periventricular and juxtacortical regions [Golden and Woody, 1987; Selcen et al., 1996] (Fig. 60-1). Conventional mildly T2-weighted spin-echo MRI studies have shown the greatest efficacy to date for identifying multiple sclerosis lesions in brain [Gawne-Cain et al., 1997]. Cerebrospinal fluid immunoglobulin G index and oligoclonal bands are positive in as many as 75% of children with multiple sclerosis [Selcen et al., 1996]. The immunoglobulin G index

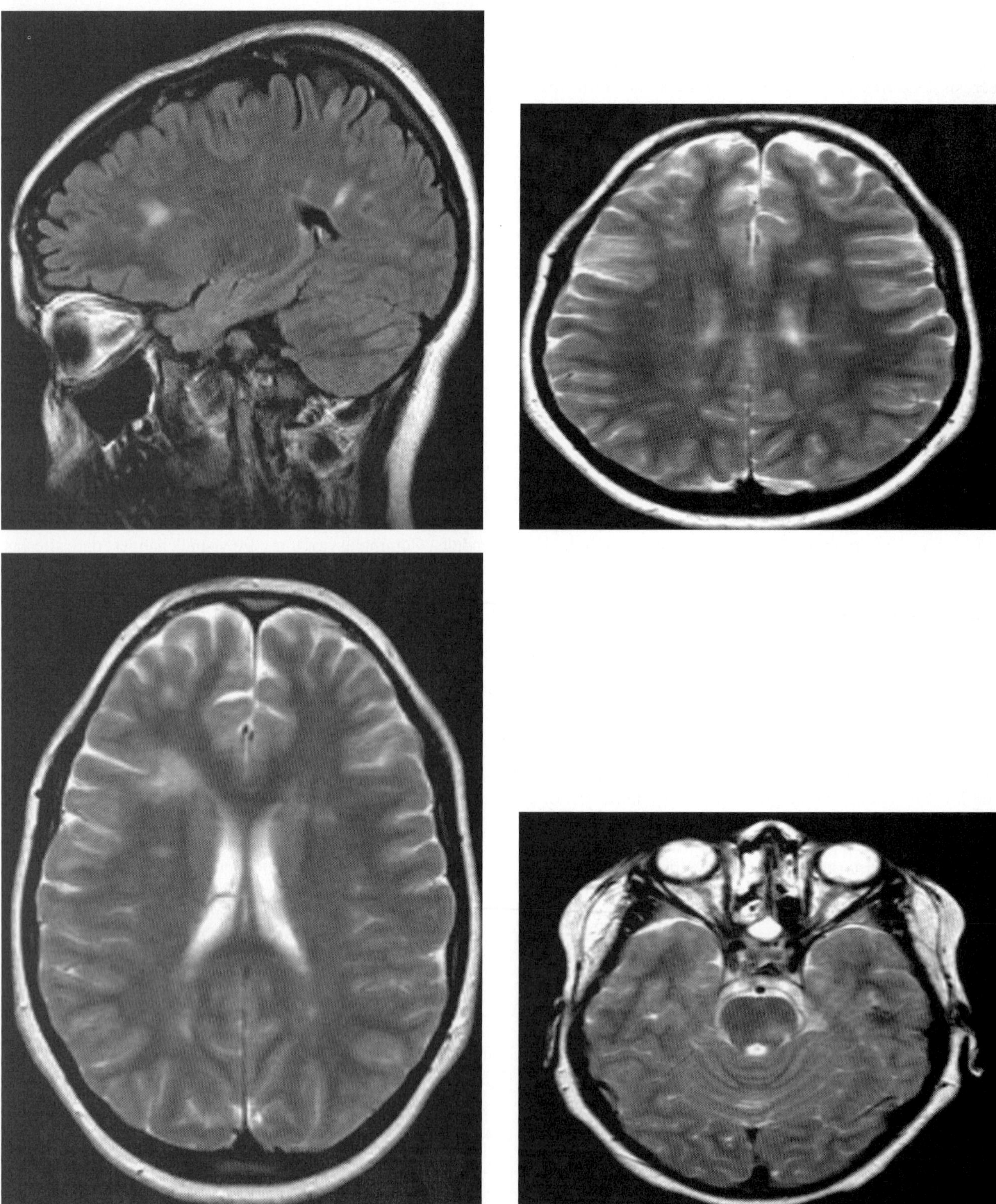

FIGURE 60-1 Sagittal fluid-attenuated inversion recovery and T2-weighted magnetic resonance images in a 12-year-old female with multiple sclerosis. The images show multiple small white matter lesions in the periventricular and juxtacortical regions. The sagittal image shows the typical ovoid shape of the periventricular lesions, so-called Dawson fingers. There is also a brainstem lesion.

is derived from the ratio of cerebrospinal fluid immunoglobulin G–albumin to serum immunoglobulin G–albumin, which should be greater than 0.65 [Hershey and Trotter, 1980]. The use of evoked potentials, such as visual-evoked potential and brainstem auditory-evoked potential, for the diagnosis of multiple sclerosis has increased over the years. An increased latency in the P100 potential of the visual evoked potential or an increase in the interpeak latency (I-III or I-V) on brainstem auditory-evoked potential often gives evidence of clinically silent lesions in the nervous system.

Pathology

The characteristic lesion noted in multiple sclerosis is the white matter plaque, which is a sharply delineated, irregularly shaped, gray or pink region characterized by complete loss of myelin, reduced numbers of oligodendrocytes, but relative sparing of axons. These plaques may occur anywhere in the brain or spinal cord but have a predilection for the periventricular regions, corpus callosum, periaqueductal region, floor of the fourth ventricle, optic nerves and tracts, corticomedullary areas, and cervical spinal cord. The plaques are frequently macroscopic, ranging from 1 mm to 4 cm [McFarlin and McFarland, 1982a, 1982b]. In acute multiple sclerosis lesions, there is perivascular and parenchymal infiltration primarily with T cells and macrophages, although some B cells are also present. As the plaques mature, axonal degeneration, astrocytic proliferation, and lipid-laden macrophages become prominent. The final evolution of the plaque is the development of pronounced gliosis, which is much more dramatic in multiple sclerosis than in other diseases affecting white matter.

Genetics

The prevalence of multiple sclerosis can vary according to region with as many as 250 cases per 100,000 population in the Orkney Islands north of the mainland of Scotland to 2 per 100,000 population in Japan [Kurtzke, 1995]. The best information available about possible genetic influences on the development of multiple sclerosis comes from monozygotic twin studies. It appears that a monozygotic twin may have up to a 25% risk for developing multiple sclerosis after the identical sibling is diagnosed with this disorder.

The most information about genetic linkage concerns the major histocompatibility locus. The human leukocyte antigen type best studied in multiple sclerosis is the DR2 haplotype. Results have demonstrated that the DR2 allele itself or a closely related gene linked to this region may be associated with the development of multiple sclerosis [Hauser et al., 1989]. Although the major histocompatibility complex is the only region that clearly and consistently demonstrates linkage and association in multiple sclerosis studies, there is substantial evidence for polygenic inheritance of the disease [Kenealy et al., 2004; Sawcer et al., 2002]. In addition to genomic screens, a number of candidate genes have been evaluated for possible linkage to the development of multiple sclerosis. The diverse list of candidates has included genes encoding myelin proteins, cytokines and chemokines, T-cell receptors and costimulatory molecules, and matrix metalloproteinases, and some involved in viral pathogenesis. Further strategies such as high-density genome scanning may eventually unravel the complex inheritance of multiple sclerosis.

Treatment

The drugs currently available to treat adult multiple sclerosis have not been extensively studied in children and adolescents. Information on treatment of childhood multiple sclerosis has been gleaned mostly from studies of adults with the disease and from pediatric case reports or small case series. However, interferon-β and glatiramer acetate have been in used in children with no unexpected negative effects, and they appear to provide the same benefits as seen in adults with multiple sclerosis.

Evidence-based clinical practice guidelines have been developed for the treatment of adult multiple sclerosis [Goodin et al., 2002]. In North America, the National Multiple Sclerosis Society has issued consensus recommendations regarding use of the current multiple sclerosis disease-modifying agents (http://www.nationalmssociety.org/pdf/forpros/Exp_Consensus.pdf) and when to consider changing therapy (http://www.nationalmssociety.org/pdf/forpros/Exp_ChangTherapy.pdf).

TREATMENT OF ACUTE EXACERBATIONS

Acute exacerbations of multiple sclerosis are generally treated with corticosteroids, administered as a short course of oral or parenteral therapy, which appear to shorten the course of the relapse. It is less certain whether steroid treatment favorably influences the extent of recovery. In the Optic Neuritis Treatment Trial [Beck et al., 1992], the group receiving intravenous methylprednisolone, 1 gram daily for 3 days, had a faster recovery of visual function than the placebo group in the first month, but by 6 months, the two groups were not statistically different with respect to visual recovery. However, the group that received methylprednisolone followed by oral steroids had a lower rate of developing multiple sclerosis in the first 2 years [Beck et al., 1993]. In the United States, intravenous methylprednisolone is the preferred treatment, although there is controversy about whether its superiority over high-dose oral steroids has been definitively established. Some practitioners provide a tapering dose of oral corticosteroids to follow the intravenous treatment, but there are limited clinical data to guide decision making on this point.

Patients with severe, acute episodes of demyelination that have not responded to corticosteroid therapy with a recent (within about 2 months) severe exacerbation may benefit from a series of plasma exchanges involving 1.1 plasma volumes (54 mL/kg) every other day for 14 days [Weinshenker et al., 1999]. Intriguing data from a small series suggest that only patients with type II pathology (i.e., with immunoglobulin-mediated demyelination and activated complement deposition) will respond favorably to plasma exchange, but that all or most such patients will respond [Keegan et al., 2004].

APPROVED DISEASE-MODIFYING THERAPIES

In 1993, interferon-β-1b (Betaseron or Betaferon) became the first medication approved by the U.S. Food and Drug Administration for the treatment of relapsing-remitting multiple sclerosis and offered a 31% reduction in exacerbation rate compared with placebo [IFNB Multiple Sclerosis Study Group, 1993]. Subsequently, other interferon-β products (Avonex, Rebif) were approved that offer lower immunogenicity and greater convenience. The relative safety and efficacy of these drugs is a highly contentious issue beyond the scope of this review. Administration of all interferon-β products requires frequent parenteral injection, either subcutaneous or intramuscular, depending on the product. All interferon-β formulations commonly cause a flulike syndrome upon initial administration, but this problem can be minimized by gradual dose escalation and pretreatment with ibuprofen or other nonsteroidal anti-inflammatory drugs. In most cases, the flulike syndrome lessens with continued use, and these drugs are generally well tolerated for long-term administration. Hepatotoxicity may occur particularly during the initial 6 months of therapy, and liver function tests are recommended for all patients taking interferon-β.

Glatiramer acetate (Copaxone, copolymer-1) is chemically unrelated to the interferons but is roughly comparable in efficacy. A synthetic random copolymer of L-alanine, L-glutamic acid, L-lysine, and L-tyrosine, it also requires frequent subcutaneous administration but does not cause a flulike syndrome. Clinical trials with glatiramer acetate have shown a 29% reduction in relapse rate in relapsing-remitting multiple sclerosis, with a low-side effect profile [Johnson et al., 1995].

The product label for mitoxantrone (Novantrone [Serona, Inc., Rockland, MA]) says that it is "indicated for reducing neurologic disability and/or the frequency of clinical relapses in patients with secondary progressive, progressive relapsing, or worsening relapsing-remitting multiple sclerosis." The drug is an immunosuppressive anthracenedione, chemically related to anthracyclines such as doxorubicin (Adriamycin). Mitoxantrone has been found in vitro to inhibit B-cell, T-cell, and macrophage proliferation and impair antigen presentation, as well as the secretion of interferon-γ, tumor necrosis factor-α, and interleukin-2. In clinical trials, mitoxantrone has demonstrated strong efficacy for reducing relapses, new MRI lesions, and accrual of disability. It appears more effective than the interferons and glatiramer but also carries a greater risk for adverse effects. A dose-dependent cardiotoxicity has led regulators to limit the lifetime cumulative dose to 140 mg/m^2, effectively limiting patients to a 2- or 3-year course of therapy. The cardiotoxicity is manifested by reduced left ventricular ejection fraction and can lead to irreversible congestive heart failure. There is also a risk for inducing malignancy; acute myelogenous leukemia is a recognized complication of anthracycline therapy and has also been reported in patients receiving mitoxantrone.

INVESTIGATIONAL THERAPIES

In view of the limited efficacy, inconvenience, toxicities, and high cost of the five approved disease-modifying drugs discussed previously, there is a clear need for new multiple sclerosis therapies. As of this writing, more than a dozen treatments are in clinical trials to evaluate their safety and effectiveness in multiple sclerosis patients. A review of these studies is beyond the scope of this chapter. However, a few of these therapies merit mention here because they are already commercially available (for other indications) or nearing regulatory approval.

Natalizumab (Tysabri) is a monoclonal antibody that disrupts the interaction between lymphocytes and CNS vascular endothelial cells and thereby reduces the entry of inflammatory cells into the CNS. The target antigen is a_4 integrin, a component of the very late, appearing antigen 4 membrane protein on the surface of T lymphocytes. Antegren is administered by monthly intravenous injection. In a phase II clinical trial lasting 6 months, this compound reduced exacerbation rate by 50% compared with a placebo in subjects with relapsing-remitting multiple sclerosis, and effected an even more marked reduction in new MRI lesions [Miller et al., 2003]. Two large phase III trials demonstrated efficacy in multiple sclerosis, and approval by the U.S. Food and Drug Administration occurred in 2004. In February 2005, the drug was suspended from marketing in the United States after the discovery of two patients with progressive multifocal leukoencephalopathy. Further clinical trials are expected to advance an understanding of the toxicity of the drug.

Alemtuzumab (Campath-1H, MabCampath) is a lymphocyte-depleting humanized monoclonal antibody that is approved in many jurisdictions for the treatment of certain leukemias. In a pilot study of patients with relapsing-remitting or secondary progressive multiple sclerosis, a single 5-day course of intravenous therapy led to a profound reduction in both relapses and new MRI lesions that was sustained for at least a year [Coles et al., 1999a]. Curiously, 30% of treated subjects in this study developed autoimmune thyroid disorders (Graves' disease, thyroiditis), a toxicity not reported among patients receiving alemtuzumab for treatment of cancers or for other indications [Coles et al., 1999b]. A phase II study is underway that should help to establish the efficacy and safety of alemtuzumab. This 3-year study involves 300 subjects with early multiple sclerosis who were randomized to receive either 60 or 120 mg of Campath or treatment with an interferon-β product, Rebif, 44 μg, for subcutaneous injection. Results are expected by 2007.

Daclizumab (Zenapax) is an immunosuppressive humanized monoclonal antibody that is approved for prophylaxis of acute renal transplant rejection. Daclizumab binds to a component of the receptor for interleukin-2 on activated T lymphocytes and thereby blocks binding of interleukin-2. In preliminary results from small phase II studies, both relapsing-remitting and secondary-progressive volunteers stabilized or improved following treatment. The phase II studies are continuing.

Mycophenolate mofetil (Cellcept) is an immunosuppressive agent approved for prophylaxis of organ transplant rejection. Its mechanism of action is inhibition of inosine 5′-monophosphate dehydrogenase type II, the enzyme responsible for the de novo synthesis of the purine nucleotide guanine within activated T and B lymphocytes and macrophages. Open-label pilot studies of Cellcept in the treatment of multiple sclerosis have reported that the clinical course of multiple sclerosis was either unchanged or subjectively improved in many of the treated patients. Small randomized trials are underway.

Schilder's Disease

The term *Schilder's disease* has been a source of confusion in the neurologic literature because the three cases, reported by Schilder between 1912 and 1924, were actually three different diseases [Poser et al., 1986]. One case, described in 1924, likely was a postinfectious encephalitis (subacute sclerosis panencephalitis); another case published in 1913 appears to have been X-linked adrenoleukodystrophy; and the third case, documented by Schilder in 1912, was a 14-year-

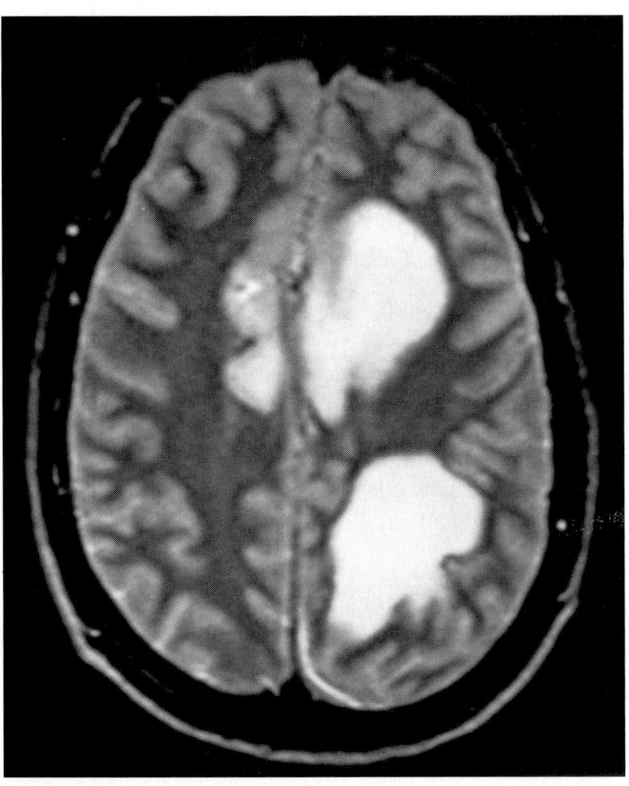

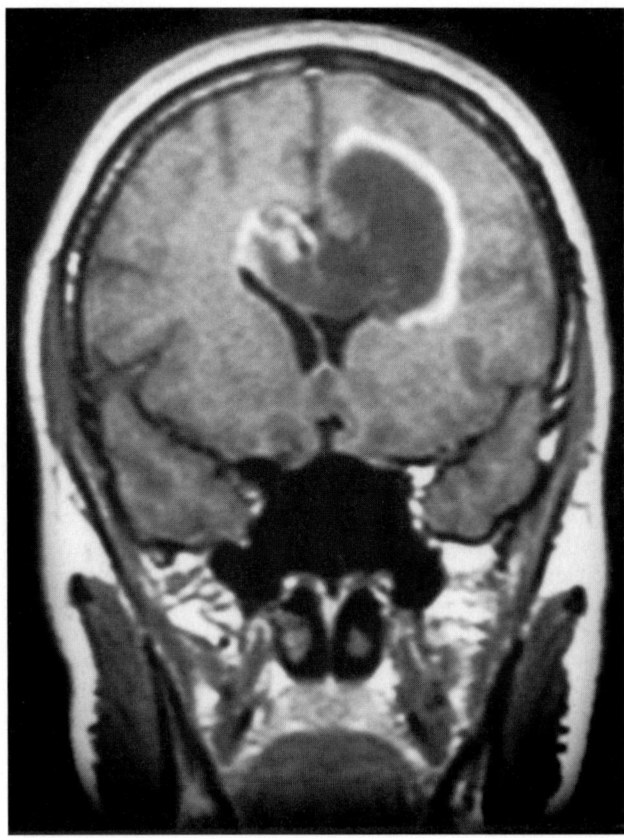

FIGURE 60-2 Axial T2-weighted (**A**) and coronal contrast-enhanced T1-weighted images (**B**) in a young adult male with Schilder's disease. Note the bilateral large, swollen lesions in the cerebral white matter, connected through a lesion in the corpus callosum. The peripheral rim of the lesion enhances.

old female with multifocal demyelination in the cerebrum associated with increased intracranial pressure and rapidly progressive neurologic signs. The last case is now considered an example of true Schilder's disease.

Clinical Characteristics and Subclassification

Schilder's disease (myelinoclastic diffuse sclerosis) is a sporadic disease of unknown etiology, but it appears to be immune mediated with pathologic features identical to those of multiple sclerosis. It is likely that Schilder's disease represents a more acute form of multiple sclerosis in children and adults [Poser et al., 1986]. The disease affects children usually between the ages of 5 and 14 years. The most common manifestation of this disease is an acute hemiplegia with headache, vomiting, behavioral deterioration, and ataxia. The clinical examination often reveals hemiplegia, aphasia, abnormal swallowing, ataxia, and increased reflexes. Some children may develop papilledema that may mimic a space-occupying mass or tumor [Kotil et al., 2002].

Clinical Studies

The CT and MRI scans are remarkable for revealing usually one to three well-demarcated large areas of abnormal density or signal, with rim enhancement frequently noted in the frontal regions (Fig. 60-2). Unlike multiple sclerosis, the remainder of the CNS is normal on imaging studies. Cerebrospinal fluid studies may indicate a pleocytosis and at times oligoclonal bands, increased synthesis of immunoglobulin G, and increased protein. The clinical diagnosis usually depends on the imaging studies once other entities have been excluded.

An important differential diagnostic possibility to be considered in all cases of Schilder's disease is X-linked adrenoleukodystrophy. In the case of doubt, very long chain fatty acids should be studied. X-linked adrenoleukodystrophy will have an elevation in the C26 fatty acids and an increase in the C26/C22 ratio. On MRI, there is usually symmetric posterior white matter involvement. Whereas the enhancement in Schilder's disease affects the border of the lesion, the enhancement in X-linked adrenoleukodystrophy involves a rim inside the lesion.

Treatment

The natural history of Schilder's disease is variable, but sequelae are frequent. Five patients reported by Aicardi did not have any recurrences over 9 years, but other studies have shown relapses [Aicardi, 1992; Lyon et al., 1996]. Steroids bring a dramatic improvement in the neuroradiologic appearance of the cerebral lesion [Aicardi, 1992].

Acute Disseminated Encephalomyelitis

Acute disseminated encephalomyelitis is usually a monophasic illness that may follow many infections or immunizations. The common infections include rubeola, rubella, varicella, herpes zoster, mumps, upper respiratory tract infections, and *Mycoplasma pneumoniae* infection [Johnson et al., 1985]. Acute disseminated encephalomyelitis commonly presents after a latent period after the infection, which may only be a few days. The clinical features in children include multifocal neurologic signs, lethargy, coma, and seizures that often implicate widespread areas of the brain, spinal cord, and optic nerves [Kesselring et al., 1990]. The optic neuritis in acute disseminated encephalomyelitis is usually bilateral, and the myelopathy is often complete, associated with areflexia. The laboratory studies, such as cerebrospinal fluid examination, often do not help differentiate acute disseminated encephalomyelitis from multiple sclerosis because pleocytosis, oligoclonal bands, and increased immunoglobulin G synthesis may be seen in both disorders [Kesselring et al., 1990]. The MRI abnormalities in acute disseminated encephalomyelitis are often more extensive, and lesions tend to be larger than multiple sclerosis lesions. The MRI findings in acute disseminated encephalomyelitis frequently include gray matter structures (cortex, basal ganglia, thalamus), as well as the brainstem, cerebellar peduncles or cerebellar hemispheres (Fig. 60-3). These features help differentiate acute disseminated encephalomyelitis from multiple sclerosis [Kesselring et al., 1990]. CT scan may be normal in many patients, and MRI is usually required to confirm the diagnosis [Leake et al., 2004]. The MRI lesions may persist even after a clinical recovery has occurred [Anlar et al., 2003].

Pathology

The pathologic appearance of acute disseminated encephalomyelitis is very similar to what is seen in animal models of experimental allergic encephalomyelitis, which suggests a hypersensitivity reaction to a viral product or immune dysregulation. The appearance histologically is a periventricular demyelination and inflammation with lymphocytes and macrophages.

Treatment

Medical management in these cases usually consists of high-dose steroids or intravenous immunoglobulins, which may result in clinical improvement and resolution of the neuroimaging findings. About 71% of patients with childhood-onset acute disseminated encephalomyelitis recovered completely after 12 months of follow-up in one study involving 39 patients; however, there was a 33% incidence of relapse [Anlar et al., 2003].

Acute Hemorrhagic Leukoencephalitis

In 1941, E. Weston Hurst described three young adults who developed an acute fatal encephalopathy after respiratory illnesses [Hurst, 1941]. These three individuals developed focal neurologic signs, confusion, and aphasia and died within a few days of the onset of the illness. The

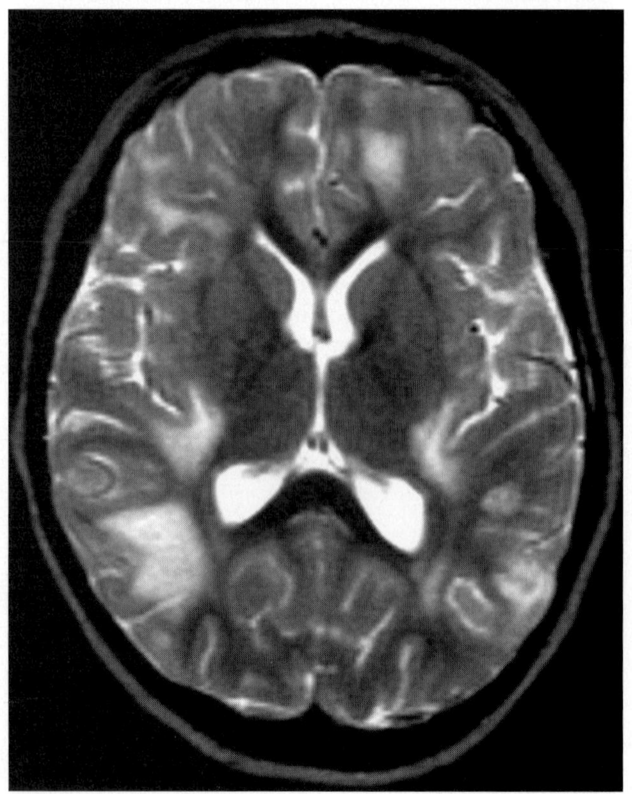

A

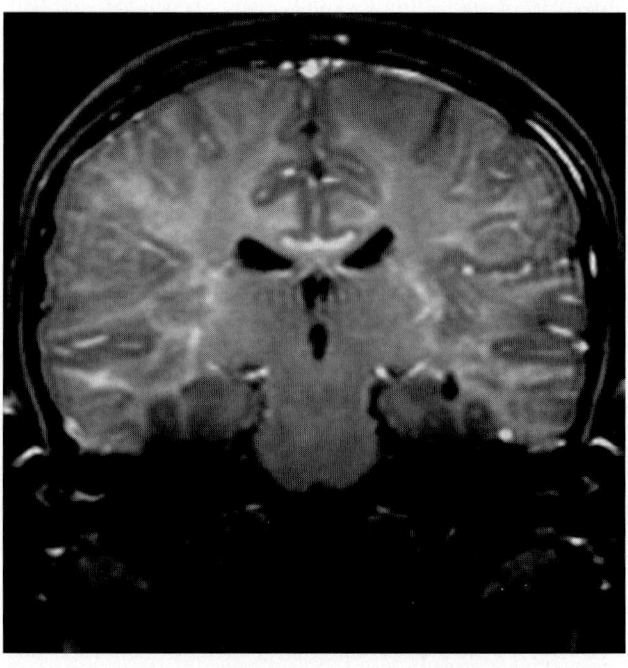

B

FIGURE 60-3 Axial T2-weighted (**A**) and coronal contrast-enhanced T1-weighted (**B**) images in a 6-year-old female with acute disseminated encephalomyelitis. Note the multifocal white matter lesions, which have an asymmetric distribution over the cerebral white matter. The cortex and basal ganglia are not entirely spared. Contrast enhancement is usually subtle in acute disseminated encephalomyelitis.

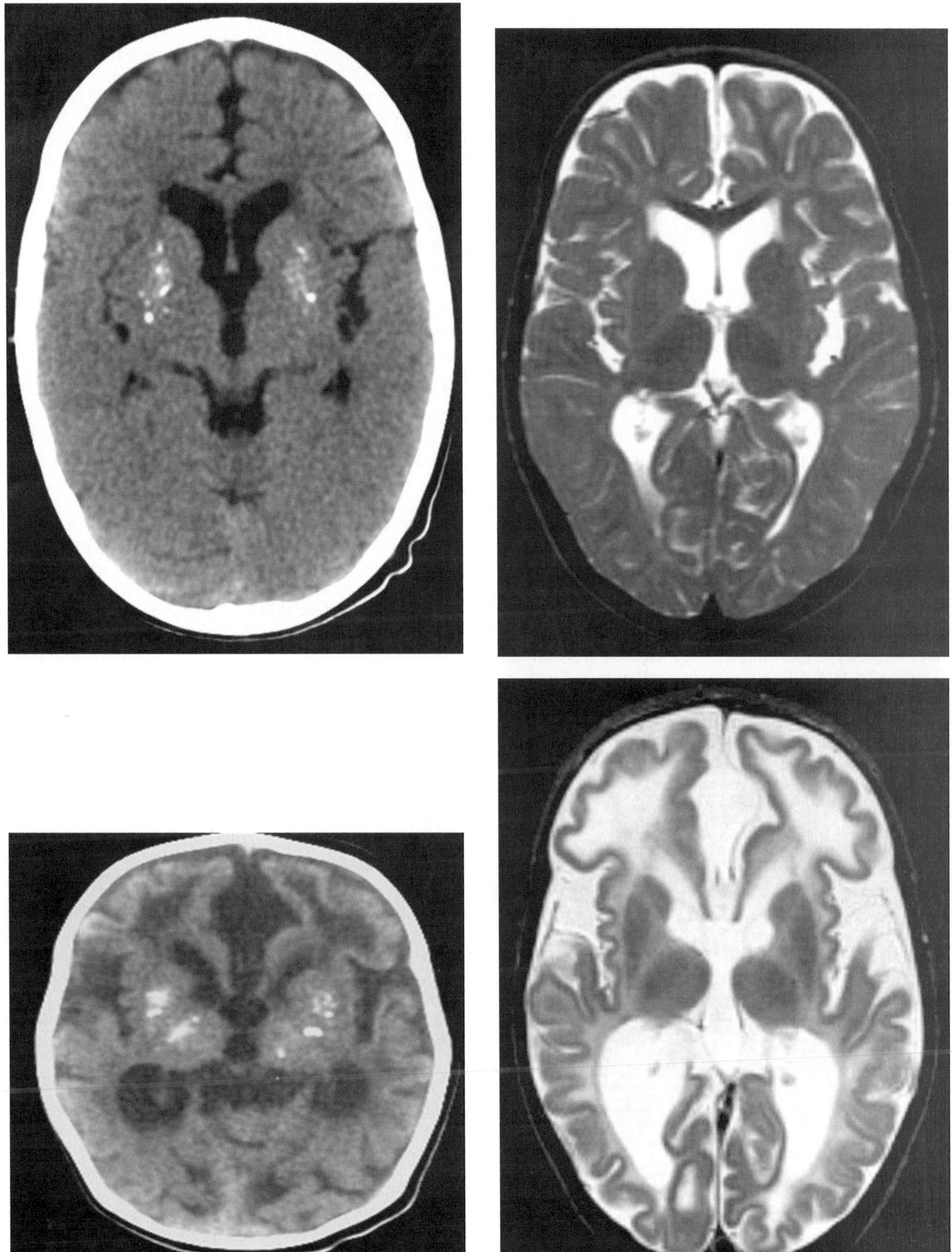

FIGURE 60-4 The two images of the *top row* originate from a 5-year-old female with Aicardi-Goutières syndrome; the two images of the *bottom row* originate from her clinically more severely affected brother of 4 months. Note the dotlike calcium deposits in the basal ganglia in both patients. The cerebral white matter disease is mild in the female, severe in her brother. The cerebral atrophy is also much more severe in the male.

pathologic findings in two cases included edema and hemorrhage in the centrum semiovale with microscopic evidence of perivascular demyelination, necrosis, and infiltration with polymorphonuclear cells. The clinical picture of acute hemorrhagic leukoencephalitis includes an abrupt onset, usually after an infection with fever, with headache, meningismus, focal neurologic signs, altered sensorium, and occasionally seizures [Rosman et al., 1997]. The cerebrospinal fluid examination in acute hemorrhagic leukoencephalitis demonstrates a polymorphonuclear pleocytosis with an elevated protein and normal glucose. This entity is considered by most investigators to be a more severe and rapidly fulminant form of acute disseminated encephalomyelitis and probably should not be separated from acute hemorrhagic leukoencephalitis on an etiologic basis until a clear understanding of the pathophysiology of the disorder becomes available.

Treatment consists of aggressive use of corticosteroids, which has been associated with a favorable outcome in some cases, although severe neurologic injury and death frequently occur [Rosman et al., 1997].

Aicardi-Goutières Syndrome

In 1984, Aicardi and Goutières reported eight infants from five families who suffered from an early-onset familial encephalopathy with chronic cerebrospinal fluid lymphocytosis and basal ganglia calcifications mimicking an intrauterine infectious process but with negative TORCH (toxoplasmosis, other infections, rubella, cytomegalovirus infection, and herpes simplex) associations [Aicardi and Goutières, 1984]. Clinically, the patients revealed bilateral spasticity, dystonia, ocular jerks, and acquired progressive microcephaly with a rapid course toward profound deterioration and death. In addition, CT scan showed diffuse and progressive brain atrophy and deep white matter hypodensities. The authors suggested a probable genetic condition with autosomal recessive inheritance.

Leukoencephalopathy is often noted on MRI, which may lead to diagnostic confusion if no CT scan is available to indicate the calcium deposits. CT scan also shows white matter hypodensities located mainly around the ventricles (Fig. 60-4). These hypodense lesions appear as hyperintense on MRI T2-weighted sequences, but they are not constant (see Fig. 60-4), and a diffuse leukodystrophic appearance is uncommon [Goutières et al., 1998]. Signs of severe and progressive brain atrophy with enlarged ventricles and sulci increasing on successive examinations are an almost constant finding on CT and MRI.

The diagnosis is confirmed by the clinical picture, identification of cerebrospinal fluid lymphocytosis, and MRI and CT findings, especially basal ganglia calcifications. A systemic sign that can occasionally be noted in patients is vascular necrotic cutaneous lesions on the toes, which appear similar to chilblains with acrocyanosis [Goutières et al., 1998]. Many of the patients studied have had elevated serum and cerebrospinal fluid levels of interferon-α, which has been used as a diagnostic marker for the disease and may be implicated in the pathophysiology for the disorder [Goutières et al., 1998; Lebon et al., 2002].

Interferons constitute a family of signal proteins. Upon binding to specific receptors, they induce activation of a signal transduction pathway that activates a broad range of genes, which are involved in antiviral, immunomodulatory, and antiproliferative activities. Transgenic mice with astrocyte-targeted chronic overproduction of interferon-α develop a progressive inflammatory encephalopathy with angiopathy and calcifications in the basal ganglia [Campbell et al., 1999]. These neuropathologic features are very similar to those found in Aicardi-Goutières syndrome, suggesting a causal relationship between the elevated levels of interferon-α and the disease. The inheritance of Aicardi-Goutières syndrome is presumed to be autosomal recessive, but no gene has been identified.

HYPOMYELINATING AND DYSMYELINATING DISORDERS

Pelizaeus-Merzbacher Disease

Classic Pelizaeus-Merzbacher disease is an X-linked disorder of proteolipid protein expression. The disease was first described clinically by Pelizaeus in 1885, and later in 1910 the clinical and pathologic features of the same family were documented by Merzbacher [Merzbacher, 1910; Pelizaeus, 1885]. The classification of Pelizaeus-Merzbacher disease as a hypomyelinating disorder was proposed by Zeman and co-workers in 1964, and they perspicaciously predicted proteolipid protein as being involved in this disease [Zeman et al., 1964]. Previous reports had divided Pelizaeus-Merzbacher disease into types I to VI based on neuropathologic and hypomyelinating features, but recent molecular genetic information more accurately defines Pelizaeus-Merzbacher disease as an X-linked disease consisting of hypomyelination that is linked to the *PLP* gene [Gencic et al., 1989; Hudson et al., 1989; Seitelberger, 1970]. The nosology of Pelizaeus-Merzbacher disease has been further complicated by the discovery that a form of X-linked spastic paraplegia and Pelizaeus-Merzbacher disease are allelic conditions [Saugier-Veber et al., 1994].

Clinical Characteristics and Subclassification

The clinical features of Pelizaeus-Merzbacher disease are slowly progressive and consist of peculiar pendular eye movements, head shaking, hypotonia, mental retardation, choreoathetosis, dystonia, cerebellar ataxia, and pyramidal signs [Adams et al., 1996; Boulloche and Aicardi, 1986]. There is a spectrum, however, in the ages of presentation and progression of symptoms that is somewhat arbitrarily divided into three types [Seitelberger et al., 1996]. A fourth type of Pelizaeus-Merzbacher disease, X-linked spastic paraplegia type 2, can also be considered as a later manifestation of proteolipid protein expression difficulties because X-linked spastic paraplegia has been described in one family in which a classic form of Pelizaeus-Merzbacher disease was also noted [Seitelberger et al., 1996].

TYPE I—CLASSIC

The classic form of Pelizaeus-Merzbacher disease begins in the first months of infancy with abnormal eye movements consisting of rapid, irregular, small- or large-amplitude oscillations that can occur in either a horizontal or vertical direction [Adams et al., 1996; Boulloche and Aicardi, 1986]. A head tremor is also noted at this time. Motor development progresses very slowly, with the eventual onset of spasticity, ataxia, and involuntary movements. Pelizaeus-Merzbacher disease is frequently misdiagnosed as cerebral palsy at this stage because of the slow onset of symptoms. Later, optic atrophy and seizures may occur. Although the physical handicaps are severe, mental abilities are usually better preserved. Typically, the progression of the disease slows towards the middle or end of the first decade, with death occurring in the adolescent or early adult ages.

TYPE II—CONNATAL

The connatal type, which presents shortly after birth, has a more aggressive clinical course consisting of severe hypotonia, extrapyramidal signs, stridor, and feeding difficulties [Boulloche and Aicardi, 1986; Seitelberger et al., 1996]. The laryngeal stridor may be a frequently overlooked presenting feature in these early-onset cases [Boulloche and Aicardi, 1986]. The marked hypotonia in the connatal form of this disease can mimic spinal muscular atrophy, although pathologic studies do not confirm an abnormality in anterior horn cells or peripheral nerve [Kaye et al., 1994]. Optic atrophy can usually be identified early, and death may occur within months to years.

TYPE III—TRANSITIONAL

Transitional forms of Pelizaeus-Merzbacher disease have a clinical presentation that often combines features from both the classic and connatal types but with quite a variable progression [Seitelberger et al., 1996]. Included in this subtype are patients with null mutations in the *PLP1* gene. These mutations prevent expression of both *PLP1* and *DM20* and are typically associated with a complicated phenotype that includes a slowly spastic paraplegia with a loss of ambulation and impaired cognitive function [Garbern et al., 2002]. These patients also have electrophysiologic evidence of mild, nonuniform demyelinating peripheral neuropathy [Shy et al., 2003].

SPASTIC PARAPLEGIA

Spastic paraplegia type 2 had been known to be an X-linked form of spastic paraplegia that could occur in a pure form consisting of a slowly progressive spastic paraplegia involving only lower limbs or a complicated form with other features of Pelizaeus-Merzbacher disease such as nystagmus, dysarthria, and ataxia. Spastic paraplegia type 2 is considered an allelic variant of Pelizaeus-Merzbacher disease with defects in the *PLP* gene identified [Saugier-Veber et al., 1994].

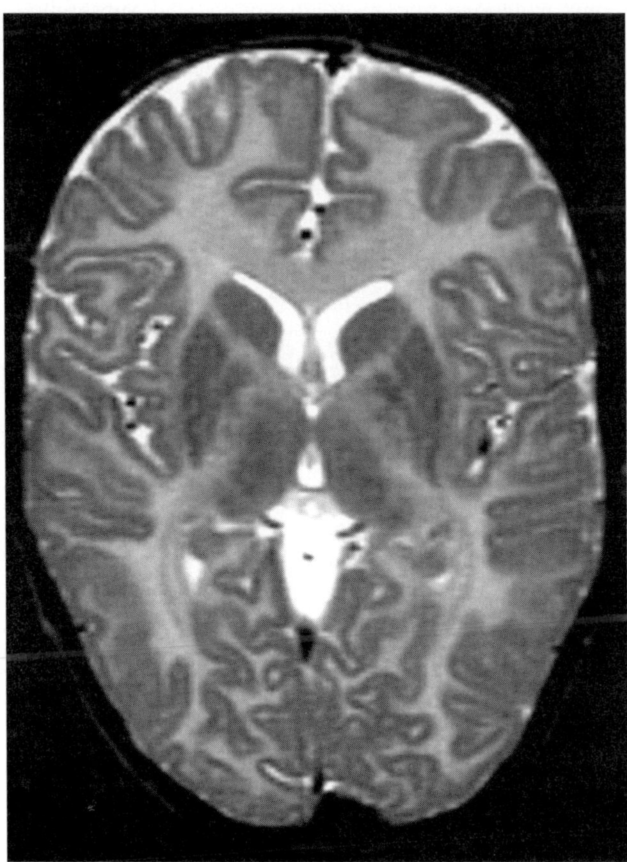

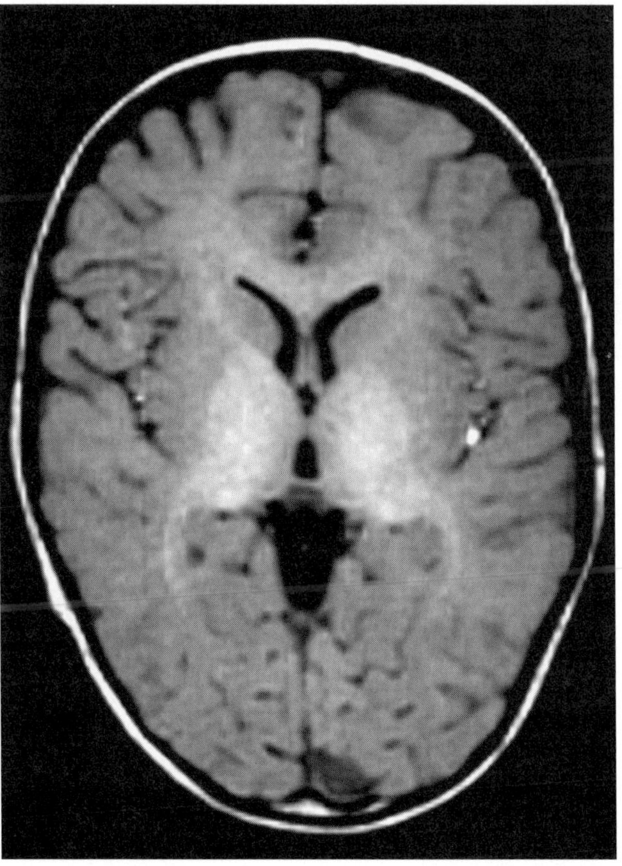

FIGURE 60-5 T2- and T1-weighted images in a 6-year-old male with Pelizaeus-Merzbacher disease. The degree of myelination would be normal for a neonate. Repeated follow-up magnetic resonance images indicated an unchanged pattern of myelin deposition in this male, indicative of an arrest of myelination early in life.

Clinical Studies

CT scan of the brain is frequently unrevealing, but MRI is helpful in demonstrating the hypomyelination that is characteristic of the disorder. The MRI shows a decrease on T1-weighted signal and an increase on T2-weighted signal in white matter regions demonstrating deficient myelin development [Kendall, 1993] (Fig. 60-5). Repeated MRI head studies from early infancy demonstrate the lack of the expected maturational decrease in the T2-weighted signal, suggesting the diagnosis of Pelizaeus-Merzbacher disease [Ono et al., 1993]. Brainstem auditory-evoked responses and somatosensory-evoked potentials are consistently abnormal. Electrophysiologic evidence of motor neuron dysfunction has been reported in infants, and a mild, nonuniform demyelinating peripheral neuropathy has been noted in adolescents with a more slowly progressive disease [Kaye et al., 1994; Shy et al., 2003].

Pathology

The gross morphologic examination of brain demonstrates cerebral and cerebellar atrophy, which is especially prominent in the early-onset forms of the disease [Seitelberger, 1970]. The characteristic neuropathologic appearance of Pelizaeus-Merzbacher disease consists of a marked deficiency of CNS myelin except for preserved islands of myelin surrounding blood vessels (tigroid appearance) [Boulloche and Aicardi, 1986; Zeman et al., 1964]. Myelin staining reveals a marked deficiency of myelin, especially in the deeper cerebral structures. Oligodendrocytes are reduced in number, whereas astrocytes are markedly increased [Seitelberger, 1995]. The nerve cells are typically normal, but heterotopic neurons can be found. There is increasing evidence of axonal pathology in Pelizaeus-Merzbacher disease, in particular in the milder variants [Garbern et al., 2002]. Myelin appearance, both macroscopically and microscopically, in peripheral nerves is normal [Boulloche and Aicardi, 1986; Zeman et al., 1964].

Biochemistry

The biochemical studies in CNS myelin led to the discovery of a defect in the metabolism of proteolipid protein. Myelin basic protein and proteolipids were reduced in Pelizaeus-Merzbacher disease [Bourre et al., 1978]. The absence of proteolipid protein, demonstrated by immunocytochemistry and enzyme-linked immunosorbent assay, was compared with the proteolipid protein defect in the jimpy mouse [Koeppen et al., 1987]. The fact that proteolipid protein is not normally found in peripheral myelin was thought to explain the sparing of peripheral nerve myelin in this disorder.

Genetics

The *PLP* gene has been linked to the Xq21-22 region [Mattei et al., 1986; Willard and Riordan, 1985] and found to be about 17 kilobases in length and to contain 7 exons [Diehl et al., 1986]. The gene encodes two protein isoforms, PLP and DM20 proteins, by means of alternative splicing [Nave et al., 1987]. The *PLP/DM20* gene is similar to some other genes, such as those encoding the neuron-specific membrane glycoprotein M6 and shark proteolipid myelin proteins, which are expressed early in development and have a broad functional range [Kittagawa et al., 1993; Yan et al., 1993]. Studies of animal models have tried to define the functions of these two myelin proteins. Based on numerous clinical and histopathologic analyses, it is clear that proteolipid protein gene products have an important structural role in the CNS myelin sheath, but these gene products also play a role in the development of oligodendrocytes. For example, the dysmyelinating proteolipid protein animal mutants such as the jimpy mouse (a splice acceptor site mutation resulting in deletion of exons and a frameshift) and the shaking pup (a His75Pro substitution) are also associated with a block in oligodendrocyte development [Hudson et al., 1987; Nadon et al., 1990]. The nonlethal mouse model for Pelizaeus-Merzbacher disease, rumpshaker (a Ile86Thr substitution), is associated with myelin deficiency but normal numbers and appearance of oligodendrocytes, suggesting potentially independent roles for proteolipid protein gene products in oligodendrocyte maturation and CNS myelin assembly [Schneider et al., 1992]. DM20 is expressed earlier than PLP in the developing CNS, but at later time points, proteolipid protein is the predominant protein, suggesting that DM20 and PLP may play different roles during CNS development [Macklin et al., 1990]. DM20 mRNA but not PLP mRNA can be detected in the peripheral nervous system, but no function for the DM20 protein in the peripheral nervous system has yet been demonstrated.

In people affected with Pelizaeus-Merzbacher disease, point mutations that result in amino acid substitutions, frameshift deletion and insertion mutations, or complete deletions of the PLP protein have been identified, but mutations in the coding region have been identified in only 25% of these cases [Nave and Boespflug-Tanguy, 1996]. Mutations that disrupt the *PLP1* gene-specific domain (residues 116 to 150), as well as null mutations, cause mild, demyelinating peripheral neuropathy [Shy et al., 2003]. It appears that up to 50% of children with Pelizaeus-Merzbacher disease may have a duplication in the PLP gene, similar to the 1.5-kilobase duplication in the *PMP22* gene identified in Charcot-Marie-Tooth disease, which results in a defect in PLP gene expression [Cailloux et al., 2000]. Also, even families without identified mutations in the *PLP* gene may demonstrate linkage to the PLP gene region on Xq22, suggesting that the molecular defect resides in the PLP genomic region, perhaps affecting gene expression [Boespflug-Tanguy et al., 1994]. In two brothers with Pelizaeus-Merzbacher disease, increased PLP gene expression was also identified without duplication of the gene [Carango et al., 1995].

There appears to be at least one other X locus for a Pelizaeus-Merzbacher–like disease because a family with a clinical appearance very similar to classic Pelizaeus-Merzbacher disease was noted to have linkage not to the *PLP* gene but to a new locus on Xq [Lazzarini et al., 1997]. In addition, there appear to be several autosomal loci, one of which contains the gene encoding alpha 12 (connexin 46.6) [Uhlenberg et al., 2004].

Alexander's Disease

Alexander's disease was first described in 1949 in a child with macrocephaly [Alexander, 1949]. This disorder is an uncommon degenerative disorder of the CNS occurring most often in children. It leads to relentless cognitive and motor decline. The pathologic hallmark of the disorder is the presence of Rosenthal fibers located within astrocytes. The genetic inheritance has been identified as a spontaneous de novo, dominant mutation in one of the alleles of the gene for the astrocytic intermediate filament protein: glial fibrillary acidic protein (GFAP) [Brenner et al., 2001; Rodriguez et al., 2001]. In several families with later-onset disease, autosomal-dominant inheritance has been documented [Namekawa et al., 2002; Stumpf et al., 2003; Thyagarajan et al., 2004].

Clinical Features and Subclassification

Alexander's disease has been classified into three distinct types; although without a biochemical or molecular genetic assay to verify the diagnosis, this distinction may be somewhat arbitrary, with progression of disease not always dependent on the age of onset [Pridmore et al., 1993]. These variants have an infantile, juvenile, and adult onset [Russo et al., 1976].

INFANTILE ONSET

The first case, which was described by Alexander, occurred in a 15-month-old child with megalencephaly, hydrocephalus, and psychomotor retardation [Alexander, 1949]. This child died 8 months after the onset of the illness and was noted on postmortem examination of the brain to have refractile bodies in the subependymal, subpial, and perivascular regions throughout the neuraxis. These refractile bodies were subsequently found to be identical to Rosenthal fibers [Schlote, 1966]. Subsequent reports confirmed the clinical features as consisting of psychomotor retardation, megalencephaly or hydrocephalus, spastic quadriparesis, and seizures. The head circumference in these children frequently exceeds the 98th percentile within 6 to 18 months [Johnson, 1996]. In children who present at a later age, the megalencephaly may not be apparent. The disease may start in the neonatal period, and some infants appear unresponsive, never even learning to smile. The ventricular system is often enlarged, with some children developing an obstructive hydrocephalus, which appears to be due to subependymal Rosenthal fibers that accumulate and obstruct the aqueduct of Sylvius [Garcia et al., 1992]. The progression of the disease is unremitting, with death occurring anywhere from age 1 to 10 years, although rarely children may survive until their teens. There appears to be an equal sex distribution for the disease, although earlier studies based on small sample sizes and ascertainment biases demonstrated a male preponderance [Reichard et al., 1996].

JUVENILE ONSET

Children who present after early childhood typically have an average onset of symptoms at age 3 to 4 years with a reported range of 3 months to 12 years [Reichard et al., 1996]. The clinical symptoms are distinct from the infantile-onset form, with progressive paresis, bulbar involvement, increased deep tendon reflexes, ataxia, and preservation of sensory and mental functions [Russo et al., 1976]. The duration of the illness is much longer, with the possibility of survival as long as 8 to 15 years after onset of symptoms.

ADULT ONSET

The adult-onset disease is an allelic variant of the infantile- and juvenile-onset disorder with mutations in the *GFAP* gene. The cases described in adults have been divided into those with a relapsing-remitting course similar to that of multiple sclerosis or asymptomatic individuals who have developed the disease in the setting of a prolonged medical illness [Russo et al., 1976]. Upon postmortem examination of the brain, Rosenthal fibers are present, but demyelination is variable, which may make the distinction from other diseases difficult because Rosenthal fibers may also be present in disorders such as multiple sclerosis. However, reports on these patients were published before the gene for Alexander's disease was found. A more recent report described three sisters and their father who had a progressive neurologic disease that consisted of palatal myoclonus, spastic paraparesis, and cerebellar ataxia starting in the adult years associated with Rosenthal fibers on postmortem examination [Schwankhaus et al., 1995]. The adult patients with Alexander's disease and documented *GFAP* mutations have a chronic progressive disease dominated by bulbar symptoms [Namekawa et al., 2002; Stumpf et al., 2003; Thyagarajan et al., 2004].

Clinical Studies

The MRI and CT scans are usually highly suggestive of the disorder. The CT scan early in the course of the disease reveals prominent low density in the frontal deep white matter that may become cystic over time [Johnson, 1996]. The areas immediately adjacent to the ventricles may demonstrate increased density, with enhancement noted in the periventricular, thalamic, and basal ganglia regions [Farrell et al., 1984] (Fig. 60-6). The MRI is more sensitive than CT scan and demonstrates similar findings with extensive cerebral white matter changes with frontal predominance, a periventricular rim with high signal on T1-weighted images and low signal on T2-weighted images, and abnormalities of basal ganglia, thalami, and brainstem, which may be used to make a presumptive diagnosis of Alexander's disease [van der Knaap et al., 2001] (see Fig. 60-6). Neurophysiologic studies performed on these patients have included electroencephalograms, which demonstrated slow activity and sharp waves at times localized over one or another frontal or frontocentral brain region [Pridmore et al., 1993]. The brainstem auditory-evoked responses have shown slowing after wave I [Pridmore et al., 1993].

Pathology

The two major pathologic features of Alexander's disease are a progressive failure of central myelination and the widespread presence of Rosenthal fibers within structural and reactive astrocytes [Reichard et al., 1996]. The cortical neurons appear unaffected. Over time, white matter throughout the brain is affected, with demyelination occurring in the centrum semiovale, although there is frequent sparing of the subcortical white matter. Rosenthal fibers are present in

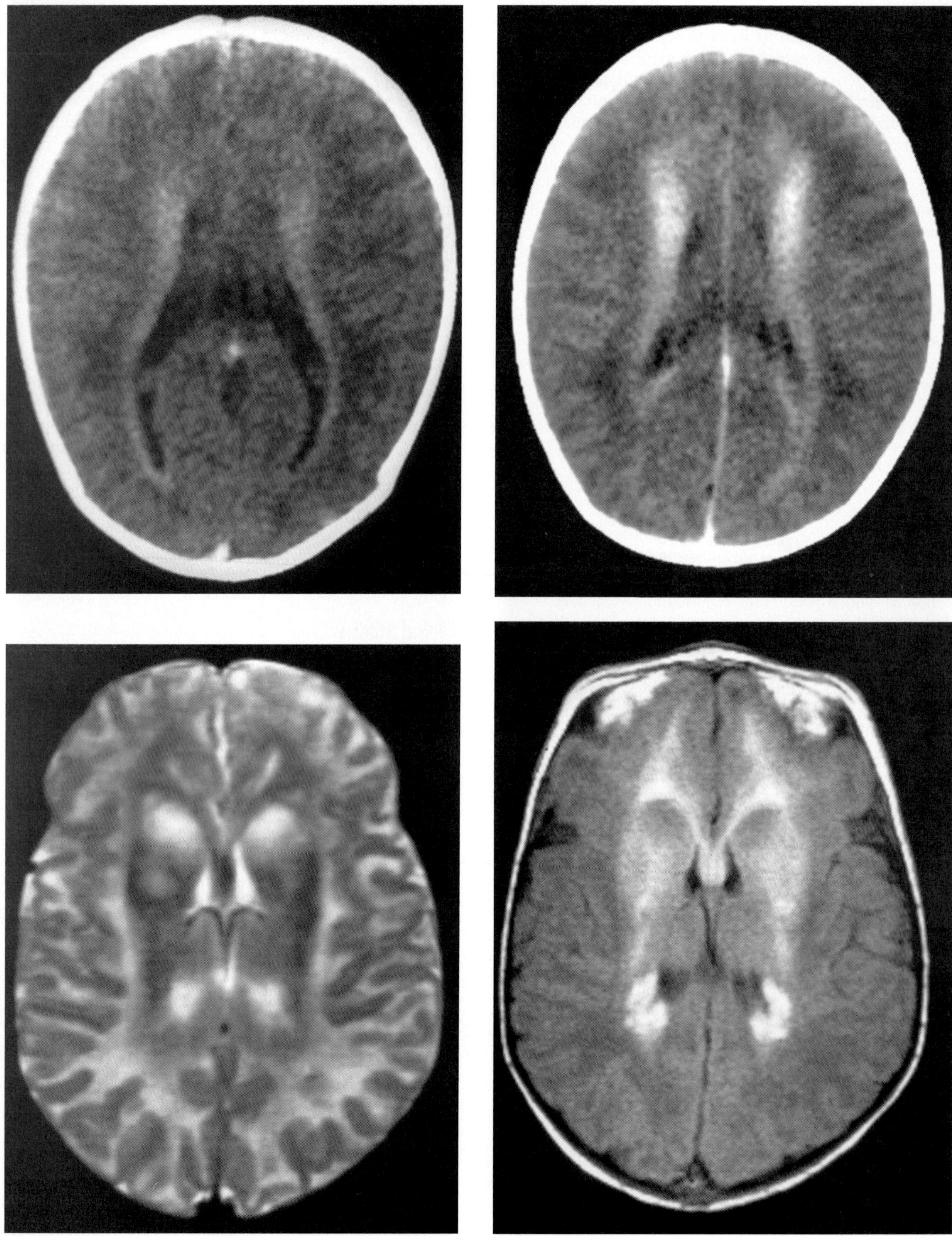

FIGURE 60-6 A, Computed tomography scan (*top row*) in a 1-month-old male with Alexander's disease demonstrates increased density of the periventricular rim (*left*), which enhances after contrast (*right*). Magnetic resonance images (*bottom row*) demonstrate a periventricular rim of low signal intensity on the T2-weighted image (*left*), which shows prominent enhancement after contrast on the T1-weighted image (*right*). There are signal abnormalities in the basal ganglia. Because both unmyelinated white matter and abnormal white matter have a high signal on T2-weighted images and a low signal on T1-weighted images, it is difficult or impossible to appreciate white matter abnormalities in a young infant.

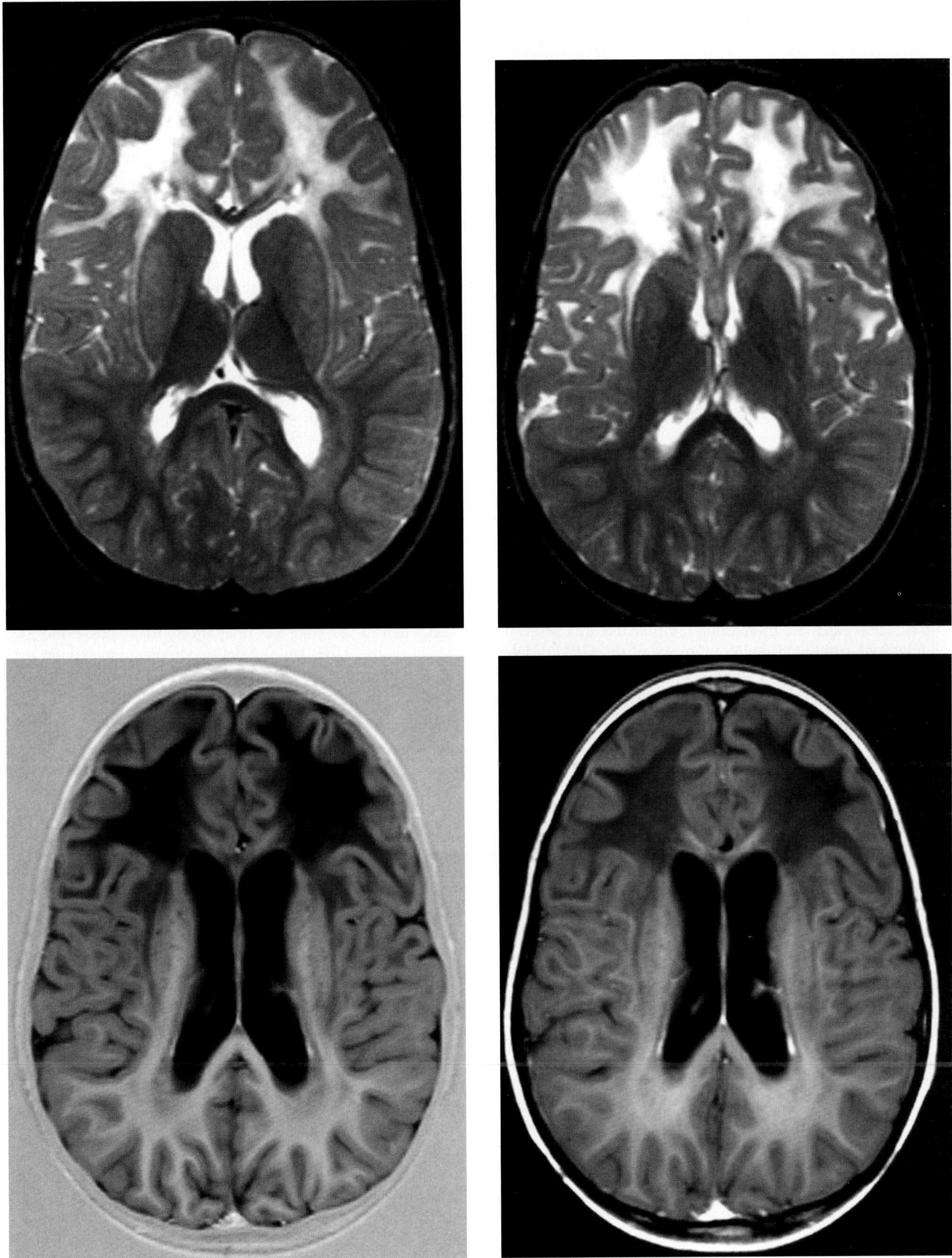

B

FIGURE 60-6 **B**, T2-weighted images (*top row*) in a male with Alexander's disease at the ages of 6 (*left*) and 10 years (*right*). Note the mild signal abnormalities and slight swelling of the basal ganglia at the age of 6. At the age of 10, the basal ganglia have become atrophic. The T1-weighted images at the age of 10 years (*bottom row*) show a discontinuous thin rim of high signal on the unenhanced image (*left*) and some enhancement of this rim after contrast (*right*). (**A,** Courtesy of Dr. S. Blaser, Department of Diagnostic Imaging, Hospital for Sick Children, Toronto.)

astrocytes throughout the neuraxis in both gray and white matter regions. There is a preponderance of Rosenthal fibers in subpial regions, subependymal zones, and perivascular cuffs [Alexander, 1949]. On the ultrastructural examination, the Rosenthal fibers appear as a dense mass of finely granular osmophilic material, enmeshed in glial filaments, located in the footplates and in the perikaryon of cells [Reichard et al., 1996]. The degree of demyelination does not always correlate with the density of Rosenthal fibers [Johnson, 1996].

Biochemistry

There has been no biochemical defect consistently described in Alexander's disease. A stress protein, alpha B crystallin, has been elevated in Alexander's disease, but this may be a nonspecific finding because no defect has been found in the gene for alpha B crystallin [Iwaki et al., 1992]. One report described elevation of tiglylglycine in urine of patients with Alexander's disease [Johnson, 1996].

Genetics

Almost all cases of childhood Alexander's disease (infantile and juvenile) are sporadic and are believed to be caused by a spontaneous de novo, heterozygous, dominant mutation in one of the alleles of the gene for the astrocytic intermediate filament protein, GFAP [Brenner et al., 2001; Gorospe et al., 2002; Li et al., 2002; Rodriguez et al., 2001; Shiroma et al., 2003]. Adult cases are more often familial and are caused by an inherited, dominant mutation in one of the *GFAP* alleles [Namekawa et al., 2002; Stumpf et al., 2003; Thyagarajan et al., 2004]. At least 21 different mutations at 15 sites (often in exons 1, 4, or 8) have been identified in more than 50 patients, many of which are predicted to cause the substitution of an arginine by another amino acid [Johnson and Brenner, 2003]. The clinical phenotype cannot be completely predicted by the genotype, although mutations in the adult-onset patients tend to occur at different locations on the gene. The severity of disease also does not strictly parallel the particular mutation present, but in some instances, a general correlation exists [Rodriguez et al., 2001]. The mutations in the *GFAP* gene have been found in the United States, Europe, and Japan [Shiroma et al., 2003]. The genetic testing for Alexander's disease has replaced the cerebral biopsy as the major tool for diagnosis. However, in two infantile cases, no *GFAP* mutation was found by sequencing despite a pathologically proven diagnosis of Alexander's disease [Brenner et al., 2001; Rodriguez et al., 2001], suggesting that there may be additional genes that are responsible for Alexander's disease.

A transgenic mouse was created that overexpressed the *GFAP* gene. This mouse model died within 10 days of birth and was noted to have widespread Rosenthal fibers throughout the CNS [Messing et al., 1998]. Although this does not necessarily provide an exact model for Alexander's disease, it provides a means to study the formation of Rosenthal fibers.

Treatment

At this time, no treatment other than supportive care and treatment of possible seizures is available to these children.

Myelin Basic Protein Deficiency

A deficiency of myelin basic protein has been described, caused by a deletion of the 18q 22.3-qter region, which contains the locus for myelin basic protein, in a 25-year-old woman who had symptoms of involuntary movements, ataxia, and mild mental retardation [Lyon et al., 1996]. The MRI demonstrated deficient and abnormal myelination. The woman's 18-month-old son was also affected. It is probably not surprising that a deficiency of myelin basic protein has been identified in humans because a mouse model, the shiverer mouse, has been recognized for some time.

A relatively frequent chromosomal deletion syndrome, the $18q^-$ syndrome, is caused by the loss of the distal part of the long arm of chromosome 18. Children with this syndrome have short stature because of growth hormone deficiency, narrow or atretic external ear canals with hearing loss, midfacial hypoplasia, microcephaly, and frequently mental retardation. MRI scans demonstrate a diffuse decrease in central white matter that is thought to be related to a reduction in the *MBP* gene [Gay et al., 1997; Lyon et al., 1996]. White matter T1 and T2 relaxation times were significantly prolonged in patients compared with controls at all ages studied, suggesting incomplete myelination. Chromosome analysis using fluorescence in situ hybridization techniques showed that all patients with abnormal MRI scans and prolonged white matter T1 and T2 relaxation times were missing one copy of the *MBP* gene [Gay et al., 1997]. The one patient with normal-appearing white matter and normal white matter T1 and T2 relaxation times possessed two copies of the *MBP* gene. MRI and molecular genetic data suggest that incomplete cerebral myelination in $18q^-$ is associated with haplo-insufficiency of the *MBP* gene [Gay et al., 1997].

SPONGIFORM LEUKOENCEPHALOPATHIES

Canavan's Disease

The first neuropathologic observation of a form of leukodystrophy known as *spongy degeneration of brain* was published by Myrtelle Canavan in 1931, although at the time, this pathology was attributed to Schilder's disease [Canavan, 1931]. Because of this classic description, however, the most commonly recognized name for spongy degeneration of brain is the eponym *Canavan's disease*. The clinical and inherited delineation of Canavan's disease was first recognized by van Bogaert and Bertrand in 1949 [van Bogaert and Bertrand, 1949]. In this report, five Jewish patients developed macrocephaly and severe mental retardation associated with spongy degeneration of brain. In 1988, Canavan's disease was identified as caused by a deficiency of aspartoacylase, which leads to an increase in *N*-acetylaspartic acid in brain and urine. The gene encoding aspartoacylase was cloned in 1993 [Matalon et al., 1988, 1993].

Clinical Characteristics and Subclassification

Canavan's disease is a relentlessly progressive autosomal-recessive leukodystrophy, which is frequently fatal within the first decade. There are three recognized clinical variants:

the most common infantile variant and two unusual presentations consisting of congenital and juvenile-onset forms. Although separating Canavan's disease into these categories is useful in terms of diagnosis, it is likely that they represent merely a spectrum of clinical manifestations.

INFANTILE ONSET

The classic presentation in infancy consists of a period of normal development followed by lethargy and significant hypotonia, especially manifested as a head lag. Frequently by 4 months of life, the head growth exceeds the 90th percentile, and by 6 months, the development is clearly delayed. The macrocephaly may not always exceed the 95%, but there is invariably a relative increase in the head size compared with the percentiles for height and weight [Gascon et al., 1990]. The diagnosis of Canavan's disease should be considered in any infant who presents with signs of hypotonia, head lag, and macrocephaly. In the later half of the first year, the children develop hyperextension of the extremities and eventually develop spasticity. Irritability and difficulty sleeping usually manifest by the end of the first year. Optic atrophy and seizures are typically apparent by the second year. Feeding inevitably becomes a major problem requiring the placement of a nasal or gastric feeding tube. The life span is limited, with most patients dying within the first decade

CONGENITAL TYPE

Children with congenital Canavan's disease begin in the first weeks of life with hypotonia and poor feeding. This congenital variant is uncommon, with only 2 of 165 biochemically confirmed cases occurring in children with symptoms during the first weeks of life [Matalon et al., 1993]. Early in the disease, the children appear to have severe visual problems despite a frequently normal-appearing funduscopic examination. Coarse pendular nystagmus or strabismus is usually noted, and optic atrophy develops later. This disease progresses to cause severe difficulty with sucking and swallowing, loss of motor control, and spasticity [Adachi et al., 1973]. Seizures, associated with hypotonia and developmental delay, may begin very early in the congenital variant, which often makes the diagnosis difficult until white matter abnormalities or macrocephaly can be appreciated.

JUVENILE VARIANT

Only a few cases of the juvenile variant of Canavan's disease have been described. These children may appear normal until as late as 4 or 5 years of age. Many of the juvenile patients had been described before the biochemical characterization of Canavan's disease [Adachi et al., 1973], but some confirmed juvenile cases have been recognized [Toft et al., 1993]. These children have a much slower progression of the disease, with dysarthria, seizures, and developmental delay as prominent features.

Clinical Studies

The CT scan early in the course of the disease is associated with a diffusely decreased attenuation of the white matter

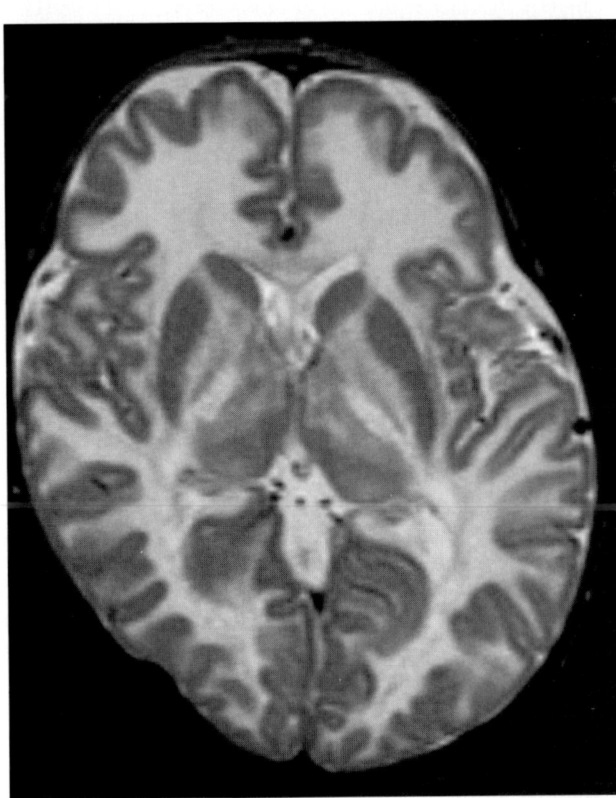

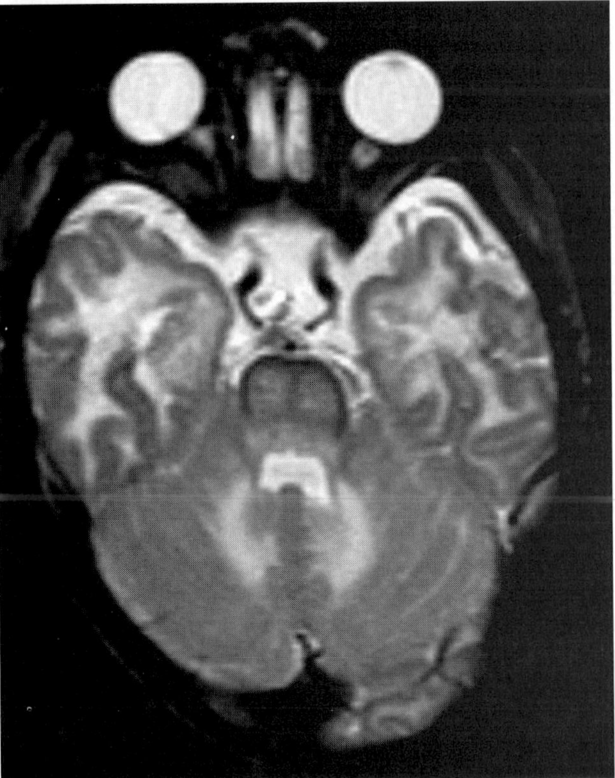

FIGURE 60-7 Axial T2-weighted images in a 12-month-old male with infantile Canavan's disease. Note the diffusely abnormal cerebral and cerebellar white matter and brainstem. There are signal abnormalities in the thalamus and globus pallidus, whereas the putamen and caudate nucleus are spared.

that affects subcortical white matter [Rushton et al., 1981]. The MRI scan is remarkable for an increased signal on T2-weighted images and decreased signal on the T1-weighted images in white matter, primarily affecting the cerebral white matter, thalamus, and globus pallidus, with sparing of the putamen and caudate nucleus [Engelbrecht et al., 1995] (Fig. 60-7). Initially, especially in the congenital variant, the MRI or CT scans may appear normal [Matalon et al., 1990]. Magnetic resonance spectroscopy may be diagnostic revealing an elevated *N*-acetylaspartate–to-creatine ratio. The electroencephalogram may also be normal despite the presence of seizures, with slowing of the background and abnormal sleep spindles at times being the only abnormality [Gascon et al., 1990]. Brainstem auditory-evoked potentials are frequently associated with slowing after wave I or slowing of the waves III to V or I to V latency [Gascon et al., 1990]. Visual-evoked potentials are usually absent or have a delayed latency of the P100 wave [Gascon et al., 1990]. Because Canavan's disease does not affect the peripheral nerve myelin, the nerve conduction velocities are normal.

Since 1988, the standard for diagnosis of Canavan's disease has been the measurement of urinary *N*-acetylaspartic acid in urine, with Canavan's disease patients typically having values at least 5- to 10-fold higher than control urine samples [Matalon et al., 1995]. Other leukodystrophies tested do not demonstrate an increase in *N*-acetylaspartic acid levels [Matalon et al., 1989]. The serum, cerebrospinal fluid, and brain also typically have elevated *N*-acetylaspartic acid levels [Matalon et al., 1990].

The deficiency of the enzyme aspartoacylase results in the accumulation of *N*-acetylaspartic acid. This enzyme is measured in fibroblasts because plasma or blood cells do not have measurable levels [Matalon et al., 1989]. Obligate heterozygotes have been found to have about a 50% level of aspartoacylase enzyme activity compared with controls, which makes carrier detection possible [Matalon et al., 1995].

Pathology

The prominent pathology noted on light microscopy is the presence of multiple vacuoles (spongy degeneration) seen in the deeper cortical regions but to a greater extent in the subcortical white matter [Adachi et al., 1973] (Fig.60-8). There is evidence of demyelination without evidence of breakdown products and sparing of axonal fibers and oligodendroglial cells early in the disease course. At a cellular level, type II Alzheimer cells are present, and there is a relative absence of microglial and inflammatory cells [Luo and Huang, 1984]. The electron microscopic appearance is noteworthy for splitting of myelin lamellae and swelling of the astrocytic cytoplasm and processes, but the neurons and their processes and synaptic complexes appear unchanged [Adachi et al., 1973].

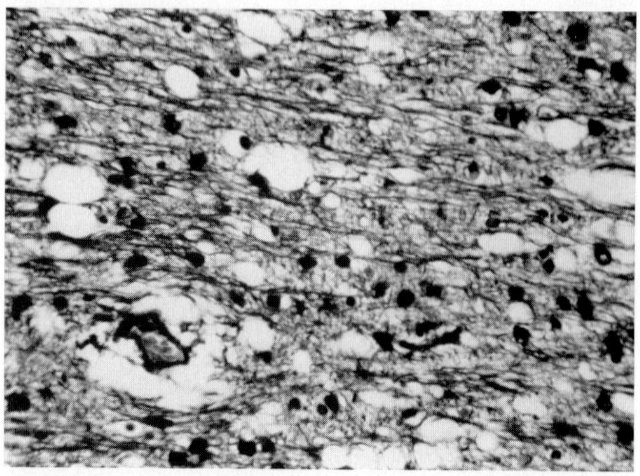

FIGURE 60-8 Light microscopy from infant with Canavan's disease demonstrating the dysmyelination with vacuoles but sparing of axons on the Bodian stain.

Biochemistry

The synthesis of *N*-acetylaspartic acid is performed exclusively in brain by the enzyme L-aspartate-*N*-acetyltransferase [Goldstein, 1959]. Despite the relative abundance of this amino acid, which is second only to glutamic acid, little is known about the functional significance of *N*-acetylaspartic acid in brain. Postulates to explain the purpose of *N*-acetylaspartic acid have suggested that it may function as a neurotransmitter [Miyake et al., 1981] or perhaps as a necessary factor for the conversion of fatty acids, which are components of myelin [Shigematsu et al., 1983]. The enzyme required to hydrolyze *N*-acetylaspartic acid into aspartate and acetate is aspartoacylase. This enzyme can be found in several tissues, including brain, but aspartoacylase activity is localized within white matter and not cortical brain tissue [Kaul et al., 1991]. The biologic function of *N*-acetylaspartic acid is not understood, but its accumulation in Canavan's disease suggests that the breakdown of *N*-acetylaspartic acid by aspartoacylase is essentially for the normal maintenance of myelin or other white matter components.

Genetics

Canavan's disease is inherited as an autosomal-recessive disorder. The molecular basis of Canavan's disease was elucidated in 1993 with the cloning of the gene and the identification of a common missense mutation [Kaul et al., 1993]. This gene for human aspartoacylase is localized to the 17p13-ter region and spans 29 kb of the genome [Kaul et al., 1994]. The transcript is 1.8 kb in length and contains an open reading frame on the complementary DNA that is 939 bases long and predicts a 313–amino acid residue [Matalon et al., 1993]. The identified mutations can be divided according into Ashkenazi Jewish and non-Jewish mutations. Two mutations account for 97% of the mutant alleles in Jewish families. These two mutations include the most frequent mutation, which causes a substitution of glutamic acid for alanine at codon 285 (Glu285Ala), and another common mutation, which results in a nonsense mutation changing a tyrosine at codon 231 to a stop codon (Tyr231ter) [Matalon et al., 1995]. Based on carrier detection frequency in the Ashkenazi Jewish population, the overall incidence of the disease in this specific population is estimated to be 1 in 5000 [Matalon, 1997]. In the non-Jewish families, an alanine to glutamic acid substitution at codon 305 (Ala305glu) occurs in about 36% of identified mutations. In the non-Jewish families, only 70% of mutations have been identified so far, with a total of 24 additional mutations being characterized [Matalon et al., 1995]. If a mutation has been identified for a pregnancy at risk for the disease, mutational analysis can be performed on chorionic villus sampling to aid in diagnosis. Prenatal diagnosis of Canavan's disease is complicated because cultured amniocytes or chorionic villus samples have low levels of aspartoacylase activity, making enzyme analysis unsatisfactory for disease detection in the fetus [Matalon et al., 1992].

Treatment

At present, there is no treatment available for children with Canavan's disease. Management is symptomatic and palliative. Physical therapy may help prevent contractures. Seizures need to be controlled, and one small study suggested the use of topiramate for treatment of megal-

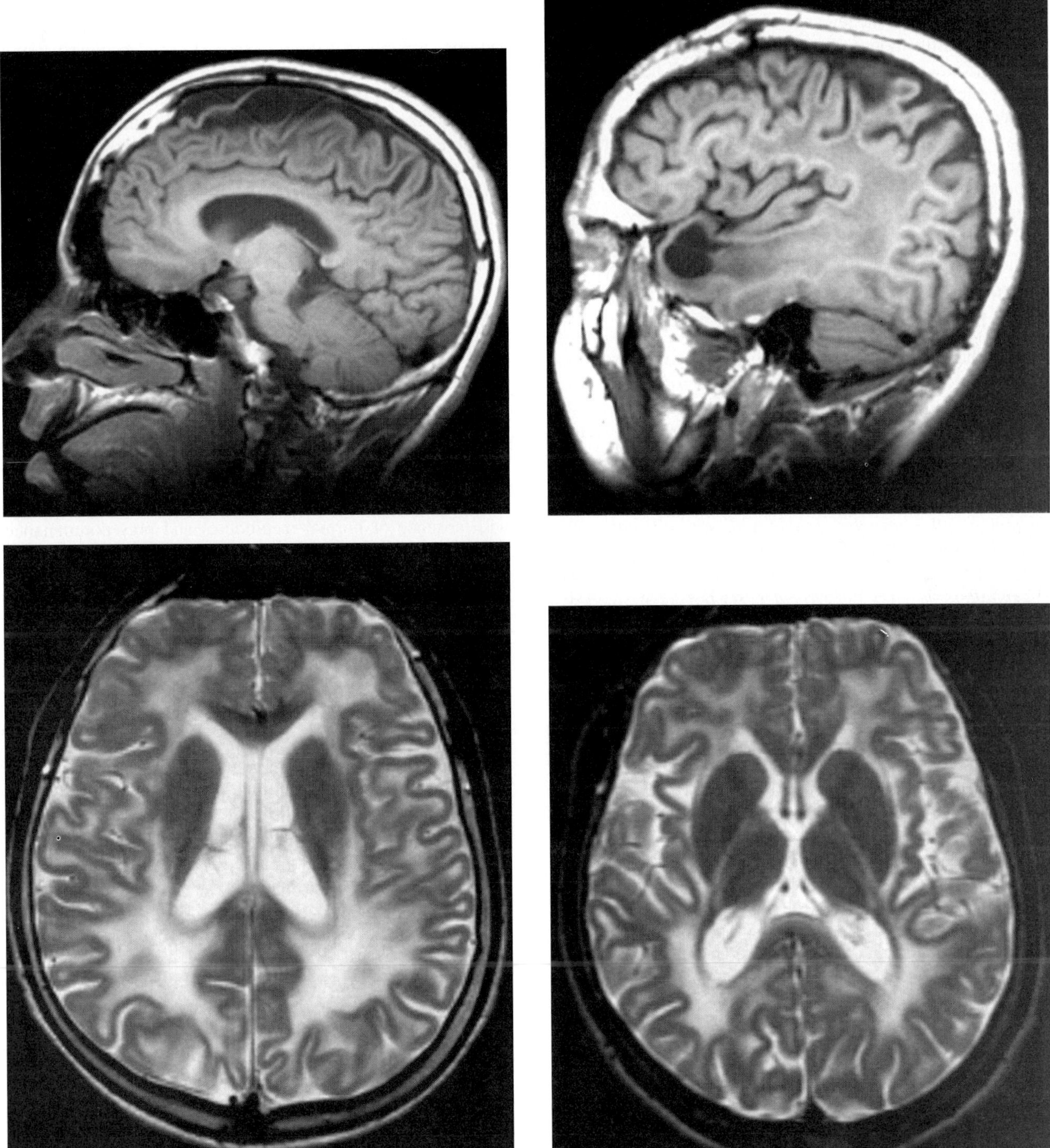

FIGURE 60-9 Sagittal T1-weighted images (*top row*) and axial T2-weighted images (*bottom row*) of a 14-year-old male with megaloencephalic leukoencephalopathy. The sagittal images show subcortical cysts in the anterior temporal and frontal areas. The T2-weighted images show diffusely abnormal and slightly swollen cerebral white matter. The corpus callosum is spared.

encephaly [Topcu et al., 2004]. Special care is needed to avoid aspiration with feedings. Nasogastric feeding or gastrostomy feeding will be needed in many of these children. There is a current clinical protocol to study the gene therapy of Canavan's disease using adeno-associated virus type 2 as a vector for aspartoacylase [Janson et al., 2002], but there are no data available yet from that trial. One previous study reported transfer of the aspartoacylase gene to two children with Canavan's disease [Fink, 2000; Leone et al., 2000]. More evaluation of these experiments will be required over time to assess the efficacy and safety of these trials.

A knockout mouse for Canavan's disease has been created [Matalon et al., 2000] that should be helpful in exploring the possibilities of gene therapy in humans. A report of a naturally occurring tremor rat may also be a model for Canavan's disease [Kitada et al., 2000]. Baslow and colleagues [Baslow et al., 2002] used lithium chloride for 5 days and showed a 13% reduction of *N*-acetylaspartic acid in the brains of these tremor rats.

Megaloencephalic Leukoencephalopathy with Subcortical Cysts

Megaloencephalic leukoencephalopathy with subcortical cysts is a recently described disease that includes the triad of leukoencephalopathy, megalencephaly, and mild clinical course. The disorder has initially described as "leukoencephalopathy with swelling and discrepantly mild clinical course" [van der Knaap et al., 1995] but has also been referred to as *vacuolating leukoencephalopathy* and *leukoencephalopathic megalencephaly with mild clinical course* [Goutières et al., 1996]. Because of the number of names for this disease, the term *megaloencephalic leukoencephalopathy with subcortical cysts* has been suggested because it correlates with neuropathologic changes seen in this disorder [van der Knaap et al., 1996]. The first description was likely by Harbord and associates when two siblings with megalencephaly and dysmyelination were reported, but van der Knaap and colleagues, Singhal and associates, and Goutières and co-workers have characterized the clinical and radiographic aspects of this disease [Goutières et al., 1996; Harbord et al., 1990; Singhal et al., 1996; van der Knaap et al., 1995]. The clinical features consist of macrocephaly occurring in the first year of life with a delayed onset of relatively mild neurologic symptoms consisting of cerebellar ataxia, pyramidal signs, and seizures [Goutières et al., 1996; van der Knaap et al., 1995]. The MRI demonstrates diffuse supratentorial white matter increased signal on T2-weighted images and decreased signal on T1-weighted images and mild swelling of the abnormal white matter (Fig. 60-9). Cysts are invariably present in the subcortical temporal region and often also in the parietal region. The brainstem and cerebellum appear largely unaffected.

The disease is inherited in an autosomal recessive pattern. Mutations in the gene *MLC1* have been identified as the cause [Leegwater et al., 2001b], but there is likely at least one other gene also responsible for the clinical features in some patients with megaloencephalic leukoencephalopathy with subcortical cysts [Blattner et al., 2002; Patrono et al., 2003].

Leukoencephalopathy with Subcortical Cysts without Megalencephaly

There appears to be a similar but distinct clinical syndrome associated with a leukoencephalopathy and subcortical cysts, but instead of the megalencephaly seen in megaloencephalic leukoencephalopathy with subcortical cysts, the head size is normal or small [Olivier et al., 1998]. This is apparently inherited in an autosomal recessive manner and does not have a mutation in the *MLC* gene. The MRI in these patients demonstrates bilateral cysts in the anterior temporal regions, with the signal intensity of the cysts being isointense with cerebrospinal fluid. Signal changes were present on MRI in the periventricular regions, but there was a characteristic sparing of the central white matter and cerebellar white matter. Although the disease is associated with delayed development in most children, the course appears to be rather static or slowly progressive.

CYSTIC LEUKOENCEPHALOPATHIES

Vanishing White Matter Disease and Childhood Ataxia with Cerebral Hypomyelination

Vanishing white matter disease and childhood ataxia with cerebral hypomyelination has been characterized in the past few years by a number of groups of investigators. In 1993, Hanefeld and colleagues reported three patients with a diffuse leukoencephalopathy and an unusual proton magnetic resonance spectrum of the affected white matter with absence of normal metabolites and presence of small glucose and lactate resonances [Hanefeld et al., 1993]. This disorder was further clarified by Schiffmann and co-workers in 1994, who described four girls with ataxia and spasticity but without peripheral nerve or cognitive involvement [Schiffmann et al., 1994]. The MRI demonstrated a diffuse confluent abnormality of the cerebral white matter, which was noted early in the course of the disease. On proton magnetic resonance spectroscopy, these girls were also noted to have a reduction of *N*-acetylaspartic acid, choline, and creatine in white matter only. The brain biopsy from two of the girls revealed a generalized reduction in myelin specific proteins and lipids but no evidence of any storage material. In 1997, nine other children were identified by van der Knaap and associates, and the term *vanishing white matter* was used to describe the entity [van der Knaap et al., 1997]. The MRI findings were similar to previous reports, but on proton density and fluid-attenuated inversion recovery studies, the white matter was noted to have signal intensity similar to that of cerebrospinal fluid (Fig. 60-10). Magnetic resonance spectroscopy also found severe reduction in *N*-acetylaspartic acid, choline, and creatine; and again, lactate and glucose peaks were observed in white matter that were suggested to originate from the cerebrospinal fluid replacing the white matter. On one postmortem examination from this series of children, the histopathology demonstrated a cavitating leukoencephalopathy with replacement of white matter between ependyma and U fibers by cerebrospinal fluid. In areas with some preservation of white matter, astrogliosis and macrophage proliferation were present.

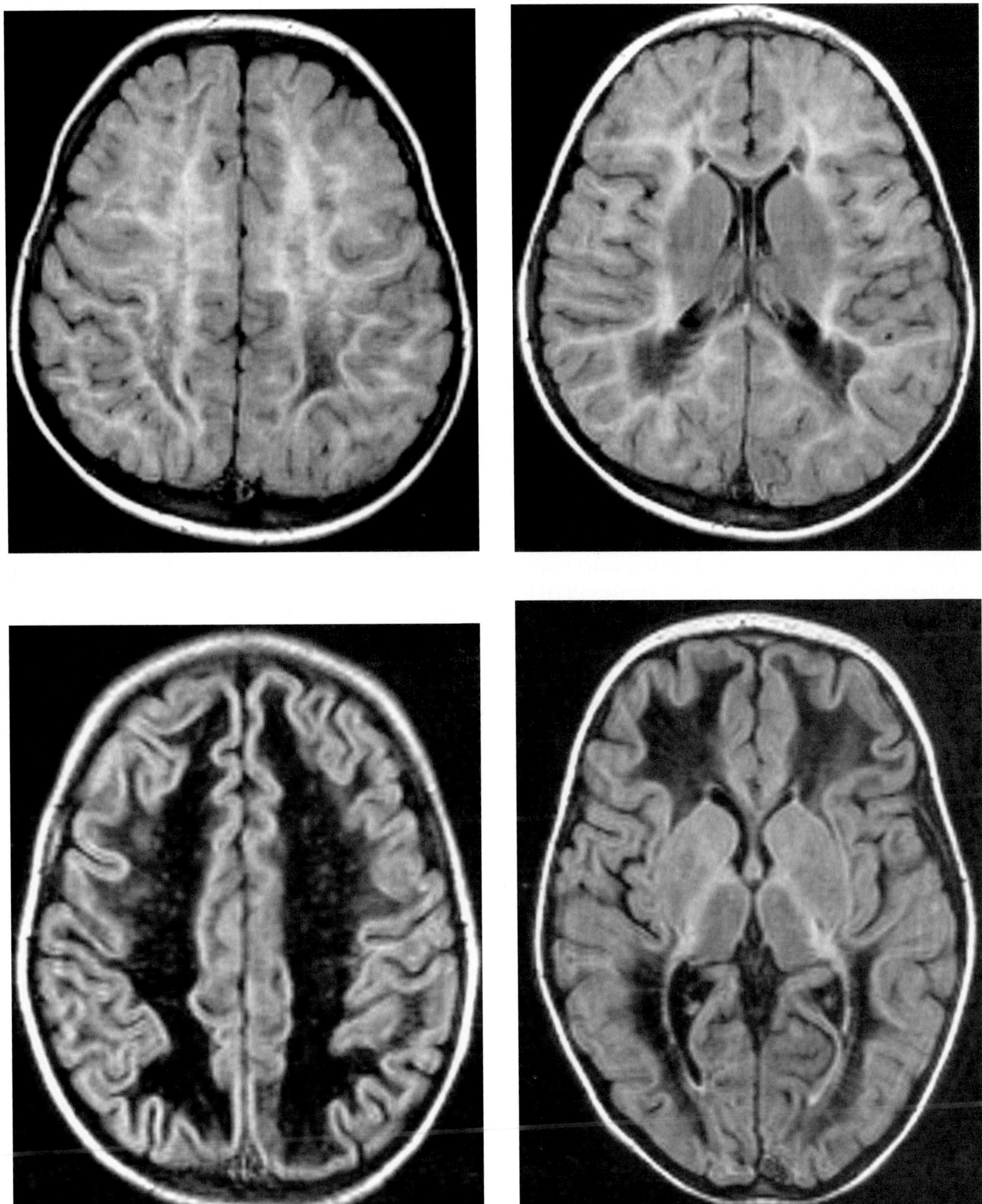

FIGURE 60-10 Axial fluid-attenuated inversion recovery images of $3^1/_2$-year-old female with classic vanishing white matter disease and childhood ataxia with cerebral hypomyelination (VWM/CACH) (*top row*), and a severely affected $3^1/_2$-year-old female with a severe form of VWM/CACH (*bottom row*). The *top row* images show the typical white matter rarefaction and vanishing of the cerebral white matter, with many small stripes and dots within the cystic white matter indicative of remaining tissue strands. The *bottom row* images show that the cerebral white matter is much more cystic. Still, the dots and radiating stripes of remaining tissue strands are visible.

A set of criteria were suggested by van der Knaap and associates [van der Knaap et al., 1997] to identify children with this disease:

- Normal or mildly delayed initial psychomotor development
- Onset in early childhood with an episodic and chronic progressive course
- Deterioration that may follow infection or minor head trauma
- Cerebellar ataxia and spasticity with relative preservation of mental function
- Diffuse symmetric white matter involvement with all or part of cerebral white matter manifesting signal intensity on MRI similar to that of cerebrospinal fluid on proton density, fluid-attenuated inversion recovery, T2-weighted, and T1-weighted images

The molecular defect of vanishing white matter disease and childhood ataxia with cerebral hypomyelination was first elucidated when the gene for this disorder was mapped to 3q27 [Leegwater et al., 1999]. The gene responsible for this disease was found to be located in the epsilon subunit of the eukaryotic initiation factor 2B (*eIF2B*) [Leegwater et al., 2001a], which is essential in the regulation of translation initiation. The *eIF2B* gene converts the eukaryotic protein synthesis initiation factor 2 (eIF2) from an inactive guanosine diphosphate–bound form into an active eukaryotic protein synthesis initiation factor 2–guanosine diphosphate complex. It is interesting to speculate why a gene that appears to be so basic to protein synthesis should only affect cerebral white matter. Subsequently, it was determined that all five subunits (alpha, beta, gamma, delta, and epsilon) of *eIF2B* contained mutations in patients with vanishing white matter disease and childhood ataxia with cerebral hypomyelination [van der Knaap et al., 2002].

The clinical spectrum of vanishing white matter disease and childhood ataxia with cerebral hypomyelination was expanded further through molecular studies to include other leukoencephalopathies, such as Cree leukoencephalopathy reported in the Cree Indians and ovario-leukodystrophy (a later-onset white matter disease with ovarian failure) as variants of vanishing white matter disease and childhood ataxia with cerebral hypomyelination [Fogli et al., 2002, 2003]. The phenotypic expression also expanded when reports were made of fatal infantile forms due to mutations in the *eIF2B* subunits [van der Knaap et al., 2003]. Initial reports suggested that there was no genotype–phenotype correlation, but recent information suggests that for some mutations in the *eIF2B* genes, phenotypic correlation can be considered. In a study involving 93 leukoencephalopathy patients identified by MRI criteria, Fogli and co-workers [2004] identified 83 individuals from 68 families with 46 distinct *eIF2B* gene mutations. Although a clear genotype–phenotype correlation could not be made in all the mutations identified, some genetic defects, such as the R113H in the *eIF2B* epsilon subunit and the E213G substitution in the *eIF2B* beta subunit, were associated with a mild clinical course. Also, van der Knaap and co-workers [2004] confirmed that the R113H mutation is associated with a milder clinical course in adults that may not always be accompanied by clinical signs such as spasticity. Although the MRI in these patients demonstrates a diffuse leukoencephalopathy, the characteristic cavitary lesions may be missing. Finally, Ohtake and colleagues from Japan identified a patient with adult-onset vanishing white matter and a point mutation in the epsilon subunit of *eIF2B*, T182M that was associated with slowly progressive neuropsychiatric symptoms and mild spasticity [Ohtake et al., 2004].

OTHER DISEASES THAT HAVE MAJOR WHITE MATTER ABNORMALITIES

Because of the sensitivity of MRI, many diseases not thought of primarily as white matter diseases need to be included in the differential diagnosis of abnormally appearing white matter on MRI.

Sjögren-Larsson Syndrome

Sjögren-Larsson syndrome is an autosomal recessive disorder consisting of the clinical triad of spasticity, congenital ichthyosis, and mental retardation and a leukoencephalopathy on MRI [Sjögren and Larsson, 1957].

Biochemistry

The primary biochemical defect in Sjögren-Larsson syndrome is deficient activity of the fatty aldehyde dehydrogenase component of fatty alcohol:NAD$^+$ oxidoreductase [Rizzo and Craft, 1991]. Enzymatic studies may determine genetic carriers for Sjögren-Larsson syndrome [Kelson et al., 1992] and allow prenatal diagnosis [Rizzo et al., 1994]. Leukotriene B_4 is broken down by fatty aldehyde dehydrogenase and is excessively secreted in the urine of Sjögren-Larsson patients. Because it is a proinflammatory agent, leukotriene B_4 appears to be involved in some of the pathologic aspects of Sjögren-Larsson syndrome, especially the pruritus [Willemsen et al., 2001a, 2001b].

Genetics

The gene is localized to chromosome 17p11.2 [Pigg et al., 1994; Rogers et al., 1995]. The complementary DNA for fatty aldehyde dehydrogenase is cloned, and several mutations have been identified in this gene [De Laurenzi et al., 1996]. At present, more than 70 different mutations, including missense and nonsense mutations, deletions, insertions, and splice-site alterations, have been reported [Carney et al., 2004; De Laurenzi et al., 1996, 1997; Rizzo et al., 1999; Sillen et al., 1997; Tsukamoto et al., 1997]. Many patients of Swedish and northern European descent carry an identical missense mutation (943C(T; Pro315[Ser]), and haplotype studies indicate that they share a common ancestor [De Laurenzi et al., 1997; Sillen et al., 1997]. Most Swedish patients are homozygous for this mutation, which is consistent with their consanguineous history. A second deletion mutation, 1297-1298delGA, is frequently seen in European patients [Rizzo et al., 1999]. About one half of European Sjögren-Larsson syndrome patients carry 943C(T or 1297-1298delGA. Overall, there appears to be a diversity of mutations associated with different haplotypes in patients with Sjögren-Larsson syndrome [Carney et al., 2004].

Clinical Features

The clinical features of Sjögren-Larsson syndrome consist of three major signs: congenital ichthyosis, mental retardation, and spastic diplegia or tetraplegia [Sjögren and Larsson, 1957]. The neurologic features usually begin before 1 year of age and consist of motor and language delay. Spastic diplegia is more common than tetraplegia, and many patients either never walk or require leg braces [Jagell and Heijbel, 1982]. The degree of mental retardation tends to correlate with the severity of spasticity, and most patients are moderately or profoundly retarded with intelligence quotient scores of less than 50. Many patients have speech defects of various types, and one third of the patients have an associated seizure disorder [Jagell and Heijbel, 1982; Theile, 1974]. Unlike with most other lipid disorders, patients with Sjögren-Larsson syndrome generally do not demonstrate neuroregression. A loss of ambulation can occur with age, but it is usually due to progressive contractures. Most patients with Sjögren-Larsson syndrome have short stature, usually due to leg contractures and decreased leg growth. Kyphoscoliosis is not uncommon, particularly in severely spastic patients. Nerve conduction studies are normal [Jagell and Heijbel, 1982]. The ichthyosis in Sjögren-Larsson syndrome is usually apparent at the time of birth, but a small proportion of patients first develop ichthyosis after several months of age or later [Jagell and Liden, 1982]. The ichthyosis tends to be mild to moderate in severity. Scales can be fine and dandruff-like, larger and more lamellar-like, or even thick and dark brown in appearance. The ichthyosis is generalized and typically affects the flexures, trunk, abdomen, back, extremities, nape of the neck, and dorsal areas of the hands and feet. Less severely affected are the palms and soles, whereas the face is usually spared. A collodion membrane is rarely seen in this disease [Rizzo, 1996]. Ophthalmologic abnormalities of the retina have been reported in Sjögren-Larsson syndrome [Jagell et al., 1980]. The most consistent finding is the presence of glistening white dots on the fundus, usually present in the foveal and perifoveal areas. These glistening white dots were observed in all 35 Swedish patients who could be examined, including young children [Jagell et al., 1980], but they have been reported in a lower percentage of non-Swedish patients. Retinal pigmentary changes and macular degeneration have also been seen in some patients, but corneal opacities or cataracts are not associated with Sjögren-Larsson syndrome [Rizzo, 1996].

A leukoencephalopathy is evident on MRI, revealing retardation of myelination and a mild persistent myelin deficit [Willemsen et al., 2004]. The MRI shows white matter disease involving primarily the parietal and frontal lobes [Hussain et al., 1995;Miyanomae et al., 1995]. A zone of increased signal intensity is seen in the periventricular white matter on T2-weighted images [Willemsen et al., 2004]. Proton magnetic resonance spectroscopy of white matter revealed a prominent peak at 1.3 ppm, normal levels of *N*-acetyl aspartate, and elevated levels of creatine (+14%), choline (+18%), and myoinositol (+54%) [Willemsen et al., 2004].

Treatment

Patients with Sjögren-Larsson may benefit from treatment with zileuton, a drug that inhibits the synthesis of leukotriene B_4 and other leukotrienes. It is especially effective for disabling pruritus [Willemsen et al., 2001a].

Cerebrotendinous Xanthomatosis

The clinical triad of cerebrotendinous xanthomatosis includes tendon xanthomas (especially of Achilles tendons), juvenile ocular cataracts, and nervous system dysfunction. The CNS abnormalities may consist of behavioral problems, mental retardation, dementia, pyramidal weakness, cerebellar ataxia, seizures, psychiatric disorders, and, rarely, parkinsonism [Berginer et al., 1989]. Juvenile cataracts are observed in more than 90% of cerebrotendinous xanthomatosis patients and may be the presenting symptom of the disease [Cruysberg et al., 1991]. Tendon xanthomas are found in 85% to 90% of patients with cerebrotendinous xanthomatosis. There is a strong preference for the Achilles tendon, but xanthomas and tuberous xanthomas are observed also in the tendons of other extensor muscles [Berginer et al., 1989]. Typically, banana-like swellings of the Achilles tendon develop and are documented by x-ray, CT, and MRI.

Neuroimaging (CT and MRI) in patients with cerebrotendinous xanthomatosis demonstrates diffuse brain and spine atrophy, white brain matter abnormalities above and especially below the tentorium, and, in some patients, focal lesions [Barkhof et al., 2000; Bencze et al., 1990]. The white matter of the cerebellum appears to be particularly affected in cerebrotendinous xanthomatosis.

Because some patients may have only the CNS changes without the cataracts or tendon xanthomas, cerebrotendinous xanthomatosis may be frequently overlooked as a diagnosis. Patients with CNS degeneration and white matter changes on MRI primarily affecting cerebellum should be screened for cerebrotendinous xanthomatosis. Cerebrotendinous xanthomatosis may be diagnosed after finding increased plasma and tissue cholestanol concentrations and low or normal plasma cholesterol levels.

The brain of patients with cerebrotendinous xanthomatosis was discovered by Menkes and colleagues [1968] to have increased amounts of cholestanol. Cholestanol is the 5-α-dihydro derivative of cholesterol and is present in small quantities associated with cholesterol in virtually every tissue and plasma. In normal subjects, cholestanol represents about 0.1% to 0.2% of the cholesterol. In contrast, cholestanol is increased 10-fold to 100-fold in cerebrotendinous xanthomatosis. The biologic basis for cerebrotendinous xanthomatosis is a deficiency of the sterol 27-hydroxylase enzyme. This enzyme is responsible for the production of bile acids. Recently mutations in the sterol 27-hydroxylase gene on the human chromosome 2 were determined to be the cause of cerebrotendinous xanthomatosis. Many mutations in the sterol 27-hydroxylase gene have been identified [Chen et al., 1998].

Because cerebrotendinous xanthomatosis results from an inherited defect in bile acid synthesis, treatment with the bile acid chenodeoxycholic acid has been used in cerebrotendinous xanthomatosis. Chenodeoxycholic acid appears to reverse the metabolic encephalopathy before destructive xanthomas appear in the brain [Salen et al., 1994]. Long-term treatment with chenodeoxycholic acid (750 mg/day) suppresses abnormal bile acid synthesis, as evidenced by the

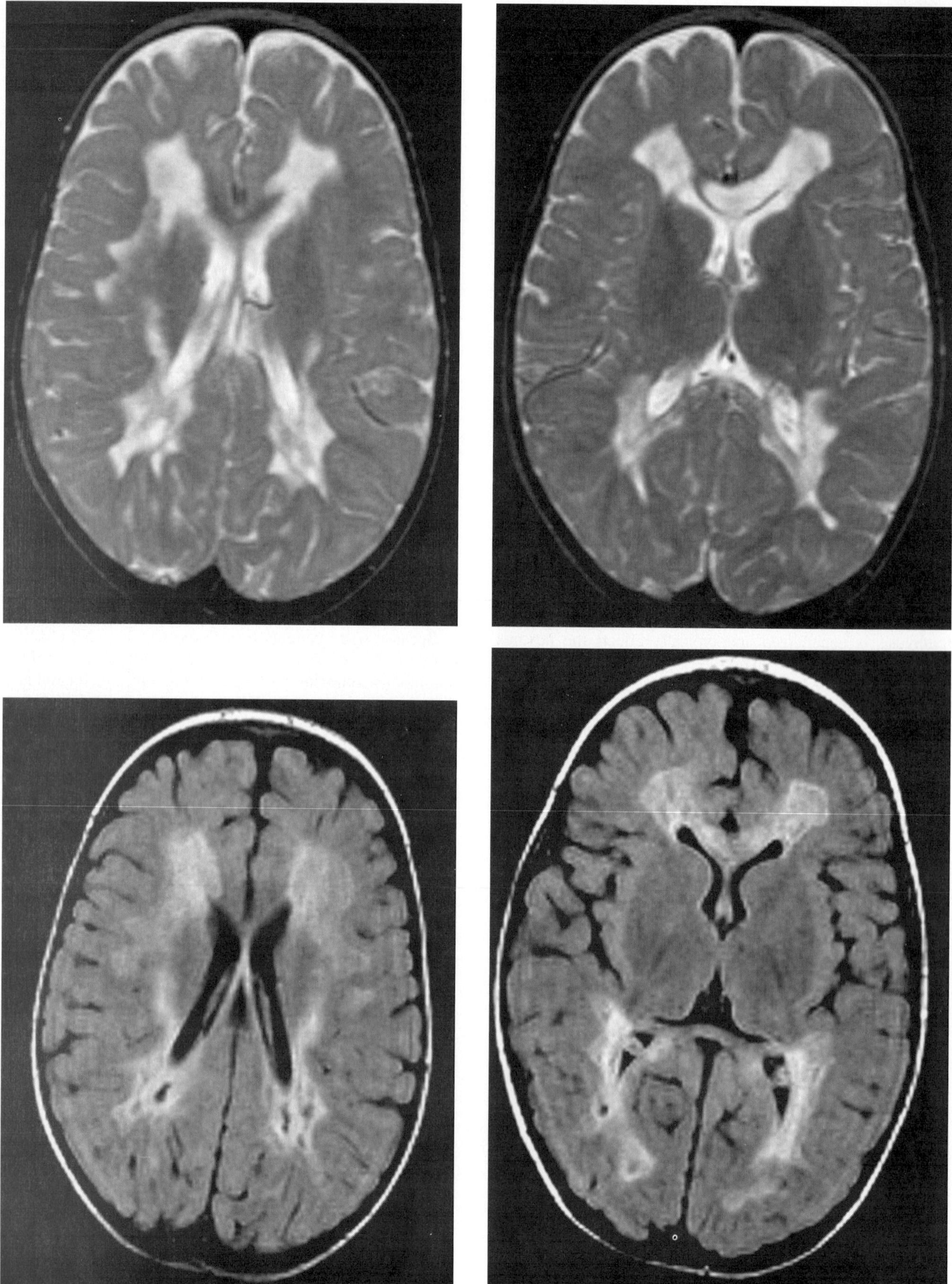

FIGURE 60-11 T2-weighted images (*top row*) and fluid-attenuated inversion recovery images (*bottom row*) in a 16-month-old female with isolated complex I deficiency. Note the extensive cerebral white matter abnormalities. The fluid-attenuated inversion recovery images show that there are multiple well-delineated cysts within the abnormal white matter.

almost total replacement of chenodeoxycholic acid in the enterohepatic pool and the disappearance of bile alcohol glucuronides from bile, plasma, and urine [Batta et al., 1987]. Plasma and cerebrospinal fluid cholestanol concentrations decline to normal levels. The neurologic improvement is better when treatment is started in young patients [van Heijst et al., 1998].

Mitochondrial Disorders

Mitochondrial disorders, diseases caused by abnormalities in mitochondrial respiratory chain function, frequently have white matter abnormalities. These include Leber's hereditary optic neuropathy, which affects optic nerve myelin, and MELAS syndrome (mitochondrial encephalomyopathy, lactic acidosis, and stroke), which has white and gray matter changes often in the parietal-occipital regions, not in a vascular distribution but probably related to a metabolic stroke. Diffuse white matter abnormalities have been noted in other mitochondrial diseases such as ubiquinone deficiency [Artuch et al., 1999] and succinate dehydrogenase deficiency [Brockmann et al., 2002]. In essence, many respiratory chain complex defects caused from mutations in either the mitochondrial or nuclear genomes may result in white matter lesions in addition to abnormalities in the gray matter [De Lonlay-Debeney et al., 2000]. The deep white matter lesions in mitochondrial diseases often appear necrotic with cystic degeneration and may occur more often in infants [Kang et al., 2002]. The white matter cysts in mitochondrial disorders tend to be multiple, small, and well delineated (Fig. 60-11). This pattern is in contrast to the white matter rarefaction and cystic degeneration in vanishing white matter disease and childhood ataxia with cerebral hypomyelination, which occurs in a melting-away pattern, usually without well-delineated cysts (see Fig. 60-10).

Cerebral Autosomal-Dominant Arteriopathy Subcortical Infarcts and Leukoencephalopathy

Cerebral autosomal-dominant arteriopathy subcortical infarcts and leukoencephalopathy (CADASIL) is a cause of leukoencephalopathy primarily affecting adults. The entity was described in 1977 as a familial multi-infarct dementia, although the disease is recognized more often because of the leukodystrophy noted on MRI [Sourander and Walinder, 1977]. The phenotypic spectrum usually begins after age 40, but asymptomatic at-risk individuals may have MRI abnormalities noted at times in childhood. The clinical manifestations consist of ischemic deficits, cognitive loss including dementia, migraine, psychiatric disturbances, and rarely seizures [Dichgans et al., 1998]. The clinical course is unrelenting and occurs very slowly over decades. Men appear to be at higher risk for the earlier loss of ambulation and life compared with women with CADASIL [Opherk et al., 2004]. The MRI pattern consists of hyperintensities on T2-weighted images in periventricular regions, deep white matter, anterior temporal lobes, basal ganglia, and infratentorial areas, which increase with age [Chabriat et al., 1998]. The cerebral pathology consists of white matter gliosis and a small vessel angiopathy with periodic acid-Schiff–positive material in the media of the vessel [Desmond et al., 1998]. Although confined to the CNS, CADASIL is a systemic vascular disease. The pathologic hallmark of the disease is a nonamyloid, nonatheroslerotic microangiopathy. Because of the ubiquitous nature of the vasculopathy, electron microscopy of skin can be used as a diagnostic tool. Electron microscopy of small arterioles in the skin demonstrates characteristic granular osmophilic material in the basement membranes, which indent the surface and appear to rise as flames of electron-dense material [Desmond et al., 1998].

The genetic basis for this autosomal-dominant disease was elucidated in 1993 when the gene was mapped to chromosome 19p13.1 and clarified further in 1996 when mutations in the *NOTCH3* were discovered [Joutel et al., 1997a]. The *NOTCH3* gene encodes a 300-kd transmembrane protein with a receptor and cell signal transduction function, which is important to embryonic development for many species. The gene contains 33 exons and contains 33 epidermal growth factor domains. As yet, the exact mechanism by which *NOTCH3* mutations cause the CADASIL phenotype is not understood. The mutations in *NOTCH3* appear to be very stereotyped, involving missense mutations with either a gain or loss of a cysteine residue [Joutel et al., 1997b]. A proposed mechanism of the disease pathology may be related to the abnormal accumulation of *NOTCH3* in the vascular smooth muscle of vessels and the abnormal *NOTCH* signaling through the RPB/JK pathway [Joutel et al., 2004]. Mutational analysis will greatly aid in diagnosis and improve the sensitivity of diagnostic testing.

Merosin Deficiency

An important cause for a leukoencephalopathy indicated on MRI is a merosin-deficient form of congenital muscular dystrophy or laminin-$\alpha 2$ deficiency [Lamer et al., 1998]. These children often have dramatic and unexpected white matter findings but no evidence of upper motor neuron signs and minimal cognitive findings. The clinical picture consists of hypotonia and gross motor delays caused by the muscle disease or at times peripheral neuropathy. The disease may be severe, with the child never able to walk, or mild, with walking occurring between the ages of 2 or 3 years. The disorder does not appear to be progressive. The MRI usually reveals a diffuse white matter signal increase on the T2-weighted image, but the cortex is not involved. The disease is associated with mutations in the laminin-2 gene, which is located on chromosome 6q2 [Hillaire et al., 1994]. Laminin-α-2 is associated with α-dystroglycan in muscle, but the protein is also found in CNS and Schwann cells within the basal lamina.

Glycogen Storage Disease Type IV (Branching Enzyme Deficiency)

Glycogen storage disease type IV (branching enzyme deficiency) usually appears in infancy with severe liver disease causing cirrhosis, portal hypertension, and early death [DiMauro et al., 1997]. Myopathy may be the presenting feature in many children, and cardiomyopathy has been reported in some individuals [Tang et al., 1994]. A late-onset variant of glycogen storage disease type IV, referred to as *adult polyglucosan storage disease*, consists of progressive weakness and spasticity of the legs, which may progress to quadriparesis, urinary incontinence, and a peripheral neuropathy. Cognitive impairments may be present, and a leukodystrophy has been noted in many patients. The branching enzyme is 1,4-glucan-6-glucosyltransferase. The gene expressing this enzyme has been identified and mapped to chromosome 3. The complementary DNA is 3 kb in length and encodes a protein of 702 amino acids [Thon et al., 1993]. One mutation (Tyr329Ser) in the gene encoding the branching enzyme has been reported in a series of Ashkenazi families with adult polyglucosan storage disease [Lossos et al., 1998].

ACKNOWLEDGMENT

The authors would like to thank David Margolin, M.D., Ph.D., for his thoughtful review and assistance on the multiple sclerosis section in this chapter.

REFERENCES

Adachi M, Schneck L, Cara J, et al. Spongy degeneration of the central nervous system (van Bogaert and Bertrand type; Canavan's disease). Hum Pathol 1973;4:331.

Adams R, Lyon G, Kolodny E. The neurology of inherited metabolic diseases. New York: McGraw-Hill, 1996.

Aicardi J. Diseases of the nervous system in childhood. Oxford: Blackwell Scientific, 1992.

Aicardi J, Goutières F. A progressive familial encephalopathy in infancy with calcifications of the basal ganglia and chronic cerebrospinal fluid lymphocytosis. Ann Neurol 1984;15:49.

Alexander WS. Progressive fibrinoid degeneration of fibrillary astrocytes associated with mental retardation in a hydrocephalic infant. Brain 1949;72:373.

Alvord EC, Jr., Jahnke U, Fischer EH, et al. The multiple causes of multiple sclerosis: The importance of age of infections in childhood. J Child Neurol 1987;2:313.

Anlar B, Basaran C, Kose G, et al. Acute disseminated encephalomyelitis in children: Outcome and prognosis. Neuropediatrics 2003;34:194.

Artuch R, Colome C, Vilaseca MA, et al. [Ubiquinone: Metabolism and functions. Ubiquinone deficiency and its implication in mitochondrial encephalopathies. Treatment with ubiquinone.] Rev Neurol 1999;29:59.

Barkhof F, Verrips A, Wesseling P, et al. Cerebrotendinous xanthomatosis: The spectrum of imaging findings and the correlation with neuropathologic findings. Radiology 2000;217:869.

Baslow MH, Kitada K, Suckow RF, et al. The effects of lithium chloride and other substances on levels of brain *N*-acetyl-L-aspartic acid in Canavan disease-like rats. Neurochem Res 2002;27:403.

Batta AK, Salen G, Shefer S, et al. Increased plasma bile alcohol glucuronides in patients with cerebrotendinous xanthomatosis: Effect of chenodeoxycholic acid. J Lipid Res 1987;28:1006.

Beck RW, Cleary PA, Anderson MM, Jr., et al. A randomized, controlled trial of corticosteroids in the treatment of acute optic neuritis. The Optic Neuritis Study Group. N Engl J Med 1992;326:581.

Beck RW, Cleary PA, Trobe JD, et al. The effect of corticosteroids for acute optic neuritis on the subsequent development of multiple sclerosis. The Optic Neuritis Study Group. N Engl J Med 1993;329:1764.

Bencze KS, Vande Polder DR, Prockop LD. Magnetic resonance imaging of the brain and spinal cord in cerebrotendinous xanthomatosis. J Neurol Neurosurg Psychiatry 1990;53:166.

Berginer VM, Salen G, Shefer S. Cerebrotendinous xanthomatosis. Neurol Clin 1989;7:55.

Bielschowsky M, Henneberg R. Über familiäre diffuse Sklerose (Leukodystrophia cerebri progressiva hereditaria). J Psychol Neurol 1928;36:131.

Blattner R, von Moers A, Leegwater PAJ, et al. Clinical and genetic heterogeneity in megalencephalic leukoencephalopathy with subcortical cysts (MLC). Neuropediatrics 2002;34:215.

Boespflug-Tanguy O, Mimault C, Melki J, et al. Genetic homogeneity of Pelizaeus-Merzbacher disease: Tight linkage to the proteolipoprotein locus in 16 affected families. PMD Clinical Group. Am J Hum Genet 1994;55:461.

Boulloche J, Aicardi J. Pelizaeus-Merzbacher disease: Clinical and nosological study. J Child Neurol 1986;1:233.

Bourre JM, Bornhoffen JH, Araoz AC, et al. Pelizaeus-Merzbacher disease: Brain lipid and fatty acid composition. J Neurochem 1978;30:719.

Brenner M, Johnson AB, Boespflug-Tanguy O, et al. Mutations in GFAP, encoding glial fibrillary acidic protein, are associated with Alexander disease. Nat Genet 2001;27:117.

Brockmann K, Bjornstad A, Dechent P, et al. Succinate in dystrophic white matter: A proton magnetic resonance spectroscopy finding characteristic for complex II deficiency. Ann Neurol 2002;52:38.

Cailloux F, Gauthier-Barichard F, Mimault C, et al. Genotype-phenotype correlation in inherited brain myelination defects due to proteolipid protein gene mutations. Clinical European Network on Brain Dysmyelinating Disease. Eur J Hum Genet 2000;8:837.

Campbell IL, Krucker T, Steffensen S, et al. Structural and functional neuropathology in transgenic mice with CNS expression of IFN-α. Brain Res 1999;835:46.

Canavan M. Schilder's encephalitis periaxialis diffusa: Report of a child aged sixteen and one half months. Arch Neurol Psychiatr 1931;25:299.

Carango P, Funanage VL, Quiros RE, et al. Overexpression of DM20 messenger RNA in two brothers with Pelizaeus-Merzbacher disease. Ann Neurol 1995;38:610.

Carney G, Wei S, Rizzo WB. Sjögren-Larsson syndrome: Seven novel mutations in the fatty aldehyde dehydrogenase gene ALDH3A2. Hum Mutat 2004;24:186.

Chabriat H, Levy C, Taillia H, et al. Patterns of MRI lesions in CADASIL. Neurology 1998;51:452.

Chen W, Kubota S, Teramoto T, et al. Genetic analysis enables definite and rapid diagnosis of cerebrotendinous xanthomatosis. Neurology 1998;51:865.

Cole GF, Auchterlonie LA, Best PV. Very early onset multiple sclerosis. Dev Med Child Neurol 1995;37:667.

Coles AJ, Wing MG, Molyneux P, et al. Monoclonal antibody treatment exposes three mechanisms underlying the clinical course of multiple sclerosis. Ann Neurol 1999a;46:296.

Coles AJ, Wing M, Smith S, et al. Pulsed monoclonal antibody treatment and autoimmune thyroid disease in multiple sclerosis. Lancet 1999b;354:1691.

Cruysberg JR, Wevers RA, Tolboom JJ. Juvenile cataract associated with chronic diarrhea in pediatric cerebrotendinous xanthomatosis [Letter]. Am J Ophthalmol 1991;112:606.

De Lonlay-Debeney P, von Kleist-Retzow JC, Hertz-Pannier L, et al. Cerebral white matter disease in children may be caused by mitochondrial respiratory chain defect. J Pediatr 2000;136:209.

De Laurenzi V, Rogers GR, Hamrock DJ, et al. Sjogren-Larsson syndrome is caused by mutations in the fatty aldehyde dehydrogenase gene. Nat Genet 1996;12:52.

De Laurenzi V, Rogers GR, Tarcsa E, et al. Sjogren-Larsson syndrome is caused by a common mutation in northern European and Swedish patients. J Invest Dermatol 1997;109:79.

Delasnerie-Laupretre N, Alperovitch A. Childhood infections in multiple sclerosis: A study of North African-born patients who migrated to France. The French Collaborative Group on Multiple Sclerosis. Neuroepidemiology 1990;9:118.

Desmond DW, Moroney JT, Lynch T, et al. CADASIL in a North American family: Clinical, pathologic, and radiologic findings. Neurology 1998;51:844.

Dichgans M, Mayer M, Uttner I, et al. The phenotypic spectrum of CADASIL: Clinical findings in 102 cases. Ann Neurol 1998;44:731.

Diehl H-J, Schaich M, Budzinski R-M, et al. Individual exons encode the integral membrane domains of human proteolipid protein. Proc Natl Acad Sci U S A 1986;83:9807.

DiMauro S, Servidei N, Tsujino S. Disorders of carbohydrate metabolism: Glycogen storage diseases. In: Rosenberg RN, Pruisner SB, DiMauro S, eds. The molecular and genetic basis of neurological disease. Boston: Butterworth-Heinemann, 1997;1067.

Duquette P, Murray TJ, Pleines J, et al. Multiple sclerosis in childhood: Clinical profile in 125 patients. J Pediatr 1987;111:359.

Engelbrecht V, Rassek M, Gartner J, et al. [Magnetic resonance tomography and localized proton spectroscopy in 2 siblings with Canavan's disease.] Rofo Fortschr Geb Rontgenstr Neuen Bildgeb Verfahr 1995;163:238.

Farrell K, Chung S, Becker LE, et al. Computed tomography in Alexander's disease. Ann Neurol 1984;15:605.
Fink DJ. Gene therapy for Canavan disease? Ann Neurol 2000;48:9.
Fogli A, Rodriguez D, Eymard-Pierre E, et al. Ovarian failure related to eukaryotic initiation factor 2B mutations. Am J Hum Genet 2003;72:1544.
Fogli A, Schiffmann R, Bertini E, et al. The effect of genotype on the natural history of eIF2B-related leukodystrophies. Neurology 2004;62:1509.
Fogli A, Wong K, Eymard-Pierre E, et al. Cree leukoencephalopathy and CACH/VWM disease are allelic at the EIF2B5 locus. Ann Neurol 2002;52:506.
Garbern JY, Yool DA, Moore GJ, et al. Patients lacking the major CNS myelin protein, proteolipid protein 1, develop length-dependent axonal degeneration in the absence of demyelination and inflammation. Brain 2002;125:551.
Garcia L, Gascon G, Ozand P, et al. Increased intracranial pressure in Alexander disease: A rare presentation of white-matter disease. J Child Neurol 1992;7:168.
Gascon GG, Ozand PT, Mahdi A, et al. Infantile CNS spongy degeneration—14 cases: Clinical update. Neurology 1990;40:1876.
Gawne-Cain ML, O'Riordan JI, Thompson AJ, et al. Multiple sclerosis lesion detection in the brain: A comparison of fast fluid-attenuated inversion recovery and conventional T2-weighted dual spin echo. Neurology 1997;49:364.
Gay CT, Hardies LJ, Rauch RA, et al. Magnetic resonance imaging demonstrates incomplete myelination in 18q– syndrome: Evidence for myelin basic protein haploinsufficiency. Am J Med Genet 1997;74:422.
Gencic S, Abuelo D, Ambler M, et al. Pelizaeus-Merzbacher disease: An X-linked neurologic disorder of myelin metabolism with a novel mutation in the gene encoding proteolipid protein. Am J Hum Genet 1989;45:435.
Ghezzi A, Deplano V, Faroni J, et al. Multiple sclerosis in childhood: Clinical features of 149 cases. Mult Scler 1997;3:43.
Golden GS, Woody RC. The role of nuclear magnetic resonance imaging in the diagnosis of MS in childhood. Neurology 1987;37:689.
Goldstein FB. Biosynthesis of N-acetyl-L-aspartic acid. Biochim Biophys Acta 1959;33:583.
Goodin DS, Frohman EM, Garmany GP Jr., et al. Disease modifying therapies in multiple sclerosis: Report of the Therapeutics and Technology Assessment Subcommittee of the American Academy of Neurology and the MS Council for Clinical Practice Guidelines. Neurology 2002;58:169.
Gorospe JR, Naidu S, Johnson AB, et al. Molecular findings in symptomatic and pre-symptomatic Alexander disease patients. Neurology 2002;58:1494.
Goutières F, Aicardi J, Barth PG, et al. Aicardi-Goutières syndrome: An update and results of interferon-alpha studies. Ann Neurol 1998;44:900.
Goutières F, Boulloche J, Bourgeois M, et al. Leukoencephalopathy, megalencephaly, and mild clinical course. A recently individualized familial leukodystrophy. Report on five new cases. J Child Neurol 1996;11:439.
Hahn CD, Shroff MM, Blaser SI, et al. MRI criteria for multiple sclerosis: Evaluation in a pediatric cohort. Neurology 2004;62:806.
Hanefeld F, Bauer HJ, Christen HJ, et al. Multiple sclerosis in childhood: Report of 15 cases. Brain Dev 1991;13:410.
Hanefeld F, Holzbach U, Kruse B, et al. Diffuse white matter disease in three children: An encephalopathy with unique features on magnetic resonance imaging and proton magnetic resonance spectroscopy. Neuropediatrics 1993;24:244.
Harbord MG, Harden A, Harding B, et al. Megalencephaly with dysmyelination, spasticity, ataxia, seizures and distinctive neurophysiological findings in two siblings. Neuropediatrics 1990;21:164.
Hauser SL, Fleischnick E, Weiner HL, et al. Extended major histocompatibility complex haplotypes in patients with multiple sclerosis. Neurology 1989;39:275.
Hershey LA, Trotter JL. The use and abuse of the cerebrospinal fluid IgG profile in the adult: A practical evaluation. Ann Neurol 1980;8:426.
Hillaire D, Leclerc A, Faure S, et al. Localization of merosin-negative congenital muscular dystrophy to chromosome 6q2 by homozygosity mapping. Hum Mol Genet 1994;3:1657.
Hohlfeld R. [Status and perspectives in the therapy of multiple sclerosis. A. Multiple sclerosis: The facts.] Krankenpfl J 1997;35:65.
Hudson L, Berndt J, Puckett C, et al. Aberrant splicing of proteolipid protein mRNA in the dysmyelinating jimpy mouse. Proc Natl Acad Sci U S A 1987;84:1454.
Hudson LD, Puckett C, Berndt J, et al. Mutation of the proteolipid protein gene PLP in a human X chromosome-linked myelin disorder. Proc Natl Acad Sci U S A 1989;86:8128.
Hurst EW. Acute haemorrhagic leukoencephalitis: A previously undefined entity. Med J Aust 1941;2:1.
Hussain MZ, Aihara M, Oba H, et al. MRI of white matter changes in the Sjögren-Larsson syndrome. Neuroradiology 1995;37:576.
IFNB Multiple Sclerosis Study Group. Interferon beta-1b is effective in relapsing-remitting multiple sclerosis. I. Clinical results of a multicenter, randomized, double-blind, placebo-controlled trial. Neurology 1993;43:655.
Iwaki A, Iwaki T, Goldman JE, et al. Accumulation of alpha B-crystallin in brains of patients with Alexander's disease is not due to an abnormality of the 5′-flanking and coding sequence of the genomic DNA. Neurosci Lett 1992;140:89.
Jagell S, Heijbel J. Sjögren-Larsson syndrome: Physical and neurological features. A survey of 35 patients. Helv Paediatr Acta 1982;37:519.
Jagell S, Liden S. Ichthyosis in the Sjogren-Larsson syndrome. Clin Genet 1982;21:243.
Jagell S, Polland W, Sandgren O. Specific changes in the fundus typical for the Sjogren-Larsson syndrome. An ophthalmological study of 35 patients. Acta Ophthalmol (Copenh) 1980;58:321.
Janson C, McPhee S, Bilaniuk L, et al. Clinical protocol. Gene therapy of Canavan disease: AAV-2 vector for neurosurgical delivery of aspartoacylase gene (ASPA) to the human brain. Hum Gene Ther 2002;13:1391.
Johnson AB. Alexander disease. In: Moser HW, ed. Neurodystrophies and neurolipidoses. Vol. 66. Amsterdam: Elsevier, 1996;701.
Johnson AB, Brenner M. Alexander's disease: Clinical, pathologic, and genetic features. J Child Neurol 2003;18:625.
Johnson KP, Brooks BR, Cohen JA, et al. Copolymer 1 reduces relapse rate and improves disability in relapsing-remitting multiple sclerosis: Results of a phase III multicenter, double-blind placebo-controlled trial. The Copolymer 1 Multiple Sclerosis Study Group. Neurology 1995;45:1268.
Johnson RT, Griffin DE, Gendelman HE. Postinfectious encephalomyelitis. Semin Neurol 1985;5:180.
Joutel A, Corpechot C, Ducros A, et al. Notch3 mutations in cerebral autosomal dominant arteriopathy with subcortical infarcts and leukoencephalopathy (CADASIL), a mendelian condition causing stroke and vascular dementia. Ann N Y Acad Sci 1997a;826:213.
Joutel A, Monet M, Domenga V, et al. Pathogenic mutations associated with cerebral autosomal dominant arteriopathy with subcortical infarcts and leukoencephalopathy differently affect Jagged1 binding and Notch3 activity via the RBP/JK signaling pathway. Am J Hum Genet 2004;74:338.
Joutel A, Vahedi K, Corpechot C, et al. Strong clustering and stereotyped nature of Notch3 mutations in CADASIL patients. Lancet 1997b;350:1511.
Kang PB, Hunter JV, Melvin JJ, et al. Infantile leukoencephalopathy owing to mitochondrial enzyme dysfunction. J Child Neurol 2002;17:421.
Kaul R, Balamurugan K, Gao GP, et al. Canavan disease: Genomic organization and localization of human ASPA to 17p13-ter and conservation of the ASPA gene during evolution. Genomics 1994;21:364.
Kaul R, Casanova J, Johnson AB, et al. Purification, characterization, and localization of aspartoacylase from bovine brain. J Neurochem 1991;56:129.
Kaul R, Gao GP, Balamurugan K, et al. Cloning of the human aspartoacylase cDNA and a common missense mutation in Canavan disease [see Comments]. Nat Genet 1993;5:118.
Kaye EM, Doll RF, Natowicz MR, et al. Pelizaeus-Merzbacher disease presenting as spinal muscular atrophy: Clinical and molecular studies. Ann Neurol 1994;36:916.
Keegan M, Konig F, Bitsh A, et al. Multiple sclerosis pathological subtype predicts response to therapeutic plasma exchange. Neurology 2004;62:A259.
Kelson TL, Craft DA, Rizzo WB. Carrier detection for Sjogren-Larsson syndrome. J Inherit Metab Dis 1992;15:105.
Kendall BE. Inborn errors and demyelination: MRI and the diagnosis of white matter disease. J Inherit Metab Dis 1993;16:771.
Kenealy SJ, Babron MC, Bradford Y, et al. A second-generation genomic screen for multiple sclerosis. Am J Hum Genet 2004; 75:1070.
Kesselring J, Miller DH, Robb SA, et al. Acute disseminated

encephalomyelitis. MRI findings and the distinction from multiple sclerosis. Brain 1990;113(Pt 2):291.

Kitada K, Akimitsu T, Shigematsu Y, et al. Accumulation of *N*-acetyl-L-aspartate in the brain of the tremor rat, a mutant exhibiting absence-like seizure and spongiform degeneration in the central nervous system. J Neurochem 2000;74:2512.

Kittagawa K, Sinoway MP, Yang C, et al. A proteolipid gene family: Expression in sharks and rays and possible evolution from an ancestral gene encoding a pore-forming polypeptide. Neuron 1993;11:433.

Koeppen AH, Ronca NA, Greenfield EA, et al. Defective biosynthesis of proteolipid protein in Pelizaeus-Merzbacher disease. Ann Neurol 1987;21:159.

Kolodny EH. Dysmyelinating and demyelinating conditions in infancy. Curr Opin Neurol Neurosurg 1993;6:379.

Kotil K, Kalayci M, Koseoglu T, et al. Myelinoclastic diffuse sclerosis (Schilder's disease): Report of a case and review of the literature. Br J Neurosurg 2002;16:516.

Kuroda Y, Shimamoto Y. Human tumor necrosis factor-alpha augments experimental allergic encephalomyelitis in rats. J Neuroimmunol 1991;34:159.

Kurtzke JF. MS epidemiology world wide. One view of current status. Acta Neurol Scand Suppl 1995;161:23.

Lamer S, Carlier RY, Pinard JM, et al. Congenital muscular dystrophy: Use of brain MR imaging findings to predict merosin deficiency. Radiology 1998;206:811.

Lazzarini A, Schwarz KO, Jiang S, et al. Pelizaeus-Merzbacher-like disease: Exclusion of the proteolipid protein locus and documentation of a new locus on Xq. Neurology 1997;49:824.

Leake JA, Albani S, Kao AS, et al. Acute disseminated encephalomyelitis in childhood: Epidemiologic, clinical and laboratory features. Pediatr Infect Dis J 2004;23:756.

Lebon P, Meritet JF, Krivine A, et al. Interferon and Aicardi-Goutières syndrome. Eur J Paediatr Neurol 2002;6(Suppl A):A47.

Leegwater PA, Konst AA, Kuyt B, et al. The gene for leukoencephalopathy with vanishing white matter is located on chromosome 3q27. Am J Hum Genet 1999;65:728.

Leegwater PA, Vermeulen G, Könst AA, et al. Subunits of the translation initiation factor eIF2B are mutant in leukoencephalopathy with vanishing white matter. Nat Genet 2001a;29:383.

Leegwater PA, Yuan BQ, van der Steen J, et al. Mutations of MLC1 (KIAA0027), encoding a putative membrane protein, cause megalencephalic leukoencephalopathy with subcortical cysts. Am J Hum Genet 2001b;68:831.

Leone P, Janson CG, Bilaniuk L, et al. Aspartoacylase gene transfer to the mammalian central nervous system with therapeutic implications for Canavan disease. Ann Neurol 2000;48:27.

Li R, Messing A, Goldman JE, et al. GFAP mutations in Alexander disease. Int J Dev Neurosci 2002;20:259.

Lossos A, Meiner Z, Barash V, et al. Adult polyglucosan body disease in Ashkenazi Jewish patients carrying the Tyr329Ser mutation in the glycogen-branching enzyme gene. Ann Neurol 1998;44:867.

Lublin FD, Reingold SC. Defining the clinical course of multiple sclerosis: Results of an international survey. National Multiple Sclerosis Society (USA) Advisory Committee on Clinical Trials of New Agents in Multiple Sclerosis. Neurology 1996;46:907.

Luo Y, Huang K. Spongy degeneration of the CNS in infancy. Arch Neurol 1984;41:164.

Lyon G, Adams RD, Kolodny EH. Neurology of hereditary metabolic diseases. New York: McGraw-Hill, 1996.

Macklin W, Gardinier M, Obaso Z. Myelination and dysmyelination. Ann N Y Acad Sci 1990;605:183.

Matalon R. Canavan disease: Diagnosis and molecular analysis. Genet Test 1997;1:21.

Matalon R, Kaul R, Casanova J, et al. SSIEM Award. Aspartoacylase deficiency: The enzyme defect in Canavan disease. J Inherit Metab Dis 1989;12(Suppl 2):329.

Matalon R, Kaul R, Michals K. Canavan disease: Biochemical and molecular studies. J Inherit Metab Dis 1993;16:744.

Matalon R, Michals K, Gashkoff P. Prenatal diagnosis of Canavan disease. J Inherit Metab Dis 1992;15:392.

Matalon R, Michals K, Kaul R. Canavan disease: From spongy degeneration to molecular analysis. J Pediatr 1995;127:511.

Matalon R, Michals K, Kaul R, et al. Spongy degeneration of the brain: Canavan disease. Int Pediatr 1990;5:121.

Matalon R, Michals K, Sebesta D, et al. Aspartoacylase deficiency and *N*-acetylaspartic aciduria in patients with Canavan disease. Am J Med Genet 1988;29:463.

Matalon R, Rady PL, Platt KA, et al. Knock-out mouse for Canavan disease: A model for gene transfer to the central nervous system. J Gene Med 2000;2:165.

Mattei MG, Alliel PM, Dautigny A, et al. The gene encoding for the major brain proteolipid (PLP) maps to the q-22 band of the human X chromosome. Hum Genet 1986;72:352.

McDonald WI, Compston A, Edan G, et al. Recommended diagnostic criteria for multiple sclerosis: Guidelines from the international panel on the diagnosis of multiple sclerosis. Ann Neurol 2001;50:121.

McFarlin DE, McFarland HF. Multiple sclerosis (first of two parts). N Engl J Med 1982a;307:1183.

McFarlin DE, McFarland HF. Multiple sclerosis (second of two parts). N Engl J Med 1982b;307:1246.

Merzbacher L. Eine eigenartige familiare Erkrankungsform (aplasia axialis extracorticalis congenita). Z Neurol Psychiat 1910;3:1.

Messing A, Head MW, Galles K, et al. Fatal encephalopathy with astrocyte inclusions in GFAP transgenic mice. Am J Pathol 1998;152:391.

Miller DH, Khan OA, Sheremata WA, et al. A controlled trial of natalizumab for relapsing multiple sclerosis. N Engl J Med 2003;348:15.

Miyake M, Kakimoto Y, Sorimachi M. A gas chromatographic method for the determination of N-acetyl-L-aspartic acid, N-acetyl-alpha-aspartylglutamic acid and beta-citryl-L-glutamic acid and their distributions in the brain and other organs of various species of animals. J Neurochem 1981;36:804.

Miyanomae Y, Ochi M, Yoshioka H, et al. Cerebral MRI and spectroscopy in Sjögren-Larsson syndrome: Case report. Neuroradiology 1995;37:225.

Nadon NL, Duncan ID, Hudson LD. A point mutation in the proteolipid protein gene of the "shaking pup" interrupts oligodendrocyte development. Development 1990;110:529.

Namekawa M, Takiyama Y, Aoki Y, et al. Identification of GFAP gene mutation in hereditary adult-onset Alexander's disease. Ann Neurol 2002;52:779.

Nave K-A, Lai C, Bloom FE, et al. Splice site selection in the proteolipid protein (PLP) gene transcript and primary structure of the DM-20 protein of central nervous system myelin. Proc Natl Acad Sci U S A 1987;84:5665.

Nave KA, Boespflug-Tanguy O. X-linked developmental defects of myelination: From mouse mutants to human genetic disease. Neuroscientist 1996;2:33.

Ohtake H, Shimohata T, Terajima K, et al. Adult-onset leukoencephalopathy with vanishing white matter with a missense mutation in EIF2B5. Neurology 2004;62:1601.

Olivier M, Lenard HG, Aksu F, et al. A new leukoencephalopathy with bilateral anterior temporal lobe cysts. Neuropediatrics 1998;29:225.

Ono J, Kodaka R, Imai K, et al. Evaluation of myelination by means of the T2 value on magnetic resonance imaging. Brain Dev 1993;15:433.

Opherk C, Peters N, Herzog J, et al. Long-term prognosis and causes of death in CADASIL: A retrospective study in 411 patients. Brain 2004;127:2533.

Patrono C, Di Giacinto G, Eymard-Pierre E, et al. Genetic heterogeneity of megalencephalic leukoencephalopathy and subcortical cysts. Neurology 2003;61:534.

Pelizaeus F. Uber eine eigentumliche form spastischer Lahmung mit Zerebralerscheinungen auf hereditarer Grundlage (multiple Sklerose). Arch Psychiatr Nervenkr 1885;16:698.

Pigg M, Jagell S, Sillen A, et al. The Sjogren-Larsson syndrome gene is close to D17S805 as determined by linkage analysis and allelic association. Nat Genet 1994;8:361.

Poser CM, Brinar VV. Diagnostic criteria for multiple sclerosis. Clin Neurol Neurosurg 2001;103:1.

Poser CM, Goutières F, Carpentier MA, et al. Schilder's myelinoclastic diffuse sclerosis. Pediatrics 1986;77:107.

Poser CM, Paty DW, Scheinberg L, et al. New diagnostic criteria for multiple sclerosis: Guidelines for research protocols. Ann Neurol 1983;13:227.

Pridmore CL, Baraitser M, Harding B, et al. Alexander's disease: Clues to diagnosis. J Child Neurol 1993;8:133.

Reichard EA, Ball WS, Bove KE. Alexander disease: A case report and review of the literature. Pediatr Pathol Lab Med 1996;16:327.

Rizzo W. Sjogren-Larsson syndrome. In: Moser HW, ed. Neurodystrophies and neurolipidoses, Vol. 22 (66). Amsterdam: Elsevier, 1996;615.

Rizzo WB, Carney G, Lin Z. The molecular basis of Sjogren-Larsson syndrome: Mutation analysis of the fatty aldehyde dehydrogenase gene. Am J Hum Genet 1999;65:1547.

Rizzo WB, Craft DA. Sjogren-Larsson syndrome. Deficient activity of the fatty aldehyde dehydrogenase component of fatty alcohol:NAD+ oxidoreductase in cultured fibroblasts. J Clin Invest 1991;88:1643.

Rizzo WB, Craft DA, Kelson TL, et al. Prenatal diagnosis of Sjogren-Larsson syndrome using enzymatic methods. Prenat Diagn 1994;14:577.

Rodriguez D, Gauthier F, Bertini E, et al. Infantile Alexander disease: Spectrum of GFAP mutations and genotype-phenotype correlation. Am J Hum Genet 2001;69:1134.

Rogers GR, Rizzo WB, Zlotogorski A, et al. Genetic homogeneity in Sjogren-Larsson syndrome: Linkage to chromosome 17p in families of different non-Swedish ethnic origins. Am J Hum Genet 1995;57:1123.

Rosman NP, Gottlieb SM, Bernstein CA. Acute hemorrhagic leukoencephalitis: Recovery and reversal of magnetic resonance imaging findings in a child. J Child Neurol 1997;12:448.

Ruddle NH, Bergman CM, McGrath KM, et al. An antibody to lymphotoxin and tumor necrosis factor prevents transfer of experimental allergic encephalomyelitis. J Exp Med 1990;172:1193.

Ruggieri M, Polizzi A, Pavone L, et al. Multiple sclerosis in children under 6 years of age. Neurology 1999;53:478.

Rushton AR, Shaywitz BA, Duncan CC, et al. Computed tomography in the diagnosis of Canavan's disease. Ann Neurol 1981;10:57.

Russo LS, Aron A, Anderson PJ. Alexander's disease: A report and reappraisal. Neurology 1976;26:607.

Salen G, Batta AK, Tint GS, et al. Comparative effects of lovastatin and chenodeoxycholic acid on plasma cholestanol levels and abnormal bile acid metabolism in cerebrotendinous xanthomatosis. Metabolism 1994;43:1018.

Saugier-Veber P, Munnich A, Bonneau D, et al. X-linked spastic paraplegia and Pelizaeus-Merzbacher disease are allelic disorders at the proteolipid protein locus. Nat Genet 1994;6:257.

Sawcer S, Maranian M, Setakis E, et al. A whole genome screen for linkage disequilibrium in multiple sclerosis confirms disease associations with regions previously linked to susceptibility. Brain 2002;125:1337.

Schiffmann R, Moller JR, Trapp BD, et al. Childhood ataxia with diffuse central nervous system hypomyelination. Ann Neurol 1994;35:331.

Schlote W. Rosenthalsche "fasern" und spongiobiasten in zentralnervensystem: II. Elektronenmikroskopische untersuchungen bedentung der Rosenthalschen "fasern." Beitr Pathol 1966;133:460.

Schneider A, Montague P, Griffiths I, et al. Uncoupling of hypomyelination and glial cell death by a mutation in the proteolipid protein gene. Nature 1992;358:758.

Schwankhaus JD, Parisi JE, Gulledge WR, et al. Hereditary adult-onset Alexander's disease with palatal myoclonus, spastic paraparesis, and cerebellar ataxia. Neurology 1995;45:2266.

Seitelberger F. Neuropathology and genetics of Pelizaeus-Merzbacher disease. Brain Pathol 1995;5:267.

Seitelberger F. Pelizaeus-Merzbacher disease. In: Vinken PJ, Bruyn GW, eds. Handbook of clinical neurology, Vol. 10. Amsterdam: Elsevier, 1970;150.

Seitelberger F, Urbanits S, Nave K-L. Pelizaeus-Merzbacher disease. In: Moser H, ed. Neurodystrophies and neurolipidoses, Vol. 66. Amsterdam: Elsevier, 1996;559.

Selcen D, Anlar B, Renda Y. Multiple sclerosis in childhood: Report of 16 cases. Eur Neurol 1996;36:79.

Shigematsu H, Okamura N, Shimeno H, et al. Purification and characterization of the heat-stable factors essential for the conversion of lignoceric acid to cerebronic acid and glutamic acid: Identification of N-acetyl-L-aspartic acid. J Neurochem 1983;40:814.

Shiroma N, Kanazawa N, Kato Z, et al. Molecular genetic study in Japanese patients with Alexander disease: A novel mutation, R79L. Brain Dev 2003;25:116.

Shy ME, Hobson G, Jain M, et al. Schwann cell expression of PLP1 but not DM20 is necessary to prevent neuropathy. Ann Neurol 2003;53:354.

Sillen A, Jagell S, Wadelius C. A missense mutation in the FALDH gene identified in Sjogren-Larsson syndrome patients originating from the northern part of Sweden. Hum Genet 1997;100:201.

Sindern E, Haas J, Stark E, et al. Early onset MS under the age of 16: Clinical and paraclinical features. Acta Neurol Scand 1992;86:280.

Singhal BS, Gursahani RD, Udani VP, et al. Megalencephalic leukodystrophy in an Asian Indian ethnic group. Pediatr Neurol 1996;14:291.

Sjögren T, Larsson T. Oligophrenia in combination with congenital ichthyosis and spastic disorders. Acta Psychiatr Neurol Scand 1957;32:1.

Sourander P, Walinder J. Hereditary multi-infarct dementia. Morphological and clinical studies of a new disease. Acta Neuropathol 1977;1:1015.

Stumpf E, Masson H, Duquette A, et al. Adult Alexander disease with autosomal dominant transmission: A distinct entity caused by mutation in the glial fibrillary acid protein gene. Arch Neurol 2003;60:1307.

Tang TT, Segura AD, Chen Y-T, et al. Neonatal hypotonia and cardiomyopathy secondary to type IV glycogenosis. Acta Neuropathol 1994;87:531.

Theile U. Larsson-Larsson syndrome. Oligophrenia—ichthyosis—di-tetraplegia. Humangenetik 1974;22:91.

Thon VJ, Khalil M, Cannon JF. Isolation of human glycogen branching enzyme cDNAs by screening complementation in yeast. J Biol Chem 1993;268:7509.

Thyagarajan D, Chataway T, Li R, et al. Dominantly-inherited adult-onset leukodystrophy with palatal tremor caused by a mutation in the glial fibrillary acidic protein gene. Mov Disord 2004;19:1244.

Toft PB, Geiss-Holtorff R, Rolland MO, et al. Magnetic resonance imaging in juvenile Canavan disease. Eur J Pediatr 1993;152:750.

Topcu M, Yalnizoglu D, Saatci I, et al. Effect of topiramate on enlargement of head in Canavan disease: A new option for treatment of megalencephaly. Turk J Pediatr 2004;46:67.

Tsukamoto N, Chang C, Yoshida A. Mutations associated with Larsson-Larsson syndrome. Ann Hum Genet 1997;61:235.

Uhlenberg B, Schuelke M, Ruschendorf F, et al. Mutations in the gene encoding gap junction protein alpha 12 (connexin 46.6) cause Pelizaeus-Merzbacher-like disease. Am J Hum Genet 2004;75:251.

van Bogaert L, Bertrand I. Sur une idiotie familiale avec degenerescence spongieuse du nevraxe. Acta Neur Psychiatr Belg 1949;49:572.

van der Knaap MS, Barth PG, Gabreels FJM, et al. A new leukoencephalopathy with vanishing white matter. Neurology 1997;48:845.

van der Knaap MS, Barth PG, Stroink H, et al. Leukoencephalopathy with swelling and a discrepantly mild clinical course in eight children. Ann Neurol 1995;37:324.

van der Knaap MS, Barth PG, Vrensen GF, et al. Histopathology of an infantile-onset spongiform leukoencephalopathy with a discrepantly mild clinical course. Acta Neuropathol 1996;92:206.

van der Knaap MS, Leegwater PA, Konst AA, et al. Mutations in each of the five subunits of translation initiation factor eIF2B can cause leukoencephalopathy with vanishing white matter. Ann Neurol 2002;51:264.

van der Knaap MS, Leegwater PA, van Berkel CG, et al. Arg113His mutation in eIF2Bepsilon as cause of leukoencephalopathy in adults. Neurology 2004;62:1598.

van der Knaap MS, Naidu S, Breiter SN, et al. Alexander disease: Diagnosis with MR imaging. AJNR Am J Neuroradiol 2001;22:541.

van der Knaap MS, van Berkel CG, Herms J, et al. eIF2B-related disorders: Antenatal onset and involvement of multiple organs. Am J Hum Genet 2003;73:1199.

van Heijst AF, Verrips A, Wevers RA, et al. Treatment and follow-up of children with cerebrotendinous xanthomatosis. Eur J Pediatr 1998;157:313.

Weinshenker BG, O'Brien PC, Petterson TM, et al. A randomized trial of plasma exchange in acute central nervous system inflammatory demyelinating disease. Ann Neurol 1999;46:878.

Willard H, Riordan J. Assignment of the gene for myelin proteolipid protein to the X chromosome: Implications for X-linked myelin disorders. Science 1985;230:940.

Willemsen MA, Lutt MA, Steijlen PM, et al. Clinical and biochemical effects of zileuton in patients with the Larsson-Larsson syndrome. Eur J Pediatr 2001a;160:711.

Willemsen MA, Rotteveel JJ, de Jong JG, et al. Defective metabolism of leukotriene B4 in the Larsson-Larsson syndrome. J Neurol Sci 2001b;183:61.

Willemsen MA, Van Der Graaf M, van der Knaap MS, et al. MR imaging and proton MR spectroscopic studies in Sjögren-Larsson syndrome: Characterization of the leukoencephalopathy. AJNR Am J Neuroradiol 2004;25:649.

Yan Y, Lagenaur C, Narayanan V. Molecular cloning of M6: Identification of a PLP/DM20 gene family. Neuron 1993;11:423.

Zeman W, DeMyer WE, Falls HF. Pelizaeus-Merzbacher disease: A study in nosology. J Neuropathol Exp Neurol 1964;23:334.

PART X

Brain Injury and Disorders of Consciousness

CHAPTER 61

Impairment of Consciousness and Coma

Donald A. Taylor and Stephen Ashwal

The study of consciousness represents one of the oldest areas of neuroscience. Multiple philosophical, metaphysical, and psychologic theories of consciousness have been elucidated [Zeman, 2001]. William James, in 1890, wrote that the cortex is the sole organ of consciousness in man [James, 1890]. Nonetheless, reconciliation of the concept of mind (consciousness and awareness) and the structure and function of the brain has long been elusive [Sperry, 1952]. Evidence that there is a neural correlate of consciousness, however, is clearly established [Crick and Koch, 1998].

An early step in the neurobiologic understanding of consciousness and its alterations was the identification of brainstem structures essential for cortical activation [Damasio, 2003; Moruzzi and Magoun, 1949; Neylan, 1995]. Recent theories that the brain's electromagnetic field is the equivalent of the conscious mind allow reconciliation of the mind-brain problem and suggest methodology to scientifically study consciousness and alteration of consciousness at the neurophysiologic level [John, 2001, 2002; John et al., 2001; McFadden, 2002a, 2002b]. Because neurobiologic processes that are realized in brain structures are responsible for consciousness [Baars et al., 2003; Neylan, 1995; Searle, 2000], neurologic disorders of the cortex and its brainstem activators result in impairment of consciousness and coma.

Understanding neurologic disease depends on the clinical assessment and interpretation of consciousness, the content of consciousness, and alterations of consciousness. The evaluation of all disorders of higher cortical function fundamentally begins with consciousness assessment, and all signs and symptoms of neurologic impairment must be interpreted based on the state of consciousness and awareness [Giacino, 1997].

Consciousness refers to the state of awareness of self and environment [James, 1890; Plum and Posner, 1982]. Evaluation of consciousness in the pediatric patient must take into account age and the appropriate developmental level. Conscious individuals may have abnormal content of consciousness, such as hallucinations, delirium, or dementia. Therefore, normal consciousness must be distinguished from abnormal consciousness as objectively as possible. Unconsciousness is unawareness of self and environment and may be physiologic (sleep) or pathologic (coma or the vegetative state). The fundamental difference between sleep and coma is that with appropriate stimulus intensity and duration, a sleeping person can be aroused to a normal state of consciousness, whereas a comatose patient cannot. Thus, the diagnosis of coma and other impairments of consciousness involves both state and reactivity. The physiologic differences between sleep and coma are actually more profound. Sleep is a biologically active state with identifiable behavioral and electroencephalographic stages, whereas coma is a state of reduced neuronal activity [Moruzzi, 1972].

Along the continuum from normal consciousness to coma or unarousable unconsciousness, many terms are used to describe mental state and reactivity. When there is doubt about the appropriate use of one of these terms, it is far better to describe the state and reactivity of the individual rather than label it. Definitions of consciousness, impairment of consciousness, coma, and related states have been proposed throughout the history of medicine and have been reviewed, refined, and stated systematically during the past several decades [Ashwal, 1996; Ashwal and Cranford, 2002; Bates, 1993; Bozza Marrubini, 1984; Medical Research Council Brain Injuries Committee, 1941; Michelson and Ashwal, 2004; Plum and Posner, 1982].

DEFINITIONS

Consciousness is the spontaneously occurring state of awareness of self and environment. Consciousness has two dimensions—wakefulness and awareness [Multi-Society Task Force on Persistent Vegetative State, 1994]. Normal consciousness requires arousal, an independent, autonomic-vegetative brain function subserved by ascending stimuli—emanating from pontine tegmentum, posterior hypothalamus, and thalamus—that activate mechanisms inducing wakefulness. Awareness is subserved by cerebral cortical neurons and their reciprocal projections to and from the major subcortical nuclei. Awareness requires wakefulness, but wakefulness can be present without awareness.

In preterm and term newborns and in infants, consciousness may require a more operational definition. Crying when uncomfortable or hungry at least suggests awareness of self, and visual alertness or soothing to an auditory stimulus (such as parent's voice) suggests environmental awareness. The presence of an appropriate socially responsive smile in the younger infant is a clear marker of consciousness. The bilateral absence of the cerebral cortex, as in anencephaly or severe hydranencephaly, may make realistic assessment of consciousness impractical.

Clouding of consciousness is the minimal reduction of wakefulness or awareness wherein the main difficulty is attention or vigilance. Clouding of consciousness is distinguished from daydreaming in that the child cannot be easily stimulated to normal consciousness. It is also distinguished from the inattention of attention-deficit–hyperactivity disorder by failure to improve with one-to-one confrontation or removal of distractions.

Confusion is the state of impaired ability to think and reason clearly at a developmentally and intellectually appropriate level. Confused children have persistent difficulty with orientation, simple cognitive processing, and acquisition of new memory. Normal suggestibility and anxiety in younger children may be misleading when assessing confusion. In newborns, infants, and younger children, clouding of consciousness and confusion are difficult to assess and are not of practical value. In the older child or adolescent, confusion may be an important indicator of drug ingestion, toxin exposure, or severity of concussion. Other definitions of impairment of consciousness states may be divided into the following categories:

- Impairment of consciousness with activated mental state
- Impairment of consciousness with reduced mental state
- Impairment of consciousness along the continuum of coma–vegetative state–minimally conscious state and related conditions

Impairment of Consciousness with Activated Mental State

Several altered states of consciousness with activated mental state can be seen in older children and may be difficult to differentiate from each other.

Hallucinations are perceptions of sensory input that are not present; *illusions* are misinterpretations of actual sensory stimuli. *Delusions* are incorrect thoughts or beliefs that do not change when challenged by contradictory evidence or logical reason. *Delirium* is an activated mental state that may include disorientation, irritability, fearful responses, and sensory misperception. Patients may be hyperactive and have signs of increased sympathetic tone. Visual hallucinations, when present, are more common than auditory hallucinations, and the patient may experience delusional thought or illusions. Delirium is more likely to involve both cerebral hemispheres than one side of the cerebrum or the brainstem alone. Search for causes of delirium, therefore, should begin with consideration of pathology of both hemispheres. In children, common causes include intoxication, infection, fever, metabolic disorders, and epilepsy. Night terrors are non–rapid-eye-movement sleep disorders that occur commonly in children and closely resemble the delirious state. Children experiencing night terrors, however, will return to normal sleep, from which they can be aroused to normal wakefulness.

Impairment of Consciousness with Reduced Mental State

Obtundation is mild to moderate alertness reduction with decreased interest in the environment and slower than normal reactivity to stimulation. Obtunded patients appear abnormally drowsy and often sleep when left alone.

Stupor is a state of unresponsiveness with little or no spontaneous movement resembling deep sleep from which the patient can only be aroused by vigorous and repeated stimulation. Communication is absent or minimal. The best responsive level of consciousness is still quite abnormal, and without continuous stimulation, the patient returns to the prestimulation state.

Coma is a state of deep, unarousable, sustained pathologic unconsciousness with the eyes closed that results from dysfunction of the ascending reticular-activating system in the brainstem or in both cerebral hemispheres [Multi-Society Task Force on Persistent Vegetative State, 1994]. Coma usually requires the period of unconsciousness to persist for at least 1 hour to distinguish coma from syncope, concussion, or other states of transient unconsciousness. The term *unconsciousness* implies global or total unawareness and applies equally to patients in coma or vegetative states. Patients in coma are unconscious because they lack both wakefulness and awareness. In contrast, patients in vegetative states are unconscious because, although they have retained wakefulness, they lack awareness. The depth of coma may be further specified by assessment of brainstem reflexes, breathing pattern, change of pulse or res-

TABLE 61-1

Severe Disorders of Consciousness and Related Conditions

CONDITION	SELF-AWARENESS	PAIN AND SUFFERING	SLEEP-WAKE CYCLES	MOTOR FUNCTION	RESPIRATORY FUNCTION	OUTCOME
Coma	Absent	No	Absent	No purposeful movement	Variably depressed	Evolves to persistent vegetative state, dies, or recovers in 2-4 weeks
Vegetative state	Absent	No	Intact	No purposeful movement	Normal	Depends on etiology
Minimally conscious state	Very limited	Yes	Intact	Severe limitation of movement	Variably depressed	Recovery unknown
Akinetic mutism	Limited	Yes	Intact	Moderate limitation of movement	Normal to variably depressed	Recovery unlikely or limited
Locked-in syndrome	Present	Yes	Intact	Quadriplegia; pseudobulbar palsy; eye movements preserved	Normal to variably depressed	Recovery unlikely; remains quadriplegic
Brain death	Absent	No	Absent	None or only reflex spinal movements	Absent	None

piratory rate to stimulation, or stimulus-induced nonspecific movement.

Vegetative State, Minimally Conscious State, and Related Conditions

Table 61-1 lists several of the major neurologic conditions that the clinician must be capable of differentiating from coma. This table was modified from the report issued by the Multi-Society Task Force on the Persistent Vegetative State [1994] and more recent work that is defining the concept of the minimally conscious state [American Congress of Rehabilitation Medicine, 1995; Giacino et al., 1997]. The principal neurologic conditions in which there may be overlap of clinical findings on examination that should be differentiated from coma are discussed in the next sections.

Vegetative State

The vegetative state can be described as a condition of complete unawareness of the self and the environment accompanied by sleep-wake cycles with either complete or partial preservation of hypothalamic and brainstem autonomic (vegetative) functions [Zeman, 1997]. Criteria to diagnose the vegetative state have been recommended for adults and children by the Multi-Society Task Force on Persistent Vegetative State and are listed in Box 61-1. Children in a vegetative state lack evidence of self-awareness or recognition of external stimuli [Feinberg and Ferry, 1984]. Rather than being in a state of "eyes-closed" coma, they remain unconscious but have irregular periods of wakefulness alternating with periods of sleeping. Vegetative patients demonstrate a variety of sounds, emotional expressions, and body movements, and they may smile or shed tears. They have inconsistent head- and eye-turning movements to sounds and inconsistent, nonpurposeful trunk and limb movements. The most objective sign is lack of sustained visual fixation or visual tracking.

It is estimated that there are about 4,000 to 10,000 children in a vegetative state in the United States [Ashwal, 1996] and about 100,000 worldwide [Ashwal, 2005]. The etiology of the vegetative state in children can be classified into the following three broad groups of disorders: (1) acute traumatic and nontraumatic brain injuries; (2) metabolic and degenerative disorders affecting the nervous system; and (3) developmental malformations. The percentage of children having these etiologies of the vegetative state is as follows: acute traumatic and nontraumatic injuries (30%), perinatal insults (17.7%), chromosomal disorders or congenital malformations (13.0%), infections (10.3%), and unknown causes (28%) [Ashwal et al., 1994].

The most common causes of acute brain injury leading to the vegetative state in children are head trauma and hypoxic-ischemic encephalopathies [Adams et al., 2000]. Severe traumatic brain injury in children is often due to non-accidental trauma but also occurs after a motor vehicle crash, particularly when infant restraints have not been used or when a pedestrian versus motor vehicle crash occurs. Hypoxic-ischemic injuries after cardiorespiratory arrest occur at birth, after episodes of near-miss sudden infant death syndrome or near drowning, and after other acute life-threatening episodes, including shock due to systemic trauma or infection.

The clinical course of evolution to a vegetative state after an acute injury usually begins with eyes-closed coma for several days to weeks followed by the appearance of sleep-wake cycles. Gillies and Seshia retrospectively determined that the transition from eyes-closed coma to the vegetative state averaged 8.6 ± 1.7 days in 17 children aged 1 month to 6 years [Gillies and Seshia, 1980]. Other responses, such as decorticate and decerebrate posturing (1.7 days), roving eye movements (1.8 days), and eye blinking (3.3 days), appeared earlier than sleep-wake cycles [Gillies and Seshia, 1980].

The progression of many metabolic and degenerative nervous system disorders in children may result in an irreversible vegetative state. In contrast to patients who become vegetative within several weeks after an acute injury, patients with metabolic or degenerative diseases slowly evolve to a vegetative state over several months or years. Severe congenital central nervous system (CNS) malformations can also result in a vegetative state. At birth, anencephaly is the only malformation in which an infant can be diagnosed as being in a vegetative state because of the absence of the cerebral cortex. Other malformations, such as hydranencephaly, may result in a vegetative state but, because of the limitations of the neurologic examination in assessing higher cortical functions and in differentiating voluntary from involuntary responses until about 3 to 6 months of age, it is recommended that such infants not be diagnosed as being vegetative until there is certainty about the diagnosis.

Diagnosis of the vegetative state is made clinically [AAN Quality Standards Subcommittee, 1995]. There are no confirmatory laboratory tests, in contrast to establishing the diagnosis of brain death. However, the absence of cortical (scalp-recorded) potentials of the somatosensory-evoked response to median nerve stimulation has been associated with the vegetative state in some studies [Beca et al., 1995; Frank et al., 1985]. Neuroimaging studies usually demonstrate diffuse or multifocal cerebral disease involving the gray and white matter or major CNS malformations (Ashwal, 1996). In patients with traumatic and nontraumatic

Box 61-1 Criteria for the Diagnosis of the Vegetative State

- No evidence of awareness of themselves or their environment; they are incapable of interacting with others
- No evidence of sustained, reproducible, purposeful, or voluntary behavioral responses to visual, auditory, tactile, or noxious stimuli
- No evidence of language comprehension or expression
- Intermittent wakefulness manifested by the presence of sleep-wake cycles
- Sufficiently preserved hypothalamic and brainstem autonomic functions to survive if given medical and nursing care
- Bowel and bladder incontinence
- Variably preserved cranial nerve (pupillary, oculocephalic, corneal, vestibulo-ocular, gag) and spinal reflexes

brain injury, serial imaging studies may demonstrate progressive atrophy. Positron emission tomography studies may demonstrate significant global reductions of cerebral glucose metabolism in infants [Larsen et al., 1993]. Proton magnetic resonance spectroscopy measurement of increased cerebral lactate in newborns, infants, and children with nervous system disease is associated with severe disability, survival in the vegetative state, or death [Ashwal et al., 1997].

Recovery from the vegetative state in children depends on the etiology and is reviewed in more detail in the Multi-Society Task Force on the Persistent Vegetative State report [1994]. In children with severe closed-head injuries who were vegetative 1 month after injury, follow-up at 1 year found that 29% remained in a vegetative state, 9% had died, and 62% recovered consciousness. Recoveries after 12 months were not reported, although one study found that 2 of 40 children with traumatic brain injury began to recover after 1 year in a vegetative state [Kriel et al., 1993]. In contrast, children in a nontraumatic vegetative state have a much poorer potential for recovery than those in a traumatic vegetative state. At 1 year, most children remained in a vegetative state (65%) or died (22%); only 13% demonstrated recovery, usually to a severe disability. It was based on this data, and consensus opinion that the Task Force came to the conclusions that in children (as well as in adults) the vegetative state could be judged permanent 12 months after traumatic brain injury and 3 months after nontraumatic injury. The chance for recovery after these time periods was exceedingly slim, and the patient almost always progressed to a severe disability. This perspective has received general acceptance, although concerns have been raised about the certainty of diagnosis and whether there is a greater potential for patients to recover than previously realized [Giacino et al., 1997; Jennett, 1997].

It is important to correctly identify children who are in a vegetative state because of the implications for continued care, family expectations, and the need for rehabilitation. Specialty programs for coma recovery are usually directed at patients who are severely disabled or are in a minimally conscious or vegetative state. Management issues are confounded by a lack of understanding of expected recovery patterns, terminology inconsistency, lack of or inappropriate use of outcome measures, and inadequate knowledge concerning medical management based on scientifically sound practices for this special patient population [Zasler et al., 1991]. Children in a vegetative state have been reported to have a considerably shorter than normal life expectancy [Ashwal et al., 1994]. Children in a vegetative state who are younger than 1 year of age had a median survival of 2.6 years, whereas the median survival of children aged 2 to 6 years was 5.2 years. In children 7 to 18 years of age, the reported median survival was 7 years.

Minimally Conscious State

Recovery from coma depends on the cause of coma, extent of brain injury, and ability of injured areas to recover or of uninjured areas to assume the functions of injured areas. Not all comatose patients recover rapidly or completely. A variety of terms have been used to define these states, and there is often confusion between recovery states and prognostic categories. The term *minimally conscious state* has been proposed to describe those patients who were in coma or a vegetative state and who are beginning to demonstrate minimal signs of awareness. Minimally conscious state may also be used to describe patients with degenerative disorders who are no longer functionally interactive but are not in the vegetative state. The minimally conscious state has been defined as a condition of severely altered consciousness in which the person demonstrates minimal but definite behavioral evidence of self- or environmental awareness [Giacino et al., 1997]. Patients in a minimally conscious state are able to do the following: (1) follow simple commands, (2) gesture or verbally give "yes" or "no" responses (regardless of accuracy), (3) verbalize intelligibly, and (4) perform movements or affective behaviors, which are not attributable to reflexive activity, in contingent relation to relevant environmental stimuli. Criteria to diagnose the minimally conscious state are in Box 61-2 [Giacino et al., 2002].

Children in the minimally conscious state are usually victims of acquired brain injury (traumatic and nontraumatic), neurodegenerative and neurometabolic disorders, or congenital or developmental disorders [Ashwal, 2003]. Based on limited literature on this disorder in adults [Giacino and Kalmar, 1999], it is possible that such children, depending on the etiology of the insult, may have a better potential for neurologic recovery and a longer life expectancy than children in the vegetative state. In a study of 5,075 children aged 3 to 15 years in a vegetative state or minimally conscious state, 564 were in the vegetative state, 705 in the minimally conscious state and immobile, and 3,806 in the minimally conscious state and mobile. The 8-year survival rates were 63% for vegetative state, 65% for

Box 61-2 Diagnostic Criteria for the Minimally Conscious State

- Simple command following
- Gestural or verbal yes-no responses (regardless of accuracy)
- Intelligible verbalization
- Purposeful behavior, including movements or effective behaviors that occur in contingent relation to relevant environmental stimuli and are not due to reflexive activity. Some behavioral examples of qualifying purposeful behaviors include the following:
  - Appropriate smiling or crying in response to the linguistic or visual content of emotional but not to neutral topics or stimuli
  - Vocalizations or gestures that occur in direct response to the linguistic content of questions
  - Reaching for objects that demonstrates a clear relationship between object location and direction of reach
  - Touching or holding objects in a manner that accommodates the size and shape of the object
  - Pursuit eye movement or sustained fixation that occurs in direct response to moving or salient stimuli

Adapted from Giacino JT, Ashwal S, Childs N, et al. The minimally conscious state. Definition and diagnostic criteria. Neurology 2002;58:349.

immobile minimally conscious state, and 81% for mobile minimally conscious state. Thus, presence of consciousness was not a critical variable in determining life expectancy in this study, and mobility was more important than consciousness in predicting survival [Strauss et al., 2000].

Locked-In Syndrome

The locked-in syndrome refers to a condition in which patients retain consciousness and cognition but are unable to move or communicate because of severe paralysis. This condition is a result of diseases involving the descending corticospinal and corticobulbar pathways at or below the pons or of severe involvement of the peripheral nervous system. By definition, patients in coma or a vegetative state are unconscious and differ from patients in a locked-in syndrome, who retain awareness, although this difference may be difficult to determine. The locked-in syndrome is quite rare in children [Habre et al., 1996; Scott et al., 1997]. Some patients with this condition can establish limited communication using eye movements.

Akinetic Mutism

Akinetic mutism is a rare condition consisting of pathologically slowed or nearly absent bodily movement accompanied by a similar loss of speech [Plum and Posner, 1982]. The original description of this condition in 1941 was in an adolescent with symptoms of intermittent depressed states of consciousness secondary to a craniopharyngioma [Cairns et al., 1941]. Since then, akinetic mutism has been seen with bacterial and viral CNS infections, other tumors of the nervous system, and hydrocephalus, and occasionally as a postoperative phenomenon [Lin et al., 1997; Melton et al., 1991]. Wakefulness and self-awareness are usually preserved in most patients, but the level of mental function is reduced. The condition characteristically accompanies gradually developing or subacute, bilateral damage to the paramedian mesencephalon, basal diencephalon, or inferior frontal lobes. The long-term outlook for children with akinetic mutism is unknown because few patients with this disorder have been reported. It is most likely related to the etiology and severity of the associated disease.

Brain Death

Brain death describes the permanent absence of all brain functions, including those of the brainstem [Task Force for the Determination of Brain Death in Children, 1987]. Brain-dead patients are irreversibly comatose and apneic, and they have absent brainstem reflexes, including the loss of all cranial nerve functions. The appearance of brain death can

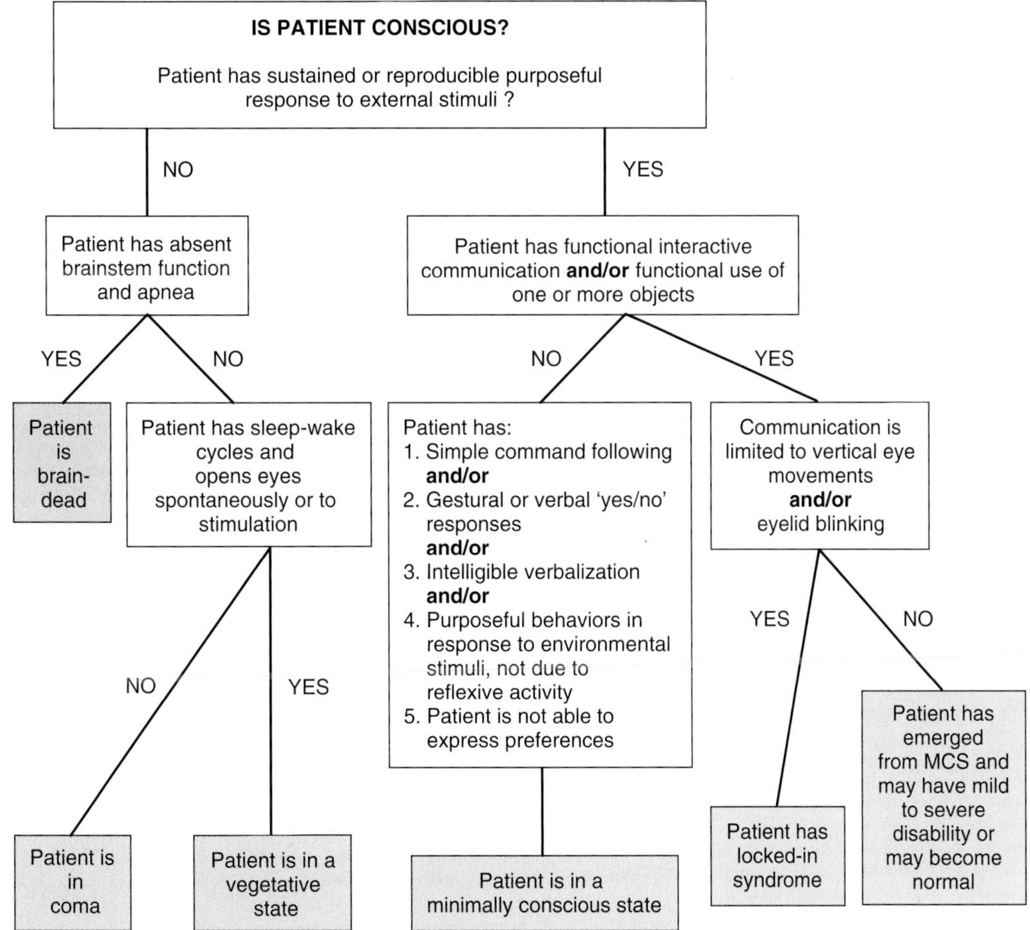

FIGURE 61-1 An algorithm useful for distinguishing among brain death, vegetative state, locked-in syndrome, and higher-order consciousness. MCS, minimally conscious state. (From Ashwal S, Cranford R. The minimally conscious state in children. Semin Pediatr Neurol 2002;9:19.)

be imitated by deep anesthesia, sedative overdose, or severe hypothermia. Patients who are brain dead differ from patients who are in a coma in that comatose patients usually have preserved brainstem functions and some degree of respiratory drive. Guidelines for the diagnosis of brain death in infants and children are well established and are reviewed in greater detail in Chapter 67. A useful algorithm for distinguishing among brain death, vegetative state, locked-in syndrome, and higher-order consciousness is presented in Figure 61-1 [Ashwal and Cranford, 2002].

CONSCIOUSNESS RATING SCALES

Because of the difficulty with imprecise use of terminology and because of the need for a truly reproducible assessment of consciousness with good inter-rater reliability, several behavior rating scales have been developed. Although typically referred to as *coma scales,* these scales have value in assessing consciousness alterations other than coma.

The best known and most widely used is the Glasgow Coma Scale, which yields a score of 3 to 15 based on best response to stimuli in the following three categories: eye opening, verbal response, and motor response (Table 61-2) [Teasdale and Jennett, 1974]. In its original form, the Glasgow Coma Scale was not developmentally suitable for assessment of newborns, infants, and younger children, and a variety of alternate scales have been proposed [Duncan et al., 1981; Hahn et al., 1988; Raimondi and Hirschauer, 1984; Reilly et al., 1988; Rubenstein, 1994; Simpson et al., 1991; Simpson and Reilly, 1982]. An ideal pediatric modification of the Glasgow Coma Scale would meet the following criteria:

1. Maintain the same maximum and minimum score as the Glasgow Coma Scale.
2. Maintain the same three categories.
3. Maintain the same numeric score range within each of the three categories.
4. Define intracategory scoring based on reasonable developmental assumptions.

The Pediatric Coma Scale [Reilly et al., 1988; Simpson et al., 1991; Simpson and Reilly, 1982] makes minor changes in the verbal scale of the Glasgow Coma Scale and redefines the "best" score based on developmental and age-appropriate norms (Table 61-3). It has the advantage of prospective evaluation and inter-rater reliability and the disadvantage of different maximum scores based on age,

TABLE 61-3

Pediatric Coma Scale

RESPONSE	SCORE
Eye Opening	
Spontaneous	4
To speech	3
To pain	2
None	1
Best Verbal Response	
Oriented	5
Words	4
Vocal sounds	3
Cries	2
None	1
Best Motor Response	
Obeys commands	5
Localizes pain	4
Flexion to pain	3
Extension to pain	2
None	1
Normal Aggregate Score	
Birth to 6 months	9
Less than 6-12 months	11
Less than 1-2 years	12
Less than 2-5 years	13
More than 5 years	14

TABLE 61-2

Glasgow Coma Scale and Modification for Children

SIGN	GLASGOW COMA SCALE	GLASGOW COMA SCALE—MODIFIED FOR CHILDREN	SCORE
Eye opening	Spontaneous	Spontaneous	4
	To command	To sound	3
	To pain	To pain	2
	None	None	1
Verbal response	Oriented	Age-appropriate verbalization, orients to sound, fixes and follows, social smile	5
	Confused	Cries, but inconsolable	4
	Disoriented	Irritable, uncooperative, aware of environment	3
	Inappropriate words	Irritable persistent cries, inconsistently consolable	2
	Incomprehensible sounds	Inconsolable crying, unaware of environment or parents, restless, agitated	1
	None	None	
Motor response	Obeys commands	Obeys commands, spontaneous movement	6
	Localizes pain	Localizes pain	5
	Withdraws	Withdraws	4
	Abnormal flexion to pain	Abnormal flexion to pain	3
	Abnormal extension	Abnormal extension to pain	2
	None	None	1
Best total score			15

TABLE 61-4

Children's Coma Scale

SIGN	SCORE
Ocular Response	
Pursuit	4
Extraocular movement intact, pupils react appropriately	3
Fixed pupils or extraocular movement impaired	2
Fixed pupils and extraocular movement paralyzed	1
Verbal Response	
Cries	3
Spontaneous respiration	2
Apneic	1
Motor Response	
Flexes and extends	4
Withdraws from painful stimuli	3
Hypertonic	2
Flaccid	1
Best Total Score	11

thus making outcome prediction and comparison difficult to study using the Glasgow Coma Scale.

The Children's Coma Scale redefines intracategory criteria and "maximum" score and changes the eye-opening category to "ocular response" [Raimondi and Hirschauer, 1984]. The Children's Coma Scale meritoriously included pupillary reflexes, extraocular movements, and apnea in its categories and is therefore substantially different from the Glasgow Coma Scale and requires different training and forms to be used (Table 61-4).

The Glasgow Coma Scale—Modified for Children maintains the same categories as the Glasgow Coma Scale and the same maximum and minimum scores, while allowing developmental and age-appropriate scoring [Hahn et al., 1988; Rubenstein, 1994]. It does, however, equate spontaneous movement with following commands to achieve 6 points in the best motor response category to allow inclusion of infants and young children (see Table 61-2). Nonetheless, the Glasgow Coma Scale—Modified for Children allows the best direct comparison with the Glasgow Coma Scale for scoring of consciousness impairment and assessment of outcome.

The Glasgow Coma Scale and its modifications for children are useful to more objectively evaluate and quantify the continuum from consciousness to coma and to allow serial reassessment that meaningfully reflects the state of the patient at a particular moment in time with good inter-rater reliability. The scores also allow a relatively large amount of information to be conveyed quickly and concisely with minimal need to remember cumbersome definitions or to write long descriptions. Their ease of use makes them even more valuable in the critical care and emergency department settings. The Glasgow Coma Scale and its pediatric modifications do not take into account the important brainstem reflexes, such as pupillary reactivity or oculocephalic, oculovestibular, or corneal reflexes. These should be a routine part of the assessment of the patient with impaired consciousness [Narayan et al., 1981].

The sum of the Glasgow Coma Scale may convey less useful information than the ocular, motor, and verbal responses individually [Teasdale et al., 1983]. In a study of 270 children aged 2 months to 12 years with acute nontraumatic coma, multivariate analysis suggests that the ocular and motor response score and not the total score were predictors of short-term survival. Additionally, the absence of one or more brainstem reflexes (oculocephalic, oculovestibular, or pupillary reactivity) predicted short-term adverse outcomes [Nayana Prabha et al., 2003].

PATHOPHYSIOLOGY

Consciousness is the result of the complex interplay between the cerebral cortex and the ascending reticular-activating system. The ascending reticular-activating system is a somewhat diffuse and poorly circumscribed group of neurons that lie in the reticular formation of the brain that extends from the lower medulla to the midbrain and diencephalon [Moruzzi and Magoun, 1949; Plum and Posner, 1982]. Coma is produced by diseases or conditions that cause bilateral cerebral cortical dysfunction, ascending reticular-activating system dysfunction, or both. Pathologically, these can be subdivided as follows [Adams et al., 1982; Gennarelli et al., 1982; Plum and Posner, 1982]:

- Metabolic, toxic, or infectious encephalopathies that diffusely affect the cerebral hemispheres, the ascending reticular-activating system, or both
- Supratentorial mass lesions that compress or displace the diencephalon or brainstem
- Subtentorial mass or destructive lesions that compress or damage the ascending reticular-activating system
- Traumatic axonal injury that affects both cerebral hemispheres, the ascending reticular-activating system, or their interconnections

Impairment of consciousness results from partial disruptions of neuronal function in these same areas. Prolonged coma after severe traumatic brain injury may be due to traumatic axonal injury or diffuse axonal injury without severe injury to the cortex or ascending reticular-activating system. This finding explains why patients with traumatic brain injury have a better potential for recovery than patients with hypoxic-ischemic injury.

CAUSES

A more relevant and practical classification for the etiology of impairment of consciousness and coma in children produces three distinct but overlapping categories: infectious or inflammatory; structural; and metabolic, nutritional, or toxic (Box 61-3).

Bacterial, viral, rickettsial, or protozoan infections of the CNS may cause conscious alteration by direct involvement of brain parenchyma, interference with blood flow, production of cerebral edema with resulting increased intracranial pressure, and increasing metabolic activity beyond metabolic substrate availability. Viral infections are more likely to involve brain parenchyma (encephalitis). The meningitis produced by bacterial infections may produce injury as a result of large blood vessel occlusion, microvascular inflammation, or disturbance of cerebral autoregulation.

Box 61-3 Etiologies of Impaired Consciousness and Coma

Infectious or Inflammatory	Structural	Metabolic, Nutritional, or Toxic
A. Infectious Bacterial meningitis Viral encephalitis Rickettsial infection Protozoan infection Helminth infestation B. Inflammatory Sepsis-associated encephalopathy Vasculitis, collagen vascular disorders Demyelination Acute disseminated encephalomyelitis Multiple sclerosis	A. Traumatic Concussion Cerebral contusion Epidural hematoma or effusion Intracerebral hematoma Diffuse axonal injury Shaken-baby syndrome B. Neoplasms C. Vascular disease Cerebral infarction Thrombosis Embolism Venous sinus thrombosis Cerebral hemorrhage Subarachnoid hemorrhage Arteriovenous malformation Aneurysm Congenital abnormality or dysplasia of vascular supply Trauma to carotid or vertebral arteries in the neck D. Focal infection Abscess Cerebritis E. Hydrocephalus	A. Hypoxic-ischemic encephalopathy Shock Cardiac or pulmonary failure Near drowning Carbon monoxide poisoning Cyanide poisoning Strangulation B. Metabolic disorders Sarcoidosis Hypoglycemia Fluid and electrolyte imbalance Endocrine disorders With acidosis Diabetic ketoacidosis Aminoacidemias Organic acidemias With hyperammonemia Hepatic encephalopathy Urea cycle disorders Disorders of fatty acid metabolism Reye's syndrome Valproic acid encephalopathy Uremia Porphyria Mitochondrial disorders Leigh's syndrome C. Nutritional Thiamine deficiency Niacin or nicotinic acid deficiency Pyridoxine dependency Folate and B_{12} deficiency D. Exogenous toxins and poisons Alcohol intoxication Over-the-counter medications Prescription medications (oral and ophthalmic) Herbal treatments Heavy-metal poisoning Mushroom and plant intoxication Illegal drugs Industrial agents E. Hypertensive encephalopathy F. Burn encephalopathy

Cerebral edema, focal mass or abscess, and hydrocephalus as a result of intracranial infection may produce injury by reducing cerebral blood flow or leading to herniation.

Structural causes of consciousness impairment or coma include intracranial neoplasm, infectious space-occupying lesion (abscess, tuberculoma), nonaccidental and accidental trauma, cerebral infarction or hemorrhage, and hydrocephalus.

Nutritional causes of alteration of consciousness or coma are relatively uncommon in the United States but represent a significant problem in other areas of the world. Wernicke's encephalopathy is related to a deficiency of thiamine. In addition to consciousness alteration, patients may have eye-movement abnormalities, ataxia, and deep tendon reflex changes. Wernicke's encephalopathy has been reported in children and adolescents as a result of systemic malignancy and because of thiamine deficiency in total parenteral nutrition, and it may occur related to anorexia nervosa, acquired immunodeficiency syndrome (AIDS), and prolonged fasting [Bruck et al., 1991; Hahn et al., 1998; Nautiyal et al., 2004; Pihko et al., 1989; Salas-Salvado et al., 2000; Vasconcelos et al., 1999].

Niacin or nicotinic acid deficiency (pellagra) with the typical features of mental changes, dermatitis, and diarrhea is rarely seen in the United States. However, disorders of the synthetic pathway from tryptophan to niacin or nicotinic acid or impaired intestinal absorption of tryptophan in Hartnup's disease may produce symptoms in children or adolescents [Clayton et al., 1991; Freundlich et al., 1981].

Metabolic and toxic causes of impaired consciousness or coma include hypoxic-ischemic injury (focal or generalized), electrolyte abnormality, endocrinopathy, hepatic or renal failure and inherited disorders, including organic and aminoacidurias, urea cycle disorders, mitochondrial disorders, and porphyria. Paroxysmal disorders such as uncontrolled seizures, nonconvulsive status epilepticus, or migraine may produce changes in consciousness that may be episodic. The diagnosis, pathophysiology, and treatment of specific disorders are reviewed elsewhere in this book.

There may be considerable overlap between these categories, and it is always necessary to consider combined causes of impaired consciousness and coma. Disorders that produce abnormalities of osmolality, such as hyponatremia, hypernatremia, and diabetic ketoacidosis, may also lead to structural complications, such as intracranial hemorrhage or stroke as a consequence of sinovenous thrombosis. Both have been reported as rare complications of diabetic ketoacidosis [Atlluru, 1986]. Cerebral edema may complicate treatment of ketoacidosis, causing alterations of consciousness or herniation [Green et al., 1990].

Children with psychiatric disorders, such as conversion, panic, or anxiety disorders, may present with neurologic symptoms including genuine or apparent impairment of consciousness. Symptoms may include dizziness, hyperventilation, paresthesias, agitation, or restlessness. The episodic and paroxysmal nature of these episodes and the complete recovery between episodes should suggest the diagnosis [Herskowitz, 1986].

EVALUATION

The clinical approach to impairment of consciousness must be comprehensive and systematic. It is especially important to evaluate the evolution of symptoms and to interview any potential witnesses to the onset of symptoms. Not all patients with impairment of consciousness progress to coma, but early recognition of the progression and intervention often yields better outcome. Coma is a medical and neurologic emergency requiring immediate consideration of key issues, including immediate life support, identification of the cause of coma, and institution of specific therapy. These critical issues will be reviewed in sequence, but all have immediate importance and significance in the comatose child. The approach to the child with impaired consciousness but not coma is similar but may be modified based on the evaluation of symptoms and clinical need.

Clinical Evaluation

The ABCs of basic life support (immediate life support—airway, breathing, and circulation) must be evaluated and managed emergently. Additionally, it is essential to assess adequacy of perfusion because children in shock may appear stable initially but then rapidly deteriorate. Glucose, the essential substrate for brain energy metabolism, must be provided through an intravenous line. Because unobserved or unreported trauma may have occurred, it is important to consider the possibility of a cervical fracture or other injury while implementing immediate life-support measures.

Identification of Cause

Accurate and rapid identification of the cause of coma is important to direct specific treatment. The history and physical examination are the basis for identification of the cause of coma. Time constraints during evaluation of symptoms and signs often require rapid transition from history and examination to diagnostic tests, such as arterial blood gas determination or computed tomography. Nonetheless, these simple steps are exceedingly important and must not be overlooked or minimized. If the eyewitness to the onset of symptoms is not with the child in the emergency department (e.g., when symptoms begin at school or day care), a member of the emergency response team (usually a physician or nurse) is assigned to interview the eyewitness by telephone, and others attend to the patient's immediate needs. If the child requires immediate resuscitation, accompanying parents, relatives, or other eyewitnesses in the emergency department are best interviewed in a quiet area to allow the most accurate elucidation of events surrounding the onset of symptoms.

History

Coma may manifest as the progression of a known underlying illness, unpredictable consequence, or complication of a known disease, or it may be the result of a totally unexpected event or illness [Bates, 1993; Michelson and Ashwal, 2004]. An accurate history of the events and circumstances before the onset of symptoms and basic information concerning past medical history and medications may be invaluable in determining the cause of coma and quickly lead to the most appropriate diagnostic testing and treatment [Bates, 1993; Plum and Posner, 1982; Vannucci and Wasiewski, 1993].

Sudden onset of coma in an otherwise normal and awake child suggests convulsions or intracranial hemorrhage. Coma preceded by sleepiness or unsteadiness suggests ingestion of a drug or toxin in an otherwise well child. Fever is typical when coma is due to an infectious process but may not be present when shock is present or if the ambient temperature is low. A history of headache may suggest elevated intracranial pressure resulting from hydrocephalus or neoplasm but may also be seen in migraine syndromes with alteration of consciousness.

When traumatic brain injury has occurred, coma may exist from the moment of impact or may be preceded by a lucid interval. The presence of a period of consciousness followed by coma warrants immediate computed tomography (CT) scanning of the head to assess for an expanding intracranial mass lesion, such as an epidural hematoma.

Evaluation of accidental versus nonaccidental trauma in children can be especially difficult. In a study of 152 children aged 2 years or younger with traumatic brain injury who died or were admitted to a pediatric intensive care unit, 80 (52.6%) had inflicted (i.e., nonaccidental) injury, and 72 (47.3%) had noninflicted traumatic brain injury [Keenan et al., 2004]. Clinical history may make the cause relatively obvious, such as a history of an automobile accident or plausible history of a fall. Retinal hemorrhage, metaphyseal fracture, rib fracture, and subdural hemorrhage are more commonly seen in children with inflicted traumatic brain injury. Skeletal survey and ophthalmologic examination alone missed 10% of inflicted traumatic brain injury cases in one recent study [Keenan et al., 2004]. When there is a high degree of suspicion of inflicted injury, CT or magnetic resonance imaging (MRI) of the head, or both, should be performed.

A history of fever or recent illness suggests an acute infectious etiology but should also lead to consideration of complications from infectious disease, such as acute disseminated encephalomyelitis, Reye's syndrome, metabolic or mitochondrial disorders. Children with diabetes may have coma because of hypoglycemia or ketoacidosis. Children with congenital heart disease may be susceptible to brain abscess or infarction. Intermittent episodes of coma should suggest ingestion, drug overdose, inborn errors of metabolism, or *Munchausen's syndrome by proxy*. Review of current medications should include use of ophthalmic drops, often overlooked as unlikely to have systemic effects. Brimonidine, an α_2-adrenergic antagonist used in the treatment of glaucoma, caused recurrent episodes of coma at home and in hospital in a 1-month-old infant [Berlin et al., 2001]. A history of the use of a kerosene stove or heater should suggest carbon monoxide poisoning.

General Physical Examination

The general physical examination begins with assessment of the vital signs, including temperature, heart rate, respiration, blood pressure, and the response to pain. Fever usually suggests infection but infrequently can be caused by an abnormality of the central control mechanisms that regulate body temperature. Fever with coma suggests sepsis, pneumonia, meningitis, encephalitis, intracranial abscess, or empyema. Very high fever and dry skin may be due to heat stroke. In children, hypothermia is most often seen with drug intoxication, especially if the ambient temperature is cold. Rapid heart rate suggests hypovolemic shock, secondary effects of fever, heart failure, or a tachyarrhythmia, such as paroxysmal atrial tachycardia. An abnormally low heart rate may reflect myocardial injury, the late effect of hypoxemia, or increased intracranial pressure. Rapid respiration suggests a primary abnormality of oxygenation, as seen in pneumonia, asthma, or pulmonary embolus, or acidosis, as in diabetic ketoacidosis and uremia. Brainstem lesions may cause central neurogenic hyperventilation. Slow, irregular, or periodic breathing patterns may indicate toxic ingestion or increased intracranial pressure. Hypotension is seen in shock, sepsis, certain drug ingestions, myocardial injury or failure, and adrenal insufficiency. Hypertension may be a primary cause of unresponsiveness, as in hypertensive encephalopathy, but may also be a compensatory mechanism to ensure brain perfusion in children with increased intracranial pressure or stroke.

Inspection of the head, scalp, and skin can be most helpful. Cyanosis suggests poor oxygenation, and jaundice is seen in liver failure. Extreme pallor may be seen in anemia and shock, and a cherry-red color suggests carbon monoxide poisoning. The presence of a cephalohematoma, boggy or swollen areas of the scalp, or head bruises suggests cranial trauma. Bleeding or clear fluid leaking from the nose or ears suggests a basilar skull fracture. Certain types of burns and multiple bruises of characteristic shape and location or varied age may suggest child abuse. Various rashes may be seen with infectious causes of coma, such as meningococcemia or rickettsial disease. The presence of neurocutaneous lesions, such as the depigmented areas of tuberous sclerosis, suggests seizures or intracranial mass as the cause of coma. Generalized increased pigmentation may be seen in Addison's disease or in adrenoleukodystrophy [Ravid et al., 2000].

The odor of exhaled breath can be characteristic in alcohol intoxication, diabetic ketoacidosis (sweet-fruity), uremia (urine-like), and hepatic coma (musty).

The cardiovascular examination may suggest congenital heart disease or endocarditis, both of which are sources of intracranial abscess dissemination. Abdominal discoloration or rigidity may suggest intra-abdominal bleeding as a source of shock. A palpable linear abdominal mass may lead to the diagnosis of intussusception encephalopathy and underscores the need to include a thorough general examination in the evaluation of the child with an altered state of consciousness or coma [Goetting et al., 1990].

Neurologic Examination

The neurologic examination is of paramount importance in the assessment of the comatose patient. In particular, examination of the optic fundi, pupillary size and reactivity, eye movement control, corneal reflexes, motor responses, body posture, and the presence or absence of meningeal signs gives important information about the potential causes and localization of brain dysfunction in the comatose patient [Bates, 1993; Plum and Posner, 1982; Vannucci and Wasiewski, 1993]. Localization may be especially aided by detailed understanding of brainstem pathways involved in the eye examination. Funduscopic examination offers important clues about the etiology of coma, including papilledema as an indicator of raised intracranial pressure and retinal hemorrhages in occult trauma. In acute increased intracranial pressure, there may not have been time for papilledema to develop at the time of presentation in the emergency department.

Passive resistance to neck flexion suggests meningeal irritation, tonsillar herniation, or craniocervical trauma. Resistance to thigh flexion with the leg extended (Kernig's sign) and thigh flexion when the neck is flexed (Brudzinski's sign) are more reliable indicators of generalized meningeal irritation. Patients with acute subarachnoid hemorrhage may not develop signs of meningeal irritation for several hours.

Pupil size and reactivity are controlled by reciprocal sympathetic and parasympathetic innervation. Sympathetic pupil innervation originates in the hypothalamus and descends to the lower cervical and upper thoracic spinal cord. After synapsing in the intermediolateral columns, preganglionic sympathetic fibers exit the spinal cord and ascend in the cervical sympathetic chain, course near the apex of the lung, and end in the superior cervical ganglion where postganglionic fibers pass along the internal carotid artery. Intracranially, the fibers travel with branches of the ophthalmic division of the trigeminal nerve to the pupil. Sympathetic innervation to sweat glands of the upper face also follows the internal carotid arteries, and other fibers innervate the smooth muscles of the eyelid. The sympathetic pathways are vulnerable at several locations, and an appropriately placed injury may produce unilateral pupillary constriction, ptosis, and facial anhidrosis (Horner's syndrome). Parasympathetic pupil innervation originates in the midbrain at or near the Edinger-Westphal nucleus and travels as a component of the oculomotor nerve to the pupils [Montgomery et al., 1986].

Pupillary reactivity can be elicited by shining a light on the eye or by opening and closing the eyelid. The afferent limb of the pupillary light reflex is through the optic nerve, and the efferent limb is through the parasympathetic fibers that travel with the oculomotor nerve. In the presence of normal visual acuity and the absence of corneal clouding, an abnormality of the pupillary light reflex suggests midbrain dysfunction. With unilateral loss of visual acuity, the opposite pupil may dilate when the light is moved from the unaffected to the affected side. This reaction results from a defect in the afferent limb of the reflex arc on the affected side.

Most metabolic disorders and drug ingestions produce symmetrically small pupils that retain some reactivity to light. Severe hypoxic-ischemic injury produces symmetric dilated pupils that may not respond to light. Structural or mass lesions of the cerebral hemispheres typically do not produce pupillary abnormalities unless herniation occurs. For example, herniation of the temporal lobe over the tentorium with compression of the parasympathetic fibers traveling with the oculomotor nerve may produce unilateral pupillary dilation because of unopposed sympathetic innervation. Hypothalamic lesions produce small pupils by interrupting sympathetic fibers at the point of origin. Structural lesions in the pons may disrupt sympathetic fibers descending from the hypothalamus. In either case, unopposed parasympathetic tone produces small or "pinpoint" pupils that may mimic those seen in metabolic disorders or in patients with toxin or drug ingestions. Midbrain injuries may interrupt both sympathetic and parasympathetic pupillary innervations, producing midposition unresponsive pupils.

Extraocular movements are controlled by the oculomotor (cranial nerve III), trochlear (cranial nerve IV), and abducens (cranial nerve VI) nuclei in the midbrain and pons. Conjugate gaze is coordinated by these cranial nerve nuclei through the medial longitudinal fasciculus. Supranuclear control of conjugate gaze resides in the two primary cerebral gaze centers found in the frontal lobes and parieto-occipital areas, respectively. The frontal gaze center produces rapid or saccadic eye movement contralateral to the side stimulated, whereas the more posterior center produces smooth pursuit or tracking movements ipsilateral to the side stimulated. The relatively large amount of cortex represented in these pathways is the basis for believing that the presence of the opticokinetic nystagmus response distinguishes coma from pseudocoma.

Unilateral stimulation of the frontal gaze center produces conjugate eye deviation to the opposite side and can be produced by seizure activity or other unilateral irritating stimuli. Unilateral injury, destruction, or metabolic exhaustion of the frontal gaze center produces conjugate deviation toward the affected side (the patient is said to look toward the lesion). This yoked system also has important input from the vestibular system, the cerebellum, and proprioceptive pathways from neck muscles. These pathways are the basis for the "doll's eyes" (oculocephalic) and caloric (oculovestibular) responses.

The oculocephalic maneuver is performed by moving the head side to side or vertically and should only be performed when there is certainty that there is no cervical spine injury or abnormality. A positive oculocephalic response consists of conjugate deviation of the eyes in the direction opposite head movement. Absence of a positive oculocephalic response may be seen in structural abnormalities of the brainstem, where it may be asymmetric, and in metabolic-toxic encephalopathies, where it is almost always symmetric. A common cause of an abnormal oculocephalic response is medication routinely given to sedate patients for procedures, tests, or critical care support. Absence of an oculocephalic response may also be seen in patients who are awake with psychogenic unresponsiveness.

Caloric or oculovestibular responses are obtained by irrigating one or both external ear canals with warm and cold water and should only be performed when the external canal is clean and the tympanic membrane intact. The usual protocol for unconscious patients involves cold-water irrigation with the head elevated 30 degrees from the horizontal, which induces convection currents in the endolymphatic fluid of the labyrinth. The resulting vestibular nuclei stimulation affects the ipsilateral paramedian pontine reticular formation–abducens nuclear complex and also the contralateral oculomotor and trochlear nuclei through the medial longitudinal fasciculus. In awake patients, cold-water irrigation produces a lateral nystagmus, with the quick phase away from the stimulated ear. Warm-water stimulation has the opposite effect. This finding gives rise to the mnemonic COWS (cold opposite, warm same). In the unconscious patient, however, the quick phase is lost, and slow tonic deviation is noted toward the irrigated ear. An intact oculovestibular response suggests functional connections from the vestibular system in the medulla to the ocular cranial nerve nuclei in the mesencephalon and pons connected by the medial longitudinal fasciculus. Unilateral or asymmetric caloric responses suggest a brainstem structural abnormality, whereas bilateral absence can be seen in metabolic, as well as structural, abnormalities. The oculocephalic response is an objective measure of lower brainstem integrity and an important addition to the neurologic examination when other medullary-controlled activities, such as respiration, are abnormal or controlled by mechanical ventilation. Caloric stimulation of the noncomatose patient may provoke nausea and vomiting, and care should be exercised to avoid the possibility of aspiration.

The corneal reflex consists of closure of the eyelid elicited by gently touching the cornea with a suitable stimulus, such as sterile gauze or cotton. The afferent or sensory limb of this reflex involves the first division of the trigeminal nerve (cranial nerve V), and the efferent or motor limb is through the facial nerve (cranial nerve VII). A normal response to unilateral corneal stimulation is bilateral blinking resulting from pontine interconnections. An absent response suggests abnormal afferent or trigeminal input or bilateral pontine involvement. A contralateral blink response suggests intact sensory input through the fifth cranial nerve, whereas an abnormal motor limb response on the ipsilateral side is more consistent with an ipsilateral structural abnormality. Metabolic lesions typically produce bilateral loss of response. Absence of the corneal reflex must be interpreted with caution in the presence of conjunctival edema or injury, or with the use of sedative or paralytic agents that are commonly used in the intensive care unit setting.

Observation of spontaneous movement and motor responses to stimulation are important clues in the assessment of coma and localization of the level of injury or lesion. Asymmetric involvement is a hallmark of structural abnormality. Unilateral cortical or subcortical structural lesions may cause contralateral weakness. Bilateral absence of movement or tone (flaccidity) occurs in metabolic-toxic encephalopathies, such as drug intoxications, and in disruption of brainstem-cortical interconnections above the pontomedullary junction. Flaccidity resulting from spinal cord injuries or neuromuscular paralysis is not associated with coma unless other injuries exist.

Posturing may occur spontaneously or in response to stimulation. Decorticate posturing involves flexion of the upper extremities and extension of the lower extremities and usually involves cortical or subcortical abnormalities with preservation of brainstem function. Decerebrate posturing involves extension of all extremities with internal rotation and may be seen with metabolic-toxic disorders or midbrain compression. Decorticate and decerebrate posturing do not have the same exquisite localizing value in clinical medicine as they do in experimentally lesioned animals. It is generally believed, however, that decerebrate posturing is "worse" than decorticate posturing and that asymmetry of posturing is more likely seen in patients with structural than with metabolic-toxic disorders. Herniation syndromes should always be considered when posturing is present.

HERNIATION SYNDROMES

The historical value of the concept of herniation syndromes was the correlation of clinical course with pathology findings to allow early identification of problems that may be progressive and life threatening and hasten appropriate early intervention. In the age of neuroimaging, the fundamental understanding of the cause of herniation symptoms is changing, but the importance of correlation of clinical signs and symptoms with intracranial pathology in vivo and in vitro remains. In this regard, an especially important concept has been the rostral-caudal deterioration—that is, that herniation proceeds from more generalized or diffuse symptoms through an orderly progression of brainstem dysfunction from diencephalon to mesencephalon to pons to medulla. That this may not always be the case does not alter the importance of critical findings, such as a unilaterally enlarged pupil in a patient with deterioration of consciousness. Whenever there is clinical evidence consistent with risk for a herniation syndrome, immediate neuroimaging and treatment to lower intracranial pressure may be life saving.

Three herniation syndromes are presented: uncal herniation, central or transtentorial downward herniation, and infratentorial herniation. Although signs and symptoms may overlap, and uncal herniation may just be a pathologically more distinct variant of transtentorial downward herniation, better understanding of the patient with consciousness alteration or coma is available to the student who studies these syndromes.

Within the skull are unique dural reflections that divide the intracranial contents into compartments. The falx cerebri lies between the cerebral hemispheres, and the tentorium cerebelli separates anterior fossa structures (cerebral hemispheres and diencephalon) from posterior structures (brainstem and cerebellum). The opening in the tentorium through which the midbrain passes is called the *tentorial notch.* Excised dura is leathery and malleable, but the dural reflections, in vivo, are relatively rigid and firm. Focal or generalized lesions, which produce mass effect or increased intracranial pressure, may produce one of the three brain herniation syndromes based on squeezing of brain structures over or through the tentorium or through the foramen magnum. It is extremely important to recognize early signs and symptoms of these herniation syndromes so that urgent and appropriate intervention can be provided.

Uncal Herniation

Uncal herniation refers to the medial displacement of the uncal gyrus of the temporal lobe over the free lateral edge of the tentorium associated with an asymmetric supratentorial mass or edema. Neuropathology-based studies presume that the uncal gyrus (uncus) comes in direct contact with the oculomotor nerve, producing ipsilateral pupillary dilation and external ophthalmoplegia. Radiologic studies, however, emphasize horizontal shift of the mesencephalon away from the lesion as the cause of early consciousness alteration because the ambient cistern and prepontine cistern are widened ipsilaterally. In this scenario, the ipsilateral pupillary dilation is due to stretch of the oculomotor nerve over the clivus rather than direct pressure from the uncus. Another early radiologic finding may be enlargement of the contralateral temporal horn of the lateral ventricle caused by compression of the ipsilateral lateral ventricle.

In either explanation, there is typically early ipsilateral pupillary dilation with sluggish reactivity to light because of interruption of parasympathetic innervation to the pupil producing unopposed sympathetic response (dilation). Parasympathetic fibers to the pupil are located peripherally along the oculomotor nerve and are therefore affected first. Further, horizontal displacement of the upper brainstem may cause the contralateral cerebral peduncle to be pressed against the opposite tentorial edge and produce hemiparesis ipsilateral to the lesion (and ipsilateral to the enlarged pupil). This finding is consistent with the often-seen pathologic finding of a hemorrhagic lesion in the contralateral cerebral peduncle, the Kernohan notch phenomenon.

False localization may occur if the uncus compresses the ipsilateral cerebral peduncle, producing contralateral hemiparesis, or if the contralateral oculomotor nerve is caught between the mesencephalon and the edge of the tentorium, producing contralateral pupillary dilation and external ophthalmoplegia.

Consciousness alteration or coma associated with unilateral pupillary dilation and ultimately external ophthalmoplegia and unilateral hemiparesis are early signs of uncal herniation and should lead to urgent evaluation for causes of increased intracranial pressure and intracranial mass lesion. Unilateral pupillary dilation is most likely to indicate ipsilateral mass lesion or asymmetric cerebral edema. However, because of the variability of normal anatomy and the possibility of progression such that the primary clinical signs may be on either side, cerebral imaging is required to make the diagnosis.

Uncal herniation is often ultimately associated with the central or transtentorial downward herniation syndrome.

Central or Transtentorial Downward Herniation

With generalized increases in intracranial pressure, there is gradual downward displacement of the diencephalon (thalamus and hypothalamus) through the tentorium cerebelli, producing progressive compression and ischemia of the brainstem from mesencephalon (rostral brainstem) to medulla (caudal brainstem). The traditional clinical-pathologic correlation is progressive deterioration of consciousness and brainstem function in a rostral to caudal direction [Plum and Posner, 1982; Young et al., 1998]. In the diencephalic stage, patients do not follow instructions but will localize to noxious stimuli and have small reactive pupils and preserved oculocephalic and oculovestibular reflexes. Respiration may be regular with yawns or sighs, or Cheyne-Stokes respirations may appear. Cheyne-Stokes respirations consist of a cyclical gradual buildup and decrease in the volume of air inhaled with each breath. Increased rigidity or decorticate posturing may appear. In the midbrain–upper pons stage, patients have decerebrate rigidity or no movement, midposition pupils that may be irregular in shape and demonstrate no reactivity, and abnormal or absent oculocephalic and oculovestibular reflexes. Patients usually hyperventilate, although Cheyne-Stokes respirations may still be noted. In the lower pontine–medullary stage, there is no spontaneous motor activity or activity in response to stimuli, midposition fixed pupils, absent oculocephalic and oculovestibular reflexes, and shallow and rapid or slow and irregular (ataxic) respirations. The lower extremities may withdraw to plantar stimulation. Finally, in the medullary stage, there is generalized flaccid tone, absence of pupillary reflexes and ocular movements, further slowing and irregularity of respiration, and ultimately death.

Clinical-radiologic correlation studies have indicated that horizontal brainstem displacement may be likely to produce progressive impairment of consciousness and coma [Fisher, 1995; Ropper, 1986; Ross et al., 1989]. Horizontal shift of midline structures may be greater than their downward vertical displacement in patients who are in coma [Ropper, 1993]. Additionally, significant downward displacement of brainstem structures may be seen in individuals with low spinal fluid pressure syndromes without consciousness alteration [Reich et al., 1993]. Other studies have found downward herniation of the diencephalon in consciousness alteration and coma by MRI, seeming to confirm the traditional clinical-pathologic correlation [Feldmann et al., 1988; Wijdicks and Miller, 1997].

In addition, downward transtentorial herniation may be associated with unilateral findings similar to those seen in uncal herniation. Recognition of the typical progressive deterioration may further be confounded by partial or total ischemia of the brainstem due to downward displacement of perforating branches of the basilar artery leading to all-at-once brainstem dysfunction at multiple levels.

In central or transtentorial downward herniation, early recognition of higher or more rostral brainstem dysfunction (e.g., abnormal pupil size or response) before lower or more caudal brainstem dysfunction (irregular or absent breathing), with or without, but generally without, focal findings suggests central herniation. Early recognition of the clinical signs may allow more effective intervention.

Infratentorial (Cerebellar) Herniation Syndromes

Space-occupying lesions in the posterior fossa can produce upward herniation of brainstem structures through the tentorial notch and may result in obstructive hydrocephalus, brainstem ischemia, and death. Progressive alteration of consciousness or coma associated with miotic pupils, gaze paresis, decerebrate posturing, and asymmetric or absent caloric response with relative preservation of respiration suggest upward transtentorial herniation in the setting of posterior fossa tumor, hemorrhage, stroke, or cerebellar edema [Cuneo et al., 1979].

Downward herniation of the cerebellum and medulla at the foramen magnum may cause apnea and death because of pressure on medullary respiratory centers. The impressive shape of the lower cerebellum at postmortem examination is often referred to as the cerebellar pressure cone. Rapid onset of respiratory deterioration and apnea in the setting of increased posterior fossa pressure (with or without supratentorial pressure) is often called *coning*.

The lesions that cause upward or downward cerebellar herniation in children are often subacute or chronic and are discovered before herniation as a result of widespread use of neuroimaging. However, some acute illnesses such as meningitis or encephalitis may be associated with either cerebellar herniation syndrome [Gohlich-Ratmann et al., 1998; Roulet Perez et al., 1993]. Early identification of impending herniation by CT or MRI criteria may allow effective treatment and improved outcome [Karantanas et al., 2002].

However, in children with meningitis, the cerebellar pressure cone effect has been implicated as a cause of death after lumbar puncture even with a normal CT scan of the head. In cases of suspected bacterial meningitis, lumbar puncture should be avoided if there is evidence of increased intracranial pressure or early coning. When lumbar puncture is performed, measurement of opening pressure is essential to allow early treatment if increased intracranial pressure persists. In all such cases, concern about risks for lumbar puncture should not delay appropriate antibiotic treatment [Oliver et al., 2003; Rennick et al., 1993; Shetty et al., 1999].

The practice of placing preoperative ventriculostomy or ventriculoperitoneal shunt before surgery for posterior fossa tumor with hydrocephalus has fallen out of favor in most situations because of the risk for precipitation of upward transtentorial herniation [Cuneo et al., 1979; Epstein and Murali, 1978; Raimondi and Tomita, 1981].

Infratentorial herniation, either upward transtentorial herniation or downward cerebellar pressure coning, should be considered in the clinical setting of deterioration of consciousness or coma associated with posterior fossa mass lesion, cerebellar edema, or cerebrospinal fluid drainage whether by ventriculostomy, ventriculoperitoneal shunt, or lumbar puncture. Cerebellar herniation associated with lumbar puncture in the clinical setting of a child with meningitis and with evidence of increased intracranial pressure is an especially important consideration.

Herniation Syndromes, Summary

That brain tissue deforms intracranially and moves from higher to lower pressure when there is asymmetric, unilateral, or generalized increased intracranial pressure is not disputed. The importance of the phenomenon is that associated symptoms, which begin with alteration of consciousness or coma and progress to involve brainstem areas from more rostral to caudal distribution, give important clues to the etiology of the deterioration and, thus, lead to more rapid and appropriate treatment.

DIAGNOSTIC TESTING

All patients with significant impairment of consciousness or coma should have immediate blood glucose finger stick determination by Chemstrip or Dextrostix and should have blood drawn for a chemistry profile and complete blood count. The blood chemistry profile should minimally include glucose, sodium, potassium, blood urea nitrogen, calcium, magnesium, and ammonia. Hypoglycemia, derangements of osmolality (hyponatremia, hypernatremia), and ketoacidosis are important causes of mental status change in children. Uremia with encephalopathy may be seen in patients with acute renal failure with evolution over hours to days. It may also be the presenting feature in the hemolytic-uremic syndrome. Disorders of calcium metabolism may impair consciousness and cause peripheral symptoms. Abnormalities of calcium or magnesium may precipitate unexpected seizures, especially in infants and young children. Hyperammonemia may alter consciousness, particularly in conjunction with hepatotoxicity resulting from valproic acid or other agents, Reye's syndrome, inborn errors of metabolism, or other disorders. A complete blood count assists in determining the presence of infection, anemia, or toxin exposure, such as lead poisoning. A urine specimen should be sent for toxicology screening (see Chapter 87). Arterial blood gas determination is often necessary, as is pulse oximetry. When infection is suspected, blood and urine cultures should be obtained.

Additional blood and urine studies that may be worth obtaining when the patient is first seen but are not usually immediately available, include urine and blood specimens for amino and organic acid disorders, thyroid function studies, plasma cortisol, free fatty acid, very-long-chain fatty acids and total and free carnitine levels, comprehensive drug testing, and screening for disorders of porphyrin metabolism.

Lumbar puncture should be performed when there is a suggestion of infection of the CNS with or without fever. Depending on the clinical findings and evaluation, CT needs to be performed before the lumbar puncture. When medically stable, all patients in coma and most, if not all, patients with impairment of consciousness of undetermined etiology should have a CT performed as rapidly as possible. In children with closed-head injury, CT or preferably MRI may be critical in identifying the specific cause of impaired loss of consciousness [Ashwal and Holshouser, 1997]. MRI is also invaluable in identifying evidence of herpes simplex encephalitis or an acute demyelinating process, such as acute disseminated encephalomyelitis.

The electroencephalogram is essential to diagnose clinically inapparent status epilepticus (i.e., nonconvulsive status epilepticus). Certain electroencephalogram patterns, such as periodic lateralized epileptiform discharges, may suggest herpes simplex encephalitis, especially in the setting of a febrile illness [Misra and Kalita, 1998]. In addition, the electroencephalogram is useful in the serial reassessment and evaluation of patients in status epilepticus or persistent coma, as well as in patients requiring pharmacologic paralysis or sedation.

TREATMENT

Treatment of the child with impaired consciousness or coma requires scrupulous attention to certain basic principles while definitive diagnostic tests are obtained and therapy initiated. Specific etiologies of many individual causes of disordered consciousness are listed in Box 61-3 and are reviewed by specific diagnostic category in other sections of this book. The following principles of management are similar in most patients and are outlined in Box 61-4.

1. *Ensure oxygenation.* Maintenance of an adequate airway remains one of the most important principles in the management of children with altered states of consciousness and coma. When necessary, an artificial airway should be established and artificial ventilation provided, even if this necessitates the use of sedative or paralytic agents. It is important, however, to ensure that cervical spine injuries are not worsened in the process of managing a patient's respiratory problems.
2. *Maintain circulation.* The second important principle in the management of these patients is to maintain cardiovascular function. Intravascular access is critical and should be provided by an appropriate intravenous line or through intraosseous access.
3. *Administer glucose.* Glucose is the essential source of adenosine triphosphate for cerebral energy metabolism. Once the initial glucose level is ascertained, glucose administration is recommended if the results reveal an abnormally low level. All other therapies are superfluous when oxygen and essential metabolic substrates (e.g., glucose) are not delivered to neurons and toxic metabolites are not removed.

Box 61-4 Treatment Goals for Patients with Impaired Consciousness and Coma

- Ensure oxygenation
- Maintain circulation
- Give glucose
- Correct acid-base and electrolyte imbalance
- Consider specific antidotes
- Reduce increased intracranial pressure
- Stop seizures
- Treat infection
- Adjust body temperature
- Manage agitation

4. *Correct acid-base and electrolyte imbalance.* Electrolyte imbalance seen after CNS insults is often mediated by inappropriate antidiuretic hormone secretion. Inappropriate administration of fluids may worsen this situation. More commonly, hyponatremia, hypernatremia, hypocalcemia, or hypomagnesemia may occur in conjunction with systemic illness and be the cause of coma. Metabolic or respiratory acidosis or alkalosis should also be corrected.
5. *Consider specific antidotes.* Naloxone is available for treatment when an opiate overdose is suspected. Although opiate overdosage is rare in children, the risks of naloxone are minimal, and administration should always be considered. Physostigmine may reverse CNS and cardiac effects of anticholinergic agents. However, physostigmine may cause nonspecific CNS stimulation or seizures. Flumazenil, a benzodiazepine receptor antagonist, may be valuable in such patients.
6. *Reduce increased intracranial pressure.* Increased intracranial pressure may exist for a variety of structural, metabolic, or toxic reasons. It is essential to identify surgically treatable causes of elevated intracranial pressure quickly to allow appropriate intervention. Head CT should be performed in all children with coma resulting from closed-head injuries and in all children in whom the cause of coma is not immediately apparent or in whom the onset was not observed or is unknown.

   When intracranial pressure elevation is not caused by a surgically treatable lesion, a variety of therapeutic interventions can be considered. Fluid administration can be limited to half or two thirds of maintenance, provided that cardiovascular function and systemic blood pressure are maintained. Fluid restriction as a treatment for increased intracranial pressure should only be used when cerebral perfusion is deemed adequate. Positioning of the head at 30 degrees above the horizontal to maximize venous outflow from the head has merit so long as cerebral perfusion pressure is not harmed. Hyperventilation through mechanical ventilation reduces intracranial pressure by lowering cerebral blood flow and may have short-term merit if cerebral perfusion pressure and delivery of metabolic substrate is maintained. Reduction of intracranial volume by reduction of brain water content using mannitol, furosemide, or hypertonic saline may be beneficial. Sedation is valuable to reduce Valsalva response and resulting reduction in brain venous outflow during noxious, but necessary, critical care such as suctioning. Barbiturate therapy to reduce cellular metabolic demand may help control intracranial pressure but does not seem to influence outcome. Reduction of fever, however, may be valuable in lowering brain metabolic demands. High-dose corticosteroid therapy may have a role in treating increased intracranial pressure due to brain tumors and in some infections but is not useful in managing traumatic brain injury, infarction, and hemorrhage [Smith and Madsen, 2004a].

   Optimal treatment of increased intracranial pressure must take into consideration that metabolic substrate supply must equal critical metabolic requirement to prevent secondary brain injury. Simply controlling intracranial pressure and cerebral perfusion pressure by using diuretics to reduce brain water content and hyperventilation to reduce cerebral blood flow and volume does not adequately take into account strategies to prevent secondary injury [Meyeret al., 2001]. Therefore, monitoring of intracranial pressure is essential, and monitoring cerebral blood flow and brain tissue Po_2 adds monitoring power.

   Decompressive craniectomy, with or without opening the dura, lowers intracranial pressure and is increasingly used for refractory increased intracranial pressure in certain situations [Figaji et al., 2003; Smith and Madsen, 2004b; Taylor et al., 2001].
7. *Stop seizures.* Treatment of status epilepticus and other seizure emergencies is discussed elsewhere. It is always important to consider seizures even when there are no obvious outward seizure manifestations. Electroencephalography is essential in identifying subclinical nonconvulsive status epilepticus or other forms of seizure activity.
8. *Treat infection.* Underlying infectious processes should be treated if specific treatment is available. Usually, the diagnosis of infectious diseases that involve the CNS requires lumbar puncture. When there is concern about elevated intracranial pressure, it may be appropriate to start antibiotic therapy for meningitis or antiviral therapy for encephalitis before lumbar puncture. In certain clinical situations, treatment can be initiated and the lumbar puncture deferred.
9. *Adjust body temperature.* Usually, normal body temperature is best for recovery and prevention of acidosis. Patients with fever should have appropriate antipyretic agents administered. The use of hypothermia is being re-evaluated as a potential treatment for coma [Bernard et al., 1997; Biagas and Gaeta, 1988; Clifton, 1995; Safar and Kochanek, 2002]. This is discussed in more detail in Chapters 62 and 63.
10. *Manage agitation.* It is particularly important to prevent agitation because of the problems it may

present in the critical care management of patients with altered consciousness or coma. Agitation may increase intracranial pressure and make it difficult to control respiration with mechanical ventilation. The decision to sedate, however, may make serial neurologic examination as a measure of change in a patient's status difficult. In these circumstances, additional serial neurodiagnostic tests, such as electroencephalography, may be valuable.

MONITORING OF THE COMATOSE PATIENT

After initiation of treatment, it is necessary to serially re-evaluate the patient's condition and effectiveness of intervention. The neurologic examination is the gold standard for evaluation and re-evaluation but often is significantly modified by iatrogenic intervention such as mechanical ventilation, sedation, and paralysis. Many clinical neurophysiology monitors are available to improve critical care monitoring; some are in more widespread use than others. All clinical neurophysiology monitors are used in one or more of the following situations:

- As extension of the neurologic examination to identify nonconvulsive status epilepticus or electroencephalographic patterns that suggest a diagnosis and to evaluate the integrity of certain neural pathways
- To improve assessment of the neurologic condition of patients who are sedated or sedated and paralyzed and on mechanical ventilation
- To assist in assessment of availability of metabolic substrate critical to maintain brain integrity and function
- To evaluate treatment effect in status epilepticus
- To improve outcome assessment

Traditionally, the electroencephalogram has been used to identify presence of or risk for seizures and has additive value in that certain patterns may suggest specific pathology such as triphasic waves in metabolic causes of coma and periodic lateralized epileptiform discharges in focal injury and infection. Electroencephalographic reactivity to sensory stimulation is considered a favorable sign in coma recovery [Young, 2000]. Electroencephalography has the advantage of ready availability in most centers and is usually definitive in the evaluation for ongoing seizures. However, there is not universal agreement about criteria to diagnose nonconvulsive status epilepticus in obtunded or comatose patients [Brenner, 2002]. Other drawbacks to the use of long-term electroencephalographic monitoring include technical training necessary to apply and maintain the electrode-scalp interface, specialized training necessary for interpretation, and electroencephalographic susceptibility to artifact in the critical care setting. Processed derivations of electroencephalographic activity, therefore, have been successfully used to monitor brain activity.

The Bispectral Index monitor is a recorder that uses processed electroencephalogram data to measure sedation depth on a scale from 0 to 100 (0, coma; 40-60, general anesthesia; 60–90, sedated; 100, awake). The Bispectral Index monitor is useful in monitoring depth of sedation during conscious sedation [Agrawal et al., 2004] and neurologic status in critically ill unsedated patients. It is also easily applied to children in critical care settings and has been used to monitor children in barbiturate coma, sedation to assist mechanical ventilation, and procedural sedation and to evaluate sedation effects of multiple medications [Grindstaff and Tobias, 2004].

Although the Bispectral Index Scale does not have the monitoring power of a full-montage electroencephalogram, it has the advantage of easier electrode application and more ready interpretation. In a study of 16 patients between 10 and 192 months of age with consciousness alteration admitted to a pediatric intensive care unit, the Bispectral Index Scale correlated well with the Glasgow Coma Scale [Hsia et al., 2004]. Amplitude-integrated electroencephalography is an alternative methodology that has been used for the evaluation of the neonate but is now being used in older children and adults to assess the severity of neurologic injury [Scheuer and Wilson, 2004; ter Horst et al., 2004].

Sensory-evoked potentials allow assessment of the integrity of visual, auditory, and somatosensory pathways in the unconscious patient. Somatosensory-evoked potentials have been especially valuable because their neural pathways extend from brainstem through thalamus and subcortical white matter to cortex. Somatosensory-evoked potentials are relatively resistant to sedation effect and are useful in predicting outcome in comatose patients. Visual-evoked potentials have not been as valuable as somatosensory-evoked potentials for outcome prediction in comatose children [Shewman, 2000a, 2000b; Taylor and Farrell, 1989]. Brainstem auditory-evoked potentials are valuable for monitoring brainstem function but do not predict cortical function [Shewman, 2000a, 2000b]. The presence of normal brainstem auditory-evoked potentials with abnormal somatosensory-evoked potentials is seen on patients who are in a vegetative state [Frank et al., 1985]. Middle latency auditory-evoked potentials have cortical representation and have been shown to improve coma outcome prediction in adults, although they may be less resistant to environmental artifact and sedation than somatosensory-evoked potentials. Event-related potentials (auditory P_{300} response) may assist in evaluating severity of injury and may correlate with closed-head injury outcome in adults [Fischer et al., 2004; Keren et al., 1998; Litscher, 1985; Logi et al., 2003].

Motor-evoked potentials have limited value in evaluation of the comatose patient and have not been studied in children for this purpose. Adult studies have found that electrically elicited but not magnetoelectrically elicited motor-evoked potentials may predict postcoma pyramidal motor deficit but do not allow prediction of severity of motor deficit. Motor-evoked potentials do not have the predictive value of somatosensory-evoked potentials for coma outcome. Motor-evoked potentials may be valuable in evaluating clinical deterioration in the acute phase of coma [Rohde et al., 1999; Zentner and Rohde, 1992, 1994].

Measurement of cerebral blood flow is a direct way to determine delivery of essential metabolic substrate to the brain but is not useful for continuous monitoring. Brain tissue Po_2 measurement, however, is suitable for continuous monitoring. In 25 patients older than 16 years with severe traumatic brain injury (Glascow Coma Scale value less than 8), it was found that intraparenchymal brain Po_2 favorably compared with stable xenon CT for measurement of cerebral blood flow and allowed continuous monitoring of this critical substrate [Doppenberg et al., 1998]. Another study of 22 severe head injury patients aged 11 to 52 years found that continuous monitoring of partial pressure of brain tissue oxygen was practical and safe, allowed monitoring of ischemia on a continuous basis, allowed demonstration of abnormalities of oxygen autoregulatory mechanisms, and was superior to jugular oximetry [Van Santbrink et al., 1996]. Low brain tissue Po_2, as a measure of cerebral hypoxia, is predictive of poor neurologic outcome and is an important independent measurement parameter in adults with severe traumatic brain injury [Bardt et al., 1998]. Monitoring of brain tissue Po_2 may also allow early detection of critical and potentially irreversible worsening and allow measurement of intervention effect on a continuous basis. This is exemplified in a case report of a 15-year-old patient with severe traumatic brain injury and uncontrollable intracranial hypertension who developed bilateral fixed and dilated pupils and critically low brain tissue Po_2 on the third day after injury, and who underwent bilateral decompressive craniotomy with immediate normalization of intracranial pressure and complete recovery of brain tissue Po_2 to normal level [Kiening et al., 1997].

Local sampling of energy substrates by microdialysis during ischemia is feasible and allows measurement of glucose, lactate, pyruvate, and glutamate in brain tissue serially over time. Glucose concentration closely follows brain tissue Po_2, lactate concentration significantly increases when brain tissue O_2 falls below critical level, and glutamate is significantly elevated with very low brain tissue Po_2 levels in adult head trauma patients [Hlatky et al., 2004]. Microdialysis measurements have thus far only been applied in children for monitoring of severe traumatic brain injury. In one study of nine children aged 2 to 14 years, a low glutamine-to-glutamate ratio was associated with increased morbidity [Tolias et al., 2002].

Near-infrared spectroscopy noninvasively monitors brain tissue oxygenation by measuring the distinct absorption spectra of oxygenated and deoxygenated hemoglobin in the frontal cortex. Near-infrared spectroscopy compares favorably to brain tissue Po_2 monitoring in adults with severe traumatic brain injury or aneurysmal subarachnoid hemorrhage [Brawanski et al., 2002]. Additionally, in a study of 43 children monitored after corrective surgery for noncyanotic congenital heart defects, noninvasive measurement of the cerebral tissue oxygenation index by near-infrared spectroscopy correlated with central venous oxygen saturation measured with a catheter placed in the right atrium [Nagdyman et al., 2004]. At least one commercially available device for near-infrared spectroscopy monitoring is approved by the U.S. Food and Drug Administration for children [Andropoulos et al., 2004] and has been used extensively to monitor brain tissue oxygenation during surgery for congenital heart disease. In a study of 26 infants and children having heart surgery with bypass and deep hypothermic circulatory arrest, low cerebrovascular hemoglobin oxygen saturation was associated with postoperative neurologic complications in 3 children (1 with seizure and 2 with prolonged coma) [Kurth et al., 1995].

Cerebral oxygenation measured by near-infrared spectroscopy has been found to be valuable in two pediatric patients (ages 4 months and 16 years) being monitored for seizures in the pediatric intensive care unit and the epilepsy monitoring unit and demonstrated preictal increase in cerebral oxygenation and suggested perfusion-metabolism mismatch during seizure activity. Thus, the monitoring of cerebral oxygenation by near-infrared spectroscopy has value in the critical care setting for continuous monitoring of dynamic changes in cerebral oxygenation in relation to changes in metabolic need [Adelson et al., 1999]. Nonetheless, use of near-infrared spectroscopy to monitor brain tissue oxygenation has not been studied extensively in children, except in surgery for congenital heart defects, and a recent study in children indicated a poor agreement between two commercially available cerebral oximeters using near-infrared spectroscopy [Dullenkopf et al., 2003].

Transcranial Doppler ultrasonography measures real-time cerebral blood flow velocity and is useful for monitoring middle cerebral artery flow velocity transcranially in all ages and through the anterior fontanel in infants. Transcranial Doppler has been used in pediatric cardiac surgery to evaluate cerebrovascular response to cardiopulmonary bypass, hypothermia, and deep hypothermia circulatory arrest [Andropoulos et al., 2004]. It has also been used to evaluate detectable cerebral perfusion threshold in low-flow cardiopulmonary bypass in neonates [Zimmerman et al., 1997]. It is important to note, however, that cerebral blood flow velocity depend on vessel diameter and is not the same measurement as cerebral blood flow, which depends on cerebral vascular resistance and varies with temperature, CO_2 pressure, cerebral perfusion pressure, and bypass flow. Therefore, cerebral blood flow velocity may correlate best with cerebral blood flow in deep hypothermia when autoregulation is lost and blood vessel diameter does not change.

Brain tissue Po_2 monitoring and microdialysis to evaluate energy substrates are complementary, and both monitoring probes require neurosurgical installation into brain parenchyma. Therefore, they are primarily used clinically to evaluate and monitor victims of severe traumatic brain injury. Near-infrared spectroscopy and transcranial Doppler are currently used to monitor brain oxygenation in children during and after cardiac surgery. The devices are small and relatively portable and can be used in the pediatric critical care environment safely, effectively, and continuously. Their ultimate value in monitoring of children in coma and guiding therapeutic interventions has yet to be delineated. However, in a prospective study of 250 patients undergoing pediatric cardiac surgery, it was found that interventions based on neurophysiologic monitoring (electroencephalography, transcranial Doppler, near-infrared spectroscopy) appeared to decrease the incidence of postoperative neurologic sequelae and reduce length of stay [Austin et al., 1997].

OUTCOME MEASUREMENT

When consciousness is impaired, outcome is related to the etiology of the insult and rapid identification and treatment of the underlying cause. Early appropriate treatment may prevent further deterioration of the mental state and injury to the nervous system and improve outcome. Outcome studies in childhood coma are available for traumatic and nontraumatic causes and typically emphasize predictive value of signs and symptoms at the time of initial medical intervention.

A commonly used and widely accepted measurement of outcome after severe closed-head injury is the Glasgow Outcome Scale [Jennett and Bond, 1975]. The Glasgow Outcome Scale has the following five broad outcome categories: (1) death; (2) persistent vegetative state; (3) severe disability (conscious but disabled); (4) moderate disability (disabled but independent); and (5) good recovery. The Glasgow Outcome Scale heavily emphasizes functional independence in mobility, transportation, and self-care. Significant functional improvement can be seen within the first three categories. The Glasgow Outcome Scale is limited in its ability to quantify impairments related to social skills and emotional and cognitive dysfunction; it does not take into account special issues of injury and recovery during the developmental period. A modified form of the Glasgow Outcome Scale for children, the Pediatric Cerebral Performance Category Scale, was published by Fiser in 1992. This six-point outcome scoring system was validated in 1469 pediatric patients suffering acute CNS injuries. It has also been correlated with neuropsychological test scores [Fiser et al., 2000]. The score includes the following outcomes: (1) normal—able to perform all age-appropriate activities; (2) mild disability—conscious, alert, and able to interact at an age-appropriate level but may have a mild neurologic deficit; (3) moderate disability—conscious, sufficient cerebral function for most age-appropriate independent activities; (4) severe disability—conscious, dependent on others for daily support because of impaired brain function; (5) persistent vegetative state; and (6) death. This scale has been used in outcome prediction studies after acute brain injury in children who were acutely evaluated with proton magnetic resonance spectroscopy [Ashwal et al., 2000; Brenner et al., 2003; Holshouser et al., 1997].

In a prospective study of 53 children less than 3 years old with severe brain injury or hypoxic-ischemic encephalopathy, the Glasgow Outcome Scale indicated good recovery in 46% of 50 children with known outcome [Robertson et al., 2002]. However, only 16% had average or above-average scores on both the mental and motor developmental sections of the Bayley Scales of Infant Development II at 18 to 36 months of age. Thus, a commonly used developmental assessment tool, the Bayley Scales of Infant Development II, provides a greater distinction between normal and delayed development than does the good recovery level of the Glasgow Outcome Scale [Robertson et al., 2002].

Early studies using the Glasgow Outcome Scale as an outcome measure after closed-head injury reported that patients advance to the highest functional level by 6 months after injury [Jennett et al., 1976, 1979; Jennett and Bond, 1975; Lange-Cossack et al., 1981]. Meaningful recovery, however, may occur for months to years after injury [Mahoney et al., 1981, 1983]. Because there may be significant functional improvement within the three highest Glasgow Outcome Scale categories (i.e., good recovery, moderate disability, and severe disability) and because long-term improvement is possible, especially when injury occurs during early childhood, alternative outcome scales have been developed.

The Disability Rating Scale consists of eight items divided into four categories: (1) arousability and awareness (best eye opening, verbal, and motor response); (2) cognitive ability for self-care activities (feeding, toileting, and grooming); (3) physical dependence on others; and (4) psychosocial adaptability for work or school [Rappaport et al., 1982]. The Disability Rating Scale is a more sensitive measure of improvement during inpatient rehabilitation than the Glasgow Outcome Scale [Hall et al., 1985] and is suitable for use in adolescents and some older children.

The Functional Independence Measure and its pediatric counterpart, the Wee Functional Independence Measure, further refine outcome assessment using six items and 18 categories [Data Management Service of the Uniform Data System of Medical Rehabilitation and the Center for Functional Assessment Research, 1989]. The Wee Functional Independence Measure items and categories are as follows: (1) self-care (eating, grooming, bathing, dressing—upper body, dressing—lower body, toileting); (2) sphincter control (bladder and bowel); (3) mobility: transfer (chair or wheelchair, toilet, tub, shower); (4) locomotion (walking, wheelchair, crawling, stairs); (5) communication (auditory and visual comprehension, verbal and nonverbal expression); and (6) social cognition (social interaction, problem solving, memory). The Wee Functional Independence Measure has good inter-rater reliability and allows serial assessment throughout the pediatric age range.

The Pediatric Evaluation of Disabilities Inventory measures both capability and performance of multiple functional activities in three areas: (1) self-care, (2) mobility, and (3) social function [Haley et al., 1992]. The Pediatric Evaluation of Disabilities Inventory is designed for use from 6 months to 7 years of age but is appropriate for older children whose functional level is within the intended age range. Specialized derivations of the Pediatric Evaluation of Disabilities Inventory specific to acquired brain injury do not improve the assessment value of the generic inventory, although further refinement may allow better functional recovery scoring in acquired brain injury [Kothari et al., 2003]. Pediatric Evaluation of Disabilities Inventory score change of about 11% has been found clinically meaningful during inpatient rehabilitation in a cohort of 53 children ages 1 to 19 years [Iyer et al., 2003].

The Wee Functional Independence Measure and the Pediatric Evaluation of Disabilities Inventory are sensitive measures of functional outcome and are suitable for inpatient rehabilitation monitoring and long-term outpatient follow-up. They are two of the most commonly used functional outcome measures in children [Ziviani et al., 2001] and are superior to the Glasgow Outcome Scale and its pediatric variants for assessment of long-term functional improvement in children across more relevant domains of recovery.

The School Functional Assessment was developed to measure performance of functional tasks that are important for participation in an elementary school level program (kindergarten through grade 6). The School Functional Assessment evaluates (1) ability to participate in major school activity settings, (2) support necessary to participate effectively in an education program, and (3) performance of specific school-related functional activities [Coster et al., 1998].

The School Functional Assessment provides for further functional assessment of short-term and long-term outcome more specific to the educational setting and may allow prediction of specialized school needs before discharge from inpatient rehabilitation.

Other standardized measures used to assess intellectual, cognitive, language, and behavioral development in children without injury are useful in evaluating and assessing outcomes in children after severe acquired brain injury. In children old enough and cooperative enough, neuropsychologic testing is the most sensitive and specific way to measure and monitor change in these domains. Valuable reviews of these issues are available [Fletcher et al., 1987; Hannay and Sherer, 1996; Levin, 1994; Ylvisaker et al., 1990]. In a retrospective analysis of 83 children aged 1 to 18 years admitted to hospital after head injury, 70% had severe head injury, and 13 died. Forty-five patients had at least one cognitive assessment, and 17 were evaluated with intelligence testing less than 4 months after injury, 5 to 15 months after injury, and 16 to 38 months after injury. Continued improvement in cognitive functioning was seen at 16 to 38 months' follow-up assessment [Campbell et al., 2004]. This improvement underscores the fact that continued cognitive recovery may progress for years and that more long-term studies are necessary.

PROGNOSIS—TRAUMATIC INJURY

Prolonged coma after global hypoxic ischemic injury as in cardiac arrest has a poor prognosis [Kirkham, 1994]. Children who survive traumatic or infectious injury may have a better prognosis depending on the specific pathophysiology and the presence of hypoxia-ischemia as a complicating variable. How prognosis is defined, however, is significant. For example, in a study of 127 children said to be in the persistent vegetative state for at least 30 days, 84% of the traumatic brain injury group, but only 55% of the hypoxic-ischemic injury group, improved beyond the vegetative state [Heindl and Laub, 1996]. This study highlights that hypoxic-ischemic injury is worse than traumatic brain injury but uses the term *persistent vegetative state* (a statement of prognosis) rather than vegetative state (a moment in time description).

It is important, therefore, to understand the operational challenges in the evaluation of coma prognosis in children. Shewman has identified and reviewed the following problems and caveats with studies of coma prognosis in children: (1) definition of coma; (2) definition of study population and outcome variables; (3) basic study design; (4) self-fulfilling nature of poor prognosis; (5) early death rate from nonneurologic causes; (6) lumping of etiologies, age groups, and outcome categories; (7) short and inhomogeneous follow-up; and (8) failure to provide confidence intervals [Shewman, 2000a, 2000b]. Lumping of etiology, age groups, and outcome categories often is an effort to compensate for low statistical power related to small total number of patients and early death rate from other causes, which further reduces sample size. Clearly, there are better outcome descriptors than the Glasgow Outcome Score and its variants. In an effort to provide a sense of the current state of outcome data in this area, several outcome studies are reviewed.

In studies of coma in children resulting from traumatic brain injury, substantially better outcome is seen in children when compared with adults [Broman and Michel, 1995]. Up to 80% to 90% of children with severe traumatic brain injury have good outcomes or recover to a moderate disability based on studies using the Glasgow Outcome Scale.

In a small retrospective review of eight survivors of severe traumatic brain injury at a mean age of 14 years, neuropsychologic evaluation was performed 1, 7, and 14 years after the injury. Three of the eight subjects went from a school situation with no adjustments to adult life without ability to be employed [Jonsson et al., 2004]. In a review of 65 children and adolescents with acquired brain injury aged 6 months to 18 years (mean age, 9.5 years), 82% were discharged home, but only 3% to 27% were deemed ready for age-expected participation in home, school, and community life [Bedell et al., 2002a]. Social behavioral activity performance at discharge explained 74% of the variance associated with participation at discharge. In the same cohort of patients, functional assessment scales of daily and social behavioral activity allowed assessment of response to treatment [Bedell et al., 2002b].

In survivors of severe traumatic brain injury, potential problems involving community re-entry including home, school, and community life can be evaluated and treatment interventions monitored serially. After school, capacity for employment may be greatly impaired by behavior and social problems, even in the individual cognitively able to be employed. Early recognition of these problems and effective intervention while in school may allow better functional outcome.

Brink and associates reported a large series of 344 pediatric patients (younger than 18 years) with severe closed-head injury and coma for a minimum of 24 hours who were admitted to a rehabilitation center between 1959 and 1977 [Brink et al., 1970, 1980]. Median coma duration was 5 to 6 weeks. One year after injury, 73% were independent in ambulation and self-care, but only 10% were physically normal. Coma duration of less than 6 weeks was associated with better outcome than coma duration of longer than 12 weeks. However, less than one third of these children had normal intelligence; about half had significant behavior problems, and most required special education services at school.

A study of 33 survivors of severe closed-head injury enrolled at 17 years of age or younger demonstrated the following Glasgow Outcome Scale distribution 5 to 7 years after injury: 27% good recovery, 55% moderate disability, and 18% severe disability. At the time of follow-up, 70% were independent in self-care, 64% in mobility, and only 24% in cognitive items on the Functional Independence Measure [Massagli et al., 1996]. More importantly, 70% received special education services, and employment histories were poor. This clearly illustrates the better specificity of the Functional Independence Measure over the Glasgow Outcome Scale when evaluating long-term quality of life and community re-entry. Moreover, most of these individuals were not involved in neurologic or rehabilitation follow-up, suggesting the need for better long-term programs of monitoring and care.

Both the Wee Functional Independence Measure and the Pediatric Evaluation of Disabilities Inventory measure functional ability taking into account amount of caregiver assistance necessary and use of special equipment. The Wee Functional Independence Measure assesses 18 variables in self-care, mobility, and cognition, whereas the Pediatric Evaluation of Disabilities Inventory evaluates 197 functional items in self-care, mobility, and social function. In a study of 205 children with disability aged 11 to 87 months, the Wee Functional Independence Measure measured similar skill areas to those assessed by the Battelle Developmental Inventory Screening Test or the Vineland Adaptive Behavior Scale. The Wee Functional Independence Measure requires less administration time than the Pediatric Evaluation of Disabilities Inventory, the Battelle Developmental Inventory Screening Test, or the Vineland Adaptive Behavior Scale and provides directly relevant functional outcome information for children and their families [Ottenbacher et al., 1999]. Further, the Wee Functional Independence Measure was an improvement over the Battelle and the Vineland scales in predicting the amount of assistance that parents or teachers must provide for basic activities of daily living [Ottenbacher et al., 2000].

PROGNOSIS—NONTRAUMATIC INJURY

Outcome after coma resulting from nontraumatic causes has been extensively reviewed and available information suggests that, as with closed-head injury, outcome in children is better than in adults. In a cohort of 104 children ranging in age from 1 month to 17 years with nontraumatic coma (average duration of coma was 3 hours to 35 days), 32% died, 50% were normal, and the remaining 18% had handicaps ranging from mild to severe. Stepwise multivariate discriminant analysis within 12 hours of onset of coma classified 75% of 102 cases correctly into one of five outcome groups and misclassified 8% of patients. When the discriminant analysis was used on data collected 24 hours after the onset of coma, 67% of the cases were correctly classified, and only 3% were misclassified. Variables that correlated best with outcome were coma severity, motor patterns, blood pressure, and seizure type. Age correlated well with outcome based on data obtained at 24 but not at 12 hours. Extraocular movements, pupillary responses, and temperature correlated with outcome at less than 12 hours but not at 24 hours. Mortality rate was highest in patients less than 1 year of age (44%), and only 24% were considered normal at follow-up. For patients aged 6 to 17 years, 24% died, and 73% were normal. Patients who died all had hypothermia, inability to maintain body temperature, and absent pupillary responses or extraocular movements [Johnston and Seshia, 1984; Seshia et al., 1983].

In a retrospective population study of nontraumatic coma in children aged 1 month to 16 years, 278 individuals were identified, representing 283 episodes of coma. The most common cause of coma was infection, and the most common cause of recurrent episodes of coma was epilepsy. Causes of nontraumatic coma were infection, 37.9%; unknown, 14.5%; intoxication, 10.3%; epilepsy, 9.6%; congenital malformation, 8.2%; other, 7.8%; accident, 6.7%; and metabolic, 5.0%. Within the unknown group, half of the cases were suspected to be due to infection because of the clinical course, but pathogens were not identified. At 12 months' follow-up, the overall mortality rate was 46%, and the etiology-specific mortality rate varied from 3% (intoxication) to 84% (accident). Most individuals were either intact (normal) at 12 months' follow-up or were deceased. Highest intact survival rates were seen in patients with epilepsy (71.4%), metabolic etiologies (60%), or unknown causes of coma (47.5%). Mortality was highest in patients in coma from accidents (84.2%), congenital malformations (72.7%), and infections (60%) [Wong et al., 2001].

In this study of 278 individuals, cognitive and adaptive outcomes were evaluated 6 weeks and 12 months after admission. Age-appropriate psychometric instruments were employed as follows: Bayley Scales of Infant Development (younger than 3.5 years); Wechsler Preschool and Primary Scale of Intelligence—Revised (3.5-6 years), and the Wechsler Intelligence Scale for Children III (older than 6 years). When appropriate, adaptive behavior was evaluated using the Vineland Adaptive Behavior Scales. Of 278 patients, 151 survived to late follow-up, and 141 (93% of survivors) completed follow-up assessment. Significant differences in outcome based on etiology could not be established, but children younger than 2 years of age at admission had no improvement, and children older than 2 years of age had improvement when evaluated 6 weeks and 12 months after initial admission. The overall incidence of moderate-to-severe disability (cognitive quotient less than 70 and moderate-to-severe behavioral disturbances) was 70%. The relation between early age at first coma episode and poor outcome was particularly evident in children with nontraumatic coma caused by epilepsy [Forsyth et al., 2001].

PROGNOSIS—CLINICAL NEUROPHYSIOLOGY

In the comatose patient, clinical neurophysiology evaluation (electroencephalogram, somatosensory-evoked potential) is the most valuable for prediction of survival, brain death, and functional recovery beyond the vegetative state [Beca et al., 1995; DeMeirleir and Taylor, 1986, 1987; Fischer et al., 2004; Goodwin et al., 1991; Mandel et al., 2002; Mewasingh et al., 2003; Shewman, 2000b; Wohlrab et al., 2001]. There are, however, a few reports of contrary findings such as normal somatosensory-evoked potentials in a child in a vegetative state following near drowning [Tsao and Ellingson, 1989]. Therefore, the clinical neurophysiology assessment is used as an adjunct to the clinical examination and other outcome predictors such as neuroimaging and cerebral blood flow. To date, there are no studies linking neurophysiologic tests to very long-term functional outcome measures such as the Wee Functional Independence Measure or the Pediatric Evaluation of Disabilities Inventory.

Several studies have indicated the prognostic value of proton magnetic resonance spectroscopy in newborns, infants, and children with CNS insult or injury of different types [Holshouser et al., 1997, 2000]. Patients with elevated cerebral lactate are more likely to die or have serious long-term disability [Ashwal et al., 1997]. Metabolic ratios of *N*-acetylaspartate/choline–containing compounds and *N*-acetylaspartate/creatine and phosphocreatine were significantly lower in patients with bad outcomes. Outcome measurement was performed at 6 to 12 months using the Pediatric Cerebral Performance Scale, and outcomes were expressed as good/moderate outcome (good, mild, moderate disability) or poor outcome (severe disability, persistent vegetative state, death). When magnetic resonance spectroscopy data were combined with clinical data and MRI scores, outcome was correctly predicted in 91% of neonates and 100% of infants and children [Ashwal et al., 1997; Auld et al., 1995; Holshouser et al., 1997; Shu et al., 1997].

In a magnetic resonance spectroscopy study of 26 infants (1 to 18 months old) and 27 children (18 months or older) with nonaccidental or other forms of traumatic brain injury, lactate was evident in 91% of infants and 80% of children with poor outcome, whereas none of the patients with good outcome had elevated lactate. Metabolic ratios were abnormal (low *N*-acetylaspartate/creatine and phosphocreatine, low *N*-acetylaspartate/choline-containing compounds, and high choline-containing compounds/creatine and phosphocreatine) in patients with poor outcome. Clinical variables alone predicted outcome in 77% of infants and 86% of children. Lactate alone predicted outcome in 96% of infants and 96% of children. Addition of metabolic ratios and clinical variables did not improve outcome prediction over lactate alone [Ashwal et al., 2000]. Myoinositol, a marker of astrocyte activity, is measurable by magnetic resonance spectroscopy, and in a study of 38 children with traumatic brain injury, aged 1.6 to 17 years, myoinositol was higher in patients with poor outcomes than in patients with good outcomes (Ashwal et al., 2004].

Susceptibility-weighted imaging, a new high-resolution gradient-echo MRI technique, is superior to conventional T2-weighted two-dimensional gradient-recalled echo imaging in identifying hemorrhagic lesions associated with diffuse axonal injury [Tong et al., 2003]. In 40 children and adolescents with traumatic brain injury and suspected diffuse axonal injury, those with Glasgow Coma Scale scores of 8 or lower, prolonged coma of more than 4 days' duration, or poor neurologic outcomes 6 to 12 months after injury had significantly increased numbers and volume of hemorrhagic lesions. More accurate evaluation of diffuse axonal damage soon after injury may provide improved prognostic information about coma duration and long-term outcome in children with traumatic brain injury [Tong et al., 2004].

CONCLUSIONS

Altered states of consciousness in pediatric patients are urgent situations, and coma is a medical emergency requiring rapid and organized intervention. Basic life support needs, evaluation of the history and physical examination, and specific laboratory and neurodiagnostic tests are of paramount importance and should proceed simultaneously in the emergency department. Specific diagnoses must be treated appropriately, but there are key general principles to impaired consciousness and coma management that apply in all situations.

The outcome for children with coma is substantially better than for adults and may be affected by the speed and appropriateness of intervention. Even with the best and most appropriate care, some children die, some survive on mechanical ventilation and become brain dead, and some survive beyond mechanical ventilation and have minimal consciousness or severe disability, or remain in a vegetative state. Decisions concerning basic life sustenance, type and location of care, and need for rehabilitation should take into consideration the type of injury, time from injury, recovery potential, family wishes, and appropriate ethical guidelines and standards [Michelson and Ashwal, 2004; Ashwal and Cranford, 2002].

REFERENCES

AAN Quality Standards Subcommittee. Practice parameters: Assessment and management of patients in the persistent vegetative state. Neurology 1995;45:1015.

Adams JH, Graham DI, Jennett B. The neuropathology of the vegetative state after an acute brain insult. Brain 2000;123:1327.

Adams JH, Graham DI, Murray LS, et al. Diffuse axonal injury due to nonmissile head injury in humans: An analysis of 45 cases. Ann Neurol 1982;12:557.

Adelson PD, Nemoto E, Scheuer M, et al. Noninvasive continuous monitoring of cerebral oxygenation periictally using near-infrared spectroscopy: A preliminary report. Epilepsia 1999;40:1484.

Agrawal D, Feldman MA, Krauss B, et al. Bispectral Index monitoring quantifies depth of sedation during emergency department procedural sedation and analgesia in children. Ann Emerg Med 2004;43:247.

American Congress of Rehabilitation Medicine. Recommendations for use of uniform nomenclature pertinent to patients with severe alterations in consciousness. Arch Phys Med Rehabil 1995;76:205.

Andropoulos DB, Stayer SA, Diaz LK, et al. Neurological monitoring for congenital heart surgery. Anesth Analg 2004;99:1365.

Ashwal S. Recovery of consciousness and life expectancy of children in a vegetative state. Neuropsychol Rehabil 2005;15:190.

Ashwal S. Medical aspects of the minimally conscious state in children. Brain Dev 2003;25:535.

Ashwal S. The persistent vegetative state in infancy and childhood. In: Frank Y, ed. Pediatric behavioral neurology. New York: CRC Press. 1996.

Ashwal S, Cranford R. The minimally conscious state in children. Semin Pediatr Neurol 2002;9:19.

Ashwal S, Eyman RK, Call TL. Life expectancy of children in a persistent vegetative state. Pediatr Neurol 1994;10:27.

Ashwal S, Holshouser BA. New neuroimaging techniques and their potential role in patients with acute brain injury. J Head Trauma Rehabil 1997;12:13.

Ashwal S, Holshouser BA, Shu SK, et al. Predictive value of proton magnetic resonance spectroscopy in pediatric closed head injury. Pediatr Neurol 2000;23:114.

Ashwal S, Holshouser BA, Tomasi LG, et al. 1H-magnetic resonance spectroscopy-determined cerebral lactate and poor neurological outcomes in children with central nervous system disease. Ann Neurol 1997;41:470.

Ashwal S, Holshouser BA, Tong K, et al. Proton spectroscopy detected myoinositol in children with traumatic brain injury. Pediatr Res 2004;56:630.

Atlluru VL. Spontaneous intracerebral hematomas in juvenile diabetic ketoacidosis. Pediatr Neurol 1986;2:167.

Auld KL, Ashwal S, Holshouser BA, et al. Proton magnetic resonance spectroscopy in children with acute central nervous system injury. Pediatr Neurol 1995;12:323.

Austin EH, Edmons HL, Auden SM, et al. Benefit of neurophysiologic monitoring for pediatric cardiac surgery. J Thorac Cardiovasc Surg 1997;114:707.

Baars BJ, Banks WP, Newman JB, eds. Essential sources in the scientific study of consciousness. Cambridge, MA: MIT Press (Bradford Books), 2003.

Bardt TF, Unterberg AW, Hartl R, et al. Monitoring of brain tissue PO_2 in traumatic brain injury: Effect of cerebral hypoxia on outcome. Acta Neurochir Suppl 1998;71:153.

Bates D. The management of medical coma. J Neurol Neurosurg Psychiatry 1993;56:589.

Beca J, Cox PN, Taylor MJ, et al. Somatosensory evoked potentials for prediction of outcome in acute severe brain injury. J Pediatr 1995;126:44.

Bedell GM, Haley SM, Coster WJ, et al. Participation readiness at discharge from inpatient rehabilitation in children and adolescents with acquired brain injuries. Pediatr Rehabil 2002a;5:107.

Bedell GM, Haley SM, Coster WJ, et al. Developing a responsive measure of change for paediatric brain injury inpatient rehabilitation. Brain Inj 2002b;16:659.

Berlin RJ, Lee UT, Samples JR, et al. Ophthalmic drops causing coma in an infant. J Pediatr 2001;138:441.

Bernard SA, Jones BM, Horne MK. Clinical trial of induced hypothermia in comatose survivors of out-of-hospital cardiac arrest. Ann Emerg Med 1997;30:146.

Biagas KV, Gaeta ML. Treatment of traumatic brain injury with hypothermia. Curr Opin Pediatr 1998;10:271.

Bozza Marrubini M. Classifications of coma. Int Care Med 1984;10:271.

Brawanski A, Faltermeier R, Rothoerl RD, et al. Comparison of near-infrared spectroscopy and tissue O_2 time series in patients after severe head injury and aneurysmal subarachnoid hemorrhage. J Cereb Blood Flow Metab 2002;22:605.

Brenner RP. Is it status? Epilepsia 2002;43(Suppl 3):103.

Brenner T, Freier MC, Holshouser BA, et al. Predicting neuropsychologic outcome after traumatic brain injury in children. Pediatr Neurol 2003;28:104.

Brink J, Garrett AL, Hale WR, et al. Recovery of motor and intellectual function in children sustaining severe head injuries. Dev Med Child Neurol 1970;12:565.

Brink JD, Umus MD, Woo-San J. Physical recovery after severe closed head trauma in children and adolescents. J Pediatr 1980;97:721.

Broman SH, Michel ME. Traumatic head injury in children. New York: Oxford University Press, 1995.

Bruck W, Christen HJ, Lakomele M, et al. Wernicke's encephalopathy in a child with acute lymphoblastic leukemia treated with polychemotherapy. Clin Neuropathol 1991;3:134.

Cairns H, Oldfield RC, Pennybacker JB, et al. Akinetic mutism with an epidermoid cyst of the third ventricle. Brain 1941;64:273.

Campbell CGN, Kuehn SM, Richards PMP, et al. Medical and cognitive outcome in children with traumatic brain injury. Can J Neurol Sci 2004;31:213.

Clayton PT, Bridges NA, Atherton DJ, et al. Pellagra with colitis due to a defect in tryptophan metabolism. Eur J Pediatr 1991;150:498.

Clifton GL. Systemic hypothermia in treatment of severe brain injury: A review and update. J Neurotrauma 1995;12:923.

Coster WJ, Deeney T, Haltiwanger J, et al. School function assessment. San Antonio, TX: The Psychology Corporation, 1998.

Crick F, Koch C. Consciousness and neuroscience. Cereb Cortex 1998;8:97.

Cuneo RA, Caronno JJ, Pitts L, et al. Upward transtentorial herniation: Seven cases and a literature review. Arch Neurol 1979;36:618.

Damasio A. Feelings of emotion and the self. Ann N Y Acad Sci 2003;1001:253.

Data Management Service of the Uniform Data System for Medical Rehabilitation and the Center for Functional Assessment. Guide for use of the functional independence measure for children (WeeFIM) of the uniform data set for medical rehabilitation. Buffalo: State University of New York at Buffalo, 1989.

DeMeirleir LJ, Taylor MJ. Evoked potentials in comatose children: Auditory brainstem responses. Pediatr Neurol 1986;2:31.

DeMeirleir LJ, Taylor MJ. Prognostic utility of SEPs in comatose children. Pediatr Neurol 1987;3:78.

Doppenberg EMR, Zauner A, Bullock R, et al. Correlations between brain tissue oxygen tension, carbon dioxide tension, pH and cerebral blood flow: A better way of monitoring the severely injured brain? Surg Neurol 1998;49:650.

Dullenkopf A, Frey B, Baenziger O, et al. Measurement of cerebral oxygenation state in anaesthetized children using the INVOS 5100 cerebral oximeter. Paediatr Anaesth 2003;13:384.

Duncan CC, Ment LR, Smith B, et al. A scale for the assessment of neonatal neurologic status. Child Brain 1981;8:299.

Epstein F, Murali RL. Pediatric posterior fossa tumors: Hazards of the "preoperative" shunt. Neurosurgery 1978;3:348.

Feinberg WM, Ferry PC. A fate worse than death, the persistent vegetative state in childhood. Am J Dis Child 1984;138:128.

Figaji AA, Fiegen AG, Peter JC. Early decompressive craniotomy in children with severe traumatic brain injury. Childs Nerv Syst 2003;19:666.

Feldmann E, Gandy SE, Becker R, et al. MRI demonstrates descending transtentorial herniation. Neurology 1988;38:697.

Fischer C, Luaute J, Adeleine P, et al. Predictive value of sensory and cognitive evoked potentials for awakening from coma. Neurology 2004;63:669.

Fiser DH. Assessing the outcome of pediatric intensive care. J Pediatr 1992;121:68.

Fiser DH, Long N, Roberson PK, et al. Relationship of pediatric overall performance category and pediatric cerebral performance category scores at pediatric intensive care unit discharge with outcome measures collected at hospital discharge and 1- and 6-month follow-up assessments. Crit Care Med 2000;28:2616.

Fisher CM. Brain herniation: A revision of classical concepts. Can J Neurol Sci 1995;22:83.

Fletcher JM, Miner ME, Ewing-Cobb SL. Age and recovery from head injury in children: Developmental issues. In: Levin HS, Grafman J, Eisenberg HM, eds. Neurobehavioral recovery from head injury. Oxford: Oxford University Press, 1987.

Forsyth RJ, Wong CP, Kelly TP, et al. Cognitive and adaptive outcomes and age at insult effects after non-traumatic coma. Arch Dis Child 2001;84:200.

Frank LM, Furgiuele TL, Etheridge JE Jr. Prediction of chronic vegetative state in children using evoked potentials. Neurology 1985;35:931.

Freundlich E, Slatter M, Yatz VS. Familial pellagra-like skin rash with neurological manifestations. Arch Dis Child 1981;56:146.

Gennarelli TA, Thibault LD, Adams JH, et al. Diffuse axonal injury and traumatic coma in the primate. Ann Neurol 1982;12:564.

Giacino JT. Disorders of consciousness: Differential diagnosis and neuropathologic features. Semin Neurol 1997;17:105.

Giacino JT, Ashwal S, Childs N, et al. The minimally conscious state. Definition and diagnostic criteria. Neurology 2002;58:349.

Giacino JT, Kalmar K. The vegetative and minimally conscious states: A comparison of clinical features and functional outcome. J Head Trauma Rehabil 1979;12:36.

Giacino JT, Zasler ND, Katz DL, et al. Development of practice guidelines for assessment of the vegetative and minimally conscious states. J Head Trauma Rehab 1997;12:79.

Gilbert TT, Wagner MR, Halukurike V, et al. Use of bispectral electroencephalogram monitoring to assess neurologic status in unsedated, critically ill patients. Crit Care Med 2001;29:1996.

Gillies JD, Seshia SS. Vegetative state following coma in childhood: Evolution and outcome. Dev Med Child Neurol 1980;22:642.

Goetting MG, Tiznado-Garcia E, Bakdash TF. Intussusception encephalopathy: An underrecognized cause of coma in children. Pediatr Neurol 1990;6:419.

Gohlich-Ratmann G, Wallot M, Baethmann M, et al. Acute cerebellitis with near-fatal cerebellar swelling and benign outcome under conservative treatment with high dose steroids. Eur J Paediatr Neurol 1988;2:157.

Goodwin SR, Friedman WA, Bellefleur M. Is it time to use evoked potentials to predict outcome in comatose children and adults? Crit Care Med 1991;19:518.

Green SA, Jefferson IG, Baum JD. Cerebral edema complicating diabetic ketoacidosis. Dev Med Child Neurol 1990;32:633.

Grindstaff RJ, Tobias JD. Applications of Bispectral Index monitoring in the pediatric intensive care unit. J Intensive Care Med 2004;19:111.

Habre W, Caffisch M, Chaves-Vischer V, et al. Locked-in syndrome in an adolescent patient with pneumococcal meningitis. Neuropediatrics 1996;27:323.

Hahn JS, Berquist W, Alcorn DM, et al. Wernicke encephalopathy and beriberi during total parenteral nutrition attributable to multivitamin infusion shortage. Pediatrics 1998;101:E10.

Hahn YS, Chyung C, Barthel MJ, et al. Head injuries in children under 36 months of age. Childs Nerv Syst 1988;4:34.

Haley SM, Coster WJ, Ludlow LM, et al. Pediatric evaluation of disability inventory: Development, standardization and administration manual, Version 1.0. Boston: Trustees of Boston University, Center for Rehabilitation Effectiveness, 1992.

Hall K, Cope N, Rappaport M. Glasgow outcome scale and disability rating scale: Comparative usefulness in following recovery in traumatic head injury. Arch Phys Med Rehabil 1985;66:35.

Hannay HJ, Sherer M. Assessment of outcome from head injury. In: Narayan RK, Wilberger JE Jr, Povlishock JT, eds. Neurotrauma. New York: McGraw-Hill, 1996.

Heindl UT, Laub MC. Outcome of persistent vegetative state following hypoxic or traumatic brain injury in children and adolescents. Neuropediatrics 1996;27:94.

Herskowitz J. Neurologic presentations of panic disorder in childhood and adolescence. Dev Med Child Neurol 1986;28:617.

Hlatky R, Valadka AB, Goodman JC, et al. Patterns of energy substrates during ischemia measured in the brain by microdialysis. J Neurotrauma 2004;21:894.

Holshouser BA, Ashwal S, Luh GY, et al. Proton MR spectroscopy after acute central nervous system injury: Outcome prediction in neonates, infants and children. Radiology 1997;202:487.

Holshouser BA, Ashwal S, Shu S, et al. Proton MR spectroscopy in children with acute brain injury: Comparison of short and long echo time acquisitions. J Magn Reson Imaging 2000;11:9.

Hsia SH, Wu CT, Wang HS, et al. The use of Bispectral Index to monitor unconscious children. Pediatr Neurol 2004;31:20.

Iyer LV, Haley SM, Watkins MP, et al. Establishing minimal clinically important differences for scores on the Pediatric Evaluation of Disability Inventory for Inpatient Rehabilitation. Phys Ther 2003;83:888.

James W. The principles of psychology. London: MacMillan, 1890.

Jennett B. A quarter century of the vegetative state: An international perspective. J Head Trauma Rehabil 1997;12:1.

Jennett B, Bond M. Assessment of outcome after severe brain damage, a practical scale. Lancet 1975;1:480.

Jennett B, Teasdale G, Brookman R, et al. Predicting outcome in individual patients after severe head injury. Lancet 1976;1:1031.

Jennett B, Teasdale G, Brookman R, et al. Prognosis of patients with severe head injury. Neurosurgery 1979;4:283.

John ER. A field theory of consciousness. Conscious Cogn 2001;10:184.

John ER. The neurophysics of consciousness. Brain Res Brain Res Rev 2002;39:1.

John ER, Prichep LS, Kox W, et al. Invariant reversible QEEG effects of anesthetics. Conscious Cogn 2001;10:165.

Johnston B, Seshia SS. Prediction of outcome in non-traumatic coma in childhood. Acta Neurol Scand 1984;69:417.

Jonsson CA, Horneman G, Emanuelson I. Neuropsychological progress during 14 years after severe traumatic brain injury in childhood and adolescence. Brain Inj 2004;18:921.

Karantanas AH, Hadjigeorgiou GM, Paterakis K, et al. Contribution of MRI and MR angiography in early diagnosis of brain death. Eur Radiol 2002;12:2710.

Keenan HT, Runyan DK, Marshall SW, et al. A population-based comparison of clinical and outcome characteristics of young children with serious inflicted and noninflicted traumatic brain injury. Pediatrics 2004;114:633.

Keren O, Ben-Dror S, Stern MJ, et al. Event-related potentials as an index of cognitive function during recovery from severe closed head injury. J Head Trauma Rehabil 1998;13:15.

Kiening KL, Hartl R, Unterberg AW, et al. Brain tissue PO_2-monitoring in comatose patients: Implications for therapy. Neurol Res 1997;19:233.

Kirkham FJ. Coma after cardiac arrest. In: Eyre JA, ed. Coma in childhood. London: Bailliere Tindall, 1994.

Kothari DH, Haley SM, Gill-Body KM, et al. Measuring functional change in children with acquired brain injury (ABI): Comparison of generic and ABI-specific scales using the Pediatric Evaluation of Disability Inventory (PEDI). Phys Ther 2003;83:776.

Kriel RL, Jrach LE, Jones-Saese C. Outcome of children with prolonged unconsciousness and vegetative states. Pediatr Neurol 1993;9:362.

Kurth CD, Steven JM, Nicolson SC. Cerebral oxygenation during pediatric cardiac surgery using deep hypothermic circulatory arrest. Anesthesiology 1995;82:74.

Lange-Cossack H, Riebel U, Grumme T, et al. Possibilities and limitation of rehabilitation after traumatic apallic syndrome in children and adolescents. Neuropediatrics 1981;12:338.

Larsen PD, Gupta NC, Lefkowitz DM, et al. PET of infants in persistent vegetative state. Pediatr Neurol 1993;9:323.

Levin HS. A guide to clinical neuropsychological testing. Arch Neurol 1994;51:854.

Lin KL, Wang HS, Chou ML, et al. Role of cavum septum pellucidum in akinetic mutism of hydrocephalic children. Pediatr Neurol 1997;16:156.

Litscher G. Middle latency auditory evoked potentials in intensive care patients and normal controls. Int J Neurosci 1995;83:253.

Logi F, Fischer C, Murri L, et al. The prognostic value of evoked responses from primary somatosensory and auditory cortex in comatose patients. Clin Neurophysiol 2003;114:1615.

Mahoney WJ, D'Souza BJ, Freeman JM. Surprising good outcome of prolonged coma after severe head injury. Ann Neurol 1981;10:286.

Mahoney WJ, D'Souza BJ, Haller JA, et al. Long-term outcome of children with severe head trauma and prolonged coma. Pediatrics 1983;71:756.

Mandel R, Martinot A, Delepoulle F, et al. Prediction of outcome after hypoxic-ischemic encephalopathy: A prospective clinical and electrophysiologic study. J Pediatr 2002;141:45.

Massagli TL, Michaud LJ, Rivara FP. Association between injury indices and outcome after severe traumatic brain injury in children. Arch Phys Med Rehabil 1996;77:125.

McFadden J. Synchronous firing and its influence on the brain's electromagnetic field: Evidence for an electromagnetic theory of consciousness. J Consciousness Studies 2002a;9:23.

McFadden J. The conscious electromagnetic field theory: The hard problem made easy. J Consciousness Studies 2002b;9:45.

McChelson D, Ashwal S. Evaluation of coma and brain death. Semin Pediatr Neurol 2004;2:105.

Medical Research Council Brain Injuries Committee. A glossary of psychological terms commonly used in cases of head injury. Medical Research Council War Memorandum Number 4. London: HM Stationery Office. 1941.

Melton AF, Appleton RE, Gardner-Medwin D, et al. Encephalitis lethargica-like illness in a five-year-old. Dev Med Child Neurol 1991;33:158.

Mewasingh LD, Christophe C, Fonteyne C, et al. Predictive value of electrophysiology in children with hypoxic coma. Pediatr Neurol 2003;28:178.

Meyer PG, Ducrocq S, Carli P. Pediatric neurologic emergencies. Curr Opin Crit Care 2001;7:81.

Michelson D, Ashwal S. Evaluation of coma and brain death. Semin Pediatr Neurol 2004;11:103.

Misra UK, Kalita J. Neurophysiological studies in herpes simplex encephalitis. Electromyogr Clin Neurophysiol 1998;38:177.

Montgomery EB, Wall M, Henderson VW. Principles of neurologic diagnosis. Boston/Toronto: Little, Brown, 1986.

Moruzzi G. The sleep-waking cycle. Rev Physiol 1972;64:1.

Moruzzi G, Magoun HW. Brainstem reticular formation and activation of the EEG. Electroencephalogr Clin Neurophysiol 1949;1:455.

Multi-Society Task Force on Persistent Vegetative State. Medical aspects of the persistent vegetative state. N Engl J Med 1994;330:1499, 1572.

Nagdyman N, Fleck T, Barth S, et al. Relation of cerebral tissue oxygenation index to central venous oxygen saturation in children. Intensive Care Med 2004;30:468.

Narayan RK, Greenberg RP, Miller JD, et al. Improved confidence of outcome prediction in severe head injury. A comparative analysis of the clinical examination, multimodality evoked potentials, CT scanning, and intracranial pressure. J Neurosurg 1981;54:751.

Nautiyal A, Singh S, Alaimo DJ. Wernicke encephalopathy: An emerging trend after bariatric surgery. Am J Med 2004;10:804.

Nayana Prabha PC, Nalini P, Tiroumouronugane Serane V. Role of Glasgow Coma Scale in pediatric nontraumatic coma. Indian Pediatr 2003;40:620.

Neylan TC. Physiology of arousal: Moruzzi and Magoun's ascending reticular activating system. J Neuropsychiatry Clin Neurosci 1995;7:250.

Oliver WJ, Shope TC, Kuhns LR. Fatal lumbar puncture: Fact versus fiction—an approach to a clinical dilemma. Pediatrics 2003;112:174.

Ottenbacher KJ, Msall ME, Lyon N, et al. Measuring developmental and functional status in children with disabilities. Dev Med Child Neurol 1999;41:186.

Ottenbacher KJ, Msall ME, Lyon N, et al. Functional assessment and care of children with neurodevelopmental disabilities. Am J Phys Med Rehabil 2000;29:114.

Panullo SC, Reich JB, Krol G, et al. MRI changes in intracranial hypotension. Neurology 1993;43:919.

Pihko H, Saarinen U, Paetau A. Wernicke encephalopathy: A preventable cause of death. Report of 2 children with malignant disease. Pediatr Neurol 1989;4:237.

Plum F, Posner JB. The diagnosis of stupor and coma, 3rd ed., revised. Philadelphia: FA Davis, 1982.

Raimondi AJ, Hirschauer J. Head injury in the infant and toddler. Coma scoring and outcome scale. Child Brain 1984;11:12.

Raimondi AJ, Tomita T. Hydrocephalus and infratentorial tumors. Incidence, clinical picture and treatment. J Neurosurg 1981;55:174.

Rappaport M, Hall KM, Hopkins K, et al. Disability rating scale for severe head trauma: Coma to community. Arch Phys Med Rehabil 1982;63:118.

Ravid S, Diamond AS, Eviatar L. Coma as an acute presentation of adrenoleukodystrophy. Pediatr Neurol 2000;22:237.

Reich JB, Sierra J, Camp W, et al. Magnetic resonance imaging measurement and clinical changes accompanying transtentorial and foramen magnum brain herniation. Ann Neurol 1993;33:159.

Reilly PL, Simpson DA, Sprod R, et al. Assessing the conscious level in infants and young children: A pediatric version of the Glasgow Coma Scale. Child Nerv Syst 1988;4:30.

Rennick G, Shann F, deCampo J. Cerebral herniation during bacterial meningitis in children. BMJ 1993;306:953.

Robertson CM, Joffe AR, Moore AJ, et al. Neurodevelopmental outcome of young pediatric intensive care survivors of serious brain injury. Pediatr Crit Care Med 2002;3:345.

Rohde V, Irle S, Hassler WE. Prediction of the post-comatose motor function by motor evoked potentials obtained in the acute phase of traumatic and non-traumatic coma. Acta Neurochir 1999;141:841.

Ropper AH. Lateral displacement of the brain and level of consciousness in patients with an acute hemispheral mass. N Engl J Med 1986;314:953.

Ropper AH. Syndrome of transtentorial herniation: Is vertical displacement necessary? J Neurol Neurosurg Psychiatry 1993;56:932.

Ross DA, Olsen WL, Ross AM, et al. Brain shift, level of consciousness and restoration of consciousness in patients with acute intracranial hematoma. J Neurosurg 1989;71:498.

Roulet Perez E, Maeder P, Cotting J, et al. Acute fatal parainfectious cerebellar swelling in two children. A rare or an overlooked situation? Neuropediatrics 1993;24:346.

Rubenstein JS. Initial management of coma and altered consciousness in the pediatric patient. Pediatr Rev 1984;15:204.

Ruf B, Heckmann M, Schroth I, et al. Early decompressive craniectomy and duraplasty for refractory intracranial hypertension in children: Results of a pilot study. Crit Care 2003;7:409.

Safar PJ, Kochanek PM. Therapeutic hypothermia after cardiac arrest. N Engl J Med 2002;346:612.

Salas-Salvado J, Garcia-Lorda P, Cuatrecasas G, et al. Wernicke's syndrome after bariatric surgery. Clin Nutr 2000;5:371.

Scheuer ML, Wilson SB. Data analysis for continuous EEG monitoring in the ICU: Seeing the forest and the trees. J Clin Neurophysiol 2004;21:353.

Scott JS, Ockey RR, Holmes GE, et al. Autonomic dysfunction associated with locked-in syndrome in a child. Am J Phys Med Rehabil 1997;76:200.

Searle JR. Consciousness. Annu Rev Neurosci 2000;23:557.

Seshia SS, Johnston B, Kasian G. Non-traumatic coma in childhood: Clinical variables in prediction of outcome. Dev Med Child Neurol 1983;25:493.

Shetty AK, Dessell BC, Craver RD, et al. Fatal cerebral herniation after lumbar puncture in a patient with a normal computed tomography scan. Pediatrics 1999;103:1284.

Shewman DA. Coma prognosis in children. Part I: Definition and methodological challenges. J Clin Neurophysiol 2000a;17:457.

Shewman DA. Coma prognosis in children. Part II: Clinical application. J Clin Neurophysiol 2000b;17:467.

Shu SK, Ashwal S, Holshouser BA, et al. Prognostic value of 1H-MRS in perinatal CNS insults. Pediatr Neurol 1997;17:309.

Simpson DA, Reilly PL. Pediatric coma scale [Letter]. Lancet 1982;2:450.

Simpson DA, Cockington RA, Heniej A, et al. Head injuries in infants and young children: The value of the pediatric coma scale. Childs Nerv Syst 1991;7:183.

Smith E, Madsen J. Cerebral pathophysiology and critical care neurology: Basic hemodynamic principals, cerebral perfusion and intracranial pressure. Semin Pediatr Neurol 2004a;11:89.

Smith E, Madsen J. Neurosurgical aspects of critical care neurology. Semin Pediatr Neurol 2004b;11:169.

Sperry RW. Neurology and the mind-brain problem. Am Scientist 1952;40:291.

Strauss DJ, Ashwal S, Day SM, et al. Life expectancy of children in vegetative and minimally conscious states. Pediatr Neurol 2000;23:312.

Task Force for the Determination of Brain Death in Children. Guidelines for the determination of brain death in children. Pediatrics 1987;80:298.

Taylor A, Butt W, Rosenfeld J, et al. A randomized trial of very early decompressive craniectomy in children with traumatic brain injury and sustained intracranial hypertension. Childs Nerv Syst 2001;17:154.

Taylor MR, Farrell EJ. Comparison of the prognostic utility of VEPs and SEPs in comatose children. Pediatr Neurol 1989;5:145.

Teasdale G, Jennett B. Assessment of coma and impaired consciousness. A practical scale. Lancet 1974;2:81.

Teasdale G, Jennett B, Murray L, et al. Glasgow coma scale: To sum or not to sum. Lancet 1983;2:678.

ter Horst HJ, Sommer C, Bergman KA, et al. Prognostic significance of amplitude-integrated EEG during the first 72 hours after birth in severely asphyxiated neonates. Pediatr Res 2004;55:1026.

Tolias CM, Richards DA, Bowery NG. Extracellular glutamate in the brains of children with severe head injuries: A pilot microdialysis study. Childs Nerv Syst 2002;18:368.

Tong KA, Ashwal S, Holshouser BA, et al. Hemorrhagic shearing lesions in children and adolescents with post-traumatic diffuse axonal injury: Improved detection and initial results. Radiology 2003;22:332.

Tong KA, Ashwal S, Holshouser BA, et al. Diffuse axonal injury in children: Clinical correlation with hemorrhagic lesions. Ann Neurol 2004;56:36.

Tsao CY, Ellingson RJ. Normal somatosensory evoked potentials in a child in persistent coma. Pediatr Neurol 1989;5:257.

Vannucci RC, Wasiewski WW. Diagnosis and management of coma in children. In: Pellock JM, Meyer ED, eds. Neurologic emergencies in infancy and childhood, 2nd ed. London: Butterworth-Heinemann, 1993;103-122.

Van Santbrink H, Maas AIR, Avezaat CJJ. Continuous monitoring of partial pressure of brain tissue oxygen in patients with severe head injury. Neurosurgery 1996;38:21.

Vasconcelos MM, Silva KP, Vidal G, et al. Early diagnosis of pediatric Wernicke's encephalopathy. Pediatr Neurol 1999;4:289.

Wijdicks EF, Miller GM. MR imaging of progressive downward herniation of the diencephalons. Neurology 1997;48:1456.

Wohlrab G, Boltshauser E, Schmitt B. Neurological outcome in comatose children with bilateral loss of cortical somatosensory evoked potentials. Neuropediatrics 2001;32:271.

Wong CP, Forsyth RJ, Kelly TP, et al. Incidence, aetiology and outcome of non-traumatic coma: A population based study. Arch Dis Child 2001;84:193.

Ylvisaker M, Chorazy AJL, Cohen SB, et al. Rehabilitation assessment following head injury in children. In: Rosenthal M, Griffith ER, Bond MR, eds. Rehabilitation of the adult and child with traumatic brain injury, 2nd ed. Philadelphia: FA Davis, 1990.

Young GB. The EEG in coma. J Clin Neurophysiol 2000;17:473.

Young GB, Ropper AH, Bolton CF. Coma and impaired consciousness: A clinical perspective. New York: McGraw-Hill, 1998.

Zasler ND, Kreutzer JS, Taylor DA. Coma stimulation and coma recovery: A critical review. NeuroRehabilitation 1991;1:33.

Zeman A. Persistent vegetative state. Lancet 1997;350:795.

Zeman A. Consciousness. Brain 2001;124:1263.

Zentner J, Rohde V. The prognostic value of somatosensory and motor evoked potentials in comatose patients. Neurosurgery 1992;31:429

Zentner J, Rohde V. SEP and MEP in comatose patients. Neurol Res 1994;16:89.

Zimmerman AA, Burrows FA, Jones RA, et al. The limits of detectable cerebral perfusion by transcranial Doppler sonography in neonates undergoing deep hypothermic low-flow cardiopulmonary bypass. J Thorac Cardiovasc Surg 1997;114:594.

Ziviani J, Ottenbacher KJ, Shephard K, et al. Concurrent validity of the Functional Independence Measure for Children (WeeFIM) and the Pediatric Evaluation of Disabilities Inventory in children with developmental disabilities and acquired brain injuries. Phys Occup Ther Pediatr 2001;22:91.

CHAPTER 62

Traumatic Brain Injury in Children

Christopher C. Giza

INTRODUCTION AND BACKGROUND

Epidemiology of Pediatric Traumatic Brain Injury

Traumatic brain injury is a leading cause of death and disability in children and has been identified as a significant public health problem in the United States and worldwide [Engberg and Teasdale, 1998; Murgio et al., 1999; Thurman, 2000; Tsai et al., 2004; Weiner and Weinberg, 2000]. Age-related incidence rates for traumatic brain injury in children have been estimated to be as high as 670 per 100,000 when head injuries of all severities are included [McCarthy et al., 2002]. When limited to traumatic brain injury resulting in hospitalization, the incidence has declined over the past 15 years, most likely because of injury prevention measures and improved motor vehicle safety. Nonetheless, traumatic brain injury is responsible for most trauma-related deaths and hospitalizations. The incidence rate of traumatic brain injury–related hospitalization remains significant, consistently around 75 to 80 per 100,000 [McCarthy et al., 2002; Reid et al., 2001]. Childhood traumatic brain injury results in an estimated 3,000 deaths, 29,000 hospitalizations, and 400,000 emergency department visits annually in the United States (children 0-14 years old) [Thurman, 2000]. Traumatic brain injury is six times more likely to cause death in childhood than acquired immunodeficiency virus and is 20 times more likely than asthma to cause death [Centers for Disease Control and Prevention, 2000]. Moderate and severe pediatric traumatic brain injury has been associated with long-standing cognitive, neurologic, and behavioral impairments [Fay et al., 1994; Massagli et al., 1996a], and the cost of these disabilities is often sustained over the person's lifetime. Fortunately, most traumatic brain injuries are mild, although recent studies suggest that even mild pediatric traumatic brain injury may have adverse long-term functional consequences [Hawley et al., 2004]. There is also increasing evidence that repeated mild traumatic brain injury, as commonly occurs in a sports-related setting, results in chronic cognitive impairment [Collins et al., 1999; Matser et al., 1999]. Despite these facts, no specific treatment standards exist for pediatric traumatic brain injury, either acutely or during recovery. A recent review of guidelines for pediatric traumatic brain injury management concluded that acute supportive therapies are often administered inconsistently or simply extrapolated from adult traumatic brain injury protocols and do not take into account the unique physiology of the immature brain [Adelson et al., 2003b].

The peak incidence of pediatric traumatic brain injury occurs during adolescence and in the young adult years, with a secondary peak in infancy [Kraus and McArthur, 2000]. The etiology of traumatic brain injury varies with age (Fig. 62-1). Adolescents sustain most head injuries in motor vehicle crashes, sports-related injuries, and assaults. Preadolescent children are also frequent victims of motor vehicle crashes, but more often as a pedestrian or while riding a bicycle. Those younger than 5 years are more prone to falls [Thurman, 2000], whereas infants are particularly vulnerable to repeated severe traumatic brain injury in the form of nonaccidental trauma (inflicted head injuries/child abuse).

Traumatic brain injury is about twice as common in boys as in girls overall, with this gender distinction becoming increasingly evident in the childhood and adolescent years [Kraus and McArthur, 2000; Rivara, 1994]. In the United States annually, about 30,000 pediatric patients incur permanent disability as a result of traumatic brain injury. These sequelae include headaches, post-traumatic epilepsy, motor disturbances, learning disabilities, cognitive impairment, and behavioral problems. Furthermore, most children suffering traumatic brain injury, even those surviving moderate or severe injury, fail to receive adequate medical, rehabilitative, or psychosocial follow-up after hospital discharge [Armstrong and Kerns, 2002; Hawley et al., 2004]. Finally, given the magnitude of recurrent head trauma as a problem of youth, it is increasingly noted that health-care providers should take every opportunity to provide important information and education to patients and their families, particularly with regard to potential sequelae of repeated injuries and effective injury prevention.

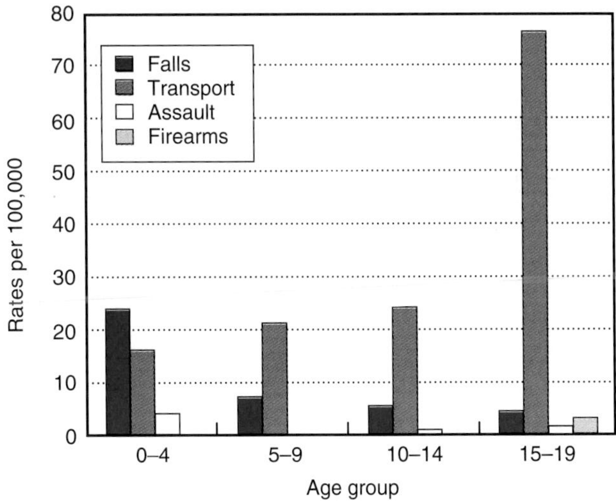

FIGURE 62-1. Etiology of pediatric traumatic brain injury by age group. (From Thurman D, for the Centers for Disease Control and Prevention. Traumatic brain injury in the U.S.: Assessing outcomes in children, Appendix B. Available at: http://www.cdc.gov.)

In this chapter, injury mechanisms and the biomechanics of injury, as well as the cellular and molecular pathophysiology of traumatic brain injury and recovery, are reviewed. In addition, a framework for the clinical evaluation and initial treatment of head trauma in children is described. Critical distinctions between traumatic injury in the developing brain and in the adult brain are also considered. Specific acute syndromes of pediatric head injury are individually described in detail, followed by discussion of appropriate management, review of published treatment guidelines, and an overview of determining prognosis after severe pediatric traumatic brain injury. Finally, this chapter describes the chronic clinical syndromes and sequelae associated with pediatric head injury.

Anatomy

To best understand the mechanisms and types of traumatic brain injury, knowledge of the basic anatomy of the brain and its coverings is essential (Fig. 62-2). The scalp is the outermost covering and is highly vascular, tending to bleed profusely when lacerated. Under the scalp is a tendinous sheath extending from the frontal to occipital regions called the *galea*. The potential space beneath this is the subgaleal compartment, an occasional site of significant bleeding after head injury. The skull is next, with the periosteum covering its outer surface. The skull is composed of three layers, the bony outer and inner tables, separated by the diploic space, which is more vascular. Between the inner table of the skull and the dura mater is the epidural space, another potential space that is a significant site for arterial bleeding, particularly after skull fracture. The dura itself is the tough outer protective layer covering the brain. Below the dura is the subdural space, which is crossed by small veins that drain into the venous sinuses and another site for post-traumatic hematomas. The next layer of brain coverings is the arachnoid, and under this, the subarachnoid space, that contains cerebrospinal fluid and into which post-traumatic bleeding is fairly common. The subarachnoid space is contiguous with the basal cisterns and the ventricular system, and cerebrospinal fluid normally flows from its site of production at the choroid plexus within the ventricles, out into the basal cisterns, over the convexities of the cerebrum, and into the venous drainage of the brain through the arachnoid villi. Subarachnoid blood can impair the flow of cerebrospinal fluid after trauma and occasionally result in hydrocephalus. The last layer is the pia mater, which lies directly over the brain surface itself.

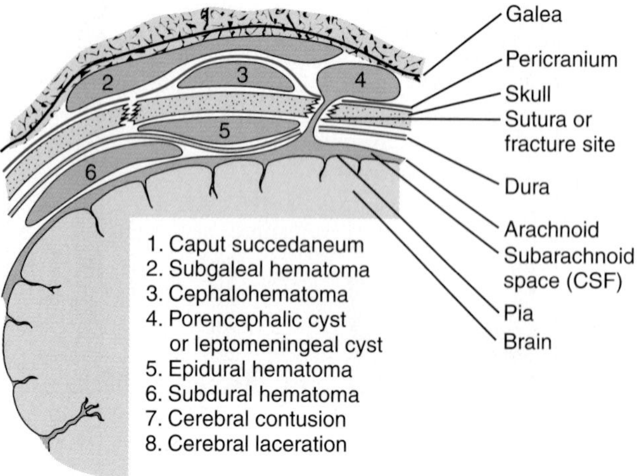

FIGURE 62-2. Schematic representation of the brain, skull, scalp, and pathologic entities related to head trauma. (From Rosman NP, Herskowitz J, Carter AP, et al. Pediatr Clin North Am 1979;26:707.)

The vascular supply of the brain originates in the great arteries of the neck (carotid and vertebral arteries; see Chapter 72). These enter the skull through foramina at its base and then arborize over the surface of the brain in fairly consistent vascular distributions. Venous drainage from the brain is routed either through deep draining veins or through small penetrating veins that traverse the subdural space, in either circumstance entering venous sinuses and eventually leaving the intracranial space through the jugular veins.

One important developmental aspect of brain and skull anatomy is the rigidity of the skull itself. Intracranial pressure is determined by the three main contents of the skull, namely, the brain itself, blood, and cerebrospinal fluid. In infancy, the skull is more pliable, with flexible sutures and open fontanels. These features provide a mechanical outlet for elevated intracranial pressure that is not present once the sutures fuse. In older infants and children, as in adults, post-traumatic brain swelling can be accommodated only by displacement of blood and cerebrospinal fluid from the intracranial space, followed in severe cases by herniation of the brain through the foramen magnum.

Biomechanics

Trauma is a unique form of brain injury, whereby a biomechanical force is imparted to the brain. In general, the forces applied to the brain may be described as linear or rotational. The clinical significance to identifying these forces is that they are often associated with particular mechanisms and types of injury. *Linear forces* refer to acceleration or deceleration forces in a straight line. As the brain "floats" in the cerebrospinal fluid, these forces often result in compression of the brain at the site of contact (i.e., "coup" injury). This injury can take the form of local hemorrhage or contusion, accompanied by overlying soft tissue swelling and occasionally skull fracture. As the intracranial contents are shifted toward the point of contact, however, a relatively low-pressure area evolves in a location opposite the coup injury. Injury in this area is termed *contrecoup* and can often be larger and more serious than the coup injury. Because of the relative irregularity of the skull floor in the anterior and middle cranial fossae, there is a propensity for focal traumatic injuries to occur in the frontal and temporal lobes. This propensity is an important consideration when evaluating a child for neurologic and cognitive impairment after injury because memory, attention, impulse control, judgment, and personality are all behavioral functions that may be localized in these brain regions and that also are undergoing rapid change during brain maturation.

Because the brain parenchyma is itself soft and deformable and brain regions are connected by fiber tracts, the brain is also prone to injury from rotational forces. This describes the forces imparted when one part of the brain is twisted in relationship to another part. In these circumstances, the underlying white matter tracts are subjected to significant shearing forces that can result in stretch injury and microhemorrhages seen clinically [Tong et al., 2004] and in experimental models [Raghupathi and Margulies, 2002]. This type of damage after trauma is referred to as *diffuse axonal injury* and can result in significant clinical disability. By its nature, diffuse axonal injury can occur throughout the brain, with a propensity for regions with major fiber tracts (e.g., corona radiata, corpus callosum, brainstem). Although the developing brain has been shown to have remarkable resilience to focal injuries such as strokes or surgical resection, its ability to recover from diffuse injuries may be much more limited.

Linear forces can play a role in collisions or falls, although it is generally difficult to separate these completely from rotational forces. Severe rotational forces are common with motor vehicle crashes. Because impact forces are offset or at an angle, the child can be injured inside a car, when thrown from a vehicle, or as a pedestrian struck by a vehicle. Rotational forces also can be seen with sports concussion, a milder but more common form of injury in older children and adolescents [Pellman et al., 2003].

Penetrating trauma, although less common, often results in enormous biomechanical forces and physical disruption of tissue along the path of the foreign object. Although the tissue destruction and surrounding necrosis, hemorrhage, and edema are major factors in determining long-term disability, the transmitted forces from the passage of the projectile to more distant parts of the brain can result in immediate death, presumably by affecting respiratory and autonomic centers [Carey, 1995]. One large series reported that younger age was associated with worse outcome from gunshot wounds [Levy et al., 1993].

Injury Types

Although specific injury types are discussed in greater detail later in the chapter, an overview of the types of injuries commonly seen in children ranges from superficial injuries to the scalp to severe diffuse cerebral edema with herniation. Scalp injuries are very common and include contusions, lacerations, and hematomas. Although scalp injuries may occur with little if any evidence of underlying brain damage, careful history and examination should be undertaken in each case to rule out the possibility of concussion or, more rarely, intracranial injury. Concussion has been redefined as any trauma-induced transient disturbance of neurologic function, even in the absence of unconsciousness [American Academy of Neurology, 1997]. A large scalp hematoma may conceal a skull fracture and, in infants, can result in significant blood loss. Skull fractures are reported after 20% of childhood traumatic brain injuries [Harwood-Nash et al., 1971], and although simple linear fractures are generally benign, the presence of any fracture greatly increases the risk for intracranial hemorrhage [Lloyd et al., 1997]. Post-traumatic intracranial bleeding may occur in the form of cerebral contusion, cerebral laceration, and epidural, subdural, or subarachnoid hemorrhage, individually or often in combination. Diffuse axonal injury represents stretch and shearing of white matter tracts and can have profound clinical consequences with prolonged unconsciousness and poor outcome. Traumatic injury at its most severe can lead to

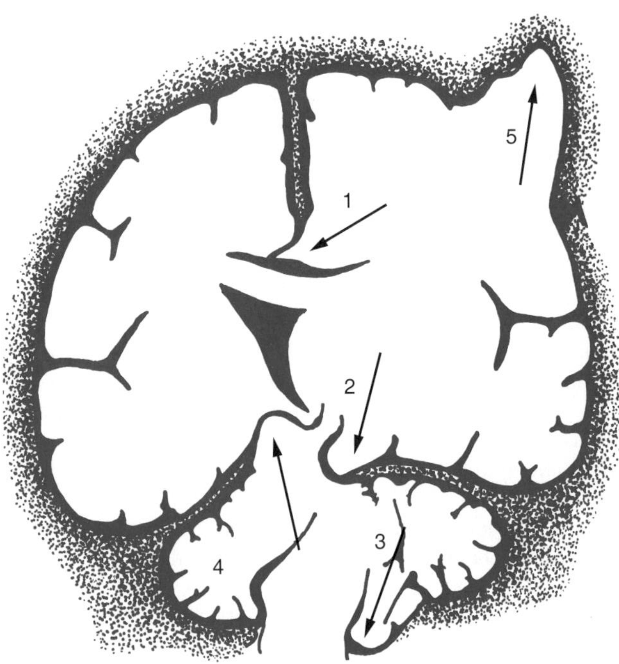

FIGURE 62-3. Different forms of brain herniation: *1*, cingulated; *2*, uncal; *3*, cerebellar tonsillar; *4*, upward cerebellar; *5*, transcalvarial. (From Fishman RA. Cerebrospinal fluid in diseases of the nervous system. Philadelphia: WB Saunders, 1980.)

cerebral swelling and elevated intracranial pressure. Although this problem may be accommodated to some degree by flexible sutures and open fontanels in infants, all ages are vulnerable to cerebral herniation. Based on location of edema or focal lesions, distinct types of herniation can occur (Fig. 62-3). Each of these injury types is discussed later in this chapter and is also reviewed in Chapter 65.

Although all the previously described injuries are associated with clinical syndromes of primary traumatic brain injury, it is important to be aware that in conjunction with the primary injury are the effects of so-called secondary injuries. Secondary injuries may be additional pathologic insults independent of the original traumatic brain injury, such as hypotension due to systemic hemorrhage, hyperthermia caused by concomitant infection, or airway occlusion by a foreign body resulting in hypoxia. In many patients, secondary injury may be directly or indirectly related to the original brain injury but occurs after it. Thus, the spectrum of secondary injury encompasses entities such as cerebral edema with reduced brain perfusion, intracranial hemorrhage, early post-traumatic seizures, respiratory compromise of neurologic origin resulting in hypoxia, and post-traumatic hydrocephalus. More general etiologies of secondary injury include ongoing excitotoxicity, free radical generation, oxidative stress, and inflammation. Clinical secondary injuries such as hypotension, hypoxia, hydrocephalus, edema, and seizures are of great clinical significance because they are generally treatable in the intensive care unit and are often independent predictors of poor outcome [Chesnut et al., 1993a; Chiaretti et al., 2002].

PATHOPHYSIOLOGY OF TRAUMATIC BRAIN INJURY

Distinctions of Injury to the Developing Brain

Biomechanical Factors

Clearly, the physics of traumatic brain injury is different in a child than in an adult. The relatively large head size, reduced muscular strength in the neck, and increased flexibility of the neck may promote a greater range of biomechanical force to be imparted to the head. On the other hand, there is less cerebrospinal fluid space around the brain, and the prominent bony ridges of the anterior and middle cranial fossae are less developed. These factors may contribute to a lower occurrence of focal lesions in pediatric traumatic brain injury [Berney et al., 1994; Bruce et al., 1979; Levi et al., 1991; Luerssen et al., 1988].

The physical properties of the developing skull also confer advantages and disadvantages. It is thinner and more prone to diffuse deformation [Margulies and Thibault, 2000]. Some investigators have reported a higher risk for skull fracture in children [Berney et al., 1994], although this finding is not universal [Levin et al., 1992]. The open fontanels and flexible sutures may serve to dampen traumatic forces and accommodate a greater degree of intracranial swelling. The brain itself, particularly in infants and young children, has a higher water content and is incompletely myelinated [Holland et al., 1986; Paus et al., 2001]. The higher water content tends to make the brain less compressible and less compliant than in the adult. The physical properties of the immature brain may thus provide unique benefits as well as potential vulnerabilities to traumatic brain injury.

Changes in Cerebral Metabolism

It is well known that cerebral metabolism changes throughout maturation. The primary source of energy for the brain changes from lactate in the perinatal period, to ketones while nursing, to glucose after weaning and on through to adulthood [Nehlig, 2004; Vannucci and Vannucci, 2000]. The ability to use alternative fuels may have important consequences on acute energy metabolism in the injured brain at different ages [Prins et al., 2004].

Even after the brain has switched to predominantly glucose metabolism, the levels of this metabolism continue to change throughout the developing years. Basal glucose metabolism rates peak at about 6 years of age, correlating with the time of maximal synaptogenesis. As synaptic pruning and dendritic rearrangement occur throughout childhood and adolescence, cerebral glucose metabolism declines, although it still remains elevated compared with the adult [Chugani et al., 1987]. Also, the brain does not mature uniformly, and brain metabolism changes have different time courses regionally.

Distinct Neurovascular Regulation

Neurovascular control may also differ in the young brain. Early studies suggested a propensity for diffuse cerebral swelling in children after closed head injury, occurring two to five times more often than in adults [Aldrich et al., 1992; Lang et al., 1994]. Recent studies report that normal children have higher baseline cerebral blood flow than adults, with significant variation across narrow age groups [Suzuki, 1990; Zwienenberg and Muizelaar, 1999]. At birth, cerebral blood flow is lower than adults but increases rapidly to peak at about age 5 years. Cerebral blood flow then appears to decline through adolescence to adult levels [Suzuki, 1990]. The effect of these developmental differences on injury-induced changes in cerebral blood flow and the mechanisms of these differences are not yet well understood. Certainly, molecular mediators of neurovascular tone, such as nitric oxide synthase, have differential expression patterns in the immature brain [Keilhoff et al., 1996; Ohyu and Takashima, 1998], and these may play a role in age-dependent changes in blood flow and response to injury.

Increased Excitatory Neurotransmission

As mentioned earlier, the number of synapses in the human brain appears to peak in early childhood and is associated with a peak in cerebral glucose metabolism. Levels of excitatory transmitter receptors are higher in the immature brain [Fosse et al., 1989; Insel et al., 1990; Miller et al., 1990]. The occurrence of early post-traumatic seizures is also noticeably higher in children, particularly infants and younger children [Annegers et al., 1980; Berney et al., 1994].

Because excessive release of excitatory neurotransmitters can result in neuronal injury (excitotoxicity) and death, the fact that the developing brain is more active might suggest that blocking excitatory transmission would be neuroprotective. However, early in development, neuronal activation also plays a critical role in both survival of immature nerve cells and proper wiring of cerebral circuitry. In fact, in animal models, use of glutamate antagonists early in postnatal development (while protective against some degrees of excitotoxic insult) resulted in a large degree of programmed cell death (apoptosis) [Bittigau et al., 1999; Ikonomidou et al., 1999; Pohl et al., 1999]. Evidence like this suggests that optimal recovery from brain injury may require a proper balance of excitation and inhibition and may also account for the relative ineffectiveness of glutamate antagonists following human brain injury [Ashwal et al., 2004b; Biegon et al., 2004; Ikonomidou and Turski, 2002].

Ongoing Cerebral Maturation

In general, the developing brain is thought to recover better after many types of brain injury, including stroke, traumatic brain injury, and even surgical resection. In fact, developmental plasticity clearly confers an advantage when the brain must recover from a focal lesion [Kennard, 1942; Kolb et al., 2000; Villablanca and Hovda, 1999] if the lesion occurs at a specific age. However, the complex task of responding to environmental stimuli and rearranging neuronal networks, a fundamental developmental principle termed *experience-dependent plasticity*, may be transiently impaired after a diffuse injury. In the mature brain, consequences of such impairment might be overcome with time; in the young brain, it is possible that reduced responsiveness at a critical window of development can result in long-term dysfunction. Furthermore, studies looking at brain development occurring after traumatic brain injury, both in experimental animals and in children, must necessarily take into account the effects of brain maturation in normal controls.

Post-traumatic Neurometabolic Cascade

Traumatic brain injury results in an immediate release of glutamate, widespread changes in ionic flux, fluctuating cerebral glucose metabolism (initially elevated, then reduced), and dynamic changes in blood flow. Later, axonal damage and disconnection, reduced responsiveness to physiologic stimuli, impaired neurotransmission, and delayed cell death occur [Giza and Hovda, 2001]. An overview of post-traumatic pathophysiology at the cellular level is summarized in Figure 62-4. Specific components of the brain's response to traumatic injury are discussed next.

Glutamate Release and Ionic Flux

After traumatic injury to the brain, there is an immediate and indiscriminate release of the excitatory neurotransmitter glutamate [Bullock et al., 1998; Katayama et al., 1990]. This release can result from widespread triggering of action potentials, synaptic neurotransmitter release, and membrane disruption. This flood of glutamate results in a massive efflux of potassium into the extracellular space [Katayama

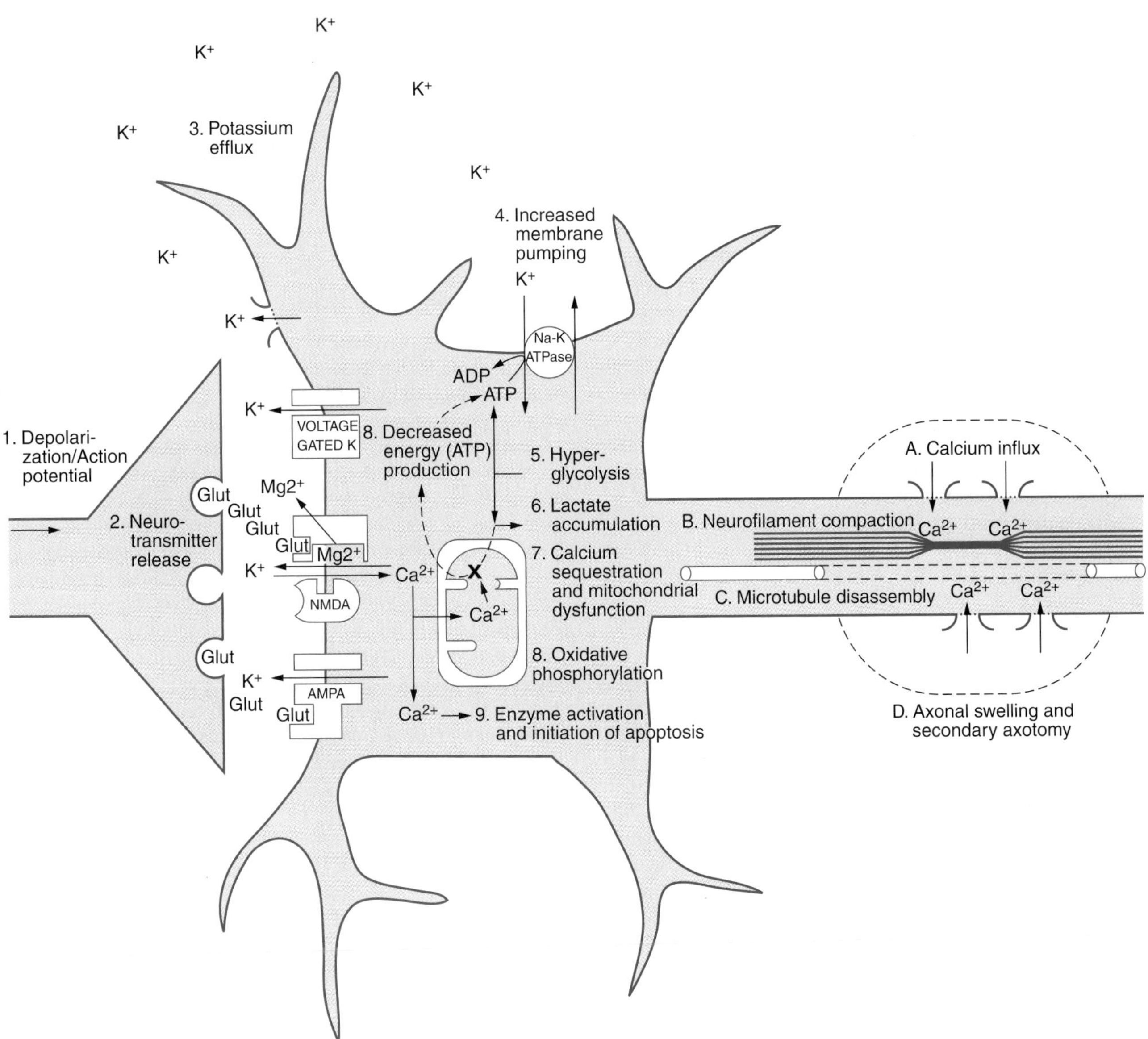

FIGURE 62-4. Neurometabolic cascade after traumatic injury. Cellular events: (1) nonspecific depolarization and initiation of action potentials; (2) release of excitatory neurotransmitters; (3) massive efflux of potassium; (4) increased activity of membrane ionic pumps to restore homeostasis; (5) hyperglycolysis to generate more adenosine triphosphate (ATP); (6) lactate accumulation; (7) calcium influx and sequestration in mitochondria leading to impaired oxidative metabolism; (8) decreased energy (ATP) production; (9) calpain activation and initiation of apoptosis. Axonal events: (A) axolemmal disruption and calcium influx; (B) neurofilament compaction via phosphorylation or sidearm cleavage; (C) microtubule disassembly and accumulation of axonally transported organelles; (D) axonal swelling and eventual axotomy. ADP, adenosine diphosphate; AMPA, alpha-amino-3-hydroxy-5-methyl-4-isoxazole propionic acid; Glut, glutamate; NMDA, *N*-methyl-D-aspartate. (From Giza CC, Hovda DA. The neurometabolic cascade of concussion. J Athl Train 2001;36:230).

et al., 1990; Nilsson et al., 1993] and an influx of sodium and calcium [Nilsson et al., 1996; Osteen et al., 2001]. Although hyperacute measures of extracellular glutamate are obviously unobtainable in human patients, microdialysis of extracellular fluid or cerebrospinal fluid samples from severely injured patients (including children) in the days after injury has demonstrated glutamate elevations and has been associated with secondary injury and possibly with poorer outcomes [Ashwal et al, 2004b; Bullock et al., 1998; Ruppel et al., 2001; Vespa et al., 1998].

Dynamic Changes in Cerebral Metabolism

As the injured cells attempt to restore ionic equilibrium after injury, membrane pumps such as the sodium-potassium adenosine triphosphatase pump are activated. An increase in cerebral glucose uptake, termed *hyperglycolysis*, is seen early after experimental traumatic brain injury and has been postulated as a mechanism of providing additional substrate to generate the energy necessary to drive these membrane ionic pumps [Kawamata et al., 1992; Yoshino et al., 1991]. Acute studies of cerebral glucose metabolism using positron emission tomography in adult patients have found increased cerebral glucose uptake [Bergsneider et al., 1997]. Interestingly, there is increasing laboratory evidence that injured neurons are capable of utilizing alternative fuels to glucose [Magistretti et al., 1999; Pellerin and Magistretti, 2004; Prins et al., 2004], and it is well known that the capacity to use alternative fuels in uninjured neurons is age specific [Vannucci and Vannucci, 2000].

After the acute period of hyperglycolysis, there is a prolonged period of diminished cerebral glucose uptake. This hypometabolism is seen in adult and immature rats, although it lasts longer in adults (7-10 days [Yoshino et al., 1991]) than in rat pups (3 days [Thomas et al., 2000]). In traumatically injured adult patients, the period of reduced glucose metabolism has been found to last weeks to months [Bergsneider et al., 2001].

Cerebral Blood Flow Hyperemia? Hypoperfusion?

Cerebral blood flow undergoes dynamic changes after injury, and the pattern of these changes may depend on the type of injury and its severity. A pattern of diffuse cerebral swelling has been reported more frequently in children than in adults [Aldrich et al., 1992; Lang et al., 1994]. This phenomenon was originally attributed to hyperemia [Bruce et al., 1981], but more recent studies suggest that the incidence of post-traumatic hyperemia has been overestimated [Muizelaar et al., 1989]. In the earlier studies of post-traumatic brain injury cerebral blood flow in children, flow values were compared with normal values from a young adult control group. Cerebral blood flow measured in normal children appears to change dramatically across development, and it is generally much higher in young children than in adults [Chiron et al., 1992; Suzuki, 1990; Zwienenberg and Muizelaar, 1999]. Subsequent studies of cerebral blood flow in children suffering traumatic brain injury, when compared with that in age-appropriate control values, have failed to demonstrate clear hyperemia [Adelson et al., 1997a; Sharples et al., 1995]. Interestingly, in an experimental model of traumatic brain injury, there is evidence for dramatically increased cerebral blood flow adjacent to a traumatic contusion; this focal hyperemia was most pronounced in immature animals [Biagas et al., 1996]. Although clinically it is important to recognize that diffuse cerebral swelling is more common in children, the mechanism of this swelling does not appear to be solely attributable to hyperemia.

The relation between cerebral blood flow and outcome appears to depend on the state of cerebral autoregulation. In the presence of intact autoregulation, increased cerebral blood flow has been associated with better perfusion and improved outcome in both children and young adults [Kelly et al., 1996; Vavilala et al., 2004]. However, after severe injuries in which autoregulation is dysfunctional and cerebral vasculature is pressure passive, increased cerebral blood flow can result in intractable elevations of intracranial pressure and poorer outcomes.

Beyond the acute phase of head injury, cerebral blood flow generally declines. Post–traumatic brain injury cerebral blood flow can decline below normal, and it is important to monitor for ischemia because this is associated with worse outcome [Bouma et al., 1991; Vespa et al., 2003]. Investigations are in progress to determine whether neurovascular coupling is intact during this period of reduced flow.

Altered Neurotransmission

Reductions in excitatory neurotransmitter systems have been reported after traumatic brain injury in experimental animals, including impairments in glutamatergic [Miller et al., 1990; Osteen et al., 2004; Sihver et al., 2001] and cholinergic [Gorman et al., 1996] transmission. These changes may correlate with the injury-induced reduction in cerebral metabolism. Furthermore, these changes may be an underlying mechanism for post–traumatic brain injury deficits in neuronal activation [Dietrich et al., 1994; Sanders et al., 2000], diminished activity-dependent molecular responsiveness [Giza et al., 2002; Griesbach et al., 2004], and impaired experience-dependent plasticity in developing animals [Fineman et al., 2000; Ip et al., 2002; Giza et al., 2005]. Activation studies using functional magnetic resonance imaging (fMRI), even after relatively mild traumatic brain injury, have shown reduced or aberrant activation patterns in traumatically injured teenagers and young adults [Jantzen et al., 2004; McAllister et al., 1999].

Axonal Disconnection

Mechanical stretch can disrupt axonal membranes, resulting in calcium influx and microtubule and neurofilament disruption. Damage to these important cytoskeletal components impairs normal axonal transport, endangering distal axonal segments and synapses. Over time, disrupted axonal transport leads to an accumulation of transported proteins and organelles at the injury site, causing axonal blebs and, eventually, disconnection [Pettus and Povlishock, 1996; Povlishock and Christman, 1995; Povlishock and Pettus, 1996]. This type of damage is seen after experimental traumatic brain injury in immature [Raghupathi and Margulies, 2002] and adult [Povlishock and Pettus, 1996] animals. In postmortem human specimens, evidence of axonal blebbing and damage has been reported long after injury

[Maxwell et al., 1997], and MRI can show abnormalities of diffuse axonal injury in pediatric and adult traumatic brain injury patients [Tong et al., 2004].

Cell Death: Necrosis and Apoptosis

Mechanisms of post–traumatic brain injury cell death occur across a spectrum from necrosis to apoptosis. Necrosis represents acute energy failure, inability to maintain ionic homeostasis, cell swelling, and eventual disruption of the plasma membrane. This type of cell death occurs when energy is depleted and does not require protein synthesis. Necrosis is seen as a direct result of traumatic injury, generally occurs acutely, and evolves in regions experiencing profound energy failure. When the cell ruptures, there is release of intracellular contents and a significant inflammatory response.

Apoptosis is characterized by nuclear condensation, DNA fragmentation, and preservation of the cell membrane. Apoptosis, also referred to as *programmed cell death*, requires energy and protein synthesis and initiates a less acute inflammatory response. Usually, apoptotic cell death takes longer to evolve after injury and continues to occur long after experimental trauma [Conti et al., 1998; Wilson et al., 2004]. Although apoptosis is seen after traumatic brain injury, it is also part of the brain's normal maturational program. Thus, apoptotic pathways are more active in the immature brain, and apoptotic cell death appears more prominently after experimental injury to the developing brain [Bittigau et al., 1999; Pohl et al., 1999].

Impaired Plasticity

An important aspect of injury in the young brain is the effect of this injury on normal neuronal responsiveness and on developmental plasticity. As mentioned earlier, increased plasticity in the immature brain results in significantly better recovery than in the adult after a focal lesion, and this has been well described in rats [Kolb and Tomie, 1988], cats [Burgess and Villablanca, 1986; Villablanca and Hovda, 1999], primates [Kennard, 1942], and humans [Hogan et al., 2000; Trauner et al., 1993]. However, the benefits of youth are less apparent when the injury is more diffuse or occurs at a critical window of brain development. Environmental enrichment is an experimental model of enhancing brain development, and animals reared in an enriched environment grow up to have larger brains [Bennett et al., 1964; Diamond et al., 1964; Rosenzweig and Bennett, 1996], increased dendritic arborization [Faherty et al.,, 2003; Greenough et al., 1973; Juraska, 1984; Volkmar and Greenough, 1972], and superior performance on neurobehavioral tasks [Tees et al., 1990; Venable et al., 1988; Williams et al., 2001]. Although injured rat pups exhibit less overt cell death and less behavioral impairment than adults [Gurkoff et al., 2005; Prins et al., 1996; Prins and Hovda, 1998], they lose the ability to benefit from being reared in an enriched environment. Specifically, they show a loss of enriched environment–induced experience-dependent plasticity: cortical thickening is blocked [Fineman et al., 2000], expansion of dendritic arbors is inhibited [Ip et al., 2002], and enriched environment–induced cognitive enhancements are absent [Giza et al., 2005]. These studies of altered developmental plasticity are also supported by findings of Prins and colleagues using a different model [Prins et al., 2003]. Following a lesion, regrowth of entorhinal cortical axons in a nontraumatically injured brain occurs in a well-characterized fashion. In juvenile rats subjected to experimental traumatic brain injury, this normal pattern of axonal regrowth was markedly disturbed, with evidence of disruption down to the synaptic level.

Studies of developmental plasticity in traumatically injured children are difficult because the effects of both age at injury and age at assessment must be considered in the control groups. However, there is growing evidence that pediatric traumatic brain injury results in altered brain development. First, although children generally have better outcome after traumatic brain injury than adults, those injured at the earliest ages (i.e., in infancy) actually have poorer outcomes [Levin et al., 1992; Luerssen et al, 1988]. Some of this may be due to different mechanisms of injury, including nonaccidental trauma (inflicted head injury), which has a very poor developmental prognosis and is predominantly an etiology seen in infancy. It is also possible that the very young brain is decidedly more vulnerable to injury, as suggested by experimental studies using hypoxia-ischemia [Ikonomidou et al., 1989] and traumatic brain injury [Bittigau et al., 1999; Pohl et al., 1999]. Second, there are anecdotal reports of cases of rare, neonatal head trauma that appear to have resulted in abnormal cortical development that was subsequently confirmed pathologically after epilepsy surgery for intractable seizures [Lombroso, 2000; Marin-Padilla et al., 2002]. Third, studies of severe pediatric traumatic brain injury show more persistent cognitive deficits when the injury was diffuse rather than focal [Levin et al, 2000]. Finally, in studies of repeated, mild sports-related traumatic brain injury sustained during adolescence or early adulthood, subtle but significant cognitive impairments are detected [Collins et al., 1999; Matser et al., 1999].

HISTORY

The clinical approach to pediatric traumatic brain injury differs based on whether the presentation is acute (e.g., emergency department, urgent care clinic) or delayed (e.g., persistent post–traumatic brain injury symptoms in regular clinic). For an acutely injured child, history taking and initial assessment begin rapidly and simultaneously. Elements of the history should be obtained from parents, witnesses, and emergency personnel. Essential information includes mechanism of injury (e.g., pedestrian struck by motor vehicle, fell 10 feet out of a tree, bicycle crash), protective factors (e.g., helmet, seatbelt), any loss of consciousness (and duration), any post-traumatic amnesia (and duration), seizure activity (with duration and description), current medications (including allergies), and any persistent neurologic signs (e.g., confusion, focal deficit). Examination, monitoring for ABCs (airway, breathing, circulation, spine), and initial management are begun simultaneously. Additional components of the history that may be relevant are sought once the patient is stabilized and include premorbid cognitive and behavioral development, prior head injuries, prior neurosurgical procedures, history of epilepsy or other neurologic disorder, and other pertinent medical conditions (e.g., coagulopathy, asthma). In older children and teenagers, the possibility of drug or alcohol use should be considered. In infants and toddlers, inconsistencies in the injury story and presence of associated injuries should raise suspicion of child abuse.

For patients presenting in clinic with persistent neurologic problems after (presumably) milder head injury, the same historical information should be sought. In addition, the child and parent should be asked about the nature of post-traumatic symptoms, including headache, neck pain, nausea, vomiting, dizziness, ataxia, visual disturbances, cognitive impairment, behavioral changes, and any focal neurologic deficits. Pain should be localized, if possible. The duration of constant symptoms should be ascertained, along with alleviating or exacerbating factors. Episodic symptoms should also be carefully investigated, including triggers, duration, pattern of episodes, and actions that result in symptom resolution.

EXAMINATION

For the acutely and severely brain injured child, physical and neurologic examination must be done expediently, with the aim of identifying immediately life-threatening signs that would direct initial management. The presence of secondary insults is a strong independent predictor of poor traumatic brain injury outcome; thus, careful assessment of airway and breathing is paramount. Pattern of breathing should be noted (e.g., irregular, tachypneic). Adequate circulation and perfusion are also critical; look for skin color, pulses, blood pressure, capillary refill, and excessive bleeding. In a hypotensive patient, bodily injuries that result in internal bleeding, such as hemothorax, liver or splenic lacerations, pelvic fracture, and long bone fractures, should be identified as soon as possible, although they may not be evident from physical examination. In infants, massive scalp hematomas may result in hypotension and shock. Spinal cord injury or cardiac injury can also result in low blood pressure. In patients who are or were unconscious, careful stabilization of the spine is necessary.

The patient's Glasgow Coma Scale score should be determined. The Glasgow Coma Scale is a quick, reproducible means of rating the severity of the patient's neurologic injury (Table 62-1) [Teasdale and Jennett, 1974] that has three components: eye opening (ranging from 1 to 4), best verbal response (ranging from 1 to 5), and best motor response (ranging from 1 to 6), for a total score from 3 (worst) to 15 (normal). There are obvious limitations to this scale in the setting of pediatric trauma, such as how to determine verbal score in infants and young children. Several Glasgow Coma Scale modifications have been proposed to make it more usable in this age group (see Chapter 61), and one modified scale is shown in Table 62-1. By convention, mild traumatic brain injury is defined by a Glasgow Coma Scale score of 13 to 15, moderate is 9 to 12, and severe is 8 or less. A patient with a Glasgow Coma Scale score of 13 to 15 who has an intracranial lesion is generally classified as having a moderate traumatic brain injury.

After the ABCs, assessment of the patient's mental state should be made, including alertness, orientation, confusion, combativeness, or unresponsiveness. Use specific descriptions of mental status (e.g., "able to follow simple commands but becomes quiet and sleepy if unstimulated") rather than vague words such as "lethargic" or "obtunded." Inspection of the head can reveal lacerations, contusions, and hematomas. Careful examination is warranted in either circumstance to identify stepoffs (i.e., palpation of a bone edge indicative of a fracture or bony separation), foreign bodies, fractures, or penetrating injuries that may underlie more superficial damage. In infants, the fontanel can be assessed quickly to look for elevated intracranial pressure. Periorbital ecchymosis ("raccoon eyes") or rhinorrhea raises concern for fracture of the anterior skull base. Retroauricular ecchymosis ("Battle's sign"), hemotympanum, and otorrhea are signs indicative of a basilar skull fracture involving the temporal bone. Ophthalmoscopic examination to detect retinal hemorrhage is very important, particularly in cases of suspected nonaccidental trauma.

Patients rendered unconscious by the injury and those who retain consciousness but report post-traumatic neck

TABLE 62-1

Glasgow Coma Scale

GLASGOW COMA SCALE		INFANT MODIFICATION	
Eye opening (E)		Eye opening (E)	
• Spontaneous	4	• Spontaneous	4
• To speech (to shout)	3	• To speech (to shout)	3
• To pain	2	• To pain	2
• None	1	• None	1
Motor response (M)		Motor response (M)	
• Obeys commands	6	• Purposeful movements	6
• Localizes pain	5	• Localizes pain	5
• Withdraws	4	• Withdraws	4
• Abnormal flexion	3	• Abnormal flexion	3
• Extensor response	2	• Extensor response	2
• None	1	• None	1
Verbal response (V)		Verbal response, modified for infants	
• Oriented	5	• Babbles, coos appropriately	5
• Confused conversation	4	• Cries, but consolable	4
• Inappropriate words	3	• Cries inconsolably	3
• Incomprehensible sounds	2	• Grunts or moans to pain	2
• None	1	• None	1

pain should have the cervical spine immobilized until it can be assessed for any significant fracture or dislocation. With the head in neutral position, the cervical spine should be carefully palpated, noting any angulation, stepoff, crepitus, or point tenderness.

The post-trauma neurologic examination is by necessity short and directed and should be able to be performed in just a few minutes. Cranial nerve testing offers rapid, objective evaluation of brainstem functions. The pupillary response tests integrity of cranial nerves II and III. Fixed midposition pupils suggest symmetric midbrain dysfunction. A unilateral fixed dilated pupil in conjunction with declining mental status is a sign of impending transtentorial herniation, usually due to a mass lesion ipsilateral to the abnormal pupil, and warrants immediate intervention. Bilateral pinpoint pupils raise the possibility of opiate ingestion, or severe pontine injury. Bilateral fixed dilated pupils are evidence of widespread injury but can also be due to systemic effects of resuscitation drugs. A pupil that fails to constrict under direct light (but does when light is presented to the opposite eye) is indicative of an afferent pupillary defect, a sign of ipsilateral optic nerve injury due to fracture of the orbit.

Integrity of nerves to the extraocular muscles (cranial nerves III, IV, and VI) and their brainstem connections can be tested in three ways. First, simply observe the eyes for spontaneous conjugate roving movements. Second is the oculocephalic response ("doll's eye" maneuver), performed by turning the child's head rapidly to one side. A normal response is for the eyes to move conjugately in the direction opposite the head turning. This test is rarely used acutely following trauma because it is not generally safe to move the head and neck until the cervical spine has been cleared. If it is absolutely necessary to assess these specific nerves, the third method is to test the vestibulo-ocular reflex (calorics). Before caloric testing, one must check for a nonoccluded ear canal, an intact tympanic membrane, and the absence of either hemotympanum or otorrhea. Then, with head positioned 30 degrees above horizontal, 30 to 60 mL of ice-cold water is irrigated rapidly into the ear. An intact response is tonic eye deviation toward the irrigated ear. After a few minutes, the response may be tested in the opposite ear.

An intact corneal response demonstrates function of cranial nerves V and VII. If, on corneal stimulation, the globe rotates upward but the eyelid does not close, this suggests an intact afferent limb but impaired motor output. Examination for other evidence of a cranial nerve VII palsy, as might be seen with a basilar skull fracture, should be performed. Tickling the inside of the nose with a wisp of cotton or administering a noxious stimulus may elicit a grimace, which should be observed for facial symmetry.

Sensorimotor examination can also be done quickly, starting with the best motor response elicited on Glasgow Coma Scale testing. Limb posture and muscle tone should be examined, and particular note should be made of any asymmetry. If the patient is unable to follow commands, then sensorimotor response may be assessed by application of a peripheral noxious stimulus (e.g., nailbed pressure) in each limb. If no response occurs, then the site of noxious stimuli can be moved centrally (e.g., sternal rub, supraorbital pressure) to distinguish between afferent and efferent impairment. Application of painful stimulus centrally allows the examiner to determine more readily whether a child can localize pain (distinction between a 4 and 5 for best motor score). If the child is awake, coordination should be assessed by observation of posture, spontaneous movements, and directed movements when the child reaches for an object or mimics the examiner. Deep tendon reflexes should be checked for asymmetry, hyperreflexia, clonus, or areflexia. Flaccid paresis with no reflexes should immediately raise suspicion of a spinal injury. An outline of the rapid trauma examination is provided in Table 62-2.

TABLE 62-2

Rapid Pediatric Trauma Exam

1. *ABCs, brief history*—mechanism of injury, loss of consciousness, amnesia, persistent neurologic symptoms
2. *Glasgow Coma Scale* score
3. *Physical examination*, particularly head and neck
   a. Scalp—depressions, stepoffs, fluid collections, lacerations
   b. Other signs of skull facture—otorrhea, hemotympanum, rhinorrhea, raccoon eyes, Battle's sign
   c. Cervical spine—deformity, point tenderness
   d. Associated severe bodily injuries—thoracic, abdominal, long bone
4. *Mental status*—describe succinctly, avoid ambiguous terms
5. *Cranial nerves*
   a. Pupillary response (CN II, III)
   b. Oculocephalic "doll's eye" response (CN III, IV, VI)
   c. Vestibulo-ocular "caloric" response (CN III, IV, VI, VIII)
   d. Corneal response, facial grimacing (CN V, VII)
   e. Gag response (CN IX, X)
6. *Sensorimotor*—asymmetry, abnormal muscle tone, coordination (if possible), movement (spontaneous, to command), movement to pain (withdrawal, decorticate, decerebrate, no movement)
7. Reflexes—asymmetry, areflexia, hyperreflexia/clonus. upgoing toes

In the mildly injured child who is conscious at the time of initial evaluation, the neurologic examination can be conducted less urgently and more completely. In such patients, mental status testing can be more extensive, starting with observation and possibly requesting the patient to repeat a series of numbers (i.e., digit span) to assess the child's attention. This assessment can be followed by evaluation of orientation, language, behavior, and memory (both anterograde, for new items, and retrograde, for past events, including events surrounding the injury). Cranial nerve, motor, coordination, and sensory examinations can include voluntary responses to the examiner's commands and subjective reports of sensory input (visual fields, tactile stimulation). Gait should be observed for signs of unsteadiness or ataxia. As with the more severely injured child, deep tendon reflexes and plantar responses should be assessed.

Neurologic reassessment is mandated based on the severity of injury. Mental status should be recorded in distinct descriptive wording such as "awake but mumbling incoherently and unable to follow commands" or "crying when approached but consolable by parent." Deterioration of the neurologic examination may be a sign of progression of the underlying injury (cerebral edema, expansion of a subdural hematoma) or may represent a new complication (hemorrhagic transformation of a contusion, seizure) and should be evaluated immediately so that appropriate treatment is instituted.

IMMEDIATE MANAGEMENT

Initial management of the child suffering from moderate or severe traumatic brain injury centers on the ABCs and avoidance of secondary insults. The airway must be secured and supplemental oxygen provided. In circumstances in which the child is unable to adequately maintain the airway, endotracheal intubation should be performed. Appropriate noninvasive monitors should be placed, including cardiac, respiratory, temperature, blood pressure, and pulse oximetry. Intubated patients should also have an end-tidal CO_2 monitor. Intravenous access must be established immediately and fluid resuscitation begun. Blood should be drawn for electrolytes, glucose, renal and hepatic function, complete blood count, prothrombin and partial thromboplastin times, type and cross-match, and, if indicated, arterial blood gas determinations and alcohol or drug screens.

ACUTE CLINICAL SYNDROMES

Because traumatic brain injury is a heterogeneous disorder with multiple manifestations, syndromes may occur in isolation but are often overlapping. For example, nonaccidental trauma is a particular etiology of infantile head trauma that can include subdural hematomas, other intracranial hematomas, cerebral edema, diffuse axonal injury, cerebral contusion, skull fracture, and early post-traumatic seizures. Epidural hematomas are often associated with skull fractures. Concussion can occur alone or as a repeated injury; it can be associated with acute seizures and, rarely, with malignant cerebral edema, second impact syndrome, herniation, and death. Fortunately, concussion can also, and almost always does, last briefly and be symptomatically self-limited.

Herniation Syndromes

Herniation is the displacement of brain tissue from one intracranial compartment to another. This injury can occur as a result of a space-occupying lesion in one region or diffuse swelling of both cerebral hemispheres (see Fig. 62-3) [Fishman, 1980; Plum and Posner, 1980]. The Cushing response is a paradoxical bradycardia with hypertension and slow irregular respiration that can be seen in the setting of elevated intracranial pressure and impending herniation. Definitive treatment for herniation requires surgical removal of the offending mass. In cases in which herniation is triggered by edema, position the head so that it is slightly elevated and in the midline (to facilitate venous drainage) and immediately initiate first tier measures to control elevated intracranial pressure: sedation, hyperventilation, and hyperosmolar therapy. Ventriculostomy with cerebrospinal fluid drainage, if feasible, should be instituted as soon as possible. Infants can tolerate elevation of intracranial pressure better because of unfused sutures and an open fontanel. These properties also allow for additional physical examination clues to the presence of increased intracranial pressure, like a tense or bulging fontanel or a steadily increasing head circumference (if chronic).

In lateral transtentorial herniation, a hemispheric mass such as an epidural or subdural hematoma can displace the medial temporal lobe structures across the tentorial notch. This displacement compresses the midbrain, resulting in impaired consciousness and ipsilateral cranial nerve III palsy with pupillary dilation and contralateral hemiparesis. Unilateral pupil dilation in an awake patient cannot be the result of herniation. Occasionally, this type of herniation compresses the posterior cerebral artery, resulting in an ipsilateral occipital lobe cerebral infarction and contralateral homonymous hemianopia.

A unilateral mass can also result in translocation of brain tissue across the midline. At first, the falx cerebri will simply be displaced away from the side of the mass. This is termed *midline shift* and can be readily seen on a computed tomography (CT) scan. When more severe, the cingulate gyrus will actually be pushed under the falx cerebri, resulting in subfalcine herniation. This herniation syndrome is associated with compression of the anterior cerebral arteries and infarction of the medial frontal lobes.

Diffuse bilateral cerebral edema or bilateral mass lesions can cause symmetric herniation of the supratentorial contents down into the posterior fossa. This result is termed *central transtentorial herniation* and is more common than the lateral syndrome. Physical examination findings consistent with the early stage of this syndrome include impaired mental status, fixed midposition pupils, impaired upward gaze, hyperventilation (central neurogenic hyperventilation), and posturing. Posturing will first take the decorticate form (arms flexed, legs extended), but as herniation progresses, decerebrate posturing (arms and legs extended) is seen. In these later stages of central herniation, pupils may become symmetrically constricted, and respirations may become irregular.

Cerebellar tonsillar herniation occurs when the posterior fossa contents are pushed down through the foramen magnum. This type of herniation usually is seen in the setting of a posterior fossa mass. Because the infratentorial compartment is smaller than the supratentorial, critical pressure effects can occur rapidly and with much smaller space-occupying lesions. Tonsillar herniation can cause head tilt, neck stiffness, and lower cranial neuropathies and can appear relatively abruptly with cardiorespiratory compromise. Posterior fossa masses can also cause herniation of cerebellar contents upward through the tentorium.

Herniation can then lead to ischemic and hemorrhagic complications (Duret's hemorrhages) in the brainstem. The final stages of herniation occur as medullary centers are compressed, resulting in apnea, cardiac collapse, and death.

Brain herniation also can occur through a traumatic or surgical defect in the skull. Transcalvarial herniation occurs when brain swelling is relieved by extrusion of brain tissue out of the cranial cavity through a fracture, burr hole, or craniotomy. In some circumstances, this type of herniation may alleviate disastrous brainstem consequences of downward herniation syndromes.

Diffuse Cerebral Swelling

Because trauma, particularly closed head trauma, is by nature a diffuse process, bilateral swelling can occur even in the absence of discrete focal lesions. In fact, diffuse cerebral swelling is more common in children [Aldrich et al., 1992; Lang et al., 1994], whereas focal cerebral damage, such as contusion, is more common in older adolescents and adults. The etiology of this swelling was originally postulated to be hyperemia [Bruce et al., 1981]. However, as discussed earlier in this chapter, original reports of post-traumatic hyperemia in children may have overestimated the frequency of this phenomenon by comparing cerebral blood flow values with those of uninjured young adult controls rather than uninjured children [Muizelaar et al., 1989; Zwienenberg and Muizelaar, 1999]. An alternative etiology could be diffuse cerebral edema. Cerebral edema is generally of two types: (1) cytotoxic, which occurs as a result of dying neurons undergoing energy failure, with loss of membrane ionic gradients and a rapid increase in intracellular water; and (2) vasogenic, which results from fluid seeping into the extracellular space across a damaged or dysfunctional blood-brain barrier. Cytotoxic edema is thought to predominate after traumatic injury. Diffuse edema can occur as a direct response to trauma but also can be due to a post-traumatic secondary insult, such as hypotension or hypoxia. At its extreme, diffuse edema can result in central transtentorial herniation and death.

Diffuse Axonal Injury

A clinical correlate to the pathophysiologic process of axonal injury and disconnection, diffuse axonal injury is thought to result from the effect of shearing and rotational forces on white matter fiber tracts [Adams et al., 1982]. These forces are usually considerable, and diffuse axonal injury is most commonly seen after a high-impact injury such as a motor vehicle crash or a high fall.

Clinically, the patient with diffuse axonal injury has a prolonged period of unresponsiveness or coma that is not explained by a mass lesion or diffuse hypoxia. Gradually, the patient recovers some movement and can initially appear to be posturing or restless. Because of brainstem involvement, autonomic symptoms may be prominent, particularly in severe cases of diffuse axonal injury.

Diffuse axonal injury can occur in the presence or absence of hypoxia-ischemia or elevated intracranial pressure but is a discrete process. The pathology of these lesions includes tearing and necrosis of nerve fibers, often with microhemorrhages. Blebs and swellings occur at points of axonal injury, locations that may subsequently become sites of axonal disconnection [Maxwell and Graham, 1997; Pettus and Povlishock, 1996; Povlishock and Christman, 1995]. These lesions are often seen at the gray-white junction of the frontal and temporal lobes, in the corpus callosum, and in the rostral brainstem. Diffuse axonal injury is rarely seen on CT, and then only if hemorrhage is present. MRI, however, is more sensitive in detecting diffuse axonal injury, which appears as areas of hypointensity on T2-weighted, two-dimensional gradient recall echo imaging (Fig. 62-5). Recently, MRI using susceptibility-weighted imaging has more clearly demonstrated and allowed quantification of hemorrhagic diffuse axonal injury lesions [Tong et al., 2004].

In general, patients with diffuse axonal injury have lasting neurologic impairments, with good outcome at 3 months ranging from 65% of mild diffuse axonal injury patients to only 15% of severely injured patients [LeRoux et al., 2000]. The aforementioned autonomic impairments may be the etiology of significant mortality in patients with diffuse axonal injury.

Nonaccidental Trauma

Child abuse has previously been termed *shaken-baby syndrome* because the etiology of the cerebral injuries was thought to be due to rapid shaking of the infant (see Chapter 63). Biomechanical studies attempting to model these injuries found that shaking alone may not be capable of generating the forces necessary to cause the severe and diffuse intracranial injuries that are typically seen [Prange et al., 2003]. It has been proposed that most injuries involve shaking and also a final impact [Duhaime

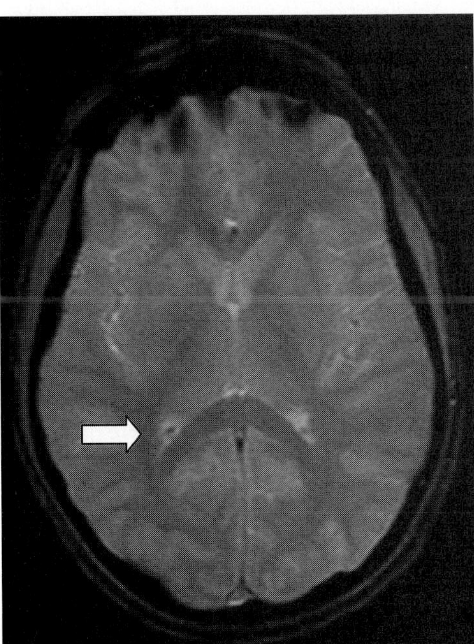

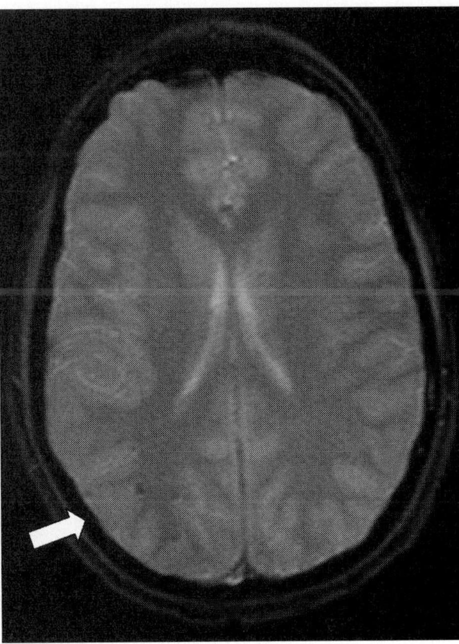

FIGURE 62-5. Areas of microhemorrhage (*arrows*) indicative of diffuse axonal injury are evident on an MRI T2-weighted, two-dimensional gradient recall echo sequence in a 15-year-old male after a motor vehicle crash.

et al., 1987]. Many experts now prefer the terms *non-accidental trauma*, *inflicted head injury*, or *shaken impact syndrome* to describe this clinical entity.

The clinical presentation is rarely straightforward because clinical signs in infants are often nonspecific, and parents may be less forthcoming about the circumstances of the infant's injury. Infants can present with lethargy, irritability, seizures, and vomiting. Physical signs include a tense or bulging fontanel, split sutures, enlarged head circumference, retinal hemorrhages, and often evidence of other inflicted bodily injuries, such as fractures, bruising in unusual locations (back, upper legs), and burns. Eventually, these infants undergo CT scanning, which may be normal on initial presentation but can reveal subdural hematomas, contusions, and other intracerebral hemorrhage. Subdural hematomas of differing ages are particularly suspicious for nonaccidental trauma and are frequently seen over the cerebral convexities or along the falx (Fig. 62-6B). Inconsistencies between the reported history and the severity of injuries should alert the physician to suspect child abuse.

Infants with nonaccidental trauma often require vigorous resuscitation, controlled ventilation, antiepileptic drug treatment, and intensive care unit management. In addition to CT neuroimaging, diagnostic evaluation should include whole-body x-rays to determine whether there are other acute or partially healing fractures. Ophthalmoscopic examination is essential to identify retinal hemorrhages (see Fig. 62-6A), as is a careful inspection for burns or excessive bruises that are often in unusual locations and in various stages of resolution. Laboratory tests should be ordered to rule out coagulopathy. Evaluation for rare inborn errors of metabolism such as glutaricaciduria and Menkes' disease needs to be considered because these disorders can manifest with bilateral subdural fluid collections, hematomas, and retinal hemorrhages.

The outcome for infants suffering nonaccidental trauma is exceedingly poor. Mortality rates range from 7% to 30%, and severe neurocognitive sequelae are reported in one third to one half [Weiner and Weinberg, 2000]. Up to 80% of deaths due to trauma before the age of 2 years are attributed to nonaccidental injury [Bruce and Zimmerman, 1989]. It is believed that these children account for the poorer prognosis reported in the very young age group, which goes against the general trend of improved outcome with younger age. Several explanations may account for this observation. The very young brain may be selectively vulnerable—it is well known to be particularly sensitive to excitotoxicity but also depends on excitatory glutamatergic stimulation for neuronal survival and development of connectivity. Second, the nature of nonaccidental trauma is such that repeated, fairly severe injuries are sustained, and the cumulative effect of this injury pattern may result in the dismal outcomes. Third, biomechanical properties of the infantile brain, including incomplete myelination and increased water content, may predispose it to shearing and disconnection types of injuries, and disconnection at this maturational stage may result in developmental failure. Finally, medical care for these children is often delayed, perhaps setting the stage for significant secondary injuries due to hypoperfusion, hypoxia-ischemia, and recurrent seizures.

Subarachnoid Hemorrhage

Subarachnoid hemorrhage occurs commonly after traumatic brain injury. Clinical symptoms of subarachnoid hemorrhage are fairly nonspecific in infants (irritability, lethargy, poor feeding), but older children present with persistent headache, nausea, vomiting, neck stiffness, and altered mental status. Blood products are irritating to the brain and the cerebral vasculature. Cortical irritation can result in seizures, and subarachnoid blood can provoke cerebral vasospasm, usually after several days. Vasospasm can be severe enough to cause cerebral ischemia or infarction. Subarachnoid hemorrhage is easily seen on CT, with hyperdense signal of acute blood visible in sulci and fissures and often in the basal cisterns (Fig. 62-7). Occasionally, when subarachnoid blood is seen in the ventricular system the risk for post-traumatic hydrocephalus is increased.

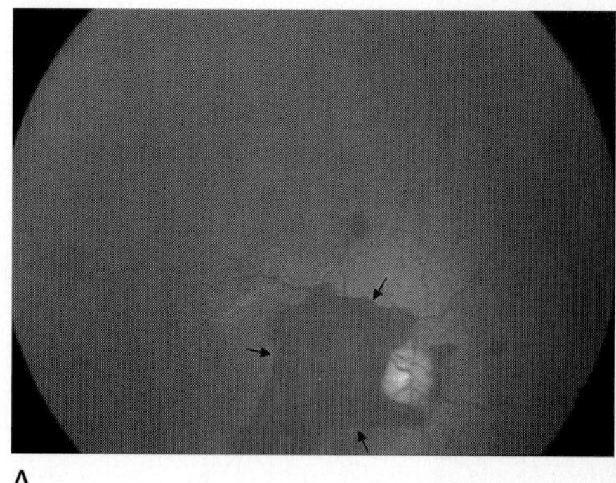
A

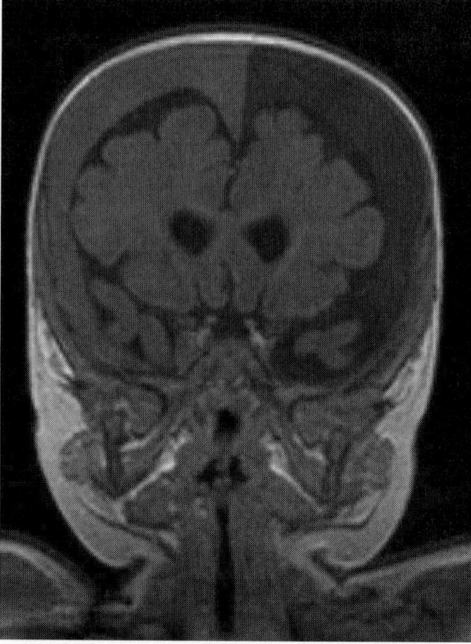
B

FIGURE 62-6. Signs suggestive of nonaccidental trauma. **A**, Retinal hemorrhage (*arrows*) on funduscopic examination. See also Color Plate. **B**, Bilateral subdural hematomas on T1-weighted MRI showing different signal intensities, indicating that the hemorrhages occurred at different times.

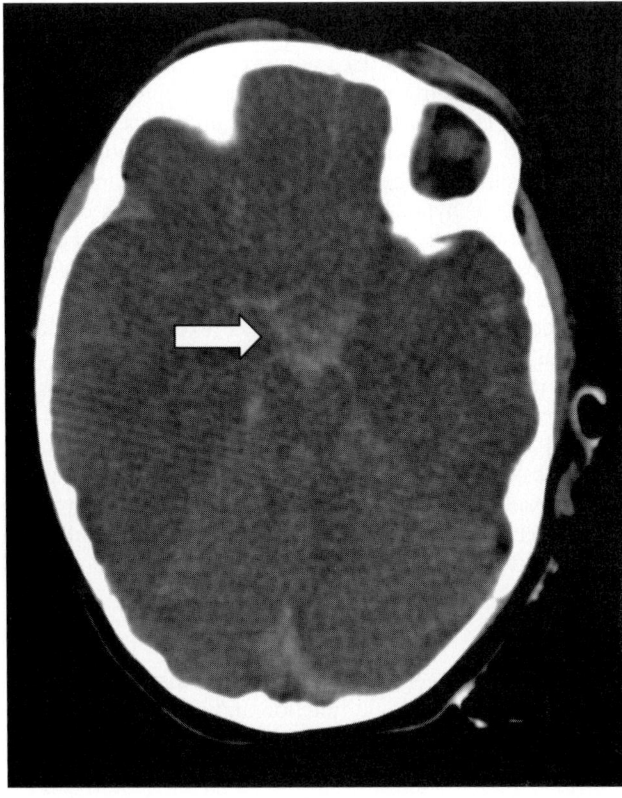

FIGURE 62-7. Post-traumatic subarachnoid hemorrhage outlining the basal cisterns (*arrow*) is clearly seen on this noncontrast head CT.

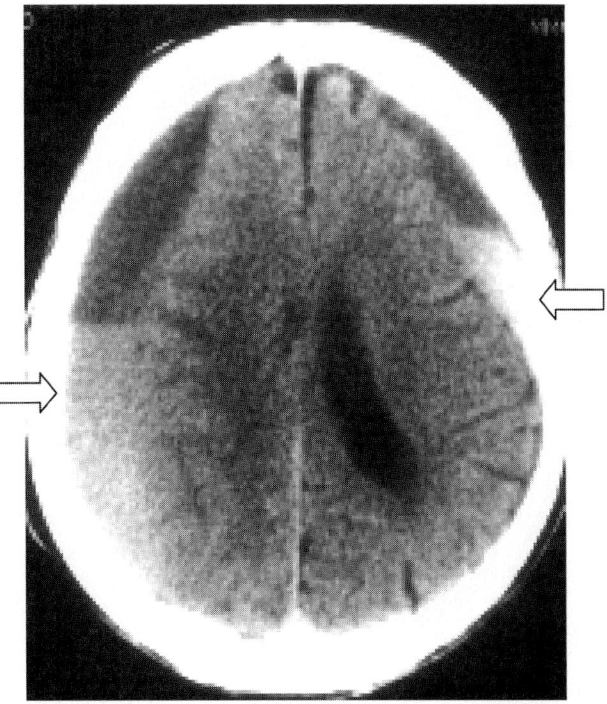

FIGURE 62-8. Bilateral subdural hematomas of mixed density are seen in this noncontrast head CT (*arrows*). Note the characteristics of subdural location, including concave morphology and extension of the hematomas across suture lines.

Subdural Hematoma

Subdural hematomas, as the name implies, occur underneath the dura mater and often result from tearing of bridging cortical veins. Subdural hematomas can be seen after significant head trauma, including accidental and nonaccidental trauma. These hemorrhages can manifest with a sudden or, more often, gradually progressive focal deficit. Mass effect can lead to neurologic symptoms of depressed mental status and, in severe cases, signs of impending herniation.

Appearance of subdural hematomas on CT scans is characteristic. An acute subdural hematoma appears as a crescent-shaped hyperdensity along the inner surface of the skull. Large subdurals may track across suture lines (Fig. 62-8). Sudural hematomas can also occur over the cerebral convexities, along the falx or tentorium, or, more rarely, in the posterior fossa. Often there is associated focal edema in the vicinity of the subdural hematoma, and midline shift can lead to subfalcine or transtentorial herniation.

Definitive treatment of an acute symptomatic subdural hematoma involves neurosurgical consultation and probable surgical evacuation. If edema is extensive, then external ventriculostomy is helpful to monitor intracranial pressure and for potentially therapeutic cerebrospinal fluid drainage. Other immediate and first-tier interventions to control elevated intracranial pressure should be instituted if necessary, including elevation of the head of the bed, maintaining the head in a neutral position, sedation, neuromuscular blockade, gentle hyperventilation, and hyperosmolar therapy. Outcome after subdural hematoma is fairly good, with up to 75% of infants having normal development. Infants with subdural hematomas due to nonaccidental trauma have a much more guarded prognosis, as mentioned earlier.

Subacute and chronic subdural hematomas appear as crescent-shaped subdural fluid collections that can be isodense and then become hypodense. In infants, a bulging fontanel and an enlarging head size may be clues in an otherwise nonspecific picture of irritability, poor feeding, lethargy, and vomiting. Seizures are frequently seen.

Chronic subdural hematomas needs to be distinguished from benign extracerebral collections of childhood, which are associated with a mildly enlarged head circumference, have a predilection for a frontal or bifrontal location, appear hypodense on CT, and occur with no history of head trauma. These collections are associated with a normal developmental prognosis and spontaneously resolve by around 18 months.

Epidural Hematoma

Epidural hematomas are acute collections of blood that occur in the potential space over the dura but beneath the calvarium. They are more commonly caused by arterial bleeding in adults, particularly underlying the pterion, where they are often due to skull fracture with tearing of the middle meningeal artery. On CT, an epidural hematoma classically appears as a convex lens–shaped hyperdensity adjacent to the skull (Fig. 62-9). Epidural hematomas generally are constrained by dural attachment to the skull and do not cross suture lines.

Although these characteristics are typical for epidural hematoma, in children there are significant distinctions.

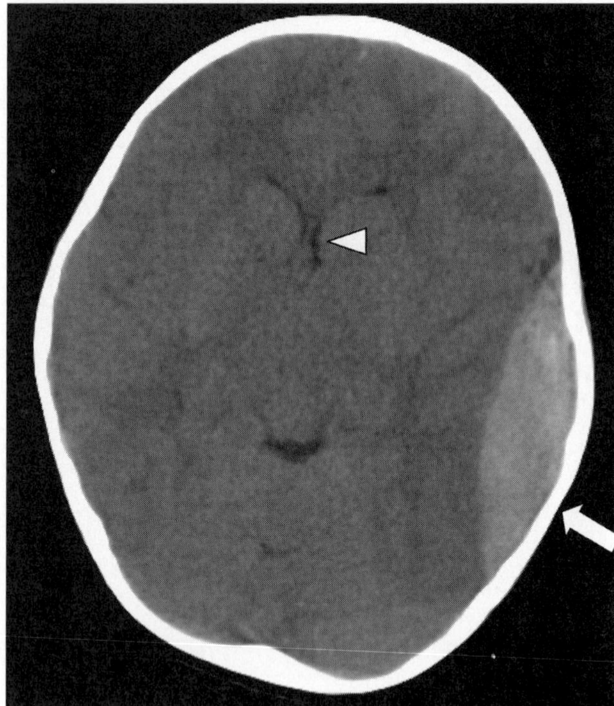

FIGURE 62-9. Typical appearance of an epidural hematoma (*arrow*), including convex shape and limitation of hematoma at suture lines. Also noted is mass effect, with shift of midline structures (septum pellucidum—*triangle*) away from the side of the hematoma.

First, epidural hematomas occur less frequently in children than in adults. Second, epidural hematomas are more likely to be due to bleeding from bridging veins or dural sinuses and thus are less commonly associated with skull fracture. Those associated with fracture in infants can occasionally push through the fracture line of the thin skull to decompress, masking symptoms and allowing the epidural hematoma to accumulate to the point at which anemia may be noted. Because they are more often venous in origin, the clinical presentation of epidural hematomas in children can be more gradual. Some reports indicate that more than 50% of children and more than 80% of infants demonstrate no alteration in mental state at the time of injury [Choux et al., 1975]. Third, although most epidural hematomas in adults or children are supratentorial, the percentage of posterior fossa epidural hematomas is higher in the pedia-tric population [Wright, 1966]. These are more often associated with occipital trauma, are venous in origin, and have delayed symptoms (ataxia, vomiting, and headache), occurring a few days after the injury. Because of the risk for compression of critical brainstem structures and potential cardiorespiratory collapse, surgical removal is preferred.

The mortality rate associated with epidural hematomas ranges from 7% to 15%. Most mortality and morbidity are due to effects of rapid enlargement of these hemorrhages with concomitant damage to underlying brain tissue. Prognosis is less certain with infants, whose nonspecific presenting symptoms increase the likelihood of diagnostic delays. If recognized and evacuated promptly, however, recovery is generally good in up to 90% of children.

Cerebral Contusion and Laceration

Cerebral contusion and laceration represent types of direct, focal damage to the brain. These types of injury are less common in children than in adults. Contusions, when they occur, tend to be frontal or temporal in location, usually along the surface of gyri (Fig. 62-10). The appearance may be as a subtle hypodensity on CT. Over time, some contusions evolve into hemorrhagic lesions (and thus become hyperdense on CT; see Fig. 62-10), and in adults, checking serial CT scans has been recommended. In severe cases with edema and mass effect, surgical excision of necrotic material has been performed.

Lacerations are also fairly rare and involve physical tearing of brain tissue. These can be associated with a depressed fracture or penetrating injury. Dura and vascular structures can be similarly torn. In infants, tearing of white matter can occur even in the setting of blunt head trauma [Calder et al., 1984]. This is due to the lack of myelin and increased water content of the very young brain.

Concussion

Concussion has been defined as any traumatically induced disturbance of neurologic function and mental state, occurring with or without actual loss of consciousness [American Academy of Neurology, 1997]. Concussion in isolation is

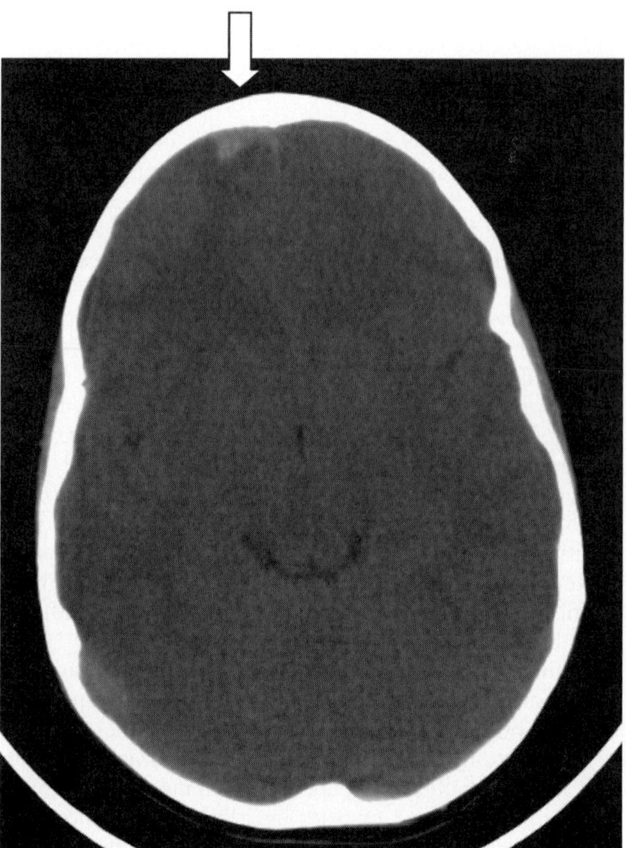

FIGURE 62-10. Typical frontopolar location of a small cerebral contusion (*arrow*), with increased density indicative of hemorrhage. If no hemorrhage is present, a contusion may simply appear as a slight hypodensity.

often referred to as *mild traumatic brain injury*, and it is important to be aware that concussive-type injuries can occur in almost every setting of head trauma, although they may be overshadowed by greater symptomatology from a skull fracture or mass lesion. Mild traumatic brain injury remains the most common form of traumatic brain injury in any age group, accounting for more than 75% to 85% of all head injuries [Kraus and McArthur, 2000].

Acute clinical symptoms are fairly consistent, including headache, transient confusion, amnesia, dizziness, unsteadiness, nausea, and vomiting. In most cases, there is no actual loss of consciousness. Signs of concussion include vacant staring, observable confusion, disorientation, memory disturbance, ataxia, incoordination, slurred speech, behavioral disturbances, and any witnessed unconsciousness. The hallmark of concussion is that the acute symptoms are self-limited and occur in the absence of demonstrable structural brain injury. Because there is little evidence of structural damage, the etiology of concussion symptoms is often ascribed to neural dysfunction that recovers over time.

Several issues regarding concussion are particularly relevant in children. There is much concern about proper evaluation of concussion or mild traumatic brain injury so as not to miss any associated intracranial injury, although exceedingly rare. This problem is addressed in the later section discussing general management of the mildly injured child. Second, duration of postacute physiologic derangement is uncertain but has significant implications for returning to normal activity. For example, a child returning to normal activity before complete physiologic recovery may have subtle cognitive or fine motor deficits that need to be considered to best integrate the child back into preinjury educational settings. Also, there is some concern that premature return to physical activity, such as contact sports, may place the individual at greater risk for a second injury. Third, although mild traumatic brain injury in adults is well described to result in persistent neurobehavioral problems, studies of a single mild traumatic brain injury in children differ with regard to the significance of long-term sequelae [Asarnow et al., 1995; Hawley et al., 2004]. Finally, there is increasing evidence that repeated mild traumatic brain injury, clinically encountered most commonly in a setting of sports-related concussion, results in a chronic accumulation of subtle deficits [Collins et al., 1999; Matser et al., 1999]. Many of these recurrent sports concussions occur in the late childhood and adolescent age groups, developmental periods where demonstrable brain maturation continues to occur, particularly in the frontal lobes [Sowell et al., 1999, 2001]. Because of the unique nature of sports concussion, with its mild, repetitive character, often occurring in brains still undergoing maturation, these issues are discussed separately.

Acute Postconcussive Syndromes

Acute behavioral change commonly occurs after mild pediatric traumatic brain injury, including lethargy, irritability, disorientation, and listlessness. These symptoms can be worrisome for worsening intracranial injury, but in the presence of a normal CT scan, they must be attributed to an undetermined physiologic dysfunction. Spreading depression, seizure activity, changes in blood flow, and even migraine have all been proposed [Ryan and Edmonds, 1988; Sanford, 1988].

Vomiting is common following childhood head injury, occurring in up to 50% of individuals [Hugenholtz et al., 1987]. Some report that frequent vomiting is actually rare in more severe head injury but is characteristic of mild traumatic brain injury [Luerssen, 1991]. However, the presence of vomiting is nonspecific, and if it is persistent or worsening, a CT scan should be performed.

Acute post-traumatic migraine is predominantly a behavioral syndrome and is diagnosed only after more serious lesions have been ruled out [Haas and Lourie, 1988]. After a mild injury, with normal postinjury behavior, the child becomes progressively more agitated, aggressive, and combative. This behavior is followed by postictal tiredness and sleep, sometimes with no recollection of the earlier events upon awakening. Headache may occur but is not invariable. A prior history or family history of migraine is not uncommon.

Cortical blindness has also been reported after mild pediatric traumatic brain injury, in the absence of intracranial pathology [Kaye and Herskowitz, 1986; Yamamoto and Bart, 1988]. Pupillary responses are preserved, and malingering may be suspected. Complete recovery usually occurs. Migraine, spreading depression, or other neurovascular changes may be responsible.

Seizure activity also may occur immediately upon impact, with no subsequent clinical or neuroimaging abnormality. Sometimes termed *impact seizure* or *immediate post-traumatic seizure*, these are generally self-limited, with complete recovery within minutes. However, seizures can also occur in response to intracranial pathology and should always be evaluated carefully.

Sports Concussion and Repeated Concussion

Sports concussion is an increasingly common problem in childhood, occurring during team play in contact sports such as football and soccer, but also in basketball, wrestling, hockey, and other sports. Children also frequently experience mild traumatic brain injury with accidents involving bicycles, rollerblades, skateboards, and scooters. Because of its association with particular recreational activities, the occurrence of sports-related concussion is more predictable than other forms of head trauma. This situation provides the opportunity to better understand this injury type by premorbid testing of at-risk individuals and by instituting postinjury clinical assessments beginning immediately after the concussion and reassessing symptoms over the range of minutes to days. Another important opportunity is the possibility of more effective prevention strategies, by using approved protective gear when engaging in these activities and by avoiding return to at-risk sports activity until recovery from injury is complete.

Epidemiology

It is estimated that more than 300,000 sports-related head injuries occur annually in the United States, most of which are mild [Thurman et al., 1998]. In high school athletes, 5% to 6% of all injuries are head injuries, most occurring during football play, but almost every sport encounters some concussions [Guskiewicz et al., 2000; Powell and Barber-Foss, 1999]. Interestingly, after sustaining a concussion, there is a threefold risk for a subsequent concussion during the same sports season [Guskiewicz et al., 2000], possibly because of a concussion-induced physiologic vulnerability, a manifestation of a particularly risky style of play in certain individuals, or perhaps subtle coordination and reaction time impairments in concussed individuals, setting them up for repeated injuries when they return to practice or play before full recovery. Most sports concussions (91%) do not involve loss of consciousness, and headache is the most common complaint (86%). Perhaps because of the mild nature of these injuries, almost one third of these players returned to play the same day [Guskiewicz et al., 2000]. There is a common mentality among both players and coaches that one can "shake it off" and "take one for the team" that sets the stage for recurrent injuries.

Pathophysiology

Physiologic studies of sports concussion have demonstrated abnormalities in brain metabolism and activation in the absence of anatomic lesions (Fig. 62-11) [Bergsneider et al., 2000; McAllister et al., 1999]. Positron emission tomography of mildly injured young adults has demonstrated dramatic reductions in cerebral glucose metabolism in walking, talking players that resemble abnormalities seen in comatose patients [Bergsneider et al., 2000]. Experimental studies of diffuse concussive injury in immature rats suggest periods of reduced glucose metabolism lasting for 2 to 3 days [Thomas et al., 2000].

More recently, functional MRI has been used to study brain activation in mildly injured patients. Even while overall performance on particular cognitive tasks was acceptable, task-associated activation patterns seen in these patients were decidedly abnormal [McAllister et al., 1999]. A general theme of functional MRI testing in concussed patients is that task-specific activation patterns become less focused and more diffuse in the injured brain [Jantzen et al., 2004]. This has been interpreted as a compensatory strategy to bypass dysfunctional circuits by using less efficient alternative routes.

Symptomatology

Symptomatology in sports concussions is similar to that described regarding concussions in general. One consideration with subjective reporting of symptoms in a sports setting is that the player, being motivated to return to play, may attempt to minimize symptoms. Many athletic teams and physicians are using a concussion checklist to assess symptoms semiquantitatively [McCrea et al., 2003]. This can be administered before injury and repeated at intervals during the recovery period. There is also increasing use of computerized neuropsychologic tests that can be administered by an athletic trainer using a laptop, shortly after injury and again repeatedly during recovery. Interestingly, there is some evidence that recovery from sports concussion is prolonged in high school compared with college athletes [Field et al., 2003]. This raises legitimate concerns about blanket return-to-play guidelines and suggests that age-specific guidelines may be more appropriate.

Sequelae

Although the long-term significance of a single mild pediatric traumatic brain injury is uncertain, several large studies have demonstrated multiple neurocognitive deficits in athletes who experienced an accumulation of lifetime concussions. One study [Collins et al., 1999] reported impairments in executive functions and information processing speed in college football players who experienced two or

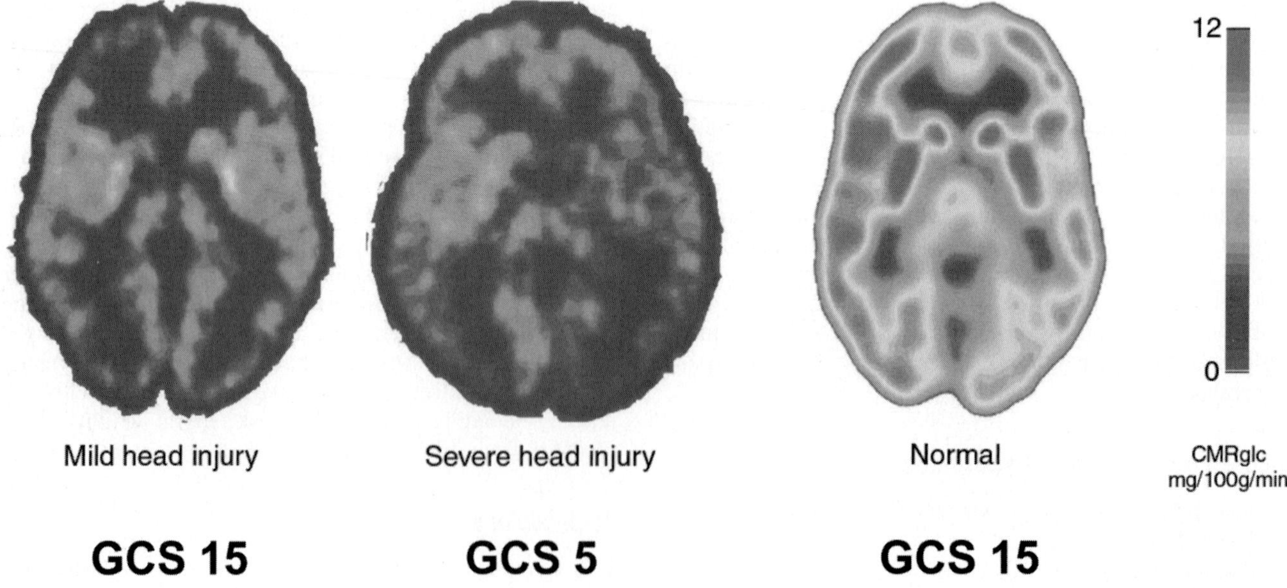

FIGURE 62-11. Reduced cerebral metabolism of glucose (CMRglc) is seen after mild or severe diffuse traumatic brain injury in human patients, suggesting a commonality in the underlying pathophysiology of different severities of traumatic injury. See also Color Plate. GCS, Glasgow Coma Scale. (From Bergsneider M, Hovda DA, Lee SM, et al. Dissociation of cerebral glucose metabolism and level of consciousness during the period of metabolic depression following human traumatic brain injury. J Neurotrauma 2000;17:389.)

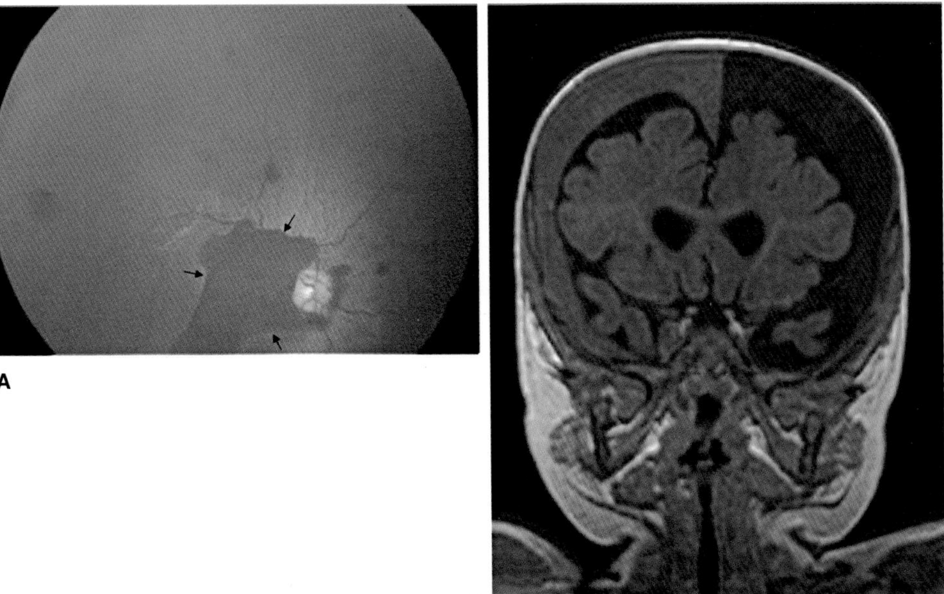

FIGURE 62-6. Signs suggestive of nonaccidental trauma. **A**, Retinal hemorrhage (*arrows*) on funduscopic examination. **B**, Bilateral subdural hematomas on T1-weighted MRI showing different signal intensities, indicating that the hemorrhages occurred at different times.

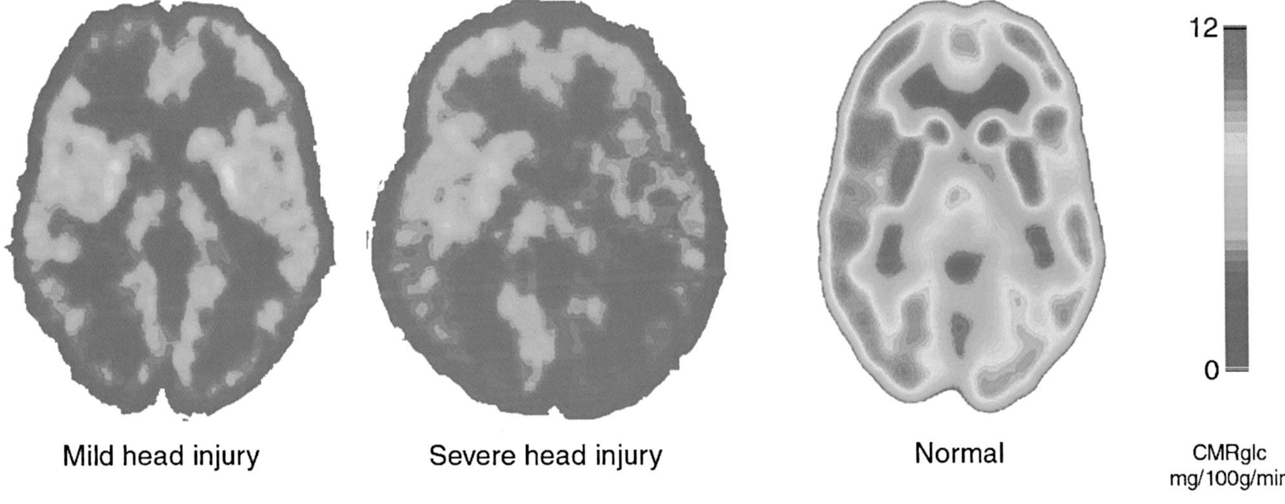

FIGURE 62-11. Reduced cerebral metabolism of glucose (CMRglc) is seen after mild or severe diffuse traumatic brain injury in human patients, suggesting a commonality in the underlying pathophysiology of different severities of traumatic injury. GCS, Glasgow Coma Scale. (From Bergsneider M, Hovda DA, Lee SM, et al. Dissociation of cerebral glucose metabolism and level of consciousness during the period of metabolic depression following human traumatic brain injury. J Neurotrauma 2000;17:389-401).

more lifetime concussions. Another study found similar neuropsychological deficits in amateur soccer players when compared with control athletes participating in noncontact sports [Matser et al., 1999]. Studies in adult rats have modeled this effect, demonstrating no significant deficit after a single mild injury, but definite impairment in spatial learning tasks after multiple repeated mild injuries [DeFord et al., 2002]. More recently, it was reported that the duration of symptoms and length of recovery from concussion was longer in patients with previous concussions [Bruce and Echemendia, 2004; Guskiewicz et al., 2003]. Further studies are needed to delineate the risk for chronic cognitive impairment and its relation to timing of injuries, number of injuries, and age at injury.

Second Impact Syndrome

Some controversy surrounds the existence of the so-called second impact syndrome [Cantu, 1998; McCrory and Berkovic, 1998]. In general, this term was invoked in circumstances in which a mild traumatic brain injury, often in a child or adolescent, resulted in catastrophic brain swelling (Fig. 62-12) and often death. On some occasions, an earlier head injury was reported, and it has been suggested that the initial injury somehow primed the brain for the dramatic and seemingly disproportionate response seen after the second injury [Kelly and Rosenberg, 1997]. A careful review of the literature raised concerns regarding poor documentation of a "first impact" in many cases [McCrory and Berkovic, 1998], and the terminology *malignant brain swelling* was proposed. Nonetheless, much of the effort to devise return-to-play guidelines is aimed at reducing the likelihood of this syndrome, as well as the chronic, apparently cumulative effects of repeated injuries.

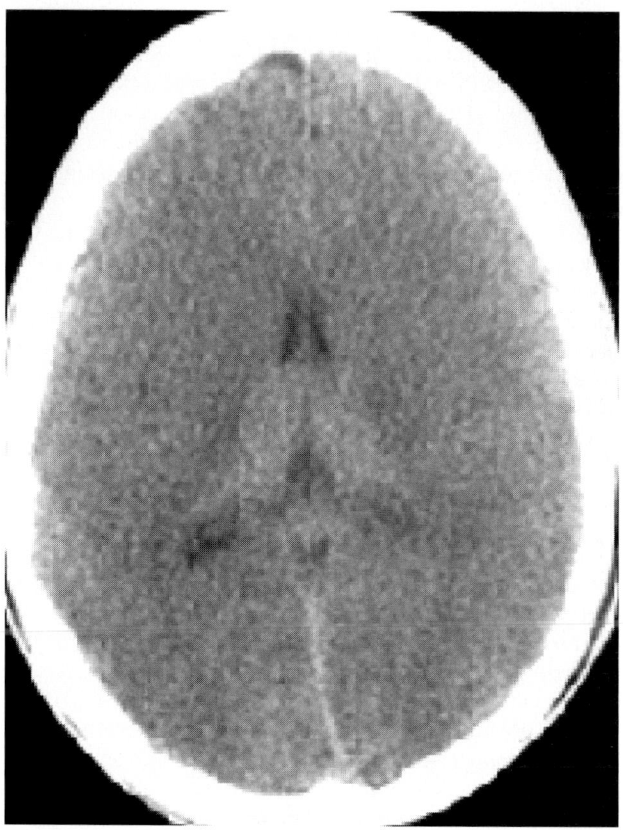

FIGURE 62-12. Diffuse cerebral edema on noncontrast head CT demonstrating sulcal effacement, constriction of lateral ventricles, and loss of gray-white distinction. When occurring after mild trauma, this clinical picture has been referred to as *second impact syndrome* or *malignant brain edema.*

Skull Fractures

Skull fractures are relatively common (20%) in the pediatric traumatic brain injury population, particularly in the youngest age groups. A main concern is their association with underlying intracranial damage such as hematomas, but fortunately, this relationship is not as strong in infants. That is, despite infants having more skull fractures than older children or adults, they are less likely to be associated with intracranial hemorrhage.

Linear fractures account for 66% to 75% of all pediatric skull fractures (Fig. 62-13). These are most commonly temporoparietal in location and can be associated with an overlying scalp injury. Although the fractures rarely require intervention, CT scanning should be performed to rule out underlying pathology.

Depressed skull fractures involve displacement of the bony skull and increase the risk for underlying cerebral contusion or laceration. In neonates, the "ping-pong" fracture is a type of depressed fracture wherein the softer infant skull is simply indented rather than broken. Scalp injuries can be a sign of an underlying depressed fracture, with pain, swelling, or contusion at the site of injury. Indications for surgical repair of depressed fractures vary, but repair is certainly indicated in patients with displaced bony fragments into brain parenchyma, dural tears, underlying large hematomas, associated focal neurologic deficits, seizures,

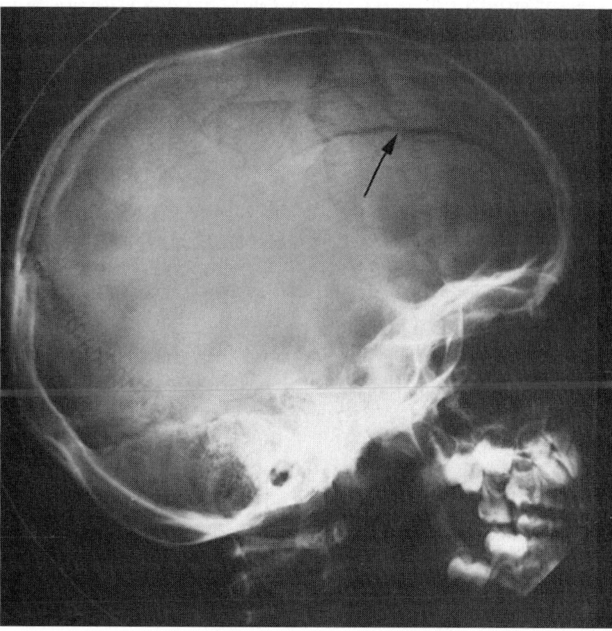

FIGURE 62-13. Lateral skull film of a 3-year-old child disclosing a linear fracture of the frontal bone (*arrow*) extending posteriorly and crossing the coronal suture. (From Rosman NP, Herskowitz J, Carter AP, et al. Pediatr Clin North Am 1979;26:707.)

and overt wound contamination. Depressions greater than 5 mm or in cosmetically unappealing locations have been considered relative indications. Surgical repair has not been shown to alter neurologic outcome or later risk for epilepsy [Braakman, 1972; Jennett et al., 1974; van den Heever and van der Merwe, 1989], presumably because any cerebral injury was likely sustained at the moment of impact.

Basal skull fractures tend to occur frontally or in the area of the petrous bone. Although these fractures can be seen on radiographs, a number of clinical signs are highly indicative of their presence. Periorbital or retroauricular ecchymosis (raccoon eyes or Battle's sign, respectively), rhinorrhea, otorrhea, and hemotympanum suggest fracture of the skull base. Traumatic cranial neuropathies are associated with these fractures, typically involving cranial nerves I, II, VII, or VIII. The presence of cerebrospinal fluid leakage (rhinorrhea or otorrhea) theoretically increases the risk for central nervous system (CNS) infection, although studies have reported conflicting results [Brown, 1990; Langley et al., 1993], and the prophylactic use of antibiotics in these patients is not universal [Einhorn and Mizrahi, 1978; Francel and Honeycutt, 2004]. Most cerebrospinal fluid leaks resolve spontaneously; however, a longer duration of the leak increases the risk for meningitis. Persistent leaks require cerebrospinal fluid diversion with a lumbar drain; if unsuccessful, surgical repair is indicated.

Compound or open skull fractures involve direct communication between the fracture and the outside environment through a scalp defect. There may be underlying brain injury, with swelling, hemorrhage, or edema that requires specific management. An open fracture represents a significant risk for infection, and surgical débridement, removal of foreign bodies, repair of any existing dural defects, and prophylactic antibiotics are indicated.

A diastatic suture represents a bony separation along suture lines. Although not necessitating acute intervention, these fractures do need to be followed to detect the development of a chronic "growing skull fracture" or leptomeningeal cyst.

Scalp Lacerations and Hematomas

Scalp injuries are one of the most common types of accidental injury in childhood. Swelling and bruising are common (sometimes referred to as a "goose egg"), even in minor head injuries in which risk for significant brain injury is minimal. Scalp lacerations, because of their propensity to bleed profusely, also tend to generate significant parental concern. Superficial injuries should be examined closely to determine whether there is any possibility of an underlying fracture. In particular, a detailed history of the accident and the child's behavior and neurologic examination after the accident should be assessed for signs and symptoms of concussion, even after a seemingly mild injury.

Treatment of scalp injuries includes proper cleansing, débridement, suturing of significant lacerations, and possibly prophylactic antibiotics. In infants, large scalp or subgaleal hematomas can sometimes result in anemia and volume loss, requiring fluid resuscitation or transfusion. It is not recommended to attempt to aspirate or drain scalp hematomas because this increases the risk for infection. Most scalp injuries resolve without significant complication.

DIAGNOSTIC EVALUATION

Neuroimaging

Neuroimaging is required for the diagnostic evaluation of children with traumatic brain injury. Although some studies have suggested that clinical variables are inconsistent in predicting the presence of intracranial pathology, certain variables warrant evaluation with neuroimaging.

Skull X-rays

Skull x-rays are still the most sensitive method to detect fractures. The presence of a skull fracture increases the likelihood of an underlying intracranial abnormality 21- to 80-fold [Quayle et al., 1997; Teasdale et al., 1990]. However, the absence of fracture on skull x-ray does not preclude intracranial pathology. The frequency of intracranial lesions discovered on CT in the absence of skull fracture on x-ray ranges from 16% to 39% [Levi et al., 1991; Lloyd et al., 1997], but these results are skewed toward more severe injuries because CT scans were obtained only in patients with "clinical indications" and in those admitted to the hospital. Of all pediatric traumatic brain injuries with CT scans positive for an intracranial lesion, 35% to 50% occurred in the absence of a skull fracture [Lloyd et al., 1997; Quayle et al., 1997; Teasdale et al., 1990]. Thus, in patients in whom underlying brain injury is already suspected, the value of screening skull radiography has been questioned [Bell and Loop, 1971; Lloyd et al., 1997].

Skull fracture does occur much more frequently in children younger than 1 or 2 years [Lloyd et al., 1997; Quayle et al., 1997; Schutzman et al., 2001] and is associated with intracranial hematomas, although less so than in older children. Nonetheless, identification of isolated skull fractures in infants is still important, with the implications of diagnosing nonaccidental trauma. Also, significant scalp injuries or hematomas may overlie a skull fracture. Skull x-rays may be warranted in evaluation of traumatic brain injury under the following circumstances: when there is a suspicion of nonaccidental trauma; in head-injured children younger than 1 or 2 years, particularly if there is scalp swelling or hematoma; or as a screening tool in older children only in areas where CT scanning is not readily available.

Computed Tomography

Noncontrast CT scanning is the neuroimaging examination of choice in the evaluation of acute head trauma. Many studies have been performed to determine clinical indications for CT after pediatric traumatic brain injury [Dunning et al., 2004; Halley et al., 2004; Homer and Kleinman, 1999; Murgio et al., 2001; Quayle et al., 1997]. Proper use of CT scanning depends on the severity of the injury sustained and the age of the child. The rationale behind use of CT is to identify intracranial complications, particularly those that would warrant urgent or emergent surgical or medical intervention to achieve optimal outcome.

In a large, prospective series of 653 children with traumatic brain injury of all severities admitted to a neurosurgical department, 34.6% demonstrated significant intracranial abnormalities [Levi et al., 1991]. Fractures were excluded, but nonsurgical pathologies such as diffuse axonal injury and contusions were included along with acute hematomas. When only acute hematomas were tabulated, 23.7% of severely injured children (Glasgow Coma Scale scores of 3 to 8) had a lesion, as compared with 12.4% of moderate (Glasgow Coma Scale scores of 9 to 12) and 5% of mild (Glasgow Coma Scale scores of 13 to 15) patients. A consecutive, prospective study of 322 children seen in an urban emergency department for "nontrivial" head injury reported an 8.3% rate of intracranial pathology. In this case, nontrivial was defined as head injury with symptoms or physical findings, except for superficial scalp injuries, that were deemed nontrivial only in infants younger than 12 months [Quayle et al., 1997]. Differences in these studies may be attributed to geographic area, inclusion criteria (neurosurgical admissions vs. emergency department visits), distribution of injury severity, and age range. In 10 studies published since 1990, each with more than 100 patients, the frequency of significant intracranial pathology in all pediatric traumatic brain injuries ranged from 1.3% [Chan et al., 1990; Teasdale et al., 1990] to 34.6% [Levi et al., 1991]. A recent meta-analysis of 16 published papers examining variables predictive of intracranial hemorrhage in pediatric traumatic brain injury reported that skull fracture was associated with a relative risk of 6.1 (i.e., the presence of a skull fracture carried a 6.1-fold increased risk for intracranial bleed) [Dunning et al., 2004]. Other variables that increased the risk for intracranial hemorrhage included focal neurologic deficits (relative risk, 9.4), Glasgow Coma Scale score less than 15 (relative risk, 5.5), and loss of consciousness (relative risk, 2.2). Seizure activity had a relative risk of 2.8 but, because of its variability between studies, did not reach statistical significance. Headache and vomiting were not predictive of Glasgow Coma Scale score. Given the high frequency of intracranial lesions in children with moderate or severe traumatic brain injury, cranial CT is warranted in patients with a Glasgow Coma Scale score of less than 13. Although the presence of risk factors listed previously should increase suspicion for an intracranial process, the absence of a factor does not mean that the risk for a lesion is reduced. Imaging recommendations are summarized in Tables 62-3 and 62-4.

Indications for CT are more controversial when only mild traumatic brain injury pediatric patients are considered. In this population, the true prevalence of intracranial injury is difficult to determine. Review of 12 studies published since 1986, each with more than 100 patients, showed that 0% [Immordino, 1986] to 19.1% [Wang et al., 2000] of mildly injured children have a significant CT abnormality. Davis and colleagues reported intracranial bleeding in 7% of 168 pediatric patients who suffered a loss of consciousness after mild traumatic brain injury; however, in a subset of 49 patients with normal neurologic examination, 0% had CT abnormalities [Davis et al., 1994]. Other studies have found less utility to clinical variables and normal neurologic examination in predicting the absence of intracranial problems in mildly injured children [Halley et al., 2004; Quayle et al., 1997]. A recent review of this question [Homer and Kleinman, 1999] concluded that only a small number of mildly injured children have significant intracranial damage but that clinical history and examination are relatively insensitive predictors of those who do. Intracranial lesions requiring surgical intervention do occur, although very rarely, even when neurologic examination is normal. The American Academy of Pediatrics consensus guideline for mild head injury states that CT imaging (in conjunction with observation) is a reasonable management option, but not required, in children older than 2 years who experience brief (less than 1 minute) loss of consciousness and have no abnormal physical or neurologic findings at the time of medical evaluation [American Academy of Pediatrics, 1999]. Currently, there are no definitive guidelines for children with mildly abnormal Glasgow Coma Scale (13 or 14) or normal Glasgow Coma Scale (15) scores with loss of consciousness for longer than 1 minute; careful observation in all children and liberal use of CT is recommended (see Table 62-3) [Dietrich et al., 1993; Halley et al., 2004; Savitsky and Votey, 2000].

Recommendations for CT scanning are even broader when children younger than 2 years are concerned. Skull fractures are more common, and abnormalities on neurologic examination may not be as easily detected as in older children [Berney et al., 1994; Dietrich et al., 1993]. A recent expert review of the literature has resulted in a proposed guideline for stratification of risk in head-injured infants

TABLE 62-3

Pediatric Traumatic Brain Injury (>2 years): Indications for Computed Tomography

Definite Indications

- Glasgow Coma Scale score <15 in emergency department
- Altered mental status
- Skull fracture (on x-ray or clinically)
- Focal neurologic signs
- Deteriorating neurologic condition
- Suspected nonaccidental trauma

Relative Indications

- Loss of consciousness or post-traumatic amnesia
- Seizure
- Known coagulopathy
- Need for anesthesia or prolonged sedation
- Persistent or worsening headache, nausea, or vomiting

TABLE 62-4

Pediatric Traumatic Brain Injury (<2 years): Indications for Computed Tomography

Definite Indications (High-Risk Patient)

- Altered mental status, irritability
- Focal neurologic signs
- Skull facture (on x-ray or clinically)
- Seizure
- Bulging fontanel
- Vomiting ≥5 times or >6 hours
- Loss of consciousness ≥1 minute
- Deteriorating neurologic condition
- Suspected nonaccidental trauma

Relative Indications (Intermediate-Risk Patient)

- Vomiting 3-4 times
- Loss of consciousness <1 minute
- Previous irritability or lethargy, now resolved
- Caregivers concerned about patient's current behavior
- High-energy mechanism of injury
- Scalp hematoma, especially if large or nonfrontal
- Known coagulopathy
- Need for anesthesia or prolonged sedation

younger than 2 years [Schutzman et al., 2001]. Indicators of high- and intermediate-risk stratification are presented in Table 62-4. In general, this algorithm recognizes that low-risk patients (low-energy mechanism of injury, no signs or symptoms, more than 2 hours since injury, and older than 12 months) may be discharged from the emergency department with-out CT scanning but with continued observation by reliable caretakers.

Magnetic Resonance Imaging

Although MRI is less able to visualize bony structures and fractures, it is better able to delineate structures in the posterior fossa and subacute hematomas that may appear isodense on CT. The ability of MRI to distinguish the approximate age of an intracranial hemorrhage makes it useful in patients with nonaccidental trauma (Table 62-5). Particular MRI sequences (i.e., T2-weighted gradient recall echoing and, more recently, susceptibility-weighted imaging) are especially good at detecting microhemorrhages that indicate foci of diffuse axonal injury [Tong et al., 2004] and that might not be seen on conventional CT. Magnetic resonance spectroscopy performed subacutely (within the first week) in patients with persistent coma has been highly accurate at predicting outcome [Ashwal et al., 2000, 2004a, 2004b; Holshouser et al., 2000].

Angiography

Angiography is useful to diagnose traumatic vascular lesions, particularly cavernous carotid fistulas and dissections of the great cervical arteries. In some cases, magnetic resonance angiography can substitute for conventional angiography.

Ultrasound

An open fontanel in younger infants provides a window for ultrasound examination. Although able to visualize more centrally located intracranial lesions, ultrasound is less sensitive in detecting epidural or subdural hematomas and is not generally used in an acute trauma setting.

TABLE 62-5

Distinguishing Age of Intracranial Hemorrhage on Magnetic Resonance Imaging

BLOOD COMPONENT	AGE	T1-WEIGHTED	T2-WEIGHTED
Oxyhemoglobin	4-6 hours (hyperacute)	Iso- or low intensity	High intensity
Deoxyhemoglobin and high protein	7-72 hours (acute)	Iso- or low intensity	Low intensity
Intracellular methemoglobin and high protein	4-7 days (subacute)	High intensity	Low intensity
Free methemoglobin and high protein	1-4 weeks (late subacute)	High intensity	High intensity with low intensity rim
Hemosiderin	Months to years (chronic)	Low intensity	Low intensity

Lumbar Puncture

Lumbar puncture in the setting of acute trauma holds the risk for precipitating herniation if cerebral edema is present and is absolutely contraindicated in the presence of a mass lesion. In a subacute or chronic setting after traumatic brain injury, lumbar puncture may be useful in diagnosing CNS infection due to a basilar skull fracture or neurosurgical complication.

Electrodiagnostic Testing

Electroencephalography (EEG) may help in the evaluation of the persistently comatose patient whose mental status is disproportionate to the documented injury. In some cases, subclinical seizures (i.e., nonconvulsive status epilepticus) may underlie prolonged unresponsiveness after traumatic brain injury [Vespa et al., 1999]. EEG and evoked potentials are more commonly used for prognostic pur-poses and are discussed with regard to this role later in this chapter.

GENERAL MANAGEMENT PRINCIPLES FOR SEVERE PEDIATRIC TRAUMATIC BRAIN INJURY

A recent expert review summarized the existing published literature regarding medical management of severe pediatric traumatic brain injury [Adelson et al., 2003b]. An evidence-based approach was used; however, the literature did not support any treatment standards. Only five recommendations achieved the level of treatment guidelines (i.e., clinical strategy or range of strategies that reflects moderate clinical certainty): (1) take children with traumatic brain injury preferentially to a pediatric trauma center; (2) avoid hypoxia—provide supplemental oxygen; (3) avoid hypotension— search for bodily injuries that may cause hypotension; (4) maintain cerebral perfusion pressure higher than 40 mm Hg; and (5) do not use antiepileptic drugs to prevent later development of post-traumatic epilepsy. However, multiple treatment options were provided, along with the rationale for their use. The following section summarizes the recommendations of this expert review and synthesizes them with traditional management strategies.

Stabilization and Prevention of Secondary Injury

Although it is clear that hypoxemia results in poorer outcome after traumatic brain injury [Ong et al., 1996; Pigula et al., 1993], studies aimed at prehospital endotracheal intubation for children have failed to prove any significant benefit in outcome [Cooper et al., 2001; Gausche et al., 2000]. After initial assessment and resuscitation, acute management is aimed primarily at avoiding or preventing secondary injuries until more definitive therapy can be instituted. Airway maintenance and provision of supplemental oxygen is crucial, and on arriving at the hospital or intensive care unit, intubation and ventilation are often necessary for the more severely injured child.

Fluid resuscitation to avoid hypotension is also essential [Luerssen et al., 1988; Pigula et al., 1993]. It is rare for pediatric head injury alone to cause systemic hypoperfusion;

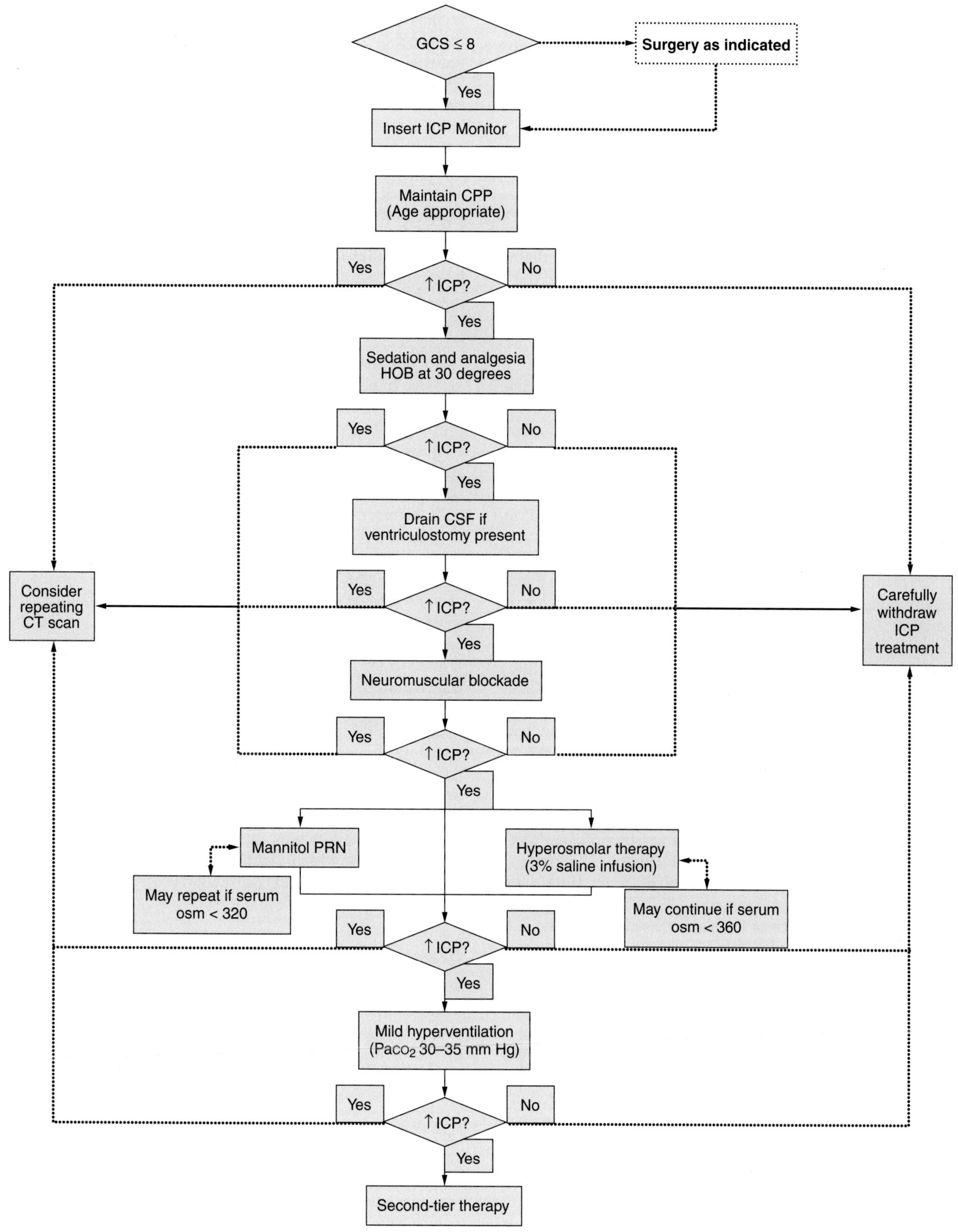

FIGURE 62-14. Algorithm for first-tier management of elevated intracranial pressure (ICP) in children after severe traumatic brain injury. CPP, cerebral perfusion pressure; CSF, cerebrospinal fluid; GCS, Glasgow Coma Scale; HOB, head of bed; ICP, intracranial pressure; OSM, osmolality; PRN, as necessary. (From Guidelines for the acute medical management of severe traumatic brain injury in infants, children, and adolescents. Pediatr Crit Care Med 2003;4[3]Supplement:S65-S67.)

an alternative cause should be sought and may include internal or external bleeding or spinal cord injury. Signs of hypoperfusion and shock include diminished pulses, prolonged capillary refill, tachycardia, and reduced urine output. Hypotension is a late sign in pediatric shock. Fluid restriction out of concern for exacerbation of cerebral edema is to be avoided in the shocky head-injured child; perfusion must be maintained.

First-Tier Intracranial Pressure Management

Intracranial pressure is determined by the brain, the cerebrospinal fluid, and blood. Management strategies targeting elevated intracranial pressure are based on the principle that to reduce intracranial pressure, the volume of one of these components must be reduced (Fig. 62-14).

Sedation and Neuromuscular Blockade

Sedatives and analgesics may be useful to reduce struggling and exacerbation of elevated intracranial pressure, promote optimal ventilation, alleviate pain, and allow for adequate nursing care (e.g., suctioning, catheter placement). A theoretical benefit of sedatives is to minimize increases in cerebral metabolic activity provoked by pain or stress. In addition, some sedatives possess antiepileptic or antiemetic properties. A potential adverse effect of sedation is hypotension, which can exacerbate poor cerebral perfusion if not addressed promptly. A recent expert literature review found insufficient evidence to recommend a specific choice of sedative medications in the setting of pediatric traumatic brain injury [Adelson et al., 2003d]. Sedatives with published reports of use in pediatric traumatic brain injury include fentanyl, morphine, sufentanil, remifentanil, diazepam, ketamine, propofol, etomidate, and barbiturates. However, most of these reports were small series, often with mixed adult and adolescent patients. There is anecdotal evidence of intracranial pressure reduction with remifentanil [Tipps et al., 2000], ketamine [Albanese et al., 1997], propofol [Farling et al., 1989; Spitzfaden et al., 1999], and barbiturates. The use of a continuous propofol infusion in children has been associated with a lethal syndrome of metabolic acidosis [Bray, 1998; Canivet et al., 1994; Cray et al., 1998; Hanna and Ramundo, 1998; Parke et al., 1992] and has not been approved for pediatric sedation by the U.S. Food and Drug Administration.

Neuromuscular blockade may aid in the management of traumatic brain injury patients by promoting ease of ventilation, reducing intracranial pressure, and stopping metabolic demands from skeletal muscle. Complications of neuromuscular blockade include an increased risk for pneumonia, cardiovascular depression, immobilization stress (if used with inadequate sedation), unnoticed seizure activity, and prolonged paralysis or myopathy. Myopathy appears to be associated with the combination of nondepolarizing agents and corticosteroids [Martin et al., 2001; Rudis et al., 1996]. When using iatrogenic paralysis, it is important to periodically monitor the depth of blockade using a "train of four" stimulation. Vecuronium, pancuronium, and doxacurium have all been used for pediatric neuromuscular blockade in the setting of traumatic brain injury.

Hyperventilation

Hyperventilation reduces blood and tissue Pco_2, resulting in vasoconstriction, decreased cerebral blood volume, and reduced intracranial pressure. These effects can be seen within minutes, making hyperventilation an important tool in managing acute neurologic deterioration or impending herniation due to edema.

Excessive hyperventilation in adults [Kiening et al., 1997; von Helden et al., 1993] and children [Skippen et al., 1997] can result in reductions in cerebral blood flow that may reach ischemic levels. The routine use of prophylactic hyperventilation (Pco_2 less than 35 mg Hg) in severe pediatric traumatic brain injury is no longer recommended.

Controlled hyperventilation (Pco_2, 30 to 35 mg Hg) may be useful to control elevated intracranial pressure that is refractory to sedation, neuromuscular blockade, cerebrospinal fluid drainage, and hyperosmolar therapy. More aggressive hyperventilation (Pco_2 less than 30 mg Hg) should be considered a second-tier therapy for intractable increased intracranial pressure. The risk for potential ischemic complications must be considered and the patient monitored appropriately for these problems. Jugular venous oxygen saturation measurements should be made through a jugular bulb catheter. This methodology provides a more global measure of cerebral tissue perfusion and can be monitored frequently as the patient's condition and treatment change. Alternative methods of determining whether ischemia is present include cerebral blood flow studies and brain tissue oxygen monitoring. Cerebral blood flow studies have the advantage of providing some regional data but are usually limited to the actual time of the testing. Brain tissue oxygen levels can be monitored continuously but are limited to measurements in the vicinity of the probe.

Despite the potential for hyperventilation to induce ischemia, hyperventilation remains a potent modulator of intracranial pressure. In the setting of acute deterioration or imminent herniation, aggressive hyperventilation may still be used for short periods of time. With the advantage of fast onset of action, hyperventilation may provide a window during which diagnostic testing can be completed and additional first-tier intracranial pressure measures optimized.

Hyperosmolar Therapy

Two agents have been recommended for hyperosmolar therapy in pediatric traumatic brain injury: mannitol and 3% saline. Hyperosmolar therapy raises the solute concentration of the serum, creating an osmotic gradient whereby free water is drawn out from the brain's extracellular space.

MANNITOL

Mannitol, an agent whose clinical use for intracranial pressure management has become almost ubiquitous, appears clearly effective in many older studies of adults [James, 1980b; Marshall et al., 1978; McGraw et al., 1978; Mendelow et al., 1985; Muizelaar et al., 1984; Schwartz et al., 1984], as well as studies including both children and adults [Nara et al., 1998; Rosner et al., 1995; Smith et al.,

1986]. Unfortunately, the pediatric component of the mixed studies was not separately defined.

Mannitol exerts its beneficial effects through several mechanisms. First, it reduces blood viscosity, improving blood flow and allowing for a reduction in cerebral blood volume [Levin et al., 1979; Muizelaar et al., 1983, 1986]. Second is the osmotic effect, drawing free water out of the brain (across an intact blood-brain barrier) and back into the bloodstream [James, 1980a]. A less well understood effect of mannitol is its ability to act as an antioxidant [Kontos and Hess, 1983]. Mannitol is administered with bolus dosing at 0.25 to 1.5 g/kg up to every 4 hours. Overall, mannitol begins to exert its intracranial pressure–reducing effects within 10 to 20 minutes, and these effects can last for several hours. In the presence of a leaky or damaged blood-brain barrier, mannitol can potentially enter the injured area and cause a rebound osmotic effect [Kaieda et al., 1989; McManus and Soriano, 1998]. Partially for this reason, bolus rather than continuous administration of mannitol is recommended.

HYPERTONIC SALINE

Hypertonic saline (3%) has been more recently investigated [Peterson et al., 2000], and several studies used prospective data collection specifically in pediatric patients to document the effectiveness of this agent in controlling refractory intracranial pressure [Khanna et al., 2000; Simma et al., 1998], yet this therapy lacks widespread clinical experience.

Hypertonic saline operates through several mechanisms. It reduces blood viscosity, osmotically draws free water from brain parenchyma, restores cell membrane potential and volume [McManus and Soriano, 1998; Nakayama et al., 1985], reduces inflammation [Qureshi and Suarez, 2000], and improves cardiovascular function. The effectiveness of hypertonic saline in pediatric patients has been demonstrated in several studies [Khanna et al., 2000; Peterson et al., 2000; Simma et al., 1998]. Despite reducing intracranial pressure, none of these studies investigated whether hypertonic saline therapy resulted in better outcomes. Dosing of hypertonic (3%) saline was on a sliding scale titrated to intracranial pressure, and serum sodium and infusion rates ranged from 0.1 to 1.0 mL/kg/hour.

Potential adverse effects of 3% saline include osmotic rebound, central pontine myelinolysis, and subarachnoid hemorrhage. For the four published pediatric 3% saline studies described, higher serum osmolalities were well tolerated (mean, 365 mOsm/L; highest, 431 mOsm/L), and none of the potential complications occurred.

With either hyperosmolar therapy, euvolemia is the goal, although serum osmolality is generally kept below 320 mOsm when using mannitol. Other osmotic agents used to treat brain edema have been less thoroughly evaluated, including urea and glycerol. Although older management schemes attempted to reduce brain edema by systemic dehydration using diuretics, this strategy is no longer supported. Hyperosmolar therapy is effective in controlling elevations in intracranial pressure, although the effects on improving cerebral perfusion pressure are not as well demonstrated. The particular agent used (mannitol or hypertonic saline) is a decision left to the treating physician.

Intracranial Pressure Monitoring: Indications and Treatment Threshold

Outcome from pediatric and adult traumatic brain injury depends on avoiding secondary insults such as ischemia and hypoperfusion [Chesnut et al., 1993a; Narayan et al., 1981]. Elevated intracranial pressure can lead to global hypoperfusion and precipitate herniation, which can cause tissue ischemia through compression and, in some situations, by impinging on cerebral arteries. Many of the specific therapies for severe traumatic brain injury are directed at preventing excessive intracranial pressure; thus, it logically follows that monitoring of intracranial pressure is an important component of traumatic brain injury management [Becker et al., 1977; Marshall et al., 1979; Narayan et al., 1982]. Although there has been no randomized clinical trial specifically validating the benefits of intracranial pressure monitoring in children, many studies have demonstrated benefits of aggressive management of elevated intracranial pressure in head-injured children [Bruce et al., 1981; Cho et al., 1995; Peterson et al., 2000; Taylor et al., 2001].

There are several commonly used intracranial pressure monitors. The mechanisms of these monitors may be divided into three distinct types. First are monitors that measure intracranial pressure through an external pressure transducer. These include ventricular catheters as well as subdural and subarachnoid catheters or bolts that measure pressure by maintaining a continuous fluid connection with the intracranial space. They are accurate and can be recalibrated, but erroneous readings can result from obstruction of the connecting line or from inconsistent placement of the external transducer in relation to the patient's head. The second type of monitor is a pressure transducer that is located at the tip of an inserted catheter. These monitors are not dependent on maintaining a long, continuous fluid connection between an external gauge and the intracranial space; however, once placed, they cannot be readily recalibrated. The third type of monitor is a fiberoptic sensor placed at the catheter tip. It has restrictions similar to the catheter-tip–mounted transducers.

A pediatric study comparing Camino fiberoptic catheters with ventricular catheters found sufficient correlation, although there were slight differences between the measured intracranial pressure from the two devices, depending on the patient's Glasgow Coma Scale score [Gambardella et al., 1993]. Several studies addressing these questions are available from the adult literature and summarized in published guidelines for traumatic brain injury management in adults [Brain Trauma Foundation et al., 2000]. A ventricular catheter with an external sensor is considered the simplest and most reliable means of measuring intracranial pressure and has the added benefit of allowing therapeutic removal of cerebrospinal fluid. Catheter-tip–mounted devices (pressure transducers or fiberoptic) are more expensive but similarly accurate when placed within the ventricular catheter. Catheter-tip devices used for intraparenchymal placement may experience measurement drift. External transducers coupled to subarachnoid, epidural, or subdural devices were thought to be less reliable; these modalities may be useful when ventricular access is problematic.

Intracranial pressure monitoring is an invasive procedure that requires a burr hole at a minimum, although suture lines or an open fontanel may be used in infants and neonates. It is important to have standard indications for children who are at greatest risk for elevated intracranial pressure following traumatic brain injury and who would be most likely to benefit from monitoring. In one series, 19 of 22 (86%) children with a Glasgow Coma Scale score of 8 or less (i.e., severely injured) who received intracranial pressure monitoring had intracranial pressure values greater than 20 mm Hg [Shapiro and Marmarou, 1982]. In a large series of 654 severely injured patients from the National Traumatic Coma Data Bank, 72% had intracranial pressure greater than 20 mm Hg during the course of their monitoring [Marmarou et al., 1991].

These studies suggest that clinical determination of severe injury (Glasgow Coma Scale score of 8 or less) delineates a group of patients at high risk for elevated intracranial pressure. Certainly, examination of less severely injured patients can provide greater sensitivity in determining clinical deterioration. This may be the situation in young children and infants, in whom the clinical examination and Glasgow Coma Scale score are less reliable than in older children or adults [Humphreys et al., 1990; Shapiro and Marmarou, 1982]. Using CT findings to predict elevated intracranial pressure is also questionable in children because they are less likely than adults to present with mass lesions. Despite the presence of open fontanels and flexible sutures, infants can still develop elevated intracranial pressure [Cho et al., 1995]. Given this information, intracranial pressure monitoring is recommended in children with a Glasgow Coma Scale score of 8 or less. In addition, intracranial pressure monitoring may be reasonable in selected patients with moderate traumatic brain injury, particularly those whose clinical examination may be clouded by concomitant sedation, paralysis, or anesthesia. Intracranial pressure monitoring also can be beneficial in infants, particularly those with severe injuries due to nonaccidental trauma.

Normative values for intracranial pressure are generally thought to be lower in children, but the consequences of exceeding particular intracranial pressure levels have only been incompletely examined (see Chapter 65). Several retrospective studies in children have shown poorer outcomes with intracranial pressure elevations above 20 mm Hg [Esparza et al., 1985; Pfenninger et al., 1983] or 30 mm Hg [Cho et al., 1995]. Other studies have indicated cerebral compliance and cerebral blood flow to be inversely proportional to intracranial pressure [Shapiro and Marmarou, 1982; Sharples et al., 1995]. It is recommended to institute intracranial pressure–lowering therapy in pediatric patients whose intracranial pressure exceeds 20 mm Hg [Adelson et al., 2003c].

Complication rates for fiberoptic monitoring in 98 children have been reported, with 7% of catheters becoming colonized (all with *Staphylococcus aureus*; average duration of catheter placement more than 7 days) and 13% having mechanical failure (on average by 9.5 days) [Jensen et al., 1997]. Complication rates were significantly different for catheters placed in the emergency department or intensive care unit. No pediatric reports of significant brain injury, hemorrhage, or seizures due to an intracranial pressure monitor placement or use were found, suggesting a very low rate of these complications.

Cerebral Perfusion Pressure

Cerebral perfusion pressure is defined as the difference between the mean arterial pressure and intracranial pressure. Reduced cerebral perfusion pressure can occur during hypotension, intracranial hypertension, or both. Retrospective pediatric studies have found a strong correlation between cerebral perfusion pressure of less than 40 mm Hg and death [Downard et al., 2000; Elias-Jones et al., 1992]. One study of 118 children with intracranial pressure monitors placed within 24 hours of traumatic brain injury found that none of the children with a mean cerebral perfusion pressure of less than 40 mm Hg survived (0 of 22) [Downard et al., 2000]. When outcome was assessed in comparison with cerebral perfusion pressure decile (e.g., 40 to 50 mm Hg, 50 to 60 mm Hg), no further relation was found. Mean cerebral perfusion pressure of less than 40 mm Hg was interpreted as a limit of survivability in severe pediatric traumatic brain injury.

Although low cerebral perfusion pressure is associated with poor outcome in children and adults, the benefits of cerebral perfusion pressure–directed therapy are uncertain. In adults, cerebral perfusion pressure of greater than 80 mm Hg was associated with better outcome in two large, retrospective studies [Changaris et al., 1987; McGraw, 1989]. Another study reported improved neurologic outcome at 6 months in patients managed for cerebral perfusion pressure and cerebral oxygen extraction (using jugular venous oxygen saturation monitoring) [Cruz, 1998]. However, a large randomized trial of 189 adults comparing cerebral perfusion pressure–directed therapy with intracranial pressure–directed therapy failed to demonstrate an outcome benefit of the former and also reported an increased risk for adult respiratory distress syndrome in the cerebral perfusion pressure group [Robertson et al., 1999].

Because systemic blood pressure varies by age, it is reasonable to assume that optimal cerebral perfusion pressure is age dependent. Based on the available evidence, maintaining cerebral perfusion pressure above 40 mm Hg at all times in pediatric traumatic brain injury patients is recommended, and the range of cerebral perfusion pressure from 40 to 65 mm Hg most likely represents a spectrum of optimal pressures across the pediatric age range. Use of vasopressors may be associated with an increased risk for pulmonary complications. Further studies are necessary to delineate optimal age-specific cerebral perfusion pressure ranges.

Cerebrospinal Fluid Drainage

Physical drainage of cerebrospinal fluid is the most direct means of reducing intracranial pressure and has been done through intraventricular or lumbar catheters. In most studies, it is difficult to separate cerebrospinal fluid drainage from other first- and second-tier means of intracranial pressure reduction. One report prospectively divided adult patients into medical management only or medical management with ventriculostomy groups after removal of surgical lesions [Ghajar et al., 1993]. The group without intracranial pressure monitoring had a fourfold higher mortality rate (53% vs. 12%), and a lower rate of independent living (20% vs. 59%).

In children, the risk for sudden increases in intracranial pressure was assessed using the pressure-volume index technique [Shapiro and Marmarou, 1982]. This method relied on the fact that brain compliance does not change linearly as fluid volume is added to the intracranial space. As the threshold for brain compliance was neared, addition of even small volumes of fluid resulted in dramatic increases in intracranial pressure. Reduced pressure-volume index (less than 80% of predicted normal) accurately predicts intracranial hypertension. All these patients were managed with cerebrospinal fluid drainage, which was found to reduce intracranial pressure and increase pressure-volume index. Cerebrospinal fluid drainage is a reasonable treatment option to reduce elevated intracranial pressure in children.

Second-Tier Intracranial Pressure Management

When elevated intracranial pressure is refractory to first-tier interventions, more intensive therapies are often instituted. These "second-tier" strategies involve methods to reduce brain metabolism and activity (e.g., barbiturates, hypothermia) or physical opening of the intracranial space to relieve pressure (craniectomy) (Fig. 62-15). In addition, more aggressive hyperventilation, in the setting of perfusion monitoring to avoid ischemia, remains an option, as does lumbar cerebrospinal fluid drainage, provided a ventriculostomy is in place and basal cisterns are open. Second-tier therapies are generally less proven or have an increased risk for potential side effects. Despite their apparent efficacy in spinal cord injury, corticosteroids have been associated with

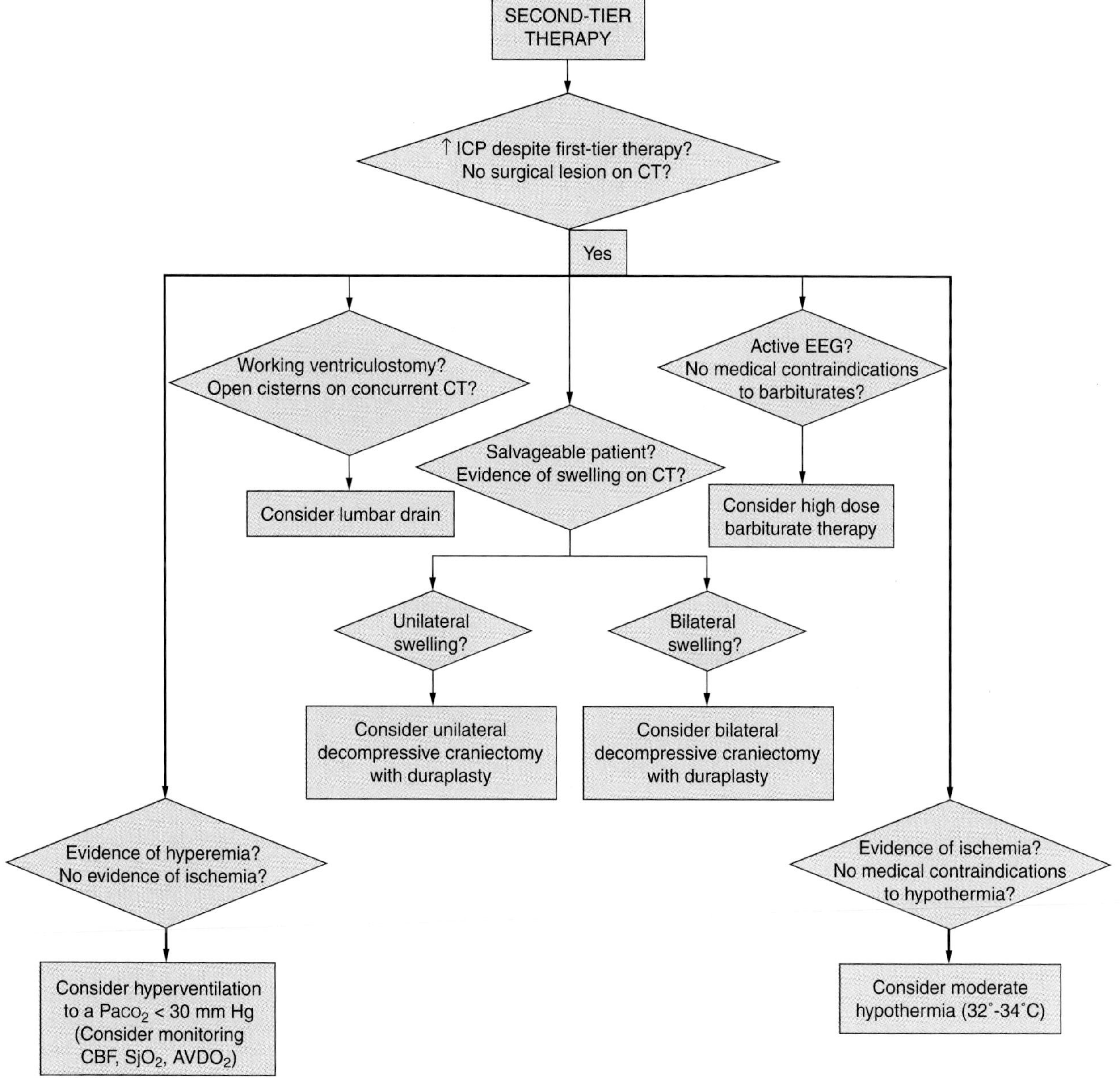

FIGURE 62-15. Algorithm for second-tier management of elevated intracranial pressure (ICP) in children following severe traumatic brain injury. CBF, cerebral blood flow; EEG, electroencephalogram.(From Guidelines for the acute medical management of severe traumatic brain injury in infants, children, and adolescents. Pediatr Crit Care Med 2003;4[3]Supplement:S65-S67.)

increased mortality in a very large, international multicenter, randomized, placebo-controlled trial of severe traumatic brain injury and are not recommended [Roberts et al., 2004].

Barbiturates

Barbiturate coma has benefit in cases of intractable intracranial pressure elevation by several potential mechanisms. Barbiturates suppress cerebral metabolism [Piatt and Schiff, 1984] and can reduce cerebral blood flow and volume, perhaps by reducing cerebral metabolic activity [Kassell et al., 1980]. Barbiturates also reduce markers of free radical–induced damage in neonates with perinatal asphyxia [Singh et al., 2004].

Evidence for the efficacy of barbiturates in refractory intracranial hypertension comes primarily from a study that included patients 15 to 50 years of age [Eisenberg et al., 1988]. In this study, intracranial pressure control was achieved in 32% of the barbiturate group, which was about twice the response rate in the conventional treatment group. The 1-month survival rate was 92% in barbiturate responders compared with 17% in nonresponders.

The use of barbiturates in children with traumatic brain injury has been described in several case series. Kasoff and associates reported cardiovascular complications and a high rate of requiring pressor support (91%) but did not mention whether there was any effect on cerebral hemodynamics or intracranial pressure [Kasoff et al., 1988]. In a different series of children with refractory intracranial pressure, addition of pentobarbital therapy achieved intracranial pressure control (less than 20 mm Hg) in 52% [Pittman et al., 1989]. Dosing of pentobarbital is best titrated to burst suppression on EEG rather than serum levels; thus, continuous EEG monitoring should be used. Intravenous loading doses of pentobarbital range from 5 to 15 mg/kg, followed by either slow continuous infusion at 1 mg/kg/hour or 5-mg/kg intermittent doses every 4 to 6 hours.

The major complications of barbiturate therapy are myocardial depression and hypotension. Infants are perhaps particularly prone to these adverse effects. There is also some experimental evidence in neonatal rat pup models that even brief blockade of synaptic activity with barbiturates can result in a significant increases in neuronal apoptosis [Bittigau et al., 2002; Ikonomidou et al., 1999; Olney et al., 2002; Pohl et al., 1999].

Use of barbiturates is an option in patients with intractable elevation of intracranial pressure. Proper EEG and cardiovascular monitoring should be used at all times. The use of barbiturate coma in traumatically injured neonates and infants should be approached with caution.

Temperature Control and Hypothermia

Temperature control can be thought of as avoidance of hyperthermia or institution of hypothermia. There is substantial experimental and adult clinical literature suggesting that hyperthermia can exacerbate brain injury by increasing metabolism, triggering seizures, elevating levels of excitotoxins, promoting inflammation, and so forth [Busto et al., 1989; Dietrich et al., 1996; Ginsberg and Busto, 1998; Wass et al., 1995]. It is recommended that fever or hyperthermia be avoided in brain-injured children.

Since the original report of hypothermia used to treat traumatic brain injury in children [Hendrick, 1959], interest in reducing temperature therapeutically has waxed and waned. Hypothermia can substantially reduce cerebral activity and has been anecdotally associated with neurologic preservation after prolonged drowning [Young et al., 1980]. In adults, several single-center studies suggested either physiologic benefits (improved cerebral perfusion pressure, reduced intracranial pressure) or trends toward better neurologic outcomes [Clifton et al., 1993; Marion et al., 1993, 1997; Shiozaki et al., 1993]. However, a more recent multicenter hypothermia trial that excluded children younger than 16 years failed to find efficacy in improving outcome [Clifton et al., 2001]. There was a trend toward better outcomes in patients who were hypothermic at presentation and in younger patients. A multicenter hypothermia trial in children is currently in progress [Adelson et al., 2005].

Surgical Management of Intracranial Pressure

Decompressive craniectomy has been used to "open the box" and relieve pressure in cases of intractable intracranial hypertension and cerebral edema. This procedure has been reported to lower intracranial pressure on average 9 to 47 mm Hg in children and adolescents [Cho et al., 1995; Polin et al., 1997; Ruf et al., 2003; Taylor et al., 2001].

One study divided 23 pediatric victims of nonaccidental trauma into a surgical group (with intracranial pressure greater than 30 mm Hg) and two medical groups (intracranial pressure greater than 30 mm Hg and less than 30 mm Hg). Children in the surgical group and the medical group with less severe intracranial pressure elevation had significantly better outcome than the medically managed patients with intracranial pressure greater than 30 mm Hg [Cho et al., 1995].

A prospective study compared 14 children with best medical management with ventricular drainage with 13 children treated with decompressive craniectomy with best medical management [Taylor et al., 2001]. Mean intracranial pressure was reduced 9 mm Hg postoperatively in the latter group, and over a 48-hour period, there were fewer episodes of intracranial pressure higher than 30 mm Hg (9 vs. 59), fewer episodes of intracranial pressure higher than 20 mm Hg (107 vs. 223), and a narrower range of intracranial pressure (11 to 25 mm Hg vs. 11 to 44 mm Hg). The surgically managed patients also tended toward a better Glasgow Outcome Scale score, although follow-up times were not standardized, and mild pre-existing cognitive impairments were identified in 2 of the medically managed patients. Other studies reporting outcome after decompressive craniectomy were case series without a control or medical-only group.

The most commonly used surgical approach for decompressive craniectomy is a combination of bilateral craniectomy and expansion duraplasty [Cho et al., 1995; Dam et al., 1996; Guerra et al., 1999; Polin et al., 1997]. The studies reported previously had another feature in common: surgery was undertaken less than 48 hours after injury. Expert review of the literature suggested that severely injured children with intractably elevated intracranial pressure who were more likely to benefit from decompressive craniectomy could be selected on the basis of meeting at least some of the criteria listed in Table 62-6. In clinical practice, unilateral craniec-

TABLE 62-6

Criteria Suggestive of Potential Benefit of Decompressive Craniectomy

1. Diffuse cerebral swelling on cranial CT
2. Within 48 hours of injury
3. No episodes of sustained intracranial pressure > 40 mm Hg before surgery
4. Glasgow Coma Scale score >3 at some point after injury
5. Secondary clinical deterioration
6. Evolving cerebral herniation syndrome

tomy has been performed ipsilateral to the hemisphere with greater edema or a surgical lesion, although there are fewer published studies using this procedure.

Early Post-traumatic Seizures and Seizure Prophylaxis

Seizures are not infrequent after traumatic brain injury. Acutely, seizures may result from stretch-induced depolarization of neurons, post-traumatic glutamate release, toxic effects of blood products, focal necrotic damage due to contusion or skull fracture, compression of neurons secondary to mass effect or cerebral edema, infection secondary to penetrating injury or skull fracture, or hypoxia-ischemia. Chronic changes after traumatic brain injury can also result in recurrent seizures. Mechanisms of post-traumatic epilepsy or seizures include neuronal death, gliosis or scarring, toxic effects of blood breakdown products, compression of neurons secondary to chronic mass lesions or post-traumatic hydrocephalus, aberrant axonal sprouting, and loss of inhibitory neurotransmission. Typically, post-traumatic seizures are divided into early and late types. Early post-traumatic seizures occur within the first week after injury and are generally reactive seizures in response to some acute or subacute insult. Late post-traumatic seizures occur after the first 7 days. They may be reactive to some subacute process, such as post-traumatic hydrocephalus; delayed infection secondary to skull fracture, cerebrospinal fluid leak, or neurosurgical complication; delayed hemorrhage or mass effect; fever; or electrolyte or metabolic disturbance. However, the main concern with late post-traumatic seizures is the development of post-traumatic epilepsy (recurrent unprovoked seizures). This development may be due to neuron death, gliosis, or scarring (e.g., mesial temporal sclerosis), development of recurrent excitatory neuronal pathways (sprouting, kindling), and loss of inhibitory γ-aminobutyric acid interneurons. In rare circumstances, neonatal head trauma has been found to result in abnormal neuronal migration, with generation of dysplastic cortical regions [Lombroso, 2000; Marin-Padilla et al., 2002].

Acute Antiepileptic Therapy

Children, particularly infants, are more prone to seizures than adults [Annegers et al., 1980; Kollevold, 1976]. Early after traumatic brain injury, an acute seizure may act as a secondary injury, increasing cerebral metabolic demand, depleting neuronal energy reserves, causing release of excitotoxins, inducing hypoxia by impairing respiration or because of aspiration, or, particularly in generalized tonic-clonic seizures, increasing body temperature and raising intracranial pressure. The incidence of early post-traumatic seizures is higher in children than in adults, and, after severe pediatric traumatic brain injury, early seizure rates of 20% to 39% have been reported [Annegers et al., 1980; Lewis et al., 1993; Ratan et al., 1999]. This risk is increased with lower Glasgow Coma Scale scores and younger age [Hahn et al., 1988a, 1988b; Hendrick and Harris, 1968; Lewis et al., 1993; Ratan et al., 1999]. Most early post-traumatic seizures in children occur within the first 24 hours.

In adults, prophylactic phenytoin and carbamazepine reduce the risk for early post-traumatic seizures [Chang et al., 2003; Glotzner et al., 1983; Temkin et al., 1990]. In children, one study determined early seizure prophylaxis based on caregiver preference [Lewis et al., 1993]. Fifty-three percent of untreated children and only 15% of treated children experienced early seizures. A larger pediatric study retrospectively described 128 severely injured children (of a total of 477) and compared treatment differences between centers. Use of prophylactic antiepileptic drugs for early seizures ranged from 10% to 35%, and the overall risk for an early post-traumatic seizure in the entire cohort was 9%. However, the risk for early seizure by treatment group or severity group was not reported. It was reported that the group treated for early seizures had an improved survival rate [Tilford et al., 2001].

Given the apparent effectiveness of prophylaxis against early post-traumatic seizure in adults, the potential risk for complications from an early seizure, the increased risk for early seizure in children, and the frequent difficulty in identifying clinical seizure activity in infants and very young children, early prophylaxis for post-traumatic seizure activity in children should be considered. Fosphenytoin can be administered intravenously more rapidly and has fewer infusion-related side effects than phenytoin. Loading doses of either drug range from 10 to 20 mg/kg, and maintenance doses are typically 5 to 7 mg/kg/day divided at least twice a day (in the case of fosphenytoin, 1 mg = 1 PE, or phenytoin equivalent). For acute seizures occurring before early prophylaxis can be initiated, or breaking through prophylaxis, intravenous bolus doses of lorazepam, 0.05 to 1.0 mg/kg/dose, may be administered until the level of fosphenytoin becomes therapeutic.

Prevention of Post-traumatic Epilepsy

Despite the effectiveness of early prevention, several prospective, randomized adult studies have revealed the inability of antiepileptic prophylaxis to prevent subsequent development of late post-traumatic epilepsy [Temkin et al., 1990; Young et al., 1983]. Given the potentially different mechanisms underlying the genesis of early and late post-traumatic epilepsy, this finding is not entirely surprising.

In a trial of antiepileptic prophylaxis for late post-traumatic epilepsy, 41 children were randomized in a double-blind placebo-controlled study [Young et al., 1983]. Phenytoin or placebo was administered; those with phenytoin sensitivity were treated with phenobarbital. Patients were then followed for 18 months, and 12% of the treated group had a late post-traumatic seizure, compared with 6% of the untreated group (not significant). Importantly, compliance with treatment was poor. Therapeutic levels were present in only 50% of treated patients at 3 months' follow-up, and by 1 year, only 10% were therapeutic.

Given the available data for adult and pediatric late posttraumatic epilepsy, antiepileptic prophylaxis cannot be recommended [Chang et al., 2003]. After the acute period, antiepileptic drugs can be gradually weaned. If a late posttraumatic seizure occurs, it should be evaluated and treated as a new-onset seizure [Adelson et al., 2003f].

Supportive Care

Management of severe traumatic brain injury includes general supportive measures to prevent complications of intensive care unit hospitalization and potentially prolonged immobilization. Aspiration precautions should be maintained, including nasogastric tube placement acutely (orogastric placement in the case of frontobasal skull fractures). Particular care should be taken shortly after a recovering patient is extubated. Meticulous skin care is necessary to prevent breakdown, decubiti, and potential infection in sedated or paralyzed critically ill children and in recovering but debilitated children after severe traumatic brain injury. Consideration should be given to prophylaxis against deep venous thromboembolism, although anticoagulants should be used cautiously if at all in a setting of acute or chronic intracranial hemorrhage. Children with hypothalamic, brainstem, or spinal cord injury are at risk for autonomic instability and should be carefully monitored and treated as needed. Pain is a common problem after traumatic injury, including head pain and bodily pain due to musculoskeletal injury. Although analgesia should not be withheld, care must be taken not to overly sedate patients when neurologic examination is necessary to observe for signs of deterioration (e.g., a more moderately injured patient without an intracranial pressure monitor). At the least, sedation and analgesia may be lightened once daily to allow for clinical assessment of mental status (see Chapter 93). Nutritional status must not be neglected. Although enteral feedings are preferred, total parenteral nutrition should be provided in individuals in whom the gastrointestinal tract is nonfunctioning. Because of the catabolic state after severe injury, nutritional calculations should attempt to provide 130% to 160% of resting metabolic needs [Adelson et al., 2003a]. Psychosocial support is also necessary for the patient and family as the patient begins to recover from injury. Children in whom nonaccidental trauma is suspected should be reported to social services for full investigation.

GENERAL MANAGEMENT OF MILD TRAUMATIC BRAIN INJURY AND CONCUSSION

Two management guidelines for children with mild traumatic brain injury and concussion have been published. The first guideline represents expert consensus guidelines developed by the American Academy of Pediatrics for the evaluation and management of the mildly head-injured child [American Academy of Pediatrics, 1999]. The second parameter was developed specifically for sports-related concussion by the American Academy of Neurology [American Academy of Neurology, 1997]. It is important to realize that the sports concussion guidelines did not specifically take into account potential age-dependent differences in symptoms or recovery.

All children with head injuries who present for medical evaluation, even those with mild traumatic brain injury or concussion, should undergo a careful history and a physical and neurologic examination. As part of this assessment, the physician should determine whether the description of the injury is consistent with the objective findings (if any) and whether the child's caregivers are capable of home observation (e.g., sufficiently educated, seemingly reliable, not intoxicated). None of these guidelines are intended for children with multiple traumatic injuries, unobserved loss of consciousness, or spinal cord injury. Other considerations that exceed the breadth of these guidelines include children with bleeding diatheses (including chronic anticoagulation) or neurologic disorders that may be worsened by traumatic brain injury (e.g., arteriovenous malformations, shunts, possibly even arachnoid cysts) and those suspected of being victims of nonaccidental trauma. In the setting of a language barrier without a reliable translator (not including the child!), these guidelines should not apply.

Mild Traumatic Brain Injury without Loss of Consciousness in Children Older than 2 Years

For children older than 2 years without loss of consciousness and in whom the physical and neurologic examination reveals no worrisome findings, careful observation is the appropriate management [American Academy of Pediatrics, 1999; Homer and Kleinman, 1999]. Neuroimaging is not generally recommended because the likelihood of a significant intracranial abnormality is exceedingly small. Observation of the child may take place in the clinic, emergency department, or home under the supervision of a competent caregiver. Observation should continue for at least 24 hours.

Signs and symptoms to be monitored include deteriorating mental status, seizure, focal neurologic signs, worsening headache, and nausea and vomiting. Postinjury instructions should be verbally explained to caregivers, who should also be provided with written instructions and a means of returning for medical care should deterioration occur.

Mild Traumatic Brain Injury with Brief Loss of Consciousness in Children Older than 2 Years

Brief loss of consciousness is defined as less than 1 minute. For children older than 2 years, the previous guidelines are applicable. The only exception is that observation alone and observation in conjunction with CT scanning are both considered acceptable strategies. The risk for an intracranial abnormality on CT remains very low in this group (reported rates range from 0% to 7% depending on the study). Clinical signs are of uncertain significance in predicting the presence of intracranial pathology. In these children (with brief loss of consciousness), the likelihood of an abnormality requiring neurosurgical intervention may be in the range of 2% to 5%. However, these percentages are likely to be overestimates owing to selection bias—most of these studies examined patients seen in emergency departments or trauma centers. Population-based studies have estimated the prevalence of a lesion requiring neurosurgical intervention after mild traumatic brain injury to be as low as 0.02%.

This management algorithm does not require immediate neuroimaging of affected children. A period of observation may be implemented first. Although clinical signs such as headache, nausea, and vomiting are probably more common in children with intracranial injury, they are not sensitive, and most children with these symptoms do not have an intracranial lesion. There are children with documented normal neurologic examination who eventually require neurosurgical intervention. Rather than obtaining a CT scan in every patient immediately, a reasonable strategy is to evaluate and observe the patient. Neuroimaging can be reserved for those with worsening symptoms and those who do not improve. If neuroimaging is warranted, CT scanning is the examination of choice (see Table 62-3). If CT scanning is not available, skull radiographs may provide useful information for triaging and assessing the risk for intracranial hemorrhage and the need for CT. If the CT scan and examination are normal, the likelihood of clinically significant late deterioration is very low, so that children in this category could be discharged home under parental observation.

Mild Traumatic Brain Injury in Children Younger than 2 Years

Because clinical assessment of the very young head-injured child can be difficult and the risk for skull fracture is particularly high in infants, special consideration needs to be given for evaluation of mild traumatic brain injury in a child younger than 2 years [Schutzman et al., 2001]. In this age group, more emphasis may be placed on the need to obtain neuroimaging depending on assessment of risk (see Table 62-4). The lowest risk group before 2 years of age includes children with low-energy mechanisms of injury (e.g., short falls) and no signs or symptoms, who have been observed for more than 2 hours.

Intermediate risk is ascribed to those infants with a more forceful mechanism of injury, repeated nausea and vomiting (three or four instances), loss of consciousness for less than 1 minute, prior history of irritability or lethargy resolved at time of evaluation, unwitnessed trauma, significant scalp hematoma, nonacute skull fracture, and parental concern about patient's behavior. Intermediate-risk infants may undergo observation or CT imaging. Following either plan, and presuming that no problems are identified, infants who meet the following criteria may be discharged home (with continued observation): (1) the patient has no significant extracranial injuries or other clinical indications (e.g., repeated vomiting), (2) the patient is easily awake and alert and with normal neurologic examination, (3) there is no suspicion of abuse or neglect, and (4) the patient lives nearby with reliable parents who can observe the child and who are ready to return if necessary.

Patients identified as high risk have one or more of the following clinical characteristics: altered mental status, focal neurologic findings, depressed or basilar skull fracture (on x-ray or just clinical signs), seizure, excessive irritability, acute skull fracture, bulging fontanel, vomiting five times or more or for more than 6 hours, and loss of consciousness for 1 minute or longer. These patients should undergo noncontrast CT scanning.

Guidelines for Return to Play after Sports Concussion

Concussion severity is determined by a simple scale [American Academy of Neurology, 1997] from grades 1 to 3 (Table 62-7). Grade 1 concussion refers to injuries for which the duration of neurologic signs or symptoms is less than 15 minutes and no loss of consciousness occurs. Grade 2 is when signs or symptoms last longer than 15 minutes. Grade 3 is used for traumatic closed head injuries with any loss of consciousness.

Return to play guidelines, based primarily on expert consensus, are listed in Table 62-8. Briefly, the athlete must be symptom free at rest and with exertion; then, the designated amount of time must elapse before the individual is cleared for return to play. The duration of time off is dependent on the "severity" of the concussion (grades 1 to 3) and whether the player has sustained more than one concussion. Remember that longer symptom duration has been linked to younger patients [Field et al., 2003] and patients with multiple concussions [Guskiewicz et al., 2003]. Be aware that these studies were published after the original guidelines were made and suggest that modifications may be necessary to adequately reflect these particular clinical scenarios. More recent sports concussion guidelines have moved toward some standardized type of premorbid cognitive testing, with return to play being determined by

TABLE 62-7

Concussion Grading Scale

Grade 1`
Transient confusion
No loss of consciousness
Symptoms or signs last <15 minutes

Grade 2
Transient confusion
No loss of consciousness
Symptoms or signs last > 15 minutes

Grade 3
Any loss of consciousness

TABLE 62-8

Return to Play Guidelines

	TIME UNTIL RETURN TO PLAY*	
CONCUSSION GRADE	**Single**	**Multiple**
1	Same day	1 week
2	1 week	2 weeks
3—Brief loss of consciousness (seconds)	1 week	≥1 month
3—Long loss of consciousness (minutes)	2 weeks	≥1 month

*Only if asymptomatic and normal neurologic examination at rest and with exercise.

resolution of symptoms and return to baseline for each individual [McCrory et al., 2005]. However, maturational differences in cognitive function in children still limit extrapolation of these strategies for those younger than 15 years [McCrory et al., 2004].

PROGNOSIS AND OUTCOME

Determining outcome after pediatric traumatic brain injury remains difficult. Despite the overall better prognosis seen in children compared with adults, there are certain characteristics worth considering during the first few days when discussing outcome with the child's parents.

Clinical Predictors of Outcome

It is important to define what is meant by outcome in assessment of the recovering traumatic brain injury patient (see Chapter 61). The most common measure of outcome from traumatic brain injury is the Glasgow Outcome Scale, which divides patients into five categories: (1) dead, (2) persistent vegetative state, (3) severe disability (conscious but disabled and dependent on others), (4) moderate disability (disabled but independent for daily activities), and (5) good recovery (back to normal). This scale was later expanded to the modified Glasgow Outcome Scale, which divided levels 3 to 5 into higher and lower levels of disability [Jennett et al., 1981]. Others report outcomes based on elaborate batteries of neuropsychologic tests. A recent review of pediatric outcome scales gives some idea of the range of potential measures currently available [Okada et al., 2003].

Demographics: Age and Gender

One of the strongest predictors of outcome after traumatic brain injury is age. Younger age has been associated with improved outcome in large series of traumatic brain injury patients. However, within the pediatric age group, younger is not always better. With regard to mortality, infants younger than 4 years had a 1-year mortality rate of 62%, as compared with only 22% in children ages 5 to 10 years, and 48% in adults [Levin et al., 1992]. Similar results were reported by other investigators [Luerssen et al., 1988]. More recently, the percentage of fatal traumatic brain injury outcome was calculated to be only 7.5% in the 0 to 4 and 5 to 9 year age groups, increasing significantly to a peak of 17.1% in 15- to 19-year-olds [Centers for Disease Control and Prevention, 2000]. Population-based death rates for traumatic brain injury suggest a nadir in the 5- to 9-year age group (about 4 per 100,000), with slight increases in younger children (8 per 100,000) and dramatic increases in adolescence (15 to 19 years, about 40 to 50 per 100,000) [Thurman, 2001].

This general reduction in mortality among pediatric head-injured patients has also been reported from an Israeli pediatric neurosurgical center and has been attributed to improved prehospital care and dedicated pediatric intensive care [Levi et al., 1998]. Overall, children 14 years old or younger admitted with traumatic brain injury had a 33% mortality rate from 1984 to 1988. This mortality was reduced to 10% during the years 1994 to 1996.

Gender plays a role in mortality rate, with males having higher mortality at all ages, although this gap is substantially greater in the 15- to 19-year age bracket (males, 40 to 50 per 100,000 vs. females, 10 per 100,000). Much of this difference can be attributed to the higher use of firearms in males [Thurman, 2001]. The issue of whether gender plays a role in outcome from traumatic brain injury is less clear, and no firm conclusions can yet be drawn.

Injury Characteristics

Injury severity as assessed by the Glasgow Coma Scale is one of the strongest predictors of mortality and outcome. In 1998, among severely injured children, a fairly strong correlation was reported between mortality and Glasgow Coma Scale score. For Glasgow Coma Scale score values of 3, 4, 5, 6, 7, and 8, mortality rates were, respectively, 100%, 47%, 22%, 14%, 7%, and 0% [Levi et al., 1998]. A similar relation was recently reported in adults [Jiang et al., 2002]. Earlier, a prospective study of 653 children with traumatic brain injury found poor outcome in 56% of those with a Glasgow Coma Scale score of 3 to 8; 3.3% of those with a score of 9 to 12, and 0% of those with a score of 13 to 15 [Levi et al., 1991]. Initial Glasgow Coma Scale score has also been correlated with cerebral blood flow and gross outcome [Sharples et al., 1995], as well as with more comprehensive neurobehavioral measurements [McDonald et al., 1994]. However, some limitations of Glasgow Coma Scale on predicting outcome have also been reported [Ong et al., 1996], with good outcomes remaining a possibility even in some pediatric patients with Glasgow Coma Scale scores of 3 to 5 [Lieh-Lai et al., 1992].

Another powerful predictor of poor outcome, generally independent of age, is the presence of secondary injuries. Secondary injuries associated with poorer outcome include hypotension [Chesnut et al., 1993a, 1993b; Jiang et al., 2002], hypoxemia [Chesnut et al., 1993a; Jiang et al., 2002; Ong et al., 1996], and possibly even hyperthermia [Jiang et al., 2002].

Physiologic Measurements

INTRACRANIAL PRESSURE

Elevations of intracranial pressure higher than 20 to 30 mm Hg have been associated with poorer outcomes in children [Cho et al., 1995; Esparza et al., 1985; Shapiro and Marmarou, 1982; Sharples et al., 1995] and adults [Miller et al., 1977]. This result is primarily because high intracranial pressure is associated with poor cerebral perfusion and inadequate substrate delivery to injured brain. It is generally accepted that intracranial pressure higher than 20 mm Hg deserves therapeutic intervention.

CEREBRAL BLOOD FLOW AND CEREBRAL PERFUSION PRESSURE

Because of the close relationship between intracranial pressure and cerebral blood flow with actual tissue perfusion and subsequent neurologic outcome, cerebral perfusion pressure has been studied with regard to predicting outcome from traumatic brain injury. In 54 adults, patients with higher cerebral blood flow on postinjury days 1 to 5 had improved outcome at 6 months by Glasgow Outcome Scale assessment and that the group with the higher average cerebral blood flow could be further divided into patients with good and poor outcomes [Kelly et al., 1997]. Patients with high cerebral blood flow and poor outcome were discovered to have severe intracranial hypertension, and this elevated intracranial pressure failed to respond to metabolic suppressive measures. It was also shown that in the presence of preserved neurovascular coupling, increased cerebral blood flow was associated with better outcome; however, when vasoreactivity was impaired, higher cerebral blood flow resulted in intractable elevations of intracranial pressure and worse outcome. Several other investigators have studied autoregulation in head-injured adults and arrived at similar conclusions [Czosnyka et al., 1996, 2000; Lam et al., 1997].

A recent study of moderately to severe pediatric traumatic brain injury found a similar relation between impaired autoregulation, hyperemia, and poor outcome [Vavilala et al., 2004]. In 36 children younger than 15 years of age, transcranial Doppler was used to measure middle cerebral artery blood velocity. Cerebral autoregulation was calculated by using the autoregulatory index, defined as the percentage change in estimated cerebrovascular resistance per percentage change in mean arterial pressure or cerebral perfusion pressure (depending on whether the patient had an intracranial pressure monitor in place). The rate of impaired autoregulation was 42% in the moderately and severely injured groups but only 17% in those more mildly injured. Hyperemia as measured by transcranial Doppler was more common in the group with impaired autoregulation and was associated with poor outcome (Glasgow Outcome Scale score of less than 4). These studies indicate the dynamic nature of blood flow changes after traumatic brain injury and how repeated assessment of cerebral perfusion can provide useful information for optimal management.

Neuroimaging and Prognosis

Computed Tomography

Several CT features have been associated with poorer short-term outcomes and mortality among head-injured children. In the Traumatic Coma Data Bank series, diffuse cerebral swelling on CT (with or without shift) and mass lesion were associated with the highest mortality rates (25% to 52.2%). The poor outcomes with these CT findings were attributed to a longer duration of time with elevated intracranial pressure. Diffuse swelling also occurred in patients with the highest rates of severe functional outcome (17.4% to 22.2%), although a high percentage (20%) of the children with diffuse axonal injury also had a severe disability [Levin et al., 1992]. These results concur with other pediatric studies that also report poorer outcome with diffuse swelling or mass lesions with shift [Bruce et al., 1978; Ong et al., 1996; Tomberg et al., 1996]. The presence of post-traumatic subarachnoid blood has also been associated with poorer outcomes in two pediatric studies [Ong et al., 1996; Pillai et al., 2001].

Structural Magnetic Resonance Imaging

Traditionally, T2-weighted gradient echo sequences have been used to visualize small hemorrhagic lesions associated with diffuse axonal injury. Using a new susceptibility-weighted imaging protocol, a recent study demonstrated a strong correlation between the number and volume of susceptibility-weighted imaging–detected hemorrhagic lesions with low initial Glasgow Coma Scale scores or coma lasting more than 4 days [Tong et al., 2004]. At 6 to 12 months' follow-up, normal or mildly disabled children had significantly fewer lesions and lower lesion volume than those in the moderate to severely disabled group. This new sequence is apparently more accurate and sensitive for detecting small hemorrhagic lesions that had a strong association with eventual outcome [Tong et al., 2003].

A study of MRI confirmed the previously reported association of diffuse cerebral edema (seen on CT) with poor outcome, at least in infants. None of 15 infants (0%) with a good outcome but 5 of 11 infants (45%) with poor outcome demonstrated diffuse edema in this series [Ashwal et al., 2000].

Magnetic Resonance Spectroscopy

Magnetic resonance spectroscopy is a method of identifying particular brain metabolites based on regional spectral patterns. When analyzing a voxel located over uninjured-appearing occipital gray matter, reduced *N*-acetylaspartate-to-creatine and *N*-acetylaspartate-to-choline ratios were associated with poorer clinical outcomes. *N*-acetylaspartate-to-creatine ratio was predictive in children and infants, whereas *N*-acetylaspartate-to-choline ratio was predictive in infants and neonates. In addition, a lactate peak was seen in a larger proportion of children with poor outcomes [Holshouser et al., 1997, 2000]. In another study from the same group, high choline-to-creatine ratios were also associated with poor outcome, as were reduced *N*-acetylaspartate-to-creatine ratios, reduced *N*-acetylaspartate-to-choline ratios, and again, the presence of lactate [Ashwal et al., 2000]. In fact, none of the patients with good outcome had a lactate peak (Fig. 62-16).

In a recent follow-up study [Brenner et al., 2003], early clinical predictors (EEG, Glasgow Coma Scale) and magnetic resonance spectroscopy predictors (*N*-acetylaspartate-to-choline ratios in infants; choline-to-creatine ratios in children; lactate in both) were compared with neuropsychologic test scores, including full-scale intelligence quotient, attention and executive function, language, sensorimotor skills, visuospatial function, and memory. Increased choline-to-creatine ratio and the presence of lactate were significantly associated with children scoring in the below-average range for each of the neuropsychologic variables tested. A decreased *N*-acetylaspartate-to-choline ratio was also associated with below-average performance on language, sensorimotor, and memory testing.

Another spectroscopy metabolite, myoinositol, has also been found to be elevated in the occipital gray matter of children with traumatic brain injury compared with controls, and was higher in those with poor outcomes than those with good neurologic outcomes [Ashwal et al., 2004a]. It was hypothesized that myoinositol, found primarily in astrocytes, was perhaps a marker for gliosis in the injured brains. Elevated levels of glutamate/glutamine have also been detected by magnetic resonance spectroscopy after pediatric traumatic brain injury and appear to be correlated with worse outcomes [Ashwal et al., 2004b]. Recent studies have also shown that a normal-appearing brain may have abnormalities detected by

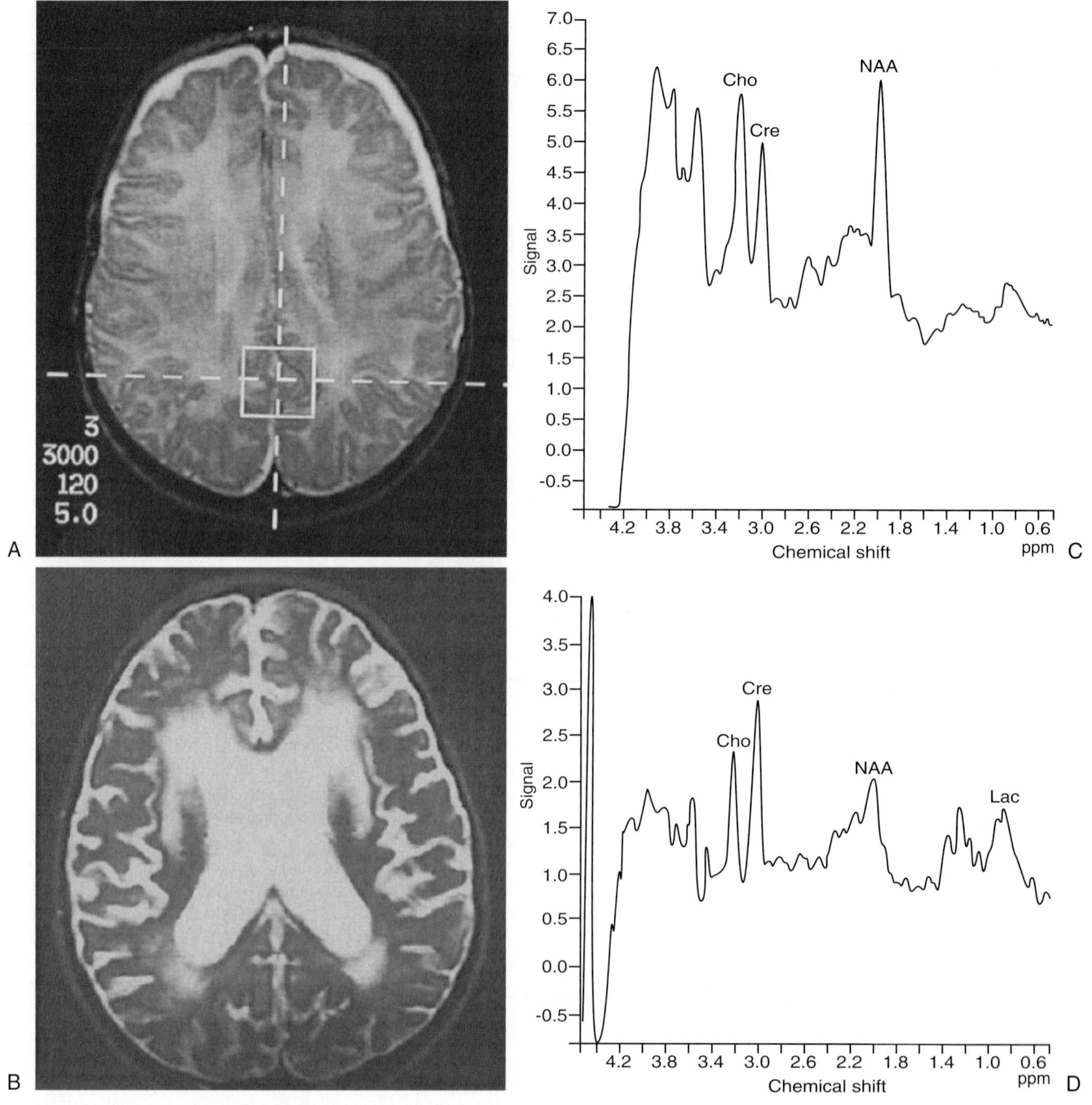

FIGURE 62-16. Examples of children after traumatic brain injury with good or bad outcomes. Anatomic MRI images (**A**, patient with good outcome; **B**, patient with poor outcome) and magnetic resonance spectroscopy (**C**, patient with good outcome; **D**, patient with poor outcome) are shown. Note the relative reduction of the *N*-acetylaspartate (NAA) peak and the presence of a lactate peak in the patient with the poor outcome. Cho, choline; Cre, creatine; Lac, lactate. (From Ashwal S, Holshouser BA, Shu SK, et al. Predictive value of proton magnetic resonance spectroscopy in pediatric closed head injury. Pediatr Neurol 2000;23:119–120.)

susceptiblity weight imaging or spectroscopy that correlate with outcomes [Holshouser et al., 2005].

Electrodiagnostic Testing and Prognosis

Electroencephalography

EEG has been loosely correlated with neurologic outcome after pediatric traumatic brain injury. Using a rating system that stratified EEG results into four categories (normal and mildly, moderately, or severely abnormal), one study reported a 73% positive predictive value for the dichotomous variable of good/moderate versus poor outcome [Ashwal et al., 2000]. It was also reported in additional studies that there was a correlation between the average EEG category score and neuropsychologic test results for full-scale intelligence quotient, attention and executive function, and memory [Brenner et al., 2003]. One caveat against using EEG to prognosticate in traumatic brain injury patients is that EEG should only be used if the patient is not sedated or anesthetized.

Somatosensory-Evoked Potentials

Median nerve somatosensory-evoked potentials have been used to help prognosticate in coma of many etiologies. A recent review and combined analysis of 41 published studies divided study patients into four groups [Robinson et al., 2003]. One group was adults and adolescents with traumatic brain injury; another group was adolescents and children with coma of any etiology (but most were traumatic brain injury). Outcomes were divided into not awakened (dead or vegetative) and awakened (severe, moderate, or no disability). In the adult and teenager traumatic brain injury group, 5% of patients with bilaterally absent somatosensory-evoked potentials eventually regained consciousness (confidence interval, 2% to 7%), as compared with 82% (confidence interval, 79% to 85%) of those with any somatosensory-evoked potential. Of the 5% who regained consciousness after having no somatosensory-evoked potentials, only 3 of 11 had better than severe disability (about 1% of total tested patients). In the child and teenager coma group, 7% of those with bilaterally absent somatosensory-evoked potentials eventually regained consciousness (confidence interval, 4% to 10%), in contrast to 80% (confidence interval, 76% to 84%) of those with any somatosensory-evoked potential. Of those 7% who awoke after absent somatosensory-evoked potentials, 10 of 16 had moderate or good recovery (4.5% of the total tested patients in this group). The authors concluded that somatosensory-evoked potentials were very good at predicting outcome from various types of coma, but that after traumatic brain injury, a small percentage of patients with absent somatosensory-evoked potentials did eventually awaken, and that after pediatric traumatic brain injury, a fairly significant number (7%) of patients with absent bilateral somatosensory-evoked potentials would eventually awaken, and more than half (4.5%) could go on to a decent recovery.

It was considered important that somatosensory-evoked potentials done within the first 24 hours after injury be interpreted with caution or repeated after the first day. There was a tendency for a few patients who had absent somatosensory-evoked potentials to eventually awaken. Somatosensory-evoked potentials, although highly sensitive, were not recommended to be used alone to determine ultimate prognosis [Beca et al., 1995; Carter et al., 1999; Robinson et al., 2003].

LATE CLINICAL SYNDROMES

Vegetative and Minimally Conscious States

After severe traumatic brain injury, children may emerge from coma into a vegetative state (see Chapter 61). This condition is characterized by the eyes being open with intact sleep-wake cycles but with no self-awareness and no purposeful movement. In the Glasgow Outcome Scale, it is given its own level (score of 2) and is generally combined with severe disability (score of 3) to describe a poor outcome. In the Traumatic Coma Data Bank series, the percentage of patients in a vegetative state at the time of discharge was relatively constant in all age groups (12% to 15% in the 0- to 4-, 5- to 10-, and 11- to 15-year and adult age ranges) [Levin et al., 1992]. However, the proportion of patients in a vegetative state declined over time in all age ranges, so that by 6 months after injury, less than 5% of any age range was classified in this category. By 1 year, the number of patients in a vegetative state declined still further, such that only about 2% of the adult group was described as having a Glasgow Outcome Scale score of 2. This percentage could have been due to death of these patients, but it is apparent that some patients in a vegetative state slowly recover and may regain self-awareness. Although patients in a vegetative state as a result of a hypoxic event are designated in a permanent vegetative state if there is no improvement by 3 months, a vegetative state secondary to traumatic brain injury is not considered "permanent" until 12 months because prolonged recoveries occur more often after traumatic brain injury. These findings are reviewed in the document prepared by the Multi-Society Task Force on Persistent Vegetative State [1994].

More recently, specific diagnostic criteria have been proposed for a distinct state of consciousness, termed the *minimally conscious state* [Giacino et al., 2002]. This is distinguished from the vegetative state by the presence of self-awareness and some limited purposeful movements, as well as the potential to experience pain and suffering, and is reviewed in Chapter 61 [Ashwal, 2003]. However, this designation has been questioned by some [Burke, 2002; Shewmon, 2002].

In a long-term follow-up of children 3 to 15 years old in a vegetative state or minimally conscious state, Strauss and colleagues [2000] found that survival in the minimally conscious state group was determined more by the degree of mobility than the level of consciousness. Mobility was defined as the ability for spontaneous or induced movements of the extremities or trunk, specifically the ability to raise one's head when prone, roll either front to back or vice versa, or sit for 5 minutes. Over 8 years of follow-up, vegetative state and immobile minimally conscious state patients had similar survival rates (63% and 65%, respectively), whereas significantly more of the mobile minimally conscious state children survived (81%) [Strauss et al., 2000]. Understanding the natural course of these states of chronically impaired consciousness is crucial to provide families with realistic expectations of outcome after severe brain injury, as well as to allow for the possibility of recovery over time.

Cognitive Impairment and Behavioral Disorders

Cognitive and behavioral impairments are some of the more debilitating sequelae of childhood traumatic brain injury and also some of the more difficult to quantify, particularly when subtle impairments follow milder injuries or when such disabilities are diagnosed years after a more severe traumatic brain injury. Nonetheless, deficits in many cognitive domains have been demonstrated after moderate-to-severe traumatic brain injury in children, including impaired executive function [Ewing-Cobbs et al., 2004], language

[Levin, 2003], memory [Levin et al., 1982, 1988, 2002], and visual-motor integration [Yeates et al., 2002]. Tests of intelligence quotient [Fay et al., 1994; Jaffe et al., 1995; Levin et al., 1982], adaptive function [Taylor et al., 2002], and academic achievement [Ewing-Cobbs et al., 1998; Taylor et al., 2002] reveal post-traumatic brain injury deficiencies. When evaluated over time, several studies demonstrate that most post-traumatic brain injury cognitive and academic recovery occurs within the first year, and the rate of improvement diminishes significantly after that [Ewing-Cobbs et al., 1998; Jaffe et al., 1995; Yeates et al., 2002]. Lower socioeconomic status has also been associated with poorer outcomes from pediatric traumatic brain injury in multiple studies [Hawley et al., 2004; Taylor et al., 2002].

Several studies suggest that the age at which the injury occurs can affect cognitive outcome and later academic performance [Ewing-Cobbs et al., 1998; Levin et al., 1982, 1988]. It has been proposed that cognitive skills under development at a particular stage of maturation are more vulnerable to injury at that age. There is some evidence that younger children may be more likely to develop later cognitive and behavioral impairments that become evident when they fail to normally acquire higher level functions [Taylor and Alden, 1997].

The presence of lasting cognitive and academic impairments after mild pediatric brain injury is controversial. Several large studies have failed to detect significant neurocognitive impairment in mildly head-injured children [Asarnow et al., 1995; Fay et al., 1993]. However, when multiple neuropsychologic outcome measures were pooled, subtle overall impairments were reported that may indicate weak injury effects across a large spectrum of measures, rather than a major effect in a single cognitive domain [Polissar et al., 1994]. More recently, several studies have reported data that suggest, at least in younger children (less than 6 years old at injury), cognitive impairment after mild traumatic brain injury may be more noticeable in particular domains at longer follow-up periods [Bijur et al., 1990; Gronwall et al., 1997]. Earlier studies with shorter follow-up periods may have underestimated impairment associated with mild traumatic brain injury.

When outcomes were assessed broadly using a parental questionnaire and an expanded outcome scale, increased symptoms and diminished outcomes were detected even in mildly injured children [Hawley et al., 2004]. Of great concern is the finding that, across all injury severities, only 30% of all head-injured children received follow-up after hospital discharge. Even in patients with identified special education needs, more than one third did not receive appropriate educational placement [Hawley et al., 2004]. Minimal medical follow-up after pediatric head injury is common despite the presence of persistent problems [Massagli et al., 1996b].

A number of animal studies have also investigated the cognitive effects of developmental traumatic brain injury. Younger animals have better behavioral outcomes than adults after traumatic brain injury [Prins and Hovda, 1998]. However, after severe traumatic brain injury with a secondary hypoxic injury, lasting motor and cognitive impairments have been reported [Adelson et al., 1997b]. Furthermore, there is evidence that experience-dependent plasticity is impaired after early traumatic brain injury. Lasting deficits in cognitive ability have been detected in animals injured early in life and subsequently reared in an enriched environment when compared with enriched but uninjured controls [Fineman et al., 2000; Giza et al., 2005].

There is also considerable evidence that pediatric traumatic brain injury results in later behavioral disturbances, including problems with impulse control, attention, and socialization [Max et al., 2004; Yeates et al., 2004]. Some investigators have suggested that many of these problems can be demonstrated premorbidly [Haas et al., 1987]. Nonetheless, a growing literature also indicates that new-onset psychiatric and behavioral disorders are more frequent following traumatic brain injury sustained during development [Bloom et al., 2001; Luis and Mittenberg, 2002; Max et al., 1997].

Spasticity and Motor Impairment

Focal or diffuse injury may affect upper motor neuron pathways, resulting in spasticity, weakness, and loss of dexterity. The resulting motor deficit will depend on the location and nature of the primary injury. Hemiparesis and quadriparesis occur depending on whether the brain injury was predominantly unilateral (focal contusion, severe hematoma with edema) or bilateral (diffuse axonal injury, bilateral hematomas, diffuse hypoxia as a secondary injury). As a general rule, focal deficits recover better than diffuse ones, and younger age appears to predict better recovery in these circumstances (except perhaps in the earliest age groups, younger than 1 to 4 years).

Passive range of motion should be instituted early enough to prevent development of contractures. Active physical and occupational therapy should be instituted when cognitive recovery sufficient to participate and follow commands has been achieved (see Chapter 92). Splints and orthotic devices (ankle-foot-orthoses, wrist splints) assist in improving function and avoiding contractures. Assistive devices to aid in ambulation should be provided when appropriate. In some cases, medical management of spasticity may also prove beneficial. Baclofen, tizanidine, dantrolene, and, rarely, benzodiazepines may be administered systemically to alleviate severe spasticity. The limiting factor for most of these medications is sedation and CNS depression. Dantrolene acts at the level of the muscle, and so avoids these central effects, but must be monitored carefully for hepatotoxicity. Botulinum toxin injections are increasingly used to locally treat spasticity in cases of cerebral palsy and brain injury. Botulinum toxin also avoids central depressive effects but can be costly. An intrathecal baclofen pump may also be considered in traumatic brain injury patients with severe spasticity who are responsive to baclofen but get limited benefits because of sedation.

Post-traumatic Hydrocephalus

Post-traumatic hydrocephalus is not a common complication but can occur after intraventricular hemorrhage and post-traumatic subarachnoid hemorrhage. Chronic headache, sometimes with nausea, vomiting, impaired vertical eye movements, and diminished level of consciousness, may be manifestations of developing hydrocephalus. Shunting may be necessary to alleviate pressure. Ventriculomegaly is perhaps more common, with enlargement of ventricular and cerebrospinal fluid spaces as brain atrophy develops over time after more severe traumatic brain injury. In the latter instance the ventricular system is not under pressure, and shunting is not warranted.

Post-traumatic Epilepsy

Epilepsy is defined as a disorder of recurrent seizures that are not reactive to an underlying metabolic derangement (e.g., electrolyte disturbance, hypoglycemia). Traumatic brain injury is responsible for about 5% of all new epilepsy cases annually in the United States [Hauser et al., 1993; Jennett, 1975]. Predictors of post-traumatic seizures include severity of traumatic brain injury, age, and type of traumatic brain injury [Annegers et al., 1980, 1998; Hahn et al., 1988b; Salazar et al., 1985; Weiss et al., 1986].

Although children are more likely than adults to experience an early post-traumatic seizure [Annegers et al., 1980, 1998], the relation between early and late post-traumatic seizures in children is unclear. Some report an increased risk for late seizures in children who experience an early one [Jennett, 1975], but this correlation has not been described in other studies [Annegers et al., 1980; Hendrick and Harris, 1968]. To some extent, the lower relative risk for post-traumatic brain injury epilepsy in children may be related to the higher spontaneous rate of developing epilepsy in the pediatric age range.

The rationale for early antiepileptic prophylaxis following pediatric traumatic brain injury was covered earlier under the guidelines for acute management. The inability of early prophylaxis to alter the subsequent development of late post-traumatic epilepsy argues against routine chronic antiepileptic prophylaxis in head-injured children, particularly given the adverse effects of antiepileptic drugs, which include sedation, cognitive impairment, behavioral disturbances, and toxicity. Recent animal studies using anticonvulsants in neonatal rodents have revealed a worrisome tendency for these drugs to trigger widespread neuronal apoptosis in the developing rat brain [Bittigau et al., 2002; Olney et al., 2002]. Such concerns necessitate clear indications and demonstration of clear benefits when considering use of these medications in the maturing brain.

Post-traumatic epilepsy includes late, recurrent, unprovoked seizures with a significant antecedent history of traumatic brain injury. Because routine prophylaxis is not generally recommended, when these patients present with their first seizure, they will likely not be taking antiepileptic drugs and should undergo a complete evaluation and workup. Evaluation includes a thorough history with a description of the prior head injury, as well as investigation for other risk factors (e.g., family history, history of other brain injury). Examination should be aimed at detecting focal neurologic impairments and determining whether these deficits are consistent with the history of the prior head injury. For example, a spastic hemiparesis on examination with a history of only a minor concussion 6 months earlier should raise suspicions for alternative etiologies. EEG is an essential part of the evaluation, with focal or multifocal abnormalities being more consistent with a diagnosis of post-traumatic epilepsy than generalized spike wave discharges. Focal findings on examination or EEG should prompt neuroimaging, with MRI being the modality of choice. MRI can identify areas suggestive of earlier traumatic brain injury, including encephalomalacia, gliosis, hemosiderin deposition, ventriculomegaly, and sulcal enlargement. Specific findings of mesial temporal sclerosis, hydrocephalus, chronic subdural fluid accumulations, prior ischemic cerebral infarction, or cerebral dysgenesis may also be revealed.

Because the specific type of post-traumatic seizure is usually one of partial onset, medication choice is generally directed toward agents with effectiveness for localization-related epilepsy (see Chapter 44). The specific choice may also take into account potential side effects of the individual drugs. Phenytoin is associated with coarsening of facial features, hirsutism, and gingival hyperplasia and thus is perhaps less desirable for chronic use in children. Phenobarbital is sedating or paradoxically activating in children, and these behavioral effects are often limiting factors. Carbamazepine, lamotrigine, valproate, topiramate, oxcarbazepine, and even gabapentin and levetiracetam may be useful. Tailoring the choice of agent to take advantage of potentially beneficial side effects is often worthwhile. For example, in a patient with coexisting migraine headaches, topiramate and valproate are logical considerations; for the obese patient, valproate and carbamazepine may be avoided in favor of topiramate or at least the weight-neutral lamotrigine. Patients with mania and seizures may benefit from the mood-stabilizing qualities of carbamazepine or valproate. Ideally, monotherapy would be attempted, with gradual increase of the medication to the therapeutic range, watching carefully for idiosyncratic or dose-related side effects. Careful attention should be given not only to parental concerns but also to school and teacher reports because chronic administration of antiepileptic drugs may result in subtle cognitive or behavioral impairments [Loring and Meador, 2004].

Subacute and Chronic Subdural Hematomas

Subacute and chronic subdural hematomas can be seen because the predominantly venous bleeding that feeds the hematoma occurs slowly over a period of time, or because of multiple repeated traumas. Clinical manifestations are those of gradually increasing intracranial pressure—recurrent vomiting, macrocrania, papilledema, seizures, slowly progressive motor deficits, and spasticity—and occasionally systemic signs such as anemia, poor appetite, or fever. Because traumas can result in subdural hematomas of differing ages, the possibility of nonaccidental trauma should be considered whenever the radiographic appearance is consistent with subdural hematomas of varying age.

Because blood products undergo a predictable pattern of breakdown visible on MRI, this remains the neuroimaging test of choice when attempting to age a subacute or chronic hematoma (see Table 62-5). In the hyperacute phase (4 to 6 hours), T1-weighted images are hypointense or isointense, and T2-weighted images are hyperintense, indicating oxyhemoglobin. Following this is a period (7 to 72 hours) during which deoxyhemoglobin becomes the predominant component. T1-weighted images are hypointense or isointense, whereas T2-weighted images become hypointense. In the early subacute period (4 to 7 days), T1-weighted images become hyperintense and T2-weighted images hypointense, representing intracellular methemoglobin. After 1 week, for the next few weeks, free or extracellular methemoglobin is present, sometimes with a thin rim of hemosiderin. T1-weighted images are hyperintense, as are T2-weighted images, with a rim of low intensity. In the chronic phase, hemosiderin is deposited and is hypointense on both T1- and T2-weighted images. Often, an inner and outer membrane may be visible.

Treatment of these hematomas often includes drainage of the offending fluid collection. In cases suspected of nonaccidental trauma, a careful search for other bodily injuries is warranted, including a whole-body x-ray series (to look for multiple fractures in varying states of healing) and skin examination (to look for bruising in unusual locations, with bruises of different ages, as well as other signs and shapes of injuries or burns) (see Chapter 63).

Post-traumatic Headache

Acute post-traumatic headache is usually self-limited. Trauma may also appear to precipitate migraines acutely or chronically. A direct causal relationship has not been proved, and it is uncertain whether this represents activation of migraines in those already predisposed to the condition. Worsening or progressive headache, particularly associated with nausea and vomiting, should warrant careful history and examination to rule out a delayed progressive intracranial complication (chronic subdural, hydrocephalus). If necessary, cranial CT can rule out the more worrisome diagnoses.

Management of chronic post-traumatic headaches is directed at the presumed underlying etiology of the headache. Chronic nonmigrainous headaches may be treated with analgesics, nonsteroidal anti-inflammatory agents, antidepressants (e.g., amitriptyline), or antiepileptic drugs (gabapentin). Narcotics should be avoided.

Migraine headaches should be treated based on their frequency, with prophylaxis considered for migraines occurring more often than once or twice every couple weeks (particularly if they result in missed school). Effective migraine prophylactic medications include topiramate, valproic acid, β blockers, amitriptyline, and possibly other medications, such as selective serotonin reuptake inhibitors, gabapentin, and calcium channel blockers. Infrequent migraines should be treated abortively using standard medications such as triptans.

Neuralgic pain may respond better to antiepileptic drugs than to analgesics. Nonpharmacologic interventions should also be considered if chronic pain becomes a significant problem. These may best be addressed in a multidisciplinary pediatric pain clinic and include acupuncture, yoga, biofeedback, and counseling.

Postconcussive Syndrome

Although most postconcussive symptoms resolve spontaneously within days to weeks after injury, persistent problems can arise. These symptoms can be difficult to quantify and even more difficult to treat and can become very disruptive to the child's daily life if they result in exclusion from school or from social or extracurricular activities.

The constellation of symptoms seen in postconcussive syndrome in children is similar to that in adults, with chronic headache, dizziness, irritability, behavior change, inattention, and listlessness being prominent. The mechanisms of postconcussive symptoms are unknown, but in general, anatomic lesions are not seen. Demonstration of brain dysfunction after mild traumatic brain injury has been performed using quantification of persistent symptoms [Collins et al., 2002; Field et al., 2003; Ponsford et al., 1999], neuropsychologic testing [Collins et al., 1999, 2003; Matser et al., 1999], functional MRI [Jantzen et al., 2004; McAllister et al., 1999], positron emission tomography [Bergsneider et al., 2000; Chen et al., 2003; Roberts et al., 1995], and single-photon emission computed tomography [Kant et al., 1997; Umile et al., 2002]. The exact relation between these physiologic abnormalities and the patient's symptoms has not been elucidated. Furthermore, other nonphysiologic factors have been implicated in the development of postconcussive symptoms, including premorbid personality traits, socioeconomic status, educational level, medicolegal compensation, and family dynamics. Most of the research into postconcussive syndrome has been performed in late adolescents and adults; thus, these findings may not be readily generalized to younger age groups.

Management of postconcussive syndrome in children should focus on a return to normalcy as much as is possible given the symptoms. Partial return to school is usually preferable to complete absence in cases in which complete return is not possible. Prolonged absence from school may soon take on a life of its own and become clouded with issues of secondary gain and avoidance.

Medical management should be aimed at identifying treatable problems and initiating appropriate interventions. Headaches may be approached as described earlier. Postconcussive behavior disturbances should be evaluated by a child psychiatrist or psychologist. Although it is uncertain whether mild traumatic brain injury results in an increased risk for new-onset behavioral diagnoses, it is clear that children with particular behavioral tendencies (attention-deficit–hyperactivity disorder, oppositional behavior) are more prone to mild traumatic brain injury, and treatment of these underlying problems is often beneficial.

Cognitive problems identified after mild traumatic brain injury may be best addressed by school assessment or neuropsychological testing. Often children with developmental delay or learning disabilities have disproportionate cognitive problems after mild traumatic brain injury. In a study of high school football players, in addition to a history of more than two prior concussions, a history of learning disability was associated with poorer results on neuropsychologic tests [Collins et al., 1999].

Late Complications of Skull Fracture

Most nondisplaced skull fractures will heal without aggressive management. However, a number of chronic complications can result from skull fracture and need to be mentioned.

"Growing skull fracture," also known as *craniocerebral erosion* or *leptomeningeal cyst*, complicates less than 1% of all skull fractures. It occurs most commonly with linear fractures of the cranial vault, usually in the parietal region in infants younger than 1 year. After a linear fracture with separation of the bony edges by 2 to 3 mm, the pulsatile nature of the intracranial contents gradually results in outward herniation of dura and underlying brain. These fractures require carefully planned surgical correction because they do not resolve spontaneously and are often associated with local brain injury in the form of degeneration, necrosis, and gliosis. Clinically, hydrocephalus, motor deficits, and seizures have been reported as sequelae.

Traumatic cranial neuropathies can also occur after fractures of the skull base, most commonly affecting olfactory, optic, facial, and vestibulocochlear nerves. Loss or impairment of olfaction can be associated with frontobasal fracture but is rarely tested and perhaps underdiagnosed. Traumatic optic neuropathies are associated with facial fractures, including fractures directly involving the optic canal. In cases in which no surgical lesion is detected, use of corticosteroids has been reported to speed recovery [Cook et al., 1996; Mahapatra and Tandon, 1993]. Complete paralysis of facial musculature suggests transection of the facial nerve in the petrous portion of the temporal bone. More often, transient facial weakness occurs, presumably because of edema and inflammation of perineural structures. Post-traumatic hearing loss may be due to cranial nerve VIII injury or direct injury to the ossicles. Again, fracture of the petrous bone should be considered. Steroids have not proved beneficial for post-traumatic facial or vestibulocochlear palsies.

In cases of basilar skull fracture, particularly with persistent cerebrospinal fluid leakage, there is an increased risk for CNS infection because of parameningeal seeding. Patients with known basilar skull fractures who present with fever, meningismus, seizures, or focal neurologic findings should be evaluated promptly for brain abscess, empyema, or meningitis.

REFERENCES

Adams JH, Graham DI, Murray LS, et al. Diffuse axonal injury due to nonmissile head injury in humans: An analysis of 45 cases. Ann Neurol 1982;12:557.

Adelson PD, Bratton SL, Carney NA, et al. Guidelines for the acute medical management of severe traumatic brain injury in infants, children, and adolescents. Chapter 18: Nutritional support. Pediatr Crit Care Med 2003a;4:S68.

Adelson PD, Bratton SL, Carney NA, et al. Guidelines for the acute medical management of severe traumatic brain injury in infants, children, and adolescents. Chapter 1: Introduction. Pediatr Crit Care Med 2003b;4:S2.

Adelson PD, Bratton SL, Carney NA, et al. Guidelines for the acute medical management of severe traumatic brain injury in infants, children, and adolescents. Chapter 6: Threshold for treatment of intracranial hypertension. Pediatr Crit Care Med 2003c;4:S25.

Adelson PD, Bratton SL, Carney NA, et al. Guidelines for the acute medical management of severe traumatic brain injury in infants, children, and adolescents. Chapter 9: Use of sedation and neuromuscular blockade in the treatment of severe pediatric traumatic brain injury. Pediatr Crit Care Med 2003d;4:S34.

Adelson PD, Bratton SL, Carney NA, et al. Guidelines for the acute medical management of severe traumatic brain injury in infants, children, and adolescents. Chapter 17: Critical pathway for the treatment of established intracranial hypertension in pediatric traumatic brain injury. Pediatr Crit Care Med 2003e;4:S65.

Adelson PD, Bratton SL, Carney NA, et al. Guidelines for the acute medical management of severe traumatic brain injury in infants, children, and adolescents. Chapter 19: The role of anti-seizure prophylaxis following severe pediatric traumatic brain injury. Pediatr Crit Care Med 2003f;4:S72.

Adelson PD, Clyde B, Kochanek PM, et al. Cerebrovascular response in infants and young children following severe traumatic brain injury: A preliminary report. Pediatr Neurosurg 1997a;26:200.

Adelson PD, Dixon CE, Robichaud P, et al. Motor and cognitive functional deficits following diffuse traumatic brain injury in the immature rat. J Neurotrauma 1997b;14:99.

Adelson PD, Ragheb J, Kanev P, et al. Phase II clinical trial of moderate hypothermia after severe traumatic brain injury in children. Neurosurgery 2005;56:740.

Albanese J, Arnaud S, Rey M, et al. Ketamine decreases intracranial pressure and electroencephalographic activity in traumatic brain injury patients during propofol sedation. Anesthesiology 1997;87:1328.

Aldrich EF, Eisenberg HM, Saydjari C, et al. Diffuse brain swelling in severely head-injured children. A report from the NIH Traumatic Coma Data Bank. J Neurosurg 1992;76:450.

American Academy of Neurology. Practice parameter: The management of concussion in sports (summary statement). Neurology 1997;48.

American Academy of Pediatrics. The management of minor closed head injury in children. Pediatrics 1999;104:1407.

Annegers JF, Grabow JD, Groover RV, et al. Seizures after head trauma: A population study. Neurology 1980;30:683.

Annegers JF, Hauser WA, Coan SP, et al. A population-based study of seizures after traumatic brain injuries. N Engl J Med 1998;338:20.

Armstrong K, Kerns KA. The assessment of parent needs following paediatric traumatic brain injury. Pediatr Rehabil 2002;5:149.

Asarnow, Satz, Light, et al. The UCLA study of mild head injury in children and adolescents. In: Bronan, Michel, eds. Traumatic head injury in children. New York: Oxford University Press, 1995.

Ashwal S. Medical aspects of the minimally conscious state in children. Brain Dev 2003;25:535.

Ashwal S, Holshouser BA, Shu SK, et al. Predictive value of proton magnetic resonance spectroscopy in pediatric closed head injury. Pediatr Neurol 2000;23:114.

Ashwal S, Holshouser B, Tong K, et al. Proton spectroscopy detected myoinositol in children with traumatic brain injury. Pediatr Res 2004a;56:630.

Ashwal S, Holshouser B, Tong K, et al. Proton MR spectroscopy detected glutamate/glutamine is increased in children with traumatic brain injury. J Neurotrauma 2004b;21:1529-1552.

Beca J, Cox PN, Taylor MJ, et al. Somatosensory evoked potentials for prediction of outcome in acute severe brain injury. J Pediatr 1995;126:44.

Becker DP, Miller JD, Ward JD, et al. The outcome from severe head injury with early diagnosis and intensive management. J Neurosurg 1977;47:491.

Bell RS, Loop JW. The utility and futility of radiographic skull examination for trauma. N Engl J Med 1971;284:236.

Bennett EL, Diamond MC, Krech D, et al. Chemical and anatomical plasticity of brain. Science 1964;164:610.

Bergsneider M, Hovda DA, Lee SM, et al. Dissociation of cerebral glucose metabolism and level of consciousness during the period of metabolic depression following human traumatic brain injury. J Neurotrauma 2000;17:389.

Bergsneider M, Hovda DA, McArthur DL, et al. Metabolic recovery following human traumatic brain injury based on FDG-PET: Time course and relationship to neurological disability. J Head Trauma Rehabil 2001;16:135.

Bergsneider M, Hovda DA, Shalmon E, et al. Cerebral hyperglycolysis following severe traumatic brain injury in humans: A positron emission tomography study [see Comments]. J Neurosurg 1997;86:241.

Berney J, Froidevaux AC, Favier J. Paediatric head trauma: Influence of age and sex. II. Biomechanical and anatomo-clinical correlations. Childs Nerv Syst 1994;10:517.

Biagas KV, Grundl PD, Kochanek PM, et al. Posttraumatic hyperemia in immature, mature, and aged rats: Autoradiographic determination of cerebral blood flow. J Neurotrauma 1996;13:189.

Biegon A, Fry PA, Paden CM, et al. Dynamic changes in N-methyl-D-aspartate receptors after closed head injury in mice: Implications for treatment of neurological and cognitive deficits. Proc Natl Acad Sci U S A 2004;101:5117.

Bijur PE, Haslum M, Golding J. Cognitive and behavioral sequelae of mild head injury in children. Pediatrics 1990;86:337.

Bittigau P, Sifringer M, Genz K, et al. Antiepileptic drugs and apoptotic neurodegeneration in the developing brain. Proc Natl Acad Sci U S A 2002;99:15089.

Bittigau P, Sifringer M, Pohl D, et al. Apoptotic neurodegeneration following trauma is markedly enhanced in the immature brain. Ann Neurol 1999;45:724.

Bloom DR, Levin HS, Ewing-Cobbs L, et al. Lifetime and novel psychiatric disorders after pediatric traumatic brain injury. J Am Acad Child Adolesc Psychiatry 2001;40:572.

Bouma GJ, Muizelaar JP, Choi SC, et al. Cerebral circulation and metabolism after severe traumatic brain injury: The elusive role of ischemia. J Neurosurg 1991;75:685.

Braakman R. Depressed skull fracture: Data, treatment, and follow-up in 225 consecutive cases. J Neurol Neurosurg Psychiatry 1972;35:395.

Brain Trauma Foundation, American Association of Neurological Surgeons, Joint Section on Neurotrauma and Critical Care. Management and prognosis of severe traumatic brain injury. J Neurotrauma 2000;17.

Bray RJ. Propofol infusion syndrome in children. Paediatr Anaesth 1998;8:491.

Brenner T, Freier MC, Holshouser BA, et al. Predicting neuropsychologic outcome after traumatic brain injury in children. Pediatr Neurol 2003;28:104.

Brown E. Antimicrobial prophylaxis for cerebrospinal fluid fistula. Br J Neurosurg 1990;4:367.

Bruce DA, Alavi A, Bilaniuk L, et al. Diffuse cerebral swelling following head injuries in children: The syndrome of "malignant brain edema." J Neurosurg 1981;54:170.

Bruce DA, Raphaely RC, Goldberg AI, et al. Pathophysiology, treatment and outcome following severe head injury in children. Childs Brain 1979;5:174.

Bruce DA, Schut L, Bruno LA, et al. Outcome following severe head injuries in children. J Neurosurg 1978;48:679.

Bruce DA, Zimmerman RA. Shaken impact syndrome. Pediatr Ann 1989;18:482.

Bruce JM, Echemendia RJ. Concussion history predicts self-reported symptoms before and following a concussive event. Neurology 2004;63:1516.

Bullock R, Zauner A, Woodward JJ, et al. Factors affecting excitatory amino acid release following severe human head injury. J Neurosurg 1998;89:507.

Burgess JW, Villablanca JR. Recovery of function after neonatal or adult hemispherectomy in cats. II. Limb bias and development, paw usage, locomotion and rehabilitative effects of exercise. Behav Brain Res 1986;20:1.

Burke WJ. The minimally conscious state: Definition and diagnostic criteria. Neurology 2002;59:1473.

Busto R, Dietrich WD, Globus MY, et al. The importance of brain temperature in cerebral ischemic injury. Stroke 1989;20:1113.

Calder IM, Hill I, Scholtz CL. Primary brain trauma in non-accidental injury. J Clin Pathol 1984;37:1095.

Canivet JL, Gustad K, Leclercq P, et al. Massive ketonuria during sedation with propofol in a 12 year old girl with severe head trauma. Acta Anaesthesiol Belg 1994;45:19.

Cantu RC. Second-impact syndrome. Clin Sports Med 1998;17:37.

Carey ME. Experimental missile wounding of the brain. Neurosurg Clin N Am 1995;6:629.

Carter BG, Taylor A, Butt W. Severe brain injury in children: Long-term outcome and its prediction using somatosensory evoked potentials (SEPs). Intensive Care Med 1999;25:722.

Centers for Disease Control and Prevention. Traumatic brain injury (TBI) in the United States: Assessing outcomes in children—background. 2000.

Chan KH, Yue CP, Mann KS. The risk of intracranial complications in pediatric head injury. Results of multivariate analysis. Childs Nerv Syst 1990;6:27.

Chang BS, Lowenstein DH, for the Quality Standards Subcommittee of the American Academy of Neurology. Practice parameter: Antiepileptic drug prophylaxis in severe traumatic brain injury. Report of the Quality Standards Subcommittee of the American Academy of Neurology. Neurology 2003;60:10.

Changaris DG, McGraw CP, Richardson JD, et al. Correlation of cerebral perfusion pressure and Glasgow Coma Scale to outcome. J Trauma 1987;27:1007.

Chen SH, Kareken DA, Fastenau PS, et al. A study of persistent post-concussion symptoms in mild head trauma using positron emission tomography. J Neurol Neurosurg Psychiatry 2003;74:326.

Chesnut RM, Marshall LF, Klauber MR, et al. The role of secondary brain injury in determining outcome from severe head injury. J Trauma 1993a;34:216.

Chesnut RM, Marshall SB, Piek J, et al. Early and late systemic hypotension as a frequent and fundamental source of cerebral ischemia following severe brain injury in the Traumatic Coma Data Bank. Acta Neurochir Suppl (Wien) 1993b;59:121.

Chiaretti A, Piastra M, Pulitano S, et al. Prognostic factors and outcome of children with severe head injury: An 8-year experience. Childs Nerv Syst 2002;18:129.

Chiron C, Raynaud C, Maziere B, et al. Changes in regional cerebral blood flow during brain maturation in children and adolescents. J Nucl Med 1992;33:696.

Cho DY, Wang YC, Chi CS. Decompressive craniotomy for acute shaken/impact baby syndrome. Pediatr Neurosurg 1995;23:192.

Choux M, Grisoli F, Peragut JC. Extradural hematomas in children: 104 Cases. Childs Brain 1975;1:337.

Chugani HT, Phelps ME, Mazziotta JC. Positron emission tomography study of human brain functional development. Ann Neurol 1987;22:487.

Clifton GL, Allen S, Barrodale P, et al. A phase II study of moderate hypothermia in severe brain injury. J Neurotrauma 1993;10:263.

Clifton GL, Miller ER, Choi SC, et al. Lack of effect of induction of hypothermia after acute brain injury. N Engl J Med 2001;344:556.

Collins MW, Field M, Lovell MR, et al. Relationship between postconcussion headache and neuropsychological test performance in high school athletes. Am J Sports Med 2003;31:168.

Collins MW, Grindel SH, Lovell MR, et al. Relationship between concussion and neuropsychological performance in college football players. JAMA 1999;282:964.

Collins MW, Lovell MR, Iverson GL, et al. Cumulative effects of concussion in high school athletes. Neurosurgery 2002;51:1175.

Conti AC, Raghupathi R, Trojanowski JQ, et al. Experimental brain injury induces regionally distinct apoptosis during the acute and delayed post-traumatic period. J Neurosci 1998;18:5663.

Cook MW, Levin LA, Joseph MP, et al. Traumatic optic neuropathy. A meta-analysis. Arch Otolaryngol Head Neck Surg 1996;122:389.

Cooper A, DiScala C, Foltin G, et al. Prehospital endotracheal intubation for severe head injury in children: A reappraisal. Semin Pediatr Surg 2001;10:3.

Cray SH, Robinson BH, Cox PN. Lactic acidemia and bradyarrhythmia in a child sedated with propofol. Crit Care Med 1998;26:2087.

Cruz J. The first decade of continuous monitoring of jugular bulb oxyhemoglobin saturation: Management strategies and clinical outcome. Crit Care Med 1998;26:344.

Czosnyka M, Smielewski P, Kirkpatrick P, et al. Monitoring of cerebral autoregulation in head-injured patients. Stroke 1996;27:1829.

Czosnyka M, Smielewski P, Piechnik S, et al. Continuous assessment of cerebral autoregulation—clinical verification of the method in head injured patients. Acta Neurochir Suppl 2000;76:483.

Dam HP, Sizun J, Person H, et al. The place of decompressive surgery in the treatment of uncontrollable post-traumatic intracranial hypertension in children. Childs Nerv Syst 1996;12:270.

Davis RL, Mullen N, Makela M, et al. Cranial computed tomography scans in children after minimal head injury with loss of consciousness. Ann Emerg Med 1994;24:640.

DeFord SM, Wilson MS, Rice AC, et al. Repeated mild brain injuries result in cognitive impairment in B6C3F1 mice. J Neurotrauma 2002;19:427.

Diamond MC, Krech D, Rosenzweig MR. The effects of an enriched environment on the histology of the rat cerebral cortex. J Comp Neurol 1964;123:111.

Dietrich AM, Bowman MJ, Ginn-Pease ME, et al. Pediatric head injuries: Can clinical factors reliably predict an abnormality on computed tomography? Ann Emerg Med 1993;22:1535.

Dietrich WD, Alonso O, Busto R, et al. Widespread metabolic depression and reduced somatosensory circuit activation following traumatic brain injury in rats. J Neurotrauma 1994;11:629.

Dietrich WD, Alonso O, Halley M, et al. Delayed posttraumatic brain hyperthermia worsens outcome after fluid percussion brain injury: A light and electron microscopic study in rats. Neurosurgery 1996;38:533.

Downard C, Hulka F, Mullins RJ, et al. Relationship of cerebral perfusion pressure and survival in pediatric brain-injured patients. J Trauma 2000;49:654.

Duhaime AC, Gennarelli TA, Thibault LE, et al. The shaken baby syndrome. A clinical, pathological, and biomechanical study. J Neurosurg 1987;66:409.

Dunning J, Batchelor J, Stratford-Smith P, et al. A meta-analysis of variables that predict significant intracranial injury in minor head trauma. Arch Dis Child 2004;89:653.

Einhorn A, Mizrahi EM. Basilar skull fractures in children. The incidence of CNS infection and the use of antibiotics. Am J Dis Child 1978;132:1121.

Eisenberg HM, Frankowski RF, Contant CF, et al. High-dose barbiturate control of elevated intracranial pressure in patients with severe head injury. J Neurosurg 1988;69:15.

Elias-Jones AC, Punt JA, Turnbull AE, et al. Management and outcome of severe head injuries in the Trent region 1985-90. Arch Dis Child 1992;67:1430.

Engberg A, Teasdale TW. Traumatic brain injury in children in Denmark: A national 15-year study. Eur J Epidemiol 1998;14:165.

Esparza J, Portillo J, Sarabia M, et al. Outcome in children with severe head injuries. Childs Nerv Syst 1985;1:109.

Ewing-Cobbs L, Fletcher JM, Levin HS, et al. Academic achievement and academic placement following traumatic brain injury in children and adolescents: A two-year longitudinal study. J Clin Exp Neuropsychol 1998;20:769.

Ewing-Cobbs L, Prasad MR, Landry SH, et al. Executive functions following traumatic brain injury in young children: A preliminary analysis. Dev Neuropsychol 2004;26:487.

Faherty CJ, Kerley D, Smeyne RJ. A Golgi-Cox morphological analysis of neuronal changes induced by environmental enrichment. Brain Res Dev Brain Res 2003;141:55.

Farling PA, Johnston JR, Coppel DL. Propofol infusion for sedation of patients with head injury in intensive care. A preliminary report. Anaesthesia 1989;44:222.

Fay GC, Jaffe KM, Polissar NL, et al. Mild pediatric traumatic brain injury: A cohort study. Arch Phys Med Rehabil 1993;74:895.

Fay GC, Jaffe KM, Polissar NL, et al. Outcome of pediatric traumatic brain injury at three years: A cohort study. Arch Phys Med Rehabil 1994;75:733.

Field M, Collins MW, Lovell MR, et al. Does age play a role in recovery from sports-related concussion? A comparison of high school and collegiate athletes. J Pediatr 2003;142:546.

Fineman I, Giza CC, Nahed BV, et al. Inhibition of neocortical plasticity during development by a moderate concussive brain injury. J Neurotrauma 2000;17:739.

Fishman RA. Cerebrospinal fluid in diseases of the nervous system. Philadelphia: WB Saunders, 1980.

Fosse VM, Heggelund P, Fonnum F. Postnatal development of glutamatergic, GABAergic, and cholinergic neurotransmitter phenotypes in the visual cortex, lateral geniculate nucleus, pulvinar, and superior colliculus in cats. J Neurosci 1989;9:426.

Francel PC, Honeycutt J. Mild brain injury in children, including skull fractures and growing fractures. In: Winn RH, ed. Youman's neurological surgery. Philadelphia: WB Saunders, 2004.

Gambardella G, Zaccone C, Cardia E, et al. Intracranial pressure monitoring in children: Comparison of external ventricular device with the fiberoptic system. Childs Nerv Syst 1993;9:470.

Gausche M, Lewis RJ, Stratton SJ, et al. Effect of out-of-hospital pediatric endotracheal intubation on survival and neurological outcome: A controlled clinical trial. JAMA 2000;283:783.

Ghajar JBG, Hariri RJ, Patterson RH. Improved outcome from traumatic coma using only ventricular cerebrospinal fluid drainage for intracranial pressure control. Adv Neurosurg 1993;21:173.

Giacino JT, Ashwal S, Childs N, et al. The minimally conscious state: Definition and diagnostic criteria. Neurology 2002;58:349.

Ginsberg MD, Busto R. Combating hyperthermia in acute stroke: A significant clinical concern. Stroke 1998;29:529.

Giza CC, Hovda DA. The neurometabolic cascade of concussion. J Athl Train 2001;36:228.

Giza CC, Griesbach GS, Hovda DA. Experience-dependent behavioral plasticity is disturbed following traumatic injury to the immature brain. Behav Brain Res 2005;157:11.

Giza CC, Prins ML, Hovda DA, et al. Genes preferentially induced by depolarization after concussive brain injury: Effects of age and injury severity. J Neurotrauma 2002;19:387.

Glotzner FL, Haubitz I, Miltner F, et al. Seizure prevention using carbamazepine following severe brain injuries. Neurochirurgia (Stuttg) 1983;26:66.

Gorman LK, Fu K, Hovda DA, et al. Effects of traumatic brain injury on the cholinergic system in the rat. J Neurotrauma 1996;13:457.

Greenough WT, Volkmar FR, Juraska JM. Effects of rearing complexity on dendritic branching in frontolateral and temporal cortex of the rat. Exp Neurol 1973;41:371.

Griesbach GS, Hovda DA, Molteni R, et al. Voluntary exercise following traumatic brain injury: Brain-derived neurotrophic factor upregulation and recovery of function. Neuroscience 2004;125:129.

Gronwall D, Wrightson P, McGinn V. Effect of mild head injury during the preschool years. J Int Neuropsychol Soc 1997;3:592.

Guerra WK, Gaab MR, Dietz H, et al. Surgical decompression for traumatic brain swelling: Indications and results. J Neurosurg 1999;90:187.

Guskiewicz KM, McCrea M, Marshall SW, et al. Cumulative effects associated with recurrent concussion in collegiate football players: The NCAA Concussion Study. JAMA 2003;290:2549.

Guskiewicz KM, Weaver NL, Padua DA, et al. Epidemiology of concussion in collegiate and high school football players. Am J Sports Med 2000;28:643.

Haas DC, Lourie H. Trauma-triggered migraine: An explanation for common neurological attacks after mild head injury. Review of the literature. J Neurosurg 1988;68:181.

Haas JF, Cope DN, Hall K. Premorbid prevalence of poor academic performance in severe head injury. J Neurol Neurosurg Psychiatry 1987;50:52.

Hahn YS, Chyung C, Barthel MJ, et al. Head injuries in children under 36 months of age. Demography and outcome. Childs Nerv Syst 1988a;4:34.

Hahn YS, Fuchs S, Flannery AM, et al. Factors influencing posttraumatic seizures in children. Neurosurgery 1988b;22:864.

Halley MK, Silva PD, Foley J, et al. Loss of consciousness: When to perform computed tomography? Pediatr Crit Care Med 2004;5:230.

Hanna JP, Ramundo ML. Rhabdomyolysis and hypoxia associated with prolonged propofol infusion in children. Neurology 1998;50:301.

Harwood-Nash DC, Hendrick EB, Hudson AR. The significance of skull fractures in children. A study of 1,187 patients. Radiology 1971;101:151.

Hauser WA, Annegers JF, Kurland LT. Incidence of epilepsy and unprovoked seizures in Rochester, Minnesota: 1935-1984. Epilepsia 1993;34:453.

Hawley CA, Ward AB, Magnay AR, et al. Outcomes following childhood head injury: A population study. J Neurol Neurosurg Psychiatry 2004;75:737.

Hendrick EB. The use of hypothermia in severe head injuries in childhood. AMA Arch Surg 1959;17.

Hendrick EB, Harris L. Post-traumatic epilepsy in children. J Trauma 1968;8:547.

Hogan AM, Kirkham FJ, Isaacs EB. Intelligence after stroke in childhood: Review of the literature and suggestions for future research. J Child Neurol 2000;15:325.

Holland BA, Haas DK, Norman D, et al. MRI of normal brain maturation. AJNR Am J Neuroradiol 1986;7:201.

Holshouser BA, Ashwal S, Luh GY, et al. Proton MR spectroscopy after acute central nervous system injury: Outcome prediction in neonates, infants, and children. Radiology 1997;202:487.

Holshouser BA, Ashwal S, Shu S, et al. Proton MR spectroscopy in children with acute brain injury: Comparison of short and long echo time acquisitions. J Magn Reson Imaging 2000;11:9.

Holshouer B, Ashwal S, Tong K. Proton magnetic resonance spectroscopic imaging detects diffuse axonal injury in pediatric traumatic brain injury. Am J Neuroradiol 2005;26:1276.

Homer CJ, Kleinman L. Technical report: Minor head injury in children. Pediatrics 1999;104:e78.

Hugenholtz H, Izukawa D, Shear P, et al. Vomiting in children following head injury. Childs Nerv Syst 1987;3:266.

Humphreys RP, Hendrick EB, Hoffman HJ. The head-injured child who "talks and dies." A report of 4 cases. Childs Nerv Syst 1990;6:139.

Ikonomidou C, Bosch F, Miksa M, et al. Blockade of NMDA receptors and apoptotic neurodegeneration in the developing brain. Science 1999;283:70.

Ikonomidou C, Mosinger JL, Salles KS, et al. Sensitivity of the developing rat brain to hypobaric/ischemic damage parallels sensitivity to N-methyl-aspartate neurotoxicity. J Neurosci 1989;9:2809.

Ikonomidou C, Turski L. Why did NMDA receptor antagonists fail clinical trials for stroke and traumatic brain injury? Lancet Neurol 2002;1:383.

Immordino FM. Management of minor head trauma. Bull Clin Neurosci 1986;51:81.
Insel TR, Miller LP, Gelhard RE. The ontogeny of excitatory amino acid receptors in rat forebrain: I. N-methyl-D-aspartate and quisqualate receptors. Neuroscience 1990;35:31.
Ip EY, Giza CC, Griesbach GS, et al. Effects of enriched environment and fluid percussion injury on dendritic arborization within the cerebral cortex of the developing rat. J Neurotrauma 2002;19:573.
Jaffe KM, Polissar NL, Fay GC, et al. Recovery trends over three years following pediatric traumatic brain injury. Arch Phys Med Rehabil 1995;76:17.
James HE. Combination therapy in brain edema. Adv Neurol 1980a;28:491.
James HE. Methodology for the control of intracranial pressure with hypertonic mannitol. Acta Neurochir (Wien) 1980b;51:161.
Jantzen KJ, Anderson B, Steinberg FL, et al. A prospective functional MR imaging study of mild traumatic brain injury in college football players. AJNR Am J Neuroradiol 2004;25:738.
Jennett B. Epilepsy after non-missile head injuries. London, Heinemann, 1975.
Jennett B, Miller JD, Braakman R. Epilepsy after nonmissile depressed skull fracture. J Neurosurg 1974;41:208.
Jennett B, Snoek J, Bond MR, et al. Disability after severe head injury: Observations on the use of the Glasgow Outcome Scale. J Neurol Neurosurg Psychiatry 1981;44:285.
Jensen RL, Hahn YS, Ciro E. Risk factors of intracranial pressure monitoring in children with fiberoptic devices: A critical review. Surg Neurol 1997;47:16.
Jiang JY, Gao GY, Li WP, et al. Early indicators of prognosis in 846 cases of severe traumatic brain injury. J Neurotrauma 2002;19:869.
Juraska JM. Sex differences in dendritic response to differential experience in the rat visual cortex. Brain Res 1984;295:27.
Kaieda R, Todd MM, Cook LN, et al. Acute effects of changing plasma osmolality and colloid oncotic pressure on the formation of brain edema after cryogenic injury. Neurosurgery 1989;24:671.
Kant R, Smith-Seemiller L, Isaac G, et al. Tc-HMPAO SPECT in persistent post-concussion syndrome after mild head injury: Comparison with MRI/CT. Brain Inj 1997;11:115.
Kasoff SS, Lansen TA, Holder D, Filippo JS. Aggressive physiologic monitoring of pediatric head trauma patients with elevated intracranial pressure. Pediatr Neurosci 1988;14:241.
Kassell NF, Hitchon PW, Gerk MK, et al. Alterations in cerebral blood flow, oxygen metabolism, and electrical activity produced by high dose sodium thiopental. Neurosurgery 1980;7:598.
Katayama Y, Becker DP, Tamura T, et al. Massive increases in extracellular potassium and the indiscriminate release of glutamate following concussive brain injury. J Neurosurg 1990;73:889.
Kawamata T, Katayama Y, Hovda DA, et al. Administration of excitatory amino acid antagonists via microdialysis attenuates the increase in glucose utilization seen following concussive brain injury. J Cereb Blood Flow Metab 1992;12:12.
Kaye EM, Herskowitz J. Transient post-traumatic cortical blindness: Brief v prolonged syndromes in childhood. J Child Neurol 1986;1:206.
Keilhoff G, Seidel B, Noack H, et al. Patterns of nitric oxide synthase at the messenger RNA and protein levels during early rat brain development. Neuroscience 1996;75:1193.
Kelly DF, Kordestani RK, Martin NA, et al. Hyperemia following traumatic brain injury: Relationship to intracranial hypertension and outcome. J Neurosurg 1996;85:762.
Kelly DF, Martin NA, Kordestani R, et al. Cerebral blood flow as a predictor of outcome following traumatic brain injury. J Neurosurg 1997;86:633.
Kelly JP, Rosenberg JH. Diagnosis and management of concussion in sports. Neurology 1997;48:575.
Kennard MA. Cortical reorganization of motor function: Studies on a series of monkeys of various ages from infancy to maturity. Arch Neurol Psych 1942;48:227.
Khanna S, Davis D, Peterson B, et al. Use of hypertonic saline in the treatment of severe refractory posttraumatic intracranial hypertension in pediatric traumatic brain injury. Crit Care Med 2000;28:1144.
Kiening KL, Hartl R, Unterberg AW, et al. Brain tissue Po_2-monitoring in comatose patients: Implications for therapy. Neurol Res 1997;19:233.
Kolb B, Cioe J, Whishaw IQ. Is there an optimal age for recovery from motor cortex lesions? I. Behavioral and anatomical sequelae of bilateral motor cortex lesions in rats on postnatal days 1, 10, and in adulthood. Brain Res 2000;882:62.
Kolb B, Tomie J. Recovery from early cortical damage in rats. IV. Effects of hemidecortication at 1, 5 or 10 days of age on cerebral anatomy and behavior. Behav Brain Res 1988;28:259.
Kollevold T. Immediate and early cerebral seizures after head injuries: Part I. J Oslo City Hosp 1976;26:99.
Kontos HA, Hess ML. Oxygen radicals and vascular damage. Adv Exp Med Biol 1983;161:365.
Kraus JF, McArthur DL. Epidemiology of brain injury. In: Cooper PR, Golfinos JG, eds. Head injury, 4th ed. New York: McGraw-Hill, 2000.
Lam JM, Hsiang JN, Poon WS. Monitoring of autoregulation using laser Doppler flowmetry in patients with head injury. J Neurosurg 1997;86:438.
Lang DA, Teasdale GM, Macpherson P, et al. Diffuse brain swelling after head injury: More often malignant in adults than children? J Neurosurg 1994;80:675.
Langley JM, LeBlanc JC, Drake J, et al. Efficacy of antimicrobial prophylaxis in placement of cerebrospinal fluid shunts: Meta-analysis. Clin Infect Dis 1993;17:98.
LeRoux PD, Choudhri HF, Andrews. Cerebral concussion and diffuse brain injury. In: Cooper PR, Golfinos JG, eds. Head injury, 4th ed. New York: McGraw-Hill, 2000.
Levi L, Guilburd JN, Bar-Yosef G, et al. Severe head injury in children: Analyzing the better outcome over a decade and the role of major improvements in intensive care. Childs Nerv Syst 1998;14:195.
Levi L, Guilburd JN, Linn S, et al. The association between skull fracture, intracranial pathology and outcome in pediatric head injury. Br J Neurosurg 1991;5:617.
Levin AB, Duff TA, Javid MJ. Treatment of increased intracranial pressure: A comparison of different hyperosmotic agents and the use of thiopental. Neurosurgery 1979;5:570.
Levin HS. Neuroplasticity following non-penetrating traumatic brain injury. Brain Inj 2003;17:665.
Levin HS, Aldrich EF, Saydjari C, et al. Severe head injury in children: Experience of the Traumatic Coma Data Bank. Neurosurgery 1992;31:435.
Levin HS, Eisenberg HM, Wigg NR, et al. Memory and intellectual ability after head injury in children and adolescents. Neurosurgery 1982;11:668.
Levin HS, Hanten G, Chang CC, et al. Working memory after traumatic brain injury in children. Ann Neurol 2002;52:82.
Levin HS, High WM, Jr., Ewing-Cobbs L, et al. Memory functioning during the first year after closed head injury in children and adolescents. Neurosurgery 1988;22:1043.
Levin HS, Song J, Chapman SB, et al. Neuroplasticity following traumatic diffuse versus focal brain injury in children: Studies of verbal fluency. In: Levin HS, Grafman J, eds. Cerebral reorganization of function after brain damage. New York: Oxford, 2000.
Levy ML, Masri LS, Levy KM, et al. Penetrating craniocerebral injury resultant from gunshot wounds: Gang-related injury in children and adolescents. Neurosurgery 1993;33:1018.
Lewis RJ, Yee L, Inkelis SH, et al. Clinical predictors of post-traumatic seizures in children with head trauma. Ann Emerg Med 1993;22:1114.
Lieh-Lai MW, Theodorou AA, Sarnaik AP, et al. Limitations of the Glasgow Coma Scale in predicting outcome in children with traumatic brain injury. J Pediatr 1992;120:195.
Lloyd DA, Carty H, Patterson M, et al. Predictive value of skull radiography for intracranial injury in children with blunt head injury. Lancet 1997;349:821.
Lombroso CT. Can early postnatal closed head injury induce cortical dysplasia? Epilepsia 2000;41:245.
Loring DW, Meador KJ. Cognitive side effects of antiepileptic drugs in children. Neurology 2004;62:872.
Luerssen TG. Head injuries in children. Neurosurg Clin N Am 1991;2:399.
Luerssen TG, Klauber MR, Marshall LF. Outcome from head injury related to patient's age. A longitudinal prospective study of adult and pediatric head injury. J Neurosurg 1988;68:409.
Luis CA, Mittenberg W. Mood and anxiety disorders following pediatric traumatic brain injury: A prospective study. J Clin Exp Neuropsychol 2002;24:270.
Magistretti PJ, Pellerin L, Rothman DL, et al. Energy on demand. Science 1999;283:496.
Mahapatra AK, Tandon DA. Traumatic optic neuropathy in children: A prospective study. Pediatr Neurosurg 1993;19:34.
Margulies SS, Thibault KL. Infant skull and suture properties: Measurements and implications for mechanisms of pediatric brain injury. J Biomech Eng 2000;122:364.

Marin-Padilla M, Parisi JE, Armstrong DL, et al. Shaken infant syndrome: Developmental neuropathology, progressive cortical dysplasia, and epilepsy. Acta Neuropathol (Berl) 2002;103:321.

Marion DW, Obrist WD, Carlier PM, et al. The use of moderate therapeutic hypothermia for patients with severe head injuries: A preliminary report. J Neurosurg 1993;79:354.

Marion DW, Penrod LE, Kelsey SF, et al. Treatment of traumatic brain injury with moderate hypothermia. N Engl J Med 1997;336:540.

Marmarou A, Anderson RL, Ward JD, et al. Impact of ICP instability and hypotension on outcome in patients with severe head trauma. J Neurosurg 1991;75:S59.

Marshall LF, Smith RW, Rauscher LA, et al. Mannitol dose requirements in brain-injured patients. J Neurosurg 1978;48:169.

Marshall LF, Smith RW, Shapiro HM. The outcome with aggressive treatment in severe head injuries. Part I: The significance of intracranial pressure monitoring. J Neurosurg 1979;50:20.

Martin LD, Bratton SL, Quint P, et al. Prospective documentation of sedative, analgesic, and neuromuscular blocking agent use in infants and children in the intensive care unit: A multicenter perspective. Pediatr Crit Care Med 2001;2:205.

Massagli TL, Jaffe KM, Fay GC, et al. Neurobehavioral sequelae of severe pediatric traumatic brain injury: A cohort study. Arch Phys Med Rehabil 1996a;77:223.

Massagli TL, Michaud LJ, Rivara FP. Association between injury indices and outcome after severe traumatic brain injury in children. Arch Phys Med Rehabil 1996b;77:125.

Matser EJ, Kessels AG, Lezak MD, et al. Neuropsychological impairment in amateur soccer players. JAMA 1999;282:971.

Max JE, Lansing AE, Koele SL, et al. Attention deficit hyperactivity disorder in children and adolescents following traumatic brain injury. Dev Neuropsychol 2004;25:159.

Max JE, Lindgren SD, Knutson C, et al. Child and adolescent traumatic brain injury: Psychiatric findings from a paediatric outpatient specialty clinic. Brain Inj 1997;11:699.

Maxwell WL, Graham DI. Loss of axonal microtubules and neurofilaments after stretch-injury to guinea pig optic nerve fibers. J Neurotrauma 1997;14:603.

Maxwell WL, Povlishock JT, Graham DL. A mechanistic analysis of nondisruptive axonal injury: A review [published erratum appears in J Neurotrauma 1997 Oct;14(10):755]. J Neurotrauma 1997;14:419.

McAllister TW, Saykin AJ, Flashman LA, et al. Brain activation during working memory 1 month after mild traumatic brain injury: A functional MRI study. Neurology 1999;53:1300.

McCarthy ML, Serpi T, Kufera JA, et al. Factors influencing admission among children with a traumatic brain injury. Acad Emerg Med 2002;9:684.

McCrea M, Guskiewicz KM, Marshall SW, et al. Acute effects and recovery time following concussion in collegiate football players: The NCAA Concussion Study. JAMA 2003;290:2556.

McCrory P, Collie A, Anderson V, et al. Can we manage sport-related concussion in children the same as in adults? Br J Sport Med 2004;38:516.

McCrory P, Johnston K, Meeuwisse W, et al. Summary and aggreement statement of the 2nd International Conference on Concussion in Sport, Prague 2004. Clin J Sport Med 2005;15:48.

McCrory PR, Berkovic SF. Second impact syndrome. Neurology 1998;50:677.

McDonald CM, Jaffe KM, Fay GC, et al. Comparison of indices of traumatic brain injury severity as predictors of neurobehavioral outcome in children. Arch Phys Med Rehabil 1994;75:328.

McGraw CP. A cerebral perfusion pressure greater than 80 mmHg is more beneficial. In: Hoff JT, Betz AL, eds. Intracranial pressure VII. Berlin: Springer-Verlag, 1989.

McGraw CP, Alexander E Jr, Howard G. Effect of dose and dose schedule on the response of intracranial pressure to mannitol. Surg Neurol 1978;10:127.

McManus ML, Soriano SG. Rebound swelling of astroglial cells exposed to hypertonic mannitol. Anesthesiology 1998;88:1586.

Mendelow AD, Teasdale GM, Russell T, et al. Effect of mannitol on cerebral blood flow and cerebral perfusion pressure in human head injury. J Neurosurg 1985;63:43.

Miller JD, Becker DP, Ward JD, et al. Significance of intracranial hypertension in severe head injury. J Neurosurg 1977;47:503.

Miller LP, Johnson AE, Gelhard RE, et al. The ontogeny of excitatory amino acid receptors in the rat forebrain. II. Kainic acid receptors. Neuroscience 1990;35:45.

Muizelaar JP, Lutz HA, III, Becker DP. Effect of mannitol on ICP and CBF and correlation with pressure autoregulation in severely head-injured patients. J Neurosurg 1984;61:700.

Muizelaar JP, Marmarou A, DeSalles AA, et al. Cerebral blood flow and metabolism in severely head-injured children. Part 1: Relationship with GCS score, outcome, ICP, and PVI. J Neurosurg 1989;71:63.

Muizelaar JP, Wei EP, Kontos HA, et al. Mannitol causes compensatory cerebral vasoconstriction and vasodilation in response to blood viscosity changes. J Neurosurg 1983;59:822.

Muizelaar JP, Wei EP, Kontos HA, et al. Cerebral blood flow is regulated by changes in blood pressure and in blood viscosity alike. Stroke 1986;17:44.

Multi-Society Task Force on Persistent Vegetative State. Medical aspects of the persistent vegetative state (2). The Multi-Society Task Force on PVS. N Engl J Med. 1994;330:1572 and 1994;330:1499.

Murgio A, Andrade FA, Sanchez Munoz MA, et al. International Multicenter Study of Head Injury in Children. ISHIP Group. Childs Nerv Syst 1999;15:318.

Murgio A, Patrick PD, Andrade FA, et al. International study of emergency department care for pediatric traumatic brain injury and the role of CT scanning. Childs Nerv Syst 2001;17:257.

Nakayama S, Kramer GC, Carlsen RC, et al. Infusion of very hypertonic saline to bled rats: Membrane potentials and fluid shifts. J Surg Res 1985;38:180.

Nara I, Shiogai T, Hara M, et al. Comparative effects of hypothermia, barbiturate, and osmotherapy for cerebral oxygen metabolism, intracranial pressure, and cerebral perfusion pressure in patients with severe head injury. Acta Neurochir Suppl 1998;71:22.

Narayan RK, Greenberg RP, Miller JD, et al. Improved confidence of outcome prediction in severe head injury. A comparative analysis of the clinical examination, multimodality evoked potentials, CT scanning, and intracranial pressure. J Neurosurg 1981;54:751.

Narayan RK, Kishore PR, Becker DP, et al. Intracranial pressure: To monitor or not to monitor? A review of our experience with severe head injury. J Neurosurg 1982;56:650.

Nehlig A. Brain uptake and metabolism of ketone bodies in animal models. Prostaglandins Leukot Essent Fatty Acids 2004;70:265.

Nilsson P, Hillered L, Olsson Y, et al. Regional changes in interstitial K+ and Ca2+ levels following cortical compression contusion trauma in rats. J Cereb Blood Flow Metab 1993;13:183.

Nilsson P, Laursen H, Hillered L, et al. Calcium movements in traumatic brain injury: The role of glutamate receptor-operated ion channels. J Cereb Blood Flow Metab 1996;16:262.

Ohyu J, Takashima S. Developmental characteristics of neuronal nitric oxide synthase (nNOS) immunoreactive neurons in fetal to adolescent human brains. Brain Res Dev Brain Res 1998;110:193.

Okada PJ, Young KD, Baren JM, et al. Neurologic outcome score for infants and children. Acad Emerg Med 2003;10:1034.

Olney JW, Wozniak DF, Jevtovic-Todorovic V, et al. Drug-induced apoptotic neurodegeneration in the developing brain. Brain Pathol 2002;12:488.

Ong L, Selladurai BM, Dhillon MK, et al. The prognostic value of the Glasgow Coma Scale, hypoxia and computerised tomography in outcome prediction of pediatric head injury. Pediatr Neurosurg 1996;24:285.

Osteen CL, Giza CC, Hovda DA. Injury-induced alterations in N-methyl-D-aspartate receptor subunit composition contribute to prolonged (45)calcium accumulation following lateral fluid percussion. Neuroscience 2004;128:305.

Osteen CL, Moore AH, Prins ML, et al. Age-dependency of 45calcium accumulation following lateral fluid percussion: Acute and delayed patterns. J Neurotrauma 2001;18:141.

Parke TJ, Stevens JE, Rice AS, et al. Metabolic acidosis and fatal myocardial failure after propofol infusion in children: Five case reports. BMJ 1992;305:613.

Paus T, Collins DL, Evans AC, et al. Maturation of white matter in the human brain: A review of magnetic resonance studies. Brain Res Bull 2001;54:255.

Pellerin L, Magistretti PJ. Neuroenergetics: Calling upon astrocytes to satisfy hungry neurons. Neuroscientist 2004;10:53.

Pellman EJ, Viano DC, Tucker AM, et al. Concussion in professional football: Reconstruction of game impacts and injuries. Neurosurgery 2003;53:799.

Peterson B, Khanna S, Fisher B, et al. Prolonged hypernatremia controls elevated intracranial pressure in head-injured pediatric patients. Crit Care Med 2000;28:1136.

Pettus EH, Povlishock JT. Characterization of a distinct set of intra-axonal ultrastructural changes associated with traumatically induced alteration in axolemmal permeability. Brain Res 1996;722:1.

Pfenninger J, Kaiser G, Lutschg J, et al. Treatment and outcome of the severely head injured child. Intensive Care Med 1983;9:13.

Piatt JH, Jr., Schiff SJ. High dose barbiturate therapy in neurosurgery and intensive care. Neurosurgery 1984;15:427.

Pigula FA, Wald SL, Shackford SR, et al. The effect of hypotension and hypoxia on children with severe head injuries. J Pediatr Surg 1993;28:310.

Pillai S, Praharaj SS, Mohanty A, et al. Prognostic factors in children with severe diffuse brain injuries: A study of 74 patients. Pediatr Neurosurg 2001;34:98.

Pittman T, Bucholz R, Williams D. Efficacy of barbiturates in the treatment of resistant intracranial hypertension in severely head-injured children. Pediatr Neurosci 1989;15:13.

Plum F, Posner JB. The diagnosis of stupor and coma, 3rd ed. Philadelphia: Davis, 1980.

Pohl D, Bittigau P, Ishimaru MJ, et al. N-methyl-D-aspartate antagonists and apoptotic cell death triggered by head trauma in developing rat brain. Proc Natl Acad Sci U S A 1999;96:2508.

Polin RS, Shaffrey ME, Bogaev CA, et al. Decompressive bifrontal craniectomy in the treatment of severe refractory posttraumatic cerebral edema. Neurosurgery 1997;41:84.

Polissar NL, Fay GC, Jaffe KM, et al. Mild pediatric traumatic brain injury: Adjusting significance levels for multiple comparisons. Brain Inj 1994;8:249.

Ponsford J, Willmott C, Rothwell A, et al. Cognitive and behavioral outcome following mild traumatic head injury in children. J Head Trauma Rehabil 1999;14:360.

Povlishock JT, Christman CW. The pathobiology of traumatically induced axonal injury in animals and humans: A review of current thoughts. J Neurotrauma 1995;12:555.

Povlishock JT, Pettus EH. Traumatically induced axonal damage: Evidence for enduring changes in axolemmal permeability with associated cytoskeletal change. Acta Neurochir Suppl (Wien) 1996;66:81.

Powell JW, Barber-Foss KD. Traumatic brain injury in high school athletes. JAMA 1999;282:958.

Prange MT, Coats B, Duhaime AC, et al. Anthropomorphic simulations of falls, shakes, and inflicted impacts in infants. J Neurosurg 2003;99:143.

Prins ML, Hovda DA. Traumatic brain injury in the developing rat: Effects of maturation on Morris water maze acquisition. J Neurotrauma 1998;15:799.

Prins ML, Lee SM, Cheng CL, et al. Fluid percussion brain injury in the developing and adult rat: A comparative study of mortality, morphology, intracranial pressure and mean arterial blood pressure. Brain Res Dev Brain Res 1996;95:272.

Prins ML, Lee SM, Fujima LS, et al. Increased cerebral uptake and oxidation of exogenous betaHB improves ATP following traumatic brain injury in adult rats. J Neurochem 2004;90:666.

Prins ML, Povlishock JT, Phillips LL. The effects of combined fluid percussion traumatic brain injury and unilateral entorhinal deafferentation on the juvenile rat brain. Brain Res Dev Brain Res 2003;140:93.

Quayle KS, Jaffe DM, Kuppermann N, et al. Diagnostic testing for acute head injury in children: When are head computed tomography and skull radiographs indicated? Pediatrics 1997;99:E11.

Qureshi AI, Suarez JI. Use of hypertonic saline solutions in treatment of cerebral edema and intracranial hypertension. Crit Care Med 2000;28:3301.

Raghupathi R, Margulies SS. Traumatic axonal injury after closed head injury in the neonatal pig. J Neurotrauma 2002;19:843.

Ratan SK, Kulshreshtha R, Pandey RM. Predictors of posttraumatic convulsions in head-injured children. Pediatr Neurosurg 1999;30:127.

Reid SR, Roesler JS, Gaichas AM, et al. The epidemiology of pediatric traumatic brain injury in Minnesota. Arch Pediatr Adolesc Med 2001;155:784.

Rivara FP. Epidemiology and prevention of pediatric traumatic brain injury. Pediatr Ann 1994;23:12.

Roberts I, Yates D, Sandercock P, et al. Effect of intravenous corticosteroids on death within 14 days in 10008 adults with clinically significant head injury (MRC CRASH trial): Randomised placebo-controlled trial. Lancet 2004;364:1321.

Roberts MA, Manshadi FF, Bushnell DL, et al. Neurobehavioural dysfunction following mild traumatic brain injury in childhood: A case report with positive findings on positron emission tomography (PET). Brain Inj 1995;9:427.

Robertson CS, Valadka AB, Hannay HJ, et al. Prevention of secondary ischemic insults after severe head injury. Crit Care Med 1999;27:2086.

Robinson LR, Micklesen PJ, Tirschwell DL, et al. Predictive value of somatosensory evoked potentials for awakening from coma. Crit Care Med 2003;31:960.

Rosenzweig MR, Bennett EL. Psychobiology of plasticity: Effects of training and experience on brain and behavior. Behav Brain Res 1996;78:57.

Rosner MJ, Rosner SD, Johnson AH. Cerebral perfusion pressure: Management protocol and clinical results. J Neurosurg 1995;83:949.

Rudis MI, Guslits BJ, Peterson EL, et al. Economic impact of prolonged motor weakness complicating neuromuscular blockade in the intensive care unit. Crit Care Med 1996;24:1749.

Ruf B, Heckmann M, Schroth I, et al. Early decompressive craniectomy and duraplasty for refractory intracranial hypertension in children: Results of a pilot study. Crit Care 2003;7:R133.

Ruppel RA, Kochanek PM, Adelson PD, et al. Excitatory amino acid concentrations in ventricular cerebrospinal fluid after severe traumatic brain injury in infants and children: The role of child abuse. J Pediatr 2001;138:18.

Ryan CA, Edmonds J. Seizure activity mimicking brainstem herniation in children following head injuries. Crit Care Med 1988;16:812.

Salazar AM, Jabbari B, Vance SC, et al. Epilepsy after penetrating head injury. I. Clinical correlates: A report of the Vietnam Head Injury Study. Neurology 1985;35:1406.

Sanders MJ, Sick TJ, Perez-Pinzon MA, et al. Chronic failure in the maintenance of long-term potentiation following fluid percussion injury in the rat. Brain Res 2000;861:69.

Sanford RA. Minor head injury in children. Semin Neurol 1988;8:108.

Savitsky EA, Votey SR. Current controversies in the management of minor pediatric head injuries. Am J Emerg Med 2000;18:96.

Schutzman SA, Barnes P, Duhaime AC, et al. Evaluation and management of children younger than two years old with apparently minor head trauma: Proposed guidelines. Pediatrics 2001;107:983.

Schwartz ML, Tator CH, Rowed DW, et al. The University of Toronto head injury treatment study: A prospective, randomized comparison of pentobarbital and mannitol. Can J Neurol Sci 1984;11:434.

Shapiro K, Marmarou A. Clinical applications of the pressure-volume index in treatment of pediatric head injuries. J Neurosurg 1982;56:819.

Sharples PM, Stuart AG, Matthews DS, et al. Cerebral blood flow and metabolism in children with severe head injury. Part 1: Relation to age, Glasgow coma score, outcome, intracranial pressure, and time after injury. J Neurol Neurosurg Psychiatry 1995;58:145.

Shewmon DA. The minimally conscious state: Definition and diagnostic criteria. Neurology 2002;58:506.

Shiozaki T, Sugimoto H, Taneda M, et al. Effect of mild hypothermia on uncontrollable intracranial hypertension after severe head injury. J Neurosurg 1993;79:363.

Sihver S, Marklund N, Hillered L, et al. Changes in mACh, NMDA and GABA(A) receptor binding after lateral fluid- percussion injury: In vitro autoradiography of rat brain frozen sections. J Neurochem 2001;78:417.

Simma B, Burger R, Falk M, et al. A prospective, randomized, and controlled study of fluid management in children with severe head injury: Lactated Ringer's solution versus hypertonic saline. Crit Care Med 1998;26:1265.

Singh D, Kumar P, Majumdar S, et al. Effect of phenobarbital on free radicals in neonates with hypoxic ischemic encephalopathy: A randomized controlled trial. J Perinat Med 2004;32:278.

Skippen P, Seear M, Poskitt K, et al. Effect of hyperventilation on regional cerebral blood flow in head-injured children. Crit Care Med 1997;25:1402.

Smith HP, Kelly DL, Jr., McWhorter JM, et al. Comparison of mannitol regimens in patients with severe head injury undergoing intracranial monitoring. J Neurosurg 1986;65:820.

Sowell ER, Thompson PM, Holmes CJ, et al. In vivo evidence for post-adolescent brain maturation in frontal and striatal regions. Nat Neurosci 1999;2:859.

Sowell ER, Thompson PM, Tessner KD, et al. Mapping continued brain growth and gray matter density reduction in dorsal frontal cortex: Inverse relationships during postadolescent brain maturation. J Neurosci 2001;21:8819.

Spitzfaden AC, Jimenez DF, Tobias JD. Propofol for sedation and control of intracranial pressure in children. Pediatr Neurosurg 1999;31:194.

Strauss DJ, Ashwal S, Day SM, et al. Life expectancy of children in vegetative and minimally conscious states. Pediatr Neurol 2000;23:312.

Suzuki K. The changes in regional cerebral blood flow with advancing age in normal children. Nagoya Med J 1990;34:159.

Taylor A, Butt W, Rosenfeld J, et al. A randomized trial of very early decompressive craniectomy in children with traumatic brain injury and sustained intracranial hypertension. Childs Nerv Syst 2001;17:154.

Taylor HG, Alden J. Age-related differences in outcomes following childhood brain insults: An introduction and overview. J Int Neuropsychol Soc 1997;3:555.

Taylor HG, Yeates KO, Wade SL, et al. A prospective study of short- and long-term outcomes after traumatic brain injury in children: Behavior and achievement. Neuropsychology 2002;16:15.

Teasdale G, Jennett B. Assessment of coma and impaired consciousness. A practical scale. Lancet 1974;2:81.

Teasdale GM, Murray G, Anderson E, et al. Risks of acute traumatic intracranial haematoma in children and adults: Implications for managing head injuries. BMJ 1990;300:363.

Tees RC, Buhrmann K, Hanley J. The effect of early experience on water maze spatial learning and memory in rats. Dev Psychobiol 1990;23:427.

Temkin NR, Dikmen SS, Wilensky AJ, et al. A randomized, double-blind study of phenytoin for the prevention of post-traumatic seizures. N Engl J Med 1990;323:497.

Thomas S, Prins ML, Samii M, et al. Cerebral metabolic response to traumatic brain injury sustained early in development: A 2-deoxy-D-glucose autoradiographic study [In Process Citation]. J Neurotrauma 2000;17:649.

Thurman DJ. Appendix B: Traumatic brain injury in children and youth as a public health problem. In: Langlios JA: Traumatic brain injury (TBI) in the United States: Assessing outcomes in children. Atlanta: National Center for Injury Prevention and Control of the Centers for Disease Control and Prevention, 2001.

Thurman DJ. Epidemiology and economics of head trauma. In: Miller LP, Hayes R, eds. Head trauma: Basic, preclinical and clinical directions. New York: Wiley-Liss, 2001.

Thurman DJ, Branche CM, Sniezek JE. The epidemiology of sports-related traumatic brain injuries in the United States: Recent developments. J Head Trauma Rehabil 1998;13:1.

Tilford JM, Simpson PM, Yeh TS, et al. Variation in therapy and outcome for pediatric head trauma patients. Crit Care Med 2001;29:1056.

Tipps LB, Coplin WM, Murry KR, et al. Safety and feasibility of continuous infusion of remifentanil in the neurosurgical intensive care unit. Neurosurgery 2000;46:596.

Tomberg T, Rink U, Pikkoja E, et al. Computerized tomography and prognosis in paediatric head injury. Acta Neurochir (Wien) 1996;138:543.

Tong KA, Ashwal S, Holshouser BA, et al. Diffuse axonal injury in children: Clinical correlation with hemorrhagic lesions. Ann Neurol 2004;56:36.

Tong KA, Ashwal S, Holshouser BA, et al. Hemorrhagic shearing lesions in children and adolescents with posttraumatic diffuse axonal injury: Improved detection and initial results. Radiology 2003;227:332.

Trauner DA, Chase C, Walker P, et al. Neurologic profiles of infants and children after perinatal stroke. Pediatr Neurol 1993;9:383.

Tsai WC, Chiu WT, Chiou HY, et al. Pediatric traumatic brain injuries in Taiwan: An 8-year study. J Clin Neurosci 2004;11:126.

Umile EM, Sandel ME, Alavi A, et al. Dynamic imaging in mild traumatic brain injury: Support for the theory of medial temporal vulnerability. Arch Phys Med Rehabil 2002;83:1506.

van den Heever CM, van der Merwe DJ. Management of depressed skull fractures. Selective conservative management of nonmissile injuries. J Neurosurg 1989;71:186.

Vannucci RC, Vannucci SJ. Glucose metabolism in the developing brain. Semin Perinatol 2000;24:107.

Vavilala MS, Lee LA, Boddu K, et al. Cerebral autoregulation in pediatric traumatic brain injury. Pediatr Crit Care Med 2004;5:257.

Venable N, Pinto-Hamuy T, Arraztoa JA, et al. Greater efficacy of preweaning than postweaning environmental enrichment on maze learning in adult rats. Behav Brain Res 1988;31:89.

Vespa PM, McArthur D, O'Phelan K, et al. Persistently low extracellular glucose correlates with poor outcome 6 months after human traumatic brain injury despite a lack of increased lactate: A microdialysis study. J Cereb Blood Flow Metab 2003;23:865.

Vespa PM, Nuwer MR, Nenov V, et al. Increased incidence and impact of nonconvulsive and convulsive seizures after traumatic brain injury as detected by continuous electroencephalographic monitoring. J Neurosurg 1999;91:750.

Vespa P, Prins M, Ronne-Engstrom E, et al. Increase in extracellular glutamate caused by reduced cerebral perfusion pressure and seizures after human traumatic brain injury: A microdialysis study. J Neurosurg 1998;89:971.

Villablanca JR, Hovda DA. Developmental neuroplasticity in a model of cerebral hemispherectomy and stroke. Neuroscience 1999;95:625.

Volkmar FR, Greenough WT. Rearing complexity affects branching of dendrites in the visual cortex of the rat. Science 1972;176:1145.

von Helden A, Schneider GH, Unterberg A, et al. Monitoring of jugular venous oxygen saturation in comatose patients with subarachnoid haemorrhage and intracerebral haematomas. Acta Neurochir Suppl (Wien) 1993;59:102.

Wang MY, Griffith P, Sterling J, et al. A prospective population-based study of pediatric trauma patients with mild alterations in consciousness (Glasgow Coma Scale score of 13-14). Neurosurgery 2000;46:1093.

Wass CT, Lanier WL, Hofer RE, et al. Temperature changes of > or = 1 degree C alter functional neurologic outcome and histopathology in a canine model of complete cerebral ischemia. Anesthesiology 1995;83:325.

Weiner HL, Weinberg JS. Head injury in the pediatric age group. In: Cooper PR, Golfinos JG, eds. Head injury, 4th ed. New York: McGraw-Hill, 2000.

Weiss GH, Salazar AM, Vance SC, et al. Predicting posttraumatic epilepsy in penetrating head injury. Arch Neurol 1986;43:771.

Williams BM, Luo Y, Ward C, et al. Environmental enrichment: Effects on spatial memory and hippocampal CREB immunoreactivity. Physiol Behav 2001;73:649.

Wilson S, Raghupathi R, Saatman KE, et al. Continued in situ DNA fragmentation of microglia/macrophages in white matter weeks and months after traumatic brain injury. J Neurotrauma 2004;21:239.

Wright RL. Traumatic hematomas of the posterior cranial fossa. J Neurosurg 1966;25:402.

Yamamoto LG, Bart RD, Jr. Transient blindness following mild head trauma. Criteria for a benign outcome. Clin Pediatr (Phila) 1988;27:479.

Yeates KO, Swift E, Taylor HG, et al. Short- and long-term social outcomes following pediatric traumatic brain injury. J Int Neuropsychol Soc 2004;10:412.

Yeates KO, Taylor HG, Wade SL, et al. A prospective study of short- and long-term neuropsychological outcomes after traumatic brain injury in children. Neuropsychology 2002;16:514.

Yoshino A, Hovda DA, Kawamata T, et al. Dynamic changes in local cerebral glucose utilization following cerebral contusion in rats: Evidence of a hyper- and subsequent hypometabolic state. Brain Res 1991;561:106.

Young B, Rapp RP, Norton JA, et al. Failure of prophylactically administered phenytoin to prevent late posttraumatic seizures. J Neurosurg 1983;58:236.

Young RS, Zalneraitis EL, Dooling EC. Neurological outcome in cold water drowning. JAMA 1980;244:1233.

Zwienenberg M, Muizelaar JP. Severe pediatric head injury: The role of hyperemia revisited. J Neurotrauma 1999;16:937.

CHAPTER 63

Inflicted Childhood Neurotrauma

Elizabeth E. Gilles and Ann-Christine Duhaime

Inflicted head injury is a form of traumatic brain injury resulting from assault. Despite increasing prevention efforts, it remains a major cause of morbidity and mortality among children [Aldrich et al., 1992; Bonnier et al., 1995; Duhaime et al., 1996b; Gilles and Nelson, 1998; Irazuzta et al., 1997]. Infants with inflicted head injuries have the most severe illness, the highest mortality risk, and the worst outcome in comparison with other forms of childhood trauma [Goldstein et al., 1993b; Gilles and Nelson, 1998; Irazuzta et al., 1997; Pfenninger and Santi, 2002; Rivara et al., 1996]. Children younger than 3 years, particularly those younger than 1 year, are at highest risk for inflicted neurotrauma [Duhaime et al., 1998]. In one study, the incidence of inflicted head injury among children younger than 2 years was 17 per 100,000 children [Keenan et al., 2003]. Other studies suggest that as many as 60% of deaths resulting from abuse or neglect are not recorded [Crume et al., 2002].

TERMINOLOGY

Inflicted and *nonaccidental childhood neurotrauma* are used in this chapter as inclusive terms to describe the range of craniospinal injuries sustained by infants and young children as a consequence of violent assault by parents or other caretakers. *Unintentional* or *accidental head injury* refers to injury sustained by chance and unrelated to specific deliberate actions of caretakers.

The terms *shaken baby syndrome* and *shaken-impact infant syndrome* imply a uniform injury event sequence, mechanism of injury, and age at time of injury that belie the actual complexity of injury and postinjury event sequences [Budenz et al., 1994; Duhaime et al., 1987; Gilles and Nelson, 1998]. Popularization of this simplistic terminology has led to at least two types of errors. First, overly simplistic analyses of clinical and imaging data can result in either overdiagnosis or underdiagnosis of abuse. Second, there is a tendency to rely on symptoms common to accidental injuries, such as the presence of impact evidence, as well as the absence of retinal hemorrhages, to prove a child was not shaken when, in fact, there is clear and convincing evidence.

HISTORICAL PERSPECTIVE

The acceptance of inflicted head injury as an age-related subtype of traumatic brain injury and of physical abuse is a relatively recent phenomenon, although descriptions of this disorder were made at least as early as the 19th century [Tardiéu, 1860]. Tardiéu was the first to document the range of injury patterns found in abused and neglected children as distinct from those in adults and to link them to caregiver actions.

Although a number of researchers independently associated fractures, subdural hematomas, and retinal hemorrhages in infants with trauma starting in the 1920s, association of these findings with caregiver actions was not made clearly until the 1950s [Caffey, 1972, 1974; Frauenberger and Lis, 1950; Guthkelch, 1971; Kempe et al., 1962; Lindenberg and Freytag, 1969; Silverman, 1952; Woolley and Evans, 1955].

Recognizing that the history offered by the caregiver was biomechanically inconsistent with the severity of injury was an important step in accepting inflicted neurotrauma as a distinct form of trauma [Billmire and Myers, 1985; Duhaime et al., 1987, 1992; Goldstein et al., 1993b; Weston, 1973]. Few authors have specifically addressed the discrepancies between initial historical data and subsequent caregiver admissions [Gilles and Nelson, 1998; Tardiéu, 1860; Weston, 1973].

John Kempe coined the term *battered child syndrome* to describe severe physical abuse with fractures, bruises, failure to thrive, brain injury, and subdural hematomas [Kempe et al., 1962]. Subsequently, Guthkelch [1971] and Caffey [1972, 1974] independently hypothesized that head injury in the absence of obvious blunt force trauma was caused by whiplash shaking of the infant's head by the caregiver. In 1974, Caffey coined the term *shaken baby syndrome* for infants who had severe head injuries but lacked signs of blunt force trauma on imaging studies.

Inflicted childhood neurotrauma has increasingly become the focus of investigation in both clinical and laboratory studies. It is important to realize that the majority of the relevant literature is observational and retrospective in nature. Most studies have failed to specify explicit inclusion or exclusion criteria and have accepted with minimal or no question histories obtained from perpetrators [Weston, 1973; Chadwick et al., 1991].

DEVELOPMENTAL DIFFERENCES PREDISPOSING THE IMMATURE NEURAXIS TO INJURY

Structural and functional changes of central and peripheral nervous system organization and function are greatest during the first 2 years of life, when nonaccidental head injury occurs most frequently [Brody et al., 1987; Duhaime et al., 1987; Kinney et al., 1988; Lenn, 1987]. A number of biologic and mechanical factors predispose the infant and young child to injury of the craniospinal axis (Box 63-1).

Box 63-1 Biologic and Mechanical Features Predisposing the Infant to Head Injury

Biomechanical Factors
- Large head-to-body ratio
- Proportionally heavy head in relation to body mass and neck strength
- Greater skull compliance
- Anatomy of inner skull table (smoother in younger infants)
- More firmly attached dura

Neuroanatomic Factors
- Immature brain (incomplete myelination)
- Increased brain water content
- Increased excitotoxicity
- Increased synaptic density
- Increased excitatory amino acid receptors
- Decreased inhibitory networks

Mechanical Factors

Although a larger head-to-body ratio than in adults and less developed neck and shoulder girdle musculature render the infant more vulnerable to significant applied forces, the immature brain is, in some ways, more resistant to injury than is the adult brain.

The smaller head requires larger rotational input for the same force as a larger brain, and the higher water content makes the brain more resistant to deformation. These features reinforce the observation that trivial trauma does not appear sufficient to cause the kinds of injuries seen in the context of abuse [Brody et al., 1987; Prange et al., 2003]. Incomplete myelination and increased percentage of brain fluid also contribute to distensibility and compliance of brain tissue during injury events [Brody et al., 1987]. The infant has a relatively smooth inner cranial table and greater skull compliance [Carter and McCormick, 1983; Courville, 1965; Duhaime et al., 1992; Lindenberg and Freytag, 1969].

Biologic Factors

Many biologic factors are important to the immediate and subsequent responses of the immature central nervous system to injury. Mechanisms initiated by mechanical brain injury may enhance vulnerability to secondary ischemic brain damage [DeWitt et al., 1995; Novack et al., 1996; Teasdale and Graham, 1998]. Some factors are age-specific differences in cerebral autoregulation, as well as differences in the structure, number, and function of neuronal synapses and receptors [Armstead and Kurth, 1994; Azzarelli et al., 1996; Herlenius and Lagercrantz, 2004; Johnston, 1996; Lea and Faden, 2001; Ruppel et al., 2001]. Synaptic density in human infants is 50% to 60% above the adult mean, and *N*-methyl-D-aspartate (NMDA) and alpha-amino-3-hydroxy-5-methyl-4-isoxazole propionic acid (AMPA) excitatory amino acid receptors are increased [Huttenlocher, 1984; Johnston, 1995; Kubova and Moshe, 1994]. These receptors are functionally and structurally different from those of adults [Johnston, 1995; McDonald et al., 1992].

The immature central nervous system has structural and organizational differences in neuronal differentiation that decrease ischemic and seizure thresholds, in comparison with the mature central nervous system, particularly after trauma and hypoxic-ischemic injury [Adelson et al., 1997; D'Souza et al., 1992; Goldstein et al., 1993b; Johnston, 1996; Kubova and Moshe, 1994; Mares et al., 2004]. Neuronal and glial injury leads to excessive release of excitatory amino acids, which in turn trigger activation of immature NMDA and AMPA receptors in the hippocampus [Hagberg et al., 1993; Mares et al., 2004]. Excessive activation triggers excitotoxic injury via intracellular calcium-mediated events [Hablitz and Lee, 1992; Johnston, 1996; Kubova and Moshe, 1994; Teasdale and Graham, 1998]. The inhibitory amino acids γ-aminobutyric acid and glycine are excitatory in the developing brain [Herlenius and Lagercrantz, 2004]. Other mediators of secondary injury include inflammatory and excitotoxic mechanisms, oxidative stress, and apoptosis [Bittigau et al., 2003; Ruppel et al., 2002].

Developmental differences alone, however, fail to explain why children with inflicted head injury have more severe illness and a higher mortality risk than do children of the same age with unintentional head injury [Bell et al., 1997; Goldstein et al., 1993b; Haviland and Russell, 1997; Irazuzta et al., 1997]. When age is removed as a confounding variable, inflicted head injury still differs substantially from unintentional head injury [Haviland and Russell, 1997]. It is still unclear which features increase or decrease vulnerability of the immature brain to the various types and combinations of traumatic insults seen in the setting of inflicted injury, but they are the focus of much ongoing research [Duhaime et al., 2000, 2003; Durham et al., 2000b; Fan et al., 2003; Tong et al., 2002].

MECHANISMS OF INJURY

Child abuse is rarely premeditated. It occurs when caregivers lose control, often when trying to stop certain behavior (such as crying) or when punishing perceived transgressions (such as toileting accidents). Although many inflicted injuries are one-time events, children may have been subjected to repeated and complex injury scenarios occurring during a single day or as a series of events over days, weeks, or months [Alexander et al., 1990; Gilles and Nelson, 1998; Weston, 1973]. The sequence of injury events is highly variable. Injury events can include shaking, throwing, hitting, slapping, gagging, strangulation, and smothering [Bonnier et al., 1995; Duhaime et al., 1987; Gilles and Nelson, 1998]. Only children with injuries severe enough to frighten the caregiver are likely to be brought to medical attention. Resuscitation delay is also a potential factor, although not a uniform finding or unique to abuse [Adelson et al., 1997]. Presumably, resuscitation delay accentuates neuronal and biochemical ischemic cascades, which contribute to the severity of secondary neuronal injury [Gilles and Nelson, 1998; Goldstein et al., 1993b; Johnson et al., 1995].

Significant forces are required to cause severe inflicted injury [Duhaime et al., 1987; Prange et al., 2003]. In general, greater applied forces result in more severe injuries, regardless of whether the injury was inflicted. As with other tissues, brain injuries occur when applied forces strain the tissue beyond its structural or functional tolerance, or both. Primary mechanisms of injury include both impact and inertial forces. Impact forces occur at the surface of the scalp, skull, and brain as a result of contact. Inertial forces arise from head movement, when the head accelerates or decelerates. Inertial forces may be translational, when the head moves in a straight line, or rotational, also known as angular, when the head rotates around its center of gravity. The exact type and the magnitude of applied forces determine the severity of injury. Most severe primary brain injuries in the clinical world result from head contact, because the forces generated are much higher than those produced by noncontact mechanisms.

In the brain, the term *primary injury* refers to immediate, irreversible damage that occurs at the time of the insult. Secondary injuries potentiate primary injuries and occur as a consequence of the initial trauma, causing further damage to tissue that may have otherwise been viable. Examples include hypoperfusion/ischemia of brain tissue (from hypotension/shock), hypoxia, seizures, and parenchymal injury sustained when brain is compressed by an expanding mass lesion (e.g., clot).

Numerous metabolic and inflammatory cascades are triggered by trauma. Infants with inflicted head injury frequently have both diffuse and focal injury as a consequence of force dynamics generated during the primary injury events and secondary hypoxic-ischemic injury [Barlow and Minns, 1999; Gilles and Nelson, 1998; Johnson et al., 1995].

In severe inflicted head injury, it is thought that secondary hypoxic-ischemic injury is a significant contributing factor in the evolution of brain swelling and deleterious outcome [Aldrich et al., 1992; Ashwal et al., 1996; Biousse et al., 2002; Chesnut et al., 1993; Geddes et al., 2003; Goldstein et al., 1993b; Johnson et al., 1995; Pigula et al., 1993; Takahashi et al., 1993]. Differences in regional cerebral blood flow, autoregulatory mechanisms, and regional sensitivity to hypoxia all contribute to the extent of hypoxic-ischemic injury [Han et al., 1990; Takahashi et al., 1993]. Imaging features include cortical laminar necrosis, border zone infarctions, and cerebral atrophy (Fig. 63-1) [Liwnicz et al., 1987; Takahashi et al., 1993].

CLINICAL FEATURES

Symptoms

Acute Presentation

Regardless of age, there is a predictable pattern of brain response to mechanical trauma, whether blunt force, primarily angular acceleration-deceleration, or both. Studies have demonstrated that severe primary brain injuries result in immediate decrease in the level of consciousness and an apneustic response, associated with apnea and initial hypertension from catecholamine surge, followed by hypotension [Atkinson, 2000; Denny-Brown and Russell, 1941; Ommaya and Gennarelli, 1974]. The apneustic response results from primary disruption of cerebral circuits between the cerebral-brainstem reticular activating system and respiratory centers or between diencephalon-brainstem connections [Atkinson et al., 1998; Ommaya and Gennarelli, 1974; Willman et al., 1997]. Preliminary data suggest a lowered threshold to disruption of respiratory and cardiovascular drive mechanisms in moderate-to-severe head injury in the younger child [Adelson et al., 1997; Biswas et al., 2000; Goldstein et al., 1996].

Trauma-induced hypoxia and hypotension are strongly associated with adverse outcome in adults and children [Chesnut et al., 1993; Gilles and Nelson, 1998; Johnson et al., 1995; Takahashi et al., 1993]. Most infants with severe head injury, inflicted or not, experience apnea or altered

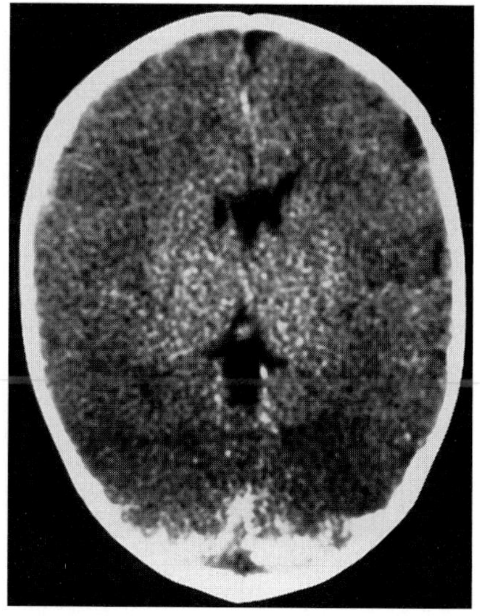
A

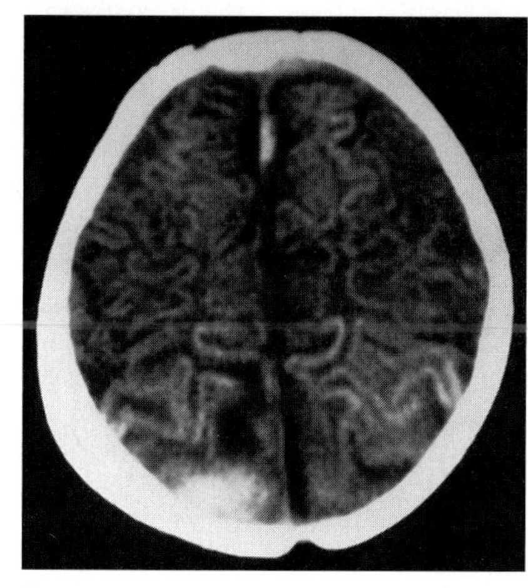
B

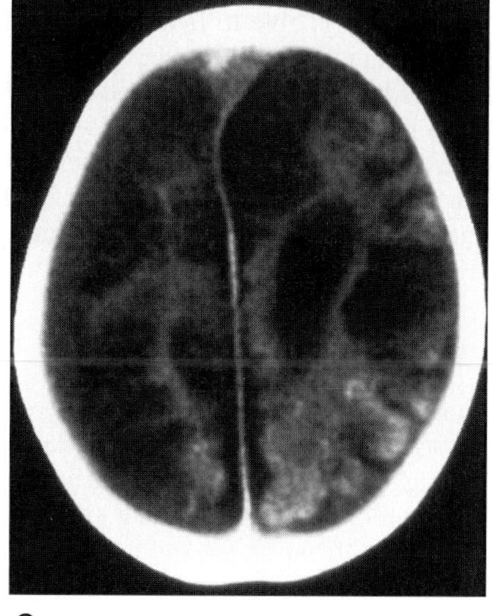
C

FIGURE 63-1. **A,** Nonenhanced computed tomographic (CT) scan of a 3-month-old child found limp and unconscious. The scan reveals diffuse cerebral hypoattenuation and thin bilateral convexity acute subdural hematoma. **B,** Nonenhanced CT scan of the same patient 10 days after admission, revealing laminar hyperdensity along the cerebral cortex, which is consistent with cortical laminar necrosis. **C,** Nonenhanced CT scan of same patient 6 months after injury. The patient is microcephalic with profound mental retardation, spastic quadriparesis, and post-traumatic epilepsy. The scan reveals diffuse cerebral atrophy.

respiration during or just after injury [Gilles and Nelson, 1998; Johnson et al., 1995; Kemp et al., 2003]. Hypotension develops frequently and is an index of neurologic insult and shock [Aldrich et al., 1992; Vavilala et al., 2003]. Apnea and hypotension can also be a response to smothering or to direct vessel compromise caused by strangulation [Bird et al., 1987, Gilles and Nelson, 1998; Glasier et al., 1987]. However, apnea or hypotension do not completely explain why one third of infants have hypodensity affecting one hemisphere, insofar as these processes would be expected to be symmetric [Duhaime et al., 1993; Gilles and Nelson, 1998] (see also "Swelling or Edema" section). Hemispheric hypodensity is generally observed subjacent to an ipsilateral subdural hematoma.

Symptoms of brain injury are nonspecific, varying by the severity of injury. The classic presentation is that of a previously healthy infant who suddenly decompensates neurologically and develops severe respiratory distress and flaccidity, with or without seizures or posturing (usually extensor) [Bonnier et al., 1995; Gilles and Nelson, 1998; Hadley et al., 1989; Johnson et al., 1995; Kemp et al., 2003]. This presentation varies considerably, however, but may be more common in younger infants.

Persistence of coma, apnea or respiratory distress, irritability, seizures, hypotonia, and vomiting reflects the severity of mechanical and physiologic disruptions and evolving secondary pathophysiologic cascades [Gilles and Nelson, 1998; Goldstein et al., 1993a; Johnson et al., 1995; Zuccarello et al., 1985]. Infants with increased intracranial pressure may have a bulging fontanel and diastatic sutures. Young children with inflicted brain injury develop the same patterns of brainstem abnormalities (pupils, eye movements, and breathing) as children and adults with severe unintentional brain injury [Atkinson et al., 1998; Gilles and Nelson, 1998; Hahn et al., 1988a; Johnson et al., 1995].

Infants who are severely injured cannot regulate behavior that requires higher cortical functions, such as coordinated action, eating, sitting, and walking. As Graham and colleagues [1989] noted, if an individual who sustains a head injury is able to talk, brain damage at the moment of injury cannot have been overwhelming. Less severely injured infants with concussive symptoms may exhibit a depressed level of consciousness, irritability, altered behavior, seizures, decreased feeding, vomiting, fever, and altered respiration. They may not appear sick enough for the perpetrator to seek medical attention. The accompanying caregiver may be unaware of the injury or may be the nondisclosing perpetrator.

EARLY POST-TRAUMATIC SEIZURES

Early post-traumatic seizures (those occurring in the first 72 to 96 hours after trauma) are more common in infants and young children with inflicted head injury than in older children or adults with unintentional head injury or cerebral infarction from other etiologies. Frequency ranges from 30% to 100% [Annegers et al., 1980; Bonnier et al., 1995; Gilles and Nelson, 1998; Goldstein et al., 1993b; Hadley et al., 1989; Hahn et al., 1988b; Johnson et al., 1995; Lewis et al., 1993; Ludwig and Warman, 1984]. Seizures correlate with age younger than 18 months, loss of consciousness, low Glasgow Coma Scale score, and abnormal computed tomographic (CT) scan [Gilles and Nelson, 1998; Hadley et al., 1989; Johnson et al., 1995; Lewis et al., 1993; Ludwig and Warman, 1984].

The majority of early post-traumatic seizures start in the first 24 hours after trauma, and although seizures can accompany injury events, extensor posturing is more common [Lewis et al., 1993]. Seizures are typically partial, partial complex, or partial with or without secondary generalization. Clinical signs may be subtle or even absent. Although the onset of symptoms generally correlates with the timing of injury, early post-traumatic seizures cannot and should not be used to time the injury events.

Early post-traumatic seizures may have potentially deleterious effects on the acute and subacute clinical course in the immature brain [Wasterlain et al., 2002]. They potentiate ischemic cascades by compromising oxygen and substrate delivery to neurons and, if unrecognized, can be the source of severe secondary injury. The high incidence of early post-traumatic seizures and the difficulties encountered in their control supports the early use of prophylactic antiepileptic medication in the child with severe inflicted closed-head injury, particularly if an infarction syndrome is suspected.

Subacute or Chronic Presentation

A child with chronic subdural hematomas may present with macrocephaly alone and look well. The true diagnosis in such children may be missed by conventional evaluation, and a level of suspicion is needed to suggest the appropriate evaluation, usually including magnetic resonance imaging (MRI) [Duhaime et al., 1998]. Other children present with a tense anterior fontanel; failure to thrive; developmental delay; and seizures, spasticity, or both [Ingraham and Heyl, 1939; Sherwood, 1930]. Anemia, recurrent vomiting, and a shrill cry are also frequent.

Sequelae of Inflicted Head Injury

Outcome data regarding inflicted childhood head injury have been accumulating since the 1950s. In contrast to the majority of children with severe unintentional head injury, who tend to be older and generally have better outcomes, infants tend to have a higher mortality rate and significant sequelae [Bonnier et al., 2003; Duhaime et al., 1987; Gilles and Nelson, 1998; Goldstein et al., 1993b; Hahn et al., 1988a; Johnson et al., 1995; Kemp et al., 2003]. Predictors of poor outcome are similar to those for other types of head injury, and include low scores on the Glasgow Coma Scale or other infant coma indexes, hyperglycemia, extensor posturing, lack of brainstem reflexes on presentation, and coma duration of more than 7 days (Box 63-2) [Durham et al., 2000a; Gjerris, 1986; Johnson et al., 1995; Prasad et al., 2002]. In inflicted head injury, the age at injury, severity of secondary insults, decreased cerebral perfusion pressure, and presence of focal lesions are other important factors [Barlow and Minns, 1999; Bonnier et al., 2003].

Visual impairment and behavioral, cognitive, and motor disabilities are common after inflicted head injury, and infants have an increased likelihood of developing post-traumatic epilepsy [Bonnier et al., 1995, 2003; Duhaime et al., 1996b; Ewing-Cobbs et al., 1999; Gilles and Nelson, 1998; Gilles et al., 2003; Haviland and Russell, 1997; Kemp et al.,

Box 63-2 Factors Affecting Severity of Injury

Types of injury events
- Biomechanical
  - Acceleration-deceleration
  - Translational
- Strangulation
- Smothering

Sequence of events
Single or multiple events
Other factors
- Duration of apnea, hypotension
- Delay in seeking medical care
- Level of consciousness at the time of the event or events
- Neuromuscular maturity of the child
- Antecedent dehydration and/or malnutrition
- Premorbid brain injury

2003]. The majority of such infants initially become macrocephalic, frequently with diastatic sutures and bulging fontanel. With time, in more severely injured children, cerebral atrophy and associated microcephaly develop with ex vacuo enlargement of the cerebrospinal fluid spaces [Bonnier et al., 2003; Gilles and Nelson, 1998; Lo et al., 2003]. On occasion, such children develop hydrocephalus. Long-term imaging anomalies include diffuse cortical atrophy, generalized white matter attenuation, multicystic encephalomalacia, porencephaly, and ulegyria [Bonnier et al., 2003; Geddes et al., 2001a; Marin-Padilla et al., 2002].

Sequelae of ocular pathology are numerous, with visual impairment found in 32% to 90% of patients [Gilles and Nelson, 1998; McCabe and Donahue, 2000; Riddoch and Goulden, 1925]. Cortical visual impairment contributes more to long-term visual deficits than do anterior visual defects [Poggi et al., 2000]. Small peripheral retinal hemorrhages resolve without compromising vision. Larger hemorrhages, however, especially those near or obscuring the macula, may affect central vision permanently [Ehrenfest, 1922].

Box 63-3 Nonaccidental Head Injury: Markers of Injury

Intracranial
- Extra-axial fluid collections
  - Subdural hematoma
  - Subarachnoid hemorrhage
  - Subdural effusions
- Brain injury
  - Brain swelling
  - Infarction syndromes
  - White matter contusional tears
  - Evidence of shearing injury
  - Diffuse axonal injury
- Skull fractures

Extracranial
- Scalp and soft tissues
  - Subgaleal hematoma
  - Cephalohematoma
  - Soft tissue swelling
  - Hair loss
  - Bruising
- Ear
  - Pinna bruising
  - Hemotympanum
  - Ruptured ear drum
- Ocular
  - Retinal hemorrhages
  - Retinal folds
  - Retinal detachment
  - Hyphema
  - Lens dislocation
- Mouth
  - Lip injury
  - Frenulum tear
  - Soft palate petechiae
  - Dental injury
- Other
  - Pattern bruising (e.g., from strangulation)
  - Long bone and rib fractures
  - Liver, kidney, or genital injury
  - Dehydration
  - Malnutrition
  - Burns
  - Excessive scarring

PATHOLOGY

About two thirds of abused children who die have lesions involving the craniospinal axis. The pathologic features parallel those found on the clinical and imaging examinations (see also "Clinical Assessment and Management" and "Radiographic Evaluation" sections). A full postmortem examination, including examination of the eyes, is mandatory for any child with an unexplained death [Case et al., 2001; Gilliland and Folberg, 1992]. This requirement is especially true in infants younger than 1 year, in whom the possibility of sudden infant death syndrome is actually stronger than that of inflicted head injury. Postmortem examination findings frequently assist in establishing an unintentional or inflicted etiology [Bass et al., 1986].

A broad range of physical findings is associated with inflicted head injury. Not all injuries have to be present to make the diagnosis, and no individual markers are pathognomonic of abusive injury. The major markers of injury are outlined in Box 63-3. In establishing the likelihood that the injuries resulted from inflicted versus unintentional mechanisms, the differential alternatives for each marker must be considered with the pattern of injuries as a whole, along with the history of injury.

Severe mechanical trauma to the developing neuraxis results in specific injuries. Particular findings that support more significant force generation are injuries to the neck and rostral spine (such as radicular avulsion), contusions or lacerations of the olfactory system (bulbs, tracts, and gyrus recti), partial or complete transection of the corpus callosum, tearing of the septum pellucidum, and acute neuronal necrosis on microscopy.

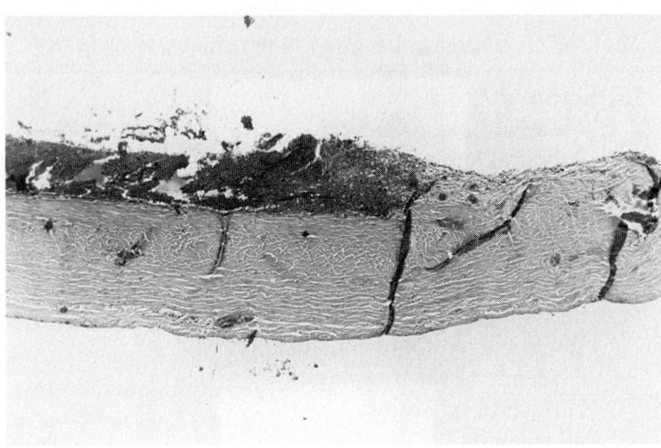

FIGURE 63-2. Gross photograph of an unstained section of retina, revealing a prominent sublaminar hemorrhage and multiple intraretinal hemorrhages.

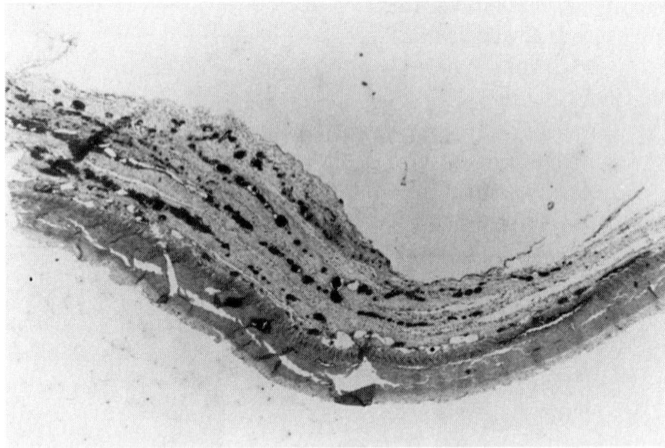

FIGURE 63-3. Retinal section stained for iron. This section came from an infant who died approximately 2 weeks after injury. Extensive resolving retinal hemorrhages are seen in multiple interretinal layers.

Aside from greatly assisting in documenting the full extent of injuries, the postmortem examination provides additional information about the pathologic timing of injury events. The presence of intra-alveolar siderophages, for instance, is suggestive of previously imposed suffocation [Becroft and Lockett, 1997]. Confirmation of specific findings, such as subdural neomembranes and positive retinal staining for hemosiderin and iron, can further assist in the timing of injuries (Figs. 63-2, 63-3, and 63-4). In instances in which the infant has been kept alive while brain death and resultant necrosis evolve, however, clinical timing of injury is typically more precise than is timing based on pathologic findings.

Ocular Pathology

Retinal Hemorrhages

A variety of injuries to the globe and optic nerve have been reported after inflicted injury, including retinoschisis, retinal folds, retinal detachment, periorbital edema and ecchymosis, subconjunctival hemorrhage, hyphema, and cataract [Buys et al., 1992; Gaynon et al., 1988; Greenwald et al., 1986; Massicotte et al., 1991; Mushin, 1971; Schloff et al., 2002]. Periorbital bleeding can result from either direct impact to the eye or a basilar fracture. Retinal and optic nerve sheath hemorrhages are the most common injuries. The frequency varies from 47% to 100% of all children with inflicted head trauma, depending on study inclusion criteria [Budenz et al., 1994; Buys et al., 1992; Duhaime et al., 1987; Elner et al., 1990; Gilliland et al., 1994; Laskey et al., 2004; Ophthalmology Child Abuse Working Party, 1999; Riffenburgh and Sathyavagiswaran, 1991; Schloff et al., 2002; Wilkinson et al., 1989].

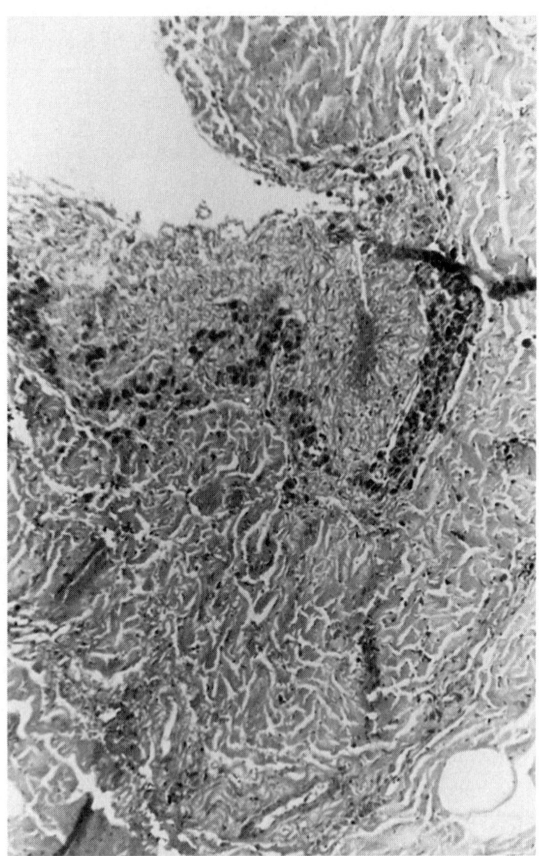

FIGURE 63-4. Hematoxylin and eosin stain photomicrograph of retina, revealing prominent hemosiderin-laden macrophages (*center*).

Retinal hemorrhages, if present, may be unilateral or bilateral, with variable appearance and distribution within the retina, and are often asymmetric (Figs. 63-5 and 63-6) [Betz et al., 1996; Elner et al., 1990; Gilles et al., 2003]. The terminology used to describe retinal hemorrhages is based on the location within the retinal layers (Table 63-1). They are most frequently found in the bipolar and nerve fiber layers [Riffenburgh and Sathyavagiswaran, 1991]. Controversy exists as to their terminology, pathogenesis, associations, and resolution.

Younger age and greater hypoxic-ischemic injury are correlated with more severe retinal hemorrhages [Gilliland et al., 1994; Matthews and Das, 1996; Riffenburgh and Sathyavagiswaran, 1991; Wilkinson et al., 1989]. Retinal hemorrhages are occasionally found in children after certain forms of nonsevere accidental head injury but are usually small and scattered hemorrhages, often occurring unilaterally, in an otherwise well-appearing child [Buys et al., 1992; Christian et al., 1999]. In four prospective studies,

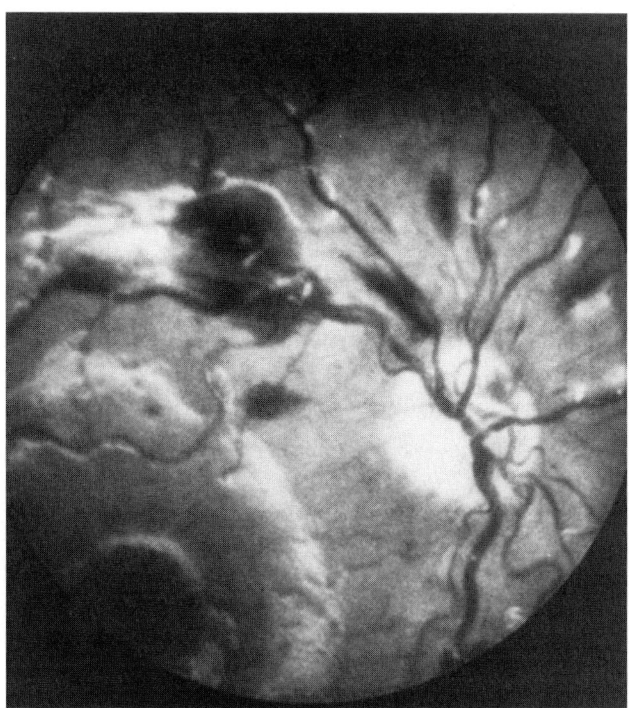

FIGURE 63-5. Nerve fiber layer and intraretinal layer retinal hemorrhages.

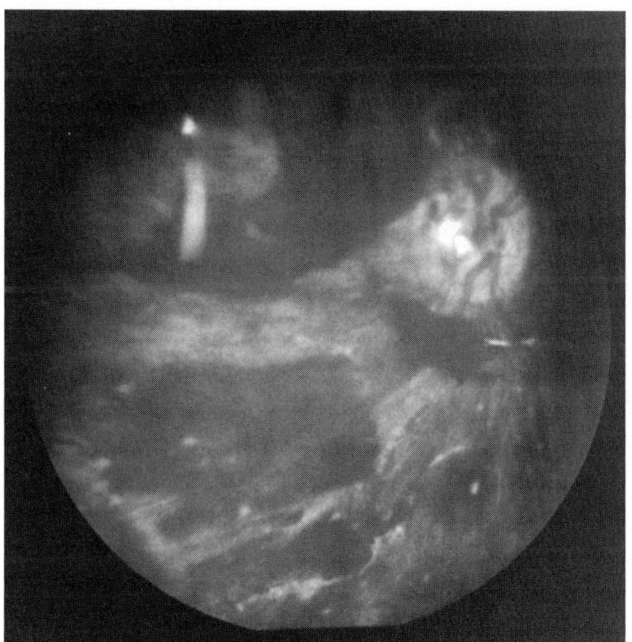

FIGURE 63-6. Extensive sublaminar and intraretinal layer retinal hemorrhages.

investigators examining a total of 290 children after accidental head injury found three children with retinal hemorrhages [Buys et al., 1992; Duhaime et al., 1992; Elder et al., 1991; Johnson et al., 1993]. Two of the three children with retinal hemorrhages were involved in side-impact car accidents [Johnson et al., 1993].

A pattern of severe, bilateral, diffuse retinal hemorrhages; retinal folds or retinoschisis; or detachment in a child with severe brain injury is highly suggestive but not pathognomonic for inflicted injury (see Fig. 63-6) [Bechtel et al., 2004; Mills, 1998; Rao et al., 1988]. This pattern is particularly suspect in the setting of a trivial mechanism of injury in an otherwise healthy child [Betz et al., 1996; Buys et al., 1992]. In contrast, these patterns have not been reported in the setting of a low-height fall in an otherwise healthy child; therefore, in this context, some workers consider these findings clearly indicative of abuse.

TABLE 63-1

Terminology for Retinal Hemorrhages

NAME	LOCATION
Vitreal	Vitreous
Subhyaloid (sublaminar or boat)	Preretinal
Intraretinal	
Flame or splinter	Nerve fiber layer
Dot (dot and blot)	Inner retinal layers (including bipolar)

The resolution rates of retinal hemorrhages after inflicted injury have not been studied systematically. The only large study is that of Pierre-Kahn and coworkers [2003], who prospectively monitored 231 children younger than 3 years who were admitted with subdural hematoma; they found that 88% of retinal hemorrhages resolved within 4 weeks. Most birth-related retinal hemorrhages are small and disappear within the first few days to 2 weeks after birth [Baum and Bulpitt, 1970; Ehrenfest, 1922; Emerson et al., 2001; Suzuki and Awaya, 1998]. Macular hemorrhages may take longer to resolve [Suzuki and Awaya, 1998].

THEORIES OF RETINAL HEMORRHAGE PATHOGENESIS

The pathogenesis of retinal and vitreal hemorrhages in infants with inflicted trauma is multifactorial and not yet understood. Several hypotheses have been proposed, with varying amounts of supportive data. These hypotheses include increased intracranial pressure, hydraulic forces, traumatic retinoschisis from deceleration forces, increased optic nerve sheath pressure, and anoxic injury [Gilles et al., 2003; Lyle et al., 1957; Massicotte et al., 1991]. Perhaps the strongest association is that with sudden intracranial hypertension, with or without intracranial hemorrhage, support for which dates back to the 1800s [de Schweinitz and Holoway, 1912; Ehrenfest, 1922; Hedges et al., 1964; Medele et al., 1998; Muller and Deck, 1974; Tureen, 1939].

Further support for the relationship between intracranial pressure and retinal hemorrhage pathogenesis comes from the observation that symmetry of retinal hemorrhages has been correlated to hemispheric intracranial pathologic processes (e.g., ipsilateral to acute subdural hematoma and regional brain swelling) in a variety of settings. The literature includes cases of unintentional and inflicted head injury in childhood and studies of adults after head injury or ruptured vascular malformations [Budenz et al., 1994; Christian et al., 1999; Drack et al., 1999; Giangiacomo et al., 1988; Gilles et al., 2003; Keane, 1979; Paviglianiti and Donahue, 1999; Shaikh et al., 2001; Shaw et al., 1977].

Cardiac compressions during cardiopulmonary resuscitation do not generate enough transmutive force to raise intracranial pressure and secondarily intraretinal pressure

[Fackler et al., 1992; Paradis et al., 1989]. Three studies documenting retinal examinations before or after death in more than 200 children who underwent either chest compressions or prolonged resuscitative efforts have failed to find an association between cardiopulmonary resuscitation and retinal hemorrhages [Budenz et al., 1994; Gilliland and Luckenbach, 1993; Kanter, 1986; Odom et al., 1997]. They do not appear to develop after seizures or Valsalva maneuvers [Herr et al., 2004; Sandramouli et al., 1997].

Optic Nerve Sheath Hemorrhage

The optic nerve sheath has dural and arachnoid components, with only the subarachnoid space in continuity with the subarachnoid spaces of the brain. Hemorrhages are found in both the subdural and potential subarachnoid space. The frequency of optic nerve sheath hemorrhages is unknown. They are found in 70% to 100% of children at postmortem examination but have not been identified accurately in the living child [Budenz et al., 1994; Elner et al., 1990; Duhaime et al., 1992; Gilliland et al., 1994; Lambert et al., 1986].

Optic nerve sheath hemorrhages are not specific to inflicted injury, having been reported secondary to sudden or prolonged increases in intracranial pressure (e.g., extensive subarachnoid hemorrhage) and, in rare cases, with unintentional head injury [de Schweinitz and Holoway, 1912; Elner et al., 1990; Muller and Deck, 1974; Munger et al., 1993; Weissgold et al., 1995]. Potential pathogenic mechanisms include local rupture of intradural vessels and bridging veins within the optic nerve sheath, injury to the optic nerve sheath with fracture of the base of the skull near the optic foramina, and spread of subarachnoid blood from the pericerebral subarachnoid space [Brinker et al., 1997; Elner et al., 1990; Muller and Deck, 1974; Munger et al., 1993].

Retinal and Optic Nerve Sheath Differential

Retinal and optic nerve sheath hemorrhages are found in numerous disorders. They have been reported most commonly in newborns but also with vascular malformations, coagulopathies, anemia, leukemia, meningitis, bacterial endocarditis, hypertension, infections, and papilledema [Carraro et al., 2001; Eisenbrey, 1979; Emerson et al., 2001; Kessler and Siegel-Stein, 1984; Marshman et al., 1999; Schloff et al., 2002; Sung et al., 2000; Weissgold et al., 1995]. Retinal hemorrhages have been reported in rare cases in children after unintentional head injury, such as high-speed motor vehicle accidents, in association with epidural hematoma, and after some falls [Buys et al., 1992; Christian et al., 1999; Elder et al., 1991; Vinchon et al., 2002]. When present in this setting, retinal hemorrhages are typically small and few in number [Betz et al., 1996]. They are not found after seizures [Mei-Zahav et al., 2002; Sandramouli et al., 1997]. Retinal hemorrhages in the presence of papilledema cannot be causally related to nonaccidental head injury. Finally, retinal hemorrhages are not usually found in the context of acute life-threatening events [Pitetti et al., 2002].

Extracranial Injuries

The most common extracranial impact injuries in inflicted injury are scalp bruising, soft tissue swelling, cephalohematoma, and subgaleal hematoma (Fig. 63-7) [Duhaime et al., 1987; Zimmerman et al., 1979]. Scalp bruising may be difficult to discern clinically [Atwal et al., 1998]. Atwal and associates found that facial and forehead bruising predominated in a series of fatal inflicted head injury, whereas limb and chest bruising were uncommon, which suggests that slapping or punching of the head, not gripping of the chest or arms and shaking, was more common. Subgaleal hematomas result from shearing injury to the scalp from impact or from a violent hair pulling [Hamlin, 1968]. At postmortem examination, evaluation of the reflected scalp allows for the identification of galeal hemorrhage and impact sites (periosteal hemorrhages). The temporalis muscle and posterior cervical muscles are additional sites where internal soft tissue injury is found.

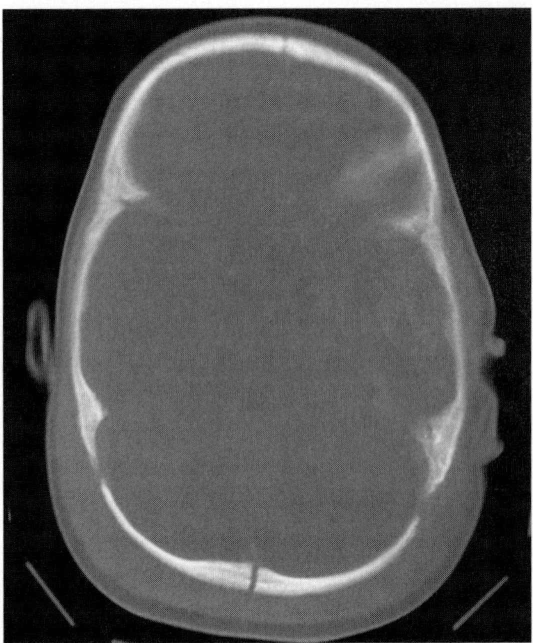

FIGURE 63-7. Occipital skull fracture extending into the foramen magnum in a 6-month-old infant. There is extensive subgaleal hematoma, seen here as soft tissue swelling around the occiput.

Skull Fractures

A variety of skull fractures have been reported after blunt trauma, regardless of etiology (see Fig. 63-7). As such, they are not specific to either unintentional or inflicted trauma [Greenes and Schutzman, 1997]. Depending on the study, between 25% and 74% of infants and children with inflicted neurotrauma sustain skull fractures [Case et al., 2001; Duhaime et al., 1992; Ewing-Cobbs et al., 2000; Geddes et al., 2001a; Rubin et al., 2003]. Simple linear fractures are the most common and tend to be parietal or occipital in location [Hobbs, 1984; Meservy et al., 1987; Rubin et al., 2003; Shane and Fuchs, 1997].

In general, fractures that are bilateral, comminuted, or multiple or that cross suture lines are more suggestive of infliction [Arnholz et al., 1998; Banaszkiewicz et al., 2002; Geddes et al., 2001a; Hobbs, 1984; Meservy et al., 1987; Shane and Fuchs, 1997]. Fractures in infants with open sutures do not usually cross suture lines. Bilateral or other multiple fractures usually indicate that more than one impact occurred but have also been reported after simultaneous, severe head compression between two unyielding surfaces or from direct occipital impacts [Arnholz et al., 1998; Hiss and Kahana, 1995]. In rare cases, complicated fractures occur after falls. Spinal trauma, although rare, has also been reported as the result of inflicted injury [Diamond et al., 1994; Ghatan and Ellenbogen, 2002; Ranjith et al., 1998; Rooks et al., 2002; Swischuk, 1969].

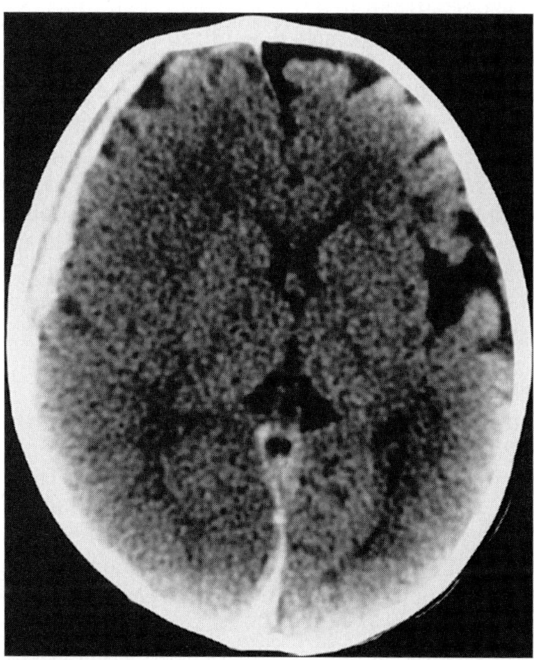

FIGURE 63-8. Nonenhanced computed tomographic scan of an 11-month-old infant admitted with acute loss of consciousness and apnea with no history of trauma. The scan, obtained shortly after arrival, demonstrates an acute right convexity subdural hematoma with ipsilateral hemispheric swelling and mild midline shift.

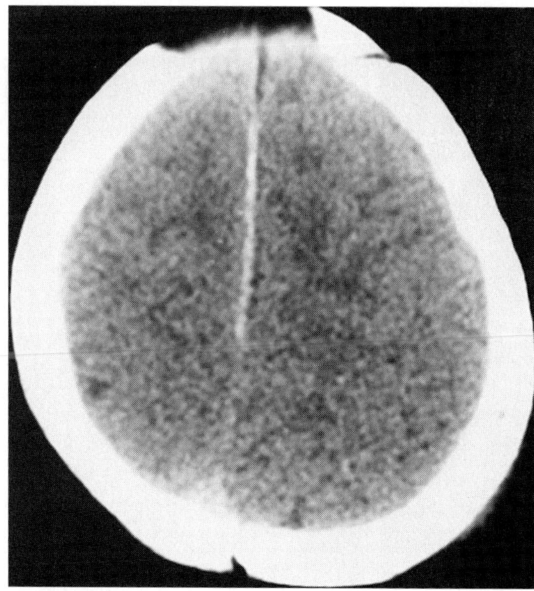

FIGURE 63-9. Nonenhanced computed tomographic scan of an acute interhemispheric subdural hematoma.

Intracranial Injuries

Extra-axial Collections

In most severely injured children, initial CT scan reveals intracranial abnormalities, most often acute subdural hematoma, cerebral hypodensity, and intraparenchymal hemorrhage (Figs. 63-8, 63-9, and 63-10; see also Figs. 63-1A and 63-15) [Cohen et al., 1985].

SUBDURAL HEMATOMA

Regardless of etiology, subdural hematomas are the most common intracranial pathologic processes in inflicted head injury observed in 38% to 100% of infants and young children with inflicted neurotrauma [Biousse et al., 2002; Dias et al., 1998; Dykes, 1986; Duhaime et al., 1992; Gjerris, 1986; Hadley et al., 1989; Hahn et al., 1983; Ludwig and Warman, 1984; Shugerman et al., 1996]. In fatal cases, some blood is almost always present in the subdural potential space.

Subdural hematomas develop from several mechanisms, alone or in combination, including the tearing of bridging veins extending from the cortex to the dural sinuses (particularly the superior sagittal sinus), injured surface vessels (about 10%), and dural lacerations [Gennarelli et al., 1982; Shenkin, 1982; Stålhammer, 1986]. Acute subdural hematomas liquefy and are resorbed, become chronic and eventually calcify, or persist as chronic subdural effusions (see the following section). These either are space occupying, in

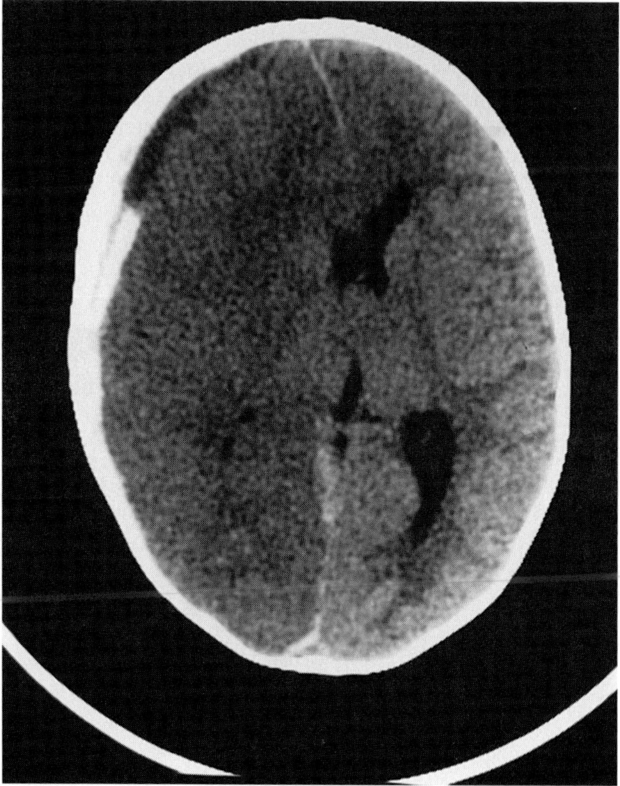

FIGURE 63-10. Nonenhanced computed tomographic scan with an acute mixed-density right subdural hematoma. Blood is layering inferiorly. There is associated subjacent hemispheric swelling and midline shift. Incidental acute post-traumatic hydrocephalus is present in the left ventricular system.

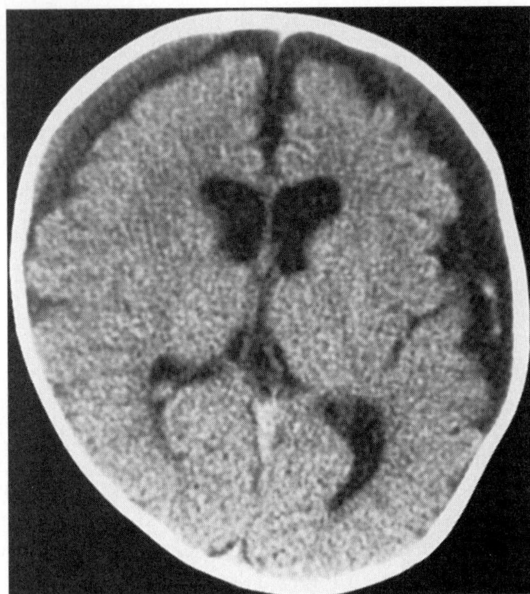

FIGURE 63-11. Nonenhanced computed tomographic scan of a 9-month-old infant admitted with macrocrania, seizures, and irritability. The scan reveals bilateral acute and chronic subdural hematoma. Ventricles are mildly enlarged.

the case of evolving cerebral atrophy, or in some cases are thought to persist as a result of abnormalities in clotting within the subdural collection. On occasion, acute subdural hematomas resolve rapidly, in 1 to 2 days [Duhaime et al., 1996a]. Extra-axial collections that mimic subdural hematoma include venous epidural collections from contact, as well as subarachnoid collections [Duhaime et al., 1996a].

Subdural hematomas associated with inflicted injuries in children are typically interhemispheric, unilateral, or bilateral over the frontoparietal convexities (see Figs. 63-1, 63-8, 63-9, 63-10, and 63-15) [Biousse et al., 2002]. Interhemispheric or falcine subdural hematomas are particularly suspect for inflicted injury and have not been reported after mild or moderate head injury, although they are observed clinically after moderate-to-severe accidental traumatic head injury (see Figs. 63-8 and 63-9) [Tzioumi and Oates, 1998]. Significant convexity or interhemispheric subdural hematomas with associated neurologic signs are extremely rare as a result of any etiology other than trauma.

Mixed-density subdural hematomas are more likely to result from a rapidly accumulating blood collection or from settling, washout, or compartmentalization of hemorrhage products than from repetitive injury events (Fig. 63-11; see also Figs. 63-10 and 63-15) [Greenberg et al., 1985; Sargent et al., 1996]. Cerebrospinal fluid mixed with blood in a subdural hematoma may also appear to be of mixed density (see Fig. 63-10) [Vinchon et al., 2002; Zouros et al., 2004]. In subdural hematomas that fail to organize, both acute and subacute components are found within the chronic hematoma. The presence of acute blood in a chronic hematoma does not necessarily mean that acute significant trauma has occurred. Chronic subdural hematomas can bleed again with minimal or no trauma [Crooks, 1991; Sargent et al., 1996]. Careful attention to the history and clinical findings is necessary in this situation.

Chronic Subdural Effusions

Proteinaceous subdural collections frequently evolve from resolving acute subdural hematomas in young infants (Figs. 63-13 and 63-14; see also Fig. 63-11). They may develop within days of the injury [Vinchon et al., 2002]. Sometimes referred to as *hygromas*, they either resolve with time or persist when there is diffuse brain injury with secondary atrophy [Hasegawa et al., 1992; Kaufman, 1993; Wetterling et al., 1988].

The use of the term *hygroma* is controversial [Wetterling et al., 1988]. Hygromas are defined as accumulations of fluid in the subdural space. They are variably attributed to resolving subdural hematomas or to abnormal collections of cerebrospinal fluid, alone or mixed with blood, in the subdural space [Zouros et al., 2004]. Analysis of attenuation coefficients on CT scan is often adequate for making the

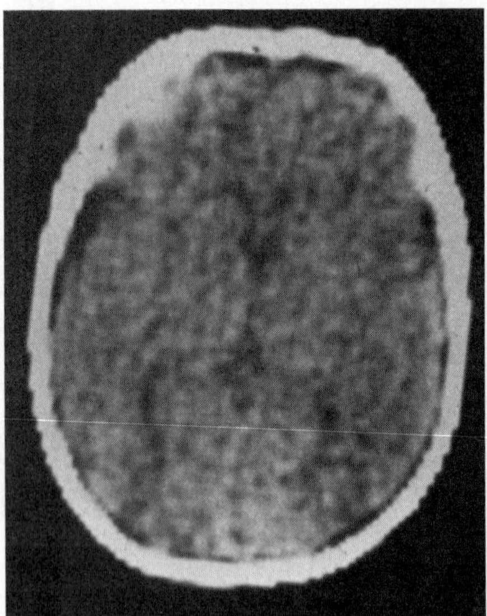

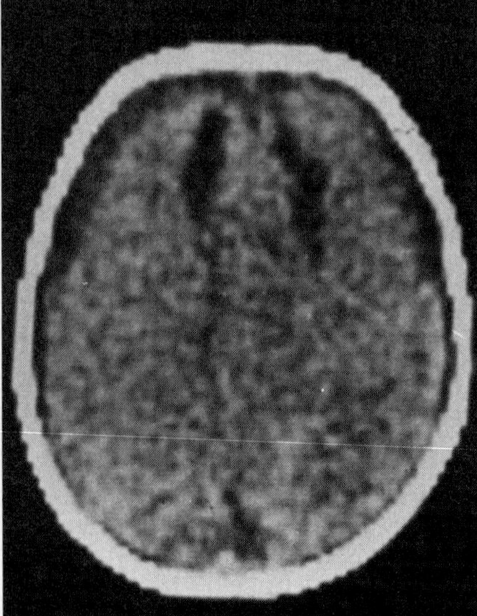

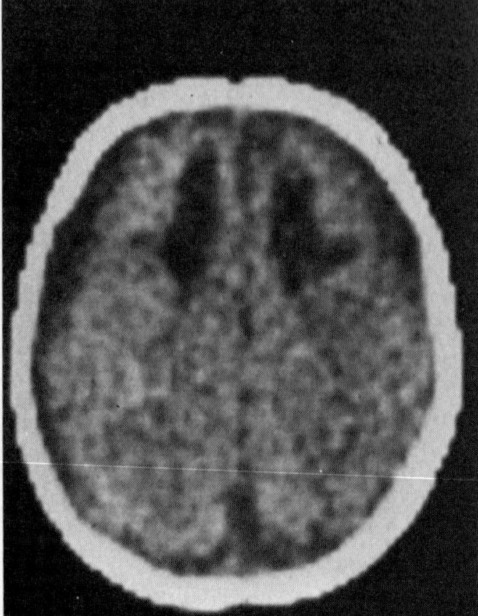

FIGURE 63-12. Computed tomographic appearance of healed white matter tears in the bifrontal regions.

diagnosis. If there is any question, MRI is the preferred technique, as it is accurate in determining whether extra-axial fluid is of cerebrospinal fluid intensity and whether fluid is in the subarachnoid or subdural space [Hasegawa et al., 1992; Wilms et al., 1993]. The majority of subdural collections resolve without intervention (see Fig. 63-14).

Enlarged subarachnoid spaces in infants (also known as *benign external hydrocephalus*) can be differentiated from subdural hygromas or subdural hematomas on MRI by sulcal prominences, prominent basilar cisterns, and normal or minimally enlarged ventricles [Aoki, 1994]. These infants, typically younger than 1 year, present with macrocrania, usually have normal growth and development, and have no history of trauma [Mori et al., 1980; Nishimura et al., 1996].

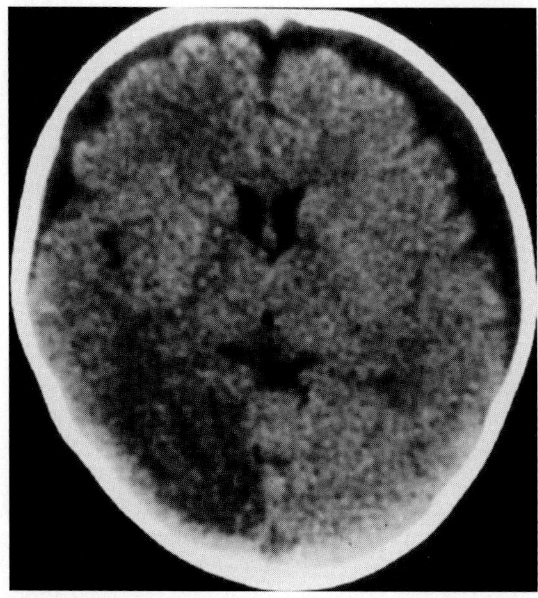

FIGURE 63-13. Nonenhanced computed tomographic scan obtained 2 weeks after admission with seizures, apnea, and left hemiparesis. There are bilateral extra-axial collections consistent with subdural hematoma and ischemia caused by right posterior cerebral artery infarction.

SUBARACHNOID HEMORRHAGE

Small patchy areas of subarachnoid hemorrhages are almost universally found at postmortem examination in infants who die from inflicted injury [Case et al., 2001]. Subarachnoid hemorrhage develops after direct surface trauma to the brain or from leakage of blood from injured cerebral vessels within the subarachnoid space. They are difficult to identify with CT scans and to differentiate from subdural hematoma, especially when interhemispheric.

Differential of Extensive Subarachnoid Hemorrhage

Among the conditions that can cause subarachnoid hemorrhages are vascular malformations, birth trauma, coagulopathy, meningitis, and unintentional trauma [Cohen et al., 1985; Govaert et al., 1990]. These are uncommon causes of subarachnoid hemorrhages, and, in the presence of extensive subarachnoid bleeding, vascular malformation is the most likely etiology. Vascular malformations, however, are an exceedingly rare cause of subarachnoid hemorrhage in young children [Crisostomo et al., 1986; Hayashi et al., 1994; Matson, 1965; Matsuzaka et al., 1989; Perret and Nishioka, 1966; Sedzimir, 1955]. Three large series, involving more than 10,000 patients with subarachnoid hemorrhages, identified no children aged 1 year or younger [Matson, 1965; Perret and Nishioka, 1966; Sedzimir, 1955].

EPIDURAL HEMATOMA

Epidural hematoma is uncommon after trauma, especially after inflicted head injury [Shugerman et al., 1996; Schutzman et al., 1993]. It is discussed here to clarify its pathogenesis and clinical course. Epidural hematoma can occur after relatively minor trauma [Schutzman et al., 1993]. The majority of such hematomas develop adjacent to the middle meningeal artery or over the cerebral convexity, but they can also occur in the posterior fossa and are usually venous, rather than arterial, in this location.

Skull fracture does not have to be present, particularly in an infant, whose increased skull compliance allows increased

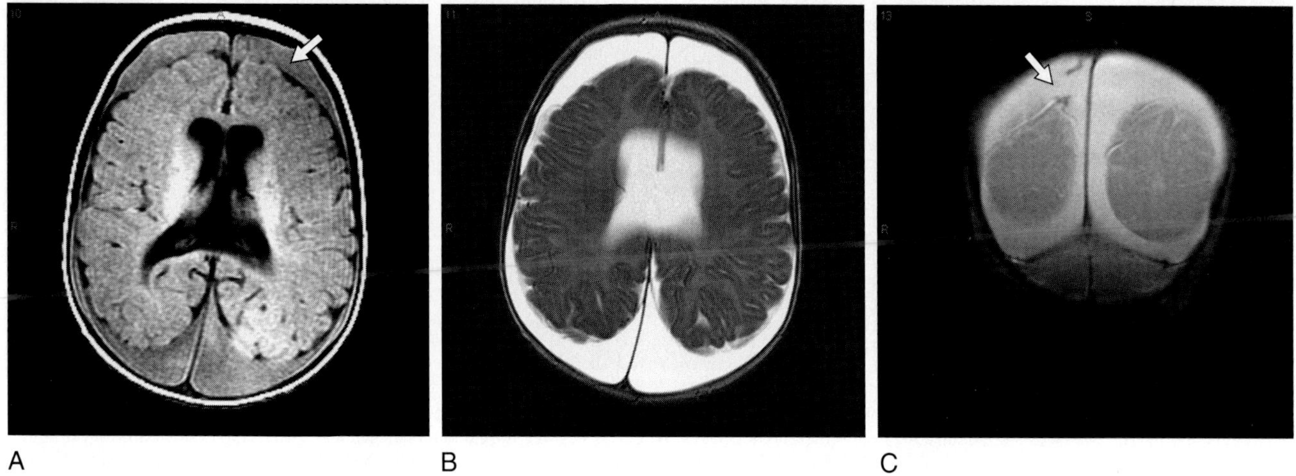

FIGURE 63-14. Images of a 3-month-old presenting with a growing head and with rib fractures. The father admitted that he had thrown the infant across the room; the mother had "no idea." Collections gradually resolved without intervention. **A,** Magnetic resonance image (MRI) with chronic subdural collections (*arrow*). **B,** T2-weighted MRI with corpus callosal tear. **C,** Gradient echo-sequence coronal MRI depicting tear of a convexity bridging vein (*arrow*).

skull deformation at the impact site [Shugerman et al., 1996]. Symptom progression varies from dramatic to more protracted, paralleling the rate of epidural accumulation.

Children with epidural hematomas are much more likely to have a lucid interval and do well clinically than are severely abused infants (see also "Timing of Injuries" section) [Schutzman et al., 1993]. This finding is congruent with the biomechanics of injury because epidural hematomas result primarily from brief linear deceleration impacts, such as falls [Shugerman et al., 1996; Schutzman et al., 1993]. Locally deforming forces do not usually injure brain parenchyma away from the impact site. Children with epidural hematomas typically do well with prompt surgical intervention when needed and aggressive supportive care.

Cerebral Injuries

SWELLING OR EDEMA

Diffuse or focal brain hypodensity is the most common parenchymal pattern found on initial CT imaging [Kazan et al., 1997; Rao et al., 1999]. Traumatic brainstem lesions are quite rare [Eder et al., 2000]. Younger infants are more likely to present with diffuse hypodensity, with or without bilateral acute subdural hematomas (see Figs. 63-1 and

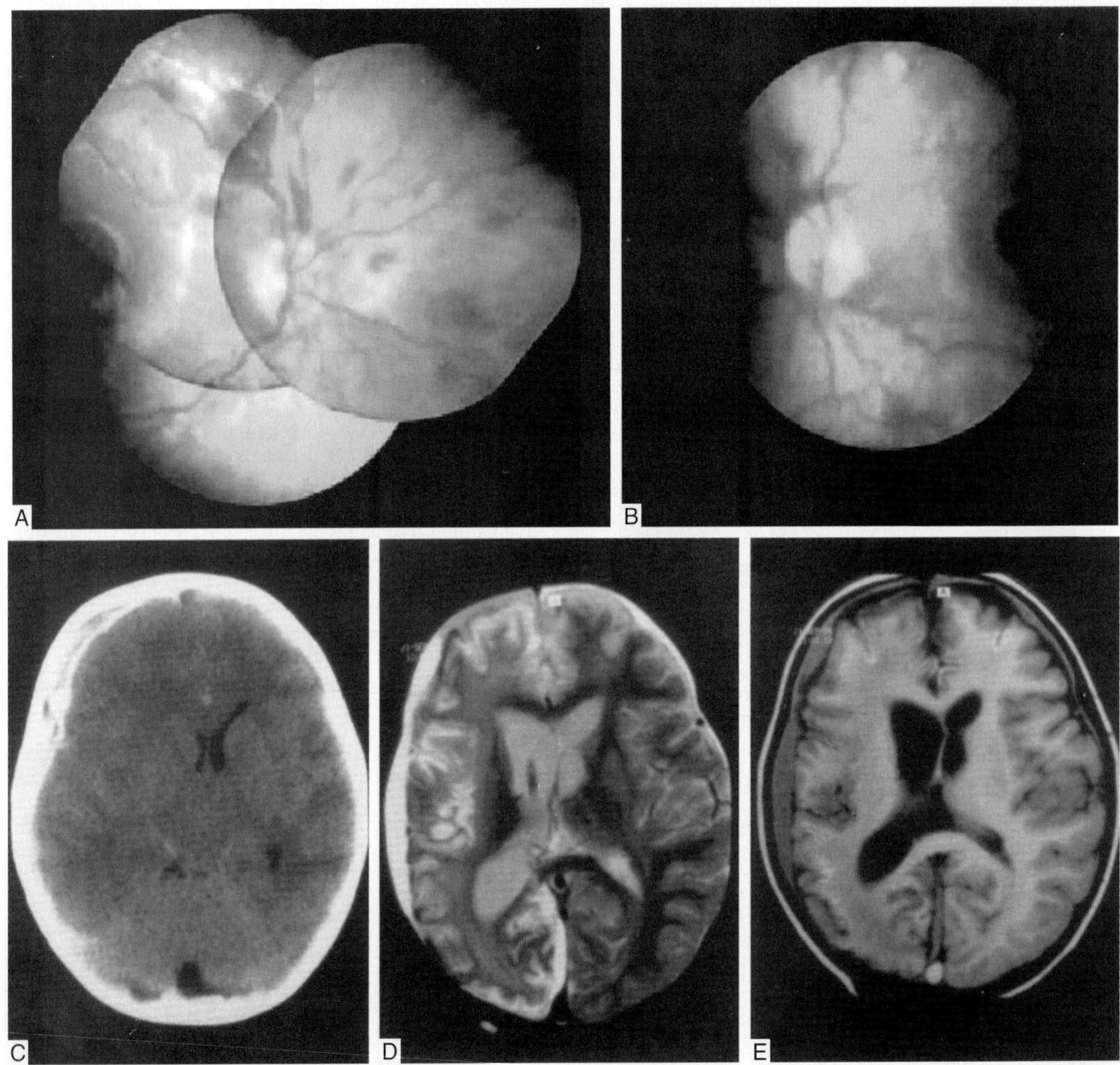

FIGURE 63-15. Images of a 4-year-old who was picked up, strangled, and thrown, hitting the occiput on a marble coffee table edge. **A,** Right eye: predominantly nerve fiber layer and three subhyaloid retinal hemorrhages. **B,** Left eye: three retinal hemorrhages less than 2 optic disc diameters from the optic nerve. **C,** Computed tomographic scan within 3 hours of the event: acute right convexity subdural hematoma with hemispheric hypoattenuation, midline shift, and early hydrocephalus of the left temporal horn. **D** and **E,** Axial T1-weighted (1.5 T; repetition time = 500 msec; echo time = 10 msec) and T2-weighted (1.5 T; recovery time = 3300 msec; echo time = 90 msec) magnetic resonance images from the same patient 3 months after injury. Scans demonstrate evolving right hemispheric and left frontal infarct and atrophy with encephalomalacia of the right hemisphere and compensatory ventriculomegaly.

63-14), whereas older infants and children more often present with focal or hemispheric brain swelling and ipsilateral acute subdural hematomas (Fig. 63-15; see also Fig. 63-10) [Aldrich et al., 1992; Bruce et al., 1981; Gilles and Nelson, 1998; Kemp et al., 2003; Rao et al., 1999]. The particular pattern of bilateral hypodensity involving the entire hemisphere is rare in adults and likely reflects a specific pathophysiologic process that is still incompletely understood [Duhaime et al., 1993; Duhaime et al., 1998; Han et al., 1990; Kazan et al., 1997; Rao et al., 1999].

Focal swelling has several patterns: hemispheric subjacent to an ipsilateral acute subdural hematoma or, less often, in a vascular distribution from an evolving infarction, or patchy scan hypodensity that is not in a vascular distribution. None of these patterns is specific for abuse [Lobato et al., 1988; Sarabia et al., 1988; Tomita et al., 1997]. Although there is a tendency to infer that focal brain swelling equates to localized brain injury, the finding of persistent coma in severely injured children in the absence of significant midline shift is supportive evidence that diffuse injury has also occurred.

The etiology of hemispheric swelling and secondary necrosis subjacent to an acute subdural hematoma is not understood, although local pressure effects in addition to compromised cerebral blood flow in the involved hemisphere are thought to contribute to evolving edema and increased intracranial pressure [Miller et al., 1990; Orlin et al., 1992; Salvant and Muizelaar, 1993; Schröder et al., 1994; Tomita et al., 1997; Tornheim et al., 1983; Xu et al., 1993].

Strangulation has been proposed as a causal mechanism of brain swelling, particularly hemispheric swelling, but corroborative clinical data are scanty (Figs. 63-16 and 63-17) [Bird et al., 1987; Bonnier et al., 1995; Drack et al., 1999; Duhaime et al., 1996b; Gilles and Nelson, 1998]. Circumferential strangulation in a young child can simultaneously compress carotid and vertebral arteries (the carotid arteries by anterior neck compression and the vertebral arteries as they pass through the scaleni muscles) [Rossen et al., 1943]. Traumatic vascular injury secondary to strangulation should be diagnosed only if there is unequivocal clinical, imaging, or postmortem examination evidence.

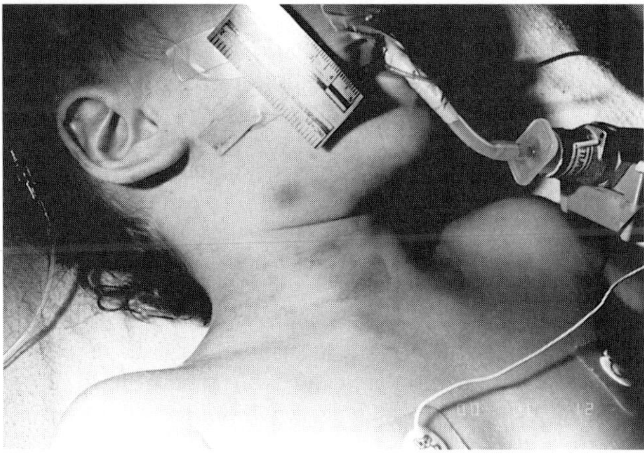

FIGURE 63-16. Strangulation injuries in a 4-year-old child. Note the thumbprints on the anterior neck and finger bruising along the mandible. Difficult to discern are the petechiae that are prominent around the neck and over the face.

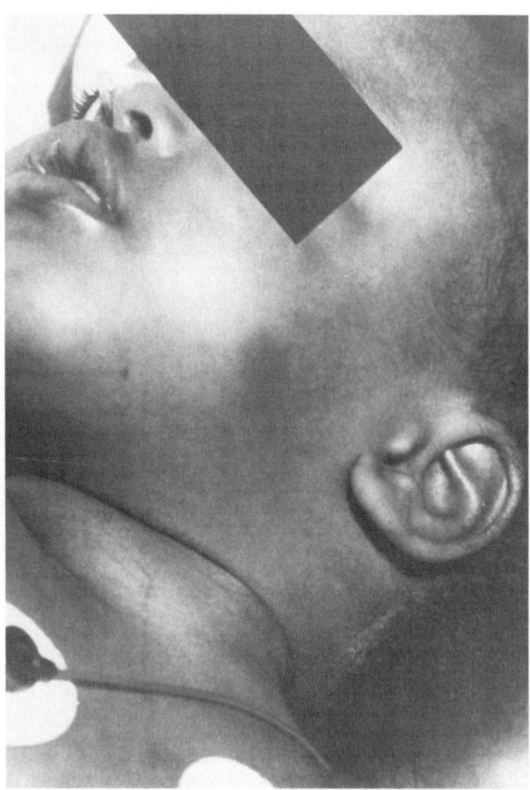

FIGURE 63-17. Three-year-old child injured because of a toileting accident. He was beaten and thrown against the wall. A unique pattern injury is present on the anterior neck consisting of the markings on the watchband.

DIFFUSE AXONAL INJURY

Diffuse axonal shear injury is an important determinant of clinical status and outcome from nonmissile head injury [Adams et al., 1982; Hammoud and Wasserman, 2002; Strich, 1961]. It is a common feature of severe traumatic brain injury in older children and adults; its frequency is not established in infants, and there is conflicting evidence about its importance in inflicted head injury [Tokutomi et al., 1997; Tong et al., 2004]. Vowles and associates [1987] described diffuse axonal shear injury in infants younger than 5 months of age. More recently, however, Geddes and coworkers [2001b] found diffuse axonal shear injury in only 2 of 37 infants younger than 9 months who died from inflicted head injury. Major angular deceleration forces are required. The most common accidental cause is a high-speed motor vehicle crash or a pedestrian struck by a high-velocity vehicle. It occurs at the moment of injury and, when severe, is associated with loss of consciousness at the moment of impact [Adams et al., 1977; Gennarelli, 1993]. Imaging findings of shear injuries include punctate hemorrhages particularly in the white matter, and tearing of the corpus callosum (see Fig. 63-14) [Mendelsohn et al., 1992].

CEREBRAL CONTUSIONS

An infant younger than 8 months is much less likely to develop cortical contusions in coup or contrecoup locations

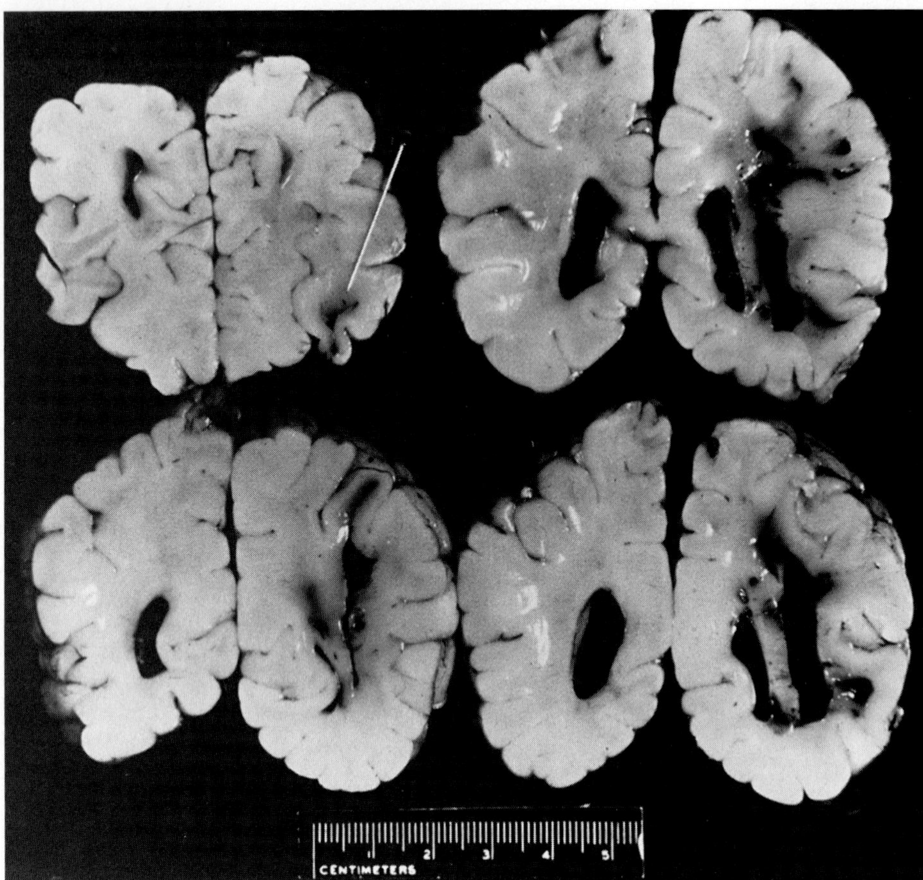

FIGURE 63-18. Gross specimens from a 2-month-old infant with multiple acute white matter contusions of the left hemisphere. One contusion is marked.

than are older children and adults [Lindenberg and Freytag, 1969]. The incidence of contrecoup injuries rises rapidly from later infancy to 3 years of age, when it begins to approximate that of the adult [Digraham et al., 1989; McLaurin and Tutor, 1961].

On occasion, young infants present with white matter tears, also referred to as *white matter contusional tears* or *gliding contusions*, which presumably are the result of rotational shearing forces [Calder et al., 1984; Jaspan et al., 1992; Lindenberg and Freytag, 1969; Vowles et al., 1987]. Contusional tears occur where shear strain is greatest: namely, deep to the gray matter–white matter junction (Fig. 63-18; see also Fig. 63-12) [Calder et al., 1984; Gentry et al., 1988; Jaspan et al., 1992; Lindenberg and Freytag, 1969]. From 1 to 3 cm in length, they are most often located in the frontal and temporal lobes, although they may be seen throughout the brain [Lindenberg and Freytag, 1969]. These tears are considerably larger than the tissue tear hemorrhages in the adult brain after closed-head injury that are punctate and are found most often in the periventricular white matter, corpus callosum, and brainstem [Wilberger et al., 1990]. When white matter tears are filled with fresh blood, they may be mistaken for parenchymal hemorrhages (rare in childhood inflicted or unintentional head injury). In an acutely swollen brain, white matter contusional tears may be difficult to visualize on CT or magnetic resonance imaging [Gentry et al., 1988]. They are more easily visualized on follow-up imaging studies, in which they appear as slitlike or oval lesions within the cerebral parenchyma (see Fig. 63-12).

CEREBRAL INFARCTION

Post-traumatic cerebral infarction develops after traumatic brain injury in both children and adults, predominantly as a result of vascular compression and herniation [Gilles and Nelson, 1998; Mirvis et al., 1990; Server et al., 2001]. The extent of infarction is correlated with poor outcome [Gilles and Nelson, 1998; Server et al., 2001]. Post-traumatic cerebral infarction after inflicted head injury has received relatively little attention [Bird et al., 1987; Gilles and Nelson, 1998; Zimmerman et al., 1979]. Posterior cerebral artery and branch anterior cerebral artery distribution infarctions predominate (see Figs. 63-13 and 63-15). Infarction in the lenticulostriate-thalamoperforating distribution leads to basal ganglia and thalamic injury. Hemispheric necrosis and border zone infarction are other prominent patterns (see Fig. 63-15). Strangulation is not a common cause of cerebral infarction in this setting [Gilles and Nelson, 1998].

DIFFERENTIAL DIAGNOSIS

The range of clinical and physical findings is unique to inflicted neurotrauma. Falls and birth trauma are the most frequently offered explanations for injury, but these are uncommon causes of severe brain injury [Duhaime et al., 1992; Feldman et al., 2001; Hobbs, 1984; Meservy et al., 1987]. It is uncommon for infants to suffer severe brain injuries from nonaccidental mechanisms. Significant applied forces are required, such as those sustained in a vertical fall greater than 10 feet or a high-speed motor vehicle accident [Meservy et al., 1987; Williams, 1991]. Birth trauma is usually excluded as a reasonable explanation by the clinical course and imaging findings.

Falls

Fall data can be grouped into short falls (less than 4 feet), falls down stairs, falls from heights, and walker falls. These data overwhelmingly support the conclusion that severe traumatic brain injury and severe retinal hemorrhages are unlikely to result from household falls, although venous or arterial extra-axial hemorrhages may occur in both younger and older children through this mechanism [Betz et al., 1996; Duhaime et al., 1992; Elder et al., 1991; Hobbs, 1984; Johnson et al., 1993; Kravitz et al., 1969; Nimityongskul and Anderson, 1987; Paret et al., 1999; Williams, 1991]. Fall data should be interpreted cautiously. The majority of data in the studies just cited were collected retrospectively without consistent evaluation protocols. Routine neuroimaging was not performed in children who were not clinically symptomatic; thus, intracranial injuries, such as small, insignificant subdural hematoma, would have been missed [Doezema et al., 1991].

Short Falls

Short falls are generally low-impact, low-velocity injuries. The most common findings are concussions, scalp contusions, some fractures, an occasional epidural hematoma, and an occasional focal subarachnoid hemorrhage. In falls of less than 2 feet that involve fracture, clavicle fractures predominate; skull fractures are more common in falls of 2 to 4 feet. In four studies, with a total of 917 short falls (ranging from 1 to 5 feet), there were seven skull fractures, four clavicle fractures, and one humerus fracture [Musemeche et al., 1991; Roshkow et al., 1990].

Except for epidural hematoma, which can be a life-threatening injury if not treated promptly, household free falls from furniture or other surfaces, with a head-to-ground distance of less than 3 feet, do not appear to result in serious injury or in significant primary brain injuries [Duhaime et al., 1992]. Falls 2 to 4 feet onto a hard surface, such as pavement, cement, linoleum, and wood, have on rare occasion resulted in complicated fractures in infants younger than 6 months [Lyons and Oates, 1993; Nimityongskul and Anderson, 1987; Reiber, 1993; Rivara et al., 1996]. Studies suggesting that serious, life-threatening injury can occur in children allegedly falling from short distances have typically relied on uncorroborated histories given by caretakers. Uncorroborated falls have a six times greater rate of serious injury, which suggests that the history was, in fact, suspect [Chadwick et al., 1991].

Small extra-axial hemorrhages can develop after simple falls. These are typically located directly under the impact site and likely result from direct injury of the surface blood vessels. Affected children have no physical injuries except those consistent with the single focal impact (e.g., soft tissue swelling, cephalohematoma, or linear nondisplaced skull fractures). In very rare cases, a complicated short fall, usually with impact to the occiput, results in more severe injury.

Falls down Stairs

Children falling down stairs (or infants dropped while being carried down stairs) most often have either no injury or fractures of the skull or extremities [Chiavello et al., 1994; Joffe and Ludwig, 1988]. Stairway falls usually are less serious than free falls of the same vertical distance [Joffe and Ludwig, 1988]. No correlation exists between the number of steps and the severity of injury. Most children who fall down stairs tumble and never develop significant acceleration, but exceptions to this general rule do exist, and the specific injuries depend on the exact mechanism and forces involved.

Falls from Heights

Children falling from heights differ from children who have been maltreated or who have had minor falls [Roshkow et al., 1990; Musemeche et al., 1991; Reiber, 1993; Williams, 1991]. Extremity injuries again outnumber head injuries, and, overall, children recover better than adults. Rare injuries from falls include superior sagittal sinus rupture after impact to the vertex of the cranium (Fig. 63-19).

The brain and skull accelerate at the same rate in a high free fall. The brain may escape major injury, and the skull may shatter with impact because the skull absorbs much of the translational energy and there is little rotational component [Lindenberg, 1973]. In infants and young children, inward deformity of the skull may cause significant surface

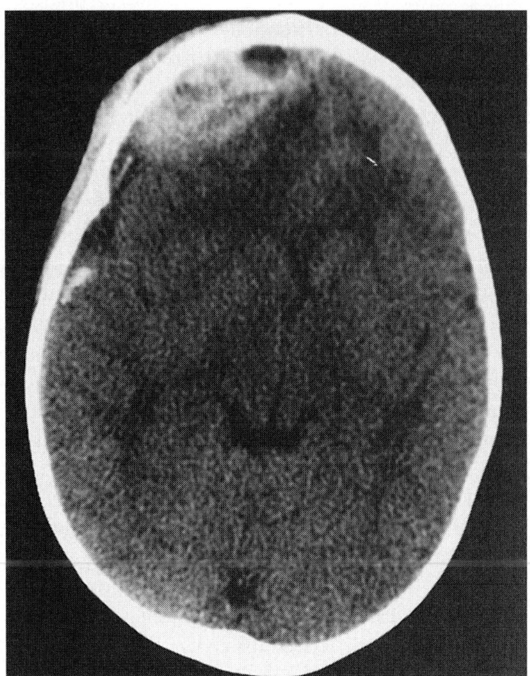

FIGURE 63-19. Seventeen-month-old child who fell from an unprotected 8-foot high porch onto a 2×4 piece of wood and suffered immediate sustained loss of consciousness and posturing. Nonenhanced computed tomographic scan is notable for a subgaleal hematoma and extensive right frontal cerebral contusion with an overlying subdural hematoma. Not well seen is an extensive right superior frontal fracture that runs into and splits the metopic suture. There is significant hemispheric swelling on the right with marked midline shift and an associated superior sagittal sinus laceration. This injury proved to be fatal.

trauma when falls are from major heights (such as out windows). Comminuted skull fracture with surface brain contusion, subarachnoid hemorrhage, or both in older children is consistent with a history of a high free fall. Venous or arterial epidural hemorrhages may occur in both older and younger children through this mechanism.

Walker Falls

Walkers continue to be widely used in this country despite the substantial amount of data detailing their risks [American Academy of Pediatrics, 2001; Chiavello et al., 1994; Emanuelson, 2003; Partington et al., 1991; Smith et al., 1997]. Mechanisms of injury include tipping over and walker falls down stairs [Ridenour, 1999]. The most common injuries are extremity trauma, bruises, skull and other fractures, and minor concussions. Some children with significant velocities can develop more significant intracranial injuries, including subdural hemorrhages and growing fractures.

Birth Trauma

Stresses applied to the cranial vault and its coverings during the birth process are an uncommon cause of a number of injuries [Shapiro and Smith, 1993]. Extracranial injuries predominate, including caput succedaneum, cephalohematomas, and subgaleal hematomas. Skull fractures, found after vaginal delivery, forceps use, or cesarean section, are generally either linear or depressed. Complicated skull fractures usually herald serious intracranial pathologic processes. Epidural and subdural hematomas, subarachnoid hemorrhage, and intracerebral hemorrhage have all been reported [Hayashi et al., 1987; Shapiro and Smith, 1993]. Subdural hematomas are usually associated with a difficult delivery or an infant large for gestational age. Approximately 70% of neonates with subdural hematoma have good outcome, which is consistent with the absence of associated primary cerebral injury [Hayashi et al., 1987].

Eleven percent to 50% of full-term newborns have retinal hemorrhages after vaginal delivery [Baum and Bulpitt, 1970; Egge et al., 1980; Emerson et al., 2001; Govind et al., 1989; O'Leary et al., 1986]. These have been hypothesized to be a consequence of molding and compression of the cavernous sinus, but exactly how they develop is unknown [Ehrenfest, 1922]. Retinal hemorrhages are more frequent after complicated or traumatic births (such as those involving vacuum extraction), protracted labor, and prematurity [Demissie et al., 2004; Egge et al., 1980; Ehrenfest, 1922; Emerson et al., 2001; O'Leary et al., 1986; Sezen, 1971; Williams et al., 1993]. Types of hemorrhage are equivalent to those in infants with inflicted injuries (flame, dot-and-blot, subhyaloid) but are rarely severe and are not usually associated with visual loss [Baum and Bulpitt, 1970; Ehrenfest, 1922; Sezen, 1971; Zwaan et al., 1997].

Infants injured during the birth process exhibit symptoms in the perinatal period, which makes the differentiation from the abused infant fairly straightforward unless the infant is just a couple of weeks old. Review of the maternal and infant birth records, as well as any pediatric records, is exceedingly helpful. This review can firmly establish any birth-related complications or other conditions that were or were not factors contributing to the acute clinical presentation.

Neurometabolic Disease

There are rare case reports of infants with metabolic disease who present with signs and symptoms that are misdiagnosed as abusive injury. Careful history taking, physical examination, and imaging characteristics usually suggest metabolic disease as a differential possibility. Infants with glutaricaciduria type 1 may present with macrocephaly, subdural effusions, and spasticity [Drigo et al., 1996; Kimura et al., 1994; Land et al., 1992; Osaka et al., 1993]. The infants in these studies had other neuroimaging features of organic acidurias: namely, widened operculae and alterations of signal intensity in the basal ganglia [Brismar and Ozand, 1994]. Menkes' disease may also manifest in infancy with subdural fluid collections and severe neurologic findings such as seizures and developmental delay [Nassogne et al., 2002]. Ganesh and coworkers [2004] reported three infants with type I osteogenesis imperfecta who presented with small subdural hematoma and retinal hemorrhages after minor trauma. These conditions are extremely rare causes of extra-axial fluid collections. Metabolic screening tests should be considered in infants presenting with somnolence, vomiting, seizures, dystonia, or dyskinesia and extra-axial fluid collections (either subdural effusion or subdural hematoma), particularly if ketoacidosis is present.

CLINICAL ASSESSMENT AND MANAGEMENT

A detailed history of the circumstances of the injury and a timeline of the infant's behavior for a minimum of the 72 hours preceding the injury is invaluable. This history should be documented in a legible summary, with quotations from caregivers as much as possible. Histories of minor injury should be closely examined, and any available caretakers should be questioned independently if at all possible.

The biomechanical history of the fall should include details such as the specific surface onto which the child fell, the location and type or types of injury, and the presence of corroborative witnesses [Duhaime et al., 1992]. It is also useful to ask about exactly what happened after the event—"What did the child look like?" "What position was he or she in?" "What did he or she do next?" "What happened then?"—and so on, until the child arrived at a medical center. Also relevant are the age of the child and the baseline gross motor and language development level (e.g., "Can the child crawl, stand, walk, or run?" "Can the child talk in words?").

General Examination

After initial coma scale scoring and resuscitative efforts, an extensive physical examination should be completed. Although the Glasgow Coma Scale is the measure most commonly used, it actually has poor interobserver variability in infants. The Infant Face Scale is a coma scale designed specifically in an attempt to correctly identify seriously injured infants who have sustained inflicted or other types of traumatic brain injuries, and it has improved interobserver variability in comparison with other impairment scales [Durham et al., 2000a].

All vital signs, including rectal temperature, should be measured. Growth parameters, including head circumference, state of hydration, and any obvious signs of neglect, need to be documented. The examiner should palpate and inspect all skin surfaces, particularly the cranium, behind the ears, and the occiput. The presence of otorrhea and rhinorrhea can be easily confirmed as cerebrospinal fluid with a Clinitest that reveals increased glucose concentration. Battle's sign (bruising over the mastoid) or "raccoon eyes" (periorbital ecchymoses) are suggestive of a basilar skull fracture. Hemotympanum can result either from direct impact over the ear or from basilar fracture. The examiner should inspect the frenula and the palate for tears and petechiae; forced feeding, smothering, and gagging can cause these injuries. Any unusual pattern of injuries should be documented (see Figs. 63-16 and 63-17).

Classic features of asphyxia are facial cyanosis, petechial hemorrhages of the eyes and face, foam in the nose and mouth, and prominent bulging eyes [Matsumura and Ito, 1996; Taff et al., 1996]. All or some of these features may be present, depending on the amount of force applied to the neck, its rate and duration, and the surface area involved. Decreased carotid pulsations ipsilateral to neck bruising are suggestive of carotid injury. The neck should also be inspected closely, particularly along the mandible, to assess for subtle signs of strangulation.

The examiner should note the location and extent of any skin lesions, including bruises and bite marks. Bruises involving skin surfaces that are fairly protected, such as inner arms and other flexor surfaces, buttocks, and lower back, are of particular concern [Pascoe et al., 1979; Roberton et al., 1982]. A history of a simple fall is incongruous with multiple bruises of the same or different age if the bruises are on multiple and different body planes. Documentation includes both a complete written record of the examiner's involvement with the child, as well as appropriate photographic documentation [Dubowitz and Bross, 1992].

Neurologic Examination

Neurologic examinations, including level of coma, should be documented sequentially (see Chapter 61). Serial funduscopic examinations are useful for documenting the final extent of retinal hemorrhage development. Particular attention needs to be given to identifying and documenting asymmetries on the examination. Children younger than 3 years are particularly at risk for spinal cord injury without radiographic findings and should also be carefully examined for possible spinal cord or vertebral injuries, with MRI if indicated [Cirak et al., 2004].

Autonomic and Neuroendocrine Responses

Traumatic brain injury and other critical illnesses are potent activators of the hypothalamic-pituitary-adrenal axis and the sympathetic efferent pathways [Chiolero and Berger, 1994; Reincke et al., 1993]. As injury severity increases, loss of adaptive negative feedback control mechanisms results in sustained activity of either or both of these pathways [Arita et al., 1993; Clifton et al., 1983; Koiv et al., 1997].

Autonomic cardiac control in children with traumatic brain injury is disrupted in proportion to the severity of injury, with autonomic uncoupling potentiated in young children [Biswas et al., 2000; Goldstein et al., 1996]. When efferent sympathetic pathways are completely interrupted, heart rate variability is lost and low-frequency heart rate power decreases; these findings are highly correlated with brain death in both children and adults [Baillard et al., 2002; Goldstein et al., 1996]. Young infants may develop evidence of hypopituitarism or adrenal insufficiency during their post-injury course.

Clinical Laboratory Evaluation

Infants who have sustained inflicted head injuries are frequently anemic and acidotic on admission. Leukocytosis is not uncommon. As in adults, hyperglycemia at presentation has been associated with a poor prognosis and more severe head injury, and it is also suggestive of more recent injury [Atkinson, 2000; Michaud et al., 1991; Paret et al., 1999]. Some data suggest that the serum glucose level is optimally maintained between 100 and 200 mg/dL, which may require an insulin infusion. As in other head-injured populations, secondary consumptive coagulopathy (disseminated intravascular coagulation) is associated with a higher mortality rate and more severe brain injury [Hulka et al., 1996]. More commonly, mild elevations of the prothrombin time or evidence of activated coagulation may be found [Hymel et al., 1997]. These abnormalities do not appear to reflect preexisting coagulation abnormalities. In situations in which a clinical index of suspicion arises or an alternative diagnosis has been proposed, such as an inherited metabolic disease, additional studies or consultation with a metabolic geneticist may be useful.

Biochemical Markers

A number of biomarkers (e.g., lactate, S-100B protein, neuron-specific enolase) have been proposed as indexes of severity of injury in several disorders, including brain injury, stroke, and neonatal encephalopathy [Ashwal et al., 2000]. Of these, S-100B protein, a glial marker, and neuron-specific enolase, a neuronal glycolytic enzyme, are most specific to traumatic brain injury.

Neuron-specific enolase is a nonspecific indicator of neuronal injury and ischemia, correlated with both reversible and irreversible damage after traumatic brain injury, stroke, cardiorespiratory arrest, and perinatal hypoxic-ischemic injury [Blennow et al., 2001; Butterworth et al., 1996; Correale et al., 1998; Fridriksson et al., 2000; Herrmann et al., 2000; Martens et al., 1998; McKeating et al., 1998; O'Regan and Brown, 1998; Raabe et al., 1998]. Transient elevations have been documented just before elevations in intracranial pressure, after cardiac surgery, after seizures, and after both convulsive and nonconvulsive status epilepticus [Correale et al., 1998; O'Regan and Brown, 1998; Schmitt et al., 1998; Woertgen et al., 1997]. Fridriksson and associates [2000] were the first to evaluate neuron-specific enolase as a biomarker in childhood traumatic brain injury. Mean neuron-specific enolase levels were significantly higher in children with an intracranial lesion (26.7 ± 21.4 versus 17.7 ± 7.8). Sensitivity of neuron-specific enolase at a level of 15.3 was 77% and specificity was 52%, with a negative predictive value of 74%.

Acute inflammatory responses to traumatic brain injury are characterized by upregulation of adhesion molecules on cerebrovascular endothelium and production of cytokines [Morganti-Kossmann et al., 2002; Woiciechowsky et al., 2002; Yakovlev and Faden, 1995]. Investigations have documented significantly greater increases in adhesion molecules (P-selectin), interleukin-8, and interleukin-10 in children younger than 4 years of age and those with inflicted head injury [Bell et al., 1997, 1999; Whalen et al., 1998, 2000]. The clinical significance of these findings is not clear.

Elevations of biomarkers do not differentiate whether an injury was inflicted or unintentional. Infants with inflicted traumatic brain injury have a greater ischemic load; greater increases in markers of neuronal and glial injury or of enhanced inflammatory and biochemical cascades likely reflect the severity of injury. Whether this is also related to patient age remains unknown [Ruppel et al., 2001].

Radiographic Evaluation

A noncontrast CT scan to include bone windows is the initial imaging study of choice [Bernardi et al., 1993]. A CT scan may miss skull fractures within the plane of the section, so skull films should be considered as part of the skeletal survey. Repeat or serial imaging is often helpful in establishing the extent of injury [Demaerel et al., 2002; Dias et al., 1998; Feldman et al., 1995]. MRI is more sensitive in defining the extent of hemorrhagic and nonhemorrhagic injury, demonstrating infarctions and delineating small extra-axial collections [Ball, 1989; Bernardi et al., 1993; Bigler, 2001; Biousse et al., 2002; Gean, 1994; Sato et al., 1989; Suh et al., 2001]. MRI is also helpful in delineating intracranial sequelae of abuse. Specific MRI sequences include diffusion-weighted imaging, T2-weighted gradient echo, T2-weighted spin echo, and susceptibility-weighted imaging [Biousse et al., 2002; Gerber et al., 2004; Huisman et al., 2003; Suh et al., 2001; Tong et al., 2004].

If carotid or vertebral injury is suspected, MRI and angiography are useful. Tong and associates [2004] described a high-resolution MRI susceptibility-weighted technique sensitive for detecting hemorrhagic diffuse axonal injury in children.

A full skeletal survey should be obtained in any child younger than 2 years or in any older child with multiple traumatic injuries suspected to be nonaccidental in origin [Demaerel et al., 2002]. A bone scan may be indicated in equivocal or negative cases with a high level of suspicion; follow-up skeletal survey may also be useful [Howard et al., 1990; Kleinman, 1990; Mandelstam et al., 2003].

There is considerable variability in the radiologic interpretation of neuroimaging data [Hymel et al., 1997]. Limited clinicopathologic studies have been published to date, and caution should be exercised in relying only on imaging to establish timing of injury. It is strongly recommended that clinicians review the neuroimaging themselves, in addition to obtaining a radiologist's interpretation.

MAKING THE DIAGNOSIS OF INFLICTED HEAD INJURY

General Considerations

Establishing the diagnosis of inflicted trauma is frequently problematic and requires a high index of suspicion. Children interface with the medical system at all points along their response curve after brain injury. It is unrealistic to expect findings in all children to be similar. Certain key questions should be asked and answered (Box 63-4). The physical findings in conjunction with historical features usually point to trauma as the most likely etiology.

Box 63-4 Key Questions in the Evaluation of the Child with Suspected Abuse

What is the distribution of injuries?
Are the injuries confined to the head?
Are the brain injuries focal, diffuse, or both?
What is the clinical timing of the injury?
Are there injuries that suggest a specific injury mechanism (slap mark, strangulation bruising, etc.)?
Are there other suspicious patterns of injury (e.g., rib fractures)?
What forces were necessary to cause such injuries?
Is the history congruent with the physical injuries?
Is there an accidental mechanism that would explain these injuries?
Is there a nonaccidental mechanism that would explain these injuries?
Is there evidence of injuries of varying ages (e.g., old bite marks)?
Was there a delay in seeking medical attention?
Was the injury witnessed?
Are there more than one history for the injury or injuries? Changing histories?
If there is suspicion of a nonaccidental etiology, has the child been reported to the hospital child abuse team and to the local child protective services?

Obvious cases are those with clear and convincing findings. The combination of acute serious brain injury, retinal hemorrhages, and posterior interhemispheric subdural hematomas appear to have greater specificity for an inflicted etiology but are not unique to inflicted injury. Evidence of impact is helpful in establishing inflicted injury when caregivers have specifically denied trauma. In the infant who survives, however, the absence of external scalp bruising, soft tissue swelling, or skull fracture does not conclusively exclude blunt-force trauma, inasmuch as evidence of impact may be found only at postmortem examination.

Severe, diffuse retinal hemorrhages, especially with retinal folds or detachments, in the setting of a trivial mechanism of injury in an otherwise healthy child is strongly suggestive of an abusive mechanism (for details, see the earlier "Retinal Hemorrhages" section) [Betz et al., 1996; Buys et al., 1992]. For example, a child with multiple skull fractures, acute subdural hematoma, brain swelling, and retinal hemorrhages with no history of trauma was abused and does not have a rare arteriovenous malformation [also see Chadwick and Krous, 1997, for additional case studies]. The presence of certain fracture patterns, such as rib fractures or metaphyseal injuries of the long bones, helps exclude accident or disease as alternative causes of the intracranial pathologic processes [Hahn et al., 1988a]. Conversely, the fewer markers of injury and the more nonspecific the history, the more difficult it is to distinguish inflicted from unintentional injury [Morris et al., 2000].

Box 63-5 Factors Associated with an Inflicted Etiology

Age younger than 1 year
Greater severity of illness
Unexplained injuries
A biomechanically inconsistent history
A changing history or one inconsistent with the child's developmental level
A delay in seeking medical attention
Parental risk factors
- History of past abuse and neglect
- Alcohol and drug use
- Previous social service intervention

Evaluating the History of the Injury or Injuries

Histories provided to clinicians typically minimize actual injury events. Most often, there is either a history of minor trauma (such as a short fall with no neurologic symptoms) or no history at all [Chadwick et al., 1991; Dykes, 1986; Shugerman et al., 1996; Weston, 1973]. Changing histories, either by the same caregiver or by multiple caregivers, should also raise concerns. Typically, the actual injury and timeline of those events are understated, whereas descriptions of the clinical behaviors of the infant are accurate [Gilles and Nelson, 1998; Hettler and Greenes, 2003]. There are a number of clues that suggest an inflicted etiology (Box 63-5) [Bechtel et al., 2004; Duhaime et al., 1998; Feldman et al., 2001; Goldstein et al., 1993b; Hettler and Greenes, 2003; Tzioumi and Oates, 1998].

Timing of Injuries

The timing of injury events in the still-living child can usually be estimated by using a combination of clinical course, physical findings, and imaging data, although best estimates are often insufficiently precise to eliminate all possible perpetrators.

Children who sustain moderate to severe traumatic brain injury are almost always immediately symptomatic, often demonstrating an immediate apneustic response to mechanical events whether abused or not [Gilles and Nelson, 1998; Nashelsky and Dix, 1995; Willman et al., 1997; Zuccarello et al., 1985]. Persistence of coma, apnea or respiratory distress, irritability, seizures, hypotonia, and vomiting reflect the severity of injury and evolving secondary pathophysiologic cascades [Aldrich et al., 1992; Gilles and Nelson, 1998; Goldstein et al., 1993b; Johnson et al., 1995; Zuccarello et al., 1985].

Xanthochromic cerebrospinal fluid supernatant with elevated protein levels suggests that subarachnoid bleeding occurred at least 4 hours previously. Timing an injury by neuroimaging findings alone is difficult. Dias and associates [1998] found that the timing of injury could be determined by imaging findings to a reasonable certainty in only 50% of infants in a series of 33 with inflicted head injury.

Lucid Interval Issues

The lucid interval consists of a period of clinical improvement after an initial loss of consciousness, followed by deterioration within minutes to hours. Lucid intervals occur in fewer than 3% of children after traumatic brain injury of all etiologies and generally imply a nonlethal injury if prompt care can be delivered [Bruce et al., 1981; Hahn et al., 1988a; Willman et al., 1997]. In Hahn and colleagues' [1988] study, only 2.2% of 738 children aged 0 to 16 years (318 younger than 36 months) with head injuries had a lucid interval. Bruce and colleagues [1981] detailed the temporal course of the lucid interval in 23 patients. Eight children with Glasgow Coma Scale scores higher than 8 had a variable period of consciousness and speech, followed by the progressive loss of speech and decreased motor activity, but none progressed to coma. All 15 children with initial Glasgow Coma Scale scores lower than 8 were unconscious after trauma, had a period of improved consciousness, and then experienced rapid secondary deterioration within minutes to hours. In a study by Willman and associates [1997] of 95 accidental childhood head injury fatalities, it was obvious in all but one child that the injury was serious from time of injury until death. Only one child (who had an epidural hematoma) had a lucid interval.

Dating of Injuries by Neuroimaging

Brain swelling may develop quite rapidly, even within 20 to 30 minutes, or more slowly [Dias et al., 1998; Gean, 1994; Kobrine et al., 1977; Waga et al., 1979]. Well-developed parenchymal abnormalities were already present on admission CT scans in nine infants whose injury had occurred within the previous 3 hours, which supports findings in the literature that evolution of cerebral parenchymal abnormalities occurs rapidly after injury [Dias et al., 1998; Duhaime et al., 1993; Lobato et al., 1988; Zimmerman et al., 1978]. In children dying from accidental head injury, Willman and associates [1997] found that head CT scans revealed cerebral hypodensity as early as 1 hour, 17 minutes after injury.

Imaging criteria for the dating of subdural hematoma are discussed in detail elsewhere [Gean, 1994]. In general, hyperdense subdural collections on noncontrast CT imaging are less than 7 days old; isointense collections, 7 to 14 days old; and hypodense collections, more than 14 days old. Subdural neomembranes, visualized with contrast CT scans, begin to develop between 7 and 10 days after injury. Subdural hematomas may appear hypodense in the very anemic infant or if there is a mixture of cerebrospinal fluid with subdural blood. The degree to which the subdural membrane has consolidated at postmortem examination and the evolution of the subdural membrane is helpful in pinpointing the age of the collection. MRI, like CT scanning, cannot precisely date injuries, and the finding of blood of different intensities does not always mean that there has been repeated trauma, inasmuch as blood in various compartments may have different signal characteristics.

Medicolegal Issues

Unlike the majority of medical diagnoses, differentiating inflicted from unintentional injury has significant medicolegal consequences, in addition to important prognostic and therapeutic implications. The diagnosis is most specific and sensitive when the event is witnessed or when there is major craniospinal trauma in the absence of any history. The diagnosis is less specific when there are particular patterns of injury that indicate a certain pathophysiologic process. Examples are strangulation evidence in the case of neck bruising and hyoid injury and white matter contusional tears in a young infant. Other pattern injuries that indicate blunt-force trauma are cord marks, bruising in unusual regions (such as abdomen or buttocks), human bites, acute genitoanal trauma, pulmonary or liver contusions, and certain rib and long bone fractures. Evidence of previous maltreatment or neglect is supportive of an inflicted etiology but does not necessarily assist in the determination of the perpetrator, unless he or she is the only caregiver.

Mandated reporting laws require physicians and other health-care professionals to report patterns of injuries and behavior when reasonable suspicion of abuse or neglect arises. Reasonable suspicion does not mean that the clinician must be certain of the diagnosis; it means only that the clinical picture warrants full investigation and protection of the injured child and any siblings. Health-care providers actually fail to diagnose or misdiagnose about a third of inflicted head injuries in infants and children during initial examinations, especially when injuries are not severe [Jenny et al., 1999; Rubin et al., 2003].

The law protects the physician if suspicion should prove erroneous but was made in good faith. Conversely, failure to report both is actionable and places children at significant risk for further harm if they are returned to the setting in which they were injured [Rubin et al., 2003]. Although there is a cross-reporting mandate between social service and law enforcement officials, it may not happen immediately. When serious physical injury is suspected to have resulted from assault, notification of both law enforcement and social services is recommended.

Translating complex information from the medical to the legal arena is a critical component of the evaluation of suspected inflicted head injury for the protection of the child, other siblings, and the alleged perpetrator [Chadwick and Krous, 1997]. This process begins with adequate written, photographic, and schematic documentation, and extends through communication with Child Protective Services, law enforcement agencies, legal counsel, and the judicial system. Investigating agencies want treating clinicians to know whether the injuries were inflicted or not, but the clinician is sometimes unable to say more than that the injuries are clearly traumatic in origin. If there is uncertainty about the significance or timing of particular findings, an expert opinion, usually from a child abuse team physician, neurosurgeon, child neurologist, or forensic neuropathologist with expertise in this area is often helpful. Ultimately, the diagnosis of inflicted injury relies on the constellation of physical findings, a history of injury that is biomechanically feasible, and the timing of injury.

CONCLUSION

Inflicted childhood neurotrauma is a complicated form of neurotrauma with a well-defined continuum of injury findings. The pathophysiology of early life traumatic brain injury needs to be systematically investigated. Neurologic, clinical, and temporal indexes need to be defined in combination with laboratory and imaging data for all children with traumatic brain injury, with secondary analysis for type of injury. The fact that inflicted neurotrauma is the most common cause of serious head injury in infancy must be kept in mind, because recognition and prevention are the best approaches to minimizing the burden of this frequent and tragic disorder.

REFERENCES

Adams J, Graham D, Murray L, et al. Diffuse axonal injury due to nonmissile head injury in humans: An analysis of 45 cases. Ann Neurol 1982;12:557.

Adams J, Mitchell D, Graham D, et al. Diffuse brain damage of immediate impact type. Brain 1977;100:489.

Adelson PD, Clyde B, Kochanek PM, et al. Cerebrovascular response in infants and young children following severe traumatic brain injury: A preliminary report. Pediatr Neurosurg 1997;26:200.

Aldrich E, Eisenberg H, Saydjari C, et al. Diffuse brain swelling in severely head-injured children. A report from the NIH Traumatic Coma Data Bank. J Neurosurg 1992;76:450.

Alexander R, Sato Y, Smith W, et al. Incidence of impact trauma with cranial injuries ascribed to shaking. Am J Dis Child 1990;144:724.

American Academy of Pediatrics Committee on Injury and Poison Prevention. Injuries associated with infant walkers. Pediatrics 2001;108:790.

Annegers JF, Grabow, JD, Groover RV, et al. Seizures after head trauma: A population study. Neurology 1980;30:683.

Aoki N. Extracerebral fluid collections in infancy: Role of magnetic resonance imaging in differentiation between subdural effusion and subarachnoid space enlargement. J Neurosurg 1994;81:20.

Arita K, Uozumi T, Oki S, et al. The function of the hypothalamic-pituitary-adrenal axis in brain dead patients. Acta Neurochir 1993;123:64.

Armstead WM, Kurth CD. Different cerebral hemodynamic responses following fluid percussion brain injury in the newborn and juvenile pig. J Neurotrauma 1994;11:487.

Arnholz D, Hymel KP, Hay TC, et al. Bilateral pediatric skull fractures: Accident or abuse? J Trauma 1998;45:172.

Ashwal S, Holshouser BA, Hinshaw D, et al. Proton magnetic resonance spectroscopy in the evaluation of children with congenital heart disease and acute central nervous system injury. J Thorac Cardiovasc Surg 1996;112:403.

Ashwal S, Holshouser BA, Shu SK, et al. Predictive value of proton magnetic resonance spectroscopy in pediatric closed head injury. Pediatr Neurol 2000;23:114.

Atkinson JL. The neglected prehospital phase of head injury: Apnea and catecholamine surge. Mayo Clin Proc 2000;75:37.

Atkinson JL, Anderson RE, Murray MJ. The early critical phase of severe head injury: Importance of apnea and dysfunctional respiration. J Trauma 1998;45:941.

Atwal GS, Rutty GN, Carter N, et al. Bruising in non-accidental head injured children: A retrospective study of the prevalence, distribution and pathological associations in 24 cases. Forensic Sci Int 1998;96:215.

Azzarelli B, Caldemeyer KS, Phillips J, et al. Hypoxic-ischemic encephalopathy in areas of primary myelination: A neuroimaging and PET study. Pediatr Neurol 1996;14:108.

Baillard C, Vivien B, Mansier P, et al. Brain death assessment using instant spectral analysis of heart rate variability. Crit Care Med 2002;30:306.

Ball WS. Nonaccidental craniocerebral trauma (child abuse): MR imaging. Radiology 1989;173:609.

Banaszkiewicz PA, Scotland TR, Myerscough EJ. Fractures in children younger than age 1 year: Importance of collaboration with child protection services. J Pediatr Orthop 2002;22:740.

Barlow KM, Minns RA. The relation between intracranial pressure and outcome in non-accidental head injury. Dev Med Child Neurol 1999;41:220.

Bass M, Kravath RE, Glass L. Death-scene investigation in sudden infant death. N Engl J Med 1986;315:100.

Baum J, Bulpitt C. Retinal and conjunctival hemorrhage in the newborn. Arch Dis Child 1970;45:344.

Bechtel K, Stoessel K, Leventhal JM, et al. Characteristics that distinguish accidental from abusive injury in hospitalized young children with head trauma. Pediatrics 2004;114:165.

Becroft D, Lockett B. Intra-alveolar pulmonary siderophages in sudden infant death: A marker for previous imposed suffocation. Pathology 1997;29:60.

Bell MJ, Kochanek PM, Doughty LA, et al. Interleukin-6 and interleukin-10 in cerebrospinal fluid after severe traumatic brain injury in children. J Neurotrauma 1997;14:451.

Bell MJ, Kochanek PM, Heyes MP, et al. Quinolinic acid in the cerebrospinal fluid of children after traumatic brain injury. Crit Care Med 1999;27:493.

Bernardi B, Zimmerman RA, Balaniuk LT. Neuroradiologic evaluation of pediatric craniocerebral trauma. Top Magn Reson Imaging 1993;5:161.

Betz P, Puschel K, Miltner E, et al. Morphometrical analysis of retinal hemorrhages in the shaken baby syndrome. Forensic Sci Int 1996;78:71.

Bigler ED. Quantitative magnetic resonance imaging in traumatic brain injury. J Head Trauma Rehabil 2001;16:117.

Billmire ME, Myers PA. Serious head injury in infants: Accident or abuse? Pediatrics 1985;75:340.

Biousse VD, Suh Y, Newman NJ, et al. Diffusion-weighted magnetic resonance imaging in shaken baby syndrome. Am J Ophthalmol 2002;133:249.

Bird R, McMahan JR, Gilles FH, et al. Strangulation in child abuse: CT diagnosis? Radiology 1987;163:373.

Biswas AK, Scott WA, Sommerauer JF, et al. Heart rate variability after acute traumatic brain injury in children. Crit Care Med 2000;28:3907.

Bittigau P, Sifringer M, Felderhoff-Muesser U, et al. Neuropathological and biochemical features of traumatic injury in the developing brain. Neurotox Res 2003;5:475.

Blennow M, Savman K, Ilves P, et al. Brain-specific proteins in the cerebrospinal fluid of severely asphyxiated newborn infants. Acta Paediatr 2001;90:1171.

Bonnier C, Nassogne M-C, Evrard P, et al. Outcome and prognosis of whiplash shaken infant syndrome: Late consequences after a symptom free interval. Dev Med Child Neurol 1995;37:943.

Bonnier C, Nassogne M-C, Saint-Martin C, et al. Neuroimaging of intraparenchymal lesions predicts outcome in shaken baby syndrome. Pediatrics 2003;112:808.

Brinker T, Ludemann W, von Rautenfeld DB, et al. Breakdown of the meningeal barrier surrounding the intraorbital optic nerve after experimental subarachnoid hemorrhage. Am J Ophthalmol 1997;124:373.

Brismar J, Ozand P. CT and MR of the brain in the diagnosis of organic acidemias. Experiences from 107 patients. Brain Dev 1994;16 (Suppl):104.

Brody B, Kinney H, Kloman A, et al. Sequence of central nervous system myelination in human infancy. I. An autopsy study of myelination. J Neuropathol Exp Neurol 1987;46:282.

Bruce DA, Alavi A, Bilaniuk L, et al. Diffuse cerebral swelling following head injuries in children: The syndrome of malignant brain edema. J Neurosurg 1981;54:170.

Budenz DL, Farber MG, Mirchandani HG, et al. Ocular and optic nerve hemorrhages in abused infants with intracranial injuries. Ophthalmology 1994;101:559.

Butterworth R, Wassif W, Sherwood RA, et al. Serum neuron-specific enolase, carnosinase, and their ratio in acute stroke. Stroke 1996;27:2064.

Buys YM, Levin AV, Enzenauer RW, et al. Retinal findings after head trauma in infants and young children. Ophthalmology 1992;99:1718.

Caffey J. On the theory and practice of shaking infants. Am J Dis Child 1972;124:161.

Caffey J. The whiplash shaken infant syndrome: Manual shaking by the extremities with whiplash-induced intracranial and intraocular bleedings, linked with residual permanent brain damage and mental retardation. Pediatrics 1974;54:396.

Calder I, Hill I, Scholtz, C, et al. Primary brain trauma in non-accidental head injury. J Clin Pathol 1984;37:1095.

Carraro MC, Rossetti L, Gerli GC. The irreplaceable image: An unexpected manifestation of anemia. Haematologica 2001;86:672.

Carter J, McCormick, A. Whiplash shaking syndrome: Retinal hemorrhages and computerized axial tomography of the brain. Child Abuse Neglect 1983;7:279.

Case ME, Graham MA, Handy TC, et al. Position paper on fatal abusive head injuries in infants and young children. Am J Forensic Med Pathol 2001;22:112.

Chadwick DL, Chin S, Salerno C, et al. Deaths from falls in children: How far is fatal? J Trauma 1991;31:1353.

Chadwick DL, Krous HF. Irresponsible testimony by medical experts in cases involving the physical abuse and neglect of children. Child Maltreat 1997;2:313.

Chesnut RM, Marshall LF, Klauber M, et al. The role of secondary brain injury in determining outcome from severe head injury. J Trauma 1993;34:216.

Chiavello C, Christoph R, Bond G, et al. Infant walker related injuries: A prospective study of severity and incidence. Pediatrics 1994;93:974.

Chiolero R, Berger M. Endocrine response to brain injury. New Horiz 1994;2:432.

Christian CW, Taylor AA, Hertle RW, et al. Retinal hemorrhages caused by accidental household trauma. J Pediatr 1999;135:125.

Cirak B, Ziegfeld S, Knight VM, et al. Spinal injuries in children. J Pediatr Surg 2004;39:607.

Clifton G, Robertson C, Kyper K, et al. Cardiovascular response to severe head injury. J Neurosurg 1983;59:447.

Cohen RA, Kaufman RA, Myers PA, et al. Cranial computed tomography in the abused child with head injury. AJNR Am J Neuroradiol 1985;6:883.

Correale J, Rabinowicz A, Heck C, et al. Status epilepticus increases CSF levels of neuron-specific enolase and alters the blood-brain barrier. Neurology 1998;50:1388.

Courville C. Contrecoup injuries of the brain in infancy: Remarks on the mechanism of fatal traumatic lesions of early life. Arch Surg 1965;90:157.

Crisostomo EA, Leaton E, Rosenblum E, et al. Features of intracranial aneurysms in infants and report of a case. Dev Med Child Neurol 1986;28:68.

Crooks DA. Pathogenesis and biomechanics of traumatic intracranial haemorrhages. Virchows Arch A Pathol Anat Histopathol 1991;418:479.

Crume TL, DiGuiseppi C, Byers T, et al. Underascertainment of child maltreatment fatalities by death certificates, 1990-1998. Pediatrics 2002;110:e18.

de Schweinitz G, Holoway T. Fracture of the skull with hemorrhage into the optic nerve-sheaths and retinas: Microscopic examination of the eyeballs. Trans Am Ophthalmol Soc 1912;13:120.

Demaerel P, Casteels I, Wilms G. Cranial imaging in child abuse. Eur Radiol 2002;12:849.

Demissie K, Rhoads GG, Smulian JC, et al. Operative vaginal delivery and neonatal and infant adverse outcomes: Population based retrospective analysis. BMJ 2004;329:24.

Denny-Brown D, Russell WR. Experimental cerebral concussion. Brain 1941;64:93.

DeWitt DS, Jenkins LW, Progh DS. Enhanced vulnerability to secondary ischemic insults after experimental traumatic brain injury. New Horiz 1995;3:376.

Diamond P, Hansen CM, Christofersen MR, et al. Child abuse presenting as a thoracolumbar spinal fracture dislocation: A case report. Pediatr Emerg Care 1994;10:83.

Dias MS, Backstrom J, Falk M, et al. Serial radiography in the infant shaken impact syndrome. Pediatr Neurosurg 1998;29:77.

Digraham D, Ford I, Adams JH, et al. Fatal head injury in children. J Clin Pathol 1989;42:18.

Distinguishing sudden infant death syndrome from child abuse fatalities. Committee on Child Abuse and Neglect, 1993-1994. Del Med J 1997;69:371.

Doezema D, King JN, Tandberg D, et al. Magnetic resonance imaging in minor head injury. Ann Emerg Med 1991;20:1281.

Drack AV, Petronio J, Capone A. Unilateral retinal hemorrhages in documented cases of child abuse. Am J Ophthalmol 1999;128:340.

Drigo P, Piovan S, Battistella PA, et al. Macrocephaly, subarachnoid fluid collection, and glutaric aciduria type I. J Child Neurol 1996;11:414.

D'Souza SW, McConnell SE, Slater P, et al. *N*-methyl-D-aspartate binding sites in neonatal and adult brain. Lancet 1992;339:1240.

Dubowitz H, Bross DC. The pediatrician's documentation of child maltreatment. Am J Dis Child 1992;146:596.

Duhaime A-C, Alario AJ, Lewander WJ, et al. Head injury in very young children: Mechanisms, injury types, and ophthalmologic findings in 100 hospitalized patients younger than 2 years of age. Pediatrics 1992;90:179.

Duhaime A-C, Balaniuk L, Zimmerman R. The big black brain: Radiographic changes after severe inflicted head injury in infancy J Neurotrauma 1993;10 (Suppl 1):S59.

Duhaime A-C, Christian C, Armonda R, et al. Disappearing subdural hematomas in children. Pediatr Neurosurg 1996a;25:116.

Duhaime A-C, Christian C, Moss E, et al. Long-term outcome in infants with the shaking-impact syndrome. Pediatr Neurosurg 1996b;24:292.

Duhaime A-C, Christian C, Rorke LB, et al. Nonaccidental head injury in infants—The shaken-baby syndrome. N Engl J Med 1998;338:1822.

Duhaime A-C, Gennarelli TA, Thibault LF, et al. The shaken baby syndrome. A clinical, pathological, and biomechanical study. J Neurosurg 1987;66:409.

Duhaime A-C, Hunter J, Grate LL, et al. Magnetic resonance imaging studies of age-dependent responses to scaled focal brain injury in the piglet. J Neurosurg 2003;99:542.

Duhaime A-C, Margulies S, Durham SR, et al. Maturation-dependent response of the piglet brain to scaled cortical impact. J Neurosurg 2000;93:455.

Durham S, Clancy R, Leuthardt E, et al. The CHOP infant coma scale (Infant Face Scale): A novel coma scale for children less than 2 years of age. J Neurotrauma 2000a;17:729.

Durham S, Raghupathi R, Helfaer MA, et al. Age-related differences in acute physiologic response to focal traumatic brain injury in piglets. Pediatr Neurosurg 2000b;33:76.

Dykes LJ. The whiplash shaken infant syndrome: What has been learned? Child Abuse Negl 1986;10:211.

Eder HG, Legat GA, Gruber W. Traumatic brain stem lesions in children. Childs Nerv Syst 2000;16:21.

Egge K, Lyng G, Maltau JM. Retinal haemorrhages in the newborn. Acta Ophthalmol (Copenh) 1980;58:231.

Ehrenfest H. Birth injuries of the child. New York: Appleton, 1922.

Eisenbrey AB. Retinal hemorrhage in the battered child. Childs Brain 1979;5:40.

Elder JE, Taylor RG, Klug G, et al. Retinal haemorrhage in accidental head trauma in childhood. J Paediatr Child Health 1991;27:286.

Elner SG, Elner VM, Arnall M, et al. Ocular and associated systemic findings in suspected child abuse. A necropsy study. Arch Ophthalmol 1990;108:1094.

Emanuelson I. How safe are childcare products, toys and playground equipment? A Swedish analysis of mild brain injuries at home and during leisure time 1998-1999. Inj Control Saf Promot 2003;10:139.

Emerson MV, Pieramici DJ, Stoessel KM, et al. Incidence and rate of disappearance of retinal hemorrhage in newborns. Ophthalmology 2001;108:36.

Ewing-Cobbs L, Prasad M, Kramer L, et al. Inflicted traumatic brain injury: Relationship of developmental outcome to severity of injury. Pediatr Neurosurg 1999;31:251.

Ewing-Cobbs L, Prasad M, Kramer L, et al. Acute neuroradiologic findings in young children with inflicted or noninflicted traumatic brain injury. Childs Nerv Syst 2000;16:25.

Fackler JC, Berkowitz ID, Green WR. Retinal hemorrhages in newborn piglets following cardiopulmonary resuscitation. Am J Dis Child 1992;146:1294.

Fan P, Yamauchi T, Noble LJ, et al. Age-dependent differences in glutathione peroxidase activity after traumatic brain injury. J Neurotrauma 2003;20:437.

Feldman KW, Bethel R, Shugerman RP, et al. The cause of infant and toddler subdural hemorrhage: A prospective study. Pediatrics 2001;108:636.

Feldman KW, Brewer DK, Shaw DW. Evolution of the cranial computed tomography scan in child abuse. Child Abuse Negl 1995;19:307.

Frauenberger G, Lis E. Multiple fractures associated with subdural hematomas in infancy. Pediatrics 1950;6:890.

Fridriksson T, Kini N, Walsh-Kelly C, et al. Serum neuron-specific enolase as a predictor of intracranial lesions in children with head trauma: A pilot study. Acad Emerg Med 2000;7:816.

Ganesh A, Jenny C, Geyer J, et al. Retinal hemorrhages in type I osteogenesis imperfecta after minor trauma. Ophthalmology 2004;111:1428.

Gaynon MW, Koh K, Marmor MF, et al. Retinal folds in the shaken baby syndrome. Am J Ophthalmol 1988;106:423.

Gean A. Imaging of head trauma. New York: Raven Press, 1994.

Geddes JF, Hackshaw AK, Vowles GH, et al. Neuropathology of inflicted head injury in children. I. Patterns of brain damage. Brain 2001a;124:1290.

Geddes JF, Tasker RC, Hackshaw AK, et al. Dural haemorrhage in non-traumatic infant deaths: Does it explain the bleeding in "shaken baby syndrome"? Neuropathol Appl Neurobiol 2003;29:14.

Geddes JF, Vowles GH, Hackshaw AK, et al. Neuropathology of inflicted head injury in children. II. Microscopic brain injury in infants. Brain 2001b;124:1299.

Gennarelli TA. Cerebral concussion and diffuse brain injuries. In: Cooper PR, ed. Head injury. Baltimore: Williams & Wilkins, 1993;137.

Gennarelli TA, Thibault LE, Adams JH, et al. Diffuse axonal injury and traumatic coma in the primate. Ann Neurol 1982;12:564.

Gentry LR, Godersky JC, Thompson B. MR imaging of head trauma: Review of the distribution and radiopathologic features of traumatic lesions. AJR Am J Roentgenol 1988;50:663.

Gerber DJ, Weintraub AH, Cusick CP, et al. Magnetic resonance imaging of traumatic brain injury: relationship of T2*SE and T2GE to clinical severity and outcome. Brain Inj 2004;18:1083.

Ghatan S, Ellenbogen RG. Pediatric spine and spinal cord injury after inflicted trauma. Neurosurg Clin North Am 2002;13:227.

Giangiacomo J, Khan JA, Levine C, et al. Sequential cranial computed tomography in infants with retinal hemorrhages. Ophthalmology 1988;95:295.

Gilles EE, McGregor ML, Levy-Clarke G. Retinal hemorrhage asymmetry in inflicted head injury: A clue to pathogenesis? J Pediatr 2003;143:494.

Gilles EE, Nelson MD. Cerebral complications of nonaccidental head injury in childhood. Pediatr Neurol 1998;19:119.

Gilliland MG, Folberg R. Retinal hemorrhages: Replicating the clinician's view of the eye. Forensic Sci Int 1992;56:77.

Gilliland MG, Luckenbach MW. Are retinal hemorrhages found after resuscitation attempts? A study of the eyes of 169 children. Am J Forensic Med Pathol 1993;14:187.

Gilliland MG, Luckenbach MW, Chenier TC. Systemic and ocular findings in 169 prospectively studied child deaths: Retinal hemorrhages usually mean child abuse. Forensic Sci Int 1994;68:117.

Gjerris F. Head injuries in children—Special features. Acta Neurochir Suppl (Wien) 1986;36:155.

Glasier CM, Seibert JJ, Williamson SL. Cerebral infarction in child abuse. Diagnosis by technetium-99m methylene diphosphonate skeletal scintigraphy. Clin Nucl Med 1987;12:897.

Goldstein B, DeKing D, Delong DJ, et al. Autonomic cardiovascular state after severe brain injury and brain death in children. Crit Care Med 1993a;21:228.

Goldstein B, Kelly MM, Bruton D, et al. Inflicted versus accidental head injury in critically injured children. Crit Care Med 1993b;21:1328.

Goldstein B, Kempski MH, DeKing D, et al. Autonomic control of heart rate after brain injury in children. Crit Care Med 1996;24:234.

Govaert P, Van De Velde E, Vanhaesebrouck P, et al. CT diagnosis of neonatal subarachnoid hemorrhage. Pediatr Radiol 1990;20:139.

Govind A, Kumari S, Lath NK. Retinal hemorrhages in newborn. Indian Pediatr 1989;26:150.

Graham DI, Ford I, Adams JH, et al. Fatal head injury in children. J Clin Pathol 1989;42:18.

Greenberg J, Cohen WA, Cooper PR. The hyperacute extra-axial intracranial hematoma: Computed tomographic findings and clinical significance. Neurosurgery 1985;17:48.

Greenes DS, Schutzman SA. Infants with isolated skull fracture: What are their clinical characteristics, and do they require hospitalization? Ann Emerg Med 1997;30:253.

Greenwald MJ, Weiss A, Oesterle CS, et al. Traumatic retinoschisis in battered babies. Ophthalmology 1986;93:618.

Guthkelch A. Infantile subdural hematoma and its relationship to whiplash injuries. BMJ 1971;2:430.

Hablitz JJ, Lee WL. NMDA receptor involvement in epileptogenesis in the immature neocortex. Epilepsy Res Suppl 1992;8:139.

Hadley MN, Sonntag VK, Rekate HL, et al. The infant whiplash-shake injury syndrome: A clinical and pathological study. Neurosurgery 1989;24:536.

Hagberg H, Thornberg E, Blennow M, et al. Excitatory amino acids in the cerebrospinal fluid of asphyxiated infants: Relationship to hypoxic-ischemic encephalopathy. Acta Paediatr 1993;82:925.

Hahn YS, Chyung C, Barthel MJ, et al. Head injuries in children under 36 months of age. Demography and outcome. Childs Nerv Syst 1988a;4:34.

Hahn YS, Fuchs S, Flannery AM, et al. Factors influencing posttraumatic seizures in children. Neurosurgery 1988b;22:864.

Hahn YS, Raimondi AJ, McLone DG, et al. Traumatic mechanisms of head injury in child abuse. Childs Brain 1983;10:229.

Hamlin H. Subgaleal hematoma caused by hair pull. JAMA 1968;204:339.

Hammoud DA, Wasserman BA. Diffuse axonal injuries: Pathophysiology and imaging. Neuroimaging Clin North Am 2002;12:205.

Han BK, Towbin RB, De Courten-Myers G, et al. Reversal sign on CT: Effect of anoxic/ischemic cerebral injury in children. AJNR Am J Neuroradiol 1990;10:1191.

Hasegawa M, Yamashima T, Yamashita J, et al. Traumatic subdural hygroma: Pathology and meningeal enhancement on magnetic resonance imaging. Neurosurgery 1992;31:580.

Haviland J, Russell RI. Outcome after severe non-accidental head injury. Arch Dis Child 1997;77:504.

Hayashi N, Endo S, Oka N, et al. Intracranial hemorrhage due to rupture of an arteriovenous malformation in a full-term neonate. Childs Nerv Syst 1994;10:344.

Hayashi T, Hashimoto T, Fukuda S, et al. Neonatal subdural hematoma secondary to birth injury. Clinical analysis of 48 survivors. Childs Nerv Syst 1987;3:23.

Hedges TR, Weinstein JD, Crystle CD. Orbital vascular response to acutely increased intracranial pressure in the rhesus monkey. Arch Ophthalmol 1964;71:226.

Herlenius E, Lagercrantz H. Development of neurotransmitter systems during critical periods. Exp Neurol 2004;190 (Suppl 1):8.

Herr S, Pierce M-C, Berger RP, et al. Does Valsalva retinopathy occur in infants? An initial investigation in infants with vomiting caused by pyloric stenosis. Pediatrics 2004;113:1658.

Herrmann M, Jost S, Kutz S, et al. Temporal profile of release of neurobiochemical markers of brain damage after traumatic brain injury is associated with intracranial pathology as demonstrated in cranial computerized tomography. J Neurotrauma 2000;17:113.

Hettler J, Greenes DS. Can the initial history predict whether a child with a head injury has been abused? Pediatrics 2003;111:602.

Hiss J, Kahana T. The medicolegal implications of bilateral cranial fractures in infants. J Trauma 1995;38:32.

Hobbs C. Skull fracture and the diagnosis of abuse. Arch Dis Child 1984;59:246.

Howard JL, Barron BJ, Smith GG. Bone scintigraphy in the evaluation of extraskeletal injuries from child abuse. Radiographics 1990;10:67.

Huisman TA, Sorensen AG, Hergan K, et al. Diffusion-weighted imaging for the evaluation of diffuse axonal injury in closed head injury. J Comput Assist Tomogr 2003;27:5.

Hulka F, Mullins RJ, Frank EH. Blunt brain injury activates the coagulation process. Arch Surg 1996;131:923.

Huttenlocher PR. Synapse elimination and plasticity in developing human cerebral cortex. Am J Ment Defic 1984;88:488.

Hymel KP, Abshire TC, Luckey D, et al. Coagulopathy in pediatric abusive head trauma. Pediatrics 1997;99:371.

Ingraham F, Heyl H. Subdural hematoma in infancy and childhood. JAMA 1939;112:198.

Irazuzta J, McJunkin J, Danadian K, et al. Outcome and cost of child abuse. Child Abuse Negl 1997;21:751.

Jaspan T, Narborough G, Punt J, et al. Cerebral contusional tears as a marker of child abuse—Detection by cranial sonography. Pediatr Radiol 1992;22:237.

Jenny C, Hymel KP, Ritzen A, et al. Analysis of missed cases of abusive head trauma. JAMA 1999;281:621.

Joffe M, Ludwig S. Stairway injuries in children. Pediatrics 1988;82:457.

Johnson DL, Boal D, Baule R, et al. Role of apnea in nonaccidental head injury. Pediatr Neurosurg 1995;23:305.

Johnson DL, Braun D, Friendly D. Accidental head trauma and retinal hemorrhage. Neurosurgery 1993;33:231.

Johnston MV. Neurotransmitters and vulnerability of the developing brain. Brain Dev 1995;17:301.

Johnston MV. Developmental aspects of epileptogenesis. Epilepsia 1996;37 (Suppl 1):S2.

Kanter RK. Retinal hemorrhage after cardiopulmonary resuscitation or child abuse. J Pediatr 1986;108:430.

Kaufman HH. Traumatic subdural hygroma: Pathology and meningeal enhancement on magnetic resonance imaging. Neurosurgery 1993;32:149.

Kazan S, Tuncer R, Karasoy M, et al. Post-traumatic bilateral diffuse cerebral swelling. Acta Neurochir (Wien) 1997;139:295.

Keane JR. Retinal hemorrhages. Its significance in 100 patients with acute encephalopathy of unknown cause. Arch Neurol 1979;36:691.

Keenan HT, Runyan DK, Marshall SW, et al. A population-based study of inflicted traumatic brain injury in young children. JAMA 2003;290:621.

Kemp AM, Stoodley N, Cobley C, et al. Apnoea and brain swelling in non-accidental head injury. Arch Dis Child 2003;88:472.

Kempe C, Silverman F, Steele B, et al. The battered child syndrome. JAMA 1962;181:17.

Kessler DB, Siegel-Stein F. Retinal hemorrhage, meningitis, and child abuse. N Y State J Med 1984;84:59.

Kimura S, Hara M, Nezu A, et al. Two cases of glutaric aciduria type 1: Clinical and neuropathological findings. J Neurol Sci 1994;123:38.

Kinney H, Brody B, Kloman A, et al. Sequence of central nervous system myelination in human infancy. II. Patterns of myelination in autopsied infants. J Neuropathol Exp Neurol 1988;47:217.

Kleinman P. Diagnostic imaging in infant abuse. Am J Radiology 1990;155:703.

Kobrine AI, Timmins E, Rajjoub RK, et al. Demonstration of massive traumatic brain swelling within 20 minutes after injury. Case report. J Neurosurg 1977;46:256.

Koiv L, Merisalu E, Zilmer K, et al. Changes in sympatho-adrenal and hypothalamic-pituitary-adrenocortical system in patients with head injury. Acta Neurol Scand 1997;96:52.

Kravitz H, Driessen G, Gomberg R, et al. Accidental falls from elevated surfaces in infants from birth to one year of age. Pediatrics 1969;44:869.

Kubova H, Moshe SL. Experimental models of epilepsy in young animals. J Child Neurol 1994;9 (Suppl 1):S3.

Lambert SR, Johnson TE, Hoyt CS. Optic nerve sheath and retinal hemorrhages associated with the shaken baby syndrome. Arch Ophthalmol 1986;104:1509.

Land J, Goulder P, Johnson A, et al. Glutaric aciduria type 1: An atypical presentation together with some observations upon treatment and the possible cause of cerebral damage. Neuropediatrics 1992;23:322.

Laskey AL, Holsti M, Runyan DK, et al. Occult head trauma in young suspected victims of physical abuse. J Pediatr 2004;144:719.

Lea PMT, Faden AI. Traumatic brain injury: Developmental differences in glutamate receptor response and the impact on treatment. Ment Retard Dev Disabil Res Rev 2001;7:235.

Lenn N. Neuroplasticity and the developing brain: Implications for therapy. Pediatr Neurosci 1987;13:176.

Lewis RJ, Yee L, Inkelis SH, et al. Clinical predictors of post-traumatic seizures in children with head trauma. Ann Emerg Med 1993;22:1114.

Lindenberg R. Mechanical injuries of brain and meninges. In: Spitz WU, Fisher RS, eds. Medicolegal investigation of death: Guidelines for the application of pathology to crime investigation. Springfield, IL: Charles C Thomas, 1973;420.

Lindenberg R, Freytag E. Morphology of brain lesions from blunt trauma in early infancy. Arch Pathol 1969;87:298.

Liwnicz BH, Mouradian MD, Ball J, et al. Intense brain cortical enhancement on CT in laminar necrosis verified by biopsy. AJNR Am J Neuroradiol 1987;8:157.

Lo TY, McPhillips M, Minns RA, et al. Cerebral atrophy following shaken impact syndrome and other non-accidental head injury (NAHI). Pediatr Rehabil 2003;6:47.

Lobato R, Sarabia R, Cordobes F, et al. Posttraumatic cerebral hemispheric swelling. J Neurosurg 1988;68:417.

Ludwig S, Warman M. Shaken baby syndrome: A review of 20 cases. Ann Emerg Med 1984;13:104.

Lyle DJ, Stapp JP, Button RR, et al. Ophthalmologic hydrostatic pressure syndrome. Am J Ophthalmol 1957;44:652.

Lyons T, Oates R. Falling out of bed: A relatively benign occurrence. Pediatrics 1993;92:125.

Mandelstam SA, Cook D, Fitzgerald M, et al. Complementary use of radiological skeletal survey and bone scintigraphy in detection of bony injuries in suspected child abuse. Arch Dis Child 2003;88:387.

Mares P, Folbergrova J, Kubova H. Excitatory amino acids and epileptic seizures in immature brain. Physiol Res 2004;53 (Suppl 1):S115.

Marin-Padilla M, Parisi JE, Armstrong DL, et al. Shaken infant syndrome: Developmental neuropathology, progressive cortical dysplasia, and epilepsy. Acta Neuropathol (Berl) 2002;103:321.

Marshman WE, Adams GG, Ohri R. Bilateral vitreous hemorrhages in an infant with low fibrinogen levels. J AAPOS 1999;3:255.

Martens P, Raabe A, Johnsson P. Serum S-100 and neuron-specific enolase for prediction of regaining consciousness after global cerebral ischemia. Stroke 1998;29:2363.

Massicotte SJ, Folberg R, Torczynski E, et al. Vitreoretinal traction and perimacular retinal folds in the eyes of deliberately traumatized children. Ophthalmology 1991;98:1124.

Matson D. Intracranial arterial aneurysms in children. J Neurosurg 1965;23:578.

Matsumura F, Ito Y. Petechial hemorrhage of the conjunctiva and histological findings of the lung and pancreas in infantile asphyxia—Evaluation of 85 cases. Kurume Med J 1996;43:259.

Matsuzaka T, Yoshinaga M, Tsuji Y, et al. Incidence and causes of intracranial hemorrhage in infancy: A prospective surveillance study after vitamin K prophylaxis. Brain Dev 1989;11:384.

Matthews GP, Das A. Dense vitreous hemorrhages predict poor visual and neurological prognosis in infants with shaken baby syndrome. J Pediatr Ophthalmol Strabismus 1996;33:260.

McCabe CF, Donahue SP. Prognostic indicators for vision and mortality in shaken baby syndrome. Arch Ophthalmol 2000;118:373.

McDonald JW, Trescher WH, Johnston MV. Susceptibility of brain to AMPA induced excitotoxicity transiently peaks during early postnatal development. Brain Res 1992;583:54.

McKeating EG, Andrews PJ, Mascia L. Relationship of neuron specific enolase and protein S-100 concentrations in systemic and jugular venous serum to injury severity and outcome after traumatic brain injury. Acta Neurochir Suppl (Wien) 1998;71:117.

McLaurin RL, Tutor FT. Acute subdural hematoma. A review of ninety cases. J Neurosurg 1961;18:61.

Medele RJ, Stummer W, Mueller AJ, et al. Terson's syndrome in subarachnoid hemorrhage and severe brain injury accompanied by acutely raised intracranial pressure. J Neurosurg 1998;88:851.

Mei-Zahav M, Uziel Y, Raz J, et al. Convulsions and retinal haemorrhage: Should we look further? Arch Dis Child 2002;86:334.

Mendelsohn DB, Levin HS, Harward H, et al. Corpus callosum lesions after closed head injury in children: MRI, clinical features and outcome. Neuroradiology 1992;34:384.

Meservy CJ, Towbin R, McLaurin RL, et al. Radiographic characteristics of skull fractures resulting from child abuse. AJR Am J Roentgenol 1987;149:173.

Michaud LJ, Rivara FP, Longstreth W, et al. Elevated initial blood glucose levels and poor outcome following severe brain injuries in children. J Trauma 1991;31:1356.

Miller JD, Bullock R, Graham DI, et al. Ischemic brain damage in a model of acute subdural hematoma. Neurosurgery 1990;27:433.

Mills M. Funduscopic lesions associated with mortality in shaken baby syndrome. J AAPOS 1998;2:67.

Mirvis SE, Wolf AL, Numaguchi Y, et al. Posttraumatic cerebral infarction diagnosed by CT: Prevalence, origin, and outcome. AJNR Am J Neuroradiol 1990;11:355.

Morganti-Kossmann MC, Rancan M, Stahel PF, et al. Inflammatory response in acute traumatic brain injury: A double-edged sword. Curr Opin Crit Care 2002;8:101.

Mori K, Handa H, Itoh M, et al. Benign subdural effusion in infants. J Comput Assist Tomogr 1980;4:466.

Morris MW, Smith S, Cressman J, et al. Evaluation of infants with subdural hematoma who lack external evidence of abuse. Pediatrics 2000;105:549.

Muller PJ, Deck JHN. Intraocular and optic nerve sheath hemorrhage in cases of sudden intracranial hypertension. J Neurosurg 1974;41:160.

Munger CE, Peiffer RL, Bouldin TW, et al. Ocular and associated neuropathologic observations in suspected whiplash shaken infant syndrome. A retrospective study of 12 cases. Am J Forensic Med Pathol 1993;14:193.

Musemeche CA, Barthel M, Costentino C, et al. Pediatric falls from heights. J Trauma 1991;31:1347.

Mushin AS. Ocular damage in the battered-baby syndrome. BMJ 1971;3:402.

Nashelsky MB, Dix JD. The time interval between lethal infant shaking and onset of symptoms. A review of the shaken baby syndrome literature. Am J Forensic Med Pathol 1995;16:154.

Nassogne MC, Sharrard M, Hertz-Pannier L, et al. Massive subdural haematomas in Menkes disease mimicking shaken baby syndrome. Childs Nerv Syst 2002;18:729.

Nimityongskul P, Anderson LD. The likelihood of injuries when children fall out of bed. J Pediatr Orthop 1987;7:184.

Nishimura K, Mori K, Sakamoto T, et al. Management of subarachnoid fluid collection in infants based on a long-term follow-up study. Acta Neurochir (Wien) 1996;138:179.

Novack TA, Dillon MC, Jackson WT. Neurochemical mechanisms in brain injury and treatment: A review. J Clin Exp Neuropsychol 1996;18:685.

Odom A, Christ E, Kerr N, et al. Prevalence of retinal hemorrhages in pediatric patients after in-hospital cardiopulmonary resuscitation: A prospective study. Pediatrics 1997;99:E3.

O'Leary JA, Ferrell RE, Randolph CR. Retinal hemorrhage and vacuum extraction delivery. J Perinat Med 1986;14:197.

Ommaya A, Gennarelli T. Cerebral concussion and traumatic unconsciousness. Correlation of experimental and clinical observations on blunt head injuries. Brain 1974;97:633.

Ophthalmology Child Abuse Working Party. Child abuse and the eye. Eye 1999;13:3.

O'Regan ME, Brown JK. Serum neuron specific enolase: A marker for neuronal dysfunction in children with continuous EEG epileptiform activity. Eur J Paediatr Neurol 1998;2:193.

Orlin JR, Zwetnow NN, Bjorneboe A. Changes in CSF pressures during experimental acute arterial subdural bleeding in pig. Acta Neurochir (Wien) 1992;118:146.

Osaka H, Kimura S, Nezu A, et al. Chronic subdural hematoma, as an initial manifestation of glutaric aciduria type-1. Brain Dev 1993;15:125.

Paradis N, Martin G, Goetting M, et al. Simultaneous aortic, jugular bulb, and right atrial pressures during cardiopulmonary resuscitation in humans. Insights into mechanisms. Circulation 1989;80:361.

Paret G, Tirosh R, Lotan D, et al. Early prediction of neurological outcome after falls in children: Metabolic and clinical markers. J Accid Emerg Med 1999;16:186.

Partington M, Swanson J, Meyer FB. Head injury and the use of baby walkers: A continuing problem. Ann Emerg Med 1991;20:652.

Pascoe JM, Hildebrandt HM, Tarrier A, et al. Patterns of skin injury in nonaccidental and accidental injury. Pediatrics 1979;64:245.

Paviglianiti JC, Donahue SP. Unilateral retinal hemorrhages and ipsilateral intracranial bleeds in nonaccidental trauma. J AAPOS 1999;3:383.

Perret G, Nishioka H. Report on the cooperative study of intracranial aneurysms and subarachnoid hemorrhage. IV. Cerebral angiography. An analysis of the diagnostic value and complications of carotid and vertebral angiography in 5,484 patients. J Neurosurg 1966;25:98.

Pfenninger J, Santi A. Severe traumatic brain injury in children—Are the results improving? Swiss Med Wkly 2002;132:116.

Pierre-Kahn V, Roche O, Dureau P, et al. Ophthalmologic findings in suspected child abuse victims with subdural hematomas. Ophthalmology 2003;110:1718.

Pigula F, Wald S, Shackford SR, et al. The effect of hypotension and hypoxia on children with severe head injuries. J Pediatr Surg 1993;28:310.

Pitetti RD, Maffei F, Chang K, et al. Prevalence of retinal hemorrhages and child abuse in children who present with an apparent life-threatening event. Pediatrics 2002;110:557.

Poggi G, Calori G, Mancarella G, et al. Visual disorders after traumatic brain injury in developmental age. Brain Inj 2000;14:833.

Prange M, Coats B, Duhaime A-C, et al. Anthropomorphic simulations of falls, shakes, and inflicted impacts in infants. J Neurosurg 2003;99:143.

Prasad MR, Ewing-Cobbs L, Swank PR, et al. Predictors of outcome following traumatic brain injury in young children. Pediatr Neurosurg 2002;36:64.

Raabe A, Grolms C, Keller M, et al. Correlation of computed tomography findings and serum brain damage markers following severe head injury. Acta Neurochir (Wien) 1998;140:787.

Ranjith RK, Mullett JH, Burke TE. Hangman's fracture caused by suspected child abuse. A case report. J Pediatr Orthop B 2002;11:329.

Rao N, Smith RE, Choi JH, et al. Autopsy findings in the eyes of fourteen fatally abused children. Forensic Sci Int 1988;39:293.

Rao P, Carty H, Pierce A. The acute reversal sign: Comparison of medical and non-accidental injury patients. Clin Radiol 1999;54:495.

Reiber GD. Fatal falls in childhood. How far must children fall to sustain fatal head injury? Report of cases and review of the literature. Am J Forensic Med Pathol 1993;14:201.

Reincke M, Allolio B, Wurth G, et al. The hypothalamic-pituitary-adrenal axis in critical illness: Response to dexamethasone and corticotropin-releasing hormone. J Clin Endocrinol Metab 1993;77:151.

Riddoch G, Goulden C. On the relationship between subarachnoid and intraocular haemorrhage. Br J Ophthalmol 1925;98:1519.

Ridenour MV. Ages of young children who fall down stairs. Percept Mot Skills 1999;88:669.

Riffenburgh RS, Sathyavagiswaran L. The eyes of child abuse victims: Autopsy findings. J Forensic Sci 1991;36:741.

Rivara JM, Jaffe KM, Polissar N, et al. Predictors of family functioning and change 3 years after traumatic brain injury in children. Arch Phys Med Rehabil 1996;77:754.

Roberton DM, Barbor P, Hull D. Unusual injury? Recent injuries in normal children and children with suspected non-accidental injury. BMJ (Clin Res Ed) 1982;285:1399.

Rooks VJ, Sisler C, Burton B. Cervical spine injury in child abuse: Report of two cases. Pediatr Radiol 1998;28:193.

Roshkow JE, Haller JO, Hotson GC, et al. Imaging evaluation of children after falls from a height: Review of 45 cases. Radiology 1990;175:359.

Rossen R, Kabat H, Anderson JP, et al. Acute arrest of cerebral circulation in man. Arch Neurol Psych 1943;50:510.

Rubin DM, Christian CW, Bilaniuk LT, et al. Occult head injury in high-risk abused children. Pediatrics 2003;111:1382.

Ruppel RA, Clark RS, Bayir H, et al. Critical mechanisms of secondary damage after inflicted head injury in infants and children. Neurosurg Clin North Am 2002;13:169.

Ruppel RA, Kochanek P, Adelson PD, et al. Excitatory amino acid concentrations in ventricular cerebrospinal fluid after severe traumatic brain injury in infants and children: The role of child abuse. J Pediatr 2001;138:18.

Salvant JB, Muizelaar JP. Changes in cerebral blood flow and metabolism related to the presence of subdural hematoma. Neurosurgery 1993;33:387.

Sandramouli S, Robinson R, Tsaloumas M, et al. Retinal haemorrhages and convulsions. Arch Dis Child 1997;76:449.

Sarabia R, Lobato R, Rivas JJ, et al. Cerebral hemisphere swelling in severe head injury patients. Acta Neurochir 1988;42 (Suppl):40.

Sargent S, Kennedy JG, Kaplan J, et al. Hyperacute subdural hematoma: CT mimic of recurrent episodes of bleeding in the setting of child abuse. J Forensic Sci 1996;41:314.

Sato Y, Yuh W, Smith W, et al. Head injury in child abuse: Evaluation with MR imaging. Radiology 1989;173:653.

Schloff S, Mullaney PB, Armstrong DC, et al. Retinal findings in children with intracranial hemorrhage. Ophthalmology 2002;109:1472.

Schmitt B, Bauersfeld U, Schmid ER, et al. Serum and CSF levels of neuron-specific enolase (NSE) in cardiac surgery with cardiopulmonary bypass: A marker of brain injury? Brain Dev 1998;20:536.

Schröder ML, Muizelaar JP, Kuta AJ. Documented reversal of global ischemia immediately after removal of an acute subdural hematoma. Report of two cases. J Neurosurg 1994;80:324.

Schutzman S, Barnes P, Mantello M, et al. Epidural hematomas in children. Ann Emerg Med 1993;22:535.

Sedzimir C. Head injury as a cause of internal carotid thrombosis. J Neurol Neurosurg Psychiatry 1955;18:293.

Server A, Dullerud R, Haakonsen M, et al. Post-traumatic cerebral infarction. Neuroimaging findings, etiology and outcome. Acta Radiol 2001;42:254.

Sezen F. Retinal haemorrhages in newborn infants. Br J Ophthalmol 1971;55:248.

Shaikh S, Fishman ML, Gaynon M, et al. Diffuse unilateral hemorrhagic retinopathy associated with accidental perinatal strangulation. A clinicopathologic report. Retina 2001;21:252.

Shane SA, Fuchs SM. Skull fractures in infants and predictors of associated intracranial injury. Pediatr Emerg Care 1997;13:198.

Shapiro K, Smith L. Special considerations for the pediatric age group. In: Cooper P, ed. Head injury. Baltimore: Williams & Wilkins, 1993;427.

Shaw HE, Landers MB, Sydnor CF. The significance of intraocular hemorrhages due to subarachnoid hemorrhage. Ann Ophthalmol 1977;9:1403

Shenkin H. Acute subdural hematoma. Review of 39 consecutive cases with high incidence of cortical artery rupture. J Neurosurg 1982;57:254.

Sherwood D. Chronic subdural hematoma in infants. Am J Dis Child 1930;39:980.

Shugerman R, Paez A, Grossman DC, et al. Epidural hemorrhage: Is it abuse? Pediatrics 1996;97:664.

Silverman F. The roentgen manifestation of unrecognized skeletal trauma in infants. Am J Roentgenol Radium Ther Nucl Med 1952;69:413.

Smith GA, Bowman MJ, Luria JW, et al. Babywalker-related injuries continue despite warning labels and public education. Pediatrics 1997;100:E1.

Stålhammer DA. Experimental models of head injury. Neurochir Suppl 1986;36:33.

Strich S. Shearing of nerve fibers as a cause of brain damage due to head injury. Lancet 1961;2:443.

Suh DY, Davis PC, Hopkins KL, et al. Nonaccidental pediatric head injury: Diffusion-weighted imaging findings. Neurosurgery 2001;49:309.

Sung VC, Murray DC, Price NJ. Subhyaloid or subinternal limiting membrane haemorrhage in meningococcal meningitis. Br J Ophthalmol 2000;84:1206.

Suzuki Y, Awaya S. Long-term observation of infants with macular hemorrhage in the neonatal period. Jpn J Ophthalmol 1998;42:124.

Swischuk L. Spine and spinal cord trauma in the battered child syndrome. Radiology 1969;92:733.

Taff ML, Boglioli LR, DeFelice JF. Controversies in shaken baby syndrome. J Forensic Sci 1996;41:729.

Takahashi S, Higano S, Ishii K, et al. Hypoxic brain damage: Cortical laminar necrosis and delayed changes in white matter at sequential MR imaging. Radiology 1993;189:449.

Tardiéu A. Etude médico-légale sur les services et mauvais traitements exercés sur des enfants. Ann Hyg Pub Méd Lég 1860;13:361.

Teasdale GM, Graham DI. Craniocerebral trauma: Protection and retrieval of the neuronal population after injury. Neurosurgery 1998;43:723.

Tokutomi T, Hirohata M, Miyagi T, et al. Posttraumatic edema in the corpus callosum shown by MRI. Acta Neurochir Suppl 1997;70:80.

Tomita H, Tone O, Ito U. Hemispheric cerebral atrophy after traumatic extra-axial hematoma in adults. Neurol Med Chir (Tokyo) 1997;37:819.

Tong KA, Ashwal S, Holshouser BA, et al. Diffuse axonal injury in children: Clinical correlation with hemorrhagic lesions. Ann Neurol 2004;56:36.

Tong W, Igarashi T, Ferriero DM, et al. Traumatic brain injury in the immature mouse brain: Characterization of regional vulnerability. Exp Neurol 2002;176:105.

Tornheim PA, Liwnicz BH, Hirsch CS, et al. Acute responses to blunt head trauma. Experimental model and gross pathology. J Neurosurg 1983;59:431.

Tureen L. Lesions of the fundus associated with brain hemorrhage. Arch Neurol Psych 1939;42:664.

Tzioumi D, Oates RK. Subdural hematomas in children under 2 years. Accidental or inflicted? A 10-year experience. Child Abuse Negl 1998;22:1105.

Vavilala MS, Bowen A, Lam AM, et al. Blood pressure and outcome after severe pediatric traumatic brain injury. J Trauma 2003;55:1039.

Vinchon M, Noizet O, Defoort-Dhellemmes S, et al. Infantile subdural hematomas due to traffic accidents. Pediatr Neurosurg 2002;37:245.

Vowles G, Scholtz C, Cameron J. Diffuse axonal injury in early infancy. J Clin Pathol 1987;40:185.

Waga S, Tochio H, Sakakura M, et al. Traumatic cerebral swelling developing within 30 minutes after injury. Surg Neurol 1979;11:191.

Wasterlain CG, Niquet J, Thompson KW, et al. Seizure-induced neuronal death in the immature brain. Prog Brain Res 2002;135:335.

Weissgold DJ, Budenz DL, Hood I, et al. Ruptured vascular malformation masquerading as battered/shaken baby syndrome: A nearly tragic mistake. Surv Ophthalmol 1995;39:509.

Weston J. Guidelines for the application of pathology to crime investigation. In: Spitz W, Fisher R, eds. Medicolegal investigation of death. Springfield, IL: Charles C Thomas, 1973;***.

Wetterling T, Demierre B, Rama B, et al. Protein analysis of subdural hygroma fluid. Acta Neurochir (Wien) 1988;91:79.

Whalen MJ, Carlos TM, Kochanek PM, et al. Soluble adhesion molecules in CSF are increased in children with severe head injury. J Neurotrauma 1998;15:777.

Whalen MJ, Carlos TM, Kochanek PM, et al. Interleukin-8 is increased in cerebrospinal fluid of children with severe head injury. Crit Care Med 2000;28:929.

Wilberger JE, Rothfus WE, Tabas J, et al. Acute tissue tear hemorrhages of the brain: Computed tomography and clinicopathological correlations. Neurosurgery 1990;27:208.

Wilkinson WS, Han DP, Rappley MD, et al. Retinal hemorrhage predicts neurologic injury in the shaken baby syndrome. Arch Ophthalmol 1989;107:1472.

Williams MC, Knuppel RA, O'Brien WF, et al. Obstetric correlates of neonatal retinal hemorrhage. Obstet Gynecol 1993;81:688.

Williams R. Injuries in infants and small children resulting from witnessed and corroborated free falls. J Trauma 1991;31:1350.

Willman KY, Bank DE, Senac M, et al. Restricting the time of injury in fatal inflicted head injuries. Child Abuse Negl 1997;21:929.

Wilms G, Vanderschueren G, Demaerel P, et al. CT and MR in infants with pericerebral collections and macrocephaly: Benign enlargement of the subarachnoid spaces versus subdural collections. AJNR Am J Neuroradiol 1993;14:855.

Woertgen C, Rothoerl R, Holzschuh M, et al. Comparison of serial S-100 or NSE serum measurements after severe head injury. Acta Neurochir (Wien) 1997;139:1161.

Woiciechowsky C, Schoning B, Cobanov J, et al. Early IL-6 plasma concentrations correlate with severity of brain injury and pneumonia in brain-injured patients. J Trauma 2002;52:339.

Woolley P, Evans W. Significance of skeletal lesions in infancy resembling those of traumatic origin. JAMA 1955;158:539.

Xu BN, Yabuki A, Mishina H, et al. Pathophysiology of brain swelling after acute experimental brain compression and decompression. Neurosurgery 1993;32:289.

Yakovlev AG, Faden AI. Molecular biology of CNS injury. J Neurotrauma 1995;12:767.

Zimmerman RA, Balaniuk LT, Bruce D, et al. Computed tomography of pediatric head trauma: Acute general cerebral swelling. Radiology 1978;126:403.

Zimmerman RA, Bilaniuk LT, Bruce D, et al. Computed tomography of craniocerebral injury in the abused child. Radiology 1979;130:687.

Zouros A, Bhargava R, Hoskinson M, et al. Further characterization of traumatic subdural collections of infancy. Report of five cases. J Neurosurg Spine 2004;100:512.

Zuccarello M, Facco E, Zampieri P, et al. Severe head injury in children: Early prognosis and outcome. Childs Nerv Syst 1985;1:158.

Zwaan J, Cardenas R, O'Connor PS. Long-term outcome of neonatal macular hemorrhage. J Pediatr Ophthalmol Strabismus 1997;34:286.

CHAPTER 64

Hypoxic-Ischemic Encephalopathy in Infants and Older Children

Ronald M. Perkin and Stephen Ashwal

Cardiopulmonary arrest in infants and children remains a significant cause of morbidity and mortality [Fink et al., 2004; Young et al., 2004]. The principal factor that influences outcome in survivors of cardiopulmonary arrest is the neurologic sequelae resulting from hypoxic-ischemic injury [Robertson et al., 2002]. This chapter reviews the pathophysiologic and clinical aspects of this disorder.

Unfortunately, there are currently no interventions to reverse the cellular consequences of hypoxic-ischemic injury [Fink et al., 2004; Kochanek et al., 2001]. Therefore, most children surviving out-of-hospital cardiopulmonary arrest have serious neurologic sequelae [Michelson and Ashwal, 2003; Morris and Nadkarni, 2003; Schindler et al., 1996; Thompson et al., 1990; Young et al., 2004]. In addition, deaths of approximately 40% of infants and children with diagnoses of brain death are caused by severe asphyxial central nervous system (CNS) injury [Ashwal and Schneider, 1991; Parker et al., 1995].

In the United States, it is estimated that 16,000 children die annually of unexpected cardiopulmonary arrest [Fink et al., 2004]. In a review summarizing the results from 44 studies totaling 3094 pediatric patients after cardiopulmonary arrest, the overall rate of survival after cardiopulmonary arrest was 13% (24% of those with in-hospital arrest, 9% with out-of-hospital arrest), with unfavorable neurologic outcome in survivors for whom outcome was reported [Young and Seidel, 1999]. Fewer than 10% of patients were found to have ventricular tachycardia or fibrillation; most had asystole, bradycardia, or pulseless electrical activity as a consequence of asphyxia [Young et al., 2004; Young and Seidel, 1999]. In addition to physical debilitation in pediatric survivors of cardiopulmonary arrest and the emotional burden to family, there are also significant monetary and psychosocial burdens [Fink et al., 2004]. The lifelong cost for continued care of a moderately to severely disabled child can easily exceed $1 million [Ronco et al., 1995].

Asphyxial cardiac arrest in infants and children most commonly results from submersion accidents, airway obstruction, aspiration, severe acute asthma, and inhalation injury (Table 64-1 and Box 64-1). In asphyxia-induced cardiac arrest, cardiac standstill or pulseless electrical activity is preceded and precipitated by a period of anoxic or hypoxic perfusion. Ventricular fibrillation is a common cause of cardiopulmonary arrest in adults. In ventricular fibrillation–induced cardiac arrest, respiration ceases as a result of the loss of perfusion (ischemic hypoxia). Although ventricular fibrillation can occur in children, asphyxia is the most common cause of cardiopulmonary arrest and the primary cause of hypoxic-ischemic encephalopathy in children [O'Rourke, 1986; Torphy et al., 1984]. Ventricular fibrillation–induced and asphyxia-induced cardiac arrest differ in pathophysiology despite having been traditionally grouped as cardiopulmonary arrests.

Results of clinical trials in adult patients suggest that some degree of hypoxic-ischemic injury can be prevented if treatment is initiated early after cardiac arrest [Bernard et al., 2002]. However, whereas a cardiac etiology is the principal cause of cardiopulmonary arrest in adults, asphyxia is the principal cause of cardiopulmonary arrest in infants and children; it results in systemic hypoxemia, hypercapnia, acidosis, and, ultimately, hypotension and bradycardia, culminating in complete cardiovascular collapse [Young and Seidel, 1999]. Until recently, there was no contemporary age-appropriate pediatric model of hypoxic-ischemic injury for the evaluation of prolonged neurodegeneration and long-term neurologic outcome [Fink et al., 2004]. Such a model may be useful for the preclinical testing of novel and currently available interventions aimed at improving neurologic outcome in infants and children after cardiopulmonary arrest.

RESPONSE TO INADEQUATE OXYGEN DELIVERY: MECHANISMS OF INJURY

In an attempt to explain the mechanisms involved in hypoxic-ischemic injury after cardiopulmonary arrest, several modes of injury that occur during ischemia and reperfusion must be considered: (1) brain energy failure, (2) calcium-mediated injury, (3) excitotoxic injury, (4) activation of intracellular proteases, (5) release of free fatty acids, (6) activation of nitric oxide synthesis, (7) formation of oxygen radicals, (8) reperfusion injury, and (9) genetic damage and regulation. In addition, there is accruing evidence that local inflammatory responses of microglia, macrophages, neutrophils, and prostaglandins are responsible for some of the neuronal injury after hypoxia-ischemia.

Brain Energy Failure

The brain depends on large amounts of exogenous substrate (oxygen and glucose) because of its high metabolic demands, limited energy stores, and reliance on oxidative metabolism. Cellular energy depletion is postulated to be the triggering event that initiates the many cascades of injury that occur during ischemia [Krause et al., 1988]. Adenosine 5-triphosphate (ATP) is the energy source that drives all cellular physiologic processes [Bellamy et al., 1996; Sweeney et al., 1995]. One of the most vital processes performed is the preservation of ATP to maintain membrane ionic gradients [Ackerman and Clapham, 1997]. Under nor-

TABLE 64-1

Etiology of Cardiac Arrest in Children

ETIOLOGY	PATIENTS (%)
Submersion	27
Sudden infant death syndrome	20
Trauma	15
Respiratory	9
Sepsis	9
Heart disease/arrhythmia	6
Other/unknown	14

Data from Hickey et al., 1995, and Schindler et al., 1996.

Box 64-1 Major Causes of Pediatric Cardiopulmonary Arrest

- Upper airway obstruction
  - Croup
  - Foreign body obstruction
  - Supraglottitis
  - Angioedema
  - Trauma (blunt and penetrating)
  - Abscess, bacterial infection
- Lower airway disease
  - Drowning
  - Inhalation injury
  - Asthma
  - Pneumonia
  - Bronchiolitis
  - Bronchopulmonary dysplasia
  - Chest trauma
  - Foreign body obstruction
- Neurologic
  - Head trauma
  - Central nervous system infection
  - Botulism
  - Cervical spine trauma
  - Increased intracervical pressure
  - Ventriculoperitoneal shunt obstruction
  - Status epilepticus
- Cardiovascular
  - Hypovolemic shock
  - Septic shock
  - Congenital heart defect
  - Cardiogenic shock
  - Dysrhythmias
  - Myocarditis
  - Pericardial effusion
- Other
  - Sudden infant death syndrome
  - Coronary artery disease
  - Burns
  - Intoxications
  - Metabolic disorders

mal conditions, maintenance of ionic gradients across the cell membrane accounts for nearly 50% of total cellular expenditure [Erecinska and Silver, 1989]. Interruption of cerebral blood flow results in loss of consciousness and reductions in electroencephalographic activity within seconds. Within 5 to 7 minutes, complete energy failure occurs, accompanied by disturbances of neuronal and glial ion homeostasis, including sodium and water influx and efflux of potassium (Fig. 64-1). When the extracellular potassium concentration reaches a critical threshold, voltage-gated channels undergo depolarization, precipitating extracellular calcium influx [Sweeney et al., 1995]. If flow remains inadequate and energy failure persists, calcium-mediated events such as phospholipase and protease activation can lead to irreversible cellular injury and necrosis, as well as cerebral acidosis with elevated lactate levels and decreased hydrogen ion concentration (pH). If blood flow is restored, recovery of basal cellular metabolism (ATP levels, protein synthesis, oxygen consumption) and normal pH occurs if the ischemic injury is of limited duration [Ljunggren et al., 1974].

Certain neurons have long been known to be especially vulnerable to global hypoxic-ischemic insults, particularly the hippocampal CA1 and CA4 zones and cortical layers III and V [Krause et al., 1988; White et al., 1996]. Five minutes of complete global brain ischemia produces cell death in these regions within 48 to 72 hours. This time interval between ischemia and cell death consists of an early postischemic period when ATP and lactate levels recover, followed after 24 hours by a decrease in ATP levels and lactate reaccumulation [Kochanek, 1993; Siesjo et al., 1995].

After anoxia or ischemia, restoration of aerobic metabolism is essential but not sufficient for recovery. Despite global metabolic recovery, certain neurons progress to cell death. Restoration of blood flow and oxidative metabolism after energy failure in the brain leads to specific cellular and molecular dysfunction because of two related processes, cell necrosis and programmed cell death (i.e., apoptosis), both of which evolve during and after resuscitation [Hockenbery, 1995; Schnaper, 1994]. These processes, coupled with the need to restore highly integrated functions, explain the unfortunate clinical scenario of the vegetative state despite restoration of normal function in other organ systems. The relation of these two forms of cell death to selective vulnerability of neurons in the brain is beginning to emerge. A clinically relevant model of pediatric cardiopulmonary arrest that has been developed may prove useful for investigating mechanisms resulting in hypoxic-ischemic encephalopathy in the developing brain [Fink et al., 2004].

Cell necrosis, which is characterized by denaturation and coagulation of cellular proteins, is the basic pattern of pathologic cell death that results from progressive reduction in cellular ATP content [Buja et al., 1993; Sweeney et al., 1995]. Necrosis involves progressive derangements in energy and substrate metabolism that are followed by a series of morphologic alterations, including swelling of cells and organelles, development of subsurface cellular blebs, amorphous deposits in mitochondria, condensation of nuclear chromatin, and breaks in plasma and cell organelle membranes [Brierley et al., 1973]. It was traditionally assumed that all ischemic cell death occurred through this process and that selective vulnerability represented a specific predilection for the development of necrosis in certain neurons after transient ischemic insults.

It has been demonstrated, however, that cell death after hypoxic-ischemic insults can occur by a second pathway: programmed cell death. Apoptosis has emerged as a mech-

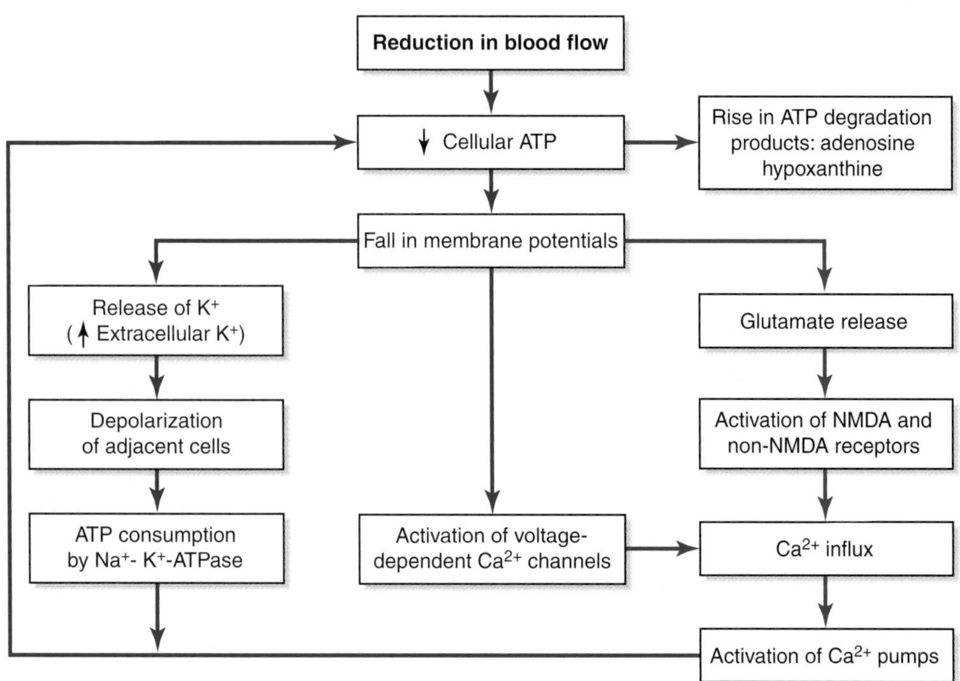

FIGURE 64-1. Global ischemia results in a cascade of events, including reduction in adenosine triphosphate (ATP), loss of cellular ionic gradients, increases in extracellular K^+ concentration, glutamate release with activation of *N*-methyl-D-aspartate (NMDA) and non-NMDA receptors, calcium influx and release of intracellular calcium, and activation of secondary messenger systems and a variety of destructive enzymatic processes.

anism of cell death that plays an important role during development, in normal physiology, and in the pathogenesis of disease [Schnaper, 1994]. Apoptosis has been described as directed cell suicide [Hockenbery, 1995]. Its unique feature is that, although external events may trigger apoptosis, all of the machinery for the process is contained within the cell. Activation of this machinery may result from toxicity of the extracellular milieu, binding to a specific cell receptor, or removal of a factor that prevents apoptosis from occurring. Apoptosis is thus clearly distinct from necrosis (Box 64-2). Necrosis occurs despite the cell's effort to survive. The development of programmed cell death involves new protein synthesis and the activation of endonucleases with a resultant characteristic cleavage of DNA at linkage regions between nucleosomes to form fragments of double-stranded DNA [Mackey et al., 1997].

Programmed cell death was classically described as associated with cell death during embryogenesis. The stimuli triggering programmed cell death are not clearly defined, although protease activation or oxidant injury to DNA has been proposed. Similarly, apoptosis may be involved in the pathophysiology of shock, trauma, and end-stage heart disease, in addition to ischemia [Narula et al., 1996; Rink et al., 1995]. Reports indicate that cell death in selectively vulnerable brain regions, such as the CA1 region of the hippocampus, after transient global brain ischemia, occurs by an apoptotic mechanism. After a global ischemic insult, DNA fragmentation is most pronounced in neurons of the CA1 region of the hippocampus, which suggests that apoptosis may play a role in both selective neuronal necrosis and delayed neuronal death [Nitatori et al., 1995]. The concept of delayed neuronal death is important because it implies that there is a window of opportunity for treatment after global ischemia.

Box 64-2 Cell Death Mechanisms

- Necrosis
  - Alterations of the extracellular environment
  - Compromised membrane integrity due to adenosine triphosphate (ATP) depletion
  - Nonspecific DNA degradation
- Apoptosis
  - Gene-directed cellular self-destruction
  - Protein synthesis is required
  - Apoptotic cells require energy
  - Specific DNA cleavage
- Multiple triggers

Programmed cell death in the post-ischemic brain is not limited to scattered neuronal death in what has traditionally been deemed selectively vulnerable regions; it is also seen in penumbral regions around evolving cerebral infarctions [Li et al., 1995]. The severity of the ischemic insult and other local factors likely determine whether an injured neuron recovers, undergoes programmed cell death, or dies a necrotic death. It is quite possible, although only a speculative notion, that after cardiopulmonary arrest and resuscitation, a continuum exists in neurons from recovery to necrosis that depends on the duration of the insult, the local milieu, and the given brain region. Nonetheless, in any given brain region, whether neuronal death is produced by necrosis, apoptosis, or both, a highly complex series of events is involved during the arrest and after restoration of spontaneous circulation. Because programmed cell death occurs in stages, there exist several potential strategies for reducing cell death [Kochanek et al., 2001].

Calcium-Mediated Injury

Calcium plays a strategic role in the regulation of many cellular metabolic processes; therefore, the concentration of cytosolic free calcium is tightly controlled. Hypoxic-ischemic injury interrupts intracellular calcium homeostasis, which

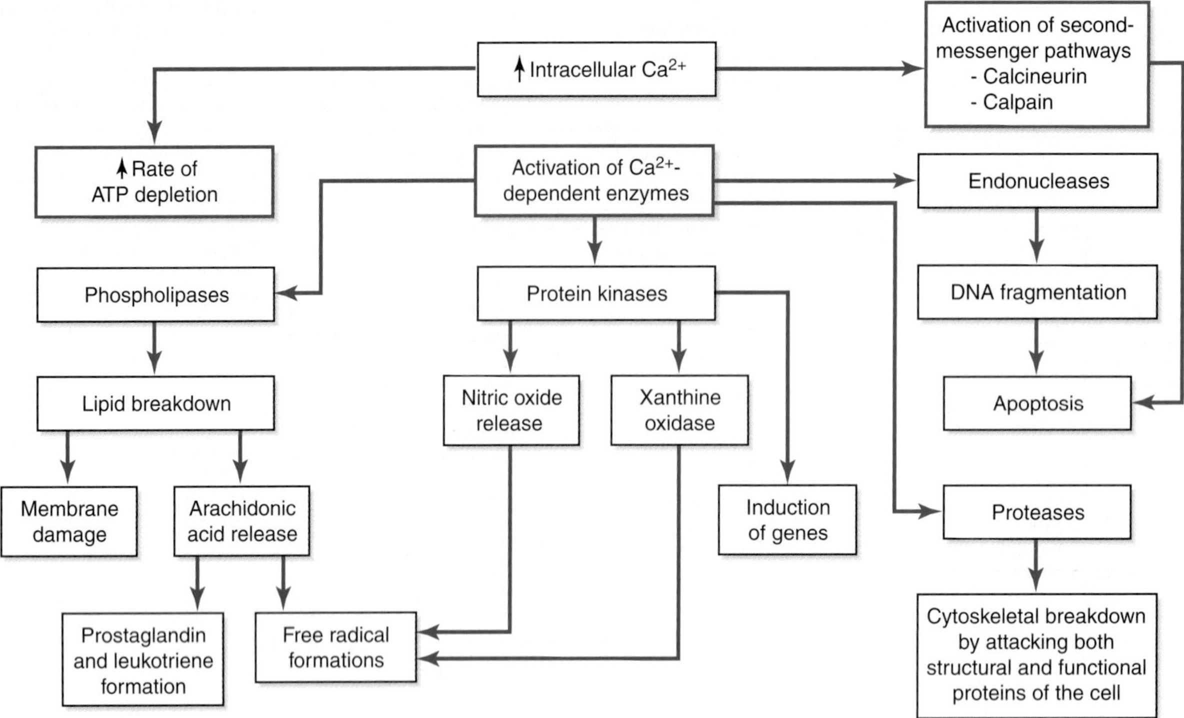

FIGURE 64-2. Increases in intracellular Ca^{2+} mediate several enzymatic pathways that cause cell injury, including those of protein kinases, proteases, phospholipases, nitric oxide synthase, other free radical synthesis, and endonucleases, as well as other second-messenger systems. The net effect is related to the severity and duration of ischemia and a series of complex events that results in cell necrosis and apoptosis, as well as other forms of partial injury that remain poorly understood. ATP, adenosine triphosphate.

results in massive increases in the intracellular concentration of calcium. This calcium accumulation is believed to promote irreversible cellular injury [Bellamy et al., 1996; Lipton et al., 1994] (Fig. 64-2).

Transient calcium accumulation occurs in all cells during ischemia, but secondary irreversible accumulation occurs in the selectively vulnerable zones many hours later. Electrophysiologic studies demonstrate that delayed neuronal death is preceded by neuronal hyperactivity. It is hypothesized that ischemic and early post-ischemic calcium accumulation leads to complex series of derangements in cellular metabolism [Morgenstern and Pettigrew, 1997; Sweeney et al., 1995]. The intracellular accumulation of calcium (1) activates proteases, lipases, and endonucleases, which results in the breakdown of membrane phospholipids; (2) activates neuronal nitric oxide synthase, which results in nitric oxide production and, in the presence of superoxide, peroxynitrate formation; (3) damages mitochondria and uncouples oxidative phosphorylation; and (4) disrupts nucleic acid sequences. The disturbance of intracellular calcium homeostasis is recognized as a final common pathway of neuronal death, either necrotic or apoptotic. These conditions, in concert with excessive release of calcium-dependent excitatory neurotransmitters (glutamate, aspartate), lead to uncontrolled excitotoxicity and cell death.

Excitotoxic Injury

During hypoxic-ischemic damage, pathologically prolonged membrane depolarization occurs and, in certain neuronal populations, leads to excessive release of neurotransmitters into the synaptic cleft [Lipton and Rosenberg, 1994; Rogers and Kirsch, 1989]. The effect of these neurotransmitters is prolonged by failure of the ATP-dependent presynaptic re-uptake mechanisms. Glutamate and aspartate are the major excitatory amino acid neurotransmitters in the mammalian CNS; both also have neurotoxic properties [Rogers and Kirsch, 1989]. Hypoxia-induced neuronal death is mediated by synaptic activity. Inhibition of synaptic glutamate release or blockade of glutamate receptors may prevent hypoxic neuronal injury. Glutamate is the major neurotransmitter in the selectively vulnerable zones and accumulates extracellularly in these regions after hypoxic or ischemic insults. The mechanisms by which glutamate may harm neurons during ischemia and reperfusion are becoming more clearly defined.

Glutamate is released at the presynaptic terminal in response to neuronal stimulation and acts by binding to postsynaptic dendritic receptors. Two main classes of excitatory neurotransmitter receptors have been identified. One class consists of the ligand-gated ion channels (ionotropic receptors) and includes *N*-methyl-D-aspartate (NMDA); alpha-amino-3-hydroxy-5-methyl-4-isoxazole propionic acid (AMPA), or quisqualate; and kainate receptor types [Rogers and Kirsch, 1989; Sweeney et al., 1995]. Toxicity caused by NMDA receptor activation is usually rapid, whereas AMPA or kainate receptor–mediated cell death is slower to develop [Dugan and Choi, 1994]. The current understanding of the glutamate receptor subtypes is that the NMDA receptor is more complex and contains more modulatory sites than does the kainate receptor [Lipton and Rosenberg, 1994]. The other class of excitatory neurotransmitter receptors includes the metabotropic receptors that are coupled with G proteins and modulate intracellular second messengers such as calcium, cyclic nucleosides, and inositol triphosphate. Seven subtypes of the metabotropic glutamate receptor have been identified [Nakanishi, 1992].

When activated, the inotropic glutamate receptors open sodium channels and may also have an important role in initiation and propagation of membrane depolarization and spreading depression. With inotropic receptor activation, rapid excitatory amino acid–mediated calcium accumulation occurs [Sweeney et al., 1995]. In the presence of ischemia, this calcium accumulation is exacerbated by cellular energy failure, which disables the Na^+/K^+-ATPase membrane pump and results in further calcium accumulation. Altered calcium homeostasis leads to activation of many deleterious processes, including activation of phospholipases, proteases, endonucleases, protein kinases, and calmodulin-regulated enzymes such as nitric oxide synthase. There is evidence that nitric oxide is an important mediator of glutamate neurotoxicity [Dawson, 1994]. Re-establishment of the energy supply can reverse these changes. Delayed glutamate-related neuronal injury is most likely caused by activation of inotropic receptors and subsequent calcium influx.

Intracellular free calcium may increase during ischemia either by influx of extracellular calcium or by release of bound or sequestered intracellular calcium [Morgenstern and Pettigrew, 1997]. Cerebral ischemia is accompanied by a significant decrease in extracellular calcium concentration, which is consistent with an intracellular shift of calcium. Energy failure during ischemia results in membrane depolarization, which allows calcium influx via voltage-sensitive calcium channels and causes glutamate release. Glutamate can promote calcium influx by three different mechanisms [Haun et al., 1996]. The first and most obvious mechanism is by opening the NMDA receptor-gated calcium channel. Second, stimulation of non-NMDA receptors opens sodium channels and results in massive influx of sodium and subsequent membrane depolarization, which then allows calcium entry via voltage-sensitive calcium channels. Third, the ion channel gated by non-NMDA receptors allows direct influx of calcium. Three additional possibilities exist for calcium entry during ischemia: (1) reversal of sodium/calcium exchanger mechanisms, (2) nonspecific membrane leakage of calcium, and (3) release of bound or sequestered intracellular calcium. Massive influx of sodium during ischemia creates conditions that inhibit or even reverse sodium/ calcium exchange, leading to further calcium influx. It is also possible that calcium enters through areas of the cell membrane that have been damaged by the ischemic insult. Release of bound or sequestered calcium likely occurs through two different mechanisms. First, hydrogen ion, which accumulates during ischemia, can directly displace bound calcium. Second, sequestered intracellular calcium may be mobilized by inositol-1,4,5-triphosphate, which is produced by glutamate-stimulated hydrolysis of polyphosphoinositides, mediated by the metabotropic receptor [Berridge and Irvine, 1984; Sugiyama et al., 1987].

Although most work has centered on the role of calcium influx, some investigations have focused on the importance of the release of sequestered calcium. Mitani and colleagues [1993] demonstrated that two thirds of the increase in intracellular concentration of calcium seen in cultures of hippocampal neurons subjected to glucose and oxygen deprivation is caused by release of sequestered calcium, whereas only one third is caused by influx of extracellular calcium. Although the relative contribution of influx and release from internal stores is still unclear, there is accumulating evidence that release from internal stores does indeed play a role.

Activation of Intracellular Enzymes

The marked increase in intracellular calcium concentration activates at least four classes of enzymes [Morgenstern and Pettigrew, 1997; Sweeney et al., 1995]. Phospholipases break down the lipid cellular membrane, releasing arachidonic acid that generates prostaglandins and free radicals. Protein kinases activate enzymes in an unordered manner, including nitric oxide synthase and xanthine oxidase, which are also generators of free radicals. Proteases begin the uninhibited breakdown of the cytoskeleton, and endonucleases initiate DNA fragmentation.

Protease activation may play a central role in mediating both necrosis and programmed cell death. With regard to necrosis, numerous calcium-dependent enzymes become activated during ischemia and produce important neuronal structural injury. One class of calcium-dependent proteases, calpains, has received the greatest amount of attention. Calpains are cytosolic thiol proteases that degrade numerous cytoskeletal proteins such as neurotubules and neurofilaments, as well as activate protein kinase C and phospholipases. Inhibition of calpain activation has produced marked reduction in ischemic brain injury, particularly after focal ischemia [Bartus et al., 1994]. Proteases may also play a pivotal role in the initiation of programmed cell death.

Phospholipase Release of Free Fatty Acids

Metabolism of membrane phospholipids through activation of phospholipases is postulated to play a key role in the pathophysiology of ischemic brain injury (Fig. 64-3).

Free fatty acids are released from neuronal membranes during ischemia; the amount of release is proportional to the duration of ischemia. Free fatty acid release is the only known cerebral metabolic indicator that continues to increase

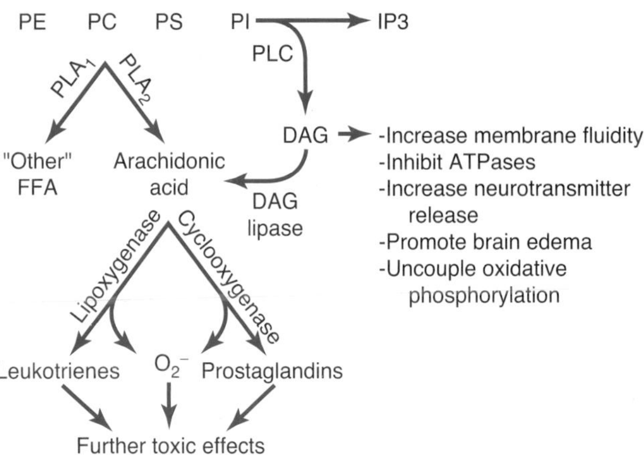

FIGURE 64-3. Membrane phospholipids are hydrolyzed by two pathways: the PLA_1/PLA_2 pathway and the PLC/DAG lipase pathway. Arachidonic acid produced by phospholipid hydrolysis is the substrate for eicosanoid synthesis and oxygen radical production. DAG, diacylglycerol; FFA, free fatty acids; IP3, inositol 1,4,5-trisphosphate; PC, phosphatidylcholine; PE, phosphatidylethanolamine; PI, phosphatidylinositol; PLA_1, phospholipase A_1; PLA_2, phospholipase A_2; PLC, phospholipase C; PS, phosphatidylserine.

in proportion to the duration of ischemia after completion of energy failure [Shin et al., 1983]. Free fatty acids are released by two distinct but related processes. First, phosphatidylinositol is hydrolyzed by phospholipase C with the production of diacylglycerol and inositol phosphates [Abe et al., 1987]. Phospholipase C–mediated hydrolysis begins during the initial moments of ischemia and is related to the magnitude of neurotransmitter receptor stimulation. Diacylglycerol is then hydrolyzed by lipases to free fatty acids, predominantly arachidonic acid and stearic acid. Second, other brain glycerophospholipids are hydrolyzed by phospholipase A_2, which is activated by increases in intracellular calcium concentration. The process of free fatty acid release and metabolism is not a generalized process in the neuronal membrane but is concentrated in synaptic regions and is thus related to excitotoxicity.

The free fatty acids released have potential detrimental effects through at least three mechanisms. First, free fatty acid metabolism via the cyclooxygenase pathway contributes to oxygen radical production during reperfusion [Kontos, 1987]. Second, free fatty acid and diacylglycerol directly increase membrane fluidity, inhibit ATPases, increase neurotransmitter release, promote brain edema, and uncouple oxidative phosphorylation. Third, enzymatic oxidation of arachidonic acid during reperfusion by cyclooxygenase, lipoxygenase, or cytochrome P-450 produces a large number of bioactive lipids (prostaglandins, thromboxanes, leukotrienes, and hydroxyl acids), many of which have detrimental effects. Ischemia induces a proinflammatory state that increases tissue vulnerability to further injury on reperfusion [Collard and Gelman, 2001].

Activation of Nitric Oxide Synthesis

Nitric oxide plays a multifaceted role in the brain as a neurotransmitter and a regulator of cerebral blood flow [Bhardwaj et al., 1997; Dawson and Dawson, 1995; Dawson et al., 1992]. Sites of nitric oxide production include neurons, vascular endothelium, perivascular neurons, and astrocytes [Bhardwaj et al., 1997]. If present in abnormally high concentrations, nitric oxide may exert neurotoxic effects [Dawson, 1994; Moncada and Higgs, 1993].

Nitric oxide is produced in a reaction catalyzed by nitric oxide synthase in which oxygen and L-arginine are converted into L-citrulline and nitric oxide. Three isoforms of nitric oxide synthase have been described [Samdani et al., 1997] (Table 64-2). There are two constitutive isoforms: neuronal and endothelial. An inducible isoform has also been described and has been demonstrated in macrophages, microglia, and astrocytes. The constitutive enzymes are calcium-calmodulin–dependent enzymes. Inducible nitric oxide synthase is calcium independent, is induced by endotoxin and cytokines, and, when stimulated, produces large amounts of nitric oxide in a sustained manner [Clark et al., 1996]. Neuronal nitric oxide synthase is present in highest concentration in the cerebellum, and its lowest concentration is in the medulla. There are neurons that express nitric oxide synthase in all brain regions.

In some neurons, nitric oxide synthase activity is regulated by the NMDA receptor. NMDA receptor stimulation results in calcium influx and activation of nitric oxide synthase. Nitric oxide is produced and then diffuses to target cells and stimulates guanylate cyclase, which leads to the production of cyclic guanosine monophosphate. Cyclic guanosine monophosphate then produces the physiologic effect (e.g., vasorelaxation, cell signaling). Inducible nitric oxide synthase is expressed by several cell types (including macrophages, microglia, and astrocytes) in response to stimulation by cytokines. Nitric oxide produced by this nitric oxide synthase isoform is involved in cell-mediated cytotoxicity [Samdani et al., 1997]. The mechanism of this cytotoxicity is not yet fully understood but may involve inhibition of key enzymes necessary for DNA replication and mitochondrial energy production.

As part of the excitotoxic cascade of injury, glutamate release activates both endothelial and neuronal nitric oxide synthase, which increase nitric oxide production during focal and global ischemia [Bari et al., 1997; Samdani et al., 1997]. During ischemia, endothelial nitric oxide synthase production may be protective by increasing cerebral blood flow, whereas during ischemia, and more so during reperfusion, neuronal nitric oxide release synthase production may cause additional neurotoxicity. Nitric oxide produced under conditions of ischemia contributes to the cytotoxicity of glutamate, presumably through hydroxyl radical production (Fig. 64-4). Nitric oxide contributes to hydroxyl radical production through its reaction with the superoxide radical. Nitric oxide and superoxide radical react to form peroxynitrite. Peroxynitrite then decomposes to yield nitrogen dioxide and the toxic hydroxyl radicals. Several days after focal ischemia, activation of inducible nitric oxide synthase from phagocytic cells may contribute to delayed injury. The majority of evidence suggesting a role for nitric oxide has been demonstrated in models of focal ischemia.

TABLE 64-2

Nitric Oxide Synthase (NOS) Isoforms

TYPE I: NEURONAL NOS	TYPE II: INDUCIBLE NOS	TYPE III: ENDOTHELIAL NOS
Activity depends on elevated Ca^{2+}	Activity is independent of Ca^{2+}	Activity depends on elevated Ca^{2+}
First identified in neurons	First identified in macrophages	First identified in endothelial cells
Constitutively expressed, but inducible under pathologic conditions	Inducible under pathologic conditions	Constitutively expressed, but inducible under pathologic conditions
Plays a prominent role in the early stage of neuronal injury after cerebral ischemia	Plays a role in the later stages of neuronal injury after cerebral ischemia	Plays a protective role in cerebral ischemia by maintaining cerebral blood flow
Protein and catalytic activity are upregulated within 10 minutes and peak 3 hours after cerebral ischemia	Protein and catalytic activity are upregulated within 12 hours and peak 48 hours after cerebral ischemia	Protein and catalytic activity are upregulated within 1 hour and peak 24 hours after cerebral ischemia

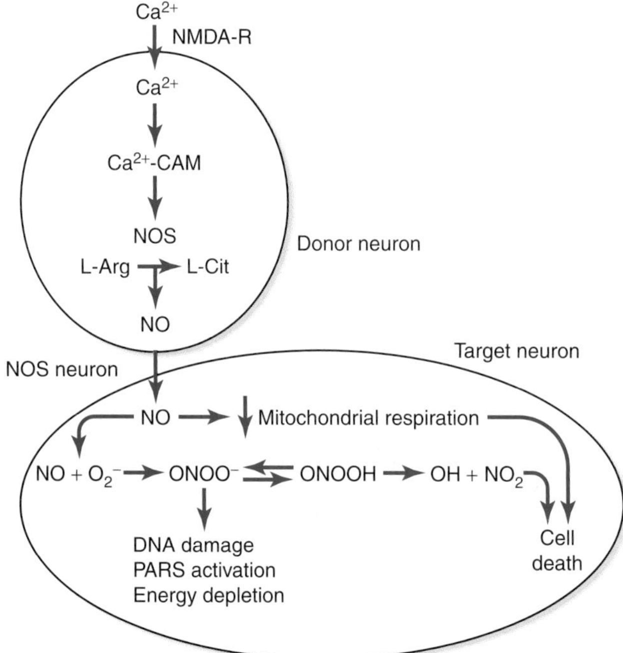

FIGURE 64-4. Excessive nitric oxide is formed on sustained glutamate stimulation of *N*-methyl-D-aspartate receptors (NMDA-R). Nitric oxide (NO) freely diffuses to adjacent target neurons, in which it combines with the superoxide anion (O_2^-) produced by mitochondria and xanthine oxidase to yield the peroxynitrite anion ($ONOO^-$), which is an extremely potent oxidant. $ONOO^-$ also is protonated and decomposes to the hydroxyl (OH) free radical and the nitrogen dioxide (NO_2) free radical, which are potent activators of lipid peroxidation. Damaged DNA activates the nuclear enzyme poly–adenosine diphosphate (ADP)–ribose synthetase (PARS). PARS transfers ADP-ribose units to nuclear proteins by using nicotinamide adenine dinucleotide (NAD) as the source of ADP-ribose. For every mole of NAD consumed in this reaction, it takes four energy equivalents of adenosine triphosphate to regenerate NAD from nicotinamide. PARS can transfer more than 100 ADP-ribose units/protein in a matter of seconds. This rapid consumption of energy can deplete a cell of its energy stores. It is hypothesized that if there is sufficient DNA damage and free radical production, the activation of PARS initiates a futile cycle, resulting in the complete depletion of cellular energy stores, impairment of the ability to regenerate those energy stores, and, subsequently, cell death. CaM, calmodulin; L-arg, L-arginine; L-cit, L-citrulline; NOS, nitric oxide synthase; ONOOH, peroxynitrous acid.

Less convincing but definite evidence exists for a potential neurotoxic role during global ischemia. Although one of the major effects of nitric oxide is to increase cyclic guanosine monophosphate, multiple mechanisms have been proposed to define its neurotoxic effects

An established pathway of nitric oxide–mediated neuronal cell death is nitric oxide activation of the nuclear enzyme poly-adenosine diphosphate (ADP)-ribose-synthetase (PARS) [Dawson and Dawson, 1995; Samdani et al., 1997]. Nitric oxide activates PARS by damaging DNA. PARS participates in DNA repair by catalyzing the transfer of ADP-ribose units from nicotinamide adenine dinucleotide (NAD) to nuclear proteins. For every mole of ADP-ribose transferred, 1 mol of NAD is consumed, and four free energy equivalents of ATP are necessary to regenerate NAD. Therefore, overactivation of PARS can rapidly deplete cellular energy stores.

Depending on its source, nitric oxide may be toxic to or protective of the brain under ischemic conditions. Overproduction of nitric oxide from either neuronal or inducible nitric oxide synthase leads to neurotoxicity; however, nitric oxide production from endothelial nitric oxide synthase protects brain tissue by maintaining regional cerebral blood flow. Studies emphasize the necessity of developing truly selective inhibitors for neuronal and inducible nitric oxide synthase to protect the brain adequately from ischemic injury caused by overproduction of nitric oxide and simultaneously to maintain or enhance regional cerebral blood flow [Samdani et al., 1997].

Formation of Oxygen Radicals

Toxic oxygen radical species, produced during postischemic reperfusion, have been implicated as important contributors to reperfusion injury and delayed cell death [Siesjo et al., 1989]. Oxygen free radicals are not one specific compound. They are a group of substances that are formed during ischemia, when oxygen becomes unavailable as the terminal electron acceptor in the electron transport chain. A free radical is any molecule that has an unpaired electron in its outermost orbit; such molecules are short-lived and highly reactive. They include nitric oxide, superoxide anion, hydrogen peroxide (not itself a free radical), hydroxyl radical, and peroxynitrite. The lone electron results in molecular instability and the tendency to initiate and propagate chain reactions.

Oxygen free radicals are generated during arachidonic acid metabolism to prostaglandins, as a byproduct of xanthine oxidase–catalyzed production of uric acid through catecholamine oxidation, through a mitochondrial leak during the oxidation of hemoglobin, and through the action of nitric oxide synthase [Kontos, 1987; Siesjo et al., 1995; Traystman et al., 1991] (Fig. 64-5). Free radicals are quite destructive to cellular components such as membrane lipids, especially in the presence of iron. Iron is normally transported in the blood, tightly bound to transferrin and stored inside the cell bound to ferritin. In ischemic conditions with accompanying acidosis, iron may be displaced from its normal binding sites and can catalyze reactions that promote oxygen radical formation [Komara et al., 1986]. Most com-

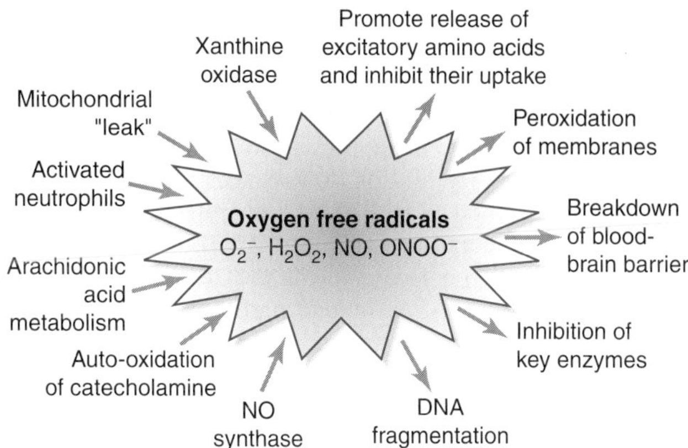

FIGURE 64-5. Sources and physiologic effects of oxygen free radicals. Reperfusion of ischemic neurons and glia produces several highly destructive free radicals, including nitric oxide (NO), peroxynitrite ($ONOO^-$), hydrogen peroxide (H_2O_2), and superoxide (O_2^-). These free radical species peroxidize cell membranes, alter the blood-brain barrier, and disrupt DNA.

monly implicated is the Haber-Weiss/Fenton reaction, whereby potent hydroxyl radicals are produced from superoxide anions and hydrogen peroxide in the presence of free iron.

The impact of the liver and the intestines in producing dysfunction in other organ systems needs further clarification. The liver and intestines have a great deal of xanthine dehydrogenase, which during ischemia can be converted to xanthine oxidase [Bellamy et al., 1996; Nielson et al., 1997]. The latter could enter the systemic circulation, generate free radicals, and cause additional dysfunction and injury at distant sites.

The brain may be particularly vulnerable to free radical injury for several reasons. One is the high concentration of polyunsaturated fatty acids, especially arachidonic acid. As noted previously, free fatty acids are released throughout ischemia. On exposure to oxygen radical species, these free fatty acids are vulnerable to lipid peroxidation [Krause et al., 1988]. Cerebrospinal fluid has low concentrations of iron-binding proteins; therefore, iron released from injured neurons or glia is likely to contribute to these peroxidation reactions. Byproducts of these reactions—for example, malondialdehyde and conjugated dienes—have been used as markers of the extent of lipid peroxidation after brain injury [Schmidley, 1990]. Lipid peroxides accumulate in the selectively vulnerable zones during reperfusion after transient forebrain ischemia [Bromont et al., 1989; Komara et al., 1986]. The peroxides do not accumulate during the ischemic period itself or in areas that are not reperfused and thus are implicated in reperfusion injury [Oliver et al., 1990].

Lipid membranes are a natural target of free radicals, especially in the brain, because they are abundant, and their polyunsaturated nature makes them easy to oxidize [Schmidley, 1990]. The effects of free radicals on membranes include changes in membrane fluidity and alteration of ion channels and transport proteins. In addition to disruption of the cell membrane, fragmentation of the mitochondrial membrane results in a decrease in cellular energy production.

The ability of the cell to defend itself against free radicals is limited, and free radical scavenging enzymes such as superoxide dismutase and catalase may be overwhelmed after an ischemic area is reperfused [Vannucci and Perlman, 1997]. Surprisingly, restoration of blood flow to hypoxic-ischemic areas is potentially detrimental because the influx of oxygen can be used as a source of oxygen free radicals through the processes noted previously. Stimulated by high tissue carbon dioxide tension, low oxygen tension, and low pH, restored blood flow to an ischemic area is often increased above normal (luxury perfusion). In experimental preparations, oxygen free radicals are detected primarily during reperfusion. After luxury perfusion, there is prolonged hypoperfusion and an associated decrease in cerebral metabolism. In animal experiments, these decreases are not seen with pretreatment with oxygen free radical scavengers.

Reperfusion Injury

Cerebral reperfusion injury is a complex series of interactions between the brain parenchyma and microcirculation that results in detrimental effects that negate some of the benefits of reperfusion [Becker, 1997]. Many of the mechanisms previously discussed contribute to additional injury during reperfusion, particularly those associated with release of free radicals. Some may be accelerated or accentuated. With circulatory return, substrate availability increases, as does the function of potentially toxic oxygen-dependent enzymes, and, separately or in combination, this may worsen injury. After focal insults, progressive microcirculatory failure is also thought to be an important aspect of reperfusion injury.

Loss of blood flow to the brain results in neuronal injury as a result of both the cessation of blood flow, leading to oxygen and nutrient deprivation, and the initiation of a cascade of secondary mechanisms [Vaagenes et al., 1996]. This neurotoxic cascade involves derangements in normal metabolic and physiologic functions, as well as initiation of cell death processes. Thus, both restoration of blood supply and control of secondary neurotoxic cascades are necessary to limit ischemic neuronal damage [Sweeney et al., 1995].

Genetic Damage and Regulation

Two aspects related to global asphyxial injury and genetic regulation are emerging as critical components of the injury cascade. The first concerns mechanisms associated with injury and repair of the genetic material itself, and the second concerns regulation of multiple genes and the proteins that they in turn regulate in response to hypoxia-ischemia.

Studies have demonstrated that ischemia and reperfusion can induce gene damage in the CNS. Reactive oxygen species generated by cerebral oxidative stress interact with nucleic acids and cause the formation of oxidative DNA and RNA lesions that result from DNA base modifications or single-stranded breaks in neurons or astrocytes [Liu and Arora, 2002; Liu et al., 2001]. Oxidative DNA lesions cause a change in coding properties during DNA and RNA synthesis (replication and transcription) or may terminate chain elongation during transcription and translation. Either process can affect protein synthesis.

The development of microarray systems for gene expression profiling since the mid-1990s has provided insights into the mechanisms of the brain's response to global hypoxic injury [Jin et al., 2001; Papadopoulos et al., 2000; Tang et al., 2002]. Future studies should not only increase the understanding of the molecular basis of ischemic injury but also suggest potential therapies. Because investigators in such studies frequently use several thousand gene transcripts, using different animal models with varying degrees of severity and duration of global hypoxia-ischemia, as well as varying time periods of reperfusion, it will be some time before a unified or general understanding of the underlying mechanisms of injury are more clearly appreciated.

Early during hypoxia-ischemia, overall gene expression in the brain is reduced or ceases to maintain energy metabolism to support essential cell activities. Immediate early genes undergo rapid induction after global ischemia [Kogure and Kato, 1993]. Some of the immediate early gene products that have been identified include c-fos, c-jun, and the zinc finger family of proteins; heat-shock proteins; and amyloid precursor protein. Immediate early genes are transcription factors that bind to target genes and alter their expression. These stress response proteins may directly affect neuronal death and survival after ischemia. However, despite much research into their expression, it remains unclear which ones contribute to the outcome of hypoxic-ischemic injury [Papadopoulos et al., 2000]. This confusion occurs partly because some are upregulated, whereas others are downregulated, and their respective neurotoxic or neuroprotective roles remain to be defined.

Another early expressed group of proteins are the heat shock proteins that are molecular chaperones, which bind intracellular proteins and prevent their inappropriate folding [Papadopoulos et al., 2000]. Hsp-70 is markedly induced by hypoxia and is neuroprotective. Hsp-32 is another heat shock protein that may be neuroprotective after hypoxia. It encodes heme-oxygenase-1, which after induction has been found to protect neurons in models of transient forebrain ischemia, possibly by producing bile pigments that are strong antioxidants, as well as carbon monoxide, which can cause vasodilation and inhibits platelet aggregation.

Growth factors are also released within hours after ischemia and may also serve a neuroprotective role. They are polypeptides and the major types of growth factors include nerve growth factor; brain-derived neurotrophic factor; neurotrophins-3, -4, -5; and basic fibroblast growth factor [Papadopoulos et al., 2000]. Nerve growth factor, brain-derived neurotrophic factor, and neurotrophin-3 bind receptors on the cell surface that have tyrosine kinase activity, and activation of tyrosine kinase is associated with neuronal survival.

Hours later, cytokines, adhesion molecules, isoforms of nitric oxide synthase, and gene products involved in apoptosis are upregulated. Some of these genes protect the cells from dying; some promote the death of injured cells; and others have no known effects on cell survival. Cytokines are produced by activated lymphocytes, macrophages, and astrocytes and include tumor necrosis factor α, transforming growth factor β, and interleukin-1β. Cytokines participate in the inflammatory response and accelerate entry of inflammatory cells from the circulation into the brain. Certain cytokines (e.g., tumor necrosis factor α and interleukin-1β) may also induce the expression of glycoproteins known as adhesion molecules on endothelial cells, which also facilitate recruitment of inflammatory cells into the ischemic brain [Papadopoulos et al., 2000].

Neuronal degeneration can also be promoted by induction of apoptosis genes or genes that cause a stress to the cells, such as those related to free radical production or to the production of various nitric oxide synthase isoforms [Koistinaho and Hokfelt, 1997]. Cells that undergo apoptosis shrink down and ultimately are phagocytosed by neighboring cells. Genes that accelerate apoptosis include members of the bax and bad families, p53, and Fas; those that inhibit apoptosis are associated with bcl-2, bcl-x (L), and DAD1 families [Papadopoulos et al., 2000]. When apoptosis is initiated, cytochrome c is released from damaged mitochondria and, in concert with apoptotic protease–activating factor, induce members of the caspase family, including interleukin-1–converting enzyme. As apoptosis proceeds, nuclear components and the cell skeleton are destroyed, detach other cell constituents and from neighboring cells, and are phagocytosed.

Two studies demonstrated both the elegance of the application of microarray technology and the dilemmas in synthesizing the results. In one study, 15 minutes of global cerebral ischemia in rats was associated with 1.7-fold or greater increased expression of 57 genes and 1.7-fold or greater decreased expression of 34 genes studied up to 72 hours after hypoxia [Jin et al., 2001]. Induced genes included those involved in protein synthesis, proapoptotic genes, antiapoptotic genes, injury-response genes, receptors, ion channels, and enzymes. Transcriptional induction of several genes was also reported, as was co-induction of several groups of related genes (e.g., vascular endothelial growth factor and its receptor, neuropilin-1). A second study examined 8000 transcripts in rat brains 24 hours after exposure to 6 hours of hypoxia (8% oxygen) and found very little gene induction (15 upregulated genes and 11 downregulated genes) [Tang et al., 2002]. In contrast, the same investigators found that in a model of permanent focal ischemia, 415 genes were upregulated and 158 were downregulated. Presumably the differences between global hypoxia and ischemia were attributable to greater tissue injury in the ischemic model, but there is no apparent explanation of the differences in the response to global hypoxia in these two groups of studies.

CLINICAL PATHOPHYSIOLOGY

The complex metabolic changes that occur after cardiopulmonary arrest have a direct relationship with the physiologic variables that are monitored both in animal studies and in patients.

Cerebral Blood Flow and Metabolism after Resuscitation

The pioneering studies in which global cerebral blood flow and cerebral metabolic rate for oxygen were measured in animal models of global ischemia or cardiac arrest focused on the early postresuscitation period. In their classic study, Snyder and associates [1975] demonstrated that after 15 minutes of global brain ischemia in dogs, cerebral blood flow transiently increased to levels well above baseline. After 15 to 30 minutes, cerebral blood flow progressively decreased to a level below normal for the rest of the monitoring period (90 minutes). This pattern of early transient post-ischemic hyperemia and subsequent delayed post-ischemic hypoperfusion has been observed almost universally in global cerebral ischemia models, including asphyxia-induced cardiac arrest. The level of hyperemia and subsequent hypoperfusion varies in relation to the duration of the insult. Although these phases of increased and decreased cerebral blood flow characterize the net global effect, regional cerebral blood flow is often heterogeneous, particularly during post-ischemic hypoperfusion, when areas of decreased and increased perfusion may coexist. Metabolism, as assessed by cerebral metabolic rate for oxygen, is reduced during the early post-ischemic period and then progressively recovers to a level that varies, depending on the model used and the duration of ischemia. In some models, including ventricular fibrillation in dogs, significant recovery of cerebral metabolic rate for oxygen may occur during the first few hours, despite persistent post-ischemic hypoperfusion, creating the potential for a secondary ischemic insult during reperfusion. Whether this increase in cerebral metabolic rate for oxygen represents appropriate synaptic activity, seizures, or changes in the basal metabolic rate is uncertain. In other models, global cerebral blood flow and cerebral metabolic rate for oxygen are matched during the first few hours after ischemia. In such cases, post-ischemic cerebral blood flow appears to be determined by the metabolic needs of the brain, and delayed hypoperfusion may not be a significant cause of neuronal injury. Thus, delayed hypoperfusion is likely the result of brain injury rather than the cause [Michenfelder and Milde, 1990].

Of historic interest is the concept of "no reflow," which was suggested in the 1960s by Ames and co-workers [1968]. These investigators noted that after a period of global cerebral ischemia, reflow could not be re-established. Early attempts at brain resuscitation were based on the concept that preventing "no reflow" would improve neurologic outcome. However, the relationship between delayed hypoperfusion and brain injury remains unclear, and therapies to improve blood flow such as hypertension and hemodilution remain controversial.

Drugs such as nimodipine can increase cerebral blood flow during the early post-ischemic hypoperfusion phase after global cerebral ischemia. Cerebral metabolic rate for oxygen recovery generally is not increased by treatment, even though nimodipine improves neurologic outcome after global ischemia in some models. Safar and associates [1996] reported that a multifaceted flow-promotion treatment strategy to increase cerebral blood flow and reduce cerebral metabolic rate for oxygen early after ventricular fibrillation in dogs improved outcome. This improvement was accomplished with brief cardiopulmonary bypass, mild hypothermia, hemodilution, and transient hypertension.

Studies in which investigators measured cerebral blood flow and cerebral metabolic rate for oxygen in humans after cardiac arrest shed interesting light on these data from animals. Whereas cerebral blood flow and cerebral metabolic rate for oxygen typically are measured early (0 to 2 hours after arrest) in experimental animal studies, such measurements in humans are obtained beginning 6 to 12 hours after arrest. Beckstead and associates [1978] measured global cerebral blood flow and cerebral metabolic rate for oxygen in 25 adults after cardiac arrest. In all, 21 of these patients had a vegetative outcome. In agreement with the experimental animal studies, Beckstead and associates observed hypoperfusion and hypometabolism with coupling of cerebral blood flow and cerebral metabolic rate for oxygen. During the subsequent 2 days, however, global cerebral blood flow increased to levels equal to or greater than normal, whereas metabolism failed to recover. Thus, in humans with poor neurologic outcome after cardiac arrest, absolute or relative delayed hyperemia followed the hypoperfusion phase. Results of two more studies in adults have confirmed these findings. Using xenon-133 washout, Cohan and colleagues [1989] observed that patients regaining consciousness had normal cerebral blood flow between 6 and 46 hours after arrest, whereas patients who died without regaining consciousness had increased cerebral blood flow (hyperemia) within 24 hours. Similarly, Love and associates [1989] used stable xenon-enhanced computed tomography (CT) and discovered that the combination of diffuse hyperemia and loss of reactivity of cerebral blood flow to changes in $Pa{CO_2}$ was seen 100 hours after arrest in adults who never regained consciousness.

Thus, immediately after cardiac arrest accompanied by restoration of systemic hemodynamic stability, transient global brain hyperemia occurs and is followed by a period of patchy hypoperfusion. The magnitude and duration of these alterations in flow appear to be related to the duration of the insult. In patients with good outcomes, global cerebral blood flow recovers over the subsequent 24 to 72 hours, and CO_2 reactivity remains intact. In patients who do not regain consciousness or progress to brain death, absolute or relative cerebral blood flow hyperemia develops with impaired CO_2 reactivity [Prough and Zornow, 1997]. It must be recognized that the measurement of metabolism in these studies has traditionally been cerebral metabolic rate for oxygen. Bergsneider and co-workers [1995] used positron emission tomography in humans after traumatic brain injury and reported the occurrence of delayed hyperglycolysis in some comatose patients. Studies of cerebral glucose utilization with positron emission tomography after cardiac arrest are needed.

Results from clinical studies of asphyxia-induced cardiac arrest in children are scarce and somewhat conflicting with regard to the prognostic implications. Normal values of post–cardiac arrest cerebral blood flow with loss of responsivity to $Pa{CO_2}$ were observed in children with poor outcome at 24 hours after asphyxia-induced cardiac arrest by strangulation, as studied with stable-xenon CT [Ashwal et al., 1991]. Similarly, in studies of subjects between 24 and 48 hours after near-drowning, Ashwal and colleagues [1990] observed low cerebral blood flow and no relationship between cerebral blood flow and $Pa{CO_2}$ in the seven nonsurvivors, which again suggests loss of cerebral blood flow reactivity to changes in $Pa{CO_2}$. In this study, hyperemia was not routinely observed in either vegetative survivors or children who died, but only a single cerebral blood flow measurement was made. Beyda [1987] obtained serial measurements of post–cardiac arrest cerebral blood flow with xenon-enhanced CT in a series of children who had suffered asphyxia-induced cardiac arrest from submersion accidents. Children with good neurologic outcomes had slightly decreased cerebral blood flow values at 12 hours that increased to normal during the subsequent 24 to 60 hours. In these children, cerebral blood flow reactivity to CO_2 was intact. Children with an eventual vegetative outcome or brain death exhibited hyperemia with loss or attenuation of CO_2 reactivity. This hyperemia progressed to low or normal flow over the next 12 to 72 hours in children with vegetative outcome and progressed to low and then no flow, with the development of brain death.

CLINICAL OUTCOME AFTER CARDIAC ARREST

The incidence of death and neurologic impairment from cardiac arrest in children is alarmingly high. Also dismaying is the suggestion that current approaches to resuscitation of these children may increase the number of successful cardiovascular resuscitations without equal neurologic recovery. Current medical literature has examined the mortality and neurologic morbidity resulting from prehospital cardiac arrest in pediatric patients (Table 64-3).

TABLE 64-3

Results of Resuscitation in Prehospital Pediatric Cardiac Arrest*

STUDY	TOTAL NO. OF PATIENTS	LONG-TERM SURVIVORS	COMMENTS
O'Rourke [1986]	34	7	All survivors sent to chronic care facility
Zaritsky et al. [1987]	11	1	Outcome of surviving patient not reported
Torphy et al. [1984]	77	3	All survivors neurologically impaired
Nichols et al. [1986]	10	0	No survivors among 10 of 13 patients asystolic on arrival to emergency department
Rosenberg [1984]	24	3	Neurologic outcome not reported for survivors
Eisenberg et al. [1983]	119	8	Neurologic outcome not reported for survivors
Friesen et al. [1982]	44	1	Outcome poor after asystole
Thompson et al. [1990]	70	3	All survivors had serious sequelae
Applebaum [1985]	22	0	18 of 22 were asystolic
Schindler et al. [1996]	80	6	All survivors had neurologic sequelae
Hickey [1995]	33	1	Severe neurologic injury in the survivor
Ronco et al. [1995]	60	6	All survivors had severe deficits; 60 of 63 children were asystolic
Dieckmann and Vardis [1995]	62	0	Study reports 62 of 65 children were asystolic at emergency department
Hazinski et al. [1994]	22	0	Trauma patients pulseless on emergency department evaluation
Sheikh and Brogan [1994]	27	0	CPR after blunt trauma; comparison of open- versus closed-chest CPR
Total	695	39	5.6% survival, none described as neurologically normal

*All patients were asystolic or pulseless on arrival to the emergency department.
CPR, cardiopulmonary resuscitation.

Interpretation of these studies' results and comparisons among them are made difficult by several factors [Perkin and van Stralen, 1992]. In some reports, cardiac arrest is not clearly differentiated from respiratory arrest. Because the outcome of resuscitation is better after respiratory than cardiac arrest, failure to clearly distinguish the two groups results in falsely optimistic outcomes. Second, the time and location of arrest vary in these studies; some investigators evaluated prehospital arrests, some assessed in-hospital arrests, and others combined the two groups. Mortality and neurologic morbidity may occur at a higher rate among patients with prehospital cardiac arrest than among emergency department and in-hospital patients as a result of the lack of emphasis on pediatric basic and advanced life support, as well as the delay in discovery of the patient. Therefore, each group should be analyzed separately. Finally, successful resuscitation is often defined as the patient's being discharged from the emergency department or hospital, without the consideration of residual neurologic damage.

Review of evaluations of outcomes of pediatric prehospital cardiac arrest reveals the following:

- Children who survived neurologically intact had cardiac activity on arrival in the emergency department. The combined rates of mortality and severe morbidity in children arriving pulseless in the emergency department approached 100%.
- Children who had a delayed response to resuscitation had little chance for neurologically intact survival. Those with resuscitation times of less than 15 minutes had a far better outcome than did those whose resuscitation times were longer [Gillis et al., 1986; Nichols et al., 1986]. Resuscitation efforts lasting more than 25 minutes were uniformly unsuccessful [Quan et al., 1990; Rosenberg, 1984].
- The extent of the resuscitation attempt, which is obviously related to the rapidity of the response to initial therapy, was another predictor of outcome in pediatric resuscitation. Many studies suggest that no pediatric patient with cardiac arrest who receives more than two doses of epinephrine survives to discharge [Nichols et al., 1986; Zaritsky et al., 1987].

Many explanations have been proposed for the poor outcome of pediatric cardiac arrest patients. Primary respiratory disorders and those that result in respiratory arrest account for the majority of cardiopulmonary arrests in children. Hypoxemia and acidosis, which occur because of the respiratory difficulty, result in bradycardia or asystole. Restoration of a cardiac rhythm is difficult, and even if it is restored, the victim is likely to suffer neurologic impairment [Goetting, 1994; O'Rourke, 1986]. Because most pediatric cardiac arrests are secondary to hypoxemia, it is logical to assume that if the hypoxemia lasts long enough and is severe enough to stop the heart, it will also have devastating neurologic effects.

Additional reasons for poor survival from prehospital pediatric cardiac arrest include unwitnessed cardiac arrest, such as that seen with sudden infant death syndrome or near-drowning, which delays resuscitation; ineffective basic cardiopulmonary resuscitation; and delays in providing advanced life support [Gausche, 1997; Kumar et al., 1997]. Unwitnessed cardiac arrest is associated with a high mortality rate, especially when the initial rhythm is bradycardia or asystole, and prehospital resuscitation is inadequate because of unavailable skills or no return to rhythm. In pediatric patients, sudden infant death syndrome is a leading cause of death in infants 1 month to 1 year of age and is an example of the futility of resuscitating patients who have suffered unwitnessed cardiac arrest [Goyco and Beckerman, 1990]. It is important to note that sudden infant death syndrome is diagnosed only after a postmortem examination reveals no physiologic cause for the sudden death of the infant. Numerous studies have demonstrated no successful resuscitations in children with confirmed diagnoses of sudden infant death syndrome [Dolan et al., 1988; O'Rourke, 1986]. In fact, in infants younger than 1 year who are found pulseless and apneic at home and are documented to be pulseless and apneic in the emergency department, the likelihood of successful resuscitation is low enough to suggest that vigorous resuscitation efforts are unwarranted.

Similarly, warm-water near-drowning victims who arrive in the emergency department with no spontaneous respirations and no perfusing heartbeat do poorly. Data from many studies confirm that all near-drowning victims who were not hypothermic (core body temperature of less than 30° C) and who were asystolic when they arrived at the first medical facility either died or survived with severe neurologic damage [Biggart and Bohn, 1990; Habib et al., 1996]. In view of these data, some experts recommend that nonhypothermic near-drowning pediatric victims who arrive in the emergency department without perfusing cardiac rhythms should not undergo prolonged and aggressive resuscitation or intensive care management [Biggart and Bohn, 1990; Habib et al., 1996; Spack et al., 1997].

Cardiopulmonary resuscitation and advanced life support that are ineffective or delayed are other variables that explain the poor outcome of prehospital pediatric resuscitation. Although paramedics may provide sophisticated advanced life support care to adults, they may not be adequately trained to establish an open and protected airway, initiate positive pressure ventilation, defibrillate, or start intravenous infusions in or give drugs to pediatric patients in cardiac arrest. In summary, a review of literature supports the following points:

- Children who are asystolic or who experience a delay in resuscitation have little chance for neurologically intact survival.
- Unsuccessful resuscitations of children are currently the rule rather than the exception.
- Serious neurologic damage is common in survivors of cardiac arrest.
- Recovery is much better in children who experienced witnessed cardiac arrests, cold water submersion, or isolated respiratory arrest; intact survival rates as high as 44% to 75% after these events have been reported [Lewis et al., 1983; O'Rourke, 1986; Torphy et al., 1984; Zaritsky et al., 1987]. Nevertheless, these clinical data seem to bear out the severe neuropathology observed in asphyxia-induced arrest in animal models because asphyxia-induced cardiac arrest is the most common mode of cardiac arrest in all of the clinical pediatric series.

MAJOR DISORDERS CAUSING CARDIAC ARREST

Table 64-1 and Box 64-1 list the common causes, by category, of pediatric cardiorespiratory arrest taken from major published pediatric cardiac arrest series. Common specific disease entities resulting in cardiac arrest are sudden infant death syndrome, drowning, strangulation, nonaccidental trauma, and lightning/electrical injury.

Sudden Infant Death Syndrome

Sudden infant death syndrome is defined as the sudden death of an infant younger than 1 year that remains unexplained after a thorough case investigation, including performance of a complete postmortem examination, examination of the death scene, and review of the medical history [Willinger et al., 1991]. The addition of requirements for examining the death scene and reviewing the history give greater precision to the diagnosis, but it remains one of exclusion, based on the absence of any specific findings on routine postmortem examination. In many unresolved cases, the history, investigation, or postmortem examination reveals information that excludes the diagnosis of sudden infant death syndrome but does not explain the cause of death: Suspected abuse, neglect, or accidental suffocation; vomiting or diarrhea without evidence of infection; unreliable information; or findings such as mild bronchopneumonia, supraglottitis, or maternal drug abuse are not sufficient to explain death [Gilbert-Barness and Barness, 1995]. Even though almost all cases of sudden unexpected death in infants continue to be ascribed to sudden infant death syndrome, the uncritical certification of the syndrome as a diagnosis, without a postmortem examination, death scene investigation, and careful history, prevents accurate diagnosis of the cause of death [Bass et al., 1986; Valdes-Dapena, 1995].

Epidemiology

INCIDENCE AND AGE AT DEATH

After the neonatal period, sudden infant death syndrome is the leading cause of death during the first year of life. Although sudden infant death syndrome may occur during the first month of life, most neonatal deaths can be accounted for by specific perinatal factors, including prematurity, infection, and congenital diseases.

The incidence of sudden infant death syndrome peaks between 2 and 4 months of age; 95% of all deaths from the syndrome occur by 6 months of age [Hunt, 1992]. Sudden infant death syndrome, therefore, is primarily a disorder that strikes children between the ages of 1 and 6 months. It is so rare outside those age limits that the diagnosis in such cases should be made with caution and only after all possible causes, including metabolic diseases, are excluded [Gilbert-Barness and Barness, 1995]. The age-at-death distribution of sudden infant death syndrome is the most consistent, unique, and provocative characteristic identified [Peterson, 1988].

Box 64-3 Epidemiologic Factors Associated with Increased Risk for Sudden Infant Death Syndrome

Maternal and prenatal risk factors
- Intrauterine hypoxia
- Fetal growth retardation
- Smoking
- Anemia
- Drug exposure (cocaine and heroin)
- Low socioeconomic status
- Decreased maternal age and education
- Increased parity and shorter interpregnancy interval

Postnatal risk factors
- Growth failure
- Perinatal asphyxia
- Prematurity and low birth weight
- Male gender
- Postnatal age of 2 to 4 months
- Formula feeding
- Thermal stress (overheating)
- Co-sleeping
- Recent (febrile) illness
- Passive smoking
- Soft bedding
- Prone sleeping position
- Ethnicity (black or Native American)

IDENTIFICATION OF RISK FACTORS

An ambitious study designed to investigate risk factors for sudden infant death syndrome was the National Institute of Child Health and Human Development Cooperative Epidemiological Study of Sudden Infant Death Syndrome Risk Factors [Hoffman et al., 1988]. This study revealed an incidence of the syndrome of 1.7 per 1000 live births. In the study, sudden infant death syndrome was ruled as the cause of death after a detailed review of microscopic slides, gross postmortem examination review, and death investigation reports by a panel of expert pathologists.

No epidemiologic differences have been of sufficient sensitivity and specificity to permit prospective identification [Hoffman and Hillman, 1992]. Maternal and prenatal factors (Box 64-3) suggest that the in utero environment of future victims of sudden infant death syndrome is suboptimal [Carroll and Loughlin, 1993]. Some of the postnatal risk factors suggest that the postnatal care is also suboptimal. A number of epidemiologic studies have documented that smoking during pregnancy and after birth are two major and independent risk factors for sudden infant death syndrome [Perkin, 2004]. With the reduction in the incidence of infants being put to sleep prone, maternal smoking has become the major modifiable risk factor for sudden infant death syndrome [Horne et al., 2002]. It has been argued that 30% of deaths from sudden infant death syndrome are preventable by not exposing infants to cigarette smoke [Chang et al., 2003].

Since the inception of infant monitoring, investigators have tried to define populations at increased risk for sudden infant death syndrome, even though it has not been demonstrated that monitoring prevents infant deaths or morbidity associated with apnea, such as neurodevelopmental delays. Four major groups could be considered to be at a high risk for sudden infant death syndrome (Box 64-4).

Box 64-4 Groups at High Risk for Sudden Infant Death Syndrome (SIDS)

- Survivors of apparent life-threatening event (ALTE)
- Subsequent siblings of SIDS victims
- Preterm infants, including those with bronchopulmonary dysplasia
- Infants of drug-dependent mothers

Sleeping in the prone position (on the stomach) by infants has been one of the most consistent risk factors for sudden infant death syndrome, and avoidance of prone sleeping has been the focus of several national campaigns to prevent the syndrome. The evidence that prone sleeping is a risk factor for sudden infant death syndrome has been so compelling that the American Academy of Pediatrics Task Force on Infant Positioning and sudden infant death syndrome [1992] recommended the supine sleeping position for infants. The fear that aspiration would occur if an infant vomited or regurgitated while sleeping in the supine position appears to be unwarranted; in fact, the incidence of death from aspiration has actually decreased among infants sleeping in the supine position [Gilbert-Barness and Barness, 1995]. Although the lateral position for sleeping has also been recommended, positioning infants on their sides may not be as safe, because the infant may roll over into the prone position.

The recommendation for sleep in a nonprone or supine position is for healthy infants only. Gastroesophageal reflux and certain upper airway anomalies that predispose to airway obstruction and perhaps some other illnesses may be indications for a prone sleeping position ["Positioning and sudden infant death syndrome (SIDS)," 1996].

There is evidence that the danger of the prone position is compounded by soft, yielding bedding [Gilbert-Barness and Barness, 1995]. Infants sleeping face down on thick, soft, cushiony surfaces such as lamb's wool, pillows, cushions filled with synthetic material, or beanbags stuffed with polystyrene pellets may hollow out a "pocket" in the soft surface. In that position, infants may rebreathe their own expired air, which is high in carbon dioxide. An infant who cannot, for any reason, lift the head out of the pocket may suffocate.

Scientific studies have demonstrated that bed sharing by mother and infant can alter and synchronize sleep patterns of the two. These studies have led to speculation in the lay press that bed sharing, sometimes referred to as *co-sleeping*, may also reduce the risk of sudden infant death syndrome. Although bed sharing may have certain benefits (such as encouraging breast-feeding), no scientific studies demonstrate that bed sharing reduces the incidence of sudden infant death syndrome. Conversely, there are studies suggesting that bed sharing, under certain conditions, may actually increase the risk of the syndrome ["Does bed sharing affect the risk of sudden infant death syndrome?" 1997].

Pathophysiology

The most compelling hypothesis to explain sudden infant death syndrome is that of a brainstem abnormality in cardiorespiratory control [Hunt, 1992]. Both the pathologic data derived from postmortem examination studies and the clinical data obtained in infants at increased epidemiologic risk for sudden infant death syndrome support this hypothesis. The postmortem findings, although subtle, are consistent with a maturational or developmental abnormality associated with the brainstem areas relevant to autonomic control of cardiorespiratory regulation. The clinical data to support the cardiorespiratory control hypothesis were initially obtained from assessments of patients with apnea of infancy and of asymptomatic infants at increased epidemiologic risk for sudden infant death syndrome.

Respiratory pattern abnormalities have been observed in infants at increased risk for sudden infant death syndrome [Goyco and Beckerman, 1990]. Because of the extent of overlap between control infants and infants who later died of sudden infant death syndrome, however, overnight recordings of respiratory pattern and heart rate have been unable to identify accurately either future victims of the syndrome or infants who will develop apnea of infancy. Consequently, the practice of performing a pneumogram or polysomnogram in early infancy to assess later risk for sudden infant death syndrome, or for apparently life-threatening events, has no identifiable predictive validity. Respiratory pattern abnormalities are just one category of cardiorespiratory control and are perhaps not one of the more important categories.

Infants at increased risk for sudden infant death syndrome have diminished ventilatory responsiveness to hypercarbia and hypoxia [Hunt, 1992]. The extent of overlap between control infants and at-risk infants, however, precludes the use of hypercarbic or hypoxic ventilatory responsiveness, or both, as a test to predict risk for the syndrome. Because of overlapping values, an individual infant cannot be classified as normal or abnormal. In addition, these tests are too time consuming and costly to be useful for large-scale application. Such tests, therefore, have no role in the routine clinical management of apnea of infancy or in the evaluation of any asymptomatic infants at increased epidemiologic risk for sudden infant death syndrome.

Respiratory pattern abnormalities and diminished ventilatory responsiveness are not inherently life threatening. A deficiency in arousal responsiveness, however, would be life threatening because the infant is thereby rendered incapable of responding effectively to progressive sleep-related asphyxia, regardless of its cause. Infants with apnea of infancy and diminished ventilatory responsiveness to hypercarbia, hypoxia, or both also have a concomitant abnormality in hypercarbic hypoxic arousal responsiveness, or both [Carroll and Loughlin, 1993]. A deficit in arousal responsiveness is likely necessary for sudden infant death syndrome to occur, but it may well be insufficient to cause the syndrome unless or until another factor that can permit or cause sleep-related asphyxia occurs.

One of the most tenable hypotheses of sudden infant death syndrome is that the sequence of events is initiated by a period of airway obstruction resulting from one of several causes, among them upper airway obstructions, edema secondary to a respiratory tract infection, or pharyngeal hypotonia during sleep. Hypoxia, acidosis, and hypercarbia follow the obstructive event. These metabolic changes usually produce arousal during active sleep; however, inappropriately weak efforts, poor coordination, or diaphragmatic fatigue associated with the event may result in atelectasis at the lung bases, increased firing of airway stretch receptors, and secondary apnea from the Hering-Breuer reflex. Because the infant fails to become aroused adequately to stimulate the respiratory control centers in the brainstem, an episode of central apnea may occur, producing more severe hypoxia and acidosis. If the sequence of events is uninterrupted, respiratory arrest, cardiac dysrhythmia, shock, and death can occur.

A strong history of sudden infant death syndrome, apparent life-threatening events, and obstructive sleep apnea in family members predisposes an infant to obstructive sleep apnea during the first year of life [McNamara and Sullivan, 2000]. The potential link among sudden infant death syndrome, apparent life-threatening events, and obstructive sleep apnea in infants is unclear; however, an increased incidence of obstructive sleep apnea in subsequent siblings of infants who died of sudden infant death syndrome and infants with apparent life-threatening events has been described. In addition, studies have documented obstructive events during sleep in infants who subsequently became victims of sudden infant death syndrome [Kato et al., 2001]. These findings suggest that sudden infant death syndrome and apparent life-threatening events are related to obstructive sleep apnea. Sleep studies should be obtained in young infants with multiple family histories of sudden infant death syndrome, apparent life-threatening events, and obstructive sleep apnea.

Studies in normal infants, subsequent siblings of victims of sudden infant death syndrome, and patients with apnea of infancy indicate that arousal responsiveness to hypoxia normally decreases with maturation, reaching a low at 2 to 3 months, the age for peak vulnerability to sudden infant death syndrome [van der Hal et al., 1985]. As is the case with respiratory pattern abnormalities and ventilatory responses, unfortunately, there is again too much overlap between normal and abnormal infants to permit use of arousal responsiveness as a means of classifying an individual infant as normal or abnormal. In addition, arousal response assessments are too time consuming and costly for routine clinical use.

Decreased heart rate variability has been reported in infants with apnea. Infants with sudden infant death syndrome have been reported to differ from control infants with regard both to higher overall heart rate in all sleep-waking states and to diminished heart rate during wakefulness [Schectman and Harper, 1993]. Through spectral analysis, it has become apparent that future victims of sudden infant death syndrome also differ from control infants in that cardiac and respiratory activity are coupled. Overall, these studies of diminished heart rate variability in infants who later died of sudden infant death syndrome indicate an abnormality of autonomic control that is consistent with the overall hypothesis of a brainstem abnormality involving, but not restricted to, cardiac control. Maturational studies indicate that the period immediately after the neonatal age is a time of increased vulnerability.

Event recordings of the terminal episode have documented early and rapid development of severe bradycardia;

it develops too soon to be explained by the progressive desaturation of prolonged apnea [Meny et al., 1994]. Although this finding lends support to the idea of an abnormality in cardiac control, it is also possible that the hypoxemia or obstructive apnea, or both, may, in at least some instances, be the underlying pathophysiologic mechanism for the terminal bradycardia.

Prediction

Potential victims of sudden infant death syndrome cannot be identified by any method before death. No test, including pneumography and polysomnography, or any risk profile can identify a specific infant destined to die of the syndrome. In addition, no test that can be performed in parents or in siblings is predictive of sudden infant death syndrome in a family. Pneumography and polysomnography can be useful in the management of selected patients, but they are not predictive for the syndrome. More work is needed, for example, in the area of metabolic defects to identify means of predicting and preventing at least some deaths resulting from sudden infant death syndrome.

Management

After a sudden infant death syndrome event, management involves the surviving parents (and the extended family), surviving siblings, and subsequent siblings.

Drowning and Near-Drowning (Submersion Injury)

Drowning is defined as death by suffocation after submersion in a liquid medium. *Near-drowning* is a term used when a patient recovers, at least temporarily, from the drowning episode. Most investigators include loss of consciousness while submerged to complete the criteria of near-drowning. Patients who are initially resuscitated after submersion but who die within 24 hours are ultimately classified as drowning victims. *Secondary drowning* refers to patients who have recovered uneventfully from a submersion injury and are asymptomatic for a period of time but who later die from respiratory failure secondary to the episode. The existence of secondary drowning has been questioned in the literature, and the term should not be used [DeNicola et al., 1997]. Patients with so-called secondary drowning have subtle but clearly manifested respiratory compromise immediately after submersion [Pratt and Haynes, 1986]. As many as 15% to 20% of near-drowning victims who ultimately die do so with severe respiratory failure. Nonetheless, the term *secondary drowning* is misleading because most of these patients have secondary pulmonary infections and concomitant severe neurologic dysfunction.

From 1990 to 2000, drowning was the second leading cause of unintentional injury death among U.S. children between 1 and 19 years of age [American Academy of Pediatrics Committee on Injury, Violence, and Poison Prevention, 2003]. In 2000, more than 1400 U.S. children younger than 20 years drowned. Rates of drowning vary with age, gender, and race. Drowning rates are the highest among children aged 1 to 2 years. In Arizona, California, Florida, and Texas, drowning is the leading cause of death in this age group (Swimming programs for infants and toddlers, 2000].

Near-drowning events, in which the victim survives at least 24 hours, also result in significant numbers of injuries in children. It is estimated that for each drowning death, there are 1 to 4 nonfatal submersions serious enough to result in hospitalization [American Academy of Pediatrics Committee on Injury, Violence, and Poison Prevention, 2003]. Children who still require cardiopulmonary resuscitation at the time they arrive at the emergency department have a poor prognosis; at least half of survivors suffer significant neurologic impairment [Kyriacou et al., 1994].

Epidemiology

Most immersions occur in privately owned swimming pools. Toddler drownings tend to occur because of a lapse in parental or adult supervision. A responsible supervising adult can be identified in 84% of toddler drownings, but only 18% of the incidents are actually witnessed [Quan et al., 1989; Wintemute, 1990].

Individuals with seizure disorders are at four times higher risk for submersion accidents regardless of age [Orlowski, 1979]. This threat extends to the bathtub as well, and some investigators have suggested that children with seizure disorders not bathe without supervision or shower instead.

In all, 60% to 90% of drownings in children younger than 5 years occur in residential swimming pools; nearly two thirds occur in the child's home pool. An additional third occur in the pools of relatives or neighbors. In most cases, the child has been unsupervised for less than 5 minutes. Bathtubs are the second most common site of drowning in young children. Bathtubs are a particular threat to children 6 to 12 months of age, who can sit but may not be able to right themselves if submerged.

Bathtubs are a source of potential submersion injuries in the home as a result of inadequate adult supervision [Lavelle et al., 1995]. In a Seattle study, all of the bathtub drowning victims were left unattended or under the supervision of another sibling who was younger than 5 years. Four of the five victims older than 5 years had known seizure disorders. This same study reported that for 19% of the bathtub drowning victims, there was evidence of child abuse or neglect, lack of parental supervision, and delays in obtaining help [Quan et al., 1989]. More recent studies have demonstrated that many submersion accidents are inflicted (8% in one study) and that bathtubs were the most common site for inflicted submersions [Gillenwater et al., 1996].

Hot tubs and spas have been recognized as drowning sites because of the opportunity for entrapment under the heavy spa cover or in the suction drain apparatus. The high temperature of the spas and the risk for enhanced exposure to bacterial agents, such as *Pseudomonas* species, have been implicated as additional risk factors for poor outcomes.

Jumbelic and Chambliss [1990] reported a new drowning hazard: the large 5-gallon industrial bucket. These buckets are constructed of rigid plastic and are difficult for a toddler to invert even when empty. Young toddlers, who have relatively large heads and a high center of gravity, fall into these buckets without tipping them and drown even in small amounts of liquid. The average number of young children who drowned in bucket-related injuries, 27 per year, is considerably lower than the number of drownings attributed to bathtubs for this age group. Nevertheless, it is higher than estimates of drowning in other in-home water sources (e.g., toilets or basins) [Mann et al., 1992].

Pathophysiology

Drowning may be subdivided into wet and dry drowning. As the victim becomes submerged, breath holding occurs and panic ensues. In approximately 15% of drowning victims, severe larynogospasm prevents the aspiration of the liquid medium (dry drowning) [DeNicola et al., 1997]. In the majority of cases, however, wet drowning occurs, in which the patient aspirates the water in which he or she is submerged.

In the 1970s, a large amount of literature made the distinction between fresh and salt water wet drowning. It was believed that the hypertonicity of seawater would result in an osmotic gradient, drawing plasma volume into the pulmonary interstitial space. Drowning in fresh water, on the other hand, was believed to create the opposite effect [Cohen et al., 1992; Conn and Barker, 1984]. Fresh water drowning would lead to hypervolemia and dilutional hyponatremia, with dilution of other serum electrolytes as well. Later experimental studies suggested that volumes far greater than is normally aspirated in a drowning victim are required to create the necessary proposed blood volume changes [Modell, 1985]. In a series of 91 victims of severe near-drowning, no serious fluid or electrolyte abnormalities were detected. It also became clear that both fresh water and salt water have the effect of washing out surfactant and creating the potential for the development of pulmonary edema. Today, the differences between salt water and fresh water drowning are downplayed. Rather, the temperature of the water and the possible contaminants contained therein appear more important. Home swimming pools that are well kept tend to have a paucity of bacteria, but the effect of chlorine on pulmonary tissues may be deleterious. Fresh water lakes may contain bacteria and various protozoan pathogens. Seawater tends to be contaminated with bacteria, algae, sand, and other particulate matter.

Cerebral hypoxia is the final common pathway in all victims of drowning, both wet and dry, fresh water or salt water [Orlowski and Szpilman, 2001]. Sophisticated critical care management of the respiratory insult in the late 1970s and 1980s made death from isolated respiratory failure after near-drowning less frequent. Some patients develop secondary bacterial pneumonia, but the majority of patients who die of respiratory failure also have severe CNS injury. On the other hand, neurologic insult secondary to hypoxia and ischemia remains the limiting factor in physicians' ability to successfully resuscitate near-drowning victims.

Neurologic care of victims of severe near-drowning remains a controversial subject. The majority of physicians, however, believe there is no advantage of cerebral resuscitation techniques over routine supportive care in near-drowning victims [DeNicola et al., 1997; Spack et al., 1997]. This belief is based on the notion that anoxic injury with cytopathic cerebral edema is determined by the extent of the injury and is not substantially affected by postinjury interventions. Indeed, poor outcome and neurologic death occur commonly in patients in whom intracranial pressure and cerebral perfusion pressures are maintained within the normal range [Spack et al., 1997]. This result is consistent with the general experience in the cerebral resuscitation literature, which also appears to indicate a lack of efficacy of interventions, such as intracranial pressure monitoring, barbiturate coma therapy, or hypothermia, for global cerebral anoxic injury.

Submersion in ice water has long been thought to be associated with better chances of survival, especially in the pediatric population. Pediatric patients tend to have large ratios of surface area to body weight and therefore cool quickly in cold water. The so-called diving reflex, which in mammals tends to shunt blood flow to the brain and heart preferentially after submersion in cold water, and the reduction in metabolic needs because of hypothermia may play a role in protecting the submerged brain from injury in such cases [Gooden, 1972]. There are more than 17 reported cases in the world literature in which prolonged submersion in ice water (water temperature less than 45° to 50° F) was associated with survival and good neurologic recovery, despite the presence of coma and other poor prognostic signs in the emergency department [Orlowski, 1987]. Paradoxically, in victims of warm water near-drowning, the presence of hypothermia is a negative prognostic sign, because hypothermia in these patients is correlated with a longer time of submersion and absence of perfusion [DeNicola et al., 1997; Kyriacou et al., 1994]. As cerebral injury progresses, the victim becomes poikilothermic. Other organ systems besides the CNS and pulmonary system are affected by severe near-drowning episodes; complications include renal failure and disseminated intravascular coagulation [Fields, 1992].

The advisability of continuing cardiopulmonary resuscitation efforts and the duration that these efforts are continued represent ongoing and perplexing dilemmas for the emergency and critical care physician. Although most people would never want to cease resuscitative efforts in a patient who has an opportunity for neurologic recovery, the potential for resuscitating drowning victims to the level of only a persistent vegetative state is very real. Despite efforts to develop prognostic criteria, there is no consensus in the literature with regard to prognostic indexes that preclude meaningful survival [Christensen et al., 1997].

Prognosis

Prognostic variables are best discussed in terms of prehospital (on-site) factors and postresuscitation (in-hospital) factors. The on-site factors affecting outcome are water temperature, duration of submersion, and duration of resuscitation. There is no doubt that near-drowning in icy water (less than 50° F) carries a higher chance of survival than that in warmer water.

The duration of submersion may also influence outcome; however, this factor is sometimes difficult to ascertain. In addition, it is difficult to separate the effect of submersion times from all other confounding variables, such as water temperature and efficacy of initial resuscitation efforts. Although Frates [1981], using multivariate analysis on warm-water drownings, could not find any correlation between duration of submersion and survival, Quan and Kinder [1992] found that duration of submersion longer than 10 minutes resulted in death or severe neurologic impairment in six of six children. These investigators also found that field resuscitation duration longer than 25 minutes ended in poor outcome or death in 17 of 17 patients. In summary, short-term submersion in icy water offers the best chance of intact neurologic survival, whereas longer submersion and field resuscitation times are associated with poor outcomes.

Predictors of outcome in the emergency department have been reported by several investigators [Habib et al., 1996]. One retrospective review revealed that age, sex, duration of submersion, core temperature, pH, absence of spontaneous respirations, lack of response to pain, and pupillary nonreactivity were unreliable predictors of outcome [Nichter and Everett, 1989]. However, use of cardiotonic medications to establish a cardiac rhythm in the initial resuscitation attempt was associated with an eventual outcome of death or severe neurologic damage in all instances. Another retrospective review of 44 admissions to the intensive care unit revealed that nonreactive pupils in the emergency department and a Glasgow Coma Scale score of less than 5 on arrival were the best independent predictors of poor neurologic outcome [Lavelle and Shaw, 1993]. No predictor was absolute, and two nonhypothermic patients who arrived at the emergency department in full cardiac arrest, requiring cardiopulmonary resuscitation and cardiotonic medications, had full neurologic recovery. Most investigators agree that the absence of a heartbeat on admission to the emergency department is a poor prognostic sign and is associated with a mortality rate greater than 90% unless there is significant hypothermia [Biggart and Bohn, 1990; Frewen et al., 1985]. Graf and colleagues [1995] reported that among comatose children, unfavorable outcomes could be predicted by a combination of absence of pupillary light reflex, increased initial blood glucose concentration, and male sex (specificity of 100% and sensitivity of 65%). These data indicate that all near-drowning victims who present to the emergency department should receive full attempts at cardiopulmonary resuscitation. If cardiovascular stability cannot be achieved in the emergency department after rewarming of hypothermic victims, the patient cannot be resuscitated and is considered a drowning victim. If cardiovascular stability can be accomplished in the emergency department, the patient should be transferred to the intensive care unit for further management. In summary, there is no medically practical index or score, applied at the scene or during emergency resuscitation, that predicts with 100% accuracy which patients will or will not survive normally. All near-drowning victims should therefore be treated initially unless rigor mortis is present. Whether treatment should be discontinued, however, is a judgment decision that has to be made by the physician in attendance.

In the pediatric critical care unit, the prognosis for neurologic outcome has proved difficult to evaluate. Accurate predictors of the prognosis are necessary for limiting or withdrawing therapy. Several scoring systems have been devised to predict outcome. Conn and Barker [1984] and Modell and associates [1980] devised a scoring system based on whether the child (1) is awake, (2) has a blunted sensorium, or (3) is comatose. All patients in the first group survived intact, whereas among those in the second and third groups, the mortality rates were 10% and 34%, respectively. Dean and Kaufman [1981], using a retrospectively assigned Glasgow Coma Scale score, found a score of less than 5 to be associated with an 80% rate of mortality or severe brain damage. Orlowski [1979] devised a scoring system for pediatric near-drowning victims, using patient's age, initial pH, submersion time, pupillary response, and the effectiveness of resuscitation. Other investigators have found that induced hypothermia, barbiturate therapy, and intracranial pressure monitoring, as well as control of intracranial pressure and maintenance of cerebral perfusion pressure, were not associated with improved outcomes. The use of brainstem auditory-evoked potentials, cerebral blood flow, and metabolic rate in combination with initial blood glucose values have all demonstrated some promise but are not available for widespread use [Ashwal et al., 1990; Fisher et al., 1992].

Studies involving xenon cerebral blood flow measurements revealed that total frontal gray and white matter and temporal and parietal gray matter flows were significantly decreased in patients who ultimately died, in comparison with those who were normal or survived in a vegetative state [Ashwal et al., 1990]. Cerebral blood flow measurements were not useful in discriminating the quality of life in those who survived.

Proton magnetic resonance spectroscopy and magnetic resonance imaging are useful in predicting outcome in near-drowning victims [Auld et al., 1995; Dubowitz et al., 1998; Holshouser et al., 1997; Kreis et al., 1996]. When performed sequentially in occipital gray matter, proton magnetic resonance spectroscopy provides useful objective information that can significantly enhance the ability to establish prognosis after near-drowning. Patients with poor outcomes appear to have increasing lactate and lower metabolic ratios, specifically the *N*-acetylaspartate (NAA)/creatine and NAA/choline ratios.

It seems that the clinical examination, particularly after a stabilization period of 12 to 24 hours, provides the best estimate of long-term outcome. In children who manifest no neurologic improvement within the first 3 to 6 hours after admission to the intensive care unit (i.e., remain comatose, flaccid, without pupillary response), survival is extremely unlikely. Continuation of aggressive care beyond this point should be considered on a case-by-case basis. Evaluation at 12 to 24 hours has revealed that failure of return of spontaneous respiration after resuscitation is associated with a 100% rate of mortality [Jacobsen et al., 1983]. In addition, abnormal posturing or seizures persisting beyond 12 hours may also indicate a poor prognosis.

In a retrospective investigation of 44 children, Bratton and colleagues [1994] found that the neurologic examination 24 hours after warm water near-drowning distinguished satisfactory outcome from unsatisfactory outcome (death or dependence on total custodial care). All survivors who were normal or had only mild deficits were awake and initiated spontaneous, purposeful movements within 24 hours after submersion. All children who survived with severe deficits or who died remained comatose 24 hours after submersion.

Christensen and associates [1997], in a retrospective review of 274 near-drowning patients, demonstrated that an observation period of 48 hours was necessary to avoid loss of intact survivors. They suggested the following strategies to maximize the number of intact survivors while minimizing the personal, hospital, and social costs of poor outcome:

- Prehospital resuscitation, including early intubation, ventilation, vascular access, and administration of advanced life support medications.
- Continued resuscitation and stabilization in the emergency department.
- Consideration of withdrawal of support if no neurologic improvement is detected after 48 hours.

Ancillary testing such as evoked responses, electroencephalography, and magnetic resonance spectroscopy may prove helpful to corroborate the neurologic examination.

Prevention

Quan and colleagues [1989], in a 10-year study of drowning and near-drowning in Kings County, Washington, found that 89% of all victims had no supervision, regardless of whether in a bathtub, pool, or ocean. Adults should be assigned specifically as observers without additional duties or distractions. Home pools should have accessible portable telephones so adults do not have to leave the poolside. If duties call the supervising adult into the house, children should leave the pool and preferably be barred from the area until the adult returns. Most toddlers who drown gain access to the pool from inside the house through doors to the pool area rather than being engaged in water activities. Fences are the only intervention that has proved effective, reducing pool immersion incidents by 50% to 70% [Present, 1987]. Risk of drowning or near-drowning involving unintended access to an unfenced pool is 3.76 times higher than the risk associated with a fenced pool [Pitt and Balanda, 1991]. There should be four-sided fencing immediately surrounding pools, not at the property line. This kind of fencing allows children access to their yards but isolates the pool.

Cardiopulmonary resuscitation may produce acceptable outcomes if immersion times are less than 5 minutes and resuscitation time is less than 10 minutes; however, 42% of children who drowned in their own home pools were retrieved by a layperson, usually a family member, and cardiopulmonary resuscitation was not instituted until emergency personnel arrived [Wintemute et al., 1987]. Immediate resuscitation before the arrival of paramedical personnel is associated with a better neurologic outcome [Kyriacou et al., 1994]. Swimming lessons and water safety courses may be useful when instituted at 4 to 5 years of age. Adults should not, however, rely on a young child's swimming ability to prevent drowning. Roughhousing, risk taking, diving, and other challenging activities increase the risk even for older children. It is highly recommended that swimming competence and basic life support certification be taught in elementary school and reinforced in middle school and high school. The American Academy of Pediatrics Committee on Injury, Violence, and Poison Prevention [2003] has produced a list of 23 recommendations to reduce the incidence of drowning in infants, children, and adolescents. Undoubtedly, the most effective and best proven intervention to prevent swimming pool drowning is four-sided fencing with self-closing, self-latching gates. Every coalition and municipality should work with pool contractors, public health officials, and local media to encourage isolation fencing on all new pools, particularly for families with young children. Institution of pool safety upgrades should be encouraged when older homes with pools are sold. Industries should continue to explore aesthetically acceptable fencing and effective self-closures for gates, doors, and sliding doors that lead into pool areas.

Child health practitioners should incorporate drowning prevention in their anticipatory guidance during well-child visits. This should include admonitions about unsupervised infant bathing, access to water-filled buckets, and open toilets, as well as the need for surveillance, isolation fencing, and door closures and locks. It is hoped that a concerted effort by parents, health workers, industry, and government can reduce the overwhelming losses caused by childhood drownings.

Strangulation Injury

Strangulation injuries result from external compression of the neck. Several forms have been described according to the method of application of compression, including hanging, postural strangulation, manual strangulation, and ligature strangulation [Scott and Wiebe, 1997]. Hanging is "complete" when the suspension point is above the height of the victim and the body is totally suspended in air and is "incomplete" when the suspension point is below the height of the victim and a part of the body is supported by the floor or other object. Complete hangings are most commonly seen in judicial executions and, although rarely performed today, were a common method of execution in the United States before 1965. Incomplete hangings are more common. The cause of hanging varies with age. For children younger than 5 years, hanging is almost exclusively accidental [Sabo et al., 1996]. These occur secondary to getting heads caught in crib slats, curtain cords, electric windows, Venetian blinds, or hammock cords and when clothing or a pacifier ribbon becomes caught on an object. However, homicides in infants have been reported. From ages 5 to 12, hangings are both accidental and suicidal. After the age of 12, most hangings are suicidal or accidental during autoerotic actions [Krol and Wolfe, 1994; Sabo et al., 1996]. Suicide is the third leading cause of death in adolescents in North America, and hanging is the second most common method of suicide in this age group.

Postural strangulation results when the neck of the victim is over an object and the weight of the body causes external compression of the neck. Manual and ligature strangulation is caused by an external mechanism, with the weight of the victim not contributing to the mechanism of injury. The most common ligature injuries are associated with ropes and extension cords. Nonintentional strangulation is seen in both adults and children. Infants are strangled when the neck is wedged between the slats of a crib or the infant becomes lodged between the mattress and crib. Toddlers and preschool-aged children are sometimes caught beneath garage doors.

The mechanism of injury in strangulation and hangings is influenced by the amount of physical force used, how the force was applied, and the duration of the force. Death is a consequence of direct injury to the CNS, immediate cardiac arrest, or compression and injury to the structures of the neck. Direct injury to the CNS results from the drop force when the victim is completely suspended, as in complete hangings. The cervical spinal cord or brainstem is disrupted, and death is instantaneous. In complete or judicial hangings, the ligature knot is located centrally over the occiput with the ligature curved symmetrically around the anterior portion of the neck. This placement may result in partial or complete avulsion of the carotid arteries, laryngeal fractures, and fractures of the vertebral bodies and base of the skull. Death from immediate cardiac arrest is thought to be secondary to a massive vagal reflex from bilateral carotid body or vagal sheath stimulation [Scott and Wiebe, 1997].

Compression of neck structures and its sequelae are the most common mechanisms of injury in strangulation and incomplete hangings. The venous drainage of the head and neck is through the jugular system and a series of intercommunicating veins related to the spinal column. Because of their superficial location, minimal external pressure results in occlusion of internal and external jugular veins, with obstruction of venous outflow from the head and neck. Venous obstruction results in ischemia, hypoxia, and loss of consciousness. The victim becomes flaccid, and with loss of muscle tone, compression of the carotid arteries occurs, resulting in increasing ischemia and hypoxia. Depending on the severity and duration of the insult, neuronal damage occurs with cerebral edema and elevated intracranial pressure [Sabo et al., 1996]. In contrast to other injuries, such as near-drowning, increased intracranial pressure occurs more frequently in childhood strangulation [Ashwal et al., 1991]. As the glottis and tongue are lifted into the pharynx, loss of muscle tone results in airway occlusion. The carotid arteries above the level of the cricoid cartilage are separated from the surface of the skin by the platysma and sternocleidomastoid muscles and deep cervical fascia. These vessels are not easily occluded by external pressure, but traction injuries can occur, ranging from small intimal tears to total disruption.

The laryngeal skeleton includes the hyoid bone and thyroid and cricoid cartilages. These structures in children are semirigid, and calcification is not complete until the third decade. Laryngeal fractures are rare in childhood, but the prevalence of fractures increases with age, coincidentally with calcification of the laryngeal skeleton. The most common laryngeal injuries in childhood are mild and include endolaryngeal edema, hematomas, and mucosal tears. More severe injuries result in extensive edema, hematomas and lacerations, cartilage fractures, and vocal cord paralysis. These injuries may cause airway discontinuity and obstruction. Cervical fractures are also rare in children [Krol and Wolfe, 1994]. A 3.5- to 4.0-mm pseudosubluxation of C2 on C3 has been demonstrated in as many as 15% of healthy children, and it is believed that laxity of the ligaments and musculature is protective. Feldman and Simms [1980] reviewed 233 childhood strangulations and did not find cervical or laryngeal fractures or evidence of airway compromise.

Cerebrovascular hemodynamic profiles have been obtained in children with hypoxic-ischemic injuries after strangulation [Ashwal et al., 1991; Hanigan et al., 1996]. In general, the profiles reveal cerebral hyperemia, loss of autoregulation, and intact but blunted vascular response to $Paco_2$. Not unexpectedly, the accumulated data demonstrate that absolute values of CO_2 reactivity vary considerably, and single-point determinations encompassing wide epochs may not reflect the continuous changes in hemodynamics of the cerebrovascular bed to hypoxic-ischemic injury and subsequent treatment. Many patients manifest negative CO_2 reactivities in various deep and cortical regions, which may represent redistribution of flow from responsive to nonresponsive vascular beds.

The findings of cerebral hyperemia, loss of autoregulation, and the presence of vascular steal phenomenon during hypocarbia suggest that therapies such as flow promotion or hyperventilation are not indicated and are potentially dangerous in strangulation injuries.

Nonaccidental Trauma

Patients with severe traumatic head injury experience immediate alterations in cerebral and systemic physiology that substantially influence neurologic outcome [Atkinson, 2000]. Two immediate pathophysiologic events occur with the onset of severe head injury that substantially affect subsequent outcome: head injury–induced apnea and a stress-related massive sympathetic discharge. The combined effects of hypoxia, hypercarbia, and acidosis and a surge in blood pressure, as well as the direct effects of catecholamines on tissue, lead to a synergistic injury effect in the patient.

The extent of apnea and catecholamine surge after severe head injury is directly related to the amount of energy transmitted to the brainstem [Atkinson, 2000]. As a result, many patients with severe head injury live or die at the scene, depending on whether they resume breathing. In patients who resume spontaneous respiration, apnea-induced hypoxic brain and cardiac injury augmented by elevated stress hormones may result in serious morbidity.

Johnson and co-workers [1995] examined intentional closed-head injury (i.e., child abuse) in 28 children and found that 57% had a verifiable history of apnea before hospitalization. They concluded that trauma-induced apnea causes cerebral hypoxia and ischemia, and these were more important in modulating outcome than was the mechanism of primary brain injury (i.e., subdural hematoma, subarachnoid hemorrhage, diffuse axonal injury, or contusions).

Geddes and colleagues [2001] identified a high incidence of widespread microscopic neuronal hypoxic brain damage in a cohort of children with nonaccidental head injury. In a proportion of infants, they found significant microscopic changes of focal axonal damage to the craniocervical junction on the cervical cord. For infants who presented with a history of apnea and hypoxic brain damage, they proposed a mechanism of cervical hyperextension and flexion during shaking, which led to damage of the brainstem respiratory centers with a consequent bad outcome from severe hypoxic brain damage.

More recent evidence further confirms that in nonaccidental head injury, hypoxic-ischemic injury is of greater importance with regard both to signs and symptoms at presentation and to long-term outcome [Kemp et al., 2003].

Lightning and Electrical Injuries

Lightning is a fascinating, albeit uncommon, form of electrical injury. Only 150 to 300 people die each year in the United States of injury secondary to lightning strike; the death rate is highest in adolescents [Fontanarosa, 1993; Volinsky et al., 1994]. Nearly two thirds of people struck by lightning survive, although many have significant sequelae.

The lightning strike is a direct-current electrical discharge with a high magnitude of energy and short duration of exposure. When the electrical discharge in a cloud is greater than the air resistance (30,000 to 50,000 V), energy is discharged to the ground. Lightning energy is estimated to be about 25,000 to 200,000 A, or 100 million to 2 billion V. The duration of the electrical discharge is from 0.00001 to 0.001 second. The estimated heat generated from the electrical discharge is between 8000° and 30,000° C at the contact area [Patten, 1992]. Survival from lightning strikes is possibly related to the short duration of electrical contact. With the presence of metal objects on the body, however, the electrical contact time is increased, resulting in a deeper burn and increased rates of morbidity and mortality. Thermal forces generated by lightning are capable of producing tremendous pressure waves from the rapid expansion and cooling of the air around the lightning strike. These pressure waves are significant enough to cause serious blunt-force trauma.

Lightning strikes produces a variety of injury patterns. A lightning strike that directly contacts the victim results in the most serious injuries. A side flash or splash injury occurs when lightning strikes a primary object and the electrical charge leaps from the object to the victim. This type of strike may seem less dangerous but can also be fatal. Lightning striking one person may be splashed to another person and has resulted in death in the second person.

Lightning strike may cause injury as a result of one of three types of energy transfer: electrical, thermal, or mechanical. The electrical injury depends on the voltage, amperage, degree of resistance, and anatomic pathway. Electrical energy follows the path of least resistance. The decreasing order of resistance for human tissues is bone, fat, tendon, skin, muscle, blood vessels, and nerves [Fontanarosa, 1993; Patten, 1992]. When the skin is dry, the electrical path is deflected over the body because of the higher resistance of the skin. The thermal energy produced may cause a break in the skin, forming a pathway for the electrical charge to pass through to less resistant tissues such as muscle, nerves, and blood vessels.

The primary effect of lightning results from a massive direct-current insult to the entire myocardium and CNS. This insult results in asystole and loss of function of the medullary respiratory centers. Lightning effects on the respiratory center last longer than the cardiac effects. Cardiac rhythm returns if apnea is corrected; if apnea is not corrected, secondary hypoxic cardiac arrest ensues. The mortality from lightning is related to the effects of apnea, not asystole. Resuscitation attempts in lightning victims have resulted in higher success rates than in victims of other cardiac dysrhythmias. The direct current of lightning causes a single countershock to the entire myocardium, as opposed to alternating current, which distributes a repetitive fibrillating stimulus to the heart. The resumption of spontaneous electrical activity may be secondary to the automaticity of the myocardium. Patients with initial rhythms associated with a poor prognosis may completely recover with prompt institution of respiratory and cardiac support. Aggressive and persistent resuscitation efforts should be continued until cerebral function can be assessed.

Anoxic cardiac and cerebral injury may be reduced in lightning injuries by causing a delay in anoxic cellular destruction. Several authors have suggested that the reason for possible recovery after prolonged cardiac arrest is that lightning causes cellular metabolism to cease instantly, thereby delaying the onset of anoxic tissue destruction and reducing the potential for anoxic cardiac and cerebral injury [Fontanarosa, 1993]. However, the metabolic basis for this concept has not been verified, and available clinical evidence does not support the concept that lightning strike confers any cellular protective mechanism.

The CNS is highly sensitive to electrical injury. Injury to the CNS may result from direct electrical injury or anoxia or may be secondary to vascular injury [Patten, 1992]. The pathophysiologic mechanism of CNS injury includes coagulation in the cortex, formation of epidural or subdural hematomas, paralysis of the respiratory center, and intraventricular hemorrhage. Symptoms of CNS injury include loss of consciousness, confusion, transient disorientation, seizures, restlessness, retrograde amnesia, and varying degrees of transient paralysis. Coma and symptoms of cerebral edema are not unusual. Transient paralysis may involve the lower extremities in two thirds of victims and the upper extremities in one third. Late sequelae include amnesia, paraplegia, neuropathy, decreased reflexes, and chronic subdural hematomas. The presence of sequelae may be related to hypoxic or blunt-force CNS injury.

Lightning strikes may also cause transient autonomic dysfunction, which may result in fixed and dilated pupils, mydriasis, anisocoria, loss of the red reflex, and Horner's syndrome. Pupillary responses cannot be used reliably as an indicator of brainstem function.

Electrical Shock

Victims of electrical shock sustain a wide spectrum of injuries ranging from a transient unpleasant sensation from brief exposure to low-intensity current to instantaneous sudden death from accidental electrocution.

Electrical shock is associated with a fatality rate of 0.5 per 100,000 per year in the United States and accounts for approximately 1000 deaths annually. Electrical injuries cause an additional 5000 patients to require emergency treatment and constitute 4% to 7% of burn center admissions.

More than 20% of all electrical injuries occur in children [Fontanarosa, 1993; Thompson and Ashwal, 1983]. Risk-taking behavior among adolescent boys, such as climbing utility poles, playing near electrical railway lines, and trespassing through transformer substations, can expose them to high-tension electrical sources. The inquisitive nature of toddlers and their habit of exploring their environment with their mouths contribute directly to the most common electrical injury in childhood, the perioral burn, which affects 4000 children per year.

Electrical injuries result from the direct effects of current and from the conversion of electrical energy into thermal energy as current passes through body tissues. Factors that determine the severity of electrical shock include the magnitude of energy delivered, resistance to current flow, type of current, duration of contact, and current pathway.

Systemic effects and tissue damage resulting from electrical shock are proportional to the magnitude and intensity of current delivered to the victim. Current flow is directly related to voltage and inversely related to resistance in the current path. Body tissues differ in their resistance to the passage of electricity. Tissues with high fluid and electrolyte content conduct current better than others. Bone is most resistant to the passage of electrical energy, followed in decreasing order of resistance by fat, tendon, skin, muscle, blood vessels, and nerves. Skin resistance is the most important factor impeding current flow. High skin resistance and a small area of contact usually concentrate electrical energy in a relatively small area and produce a severe local skin wound, limiting internal current flow. Once the skin becomes charred, the external barrier to flow is removed, allowing the current easy internal access. Skin resistance also can be reduced substantially by moisture, sweat, or skin contaminants, which decrease the impediment to current flow and convert what ordinarily may be a minor low-voltage injury into a life-threatening shock.

Alternating current at 60 cycles per second, the frequency used in most household and commercial sources of electricity, is substantially more dangerous than direct current of the same magnitude. Contact with alternating current may cause tetanic skeletal muscle contractions, preventing the victim from releasing hold of the electrical source and leading to increased current delivery. In contrast, direct current usually causes a single strong flexion of skeletal muscle and often thrusts the victim away from the current source.

Low-voltage alternating current (60 Hz) has a narrow margin of safety [Fontanarosa, 1993]. Low-intensity current at 1 to 4 mA is perceived as an unpleasant tingling sensation. Contact with alternating current at 10 to 20 mA causes repetitive stimulation of muscle fibers, produces tetanic skeletal muscle contractions, which may prevent the victim's hand from releasing its grasp from the current source, and lengthens the duration of contact with the energized source. Thoracic muscle tetany involving the diaphragm and intercostal muscles occurs at 30 to 50 mA and can result in respiratory arrest. Prolonged contact leads to sustained apnea with hypoxemia and secondary cardiac arrest. Ventricular fibrillation may occur with exposure to as little as 50 to 100 mA. The repetitive frequency of alternating current increases the likelihood of current delivery to the myocardium during the vulnerable recovery period of the cardiac cycle and can precipitate ventricular fibrillation.

Cardiopulmonary arrest is the primary cause of immediate death from electrical injury. The initial dysrhythmia producing sudden death is a function of the magnitude of current. Alternating current (100 mA to 1 A) generally causes ventricular fibrillation, whereas higher intensity current (>10 A) may cause asystole. Respiratory arrest may occur immediately after electrical shock and results from one or a combination of the following mechanisms: (1) electrical current passing through the brain may cause inhibition of medullary respiratory center function, (2) tetanic contraction of the diaphragm and chest wall musculature may occur during current exposure, (3) prolonged paralysis of respiratory muscles may continue after contact with the electrical current has terminated, or (4) respiratory arrest may accompany cardiac arrest in patients with ventricular fibrillation or asystole.

Respiratory arrest may last minutes to hours after the electrical shock terminates and may persist after restoration of spontaneous circulation. In some patients, cardiac activity may be maintained in the absence of spontaneous ventilation. If respiratory arrest is not corrected promptly by artificial ventilation and oxygenation, secondary hypoxic cardiac arrest may occur.

Neurologic complications are reported frequently and include coma, seizures, agitation, myelopathy, and peripheral nerve damage. Vascular complications include arterial spasm, thrombosis and rupture, and venous thrombosis. Depending on the extent of injury, electrically injured extremities may appear edematous or, in cases of underlying coagulation necrosis, can be mummified. Arterial damage may cause peripheral pulses to be absent or difficult to palpate, and thrombosis of peripheral veins precludes their use for intravenous access.

Sudden Cardia Arrest in Children and Adolescents

Sudden cardiac arrest is the sudden cessation of cardiac activity so that the victim becomes unresponsive with no normal breathing and no signs of circulation. Unless the victim receives immediate cardiopulmonary resuscitation and other treatment to restore normal cardiac activity, he or she will die. Although the precise incidence of sudden cardiac arrest in children is unknown, it is not a leading cause of death [Hazinski et al., 2004].

When sudden cardiac arrest does occur in children and adolescents, it may be precipitated by ventricular fibrillation or rapid ventricular tachycardia (pulseless ventricular tachycardia). These abnormal heart rhythms in children are typically caused by inherited or congenital cardiac conditions or by acute medical problems that cause inflammation of the heart. Examples of such conditions include long QT syndrome, hypertrophic cardiomyopathy, abnormal development of the coronary arteries, aortic dissection, myocarditis, coronary artery aneurysm associated with Kawasaki's disease, and congenital aortic stenosis [Liberthson, 1996]. Many of these conditions are not detected during routine screening for school physical examinations or sports activities; thus, sudden cardiac arrest may be the first sign of these conditions [Maron, 2003].

Sudden cardiac arrest may also result from *commotio cordis,* a condition resulting from a blow to the chest that causes ventricular tachycardia or fibrillation. Each year approximately 10 cases of *commotio cordis* are reported in the United States for victims of all ages [Maron et al., 2002].

If a child develops sudden cardiac arrest caused by ventricular fibrillation or pulseless ventricular tachycardia, immediate cardiopulmonary resuscitation by a bystander and early defibrillation are needed. Automatic external defibrillators are computerized defibrillators designed for use by lay rescuers to treat sudden cardiac arrest. The automatic external defibrillator provides voice and visual prompts to guide the rescuer. When attached to an unresponsive victim in cardiac arrest, the automatic external defibrillator analyzes the victim's heart rhythm and determines whether a shock is needed, charges to an appropriate shock dose, and prompts the rescuer to deliver a shock. The automatic external defibrillator delivers a shock only if ventricular fibrillation or ventricular tachycardia is present [Hazinski et al., 2004].

The U.S. Food and Drug Administration has cleared automatic external defibrillators for use in children younger than

8 years. Two of these devices have accurately identified ventricular fibrillation and rapid ventricular tachycardia in young children [Atkinson et al., 2003]. The American Heart Association states that automatic external defibrillators may be used with cardiopulmonary resuscitation for treatment of prehospital cardiac arrest in children 1 to 8 years of age [Hazinski et al., 2004]. The American Heart Association continues to recommend the use of cardiopulmonary resuscitation with automatic external defibrillators for treatment of cardiac arrest in children 8 years of age and older and in adults.

NEUROLOGIC EXAMINATION AFTER CARDIAC ARREST

Features of the neurologic examination of infants and children who have experienced prolonged cardiac arrest and global hypoxic-ischemic encephalopathy are reviewed in Chapter 61 on impairment of consciousness and coma. Several points need re-emphasis including the following:

- Careful monitoring of brainstem reflexes, particularly pupillary and oculocephalic
- Determination of whether the patient is apneic and assessment of the patterns of respiration present
- Evidence of increasing intracranial pressure
- Evidence of the development of worsening alterations of tone, either (1) severe hypotonia or flaccidity, suggestive of deteriorating cortical and brainstem function, or (2) severe increases in tone including posturing, suggestive of worsening white matter function as a result of edema, osmotic demyelination, or secondary degeneration

NEUROLOGIC COMPLICATIONS AFTER CARDIAC ARREST

Delayed Posthypoxic Injury

Delayed posthypoxic injury may occur 24 to 48 hours after the initial recovery of consciousness after coma. In children, this injury occurs most frequently after near-drowning accidents or cardiac surgery in which profound hypothermia and either low-flow bypass or circulatory arrest was used. Magnetic resonance imaging studies may reveal evidence suggestive of edema or demyelination, which may be postanoxic or osmotic in etiology. In addition, diffusion-weighted imaging may reveal restricted diffusion, typically in the basal ganglia, cerebellum, and cortex. These changes are seen initially in gray matter and later in white matter [Arbelaez et al., 1999; Bydder and Rutherford, 2001].

Experience has revealed that early extubation of patients with post-ischemic injury is potentially dangerous. Even though the condition of these children may appear to have improved, development of a posthypoxic encephalopathy may result in inadequate airway control and ventilatory drive, which could add secondary injury.

Post-ischemic Seizures

Excessive excitatory transmitter release during brain ischemia can lead to paroxysmal discharges in the cerebrum, especially in the hippocampus, beginning within minutes and lasting several hours despite cerebral reperfusion. Repetitive discharges may progress to clinically overt seizures, and suppression is then necessary to prevent further injury. Seizures, including episodes of convulsive and nonconvulsive status epilepticus, frequently follow cerebral anoxia. Status epilepticus after anoxic injury is associated with poor outcome and persistent unconsciousness [Jumas and Brenner, 1990; Krumholz et al., 1988]. In addition, electrographically documented status epilepticus without somatic motor manifestations has also been suggestive of poor outcome [Simon and Aminoff, 1986].

Status epilepticus can itself result in permanent anoxic brain damage and necessitates immediate attention. Clinical seizures should be treated aggressively with benzodiazepines and phenytoin. If these agents are unsuccessful, barbiturates may be added. The disadvantage of barbiturates in this setting is that they will further depress the sensorium and make prognostication difficult.

Post-ischemic seizures account for 5% to 10% of cases of childhood status epilepticus [Pellock, 1994]. Children who have these seizures should be treated aggressively; electroencephalography is indicated to guarantee that seizure activity is ablated. Nonconvulsive status epilepticus may exist after apparent successful treatment of convulsive status epilepticus [Perkin et al., 1996]. A potential risk of intensive care unit therapy is failure to recognize status epilepticus in the critically ill, paralyzed patient with injury [Michelson and Ashwal, 2004; Weise and Bleck, 1997]. This clinical setting may pose significant risk for increased morbidity in the already compromised patient; continuous encephalographic monitoring may be warranted if paralysis is truly required for cardiorespiratory management.

Delayed Postanoxic Myoclonic Seizures

Delayed postanoxic myoclonic seizures may occur after severe anoxic brain injury. Myoclonus usually appears within the first 24 to 48 hours after cardiac arrest and is generalized, involving all voluntary muscles. The electroencephalogram (EEG) is usually abnormal, with generalized synchronous spike discharges or burst-suppression activity. Control of the myoclonic seizure activity is difficult with phenytoin or phenobarbital, and treatment with intravenous benzodiazepines is frequently necessary. The presence of postanoxic myoclonus is usually indicative of a high risk for long-term neurologic sequelae [Krumholz et al., 1988].

In one study of comatose adult patients after cardiac resuscitation, myoclonic seizures developed in 37%, and all of those patients died [Wijdicks et al., 1994]. The authors concluded that myoclonic status epilepticus in comatose survivors after cardiac resuscitation indicates devastating anoxic brain injury. Myoclonic status epilepticus should be considered an agonal phenomenon, and its presence should strongly influence the decision to withdraw life support.

LABORATORY TESTS USED TO PREDICT OUTCOME

The clinical course and prognosis of coma after resuscitation from pediatric cardiac arrest must be clearly defined, and full documentation of the resulting morbidity must be made. Early, accurate predictors of outcome are important for guiding the difficult ethical, medical, and economic decisions involved in treating these children. Furthermore, such information is useful for counseling families, collaborating with organ transplant teams, evaluating experimental resuscitative therapies, and planning further therapies. Physicians are obligated to keep abreast of clinical, laboratory, and neurophysiologic markers that could help to determine how much neurologic damage a child might have sustained in a hypoxic-ischemic event.

Currently, the most powerful individual predictor of neurologic outcome after cardiorespiratory arrest is the neurologic examination. Sequential observations of a patient's breathing pattern, eye movements, body posture, and reflexes provide essential information to help establish expectation of outcome [Trubel et al., 2003]. Levy and co-workers [1985] applied multivariate analysis to variables from the neurologic examination in a series of 210 comatose adults studied after hypoxic-ischemic insults. Of the 15 patients who were vegetative at 1 month, none regained independent function. The oculocephalic response and the 3-day motor response enabled the investigators to identify all patients who gained independent function. This identification was true even for the 2 of 57 patients who remained in eyes-closed coma for 3 days and then ultimately regained independent function. Edgren and associates [1987] applied the Glasgow Coma Scale score to assess outcome in 262 adult comatose survivors of cardiac arrest. Glasgow Coma Scale scores of less than 6 at 3 days after cardiac arrest were predictive of poor outcome at 6 months, with no false-negative results. In a similar study of 216 adults after out-of-hospital cardiac arrest, Mullie and co-workers [1988] found that a best Glasgow Coma Scale score of less than 4 as early as 2 days after cardiac arrest was predictive of death or vegetative outcome in all but one patient. The one exception progressed from vegetative state to severe disability. A study involving 109 comatose children with hypoxic-ischemic encephalopathy documented that the absence of a motor response on the third day after admission was associated with an unfavorable outcome [Beca et al., 1995]. Nevertheless, in 23% of the children, clinical evaluation was difficult because of neuromuscular paralysis or heavy sedation. This reinforces the relevance of other early prognostic factors, such as electrophysiologic data.

Although a few patients are thought to "defy the textbooks," they likely represent cases of asphyxia without cardiac arrest, coma of an origin other than asphyxia-induced cardiac arrest, unrecognized hypothermia, or an associated overdose of a cerebrally protective drug. Although the Glasgow Coma Scale score was not predictive of outcome when applied after asphyxia-induced cardiac arrest in pediatric patients, its predictive power was tested with only a single score on initial presentation [Dean and Kaufman, 1981]. Careful studies to determine which components of the neurologic examination in children after hypoxic injury correlate best with outcome have not been done [Jacinto et al., 2001; Kriel et al., 1994; Trubel et al., 2003].

Electroencephalography

The EEG also can provide prognostic information after cardiopulmonary arrest. Chen and associates [1996] retrospectively examined the relation between first post–cardiac arrest EEG and clinical outcome in 408 adult cases. A five-grade classification was used to categorize EEGs. Although permanent severe neurologic damage was observed in some patients with grade I EEG, none of the 208 patients with grade IV or V (i.e., severely abnormal) EEGs had a good neurologic recovery. Adjunctive prognostic information also can be derived from cerebrospinal fluid enzyme elevations of the brain isoenzyme of creatine phosphokinase or neuron-specific enolase. The neurologic examination, EEG, and cerebrospinal fluid neuron-specific enzyme levels used together could provide powerful prognostic information as early as 48 to 72 hours after resuscitation.

Before a study by Mandel and co-workers [2002], there were no prospective studies on the pediatric population in which the relationship between early electroencephalographic criteria and long-term outcome was analyzed. In their study, the first EEG was obtained within the first 24 hours after admission. Among their population of children who were still comatose at 24 hours, the presence of a discontinuous tracing and the absence of reactivity were indicative of an unfavorable outcome, as was also observed by Chen and associates [1996]. The presence of spikes or epileptiform discharges was always associated with an unfavorable outcome. Electroencephalographic findings must be interpreted cautiously because they may be altered by sedative medication.

Somatosensory- and Auditory-Evoked Potentials

Evoked potential monitoring has been used in an attempt to provide early prognostic information about outcome after cardiopulmonary resuscitation. Evoked potentials are inexpensive and can be obtained within the intensive care unit; their advantages over electroencephalography are that the responses are not affected by sedative administration and they are insensitive to electrical noise in the environment. Madl and colleagues [1996] tested somatosensory-evoked potentials in 441 adults after successful resuscitation from cardiac arrest. They reported that 20% of the patients had no N_{20} response and observed that the presence or absence and the latency of the cortical N_{20} peak reliably differentiated between bad and favorable outcome with 100% predictive ability. They also found that a preserved N_{20} peak was not useful for discriminating whether an individual patient would survive. Testing was performed within 48 hours of resuscitation, which is a clinically relevant time frame. Beca and associates [1995] used somatosensory-evoked potentials in children within 48 hours after different neurologic injuries (e.g., trauma, ischemia, meningitis). They demonstrated predictive power of 100% for good outcome in patients with normal somatosensory-evoked potentials and 100% prediction for poor outcome with absence of somatosensory-evoked potentials in 99 children tested, when they excluded certain cases in which there was a physical barrier that impeded cutaneous reception of the electrical impulse (e.g., subdural effusions).

A systematic review of studies of somatosensory-evoked potential results in comatose patients enables estimation of outcomes with a higher degree of certainty than is available from individual studies [Robinson et al., 2003]. Adults in coma from hypoxic-ischemic injury with absence of somatosensory evoked potential responses have less than a 1% chance of awakening. However, in children, exceptions to this rule occur; of the 7% who awaken despite absence of evoked responses, the majority have an outcome better than a severe disability [Robinson et al., 2003].

Brainstem auditory-evoked potential testing has been used in children who experienced cardiac arrest after submersion accidents [Fisher et al., 1992]. Normal evoked responses were observed in all children who recovered neurologically intact. Children who recovered with significant handicaps demonstrated reduction in wave V amplitude over time and prolonged wave I-V interpeak latencies. Other reports, however, have not found brainstem auditory-evoked potentials to be that reliable for outcome prediction after anoxic coma, although they were useful in comatose patients with traumatic brain injury [Guerit et al., 1993].

The predictive powers of the clinical examination, EEG, and somatosensory-evoked potentials in determining the prognosis of patients in anoxic coma have been evaluated and compared in adult patients to identify combinations that may improve the accuracy of prediction. In one study, clinical examination correctly predicted outcome in 58% of patients, somatosensory-evoked potentials in 59%, and EEG in 41% [Basetti et al., 1996]. The combination of clinical

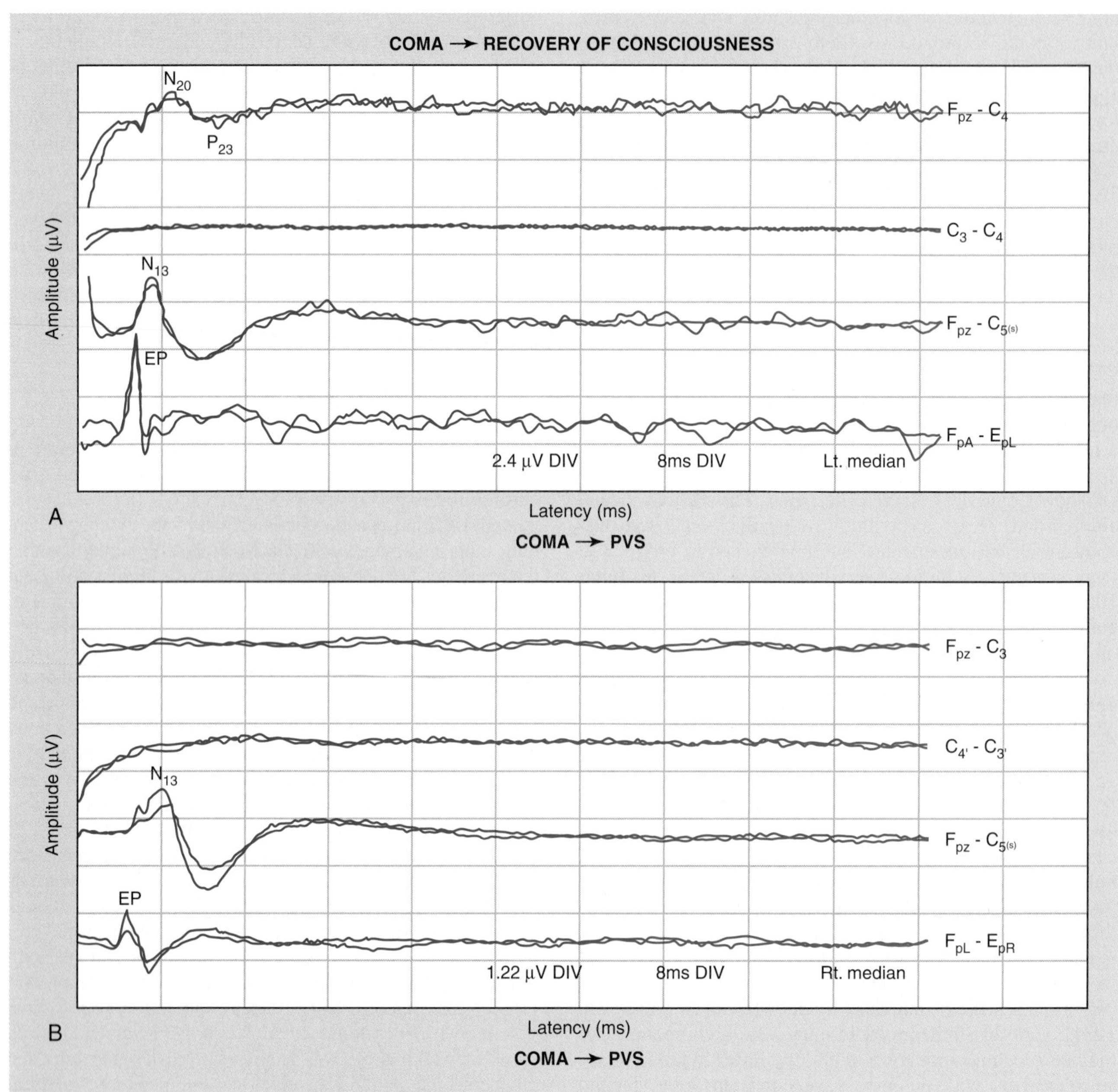

FIGURE 64-6. Usefulness of somatosensory evoked response (SER) studies for outcome prediction after acute brain injury. Median nerve SERs in two children. **A,** SER in a 2½-year-old child who was in a coma secondary to a near-drowning accident. His SER demonstrated an intact thalamocortical response (N_{20}-P_{23}), which is usually predictive of recovery from coma to a conscious state. He slowly recovered consciousness over several weeks. **B,** SER in a 6-month-old boy with medium-chain acetyl coenzyme A dehydrogenase deficiency who presented in coma and status epilepticus. The SER could be elicited at the level of the cervical spinal cord and brachial plexus. The thalamocortical response was absent; his condition evolved over 2 weeks to a persistent vegetative state (PVS), and as of 1 year later, he remained in this condition.

examination, somatosensory-evoked potentials, and EEG raised the percentage of correct predictions to 82%. Another report of 34 adult patients with anoxic coma revealed that patients with extensor posturing to painful stimulation and a "malignant" EEG or those with flexed posturing and bilateral absence of somatosensory-evoked potentials on day 3 or later had poor outcomes [Chen et al., 1996]. These findings are important and suggest that evoked response measurement can provide important adjunctive information to aid in decision making after asphyxia-induced cardiac arrest (Fig. 64-6). However, decisions regarding continuation or forgoing of life-sustaining therapies should be based on all of the available clinically relevant information.

The objective of establishing the most accurate information possible is essential in the discussion with the family. It is currently recommended that maximal support be given to the child for the first 24 hours. After this time, the association of the clinical factors (Glasgow Coma Scale score <5, absence of spontaneous respirations and pupillary reflexes) and the presence of electrophysiologic factors (discontinuous activity in the EEG, absence of electroencephalographic reactivity, and abolition of the N_{20} wave) are highly predictive of death or severe long-term disability [Mandel et al., 2002].

Biochemical Markers

Biochemical variables in the cerebrospinal fluid, such as lactate, creatine phosphokinase BB-isoenzyme, lactate dehydrogenase, and neuron-specific enolase, have been investigated as early prognostic markers of neurologic outcome after cardiac arrest [Fogel et al., 1997; Garcia et al., 1994; Karkela et al., 1992]. Examination of the cerebrospinal fluid in the early phase after cardiac arrest may be hazardous, particularly if there is the possibility of an intracranial mass lesion. Moreover, serial examinations of cerebrospinal fluid might be difficult to justify. Therefore, valid biochemical markers of outcome in serum must be established.

Several proteins synthesized in astroglial cells or neurons have been proposed as serum biochemical markers of cell damage in the CNS [Qureshi, 2002]. The ideal serum markers should have high specificity and sensitivity for brain injury, be released only after irreversible destruction of brain tissue, have a rapid appearance in serum, and have temporal correlation with the onset of injury. The variability in measurement should be low, to ensure a predictable relationship between the serum concentration and the amount of brain injury. The marker should be able to provide prognostic information regarding brain injury. Furthermore, reliable assays for immediate analyses should be available [Qureshi, 2002].

With regard to reliable biochemical markers of brain injury, increased serum levels of the low-molecular-weight protein S-100B have been reported in cases of cardiac arrest and traumatic brain injury [Mussack et al., 2002; Spinella et al., 2003]. Urinary S-100B protein concentrations are used as a marker for brain damage in asphyxiated infants [Gazzolo et al., 2004].

The biologic role of S-100B protein, a calcium-binding protein found in the nervous system, is still unclear [Dennery, 2003]. Its half-life is about 1 hour, and it is excreted mainly in the urine [Gazzolo et al., 2004]. Increased S-100B concentrations in biologic fluids are a reliable marker of brain damage in adults, infants, and fetuses [Gazzolo et al., 2004]. The short half-life of S-100B protein makes it an interesting marker for longitudinal monitoring. Elevated S-100B levels 12 hours after cardiac arrest are suggestive of severe global cellular brain damage, which is correlated with an unfavorable outcome after 12 months [Mussack et al., 2002].

In one analysis, neuron-specific enolase concentrations in serum samples were correlated with patient outcome after cardiac arrest [Fogel et al., 1997]. A serum neuron-specific enolase concentration of 33 ng/mL determined up to day 3 after cardiac arrest can predict poor neurologic outcome.

Neuroimaging

Studies have indicated that normal results of head CT performed immediately after anoxic injury are not correlated with outcome [Han et al., 1990; Romano et al., 1993]. However, abnormal results obtained in the initial hours after injury are associated with a poor prognosis.

Patients with anoxic-ischemic insults may exhibit a variety of findings on CT of the brain. In a study of 53 patients (all ages) scanned 3 days after an out-of-hospital cardiac arrest, clinical differences were found between patients who had cerebral edema and those who did not [Morimoto et al., 1993]. In all, 23 of 25 patients with cerebral edema had cardiac arrest as a result of respiratory distress, whereas this finding was true in only 5 of 28 patients without cerebral edema. Initial arterial pH was significantly lower in patients with cerebral edema, and significantly more of these patients remained comatose or were diagnosed as brain dead. Cerebral edema was apparent in 9 of these 25 patients when scanned the first day of hospitalization. Over the next 2 days, low-density areas involving the basal ganglia, midbrain, and thalamus developed in 22 of the 25 patients. Eventually, loss of the normal gray-white matter differentiation was seen in all patients. It was suggested that brain swelling in the early postresuscitation period might be one of the predictors of a poor neurologic outcome in patients who experience an out-of-hospital cardiac arrest [Morimoto et al., 1993].

Although basal ganglia injury is a well-known cerebral effect of hypoxic-ischemic injury, documentation comes from postmortem studies, with only sporadic reports in live patients [Jacobs et al., 1990]. Magnetic resonance imaging makes it possible to detect lesions in the basal ganglia after cardiopulmonary arrest, which are correlated with the development of movement disorder. The course of the clinical signs is correlated with the presence of abnormalities on magnetic resonance imaging [Jacobs et al., 1990; Wallays et al., 1995], as well as with the results of diffusion-weighted imaging [Arbelaez et al., 1999].

Magnetic Resonance Spectroscopy

Proton magnetic resonance spectroscopy is clinically useful for identifying noninvasively the biochemical state of the CNS, as reviewed in Chapter 11. Proton magnetic resonance spectroscopy has been used to study patients after acute nontraumatic and traumatic injuries [Ashwal et al., 1995, 1997; Ross and Michaelis, 1994]. Pediatric patients with severe closed-head injuries or strokes with severe long-term neurologic sequelae exhibit reduced NAA peaks and reduced NAA/creatine ratios [Ashwal et al., 2000]. Adults with cardiac arrest, elevated brain lactate levels on proton magnetic resonance spectroscopy, and absence of N_{20} somatosensory-evoked responses had a poor prognosis if they were still alive 4 weeks after injury [Berek et al., 1995].

Several studies have addressed the metabolic changes in response to acute cerebral injury in children through the use of proton spectroscopy [Holshouser et al., 1997]. Proton magnetic resonance spectroscopy has been used to evaluate the prognosis of pediatric near-drowning victims [Dubowitz et al., 1998; Kreis et al., 1996]. Of 16 children reported, those with excessive lactate levels universally had a poor

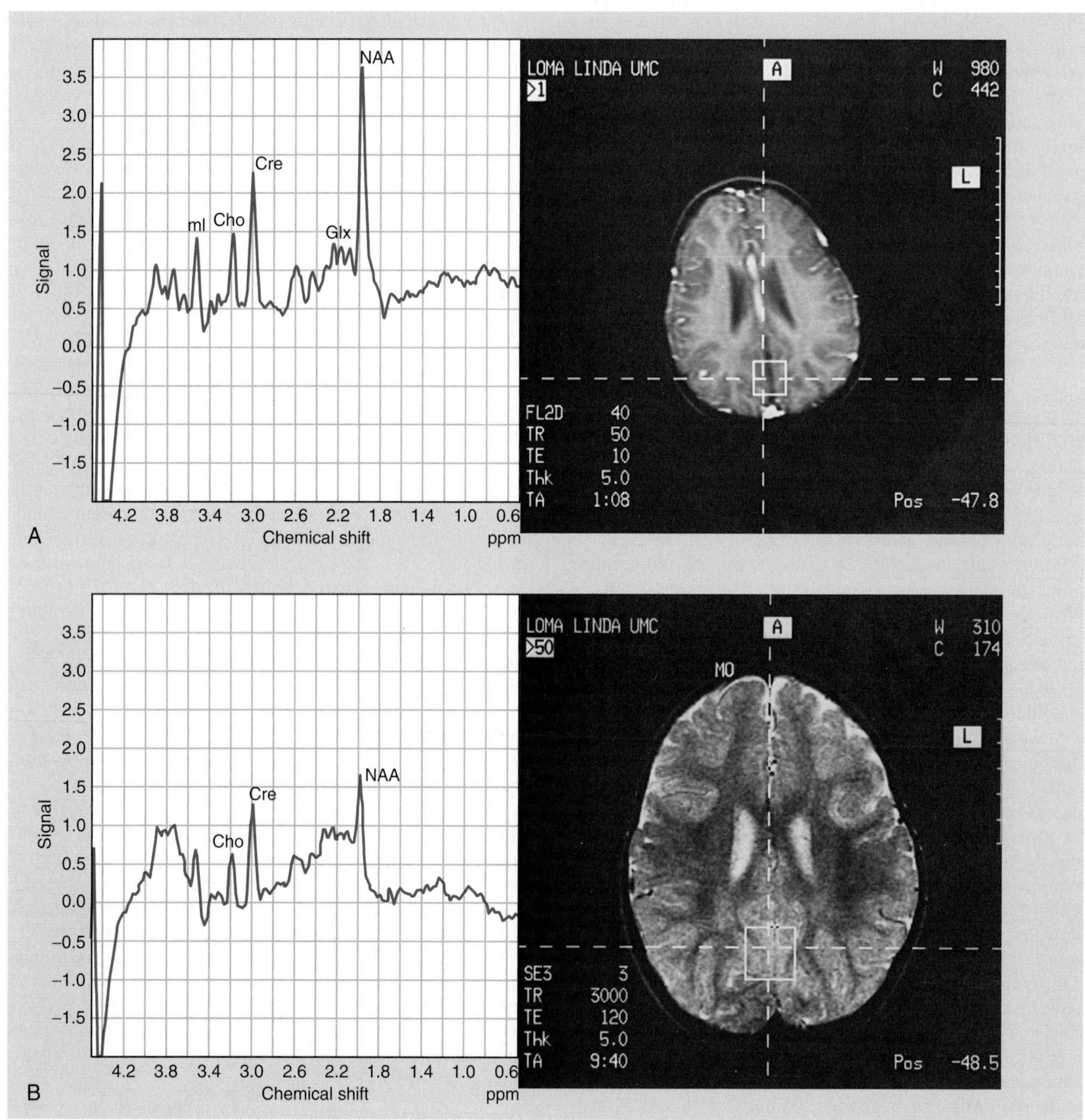

FIGURE 64-7. Proton magnetic resonance spectrum studies in a child without brain injury and in two children with acute global ischemic central nervous system insults. **A,** Spectra from occipital cortex in a normal 21-month-old female, displaying the increases in *N*-acetyl aspartate (NAA) and in creatine-phosphocreatine (Cre), with decreases in choline (Cho) and myoinositol (mI) that is seen in comparison with younger patients (see Chapter 11 for spectra in younger children). Glx, glutamine. **B,** Spectra from the occipital cortex in an 18-month-old female with severe post–hypoxic-ischemic injury on day 4 after a near-drowning injury with a normal T_2-weighted magnetic resonance image (MRI) at the same time. The decreases in NAA and Cre with increase in Glx are apparent (echo time [TE] = 20 milliseconds, repetition time [TR] = 3 seconds). This child made some recovery to a moderate-to-severe disability. (Courtesy of Dr. Barbara Holshouser, Department of Radiology, Loma Linda University Medical Center.)

outcome, usually surviving in a vegetative state. Lactate level was also more likely to peak by day 4 rather than immediately after injury. Holshouser and colleagues [1997] demonstrated the potential value of proton magnetic resonance spectroscopy in predicting outcome after acute CNS injuries in 82 infants and children. In this study, changes in metabolite ratios and the presence or absence of lactate in combination with clinical and magnetic resonance imaging score data predicted outcome correctly in 91% of CNS-injured neonates and in 100% of CNS-injured infants and children. Poor-outcome groups had lower Glasgow Coma Scale scores, longer periods of unconsciousness, and lower NAA/creatine and NAA/choline ratios and were more likely to have lactate. Several clinical examples of children with acute brain injuries and abnormal proton spectra that demonstrate the clinical utility of magnetic resonance spectroscopy are depicted in Figure 64-7.

TREATMENT

Treatment of children with global hypoxic-ischemic brain injuries involves multiple specialties and a systematic approach to initially providing emergency care in the field, emergency department, and intensive care unit. Urgent neuroimaging studies and early neurologic evaluation are helpful in the initial evaluation to determine the presence of a neurosurgical condition that necessitates immediate treatment, the etiology of injury, and the appropriate course of treatment.

Prehospital Care

Currently, aggressive hospital treatment does not lead to intact survival for children who have out-of-hospital cardiopulmonary arrests and present to the pediatric emergency department with a preterminal rhythm (asystole, idioventricular rhythm, electromechanical dissociation) and absence of spontaneous circulation. Resuscitation efforts in the emergency department, although commonly successful, lead to severe neurologic sequelae or death at discharge with extremely high costs of care. Prehospital emergency medical services are capable of providing the earliest medical interventions and hold the greatest promise for improving outcome from prehospital pediatric cardiopulmonary arrest. Emergency medical services have developed sophisticated methods for dispatch and transport, and personnel have been trained to perform advanced cardiac life support. However, for children in cardiopulmonary arrest, prehospital providers successfully perform endotracheal intubation, establish intravascular access, and administer epinephrine significantly less frequently than in their adult counterparts [Kumar et al., 1997]. Basic approaches likely have the greatest opportunity to affect outcome by simply opening the airway and providing adequate ventilation to prevent cardiac arrest. It is also likely that once asphyxia has led to cardiac arrest, novel therapies, to be effective, almost certainly need to be initiated in the field.

In many animal models, high-dose epinephrine has improved resuscitation rates [Becker, 1997; Berg et al., 1996; Brown and Werman, 1990]. What have not been established are the effects of high-dose epinephrine on long-term survival and neurologic outcome in humans. A small study in children with previous victims used as control subjects demonstrated a beneficial effect on resuscitation and outcome in patients receiving high-dose epinephrine [Goetting and Paradis, 1991].

Subsequent studies in adult populations, however, have failed to reveal a significant benefit in terms of neurologic

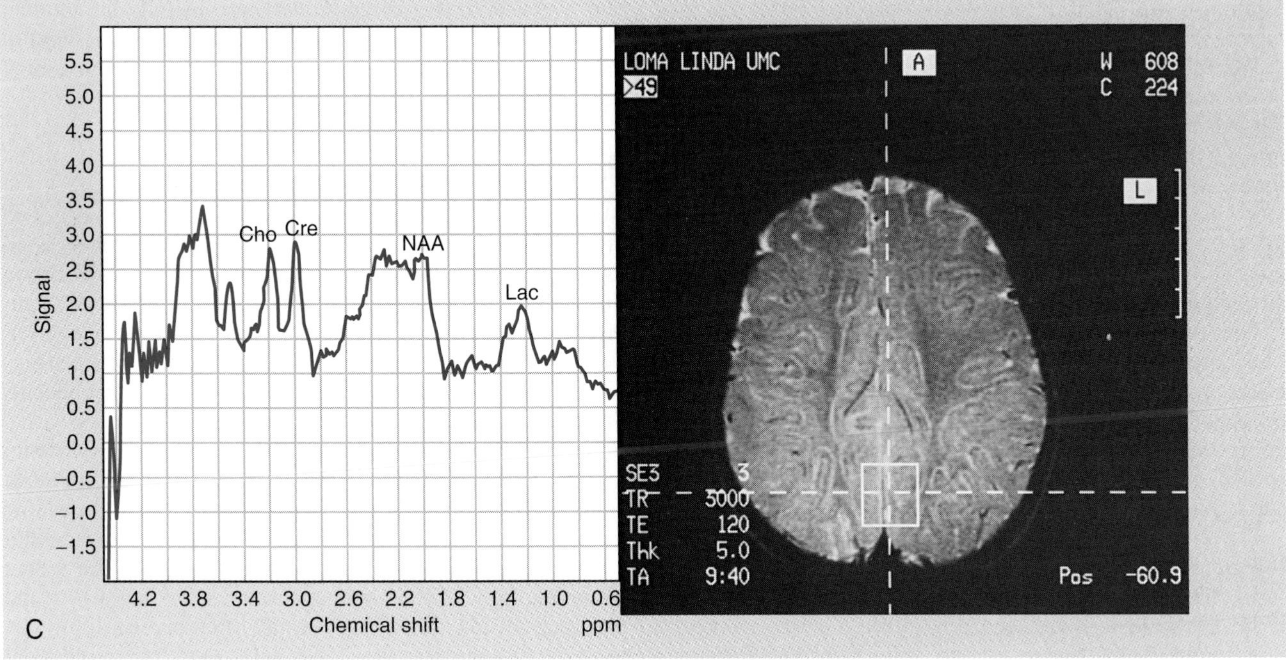

FIGURE 64-7. *(continued)* **C,** Spectra from occipital cortex in a 17-month-old female in a permanent vegetative state resulting from a near-drowning accident. Her spectrum discloses a low NAA peak, which was difficult to measure because of the greatly increased Glx with reversal of the Cho/Cre peaks and the presence of lactate, all of which suggest a poor prognosis (TE = 20 milliseconds, TR = 3 seconds). T_2-weighted MRI demonstrates diffuse edema.

outcome and survival to discharge, and some authors have questioned the advisability of routine use of high-dose epinephrine in resuscitation protocols [Brown et al., 1992; Callahan et al., 1992; Frank, 1994; Stiell et al., 1992]. Studies in pediatric patients with out-of-hospital and in-hospital cardiopulmonary arrest have failed to demonstrate benefits from the use of high-dose epinephrine in terms of either the rate of resuscitation or eventual outcome [Carpenter and Stenmark, 1997; Dieckmann and Vardis, 1995; Ronco et al., 1995].

Contrary to the conventional wisdom that if a little is good, more is better, evidence has been accumulating that high-dose epinephrine is not beneficial and may even impair organ function and survival after the arrest [Lister and Fontan, 2004; Perondi et al., 2004]. The key to understanding this adverse influence of high-dose epinephrine on survival may reside in the calorigenic effects of epinephrine on various tissues, including the myocardium. Epinephrine may increase myocardial and cerebral perfusion during resuscitation, but in the process, it also increases oxygen use for a given measure of mechanical work by the heart and for the delivery of a given amount of oxygen to many other organs [Lister and Fontan, 2004].

Therefore, although epinephrine has been used during cardiopulmonary resuscitation for more than 100 years, its use has become controversial because it is associated with myocardial dysfunction during the period after resuscitation [Paradis et al., 2002]. Because it was found that endogenous vasopressin levels in successfully resuscitated patients were significantly higher than levels in patients who died, it was postulated that it might be beneficial to administer vasopressin during cardiopulmonary resuscitation [Lindner et al., 1992]. Laboratory studies of cardiopulmonary resuscitation revealed that vasopressin administration was associated with better blood flow to vital organs, better delivery of cerebral oxygen, better chances of resuscitation, and better neurologic outcome than was epinephrine [Wenzel et al., 2004].

Wenzel and co-workers [2004] demonstrated the success of vasopressin alone and vasopressin followed by epinephrine in refractory asystolic cardiac arrest—an important breakthrough in the science of resuscitation. Epinephrine consumes oxygen, whereas vasopressin increases coronary blood flow and the availability of oxygen to the myocardium [McIntyre, 2004]. These dynamics may contribute to the success of vasopressin therapy in asystolic cardiac arrest and the lack of success of epinephrine therapy.

The American Heart Association and International Liaison Committee on Resuscitation engaged in an evidence-based review of the literature on resuscitation, which culminated in an international consensus conference in January 2005, followed by treatment recommendations [Nolan et al., 2004]. Perhaps vasopressin will be incorporated into the new recommendations.

The efficacy of pharmacologic therapy during cardiopulmonary resuscitation is likely limited by the minimal perfusion provided by this procedure [Goetting, 1994; Safar, 1996]. New methods are needed to increase perfusion pressure during cardiac arrest to allow delivery of these agents to the target organs [Halperin et al., 1996]. Debate continues regarding the use of open-chest cardiac massage during cardiac arrest, but social and technical limitations currently prevent its application in the prehospital setting [Dizon and Santanello, 2003; Sheikh and Brogan, 1994]. Established mechanical methods such as cardiopulmonary bypass and mechanical ventricular assistance can restore cardiac and cerebral perfusion to near-normal values during cardiac arrest, but these present great technical problems for application, particularly in children. Development and implementation of improved perfusion techniques would provide an increased therapeutic window and a better chance of reducing long-term neurologic morbidity.

Preventing brain damage after cardiac arrest requires minimizing normothermic no-flow times through early (automatic) defibrillation and early initiation of cooling [Safar et al., 2002]. Rapid induction of mild cerebral hypothermia requires novel cooling methods for use by paramedics and emergency physicians. The objective of the ongoing Smart aortic arch catheter research and development program is to engineer "smart" catheter systems for enabling rapid vascular access and catheter placement, primarily within the aorta, for emergency induction of hypothermia and suspended animation [Yaffe et al., 2004]. According to initial design developments and prototype demonstrations, moving suspended animation from the laboratory to the field is fully feasible and achievable in the near future.

Hospital Care

The underlying foundation of neurointensive care is excellent supportive care. Until a neuroprotective agent is developed, state-of-the-art care for a patient who has suffered a hypoxic-ischemic injury consists of maintenance of adequate blood pressure; oxygenation; ventilation; electrolyte homeostasis; nutritional supplementation; and prevention of hyperglycemia, hyperthermia, and seizures [Gisvold et al., 1996].

Several features of supportive post-ischemic intensive care warrant further discussion. These include intracranial pressure monitoring and control, glucose homeostasis, cardiovascular support, temperature regulation, and reduction of metabolic rate.

Intracranial Pressure Monitoring and Control

Improvements in outcome with appropriate monitoring and control of increased intracranial pressure in Reye's syndrome and cerebral trauma fostered the routine application of intracranial pressure monitoring and intracranial pressure-directed therapy in the post–cardiac arrest setting. However, published studies in both clinical and laboratory settings have raised questions about both the rationale and the benefits of these maneuvers.

Results of clinical studies suggest that intracranial pressure elevation is more common after asphyxia-induced cardiac arrest than after isolated global brain ischemia or ventricular pressure arrest [Scollo-Lavizzari and Bassetti, 1987]. This finding is not surprising in view of the severe histopathology of the asphyxia-induced cardiac arrest and the long insult times from which the myocardium can recover in children. Sustained elevation of intracranial pressure (>20 mm Hg) was a predictor of poor outcome in a series of pediatric submersion accidents [Dean and McComb, 1981; Frewen et al., 1985; Nussbaum and Galant, 1983; Sarnaik et al., 1985]. Unfortunately, as in ventricular fibrillation– induced cardiac arrest, the threshold for poor outcome from asphyxia-induced cardiac arrest appears to be below the threshold for the occurrence of intracranial hypertension because many patients experience poor outcome despite normal intracranial pressure. Although there are anecdotal cases of asphyxia-induced cardiac arrest in patients with intact neurologic outcome despite elevated intracranial pressure, the ability to control intracranial pressure elevation does not result in meaningful survival. Routine monitoring and treatment of intracranial pressure are not currently recommended after asphyxia-induced cardiac arrest.

Hyperventilation has been advocated after cerebral injury as a means of decreasing intracranial pressure. However, the use of hyperventilation, even after traumatic brain injury, is being re-evaluated [Muizelaar et al., 1991; Skippen et al., 1997; Yundt and Diringer, 1997]. There is no evidence of any sustained beneficial effect of hyperventilation after hypoxic-ischemic brain injury, and its use should be avoided [Hickey and Zuckerbraun, 2003]. The failure of intracranial pressure–directed therapy to improve outcome after cardiopulmonary arrest and the commonly observed period of hypoperfusion in the first hours to days after the arrest raises serious questions about the blind application of an intervention with the potential to further reduce cerebral blood flow. Thus, hyperventilation should be reserved for patients with signs of cerebral herniation or suspected pulmonary hypertension [Hickey and Zuckerbraun, 2003].

The traditional approach to cerebral resuscitation has also recommended the use of mannitol in the post–cardiac arrest period. Again, studies in the setting of cardiopulmonary arrest are lacking. In dogs subjected to 6 minutes of global ischemia, mannitol (2 g/kg) further reduced cerebral blood flow during the post-ischemic hypoperfusion phase [Arai et al., 1986]. This unwanted effect of mannitol likely represents a result of dehydration. A theoretically beneficial oxygen radical–scavenging effect of mannitol has also been proposed, but if significant oxygen radical–induced brain injury occurs, significantly more potent oxygen radical scavengers are available.

Glucose Homeostasis

Observations in animals and humans have suggested that an elevated serum glucose level at or about the time of an ischemic insult is associated with enhanced post-ischemic damage of cerebral tissue [Kushner et al., 1990]. Preexisting hyperglycemia worsens the outcome from global hypoxic-ischemic injury in adult and juvenile animals [Chopp et al., 1988; Combs et al., 1990; Kalimo et al., 1981; Lanier et al., 1987; Pulsinelli et al., 1982]. Outcome from out-of-hospital cardiac arrest is worse in adults with elevated glucose concentrations at admission [Longstreth, 1987] and in hyperglycemic children after submersion injury [Ashwal et al., 1990]. Hyperglycemia has also been described as increasing brain damage when traumatic brain injury is complicated by secondary ischemia [Cherian et al., 1997]. As a mechanism for the adverse effect of hyperglycemia, most attention has focused on the neuronal effects of increased tissue lactate production and lowered tissue pH [Cherian et al., 1997; Kawai et al., 1997].

Several studies have demonstrated that (1) lactate production during ischemia is directly related to pre-ischemic stores of glucose and glycogen and (2) pre-ischemic hyperglycemia results in a more pronounced fall in both intracellular and extracellular brain pH during ischemia [Ljunggren et al., 1974; Smith et al., 1986]. In addition, researchers have demonstrated that when subjected to the same ischemic insult, hyperglycemic animals have a more pronounced histopathologic injury than do normoglycemic animals [Kalimo et al., 1981]. In children, increased brain lactate level, as detected by magnetic resonance spectroscopy, has been associated with poorer long-term neurologic outcomes [Ashwal et al., 1997].

The mechanisms by which lactate and acidosis may augment cellular injury during ischemia remain unclear [Kim et al., 1996; Steingrub and Mundt, 1996]. Direct cytotoxicity, cellular swelling, oxygen radical–mediated damage, and alterations in intracellular calcium homeostasis have been proposed as mechanisms of acidosis-induced injury [Kim et al., 1996; Siesjo et al., 1993]. Lactate induces alterations in calcium homeostasis and may contribute to synaptic dysfunction.

Other mechanisms by which hyperglycemia may enhance cerebral ischemic injury include effects on cerebral vasculature and cerebral blood flow [Cipolla et al., 1997; Kawai et al., 1997], alteration in the modulation of protein synthesis in the post-ischemic period [Lin et al., 1997], decreased adenosine production [Hsu et al., 1991], blood-brain barrier breakdown [Dietrich et al., 1993], and hyperosmolality [Gisselsson et al., 1992].

On the basis of these findings, it has also been suggested that in the presence of impaired oxygen delivery, ongoing delivery of glucose may be detrimental. The administration of glucose, once performed in every comatose patient, is questioned, and protocols involving glucose-free solutions are suggested [Sieber and Traystman, 1991].

The prospect of withholding glucose-containing solutions from patients should be considered in view of the following: (1) There is evidence that acidosis is not as harmful as previously thought and that mild acidosis may be neuroprotective via its modulating effect on the excitotoxic component of ischemic injury [Tombaugh and Sapolski, 1990]; (2) current investigations have raised questions about the association between the concentration of glucose after resuscitation and neurologic outcome [Steingrub and Mundt, 1996]; and (3) the influence of serum glucose levels on hypoxic-ischemic neuronal injury appears to depend on the age of the patient [Loepke and Spaeth, 2004].

In summary, the optimal level of blood glucose after resuscitation from either a global or focal hypoxic-ischemic event has not been determined. From a practical point, it seems wise to avoid hypoglycemia in a neonate with hypoxic-ischemic injury and to avoid hyperglycemia in older patients. There is evidence that hyperglycemia is common in acutely ill children and that time of onset, duration, and intensity of hyperglycemia are associated with mortality [Srinivasan et al., 2004].

Cardiovascular Support

Although the optimal cerebral perfusion pattern for neuronal recovery remains to be defined, blood pressure fluctuations, both high and low, adversely affect outcome. In several important reviews, investigators have suggested a benefit of transient hypertension during the immediate postresuscitation period, hypothesizing that this improves flow in areas with microvascular sludging. Safar and associates [1996] suggested that transient hypertension was beneficial after cardiac arrest in dogs. However, it was used as part of a multifaceted treatment protocol, and its specific benefit is controversial.

Shock after a generalized hypoxic-ischemic episode is frequently encountered in infants and children without preexisting cardiovascular or pulmonary disease. The shock state after hypoxic-ischemic events is cardiogenic and is characterized by low flow and high resistance [Lucking et al., 1986]. The cardiac index is depressed in the early stages, with elevated systemic and pulmonary vascular resistance indexes and with elevated filling pressures of both the right and left sides of the heart. Investigators have documented systolic and diastolic myocardial dysfunction immediately after successful cardiac resuscitation with restoration of spontaneous circulation [Gazmuri et al., 1996; Tang et al., 1993]. In young children, these cardiopulmonary derangements resolve over time as the cardiac index increases and systemic and pulmonary vascular resistances decrease.

The systemic vascular resistance after hypoxic-ischemic events in children is often inappropriately elevated. Although it is possible that this effect is secondary to the therapies given to these patients, it is also possible that other pathophysiologic mechanisms account for the elevated blood pressures. Renin-mediated hypertension may follow ischemic injury, or CNS injury can cause increases in vascular tone by increasing adrenergic tone.

Because of the multiple influences on cardiac output, cardiac support can be difficult to manage. Careful use of fluids, inotropic agents, and vasoactive drugs is indicated. Vasodilators may result in profound reductions in blood pressure. In a retrospective human study, postresuscitative hypertension was associated with a better neurologic outcome [Morris and Nadkarni, 2003].

Temperature Control

The effectiveness of hypothermia as a cerebral protective intervention (i.e., before cardiopulmonary arrest) is unquestioned. Hypothermia has been successfully applied during cerebrovascular and cardiovascular surgery for decades [Marion et al., 1996]. The beneficial effects of hypothermia applied immediately before and during cardiopulmonary arrest are clearly demonstrated by the clinical experience with victims of cold-water submersion accidents [Biggart and Bohn, 1990] and with victims of accidental deep hypothermia [Walpoth et al., 1997].

When considering hypothermia (defined as a core temperature <35° C), the clinician should distinguish between uncontrolled (i.e., spontaneous, accidental) and controlled hypothermia induced by artificial cooling, which is used to prevent or attenuate various forms of neurologic injury [Polderman, 2004]. There is growing evidence that induced hypothermia can have neuroprotective effects in some patients with neurologic injury.

Class I evidence (from animal experiments, two randomized controlled trials, and various nonrandomized trials) supports the use of hypothermia in selected categories of patients after cardiopulmonary resuscitation [Bernard and Buist, 2003; Bernard et al., 2002; The Hypothermia after Cardiac Arrest Group, 2002; Sessler, 1997]. Cooling should be initiated as soon as possible but should not be withheld even if delays of up to 8 hours occur [Polderman, 2004]. Treatment should be continued for 12 to 24 hours, with target temperatures of 32° to 33° C. Patients should be rewarmed slowly, because there is evidence that quick rewarming may have deleterious effects [Hickey et al., 2003; Safar and Kochanek, 2002].

The effect of hypothermia on the injured brain is complex. For each 1° C decrease in temperature, the cerebral metabolic rate for oxygen decreases by 6% to 7% [Bernard and Buist, 2003]. However, hypothermia's main beneficial effect is to provide protection against numerous deleterious biochemical mechanisms [Safar and Kochanek, 2002]. Over a period of days after the restoration of spontaneous circulation, these mechanisms—which include calcium shifts, excitotoxicity, lipid peroxidation and other free radical reactions, DNA damage, mitochondrial injury, and inflammation—lead to death of neurons in vulnerable regions of the brain [Safar and Kochanek, 2002].

Potential mechanisms for the protective effect of hypothermia include inhibition of glutamate release, inhibition of adenine nucleotide depletion, prevention of brain acidosis, and preservation of protein kinase activity [Cardell et al., 1991; Chen et al., 1992; Duhaime and Ross, 1990; Sutton et al., 1991]. Hypothermia also may inhibit free radical mechanisms by decreasing free fatty acid release, preserving endogenous antioxidants, and antagonizing free radical insults [du Plessis and Johnston, 1997]. The marked amelioration of delayed energy failure and specific inhibition of apoptosis (demonstrated in a piglet model) suggest that hypothermia may delay apoptotic commitment, allowing endogenous protective mechanisms to restore cellular integrity [Thoresen and Wyatt, 1997].

The use of induced mild hypothermia should be considered in patients after cardiopulmonary resuscitation, provided that there are no significant contraindications (such as ongoing hemorrhage) and that the prognosis does not appear hopeless for other reasons (e.g., presence of malignancies, severe chronic diseases). Temperature levels are important; mild hypothermia (33° to 36° C) may be most effective, and it is simple and safe. Moderate hypothermia (28° to 32° C) can cause dysrhythmias, coagulopathy, and infection [Safar and Kochanek, 2002].

Reduction of Metabolic Rate

The observation in certain animal models that hypermetabolism accompanies post-ischemic hypoperfusion formed the basis for early clinical cerebroprotective strategies in the post–cardiac arrest setting. Therapies directed at attenuating active cerebral metabolism (rate of cerebral O_2 metabolism attributable to synaptic transmission) were applied in the hope of reducing this secondary insult of hypoperfusion plus hypermetabolism. The cerebral protective effects of interventions that decrease cerebral metabolic rate before the onset of ischemia, such as barbiturates and hypothermia, are well established and clinically important [Kuroiwa et al., 1990; Steen and Michenfelder, 1980]. The selective inhibitory effect of barbiturates on active cerebral metabolic rate of O_2 was particularly attractive. However, therapeutic reductions in brain metabolism when applied after the insult, as in the "HYPER" therapy of the 1970s, did not improve outcome [Abramson et al., 1986]. This result may have arisen from the relative lack of post–cardiac arrest hypermetabolism in humans. In addition, adverse hemodynamic consequences of barbiturates and the ill effects of sustained deep hypothermia on immune function and blood rheology may have masked any beneficial effects [Biggart and Bohn, 1990].

The ability of barbiturates to protect against multifocal incomplete ischemia in selected cases of cardiac or neurologic surgery, to control seizures, and to aid in the reduction of intracranial hypertension is better confirmed than are their potential effects after cardiac arrest [Safar, 1993].

Potential Therapies

Modulation of Endogenous Defenses

The potential mechanisms involved in cell death after cardiac arrest and restoration of circulation are complex. An evolving understanding of these mechanisms may allow clinicians to take advantage of these endogenous neuroprotectants as future therapies to improve neuronal survival after cardiac arrest. Several events are essential if neurons are to recover. First and foremost, ATP levels must be restored and maintained. Reperfusion is essential, although not the sole requirement for neuronal rescue, inasmuch as the cells require energy sources and the means to eliminate their waste. Therefore, a second factor that is critical is that the cells must not be subject to overwhelming cytosolic calcium burdens; therefore, not only must ATP levels be maintained but also excitotoxicity should be minimized [Sweeney et al., 1995]. Other factors thought to be important include avoiding excessive formation of free radicals and metabolism of free fatty acids. In response to the complex sequence of pathophysiologic events that evolve after brain injury, several biochemical and molecular mediators that may have neuroprotective roles are present. These endogenous neuroprotectants are produced, induced, or activated after ischemia, and their postulated or proven functions improve cell (specifically neuronal) survival in in vivo, in vitro, or both models.

HEAT SHOCK PROTEINS

Heat shock proteins are one family of candidate neuroprotectants that are highly conserved among biologic species and are induced in cells after a variety of stimuli. Heat stress is the classic example; however, any insult that damages protein structure, including ischemic and traumatic brain injury, can produce a heat shock protein response [Raghupathi et al., 1995; Simon et al., 1991]. Heat shock proteins have generated major interest as potential neuroprotectants because their prior induction by a sublethal stress can afford protection from subsequent injury. Transient entire-body hyperthermia reduces subsequent ischemic brain injury in rats [Chopp, 1989].

Heat shock proteins likely play an important role in cellular defense against environmental stresses [Kogure and Kato, 1993]. The HSP70 gene is the heat shock gene that has been best characterized after cerebral ischemia. Numerous studies have demonstrated increased transcription of HSP70 messenger RNA and increased synthesis of HSP70 and HSP72 after global cerebral ischemia [Gonzalez et al., 1991; Nowak et al., 1993; Vass et al., 1988]. This gene appears to be expressed in proportion to the duration of ischemia. Increasing durations of ischemia lead to HSP70 expression, first in neurons from selectively vulnerable regions, next in relatively resistant neurons, then in glia, and, finally, in endothelial cells [Sharp et al., 1993; Simon et al., 1991]. Although a direct cause-and-effect relationship between heat shock proteins and neuroprotection in vivo has not been established, novel techniques to specifically increase heat shock proteins in neurons after injury should help in answering this question.

ADENOSINE

An endogenous biochemical mediator that may serve a protective role after cerebral ischemia, particularly early after injury, is adenosine. Adenosine levels are increased in brain tissue after experimental ischemia and in response to hypoxia, hypotension, and hypoglycemia [Laudignon et al., 1991; Morii et al., 1987; Ruth et al., 1993]. The bulk of the extracellular adenosine derives from the intracellular catabolism of ATP. The release of adenosine after ischemia could afford neuroprotection by a combination of several mechanisms. When bound to A_2 receptors, adenosine is a cerebrovasodilator [Sweeney et al., 1995]. When bound to A_1 receptors, adenosine reduces neuronal metabolism and excitatory amino acid release, stabilizes postsynaptic membranes, and inhibits platelet activation and neutrophil function [Miller and Hsu, 1992]. Thus, the beneficial effects of adenosine after cerebral ischemia include improved regional blood flow, reduced local oxygen demand, attenuation of excitotoxicity, increases in intracellular calcium, and anti-inflammatory and rheologic effects.

The effects of adenosine and synthetic adenosine derivatives on ischemic, hypoxic, or traumatic CNS damage, when given before or after the insult, protect against neuronal damage [Rudolphi and Schubert, 1996]. The therapeutic value of the agonist approach is questionable because most adenosine derivatives have prohibitive CNS and cardiovascular side effects, such as strong sedation, hypotension, cardiodepression, and renal vasoconstriction.

Targeting Delayed Neuronal Death

Although a portion of neuronal death occurs immediately after acute brain injury, it is clear that some portion of neurons die in a delayed manner by programmed cell death. The completion of programmed cell death leads to a distinct cell morphologic process termed *apoptosis* [Kochanek et al., 2001].

Because programmed cell death occurs in stages, there exist several potential strategies for reducing cell death. Targeting upstream regulators of the programmed cell death cascade, such as bcl-2 family proteins and cell death receptors is one such strategy [Kochanek et al., 2001]. Regulation of cell death may depend on the proportion of pro-apoptotic versus anti-apoptotic bcl-2 proteins in the cell after injury.

Another potential anti-apoptotic strategy is to target the final common pathway of the programmed cell death cascade. Activation of caspase-8, caspase-9, and other caspases is the key committed step in the programmed cell death cascade [Clark et al., 2000]. Caspase-3 activates endonucleases and other proteases, inactivates enzymes important in DNA repair, and cleaves cytoskeletal proteins, culminating in morphologic features of apoptosis [Kochanek et al., 2001]. Pan-caspase and relatively selective peptide inhibitors of many caspases are available and undergoing experimental trials.

Several contemporary strategies used for ischemic injury may reduce programmed cell death. Hypothermia, antioxidants, and anti-excitotoxic strategies may prevent programmed cell death and are discussed elsewhere in this chapter.

Reduction of Excitotoxicity

Death of selectively vulnerable neurons is mediated by local release of excitatory neurotransmitters with hypermetabolism and calcium accumulation. This process has led to attempts to attenuate post-ischemic excitotoxicity more selectively by administering specific receptor antagonists. NMDA and non-NMDA receptor antagonists have been studied extensively in numerous animal models.

Competitive antagonists at NMDA binding sites have been disappointing in animal studies because of the large doses (and hence systemic adverse effects) necessary to penetrate the blood-brain barrier and reduce the high ischemic levels of glutamate at the NMDA receptor. These factors limit the therapeutic index and clinical utility of competitive antagonists [du Plessis and Johnston, 1997].

Noncompetitive antagonism can be mediated at several sites within the NMDA ion channel. This discussion is confined to magnesium blockade and agents acting at the phencyclidine channel site, such as the experimental agent MK-801 (dizocilpine), and several agents already in clinical use, such as dextromethorphan and ketamine. These agents are not likely to be subjected to clinical trials because of concerns regarding their psychomimetic effects and potential toxicity.

MK-801 is a noncompetitive NMDA antagonist; that is, it does not compete with glutamate for binding to the NMDA receptor but instead blocks influx of extracellular calcium by binding to a site within the NMDA receptor–gated calcium channel. Results of numerous studies suggest that this agent is neuroprotective in the setting of focal ischemia [McCulloch, 1992; Pulsinelli et al., 1993]; however, results of MK-801 treatment in the setting of global brain ischemia are discouraging.

Sterz and co-workers [1989] gave MK-801 either before or after a 17-minute ventricular fibrillation–induced cardiac arrest in dogs and found that it did not improve neurologic or histologic outcome at 96 hours. In a similar study, MK-801 administered after cardiac arrest in cats had no beneficial effect on neurologic outcome at 7 days [Fleischer et al., 1989]. Lanier and associates [1990] found comparable results of no benefit in a primate model of global brain ischemia.

Blockade of non-NMDA receptors (i.e., AMPA and kainate receptors) with quinoxalinedione compounds has most consistently prevented delayed neuronal cell loss in the hippocampal CA1 region in animal models of global cerebral ischemia. NBQX (2,3-dihydroxy-6-nitro-7-sulfamoyl-benzoquinoxaline) is a non-NMDA receptor antagonist that appears to provide histologic protection in the cortex, hippocampus, or both in rat models of global ischemia [Buchan et al., 1991; Diemer et al., 1993; Nellgard and Wicloch, 1992]. Of interest, delayed treatment with NBQX appears to be effective. Treatment 12 hours after global ischemia in the rat [Li and Buchan, 1993] and 24 hours after global ischemia in the gerbil [Sherdown et al., 1993] resulted in significantly decreased delayed neuronal death in the CA1 region of the hippocampus.

The protective efficacy of AMPA-receptor antagonists against delayed neuronal death may be explained in the following ways. First, in the post-ischemic phase, AMPA receptors may become upregulated and more responsive [du Plessis and Johnston, 1997]. Furthermore, NMDA antagonists increase and AMPA antagonists decrease glucose metabolism. Consequently, during the period of disturbed metabolism after ischemia, a decrease in glucose metabolism, as occurs with AMPA antagonists, promotes neuronal survival [du Plessis and Johnston, 1997].

The divalent cation Mg^{2+} acts as a glutamate receptor antagonist to the extent that it blocks the neuronal influx of Ca^{2+} within the ion channel. In this regard, magnesium sulfate has reduced the severity of hypoxic-ischemic brain damage in immature rats [Vannucci and Perlman, 1997]. Clinical trials have revealed variable effects [Christensen et al., 1996; Gisvold et al., 1996].

Inhibition of Calcium Accumulation

Calcium accumulation in neurons and release of stored intracellular calcium are pivotal events leading to irreversible cellular damage during the reperfusion phase after an ischemic insult. Calcium accumulation occurs through receptor-operated channels such as the NMDA receptor–activated channels, voltage-operated calcium channels, nonspecific membrane channels, and release of intracellular calcium via the inositol second-messenger pathway. Conflicting results regarding the ability of the voltage-operated calcium channel antagonists (lidoflazine, nimodipine, nicardipine, flunarizine) to attenuate calcium accumulation in brain cells after ischemia have been obtained [Grotta et al., 1990]. The contribution of the voltage-gated channels to post-ischemic calcium accumulation is apparently less than that of the NMDA-operated channels in selectively vulnerable zones. Nevertheless, clinical experience with the voltage-operated calcium channel antagonists and their cerebral vasodilatory effects prompted laboratory and clinical evaluations.

Calcium channel blockers have been studied in a variety of animal models of global ischemia and have been subjected to clinical trials. Despite some encouraging findings in animal models, the clinical trials have failed to yield positive results [Morgenstern and Pettigrew, 1997].

Nimodipine, a dihydropyridine compound that selectively blocks the L-type calcium channel, has been studied in animal models of global cerebral ischemia and in human survivors of cardiac arrest. Using a canine model, Steen and colleagues [1983] demonstrated that pre-ischemic treatment with nimodipine resulted in increased cerebral blood flow and improved neurologic outcome after 10 minutes of global ischemia. However, when the drug was administered after ischemia, the results were intermediate; cerebral blood flow was improved, but outcome was unchanged [Steen et al., 1984]. Subsequently, Milde and co-workers [1986] studied the effect of post-ischemic treatment with nimodipine on cerebral blood flow in the early reperfusion period. Nimodipine-treated dogs had significantly higher cerebral blood flow, but nimodipine treatment had no effect on cerebral metabolism. Again, this raises the question of whether improving blood flow in the early reperfusion period has any effect on neurologic outcome. These results culminated in a clinical trial of nimodipine treatment in survivors of cardiac arrest (ventricular fibrillation) [Roine et al., 1990]. There was no difference in neurologic outcome or survival at 3 or 12 months after cardiac arrest.

Lidoflazine is a nonselective voltage-sensitive calcium channel antagonist that in early animal studies appeared to ameliorate hypoxic-ischemic brain injury. However, later studies, including a large clinical trial, failed to substantiate the results of the early experiments [Brain Resuscitation Clinical Trial II Study Group, 1991].

Antioxidants

Free radicals can damage membrane lipids, cellular proteins, enzymes, and DNA. The importance of damage to each brain component and subsequent contribution to triggering or mediating the final pathway of neuronal death remain to be defined. As a result, a variety of approaches to preventing oxidative free radical–mediated brain injury have been devised. Most cerebral ischemia literature refers to antioxidants and agents that block the chain reaction of lipid peroxidation; however, other agents prevent oxidation of substances other than lipids and by multiple mechanisms.

Because all biologic systems generate oxygen free radicals even under physiologic conditions, enzymes are present within the cell to protect its constituents from the oxidizing effect of hydrogen peroxide and its metabolic products; these enzymes include superoxide dismutase, endoperoxidase, and catalase, which convert hydrogen peroxide to either water or stable oxygen. Additional defenses are provided by endogenous scavengers, which include cholesterol, alpha-tocopherol (vitamin E), ascorbic acid (vitamin C), and thiol-containing compounds, notably glutathione. Thus, cells that include neurons are capable of rapidly destroying free radicals, once formed, through both enzymatic and nonenzymatic quenching. Free radicals and reactive oxygen species (superoxide and hydrogen peroxide) cause tissue injury only when the radicals overpower the brain's endogenous antioxidant defenses.

There are two distinct types of superoxide dismutases in mammalian cells: copper-zinc and manganese [Tainer et al., 1983]. Copper-zinc superoxide dismutase is located in the cytosol, whereas manganese superoxide dismutase is located in the mitochondria. Superoxide dismutases are widely distributed throughout the body, but plasma levels are very low as a result of efficient renal clearance [Marklund, 1984].

Copper-zinc superoxide dismutase has been proposed as a therapeutic agent for reperfusion injury because of its ability to scavenge oxygen radicals. Superoxide dismutase has two drawbacks as a therapeutic agent. First, it is cleared rapidly by the kidney and has a circulatory half-life of approximately 8 minutes [Turrens et al., 1984]. Second, and more important, copper-zinc superoxide dismutase is a large, water-soluble molecule and therefore cannot readily penetrate cell membranes or cross the blood-brain barrier in significant quantities after intravenous administration [Beckman et al., 1988; Freeman et al., 1983]. Thus, if access to intracellular compartments is required for therapeutic efficacy, it appears unlikely that copper-zinc superoxide dismutase would provide a protective effect.

Investigators have tried two different modifications in the delivery of superoxide dismutase in an effort to increase the circulatory half-life and intracellular access of the intravenously administered enzyme: liposome-entrapped superoxide dismutase and polyethylene glycol–conjugated superoxide dismutase. Superoxide dismutase delivered in positively charged liposomes has a circulatory half-life of approximately 4 hours and has dramatically increased access into cultured endothelial cells [Freeman et al., 1983; Turrens et al., 1984]. Administration of liposome-entrapped superoxide dismutase produces both increased brain superoxide dismutase activity and reduced extent of infarctions in a rat model of global ischemia [Imaizumi et al., 1990]. Conjugation of polyethylene glycol monomers to superoxide dismutase increases its circulatory half-life to approximately 37 hours and increases its uptake into cultured endothelial cells [Beckman et al., 1988]. However, polyethylene glycol–conjugated superoxide dismutase does not appear to increase brain superoxide dismutase activity [Haun et al., 1991].

Multiple endogenous substances in the brain are capable of scavenging free radicals. The predominant lipid-soluble endogenous free radical scavenger in the brain is alpha-tocopherol. Alpha-tocopherol is incorporated directly into cell membranes and blocks the propagation of lipid peroxidation by interacting with intermediate peroxyl radicals, thus preventing further destruction of other lipids in the cell membrane. There is controversy over whether alpha-tocopherol levels are depleted during brain ischemia and reperfusion.

The amount of oxygen administered during resuscitation also appears to influence the severity of the free radical damage, and the practice of using 100% oxygen during cardiac arrest needs to be re-examined [Feet et al., 1997; Lipinski et al., 1999; Liu et al., 1998; Zwemer et al., 1994].

Interventions directed at pathways indirectly related to free radical generation may be beneficial for reducing oxidative stress in the brain. Hypothermia reduces lipid peroxidation and maintains endogenous antioxidant activity during reperfusion from global brain ischemia [Baiping et al., 1994]. Acidosis during ischemia increases free radical production and may inactivate endogenous antioxidants [Links, 1988]; however, the role of buffer therapy is controversial.

Reduction of Lipid Peroxidation

Lipid-soluble agents rapidly cross the blood-brain barrier, a beneficial property for cerebral resuscitation. Administration of alpha-tocopherol after cerebral ischemia reduces ischemic neuronal damage in gerbils.

Lipid-soluble compounds termed *lazaroids* have been developed to reduce iron-dependent lipid peroxidation after cerebral ischemia. The 21-aminosteroid lazaroids are potent inhibitors of lipid peroxidation but lack classic steroidal activities [Braughler et al., 1987]. The 21-aminosteroids are potent inhibitors of free radical–induced lipid peroxidation, and they have multiple antioxidant actions: (1) scavenging of lipid peroxyl, (2) decreasing formation or scavenging of hydroxyl radicals, (3) reducing lipid peroxidation–induced arachidonic acid release, (4) maintaining the levels of endogenous vitamin E, and (5) membrane stabilization by decreasing membrane fluidity [Hall et al., 1994; Schmid-Elsaesser et al., 1997]. The most extensively studied 21-aminosteroid, U74006F (tirilazad mesylate), appears to possess multiple antioxidant properties; however, preliminary studies of the use of this agent in global cerebral ischemia have yielded mixed results [Sweeney et al., 1995]. An explanation for the limited effect in global ischemia is that tirilazad is lipophilic and therefore accumulates in cell membranes with a high affinity for vascular endothelium. Tirilazad may protect the vascular endothelium from peroxidative damage but is not expected to cross the blood-brain barrier [Schmid-Elsaesser et al., 1997].

Recent experimental study has demonstrated that the lazaroid compound U74389G, administered during cardiac arrest, mitigated postresuscitation myocardial dysfunction and improved survival rates [Wang et al., 2004].

It has been proposed that free radical injury of the brain mainly involves the microvasculature, although both brain parenchyma and vascular endothelium have the potential to generate free radicals [Grammas et al., 1993; Siesjo et al., 1995]. One newly discovered group of antioxidants, the pyrrolopyrimidines, have a significantly greater potential to enter the brain parenchyma. Results of early investigations suggest that these compounds, which are able to cross the blood-brain barrier, may have a greater potential to treat cerebral ischemia [Schmid-Elsaesser et al., 1997].

Iron Chelation

An alternative approach to reducing the production of free radicals is to interfere with intermediates in the formation of free radicals. Transitional metals such as ferrous iron and possibly copper are involved with the formation of free radicals in the brain. A chelating agent such as hydroxyl starch–conjugated deferoxamine, which penetrates the blood-brain barrier and interacts with these metals, can reduce free radical production and may decrease brain injury.

Nitric Oxide Inhibition

As described earlier, nitric oxide could be both beneficial and detrimental to the brain during ischemia and reperfusion. Possible beneficial effects include vasodilation, inhibition of platelet aggregation, and downregulation of NMDA receptors, whereas possible detrimental effects include production of hydroxyl radicals, increased inflammatory effects mediated through inducible nitric oxide synthase, and inhibition of key enzymes necessary for DNA replication and mitochondrial energy production [Choi, 1993]. It is therefore not surprising that animal studies in which nitric oxide synthase inhibitors were used for treatment of cerebral ischemia have yielded both positive and negative results. Nitric oxide synthase inhibitors are analogs of L-arginine, the substrate for nitric oxide synthase. These analogs competitively inhibit the conversion of L-arginine to L-citrulline and nitric oxide.

In animal models, inhibitors of nitric oxide synthesis, including desmethyl tirilazad [Fernandez et al., 1997], 7-nitroindazole [O'Neill et al., 1996], and *N*-omega-nitro-L-arginine [Kohno et al., 1997], have all reduced the effects of global hypoxic-ischemic injury. However, because the competing neurotoxic versus neuroprotective vasodilator effects of nitric oxide remain poorly understood in focal and global ischemic injury, extensive animal and subsequent human clinical research is needed.

Blood Flow Promotion

Cerebral hypoperfusion follows cardiac arrest, including asphyxia-induced cardiac arrest. A brief period of systemic hypertension may improve cerebral blood flow after cardiac arrest. Hypertension early after cardiac arrest is associated with favorable outcome and was reviewed earlier [Sasser et al., 1999].

Modulation/Protein Synthesis

Protein synthesis is essential for cell survival. Proteins are involved in nearly every process in the cell (e.g., enzymatic reactions, transport, storage, intracellular signaling, intercellular signaling, and cytoskeletal support). Obviously, intact protein synthesis is important for cellular recovery after hypoxic-ischemic injury. However, total protein synthesis is impaired after cerebral ischemia [Kleihues and Hossmann, 1971; Nowak et al., 1985]. Inhibition of protein synthesis is slow to recover, requiring hours to days to return to normal levels. The inhibition of protein synthesis is not regionally homogeneous; inhibition is more severe and prolonged in the cortex, hippocampus, and caudate [Bodsch et al., 1986; Widmann et al., 1991]. Failure of protein synthesis to recover after ischemia is the biochemical correlate of cell death. Protein synthesis in neurons of the vulnerable CA1 region of the hippocampus fails to recover after even short periods of ischemia. The inhibition of protein synthesis, which appears to be reperfusion-specific, prevents cells from responding to free radical damage by synthesizing the enzymes necessary to detoxify radicals and repair membrane damage [White et al., 1996].

Although total protein synthesis is decreased after cerebral ischemia, the synthesis of some proteins is actually increased. It is enticing to postulate that these proteins may play an important role in reparative processes after cerebral ischemia; however, it is equally plausible that the selective expression of some genes may contribute to delayed neuronal death, possibly through apoptotic mechanisms [Akins et al., 1996]. Ischemia appears to cause dramatic changes in gene expression [Kogure and Kato, 1993; Sharp et al., 1993]. Genes that have received the most attention in models of cerebral ischemia include the immediate early genes (c-*fos* and c-*jun*), heat shock protein genes, and trophic factor genes. Immediate early genes code for proteins (*fos, jun,* and others) that function as transcription factors and control the expression of many genes in the CNS [Nowak et al., 1993]. Increased expression of c-*fos* and c-*jun* has been demonstrated after global cerebral ischemia [Akins et al., 1996].

Trophic factors appear to be produced in the CNS after ischemic brain injury and may contribute to the repair of damaged cells [Kogure and Kato, 1993]. Fibroblast growth factor and nerve growth factor are two growth factors elaborated in the CNS that appear to be important for the survival and development of neurons. Takami and colleagues [1992] demonstrated increased production of fibroblast growth factor messenger RNA and fibroblast growth factor after global ischemia in the rat. Nerve growth factor levels have also been demonstrated to increase after cerebral ischemia. Both fibroblast growth factor and nerve growth factor, administered by injection into the lateral ventricle, decrease neuronal injury after cerebral ischemia in gerbils [Shigeno et al., 1991; Wen et al., 1995]. Thus, increased expression of growth factors after ischemia appears to be an attempt by the injured brain to prevent further injury and promote repair. Use of neurotrophic factors or novel brain-penetrating neurotrophic factor receptor agonists to prevent neuronal death or to promote regeneration and rewiring of injured brain represents an exciting area of study.

Vascular endothelial growth factor is an angiogenic and neurotrophic peptide whose expression is transcriptionally induced in hypoxic tissues through the action of hypoxia-inducible factor-1a [Jin et al., 2001]. Experimental studies have demonstrated initial upregulation of this factor, followed by increased vascular endothelial growth factor [Pichiule et al., 2003]. These findings suggest that cardiac arrest and resuscitation triggers hypoxia-inducible factor-1a induction, which might be partly responsible for the stimulation of vascular endothelial growth factor expression and the subsequent downstream adaptive mechanisms that might promote recovery.

Insulin is a member of an important group of growth factors that includes insulin-like growth factor-1 and nerve growth factor. There is evidence that members of the insulin growth factor family, when delivered to the brain in the 2 hours after reperfusion, can salvage a percentage of the neurons that would otherwise die [White et al., 1996].

Gene expression after cerebral ischemia is incompletely understood but exciting in that it may provide a mechanism to improve outcome. In animal studies in which gene regulation was examined in a model of hypoxic conditioning in the newborn, preliminary data revealed the potential of manipulating gene regulation after hypoxic insults [Bernaudin et al., 2002].

Anti-inflammatory Therapy

There is evidence of an important role of the inflammatory response after focal and global ischemic injury; this evidence provides alternative approaches directed at the "delayed" onset of treatment of such patients in a hospital setting [Becker, 1998; Lipton et al., 1998; Saikumar et al., 1998].

Inhibition of Arachidonic Acid Metabolism

Although many avenues exist for manipulation of phospholipid-derived mediator formation after global cerebral ischemia or cardiorespiratory arrest, most studies have focused on the arachidonic acid cascade. Pretreatment with cyclooxygenase inhibitors (indomethacin, piroxicam, diclofenac, or ibuprofen) before 5 minutes of global brain ischemia in gerbils attenuated selectively vulnerable cell death [Nakagomi et al., 1989; Sasaki et al., 1988]. In contrast, inhibition of the lipoxygenase pathway did not prevent selectively vulnerable cell death. Prostaglandins potentiate the effects of excitatory amino acids, and inhibition of this effect may explain the protection afforded by these agents. Similarly, inhibition of superoxide anion synthesis during the metabolism of arachidonic acid also may be an important mechanism for this effect. Alternatively, cyclooxygenase metabolites of arachidonic acid are important regulators of normal cerebral blood flow, especially in the immature brain, and cyclooxygenase inhibitors increase cerebral blood flow after global ischemia. However, indomethacin administration after ischemia does not increase cerebral blood flow, and the effect of resuscitation with cyclooxygenase inhibitors on cerebral blood flow after cardiorespiratory arrest has not been studied. A limit to the clinical effectiveness of cyclooxygenase inhibitors may be that a burst of cyclooxygenase product formation occurs within seconds of reperfusion.

Some studies have suggested that an inducible form of cyclooxygenase, cyclooxygenase II, is found after tissue injury [Szczepanski et al., 1994]. This enzyme may be a more appropriate therapeutic target, if prostanoids or arachidonic acid metabolites play an important role in ischemic brain injury.

Glucocorticoids

Glucocorticoids inhibit phospholipase A_2 activity and have a history of use in cerebral resuscitation. The use of corticosteroids as a therapy after cardiorespiratory arrest, however, is unsupported. Pretreatment with dexamethasone in global ischemia models worsened neuronal survival, perhaps because of steroid-induced hyperglycemia. Corticosteroid treatment after global cerebral ischemia in animal models has produced effects ranging from very detrimental to minimally protective. Jastremski and associates [1989] retrospectively assessed the impact of steroid use in the 262 patients who did not receive thiopental in the Brain Resuscitation Clinical Trial I. Four groups (receiving no, low-dose, medium-dose, or high-dose steroid) were compared. No effect on mortality or neurologic outcome was seen.

Hyperbaric Oxygen Treatment

Hyperbaric oxygen treatment has been demonstrated to prolong survival [Krakovsky et al., 1998] and have some neuroprotective properties when used in acute settings in models of global ischemia [Kapp et al., 1982; Takahashi et al., 1992; Zhou et al., 2003]. However, clinical reviews of patients with traumatic brain injury [Longhi and Stochen, 2004] or stroke [Rusyniak et al., 2003] have suggested that it is unlikely to be of benefit, but clinical trials examining the potential benefits versus risk of hyperbaric oxygen treatment have not yet been performed.

Albumin

Albumin treatment has been revealed to have some neuroprotective properties when used acutely in models of global ischemia [Belayev et al., 1999]. Further research is needed to determine whether this would be clinically applicable in studies of adults, as well as of children. Currently, high-dose albumin is being investigated in adult patients with strokes to determine whether it is neuroprotective.

DILEMMA OF NEUROLOGIC MORBIDITY

The CNS is particularly vulnerable to injury from cardiac arrest. Although young children are considered more likely than adults to survive anoxic-ischemic events, much of this pediatric survival appears to result from brainstem recovery. Thus, after prolonged ventilatory support, a child may be more likely to recover the ability to breathe and survive, but there will be little or no return of cortical functions.

Major efforts have been made to discover therapies that improve neurologic recovery after severe brain injuries; much research has been accomplished in the field of brain resuscitation since the mid-1990s. Nevertheless, there currently exists no specific therapy to lessen the incidence of post–cardiac arrest brain damage.

It appears that the duration of hypoxia (from respiratory arrest leading to cardiac arrest), the duration of complete global ischemia (from the beginning of cardiac arrest until resuscitation begins), the duration of incomplete global ischemia (from resuscitation until perfusion is re-established), and the effect of reperfusion injury are the major determinants of brain damage after cardiac arrest. Currently, the outcome of these insults cannot be changed, but as more is learned about the pathophysiology of brain ischemia, ways of preventing secondary brain damage may be found. Because of the tremendous emotional and financial burdens associated with acute and chronic care of children who are severely disabled, minimally conscious, or in a vegetative state after cardiac arrest, the efficiency of resuscitative efforts must be continually evaluated.

Physicians are often faced with decisions about the degree of continued medical support to be given to patients who do not awaken after cardiac arrest and, to a lesser degree, with decisions about specific treatment modalities. The degree of medical support that a patient needs after cardiac arrest is straightforward and is based on medical indications. Certain treatment modalities, such as mechanical ventilation, pharmacologic support of the heart, and intravenous nutrition, however, may be considered heroic or futile by the physician or the family.

Brain damage in these severely injured survivors is typically profound, and long-term improvement is limited. Children in such situations require long-term intensive care, which is financially expensive whether supported at home or in long-term care facilities. In addition to issues of the child's well-being and the financial burden, the effect on the family's quality of life is profound, although difficult to quantify.

Finally, there is evidence that almost one third of cardiac arrest survivors suffer from post-traumatic stress disorder and that the occurrence of this disorder seriously compromises an otherwise satisfying outcome of cost- and resource-intensive medical procedures [Gamper et al., 2004]. Post-traumatic stress disorder leads to an incapacitation that is well beyond the limitations imposed by the organic disease, and it may persist for a long time. This condition may be especially important because it affects predominantly younger patients, seriously compromising their social life [Gamper et al., 2004].

REFERENCES

Abe K, Kogure K, Yamamoto H, et al. Mechanisms of arachidonic acid liberation during ischemia in gerbil brain cerebral cortex. J Neurochem 1987;48:503.

Abramson NS, Safar P, Detre KM, et al. Randomized clinical study of cardiopulmonary cerebral resuscitation: Thiopental loading of comatose cardiac arrest survivors. N Engl J Med 1986;314:397.

Ackerman MJ, Clapham DE. Ion channels—basic science and clinical disease. N Engl J Med 1997;336:1575.

Akins PT, Lin PK, Hsu CY. Immediate early gene expression in response to cerebral ischemia. Stroke 1996;27:1682.

American Academy of Pediatrics AAP Task Force on Infant Positioning and sudden infant death syndrome. Positioning and SIDS. Pediatrics 1992;89:1120.

American Academy of Pediatrics Committee on Injury, Violence, and Poison Prevention. Prevention of drowning in infants, children, and adolescents. Pediatrics 2003;112:437-445.

Ames AI, Wright RL, Kowada M, et al. Cerebral ischemia II. The no-reflow phenomenon. Am J Pathol 1968;52:437.

Andres Arbelaez A, Castillo M, Mukherji SK. Diffusion-weighted MR imaging of global cerebral anoxia. AJNR Am J Neuroradiol 1999;20:999.

Applebaum D. Advanced prehospital care for pediatric emergencies. Ann Emerg Med 1985;14:656.

Arai T, Tsukalara I, Nitta K, et al. Effects of mannitol on cerebral circulation after transient complete cerebral ischemia in dogs. Crit Care Med 1986;14:634.

Ashwal S, Holshouser B, Perkin R, et al. ^{1}H-MRS obtained 3 to 5 days after acute CNS injury predicts outcome in children 18 months or older. Ann Neurol 1995;38:552.

Ashwal S, Holshouser BA, Shu SK, et al. Predictive value fo proton magnetic resonance spectroscopy in pediatric closed head injury. Pediatr Neurol 2000;23:114-125.

Ashwal S, Holshouser BA, Tomasi LG. ^{1}H–magnetic resonance spectroscopy-determined cerebral lactate is associated with poor neurologic outcomes in children with central nervous system disease. Ann Neurol 1997;41:470.

Ashwal S, Perkin RM, Thompson JR, et al. CBF and CBF/P_{CO_2} reactivity in childhood strangulation. Pediatr Neurol 1991;7:369.

Ashwal S, Schneider S, Tomasi L, et al. Prognostic implications of hyperglycemia and reduced cerebral blood flow in childhood near-drowning. Neurology 1990;40:820.

Ashwal S, Schneider S. Pediatric brain death: Current perspectives. In: Barness LA, ed. Advances in pediatrics. Chicago: Mosby–Year Book, 1991;181.

Atkinson E, Mikysa B, Conway JA, et al. Specificity and sensitivity of automated external defibrillator rhythm analysis in infants and children. Ann Emerg Med 2003;42:185.

Atkinson JLD. The neglected prehospital phase of head injury: Apnea and catecholamine surge. Mayo Clin Prac 2000;75:37.

Auld KL, Ashwal S, Holshouser BA, et al. Proton magnetic resonance spectroscopy in children with acute central nervous system injury. Pediatr Neurol 1995;12:323.

Baiping L, Xiujuan T, Hongwei C, et al. Effect of moderate hypothermia on lipid peroxidation in canine tissue after cardiac arrest and resuscitation. Stroke 1994;25:147.

Bari F, Louis TM, Busija DW. Kainate-induced cerebrovascular dilation is resistant to ischemia in piglets. Stroke 1997;28:1272.

Bartus RT, Baker KL, Heiser AD, et al. Postischemic administration of AK275, a calpain inhibitor, provides substantial protection against focal ischemic brain damage. J Cereb Blood Flow Metab 1994;14:537.

Basetti C, Bomio F, Mathis J, et al. Early prognosis in coma after cardiac arrest. J Neurol Neurosurg Psychiatry 1996;61:610.

Bass M, Kravath RE, Glass L. Death-scene investigation in sudden infant death. N Engl J Med 1986;315:100.

Beca J, Cox PN, Taylor MJ, et al. Somatosensory evoked potentials for prediction of outcome in acute severe brain injury. J Pediatr 1995;126:44.

Becker KJ. Inflammation and acute stroke. Curr Opin Neurol 1998;11:45.

Becker LB. Minimizing hypoxic injury during cardiac arrest. New Horiz 1997;5:145.

Beckman JS, Minor RL, White CW, et al. Superoxide dismutase and catalase conjugated to polyethylene glycol increases endothelial enzyme activity and oxidant resistance. J Biol Chem 1988;263:6884.

Beckstead JE, Tweed WA, Lee J, et al. Cerebral blood flow and metabolism in man following cardiac arrest. Stroke 1978;9:569.

Belayev L, Saul I, Huh PW, et al. Neuroprotective effect of high-dose albumin therapy against global ischemic brain injury in rats. Brain Res 1999;845:107.

Bellamy R, Safar P, Tisherman SA, et al. Suspended animation for delayed resuscitation. Crit Care Med 1996;24:S24.

Berek K, Lechleitner P, Luet G, et al. Early determination of neurological outcome after prehospital cardiopulmonary resuscitation. Stroke 1995;26:543.

Berg RA, Otto CW, Kern KB, et al. A randomized, blinded trial of high-dose epinephrine versus standard-dose epinephrine in a swine model of pediatric asphyxial cardiac arrest. Crit Care Med 1996;24:1695.

Bergsneider M, Kelly DF, Shannon E, et al. Early hyperglycolysis following severe human traumatic brain injury: A positron emission tomography study. J Neurotrauma 1995;12:371.

Bernard SA, Buist M. Induced hypothermia in critical care medicine: A review. Crit Care Med 2003;31:2041.

Bernard SA, Gray TW, Buist MD, et al. Treatment of comatose survivors of out-of-hospital cardiac arrest with induced hypothermia. N Engl J Med 2002;346:557.

Bernaudin M, Tang Y, Reilly M, et al. Brain genomic response following hypoxia and re-oxygenation in the neonatal rat. Identification of genes that might contribute to hypoxia-induced ischemic tolerance. J Biol Chem 2002;277:39728.

Berridge MJ, Irvine RF. Inositol triphosphate, a novel second messenger in cellular signal transduction. Nature 1984;312:315.

Beyda DH. The prognostic value of measuring regional cerebral blood flow in the neuro-compromised pediatric patient. In: Wade J, ed. Current problems in neurology: Impact of functional imaging in neurology and psychiatry. London: J. Libbey, 1987;212.

Bhardwaj A, Northington FJ, Ichord RN, et al. Characterization of inotropic glutamate receptor–mediated nitric oxide production in vivo in rats. Stroke 1997;28:850.

Biggart MJ, Bohn DJ. Effect of hypothermia and cardiac arrest on outcome of near-drowning accidents in children. J Pediatr 1990;117:179.

Bodsch W, Barbier A, Ochmichen M, et al. Recovery of monkey brain after prolonged ischemia. II. Protein synthesis and morphological alterations. J Cereb Blood Flow Metab 1986;6:22.

Brain Resuscitation Clinical Trial II Study Group. A randomized clinical study of a calcium-entry blocker (lidoflazine) in the treatment of comatose survivors of cardiac arrest. N Engl J Med 1991;324:1225.

Bratton SL, Jardine DS, Morray JP: Serial neurologic examinations after near drowning and outcome. Arch Pediatr Adolesc Med 1994;148:167.

Braughler JM, Pregenzer JF, Chase RL, et al. Novel 21-amino steroids as potent inhibitors of iron-dependent lipid peroxidation. J Biol Chem 1987;262:10438.

Brierley JB, Meldrum BJ, Brown AW. The threshold and neuropathology of cerebral "anoxic-ischemic" cell change. Arch Neurol 1973;29:367.

Bromont C, Marie C, Bralet J. Increased lipid peroxidation in vulnerable brain regions after transient forebrain ischemia in rats. Stroke 1989;20:918.

Brown CG, Martin DR, Pepe PN, et al. A comparison of standard-dose and high-dose epinephrine in cardiac arrest outside the hospital. N Engl J Med 1992;327:1051.

Brown CG, Werman HA. Adrenergic agonists during cardiopulmonary resuscitation. Resuscitation 1990;19:1.

Buchan AM, Li H, Cho S, et al. Blockade of the AMPA receptor prevents CA1 hippocampal injury following severe but transient forebrain ischemia in adult rats. Neurosci Lett 1991;132:255.

Buja LM, Eigenbrodt ML, Eigenbrodt EH. Apoptosis and necrosis: Basic types and mechanisms of cell death. Arch Pathol Lab Med 1993;117:1208.

Bydder GM, Rutherford MA. Diffusion-weighted imaging of the brain in neonates and infants. Magn Reson Imaging Clin North Am 2001;9:83.

Callahan M, Madsen CD, Barton CW, et al. A randomized clinical trial of high-dose epinephrine and norepinephrine vs. standard-dose epinephrine in prehospital cardiac arrest. JAMA 1992;268:2667.

Cardell M, Boris-Moller F, Wieloch T. Hypothermia prevents the ischemia-induced translocation and inhibition of protein kinase C in rat striatum. J Neurochem 1991;57:1814.

Carpenter TC, Stenmark KR. High-dose epinephrine is not superior to standard-dose epinephrine in pediatric in-hospital cardiopulmonary arrest. Pediatrics 1997;99:403.

Carroll JL, Loughlin GM. Sudden infant death syndrome. Pediatr Rev 1993;14:83.

Chang AB, Wilson SJ, Masters JB, et al. Altered arousal response in infants exposed to cigarette smoke. Arch Dis Child 2003;88:30.

Chen H, Chopp M, Vande Linde AM, et al. The effects of post-ischemic hypothermia on the neuronal injury and brain metabolism after forebrain ischemia in the rat. J Neurol Sci 1992;107:191.

Chen R, Bolton CF, Young GB. Prediction of outcome in patients with anoxic coma: A clinical and electrophysiologic study. Crit Care Med 1996;24:672.

Cherian L, Goodman JL, Robertson CS. Hyperglycemia increases brain injury caused by secondary ischemia after cortical impact injury in rats. Crit Care Med 1997;25:1378.

Choi DW. Nitric oxide: Foe or friend to the injured brain? Proc Natl Acad Sci U S A 1993;90:9741.

Chopp M. Transient hyperthermia protects against subsequent forebrain ischemia damage in the rat. Neurology 1989;39:1396.

Chopp M, Welch KMA, Tidwell CD, et al. Global cerebral ischemia and intracellular pH during hyperglycemia and hypoglycemia in cats. Stroke 1988;19:1383.

Christensen DW, Ashwal S, Perkin RM. Magnesium treatment in childhood near drowning. Proceedings of the Magnesium in Biochemical Process Conference, Ventura, CA, 1996.

Christensen DW, Jansen P, Perkin RM: Outcome and acute care hospital costs after warm water near drowning in children. Pediatrics 1997;99:715.

Cipolla MJ, Porter JM, Osol G. High glucose concentrations dilate cerebral arteries and diminish myogenic tone through an endothelial mechanism. Stroke 1997;28:405.

Clark RS, Kochanek PM, Obrist WD, et al. Cerebrospinal fluid and plasma nitrate and nitrate concentrations after head injury in humans. Crit Care Med 1996;24:1243.

Clark RSB, Kochanek PM, Watkins SC, et al. Caspase-3 mediated neuronal death after traumatic brain injury in rats. J Neurochem 2000;74:740-753.

Cohan SL, Mun SK, Petite J, et al. Cerebral blood flow in humans following resuscitation from cardiac arrest. Stroke 1989;20:761.

Cohen DS, Matthay MA, Cogan MG, et al. Pulmonary edema associated with salt water near-drowning. Am Rev Respir Dis 1992;146:794.

Collard CD, Gelman S. Pathophysiology, clinical manifestations, and prevention of ischemia-reperfusion injury. Anesthesiology 2001;94:1133.

Combs DJ, Dempsey RT, Maley M, et al. Relationship between plasma glucose, brain lactate, and intracellular pH during cerebral ischemia in gerbils. Stroke 1990;21:936.

Conn AN, Barker GA. Fresh water drowning and near-drowning—An update. Can J Anaesth 1984;31:S38.

Dawson DA. Nitric oxide and focal cerebral ischemia: Multiplicity of actions and diverse outcomes. Cerebrovasc Brain Metab Rev 1994;6:299.

Dawson TM, Dawson VL. ADP-ribosylation as a mechanism for the action of nitric oxide in the nervous system. New Horiz 1995;3:86.

Dawson TM, Dawson VL, Snyder SH. A novel neuronal messenger molecule in brain: The free radical nitric oxide. Ann Neurol 1992;32:297.

Dean JM, Kaufman ND. Prognostic indicators in pediatric near-drowning: The Glasgow Coma Scale. Crit Care Med 1981;9:536.

Dean JM, McComb JG. Intracranial pressure monitoring in severe pediatric near-drowning. Neurosurgery 1981;9:627.

DeNicola LK, Falk JL, Swanson ME, et al. Submersion injuries in children. Crit Care Clin 1997;13:477.

Dennery PA. Predicting neonatal brain injury: Are we there yet? Arch Pediatr Adolesc Med 2003;157:1151.

Dieckmann RA, Vardis R. High-dose epinephrine in pediatric out-of-hospital cardiopulmonary arrest. Pediatrics 1995;95:901.

Diemer NH, Valente E, Bruhn T, et al. Glutamate receptor transmission and ischemic nerve cell damage: Evidence for involvement of excitotoxic mechanisms. Prog Brain Res 1993;96:105.

Dietrich WD, Alonso O, Busto R. Moderate hyperglycemia worsens acute blood-brain barrier injury. Stroke 1993;24:111.

Dizon VV, Santanello SA. ED thoracotomy revisited: A complete reassessment of its past, present, and future. Trauma Rep 2003;4(6):1-12.

Does bed sharing affect the risk of SIDS? American Academy of Pediatrics. Task Force on Infant Positioning and SIDS. Pediatrics 1997;100:272.

Dolan MA, Sharma V, Forgue D. SIDS resuscitation: When to stop? Pediatr Emerg Care 1988;4:292.

Dubowitz DJ, Bluml S, Arcinue E, et al. MR of hypoxic encephalopathy

in children after near drowning: Correlation with quantitative proton MR spectroscopy and clinical outcome. Am J Neuroradiol 1998;19:1617.
Dugan LL, Choi DW. Excitotoxicity, free radicals, and cell membrane changes. Ann Neurol 1994;35:S17.
Duhaime AC, Ross DT. Degeneration of hippocampal CA1 neurons following transient ischemia due to raised intracranial pressure: Evidence for a temperature-dependent excitotoxic process. Brain Res 1990;512:169.
du Plessis AJ, Johnston MV. Hypoxic-ischemic brain injury in the newborn. Clin Perinatol 1997;24:627.
Edgren E, Hedstrand U, Nordin M, et al. Prediction of outcome after cardiac arrest. Crit Care Med 1987;15:820.
Eisenberg M, Bergner L, Hallstrom A. Epidemiology of cardiac arrest and resuscitation in children. Ann Emerg Med 1983;12:672.
Erecinska M, Silver IA. ATP and brain function. J Cereb Blood Flow Metab 1989;9:2.
Feet BA, Yu X, Rootwelk T, et al. Effects of hypoxemia and reoxygenation with 21% or 100% oxygen in newborn piglets: Extracellular hypoxanthine in cerebral cortex and femoral muscle. Crit Care Med 1997;25:1384.
Feldman KW, Simms RJ. Strangulation in childhood: Epidemiology and clinical course. Pediatrics 1980;65:1079.
Fernandez MP, Belmonte A, Meizoso MJ, et al. Desmethyl tirilazad reduces brain nitric oxide synthase activity and cyclic guanosine monophosphate during cerebral global transient ischemia in rats. Res Commun Mol Pathol Pharmacol 1997;95:33.
Fields AI. Near-drowning in the pediatric population. Crit Care Clin 1992;8:113.
Fink EL, Alexander H, Marco CD, et al. Experimental model of pediatric asphyxial cardiopulmonary arrest in rats. Pediatr Crit Care Med 2004;5:139.
Fisher B, Peterson B, Hicks G. Use of brain stem auditory evoked response testing to assess neurological outcome following near-drowning in children. Crit Care Med 1992;20:578.
Fleischer JE, Tateishi A, Drummond JL, et al. MK-801, an excitatory amino acid antagonist, does not improve neurologic outcome following cardiac arrest in cats. J Cereb Blood Flow Metab 1989;9:795.
Fogel W, Krieger D, Veith M, et al. Serum neuron-specific enolase as early predictor of outcome after cardiac arrest. Crit Care Med 1997;25:1133.
Fontanarosa PB. Electrical shock and lightning strike. Ann Emerg Med 1993;22:378.
Frank SE. High-dose epinephrine in cardiopulmonary resuscitation: Are we missing the question? Crit Care Med 1994;22:2030.
Frates RC. Analysis of predictive factors in the assessment of warm water near-drowning in children. Am J Dis Child 1981;135:1006.
Freeman BA, Young SL, Crapo ID. Liposome-mediated augmentation of superoxide dismutase in endothelial cells prevents oxygen injury. J Biol Chem 1983;258:12534.
Frewen TC, Sumabat WO, Han K, et al. Cerebral resuscitation therapy in pediatric near-drowning. J Pediatr 1985;106:615.
Friesen RM, Duncan P, Tweed WA, et al. Appraisal of pediatric cardiopulmonary resuscitation. Can Med Assoc J 1982;126:1055.
Gamper G, Willeit M, Sterz F, et al. Life after death: Posttraumatic stress disorder in survivors of cardiac arrest—Prevalence, associated factors, and the influence of sedation and analgesic. Crit Care Med 2004;32:378.
Garcia AA, Cabanas F, Pellicer A, et al. Neuron-specific enolase and myelin basic protein: Relationship of cerebrospinal fluid concentrations to the neurologic condition of asphyxiated full-term infants. Pediatrics 1994;93:234.
Gausche M. Differences in the out-of-hospital care of children and adults: More questions than answers. Ann Emerg Med 1997;29:776.
Gazmuri RJ, Weil MH, Bisera J, et al. Myocardial dysfunction after successful resuscitation from cardiac arrest. Crit Care Med 1996;24:992.
Gazzolo D, Marinoni E, Dilorio R, et al. Urinary S-100B protein measurements: A tool for the early identification of hypoxic-ischemic encephalopathy in asphyxiated full-term infants. Crit Care Med 2004;32:131.
Geddes JF, Vowles GH, Hackshaw AK, et al. Neuropathology of inflicted head injury in children II. Microscopic brain injury in infants. Brain 2001;124:1299.
Gilbert-Barness E, Barness L. Sudden infant death: A reappraisal. Contemp Pediatr 1995;12:88.
Gillenwater JM, Quan L, Feldman KW: Inflicted submersion in childhood. Arch Pediatr Adolesc Med 1996;150:298.
Gillis J, Dickson D, Rieder M, et al. Results of inpatient pediatric resuscitation. Crit Care Med 1986, 14:469.
Gisselsson L, Smith ML, Siesjo BK. Influence of preischemic hyperglycemia on osmolality and early postischemic edema in the rat. J Cereb Blood Flow Metab 1992;12:809.
Gisvold S, Sterz F, Abramson NS, et al. Cerebral resuscitation from cardiac arrest: Treatment potentials. Crit Care Med 1996;24:S69.
Goetting MG. Mastering pediatric cardiopulmonary resuscitation. Pediatr Clin North Am 1994;41:1147.
Goetting MG, Paradis NA. High-dose epinephrine improves outcome from pediatric cardiac arrest. Ann Emerg Med 1991;20:22.
Gonzalez MF, Lowenstein D, Fernyak S, et al. Induction of heat shock protein 72–like immunoreactivity in the hippocampal formation following transient global ischemia. Brain Res Bull 1991;26:241.
Gooden B. Drowning and the diving reflex in man. Med J Aust 1972;2:583.
Goyco PG, Beckerman RC. Sudden infant death syndrome. Curr Probl Pediatr 1990;6:299.
Graf WD, Cummings P, Quan L, et al. Predicting outcome in pediatric submersion victims. Ann Emerg Med 1995;26:312.
Grammas P, Liu GJ, Wood K, et al. Anoxia/reoxygenation induces hydroxyl free radical formation in brain microvessels. Free Radic Biol Med 1993;14:553.
Grotta JL, Picone CM, Earls R, et al. Calcium-calmodulin binding in ischemic rat neurons after calcium channel blocker therapy. Stroke 1990;21:948.
Guerit JM, de Tourtchaninoff M, Soveges L, et al. The prognostic value of three-modality evoked potentials (TMEPs) in anoxic and traumatic comas. Neurophysiol Clin 1993;23:209.
Habib DM, Tecklenburg FW, Webb SA, et al. Prediction of childhood drowning and near-drowning morbidity and mortality. Pediatr Emerg Care 1996;12:255.
Hall ED, McCall JM, Means ED. Therapeutic potential of the lazaroids (21-aminosteroids) in acute central nervous system trauma, ischemia and subarachnoid hemorrhage. Adv Pharmacol 1994;28:221.
Halperin HR, Chandra NL, Levin HR, et al. Newer methods of improving blood flow during CPR. Ann Emerg Med 1996;27:553.
Han BK, Towbin RB, De Courten Myers G, et al. Reversal sign on CT: Effect of anoxic/ischemic cerebral injury in children. AJR Am J Roentgenol 1990;154:361.
Hanigan WC, Aldag J, Sabo RA, et al. Strangulation injuries in children. Part 2. Cerebrovascular hemodynamics. J Trauma 1996;40:73.
Haun SE, Kirsch JR, Dean JM. Theories of brain resuscitation. In: Rogers MC, ed. Textbook of pediatric intensive care. Baltimore: Williams & Wilkins, 1996;699.
Haun SE, Kirsch JR, Helfaer MA, et al. Polyethylene glycol-conjugated superoxide dismutase fails to augment brain superoxide dismutase activity in piglets. Stroke 1991;22:655.
Hazinski MF, Chahine AA, Holcomb GW, et al. Outcome of cardiovascular collapse in pediatric blunt trauma. Ann Emerg Med 1994;23:1229.
Hazinski MF, Markenson D, Neish S, et al. Response to cardiac arrest and selected life-threatening medical emergencies: The medical emergency response plan for schools. Pediatrics 2004;113:155.
Hickey RW, Cohen DM, Strausbaugh S, et al. Pediatric patients requiring CPR in the prehospital setting. Ann Emerg Med 1995;25:495.
Hickey RW, Kochanek PM, Ferimer H, et al. Induced hyperthermia exacerbates neurologic neuronal histologic damage after asphyxial cardiac arrest in rats. Crit Care Med 2003;31:531.
Hickey RW, Zuckerbraun NS. Pediatric cardiopulmonary arrest: Current concepts and future directions. Pediatr Emerg Med Rep 2003;8:1.
Hockenbery D. Defining apoptosis. Am J Pathol 1995;146:16.
Hoffman HJ, Damus K, Hillman L, et al. Risk factors for SIDS: Results of the National Institute of Child Health and Human Development SIDS Cooperative Epidemiological Study. Ann N Y Acad Sci 1988;533:13.
Hoffman HJ, Hillman LS. Epidemiology of the sudden infant death syndrome: Maternal, neonatal, and post neonatal risk factors. Clin Perinatol 1992;19:717.
Holshouser BA, Ashwal S, Luh GY, et al. Proton MR spectroscopy after acute central nervous system injury: Outcome prediction in neonates, infants and children. Radiology 1997;202:487.
Horne RSC, Ferens D, Watts AM, et al. Effects of maternal tobacco smoking, sleeping position, and sleep state on arousal in healthy term infants. Arch Dis Child Fetal Neonatal Ed 2002;87:F100.

Hsu SS, Meno JR, Ahou JG, et al. Influence of hyperglycemia on cerebral adenosine production during ischemia and reperfusion. Am J Physiol 1991;261:H398.

Hunt CE. The cardiorespiratory control hypothesis for SIDS. Clin Perinatol 1992;19:757.

Hypothermia after Cardiac Arrest Group. Mild therapeutic hypothermia to improve the neurologic outcome after cardiac arrest. N Engl J Med 2002;346:549.

Imaizumi S, Woolworth V, Fishman RA, et al. Liposome-entrapped superoxide dismutase reduces cerebral infarction in cerebral ischemia in rats. Stroke 1990;21:1312.

Jacinto SS, Gieron-Korthals M, Ferreira JA. Predicting outcome in hypoxic-ischemic brain injury. Pediatr Clin North Am 2001;48:647.

Jacobs MB, Gieron MA, Martinez CR, et al. Basal ganglia injury after cardiopulmonary arrest: Clinical and magnetic resonance imaging correlation. Am J Dis Child 1990;144:937.

Jacobsen WK, Mason LJ, Briggs BA, et al. Correlation of spontaneous respiration and neurological damage in near-drowning. Crit Care Med 1983;11:487.

Jastremski M, Sutton-Tyrell K, Vaagenes P, et al. Glucocorticoid treatment does not improve neurological recovery following cardiac arrest. JAMA 1989;262:3427.

Jin K, Mao XO, Eshoo MW, et al. Microarray analysis of hippocampal gene expression in global cerebral ischemia. Ann Neurol 2001;50:93.

Johnson DL, Boal D, Baule R. Role of apnea in nonaccidental head injury. Pediatr Neurosurg 1995;23:305.

Jumas A, Brenner RP. Myoclonic status epilepticus: A clinical and electroencephalographic study. Neurology 1990;40:1199.

Jumbelic M, Chambliss M. Accidental toddler drowning in 5-gallon buckets. JAMA 1990;263:1952.

Kalimo H, Rehncrone S, Soderfeldt B, et al. Brain lactic acidosis and ischemic cell damage: 2. Histopathology. J Cereb Blood Flow Metab 1981;1:313.

Kapp JP, Phillips M, Markov A, et al. Hyperbaric oxygen after circulatory arrest: Modification of postischemic encephalopathy. Neurosurgery 1982;11:496.

Karkela J, Pasanen M, Kaukinen S, et al. Evaluation of hypoxic brain injury with spinal fluid enzymes, lactate, and pyruvate. Crit Care Med 1992;20:378.

Kato I, Groswasser J, Franco P, et al. Developmental characteristics of apnea in infants who succumb to sudden infant death syndrome. Am J Respir Crit Care Med 2001;164:1461.

Kawai N, Keep RF, Betz AL. Hyperglycemia and the vascular effects of cerebral ischemia. Stroke 1997;28:149.

Kemp AM, Stoodley N, Cobley C, et al. Apnea and brain swelling in nonaccidental head injury. Arch Dis Child 2003;88:472.

Kim H, Koehler RL, Hurn PD, et al. Amelioration of impaired cerebral metabolism after severe acidotic ischemia by tirilazad post-treatment in dogs. Stroke 1996;27:114.

Kleihues P, Hossmann KA. Protein synthesis in the cat brain after prolonged cerebral ischemia. Brain Res 1971;35:409.

Kochanek PM. Ischemic and traumatic brain injury: Pathobiology and cellular mechanisms. Crit Care Med 1993;21:S333.

Kochanek PM, Clark RS, Ruppel RA, et al: Cerebral resuscitation after traumatic brain injury and cardiopulmonary arrest in infants and children in the new millennium. Pediatr Clin North Am 2001;48:661.

Kogure K, Kato H. Altered gene expression after brain ischemia. Stroke 1993;24:2121.

Kohno K, Higuchi T, Ohta S, et al. Neuroprotective nitric oxide synthase inhibitor reduces intracellular calcium accumulation following transient global ischemia in the gerbil. Neurosci Lett 1997;224:17.

Koistinaho J, Hokfelt T. Altered gene expression in brain ischemia. Neuroreport 1997;8(2):i.

Komara JS, Nayini NR, Bialick HA, et al. Brain iron delocalization and lipid peroxidation following cardiac arrest. Ann Emerg Med 1986;15:384.

Kontos HA. Oxygen radicals from arachidonate metabolism in abnormal vascular responses. Am Rev Respir Dis 1987;136:474.

Krakovsky M, Rogatsky G, Zarchin N, Mayevsky A. Effect of hyperbaric oxygen therapy on survival after global cerebral ischemia in rats. Surg Neurol 1998;49:412.

Krause GS, White BC, Aust SD, et al. Brain cell death following ischemia and reperfusion: A proposed biochemical sequence. Crit Care Med 1988;16:714.

Kreis R, Arcinue E, Ernst T, et al. Hypoxic encephalopathy after near-drowning studied by quantitative 1H–magnetic resonance spectroscopy. J Clin Invest 1996;97:1142.

Kriel RL, Krach LE, Luxenberg MG, et al. Outcome of severe anoxic/ischemic brain injury in children. Pediatr Neurol 1994;10:207.

Krol LV, Wolfe R. The emergency department management of near-hanging victims. J Emerg Med 1994;12:285.

Krumholz A, Stern BJ, Weiss HD. Outcome from coma after cardiopulmonary resuscitation: Relation to seizures and myoclonus. Neurology 1988;38:401.

Kumar VR, Bachman DT, Kiskaddon RT. Children and adults in cardiopulmonary arrest: Are advanced life support guidelines followed in the prehospital setting? Ann Emerg Med 1997;29:743.

Kuroiwa T, Bonnekoh P, Hossmann KA. Therapeutic window of CA1 neuronal damage defined by an ultra short-acting barbiturate after brain ischemia in gerbils. Stroke 1990;21:1489.

Kushner M, Nencini P, Reivich M, et al. Relation of hyperglycemia early in ischemic brain infarction to cerebral anatomy, metabolism, and clinical outcome. Ann Neurol 1990;28:129.

Kyriacou DN, Arcinue EL, Peck C, Kraus JF. Effect of immediate resuscitation on children with submersion injury. Pediatrics 1994;94:137.

Lanier WL, Perkins WJ, Karlsson BR, et al. The effects of dizocilpine maleate (MK-801), an antagonist of *N*-methyl-D-aspartate receptor, on neurologic recovery and histopathology following complete cerebral ischemia in primates. J Cereb Blood Flow Metab 1990;10:252.

Lanier WL, Stangland KJ, Scheithaur BW, et al. The effects of dextrose infusion and head position on neurologic outcome after complete cerebral ischemia in primates: Examination of a model. Anesthesiology 1987;66:39.

Laudignon N, Beharry K, Farri E, et al. The role of adenosine in the vascular adaptation of neonatal cerebral blood flow during hypotension. J Cereb Blood Flow Metab 1991;11:424.

Lavelle JM, Shaw KN. Near drowning: Is emergency department cardiopulmonary resuscitation or intensive care unit cerebral resuscitation indicated? Crit Care Med 1993;21:368.

Lavelle JM, Shaw KN, Seidl T, Ludwig S. Ten-year review of pediatric bathtub near-drownings: Evaluation for child abuse and neglect. Ann Emerg Med 1995;25:344.

Levy DE, Caronna JJ, Singer BH, et al. Predicting outcome from hypoxic-ischemic coma. JAMA 1985;253:1420.

Lewis J, Minter M, Eshlman L, et al. Outcome of pediatric resuscitation. Ann Emerg Med 1983;12:297.

Li H, Buchan AM. Treatment with an AMPA antagonist 12 hours following severe normothermic forebrain ischemia prevents CA1 neuronal injury. J Cereb Blood Flow Metab 1993;13:933.

Li Y, Chopp M, Jiang N, et al. Temporal profile of in situ DNA for augmentation after transient middle cerebral artery occlusion in the rat. J Cereb Blood Flow Metab 1995;15:389.

Liberthson RR. Sudden death from cardiac conditions in children and young adults. N Engl J Med 1996;334:1039.

Lin TN, Te J, Huang HC, et al. Prolongation and enhancement of postischemic c-fos expression after fasting. Stroke 1997;28:412.

Lindner KH, Strohmenger HU, Ensinger H, et al. Stress hormone response during and after cardiopulmonary resuscitation. Anesthesiology 1992;77:662.

Links E. The mechanism of pH-dependent hydrogen peroxide cytotoxicity in vitro. Arch Biochem Biophys 1988;265:362.

Lipinski CA, Hicks SD, Callaway CS. Normoxic ventilation during resuscitation and outcome from asphyxial cardiac arrest in rats. Resuscitation 1999;42:221.

Lipton JM, Catania A, Delgado R. Peptide modulation of inflammatory processes within the brain. Neuroimmunomodulation 1998;5:178.

Lipton SA, Rosenberg PA. Excitatory amino acids as a final common pathway for neurologic disorders. N Engl J Med 1994;330:613.

Lister G, Fontan JJP. Can resuscitation jeopardize survival? N Engl J Med 2004;305:1708.

Liu PK, Arora T. Transcripts of damaged genes in the brain during cerebral oxidative stress. J Neurosci Res 2002;70:713.

Liu PK, Grossman RG, Hsu CY, Robertson CS. Ischemic injury and faulty gene transcripts in the brain. Trends Neurosci 2001;24:581.

Liu Y, Rosenthal RE, Haywood Y, et al. Normoxic ventilation after cardiac arrest reduces oxidation of brain lipids and improves neurological outcome. Stroke 1998;29:1679.

Ljunggren B, Norbery K, Siesjo BK. Influence of tissue acidosis upon restitution of brain energy metabolism following total ischemia. Brain Res 1974;77:173.

Loepke AW, Spaeth JP. Glucose and heart surgery: Neonates are not just small adults. Anesthesiology 2004;100:1339.

Longhi L, Stocchetti N. Hyperoxia in head injury: Therapeutic tool? Curr Opin Crit Care 2004;10:105.

Longstreth WT. The neurologic sequelae of cardiac arrest. West J Med 1987;147:175.

Love T, Darby J, Yonas H, et al. CO_2 reactivity and CBF in comatose survivors of cardiac arrest. Crit Care Med 1989;17:346.

Lucking SE, Pollack MM, Fields AI. Shock following generalized hypoxic-ischemic injury in previously healthy infants and children. J Pediatr 1986;108:359.

Mackey ME, Win Y, Hu R, et al. Cell death suggestive of apoptosis after spinal cord ischemia in rabbits. Stroke 1997;28:2012.

Madl C, Kramer L, Yeganehfar W, et al. Detection of nontraumatic comatose patients with no benefit of intensive care treatment by recording of sensory evoked potentials. Arch Neurol 1996;53:512.

Mandel R, Martinot A, Delepoulle F, et al. Prediction of outcome after hypoxic-ischemic encephalopathy: A prospective clinical and electrophysiologic study. J Pediatr 2002;141:45.

Mann NC, Weller SC, Ranchschwalbe R: Bucket-related drownings in the United States, 1984 through 1990. Pediatrics 1992;89:1068.

Marion DW, Leonov Y, Ginsberg M, et al. Resuscitative hypothermia. Crit Care Med 1996;24:S81.

Marklund SL. Extracellular superoxide dismutase in human tissues and human cell lines. J Clin Invest 1984;74:1398.

Maron BJ. Sudden death in young athletes. N Engl J Med 2003;349:1064.

Maron BJ, Gohman TE, Kyle SB, et al. Clinical profile and spectrum of commotio cordis. JAMA 2002;287:1142.

McCulloch J. Excitatory amino acid antagonists and their potential for the treatment of ischaemic brain damage in man. Br J Clin Pharmacol 1992;34:106.

McIntyre KM. Vasopressin in asystolic cardiac arrest. N Engl J Med 2004;350:179.

McNamara F, Sullivan CE. Obstructive sleep apnea in infants: Relation to family history of sudden infant death syndrome, apparent life-threatening events, and obstructive sleep apnea. J Pediatr 2000;136:318.

Meny RG, Carroll JL, Carbone MT, et al. Cardiorespiratory recordings from infants dying suddenly and unexpectedly at home. Pediatrics 1994;93:44.

Michelson DJ, Ashwal S. Evaluation of coma and brain death. Semin Pediatr Neurol 2004;11:105.

Michenfelder JD, Milde JH. Postischemic canine cerebral blood flow appears to be determined by cerebral metabolic needs. J Cereb Blood Flow Metab 1990;10:71.

Milde LN, Milde JH, Michenfelder JD. Delayed treatment with nimodipine improves cerebral blood flow after complete cerebral ischemia in the dog. J Cereb Blood Flow Metab 1986;6:332.

Miller LP, Hsu C. Therapeutic potential for adenosine receptor activation in ischemic brain injury. J Neurotrauma 1992;9:S563.

Mitani A, Yanase H, Sakai K, et al. Origin of intracellular Ca^{2+} elevation induced by in vitro ischemia-like condition in hippocampal slices. Brain Res 1993;601:103.

Modell JH. Serum electrolyte changes in near-drowning victims. JAMA 1985;253:253.

Modell JH, Graves SA, Kuch EJ. Near-drowning: Correlation of level of consciousness and survival. Can J Anaesth 1980;27:211.

Moncada S, Higgs A. The L-arginine-nitric oxide pathway. N Engl J Med 1993;329:2002.

Morgenstern LB, Pettigrew LC. Brain protection: Human data and potential new therapies. New Horiz 1997;5:397.

Morii S, Ngai AC, Ko KR, et al. Role of adenosine in regulation of cerebral blood flow: Effects of theophylline during normoxia and hypoxia. Am J Physiol 1987;253:H165.

Morimoto Y, Kemmotsu O, Kitami K, et al. Acute brain swelling after out-of hospital cardiac arrest: Pathogenesis and outcome. Crit Care Med 1993;21:104.

Morris ML, Nadkarni VM. Pediatric cardiopulmonary-cerebral resuscitation: An overview and future directions. Crit Care Clin 2003;19:337.

Muizelaar JP, Marmaron A, Ward JD, et al. Adverse effects of prolonged hyperventilation in patients with severe head injury: A randomized clinical trial. J Neurosurg 1991;75:731.

Mullie A, Baylaert W, Michum N, et al. Predictive value of Glasgow coma score for awakening after out-of-hospital arrest. Lancet 1988;1:137.

Mussack T, Biberthaler P, Kanz K, et al. Serum S-100B and interleukin-8 as predictive markers for comparative neurologic outcome analysis of patients after cardiac arrest and severe traumatic brain injury. Crit Care Med 2002;30:2669.

Nakagomi T, Saski T, Kirino T, et al. Effect of cyclooxygenase and lipoxygenase inhibitors on delayed neuronal death in the gerbil hippocampus. Stroke 1989;20:925.

Nakanishi S. Molecular diversity of glutamate receptors and implications for brain function. Science 1992;258:597.

Narula J, Haider N, Virmani R, et al. Apoptosis in myocytes in end-stage heart failure. N Engl J Med 1996;335:1189.

Nellgard B, Wicloch T. Postischemic blockade of AMPA but not NMDA receptors mitigates neuronal damage in the rat brain following transient severe cerebral ischemia. J Cereb Blood Flow Metab 1992;12:2.

Nichols DG, Kettrick RG, Swedlow DB, et al. Factors influencing outcome of cardiopulmonary resuscitation in children. Pediatr Emerg Care 1986;2:1.

Nichter MA, Everett PB. Childhood near-drowning: Is cardiopulmonary resuscitation always indicated? Crit Care Med 1989;17:993.

Nielsen VG, Tan S, Baird MS, et al. Xanthine oxidase mediates myocardial injury after hepatoenteric ischemia-reperfusion. Crit Care Med 1997;25:1044.

Nitatori T, Sato N, Waguri S, et al. Delayed neuronal death in the CA1 pyramidal cell layer of the gerbil hippocampus following transient ischemia in apoptosis. J Neurosci 1995;15:100.

Nolan JP, Nadkarni V, Montgomery WH. Vasopressin versus epinephrine for cardiopulmonary resuscitation. N Engl J Med 2004;350:2206.

Nowak TS Jr, Fried RL, Lust WD, et al. Changes in brain energy metabolism and protein synthesis following transient bilateral ischemia in the gerbil. J Neurochem 1985;44:487.

Nowak TS Jr, Osborne OC, Suga S. Stress protein and proto-oncogene expression as indicators of neuronal pathophysiology after ischemia. Prog Brain Res 1993;96:195.

Nussbaum E, Galant SP: Intracranial pressure monitoring as a guide to prognosis in the nearly drowned, severely comatose child. J Pediatr 1983;102:215.

Oliver CN, Starke-Reed PE, Stadtman E, et al. Oxidative damage to brain proteins, loss of glutamine synthetase activity, and production of free radicals during ischemia/reperfusion injury to gerbil brain. Proc Natl Acad Sci U S A 1990;87:5144.

O'Neill MJ, Hicks C, Ward M. Neuroprotective effects of 7-nitroindazole in the gerbil model of global cerebral ischemia. Eur J Pharmacol 1996;310:115.

Orlowski JP. Prognostic factors in pediatric cases of drowning and near-drowning. J Am Coll Emerg Phys 1979;8:176.

Orlowski JP. Drowning, near-drowning, and ice-water submersions. Pediatr Clin North Am 1987;34:75.

Orlowski JP, Szpilman D. Drowning: Rescue, resuscitation, and reanimation. Pediatr Clin North Am 2001;48:627.

O'Rourke PP. Outcome of children who are apneic and pulseless in the emergency room. Crit Care Med 1986;14:466.

Paradis NA, Wenzel V, Southall J. Pressor drugs in the treatment of cardiac arrest. Cardiol Clin 2002;20:61.

Parker BL, Frewen TC, Levin SD, et al. Declaring pediatric brain death: Current practice in a Canadian pediatric critical care unit. Can Med Assoc J 1995;153:909.

Papadopoulos MC, Giffard RG, Bell BA. An introduction to the changes in gene expression that occur after cerebral ischaemia. Br J Neurosurg 2000;14:305.

Patten BM. Lightning and electrical injuries. Neurol Clin 1992;10:1047.

Pellock JM. Status epilepticus in children: Update and review. J Child Neurol 1994;9:2S27.

Perkin RM. Sudden infant death syndrome: What it is, and what it is not. Pediatr Emerg Med Rep 2004;9(2):13.

Perkin RM, Jansen P, Ashwal S. Status epilepticus in 149 consecutive pediatric patients. Pediatrics 1996;98:547.

Perkin RM, van Stralen DW. Facts and dilemmas: Resuscitating pediatric cardiac arrest victims. J Emerg Med Serv 1992;17:68.

Perondi MBM, Reis AG, Paiva EF, et al. A comparison of high-dose and standard-dose epinephrine in children with cardiac arrest. N Engl J Med 2004;350:1722.

Peterson DR. The epidemiology of sudden infant death syndrome. In: Culbertson JL, Krons HF, Bendell RD, eds. Sudden infant death syndrome: Medical aspects and psychological management. Baltimore: Johns Hopkins University Press, 1988.

Pichiule P, Agani F, Chavez JC, et al. HIF-1 alpha and VEGF expression after transient global cerebral ischemia. Adv Exp Med Biol 2003;530:611.

Pitt WR, Balanda KP. Childhood drowning and near-drowning in Brisbane: The contribution of domestic pools. Med J Aust 1991;154:661.

Polderman KH. Application of therapeutic hypothermia in the ICU: Opportunities and pitfalls of a promising treatment modality. Part 1: Indications and evidence. Intensive Care Med 2004;30:556.

Positioning and sudden infant death syndrome (SIDS): Update. American Academy of Pediatrics Task Force on Infant Positioning and SIDS. Pediatrics 1996;98:1216.

Pratt FD, Haynes BE. Incidence of secondary drowning after saltwater submersion. Ann Emerg Med 1986;15:1084.

Present P. Childhood drowning study, a report on the epidemiology of drowning in residential pools in children under age five. Washington, DC: Consumer Product Safety Commission, 1987.

Prough DS, Zornow MH. Global cerebral ischemia in humans: How long is too long? Crit Care Med 1997;25:1776.

Pulsinelli W, Sarokin A, Buchan A. Antagonism of the NMDA and non-NMDA receptors in global versus focal ischemia. Prog Brain Res 1993;96:125.

Pulsinelli WA, Waldman S, Rawlinson D, et al. Moderate hyperglycemia augments ischemic brain damage: A neuropathological study in the rat. Neurology 1982;32:1239.

Quan L, Gure EJ, Wentz K, et al. Ten-year study of pediatric drownings and near-drownings in Kings County, Washington: Lessons in injury prevention. Pediatric 1989;83:1035.

Quan L, Kinder D. Pediatric submersions: Prehospital predictors of outcome. Pediatrics 1992;90:909.

Quan L, Wentz KR, Gore EJ, et al. Outcome and predictors of outcome in pediatric submersion victims receiving prehospital care in King County, Washington. Pediatrics 1990;86:586.

Qureshi AI. Evaluation of brain injury using a blood test: Is there a role in clinical practice? Crit Care Med 2002;30:2778.

Raghupathi R, Welsh FA, Lowenstein DH, et al. Regional induction of c-fos and heat shock protein-72 mRNA following fluid-percussion brain injury in the rat. J Cereb Blood Flow Metab 1995;15:467.

Rink AD, Fung KM, Perri BR, et al. Traumatic brain injury induces apoptosis. J Neurotrauma 1995;12:424.

Robertson CM, Joffe AR, Moore AJ, et al: Neurodevelopmental outcome of young pediatric intensive care unit survivors of serious brain injury. Pediatr Crit Care Med 2002;3:345.

Robinson LR, Mickleson PJ, Tirschwell DL, et al. Predictive value of somatosensory evoked potentials for awakening from coma. Crit Care Med 2003;31:960.

Rogers MC, Kirsch JR. Current concepts in brain resuscitation. JAMA 1989;261:3143.

Roine RO, Kaste M, Kinnunen A, et al. Nimodipine after resuscitation from out-of-hospital ventricular fibrillation. A placebo-controlled, double-blind, randomized trial JAMA 1990;264:3171.

Romano C, Brown T, Freuson TC. Assessment of pediatric near-drowning victims: Is there a role for cranial CT? Pediatr Radiol 1993;23:261.

Ronco R, King W, Donley DK, et al. Outcome and cost at a children's hospital following resuscitation for out-of-hospital cardiorespiratory arrest. Arch Pediatr Adolesc Med 1995;149:210.

Rosenberg NM. Pediatric cardiopulmonary arrest in the emergency department. Am J Emerg Med 1984;2:497.

Ross B, Michaelis T. Clinical applications of magnetic resonance spectroscopy. Magn Reson Q 1994;10:191.

Rudolphi KA, Schubert P. Purinergic interventions in traumatic and ischemic injury. In: Peterson PL, Phillis JW, eds. Novel therapies for CNS injuries: Rationales and results. Boca Raton, FL: CRC Press, 1996;112.

Rusyniak DE, Kirk MA, May JD, et al. Hyperbaric oxygen therapy in acute ischemic stroke: Results of the Hyperbaric Oxygen in Acute Ischemic Stroke Trial Pilot Study. Stroke 2003;34:571.

Ruth VJ, Park TS, Gonzales ER, et al. Adenosine and cerebrovascular hyperemia during insulin-induced hypoglycemia in newborn piglets. Am J Physiol (Heart Circ Physiol) 1993;267:H1762.

Sabo RA, Hanigan WC, Flessner K, et al. Strangulation injuries in children. Part 1. Clinical analysis. J Trauma 1996;40:68.

Safar P. Cerebral resuscitation after cardiac arrest: Research initiatives and future directions. Ann Emerg Med 1993;22:324.

Safar P. Resuscitation medicine research: Quo vadis. Ann Emerg Med 1996;27:542.

Safar PJ, Kochanek PM. Therapeutic hypothermia after cardiac arrest. N Engl J Med 2002;346:612.

Safar P, Xiao F, Radovsky A, et al. Improved cerebral resuscitation from cardiac arrest in dogs with mild hypothermia plus blood flow promotion. Stroke 1996;27:105.

Saikumar P, Dong Z, Weinberg JM, et al. Mechanisms of cell death in hypoxia/reoxygenation injury. Oncogene 1998;17:33.

Samdani AF, Dawson TM, Dawson VL. Nitric oxide sÿnthase in models of focal ischemia. Stroke 1997;28:1283.

Sarnaik AP, Preston G, Lich-Lai M, et al. Intracranial pressure and cerebral perfusion pressure in near-drowning. Crit Care Med 1985;13:224.

Sasaki T, Nakagomi T, Kirino T, et al. Indomethacin ameliorates ischemic neuronal damage in the gerbil hippocampal CA1 sector. Stroke 1988;19:1399.

Sasser HC, Safar P, Kelsey SF, et al. Arterial hypertension after cardiac arrest is associated with good cerebral outcome in patients. Crit Care Med 1999;27:A29.

Schectman VL, Harper RM. Minute-by-minute association of heart rate variation with basal heart rate in developing infants. Sleep 1993;16:23.

Schindler MB, Bohn D, Cox PN, et al. Outcome of out-of-hospital cardiac or respiratory arrest in children. N Engl J Med 1996;335:1473.

Schmid-Elsaesser R, Zansinger S, Hungerhuber E, et al. Superior neuroprotective efficacy of a novel antioxidant with improved blood-brain barrier permeability in focal cerebral ischemia. Stroke 1997;28:2018.

Schmidley JW. Free radicals in central nervous system ischemia. Curr Concepts Cerebrovasc Dis Stroke 1990;25:7.

Schnaper HW. Apoptosis: Death as a vital biological function. Pediatr Nephrol 1994;8:377.

Scollo-Lavizzari G, Bassetti C. Prognostic value of EEG in postanoxic coma after cardiac arrest. Eur Neurol 1987;26:161.

Scott SM, Wiebe RA. Near-hanging and choking injury. In: Levin DL, Moriss FL, eds. Essentials of pediatric intensive care. New York: Churchill Livingstone, 1997;999.

Sessler DI. Mild perioperative hypothermia. N Engl J Med 1997;336:1730.

Sharp FR, Kinouchi H, Koistinaho J, et al. HSP 70 heat shock gene regulation during ischemia. Stroke 1993;24:172.

Sheikh A, Brogan T. Outcome and cost of open- and closed-chest cardiopulmonary resuscitation in pediatric cardiac arrests. Pediatrics 1994;93:392.

Sherdown MJ, Suzdak PD, Nordholm L. AMPA, but not NMDA, receptor antagonism is neuroprotective in gerbil global ischemia, even when delayed 24 hours. Eur J Pharmacol 1993;236:347.

Shigeno T, Mima T, Takakura K, et al. Amelioration of delayed neuronal death in the hippocampus by nerve growth factor. J Neurosci 1991;11:2914.

Shin GJ, Nemmer JP, Nemoto EM. Reassessment of brain free fatty acid liberation during global ischemia and its attenuation by barbiturate anesthesia. J Neurochem 1983;40:880.

Sieber FE, Traystman RJ. Glucose and the brain. Crit Care Med 1991;20:104.

Siesjo BK, Agardh CD, Bengtsson F: Free radicals and brain damage. Cerebrovasc Brain Metab Rev 1989;1:165.

Siesjo BK, Katsura K, Mellergard P, et al. Acidosis-related brain damage. Prog Brain Res 1993;96:23.

Siesjo BK, Zhao Q, Pahlmark K, et al. Glutamate, calcium, and free radicals as mediators of ischemic brain damage. Ann Thorac Surg 1995;59:1316.

Simon RP, Aminoff MJ. Electroencephalographic status epilepticus in fatal anoxic coma. Ann Neurol 1986;20:351.

Simon RP, Cho H, Gwinn R, et al. The temporal profile of 72-kDa heat-shock protein expression following global ischemia. J Neurosci 1991;11:881.

Skippen P, Seear M, Poskitt K, et al. Effect of hyperventilation on regional cerebral blood flow in head-injured children. Crit Care Med 1997;25:1402.

Smith MC, von Hanwehr R, Siesjo BK. Changes in extra- and intracellular pH in the brain during and following ischemia in hyperglycemic and in moderately hypoglycemic rats. J Cereb Blood Flow Metab 1986;6:574.

Snyder JV, Nemoto EM, Carroll RG, et al. Global ischemia in dogs: Intracranial pressures, brain blood flow and metabolism. Stroke 1975;6:21.

Spack L, Gedeit R, Splaingard M, Havens PL. Failure of aggressive therapy to alter outcome in pediatric near-drowning. Pediatr Emerg Care 1997;13:98.

Spinella PC, Dominquez T, Brott HR, et al. S-100B Protein-serum levels in healthy children and its association with outcome in pediatric traumatic brain injury. Crit Care Med 2003;31:939.

Srinivasan V, Spinella PC, Drott HR, et al. Association of timing, duration, and intensity of hyperglycemia with intensive care unit mortality in critically ill children. Pediatr Crit Care Med 2004;5:329.

Steen PA, Michenfelder JD. Mechanisms of barbiturate protection. Anesthesiology 1980;53:183.

Steen PA, Newberg CA, Milde JH, et al. Nimodipine improves cerebral blood flow and neurologic recovery after complete cerebral ischemia in the dog. J Cereb Blood Flow Metab 1983;3:38.

Steen PA, Newberg CA, Milde JH, et al. Cerebral blood flow and neurologic outcome when nimodipine is given after complete cerebral ischemia in the dog. J Cereb Blood Flow Metab 1984;4:82.

Steingrub JS, Mundt DJ. Blood glucose and neurologic outcome with global brain ischemia. Crit Care Med 1996;24:802.

Sterz F, Leonov Y, Safar P, et al. Effect of excitatory amino acid receptor blocker MK-801 on overall neurologic and morphologic outcome after prolonged cardiac arrest in dogs. Anesthesiology 1989;71:907.

Stiell IG, Herbert PC, Weitzman BN, et al. High-dose epinephrine in adult cardiac arrest. N Engl J Med 1992;327:1045.

Sugiyama H, Ito I, Hirono C. A new type of glutamate receptor linked to inositol phospholipid metabolism. Nature 1987;325:531.

Sutton LN, Clark BJ, Norwood CR, et al. Global cerebral ischemia in piglets under conditions of mild and deep hypothermia. Stroke 1991;22:1567.

Sweeney MI, Yager JY, Walz W, et al. Cellular mechanisms involved in brain ischemia. Can J Physiol Pharmacol 1995;73:1525.

Swimming programs for infants and toddlers. Committee on Sports Medicine and Fitness and Committee on Injury and Poison Prevention. American Academy of Pediatrics. Pediatrics 2000;105:868.

Szczepanski A, Moatter T, Carley WW, et al. Induction of cyclooxygenase II in human synovial microvessel endothelial cells by interleukin-1: Inhibition by glucocorticoids. Arthritis Rheum 1994;37:495.

Tainer J, Getzoff ED, Richardson JS, et al. Structure and mechanism of copper, zinc superoxide dismutase. Nature 1983;306:284.

Takahashi M, Iwatsuki N, Ono K, et al. Hyperbaric oxygen therapy accelerates neurologic recovery after 15-minute complete global cerebral ischemia in dogs. Crit Care Med 1992;20:1588.

Takami K, Iwane M, Kiyota Y. Increase of basic fibroblast growth factor immunoreactivity and its mRNA level in rat brain following transient forebrain ischemia. Exp Brain Res 1992;90:1.

Tang W, Weil MH, Sun S, et al. Progressive myocardial dysfunction after cardiac resuscitation. Crit Care Med 1993;21:1046.

Tang Y, Lu A, Aronow BJ, et al. Genomic responses of the brain to ischemic stroke, intracerebral haemorrhage, kainate seizures, hypoglycemia, and hypoxia. Eur J Neurosci 2002;15:1937.

Thompson JC, Ashwal S. Electrical injuries in children. Am J Dis Child 1983;137:231.

Thompson JE, Bonner B, Lower GM. Pediatric cardiopulmonary arrests in rural populations. Pediatrics 1990;86:302.

Thoresen M, Wyatt J. Keeping a cool head, post-hypoxic hypothermia—An old idea revisited. Acta Paediatr 1997;86:1029.

Tombaugh GC, Sapolsky RM. Mild acidosis protects hippocampal neurons from injury induced by oxygen and glucose deprivation. Brain Res 1990;343.

Torphy DE, Minter MG, Thompson BM. Cardiopulmonary arrest and resuscitation of children. Am J Dis Child 1984;138:1099.

Traystman R, Kirsch J, Koehler C. Oxygen radical mechanisms of brain injury following ischemia and reperfusion. J Appl Physiol 1991;71:1185.

Trubel HK, Novotny E, Lister G. Outcome of coma in children. Curr Opin Pediatr 2003;15:283.

Turrens JF, Crapo JD, Freeman BA. Protection against oxygen toxicity by intravenous injection of liposome-entrapped catalase and superoxide dismutase. J Clin Invest 1984;73:87.

Vaagenes P, Ginsberg M, Ebmeyer U, et al. Cerebral resuscitation from cardiac arrest: Pathophysiologic mechanisms. Crit Care Med 1996;24:S57.

Valdes-Dapena M. The postmortem examination. Pediatr Ann 1995;24:365.

van der Hal AL, Rodriguez AM, Sargent CW, et al. Hypoxic and hypercapneic arousal responses and prediction of subsequent apnea in apnea of infancy. Pediatrics 1985;75:848.

Vannucci RL, Perlman JM. Interventions for perinatal hypoxic-ischemic encephalopathy. Pediatrics 1997;100:1004.

Vass K, Welch WJ, Nowak TX. Localization of 70-KDa stress protein induction in gerbil brain after ischemia. Acta Neuropathol (Berl) 1988;77:128.

Volinsky JB, Hanson JB, Lustig JV, et al. Clinical picture. Lightning burns. Arch Fam Med 1994;3:657.

Wallays C, Feve A, Bondghene F, et al. Hypoxic cerebral lesions: X-ray computed tomography and MRI aspects. J Neuroradiol 1995;22:77.

Walpoth BH, Walpoth-Aslan BN, Mattle HP, et al. Outcome of survivors of accidental deep hypothermia and circulatory arrest treated with extra-corporeal blood warming. N Engl J Med 1997;337:1500.

Wang J, Weil MH, Kamohara T, et al. A lazaroid mitigates postresuscitation myocardial dysfunction. Crit Care Med 2004;32:553.

Weise KL, Bleck TP. Status epilepticus in children and adults. Crit Care Clin 1997;13:629.

Wen TC, Matsuda S, Yoshimura H, et al. Protective effect of basic fibroblast growth factor–heparin and neurotoxic effect of platelet factor 4 on ischemic neuronal loss and learning disabilities in gerbils. Neuroscience 1995;65:513.

Wenzel J, Krismer AC, Arntz HR, et al. A comparison of vasopressin and epinephrine for out-of-hospital cardiopulmonary resuscitation. N Engl J Med 2004;350:105.

White BC, Grossman LI, O'Neil BJ, et al. Global brain ischemia and reperfusion. Ann Emerg Med 1996;27:588.

Widmann R, Kuroiwa T, Bonnckoh P, et al. [14C] Leucine incorporation into brain proteins in gerbils after transient ischemia: Relationship to selective vulnerability of hippocampus. J Neurochem 1991;55:789.

Wijdicks EFM, Parisi JE, Sharbrough FW. Prognostic value of myoclonus status in comatose survivors of cardiac arrest. Ann Neurol 1994;35:239.

Willinger M, James LS, Catz C. Defining the sudden infant death syndrome (SIDS): Deliberations of an expert panel convened by the National Institute of Child Health and Human Development. Pediatr Pathol 1991;11:677.

Wintemute GJ. Childhood drowning and near-drowning in the United States. Am J Dis Child 1990;144:663.

Wintemute GJ, Kraus JF, Teret SP, et al. Drowning in childhood and adolescence: A population-based study. Am J Public Health 1987;77:830.

Yaffe L, Abbott D, Schulte B. Smart aortic arch catheter: Moving suspended animation from the laboratory to the field. Crit Care Med 2004;32 (Suppl):S51.

Young KD, Gausche-Hill M, McClung CD, et al. A prospective, population-based study of the epidemiology and outcome of out-ot-hospital pediatric cardiopulmonary arrest. Pediatrics 2004;114:157.

Young KD, Seidel JS: Pediatric cardiopulmonary resuscitation: A collective review. Ann Emerg Med 1999;33:195.

Yundt KD, Diringer MN. The use of hyperventilation and its impact on cerebral ischemia in the treatment of traumatic brain injury. Crit Care Clin 1997;13:163.

Zaritsky A, Nadkarni V, Getson P, et al. CPR in children. Ann Emerg Med 1987;16:1107.

Zhou C, Li Y, Nanda A, Zhang JH. HBO suppresses Nogo-A, Ng-R, or RhoA expression in the cerebral cortex after global ischemia. Biochem Biophys Res Commun 2003;309:368.

Zwemer C, Whitesall S, D'Alecy L. Cardiopulmonary-cerebral resuscitation with 100% oxygen exacerbates neurological dysfunction following nine minutes of normothermic cardiac arrest in dogs. Resuscitation 1994;27:267.

CHAPTER 65

Increased Intracranial Pressure

Suresh Kotagal

Increased intracranial pressure (ICP) is seen in a diverse group of neurologic disorders. It may develop acutely over hours or have a subacute course that evolves over days to weeks. The clinical manifestations vary according to the age of the child, the nature of the disorder, and the rapidity of its progression. Common etiologies for raised ICP are listed in Box 65-1. Intracranial hypertension is eminently treatable in its early stages, but delay in recognition and treatment can have disastrous consequences for the patient. This chapter reviews some relevant basic concepts and clinical issues.

NORMAL INTRACRANIAL PRESSURE

The normal value for ICP in newborns is about 82 mm H_2O, or 6 mm Hg [Welch, 1980]. It rises gradually from 82 to 176 mm H_2O in 1- to 7-year-olds to 136 to 204 mm H_2O in adolescents. Minor fluctuations in the physiologic ICP occur with heartbeats, breathing, the Valsalva maneuver, and rapid eye movement sleep. Brief, sharp increases of up to 1000 mm H_2O may occur transiently during sneezing and coughing. The normal brain is capable of adapting to these transient changes.

In the first 3 years of life, subacute or chronically elevated ICP leads to the separation of cranial sutures, followed by excessive cranial enlargement. Serial measurements of head circumference that are plotted on an appropriate growth chart are a useful index against which to measure subacute or chronically elevated ICP in infancy and early childhood. The normal rate of growth of head circumference in infants born at full term is 2 cm per month for the first 3 months, 1 cm per month for the next 3 months, and 0.5 cm per month for the subsequent 3 months [Bray et al., 1969].

PATHOPHYSIOLOGY OF RAISED INTRACRANIAL PRESSURE

According to the Monroe-Kellie doctrine, the skull is a rigid cavity and its contents are relatively noncompressible, consisting of the brain parenchyma, intravascular blood, and cerebrospinal fluid [Kellie, 1824; Monro, 1783]. Expansion in the volume of any one compartment is at the expense of the other two; for example, an increase in the volume of the brain parenchyma because of a neoplasm is compensated for by the expression of cerebrospinal fluid out of the brain compartment into the spinal subarachnoid space and a decrease in blood volume because of compression of the dural venous sinuses. Because each compartment is relatively noncompressible, its volume is directly proportional to its intrinsic pressure. The global ICP represents the sum of the partial pressures of the individual compartments. Although the Monroe-Kellie doctrine is a useful concept, it is not as consistently applicable to infants as it is to adults [Luerssen, 1997] because of the inherent compressibility of the brain parenchyma, inasmuch as a neoplasm can expand locally in the relatively pliable, unmyelinated brain of an infant, exerting localized pressures that are not uniformly transmitted to the entire brain. Also, the cranial cavity is not a rigid container in infants, as it can continue to enlarge by separation of the cranial sutures. The pressure-volume relationships in the brain may be described by the following equation:

$$C \sim dV/dp$$

where C represents compliance and dV represents the change in volume that accompanies a change in pressure (dp) [Friden and Ekstedt, 1983; Trauner, 1989]. Compliance is the ability of the brain to accommodate increases in intracranial volume without changes in ICP. It follows a hyperbolic curve (Fig. 65-1). As ICP rises, compliance decreases. Along the horizontal segment of the curve, increases in intracranial volume raise the pressure only slightly because compensatory mechanisms maintain a physiologic state. Beyond a certain point, however, even minor increases in volume lead to a disproportionately greater rise in ICP. In the healthy brain, compliance is along the horizontal segment of the curve, whereas in a damaged, swollen brain, compliance is located along the vertical segment of the curve. The overall slope of the pressure-volume curve is steeper in infancy than in older children (Fig. 65-2). An increase in intracranial volume by 10 mL is not likely to cause as much of an increase in ICP in an adolescent as in an infant [Shapiro et al., 1994]. This steeper volume-pressure curve persists in infancy until the point of separation of the cranial sutures. Thereafter, the infant's cranial cavity is able to accommodate relatively more volume than is the adult skull. An alternative measure of compensatory reserve in patients with brain edema is the correlation (R) between amplitude (A) and mean pressure (P) (RAP). This index is derived by calculating the linear correlation between consecutive, time-averaged data points of ICP waveform amplitude and mean ICP over a short time, such as 4 minutes. A RAP coefficient close to 0 is physiologic and indicates a good pressure-volume compensatory reserve. In other words, when intracranial volume increases, there is no corresponding rise in ICP. When RAP rises to 1+, the working point of the pressure-volume curve shifts to the right, and increases in intracranial volume start becoming linked to ICP [Czosnyka and Pickard, 2004].

Brain edema occurs consistently in patients with increased ICP. It can be vasogenic, cytotoxic, or hydrostatic

Box 65-1 Common Causes of Raised Intracranial Pressure

Extracerebral disorders
- Primary craniosynostosis
- Crouzon's disease
- Apert's syndrome
- Kleeblattschädel deformity
- Extradural hemorrhage
- Chronic subdural hematoma

Subarachnoid space lesions
- Communicating hydrocephalus

Parenchymal/ventricular disorders
- Neoplasms
- Pseudotumor cerebri
- Obstructive hydrocephalus
- Communicating hydrocephalus
- Bacterial meningitis
- Viral meningoencephalitis
- Head injury
- Hypoxic-ischemic encephalopathy
- Reye's syndrome
- Inborn errors of metabolism
- Diabetic ketoacidosis
- Hepatic coma

in nature. Vasogenic cerebral edema is related to opening of the tight junctions in the blood-brain capillaries and transudation of fluid into the extracellular space. It is commonly observed in head trauma, neoplasms, inflammatory disorders, and lead encephalopathy and is responsive to glucocorticoids. More recently, the brain swelling associated with head injury has been thought to be related to a combination of vasogenic and cytotoxic edema [Marmarou, 2003]. Neurogenic inflammation linked to the release of peptides such as substance P and calcitonin gene–related peptide may also play a major in the pathogenesis of posttraumatic brain edema [Nimmo et al., 2004]. Diffusion-weighted magnetic resonance imaging reveals increased signal intensities in the T2 sequences in patients with vasogenic edema, which helps differentiate it from cytotoxic brain edema [Schaefer et al., 1997]. Endothelial damage triggered by the local release of cytokines such as tumor necrosis factor α, interleukin-1β, interleukin-6, histamine, and arachidonic acid may play a role in the development of vasogenic edema [Gourin and Schackford, 1997; Schilling and Wahl, 1997]. Cytotoxic edema results from processes, usually toxic or metabolic, that affect the integrity of cell membranes of neurons and glial cells so that they are unable to maintain a stable pump mechanism and internal milieu, leading to hydropic swelling. It commonly occurs during hypoxic-ischemic encephalopathy and is not steroid responsive. Interstitial edema is characterized by transependymal transudation of cerebrospinal fluid into the adjacent white matter and is generally seen in patients with hydrocephalus. The various forms of edema are not mutually exclusive and may coexist to varying degrees.

Impact on Cerebral Perfusion

The normal cerebral blood flow rate in newborns is about 40 mL/100 grams/minute and 53 mL/100 grams/minute in older children and adults [Shapiro et al., 1994]. Increased ICP reduces cerebral blood flow. The primary objective in controlling brain swelling is therefore the prevention of brain ischemia [Luerssen, 1997]. This relationship between ICP and blood flow is best expressed by the following equations:

$$CPP \cong \underline{MAP} - ICP$$

or

$$CPP \cong \frac{SAP + 2DAP}{3} - ICP$$

where:
CPP = cerebral perfusion pressure,
MAP = mean arterial pressure,
SAP = systolic arterial pressure, and
DAP = diastolic arterial pressure.

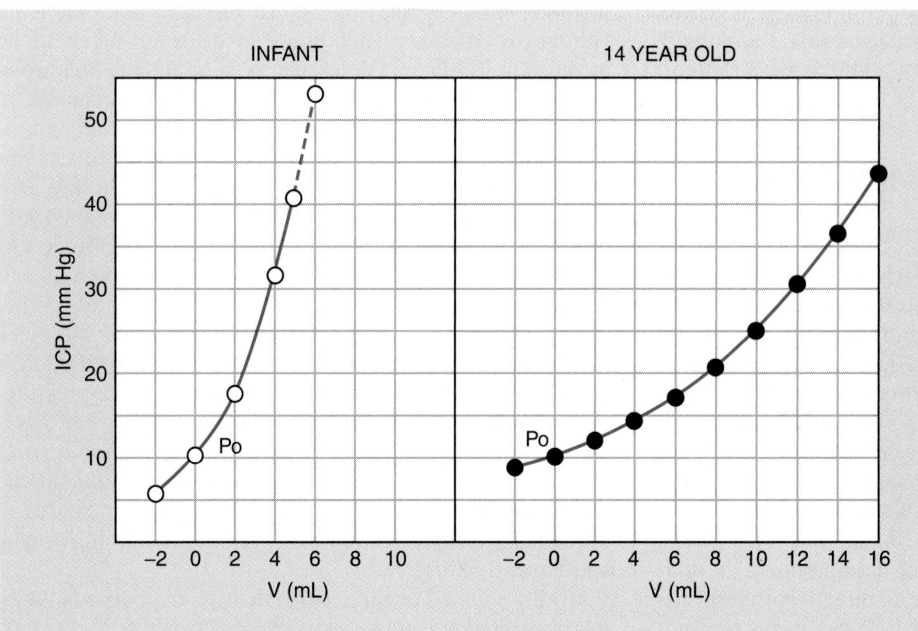

FIGURE 65-1. Pressure-volume curves of an infant and a 14 year old, generated by injecting and withdrawing cerebrospinal fluid into the ventricular system. Note that the curve is steeper in the infant than in the 14 year old; this reflects the infant's lesser ability to buffer increases in intracranial volume. ICP, intracranial pressure. (Adapted with permission from Shapiro K, Morris WJ, Teo C. Intracranial hypertension: Mechanisms and management. In: Cheek WR, Marlin AE, McLone DJ, et al., eds. Pediatric neurosurgery. Surgery of the developing nervous system. Philadelphia: WB Saunders, 1994;310.)

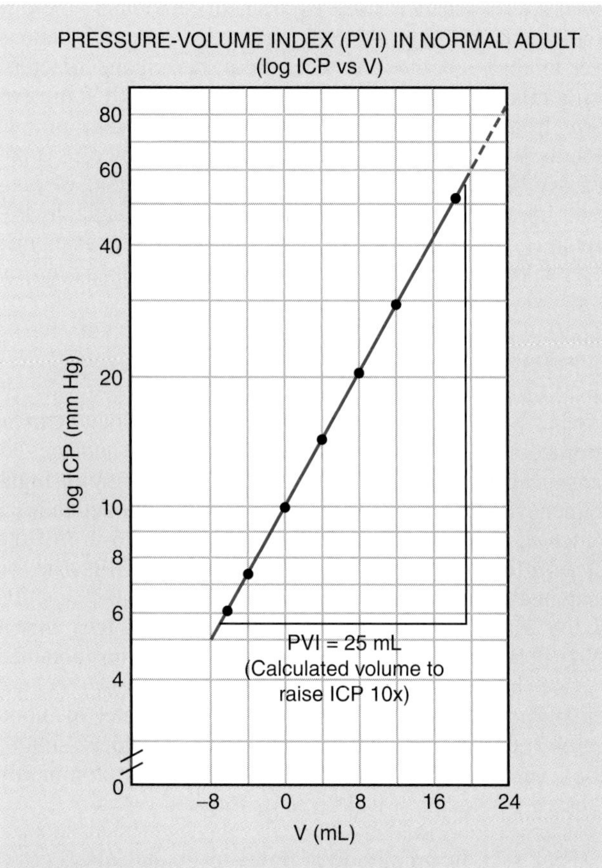

FIGURE 65-2. Pressure-volume index (PVI) in a normal adult. The PVI is the calculated volume (in milliliters) needed to raise the cerebrospinal fluid pressure by a factor of 10. The concept is identical in children. The normal PVI of an infant is around 10, whereas that of a normal adult is around 25. When compliance is reduced, the PVI diminishes. (Adapted with permission from Shapiro K, Morris WJ, Teo C. Intracranial hypertension: Mechanisms and management. In: Cheek WR, Marlin AE, McLone DJ, et al, eds. Pediatric neurosurgery. Surgery of the developing nervous system. Philadelphia: WB Saunders, 1994.)

The normal cerebral perfusion pressure varies between 20 mm Hg in preterm infants at birth to 80 mm Hg at 12 months [Sato et al., 1988]; the value in young adults is 50 to 55 mm Hg. A drop in the cerebral perfusion pressure below the physiologic level may be associated with ischemic brain injury. When cerebral perfusion pressure decreases to 40% of normal, electrophysiologic function in the brain fails, and neuronal ischemia ensues [Trauner, 1989]. This underscores the importance of avoiding hypotension in any patient with increased ICP from overzealous fluid restriction or excessive use of volume-depleting, hyperosmolar agents.

Autoregulation is the ability of the brain to maintain stable blood flow in the presence of fluctuations in the cerebral perfusion pressure. It is accomplished through regional vasoconstriction or vasodilation. Autoregulation is frequently compromised in patients with raised ICP, and this creates a "pressure-passive" system wherein systemic hypotension can provoke additional ischemic injury. The mediators of metabolic autoregulation are changes in tissue pH, potassium, and calcium ions [Siesjo, 1984]. The cerebral vasculature is also responsive to changes in arterial oxygen and carbon dioxide tension. Small fluctuations in arterial oxygen tension do not alter cerebral blood flow, but there is an inverse relationship between cerebral blood flow and oxygen tension when the arterial oxygen tension drops below 50 mm Hg. The vascular response to changes in arterial carbon dioxide tension is even more sensitive. For each 1-mm Hg change in arterial carbon dioxide tension, cerebral blood flow changes in the same direction by 3% to 4% [Siesjo, 1984]. The lower limit for this response is about 20 mm Hg in adults and about 15 mm Hg in children [Trauner, 1989]. When compliance is impaired and shifted to the steep segment of the pressure-volume curve, autoregulation is also impaired, and even minor increases in cerebral blood flow—for example, because of hypercarbia—can lead to significant rises in ICP.

INTRACRANIAL PRESSURE MONITORING

Rationale

Increased ICP is difficult to verify on clinical grounds alone. In comatose patients, the yield of the clinical examination may also be compromised by sedative agents or skeletal muscle paralytic agents that have been administered for ventilator management. The objective of management is to recognize and reduce ICP well before it leads to irreparable brain damage. The decision to monitor ICP in any given patient is based on the premise that the ICP elevation is going to persist for some time (more than a few hours). It should be combined with accurate measurements of systemic blood pressure and fluid balance through intra-arterial and central venous pressure lines.

Methodology

ICP monitoring requires the placement of a pressure-sensing device into the cranial cavity. Initial work on the direct monitoring of ICP after ventricular puncture was carried out by Guillaume and Janny [1951] and Lundberg [1960]. The following three basic patterns of ICP were described by Lundberg:

- Plateau or A waves: increases of ICP in the range of 540 to 650 mm H_2O (40 to 50 mm Hg) that are sustained for 2 to 10 minutes, followed by a return to a higher baseline than before. They are indicative of a significant decrease in brain compliance.
- B waves: brief elevations of a moderate degree (range of 272 to 408 mm H_2O [20 to 30 mm Hg]); related to fluctuations in respiration and also indicative of decreased compliance.
- C waves: small-amplitude fluctuations related to intracranial transmission of arterial pulses.

ICP is most reliably monitored by the placement of an intraventricular catheter that is connected to a pressure transducer and a recording device or continuous strip chart. Placement of an intraventricular catheter can be technically difficult when severe brain swelling leads to compression of the ventricles or, in some instances, to ventricular displacement. On the other hand, it has the advantage of facilitating a decrease in intracranial volume and pressure by withdrawing small amounts of cerebrospinal fluid (1 to 2 mL). Compliance can also be studied in patients with the intraventricular cannula by determining the pressure-volume index, which consists of plotting the ICP logarithmically against volume [Marmarou and Shulman, 1976]. A small amount of saline (0.5 to 1 mL) is instilled into the intraventricular catheter. The pressure-volume index is the volume (in milliliters) needed to raise the ICP by a factor of 10 (see Fig. 65-2). The normal pressure-volume index is approximately 25 mL in adults and approximately 10 mL in infants. Adult values are reached at approximately age 14 years. A decrease in compliance leads to a decrease in the pressure-volume index.

The risks associated with the use of ventricular catheters include hemorrhage and infection. The overall risk of ventriculitis is 1% to 5% [Rosner and Becker, 1976] and rises when the catheter has been left in place for more than 3 to 4 days. Other ICP monitoring devices include the subarachnoid bolt, the epidural transducer, and the fiberoptic intraparenchymal catheter-transducer. One advantage of the intraparenchymal monitor is the ease of insertion. The disadvantage is that measurements may drift over time, because there is no way to recalibrate the system [Adelson et al., 2003].

The normal ICP in children between 1 and 7 years of age ranges from 82 to 176 mm of cerebrospinal fluid (5 to 15 mm Hg), and the generally acceptable threshold for treatment of raised ICP is over 200 to 240 mm (15 to 18 mm Hg). The cerebral perfusion pressure should also be monitored and kept well over 50 to 55 mm Hg; the normal cerebral perfusion pressure is 70 to 73 mm Hg in infants and 73 to 77 mm Hg in children [Shapiro et al., 1994]. Raised ICP is seen in 40% to 60% of patients with severe head injury and in 50% of those who die from it [Narayan et al., 1982].

Utility

ICP monitoring is definitely indicated in all comatose head-injured patients with a Glasgow Coma Scale score of 8 or less, because studies have demonstrated that monitoring may contribute to enhancing the outcome in this group [Narayan et al., 1982]. It may also be beneficial in the management of patients with brain tumors, slit-ventricle syndrome, craniosynostosis, hepatic encephalopathy, and Reye's syndrome. Its use does not, however, lead to improvement in the outcome in coma related to severe hypoxic-ischemic encephalopathy, as occurs in near-drowning, acute encephalitis, or hepatic failure [Luerssen, 1997].

Monitoring of Intracranial Pressure from the Anterior Fontanel

The tension over the anterior fontanel can be used as a gauge of ICP in newborns and infants. A helpful review is provided by Volpe [2000]. The basis for all the available devices is the applanation principle [Menke et al., 1982; Salmon et al., 1977], which is that when the anterior fontanel is maintained in the flat position, pressure on either side is equal. A hand-held pressure-sensing device is pressed over the anterior fontanel, and the pressure necessary to eliminate bulging of the skin is determined; this corresponds to the ICP. The manner of placement of each device over the fontanel is a key issue. When it is used by trained individuals, there is excellent correlation between pressure readings obtained after lumbar puncture and those from the fontanellometers. Using this device, Volpe et al. [2000] found the ICP in newborns free of intracranial pathology was 40 to 50 mm H_2O (2.9 to 3.6 mm Hg). Serial measurements by this noninvasive technique may help in the management of neonatal intraventricular hemorrhage, posthemorrhagic hydrocephalus, bacterial meningitis, and hypoxic-ischemic encephalopathy.

Blood-Flow Velocity Measurement by Doppler Devices and Intracranial Pressure

Doppler assessments of cerebral blood flow velocity can be obtained serially at the bedside in critically ill neonates. A transducer placed over the anterior fontanel emits high-frequency sound waves that are directed at the pericallosal branch of the anterior cerebral artery. After closure of the anterior fontanel, vessels in the circle of Willis can be insonated through the temporal bone. The frequency shifts of the back-scattered echoes are converted into visual images. Blood-flow velocity measurements thus obtained provide indirect information about blood flow because velocity is inversely proportional to the diameter of blood vessels, and severe cerebral edema leads to compression of blood vessels. The resistive index is the most commonly assessed parameter. It is derived as follows:

$$\frac{\text{(Peak systolic amplitude of flow − peak diastolic amplitude of flow)}}{\text{Peak systolic amplitude of flow}}$$

The resistive index is a useful index of blood flow velocity. Although isolated resistive index values are of not much significance, serial increases over time are correlated with rising ICP. Improvements in technology have made it easy to determine the resistive index in dural venous sinuses through transcranial color-coded duplex sonography [Mursch et al., 1999]. Blood flow velocity measurements from over the large venous sinuses are helpful in evaluating raised ICP secondary to venous sinus thrombosis.

CLINICAL MANIFESTATIONS OF RAISED INTRACRANIAL PRESSURE

Headache

Supratentorial mass lesions frequently lead to traction on the dura, which is innervated by the trigeminal nerve, thus causing pain that is referred to the frontal and temporal regions, whereas lesions of the infratentorial structures might lead to pain localized over the occipital regions. The headache is frequently exacerbated by measures that increase ICP, such as coughing, bending, and sneezing. It might also be worsened by the recumbent position, and patients frequently have a history of headache on awakening in the morning. The duration of the headache is generally brief, lasting days to weeks. Sutures can split in children younger than 10 years of age, thus providing temporary relief from symptoms, except that the headache returns within a few days because of further increases in

ICP. Analgesics provide little to no relief. Patients with third ventricular tumors may sometimes find relief by assuming a kneeling position and flexing their necks forward. Headache from brain tumors is more likely to be recognized in children older than 2 years [Dobrovoljac et al., 2002] and is generally of only short duration (4 to 6 weeks).

Diplopia

Of all the cranial nerves, the sixth cranial nerve is the longest, thus making it susceptible to displacement and traction from an enlarging mass lesion. Traction on cranial nerve VI can lead to its unilateral or bilateral paresis, thus causing a "false localizing sign" because there is no intrinsic pontine lesion. The patient presents with binocular diplopia, made worse in the direction of gaze of the paretic muscle. There is no relation of the paresis with the level of ICP.

Decreased Sensorium

Stupor begins to appear in adults when the ICP reaches the 204 to 540 mm H_2O (15 to 40 mm Hg) range [Ropper, 1984]. Comparable data are not available for children. The mechanisms postulated include one swollen hemisphere compressing the contralateral hemisphere and creating "bihemispheral coma" and compression of the ascending reticular formation in the mesencephalic-diencephalic regions.

Impaired Upward Gaze

Pressure over the pretectal region of the midbrain from supratentorial mass lesions impairs upward gaze. Patients exhibit mild retraction of the upper eyelids because of sympathetic overactivity. These two elements combine to produce the sunset sign, which is especially obvious in infants in the form of prominent eyes with downward deviation of gaze.

Change in Personality

Nonspecific manifestations such as irritability, mood swings, apathy, and lethargy are common in infants and children with subacute, progressive increases in ICP.

Excessive Cranial Enlargement

Increasing intracranial volume in infants and toddlers from subacute or chronic mass lesions frequently leads to tenseness and bulging of the anterior fontanel, prominence of the scalp veins, splitting of the cranial sutures, and macrocephaly. Serial measurements of the head circumference plotted on a head growth chart might demonstrate an upward shift to higher percentiles. In addition, it may be possible to palpate splitting of the sutures. Closure of the anterior fontanel, which generally occurs between 8 to 18 months, might also be delayed.

Papilledema

Papilledema is the most reliable sign of increased ICP; it is caused by edema in the nerve fiber layer of the retina that arises because of impaired retinal venous return as a result of the increased ICP. It may be unilateral or bilateral with supratentorial mass lesions but is bilateral with infratentorial lesions. Most patients do not complain of visual symptoms, but in the late stages of papilledema, there might be "transient visual obscurations," which are fleeting episodes of vision loss lasting seconds. Early papilledema is characterized by a loss of retinal venous pulsations (however, about 20% of normal children also do not demonstrate venous pulsations). This loss is followed by elevation and blurring of the optic disc margins, tortuosity of the retinal veins, hemorrhages, and exudates (Fig. 65-3). In contrast to papillitis, visual acuity remains normal in papilledema until the late stages. Although papilledema reliably indicates increased ICP, its absence does not exclude its possibility. In a population of 120 children with craniosynostosis (premature closure of the sutures), the presence of papilledema was 98% specific as an indicator for raised ICP, but its sensitivity was age dependent [Tuite et al., 1996]. It was a reliable indicator of raised ICP in children older than 5 years but not in preschool-aged children. Papilledema is generally also not seen in infants because of compensation for raised ICP by splitting of the sutures and cranial enlargement. A false impression of papilledema can be created by "drusen," alternatively termed *colloid* or *hyaline bodies.* They are located over the optic nerve head, dominantly inherited [Fenichel, 2001] more common in white persons, and generally seen after the age of 11 years [Glaser, 1978].

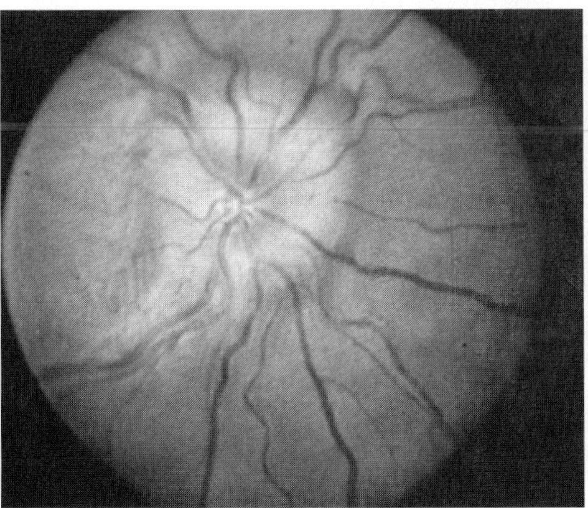

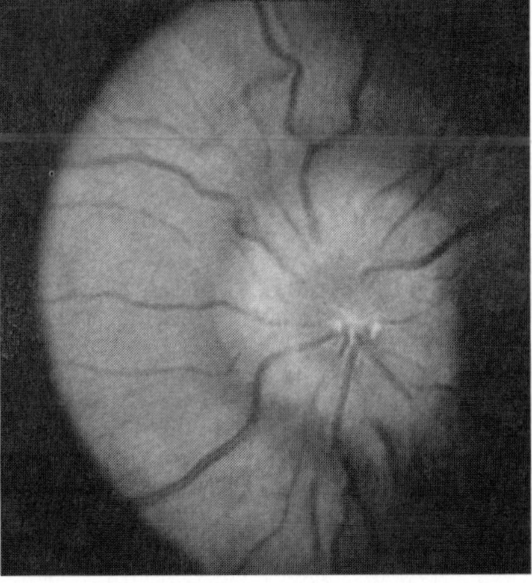

FIGURE 65-3. Fundoscopy illustrating moderate papilledema, with slightly increased tortuosity of vessels, blurring, and elevation of the optic disc margins. (Reproduced with the kind permission of Dr. John B. Selhorst, St. Louis University, St. Louis, MO.)

Cushing Response

Compression of the brainstem may lead to slowing of the respiratory rate, bradycardia, and elevation of the blood pressure. It may be a beneficial, adaptive response that is designed to maintain adequate cerebral perfusion pressure in the presence of moderate intracranial hypertension [Barbiro-Michaely et al., 2003]. It is observed inconsistently, however, and only in one fifth to one third of patients with documented ICP elevations [Marshall et al., 1979]. In fact, tachycardia is seen with raised ICP as often as is bradycardia.

Acute Pulmonary Edema

Acute pulmonary edema is a rare but significant complication of cerebral edema [Ducker et al., 1969]. It is triggered by an excessive autonomic discharge, which leads to increased pulmonary vascular permeability; it is reversible on reduction of ICP.

Brain Herniation Syndromes

Severe cerebral edema (Fig. 65-4) ultimately leads to brain herniation, during which portions of the swollen brain become impacted in abnormal locations (e.g., the tentorial notch or the foramen magnum) [Plum and Posner, 2000]. The displaced brain tissue impinges on vessels, leading to impairment of venous return, additional swelling, and tissue injury. The following vicious cycle develops, which, if untreated, can be fatal:

Cerebral edema → Vascular occlusion
↑ ↓
Cellular injury ← Brain ischemia

Transtentorial Herniation

Transtentorial herniation is characterized by the swollen, uncal portion of the temporal lobe's becoming displaced in a medial and caudal direction and becoming impacted in the tentorial notch, thus compressing the ipsilateral third cranial nerve, midbrain, ipsilateral cerebral peduncle, and posterior cerebral artery. The initial clinical manifestations include an ipsilateral dilated pupil (resulting from extrinsic compression of the pupilloconstrictor fibers in the outer core of the third nerve), progressive decline in consciousness, loss of oculocephalic (doll's-eye) reflexes, and the appearance of decorticate posturing. At times, there can also be pressure on the contralateral cerebral peduncle, leading to hemiparesis that is ipsilateral to the mass lesion.

Central Herniation

Central herniation is seen when both diffusely swollen cerebral hemispheres compress the diencephalic structures and midbrain from above. In its early stages, central herniation is characterized by a progressive decline in the level of consciousness, constricted pupils (resulting from diencephalic sympathetic dysfunction), and Cheyne-Stokes respiration. With further progression, there is loss of oculocephalic reflexes, central neurogenic hyperventilation, and decerebrate posturing that ultimately progresses to complete loss of brainstem function.

Tonsillar Herniation

The cerebellar tonsils become impacted in the foramen magnum, thus compressing the medulla oblongata and the upper cervical spinal cord. This type of herniation can occur with either supratentorial or infratentorial mass lesions, although it is encountered more often with posterior fossa mass lesions. It is characterized by an abrupt loss of consciousness, opisthotonic posturing, stiff neck, irregular respiration, and apnea.

The late stages of uncal, central, and tonsillar herniation are indistinguishable, with the presence of flaccid limbs, unresponsive midsize pupils, loss of caloric and oculocephalic reflexes, and irreversible apnea that leads to death.

Cingulate Herniation

Cingulate herniation is characterized by shifting of the swollen cingulate gyrus underneath the free edge of the falx

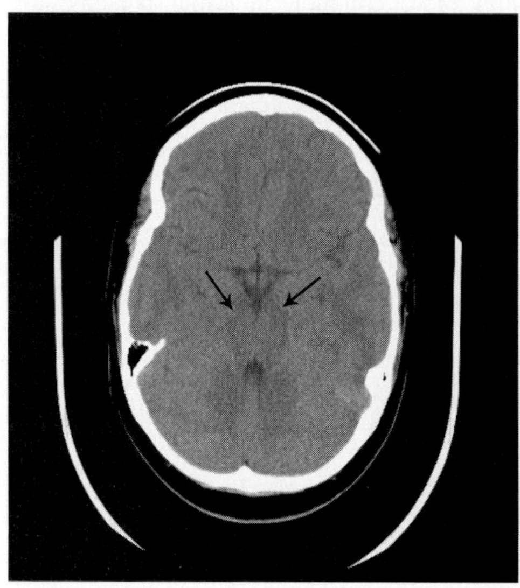

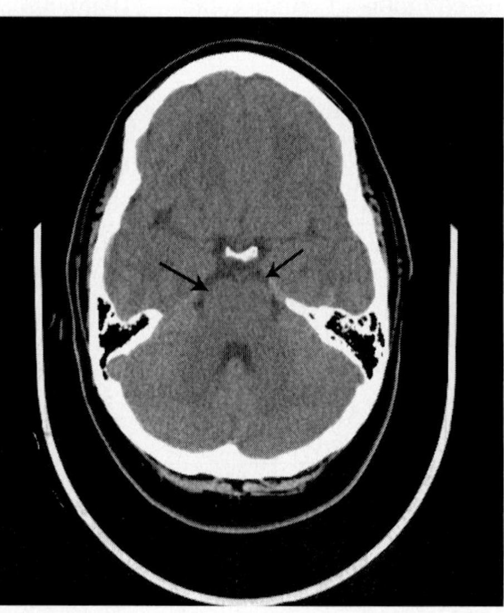

FIGURE 65-4. Noncontrast head computed tomographic scan in a child with severe closed-head injury, demonstrating severe, diffuse cerebral edema. Note that the brain swelling is leading to loss of gray-white matter junction differentiation, compression of the frontal horns of lateral ventricles (*arrowhead*), and obliteration of the cisterna ambiens (*arrows*).

cerebri, causing compression of the ipsilateral or bilateral anterior cerebral arteries and the internal cerebral vein. This leads to infarction of the paracentral lobules.

LUMBAR PUNCTURE IN PATIENTS WITH RAISED INTRACRANIAL PRESSURE

Lumbar puncture is contraindicated in patients with raised ICP because of the risk of precipitating brain herniation. The ocular fundi should be carefully assessed for papilledema in every patient before a lumbar puncture is initiated. If the fundi cannot be visualized and symptoms are suspect for increased ICP, pertinent diagnostic information may be obtained by computed tomographic or magnetic resonance image scanning. For suspected acute encephalitis and bacterial meningitis, cerebrospinal fluid sampling is still crucial to diagnosis and management, but the least amount of cerebrospinal fluid necessary should be withdrawn. A post-lumbar puncture prophylactic dose of mannitol, 0.25 to 1 gram/kg, may also be administered.

If the cerebrospinal fluid opening pressure exceeds 200 mm H_2O, it is important to complete the measurement of the ICP and then carefully monitor the patient. In most clinical situations, the patient remains clinically stable, and so an individualized decision can be made in regard to the need for treatment with furosemide (Lasix), mannitol, or hypertonic saline for ICP monitoring or placement of a lumbar cerebrospinal fluid drain, additional treatment of the underlying disease, neurosurgical consultation or transfer to a critical care unit, and other measures. It is not uncommon for patients with elevated ICP (e.g., patients with idiopathic intracranial hypertension [IIH]) to feel better after a lumbar puncture. However, patients must be monitored for signs of neurologic deterioration if the ICP is increased.

MANAGEMENT OF ACUTELY ELEVATED INTRACRANIAL PRESSURE

Whenever possible, treatment should be directed toward the underlying cause of the raised ICP, such as acute encephalitis or abscess. Supportive measures outlined in the following sections are also indicated. An algorithm for the evaluation of the child with suspected increased ICP is presented in Figure 65-5. This algorithm is intended to assist in the evaluation and management of raised ICP in childhood. It does not address each and every possible clinical scenario; rather, it serves as a broad road map. As is true for any medical emergency, there must be a high index of suspicion of the various possible disorders, as well as efficient team work between the emergency room physician/intensivist, nursing staff, neurologist, and neurosurgeon, as well as the family.

Respiratory Management

Children with increased ICP require sedation, analgesia, and skeletal muscle paralytic agents. These measures help suppress pain, coughing, and gagging, which might provoke reflex increases in ICP [Palmer, 2000]. These therapeutic measures also necessitate endotracheal intubation and placement on a ventilator. Hyperventilation with maintenance of arterial carbon dioxide tension between 25 and 30 mm Hg effectively reduces ICP by causing cerebral vasoconstriction, thus decreasing intracranial volume. For the purpose of endotracheal intubation, a topical anesthetic should be sprayed over the vocal cords to minimize procedural trauma, which may provoke a rise in ICP. In such instances, it is also advisable to lower the ICP by infusing hyperosmolar agents such as mannitol before the intubation. A drop in ICP occurs within 1 to 5 minutes of initiation of hyperventilation [Ropper, 1984]. ICP can be satisfactorily controlled in two thirds of patients by a combination of a hyperosmolar agent and hyperventilation. Failure to reduce ICP despite hyperventilation is a grave prognostic sign. Hyperventilation should be discontinued gradually over 24 to 48 hours, because abrupt cessation can lead to a rebound increase in ICP. A rise in ICP from indirect transmission of elevated intrathoracic pressure to intracranial vessels can be avoided by sedation and decreasing the inspiratory phase of the respirator [Ersson et al., 1990]. Positive end-expiratory pressure could also theoretically raise the ICP, but this does not appear to be an issue in clinical practice [Frost, 1977; Shapiro et al., 1994].

Positioning of the Head

Elevation of the head by 15 to 30 degrees facilitates venous return from the head, thus helping to reduce ICP. This degree of head elevation does not lower the cerebral perfusion pressure [Rosner and Coley, 1986]. Hyperextension, twisting of the neck, and traction on the endotracheal tube should be avoided. The head should not be elevated in hypotensive patients.

Fluid Management

A central venous pressure catheter should be placed in patients with significantly raised ICP to help manage fluid balance. Hypotonic intravenous fluids should be avoided because they can precipitate a fluid shift into the brain compartment and exacerbate cerebral edema. A 5% dextrose solution with half normal saline, normal saline, or Ringer's lactate is preferred. The patient should be monitored closely for the syndrome of inappropriate secretion of antidiuretic hormone, with measurements of serum and urine osmolality. Fluid intake should be kept at maintenance levels but lowered if this syndrome develops. Hypovolemia should be avoided.

Hyperosmolar Agents

Mannitol, urea, glycerol, and hypertonic saline are the most commonly recommended hyperosmolar agents. They produce an abrupt rise in intravascular osmolality in relation to the brain compartment. The rise in intravascular osmolality facilitates fluid shift from the brain into the vascular space [Bell et al., 1987]. Mannitol is most commonly used. Its intravascular and brain concentrations do not equilibrate as rapidly as those of glycerol or urea [Shapiro et al., 1994]. It is available as a 20% solution. The dose is 0.25 to 1 gram/kg, given intravenously over 10 to 15 minutes as a bolus. The lower end of the dose range is recommended for infants and young children. The onset of mannitol action occurs within 1 to 5 minutes, and the duration of action is 2 to 3 hours. Serum osmolality should be maintained below 320 mOsm/ liter. Despite the popularity of mannitol, evidence of its efficacy consists of only two class III studies [The Society of Critical Care Medicine and the World Federation of Pediatric Intensive and Critical Care Societies, 2003]. Furosemide has synergistic effect with mannitol in terms of reducing the ICP by virtue of decreasing free water. It might also lower the rate of formation of cerebrospinal fluid, but this effect is not significant in the clinical setting [Shapiro, 1994]. Glycerol is available as a 10% solution, given intravenously in a dose of 1 gram/kg, three to four times a day. Its onset of action occurs within 30 minutes. Hypertonic saline is a promising alternative for the reduction of ICP. The recommended dose of 3% saline is 0.1 to 1.0 mL/kg of body weight per hour, administered as a continuous infusion on a sliding scale, and serum osmolality should be maintained below 360 mOsm/liter. Evidence supporting the use of hypertonic saline consists of three class II studies and one class III study [The Society of Critical Care Medicine and the World Federation of Pediatric Intensive and Critical Care Societies, 2003]. There have been no "head-to-head" studies comparing the efficacy of mannitol with that of hypertonic saline in reducing ICP in

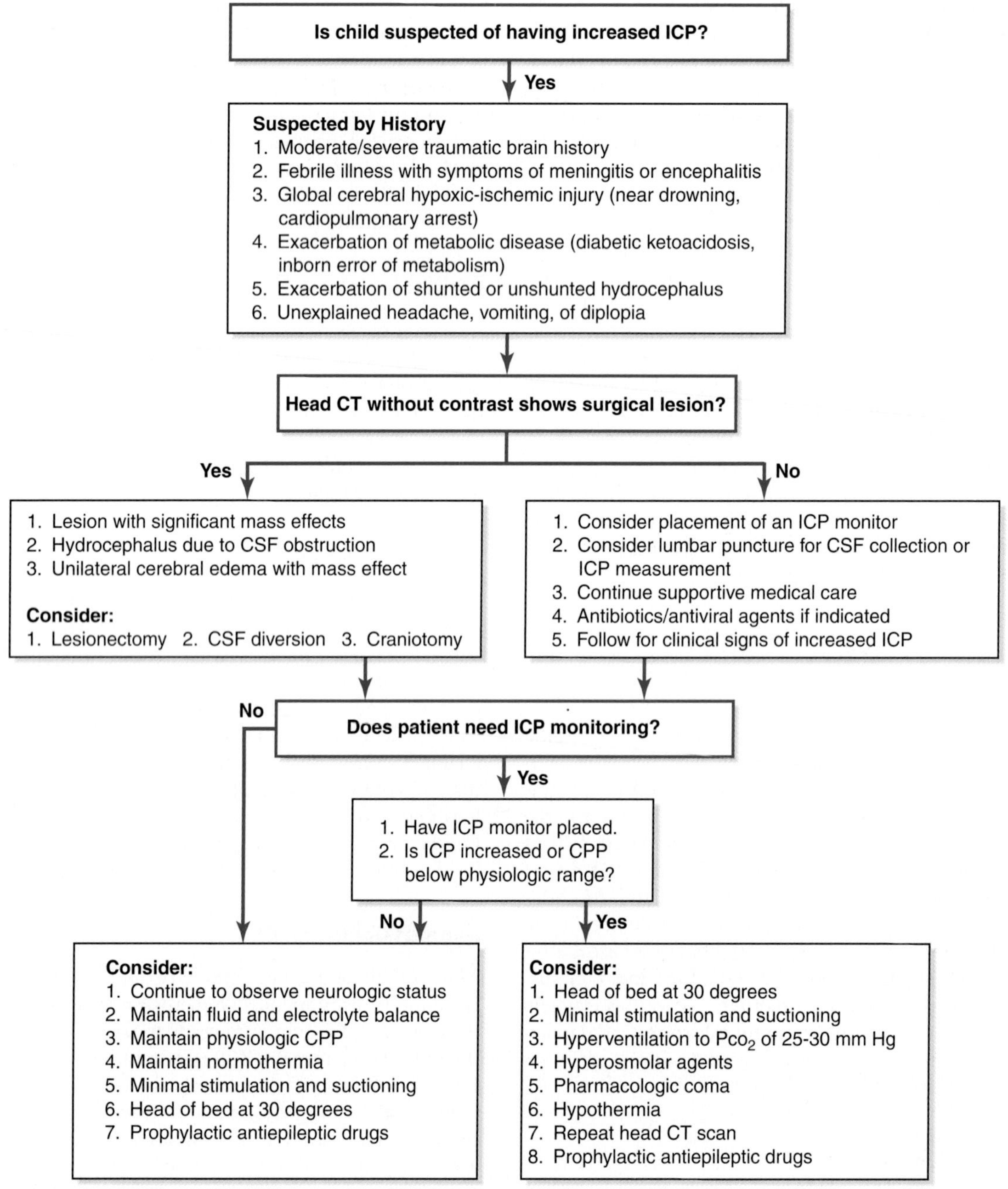

FIGURE 65-5. Algorithm for the evaluation of the child with suspected increased intracranial pressure (ICP). CPP, cerebral perfusion pressure; CSF, cerebrospinal fluid; CT, computed tomography; Pco_2, carbon dioxide tension. Algorithm developed by Drs. Suresh Kotagal, David Michelson, and Stephen Ashwal.

children or, for that matter, regarding the long-term outcome of children receiving these agents. Complications from the use of osmotic agents include dehydration, central pontine myelinolysis, and electrolyte imbalance, especially hypernatremia. Moreover, the administration of repeated doses of any osmotic agent over a short period of time, such as four to five doses over 24 hours, may lead to a rebound increase in ICP [Node and Nakazawa, 1990]. Placement of a central venous catheter to assess fluid balance and of an ICP monitor is vital in any subject receiving repeated infusions of intravenous osmotic agents.

Corticosteroids

Lipid hydrolysis and free radical–induced lipid peroxidation are inhibited by corticosteroids [Hall and Braughler, 1982]. This inhibition might indirectly limit the development of vasogenic edema, but the exact mechanism of action of steroids has not been fully established. Although the efficacy of steroids in the treatment of brain edema associated with neoplasms is unquestionable, there is no clear proof that they alleviate edema seen with post-traumatic, metabolic, and inflammatory disorders. The recommended dose of dexamethasone in infants and young children is 0.4 to 1 mg/kg/day in four divided doses; the dose in adolescents is 4 mg every 6 hours. Onset of action may take 12 to 24 hours.

Hypothermia

Medically induced hypothermia to 34° C may be used in comatose head-injured children for decreasing the cerebral metabolic rate and blood flow and thus the ICP. There are no data that hypothermia necessarily improves outcome in children, however. It may be induced through use of tepid water sponging or a cooling blanket. Shivering should be avoided, because it inhibits cooling. Complications of cooling include cardiac dysrhythmias, neutropenia, diminished myocardial contractility, and clotting abnormalities. Rewarming should be gradual, with monitoring for hyperkalemia resulting from a sudden shift in potassium from the intracellular space into the extracellular compartment [Palmer, 2000].

Intracranial Pressure Monitoring Device

Bedside neurologic examination is of limited value in a patient who is comatose or pharmacologically paralyzed for ventilatory management, especially when two or more doses of an osmotic agent have already been administered for control of suspected increased ICP. Placement of an ICP monitor should be considered for such patients.

Barbiturates

Pentobarbital is more effective than phenobarbital in sharply reducing cerebral metabolism, which in turn leads to reduced cerebral blood flow and lowering of intracranial volume and, thus indirectly, of the ICP. Barbiturates are generally used only when standard therapy consisting of osmotic agents, hyperventilation, and head positioning has failed to control the ICP. An initial bolus of 5 to 10 mg/kg of pentobarbital given over 30 minutes is followed by its infusion at a rate of 1 to 5 mg/kg/hour to maintain the serum pentobarbital level between 35 to 45 mg/mL. The electroencephalogram should also be monitored continuously to ensure that the lowering of cerebral metabolism is sufficient enough to create a suppression-burst pattern, as well as to monitor for electrographic seizures. Barbiturates should be used only in the intensive care setting, with close monitoring of the mean arterial pressure, ICP, cardiac index, and pulmonary artery wedge pressures. Hypotension, mostly from depressed cardiac contractility, develops in 50% of subjects despite adequate volume replacement. It may necessitate correction with dopamine or dobutamine. Other complications of barbiturate-induced coma include pneumonia and hyponatremia. Although barbiturates are effective in lowering the ICP in patients whose condition is refractory to standard therapy [Eisenberg et al., 1988], they do not improve the outcome in severe head injury [Ward et al., 1985], metabolic disorders [Ward et al., 1987], or stroke [Ropper, 1984].

Relief of Acute Hydrocephalus

An emergency ventriculostomy can temporarily relieve raised ICP in patients with acute hydrocephalus. This procedure is especially useful in patients with brain tumors because hydrocephalus in some of these patients might be transient, and placement of a permanent ventriculoperitoneal shunt may be avoided. The pressure is monitored continuously and, if it exceeds a certain threshold, cerebrospinal fluid is drained. In other instances, however, on the basis of etiology, the neurosurgeon might well consider placement of a permanent ventriculoperitoneal shunt.

Control of Seizures

The abrupt onset of seizures in a patient with raised ICP may indicate deterioration in neurologic function. Seizures provoke further rises in ICP by increasing cerebral blood flow. The seizures may develop as a consequence of the underlying cerebral insult, fluid and electrolyte imbalance, or infection. Unfortunately, they may be particularly difficult to recognize in a pharmacologically paralyzed and heavily sedated patient. A high index of suspicion and continuous electroencephalographic monitoring are needed. The ICP monitor may limit electrode application. There should be a low threshold for adding prophylactic antiseizure medications such as phenytoin, phenobarbital, lorazepam, or valproic acid.

Decompressive Surgery

There is emerging literature on the value of decompressive craniotomy with durotomy or decompressive craniectomy in children who have refractory intracranial hypertension, specifically those with ICP greater than 20 mm Hg for more than 30 minutes. In traumatic brain injury, decompressive surgery seems to more effective when carried out early (within 48 hours of trauma) rather than later [Ruf et al., 2003]. The procedure may decrease the midline shift. Long-term outcome has not been adequately studied, but case reports with small numbers of patients suggest that half the subjects are free of major neurologic deficits [Figaji et al., 2003; Ruf et al., 2003].

IDIOPATHIC INTRACRANIAL HYPERTENSION

IIH, or primary idiopathic intracranial hypertension (previously termed pseudotumor cerebri), may develop at any age. To some extent, it is a diagnosis of exclusion, dependent on excluding identifiable causes of raised ICP [Friedman and Jacobson, 2002]. If untreated, the patient may experience progressive visual loss from ischemic optic neuropathy. The nomenclature remains a bit unclear. *Benign intracranial hypertension* has been discarded as patients may develop significant long-term visual deficits. The term *pseudotumor cerebri* is also not used as often because it leaves an impression that the disorder is not a real disease (Friedman and Jacobson, 2004). For those in whom an appropriate cause is found, the diagnosis should be "intracranial hypertension secondary to—."

IIH presents subacutely with daily headache that is made worse by maneuvers that raise ICP, such as coughing and bending. Infants may manifest irritability, the sunset sign, and a bulging anterior fontanel. Cranial nerve VI paresis from traction on the nerve caused by raised ICP may lead to diplopia that worsens with lateral gaze [Bergman, 1994]. Other manifestations of IIH include tinnitus, blurring of vision, vertigo, decreased visual acuity, and transient visual obscurations. Patients remain alert and fully oriented. Adolescents with IIH may be obese; among adolescents, IIH is slightly more common in girls than in boys, but there is no specific gender predilection during infancy and early childhood. The retinal examination discloses papilledema. Bedside and formal visual field testing may demonstrate enlargement of the blind spot but, in general, only in the advanced stages. Magnetic resonance imaging, magnetic resonance venographic, and computed tomographic studies usually yield normal results. Infrequently, the ventricles may appear slitlike. Lumbar puncture is needed to establish a definitive diagnosis. It reveals significantly raised opening and closing pressures, normal white blood cell count, protein, and glucose.

Disorders associated with secondary intracranial hypertension are listed in Box 65-2 [Geenen et al., 1996; Gironell et al., 1997; Kone-Paut et al., 1997; Lombaert and Carton, 1976; Raghavan et al., 1997; Selhorst et al., 1984]. Dural venous sinus thrombosis is a significant cause of secondary intracranial hypertension. It is now being detected more often because magnetic resonance venography is increasingly used in the investigation of patients with headache and papilledema (Fig. 65-6). Lumbar puncture might show increases in opening pressure, red blood cells, and protein content. Before the advent of magnetic resonance venography, many affected patients received mistaken diagnoses of IIH. Sickle cell anemia with normal venous flow has also been linked to secondary intracranial hypertension or pseudotumor cerebri [Henry et al., 2004].

The treatment of IIH depends on whether visual function is compromised. In patients with unimpaired visual function, the treatment consists of agents that decrease the formation of cerebrospinal fluid (acetazolamide, 20 mg/kg/day in two divided doses) or diuretics such as furosemide (1 mg/kg/day in two divided doses). Patients receiving acetazolamide should be monitored for side effects such as drowsiness; anorexia; nausea; numbness of the hands, feet,

Box 65-2 Disorders Associated with "Idiopathic" Intracranial Hypertension

- Drugs
  - Use of corticosteroids and corticosteroid withdrawal
  - Tetracyclines
  - Oral contraceptives
  - Hypervitaminosis A
  - Nalidixic acid
  - Phenothiazines
- Systemic disorders
  - Iron deficiency anemia
  - Guillain-Barré syndrome
  - Leukemia
  - Non-Hodgkin's lymphoma
  - Polycythemia
  - Chronic otitis media or sinusitis
  - Behçet's disease
  - Antiphospholipid antibody syndrome
  - Familial deficiency of antithrombin III
  - Systemic lupus erythematosus
  - Other systemic infections
- Metabolic/endocrine disorders
  - During initiation of treatment of hypothyroidism
  - Hyperthyroidism
  - Hypoparathyroidism
  - Adrenal insufficiency
  - Hyperadrenalism
  - Obesity, menarche, pregnancy
  - Hypophosphatasia

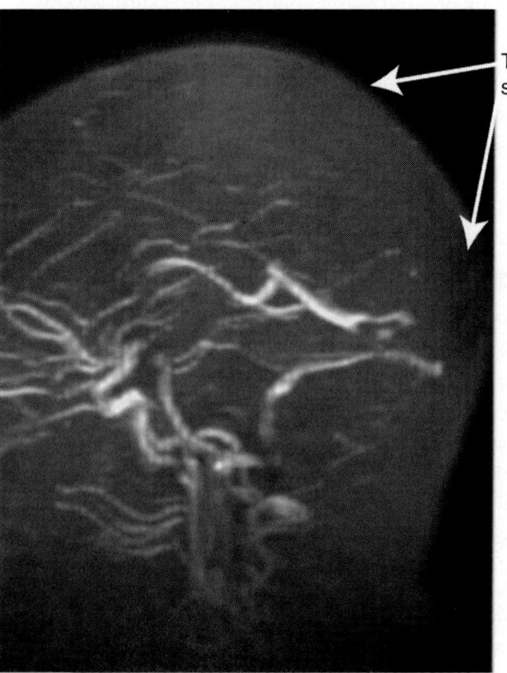

FIGURE 65-6. Magnetic resonance venogram in a 10-year-old girl with acute lymphocytic leukemia who developed headache and papilledema during the course of chemotherapy with L-asparaginase. Note lack of flow signal in the superior and inferior sagittal sinuses and the sigmoid sinuses (*arrows*), which is consistent with sinus thrombosis.

or face; and renal calculi. Patients taking furosemide should be monitored for hypokalemia. There are no data on the comparative efficacy of acetazolamide and furosemide. Weight reduction measures are also recommended for obese subjects. A 2- to 3-week course of dexamethasone may also be beneficial [Fenichel, 2001], but there is a risk of weight gain from steroid use. The discontinuation of steroids might also exacerbate the pseudotumor. Serial lumbar punctures, carried out every 5 to 7 days, with drainage of 20 to 25 mL of cerebrospinal fluid on each tap, are also helpful in lowering the closing pressure below 200 mm Hg. Pain at the lumbar puncture site and post–lumbar puncture headache are potential complications. Simple analgesics such as acetaminophen and ibuprofen, combined with bed rest, are used to treat these complications. A careful examination of the visual acuity and formal visual fields should be performed every 1 to 3 months. Patients who demonstrate compromise of visual function despite medical therapy may need optic nerve sheath fenestration, a surgical procedure that reduces pressure around the nerve. Medical therapy should continue. In a study of 29 eyes of patients with IIH who were subjected to optic nerve sheath fenestration and monitored for a mean of 15.7 months [Goh et al., 1997], the visual acuity improved in 4 eyes (13.8%), stabilized in 22 eyes (76%), and deteriorated in 3 eyes (10.3%). A lumboperitoneal shunt [Johnston et al., 1988] may also be used when IIH is refractory to standard medical therapy.

The treatment of secondary intracranial hypertension is similar to that of IIH but additionally includes removal of the underlying precipitant, such as discontinuation of tetracycline or vitamin A, and the use of low-molecular-weight heparin for dural venous sinus thrombosis [DeVeber et al., 1998; Johnson et al., 2003; Stam et al., 2002].

CEREBRAL EDEMA IN DIABETIC KETOACIDOSIS

A mild degree of cerebral edema, characterized by effacement of the cortical sulci and mild compression of the lateral ventricles on computed tomographic scans, is a common finding in juvenile diabetic ketoacidosis [Krane et al., 1985]. Most patients, however, remain clinically asymptomatic from the standpoint of raised ICP. Severe cerebral edema, in contrast, is a rare but potentially lethal complication, with a mortality rate of 90% [Dunger et al., 2004; Krane et al., 1985]. Paradoxically, it becomes apparent 6 to 10 hours after initiation of therapy for diabetic ketoacidosis with intravenous fluids and insulin—at a time when the blood glucose levels are falling and adequate peripheral circulation has been restored [Krane et al., 1985].

The pathogenesis is not fully understood, but it may include osmotic dysequilibrium between the intravascular and intracerebral contents. Diabetic ketoacidosis is associated with accumulation in the brain of polyols (sorbitol, xylitol, and dulcitol) and other unidentified, osmotically active substrates termed *idiogenic osmoles.* An osmotic dysequilibrium may develop when the intravascular hyperosmolality is corrected sooner than the brain hyperosmolality, which results in a large fluid shift into the brain and cerebral edema [Arieff and Kleeman, 1973; Prockop, 1971]. However, Hale and colleagues [1997] believed that the syndrome is more likely to develop in patients with low initial serum sodium levels and low serum osmolality. Other series of investigators have believed that the syndrome is related primarily to rapid correction of serum glucose and that a rapid movement of sodium into the brain is not the cause. It appears that acidosis does not play any significant role in the pathogenesis. There is active debate about whether this potentially fatal complication can be predicted or prevented [Dunger et al., 2004].

Once the massive brain swelling has begun, it leads to an abrupt deterioration in the level of consciousness in a patient who was otherwise becoming gradually more alert. Central or uncal herniation may develop, heralded by changes in pupillary size, tonic posturing, loss of oculocephalic reflexes, and respiratory arrest.

The management calls for immediate intravenous administration of mannitol (0.25 to 1 gram/kg), followed by endotracheal intubation and hyperventilation if necessary.

CRANIOSYNOSTOSIS

Secondary craniosynostosis is linked to micrencephaly, premature suture closure resulting from lack of brain growth. It does not lead to increased ICP. Primary premature closure of the cranial sutures (incidence about 0.4 per 1000) can, however, lead to raised ICP. Most cases of primary craniosynostosis are sporadic, although both autosomal-recessive and autosomal-dominant forms can also occur. At least 50 syndromic conditions have been linked to primary craniosynostosis (see Chapter 19) [Shapiro et al., 1994]. Sagittal synostosis is the most common type, leading to scaphocephaly, followed by coronal synostosis that leads to brachycephaly/plagiocephaly. Premature closure of one suture usually causes only a cosmetic deformity. Increased ICP is more likely to occur with premature closure of multiple sutures. Raised ICP has been documented in 33% [Reiner et al., 1982] to 73% [Thompson et al., 1995] of patients with primary craniosynostosis. Both reduced intracranial volume and deformation of the intracranial venous sinuses play a role in the development of raised ICP [Mursch et al., 1999]. This is manifested as irritability, opisthotonic posturing, headache, vomiting, or papilledema.

There are probably multiple mechanisms underlying the premature closure of the sutures, including genetic factors, teratogens, metabolic bone disease, intrauterine positioning, and molding [Cohen, 2005]. Intracranial abnormalities such as septo-optic dysplasia and ventriculomegaly can also coexist. Crouzon's disease is an autosomal-dominant disorder caused by mutations in the fibroblast growth factor receptor 2 gene. It is characterized by early closure of any or all sutures in association with midface hypoplasia [Theone, 1995]. Patients manifest hypertelorism, exophthalmos, a parrot-beaked nose, hypoplastic maxilla, and prognathism. Progressive visual and hearing loss occur in half the patients, and mental retardation in a third. Apert's syndrome is characterized by coronal synostosis and syndactyly, hypertelorism, exophthalmos, cataracts, a high pointed palate, and normal intelligence [Theone, 1995]. Above-average parental age has been reported in sporadic cases. Mutations involving the fibroblast growth factor receptor 2 gene have also been observed. The kleeblattschädel (cloverleaf) deformity is seen with primary craniosynostosis involving all sutures. It may be inherited as a recessive or dominant trait.

Skull radiographs in patients with craniosynostosis reveal obliteration of the sutures and sclerosis along their margins and a "beaten silver" appearance. Computed tomography is helpful in excluding associated intraparenchymal lesions. Elevated ICP can be established by lumbar puncture or by epidural or intraparenchymal ICP monitors. Serial measurements of the resistive index with transcranial color-coded duplex sonography of the superior sagittal sinus are also useful in the preoperative and postoperative assessment of ICP [Mursch et al., 1999]. Surgical treatment, whether for cosmetic reasons alone or for alleviation of increased ICP, requires a team approach, entailing the expertise of a primary care physician, a neurosurgeon, a craniofacial plastic surgeon, a neuro-ophthalmologist, an anesthesiologist, and a social worker. The operative procedure may vary from strip craniectomy along the suture margins to more extensive plastic procedures. There is a high incidence of recurrence of increased ICP in patients with syndromic craniosynostosis. In a study of 22 consecutive infants with syndromic craniosynostosis who underwent initial surgery between 6 to 18 months, Pollack and associates [1996] found that 8 (36%) of the infants developed asymptomatic increases in ICP at a median of 16.5 months after the initial surgery.

CONCLUSION

In infants and children, a high index of suspicion should be maintained for raised ICP. The symptom is of diverse etiology. The presentation may be acute or subacute. Acutely elevated ICP may be life threatening and necessitates a team approach for management, with involvement of the family, nursing staff, pediatric intensivist, neurosurgeon, and child neurologist. The algorithm shown in Figure 65-5 may help in management.

REFERENCES

Adelson PD. Bratton SL, Carney NA, et al. Guidelines for the acute medical management of severe traumatic brain injury in infants, children, and adolescents. Pediatr Crit Care Med 2003;4:S28.

Arieff AI, Kleeman CR. Studies on mechanisms of cerebral edema in diabetic coma: Effects of hyperglycemia and rapid lowering of plasma glucose in normal rabbits. J Clin Invest 1973;52:571.

Barbiro-Michaely E, Mayevsky A. Effects of elevated ICP on brain function: Can the multiparametric monitoring system detect the "Cushing response?" Neurol Res 2003;25:42.

Bell BA, Smith MA, Kean DM. Brain water measured by magnetic resonance imaging: Correlation with direct estimation and changes after mannitol and dexamethasone. Lancet 1987;1:66.

Bergman I. Increased intracranial pressure. Pediatr Rev 1994;15:241.

Bray PF, Shields WD, Wolcott GJ, et al. Occipito-frontal head circumference—An accurate measurement of intracranial volume. J Pediatr 1969;75:303.

Cohen MM. Editorial: Perspectives on craniosynostosis. Am J Med Genet 2005;136A:313.

Czosnyka M, Pickard JD. Monitoring and interpretation of intracranial pressure. J Neurol Neurosurg Psychiatry 2004;75:813.

DeVeber G, Chan A, Monagle P, et al. Anticoagulation therapy in pediatric patients with sinovenous thrombosis: A cohort study. Arch Neurol 1998;55:1533.

Dobrovoljac M, Hengartner H, Bolthauser E, et al. Delay in the diagnosis of pediatric brain tumors. Eur J Pediatr 2002;161:663.

Ducker TB, Simmons RL, Martin AM. Pulmonary edema as a complication of intracranial disease. Am J Dis Child 1969;118:638.

Dunger DB, Sperling MA, Acerini CL, et al. ESPE/LWPES consensus statement on diabetic ketoacidosis in children and adolescents. Arch Dis Child 2004;89:188.

Eisenberg HM, Frankowski RF, Contant CF, et al. High-dose barbiturate control of elevated intracranial pressure in patients with severe head injury. J Neurosurg 1988;69:15.

Ersson U, Carlson H, Mellstrom A, et al. Observations on intracranial dynamics during respiratory physiotherapy in unconscious neurosurgical patients. Acta Anesthesiol Scand 1990;34:99.

Fenichel GM. Increased intracranial pressure. In: Fenichel GB, ed. Clinical pediatric neurology. A signs and symptoms approach, 4th ed. Philadelphia: WB Saunders, 2001;91.

Feske SK. Coma and confusional states: Emergency diagnosis and management. Neurol Clin 1998;16:237.

Figaji AA, Fieggen AG, Peter JC. Early decompressive craniotomy in children with severe traumatic brain injury. Child's Nerv System 2003;19:666.

Friden HG, Ekstedt J. Volume/pressure relationship of the cerebrospinal space in humans. Neurosurgery 1983;13:351.

Friedman D, Jacobson D. Diagnostic criteria for idiopathic intracranial hypertension. Neurology 2002;59:1492.

Friedman D, Jacobson DM. Idiopathic intracranial hypertension. J Neuro-ophthalmol 2004;24:138.

Frost EAM. Effects of positive end-expiratory pressure on intracranial pressure and compliance in brain-injured patients. J Neurosurg 1977;47:195.

Geenen C, Tein I, Ehrlich RM. Addison's disease presenting with cerebral edema. Can J Neurol Sci 1996;23:141.

Gironell A, Marti-Fabregas J, Bello J, et al. Non-Hodgkin's lymphoma as a new cause of non-thrombotic superior sagittal sinus occlusion. J Neurol Neurosurg Psychiatry 1997;63:121.

Glaser, JS. Topical diagnosis: Prechiasmal visual pathways. In: Glaser JS, ed. Neuro-ophthalmology. Hagerstown, MD: Harper & Row, 1978;61.

Goh KY, Schatz NJ, Glaser JS. Optic nerve sheath fenestration for pseudotumor cerebri. J Neuroophthalmol 1997;17:86.

Gourin CG, Shackford SR. Production of tumor necrosis factor-alpha and interleukin-1-beta by human cerebral microvascular endothelium after percussive trauma. J Trauma 1997;42:1101.

Guillaume J, Janny P. Manometrie intracranienne continue; interet physio-pathologique et clinique de la methode [Continuous intracranial manometry; physiopathologic and clinical significance of the method]. Presse Med 1951;59:953.

Hale PM, Rezvani I, Braunstein AW, et al. Factors predicting cerebral edema in young children with diabetic ketoacidosis and new onset type I diabetes. Acta Pediatr 1997;86:626.

Hall ED, Braughler JM. Effects of intravenous methylprednisolone on spinal cord lipid peroxidation and Na-K ATPase activity. Dose-response analysis during 1st hour after contusion injury in the cat. J Neurosurg 1982;57:247.

Henry M, Driscoll MC, Miller M, et al. Pseudotumor cerebri in children with sickle cell disease: A case series. Pediatrics 2004;113:e265.

Johnson MC, Parkerson N, Ward S, et al. Pediatric sinovenous thrombosis. J Pediatr Hematol Oncol 2003;25:312.

Johnston I, Besser M, Morgan MK. Cerebrospinal fluid diversion in the treatment of benign intracranial hypertension. J Neurosurg 1988;69:195.

Kellie G. The account of the appearances observed in the dissection of two of the three individuals presumed to have perished in the storm of the 3rd, and whose bodies were discovered in the vicinity of Leith on the morning of 4th November, 1821, with some reflections on the pathology of the brain. Trans Med Chir Sci Edinburgh 1824;1:84.

Kone-Paut I, Chabrol B, Riss JM, et al. Neurologic onset of Behçet's disease: A diagnostic enigma in childhood. J Child Neurol 1997;12:237.

Krane EJ, Rockoff MA, Wallman JK. Subclinical brain swelling in children during the treatment of diabetic ketoacidosis. N Engl J Med 1985;312:1147.

Lombaert A, Carton H. Benign intracranial hypertension due to A-hypervitaminosis in adults and adolescents. Eur Neurol 1976;14:340.

Luerssen TG. Intracranial pressure: Current status in monitoring and management. Semin Pediatr Neurol 1997;4:146.

Lundberg N. Continuous recording and control of ventricular fluid pressure in neurosurgical practice. Acta Psychiatr Neurol Scand

1960;36 (Suppl 149):S1.
Marmarou A. Pathophysiology of traumatic brain edema: Current concepts. Acta Neurochir Suppl 2003;86:7.
Marmarou A, Shulman K. Pressure-volume relationships—Basic aspects. In: McLaurin RL, ed. Head injuries. New York: Grune & Stratton, 1976;5.
Marshall LF, Smith RW, Shapiro HM. The outcome with aggressive treatment in severe head injuries. Part I. The significance of intracranial pressure monitoring. J Neurosurg 1979;50:20.
Menke JA, Miles R, McIlhany M, et al. The fontanelle tonometer: A non-invasive method for measurement of intracranial pressure. J Pediatr 1982;100:960.
Monro A. Observations on the structure and function of the nervous system. Edinburgh: Creech and Johnston, 1783.
Mursch K, Enk T, Christen HJ, et al. Venous intracranial hemodynamics in children undergoing operative treatment for the repair of craniosynostosis. Childs Nerv Syst 1999;15:110.
Narayan RK, Kishore PR, Becker DP, et al. Intracranial pressure: To monitor or not to monitor? A review of our experience with severe head injury. J Neurosurg 1982;56:650.
Nimmo AJ, Cernak I, Heath DL, et al. Neurogenic inflammation is associated with development of edema and functional deficits following traumatic brain injury in rats. Neuropeptides 2004;38:40.
Node Y, Nakazawa S. Clinical study of mannitol and glycerol on raised intracranial pressure and on their rebound phenomenon. Adv Neurol 1990;52:359.
Palmer J. Management of raised intracranial pressure in children. Intensive Crit Care Nurs 2000;16:319.
Plum F, Posner JB. Supratentorial lesions. In: Plum F, Posner JB, eds. The diagnosis of stupor and coma. New York: Oxford University Press, 1980;109.
Pollack IF, Losken HW, Biglan AW. Incidence of increased intracranial pressure after early surgical treatment of syndromic craniosynostosis. Pediatr Neurosurg 1996;24:202.
Prockop LD. Hyperglycemia, polyol accumulation, and increased intracranial pressure. Arch Neurol 1971;25:126.
Raghavan S, DiMartino-Nardi J, Saenger P, et al. Pseudotumor cerebri in an infant after L-thyroxine therapy for transient neonatal hypothyroidism. J Pediatr 1997;130:478.
Reiner D, Sainte-Rose C, Marchac D, et al. Intracranial pressure in craniosynostosis. J Neurosurg 1982;57:370.
Ropper AH. Raised intracranial pressure in neurologic disease. Semin Neurol 1984;4:5.
Rosner MJ, Becker DP. ICP monitoring: Complications and associated factors. Clin Neurosurg 1976;23:494.
Rosner MJ, Coley IB. Cerebral perfusion pressure, intracranial pressure, and head elevation. J Neurosurg 1986;60:636.
Ruf B, Heckmann M, Schorth I, et al. Early decompressive craniectomy and duroplasty for refractory intracranial hypertension in children: Results of a pilot study. Crit Care 2003;7:409.
Salmon JH, Hajjar W, Bada HS. The fontogram: A non-invasive intracranial pressure monitor. Pediatrics 1977;60:721.
Sato H, Sato N, Tamaki N, et al. Threshold of cerebral perfusion pressure as a prognostic factor in hydrocephalus during infancy. Childs Nerv Syst 1988;4:274.
Saul TG, Ducker TB. The effect of intracranial pressure monitoring and aggressive treatment on mortality in severe head injury. J Neurosurg 1982;56:498.
Schaefer PW, Buonanno FS, Gonzalez RG, et al. Diffusion-weighted imaging discriminates between cytotoxic and vasogenic edema in a patient with eclampsia. Stroke 1997;28:1082.
Schilling L, Wahl M. Brain edema: Pathogenesis and therapy. Kidney Int Suppl 1997;59:S69.
Selhorst JB, Waybright EA, Jennings S, et al. Liver lover's headache: Pseudotumor cerebri and vitamin A intoxication. JAMA 1984;252:3365.
Shapiro K, Morris WJ, Teo C. Intracranial hypertension: Mechanisms and management. In: Cheek WR, Marlin AE, McLone DJ, et al., eds. Pediatric neurosurgery. Surgery of the developing nervous system. Philadelphia: WB Saunders, 1994;307.
Shapiro S, Bowman R, Callahan J, et al. The fiberoptic cerebral pressure monitor in 244 patients. Surg Neurol 1996;45:278.
Siesjo BK. Cerebral circulation and metabolism. J Neurosurg 1984;60:883.
Society of Critical Care Medicine and The World Federation of Pediatric Intensive and Critical Care Societies. 2003;4(3, suppl):SD40.
Stam J, De Bruijn SF, DeVeber G. Anticoagulation for cerebral sinus thrombosis. Cochrane Database Syst Rev 2002;(4):CD002005.
Theone JG, ed. Physician's guide to rare diseases, 2nd ed. Montvale, NJ: Dowden, 1995.
Thompson DN, Harkness WJ, Jones B, et al. Subdural intracranial pressure monitoring in craniosynostosis: Role in surgical management. Childs Nerv Syst 1995;11:269.
Trauner DA. Increased intracranial pressure. In: Swaiman KF, ed. Pediatric neurology. Principles and practice, 2nd ed. St. Louis: CV Mosby, 1989.
Tuite GF, Chong WK, Evanson J, et al. The effectiveness of papilledema as an indicator of raised intracranial pressure in children with craniosynostosis. Neurosurgery 1996;38272.
Volpe JJ. Specialized studies in the neurological evaluation. In: Volpe JJ, ed. Neurology of the newborn, 4th ed. Philadelphia: WB Saunders, 2000;134.
Ward JD, Becker DP, Miller JD, et al. Failure of prophylactic barbiturate coma in the treatment of severe head injury. J Neurosurg 1985;62:383.
Welch K. The intracranial pressure in infants. J Neurosurg 1980;52:693.

CHAPTER 66

Spinal Cord Injury

N. Paul Rosman and Chellamani Harini

In the United States and Canada, the annual incidence of traumatic spinal cord injury is 30 to 46 cases per 1 million population [Decker and Hergenroeder, 2004]. In the United States, 8000 to 12,000 new spinal cord injuries occur each year. Less than 10% of these patients die from their acute injuries [Walker, 1991], with 200,000 to 250,000 persons now living in the United States with sequelae of spinal cord trauma [Green and Eismont, 1984; Meyer et al., 1991; Oliver, 1992; Walker, 1991]. Pediatric patients constitute 0.3% to 10% of that number [Dias, 2004; Hadley et al., 1988; Hill et al., 1984; Proctor, 2002], with 3% to 5% of the spinal cord injuries that occur each year in the United States occurring in persons younger than 15 years of age and 20% occurring in persons younger than 20 years of age [Vogel and Anderson, 2003]. The risk of spinal cord injury is equal for males and females from birth to age 3 years; the male-to-female ratio is 6:4 from age 4 to 8 years, 7:3 from age 9 to 15 years, and 8.5:1.5 from age 16 to 20 years [Massagli, 2000]. Half of the spine injuries in children 0 to 3 years old occur at the C1 to C2 level, whereas only 8% affect this level in children age 4 to 12 years. These differences are probably explained by the higher fulcrum of motion in younger children and perhaps by weakness of C2 as a result of incomplete ossification of its synchondrosis [Proctor, 2002].

Motor vehicle accidents, including lap belt injuries to the lumbar spine, are the principal cause of spinal cord injuries, followed in decreasing order of frequency by falls, recreational or sports activities (especially diving accidents and football injuries), and penetrating injuries of the spinal column (e.g., gunshot, knife) [Gibson, 1992; Maroon et al., 1980; Massagli, 2000; Meyer et al., 1991; Mueller and Blyth, 1987; Schneider, 1964; Vogel and Anderson, 2003]. Since the 1980s, violence has increased from 10% to 30% as a cause of spinal cord injury in patients ages 16 to 20 years [Vogel et al., 1997]. Traumatic birth injury accounts for only 10% to 15% of all cases [Hadley, 1992]. Determinants of the severity of injury occurring after spinal cord trauma include the following: (1) nature, direction, and degree of the traumatic insult; (2) site of injury; (3) presence of any preexisting spine anomaly; (4) extent of tissue damage; (5) degree of vascular compromise complicating the spinal trauma; and (6) rapidity and efficacy of treatment [Rosman and Herskowitz, 1982]. The mortality from spinal cord injury in children is more than twice that seen in adults [Hamilton and Myles, 1992].

ANATOMY

Bony Spine and Ligaments

The structure of the bony spine provides protection for and prevents excessive movement of the underlying spinal cord. Major ligaments that functionally divide the spine into anterior and posterior compartments maintain stability of the bony spinal column during movement [Chilton and Dagi, 1985]. Anteriorly, these ligaments are the anterior and posterior longitudinal ligaments; posteriorly, the ligaments include the ligamentum flavum and the interspinous, intertransverse, supraspinous, and facet capsular ligaments. Additionally the transverse or cruciate ligament provides important stability between the atlas and axis. Stability of the spine as a whole is ensured if all of the anterior ligaments or if all of the posterior ligaments plus one anterior ligament are intact [Chilton and Dagi, 1985].

The most mobile portion of the spinal column is the cervical region, making that area the most common site of spinal cord injury [Green and Eismont, 1984; Hill et al., 1984]. Younger children are particularly susceptible to injuries of the high cervical cord [Davis et al., 1993; Piper and Menezes, 1996; Vogel et al., 1997]. Factors predisposing the upper cervical spine to injury in the young child include a proportionally larger and heavier head, relative underdevelopment of the neck muscles and ligaments, incomplete ossification of the vertebral bodies with relative anterior wedging [Massagli, 2000], incomplete development of the uncinate processes, smaller vertebral bodies of C1 to C2 compared with C3 to C5, and the more horizontal orientation of the articular surfaces of the cervical facet joints [Glasser and Fessler, 1996; Hadley et al., 1988; White and Panjabi, 1990]. Approximately 55% of spinal cord injuries involve the cervical spine, 30% involve the thoracic spine, and 15% involve the lumbar spine [Marion, 1998]. With birth trauma, spinal cord injuries are most common in the high cervical region (usually during an instrumental cephalic delivery) and in the lower cervical and upper thoracic regions (usually during a breech delivery). With increased use of cesarean sections to avoid potentially problematic vaginal deliveries, the frequency of spinal cord injury incurred during delivery has lessened appreciably [Morgan and Newell, 2001]. Between infancy and 8 years of age, 75% of spinal injuries occur in the cervical spine, particularly in its upper portion. Between age 8 and 14 years, 60% of injuries occur in the cervical spine, and 20% occur in the thoracic region, with the remainder at lower spinal levels [Menezes et al., 1989]. Conditions predisposing to cervical spinal cord injury in children include Down syndrome (15% have atlantoaxial instability), Klippel-Feil syndrome, Morquio's syndrome, Larsen's syndrome, achondroplasia, and previous cervical spine surgery [Caviness, 2004; Massagli, 2000].

The most common causes of cervical spine trauma in persons 18 years old and younger were motor vehicle accidents (45%), diving (23%), falls (11%), gymnastics

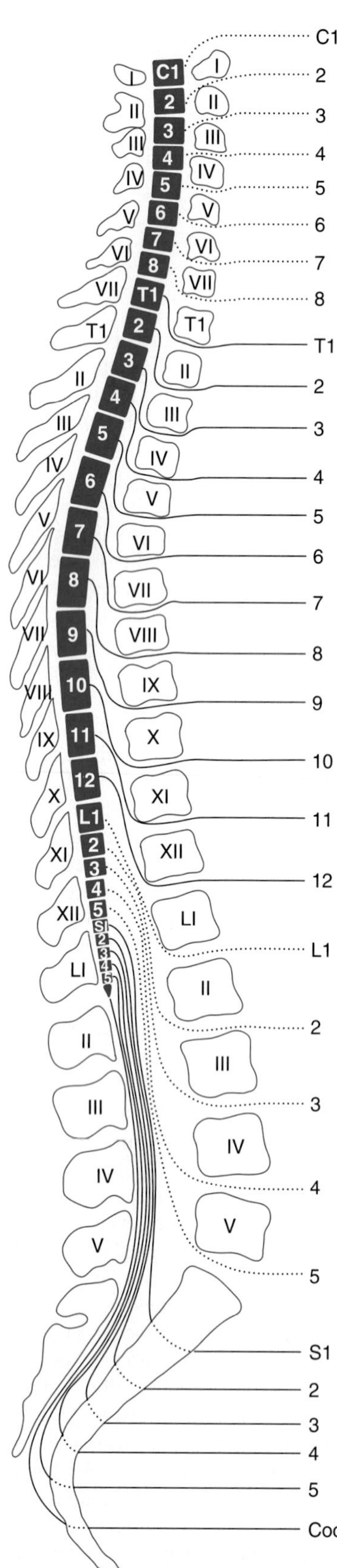

FIGURE 66-1. Spinal cord root levels in relation to the vertebral bodies. (From Haymaker W, Woodhall B. Peripheral nerve injuries, 2nd ed. Philadelphia: WB Saunders, 1953.)

(7%), football (5%), and other miscellaneous causes (8%) [Hill et al., 1984]. The second most mobile portion of the spine is the thoracolumbar region. It also is the second most commonly injured area, with T10 the site most frequently fractured [Ruge et al., 1988]. Regardless of the mechanism of injury, the thoracic spine (T2 through T10) is the most common site of fracture in pediatric trauma patients [Reddy et al., 2003]. The thoracic and lumbosacral regions are the portions of the cord least often injured after trauma [Green and Eismont, 1984].

Spinal Cord

A disparity exists between vertebral and segmental cord levels that changes with age. Early in fetal life, the spinal cord extends throughout the bony vertebral column, but during later development, the vertebral column becomes longer than the spinal cord. The caudal end of the cord comes to lie at successively higher vertebral levels; at birth, it is at the level of the second lumbar vertebra, and in adulthood, it is at the first lumbar level. Disparity also exists between the levels of exit of nerve roots from the spinal canal and corresponding spinal segmental levels from which they originate, with the nerve roots emerging below their sites of origin (see Chapter 2). Below the first lumbar segment, there is no spinal cord, only the lumbosacral roots composing the cauda equina (Fig. 66-1).

Blood Supply

The anterior spinal artery is an unpaired vessel formed by junction of a branch from the two vertebral arteries. It descends the entire length of the spinal cord ventrally in the anterior median sulcus. Between C3 and L3, the anterior spinal artery receives additional blood supply from anterior radicular arteries derived from lateral spinal arteries. Branches from the anterior spinal artery supply the entire anterior columns and most of the lateral columns of the spinal cord. The two posterior spinal arteries communicate with posterior radicular branches of the lateral spinal arteries to form a rich plexus of collaterals that supply the entire posterior columns and the remainder of the lateral columns of the spinal cord [Herren and Alexander, 1939; Suh and Alexander, 1939].

PATHOGENESIS: MECHANISMS OF SPINAL CORD INJURY

When the spinal cord sustains traumatic injury, the forces applied to the spine usually have been sufficient to cause displacement of vertebral ligaments and bones [Kakulas, 1984]. There are five major ways in which trauma to the spine can result in injury to the spinal cord: forward flexion, lateral flexion, rotation, axial compression, and hyperextension [Chilton and Dagi, 1985]. The forces generated by these movements can result in vertebral distraction, dislocation, fracture, and disk herniation. Often, as is the case in motor vehicle accidents and birth trauma, several forces act at the same time to injure the spine [Glasser and Fessler, 1996]. Osseous disruption (fracture or displacement) is the most common cause of spinal cord injury. Ligamentous injury, without osseous disruption, causing spinal cord injury

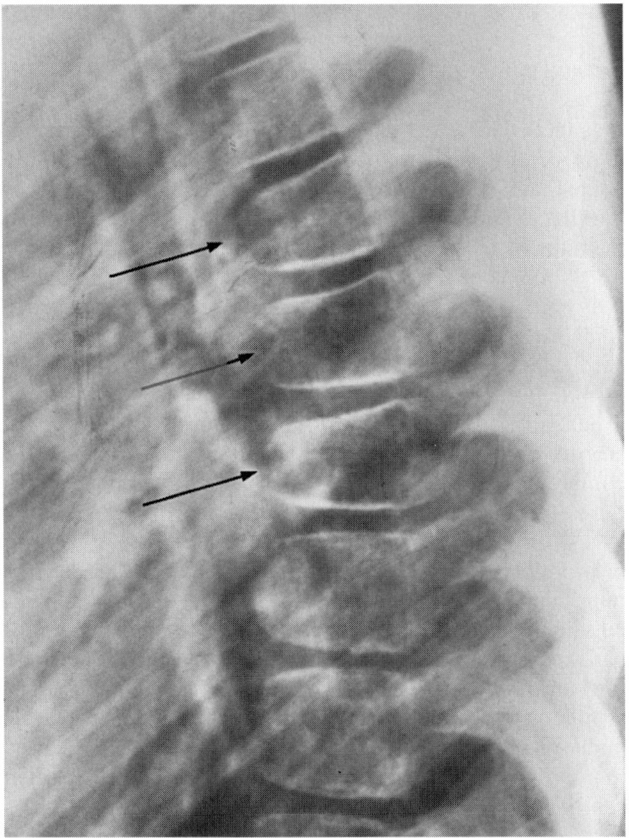

FIGURE 66-2. Plain lateral view of the thoracic spine in an 8-year-old female who sustained a hyperflexion injury after a fall from a height of 10 feet. There is anterior wedging of the bodies of T4 and T6 *(arrows)*.

is common in children, resulting in spinal cord injury without radiographic abnormality (SCIWORA). Disk herniation occurs in approximately 50% of spinal cord–injured patients [Flanders et al., 1990].

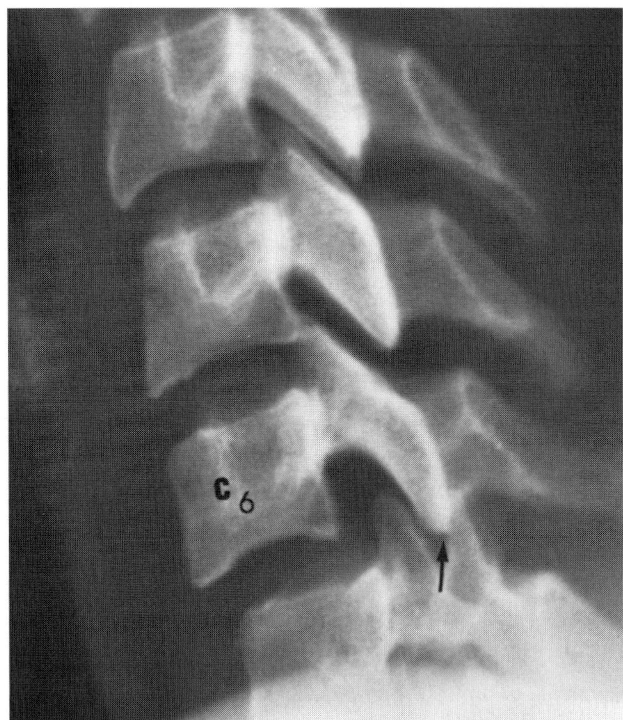

FIGURE 66-3. Plain lateral view of the cervical spine disclosing anterior dislocation of C6, resulting in one of its inferior facets *(arrow)* locking into a superior facet of C7 immediately below. Both superior facets of C7 are visible because of rotation of that vertebra.

Forward flexion can lead to wedge or teardrop fractures, which usually begin at or near the intervertebral disk (Fig. 66-2). These fractures are often encountered in motor vehicle accidents in passengers not wearing seat belts, but

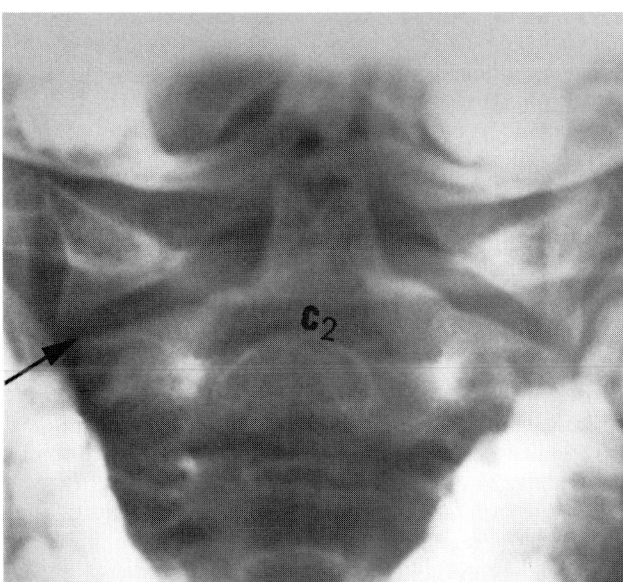

A

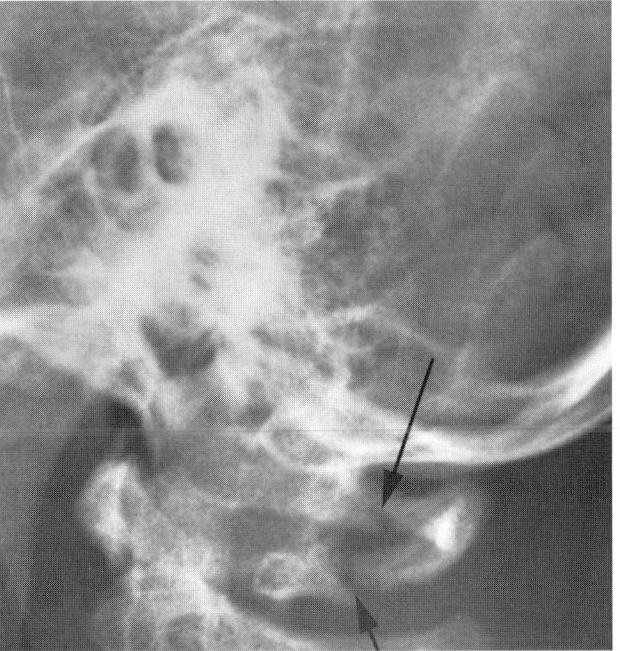

B

FIGURE 66-4. A, Plain anteroposterior view of upper cervical spine indicates a Jefferson fracture of the atlas (C1) with a lateral mass of C1 displaced laterally on the body of C2 *(arrow)*. **B,** Plain lateral view of the skull and upper cervical spine in the same patient. Accompanying the Jefferson fracture are fractures *(arrows)* through the posterior arch of C1.

also can be seen in children wearing ill-fitting adult types of lap-sash belts (cervical seat-belt syndrome) [Hoy and Cole, 1993]. Excessive lateral flexion of the cervical spine is always accompanied by rotation and can cause a unilateral locked facet (Fig. 66-3). This locked facet occurs when the inferior facet contralateral to the side of flexion rotates too far anteriorly and locks into the superior facet of the vertebral body below [Panjabi and White, 1980]. Simple flexion alone usually causes little damage, but with the addition of rotation, ligaments can rupture, rendering the spine unstable and prone to distraction and dislocation. Rotation and flexion, accompanied by posterior ligamentous tear, also can cause vertebral body shear fractures.

Axial compression typically occurs in diving accidents, falls, and sports injuries. Axial compression can result in a burst fracture in which the vertebral end plate is injured, allowing the intervertebral disk to rupture into the vertebral body, which then bursts. In the Jefferson fracture, a direct blow to the top of the head results in axial compression that is transmitted through the occipital condyles to the atlas, the arch of which bursts, allowing fragments to be displaced outward (Fig. 66-4) [Shapiro et al., 1973]. Severe hyperextension is often encountered in rear-end motor vehicle accidents (whiplash injury) and in the head-shaking injury of child abuse. This hyperextension can result in transverse fractures of the neural arches of the cervical spine, usually accompanied by tearing of the anterior longitudinal ligament [Caffey, 1974; Janes and Hooshmand, 1965; Ommaya, 1969]. The so-called hangman's fracture occurs from a hyperextension injury through the synchondrosis between the odontoid and the arch of C2 [Reynolds, 2000]. Because the vertebral arteries lie in the transverse processes of these vertebrae, they can be torn or thrombosed after such injuries with resultant ischemia to the anterior two-thirds of the spinal cord. Such injuries have been reported after neck hyperextension in football games and in infants with C1 to C2 instability [Gilles et al., 1979; Schneider et al., 1970]. Displacement of the vertebrae during spinal trauma can compress the arteries of the spinal cord, resulting in ischemic injury, often without radiographic abnormalities.

NEUROPATHOLOGY

The nature and severity of traumatic injury to the spinal cord are related to the type and location of vertebral damage, the presence of any preexisting disorder affecting the size of the spinal canal or mobility of the spinal cord (e.g., spinal stenosis, spondylitis, prolapsed disk), and the occurrence of concomitant vascular injury [Braakman and Penning, 1976; Chilton and Dagi, 1985]. Pathologic examination after spinal cord trauma has disclosed injuries that are either intraspinal intramedullary (affecting the spinal cord primarily) or, less often, intraspinal extramedullary (affecting the spinal cord secondarily). Intraspinal intramedullary pathologies include concussion, ischemia, contusion, compression, laceration, and intramedullary hemorrhage [Jellinger, 1976]. Intraspinal extramedullary injuries include epidural, subdural, and subarachnoid hemorrhages; epidural abscess; arachnoid cyst; epidermoid tumor; herniation of the nucleus pulposus; and cauda equina injuries.

Intraspinal Intramedullary Lesions

Pathogenesis and Pathologies

In spinal concussion, there is a functional rather than pathologic disturbance, usually with return of function within hours [Tator, 1996]. Extravasation of potassium from neurons into the extracellular space, after direct injury of nerve cell membranes or secondary nerve cell damage from vascular disruption, is the most likely mechanism of spinal cord concussion. Ischemia of the spinal cord can occur from anterior spinal artery or other vascular compression during spinal cord trauma, but also can occur when the trauma does not involve the spinal cord directly. Hypotension, systemic shock, and vascular injury to the aorta or a vertebral artery are the most common causes of this type of injury. With compression of the anterior spinal artery, the anterior two thirds of the spinal cord is affected, causing weakness and loss of pain and temperature perception, with preservation of proprioception and light touch. Contusion results from a blunt injury of the spinal cord without continued compression or disruption of nerve tissue, resulting in transient paresthesias and dysesthesias in the upper limbs, especially the hands (burning hands syndrome), accompanied by transient long tract signs. Recovery is incomplete, however, distinguishing contusion from concussion. Central cord necrosis (hemorrhagic or ischemic) is a common sequela that often can be seen on magnetic resonance imaging (MRI) [Bailes et al., 1991; Jellinger, 1976]. Compression of the spinal cord can be caused by vertebral dislocation or by pressure from bony fragments, a herniated disk, or extramedullary bleeding [Jellinger, 1976]. Laceration occurs when there is interruption of spinal cord tissue by bony fragments, knife or bullet wounds, fracture-dislocation, or severe stretching. In older children, the most frequent cause of laceration is a penetrating agent, whereas in newborns, hyperextension of the neck during breech delivery is the most likely cause [Allen et al., 1969; Bresnan and Abroms, 1974; Byers, 1975; Crothers, 1923]. Intramedullary hemorrhage, which can extend over several spinal cord segments (hematomyelia), is believed to result from direct injury to blood vessels or from altered vascular permeability, as from acidosis.

The pathology of intraspinal intramedullary injuries has been studied in detail in experimental animals and in human postmortem examination material [DeLaTorre, 1981; Dumont et al., 2001a; Jellinger, 1976; Kakulas, 1984; Norenberg et al., 2004; Park et al., 2004; Profyris et al., 2004]. To mimic most events that lead to various forms of human spinal cord injury, several experimental models have been developed, the most common being *transection, compression,* or *contusion* [Rosenzweig and McDonald, 2004]. Because there are striking pathophysiologic similarities between human spinal cord injury and experimental models of spinal cord injury, particularly in the rat, findings in experimental spinal cord injury are commonly extrapolated to human injury. Such extrapolation requires caution, however, because regulation of secondary events after spinal cord injury varies greatly among different animal species and strains [Profyris et al., 2004]. The pathologic changes observed in the spinal cord after trauma can be subdivided into early, late, and very late.

EARLY CHANGES

Fifteen to 30 minutes after cord injury, erythrocytes leak predominantly into the central gray matter owing to the region's soft consistency, rich vascularity, and high metabolic demand [Dumont et al., 2001a; Profyris et al., 2004]. These small hemorrhages aggregate and within 1 to 2 hours spread outward; petechial hemorrhages appear, and edema develops, with spread to involve adjacent white matter. Coagulation necrosis, which can involve the entire cross-section of the cord, may develop within the next few hours (Fig. 66-5). Hemorrhage still evident by 3 days is totally gone by day 8. Liquefaction occurs, with formation of cavitations by 21 days; these coalesce, and by 14 weeks they form a large cystic region surrounded by gliotic scar tissue [Profyris et al., 2004; Silver and Miller, 2004].

Necrosis and Apoptosis

A barrage of pathophysiologic events that cause necrosis and apoptosis governs the biology of secondary injury after acute spinal cord injury.

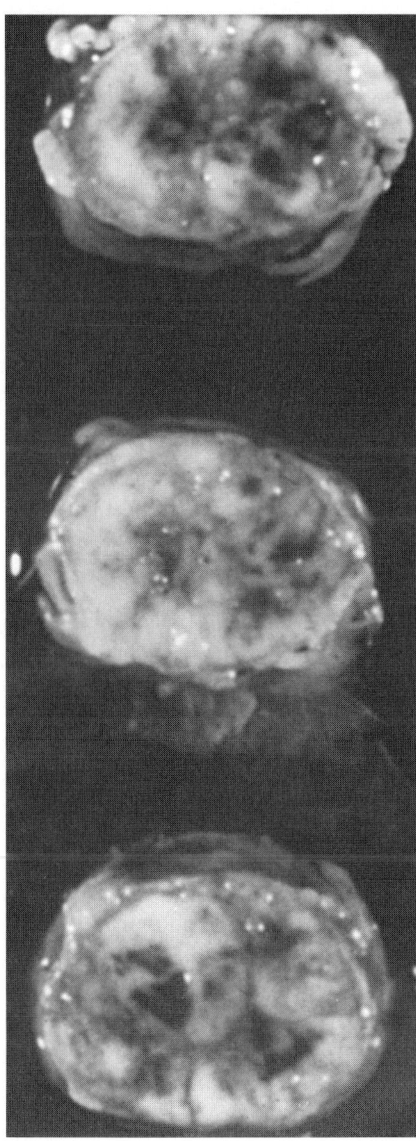

FIGURE 66-5. Severe traumatic injury to the spinal cord with secondary hemorrhage and coagulation necrosis.

NECROSIS. After acute spinal cord injury, a centripetal and rostrocaudal necrotic wave develops that originates at the site of primary injury and that may spread two vertebral levels above and two below the initial lesion; by 8 hours, these changes are irreversible. Contributors to this necrosis include (1) infarction, (2) excitotoxicity, and (3) reperfusion injury. *Infarction* is caused by vascular damage to small vessels (arterioles, capillaries, and venules), vasospasm, thrombosis, and neurogenic shock. At a cellular level, infarction results in a loss of oxidative phosphorylation and glycolysis, resulting in ATP depletion, which triggers several necrotic mechanisms. Also, after spinal cord injury, there is an increase in extracellular glutamate. Excess of this excitatory neurotransmitter overstimulates *N*-methyl-D-aspartate, α-amino-3-hydroxy-5-methyl-4-isoxazole-propionate (AMPA), and kainate to trigger waves of *excitotoxic cell death*. This cell death is caused by an influx of intracellular sodium and water, resulting in cell lysis, and by an accompanying increase in intracellular calcium, which stimulates an array of calcium-depleted proteases and lipases, including calpains (which can degrade structural proteins of the myelin-axon unit) and cyclooxygenase-1 (injurious to cell membranes) [Dumont et al., 2001a]. Glutamate excitotoxicity plays a key role not only in neuronal cell death, but also in oligodendrocyte apoptosis, with the latter attributable to activation of specific caspases and an increase in intracellular calcium [Kim et al., 2003; Park et al., 2004]. *Reperfusion* of tissue within the first few days after spinal cord injury also exacerbates the ensuing tissue damage by generating deleterious free radicals and other toxic by-products, including oxygen-derived free radicals (superoxide, hydroxyl radicals, nitric oxide) [Dumont et al., 2001a]. Reexposure of endothelial cells to oxygen after an earlier ischemic insult also triggers an enzymatic reaction that gives rise to reactive oxygen species (ROS), a potent stimulus for cell death by modifying cellular lipids, proteins, and nucleic acids [Profyris et al., 2004].

APOPTOSIS. Apoptosis is the other important mediator of secondary damage after acute spinal cord injury. Apoptosis occurs in two phases. It initially begins 6 hours after injury at the lesion center, and for several days thereafter, the number of apoptotic cells in this region increases steadily, with death of multiple cell types. By 1 week, the central apoptotic count decreases, but there is now an increase in apoptotic death away—sometimes far away—from the site of the primary injury center; this second phase of cell death is localized predominantly in spinal cord white matter [Profyris et al., 2004].

Oligodendrocyte apoptosis is a widely dispersed phenomenon in spinal cord injury that leads to long-term and persisting demyelination. This denudement of axons, with resultant deterioration of their conductive abilities, adds significantly to functional decline. The high concentration of tumor necrosis factor-α in the central nervous system after spinal cord injury, together with its ability to induce apoptosis, makes it a likely instigator of oligodendrocyte apoptosis, although other factors also play a role [Profyris et al., 2004].

Immunopathology

Inflammatory responses are of central importance in the pathogenesis of acute and chronic spinal cord injury. During both phases, the injured spinal cord recruits *innate immunity* and *adaptive immunity*.

INNATE IMMUNITY. The injured environment during the acute phase of spinal cord injury is dominated by the presence of proinflammatory cytokines (tumor necrosis factor-α, interleukin-1, and interleukin-6). Binding of tumor necrosis factor-α and interleukin-1 to their receptors causes them to induce an inflammatory response by signaling through the nuclear factor-κB pathway. This response stimulates the production of inflammatory mediators (reactive oxygen species, cytokines, inducible nitric oxide synthase, and prostaglandin). The anti-inflammatory agent methylprednisolone, the most effective therapy in spinal cord injury (see later section on drug therapy) has been shown to inhibit the nuclear factor-κB pathway. Spinal cord injury also induces the expression of the anti-inflammatory cytokine transforming growth factor-β, which counteracts the effects of proinflammatory cytokines. After acute spinal cord injury, neutrophils are recruited to the site of primary injury, and by 24 hours they migrate into the lesion to phagocytose debris. As the numbers of neutrophils decline, increased numbers of monocytes appear in the injured parenchyma, which by 72 hours go on to differentiate into microglia and macrophages. When activated, microglia and macrophages phagocytose necrotic and apoptotic debris, but in contrast to neutrophils, their activity is sustained longer. In rat models of spinal cord injury, microglia and macrophages do not decrease until 1 week after injury, whereas the microglial/macrophage presence in degenerating tracts does not plateau until 2 to 4 weeks.

Given the wide array of noxious mediators that are secreted by neutrophils, microglia, and macrophages, treatments to reduce their presence have been widely used in models of spinal cord injury. Decreasing the numbers of these cells at the locus of primary injury may be potentially harmful, however, because microglia and macrophages also facilitate the release of mediators that promote central nervous system repair (ciliary neurotrophic factor, insulin-like growth factor-1, nerve growth factor, and brain-derived growth factor). After contributing to the acute phase of injury, these phagocytes potentially may aid regeneration at more chronic stages by secreting neuronal survival and regeneration factors [Profyris et al., 2004].

ADAPTIVE IMMUNITY. It is likely that most T helper cells activated in spinal cord injury are activated by macrophages. Silencing this adaptive immune response may impede functional recovery after spinal cord injury, however, because activated T helper cells secrete significant amounts of several neurotrophins (nerve growth factor, brain-derived growth factor, neurotrophins NT-3 and NT-4/5) potentially important in enhancing spinal cord repair [Profyris et al., 2004].

Molecular Mechanisms

After spinal cord injury, the proximal ends of cut axons reseal and form a growth cone, a structure that on elongation gives rise to an axon. From the midpoint of the growth cone, processes termed *filopodia* project to probe the surrounding environment and deduce whether axonal extension is feasible or, conversely, deterrent to axonal elongation. The principal axonal regrowth inhibitor in the acute phase of spinal cord injury is central nervous system myelin, which contains numerous inhibitory components (myelin-associated glycoprotein, Nogo-A, and oligodendrocyte myelin glycoprotein). Growth cone "lipid rafts," enriched in cholesterol and sphingolipids, provide an ordered platform for signal transduction. Concentrated in these rafts is the Nogo-66 receptor (NgR), which plays a central role because of its ability to bind all three myelin inhibitory molecules. With the recent finding of two novel proteins that are homologous both structurally and biochemically to NgR [NgR homologues 1 and 2 (NgR H1 and NgR H2)], it is likely that there is added complexity to membrane signaling by myelin-associated inhibitory molecules [Profyris et al., 2004].

LATE CHANGES

In patients who have survived spinal cord injury for 3 to 6 months, the central portion of the spinal cord is replaced by a cystic cavity extending for several segments above and below the point of impact, resulting in *post-traumatic syringomyelia*; this extension can continue over many years, significantly increasing the patient's neurologic deficit [Barnett and Jousse, 1976; Profyris et al., 2004]. Wallerian degeneration of ascending and descending tracts occurs within 6 to 12 months [Kakulas, 1999], and nerve roots at the level of the lesion become atrophic. The cord becomes thin in the area of injury, with fibrosis and thickening of the overlying meninges [Kakulas, 1984]. In 3% of such spinal cord injuries, a progressive syndrome develops, months to years later, characterized by causalgic pain followed by proprioceptive sensory loss and weakness [Tator, 1996].

VERY LATE CHANGES

Enlarging traumatic neuromas and spinal stenosis (from accelerated osteoarthritis) are effects of spinal cord injury that can occur 5 or more years after the initial impact [Kakulas, 1984]. They are probably responsible for the late clinical deterioration encountered in some long-term survivors.

Intraspinal Extramedullary Lesions

Pathogenesis and Pathologies

The mode of spinal cord injury from intraspinal extramedullary conditions is primarily by spinal cord compression, although secondary vasospasm and ischemia also play a role. The causative pathologies include hemorrhage, infection, cystic fluid, and solid tissues. The degree of resultant injury to cord depends on the location and size of the mass and the duration of cord compression. Post-traumatic intraspinal extramedullary mass lesions occur relatively infrequently and, when present, are often small, causing little, if any, cord compression. Included among these disorders are spinal epidural, subdural, and subarachnoid hemorrhages; spinal epidural abscess; arachnoid cyst; epidermoid tumor; and herniation of the nucleus pulposus and cauda equina injuries.

CLINICAL ASSESSMENT

History

A detailed history of the circumstances of the spinal cord injury should be sought from the child and observers of the episode. The history often discloses the additional occurrence of head trauma, which complicates the evaluation of the child, particularly when there has been alteration of consciousness. Details concerning the mechanism of injury, the activity of the child at that time, and the use of restraining devices, such as seat belts, car seats, head rests, and air bags, should be ascertained. One should inquire about the possible presence of any genetic disorders (e.g., Down syndrome), congenital abnormalities of the bony spine (e.g., hemivertebrae), or blood dyscrasias (e.g., hemophilia) that may render a child more vulnerable to spinal cord injury, which in such circumstances can occur after relatively minor trauma. The condition of the child at the scene of the injury and any subsequent changes should be carefully documented.

General Physical Examination

It is crucial to assess the *entire child,* even in the presence of an obvious spinal injury. Particular attention should be directed to the vital signs. Respiratory difficulty may be caused by a traumatic pneumothorax or by diaphragmatic paralysis consequent to injury of the mid cervical spinal cord. Hypotension with tachycardia may result from intra-abdominal bleeding from a ruptured spleen. Temperature instability may accompany spinal shock. The entire spine, particularly the cervical portion, should be examined with great care. One should look for overlying bruising and any spinal deformity. While in-line immobilization of the spine, with particular attention to the neck, is maintained, the entire spine should be palpated for any point tenderness, deformities, crepitus, or muscle spasm [Kadish, 2001].

Neurologic Examination

The diagnosis of spinal cord injury is often overlooked in children with multiple injuries, unless constant vigilance to detect such injury is maintained. Spinal cord trauma should be suspected in cases of breech or otherwise difficult delivery; multiple trauma; child abuse; and certain sports injuries, such as football, gymnastics, and ice hockey [Braakman and Penning, 1976; Torg et al., 1979]. Patients with spinal cord injury can present with any combination of the following symptoms and signs: neck or back pain, weakness, sensory loss, decrease in deep tendon reflexes, loss of bladder or bowel control, autonomic dysfunction, and meningismus. Such symptoms may be classified further as acute, subacute, chronic, intermittent, delayed or late, or progressive. After the initial neurologic deficit in acute spinal cord injury, secondary deterioration is sometimes seen. Such worsening can be (1) early (<24 hours) (e.g., from spinal immobilization and traction), (2) delayed (1 to 7 days) (e.g., from hypotension complicating fracture-dislocation, or (3) late (>7 days) (e.g., from vertebral artery injury) [Harrop et al., 2001]. Signs of spinal cord injury usually include impairment of motor and sensory function. The degree of motor involvement can vary from subtle weakness to complete paraplegia or quadriplegia. Loss of sensation is often ascertainable at an obvious dermatomal level. In 1992, the American Spinal Injury Association (ASIA) and the International Medical Society of Paraplegia (IMSOP) published a Standard Neurological Classification of Spinal Cord Injury (Fig. 66-6). Such a classification offers a systematic documentation of motor, sensory, and sphincter function for the accurate classification and scoring of acute spinal cord injuries. Ten key muscle groups are tested for motor function, using the Medical Research Council 0-to-5 muscle grading system, and sensation is tested over 28 dermatomes on both sides of the body. The neurologic levels and completeness or incompleteness (partial preservation) of spinal cord involvement are documented [American Spinal Injury Association, 1992].

Box 66-1 ASIA/IMSOP Spinal Cord Impairment Scale*

A. Complete: No motor or sensory function is preserved in sacral segments S4 to S5.

B. Incomplete: Sensory but not motor function is preserved below the neurologic level and includes sacral segments S4 to S5.

C. Incomplete: Motor function is preserved below the neurologic level, and more than half of key muscles below the neurologic level have a muscle grade less than 3.

D. Incomplete: Motor function is preserved below the neurologic level, and at least half of key muscles below the neurologic level have a muscle grade of 3 or more.

E. Normal: Motor and sensory function is normal.

*This scale distinguishes complete spinal cord injury and three degrees of incomplete injury from an absence of injury with normal motor and sensory function.

ASIA, American Spinal Injury Association; IMSOP, International Medical Society of Paraplegia.

In 1992, the ASIA with the IMSOP developed the ASIA/IMSOP Spinal Cord Impairment Scale (Box 66-1) [Tator, 1996]. The ASIA/IMSOP scale incorporates the Medical Research Council muscle grading and pinprick/light touch sensory testing into a system differentiating complete and incomplete spinal cord deficit. Complete injury is defined as loss of all motor and sensory function in all segments below the neurologic level, including the sacral dermatomes (S4 to S5). To make this determination, perineal and deep anal sensation and digital sphincter tone and contraction must be totally lacking. If there is preservation of any sensory or motor function below the neurologic level, the injury is classified as incomplete (see Fig. 66-6). Using this classification system, the examiner identifies the sensory and motor levels, defined as the most caudal spinal cord segment with normal sensory and motor function, on both sides. The zone of partial preservation is defined as the dermatomes caudal to the neurologic level with partial preservation of function in an otherwise complete injury. A zone of partial preservation implies injury of multiple spinal cord segments, whereas its absence implies injury at only one level.

Occasionally, brachial or lumbosacral plexus injuries causing weakness and sensory loss in a radicular distribution may coexist with a spinal injury, complicating the clinical picture. After injury to the spinal cord, the deep tendon reflexes are depressed or absent, with this lack of response persisting until the phase of spinal shock has resolved (1 to 12 weeks) [Green and Eismont, 1984; Guttmann, 1976; Meinecke, 1976]. Thereafter, hyperreflexia and extensor posturing are evident below the level of the lesion. Accompanying autonomic dysfunction can be manifested by

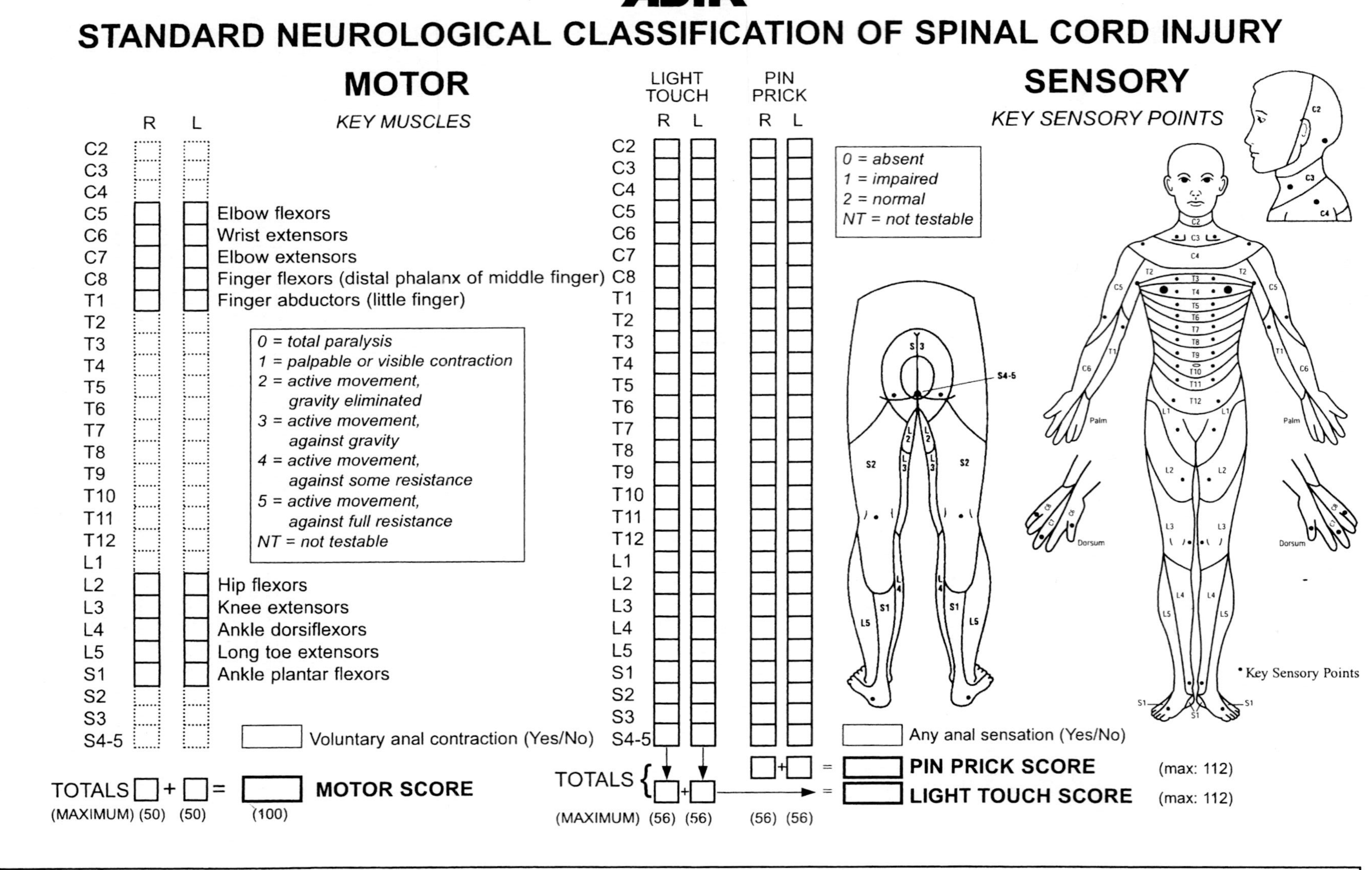

FIGURE 66-6. American Spinal Injury Association (ASIA) and International Medical Society of Paraplegia (IMSOP) Standard Neurological Classification of Spinal Cord Injury. This classification provides quantitative assessment of motor, sensory, and sphincter function; neurologic level of dysfunction; and whether any loss is complete or incomplete. (Available at: http://www.asia-

Horner's syndrome, hypertension, bowel and bladder atonia, and disturbances in temperature regulation.

Laboratory Studies

Radiographic Evaluation

Radiographic evaluation of the child suspected to have spinal cord injury should begin in the emergency department with plain films of the entire spine. The purpose of the evaluation is to look for evidence of unstable fractures or vertebral dislocations that may require emergency surgical intervention. Radiography of the entire spine is important because approximately 15% of patients have injury at multiple sites [Hadley, 1992; Hadley et al., 1988]. Radiologic evaluation of the spine is often neither possible nor desirable in an emergency situation, however, and may need to be deferred until the spine is stabilized. In such circumstance, only the spinal area clinically involved needs immediate imaging. In cases in which the patient cannot be assessed adequately by plain radiography, MRI may be required early in the evaluation. Stringer and Andersen suggested a diagnostic algorithm for spinal injury combining the findings on neurologic examination and results of radiographic studies [Andersen and Stringer, 1996; Stringer and Andersen, 1996].

Children with spinal cord injury routinely have sandbag and tape fixation of the head and neck, making optimal radiographic examination more difficult. Nonetheless, it is crucial to obtain anteroposterior, lateral, and oblique views of the spine. All seven cervical vertebrae and the C7 to T1 interspace must be visualized. Swimmer's views are often necessary to visualize all of the lower cervical vertebrae, and an open-mouth view may be needed to visualize the odontoid process [Goldberg et al., 1990], although the open-mouth view can be safely omitted if the other views are normal [Dias, 2004]. Flexion/extension cervical x-rays and fluoroscopy are sometimes indicated to exclude ligamentous instability when there is still suspicion of cervical spine instability after static x-rays have been obtained [Hadley, 2002b]. Care must be taken not to misinterpret normal variations in cervical spine films of a child. These variations include pseudosubluxation of C2 on C3 (seen in 20% of normal children age 1 to 7 years) and the cartilaginous plate at the base of the odontoid (normally seen in children <3 years old and often mistaken for a recent fracture) [Cattell and Filtzer, 1965].

In spine-injured children, the upper cervical spine is especially susceptible to injury. Specific injuries to this region include (1) occipitoaxial dislocations, (2) atlantoaxial instability, (3) fractures of the atlas (Jefferson fracture), (4) odontoid fractures, and (5) "hangman's fractures" [Piper and Menezes, 1996]. Occipitoaxial dislocations can be identified on plain radiographs in some patients using the Powers ratio (distance of the basion [midpoint of the anterior border of the foramen magnum] to the posterior arch of C1, divided by the distance of the opisthion [midpoint of the lower border of the foramen magnum] to the anterior arch of C1). This ratio is usually 0.77. Ratios greater than 1 are abnormal. Most often, MRI is needed to identify occipitoaxial dislocations. Instability of the atlantoaxial region is suspected when the preodontoid space exceeds 5 mm in a child or 3 mm in an adult. Fractures of the atlas often can be stabilized by using a rigid (Philadelphia) collar [Alker et al., 1975]. Odontoid fractures and hangman's fractures are rare in childhood and, if present, usually can be treated nonoperatively (halo brace) [Anderson and D'Alonzo, 1974].

Measurements made to assess alignment of the spinal column follow the "rule of 2," that is, the allowable displacement between vertebrae in any direction should not exceed 2 mm in adults, with a greater allowance in children. The evaluation of bony integrity can be difficult at times, especially of the odontoid process and C1. If adequate quality cannot be obtained by plain radiographs, computed tomography (CT) is indicated [Andersen and Stringer, 1996; Stringer and Andersen, 1996].

Further limitations of plain radiographs of the spine include 40% false-positive and 20% false-negative interpretations. Also, significant spinal cord injury frequently occurs in children without radiographic abnormality (e.g., vertebral fracture or dislocation) (SCIWORA) [Burke, 1974; Pang and Wilberger, 1982], with this discrepancy observed in 15% to 70% of all pediatric spinal cord injuries [Hadley et al., 1988; Menezes et al., 1989; Pang and Wilberger, 1982]. Based on radiographic findings, spinal column injuries can be classified as follows: (1) isolated fractures (40% of cases), (2) fractures and subluxations (most common in adolescents), (3) subluxation without fractures (more common in younger patients), and (4) SCIWORA (more common in children <8 years old). SCIWORA, as first described, referred to cases of spinal cord injury with objective signs of myelopathy in the absence of abnormalities on standard radiographs, flexion/extension views, and cervical CT. With modern MRI, many such cases show radiologic evidence of injury to the spinal cord or spinal cord ligaments [Caviness, 2004; Davis et al., 1993; Matsumura et al., 1990; Proctor, 2002], with MRI abnormalities seen in about two thirds of cases [Massagli, 2000].

In a series of 20 pediatric cases of SCIWORA, in 19 of whom a spinal MRI was done, the MRI was normal in 17 of 19. The spinal injuries in all 17 cases were partial, whereas in the two cases with abnormal MRI scans, the spinal injuries were complete. In 14 of the 18 cases with partial injuries, the neurologic deficits resolved, suggesting that in this series of SCIWORA cases, the spinal trauma was milder than in many other reported cases [Dare et al., 2002]. Because the vertebral column in early life is quite elastic, allowing for significant flexion, hyperextension, and vertebral distraction without accompanying fracture or dislocations, SCIWORA is seen most often in infants and young children, in whom the frequency is three times greater than in children older than 10 years of age [Massagli, 2000]. Also predisposing to SCIWORA in young children is the greater elasticity of the spinal column than of the spinal cord; the bony spine can tolerate 5 cm of distraction, whereas the spinal cord can tolerate only 5 mm before disruption [Caviness, 2004]. SCIWORA most often affects the cervical spine, typically producing signs of a central cord syndrome [Babcock, 1975]. In some cases, transient neurologic symptoms may be the only indication that the cervical spinal cord has been injured; in other cases, permanent deficits may result, reflecting more severe spinal cord injuries that can be partial or complete [Caviness, 2004; Massagli, 2000]. In one study, 52% of children with SCIWORA had delayed onset of paralysis

4 days after their injury [Pang and Wilberger, 1982]. Children with spinal trauma must be examined frequently for signs of clinical deterioration in the days after their injury, even when plain radiographs of the spine are normal. Children with SCIWORA should be treated with immobilization of the spine until (1) spine tenderness clears; (2) the neurologic examination has normalized; and (3) radiographic evaluation is negative for instability or for 12 weeks, whichever is longer. Avoidance of high-risk activities for 6 months is recommended [Gunnarsson and Fehlings, 2003].

CT is the best means of detecting subtle spinal fractures and clarifying equivocal areas seen on plain films. CT also should be used when plain films are normal, but clinical suspicion of instability or fracture still exists [Andersen and Stringer, 1996; Stringer and Andersen, 1996] or when fracture/displacement is seen on plain radiography [Caviness, 2004].

More recently, MRI of the spine has replaced CT and myelography as the preferred means of imaging the injured spinal cord (Fig. 66-7) [Goldberg et al., 1988; Hyman and Gorey, 1988; Greenberg, 1991]. Many MRI sequences can be used, depending on the type of injury and the spinal cord area of concern, including spin-echo, fast-spin-echo, gradient-recall-echo, and inversion-recovery sequences. Excellent review articles on the use of these different sequences in specific situations are available [Andersen and Stringer, 1996; Stringer and Andersen, 1996]. MRI can distinguish intramedullary lesions from extramedullary ones and early pathologic changes from later ones [Davis et al., 1993; Kalfas et al., 1988; Levitt and Flanders, 1991; Sett and Crockard, 1991]. In general, findings on MRI correlate well with the degree of deficit found on neurologic examination [Bondurant et al., 1990; Davis et al., 1993; Flanders et al., 1990]. Additionally, the type and severity of spinal cord injury seen on MRI correlate well with the degree of recovery. In one study, MRI findings were classified into the following three categories: type I, inhomogeneous on T1-weighted image, large central hypointensity with thin hyperintense rim on T2-weighted image; type II, normal T1-weighted image, hyperintense cord on T2-weighted image; type III, normal T1-weighted image, isointense center with thick hyperintense rim on T2-weighted image. These findings correlated with a poor, intermediate, and good outcome [Kulkarni et al., 1987].

In general, spinal cord injuries in which there is no identifiable MRI abnormality carry a better prognosis for recovery than injuries in which MRI abnormalities are found [Davis et al., 1993]. The usefulness of MRI in visualizing spinal cord injury in neonates, in whom neurologic abnormalities can be difficult to find and in whom significance can be difficult to interpret, has been documented [Lanska et al., 1990]. MRI also is useful in showing abnormalities that may not be seen with other imaging modalities, including ligamentous instability and disruptions, other soft tissue injuries, disk herniations, intraspinal hemorrhage, and nerve root injuries [Kadish, 2001; Proctor, 2002]. In some cases, it may be necessary to use a combination of MRI and CT to identify coexisting injuries of the spinal cord and bony spine [Levitt and Flanders, 1991; Wittenberg et al., 1990]. MRI can be useful in predicting outcome in intramedullary lesions because it can differentiate hematoma (which often has a

A

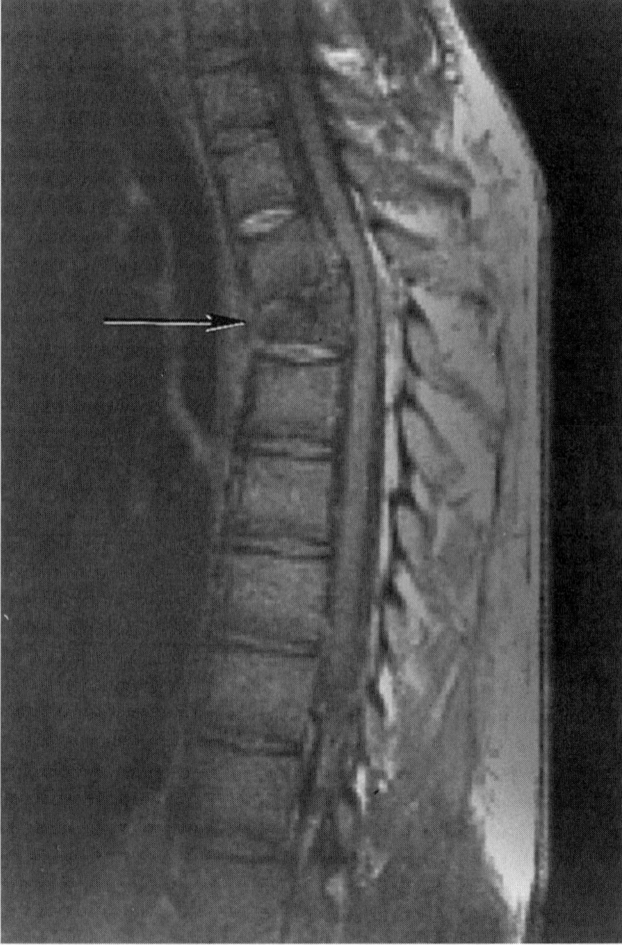

B

FIGURE 66-7. A, CT of thoracic spine in a 19-year-old male after a car accident in which he was an unrestrained passenger. There is a fracture of the right lamina of T3, with a burst fracture of the body of T4, causing deformity and anteroposterior narrowing of the spinal canal. **B,** MRI of thoracic spinal cord in the same patient, obtained the same day (T1-weighted image). There is a wedge fracture of T4 *(arrow)*, producing compression of the underlying spinal cord.

poor prognosis) from spinal cord edema, which usually has a better outcome [Schaefer et al., 1992]. In 49 patients who underwent MRI within 72 hours of sustaining a cervical spinal cord injury, the imaging features that correlated with a poor functional recovery included hemorrhage, long segments of edema, and high cervical lesions [Flanders et al., 1999].

Functional MRI has been used to assess the degree of spinal cord damage in 27 patients with complete and incomplete cervical and thoracic spinal cord injuries. With thermal stimuli applied to the inner calf (L4 sensory dermatome), activity in ipsilateral dorsal gray matter was diminished with complete and incomplete injuries; in the ventral regions, however, activity was increased with complete injuries, but with incomplete lesions, it was similar to or diminished compared with healthy subjects (i.e., it was notably less than in subjects with complete spinal cord injuries) [Stroman et al., 2004].

Serial MRI studies also can be helpful in following the evolution of traumatic spinal cord lesions [Sett and Crockard, 1991; Sato et al., 1994]. The need for metrizamide CT, used previously in evaluating post-traumatic spinal cord cysts and syringomyelia [Quencer et al., 1983; Rossier et al., 1983; Mace, 1985], has diminished substantially with the accuracy of MRI in showing these lesions. Also, because of the availability of MRI, the need for myelography to identify surgically remediable spinal cord injuries (e.g., extramedullary hematomas and major fracture-dislocations) has diminished greatly. When the patient's clinical condition permits, most centers currently advocate early MRI for acute spinal trauma.

Electrophysiologic Evaluation

The usefulness of somatosensory-evoked potentials and electromyography in evaluating the level of spinal cord injury and predicting clinical outcome is controversial. Somatosensory-evoked potentials are often useful in identifying the level of spinal cord injury [Louis et al., 1985] and in identifying areas of spinal cord damage that have been clinically unapparent [Toleikis and Sloan, 1987]. This test can be especially helpful in infants and young children in whom the degree of deficit often cannot be determined confidently by clinical examination [Kamimura et al., 1988]. It is unknown, however, whether somatosensory-evoked potentials are superior to MRI in identifying the extent of a spinal cord injury and predicting clinical outcome. Some investigators have noted a high degree of correlation between abnormal somatosensory-evoked potentials and potential for neurologic recovery [Li et al., 1990; Perot, 1973; Rowed et al., 1976; Ziganow, 1986], but others have not [Katz et al., 1991; York et al., 1983]. One study of experimental spinal cord injury revealed no correlation between the absence of somatosensory-evoked potential waveforms and the degree of spinal cord injury [Singer et al., 1977]. In that study, animals demonstrated good return of function at 8 to 9 days, even though somatosensory-evoked potential waveforms were not recordable 3 to 19 days after injury. Other studies have suggested, however, that patients with absent somatosensory-evoked potentials after spinal cord injury are unlikely to have any meaningful recovery of neurologic function [Shurman et al., 1996].

The presence of F-waves and H-reflexes depends on the integrity of the motor neuron pool. H-reflexes disappear in the first 24 hours of spinal shock, but return thereafter; F-waves disappear below the level of injury during spinal shock and reappear with its resolution [Horowitz and Patel, 2003]. F-wave and H-reflex latencies and electromyogram can show lower motor neuron unit abnormalities three to four myotome levels beyond the site of a spinal cord lesion [Shefner and Tun, 1991]. Based on such electrophysiologic findings, the extent of deficit, whether functional or anatomic, is often found to be more extensive than indicated by clinical examination. As with somatosensory-evoked potentials, it is uncertain whether abnormalities on electromyogram can increase significantly the predictability of clinical outcome in spinal cord injury.

Lumbar Puncture

Lumbar puncture can provide useful diagnostic information in certain types of spinal injury. The presence of extramedullary hematomas should be suspected with bloody or xanthochromic cerebrospinal fluid. Conversely, spinal epidural abscess usually causes a mild cerebrospinal fluid pleocytosis with an elevated cerebrospinal fluid protein concentration and a normal glucose concentration. Very low cerebrospinal fluid pressure at the time of lumbar puncture suggests the presence of a spinal block.

CLINICAL SYNDROMES

Intraspinal Intramedullary Injuries

Intraspinal intramedullary injuries can cause complete or incomplete loss of spinal cord function [Chilton and Dagi, 1985; Tator, 1983; Tator et al., 1993]. With complete loss, there is absence of all motor, sensory, and reflex function below the level of injury. With incomplete loss, some motor, sensory, and reflex function persists (see Box 66-1).

Complete Spinal Cord Injuries

Complete loss of spinal cord function, as defined by the ASIA/IMSOP Spinal Cord Impairment scale, can be either physiologic or pathologic. In physiologic loss, there is no morphologic alteration of the spinal cord, which becomes dysfunctional after impact. This dysfunction may occur with transient compression of the cord by a dislocated vertebra. With more sustained compression of the spinal cord, anatomic disruption of spinal cord elements may result, with accompanying pathologic loss of function. The frequency of complete spinal cord injury in pediatric patients varies widely, depending on the series reviewed, ranging from 20% to 95% of all pediatric spinal cord injuries [Anderson and Shutt, 1980; Burke, 1974].

The initial phase of complete loss of spinal cord function is characterized by spinal shock [Green and Eismont, 1984; Kiss and Tator, 1993]. The truncal and extremity muscles below the level of the lesion are flaccid, deep tendon and superficial reflexes are depressed or lost, plantar responses are absent, anesthesia is present to all modalities, and autonomic dysfunction (hypotension and bradycardia) is present. The mechanism of spinal shock is unknown, but its physiologic effects must be differentiated from the more permanent pathologic effects of spinal cord injury. Motor and sensory deficits resulting from spinal shock alone resolve within 1 hour. Persistence of motor and sensory deficits beyond 1 hour implies that pathologic, more permanent injury has occurred. After 6 to 13 weeks in adults and within 1 week in children, tendon reflexes return, and muscle tone improves. The reflexes later become pathologically active, and spasticity ensues if the injury is more permanent, and there usually is no significant return of motor or sensory function. A four-phase model of the sequential clinical changes seen in spinal shock and the neuronal mechanisms that may underlie those changes has been described: phase 1 (0 to 1 day), areflexia/hyporeflexia (from loss of descending facilitation); phase 2 (1 to 3 days), initial reflex return (from denervation supersensitivity); phase 3 (1 to 4 weeks), initial hyperreflexia (from axon-supported synapse growth); and phase 4 (1 to 2 months), final hyerreflexia (from soma-supported synapse growth) [Ditunno et al., 2004].

Autonomic dysfunction can persist for weeks to months. Also, ventilation may be compromised if the intercostal muscles are involved. Flaccid paralysis of the bladder can develop, with urinary retention and overflow incontinence. The gastrointestinal tract can be atonic. Vasomotor dysfunction can develop, with orthostatic hypotension, impaired shivering, sweating, and disturbances in temperature regulation persisting for weeks to months.

After complete injury of the cervical or upper thoracic spinal cord, an acute syndrome of bradycardia, hypotension, and hypothermia can occur, probably because of disturbed sympathetic outflow at the cervical and upper thoracic levels; most patients with quadriplegia after spinal cord injury have chronic hypothermia with poor temperature control related to loss of sympathetic peripheral vascular control [Green and Eismont, 1984]. Recovery from complete spinal cord injury is rare. The prognosis is poor. Tator estimated that less than 2% of patients with complete injury recover some distal cord function [Tator, 1996]. More encouraging was a comprehensive review of several large series of patients with complete spinal cord injury that found that about 2% of the patients became ambulatory [Hansebout, 1982].

Incomplete Spinal Cord Injuries

Incomplete spinal cord injuries warrant special attention because children with these injuries often demonstrate significant recovery of function with a relatively good prognosis. Included among incomplete spinal cord injuries are the cervicomedullary syndrome, central spinal cord syndrome, syndromes of the anterior spinal cord and posterior spinal cord, Brown-Séquard syndrome, and conus medullaris syndrome.

CERVICOMEDULLARY SYNDROME

With upper cervical injury, there is often injury to the medulla as well, causing respiratory arrest, hypotension, quadriparesis, and facial and upper cervical (C1 to C4) anesthesia. The facial anesthesia is of onionskin or Dejerine type. It is important that facial sensation be tested carefully in all patients with spinal cord injury. As in the central spinal cord syndrome (see later), there often can be more weakness in the arms than in the legs. This pattern of weakness is due to the crossing of fibers subserving the arms in the pyramidal decussation so that they come to be located more centrally than the leg fibers, which cross at a lower (C1 to C2) level [Tator, 1996]. There often is selective arm weakness with little, if any, weakness of the legs [Bell, 1970]. Several authors have challenged this concept, pointing to evidence that the fibers of the corticospinal tract may not be layered but are intermingled and that pathologically there is little evidence of central necrosis or hydromyelia in such patients [Quencer et al., 1992]. The mechanisms of injury causing cervicomedullary syndrome include atlantoaxial dislocation, atlanto-occipital dislocation, odontoid fracture, burst fracture of C1, and a ruptured C1 to C2 disk [Baskin, 1996; Donahue et al., 1994; Tator, 1996].

CENTRAL SPINAL SYNDROME

Central spinal syndrome can complicate hyperextension injury, particularly when there is a preexisting spinal abnormality, such as spinal canal stenosis, disk herniation, bony spurs, or compression by an abnormal ligamentum flavum [Rand and Crowdall, 1962; Quencer et al., 1992]. Conversely, this syndrome often can occur, particularly in young children, without an accompanying radiographic abnormality [Osenbach and Menezes, 1989, 1992; Ruge et al., 1988]. Here the central portion of the cord (usually cervical) is damaged, probably from ischemia because the central cord is perfused by end arteries from the anterior spinal artery, making it vulnerable to states of low perfusion [Schneider et al., 1973]. Neurologically, motor and sensory deficits are partial and are greater in the arms than in the legs, with the greatest impairment in the distal upper limbs [Green and Eismont, 1984]. Bowel and bladder function can be lost early, but usually return. Patients are generally ambulatory with a spastic gait; painful dysesthesias in the arms may persist for years. There is still debate whether early surgery is warranted in this condition because many patients recover spontaneously [Schneider et al., 1973; Sonntag and Francis, 1995].

ANTERIOR SPINAL CORD SYNDROME

Anterior spinal cord syndrome, which can follow hyperflexion injury of the spine, is characterized by analgesia and paresis below the level of the lesion, with preservation of proprioception, light touch, and vibration [Schneider, 1955]. This condition is usually caused by direct compression of the anterior and lateral white matter tracts by a herniated disk or by a fractured vertebra with posterior dislocation [Schneider, 1951]. The posterior columns are spared. There is no evidence for compression of the anterior spinal artery in this disorder [Tator, 1996]. Early surgery is probably warranted in all cases.

POSTERIOR SPINAL CORD SYNDROME

Posterior spinal cord syndrome is an extremely rare disorder (some doubt its existence), characterized by major damage to the posterior spinal cord (resulting in loss of movement and proprioception), with some residual function of the anterior cord (with retained perception of pain and temperature) [Tator, 1996].

BROWN-SÉQUARD SYNDROME

Brown-Séquard syndrome is caused by injury of the lateral half of the spinal cord (usually cervical) and is characterized by ipsilateral motor paralysis, ipsilateral loss of touch and proprioception, and contralateral loss of pain and temperature sensation below the level of the lesion [DeMyer, 1985]. Although this syndrome is often caused by penetrating trauma to the spine, cases also have been caused by hyperextension injury, compression fractures, and disk herniation. Blunt trauma with central cord injury sometimes can result in asymmetric pareses and sensory impairment that can mimic the true syndrome [Chilton and Dagi, 1985]. Recovery is variable.

CONUS MEDULLARIS SYNDROME

Conus medullaris syndrome produces paralysis of the lower extremities and the anal sphincter. Such a lesion, by definition, would be a form of complete spinal cord injury [Tator, 1983]. There is sacral sparing in many cases, however, making the injuries frequently of the incomplete type. The lumbar cord is positioned opposite the T12 vertebra, and the sacral cord is opposite L1. Dislocation, displaced fractures, and disk herniation of T12 and L1 can produce this injury. Prognosis for recovery is poor [Tator, 1983].

Intraspinal Extramedullary Injuries

Intraspinal extramedullary injuries include hemorrhage into the epidural, subdural, and subarachnoid spaces; spinal epidural abscess; spinal arachnoid cyst; spinal epidural tumors; herniation of the nucleus pulposus; and cauda equina injuries.

Spinal Epidural Hematoma

Spinal epidural hematoma can occur with substantial trauma to a normal spine, particularly in a newborn after breech delivery, or with mild trauma to the spine in a patient with a bleeding diathesis, with a spinal epidural hemangioma, or after multiple lumbar punctures [Bruyn and Bosma, 1976; Hehman and Norrell, 1968; Robertson et al., 1979]. In contrast to most intracranial epidural hematomas, spinal epidural hemorrhage is of venous (not arterial) origin [Bruyn and Bosma, 1976]. The main venous structure within the spinal epidural space lies ventrolateral to the cord and comprises a "rope ladder" plexus of thin-walled veins lacking true valves. This internal plexus connects with an external plexus of veins around the spinal column, with segmental spinal veins draining into the inferior vena cava, and with intracranial dural sinuses [Bruyn and Bosma, 1976]. Signs of spinal epidural hematoma can be acute, chronic, or intermittent. A newborn with acute spinal epidural hematoma typically manifests respiratory depression, hypotonia, areflexia, and other signs of spinal shock [Francisco, 1970; Towbin, 1964]. The occurrence of clinically significant traumatic spinal epidural bleeding is uncommon after infancy. When it occurs in older children (as with minor trauma complicating a blood dyscrasia), there is usually severe back pain that is worsened by pressure over the spine, neck flexion, or the Valsalva maneuver. Over the ensuing hours to weeks, signs of spinal cord compression usually develop [Bruyn and Bosma, 1976].

Spinal Subdural Hematoma

Spinal subdural hematoma occurs much less commonly; the source of bleeding in this hematoma is unclear. Similar to spinal epidural hematoma, it occurs mainly in the neonatal period, although it too is occasionally observed in children and adolescents with bleeding diatheses who sustain an otherwise insignificant injury to the spine, such as that occurring at the time of lumbar puncture [Edelson, 1976; Edelson et al., 1974; Towbin, 1964; Walter and Tedeschi, 1970]. Clinical features include back and radicular pain [Edelson, 1976].

Spinal Subarachnoid Hemorrhage

Traumatic subarachnoid hemorrhage caused by injury to the spine also is uncommon. This hemorrhage can occur after penetrating injury, but most often occurs after birth trauma (often with accompanying epidural, subdural, or intraspinal hemorrhage) [Plotkin et al., 1966; Towbin, 1964]. The amount of blood that accumulates is usually not great, and significant compression of the cord is rare. Signs of spinal subarachnoid hemorrhage are difficult to distinguish from signs of other spinal hemorrhages (e.g., epidural) that often coexist. Spinal subarachnoid hemorrhage should be suspected when back pain, meningismus, or fever occurs. The diagnosis is indicated by the presence of blood in the spinal fluid or by cerebrospinal fluid xanthochromia. Occasionally the blood obstructs the subarachnoid space, resulting in a "dry tap." Spinal subarachnoid hemorrhage must be differentiated from subarachnoid bleeding of intracranial origin and from blood caused by a traumatic lumbar puncture.

Spinal Epidural Abscess

Infections of the skin overlying the spine or of the bony spine itself (osteomyelitis) can occur after spinal trauma and may result in a spinal epidural abscess [Baker et al., 1975; Browder and Meyers, 1941; Hancock, 1976; Heusner, 1948]. *Staphylococcus aureus* is the organism most often responsible for such infections [Joshi et al., 2003; Pereira and Lynch, 2005]. The signs and symptoms of spinal epidural abscess are difficult to differentiate from the signs and symptoms of spinal epidural hematoma. Usually, other signs of inflammation and local infection of the overlying skin or bone can be identified.

Spinal Arachnoid Cyst

Spinal arachnoid cyst can develop after spinal trauma or may appear idiopathically and can cause significant spinal cord compression [Elsberg et al., 1934; Herskowitz et al., 1978; Nugent et al., 1959; Swanson and Fincher, 1947]. These cysts produce progressive signs with lower limb weakness in neonates and recurrent gait and sensory difficulties in older children. Scoliosis may accompany these cysts. The diagnosis is suggested on plain films by widening of the interpeduncular distances [Elsberg et al., 1934; Herskowitz et al., 1978; Nugent et al., 1959; Swanson and Fincher, 1947].

Spinal Epidermoid Tumor

Epidermoid tumors are infrequent complications of lumbar puncture [Batnitzky et al., 1977; Gibson and Norris, 1958; Manno et al., 1962; Shaywitz, 1972]. These tumors may develop 1 to 20 or more years after a lumbar puncture and have been attributed to skin and subcutaneous tissues implanted intraspinally at the time of a spinal tap. The symptoms are slowly progressive and usually manifest by back and leg pain followed by gait difficulties [Batnitzky et al., 1977; Gibson and Norris, 1958; Manno et al., 1962; Shaywitz, 1972].

Herniation of the Nucleus Pulposus

Herniation of the nucleus pulposus (protrusion of central intervertebral disk tissue) can result from severe flexion/compression of the spine and can cause compression of the underlying spinal cord [Burke, 1976; Herkowitz and Samberg, 1978; Swischuk, 1969]. The symptoms and signs are similar to those of any intraspinal extradural mass: pain and dysesthesias in radicular distribution, loss of tendon reflexes, muscle weakness, and atrophy [Burke, 1976; Herkowitz and Samberg, 1978; Swischuk, 1969].

Cauda Equina Injuries

A special category of extramedullary injury comprises injury involving the cauda equina, which is technically not a spinal cord injury. The level of spinal column and ligament displacement in these injuries varies with age, depending at which vertebral level the spinal cord terminates (L2 in infancy and L1 in adulthood). When any of the extramedullary pathologies just discussed are localized below the spinal cord, they can cause injury to the cauda equina. In incomplete injuries of the cauda equina, there is always preservation of sensation, often with only a partial motor deficit [Tator, 1996]. Bowel and bladder involvement is common. The prognosis in cauda equina injury is better than the prognosis in spinal cord injury because the lower motor neuron apparently has a greater capacity to recover than the upper motor neuron [Tator, 1996].

MANAGEMENT

Medical management of spinal cord injury includes measures aimed at treating the acute cord injury and more long-term management.

Short-Term Management

Spine Immobilization and Supportive Care

The treatment of acute spinal cord injury must include stabilization of the spine to prevent further injury, in addition to maintenance of vital signs. First aid at the scene of the accident should include placement of the child on a rigid stretcher or firm backboard and fixation of the head by sandbags or towel rolls with tape over the forehead to prevent movement of the head on the spine. A cervical collar alone does not accomplish this goal adequately [Green and Eismont, 1984]. Restriction of movement manually with the arm on the chest and hand on the mandible, exerting slight extension and traction on the head, can help stabilize the cervical spine until the head is taped. Care must be taken not to exert too much spinal distraction with this maneuver [Benzel and Doezema, 1996]. The disproportionately large head of a young child places the child into flexion when he or she is put on a neutral board. Because the high cervical region is the most likely level of injury, neck flexion is particularly dangerous. Flexion can be avoided with a special board with a recess for the occiput, allowing the head to rest in line with the body, or by placing something under the child's shoulders to elevate the neck in line with the head [Proctor, 2002]. It has been estimated that careful attention to stabilization of the spine before mobilization at the scene has reduced occurrence of complete spinal cord injury by approximately 10% [Gunby, 1981]. More recently, it has been suggested that this type of immobilization is painful and potentially harmful (restricted breathing, tissue ischemia, decubiti, intracranial hypertension), offering little, if any, benefit. Although a spine board eases transfer of a patient with a potentially unstable spinal injury to and from an ambulance stretcher, when the patient arrives at the hospital, a hard cervical collar and a firm mattress adequately immobilize the patient before application of traction or definitive stabilization [Hauswald and Braude, 2002].

A patent airway must be established, which may necessitate endotracheal intubation, which is frequently required in complete cervical cord injury (with impairment of diaphragmatic and intercostal muscle function). Intubation should be accomplished by chin lift without or with minimal neck extension. Tracheostomy and cricothyroidotomy should be avoided. Cardiac rate and rhythm should be monitored, and intravenous, central venous, and arterial lines should be placed. Cervical spinal cord trauma is often associated with significant hemodynamic deficits, including hypotension. In addition, injury to other organs (e.g., a ruptured liver or spleen) can cause significant blood loss and hypotension, which must be treated promptly by intravenous crystalloid or blood. Intravenous atropine, glycopyrrolate, phenylephrine, or dopamine may be needed to maintain normal blood pressure after volume depletion is corrected. Aggressive treatment of hypotension after spinal cord injury may improve outcome significantly [Levi et al., 1993; Vale et al., 1997]. The stomach should be emptied by a nasogastric tube. With urinary retention, the bladder should be catheterized. Radiologic studies usually should be performed (see section on radiologic evaluation earlier). In the case of cervical spine trauma, if the child is alert and interactive and has no neurologic deficit, no midline cervical tenderness, no painful distracting injury, and no evidence of intoxication, cervical spine films are probably not needed [Hadley, 2002b]. Spinal alignment is an important next step that usually can be accomplished with skeletal traction [Ducker et al., 1983] (see section on long-term management later).

Drug Therapy

Based on results of experimental models of spinal cord injury and its treatment (see section on leading investigational treatments later), a variety of therapies have been shown to be of proven or potential benefit in improving outcome after spinal cord injury.

BENEFICIAL TREATMENTS

Methylprednisolone, Naloxone, and Tirilazad

Steroids have often been used in treatment of acute spinal cord injury in an attempt to reduce cord swelling and limit central cord necrosis [Babcock, 1975; Ducker and Hamit, 1969]. In experimental models of spinal cord injury, methylprednisolone, given within hours of the injury, has been found to affect the cascade of inflammatory responses after spinal cord injury, mainly by scavenging damaging free radicals but also by influencing excessive calcium influx into cells and inhibiting the release of eicosanoids and cytokines. When methylprednisolone has been given later in such models, it has been found to block regenerative mechanisms. Other potential mechanisms of action of steroids include stabilizing membranes, maintaining the blood-spinal cord barrier, reducing vasogenic edema, enhancing spinal cord blood flow, altering electrolyte concentrations at the site of injury, blocking endorphin release, inhibiting lipid peroxidation, and limiting inflammation after injury [Ball and Nockels, 2001; Hadley, 2002a].

Until 1990, steroid treatment had shown no apparent benefit in humans, possibly related to the size and the timing of the steroid dose. In a randomized controlled study, a methylprednisolone bolus of 30 mg/kg given intravenously after an acute spinal cord injury and followed by methylprednisolone infusion at 5.4 mg/kg/hr for the next 23 hours was compared with naloxone and placebo, both also given by bolus followed by a 23-hour infusion (National Acute Spinal Cord Injury Study [NASCIS] 2 protocol). Naloxone, an opiate-receptor antagonist, has been used with apparent success after spinal cord trauma in animals demonstrating short-term motor function improvement [Baskin et al., 1993], suggesting that endorphins might influence outcome in spinal cord injury [Faden, 1996]. Administration of methylprednisolone within 8 hours of injury was associated with a significant improvement in motor function and sensation at a 6-month follow-up examination compared with patients receiving methylprednisolone more than 8 hours after injury and with patients receiving naloxone or placebo. This difference was found with complete and incomplete spinal cord lesions. Reanalysis of the data indicated, however, some benefit from the use of naloxone with injuries that were incomplete [Bracken and Holford, 1993]. At 1-year follow-up, patients who had received methylprednisolone within 8 hours of injury still exhibited significantly improved motor scores, but there were no significant differences in sensory scores among the three groups [Bracken et al., 1990, 1992]. The improvements noted were small, however, and the functional significance of these gains has been questioned [Wilberger, 1996]. Also, wound infections and gastrointestinal bleeding occurred more often in the patients given methylprednisolone than in the other two groups. A similar beneficial effect of methylprednisolone was not found when it was given in an identical fashion to patients after penetrating spinal cord injury [Levy et al., 1996]. In an earlier study by Bracken and colleagues (NASCIS 1), high-dose methylprednisolone (1000-mg bolus [14.3 mg/kg for a 70-kg patent] followed by 1000 mg/day for 10 days) was com-pared with standard-dose methylprednisolone (100-mg bolus [1.4 mg/kg for a 70-kg patient] followed by 100 mg/day for 10 days). No significant difference was found between the two groups in recovery of motor or sensory function 1 year after injury. There were no placebo control subjects in the study [Bracken et al., 1984].

A 1997 study by Bracken and colleagues compared the efficacy of methylprednisolone given for 24 hours with that of methylprednisolone given for 48 hours and with tirilazad, a 21-amino steroid lipid peroxidation inhibitor, given for 48 hours; there was no placebo control group (NASCIS 3). When treatment was begun 3 to 8 hours after injury, the patients who received methylprednisolone for 48 hours demonstrated significantly better motor function at 6 weeks and 6 months after injury than the other two groups. Also, at 6 months, the 48-hour methylprednisolone patients had significantly better functional recovery (self-care, sphincter control) than the other two groups. The 48-hour methylprednisolone patients also had more severe sepsis and severe pneumonia. When treatment was begun within 3 hours of injury, the rates of motor recovery were identical in the two groups given methylprednisolone and the one given tirilazad, confirming reports of tirilazad's benefit in experimental spinal cord injury [Bracken et al., 1997; Francel et al., 1993]. One year after injury, when treatment had been started within 3 hours of the injury, neurologic and functional recovery was again equal among the three treatment groups. When treatment had not been started until 3 to 8 hours after injury, patients who had received methylprednisolone for 48 hours had greater motor recovery at 1 year, whereas motor recovery was diminished in patients who had received only 24 hours of methylprednisolone [Bracken et al., 1998]. Based on this study, it was concluded that patients who receive methylprednisolone within 3 hours of injury should be maintained on the drug for 24 hours, but when methylprednisolone is begun 3 to 8 hours after injury, it should be continued for 48 hours unless there are complicating medical factors.

Many investigators have disagreed with this recommendation, citing largely insignificant differences in motor recovery scores and in functional outcome measures among study patients, while also detailing methodologic, scientific, and statistical flaws in the NASCIS 2 and 3 studies. The role of steroids as neuroprotective agents with acute spinal cord injury remains controversial [Ball and Nockels, 2001; Hadley, 2002a; Nesathurai, 1998]. Although neurologic outcome is improved by high-dose methylprednisolone, the benefit seems to be modest at best, and against this one needs to weigh the risk of potentially serious complications of high-dose steroid therapy [Galandiuk et al., 1993; Hadley, 2002a].

G_{M1} Ganglioside

Based on experimental studies that have shown G_{M1} ganglioside to induce the regeneration of damaged neurons, a randomized, placebo-controlled trial of G_{M1} was performed on 34 patients after spinal cord injury [Geisler et al., 1991]. Subjects were given 100 mg of either G_{M1} or placebo intravenously within 72 hours of injury and continued daily for a mean duration of 26 days. No untoward neurologic events related to G_{M1} administration were seen, and better recovery occurred in the G_{M1}-treated patients than in the controls after 1 year of follow-up. The number of patients treated was small (16 G_{M1}, 18 placebo), and there was a maldistribution between the two groups, with a smaller number of patients with the most severe injuries (complete spinal cord injury) randomized to the G_{M1} group (38% of G_{M1}-treated patients versus 56% of the placebo group) [Landi and Ciccone, 1992]. Functional outcomes of patients were considered to be equivalent in the two groups.

A multicenter G_{M1} ganglioside study in patients with acute nonpenetrating spinal cord injury of at least moderate severity was initiated in 1992. The study was prospective, double-blind, randomized, and stratified. By the study's end in 1997, 797 patients had been enrolled (a primary efficacy analysis was done in 760 of the patients). All patients first received intravenous methylprednisolone within 8 hours of injury and following the NASCIS 2 protocol. The patients were randomized into three study groups: placebo, low-dose G_{M1} (300-mg loading dose followed by 100 mg/day for 56 days), and high-dose G_{M1} (600-mg loading dose followed by 200 mg/day for 56 days). A planned interim analysis resulted in discontinuation of the high-dose G_{M1} treatment strategy because of an early trend for higher mortality. There was no significant difference in mortality between treatment groups. Although the data suggested improved neurologic recovery in patients with acute spinal cord injury given G_{M1} ganglioside for 56 days after the administration of methylprednisolone within 8 hours of an acute spinal cord injury, the primary analysis failed to prove this difference to be statistically significant. Nonetheless, because numerous secondary analysis indicated that G_{M1} was beneficial in the treatment of acute spinal cord injury, the use of low-dose G_{M1} after initial intravenous methylprednisolone remains a therapeutic option. The authors could not confirm the NASCIS 2 and NASCIS 3 findings indicating that the timing of methylprednisolone therapy had an impact on spinal cord recovery [Geisler et al., 2001; Hadley, 2002a].

ADDITIONAL POTENTIALLY BENEFICIAL TREATMENTS

Patients with hyperextension spinal cord injury without accompanying bone injury given hyperbaric oxygen seemed to do better than patients not given hyperbaric oxygen, but no data were provided to indicate whether or not that improvement was sustained [Asamoto et al., 2000]. Oral 4-aminopyridine, a voltage-gated fast potassium channel blocker, has been found to improve axonal conduction by facilitating the propagation of action potentials in demyelinated nerve fibers [Segal et al., 1999]. Although some studies have indicated that 4-aminopyridine given to patients with spinal cord injury enhances their motor and sensory function [Grijalva et al., 2003; Segal et al., 1999], improves their pulmonary function [Segal et al., 1999], lessens their spasticity [Segal et al., 1999], and results in functional gains [Grijalva et al., 2003], other studies have failed to show any significant benefit from the drug [Dumont et al., 2001b].

Other agents believed to be promising in experimental spinal cord injury, including thyrotropin-releasing hormone [Pitts et al., 1995], calcium channel blockers (e.g., nimodipine), sodium channel blockers (e.g., riluzole), and cyclosporine [Dumont et al., 2001b], have demonstrated lack of efficacy, inconclusive efficacy, or inadequate study in humans [Dumont et al., 2001b]. In experimental spinal cord injury, neurotrophic factors have been used to augment the poor intrinsic regenerative capacity of central nervous system neurons, and the need for sophisticated delivery of such trophic agents has stimulated the application of gene therapy [Kwon and Tetzlaff, 2001]. This work is summarized in the next section. Before such treatments can be studied clinically, it is first necessary to resolve safety issues, including side effects of neurotrophic factor infusion and potential hazards accompanying the use of viral vectors [Kwon and Tetzlaff, 2001]. There is one report from Taiwan of fibroblast growth factor given to a patient with chronic paraplegia 4 years after a stabbing injury that resulted in a spinal cord gap at T11. The gap was bridged with four sural nerve grafts, stabilized with fibrin glue containing acidic fibroblast growth factor. After the procedure, there was a remarkable change in the patient's functional status, which improved from his being wheelchair bound to being able to ambulate independently with a walker 2.5 years after the surgery [Cheng et al., 2004].

In an effort to overcome the inhibitory environment into which regenerating axons must grow in spinal cord injury, strategies have been developed to bridge the injury site and facilitate axonal growth across the site with a variety of cellular substrates. These include fetal tissue transplants and implants of stem cells, Schwann cells, and olfactory ensheathing glial cells [Dobkin and Havton, 2004; Kwon and Tetzlaff, 2001; Rabinovich et al., 2003]. In safety trials, patients with multiple sclerosis received autologous Schwann cells and olfactory ensheathing glial cells placed into plaques, and in another safety trial in patients with spinal cord injury, oligodendrocyte precursors from pigs were implanted into the lesion bed. The results of these trials are pending [Dobkin and Havton, 2004]. In a study in China, fetal olfactory ensheathing glial cells were injected above and below the lesion site in patients 6 or more months after a traumatic spinal cord injury; this reportedly resulted in improved sensation over a few levels and in increased motor function for two levels below the lesion [Dobkin and Havton, 2004]. In a study from Russia, cells from fetal neurons and hematopoietic tissues were implanted subarachnoidally into five patients with traumatic spinal cord injury. All of the injuries were cervical or thoracic in location, and all were severe, with complete motor and sensory loss (Frankel score A: a standardized grading scale of neurologic function [Frankel et al., 1969]). The times after spinal cord injury ranged from 1 month to 6 years, and each patient underwent one to four cell transplantations. Eleven of the 15 patients improved; 6 improved to a Frankel score of C (incomplete restoration of motor and sensory function), and 5 improved to a Frankel score of B (incomplete restoration of sensory function and contraction of some muscles). No improvement occurred in the remaining four patients. There were no serious complications to the cellular transplants [Rabinovich et al., 2003].

Leading Investigational Treatments

Research into the repair of spinal cord injury has grown rapidly in the years since the groundbreaking work in which a peripheral nerve graft was used as a bridge across a spinal cord injury site [Rosenzweig and McDonald, 2004]. Advances in treatment of spinal cord injury have accelerated as factors inhibiting or limiting spinal cord regeneration have been identified, and interventions have been developed to counteract those factors. Particularly encouraging progress has been made in limiting the occurrence and progression of secondary damage often seen after spinal cord injury [Rosenzweig and McDonald, 2004].

Most experimental work on spinal cord injury repair has been carried out in rodents. At least seven overlapping approaches to spinal cord injury repair have been studied [Rosenzweig and McDonald, 2004; Dobkin and Havton, 2004].

1. *Bridging the gap*. An exogenous, growth-permissive matrix is placed across the injury site to allow regrowing axons to cross. Substances used have included biodegradable polymers, peripheral nerve, fetal spinal cord tissue, Schwann cells, olfactory ensheathing cells, fibroblasts, bone marrow stromal/stem cells, stem/progenitor cells, and skin [Dobkin and Havton, 2004; Kwon and Tetzlaff, 2001; Rosenzweig and McDonald, 2004].
2. *Constructing new spinal cord circuitry*. This has been attempted with stem cells [Rosenzweig and McDonald, 2004].
3. *Remyelinating demyelinated axons*. Such axons are frequently found in spinal cord injury, and neural stem cells, oligodendrocyte precursors, Schwann cells and olfactory ensheathing cells have been used in attempts to remyelinate these axons [Dobkin and Havton, 2004; Rosenzweig and McDonald, 2004].
4. *Providing neurotrophic support*. A variety of neurotrophic factors have been given in an attempt to stimulate the sprouting of spared axons or the regeneration of axotomized axons. These include brain-derived neurotrophic factor, neurotrophin-3, nerve growth factor, glia-derived neurotrophic factor, ciliary neurotrophic factor, fibroblastic growth factor, vascular endothelial growth factor, and insulin growth factor-1 [Dobkin and Havton, 2004; Rosenzweig and McDonald, 2004]. Trophic factors are diffusible. They can be provided orally, injected or pumped into the cerebrospinal fluid, or infused near the lesion site [Dobkin and Havton, 2004; Rosenzweig and McDonald, 2004]. Many of the cells that have been used for transplantation either secrete neurotrophins or can be engineered to do so. An advance in this area is gene therapy, employing the use of adenoviruses, adeno-associated viruses, or lentiviruses to transfer neurotrophin-encoded genes (e.g., nerve growth factor, fibroblastic growth factor, brain-derived neurotrophic factor, glia-derived neurotrophic factor, neurotrophin-3) directly to central nervous system cells [Hidaka et al., 2002; Rosenzweig and McDonald, 2004]. Neurotrophic factors have emerged as leading candidates for enhancing central nervous system regeneration because of their stimulation of numerous genes shown to be upregulated or constitutionally expressed in association with axonal growth; these collectively have been termed *regeneration-associated genes*. The products of these genes include cytoskeletal proteins (involved in axonal extension), cytoplasmic growth cone proteins (involved in mediating signal transduction), and cell adhesion molecules (involved in growth cone guidance) [Kwon and Tetzlaff, 2001].
5. *Overcoming myelin-associated growth inhibitors*. Antibodies, peptides, genetic mutations, and elevations of cyclic adenosine monophosphate (cAMP) have been used to overcome myelin-associated growth inhibitors. Such inhibitors are produced by oligodendrocytes, including Nogo-A, myelin-associated glycoprotein, and oligodendrocyte myelin glycoprotein [Dobkin and Havton, 2004; Rosenzweig and McDonald, 2004]. A GTPase called *Rho,* which interferes with growth cone support, is inactivated by cAMP, rendering the growth cone less sensitive to Nogo-A, myelin-associated glycoprotein, and oligodendrocyte myelin glycoprotein [Dobkin and Havton, 2004].
6. *Overcoming glial scar–associated growth inhibition*. Chondroitin sulfate proteoglycans and other extracellular matrix molecules associated with the glial scar seem to inhibit neurite outgrowth. The enzymatic digestion of chondroitin sulfate proteoglycan glycosaminoglycan chains is a promising means of overcoming this barrier to spinal cord regeneration [Dobkin and Havton, 2004; Rosenzweig and McDonald, 2004].
7. *Protecting neurons and glia from secondary cell death*. Much research has focused on neural and glial protection—preventing the cascade of secondary cell death that follows spinal cord injury, a cascade caused by combinations of inflammation, excitotoxicity, apoptosis, ischemia, and delayed oligodendrocyte death [Dobkin and Havton, 2004].

Other Investigational Treatments

A variety of additional therapies have provided encouraging results in experimental spinal cord injury, particularly in rats, by lessening the degree of spinal cord damage, improving functional outcome, or both. These therapies include hyperbaric oxygen [Huang et al., 2003]; erythropoietin [Kaptanoglu et al., 2004]; quercetin, an iron-chelating flavonoid [Schultke et al., 2003]; riluzole, a sodium-channel blocker [Schwartz and Fehlings, 2001, 2002]; and induction of manganese superoxide dismutase [Earnhardt et al., 2002].

Long-Term Management

Cervical Spine Immobilization

In spine and spinal cord injuries in children the main imperatives are to decompress the neural elements and to stabilize the spine to prevent further injury [Proctor, 2002]. Cervical traction serves to immobilize the spine and reduce fractures. Reduction of fractures or subluxation must be undertaken with care in young patients because over-distraction can worsen the patient's neurologic dysfunction. Manual positioning under fluoroscopy often is required in cases of cervical ligamentous injury. Crown halo rings can be applied in younger patients at a pressure of 2 inches/

pound of torque per pin [Pang and Hanley, 1990]. In older patients, cervical traction can be used with relative safety. Many spine-injured children can be managed with external stabilization without a need for later surgery [Hadley, 1992; Proctor, 2002]. Various devices can be used, depending on the level and severity of injury, including the Philadelphia cervical collar, Yale braces, SOMI braces, four-poster braces, halo rests, crown halo rings, and thoracolumbar orthoses. When such devices are used, frequent radiographic reevaluations are needed to ensure continuing proper alignment of spinal elements because adequate external (and internal) fixation can be difficult to achieve in a young child [Proctor, 2002]. Specific recommendations for the management of SCIWORA were discussed earlier [Gunnarsson and Fehlings, 2003].

Supportive Medical Care

For patients with mid cervical or upper cervical spinal cord injuries, there is a high risk of respiratory failure. Because the lower motor neurons for the phrenic nerve are at cervical levels 3 through 5, patients with severe spinal cord injuries above this level require permanent mechanical ventilation. Although patients with mid cervical spinal cord injuries initially may have adequate spontaneous ventilation, their ventilatory ability may deteriorate within a few days consequent to ascending spinal cord edema [Marion, 1998]. Children with high cervical lesions who are ventilator dependent may be candidates for phrenic nerve pacing [Massagli, 2000].

In addition to causing respiratory difficulties, spinal cord trauma can result in a variety of other medical problems requiring ongoing care [Luce, 1985]. Cardiovascular function can be altered by the trauma and its acute management. In one study, four of nine patients developed pulmonary edema after spinal cord injury, probably from overhydration during acute resuscitation [Meyer et al., 1971]. Patients with spinal cord lesions above T7 requiring long-term management have decreased cardiac output, hypotension, and problems with temperature regulation, limiting adaption to exercise. Nasogastric tube feeding after restoration of normal intestinal activity, antacids, hyperalimentation when bowel atonia persists, and digital stimulation, especially in young children, may be needed [Goetz et al., 1998]. In some children, gentle disimpaction is indicated. The use of enema continence catheters for bowel dysfunction after spinal cord trauma may significantly facilitate bowel care in such patients [Liptak and Revell, 1992]. Intermittent catheterization of the bladder is preferred to placement of an indwelling catheter to reduce the risk of urinary tract infection and renal failure [Luce, 1985; Nygaard and Kreder, 1996; Pannek et al., 1997].

Renal failure is a major cause of mortality in patients with chronic spinal cord injury [Hackler, 1984]. Anticholinergic and botulinum toxin therapy can reduce the effects of detrusor hyperreflexia (neurogenic bladder), present in approximately 60% of patients rendered quadriparetic from spinal cord injuries [Curt et al., 1997; Schurch et al., 1997]. Hyperhidrosis, fever, and disrupted temperature regulation are additional autonomic dysfunctions frequently encountered in patients with spinal cord injury. Anticholinergic treatment may help [Canaday and Stanford, 1995].

Other general measures include chest physiotherapy to prevent pneumonia, frequent repositioning of the patient and the use of spinal beds (Stryker frame RotaBed) to avoid decubiti, and the use of Jobst stockings to minimize the risk of deep vein thromboses and the attendant potential for pulmonary emboli. Occasionally, ventilation-perfusion scanning and pulmonary angiography are needed to establish the diagnosis of pulmonary emboli. It is estimated that one third of the deaths within the first weeks of spinal cord injury are due to pulmonary embolism. The use of mini-heparin treatment (1 μg/kg/hr, continuous infusion) or intermittent low-dose heparin therapy may reduce the risk of pulmonary embolism [Borow and Goldson, 1983]. In patients for whom anticoagulant therapy is contraindicated, placement of an inferior vena cava filter may be necessary. The healing of decubitus ulcers is aided by treatment with vitamin C (15 to 20 mg/kg/day) [Taylor et al., 1974]. Muscle relaxants, such as diazepam, baclofen, cyclobenzaprine, and intravenous orphenadrine citrate [Casale et al., 1995], may be helpful in the long-term management of spasticity after spinal cord injury. Additional antispasmodic treatments include intrathecal baclofen and tizanidine [Abel and Smith, 1994; Lewis and Mueller, 1993; Nance et al., 1994]. Progressive spinal deformity is common in children after spinal cord injury, particularly after laminectomy [Lonstein, 1995]. Chronic pain is also common, and its management can be difficult, necessitating intervention by pain management specialists [Chiou-Tan et al., 1996; Drewes et al., 1994; Siddall et al., 1995; Yezierski, 1996]. In patients in whom there is delayed deterioration of neurologic functioning, the presence of a syrinx should be sought; if one is found, the syrinx may need to be shunted [Proctor, 2002].

Physical Therapy

Physical therapy is an important component in the long-term care of all patients with spinal cord injury [Jacobs and Nash, 2004]. Physical therapy should begin early and continue indefinitely. Measures such as proper limb positioning and passive muscle stretching can be instituted when the patient is medically and surgically stable. Later, after spinal shock has resolved, and early spasticity is evident, inhibitive casting can be used to minimize the development of limb contractures. Despite such measures, many patients later require phenol blocks, botulinum toxin injections, tendon lengthenings, and tendon transfers. As an alternative to long leg bracing for upright mobility, lower limb functional electric stimulation has proved effective in children and adolescents rendered paraplegic after a spinal cord injury. Electrodes were placed in nine such patients to provide constant stimulation to their hip and knee extensors and hip abductors and adductors; the seven who were able to complete their training all gained increased functional abilities over traditional long leg braces and a decreased need for physical assistance by a caregiver [Johnston et al., 2003]. Functional electric stimulation has been used to augment function of the lower limbs, upper limbs, bladder, bowel, respiration, and erection/ejaculation [Creasey et al., 2004; Kirshblum, 2004]. Short-term stimulation can be provided by electrodes on the skin or by percutaneous fine wires, but implanted systems are preferable for long-term use [Creasey et al., 2004].

Psychologic Therapy

Counseling should be provided, beginning early in the postinjury period and continuing throughout all stages of rehabilitation to provide maximal, ongoing support for the child and family [Talbot, 1971; Geller and Greydanus, 1979]. Health professionals from many disciplines can assist in providing such support.

Surgical Management

The surgical treatment of acute spinal cord injury may include traction, later immobilization by casting, reduction of dislocated vertebrae, removal of compressive substances (e.g., vertebral fragments, extramedullary hemorrhage), and bony spinal fusion. If surgery is necessary, a variety of surgical approaches and techniques are used, depending on

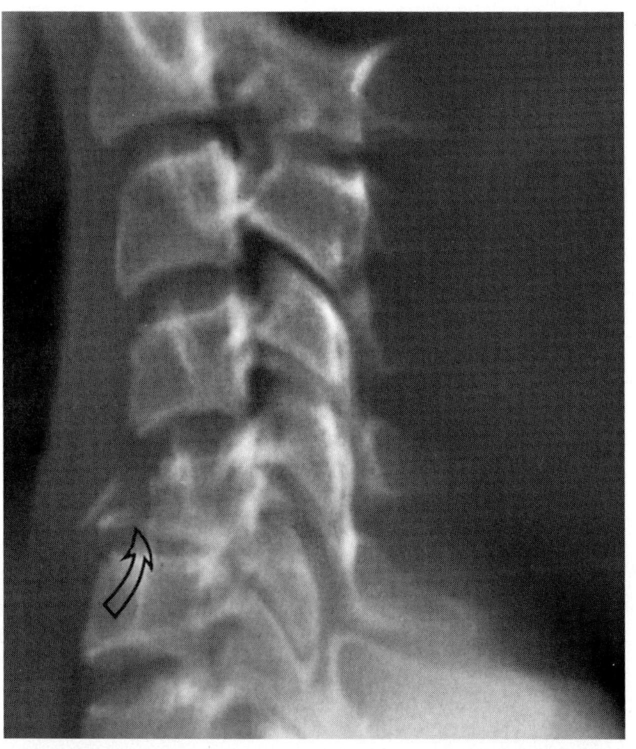

A

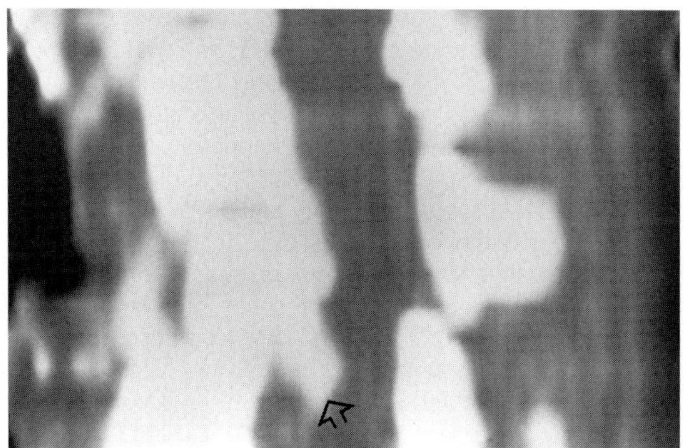

B

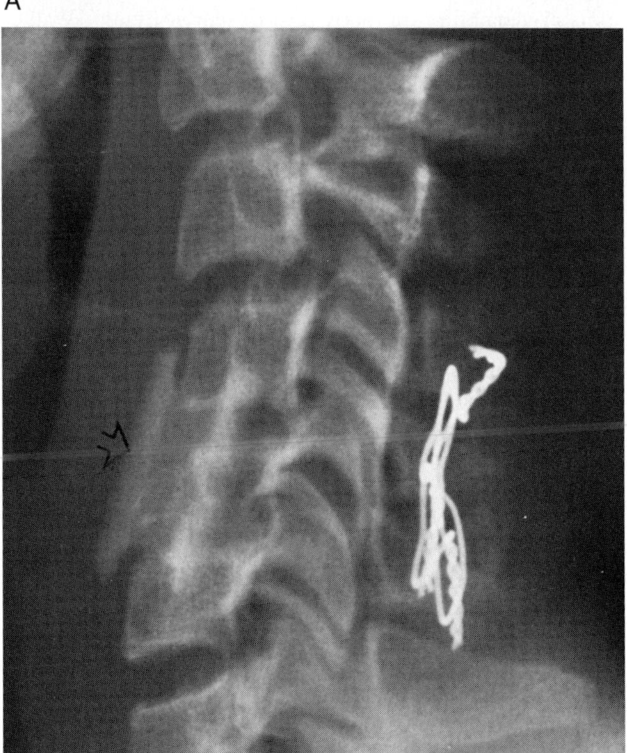

C

FIGURE 66-8. **A,** Plain lateral film of the cervical spine in a 12-year-old female. There is a wedge-shaped fracture of C5 *(arrow)* with posterior dislocation of C5 on C6 and loss of the disk space between those two vertebrae. **B,** CT sagittal reconstruction from 2-mm axial scans through the C4 to C6 level (unenhanced study) in the same patient as in Figure 66-7. Posterior dislocation of a fracture fragment *(arrow)* from the inferoposterior margin of C5 has resulted in narrowing of the anteroposterior diameter of the spinal canal. **C,** Plain lateral film of the cervical spine in the same patient as in Figure 66-7. The spine has been stabilized by anterior bony fusion *(arrow)* and posterior wiring to prevent further narrowing of the spinal canal.

the nature and level of the injury and individual surgeon preference [Chilton and Dagi, 1985]. An anterior approach is often used for removal of displaced fragments of a fractured vertebra or a herniated intervertebral disk. Posterior laminectomy usually is preferred for the removal of intraspinal extramedullary masses, such as epidural and subdural hematomas, and for the relief of spinal cord swelling. Surgical interventions include decompression, stabilization, and fusion. Surgical procedures usually are preceded by MRI; metrizamide CT (Fig. 66-8B) and myelography are less often used.

The indications for and timing of surgical treatment for spinal cord injury continue to be debated [Chesnut, 2004; Tator et al., 1999]. Some authors maintain that early treatment of compressive lesions before central myelomalacia has occurred (at about 24 hours) favorably affects outcome [Baskin, 1996; Bruyn and Bosma, 1976]. Support for this view is found in experimental studies in animals indicating that there is a window of 4 to 8 hours after injury when decompression of the injured spinal cord can improve recovery [Fehlings et al., 2001]. In a retrospective review of 50 patients with traumatic central cord syndrome who underwent early (≤24 hours after injury) or late (>24 hours after injury) surgery, patients who underwent early surgery and had an underlying acute disk herniation or a fracture-dislocation had significantly greater overall motor improvement than patients who underwent late surgery [Guest et al., 2002]. Other authors claim, however, that there is no difference in outcome when comparing early surgical, late surgical, and nonsurgical management in complete and incomplete spinal cord injury, arguing that maximal injury to the cord already has occurred at impact [Asazuma et al., 1996; Guttmann, 1963; Hadley et al., 1988; Kakulas, 1984; Katoh et al., 1996; Kewalramani and Tori, 1980; Levi et al., 1991].

Using data from NASCIS 2, the effectiveness of surgery on the treatment of acute spinal cord injury and its relation to pharmacologic treatment was studied. Three, nonrandomized study groups comprising 487 patients from 10 medical centers were recruited: (1) patients who underwent anterior surgery, (2) patients who underwent posterior surgery, and (3) patients who did not have surgery. Patients who did not undergo surgery had more severe spinal cord injuries initially than the surgical groups, yet there were no differences in neurologic improvement at 1-year follow-up between patients who underwent surgery and patients who did not. The data suggested that either early surgery (≤25 hours) or late surgery (>200 hours) might be followed by a better motor outcome. Surgery was not shown to influence the efficacy of drug treatment. As the authors themselves stated, a randomized study is needed to obtain valid comparisons of the effectiveness of different surgical treatments and of the timing of those interventions (Duh et al., 1994). More recently, 91 consecutive patients with acute traumatic spinal cord injury were studied prospectively; 66 patients (protocol group) underwent emergency MRI to determine the presence of persistent spinal cord compression, followed, if indicated, by immediate operative decompression and stabilization; the other 25 patients, for several different reasons, were managed outside the treatment protocol (reference group). Clinically the two groups were comparable. On follow-up, twice as many of the protocol patients (50%) as the reference patients (24%) demonstrated improvement in their admitting Frankel grade. These findings further underscored the need for a prospective randomized, multicenter study to determine the true efficacy of immediate surgical intervention in the management of patients with acute spinal cord injury [Papadopoulos et al., 2002].

One reasonable approach to spinal surgery in acute spinal cord injury might be to limit surgery to patients with partial cord injuries and a progressing neurologic deficit and patients with an unstable fracture or dislocation; surgery in the latter group would minimize the risk of curvature of the spine developing later. Additional appropriate indications for surgery might include the following: (1) inadequate reduction of a spinal fracture by traction alone, (2) epidural hematoma, (3) traumatic disk herniation, and (4) spinal cord compression by bony fragments [Duh et al., 1994; Pang and Hanley, 1990; Parisini et al., 2002; Weinshel et al., 1990]. Other authors believe, however, that decompressive surgery should be done only when there is proven residual compression of neural elements after spinal alignment [Ducker et al., 1983]. Evidence indicating a clear relationship between the timing of spinal surgery and neurologic outcome is still lacking [Duh et al., 1994].

PROGNOSIS

The most widely used rating scale to assess the severity of spinal cord injury and to quantify spinal cord function during recovery is the ASIA/IMSOP scale, a modification of the older Frankel scale. Other rating scales that have been used include the University of Miami Neurospinal Index and the Barthel Index [Klose et al., 1980; Mahoney and Barthel, 1965]. The disadvantage of such scoring systems is the difficulty in translating numerical scores into descriptions of clinical capability or activities of daily living [Walker, 1991]. A variety of functional scales have been used to measure changes that correlate highly with activity level and lifestyle [Geisler et al., 1991; Piepmeier and Collins, 1992].

Despite modern intensive care management and advances in therapy, mortality from spinal cord injury remains high, averaging 10% to 15%, with higher mortalities in patients rendered quadriplegic [Bracken et al., 1981; Ducker et al., 1983; Krause et al., 1997; Michaelis, 1976]. Two-year survival rates are better in younger patients (16 to 30 years old) than in older ones (61 to 86 years old), 95% versus 59% [DeVivo et al., 1990]. Overall morbidity (gastrointestinal hemorrhage, pulmonary emboli, and renal stones) also is lower in younger age groups. Limited recovery of neurologic function is possible after complete spinal cord injury, especially when there has been some improvement within the first 24 hours [Chilton and Dagi, 1985]. Nonetheless, approximately 70% to 95% of patients with complete lesions exhibit no improvement on long-term follow-up. Patients with complete injury persisting for longer than 1 week usually do not recover neurologic function, although some improvement may occur if there is a zone of partial preservation [Ditunno, 1996]. In general, recovery from thoracolumbar lesions is better than with higher lesions. Patients with partial spinal cord lesions can recover 25% of their power, and in patients with central cord lesions, recovery of power can be 80% [Ducker et al., 1983].

Additionally, patients with complete paralysis but with preserved sensation (ASIA/IMSOP grade B) have substantially greater improvement than patients with complete loss of motor and sensory function (ASIA/IMSOP grade A) [Landi and Ciccone, 1992].

Age at time of injury also influences recovery from spinal cord trauma. In one study, 90% of younger patients (<50 years old) with incomplete injury and preserved motor function (but with a muscle grade <3; ASIA/IMSOP grade C) became ambulatory compared with 42% of older patients. All patients with incomplete ASIA/IMSOP grade D lesions (muscle grade ≥3) developed independent ambulation [Burns et al., 1997]. Similar poor outcome in older patients with complete and incomplete spinal cord injury was noted in another study in which only 14% of complete injury and 50% of incomplete injury patients survived beyond 1 year [Alander et al., 1997]. Recovery from spinal injury is not only better in children than in adults, but also in children improvement can continue for many months after the injury [Wang et al., 2004].

As mentioned earlier, MRI, somatosensory-evoked potentials, and electromyography have been the main laboratory tests used to assist prediction of outcome after spinal cord injury. Of the three, MRI is the most helpful. MRI can distinguish intramedullary hematomas (poorer prognosis) from spinal cord edema (better prognosis). Patients in whom the edema is restricted to a single spinal segment or less have the best prognosis [Schaefer et al., 1992]. The clinical and prognostic value of emergency MRI was studied in 55 patients with acute cervical spinal cord injuries. Although the best single predictor of long-term improvement in neurologic function was the initial neurologic examination, four MRI characteristics provided additional prognostic information—the presence of intra-axial hematoma; the sagittal length of spinal cord hematoma; the extent of spinal cord edema; and spinal cord compression by extra-axial hematoma [Selden et al., 1999]. Conclusions about the usefulness of different laboratory investigations in aiding the prediction of neurologic outcome must be viewed with some circumspection, however, because in most series relatively few patients of different ages have been studied.

Data comparing surgical and nonsurgical management in acute spinal trauma come mainly from adult studies. In patients with complete spinal cord lesions treated conservatively, 27% to 34% showed some improvement [Frankel et al., 1969; Guttmann, 1963]. Of 27 patients with complete lesions who were managed surgically, 25 improved, but this improvement was seen only in nerve root function at the site of the injury [Stauffer, 1984]. In patients with incomplete spinal cord lesions, 64% to 90% have improved with conservative treatment [Guttmann, 1963; Meinecke, 1964]. Surgical treatment of such patients had resulted in improvement in 82% [Forsyth et al., 1959]. In incomplete and complete spinal cord lesions, there are no clear differences in neurologic outcome between surgical and nonsurgical management.

The mechanism of recovery after spinal cord injury is suggested by studies indicating reorganization of motor pathways rostral to the injury site (cortical or spinal or both), with these motor pathways facilitating later recovery [Topka et al., 1991]. There is considerable experimental evidence to indicate that neurons of the mammalian nervous system maintain an ability to regenerate and regain function. In spinal cord injury, however, environmental factors, such as nerve growth inhibitors (released at the time of spinal cord injury) and apoptosis or programmed cell death (occurring in areas of spinal cord injury), interfere with such regeneration. Much work is ongoing to try to develop methods to combat these and other adverse environmental factors found in acute spinal cord injury (see earlier section on leading investigational treatments).

PREVENTION

Spinal cord injuries are devastating at any age, but are especially tragic and expensive in children. Preventing these injuries is probably the greatest challenge in dealing with spinal cord injuries. Continued investment in educational programs, with ongoing efforts to heighten public awareness of the risks and consequences of spinal cord injuries, is crucial. People who drink alcohol should not drive. Risk-taking behavior must be minimized, particularly in people taking sedating medications or illicit drugs. The need for protective helmets, in sports such as skiing, snowboarding, and bicycling, cannot be overstressed. Diving into unfamiliar waters must be avoided. Certain sports, particularly tackle football, carry with them a substantial risk of spinal injury, and this needs to be recognized. Appropriate seat-belt designs, proper use of child restraints, and positioning small children in the rear seats of automobiles fitted with airbags save lives and neurologic function. Finally, any efforts that can result in reduction of societal violence, particularly involving guns and knives, can be expected to result in a corresponding reduction in spinal cord injuries [Ackery et al., 2004; Rekate et al., 1999]. A valuable resource for parents is the web site of the ASIA at http://www.asia-spinalinjury.org/home/index.html.

REFERENCES

Abel NA, Smith RA. Intrathecal baclofen for treatment of intractable spinal spasticity. Arch Phys Med Rehab 1994;75:54.

Ackery A, Tator C, Krassioukov A. A global perspective on spinal cord injury epidemiology. J Neurotrauma 2004;21:1355.

Alander DH, Parker J, Stauffer ES. Intermediate-term outcome of cervical spinal cord-injured patients older than 50 years of age. Spine 1997;22:1189.

Alker GJ, Oh YS, Leslie EV, et al. Postmortem radiology of head and neck injuries in fatal traffic accidents. Radiology 1975;14:611.

Allen JP, Myers GG, Condon VR. Laceration of the spinal cord related to breech delivery. JAMA 1969;208:1019.

American Spinal Injury Association, International Medical Society of Paraplegia (ASIA/IMSOP). International standards for neurological and functional classification of spinal cord injury. Revised, 1992.

Andersen BJ, Stringer WA. Imaging after spinal injury. In: Narayan RK, Wilberger JE, Povlishock JT, eds. Neurotrauma. New York: McGraw-Hill, 1996.

Anderson JM, Shutt AH. Spinal injury in children: A review of 156 cases seen from 1950 through 1978. Mayo Clin Proc 1980;55:499.

Anderson LD, D'Alonzo RT. Fractures of the odontoid process of the axis. J Bone Joint Surg Am 1974;56:1663.

Asamoto S, Sugiyama H, Doi H, et al. Hyperbaric oxygen (HBO) therapy for acute traumatic cervical spinal cord injury. Spinal Cord 2000;38:538.

Asazuma T, Satomi K, Suzuki N, et al. Management of patients with an incomplete cervical spinal cord injury. Spinal Cord 1996;34:620.

Babcock JL. Spinal injuries in children. Pediatr Clin North Am 1975;22:487.

Bailes JE, Hadley MN, Quigley MR, et al. Management of athletic injuries of the cervical spine and spinal cord. Neurosurgery 1991;29:491.

Baker AS, Ojemann RG, Swartz MN, et al. Spinal epidural abscess. N Engl J Med 1975;293:463.

Ball PA, Nockels RP. Summary statement: Nonoperative management and critical care of acute spinal cord injury. Spine 2001;26:S38.

Barnett HJM, Jousse AT. Posttraumatic syringomyelia (cystic myelopathy). In: Vinken PJ, Bruyn CH, Braakman R, eds. Injuries of the spine and spinal cord, II, Vol. 26. Handbook of clinical neurology. Amsterdam: North Holland Publishing Company, 1976.

Baskin DS. Spinal cord injury. In: Evans RW, ed. Neurology and trauma. Philadelphia: WB Saunders, 1996.

Baskin DS, Simpson RK Jr, Browning JL, et al. The effect of long-term high-dose naloxone infusion in experimental blunt spinal cord injury. J Spin Dis 1993;6:38.

Batnitzky S, Keucher TR, Mealey J Jr, et al. Iatrogenic intraspinal epidermoid tumors. JAMA 1977;237:148.

Bell HS. Paralysis of both arms from injury of the upper portion of the pyramidal decussation: "cruciate paralysis." J Neurosurg 1970;33:376.

Benzel EC, Doezema D. Prehospital management of the spinally injured patient. In: Narayan RK, Wilberger JE, Povlishock JT, eds. Neurotrauma. New York: McGraw-Hill, 1996.

Bondurant FJ, Cotler HB, Kulkarni MV, et al. Acute spinal cord injury: A study using physical examination and magnetic resonance imaging. Spine 1990;15:161.

Borow M, Goldson HJ. Prevention of postoperative deep venous thrombosis and pulmonary emboli with combined modalities. Am Surg 1983;49:599.

Braakman R, Penning L. Injuries of the cervical spine. In: Vinken PJ, Bruyn GW, eds. Handbook of clinical neurology, Vol. 25. Amsterdam: North Holland, 1976.

Bracken MB, Collins WF, Freeman DF, et al. Efficacy of methylprednisolone in acute spinal cord injury. JAMA 1984;251:45.

Bracken MB, Freeman DH, Hellenbrand K. Incidence of acute traumatic hospitalized spinal cord injury in the United States, 1970-1977. Am J Epidemiol 1981;113:615.

Bracken MB, Holford TR. Effects of timing of methylprednisolone or naloxone administration on recovery of segmental and long-tract neurological function in NASCIS 2. J Neurosurg 1993;79:500.

Bracken MB, Shepard MJ, Collins WF, et al. A randomized, controlled trial of methylprednisolone or naloxone in the treatment of acute spinal-cord injury: Results of the second national acute spinal cord injury study. N Engl J Med 1990;322:1405.

Bracken MB, Shepard MJ, Collins WF, et al. Methylprednisolone or naloxone treatment after acute spinal cord injury: 1-Year follow-up data—results of the Second National Acute Spinal Cord Injury Study. J Neurosurg 1992;76:23.

Bracken MB, Shepard MJ, Holford TR, et al. Administration of methylprednisolone for 24 or 48 hours or tirilazad mesylate for 48 hours in the treatment of acute spinal cord injury: Results of the Third National Spinal Cord Injury Randomized Control Trial. National Acute Spinal Cord Injury Study. JAMA 1997;277:1597.

Bracken MB, Shepard MJ, Holford TR, et al. Methylprednisolone or tirilazad mesylate administration after acute spinal cord injury: 1-Year follow up. J Neurosurg 1998;89:699.

Bresnan MJ, Abroms IF. Neonatal spinal cord transection secondary to hyperextension of the neck in breech presentation. J Pediatr 1974;84:734.

Browder J, Meyers R. Pyogenic infections of the spinal epidural space. Surgery 1941;10:296.

Bruyn GW, Bosma MJ. Spinal extradural haematoma. In: Vinken PJ, Bruyn GW, eds. Handbook of clinical neurology, Vol. 25. Amsterdam: North Holland, 1976.

Burke DC. Traumatic spinal paralysis in children. Paraplegia 1974;11:268.

Burke DC. Injuries of the spinal cord in children. In: Vinken PJ, Bruyn GW, eds. Handbook of clinical neurology, Vol. 25. Amsterdam: North Holland, 1976.

Burns SP, Golding DG, Rolle WA Jr, et al. Recovery of ambulation in motor-incomplete tetraplegia. Arch Phys Med Rehab 1997;78:1169.

Byers RK. Spinal-cord injuries during birth. Dev Med Child Neurol 1975;17:103.

Caffey J. The whiplash shaken infant syndrome. Pediatrics 1974;54:396.

Canaday BR, Stanford RH. Propantheline bromide in the management of hyperhidrosis associated with spinal cord injury. Ann Pharmacother 1995;29:489.

Casale R, Glynn CJ, Buonocore M. Reduction of spastic hypertonia in patients with spinal cord injury: A double-blind comparison of intravenous orphenadrine citrate and placebo. Arch Phys Med Rehab 1995;76:660.

Cattell HS, Filtzer DL. Pseudosubluxation and other normal variations in the cervical spine in children. J Bone Joint Surg Am 1965;47:1295.

Caviness AC. Evaluation of cervical spine injuries in children and adolescents. UpToDate, Version 12.3, 2004.

Cheng H, Liao KK, Liao SF, et al. Spinal cord repair with acidic fibroblast growth factor as a treatment for a patient with chronic paraplegia. Spine 2004;29:E284.

Chesnut RM. Management of brain and spine injuries. Crit Care Clin 2004;20:25.

Chilton J, Dagi TF. Acute cervical spinal cord injury. Am J Emerg Med 1985;3:340.

Chiou-Tan FY, Tuel SM, Johnson JC, et al. Effect of mexiletin on spinal cord injury dysesthetic pain. Am J Phys Med Rehab 1996;75:84.

Creasey GH, Ho CH, Triolo RJ, et al. Clinical applications of electrical stimulation after spinal cord injury. J Spinal Cord Med 2004;27:365.

Crothers B. Injury of the spinal cord in breech extraction as an important cause of fetal death and of paraplegia in childhood. Am J Med Sci 1923;165:94.

Curt A, Nitsche B, Rodic B, et al. Assessment of autonomic dysreflexia in patients with spinal cord injury. J Neurol Neurosurg Psychiatry 1997;62:473.

Dare AO, Dias MS, Li V. Magnetic resonance imaging correlation in pediatric spinal cord injury without radiographic abnormality. J Neurosurg (Spine 1) 2002;97:33.

Davis PC, Reisner A, Hudgins PA, et al. Spinal injuries in children: Role of MR. AJNR Am J Neuroradiol 1993;14:607.

Decker JE, Hergenroeder AC. Overview of cervical spinal cord and cerivcal peripheral nerve injuries in the young athlete. UpToDate, Version 12.3, 2004.

DeLaTorre JC. Spinal cord injury: Review of basic and applied research. Spine 1981;6:315.

DeMyer W. Anatomy and clinical neurology of the spinal cord. In: Baker AB, Joynt RJ, eds. Clinical neurology, Vol. 3. Philadelphia: Harper & Row, 1985.

DeVivo MJ, Kurtus PL, Rutt RD, et al. The influence of age at time of spinal cord injury on rehabilitation outcome. Arch Neurol 1990;47:687.

Dias MS. Traumatic brain and spinal cord injury. Pediatr Clin North Am 2004;51:271.

Ditunno JF. Rehabilitation assessment and management in the acute spinal cord injury (SCI) phase. In: Narayan RK, Wilberger JE, Povlishock JT, eds. Neurotrauma. New York: McGraw-Hill, 1996.

Ditunno JF, Little JW, Tessler A, et al. Spinal shock revisited: A four-phase model. Spinal Cord 2004;42:383.

Dobkin BH, Havton LA. Basic advances and new avenues in therapy of spinal cord injury. Annu Rev Med 2004;55:255.

Donahue DJ, Muhlbauer MS, Kaufman RA, et al. Childhood survival of atlantooccipital dislocation: Underdiagnosis, recognition, treatment, and review of the literature. Pediatr Neurosurg 1994;21:105.

Drewes AM, Andreasen A, Poulsen LH. Valproate for treatment of chronic central pain after spinal cord injury: A double-blind cross-over study. Paraplegia 1994;32:565.

Ducker TB, Hamit HF. Experimental treatments of acute spinal cord injury. J Neurosurg 1969;30:693.

Ducker TB, Lucas JT, Wallace CA. Recovery from spinal cord injury. Clin Neurosurg 1983;30:495.

Duh M, Shepard MJ, Wilberger JE, et al. The effectiveness of surgery on the treatment of acute spinal cord injury and its relation to pharmacological treatment. Neurosurgery 1994;35:240.

Dumont RJ, Okonkwo DO, Verma S, et al. Acute spinal cord injury, part I: Pathophysiologic mechanisms. Clin Neuropharmacol 2001a;24:254.

Dumont RJ, Verma S, Okonkwo DO, et al. Acute spinal cord injury, part II: Contemporary pharmacotherapy. Clin Neuropharmacol 2001b;24:265.

Earnhardt JN, Streit WJ, Anderson DK, et al. Induction of manganese superoxide dismutase in acute spinal cord injury. J Neurotrauma 2002;19:1065.

Edelson RN. Spinal subdural hematoma. In: Vinken PJ, Bruyn GW, eds. Handbook of clinical neurology, Vol. 26. Amsterdam: North Holland, 1976.

Edelson RN, Chernik NL, Posner JD. Spinal subdural hematomas complicating lumbar puncture. Arch Neurol 1974;31:134.

Elsberg CA, Dyke CG, Brewer ED. The symptoms and diagnosis of extradural cysts. Bull Neurol Inst N Y 1934;3:39.

Faden AI. Pharmacological treatment approaches for brain and spinal cord trauma. In: Narayan RK, Wilberger JE, Povlishock JT, eds. Neurotrauma. New York: McGraw-Hill, 1996.

Fehlings MG, Sekhon LH, Tator C. The role and timing of decompression in acute spinal cord injuries: What do we know? What should we do? Spine 2001;26 (24 Suppl):S101.

Flanders AE, Schaefer DM, Doan HT, et al. Acute cervical spine trauma: Correlation of MR imaging findings with degree of neurologic deficit. Radiology 1990;177:25.

Flanders AE, Spettell CM, Friedman DP, et al. The relationship between the functional abilities of patients with cervical spinal cord injury and the severity of damage revealed by MRI imaging. AJNR Am J Neuroradiol 1999;20:926.

Forsyth HF, Alexander E, Underal R. The advantages of early spine fusion in the treatment of fracture-dislocation of the cervical spine. J Bone Joint Surg 1959;41:17.

Francel PC, Long BA, Malik JM, et al. Limiting ischemic spinal cord injury using a free radical scavenger 21-aminosteroid and/or cerebrospinal fluid drainage. J Neurosurg 1993;79:742.

Francisco JT. Smothering in infancy: Its relationship to the "crib death syndrome." South Med J 1970;63:1110.

Frankel HL, Hancock DO, Hyslop G, et al. The value of postural reduction in the initial management of closed injuries of the spine with paraplegia and tetraplegia. Paraplegia 1969;7:179.

Galandiuk S, Raque G, Appel S, et al. The two-edged sword of large-dose steroids for spinal cord trauma. Ann Surg 1993;218:419.

Geisler FH, Coleman WP, Grieco G, et al. The Sygen Study Group: The GM1 ganglioside multicenter acute spinal cord injury study. Spine 2001;26 (24 Suppl):S87.

Geisler FH, Dorsey FC, Coleman WP. Recovery of motor function after spinal-cord injury—a randomized, placebo-controlled trial with GM-1 ganglioside. N Engl J Med 1991;324:1829.

Geller B, Greydanus DE. Psychological management of acute paraplegia in adolescence. Pediatrics 1979;63:562.

Gibson CJ. An overview of spinal cord injury. Phys Med Rehab Clin N Am 1992;3:699.

Gibson T, Norris W. Skin fragments removed by injection needles. Lancet 1958;2:983.

Gilles FH, Bina M, Sotrel A. Infantile atlanto-occipital instability. Am J Dis Child 1979;133:30.

Glasser RS, Fessler RG. Biomechanics of cervical spine trauma. In: Narayan RK, Wilberger JE, Povlishock JT, eds. Neurotrauma. New York: McGraw-Hill, 1996.

Goetz LL, Hurvitz EA, Nelson VS, et al. Bowel management in children and adolescents with spinal cord injury. J Spinal Cord Med 1998;21:335.

Goldberg AL, Daffner RH, Schapiro RL. Imaging of acute spinal trauma: An evolving multi-modality approach. Clin Imaging 1990;14:11.

Goldberg AL, Rothfus WE, Deeb ZL, et al. The impact of magnetic resonance on the diagnostic evaluation of acute cervicothoracic spinal trauma. Skeletal Radiol 1988;17:89.

Green BA, Eismont FJ. Acute spinal cord injury: A systems approach. Cent Nerv Syst Trauma 1984;1:173.

Greenberg JO. Neuroimaging of the spinal cord. Neurol Clin North Am 1991;9:679.

Grijalva I, Guizar-Sahagun G, Castaneda-Hernandez G, et al. Efficacy and safety of 4-aminopyridine in patients with long-term spinal cord injury: A randomized, double-blind, placebo-controlled trial. Pharmacotherapy 2003;23:823.

Guest J, Eleraky MA, Apostolides PJ, et al. Traumatic central cord syndrome: Results of surgical management. J Neurosurg (Spine 1) 2002;97:25.

Gunby P. New focus on spinal cord injury. JAMA 1981;245:1201.

Gunnarsson T, Fehlings MG. Acute neurosurgical management of traumatic brain injury and spinal cord injury. Curr Opin Neurol 2003;16:717.

Guttmann L. Early management of the paraplegic: Symposium on spinal injuries. J Roy Coll Surg 1963;43:133.

Guttmann L. Spinal shock. In: Vinken PJ, Bruyn GW, eds. Handbook of clinical neurology, Vol. 26. Amsterdam: North Holland, 1976.

Hackler RH. Urologic care of the spinal cord injured patient. AUA Update Series 1984;3:1.

Hadley MN. Pediatric spine injuries. In: Camins MB, O'Leary PF, eds. Disorders of the cervical spine. Baltimore: Williams & Wilkins, 1992.

Hadley MN. Pharmacological therapy after acute cervical spinal cord injury. Neurosurgery 2002a;50:S63.

Hadley MN. Management of pediatric cervical spine and spinal cord injuries. Neurosurgery 2002b;50:S85.

Hadley MN, Zabramski JM, Browner CM, et al. Pediatric spinal trauma: Review of 122 cases of spinal cord and vertebral column injuries. J Neurosurg 1988;68:18.

Hamilton MG, Myles ST. Pediatric spinal injury: A review of sixty-one deaths. J Neurosurg 1992;77:705.

Hancock DO. Spinal extradural abscess. In: Vinken PJ, Bruyn GW, eds. Handbook of clinical neurology, Vol. 26. Amsterdam: North Holland, 1976.

Hansebout RR. A comprehensive review of methods of improving cord recovery after acute spinal cord injury. In: Tator CH, ed. Early management of acute spinal cord injury. New York: Raven Press, 1982.

Harrop JS, Sharan AD, Vaccaro AR, et al. The cause of neurologic deterioration after acute cervical spinal cord injury. Spine 2001;26:340.

Hauswald M, Braude D. Spinal immobilization in trauma patients: is it really necessary? Curr Opin Crit Care 2002;8:566.

Hehman K, Norrell H. Massive chronic spinal epidural hematoma in a child. Am J Dis Child 1968;116:308.

Herkowitz HN, Samberg LC. Vertebral column injuries associated with tobogganing. J Trauma 1978;18:806.

Herren RY, Alexander L. Sulcal and intrinsic blood vessels of human spinal cord. Arch Neurol Psychiatry 1939;41:678.

Herskowitz J, Bielawski MA, Venna N, et al. Anterior cervical arachnoid cyst simulating syringomyelia. Arch Neurol 1978;35:57.

Heusner AP. Non-tuberculous spinal epidural infections. N Engl J Med 1948;239:845.

Hidaka C, Khan SN, Farmer JC, et al. Gene therapy for spinal applications. Orthop Clin North Am 2002;33:439.

Hill SA, Miller CA, Kosnik EJ, et al. Pediatric neck injuries: A clinical study. J Neurosurg 1984;60:700.

Horowitz SH, Patel N. Peripheral neurophysiology of acute distal spinal cord infarction. Pediatr Neurol 2003;28:64.

Hoy GA, Cole WG. The paediatric cervical seat belt syndrome. Injury 1993;24:297.

Huang L, Mehta MP, Nanda A, et al. The role of multiple hyperbaric oxygenation in expanding therapeutic windows after acute spinal cord injury in rats. J Neurosurg Spine 2003;99:198.

Hyman RA, Gorey MT. Imaging strategies for MR of the spine. Radiol Clin North Am 1988;26:505.

Jacobs PL, Nash MS. Exercise recommendations for individuals with spinal cord injury. Sports Med 2004;34:727.

Janes JM, Hooshmand H. Severe extension-flexion injuries of the cervical spine. Mayo Clin Proc 1965;40:353.

Jellinger K. Neuropathology of cord injury. In: Vinken PJ, Bruyn GW, eds. Handbook of clinical neurology, Vol. 25. Amsterdam: North Holland, 1976.

Johnston TE, Betz RR, Smith BT, et al. Implanted functional electrical stimulation: An alternative for standing and walking in pediatric spinal cord injury. Spinal Cord 2003;41:144.

Joshi SM, Hatfield RH, Martin J, et al. Spinal epidural abscess: A diagnostic challenge. Br J Neurosurg 2003;17:160.

Kadish HA. Cervical spine evaluation in the pediatric trauma patient. Clin Pediatr Emerg Med 2001;2:41.

Kakulas BA. Pathology of spinal injuries. Cent Nerv Syst Trauma 1984;1:117.

Kakulas BA. A review of the neuropathology of human spinal cord injury with emphasis on special features. J Spinal Cord Med 1999;22:119.

Kalfas I, Wilberger J, Goldberg A, et al. Magnetic resonance imaging in acute spinal cord trauma. Neurosurgery 1988;23:295.

Kamimura N, Shichida K, Tomita Y, et al. Spinal somatosensory evoked potentials in infants and children with spinal cord lesions. Brain Dev 1988;10:355.

Kaptanoglu E, Solaroglu I, Okutan O, et al. Erythropoietin exerts neuroprotection after acute spinal cord injury in rats: Effect on lipid peroxidation and early ultrastructural findings. Neurosurg Rev 2004;27:113.

Katoh S, el Masry WS, Jaffray D, et al. Neurologic outcome in conservatively treated patients with incomplete closed traumatic cervical spinal cord injuries. Spine 1996;21:2345.

Katz RT, Toleikis RJ, Knuth AE. Somatosensory-evoked and dermatomal-evoked potentials are not clinically useful in the prognostication of acute spinal cord injury. Spine 1991;16:730.

Kewalramani LS, Tori JA. Spinal cord trauma in children: Neurological patterns, radiologic features, and pathomechanics of injury. Spine 1980;5:11.

Kim DH, Vaccaro AR, Henderson FC, et al. Molecular biology of cervical myelopathy and spinal cord injury: Role of oligodendrocyte apoptosis. Spine J 2003;3:510.

Kirshblum S. New rehabilitation interventions in spinal cord injury. J Spinal Cord Med 2004;27:342.

Kiss ZHT, Tator CH. Neurogenic shock. In: Geller ER, ed. Shock and resuscitation. New York: McGraw-Hill, 1993.

Klose KJ, Green BA, Smith RS, et al. University of Miami Neuro-Spinal Index (UMNI): A quantitative method for determining spinal cord function. Paraplegia 1980;18:331.

Krause JS, Sternberg M, Lottes S, et al. Mortality after spinal cord injury: An 11-year prospective study. Arch Phys Med Rehab 1997;78:815.

Kulkarni MV, McArdle CB, Kopanicky D, et al. Acute spinal cord injury: MR imaging at 1.5T. Radiology 1987;164:837.

Kwon BK, Tetzlaff W. Spinal cord regeneration from gene to transplants. Spine 2001;26:S13.

Landi G, Ciccone A. GM-1 ganglioside for spinal-cord injury. [Letter to the editor]. N Engl J Med 1992;326:493.

Lanska MJ, Roessmann U, Wiznitzer M. Magnetic resonance imaging in cervical cord birth injury. Pediatrics 1990;85:760.

Levi L, Wolf A, Belzberg H. Hemodynamic parameters in patients with acute cervical cord trauma: Description, intervention, and prediction of outcome. Neurosurgery 1993;33:1007.

Levi L, Wolf A, Rigamonti D, et al. Anterior decompression in cervical spine trauma: Does the timing of surgery affect the outcome? Neurosurgery 1991;29:216.

Levitt MA, Flanders AE. Diagnostic capabilities of magnetic resonance imaging and computed tomography in acute cervical spinal column injury. Am J Emerg Med 1991;9:131.

Levy ML, Gans W, Wijesinghe HS, et al. Use of methylprednisolone as an adjunct in the management of patients with penetrating spinal cord injury: Outcome analysis. Neurosurgery 1996;39:1141.

Lewis KS, Mueller WM. Intrathecal baclofen for severe spasticity secondary to spinal cord injury. Ann Pharmacother 1993;27:767.

Li C, Houlden DA, Rowed DW. Somatosensory evoked potentials and neurological grades as predictors of outcome in acute spinal cord injury. J Neurosurg 1990;72:600.

Liptak GS, Revell GM. Management of bowel dysfunction in children with spinal cord disease or injury by means of the enema continence catheter. J Pediatr 1992;120:190.

Lonstein JE. Post-laminectomy spine deformity. In: Lonstein JE, Bradford DS, Winter RB, et al, eds. Moe's textbook of scoliosis and other spinal deformities, 3rd ed. Philadelphia: WB Saunders, 1995:506.

Louis AA, Gupta P, Perkash I. Localization of sensory levels in traumatic quadriplegia by segmental somatosensory evoked potentials. Electroencephalogr Clin Neurophysiol 1985;62:313.

Luce JM. Medical management of spinal cord injury. Crit Care Med 1985;13:6.

Mace SE. Emergency evaluation of cervical spine injuries: CT versus plain radiographs. Ann Emerg Med 1985;14:973.

Mahoney FI, Barthel DW. Functional evaluation: The Barthel index. Maryland Med J 1965;14:61.

Manno NJ, Uhlein A, Kernohan JW. Intraspinal epidermoids. J Neurosurg 1962;19:754.

Marion DW. Head and spinal cord injury. Neurol Clin North Am 1998;16:485.

Maroon JC, Steele PB, Berlin R. Football head and neck injuries—an update. Clin Neurosurg 1980;27:414.

Massagli TL. Medical and rehabilitation issues in the care of children with spinal cord injury. Physical Med Rehab Clin N Am 2000;11:169.

Matsumura A, Meguro K, Tsurushima H, et al. Magnetic resonance imaging of spinal cord injury without radiographic abnormality. Surg Neurol 1990;33:281.

Meinecke FW. Early treatment of traumatic paraplegia. Paraplegia 1964;1:262.

Meinecke FW. Initial clinical appraisal. In: Vinken PJ, Bruyn GW, eds. Handbook of clinical neurology, Vol. 26. Amsterdam: North Holland, 1976.

Menezes AH, Godersky JC, Smoker WRK. Spinal cord injury. In: McLaurin RL, Venes JL, Schut L, et al, eds. Pediatric neurosurgery: Surgery of the developing nervous system, 2nd ed. Philadelphia: WB Saunders, 1989.

Meyer GA, Berman IR, Doty DB, et al. Hemodynamic responses to acute quadriplegia with or without chest trauma. J Neurosurg 1971;34:168.

Meyer PR, Cybulski GR, Rusin JJ, et al. Spinal cord injury. Neurol Clin North Am 1991;9:625.

Michaelis LS. Prognosis of spinal cord injury. In: Vinken PJ, Bruyn GW, eds. Handbook of clinical neurology, Vol. 26. Amsterdam: North Holland, 1976.

Morgan C, Newell SJ. Cervical spinal cord injury following cephalic presentation and delivery by Caesarean section. Dev Med Child Neurol 2001;43:274.

Mueller FO, Blyth CS. Fatalities from head and cervical spine injuries occurring in tackle football: 40 years' experience. Clin Sports Med 1987;6:185.

Nance PW, Bugaresti J, Shellenberger K, et al. Efficacy and safety of tizanidine in the treatment of spasticity in patients with spinal cord injury. North American Tizanidine Study Group. Neurology 1994;44 (11 Suppl 9):S44.

Nesathurai S. Steroids and spinal cord injury: Revisiting the NASCIS 2 and NASCIS 3 trials. J Trauma Injury Infect Crit Care 1998;45:1088.

Norenberg MD, Smith J, Marcillo A. The pathology of human spinal cord injury: Defining the problems. J Neurotrauma 2004;21:429.

Nugent GR, Odom GL, Woodhall B. Spinal extradural cysts. Neurology 1959;9:397.

Nygaard IE, Kreder KJ. Spine update: Urological management in patients with spinal cord injuries. Spine 1996;21:128.

Oliver NJ. Annual estimates: Stroke and central nervous system trauma. Bethesda, MD: NINDS Office of Scientific and Health Reports, 1992.

Ommaya AK. Whiplash injury: A review of clinical and experimental observations. Pak Med Rev 1969;4:13.

Osenbach RK, Menezes AH. Spinal cord injury without radiographic abnormality in children. Pediatr Neurosci 1989;15:168.

Osenbach RK, Menezes AH. Pediatric spinal cord and vertebral column injury. Neurosurgery 1992;30:385.

Pang D, Hanley EN. Special problems of spinal stabilization in children. In: Cooper PR, ed. Management of post-traumatic spinal instability. Park Ridge, IL: AANS, 1990.

Pang D, Wilberger JE. Spinal cord injury without radiographic abnormalities in children. J Neurosurg 1982;57:114.

Panjabi M, White A. Basic biomechanics of the spine. Neurosurgery 1980;7:76.

Pannek J, Diederichs W, Botel U. Urodynamically controlled management of spinal cord injury in children. Neurourol Urodyn 1997;16:285.

Papadopoulos SM, Selden NR, Quint DJ, et al. Immediate spinal cord decompression for cervical spinal cord injury: Feasibility and outcome. J Trauma Injury Infect Crit Care 2002;52:323.

Parisini P, Di Silverstre M, Greggi T. Treatment of spinal fractures in children and adolescents: Long-term results in 44 patients. Spine 2002;27:1989.

Park E, Velumian AA, Fehlings MG. The role of excitotoxicity in secondary mechanisms of spinal cord injury: A review with an emphasis on the implications for white matter degeneration. J Neurotrauma 2004;21:754.

Pereira CE, Lynch JC. Spinal epidural abscess: An analysis of 24 cases. Surg Neurol 2005;63:S26.

Perot PL. The clinical use of somatosensory evoked potentials in spinal cord injury. Clin Neurosurg 1973;20:367.

Piepmeier JM, Collins WF. Recovery of function following spinal cord injury. In: Vinken PJ, Bruyn GW, Klawans HL, eds. Handbook of clinical neurology, Vol. 61 (RS 17). Amsterdam: Elsevier Science, 1992.

Piper JG, Menezes AH. Pediatric spinal cord injury. In: Narayan RK, Wilberger JE, Povlishock JT, eds. Neurotrauma. New York: McGraw-Hill, 1996.

Pitts LH, Ross A, Chase GA, et al. Treatment with thyrotropin-releasing hormone (TRH) in patients with traumatic spinal cord injuries. J Neurotrauma 1995;12:235.

Plotkin R, Ronthal M, Froman C. Spontaneous spinal subarachnoid haemorrhage: report of 3 cases. J Neurosurg 1966;25:443.

Proctor MR. Spinal cord injury. Crit Care Med 2002;30 (Suppl):S489.

Profyris C, Cheema SS, Zang D, et al. Degenerative and regenerative mechanisms governing spinal cord injury. Neurobiol Dis 2004;15:415.

Quencer RM, Bunge RP, Egnor M, et al. Acute traumatic central cord syndrome: MRI-pathological correlations. Neuroradiology 1992;34:85.

Quencer RM, Green BA, Eismont FJ. Post-traumatic spinal cord cysts: Clinical features and characterization with metrizamide computed tomography. Radiology 1983;146:415.

Rabinovich SS, Seledtsov VI, Poveschenko OV, et al. Transplantation treatment of spinal cord injury patients. Biomed Pharmacother 2003;57:428.
Rand RW, Crowdall PH. Central spinal cord syndrome in hyperextension injuries of the cervical spine. J Bone Joint Surg 1962;44:1415.
Reddy SP, Junewick JJ, Backstrom JW. Distribution of spinal fractures in children: Does age, mechanism of injury, or gender play a significant role? Pediatr Radiol 2003;33:776.
Rekate HL, Theodore N, Sonntag VKH, et al. Pediatric spine and spinal cord trauma: State of the art for the third millennium. Child Nerv Syst 1999;15:743.
Reynolds R. Pediatric spinal injury. Curr Opin Pediatr 2000;12:67.
Robertson WC Jr, Lee YE, Edmonson MB. Spontaneous spinal epidural hematoma in the young. Neurology 1979;29:120.
Rosenzweig ES, McDonald JW. Rodent models for treatment of spinal cord injury: research trends and progress toward useful repair. Curr Opin Neurol 2004;17:121.
Rosman NP, Herskowitz J. Spinal cord trauma. In: Swaiman KF, Wright FS, eds. Practice of pediatric neurology, 2nd ed. St. Louis: Mosby, 1982.
Rossier AB, Foo D, Nabeedy MH, et al. Radiography of posttraumatic syringomyelia. AJNR Am J Neuroradiol 1983;4:637.
Rowed DW, McLean JA, Tator CH. Somatosensory evoked potentials in acute spinal cord injury: Prognostic value. Surg Neurol 1976;9:203.
Ruge JR, Sinson GP, McLone DG, et al. Pediatric spinal injury: The very young. J Neurosurg 1988;68:25.
Sato T, Kokubun S, Rijal KP, et al. Prognosis of cervical spinal cord injury in correlation with magnetic resonance imaging. Paraplegia 1994;32:81.
Schaefer DM, Flanders AE, Osterholm JL, et al. Prognostic significance of magnetic resonance imaging in the acute phase of cervical spine injury. J Neurosurg 1992;76:218.
Schneider RC. A syndrome in acute cervical injuries for which early operation is indicated. J Neurosurg 1951;8:360.
Schneider RC. The syndrome of acute anterior spinal cord injury. J Neurosurg 1955;12:95.
Schneider RC. Serious and fatal neurosurgical football injuries. Clin Neurosurg 1964;12:226.
Schneider RC, Crosby EC, Russo RH, et al. Traumatic spinal cord syndromes and their management. Clin Neurosurg 1973;20:424.
Schneider RC, Gosch HH, Norrell H, et al. Vascular insufficiency and differential distortion of brain and cord caused by cervicomedullary football injuries. J Neurosurg 1970;33:363.
Schultke E, Kendall E, Kamencic H, et al. Quercetin promotes functional recovery following acute spinal cord injury. J Neurotrauma 2003;20:583.
Schurch B, Hodler J, Rodic B. Botulinum A toxin as a treatment of detrusor-sphincter dyssynergia in patients with spinal cord injury: MRI controlled transperineal injections. J Neurol Neurosurg Psychiatry 1997;63:474.
Schwartz G, Fehlings MG. Evaluation of the neuroprotective effects of sodium channel blockers after spinal cord injury: Improved behavioral and neuroanatomical recovery with riluzole. J Neurosurg 2001;94:245.
Schwartz G, Fehlings MG. Secondary injury mechanisms of spinal cord trauma: A novel therapeutic approach for the management of secondary pathophysiology with the sodium channel blocker riluzole. In: McKerracher L, Doucet G, Rossignol S, eds. Progress in brain research, Vol. 137. Amsterdam: Elsevier Science, 2002.
Segal JL, Pathak MS, Hernandez JP, et al. Safety and efficacy of 4-aminopyridine in humans with spinal cord injury: A long-term, controlled trial. Pharmacotherapy 1999;19:713.
Selden NR, Quint DJ, Patel N. Emergency magnetic resonance imaging of cervical spinal cord injuries: Clinical correlation and prognosis. Neurosurgery 1999;44:785.
Sett P, Crockard HA. The value of magnetic resonance imaging (MRI) in the follow-up management of spinal injury. Paraplegia 1991;29:396.
Shapiro R, Youngberg A, Rothman S. The differential diagnosis of traumatic lesions of the occipito-atlanto-axial segment. Radiol Clin North Am 1973;11:505.
Shaywitz BA. Epidermoid spinal cord tumors and previous lumbar punctures. J Pediatr 1972;80:638.
Shefner JM, Tun C. Clinical neurophysiology of focal spinal cord injury. Neurol Clin North Am 1991;9:671.
Shurman G, Lobaugh P, Wilberger JE. Application of evoked potential monitoring in spinal cord injury. In: Narayan RK, Wilberger JE, Povlishock JT, eds. Neurotrauma. New York: McGraw-Hill, 1996.
Siddall PJ, Taylor D, Cousins MJ. Pain associated with spinal cord injury. Curr Opin Neurol 1995;8:447.
Silver J, Miller JH. Regeneration beyond the glial scar. Nature 2004;5:146.
Singer PA, Prokop LD, Anderson DK. Somatosensory cortical evoked responses after feline experimental spinal cord injury. Paraplegia 1977;15:160.
Sonntag VKH, Francis PM. Patient selection and timing of surgery in contemporary management of spinal cord injury. Park Ridge, IL: AANS Publication Committee, 1995.
Stauffer ES. Neurologic recovery following injuries to the cervical spinal cord and nerve roots. Spine 1984;9:532.
Stringer WA, Andersen BJ. Imaging after spine trauma. In: Evans RW, ed. Neurology and trauma. Philadelphia: WB Saunders, 1996.
Stroman PW, Kornelsen J, Bergman A, et al. Noninvasive assessment of the injured human spinal cord by means of functional magnetic resonance imaging. Spinal Cord 2004;42:59.
Suh TH, Alexander L. Vascular system of the human spinal cord. Arch Neurol Psychiatry 1939;41:659.
Swanson HS, Fincher EF. Extradural arachnoidal cysts of traumatic origin. J Neurosurg 1947;4:530.
Swischuk LE. Spine and spinal cord trauma in the battered child syndrome. Radiology 1969;92:733.
Talbot HS. Psycho-social aspects of sexuality in spinal cord injury patients. Paraplegia 1971;9:37.
Tator CH. Spine-spinal cord relationships in spinal cord trauma. Clin Neurosurg 1983;30:479.
Tator CH. Classification of spinal cord injury based on neurological presentation. In: Narayan RK, Wilberger JE, Povlishock JT, eds. Neurotrauma. New York: McGraw-Hill, 1996.
Tator CH, Duncan EG, Edmonds VE, et al. Changes in epidemiology of acute spinal cord injury from 1947 to 1981. Surg Neurol 1993;40:207.
Tator CH, Fehlings MG, Thorpe K, et al. Current use and timing of spinal surgery for management of acute spinal cord injury in North America: Results of a retrospective multicenter study. J Neurosurg (Spine 1) 1999;91:12.
Taylor TV, Rimmer S, Day B, et al. Ascorbic acid supplementation in the treatment of pressure sores. Lancet 1974;2:544.
Toleikis JR, Sloan TB. Comparison of major nerve and dermatomal somatosensory evoked potentials in the evaluation of patients with spinal cord injury. In: Barber C, Blum T, eds. Evoked potentials III. The Third International Evoked Potentials Symposium. Boston: Butterworth, 1987.
Topka H, Cohen LG, Cole RA, et al. Reorganization of corticospinal pathways following spinal cord injury. Neurology 1991;41:1276.
Torg JS, Truex R, Quedenfeld TC, et al. The national football head and neck injury registry: Report and conclusions. 1978. JAMA 1979;241:1477.
Towbin A. Spinal cord and brain stem injury at birth. Arch Pathol 1964;77:620.
Vale FL, Burns J, Jackson AB, et al. Combined medical and surgical treatment after acute spinal cord injury: Results of a prospective pilot study to assess the merits of aggressive medical resuscitation and blood pressure management. J Neurosurg 1997;87:239.
Vogel L, Mulcahy MJ, Betz RR. The child with a spinal cord injury. Dev Med Child Neurol 1997;39:202.
Vogel LC, Anderson CJ. Spinal cord injuries in children and adolescents: a review. J Spinal Cord Med 2003;26:193.
Walker MD. Acute spinal-cord injury. N Engl J Med 1991;324:1885.
Walter CE, Tedeschi LG. Spinal injury and neonatal death. Am J Obstet Gynecol 1970;106:272.
Wang MY, Hoh DJ, Leary SP, et al. High rates of neurological improvement following severe traumatic pediatric spinal cord injury. Spine 2004;29:1493.
Weinshel SS, Maiman DJ, Baek P, et al. Neurologic recovery in quadriplegia following operative treatment. J Spinal Disord 1990;3:244.
White AA, Panjabi M. Clinical biomechanics of the spine. 2nd ed. Philadelphia: JB Lippincott, 1990.
Wilberger JE. Pharmacological resuscitation for spinal cord injury. In: Narayan RK, Wilberger JE, Povlishock JT, eds. Neurotrauma. New York: McGraw-Hill, 1996.
Wittenberg RH, Boetel U, Beyer HK. Magnetic resonance imaging and computer tomography of acute spinal cord trauma. Clin Orthop 1990;260:176.

Yezierski RP. Pain following spinal cord injury: The clinical problem and experimental studies. Pain 1996;68:185.

York DH, Watts C, Raffensberger M, et al. Utilization of somatosensory evoked cortical potentials in spinal cord injury, prognostic limitations. Spine 1983;8:832.

Ziganow S. Neurometric evaluation of the cortical somatosensory evoked potential in acute incomplete spinal cord injuries. Electroencephalogr Clin Neurophysiol 1986;65:86.

CHAPTER 67

Determination of Brain Death in Infants and Children

Stephen Ashwal

The diagnosis of brain death in infants and children can be established after careful review of the medical history and performance of a detailed neurologic examination. Although criteria in children follow those established in adults, there are no universally accepted worldwide criteria for brain death determination in adults [Haupt and Rudolf, 1999; Wijdicks, 2001, 2002]. In the United States and in most countries the 1987 pediatric guidelines have been employed with general agreement regarding their usefulness [Banasiak and Lister 2003; Farrell and Levine, 1993; Kaufman, 1989], although criticisms about their validity and specificity, particularly in young infants, have been raised [Freeman and Ferry, 1988; Shewmon, 1988; Volpe, 1987]. In some countries, such as Japan, criteria for brain death in children have been established only more recently [Miyasaka et al., 2001].

HISTORICAL PERSPECTIVE

A state beyond coma, or *coma depassé,* was proposed in 1959 by Mollaret and Goulon to describe a premorbid clinical condition with loss of sensation, motor activity, consciousness, and vegetative functions [Mollaret and Goulon, 1959]. In 1968, an ad hoc committee of the Harvard Medical School faculty recommended clinical guidelines that subsequently shaped development of brain death concepts [Beecher, 1968]. The committee proposed that brain death could be defined by coma, apnea, lack of spontaneous or purposeful movements, and loss of selective cranial nerve functions, including the corneal reflex, pupillary response to light, pharyngeal gag and swallowing, yawning, vocalization, and failure of eye deviation to caloric stimulation of the tympanic membranes. Failure of improvement, sustained over 24 hours of observation, established a diagnosis of brain death. Two caveats were that the patient was normothermic and drugs capable of maintaining coma were excluded. Two isoelectric electroencephalograms (EEGs) performed 24 hours apart were considered confirmatory, but not essential in the declaration of brain death. The neurologic examination of brainstem function, an observation period, and ancillary neurodiagnostic tests when diagnostic doubt exists remain fundamental to a present-day diagnosis of brain death. In 1971, Mohandas and Chou emphasized the importance of determining the etiology of coma and documenting the persistence of apnea [Mohandas and Chou, 1971].

The Conference of Medical Royal College and Faculties in the United Kingdom in 1976 proposed the following definition: "Permanent functional death of the brainstem constitutes brain death" [Conference, 1976]. Irreversible structural brainstem damage was defined carefully and believed to be clinically diagnosable without confirmatory EEG recordings. A follow-up report in 1979 recommended that brainstem death be considered death [Conference, 1979]. Subsequently a working group convened by the Royal College of Physicians further defined the criteria of brainstem death [Criteria, 1995].

In 1980, the National Institute of Neurologic and Communicative Disorders and Stroke (NINCDS) Collaborative Study of Brain Death reported on the outcome of 503 adult comatose and apneic patients, including neuropathologic brain studies and EEGs [NINCDS, 1980]. The combination of loss of pupillary light reflex, corneal reflex, oculocephalic reflex (doll's eye phenomenon), and oculovestibular reflex (caloric eye deviation) was highly predictive of death. Apnea, coma, and absence of brainstem reflexes, combined with an electrocerebral silent EEG, were highly associated with pathology in a brain that had experienced long-term respirator exposure ("respirator brain"). Exceptions were rarely noted. A few respirator brains occurred in patients with persistent biologic EEG activity, and several brain specimens did not show the neuropathologic features of a respirator brain despite electrocerebral silence. EEG use was recommended in confirming brain death when the clinical neurologic examination was equivocal. An isoelectric EEG, despite its rare failure always to diagnose brain destruction, was predictive of a fatal outcome except in two patients with drug intoxication. The report emphasized that a patient was not considered brain dead if the EEG was not isoelectric. About 30% of the population had drug toxicity despite the absence of a history of ingestion; 28% had measurable amounts of drugs that would suppress EEG activity. The report concluded that drug screening and EEG monitoring were mandatory before declaring brain death. Subsequent reports in adults [Grigg et al., 1987] and children [Ashwal and Schneider, 1979] documented that EEG activity could persist in unequivocally brain dead patients.

In 1981, a U.S. presidential commission was convened to establish guidelines for the determination of brain death [President's Commission, 1981]. These guidelines, outlined in Box 67-1, emphasized diagnosis based on the irreversible cessation of function of the entire brain. This report recognized that adult criteria might not be applicable to children because of developmental factors, a possible greater tolerance to asphyxia, and the recognition that infants and children occasionally exhibited significant recovery despite prolonged coma. The age of 5 years was selected as the earliest age suitable for the application of adult criteria, although this age selection reflected no known biologic phenomena.

Seeking to remedy this exclusion of infants and children, multiple professional neurologic and pediatric societies in 1987 convened a task force to propose a pediatric standard

Box 67-1 President's Commission Guidelines for the Determination of Brain Death

An individual presenting with the findings in section A (cardiopulmonary) or section B (neurologic) is dead. A diagnosis of death requires that cessation of functions (subsection 1) and irreversibility (subsection 2) be shown.

(A) An individual with irreversible cessation of circulatory and respiratory functions is dead.

(1) Cessation is recognized by an appropriate examination.

(2) Irreversibility is recognized by persistent cessation of functions during an appropriate period of observation or trial of therapy or both.

(B) An individual with irreversible cessation of all functions of the entire brain, including the brainstem, is dead.

(1) Cessation is recognized when evaluation discloses findings of (a) and (b).

(a) Cerebral functions are absent.

(b) Brainstem functions are absent.

(2) Irreversibility is recognized when evaluation discloses findings of (a), (b), and (c).

(a) The cause of coma is established and sufficient to account for loss of brain functions.

(b) The possibility of recovery of any brain function is excluded.

(c) Cessation of all brain functions persists for an appropriate period of observation or trial of therapy or both.

Other Factors:

1. Complicating conditions, such as drug and metabolic intoxication and hypothermia (core temperature <32.2° C), should be excluded.
2. The presence of shock should alert the physician to be particularly cautious in applying neurologic criteria to determine death.
3. *Children:* The brains of infants and young children have increased resistance to damage and may recover substantial functions even after exhibiting unresponsiveness on neurologic examination for longer periods compared with adults. Physicians should be particularly cautious in applying neurologic criteria to determine brain death in children <5 years old.

Adapted from the President's Commission report for the study of ethical problems in medicine and biomedical and behavioral research. JAMA 1981;246:2184.

for brain death determination [Guidelines, 1987]. History of the etiology and reversibility of coma was emphasized, as was the loss of brainstem function and apnea (Box 67-2). Age-dependent observation periods of 12 to 48 hours were recommended. Ancillary EEG or radionuclide scanning was recommended in children younger than 1 year of age. Infants less than 7 days of age were excluded because of a lack of supportive literature. Later studies confirmed the validity of applying these specific guidelines in newborns greater than 34 weeks of conceptual life [Ashwal and Schneider, 1989].

Box 67-2 Guidelines for the Determination of Brain Death in Children

A. History: Determine cause of coma to eliminate remediable or reversible conditions

B. Physical examination criteria

1. Coma and apnea
2. Absence of brainstem function
   (a) Midposition or fully dilated pupils
   (b) Absence of spontaneous oculocephalic (doll's eye) and caloric-induced eye movements
   (c) Absence of movement of bulbar musculature, corneal, gag, cough, sucking, and rooting reflexes
   (d) Absence of respiratory effort with standardized testing for apnea
3. Patient must not be hypothermic or hypotensive
4. Flaccid tone and absence of spontaneous or induced movements excluding activity mediated at spinal cord level
5. Examination should remain consistent for brain death throughout the predetermined period of observation

C. Observation period according to age

1. *7 days to 2 months:* Two examinations and EEGs 48 hours apart
2. *2 months to 1 year:* Two examinations and EEGs 24 hours apart or one examination and an initial EEG showing electrocerebral silence combined with a radionuclide angiogram showing no cerebral blood flow, or both
3. *>1 year:* Two examinations 12 to 24 hours apart; EEG and isotope angiography are optional

EEG, electroencephalogram.

From Report of special task force. Guidelines for the determination of brain death in children. Ad Hoc Task Force consisting of representatives from the American Academy of Pediatrics, American Academy of Neurology, Child Neurology Society, American Neurological Association, American Bar Association, and the NINCDS. Pediatrics 1987;80:298.

LEGAL DEFINITION OF BRAIN DEATH

The American Medical Association and the American Bar Association supported universal enactment of the Uniform Determination of Death Act published in 1980 [Uniform, 1980]. The Act defined death stating that "an individual who has sustained either (1) irreversible cessation of circulatory and respiratory functions; or (2) irreversible cessation of all functions of the brain including the brainstem is dead." Subsequently, all states of the United States have enacted legislation accepting death by this definition. Brain death can be declared despite heart-lung respirator maintenance.

EPIDEMIOLOGY

Incidence of Brain Death

The overall incidence of brain death in children is unknown. In the United States, data are available concerning the number of brain dead children who become organ donors (see United Network Organ Sharing [UNOS] web site at http://www.unos.org/), and more recent studies have suggested that approximately 55% of children declared brain dead become organ donors [Sheehy et al., 2003]. Combining such data suggests there are approximately 1800 children per year in the United States declared brain dead, with most being between 11 and 17 years of age (Fig. 67-1). Accurate data for neonates and infants younger than 1 year of age are not available. There also was a decrease between 1993 and 2003 in the number of brain dead children who were organ donors (from 1137 to 886 [22%]), suggesting that the total number of children who are annually being declared brain dead has decreased (see UNOS web site). This decrease likely is due to the 26% decline in the total number of pediatric deaths since the 1990s (data from the National Center for Health Statistics web site at http://www.cdc.gov/nchs/).

Studies from pediatric intensive care units in the 1990s reported that the incidence of brain death in older infants and children ranges from 0.65% to 1.2% of admissions [Ashwal and Schneider, 1999]. In one study, the mortality rate in the pediatric intensive care unit was 8.7%, with 22% of these children declared brain dead [Ryan et al., 1993]. The mortality rate in the neonatal intensive care unit was 5.6%, with none of the infants declared brain dead. Another study reported the percentage of brain deaths to overall deaths to be 31.4% in children older than 1 month of age and 6.3% in neonates [Parker et al., 1995]. Similar findings from other countries have been reported [Goh et al., 1999; Gotay-Cruz and Fernandez-Sein, 2002; Lopez-Herce et al., 2000; Martinot et al., 1998]. Data from Loma Linda University Children's Hospital indicate that the percentage of brain deaths to overall deaths is 28% and 2.1% in the pediatric and neonatal intensive care units. In some pediatric intensive care units, the percentage of patients diagnosed as brain dead compared with all deaths is even higher (37% to 38%) [Martinot et al., 1995; Mejia and Pollack, 1995].

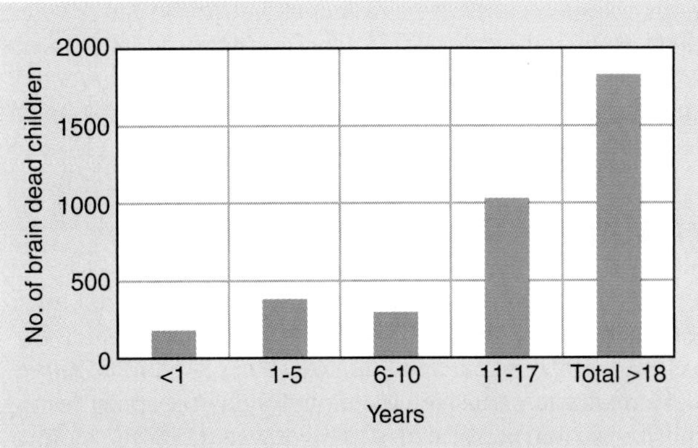

FIGURE 67-1. Number of children declared brain dead by age in the United States. Data based on the number of children who are brain dead who become organ donors and the assumption that approximately 55% of children who are brain dead become donors. (Data from the United Network Organ Sharing web site: http://www.unos.org/.)

Etiologies of Brain Death

Table 67-1 provides information on the age distribution of infants and children in whom brain death has been diagnosed and characterization by disease categories that were responsible for the cerebral insult. Brain death most commonly occurs in adolescents and is less common in infants younger than 1 year of age. Closed head injury was the most common clinical presentation leading to brain death (50%), followed by intracranial hemorrhage and stroke (12%). Asphyxial injury usually occurred as a complication of septic or hemorrhagic shock, with unexplained out-of-hospital cardiac arrest or from strangulation or suffocation. Sudden infant death syndrome was a rare cause of brain death. Brain death secondary to meningitis was seen in patients who developed massive cerebral edema with herniation within 2 to 24 hours of admission. Miscellaneous causes of brain death involve rare metabolic diseases, perioperative insults to the central nervous system, acute hydrocephalus, and a variety of other rare disorders that ultimately affect the brain.

Outcome after Diagnosis of Brain Death

Most children are removed from life support or are used for organ donation within a 2-day time period when the diagnosis of brain death is confirmed [Ashwal and Schneider, 1988]. Some children are continued on ventilator support until cardiac arrest occurs, and their "survival" has averaged about 17 days. In rare cases, children have been maintained on ventilator support for periods ranging from 6 months to 5 years [Shewmon, 1998]. There have been no reports of children recovering neurologic function who met adult brain

TABLE 67-1

Age Distribution and Etiologies of Brain Death in Children

AGE	PERCENT PATIENTS (n = 219)*	ETIOLOGY	PERCENT PATIENTS (n = 4794)†
Term	6	Traumatic brain injury	50
0–4 mo	12	Intracranial hemorrhage/stroke	12
4–12 mo	15	Gunshot wound	10
1–2 yr	17	Unknown/other	8
2–5 yr	32	Asphyxia	7
5–10 yr	8	Cardiovascular disease	6
10–18 yr	10	Drowning	4
		Seizure/status epilepticus	1
		Drug associated	1
		Sudden infant death syndrome	1

*Data from Ashwal S, Schneider S. Brain death in children: Part I and part II. Pediatr Neurol 1988;3:69.

†Data from UNOS web site: http://www.unos.org/.

death criteria on neurologic examination [Moshe and Alvarez, 1986; Rowland et al., 1983]. These criteria include an absence of spontaneous activity; specific cranial nerve dysfunction; and cardiac response to ocular compression, decerebrate or decorticate posturing, and apnea.

NEUROLOGIC EVALUATION

Reports indicate that a marked variability exists in the knowledge and use of the 1987 pediatric brain death guidelines [Ashwal, 1991; Mejia and Pollack, 1995]. A national survey of 16 pediatric intensive care units found that apnea testing either was not performed (25%) or was deemed "controversial" (22%) in children diagnosed as brain dead, and in many of these infants and children, appropriate confirmatory testing was not done [Mejia and Pollack, 1995]. Similar findings were noted in a survey of neurosurgeons and the criteria they employed in evaluating children with head injury for brain death [Chang et al., 2003]. Likewise, a survey of pediatric attending physicians and residents in the United States found a high percentage (39% to 58%) who could not define brain death correctly or recognize that brain death could be diagnosed without confirmatory testing in children older than 1 year of age [Harrison and Botkin, 1999].

Clinical Examination

Cerebral Unresponsivity

The neurologic evaluation for brain death is difficult in a comatose patient, particularly in infants and children. It is necessary to standardize the basal conditions under which the patient is examined. The patient should be normothermic, and pharmacologic agents capable of producing coma or neuromuscular blocking agents must be excluded [Kennedy and Kiloh, 1996; Tobin, 1996]. Assessment for cerebral unresponsivity, loss of cranial nerve function, and determination of apnea (tested with a hypercapneic stimulus) must be performed and documented. Confounding circumstances always increase the complexity of the evaluation. Cerebral unresponsivity or coma can be quantitated using the Glasgow Coma Scale score, which ranges from 3 (no response) to 15 (normal) using assigned scores for eye opening, motor activity, and vocalization (see Chapter 61) [Jennett and Bond, 1975]. The scale should be modified substituting socialization for verbalization for infants and children who are too young to have developed speech.

The predictive value of the duration of unresponsivity in infants and young children may be less trustworthy than in adults. In young children, recovery may occur when unresponsiveness has occurred for prolonged periods and even when serious structural nervous system dysfunction is present. If the neurologic evaluation is uncertain or inconsistent in children younger than 1 year of age, supportive laboratory documentation, including EEG and cerebral blood flow determinations, should be considered.

Brainstem Examination

Cessation of brainstem reflexes is generally accepted as the hallmark of brain failure. The NINCDS reported, however, that 141 of 459 comatose patients who died retained one or more brainstem reflexes [NINCDS, 1980]. No single preserved brainstem reflex could discriminate the preservation of any other brainstem reflex. The combination of pupillary light response and oculocephalic and vestibular reflexes had the greatest specificity, but this combination included 4% of patients who retained other brainstem reflexes. Box 67-3 outlines the procedures used to assess the caloric response.

Premature infants less than 32 weeks' conceptual age do not have completely developed cranial nerve function. Neurologists examining these infants should be aware of the development of the different cranial nerve reflexes during gestation (Table 67-2). Newborns often present obstacles to examination. Ear canals are frequently small and may be plugged, pupils are small, adhesive tape obscures the face and extremities, and neuromuscular blocking agents alter the examination.

Apnea

Documentation of apnea, under controlled conditions, is the most important determination in clinically evaluating brain

Box 67-3 Cold Water Caloric Tympanic Membrane Stimulation

Equipment
400 mL of tap water/ice cubes
25- or 50-mL disposable syringe
Large-bore intravenous catheter (shortened 2 to 3 inches from hub)

Preparation
Check ear canals for patency and integrity of drum
Patient's head flat

Test
Irrigate each drum with 80 mL of cold water over minimum of 3 minutes
Repeat with head at 45-degree angle

Positive Result in Coma
Head level: Eyes deviate to side of irrigation
Head at 45-degree angle: Eyes vertically depressed

TABLE 67-2

Reflex Development in Preterm Infants

DEVELOPMENTAL REFLEX	GESTATIONAL AGE (WEEKS) WHEN REFLEX IS ELICITABLE
Suck, root, gag	32–34
Auditory response	30–32
Pupillary response to light	30–32
Oculocephalic response	28–32
Corneal response	28–32
Moro response	28–32
Grasp response (palmar)	30–32
Alertness	30–32
Apnea response to $Paco_2$ stimulus	33

Data from Fanaroff et al., 1987; Swaiman, 1994.

death. Virtually all protocols recommend a period of unassisted ventilation, allowing hypercapnia maximally to stimulate the respiratory effort. The first formal observation period (3 minutes) was recommended by the Ad Hoc Harvard Medical School Faculty [Beecher, 1968]. The Conference of Royal Colleges and Faculties suggested administering a mixture of 5% carbon dioxide and 95% oxygen for 5 minutes while withholding respirator support and then supplying 100% tracheal oxygen [Conference, 1976]. The President's Commission recommended 100% oxygen ventilation for 10 minutes followed by passive 100% tracheal oxygen for a period long enough to achieve a Pco_2 of at least 60 mm Hg [President's Commission, 1981].

The normal physiologic apneic threshold (minimum Pco_2 at which respiration begins) depends on many factors and can be altered by anesthetic agents, narcotics, sedatives, and certain disease states. Schafer and Caronna described three patients, suspected to be brain dead, who developed spontaneous respiration at Pco_2 levels between 45 mm Hg and 50 mm Hg, which suggested a maximal end point of 60 mm Hg [Schafer and Caronna, 1978]. Ropper and coworkers studied seven brain dead patients and reported a Pco_2 of 44 mm Hg as a maximal excitatory end point [Ropper et al., 1981], but this has not been studied in children.

The maximal Pco_2 apneic threshold in children is probably similar to adults. Outwater and Rockoff studied 10 patients, age 10 months to 15 years, in whom they increased mean Pco_2 from 34.4 mm Hg to 59.5 mm Hg over 5 minutes while supplying 100% tracheal oxygen [Outwater and Rockoff, 1984]. The Po_2 exceeded 200 mm Hg during the test period. Rowland and colleagues performed 16 apnea tests on nine patients, age 4 months to 13 years, four of whom had detectable phenobarbital levels between 10 and 25 mg/dL [Rowland et al., 1984]. These patients received 100% oxygen for 10 minutes. Oxygen then was delivered at 6 liters/min through a catheter into the length of the endotracheal tube with the ventilator turned off during the 15-minute study period. These patients were moderately hyperventilated before the apnea test with a mean Pco_2 of 28 mm Hg. The Pco_2 increased 4.4 mm Hg, 3.4 mm Hg, and 2.6 mm Hg per minute at 5, 10, and 15 minutes. Arterial Pco_2 at the end of 15 minutes ranged from 40 to 116 mm Hg, and by 15 minutes, 14 of 16 patients had Pco_2 levels greater than 60 mm Hg. Two patients had Pco_2 levels of 100 mm Hg and 116 mm Hg with pH determinations of 6.92 and 6.98. Arterial Po_2 remained greater than 100 mm Hg, and in 12 of 16 patients it was greater than 200 mm Hg. Mild alterations of pulse or blood pressure or both also were observed in six patients but were reversible. Both studies concluded that apnea test periods of 5 to 10 minutes would result in Pco_2 levels exceeding 60 mm Hg without danger of hypoxemia.

Apnea challenges (Box 67-4), when initiated at Pco_2 levels of 40 to 50 mm Hg, have a predictive Pco_2 linear increase [Paret and Barzilay, 1995]. When the initial Pco_2 was 40 to 51 mm Hg in 11 patients, the minute Pco_2 increase was 5.1 to 6.7 mm Hg. During the pretest period, the Pco_2 was stabilized for 10 minutes. Most studies recommend that Pco_2 levels be determined at 5-minute intervals and continued out to 15 minutes if the Pco_2 has not reached 60 mm Hg and the Po_2 has not decreased to less than 50 mm Hg.

Apnea testing of patients who are hypothermic or receiving medications that suppress respiration is not valid for documenting brainstem failure. It still can be performed under such circumstances, however, because the presence of respiratory effort would eliminate brain death as a diagnosis.

Box 67-4 Apnea Challenge Test

Patient normothermic and normotensive

No central nervous system pharmacodepressants or neuromuscular blocking agents

Patient maintained at arterial Pco_2 30 to 40 mm Hg

Ventilate at constant rate with 100% oxygen for 20 minutes

Endotracheal catheter delivering 8 L of oxygen (adult) after disconnecting respirator

Pulse oximeter in place (or measure arterial Po_2)

Measure arterial Pco_2 every 3 minutes until Pco_2 >60 mm Hg or patient attempts periodic breathing

Several case reports involving only a few patients have raised related issues concerning apnea testing in young infants and children that also apply to newborns. Ammar and coworkers reported five children, age 9 months to 7 years, with severe brainstem dysfunction, including loss of pupillary reflexes and apnea, that was due to surgically resectable brainstem lesions with return of spontaneous respirations and substantial neurologic function [Ammar et al., 1993]. None of these children were considered brain dead before surgery, although they were severely compromised. These investigators correctly pointed out that treatment of compressive brainstem lesions might reverse severe neurologic deficits that mimic brain death. A second report concerns a 3-month-old infant who met the task force criteria for brain death, but who, on day 43 after admission, developed two to three breaths per minute [Okamoto and Sugimoto, 1995]. The infant died 71 days after presentation. At issue is whether this case should be considered a return of respiratory function. An editorial commentary on this case by Fishman stated, "The return of no clinical neurologic function other than two to three ineffectual respirations/minute due to the survival of only a small group of neurons in the medulla should not be considered an example of reversible deficits and failure of current brain death criteria" [Fishman, 1995]. A third case report described a 4-year-old male with a posterior fossa mass who became brain dead 4 days after admission [Vardis and Pollack, 1998]. His first apnea test had a Pco_2 of 91 mm Hg, at which time he developed spontaneous respirations. A repeat apnea test the following day found an initial Pco_2 of 67 mm Hg, but no respiratory effort was detected; he began to breathe spontaneously when challenged again, and the Pco_2 was 71 mm Hg. This last patient raises the question as to whether the carbon dioxide threshold may be age dependent or disease dependent. Because of the limited number of patients in these few case reports, additional research into these issues is required.

Apnea testing should be performed in children only after a full explanation to the parents is provided, and permission for the procedure is obtained. Rarely, parents refuse to allow an apnea challenge. On these rare occasions, carbon dioxide augmentation at 1 liter/min, preceded by 100% preoxygenation, increases the Pco_2 to 60 mm Hg within 2 minutes. At this time, a respirator can be interrupted for 3 to 5 minutes as a substitute test of apnea [Lang, 1995].

ANCILLARY NEURODIAGNOSTIC STUDIES

Virtually all guidelines have stressed that the historical events leading to coma, when combined with the clinical triad of coma, absence of brainstem reflexes, and a failed apnea challenge, are fundamental to brain death diagnosis. Many physicians are uncomfortable with a clinical diagnosis and have sought an absolute laboratory test to confirm brain death. A universally applicable, valid, and reliable study is a laudable, but probably unattainable goal [Shewmon, 1987]. All brain cells do not die simultaneously; highly selective tests lack the sensitivity to report absolutely that the brain has failed and such failure is permanent. The combination of clinical evaluation and pertinent diagnostic studies (EEG, cerebral blood flow studies) can yield a sound clinical decision, however.

Electroencephalogram

Despite limitations of the EEG, especially in regard to measurement of brainstem activity, many physicians tend to equate an isoelectric EEG (electrocerebral silence) with brain death. Despite the obvious dangers in depending only on the EEG, the isoelectric EEG, combined with the clinical triad of coma, absent brainstem reflexes, and apnea, remains the best documented tool for determining brain death. It is widely available, has bedside portability, is noninvasive, is relatively inexpensive, and can be interpreted by most neurologists. The American Electroencephalographic Society Guidelines has developed criteria for brain death recordings [American Electroencephalographic Society, 1986, 1994]. The recording should be isoelectric for a minimum of 30 minutes and show no electrical activity beyond 2 μV at a sensitivity of 2 μV/mm, with filter settings at 0.1 or 0.3 second at 70 Hz. Telephone transmission of EEGs is unacceptable for brain death determinations. Technical problems in performing EEGs have been reviewed previously [Bennett et al., 1976; Chatrian, 1986; Moshe, 1989; Schneider, 1989] and summarized here.

Electroencephalogram in Pediatric Brain Death

Pediatric patients present unique difficulties in interpretation of the EEG because of shorter interelectrode distances, greater electrocardiogram contamination, reduced cortical potentials in premature infants, and delayed metabolism of barbiturates. Reversible electrocerebral silence may occur with the use of central nervous system–depressant drugs, hypothermia, cardiovascular shock, or metabolic encephalopathies. In children, the most common medications causing the reversible loss of brain electrocortical activity include barbiturates, benzodiazepines, narcotics, and certain intravenous (thiopental, ketamine, midazolam) and inhalation (halothane and isoflurane) anesthetics. Phenobarbital is the most common drug responsible for reversible electrocerebral silence because it is widely used for seizure control. Previous studies have suggested that phenobarbital levels greater than 25 μg/mL might suppress EEG activity to the point of electrocerebral silence and that levels less than 20 to 25 μg/mL are unlikely to cause electrocerebral silence or affect apnea testing or the examination of brainstem reflexes [Ashwal and Schneider, 1989]. A study in 92 children reported data suggesting that therapeutic levels of phenobarbital (i.e., 15 to 40 μg/mL) do not affect the EEG [LaMancusa et al., 1991]. The authors also recommended that physicians and families do not have to wait the 3.7 days for subtherapeutic (<15 mg/mL) or the 6 days for therapeutic (15 to 40 μg/mL) barbiturate levels to be completely metabolized to consider withdrawal of life support. Others have reported that absent brainstem reflexes could not be correlated to thiopentone levels [Grattan Smith and Butt, 1993]. A study performed in adults found residual postmortem toxic brain levels of barbiturates despite absent premorbid serum levels [Saito et al., 1995].

A core temperature greater than 32.2° C (>90° F) has been regarded as a prerequisite for reliably determining brain death by EEG [Hicks and Poole, 1981]. In adults, electrocerebral silence does not occur until the temperature decreases to less than 20° C (68° F). In children, suppression of EEG activity does not appear until 24° C (75.2° F), and complete loss of EEG activity does not occur until the temperature is less than 18° C (<64.4° F) [Jorgensen and Malchow-Moller, 1978]. The average temperature when EEGs are obtained for confirmation of brain death is 97.3° F ± 1.4° F. This finding suggests that hypothermia is not likely to be a significant problem for pediatric EEG interpretation.

Reversible electrocerebral silence may occur soon after a child has had a cardiac arrest [Schmitt et al., 1993]. Several infants in whom the initial EEG was observed 8 to 10 hours after a cardiac arrest had electrocerebral silence, but a repeat study 12 to 24 hours later demonstrated diffuse low-voltage activity. Several of these infants survived in a vegetative or minimally conscious state; most died as a result of other complications of the acute catastrophic insult. Similar observations have been reported in adults [DeOliveira et al., 1984].

Although not well documented, electrolyte, acid-base, and blood-gas abnormalities; severe hepatic and renal dysfunction; and certain inborn errors of metabolism all have been considered capable of decreasing brain electrocortical activity to the point of causing complete cortical inactivity. In selected children in whom the etiology of brain death is uncertain, evaluation for metabolic diseases, including urea cycle enzyme defects; disorders of lactate, amino acid, and organic acid metabolism; and mitochondrial diseases, should be considered.

Extensive literature exists documenting persistent EEG activity in brain dead infants, children, and adults [Ashwal and Schneider, 1979; Grigg et al., 1987]. Of patients meeting brain death criteria in the NINCDS report, 8% to 40% maintained EEG activity for brief periods. Conversely, 20 premature infants recovered from electrocerebral silence; however, 15 of these patients had clinical evidence of brain function during electrocerebral silence [Sher et al., 1996].

Since Green and Lauber's report in 1972 of two infants who had return of some EEG activity after an initial electrocerebral silence recording [Green and Lauber, 1972], there have only been a few additional infants reported in whom EEG activity returned [Ashwal, 1997; Ashwal et al., 1977; DeOliveria et al., 1984; Juguilon and Reilly, 1982; Kohrman and Spivack, 1990; Pezzani et al., 1986; Toffol et al., 1987]. A previous report, based on most of these cases, estimated that the return of EEG activity when the initial study was isoelectric was approximately 0.02% [Ashwal, 1997]. There are presumably additional unreported cases in which EEG activity returned, but these additional cases are unlikely to

TABLE 67-3

Principal Methods to Assess Cerebral Blood Flow in Brain Dead Patients

METHOD	MEASUREMENT	ABSENT CIRCULATION INDICATED BY
Cerebral angiography	High pressure and rapid, intra-arterial injection of contrast agent	Absence of intracranial filling of large cerebral arteries and their major branches
Radionuclide imaging	Intravenous rapid bolus injection of radionuclide isotope	Absence of radionuclide detection in distribution of large vessels and in brain parenchyma
HMPAO SPECT	Similar to radionuclide imaging but with different detection system and isotope	Absence of activity on dynamic scintigraphy or by delayed isotope uptake
Transcranial Doppler	Measures blood velocity from large intracranial vessels during diastole and systole	Serial changes with loss of diastolic flow, flow reversal, and loss of systolic flow
Digital subtraction angiography	Imaging that provides visualization of cerebral vessels	Absence of contrast material within large cerebral vessels
Xenon CT	Provides quantitative measure of cerebral blood flow by inhalation of xenon gas detected with cranial CT	Cerebral blood flow values <5-10 mL/min/100 g indicate absence of cerebral circulation

CT, computed tomography; HMPAO, hexamethylpropyleneamine oxime; SPECT, single-photon emission computed tomography.

affect substantially this extremely low ratio. Concerns about the return of EEG activity have been overemphasized. In addition, if one considers issues related to subsequent clinical recovery of the patients in whom EEG activity returned, none of the patients made significant clinical recoveries.

The lack of absolute correlation between EEG findings and other supportive ancillary brain death tests limits reliance on the EEG as a single confirmatory test [Paolin et al., 1995]. Despite these well-documented drawbacks, the EEG remains extremely valuable when combined with the neurologic examination and other confirmatory studies [Schneider, 1989]. The EEG continues as the most widely used ancillary study in brain death determinations.

Measurements of Cerebral Perfusion

Several technologies are available for estimating or measuring cerebral blood flow (Table 67-3), cerebral perfusion, or cerebral blood velocity. Their use in children has followed after application and testing in adults. New and older technologies have been applied in the search for an ideal test. Each advance in technology needs to be carefully scrutinized in terms of availability, cost, 24-hour accessibility, portability, patient risk, invasiveness, and simultaneous outcomes comparison with established techniques. The neurologist who is requested to perform brain death determinations should be aware of individual institutional resources. Concerns exist about the validity and reliability of several of these methods in preterm and newborn infants, in whom cerebral blood flow values are quite low, and whether these methods possess the sensitivity to detect very low flow values [Altman et al., 1988; Greissen, 1986].

Cerebral Angiography

Direct visualization of the cerebral circulation with angiography that shows the complete cessation of cerebral blood flow has long been accepted as the standard for comparing all other neuroimaging modalities for brain death confirmation. Near-simultaneous comparisons of multiple techniques confirm the sensitivity of this long-held but seldom challenged concept [Bradac and Simon, 1974; Conrad and Sinha, 2003; Paolin et al., 1995]. The technique should be considered only for unresolvable clinical situations, however, because of its limitations, which include patient transfer, invasiveness, limited radiologic personnel, and prolonged study time. Few cases have been reported in which this invasive method has been performed in brain dead children to validate the absence of cerebral circulation [Ashwal and Schneider, 1979].

Radionuclide Imaging

Several radionuclide techniques have been used in brain dead patients since the 1970s to determine noninvasively whether there has been cessation of cerebral circulation [Conrad and Sinha, 2003]. With most methods, circulation was assessed during an early "dynamic" phase and later by examining static images for cerebral uptake of the specific radionuclide (usually technetium-99m pertechnetate, technetium-99m glucoheptonate, or technetium-99m DTPA) (Fig. 67-2). During the dynamic phase, a bolus of the radionuclide was injected rapidly, and isotopic cranial images were obtained similar to that of a carotid arteriogram. Usually in the arterial phase, cerebral activity was detectable within several seconds, and from the time of peak cerebral activity, sagittal sinus activity was observed within 6 to 8 seconds [Thompson et al., 1987]. Various terms have been used to describe the early phase of this study, including *radioisotopic bolus angiography* and *dynamic brain scintigraphy*. If activity was not detectable in this early phase, cerebral blood flow was considered absent resulting from either low cardiac output or very high intracranial pressure (as is seen with brain death). Because most tracers have a half-life of several hours, the static phase of a radionuclide imaging study usually was done later, looking for the absence or presence of diffuse parenchymal isotopic uptake. Currently, most centers are using single-photon emission computed tomography scanning and technetium-99m hexamethylpropylene amine oxime (HMPAO) as the isotopic agent [Abdel Dayem et al., 1989; Bonetti et al., 1995; Galaske et al., 1988; Mrhac et al., 1995; Spieth et al., 1995; Valle et al., 1993; Wieler et al., 1993; Wilson et al., 1993]. This agent is more lipophilic, is not dependent on the quality of the bolus injection, and enables more precise static imaging of parenchymatous brain perfusion in contrast to conventional dynamic imaging because of retention in the intact brain parenchyma. With this technology, the isotope can be injected in the intensive care

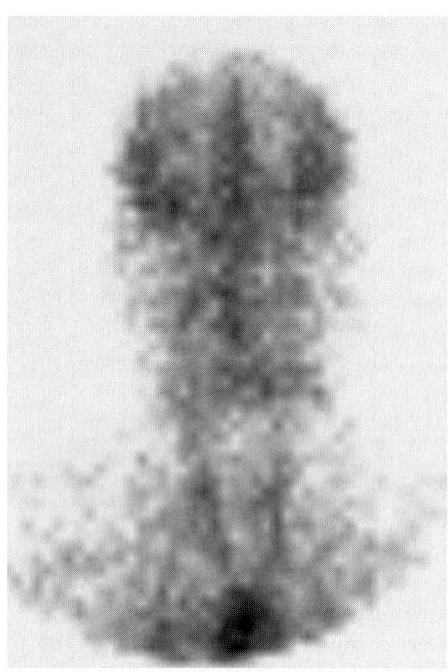
A

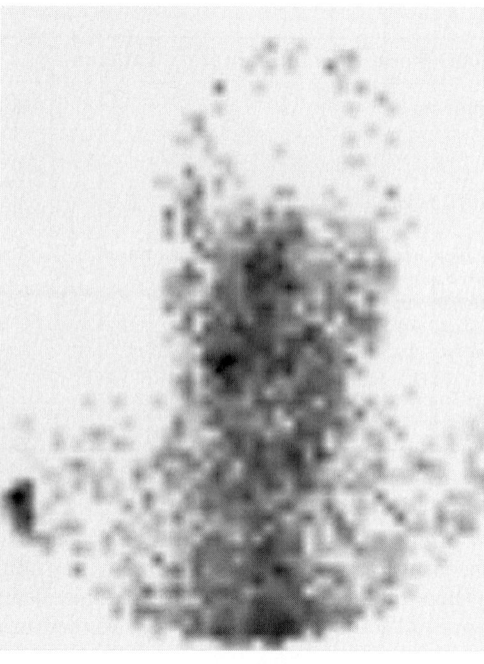
B

FIGURE 67-2. Technetium cerebral blood flow study. This 13-year-old female was suspected of being brain dead after a cardiac arrest associated with exacerbation of an asthma attack. Her first study **(A)**, using 1-second images selected from the dynamic cerebral blood flow studies done with 20 mCi of technetium-99m pertechnetate, showed normal intracranial circulation. A repeat study **(B)** the following day showed a "light bulb sign"—no intracranial circulation. Also noted is the "hot nose sign" resulting from vasodilation around the cribriform plate in an attempt to develop collateral circulation. (Courtesy of Dr. Eloy Schulz, Department of Radiology, Loma Linda University Medical Center.)

unit, and better planar images can be obtained at a later time using a mobile camera or whenever the patient can be moved to the nuclear medicine department.

Multiple studies in adults and children have documented radionuclide imaging to be accurate and reproducible, and it has been compared favorably with other methods of detecting the presence or absence of cerebral blood flow [Conrad and Sinha, 2003; Drake et al., 1986; Goodman et al., 1985; Holtzman et al., 1983; Kaukinen et al., 1995; Parker et al., 1995; Ruiz-Garcia et al., 2000; Schneider, 1989; Schwartz et al., 1984; Wieler et al., 1993]. This technique is particularly useful when hypothermia or elevated barbiturate levels prevent valid EEG interpretation [Holtzman et al., 1983]. Premature and full-term newborns, despite having extremely reduced cerebral blood flow compared with older children, can be readily evaluated using radionuclide measurements [Ashwal et al., 1989; Greissen, 1986]. Hospital nuclear medicine departments should be aware of improved advances in radiopharmaceuticals [Spieth et al., 1995; Wilson et al., 1993] and the ability to detect flow in the posterior fossa circulation [Spieth et al., 1995] and that ventricular drainage procedures may give a false-negative indication that cerebral blood flow is absent [Hansen et al., 1993].

Transcranial Doppler

Transcranial Doppler ultrasonography has advocates because of its obvious portability and noninvasiveness and isolette accessibility [Ahmann et al., 1987; Feri et al., 1994; Manno, 1997; McMenamin and Volpe, 1983]. More recent studies document a high rate of false-negative test results and lower levels of specificity and sensitivity, which suggest significant limitations for use of this technique for brain death confirmation [Chiu et al., 2003; de Freitas et al., 2003; Dosemeci et al., 2004; Rodriguez et al., 2002].

With the pulsed transcranial Doppler technique, characteristic blood velocity waveforms are detected during systole and diastole, usually from the anterior cerebral and common carotid arteries [Petty et al., 1990]. McMenamin and Volpe reported six brain dead infants, 28 to 40 weeks' gestation, who had the characteristic progression of velocity changes as cerebral edema and intracranial pressure increased [McMenamin and Volpe, 1983]. Changes included the loss of diastolic flow, the appearance of retrograde diastolic flow, the diminution of systolic flow in the anterior cerebral artery with unchanged flow in the common carotid artery, and the loss of any detectable flow in these vessels. Intracranial pressure in four of six infants was elevated, and EEGs in three infants revealed electrocerebral silence. Although cerebral and isotopic angiography was not performed to verify the Doppler results, postmortem examination revealed severe brain injury consistent with but not necessarily typical of injuries reported with brain death. In other studies with pulsed Doppler ultrasound, 19 of 23 brain dead children older than 4 months had a characteristic velocity pattern with a single sharp systolic peak followed by a rapid negative deflection below baseline, sharply rebounding to forward flow in early to mid diastole with gradual tapering at the end of diastole to the zero baseline or below [Ahmann et al., 1987]. Eight of the 19 patients with this waveform also exhibited absent cerebral blood flow by radionuclide angiography. Infants younger than 4 months who were studied had atypical waveforms, suggesting that use of the pulsed Doppler technique in the newborn period may not be as reliable. Another study in 17 comatose children found Doppler velocity changes similar to those reported by McMenamin and Volpe in 11 children who progressed to brain death [Messer et al., 1990].

Other investigations have indicated the limitations of this technique. In one study, only five of seven (71%) patients with the diagnosis of brain death had bilateral reversal of flow (characteristic of increased cerebrovascular resistance and absent cerebral circulation), yielding a specificity of 100% and sensitivity of only 71.4% [Jalili et al., 1994]. An earlier report by Bode and colleagues examined nine brain dead children, and in eight, typical findings were reported [Bode et al., 1989]. One newborn exhibited normal systolic and end-diastolic flow velocities in the basal cerebral arteries for 2 days despite clinical and EEG signs of brain death. Other authors also have encountered individual cases that did not follow a similar progression as that originally described [Glasier et al., 1989]. In one case study of an infant with sudden infant death syndrome declared brain dead, transcranial Doppler sonography indicated nearly normal cerebral perfusion, which increased day by day notwithstanding the persistence of other signs of brain death [Sanker et al., 1992]. In most of the more recently reported series, several patients who had Doppler findings typically seen with brain death recovered, and patients who were brain dead frequently did not have the previously described progression of Doppler abnormalities [Chiu et al., 2003; de Freitas et al., 2003; Dosemeci et al., 2004; Rodriguez et al., 2002]. Doppler studies have been used on at least one occasion to confirm the diagnosis of fetal brain death in a 23-week gestational age infant [Otsubo et al., 1999].

Digital Subtraction Angiography

Digital subtraction angiography is another technique that has been used to assess the intracranial circulation. This technique can be performed intravenously [Van Bunnen et al., 1989] or by intra-arterial injection [Albertini et al., 1993]. A small amount of nonionic contrast material is injected while digital subtraction imaging of the cerebral vasculature is done similar to conventional cerebral angiography. This procedure allows visualization of contrast within the major intracranial vessels; lack of such visualization indicates absence of cerebral blood flow. There are few reports of this technique in children and only one case report in a neonate diagnosed with brain death [Albertini et al., 1993]. A report using intravenous digital subtraction angiography in 110 patients with clinical signs of brain death observed that the first study documented absent contrast enhancement in 105 patients [Van Bunnen et al., 1989]. Repeat studies in the remaining five patients within several hours also confirmed the cessation of cerebral blood flow.

Xenon Computed Tomography

Stable xenon computed tomography (CT) and 133-xenon CT are examples of useful, reliable, and well-documented tests that are seldom available because of cost and limited personnel [Pistoia et al., 1991]. Xenon CT allows quantitative and regional measurement of cerebral blood flow. In brain dead adults, cerebral blood flow values of 1.6 ± 2 mL/min/100 grams have been reported [Darby et al., 1987]. Previous studies found an average cerebral blood flow of 1.3 ± 1.6 mL/min/100 grams in 10 brain dead children compared with 33.5 ± 16.3 mL/min/100 grams in 11 profoundly comatose children [Ashwal et al., 1989]. This finding compares favorably with average cerebral blood flow values of 12 mL/min/100 grams using 133-xenon CT [Greissen, 1986] and 7 to 11 mL/min/100 grams using positron emission tomography in preterm infants who were not brain dead [Altman et al., 1988].

Positron Emission Tomography

The results of positron emission tomography (see Chapter 11) have been reported in only a few brain dead patients [Medlock et al., 1993; Meyer, 1996; Vander Borght et al., 2001]. Because of limited availability, cost, and lack of comparison studies, positron emission tomography offers no advantages over the more standardized methods previously discussed. Meyer reported an 18-year-old brain dead adolescent whose dynamic positron emission tomography study, performed 7 days after a severe post-traumatic closed-head injury, found no intracerebral uptake or retention of tracer and was considered consistent with the diffuse absence of brain metabolism [Meyer, 1996]. Medlock and associates reported a 2-month-old brain dead infant with preserved cerebral blood flow whose positron emission tomography scan on the 11th day after injury revealed a normal glucose metabolic gradient between gray and white matter [Medlock et al., 1993]. Postmortem examination revealed widespread necrosis with mononuclear cell infiltrates throughout all cerebral cortical layers. The persistence of glucose metabolism was thought to be associated with the presence of inflammatory microglial cells and suggested that the persistence of cerebral blood flow and glucose metabolism in brain dead children might not indicate neuronal survival.

Magnetic Resonance Imaging

Magnetic resonance imaging (MRI) also has been reported in small series of brain dead patients [Karantanas et al., 2002]. Characteristic features seen in most brain dead (but not comatose) patients include the following: (1) transtentorial and foramen magnum herniation, (2) absent intracranial vascular flow void, (3) poor gray-white matter differentiation, (4) no intracranial contrast enhancement, (5) carotid artery enhancement (intravascular enhancement sign), and (6) prominent nasal and scalp enhancement (MRI hot-nose sign) [Orrison et al., 1994]. Similar findings have been described by other investigators, although the loss of gray-white matter differentiation is not a consistent finding [Lee et al., 1995; Matsumura et al., 1996]. In another study, magnetic resonance angiography also was performed, and nonvisualization above the level of the supraclinoid portion of the internal carotid arteries was found [Ishii et al., 1996]. Abnormalities of diffusion-weighted imaging also have been observed in adult patients who are brain dead [Lovblad et al, 2000]. Presumably, similar neuroimaging findings would be present in children, but this has not yet been reported.

Magnetic Resonance Spectroscopy

In the 1980s and 1990s, phosphorus (^{31}P) and proton (^{1}H) magnetic resonance spectroscopy (MRS) have been used to measure noninvasively aspects of brain metabolic activity (see Chapter 11). Studies in neonates, older infants, and children have reported significant abnormalities using these techniques with loss of metabolic activity associated with severe acute central nervous system insults and with poor long-term outcomes [Holshouser et al., 1997; Martin et al., 1996]. ^{31}P-MRS has been reported in 3 infants, 4 children, and 17 adults who met adult criteria for brain death. Spectra in these patients indicated the absence of adenosine triphosphate (ATP) and phosphocreatine. The inorganic phosphate and phosphodiester peaks were still detectable [Kato et al., 1991]. Another ^{31}P-MRS study involving three brain dead adults found similar spectral abnormalities [Aichner, 1992]. These findings suggest that MRS could provide another technique to assess objectively the complete loss of cerebral function. The advantage of MRS is that it can be done in conjunction with MRI, which allows acquisition of anatomic and metabolic data that could clarify the etiology of the central nervous system insult and determine whether there is irreversible neuronal loss. Terk and colleagues reported a term brain dead infant whose ^{31}P spectra on days 11 and 18 demonstrated three distinct ATP peaks and several other peaks, however, which suggested the persistence of metabolic activity [Terk et al., 1992]. Although no definite reasons could be ascertained for this finding compared with the study of Kato and associates, they suggested that any proposed spectral signature for brain death would need to be modified.

There are no published case reports concerning proton MRS and brain death in children. At Loma Linda University Children's Hospital, 10 brain dead children were studied with proton MRS. All spectra were markedly abnormal with severe reductions or loss of the metabolite peaks (*N*-acetyl-aspartate, choline, creatinine) and a clearly identifiable and elevated lactate peak. These findings were similar to other patients, however, who ultimately were vegetative or severely disabled, suggesting that the specificity for brain death of MRS is insufficient.

Evoked Potentials

Brainstem auditory potentials have been studied extensively as a brain death determinant [Guerit, 1992; Litscher et al., 1995; Lutschg et al., 1983; Machado et al., 1991; Ruiz-Garcia et al., 2000; Ruiz-Lopez et al., 1999; Steinhart and Weiss, 1985]. The portability, rapidity, and noninvasiveness seem ideal, but multiple studies have raised significant doubts as to the reliability of brainstem auditory responses in brain death determinations [Dear and Godfrey, 1985; De Merlier and Taylor, 1986; Flannery, 1999; Schmitt et al., 1993; Steinhart and Weiss, 1985; Taylor et al., 1983]. Somatosensory-evoked potentials also have been used for the confirmation of brain death [Beca et al., 1995; Ruiz-Garcia et al., 2000; Ruiz-Lopez et al., 1999; Wagner, 1996; Ying et al., 1992], but there are insufficient data to assess whether it is superior to brainstem-evoked responses for brain death determination.

BRAIN DEATH IN NEWBORNS

Because there are no consensus-approved criteria, the ability to diagnose brain death in newborns is unresolved [Ashwal, 1997]. Not only have individual physicians expressed misgivings about being able to diagnose brain death in this age group, but also many institutions have had difficulty developing policies for the diagnosis of brain death. This problem is primarily due to the small number of brain dead neonates (i.e., <100) reported in the literature.

As previously noted, preterm infants and term infants less than 7 days of age were excluded from the 1987 pediatric brain death guidelines. Several years after the publication of these guidelines, data on 18 brain dead neonates were published, and it was suggested that brain death could be diagnosed in full-term newborn infants and preterm infants greater than 34 weeks gestational age within the first week of life [Ashwal and Schneider, 1989]. Because a newborn has patent sutures and an open fontanel, increases in intracranial pressure after acute injury are not as significant as in older patients. The usual cascade of events in older patients after acute brain injury that results in increasing intracranial pressure and reduced cerebral perfusion is less likely to occur in a newborn. Consequently, absent cerebral blood flow is less likely, as is the development of electrocerebral silence. The use of whole-brain death criteria might not be appropriate in a newborn. It might be more medically justifiable to use brainstem death as the major criterion for brain death in newborns. In many situations, the issue of whether a neonate is brain dead or just catastrophically and irreversibly brain injured is resolved by the decision of physicians caring for the neonate with the understanding and agreement of the family to withdraw ventilatory support.

Epidemiology

It has been estimated that there are about 550 newborns diagnosed each year as brain dead out of a total of 3,900,089 live births [Ashwal, 1997]. Etiologies of brain death based on data from 88 newborns less than 1 month of age included hypoxic-ischemic encephalopathy (61%), birth trauma (8%), central nervous system malformations (6%), central nervous system hemorrhage (6%), infection (7%), sudden infant death syndrome (7%), nonaccidental trauma (4%), and metabolic disorders (1%).

Duration of Observation

This section reviews the time period in newborns required to confirm the diagnosis of brain death. Additional aspects of the neurologic examination are discussed later. Discussions of specific issues regarding certainty of diagnosis, immaturity of the nervous system, and the effects of development on the pathophysiology and diagnosis of brain death in preterm and term infants have been published previously [Coulter, 1987; Freeman and Ferry, 1988; Kohrman, 1993; Volpe, 1987] and updated [Ashwal, 1997]. For the most part, the task force recommendations concerning the duration of observation of brain death in children of different ages were based on expert opinion and consensus rather than being evidence based. Data from 87 newborns allowed an estimation of the duration of coma after the insult until brain death was initially diagnosed (37 hours), duration of time before brain death confirmation (75 hours), and duration of time to transplantation (20 hours) [Ashwal, 1997]. The average duration of brain death in these patients was about 95 hours (i.e., 4 days). Recovery of brainstem function was not observed in any of the patients despite a variety of EEG and cerebral blood flow results. Further analysis examining the duration of brain death was done on the 53 neonates whose organs were donated for transplantation. The total duration of brain death (including time to transplantation) averaged 2.8 days in neonates less than 7 days of age. In neonates 1 to 3 weeks old, the duration was approximately 5.2 days. The data suggest that a 24- to 48-hour observation period in neonates less than 7 days of age should be sufficient to confirm the diagnosis of brain death.

Neurodiagnostic Testing

EEG and radionuclide imaging techniques, as in older infants, children, and adults, remain the most commonly used ancillary studies to confirm the diagnosis of brain death. The 1987 task force guidelines on pediatric brain death did recommend two examinations and EEGs 48 hours apart in neonates 7 days to 2 months old, but made no statement concerning the use of cerebral perfusion techniques because of limited data. Likewise, no recommendations were made for infants less than 7 days old or preterm infants. These recommendations frequently have been misinterpreted to mean that such testing should not be done or is unreliable or that brain death cannot be declared in infants less than 7 days of age. None of these conclusions were intended by the criteria set forth by the task force [Report of special task force, 1987].

Because of the significant physiologic and cerebrovascular differences in the neonatal response to injuries resulting in brain death, previous studies have observed a much higher incidence of newborns with EEG activity or cerebral perfusion [Ashwal, 1989]. In addition, some newborns with electrocerebral silence demonstrated preserved cerebral blood flow, and conversely, others without cerebral blood flow showed EEG activity. In neonates, even though cerebral blood flow and mean arterial blood pressures are much lower, increases in intracranial pressure after acute injury are less dramatic. In a neonate in whom the cerebral metabolic rate is lower, cerebral perfusion is likely to persist to the extent that even when the neonate is brain dead, cerebral blood flow can be detected, and some neuronal viability persists because of this low flow state. Data on 30 newborns who had EEGs and radionuclide perfusion studies found that one third (4 of 12) with electrocerebral silence showed evidence of cerebral blood flow, and 58% (11 of 19) of newborns with absent cerebral blood flow had evidence of EEG activity [Ashwal, 1997]. These data suggest that in this age group, clinical rather than laboratory data may be more appropriate, provided that a sufficient period of observation is allowed.

Data on 37 of 53 brain dead newborns in whom EEGs were performed revealed the following: electrocerebral silence ($n = 21$), very low voltage ($n = 13$), burst suppression ($n = 1$), seizure activity ($n = 1$), and normal ($n = 1$) [Ashwal, 1997]. Almost all patients whose first EEG demonstrated electrocerebral silence had electrocerebral silence on the second study, and most of the patients who initially did not have electrocerebral silence on their first EEG did so on a repeat study. The data suggested that for confirmation of brain death only, one EEG demonstrating electrocerebral silence is necessary, provided that the examination remains unchanged. Also, if the first EEG indicates activity, a second EEG is likely to be isoelectric and confirm brain death. In the remaining newborns in whom a second EEG reveals activity, continued observation for a total period of at least 2 days is warranted. If the clinical examination is unchanged, brain death can be confirmed.

Data from radionuclide imaging studies also suggest that not all newborns who are clinically brain dead have an absence of cerebral blood flow for the reasons discussed previously [Ashwal, 1997]. Only 13 of 18 patients showed absence of cerebral blood flow. No significant differences were observed, however, in the median duration of brain death for the neonates without cerebral blood flow compared with the neonates with cerebral blood flow. These findings emphasize the limitations of cerebral blood flow determinations for brain death confirmation in neonates.

Brain death in a newborn can be diagnosed as long as the physician is aware of the limitations of the clinical examination and laboratory testing. It is important to examine these infants carefully and repeatedly with particular attention to the examination of brainstem reflexes and apnea testing. Brain death can be diagnosed in a term infant, even when less than 7 days of age. An observation period of 48 hours is recommended to confirm the diagnosis. If an EEG is isoelectric, or if a cerebral blood flow study reveals no flow, the observation period can be shortened to 24 hours. Although there are few cases of preterm infants who are brain dead, it is likely that the same time frame would be applicable. Based on available data, the risk of misdiagnosis seems exceedingly low. There have been a few instances of neonates or older infants who exhibited minimal transient clinical or EEG recovery, but none seem to have regained meaningful neurologic function; all died within a brief time [Goh and Mok, 2004].

Determination of Brain Death in the Comatose Pediatric Patient

An algorithmic approach to the evaluation of a comatose child to determine whether the child is brain dead is presented in Figure 67-3. The question of whether a comatose child is brain dead arises within the first days of hospitalization. Occasionally, this issue occurs later because the long-term use of sedative and paralytic agents do not permit the necessary screening to assess for the presence of coma and loss of brainstem function, especially the loss of pupillary reflexes that triggers the question as to whether a child is brain dead. Neurologic or neurosurgical consultation usually is requested at this time by the intensive care unit staff for brain death determination. This assessment must include determination of the proximate cause of coma with review of all neuroimaging, neurophysiologic, metabolic, and toxicology screening studies that were performed to determine the etiology of the global cerebral insult and to determine whether the insult is or is not irreversible. Serum and urine studies should include toxicology screens and serum electrolytes, glucose, calcium, urea nitrogen, creatinine, liver enzymes, lactate, pyruvate, and ammonia determinations (see also Chapter 87) [Kennedy and Kiloh, 1996; Tobin, 1996]. If the history suggests a metabolic disorder, serum amino acid and urine organic acid studies should be considered. Neuromuscular blocking agents and all sedative agents also should be discontinued.

As part of the examination, it is necessary to ensure that the core body temperature (i.e., 36.1° C [97° F] to 37.2° C [99° F]) and blood pressure are within the normal range. The presence of purposeful movements in response to external stimuli or spontaneous (not spinal related) movements, postur-

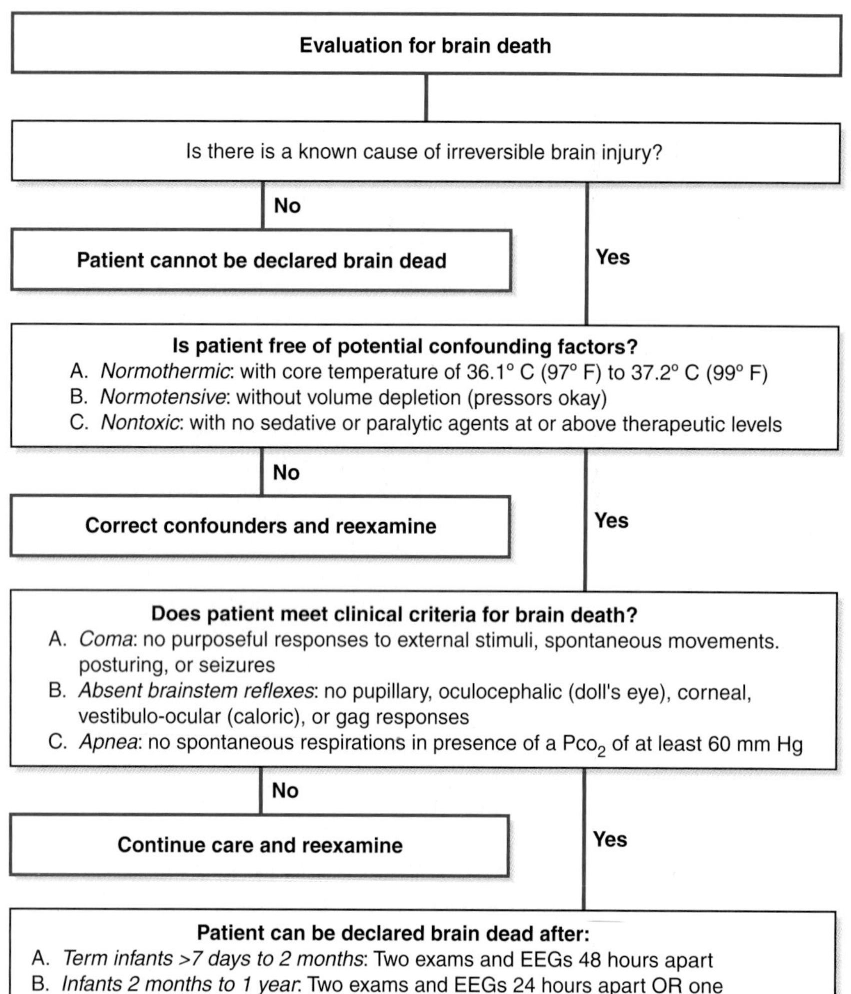

FIGURE 67-3. Algorithm for the evaluation for brain death in a comatose child. It is assumed that patients have had an extensive clinical and laboratory evaluation to determine the etiology of coma, including toxicology testing and, if indicated, evaluation for structural, infectious, and metabolic diseases. This algorithm suggests the process for confirmation of brain death in patients in whom this condition is suspected. CBF, cerebral blood flow; EEG, electroencephalogram. (Algorithm prepared by Dr. David Michelson and Dr. Stephen Ashwal, Loma Linda University School of Medicine.)

ing, or occurrence of seizures would obviate the diagnosis of brain death. A careful examination and documentation of the absence of brainstem reflexes is crucial and may be difficult to perform, particularly in an intubated neonate or young infant. Generally, parents should be allowed to observe the process, and nursing and respiratory therapy staff should be informed of the findings. As previously discussed (see Box 67-2), the duration of observation to confirm the diagnosis of brain death depends on the child's age, as do recommendations for confirmatory testing (see Fig. 67-3). Children younger than age 2 months require 48 hours of observation, infants 2 months to 1 year require 24 hours, and children older than 1 year require 12 to 24 hours to confirm the diagnosis of brain death. There are no consensus criteria for term or preterm neonates, but recommendations based on available data suggest that 48 hours of observation (with EEGs) in term infants less than 7 days old and 72 hours of observation (with EEGs) in preterm infants are reasonable guidelines [Ashwal and Schneider, 1989].

Confirmatory studies, depending on the child's age, are recommended as outlined in Box 67-2 and Figure 67-3. These tests are readily available in all hospitals and are helpful in establishing the diagnosis of brain death. Results of these tests provide physicians with an opportunity to discuss with the child's family the concept of brain death and the loss of electrocortical activity and cerebral blood flow. The tests also allow the physician to explain how the cause of injury ultimately caused brain death to develop.

Discussions with Family Members and Staff

Most pediatric brain death determinations are done on patients who were normal children just hours or days before the injury, and even after extensive discussions with family members the concept of brain death remains unclear for many [Siminoff et al., 2003]. Grieving parents may not understand the futility of continued respirator support and may not accept that continuing care cannot benefit the child. Without being confrontational, physicians caring for the child should discuss the prognosis with parents. Frequently a conference with family members and members from the health-care team (e.g., physicians, nurses, therapists, social workers, clergy) is helpful in educating the family and assuring them that the health-care professionals are in agreement with the diagnosis and recommendations. Caregivers, particularly nursing and respiratory technicians, can be overlooked regarding their own need for emotional support and the grief they share with parents [House and Benitez, 1992; Stoyles, 1995].

Organ Donation

The National Organ Transplant Act of 1987 requires that every hospital in the United States develop a protocol for requesting organ donation. After declaration of brain death, parents of a potential donor should be approached regarding donation [Williams et al., 2003]. Refusal from parents with whom donation has been explored should be respected. If the child is not a potential donor (sepsis, severe ischemia), it is important to discuss the reason why donation is not suitable so that parents do not believe donation was neglected.

Strategies for retrieval of organs should be in place in the pediatric intensive care unit [Dutie et al., 1993; Tsai et al., 2000]. In many centers, the intensivist caring for the patient is the individual who may first declare the patient brain dead and initiate the discussion regarding organ donation, so it is important and prudent to have independent confirmation of brain death by a second physician. Brain dead child abuse victims represent a significant percentage of brain death diagnoses and as such require medicolegal evaluation before organ donation can proceed [Zenel and Goldstein, 2002].

Maintenance of brain dead patients requires careful management in anticipation of organ donation [Lutz-Dettinger et al., 2001]. Maintenance of temperature [Goldstein et al., 1993] and providing adequate fluids and supplemental oxygen to achieve satisfactory perfusion are necessary, as is consideration for hormone replacement [Rosendale et al., 2003] with corticosteroids [Arita et al., 1993], vasopressin [Pennefather et al., 1995], and thyroxine [Roels et al., 2000]. Diabetes insipidus, hypernatremia, hyperglycemia, and coagulopathies commonly occur in brain dead children and require special management if transplantation is being considered [Lutz-Dettinger et al., 2001]. By developing a careful balance between the care of a child who is brain dead and the desire to retrieve organs for donation, physicians can help grieving families and improve the opportunity to increase the number of organs that are being donated to save the lives of children with many different forms of severe, disabling, and life-threatening diseases.

ACKNOWLEDGMENT

This chapter is based on Chapter 62 in the third edition of this book, which was coauthored with Dr. Sanford Schneider.

REFERENCES

Abdel Dayem HM, Bahar RH, Sigurdsson GH, et al. The hollow skull: A sign of brain death in Tc-99m HM-PAO brain scintigraphy. Clin Nucl Med 1989;14:912.

Ahmann PA, Carrigan TA, Carlton D, et al. Brain death in children: Characteristic common carotid arterial velocity patterns measured with pulsed Doppler ultrasound. J Pediatr 1987;110:723.

Aichner F, Felber S, Birbamer G, et al. Magnetic resonance: A noninvasive approach to metabolism, circulation, and morphology in human brain death. Ann Neurol 1992;32:507.

Albertini A, Schonfeld S, Hiatt M, et al. Digital subtraction angiography—a new approach to brain death determination in the newborn. Pediatr Radiol 1993;23:195.

Altman DI, Powers WJ, Perlman JM, et al. Cerebral blood flow requirements for brain viability in newborn infants is lower than in adults. Ann Neurol 1988;24:218.

American Electroencephalographic Society. Guidelines in EEG 1-7 (revised 1985). J Clin Neurophysiol 1986;3:131.

American Electroencephalographic Society. Guideline three: Minimum technical standards for EEG recording in suspected cerebral death. J Clin Neurophysiol 1994;11:10.

Ammar A, Awada A, Al-Luwami I. Reversibility of severe brain stem dysfunction in children. Acta Neurochir 1993;124:86.

Arita K, Uozumi T, Oki S, et al. The function of the hypothalamo-pituitary axis in brain dead patients. Acta Neurochir Wien 1993;123:64.

Ashwal S. Brain death in the newborn. Clin Perinatol 1989;16:501.

Ashwal S. Are we diagnosing brain death in newborns accurately? J Heart Lung Transplant 1991;10:863.

Ashwal S. Brain death in the newborn. Clin Perinatol 1997;24:859.

Ashwal S, Schneider S. Failure of electroencephalography to diagnose brain death in comatose patients. Ann Neurol 1979;6:512.

Ashwal S, Schneider S. Brain death in children: Part I and part II. Pediatr Neurol 1988;3:69.

Ashwal S, Schneider S. Brain death in the newborn: Clinical, EEG and blood flow determinations. Pediatrics 1989;84:429.

Ashwal S, Schneider S. Determination of brain death in infants and children. In: Swaiman KF, Ashwal S, eds. Pediatric neurology: Principles and practice. St. Louis: Mosby, 1999;969.

Ashwal S, Schneider S, Thompson J. Xenon computed tomography cerebral blood flow in determination of brain death in children. Ann Neurol 1989;25:539.

Ashwal S, Smith AJK, Torres F, et al. Radionuclide bolus angiography: A technique for verification of brain death in infants and children. J Pediatr 1977;91:722.

Asmundsson P. Status of organ donation in Iceland. Nord Med 1994;109:320.

Banasiak KJ, Lister G. Brain death in children. Curr Opin Pediatr 2003;15:288.

Beca J, Cox PN, Taylor MJ, et al. Somatosensory evoked potentials for prediction of outcome in acute severe brain injury. J Pediatr 1995;126:44.

Beecher HK. A definition of irreversible coma: Report of the ad hoc committee of Harvard Medical School to examine the definition of brain death. JAMA 1968;205:337.

Bennett DR, Hughes JR, Korein J, et al. Atlas of electroencephalography in coma and cerebral death. New York: Raven Press, 1976.

Bode H, Sauer M, Pringsheim W. Diagnosis of brain death by transcranial Doppler sonography. Arch Dis Child 1989;63:1474.

Bonetti MG, Ciritella P, Valle G, et al. 99mTc HM-PAO brain perfusion SPECT in brain death. Neuroradiology 1995;37:365.

Bradac GB, Simon RS. Angiography in brain death. Neuroradiology 1974;7:25.

Chang MY, McBride LA, Ferguson MA. Variability in brain death declaration practices in pediatric head trauma patients. Pediatr Neurosurg 2003;39:7.

Chatrian GE. Electrophysiologic evaluation of brain death: A critical appraisal. In: Aminoff MJ, ed. Electrodiagnosis in clinical neurology. New York: Churchill-Livingstone, 1986.

Chiu NC, Shen EY, Ho CS. Outcome in children with significantly abnormal cerebral blood flow detected by Doppler ultrasonography: Focus on the survivors. J Neuroimaging 2003;13:53.

Conference of Medical Royal Colleges and their Faculties in the UK. Diagnosis of death. BMJ 1976;2:1187.

Conference of Medical Royal Colleges and their Faculties in the UK. Diagnosis of death. BMJ 1979;1:332.

Conrad GR, Sinha P. Scintigraphy as a confirmatory test of brain death. Semin Nucl Med 2003;33:312.

Coulter DL. Neurologic uncertainty in newborn intensive care. N Engl J Med 1987;316:840.

Criteria for the diagnosis of brain stem death. Review by a working group convened by the Royal College of Physicians and endorsed by the Conference of Medical Royal Colleges and their Faculties in the United Kingdom. J R Coll Physicians Lond 1995;29:381.

Darby JM, Yonas H, Gur D, et al. Xenon-enhanced computed tomography in brain death. Arch Neurol 1987;44:551.

Dear PRF, Godfrey DJ. Neonatal auditory brainstem response cannot reliably diagnose brainstem death. Arch Dis Child 1985;60:17.

de Freitas GR, Andre C, Bezerra M, et al. Persistence of isolated flow in the internal carotid artery in brain death. J Neurol Sci 2003;210:31.

De Merlier JL, Taylor MJ. Evoked potentials in comatose children:

Auditory brain stem responses. Pediatr Neurol 1986;2:31.
DeOliveira WM, DeOliveira MLJ, Pereira IE, et al. Reavaliacao dos criterios clinicos e electroencefalograficos de determinacao da morte cerebral na crianca. Arq Neuropsiquiatr 1984;42:25.
Dosemeci L, Dora B, Yilmaz M, et al. Utility of transcranial Doppler ultrasonography for confirmatory diagnosis of brain death: Two sides of the coin. Transplantation 2004;77:71.
Drake B, Ashwal S, Schneider S. Determination of cerebral death in the pediatric intensive care unit. Pediatrics 1986;78:107.
Dutie SE, Peterson BW, Cutler J, et al. Successful organ donation in victims of child abuse. Clin Transplant 1993;9:415.
Fanaroff A, Martin RJ, Miller MJ. The respiratory system. In: Fanaroff A, Martin RJ, eds. Neonatal-perinatal medicine: Diseases of the fetus and newborn. St. Louis, Mosby, 1987.
Farrell MM, Levine DL. Brain death in the pediatric patient: Historical, sociological, medical, religious, cultural, legal, and ethical considerations. Crit Care Med 1993;21:1951.
Feri M, Ralli L, Felici M, et al. Transcranial Doppler and brain death diagnosis. Crit Care Med 1994;22:1120.
Fishman MA. Validity of brain death criteria in infants. Pediatrics 1995;96:513.
Flannery AM. Brain death and evoked potentials in pediatric patients. Crit Care Med 1999;27:264.
Freeman JM, Ferry PC. New brain death guidelines in children: Further confusion. Pediatrics 1988;81:301.
Galaske RG, Schober O, Heyer R. 99mTc-HM-PAO and 1231-amphetamine cerebral scintigraphy: A new, noninvasive method in determination of brain death in children. Eur J Nucl Med 1988;14:446.
Glasier CM, Seibert JJ, Chadduck WM, et al. Brain death in infants: Evaluation with Doppler US. Radiology 1989;172:377.
Goh AY, Lum LC, Chan PW, et al. Withdrawal and limitation of life support in paediatric intensive care. Arch Dis Child 1999;80:424.
Goh AY, Mok Q. Clinical course and determination of brainstem death in a children's hospital. Acta Paediatr 2004;93:47.
Goldstein B, DeKing D, DeLong DJ, et al. Autonomic cardiovascular state after severe brain injury and brain death in children. Crit Care Med 1993;21:228.
Goodman JM, Heck LL, Moore BD. Confirmation of brain death with portable isotope angiography: A review of 204 consecutive cases. Neurosurgery 1985;16:492.
Gotay-Cruz F, Fernandez-Sein A. Pediatric experience with brain death determination. P R Health Sci J 2002;21:11
Grattan Smith PJ, Butt W. Suppression of brainstem reflexes in barbiturate coma. Arch Dis Child 1993;69:151.
Green R, Lauber A. Recovery of activity in young children after ECS. J Neurol Neurosurg Psychiatry 1972;35:103.
Greissen G. Cerebral blood flow in preterm infants during the first week of life. Acta Paediatr Scand 1986;75:43.
Grigg G, Kelly M, Celesia G, et al. Electroencephalographic activity after brain death. Arch Neurol 1987;44:948.
Guerit JM. Evoked potentials: A safe brain-death confirmatory tool? Eur J Med 1992;1:233.
Hack M. The sensorimotor development of the preterm infant. In: Fanaroff A, Martin RJ, eds. Neonatal-perinatal medicine: Diseases of the fetus and newborn. St. Louis: Mosby, 1987.
Hansen AV, Lavin PJ, Moody EB, et al. False-negative cerebral radionuclide flow study, in brain death, caused by a ventricular drain. Clin Nucl Med 1993;18:502.
Harrison AM, Botkin JR. Can pediatricians define and apply the concept of brain death? Pediatrics 1999;103:e82.
Haupt WF, Rudolf J. European brain death codes: a comparison of national guidelines. J Neurol 1999;246:432.
Hicks RC, Poole JL. Electroencephalographic changes with hypothermia and cardiopulmonary bypass in children. J Thorac Cardiovasc Surg 1981;81:781.
Holtzman BH, Curless RG, Seakianakis GN, et al. Radionuclide cerebral perfusion scintigraphy in determination of brain death in children. Neurology 1983;33:1027.
Holshouser BA, Ashwal S, Luh GY, et al. Proton MR spectroscopy after acute central nervous system injury: outcome prediction in neonates, infants and children. Radiology 1997;202:487.
House MA, Benitez N. Multiple organ retrieval: Impact on staff and institutions. Semin Perioper Nurs 1992;1:51.
Huet H, Leroy G, Toulas P. Radiological confirmation of brain death: Digitized cerebral parenchymography: Preliminary report. Neuroradiology 1996;38(Suppl 1):S42.
Ishii K, Onuma T, Kinoshita T, et al. Brain death: MR and MR angiography. AJNR Am J Neuroradiol 1996;17:731.
Jalili M, Crade M, Davis AL. Carotid blood-flow velocity changes detected by Doppler ultrasound in determination of brain death in children: A preliminary report. Clin Pediatr Phila 1994;33:669.
Jastremski MS, Powner D, Snyder J, et al. Spontaneous decerebrate movement after declaration of brain death. Neurosurgery 1991;29:479.
Jennett B, Bond M. Assessment of outcome after severe brain damage, a practical scale. Lancet 1975;1:480.
Jorgensen EO, Malchow-Moller A. Cerebral prognostic signs during cardiopulmonary resuscitation. Resuscitation 1978;6:217.
Juguilon AC, Reilly EL. Development of EEG activity after ten days of electrocerebral inactivity: Ten days of electrocerebral inactivity: A case report in a premature neonate-hydranencephaly or massive ventricular enlargement. Clin Electroencephalogr 1982;13:233.
Karantanas AH, Hadjigeorgiou GM, Paterakis K, et al. Contribution of MRI and MR angiography in early diagnosis of brain death. Eur Radiol 2002;12:2710.
Kato T, Tokumaru A, O'uchi T, et al: Assessment of brain death in children by means of P-31 MR spectroscopy: Preliminary note. Radiology 1991;179:95.
Kaufman HH. Pediatric brain death and organ/tissue retrieval: Medical, ethical, and legal aspects. New York: Plenum, 1989.
Kaukinen S, Makela K, Hakkinen VK, et al. Significance of electrical brain activity in brain-stem death. Intensive Care Med 1995;21:76.
Kennedy M, Kiloh N. Drugs and brain death. Drug Saf 1996;14:171.
Kohrman MH. Brain death in neonates. Semin Neurol 1993;13:116.
Kohrman MH, Spivack BS. Brain death in infants: Sensitivity and specificity of current criteria. Pediatr Neurol 1990;6:47.
Korein J, Braunstein P, George A, et al. Brain death: I. Angiographic correlation with a radioisotope bolus technique for evaluation of cerebral blood flow. Ann Neurol 1977;2:195.
LaMancusa J, Cooper R, Vieth R, et al. The effects of the falling therapeutic and subtherapeutic barbiturate blood levels on electrocerebral silence in clinically brain-dead children. Clin Electroencephalogr 1991;22:112.
Lang CJ. Apnea testing by artificial CO_2 augmentation. Neurology 1995;45:966.
Lee DH, Nathanson JA, Fox AJ, et al. Magnetic resonance imaging of brain death. Can Assoc Radiol J 1995;46:174.
Litscher G, Schwartz G, Kleinert R. Brainstem auditory evoked potential monitoring: Variations of stimulus artifact in brain death. Electroencephalogr Clin Neurophysiol 1995;96:413.
Lock M. Death in technological time: Locating the end of meaningful life. Med Anthropol Q 1996;10:575.
Lopez-Herce J, Sancho L, Martinon JM. Study of paediatric intensive care units in Spain. Spanish Society of Paediatric Intensive Care. Intensive Care Med 2000;26:62.
Lovblad KO, Bassetti C, Basssetti C. Diffusion-weighted magnetic resonance imaging in brain death. Stroke 2000;31:539.
Lutschg J, Pfenninger J, Lundin HP, et al. Brainstem auditory evoked potentials and early somatosensory evoked potentials in neuro-intensively treated comatose children. Am J Dis Child 1983;137:421.
Lutz-Dettinger N, de Jaeger A, Kerremans I. Care of the potential pediatric organ donor. Pediatr Clin North Am 2001;48:715.
Machado C, Valdes P, Garcia Tigera J, et al. Brain-stem auditory evoked potentials and brain death. Electroencephalogr Clin Neurophysiol 1991;80:392.
Manno EM. Transcranial Doppler ultrasonography in the neurocritical care unit. Crit Care Clin 1997;13:79.
Martin E, Buchli R, Ritter S, et al. Diagnostic and prognostic value of cerebral ^{31}P magnetic resonance spectroscopy in neonates with perinatal asphyxia. Pediatr Res 1996;40:749.
Martinot A, Grandbastien B, Leteurtre S, et al. No resuscitation orders and withdrawal of therapy in French paediatric intensive care units. Groupe Francophone de Reanimation et d'Urgences Pediatriques. Acta Paediatr 1998;87:769.
Martinot A, Lejeune C, Hue V, et al. Modality and causes of 259 deaths in a pediatric intensive care unit. Arch Pediatr 1995;2:735.
Matsumura A, Meguro K, Tsurushima H, et al. Magnetic resonance imaging of brain death. Neurol Med Chir (Tokyo) 1996;36:166.
McMenamin JB, Volpe JJ. Doppler ultrasonography in the determination of neonatal brain death. Ann Neurol 1983;14:302.

Medlock MD, Hanigan WC, Cruse RP. Dissociation of cerebral blood flow, glucose metabolism, and electrical activity in pediatric brain death: Case report. J Neurosurg 1993;79:752.

Mejia RE, Pollack MM. Variability in brain death determination practices in children. JAMA 1995;274:550.

Messer J, Burtscher A, Haddad J, et al. Contribution of transcranial Doppler sonography to the diagnosis of brain death in children. Arch Fr Pediatr 1990;47:647.

Meyer MA. Evaluating brain death with positron emission tomography: Case report on dynamic imaging of 18F-fluorodeoxyglucose activity after intravenous bolus injection. J Neuroimaging 1996;6:117.

Miyasaka K, Takeuchi K, Takeshita H. Paediatric brain death in Japan. Lancet 2001;357(9268):1625.

Mohandas A, Chou SN. Brain death: A clinical pathological study. J Neurosurg 1971;35:211.

Mollaret P, Goulon M. Le coma depasse. Rev Neurol 1959;101:3.

Moshe SL. Usefulness of EEG in the evaluation of brain death in children: The pros. Electroencephalogr Clin Neurophysiol 1989;73:272.

Moshe SK, Alvarez LA. Diagnosis of brain death in children. J Clin Neurophysiol 1986;3:239.

Mrhac L, Zakko S, Parikh Y. Brain death: The evaluation of semi-quantitative parameters and other signs in HMPAO scintigraphy. Nucl Med Commun 1995;16:1016.

National Institute of Neurologic and Communicative Disorders and Stroke. The NINCDS collaborative study of brain death. Monograph No. 24, NIH Pub. No. 81-2286. Bethesda, MD: NINCDS, 1980.

Okamoto K, Sugimoto T. Return of spontaneous respiration in an infant who fulfilled current criteria to determine brain death. Pediatrics 1995;96:518.

Orrison WW Jr, Champlin AM, Kesterson OL, et al. MR "hot nose sign" and "intravascular enhancement sign" in brain death. AJNR Am J Neuroradiol 1994;15:913.

Otsubo Y, Yoneyama Y, Sawa R, et al. Fetal brain death and Dandy-Walker malformation. Prenat Diagn 1999;19:777.

Outwater KM, Rockoff MA. Apnea testing to confirm brain death in children. Crit Care Med 1984;12:357.

Paolin A, Manuali A, Di Paola F, et al. Reliability in diagnosis of brain death. Intensive Care Med 1995;21:657.

Paret G, Barzilay Z. Apnea testing in suspected brain dead children—physiological and mathematical modelling. Intensive Care Med 1995;21:247.

Parker BL, Frewen TC, Levin SD, et al. Declaring pediatric brain death: Current practice in a Canadian pediatric critical care unit. Can Med Assoc J 1995;153:909.

Penchas S, Roll M. Organ transplantation: Evolving a national transplantation policy and methodology in Israel. Transplant Proc 1996;28:2345.

Pennefather SH, Bullock RE, Mantle D, et al. Use of low dose arginine vasopressin to support brain-dead organ donors. Transplantation 1995;59:58.

Petty GW, Mohr JP, Pedley TA, et al. The role of transcranial Doppler in confirming brain death: Sensitivity, specificity, and suggestions for performance and interpretation. Neurology 1990;40:300.

Pezzani C, Radvanyi-Bouvet MF, Relier JP, Monod N. Neonatal electroencephalography during the first twenty-four hours of life in full-term newborn infants. Neuropediatrics 1986;17:11.

Pistoia F, Johnson DW, Darby JM, et al. The role of xenon CT measurements of cerebral blood flow in the clinical determination of brain death. AJNR Am J Neuroradiol 1991;12:97.

President's Commission for the Study of Ethical Problems in Medicine and Biomedical and Behavioral Research. Guidelines for the determination of death. JAMA 1981;246:2184.

Report of special task force. Guidelines for the determination of brain death in children. Ad Hoc Task Force consisting of representatives from the American Academy of Pediatrics, American Academy of Neurology, Child Neurology Society, American Neurological Association, American Bar Association, and the NINCDS. Pediatrics 1987;80:298.

Rodriguez RA, Cornel G, Alghofaili F, et al. Transcranial Doppler during suspected brain death in children: Potential limitation in patients with cardiac "shunt." Pediatr Crit Care Med 2002;3:153.

Roels L, Pirenne J, Delooz H, et al. Effect of triiodothyronine replacement therapy on maintenance characteristics and organ availability in hemodynamically unstable donors. Transplant Proc 2000;32:1564.

Ropper AH, Kennedy SK, Russell L. Apnea testing in the diagnosis of brain death. J Neurosurg 1981;55:942.

Rosendale JD, Kauffman HM, McBride MA, et al. Hormonal resuscitation yields more transplanted hearts, with improved early function. Transplantation 2003;75:1336.

Rowland TW, Donnelly JH, Jackson AH. Apnea documentation for determination of brain death in children. Pediatrics 1984;74:505.

Rowland RW, Donnelly JH, Jackson AH, et al. Brain death in the pediatric intensive care unit. Am J Dis Child 1983;137:547.

Ruiz-Garcia M, Gonzalez-Astiazaran A, Collado-Corona MA, et al. Brain death in children: Clinical, neurophysiological and radioisotopic angiography findings in 125 patients. Childs Nerv Syst 2000;16:40.

Ruiz-Lopez MJ, Martinez de Azagra A, Serrano A, et al. Brain death and evoked potentials in pediatric patients. Crit Care Med 1999;27:412.

Ryan CA, Byrne P, Kuhn S, et al. No resuscitation and withdrawal of therapy in a neonatal and a pediatric intensive care unit in Canada. J Pediatr 1993;123:534.

Saito T, Takeichi S, Nakajima Y, et al. Influence of antemortem medication on the determination of brain death. Nippon Hoigaku Zasshi 1995;49:484.

Sanker P, Roth B, Frowein RA, et al. Cerebral reperfusion in brain death of a newborn: Case report. Neurosurg Rev 1992;15:315.

Schafer JA, Caronna JJ. Duration of apnea needed to confirm brain death. Neurology 1978;28:661.

Schmitt B, Simma B, Burger R, et al. Resuscitation after severe hypoxia in a young child: Temporary isoelectric EEG and loss of BAEP components. Intensive Care Med 1993;19:420.

Schneider S. Usefulness of EEG in the evaluation of brain death in children: The cons. Electroencephalogr Clin Neurophysiol 1989;73:276.

Schwartz JA, Baxter J, Brill DR. Diagnosis of brain death in children by radionuclide cerebral imaging. Pediatrics 1984;73:14.

Sheehy E, Conrad SL, Brigham LE, et al. Estimating the number of potential organ donors in the United States. N Engl J Med 2003;349:667.

Sher MS, Barabas RE, Barmada MA. Clinical examination findings in neonates with the absence of electrocerebral activity: An acute or chronic encephalopathic state? J Perinatol 1996;16:455.

Shewmon DA. The probability of an inevitability: The inherent impossibility of validating criteria for brain death or "irreversibility" through clinical studies. Stat Med 1987;6:535.

Shewmon DA. Commentary on guidelines for the determination of brain death in children. Ann Neurol 1988;24:789.

Shewmon DA. Chronic "brain death": Meta-analysis and conceptual consequences. Neurology 1998;51:1538.

Siminoff LA, Mercer MB, Arnold R. Families' understanding of brain death. Prog Transplant 2003;13:218.

Spieth M, Abella E, Sutter C, et al. Importance of the lateral view in the evaluation of suspected brain death. Clin Nucl Med 1995;20:965.

Spieth ME, Ansari AN, Kawada TK, et al. Direct comparison of Tc-99m DTPA and Tc-99m HMPAO for evaluating brain death. Clin Nucl Med 1994;19:867.

Staworn D, Lewison L, Marks J, et al. Brain death in pediatric intensive care unit patients: Incidence, primary diagnosis, and the clinical occurrence of Turner's triad. Crit Care Med 1994;22:1301.

Steinhart CM, Weiss IP. Use of brainstem auditory evoked potentials in pediatric brain death. Crit Care Med 1985;13:560.

Stoyles HA. Management of multi organ donor. Axone 1995;16:97.

Swaiman KF. Neurological examination of the preterm infant. In: Swaiman KF, ed. Pediatric neurology: Principles and practice, 2nd ed. St. Louis: Mosby, 1994.

Taylor MJ, Houston BD, Lowry NJ. Recovery of auditory brainstem responses after a severe hypoxic ischemic insult. N Engl J Med 1983;309:1169.

ten Velden GH, van Huffelen AC. Brain death criteria: Guidelines by the Public Health Council. Ned Tijdschr Geneeskd 1997;141:77.

Terk MR, Gober JR, DeGiorgio C, et al. Brain death in the neonate: Assessment with P-31 MR spectroscopy. Radiology 1992;182:582.

Thompson JR, Ashwal S, Schneider S, et al. Comparison of cerebral blood flow measurements by xenon computed tomography and dynamic brain scintigraphy in clinically brain dead children. 13th Symposium Neuroradiologicum. Acta Radiol Suppl (Stockh) 1987;369:675.

Tobin B. Drugs and brain death: A matter of "practical certainty." Clin Exp Pharmacol Physiol 1996;23:S44.

Toffol GJ, Lansky LL, Hughes JR, et al. Pitfalls in diagnosing brain death in infancy. J Child Neurol 1987;2:134.

Tsai E, Shemie SD, Cox PN, et al. Organ donation in children: Role of the pediatric intensive care unit. Pediatr Crit Care Med 2000;1:156.

Uniform determination of death act #7180 of the health and safety code. Uniform Law Annotated 1980;12:310.

Valle G, Ciritella P, Bonetti MG, et al. Considerations of brain death on a SPECT cerebral perfusion study. Clin Nucl Med 1993;18:953.

Van Bunnen Y, Delcour C, Wery D, et al. Intravenous digital subtraction angiography: A criteria of brain death. Ann Radiol Paris 1989;32:279.

Vander Borght T, Laloux P, Maes A, et al. Guidelines for brain radionuclide imaging: Perfusion single photon computed tomography (SPECT) using Tc-99m radiopharmaceuticals and brain metabolism positron emission tomography (PET) using F-18 fluorodeoxyglucose. The Belgian Society for Nuclear Medicine. Acta Neurol Belg 2001;101:196.

Vardis R, Pollack MM. Increased apnea threshold in a pediatric patient with suspected brain death. Crit Care Med 1998;26:1917.

Vernon DD, Dean JM, Timmons OD, et al. Modes of death in the pediatric intensive care unit: Withdrawal and limitation of supportive care. Crit Care Med 1993;21:1798.

Vernon DD, Holzman BH. Brain death: considerations for pediatrics. J Clin Neurophysiol 1986;3:251.

Volpe JJ. Commentary on brain death determination in the newborn. Pediatrics 1987;80:293.

Wagner W. Scalp, earlobe and nasopharyngeal recordings of the median nerve somatosensory evoked p14 potential in coma and brain death: Detailed latency and amplitude analysis in 181 patients. Brain 1996;119:1507.

Wieler H, March K, Kaisar KP, et al. Tc-99m HmPAO cerebral scintigraphy: A reliable, noninvasive method for determination of brain death. Clin Nucl Med 1993;18:104.

Wijdicks EF. Determining brain death in adults. Neurology 1995;45:1003.

Wijdicks EF. Brain death worldwide: Accepted fact but no global consensus in diagnostic criteria. Neurology 2002;58:20.

Wijdicks EFM, ed. Brain death. Philadelphia: Lippincott, 2001.

Williams MA, Lipsett PA, Rushton CH, et al. The physician's role in discussing organ donation with families. Crit Care Med 2003;31:1568.

Wilson K, Gormon L, Seeby JB. The diagnosis of brain death with Tc-99m HmPAO. Clin Nucl Med 1993;18:428.

Ying Z, Schmid UD, Schmid J, Hess CW. Motor and somatosensory evoked potentials in coma: Analysis and relation to clinical status and outcome. J Neurol Neurosurg Psychiatry 1992;55:470.

Zenel J, Goldstein B. Child abuse in the pediatric intensive care unit. Crit Care Med 2002;30(11 Suppl):S515.

PART XI

Infections of the Nervous System

CHAPTER 68

Bacterial Infections of the Nervous System

Martin G. Täuber and Urs B. Schaad

The brain is normally a sterile site that is protected from infection by specialized barriers, including the bony skull and the blood-brain barrier. Consequently, infections of the central nervous system (CNS) are comparatively rare. In the United States, the incidence of bacterial meningitis, the most frequent bacterial infection of the CNS, was 3 to 5 cases per 100,000 population in 1995 [Schuchat et al., 1997], in stark contrast to the incidence of sepsis, which was more than 200 cases per 100,000 in in 1995 [Martin et al., 2003].

Bacterial infections of the CNS are often devastating, leading to death or significant neurologic sequelae that can have a major negative impact on the development and well-being of affected children. The exquisite vulnerability of the brain to infection is related to deficient local host defenses that do not suppress the multiplication of pathogens, detrimental effects of cerebral blood flow alterations when the infection involves the cerebral vasculature, harmful effects of increased intracranial pressure caused by brain swelling and mass lesions, the destruction of brain tissue by the inflammatory process, and limited repair mechanisms of neuronal tissue. In many infections, such as bacterial meningitis, damage to the brain is a consequence not primarily of the invasion by the pathogen, but rather of the ensuing overwhelming inflammatory response. This chapter reviews pertinent information on the pathogenesis, clinical features, treatment, and prevention of bacterial infections of the nervous system.

ACUTE BACTERIAL MENINGITIS

Bacterial meningitis is an inflammation of the leptomeninges triggered by bacteria present in the subarachnoid space. Children still die or suffer permanent neurologic sequelae as a result of meningitis [Klein et al., 1986]. Prevention or prompt diagnosis and aggressive management are the goals [Schaad, 1997]. Before the discovery of antibiotics, therapy consisted of withdrawal of cerebrospinal fluid through repeated lumbar puncture and intrathecal or intravenous administration of antimeningococcal antiserum raised in horses. More recent milestones include the introduction of new, potent bactericidal antibiotics, active vaccination, and anti-inflammatory therapy [Rockowitz and Tunkel, 1995].

Epidemiology

Bacterial meningitis has a unique epidemiologic profile. The disease has a worldwide distribution, the typical host is a previously healthy patient, the typical symptoms usually develop rapidly, there are numerous and severe sequelae, and the disease is increasingly preventable [Schuchat et al., 1997]. Bacterial meningitis occurs in people of all ages, but there are striking age-related differences in the predominant etiologic agents. Differences relate to immunologic maturation, social or behavioral influences, and the coexistence of other chronic or acute clinical conditions.

Neonatal meningitis typically follows obstetric complications, and the predominant bacteria are group B streptococcus, *Listeria monocytogenes,* and gram-negative enteric bacteria. Older infants have substantial risk of meningitis caused by *Haemophilus influenzae* type b and *Streptococcus pneumoniae,* although where *H. influenzae* conjugate vaccines are in use, *H. influenzae* type b meningitis has been virtually eliminated. School-age children are at greatest risk of meningococcal disease, which occurs in outbreaks throughout the world and causes major epidemics in sub-Saharan Africa and parts of Asia. *S. pneumoniae* is the leading cause of bacterial meningitis in adults, and the emergence of antimicrobial-resistant pneumococci has complicated pediatric meningitis worldwide [Schuchert et al., 1997].

Bacterial meningitis occurs with increased frequency in certain population groups. Native Americans and aboriginal populations are at particular risk for *H. influenzae* type b disease [Coulehan et al., 1984; Ward et al., 1986]. Risk of group B streptococcal disease is substantially higher among African-Americans than other racial or ethnic groups in the United States [Zangwill et al., 1992].

Immunologic defenses against bacterial infection are reduced in certain chronic illnesses. Persons with sickle cell disease or other states of functional asplenia have increased susceptibility to encapsulated bacteria, especially the pneumococcus. Terminal complement deficiency predisposes these persons to meningococcal disease. Patients with human immunodeficiency virus infection are at substantially increased risk of invasive infection with *S. pneumoniae* and *L. monocytogenes.* Cell-mediated immunity is crucial for defense against listeriosis.

Variation in the incidence of bacterial meningitis reported from different regions may relate to differences in diagnosis and reporting (surveillance artifact) but also may be caused by true environmental or population differences in risk of disease. The best example of geographic variation in meningitis is recurrent epidemic meningococcal disease in the meningitis belt of sub-Saharan Africa.

Institutional settings, such as daycare centers, provide opportunities for enhanced transmission of respiratory pathogens, including *H. influenzae* type b, meningococcus, and pneumococcus. Transmission of antimicrobial-resistant infections among daycare center attendees is an emerging problem [Reichler et al., 1992]. Meningococcal meningitis clusters have been described in schools, on college campuses, and in refugee settings.

Seasonal fluctuations in bacterial meningitis occur in some areas. Pneumococcal disease is most common in winter, when other respiratory infections predominate. The role of viral and bacterial respiratory cofactors in the risk of bacterial meningitis may explain some of the increased disease prevalence in winter months [Krasinski et al., 1987].

Most bacterial meningitis occurs as sporadic or isolated cases. After single cases of meningitis caused by *H. influenzae* type b and meningococcus, secondary cases can occur. Despite a high prevalence of pneumococcal colonization among young children, secondary cases of invasive pneumococcal disease are extremely rare.

Pathogenesis

To establish bacterial meningitis, pathogens have to gain access to the subarachnoid space. Most cases of bacterial meningitis likely arise from bacteremia, which is caused by invasion of the bloodstream by the pathogen after colonization of the nasopharyngeal mucosa. Most meningeal pathogens are transmitted person to person by the respiratory route. In neonates, transmission usually occurs vertically during birth. Predisposing factors include maternal infection, premature rupture of maternal membranes, prolonged labor, obstetric trauma, and fetal distress. In the postnatal phase, premature or hospitalized infants are at increased risk for bacteremia and subsequent meningitis as a result of arterial and intravenous lines and mechanical ventilation.

Adherence to the nasopharyngeal epithelium is mediated by specialized surface components (e.g., the polysaccharide capsule with specific epitopes and fimbriae or pili) of meningeal pathogens. These factors also are crucial for evasion of local host defense mechanisms and subsequent invasion of the bloodstream. The lack of specific mucosal antibodies correlates with an increased risk of invasive disease. Viral infection of the respiratory tract also may promote invasive disease.

From the nasopharyngeal surface, encapsulated organisms cross the epithelial cell layer and invade the small subepithelial blood vessels. In the bloodstream, pathogens are protected from complement-mediated bactericidal mechanisms and neutrophil phagocytosis by their capsule. Impairment of the alternative complement pathway occurs in patients with sickle cell disease and in patients who have undergone splenectomy, and these patients are predisposed to the development of pneumococcal meningitis. Similarly, functional deficiencies of components involved in activation and function of complement-mediated defenses (i.e., mannose binding lectin, properdin, lack of terminal complement components) increase the susceptibility for invasive meningococcal infections [Van Deuren et al., 2000]. Neonates are at an increased risk of bacterial meningitis because of impaired nonspecific immunity. This impaired immunity includes defects in leukocyte chemotaxis, phagocytosis, bactericidal activity, and low levels of immunoglobulin M (IgM) antibodies and complement, which are not transferred across the placenta but are important in defense against gram-negative organisms [Mariscalco et al., 2002].

Studies in models of bacterial meningitis indicate that cells of the choroid plexus and cerebral capillaries possess receptors for meningeal pathogens and that the choroid plexus is the preferential site of primary invasion of the cerebrospinal fluid space. For *Escherichia coli,* a complex interplay between endothelial factors and microbial genes orchestrates the crossing of the blood-brain barrier by bacteria [Hoffman et al., 2000]. Pneumococci are thought to enter the CNS by crossing the blood-brain barrier or the blood–cerebrospinal fluid barrier either by local tissue damage or by transcytosis through microvascular endothelial cells [Ring et al., 1998].

Not all bacterial infections of the CNS are the result of bacteremia. Nonhematogenous invasion of the cerebrospinal fluid by bacteria occurs in situations of compromised integrity of the barriers surrounding the brain (e.g., in otitis media, mastoiditis, sinusitis). Direct communication between the subarachnoid space and the skin or mucosal surfaces as a result of malformation or trauma gives rise to meningeal infection. Bacteria also can reach the cerebrospinal fluid as a complication of neurosurgery, spinal anesthesia, or ventriculostomy placement [Alleyne et al., 2000]. Infections of cerebrospinal fluid shunts are another cause of meningitis. Most cases occur shortly after implantation of the shunt and are attributed to intraoperative inoculation, but late shunt infections can occur several years after implantation [Vinchon et al., 2002]. Staphylococci, in particular coagulase-negative staphylococci, are the major pathogens in shunt infections [Filka et al., 1999]. These organisms have unique capabilities to colonize the surface of foreign bodies because of specialized surface proteins (e.g., clumping factor, fibronectin binding protein) that allow the organism to adhere to the catheters, in particular after they are coated with host-derived proteins, such as fibrin and fibronectin [Ziebuhr et al., 2000]. Adhering organisms rapidly develop into a biofilm, characterized by bacteria embedded in an extracellular matrix. Elimination of bacterial biofilms from the surface of foreign bodies by antibiotics or host defenses is notoriously difficult [Ziebuhr et al., 2000]. Colonization of cerebrospinal fluid shunts with coagulase-negative staphylococci leads to clinically apparent meningitis or ventriculitis in only approximately 30% [Odio et al., 1984; Vinchon et al., 2002].

Pathogens reaching the cerebrospinal fluid are likely to survive because of a paucity of resident macrophages and deficient opsonization caused by low concentrations of capsule-specific immunoglobulins and complement in the cerebrospinal fluid. Lack of opsonization greatly reduces the effectiveness of incoming granulocytes and allows largely unrestricted multiplication of the meningeal pathogens. Bacterial multiplication is associated with the release of bacterial products (fragments of cell wall, lipopolysaccharide) that trigger the inflammatory response in the subarachnoid space by inducing the production and release of inflammatory cytokines and chemokines. Cytokines, including tumor necrosis factor-α, interleukin-1, and interleukin-6; chemokines, such as interleukin-8, growth-related protein-α, and monocyte chemotactic protein-1; and lipid inflammatory mediators, such as platelet activation factor, upregulate adhesion molecules on brain vascular endothelial cells and promote the recruitment of granulocytes into the cerebrospinal fluid. Matrix metalloproteases contribute to the inflammatory process by mediating breakdown of blood-brain barrier and activating cytokines [Kieseier et al., 1999]. This granulocytic inflammation is primarily responsible for the complex pathophysiologic CNS alterations and clinical manifestations of bacterial meningitis [Meli et al., 2002].

Diagnosis

Prompt diagnosis is crucial for a life-threatening illness such as bacterial meningitis. Routine early diagnosis requires educated suspicion of meningitis and immediate performance of lumbar puncture and adequate tests when the cerebrospinal fluid has been obtained [Schaad, 1995].

Clinical Features

The sudden onset of a stiff neck with fever in a child who appears ill usually indicates the presence of meningitis (Table 68-1). In these cases, a lumbar puncture is a crucial part of the initial evaluation.

MENINGISMUS

Meningismus reflects tense neck and back muscles as a reflex to avoid painful extension of inflamed meninges. Clinical findings of meningeal irritation include Kernig's sign (passive extension of the knee from the flexed thigh position elicits pain in the back), Brudzinski's sign (passive flexion of the neck elicits spontaneous flexion of the lower extremities), tripod sign (while sitting the patient holds the back erect by placing both extended arms behind the buttock), and knee-kissing sign (the patient is unable to kiss his or her own knees). Nuchal rigidity is absent throughout the course of meningitis in only 1% to 2% of infants and children; generally the younger the patient, the less prominent nuchal rigidity [Geiseler and Nelson, 1982].

Nuchal rigidity is not always the result of meningeal irritation secondary to infection. The patient's history and physical examination usually lead to the consideration of other possibilities, such as other sites of infection (e.g., cervical adenitis, tonsillopharyngitis, retropharyngeal abscess, and cervical spine osteomyelitis), vascular abnormalities (e.g., subarachnoid hemorrhage), neoplasms (e.g., brain tumor and meningeal leukemia), or bony and muscular disorders (e.g., fracture, torticollis, and myositis).

INITIAL PRESENTATION

Fever (94%), vomiting (82%), and nuchal rigidity (77%) are the most common presenting symptoms of meningitis in children 1 to 4 years old. Many children also experience lethargy, irritability, anorexia, and photophobia [Ashwal et al., 1993]. Seizures, bulging fontanel, and coma occur less commonly and usually occur later in the course of the illness. Older patients report headache and neck pain.

TABLE 68-1

Signs and Symptoms of Bacterial Meningitis

Fever, acute course
Vomiting, anorexia
Nuchal rigidity
Meningismus
Kernig's sign
Brudzinski's sign
Tripod and knee-kissing sign
Depression of consciousness, coma
Irritability, photophobia, headache
Seizures, focal neurologic deficits

TWO MODES OF PRESENTATION

The first pattern develops over several days with fever and nonspecific manifestations suggesting viral infection without or with localization (e.g., upper respiratory or gastrointestinal tract). In these patients, it is difficult to pinpoint the exact onset of meningitis. The second pattern is acute, sometimes fulminant, and the symptoms and signs of sepsis (e.g., cardiovascular instability, cutaneous manifestations such as an erythematous, maculopapular, or petechial rash) and meningitis evolve rapidly over a few hours.

NEUROLOGIC FINDINGS

Seizures occur before hospital admission or within the first 2 days of hospitalization in 20% to 30% of pediatric patients with bacterial meningitis [Feigin et al., 1992]. Generalized seizures usually are not a predictor of poor outcome. In contrast, focal neurologic signs, such as paresis, cranial nerve palsy, and focal seizure activity, often precede more adverse outcomes of irreversible brain damage. Severely depressed consciousness at the time of hospital admission usually signals a poor prognosis because of the likelihood of extensive encephalitic involvement or massively increased intracranial pressure in both of these patients [Tunkel and Scheld, 1995].

ARTHRITIS AND OTHER SYSTEMIC MANIFESTATIONS

Arthritis can precede or follow *H. influenzae* and *Neisseria meningitidis* meningitis and confuses the neurologic examination by producing the superficial appearance of a monoparesis. Knees and elbows are common sites for arthritis. Of patients with *H. influenzae* type b septic arthritis, approximately 30% have concurrent meningitis [Rotbart and Glode, 1985]. Periorbital cellulitis occurs in *H. influenzae* meningitis.

DIFFERENTIAL DIAGNOSIS

The differential diagnosis of bacterial meningitis includes aseptic meningitis, encephalitis, brain abscess, febrile seizure, head trauma, intracranial hemorrhage, and neoplastic meningitis. In addition, unusual infectious agents, such as fungus, rickettsia, or tuberculosis, must be considered. A fever with a simple seizure is unlikely to be bacterial meningitis [Green et al., 1993].

NEONATAL MENINGITIS

The traditional clinical signs of meningitis are usually lacking in neonates. Nuchal rigidity rarely occurs. Fever and a full fontanel may be absent. An associated sepsis is common. Bacterial meningitis should be considered at any age (so-called early and late onset) in any newborn who fails to thrive and has irritability, apnea, seizures, a tendency to opisthotonos, poor feeding, emesis, hypothermia or hyperthermia, hypotonia or hypertonia, a gray appearance, jaundice, or other evidence of sepsis. Apnea may be the only sign of meningitis in a neonate [Heath et al., 2003; Schaad, 1992].

SHUNT INFECTIONS

Infections of CNS shunt occur in approximately 5% to 10% of patients, usually within 1 to 2 months of surgical insertion [McGirt et al., 2003; Ronan et al., 1995]. Most of these infections are due to coagulase-negative *Staphylococcus* or *Staphylococcus aureus*; however, a variety of other organisms, including gram-negative bacteria and other skin flora, can be causative.

Diagnosis of CNS shunt infection versus CNS shunt malfunction often represents a dilemma in children who present with constitutional signs and symptoms [McClinton et al., 2001]. Clinical manifestations of CNS shunt infection usually include low-grade fever, vomiting, irritability or lethargy, and other signs of increased intracranial pressure. The onset is often insidious but can be more acute, particularly if shunt malfunction also is present. Neck stiffness is uncommon. Shunt infection should be suspected in any child with an indwelling CNS drainage system and fever.

The symptoms and signs of shunt infection are referable to the age of the patient, the infecting microorganisms, the degree of surgical trauma, and other underlying conditions of the host. Ventriculoperitoneal shunt infections may present with signs of acute peritonitis. Symptoms associated with bacteremia can range from general malaise to shock.

A percutaneous aspiration of cerebrospinal fluid from the shunt reservoir should be performed. Treatment of shunt infections needs to be tailored to meet the specific susceptibilities of the infecting microorganism and to obtain high concentrations of antibiotics within the cerebrospinal fluid and shunt system. This goal most commonly is achieved by a combination of systemic and intraventricular antibiotics.

MENINGITIS AFTER COCHLEAR IMPLANTS

Cochlear implant is the standard treatment for patients with severe-to-profound hearing loss in which well-fit hearing aids fail to permit effective oral communication. The implant is a neural stimulator whose electrode array is placed surgically in the lumen of the cochlea, near the auditory nerve. An external microphone picks up speech signals, and the signal processor transforms these signals into digital impulses that a radiofrequency carrier transmits percutaneously into the internal receiver-stimulator and electrode array. The auditory cortex is stimulated by the implant, permitting the perception of the digitally processed information as speech [Gates and Miyamoto, 2003].

Complications from cochlear implantation are unusual. Reports of postoperative meningitis have called attention to a previously unrecognized risk [Arnold et al, 2002; Reefhuis et al., 2003]. Most cases of meningitis occur in children with a typical presentation. Available information indicates that the mode for infection is a time-limited or, rarely, persistent cerebrospinal fluid leak into the middle ear. Bacteria from the middle ear—usually causing otitis media—may enter the meninges. The most common offending pathogens are *S. pneumoniae* and *H. influenzae*.

Most meningitis cases were associated with a two-component electrode that has been withdrawn from the market. Prevention by active immunization against *S. pneumoniae* and *H. influenzae* type b, meticulous sealing of the cochleostomy site, and urgent treatment of otitis media are recommended. The role of perioperative antimicrobial prophylaxis needs to be determined.

On the first symptoms of meningitis, prompt antibiotic treatment in accordance with the guidelines described subsequently must be started, and high-resolution computed tomography (CT) and magnetic resonance imaging (MRI) must be performed. In most cases of otogenic meningitis in a cochlear implant patient, a surgical revision of the middle ear and mastoid is mandatory.

Lumbar Puncture

The diagnosis of bacterial meningitis is based on examination of cerebrospinal fluid [Feigin et al., 1992]. A lumbar puncture should be performed whenever the diagnosis of meningitis is suspected on the basis of clinical signs. Rarely, other sites may be used to obtain cerebrospinal fluid, including ventricles or shunts installed to divert cerebrospinal fluid. Minimizing sequelae of bacterial meningitis depends on the prompt initiation of effective antibiotic therapy. Lumbar puncture is indicated whenever there is even minimal clinical evidence for meningitis. Such an approach in the ambulatory clinical setting results in the diagnosis of approximately 1 case of aseptic or bacterial meningitis for every 10 lumbar punctures [Feigin et al., 1992].

Lumbar puncture is a safe procedure for most patients. Minor discomfort may occur, but serious consequences are rare. Headache 1 to 6 hours after lumbar puncture is a troublesome but benign complication. When present, the headache is frontal and is exaggerated by movement from a lying to a sitting or standing position. Headache after lumbar puncture seems to be caused by continued leak of cerebrospinal fluid from the site of the lumbar puncture with resulting low cerebrospinal fluid pressure and traction on pain-sensitive structures. The problem can be mitigated by removal of a minimal amount of fluid and use of a small-bore needle [Lynch et al., 1992]. Pain in the low back or legs occurs occasionally after lumbar puncture; this pain is of uncertain etiology and resolves spontaneously in several days.

Herniation of the brainstem and cerebellar tonsils into the foramen magnum is extremely rare in children [Marton and Gean, 1986]. A risk of hernation is clearly related to substantially increased intracranial pressure [Richards and Towu-Aghantse, 1986]. The risk of producing meningitis by performing a lumbar puncture in a child with septicemia is insignificant and is not a contraindication to the test [Shapiro et al., 1986].

Repeated lumbar puncture is indicated only when delayed cerebrospinal fluid sterilization or relapse or recurrence of meningitis is clinically suspected. Lumbar puncture should not be repeated, unless the expected findings would make a difference in management. Most patients with bacterial meningitis require just one initial diagnostic lumbar puncture.

LABORATORY TESTS

As mentioned before, the initial diagnosis of meningitis is based on examination of cerebrospinal fluid. Bacterial infection is suggested by increased opening and closing pressure; a cloudy (i.e., not clear) cerebrospinal fluid; or a cerebro-

TABLE 68-2

Cerebrospinal Fluid in Neurologic Infections

DISEASE	PRESSURE	ASPECT	TOTAL WBC	PNC (%)	MNC (%)	PROTEIN	GLUCOSE	GRAM STAIN/ RAPID TEST
Bacterial meningitis	↑↑	Cloudy	>1000	+++	+	↑↑	↓↓	Positive
Aseptic meningitis	Normal/(↑)	Clear	10–1000	(+)	+++	Normal/(↑)	Normal	Negative
Encephalitis	↑	Clear	10–500	(+)	++	Normal/(↑)	Normal	Negative
Encephalopathy	↑	Clear	<10	–	–	Normal	Normal	Negative
Brain abscess				Not indicated				

MNC, mononuclear cells; PNC, polymorphonuclear cells; WBC, white blood cells; ↑, mildly elevated to normal; (+), few to none.

spinal fluid pleocytosis with polymorphonuclear predominance, increased protein concentration, or decreased glucose concentration. Details and normal values have been described previously (Table 68-2) [Ahmed et al, 1996; Bonadio, 1992].

Confirmation of the diagnosis requires the detection in the cerebrospinal fluid of a specific bacterial pathogen by microscopy or a positive culture, polymerase chain reaction, or rapid antigen-detection test of cerebrospinal fluid. Smears of cerebrospinal fluid should be examined by Gram stain (acid-fast stain if tuberculosis is suspected). In experienced hands, Gram-stained smears of the cerebrospinal fluid sediment reveals bacteria in more than 90% of cases of pediatric bacterial meningitis [Stahelin-Massik et al., 1994]. The cerebrospinal fluid should be cultured on a blood agar plate, on a chocolate agar plate (or on Fildes or Leventhal medium), and in broth. Special cultures for mycobacteria, fungi, or other microorganisms should be undertaken if clinically indicated. In an area of increasing antimicrobial resistance, adequate in vitro susceptibility testing must be routine for any cultured neonatal pathogen. Various antigen-detection tests have become available (e.g., countercurrent immunoelectrophoresis, latex particle agglutination, enzyme-linked immunosorbent assay) and may be helpful in establishing an etiologic diagnosis rapidly.

Polymerase chain reaction and other sequence-based microbial detection methods are being used increasingly in the clinical microbiology laboratory [Fredricks and Relman, 1999]. Polymerase chain reaction–based assays detect microbial nucleic acid in clinical samples including cerebrospinal fluid and do not require growth of the organism. Polymerase chain reaction–based assays can be fast, sensitive, and specific but also may be associated with technical problems, such as false-positive reactions secondary to sample contamination, and false-negative reactions secondary to the presence of polymerase chain reaction inhibitors in the sample.

Many other nonspecific parameters have been studied in the cerebrospinal fluid to establish or exclude a bacterial etiology rapidly, including various indices of inflammation (e.g., cytokines, C-reactive protein, and lactate) and measurement of various enzyme activities [Gray et al., 1986; Lutsar et al., 1994]. Further refinements are needed to confirm the usefulness of these tests in unselected populations and different centers.

CONTRAINDICATIONS

Four contraindications to lumbar punctures are as follows: (1) obvious signs of increased intracranial pressure identified by either clinical or neuroimaging examination; (2) clinically relevant cardiorespiratory compromise, especially in neonatal or older extremely sick patients; (3) history or signs of a bleeding disorder; and (4) signs of infection at puncture sites (e.g., pyoderma, cellulitis, erysipelas). In such cases, lumbar punctures should be withheld only until the condition has been corrected or excluded as a possibility. If lumbar puncture is withheld in a patient with suspected meningitis, appropriate age-specific antimicrobial and anti-inflammatory treatment for meningitis should be started without delay (see later). A short period of antibiotic and corticosteroid therapy before lumbar puncture would not cause significant alteration in cerebrospinal fluid findings.

Other Tests

Most pediatric patients with bacterial meningitis are initially bacteremic as might be expected based on the hematogeneous pathogenesis of the disease. Blood cultures taken at hospital admission are valuable and are positive in 80% to 90% of cases of bacterial meningitis [Feigin et al., 1992].

Cultured bacteria from skin or mucosal surfaces, including throat and nose, are neither sensitive (organisms causing the meningitis may not be present) nor specific (other organisms are often present) and are not helpful. The culture of appropriate sites of primary or concomitant infected foci, such as cellulitis (e.g., periorbital and buccal), middle ear effusions, sinusitis, and mastoiditis, and urine in young infants may yield the meningitis-causing pathogen. Petechiae often represent microemboli, with bacteria (e.g., meningococci) present in the lesion. Gram-stained smears made from petechiae may provide immediate clues as to the identity of the invading microorganisms.

Tests of inflammatory responses, such as a total and differential peripheral white blood cell count, erythrocyte sedimentation rates, and measurement of C-reactive protein concentration, may be helpful diagnostically and during the treatment of invasive bacterial disease. Such tests are not useful, however, in making or excluding a diagnosis of bacterial meningitis.

Brain Imaging

Neuroimaging studies, such as CT, MRI, and cranial sonography (in young infants with access through open fontanel), should be used in patients with signs of increased intracranial pressure (e.g., depressed consciousness, sluggishly reactive or dilated pupils, ophthalmoplegia, retinal changes, abnormal respiratory patterns, and cardiovascular

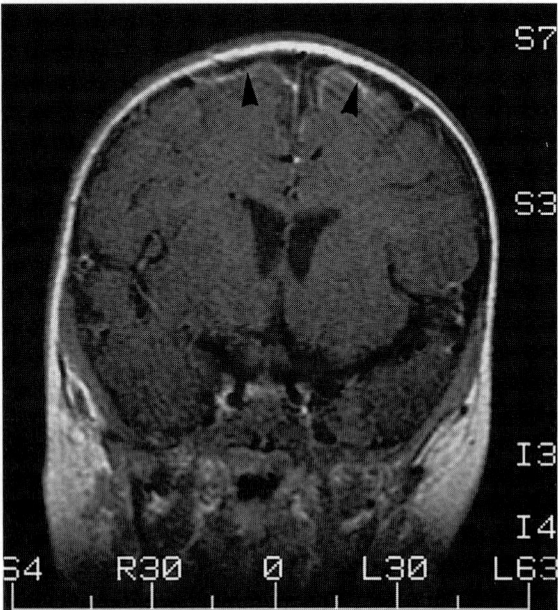

FIGURE 68-1. Postcontrast coronal magnetic resonance image of a 6-month-old infant with *Streptococcus pneumoniae* meningitis. Meningeal enhancement is visible *(arrowheads)*. (Courtesy of Blaine Hart, MD.)

instability). Increased intracranial pressure usually is caused by fulminant cerebral edema or other intracranial complications, such as subdural collection, thrombosis, infarction, brain abscess, and hydrocephalus [Ashwal, 1995; Tunkel and Sheld, 1995].

MRI has improved resolution compared with CT, provides additional insights into the pathogenesis of neurologic complications, and eventually may replace CT in most situations [Smith and Caldemeyer, 1999]. Cortical enhancement may be identified and is presumed to indicate cerebritis. Repeat imaging is useful in following the evolution of abnormalities [Bodino et al., 1982] and in determining the need for subsequent intervention. Abnormalities on imaging are associated with an unfavorable outcome [Packer et al., 1982]. Contrast MRI, although not usually considered a diagnostic test for meningitis, can show meningeal enhancement (Fig. 68-1) [Kioumehr et al., 1995; Runge et al., 1995].

Complications

Pathophysiologic Changes

BLOOD-BRAIN BARRIER DISRUPTION

The permeability of the blood-brain barrier increases in meningitis as a result of disrupted intercellular tight junctions and increased transendothelial pinocytosis [Quagliarello et al., 1986]. Inflammatory components, including granulocytes and matrix metalloproteinases, contribute to the increased permeability of the blood-brain barrier [Leppert et al., 2001]. This increased permeability results in increased extravasation of serum components and contributes to vasogenic brain edema but also allows for approximately fivefold higher concentrations of antibiotics in the cerebrospinal fluid during therapy compared with the uninfected state.

BRAIN EDEMA

Brain edema during meningitis has vasogenic, cytotoxic, and interstitial components. Vasogenic cerebral edema is primarily a consequence of increased blood-brain barrier permeability (see earlier). Cytotoxic edema results from an increase in intracellular water after alterations of the cell membrane and loss of cellular homeostasis with influx of sodium and calcium into the cell. Cytotoxic mechanisms include ischemia and the effect of excitatory amino acids [Derugin et al., 2000]. Interstitial edema occurs as a result of an increase in cerebrospinal fluid volume, through either increased cerebrospinal fluid production (increased blood flow in the choroid plexus) or decreased resorption secondary to increased cerebrospinal fluid outflow resistance across the arachnoid villi system of the sagittal sinus [Scheld et al., 1980]. The major dangers of extensive brain edema during meningitis are herniation of brain tissue and compression of the brainstem secondary to increased intracranial pressure, which can cause complete cessation of cerebral circulation (Table 68-3). Brain edema contributes substantially to the acute fatal outcome of bacterial meningitis [Winkler et al., 2002].

HYPONATREMIA, DEHYDRATION, AND INAPPROPRIATE SECRETION OF ANTIDIURETIC HORMONE

Patients with acute meningitis often present with hypovolemia secondary to dehydration, and some develop hyponatremia. Based on clinical signs, it is impossible to distinguish between hyponatremia secondary to dehydration and the syndrome of inappropriate antidiuretic hormone secretion (SIADH) in patients with meningitis. It also is unclear how frequently the hyponatremia is related to SIADH with secondary fluid retention [Moller et al., 2001]. SIADH results in hypotonicity of extracellular fluid, which in meningitis may contribute to cytotoxic edema [Kaplan and Feigin, 1978]. The overall risk of worsened clinical outcome owing to SIADH seems small, however, and does not justify routine fluid restrictions in patients with meningitis and hyponatremia because fluid restriction may have harmful effects on systemic blood pressure and cerebral perfusion. In cases of severe or persistent hyponatremia, SIADH should be excluded with appropriate laboratory tests.

INTRACRANIAL HYPERTENSION

Increased intracranial pressure is present early in most patients with bacterial meningitis. In infants with open fon-

TABLE 68-3

Common Neurologic Sequelae after Bacterial Meningitis

DEFICIT	APPROXIMATE FREQUENCY (%)
Hearing loss	15–30
Parenchymal damage	5–30
Cerebral palsy	5–10
Learning disabilities	5–20
Seizure disorders	<5
Cortical blindness	<5
Cerebral herniation	3–20
Hydrocephalus	2–3

tanels and symptoms compatible with meningitis, the full fontanel may lead to the correct diagnosis. Early in the course of meningitis, cerebral hyperemia may be the most important mechanism of intracranial pressure elevation. In more advanced stages, brain edema is probably the most important factor contributing to increased intracranial pressure, but obstructive hydrocephalus, cerebritis, cerebral infarction, cerebral venous thrombosis, status epilepticus, and SIADH also contribute to increases in intracranial pressure [Brown and Feigin, 1994].

Markedly elevated intracranial pressure during meningitis contributes to brain injury by compromising cerebral blood flow and leading to cerebral herniation in the most severe cases. The symptoms of massively increased intracranial pressure in meningitis are seizures and coma. In very advanced disease, signs of critical impairment of cerebral blood flow or impending herniation are observed, such as unresponsive pupils, decorticate or decerebrate posturing, abnormal respiratory patterns, bradycardia, elevated blood pressure, and irregular vital signs.

CEREBRAL BLOOD FLOW CHANGES

In the early phase of bacterial meningitis, an increase in cerebral blood flow is observed, which seems to be mediated by nitric oxide and oxidative radicals resulting from the inflammation in the cerebrospinal fluid space. As the disease progresses, cerebral blood flow reductions are observed globally and focally [Pfister et al., 1992]. Global cerebral blood flow reduction is the result of reduced cerebral perfusion pressure because of increased intracranial pressure, systemic hypotension, or both, in the setting of impaired cerebral blood flow autoregulation. Focal ischemia is the result of vascular involvement of cerebral arteries and veins by the subarachnoid space inflammation [Pfister et al., 1992]. Reactive oxygen radicals and endothelins, a family of vasoactive peptides released into the cerebrospinal fluid during bacterial meningitis, contribute to reductions of cerebral blood flow [Koedel et al., 1997; Pfister et al., 2000]. Several clinical studies have found an association between severe cerebral blood flow reduction and adverse outcome in children and adults with meningitis, making ischemia an important mediator of brain damage in meningitis [Ashwal et al., 1992; Förderreuther et al., 1992; Odio et al., 1991].

Seizures

Seizures complicate 20% to 30% of cases of childhood bacterial meningitis. Patients with severe illness are more likely to have seizures. They occur most frequently 2 to 3 days into the illness and cease 1 to 3 days later. Seizures may be focal or generalized, and the electroencephalogram may be normal or may show generalized or focal epileptiform abnormalities, focal slowing, or only background slowing. The functional and structural alterations of the brain resulting from the meningitic process that may induce seizures include vasculitis and infarction, fever, electrolyte imbalances, and metabolic changes. Chronic seizures after recovery from meningitis are approximately threefold more common in patients than in age-matched control children [Bedford et al., 2001].

Deafness and Cranial Nerve Damage

Deafness is the most frequent neurologic sequela of bacterial meningitis. Of patients with bacterial meningitis, 5% to 30% develop clinical deafness (see Table 68-3), and the risk is highest when meningitis is caused by *S. pneumoniae*. Low cerebrospinal fluid glucose concentrations are another risk factor for hearing loss [Eisenhut et al., 2003]. Hearing impairment after meningitis can improve for several months, but many children have severe, permanent, and bilateral hearing loss [Wellman et al., 2003]. Typically, sensorineural hearing loss in both ears is found; rarely a conductive hearing loss associated with a middle ear infection may be present. Hearing should be assessed in children with bacterial meningitis before discharge. Audiometry is an appropriate test in older children. In young infants, brainstem auditory-evoked responses or transient otoacoustic emissions can be used to detect hearing loss early [Cohen et al., 1988; Francois et al., 1997]. When hearing loss occurs, early intervention by a team that is knowledgeable in the management of this problem in infants and children should be encouraged. Cochlear implants are a consideration in the most severe cases.

Experimental studies suggest that bacteria reach the cochlea primarily via the cochlear aqueduct [Bhatt et al., 1993]. The deafness is caused by infection and inflammation in the cochlea [Klein et al., 2003]. Nitric oxide, other inflammatory mediators, and bacterial products, specifically the pneumococcal toxin pneumolysin, contribute to the loss of hairy cells in the cochlea [Amaee et al., 1995].

Other cranial nerve abnormalities develop in bacterial meningitis because of the involvement of the cranial nerves by the inflammatory process in the subarachnoid space. Increased intracranial pressure also can cause cranial nerve dysfunction by pressure or stretching. Cranial nerves VI and III are involved relatively frequently. Ocular palsies are usually reversible.

Neuronal Damage

The neurologic sequelae after meningitis, in addition to hearing loss (see previously), include focal sensorimotor deficits, mental retardation, seizure disorders, and cortical blindness (see Table 68-3). Detailed studies of the neurologic outcome after bacterial meningitis have led to an appreciation of the significant long-term functional impairment resulting from the disease [Grimwood et al., 1995; Bedford et al., 2001; Oostenbrink et al., 2002]. In a cohort of 5-year-old children who had survived bacterial meningitis during their first year of life, there was a 10-fold increase in the risk of moderate-to-severe disabilities, with 7.5% demonstrating learning difficulties; 8.1%, neuromotor disabilities; 7.3%, seizure disorders; 25.8%, hearing problems; and 11.9%, behavioral problems [Bedford et al., 2001]. Neurologic sequelae of childhood meningitis can persist at least into young adulthood, impairing learning during the entire time that children go to school [Grimwood et al., 2000]. *S. pneumoniae* consistently was associated with higher rates of disabilities than infection with *H. influenzae* or *N. meningitidis* [Grimwood et al., 1996].

Meningitis causes brain damage of cortical and subcortical structures (Fig. 68-2). For much of the brain damage,

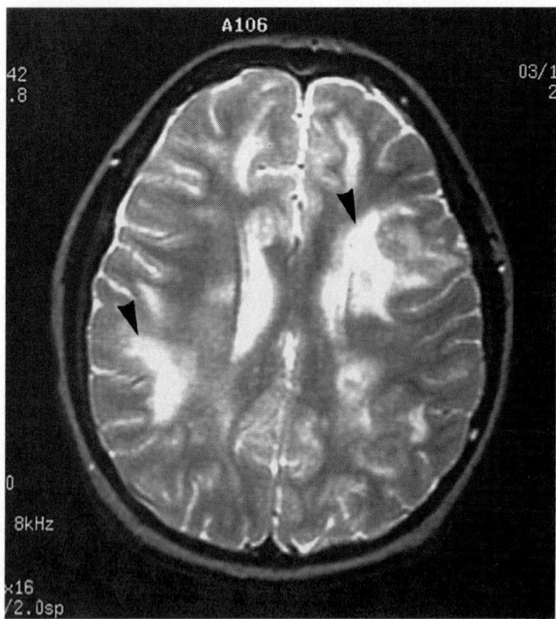

FIGURE 68-2. Axial T2-weighted MRI of 13-year-old child with *Neisseria meningitidis* meningitis complicated by multiple areas of cerebritis (*arrowheads* and other locations). (Courtesy of Blaine Hart, MD.)

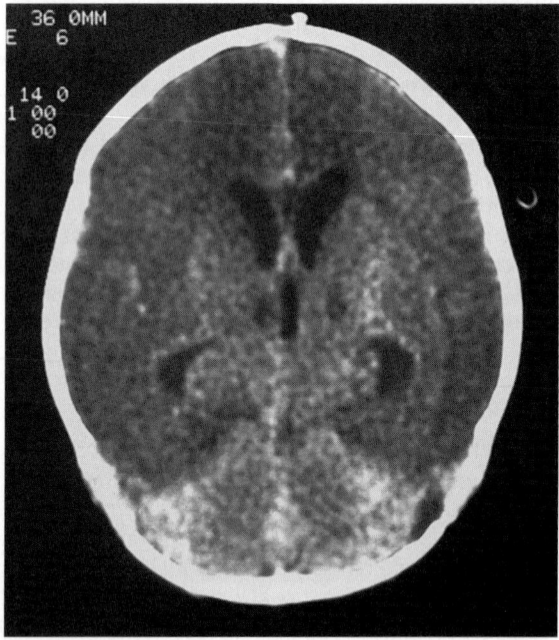

FIGURE 68-3. Computed tomography scan of 16-day-old neonate with group B streptococcal meningitis. There is massive infarction of anterior circulation. (Courtesy of Blaine Hart, MD.)

particularly in the cortex, ischemia represents an important mechanism of injury (Fig. 68-3) [Pfister et al., 2000]. In keeping with this notion, inhibition of excitatory amino acids and preservation of cerebral blood flow through inhibition of reactive oxygen radicals or endothelins are protective in experimental meningitis [Meli et al., 2002]. Matrix metalloproteinases, in addition to their effect on the blood-brain barrier and on cytokine release, also may contribute directly to ischemic changes in the brain.

A structure frequently damaged during meningitis is the dentate gyrus of the hippocampus. This structure is important for learning and memory acquisition and represents one of the few areas of the brain where neurogenesis is ongoing throughout life. Within this structure, pathology studies in humans dying from meningitis and animal models of meningitis consistently have documented damage to neurons [Gianinazzi et al., 2003; Nau et al., 1999]. Two forms of injury seem to affect the dentate gyrus neurons [Bifrare et al., 2003]. One is mediated by activation of caspase-3 and corresponds to classic apoptosis. This form of injury preferentially affects immature, postmitotic neurons, is associated with learning deficits in experimental animals surviving meningitis, and may represent an anatomic substrate for cognitive impairment and learning disabilities after meningitis [Bifrare et al., 2003; Leib et al., 2003]. The other form of dentate gyrus injury exhibits no obvious selectivity for a subset of neuronal cells and is associated with translocation of apoptosis-inducing factor. At least in the infant rat model, *S. pneumoniae* primarily induces apoptotic damage in immature neurons, whereas group B streptococcal meningitis leads to apoptosis-inducing factor–associated meningitis [Bifrare et al., 2003]. For both forms of dentate gyrus injury, the exact molecular triggers are unknown, but ischemia does not seem to be important. Potential mediators include pneumococcal products (pneumolysin and hydrogen peroxide), inflammatory mediators (e.g., tumor necrosis factor-α), matrix metalloproteinases, excitatory amino acids, reactive oxygen species, and others [Meli et al., 2002].

Hydrocephalus

Meningitis leads to disturbances of cerebrospinal fluid homeostasis with increased cerebrospinal fluid production and reduced cerebrospinal fluid absorption across the sagittal sinus–arachnoid villi system [Scheld et al., 1980]. In the acute phase, these disturbances can lead to ventriculomegaly associated with intracranial hypertension. This form of ventriculomegaly is frequently transient. Chronic hydrocephalus occurs as a long-term sequela of bacterial meningitis in infants and children (see Table 68-3). Its pathogenesis is either obstructive secondary to inflammatory changes of cerebrospinal fluid drainage pathways or ex vacuo secondary to loss of brain parenchyma. Chronic internal shunting with internal drainage is necessary in patients with persistent obstructive hydrocephalus.

Septic Shock and Disseminated Intravascular Coagulation

Bacterial meningitis can be complicated by sepsis and septic shock independent of the infecting organism. All patients with bacterial meningitis need to undergo close cardiovascular monitoring until they are clinically stabilized with antimicrobial and supportive therapy. The association of sepsis and extensive disseminated intravascular coagulation suggests infection caused by *N. meningitidis* [Yung and McDonald, 2003]. A similarly fulminant and devastating course can be seen with *S. pneumoniae* in patients without a functional spleen. These patients present with rapidly progressive signs of severe illness, rigors, severe muscular pain, and skin lesions that progress from an early maculopapular rash to petechiae to enlarging purpuric lesions [Yung and McDonald, 2003]. The organism sometimes can be visualized on Gram stain of scrapings from purpuric lesions. Signs and symptoms of meningitis often are not prominent in patients with disseminated meningococcal sepsis. Laboratory abnormalities include thrombocytopenia, hypofibrinogenemia, and massively elevated D-dimers. Overt adrenal insufficiency seems to be relatively rare in children with meningococcal disease [Riordan et al., 1999]. The most fulminant form of sepsis and disseminated intravascular coagulation is the Waterhouse-Friderichsen syndrome, which leads to sudden cardiovascular collapse associated with adrenal hemorrhage.

Extra-axial Fluid Collections

The subdural space is a potential intracranial space situated between the arachnoid and dura. Fluid can collect in the subdural space and in the subarachnoid space. The collection in the subarachnoid space may represent loculated cerebrospinal fluid, widening of the subarachnoid space in response to inflammation, or loss of brain parenchyma. Because imaging often cannot distinguish between a fluid collection and a widened subarachnoid space, the fluid collection as seen on imaging is referred to as an *extra-axial fluid collection.* Extra-axial fluid collections are found in 50% of children with bacterial meningitis who have cranial CT performed [Syrogiannopoulos et al., 1986].

Extra-axial fluid collections occur more commonly in bacterial meningitis during the first year of life and often are recognized during the first week of illness. The extra-axial fluid is preferentially situated over the convexities, may accumulate bilaterally, is serosanguineous with granulocytes and high protein concentrations, and is usually sterile (Fig. 68-4) [Snedeker et al., 1990]. Extra-axial fluid collections are detected often on imaging studies performed because of persistent fever, clinical signs of meningitis, seizures, or focal neurologic deficits. They may be the cause of persistent increase in intracranial pressure or focal neurologic deficits. More commonly, fluid collections represent a coincidental finding, and their causative role for the symptoms prompting the imaging studies is doubtful.

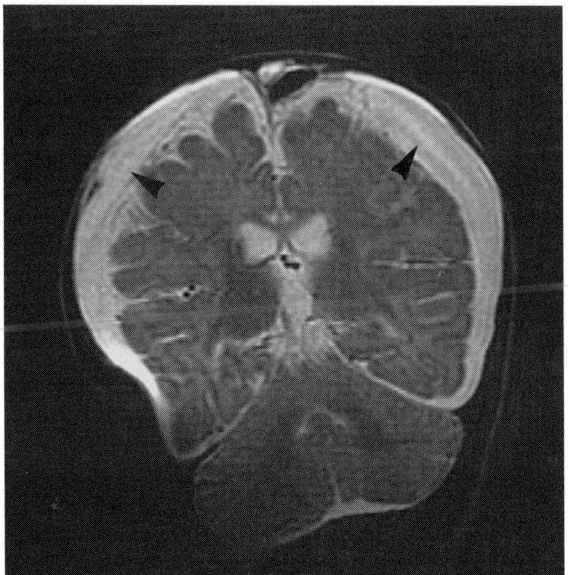

FIGURE 68-4. Coronal T2-weighted MRI of 6-month-old infant with *Streptococcus pneumoniae* meningitis. Massive extra-axial fluid collections are visible *(arrowheads).* (Courtesy of Blaine Hart, MD.)

Pathology

Subarachnoid space inflammation appears as a grayish yellow to green exudate covering the base and convexities of the brain. Histologic examination indicates that the exudate in acute bacterial meningitis consists predominantly of granulocytes; there is a mixture of lymphocytes, macrophages, and granulocytes in subacute to chronic forms of meningitis. Cerebral arteries and veins have focal infiltration of the vessel walls by the inflammatory cells. The inflammation of the vessel wall may be associated with thrombosis and vascular occlusion [Cairns and Russell, 1946]. In fatal cases of neonatal meningitis, inflammatory vasculitis is uniformly present, possibly indicating that the cerebral vasculature of the neonate is particularly susceptible to inflammatory damage [Berman and Banker, 1966]. Some of the severe structural damage in the neonatal brain after meningitis may be related to this susceptibility of the vasculature to inflammatory damage.

Damage to the brain parenchyma is manifested by signs of brain edema and frequently cerebral herniation (see later) and by areas of cerebral infarction resulting from ischemia [Arseni and Nereantiu, 1972; Berman and Banker, 1966]. Throughout the brain, there is loss of neurons, usually in a focal pattern, most extensively in patients who survived the acute meningitis for several days before succumbing to the disease. Neuronal loss is associated with a marked reaction of astrocytes and microglia.

In the dentate gyrus of the hippocampus, evidence of cell death of neurons seems common in meningitis based on limited pathologic studies in humans and extensive work in animal models [Nau et al., 1999]. Apoptotic neuronal cell death can be detected primarily in the subgranular zone of the dentate gyrus and is characterized morphologically by condensed, fragmented nuclei. The apoptotic nature of this form of cell death has been confirmed by the detection of fragmented DNA (i.e., TUNEL-stain) and activation of caspase-3 [Gianinazzi et al., 2003]. The second form of hippocampal neuronal damage is characterized by the appearance of uniformly shrunken, pyknotic nuclei forming clusters of damaged cells predominantly in the lower blade of the dentate gyrus [Leib et al., 1996]. This form of injury has been characterized primarily in animal models, and it is not clear to what extent it is found in humans.

Treatment

Antibiotics

Effective eradication of the infecting pathogen requires that antibiotics display bactericidal activity in the cerebrospinal fluid. Experimental studies have documented that cerebrospinal fluid concentrations that exceed the in vitro minimal inhibitory concentration severalfold (>10-fold for most antibiotics) are required to achieve maximal bacterial killing rates. Cerebrospinal fluid concentrations of antibiotics even with inflamed meninges are only a fraction of simultaneous serum concentration (usually between 5% and 25%), and antibiotics must be dosed higher for the treatment of meningitis than for most other infections [Täuber and Sande, 1990].

Empiric therapy should be instituted rapidly in all children with suspected bacterial meningitis. The progressive pathophysiologic alterations during meningitis, which rapidly lead to brain damage and death in most untreated patients, strongly suggest that any delay in antibiotic treatment may be harmful and should be avoided [Aronin et al., 1998]. In practice, the appropriate sequence of obtaining cerebrospinal fluid and blood for cultures and other tests, instituting antibiotics, and obtaining imaging studies to exclude mass lesions and other pathologies needs to be adapted to the individual patient. The sicker the patient and the more rapidly progressive the disease, the more urgent is the start of antibiotic therapy. Antibiotic therapy should not be delayed by more than approximately 15 minutes in critically ill patients for an attempt to obtain cerebrospinal fluid or blood, despite the reduced yield of bacterial cultures if the samples are obtained after initiation of antibiotics. A CT scan is required before the lumbar puncture in all patients in whom there is suspicion of important CNS alterations, particularly if a mass lesion is suspected, and the patient has signs of increased intracranial pressure. In adults, criteria have been established to identify patients with suspected meningitis in whom a lumbar puncture can be performed safely [Hasbun et al., 2001]. Whether these criteria are valid in children has not been established. The contraindications for lumbar puncture were discussed earlier.

The choice of empiric antibiotics depends on the suspected pathogens and their antibiotic susceptibilities, which may display regional differences. All pathogens commonly encountered in a particular patient population should be covered empirically, and rare pathogens should be empirically targeted in patients with corresponding risk factors (Tables 68-4 and 68-5). Recommended empiric treatment regimens adequate for patients without additional risk factors are shown in Table 68-6. When the causative pathogen has been isolated, and antibiotic sensitivities are known, therapy should be adjusted to cover the respective pathogen optimally (see later).

TABLE 68-4

Common Causes of Acute Bacterial Meningitis According to Age

AGE	PATHOGEN
0–4 wk	*Streptococcus agalactiae* *Escherichia coli* *Listeria monocytogenes* *Streptococcus pneumoniae*
1–3 mo	*E. coli* *L. monocytogenes* *Neisseria meningitidis* *S. agalactiae* *S. pneumoniae* *Haemophilus influenzae*
3 mo–18 y	*N. meningitidis* *S. pneumoniae* *H. influenzae*

TABLE 68-5

Rare Causes of Bacterial Meningitis in Infants and Children

PATHOGEN	PREDISPOSING FACTORS
Staphylococcus aureus	Trauma, neurosurgery, shunt
Staphylococcus epidermidis	Trauma, neurosurgery, shunt
Enterococcus faecalis	Neonatal period
Group A streptococcus	Pharyngitis, sepsis
Viridans streptococci	Endocarditis, anatomic defect
Moraxella	Otitis media
*Escherichia coli**	Urinary tract infection, immunosuppression
Klebsiella pneumoniae	Immunosuppression
Salmonella	Sickle cell disease, immunosuppression
Proteus	Neonatal period, immunosuppression
Citrobacter	Neonatal period, immunosuppression
Other Enterobacteriaceae	Immunosuppression
Pseudomonas aeruginosa	Immunosuppression
Pasteurella multocida	Animal bites
Francisella tularensis	Wild animal contacts
Propionibacterium acnes	Shunt
Nocardia	Chronic pulmonary disease

*Rare past the neonatal period.

TABLE 68-6

Recommendations for Empiric Antibiotic Therapy of Bacterial Meningitis

PATIENTS AND SPECIAL MODIFYING CIRCUMSTANCES	ANTIBIOTIC	DOSAGE (IV)
Neonate/infant <3 mo	Ampicillin *plus*	50-100 mg/kg q6-8h
	Cefotaxime *or*	100 mg/kg q8h
	Gentamicin	2.5 mg/kg q8h
Neonate preterm, low birth weight	Vancomycin *plus*	15 mg/kg q8-24h
	Ceftazidime	100 mg/kg q8-12h
>3 mo to <50 yr	Ceftriaxone *or*	100 mg/kg q24h (max. 4 g q24h)
	Cefotaxime	100 mg/kg q8h (max. 12 g per day)
Drug-resistant *Streptococcus pneumoniae*	Ceftriaxone *plus*	100 mg/kg q24h (max. 4 g q24h)
	Rifampin *or*	10–20 mg/kg q24h (max. 600 mg q24h)
	Vancomycin	15 mg/kg q6h (max. 500 mg q6h)
Neurosurgery, CSF shunt, or head trauma	Ceftazidime *plus*	100 mg/kg q8h (max. 12 g per day)
	Nafcillin *or* Flucloxacillin	50 mg/kg q6h (max. 12 g per day)
	(or Vancomycin *plus*	15 mg/kg q6h (max. 500 mg q6h)
	Aminoglycoside)	2.0-2.5 mg/kg q8h

CSF, cerebrospinal fluid.

The proper duration of therapy is not well defined. Meningitis caused by *N. meningitidis* can be treated for 5 to 7 days, and even shorter durations have been found to be effective [Viladrich et al., 1986]. For *S. pneumoniae* or *H. influenzae,* 10 to 14 days is deemed appropriate. Meningitis caused by Enterobacteriaceae, *L. monocytogenes,* or other unusual pathogens may require treatment courses of 3 weeks. Antibiotic therapy should not be prolonged past the recommended durations because of a persistent fever in a child who has otherwise displayed a favorable clinical response. Other causes for fever, such as drug fever, intravenous line infections, other undiagnosed infections, and extra-axial fluid collections, should be considered.

STREPTOCOCCUS PNEUMONIAE

For sensitive *S. pneumoniae,* penicillin G remains the drug of choice, and third-generation cephalosporins (ceftriaxone or cefotaxime) are effective alternatives. Increasing resistance against β-lactam antibiotics is observed worldwide, regarding the prevalence of resistant strains and increasing levels of resistance [Jones et al., 2004]. Penicillin and chloramphenicol are ineffective against strains displaying any degree of resistance, whereas third-generation cephalosporins may fail in highly penicillin-resistant strains. A combination of a third-generation cephalosporin with vancomycin is most commonly recommended for these strains [Bradley and Scheld, 1997]. Dexamethasone reduces cerebrospinal fluid concentrations of vancomycin in adults but apparently not in children. Rifampicin can be used instead of vancomycin, if the strain is sensitive. There is currently limited clinical experience with newer quinolones [Saez-Llorens et al., 2002], which look promising in experimental meningitis [Cottagnoud and Täuber, 2004]. In these models, the newer quinolones display strong synergism with β-lactams or vancomycin, and these combinations may provide a treatment option in cases caused by high-level resistant pneumococci.

HAEMOPHILUS INFLUENZAE

Ampicillin is the drug of choice for sensitive *H. influenzae,* but 5% to 30% of strains worldwide are resistant to ampicillin owing to a β-lactamase. These strains are best treated with a third-generation cephalosporin. Rapid spread of non–β-lactamase–producing, ampicillin-resistant *H. influenzae* type b strains has been reported from Japan [Hasegawa et al., 2004]. These strains exhibit mutations in their penicillin-binding proteins and increased minimal inhibitory concentration to cephalosporins. Optimal treatment of these strains may require the combination of high-dose third-generation cephalosporins with meropenem or possibly a fluoroquinolone [Hasegawa et al., 2004].

NEISSERIA MENINGITIDIS

Most strains of *N. meningitidis* are sensitive to penicillin G, which continues to be the drug of choice. An increase in penicillin minimal inhibitory concentration has been documented in occasional strains, but the third-generation cephalosporins remain universally active and are a reliable alternative to penicillin [Canica et al., 2004].

GROUP B STREPTOCOCCI

Group B streptococcal meningitis in neonates is treated with penicillin G, to which the streptococci have retained universal sensitivity. Third-generation cephalosporins also are active. Whether addition of an aminoglycoside results in a clinical benefit has not been resolved in controlled studies.

LISTERIA MONOCYTOGENES

The best treatment of *L. monocytogenes* meningitis is an aminopenicillin. Based on data in rabbits, which indicated increased bactericidal activity of the combination of penicillin with gentamicin [Scheld et al., 1979], an aminoglycoside usually is added to penicillin. Trimethoprim-sulfamethoxazole is used in patients who cannot tolerate penicillin.

GRAM-NEGATIVE BACILLI

E. coli, Klebsiella, and *Pseudomonas aeruginosa* are among the more frequent causes of gram-negative bacillary meningitis. Treatment options include third-generation cephalosporins, fluoroquinolones, aminoglycosides, and meropenem. Given the unpredictability of resistance in these organisms, treatment has to be based on sensitivity testing. In severe and difficult-to-treat cases, the combination of a β-lactam with an aminoglycoside can be used. The aminoglycoside can be administered intrathecally in desperate cases.

STAPHYLOCOCCI

Most *S. aureus* strains express a penicillinase, and a penicillinase-resistant penicillin (nafcillin or flucloxacillin, depending on availability) is used to treat meningitis. If the infecting strain is methicillin resistant, vancomycin must be used. Experiences with newer drugs active against gram-positive pathogens (linezolide, streptogramins, lipopeptides) in the treatment of meningitis do not support their routine use for meningitis [Cottagnoud and Täuber, 2004]. *Staphylococcus epidermidis* is encountered mostly in shunt infections. The organism is often resistant to β-lactams, in which case it has to be treated with vancomycin. The combination of systemic and intraventricular administration of vancomcycin may achieve the highest concentrations at the site of infection. Whenever possible, the infected shunt should be removed and, if necessary, replaced by a temporary external drainage until the infection is cleared, and a new permanent shunt can be placed. Addition of rifampicin, if active against the infecting pathogen, can help clear the infection when the infected shunt cannot be removed.

Corticosteroids

In studies of experimental meningitis, corticosteroids reduce brain edema, reduce intracranial pressure, and stabilize the blood-brain barrier [Täuber et al., 1985]. The last effect is associated with a reduction of antibiotic concentrations in the cerebrospinal fluid to a degree that does not, with the possible exception of vancomycin, jeopardize antibacterial effectiveness. Corticosteroids, when given at the time of the first antibiotic dose, reduce the increase in inflammation in the cerebrospinal fluid that follows the release of proinflammatory bacterial products induced by the antibiotics [Saez-Llorens et al., 1991]. As a potential risk, dexamethasone increased the number of apoptotic cells in the dentate gyrus of animals with experimental meningitis and was associated with impaired learning in infant rats 3 weeks after pneumococcal meningitis [Leib et al., 2003]. The relevance of this observation for humans is currently unknown.

Dexamethasone has been tested in several controlled trials in patients with bacterial meningitis. Although some studies failed to prove a significant benefit, most studies found some beneficial effect on outcome with little toxicity and no adverse effect on clearing of bacteria from the cerebrospinal fluid [Van de Beek et al., 2003]. Based on a meta-analysis, dexamethasone reduces hearing loss in children with *H. influenzae* and possibly *S. pneumoniae* meningitis. Overall neurologic outcome also is improved in children with *H. influenzae* meningitis [Van de Beek et al., 2003]. A controlled study in adults found improved survival and overall outcome in patients with pneumococcal meningitis [De Gans et al., 2002].

Based on the available data, it seems reasonable to administer dexamethasone to all patients with strong clinical evidence of bacterial meningitis. Because the drug mitigates the inflammatory response after institution of antibiotics, it is best given shortly before or simultaneously with the first antibiotic dose [Odio et al., 1991]. The recommended dose is 0.15 mg/kg every 6 hours for a maximum of 4 days; 2 days is equally effective [Schaad et al., 1993]. It is not clear that the risk for major gastrointestinal bleeding is increased with dexamethasone, but patients should be examined for evidence of gastrointestinal blood loss. The course of nonbacterial meningitis is not adversely affected by dexamethasone [Waagner et al., 1990], but the drug temporarily reduces symptoms even if the empiric antimicrobial therapy is ineffective. Little experience exists with dexamethasone in the neonatal period, and the drug should not be used routinely in this patient population.

Approach to Seriously Ill Patients

The approach to the treatment of a seriously ill patient with meningitis is based on a careful clinical assessment, with special attention to the presence of complications such as seizures, sepsis, or dehydration; on an estimate of intracranial pressure at the time of lumbar puncture; and on neuroimaging studies, which can be categorized as follows: (1) normal scan, (2) cerebral edema, (3) hydrocephalus, (4) subdural effusions, and (5) cerebral infarction [Ashwal, 1995].

SEIZURES

Adequate ventilation and cardiovascular support must be ensured. There is no seizure treatment specific for meningitis-associated seizures. Drugs such as phenobarbital, fosphenytoin, diazepam, and lorazepam, individually or in combination, are used to control seizures.

SHOCK AND DISSEMINATED INTRAVASCULAR COAGULATION

Standard support for all vital systems in an intensive care setting must be provided to critically ill patients who have signs of sepsis, organ failure, and disseminated intravascular coagulopathy. A detailed discussion of these complex therapies is beyond the scope of this chapter. Attempts have been made to develop specific therapies for sepsis that are based on interfering with microbial mediators, host defense pathways, or coagulation pathways involved in the pathogenesis of sepsis. Although most of these attempts have failed in clinical trials, activated protein C (drotrecogin alfa) was found to improve organ failure, including disseminated intravascular coagulation, and survival in a large controlled trial [Bernard et al., 2001]. The limited data in children treated with drotrecogin alfa suggest that the drug can improve outcome in children with meningitis complicated by severe sepsis and disseminated intravascular coagulation. Contraindications include severe coagulopathy, trauma, and recent or impending invasive procedures, in particular procedures involving major vessels of the brain [Bernard et al., 2001].

FLUID BALANCE AND ELECTROLYTES

In bacterial meningitis, a balanced fluid status should be established and maintained. Fluid restriction does not improve outcome and should be limited to a subset of patients with specific indications [Singhi et al., 1995]. Dehydration is potentially harmful because of hypotension and intravascular sludging and thrombosis, all of which can adversely affect cerebral perfusion and increase ischemia [Moller et al., 2001; Tureen et al., 1992]. Many meningitis patients are dehydrated at diagnosis. Their fluid deficit should be corrected promptly, and appropriate maintenance fluid should be administered subsequently [Powell et al., 1990]. Usually the fluid is given as one quarter to one third normal saline in 5% dextrose. Substantial overhydration should be avoided, but its potential to exacerbate brain edema probably has been overestimated in the past [Täuber et al., 1993].

Treatment of SIADH secretion is fluid restriction. It is recommended that fluid restriction be instituted only when SIADH has been documented by appropriate laboratory tests, and the serum sodium concentration has declined to less than 125 mEq/liter. Rapid correction of severe hyponatremia may be harmful.

INTRACRANIAL HYPERTENSION

Invasive monitoring of intracranial pressure may be helpful in patients who have signs of severe meningitis, in particular patients with markedly reduced Glasgow Coma Scale and very high opening pressure on initial lumbar puncture. These patients usually must be mechanically ventilated. The P_{CO_2} should be maintained at the lower range of normal, but pronounced hyperventilation must be avoided because it can worsen cerebral ischemia [Ashwal et al., 1990]. Sedation or administration of a neuromuscular blocking agent may be necessary to enhance controlled ventilation. A paradigm for the management of seriously ill patients with bacterial meningitis using the results of intracranial pressure measurements and neuroimaging has been published [Ashwal, 1995].

In patients with cerebral edema on CT or MRI, administration of dexamethasone is indicated given its beneficial effects on brain edema and intracranial hypertension [Odio et al., 1991; Täuber et al., 1985]. Mannitol, 0.25 to 1 g/kg, can be administered intravenously over 20 to 30 minutes. This dose can be repeated every 2 to 4 hours, but the effect of subsequent doses progressively diminishes. Use of diuretics, such as furosemide (Lasix), 0.5 to 1 mg/kg, should be restricted to patients with evidence of fluid overload to avoid the adverse effects of fluid depletion and hypotension.

An alternative approach to lower severely increased intracranial pressure during meningitis has been pioneered by Scandinavian groups. Their protocol consists of a combination of (1) normalizing plasma colloidal osmotic pressure and blood volume with blood transfusions and albumin infusions; (2) antihypertensive therapy with β_1-antagonists and α_2-agonists; and (3) "antistress" therapy with a combination of thiopental, clonidine, and fentanyl. Although randomized controlled trials have not been performed, the published case series, which included children, documented pronounced effects on intracranial pressure and outcome, including the reversal of impending cerebral herniation, in most patients [Grande et al., 2002; Lindvall et al., 2004].

If the intracranial pressure is elevated in the presence of a normal CT scan or MRI, this may be due to increased intracranial blood or cerebrospinal fluid volume. Controlled ventilation and dexamethasone therapy should be applied in these patients. Whether other means to lower intracranial pressure are necessary in this situation must be decided based on the severity of intracranial hypertension and the response to therapy with dexamethasone.

CEREBRAL INFARCTION

In patients in whom neuroimaging studies reveal infarction, the treatment guidelines outlined earlier for increased intracranial pressure and fluid balance should be applied with particular care. Alternative therapies, such as use of barbiturates or hypothermia, have not been systematically studied in patients with stroke secondary to meningitis. The risk of severe intracranial bleeding seems to preclude the use of thrombolytic agents.

HYDROCEPHALUS

Patients with increased cerebrospinal fluid volume and normal intracranial pressure do not require treatment because spontaneous resolution of this abnormality occurs as the infection resolves. In patients with markedly elevated intracranial pressure as manifested by full fontanel, depressed consciousness, or signs of acutely jeopardized cerebral perfusion (i.e., new-onset focal neurologic deficits), ventricular drainage should be considered to reduce intracranial hypertension and improve cerebral perfusion pressure rapidly. The drainage should be to an external collection device because it is needed only transiently in most cases. In less acute situations, decreasing cerebrospinal fluid volume and pressure by one or more conventional therapies (furosemide, mannitol, dexamethasone) may be attempted.

SUBDURAL EFFUSION

Most extra-axial fluid collections resolve without intervention. If fever and clinical signs persist despite antibiotic therapy or if the fluid accumulates and acts as a mass, puncture of the fluid is indicated to exclude an empyema and to reduce possible mass effect.

Prognosis

Knowledge about factors associated with a poor prognosis is important in selecting patients for more intensive surveillance and treatment and in identifying candidates for new preventive or therapeutic strategies. Various studies have reported different and partially conflicting risk factors [Algren et al., 1993; Baraff et al., 1993; Kaaresen and Flaegstad, 1995; Kornelisse et al., 1995]. Table 68-7 summarizes the major prognostic factors.

Bacterial etiology has a substantial impact on outcome. A meta-analysis found a fourfold higher mortality from *S. pneumoniae* (15.3%) compared with *H. influenzae* (3.8%) and a corresponding twofold to threefold higher rate of neurologic sequelae (*S. pneumoniae* 15% to 30% versus *H. influenzae* 5% to 20%) [Kaaresen and Flaegstad, 1995; Kornelisse et al., 1995]. Although the mortality from *N. meningitidis* meningitis (7.5%) is midway between the other two principal etiologies of bacterial meningitis, sequelae from this infection are much less frequent (2% to 5%). This discrepancy is explained by the relatively frequent presence of sepsis with diffuse coagulopathy in patients with meningococcal meningitis [Algren et al., 1993]. The quantity of antigen in the initial cerebrospinal fluid specimen and the number of bacteria present (bacteriorrhachia) also are correlated significantly with sequelae of meningitis [Feldman et al., 1982].

Bacterial meningitis in newborns is associated with high mortality (15% to 30%), and 20% to 40% of survivors have permanent neurologic sequelae. Factors contributing to this poor prognosis are specific etiologies (e.g., gram-negative enteric bacilli), immaturity, delayed diagnosis, and concomitant disease [Schaad, 1992; Stevens et al., 2003].

Other indicators of poor outcome are focal neurologic findings (e.g., seizures), coma, cardiovascular compromise (e.g., peripheral vasoconstriction, shock), absence of fever, and less than 1000×10^6/liter leukocytes in cerebrospinal

TABLE 68-7

Risk Factors Associated with Poor Prognosis of Bacterial Meningitis

Etiology	*Streptococcus pneumoniae*
	Gram-negative enteric bacteria
	High bacterial titers
Patient	Newborn infant
	Decreased immune defense
Severity of disease on admission	Advanced disease
	Focal neurologic finding
	Coma
	Cardiovascular compromise
	Absence of fever
	$<1000 \times 10^6$/L leukocytes in CSF
Type of management	Need for intensive care
	Inadequate antibacterial therapy
	Lack of anti-inflammatory therapy
Course of meningitis	Delayed CSF sterilization
	High number/severity of complications

CSF, cerebrospinal fluid.

fluid at the time of admission. There is no clear association between duration of symptoms before diagnosis and outcome [Kaaresen and Flaegstad, 1995; Kilpi et al., 1993]. Relevant for the prognosis after diagnosis are management (e.g., intensive care, antibacterial and anti-inflammatory therapies); time to cerebrospinal fluid sterilization; and number and severity of complications such as seizures, cranial nerve palsies, coma, subdural effusion, and cerebral herniation (see Table 68-3) [Schaad, 1997].

Prevention

The goals of immunoprophylaxis and chemoprophylaxis are prevention of specific types of bacterial meningitis and limitation of the spread of disease when infection occurs.

Immunoprophylaxis

The available conjugate vaccines against *H. influenzae* type b are dramatically effective and extremely safe [Feigin et al., 1992; Rockowitz and Tunkel, 1995]. The vaccine prevents all invasive diseases resulting from bacteremia, including meningitis and epiglottitis. Concerted efforts to vaccinate all infants in all countries must continue.

Meningococcal disease remains a substantial problem worldwide, with approximately 1.2 million cases per year [Balmer and Miller, 2002]. Vaccines comprising the polysaccharide capsule of serogroups A, C, W-135, and Y have been available for approximately 25 years. These polysaccharide vaccines are not immunogenic in young children, however, and induce only short-lived protection. To improve the immunogenicity of the meningococcal serogroup C polysaccharide vaccine, a carrier protein was covalently attached, converting the vaccine to a T cell–dependent antigen, which can stimulate long-term immunity. This vaccine has proved to be successful in reducing the incidence of serogroup C meningococcal disease in various countries, including the United Kingdom [Miller et al., 2001], Spain [Salleras et al., 2001], and Canada [De Wals et al., 2001].

A comprehensive vaccine conferring protection against all disease-associated serogroups remains elusive. The major challenge in the prevention of meningococcal disease by vaccination is the development of an effective serogroup B meningococcal vaccine. Serogroup B disease is endemic in most industrialized countries, with the burden of disease occurring mainly in young children. The serogroup B capsular polysaccharide is poorly immunogenic, possibly because it shares homology with glycopeptides of neural cell adhesion molecules [Pon et al., 1997]. Advances in bacterial genomics and proteomics have provided new and promising approaches in the identification of novel vaccine candidates [Rappuoli, 2001; Pollard and Levin, 2000].

As is true for all meningeal pathogens, the polysaccharide capsule of *S. pneumoniae* is a critical virulence factor, helping the organism to avoid phagocytosis. Ninety different capsular serotypes have been identified. Vaccine development throughout most of the 20th century focused on using combinations of polysaccharides as the key vaccine components [Whitney, 2002].

As mentioned before, vaccines composed of polysaccharide antigens alone produce weak and short-lived immune responses in infants and toddlers. Conjugating pneumococcal polysaccharide to a carrier protein induces a T cell–dependent response that can occur even in early infancy. The first protein-polysaccharide conjugate pneumococcal vaccine that is safe and effective in infants and toddlers was approved in February 2000 in the United States and is now licensed for use in many other countries. The vaccine includes polysaccharide antigens for the seven most common serotypes occurring in children in the United States and in many other countries [Pelton and Klein, 2002]. Other conjugate vaccine formulations are being tested in young children. Clinical trials indicate that conjugate vaccines are highly efficacious against invasive pneumococcal disease, including meningitis, and modestly efficacious against otitis media and pneumonia [Giebink, 2001]. In carriage studies, conjugate vaccines reduced vaccine-type carriage but usually led to an increase in carriage of other serotypes. Remaining questions include whether less frequent transmission of vaccine serotypes would mean less disease in unvaccinated children and adults or conversely nonvaccine serotypes would begin to cause more disease. The seven-valent pneumococcal conjugate vaccine is now part of routine infant immunization in the United States and some other countries.

Chemoprophylaxis

Many studies have documented increased risk of disease in close contacts of index patients with invasive disease caused by *N. meningitidis* and *H. influenzae* type b [Feigin et al., 1992]. The risk is age dependent, and disease among unvaccinated household contacts younger than 4 years old is increased. The spread of such strains is a particular concern in daycare centers.

Chemoprophylactic regimens are aimed at eradicating nasopharyngeal carriage of potentially invasive bacteria, preventing further transmission and development of disease in people already colonized. The preferred drug is rifampicin (20 mg/kg/day, maximum daily dose 600 mg) for either 2 days (*N. meningitidis*) or 4 days (*H. influenzae*). Alternatives for the elimination of nasopharyngeal carriage of *N. meningitidis* include single doses of either ciprofloxacin or ceftriaxone. Because treatment for bacterial meningitis with β-lactam antibiotics does not eradicate the organism from the nasopharynx, chemoprophylaxis also is recommended for the index patient before discharge.

Careful observation of exposed persons is essential for identifying early signs of disease and initiating therapy, independent of whether they received chemoprophylaxis or not because chemoprophylaxis is far from being 100% effective. Cultures of the upper respiratory tract in contacts are not useful in the care of exposed persons and are valuable only in epidemiologic investigations.

Numerous studies have found that maternal intrapartum chemoprophylaxis can prevent maternal febrile morbidity and early-onset neonatal group B streptococcal disease, including meningitis [Krohn et al, 1999]. Guidelines recommend the use of a risk-based or a screening-based approach to identify candidates for intrapartum prophylaxis with amoxicillin [Schrag et al, 2000]. Alternative algorithms combining the two strategies are also in use [Boyer and Gotoff, 1998].

Recurrent Acute Bacterial Meningitis

Recurrent bacterial meningitis is rare and must prompt a careful evaluation for either an anatomic defect facilitating access of bacteria to the cerebrospinal fluid space or an immunologic deficit. Anatomic defects can be acquired or developmental [Schick et al., 1997] and typically lead to meningitis caused by *S. pneumoniae* or rarely *H. influenzae*. Defects may involve the temporal bone or the anterior skull base and are not always associated with cerebrospinal fluid rhinorrhea or otorrhea. Developmental defects include meningomyelocele, dermal sinus, or neurenteric cyst and malformations of the inner ear. Contrast-enhanced high-resolution CT, MRI cisternography, and search for cerebrospinal fluid leakage into the nose or middle ear can help identify an anatomic defect [Drummond et al., 1999; Meco and Oberascher, 2004]. If such a defect is found, surgical correction is indicated.

Among the immunologic conditions predisposing to recurrent meningitis, deficiencies of the latter components of the complement pathway (C5 through C9) or properdin (alternative pathway) have been associated with recurrent infections caused by *Neisseria* [Overturf, 2003]. Functional or anatomic asplenia, agammaglobulinemia, and deficiencies of the early components of complement (C1 through C3) have been associated with recurrent episodes of meningitis caused by *S. pneumoniae, H. influenzae,* and *N. meningitidis* [Overturf, 2003]. Commonly, children with congenital immunodeficiencies have a history of frequent infections other than meningitis. After a second episode of bacterial meningitis, immunoglobulin levels, total complement activity (CH50), and possibly individual complement components should be determined. Splenic function should be assessed, if there is a risk for splenic dysfunction (e.g., sickle cell anemia) or congenital asplenia (e.g., congenital heart disease). Identified deficiencies should be corrected where possible, and chronic antibiotic prophylaxis must be considered in children at high risk for recurrent, severe infections (e.g., in children with asplenia).

Conditions other than bacterial meningitis are frequently the cause of recurrent meningitis, but these are rare in children. They include Behçet's syndrome, sarcoidosis, and Mollaret's meningitis associated with recurrent herpes simplex infection [Ginsberg, 2004]. Acute meningitis indistinguishable clinically from bacterial meningitis can result from an allergic reaction to drugs (e.g., trimethoprim-sulfamethoxazole, nonsteroidal anti-inflammatory drugs, and intravenous immunoglobulins).

CHRONIC BACTERIAL MENINGITIS

Chronic bacterial meningitis evolves over days to weeks. Patients complain of headaches, often associated with constitutional signs of infection (fever, anorexia). Nuchal rigidity may be subtle or absent in cases of chronic meningitis. Many forms of chronic meningitis involve the base of the brain and lead to cranial nerve palsies. As the syndrome progresses, signs of brain involvement with seizures, mental status changes such as confusion or hallucinations, and focal neurologic deficits may develop. Hydrocephalus and increased intracranial pressure also may accompany the syndrome. The bacterial causes of chronic meningitis include tuberculosis, Lyme borreliosis, syphilis, and leptospirosis. Other etiologies of chronic meningitis include fungal infections, such as *Cryptococcus neoformans* or *Coccidioides immitis*, viral infections (e.g., cytomegalovirus, human immunodeficiency virus), and noninfectious causes (e.g., neoplasms, sarcoidosis).

Tuberculous Meningitis

Epidemiology and Pathogenesis

Tuberculosis remains one of the most prevalent infections worldwide. *Mycobacterium tuberculosis* is transmitted by respiratory aerosols and frequently infects infants and children, particularly in developing countries. CNS involvement is a life-threatening extrapulmonary manifestation of tuberculosis, and 1% to 2% of children with untreated tuberculosis develop meningitis [Starke, 1999]. Tuberculous meningitis is rare before 3 months of age but increases during the first 5 years of life. A history of close contact with a known case of tuberculosis is often found in children with CNS tuberculosis.

Tuberculosis of the CNS follows the dissemination of tuberculosis after primary infection, usually in the lung. During the primary disease, or on reactivation later in life, tubercle bacilli can be discharged into the subarachnoid space from a caseous subependymal lesion. Multiplying organisms induce basilar meningitis but also can cause focal parenchymal infections (tuberculomas). The inflammatory exudate in the subarachnoid space affects cerebral vessels and cranial nerves, resulting in ischemic changes and cranial nerve palsies. Hydrocephalus is often present already at the time of diagnosis and can be communicating or noncommunicating.

Clinical Characteristics

Tuberculous meningitis usually evolves over several days to a few weeks, although an acute onset is found in about half of the affected children. Initial symptoms are vague and consist of generally poor health, irritability, and apathy (stage I). In young infants, fever, cough, altered consciousness, bulging anterior fontanel, and generalized tonic-clonic seizures are presenting symptoms [Tung et al., 2002]. In older children, low-grade fever, nausea, vomiting, headache, and abdominal pain occur [Farinha et al., 2000]. Nuchal rigidity is not prominent. In stage II, unilateral or bilateral cranial nerve deficits result from the basilar meningitis. Neuro-ophthalmologic changes, including retrobulbar neuritis, gaze palsies, and lesions of the chorioretina, are common [Amitava et al., 2001]. As the disease progresses to stage III, the patient develops depression of consciousness, convulsions, possibly papilledema, and major neurologic deficits. Tuberculosis can involve the spinal cord directly, by pressure from vertebral abscess, and by the production of arachnoiditis [Hernandez-Albujar et al., 2000]. Many patients present with hyponatremia, either on the basis of SIADH or, less commonly, as a cerebral salt-wasting syndrome [Farinha et al., 2000].

Diagnosis

Head CT and MRI document findings similar to those of bacterial meningitis, especially around the base of the brain,

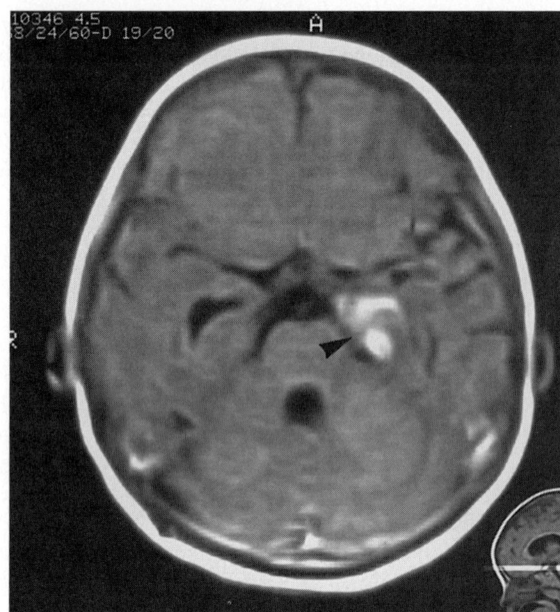

FIGURE 68-5. Postcontrast coronal low-field MRI of 16-month-old child with *Mycobacterium tuberculosis* meningitis. A tuberculoma is present *(arrowhead)*. (Courtesy of Blaine Hart, MD.)

and may reveal parenchymal lesions, infarction, and tuberculomas (Fig. 68-5). Hydrocephalus is found in most patients [Farinha et al., 2000]. Intracranial tuberculomas, which continue to be found frequently in countries with a high prevalence of tuberculosis, present with symptoms of a space-occupying lesion with headache, seizures, and other focal neurologic symptoms. Imaging is essential in the diagnosis of spinal involvement [Bernaerts et al., 2003]. CT or MRI of the spine is indicated in a child with suspected tuberculosis and neurologic signs of cord involvement. Chest radiographs are commonly abnormal with lymphadenopathy or pulmonary infiltrates but can be normal [Yaramis et al., 1998]. Fifty percent of patients with tuberculous meningitis have a negative tuberculin skin test [Starke, 1999].

The cerebrospinal fluid opening pressure is often elevated. The cerebrospinal fluid seldom contains more than 500 cells/mm^3, most of which are lymphocytes. Protein content is elevated but rarely greater than 500 mg/dL. Glucose concentration usually is decreased to varying degrees [Farinha et al., 2000]. Detection of the infecting organism in cerebrospinal fluid is notoriously difficult. Large quantities of cerebrospinal fluid (10 mL, if possible) should be collected and examined for acid-fast bacilli. Culture and detection of the *M. tuberculosis* genome may yield the diagnosis, but in a substantial proportion of cases, all tests remain negative [Farinha et al., 2000]. Repeated cerebrospinal fluid studies may allow the diagnosis to be established.

Treatment

The appearance of organisms resistant to antituberculous drugs is an increasing problem in several areas of the world. Isoniazid, rifampin, ethambutol, pyrazinamide, and streptomycin remain the first-line drugs for the treatment for tuberculous meningitis caused by sensitive organisms. Newer fluoroquinolones also are highly active against tuberculosis, and although their role for the treatment of tuberculous meningitis has not been clearly delineated, they may represent a backup option in difficult-to-treat cases. Initial therapy is started with four drugs for 2 months (isoniazid, rifampicin, pyrazinamide, and ethambutol or streptomycin), particularly when strains resistant to first-line drugs are a possibility. After 2 months, treatment is reduced to two active drugs based on sensitivity testing, with rifampin and isoniazid as first choices [Shingadia and Novelli, 2003]. Pyridoxine is recommended in malnourished children to prevent isoniazid-induced peripheral neuropathy [Shingadia and Novelli, 2003]. Response to antituberculous treatment usually is evident within 2 weeks. Therapy should be continued for at least 9 to 12 months, and in patients with slow responses, extensive disease or resistant organisms necessitating treatment with second-line drugs, for 18 to 24 months. Treatment of pulmonary tuberculosis in children reduces the incidence of CNS infection. Surgical shunting procedures may be necessary for hydrocephalus, particularly in cases of noncommunicating hydrocephalus [Schoeman et al., 2002].

Corticosteroids seem to reduce the mortality and the morbidity from inflammation and subsequent fibrosis in patients with tuberculous meningitis [Schoeman et al., 1997]. Their use is advocated, particularly in patients with a decreased level of consciousness, papilledema, focal deficits, or elevated intracranial pressure. A course of prednisone or dexamethasone for 6 weeks with subsequent tapering over several weeks is the most common regimen recommended.

The mortality of tuberculous meningitis is 10% to 20%. Major sequelae occur and are most common in children in stage III. Visual and auditory impairments are common, as are hemiparesis, mental retardation, and seizures [Schoeman et al., 2002]. Involvement of the hypothalamus and basal cisterns leads to endocrinopathies, such as diabetes insipidus, growth retardation, sexual precocity, and obesity.

Syphilis

Epidemiology and Pathogenesis

Syphilis, which is caused by the spirochete *Treponema pallidum,* remains an important and prevalent sexually transmitted disease worldwide. The introduction of penicillin led to a decline of the disease, but its prevalence has increased in more recent years. In developed countries, syphilis in children is rare, but it is disproportionately frequent in underprivileged segments of the population and in the setting of drug abuse [Sison et al., 1997]. In countries with few resources, congenital syphilis remains an important health issue. Transmission occurs across the placenta after the fifth month of gestation or rarely at birth by contact with infectious maternal lesions. Congenital syphilis can be prevented by screening and treating pregnant women [Walker and Walker, 2002]. When older children acquire syphilis, this is the result of either sexual abuse or precocious sexual activity. *T. pallidum* disseminates widely in the body in congenital and acquired syphilis and can cause disease in various organs, including the CNS. Pathologic lesions involve endothelial cell proliferation and perivascular inflammation with lymphocytes and plasma cells.

Clinical Characteristics

Congenital syphilis is associated with stillbirth or perinatal death in half of the cases [Darville, 1999]. Early congenital syphilis, which includes all manifestations in the first 2 years of life, manifests at birth or within the first weeks of life. Early signs include prematurity and low birth weight, skin and mucous membrane lesions, hepatosplenomegaly, and skeletal abnormalities (osteochondritis), which can be painful and prevent the child from moving affected limbs. Snuffles consist of a thick nasal discharge rich with spirochetes. The eyes (chorioretinitis, uveitis) and CNS (meningitis, meningovascular syphilis, hydrocephalus) are commonly involved, but clinical signs of neurosyphilis are rare in neonates [Parish, 2000].

In late congenital syphilis, clinical findings do not appear until several years of age. Interstitial keratitis occurs typically in the second decade. Usually, both eyes are involved. Bone lesions result in destruction of the palate and nasal septum, with depression of the nose (saddle nose). Scars appear about the mouth from earlier fissures (rhagades). The tibia may become bowed (saber shins), and the knee joint can be affected with hydrarthrosis (Clutton's joints). Permanent dentition is abnormal, especially the upper central incisors, which are dwarfed and notched (Hutchinson's teeth), and the first lower molars, which have poorly developed cusps (mulberry molars). CNS involvement can manifest with multiple defects. Meningovascular syphilis leads to findings of chronic meningoencephalitis, such as intellectual decline (juvenile paresis), which may begin by 4 to 5 years of age, headache, seizures, blindness, cranial nerve VIII deafness, other cranial nerve involvement, hemiparesis, and hydrocephalus. Hutchinson's triad consists of Hutchinson's teeth, interstitial keratitis, and nerve deafness [Parish, 2000].

Acquired syphilis, which resembles the disease in adults, can occur in children and adolescents. The primary stage with chancre appears 2 to 4 weeks after exposure, but the chancre may go unnoticed. The cutaneous eruptions of the second stage follow usually within 2 months and can be associated with mucous membrane patches, condylomata lata, and patchy alopecia. Mild constitutional symptoms, such as fever, malaise, arthralgias, rhinorrhea, and lymphadenopathy, occur as a result of the disseminating infection. Rarely, secondary syphilis is associated with meningitis, leading to headache, meningism, nausea, and vomiting. If the condition is not treated, the tertiary stage of neurosyphilis (tabes dorsalis) may develop after an asymptomatic period of many years; this is extremely rare in pediatric patients.

Diagnosis

The diagnosis of syphilis relies on clinical suspicion, serologic testing, and visualization of the organism from infected superficial lesions. Tissue biopsy specimens and attempts to culture the organism do not play a role in clinical practice. Serology relies on nontreponemal tests (Venereal Disease Research Laboratory [VDRL]), which are useful for screening and monitoring of treatment, and treponemal tests, such as the microhemagglutination–*T. pallidum* (MHA-TP) and fluorescent treponemal antibody absorption (FTA-ABS) tests, which are used to confirm the diagnosis. Suspected infections should be investigated by serologic testing of the mother and child. The tests can be negative in a newborn if the mother acquired the disease late in pregnancy, whereas passive transfer of maternal antibodies can result in a false-positive test in an unaffected newborn. Microscopic examination by darkfield microscopy or direct fluorescence antibodies can identify organisms in mucocutaneous lesions. If acquired syphilis is diagnosed in a child, the possibility of sexual abuse must be investigated [Connors et al., 1998].

Laboratory diagnosis of CNS involvement depends on cerebrospinal fluid examination. CNS involvement is assumed if the cerebrospinal fluid has increased cell counts (mostly mononuclear cells), elevated protein, and a positive VDRL result. Cerebrospinal fluid VDRL results can be false-negative, however, and reliable exclusion of CNS involvement in neonates may be difficult. If clinically indicated, radiographs of the chest and bones and ophthalmologic and audiometric examinations should be performed.

Treatment

Penicillin remains the treatment of choice for all clinical forms of syphilis. For early stages of acquired syphilis, one injection of benzathine penicillin is sufficient. For neurosyphilis and congenital syphilis, high-dose treatment with intravenous penicillin G is recommended [Workowski and Berman, 2002]. In allergic patients, desensitization should be attempted because penicillin is more effective than alternative treatments that can be given in children.

Lyme Borreliosis

Clinical Characteristics

Lyme disease is caused by the spirochetes *Borrelia burgdorferi.* They are transmitted in endemic areas by the bite of *Ixodes* ticks during the warm season, and children frequently are affected. The species of Lyme *Borrelia* differ between the United States and Europe. The disease occurs in three stages: early localized disease (erythema chronicum migrans), early disseminated disease, and persistent late disease. Extracutaneous manifestations involve the heart, the joints, and the CNS.

Neurologic manifestations of Lyme disease are observed in 10% of patients and include lymphocytic meningitis, radiculitis and neuritis, encephalomyelitis, peripheral neuropathy, and subtle encephalopathic syndromes with memory and cognitive dysfunctions [Gerber et al., 1996]. Neurologic symptoms develop within weeks after onset of erythema chronicum migrans and tend to be more frequent and severe in Europe than in the United States, likely as a result of the increased neurotropism of *Borrelia garinii,* which is found only in Europe. In children, meningitis and peripheral palsy of cranial nerve VII are the most common neurologic manifestations of Lyme disease [Christen, 1996]. Rare manifestations of neuroborreliosis in children include cerebrovascular disease with sensorimotor deficits, optic nerve impairment caused by inflammation, and increased intracranial pressure. Chronic neuroborreliosis is manifested as a failure to thrive, headaches, and pseudotumor cerebri [Rothermel et al., 2001; Wilke et al., 2000].

Diagnosis

The diagnosis of erythema chronicum migrans is clinical and does not require laboratory confirmation. Serologic tests are used to diagnose later or disseminated manifestations of Lyme disease. Enzyme-linked immunosorbent assay or immunofluorescence tests with high sensitivity serve as screening tests in patients with symptoms compatible with Lyme disease. Positive or equivocal tests must be confirmed by a more specific Western blot test. With these tests, IgM and IgG can be measured. Chronic forms of Lyme disease elicit an IgG response, whereas the IgM response can persist at the same time for months or years. Isolated IgM responses in chronic conditions are usually false-positive. Neurologic involvement is diagnosed based on suggestive symptoms combined with cerebrospinal fluid signs of inflammation (lymphocytic pleocytosis, increased protein concentrations). Antibodies (IgM, IgG, and IgA) can be detected in the cerebrospinal fluid as a result of intrathecal antibody production. Direct demonstration of spirochetes in the cerebrospinal fluid is not feasible in most cases, whereas polymerase chain reaction may be positive in early stages of CNS involvement.

Treatment

In early stages of the disease, doxycycline or amoxicillin is recommended. The latter is preferred in children younger than 8 years old; in the late stage with CNS or peripheral nervous system involvement, intravenous therapy with a cephalosporin (ceftriaxone or cefotaxime) or penicillin is the recommended therapy [Wormser et al., 2000]. The prognosis is excellent for children with early Lyme disease who are treated with appropriate antimicrobial therapy [Gerber et al., 1996].

Leptospirosis

Leptospirosis, caused by spirochetes of the species *Leptospira,* is acquired through the skin in water infested by rats but also can be transmitted to children by dogs. After an incubation period of 1 to 2 weeks, the acute, septicemic illness manifests itself by high fevers and constitutional symptoms, headaches, gastrointestinal symptoms, muscle pain, and conjunctivitis. After a period of apparent recovery, a second, immunologically mediated phase occurs. During this second phase, the liver, kidney, and nervous system may be affected. Nervous system involvement takes the form of meningitis, encephalitis, or neuritis. Meningitis is documented in approximately 10% to 20% of cases [Rajajee et al., 2002]. Meningitis and encephalitis rarely may become chronic. Neuritis tends to involve the brachial plexus or cranial nerves.

Pleocytosis is found in the cerebrospinal fluid, which in the initial phase is polymorphonuclear, whereas lymphocytes are found in the second phase. The protein is elevated with normal glucose concentrations. The diagnosis usually is established by documenting rising antibody titers in serum, but the organism also can be visualized by dark-field microscopy in blood, urine, and occasionally cerebrospinal fluid (in the early phase) and can be cultured using Fletcher medium. Polymerase chain reaction facilitates early diagnosis [Gerke and Rump, 2003]. Penicillin is the treatment of choice [Marotto et al., 1997], although proof of its benefit is lacking. Patients with encephalitis may be left with sequelae even when treated with antibiotics.

TABLE 68-8

Signs and Symptoms of Brain Abscess
Fever, subacute course, headache
Depressed consciousness, confusion
Nuchal rigidity, papilledema
Seizures, hemiparesis, dysphagia

BRAIN ABSCESS

With refinement in diagnostic techniques, brain abscesses are being recognized more promptly and at earlier stages in their evolution [Mathisen and Johnson, 1997].

Clinical Characteristics

The initial clinical appearance of bacterial brain abscess is seldom dramatic, and the history and clinical findings are typically vague (Table 68-8). The diagnosis of brain abscess is suggested by the subacute development of fever, headache, vomiting, confusion, depressed consciousness, seizures, papilledema, and focal neurologic signs. Nuchal rigidity may occur in a few patients. Multiple brain abscesses do not have a unique presentation [Basit et al., 1999].

A brain abscess behaves as an expanding intracranial mass that can obstruct cerebrospinal fluid flow and produce hydrocephalus. Papilledema, a distinctly uncommon finding with bacterial meningitis, occurs with brain abscess if cranial sutures have closed. Multiple abscesses are found especially in patients with cyanotic congenital heart disease [Basit et al, 1989]. The differential diagnosis includes neoplasm, subdural hematoma, and focal encephalitis, such as herpes simplex. Brain abscess is rare before 2 years of age except in neonates [Daniels et al., 1985; Wessalowksi et al., 1993].

Brain Imaging

MRI and CT are appropriate tests during the stage of cerebritis. Enhanced MRI and CT are the definitive tests in a mature abscess, revealing a characteristic capsular ring. Magnetic resonance spectroscopy may be useful in differentiating an abscess from a neoplasm [Martinez-Perez et al., 1997]. The electroencephalogram may be normal, may display focal abnormalities in the region of the abscess as either slowing or spikes, may contain periodic lateralized epileptiform discharges, or may be diffusely slow.

Lumbar Puncture

Lumbar puncture should be approached extremely cautiously in any patient with suspected brain abscess because of the risk of herniation secondary to elevated intracranial pressure. Brain abscess documented by imaging contraindicates lumbar puncture. The yield for recovery of causative bacteria is higher with stereotactic biopsy than with blood culture.

Pathogenesis and Pathology

Either hematogenous or direct spread of the organism can lead to a brain abscess. Brain abscess occurs in children in association with cyanotic congenital heart disease, in association with lung infection, after neurosurgical procedures, after penetrating head trauma, secondary to infections about the sinuses and orbits, and spontaneously [Anderson, 1993; Mathisen and Johnson, 1997]. Abscesses also occur in immunosuppression; in chronic pulmonary disease, especially in patients with cystic fibrosis; and in association with a continuing focus of infection, such as chronic otitis [Tekkok and Erbengi, 1992]. Brain abscess is rare as a complication of bacterial meningitis except in neonates (typically caused by *Citrobacter* and other gram-negative organisms) [Renier et al., 1998; Schaad, 1992].

An abscess of hematogenous origin localizes at the border of the gray and white matter. The lesion is initially a cerebritis, which may persist for several weeks. Edema surrounds the cerebritis, leading to increasing mass effect. Progressing from the cerebritis phase, a capsule of inflammatory granulation tissue develops over a variable period around a necrotic infected area. Abscesses are usually in the hemispheres, but may occur in the brainstem or cerebellum. A wide spectrum of unusual aerobic and anaerobic organisms has been isolated from brain abscesses [Brook, 1992].

Treatment

Anaerobic bacteria are found in 90% of brain abscesses. Multiple organisms may be present. *Streptococcus, Staphylococcus,* and *Bacteroides fragilis* are common in abscesses. In neonates, the offending pathogen is often *Proteus*. Surgical drainage or excision and appropriate antibiotics constitute appropriate treatment [Stephanov, 1988]. Surgery provides an opportunity to culture the organisms and hastens the resolution of abscesses.

Empiric therapy usually consists of vancomycin, ceftriaxone, and metronidazole for 3 to 6 weeks. Brain abscesses have been cured by antibiotics without surgical drainage [Aebi et al., 1991; Wong et al., 1989]. Medical management with or without needle aspiration should be considered when abscess formation is still in the cerebritis stage, when there are multiple abscesses or when the abscess is located in a critical area [Aebi et al., 1991; Brook, 1995]. Serial CT or MRI can be used to determine when medical therapy is failing. Increased intracranial pressure rarely may indicate controlled hyperventilation, osmotic agents such as mannitol, corticosteroids, or surgical drainage.

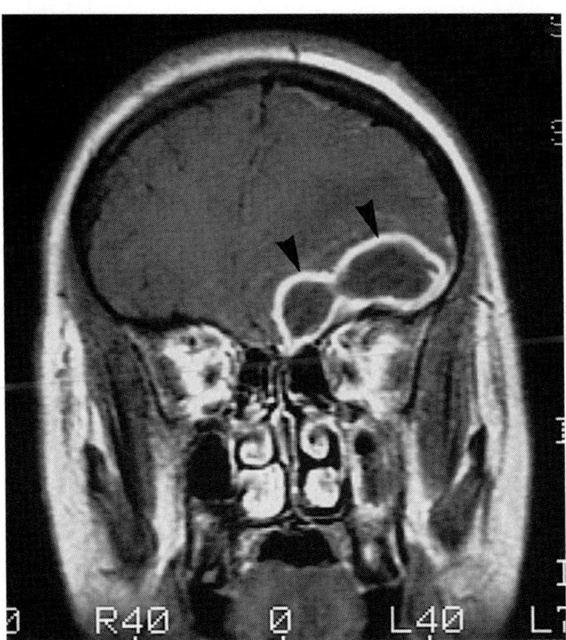

FIGURE 68-6. Postcontrast coronal MRI of 15-year-old child with subdural empyema *(arrowheads)* and midline shift. (Courtesy of Blaine Hart, MD.)

Prognosis

Because of difficulty in diagnosis and management of brain abscess, mortality is still high, and sequelae are frequent [Aebi et al., 1991; Saez-Llorens et al., 1989]. Imaging improves the ability to follow brain abscess and may reduce morbidity and mortality. The outlook is poor when multiple abscesses are present [Basit et al., 1989] and when age is less than 1 year [Wong et al., 1989]. Mortality in infants approaches 50% [Tekkok and Erbengi, 1992]. Chronic seizure disorders are common after brain abscess [Hegde et al., 1986].

CRANIAL AND SPINAL EPIDURAL ABSCESS

Cranial Epidural Abscess

The terms *epidural* and *extradural* are interchangeable terms and are used to describe a suppurative infection between the dura and cranium. Such infections are usually a complication of trauma, neurosurgery, or spread of infection from contiguous structures. The condition is rare in childhood [Auletta and John, 2001]. *S. aureus, S. epidermidis, Streptococcus,* and *B. fragilis* are some of the organisms found. Symptoms may be subtle and include fever, headache, stiff neck, focal seizures, and focal neurologic deficits, such as hemiparesis. The abscess acts as an enlarging mass. Lumbar puncture usually is contraindicated.

Imaging of cranial epidural abscess typically reveals a lenticular collection of fluid between the bone and CNS of variable appearance and enhancement characteristics (Fig. 68-6). MRI is preferred to CT [Weingarten et al., 1989]. Treatment consists of antibiotics (see discussion on treatment of meningitis for appropriate choices) and surgical drainage [Auletta and John, 2001]. Delay in diagnosis and treatment is associated with an unfavorable outcome.

Spinal Epidural Abscess

Spinal epidural abscess is usually secondary to bacteremia. The condition is rare as a complication of lumbar puncture. *S. aureus* is the most common organism recovered, although *M. tuberculosis* is always a consideration. Presentation is a "painful, febrile, spinal syndrome" [Hancock, 1973]. Progression can be rapid with motor and sphincter involvement and a clinical picture resembling acute transverse myelitis. Children often have no clear-cut presentation.

With a suspicion of spinal epidural abscess, immediate MRI with gadolinium is indicated, and lumbar puncture usually is contraindicated. Surgical treatment with appropriate antibiotic coverage is the mainstay of therapy [Hlavin et al., 1990; Rosenfeld and Rowley, 1994]. Antibiotics alone may be appropriate in selected cases [Slade and Lonano, 1990].

OTHER BACTERIAL INFECTIONS OF THE NERVOUS SYSTEM

Bartonella

Bartonella species include, among others, *B. henselae,* an organism that is endemic in cats and transmitted to humans by cat scratches and fleas, and *B. quintana,* which is spread among humans under poor sanitary conditions by the human body louse. *B. henselae* is the agent of cat-scratch disease, a common disease in children characterized by a cutaneous papule at the inoculation site, regional lymphadenopathy, low-grade fever, malaise, and anorexia; a subset of patients present with Parinaud's syndrome (oculoglandular disease). *B. quintana* causes the trench fever observed during World War I, a febrile illness associated with headaches, conjunctivitis, rash, myalgias, and bone pain. Both species can cause severe systemic diseases in immunocompromised patients, notably bacillary angiomatosis and peliosis hepatis.

B. henselae causes CNS involvement in the form of encephalitis, cerebral vasculitis, or radiculitis. It is estimated that 2% to 10% of cases of cat-scratch disease are complicated by encephalitis. Typical symptoms include generalized tonic-clonic seizures and other deficits attributable to encephalitis [Carithers and Margileth, 1991]. Onset of the disease is usually subacute over days to weeks but may be acute if seizures are the primary manifestation. Imaging studies usually are normal, and cerebrospinal fluid indicates no signs of inflammation [Lewis and Tucker, 1986]. More recently, cases of encephalitis or focal cerebral lesions caused by *B. quintana* have been described [Parrott et al., 1997]. The diagnosis is based on serology, which does not discriminate reliably between the two species (cross-reactivity), and polymerase chain reaction, which can differentiate between them [Parrott et al., 1997]. The fastidious pleomorphic rods are difficult to culture, but can be detected in tissue by Warthin-Starry silver stain.

Uncomplicated cat-scratch disease is self-limiting and does not require antimicrobial therapy. In patients with encephalitis or focal brain lesions associated with *Bartonella* infection, antibiotics may be prescribed, although their benefit is uncertain. Anecdotal reports indicate that trimethoprim-sulfamethoxazole, macrolides, doxycycline, or quinolones, sometimes combined with rifampin, may be effective.

Mycoplasma pneumoniae

Although *Mycoplasma pneumoniae,* a small bacterium without a cell wall, is primarily a respiratory tract pathogen causing pneumonia, it is prone to induce immune-mediated secondary clinical manifestations, such as hemolytic anemia, and has been implicated in diseases affecting the CNS. Of cases of encephalitis in children, 10% have been attributed to *M. pneumoniae* [Bitnun et al., 2001]. After a prodromal respiratory illness in about two thirds of patients, a variety of neurologic syndromes, such as meningitis, acute disseminated encephalomyelitis, hemorrhagic encephalitis, transverse myelitis, radiculitis, and an ascending paralysis similar to Guillain-Barré syndrome, have been described [Lin et al., 2002]. In 11 children with probable CNS involvement secondary to *M. pneumoniae,* the most common neurologic manifestations were seizures in 7 children and focal motor deficits and ataxia in 4 each. Half of the children had cerebrospinal fluid abnormalities, primarily a mononuclear pleocytosis, and pathologic imaging studies, whereas 80% had abnormal findings on electroencephalogram [Bitnun et al., 2001].

The diagnosis of CNS involvement secondary to *M. pneumoniae* is difficult. Serology may indicate false-negative and false-positive results and should not be used as sole evidence to support the diagnosis. The organism can be cultured in cerebrospinal fluid or nervous tissue, but polymerase chain reaction seems to be more sensitive and provides the most compelling evidence for CNS invasion by the organism [Bitnun et al., 2001]. The mechanisms by which *M. pneumoniae* causes damage to nervous tissue have not been clearly delineated. Direct invasion of nervous tissue and immune-mediated mechanisms may play a role, possibly depending on the type of neurologic manifestions.

In suspected cases, antimicrobial therapy with drugs that penetrate into the CNS and have activity against *M. pneumoniae* (e.g., doxycycline, quinolones) should be instituted despite the lack of firm evidence of a beneficial effect [Bitnun et al., 2003]. The role of immune modulation (corticosteroids, immunoglobulins, plasmapheresis) is also of uncertain benefit [Sakoulas, 2001]. Recovery is prolonged, and permanent deficits are common, although children display a more favorable outcome than adults [Carstensen and Nilsson, 1987].

Leprosy

Despite increasing efforts to control leprosy (Hansen's disease), it is still prevalent in some countries of Asia, Africa, and South America. The disease should be considered in patients with persistent skin lesions and peripheral neuropathy who have lived in countries with warm climates and limited resources. Children comprise only a small proportion of patients presenting with leprosy (2% in India, the country with currently the highest prevalence) [Britton and Lockwood, 2004].

The disease is caused by *Mycobacterium leprae,* an obligatory intracellular bacillus with tropism for macrophages and Schwann cells. It is a chronic disease with incubation periods varying from months to many years. The clinical manifestations are determined by the host's immune reaction based on genetic traits. On one extreme, tuberculous leprosy is characterized by limited disease, few bacilli, and a vigorous host defense driven by Th1 CD4 T cells. The other extreme is lepromatous leprosy, with extensive multibacillary disease of the skin and mucous membranes; many patients, including children, have intermediary forms.

Leprosy affects only peripheral nerves and spares the CNS, probably because *M. leprae* binds to a form of laminin that is found only in the basal lamina of Schwann cells of peripheral nerves [Rambukkana et al., 1998]. The disease affects peripheral nerve trunks in fibro-osseus tunnels (e.g., ulnar, median, lateral popliteal, and posterior tibial nerves) and small dermal nerves. The symptoms are sensory and motor loss, hypesthesia, and anhydrosis. The diagnosis is made clinically based on the presence of one or more of the following signs: hypopigmented or reddish patches with reduced sensation, thickening of peripheral nerves, or acid-fast bacilli on skin smears or biopsy material. Polymerase chain reaction methods are in development, but their clinical role has not been defined [Santos et al., 1997].

Treatment depends on the form of disease and uses multi-drug approaches consisting of dapsone, clofazimine, rifampin, ofloxacin, and minocycline [Britton and Lockwood, 2004]. Guidelines issued by the World Health Organization should be consulted. Neuritis (painful peripheral nerves, new anesthesia, or motor loss) and inflamed skin lesions should be treated with corticosteroids in addition to antimicrobial therapy [Britton, 1998].

REFERENCES

Aebi C, Kaufmann F, Schaad UB. Brain abscess in childhood—long-term experiences. Eur J Pediatr 1991;150:282.

Ahmed A, Hickey SM, Ehret S, et al. Cerebrospinal fluid values in the term neonate. Pediatr Infect Dis J 1996;15:298.

Algren JT, Lal S, Cutliff SA, Richman BJ. Predictors of outcome in acute meningococcal infection in children. Crit Care Med 1993;21:447.

Alleyne CH, Hassan M, Zabramski JM. The efficacy and cost of prophylactic and perioprocedural antibiotics in patients with external ventricular drains. Neurosurgery 2000;47:1124.

Amaee FR, Comis SD, Osborne MP. N^{G}-methyl-L-arginine protects the guinea pig cochlea from the cytotoxic effects of pneumolysin. Acta Otolaryngol 1995;115:386.

Amitava AK, Alarm S, Hussain R. Neuro-ophthalmic features in pediatric tubercular meningoencephalitis. J Pediatr Ophthalmol Strabismus 2001;38:229.

Anderson M. Management of cerebral infection. J Neurol Neurosurg Psychiatry 1993;56:1243.

Arnold W, Bredberg G, Gstöttner W, et al. Meningitis following cochlear implantation: Pathomechanisms, clinical symptoms, conservative and surgical treatments. Otorhinolaryngology 2002;64:382.

Aronin SI, Peduzzi P, Quagliarello VJ. Community-acquired bacterial meningitis: Risk stratification for adverse clinical outcome and effect of antibiotic timing. Ann Intern Med 1998;129:862.

Arseni C, Nereantiu F. Multiple vascular thrombosis with vasculogenic lesions in the course of meningoencephalitis. Confin Neurol 1972;34:339.

Ashwal S. Neurologic evaluation of the patient with acute bacterial meningitis. Neurol Clin 1995;13:549.

Ashwal S, Perkin RM, Thompson JR, et al. Bacterial meningitis in children: Current concepts of neurologic management. Adv Pediatr 1993;40:185.

Ashwal S, Stringer W, Tomasi L, et al. Cerebral blood flow and carbon dioxide reactivity in children with bacterial meningitis. J Pediatr 1990;117:523.

Ashwal S, Tomasi L, Schneider S, et al. Bacterial meningitis in children: Pathophysiology and treatment. Neurology 1992;42:739.

Auletta JJ, John CC. Spinal epidural abcesses in children: A 15-year experience and review of the literature. Clin Infect Dis 2001;32:9.

Balmer P, Miller E. Meningococcal disease: How to prevent and how to manage. Curr Opin Infect Dis 2002;15:275.

Baraff LJ, Lee SI, Schriger DL. Outcomes of bacterial meningitis in children: A meta-analysis. Pediatr Infect Dis J 1993;12:389.

Basit AS, Ravi B, Banerji AK, et al. Multiple pyogenic brain abscesses: An analysis of 21 patients. J Neurol Neurosurg Psychiatry 1989;52:591.

Bedford H, De Louvois J, Halket S, et al. Meningitis in infancy in England and Wales: Follow up at age 5 years. BMJ 2001;323:533.

Berman PH, Banker BQ. Neonatal meningitis: A clinical and pathological study of 29 cases. Pediatrics 1966;38:6.

Bernaerts A, Vanhoenacker FM, Parizel PM, et al. Tuberculosis of the central nervous system: Overview of neuroradiological findings. Eur Radiol 2003;13:1876.

Bernard GR, Vincent JL, Laterre PF, et al. Efficacy and safety of recombinant human activated protein C for severe sepsis. N Engl J Med 2001;344:699.

Bhatt SM, Lauretano A, Cabellos C, et al. Progression of hearing loss in experimental pneumococcal meningitis: Correlation with cerebrospinal fluid cytochemistry. J Infect Dis 1993;167:675.

Bifrare YD, Gianinazzi C, Imboden H, et al. Bacterial meningitis causes two distinct forms of cellular damage in the hippocampal dentate gyrus in infant rats. Hippocampus 2003;13:481.

Bitnun A, Ford-Jones E, Blaser S, Richardson S. *Mycoplasma pneumoniae* encephalitis. Semin Pediatr Infect Dis 2003;14:96.

Bitnun A, Ford-Jones EL, Petric M, et al. Acute childhood encephalitis and *Mycoplasma pneumoniae*. Clin Infect Dis 2001;32:1674.

Bodino J, Lylyk P, de Valle M, et al. Computed tomography in purulent meningitis. Am J Dis Child 1982;136:495.

Bonadio WA. The cerebrospinal fluid: Physiologic aspects and alterations associated with bacterial meningitis. Pediatr Infect Dis J 1992;11:423.

Boyer KM, Gotoff SP. Alternative algorithms for prevention of perinatal group B streptococcal infections. Pediatr Infect Dis J 1998;17:973.

Bradley JS, Scheld WM. The challenge of penicillin-resistant *Streptococcus pneumoniae* meningitis: Current antibiotic therapy in the 1990s. Clin Infect Dis 1997;24 (Suppl 2):S213.

Britton WJ. The management of leprosy reversal reactions. Lepr Rev 1998;69:225.

Britton WJ, Lockwood DN. Leprosy. Lancet 2004;363:1209.

Brook I. Aerobic and anaerobic bacteriology of intracranial abscesses. Pediatr Neurol 1992;8:210.

Brook I. Brain abscess in children: Microbiology and management. J Child Neurol 1995;10:283.

Brown LW, Feigin RD. Bacterial meningitis: Fluid balance and therapy. Pediatr Ann 1994;23:93.

Cairns H, Russell DS. Cerebral arteritis and phlebitis in pneumococcal meningitis. J Pathol Bacteriol 1946;58:649.

Canica M, Dias R, Ferreira E. *Neisseria meningitidis* C:2b:P1.2,5 with intermediate resistance to penicillin, Portugal. Emerg Infect Dis 2004;10:526.

Carithers HA, Margileth AM. Cat-scratch disease: Acute encephalopathy and other neurologic manifestations. Am J Dis Child 1991;145:98.

Carstensen H, Nilsson KO. Neurological complications associated with *Mycoplasma pneumoniae* infection in children. Neuropediatrics 1987;18:57.

Christen HJ. Lyme neuroborreliosis in children. Ann Med 1996;28:235.

Cohen BA, Schenk VA, Sweeney DB. Meningitis-related hearing loss evaluated with evoked potentials. Pediatr Neurol 1988;4:18.

Connors JM, Schubert C, Shapiro R. Syphilis or abuse: Making the diagnosis and understanding the implications. Pediatr Emerg Care 1998;14:139.

Cottagnoud PH, Täuber MG. New therapies for pneumococcal meningitis. Expert Opin Investig Drugs 2004;13:393.

Coulehan JL, Michaels RH, Hallowell C, et al. Epidemiology of *Haemophilus influenzae* type b disease among Navajo Indians. Public Health Rep 1984;99:404.

Daniels SR, Price JK, Towbin RB, et al. Nonsurgical cure of brain abscess in a neonate. Childs Nerv Syst 1985;1:346.

Darville T. Syphilis. Pediatr Rev 1999;20:160.

De Gans J, Van de Beek D, for the European Dexamethasone in Adulthood Bacterial Meningitis Study Investigators. Dexamethasone in adults with bacterial meningitis. N Engl J Med 2002; 347:1549.

Derugin N, Wendland M, Muramatsu K, et al. Evolution of brain injury after transient middle cerebral artery occlusion in neonatal rats. Stroke 2000;31:1752.

De Wals P, de Serres G, Niyonsenga T. Effectiveness of a mass immunization campaign against serogroup C meningococcal disease in Quebec. JAMA 2001;285:177.

Drummond DS, de Jong AL, Giannoni C, et al. Recurrent meningitis in the pediatric patient—the otolaryngologist's role. Int J Pediatr Otorhinolaryngol 1999;48:199.

Eisenhut M, Meehan T, Batchelor L. Cerebrospinal fluid glucose levels and sensorineural hearing loss in bacterial meningitis. Infection 2003;31:247.

Farinha NJ, Razali KA, Holzel H, et al. Tuberculosis of the central nervous system in children: A 20-year survey. J Infect 2000;41:61.

Feigin RD, McCracken GH Jr, Klein JO. Diagnosis and management of meningitis. Pediatr Infect Dis J 1992;11:785.

Feldman WE, Ginsburg CM, McCracken GH Jr, et al. Relation of concentrations of *Haemophilus* type b in cerebrospinal fluid to late sequelae of patients with meningitis. J Pediatr 1982;100:209.

Filka J, Huttova M, Tuharsky J, et al. Nosocomial meningitis in children after ventriculoperitoneal shunt insertion. Acta Paediatr 1999;88:576.

Förderreuther S, Tatsch K, Einhäupl KM, Pfister HW. Abnormalities of cerebral blood flow in the acute phase of bacterial meningitis in adults. J Neurol 1992;239:431.

Francois M, Laccourreye L, Huy ET, Narcy P. Hearing impairment in infants after meningitis: Detection by transient evoked otoacoustic emissions. J Pediatr 1997;130:712.

Fredricks DN, Relman DA. Application of polymerase chain reaction to the diagnosis of infectious diseases. Clin Infect Dis 1999;29:475.

Gates GA, Miyamoto T. Cochlear implants. N Engl Med 2003;349:421.

Geiseler PJ, Nelson KE. Bacterial meningitis without clinical signs of meningeal irritation. South Med J 1982;75:448.

Gerber MA, Shapiro ED, Burke GS, et al. Lyme disease in children in southeastern Connecticut. Pediatric Lyme Disease Study Group. N Engl J Med 1996;335:1270.

Gerke P, Rump LC. Leptospirosis—3 cases and a review. Clin Nephrol 2003;60:42.

Gianinazzi C, Grandgirard D, Imboden H, et al. Caspase-3 mediates hippocampal apoptosis in pneumococcal meningitis. Acta Neuropathol (Berl) 2003;105:499.

Giebink GS. The prevention of pneumococcal disease in children. N Engl J Med 2001;345:1177.

Ginsberg L. Difficult and recurrent meningitis. J Neurol Neurosurg Psychiatry 2004;75 (Suppl 1):i16.

Grande PO, Myhre EB, Nordstrom CH, Schliamser S. Treatment of intracranial hypertension and aspects on lumbar dural puncture in severe bacterial meningitis. Acta Anaesthesiol Scand 2002;46:264.

Gray BM, Simmons DR, Mason H, et al. Quantitative levels of C-reactive protein in cerebrospinal fluid in patients with bacterial meningitis and other conditions. J Pediatr 1986;108:665.

Green SM, Rothrock SG, Clem KJ, et al. Can seizures be the sole manifestation of meningitis in febrile children? Pediatrics 1993;92:527.

Grimwood K, Anderson P, Anderson V, et al. Twelve year outcomes following bacterial meningitis: Further evidence for persisting effects. Arch Dis Child 2000;83:111.

Grimwood K, Anderson VA, Bond L, et al. Adverse outcomes of bacterial meningitis in school-age survivors. Pediatrics 1995;95:646.

Grimwood K, Nolan TM, Bond L, et al. Risk factors for adverse outcomes of bacterial meningitis. J Paediatr Child Health 1996;32:457.

Hancock DO. A study of 49 patients with acute spinal extradural abscess. Paraplegia 1973;10:285.

Hasbun R, Abrahams J, Jekel J Quagliarello VJ. Computed tomography of the head before lumbar puncture in adults with suspected meningitis. N Engl J Med 2001;345:1727.

Hasegawa K, Chiba N, Kobayashi R, et al. Rapidly increasing prevalence of beta-lactamase-nonproducing, ampicillin-resistant *Haemophilus influenzae* type b in patients with meningitis. Antimicrob Agents Chemother 2004;48:1509.

Heath PT, Nik NK, Baker CJ. Neonatal meningitis. Arch Dis Child Fetal Neonatal Educ 2003;88:F173.

Hegde AS, Venkataramana NK, Das BS. Brain abscess in children. Child Nerv Syst 1986;2:90.

Hernandez-Albujar S, Arribas JR, Royo A, et al. Tuberculous radiculomyelitis complicating tuberculous meningitis: Case report and review. Clin Infect Dis 2000;30:915.

Hlavin ML, Kaminski HJ, Ross JS, et al. Spinal epidural abscess: A ten-year perspective. Neurosurgery 1990;27:177.

Hoffman JA, Badger JL, Zhang Y, et al. *Escherichia coli* K1 aslA contributes to invasion of brain microvascular endothelial cells in vitro and in vivo. Infect Immun 2000;68:5062.

Jones ME, Draghi DC, Karlowsky JA, et al. Prevalence of antimicrobial resistance in bacteria isolated from central nervous system specimens as reported by U.S. hospital laboratories from 2000 to 2002. Ann Clin Microbiol Antimicrob 2004;3:3.

Kaaresen PI, Flaegstad T. Prognostic factors in childhood bacterial meningitis. Acta Pediatr 1995;84:873.

Kaplan SL, Feigin RD. The syndrome of inappropriate secretion of antidiuretic hormone in children with bacterial meningitis. J Pediatr 1978;92:758.

Kieseier BC, Paul R, Koedel U, et al. Differential expression of matrix metalloproteinases in bacterial meningitis. Brain 1999;122:1579.

Kilpi T, Anttila M, Kallio MJT, Peltola H. Length of prediagnostic history related to the course and sequelae of childhood bacterial meningitis. Pediatr Infect Dis 1993;12:184.

Kioumehr F, Dadsetan MR, Feldman N, et al. Postcontrast MRI of cranial meninges: Leptomeningitis versus pachymeningitis. J Comput Assist Tomogr 1995;19:713.

Klein JO, Feigin RD, McCracken GH Jr. Report of the Task Force on Diagnosis and Management of Meningitis. Pediatrics 1986;78:959.

Klein M, Koedel U, Pfister HW, Kastenbauer S. Morphological correlates of acute and permanent hearing loss during experimental pneumococcal meningitis. Brain Pathol 2003;13:123.

Koedel U, Gorriz C, Lorenzl S, Pfister HW. Increased endothelin levels in cerebrospinal fluid samples from adults with bacterial meningitis. Clin Infect Dis 1997;25:329.

Kornelisse RF, Westerbeek CML, Spoor AB, et al. Pneumococcal meningitis in children: Prognostic indicators and outcome. Clin Infect Dis 1995;21:1390.

Krasinski K, Nelson JD, Butler S, et al. Possible association of mycoplasma and viral respiratory infections with bacterial meningitis. Am J Epidemiol 1987;125:499.

Krohn MA, Hillier SL, Baker CJ. Maternal peripartum complications associated with vaginal group B streptococci colonization. J Infect Dis 1999;179:1410.

Leib SL, Heimgartner C, Bifrare YD, et al. Dexamethasone aggravates hippocampal apoptosis and learning deficiency in pneumococcal meningitis in infant rats. Pediatr Res 2003;4:4.

Leib SL, Kim YS, Chow LL, et al. Reactive oxygen intermediates contribute to necrotic and apoptotic neuronal injury in an infant rat model of bacterial meningitis due to group B streptococci. J Clin Invest 1996;98:2632.

Leppert D, Lindberg RL, Kappos L, Leib SL. Matrix metalloproteinases: Multifunctional effectors of inflammation in multiple sclerosis and bacterial meningitis. Brain Res Brain Res Rev 2001;36:249.

Lewis DW, Tucker SH. Central nervous system involvement in cat scratch disease. Pediatrics 1986;77:714.

Lin WC, Lee PI, Lu CY, et al. *Mycoplasma pneumoniae* encephalitis in childhood. J Microbiol Immunol Infect 2002;35:173.

Lindvall P, Ahlm C, Ericsson M, et al. Reducing intracranial pressure may increase survival among patients with bacterial meningitis. Clin Infect Dis 2004;38:384.

Lutsar I, Haldre S, Topman M, Talvik T. Enzymatic changes in the cerebrospinal fluid in patients with infections of the central nervous system. Acta Pediatr 1994;83:1146.

Lynch J, Arhelger S, Krings-Ernst I. Post-dural puncture headache in young orthopaedic in-patients: Comparison of a 0.33 mm (29-gauche) Quincke-type with a 0.7 mm (22-gauche) Whitacre spinal needle in 200 patients. Acta Anaesthesiol Scand 1992;36:58.

Mariscalco MM, Vergara W, Mei J, et al. Mechanisms of decreased leukocyte localization in the developing host. Am J Physiol Heart Circ Physiol 2002;282:H636.

Marotto PC, Marotto MS, Santos DL, et al. Outcome of leptospirosis in children. Am J Trop Med Hyg 1997;56:307.

Martin GS, Mannino DM, Eaton S, Moss M. The epidemiology of sepsis in the United States from 1979 through 2000. N Engl J Med 2003;348:1546.

Martinez-Perez I, Morena A, Alonso J, et al. Diagnosis of brain abscess by magnetic resonance spectroscopy: Report of 2 cases. J Neurosurg 1997;86:708.

Marton KI, Gean AD. The diagnostic spinal tap. Ann Intern Med 1986;104:880.

Mathisen GE, Johnson JP. Brain abscess. Clin Infect Dis 1997;25:763.

McClinton D, Carraccio C, Englander R. Predictors of ventriculoperitoneal shunt pathology. Pediatr Infect Dis J 2001;20:593.

McGirt MJ, Zaas A, Fuchs HE, et al. Risk factors for pediatric ventriculoperitoneal shunt infection and predictors of infectious pathogens. Clin Infect Dis 2003;36:858.

Meco C, Oberascher G. Comprehensive algorithm for skull base dural lesion and cerebrospinal fluid fistula diagnosis. Laryngoscope 2004;114:991.

Meli DN, Christen S, Leib SL, Täuber MG. Current concepts in the pathogenesis of meningitis caused by *Streptococcus pneumoniae*. Curr Opin Infect Dis 2002;15:253.

Miller E, Salisbury D, Ramsay M. Planning, registration, and implementation of an immunisation campaign against meningococcal serogroup C disease in the UK: A success story. Vaccine 2001; 20 (Suppl 1):S58.

Moller K, Larsen FS, Bie P, Skinhoj P. The syndrome of inappropriate secretion of antidiuretic hormone and fluid restriction in meningitis—how strong is the evidence? Scand J Infect Dis 2001;33:13.

Nau R, Soto A, Bruck W. Apoptosis of neurons in the dentate gyrus in humans suffering from bacterial meningitis. J Neuropathol Exp Neurol 1999;58:265.

Odio C, McCracken GH Jr, Nelson JD. CSF shunt infections in pediatrics: A seven-year experience. Am J Dis Child 1984;138:1103.

Odio CM, Faingezicht I, Paris M, et al. The beneficial effects of early dexamethasone administration in infants and children with bacterial meningitis. N Engl J Med 1991;324:1525.

Oostenbrink R, Maas M, Moons KG, Moll HA. Sequelae after bacterial meningitis in childhood. Scand J Infect Dis 2002;34:379.

Overturf GD. Indications for the immunological evaluation of patients with meningitis. Clin Infect Dis 2003;36:189.

Packer RJ, Bilaniuk LT, Zimmerman RA. CT parenchymal abnormalities in bacterial meningitis: Clinical significance. J Comput Assist Tomogr 1982;6:1064.

Parish JL. Treponemal infections in the pediatric population. Clin Dermatol 2000;18:687.

Parrott JH, Dure L, Sullender W, et al. Central nervous system infection associated with *Bartonella quintana*: A report of two cases. Pediatrics 1997;100:403.

Pelton SI, Klein JO. The future of pneumococcal conjugate vaccines for prevention of pneumococcal diseases in infants and children. Pediatrics 2002;110:805.

Pfister HW, Borasio GD, Dirnagl U, et al. Cerebrovascular complications of bacterial meningitis in adults. Neurology 1992;42:1497.

Pfister LA, Tureen JH, Shaw S, et al. Endothelin inhibition improves cerebral blood flow and is neuroprotective in pneumococcal meningitis. Ann Neurol 2000;47:329.

Pollard AJ, Levin M. Vaccines for prevention of meningococcal disease. Pediatr Infect Dis J 2000;19:333.

Pon RA, Lussier M, Yang QL, Jennings HJ. *N*-propionylated group B meningococcal polysaccharide mimics a unique bactericidal capsular epitope in group B *Neisseria meningitidis*. J Exp Med 1997;185:1929.

Powell KR, Sugarman LI, Eskenazi AE, et al. Normalization of plasma arginine vasopressin concentrations when children with meningitis are given maintenance plus replacement fluid therapy. J Pediatr 1990;117:515.

Quagliarello VJ, Long WJ, Scheld WM. Morphologic alterations of the blood-brain barrier with experimental meningitis in the rat: Temporal sequence and role of encapsulation. J Clin Invest 1986;77:1084.

Rajajee S, Shankar J, Dhattatri L. Pediatric presentations of leptospirosis. Indian J Pediatr 2002;69:851.

Rambukkana A, Yamada H, Zanazzi G, et al. Role of alpha-dystroglycan as a Schwann cell receptor for *Mycobacterium leprae*. Science 1998;282:2076.

Rappuoli R. Reverse vaccinology, a genome-based approach to vaccine development. Vaccine 2001;19:2688.

Reefhuis J, Honein MA, Whitney CG, et al. Risk of bacterial meningitis in children with cochlear implants. N Engl J Med 2003;349:435.

Reichler MR, Allphin AA, Breimann RF, et al. The spread of multiply-resistant *Streptococcus pneumoniae* at a day care center in Ohio. J Infect Dis 1992;166:1346.

Renier D, Flandin C, Hirsch E, et al. Brain abscess in neonates: A study of 30 cases. J Neurosurg 1988;69:877.

Richards PG, Towu-Aghantse E. Dangers of lumbar puncture. BMJ 1986;292:605.

Ring A, Weiser JN, Tuomanen EI. Pneumococcal trafficking across the blood-brain barrier: Molecular analysis of a novel bidirectional pathway. J Clin Invest 1998;102:347.

Riordan FF, Thomson AP, Ratcliffe JM, et al. Admission cortisol and adrenocorticotrophic hormone levels in children with meningococcal disease: Evidence of adrenal insufficiency? Crit Care Med 1999;27:2257.

Rockowitz J, Tunkel AR. Bacterial meningitis—practical guidelines for management. Drugs 1995;50:838.

Ronan A, Hogg GG, Klug GL. Cerebrospinal fluid shunt infections in children. Pediatr Infect Dis J 1995;14:782.

Rosenfeld EA, Rowley AH. Infectious intracranial complications of sinusitis, other than meningitis, in children: 12-Year review. Clin Infect Dis 1994;18:750.

Rotbart HA, Glode MP. *Haemophilus influenzae* type b septic arthritis in children: Report of 23 cases. Pediatrics 1985;75:75.

Rothermel H, Hedges TR 3rd, Steere AC. Optic neuropathy in children with Lyme disease. Pediatrics 2001;108:477.

Runge VM, Wells JW, Williams NM, et al. Detectability of early brain meningitis with magnetic resonance imaging. Invest Radiol 1995;30:484.

Saez-Llorens X, Jafari HS, Severien C, et al. Enhanced attenuation of meningeal inflammation and brain edema by concomitant administration of anti-CD18 monoclonal antibodies and dexamethasone in experimental *Haemophilus* meningitis. J Clin Invest 1991;88:2003.

Saez-Llorens X, Mccoig C, Feris JM, et al. Quinolone treatment for pediatric bacterial meningitis: A comparative study of trovafloxacin and ceftriaxone with or without vancomycin. Pediatr Infect Dis J 2002;21:14.

Saez-Llorens XJ, Umana MA, Odio CM, et al. Brain abscess in infants and children. Pediatr Infect Dis J 1989;8:449.

Salleras L, Dominguez A, Prats G, et al. Dramatic decline of serogroup C meningococcal disease incidence in Catalonia (Spain) 24 months after a mass vaccination programme of children and young people. J Epidemiol Commun Health 2001;55:283.

Sakoulas G. Brainstem and striatal encephalitis complicating *Mycoplasma pneumoniae* pneumonia: Possible benefit of intravenous immunoglobulin. Pediatr Infect Dis J 2001;20:543.

Santos AR, Nery JC, Duppre NC, et al. Use of the polymerase chain reaction in the diagnosis of leprosy. J Med Microbiol 1997;46:170.

Schaad UB. Etiology and management of neonatal bacterial meningitis. Antibiot Chemother 1992;45:192.

Schaad UB. Current concepts of bacterial meningitis. Eur J Pediatr 1995;154:S20.

Schaad UB. Management of bacterial meningitis in childhood. Rev Med Microbiol 1997;8:171.

Schaad UB, Lips U, Gnehm HE, et al. Dexamethasone therapy for bacterial meningitis in children. Swiss Meningitis Study Group. Lancet 1993;342:457.

Scheld WM, Dacey RG, Winn HR, et al. Cerebrospinal fluid outflow resistance in rabbits with experimental meningitis: Alterations with penicillin and methylprednisolone. J Clin Invest 1980;66:243.

Scheld WM, Fletcher DD, Fink FN, Sande MA. Response to therapy in an experimental rabbit model of meningitis due to *Listeria monocytogenes*. J Infect Dis 1979;140:287.

Schick B, Draf W, Kahle G, et al. Occult malformations of the skull base. Arch Otolaryngol Head Neck Surg 1997;123:77.

Schoeman J, Wait J, Burger M, et al. Long-term follow up of childhood tuberculous meningitis. Dev Med Child Neurol 2002;44:522.

Schoeman JF, Van Zyl LE, Laubscher JA, Donald PR. Effect of corticosteroids on intracranial pressure, computed tomographic findings, and clinical outcome in young children with tuberculous meningitis. Pediatrics 1997;99:226.

Schrag SJ, Zywicki S, Farley MM, et al. Group B streptococcal disease in the era of intrapartum antibiotic prophylaxis. N Engl J Med 2000;342:15.

Schuchat A, Robinson K, Wenger JD, et al. Bacterial meningitis in the United States in 1995. Active Surveillance Team. N Engl J Med 1997;337:970.

Shapiro ED, Aaron NH, Wald ER, et al. Risk factors for development of bacterial meningitis among children with occult bacteremia. J Pediatr 1986;109:15.

Shingadia D, Novelli V. Diagnosis and treatment of tuberculosis in children. Lancet Infect Dis 2003;3:624.

Singhi SC, Singhi PD, Srinivas B, et al. Fluid restriction does not improve the outcome of acute meningitis. Pediatr Infect Dis J 1995;14:495.

Sison CG, Ostrea EM Jr, Reyes MP, Salari V. The resurgence of congenital syphilis: A cocaine-related problem. J Pediatr 1997;130:289.

Slade WR, Lonano F. Acute spinal epidural abscess. J Natl Med Assoc 1990;82:713.

Smith RR, Caldemeyer KS. Neuroradiologic review of intracranial infection. Curr Probl Diagn Radiol 1999;28:1.

Snedeker JD, Kaplan SL, Dodge PR, et al. Subdural effusion and its relationship with neurologic sequelae of bacterial meningitis in infancy: A prospective study. Pediatrics 1990;86:163.

Stahelin-Massik J, Levy F, Friderich P, Schaad UB. Meningitis caused by *Ureaplasma urealyticum* in a full term neonate. Pediatr Infect Dis J 1994;13:419.

Starke JR. Tuberculosis of the central nervous system in children. Semin Pediatr Neurol 1999;6:318.

Stephanov S. Surgical treatment of brain abscess. Neurosurgery 1988;22:724.

Stevens JP, Eames M, Kent A, et al. Long term outcome of neonatal meningitis. Arch Dis Child Fetal Neonatal Educ 2003;88:F179.

Syrogiannopoulos GA, Nelson JD, McCracken GH Jr. Subdural collections of fluid in acute bacterial meningitis: A review of 136 cases. Pediatr Infect Dis 1986;5:343.

Täuber MG, Khayam-Bashi H, Sande MA. Effects of ampicillin and corticosteroids on brain water content, cerebrospinal fluid pressure, and cerebrospinal fluid lactate levels in experimental pneumococcal meningitis. J Infect Dis 1985;151:528.

Täuber MG, Sande E, Fournier MA, et al. Fluid administration, brain edema, and cerebrospinal fluid lactate and glucose concentrations in experimental *Escherichia coli* meningitis. J Infect Dis 1993;168:473.

Täuber MG, Sande MA. General principles of therapy of pyogenic meningitis. Infect Dis Clin North Am 1990;4:661.

Tekkok IH, Erbengi A. Management of brain abscess in children: Review of 130 cases over a period of 21 years. Child Nerv Syst 1992;8:411.

Tung YR, Lai MC, Lui CC, et al. Tuberculous meningitis in infancy. Pediatr Neurol 2002;27:262.

Tunkel AR, Scheld WM. Acute bacterial meningitis. Lancet 1995;346:1675.

Tureen JH, Täuber MG, Sande MA. Effect of hydration status on cerebral blood flow and cerebrospinal fluid lactic acidosis in rabbits with experimental meningitis. J Clin Invest 1992;89:947.

Van de Beek D, de Gans J, Mcintyre P, Prasad K. Corticosteroids in acute bacterial meningitis. Cochrane Database Syst Rev 2003;CD004305.

Van Deuren M, Brandtzaeg P, van der Meer JW. Update on meningococcal disease with emphasis on pathogenesis and clinical management. Clin Microbiol Rev 2000;13:144.

Viladrich PF, Pallares R, Ariza J, et al. Four days of penicillin therapy for meningococcal meningitis. Arch Intern Med 1986;146:2380.

Vinchon M, Lemaitre MP, Vallee L, Dhellemmes P. Late shunt infection: Incidence, pathogenesis, and therapeutic implications. Neuropediatrics 2002;33:169.

Waagner DC, Kennedy WA, Hoyt MJ, McCracken GH Jr. Lack of adverse effects of dexamethasone therapy in aseptic meningitis. Pediatr Infect Dis J 1990;9:922.

Walker DG, Walker GJ. Forgotten but not gone: The continuing scourge of congenital syphilis. Lancet Infect Dis 2002;2:432.

Ward JI, Lum MK, Hall DB, et al. Invasive *Haemophilus influenzae* type b disease in Alaska: Background epidemiology for a vaccine efficacy trial. J Infect Dis 1986;153:17.

Weingarten K, Zimmerman RD, Becker RD, et al. Subdural and epidural empyemas: MR imaging. AJR Am J Roentgenol 1989;152:615.

Wellman MB, Sommer DD, Mckenna J. Sensorineural hearing loss in postmeningitic children. Otol Neurotol 2003;24:907.

Wessalowski R, Thomas L, Kivit J, Voit TH. Multiple brain abscesses caused by *Salmonella enteritidis* in a neonate: Successful treatment with ciprofloxacin. Pediatr Infect Dis J 1993;12:683.

Whitney CG. The potential of pneumococcal conjugate vaccines for children. Pediatr Infect Dis J 2002;21:961.

Wilke M, Eiffert H, Christen HJ, Hanefeld F. Primarily chronic and cerebrovascular course of Lyme neuroborreliosis: Case reports and literature review. Arch Dis Child 2000;83:67.

Winkler F, Kastenbauer S, Yousry TA, et al. Discrepancies between brain CT imaging and severely raised intracranial pressure proven by ventriculostomy in adults with pneumococcal meningitis. J Neurol 2002;249:1292.

Wong T, Lee L, Wang H, et al. Brain abscesses in children—a cooperative study of 83 cases. Child Nerv Syst 1989;5:19.

Workowski KA, Berman SM. CDC sexually transmitted diseases treatment guidelines. Clin Infect Dis 2002;35:S135.

Wormser GP, Nadelman RB, Dattwyler RJ, et al. Practice guidelines for the treatment of Lyme disease. The Infectious Diseases Society of America. Clin Infect Dis 2000;31 (Suppl 1):1.

Yaramis A, Gurkan F, Elevli M, et al. Central nervous system tuberculosis in children: A review of 214 cases. Pediatrics 1998;102:E49.

Yung AP, McDonald MI. Early clinical clues to meningococcaemia. Med J Aust 2003;178:134.

Zangwill KM, Schuchat A, Wenger JD. Group B streptococcal disease in the United States, 1990: Report from a multistate active surveillance system. MMWR CDC Surveill Summ 1992;41:25.

Ziebuhr W, Dietrich K, Trautmann M, Wilhelm M. Chromosomal rearrangements affecting biofilm production and antibiotic resistance in a *Staphylococcus epidermidis* strain causing shunt-associated ventriculitis. Int J Med Microbiol 2000;290:115.

CHAPTER 69

Viral Infections of the Nervous System

James F. Bale, Jr.

Throughout recorded history, viral infections have caused considerable human suffering [Hughes, 1977]. Approximately 100 viral species from 13 different families have been associated directly or indirectly with disorders of the central or peripheral nervous systems (Box 69-1) [Johnson, 1998; McKendall and Stroop, 1994]. Although several viral infections have become infrequent because of immunization programs (Fig. 69-1), others remain potential threats to the well-being of children throughout the world. This chapter describes virus-induced neurologic disorders, emphasizing pathogenesis, clinical manifestations, epidemiology, and prevention.

GENERAL CONSIDERATIONS

The pathogenesis of viral neurologic infections reflects the complex interactions of viral pathogens and host cells. Virus-induced neurologic disorders begin with virus entry and replication at extraneural locations, such as the skin, conjunctiva, or mucosal surfaces of the gastrointestinal, respiratory, and genital tracts [Fields and Knipe, 1990; Johnson, 1998; McKendall and Stroop, 1994]. Consequently, several factors, such as the gastric pH, local immune responses, integrity of the skin or mucosal barriers, or enzymes that inactivate viruses, influence whether viral pathogens successfully invade human tissues.

Viruses, among the smallest microorganisms causing human disease, consist of an outer capsid, composed of glycoproteins and lipids, and an inner core, composed of RNA or DNA [Fields and Knipe, 1990]. Virus attachment and penetration of host cells depend on the virus encountering and attaching to receptors located on the surface of these cells. The molecular components of this interaction consist of the viral surface glycoproteins and the host cell surface proteins, such as preexisting cellular receptors that mediate certain essential cell functions [Fields and Knipe, 1990; Johnson, 1998; McKendall and Stroop, 1994]. An example of the virus-host interaction that leads to successful viral replication is the attachment of glycoprotein 120 of the human immunodeficiency virus (HIV) to the CD4 molecule and chemokine receptors of host cells [Deng et al., 1996].

Viruses enter host cells by endocytosis, release of genomic material, or fusion of the virus envelope with the cell membrane. Viruses use host cell synthetic pathways to uncoat their nucleic acid and to produce virus-encoded nucleic acids and proteins. Replicative strategies vary among viruses [Fields and Knipe, 1990]. The double-stranded DNA herpesviruses use RNA polymerases in the host cell nucleus to transcribe viral DNA into viral mRNA. The RNA of positive-strand RNA viruses serves as the viral mRNA, whereas negative-strand RNA viruses first must be transcribed into an mRNA strand. By contrast, RNA-containing retroviruses, such as HIV, replicate via a DNA intermediary synthesized in the host cell cytoplasm by a viral-encoded reverse transcriptase [Fields and Knipe, 1990; McKendall and Stroop, 1994].

Next, virus-encoded immediate-early and early proteins facilitate the production of additional viral proteins and assembly of mature virus particles, called *virions*. Viral replication occurs within the nucleus or cytoplasm of the host

Box 69-1 Selected Viruses Associated with Human Neurologic Disease

Family	Examples
DNA viruses	
Herpesviridae	Herpes simplex viruses; cytomegalovirus; varicella-zoster virus; Epstein-Barr virus; human herpesviruses 6, 7, and 8
Adenoviridae	Adenovirus
RNA viruses	
Picornaviridae	Poliovirus types 1 to 3; nonpolio enteroviruses, including enteroviruses 70 and 71
Togaviridae	Eastern and western equine encephalitis viruses, Venezuelan equine encephalitis virus, rubella virus (non–arthropod borne)
Flaviviridae	Japanese and St. Louis encephalitis viruses, West Nile virus
Bunyaviridae	La Crosse encephalitis virus (California encephalitis virus group)
Reoviridae	Colorado tick fever virus, rotavirus
Paramyxoviridae	Mumps and measles viruses, parainfluenza virus, respiratory syncytial virus
Orthomyxoviridae	Influenza viruses
Rhabdoviridae	Rabies virus
Arenaviridae	Lymphocytic choriomeningitis virus
Retroviridae	Human T-cell lymphotropic virus type I, human immunodeficiency viruses type 1 and 2

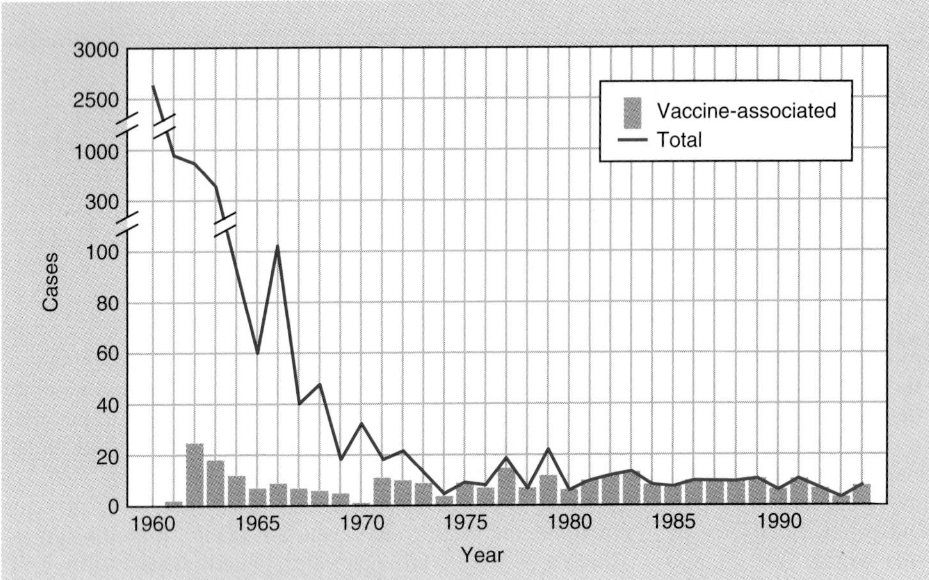

FIGURE 69-1. Data for paralytic poliomyelitis in the United States from 1960 to 1994 illustrate the dramatic decline in cases in the 1960s and the emergence of vaccine-related cases when oral polio vaccines were widely used [CDC, 1997b].

cell, depending on the viral species, and final assembly of viral particles uses existing host cell structures, such as the nuclear membrane or the Golgi apparatus [Fields and Knipe, 1990; McKendall and Stroop, 1994]. Mature virus particles are released from host cells by budding or lysis. Effective replication ultimately releases large quantities of infectious virions into the lymphatics and peripheral circulation of the infected host.

Most viruses, including HIV and the enteroviruses, reach the central nervous system (CNS) hematogenously and penetrate the blood-brain barrier via the choroid plexus or through the vascular endothelium [Johnson, 1998; McKendall and Stroop, 1994]. CNS infection depends on the magnitude and duration of viremia, which reflect the efficiency of systemic viral replication and the ability of the virus to evade host defense mechanisms. Viral infections associated with transient viremia or low viral loads are less likely to lead to CNS invasion.

A few viruses, notably the rabies virus and certain herpesviruses, reach the CNS predominantly through neural routes [Johnson, 1998; McKendall and Stroop, 1994]. Rabies virus, a negative-strand RNA virus, infects neuromuscular junctions, enters nerve endings, and travels by retrograde axonal transport to the neurons of the spinal cord. The virus then ascends to the brain. Transmission via nerve pathways also mediates the pathogenesis of herpes simplex virus type 1 encephalitis and the mucocutaneous reactivations of herpes simplex virus type 1, herpes simplex virus type 2, and varicella-zoster virus.

Viruses induce neurologic signs and symptoms by damaging neural cells directly or by stimulating host-dependent immune responses that perturb neural cell function [Johnson, 1998; McKendall and Stroop, 1994]. The spectrum and severity of neurologic signs or symptoms depend on several factors, including neurovirulence (the capacity of the virus to cause disease within the nervous system), neurotropism (the propensity of the virus to infect specific cell groups of the CNS), and the nature of the host immune responses.

Certain viruses, such as herpes simplex virus type 1, produce lytic infection of neuronal cells and cause hemorrhagic necrosis within the brain, whereas other viruses, such as the La Crosse encephalitis virus, produce minimal cellular damage despite infection of neural cells. The JC virus, the cause of progressive multifocal leukoencephalopathy, selectively infects oligodendrocytes, causing demyelination [Johnson, 1998; McKendall and Stroop, 1994]. Some viruses may not infect neural cells directly, but induce immune-mediated processes, such as *acute disseminated encephalomyelitis,* a condition that accounts for approximately 10% to 15% of acute encephalitis cases in the United States [Gendelman et al., 1984; Johnson, 1996].

Cellular and humoral host immune responses and responses mediated by inflammatory cytokines (e.g., tumor necrosis factor and the interleukins) have major roles in inhibiting viral infections of the CNS [McKendall and Stroop, 1994]. The immune responses to viral infection also can provoke neurologic disorders, such as Guillain-Barré syndrome, Bell's palsy, transverse myelopathy, or acute disseminated encephalomyelitis. These illnesses potentially complicate several childhood infections, including relatively benign viral syndromes [Johnson, 1996, 1998].

CLINICAL MANIFESTATIONS OF VIRAL NEUROLOGIC DISORDERS

Neurologic disorders induced by viruses frequently begin with nonspecific, systemic features, such as malaise, anorexia, chills, fever, myalgias, vomiting, or headache. Certain viral infections produce rash, diarrhea, arthralgia, pharyngitis, cough, nausea, or abdominal pain during the prodrome. These prodromal symptoms and signs reflect viral invasion, replication in systemic tissues, and viremia.

Aseptic Meningitis

Aseptic meningitis, the most frequent CNS disorder associated with viral infections (Box 69-2), produces headache, vomiting, irritability, and neck or back pain. Children appear moderately ill with photophobia and signs of meningeal

Box 69-2 Viruses Associated with Aspetic Meningitis and Encephalitis in Children

Meningitis
- Nonpolio enteroviruses
- Herpes simplex virus types 1 and 2
- Adenoviruses
- Colorado tick fever virus
- Polioviruses
- Lymphocytic choriomeningitis virus
- Epstein-Barr virus
- Human immunodeficiency virus
- St. Louis encephalitis virus
- Tick-borne encephalitis viruses
- Mumps virus

Encephalitis
- Herpes simplex virus types 1 and 2
- Eastern and western equine encephalitis viruses
- St. Louis encephalitis virus
- Japanese encephalitis virus
- West Nile virus
- La Crosse encephalitis virus
- Epstein-Barr virus
- Rabies virus
- Human immunodeficiency virus
- Tick-borne encephalitis viruses
- Varicella-zoster virus
- Cytomegalovirus
- Powassan virus
- Enterovirus 71
- Mumps virus

irritation, including Kernig's sign (involuntary spasm of the hamstring muscle provoked by knee extension in a supine patient) or Brudzinski's sign (flexion of the knees provoked by forced flexion of the neck). In a young infant, signs of meningeal irritation are often absent, and the features of CNS infection in general can be quite subtle.

Systemic features in children with aseptic meningitis, such as skin rash, lymphadenopathy, hepatosplenomegaly, or parotid gland enlargement, can provide useful etiologic clues. The nonpolio enteroviruses, agents associated with the greatest proportion of aseptic meningitis cases in most regions, produce erythematous skin rashes or oral lesions. Hepatosplenomegaly or lymphadenopathy suggests infection with Epstein-Barr virus, cytomegalovirus, or possibly HIV. Children with aseptic meningitis have brief, self-limited illnesses and recover without sequelae.

Encephalitis

Numerous viruses, including members of the arthropod-borne and herpesvirus groups (see Box 69-2), have been associated with encephalitis in childhood. In addition to the headache, vomiting, and systemic features common in aseptic meningitis, children with viral encephalitis have seizures and altered sensorium, ranging from somnolence, or irritability, to coma [Whitley, 1990; Johnson, 1996]. Fever, a common but not invariable feature, ranges from low grade to 40° C or higher.

Seizures affect 15% to 60% of infants or children with encephalitis and can be partial or generalized. Although partial seizures increase the probability of herpes simplex virus encephalitis, partial seizures can accompany several forms of viral encephalitis, including relatively mild cases resulting from the nonpolio enteroviruses or from the La Crosse encephalitis virus, the agent causing most cases of California encephalitis. Neurologic examination of children or adolescents with encephalitis reveals hyperreflexia, ataxia, cognitive disturbances, or focal deficits, such as aphasia or hemiparesis. Severely affected patients may exhibit signs of increased intracranial pressure, including pupillary, respiratory, and postural abnormalities. Outcome of viral encephalitis varies considerably, depending on the virulence of the pathogen, the immune competence of the infected host, and the availability of specific antiviral therapy.

Other Neurologic Disorders

Myelitis, Guillain-Barré syndrome, Bell's palsy, acute cerebellar ataxia, myositis, and poliomyelitis-like disorders are additional neurologic conditions that can be associated with antecedent childhood viral infections (Box 69-3). Myelitis and Guillain-Barré syndrome frequently begin with vague sensory phenomena, but flaccid weakness and areflexia become the predominant neurologic signs. Marked sensory dysfunction, such as a sensory loss corresponding to a spinal level, indicates spinal cord involvement, whereas facial paralysis favors Guillain-Barré syndrome. Autonomic nervous system dysfunction also can be a major complication of the latter condition, producing life-threatening cardiac dysrhythmias or blood pressure fluctuations. Children with myelitis or Guillain-Barré syndrome can have permanent neurologic deficits despite appropriate medical management.

Cerebellar ataxia (see Chapter 58), as summarized by Connolly and associates, can complicate systemic infections with several different viruses [Connolly et al., 1994]. Varicella-associated ataxia typically begins 5 to 14 days after the onset of the characteristic rash, although occasional cases can appear during the preeruptive phase of infection. Virus-induced ataxia and the associated behavioral disturbance peak in severity at onset or within 1 to 2 weeks, then improve during the ensuing 4 to 8 weeks. Most children with ataxia after varicella recover completely [Connolly et al., 1994], but some children with virus-induced ataxia have residual cerebellar or behavioral deficits.

Before widespread immunization, the polioviruses (usually type 1) could infect the anterior horn cells of the spinal cord and cause asymmetric paralysis of the extremities (infantile paralysis) and often respiratory failure [Johnson, 1998]. Currently, several viruses, including West Nile virus, enterovirus 71, and other nonpolio enteroviruses, produce disorders that can mimic classic poliomyelitis [Cheng-Yu et al., 2001; Huang et al., 1999; Li et al., 2003]. The features of these disorders consist of symmetric or asymmetric paralysis and magnetic resonance imaging (MRI) evidence of anterior horn cell damage [Maschke et al., 2004].

Intrauterine and Perinatal Viral Infections

Intrauterine infections with certain viruses (and several nonviral pathogens) (see Box 69-3) can seriously damage the

Box 69-3 Viruses Associated with Myelopathy, Guillain-Barré Syndrome, Acute Cerebellar Ataxia, and Intrauterine Infection

Myelopathy
- Varicella-zoster virus
- Herpes simplex viruses
- Nonpolio enteroviruses
- Human T-cell lymphotropic virus type I
- Human immunodeficiency virus
- Cytomegalovirus
- West Nile virus

Guillain-Barré Syndrome
- Epstein-Barr virus
- Cytomegalovirus
- Nonpolio enteroviruses
- Mumps virus
- Human immunodeficiency virus

Acute Cerebellar Ataxia
- Varicella-zoster virus
- Enteroviruses
- Epstein-Barr virus
- Mumps virus
- Measles virus

Intrauterine Infection
- Cytomegalovirus
- Herpes simplex viruses (especially type 2)
- Rubella virus
- Lymphocytic choriomeningitis virus
- Varicella-zoster virus
- Human immunodeficiency virus
- Venezuelan equine encephalitis virus
- West Nile virus

developing CNS, causing hydrocephalus, cerebral atrophy, intracranial calcifications, schizencephaly, porencephaly, or hydranencephaly [Bale, 1994]. Linked conceptually by the *TORCH* (*to*xoplasmosis, *r*ubella, *c*ytomegalovirus, and *h*erpes simplex virus) acronym, these viruses produce similar neonatal symptoms and signs consisting of intrauterine growth retardation, hepatosplenomegaly, jaundice, and petechial or purpuric rash [Bale and Murph, 1992]. Neurologic features include microcephaly, chorioretinitis, macrocrania, sensorineural hearing loss, seizures, hypotonia, and focal deficits. Infants with intrauterine infections have varied prognoses, depending on the virus, the timing of intrauterine infection, and the extent of CNS damage.

Infants with perinatal viral infections involving the CNS challenge the clinician because the historical and clinical features can be vague during the initial phase of the illness. Early symptoms of serious viral CNS disease, including neonatal herpes simplex virus encephalitis, may consist only of poor feeding or fussiness, and the physical examination often reveals few signs localizing to the CNS [Bale and Murph, 1997]. Consequently the physician examining an ill-appearing young infant must consider the possibility of a CNS infection. Infants with perinatal viral infections have varied prognoses, depending on the agent, extent of disease, and availability of specific antiviral therapy.

Slow Viral Infections

Conventional viral pathogens have been associated with several unusual chronic disorders of the CNS, historically termed *slow viral infections.* These include subacute sclerosing panencephalitis [Dyken and Cunningham, 1989], post-rubella panencephalitis, chronic nonpolio enterovirus infection, and progressive multifocal leukoencephalopathy caused by the JC virus (a polyomavirus unrelated to Creutzfeldt-Jakob disease, but named for the initials of the patient from whom the virus initially was isolated). Children with these disorders generally lack systemic signs of infection and have clinical signs restricted to the CNS, including dementia, spasticity, paralysis, vision loss, and seizures. These slow viral disorders typically cause progressive debility and death.

Prions (transmissible proteinaceous particles), novel agents with biologic characteristics distinct from conventional viral pathogens, produce several progressive, degenerative neurologic disorders, including kuru, Creutzfeldt-Jakob disease, Gerstmann-Sträussler-Scheinker syndrome, fatal familial insomnia, and a Creutzfeldt-Jakob disease variant linked to bovine spongiform encephalopathy [Prusiner, 1997]. These disorders typically affect adults and manifest with progressive dementia, myoclonus, cerebellar ataxia, or sleep disturbances [Prusiner, 1997; Prusiner and Hsiao, 1994]. Adolescents have been described with variant Creutzfeldt-Jakob disease and with classic Creutzfeldt-Jakob disease acquired by contact with prion-contaminated cortical electrodes or human growth hormone extracts [Brown, 1988; Brown et al., 1985, 1994; Koch et al., 1985; Monreal et al., 1981]. Creutzfeldt-Jakob disease and other prion-induced disorders cannot be treated with specific antimicrobial agents and invariably lead to death.

EPIDEMIOLOGY OF VIRAL INFECTIONS

Worldwide statistics suggest that viral encephalitis develops in several thousand persons annually, and that many thousands more experience aseptic meningitis. The rates of encephalitis range from 3 to 8 cases per 100,000 persons [Johnson, 1996; Nicolosi et al., 1986] to 33 per 100,000 person-years, with rates highest among children [Koskiniemi et al., 1991, 2001]. Japanese encephalitis, a disease of young children, accounts for several thousand cases of encephalitis annually in the endemic regions of India and eastern Asia [CDC, 1993a].

Until the emergence of West Nile virus in the United States in 1999, the Centers for Disease Control and Prevention received reports of 200 to 500 cases of arboviral encephalitis and several thousand cases of aseptic meningitis every year (Fig. 69-2) [CDC, 1993a]. In 2003, the Centers for Disease Control and Prevention recorded more than 2800 human cases of neuroinvasive disease caused by West Nile virus [CDC, 2004a]. Because of mandatory vaccination of domestic dogs, the United States has fewer than five indigenous cases of human rabies per year [Krebs et al., 2002; Plotkin, 2000]. By contrast, rabies cases average

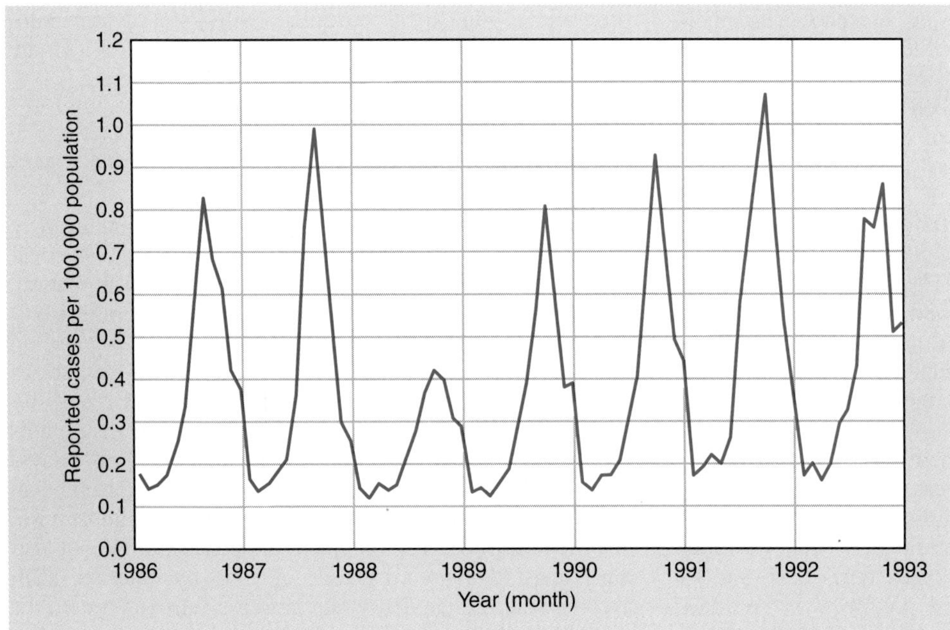

FIGURE 69-2. Data regarding the incidence of aseptic meningitis in the United States as reported to the Centers for Disease Control and Prevention from 1986 to 1992 [CDC, 1993a].

between 1 per 1 million and 1 per 100,000 persons annually in Africa and Asia, causing several thousand deaths per year [Dutta, 1999; Fishbein and Robinson, 1993; Haupt, 1999].

Some viruses, such as arthropod-borne and rabies viruses, are maintained in environmental reservoirs and transmitted by animals or insect vectors, whereas others, such as members of the herpesvirus family, are harbored by humans and transmitted by contact with human blood, tissues, or body fluids [Bale, 2003]. This distinction, environmental versus human etiology, provides a useful paradigm for understanding the epidemiology of most viral infections of the CNS. Several additional factors, including the age and immunocompetence of the host and the availability of vaccines or other preventive measures, influence the probability or severity of viral neurologic diseases.

Environmentally derived viral pathogens display relatively uniform epidemiologic characteristics. Mosquitoes, ticks, and biting flies serve as the vectors for most human viral diseases, aside from rabies. Human disease occurs most commonly when vectors are active, typically in spring, summer, and fall in temperate climates. Human disease also exhibits geographic distributions that correspond to the habitat of the vector. Hiking, camping, and outdoor professions facilitate vector contact and enhance the probability of infections with vector-borne diseases.

By contrast, human-derived viral pathogens require direct contact with the infected host, either by exposure to aerosols that contain infectious viruses or by contact with tissues or body fluids from infected individuals. Herpes simplex virus type 1 can be acquired by oral-oral or oral-genital contact, whereas

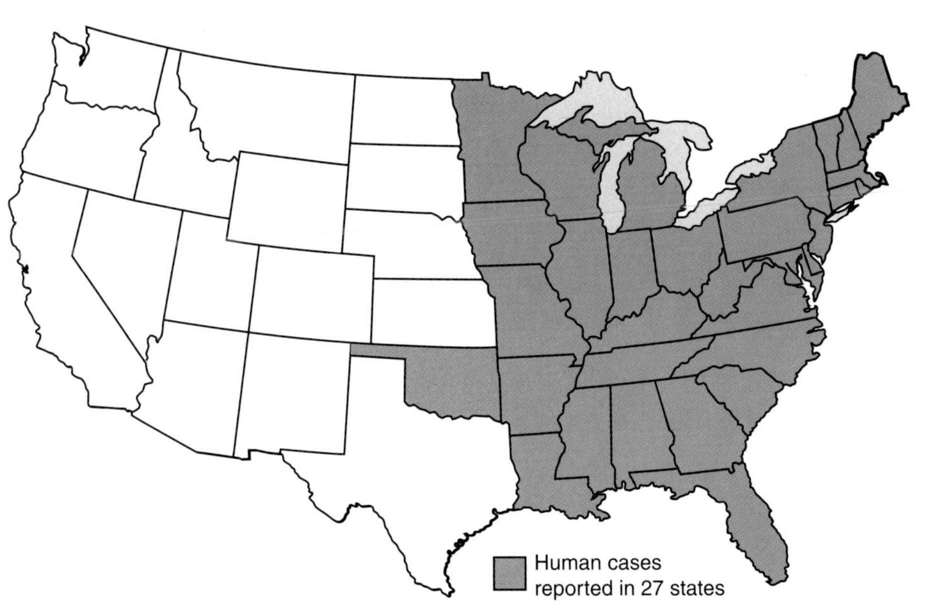

FIGURE 69-3. Map showing the geographic distribution of California (La Crosse) encephalitis cases reported to the Centers for Disease Control and Prevention from 1964 to 1997. An average of 73 cases was reported annually. (Adapted from the Centers for Disease Control and Prevention. Available at: www.cdc.gov/ncidod/dvbid/arbor/lac_map_sm.htm.)

varicella-zoster virus (the virus causing chickenpox) usually is transmitted by exposure to aerosolized particles that contain varicella-zoster virus. Cytomegalovirus can be acquired by direct contact with infected secretions or by transfusion of blood products or transplantation of organs or tissues from cytomegalovirus-seropositive persons [Bale, 1999].

La Crosse virus encephalitis, a frequently recognized arthropod-borne neurologic infection in the United States, illustrates the epidemiologic characteristics of environmentally derived agents [Balfour, 1974]. The disorder affects children who reside in the East and Midwest (Fig. 69-3), prime habitat for the *Aedes triseriatus* mosquito, a species that breeds preferentially in water that collects in tree trunks ("tree-holes") and discarded automobile tires. Cases occur from June to early October, reflecting the seasonal activity of the mosquito vector, and frequently involve males 5 to 15 years old who enter wooded areas to hunt or play.

Members of the herpesvirus family (herpes simplex virus types 1 and 2; cytomegalovirus; Epstein-Barr virus; varicella-zoster virus; and human herpesviruses types 6, 7, and 8) display few seasonal or geographic predilections [Whitley et al., 1982]. When Whitley and colleagues reviewed the epidemiology of herpes simplex virus encephalitis, they observed no unique characteristics with regard to race, sex, age, season, or geographic location [Whitley et al., 1982]. Epidemiologic data indicate, however, that herpes simplex virus type 1 is the most common cause of nonepidemic encephalitis in persons older than age 50 years. These data reflect the current opinion that most cases of herpes simplex virus encephalitis in older individuals result from reactivated herpes simplex virus infections rather than primary exposures to the virus.

Infection with HIV illustrates the potential effects that host behaviors and immune competence have on the epidemiology and spectrum of disease resulting from neurotropic viral agents. Early in the epidemic of acquired immunodeficiency syndrome (AIDS) in the United States, intravenous drug use, homosexuality, and sexual contact with persons in these groups increased substantially the probability of HIV infection. When $CD4^+$ cell counts decrease to less than 200/mL in persons infected with HIV, opportunistic infections, including infections resulting from other neurotropic viruses, become more likely. The latter conditions include progressive multifocal encephalopathy and cytomegalovirus retinitis and encephalitis [Jacobson, 1997], which are uncommon disorders in immunocompetent persons.

DIAGNOSTIC EVALUATION

An infant, child, or adolescent with fever and neurologic signs or symptoms requires a thorough neurodiagnostic evaluation that may include a cerebrospinal fluid examination, electrophysiologic studies (e.g., electroencephalogram [EEG] or electromyography/nerve conduction velocities), and an imaging study of the brain or spinal cord. The precise sequence of these studies depends on the nature and severity of the child's condition and the clinician's concerns regarding the presence of increased intracranial pressure or systemic conditions requiring specific interventions. The clinician must remain alert for signs that suggest a treatable viral disorder, such as herpes simplex virus encephalitis, but also must consider nonviral causes of CNS dysfunction, such as bacterial meningitis, brain abscess, stroke, tumor, or noninfectious, inflammatory conditions.

Cerebrospinal Fluid

The cerebrospinal fluid in viral meningitis or encephalitis typically has a lymphocytic pleocytosis (5 to 500 cells/mL), mildly elevated protein content (usually <200 mg/dL), and normal or slightly depressed glucose content (Table 69-1). The cerebrospinal fluid profile can vary, however, depending on the specific viral pathogen and the timing of the lumbar puncture. Many patients (5% to 15%) with herpes simplex virus encephalitis have an entirely normal initial cerebrospinal fluid examination [Koskiniemi, 1984; Whitley et al., 1982], and 10% or more of children with California encephalitis have normal cerebrospinal fluid parameters [Balfour, 1974].

Early in the course of viral CNS infections, the cerebrospinal fluid frequently has a preponderance of neutrophils, mimicking bacterial disease, but typically shifts to a lymphocytic pleocytosis over time [Feigin and Shackelford, 1973]. Protein elevations in viral meningitis and encephalitis tend to be modest (often <100 mg/dL), and glucose

TABLE 69-1

Cerebrospinal Fluid Profiles in Central Nervous System Infections

	ORGANISM			
PARAMETER	Virus	Bacterium	Mycobacterium	Fungus
Cell number*	N to ↑↑	↑ to ↑↑↑	↑ to ↑↑	N to ↑↑
Cell type†	Lymph	PMN	Lymph	Mixed
Protein content‡	N to ↑	↑ to ↑↑↑	N to ↑↑	N to ↑↑
Glucose content§	N to ↓	↓ to ↓↓↓	N to ↓	N to ↓

*Cell number: N, <5; ↑, 10-100/mm^3; ↑↑, 100-1000/mm^3; ↑↑↑, >1000/mm^3.

†Dominant cell type. Lymph, lymphocyte; PMN, polymorphonuclear leukocyte; Mixed, variable mix of PMNs and lymphocytes depending on the organism. PMNs can be the dominant cerebrospinal fluid leukocyte during the early phase of viral central nervous system infections, and meningitis with certain bacteria, notably *Listeria monocytogenes,* can be associated with a predominance of lymphocytes. Eosinophils occasionally can be observed in viral, fungal, or parasitic central nervous system infections.

‡Protein content: N, <50 mg/dL; ↑, 50-100 mg/dL; ↑↑, 100-500 mg/dL; ↑↑↑, >500 mg/dL.

§Glucose content: N, cerebrospinal fluid–to-serum ratio of >0.6; ↓, cerebrospinal fluid–to-serum ratio of <0.4; ↓↓↓, 0. Virus-associated reductions in the cerebrospinal fluid glucose content are usually modest, with levels ranging from 25 to 50 mg/dL in herpes simplex, lymphocytic choriomeningitis, and mumps viruses.

content in viral diseases, although modestly depressed in some cases (30 to 50 mg/dL), rarely reaches the low levels (e.g., <20 mg/dL) common in acute bacterial meningitis. Nonetheless, some viral infections, such as eastern equine encephalitis, may have cerebrospinal fluid parameters that seem more "bacterial" than "viral" [Przelomski et al., 1988].

The cerebrospinal fluid in viral myelitis can be normal or have features similar to those of aseptic meningitis (lymphocytic or mixed pleocytosis, normal glucose content, and normal or mildly elevated protein content). Children with Guillain-Barré syndrome frequently display an albuminocytologic dissociation (elevated protein content and no or few white blood cells), but the cerebrospinal fluid may be entirely normal early in the course of Guillain-Barré syndrome. Children with acute disseminated encephalitis frequently have cerebrospinal fluid profiles that mimic cerebrospinal fluid profiles of viral encephalitis or meningitis.

Electrodiagnostic Studies

The EEG has an important role in evaluating pediatric patients with suspected viral encephalitis. Although the EEG occasionally can be normal in such patients, infants or children with encephalitis usually have abnormal studies consisting of slowing or epileptiform discharges that can be diffuse or focal. Because herpes simplex virus encephalitis of children or adults frequently produces focal EEG features [Whitley et al., 1982], consisting of slowing, sharp-wave discharges, or periodic lateralizing epileptiform discharges, the EEG has considerable value in suspected herpes simplex virus encephalitis. Although these abnormalities usually localize to the temporal lobes in children, atypical cases of herpes simplex virus encephalitis with other cortical localizations have been confirmed by MRI and polymerase chain reaction detection of herpes simplex virus DNA in the cerebrospinal fluid [Schlesinger et al., 1995]. Neonates also may have early EEG abnormalities that alert clinicians to the possibility of herpes simplex virus encephalitis [Mikati et al., 1990; Mizrahi and Tharp, 1982].

The EEG has modest sensitivity and specificity in several other forms of encephalitis. Of patients with La Crosse encephalitis or eastern equine encephalitis, 40% to 50% have lateralizing EEG abnormalities that suggest focal brain disease [Hilty et al., 1972; Przelomski et al., 1988]. In many cases the EEG shows only diffuse slowing of variable severity.

Electrophysiologic studies, such as electromyography and nerve conduction velocities, have utility in children with suspected postinfectious polyneuropathies. Although nerve conduction velocities can be normal early in Guillain-Barré syndrome, children have conduction block or absent F waves, a neurodiagnostic measure of the integrity of spinal reflex arcs. Within 3 weeks of disease onset, most patients with Guillain-Barré syndrome have reduced nerve conduction velocities, indicating segmental demyelination and differentiating Guillain-Barré syndrome from other causes of acute weakness, such as myelitis. Electrophysiologic studies of peripheral nerves also have diagnostic value in selected patients with Bell's palsy or postinfectious lumbar or brachial plexopathies.

Neuroimaging

Computed tomography (CT) and MRI have major roles in evaluating infants and children with CNS viral infections [Bale, 1999; Barkovich, 1995; Kimberlin, 2004]. Depending on their clinical status, patients with suspected viral encephalitis should undergo a neuroimaging study early in the course of their illnesses. Although large mass lesions, such as tumors or brain abscess, can be detected reliably by CT, especially when obtained with contrast enhancement, MRI has sensitivity that exceeds CT, especially in patients with herpes simplex encephalitis [Domingues et al., 1998; Schroth et al., 1987]. Because of the sensitivity of MRI for the early changes of herpes simplex encephalitis, MRI is the preferred imaging modality in children with suspected viral encephalitis.

MRI in non-neonatal herpes simplex encephalitis reveals T2 prolongation in the medial temporal lobe, orbitofrontal region, or cingulate gyrus and cortical enhancement in these regions when the paramagnetic agent, gadolinium, is administered intravenously [Barkovich, 1995]. Atypical features can be observed, however, including parieto-occipital localization of T2 prolongation and abnormalities of diffusion-weighted images [Leonard et al., 2000; Maschke et al., 2004].

Neuroimaging frequently reveals diffuse or focal brain edema in infants with neonatal herpes simplex encephalitis, a disease that differs pathogenetically from herpes simplex encephalitis of older children [Bale, 2004; Kimberlin, 2004]. Neonatal herpes simplex encephalitis results from hematogenous transmission of the virus to brain, whereas herpes simplex encephalitis in older individuals usually reflects reactivation and neural transmission of herpes simplex virus.

MRI can detect focal abnormalities of the basal ganglia in children with Japanese or Epstein-Barr virus encephalitis [Maschke et al., 2004], and patients with neuroinvasive West Nile virus infections can have imaging abnormalities of the substantia nigra, brainstem, or spinal cord [Maschke et al., 2004]. The sensitivity of MRI exceeds that of CT in detecting the lesions of acute disseminated encephalomyelitis, a condition that mimics the clinical features of viral encephalitis [Dunn et al., 1986; Rust, 2000] and often responds to corticosteroids. In this condition, MRI reveals multifocal areas of T2 prolongation involving the white matter of the cerebrum, cerebellum, and brainstem. MRI in other forms of viral encephalitis can be normal; reveal diffuse, nonspecific changes of edema or inflammation; or have focal abnormalities that mimic herpes simplex virus encephalitis [Barkovich, 1995]. Children with aseptic meningitis typically have normal brain parenchyma when studied by CT or MRI.

Infants with suspected intrauterine viral infections should be evaluated by CT initially because small intracranial calcifications, a common feature of intrauterine infection, are detected better by this imaging modality than by MRI or ultrasonography [Bale and Murph, 1992; Barkovich, 1995]. These infants may benefit from a subsequent MRI study, however, to identify coexisting brain abnormalities, such as lissencephaly-pachygyria, periventricular leukomalacia, or cortical dysplasia. CT or MRI may reveal hydrocephalus, hydranencephaly, or cystic encephalomalacia in infants with intrauterine or perinatal viral infections.

TABLE 69-2

Preferred Diagnostic Methods for Selected Viral Infections of the Nervous System

AGENT	NEONATAL INFECTION	NON-NEONATAL INFECTION
HSV	Cultures of CSF; swabs of nasopharynx, conjunctivae, and skin lesions; CSF PCR	CSF PCR
CMV	Cultures of urine and saliva	Cultures of urine, saliva, or circulating leukocytes; serum and CSF PCR
VZV	Difficult by any method	Culture of skin vesicle fluid, immunohistology, CSF PCR
EBV	—	Acute and convalescent sera, CSF PCR
HHV 6, HHV 7, HHV 8	—	CSF PCR
Enteroviruses	Cultures of swabs of rectum and nasopharynx; serum and CSF PCRs	Serum and CSF PCR
Arthropod-borne encephalitis viruses	Virus-specific IgM	Virus-specific CSF or serum IgM; CSF PCR; acute and convalescent sera
Rabies virus	—	Virus culture, serum IgG after day 15; immunohistology of skin biopsy
Lymphocytic choriomeningitis virus	Serologic studies of infant and mother	Acute and convalescent sera; CSF PCR
HIV	Plasma PCR	Serologic studies; Western blot; plasma and CSF PCR

CMV, cytomegalovirus; CSF, cerebrospinal fluid; EBV, Epstein-Barr virus; HHV, human herpesvirus; HIV, human immunodeficiency virus; HSV, herpes simplex virus; PCR, polymerase chain reaction; VZV, varicella-zoster virus.

Microbiologic Evaluation

The diagnostic techniques available to the clinician include serology, cell culture, immunohistology, and molecular methods, such as polymerase chain reaction (Table 69-2) [Gleaves et al., 1994]. Serology provides indirect evidence of infection because it depends on the host to mount an antibody response specific to the etiologic agent. Certain infections, such as infections resulting from Epstein-Barr, lymphocytic choriomeningitis, and West Nile viruses, usually are identified by serologic studies, and others, such as La Crosse, eastern and western equine, St. Louis, and Japanese encephalitis viruses, can be diagnosed rapidly by immunoglobulin M (IgM) antibody capture methods.

Cell culture provides direct evidence of infection by detecting viral pathogens in cerebrospinal fluid, blood, or other body fluids. Viruses that lend themselves to this diagnostic approach include the herpesviruses (especially cytomegalovirus and certain herpes simplex virus infections), enteroviruses, adenoviruses (a rare cause of CNS infection), HIV, and rabies virus. Cultures of cerebrospinal fluid or mucosal surfaces often yield virus in neonatal herpes simplex virus infections [Kimberlin, 2004], but infectious virus can be detected in the cerebrospinal fluid in less than 5% of cases of non-neonatal herpes simplex virus encephalitis. Consequently, polymerase chain reaction has become the standard for evaluation of infants and children with suspected herpes simplex virus encephalitis or meningitis, especially as laboratories establish polymerase chain reaction protocols with high sensitivity and specificity [Mitchell et al., 1997; Whitley and Gnann, 2002]. Specific immunohistologic detection of herpes simplex virus and varicella-zoster virus has supplanted the nonspecific and insensitive Tzanck preparation.

Polymerase chain reaction detects herpes simplex virus DNA in the cerebrospinal fluid in most neonatal or non-neonatal cases of herpes simplex virus encephalitis or meningitis [Domingues et al., 1998; Kimberlin et al., 1996; Lakeman and Whitley, 1995; Mitchell et al., 1997; Read et al., 1997]. The specificity of polymerase chain reaction in herpes simplex virus encephalitis approaches 100%, whereas the sensitivity ranges from 75% in neonates to greater than 95% in children or adolescents [Johnson, 1996; Kimberlin, 2004]. Because polymerase chain reaction-negative cases of herpes simplex virus encephalitis occur, however, clinicians must use sound clinical judgment when making treatment decisions. Polymerase chain reaction also affords rapid diagnosis of infections with cytomegalovirus, enteroviruses, JC virus, human herpesvirus 6, varicella-zoster virus, and HIV and can be used to detect nonviral agents that cause intrauterine infection, encephalitis, or aseptic meningitis [Read et al., 1997; Souza and Bale, 1995].

OVERVIEW OF TREATMENT

Therapy for CNS viral infections must be tailored to illness severity, the suspected agent, and the availability of specific antiviral medications. Numerous nonviral and noninfectious conditions can produce clinical signs that mimic signs of CNS infection. Children with life-threatening viral diseases, such as herpes simplex virus encephalitis, require hospitalization in a skilled nursing unit, such as a pediatric intensive care unit, which can provide frequent assessment of the child's responsiveness and anticipatory monitoring for seizures and increased intracranial pressure. Outcome of CNS viral infection varies according to the viral pathogen, the child's age, and availability of specific antiviral therapy (Table 69-3).

Antiviral Chemotherapy

An increasing number of viral CNS infections, including herpes simplex virus encephalitis, varicella-zoster virus encephalitis, systemic or neurologic HIV infections, and invasive cytomegalovirus infections, can be treated with specific antiviral drugs. In general, the available agents inhibit viral infection by binding with viral nucleic acid and

TABLE 69-3

Outcome of Selected Viral Central Nervous System Disorders

DISORDER	MORTALITY (%)	MORBIDITY (%)
Herpes simplex virus*		
Congenital infection	10	100
Neonatal encephalitis	<10	40
Non-neonatal encephalitis	<10	40
Cytomegalovirus		
Symptomatic congenital	5	95
Encephalitis-AIDS	>50	High
Enterovirus		
Aseptic meningitis	Negligible	Negligible
Encephalitis	Negligible	Low
Togaviruses		
Eastern equine encephalitis	40	50
Western equine encephalitis	10	15
Rubella virus		
Symptomatic congenital	5	90
Flaviviruses		
Japanese encephalitis	40	50
St. Louis encephalitis	10	20
West Nile virus	5	33
Bunyaviruses		
La Crosse encephalitis	Negligible	15
Paramyxoviruses		
Measles encephalomyelitis	20	50
Subacute measles encephalitis	80	100
SSPE	100	—
Rabies virus†	100	—
Lymphocytic choriomeningitis virus		
Symptomatic congenital	40	80
Aseptic meningitis	Negligible	Negligible
Retroviruses‡		
HTLV-I	Negligible	100
HIV	Variable	Variable

*Assumes appropriate management with acyclovir. Rates for untreated cases are higher.

†Survival reported in <10 persons (total) with symptomatic rabies [American Academy of Pediatrics, 2003].

‡Outcomes related to current management.

AIDS, acquired immunodeficiency syndrome; HIV, human immunodeficiency virus; HTLV-I, human T-cell lymphotropic virus type I; SSPE, subacute sclerosing

preventing successful DNA or RNA replication. Acyclovir, a drug effective against herpes simplex virus and varicella-zoster virus, has few side effects and should be initiated as soon as the possibility of herpes simplex virus infection is considered. Additional useful antiviral agents include ganciclovir and foscarnet, effective in cytomegalovirus infections; ribavirin, potentially useful in RNA virus infections; inosine pranobex, potentially beneficial in subacute sclerosing panencephalitis; and several potent antiretroviral drugs, including zidovudine, didanosine, ritonavir, and others.

Supportive Care

Many viral CNS infections, including West Nile encephalitis and other infections with arthropod-borne viruses, cannot be treated with specific therapy. Several other disorders, such as enteroviral meningitis or postvaricella ataxia, resolve spontaneously with conservative management. Children may require adjunctive therapies, consisting of antipyretics, intravenous fluids, antiepileptic drugs, and occasionally corticosteroids.

Seizures, a frequent complication of viral encephalitis, can be treated acutely with lorazepam and may require maintenance therapy with phenobarbital or phenytoin in standard doses. Occasionally, high-dose, intravenous barbiturate or benzodiazepine therapy is required to inhibit seizure activity refractory to standard therapies. Several of the newer antiepileptic drugs may also be used, although these have not been studied specifically for postencephalitic epilepsy. Increased intracranial pressure, another potentially life-threatening complication of encephalitis, may require osmotic diuretic therapy, cautious fluid restriction, and hyperventilation. Critically ill patients require referral to tertiary medical centers for intensive monitoring and evaluation by specialists in neurology, critical care, neurosurgery, and infectious disease.

Children or adolescents with optic neuritis, myelitis, inflammatory vasculitis, and acute disseminated encephalomyelitis may benefit from corticosteroid therapy. Regimens can be modeled after the successful treatment of optic neuritis in adults. Children can receive 2 weeks of daily corticosteroids, beginning with a short course of high-dose methylprednisolone intravenously (e.g., 15 mg/kg/day divided equally every 6 hours for 3 to 5 days) and followed by prednisone orally (e.g., 1 to 2 mg/kg/day for 7 to 10 days). Children with postviral Guillain-Barré syndrome do not benefit from corticosteroids but may improve after intravenous immunoglobulin [Abd-Allah et al., 1997; Jansen et al., 1992; Ropper, 1992].

SPECIFIC VIRAL INFECTIONS

Herpesviridae

The human herpesviruses, a family of DNA viruses, commonly produce neurologic disease after infections in utero, perinatally, or postnatally. Important members of this family are herpes simplex virus types 1 and 2, both of which cause neonatal infection and focal encephalitis; cytomegalovirus, a major cause of intrauterine viral infection and opportunistic infections in immunocompromised hosts; Epstein-Barr virus, a cause of Guillain-Barré syndrome and encephalitis; human herpesvirus 6 and human herpesvirus 7, the agents of roseola and a frequent cause of febrile convulsions; and varicella-zoster virus, often associated with postinfectious ataxia. Other neurologic conditions linked to the herpesviruses include aseptic meningitis, myelitis, optic neuritis, Bell's palsy, and postinfectious neuritis.

Herpes Simplex Virus

CLINICAL FEATURES

Most humans acquire herpes simplex virus type 1 by oral transmission during childhood [Corey and Spear, 1986]. Primary herpes simplex virus infections are frequently asymptomatic, although some children experience vesicular pharyngitis or gingivostomatitis, a condition associated with fever, diminished oral intake, drooling, and herpetic lesions of the face and mouth. By contrast, herpes simplex virus type 2, usually acquired by sexual contact, causes genital lesions in young adults. In children, herpes simplex virus-induced neurologic infections can be due to primary or reactivated infections, whereas most herpes simplex virus–induced disease after age 30 years, whether due to herpes simplex virus type 1 or type 2, reflects reactivated infection.

Neonatal herpes simplex virus infection, most often due to herpes simplex virus type 2, can be categorized as (1) skin, eyes, and mouth disease; (2) disseminated disease; or (3) encephalitis and can affect approximately 43%, 23%, and 34% of herpes simplex virus–infected infants [Kimberlin, 2004; Whitley et al., 1988]. In addition, a small proportion (5%) of herpes simplex virus–infected infants have intrauterine infections [Hutto et al., 1987]. Neonatal herpes simplex encephalitis can be accompanied by pneumonitis, hepatitis, or disseminated intravascular coagulopathy, but one third of infants with neonatal herpes simplex virus encephalitis have disease restricted to the CNS [Koskiniemi et al., 1989]. Neonatal herpes simplex virus disease usually begins with nonspecific clinical features (poor oral intake, behavioral change, or fever) during the second or third weeks of life [Kimberlin, 2004]. Neonatal herpes simplex virus disease can begin as early as the first day of life, however [Koskiniemi et al., 1989].

Neonatal herpes simplex encephalitis produces focal or generalized seizures, paralysis, apnea, and lethargy or coma [Kimberlin, 2004; Koskiniemi et al., 1989; Whitley et al., 1988]. Vesicular rash is present in approximately two thirds of infants. The infection can be rapidly fatal with multiorgan system failure or be associated with apnea, impaired bulbar function, and intractable seizures. Approximately 5% of infants infected with herpes simplex virus acquire the virus in utero and have a relatively characteristic disorder manifested by microcephaly, cataracts, intracranial calcifications (Fig. 69-4), intrauterine growth retardation, and vesicular rash [Grose, 1994; Hutto et al., 1987].

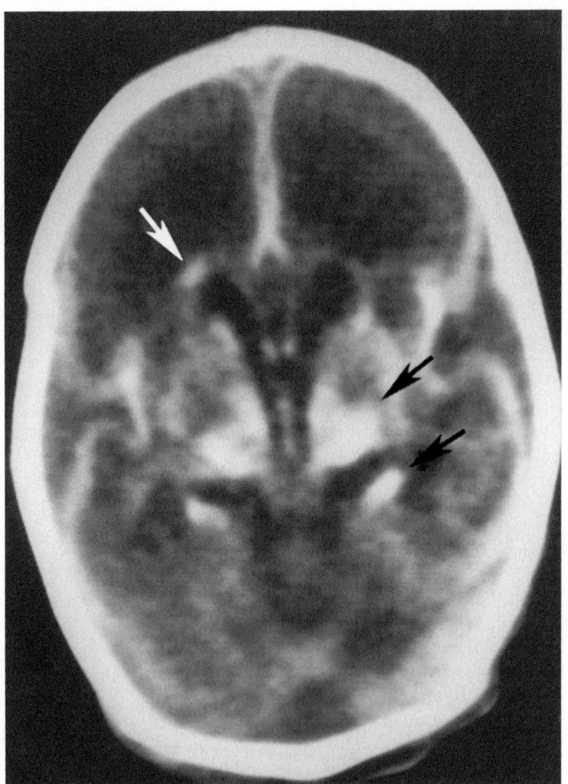

FIGURE 69-4. Unenhanced CT scan of an infant with congenital herpes simplex virus infection reveals dense thalamic and periventricular calcifications *(dark arrows)*, an additional periventricular density that may be calcium or hemorrhage *(white arrow)*, and abnormal cerebral parenchyma. (From Souza IE, Bale JF. The diagnosis of congenital infections: Contemporary strategies. J Child Neurol 1995;10:271.)

In older children or adolescents, herpes simplex encephalitis, typically herpes simplex virus type 1, begins nonspecifically with headache, fever, malaise, vomiting, and behavioral changes. Focal neurologic signs, such as hemiparesis, dysphasia, or visual field defects, appear subsequently in most patients. Seizures can occur in approximately 40% of patients with biopsy-confirmed herpes simplex encephalitis and may be generalized or partial [Whitley et al., 1982]. Focal abnormalities reflect the predilection of herpes simplex virus to infect frontotemporal brain regions, but other areas of the brain can be affected [Leonard et al., 2000]. The clinical course of herpes simplex encephalitis can be rapidly progressive, with refractory seizures, coma, increased intracranial pressure, and death within 2 weeks, or more indolent with memory loss and behavioral disturbances.

In addition to causing necrotizing encephalitis, herpes simplex virus has been linked to Bell's palsy by detecting herpes simplex virus type 1 DNA in facial nerve tissues or in the geniculate ganglia [Burgess et al., 1994]. Herpes simplex virus also has been associated with primary or recurrent aseptic meningitis (Mollaret's meningitis) [Bergström et al., 1990]. Common clinical manifestations of herpes simplex virus-associated aseptic meningitis include fever, photophobia, vomiting, and headache, but children with herpes simplex virus–induced meningitis usually lack herpetic lesions of the skin or mucosal surfaces [Rathore et al., 1996]. The diagnosis can be established by assaying cerebrospinal fluid by culture or polymerase chain reaction. Although children with herpes simplex virus type 1 meningitis can recover uneventfully without therapy [Rathore et al., 1996], acyclovir therapy should be considered. Herpes simplex virus infection also has been associated with a necrotizing myelopathy in childhood, although it more commonly occurs in adults with reactivated herpes simplex virus infections [Ellstein-Shturman et al., 1976].

DIAGNOSIS

Neonates with herpes simplex virus infections may have elevated serum transaminases, direct hyperbilirubinemia, and laboratory features of disseminated intravascular coagulopathy [Kimberlin, 2004; Koskiniemi et al., 1989]. The cerebrospinal fluid in neonatal herpes simplex encephalitis reveals a lymphocytic pleocytosis and elevations of the protein content. MRI and CT usually reveal diffuse edema during the acute stage and later exhibit atrophy, parenchymal calcification, or cystic encephalomalacia [Tien et al., 1993]. EEGs are frequently abnormal in infants with encephalitis, revealing slow background activity and paroxysmal discharges that occasionally are periodic [Mikati et al., 1990].

Herpes simplex virus infection can be confirmed by isolating virus from cerebrospinal fluid, skin lesions, or mucosal surfaces of the eye, oropharynx, or rectum or by detecting herpes simplex virus DNA in cerebrospinal fluid by using polymerase chain reaction. In a retrospective analysis of cerebrospinal fluid samples accumulated by the National Institutes of Health–Collaborative Antiviral Study Group, herpes simplex virus DNA was detected by polymerase chain reaction in the cerebrospinal fluid of 93% of the infants with disseminated infection, 76% of infants with encephalitis, and only 24% of infants with skin-eyes-mouth disease [Kimberlin et al., 1996]. In other National Institutes of Health–Collaborative Antiviral Study Group studies, herpes simplex virus DNA was detected in the cerebrospinal fluid of 98% of patients with biopsy-proven herpes simplex virus encephalitis, whereas only 6% of biopsy-negative patients had herpes simplex virus DNA in cerebrospinal fluid [Lakeman and Whitley, 1995]. These results and results from other laboratories indicate that the sensitivity and specificity of polymerase chain reaction for herpes simplex encephalitis are 90% to 95% [Mitchell et al., 1997; Read et al., 1997]. Cerebrospinal fluid analysis by polymerase chain reaction is the current standard for the diagnosis of encephalitis, as well as meningitis, resulting from herpes simplex virus.

Because older infants, children, and adolescents with herpes simplex virus encephalitis rarely have systemic signs of infection, neurodiagnostic and cerebrospinal fluid polymerase chain reaction studies have major roles in establishing the diagnosis [Mitchell et al., 1997; Whitley and Lakeman, 1995; Whitley et al., 1982]. MRI may indicate unilateral or bilateral abnormalities consisting of T2 prolongation in the temporal lobe or insula and enhancement of the insula, temporal cortex, and cingulate gyrus on T1-weighted, gadolinium-enhanced images [Schroth et al., 1987; Tien et al., 1993]. Focal abnormalities involving other cortical regions, including parietal or occipital lobes, can be observed, however, in atypical cases of herpes simplex encephalitis [Schlesinger et al., 1995]. EEGs, abnormal in approximately 80% or more of patients, reveal focal or diffuse slowing and epileptiform discharges that can be periodic and lateralizing.

TREATMENT AND OUTCOME

Infants with herpes simplex virus infections should receive acyclovir, 20 mg/kg every 8 hours for 21 days, and older children should be treated with 20 mg/kg every 8 hours for at least 21 days [Bale, 2004; Kimberlin et al., 2001b; Whitley et al., 1986, 1991a, 1991b]. Adolescents can receive 1500 mg/m^2 for 21 days. Potential side effects include tremulousness, hematuria, and reversible nephropathy. Although the drug is well tolerated, complete blood counts and serum creatinine levels should be monitored during prolonged courses of acyclovir. Although favorable outcome after neonatal or childhood herpes simplex virus infections correlates with the early initiation of acyclovir, sequelae are common even after appropriate medical management.

Fewer than 40% of the survivors of neonatal or childhood herpes simplex virus encephalitis recover to their baseline levels of function [Kimberlin et al., 2001a, 2001b; Whitley et al., 1991b]. Potential sequelae consist of partial and generalized seizure disorders, developmental delay, cerebral palsy, language dysfunction, behavioral abnormalities, and motor deficits. All acyclovir-treated infants with skin, eye, and mouth infections survive, and nearly all such infants have no long-term sequelae of their infections, other than the propensity to have occasional recurrences of skin lesions

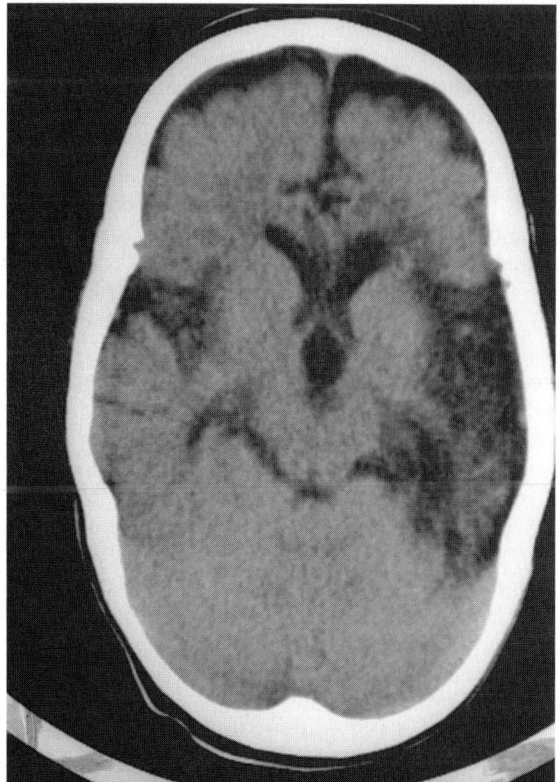

FIGURE 69-5. Unenhanced CT scan of a young child who survived herpes simplex virus encephalitis reveals cerebral atrophy and destructive changes of the insular cortex bilaterally. Despite treatment with acyclovir, the infant sustained extensive damage to both opercular areas and manifested severe pseudobulbar palsy.

[Kimberlin et al., 2001a]. Approximately 30% of the infants with disseminated neonatal herpes simplex virus infections die despite appropriate therapy, and 20% to 30% of the survivors have sequelae ranging from mild (speech delay or mild motor delay) to severe (spastic quadriparesis or severe developmental delay). Neonates with encephalitis have less than 10% mortality, but 40% of the surviving infants have severe sequelae despite acyclovir therapy [Kimberlin et al., 2001b]. Infants who survive herpes simplex virus encephalitis can have permanent pseudobulbar palsy with mutism and feeding difficulties (Fig. 69-5) [Grattan-Smith et al., 1989]. Infants with congenital herpes simplex virus infections have a uniformly poor prognosis [Hutto et al., 1987].

Relapse or persistence of symptoms in herpes simplex virus encephalitis, associated with fever, lethargy, headache, and movement disorder, can develop despite appropriate initial management and acyclovir therapy [Carpentier-Barthez et al., 1995; Gutman et al., 1986]. Such children require repeat cerebrospinal fluid polymerase chain reaction for herpes simplex virus, MRI, repeat treatment with acyclovir, and corticosteroid therapy if imaging suggests acute disseminated encephalitis. Because of the substantial morbidity associated with neonatal and childhood herpes simplex virus encephalitis, ongoing studies are evaluating the role for prolonged suppressive therapy with acyclovir in neonates with herpes simplex virus infections [Kimberlin, 2004].

Cytomegalovirus

CLINICAL FEATURES

Infection with cytomegalovirus, a ubiquitous member of the herpesvirus family, has been associated with several childhood neurologic conditions, including intrauterine infection; infantile spasms; Guillain-Barré syndrome; and encephalitis, myelitis, or retinitis in immunosuppressed hosts, especially persons with acquired immunodeficiency syndrome (AIDS) [Bale, 1984; McCuthan, 1995]. Approximately 1% of infants excrete cytomegalovirus at birth, and the virus is acquired steadily thereafter throughout life. Young children who attend daycare centers, adults who have contact with young children, and persons with multiple sexual partners acquire cytomegalovirus at annual rates of 8% to 25% or more, considerably higher than the background infection rates of 2% to 5% per year [Demmler, 1991; Murph and Bale, 1988]. Children acquire cytomegalovirus by contact with persons who shed cytomegalovirus in urine or saliva and by transfusion of blood products or transplantation of organs from cytomegalovirus-seropositive donors [Demmler, 1991].

At birth, 0.4% to 2.5% of newborns shed cytomegalovirus in urine or saliva, indicating congenital infection [Bale, 1984; Demmler, 1991]. Approximately 90% of cytomegalovirus-infected infants are asymptomatic at birth. Although sensorineural hearing loss develops subsequently in 7% to 10% of these infants [Fowler et al., 1997], they rarely have other CNS complications. The remaining 10% of infants with congenital cytomegalovirus infection have hepatomegaly, splenomegaly, jaundice, petechial or purpuric skin rash, intrauterine growth retardation, microcephaly, or chorioretinitis [Bale, 1984; Boppana et al., 1997; Demmler, 1991; Istas et al., 1995].

Cytomegalovirus has been linked to infantile spasms, usually in infants with intrauterine infection [Riikonen, 1978]. Immunocompetent children or adolescents with cytomegalovirus infections can have a mild, self-limited encephalitis [Studahl et al., 1992] or Guillain-Barré syndrome [Dowling and Cook, 1981]. The latter disorder begins with paresthesias and causes weakness that usually begins in the lower extremities. Affected children can have bilateral facial paresis, respiratory failure, or cardiac dysrhythmias [Ropper, 1992]. Symptoms of a cytomegalovirus-induced mononucleosis syndrome [Horwitz et al., 1986]—malaise, low-grade fever, or headache—may precede or accompany the onset of Guillain-Barré syndrome.

Patients immunocompromised by AIDS, malignancy, transplantation, or immunosuppressive therapy are at risk for cytomegalovirus-induced retinitis, encephalitis, myelopathy, and Guillain-Barré syndrome–like disorders. Given the demographics of AIDS, most reported patients with cytomegalovirus retinitis, encephalitis, or myelitis are adults between the ages of 20 and 50 years [Holland et al., 1994; Jacobson, 1997; Morgello et al., 1987; Palestine et al., 1984]. Immunocompromised infants or children, especially those with HIV infection, are at risk for retinitis, colitis, pneumonitis, and CNS complications of cytomegalovirus infections [Chandwani et al., 1996; Darin et al., 1994].

DIAGNOSIS

The diagnosis of intrauterine cytomegalovirus infection is established by assaying urine or saliva using shell vial methods. Polymerase chain reaction can be used to detect cytomegalovirus DNA in urine, saliva, or serum, but the shell vial assay is sensitive and cost-effective [Demmler et al., 1988]. Common, nonspecific laboratory features of congenital cytomegalovirus infections include thrombocytopenia, direct hyperbilirubinemia, and elevated serum transaminases [Istas et al., 1995]. CT scans reveal intracranial calcifications (Figs. 69-6 to 69-8) in 25% to 50% of symptomatic infants [Boppana et al., 1997; Pass et al., 1980]. Hydranencephaly, atrophy, lissencephaly, schizencephaly, and cerebellar hypoplasia also can accompany congenital cytomegalovirus infections [Hayward et al., 1991; Iannetti et al., 1998]. Approximately 50% of symptomatic infants have abnormal auditory-evoked responses indicating sensorineural hearing loss [Boppana et al., 1997; Pass et al., 1980; Rivera et al., 2002].

Infection in older infants or children can be established by isolating cytomegalovirus from urine, saliva, or circulating leukocytes; by detecting cytomegalovirus-specific antigens in circulating leukocytes; or by detecting cytomegalovirus-specific DNA in cerebrospinal fluid, serum, or urine [Clifford et al., 1993]. Some patients with cytomegalovirus infection have elevated serum transaminases or hematologic abnormalities, such as leukopenia, anemia, or thrombocytopenia. CT or MRI may reveal abnormalities of the brain or spinal cord consisting of demyelination or inflammation involving cortical or periventricular regions [Miller et al., 1997; Post et al., 1986].

TREATMENT AND OUTCOME

Most infants who survive symptomatic, intrauterine cytomegalovirus infections have permanent neurodevelopmental sequelae consisting of mental retardation, seizure disorders,

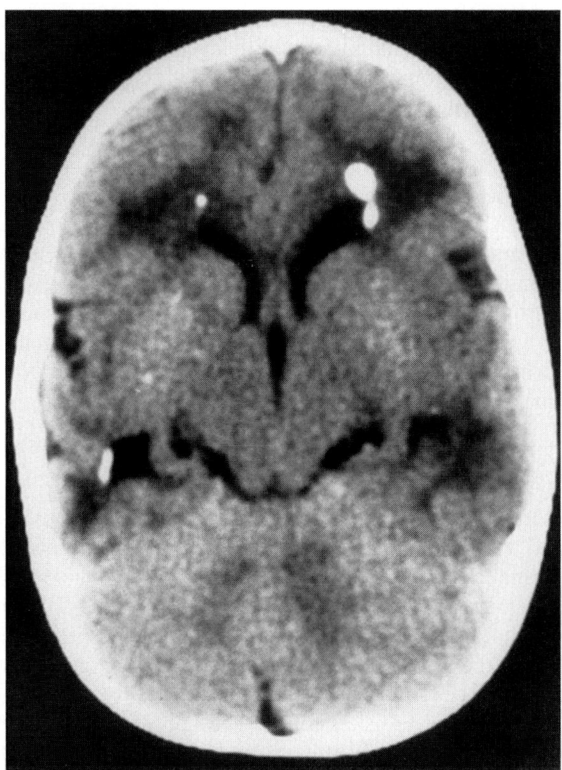

FIGURE 69-6. Unenhanced CT scan of an infant with symptomatic congenital cytomegalovirus infection reveals dense periventricular calcifications and bilateral periventricular leukomalacia. (From Souza IE, Bale JF. The diagnosis of congenital infections: Contemporary strategies. J Child Neurol 1995;10:271.)

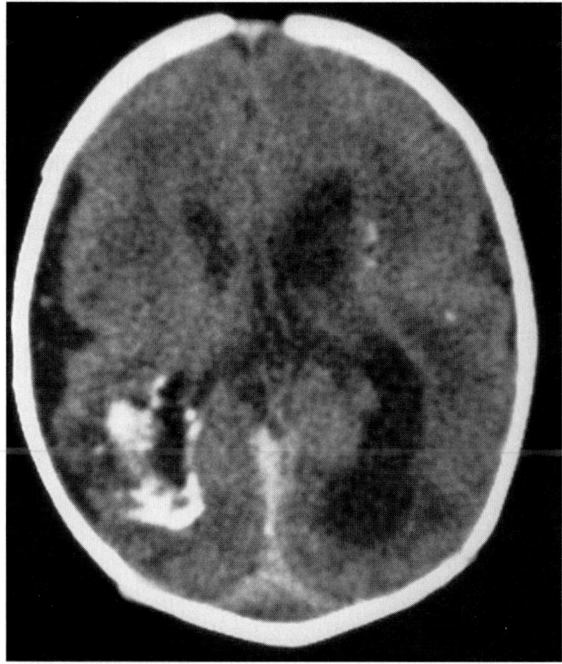

FIGURE 69-7. Unenhanced CT scan of an infant with symptomatic congenital cytomegalovirus infection reveals dense periventricular calcifications surrounding the occipital horn of the left lateral ventricle and bilateral cortical abnormalities suggesting lissencephaly/pachygyria.

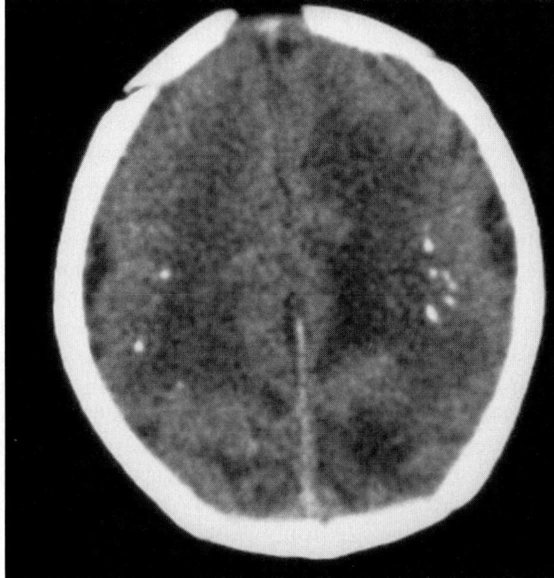

FIGURE 69-8. A higher CT section from the same infant in Figure 69-7 reveals diffuse parenchymal calcifications bilaterally and an abnormal-appearing cortex.

behavioral disturbances, visual impairment, and sensorineural hearing loss [Bale, 1984; Boppana et al., 1997; Pass et al., 1980]. Because hearing loss can be progressive, even after silent, intrauterine cytomegalovirus infection, infants with known congenital cytomegalovirus infection require serial audiometry at frequent intervals during infancy and childhood [Williamson et al., 1992]. Infants with abnormal CT scans are more likely to have adverse neurodevelopmental outcomes [Boppana et al., 1997; Noyola et al., 2001]. At present, intrauterine cytomegalovirus infection cannot be prevented by vaccination. Ganciclovir, an antiviral drug closely related to acyclovir, may provide modest benefit to infants with congenital cytomegalovirus disease [Nigro et al., 1994]. A controlled trial of ganciclovir indicates that prolonged courses of ganciclovir, 10 to 12 mg/kg/day for 42 days, can improve hearing outcomes [Kimberlin et al., 2003]. Bone marrow suppression is a potentially serious side effect.

Immunocompromised children with invasive cytomegalovirus disease, especially retinitis, should receive ganciclovir, beginning with 5 mg/kg intravenously twice daily for approximately 14 days. Long-term maintenance therapy, using 5 to 10 mg/kg/day, is required in persons with cytomegalovirus retinitis and HIV infection [Jacobson, 1997]. Complete blood counts and renal function should be monitored frequently. Outcome of acquired cytomegalovirus infection depends greatly on the immunocompetence of the infected host. Patients who are immunosuppressed by AIDS or transplantation have increased risks of death. By contrast, most children with normal immune systems generally recover from acquired cytomegalovirus infections. The prognosis of cytomegalovirus-induced Guillain-Barré syndrome in immunocompetent children is comparable with that of Guillain-Barré syndrome resulting from other causes.

Varicella-Zoster Virus

CLINICAL FEATURES

Varicella-zoster virus, the cause of chickenpox (varicella) and shingles (zoster), has been associated with several neurologic conditions in children, including acute ataxia, myelitis, stroke, postherpetic neuralgia, Bell's palsy, Ramsay-Hunt syndrome, aseptic meningitis, encephalitis, congenital varicella syndrome, and Reye's syndrome [Fleisher et al., 1981; Gilden, 2004; Huder, 1997; McKendall and Stroop, 1994; Weller, 1983]. These conditions affect immunocompetent or immunocompromised hosts, although immunosuppressed hosts, such as patients with AIDS or hematologic malignancies, have greater risks of severe, invasive infections. Certain conditions, such as varicella-induced ataxia or Reye's syndrome (rarely seen, currently), occur almost exclusively in immunocompetent children.

Chickenpox, the illness associated with primary varicella-zoster virus infection, peaks among children between the ages of 5 and 9 years and occurs more often in winter months. The virus spreads by aerosolization and respiratory transmission; children are contagious 2 days before and 5 days after the onset of the chickenpox rash. The incubation period averages 14 days. After primary infection, the virus enters a latent stage in sensory ganglia and can reactivate, causing zoster or shingles [Gilden, 2004]. Consequently, zoster more commonly affects the elderly or persons with immunocompromising conditions. Zoster can occur in otherwise healthy children or adolescents, however [Fleisher et al., 1981; Guess et al., 1985]. Zoster in persons without obvious risk factors should be considered a potential harbinger of HIV infection [Gnann and Whitley, 1991].

Less than 0.1% of otherwise healthy children with chickenpox experience neurologic complications. Acute cerebellar ataxia, the most common complication, begins approximately 10 days after the onset of the rash. Ataxia preceding the rash or after varicella vaccination has been reported [Johnson and Milbourn, 1970; Sunaga, et al., 1995]. Truncal ataxia, dysmetria, vomiting, and irritability are common clinical features. The ataxia, often maximum at onset, frequently inhibits independent ambulation, and nystagmus can be present [Connolly et al., 1994]. The pathogenesis of ataxia after varicella remains undetermined.

Other varicella-zoster virus–related neurologic complications are uncommon. Reye's syndrome, a now rare disorder characterized by pernicious vomiting, coma, and increased intracranial pressure, can be prevented by avoiding aspirin therapy in children or adolescents with varicella or influenza. Varicella encephalitis, another rare complication of either varicella or zoster, usually appears 3 to 7 days after the onset of the rash and produces headache, fever, seizures, coma, or paralysis [Appelbaum et al., 1953; Gilden, 2004; Hausler et al., 2002]. Myelitis causes urinary retention or incontinence, paraparesis, and sensory abnormalities [Rosenfield et al., 1993]. Ramsay-Hunt syndrome, an uncommon complication of zoster in childhood, consists of acute facial palsy, pain, unilateral hearing loss, and occasionally other cranial palsies in association with zoster of the ear or neck [Grose et al., 2002; Huder, 1997]. Children infrequently have postherpetic neuralgia [Kost and Strauss, 1996].

Stroke [Bodensteiner et al., 1992; Askalan et al., 2001; Sebire et al., 1999] or, rarely, herpes zoster ophthalmicus [Gilden, 2004; Leis and Butler, 1987] has been reported in children after varicella. Usually occurring within 4 to 8 weeks of varicella or zoster infection, these disorders are characterized by headache, focal deficits, lethargy or somnolence, and occasionally seizures. The pathogenesis of stroke in these pediatric cases seems to reflect vasculopathy mediated by varicella-zoster virus and is analogous to that of herpes zoster ophthalmicus and delayed infarction, a potential complication of varicella-zoster virus reactivation in adults [Hilt et al., 1983].

The intrauterine varicella syndrome affects approximately 2% to 3% of the offspring of women who have chickenpox during their first or second trimesters of pregnancy [Alkaly et al., 1987; Brunnell, 1992; Grose, 1994]. The characteristics of this disorder include intrauterine growth retardation, cicatricial skin lesions in a dermatomal distribution, eye abnormalities (chorioretinitis, cataracts, optic atrophy), limb hypoplasia, and neurologic abnormalities (hydrocephalus, microcephaly, seizures, or Horner's syndrome) [Alkaly et al., 1987; Grose, 1994].

DIAGNOSIS

Children or adolescents with neurologic conditions associated with varicella-zoster virus have cerebrospinal fluid abnormalities consisting of a lymphocytic pleocytosis and elevated protein content. Approximately 50% of children with ataxia after varicella have a lymphocytic pleocytosis, although the total leukocyte count and protein content rarely exceed 100 cells/mm^3 and 40 mg/dL [Connolly et al., 1994]. Varicella-zoster virus infection is suspected when characteristic skin lesions are present and confirmed by detecting infectious virus in skin lesions or varicella-zoster virus-specific antibodies or varicella-zoster virus DNA in cerebrospinal fluid using polymerase chain reaction [Dangond et al., 1993; Gilden, 2004; Kido et al., 1991]. Some adults and, presumably, children or adolescents with varicella-zoster virus–related neurologic complications lack cutaneous manifestations of varicella-zoster virus [Gilden, 2004]. This is especially true when remote complications of varicella-zoster virus, such as childhood stroke, occur [Askalan et al., 2001].

The results of neuroimaging studies vary, depending on the disorder and immune status of the child. Children with ataxia or encephalitis after varicella often have normal imaging studies, although MRI occasionally can detect edema or white matter lesions compatible with demyelination. Occasionally, features suggesting acute disseminated encephalitis are observed. MRI indicates focal cerebral or cerebellar lesions in children with stroke [Bodensteiner et al., 1992; Leis and Butler, 1987; Sunaga et al., 1995] and hydrocephalus, cortical atrophy, hydranencephaly, or intracranial calcifications in infants with congenital varicella-zoster virus embryopathy [Alkaly et al., 1987; Cuthbertson et al., 1987; Grose, 1994].

TREATMENT AND OUTCOME

Children with varicella-zoster virus–related ataxia recover without antiviral or corticosteroid therapy [Connolly et al., 1994], indicating that conservative management of these children is warranted. Virtually all children with varicella-induced ataxia recover completely within 8 weeks of onset, although behavioral disturbances may persist longer. In contrast, children or adolescents with encephalitis or myelitis should receive acyclovir, 1500 mg/m^2/day in three equally divided doses for at least 10 days, especially if immunocompromised by AIDS, transplantation, or chemotherapy [Gilden, 2004]. Children with Ramsay-Hunt syndrome also may benefit from acyclovir [Huder, 1997].

Corticosteroid therapy (e.g., intravenous methylprednisolone) should be considered in children or adolescents with myelitis, acute disseminated encephalitis, or stroke secondary to varicella-zoster virus vasculitis. Outcome of varicella-related stroke in children seems to be more favorable than the outcome in adults [Bodensteiner et al., 1992]. Infants with intrauterine infections have variable outcomes with high rates of permanent neurodevelopmental sequelae [Grose, 1994]. Varicella can be prevented by vaccination [CDC, 1996], suggesting that certain neurologic complications also may be preventable.

Epstein-Barr Virus

CLINICAL FEATURES

Epstein-Barr virus, the cause of infectious mononucleosis, has been associated with several neurologic disorders of children and adults, including encephalitis, Guillain-Barré syndrome, optic neuritis, Bell's palsy, acute ataxia, chronic daily headaches, acute chorea, and "Alice in Wonderland" syndrome [Connelly and DeWitt, 1994; Dowling and Cook, 1981; Volpi, 2004]. Epstein-Barr virus, transmitted by contact with oral secretions, commonly infects children before the age of 5 years, children and adolescents after age 10 years, and young adults. Most primary infections are asymptomatic, although infected individuals can experience infectious mononucleosis, an illness associated with fever, malaise, headache, sore throat, lymphadenopathy, splenomegaly, and rash [Sumaya and Ench, 1985a].

Epstein-Barr virus encephalitis accounts for 5% of cases of acute encephalitis and produces fever, headache, altered consciousness, and seizures, including acute status epilepticus [Connelly and DeWitt, 1994; Domachowske et al., 1996; Hung et al., 2000]. In the National Institutes of Health-Collaborative Antiviral Study Group studies, Epstein-Barr virus was the most common infectious agent mimicking herpes simplex virus encephalitis [Whitley et al., 1989]. "Alice in Wonderland" syndrome, another cerebral manifestation of Epstein-Barr virus infection, causes personality changes and illusions of distorted size, shape, or distance (metamorphopsia) [Liaw and Shen, 1991].

Other neurologic conditions attributed to Epstein-Barr virus, such as optic neuritis [Frey, 1973], Guillain-Barré syndrome [Grose and Feorino, 1972], acute hemiplegia [Baker et al., 1983], and acute ataxia [Connolly et al., 1994], lack distinguishing features that allow the clinical diagnosis of Epstein-Barr virus. The association of Epstein-Barr virus with these disorders often has been established retrospectively by serologic studies and exclusion of other potential causative factors. The lymphoproliferative syndrome associated with Epstein-Barr virus in transplant patients may cause seizures or altered sensorium as a consequence of intracranial mass lesions or lymphomatous meningitis [Boyle et al., 1997].

DIAGNOSIS, TREATMENT, AND OUTCOME

Children with Epstein-Barr virus infection frequently have elevated serum transaminases and hematologic abnormalities, including thrombocytopenia, leukopenia, and an atypical lymphocytosis [Sumaya and Ench, 1985a]. A positive heterophil response supports recent Epstein-Barr virus infection, although children younger than age 4 years frequently have false-negative results [Sumaya and Ench, 1985b]. The diagnosis of Epstein-Barr virus infection can be established specifically by a serologic panel that assays Epstein-Barr virus–specific antibody responses to viral capsid, early, and

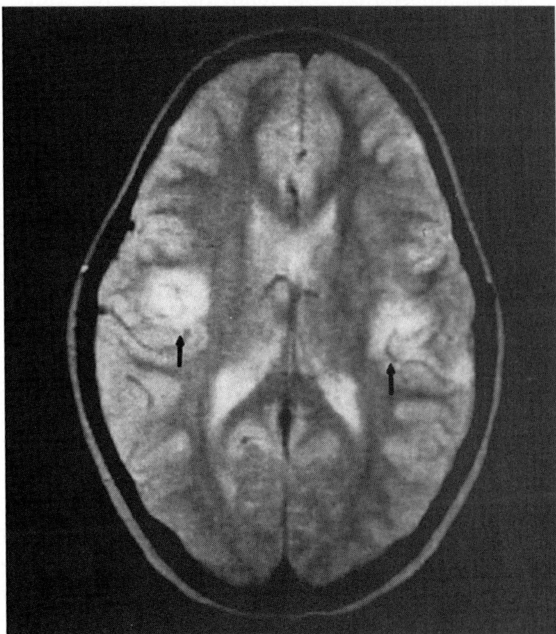

FIGURE 69-9. T2-weighted MRI from a child with Epstein-Barr virus encephalitis reveals bilateral areas of T2 prolongation *(arrows)* reminiscent of acute disseminated encephalomyelitis. (From Bale JF, Andersen RA, Grose C. Magnetic resonance imaging of the brain in childhood herpesvirus infections. Pediatr Infect Dis J 1987;6:644.)

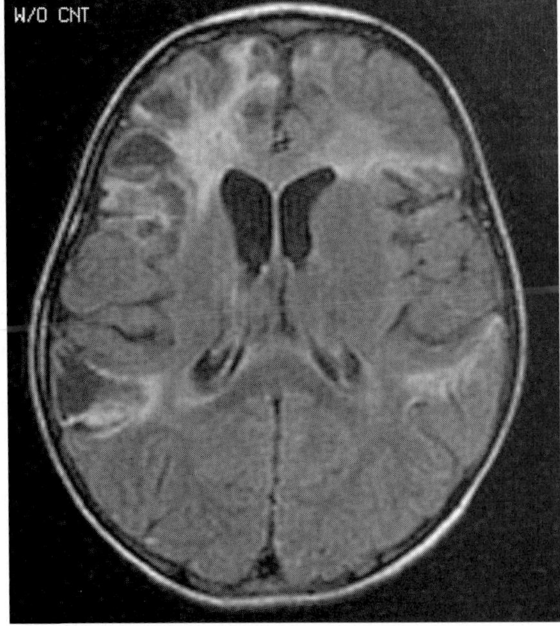

FIGURE 69-10. T1-weighted MRI from a child with neurologic sequelae from Epstein-Barr virus encephalitis shows cystic encephalomalacia and gliosis.

nuclear antigens [Sumaya, 1985]. Acute infection is suggested by the presence of viral capsid antigen IgM or IgG and the absence of Epstein-Barr nuclear antigen IgG [Sumaya and Ench, 1985b]. Epstein-Barr virus infection of the CNS also can be diagnosed by detecting Epstein-Barr virus DNA in cerebrospinal fluid [Halsted and Chang, 1979; Landgren et al., 1994; Volpi, 2004]. EEG may indicate slowing or epileptiform discharges during acute Epstein-Barr virus encephalitis or "Alice in Wonderland" syndrome. Neuroimaging studies occasionally can be abnormal (Fig. 69-9) [Bale et al., 1987; Domachowske et al., 1996; Ono et al., 1998]. Current antiviral medications have minimal effect on Epstein-Barr virus, but most children recover completely with supportive care. Neurologic sequelae of Epstein-Barr virus encephalitis can occur, however (Fig. 69-10) [Domachowske et al., 1996].

Human Herpesviruses Types 6, 7, and 8

Human herpesviruses type 6 and type 7, discovered in 1986 and 1990, cause roseola (exanthem subitum) in young children and occasionally neurologic complications in children or adults [Leach et al., 1992; Torigoe et al., 1996]. These viruses commonly infect infants and toddlers such that virtually all children have serologic evidence of infection by 5 years of age. Although primary infections are frequently asymptomatic, human herpesvirus type 6 and human herpesvirus type 7 produce roseola, an acute childhood illness with high fever (often >40°C), lymphadenopathy, and an erythematous rash that characteristically appears after the fever. By causing high fever at a vulnerable age, these viruses account for a substantial proportion of febrile seizures of childhood [Barone et al., 1995; Hall et al., 1994].

In addition to inducing febrile seizures, human herpesvirus type 6 and human herpesvirus type 7 have been linked with acute encephalopathy or encephalitis in young children and myelitis or encephalitis in adults [Barone et al., 1995; Drobyski et al., 1994; Hall et al., 1994; Leach et al., 1992; Suga et al., 1993; Torigoe et al., 1996; Yoshikawa et al., 1992]. Young children with symptomatic infections have high fevers and seizures that are usually generalized. Transient or permanent hemiparesis and coma are additional clinical features. The diagnosis can be established serologically or by polymerase chain reaction [Yoshikawa et al., 2000].

Human herpesvirus type 8, a herpesvirus that was linked initially to Kaposi's sarcoma in 1994, is acquired after adolescence in the United States and Europe, an epidemiologic feature that suggests sexual transmission [Chang et al., 1994; Martin et al., 1998]. Nonsexual modes contribute to the transmission of human herpesvirus type 8 in endemic regions of the developing world, however [Andreoni et al., 1999]. Although neurologic complications of human herpesvirus type 8 are rare, human herpesvirus type 6, human herpesvirus type 7, and human herpesvirus type 8 can be opportunistic CNS pathogens in persons with impaired cell-mediated immunity [Volpi, 2004].

Treatment of these infections consists of supportive care. Acyclovir, a potent inhibitor of herpes simplex virus and varicella-zoster virus, seems to be ineffective. Although most children recover uneventfully, permanent neurologic sequelae and death have been reported after human human herpesvirus type 6 or human herpesvirus type 7 CNS infections.

Adenoviridae

Adenoviruses, important causes of mild upper respiratory illnesses, pneumonia, and keratoconjunctivitis, have been associated occasionally with encephalitis or aseptic meningitis [Chany et al., 1958; Chuang et al., 2003; Kim and Gold, 1983]. Acquired by contact with infected respiratory or conjunctival secretions, childhood adenoviral infections produce low-grade fever, cough, coryza, and conjunctivitis. Adenovirus infections usually remit spontaneously. Infrequently, they can cause coma, seizures, and meningeal signs. The diagnosis can be established by isolating adenoviruses from cerebrospinal fluid, respiratory secretions, or urine. Treatment consists of supportive care. Although fatal cases have been described, most children recover uneventfully.

Picornaviridae

CLINICAL FEATURES

Members of the picornavirus family, especially the enteroviruses, are important potential causes of neurologic infections worldwide. Although paralytic poliomyelitis has been eliminated from nearly all regions of the world, nonpolio enteroviruses continue to be associated with a spectrum of neurologic disease that includes aseptic meningitis, acute ataxia, acute hemiplegia, opsoclonus-myoclonus, encephalitis, Guillain-Barré syndrome, and polio-like paralysis [Alexander et al., 1994; Berg and Jelke, 1965; Cheng-Yu et al., 2001; Cramblett et al., 1964; Huang et al., 1999; Kuban et al., 1983; Modlin et al., 1991; Rorabaugh et al., 1993; Rotbart, 1995; Sawyer, 2002]. The last case of wild poliomyelitis in the United States occurred in 1979 (see Fig. 69-1), and the World Health Organization has certified that the Americas, Europe, and the Western Pacific regions are free of polio [CDC, 1994a, 2004b]. Eradicating poliomyelitis from the remaining six endemic locations (Afghanistan, Egypt, India, Niger, Nigeria, and Pakistan) remains the objective of the World Health Organization. Before the use of the inactivated poliovirus vaccine for the complete childhood immunization series, vaccine-related poliomyelitis occurred occasionally in the United States [CDC, 1997b].

Spread by the fecal-oral route, the nonpolio enteroviruses, coxsackieviruses, and echoviruses produce several distinct systemic syndromes, including pharyngitis, herpangina, gastroenteritis, hand-foot-and-mouth syndrome, neonatal sepsis, and neurologic disorders. Data from the Centers for Disease Control and Prevention indicate that approximately 30 million cases of nonpolio enteroviral infections occur annually in the United States [CDC, 1997c]. More than 10,000 cases of nonpolio enterovirus aseptic meningitis are reported to the Centers for Disease Control and Prevention annually [Sawyer, 2002].

Aseptic meningitis, the most common neurologic manifestation of nonpolio enteroviral infection, appears epidemically during the late summer and early fall, although cases can be observed throughout the year. Affected children have fever, irritability, headache, photophobia, nausea, vomiting, meningeal signs, and other signs of enteroviral disease, including diarrhea, abdominal discomfort, and a maculopapular or petechial rash [Rorabaugh et al., 1993; Rotbart, 1995; Sawyer, 2002]. Signs of aseptic meningitis in a young infant may be remarkably subtle, consisting only of fussiness or poor oral intake. Fever is an inconsistent feature.

Occasionally, children with nonpolio enteroviral infections have an acute encephalitic presentation with fever, seizures, somnolence, coma, or focal deficits [Modlin et al., 1991]. Such children may have focal clinical, EEG, or neuroimaging abnormalities that resemble herpes simplex encephalitis. Children with acute opsoclonus-myoclonus, a syndrome associated more commonly with occult neural crest tumors, have involuntary, chaotic eye movements and random myoclonus of the extremities [Kuban et al., 1983]. Enterovirus 71, in addition to being associated with encephalitis and aseptic meningitis, causes an acute neurologic disorder with unilateral or bilateral flaccid paralysis that can resemble poliomyelitis or Guillain-Barré syndrome [Alexander et al., 1994; Cheng-Yu et al., 2001; Huang et al., 1999].

Children with poliomyelitis have a biphasic illness; the initial, nonspecific phase consists of fever, malaise, vomiting, or diarrhea, and the second, neurologic phase consists of aseptic meningitis or paralytic disease, usually more severe in the lower extremities [CDC, 1997b]. Mild or inapparent poliovirus infections greatly exceed the number of paralytic cases. Although the pathogenesis of their condition remains uncertain, persons with paralytic poliomyelitis may experience muscle pain, weakness, and fatigue after many years, a condition that has been labeled *postpolio syndrome* [Windebank et al., 1991].

Infants with nonpolio enteroviral infections can have a disseminated illness that resembles bacterial sepsis or herpes simplex virus infection. Clinical features of this condition include fever, respiratory distress, seizures, lethargy, shock, or disseminated intravascular coagulopathy [Morens, 1978]. During community enteroviral outbreaks, 10% to 15% of young infants acquire enteroviruses, usually asymptomatically [Jenista et al., 1984]. Children with agammaglobulinemia can have a persistent, often fatal neurologic condition caused by chronic nonpolio enterovirus infection of the CNS [Mease et al., 1981; Wilfert et al., 1977]. Patients with this rare disorder exhibit a dermatomyositis-like disorder and neurologic signs, which may include seizures, mental status changes, hemiparesis, and headache.

DIAGNOSIS

Infants with disseminated enteroviral infections can have leukocytosis, elevated serum transaminases, and thrombocytopenia, whereas infants or children with aseptic meningitis have mild cerebrospinal fluid changes, consisting of a lymphocytic pleocytosis and protein elevation [Negrini et al., 2000] and occasionally laboratory abnormalities consistent with the syndrome of inappropriate antidiuretic hormone secretion [Chemtob et al., 1985]. The diagnosis of enteroviral infection can be established by isolating enteroviruses from cerebrospinal fluid or stool or throat swabs or by detecting enteroviral RNA in stool, serum, or cerebrospinal fluid by using reverse transcriptase polymerase chain

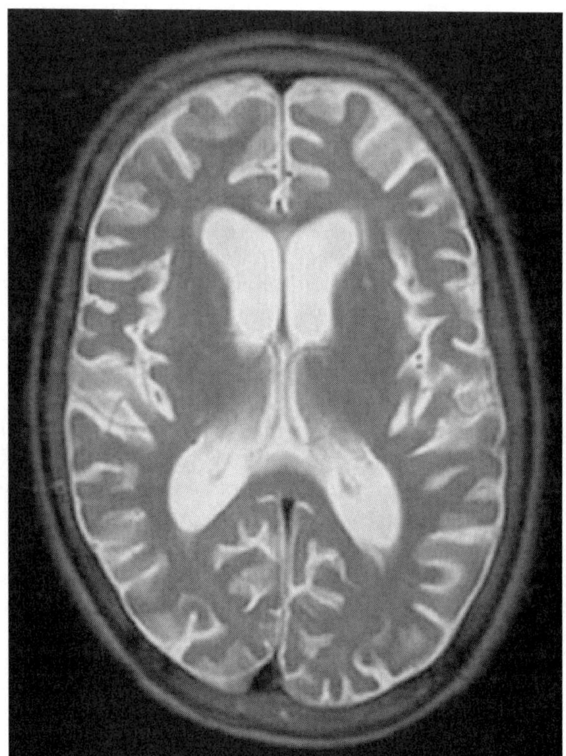

FIGURE 69-11. Axial T2-weighted MRI from a child with agammaglobulinemia and presumed progressive nonpolio enterovirus encephalopathy shows ventriculomegaly and diffuse cortical atrophy.

reaction [Hamilton et al., 1999; Rotbart, 1995; Sawyer, 2002; Schlesinger et al., 1994]. Imaging studies are normal in nonpolio enterovirus aseptic meningitis. Children with progressive nonpolio enterovirus infections have progressive cortical atrophy (Fig. 69-11).

TREATMENT AND OUTCOME

In most instances, children with enteroviral CNS infections require supportive care only. Children with severe nonpolio enteroviral infections may benefit from pleconaril, a novel antiviral drug with efficacy against several RNA viruses [Abzug et al., 2003; Sawyer, 2002]. Children with agammaglobulinemia and persistent echovirus infections may improve during immunoglobulin replacement therapy [Mease et al., 1981]. Infants with enteroviral aseptic meningitis recover uneventfully [Bergman et al., 1987], whereas the outcome in infants with myocarditis or children with encephalitis or enterovirus 71 infections can be less favorable [Modlin et al., 1991; Morens, 1978; Sawyer, 2002]. Persistent enterovirus infections in children with agammaglobulinemia are often fatal.

Togaviridae

Togaviridae includes the alphaviruses—eastern equine encephalitis virus, western equine encephalitis virus, and Venezuelan equine encephalitis virus—potential causes of encephalitis among humans living in the Western hemisphere, and the rubiviruses—rubella virus—a cause of the congenital rubella syndrome worldwide. The alphaviruses, maintained in bird–mosquito–wild vertebrate cycles, infect equines and humans as dead-end hosts and typically cause human disease between June and October, when the mosquito vectors are active. Most exposures are asymptomatic, although attack rates have been highest historically among infants and young children. As their names imply, eastern equine encephalitis, western equine encephalitis, and Venezuelan equine encephalitis occur in the eastern United States, western United States and Canada, and Latin America. Rubella virus, a nonarthropod member of this family, causes an exanthematous illness that has become rare in many regions because of immunization.

Eastern Equine Encephalitis Virus

Although having the lowest incidence of the major North American arthropod-borne encephalitides, with only 163 human cases reported to the Centers for Disease Control and Prevention during the 30-year interval from 1956 to 1985, eastern equine encephalitis has the highest mortality rate, ranging from 30% to 50% during the past several decades [Deresiewicz et al., 1997; Przelomski et al., 1988]. Cases among equines and humans, usually adults, appear during the summer months in states bordering the Atlantic Ocean and the Gulf of Mexico. Indigenous cases have been observed as far west as Michigan and Wisconsin.

The disorder usually begins abruptly with high fever, lethargy, vomiting, and convulsions, although some patients have a prodromal phase lasting several days characterized by fever, headache, malaise, and myalgias. Signs are usually diffuse, but patients may have focal findings, raising consideration of herpes simplex virus encephalitis [Morse et al., 1992]. EEGs usually exhibit diffuse slowing, and neuroimaging studies can be normal or indicate diffuse edema or focal lesions involving the thalami or basal ganglia [Deresiewicz et al., 1997; Morse et al., 1992; Przelomski et al., 1988]. The diagnosis can be confirmed by detecting eastern equine encephalitis virus–specific IgM in serum or cerebrospinal fluid and by detecting eastern equine encephalitis virus RNA using reverse transcriptase polymerase chain reaction. Treatment consists of supportive care.

Western Equine Encephalitis Virus

Although the western equine encephalitis virus can be detected in bird and mosquito reservoirs throughout the Americas, most human cases occur in the western United States or Canada, peaking in July and August [Calisher, 1994]. The incidence of western equine encephalitis varies considerably from year to year; however, epidemics appear at approximately 10-year intervals, with the largest affecting more than 3000 persons in 1941 [CDC, 1987]. The Centers for Disease Control and Prevention received reports of nearly 300 cases in 1975 and 37 cases in 1987, the largest more recent outbreaks. Residing in rural areas or engaging in outdoor occupations are risk factors associated with acquiring western equine encephalitis. Adults constitute most cases.

The clinical features of western equine encephalitis consist of fever, headache, somnolence, stiff neck, nausea, vomiting, and myalgias [Leech et al., 1981]. Coma, paralysis, seizures, and other more severe neurologic complications, although infrequent in adults, were common in infants affected during the 1941 epidemic [Medovy, 1943]. Infants can acquire the virus transplacentally and become symptomatic during the neonatal period [Shinefield and Townsend, 1953]. The diagnosis can be established by detecting western equine encephalitis virus–specific IgM in serum or cerebrospinal fluid or by using polymerase chain reaction [Calisher et al., 1986; Lambert et al., 2003]. Despite few reports of neurodiagnostic studies, EEG slowing and normal or nonspecific neuroimaging findings can be anticipated. Most children with western equine encephalitis recover completely, although developmental delay, an increased risk for seizures, and behavioral disturbance are potential sequelae [Earnest et al., 1971].

Venezuelan Equine Encephalitis Virus

Venezuelan equine encephalitis virus causes influenza-like disease, encephalitis, and intrauterine infection among inhabitants of Latin America [CDC, 1993a, 1995a]. During major epidemics, equine and human cases have been observed as far north as the southern United States. A major outbreak of Venezuelan equine encephalitis occurred in 1995, affecting 75,000 persons in Colombia, but this epidemic did not spread to North America [Rivas et al., 1997]. Encephalitis affects approximately 10% of infected persons and tends to be mild with headache, somnolence, and occasionally convulsions. Intrauterine infection, a rare complication of maternal Venezuelan equine encephalitis virus infection, can cause fetal death or severe, encephaloclastic CNS lesions, including hydranencephaly [Wenger, 1977]. The diagnosis can be established serologically or by virus isolation.

Rubella Virus

CLINICAL FEATURES

Rubella virus causes neurologic dysfunction during acute childhood infection and in the offspring of women who are infected with rubella virus during the first trimester. These complications are rare in the United States and other regions with compulsory vaccination against rubella virus (Fig. 69-12). Before vaccine licensure in 1969, rubella epidemics occurred at 6- to 9-year intervals, and during the last major pandemic in the mid-1960s, 20,000 cases of congenital rubella syndrome were reported. Ten percent to 20% of adults living in regions with compulsory immunization remain susceptible to rubella [CDC, 1997f], however, and outbreaks of rubella and congenital rubella syndrome [CDC, 1997d; Panagiotopoulos and Georgakopoulou, 2004] indicate that the rubella virus continues to pose a real threat in many regions of the world [Spika et al., 2003]. Rarely, maternal reinfection with rubella virus causes fetal infection [Robinson et al., 1994].

Rubella virus produces fever, coryza, lymphadenopathy of the posterior auricular and occipital nodes, and a maculopapular rash involving the face and trunk. Rare neurologic complications after acquired rubella virus infection consist of headache, seizures, or Guillain-Barré syndrome. The clinical features of intrauterine rubella virus infection, recognized first by Gregg in 1941, include cataracts, congenital heart disease, sensorineural hearing loss, microcephaly, intrauterine growth retardation, hepatosplenomegaly, petechial rash, osteopathy, jaundice, and pneumonitis [Dudgeon,

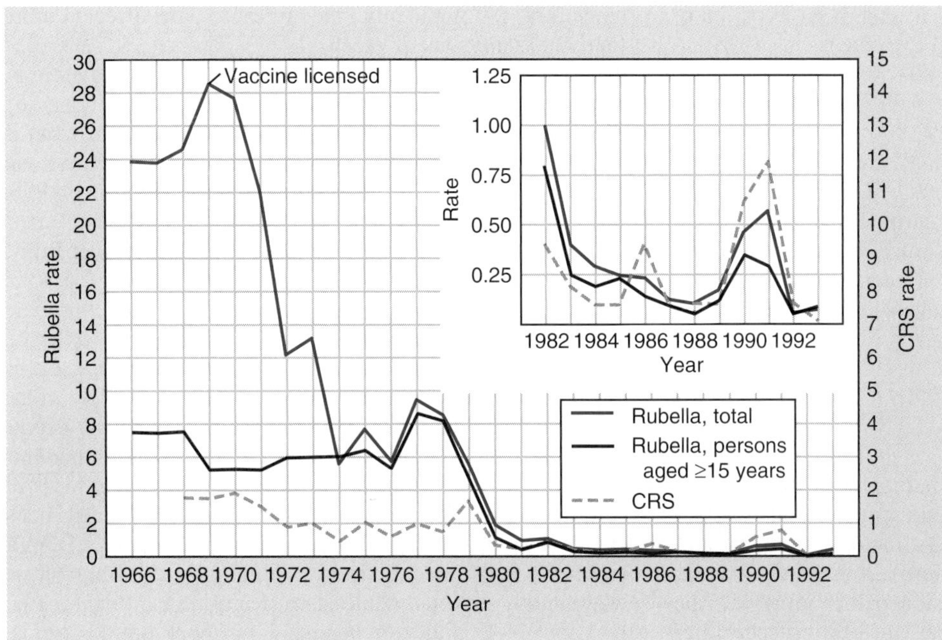

FIGURE 69-12. Data regarding the incidence of rubella and congenital rubella syndrome (CRS) in the United States from 1966 to 1992, as reported to the Centers for Disease Control and Prevention, show the dramatic decline in rubella and CRS. The inset depicts the resurgence of CRS that was observed in the early 1990s. Cases of rubella reported to the National Notifiable Diseases Surveillance System per 100,000 population; cases of congenital rubella reported to the National CRS Registry per 100,000 live births. (From Rubella and congenital rubella syndrome—United States. MMWR Morb Mortal Wkly Rep 1994;43:391, 397.)

1975]. Sequelae relate directly to the gestational timing of maternal infections, with severe defects common before 12 weeks, when the risk of congenital rubella syndrome approaches 90% [Ueda et al., 1979]. By contrast, maternal infections after 24 weeks of gestation tend to be benign.

DIAGNOSIS

The diagnosis of rubella virus infection can be established serologically by isolating the rubella virus from urine or nasopharyngeal secretions or by detecting rubella virus RNA in cerebrospinal fluid or other fluids by using reverse transcriptase polymerase chain reaction [Bosma et al., 1995]. Direct hyperbilirubinemia, elevated serum transaminases, and thrombocytopenia are potential laboratory abnormalities after intrauterine infection. Imaging of infants with congenital rubella syndrome reveals cerebral atrophy, intracranial calcifications, periventricular cysts, or leukomalacia [Yamashita et al., 1991].

TREATMENT AND OUTCOME

At present, therapy for rubella virus infections, including intrauterine infection, consists of supportive care. Survivors of intrauterine rubella virus infection have high rates of sequelae affecting vision, hearing, cardiac function, and intellect [Forrst et al., 2002; Givens et al., 1993]. Potential delayed sequelae of congenital rubella syndrome include endocrinopathies (diabetes mellitus, thyroid dysfunction, and growth hormone deficiency), progressive hearing loss, glaucoma, vascular abnormalities, and postrubella panencephalitis [Sever et al., 1985; Townsend et al., 1975].

Flaviviridae

Flaviviridae, another large family of arthropod-borne viruses, include Japanese encephalitis virus; St. Louis encephalitis virus; West Nile virus; and several agents associated with tick-borne encephalitis in Europe, Asia, and North America [Kunz, 1992; Tsai, 1991]. Japanese encephalitis, the most common arthropod-borne encephalitis worldwide, causes several thousand encephalitis cases annually in endemic areas of eastern Asia, although vaccine programs have reduced the incidence of Japanese encephalitis in some regions [CDC, 1993b]. Tick-borne encephalitides are infrequent in the United States and Canada but are relatively common in Europe and Asia [Kunz, 1992]. The Centers for Disease Control and Prevention received reports of nearly 5000 cases of St. Louis encephalitis between 1956 and 1985 [CDC, 1986], and nearly half of these were observed during the massive epidemic of 1975 involving 29 states and the District of Columbia [Creech, 1977]. Beginning in 1999, West Nile virus spread throughout the United States, causing systemic and neurologic illness among adults and children [Hayes and O'Leary, 2004].

Japanese Encephalitis Virus

CLINICAL FEATURES

Japanese encephalitis, a mosquito-borne virus endemic throughout much of eastern Asia, causes 50,000 or more cases of encephalitis each year, usually in children younger than 15 years of age [CDC, 1993b]. Disease activity peaks from May to October, although some countries, such as Indonesia, Malaysia, and India, experience cases year-round. The virus is maintained in a bird-vertebrate cycle involving *Culex* mosquitoes, domestic pigs, and wading birds [Fields, 1990; CDC, 1993b].

Children with Japanese encephalitis have an abrupt, fulminant illness with fever, convulsions, and coma [Burke et al., 1985; Kumar et al., 1990]. Headache, vomiting, increased muscle tone, breathing irregularities, and occasionally focal neurologic deficits are additional clinical manifestations [Kumar et al., 1990]. Although the prodromal phase is less than 24 hours long in most children with Japanese encephalitis, it can last 7 or more days.

DIAGNOSIS

The diagnosis of Japanese encephalitis can be confirmed by isolating the virus from cerebrospinal fluid or brain tissue, detecting serologic responses to the virus [Burke et al., 1982], or detecting Japanese encephalitis virus RNA in cerebrospinal fluid using reverse transcriptase polymerase chain reaction [Meiyu et al., 1997]. MRI can reveal bilateral lesions of the thalami or basal ganglia [Kalita and Misra, 2000; Kumar et al., 1997].

TREATMENT AND OUTCOME

Mortality rates for Japanese encephalitis range from 25% to 40%; most survivors have neurologic sequelae consisting of mental retardation, seizure disorders, motor deficits, or subtle behavioral and intellectual abnormalities [Kumar et al., 1993]. An inactivated Japanese encephalitis virus vaccine prevents infection. The vaccine has an 80% efficacy after two doses [CDC, 1993b]; adverse reactions occur at a rate of approximately 15 per 100,000 doses [Berg et al., 1997; Takahashi et al., 2000].

St. Louis Encephalitis Virus

CLINICAL FEATURES

St. Louis encephalitis virus, a mosquito-borne virus endemic to the midwestern United States, occasionally causes epidemics of aseptic meningitis, encephalitis, and influenza-like illness, often involving older adults in urban or suburban areas. The 1975 epidemic, the largest to date, affected more than 2000 persons [Creech, 1977]. The attack rates and disease severity of St. Louis encephalitis virus infections, similar to those of West Nile virus, increase with advancing age [Luby et al., 1969; Meehan et al., 2000]. The virus is maintained in a cycle involving *Culex* mosquitoes and pigeons, sparrows, doves, and other birds [Johnson, 1998; Luby et al., 1969].

Clinical syndromes associated with St. Louis encephalitis virus infection include nonspecific febrile illnesses, aseptic meningitis, and encephalitis, although most infections are asymptomatic [Creech, 1977; Riggs et al., 1965]. After an incubation period of 21 days, children with St. Louis encephalitis may have a biphasic illness, with low-grade fever, diarrhea, vomiting, and malaise preceding the neurologic signs and symptoms [Kaplan et al., 1978]. In patients with encephalitis, representing approximately two thirds of symptomatic infections, headache, vomiting, fever, neck stiffness, and lethargy or agitation begin abruptly. Tremor can be present; focal neurologic findings are infrequent, at least among reported adult cases [Riggs et al., 1965]. Fever may be 41°C and can persist 7 or more days. Clinical improvement usually begins within 7 to 10 days of disease onset [Riggs et al., 1965].

DIAGNOSIS, TREATMENT, AND OUTCOME

The cerebrospinal fluid reveals a pleocytosis in most patients with St. Louis encephalitis. Neuroimaging studies are normal or nonspecifically abnormal, and EEGs may indicate diffuse slowing. The diagnosis can be established by detecting serologic responses in serum or cerebrospinal fluid [Monath et al., 1984]. Treatment consists of supportive care. Mortality, ranging from 8% to 20% [Creech, 1977; Meehan

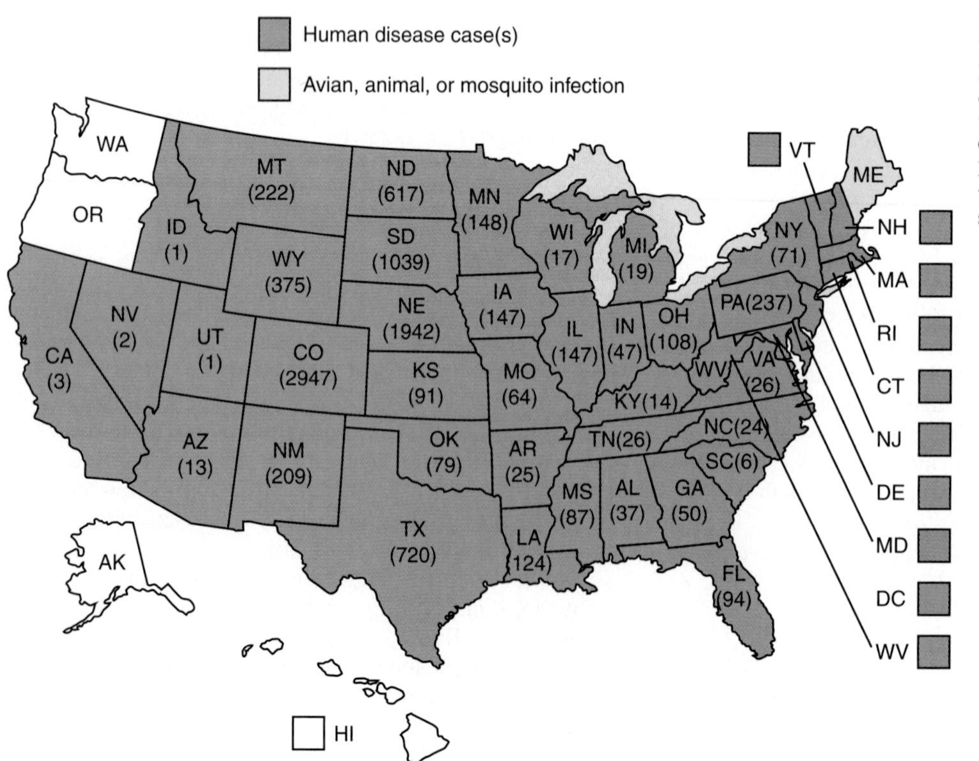

FIGURE 69-13. A map of the United States showing Centers for Disease Control and Prevention data regarding human West Nile virus cases in 2003. (From the Centers for Disease Control and Prevention. Available at: www.cdc.gov/ncidod/dvbid/westnile/surv&control03Maps.htm.)

et al., 2000; Riggs et al., 1965], is highest among persons older than age 50 years. Potential sequelae include seizures, parkinsonism, and intellectual deficits.

West Nile Virus

CLINICAL FEATURES

First identified in Uganda in 1937, West Nile virus later appeared in Egypt and Israel in the 1950s [Marberg et al., 1956]. Beginning in the mid-1990s, human outbreaks became more frequent and severe, causing meningitis, encephalitis, and fatalities among persons living in Israel, Algeria, and Romania [Hubalek and Halouzka, 1999]. In 1999, cases of West Nile virus infection occurred in the United States, marking the first appearance of the virus in the Western hemisphere. An encephalitis outbreak in the New York City metropolitan area, linked to a West Nile virus strain closely related to a strain identified in Israel in 1998, caused seven deaths among adults [Lanciotti et al., 1999; Nash et al., 2001].

In 2000, West Nile virus activity was detected in 12 states surrounding New York State, and by the end of 2001, 27 states and the District of Columbia reported the presence of West Nile virus [Petersen, et al., 2002]. The rapid spread of West Nile virus among North American birds and mosquitoes heralded an enormous human outbreak in 2003 that affected more than 4000 inhabitants of 45 states from New York to California (Fig. 69-13). Only two western states (Oregon and Washington) did not report West Nile virus activity [CDC, 2004a, 2004c]. West Nile virus is maintained in a bird-mosquito cycle, involving rural and urban wild birds and *Culex* and *Aedes* mosquitoes.

Asymptomatic infections with West Nile virus outnumber symptomatic cases by approximately 5 to 1 [CDC, 2004c]. Neurologic manifestations, including meningitis, encephalitis, myelitis, polio-like illness, and others, occur in approximately 1 of every 150 infected persons. Adults constitute most cases. After an incubation period of 2 to 14 days, systemic symptoms of fever, malaise, headache, nausea, and vomiting occur in symptomatic infections. Of symptomatic patients, 50% have a maculopapular rash and lymphadenopathy.

To date, most patients with the neurologic complications of West Nile virus infections have been older than age 25 years. Approximately 60% of persons with West Nile virus-induced neurologic disease have encephalitis [Sejvar et al., 2003]. Encephalitis can begin with the usual systemic prodrome or more abruptly with high fever and coma [Campbell et al., 2002]. Typical abnormalities in West Nile virus encephalitis include altered mental status, coma, diffuse muscle weakness (proximal greater than distal), respiratory paralysis, and hyporeflexia. Tremor, myoclonus, and parkinsonian features are additional components of the acute illness [Sejvar et al., 2003].

Less frequent neurologic manifestations of West Nile virus infection include aseptic meningitis, myelitis, optic neuritis, and Guillain-Barré syndrome [Campbell et al., 2002; Sejvar et al., 2003]. Involvement of the anterior horn cells can produce a poliomyelitis-like disorder with asymmetric paralysis of the upper or lower extremities [Li et al., 2003; Heresi et al., 2004; Sejvar, 2004]. This disorder produces clinical, histopathologic, and electrophysiologic abnormalities comparable to those of classic poliomyelitis [Sevjar, 2004]. Although patients with West Nile virus–induced meningitis and encephalitis gradually recover, patients with limb paralysis usually have permanent deficits [Li et al., 2003; Sejvar et al., 2003].

A single case report indicates that West Nile virus can be transmitted to the fetus, causing intrauterine infection of the CNS [CDC, 2002]. In late 2002, an infant was born to a woman who had experienced meningoencephalitis during her pregnancy. At birth, the infant was found to have bilateral chorioretinitis and cystic encephalomalacia. Studies for the conventional causes of intrauterine infection, including cytomegalovirus, herpes simplex virus, lymphocytic choriomeningitis virus, and *Toxoplasma gondii,* were negative, but serologic studies of the mother and infant confirmed West Nile virus infection.

DIAGNOSIS, TREATMENT, AND OUTCOME

Laboratory abnormalities include mild anemia and peripheral leukocytosis or leukopenia. The cerebrospinal fluid of West Nile virus encephalitis resembles that of most arboviral infections, consisting of a mild, lymphocytic pleocytosis (30 to 100 cells/mm^3); elevated protein content (80 to 100 mg/dL); and normal glucose content. Cranial CT is normal, whereas MRI can reveal leptomeningeal enhancement, periventricular inflammation, or abnormalities of the spinal cord [Campbell et al., 2002]. The diagnosis of West Nile virus infection can be confirmed by serologic studies that detect neutralizing antibodies to the virus in acute or convalescent serum samples or West Nile virus–specific IgM in serum or cerebrospinal fluid. West Nile virus–specific IgM persists in serum for at least 16 months in more than half of infected persons [Campbell et al., 2002]. Infected patients experience brief periods of viremia, but infectious virus is rarely isolated from serum or cerebrospinal fluid. Reverse transcriptase polymerase chain reaction can be used to detect West Nile virus in clinical samples [Lanciotti and Kersat, 2001]. A Centers for Disease Control and Prevention protocol guides the evaluation of infants with suspected intrauterine West Nile virus infection [CDC, 2004f].

Therapy for the neurologic complications of West Nile virus infection currently consists of supportive care with close observation for respiratory decompensation. Ribavirin possesses activity against the West Nile virus in vitro, but there are no controlled trials on which to base management decisions. There were 284 deaths among the 4156 cases reported to the Centers for Disease Control and Prevention in 2003, corresponding to a mortality rate of slightly less than 7% [CDC, 2004a]. Deaths have been more common among the elderly. Approximately one third of survivors have permanent sequelae affecting cognition, behavior, or motor function.

Tick-Borne Flaviviruses

Several closely related, tick-borne flaviviruses of Europe, Asia, and North America produce encephalitis or aseptic meningitis in children and adults [Kunz, 1992; Lesnicar et al., 2003]. Tick-borne encephalitis represents a major public health concern among unvaccinated persons in eastern Europe and Asia. Patients with European tick-borne encephalitis often have a biphasic illness, experiencing headache, malaise, myalgia, and low-grade fever during the initial, nonspecific phase. Approximately 20% of symptomatic patients have a second, neurologic phase with severe headache, high fever, somnolence, coma, convulsions, cranial nerve palsies, or paralysis that mimics Guillain-Barré syndrome [Kunz, 1992]. Cases of tick-borne encephalitis have been described after consumption of unpasteurized, virus-contaminated milk or in travelers to endemic regions [Cruse et al., 1979]. Immunization can prevent infection among children inhabiting or visiting endemic regions [Kunze et al., 2004].

In North America, the tick-borne Powassan virus, maintained in a vertebrate-mosquito cycle in eastern Canada and the northeastern United States, has been associated with cases of encephalitis, sometimes in children [Embil et al., 1983; McLean and Donohue, 1959; Smith et al., 1974]. Clinical features consist of seizures, somnolence, or coma; occasionally children can have focal features suggesting herpes simplex virus [Embil et al., 1983]. Cerebrospinal fluid examination usually reveals a mixed pleocytosis; EEGs may be slow or epileptiform. The diagnosis is established serologically. Children generally recover completely with supportive care, although sequelae and death have been described.

Bunyaviridae

La Crosse Virus

CLINICAL FEATURES

La Crosse virus, a California serogroup virus maintained in the wild through a mosquito-vertebrate animal, causes encephalitis—known as *California* or *La Crosse encephalitis*—among children living in the midwestern United States [Balfour, 1974]. Before the emergence of West Nile virus in the United States, La Crosse encephalitis represented the most common arthropod-borne encephalitis in America (see Fig. 69-3), accounting for approximately 100 reported cases among children per year [Bale, 2003; McJunkin et al., 2001; Rust et al., 1999].

Nonspecific clinical features, consisting of fever, vomiting, headache, abdominal pain, and malaise, begin 3 to 7 days after exposure to the virus. Neurologic features appear 2 to 4 days later and consist of seizures (60%), lethargy or coma (50%), and focal deficits (20%) [Balfour, 1974; Balfour et al., 1973; Hilty et al., 1972; McJunkin et al., 2001; Rust et al., 1999]. Neurologic symptoms usually resolve during the subsequent week.

DIAGNOSIS

Laboratory findings include a peripheral leukocytosis (often with a neutrophil predominance) and mixed cerebrospinal fluid pleocytosis ranging from 10 to 500 leukocytes/mL in approximately 90% of children. Some children have normal cerebrospinal fluid profiles [Hilty et al., 1972]. EEGs can be diffusely or focally slow, whereas CT and MRI are usually normal. The diagnosis of California encephalitis can be established serologically using IgM capture assays of serum or cerebrospinal fluid [Dykers et al., 1985; McJunkin et al., 2001]. The diagnosis also has been established by brain biopsy and immunofluorescence staining [McJunkin et al., 1997], but invasive diagnostic procedures, such as brain biopsy, are rarely necessary. Reverse transcriptase polymerase chain reaction can detect the RNA of California group viruses [Kuno et al., 1996].

TREATMENT AND OUTCOME

Because most cases of La Crosse encephalitis are mild, and current antiviral agents, with the possible exception of ribavirin [McJunkin et al., 1997], lack anti–California encephalitis virus activity, therapy consists of supportive care. Focal EEG or clinical manifestations of La Crosse encephalitis mimic herpes simplex virus and necessitate acyclovir therapy while awaiting the results of microbiologic studies. Most children with California encephalitis recover completely, although residual behavioral changes, seizure tendencies, or EEG abnormalities have been reported in 10% to 15% of children with proven California encephalitis [Balfour, 1974; Balkhy and Schreiber, 2000; Grabow et al., 1969; McJunkin et al., 2001; Rust et al., 1999].

Reoviridae

Colorado Tick Fever Virus

Colorado tick fever, a disorder endemic in the western United States, causes an influenza-like illness that begins approximately 5 days after exposure to Colorado tick fever–infected Rocky Mountain wood ticks, *Dermacentor andersoni* [Goodpasture et al., 1978]. The disorder usually appears in May through July in young adults who engage in outdoor recreational activities and often report tick exposure. Typical signs and symptoms include fever, headache, malaise, myalgia, abdominal pain, and vomiting. CNS manifestations, consisting of meningitis or mild encephalitis, affect less than 5% of children with Colorado tick fever [Goodpasture et al., 1978; Spruance and Bailey, 1973]. Such patients may have peripheral leukocytosis, a mixed cerebrospinal fluid pleocytosis, and diffusely slow EEGs [Spruance and Bailey, 1973]. The diagnosis can be established by virus isolation during the prolonged viremic phase [Goodpasture et al., 1978] or serologic studies. Reverse transcriptase–polymerase chain reaction holds promise as a rapid, specific diagnostic method [Johnson et al., 1997]. Patients require supportive care and usually recover without sequelae.

Rotavirus

Rotavirus commonly infects infants or young children during the winter months and causes fever, diarrhea, vomiting, and dehydration [Blacklow and Cukor, 1981; McCormack, 1982]. Rarely, children with rotavirus gastroenteritis experience seizures or altered sensorium [Salmi et al., 1978; Schumacher and Forster, 1999; Yoshida et al., 1995]. Cerebrospinal fluid findings in children with rotavirus-associated CNS complications include a normal glucose content, normal protein content, and normal or elevated cerebrospinal fluid white blood cell count [Yoshida et al., 1995]. The EEG may reveal diffuse, nonspecific slowing, whereas neuroimaging studies are usually normal. Rotavirus gastroenteritis can be diagnosed by detecting rotavirus antigen in stool samples, and CNS involvement can be established by detecting rotavirus RNA in cerebrospinal fluid by using reverse transcriptase polymerase chain reaction [Yoshida et al., 1995]. Children with rotavirus infections have benign, self-limited illnesses, although fluid status must be monitored carefully.

Paramyxoviridae

The paramyxovirus family, containing the mumps and measles viruses, has contributed historically to considerable mortality and neurologic morbidity [CDC, 1997f; Fields and Knipe, 1990; Hughes, 1977; Johnson, 1998]. Consequently, vaccines were developed for these viruses and introduced in the late 1960s. Although measles cases have declined in the United States and other countries with compulsory immunization programs, measles still caused 777,000 deaths worldwide in 2000 [CDC, 1997f; Henao-Restrepo et al., 2003]. Measles caused 5% of all deaths in children younger than age 5 years in 2000. Other members of the paramyxovirus family, parainfluenza viruses and respiratory syncytial virus, cause neurologic disease infrequently. Members of the closely related orthomyxovirus family, the influenza viruses, have been associated with Reye's syndrome, a postinfectious disorder, and meningoencephalitis, albeit rarely.

Measles Virus

CLINICAL FEATURES

Despite the availability of the measles vaccine, a safe and effective live-virus preparation, measles remains a major worldwide public health concern [CDC, 1997f; Henao-Restrepo et al., 2003]. Measles virus spreads via the respiratory route, with contagion highest during the prodromal, catarrhal stage that precedes the rash. Before vaccine availability, measles typically caused disease in infants and young children during the winter and spring [Morgan and Rapp, 1977]. In the United States, only 216 cases of measles were reported to the Centers for Disease Control and Prevention between 2001 and 2003, a nearly 100% reduction compared with the number in the prevaccine era. Approximately 50% of the cases were imported, and a substantial proportion of the remainder was "import-linked" [CDC, 2004d]. The World Health Organization and other organizations have targeted measles for eradication worldwide by 2010.

Symptoms of measles infection include fever, cough, coryza, and conjunctivitis, beginning approximately 12 days after exposure in susceptible persons. The characteristic maculopapular exanthem appears on the face and spreads centrifugally to involve the trunk and extremities. Neurologic complications consist of three distinct disorders: (1) measles encephalomyelitis, a postinfectious demyelinating disorder of immunocompetent hosts; (2) subacute measles virus encephalopathy (also known as *subacute measles encephalitis* or *measles inclusion-body encephalitis*), a disorder of immunocompromised hosts; and (3) subacute sclerosing panencephalitis, a neurodegenerative disorder of complex pathogenesis occurring several years after measles virus infection in otherwise healthy hosts. Subacute sclerosing panencephalitis, with an incidence of approximately 1 case per 1 million cases of measles [Modlin et al., 1979; Payne et al., 1969], has virtually disappeared in many regions as a consequence of measles vaccination [Dyken et al., 1989]. Because of the rarity of subacute sclerosing panencephalitis in the United States, however, the disorder is often unsuspected during the early stages [Honarmand et al., 2004].

Measles encephalomyelitis, an immune-mediated disorder with an incidence of approximately 1 case per 1000 cases of measles, begins within 7 days after the onset of the measles rash [Johnson et al., 1984; LaBoccetta and Tornay, 1964], and children younger than age 10 years constitute most cases. Clinical manifestations include headache, irritability, somnolence, coma, and seizures, although some children have ataxia, choreoathetosis, or focal deficits [Johnson et al., 1984; LaBoccetta and Tornay, 1964].

Subacute measles encephalopathy, first reported in the 1970s [Murphy and Yunis, 1976], begins 1 to 7 months after measles infection or immunization in an immunocompromised host, often a child with acute leukemia [Mustafa et al., 1993]. Altered consciousness and generalized or focal seizures, including epilepsia partialis continua, are typical clinical signs; 15% to 40% of patients have hemiparesis, hemiplegia, ataxia, aphasia, or visual symptoms [Mustafa et al., 1993].

Subacute sclerosing panencephalitis, a rare disease currently, affects young children; the age at onset averages approximately 7 years, and the disorder begins 5 to 10 years after measles infection [Anlar et al., 2001; Honarmand et al., 2004; Modlin et al., 1979]. The disorder displays relatively stereotyped clinical stages, beginning with insidious declines in behavior and cognition that may mimic a psychiatric disorder. Myoclonus, a prominent component of the next phase of subacute sclerosing panencephalitis, involves the extremities, trunk, or head, and generalized or focal seizures may begin concurrently [Risk and Haddad, 1979]. As the disorder progresses, speech and intellectual function deteriorate; myoclonus intensifies; and other neurologic abnormalities, such as choreoathetosis, bradykinesia, or rigidity, appear. The typical course ends in debility, coma, and death. Approximately half of patients have chorioretinitis and visual impairment. A small proportion of patients with subacute sclerosing panencephalitis have atypical infections with rapid deterioration and death [Silva et al., 1981].

DIAGNOSIS

The diagnosis of measles encephalomyelitis can be established by detecting measles virus IgG titer elevations in acute and convalescent serum or measles-specific IgM in serum or cerebrospinal fluid. Measles virus also can be detected in clinical samples by using reverse transcriptase polymerase chain reaction [Shimizu et al., 1993]. MRI may reveal white matter lesions compatible with acute demyelination. In subacute measles encephalopathy, the cerebrospinal fluid, although usually normal, may reveal a lymphocytic pleocytosis. EEGs typically reveal focal or generalized slowing or epileptiform discharges. CT is usually normal, but MRI can detect nonspecific changes involving the cortex, white matter, or deep nuclei (Fig. 69-14) [Chen et al., 1994]. Paramyxovirus particles or measles virus RNA can be detected in brain tissue.

The pathogenesis of subacute sclerosing panencephalitis, although still obscure, reflects defective replication of the

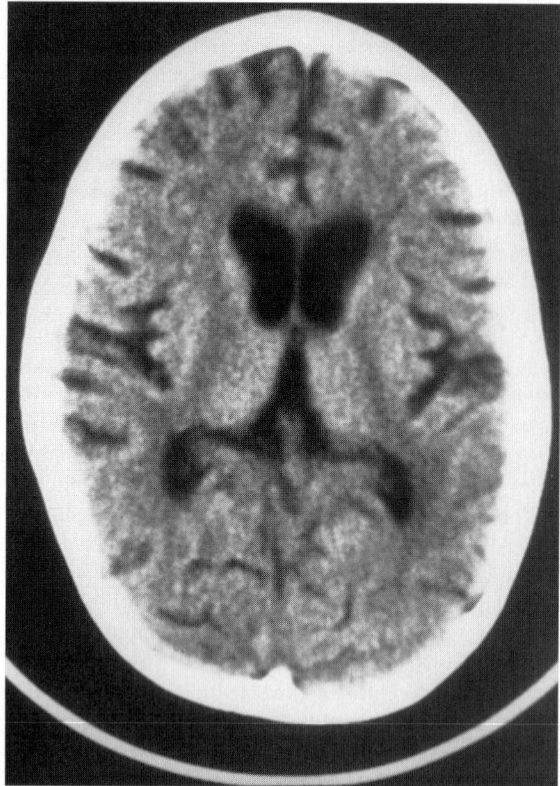

FIGURE 69-14. T1-weighted MRI from an immunocompromised child with measles encephalitis reveals diffuse cortical atrophy; patchy, hypointense areas at the gray-white matter interface; and subtle basal ganglia calcifications.

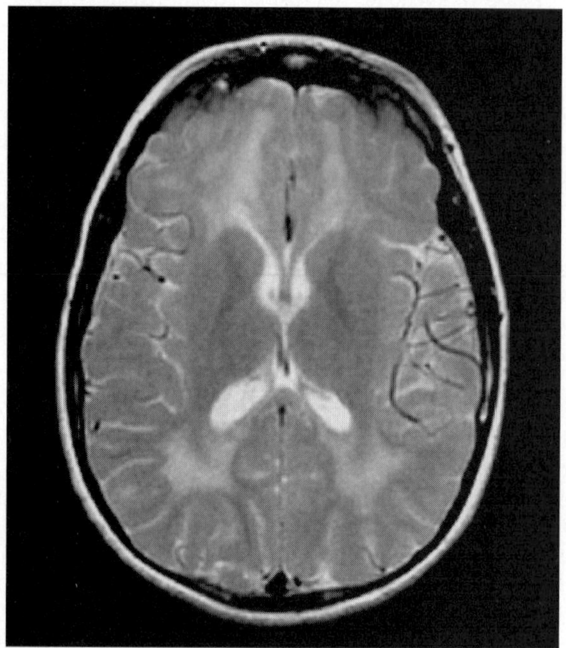

FIGURE 69-15. T2-weighted MRI from an adolescent with subacute sclerosing panencephalitis shows demyelination and early cortical atrophy.

measles virus in neural tissues. Patients with subacute sclerosing panencephalitis have elevated cerebrospinal fluid immunoglobulin levels, oligoclonal bands, and increased IgG synthesis rates, indicating massive production of measles-specific IgG. High cerebrospinal fluid titers of measles-specific IgG establish the diagnosis of subacute sclerosing panencephalitis, and measles virus RNA can be detected in cerebrospinal fluid or plasma by reverse transcriptase–polymerase chain reaction [Nakayama et al., 1995]. EEGs show bilaterally synchronous spike-wave or slow-wave bursts that assume a suppression-burst pattern over time. MRI commonly exhibits T2 prolongation of subcortical and periventricular white matter and eventually cortical atrophy (Fig. 69-15) [Lum et al., 1986; Anlar et al., 1996].

TREATMENT AND OUTCOME

Treatment of measles encephalomyelitis consists of supportive care. Outcome varies, ranging from complete recovery to survival with impaired intellectual function, motor deficits, or death. Although one report suggests transient improvement after ribavirin therapy [Mustafa et al., 1993], most persons with subacute measles encephalopathy die or have severe neurologic sequelae. Subacute sclerosing panencephalitis progresses to death in 1 to 3 years in most cases, although some patients have extended plateau phases, either spontaneously or coincident with inosine pranobex or interferon alfa therapy or both [Risk and Haddad, 1979; Yalaz et al., 1992]. A multinational trial indicated that approximately 35% of patients with subacute sclerosing panencephalitis stabilize during inosine pranobex therapy, but found no added benefit from interferon alfa [Gascon, 2003].

Mumps Virus

CLINICAL FEATURES

Before vaccine licensure, mumps virus infection accounted for most cases of aseptic meningitis and mild encephalitis in the United States and many other regions. More than 150,000 cases of mumps were reported in the United States in 1968, with aseptic meningitis in 10% and encephalitis in 0.2%, whereas less than 2000 cases of mumps were reported in 1993, a 99% decrease [CDC, 1995b]. The Finnish epidemiologic survey [Koskiniemi et al., 1991] documented the dramatic decline in mumps meningoencephalitis and measles encephalomyelitis after vaccine licensure. By the early 1980s, mumps meningoencephalitis had disappeared in many regions of the world.

Clinical features appear 2 weeks after acquisition and consist of anorexia, malaise, and low-grade fever; parotitis is a cardinal clinical feature. One third or more of mumps virus infections are asymptomatic. Aseptic meningitis or encephalitis, heralded by headache, vomiting, and high fever, is associated with stiff neck, somnolence, and occasionally seizures, coma, or focal deficits [Koskiniemi et al., 1983]. Additional neurologic complications of mumps include acute cerebellar ataxia and hydrocephalus secondary to mumps virus–induced ependymitis [Bray, 1972; Herndon et al., 1974; Ichiba et al., 1988].

DIAGNOSIS, TREATMENT, AND OUTCOME

Cerebrospinal fluid pleocytosis is the rule in mumps virus meningitis or encephalitis. Cerebrospinal fluid protein content is usually normal, and the glucose content can be slightly reduced [Koskiniemi et al., 1983]. The diagnosis can be confirmed by detecting mumps virus–specific IgM or IgG. EEGs in children with encephalitis may reveal generalized or focal slowing. Children require supportive care; most recover completely.

Nipah Virus

In fall 1998, an outbreak of severe encephalitis appeared in Malaysia [Chua, 2003; Chua et al., 2000; Johnson, 2003]. Electron microscopic studies of infected tissues identified a paramyxovirus, named *Nipah virus* after Kampung Sungei Nipah, the Malaysian village in which the virus was first detected. Fruit bats (genus *Pteropus*) serve as the natural reservoir of the virus. During the first outbreak, 265 cases of encephalitis occurred in humans ranging in age from 10 years to nearly 70 years. The clinical features included fever, headache, vomiting, cough, cerebellar signs, pupillary abnormalities, seizures, autonomic dysfunction, and coma [Goh et al., 2000]. Among the 265 human cases, there were 105 deaths, corresponding to a mortality rate of nearly 40%; ribavirin therapy was associated with reduced mortality [Chong et al., 2001]. Case-control studies indicated that Nipah encephalitis in humans resulted from contact with pigs or with pig excrement [Parashar, et al., 2000], and after slaughter and disposal of pigs, the initial outbreak ended [Chua et al., 2000].

Rhabdoviridae

Rabies Virus

CLINICAL FEATURES

Dreaded since antiquity, rabies poses a threat to individuals in many regions of the world, especially in the developing countries of Africa and Asia, where the incidence of 1 in 100,000 to 1 in 1 million inhabitants corresponds to approximately 50,000 deaths annually [Fishbein and Robinson, 1993; Plotkin, 2000]. In these regions, domestic dogs or wild canines transmit rabies, and children constitute most human rabies cases. By contrast, human and animal rabies has been eradicated in a few regions as a result of quarantine and vaccination of domestic animals [CDC, 1997a; Haupt, 1999; Johnson, 1998].

In the United States, rabies remains endemic in certain wild animals, including raccoons, skunks, foxes, and bats. In the northeastern states, the number of infected raccoons has increased steadily since the 1970s [CDC, 1997e; Fishbein and Robinson, 1993; Krebs, et al., 2002; Rupprecht et al., 1995]. This epizootic constitutes a potential health hazard and an economic burden for postexposure prophylaxis [CDC, 1993b]. The cost of human rabies prophylaxis in the United States exceeds $40 million annually. The Centers for Disease Control and Prevention receives reports of one to three indigenous cases of human rabies annually in the United States. Many cases have no apparent history of animal bites and have been linked by molecular analysis to the rabies virus strain carried by the insectivorous silver-haired bat [CDC, 1993b].

Rabies, similar to many viral CNS infections, begins nonspecifically, mimicking upper respiratory or gastrointestinal disorders. After a variable incubation period averaging 20 to 60 days, human rabies begins with chills, fever, headache, sore throat, malaise, nausea, or abdominal pain [Anderson et al., 1984; Johnson, 1998; Plotkin, 2000]. Pain or itching corresponding to the site of inoculation is common. Neurologic symptoms and signs begin thereafter; symptoms and signs are cerebral in 80% and Guillain-Barré syndrome–like in the remainder.

Patients with cerebral symptoms have marked behavioral changes with agitation, hypersalivation, delirium, and occasionally opisthotonic posturing [Dupont and Earle, 1966; Warrell, 1976]. Hydrophobia, present in 20% to 50% of patients, produces spasms of the laryngeal muscles, diaphragm, and accessory respiratory muscles, which can lead to respiratory arrest and death [Warrell, 1976]. Seizures ensue in many cases. Eventually, patients with rabies encephalitis lapse into a fatal coma. Rabies-induced Guillain-Barré syndrome–like disease produces bulbar dysfunction, facial diplegia, and often respiratory arrest [Chopra et al., 1980]. Cardiac dysrhythmias and irreversible coma are additional causes of death in paralytic cases.

DIAGNOSIS

Because of its rarity in the United States and Canada, human rabies is often unsuspected [Noah et al., 1998], especially during the early, nonspecific phase. Consequently, rabies usually is identified at postmortem examination. Premortem diagnosis can be established by immunofluorescence examination of skin from the nape of the neck, detection of rabies virus antibody in cerebrospinal fluid or serum (assuming the patient was not vaccinated previously), or isolation of rabies virus from saliva or cerebrospinal fluid [Plotkin, 2000; Smith, 1996]. Reverse transcriptase polymerase chain reaction can be used to detect rabies virus and determine the molecular profile and animal origin of the rabies virus strain. Cerebrospinal fluid may be normal or reveal nonspecific changes with a mixed or lymphocytic pleocytosis and mild protein elevation [Chopra et al., 1980; Plotkin, 2000]. CT is normal; MRI can demonstrate signal abnormalities of the basal ganglia or thalami [Awasthi et al., 2001].

TREATMENT AND OUTCOME

Current antiviral drugs do not benefit patients with rabies, and virtually all patients die despite supportive care. The few reported survivors of rabies had received postexposure prophylaxis or had been immunized previously. A recent survivor of symptomatic rabies was treated with ribavirin, amantadine, and drug-induced coma [Willoughby et al., 2005]. Children with suspected rabies exposures should receive postexposure prophylaxis in accordance with Centers for Disease Control and Prevention and local public health guidelines, taking into account the animal species and the nature of the exposure. All postexposure treatment should begin with immediate and thorough cleansing of the wound with soap and water [Plotkin, 2000]. Bites are more likely to transmit the virus than scratches or other encounters [Fishbein and Robinson, 1993].

Because of the strong epidemiologic relationship between bat rabies strains and human rabies, prophylaxis should be administered after contact with bats, unless testing of the bat proves negative for rabies [CDC, 1997f]. Human-to-human transmission of rabies virus has been reported after corneal and organ transplantation [CDC, 2004e; Houff et al., 1979], but transmission by body fluids has not been described. Nonetheless, persons with suspected rabies should be maintained in strict isolation to minimize contact with rabies virus-contaminated fluids and to reduce the number of health-care workers who require postexposure prophylaxis. An average of 54 persons (family members and heath-care workers) per patient have required postexposure prophylaxis after contact with U.S. human rabies cases [Noah et al., 1998].

Arenaviridae

Lymphocytic choriomeningitis virus, a rodent-borne arenavirus, infects humans in temperate regions throughout Europe and North America, and outbreaks of human lymphocytic choriomeningitis virus disease have been linked to hamsters and wild or laboratory mice [Deibel et al., 1975; Dykewicz et al., 1992; Peters et al., 1996]. Although many infections occur without symptoms, lymphocytic choriomeningitis virus can induce a nonspecific, influenza-like disorder with fever, headache, myalgia, nausea, vomiting, backache, and cough [Dykewicz et al., 1992]. Occasional patients, including children, have prominent CNS symptoms with aseptic meningitis or mild meningoencephalitis [Deibel et al., 1975]. Cerebrospinal fluid findings include a mixed pleocytosis, sometimes including eosinophils, normal or elevated protein content, and a normal or depressed glucose content [Hirsch et al., 1974]. CT reveals hydrocephalus secondary to the meningeal and ependymal inflammation.

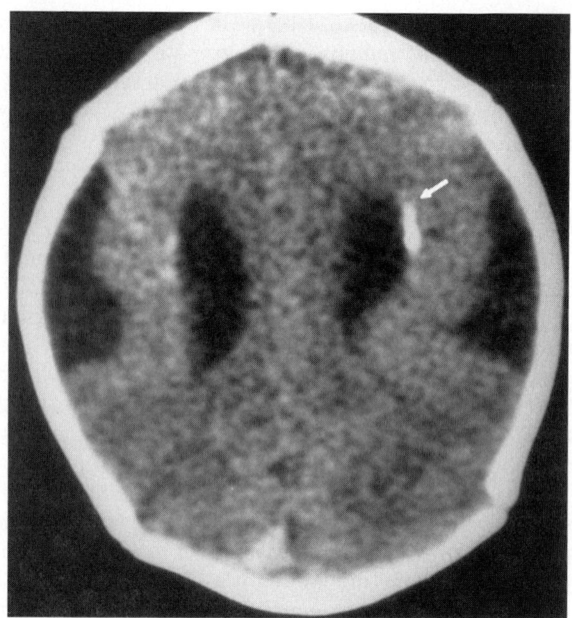

FIGURE 69-17. Unenhanced CT scan of another infant with congenital lymphocytic choriomeningitis virus infection reveals periventricular calcifications *(arrow)* and an abnormal cortex compatible with a disorder of neuronal migration. (From Wright R, Johnson D, Neumann M, et al. Congenital lymphocytic choriomeningitis virus syndrome: A disease that mimics congenital toxoplasmosis or cytomegalovirus infection. Pediatrics 1997;100:1.)

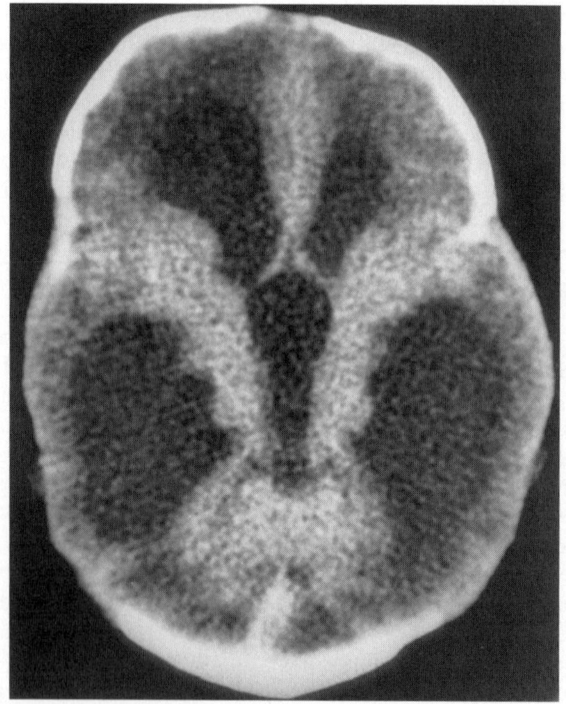

FIGURE 69-16. Unenhanced CT scan of an infant with congenital lymphocytic choriomeningitis virus infection reveals massive ventriculomegaly compatible with aqueductal obstruction. (From Wright R, Johnson D, Neumann M, et al. Congenital lymphocytic choriomeningitis virus syndrome: A disease that mimics congenital toxoplasmosis or cytomegalovirus infection. Pediatrics 1997;100:1.)

Lymphocytic choriomeningitis virus causes an intrauterine infection with clinical and radiographic features that resemble intrauterine cytomegalovirus disease or intrauterine toxoplasmosis [Barton and Mets, 2001; Barton et al., 1993; Wright et al., 1997]. Infants with this disorder frequently display chorioretinitis, microcephaly, or macrocephaly [Barton and Mets, 2001; Wright et al., 1997], and imaging studies reveal hydrocephalus, cerebral atrophy, or intracranial calcifications (Figs. 69-16 and 69-17). The diagnosis of congenital lymphocytic choriomeningitis virus infection can be established by detecting lymphocytic choriomeningitis virus–specific antibodies in cerebrospinal fluid or serum and potentially by detecting lymphocytic choriomeningitis virus RNA in cerebrospinal fluid with reverse transcriptase polymerase chain reaction [Read et al., 1997]. Patients with acquired infections recover completely, whereas congenitally infected infants have high rates of neurodevelopmental sequelae [Barton and Mets, 2001; Wright et al., 1997]. Current antiviral drugs do not possess clinically useful antilymphocytic choriomeningitis virus activity.

Retroviridae

HIV and human T-cell lymphotropic virus type I, linked in the 1980s to AIDS and progressive myelopathy, contribute to considerable neurologic morbidity among humans worldwide [Varmus, 1988]. Maintained in human reservoirs and transmitted via virus-contaminated human fluids or blood products, these retroviruses chronically infect the host, producing neurologic disease coincident with primary infection or subsequently during virus reactivation. Although antiretroviral therapy has advanced considerably since the 1990s, vaccines to prevent these infections are not yet available.

Human Immunodeficiency Virus

CLINICAL FEATURES

Cases of AIDS in children first appeared in the early 1980s before the causative agent, HIV, was identified [Falloon et al., 1989]. Early cases of childhood AIDS were traced epidemiologically to blood transfusions, hemophilia requiring factor replacement, or having a parent with AIDS or an AIDS-related condition. Subsequently, most HIV infections in infants and children were linked to mothers harboring HIV. The offspring of untreated, HIV-infected women have a 15% to 30% risk of acquiring the virus, whereas current combined antiretroviral treatment and management strategies in HIV-infected mothers and their infants can reduce the risk of perinatal transmission to 2% or less [American Academy of Pediatrics, 2003; CDC, 1994b, 1997g; Connor et al., 1994; Havens and Waters, 2004].

By the late 1980s, AIDS cases had been identified in more than 100 countries or territories, and the total number of AIDS cases worldwide rose exponentially from approximately 12,000 in 1984 to greater than 100,000 by 1989. Although the rates of HIV infection plateaued or declined in the United States and other regions of the developed world during the 1990s, HIV infection remains a major threat to the world's population [De Cock et al., 2000; UNAIDS, 2002]. Currently, more than 90% of new HIV infections occur among persons living in Asia and Africa. More than 800,000 Chinese were living with HIV/AIDS in 2001 [UNAIDS, 2002]. Globally the number of people living with HIV continues to grow—from 35 million in 2001 to 38 million in 2003. The World Health Organization estimates that 16,000 new cases of HIV infection occur daily and that 100 million persons worldwide will be infected with HIV by 2010 [UNAIDS, 2002]. More than 20 million infants, children, and adults have died since the first cases of AIDS were identified in 1981.

Infants infected with HIV vertically become symptomatic after the third month of life, manifesting hepatomegaly, lymphadenopathy, failure to thrive, interstitial pneumonitis, opportunistic infections (especially with *Pneumocystis carinii* or cytomegalovirus), or neurologic disease [Falloon et al., 1989]. The severity and spectrum of the clinical manifestations are modified, however, by antiparasitic, antiviral, and antiretroviral therapies. In some children, HIV can remain dormant, and 10 or more years may elapse before symptoms of HIV infection appear. Before current therapies, a child infected vertically with HIV had a 50% probability of severe HIV-related disease by age 5 years [Barnhart et al., 1996].

Neurologic complications were noted among adults early during the AIDS epidemic, and by the mid-1980s, similar disorders were reported in children [Belman et al., 1985; Epstein et al., 1985]. These early reports emphasized the dramatic, progressive decline in motor and intellectual skills in HIV-infected children, sometimes coinciding with the appearance of opportunistic infections with cytomegalovirus, *P. carinii, Toxoplasma gondii,* or other microorganisms. Early studies suggested that HIV-associated progressive encephalopathy develops in approximately 50% of children with advanced HIV disease, whereas improved antiretroviral therapies have modified the natural history of encephalopathy in HIV-infected children [Belman, 1992, 2002]. In utero exposure to HIV without evidence of perinatal infection does not adversely affect early neurologic development [Belman et al., 1996].

Before the availability of antiretroviral therapies, infants and children with HIV encephalopathy exhibited progressive motor dysfunction, cognitive abnormalities, developmental delay, and acquired microcephaly [Belman et al., 1985, 1986, 1988; Epstein et al., 1985]. Typical neurologic findings, attributable to the direct CNS effects of HIV, consist of apathy, dementia, ataxia, hyperreflexia, weakness, seizures, or myoclonus. Current antiretroviral therapies prevent or delay the onset of certain HIV-related neurologic complications [Gavin and Yogev, 1999; Belman, 2002].

The pathogenesis of brain abnormalities in infected infants and children has yet to be elucidated fully. HIV invades the CNS early after intrauterine or postnatal infection and displays tropism for microglia, macrophages, and astrocytes [Epstein and Gendelman, 1993; Epstein and Sharer, 1994; Ho et al., 1985]. Certain CNS cell populations, including neurons and oligodendrocytes, contain little or no HIV, suggesting that HIV causes dysfunction of these cell populations indirectly through cytokines or excitotoxins [Belman, 1997; Epstein and Sharer, 1994]. CNS disease parallels immunodeficiency [Belman, 1997, 2002] and reflects the viral load of infected persons.

Additional disorders linked directly to HIV infection of the CNS or peripheral nervous system are aseptic meningitis, meningoencephalitis, myopathy, and Guillain-Barré syndrome–like conditions [Raphael et al., 1991; Srugo et al., 1992]. HIV infection and AIDS also produce numerous secondary CNS complications, including stroke [Park et al., 1990], primary CNS lymphoma [Epstein et al., 1988], and CNS infections with *T. gondii,* cytomegalovirus, varicella-zoster virus, *Mycobacterium tuberculosis,* fungi, and JC virus, the cause of progressive multifocal leukoencephalopathy [Wrzolek et al., 1995]. The last-mentioned condition occurs in approximately 4% of adults with AIDS and some children and causes weakness, visual loss, cognitive decline, gait abnormalities, and sensory disturbances [Berger et al., 1987, 1992]. Polymerase chain reaction can be used to detect JC virus in clinical samples [McGuire et al., 1995].

DIAGNOSIS

Passive transfer of maternal antibody complicates detection of HIV infection during the first 18 months of life, and 30% or more of exposed infants serorevert [American Academy of Pediatrics, 2003]. Consequently, detection of HIV nucleic acid by polymerase chain reaction is necessary to diagnose HIV infection in young infants [American Academy of Pediatrics, 2003; Belman, 1997, 2002; Bremer et al., 1996]. HIV infection in infants can be confirmed by serial serum polymerase chain reaction assays, with the first test in the immediate newborn period, a second test during the first or second month of life, and a third test after 4 months of age. If two samples are positive for HIV, the infant is considered infected; two successive negative tests indicate infection is

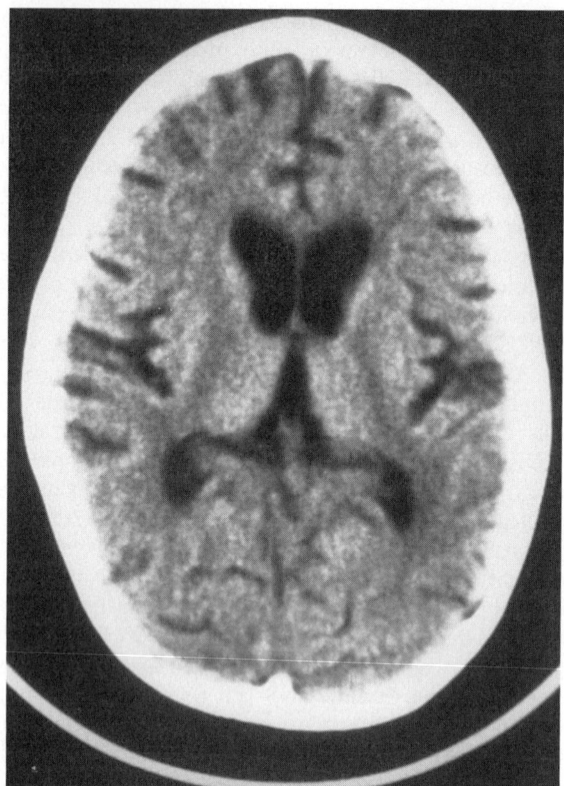

FIGURE 69-18. Unenhanced CT scan of a male with hemophilia and progressive encephalopathy resulting from human immunodeficiency virus infection reveals diffuse cortical atrophy. (From Bale JF. Encephalitis and other virus induced disorders of the nervous system. In: Joynt RJ, Griggs RC, eds. Clinical neurology. New York: Lippincott-Raven, 1996.)

unlikley [American Academy of Pediatrics, 2003]. In children and adolescents, serologic studies using enzyme-linked immunosorbent assay and Western blotting can identify HIV infection. Reverse transcriptase–polymerase chain reaction monitoring of virus loads guides the treatment of HIV-infected infants, children, and adolescents [American Academy of Pediatrics, 2003; Nielsen and Bryson, 2000].

The cerebrospinal fluid is usually normal in HIV-associated progressive encephalopathy, whereas the EEG may exhibit diffuse slowing. Neuroimaging studies reveal cortical atrophy in vertically or horizontally acquired infections (Fig. 69-18). Calcifications of the basal ganglia or frontal white matter—best detected by CT—and nonspecific abnormalities of white or gray matter—most evident by MRI—also have been reported in vertically acquired HIV infections [DeCarli et al., 1993; Belman et al., 1986]. CT, MRI, and studies of cerebrospinal fluid or blood can identify secondary infectious and neoplastic complications in HIV-infected children. Highly active antiretroviral therapy (HAART) has improved the prognosis for many of the opportunistic infections in persons with AIDS [Belman, 2002; Clifford et al., 1999].

TREATMENT AND OUTCOME

HAART and refined treatments for the infectious or neoplastic complications of AIDS have enhanced greatly the survival of HIV-infected persons [American Academy of Pediatrics, 2003; Belman, 1997, 2002; Melvin, 1997; van Rossum et al., 2002]. The mean survival time for children with AIDS exceeds 9 years, which is substantially greater than that of children treated for HIV infection in the early 1990s [Palumbo, 2000; Pizzo et al., 1988]. Several infectious disorders, including cytomegalovirus retinitis, cerebral toxoplasmosis, *P. carinii,* herpes zoster, and CNS or systemic fungal infections, respond favorably to current antiviral, antiparasitic, and antifungal therapies. Intravenous immunoglobulin also benefits selected children with hypogammaglobulinemia or recurrent, serious bacterial infections [Spector et al., 1994]. Certain complications, such as progressive multifocal leukoencephalopathy or primary CNS lymphoma, remain poorly responsive to the available therapies, however; the prolonged survival of HIV-infected patients seems to increase their lifetime risk of developing progressive multifocal leukoencephalopathy or CNS lymphoma.

HAART uses combinations of nucleoside/nucleotide reverse transcriptase inhibitors, such as zidovudine and didanosine; protease inhibitors, such as ritonavir and indinavir; and non-nucleoside reverse transcriptase inhibitors, such as nevirapine and efavirenz. The goal of therapeutic strategies is to reduce the HIV viral load to undetectable levels and to restore immunologic function. HAART produces immunologic and neurocognitive improvement, even in advanced HIV infection [Essajee et al., 1999; Tozzi et al., 1999]. Measurement of virus loads by quantitative reverse transcriptase–polymerase chain reaction has an essential role in monitoring the efficacy of therapy in HIV-infected children.

The development of drug resistance remains a serious, potential threat for HIV-infected patients [Boden et al., 1999]. In addition, HAART-associated immune reconstitution in patients with AIDS can lead to immune restoration disease, a condition characterized by paradoxical exacerbation of secondary infections during the initial 6 months of HAART [French et al., 2004; Stoll and Schmidt, 2003]. Immune restoration disease may occur in 30% of AIDS patients with low $CD4^+$ cell counts who begin HAART. Children who undergo HAART can experience lipodystrophy, insulin resistance, osteopenia, and growth failure [Leonard and McComsey, 2003]. Secondary infectious complications of AIDS, such as cytomegalovirus retinitis, *Toxoplasma* encephalitis, and cryptococcal or tuberculous meningitis, require therapy with appropriate antimicrobial agents. Treatment of primary CNS lymphoma in persons with AIDS remains problematic [Belman, 1997; Epstein et al., 1988].

Because treatment of HIV infection continues to evolve, centers experienced in HIV treatment should be consulted regarding current therapeutic approaches (for information regarding the available antiretroviral therapies and current treatment guidelines, see www.aidsinfo.nih.gov). Despite the remarkable success of HAART, current therapies do not eradicate HIV from infected persons [Lambotte et al., 2003]. Persons who reach end-stage AIDS despite HAART frequently experience AIDS-defining conditions, such as HIV dementia/encephalopathy, progressive multifocal leukoencephalopathy, lymphoma, or invasive cytomegalovirus infections, during the 12 months before death [Welch and Morse, 2002]. Vaccines to prevent HIV infection and AIDS are not yet available.

Human T-Cell Lymphotropic Virus Type I

Human T-cell lymphotropic virus type I, originally detected in adults with T-cell leukemia, causes a progressive myelopathy known as *human T-cell lymphotropic virus type I–associated myelopathy/tropical spastic paraparesis,* an endemic disorder in Japan, certain Caribbean Islands, the Seychelles, Africa, India, and certain regions of Latin America [Levin and Jacobson, 1997; Osame et al., 1987; Román et al., 1987]. Transmission of human T-cell lymphotropic virus type I parallels that of HIV, involving vertical (mother-to-child) and horizontal (person-to-person or transfusion of blood products) routes. Infection during childhood occurs commonly in endemic regions. Although most reported patients have been adults, a few have had onset of symptoms during late childhood or early adolescence [de Oliveira et al., 2004; Janssen et al., 1991; LaGrenade et al., 1995]. Clinical manifestations of human T-cell lymphotropic virus type I–associated myelopathy/tropical spastic paraparesis are those of a chronic, progressive myelopathy with spastic paraparesis, lower extremity hyperreflexia, sensory dysfunction, and bladder dysfunction. Although some patients respond temporarily to corticosteroid therapy, no curative antiviral therapy is currently available.

REFERENCES

Abd-Allah SA, Jansen PW, Ashwal S, et al. Intravenous immunoglobulin as therapy for pediatric Guillain-Barré syndrome. J Child Neurol 1997;12:376.

Abzug MJ, Cloud G, Bradley J, et al. Double blind placebo-controlled trial of pleconaril in infants with enterovirus meningitis. Pediatr Infect Dis J 2003;22:335.

Alexander JP, Baden L, Pallansch MA, et al. Enterovirus 71 infections and neurologic disease—United States, 1977-1991. J Infect Dis 1994;169:905.

Alkaly AL, Pomerance JJ, Rimoin DL. Fetal varicella syndrome. J Pediatr 1987;111:320.

American Academy of Pediatrics. 2003 Red Book: Report of the Committee on Infectious Diseases, 26th ed. Elk Grove Village, IL: American Academy of Pediatrics, 2003.

Anderson LJ, Nicholson KG, Tauxe RV, et al. Human rabies in the United States, 1960 to 1979: Epidemiology, diagnosis, and prevention. Ann Intern Med 1984;100:728.

Andreoni M, El-Sawaf G, Rezza G, et al. High seroprevalence of antibodies to human herpesvirus-8 in Egyptian children: Evidence of nonsexual transmission. J Natl Cancer Inst 1999;91:465.

Anlar B, Köse G, Gürer Y, et al. Changing epidemiologic features of subacute sclerosing panencephalitis. Infection 2001;29:192.

Anlar B, Saatçi I, Köse G, et al. MRI findings in subacute sclerosing panencephalitis. Neurology 1996;47:1278.

Appelbaum E, Rachelson JH, Dolgopol VB. Varicella encephalitis. Am J Med 1953;15:223.

Askalan R, Laughlin S, Mayank S, et al. Chickenpox and stroke in childhood: A study of frequency and causation. Stroke 2001;32:1257.

Awasthi M, Parmar H, Patankar T, et al. Imaging findings in rabies encephalitis. AJNR Am J Neuroradiol 2001;22:677.

Baker FJ, Kotchman GS, Foshee MS, et al. Acute hemiplegia of childhood associated with Epstein-Barr virus infection. Pediatr Infect Dis J 1983;2:136.

Bale JF. Human cytomegalovirus infection and disorders of the nervous system. Arch Neurol 1984;41:310.

Bale JF, ed. Congenital infections of the central nervous system. Semin Pediatr Neurol 1994;1.

Bale JF. Human herpesviruses and neurological disorders of childhood. Semin Pediatr Neurol 1999;4:278.

Bale JF. Virus induced disorders of the nervous system. In: Joynt RJ, Griggs RC, eds. Clinical neurology. New York: Lippincott-Raven, 2003.

Bale JF, Miner LJ. Herpes simplex virus infections of the newborn. Curr Treat Options Neurol 2005;7:151.

Bale JF, Andersen RA, Grose C. Magnetic resonance imaging of the brain in childhood herpesvirus infections. Pediatr Infect Dis J 1987;6:644.

Bale JF, Murph JR. Congenital infections and the nervous system. Pediatr Clin North Am 1992;39:669.

Bale JF, Murph JR. Infections of the central nervous system in the newborn. Clin Perinatol 1997;24:787.

Balfour HH. California (La Crosse virus) encephalitis in Minnesota. Minn Med 1974;57:876.

Balfour HH, Siem RA, Bauer H, et al. California arbovirus (LaCrosse) infections. Pediatrics 1973;52:680.

Balkhy HH, Schreiber JR. Severe La Crosse encephalitis with significant neurologic sequelae. Pediatr Infect Dis J 2000;19:77.

Barkovich J. Pediatric neuroimaging, 2nd ed. New York: Raven Press, 1995.

Barnhart HX, Caldwell MB, Thomas P, et al. Natural history of human immunodeficiency virus disease in perinatally infected children: An analysis from the Pediatric Spectrum of Disease Project. Pediatrics 1996;97:710.

Barone SR, Kaplan MH, Krilov LR. Human herpesvirus-6 infection in children with first febrile seizures. J Pediatr 1995;127:95.

Barton LL, Budd SC, Morfitt WS, et al. Congenital lymphocytic choriomeningitis virus infection in twins. Pediatr Infect Dis J 1993;12:942.

Barton LL, Mets MB. Congenital lymphocytic choriomeningitis virus infection: Decade of rediscovery. Clin Infect Dis 2001;33:370.

Belman AL. Central nervous system involvement in pediatric HIV-1 infection. Int Pediatr 1992;7:126.

Belman AL. Neurologic disorders associated with human immunodeficiency virus infections in children. In: Roos KL, ed. Central nervous system infectious diseases and therapy. New York: Marcel Dekker, 1997.

Belman AL. HIV infection and AIDS. Neurol Clin 2002;20:983.

Belman AL, Diamond G, Dickson D, et al. Pediatric acquired immunodeficiency syndrome: Neurologic syndromes. Am J Dis Child 1988;142:29.

Belman AL, Lantos G, Horoupian D, et al. AIDS: Calcifications of the basal ganglia in infants and children. Neurology 1986;36:1192.

Belman AL, Muenz LR, Marcus JC, et al. Neurologic status of human immunodeficiency virus 1-infected infants and their controls: A prospective study from birth to 2 years. Pediatrics 1996;98:1109.

Belman AL, Ultmann MH, Horoupian D, et al. Neurological complications in infants and children with acquired immune deficiency syndrome. Ann Neurol 1985;18:560.

Berg R, Jelke H. Acute cerebellar ataxia in children associated with Coxsackie viruses group B. Acta Paediatr Scand 1965;54:497.

Berg SW, Mitchell BS, Hanson RK, et al. Systemic reactions in U.S. Marine Corps personnel who received Japanese encephalitis vaccine. Clin Infect Dis 1997;24:265.

Berger J, Albrecht J, Belman AL, et al. Progressive multifocal leukoencephalopathy in children with HIV infection. AIDS 1992;6:837.

Berger JR, Kaszovitz B, Post JD, et al. Progressive multifocal leukoencephalopathy associated with human immunodeficiency virus infection. Ann Intern Med 1987;107:78.

Bergman I, Painter MJ, Wald ER, et al. Outcome in children with enteroviral meningitis during the first year of life. J Pediatr 1987;110:705.

Bergström T, Vahlne A, Alestig K, et al. Primary and recurrent herpes simplex virus type 2 induced meningitis. J Infect Dis 1990;162:322.

Blacklow NR, Cukor G. Viral gastroenteritis. N Engl J Med 1981;304:397.

Boden D, Hurley A, Zhang L, et al. HIV-1 drug resistance in newly infected individuals. JAMA 1999;282:1135.

Bodensteiner JB, Hille MR, Riggs JE. Clinical features of vascular thrombosis following varicella. Am J Dis Child 1992;146:100.

Boppana SB, Fowler KB, Vaid Y, et al. Neuroradiographic finding in the newborn period and long-term outcome in children with symptomatic congenital cytomegalovirus infection. Pediatrics 1997;99:409.

Bosma TJ, Corbett KM, Eckstein MB, et al. Use of PCR for prenatal and postnatal diagnosis of congenital rubella. J Clin Microbiol 1995;33:2881.

Boyle GJ, Michaels MG, Webber ST, et al. Posttransplantation lymphoproliferative disorders in pediatric thoracic organ recipients. J Pediatr 1997;131:309.

Bray PF. Mumps—a cause of hydrocephalus? Pediatrics 1972;49:446.

Bremer JW, Lew JF, Cooper E, et al. Diagnosis of infection with human immunodeficiency virus type 1 by a DNA polymerase chain reaction assay among infants enrolled in the Women and Infant's Transmission Study. J Pediatr 1996;129:198.
Brown P. Human growth hormone therapy and Creutzfeldt-Jakob disease: A drama in three acts. Pediatrics 1988;81:85.
Brown P, Cervenakova L, Goldfarb LG, et al. Iatrogenic Creutzfeldt-Jakob disease: An example of the interplay between ancient genes and modern medicine. Neurology 1994;44:291.
Brown P, Gajdusek DC, Gibbs CJ Jr, et al. Potential epidemic of Creutzfeldt-Jakob disease from human growth hormone therapy. N Engl J Med 1985;313:728.
Brunnell P. Varicella in pregnancy, the fetus, and the newborn: Problems in management. J Infect Dis 1992;166:S42.
Burgess RC, Michaels L, Bale JF, et al. Polymerase chain reaction amplification of herpes simplex viral DNA from the geniculate ganglion of a patient with Bell's palsy. Ann Otol Rhinol Laryngol 1994;103:775.
Burke DS, Lorsomrudee W, Leake CJ, et al. Fatal outcome in Japanese encephalitis. Am J Trop Med Hyg 1985;34:1203.
Burke DS, Nisalak A, Ussery MA. Antibody capture immunoassay detection of Japanese encephalitis virus immunoglobulin M and G antibodies in cerebrospinal fluid. J Clin Microbiol 1982;16:1034.
Calisher CH. Medically important arboviruses of the United States. Clin Microbiol Rev 1994;7:89.
Calisher CH, Berardi VP, Muth DJ, et al. Specificity of immunoglobulin M and G antibody response in humans infected with eastern and western equine encephalitis viruses: Applications to rapid serodiagnosis. J Clin Microbiol 1986;23:369.
Campbell GL, Marfin AA, Lanciotti RS, et al. West Nile virus. Lancet 2002;20:519.
Carpentier-Barthez MA, Rozenberg F, Dussaix E, et al. Relapse of herpes simplex encephalitis. J Child Neurol 1995;10:363.
Centers for Disease Control and Prevention. Arboviral infections of the central nervous system. MMWR Morb Mortal Wkly Rep 1986;35:342.
Centers for Disease Control and Prevention. Western equine encephalitis in the United States and Canada, 1987. Morb Mortal Wkly Rep 1987; 36:655.
Centers for Disease Control and Prevention. Human rabies—New York, 1993. MMWR Morb Mortal Wkly Rep 1993a;42:799
Centers for Disease Control and Prevention. Inactivated Japanese encephalitis virus vaccine. MMWR Morb Mortal Wkly Rep 1993b;42(RR-1):1.
Centers for Disease Control and Prevention. Certification of poliomyelitis eradication—the Americas, 1994. MMWR Morb Mortal Wkly Rep 1994a;43:720.
Centers for Disease Control and Prevention. Recommendations of the U.S. Public Health Service task force on the use of zidovudine to reduce perinatal transmission of human immunodeficiency virus. MMWR Morb Mortal Wkly Rep 1994b;43(RR-11):1.
Centers for Disease Control and Prevention. Venezuelan encephalitis—Colombia, 1995. MMWR Morb Mortal Wkly Rep 1995a;44:721.
Centers for Disease Control and Prevention. Mumps surveillance—United States, 1988-1993. MMWR Morb Mortal Wkly Rep 1995b;44(SS-3):1.
Centers for Disease Control and Prevention. Prevention of varicella. MMWR Morb Mortal Wkly Rep 1996;45(RR-11):1.
Centers for Disease Control and Prevention. Update: Raccoon rabies epizootic—United States, 1996. MMWR Morb Mortal Wkly Rep 1997a;45:1117.
Centers for Disease Control Prevention. Paralytic poliomyelitis—United States, 1980-1994. MMWR Morb Mortal Wkly Rep 1997b;46:79.
Centers for Disease Control and Prevention. Nonpolio enterovirus surveillance—United States, 1993-1996. MMWR Morb Mortal Wkly Rep 1997c;46:748.
Centers for Disease Control and Prevention. Rubella and congenital rubella syndrome—United States, 1994-1997. MMWR Morb Mortal Wkly Rep 1997d;46:350.
Centers for Disease Control and Prevention. Human rabies—Montana and Washington, 1997. MMWR Morb Mortal Wkly Rep 1997e;46:770.
Centers for Disease Control and Prevention. Measles eradication: Recommendations from a meeting cosponsored by the World Health Organization, the Pan American Health Organization, and CDC. MMWR Morb Mortal Wkly Rep 1997f;46(RR-11):1.
Centers for Disease Control and Prevention. Update: Perinatally acquired HIV/AIDS—United States, 1997. MMWR Morb Mortal Wkly Rep 1997g;46:1086.
Centers for Disease Control and Prevention. Intrauterine West Nile Virus infection—New York, 2002. MMWR Morb Mortal Wkly Rep 2002;51:1135.
Centers for Disease Control and Prevention. Available at: www.cdc.gov/ncidod/dvbid/westnile/surv&controlCaseCount03_detailed.htm. 2004a.
Centers for Disease Control and Prevention. Progress toward poliomyelitis eradication—Nigeria, January 2003-March 2004. MMWR Morb Mortal Wkly Rep 2004b;53:343.
Centers for Disease Control and Prevention. Available at: www.cdc.gov/ncidod/dvbid/westnile/background.html. 2004c.
Centers for Disease Control and Prevention. Epidemiology of measles—United States, 2001-2003. MMWR Morb Mortal Wkly Rep 2004d;53:713.
Centers for Disease Control and Prevention. Update: Investigation of rabies infections in organ donor and transplant recipients—Alabama, Arkansas, Oklahoma, and Texas, 2004. MMWR Morb Mortal Wkly Rep 2004e;53:615.
Centers for Disease Control and Prevention. Interim guidelines for the evaluation of infants born to mothers infected with West Nile virus during pregnancy. MMWR Morb Mortal Wkly Rep 2004f;53:154.
Chandwani S, Kaul A, Bebenroth D, et al. Cytomegalovirus infection in human immunodeficiency virus type 1-infected children. Pediatr Infect Dis J 1996;15:310.
Chang Y, Cesarman E, Pessin MS, et al. Identification of herpesvirus-like DNA sequences in AIDS-associated Kaposi's sarcoma patients. Science 1994;266:1865.
Chany C, Lepine P, Lelong M, et al. Severe and fatal pneumonia in infants and young children associated with adenovirus infections. Am J Hyg 1958;67:367.
Chemtob S, Reece ER, Mills EL. Syndrome of inappropriate secretion of antidiuretic hormone in enteroviral meningitis. Am J Dis Child 1985;139:292.
Chen RE, Ramsay DA, deVeber LL, et al. Immunosuppressive measles encephalitis. Pediatr Neurol 1994;10:325.
Cheng-Yu Ch, Ying-Chao C, Chao-Ching H, et al. Acute flaccid paralysis in infants and young children with enterovirus 71 infections: MR imaging findings and clinical correlates. AJNR Am J Neuroradiol 2001;22:200.
Chong HT, Kamarulzaman A, Tan CT, et al. Treatment of acute Nipah encephalitis with ribavirin. Ann Neurol 2001;49:810.
Chopra JS, Banerjee AK, Murthy JMK, et al. Paralytic rabies: A clinic—pathological study. Brain 1980;103:789.
Chua KB. Nipah virus outbreak in Malaysia. J Clin Virol 2003;26:265.
Chua KB, Bellini WJ, Rota PA, et al. Nipah virus: A recently emergent deadly paramyxovirus. Science 2000;288:1432.
Chuang YY, Chiu CH, Wong KS, et al. Severe adenovirus infection in children. J Microbiol Immunol Infect 2003;36:37.
Clifford DB, Buller RS, Mohammed S, et al. Use of polymerase chain reaction to demonstrate cytomegalovirus DNA in CSF of patients with human immunodeficiency virus infection. Neurology 1993;43:75.
Clifford DB, Yiannoutsos C, Glicksman M, et al. HAART improves prognosis in HIV-associated progressive multifocal leukoencephalopathy. Neurology 1999;52:623.
Connelly KP, DeWitt LD. Neurology complications of infectious mononucleosis. Pediatr Neurol 1994;10:181.
Connolly AM, Dodson W, Prensky AL, et al. Course and outcome of acute cerebellar ataxia. Ann Neurol 1994;35:673.
Connor EM, Sperling RS, Gelber R, et al. Reduction of maternal-infant transmission of human immunodeficiency virus type 1 with zidovudine treatment. N Engl J Med 1994;331:1173.
Corey L, Spear PG. Infections with herpes simplex viruses. N Engl J Med 1986;314:686.
Cramblett HG, Moffett HL, Black JP, et al. Coxsackie virus infections. J Pediatr 1964;64:406.
Creech WB. St. Louis encephalitis in the United States, 1975. J Infect Dis 1977;135:1014.
Cruse RP, Rothner AD, Erenberg G, et al. Central European tick-borne encephalitis: An Ohio case with a history of foreign travel. Am J Dis Child 1979;33:1070.
Cuthbertson G, Weiner CP, Giller RH, et al. Prenatal diagnosis of second trimester congenital varicella syndrome by virus-specific immunoglobulin M. J Pediatr 1987;111:592.
Dangond R, Engel E, Yessayan L, et al. Pre-eruptive varicella cerebellitis confirmed by PCR. Pediatr Neurol 1993;9:491.
Darin N, Bergstrom T, Fast A, et al. Clinical, serological, and PCR

evidence of cytomegalovirus infection in the central nervous system of childhood. Neuropediatrics 1994;25:316.

DeCarli C, Civitello LA, Brouwers P, et al. The prevalence of computed tomographic abnormalities of the cerebrum in 100 consecutive children symptomatic with human immune deficiency virus. Ann Neurol 1993;34:198.

De Cock KM, Fowler MG, Mercier E, et al. Prevention of mother-to-child HIV transmission in resource-poor countries: Translating research into policy and practice. JAMA 2000;283:1175.

Deibel R, Woodall JP, Decher WJ. Lymphocytic choriomeningitis virus in man. JAMA 1975;232:501.

Demmler GJ. Summary of a workshop on surveillance for congenital cytomegalovirus disease. Rev Infect Dis 1991;13:315.

Demmler GJ, Buffone GJ, Schimbor CM, et al. Detection of cytomegalovirus in urine from newborns by using polymerase chain reaction DNA amplification. J Infect Dis 1988;158:1177.

Deng H, Liu R, Ellmeier W, et al. Identification of a major co-receptor for primary isolates of HIV. Nature 1996;381:661.

de Oliveira MF, Bittencourt AL, Brites C, et al. HTLV-I associated myelopathy/tropical spastic paraparesis in a 7-year-old boy associated with infective dermatitis. J Neurol Sci 2004;222:35.

Deresiewicz RL, Thaler SJ, Hsu L, et al. Clinical and neuroradiographic manifestations of eastern equine encephalitis. N Engl J Med 1997;336:1867.

Domachowske JB, Cunningham CK, Cummings DL, et al. Acute manifestations and neurologic sequelae of Epstein-Barr virus encephalitis in children. Pediatr Infect Dis J 1996;15:871.

Domingues RB, Fink MC, Tsanaclis SM, et al. Diagnosis of herpes simplex encephalitis by magnetic resonance imaging and polymerase chain reaction assay of cerebrospinal fluid. J Neurol Sci 1998;157:148.

Dowling PC, Cook SD. Role of infection in Guillain-Barré syndrome: Laboratory confirmation of herpesviruses in 41 cases. Ann Neurol 1981;9:44.

Drobyski WR, Knowx KK, Majewski D, et al. Brief report: Fatal encephalitis due to variant B human herpesvirus-6 infection in a bone marrow transplant recipient. N Engl J Med 1994;330:1356.

Dudgeon JA. Congenital rubella. J Pediatr 1975;87:1078.

Dunn V, Bale JF, Zimmerman RA, et al. MRI in children with postinfectious disseminated encephalomyelitis. MRI 1986;4:25.

Dupont JR, Earle KM. Human rabies encephalitis. Neurology 1966;15:1023.

Dutta JK. Human rabies in India: Epidemiologic features, management and current methods of prevention. Trop Doct 1999;29:196.

Dyken PR, Cunningham SC, Ward LC. Changing character of subacute sclerosing panencephalitis in the United States. Pediatr Neurol 1989;5:339.

Dykers TI, Brown KL, Gundersen CB, et al. Rapid diagnosis of LaCrosse encephalitis: Detection of specific immunoglobulin M in cerebrospinal fluid. J Clin Microbiol 1985;22:740.

Dykewicz CA, Dato VM, Fisher-Hoch SP, et al. Lymphocytic choriomeningitis outbreak associated with nude mice in a research institute. JAMA 1992;267:1349.

Earnest MP, Goolishian HA, Calverley JR, et al. Neurologic, intellectual and psychologic sequelae following western encephalitis. Neurology 1971;21:969.

Ellstein-Shturman R, Borkowsky W, Fish I, et al. Myelitis associated with genital herpes in a child. J Pediatr 1976;88:523.

Embil JA, Camfield P, Artsob H, et al. Powassan virus encephalitis resembling herpes simplex encephalitis. Arch Intern Med 1983;143:341.

Epstein LG, DiCarlo FJ, Joshi VV, et al. Primary lymphoma of the central nervous system in children with the acquired immunodeficiency syndrome. Pediatrics 1988;82:355.

Epstein LG, Gendelman HE. Human immunodeficiency virus type 1 infection of the central nervous system: Pathogenetic mechanisms. Ann Neurol 1993;33:429.

Epstein LG, Sharer LR. Neurological manifestations of perinatally acquired HIV-1 infection. Semin Pediatr Neurol 1994;1:50.

Epstein LG, Sharer LR, Joshi VV, et al. Progressive encephalopathy in children with acquired immune deficiency syndrome. Ann Neurol 1985;17:488.

Essajee SM, Kim M, Gonzalez C, et al. Immunologic and virologic responses to HAART in severely immunocompromised HIV-1-infected children. AIDS 1999;13:2523.

Falloon J, Eddy J, Wiener L, et al. Human immunodeficiency virus infection in children. J Pediatr 1989;114:1.

Feigin RD, Shackelford PG. Value of repeat lumbar puncture in the differential diagnosis of meningitis. N Engl J Med 1973;289:571.

Fields BN, Knipe DM. Fields virology. New York: Raven Press, 1990.

Fishbein DB, Robinson LE. Rabies. N Engl J Med 1993;329:1632.

Fleisher G, Henry W, McSorley M, et al. Life-threatening complications of varicella. Am J Dis Child 1981;135:896.

Forrst JM, Turnbull FM, Sholler GF, et al. Gregg's congenital rubella patients 60 years later. Med J Aust 2002;177:664.

Fowler KB, McCollister FP, Dahle AJ, et al. Progressive and fluctuating sensorineural hearing loss in children with asymptomatic congenital cytomegalovirus infection. J Pediatr 1997;130:624.

French MA, Price P, Stone SF. Immune restoration disease after antiretroviral therapy. AIDS 2004;18:1615.

Frey T. Optic neuritis in children: Infectious mononucleosis as an etiology. Doc Ophthalmol 1973;34:183.

Gascon GG. International Consortium on Subacute Sclerosing Panencephalitis. Randomized treatment study of inosiplex versus combined inosiplex and intraventricular interferon-alpha in subacute sclerosing panencephalitis (SSPE): International multicenter study. J Child Neurol 2003;18:819.

Gavin P, Yogev R. Central nervous system abnormalities in pediatric human immunodeficiency virus infection. Pediatr Neurosurg 1999;31:115.

Gendelman HE, Wolinsky JS, Johnson RT, et al. Measles encephalomyelitis: Lack of evidence viral invasion of the central nervous system and quantitative study of the demyelination. Ann Neurol 1984;15:353.

Gilden D. Varicella zoster virus and central nervous system syndromes. Herpes 2004;11(Suppl 2):89a.

Givens KT, Lee DA, Jones T, et al. Congenital rubella syndrome: Ophthalmic manifestations and associated systemic disorders. Br J Ophthalmol 1993;77:358.

Gleaves CA, Hodknka RL, Johnston SLG, et al. Laboratory diagnosis of viral infections: CUMITECH. Am Soc Microbiol 1994;15A.

Gnann JW, Whitley RJ. Natural history and treatment of varicella-zoster in high-risk populations. J Hosp Infect 1991;18:317.

Goh KJ, Tan CT, Chew NK, et al. Clinical features of Nipah virus encephalitis among pig farmers in Malaysia. N Engl J Med 2000;342:1229.

Goodpasture HC, Poland JD, Francy DB, et al. Colorado tick fever: Clinical, epidemiologic, and laboratory aspects of 228 cases in Colorado in 1973-1974. Ann Intern Med 1978;88:303.

Grabow JD, Matthews CG, Chun RW, et al. The electroencephalogram and clinical sequelae of California arbovirus encephalitis. Neurology 1969;19:394.

Grattan-Smith J, Hopkins IJ, Shield LK, et al. Acute pseudobulbar palsy due to bilateral focal cortical damage: The opercular syndrome of Foix-Chavany-Marie. J Child Neurol 1989;4:131.

Grose C: Congenital infections caused by varicella zoster virus and herpes simplex virus. Semin Pediatr Neurol 1994;1:43.

Grose C, Bonthius D, Afifi AK. Chickenpox and the geniculate ganglion: Facial nerve palsy, Ramsay Hunt syndrome and acyclovir treatment. Pediatr Infect Dis J 2002;21:615.

Grose C, Feorino PM. Epstein-Barr virus and Guillain-Barré syndrome. Lancet 1972;2:1285.

Guess HA, Broughton DD, Melton LJ, et al. Epidemiology of herpes zoster in children and adolescents. Pediatrics 1985;76:512.

Gutman LT, Wilfert CM, Eppes S. Herpes simplex virus encephalitis in children: Analysis of cerebrospinal fluid and progressive neurodevelopmental deterioration. J Infect Dis 1986;154:415.

Hall CB, Long CE, Schnabel KC, et al. Human herpesvirus-6 infection in children. N Engl J Med 1994;331:432.

Halsted CC, Chang RS. Infectious mononucleosis and encephalitis: Recovery of EB virus from spinal fluid. Pediatrics 1979;64:257.

Hamilton MS, Jackson MA, Abel D. Clinical utility of polymerase chain reaction testing for enteroviral meningitis. Pediatr Infect Dis J 1999;18:533.

Haupt W. Rabies: Risk of exposure and current trends in prevention of human cases. Vaccine 1999;17:1742.

Hausler M, Schaade L, Kemeny S, et al. Encephalitis related to primary varicella-zoster virus infection in immunocompetent children. J Neurol Sci 2002;195:111.

Havens PL, Waters D. Management of the infant born to a mother with HIV infection. Pediatr Clin North Am 2004;51:909.

Hayes EB, O'Leary DR. West Nile virus: A pediatric perspective. Pediatrics 2004;113:1375.

Hayward JC, Titelbaum DS, Clancy RR, et al. Lissencephaly-pachygyria associated with congenital cytomegalovirus infection. J Child Neurol 1991;6:109.

Henao-Restrepo AM, Strebel P, Hoekstra EJ. Experience in global measles control, 1990-2001. J Infect Dis 2003;187 (Suppl 1):S-15.

Heresi GP, Mancias P, Mazur LJ, et al. Poliomyelitis-like syndrome in a child with West Nile virus infection. Pediatr Infect Dis J 2004;23:788.

Herndon RM, Johnson RT, Davis LE, et al. Ependymitis in mumps virus meningitis. Arch Neurol 1974;30:475.

Hilt DC, Buchholz D, Krumholz A, et al. Herpes zoster ophthalmicus and delayed contralateral hemiparesis caused by cerebral angiitis: Diagnosis and management approaches. Ann Neurol 1983;14:543.

Hilty MD, Haynes RE, Azimi PH, et al. California encephalitis in children. Am J Dis Child 1972;124:530.

Hirsch MS, Moellering RC, Pope HG, et al. Lymphocytic choriomeningitis virus infection traced to a pet hamster. N Engl J Med 1974;291:610.

Ho DD, Rota TR, Schooley RT, et al. Isolation of HTLV-III from cerebrospinal fluid and neural tissues of patients with neurologic syndromes related to the acquired immunodeficiency syndrome. N Engl J Med 1985;313:1493.

Holland NR, Power C, Mathews V, et al. Cytomegalovirus encephalitis in acquired immunodeficiency syndrome (AIDS). Neurology 1994;44:507.

Honarmand S, Glaser CA, Chow E, et al. Subacute sclerosing panencephalitis in the differential diagnosis of encephalitis. Neurology 2004;63:1489.

Horwitz CA, Henle W, Henle G, et al. Clinical and laboratory evaluation of cytomegalovirus-induced mononucleosis in previously healthy individuals. Medicine 1986;66:124.

Houff SA, Burton RC, Wilson RW, et al. Human-to-human transmission of rabies virus by corneal transplant. N Engl J Med 1979;300:603.

Huang CC, Liu CC, Chang YC, et al. Neurologic complications in children of enterovirus 71 infection. N Engl J Med 1999;341:936.

Hubalek Z, Halouzka J: West Nile fever-a reemerging mosquito-borne viral disease in Europe. Emerg Infect Dis 1999;5:643.

Huder SW. Infectious etiologies of facial palsy. In: Roos KL, ed. Central nervous system infectious diseases and therapy. New York: Marcel Dekker, 1997.

Hughes SS. The virus: A history of the concept. London: Heinemann Educational Books, 1977.

Hung KL, Liao HT, Tsai ML. Epstein-Barr virus encephalitis in children. Acta Paediatr Taiwan 2000;41:140.

Hutto C, Arvin A, Jacobs R, et al. Intrauterine herpes simplex virus infections. J Pediatr 1987;110:97.

Iannetti P, Nigro G, Spalice A, et al. Cytomegalovirus infection and schizencephaly: Case reports. Ann Neurol 1998;43:123.

Ichiba N, Miyake Y, Sato K, et al. Mumps-induced opsoclonus-myoclonus and ataxia. Pediatr Neurol 1988;4:224.

Istas AS, Demmler GJ, Dobbins JG, et al. Surveillance for congenital cytomegalovirus disease: A report from the national congenital cytomegalovirus disease registry. Clin Infect Dis 1995;20:665.

Jacobson MA. Treatment in cytomegalovirus retinitis in patients with the acquired immunodeficiency syndrome. N Engl J Med 1997;337:105.

Jansen PW, Perkin RM, Ashwal S. Guillain-Barré syndrome in childhood: Natural course and efficacy of plasmapheresis. Pediatr Neurol 1992;9:1.

Janssen RS, Kaplan JE, Khabbaz RF, et al. HTLV-I associated myelopathy/tropical spastic paraparesis in the United States. Neurology 1991;41:1355.

Jenista JA, Powell KA, Menegus MA. Epidemiology of neonatal enterovirus infections. J Pediatr 1984;104:685.

Johnson AJ, Karabatsos N, Lanciotti RS. Detection of Colorado tick fever virus by using reverse transcriptase PCR and application of the technique in laboratory diagnosis. J Clin Microbiol 1997;35:1203.

Johnson R, Milbourn PE. Central nervous system manifestations of chickenpox. Can Med Assoc J 1970;102:831.

Johnson RT. Acute encephalitis. Clin Infect Dis 1996;23:219.

Johnson RT. Viral infections of the nervous system, 2nd ed. New York: Lippincott-Raven, 1998.

Johnson RT. Emerging infections of the nervous system. J Neurovirol 2003;9:140.

Johnson RT, Griffin DE, Hirsch RL, et al. Measles encephalomyelitis—clinical and immunologic studies. N Engl J Med 1984;310:137.

Kalita J, Misra UK. Comparison of CT scan and MRI findings in the diagnosis of Japanese encephalitis. J Neurol Sci 2000;174:3.

Kaplan AM, Longhurst WL, Randall DL. St. Louis encephalitis in children. West J Med 1978;128:279.

Kido S, Ozaki T, Asada H, et al. Detection of varicella-zoster virus (VZV) DNA in clinical samples from patients with VZV by the polymerase chain reaction. J Clin Microbiol 1991;29:76.

Kim KW, Gold RS. Acute encephalopathy in twins due to adenovirus type 7 infection. Arch Neurol 1983;40:58.

Kimberlin DW. Herpes simplex virus, meningitis, and encephalitis in neonates. Herpes 2004;11 (Suppl 2):65A.

Kimberlin DW, Lakeman FD, Arvin AM, et al. Application of the polymerase chain reaction to the diagnosis and management of neonatal herpes simplex virus disease. J Infect Dis 1996;174:1162.

Kimberlin DW, Lin C-Y, Jacobs RF, et al. Natural history of neonatal herpes simplex virus infections in the acyclovir era. Pediatrics 2001a;108:223.

Kimberlin DW, Lin CY, Jacobs RF, et al. Safety and efficacy of high-dose intravenous acyclovir in the management of neonatal herpes simplex virus infections. Pediatrics 2001b;108:230.

Kimberlin DW, Lin CY, Sanchez PJ, et al. Effect of ganciclovir therapy on hearing in symptomatic congenital cytomegalovirus disease involving the central nervous system: A randomized, controlled trial. J Pediatr 2003;143:16.

Koch TK, Berg BO, DeArmond SJ, et al. Creutzfeldt-Jakob disease in a young adult with idiopathic hypopituitarism: Possible relation to the administration of cadaveric growth hormone. N Engl J Med 1985;313:73.

Koskiniemi M. Cerebrospinal fluid alterations in herpes simplex virus encephalitis. Rev Infect Dis 1984;6:608.

Koskiniemi M, Donner M, Pettay O. Clinical appearance and outcome in mumps encephalitis in children. Acta Paediatr Scand 1983;72:603.

Koskiniemi M, Happonen JM, Järvenpää AJ, et al. Neonatal herpes simplex virus infection: A report of 43 patients. Pediatr Infect Dis J 1989;8:830.

Koskiniemi M, Rantalaiho T, Piiparinen H, et al. Infections of the central nervous system of suspected viral origin: A collaborative study from Finland. J Neurovirol 2001;7:400.

Koskiniemi M, Rautonen J, Lehtokoski-Lehtiniemi E, et al. Epidemiology of encephalitis in children: A 20 year survey. Ann Neurol 1991;29:492.

Kost RG, Strauss SE. Post-herpetic neuralgia—pathogenesis, treatment, and prevention. N Engl J Med 1996;335:32.

Krebs JW, Noll HR, Rupprecht CE, et al. Rabies surveillance in the United States during 2001. J Am Vet Med Assoc 2002;221:1690.

Kuban KC, Ephros MA, Freeman RL, et al. Syndrome of opsoclonus-myoclonus caused by Coxsackie B3 infection. Ann Neurol 1983;13:69.

Kumar R, Mathur A, Kumar A, et al. Clinical features and prognostic indicators of Japanese encephalitis in children in Lucknow (India). Indian J Med Res 1990;91:321.

Kumar R, Mathur A, Singh KB, et al. Clinical sequelae of Japanese encephalitis in children. Indian J Med Res 1993;97:9.

Kumar S, Misra UK, Kalita J, et al. MRI in Japanese encephalitis. Neuroradiology 1997;39:180.

Kuno G, Mitchell CJ, Chang GJ, et al. Detecting bunyaviruses of the Bunyamwera and California serogroups by a PCR technique. J Clin Microbiol 1996;34:1184.

Kunz CH. Tick-borne encephalitis in Europe. Acta Leidensia 1992;60:1.

Kunze U, Asokliene L, Bektimirov T, et al. Tick-borne encephalitis in childhood—consensus 2004. Wien Med Wochenschr 2004;154:242.

LaBoccetta AC, Tornay AS. Measles encephalitis. Am J Dis Child 1964;107:247.

Lambotte O, Deiva K, Tardieu M. HIV-1 persistence, viral reservoir, and the central nervous system in the HAART era. Brain Pathol 2003;13:95.

LaGrenade L, Morgan C, Carberry C, et al. Tropical spastic paraparesis occurring HTLV-I associated infective dermatitis: Report of two cases. West Indian Med J 1995;44:34.

Lakeman FD, Whitley RJ. Diagnosis of herpes simplex encephalitis: Application of polymerase chain reaction to cerebrospinal fluid from brain biopsied patients and correlation with disease. J Infect Dis 1995;171:857.

Lambert AJ, Martin DA, Lanciotti RS. Detection of North American eastern and western equine encephalitis viruses by nucleic acid amplification assays. J Clin Microbiol 2003;41:379.

Lanciotti RS, Kersat AJ. Nucleic acid sequence-based amplifications assays for rapid detection of West Nile and St. Louis encephalitis viruses. J Clin Microbiol 2001;39:4506.

Lanciotti RS, Roehrig JT, Deubel V, et al. Origin of the West Nile virus responsible for an outbreak of encephalitis in the northeastern United States. Science 1999;286:2333.

Landgren M, Kyllerman M, Bergström T, et al. Diagnosis of Epstein Barr virus-induced central nervous system infections by DNA amplification from cerebrospinal fluid. Ann Neurol 1994;35:631.

Leach CT, Sumaya CV, Brown NA. Human herpesvirus-6: Clinical implications of a recently discovered, ubiquitous agent. J Pediatr 1992;121:173.

Leech RW, Harris JC, Johnson RH. 1975 encephalitis epidemic in North Dakota and Western Minnesota. Minn Med 1981;64:545.

Leis AA, Butler IJ. Infantile herpes zoster ophthalmicus and acute hemiparesis following intrauterine chickenpox. Neurology 1987;37:1537.

Leonard EG, McComsey GA. Metabolic complications of antiretroviral therapy in children. Pediatr Infect Dis J 2003;22:77.

Leonard JR, Moran CJ, Cross DT, et al. MR imaging of herpes simplex type 1 encephalitis in infants and young children: A separate pattern of findings. AJR Am J Roentgenol 2000;174:1651.

Lesnicar G, Poljak M, Seme K, et al. Pediatric tick-borne encephalitis in 371 cases from an endemic region in Slovenia, 1959 to 2000. Pediatr Infect Dis J 2003;22:612.

Levin MC, Jacobson S. HTLV-I associated myelopathy/tropical spastic paraparesis (HAM/TSP): A chronic progressive neurologic disease associated with immunologically mediated damage to the central nervous system. J Neurovirol 1997;3:126.

Li J, Loeb JA, Shy ME, et al. Asymmetric flaccid paralysis: A neuromuscular presentation of West Nile virus infection. Ann Neurol 2003;53:703.

Liaw S-B, Shen E-Y. Alice in Wonderland syndrome as presenting symptom of EBV infection. Pediatr Neurol 1991;7:464.

Luby JP, Sulkin SE, Sanford JP. The epidemiology of St. Louis encephalitis: A review. Ann Rev Med 1969;20:329.

Lum GB, Williams JP, Dyken PR, et al. Magnetic resonance and CT imaging correlated with clinical status in SSPE. Pediatr Neurol 1986;2:75.

Marberg K, Goldblum N, Sterk VV, et al: The natural history of the West Nile fever: 1. Clinical observations during an epidemic in Israel. Am J Hyg 1956;64:259.

Martin JN, Ganem DE, Osmond DH, et al. Sexual transmission and the natural history of human herpesvirus 8 infection. N Engl J Med 1998;338:948.

Maschke M, Kastrup O, Forsting M, et al. Update on neuroimaging of infectious central nervous system disease. Curr Opin Neurol 2004;17:475.

McCormack JG. Clinical features of rotavirus gastroenteritis. J Infect 1982;4:167.

McCutchan JA. Clinical impact of cytomegalovirus infections of the nervous system in patients with AIDS. Clin Infect Dis 1995;21:S196.

McGuire D, Barhite S, Hollander H, et al. JC virus DNA in cerebrospinal fluid in human immunodeficiency virus-infected patients: Predictive value for progressive multifocal leukoencephalopathy. Ann Neurol 1995;37:395.

McJunkin JE, Khan R, de-los Reyes EC, et al. Treatment of severe La Crosse encephalitis with intravenous ribavirin following diagnosis by brain biopsy. Pediatrics 1997;99:261.

McJunkin JE, de los Reyes EC, Irazuzta JE, et al. La Crosse encephalitis in children. N Engl J Med 2001;344:801.

McKendall RR, Stroop WG. Handbook of neurovirology. New York: Marcel Dekker, 1994.

McLean DM, Donohue WL. Powassan virus: Isolation of virus from a fatal case of encephalitis. Can Med Assoc J 1959;80:708.

Mease PJ, Ochs HD, Wedgwood RJ. Successful treatment of meningoencephalitis and myositis-fasciitis with intravenous immune globulin therapy in a patient with X-linked agammaglobulinemia. N Engl J Med 1981;304:1278.

Medovy H. Western equine encephalomyelitis in infants. J Pediatr 1943;22:308.

Meehan PJ, Wells DL, Paul W, et al. Epidemiological features of and public health response to a St. Louis encephalitis epidemic in Florida, 1990-1. Epidemiol Infect 2000;125:181.

Meiyu F, Huosheng C, Cuihua C, et al. Detection of flaviviruses by reverse transcriptase-polymerase chain reaction with the universal primer set. Microbiol Immunol 1997;41:209.

Melvin A. Clinical, virological, and immunologic responses of children with advanced human immunodeficiency virus type 1 disease treated with protease inhibitors. Pediatr Infect Dis J 1997;16:968.

Mikati MA, Feraru E, Krishnamoorthy K, et al. Neonatal herpes simplex meningoencephalitis. Neurology 1990;40:1433.

Miller RF, Lucas SB, Hall-Craggs MA, et al. Comparison of magnetic resonance imaging with neuropathological findings in the diagnosis of HIV and CMV associated CNS disease in AIDS. J Neurol Neurosurg Psychiatry 1997;62:346.

Mitchell PS, Epsy MJ, Smith TE, et al. Laboratory diagnosis of central nervous system infections with herpes simplex virus by PCR performed in cerebrospinal fluid specimens. J Clin Microbiol 1997;35:2873.

Mizrahi EM, Tharp BR. A characteristic EEG pattern in neonatal herpes simplex encephalitis. Neurology 1982;32:1215.

Modlin JF, Dagan R, Berlin LE, et al. Focal encephalitis with enterovirus infections. Pediatrics 1991;88:841.

Modlin JF, Halsey NA, Eddins DL, et al. Epidemiology of subacute sclerosing panencephalitis. J Pediatr 1979;94:231.

Monath TP, Nystrom RR, Bailey RE, et al. Immunoglobulin M antibody capture enzyme-linked immunosorbent assay for diagnosis of St. Louis encephalitis. J Clin Microbiol 1984;20:784.

Monreal J, Collins GH, Masters CL, et al. Creutzfeldt-Jakob disease in an adolescent. J Neurol Sci 1981;52:341.

Morens DM. Enteroviral disease in early infancy. J Pediatr 1978;92:374.

Morgan EM, Rapp F. Measles virus and its associated disease. Bacteriol Rev 1977;41:636.

Morgello S, Cho E-S, Nielsen S, et al. Cytomegalovirus encephalitis in patients with acquired immunodeficiency syndrome. Hum Pathol 1987;18:289.

Morse RP, Bennish ML, Darras BT. Eastern equine encephalitis presenting with a focal brain lesion. Pediatr Neurol 1992;8:473.

Murph JR, Bale JF. The natural history of acquired cytomegalovirus infection among children in group day care. Am J Dis Child 1988;142:843.

Murphy JV, Yunis EJ. Encephalopathy following measles infection in children with chronic illness. J Pediatr 1976;88:937.

Mustafa MM, Weitman SD, Winick NJ, et al. Subacute measles encephalitis in the young immunocompromised host: Report of two cases diagnosed by polymerase chain reaction and treated with ribavirin and review of the literature. Clin Infect Dis 1993;16:654.

Nakayama NT, Mori T, Yamaguchi S, et al. Detection of measles virus genome directly from clinical samples by reverse-transcriptase-polymerase chain reaction and genetic variability. Virus Res 1995;35:1.

Nash D, Mostashari F, Fine A, et al. The outbreak of West Nile virus infection in the New York City area in 1999. N Engl J Med 2001;344:1807.

Negrini B, Kelleher KJ, Wald ER. Cerebrospinal fluid findings in aseptic versus bacterial meningitis. Pediatrics 2000;105:316.

Nicolosi A, Hauser WA, Beghi E, et al. Epidemiology of central nervous system infections in Olmstead County, Minnesota, 1950-1981. J Infect Dis 1986;154:399.

Nielsen K, Bryson YJ. Diagnosis of HIV infection in children. Pediatr Clin North Am 2000;47:39.

Nigro G, Scholz H, Bartmann U. Ganciclovir therapy for symptomatic congenital cytomegalovirus infection in infants: A two-regimen experience. J Pediatr 1994;124:318.

Noah DL, Drenzek CL, Smith JS, et al. Epidemiology of human rabies in the United States, 1980 to 1996. Ann Intern Med 1998;128:922.

Noyola DE, Demmler GJ, Nelson CT, et al. Early predictors of neurodevelopmental outcome in symptomatic congenital cytomegalovirus infection. J Pediatr 2001;138:325.

Ono J, Shimizu K, Harada K, et al. Characteristic MR features of encephalitis caused by Epstein-Barr virus: A case report. Pediatr Radiol 1998;28:569.

Osame M, Matsumoto M, Usuku K, et al. Chronic progressive myelopathy associated with elevated antibodies to human T-lymphotropic virus type I and adult T-cell leukemia-like cells. Ann Neurol 1987;21:117.

Palestine AG, Rodrigues MM, Macher AM, et al. Ophthalmic involvement in acquired immunodeficiency syndrome. Ophthalmology 1984;91:1092.

Palumbo PE. Antiretroviral therapy of HIV infection in children. Pediatr Clin North Am 2000;47:155.

Panagiotopoulos T, Georgakopoulou T. Epidemiology of rubella and congenital rubella syndrome in Greece, 1994-2003. Eur Surveill 2004;1:9.

Parashar UD, Sunn LM, Ong F, et al. Case-control study of risk factors for human infection with a new zoonotic paramyxovirus, Nipah virus during 1998-1999 outbreak of severe encephalitis in Malaysia. J Infect Dis 2000;181:1755.

Park YD, Belman AL, Kim TS, et al. Stroke in pediatric acquired immunodeficiency syndrome. Ann Neurol 1990;28:303.

Pass RF, Stagno S, Myers GJ, et al. Outcome of symptomatic congenital cytomegalovirus infection: Results of long-term longitudinal follow-up. Pediatrics 1980;66:758.

Payne FE, Baublis JV, Itabashi HH. Isolation of measles virus from cell culture of brain of a patient with subacute sclerosing panencephalitis. N Engl J Med 1969;281:585.

Peters CJ, Buchmeir M, Rollin PE, et al. Arenaviruses. In: Fields BN, Knipe DM, Howley PM, et al, eds. Fields virology. Philadelphia: Lippincott-Raven, 1996.

Petersen LR, Roehrig JT, Hughes JM. West Nile virus encephalitis. N Engl J Med 2002;347:1225.

Pizzo PA, Eddy J, Falloon J, et al. Effect of continuous intravenous infusion of zidovudine (AZT) in children with symptomatic HIV infection. N Engl J Med 1988;319:889.

Plotkin SA. Rabies. Clin Infect Dis 2000;30:4.

Post MJD, Hensley GT, Moskowitz LB, et al. Cytomegalic inclusion virus encephalitis in patients with AIDS: CT, clinical, and pathologic correlation. AJNR Am J Neuroradiol 1986;7:275.

Prusiner SB. Prion disease and the BSE crisis. Science 1997;278:245.

Prusiner SB, Hsiao KK. Human prion diseases. Ann Neurol 1994;35:385.

Przelomski MM, O'Rourke E, Grady GF, et al. Eastern equine encephalitis in Massachusetts. Neurology 1988;38:736.

Raphael SA, Price ML, Lischner HW, et al. Inflammatory demyelinating polyneuropathy in a child with symptomatic human immunodeficiency virus infection. J Pediatr 1991;118:242.

Rathore MH, Mercurio K, Halstead D. Herpes simplex type 1 meningitis. Pediatr Infect Dis J 1996;15:824.

Read SJ, Jeffery KJ, Bangham CR. Aseptic meningitis and encephalitis: The role of PCR in the diagnostic laboratory. J Clin Microbiol 1997;35:691.

Riggs S, Smith DL, Phillips CA. St. Louis encephalitis in adults during the 1964 epidemic. JAMA 1965;93:104.

Riikonen R. Cytomegalovirus infection and infantile spasms. Dev Med Child Neurol 1978;20:570.

Risk WS, Haddad FS. The variable natural history of subacute sclerosing panencephalitis. Arch Neurol 1979;36:610.

Rivas F, Diaz LA, Cardenas VM, et al. Epidemic Venezuelan equine encephalitis in La Guajira, Colombia, 1995. J Infect Dis 1997;175:828.

Rivera LB, Boppana SB, Fowler KB, et al. Predictors of hearing loss in children with symptomatic congenital cytomegalovirus infection. Pediatrics 2002;110:762.

Robinson J, Lemay M, Vaudry WL. Congenital rubella after anticipated maternal immunity: Two cases and a review of the literature. Pediatr Infect Dis J 1994;13:812.

Román GC, Schoenberg BS, Madden DL, et al. Human T-lymphotrophic virus type I antibodies in the serum of patients with tropical spastic paraparesis in the Seychelles. Arch Neurol 1987;44:605.

Ropper AH. The Guillain-Barré syndrome. N Engl J Med 1992;326:1130.

Rorabaugh ML, Berlin LE, Heldrich F, et al. Aseptic meningitis in infants younger than 2 years of age: Acute illness and neurologic complications. Pediatrics 1993;92:206.

Rosenfield J, Taylor CL, Atlas SW. Myelitis following chickenpox: A case report. Neurology 1993;43:1834.

Rotbart HA. Enteroviral infections of the central nervous system. Clin Infect Dis 1995;20:971.

Rupprecht CE, Smith JS, Fekadu M, et al. The ascension of wildlife rabies: A cause for public concern or intervention? Emerg Infect Dis 1995;4:107.

Rust R. Multiple sclerosis, acute disseminated encephalomyelitis, and related conditions. Semin Pediatr Neurol 2000;7:66.

Rust R, Thompson WH, Mathews CG, et al. La Crosse and other forms of California encephalitis. J Child Neurol 1999;14:1.

Salmi TT, Arstila P, Koivikko A, et al. Central nervous system involvement in patients with rotavirus gastroenteritis. Scand J Infect Dis 1978;10:29.

Sawyer MH. Enterovirus infections: Diagnosis and treatment. Semin Pediatr Infect Dis 2002;13:40.

Schlesinger Y, Buller RS, Brunstrom JE, et al. Expanded spectrum of herpes simplex encephalitis in childhood. J Pediatr 1995;126:234.

Schlesinger Y, Sawyer MH, Storch GA. Enteroviral meningitis in infancy: Potential role for polymerase chain reaction in patient management. Pediatrics 1994;94:157.

Schroth G, Gawehn J, Thron A, et al. Early diagnosis of herpes simplex encephalitis by MRI. Neurology 1987;37:179.

Schumacher RF, Forster J. The CNS symptoms of rotavirus infections under the age of two. Klin Padiatr 1999;211:61.

Sebire G, Meyer L, Chabrier S. Varicella as a risk factor for cerebral infarction in childhood: A case-control study. Ann Neurol 1999;45:679.

Sejvar JJ. West Nile and "poliomyelitis." Neurology 2004;63:206.

Sejvar JJ, Haddad MB, Tierney BC, et al. Neurologic manifestations and outcome of West Nile virus infection. JAMA 2003;290:511.

Sever JL, South MA, Shaver KA. Delayed manifestations of congenital rubella. Rev Infect Dis 1985;7:S164.

Shimizu H, McCarthy CA, Smaron MF, et al. Polymerase chain reaction for detection of measles virus in clinical samples. J Clin Microbiol 1993;31:1034.

Shinefield HR, Townsend TE. Transplacental transmission of western equine encephalomyelitis. J Pediatr 1953;43:21.

Silva CA, Paula-Barbosa MM, Pereira S, et al. Two cases of rapidly progressive subacute sclerosing panencephalitis. Arch Neurol 1981;38:109.

Smith JS. New aspects of rabies with emphasis on epidemiology, diagnosis and prevention of disease in the United States. Clin Microbiol Rev 1996;9:166.

Smith R, Woodall JP, Whitney E, et al. Powassan virus infection: A report of three human cases of encephalitis. Am J Dis Child 1974;127:691.

Souza IE, Bale JF. The diagnosis of congenital infections: Contemporary strategies. J Child Neurol 1995;10:271.

Spector SA, Gelber RD, McGrath N, et al. A controlled trial of intravenous immune globulin for the prevention of serious bacterial infections in children receiving zidovudine for advanced human immunodeficiency virus infection. Pediatric AIDS Clinical Trials Group. N Engl J Med 1994;331:1181.

Spika JS, Wassilak S, Pebody R. Measles and rubella in the world health organization European region: Diversity creates challenges. J Infect Dis 2003;187 (Suppl):S191.

Spruance SL, Bailey A. Colorado tick fever. Arch Intern Med 1973;131:288.

Srugo I, Wittek AE, Israele V, et al. Meningoencephalitis in a neonate congenitally infected with human immunodeficiency virus type 1. J Pediatr 1992;120:93.

Stoll M, Schmidt RE. Immune restoration inflammatory syndromes: The dark side of successful antiretroviral treatment. Curr Infect Dis Rep 2003;5:266.

Studahl M, Ricksten A, Sandberg T, et al. Cytomegalovirus encephalitis in four immunocompetent patients. Lancet 1992;340:1045.

Suga S, Yoshikawa T, Asano Y, et al. Clinical and virological analyses of 21 infants with exanthem subitum (roseola infantum) and central nervous system complications. Ann Neurol 1993;33:597.

Sumaya CV. Serologic testing for Epstein-Barr virus—developments in interpretation. J Infect Dis 1985;151:984.

Sumaya CV, Ench Y. Epstein-Barr virus infectious mononucleosis in children: I. Clinical and general laboratory findings. Pediatrics 1985a;75:1003.

Sumaya CV, Ench Y. Epstein-Barr virus infectious mononucleosis in children: II. Heterophil antibody and viral specific responses. Pediatrics 1985b;75:1011.

Sunaga Y, Hikima A, Ostuka T, et al. Acute cerebellar ataxia with abnormal MRI lesions after varicella infection. Pediatr Neurol 1995;13:340.

Takahashi H, Pool V, Tsail TF, Chen RT. Adverse events after Japanese encephalitis vaccination: Review of post-marketing surveillance data from Japan and the United States. The VAERS Working Group. Vaccine 2000;18:2963.

Tien RD, Felsberg GJ, Osumi AK. Herpesvirus infections of the CNS: MR findings. Am J Radiol 1993;161:167.

Torigoe S, Koide W, Yamada M, et al. Human herpesvirus 7 infection associated with central nervous system manifestations. J Pediatr 1996;129:301.

Townsend JJ, Baringer JR, Wolinsky JS, et al. Progressive rubella panencephalitis. N Engl J Med 1975;292:990.

Tozzi V, Balestra P, Galgani S, et al. Positive and sustained effects of highly active antiretroviral therapy on HIV-1 associated neurocognitive impairment. AIDS 1999;13:1889

Tsai T. Arboviral infections in the United States. Infect Dis Clin N Am 1991;5:73.

Ueda K, Nishida Y, Oshima K, et al. Congenital rubella syndrome: Correlation of gestational age at time of maternal rubella with type of defect. J Pediatr 1979;94:763.

UNAIDS. A global overview of the epidemic. Barcelona Report 2002:22.

van Rossum AM, Fraaij PL, de Groot R. Efficacy of highly active antiretroviral therapy in HIV-1 infected children. Lancet Infect Dis 2002;2:93.

Varmus H. Retroviruses. Science 1988;240:1427.

Volpi A. Epstein-Barr virus and human herpesvirus type 8 infections of the central nervous system. Herpes 2004;11 (Suppl 2):120A.

Warrell DA. The clinical picture of rabies in man. Trans Royal Soc Trop Med Hyg 1976;70:188.

Welch K, Morse A. Adult Spectrum of Disease Project in New Orleans. The clinical profile of end-stage AIDS in the era of highly active antiretroviral therapy. AIDS Patient Care STDS 2002;16:75.

Weller TH. Varicella and herpes zoster. N Engl J Med 1983;309:1362.

Wenger F. Venezuelan equine encephalitis. Teratology 1977;16:359.

Whitley RJ. Virus encephalitis. N Engl J Med 1990;323:242.

Whitley RJ, Alford CA, Hirsch MS, et al. Vidarabine versus acyclovir therapy in herpes simplex encephalitis. N Engl J Med 1986;314:144.

Whitley RJ, Arvin A, Prober C, et al. A controlled trial comparing vidarabine with acyclovir in neonatal herpes simplex virus infection. N Engl J Med 1991a;324:444.

Whitley RJ, Arvin A, Prober C, et al. Predictors of mortality in neonates with herpes simplex virus infections. N Engl J Med 1991b;324:450.

Whitley RJ, Cobbs CG, Alford CA, et al. Diseases that mimic herpes simplex encephalitis. JAMA 1989;262:234.

Whitley RJ, Corey L, Arvin A, et al. Changing presentation of herpes simplex virus infection in neonates. J Infect Dis 1988;158:109.

Whitley RJ, Gnann JW. Viral encephalitis: Familiar infections and emerging pathogens. Lancet 2002;359:507.

Whitley RJ, Lakeman F. Herpes simplex virus infections of the central nervous system: Therapeutic and diagnostic considerations. Clin Infect Dis 1995;20:414.

Whitley RJ, Soong SJ, Linneman C, et al. Herpes simplex encephalitis. JAMA 1982;247:317.

Wilfert CM, Buckley RH, Mohanakumar T, et al. Persistent and fatal central nervous system echovirus infections in patients with agammaglobulinemia. N Engl J Med 1977;296:1485.

Williamson WD, Demmler GJ, Percy AK, et al. Progressive hearing loss in infants with asymptomatic congenital cytomegalovirus infection. Pediatrics 1992;90:862.

Willoughby RE Jr, Tieves KS, Hoffman GM, et al. Survival after treatment of rabies with induction of coma. N Engl J Med 2005;352:2508.

Windebank AJ, Litchy WJ, Daube JR, et al. Late effects of paralytic poliomyelitis in Olmstead County, Minnesota. Neurology 1991;41:501.

Wright R, Johnson D, Neumann M, et al. Congenital lymphocytic choriomeningitis virus syndrome: A disease that mimics congenital toxoplasmosis or cytomegalovirus infection. Pediatrics 1997;100:1.

Wrzolek MA, Brudkowska J, Kozlowski PB, et al. Opportunistic infections of the central nervous system in children with HIV infection: Report of 9 cases and review of the literature. Clin Neuropathol 1995;14:187.

Yalaz K, Anlar B, Oktem F, et al. Intraventricular interferon and oral inosiplex in the treatment of subacute sclerosing panencephalitis. Neurology 1992;42:488.

Yamashita Y, Matsuishi T, Murakami Y, et al. Neuroimaging findings (ultrasonography, CT, MRI) in 3 infants with congenital rubella syndrome. Pediatr Radiol 1991;21:547.

Yoshida A, Kawamitu T, Tanaka R, et al. Rotavirus encephalitis: Detection of the virus genomic RNA in the cerebrospinal fluid of a child. Pediatr Infect Dis J 1995;14:914.

Yoshikawa T, Ihira M, Suzuki K, et al. Invasion by human herpesvirus 6 and human herpesvirus 7 of the central nervous system in patients with neurological signs and symptoms. Arch Dis Child 2000;83:170.

Yoshikawa T, Nakashima T, Suga S, et al. Human herpesvirus-6 DNA in cerebrospinal fluid of a child with exanthem subitum and meningoencephalitis. Pediatrics 1992;89:888.

CHAPTER 70

Fungal, Rickettsial, and Parasitic Diseases of the Nervous System

Carol A. Glaser, Paul F. Lewis, and Frederick L. Schuster

FUNGAL DISEASES

The importance of fungal infections has risen because progress in medicine has enabled more immunocompromised patients, including preterm infants, to survive. Patients, including children, with congenital immunodeficiency or poorly controlled human immunodeficiency virus infection are also at risk for invasive fungal infection as are diabetic, aplastic anemia, and oncology patients. The normal host is also susceptible to fungal infections, albeit to a smaller spectrum of organisms [Chimelli and Mahler-Araujo, 1997]. Fungal diseases involving the brain are usually secondary to systemic or pulmonary infection, and, in most patients, spread hematogenously. Occasionally, they arise from local direct extension from adjacent sinuses or the cranial vault.

With the exception of *Candida* meningitis in premature neonates and *Aspergillus* brain abscess in hematologic malignancy/hematopoietic stem cell transplant recipients, the individual fungal infections of the central nervous system (CNS) in children are rare. A review from a large university children's hospital found that in a 6-year period, 2% of 1498 positive cerebrospinal fluid cultures recovered fungal isolates [Arisoy et al., 1994]. *Candida* species accounted for 94.5% of all positive fungal cerebrospinal fluid cultures. About 39% of all patients were neonates, almost all of whom were low-birth-weight infants. For children beyond the newborn period, risk factors were prior antimicrobial therapy, chronic systemic or CNS disease, and central venous catheterization. Disseminated fungal infection was documented in 40% of all patients with positive cerebrospinal fluid cultures but, surprisingly, in 35% of patients the fungi recovered in the cerebrospinal fluid were considered contaminants. Such findings demonstrate that the clinician must always consider fungal CNS infections, particularly in certain high-risk groups, but results of positive cerebrospinal fluid cultures need careful interpretation. Table 70-1 provides a more extensive list of risk factors associated with fungal infections of the nervous system. Clinical manifestations of fungal infections can be subtle, and errors or delays in diagnosis are common. Fungi may cause meningitis, brain abscesses, granulomas, and spinal cord disease, and may invade and occlude the cerebral vasculature [Salake et al., 1984].

FUNGAL INFECTIONS IN NORMAL HOSTS

For purposes of discussion, separating fungi that infect normal hosts from those that infect immunologically compromised hosts is useful. Fungal infections in normal hosts include the following: *Cryptococcus neoformans, Coccidioides immitis, Blastomyces dermatitidis, Paracoccidioides brasiliensis, Histoplasma capsulatum*, and *Nocardia asteroides*. Compromised hosts may encounter the same pathogens as normal hosts but are especially susceptible to a wide range of opportunistic fungal pathogens including molds, such as *Aspergillus* and *Rhizopus*.

Cryptococcosis

Cryptococcosis is globally distributed and is most commonly seen in patients with acquired immunodeficiency syndrome (AIDS) and in those receiving systemic corticosteroids; infection also occurs in those without apparent predisposition, but at a lower frequency [Wendisch et al., 1996]. Although children are less frequently infected than adults, infants have contracted the disease [Hung et al., 1995; Littman and Walter, 1968; Wang et al., 1996] and vertical transmission has been reported from a mother with advanced AIDS [Sirinavin et al., 2004]. *C. neoformans* is an encapsulated yeast that reproduces by budding and has a sexual stage (Fig. 70-1). Bird feces, particularly from pigeons, harbor numerous cryptococcal organisms. The mode of entry in humans is probably through inhalation or ingestion. Hematogenous dissemination to the nervous system is usually preceded by pulmonary infection.

Clinical Characteristics, Clinical Laboratory Tests, and Diagnosis

Cryptococcus causes a meningoencephalitis often characterized by typical features, including nausea, vomiting, headache, and fever, all of which may fluctuate. Caution is urged in ruling out the diagnosis based on history and physical examination alone because many patients are afebrile (40%), have no meningeal signs [Sabetta and Andriole, 1985], and presenting symptoms such as somnolence, clumsiness, poor memory, and confusion can be nonspecific. Ocular palsies and personality changes may also occur. In AIDS patients, CNS cryptococcosis tends to be acute with fever and headache in 70%, meningismus, photophobia, or mental status changes in 20% to 25%, and focal deficits in a small percentage [Daar and Meyer, 1992]. Most patients with cryptococcal meningitis have an abnormal chest radiograph (e.g., bilateral alveolar or interstitial pneumonitis). Some of these patients may have a second opportunistic infection as well, particularly *Pneumocystis jiroveci* (formerly known as *Pneumocystis carinii*) [Clark et al., 1990].

C. neoformans most often causes meningoencephalitis but can also cause brain abscesses and granulomas. Granulomas may result in findings associated with mass lesions,

TABLE 70–1

Fungal Infections

ORGANISM	DISEASE	GEOGRAPHIC DISTRIBUTION	RISK FACTORS	MOST COMMON CNS SYNDROME(S)	DIAGNOSTIC TECHNIQUES	ANTIMICROBIAL THERAPY*
Cryptococcus neoformans	Cryptococcosis	Worldwide	HIV/AIDS, contact with pigeon droppings	Meningoencephalitis, abscesses, granulomas	Cultivation of CSF, latex agglutination	AMB, fiuconazole
Coccidiodes immitis	Coccidioidomycosis	Southwest US, Latin America	Dark-skinned individuals (Hispanic, black, Filipino), HIV/AIDS, dry periods with airborne soil	Meningitis, meningoencephalitis	Cultivation and/or microscopic examination of CSF, CF, neuroimaging	Fluconazole, itraconazole, AMB
Blastomyces dermatitidis	North American blastomycosis	Worldwide, endemic in parts of US (Great Lakes region)	Black ethnicity; more common in males, diabetes	Meningitis, intracranial mass, spinal mass	Cultivation of ventricular fluid, neuroimaging, biopsy	AMB, fiuconazole
Paracoccidioides brasiliensis	South American blastomycosis	Mexico, South America (particularly Brazil)	Age >30 years, poor nutrition, more common in males	Granulomatous lesions in CSF (cerebellum), meningeal involvement	Microscopic examination of mucosal lesions, sputum, cultivation	AMB, itraconazole, ketoconazole, TMP-SMX
Histoplasma capsulatum	Histoplasmosis	Worldwide: Mississippi River basin, Latin America	Living in an endemic region; contact with chicken coops, soil; inhalation of coal dust	Meningitis, brain/spine abscess, encephalitis, CVA	Cultivation of sputum, stomach aspirate, CSF, blood; radiography, CF, skin test, antigen in serum or urine	AMB
Nocardia spp.	Nocardiosis	Worldwide	Immunocompromised hosts, more common in males	Brain abscess, meningitis	Cultivation from CSF	Ceftriaxone, amikacin plus imipenem, TMP-SMX
Actinomyces spp.	Actinomycosis	Worldwide	Age between 10 and 60 years; males more affected; congenital heart disease	Meningitis, brain abscess	Identification of the organism from drained abscess, neuroimaging	Penicillin, cefotaxime, ceftriaxone
Aspergillus fumigatus	Aspergillosis	Worldwide (organism in soil/decaying vegetation)	Leukemia, lymphoma	Brain abscess, CVA, intracranial invasion via sinuses	Cultivation from biopsy material	AMB, voriconazole, caspofungin
Candida spp.	Candidiasis	Worldwide (organism part of normal microflora)	Diabetes, neutropenia, HIV/AIDS, nosocomial medical procedures	Meningitis, brain abscesses (often multiple microabscesses)	Cultivation of organisms from CSF	Speciation essential, AMB, fiucytosine, fiuconazole
Rhizopus spp. *Mucor* spp.	Phycomycosis (mucormycosis, zygomycosis)	Worldwide	Diabetes, chronic illness, IV drug use, immunocompromised	Intracranial invasion via sinuses	NP biopsy	AMB, surgery
Pseudoallescheria boydii	Allescheriosis	Worldwide	Severe immunocompromised Survival of near drowning	Brain abscess	Brain biopsy, cultivation of organism	Voriconazole

*Note that optimal treatment for CNS fungal infections should be done with input from infectious disease consultant.
AIDS, acquired immunodeficiency virus; AMB, amphotericin B; CF, complement fixation; CNS, central nervous system; CSF, cerebrospinal fiuid; CVA, cerebrovascular accident; HIV, human immunodeficiency virus; IV, intravenous; NP, nasopharyngeal; TMP-SMX, trimethoprim-sulfamethoxazole.

including papilledema, cranial neuropathies, and hemiparesis [Hung et al., 1995]. The disease course may be indolent but if untreated, the mortality is high. Hydrocephalus occurs regularly and often necessitates shunting [Richardson et al., 1976]. Definitive identification of cryptococcal disease is made by culturing cerebrospinal fluid on Sabouraud's agar; large volume culture on more than one occasion may be needed. Latex agglutination detection of cryptococcal antigen is a rapid and useful test for both serum and cerebrospinal fluid specimens. In the cerebrospinal fluid, the antigen detection has an estimated sensitivity of 90% [Sabetta and Andriole, 1985]. *C. neoformans* can also frequently be cultured from urine or sputum in patients with disseminated disease. Cranial computed to-

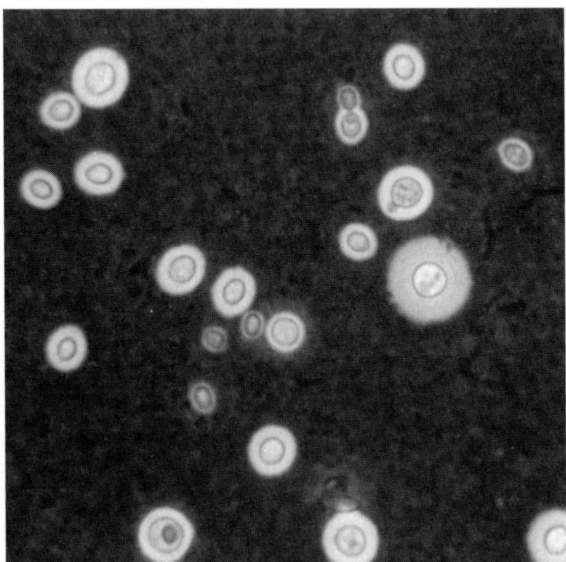

FIGURE 70-1. Capsulated budding yeast cells of *Cryptococcus neoformans* mounted in India ink.

mography (CT) and magnetic resonance imaging (MRI) scans reveal mass lesions and hydrocephalus caused by *C. neoformans*. Children with indolent CNS cryptococcal infection may have a modest increase in the cerebrospinal fluid ferritin levels despite traditional cerebrospinal fluid markers being normal [Katnik, 1995].

Management

The initial combination of amphotericin B and flucytosine is the best therapeutic regimen for cryptococcal meningitis in both AIDS and non-AIDS patients [Bennett et al., 1979; Gilbert et al, 2004; van der Horst et al., 1997]. Fluconazole orally is an alternative to amphotericin B as the primary treatment of cryptococcal meningitis and is used for the prolonged, sometimes indefinite, suppressive therapy needed for this disease. Oral fluconazole is superior to weekly intravenous therapy with amphotericin B in preventing relapse after primary treatment with amphotericin B [Powderly et al., 1992; Saag et al., 1992]. In AIDS patients treated successfully for both cryptococcus and human immunodeficiency virus (HIV), clinicians may consider stopping fluconazole if the CD4 count remains greater than 100 cells/mm^3. All cases of CNS cryptococcal disease should be managed in consultation with an infectious disease specialist.

Coccidioidomycosis

Epidemiology, Microbiology, Pathology

Coccidioidomycosis is caused by the fungus *C. immitis,* a dimorphic fungus that grows as either a mycelium or a unique structure called a *spherule*. Disease caused by *C. immitis* most commonly occurs in endemic areas of the southwestern United States, northern Mexico, and portions of Central and South America. The San Joaquin Valley in California is the most notorious endemic zone, giving rise to the terms *valley fever* and *desert fever*, but infection is also common in parts of Arizona, New Mexico, and Texas. Most infections occur during the dry season when spores are borne by dust. Most often, *C. immitis* infection is unnoticed or causes a self-limited respiratory tract infection; dissemination (discussed later) is uncommon, but the risk is higher in patients of black, Filipino, and Hispanic backgrounds [Einstein, 1993] and especially in the setting of immunocompromise, such as HIV infection, organ transplantation, or prolonged use of corticosteroids. Coccidioidomycosis is acquired by inhalation of spore-laden dust or transcutaneously after skin abrasion. Because most (60%) infections are asymptomatic or mildly symptomatic, reported cases represent only a small fraction of the total burden of disease. Central nervous system infection in children is rarely reported, so the true frequency is unknown. The disease is not spread person to person, and there is no need for special infection control measures. Paranasal skin lesions may predispose a person to CNS infections [Salake et al., 1984].

The spectrum of neuropathologic change ranges from meningitis to meningoencephalitis and meningomyelitis with extensive parenchymal destruction, sometimes as a result of an associated endarteritis obliterans [Mischel et al., 1995]. Microscopic examination of the thickened leptomeninges demonstrates widespread infiltration with inflammatory cells (e.g., plasma cells, lymphocytes, macrophages). Polymorphonuclear leukocytes are present during the acute phases. In more chronic infections, early fibrosis indicated by collagen fiber formation may be present. Parenchymal brain lesions have been reported in fewer than 40 cases during the 20th century and may occur in the absence of meningitis [Banuelos et al., 1996]. The infection produces both obstructive and communicating hydrocephalus, which may require shunting, by blocking cerebrospinal fluid flow and absorption.

Clinical Characteristics, Clinical Laboratory Tests, and Diagnosis

Studies done on military recruits in the 1940s using skin testing demonstrated that many patients with acute coccidioidomycosis are asymptomatic; only 40% experience acute respiratory symptoms [Smith et al., 1946]. Pulmonary infection is evident within 3 weeks after exposure and is marked by fever, chills, night sweats, cough, anorexia, and weight loss. Chest pain occurs in approximately 40% of symptomatic patients and can be severe. Erythema nodosum or erythema marginatum is manifest in 5% of males and 10% or more of females. The painful subcutaneous nodules of erythema nodosum occur most often along the anterior shins and are considered pathognomonic of coccidioidomycosis in endemic areas [Hedges and Miller, 1990]. A fine macular skin rash and conjunctivitis sometimes occur. Chest radiographs often indicate unilateral infiltrates, pleural effusions, and hilar adenopathy; nodules (4%) or cavities (8%) in adult patients are less common findings. Diffuse infiltrates and a septic shocklike presentation can occur, usually in immunocompromised hosts. Dissemination of the infection from the pulmonary focus to distant sites occurs in approximately 0.5% of cases, half of which involve the CNS, usually as meningitis [Banuelos et al., 1996]. Other sites include skin, lymph nodes, bones, and joints. Dissemination usually occurs 1 to 6 months after primary infection but can be delayed for a number of years.

The clinical characteristics of coccidioidal meningitis are nonspecific. Prompt diagnosis often proves difficult [Caudill et al., 1970]. The most prevalent manifestations are headache, fever, malaise, and weight loss; meningismus may be absent [Saitoh, 2000]. Mental aberrations, such as confusion, personality changes, and decreased level of consciousness, may ensue. Neurologic findings include focal defects, ataxia, obtundation, and coma. Brain and spinal cord abscesses can occur with or without concurrent meningitis [Banuelos et al., 1996]. Spinal cord involvement may occur in conjunction with coccidioidal osteomyelitis of the cervical vertebra [Jackson et al., 1964].

Cerebrospinal fluid abnormalities include mononuclear pleocytosis, increased protein content, increased chloride concentration, and normal or decreased glucose concentration. Diagnostic confirmation can be made by either direct microscopic study or culture of the cerebrospinal fluid (Fig. 70-2). Unfortunately cerebrospinal fluid cultures are often negative in *C. immitis* meningitis and serologic testing of serum and cerebrospinal fluid may be required for diagnosis. Complement fixation and precipitin tests are dependable and provide accurate diagnosis in more than 99% of patients with disseminated infection [Pappagianis, 1976]. Any discernible titer of complement fixation antibody in spinal fluid is considered diagnostic [Lyons and Andriole, 1986]. The coccidioidin skin test is not used for diagnosis of acute disease.

Imaging by CT or MRI scan may reveal widespread cisternal and cervical subarachnoid meningeal involvement in patients with coccidioidal meningitis [Wrobel et al., 1992] and may demonstrate the need for serial imaging to detect developing hydrocephalus.

Management

Until recently, amphotericin B administered intravenously and intrathecally was considered the recommended treatment [Galgani, 1997; Wright, 1978]. The drug must be given intrathecally because it is absorbed so poorly from the circulation into the cerebrospinal fluid and a subcutaneous reservoir for direct intraventricular instillation can be used [Diamond and Bennett, 1973]. Relapses can occur in all forms of disseminated coccidioidomycosis and especially in meningitis, even after prolonged treatment with amphotericin B. Fluconazole and itraconazole also are effective in the treatment of coccidioidal meningitis [Taylor et al., 1990; Tucker et al., 1992; Wheat, 1994], and high-dose fluconazole is now recommended for primary therapy. Fluconazole is well tolerated in both children and adults and the oral form is highly bioavailable. In adults, the dose of 400 mg per day resulted in a 70% response rate [Galgani, 1997]; in children most authorities recommend using the high end of the 3- to 12-mg/kg/day dose range, but data on response rate are lacking. Patients with *C. immitis* meningitis must be treated indefinitely with fluconazole to prevent relapse.

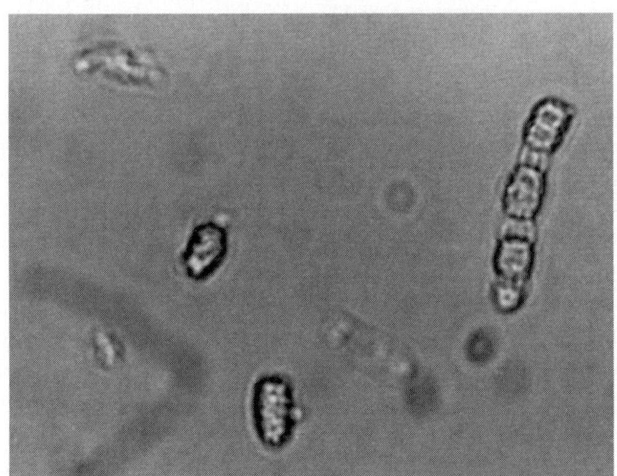

FIGURE 70-2. Infectious fragmentation spores of *Coccidioides immitis.*

North American Blastomycosis

Blastomycosis is caused by inhalation of airborne spores from *B. dermatitidis,* a dimorphic fungus found in soil [Bradsher, 1996]. The spectrum of clinical manifestations in adults includes acute pulmonary disease, subacute and chronic pulmonary disease, and disseminated extrapulmonary disease. Lung and skin involvement is most common, followed by bone, the genitourinary tract, and the CNS. Children, who are infrequently affected, suffer a similar spectrum of illness as adults [Schutze et al., 1996] and may be at increased risk if they play near beaver dams [Dismukes, 1986; Klein et al., 1986]. The three major CNS clinical manifestations are meningitis, intracranial mass, and spinal mass [Gonyea, 1978]. In the past decade, the incidence of blastomycosis has increased because of its prevalence in patients with AIDS, in whom it is associated with a high and early mortality [Witzig et al., 1994].

Skin tests and serologic tests are not helpful in the diagnosis of North American blastomycosis. The organisms may be identified by culture of ventricular and cisternal fluid; lumbar cerebrospinal fluid cultures are rarely positive. Neuroimaging and myelography demonstrate brain, spinal cord, or extradural lesions [Ward et al., 1995]. Microscopic study of biopsy material provides positive identification of the fungus.

Management

Amphotericin B is the most efficacious drug and may be used intraventricularly and intravenously [Morgan et al., 1979]. Early and aggressive therapy with amphotericin B is indicated for most immunocompromised patients with blastomycosis [Pappas et al., 1993]. Infectious Disease Society of America guidelines for CNS infection recommend conventional or liposomal amphotericin B as first-line therapy, with fluconazole at a high dose as an alternative in special circumstances [Chapman, 2000]. Surgery may be indicated in patients with mass lesions, those with a need for a diagnostic biopsy, or those with osteomyelitis refractory to pharmacotherapy [Ward et al., 1995].

South American Blastomycosis

South American blastomycosis is caused by the fungus *P. brasiliensis* [Lutz, 1908]. The organism is a dimorphic fungal saprophyte found in soil and plants that grows as a yeast at body temperature. Acquisition of disease is restricted to people living in latitudes between Mexico and Argentina, with most patients reported from Brazil. Most disease occurs in people older than the age of 30 years with a striking male preponderance; among the rare childhood cases the gender distribution is equal [Restrepo, 2000].

The organism first invades the lymph nodes, and then bilateral pulmonary infection or a buccopharyngeal granulomatous lesion develops. The latter must be distinguished from mucocutaneous leishmaniasis. Nervous system involvement is generally thought to be rare but may follow disseminated infection. One review from Brazil found CNS involvement in 14% of symptomatic patients [de Almeida et al., 2004]. Osteomyelitis of the cranium without other lesions has been reported [Krivoy et al., 1978].

Clinical Characteristics, Clinical Laboratory Tests, and Diagnosis

The most common presenting complaints and findings in a series of 24 cases included seizures, hemiparesis, cerebellar signs, headache, and hydrocephalus [de Almeida et al., 2004]. CNS granulomas can be solitary or multiple and are located supratentorially or in the cerebellum. Brain CT scan with contrast shows solitary or multiple hypodensities with contrast enhancement. The abscesses contain a necrotic core in which inflamed blood vessels are found. The abscesses may cause focal neurologic signs, increased intracranial pressure, and symptoms of meningeal involvement.

The diagnosis of South American blastomycosis is suggested by simultaneous involvement of several organs or by characteristic oral and skin lesions in patients who reside in endemic areas. Microscopic study of scrapings from mucous lesions, sputum, gastric contents, lymph nodes, or surgical specimens is most helpful. Typical morphology consists of round cells bearing many small buds at the periphery and affixed by slim openings to the surface of the parent cell. The etiology of brain lesions must be deduced from culture results outside the CNS or via brain biopsy. Cerebrospinal fluid findings are normal except for slightly elevated protein, and cerebrospinal fluid microscopy and culture are typically negative (de Almeida et al., 2004).

Management

Sulfamethoxypyridazine therapy is one low-cost therapeutic option, although the treatment must be continued for 3 to 5 years. Amphotericin B is faster acting but more expensive, more difficult to administer, and more toxic [Araujo et al., 1978]. Itraconazole and ketoconazole, although effective for disease not involving the CNS, cannot be recommended because of poor penetration into the brain and spinal fluid. Authorities currently recommend trimethoprim-sulfamethoxazole at high dose (480 mg/day of trimethoprim in three divided doses for adults); voriconazole is considered a promising but unproven alternative (de Almeida et al., 2004).

Histoplasmosis

Epidemiology, Microbiology, and Pathology

Histoplasmosis was first described by Darling in the Panama Canal Zone in a 27-year-old Martinique man [Darling, 1906] originally thought to have tuberculosis. Darling believed the disease was similar to the condition kala-azar reported by Leishman and Donovan. He named the disease *histoplasmosis*: "*histo*" signifying "histocyte" and "*plasma*" signifying "plasmodium-like organisms." Not until 1934 did DeMonbreum definitively demonstrate the fungal association with histoplasmosis [DeMonbreum, 1934].

Histoplasmosis is globally distributed. Among the endemic zones are the Mississippi River basin, Mexico, and Central and South America [Loosli, 1957]. In these regions, as many as 80% of children manifest positive histoplasmosis skin test results by age 5 years [Rogers, 1967]. Humans and many wild and domestic animals are targets of infection. No racial predilection exists for skin test reactivity. With rare exception the condition is benign and self-limiting. About 10% of those infected with *H. capsulatum* have pulmonary disease to a degree prompting medical evaluation; those younger than the age of 2 years, the elderly, and those with immunocompromising conditions are more likely to be symptomatic. Overall, males are more likely to have symptomatic pulmonary disease, whereas the disseminated form of the disease affects males and females equally. Only a small subset of individuals with primary histoplasmosis develop disseminated disease, and an even smaller group develop a CNS infection. A review of 235 cases of histoplasmosis reported between 1952 and 1960 revealed that of the one third of the patients who had disseminated disease, one fourth exhibited CNS impairment [Cooper and Goldstein, 1963]. In contrast, a review of histoplasmosis among pediatric oncology patients from an endemic area found disseminated disease twice as common as pulmonary disease, but CNS infection was not described.

Histoplasma capsulatum is found in the Americas, *H. duboisii* in Africa. This dimorphic fungus grows as a yeast at body temperature, whereas mycelia form at room temperature. The mycelia phase contains macroconidia (8 to 15 mm) and microconidia (2 to 5 mm); the later may be essential for human infectivity because they are small enough to reach the alveoli. The organism grows as a saprophyte in the soil. Dampness and nutrients from bird and bat droppings encourage growth in aviaries, chicken coops, mines, caves, and open fields [Ajello and Zeidberg, 1951]. During dry spells, the organism may become airborne and the spores inhaled. No evidence of person-to-person or animal-to-human transmission exists.

The gross features at postmortem examination are primarily those of a granulomatous disease similar to miliary tuberculosis that affects the lungs and reticuloendothelial system. Biopsy of infected tissue, such as lymph nodes or liver, demonstrates granulomas that superficially resemble lymphoma, tuberculosis, sarcoidosis, Hodgkin's disease, and leishmaniasis. The predominant pathologic alterations that occur within the CNS include perivenous miliary granulomatosis, parenchymatous granulomatosis, meningitis, histoplasmoma, and histiocytic histoplasmosis.

Clinical Characteristics, Clinical Laboratory Tests, and Diagnosis

Respiratory infection follows inhalation of spore-laden soil or dust. Most children remain asymptomatic or experience little clinical difficulty [Ibach et al., 1954]. A nonspecific mild lung infection may follow exposure after 5 to 15 days. Fever, chills, and a productive cough are common features, but more severe symptoms may occur, including chest pain, dyspnea, and, rarely, prostration. The initial chest radiograph may document a nodular or more dispersed infiltrate. Cultures of the sputum or stomach aspirate may grow the organism. After several years, chest radiographs demonstrate characteristic calcification in the central lymph nodes and peripheral lung fields. If untreated, the infection lasts 2 to 12 weeks. The histoplasmin skin test converts to positive during the course of the acute infection but this test is not used diagnostically. Complement fixation titers can be used to detect infection by detecting a fourfold rise between acute and convalescent specimens or finding a single elevated titer in the correct clinical setting. A rise in complement fixation titers after treatment suggests relapse.

Progressive disseminated histoplasmosis is rare in normal children. In one report of 10 children with disseminated disease, most had fever, anemia, and hepatosplenomegaly. Only two children had neurologic involvement: one had nuchal rigidity, and the other had positive Babinski's sign and tetany [Cooper and Goldstein, 1963]. Signs and symptoms associated with CNS involvement in children include intracranial hypertension, memory impairment, confusion, seizures, and urinary incontinence [Machado et al., 1993]. Reported CNS complications in children include hydrocephalus [Enarson et al., 1978], meningitis [Couch et al., 1978], ataxia, seizures, and cranial nerve palsy [Rivera et al., 1992]. Approximately 5% of adult patients with disseminated histoplasmosis will have CNS involvement [Borges et al., 1997] with the median time to diagnosis of 36 months [Machado et al., 1993].

Directed laboratory studies include culture of cerebrospinal fluid, blood, and bone marrow; biopsy of liver, bone marrow, and lymph nodes; and detection of *Histoplasma* antigen in serum or urine. [Wheat et al., 1986]. *Histoplasma* antigen is present in the cerebrospinal fluid of some patients with chronic *Histoplasma* meningitis, but its measurement and diagnostic precision are unreliable [Wheat et al., 1989]. All patients with disseminated histoplasmosis should be evaluated for adrenal insufficiency. In one series, half of the patients, regardless of treatment, had adrenal insufficiency, which was the most common cause of death [Sarosi et al., 1971]. Because *Histoplasma* can remain quiescent in the lungs or the adrenal glands for more than 40 years before dissemination, it needs to be considered in unexplained neurologic disease, particularly in people who lived in endemic areas as children [Tan et al., 1992].

Management

Non-CNS *Histoplasma* infections are usually treated with itraconazole unless the disease is severe or occurs in immunocompromised hosts, in which case an amphotericin preparation is preferred [Bradsher, 1996; Carpentier et al., 1996; Wheat et al., 1995]. There are no prospective data comparing different treatments for *Histoplasma* meningitis or brain or spine disease. Current Infectious Disease Society of America guidelines recommend that *Histoplasma* disease involving the CNS initially be treated with conventional or lipid formulation of amphotericin B followed by fluconazole for a prolonged period [Wheat et al., 2000]. Neither itraconazole nor fluconazole is ideal for CNS histoplasmosis; itracona zole has excellent antifungal activity but poor CNS penetration, whereas fluconazole has inferior antifungal activity but excellent CNS penetration. The prognosis of *Histoplasma* CNS infections is guarded: 20% to 40% of patients die despite treatment, and relapse among survivors is common [Wheat et al., 2000]. The role of the most recently released azole antifungal agent, voriconazole, in the treatment of histoplasmosis has not been defined.

Nocardiosis

Nocardia spp. are ubiquitous in the environment. *Nocardia asteroides, N. farcinica, and N. brasiliensis* are the species most often responsible for nocardiosis. Nocardiosis is considered a bacterial infection but is included in this section for the sake of completeness [Threlkeld and Hooper, 1997]. Nocardial disease during childhood is relatively uncommon, and nocardial involvement of the CNS is rare [Stites and Glezen, 1967]. Risk factors for pediatric CNS infections include malignancy, chronic granulomatous disease, lupus, human immunodeficiency virus infection, organ transplantation, and surgery [Marlowe et al., 2000].

Pulmonary manifestations are most common in nocardiosis and include pneumonia, lung abscess, and empyema that may be present concurrently with brain disease. The CNS is involved in a substantial minority of *Nocardia* infections, many of which occur in those without immune suppression. In those with disseminated infection, CNS involvement should be viewed with concern because it is associated with mortality rates of 80% [Beaman and Beaman, 1994; Threlkeld and Hooper, 1997]. CNS disease may be the only manifestation of nocardiosis suggesting that inapparent pulmonary disease has resolved. Abscesses are the most frequently reported CNS complication, but meningitis accounts for one third.

CNS disease caused by *Nocardia* often has a subacute or chronic course. A variety of neurologic and behavioral or psychiatric presentations occur. Although uncommon, nocardiosis should be considered in the differential diagnosis of subacute meningitis, especially when the cerebrospinal fluid contains a high concentration of neutrophils, elevated protein levels, and a low glucose level. Nocardial pulmonary disease or cerebral abscesses confirm the diagnosis, as do positive cultures from cerebrospinal fluid [Bross and Gordon, 1991]. Neuroimaging can detect abscess formation, hydrocephalus, and, in some patients, the presence of small subependymal nodules [LeBlang et al., 1995].

Parenteral therapy with amikacin plus imipenem or ceftriaxone is the currently recommended treatment [Gilbert et al., 2004]. A review of antibiotic treatment for nocardial infections has been published [Threlkeld and Hooper, 1997]. Serial neuroimaging studies during treatment are also helpful in monitoring resolution of the abscesses [Kirmani et al., 1978]. In selected patients, surgical extirpation of multiple abscesses can be successfully accomplished [Rosenblum and Rosegay, 1979].

FUNGAL AND OTHER INFECTIONS IN THE IMMUNOCOMPROMISED HOST

Actinomycosis

Epidemiology, Microbiology, and Pathology

Actinomyces spp. are anaerobic or microaerophilic gram positive, non–spore forming branching bacilli that normally colonize the mouth, intestine, and female genital tract. Invasive disease, usually caused by *Actinomyces isralei*, is most common in those ages 10 to 60 years; males are more frequently affected than females. Risk factors include untreated focal infections, immunosuppression, and congenital heart disease with right-to-left shunts [Olah et al., 2004]. CNS disease is rare but can result from direct extension from a contiguous focus or by hematogenous spread from another site.

Clinical Characteristics, Clinical Laboratory Tests, and Diagnosis

Actinomycosis is a chronic, slow-growing, inflammatory mass most frequently affecting the lungs, cervicofacial region, abdomen, and pelvis (in association with intrauterine devices) [Vinard et al., 1992; Winking et al., 1996]. The mass has a tough, fibrous capsule, does not respect tissue planes, and develops sinus tracts. Concurrent chronic infections and other debilitating conditions predispose patients to dissemination.

A review of 181 cases of actinomycosis revealed that less than 2% of patients had cerebral involvement as manifested by meningitis or abscess (solitary or multiple) [Brown, 1973; Fetter et al., 1967]. Neurologic involvement includes meningeal, granulomatous, and pseudotumoral forms [Winking et al., 1996]. Abscesses have been reported in the cerebrum, cerebellum, optic chiasm, parasellar region, and subdural space [Bebrova et al., 1994; Brown, 1973]. Osteomyelitis of the spine may be the origin of spinal cord abscess and compression [Fetter et al., 1967]. Neuroimaging demonstrates abscess easily, but microbiologic diagnosis of CNS disease can be challenging because the organism may be difficult to recover if antibiotics have been given. In addition, infections involving *Actinomyces* spp. are often polymicrobial, clouding the role of individual species. The etiology of CNS disease may be inferred if *Actinomyces* spp. are isolated at another site, particularly the lung.

Management

Recommendations for treatment of actinomycosis at any site are based on experience and in vitro susceptibility testing rather than clinical trials. Standard recommended treatment for CNS disease is penicillin for at least 6 months. Recently, successful shorter courses of treatment with drugs other than penicillin such as ceftriaxone and cefotaxime for CNS and non-CNS disease have been reported [Olah, 2004; Sudhakar, 2004]. Surgical drainage of the abscess frequently is indicated [Jamjoom et al., 1994; Winking et al., 1996] and may be needed for definitive diagnosis of CNS disease.

Aspergillosis

Epidemiology, Microbiology, and Pathology

Aspergillus spp. (most commonly *fumigatus*) affecting humans (Fig. 70-3), like many fungal pathogens, initially gain entrance to the lung after inhalation. The name of this fungus was established because of the similarity of its fruiting head to the aspergillum, a perforated globe used to sprinkle holy water during religious ceremonies. Dissemination and CNS infection are nearly always accompanied by an underlying debilitating condition.

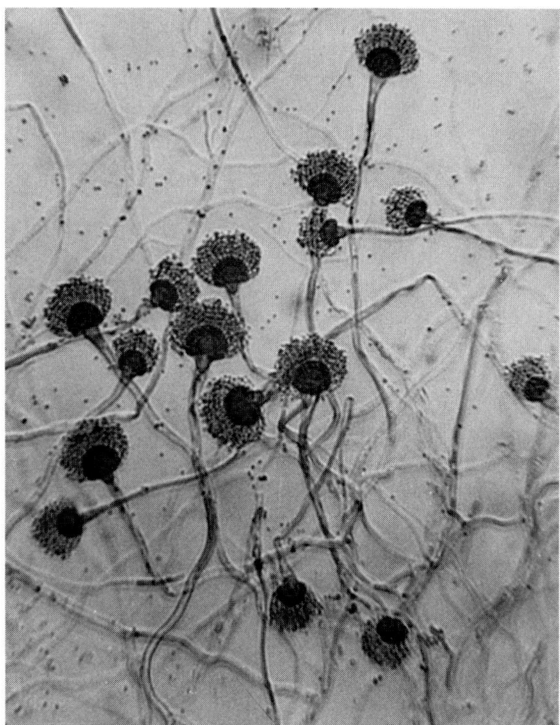

FIGURE 70-3. Spore heads of *Aspergillus fumigatus* in culture.

Aspergillosis of the CNS was rare until the large increase in immunocompromised hosts, including children, in the past two decades [Carpentier et al., 1996; Sparano et al., 1992; Torre Cisneros et al., 1993; Wright et al., 1993]. Among compromised hosts, the highest frequency of invasive aspergillosis is in heart and lung transplant recipients (19% to 26%) followed by those with chronic granulomatous disease (24% to 40%), acute leukemia (5% to 24%), bone marrow or hematopoietic stem cell recipients (0.5% to 9%), AIDS (0% to 12%), and solid organ transplant recipients (0.5% to 10%) [Denning, 1998]. Central nervous system disease complicates 10% to 20% of invasive disease and is nearly universally accompanied by concurrent infection at other sites.

More than 150 species of *Aspergillus* have been identified. Pathogenic isolates grow quickly on both mycological media and standard bacteriologic plates at 37° C and the genus is identified quickly using microscopy. Disease occurs after spores evade local defenses in the respiratory tract, skin, or wounds weakened by underlying disease or treatment. After an incubation period that may range from days to months, pulmonary infection begins and may be followed by the dissemination to brain, eye, heart, kidney, liver, and bone. A frequent feature of invasive disease is vascular invasion leading to tissue necrosis. Hyphae are abundant and are best seen with silver stains; hyphae in tissue are characterized by frequent septae and branching at 45 degrees.

Clinical Characteristics, Clinical Laboratory Tests, and Diagnosis

The following three distinctive types of clinical presentation have been reported with CNS aspergillosis: (1) an intracranial form, the most common, presenting like a space-occupying lesion; (2) a rhinocerebral form with primary involvement of the sinuses and secondary involvement of the skull base, cranial nerves, and brain; and (3) a vascular form with strokelike symptoms [Haran and Chandy, 1993]. In addition to brain abscess, aspergillosis can also cause meningitis, meningoencephalitis, hemorrhagic or ischemic necrosis, solitary granulomas, and invasive fungal arteriitis [Torre Cisneros et al., 1993]. The clinical presentation is variable and depends on the host. Highly immunocompromised patients may have altered mental status and seizures, whereas more competent hosts may have headache and focal complaints. In one series, the most frequent neurologic symptoms included altered mental status (86%), seizures (41%), and focal neurologic deficits (32%) [Torre Cisneros et al., 1993]. Neuroimaging may reveal sinus invasion, enhancing or nonenhancing hypodense lesions indicative of abscess [Sparano et al., 1992], or prominent ischemic lesions in the basal ganglia [Miaux et al., 1995]; concurrent chest radiography or CT scan usually indicates multiple nodular lesions.

Definitive diagnosis is made by smear and culture of biopsy material. A presumptive diagnosis can be made if cranial imaging is typical and aspergillus is demonstrated at another site. Serum galactomannan testing for invasive aspergillosis is available [Herbrecht et al., 2002] and provides a noninvasive alternative to support the diagnosis; however, published cutoffs of sensitivity and specificity are variable [Marr et al., 2004].

Management

Cerebral aspergillosis has a poor prognosis, particularly in the immunocompromised host. Surgical drainage and removal of abscesses and granulomas are often performed but are usually of little value [Casey et al., 1994; Haran and Chandy, 1993]. Similarly, treatment with high-dose conventional amphotericin B contributes toxicity yet little efficacy. The availability of lipid formulations of amphotericin, voriconazole, and caspofungin may improve the prognosis. Case reports and one retrospective review suggest that a subset of patients will respond and some may be cured [Damaj et al., 2004; de Lastours et al., 2003; Schwartz and Thiel, 2004].

Candidiasis

Candida spp. are responsible for the most common invasive fungal infections in infants and children [Arisoy et al., 1994]. Cerebral candidiasis is a rare sequela of disseminated disease in a debilitated patient. Predisposing factors include prematurity and its complications, use of broad-spectrum antibiotics, total parenteral nutrition, central venous catheterization, immunosuppression, immunodeficiency (congenital or acquired), chronic renal disease, diabetes, neutropenia, and ventriculoperitoneal shunts [Arisoy et al., 1994; Chiou et al., 1994; McAbee et al., 1995]. Historically, *Candida albicans* has been the most common species identified in CNS disease. Other species, including *Candida tropicalis*, *Candida lusitaniae*, and *Candida parapsilosis*, have also been reported. One series comprising pediatric oncology patients found that 11 of 12 cases of meningitis were caused by *C. tropicalis* [McCullers et al., 2000].

Clinical Characteristics, Clinical Laboratory Tests, and Diagnosis

Meningitis (most common), abscesses, and granulomas occur independently and in combination (Fig. 70-4). Typically, multiple microabscesses are found rather than a solitary abscess, and reflect the hematogenous dissemination of *Candida* [Incesu et al., 1994]. Intracerebral abscess after candida septicemia is illustrated in Figure 70-4B. The clinical presentation of meningitis may be subtle because many patients are seriously ill from other medical problems or primary infections. Hemiparesis, cranial nerve palsies, or signs of hydrocephalus may be found [Coker and Beltran, 1988]. Fungal arterial and venous involvement can cause serious complications as can the development of intracranial mycotic aneurysms [Goldman et al., 1979]. Diagnosis can be confirmed by identification of the organism in spinal fluid or infected neural tissue [McGinnis, 1983]. Pleocytosis or reduced cerebrospinal fluid glucose occurs in only about half of the patients who are culture positive [Hughes, 1992].

Management

There are no comparative trials to permit definitive antifungal recommendations. Prompt speciation and susceptibility testing may help optimize empiric antifungal therapy. Standard of care suggests that initial combined treatment with amphotericin B (conventional or liposomal) and 5-fluorocytosine or fluconazole may be successful [Lisch and Steudel, 1994; Smego et al., 1984], although amphotericin is often used alone [Incesu et al., 1994]. The role of voriconazole and caspofungin for this uncommon disease is not yet defined, and consultation with an infectious disease specialist is recommended. If feasible, use of antibacterials and immunosuppressive agents should be avoided during treatment of candidal infection.

Phycomycosis

Extension of a phycomycotic infection from the nose and nasopharynx through the sinuses or cribriform plate into the meninges and CNS is termed *rhinocerebral phycomycosis.* The term *mucormycosis* is frequently used interchangeably with phycomycosis, although Mucoraceae represent only one of the subfamilies of the class Phycomycetes. Spread of infection into the orbit by way of the nasolacrimal duct is accompanied by proptosis and panophthalmitis.

Clinical Characteristics, Clinical Laboratory Tests, and Diagnosis

Diabetes mellitus is frequently associated with this fungal infection, but intravenous drug use, renal transplantation, and other immunocompromised conditions are additional risk factors; this infection rarely occurs in the immunocompetent individuals or in children [Hussain et al., 1995]. Fever, facial and ocular pain, or CNS symptoms may herald the onset, and a black eschar-like plaque may be seen in the oro- or nasopharynx. Etiology of CNS disease seen in MRI or CT imaging can be inferred from biopsy of nasopharyngeal or sinus specimens. Hyphae can be seen with conventional and special stains and are distinguished by their lack of septae, 90-degree branching, and breadth (10 to 20 μM).

Prognosis is usually poor; however, several case reports describe survival of well-controlled diabetic patients treated with surgical debridement plus local and systemic administration of amphotericin B [Hamilton et al., 2003; Moll et al., 1994; Sandler et al., 1971].

Management

The fungus tends to infect and obstruct cranial blood vessels, and thus, thwart drug treatment. General principles of

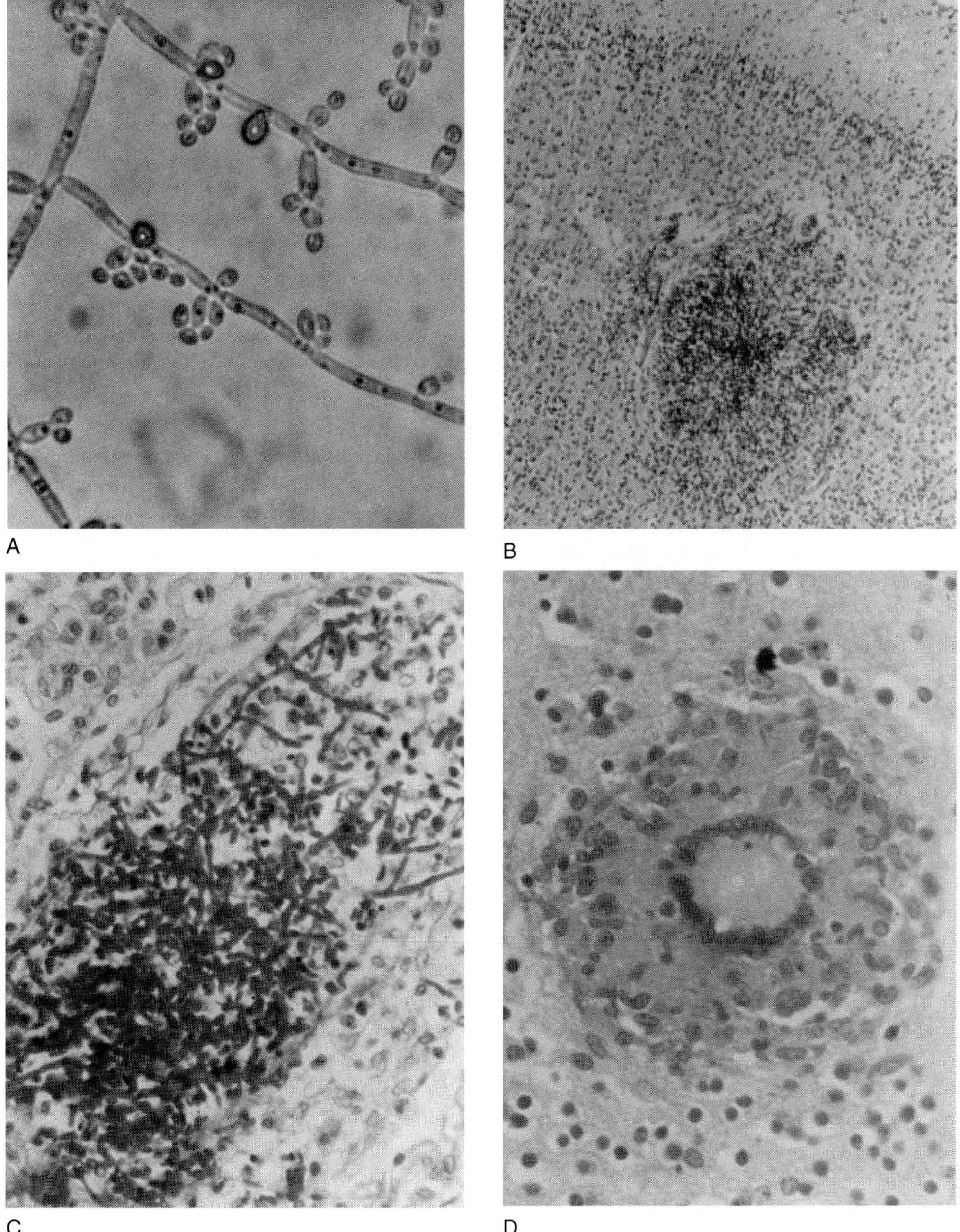

FIGURE 70-4. **A**, Pseudohyphae and budding yeast cells of *Candida albicans*. **B**, Candidal abscess. **C**, Cerebral vein clogged with *Candida* organism. **D**, Giant cell granuloma.

management include correcting diabetic ketoacidosis, discontinuing immunosuppressive therapy, if possible, and removing infected tissue surgically. Standard treatment includes extensive debridement inside and outside of the CNS, in addition to amphotericin treatment [Cuadrado et al., 1988; Galetta et al., 1990; Hussain et al., 1995]. The rapid escalation of amphotericin dose is advocated because of the poor prognosis; renal toxicity should prompt use of lipid formulations of amphotericin and many experts would initiate therapy with a lipid formulation of amphotericin B. The recently available agents voriconazole and caspofungin are not typically active against phycomycosis. Some authors have advocated less radical surgery combined with systemic and local (via Omaya reservoir) amphotericin augmented by hyperbaric oxygen therapy (Hamilton et al., 2003).

Pseudallescheria boydii (Scedosporium angiospermum) Infection

Allescheriosis is a rare cause of human disease, but when disseminated in compromised hosts, CNS involvement occurs. Risk groups include compromised hosts as well as survivors of near drowning in unclean water. A comprehensive review of CNS disease of 38 cases, the youngest reported case being 24 months, was recently published [Nesky et al., 2000].

Clinical Characteristics, Clinical Laboratory Tests, and Diagnosis

P. boydii can cause a chronic subcutaneous infection (mycetoma) or invasive lung, bone, joint, and CNS disease. Brain abscess is the typical CNS manifestation and can be solitary [Bell and Myers, 1978] or multiple [Rosen et al., 1965]. Definitive diagnosis is through brain biopsy, although culture of the organism from a nonsterile site can support the diagnosis. There are no available noninvasive or antigen detection tests. On biopsy, this organism can be confused with *Aspergillus* or *Fusarium* spp., but it is easily distinguished once cultured.

Management

Surgical resection of brain abscesses along with antifungal therapy have been used, but this organism is notoriously resistant to antifungal therapy, and most cases succumb. The availability of voriconazole, which has in vitro activity, and case reports of success may change this grim prognosis when combined with surgical drainage [Nesky et al., 2000; Poza et al., 2000].

RICKETTSIAL DISEASES

Rickettsiae are pleomorphic coccobacilli that are obligate intracellular bacteria whose arthropod vectors include ticks, mites, fleas, or lice [Kim and Durack, 1997]. Rickettsial diseases include the spotted fevers, typhus fevers, scrub typhus, Q fever, and ehrlichioses [Marrie and Raoult, 1992; Pai et al., 1997]. Rickettsial infections often have an accompanying skin eruption. *Coxiella burnetii*, the rickettsia causing Q fever, differs from the other organisms because it does not require a vector and rarely causes a skin rash.

CNS involvement can occur in all forms of rickettsial infections [Marrie and Raoult, 1992]. Pathologic changes may be extensive and, in some infections, systemic and cerebral vasculitis may be prominent. The clinical and pathologic response of the CNS to different infections caused by *Rickettsia* spp. is generally similar and differs only in severity [Harrell, 1953b; Woodward and Osterman, 1984]. Headache is often the earliest and most frequent symptom in all rickettsial infections [Harrell, 1953b].

Diagnostic testing is similar for most rickettsial infections. Isolation in cell culture, localization in patient tissues by immunohistochemical stains, or detection of the rickettsial agent in blood or tissues by molecular assays (e.g., polymerase chain reaction) may be useful for diagnosis of acute infection; however, these tests are often available only at specialized research laboratories. Serology is the most generally available and widely used method to establish a diagnosis of rickettsial infection. The indirect fluorescent antibody assay is considered the gold standard. However, because most patients with rickettsial diseases do not develop antibodies reactive with these agents in the first week of illness, serologic tests are often negative during the acute phase of the illness. Confirmation of disease is best accomplished by evaluation of paired serum specimens collected during the acute and convalescent phases of the illness for a fourfold or greater change in antibody titer. Extensive cross-reactivity exists among antigens of the spotted fever group rickettsiae (e.g., *Rickettsia rickettsii, Rickettsia akari*, and *Rickettsia conorii*), and among antigens in the typhus group (*Rickettsia prowazekii* and *Rickettisa typhi*). In this context, most indirect fluorescent antibody assays are group-specific rather than species-specific tests for rickettsial infection.

Recommended treatment of rickettsial diseases in almost all clinical situations includes tetracyclines. Most broad-spectrum antibiotics such as penicillins, cephalosporins, and penems are ineffective. Doxycycline is considered the drug of choice in almost all clinical situations for both pediatric and adult patients [Dalton et al., 1995; Kirkland et al., 1995]. The dosage is 100 mg twice per day for adults and 4 mg/kg/day, divided twice daily, intravenously or orally, for 10 to 14 days [Schutz and Jacobs, 1997]. Because tetracyclines are contraindicated during pregnancy, chloramphenicol is used as an alternate drug in this patient population; however, this drug has questionable efficacy for patients with ehrlichiosis and Q fever [Markley et al., 1998]. Empiric treatment with doxycycline should be initiated early in the course if clinical and epidemiologic findings are suggestive of a rickettsial infection because delays in treatment can lead to adverse outcomes. Tetracycline use in pediatric patients is often discouraged because of the potential association with tooth discoloration. For suspected cases of rickettsial illnesses, however, it is important to use a tetracycline. Tetracycline tooth staining is dose related and studies have found that perceptible tooth staining does not occur until multiple courses have been used [Grossman et al., 1971; Lochary et al., 1998].

Table 70-2 lists rickettsial diseases, organisms, vectors, reservoirs, and geographic distribution. Rocky Mountain spotted fever is the prototypic condition for these infections.

TABLE 70–2

Rickettsia Infections

AGENT	DISEASE	CASES/ YEAR (US)	GEOGRAPHY	MODE OF INFECTION/ VECTOR	RESERVOIR	INCUBATION PERIOD	CLINICAL	LABORATORY STUDIES	TREATMENT	COMMENT
Rickettsia rickettsii	Rocky Mountain spotted fever	250–1000	North, Central, and South America	Tick	Rodents	2–14 days	HA, F, lethargy, periorbital edema, ARF, rash initially maculopapular then petechial (often begins on ankles or wrists) CNS; vasculitis, cerebral edema	Hyponatremia, thrombocytopenia DIC Serology: IFA DFA on skin biopsy PCR—limited availability	Doxycyline	Important to treat early; most common fatal tick-borne disease in the US
Rickettsia prowazekii	Epidemic typhus (louse-borne typhus fever)	Imported cases only	North America, Europe, some Asian and Southeast Asian countries, mountainous regions of Africa, Central and South America, and Mexico	Human louse, rat louse	Humans, eastern flying squirrels (US)	7–14 days	HA, F, cough, arthralgia MP rash (often begins on trunk) CNS: confusion, prostration, photophobia	Anemia, thrombocytopenia, hyponatremia, low albumin, increased LFTs Serology; IFA, EIA, CF, latex agglutination PCR	Doxycycline	Epidemics can occur, especially under poor hygienic conditions
	Brill-Zinsser					Generally years	Relapsing form of louse-borne; symptoms milder			Can occur years to decades after primary infection
Rickettsia typhi	Murine or endemic typhus	<50	Worldwide; in US, endemic foci southern California, Texas	Rat flea	Rodents, cats, opossums, raccoons, skunks	7–14 days	Same as epidemic typhus although may not be as severe	Same as epidemic typhus	Same as epidemic typhus	Usually less severe than epidemic typhus
Orientia tsutsu-gamushi	Scrub typhus	Imported cases only	Southwest Pacific, Southeast Asia, Asia, Australia, India, Sri Lanka	Mite (chigger)	Mites, rodents (secondary reservoir)	7–21 days	F, HA, conjunctival injection, adenopathy, respiratory distress, eschar, rash (often begins on trunk) CNS: meningitis, encephalitis	Leukopenia, thrombocytopenia, anemia Serology; ELISA	Doxycycline	
Coxiella burnetti	Q fever	61	Worldwide, most common in rural	Inhalation of infectious aerosols from milk, urine, feces, amniotic fluids of infected animals	Cattle, sheep, goats, cats,dogs, wildlife	2–3 weeks	F, HA, malaise, sore throat, chills, sweats, non-productive cough, nausea, vomiting, diarrhea, abdominal pain, chest pain, weight loss, pneumonia, hepatitis	Elevated LFTs, thrombcytopenia, Serology; IFA IHC staining, PCR	Doxycycline	Complication of chronic disease include myocarditis and endocarditis
Ehrlichia chaffeensis	Human monocytic ehrlichia	200	Western Hemisphere, Europe, Asia, Southeast Asia, Africa, Israel	Lone Star tick (American dog tick)	Deer, canines, rodents	5–10 days	F, HA, malaise, nausea, occasionally rash, cough, arthralgia ARDS, renal failure, DIC in severe cases CNS: meningoencephalitis (20%)	Leukopenia, thrombocytopenia, neutropenia, anemia, elevated LFTs Serology; IFA blood smears for morulae in mononuclear cells, culture PCR on blood/CSF	Doxycycline, chloramphenicol only in pregnant women (see text)	Treatment failure seen with chloramphe-nicol; IFA test most sensitive for diagnosis, but may be negative acute sera
Anaplasma phago-cytophilum	Human granulocytic ehrlichia	500	US, Europe, China	Blacklegged ticks (*Ixodes scapularis* and *Ixodes pacificus*)	Deer, rodents	5–10 days	F, HA, arthralgias, nausea, vomiting, rash (<10%), cough, pharyngitis, lymphadenopathy, respiratory and renal insufficiency, myocardial involvement in severe cases CNS: confusion, seizures, coma, stiff neck (20%), demyelinating polyneuropathy	Same as HME, except morulae in granulocytes	Doxycycline	
Ehrlichia ewingii		25	US	Lone Star tick (American dog tick)	Humans, deer, canines	5–10 days	Same as HME	Thrombocytopenia, leukopenia, elevated LFTs, morulae in granulocytes Serology: IFA	Doxycycline	Occurs especially in patients with underlying immuno-suppression

ARDS, acute respiratory distress syndrome; ARF, acute renal failure; CF, complement fixation; CNS, central nervous system; DIC, disseminated intravascular coagulation; DFA, direct fluorescent antibody; EIA, enzyme immunoassay; ELISA, enzyme-linked immunosorbent assay; F, fever; HA, headache; HME, human monocytic ehrlichiosis; IFA, indirect fluorescent antibody; IHC, immunohistochemical; LFT, liver function test; MP, maculopapular; PCR, polymerase chain reaction.

Rocky Mountain Spotted Fever

Rocky Mountain spotted fever is caused by *R. rickettsii* and is the most common fatal tick-borne illness in the United States [CDC, 2004]. Early missionaries and settlers discerned the association of tick bites with the disease and called the disease tick fever [Aikawa, 1966]. Howard Ricketts identified the etiologic organism in 1906 and established the tick as the vector in transmitting the organism to humans.

The disease is prevalent in wide geographic areas. Rocky Mountain spotted fever has been reported throughout the United States with the exception of Hawaii and Vermont [Walker, 1995]. Between 1981 and 1991, the states with the highest incidence of Rocky Mountain spotted fever were Oklahoma, North Carolina, Virginia, Maryland, Georgia, Missouri, Arkansas, Montana, and South Dakota [CDC, 1990]. Approximately 200 to 1000 cases are reported annually in the United States. Outside the United States, it has been described in Canada and several countries of Central and South America [Heldrich, 1987]. In the Northern Hemisphere, the incidence of the disease is greatest from April to September, when tick bites are most likely to occur. The American dog tick *(Dermacentor variabilis)* is the primary vector responsible for the transmission of *R. rickettsii* along the southern Atlantic coast and southeastern and south-central United States. In the western region of the United States, the vector is usually the wood tick *(Dermacentor andersoni)* (Fig. 70-5). Given the habitat preferences of the vector, rural and suburban populations are more likely to be infected than urban residents.

Children have a higher risk of infection (half of the cases are younger than 19 years of age [Kamper, 1991]) because they are exposed to tick bites during outdoor play. Rocky Mountain spotted fever should be considered in the differential diagnosis of anyone with compatible clinical features and exposure to a grassy or wooded area where ticks may be present [Walker, 1995]. Dogs may carry ticks into households and yards and are a risk factor for infection [Paddock et al., 2002; Walker, 1995]. The absence of a reported tick bite history should not dissuade a clinician from suspecting Rocky Mountain spotted fever.

The incubation period ranges from 2 to 14 days (mean 7 days) after a tick bite [Thorner et al., 1998]. Transmission of rickettsiae occurs as a tick feeds on the blood of its host. After entering the body, rickettsiae multiply and disrupt the endothelial cells of capillaries and arterioles. In Rocky Mountain spotted fever, the rickettsiae may also infect the smooth muscle cells of the tunica media. Loss of integrity of the small vessels in the brain results in hemorrhage into the subarachnoid space. Subsequent meningeal irritation and an accompanying perivascular mononuclear infiltrate develop. The brain parenchyma is studded with areas of microscopic infarctions. In the healing phase, a proliferative fibroblastic and gliotic response is evident; the ensuing focal nodules develop more often in white matter in spotted fever and more often in gray matter in typhus.

Clinical Characteristics, Clinical Laboratory Tests, and Diagnosis

Symptoms of Rocky Mountain spotted fever vary in severity from mild to severe; the course may rapidly lead to death. Initial symptoms are nonspecific and include fever, malaise, lethargy, and headache. The headache is usually intense and refractory to most analgesics. Progressive restlessness, irritability, confusion, and delirium may also occur. By day 5 of the illness, 85% of patients develop a rash. The rash often begins with a maculopapular appearance and becomes more defined as petechiae as the rash evolves. The rash often begins around the ankles or wrists and then spreads to other parts of the body (Fig. 70-6). Acute renal failure, coagulopathy and cerebral edema are well-recognized complications. Edema, usually periorbital at first and then generalized, is characteristic of and may suggest the diagnosis. Hepatosplenomegaly accompanied by liver dysfunction, including coagulation defects, may confound the diagnostic process. In fulminating disease, shock, coma, and general or focal neurologic impairment, including vertigo, seizures, hemiparesis and ataxia may dominate the clinical manifestations [Marrie, 1992]. Skin necrosis and gangrene can be a late complication (Fig. 70-7). Rocky Mountain spotted fever may manifest as a skeletal muscle disease. Muscle weakness may be overwhelming; therefore, Guillain-Barré syndrome, viral myositis, and collagen disease may be erroneously diagnosed. Conversely, a case of Guillain-Barré syndrome associated with Rocky Mountain spotted fever has been documented [Toerner et al., 1996]. Muscle biopsy

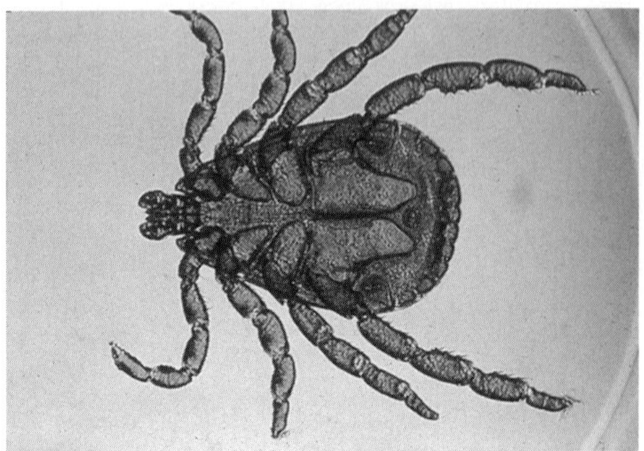

FIGURE 70-5. *Dermacentor andersoni,* the tick responsible for transmission of Rocky Mountain spotted fever in western regions of the United States.

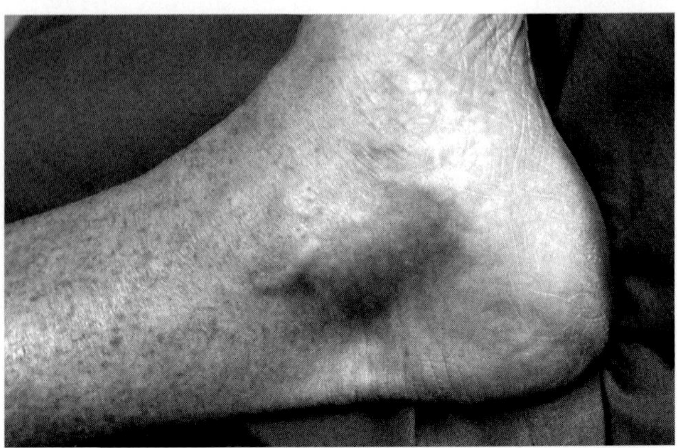

FIGURE 70-6. Petechial rash of Rocky Mountain spotted fever involving the ankle. (Courtesy Dr. Daniel J. Sexton.)

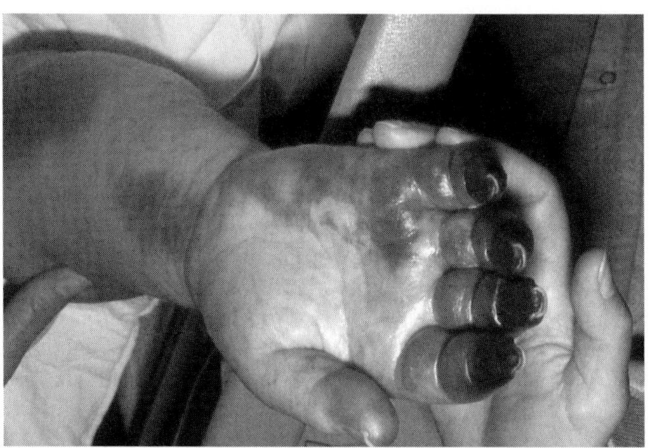

FIGURE 70-7. Necrosis and gangrene of digits is a late complication of Rocky Mountain spotted fever. (Courtesy Dr. Daniel J. Sexton.)

reveals perivascular infiltrates of chronic inflammatory cells and focal chronic interstitial myositis [Krober, 1978]. Other organs, including kidneys, heart, lungs, spleen, and epididymis may also be affected [Green et al., 1978].

Acute temporary hearing impairment has been described, but permanent auditory disruption is uncommon [Kelsey, 1979]. Ophthalmic features in all rickettsial disorders are virtually identical [Raab et al., 1969; Smith and Burton, 1977] and may include photophobia, conjunctivitis, petechiae on the bulbar conjunctiva, exudates and retinal venous engorgement, papilledema, and ocular palsies.

Laboratory abnormalities are common in severe disease and often include hyponatremia and thrombocytopenia. Spinal fluid may indicate a lymphocytic pleocytosis and the protein is elevated in about 30% to 50% of patients [Kim and Durack, 1997]. The cellular response in cerebrospinal fluid may suggest bacterial meningitis, and the dermal petechiae may mimic those in meningococcemia. Magnetic resonance imaging of the brain reveals increased signal intensity in the distribution of perivascular spaces, which resolves in relation to clinical improvement [Baganz et al., 1995]. Postmortem examination of Rocky Mountain spotted fever cases has demonstrated that rickettsial vasculitis can result in focal neurologic damage in the brain and spinal cord as well as myocarditis and vasculitis in the lungs, kidney, and spleen [Walker and Mattern, 1980].

The most widely used and best serologic test for Rocky Mountain spotted fever is the indirect fluorescent antibody assay and is available through commercial labs and most state health departments [Lochary et al., 1998; Sexton et al., 2002]. Immunofluorescent antibody for immunoglobulin M or immunoglobulin G antibodies can be used to make a presumptive diagnosis of acute infection, although these antibodies are often undetectable in the early phase of the illness. Confirmatory indirect fluorescent antibody testing requires demonstration of a fourfold or greater rise in immunoglobulin G or immunoglobulin M antibody titer between paired serum specimens, and is generally considered as a retrospective diagnosis [Thorner et al., 1998]. Direct immunofluorescence antibody or immunohistochemical staining of skin biopsies is 70% to 90% sensitive for patients with a rash. For patients without a rash, diagnosis by direct immunofluorescence antibody can be problematic. The use of polymerase chain reaction testing for *R. rickettsii* DNA can be applied to serum, whole blood, or tissue specimens but is generally available only at specialized research labs, and the sensitivity of the assay is directly related to the severity of the illness [Sexton et al., 1994].

Management

Early therapy with doxycycline for at least 7 days is recommended. The case fatality is 2% to 10% in treated patients and may be as high as 30% in untreated patients [Dalton et al., 1995]. Serologic confirmation may be delayed for 2 to 3 weeks; therefore, therapy should be administered when the diagnosis is suspected based on clinical and epidemiologic findings. A history of tick bite is a useful epidemiologic clue in making a presumptive diagnosis. With early treatment, the prognosis for full recovery from Rocky Mountain spotted fever is excellent. Neurologic sequelae may occur when therapy is postponed [Miller and Price, 1972]; mild intellectual impairment has been described [Wright, 1972].

TYPHUS FEVER GROUP

The typhus fever group consists of epidemic (louse-borne typhus), Brill-Zinsser disease, and murine (flea-borne) typhus. Louse-borne typhus fever, caused by *Rickettsia prowazekii,* is distributed worldwide. Epidemics of typhus fever occur by human-to-louse-to-human transmission, typically after rubbing skin that is contaminated with infective louse feces. Epidemics of typhus fever are often associated with war, movements of large numbers of people, and squalid living conditions [Zinsser, 1935]. Systemic and neurologic symptoms are similar to Rocky Mountain spotted fever. A severe headache is almost always present. More severe CNS features such as neck stiffness, seizures, delirium, and coma can also be present. Treatment (e.g., with doxycycline) is the same as that used for the spotted fever group of infections.

Brill-Zinsser disease is a relapsing form of louse-borne typhus that may occur years to decades after the primary attack [Feigin et al., 1992]. Presumably the rickettsiae remain dormant in the reticuloendothelial system until a subsequent reactivation occurs. Symptoms are similar to the primary attack although generally milder, and doxycycline is the recommended therapy.

Murine, or flea-borne typhus, caused by *R. typhi,* is one of the most prevalent rickettsial diseases in humans throughout the world [Azad, 1990]. Before World War II, murine typhus was widespread in the United States and approximately 42,000 cases were reported between 1931 and 1946 [Azad, 1990; Pratt, 1958]. During the Vietnam War, murine typhus was one of the most common causes of acute febrile illness in American military personnel [Berman and Kundin, 1973; Miller, 1946]. Currently, endemic foci often exist around port cities and adjacent coastal areas [Azad, 1990]. *R. typhi* is transmitted from rat to rat by the rat flea. In addition to rats, many animals such as other rodents, skunks, opossums, shrews, and cats can serve as hosts for *R. typhi* and arthropod vectors. Human infection occurs after exposure of abraded or flea-bitten skin to infective flea feces [Feigin et al., 1992]. Unlike many other arthropod-borne infections, murine typhus can be acquired in households because the transmission cycle includes commensal rats and fleas [Azad, 1990]. Symptoms of murine typhus are similar to but generally milder than those occurring in Rocky Mountain spotted fever. *R. typhi* infections are likely underdiagnosed because the clinical and laboratory features are similar to viral infections. The illness is often characterized by fever (often prolonged), headache, myalgia, and sometimes a maculopapular or petechial rash [Gelston and Jones, 1977]. Lymphadenopathy was reported as a common manifestation in a study in children [Bitsori et al., 2002]. When present, the rash often occurs on the trunk. The infection may resemble Kawasaki's disease [Bitsori et al., 2002]. There is considerable variability in the frequency of reports of neurologic manifestations of murine typhus ranging from 2% to 20% of cases [Allen and Saltz, 1945; Bitsori, 2002]. Meningitis and encephalitis are occasionally reported [Bitsori, 2002; Galanakis et al., 2002; Gelston, 1977]. Less commonly, focal symptoms such as papilledema, focal seizure, and hemiparesis have also been described [Masalha et al., 1998]. Diagnostic evaluation and treatment are similar to other diseases of the typhus group.

Scrub Typhus

Scrub typhus, caused by *Orientia tsutsugamushi,* is a systemic illness that causes a generalized vasculitis [Pai, 1997]. *O. tsutsugamushi* was formerly a member of the spotted fever group of *Rickettsia* spp. but was placed in its own genus based on molecular phylogenetic studies [Tamura et al., 1995]. Trombiculid (chigger) mites serve as reservoirs and vectors of this disease, and human infection occurs after a chigger bite in endemic areas primarily in the southwest Pacific and Southeast Asia [Feigin et al., 1992]. An eschar, a characteristic feature of the disease, is seen in 60% to 80% of cases [Jelinek and Loscher, 2001] [Fig. 70-8]. Fever, headache, and rash are also common clinical manifestations. Complications include renal failure, pneumonitis, acute respiratory distress syndrome, and myocarditis. CNS complications include meningitis or meningoencephalitis [Fang et al., 1997; Pai, 1997]. Brachial plexus neuropathy has been described in one case report [Ting et al., 1992]. Approximately 50% of patients will have a mild cerebrospinal fluid monocytic pleocytosis or an increase in protein concentration [Pai, 1997]. Doxycycline is considered the most effective treatment.

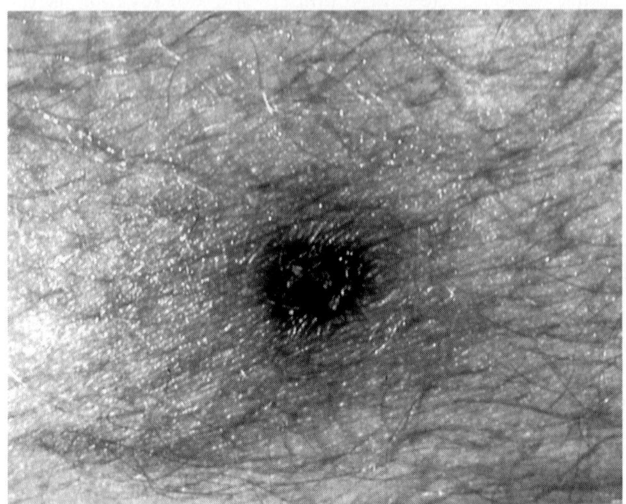

FIGURE 70-8. Eschar seen in scrub typhus. (Courtesy Dr. Daniel J. Sexton.)

Q Fever

Q fever, caused by *Coxiella burnetii,* is a worldwide zoonosis. Infection in humans occurs from inhalation of the organism in areas where infected livestock are kept and, on occasion, from ingestion of contaminated dairy products. Occasional outbreaks in research laboratories that use sheep or cattle have also been reported [Feigin et al., 1992]. Prominent symptoms include fever, headache, and pneumonia. A rash rarely, if ever, occurs. Cases of encephalitis have been reported to occur with Q fever and may occur late in the course [Maurin and Raoult, 1999].

Other Rickettsiae

Several new rickettsiae have been described since the early 1990s: *Rickettsia japonica* in Japan, *Rickettsia honei* on Flinders Island, *Rickettsia africae* in Africa and the West Indies, *Rickettsia slovaca* in Europe, *Rickettsia aeschlimannii* in Africa and Europe, *Rickettsia heilongjanghensis* in Asia, and *Rickettsia parkeri* in the United States [Raoult, 2004]. The extent of neurologic involvement with these emerging infections is unknown.

Ehrlichiosis

Ehrlichia are obligate intracellular bacteria and belong to the family Rickettsiaceae. Emerging infections, akin to those caused by other rickettsial agents, have been increasingly reported in recent years [Walker et al., 1996].

The term *ehrlichiosis* was initially used to described veterinary infections with rickettsia-like bacteria that infected leukocytes. Human infection with *Ehrlichia* in the United States was first identified in a 51-year-old male with a history of a tick bite, fever, leukopenia, thrombocytopenia, and elevated liver enzymes [Maeda et al., 1987]. The patient was initially diagnosed with Rocky Mountain spotted fever. Cytoplasmic inclusions were observed in peripheral lymphocytes, and the patient was subsequently diagnosed with an *Ehrlichia* species. Since then, two additional *Ehrlichia* infections have been described in humans caused by *Ehrlichia ewingii* and *Anaplasma* (formerly *Ehrlichia*) *phagocytophilum.* All *Ehrlichia* are transmitted by ticks, and the interval from tick exposure to onset of illness is between 2 and 21 days [Harkess, 1991]. *Ehrlichia chaffeensis* infects mononuclear cells and causes human monocytic ehrlichiosis. The incidence of human monocytic ehrlichiosis is equal to or higher than Rocky Mountain spotted fever [Fishbein et al., 1990]. *Anaplasma phagocytophilum* causes human anaplasmosis (formerly human granulocytic ehrlichiosis) and infects neutrophils. *E. ewingii* also infects neutrophils and has serologic cross-reactivity with *E. chaffeensis.* Rashes are generally less common with the ehrlichioses compared with rickettsial infections [CDC, 1988].

Human Monocytic Ehrlichiosis

Human monocyctic ehrlichiosis generally causes an acute febrile illness occurring after *E. chaffeensis* is inoculated by the Lone Star tick *(Amblyomma americanum).* Fever, headache, and malaise are commonly described. A skin rash, appearing macular or maculopapular, occurs more commonly in children than adults and is often on the trunk or extremities [Everett et al., 1994; Fishbein et al.,1994; Ratnasamy, 1996]. Nausea, vomiting, abdominal pain, and cough are other frequent manifestations. Approximately 20% of infections result in meningoencephalitis. Long-term neurologic sequelae have been reported in a limited number of children, including a 7 year old with reading problems and impairment of fine motor skills and an 11-year-old with bilateral footdrop and speech impairment [Schutze, 1997].

Laboratory testing often reveals leukopenia, thrombocytopenia, anemia, and increases in hepatic transaminases. Peripheral blood examination can reveal intracytoplasmic inclusions (termed *morulae*) in white blood cells in a small percentage of cases (Fig. 70-9). Cerebrospinal fluid abnormalities often include lymphocytic pleocytosis (73%) and high protein (76%) [Ratnassamy, 1996]. Serologic testing can sometimes be helpful but is often negative during the early stages of the illness. Evaluation of paired serum samples is generally the optimal method of establishing the diagnosis but provides only retrospective confirmation. Molecular testing (e.g., polymerase chain reaction) is available in some settings and can be helpful during the acute phases of infection (particularly before antibiotic use) [Dumler, 2003]; however, the clinical sensitivity of polymerase chain reaction for human monocytic ehrlichiosis is unknown.

Human Anaplasmosis

Human anaplasmosis was identified in humans in the 1990s. The organism in humans was initially believed to be the same organism that causes disease in horses *(Ehrlichia equi)* and ruminants *(Ehrlichia phagocytophila)* [Chen et al., 1994; Madigan et al., 1995]. Molecular analysis of these organisms resulted in a taxonomic reassignment of human anaplasmosis so that the organism is now considered to belong in the family Anaplasmataceae rather than family Rickettsiaeceae. Current terminology often refers to this disease as *human anaplasmosis. Anaplasma phagocytophilum*, the organism causing *human anaplasmosis*, is transmitted by blacklegged ticks (*Ixodes scapularis* and *Ixodes pacificus*).

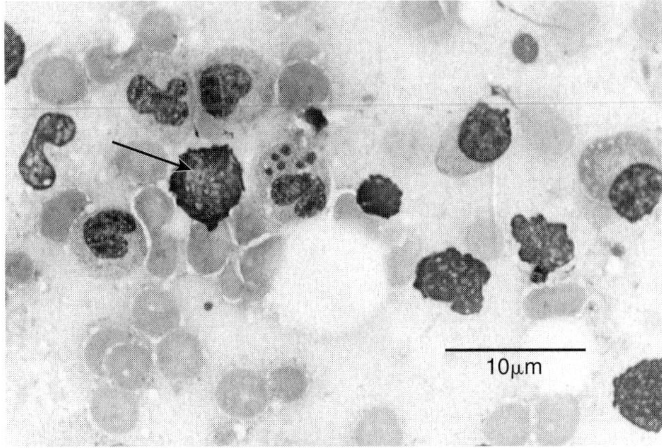

FIGURE 70-9. Intracytoplasmic inclusion (morulae) of *Ehrlichia morula* seen in the white blood cells from a bone marrow aspirate. Bar measures 10 μm. (Courtesy Dr. Christopher Paddock.)

The clinical features of human anaplasmosis are similar to human monocytic ehrlichiosis, including fever, headache, and myalgias. Gastrointestinal symptoms are seen in about 25% and a rash in 10%. Unlike human monocytic ehrlichiosis, there are few data to support invasion of the CNS by *A. phagocytophilum;* however, neck stiffness [Dumler, 2003] and brachial plexopathy and demyelinating polyneuropathy have been described [Horowitz et al., 1996]. Severe clinical manifestations include septic shock manifestations, toxic shock syndrome, acute respiratory distress syndrome, myocarditis, and rhabdomyolysis.

Laboratory testing often reveals leukopenia, thrombocytopenia, and mild increases in serum transaminases. Diagnostic testing during the active phase includes checking for morulae in a blood smear, polymerase chain reaction on blood, culture, and possibly serology. Serologic testing with paired sera is helpful for confirmation but not always helpful during the acute stage of infection. When found, morulae are helpful in making a rapid diagnosis, but this is considered to be an insensitive method.

Ehrlichia ewingii Ehrlichiosis

In the late 1990s, another *Ehrlichia* species emerged in the United States: *E. ewingii* [Buller et al., 1999]. Similar to *E. chaffeensis*, *E. ewingii* is transmitted by the Lone Star tick. Of the few cases reported to date, clinical symptoms are similar to human monocytic ehrlichiosis and human anaplasmosis but are generally milder. Laboratory abnormalities such as leukopenia, thrombocytopenia, and elevated transaminases are seen in cases as in other *Ehrlichia* infections. Morulae can be identified in neutrophils, yet there can be serologic cross-reactivity to *E. chaffeensis.*

PARASITIC DISEASES

Human parasitic infestation occurs worldwide [Bia and Barry, 1986; Markell et al., 1992; Warren and Mahmoud, 1984]. Parasites infect humans in tropical, temperate, and cold climates. Parasitic infections impair the CNS [Brown and Voge, 1982] by a variety of mechanisms, including the following: (1) direct invasion from the circulation or lymphatic system may cause local changes, such as inflammation and edema, (2) granuloma development may result in disturbances associated with mass lesions, (3) remote effects associated with nutrient deprivation of the CNS may cause diffuse or focal CNS symptomatology, and (4) immunologic or hypersensitivity effects may develop.

Changes in society have spread what were once exotic diseases largely restricted to developing countries into the developed world. Ease and frequency of travel require that all clinicians have general familiarity of these infections when considering differential diagnoses. Population shifts, whether due to immigration or social unrest, have brought unfamiliar parasitic infections into urban and other areas. The following are some examples of the need for increased awareness of parasitic diseases: Peace Corps volunteers returning to the United States may bring with them parasitic worm infestations; malaria has developed in airport workers and people living in the vicinity of airports perhaps because of inadvertent importation of mosquitoes in airplane cabins;

sleeping sickness should be considered in the differential of patients presenting with a neuropathology or encephalopathy and a recent travel history to west and central Africa.

Many different classifications of parasitic disease have been proposed [Garcia, 1992; Markell et al., 1992], but none is completely satisfactory because of the complexity, widespread distribution, and incredible variety of infectious agents that are known. Modified or even new classification systems for parasites are being proposed based on data from DNA sequencing studies, which has become an important tool in the understanding of phylogeny and taxonomy of these organisms. Table 70-3 lists the most common parasitic diseases that are known to cause serious neurologic disease and are reviewed in this section. Another large group of parasites includes the helminths. The helminths (worms) are subdivided into three categories: nematodes, cestodes, and trematodes. Nematodes are cylindrical and nonsegmented worms. *Trichinella, Angiostrongylus,* and *Toxocara* are genera in this class that infect the CNS. Cestodes that infect humans belong to the subclass *Eucestoda,* the true tapeworms. These endoparasites have no epidermis or digestive tract and have elongated segmented bodies. Adults have a multihook organ of attachment at the anterior end called the *scolex*. Genera of cestodes associated with CNS infection in the larval stage include *Dibothriocephalus (Diphyllobothrium), Taenia, Multiceps,* and *Echinococcus.* Trematodes (flukes) are nonsegmented worms that possess a digestive tract. Trematodes infecting the nervous system include the genera *Schistosoma* and *Paragonimus.*

Isolation and growth are important for accurate identification of etiologic agents, preparation of antibodies for serology, testing for efficacy of antimicrobial agents, and as a source of DNA for diagnostic and molecular biologic procedures [Visvesvara and Garcia, 2002]. Cultivation of parasitic protozoa is often demanding and may require complex media that are not readily available to most diagnostic laboratories or in the field. For this reason, in vitro cultivation of protozoal parasites is relegated to research or reference laboratories. In the United States, in vitro growth of these parasites is done primarily by the Centers for Disease Control and Prevention (CDC), specific (usually academic) research laboratories, or at state public health laboratories [Lowichik and Siegel, 1995]. In such cases, consulting with and sending specimens to these laboratories is usually helpful for early diagnosis and treatment. For the parasitic worms, in vitro cultivation has yet to be realized.

Microsporidial infections in humans were once a rarity but are now one of the major infections, and often a cause of death, of AIDS patients. Similarly, systemic infections with *Acanthamoeba* occur almost exclusively in AIDS and organ transplant patients. Reactivated toxoplasmosis has also become an important disease of immunocompromised hosts. Baylisascariasis, caused by a nematode worm infecting raccoons, has been recognized to cause human illness, especially in children.

The sequencing of genomes of parasites is another new contribution to developing new and effective controls. The sequencing of the *Plasmodium falciparum* genome opens the door to development of antimicrobials targeted to specific gene products. Progress has been made in the sequencing of the genome of the African trypanosome, the etiologic agent of sleeping sickness, leading to a better understanding of the mechanisms of immune evasion of the parasite.

The polymerase chain reaction was not considered a practical diagnostic tool at the time the previous edition appeared, but is now used in identification of many protozoal and other parasitic organisms. Its use, however, is restricted to reference and research laboratories. A drawback of polymerase chain reaction is that it cannot differentiate between DNA from viable and nonviable disease agents, perhaps leading to inappropriate or unnecessary additional therapy in a setting where antimicrobial therapy has been used successfully to combat infection.

PROTOZOAL INFECTIONS OF THE CENTRAL NERVOUS SYSTEM

The major protozoal diseases that affect the nervous system include the amebic infections, toxoplasmosis, malaria, babesiosis, and trypanosomiasis. These diseases differ from one another in many respects, including the nature of the etiologic agents, mode of transmission of the parasites, mechanisms of pathogenesis, and responses to antimicrobials.

AMEBIC INFECTIONS OF THE CENTRAL NERVOUS SYSTEM

Disease-causing amebas are a mixed group of organisms. *Entamoeba histolytica* is an obligate parasite, generally associated with enteric disease. The free-living amebas (*Naegleria fowleri*, *Acanthamoeba* spp., *Balamuthia mandrillaris*) are facultative parasites, with some acting as opportunistic pathogens.

E. histolytica is an anaerobic protozoon found in nature only in the dormant cystic stage. The typical mode of infection is the fecal-oral route by ingestion of cysts, either from water or uncooked foods contaminated with fecal matter. Person-to-person spread of cysts, as by infected food handlers, is the main mode of transmission. The disease is more likely to occur in developing areas of the world where drinking water is not carefully monitored for sewage contamination. The pathogenic free-living amebas *(Naegleria, Acanthamoeba, Balamuthia)* are globally dispersed in soil and water, with many opportunities for contact between them and humans. Human-to-human spread does not occur. *Acanthamoeba* spp. cause infections chiefly in immunocompromised hosts, *N. fowleri* infects immunocompetent hosts, and *B. mandrillaris* infections have occurred in both groups of individuals. Because of the ubiquitous dispersal of free-living amebas, many are exposed to them as indicated by studies of antibody titers in healthy individuals, but clinical disease is a rarity. When infection results in disease, the difficulty in diagnosis of the infections and the lack of optimal antimicrobial therapy are responsible for a high mortality.

Cerebral Amebiasis: *Entamoeba histolytica*

Epidemiology, Microbiology, and Pathology

Amebiasis results from gastrointestinal infection by the protozoon *E. histolytica.* Amebic dysentery was described in

TABLE 70–3

Parasite Infections

CLASSIFICATION	ORGANISM	DISEASES	GEOGRAPHIC DISTRIBUTION	RISK FACTORS	MODE OF INFECTION	NEUROPATHOLOGY	PREDOMINANT SYMPTOMS	DIAGNOSTIC TECHNIQUE	ANTIMICROBIAL THERAPY
Amebas	*Entamoeba histolytica*	Amebiasis	Worldwide	Living in regions with poor sewage treatment	Ingestion of cysts with water or food	Cyst formation in cerebrum	Diarrhea	MRI/CT	Metronidazole, paromomycin
	Naegleria fowleri	Primary amoebic meningo-encephalitis	Worldwide	Swimming in fresh water	Amebas entering nostrils	Hemorrhagic necrosis of frontal lobes	F, HA, stiff neck, fulminant disease	Detection of amebas in CSF, IIF of tissue	Amphotericin B
	Acanthamoeba spp.	Granulomatous amebic encephalitis	Worldwide	Immuno-compromised status, immuno-competent children	Inhalation of windblown soil, contamination of wound with soil	Hemorrhagic necrosis of cerebrum, cerebellum, granuloma formation	F, mass effect	Biopsy, MRI/CT, IIF staining of serum or tissue	Combination drug therapy: fluconazole, 5-fluo-cytosine, pentamidine, azithromycin
	Balamuthia mandrillaris	Granulomatous amebic encephalitis	Worldwide	Same as *Acanth-amoeba* spp.	Same as *Acanth-amoeba* spp.	Same as *Acanth-amoeba* spp.	Same as *Acanth-amoeba* spp.	Same as *Acanth-amoeba* spp.	Same as *Acanth-amoeba* spp.
Flagellates	*Trypanosoma brucei*	Sleeping sickness	Africa	Exposure to vector	Tsetse fly bites	Cerebral edema (early), cerebral and cerebellar atrophy (late)	Somnolence	Blood smear	Suramin, meltefosin, melarsoprol, eflornithine
	Trypanosoma cruzi	Chagas' disease	Latin America, southwestern US	Exposure to vector	Reduviid bug bites	Cerebral edema, destruction of autonomic ganglia, nodules in brain and spinal cord	Often acute in children: muscle/bone pain, neural disorders	Blood/CSF smears serology; ELISA cultivation	Benznidazole, nifurtimox
Apicomplexa	*Plasmodium falciparum*	Malaria	Southern Asia, Southeast Asia, Africa, South America	Exposure to vector	Mosquito bites	Cerebral malaria, hemorrhagic necrosis	Fulminant in children; mental deterioration, delirium, coma	Blood smear, serology; IFA	Chloroquine, quinidine gluconate artemesinin
	Babesia spp.	Babesiosis	Europe, north and south Africa, Middle East, US, Asia	Exposure to vector, splenectomy	Tick bites		F, sweating, myalgia, depression	Blood smear	Quinine, clindamycin, atovaquone and azithromycin
	Toxoplasma gondii	Toxoplasmosis	Worldwide	Exposure to source of oocysts, particularly during pregnancy	Ingestion of oocysts in undercooked meat; oocysts present in cat feces	Necrotic cerebral lesions, cerebral calcification	Focal neurologic deficits, seizures	Serology; ELISA/IFA PCR	Sulfadiazine, pyrimethamine, folinic acid
Microsporidia	*Encephalito-zoon cuniculi*	Microsporidiosis	Worldwide	Immuno-compromised status				CSF smears, sputum and urinary samples	Albendazole
Nematode	*Trichinella spiralis* (and other *Trichinella* sp.)	Trichinosis	Worldwide, especially in Balkans, Baltic Republics, Russia, China and Argentina	Dietary habits	Ingestion of uncooked meat (especially pork, bear, horse)	CNS inflammatory infiltration	Gastroenteritis myositis, facial/ periorbital edema, myocarditis, encephalitis	Serology; ELISA, IFA muscle biopsy, eosinophilia	Mebendazole, thiabendazole, corticosteroids, albendazole
	Angiostrongylus cantonensis	Angiostrongyliasis	SE Asia, South Pacific, Taiwan Caribbean, Africa, Australia US: Hawaii, Louisiana	Dietary habits of ingestion of under-cooked mollusks, or unwashed vegetables	Ingestion of larvae in raw prawns, snails, or shrimp	Leptomeningitis Small worm tracks	Eosinophilic meningitis, paresthesias	CSF eosinophilia serology (ELISA)	Supportive measures; steroids, analgesics, lumbar punctures
	Gnathostoma spp.	Gnathostomiasis	Southeast Asia, particularly Thailand and Japan, Latin America	Dietary habits	Ingestion of undercooked fish (e.g. cerviche), frogs, snakes, chickens, ducks	Myeloencephalitis	Cutaneous larvans and visceral pain CNS, HA; radicular pain with later paralysis and bladder incontinence	Identification of worm in tissues, eosinophilia	Albendazole, ivermectin
	Baylisascaris procyonis	Baylisascariasis	North America, Europe, parts of Asia	Young children or develop-mentally disabled people, pica	Ingestion of raccoon roundworm eggs	Worm tracts with inflammatory cells	Eosinophilic meningo-encephalitis	Serology (IFA), eosinophilia and blood	No known effective treatment but albendazole and steroids have been used in some cases

Continued

TABLE 70–3, cont'd

Parasite Infections

CLASSIFICATION	ORGANISM	DISEASES	GEOGRAPHIC DISTRIBUTION	RISK FACTORS	MODE OF INFECTION	NEUROPATHOLOGY	PREDOMINANT SYMPTOMS	DIAGNOSTIC TECHNIQUE	ANTIMICROBIAL THERAPY
Cestodes	*Diphyllobothrium latum*	Diphyllobothriasis	Worldwide, especially in temperate and subarctic zones in Northern Hemisphere	Dietary habits	Eating undercooked freshwater fish contaminated with the tapeworm	Optic atrophy, spinal cord degeneration	Usually minimal unless prolonged infection	Blood smear: megaloblastic anemia	Adult worms: niclosamide, praziquantel
	Taenia solium	Cysticercosis	Worldwide, especially in Latin America, Southeast Asia, Africa, eastern Europe	Areas with poor sanitation	Adult tapeworms: Ingestion of pork tapeworm NC: ingestion of ova shed by tapeworm carrier	Cysts in varying stages of inflammation, cerebral edema, encephalitis	Signs of ICP	Serology; CF, HI, ELISA, eosinophilia CT/MRI	Adult tapeworms: praziquantel or niclosamide NC: individualized for each case depending on presentation, number and location of cysts: steroids, antiseizure medications, and anthelmintic drugs
	Taenia multiceps	Coenurosis	Americas, Europe, Africa	Rarely reported: unknown	Ingestion of food/water contaminated with dog feces	Similar to cysticercosis	Similar to cysticercosis; seizures, meningitis	CT/MRI	Because rarely seen, limited information, may be similar to above
	Echinococcus spp.	Echinococcosis	Worldwide	Sheep or cattle herding	Ingestion of food/water contaminated with feces from infected dogs	Cyst formation common in liver, but also may be found in lungs and CNS, typically in white matter extending to meninges and ventricles	RUQ pain/ jaundice (if liver affected) chest pain, cough, fever, hemoptysis (if lungs affected) neurologic: signs of ICP	CT/MRI serology	Albendazole, mebendazole

CF, complement fixation; CNS, central nervous system; CSF, cerebrospinal fluid; CT, computed tomography; ELISA, enzyme-linked immunosorbent assay; F, fever; HA, headache; HI, hemagglutination; ICP, intracranial pressure; IFA, indirect fluorescent antibody; MRI, magnetic resonance imaging; NC, neurocysticercosis; PCR, polymerase chain reaction; RUQ, right upper quadrant.

ancient times by Galen and Hippocrates, and even earlier descriptions of dysentery-like illness were found in Assyrian and Babylonian writings [Cox, 2002]. The role of *E. histolytica* in causing pathogenic intestinal and hepatic lesions was described definitively by Kartulis [1886] and Councilman and Lafleur [1891]. Its distribution is global, although it is more common in regions that have hot, humid climates. Despite its partiality for tropical climates, the organism was first isolated from a stool sample by Lösch in St. Petersburg, Russia, in 1873, and an outbreak of amebiasis occurred at a Chicago hotel at the time of the 1933 World's Fair, resulting in about 100 deaths.

Gross postmortem examination of the brain reveals abscesses, petechiae, and suppurative meningitis. Necrotic areas are distributed throughout the brain but are concentrated in the basal ganglia and frontal lobes. Cerebral edema and transtentorial herniation are often seen. Microscopic study demonstrates a zone of disruption; necrotic areas are more common than areas of inflammation. The inflammatory response is attended by mononuclear cells [Lombardo et al., 1964].

Clinical Characteristics, Clinical Laboratory Tests, and Diagnosis

From the intestine, the liver, lungs, and brain are secondarily affected. Cerebral amebiasis is the most unusual condition and principally occurs in patients with hepatic or pulmonary infections. Most patients with cerebral amebiasis have symptoms that accompany the effects of systemic disease, such as fever, weight loss, and anorexia. Cerebral amebiasis is rare, and many of the patients who have this disorder do not manifest neurologic symptoms. In one series, only 5 of 17 patients had neurologic manifestations consisting of increased intracranial pressure, hemiplegia, meningeal irritation, nuchal rigidity, confusion, and headache [Lombardo et al., 1964]. The presence of a focal CNS lesion in a febrile patient with hepatic or intestinal disease should suggest amebiasis, particularly if there is a history of travel to an endemic area and if more common causes, such as bacterial brain abscesses or tumors, have been ruled out [Durack, 1997].

The diagnosis of cerebral amebiasis can usually be confirmed by serologic evaluation using an indirect hemagglutination assay or indirect immunofluorescent staining. Commercial kits are available for detection of ameba antigen, and the polymerase chain reaction has been used for detecting *Entamoeba* DNA [Leber and Novak, 1999; Tanyuksel and Petri, 2003]. Cerebrospinal fluid evaluation is usually not helpful; cultures are usually sterile, and cytology or changes in the protein or glucose concentrations are nonspecific. The polymerase chain reaction applied to fluid drained from a brain abscess in an adult detected *E. histolytica* DNA, though intact amebas were not seen [Ohnishi et al., 1994]. In a pediatric case, intact amebas were recovered in fluid aspirated from the thorax but were not detected in the child's stool [Hughes et al., 1975]. Stool cultures are usually negative when nervous system involvement appears. Neuroimaging may reveal abscess formation with perilesional edema [Tikly et al., 1988]. General testing for amebic colitis and liver abscess is reviewed in Tanyuksel and Petri [2003].

Management

Cerebral amebiasis is rarely treated successfully. Metronidazole is currently the preferred drug (15 mg/kg initially followed by 30 mg/kg/day divided into four doses) [Strickland, 1992], although trinidazole may be more effective than metronidazole [Medical Letter, 2004]. Emetine and chloroquine are alternative medications.

A combination of metronidazole and chloroquine was used successfully in treating a pediatric case of cerebral amebiasis with three abscesses [Hughes et al., 1975]. Amebiasis in an adult was treated with metronidazole and dehydroemetine after drainage of a brain abscess [Ohnishi et al., 1994]; the patient recovered with minor neurologic impairment. An adult male in a stuporous state with signs of encephalitis and hepatic abscesses had a low titer for *E. histolytica* by indirect hemagglutination, but countercurrent immunoelectrophoresis was positive [Schmutzhard et al., 1986]. CT scans of the brain exhibited approximately 40 small ringlike lesions, mostly in the white matter of both hemispheres. Treatment with metronidazole, chloroquine, and tetracycline effected a partial recovery; further regression of the lesions and recovery occurred after a course of dehydroemetine treatment. Paromomycin has been used for asymptomatic cases [Medical Letter, 2004].

Primary Amebic Meningoencephalitis: *Naegleria fowleri*

Epidemiology, Microbiology, and Pathology

Primary amebic meningoencephalitis is a fulminant disease occurring in children and young adults. The disease was first reported from Australia and was initially attributed to *Acanthamoeba* [Fowler and Carter, 1965], which had been previously found to cause death of mice inoculated intranasally with amebas [Culbertson et al., 1958]. The disease was soon reported from Florida and was then characterized as primary amebic meningoencephalitis [Butt, 1966]. *N. fowleri* is a free-living, facultative parasite, with a life cycle that includes an ameboid trophic (feeding) stage, a transitory flagellate stage, and a double-walled cyst able to withstand desiccation. The amebas measure about 15 to 30 µm, and cysts from 7 to 15 µm in diameter. The ameba is found in water, soil, sewage, or other decaying organic material where there is a bacterial food source [Marshall et al., 1997], and grows optimally at elevated temperatures (37° C to 45° C). Of an estimated 200 cases since the first descriptions of primary amebic meningoencephalitis, more than 90% of the patients have died. The disease has been reported from Australia, Belgium, Czech Republic, Great Britain, Mexico, India, New Zealand, Nigeria, and the United States. Extended descriptions of the organism and the disease can be found in several review articles [Barnett et al., 1996; Duma, 1984; John, 1993].

In the United States, most of the cases have developed in the southern tier of the country, where warm water conditions are more likely to be encountered. In Florida, where a number of cases have been reported after swimming in lakes, the probability of infection was estimated to be 1 case per 2.6 million exposures [Wellings, 1977]. No cases have resulted from drinking water containing amebas.

Typically, infection with *N. fowleri* occurs while swimming or washing in warm, fresh water containing the amebas, and early manifestations of the disease ensue. Bodies of water associated with amebic infections have included ponds, man-made lakes, hot springs, wading pools, irrigation canals, thermally polluted streams, and inadequately chlorinated swimming pools. Those affected are children or young adults without underlying disease. Infection has been associated with prolonged immersion in water, diving, underwater swimming, or other activities that allow water to enter the nostrils. Acute meningoencephalitis ensues usually within 2 to 3 days.

Amebas enter the nasal passages and gain access to the nervous system by penetrating the olfactory mucosa, entering the submucosal nervous plexus, migrating along the olfactory nerves, and traversing the cribriform plate. Hemorrhagic destruction of gray matter and devastation of the olfactory bulbs follow sanguinopurulent meningitis and pronounced brain edema [Martinez et al., 1973]. Spinal cord involvement is signaled by similar gray matter disruption. Perivascular infiltrates include leukocytes and amebas (Fig. 70-10). Numerous eosinophils may be present. Simultaneous bronchopneumonia and pulmonary edema, myocarditis, and splenitis may occur.

Clinical Characteristics, Clinical Laboratory Tests, and Diagnosis

Among the most common symptoms of primary amebic meningoencephalitis are severe headache, stiff neck, nausea, vomiting, fever (39° C to 40° C), behavioral changes, seizures, diplopia, and coma [Duma, 1984; Martinez, 1985]. One patient complained of a violent headache and foul odors before becoming unconscious [Duma, 1984]. Distortion of taste has also been reported [Martinez, 1993]. Cerebrospinal fluid is typically cloudy with a slightly decreased glucose concentration, increased protein content (75 to 970 mg/dL), and innumerable white blood cells

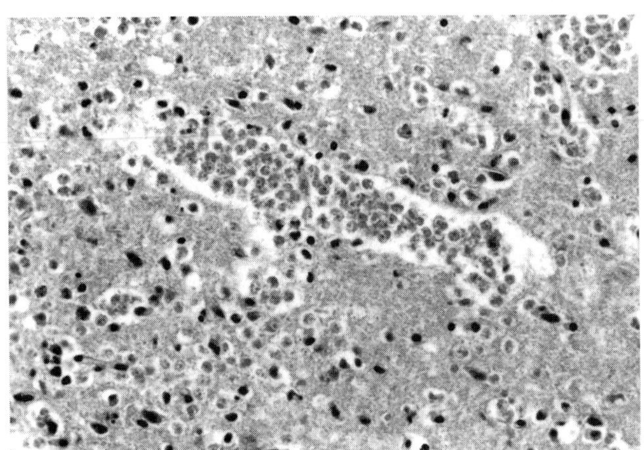

FIGURE 70-10. Section through cerebral cortex of an individual with primary amebic meningoencephalitis, with large numbers of *Naegleria fowleri* amebas in the perivascular space. (Hematoxylin-eosin)

(300 to 24,600/mm^3) and erythrocytes [Martinez, 1985]. Polymorphonuclear cells make up 52% to 99%, lymphocytes 1% to 48%, and monocytes 1% to 2% of the white blood cells in the cerebrospinal fluid. High opening pressures may be observed.

Differential diagnosis for primary amebic meningoencephalitis is bacterial meningitis, but the cerebrospinal fluid is sterile in primary amebic meningoencephalitis [Martinez, 1993]. A Gram stain of the cerebrospinal fluid is not particularly helpful in diagnosis because the amebas may lyse during preparation of the slide. In freshly obtained spinal fluid, motile *Naegleria* amebas can usually be seen in wet-mount preparations [Lowichik and Ruff, 1995a], which are best viewed with a phase-contrast microscope. The cerebrospinal fluid should not be refrigerated or frozen before examination. Low-speed centrifugation of the sample may help concentrate the amebas and make them easier to find. In cerebrospinal fluid from three primary amebic meningoencephalitis patients, amebas numbered from 26 to 118/mm^3, as compared with 330 to more than 9000 leukocytes/mm^3 [Duma et al., 1971]. The amebas can be recognized by their relatively swift movement with an anterior, eruptive pseudopod (Fig. 70-11), contrasting with the sluggish motility of the leukocytes with indistinct pseudopodal activity. As an aid in diagnosis, amebas can be readily cultured on non-nutrient agar plates spread with a suspension of *Escherichia coli* as a food source [Visvesvara, 1999]. Immunofluorescent staining for *Naegleria* antibodies in acute phase serum is of little diagnostic value because of the fulminant nature of the disease and a delayed humoral response.

Neuroimaging is not particularly helpful in diagnosis, with results being nonspecific. CT and MRI scans of a 9-year-old child hospitalized with what was diagnosed upon postmortem examination as primary amebic meningoencephalitis showed no abnormalities at time of admission [Kidney and Kim, 1998]. Three days later, one day before the child died, a CT scan indicated developing hydrocephalus and brain edema but no focal lesions.

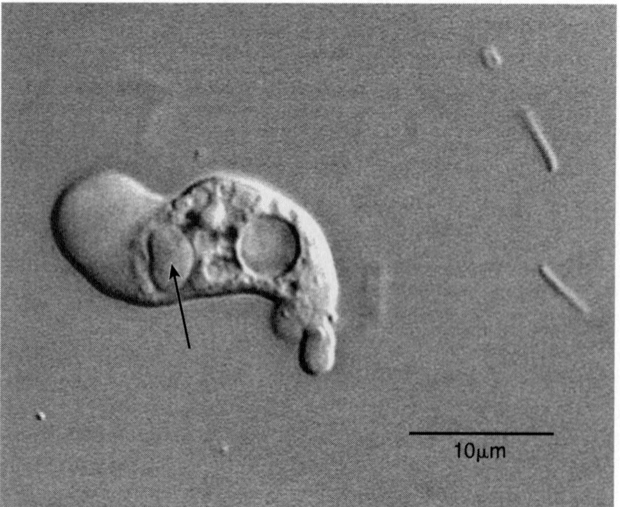

FIGURE 70-11. *Naegleria* ameba from culture in wet mount. An ectoplasmic pseudopod is present at the anterior end of the ameba. When seen in cerebrospinal fluid samples, the clear pseudopod and rapid movement (~1μm/second) distinguishes *Naegleria* amebas from sluggishly motile leukocytes that may also be present in the cerebrospinal fluid. The nucleus is indicated by an *arrow;* some rod-shaped bacteria *(Escherichia coli)* can also be seen. Bar measures 10 μm. (Interference-contrast)

Management

The high mortality from primary amebic meningoencephalitis is largely a consequence of delays in diagnosis and initiation of antimicrobial therapy. Early diagnosis and intensive care may improve the small chance of recovery [Seidel, 1985b]. Differences in virulence of primary amebic meningoencephalitis ameba isolates, when tested by mouse inoculations, indicate that this may be a factor affecting survival. *Naegleria* amebas are sensitive to amphotericin B, the drug of choice in treating primary amebic meningoencephalitis. In a well-documented primary amebic meningoencephalitis case, the patient, a 9-year-old female, had been swimming in a California hot spring before developing symptoms of meningoencephalitis. She was given intravenous and intrathecal amphotericin B and miconazole, oral rifampin, and sulfisoxazole, and recovered with minimal neurologic sequelae [Seidel et al., 1982]. Other successful treatments have been reported [Apley et al, 1970; Brown, 1991; Jain et al, 2002; Wang et al, 1993]. The macrolide azithromycin has demonstrated amebacidal activity in vitro and in the mouse model and may have potential for treating primary amebic meningoencephalitis [Goswick and Brenner, 2003]. Although azithromycin penetrates the brain, its low concentration in cerebrospinal fluid may render it less effective in primary amebic meningoencephalitis [Jaruratanasirikul et al., 1996]. Despite a small number of successful treatments, most cases are fatal [Seidel, 1985a].

Granulomatous Amebic Encephalitis: *Acanthamoeba* spp.

Epidemiology, Microbiology, and Pathology

It was largely through the observations of Culbertson that free-living amebas were recognized as potentially pathogenic organisms. He detected acanthamoebas in monkey kidney cell cultures used for growing poliovirus, and demonstrated their pathogenicity in mice [Culbertson et al., 1958]. It was *N. fowleri,* however, that was the first free-living ameba recognized in human infections.

Two different, although closely related amebas, cause granulomatous encephalitis: *Acanthamoeba* spp. and *Balamuthia mandrillaris*. *Acanthamoeba* granulomatous encephalitis is an opportunistic, chronic disease that may have a prodromal period of weeks to months, with most patients being immunocompromised [Martinez, 1980]. A sharp increase in the number of cases followed the appearance of HIV/AIDS, but there have been non-AIDS cases reported in individuals on immunosuppressive medication after organ transplants. Among predisposing factors to acanthamebiasis, ordered in relative frequency, are antibiotic or steroid treatments, chemotherapy, radiation therapy, alcoholism, and pregnancy [Martinez, 1980]. A small number of *Acanthamoeba* granulomatous encephalitis cases have been described in immunocompetent children.

Acanthamoeba is perhaps the most common ameba found in soil, which is often the source of infection. It is remarkably tolerant of a range of environmental conditions and can be isolated from seawater and fresh water, and from Arctic soils and beach sands. *Acanthamoeba* is also found in the home in aquaria, flowerpot soil, humidifiers, and sink taps and drains. It has been isolated from hot tubs, hydrotherapy baths, dental irrigation equipment, and laboratory eye wash stations. The life cycle consists of alternating ameboid and cyst stages. Cysts are particularly resistant to both physical (heat, desiccation, drying) and chemical (chlorine, antimicrobials) agents, and have remained viable in the laboratory in excess of 20 years. Infection may be through breaks in the skin that are contaminated with soil, or by inhalation of airborne ameba cysts originating from soil. In surveys of healthy groups of individuals (students, military recruits), *Acanthamoeba* has been cultured from the nasal passages, indicating exposure and infection but not disease [Badenoch et al., 1988; Cerva et al., 1973].

Clinical Characteristics, Clinical Laboratory Tests, and Diagnosis

In addition to encephalitis, *Acanthamoeba* can cause nasopharyngeal, cutaneous, and disseminated infections. Nasopharyngeal and cutaneous infections can be precursors to disseminated amebiasis or encephalitis, as amebas spread from their initial portal of entry. The CNS becomes infected by hematogenous transport of amebas, either from the lungs or from cutaneous lesions. A granulomatous reaction occurs, which can be seen in histopathologic slide preparations, but this reaction may be absent in immunocompromised hosts [Martinez, 1980]. Areas of the brain affected are usually the cerebrum, cerebellum, and brainstem, where the amebas produce hemorrhagic necrotic lesions. Large numbers of amebas can be found in the perivascular areas of brain tissue. Cysts of *Acanthamoeba* may be seen in histopathologic sections; *Naegleria* amebas do not form cysts in tissue. Reports of detecting amebas in cerebrospinal fluid are rare. Because of the absence of clear pathognomonic symptoms, *Acanthamoeba* granulomatous encephalitis is often unrecognized and diagnoses are often made postmortem.

Unrelated to its role as etiologic agent of *Acanthamoeba* granulomatous encephalitis, *Acanthamoeba* can also cause amebic keratitis as a result of corneal trauma or wearing contact lenses. Ophthalmic solutions prepared from nonsterile tap water, and lens cases that harbor bacterial biofilms can support growth of the amebas. Keratitis has not been reported to develop into encephalitis; however, a child diagnosed with uveitis and pharyngitis caused by *Acanthamoeba* went on to develop fatal encephalitis [Jones et al., 1975]. Because the disease is chronic, an antibody response develops over time and the infection can be diagnosed by indirect immunofluorescence staining of the patient's serum. Surveys of human populations for *Acanthamoeba* antibodies have found that many healthy people have elevated antibody titers, probably resulting from exposure to the amebas through contact with soil or water [Cerva, 1989; Cursons et al., 1980].

Diagnosis of *Acanthamoeba* granulomatous encephalitis is difficult and the disease mimics other types of encephalitis. Children infected with *Acanthamoeba* have exhibited headache, stiff neck, vomiting, abnormal behavior, seizures, fever, ataxia, and tonic-clonic seizures [Karande et al., 1991; Sharma et al., 1993; Singhal et al., 2001]. Hydrocephalus may also develop [Karande et al., 1991]. Differential diagnoses are neurotuberculosis, tuberculoma, and neurocysticercosis. Although the amebas are generally not recovered from cerebrospinal fluid, several cases were reported in which the amebas were seen in wet-mount preparations of spinal fluid, and/or were cultured from cerebrospinal fluid [Callicot et al., 1968; Karande et al., 1991; Kidney and Kim, 1998; Sharma et al., 1993]. In wet-mount slide preparations, trophic *Acanthamoeba* have radiating finger-like pseudopodia over the surface and are relatively slow-moving amebas. More often, amebas are cultured from biopsied brain tissue or skin ulcers onto plates of non-nutrient agar coated with *E. coli* and incubated at 37° C [Visvesvara, 1999]. Cerebrospinal fluid protein is elevated (range of 31 to 500 mg/dL), as is the white blood cell count (14 to 750 cells/μL) and glucose level (17 to 240 mg/dL); among the white blood cells are lymphocytes (19% to 100%) and polymorphonuclear leukocytes (2% to 70%) [Martinez, 1980; 1985]. The cerebrospinal fluid protein in an 8-year-old female with *Acanthamoeba* meningitis increased from 200 mg/dL at onset to a high of 500 mg/dL and then decreased to 41 mg/dL after completion of drug therapy 5 months after the patient was first seen [Singhal et al., 2001]. Neuroimaging by MRI of an adult male diagnosed with acanthamebiasis revealed punctate focal lesions mainly in the cerebellar hemispheres and fewer lesions in the cerebral hemispheres and the corpus callosum [Kidney and Kim, 1998].

Management

There are several reported cases of acanthamebiasis in pediatric HIV/AIDS patients. An 8-year-old patient developed cutaneous and sinus lesions, in which *Acanthamoeba* cysts and trophozoites were seen, along with a weak granulomatous response [Friedland et al., 1992]. The infection progressed after about 3 months to disseminated disease with CNS involvement (multiple lesions within the right basal ganglia by MRI) and ultimately proved fatal, despite treatment with ketoconazole, fluconazole, sulfadiazine, and trimethoprim-sulfamethoxazole. Acanthamebiasis in another pediatric case with congenital HIV/AIDS developed as osteomyelitis and subcutaneous abscesses without neural involvement [Selby et al., 1998]. Initial treatment was with oral fluconazole but was subsequently changed to intravenous pentamidine, oral flucytosine (5-fluorocytosine), and oral itraconazole, and disease progression was successfully halted. In both adult and pediatric acanthamebiasis, death is usually a consequence of multiple AIDS-related infections rather than from the amebic infection per se.

Acanthamoeba infections of the CNS are almost always fatal, although some reports of successful antimicrobial treatment are known. Often, however, the same antimicrobial agents used successfully in one case are unsuccessful in other acanthamebiasis cases. Response to therapy depends, to a large extent, on infective dose of amebas, virulence of the infecting strain, the time at which diagnosis is made, the extent of dissemination of the infection, and the immune status of the patient. As yet, there is no optimal antimicrobial therapy for treatment of *Acanthamoeba* encephalitis. Most recoveries have been treated successfully with combinations of antimicrobials: sulfadiazine, pyrimethamine, and fluconazole in an adult HIV/AIDS patient [Martinez et al., 2000], and with ketoconazole, rifampin, and trimethoprim-sulfamethoxazole in two pediatric patients [Singhal et al., 2001]. Isolates from patients vary in their virulence, as can be demonstrated by intranasal inoculation in a mouse model of encephalitis, or assessing cytopathology caused by amebas in tissue cultures. Variation is also seen among *Acanthamoeba* isolates in antimicrobial sensitivity, reflecting different strains isolated from clinical specimens.

Granulomatous Amebic Encephalitis: *Balamuthia mandrillaris*

Epidemiology, Microbiology, and Pathology

Balamuthia granulomatous encephalitis was initially described in immunocompromised humans [Anzil et al., 1991; Visvesvara et al., 1990], but more recent cases have occurred in immunocompetent children [Bakardjiev et al., 2003; Duke et al., 1997; Reed et al., 1997; Rowen et al., 1995]. The life cycle comprises trophic and cystic stages; the cyst is a triple-layered structure without pores. Little is known about the ecology of the ameba, other than that it is found in soil. Like *Acanthamoeba,* it is likely to enter the body by inhalation of cysts in windblown soil, or through breaks in the skin contaminated by soil, followed by hematogenous spread. Balamuthiasis can develop as cutaneous, nasopharyngeal, or CNS lesions. In a review of 30 cases reported from Peru, all developed initially as cutaneous lesions, mostly on the nose or the central region of the face, and progressed to infections of the CNS [Bravo and Sanchez, 2003]. The disease may be chronic with a prodrome that can extend as long as 2 years, but it often presents in an acute form [Bakardjiev et al., 2003]. The long incubation period makes it difficult to pinpoint the source and time of infection. A 3-year-old female may have become infected through playing with soil in a flowerpot, from which *Balamuthia* was subsequently isolated (Fig. 70-12) [Schuster et al., 2003]. Evidence of exposure to *Balamuthia* among healthy individuals is seen in elevated serum antibody titers in studies performed in Australia and the United States [Huang et al., 1999; Schuster et al., 2001]. The relative prevalence of *Balamuthia* granulomatous encephalitis in Hispanics is high [Schuster et al., 2004]: In the United States, about 50% of cases occurred in Hispanic Americans (who comprise ~12% of the U.S. population), and almost half of the number of cases worldwide have been described from Latin America and Mexico [Bravo and Sanchez, 2003; Galarza et al., 2002; Martinez et al., 1994; Recavarren-Arce et al., 1999; Taratuto et al., 1991; Uribe-Uribe et al., 2001]. The reasons for the high proportion of Hispanics with balamuthiasis could be because of genetic susceptibility or environmental or sociologic factors or a combination of these factors.

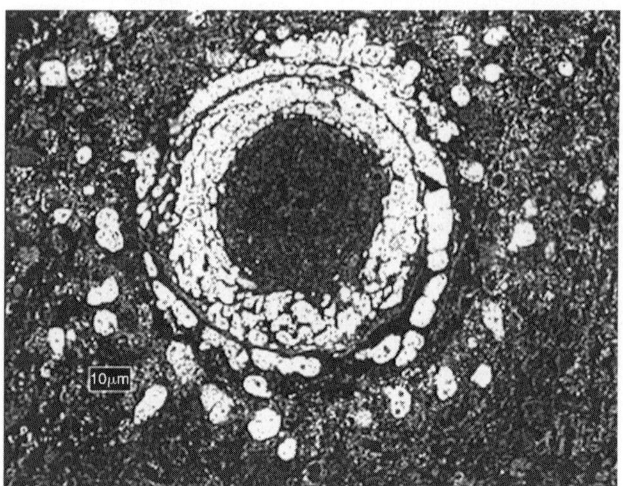

FIGURE 70-12. Indirect immunofluorescent antibody–stained section of the brain of a 3-year-old child with *Balamuthia* granulomatous encephalitis. The amebas are clustered in a pavement-like arrangement around a blood vessel. Other amebas have moved away from the perivascular region into the brain tissue. (Fluoresence microscope) (Courtesy Dr. G.S. Visvesvara.)

Clinical Characteristics, Clinical Laboratory Tests, and Diagnosis

Symptoms of *Balamuthia* granulomatous encephalitis include fever, headache, vomiting, ataxia, hemiparesis, tonic-clonic seizures, cranial nerve palsies (third and sixth cranial nerves), and diplopia [Bakardjiev et al., 2003; Martinez and Visvesvara, 2001]. Areas of the brain that are typically infected are the basal ganglia, midbrain, brainstem, and cerebral hemispheres [Martinez and Visvesvara, 1997]. Otitis media has preceded the onset of *Balamuthia* granulomatous encephalitis in several pediatric cases [Bakardjiev et al., 2003; Kodet et al., 1998; Rowen et al., 1995]. Cerebrospinal fluid may have mild to markedly elevated protein (>1000 mg/dL), and leukocyte levels but normal or slightly decreased glucose. Hydrocephalus develops in many cases [Duke et al., 1997; Kodet et al., 1998]. Because of its vague symptomatology, diagnosis of balamuthiasis requires a high index of suspicion by the physician, and differential diagnoses are bacterial or viral encephalitis, neurotuberculosis, tuberculoma, or neurocysticercosis [Bakardjiev et al., 2003]. What was initially identified as brainstem glioma in an infant was, at postmortem examination, recognized as a *Balamuthia* infection [Lowichik et al., 1995]. *Balamuthia* granulomatous encephalitis should also be considered in patients with suspected herpes simplex virus encephalitis when testing for the virus yields negative results [Deetz et al., 2003; Reed et al., 1997].

Most diagnoses of the disease are made at postmortem examination. In histopathologic sections of brain tissue, the amebas are found in large numbers within perivascular areas. Because of the chronic nature of the disease, an antibody response to *Balamuthia* develops over the course of the infection and is the basis for indirect immunofluorescent staining as a diagnostic aid. Likewise, immunohistopathology is useful for visualizing amebas in brain and other tissues. Neuroimaging is helpful in making a diagnosis [Deetz et al., 2003; Healy, 2002]; the presence of single or multiple space-occupying or ring-enhancing lesions in the brain on MRI may be indicative of balamuthiasis (Fig. 70-13). In brain and other tissue sections, the ameba is difficult to distinguish from *Acanthamoeba* because the organisms have similar morphologies. Trophic *Acanthamoeba* are somewhat smaller (~20 µm) than *Balamuthia* (~50 µm), though multiple nucleoli are sometimes seen in *Balamuthia* nuclei in situ. Both amebas form cysts in tissue, but *Balamuthia* cysts are larger (up to 30 µm) and have a wrinkled wall

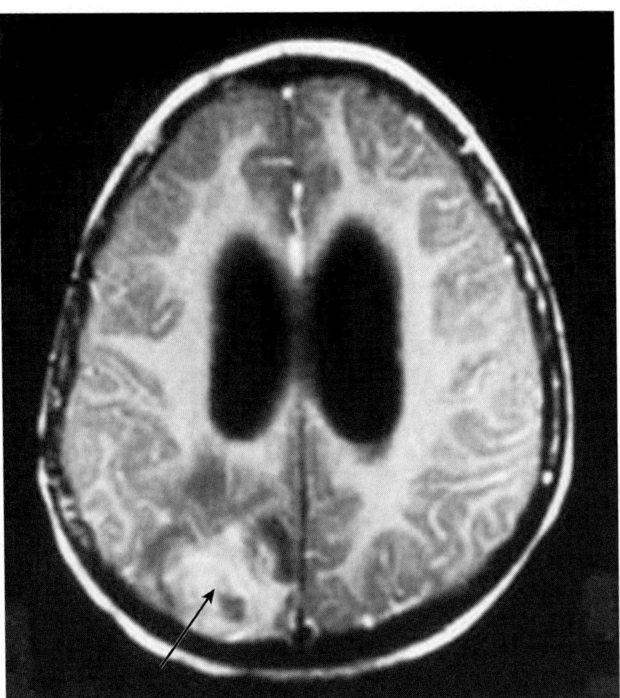

FIGURE 70-13. Magnetic resonance image of the brain of a 2 year old with *Balamuthia* amebic encephalitis. *Arrow* points to space-occupying lesion in the right occipitoparietal region of the brain.

without pores. Immunofluorescent staining, however, can distinguish between the two amebas. *Balamuthia* cannot be readily cultured from biopsied tissues because the organism grows slowly and requires tissue culture cells as a feeder layer. Attempts to culture from macerated brain tissue have taken from 10 to about 30 days at 37° C. Polymerase chain reaction technology is available for identification of *Balamuthia* DNA in tissues and in cerebrospinal fluid but is largely limited to research laboratories (e.g., the California Department of Health Services, Viral and Rickettsial Disease Laboratory, Richmond; The Ohio State University, Department of Molecular Genetics, Columbus).

Management

Of the approximately 100 recognized *Balamuthia* cases, successful outcomes have been reported in 3 individuals [Deetz et al., 2003; Jung et al, 2004], one of them a 5-year-old female. Successful therapy was based on antimicrobial combinations: flucytosine, pentamidine isethionate, fluconazole, sulfadiazine, and a macrolide antibiotic (azithromycin or clarithromycin). In vitro testing of antimicrobials on clinical isolates indicates varied sensitivity to some of the drugs. Pentamidine, however, is particularly effective against all isolates in vitro [Schuster and Visvesvara, 2004], but the drug is slow to cross the blood-brain barrier [Donnelly et al., 1988].

Other Central Nervous System Amebic Infections

A single case of encephalitis due to *Sappinia diploidea,* previously described in the feces of large herbivores but never associated with disease in humans or otherwise, has been reported from an immunocompetent adult male [Gelman et al., 2003]. A mass detected by MRI in the left temporal lobe was excised and, upon histopathologic examination, was found to contain an ameba with two closely apposed nuclei characteristic of *Sappinia*. The patient recovered after treatment with a combination of antimicrobials similar to those used for balamuthiasis. The infection had been preceded by a sinus infection, suggesting that the portal of entry into the body was the respiratory tract, with subsequent transport to the CNS. The recognition of *Sappinia* as an etiologic agent of human encephalitis suggests that it and other amebas previously regarded as innocuous might also be potential pathogens.

Other amebas have been implicated as etiologic agents of neural disease. The soil ameba, *Hartmannella,* was isolated from the cerebrospinal fluid of a patient with meningoencephalitis, but the ameba was most likely a secondary invader of an existing lesion or possibly a contaminant of clinical specimens [Centeno et al., 1996]. Because of the ubiquity of these free-living amebas, caution is advised when assigning them an etiologic role based on results from cultivation of clinical specimens.

MICROSPORIDIAL INFECTIONS OF THE NERVOUS SYSTEM

Interest in the microsporidia developed in the 19th century largely because of their role in diseases of insects. Pébrine, a disease of silkworms that threatened the industry in France, was studied by Pasteur [Cox, 2002], but the role of microsporidia as etiologic agents of human disease was only recognized in the 20th century, during the HIV/AIDS epidemic. There are about 150 genera and 1400 species, of which 8 genera and 14 species are human parasites. Host specificity for the group is low and a number of the species that infect humans also parasitize other mammals. Evidence from genome sequencing, beta-tubulin gene analysis, and similarity in the types of mitotic figures, point to fungal affinities for this group [Katinka et al., 2001; Weiss, 2003]. In humans, microsporidia are responsible for a range of infections, including diarrhea, bronchitis, sinusitis, keratitis, keratoconjunctivitis, myositis, interstitial nephritis, CNS vasculitis, and disseminated infections. They are opportunistic pathogens and the majority of these infections have been reported from HIV/AIDS patients. Cases in immunocompetent individuals are rare.

Microsporidiosis

Epidemiology, Microbiology, and Pathology

The microsporidia are obligate intracellular parasites that cause infections in invertebrates and vertebrates, including humans [Weber et al., 1994]. The life cycle consists of an infective spore stage, in which the spore may be as small as a bacterium (typically 1 to 2 μm by 2 to 5 μm), and an intracellular proliferative stage that ultimately develops into spores. On release from infected cells, spores may be found in urine, sputum, conjunctival fluid, feces, and cerebrospinal fluid, depending on the site of infection. Spores discharged in urine can contaminate ground water, which is a possible source of infection. Ingestion of spores is the most common route of infection for all species, although transplacental infection is known for nonhuman mammals, particularly carnivores [Didier and Bessinger, 1999; Weber et al., 1994]. Other routes of infection include zoonotic transmission and aerosol dispersal. Depending on species, spore germination and discharge occur in the presence of enterocytes, respiratory and nasal epithelial cells, corneal epithelial cells or stroma, and macrophages as primary sites of infection. Infection may be secondarily spread to the kidneys and the CNS by macrophages.

Clinical Characteristics, Clinical Laboratory Tests, and Diagnosis

Human microsporidial infections of the neural system occur principally in HIV/AIDS adults. Pediatric cases are rare. The first recognized case of human microsporidiosis was in a 9-year-old Japanese male with severe headache, vomiting, and convulsions, and was suspected of having Japanese encephalitis or epilepsy (Matsubayashi et al., 1959). *Toxoplasma*-like bodies were seen in cerebrospinal fluid following staining and were also observed in the urine. The infection was transferable to mice by intraperitoneal injection of the patient's cerebrospinal fluid, urine, or blood. Based on morphologic distinctions from *Toxoplasma,* the infective agent was tentatively identified as *Encephalitozoon* sp. The child, who had been treated for toxoplasmosis with penicillin and sulfisoxazole, recovered. The child lived on a farm and had contact with a variety of farm animals, and an animal reservoir is likely to have been the source of the infection. In another case of apparent zoonotic transmission, an adult male HIV/AIDS patient infected with *Encephalitozoon cuniculi*, a species found in rabbits, had handled rabbits while living on a farm [Weber et al., 1997].

Diagnosis of infections is by microscopic examination of tissues or body fluids [Weber et al., 1999]. The Gram and Giemsa stains are good for detection of spores, as is hematoxylin-eosin staining. Spores are gram-positive (purple) or stain blue with Giemsa. The polarization microscope is helpful in visualizing spores because of their birefringence due to the presence of chitin in the spore wall. Body fluids (urine, cerebrospinal fluid) containing spores can be inoculated into tissue culture monolayers for cultivation of the parasite [Visvesvara et al., 1999; Weber and Canning, 1999]. Definitive identification of microsporidial species is done by electron microscopy or polymerase chain reaction, or both. Magnetic resonance imaging reveals multiple ring-enhancing lesions in the brain. A comprehensive review of techniques for identification of microsporidia in clinical specimens is available [Garcia, 2002].

A child from Colombia who was adopted by a Swedish family developed convulsions. Serologic studies detected the presence of immunoglobulin G and immunoglobulin M antibodies against *E. cuniculi* [Bergquist et al., 1984]. Examination and staining of sediment from his urine revealed small bodies, either dispersed or in aggregates. The infection was transferable to mice by intraperitoneal injection of the bodies or to cultures of canine kidney cells. The child was successfully treated with carbamazepine and an anticonvulsive drug, and, aside from later minor arthritic symptoms that may have been sequelae of the microsporidial infection, remained in good health.

A 9-year-old black female with congenital HIV/AIDS and a CNS tumor developed tonic-clonic seizures and died after 8 days in the hospital [Yachnis et al., 1996]. Her symptoms, before hospitalization, included aphasia, hallucinations, inability to walk, and reduced consciousness. A CT scan exhibited multiple lesions in the cortical gray matter and at the gray-white junction. At postmortem examination, necrotic lesions were found in the cerebral cortex, cerebellum, pons, and medulla. Macrophages and astrocytes in histopathologic sections were filled with spores located in vesicles. Free spores released from destroyed cells were seen in the perivascular spaces. Spores were recognized in hematoxylin-eosin sections, in Gram- and Giemsa-stained preparations, and by polarization microscopy, and were later identified as *Trachipleistophora anthropophthera*.

Management

Albendazole and other benzamidazoles, such as ebendazole and thiabendazole, are currently the recommended antimicrobials for treatment of microsporidiosis, although they may not be effective against mature spores [Weber et al., 2000]. The drugs act by binding to tubulin and inhibiting microsporidial divisions. Disseminated infections caused by *E. cuniculi* are treated in adults with a dose of 400 mg twice a day [Medical Letter, 2004].

APICOMPLEXAN INFECTIONS OF THE CENTRAL NERVOUS SYSTEM

Apicomplexans are parasitic protozoa that contain an organelle at the anterior end of the organism called the *apical complex*. Components of the complex aid in locomotion of the parasite and penetration into host cells by the release of enzymes. Typical organelles of locomotion such as cilia, flagella, or pseudopods are absent. The Apicomplexa contains some of the most important and destructive parasites of humans, including the agents of toxoplasmosis, malaria, and babesiosis.

Toxoplasmosis

Epidemiology, Microbiology, and Pathology

The causal agent of toxoplasmosis was described from a desert rodent, the gondi, in 1908, but it was 1923 before the association with human disease was reported, and 1937 when its role in congenital infections was recognized [Cox, 2002; Remington et al., 2001]. It then became apparent that the main threat of toxoplasmosis was during gestation. *Toxoplama gondii* is a protozoon that reproduces only after gaining access to a host cell. The organism is found worldwide in a variety of mammals and birds. Toxoplasmosis is a major public health problem in both developed and developing countries. Approximately 20% to 40% of the adult population in the United States is seropositive. Factors that increased risk of infection in the United States were foreign birth, soil-related occupation, and little or no formal education [Jones et al., 2001]. The domesticated cat, the major reservoir and definitive host of the parasite, excretes oocysts in the feces. Ingestion of the oocyst by animals and humans continues the cycle [Frenkel, 1985]. After being ingested by the host, the oocyst releases sporozoites that invade cells, either by active penetration or by phagocytosis, giving rise to rapidly reproducing trophozoites, or tachyzoites. These tachyzoites proliferate within a parasitophorous vacuole, causing lysis of the host cell and release of more tachyzoites. Tachyzoites eventually transform into slower-growing bradyzoites that form intracellular tissue cysts and may remain quiescent for years in the host, particularly in muscle and brain tissues. Cyst formation is triggered by the host's developing immune response, and the continued release of bradyzoites from tissue cysts stimulates the immune system, resulting in lasting immune protection.

Humans are infected by ingestion of raw or inadequately cooked meat (particularly pork and lamb, and, to a lesser extent, beef) containing tissue or by ingestion of oocysts shed in cat feces. Of the two possible sources of infection, undercooked meat is the more likely vehicle of transmission. Through dissemination of the parasite by tissue cysts in undercooked meats, *Toxoplasma* has effectively bypassed the need for the cat as an intermediate host, relying entirely upon food as a vehicle for direct transmission [Su et al., 2003]. Bradyzoites, either free or within tissue cysts, are resistant to pepsin and trypsin digestion, whereas tachyzoites can withstand trypsin, but less so pepsin, and are destroyed in the stomach. Transfusion of whole blood from asymptomatic carriers can also serve as a mode of transmission. Reactivation of a latent infection can be triggered by the host becoming immunodeficient or immunocompromised.

Studies of the *Toxoplasma* genome have revealed a clonal structure of the populations with recognition of three different genotypic patterns: types I, II, and III [Dardé, 2004; Howe and Sibley, 1995]. These have different virulence phenotypes, host specificity, and geographic distribution. Type I parasites are highly virulent for mice but rare in humans; type II is the type most commonly detected in humans and some domestic animals (pigs, sheep) with low virulence for mice; and type III is usually encountered in wild animals and some human populations with intermediate virulence [Dardé, 2004]. Type I parasites, however, have been detected in cases of congenital toxoplasmosis, suggesting that the virulence phenotype may also be expressed in humans [Fuentes et al., 2001].

Intrauterine or congenital toxoplasmosis may develop in the fetus if the mother is infected during pregnancy. The placenta is invaded by parasites from the maternal circulatory system that eventually pass into fetal circulation. Infection may be asymptomatic in the mother; however, the fetus develops a generalized infection involving spleen, liver, eyes, and CNS [Desmonts and Couvreur, 1974; Lowichik and Siegel, 1995]. The incidences of maternal and fetal infection in the United States are 6 and 2 per 1000, respectively [Wilson and Remington, 1992]. The risk of fetal infection increases as the pregnancy progresses: 25% in the first trimester, 54% in the second trimester, and 65% in the third trimester. However, severity of infection is inversely related to when infection occurs during pregnancy. When disseminated, acquired toxoplasmosis produces systemic manifestations consisting of multiple organ infection, including the brain. Calcium is deposited in necrotic cerebral lesions; cerebral calcification is often seen in CT or MRI scans and plain radiographs of neonates (Fig. 70-14).

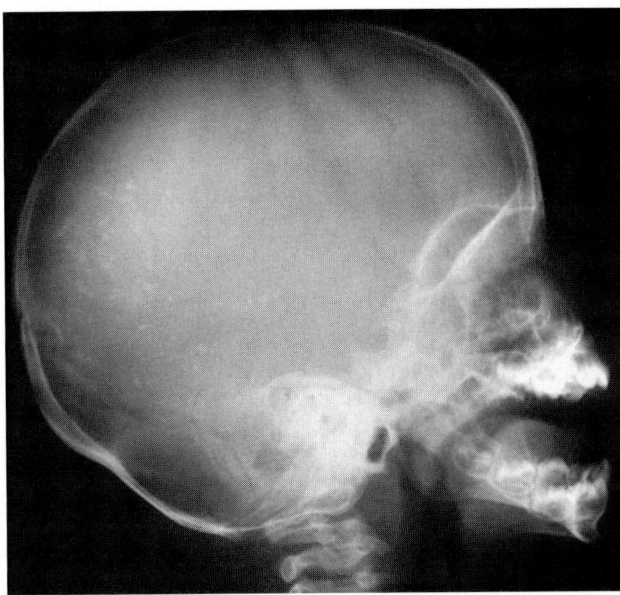

FIGURE 70-14. Toxoplasmosis. Radiograph of infant skull demonstrates fine intracranial calcifications.

Postmortem examination of brain tissue in the congenital form of the disease reveals pseudocysts or the organism itself. Severe fibrosis of the meninges develops with resultant thickening. The cortex contains many regions of encephalomalacia. Hydrocephalus occurs often. Microscopic study demonstrates that the numerous lesions comprise large or small granulomas accompanied by glial proliferation and inflammatory infiltrate; areas of nonspecific necrosis are usually present. Giemsa staining delineates the parasite. The acquired form of toxoplasmosis causes meningoencephalitis and pathologic changes similar to those associated with the congenital form (i.e., necrosis, cyst formation) [Townsend et al., 1975].

Long-term sequelae are common. The approximate incidence of abnormalities in 180 cases of intrauterine toxoplasmosis was as follows: microcephaly (20%), hydrocephalus (25%), microphthalmia (35%), seizures (40%), psychomotor retardation (45%), cerebral calcification (60%), and chorioretinitis (95%) [Feldman, 1969]. More recent studies have reported similar percentages [Lowichik and Siegel, 1995; Wilson and Remington, 1992]. Approximately 80% to 90% of survivors of overt congenital toxoplasmosis have mental retardation, cerebral palsy, epilepsy, or visual impairment [Stern et al., 1969]. Asymptomatic congenital toxoplasmosis may be associated with minimal intellectual impairment. Although the manifestations of some cases have been similar to those of congenital cytomegalic inclusion disease, CNS involvement is usually more common and extensive in toxoplasmosis. Hydrocephalus with a tense or bulging fontanel, vomiting, a high-pitched cry, and opisthotonic posturing may dominate the neonatal period (Fig. 70-15). Skull radiographs and ultrasound document punctate, scattered calcifications and separated cranial sutures. Hydranencephaly rather than hydrocephalus has been reported [Altshuler, 1973], as has infantile diabetes insipidus [Silver and Dixon, 1954] and growth hormone deficiency [Massa et al., 1989]. Delayed onset with hydrocephalus, seizures, chorioretinitis, and mental retardation can also occur [Miller et al., 1971]. Up to 85% of children

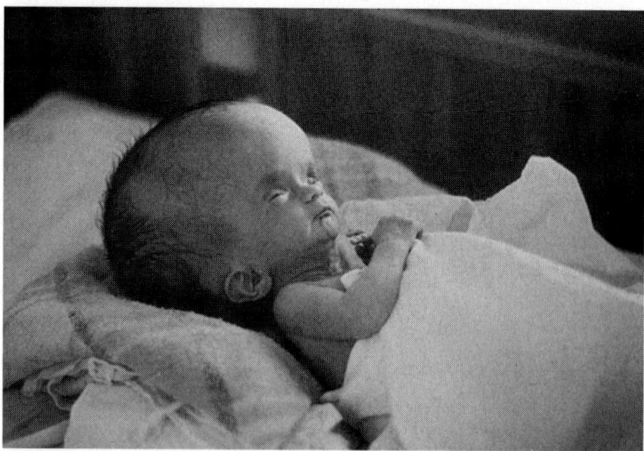

FIGURE 70-15. Hydrocephalus in congenital toxoplasmosis.

with congenital toxoplasmosis will develop retinal and choroidal involvement [Wilson et al., 1980]. Lesions initially are edematous with hemorrhage, and a yellowish exudate gives rise to areas of peripheral irregular hyperpigmentation with a pale atrophic center. Even in those infants with toxoplasmosis who are asymptomatic at birth, up to 85% may develop chorioretinitis or serious neurologic disability by 8.3 years [Wilson et al., 1980]. Toxoplasmosis in the fetus and newborn is reviewed by Remington and colleagues [2001], and methods for diagnosis of the disease are discussed by Wilson and McAuley [1999] and Wilson and associates [2002].

Clinical Characteristics, Clinical Laboratory Tests, and Diagnosis

There have been reports of disseminated generalized toxoplasmosis after immunosuppressive therapy in patients receiving transplantation [Ghatak et al., 1970; Khan and Correa, 1997; Seong et al., 1993] and, to a lesser extent, in those with malignancy [Israelski and Remington, 1993]. Immunodeficiency can lead to reactivation of dormant tissue cysts and the release of bradyzoites. Meningoencephalitis, often fatal, is a major complication. Optic neuritis has also been reported in children [Roach et al., 1985]. Although cerebral toxoplasmosis is an important complication of AIDS in adults [Bertoli et al., 1995], it is not common in neonates or older children [Lowichik and Ruff, 1995a; Miller and Remington, 1990]. When present, children appear to have similar clinical and neuroimaging findings (although less severe) than adults. Maternal HIV infection appears to reactivate a latent toxoplasmosis, which can be transmitted to the fetus. These infants with both HIV and toxoplasmosis usually present at 3 to 4 months of age with similar symptoms as those seen in infants with severe intrauterine toxoplasmosis infection [Lowichik and Ruff, 1995a]. Neuroimaging studies in infants with both infections are similar to those in infants with just toxoplasmosis. Overall, MRI appears more sensitive in detecting lesions than CT. However, in older patients, it is frequently difficult to correlate neuroimaging abnormalities in gray-white matter regions or basal ganglia with either infection or the presence of lymphoma [Ciricillo and Rosenblum, 1990]. This subject has recently been reviewed, and there are recommended treatment protocols for children infected with HIV and CNS toxoplasmosis [Khan and Correa, 1997].

Immunologic diagnosis of toxoplasmosis relies on the Sabin-Feldman dye test (which detects live parasites), the direct hemagglutination test, the double-sandwich enzyme-linked immunosorbent assay, the immunosorbent agglutination assay, the complement fixation test, the evaluation of immunoglobulin M levels, and the indirect fluorescent antibody test. Comparative information on commercially available kits for detecting immunoglobulin M in serum samples is available [Wilson et al., 1997]. The antibody test may be the most dependable, but the hemagglutination test is used most often (see Table 70-2). Examination of body fluids for parasites is problematic. Body fluids or macerated or digested tissue samples (with trypsin or pepsin), if inoculated into mice, can produce symptoms within 5 to 10 days [Wilson and McAuley, 1999]. Tissue cultures (human embryonic fibroblasts) inoculated with similar materials will exhibit cell destruction by parasites in about a week [Remington et al., 2001]. Prenatal diagnosis of congenital toxoplasmosis with a polymerase chain reaction test on amniotic fluid is possible and cost effective [Hohlfeld et al., 1994; Sahai and Onyett, 1996].

Neospora caninum is a parasite related to *Toxoplasma* that causes encephalitis and abortion in cattle and has been transmitted to monkeys. It has a similar pathology and clinical course as *Toxoplasma*. The dog, which passes oocysts in its feces, is the definitive host of the parasite rather than the cat. In a California population sample of more than 1000 humans tested for *Neospora* antibodies, approximately 7% tested positive by indirect fluorescent antibody staining, raising the possibility that some cases diagnosed as toxoplasmosis may, in reality, be neosporosis [Tranas et al., 1999]. A polymerase chain reaction technique has been developed to distinguish between the two parasites [Kaufmann et al, 1996].

Management

The value of therapy for congenital toxoplasmosis has recently been demonstrated. Early treatment with spiramycin for the mother and sulfadiazine, pyrimethamine, and folinic acid for the infant is beneficial and 70% effective [Lowichik and Siegel, 1995; Roizen et al., 1995; Wilson and Remington, 1992]. In the acquired form of the disease, treatment is required. Again, sulfadiazine, pyrimethamine, and folinic acid (to counteract the folate-inhibiting effects of pyrimethamine) are most effective [Jones, 1979; Remington, 2001]. Duration of treatment, usually for 2 to 6 weeks after signs and symptoms have resolved, will depend on the severity of infection and the immunologic status of the patient. In the immunocompromised patient or in those patients whose symptoms do not resolve or recur, treatment for up to 1 year may be necessary [Mitchell et al., 1990].

Malaria

Epidemiology, Microbiology, and Pathology

Malaria is caused by protozoal parasites of the genus *Plasmodium* with life cycle stages alternating between the mosquito and a variety of mammals and birds. Several species of *Plasmodium* cause malaria in humans—*Plasmodium falciparum, Plasmodium vivax, Plasmodium malariae*—

but *P. falciparum* is the only member of the genus that affects the host's nervous system. Awareness of the disease dates back some 5000 years, with the description of malaria-like symptoms in writings from China, and later in texts from India, Sumer, Egypt, and ancient Greece [Carter and Mendis, 2002]. Hippocrates (ca. 400 BC) recognized the regular occurrence of febrile episodes of the disease, and used the terms "*quotidian*" (daily), "*tertian*" (every 3 days), and "*quartan*" (every 4 days) to characterize them. The disease derives it name from the misplaced belief that it was caused by miasmas, or "bad air." The recent sequencing of the *P. falciparum* genome presents opportunities for development of drugs and vaccines targeted to specific gene products of the parasite [Gardner et al., 2002].

As early as 1640, long before the etiologic agent was demonstrated, the therapeutic attributes of cinchona (quinine, quinidine) for treatment of malaria were generally recognized. The mainstay of current therapy is chloroquine, whose efficacy has been compromised in many parts of the world by the appearance of drug-resistant strains of the parasite. Other factors, including insecticide-resistant species of mosquitoes, ecologic and practical constraints on drainage of swamps, and limits on widespread use of insecticides, make it likely that malaria will persist as a major public health problem throughout the world. From 200 to 500 million people are affected annually, particularly in many developing tropical and subtropical regions. Children younger than 5 years of age account for about 90% of the more than 2 million deaths that occur each year. Much of the knowledge gained about pediatric malaria has come from studies of children in the nations of sub-Saharan Africa: Kenya, Zambia, Nigeria, The Gambia, Malawi, and so on, comprising some 30 different countries. Malaria acquired by recipients of blood transfusions from infected but asymptomatic carriers is also a major problem in endemic regions of the world. Because of increased international travel, increasing numbers of cases in adults and children are being recognized in the United States [Emanuel et al., 1993]. Close to 100 cases have appeared in individuals living in the vicinity of or working at airports, probably as the result of inadvertent import of mosquitoes from malarial areas of the world in airplane cabins or luggage [Lusina et al., 2000; Thang et al., 2002]. The malaria literature is voluminous and is frequently reviewed, reflecting the importance of the disease [Birbeck, 2004; Maitland and Marsh, 2004; Newton and Krishna, 1998; Newton et al., 2000; Satpathy et al., 2004].

The definitive host and vector, the female *Anopheles* mosquito, is the site of sexual reproduction of plasmodia. The mosquito injects the organism as sporozoites when it bites humans, who are the intermediate hosts; in humans the organism undergoes asexual reproduction. The hepatic cells are the first location of asexual reproduction during the pre-erythrocytic phase. Reproduction in hepatic cells is followed by release of parasites that invade erythrocytes during the prepatent period, which lasts 5 or 6 days. The erythrocytic phase, which produces merozoites by schizogony, commences subsequent to the entry of the parasite into the erythrocyte and continues synchronously for 1 to 3 weeks, which is the incubation period. In its early stages of schizogony, the parasite appears as a ringlike structure within the parasitized erythrocyte. Hemozoin, the product of hemoglobin degradation by the parasite, accumulates in the erythrocyte. Hemolysis of the parasitized blood cells is signaled by chills and fever, with synchrony and periodicity typical for the different *Plasmodium* spp. For *falciparum* (subtertian) malaria, the period is about 48 hours. In the bloodstream of the host, some merozoites differentiate into gamete precursors. When the human host is bitten, infected erythrocytes enter the mosquito carrying micro- and macrogametocytes (male and female gamete precursors), and the cycle begins anew.

The most serious consequence of *falciparum* malaria and the CNS develops when the parasitized erythrocytes lodge in the brain vasculature. Cerebral involvement follows binding of infected red blood cells to the microvascular endothelium. Sequestration and hemolysis follow and cause obstruction of blood vessels [Sein et al., 1993]. Parasite-induced knobby projections on the surface of infected erythrocytes bind to the endothelial cells in brain, heart, liver, and lungs, causing capillary congestion. By attaching to the endothelial lining of blood vessels, the parasitized erythrocytes effectively avoid destruction that might otherwise occur upon passage through the spleen. This is accompanied by a change in the erythrocyte from a readily pliant state to one of rigidity, which further contributes to blood vessel occlusion. Additionally, rosette formation resulting from clustering of parasitized and nonparasitized blood cells may facilitate transfer of parasites from hemolyzed cells to uninfected red blood cells. Rosette formation can be reversed by heparin. Local hypoxia, microinfarction, necrosis, hemorrhage, and inflammation subsequently occur. The sequestration and resulting occlusion may deplete the oxygen level in cerebral vasculature, providing a more optimal environment for metabolism and replication of the parasites [Chen et al., 2000]. Thrombi may form and be associated with clotting aberrations, including disseminated intravascular coagulation [Butler et al., 1973]. The blood-brain barrier is disrupted by changes in endothelial cell junctional permeability leading to cerebral edema, more commonly encountered in children than adults [Adams et al., 2002].

A number of theories have been proposed to explain the pathology of cerebral malaria. Hypoxia is one such theory based on the impedance of blood flow to the brain and the consequent oxygen deficiency. On recovery, however, there is no evidence of neuronal damage that might be expected to occur as a result of oxygen deprivation. Another explanation is that the surge of mediators that occurs in the CNS may be responsible for the pathology of cerebral malaria [Medana et al., 2001]. Release of proinflammatory cytokines and interleukins (tumor necrosis factor-α, IL-1, IL-6, nitric oxide lymphotoxin) results in endothelial damage and mimics the clinical condition of sepsis [Clark et al., 2004; Maitland and Marsh, 2004]. Presence of malarial antigens stimulates release of tumor necrosis factor-α that, in turn, upregulates endothelial adhesion molecules and promotes attachment of parasitized erythrocytes to the vascular lining [Gimenez et al., 2003]. Once parasites are cleared from the blood, the effects of cerebral malaria are reversible and long-term sequelae generally do not develop [Adams et al., 2002]. The role of proinflammatory cytokines in malarial pathology has been reviewed by Clark and associates [2004] in the context of other infectious diseases and noninfectious conditions, and the molecular aspects of cerebral malaria have been reviewed by Chen and co-workers [2000].

Postmortem studies of gross specimens demonstrate fulminating cerebral edema and accompanying transtentorial herniation (Fig. 70-16). Congestion of arachnoid vessels causes the brain to appear pink or bright cherry red. Petechiae are evident on the cut surface. Microscopic examination reveals that small arterioles and capillaries are obstructed with parasitized erythrocytes. Mononuclear cells are readily discernible in meningeal and perivascular infiltrates. Microinfarction and ensuing multifocal necrosis and demyelination are widespread.

Clinical Characteristics, Clinical Laboratory Tests, and Diagnosis

Cerebral malaria is most often heralded by manifestations of mental deterioration, particularly confusion or delirium; further deterioration is signaled by progression to stupor and coma that transpires during the next 1 to 3 days. In children, cerebral involvement is more fulminant, with most becoming comatose within 2 days [Molyneux et al., 1989]. Early features include fever, anorexia, vomiting, diarrhea, and seizures, which may be confused with febrile seizures in young children [Osuntokun, 1977]. Severe hypoglycemia is also common. Elevated intracranial pressure occurs in fatal cases [Maitland and Marsh, 2004]. Lactic acidosis due to metabolic impairment is responsible for respiratory distress [Birbeck, 2004]. Extensor plantar responses, cerebellar impairment, abnormal movements, and psychosis may also occur [Daroff et al., 1967]. Children are more likely to have decreased tone compared with adults and impaired brainstem cranial nerve responses and abnormal respiratory function [Molyneux et al., 1989; Newton et al., 1991]. Children with severe illness exhibit evidence of transtentorial herniation [Newton et al., 1991]. Papilledema and extramacular retinal edema are markers of a poor prognosis [Lewallen et al., 1993]. The presence of impaired consciousness, prolonged seizure activity, hypoglycemia, or respiratory distress identifies those at high risk for death or long-term sequelae [Marsh et al., 1995; Steele et al., 1995]. In one study of 308 children with cerebral malaria, the mortality rate was 14%; of the survivors, 12% had significant long-term neurologic deficits, including language and motor deficits, ataxia, and cortical blindness [Bruster et al., 1990].

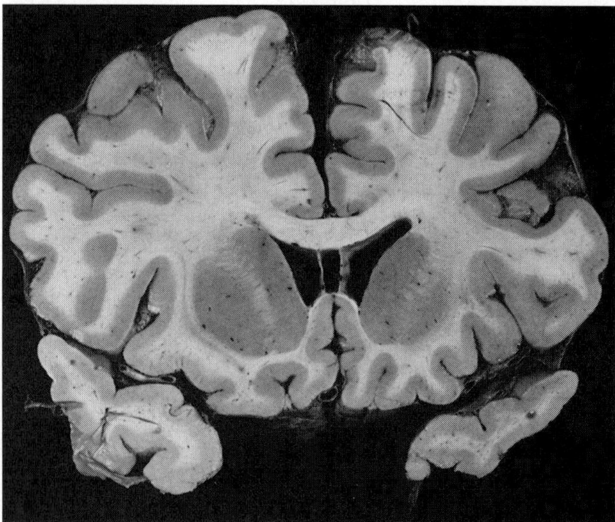

FIGURE 70-16. Cerebral malaria. Petechial hemorrhages are scattered throughout the brain.

In endemic areas such as sub-Saharan Africa, neonates are protected from infection by maternal (transplacental) immunoglobulin G and, in part, from the vestigial presence of fetal hemoglobin. Studies using transgenic mice indicate that the parasite cannot readily break down fetal hemoglobin, thus impairing intraerythrocytic development and replication [Shear et al., 1998]. This protection lasts for about 1 year, after which the infant becomes susceptible to disease. The child of 1 to 4 years of age is the most vulnerable to infection and the development of severe malaria, with a mortality of about 5%. Once this period has passed, the host and parasite exist in a state of détente, with the host exhibiting chronic asymptomatic parasitemia [Kyes et al., 2001]. Additional infections due to continued exposure to parasites from mosquito bites result either in death or the development of clinical immunity. In endemic areas, a large percentage of adults and children will be infected, but only a small number of these will go on to develop clinical disease [Kyes et al., 2001]. The immunity that develops encompasses both cellular and humoral elements. Purified immunoglobulin preparations from individuals with naturally acquired immunity have been used for protection of children from recurrent malaria infections [Sabchareon et al., 1991].

Neurologic sequelae are not uncommon in children recovering from cerebral malaria. In studies combining data on African children, sequelae develop in about 10% to 30% of patients [Birbeck, 2004; Newton and Krishna, 1998]. The occurrence of sequelae has been attributed to a number of factors, including seizures, prolonged coma, hypoglycemia, elevated intracranial pressure, and neurologic pathology. The sequelae are manifested as ataxia, epilepsy, hemiparesis, cortical blindness, impaired hearing, behavioral abnormalities, and cognitive deficits (impaired learning, reasoning, dexterity, memory, perception, etc.). In most cases, recovery occurs within weeks to 6 months, but some sequelae, such as epilepsy, may persist.

Diagnosis necessitates study of thick and thin peripheral blood films to ascertain the presence of small, ring-form trophozoites and crescent-shaped gametocytes; close scrutiny is required to ensure accuracy [Coatney et al., 1971; Lowichik and Ruff, 1995a]. In the hands of a skilled technician, thick films can detect 1 infected cell in 1000 red blood cells (0.001%), or 50 parasites/μL of blood [Moody, 2002]. Erythrocytes containing *Plasmodium* ring stages are more likely to be found in peripheral blood because the mature stages undergoing intraerythrocytic replication become sequestered in brain and other deep areas of the body. Blood smears should be prepared at 8- to 12-hour intervals, until diagnosis can be made [Birbeck, 2004]. If antimalarial therapy was started before preparation of blood smears, the smears may be negative. Polymerase chain reaction has also been used for diagnosis, with the capability of detecting 5 parasites or fewer per μL of blood a great advantage when parasites in peripheral blood samples are in low numbers. Immunochromatography in the form of a dipstick kit has also been employed for *Plasmodium* detection [Moody, 2002]. Sensitive indirect fluorescent antibody and hemagglutination tests provide further diagnostic capability [Wilson et al., 1975]. The electroencephalogram (EEG) in children with cerebral malaria reveals nonspecific generalized slowing [Molyneux et al., 1989] and may be helpful in detection of subclinical seizures that might otherwise pass unnoticed [Maitland and Marsh, 2004]. Neuroimaging may also be abnormal. Acutely, MRI may demonstrate multifocal T_2-enhancing lesions indicative of capillary occlusion and cerebral edema [Chia et al., 1992]. Computed tomography scan has been reported to demonstrate generalized and sulcal atrophy as a sequela of disease [Newton et al., 1994]. Moody [2002] has reviewed testing for malarial parasites with emphasis on methods capable of giving results in 1 hour or less.

Management

Cerebral malaria is defined as a coma without apparent etiology, inability to localize painful stimuli, and *falciparum* parasitemia as demonstrated by blood smears [Birbeck, 2004; Newton and Krishna, 1998; Warrell et al., 1982]. A coma is assessed on the basis of the Balantyre or Glasgow coma scales, taking into account eye movements and motor and verbal abilities. The scales may be of greater value in predicting mortality rather than as a diagnostic tool [Newton and Krishna, 1998].

In the management of malaria there are two considerations. One is treating an uncomplicated case of *falciparum* parasitemia, preventing it from developing into life-threatening, fulminant malaria. If the patient has already progressed to cerebral malaria, the second consideration goes beyond the use of antimalarial drugs and requires measures to treat deep coma, elevated intracranial pressure, hypovolemia, metabolic imbalance, anemia, convulsions, and other manifestations that accompany this often fatal phase of the disease.

The chemoprophylaxis and therapy of malaria are major areas of complexity. Excellent review articles are available and should be consulted when appropriate [Birbeck, 2004]. Chloroquine, primaquine, and quinine remain the mainstays of both prophylaxis and therapy. However, because of the increasing prevalence of chloroquine-resistant strains of malaria in Southeast Asia, Africa, and South America, quinidine gluconate as a continuous infusion is currently recommended (in combination with doxycycline, tetracycline, and sulfadoxine-pyrimethamine) as the agent of choice for severe *P. falciparum* infection [Jotte and Scott, 1993; Medical Letter, 2004; Phillips et al., 1985]. The clinician should be aware of side effects and obvious toxic reactions, particularly hypoglycemia and cardiac dysrhythmias, before administration. Trial administration to determine individual reactions to the drugs is recommended before long-term, large-dose therapy is instituted [Randall and Seidel, 1985]. Most patients will respond within 72 hours to intravenous quinidine and should then be switched to oral administration for an additional 3 to 7 days [CDC, 1991; Molyneux et al., 1989].

Iron chelation therapy with deferoxamine has been found to hasten the clearance of parasitemia and enhance the recovery from deep coma in Zambian children with cerebral malaria [Goerduk et al., 1992]. However, survival rates of parasitemic-comatose Zambian children treated with deferoxamine plus quinine, or placebo plus quinine were compared and no difference was reported between the two groups [Thuma et al., 1998]; children in the deferoxamine-treated group showed a somewhat higher mortality. Deferoxamine may act by binding iron and withholding it from the parasite, or by formation of toxic complexes leading to free radical production and intracellular destruction of the parasite [Mabeza et al., 1999]. Other studies point to a third mechanism of action; the chelating agent may act on interferon-γ (IFN-γ) nitric oxide, and reactive oxygen intermediates [Fritsche et al., 2001]. Nitric oxide in particular may, through interaction with IFN-γ, activate macrophages to reduce parasitemia. Alternately, nitric oxide may contribute to the pathology of cerebral malaria by causing vasodilation and increased intracranial pressure. The use of iron chelation therapy for malaria has been reviewed [Mabeza et al., 1999].

The Chinese medicinal herb qinghao *(Artemisia annua)*, also known as annual or sweet wormwood, has been used since antiquity to treat malaria. Recent efforts to understand its chemistry and pharmacology have been very fruitful. The plant yields a sesquiterpene compound called qinghaosu or artemisinin, which is active against plasmodium. Artemisinin and its derivatives have been found to cure malaria with much less toxicity than quinoline antimalarials [Hien and White, 1993], and resistance to artemisinin has not yet been encountered. Artemisinin is also effective against the gametocyte stage in the bloodstream (the stage taken up by the mosquito), thereby reducing disease transmission in malaria-endemic areas. To further lessen the chance of emergence of drug resistance, artemisinin has been coupled with other differently acting drugs in artemisinin-combination therapy [Adjuik et al., 2004]. Artemether (arthemeter), artesunate, and arteether are artemisinin derivatives that have been effective when used in combination with a second drug (e.g., artesunate-mefloquine) [Ashley, 2004; Olliaro and Taylor, 2004]. Arthemeter and artesunate, however, are not available in the United States [Birbeck, 2004].

Among other antimalarials, atovaquone-proguanil (Malarone or Malarone Pediatric) is used in areas where chloroquine resistance has been encountered [Medical Letter, 2004]. Sulfadoxine-pyrimethamine (Fansidar) has been widely used, but drug resistance is encountered, particularly in Southeast Asia and east Africa [Olliario and Taylor, 2004]. Mefloquine and quinine (available in the United States as quinidine) are other mainstays of the malaria pharmacopeia. Fosmidomycin is a phosphonic acid derivative that specifically targets a metabolic pathway in the apicoplast of malarial parasites, but not in human cells. It has been effective and is well tolerated in the treatment of uncomplicated *falciparum* malaria [Missinou et al., 2002]. The combination of chlorproguanil-dapsone (Lapdap) has been tested against sulfadoxine-pyrimethamine in treatment of uncomplicated malaria and was found to be more effective [Alloueche et al., 2004]. Halofantrine has also been used against resistant *falciparum* malaria. When given at high dosages (8 mg/kg q8h for 3 days for a total of 72 mg/kg), halofantrine compared favorably with mefloquine (25 mg/kg for one day) in treating multidrug-resistant *falciparum* malaria [Ter Kuile et al., 1993]. The drug, however, has demonstrated cardiotoxicity. Recent reviews of antimalarials emphasize increasing drug resistance and decreasing options for treatment [Kain, 1996; Ter Kuile et al., 1993; White, 1996]. The topic of antimicrobial treatment of *falciparum* malaria has been reviewed by Winstanley and colleagues [2004].

In cerebral malaria, the focus shifts from treating an infectious disease to dealing with a medical emergency. Fluid and electrolyte balance have to be restored or managed. This includes hypovolemia (remedied by hydration with saline), hypoglycemia (50% dextrose intravenously), hyponatremia and hypokalemia (hydration with saline), renal failure (peritoneal dialysis), and elevated intracranial pressure. Dexamethasone, used to relieve intracranial pressure, was found to be no better than a placebo in Thai patients (6 to 70 years); it prolongs coma, leads to complications, and is usually contraindicated [Warrell et al., 1982]. Neither heparin nor dextran has been shown to be beneficial in reducing intracranial pressure by lowering blood viscosity [Newton and Krishna, 1998]. Mannitol or glycerol can reduce intracranial pressure by creating an osmotic gradient across the blood-brain barrier and drawing fluid into the vascular system. Pentoxifylline, which acts as a vasodilator, reduces blood viscosity and reduces tumor necrosis factor-α and may be helpful in treating intracranial pressure, but additional controlled studies are needed to establish its efficacy [Birbeck, 2004; Newton and Krishna, 1998].

Fever can be controlled with antipyretics (acetaminophen, ibuprofen, aspirin). Blood problems include severe anemia (remedied by exchange transfusion), lactic acidosis (hydration, restoration of normal glucose level, improved oxygenation), and parasite load (transfusion to reduce parasitemia). Convulsions are treated with lorazepam, diazepam, and paraldehyde; recurrent seizures can be treated with phenytoin, fosphenytoin, and phenobarbital [Birbeck, 2004]. Because cerebral malaria can mimic bacterial meningitis, a lumbar puncture to obtain cerebrospinal fluid for cultivation may be advised. Caution, however, should be exercised due to the elevated intracranial pressure. Cerebrospinal fluid in cerebral malaria is clear, with protein ranging to a high of 0.4 g/L (400 mg/dL); septic cerebrospinal fluid is cloudy, with neutrophils comprising about 99% of leukocytes and protein ranging from approximately 1 to 3 g/L (1000 to 3000 mg/dL). Emergency measures for treatment of severe malaria have been described in several reviews [Birbeck, 2004; Maitland and Marsh, 2004; Newton and Krishna, 1998].

A vaccine for the prevention of malaria has yet to be realized, although several promising clinical trials are being conducted [Moorthy et al., 2004; Webster and Hill, 2003]. Development of an effective vaccine has been hampered by the presence of different stage-specific antigens displayed during the complex life cycle of the parasite. Of the 5300 genes present in the *P. falciparum* genome, approximately 4% are involved in immune evasion, including antigenic variation [Gardner et al., 2002]. Thus, it is likely that an effective vaccine will have to contain a combination of antigens able to protect against the infective sporozoite stage, the erythrocytic stage, and the transmissive gametocyte (sexual) stage. The role of antigenic variation in pathology of *falciparum* malaria has been reviewed by Kyes and associates [2001].

Babesiosis

Babesia is the etiologic agent of babesiosis, a malaria-like tick-borne disease occurring in many species of wild and domestic animals, and occasionally humans. The organism was named for Viktor Babès, who first recognized it in blood cells of cattle in the 19th century, but it was not until 1957 that the first human infection was recognized. Babesiosis is a zoonotic disease transmitted to humans from rodents and other mammals. The parasites are contained within erythrocytes and are transmitted by ixodid (hard-bodied) ticks. Human-to-human transmission can occur through blood transfusion [Gerber et al., 1994]. Unlike *Plasmodium* spp., *Babesia* does not have an exoerythrocytic stage, divides in the erythrocyte by binary fission rather than schizogony, develops within the cytoplasm of the host cell and not in a parasitophorous vacuole, and does not form hemozoin pigment from hemoglobin as do the malaria parasites. Two species of *Babesia* are important in human disease: *Babesia microti* from rodents and *Babesia divergens* from bovines. *B. microti* is the species present in the United States, whereas *B. divergens* is found in Europe. Of the two species, *B. divergens* is the more virulent with 42% mortality, compared with 5% mortality for *B. microti* [Gorenflot et al., 1998]. In the northeastern and upper midwestern United States, the transmission cycle of *B. microti* overlaps that of another well-known zoonotic agent, *Borrelia burgdorferi,* the causative agent of borreliosis, or Lyme disease [Persing and Conrad, 1995], which is reviewed in Chapter 68. Most cases of human infections have involved elderly adults [Meldrum et al, 1992]. Asplenic individuals are also at higher risk for infection; splenectomy predisposed four adult males to infection (two died) in a mini-epidemic in northern California [Persing et al., 1995]. Human infections on the West Coast of the United States have been due to *Babesia*-like parasites (the WA-1 strain, after a strain first detected in Washington state) that defy classification as either *B. microti* or *B. divergens,* and may be related to *Babesia* spp. from canines and rodents [Quick et al., 1993]. Other unusual strains have been isolated in northern California, Missouri, and Wisconsin.

Clinical Characteristics, Clinical Laboratory Tests, and Diagnosis

Clinical manifestations consist of a persistent fever, sweating, chills, myalgia, and mildly to moderately severe hemolytic anemia. Emotional depression has been reported, but severe neurologic symptoms are rare. *Babesia* in bovines can cause encephalitis, as does *P. falciparum* in humans. Parasitized red blood cells adhere to the endothelial lining of brain capillaries, thus evading destruction in the spleen [O'Connor et al., 1999; Wright et al., 1989].

Babesiosis should be suspected in patients who have spent time in tick-infested areas, had recent blood transfusions, or have undergone splenectomy [Homer et al., 2000]. The diagnosis is made by identification of the organism on thick and thin blood smears, but only if the parasitemia is high. In blood smears, the organism can be mistaken for the malaria parasite, but infected erythrocytes lack the malaria-characteristic hemozoin pigment (Fig. 70-17). Inoculation of hamsters with suspect blood samples is useful in cases with low parasitemia but may require weeks for the disease to develop. However, the development of indirect fluorescent antibody assays and the polymerase chain reaction provide more sensitive detection of the parasitemia asso-

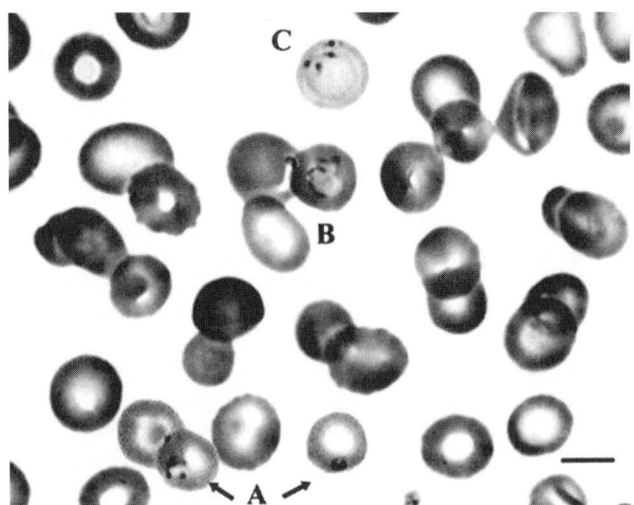

FIGURE 70-17. Blood film showing human erythrocytes, some of which are infected with *Babesia*. Although different in morphology, *Babesia* can be mistaken for *Plasmodium* in infected cells. The varied forms of the parasites can be seen: A, ring forms; B, ameboid shape; C, tetrad configuration. Bar in micrograph represents 10 μm. (Giemsa stain) (Courtesy Dr. Anne Kjemptrup. From Schuster, FL. Clin Microbiol Rev 2002;15:365. Copyright © 2002, the American Society of Microbiology. 2002.)

ciated with babesiosis [Homer et al., 2000; Pruthi et al., 1995]. Serologic confirmation of infection has been determined in asymptomatic children [Ruebush et al., 1977]. Cross-reactivity with *Plasmodium* surface antigens has been reported [Gorenflot et al., 1998].

Management

Babesiosis was described in a neonate whose mother had been bitten by a tick 1 week before giving birth [Esernio-Jenssen et al., 1987]. Treatment with clindamycin and quinine was successful in effecting recovery. Two other cases of babesiosis in pregnancy were reported; in both, the pregnancies went to term and the infants were unaffected [Feder et al., 2003; Raucher et al., 1984].

Atovaquone (for pediatric patients 20 mg/kg twice a day for 7 to 10 days) plus azithromycin (12 mg/kg daily for 7 to 10 days) are the drugs of choice in treating babesiosis [Medical Letter, 2004], with clindamycin (20 to 40 mg/kg/day orally in three doses for 7 days) plus quinine (25 mg/kg/day orally in three doses for 7 days) as alternatives [Medical Letter, 2004]. Chloroquine therapy has been ineffective [Miller et al., 1978]. In seriously ill patients, exchange transfusion in combination with the above medications was reported to be efficacious, presumably by reducing the acute parasitic load [Doan-Wiggins, 1991]. Homer and colleagues [2000] have prepared a comprehensive review of the organism and of the disease.

TRYPANOSOMAL INFECTIONS OF THE NERVOUS SYSTEM

The trypanosomes are a group of flagellated protozoa defined by the presence of the kinetoplast, a DNA-containing organelle. The parasites have morphologically distinct life cycle stages based on the length of the flagellum and the location of the kinetoplast with respect to the nucleus. They infect a variety of vertebrates but the clinically important species for humans are *Trypanosoma cruzi* (Chagas' disease or American trypanosomiasis) and *Trypanosoma brucei* (African sleeping sickness). Both species are transmitted to humans by insect vectors.

Chagas' Disease

Chagas' disease (American trypanosomiasis) is a public health problem in Latin America, from Argentina to the Mexican border with the United States. It is a disease of poverty, with the poor bearing the brunt of the disease. The disease has also crossed into the United States, mostly in the southern tier, because of immigration from Latin America, where 8% of the population is seropositive. As a result, more than 50,000 to 100,000 people living in the United States have been infected [Kirchoff, 1993]. Acute Chagas' disease occurs primarily in childhood and usually is mild [Cegielski and Durack, 1997].

The source of infection is the triatomine bug (*Triatoma* spp.), which lives in walls and roofs of houses. The disease occurs mainly in rural areas, although population movements to the cities have shifted the disease to an urban setting. Humans, cats, dogs, and other mammals serve as reservoirs from which the vector acquires the parasite. The parasite is found in the midgut and rectum of the insect. At the time the triatomine bug bites a human, it defecates on the skin surface, leaving a drop containing parasites. The parasite penetrates the broken skin when the presumptive host scratches or rubs the deposited fecal matter into the site of the insect bite, or when fecal matter is transferred by fingers onto the corneal surface of the eye or mucous membranes. Inflammation develops at the portal of entry of the trypanosomes, producing a nodule (chagoma), and causing swelling of proximal lymph nodes. Initially in the bloodstream of the host, the parasite enters macrophages and other cell types, in which replication occurs. Pseudocysts filled with trypanosomes can be found in muscle tissue. Upon lysis of the infected host cell, new cells are attacked, with some parasites entering the bloodstream, where they are acquired by the bug when it takes a blood meal. The disease can also be passed by transplacental infection or through breast-feeding, though data to distinguish this route from intrauterine transmission are not available. Blood transfusions are another source of infection in endemic areas where the blood supply is not monitored for trypanosomes.

Clinical Characteristics, Clinical Laboratory Tests, and Diagnosis

Chagas' disease in childhood can arise either as a result of congenital infection or after being bitten by the insect vector. Intrauterine Chagas' disease occurs in 2% to 4% of infants born to mothers who have acute or chronic infection with *T. cruzi* [Lowichik and Ruff, 1995a]. Such infants are usually born prematurely and are small for gestational age. Systemic symptoms are similar to other intrauterine infections and include jaundice, hepatosplenomegaly, edema, petechiae, and dysrhythmias. When meningoencephalitis is present, seizures, hypotonia, and a weak suck are characteristically present [Bittencourt, 1976]. Almost half the infants who acquire infection in utero die by age 4 months. Unilateral orbital edema is frequently present and characteristic of the disease. Lymphadenopathy, vomiting, diarrhea, and cardiac symptoms suggestive of myocarditis and dysrythmias may be present. Signs of a generalized encephalopathy with meningeal irritation and, occasionally, seizures may occur. After a latent period, more chronic forms of Chagas' disease develop, manifested by cardiovascular (cardiomyopathy) and gastrointestinal (megaesophagus and megacolon) involvement. Without treatment, infection with *T. cruzi* is lifelong.

The disease is fulminant in children younger than 5 years but chronic in adults. Neuropathologic characteristics include leptomeningeal mononuclear infiltration, cerebral edema, and other abnormalities similar to those present in African trypanosomiasis [Pentreath, 1995; Pitella, 1993]. Parasitic nodules may be evident throughout the brain and spinal cord.

T. cruzi can be isolated from cerebrospinal fluid in up to 75% of adult Chagas' patients, but there is no evidence of overt CNS clinical symptoms [Cegielski and Durack, 1997]. Rarely, a fulminant meningoencephalitis will occur and be fatal. In a series of 11 children with CNS infection from Chagas' disease, *T. cruzi* was isolated from the spinal fluid in 8 [Hoff et al., 1978]. Spasticity, mental deficiency, and cerebellar symptoms are sequelae of meningoencephalitis. Peripheral neuropathy is observed in chronic American trypanosomiasis. Stroke may complicate chronic cardiomyopathy [Spina-Franca, 1996]. The scarcity of parasites in the host and the severe nature of the disease have led to the suggestion that the pathology of the disease may be due to an autoimmune response caused by cross-reactivity between human antigens and *T. cruzi* [Brener, 1994].

The diagnosis of Chagas' disease is made by culture, direct microscopy, or histologic detection of *T. cruzi* in the blood, cerebrospinal fluid, or tissue obtained from brain biopsy. Serology is useful for diagnosis of neonatal Chagas' disease, but can also be misleading due to the presence of maternal antibodies in circulation. Positive serology in the absence of parasitemia and symptoms is probably due to antibody cross-reactivity. Cerebrospinal fluid reveals a monocytic pleocytosis with protein elevation. Neuroimaging studies may reveal nonspecific ring-enhancing lesions seen with many CNS infections [Leiguarda et al., 1990]. No EEG abnormalities were seen in children with Chagas' disease, although temporary irregularities appeared [Moya, 1994]. Sequence data on the *T. cruzi* genome are now available, which may lead to future attempts at intervention at specific genic targets [El-Sayed et al., 2005b].

Management

The intracellular location of the parasite protects it from most drug therapy. Nifurtimox (for 1 to 10 yrs: 15 to 20 mg/kg/day in four doses for 90 days), available through the CDC, is used for the treatment of Chagas' disease [Medical Letter, 2004]. Benznidazole (for ages up to 12 years, 10 mg/kg/day in two doses for 30 to 90 days) is an alternative drug [Medical Letter, 2004]. Nifurtimox has been associated with a higher risk of chromosomal abnormalities, suggesting that alternative medications might be better. Allopurinol has been found to be as effective as nifurtimox or benznidazole in treating *T. cruzi* infection at a dose of 300 mg two or three times a day for 60 days [Gallerano et al., 1990].

Resistance to the basic drug therapy is a concern, and there is interest in finding or developing new drugs that are effective in treatment of Chagas' disease. Itraconazole [McCabe et al., 1986] and ketoconazole [McCabe et al., 1987] were effective against *T. cruzi* in a mouse model of disease, but no trials have been conducted in humans. Ketoconazole combined with benznidazole demonstrated synergism when tested in the mouse model, but different strains of parasites exhibited variability in response to the drugs [Araújo et al., 2000]. Miltefosine (hexadecylphosphocholine), a phospholipid analog and anticancer drug that has been used with success in treatment of visceral leishmaniasis [Sundar et al., 2002], has been tested in vitro against intracellular stages of *T. cruzi* and has promise as an antimicrobial [Croft et al., 2003; de Castro et al., 2004]. Alkylphosphocholines, including miltefosine, in combination with ketoconazole, had in vitro activity against *T. cruzi* [Lira et al., 2001].

African Sleeping Sickness

Epidemiology, Microbiology, and Pathology

Bruce and Nabarro [1903] reported the trypanosomal etiology of African sleeping sickness and its tsetse fly vector. *Trypanosoma brucei gambiense* is often the organism isolated in patients from western and central Africa (Fig. 70-18). *Trypanosoma brucei rhodesiense* infections occur in eastern and southern Africa. In the 1960s, the disease was kept in

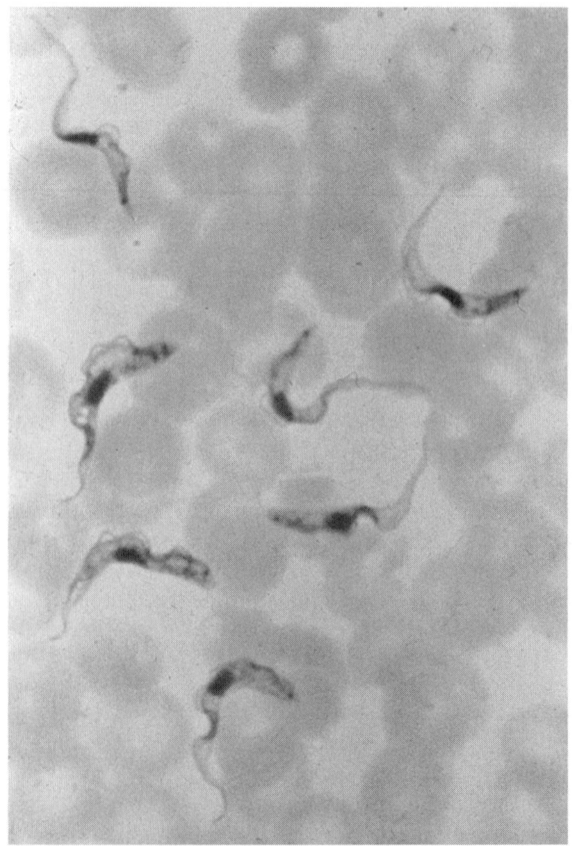

FIGURE 70-18. *Trypanosoma gambiense* in peripheral blood. (Leishman stain)

check through surveillance and insect control. The past several decades in Africa have witnessed civil strife, population shifts, development of disease-resistant trypanosomes, and inadequate funding of programs to control trypanosomiasis, with a resultant resurgence of the disease. Large areas of Africa have been rendered unsuitable for raising and grazing cattle because of the risk of sleeping sickness in domestic stock. The reservoir consists of wild game; tsetse flies (*Glossina* spp.) are the vectors. Once infected, the tsetse fly remains a vector of parasites for its entire life. After the host is bitten by an infected fly, the trypanosomes traverse the lymphatic pathways to regional lymph nodes, where they reproduce, multiply, and subsequently enter the bloodstream. Splenomegaly follows accumulation of the trypanosomes within the splenic parenchyma. Pancarditis frequently occurs. Impairment of the nervous system is the result of leptomeningitis, usually centered over the vertex. The World Health Organization estimates that about 20 to 30 cases of Gambian sleeping sickness are diagnosed annually outside of Africa [Lejon et al., 2003a]. With increasing tourism to trypanosome-endemic regions of Africa, there is a greater likelihood that physicians outside of these areas will be seeing cases of sleeping sickness. Of the two types of sleeping sickness, the Gambian form, because it can develop as a chronic disease, is more likely to be encountered than the fulminant Rhodesian form [Lejon et al., 2003a]. The disease in humans has been reviewed by Kennedy [2004] and Pentreath [1995].

Dural thickening and adhesion to surrounding structures are often present at postmortem examination. Cerebral edema and petechiae are readily seen in most fatal cases. The perivascular infiltrate in the gray and white matter is delineated so clearly that it has been called a *gray sleeve.* Obstruction of cerebrospinal fluid flow may lead to ventricular dilation. Cerebral and cerebellar atrophy may occur in the late stages of the disease. The spinal cord remains unaffected. A mononuclear infiltrate is seen in the meninges and Virchow-Robin spaces during microscopic examination. Lymphocytes are more numerous than plasma cells. Endothelial proliferation of the capillaries may be present. The characteristic morular cell, a plasma cell with immunoglobulin M–containing inclusions (Russell bodies), was first reported by Mott [1906]. Differentiating the neuropathologic changes in African sleeping sickness from Chagas' disease is relatively impossible. Endemic geographic areas of the diseases do not overlap, which is helpful in distinguishing between the two types of trypanosomiasis.

Tryptophol, the 3-indole ethanol formed by the parasite in trypanosomal sleeping sickness, produces the characteristic sleep [Cornford et al., 1979; Feldstein, 1973; Stibbs and Seed, 1973a; 1973b]. Because tryptophol also gains access to lymphoid tissues, such as spleen, thymus, and mesenteric lymph nodes, it may foster immunosuppression in sleeping sickness [Ackerman and Seed, 1976]. The trypanosome induces formation of antibodies to antigens on its surface called variable surface glycoproteins. The variable surface glycoproteins are under genic control and generate antigenic variation by activation and expression of a succession of variable surface glycoprotein genes—of which there are about 1000 in a genome containing 10,000 genes [Donelson, 2003]. Thus, host antibodies aimed at one set of surface antigens are soon rendered ineffectual by selection of bloodstream forms exhibiting newly synthesized surface glycoproteins. The recurring appearance in the bloodstream of trypanosomes with new surface antigens gives rise to periodic fluctuations in parasitemia. Development of a mechanism to modify or terminate this process appears necessary before control or eradication of this disease is feasible [Donelson and Turner, 1985]. Given the immunologic evasion conferred by antigenic switching, the availability of a vaccine in the near future appears unlikely. The trypanosome genome and, in particular, the phenomenon of antigenic variation has been reviewed by Donelson [2003]. Comparative information on trypanosomatid genomes is now available [El-Sayed et al., 2005a], as are sequence data on the *T. brucei* genome [Berriman et al., 2005].

Clinical Characteristics, Clinical Laboratory Tests, and Diagnosis

Mid-African sleeping sickness results from infection by *T. brucei gambiense* and is a less severe but more chronic illness than Rhodesian sleeping sickness. A furuncle or chancre may appear at the site of the fly bite, followed by fever of about 1 week's duration and a rash [Lejon et al., 2003a]. Regional lymphadenitis follows the bite and is the dominant feature for approximately 14 days. Fever, malaise, headache, arthralgia, erythematous and edematous cutaneous eruption, and generalized lymphadenopathy, particularly in the posterior cervical nodes (Winterbottom's sign), compose the next stage, which persists for a week to a month. In the CNS, the disease progresses insidiously from meningitis to encephalopathy through sequential stages including inflammation and cellular infiltration, alteration of EEG patterns, edema, breakdown of the blood-brain barrier, and stimulation of cytokine production [Pentreath, 1995]. Disseminated intravascular coagulation may be a consequence of complement activation by immune complexes. Production of interferon-γ and tumor necrosis factor-α contributes to the overall inflammatory response in the CNS. Autoimmunity may develop, more likely as a consequence of late-stage neuropathology. Although acute rheumatoid arthritis and rheumatic fever are included in the differential diagnosis, they are readily excluded after appearance of manifestations of nervous system impairment, including confusion, somnolence, memory loss, ataxia, and loss of sphincter control.

T. brucei rhodesiense infection causes East African sleeping sickness. The clinical course may be similar to Gambian trypanosomiasis or may appear as a fulminating infection that, if untreated, causes death within 6 to 9 months. Pancarditis with massive pericardial effusion often occurs, with death occurring before neurologic symptomatology appears.

Criteria for diagnosis of trypanosomiasis are the presence of flagellates in the cerebrospinal fluid, elevated cerebrospinal fluid leukocyte levels (5 to 20/μL), and the presence of intrathecal immunoglobulin M as shown by the card agglutination trypanosomiasis test [Lejon et al., 2003b; Truc et al., 2002]. The elevated leukocyte count and the increase of intrathecal immunoglobulin M (as much as a 40-fold rise in late-stage trypanosomiasis) are taken as evidence of an intrathecal inflammatory process [Lejon et al., 2003a; 2003b]. Increase in cerebrospinal fluid protein (≥750 mg/L [≥75 μg/dL]) is a reflection of the elevated immunoglobulin levels [Lejon et al., 2003b]. The diagnostic profile for trypanosomiasis can mimic syphilis, tuberculosis, toxoplasmosis, borreliosis with neural involvement, and mumps meningoencephalitis [Lejon et al., 2003b]. Supporting evidence of infection includes irregular EEG patterns, and nonspecific CNS abnormalities seen by MRI and CT scans [Kennedy, 2004]. Demonstration of trypanosomes in thick and thin smears of peripheral blood remains the diagnostic gold standard, but parasites are less likely to be found in Gambian disease or in early stages of infection. The polymerase chain reaction has been used to detect trypanosomal DNA in cerebrospinal fluid.

Diagnostic evidence of the parasite in the peripheral blood or cerebrospinal fluid is definitive. Spinal fluid pleocytosis and increased protein concentration are usually present but nonspecific. A sensitive and specific study results from inoculation of the patient's blood into a mouse with subsequent demonstration of the organisms in the mouse's blood. Blood stages of the trypanosomes can be cultured in a biphasic medium (blood-nutrient agar slant with an overlay of glucose-containing Locke's solution) [Tobie et al., 1950] but is best carried out in a reference laboratory. Serum immunoglobulin M content is increased greatly and, as noted above, is the basis for diagnostic testing [Lejon et al., 2003b]. The use of precipitin testing provides diagnostic proof (see Table 70-2), although complement fixation studies are reasonably reliable.

Management

Staging of the disease, either early or late, is critical because the type of therapy employed depends on whether the trypanosomes have invaded the CNS. Staging is determined by a lumbar puncture. Use of inappropriate therapy in late-stage disease can lead to relapse. Cerebrospinal fluid leukocyte counts of greater than 20/μL and high levels of immunoglobulin M (up to 100 times normal) are indicative of CNS disease [Lejon et al., 2003]. Suramin (or alternatively, pentamidine) is recommended for patients presenting before the development of CNS disease, although drug resistance is reported to both these agents. Both drugs penetrate poorly across the blood-brain barrier into the CNS, making them ineffective in late-stage disease, and both have serious side effects. The following drugs and dosages are recommended for pediatric patients: for suramin, 20 mg/kg on days 1, 3, 7, 14, and 21; for pentamidine, 4 mg/kg/day intramuscularly for 10 days [Medical Letter, 2004]. Pentamidine is reportedly less effective in treating Rhodesian than Gambian disease [Fairlamb, 2003]. A more recent alternative that is apparently less toxic and perhaps more effective is difluoromethylornithine (eflornithine) for both early- and late-stage disease [Doua and Boa Yapo, 1994; Fairlamb, 2003]. Difluoromethylornithine is not available in the United States but can be obtained through the World Health Organization [Medical Letter, 2004]. Recommended dosage is 400 mg/kg/day intravenously in four divided doses for 14 days [Fairlamb, 2003; Medical Letter, 2004]. Difluoromethylornithine is effective against the Gambian but not the Rhodesian forms of the disease. Synergy has been found in combining suramin with eflornithine [Fairlamb, 2003].

In late stages of the disease, melarsoprol is recommended and is administered intravenously (for pediatric patients, initial dose of 0.36 mg/kg, increasing to maximum of 3.6 mg/kg at intervals of 1 to 5 days for a total of 9 or 10 doses; for a total of 18 to 25 mg/kg over 1 month) [Medical Letter, 2004]. The drug can cross the blood-brain barrier. However, this agent is recognized to have serious toxicity, including seizures, psychosis, coma, and a fatal encephalopathy associated with increased intracranial pressure [Haller et al., 1986]. The drug is effective against both forms of trypanosomiasis. Mortality after melarsoprol use, however, is about 50%. Administration of corticosteroids (prednisolone) can lessen the likelihood of post-treatment sequelae and prevent arsenical encephalopathy [Pepin et al., 1995]. The clinician must be aware of the side effects of these drugs before therapy is initiated, and gradual increase in dosage is advised [Medical Letter, 2004; Seidel, 1985]. Nifurtimox, used in treating Chagas' disease, has also been used in late-stage disease, when other late-stage antimicrobials are ineffective. Antimicrobial therapy for trypanosomiasis has been reviewed by Burchmore and co-workers [2002] and Fairlamb [2003].

HELMINTHS

The helminths include a broad range of organisms and are typically grouped into three categories: nematodes, cestodes, and trematodes. The helminths are generally larger than other parasites, and many are large enough to be visible to the human eye. They are extracellular parasites, and the host response is dominated by mechanisms aimed at extracellular parasites and often results in eosinophilia. Most helminths have complex life cycles with multiple hosts. The definitive host is the host in which the sexual reproduction of the parasites takes place. The intermediate host is typically one in which there is no reproduction of the parasite. In many cases, humans are an accidental or "dead end" host and not part of the parasite life cycle. Nematodes are cylindrical and nonsegmented worms. *Trichinella, Angiostrongylus,* and *Toxocara* are genera in this class that infect the CNS. Cestodes that infect humans belong to the subclass Eucestoda, the true tapeworms. These endoparasites have no epidermis or digestive tract and elongated segmented bodies. Adults have a multihook organ of attachment at the anterior end, which is called the *scolex*. Genera of cestodes associated with CNS infection include *Dibothriocephalus (Diphyllobothrium), Taenia, Multiceps,* and *Echinococcus*. Trematodes (flukes) are nonsegmented worms that possess a digestive tract. Trematodes infecting the nervous system include the genera *Schistosoma* and *Paragonimus*.

Many helminth parasites of animals are potential causes of larva migrans. *Larva migrans* refers to the prolonged migration and persistence of helminth larvae in the tissues of humans [Beaver 1969, Kazacos 2001]. Larva migrans can be separated pathologically and clinically into visceral, ocular, neural, and cutaneous larva migrans based on the organ systems involved [Kazacos 2001]. Visceral larva migrans and neural larva migrans are usually diseases of childhood, affecting children 1 to 8 years old. These include various ascarids, hookworms, gnathostomiasis, *Angiostrongylus cantonensis*, *Spirometra*, *Alaria,* and others. Of these, the ascarids are the most important group with *Toxocara* and *Baylisascaris* accounting for the majority of cases in humans.

Toxocariasis

Epidemiology, Microbiology, and Pathology

Toxocariasis results from infection with the ascarid worm, *Toxocara,* and is widely distributed throughout the world. Toxocariasis was first described in 1921 in a patient with eosinophilia, dyspnea, and cyanosis [Aubertin and Giroux, 1921]. Central nervous system involvement with *Toxocara* was demonstrated in later case reports [Beautyman et al., 1965; Dent et al., 1956]. *Toxocara canis* and *Toxocara cati* are common ascarid infections of dogs and cats, respectively, and are found worldwide. The prevalence of *T. canis* shedding is highest in puppies, and more than 90% of dogs less than 6 months in North America shed *Toxocara* eggs in their stool [Kazacos, 1991]. As dogs mature, the shedding of eggs decreases. Cats shed *Toxocara cati,* and the prevalence may be as high as 75% in kittens [Schantz and Glickman, 1981]. Infected animals can shed millions of eggs per day. *Toxocara* eggs are able to survive for long periods, especially in warm and humid environments, and extensive contamination of the environment can occur. Up to 30% of soil samples are contaminated with *Toxocara* eggs [Arpino et al., 1990]. *Toxocara* infects humans, primarily children, through the ingestion of soil contaminated with eggs. Young children may come into contact with eggs while playing on playgrounds and sandboxes contaminated by dogs and cats. Infected children often have a history of pica and many children with toxocariasis have had a dog in their household within 1 year of illness [Huang and Schantz, 2004]. Once eggs are ingested, larvae hatch in the small intestine, penetrate the mucosa, then migrate through many organs and tissues. The liver is a common site of involvement. Because humans are an aberrant host, *Toxocara* spp. do not complete their life cycle beyond the second-stage larvae. Seroprevalence studies have found varying rates of seropositivity: 83% in Saint Lucia, 51% in Taiwan, 6.4% in the United States, and 3.6% in Japan [Schantz, 1989].

Clinical Characteristics, Clinical Laboratory Tests, and Diagnosis

Most infections with *Toxocara* are asymptomatic. Symptomatic individuals often have features of visceral larva migrans, such as fever, hepatomegaly, cough, and wheezing. Splenomegaly and lymphadenopathy may also occur. Neurologic involvement is relatively uncommon. Meningoencephalitis, encephalopathy, transverse myelitis, focal mass lesions, psychiatric disturbances, seizures, and arachnoiditis have all been described [Mikhael et al., 1974; Bachli et al., 2004]. Fatalities from the infection have been described but are rare [Schochet, 1967].

Infection of the eye generally occurs in children 8 years and older and is usually unilateral. Patients often present with visual loss, strabismus, or eye pain. The larvae can cause endophthalmitis with retinal detachment, posterior and peripheral retinochoroiditis, optic papillitis and uveitis [Hotez, 1993; Molk, 1983; Shields, 1984].

Multiple studies have documented an association between seizure disorders and *Toxocara* antibodies, but a causal relationship has not been well established [Arpino et al., 1990; Glickman et al., 1979; Woodruff et al., 1966]. Similarly, behavioral disorders and declines of cognitive ability have been correlated with *Toxocara* seropositivity but the significance is unclear [Marmor et al., 1987; Worley et al., 1984].

Laboratory features of infection often include eosinophilia, leukocytosis, anemia, elevated sedimentation rate, and hypergammaglobulinemia. The diagnosis is usually suggested by the patient's age, as well as clinical and laboratory features. Definitive diagnosis can be made when larvae are identified in affected tissue, but this has a low diagnostic yield. An enzyme-linked immunosorbent assay, available at the CDC, has a reported specificity of over 90% and can be used as supportive evidence of infection [Wilson, 2002].

Neuroimaging findings are variable. Hyperintense lesions in white matter with basilar enhancement, and ring-enhancing lesions have been described. [Bachli, 2004; Duprez, 1996; Ruttinger et al., 1991; Sommer and Hadidi, 1994]. One case report describes more than 25 lesions located in the cortical and subcortical regions with a hyperintense appearance on T2-weighted images [Ruttinger and Hadidi, 1991]. Neuropathology may reveal perivascular cuffing in the white matter, leptomeningeal inflammation, eosinophilic granulomas, or vasculitic lesions [Beautyman et al., 1965; Dent et al., 1956; Hill et al., 1985; Moore, 1962].

Management

Most patients recover without specific treatment. There is no proven therapy, especially for CNS disease, but anthelmintic and anti-inflammatory medications should be considered in cases with serious complications. Albendazole (400 mg twice a day for 5 days) or mebendazole (100 to 200 mg twice day for 5 days) is the recommended therapy [Medical Letter, 2004], but optimal duration is unknown.

Baylisascaris Procyonis Infection

Epidemiology, Microbiology, and Pathology

Baylisascaris procyonis is a roundworm of raccoons and causes a rapidly fatal eosinophilic encephalitis in humans. Raccoons are the definitive host, and humans are considered an accidental intermediate host. *B. procyonis* infection in raccoons, like *Ascaris lumbricoides* infection in humans or any ascarid infection in its respective natural definitive host, is usually asymptomatic. *B. procyonis* occurs in raccoons in North America, Europe, and parts of Asia [Kazacos, 2001]. The prevalence of *B. procyonis* in raccoons is highest in the midwestern and northeastern United States, where more than 90% of juvenile raccoons are infected [Kazacos and Boyce, 1989]. The eggs become infectious for humans and other animals about 3 to 4 weeks after they are shed by the raccoon. Humans become infected by ingesting raccoon roundworm eggs in raccoon feces, by soil or water contaminated with raccoon feces, or via contaminated hands. Small children are particularly vulnerable to infection because of their propensity to put dirt and other objects in their mouth. Once swallowed, eggs hatch into larvae, then migrate through the liver, brain, spinal cord, and other organs. Larvae are found in tissues throughout the intermediate host but cause the most damage in the CNS and eye. The combination of marked larval growth and aggressive somatic migration make *Baylisascaris* more pathogenic than *Toxocara* infection in humans.

Clinical Characteristics, Clinical Laboratory Tests, and Diagnosis

B. procyonis infection in humans was first recognized in a 10-month-old boy with eosinophilic meningoencephalitis in 1984 [Huff et al., 1984]. Many case reports have followed [Cunningham et al., 1994; Moertel et al., 2001; Park et al., 2000]. Infected humans may have classical visceral larva migrans with fever, leukocytosis, eosinophilia, hepatomegaly, and pneumonitis. If larvae reach the CNS, they produce damage and inflammation, resulting in progressive CNS disease, and the severity is often dose related [Kazacos et al., 2001]. Presenting CNS symptoms include lethargy, irritability, loss of muscle coordination, ataxia, nystagmus, loss of spontaneous movement, extensor rigidity, and ultimately result in coma and death [Fox et al., 1985; Moertel et al., 2001; Park et al., 2000].

Ocular larva migrans usually involves children seven years of age and older, with no history of pica and without marked eosinophilia. Ocular larva migrans is usually a result of an infection with a few larvae followed by chance migration [Kazacos, 1985].

The diagnosis of neural larva migrans is often suggested by a history of exposure to raccoons (or their feces) and clinical presentation. Laboratory findings of persistent eosinophilia in the blood and spinal fluid are important. Early in the course of illness neuroradiologic studies may document periventricular white matter disease. Atrophy occurs in later stages of illness [Rowley, 2000] (Fig. 70-19).

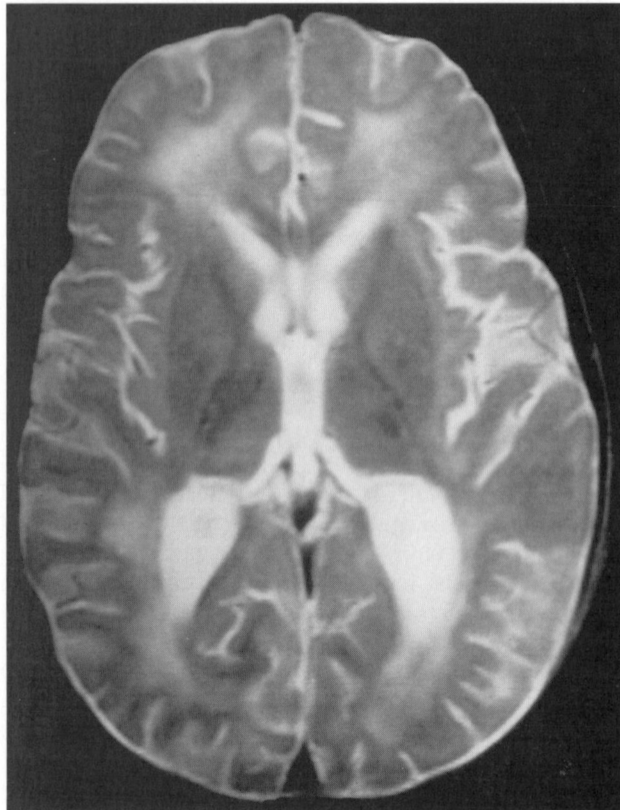

FIGURE 70-19. Magnetic resonance image (axial T2 image) showing abnormal hyperintensity in the periventricular white matter 12 days after presentation of a child with *Baylisascaris* meningoencephalitis. (Courtesy Dr. Howard Rowley.)

Larvae can sometimes be recovered from tissues or visualized in histopathology or biopsy. On pathology, larvae are generally surrounded by epithelial granulomas with a variable number of eosinophils, plasma cells, and lymphocytes. In ocular larva migrans, migrational tracks or live larvae are sometimes observed by funduscopic examination. Serologic testing is available in a limited number of laboratories throughout the world [Boyce et al., 1989].

Management

There is no known effective treatment for neurologic involvement of *Baylisascaris*. Treatment with antiparasitic agents and steroids has been attempted but with only marginal success [Cunningham et al., 1994; Park et al., 2000].

Trichinosis

Epidemiology, Microbiology, and Pathology

Trichinosis develops when raw or undercooked meat contaminated with *Trichinella* spp. larvae is ingested. *Trichinella* spp. are widely distributed throughout the world and occur in a large number of carnivorous animals. Humans are incidental hosts. Most human infections involve *Trichinella spiralis,* which is often associated with pork, but there are many other species of *Trichinella* that can infect humans. These other species have been found in many other mammals, including horses, bears, foxes, hyenas, felines, and even whales. The incidence of trichinosis is highest in the Balkans, Russia, China, Argentina, and the Baltic Republics [Dupouy-Camet, 2000]. In the United States, the national trichinellosis surveillance system has documented a steady decline in the reported incidence of this disease. From 1947 to 1951, a median of 393 cases (range 327 to 487) was reported annually, including 57 trichinellosis-related deaths [CDC, 2003]. From 1997 to 2001, the incidence decreased to a median of 12 cases annually (range 11 to 23), with no reported deaths. Although the United States has had a steady decline in cases, some European countries have had a re-emergence of the disease in the past 25 years. Infected horsemeat, rather than pork, was responsible for at least 3000 human cases in Italy and France [Dupouy-Camet, 2000].

Clinical Characteristics, Clinical Laboratory Tests, and Diagnosis

Clinical symptoms are usually biphasic. After ingestion of the encysted larvae, gastroenteritis of varying severity ensues within 5 to 15 days. Larvae develop into adult worms within the small intestine and ultimately release motile larvae that gain access to the bloodstream. From the bloodstream, larvae seed the skeletal musculature. The second phase of symptoms begins about 1 to 2 weeks after infection and is characterized by muscle invasion and prominent facial and periorbital or facial edema, fever, conjunctivitis, subconjunctival hemorrhages, eosinophilia, and myalgias. High fevers are often seen during larval tissue migration. Myalgias and myositis are usually most severe 2 to 3 weeks after infection. The most common muscles affected are the extraocular, masseters, and diaphragmatic muscles. Severe complications of trichinosis include myocarditis, pneumonitis, and encephalitis.

Neurotrichinosis occurs in only a small proportion of cases and during the late phase of illness. Meningoencephalitis is the most common manifestation. A variety of neurologic presentations have been reported, including confusion, memory loss, psychosis, flaccid monoparesis, urinary retention, cranial nerve deficits, and cerebellar ataxia [Ellrodt et al., 1987; Kreel et al., 1988; Mawhorter and Kazura, 1993]. A syndrome including both encephalopathy and acute myocardial injury has also been described [Fourestie et al., 1993]

The diagnosis of acute infection is based on a combination of the history, clinical features, and laboratory findings. Eosinophilia, the most common laboratory abnormality, usually peaks at 3 to 4 weeks after infection and may range from 10% to 90% [Markell et al., 1992]. Leukocytosis and elevated immunoglobulin E are also common signs of infection. Enzyme-linked immunosorbent assay or indirect fluorescent antibody can be used for antibody detection; however, antibody levels are often not detectable for 3 to 5 weeks after infection [Wilson et al., 2002]. Molecular tests and antigen testing have been developed but are not widely available [Huang et al., 2004; Taratuto and Venturiello, 1997b]. Skin testing is unreliable. Muscle biopsy demonstrates an inflammatory myositis. The *T. spiralis* larvae are surrounded by inflammatory mononuclear, polymorphonuclear, and eosinophilic cells. Granuloma and capsule formation with encystment of the larvae develop over several months [Taratuto and Venturiello, 1997b]. In patients with CNS involvement, cerebrospinal fluid studies may indicate pleocytosis and eosinophilia or even the presence of larvae. Cerebrospinal fluid eosinophilia or larvae are found in 8% to 28% of cases [Huang et al., 2004]. Electroencephalographic studies reflect changes expected with a diffuse encephalopathy [Ryczak et al., 1987]. If vascular involvement occurs, subacute cortical infarcts may be found on CT and MRI [Feydy et al., 1996; Fourestie et al., 1993]. CT or MRI studies may show small contrast-enhancing nodular lesions and focal calcifications [Ellrodt et al., 1987; Fourestie et al., 1993]. Neuropathology has found cortical vein thrombosis, granulomas, brain edema, and hyperemia of the meninges in these cases [Ellrodt et al., 1987; Gay et al., 1982].

Limited effective treatment is available for trichinosis. Mebendazole (200 to 400 mg three times a day for 3 days then 400 to 500 mg three times a day for 10 days) or albendazole (400 mg twice a day for 8 to 14 days) has been recommended. Corticosteroids may be helpful in reducing the risk of hypersensitivity reactions resulting from the dying parasites or the development of cerebral edema, myocarditis, or cerebritis [Ellrodt et al., 1987; Ryczak et al., 1987].

Angiostrongylus Infection

Epidemiology, Microbiology, and Pathology

Angiostrongylus cantonensis, the rat lungworm, is the principal cause of human eosinophilic meningitis worldwide. Human *A. cantonensis* was first reported in 1945 in a fatal case of eosinophilic meningitis [Beaver and Rosen, 1964]. Rodents are the definitive host of the parasite and mollusks are the intermediate host. Humans are the incidental host and become infected by ingestion of the third-stage larvae in the molluscan intermediate host (e.g., snails, crabs, freshwater prawns) or contaminated vegetables. After humans ingest infective larvae in undercooked or raw snails, the larvae penetrate the intestinal wall and reach the CNS via the bloodstream.

The infection in humans often occurs in warm climates and is well known to occur in Southeast Asia, the South Pacific, and Taiwan [Kliks and Palumbo, 1992; Punyagupta et al., 1975; Yii et al., 1975]. In some regions of the world, children are most commonly affected; in Taiwan, for example, 80% of *Angiostrongylus* cases are in the pediatric age group [Chen, 1991]. Other areas include Africa, Polynesia, and eastern Australia [Prociv et al., 2000]. In the United States, *Angiostrongylus* has occurred in Hawaii and Louisiana. Other countries of the Western Hemisphere cases include Puerto Rico, Cuba, Jamaica, and the Dominican Republic. Rats on cargo ships are the principal mode of expansion of the parasite beyond the Indo-Pacific area [Kliks and Palumbo, 1992].

Clinical Characteristics, Clinical Laboratory Tests, and Diagnosis

The onset of CNS symptoms occurs 1 to 35 days after ingestion of the infective larvae [Huang et al., 2004]. Clinical illness often consists of severe headache, photophobia, meningeal signs, hyperesthesia, and paresthesia. The presence, height, and duration of fever vary. Whereas most cases are self-limiting, severe forms of the disease occur, including coma, paralysis of extremities, and seizures [Fuller, 1993; Kuberski and Wallace, 1979; Yii et al., 1975]. Conjunctivitis, periorbital swelling, retinal hemorrhage, retinal detachment, or blindness may occur if the eye is infected [Punyagupta et al., 1975; Toma et al., 2002]. In most cases recovery occurs approximately 4 weeks after onset but may take several months. In some cases involving very young children, progressive deterioration of CNS function has been described [Cooke-Yarbourough et al., 1999; Lindo et al., 2004]. The severity of the disease is often related to the number of larvae ingested. Deaths are uncommon but have been reported [Lindo et al., 2004].

The diagnosis is often suggested by the exposure history and clinical and laboratory features. Eosinophilic pleocytosis is very common. Peripheral eosinophilia and elevated immunoglobulin E levels may also be seen. The eosinophilia may persist for months [Jindrak, 1975]. The larvae can occasionally be visualized in the cerebrospinal fluid [Hwang and Chen, 1991]. An enzyme-linked immunosorbent assay test has been developed but is not widely available [Cross and Chi, 1982; Intapan et al., 2002]. Molecular tests are under development [Chye et al., 2004]. CT scans of the brain may show areas of attenuation with surrounding hypodense areas [Ko et al., 1987]. Meningeal enhancement and high signal intensity at the subcortical white matter on T2-weighted images may also be seen [Tsai et al., 2004].

In humans, postmortem examination has found infiltration of the meninges and around intracerebral vessels of lymphocytes, eosinophils, and plasma cells [Sonakul, 1978]. Small worm tracks (0.1 to 2.0 mm in size), with and without hemorrhage, are also seen [Kanpittaya et al., 2000; Sonakul, 1978]. Live larvae are sometimes seen, and tissues around them typically have little or no reaction. In contrast, dead worms are surrounded by a zone of suppurative necrosis or granuloma [Jindrak, 1975; Sonakul, 1978].

Management

Treatment with anthelmintics has been attempted, but efficacy is questionable and may even worsen symptoms. Sequential lumbar punctures, steroids, and analgesics have been reported to improve symptoms [Chotmongkol et al., 2000; Tsai et al., 2004].

Gnathostomiasis

Epidemiology, Microbiology, and Pathology

Gnathostomiasis, most commonly caused by the nematode *Gnathostoma spinigerum,* is the cause of eosinophilic myeloencephalitis. Most cases are associated with the ingestion of raw or undercooked fish, frogs, snakes, chickens, or ducks. The disease is commonly reported from Southeast Asia, particularly Thailand and Japan, because of dietary habits in those countries. Gnathostomosis is an emerging public health problem in Peru, Ecuador, and most recently in Mexico [Pelaez and Perez-Reyes, 1970]. The consumption of cerviche is responsible for many of the cases seen in South America. The median time from ingestion of infected food to onset of symptoms may be several weeks to several months [Ogata et al., 1998].

Clinical Characteristics, Clinical Laboratory Tests, and Diagnosis

If the larva migrates to vital organs of the host, severe illness or death can occur [Rusnak and Lucey, 1993]. Common symptoms include intermittent episodes of cutaneous larva migrans ("creeping eruption") with localized pain and pruritus. These lesions may recur for several years [Ogata, 1998]. Visceral symptoms occur if larvae migrate to deep tissues.

CNS involvement is rare and occurs more frequently in adults but occasional cases occur in older children. CNS findings include the sudden onset of radicular pain or headache. Paralysis of the extremities and loss of bladder control typically follows [Boongird et al., 1977]. Cranial nerve abnormalities may also occur. Acute eosinophilic meningitis and encephalitis are also described [Chitanondh and Rosen, 1967]. Intermittent symptoms can occur for 10 to 15 years because the larvae are long-lived [Huang et al., 2004]. Deaths are usually due to direct involvement of the brainstem or secondary complications of pneumonia or sepsis [Boongrid et al., 1977]. Ocular involvement can result in iris holes, anterior uveitis, and subretinal hemorrhages [Biswas et al., 1994].

Definitive diagnosis is made when the worm is identified in biopsies of tissue, especially the skin. Patients with gnathostomiasis will often have pronounced eosinophilia, with values exceeding 50% of the total white blood count [Rusnak and Lucey, 1993]. In cases with CNS involvement, spinal fluid analysis shows eosinophilic pleocytosis and normal to increased protein. Grossly bloody spinal fluid is common secondary to hemorrhage [Punyagupta, 1975]. CT scans may demonstrate subarachnoid or intracerebral hemorrhage. If there is ocular involvement, worms can sometimes be visualized by a routine eye examination [Baquera-Heredia et al., 2002]. An enzyme-linked immunosorbent assay test has been developed but is not widely available [Tapchaisri et al., 1991].

Management

Treatment recommendations include albendazole (400 mg twice a day for 21 days) or ivermectin (0.2 mg/kg for 2 days) for dermal and subcutaneous gnathostomiasis [Nontasut et al., 2000]. Similar treatment is generally recommended for CNS disease, although data on efficacy are limited. Surgical removal is often needed if larvae are identified in the eye [Biswas et al., 1994; Funata et al., 1993].

CESTODES

Diphyllobothriasis

Epidemiology, Microbiology, and Pathology

Diphyllobothrium latum, the fish tapeworm, is found throughout the world and causes a public health problem in many regions of the temperate and subarctic zones in the Northern Hemisphere. Megaloblastic anemia and neurologic illness in humans are the result of vitamin B_{12} deficiency caused by the tapeworm; optic atrophy and subacute combined degeneration of the spinal cord result [Bjorkenheim, 1966; Nyberg, 1963].

Fish tapeworm infestation can be prevented by thorough cooking of all freshwater fish. Freezing at 10° C for 48 hours is also recommended to kill the organism before ingestion. Diphyllobothriasis can be treated with niclosamide (single dose of 50 mg/kg) or praziquantel (single dose of 5-10 mg/kg).

Echinococcosis

Epidemiology, Microbiology, and Pathology

Echinococcosis, commonly referred to as *hydatid disease*, has a worldwide distribution and is a major public health problem. The term *hydatid* refers to the fluid-filled larval stage found in the intermediate host. These bladder-like cysts, particularly in the liver, were well known in ancient times, as noted by Hippocrates as early as the 4th century BC [Cox, 2002]. The two major species of *Echinococcus* that are of public health and medical importance are *Echinococcus granulosus* and *Echinococcus multilocularis*. *E. granulosus* disease is characterized by cystic lesions found primarily in the liver and lungs and is known as *cystic hydatid disease*. *E. multilocularis* disease is less common but is a more malignant form than that caused by *E granulosus*. *E. multilocularis* is characterized by tumor-like collections of vesicular parasites found primarily in the liver and is known as *alveolar hydatid disease*.

Canines are the definitive host, and sheep are the most common intermediate host for *E. granulosus*. Dogs and other canids are the hosts to the adult tapeworm. When dogs pass eggs in their stool, sheep and other animals become infected when they ingest the eggs. After ingestion, eggs hatch in the intestine, penetrate the intestinal wall, and migrate to tissues. Humans become an inadvertent intermediate host by ingestion of food or water contaminated with feces from infected dogs. Direct contact with an infected dog may also lead to infection since *Echinoccocus* eggs can adhere to the dog's fur [Eckert and Deplaze, 2004]. A similar life cycle occurs with *E. multilocularis;* foxes and wolves are the common definitive hosts, and rodents generally serve as the intermediate host.

E. granulosus is found on all continents, and its distribution is related to sheep and cattle herding. It is particularly prevalent in the Mediterranean, Middle East, and northern and eastern regions of Africa, parts of Russia, China, Australia, and countries in South America [Eckert and Deplaze, 2004]. *E. multilocularis* is found mostly in alpine or artic regions in the Northern Hemisphere, including Central Europe, Russia, China, and North America.

Clinical Characteristics, Clinical Laboratory Tests, and Diagnosis

The clinical manifestations of hydatid disease are dependent on the number, size, and developmental stage of the parasite. During the initial stage of the infection humans are asymptomatic. The disease is often acquired in childhood, with latency periods lasting as long as 20 years. In cases of *E. granulosa*, cysts grow slowly and may ultimately contain several liters of fluid. Symptoms are frequently caused by pressure induced by the expanding cysts. The majority of hydatid cysts occur in the liver (75%) or lungs (15%) [Beggs, 1985]. Less common sites include the bone, pelvis, spleen, and CNS.

With hepatic cysts, right upper quadrant pain, jaundice, or symptoms mimicking biliary disease occur [Dhar et al., 1996]. When the lungs are involved, chest pain, cough, fever, and hemoptysis are common. Anaphylaxis or dissemination of cysts may occur if the cysts rupture.

E. granulosus infection of the CNS occurs in 2% to 5% of cases and may be primary or secondary when lesions occur in the CNS [Ciurea et al., 1995; Huang et al., 2004; Lunardi et al., 1991]). CNS disease is more common in children than adults [Carrea et al., 1975; Ersahin et al., 1993]. Most cysts are singular, intraparenchymal, and in the region of the middle cerebral artery [Gossios et al., 1997]. Patients with *E. granulosus* lesions in the CNS typically present with signs of increased cranial pressure: headache, vomiting, nausea, and papilledema [Altinros et al., 2000; Eckert and Deplaze, 2004; Taratuto et al., 1997a]. Hydatid disease involves the spine in 1% of cases and often resembles tuberculous spondylitis [Hughes and Biggs, 2002]. Extradural, intraventricular, cerebellar, thalamic, and orbital hydatid cysts have been reported in children but are rare [Copley et al., 1992; Ergun et al.,1997; Sener, 1996].

The clinical manifestation of *E. multilocularis* is characterized by invasive growth of larvae in the liver with occasional metastasis. Patients often complain of right upper quadrant pain or a palpable mass in the right upper quadrant. When metastasis to the brain occurs, the patient often presents with a mass lesion. *E. multilocularis* is almost always seen in adults.

Diagnosis of hydatid disease is usually suggested by a history of residence in an endemic area, the clinical features, and characteristic radiologic findings. Neuroimaging is extremely helpful in the diagnosis of CNS hydatid disease. In cases of *E. granulosus,* CT and MRI brain scans often demonstrate oval or spherical, homogeneous, sharply demarcated cystic lesions with smooth borders [Gossios et al., 1997; Tuzun et al., 2002]. If the protoscolex, referred to as "hydatid sand," is seen in the image, it is considered diagnostic. The cyst is often located in the white matter; as the cyst enlarges it extends toward the meninges or ventricles [Esharin et al., 1993]. Because there is little inflammation around the cysts, there is no edema or enhancement. Calcification of the wall is rarely observed [Tuzun et al., 2002]. In *E. multilocularis* of the CNS, cysts are less distinct on neuroimaging and may appear as an ill-defined mass. A cauliflower-like contrast enhancement pattern on MRI is sometimes described [Tunaci et al., 1999]. Liver involvement is almost always present in these cases and ultrasound or other imaging of the abdomen may be helpful.

Eosinophilia and elevated liver enzymes are variably present. Serology can be helpful in cases that have unclear neuroimaging studies. Enzyme-linked immunosorbent assay or indirect hemagglutination is available for screening, and immunoblot assay can help confirm the diagnosis. False-positive tests may occur in individuals with other helminth parasite infections, chronic immune disorders, and cancer [Wilson et al., 2002]. In extrahepatic disease, false negatives may occur [Huang et al., 2004].

Management

Surgical removal and an antiparasitic drug are usually the recommended treatments for CNS disease. In cases of *E. granulosus,* meticulous care must be used during surgery to prevent spillage of the cysts' contents. Intraoperative rupture rates for intracranial cysts were reported to be 17% in one recent study [Altinors et al., 2000]. Rupture of the cyst into the subarachnoid space may lead to widespread dissemination, followed by a severe inflammatory or anaphylactic reaction. Some authors have reported good outcomes with medical therapy alone [Kalaitzoglou et al., 1998; Singounas et al., 1992]. One of the newer benzoimidazoles, albendazole (15 mg/kg/ day [maximum 800 mg] for 1 to 6 months), is generally recommended [Medical Letter, 2004]. Praziquantel, in combination with albendazole, has shown utility [Anadol et al., 2001]. For *E. multilocularis,* CNS involvement is usually a consequence of advanced disease. Surgery and prolonged, often lifelong, antiparasitic medications are generally recommended [Reuter et al., 2004]. Case reports of successful outcomes using radiotherapy and interferon have also been described [Schmid et al., 1995; 1998].

Cysticercosis

Epidemiology, Microbiology, and Pathology

Cysticercosis, an infection caused by the larval form of the pork tapeworm *Taenia solium,* is the most common parasitic infection of the CNS worldwide. The encysted larvae in the

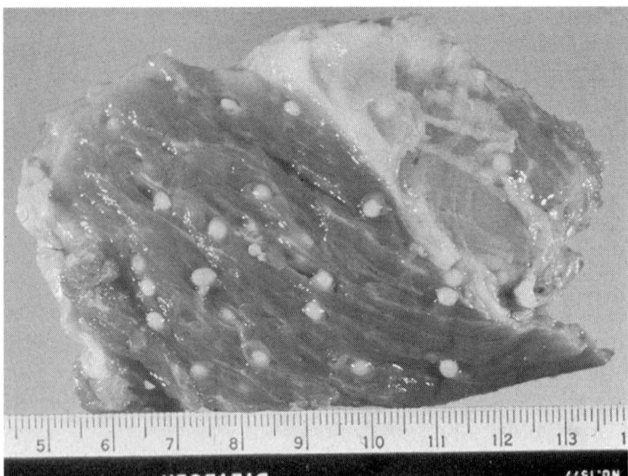

FIGURE 70-20. Pork infected with the larval form of *Taenia solium*, also know as "measly pork." (Courtesy Dr. Lawrence Ash.)

flesh of pigs, known as cysticerci, were known as "measly pork" to the ancient Greeks, although the correlation with human illness was not understood at that time (Fig. 70-20) [Cox, 2002]. There are descriptions of cysticerci in humans in the 16th century [Nieto, 1956], but the recognition that cysticerci were the larval stages of tapeworm was not made until almost 100 years later by Goeze Johann [Cox, 2004].

Cysticercosis is a disease found in areas with poor sanitation, especially in areas where pigs have access to human feces. The incidence of cysticercosis decreased in most European countries a century ago because of improvements in general sanitation. The disease is endemic in many less-developed countries and is especially prevalent in Central and South America, sub-Saharan Africa, and Southeast Asia. Epidemiology surveys for human cysticercosis report seroprevalences of 8% to 12% in parts of Latin America [Carpio et al., 1998]. It is increasingly recognized in the United States and other industrialized nations because of immigration and increased travel to endemic areas [Maguire, 2004; Schantz et al., 1992; Sorvillo et al., 1992].

The life cycle of *T. solium* requires two hosts and two different forms of the parasite. Humans serve as the definitive host for the adult intestinal tapeworm form. Humans become infected with the intestinal tapeworm by consumption of undercooked pork containing cysticerci, the so-called measly pork (see Fig. 70-20). In the small intestine, the cysticerci then develop into adult tapeworms, sometimes reaching a length of 30 feet. The adult tapeworm typically causes minimal problems for the human host and can reside in the small intestine for 10 to 20 years. Eggs are periodically shed in the stool of an infected person. *Taenia* eggs can survive for long periods in the environment. Human feces used as fertilizer contaminates the environment. Pigs eating in this area become infected with eggs and serve as the most common intermediate host.

Once the eggs are ingested, oncospheres hatch in the intestine, invade the small intestine, and invade muscle and other tissues of the body. The life cycle is complete when humans then eat pork containing cysticerci. Human cysticercosis is not acquired directly from pork but from ingestion of ova shed in human feces by a tapeworm carrier or by autoinfection.

Clinical Characteristics, Clinical Laboratory Tests, and Diagnosis

The adult stage of *T. solium* (the tapeworm) is often asymptomatic but occasionally causes mild gastrointestinal complaints, such as nausea, diarrhea, and abdominal pain. The clinical manifestations of the larval stage are extremely variable and depend on the site of infection, the number of cysts, and the host response. At the time of larval migration there may be myalgia, fever, and eosinophilia, but this stage is usually not recognized. Larval migration occurs most commonly to the muscle, liver, brain, and other tissues, where the larvae then develop into cysticerci. Cysticerci located in sites other than the CNS or eye rarely cause damage.

Neurocysticercosis occurs when larvae enter the CNS. Many individuals with neurocysticercosis have no symptoms. When CNS symptoms do occur, they often appear 5 to 7 years after the initial infection, but latencies of 6 months to 30 years have been described [Dixon and Lipscomb, 1961]. Neurocysticercosis can be either active or inactive. Inactive lesions are generally characterized by calcified foci. Active neurocysticercosis is usually associated with viable or degenerating cysticerci on CT or MRI. Seizures are the most frequent manifestations of neurocysticercosis and occur in 70% to 90% of reported cases [Shandera et al., 1994; White, 1997]. Other common clinical manifestations include headache, behavioral disturbances, and signs of increased intracranial pressure. In children, the most common presentation are focal or generalized seizures that are due to the acute reaction occurring at the time of cyst degeneration. Occasionally, children can present with acute encephalitis or cerebral edema when multiple inflammatory cysts exist. When cysts are located in the ventricular system, obstructive hydrocephalus can occur. A single cyst may also present as a space-occupying lesion and may appear as a brain tumor. A less common but severe form of neurocysticercosis occurs when cysticerci are clustered at the base of the brain and grow in subarachnoid space in grapelike clusters called the *racemose cyst*—this form is almost never seen in children. Spinal involvement may lead to cord compression.

Evidence from a number of recent studies has found that chronic calcified cysts may be a major cause of epilepsy [Nash et al., 2004] and a primary reason for the higher incidence of epilepsy in underdeveloped countries compared with industrialized countries [Nicoletti, 2002].

Accurate diagnosis of neurocysticercosis requires a thorough review of the exposure history and clinical information, as well as neuroimaging and serologic data. Routine laboratory testing is usually nonspecific. Spinal fluid analysis is often normal or may show pleocytosis or increased protein [Mitchell and Crawford, 1988; Thomson et al., 1984], and eosinophilia is variably present [Dawood and Moosa, 1984; Mitchell and Crawford, 1988]. Immunoassays, such as an enzyme-linked immunosorbent assay and enzyme immunoelectrotransfer blot assay, are available to detect antibody against *T. solium* or cysticerci. Studies have found that the immunoelectrotransfer blot assay is both more sensitive and specific than enzyme-linked immunosorbent assay for the diagnosis of neurocysticercosis [Kojic and White, 2003; Schantz et al., 1994]. Serology is more sensitive in cases with multiple cysts than in cases with a single cyst or calcified lesions [Wilson et al., 1991]. In the United States, the immunoelectrotransfer blot assay is available at the CDC. Unfortunately, serology does not differentiate asymptomatic infections from infections with overt clinical symptoms. Diagnostic criteria based on the epidemiology, clinical history, neuroimaging, and serology results have been proposed for classification of neurocysticercosis [Del Brutto, 2001].

Neuroimaging may indicate a cystic lesion with an associated scolex and is considered pathognomonic for cysticercosis [Nash, 2003]. Most neuroimaging, however, will not reveal a scolex. More typically, cystic lesions, single or multiple ringlike or nodular enhancing lesions, and parenchymal brain calcifications will be seen (Fig. 70-21). Parenchymal cysts are often round, 5 to 20 mm in diameter and often found in the cerebral cortex and basal ganglia. [Carpio and Hauser, 2002; Huang et al., 2004]. Cysts in the subarachnoid space are typically larger and may be as large as 60 mm. Ring-enhancing or nodular enhancing lesions are also highly suggestive of neurocysticercosis. Parenchymal brain calcifications are usually 2 to 100 mm in diameter and are often solid, dense, and supratentorial. As cysts die, often when the patient is symptomatic, they lose their characteristic appearance and appear as dense granuloma with surrounding edema and may mimic a cerebral tumor. MRI provides better imaging detection and definition than CT [Garcia and Del Brutto, 2003].

Cysts in the brain undergo a number of different pathologic stages. After entering the brain, cysticerci are often dormant for years. Animal data suggest that the parasite uses mechanisms to suppress the immune response. Postmortem examinations in humans have demonstrated that patients with seizures have inflammatory infiltrates present, whereas viable cysticerci are found incidentally in individuals without CNS symptoms [Huang et al., 2004]. This finding suggests that seizures are likely a result of the host response rather than the parasite itself. In animal models, the granuloma, rather than the parasite, was the cause of seizure [Stringer et al., 2001]. After months to years, the cysticerci become infiltrated and are surrounded by host inflammatory cells composed of mononuclear cells, eosinophils, and neutrophils [Escobar, 1983]. Later the walls of the cysticerci degrade, and the cyst cavity is invaded by inflammatory cells (colloid stage). The granular nodular stage occurs next, with fibrosis and collapse of the cyst cavity. The calcific stage includes further fibrosis and calcifications.

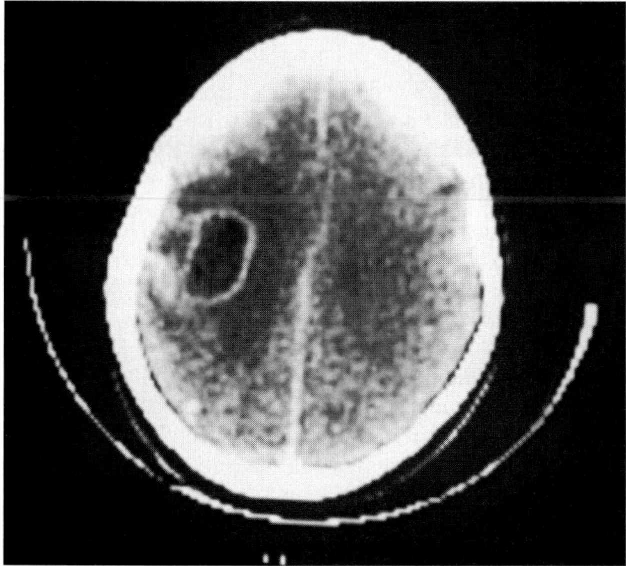

FIGURE 70-21. Cerebral cysticercosis revealed on computed tomography scan.

Management

Treatment of the adult tapeworm is routinely recommended. Praziquantel and niclosamide are highly effective for the eradication of the adult tapeworm. Treatment of neurocysticercosis should be individualized and based on clinical presentation and the number, location, and viability of cysticerci within the nervous system. Because seizures may recur for months, antiepileptic drug therapy is often recommended until there is evidence of resolution on CT or MRI, and no seizures have occurred for 1 to 2 years [Carpio and Hauser, 2002]. Considerable controversy exists about the role of antiparasitic treatment of neurocysticercosis [Proano et al., 2001]. Albendazole and praziquantel are the most common anthelmintics recommended. For individuals with multiple cysticerci or nonenhancing lesions (live parenchymal cysts) on brain scan, many experts recommend antiparasitic treatment together with steroids and an antiseizure medication [Garcia et al., 2004; St. Geme et al., 1993]. The argument in support of treatment is that the elimination of cysts reduces the risk of recurrent seizures, and the complications of cyst death can be managed better in a controlled situation (with both anti-inflammatory and anticonvulsant therapy), more than when cysts die naturally and unpredictably. The argument against treatment is that the cysts often die without causing symptoms, and there is the suggestion that antiparasitic drugs may enhance the development of scars and calcifications that lead to chronic seizures. Clinical studies have yielded conflicting results. Some studies have found evidence that the use of antiparasitic treatment gives a more favorable outcome [Del Brutto, 1992; Vasquez, 1992]. Other studies have not found an advantage with treatment [Carpio, 1995; Singhi, 2004; White, 2000]. Most recently, a large double-blind placebo controlled trial of patients with viable parenchymal cysts treated with both albendazole and steroids demonstrated a significant decrease in generalized seizures compared with individuals in the placebo group [Garcia et al., 2004]. Albendazole at 15 mg/kg/day (maximum 800 mg) in two doses for 8 to 30 days is recommended [Medical Letter, 2004]. Individuals with subarachnoid cysts or giant cysts in the fissures should be treated for at least 1 month [Proano, 2001].

No anthelmintic therapy is recommended by most experts for individuals with nonviable cysts on neuroimaging [Riley, 2003; Sotelo et al., 1985]. Furthermore, antiparasitic drugs may be contraindicated in patients with cerebral edema [Riley, 2003]. Because antiparasitic drugs may cause irreparable damage when used to treat ocular or spinal cysts, an ophthalmic examination should always precede antiparasitic treatment to rule out ocular cysts. Steroids are used in neurocysticercosis therapy to control inflammation and are particularly helpful in cases of encephalitis and subarachnoid, and spinal intramedullary diseases. Steroids are also recommended during the first few days of anthelmintic therapy to minimize the inflammation associated with the death of the parasite. In instances in which calcification of the cysts has occurred, prolonged use of antiepileptic drugs may be warranted [Nash, 2003]. Surgical intervention may be required to alleviate mass effect, remove cysts causing obstruction of the ventricles, or for shunt placement for hydrocephalus [Bale, 2000; Nash, 2003]. Ocular cysticercosis may also require surgical excision of the cyst.

Coenurosis

Coenurois is caused by the larval stage of *Taenia (Multiceps)* spp. *(T. multiceps, Taenia crassiceps,* and *Taenia serialis).* Cerebral coenurosis is exceedingly rare in humans. Most cases are reported from Africa, but cases have reported from Europe and South and North America [Ing, 1998]. In North America, dogs, coyotes, and foxes are the definitive hosts for *Taenia (Multiceps)* spp. (where the adult tapeworm of *T. serialis* is found). Squirrels, hares, and rabbits serve as the intermediate hosts (where the cystic larval form is generally found). When humans are accidentally infected they serve as an intermediate host, and the cystic larvae may develop in the CNS, eye, or subcutaneous or intramuscular tissues. Basal arachnoiditis and hydrocephalus are common. The clinical manifestations typically present with signs of increased intracranial pressure. The parents may describe an insidious increase in head circumference [Lowichik et al., 1995]. Death has been reported in early childhood [Hermos, 1970; Schellhas and Norris, 1985].

TREMATODES

Schistosomiasis

Epidemiology, Microbiology, and Pathology

Schistosoma haematobium infection was reported by Bilharz [1852], *Schistosoma mansoni* by Gonzalez-Martinez [1904], and *Schistosoma japonicum* was described as early as 1847 [Katsurada, 1904]. The history of schistosomiasis (bilharziasis) has been reviewed in detail [Mahmoud, 1984]. Schistosomiasis is a significant global public health problem; more than 200 million people are infected. *S. mansoni* is endemic in Africa, South America, and the Caribbean Islands. Highly concentrated areas of infestation are present in the Nile delta region and northeastern Brazil. *S. haematobium*, the organism that causes classic urinary tract bilharziasis, is found in Asia from Bombay to the Suez Canal and in Africa. *S. japonicum* causes illness in the Far East, including China, Japan, Indochina, the Philippines, and Indonesia. Several other species are recognized; *Schistosoma mekongi* and *Schistosoma malayensis* in Southeast Asia and *Schistosoma intercalatum* in Africa but are of lesser importance.

Flukes (flatworms) have complicated life cycles. The eggs gain access to water from feces or urine, where the ciliated miracidia are released and then invade the intermediate host, which is a mollusk (snail). Cercariae then emerge from the snail, penetrate the skin of humans, and are transported by the blood to the distal afferent veins of the liver, where further growth ensues followed by migration of the fluke. The snail hosts are specific for the different schistosome species, a restriction that determines the spread of disease.

S. haematobium is brought by the circulation to the bladder venous plexus and lower abdominal vessels. Urinary tract symptoms and complications follow. The liver and lower gastrointestinal tract are sometimes affected. This pattern of involvement differs from that of *S. mansoni* and *S. japonicum,* in which the organism preferentially enters the mesenteric portal and caval circulation before infecting the liver, intestines, and other organs (e.g., spleen, lungs, heart, CNS).

About 2% of patients have neurologic involvement during the third phase, with about 60% of cases caused by *S. japonicum* and 20% to 30% by *S. mansoni*. Of the three most common schistosome species, *S. japonicum* infections are more likely to involve the brain and meninges. *S. japonicum* is also the most prolific egg producer, with as many as 3500 eggs per day, about 10-fold more than the other two species produce. Eggs of the other species are more likely to produce lesions in the spinal cord, resulting in jacksonian epilepsy, transverse myelopathy, cord compression, and, in some cases, a massive and fatal necrosis [Liu, 1993]. Space-occupying lesions, or bilharziomas, are apparent on MRI and CT scans [Sun, 1982]. Adult worms, which can remain viable for 10 to 25 years, have also been reported in ectopic locations, such as brain tissue [Houston et al., 2004]. The pathogenesis of neurologic impairment is undetermined despite experimental efforts to reproduce the condition in primates [Jane et al., 1970].

Two types of lesions exist. One consists of isolated granulomatous masses that contain ova and can be surgically excised. The other type consists of diffuse small lesions that are located in both white and gray matter and are often asymptomatic. In one series of 97 patients with neurologic impairment from schistosomiasis, 60 patients were infected with *S. japonicum,* 11 with *S. haematobium,* and 26 with *S. mansoni* [Marcial-Rojas and Fiol, 1963].

Neurologic features include focal deficits, convulsions, vertigo, encephalitis, meningitis, tumor-like mass lesions, and transverse myelitis [Boyce, 1990; Brito et al., 1992; Liu, 1993; Pittella et al., 1996; Scrimgeour and Gajdusek, 1985]. Growth retardation in children, associated with depressed function of the pars anterior of the pituitary gland, has occurred [Jordan and Webbe, 1969; McGarvey et al., 1992]. A recent review has updated information on pathogenesis and diagnostic techniques relating to neuroschistosomiasis [Nascimento-Carvalho and Moreno-Carvalho, 2005].

Clinical Characteristics, Clinical Laboratory Tests, and Diagnosis

Clinical symptoms occur in three phases, the first being associated with cutaneous penetration and migration of the *Schistosoma* that results in an active dermatitis ("swimmer's itch"). The second phase (Katayama fever or syndrome) occurs 6 to 8 weeks later and consists of a wide variety of symptoms including chills, headache, fever, fatigue, hepatosplenomegaly, lymphadenopathy, eosinophilia, urticaria, and gastrointestinal distress. This phase of the disease coincides with production of eggs by the parasites, and the humoral response of the host's immune system [Sun, 1982]. Fibrous granulomas containing eosinophils, macrophages, lymphocytes, and fibroblasts develop around the eggs, producing pseudotubercles, which resemble the tubercles of tuberculosis. The third, or chronic, phase usually involves the liver, bladder wall, spleen, lung, and heart [Markell et al., 1992]. Bloody urine or bloody diarrhea may occur in *S. japonica* and intestinal schistosomiasis, but the chronic stage is often asymptomatic.

The diagnosis of schistosomiasis can be made by finding ova in stool or urine samples. Concentration of the specimen may be necessary (Kato technique) because of the small number of eggs that might be present in clinical samples. In chronic schistosomiasis, however, eggs may not be passed, and rectal, bladder, or liver biopsies may be required for definitive diagnosis. Immunodiagnostic techniques for antibody detection are of limited worth because of cross-reactivity with other helminth infections. Slow and diffuse alpha wave patterns have been reported in EEGs of some patients [Hayashi, 2003]. Diagnosis of schistosomiasis may be established with several tests, including an intradermal skin test, a complement fixation test, a cholesterol-lecithin cercarial slide flocculation test, and a bentonite flocculation test. The cholesterol-lecithin test has a sensitivity of 77% to 90% in parasitologically confirmed cases. Identification of the parasite in urine, feces, and tissue is diagnostic (see Table 70-3). An enzyme-linked immunosorbent assay test for circulating schistosome antigen can give both qualitative and quantitative (the parasite burden) results [Deelder et al., 1989]. Brain neuroimaging studies may reveal edema, multifocal lucencies, and atrophy in later stages of the disease [Kirchoff and Nash, 1984; Khalil et al., 1984; Pittella et al., 1996], whereas investigation of spinal cord schistosomiasis may reveal myelitis, swelling at the base of the cord (conus medullaris), or cord compression [Brito et al., 1992; van Leusen and Perquin, 2000].

In a study of patients ages 3 to 19 years living in an area endemic for *S. mansoni* and with stool or biopsy verification of infection, cerebrospinal fluid examination revealed pleocytosis (7 to 560 white blood cells/mm^3), eosinophilia (1 to 66 cells/mm^3), and elevated protein (45 to 3540 mg/dL) [Nascimento-Carvalho and Moreno-Carvalho, 2004]. Ova have not been found in cerebrospinal fluid [Hughes and Biggs, 2002]. Paraparesis, urinary retention, and paraplegia were the most common symptoms presenting by pediatric patients [Nascimento-Carvalho and Moreno-Carvalho, 2004].

Management

Schistosomiasis should be considered in individuals with neurologic impairment and a travel history to endemic areas, particularly if patients had been bathing, swimming, or wading in sewage-contaminated rivers or streams. Praziquantel (40 to 60 mg/day divided into two or three doses for pediatric and adult patients) is the drug of choice for the treatment of *S. haematobium, S. mansoni,* and *S. intercalatum* infections [Markell et al., 1992; Medical Letter, 2004]. An antiepileptic drug is recommended in cases with more than two seizures per week [Hayashi, 2003]. In vivo testing of praziquantel on mice, at a dose 5 to 10 times that used in humans, found that the drug killed mature *S. mansoni* ova, and may be useful in treating CNS infections [Richards et al., 1989]. Corticosteroid use, with and without praziquantel, was effective in lessening symptoms in some cases, though controlled studies have not been done due to the relative rarity of the disease [Fowler et al., 1999; Haribhai et al., 1991; Houston et al., 2004]. Oxamniquine (pediatric dose of 20 mg/kg in two divided doses times 1 day) is an alternative agent for *S. mansoni.* Niridazole, stibophen, and antimony potassium tartrate are also of value. Intravenous injection of tartar emetic is the recommended therapy for *S. japonicum.* Surgical intervention may prove necessary for mass lesions in the brain or spinal cord.

Paragonimiasis

Epidemiology, Microbiology, and Pathology

Paragonimiasis, a neurologic and neurosurgical condition, has a high incidence in the Far East and occurs less frequently in some regions of Africa and South America [Kusner and King, 1993]. Otani first reported cerebral paragonimiasis in 1887 [Otani, 1887]. The condition is a serious complication of the benign infection caused by the lung fluke, *Paragonimus westermani.* The ingestion of the metacercarial parasite, while residing in its crab or crayfish intermediate host, is the usual mode of human infection. The crustaceans are infected after ingestion of cercaria-laden snails that have previously been infected by miracidia. A number of carnivorous mammals may serve as reservoir hosts for humans, passing ova in feces.

Gross observation of the brain demonstrates meningeal adhesions and areas of exudate. Cortical atrophy is sometimes present. Nodules and cysts may be found in the subcortical region. Abscesses with suppurative material in their centers appear throughout the brain. Cavitation and liquefaction around the egg may be due to toxin release [Sun, 1982]. Ova are sometimes present in the abscesses and meningeal infiltrate. All types of leukocytes are seen in the areas of inflammation when examined microscopically. Granulomas with giant Langhans' cells and epithelioid cells are frequently found in chronic granulomas. Gliosis and fibrosis, appropriate to anatomic location, are widespread. Calcification of the lesion eventually occurs. If cerebrospinal fluid circulation is impeded, hydrocephalus may result [Sun, 1982]. Spinal paragonimiasis, either epidural or intradural, is usually represented by ovum-filled cysts. Spinal cord atrophy may be prominent. The microscopic pathologic abnormalities are indistinguishable from those present in the brain.

Clinical Characteristics, Clinical Laboratory Tests, and Diagnosis

After human ingestion of infected raw or poorly cooked crab or crayfish, the metacercariae excyst in the small intestine and pierce the intestinal wall as larvae, embedding in the abdominal wall. After several days the larvae re-enter the abdominal cavity and migrate to the diaphragm, pleural cavity, and lungs before maturing into adult flukes. Although the worms are hermaphroditic, they usually occur in pairs and cross-fertilize. Adult worms are reported to live for 10 to 20 years [Hughes and Biggs, 2002]. The mechanism of entrance of the immature fluke into the brain or spinal cord is not precisely known. The most widely held theory of the mechanism of brain involvement is that larvae traverse the soft tissues of the neck surrounding the jugular vein and nerve trunks and then enter the brain through the jugular foramen, causing arachnoiditis, abscesses, or granulomas [Yokogawa, 1921]. Direct invasion of larvae from the lung is assumed to cause extradural spinal involvement, and extension of infection from the brain through the subarachnoid space is believed to be the mechanism of intradural spinal infection [Oh, 1978].

Lung disease, including pleurisy, pneumothorax, and hemoptysis, constitutes the cardinal clinical feature of paragonimiasis. Cerebral infection occurs in approximately 0.8% of patients; spinal cord involvement is even less common. Less than 50% of the patients with neurologic disease are younger than 20 years of age. Prominent cerebral characteristics include meningitis, subacute progressive encephalopathy, cerebral infarction, seizures, mass lesions, and dementia. Approximately two thirds of 62 patients were reported to have seizures [Oh, 1978]. The emergence of clinical manifestations is gradual. Meningitis is the initial condition in two thirds of patients. Headache, nausea and vomiting, visual impairment, hemiplegia, and mental deterioration often occur early in the course of the illness. Neurologic evaluation frequently documents dementia, homonymous hemianopia, optic atrophy, diminished visual acuity, hemiparesis, hemihypesthesia, and meningismus [Oh, 1978]. When the condition is diagnosed and treated in a timely manner, the prognosis is excellent. The most common location of spinal involvement is in the lower thoracic area. An extradural mass may cause spastic paraplegia. More rarely an intradural lesion occurs.

Definitive diagnosis of paragonimiasis requires finding the operculated eggs in sputum or feces. Ova, however, may not be found in sputum for some species of *Paragonimus* or if adult worms are in an ectopic location. In one report, chest radiographs were abnormal in 80% of patients; they revealed pneumonia, pleural abnormalities, and cystonodular lesions. Approximately 70% of patients had abnormal cranial radiographs that indicated increased intracranial pressure (25%) and calcifications (50%). Porencephaly and cortical and subcortical atrophy were demonstrated by pneumoencephalography in several patients. Myelography proved necessary for the diagnosis of spinal cord lesions [Oh, 1978]. Newer imaging techniques may prove superior for screening purposes [Lowichik and Ruff, 1995b]. Other studies include intradermal skin injection, examination of sputum and stool for ova, and immunologic determinations. An enzyme-linked immunosorbent assay test is available. The complement fixation test is valuable and sensitive. Peripheral blood eosinophilia is often present. Pleocytosis (approximately equal numbers of polymorphonuclear cells and mononuclear cells), decreased glucose concentration, and increased protein and chloride content are frequent spinal fluid findings. Differential diagnoses are neurotuberculosis, neoplasm, encephalitis, neurocysticercosis, and cerebral hemorrhage [Sun, 1982]. A case of cerebral paragonimiasis, apparently acquired in childhood, lay dormant for about 30 years before becoming symptomatic [Kang et al., 2000].

Management

Praziquantel (75 mg/kg day divided into three doses for 2 days, for both pediatric and adult patients) is used as initial treatment [Medical Letter, 2004]. Bithionol therapy (30 to 50 mg/kg on alternate days for 10 to 15 doses) can alternatively be used for meningitic involvement. Chronic cerebral lesions or spinal cord lesions require surgical intervention accompanied by adjunctive chemotherapy [Higashi et al., 1971; Oh, 1978].

ACKNOWLEDGMENTS

The assistance of Sabrina Gilliam and Penny Savage is greatly appreciated. The comments of Dr. Chris Paddock, Peter Schantz, Kevin Kazacos, and Daniel Sexton are also appreciated.

REFERENCES

Ackerman SB, Seed JR. The effects of tryptophol on immune responses and its implications towards trypanosome induced immunosuppression. Experientia 1976;15:645.

Adams S, Brown H, Turner G. Breaking down the blood-brain barrier: Signaling a path to cerebral malaria? Trends Parasitol 2002;18:360.

Adjuik M, Babiker A, Garner P, et al. International Artemisinin Study Group. Artesunate combinations for treatment of malaria: Meta-analysis. Lancet 2004;363:9.

Aikawa JC. Rocky Mountain spotted fever. Springfield, IL: Charles C Thomas, 1966.

Ajello L, Zeidberg LD. Isolation of *Histoplasma capsulatum* and *Allescheria boydii* from soil. Science 1951;113:662.

Allen AC, Saitz S. A comparative study of the pathology of scrub typhus and other rickettsial diseases. Am J Pathol 1945:21;603.

Allouche A, Baily W, Barton S, et al. Comparison of chlorproguanil-dapsone with sulfadoxine-pyrimethamine for the treatment of uncomplicated falciparum malaria in young African children: Double-blind randomized controlled trial. Lancet 2004;363:1843.

Altinors N, Bavbek M, Caner HH, et al. Central nervous system hydatidosis in Turkey: A cooperative study and literature survey analysis of 458 cases. J Neurosurg 2000;93:1.

Altschuler G. Toxoplasmosis as the cause of hydranencephaly. Am J Dis Child 1973;125:251.

Anadol D, Ozcelik U, Kiper N, et al. Treatment of hydatid disease. Paediatr Drugs 2001;3:123.

Anzil AP, Rao C, Wrzolek MA, et al. Amebic encephalitis in a patient with AIDS caused by a newly recognized opportunistic pathogen. Arch Pathol Lab Med 1991;115:21.

Apley J, Clarke SKR, Roome APCH, et al. Primary amoebic meningoencephalitis in Britain. BMJ 1970;1:596.

Araújo JC, Werneck L, Cravo MA. South American blastomycosis presenting as a posterior fossa tumor. J Neurosurg 1978;49:425.

Araújo MSS, Martins-Filho OA, Pereira MES, Brener Z. A combination of benznidazole and ketoconazole enhances efficacy of chemotherapy of experimental Chagas' disease. J Antimicrob Ther 2000;45:819.

Arisoy ES, Arisoy AE, Dunne WM Jr. Clinical significance of fungi isolated from cerebrospinal fluid in children. Pediatr Infect Dis J 1994;13:128.

Arpino C, Gattinara GC, Piergili D, et al. *Toxocara* infection and epilepsy in children: A case control study. Epilepsia 1990;31:33.

Ashley NF. The detection and treatment of *Plasmodium falciparum* malaria: Time for change. J Postgrad Med 2004;50:35.

Aubertin C, Giroux L. Existe-t-il une leucemie Aga eosinophiles? Presse Med 1921;29:314.

Azad AF. Epidemiology of murine typhus. Annu Rev Entomol 1990;35:553.

Bächli H, Minet JC, Gratzal O. Cerebral toxocariasis: A possible cause of epileptic seizure in children. Childs Nerv Syst 2004;20:468.

Badenoch PR, Grimmond TR, Cadwgan J, et al. Nasal carriage of free-living amoebae. Microbiol Ecol Health Dis 1988;1:209.

Baganz MD, Dross PE, Reinhardt JA. Rocky Mountain spotted fever encephalitis: MR findings. Am J Neuroradiol 1995;16:919.

Bakardjiev A., Azimi PH, Ashouri N, et al. Amebic encephalitis caused by *Balamuthia mandrillaris*: Report of four cases. Pediatr Infect Dis 2003;22:447.

Bale JF Jr. Cysticercosis. Curr Treat Options Neurol 2000;2:355.

Banuelos AF, Williams PL, Johnson RH, et al. Central nervous system abscesses due to *Coccidioides* species. Clin Infect Dis 1996;22:240.

Baquera-Heredia J, Cruz-Reyes A, Flores-Gaxiola A, et al. Case report: Ocular gnathostomiasis in northwestern Mexico. Am J Trop Med Hyg 2002;66:572.

Barnett NDP, Kaplan AM, Hopkin RJ, et al. Primary amoebic meningoencephalitis with *Naegleria fowleri:* Clinical review. Pediatr Neurol 1996;15:230.

Beaman BL, Beaman L. *Nocardia* species: Host parasite relationships. Clin Microbiol Rev 1994;7:213.

Beautyman W, Beaver PC, Buckley JC, et al. Review of a case previously reported as showing an ascarid larva in the brain. J Pathol Bacteriol 1965;91:271.

Beaver PC, Rosen L. Memorandum on the first report of *Angiostrongylus* in man, by Nomura and Lin 1945. Am J Trop Med Hyg 1964;13:589.

Beaver PC. The nature of visceral larva migrans. J Parasitol 1969;55(1):3.

Bebrova E, Lochmann O, Tichy M, et al. *Actinomyces viscosus* in subdural empyema. Cesk Epidemiol Mikrobiol Imunol 1994;43:21.

Beggs I. The radiology of hydatid disease. AJR Am J Roentgenol 1985;145:639.

Bell WE, Myers MG. *Allescheria (Petriellidum) boydii* brain abscess in a child with leukemia. Arch Neurol 1978;35:386.

Bennett JE, Dismukes WE, Duma RJ, et al. A comparison of amphotericin B alone combined with flucytosine in the treatment of cryptococcal meningitis. N Engl J Med 1979;301:126.

Bergquist NR, Stintzing G, Smedman L, et al. Diagnosis of encephalitizoonosis in man by serological tests. BMJ 1984;288:902.

Berman SJ, Kundin WD. Scrub typhus in South Vietnam: A study of 87 cases. Ann Intern Med 1973;79:26.

Berriman M, Ghedin E. Hertz-Fowler C, et al. The genome of the African trypanosome *Trypanosoma brucei.* Science 2005;309:416.

Bertoli F, Espino M, Arosemena JR 5th, et al. A spectrum in the pathology of toxoplasmosis in patients with acquired immunodeficiency syndrome. Arch Pathol Lab Med 1995;119:214.

Bia FJ, Barry M. Parasitic infections of the central nervous system. Neurol Clin 1986;4:171.

Bilharz T. Ein Beitrag zur Helminthographia humana, aus brieflichen Mittheilungen des Dr. Bilharz in Cairo. Z Wiss Zool 1852; 4:53.

Birbeck GL. Cerebral malaria. Curr Treat Options Neurol 2004;6:125.

Biswas J, Gopal L, Sharma T, et al. Intraocular *Gnathostoma spinigerium:* Clinicopathologic study of two cases with review of literature. Retina 1994;14:438.

Bitsori M, Galanakis E, Gikas A, et al. *Rickettsia typhi* infction in childhood. Acta Paediatr 2002;91(1):59.

Bittencourt AL. Congenital Chagas' disease. Am J Dis Child 1976;130:97.

Bjorkenheim B. Optic neuropathy caused by vitamin B_{12} deficiency in carriers of the fish tapeworm: *Diphyllobothrium latum.* Lancet 1966;1:688.

Boongird P, Phuapradit P, Siridej N, et al. Neurological manifestations of gnathostomiasis. J Neurol Sci 1977;31:279.

Borges AS, Ferreira MS, Silvestre MT, et al. Histoplasmosis in immunodepressed patients: Study of 18 cases seen. Rev Soc Bras Med Trop 1997;30:119.

Boyce TG. Acute transverse myelitis in a 6-year-old girl with schistosomiasis. Pediat Infect Dis J 1990;9:279.

Boyce WM, Asai DJ, Wilder JK et al. Physicochemical characterization and monoclonal and polyclonal antibody recognition of *Baylisascaris procynosis* larval excretory secretory antigens. J Parasitol 1989;75:540.

Bradsher RW. Histoplasmosis and blastomycosis. Clin Infect Dis 1996;22(Suppl 2):S102.

Bravo F, Sanchez, MR. New and re-emerging cutaneous infectious diseases in Latin America and other geographic areas. Dermatol Clin 2003;21:655.

Brener A. The pathogenesis of Chagas' disease: An overview of current theories. Washington, DC. PAHO, 1994 (Scientific Publication No. 547).

Brito JC, DaSilva JA, DaSilva EB, et al. Spinal cord neuroschistosomiasis: Clinical and laboratory evaluation of 5 cases. Arq Neuropsiquiatr 1992;50:207.

Bross JE, Gordon G. Nocardial meningitis: Case reports and review. Rev Inf Dis 1991;13:160.

Brown JR. Human actinomycosis: A study of 181 subjects. Hum Pathol 1973;4:319.

Brown RL. Successful treatment of primary amebic meningoencephalitis. Arch Intern Med 1991;151:1201.

Brown WJ, Voge M. Neuropathology of parasitic infections. Oxford: Oxford University Press, 1982.

Bruce D, Nabarro D. Progress report on sleeping sickness in Uganda. Reports of the Sleeping Sickness Commission of the Royal Society 1903;1:11.

Bruster DR, Kwiatsowski D, White NJ. Neurological sequelae of cerebral malaria in children. Lancet 1990;336:1039.

Buller RS, Arens M, Hmiel SP et al. *Ehrlichia ewingii,* a newly recognized agent of human ehrlichiosis. N Eng J Med 1999;341:148.

Burchmore RJA, Ogbunde POJ, Enanga B, Barrett MP. Chemotherapy of human African trypanosomiasis. Curr Pharmaceut Design 2002;8:195.

Butler T, Tong MJ, Fletcher JR, et al. Blood coagulation studies in *Plasmodium falciparum* malaria. Am J Med Sci 1973;265:63.

Butt CG. Primary amebic meningoencephalitis. N Eng J Med 1966;274:1473.

Callicot JH, Nelson EC, Jones, MM, et al. Meningoencephaltis due to pathogenic free-living amoebae. Report of two cases. JAMA 1968;206:579.

Carpentier AF, Bernard L, Poisson M, et al. Central nervous system infections in patients with malignant diseases. Rev Neurol Paris 1996;152:587.

Carpio A, Hauser WA. Prognosis for seizure recurrence in patients with newly diagnosed neurocysticercosis. Neurology 2002;59:1730.

Carpio A, Escobar A, Hauser WA. Cysticercosis and epilepsy: A critical review. Epilepsia 1998;39:1025.

Carpio A, Santillan F, Leon P, et al. Is the course of neurocysticercosis modified by treatment with antihelminthic agents? Arch Intern Med 1995;155:1982.

Carrea R, Dowling E Jr, Guevara JA. Surgical treatment of hydatid cysts of the central nervous system in the pediatric age (Dowling's technique). Childs Brain 1975;1:4.

Carter R, Mendis KN. Evolutionary and historical aspects of the burden of malaria. Clin Microbiol Rev 2002;15:564.

Casey AT, Wilkins P, Uttley D. Aspergillosis infection in neurosurgical practice. Br J Neurosurg 1994;8:31.

Caudill RG, Smith CE, Reinarz JA. Coccidioidal meningitis, a diagnostic challenge. Am J Med 1970;49:360.

Cegielski JP, Durack DT. Trypanosomiasis. In: Scheld WM, Whitley RJ, Durack DY, eds. Infections of the central nervous system, 2nd ed. Philadelphia: Lippincott-Raven, 1997.

Centeno M, Rivera F, Cerva L, et al. *Hartmannella vermiformis* isolated from the cerebrospinal fluid of a young male patient with meningoencephalitis and bronchopneumonia. Arch Med Res 1996;27:579.

Centers for Disease Control. Epidemiologic notes and reports of human ehrlichiosis 1988;(17):275.

Centers for Disease Control. Current trends, Rocky Mountain spotted fever and human ehrlichiosis—United States, 1989. MMWR 1990;39(17):281.

Centers for Disease Control. Treatment of severe *Plasmodium falciparum* malaria with quinidine gluconate: Discontinuation of parenteral quinine from CDC drug service. MMWR 1991;40(14):240.

Centers for Disease Control. Trichinellosis surveillance—United States, 1997–2001. MMWR 2003;52 (No. SS-6):1.

Centers for Disease Control. Fatal cases of Rocky Mountain spotted fever in family clusters—three states, 2003. MMWR 2004;53:407.

Cerva L. *Acanthamoeba culbertsoni* and *Naegleria fowleri:* Occurrence of antibodies in man. J Hyg Epidemiol Microbiol 1989;33:99.

Cerva L, Serbus C, Skocil V. Isolation of limax amoebae from the nasal mucosa of man. Folia Parasitol (Praha) 1973;20:97.

Chapman SW, Bradsher RW, Campbell GD, et al Practice guidelines for the management of patients with blastomycosis. Clin Infect Dis 2000;30:679.

Chen ER. Current status of food-borne parasitic zoonoses in Taiwan. Southeast Asian J Trop Med Public Health 1991;22:62.

Chen Q, Schlichtherle M, Wahlgren M. Molecular aspects of severe malaria. Clin Microbiol Rev 2000;13:439.

Chen SM, Dumler JS, Feng HM, et al. Identification of the antigenic constituents of *Ehrlichia chaffeensis.* Am J Trop Med Hyg 1994;50:52.

Chia JKS, Nakata MM, Schenley C. Smear-negative cerebral malaria due to mefloquine-resistant *Plasmodium falciparum* acquired in the Amazon. J Infect Dis 1992;165:599.

Chimelli L, Mahler-Araujo MB. Fungal infections. Brain Pathol 1997;7:613.

Chiou CC, Wong TT, Lin HH, et al. Fungal infection of ventriculoperitoneal shunts in children. Clin Infect Dis 1994;19:1049.

Chitanondh H, Rosen L. Fatal eosinophilic encephalomyelitis caused by the nematode *Gnathostoma spinigerum*. Am J Trop Med Hyg 1967;16:638.

Chotmongkol V, Sawanyawisuth K, Thavornpitak Y. Corticosteroid treatment of eosinophilic meningitis. Clin Infect Dis 2000;31:660.

Chye SM, Lin SR, Chen YL, et al. Immuno-PCR for detection of antigen to *Angiostrongylus cantonensis* circulating fifth-stage worms. Clin Chem 2004;50:51.

Ciricillo SF, Rosenblum MI. Use of CT and MR imaging to distinguish intracranial lesions and to define the need for biopsy in AIDS patients. J Neurosurg 1990;73:720.

Ciurea AV, Vasilescu G, Nuteanu L, et al. Cerebral hydatid cyst in children. Experience of 27 cases. Childs Nerv Syst 1995;11:679.

Clark IA, Alleva LM, Mills AC, Cowden WB. Pathogenesis of malaria and clinically similar conditions. Clin Microbiol Rev 2004;17:509.

Clark RA, Greer D, Atkinson W, et al. Spectrum of *Cryptococcus neoformans* infection in 68 patients affected with human immunodeficiency virus. Rev Inf Dis 1990;12:768.

Coatney GR, Collins WE, Warren M, et al. The primary malarias. Bethesda, MD: US Department of Health, Education and Welfare, National Institutes of Health, National Institutes of Allergy and Infectious Disease, 1971.

Coker SB, Beltran RS. *Candida* meningitis: Clinical and radiographic diagnosis. Pediatr Neurol 1988;4:317.

Cooke-Yarborough CM, Lornberg AJ, Hogg GG, et al. A fatal case of angiostrongyliasis in an 11-month-old infant. Med J Aust 1999;7:517.

Cooper RA Jr, Goldstein EG. Histoplasmosis of the central nervous system. Am J Med 1963;35:45.

Copley IB, Fripp PJ, Erasmus AM, et al. Unusual presentations of cerebral hydatid disease in children. Br J Neurosurg 1992;6:203.

Cornford E, Bocash WD, Braun LD, et al. Rapid distribution of tryptophol (3-indole ethanol) to the brain and other tissues. J Clin Invest 1979;63:1241.

Couch JR, Abdou NI, Sagawa A. *Histoplasma* meningitis with hyperactive suppressor T cell in cerebrospinal fluid. Neurology 1978;28:119.

Councilman WT, Lafleur HA. Amebic dysentery. Johns Hopkins Hosp Rep 1891;2:193.

Cox FEG. History of human parasitology. Clin Microbiol Rev 2002;15:595.

Croft SL, Seifert K, Duchêne M. Antiprotozoal activities of phospholipid analogues. Mol Biochem Parasitol 2003;126:165.

Cross JH, Chi JC. ELISA for the detection of *Angiostrongylus cantonensis* antibodies in patients with eosinophilic meningitis. Southeast Asian J Trop Med Public Health 1982;13:73.

Cuadrado LM, Guerrero A, Garcia Asenjo JA, et al. Cerebral mucormycosis in two cases of acquired immunodeficiency syndrome. Arch Neurol 1988;45:109.

Culbertson CG, Smith JW, Minner JR. *Acanthamoeba*: Observations on animal pathogenicity. Science 1958;127:1506.

Cunningham CK, Kazacos K, McMillan JA, et al. Diagnosis and management of *Baylisascaris procyonis* infection in an infant with nonfatal meningoencephalitis. Clin Inf Dis 1994;18:868.

Cursons RTM, Brown TJ, Keys EA, et al. Immunity to pathogenic free-living amoebae: Role of humoral immunity. Infect Immun 1980;29:401.

Daar ES, Meyer RD. Bacterial and fungal infections. Med Clin North Am 1992;76:173.

Dalton MJ, Clarke MJ, Holman RC, et al. National surveillance for Rocky Mountain spotted fever, 1981-1992: Epidemiologic summary and evaluation of risk factors for fatal outcome. Am J Trop Med Hyg 1995;52(5):405.

Damaj G, Ivanov V, Le Brigand B, et al. Rapid improvement of disseminated aspergillosis with caspofungin/voriconazole combination in an adult leukemic patient. Ann Hematol 2004 Jun;83(6):390.

Dardé M-L. Genetic analysis of the diversity in *Toxoplasma gondii*. Ann Ist Super Sanita 2004;40:57.

Darling ST. A protozoan general infection producing pseudotubercles in the lungs and focal necrosis in the liver, spleen, and lymph nodes. JAMA 1906;202:679.

Daroff RB, Deller JJ, Kasti AJ, et al. Cerebral malaria. JAMA 1967;202:679.

Dawood AA, Moosa A. Cerebral cysticercosis in children. J Trop Pediatr 1984;30;136.

de Almeida SM, Queiroz-Telles F, Teive HA, et al Central nervous system paracoccidioidomycosis: Clinical features and laboratorial findings. J Infect 2004;48:193.

de Castro SL, Santa-Rita RM, Urbina JA, Croft SL. Antiprotozoal lysophospholipid analogues: A comparison of their activity against trypanosomal parasites and tumor cells. Mini-Rev Med Chem 2004;4:141.

Deelder AM, De Jonge N, Boerman OC, et al. Sensitive determination of circulating anodic antigen in *Schistosoma mansoni* infected individuals by an enzyme-linked immunosorbent assay using monoclonal antibodies. Am J Trop Med Hyg 1989;40:268.

Deetz TR, Sawyer MH, Billman G, et al. Successful treatment of *Balamuthia* amoebic encephalitis: Presentation of two cases. Clin Infect Dis 2003;37:1304.

de Lastours V, Lefort A, Zappa M, et al. Two cases of cerebral aspergillosis successfully treated with voriconazole. Eur J Clin Microbiol Infect Dis. 2003 May;22(5):297.

Del Brutto OH, Rajshekhar V, White AC Jr, et al. Proposed diagnostic criteria for neurocysticercosis. Neurology 2001;57:177

Del Brutto OH. Cysticercosis and cerebrovascular disease: A review. J Neurol Neurosurg Psychiatr 1992;55:252.

DeMonbreum WA. Cultivation and cultural characteristics of Darling's *Histoplasma capsulatum*. Am J Trop Med 1934;14:93.

Denning DW. Invasive aspergillosis. Clin Infect Dis 1998;26:781.

Dent JH, Nichols RL, Beaver PC, et al. Visceral larva migrans; with a case report. Am J Pathol 1956;32(4):777.

Desmonts G, Couvreur J. Congenital toxoplasmosis. N Engl J Med 1974;290:1110.

Dhar P, Chaudhary A, Desai R, et al. Current trends in the diagnosis and management of cystic hydatid disease of the liver. J Commun Dis 1996;28:221.

Diamond RD, Bennett JE. A subcutaneous reservoir for intrathecal therapy of fungal meningitis. N Engl J Med. 1973 Jan 25;288(4):186.

Didier ES, Bessinger GT. Host-parasite relationships in microsporidiosis: Animal models and immunology. In: Wittner M, Weiss, LM, eds. The microsporidia and microsporidiosis. Washington, DC: ASM Press, 1999.

Dismukes WE. Blastomycosis: Leave it to beaver. N Engl J Med 1986;314:575.

Dixon MBF, Lipscomb FM. Cysticercosis; an analysis and follow-up of 450 cases. 1961 London: Her Majesty's Stationary Service.

Doan-Wiggins L. Tick-borne diseases. Emerg Med Clin North Am 1991;9:303.

Donelson JE. Antigenic variation and the African trypanosome genome. Acta Trop 2003;85:391.

Donelson JE, Turner MJ. How the trypanosome changes its coat. Sci Am 1985;252:44.

Donnelly H, Bernard EM, Rothkotter H, et al. Distribution of pentamidine in patients with AIDS. J Infect Dis 1988;157:985.

Donovan BJ, Weber DJ, Rublein JC, et al. Treatment of tick-borne diseases. Ann Pharmachother 2002;36(10):1590.

Doua F, Boa Yapo F. Current therapy of trypanosomiasis. Bull Soc Pathol Exot 1994;87:337.

Duke BJ, Tyson RW, DeBiasi R, et al. *Balamuthia mandrillaris* meningoencephalitis presenting with acute hydrocephalus. Pediatr Neurosurg 1997;26:107.

Duma RJ. Primary amebic meningoencephalitis. In: Warren KS, Mahmoud AAD, eds. Tropical geographical medicine. New York: McGraw-Hill, 1984.

Duma RJ, Rosenblum WI, McGehee RF, et al. Primary amoebic meningoencephalitis caused by *Naegleria*. Two new cases, response to amphotericin B, and a review. Ann Int Med 1971;74:923.

Dumler JS. Molecular methods for ehrlichiosis and Lyme disease. Clin Lab Med 2003;23(4):867.

Dupouy-Camet J. Trichinellosis: a worldwide zoonosis. Vet Parasitol 2000;Dec 1;93(3-4):191.

Duprez TP, Bigaignon G, Delgrange E, et al. MRI of cervical cord lesions and their resolution in *Toxocara canis* myelopathy. Neuroradiology 1996; 38:792.

Durack DT. Amebic infections. In: Scheld WM, Whitley RJ, Durack DY, eds. Infections of the central nervous system, 2nd ed. Philadelphia: Lippincott-Raven, 1997.

Eckert J, Deplaze P. Biological, epidemiological, and clinical aspects of echinococcosis, a zoonosis of increasing concern. Clin Microbiol Rev. 2004;17:107.

Einstein, HE, Johnson, RH. Coccidioidomycosis: New aspects of epidemiology and therapy. Clin Infect Dis 1993;16:349.

Ellrodt Z, Halfon P, Le Bras P, et al. Multifocal central nervous system lesions in three patients with trichinosis. Arch Neurol 1987;44:432.

El-Sayed NM, Myler PJ, Blandin G, et al. Comparative genomics of trypanosomatid parasitic protozoa. Science 2005a;309:404.

El-Sayed NM, Myler PJ, Bartholomeu DC, et al. The genome sequence of *Trypanosoma cruzi*, etiologic agent of Chagas disease. Science 2005b;309:409.

Emanuel B, Aronson N, Shulman S. Malaria in children in Chicago. Pediatrics 1993;92:83.

Enarson DA, Keys TF, Onofrio BM. Central nervous system histoplasmosis with obstructive hydrocephalus. Am J Med 1978;64:895.

Ergun R, Okten AL, Yuksel M, et al. Orbital hydatid cysts: Report of four cases. Neurosurg Rev 1997;20:33.

Ersahin Y, Mutluer S, Guzelbag E. Intracranial hydatid cysts in children. Neurosurgery 1993;33:219.

Escobar A. The pathology of neurocysticercosis. In: Palacios E, Rodriguez-Carbajal J, Taveras J, et al. Cysticercosis of the central nervous system. Springfield, IL: Charles C Thomas, 1983;27.

Esernio-Jenssen D, Scimeca PG, Benach JL, Tenenbaum MJ. Transplacental/perinatal babesiosis. J Pediatr 1987;110:57.

Everett ED, Evans KA, Henry RB, et al. Human ehrlichiosis in adults after tick exposure: Diagnosis using polymerase chain reaction. Ann Intern Med 1994;120:730.

Fairlamb AH. Chemotherapy of human African trypanosomiasis: Current and future prospects. Trends Parasitol 2003;19:488.

Fang, CT, Ferng WF, Hwang JJ, et al. Life-threatening scrub typhus with meningoencephalitis and acute respiratory distress syndrome. J Formos Med Assoc l997;96:213.

Feder Jr HM, Lawlor M, Krause PJ. Babesiosis in pregnancy. N Eng J Med 2003;349:195.

Feigin RD, Snider RL, Edwards MS. Rickettsial diseases. In: Feigin RD, Cherry JD, eds. Textbook of pediatric infectious diseases, 3rd ed. Philadelphia: WB Saunders, 1992.

Feldman HA. Toxoplasma and toxoplasmosis. Hosp Pract 1969;4:64.

Feldstein A. Ethanol-induced sleep in relation to serotonin turnover and conversion to 5-hydroxyindole-acetaldehyde, 5-hydroxytryptophol and 5-hydroxyindole acetic acid. Ann N Y Acad Sci 1973;215:71.

Fetter BF, Klintworth GK, Hendry WS. Mycoses of the central nervous system. Baltimore: Williams & Wilkins, 1967.

Feydy A, Touze E, Miaux Y, et al. MRI in a case of neurotrichinosis. Neuroradiology 1996;38(Suppl 1):S80.

Fishbein DB, Dawson JE, Robinson LE. Human ehrlichiosis in the United States, 1985 to 1990. Ann Intern Med 1994;120:736.

Fishbein DB, Frontini MG, Giles R, et al. Fatal cases of Rocky Mountain spotted fever in the United States, 1981-1988. Ann N Y Acad Sci. 1990;590:246.

Fourestie V, Douceron H, Brugieres P, et al. Neurotrichinosis. A cerebrovascular disease associated with myocardial injury and hypereosinophilia. Brain 1993;116:603.

Fowler M, Carter RF. Acute pyogenic meningitis probably due to *Acanthamoeba* spp: A preliminary report. BMJ 1965;2:240.

Fowler R, Lee C, Keystone JS. The role of corticosteroids in the treatment of cerebral schistosomiasis caused by *Schistosoma mansoni:* Case report and discussion. Am J Trop Med Hyg 1999;61:47.

Fox AS, Kazacos KR, Gould NS, et al. Fatal eosinophilic meningoencephalitis and visceral larva migrans caused by the raccoon ascarid *Baylisascaris procyonis*. N Engl J Med 1985;312:1619.

Frenkel JK. Toxoplasmosis. Pediatr Clin North Am 1985;32:917.

Friedland LR, Raphael SA, Deutsch ES, et al. Disseminated *Acanthamoeba* infection in a child with symptomatic human immunodeficiency virus infection. Pediatr Infect Dis J 1992;11:404.

Fritsche G, Larcher C, Schennach H, Weiss G. Regulatory interactions between iron and nitric oxide metabolism for immune defense against *Plasmodium falciparum* infection. J Infect Dis 2001;183:1388.

Fuentes I, Rubio JM, Ramirez C, Alcar J. Genotypic characterization of *Toxoplasma gondii* strains associated with human toxoplasmosis in Spain: Direct analysis from clinical samples. J Clin Microbiol 2001;39:1566.

Fuller A, Munckhoff W, Kiers L, et al. Eosinophilic meningitis due to *Angiostrongylus cantonensis*. West J Med 1993;159:78.

Funata M, Custis P, de la Cruz Z, et al. Intraocular gnathostomiasis. Retina 1993;13:240.

Galanakis E, Gikas A, Bitsori M, Sbyrakis S. *Rickettsia typhi* infection presenting as subacute meningitis. J Chil Neurol 2002;17(2):156.

Galarza M, Cuccia V, Sosa FP, et al. Pediatric granulomatous cerebral amebiasis: A delayed diagnosis. Pediatr Neurol 2002;26:153.

Galetta SL, Wule AE, Goldberg HI, et al. Rhinocerebral mucormycosis: Management and survival after carotid occlusion. Ann Neurol 1990;28:103.

Galgani JN. Coccidiomycosis. In: Remington JS, Swartz MN, eds. Current clinical topics in infectious disease. Boston: Blackwell Scientific Publications, 1997.

Gallerano RH, Marr JJ, Sosa RR. Therapeutic efficacy of allopurinol in patients with chronic Chagas' disease. Am J Trop Med Hyg 1990;43:159.

Garcia HH, Del Brutto OH. Imaging findings in neurocysticercosis. Acta Trop 2003;87:71.

Garcia HH, Pretell EJ, Gilman RH, et al. A trial of antiparasitic treatment to reduce the rate of seizures due to cerebral cysticercosis. N Engl J Med 2004;350:249.

Garcia L. Parasitic diseases. In: Feigin RD, Cherry JD, eds. Textbook of pediatric infectious diseases, 3rd ed. Philadelphia: WB Saunders, 1992.

Garcia LS. Laboratory identification of the microsporidia. J Clin Microbiol 2002;40:1892.

Gardner MJ, Hall N, Fung E, et al. Genome sequence of the human malaria parasite *Plasmodium falciparum*. Nature 2002;419:498.

Gay T, Pankey G, Beckman E, et al. Fatal CNS trichinosis. JAMA 1982;247:1024.

Gelman BB, Popov V, Chaljub G, et al. Neuropathological and ultrastructural features of amebic encephalitis caused by *Sappinia diploidea*. J Neuropathol Exp Neurol 2003;62:99.

Gelston AL, Jones TC. Typhus fever: Report of an epidemic in New York City in 1847. J Infect Dis 1977;36(6):813.

Gerber MA, Shapiro ED, Krause PJ, et al. The risk of acquiring Lyme disease or babesiosis from a blood transfusion. J Infect Dis 1994;170:231.

Ghatak NR, Poon TP, Zimmerman HM. Toxoplasmosis of the central nervous system in the adult. Arch Pathol 1970;89:333.

Gilbert DN, Moellering RC, Sande MA. The Sanford guide to antimicrobial therapy 2004, 34th ed. Hyde Park, VT: Antimicrobial Therapy, Inc., 2004.

Gimenez F, Barraud de Lagerie S, Fernandez C, et al. Tumor necrosis factor alpha in the pathogenesis of cerebral malaria. Cell Mol Life Sci 2003;60:1623.

Glickman LT, Schantz PM, Cypess RH. Epidemiological characteristics and clinical findings in patients with serologically proven toxocariasis. Trans Roy Soc Trop Med 1979;73(3):254.

Goerduk V, Thuma P, Brittenham G, et al. Effect of iron chelation therapy on recovery from deep coma in children with cerebral malaria. N Engl J Med 1992;327:143.

Goldman JA, Fleischer AS, Leifer W, et al. *Candida albicans* mycotic aneurysm associated with systemic lupus erythematosus. Neurosurgery 1979;4:325.

Gonyea EF. The spectrum of primary blastomycotic meningitis: A review of central nervous system blastomycosis. Ann Neurol 1978;3:26.

Gonzalez-Martinez I. Refiriendo a un estudio de Bilharzia hematobium y bilharziosis en Puerto Rico. Rev Med Trop Habana 1904;5:193.

Gorenflot A, Moubri K, Precigout E, et al. Human babesiosis. Ann Trop Med Parasitol 1998;92:489.

Gossios KJ, Kontoyiannis DS, Dascalogiannaki M, et al. Uncommon locations of hydatid disease: CT appearances. Eur Radiol 1997;7:1303.

Goswick SM, Brenner GM. Activities of azithromycin and amphotericin B against *Naegleria fowleri* in in vitro and in a mouse model of primary amebic meningoencephalitis. Antimicrob Agents Chemother 2003a;47:524.

Green WR, Walker DH, Cain BG. Fatal viscerotrophic Rocky Mountain spotted fever. Am J Med 1978;64:523.

Grossman ER, Walcheck A, Freedman H. Tetracyclines and permanent teeth: The relationship between dose and teeth color. Pediatrics 1971;47:567.

Haller L, Adams H, Merouze F, et al. Clinical and pathological aspects of human African trypanosomiasis (T b Gambiense) with particular reference to reactive arsenical encephalopathy. Am J Trop Med Hyg 1986;35:94.

Hamilton JF, Bartkowski HB, Rock JP. Management of CNS mucormycosis in the pediatric patient. Pediatr Neurosurg 2003;38:212.

Haran RP, Chandy MJ. Intracranial *Aspergillus* granuloma. Br J Neurosurg 1993;7:383.

Haribhai HC, Bhigjee AI, Bill PLA, et al. Spinal cord schistosomiasis. A clinical, laboratory and radiological study, with a note on therapeutic aspects. Brain 1991;114:709.

Harkess JR. Ehrlichiosis. Infect Dis Clin North Am 1991;5:37.

Harrell GT. Rickettsial involvement of the nervous system. Med Clin North Am 1953;37:395.
Hayashi M. Clinical features of cerebral schistosomiasis, especially in cerebral and hepatosplenomegalic type. Parasitol Int 2003;52:375.
Healy JF. *Balamuthia* amebic encephalitis: Radiographic and pathologic findings. Am J Neuroradiol 2002;23:486.
Hedges E, Miller S. Coccidioidomycosis: Office diagnosis and treatment. Am Family Pract 1990;41:1499.
Heldrich FJ. Rocky Mountain spotted fever. In: Hoekelman RA, Seidel SB, Friedman NM, et al., eds. Primary pediatric care. St Louis: Mosby, 1987.
Herbrecht R, Letscher-Bru V, Oprea C, et al. *Aspergillus galactomannan* detection in the diagnosis of invasive aspergillosis in cancer patients J Clin Oncol 2002;20:1898.
Hermos JA, Healey GR, Schultz MG, et al. Fatal human cerebral coenurosis. JAMA 1970;213:1461.
Hien TT, White NJ. Qinghaosu. Lancet 1993;341:603.
Higashi K, Aoki H, Tatebayashi K, et al. Cerebral paragonimiasis. J Neurosurg 1971;34:515.
Hill IR, Denham DA, Scholtz CL. *Toxocara canis* larvae in the brain of a British child. Trans R Soc Trop Med Hyg 1985;79(3):351.
Hoff R, Teixeira RS, Carvalho JS, et al. *Trypanosoma cruzi* in the cerebrospinal fluid during the acute stage of Chagas' disease. N Engl J Med 1978;298:604.
Hohlfeld P, Dattos F, Costa JM, et al. Prenatal diagnosis of congenital toxoplasmosis with a polymerase-chain-reaction test on amniotic fluid. N Engl J Med 1994;331:695.
Homer MJ, Aguilar-Delfin I, Telford JR III, et al. Babesiosis. Clin Microbiol Rev 2000;13:451.
Horowitz HW, Marks SJ, Weintraub M, et al. Brachial plexopathy associated with human granulocytic ehrlichiosis. Neurology 1996;46:1026.
Hotez P. Visceral and ocular larva migrans. Semin Neurol 1993;13:175.
Houston S, Kowalewska-Grochowska K, Naik S, et al. First report of *Schistosoma mekongi* infection with brain involvement. Clin Infect Dis 2004;38:e1
Howe DK, Sibley LD. *Toxoplasma gondii* comprises three clonal lineages: Correlation of parasite genotype with human disease. J Infect Dis 1995;172:1561.
Huang DB, Schantz PS, White CA. Helminths infections In: Scheld WM, Whitley RJ, Marra CM, eds. Infections of the central nervous system, 3rd ed. Philadelphia: Lippincott Williams & Wilkins, 2004;97.
Huang ZH, Ferrante A, Carter RF. Serum antibodies to *Balamuthia mandrillaris,* a free-living amoeba recently demonstrated to cause granulomatous amoebic encephalitis. J Infect Dis 1999;179:1305.
Huff DS, Neafie RC, Binder MJ, et al. Case 4. The first fatal *Baylisascaris* infection in humans: An infant with eosinophilic meningoencephalitis. Ped Pathol 1984;2(3):345.
Hughes AJ, Biggs BA. Parasitic worms of the central nervous system: An Australian perspective. Int Med J 2002;32:541.
Hughes FB, Faehnle ST, Simon JL. Multiple cerebral abscesses complicating hepatopulmonary amebiasis. J Pediatr 1975;86:85.
Hughes WT. Candidiasis. In: Feigin RD, Cherry JD, eds. Textbook of pediatric infectious diseases, 3rd ed. Philadelphia: WB Saunders, 1992.
Hung PC, Wang HS, Chou ML, et al. Cerebral cryptococcosis in a child. Acta Paediatr Sin 1995;36:131.
Hussain S, Salahuddin N, Ahmad I, et al. Rhinocerebral invasive mycosis: Occurrence in immunocompetent individuals. Eur J Radiol 1995;20:151.
Hwang KP, Chen ER. Clinical studies on *Angiostrongylus cantonensis* among children in Taiwan. Southeast Asian J Trop Med Public Health 1991;22:194.
Ibach MJ, Larsh HW, Furcolow ML. Isolation of *Histoplasma capsulatum* from air. Science 1954;119:71.
Incesu L, Akan H, Arslan A. Neonatal cerebral candidiasis: CT findings and clinical correlation. J Belge Radiol 1994;77:278.
Ing MB, Schantz PM, Turner JA. Human coenurosis in North America: Case reports and review. Clin Infect Dis 1998;27(3):519.
Intapan PM, Maleewong W, Polsan Y, et al. Specific IgG antibody subclasses to *Angiostrongylus cantonensis* in patients with angiostrongyliasis. Asian Pac J Allery Immunol 2002;20:235.
Israelski DM, Remington JS. Toxoplasmosis in patients with cancer. Clin Infect Dis 1993;17:S423.
Jackson FE, Kent D, Clare F. Quadriplegia caused by involvement of cervical spine with *Coccidioides immitis*. J Neurosurg 1964;21:512.
Jain R, Prabhakar S, Modi M, et al. *Naegleria* meningitis: A rare survival. Neurol India 2002;50:470.
Jamjoom AB, Jamjoom ZA, al Hedaithy SS. Actinomycotic brain abscess successfully treated by burr hole aspiration and short course antimicrobial therapy. Br J Neurosurg 1994;8:545.
Jane JA, Warren KS, van den Noort S. Experimental cerebral schistosomiasis japonica in primates. J Neurol Neurosurg Psychiatr 1970;33:426.
Jaruratanasirikul S, Hortiwakkul R, Tantisarasart T, et al. Distribution of azithromycin into brain tissue, cerebrospinal fluid, and aqueous humor of the eye. Antimicrob Agents Chemother 1996;40:825.
Jelinek T, Loscher T. Clinical features and epidemiology of tick typhus in travelers. J Travel Med 2001;8:57.
Jindrak K. *Angionstrongylus cantonesis*. In: Hornabrook RW, ed. Topics on tropical neurology. Philadelphia: F.A. Davis, 1975;133.
John DT. Opportunistically pathogenic free-living amebae. In: Kreier JP, Baker JR, eds. Parasitic protozoa, Vol. 3, 2nd ed. New York: Academic Press, 1993.
Jones DB, Visvesvara GS, Robinson NM. *Acanthamoeba polyphaga* keratitis and uveitis associated with fatal meningoencephalitis. Trans Ophthal Soc U K 1975;95:221.
Jones JL, Kruszon-Moran D, Wilson M, et al. *Toxoplasma gondii* infection in the United States: Seroprevalence and risk factors. Am J Epidemiol 2001;154:357.
Jones TC. Toxoplasmosis. In: Conn HF, ed. Current therapy, 1979: Latest approved methods of treatment for the practicing physician. Philadelphia: WB Saunders, 1979.
Jordan P, Webbe G. Human schistosomiasis. London: William Heinemann Medical Books, 1969.
Jotte RS, Scott J. Malaria: Review of features pertinent to the emergency physician. J Emerg Med 1993;11:729.
Jung S, Schelper RL, Visvesvara GS, Chang HT. *Balamuthia mandrillaris* meningoencephalitis in an immunocompetent patient: An unusual clinical course and a favorable outcome. Arch Pathol Lab Med 2004;128;466.
Kain KC. Chemotherapy of drug-resistant malaria. Can J Infect Dis 1996;7:25.
Kalaitzoglou I, Drevelengas A, Petridis A, et al. Albendazole treatment of cerebral hydatid disease: Evaluation of results with CT and MRI. Neuroradiology 1998;40:36.
Kamper C. Treatment of Rocky Mountain spotted fever. J Pediatr Health Care 1991;5:216.
Kang S-Y, Kim T-K, Kim T-Y, et al. A case of chronic cerebral paragonimiasis westermani. Korean J Parasitol 2000;38:167.
Kanpittaya J, Jitpimolmard S, Tiamkao S, et al. MR findings of eosinophilic meningoencephalitis attributed to *Angiostrongylus cantonensis*. AJNR Am J Neuroradiol 2000;21:1090.
Karande SC, Lahiri KR, Sheth SS, et al. *Acanthamoeba* meningoencephalitis complicating pyogenic meningitis. Ind Pediatr 1991;28:794.
Kartulis S. Zur Aetiologie der Dysenterie aegypten. Virchows Arch (A) 1886;105:521.
Katinka MD, Duprat S, Cornillot E, et al. Genome sequence and gene compaction of the eukaryote parasite *Encephalitozoon cuniculi.* Nature 2001;414:450.
Katnik R. A persistent biochemical marker for partially treated meningitis/ventriculitis. J Child Neurol 1995;10:93.
Katsurada F. Schistosomum japonicum, ein neuer menschicher Parasit, durch welchen eine endemische Krankheit in verscheidenen Gegenden Japans verursacht wird. Annot Zool Jpn 1904;5:147.
Kaufmann H, Yamage M, Roditi I, et al. Discrimination of *Neospora caninum* from *Toxoplasma gondii* and other apicomplexan parasites by hybridization and PCR. Mol Cell Probes 1996;10:289.
Kazacos KR. Visceral and ocular larval migrans. Semin Vet Med Surg 1991;6:227.
Kazacos KR. Visceral, ocular, and neural larval migrans. In: Connor DH, Chandler FW, Schwartz PA, et al, eds. Pathology of infectious diseases, Vol. 2. Stamford, CT: Appleton and Lange, 2001;1459.
Kazacos KR, Boyce WM: *Baylisascaris* larva migrans. J Am Vet Med Assoc 1989;195:894.
Kazacos KR, Raymond LA, Kazacos EA, Vestre WA. The raccoon ascarid; a probable cause of human ocular larva migrans. Ophthalmology 1985;92:1735.

Kelsey DS. Rocky Mountain spotted fever. Pediatr Clin North Am 1979;26:367.
Kennedy PGE. Human African trypanosomiasis of the CNS: Current issues and challenges. J Clin Invest 2004;113:496.
Khalil HH, Abd el Wahab M, el Deeb A, et al. Cerebral atrophy: A schistosomiasis manifestation. Am J Trop Med Hyg 1986;35:531.
Khan EA, Correa AG. Toxoplasmosis of the central nervous system in non-human immunodeficiency virus-infected children: Case report and review of the literature. Pediatr Infect Dis J 1997;16:611.
Kidney DD, Kim SH. CNS infections with free-living amebas: Neuroimaging findings. Am J Roentgenol 1998;171:809.
Kim JH, Durack DT. Rickettsiae. In: Scheld WM, Whitley RJ, Durack DY, eds. Infections of the central nervous system, 2nd ed. Philadelphia: Lippincott-Raven, 1997.
Kirchoff LV. American trypanosomiasis (Chagas disease): A tropical disease now in the United States. N Engl J Med 1993;329:629.
Kirchoff LV, Nash TE. A case of schistosomiasis japonica: Resolution of CAT-scan detected cerebral abnormalities without specific therapy. Am J Trop Med Hyg 1984;33:1155.
Kirkland KB, Wilkinson WE, Sexton DJ. Therapeutic delay and mortality in cases of Rocky Mountain spotted fever. Clin Inf Dis 1995;20:1118.
Kirmani N, Tuazon CU, Ocuin JA, et al. Extensive cerebral nocardiosis cured with antibiotic therapy alone. J Neurosurg 1978;49:924.
Klein BS, Belfort EA, Mondolfi A, et al. Isolation of *Blastomyces dermatitidis* in soil associated with a large outbreak of blastomycosis in Wisconsin. N Engl J Med 1986;314:529.
Klein NC, Cunha BA. New uses of older antibiotics. Med Clin North Am 2001;85(1):125.
Kliks MM, Palumbo NE. Eosinophilic meningitis beyond the Pacific Basin: The global dispersal of a peridomestic zoonosis caused by *Angiostrongylus cantonensis*, the nematode lungworm of rats. Soc Sci Med 1992;34:199.
Ko RC, Chan SW, Chan KW, et al. Four documented cases of eosinophilic meningoencephalitis due to *Angiostrongylus cantonensis* in Hong Kong. Trans R Soc Trop Med Hyg 1987;81:807.
Kodet R, Nohynkova E, Tichy M, et al. Amebic encephalitis caused by *Balamuthai mandrillaris* in a Czech child: Description of the first case from Europe. Pathol Res Practice 1998;194:423.
Kojic EM, White AC Jr. A positive enzyme-linked immunoelectrotransfer blot assay result for a patient without evidence of cysticercosis. Clin Infect Dis. 2003;36:e7.
Kreel L, Poon WS, Nainby-Luxmoore JC. Trichinosis diagnosed by computed tomography. Postgrad Med J 1988;64:626.
Krivoy S, Belfort EA, Mondolfi A, et al. Paracoccidioidomycosis of the skull: Case report. J Neurosurg 1978;49:429.
Krober MS. Skeletal muscle involvement in Rocky Mountain spotted fever. South Med J 1978;71:1575.
Kuberski T, Wallace JD. Clinical manifestations of eosinophilic meningits due to *Angiostrongylus cantonensis*. Neurology 1979;29:1566.
Kusner D, King C. Cerebral paragonimiasis. Semin Neurol 1993;13:201.
Kyes S, Horrocks P, Newbold C. Antigenic variation at the infected red cell surface in malaria. Ann Rev Microbiol 2001;55:673.
Leber AL, Novak SM. Intestinal and urogenital amebae, flagellates and ciliates. In: Murray PR, Baron EJ, Pfaller MA, et al, eds. Manual of clinical microbiology, 7th ed. Washington, DC: ASM Press, 1999.
LeBlang SD, Whiteman ML, Post MJ, et al. CNS *Nocardia* in AIDS patients: CT and MRI with pathologic correlation. J Comput Assist Tomogr 1995;19:15.
Leiguarda R, Roncoroni A, Taratuto AL, et al. Acute CNS infection by *Trypanosoma cruzi* (Chagas' disease) in immunosuppressed patients. Neurology 1990;40:850.
Lejon V, Boelaert M, Jannin J, et al. The challenge of *Trypanosoma brucei gambiense* sleeping sickness diagnosis outside Africa. Lancet 2003a;3:804.
Lejon V, Reiber H, Legros, D, et al. Intrathecal immune response pattern for improved diagnosis of central nervous system involvement in trypanosomiasis. J Infect Dis 2003b;187:1475
Lewallen S, Taylor TE, Molyneux ME, et al. Ocular fundus findings in Malawian children with cerebral malaria. Ophthalmology 1993;100:857.
Lindo JF, Escoffery CT, Reid B, et al. Fatal autochthonous eosinophilic meningitis in a Jamaican child caused by *Angiostrongylus cantonensis*. Am J Trop Med Hyg 2004;70:425.
Lira R, Contreras LM, Santa Rita RM, Urbina JA. Mechanism of action of anti-proliferative lysophospholipid analogues against the protozoan parasite *Trypanosoma cruzi:* Potentiation of in vitro activity by the sterol biosynthesis inhibitor ketoconazole. J Antimicrob Chemother 2001;47:537.
Lisch S, Steudel WI. Unusual course of candidiasis of the central nervous system. Dtsch Med Wochenschr 1994;119:13.
Littman ML, Walter JE. Cryptococcosis: Current status. Am J Med 1968;45:922.
Liu I. Spinal and cerebral schistosomiasis. Semin Neurol 1993;13:189.
Lochary ME, Lockhart PB, Williams WT. Doxycycline and staining of permanent teeth. Pediatric Inf Dis J 1998;17:429.
Lombardo L, Alonso P, Arroyo LS, et al. Cerebral amebiasis. J Neurosurg 1964;21:704.
Loosli CG. Histoplasmosis. J Chronic Dis 1957;5:473.
Lowichik A, Rollins N, Delgado R, et al. Leptomyxid amebic meningoencephalitis mimicking brain stem glioma. Am J Neuroradiol 1995;16:926.
Lowichik A, Ruff AJ. Parasitic infections of the central nervous system in children. Part II: disseminated infections. J Child Neurol 1995a;10:77.
Lowichik A, Ruff AJ. Parasitic infections of the central nervous system in children. Part III: space-occupying lesions. J Child Neurol 1995b;10:177.
Lowichik A, Siegel JD. Parasitic infections of the central nervous system in children. Part I: Congenital infections and meningoencephalitis. J Child Neurol 1995;10:4.
Lunardi P, Missori P, DiLorenzo N, et al. Cerebral hydatidosis in childhood: A retrospective survey with emphasis on long-term follow-up. Neurosurgery 1991;29:515.
Lusina D, Legros F, Klerlein M, et al. Airport malaria: Four new cases in suburban Paris during summer 1999. Euro Surveill 2000;5:76.
Lutz A. Uma micose pseudococcidica localisada na boca e observada no Brasil: contribuicao ao conhecimento das hyphoblastomycoses americanos. Braz Med 1908;22:121.
Lyons RW, Andriole VT. Fungal infections of the CNS. Neurol Clin 1986;4(1):159.
Mabeza GF, Loyevsky M, Gordeuk VR, Weiss G. Iron chelation therapy for malaria: A review. Pharmacol Ther 1999;81:53.
Machado LR, Nobrega JP, Livramento JA, et al. Histoplasmosis of the central nervous system. Clinical aspects in 8 patients. Arq Neuropsiquiatr 1993;51:209.
Madigan JE, Richter PJ Jr, Kimsey RB, et.al. Transmission and passage in horses of the agent of human granulocytic ehrlichiosis. J Infect Dis 1995;172:1141.
Maeda K, Markowitz N, Hawley RC, et al. Human infection with *Ehrlichia canis,* a leukocytic rickettsia. N Engl J Med 1987; 316:853.
Maguire JH. Tapeworms and seizures—treatment and prevention. N Engl J Med 2004;350:3.
Mahmoud AA. Schistosomiasis. In: Warren KS, Mahmoud AAF, eds. Tropical and geographical medicine. New York: McGraw-Hill, 1984.
Maitland K, Marsh K. Pathophysiology of severe malaria in children. Acta Trop 2004;90:131.
Marcial-Rojas RA, Fiol RE. Neurologic complications of schistosomiasis: Review of the literature and report of two cases of transverse myelitis due to *S. mansoni.* Ann Intern Med 1963;59:215.
Markell EK, Voge M, John DT. Medical parasitology. Philadelphia: WB Saunders, 1992.
Markley KC, Levine AB, Chan Y. Rocky Mountain spotted fever in pregnancy. Obstet Gynecol 1998:91(Suppl):860.
Marlowe M, Ali-Amad D, Cherrick I, et al Central nervous system nocardiosis in an immunocompetent child. Pediatr Infect Dis J 2000;19:661.
Marmor M, Glickman L, Shofer F, et al. *Toxocara canis* infection of children: Epidemiologic and neuropsychologic findings. Am J Public Health 1987;77:554.
Marr, KA, Balajee SA, McLaughlin L, et al. Detection of galactomannan antigenemia by enzyme immunoassay for the diagnosis of invasive aspergillosis: Variables that affect performance. J Infect Dis 2004;190:641.
Marrie TJ, Raoult D. Rickettsial infections of the central nervous system. Semin Neurol 1992; 12:213.
Marsh K, Forster D, Wariuru C, et al. Indicators of life threatening malaria in African children. N Engl J Med 1995;332:1339.
Marshall MM, Naumovitz D, Ortega Y, et al. Waterborne protozoan pathogens. Clin Microbiol Rev 1997;10:67.
Martinez AJ. Is *Acanthamoeba* encephalitis an opportunistic infection? Neurology 1980;30:567.
Martinez AJ. Free-living amebas: Natural history, prevention, diagnosis,

pathology, and treatment of disease. Boca Raton, Florida: CRC Press, 1985.
Martinez AJ. Free-living amebas: Infection of the central nervous system. Mount Sinai J Med 1993;60:271.
Martinez AJ, Ahdab Barmada M. The neuropathology of liver transplantation: comparison of main complications in children and adults. Mod Pathol 1993;6:25.
Martinez AJ, Duma RJ, Nelson EC, et al. Experimental *Naegleria* meningoencephalitis in mice: Penetration of the olfactory mucosal epithelium by *Naegleria* and pathologic changes produced: A light and electron microscope study. Lab Invest 1973;29:121.
Martinez AJ, Guerra AE, García-Tamayo J, et al. Granulomatous amebic encephalitis: A review and report of a spontaneous case from Venezuela. Acta Neuropathol 1994;87:430.
Martinez AJ, Visvesvara GS. Free-living, amphizoic and opportunistic amebas. Brain Pathol 1997;7:583.
Martinez AJ, Visvesvara GS. *Balamuthia mandrillaris* infection. J Med Microbiol 2001;50:205. (Editorial)
Martinez MS, Gonzalez-Mediero G, Santiago P, et al. Granulomatous amebic encephalitis in a patient with AIDS: Isolation of *Acanthamoeba* sp. group II from brain tissue and successful treatment with sulfadiazine and fluconazole. J Clin Microbiol 2000;38:3892.
Masalha R, Merkin-Zaborsky H, Matar M, et al. Murine typhus presenting as subacute meningoencephalitis. J Neurol 1998;245(10):665.
Massa G, Vanderschueren-Lodeweyckx M, Van Vliet G, et al. Hypothalamopituitary dysfunction in congenital toxoplasmosis. Eur J Pediatr 1989;148:742.
Matsubayashi H, Koike T, Mikata I, et al. A case of *Encephalitozoon*-like body infection in man. Arch Pathol 1959;67:181.
Maurin M, Raoult D. Q Fever. Clin Microbiol Rev 1999;12:518.
Mawhorter SD, Kazura JW. Trichinosis of the central nervous system. Semin Neurol 1993;13:148.
McAbee G, Ciminera P, Knapik M, et al. Rapid and fatal neurologic deterioration due to central nervous system *Candida* infection in an HIV-1-infected child. J Child Neurol 1995;10:405.
McCabe RE, Remington JS, Araujo FG. In vitro and in vivo effects of itraconazole against *Trypanosoma cruzi.* Am J Trop Med Hyg 1986;35:280.
McCabe RE, Remington JS, Araujo FG. Ketoconazole promotes parasitological cure of mice infected with *Trypanosoma cruzi.* Trans R Soc Trop Med Hyg 1987;81:613.
McCullers JA, Vargas SL, Plynn PM, et al. Candidal meningitis in chidren with cancer. Clin Infect Dis 2000;31:451.
McGarvey ST, Alegui G, Daniel BL, et al. Child growth and schistosomiasis japonica in northeastern Leyte, the Philippines: Cross-sectional results. Am J Trop Med Hyg 1992; 46:571.
McGinnis MR. Detection of fungi in cerebrospinal fluid. Am J Med 1983;75:129.
Medana IM, Chaudhri G, Chan-Ling T, Hunt NH. Central nervous system in cerebral malaria: "Innocent bystander" or active participant in the induction of immunopathology? Immunol Cell Biol 2001;79:101.
Medical Letter: Drugs for parasitic infections. New Rochelle, NY: The Medical Letter, Inc, 2004.
Meldrum SC, Birkhead GS, White DJ, et al. Human babesiosis in New York State: An epidemiological description of 136 cases. Clin Infect Dis 1992;14:1019.
Miaux Y, Ribaud P, Williams M, et al. MR of cerebral aspergillosis in patients who have had bone marrow transplantation. Am J Neuroradiol 1995;16:555.
Mikhael NZ, Montpetil VJ, Orizaya M, et al. *Toxocara canis* infestation with encephalitis. Can J Neurol Sci 1974;1:114.
Miller ES, Beeson PB. Murine typhus fever. Medicine 1946;25:1.
Miller JQ, Price TR. The nervous system in Rocky Mountain spotted fever. Neurology 1972;22:561.
Miller LH, Neva FH, Gill F. Failure of chloroquine in human babesiosis *(Babesia microti).* Ann Intern Med 1978;88:200.
Miller LH, Reifsnyder DN, Martinez SA. Late onset of disease in congenital toxoplasmosis. Clin Pediatr 1971;10:78.
Miller MJ, Remington JS. Toxoplasmosis in infants and children with HIV positive infection or AIDS. In: Pizzo PA, Wilfert CM, eds. Pediatric AIDS: The challenge of HIV infection in infants, children and adolescents. Baltimore: Williams & Wilkins, 1990.
Mischel PS, Vinters HV. Coccidioidomycosis of the central nervous system: Neuropathological and vasculopathic manifestations and clinical correlates. Clin Infect Dis 1995;20:400.
Missinou MA, Borrmann S, Schindler A, et al. Fosmidomycin for malaria. Lancet 2002;360:1941.
Mitchell CD, Erlich SS, Mastrucci MT, et al. Congenital toxoplasmosis occurring in infants perinatally infected with human immunodeficiency virus 1. Pediatr Infect Dis J 1990;9:512.
Mitchell WG, Crawford TO. Intraparenchymal cerebral cysticercosis in children. Diagnosis and treatment. Pediatrics 1988;82:76.
Moertel CL, Kazacos KR, Butterfield JH, et al. Eosinophil-associated inflammation and elaboration of eosinophil-derived proteins in 2 children with raccoon roundworm *(Baylisascaris procynosis)* encephalitis. Pediatrics 2001;5:E93.
Molk R. Ocular toxocariasis: A review of the literature. Ann Ophthalmol 1983;15:216
Moll GW Jr, Riala FA, Liu GC, et al. Rhinocerebral mucormycosis in IDDM. Sequential magnetic resonance imaging of long-term survival with intensive therapy. Diabetes Care 1994;17:1348.
Molyneux ME, Taylor TE, Wirima JJ, et al. Clinical features and prognostic indicators in paediatric cerebral malaria: A study of 131 comatose Malawian children. Q J Med 1989;71:441.
Moody A. Rapid diagnostic tests for malaria parasites. Clin Microbiol Rev 2002;15:66.
Moore MT. Human *Toxocara canis* encephalitis with lead encephalopathy. J Neuropathol Exp Neurol 1962;21:201.
Moorthy VS, Good MF, Hill AVS. Malaria vaccine developments. Lancet 2004;363:150.
Morgan D, Young RF, Chow AW, et al. Recurrent intracerebral blastomycotic granuloma: Diagnosis and treatment. Neurosurgery 1979;4:319.
Mott FW. Histologic observations on sleeping sickness and other trypanosome infections. Reports of the Sleeping Sickness Commission 1906;7:3.
Moya PR. Chagas' disease in children: Neurological and psychological aspects. In: Pan American Health Organization. Chagas' Disease and the Nervous System. Washington, DC. PAHO, 1994 (Scientific Publication No. 547).
Nascimento-Carvalho CM, Moreno-Carvalho OA. Clinical and cerebrospinal fluid findings in patients less than 20 years old with presumptive diagnosis of neuroschistosomiasis. J Trop Pedr 2004;50:98.
Nascimento-Carvalho CM, Moreno-Carvalho OA. Neuroschistosomiasis due to *Schistosoma mansoni*. A review of pathogenesis, clinical syndromes and diagnostic approaches. Rev Inst Med Trop Sao Paulo 2005;47:179.
Nash TE. Human case management and treatment of cysticercosis. Acta Tropica 2003;87:61.
Nash TE, Del Brutto MD, Butman JA, et al. Calcific neurocysticercosis and epileptogenesis. Neurology 2004;62:1934.
Nesky MA, McDougal EC, Peacock JE. *Pseudoallescheria boydii* brain abscess successfully treated with voriconazole and surgical drainage: Case report and literature review of central nervous system pseudallescheriasis. Clin Infect Dis J 2000;31:673.
Newton CRJC, Hien TT, White N. Cerebral malaria. J Neurol Neurosurg Psychiatry 2000;69:433.
Newton CRJC, Krishna S. Severe falciparum malaria in children: Current understanding of pathophysiology and supportive treatment. Pharmacol Ther 1998;79:1.
Newton CRJC, Nirkham FJ, Winstanley PE, et al. Intracranial pressure in African children with cerebral malaria. Lancet 1991;337:573.
Newton CRJC, Peshu N, Kendall B, et al. Brain swelling and ischemia in Kenyans with cerebral malaria. Arch Dis Child 1994;70:281.
Nicoletti A, Bartoloni A, Reggio A, et al. Epilepsy, cysticercosis, and toxocariasis. A population-based case-control study in rural Bolivia. Neurology 2002;58:1256.
Nieto D. Cysticercosis of the nervous system. Neurology 1956;6:725.
Nontasut P, Bussaratid V, Chullawichit S, et al. Comparison of ivermectin and albendazole treatment for gnathostomiasis. Southeast Asian J Trop Med Public Health 2000;31:374.
Nyberg W. *Diphyllobothrium latum* and human nutrition with particular reference to vitamin B_{12} deficiency. Proc Nutr Soc 1963;22:8.
O'Connor RM, Long JA, Allred DR. Cytoadherence of *Babesia bovis*–infected erythrocytes to bovine brain capillary endotherlial cells provides an in vitro model for sequestration. Infect Immun 1999;67:3921.
Ogata K. Nawa Y, Akahane H. Short report: Gnathostomiasis in Mexico. Am J Trop Med Hyg 1998;58:316.

Oh SJ. Paragonimiasis in the central nervous system. In: Vinken PJ, Bruyn GW, eds. Handbook of clinical neurology. Infections of the nervous system, Part III, Vol. 35. New York, North-Holland: Elsevier, 1978.

Ohnishi K, Murata M, Kojima H, et al. Brain abscess due to infection with *Entamoeba histolytica*. Am J Trop Med Hyg 1994;51:180.

Olah E., Berger C., Boltshauser E, Nadal D. Cerebral actinomycosis before adolescence. Neuropediatrics 2004;35:239.

Olliaro PL, Taylor WRJ. Developing artemisinin based drug combinations for the treatment of drug resistant falciparum malaria: A review. J Postgrad Med 2004;50:40.

Osuntokun BO. Epilepsy in the African continent. In: Penry JK, ed. Epilepsy. The eighth international symposium. New York: Raven Press, 1977.

Otani SA. On the anamnesis and the postmortem examination of paragonimiasis patients. Tokyo: Igakkai Zasshi 1887;1:458.

Paddock CD, Brenner O, Vaid C, et al. Short report: Concurrent Rocky Mountain spotted fever in a dog and its owner. Am J Trop Med Hyg 2002;66:197.

Pai H, Sohn S, Seong Y, et al. Central nervous system involvement in patients with scrub typhus. Clin Infect Dis 1997;24:436.

Pappagianis D. Coccidioidomycosis. In: Top FJ, Wehrle PF, eds. Communicable and infectious diseases, 8th ed. St Louis: Mosby, 1976.

Pappas PG, Threlkeld MG, Bedsole GD, et al. Blastomycosis in immunocompromised patients. Medicine Baltimore 1993;72:311.

Park SY, Glaser CA, Murray WJ, et al. Raccoon roundworm *(Baylisascaris procyonis)* encephalitis: Case report and field investigation. Pediatrics 2000;106:E56.

Pelaez D, Perez-Reyes R. Gnatostomiasis humana en America. Rev Latinoam Microbiol 1970;12:83.

Pentreath VW. Trypanosomiasis and the nervous system. Pathology and immunology. Trans R Soc Trop Med Hyg 1995;89:9.

Pepin J, Milord F, Khonde AN, et al. Risk factors for encephalopathy and mortality during melarsoprol treatment of *Trypanosoma brucei gambiense* sleeping sickness. Trans R Soc Trop Med Hyg 1995;89:92

Persing DH, Conrad PA. Babesiosis: new insights from phylogenetic analysis. Infect Agents Dis 1995;4:182.

Persing DH, Herwaldt BL, Glaser C, et al. Infection with a *Babesia*-like organism in northern California. N Engl J Med 1995;332:298.

Phillips RE, Warrell DA, White NJ, et al. Intravenous quinidine for the treatment of severe falciparum malaria. N Engl J Med 1985;312:1273.

Pittella JE. Central nervous system involvement in Chagas' disease: An updating. Rev Inst Med Trop Sao Paulo 1993;35:111.

Pittella JE, Gusmao SN, Carvalho GT, et al. Tumoral form of cerebral schistosomiasis mansoni. A report of four cases and a review of the literature. Clin Neurol Neurosurg 1996;98:15.

Powderly WG, Saag MS, Cloud GA, et al. A controlled trial of fluconazole or amphotericin B to prevent relapse of cryptococcal meningitis in patients with the acquired immunodeficiency syndrome. N Engl J Med 1992;326:793.

Poza G, Montoya J, Redondo C, et al. Meningitis caused by *Pseudallescheria boydii* treated with voriconazole. Clin Infect Dis 2000;30:981.

Pratt HD. The changing picture of murine typhus in the United States. Ann N Y Acad Sci 1958;70:516.

Proano JV, Madrazo I, Avelar F, et al. Medical treatment for neurocysticercosis characterized by giant subarachnoid cysts. N Engl J Med 2001;345:879.

Provic P, Spratt DM, Carlisle MS. Neuro-angiostrongylus: Unresolved issues. Int J Parasitol 2000;30:1295.

Pruthi RK, Marshall WF, Wiltsie JC, et al. Human babesiosis. Mayo Clin Proc 1995;70:853.

Punyagupta S, Juttijudata P, Bunnag T. Eosinophilic meningitis in Thailand. Clinical studies of 484 typical cases probably caused by *Angiostrongylus cantonensis*. Am J Trop Med Hyg 1975;24:921.

Quick RE, Herwaldt BL, Thomford JW. Babesiosis in Washington State: A new species of *Babesia?* Ann Int Med 1993;119:284.

Raab EL, Leopold IH, Hodes HL. Retinopathy in Rocky Mountain spotted fever. Am J Ophthalmol 1969;68:42.

Randall G, Seidel JS. Malaria. Pediatr Clin North Am 1985;32:893.

Raoult D. A new rickettsial disease in the United States. Clin Infect Dis 2004;38(6):805.

Ratnasamy N, Everett ED, Roland WE, et al. Central nervous system manifestations of human ehrlichiosis. Clin Inf Dis 1996;23:314.

Raucher H, Jaffin H, Glass JL. Babesiosis in pregnancy. Obstet Gynecol 1984;63:7S.

Recavarren-Arce S, Velarde C, Gotukzzo E, Cabrera J. Amoeba angeitic lesions of the central nervous system in *Balamuthia mandrilaris* amoebiasis. Hum Pathol 1999;30:269.

Reed RP, Cooke-Yarborough CM, Jaquiery AL, et al. Fatal granulomatous amoebic encephalitis caused by *Balamuthia mandrillaris*. Med J Aust 1997;167:82.

Remington JS, McLeod R, Thulliez P, Desmonts G. Toxoplasmosis. In: Remington JS, Klein JO, eds. Infectious diseases of the fetus and newborn infant, 5th ed. Philadephia: WB Saunder, 2001.

Restrepo A. Morphological aspects of *Paracoccidioides brasiliensis* in lymph nodes: Implications for the prolonged latency of paracoccidioidomycosis? Med Mycol 2000;38(4):317.

Reuter S, Buck A, Manfras B, et al. Structured treatment interruption in patients with alveolar echinococcosis. Hepatology 2004;39:509.

Richards F Jr, Sullivan J, Ruiz-Tiben E, et al. Effect of praziquantel on the eggs of *Schistosoma mansoni,* with a note on the implications for managing central nervous system schistosomiasis. Ann Trop Med Parasitol 1989;83:465.

Richardson PM, Mohandas A, Arumugasamy N. Cerebral cryptococcosis in Malaysia. J Neurol Neurosurg Psychiatr 1976;39:330.

Riley T, White AC, Jr. Management of neurocysticercosis. CNS Drugs 2003;17:577.

Rivera IV, Curless RG, Indacochea FJ, et al. Chronic progressive CNS histoplasmosis presenting in childhood: Response to fluconazole therapy. Pediatr Neurol 1992;8:151.

Roach ES, Zimmerman CF, Troost BT, et al. Optic neuritis due to acquired toxoplasmosis. Pediatr Neurol 1985;1:114.

Rogers DE. The spectrum of histoplasmosis in man. Respir Physiol 1967;13:54.

Roizen N, Swisher CN, Stein M, et al. Neurologic and developmental outcome in treated congenital toxoplasmosis. Pediatrics 1995;95:11.

Rosen F, Deck JHN, Rewcastle NB. *Allescheria boydii:* Unique systemic dissemination to thyroid and brain. Can Med Assoc J 1965;93:1125.

Rosenblum M, Rosegay H. Resection of multiple nocardial brain abscesses: Diagnostic role of computerized tomography. Neurosurgery 1979;4:315.

Rowen JL, Doerr CA, Vogel H, et al. *Balamuthia mandrillaris:* A newly recognized agent for amebic meningoencephalitis. Pediatr Infect Dis J 1995;14:705.

Rowley HA, Uht RM, Kazacos KR, et al. Radiologic-pathologic findings in raccoon roundworm *(Baylisascaris procyonis)* encephalitis. Am J Neuroradiol 2000;21:415.

Ruebush TK II, Juranek DD, Chisholm ES, et al. Human babesiosis on Nantucket Island. N Engl J Med 1977;297:825.

Rusnak JM, Lucey DR. Clinical gnathostomiasis: Case report and review of the English-language literature. Clin Infect Dis 1993;16:33.

Ruttinger P, Hadidi H. MRI in cerebral toxocaral disease. J Neurol Neurosurg Psychiatry 1991;54:361.

Ryczak M, Sorber WA, Kandora TF, et al. Difficulties in diagnosing *Trichinella* encephalitis. Am J Trop Med Hyg 1987;36:573.

Saag MS, Powderly WG, Cloud GA, et al. Comparison of amphotericin B with fluconazole in the treatment of acute AIDS-associated cryptococcal meningitis. N Engl J Med 1992;326:83.

Sabchareon A, Burnouf T, Ouattara D, et al. Parasitologic and clinical human response to immunoglobulin administration in falciparum malaria. Am J Trop Med Hyg 1991;45:297.

Sabetta JR, Andriole VT. Cryptococcal infection of the central nervous system. Med Clin North Am 1985;69:333.

Sahai VS, Onyett H. A cost-benefit analysis of prenatal screening for toxoplasmosis. Can J Infect Dis 1996;7:259.

Saitoh, A, Homans J, Kovacs, A. Fluconazole treatment of coccidioidal meningitis in children: two case reports and a review of the literature. Pediatr Infect Dis J 2000;19(12):1204.

Salake JS, Louria DB, Chmel H. Fungal and yeast infections of the central nervous system. Medicine 1984;63:108.

Sandler R, Tallman CB, Keamy DG, et al. Successfully treated rhinocerebral phycomycosis in well controlled diabetes. N Engl J Med 1971;285:1180.

Sarosi GA, Voth DW, Dahl BA, et al. Disseminated histoplasmosis: Results of long term follow-up. Ann Intern Med 1971;75:511.

Satpathy SK, Mohanty N, Nanda P, Samal G. Severe falciparum malaria. Indian J Pediatr 2004;7:133.

Schantz, PM. *Toxocara* larva migrans now. Am J Trop Med Hyg 1989;41:21.

Schantz PM, Glickman LT. Roundworms in dogs and cats: Veterinary and public health consideration. Compend Contin Educ Pract Vet 1981;3:773.

Schantz PM, Moore AC, Munoz JL, et al. Neurocysticercosis in an Orthodox Jewish community in New York City. N Engl J Med 1992;327:692.

Schantz PM, Sarti E, Plancarte A, et al. Community-based epidemiological investigations of cystcercosis due to *Taenia solium:* Comparison of serological screening tests and clinical findings in two populations in Mexico. Clin Infect Dis 1994;18:879.

Schellhas KP, Norris GA. Disseminated human subarachnoid coenurosis: Computed tomographic appearance. Am J Neuroradiol 1985;6:638.

Schmid M, Pendl G, Samonigg H, et al. Gamma knife radiosurgery and albendazole for cerebral alveolar hydatid disease. Clin Infect Dis. 1998;26:1379.

Schmid M, Samonigg H, Stoger H, et al. Use of interferon gamma and mebendazole to stop the progression of alveolar hydatid disease: Case report. Clin Infect Dis 1995;20:1543.

Schmutzhard E, Mayr U, Rumpl E, et al. Secondary cerebral amebiasis due to infection with *Entamoeba histolytica*. A case report with computer tomographic findings. Eur Neurol 1986;25:161.

Schochet SS. Human *Toxocara canis* encephalopathy in a case of visceral larva migrans. Neurology 1967:17:227.

Schuster FL, Dunnebacke TH, Booton GC, et al. Environmental isolation of *Balamuthia mandrillaris* associated with a case of amebic encephalitis. J Clin Microbiol 2003;41:3175.

Schuster FL, Glaser C, Gilliam S, Visvesvara GS. Survey of sera from encephalitis patients for *Balamuthia mandrillaris* antibody. J Eukaryot Microbiol 2001;48;10S.

Schuster FL, Glaser C, Honarmand S, Maguire JH, Visvesvara GS. *Balamuthia* amebic encephalitis risk, Hispanic Americans. Emerg Infect Dis 2004;10:1510.

Schuster FL, Visvesvara GS. Opportunistic amoebae: Challenges in prophylaxis and treatment. Drug Resist Update 2004;7:41.

Schutze GE, Hickerson SL, Fortin EM, et al Blastomycosis in children. Clin Infect Dis 1996:224:496.

Schutze GE, Jacobs RF. Human monocytic ehrlichiosis in children. Pediatrics 1997;100:E10.

Schwartz S, Thiel E. Update on the treatment of cerebral aspergillosis. Ann Hematol. 2004;83(Suppl 1):S42.

Scrimgeour EM, Gajdusek DC. Involvement of the central nervous system in *Schistosoma mansoni* and *S. hematobium* infection. Brain 1985;108:1023.

Seidel JS. Primary amebic meningoencephalitis. Pediatr Clin North Am 1985a;32:881.

Seidel JS. Treatment of parasitic infections. Pediatr Clin North Am 1985b;32:1077.

Seidel JS, Harmatz P, Visvesvara GS, et al. Successful treatment of primary amebic meningoencephaliltis. N Eng J Med 1982;306:346.

Sein KK, Maeno Y, Thuc HV, et al. Differential sequestration of parasitized erythrocytes in the cerebrum and cerebellum in human cerebral malaria. Am J Trop Med Hyg 1993;48:504

Selby DM, Chandra RS, Rakkusan TA, et al. Amebic osteomyelitis in a child with acquired immunodeficiency syndrome. A case report. Pedtr Pathol Lab Med 1998;18:89.

Sener RN. Thalamic hydatid cyst: Contrast-enhanced MR imaging findings. Comput Med Imaging Graph 1996;20:395.

Seong DC, Przepiorka D, Bruner JM, et al. Leptomeningeal toxoplasmosis after allogeneic marrow transplantation. Case report and review of the literature. Am J Clin Oncol 1993;16:105.

Sexton DJ, Kanj SS, Wilson K, et al. The use of a polymerase chain reaction as a diagnostic test for Rocky Mountain spotted fever. Am J Trop Med Hyg 1994;50:59.

Sexton DJ, Kaye KS. Rocky mountain spotted fever. Med Clin North Am 2002;86(2):351.

Shandera WX, White AC Jr, Chen JC, et al. Neurocysticercosis in Houston, Texas. A report of 112 cases. Medicine 1994;73:37

Sharma PP, Gupta P, Murali MV, Ramachandran VG. Primary amebic meningoencephalitis caused by *Acanthamoeba*: Successfully treated with cotrimoxazole. Indian Pediatr 1993;30:1219.

Shear HL, Grinberg L, Gilman J, et al. Transgenic mice expressing human fetal globin are protected from malaria by a novel mechanism. Blood 1998;92:2520.

Shields JA. Ocular toxocariasis. A review. Surv Ophthalmol 1984;28:361.

Silver HK, Dixon MS Jr. Congenital toxoplasmosis: Report of case with cataract, "atypical" vasopressin-sensitive diabetes insipidus, and marked eosinophilia. Am J Dis Child 1954;88:84.

Singhal T, Bajpai A, Kalra V, et al. Successful treatment of *Acanthamoeba* meningitis with combination oral antimicrobials. Pediatr Infect Dis 2001;20:623.

Singhi P, Jain V, Khandelwal N. Corticosteroids versus albendazole for treatment of single small enhancing computed tomographic lesions in children with neurocysticercosis. J Child Neurol. 2004;19:323.

Singounas EG, Leventis AS, Sakas DE, et al. Successful treatment of intracerebral hydatid cysts with albendazole: Case report and review of the literature. Neurosurgery 1992;31:571.

Sirinavin S, Intusoma U, Tuntirungsee S. Mother-to-child transmission of *Cryptococcus neoformans*. Pediatr Infect Dis J. 2004;23:278.

Smego RA, Perfect JR, Durack DT. Combined therapy with amphotericin B and 5-fluorocytosine for *Candida* meningitis. Rev Infect Dis 1984;6:791.

Smith CE, Beard RR, Whiting EG, et al. Varieties of coccidiodal infection in relation to the epidemiology and control of the disease. Am J Public Health 1946;36:1394.

Smith TW, Burton TC. The retinal manifestations of Rocky Mountain spotted fever. Am J Ophthalmol 1977;84:259.

Sommer C, Ringelstein EB, Biniek R, et al. Adult *Toxocara canis* encephalitis. J Neurol Psychiatry 1994;57:229.

Sonakul D. Pathological findings in four cases of human angiostrongyliasis. Southeast Asia J Trop Med Public Health 1978;9:220.

Sorvillo FJ, Waterman SH, Richards FO, et al. Cysticercosis surveillance: Locally acquired and travel-related infections and detection of intestinal carriers in Los Angeles county. Am J Trop Med Hyg 1992;47:365.

Sotelo J, Torres B, Rubio-Donnadieu F, et al. Praziquantel in the treatment of neurocysticercosis long-term follow-up. Neurology 1985a;35:752.

Sparano JA, Gucalp R, Llena JF, et al. Cerebral infection complicating systemic aspergillosis in acute leukemia: Clinical and radiographic presentation. J Neurooncol 1992;13:91.

Spina-Franca A. American trypanosomiasis In: Skakir RA, Newman PK, Poser CM. Tropical neurology. London: WB Saunders, 1996.

Steele RW, Baffoe-Bonnie B. Cerebral malaria in children. Pediatr Infect Dis J 1995;14:281.

Stern H, Elek SD, Booth JC, et al. Microbial causes of mental retardation. Lancet 1969;2:443.

St. Geme JW 3rd, Maldonado YA, Enzmann D, et al. Consensus: Diagnosis and management of neurocysticercosis in children. Pediatr Infect Dis J 1993;12:455.

Stibbs HH, Seed JR. Chromatographic evidence of the synthesis of possible sleep-mediators in *Trypanosoma brucei gambiense.* Experientia 1973a;29:1563.

Stibbs HH, Seed JR. Further studies on the metabolism of tryptophan in *Trypanosoma brucei gambiense:* Cofactors, inhibitors, and end products. Experientia 1973b;31:275.

Stites DP, Glezen WP. Pulmonary nocardiosis in childhood. Am J Dis Child 1967;114:101.

Strickland AD. *Entamoeba histolytica*. In: Feigin RD, Cherry JD, eds. Textbook of pediatric infectious diseases, 3rd ed. Philadelphia: WB Saunders, 1992.

Stringer JL, Marks LM, White AC Jr. Epileptigenic activity of granulomas associated with murine cysticercosis. Exp Neurol 2003;183:532.

Su C, Evans D, Cole RH, et al. Recent expansion of *Toxoplasma* through enhanced oral transmission. Science 2003;299:414.

Sudhakar S, Ross J. Short-term treatment of actinomycosis: Two cases and a review. Clin Infect Dis 2004;38:444-7

Sun T. Pathology and clinical features of parasitic diseases. New York: Masson Publishing USA, Inc, 1982.

Sundar S, Jha TK, Thakur CP, et al. Oral miltefosine for Indian visceral leishmaniasis. N Eng J Med 2002;347:1739.

Tamura AN, Ohashi N, Urakami H, Miyamura S. Classification of *Rickettsia tsutsugamushi* in a new genus, *Orientia* gen. Nov., as *Orientai tsutsugamushi* comb. Nov Int J Syst Bacteriol 1995;45:589.

Tan V, Wilkins P, Badve S, et al. Histoplasmosis of the central nervous system. J Neurol Neurosurg Psychiatr 1992;55:619.

Tanyuksel M, Petri WA Jr. Laboratory diagnosis of amebiasis. Clin Microbiol Rev 2003;16:713.

Tapchaisri P, Nopparatana C, Chaicumpa W, et al. Specific antigen of *Gnathostoma spinigerum* for immunodiagnosis of human gnathostomiasis. Int J Parasitol 1991;21:315.

Taratuto AL, Monges J, Acefe JC, et al. Leptomyxid amoeba encephalitis: Report of the first case in Argentina. Trans Roy Soc Trop Med Hyg 1991;85:77

Taratuto AL, Venturiello SM. Echinococcosis. Brain Pathol 1997a;7:673.

Taratuto AL, Venturiello SM. Trichinosis. Brain Pathol 1997b;7:663.

Taylor GD, Boettger DW, Miedzinski LJ, et al. Coccidioidal meningitis acquired during holidays in Arizona. Can Med Assoc J 1990;142:1388.

Ter Kuile FO, Dolan G, Nosten F, et al. Halofantrine versus mefloquine in treatment of multidrug-resistant falciparum malaria. Lancet 1993;341:1044.

Thang HD, Elsas RM, Veenstra J. Airport malaria: Report of a case and a brief review of the literature. Neth J Med 2002;60:441.

Thomson AJ, DeVilliers JC, Moosa A, et al. Cerebral cysticercosis in children in South Africa. Ann Trop Paediatr 1984;4:62.

Thorner ST, Walker DH, Petri NA. Rocky Mountain spotted fever. Clin Infect Dis 27:1998;1353.

Threlkeld SC, Hooper DC. Update on management of patients with *Nocardia* infection. In: Remington JS, Swartz MN, eds. Current clinical topics in infectious disease. Boston: Blackwell Scientific Publications, 1997.

Thuma PE, Mabeza GF, Biemba G, et al. Effect of iron chelation therapy on mortality in Zambian children with cerebral malaria. Trans R Soc Trop Med Hyg 1998;92:214.

Tikly M, Denath FM, Hodkinson HJ, et al. Computerized tomographic findings in amoebic brain abscess. S Afr Med J 1988;73:258.

Ting KS, Lin JC, Chang MK. Brachial plexus neuropathy associated with scrub typhus: Report of a case. J Formos Med Assoc 1992;91:110.

Tobie EJ, von Brand T, Mehlman B. Cultural and physiological observations on *Trypanosoma rhodesiense* and *Trypanosoma gambiense*. J Parasitol 1950;36:48.

Toerner JG, Kumar PN, Garagusi VF. Guillain-Barré syndrome associated with Rocky Mountain spotted fever; case report and review. Clin Inf Dis 1996;22:1090.

Toma H, Matsumura S, Oshiro C, et al. Ocular angiostrongyliasis without meningitis symptoms in Okinawa, Japan. J Parasitol 2002;88:211.

Torre Cisneros J, Lopez OL, Kusne S, et al. CNS aspergillosis in organ transplantation: A clinicopathological study. J Neurol Neurosurg Psychiatr 1993;56:188.

Townsend JJ, Wolinsky JS, Baringer JR, et al. Acquired toxoplasmosis: Neglected cause of treatable nervous system disease. Arch Neurol 1975;32:335.

Tranas J, Heinzen RA, Weiss LM, McAllister MM. Serological evidence of human infection with the protozoan *Neospora caninum*. Clin Diagn Lab Immunol 1999;6:765.

Truc P, Lejon V, Magnus E, et al. Evaluation of the micro-CATT/*Trypanosoma brucei gambiense*, and LATEX/*T. b. gambiense* methods for serodiagnsosis and surveillance of human African trypanosomiasis in West and Central Africa. Bull World Health Org 2002;80:882.

Tsai HC, Lee SS, Huang CK, et al. Outbreak of eosinophilic meningitis associated with drinking raw vegetable juice in southern Taiwan. Am J Trop Med 2004;71:222.

Tucker RM, Denning DW, Dupont B, et al. Itraconazole therapy for chronic coccidioidal meningitis. Ann Int Med 1992;112:108.

Tunaci M, Tunaci A, Engin G, et al. MRI of cerebral alveolar *Echinococcus*. Neuroradiology. 1999;41:844-6.

Tuzun M, Altinors N, Arda IS, et al. Cerebral hydatid disease: CT and MR findings. Clin Imag 2002;26:353.

Uribe-Uribe NO, Becerra-Lomelí M, Alvarado-Cabrero I, et al. Granulomatous amebic encephalitis by *Balamuthia mandrillaris*. Patología 2001;39:141.

van der Horst CM, Saag MS, Cloud GA, et al. Treatment of cryptococcal meningitis associated with the acquired immunodeficiency syndrome. N Engl J Med 1997;337:15.

van Leusen H, Perquin WVM. Spinal cord schistosomiasis. J Neurol Neurosurg Psychiatry 2000;69:690.

Vasquez V, Sotelo J. The course of seizures after treatment for cerebral cysticercosis. N Engl J Med 1992;327:696.

Vinard JL, Adam G, Loubrieu G, et al. Pseudotumoral thoracic actinomycosis with lung and brain metastases. Apropos of a case. Review of one hundred thirty one cases in the literature. Ann Chir 1992;46:748.

Visvesvara GS. Pathogenic and opportunistic free-living amebae. In: Murray PR, Baron EJ, Pfaller MA, et al, eds. Manual of clinical microbiology, 7th ed. Washington, DC: ASM Press, 1999.

Visvesvara GS, Garcia LS. Culture of protozoan parasites. Clin Microbiol Rev 2002;15:327.

Visvesvara GS, Martinez AJ, Schuster FL, et al. Leptomyxid ameba, a new agent of amebic meningoencephalitis in humans and animals. J Clin Microbiol 1990;28:2750.

Visvesvara GS, Moura H, Leitch GJ, Schwartz DA. Culture and propagation of microsporidia. In: Wittner M, Weiss, LM, eds. The microsporidia and microsporidiosis. Washington, DC: ASM Press, 1999.

Walker DH. Rocky Mountain spotted fever: A seasonal alert. Clin Inf Dis 1995;20(5):1111.

Walker DH, Barbour AG, Oliver JH, et al Emerging bacterial zoonotic and vector-borne diseases. Ecological and epidemiological factors. JAMA 1996;14:275.

Walker DH, Mattern WD: Rickettsial vasculitis. Am Heart J 1980;100:896.

Wang A, Kay R, Poon WS, Ng HK. Successful treatment of amoebic meningoencephalitis in a Chinese living in Hong Kong. Clin Neurol Neurosurg 1993;95:249.

Wang LW, Lin CH, Liu CC, et al. Systemic fungal infection in very low-birth-weight infants. Acta Paediatr Sin 1996;37:272.

Ward BA, Parent AD, Raila F. Indications for the surgical management of central nervous system blastomycosis. Surg Neurol 1995;43:379.

Warrell DA, Looareesuwan S, Warell M, et al. Dexamethasone proves deleterious in cerebral malaria. A double-blind trial in 100 comatose patients. N Engl J Med 1982;306:313.

Warren KS, Mahmoud AA, eds. Tropical and geographic medicine. New York: McGraw-Hill, 1984.

Weber R, Bryan RT, Schwartz DA, Owen RL. Human microsporidial infections. Clin Microbiol Rev 1994;7:426.

Weber R, Canning EU. Microsporidia. In: Murray PR, Baron EJ, Pfaller MA, et al, eds. Manual of clinical microbiology, 7th ed. Washington, DC: ASM Press, 1999.

Weber R, Deplazes P, Flepp M, et al. Cerebral microsporidiosis due to *Encephalitozoon cuniculi* in a patient with human immunodeficiency virus infection. N Eng J Med 1997;336:474.

Weber R, Deplazes P, Schwartz D. Diagnosis and clinical aspects of human microsporidiosis. In: Petry F, ed. Cryptosporidiosis and microsporidiosis. Basel: Karger, 2000.

Weber R, Schwartz DA, Deplazes P. Laboratory diagnosis of microsporidiosis. In: Wittner M, Weiss, LM, eds. The microsporidia and microsporidiosis. Washington, DC: ASM Press, 1999.

Webster D, Hill AVS. Progress with new malaria vaccines. Bull World Health Org 2003;81:902

Weiss LM. Microsporidia 2003: IWOP 8. J Eukaryot Microbiol 2003; 50:566.

Wellings FM. Amoebic meningoencephalitis. J Florida Med Assn 1977;64:327. (Editorial).

Wendisch J, Blaschke Hellmessen R, Kaulen F, et al. Lethal meningeal encephalitis from *Cryptococcus neoformans* var. *neoformans* in a girl without serious immunodeficiency. Mycoses 1996;39(Suppl 1):97.

Wheat J. Histoplasmosis and coccidioidomycosis in individuals with AIDS. A clinical review. Infect Dis Clin North Am 1994;8:467.

Wheat J, Hafner R, Korzun AH, et al. Itraconazole treatment of disseminated histoplasmosis in patients with the acquired immunodeficiency syndrome. AIDS Clinical Trial Group. Am J Med 1995;98:336.

Wheat J, Sarosi G, McKinsey D, et al. Practice guidelines for the management of patients with histoplasmosis. Infectious Diseases Society of America. Clin Infect Dis 2000 Apr;30(4):688.

Wheat LJ, Kohler RB, Tewari RP. Diagnosis of disseminated histoplasmosis by detection of *Histoplasma capsulatum* antigen in serum and urine specimens. N Engl J Med 1986;314:83.

Wheat LJ, Kohler RB, Tewari RP, et al. Significance of histoplasma antigen in the cerebrospinal fluid of patients with meningitis. Arch Intern Med 1989;149:302.

White AC Jr. Neurocysticercosis: A major cause of neurologic disease worldwide. Clin Infect Dis 1997;24:101.

White AC Jr. Neurocysticercosis: Updates on epidemiology, pathogenesis, diagnosis, and management. Annu Rev Med. 2000;51:187.

White NJ. The treatment of malaria. N. Engl J Med 1996;335:800.

Wilson CB, Remington JS. Toxoplasmosis. In: Feigin RD, Cherry JD, eds. Textbook of pediatric infectious diseases, 3rd ed. Philadelphia: WB Saunders, 1992

Wilson CB, Remington JS, Stagno S, et al. Development of adverse sequelae in children born with subclinical congenital *Toxoplasma* infection. Pediatrics 1980;66:767.

Wilson M, Bryan RT, Fried JA, et al. Clinical evaluation of the cysticercosis enzyme-linked immunoelectrotransfer blot in patients with neurocysticercosis. J Infect Dis 1991;164(5):1007.

Wilson M, Fife EH, Mathew HM, et al. Comparison of the complement fixation, indirect immunofluorescence, and indirect hemagglutination tests for malaria. Am J Trop Med 1975;24:755.

Wilson M, McAuley JB. *Toxoplasma*. In: Murray PR, Baron EJ, Pfaller MA, et al, eds. Manual of clinical microbiology, 7th ed. Washington, DC: ASM Press, 1999.

Wilson M, Remington JS, Clavet C, et al. Evaluation of six commercial kits for detection of human immunoglobulin M antibodies to *Toxoplasma gondii*. J Clin Microbiol 1997;35:3112.

Wilson M, Schantz PM, Nutman T, Tsang VCW. Clinical immunoparasitology. In: Rose NR, Hamilton RG, Detrick B, eds. Manual of clinical immunology, 6th ed. Washington, DC: ASM Press, 2002.

Winking M, Deinsberger W, Schindler C, et al. Cerebral manifestation of an actinomycosis infection. A case report. J Neurosurg Sci 1996;40:145.

Winstanley P, Ward S., Snow R, Breckenridge A. Therapy of falciparum malaria in sub-Saharan Africa: From molecule to policy. Clin Microbiol Dis 2004;17:612.

Witzig RS, Hoadley DJ, Greer DL, et al. Blastomycosis and human immunodeficiency virus: Three new cases and review. South Med J 1994;87:715.

Woodruff AW, Bisseru B, Bowe JC. Infection with animal helminths as a factor in causing poliomelytis and epilepsy. BMJ 1966;5503:1576.

Woodward TE, Osterman J. Rickettsial diseases. In: Warren KS, Mahmoud AAF, eds. Tropical and geographical medicine. New York: McGraw-Hill, 1984.

Worley G, Green JA, Frothingham TE, et al. *Toxocara canis* infection: Clinical and epidemiological associations with seropositivity in kindergarten children. J Infect Dis 1984;149(4):591.

Wright HT Jr. Coccidioidomycosis. In: Gellis SS, Kagan BM, eds. Current pediatric therapy, Vol. 8. Philadelphia: WB Saunders, 1978.

Wright IG, Goodger BV, Buffington GD, et al. Immunopathology of babesial infections. Trans R Soc Trop Med Hyg 1989;83:11.

Wright L. Intellectual sequelae of Rocky Mountain spotted fever. J Abnorm Psychol 1972;80:135.

Wright M, Fikrig S, Haller JO. Aspergillosis in children with acquired immune deficiency. Pediatr Radiol 1993;23:492.

Wrobel CJ, Meyer S, Johnson RH, et al. MR findings in acute and chronic coccidioidomycosis meningitis. AJNR 1992;13:1241.

Yachnis AT, Berg J, Martinez-Salazar A, et al. Disseminated microsporidiosis especially infecting the brain, heart, and kidneys. Report of a newly recognized pansporoblastic species in two symptomatic AIDS patients. Clin Microbiol Infect Dis 1996;106:535.

Yii CY, Chen CY, Chen ER, et al. Epidemiologic studies of eosinophilic meningitis in southern Taiwan. Am J Trop Med Hyg 1975; 24:447.

Yokogawa S. An experimental study of the intracranial parasitism of the human lung fluke, *Paragonimus westermani*. Am J Hyg 1921;1:63.

Zinsser H. Rats, lice and history. Boston: Little, Brown, and Co, 1935.

PART XII

Tumors and Vascular Disorders of the Nervous System

CHAPTER 71

Tumors of the Brain and Spinal Cord, Including Leukemic Involvement

Michael E. Cohen and Patricia K. Duffner

Intracranial tumors of the brain and spinal cord are the second most common group of neoplasms in children, exceeded only by leukemia. The Third National Cancer Survey of the United States, in 1975, placed the incidence of central nervous system (CNS) neoplasia for children younger than 15 years of age at approximately 2.4 per 100,000 [Young and Miller, 1975]. Since this report in the mid-1970s, there is increasing evidence that the incidence of CNS neoplasia in young children may be rising (Fig. 71-1). Of interest is the observation that incidence rates of childhood brain tumors increased sharply in the mid-1980s with the concurrent introduction of magnetic resonance imaging (MRI) and have remained stable since then [Jukich et al., 2001]. To some extent the increasing incidence of childhood brain tumors has been offset by improving survivals [Davis et al., 2001; Smith 1998] (Fig. 71-2).

The most accurate sources of information regarding the incidence of brain tumors in the United States are the Surveillance, Epidemiology, End Results (SEER) Registry and the Central Brain Tumor Registry of the United States (CBTRUS). The SEER program is a population-based data reporting system that is a continuing project of the National Cancer Institute. The population covered by these registries represents slightly more than 26% of the U.S. population. Completeness of reporting in the SEER Registry is estimated at greater than 95%, and follow-up is more than 80%. The SEER Registry's areas include Connecticut, Detroit, Seattle, Hawaii, Utah, San Francisco, Iowa, Atlanta, and New Mexico. Until recently SEER data have been considered the most reliable source of incidence and survival information.

CBTRUS is a database that compiles information from state cancer registries. Unlike SEER, the CBTRUS registry includes information about both benign and malignant tumors. SEER data are limited by the lack of information regarding craniopharyngiomas and nonmedulloblastoma primitive neuroectodermal tumors. In other series, craniopharyngiomas may account for 6% to 10% of all pediatric brain tumors [Rubinstein, 1972]. A report published by the CBTRUS has placed the annual incidence of childhood brain tumors at 4 per 100,000 person-years in children 0 to 19 years of age. Thus, based on the current U.S. population, approximately 3200 newly diagnosed cases of brain tumors can be expected to be identified each year in the United States. Of these two thirds or more will be in children younger than 15. Of interest, an analysis of trends of age-adjusted cancer incidence rates (1974 to 1991) revealed a rise in astroglial tumors in children younger than 5 years of more than 4% per year. Rates of ependymomas have also increased substantially in children less than 2 years old (4.8%) [Gurney et al., 1996]. The incidence of primary brain tumors is highest in the 0 to 4 age group and lowest in the 10 to 14 age group. The rate is slightly higher in males (4.2/100,000) than females (3.8/100,000 person-years). The most common histologies are pilocytic astrocytomas (21%) and medulloblastomas (embryonal tumors) (18%) [CBTRUS, 2004] (Fig. 71-3). The majority are located within the cerebrum and cerebellum. A spinal cord tumor is much less common. The two most common intracranial sites are the cerebellum and the brainstem (Fig. 71-4). The 5-year relative survival rate in the 0 to 19 age group is approximately 64.3%. This compares with a 5-year survival rate of 6.5% to 4.7% in the 65 and older age group [CBTRUS, 2004] (Table 71-1).

Most brain tumors derive from intrinsic elements of the CNS. Bailey and Cushing [1926] are generally credited with applying the term *glioma* to that group of tumors arising from parenchymatous elements of the nervous system. Since then, clusters of histologic features have been used to assess the benign or malignant potential of a given tumor. These observations gave rise to the postulate that morphologic properties could predict the clinical course. Thus astrocytomas with cysts and Rosenthal fibers were associated with a slowly evolving course, whereas those associated with necrosis, pseudopalisading, and anaplasia were associated with a more malignant course. Unfortunately, pathol-

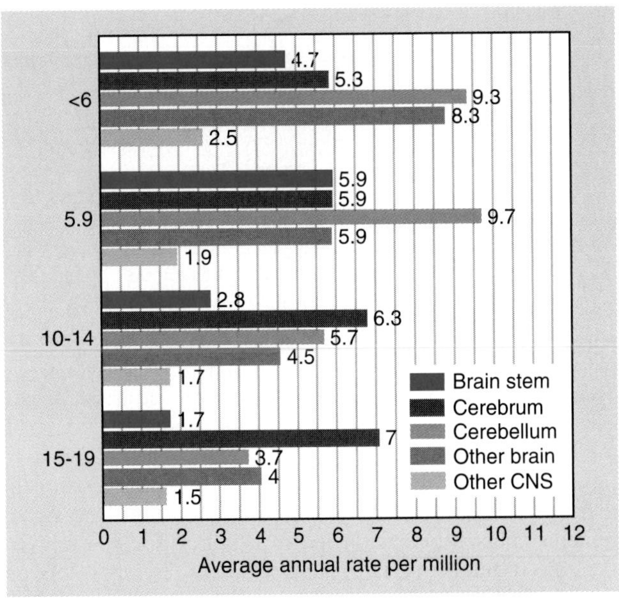

FIGURE 71-1. SEER data 1995 CBTRUS. (From 2004-2005 Statistical Report. Primary Brain Tumors in the United States Statistical Report, 1997-2001 [years data collected]. CBTRUS [2004]. Statistical Report: Primary Brain Tumors in the United States, 1997-2001. Published by the Central Brain Tumor Registry of the United States.)

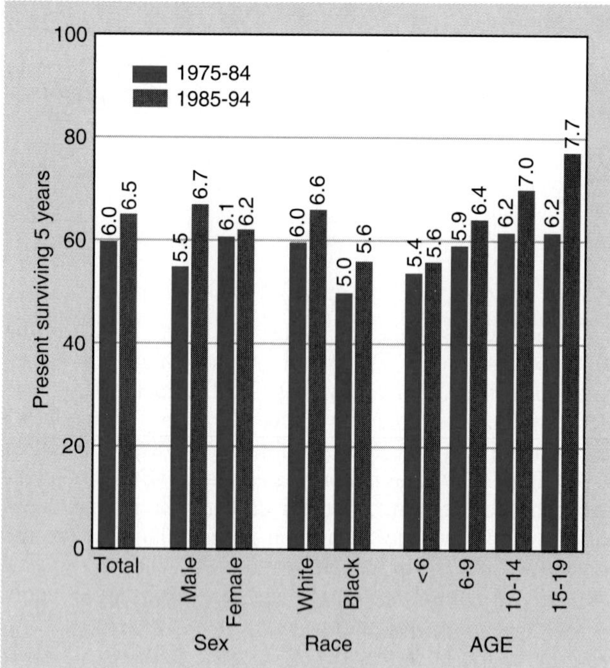

FIGURE 71-2. SEER survival data showing suggestive increase in survivals in the period 1985-1994 compared with the previous decade. (From 2004-2005 Statistical Report. Primary Brain Tumors in the United States Statistical Report, 1997-2001 [years data collected]. CBTRUS [2004]. Statistical Report: Primary Brain Tumors in the United States, 1997-2001. Published by the Central Brain Tumor Registry of the United States.)

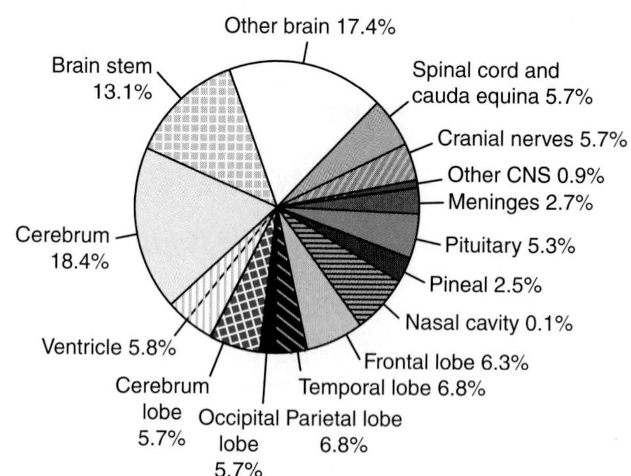

FIGURE 71-4. Distribution of all childhood primary brain and CNS tumors (0-19 years) by site. CBTRUS 1997-2001 (n = 5028). (From 2004-2005 Statistical Report. Primary Brain Tumors in the United States Statistical Report, 1997-2001 [years data collected]. CBTRUS [2004]. Statistical Report: Primary Brain Tumors in the United States, 1997-2001. Published by the Central Brain Tumor Registry of the United States.)

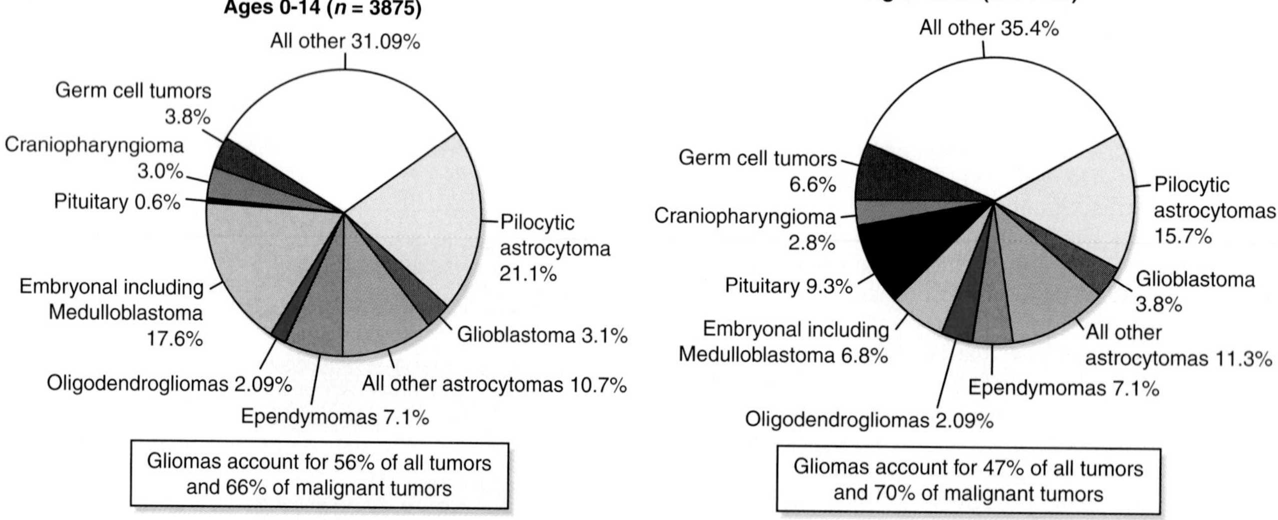

FIGURE 71-3. Distribution of childhood primary brain and CNS tumors by histology. CBTRUS 1997-2001. (From 2004-2005 Statistical Report. Primary Brain Tumors in the United States Statistical Report, 1997-2001 [years data collected]. CBTRUS [2004]. Statistical Report: Primary Brain Tumors in the United States, 1997-2001. Published by the Central Brain Tumor Registry of the United States.)

ogy cannot fully predict outcome, and much confusion in the definition of terms and the ability to prognosticate remains. This imprecision led to a search for new classifications of tumors and a general reluctance to rely solely on pathologic features for prognosis. At the turn of the 21st century, traditional approaches to histopathology have been increasingly challenged as new techniques have been added to the pathologic armamentarium. Immunohistochemistry allows the pathologist to assay for the presence of antibodies to epitopes of glial and neuronal proteins. Monoclonal technology has resulted in the identification of antibodies with specificity for various CNS tumors. Astrocytic tumors are now routinely stained for glial fibrillary acidic protein, an intermediate filament with a diameter of 10 to 12 nm observed in patients with well-differentiated astrocytomas. Glial fibrillary acidic protein reactivity is not specific because it is weakly observed in ependymomas, choroid plexus tumors, and oligodendrogliomas. Vimentin, a 57-kd fila-

TABLE 71-1

One-, Two-, Three-, Four-, Five-, and Ten-Year Relative Survival Rates* for Selected Malignant Brain and Central Nervous System Tumors† by Age Groups, Seer 1973-2001

HISTOLOGY	AGE GROUP	NO. OF CASES	1-YR	2-YR	3-YR	4-YR	5-YR	10-YR
Pilocytic astrocytoma	0-14	633	97.4	96.5	96.1	94.5	93.8	92.0
	0-19	762	97.2	96.4	96.0	94.5	93.7	92.3
	20-44	245	93.7	91.0	89.0	87.5	87.0	82.7
	45-54	43	90.4	87.9	82.1	79.3	76.0	66.8
	55-64	16	93.7	83.8	—	—	—	—
	65-74	13	—	—	—	—	—	—
	75+	7	—	—	—	—	—	—
	Total	**1086**						
Diffuse astrocytoma	0-14	106	92.4	85.4	82.2	82.2	81.2	80.0
	0-19	134	92.5	86.9	83.6	83.6	82.8	82.0
	20-44	288	89.9	82.0	73.3	63.7	57.5	39.3
	45-54	92	71.6	49.8	40.1	37.7	35.1	19.1
	55-64	85	46.5	21.8	16.0	13.7	10.2	7.6
	65-74	82	30.5	16.4	9.9	8.7	7.2	—
	75+	27	27.8	8.9	4.7	—	—	—
	Total	**708**						
Anaplastic astrocytoma	0-14	129	72.3	58.0	52.8	49.1	49.1	46.8
	0-19	172	76.3	60.1	55.6	51.6	51.6	46.9
	20-44	840	85.2	71.7	62.3	54.7	48.3	32.1
	45-54	348	63.2	43.6	32.3	26.8	25.4	18.2
	55-64	309	44.3	20.1	13.9	10.5	5.9	3.7
	65-74	338	23.7	6.5	3.8	3.2	3.2	1.3
	75+	176	12.5	4.5	2.5	1.8	—	—
	Total	**2183**						
Astrocytoma, NOS	0-14	881	87.5	82.3	80.2	78.5	78.0	74.4
	0-19	1150	87.7	81.8	79.2	77.7	76.7	73.2
	20-44	2121	86.6	75.6	68.3	61.5	54.8	38.1
	45-54	951	62.6	41.0	33.0	29.0	26.7	17.6
	55-64	1178	40.0	20.1	15.1	12.9	11.1	6.5
	65-74	1186	22.3	9.1	6.2	5.6	5.0	2.3
	75+	600	12.4	5.5	4.2	3.8	3.5	—
	Total	**7186**						
Glioblastoma	0-14	176	47.2	23.9	19.6	18.3	17.0	15.5
	0-19	265	50.5	27.7	21.3	19.6	18.8	16.2
	20-44	1787	59.4	30.0	21.1	16.5	13.6	8.9
	45-54	2517	41.9	11.7	6.0	3.9	3.5	1.7
	55-64	3918	31.1	5.9	2.6	1.7	1.4	0.5
	65-74	4125	16.6	2.6	1.0	0.6	0.4	0.2
	75+	2486	7.9	1.4	0.6	0.4	0.4	0.2
	Total	**15,098**						
Oligodendroglioma	0-14	109	93.4	90.4	89.4	88.3	87.1	79.7
	0-19	175	92.9	87.9	85.9	85.2	84.4	79.7
	20-44	886	95.7	91.9	88.3	84.4	80.6	62.6
	45-54	313	91.2	82.5	76.1	69.4	64.4	38.1
	55-64	212	81.8	67.3	58.1	47.0	44.1	29.2
	65-74	118	61.7	50.9	50.3	41.6	35.0	11.8
	75+	44	45.5	32.2	19.0	—	—	—
	Total	**1748**						
Anaplastic oligodendroglioma	0-14	7	—	—	—	—	—	—
	0-19	10	—	—	—	—	—	—
	20-44	140	91.1	75.9	71.1	64.2	55.8	37.2
	45-54	73	82.0	62.6	58.1	43.5	43.5	35.5
	55-64	56	67.1	52.6	43.7	35.7	27.2	—
	65-74	38	49.9	35.3	32.4	32.4	19.3	—
	75+	23	32.7	—	—	—	—	—
	Total	**340**						

Continued

TABLE 71-1, *cont'd*

One-, Two-, Three-, Four-, Five-, and Ten-Year Relative Survival Rates* for Selected Malignant Brain and Central Nervous System Tumors† by Age Groups, Seer 1973–2001

HISTOLOGY	AGE GROUP	NO. OF CASES	1-YR	2-YR	3-YR	4-YR	5-YR	10-YR
Ependymoma/ anaplastic ependymoma	0-14	369	84.6	70.4	61.3	54.6	50.7	45.5
	0-19	414	85.8	73.0	63.8	57.9	54.5	47.1
	20-44	403	91.3	89.3	85.4	84.3	84.1	77.2
	45-54	149	91.3	86.2	79.6	79.2	75.7	67.8
	55-64	117	80.9	76.2	72.9	71.7	66.4	50.4
	65-74	69	78.3	75.6	72.5	71.2	71.2	43.7
	75+		18	63.5	—	—	—	—
	Total	**1170**						
Mixed glioma	0-14	76	88.1	80.1	76.0	70.5	69.1	62.9
	0-19	108	86.9	80.1	77.1	72.0	71.0	65.5
	20-44	374	92.3	84.9	79.2	72.7	68.3	49.3
	45-54	118	78.9	64.7	53.1	45.9	39.3	30.6
	55-64	89	78.1	52.4	38.6	33.3	30.6	15.2
	65-74	53	50.9	37.1	27.1	17.8	15.4	6.7
	75+	12	—	—	—	—	—	—
	Total	**754**						
Glioma malignant, NOS	0-14	578	68.3	49.7	46.3	45.5	44.1	41.0
	0-19	653	69.9	52.7	49.1	48.2	46.8	42.7
	20-44	455	80.3	67.7	61.9	56.2	51.1	36.6
	45-54	250	55.2	37.5	31.0	29.7	28.3	20.0
	55-64	329	42.0	26.2	21.6	19.1	16.8	11.6
	65-74	430	23.7	13.1	11.9	8.4	7.5	5.0
	75+	456	10.4	6.6	5.6	4.2	3.3	2.9
	Total	**2573**						
Neuroepithelial	0-14	47	85.1	74.2	67.7	63.3	59.0	56.8
	0-19	63	87.3	77.6	72.6	69.3	66.0	64.3
	20-44	65	77.1	64.7	58.5	53.9	52.4	32.7
	45-54	34	53.3	32.8	24.1	21.0	21.0	11.1
	55-64	31	36.1	20.0	16.9	—	—	—
	65-74	30	20.7	14.2	11.1	—	—	—
	75+	15	—	—	—	—	—	—
	Total	**238**						
Malignant neuronal/glial, neuronal, and mixed	0-14	108	75.0	63.5	57.5	54.4	54.4	52.0
	0-19	122	75.5	65.3	58.3	54.7	52.7	50.5
	20-44	63	93.8	79.4	77.8	74.1	72.2	63.1
	45-54	48	89.3	87.3	85.1	76.2	73.1	50.2
	55-64	44	89.6	68.2	66.3	64.2	64.2	53.8
	65-74	15	—	—	—	—	—	—
	75+	15	—	—	—	—	—	—
	Total	**307**						
Embryonal/primitive/ medulloblastoma	0-14	919	78.9	68.4	62.6	56.7	54.0	47.2
	0-19	1013	80.0	69.8	64.0	58.0	54.8	47.6
	20-44	305	86.4	76.8	68.8	63.0	57.1	46.7
	45-54	38	81.5	76.1	76.1	73.6	63.0	45.2
	55-64	16	—	—	—	—	—	—
	65-74	5	—	—	—	—	—	—
	75+	6	—	—	—	—	—	—
	Total	**1383**						
Lymphoma	0-14	18	56.3	48.2	40.2	—	—	—
	0-19	35	66.7	60.1	56.8	49.7	—	—
	20-44	910	22.5	16.3	14.1	12.7	11.2	9.3
	45-54	365	41.9	34.2	31.1	28.4	25.7	16.1
	55-64	363	53.8	40.9	31.4	26.6	21.8	12.4
	65-74	461	44.6	29.9	22.7	18.3	15.3	8.2
	75+	280	33.7	20.7	15.5	12.7	11.1	2.6
	Total	**2414**						

TABLE 71-1, *cont'd*

One-, Two-, Three-, Four-, Five-, and Ten-Year Relative Survival Rates* for Selected Malignant Brain and Central Nervous System Tumors† by Age Groups, Seer 1973–2001

HISTOLOGY	AGE GROUP	NO. OF CASES	1-YR	2-YR	3-YR	4-YR	5-YR	10-YR
TOTAL: ALL BRAIN AND CNS†‡	0-14	4541	81.0	71.4	67.3	64.3	62.9	58.8
	0-19	5628	82.2	72.9	68.8	65.9	64.3	59.9
	20-44	9403	76.2	63.4	57.0	51.9	47.6	35.7
	45-54	5636	55.8	33.7	27.3	24.2	22.5	15.4
	55-64	7146	40.2	18.7	14.1	12.1	10.6	6.9
	65-74	7443	24.3	11.1	8.6	7.3	6.5	4.0
	75+	4785	14.5	7.6	6.0	5.2	4.7	3.3
	Total	**40,041**						

*Rates are an estimate of the percentage of patients alive at 1, 2, 3, 4, 5, and 10 years, respectively.
†In contrast with survival estimates reported in previous editions of the CBTRUS statistical report, brain lymphomas, olfactory tumors of the nasal cavity, and malignant tumors of the pituitary and pineal glands are included.
‡Includes histologies not listed in this table.
Abbreviations: SEER, Serveillance, Epidemiology, End Results; NOS, not otherwise specified; —, too few cases to estimate.

ment, is a neurofilament found in immature rather than differentiated glial cells. As myelination and differentiation proceed, vimentin decreases, whereas glial fibrillary acidic protein becomes more apparent. Vimentin has been found in meningiomas, schwannomas, carcinomas, sarcomas, melanomas, and lymphomas. Neurofilament markers are being used to identify neuronal tumors, such as gangliogliomas. Although these markers recognize neurons, axons, and mature neural elements, they are less helpful in identification of more primitive tumors such as medulloblastomas, primitive neuroectodermal tumors, and neuroblastomas. Conversely, synaptophysin, a glycosylated polypeptide component of the presynaptic vesicle membrane, has been used to determine neuroectodermal differentiation.

New techniques complement standard histopathology in assessing cell proliferation. Flow cytometry, a technique that measures physical or chemical characteristics of single cells, is widely used to determine deoxyribonucleic acid (DNA) content. A DNA histogram is characterized by two peaks. The majority of cells in the resting phase (G-0) or in the G-1 phase of the cell cycle contain a similar amount of DNA. Next to this dominant peak, histograms demonstrate smaller peaks composed of cells in G-2 or those undergoing mitosis. DNA of tumor cells is then compared with the DNA content of diploid standards and a DNA index is determined. A diploid sample with normal DNA content has a diploid index of 1, whereas a DNA index less than or greater than 1 is abnormal. Most malignant cells are commonly aneuploid with varying amounts of DNA, suggesting that the DNA content varies from the diploid standard [Coon et al., 1987]. Using these techniques, flow cytometry permits assessment of biologic behavior.

Proliferation antigens have been identified to assess proliferative activity. These are nuclear antigens that estimate the growth fraction of normal and neoplastic cells, thereby providing an estimate of doubling time. Ki-67, a murine monoclonal antibody is a proliferation marker, which binds to human nuclear protein in various stages of the cell cycle. The monoclonal antibody MIB-1 is a variant of Ki-67. Both markers are used to define tumors that have a high growth fraction. Another marker of DNA synthesis is the halogenated pyrimidine bromodeoxyuridine. Because it is incorporated into DNA during the S phase of the cell cycle, this marker is used as a marker of cell proliferation. After exposure to bromodeoxyuridine, a labeling index is determined and the percentage of positive staining cells is used to determine a mitotic index.

Identification of growth factors and oncogenes with tumor specificity will further add to the ability to classify tumors [Burger and Fuller, 1991; Cohen and Duffner, 1994a]. Loss of heterozygosity, fluorescein in situ hybridization, and quantitative polymerase chain reaction represent some of the newer molecular tools used to identify genetic aberrations that correlate with tumor type and degree of malignancy [Louis et al., 2001].

HISTOPATHOLOGIC GROUPINGS

Until newer techniques become routinely accepted, tumors will be graded according to the World Health Organization's system, which is based on site, histologic type, and degree of malignancy (Box 71-1) [Kleihues and Cavenee, 2000]. This classification, as well as many others that have preceded it, is somewhat arbitrary and presumptive in that classifications rely on the presence of a stem cell from which more differentiated cell types derive. For instance, medulloblastoma is believed to be a tumor of undifferentiated cells arising from putative stem cells of the developing nervous system. Similarly, a central tenet in the approach to the diagnosis of primitive neuroectodermal tumors is the assumption that these tumors, regardless of site of origin, were derived from a common precursor with the potential for glial, ependymal, neuronal, or bipolar differentiation. Objections to this approach have been raised because of the lack of a single stem cell and the tendency to fit all undifferentiated tumors into this category. Burger and associates [1991] suggested that an uncritical use of this grouping would place malignant ependymomas, pineoblastomas, glioblastomas, neurocytomas, and oligodendrogliomas into a similar grouping because of a focus on cellularity alone. It is well recognized that primitive neuroectodermal tumors, depending on site and age, have different responses to treatment and thus may suggest a different biology.

The optimal classification of brain tumors should include pathologic characteristics, tumor biology, anatomic loca-

Box 71-1 Brain Tumor Classification (Adapted from the World Health Organization)

Tumor of Neuroepithelial Tissue

Astrocytic tumors

Astrocytoma
Variants: Fibrillary
Protoplasmic
Gemistocytic
Anaplastic (malignant) astrocytoma
Glioblastoma
Variants: Giant cell glioblastoma
Gliosarcoma
Pilocytic astrocytoma
Plemorphic xanthoastrocytoma
Subependymal giant cell astrocytoma (tuberous sclerosis)

Oligodendroglial tumors

Oligodendroglioma
Anaplastic (malignant) oligodendroglioma

Ependymal tumors

Ependymoma
Variants: Cellular
Papilary
Clear cell
Anaplastic (malignant) oligoastrocytoma
Myxopapillary ependymoma
Subependymoma

Mixed gliomas

Oligoastrocytoma
Anaplastic (malignant) oligoastrocytoma
Others

Choroid plexus tumors

Choroid plexus papilloma
Choroid plexus carcinoma

Neuroepithelial tumors of uncertain origin

Astroblastoma
Polar spongioblastoma
Gliomatosis cerebri

Neuronal and mixed neuronal-glial tumors

Gangliocytoma
Dysplastic gangliocytoma of cerebellum (Lhermitte-Duclos)
Desmoplastic infantile ganglioglioma
Dysembryoplastic neuroepithelial tumor
Ganglioglioma
Anaplastic (malignant) ganglioglioma
Central neurocytoma
Paraganglioma of the filum terminate
Olfactory neuroblastoma (esthesioneuroblastoma)
Variant: Olfactory neuroepithelioma

Pineal parenchymaltumors

Pineocytoma
Pineoblastoma
Pinealoma
Mixed transitional pineal tumors

Enbryonal tumors

Medulloepithelioma
Pinealoblastoma
Neuroblastoma
Variant: Ganglioneuroblastoma
Ependymoblastoma
Primitive neuroectodermal tumors (PNETs)
Medulloblastoma
Variants: Desoplastic medulloblastoma
Medullomyoblastoma
Melanocytic medulloblastoma

Tumors of the Meninges

Tumors of meningothelial cells

Meningioma
Variants: Meningothelial
Fibrous (fibroblastic)
Transitional (mixed)
Psammomatous
Angiomatous
Microcystic
Secretory
Clear cell
Chordoid
Lymphoplasmacyte-rich
Metaplastic
Atypical meningioma
Papillary meningioma
Anaplastic (malignant) meningioma

Germ cell tumors

Germinoma
Embryonal carcinoma
Yolk sac tumor (endodermal sinus tumor)
Choriocarcinoma
Teratoma
Immature
Mature
Teratoma with malignant transformation
Mixed germ cell tumors

From Kleihues and Cavenee, 2000.

tion, patient age, and response to therapy. With this information, physicians may provide a more realistic assessment of the prognosis associated with a given diagnosis. The largest histopathologic grouping in both the SEER and CBTRUS registries is for astrocytomas. This category includes such diverse tumors as cerebellar astrocytomas, brainstem gliomas, high-grade supratentorial astrocytomas, and low-grade supratentorial astrocytomas. In the SEER database for children 0 to 15 years, astrocytomas represented 57%, medulloblastomas 23%, and ependymomas 8% of the total population. The incidence for childhood brain tumors in the CBTRUS data for the age cohort 0 to 19 is somewhat different. Astrocytomas represent 40.5 % of the series; medulloblastomas 20.5%, and ependymomas 7.6% (see Table 71-1). Although individual series report some variation, astrocytomas remain the most common grouping.

The type of tumor varies with age at diagnosis. In the age interval 0 to 4 years, glioblastomas, medulloblastomas/primitive neuroectodermal tumors, pilocytic astrocytomas, and ependymomas predominate. Brainstem gliomas are less common in infancy but are increasingly recognized throughout childhood. Excluding infancy, the most common tumors identified in children are low-grade astrocytomas, medulloblastomas, high-grade astrocytomas, and cerebellar astrocytomas. Dysembryoblastic neuroepithelial tumors, central neurocytomas, hamartomas, craniopharyngiomas, and, to some extent, choroid plexus tumors represent a less common but more benign group of neoplasms with an excellent prognosis. Germ cell and non–germ cell tumors have an intermediate prognosis. Nonmedulloblastoma primitive neuroectodermal tumors were not coded in the SEER Registry data and are combined with medulloblastomas in the CBRTUS data. Increasingly more children, particularly in the first 2 years of life, are being identified with this diagnosis.

EPIDEMIOLOGY

The causation of brain tumors is not a chance phenomenon. Proponents of causal inference generally agree on the following five criteria:

1. Biologic plausibility: Any agent implicated in the occurrence of a brain tumor should have direct access to the CNS, can interfere with intracranial cellular growth, and in some way can damage normal repair mechanisms.
2. The association between exposure and occurrence of tumor: Exposure is considered etiologically significant when the risk is increased fivefold rather than twofold. This epidemiologic axiom reflects the concept that the higher the risk, the less likely are confounding biases.
3. Consistency: The more reproducible, the more likely the association is meaningful.
4. Temporal order: Exposure occurs at a time in keeping with the known interval between tumor initiation and promotion.
5. Biologic gradient or dose-response relation: If the known factor (e.g., radiation) contributes to the risk of a brain tumor, those with the greatest exposure will have the highest risk of brain tumor development [Leviton, 1994].

There are well-known risk factors associated with the subsequent development of brain tumors. Genetic syndromes, such as neurofibromatosis, tuberous sclerosis, Lindau-von Hippel disease, Li-Fraumeni syndrome, Turcot's syndrome, and the basal cell nevus syndrome, are all associated with increased risk of brain tumor in children. Patients with Wilms' tumor and those with nevoid basal-cell carcinoma are more prone to develop medulloblastomas. It is also known that epilepsy and stroke tend to be more common in families of children with brain tumors [Schoenberg et al., 1975].

Another accepted risk factor is immunosuppression. Individuals immunosuppressed before or during renal transplantation have a 350 times greater risk of developing reticulum cell sarcoma [Schneck and Penn, 1971]. Similarly, children with ataxia-telangiectasia, who have a number of immunologic abnormalities, are also at greater risk for developing neoplasia [Swift et al., 1976].

Environmental factors are also believed to increase the risk for development of CNS tumors. These factors include exposure to aromatic hydrocarbons, *N*-nitroso compounds, triazines, and systemic hydrazines [Zeller et al., 1982]. Less well-documented associations implicated in the production of tumors are maternal consumption of barbiturates, background radiation, prenatal exposure to diagnostic x-ray studies [National Radiological Protection Board, 1981], trauma, infection, familial aggregation, and exposure to anesthetics at the time of pregnancy [Davis et al., 2001]. Ionizing radiation is a well-recognized cause of secondary oncogenesis in patients irradiated for CNS tumors. This is not exclusively a dose-related phenomenon as there are reports of low dose radiation associated with the subsequent development of meningiomas [Modan et al., 1974]. There is no accepted causal relationship however between CNS tumors and either electromagnetic field or microwave exposure.

Of the inherited syndromes, neurofibromatosis may potentially provide the most information regarding oncogenesis. The association of neurofibromatosis with a diversity and multiplicity of tumors and the ability of these tumors to produce local hypertrophy of bone, skin, and muscle implies the presence of a substance capable of initiating or promoting tissue growth. Type 1 neurofibromatosis occurs with a loss of tumor suppressor gene and maps to the 17q11.2 chromosome region. The genes in this area encode for proteins instrumental in the signaling network of the P21 ras proteins [Buchberg et al., 1990]. The area of deletion on the long arm of chromosome 17 is quite large and therefore must have multiple functions. It is postulated that the NF1 gene product downregulates the function of the *ras* oncogene product, which provides a growth stimulus for signal transduction. These findings support the premise that advances in molecular biology will eventually lead to a basic understanding of oncogenesis.

Tumors manifesting in the last half of the first decade of life, limited malignant features on histologic preparation, and long duration of symptoms before diagnosis are considered good prognostic signs. Neoplasms occurring in infancy, brainstem and thalamic location, and evidence of histologic aggressiveness are considered poor prognostic signs.

Conditional probabilities address the question of the likelihood of survival for the next period of time if an individual has survived for a specified period. The probability of 5-year conditional survival if an individual has survived 2 years is greatest in the pediatric age group younger than 21 years, and for most tumors in this age group, other than glioblastoma, it is more than 70%. This suggests that 2 years may be a reasonable period in which to judge subsequent survival [Davis et al., 1999] (Fig. 71-5).

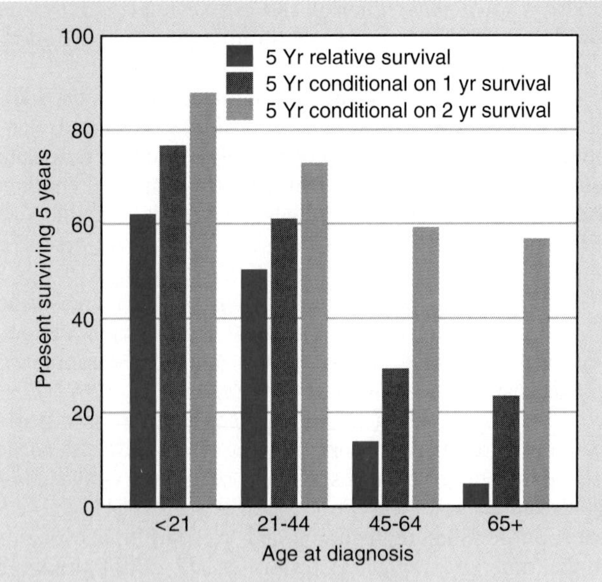

FIGURE 71-5. Relative survival rates in patients with any primary malignant brain tumors (including those that were not confirmed microscopically) ages less than 21, 21 to 44, 45 to 64, and 65 years and older compared with relative survival conditional on having survived 1 to 2 years post diagnosis. (From Davis et al., 1999.)

DIAGNOSIS

The diagnosis of a brain tumor depends on clinical suspicion, the diagnostic acumen of the physician, and the availability of MRI. Signs and symptoms of brain tumors vary, depending on age and development of the child, tumor location, and amount of neurologic integrity that is compromised. No pathognomonic features exist. The temporal course of a child with a brain tumor is usually progressive and insidious. At times, a remitting course followed by exacerbation is recognized. It is instructive to refer to Cushing's monograph, which describes the course of a young child with a cerebellar astrocytoma [Cushing, 1931]. Cushing reported that a child, apparently normal in all respects, may have a history of early morning headache and vomiting. The symptoms may resolve during the course of the day. As an expansible head enlarges to accommodate increasing pressure, symptoms may abate and the episode may be forgotten. Subsequently, the child may develop an ataxic syndrome and present with papilledema, signaling uncompensated growth of a posterior fossa mass. Thus, although the temporal history of most brain tumors is insidious and progressive, remitting and exacerbating courses are well known.

Signs and symptoms of a general nature without focal signature may reflect increased intracranial pressure. Elevation of intracranial pressure can result from obstruction of ventricular pathways or from a mass growing within a fixed cranial volume. Nonspecific symptoms of intracranial pressure include irritability, lethargy, vomiting, anorexia, headache, weight gain or weight loss, and changes in behavior, personality, or school performance.

Focal pathology may not signify focal disease. For instance, the abducens nerve, because of its long free intracranial course and proximity to bony structures, may be compromised as the result of increased pressure. Thus diplopia secondary to abducens paresis may not signal a focal pathologic condition but rather increased intracranial pressure.

It is axiomatic that papilledema always suggests increased intracranial pressure and, by extension, the possible presence of a mass lesion. When present, optic atrophy or visual loss implies either long-standing, unrecognized pressure or a focal pathologic process. The earliest sign of papilledema is an increase in either the blind spot (cecal scotoma) or loss of color vision (dyschromatopsia). These signs must be assiduously sought because most children with insidious compromise of the visual axis do not spontaneously offer visual complaints.

Obstruction of cerebrospinal fluid pathways occurs with tumors invading the midline of the cerebellum, mesencephalon, diencephalic regions, or within the ventricles. Because pontine tumors are primarily found on the ventral surface of the brainstem, they may not occlude the ventricular outflow tracts until late in their course. Hemispheric tumors tend to produce pressure by mass effect rather than by obstruction of the ventricular pathways.

Increased intracranial pressure may not produce symptoms other than headache and vomiting until pressure rises high enough to impede cerebral circulation. Acute changes in pressure have the potential for producing dynamic effects within the head. Different herniation syndromes (uncal, transtentorial, and central herniation) may occur and are reviewed in Chapter 65 [Plum and Posner, 1982]. Unlike downward herniation syndromes, posterior fossa lesions may lead to alterations of consciousness because of upward rather than downward shift. Herniation of the superior vermis of the cerebellum through the tentorium may compromise midbrain and diencephalic structures. Both downward and upward herniation can interfere with the reticular formation, resulting in alterations in the level of consciousness. Early signs of tonsillar herniation may be head tilt and stiff neck. The latter occurs as a result of irritation of cervical roots by the herniating mass. Although herniation syndromes are not common, they do represent an acute neurologic emergency and require immediate intervention.

Bailey and co-workers [1939] commented that headache was an uncommon symptom in children and, when present, suggested organic disease. Head pain is one of the most common complaints that a pediatric neurologist is asked to evaluate. This complaint involves all age groups and may not signify structural disease. Suspicion of a brain tumor should be greatest in the child with onset of headache within the past 4 to 6 months [Honig and Charney, 1982]. Location of headache is not pathognomonic. Headache associated with cerebellar tumors may be frontal or occipital in location. Focal headache, however, is more likely to imply organic disease than generalized headache and, in the absence of intracranial pressure, may suggest pathology underlying the point of pain or a referral pattern from a distant source (Fig. 71-6). Headaches that increase with coughing, sneezing, straining at stool, or other forms of Valsalva maneuvers are a reliable but often unsolicited symptom of increased intracranial pressure. Early morning headache relieved by vomiting, and headaches that awaken the child from sleep are particularly worrisome for increased intracranial pressure and mass lesions.

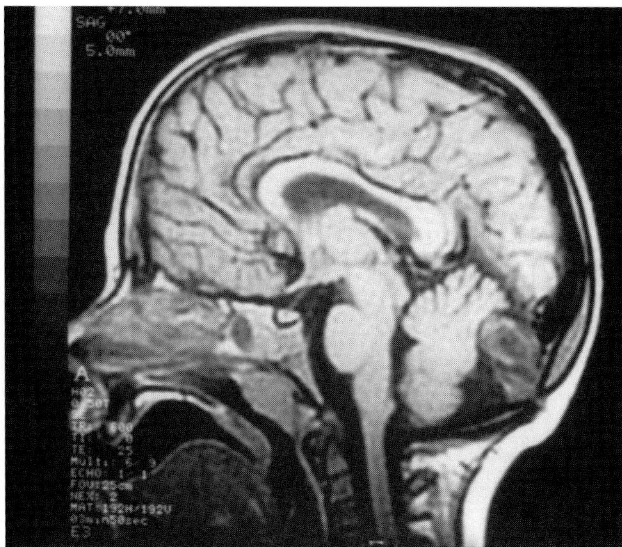

FIGURE 71-6. Focal headache in 2-year-old with dermoid. Note inner table defect in occiput.

Perhaps more than headache, changes in personality, energy level, or motivation are the harbingers of intracranial pathology. Anorexia, bulimia, abulia (i.e., lack of motivation), weight gain or loss, lethargy, sexual precocity, or autonomic abnormalities should raise the suspicion of hypothalamic or pituitary disease. Focal seizures, when accompanied by slow-wave changes in the electroencephalogram (EEG) or clinical observations of impaired neurologic function, may suggest an underlying mass.

Signs pointing to location in the cerebellar hemisphere or vermis should suggest the presence of a cerebellar tumor. The findings of ataxia, cranial neuropathies, and long tract signs without evidence of increased intracranial pressure suggest a lesion of the brainstem. Alterations in mentation, endocrinopathy, and changes in visual acuity raise the possibility of disease of the midline of the CNS. Hemisensory, hemimotor, and hemianopic abnormalities all suggest localization to specific parts of the cerebral hemispheres.

Because most brain tumors are compressive rather than destructive, neurologic signs may be subtle. Visual inattention, decreased arm swing on one side, a hint of foot drag, or suggestive flattening of the nasolabial fold may be the first indication of a cerebral hemispheric mass. Similarly, increasing clumsiness, inability to run or hop, or changes in energy level may suggest disease of the posterior fossa or midline brain structures.

On suspicion of a mass lesion, diagnosis is confirmed by neuroimaging studies. For the most part, MRIs with and without gadolinium or high-resolution computed tomography (CT) scans with contrast have replaced other forms of imaging. Although high-resolution CT scanners can provide exquisite definition of most mass lesions in the nervous system (Fig. 71-7), this technique has generally been replaced by MRI (Fig. 71-8). Because the MRI does not image bone, parts of the nervous system inaccessible by CT scan can now be readily imaged. Lesions of the parasellar area, posterior fossa, and spinal cord are easily visualized by MRI. Failure to define soft tissue density because of the presence of bone and partial volume effects is obviated by MRI. The ability to image tissue in multiple planes, as well as the many paradigms of imaging coupled with ferromagnetic contrast agents, provide unsurpassed definition in both pathology and anatomy. T1-weighted images obtained in any plane provide in vivo–like definition of anatomy, whereas T2-weighted images readily identify tumor spread and resultant edema. The time to obtain an image and the consequent need for anesthesia in the young child are limiting factors.

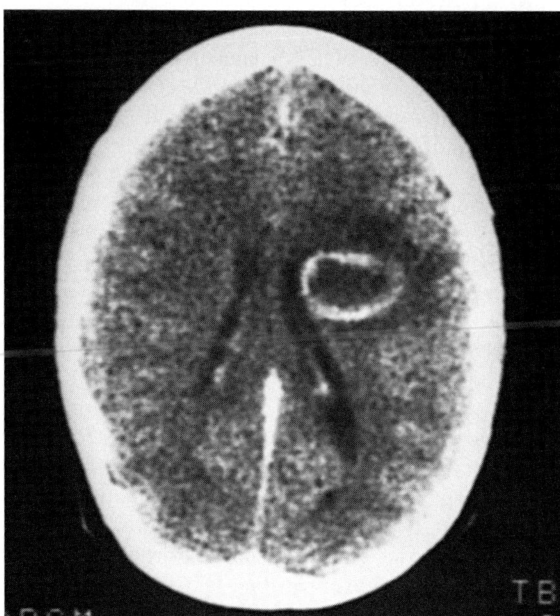

FIGURE 71-7. Axial CT of a 16-year-old with an astrocytoma demonstrating ring enhancement.

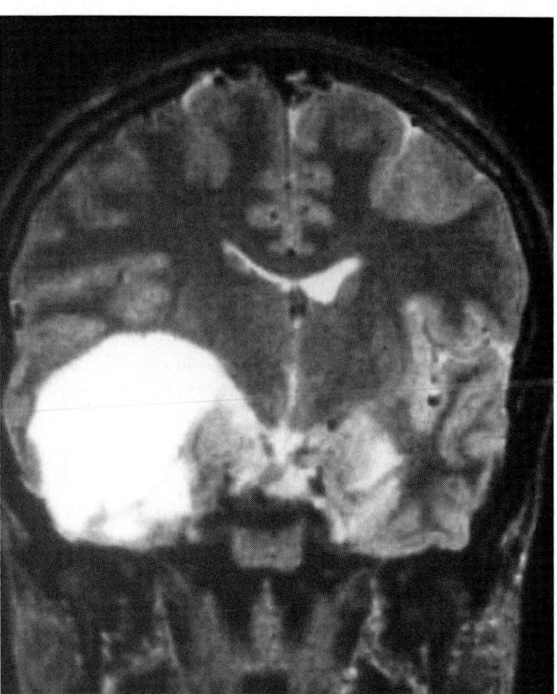

FIGURE 71-8. MRI revealing large temporal lobe mass in an 18-year-old who presented with a single seizure. Surprisingly, neurologic examination was normal.

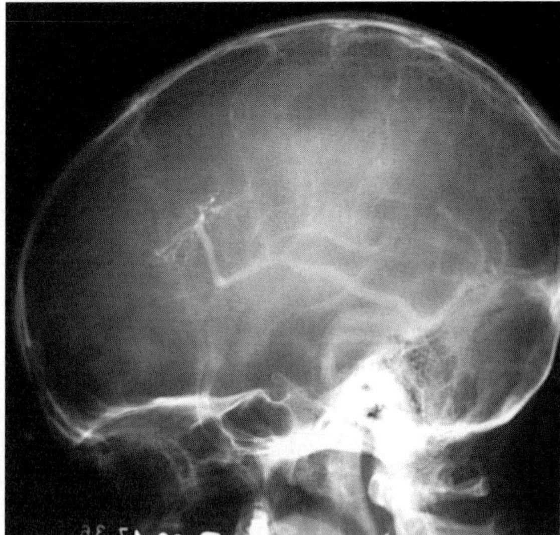

FIGURE 71-9. Angiogram of a 9-year-old male with recent onset of seizures. CT was equivocal. Simultaneous MRI revealed increased T2 signal, and angiogram demonstrated venous angioma. Patient is believed to have a venous angioma occurring in association with a hamartoma.

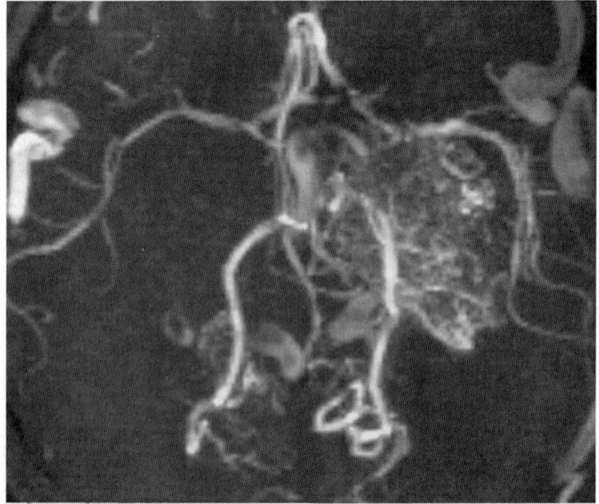

FIGURE 71-10. MRI angiogram of a patient with arteriovenous malformation. (Courtesy Siemens Medical Corporation.)

Other adjuncts to diagnosis continue to be used, although in a limited way. Arteriography provides information regarding the vascularity of the tumor and helps exclude the possibility of a vascular malformation (Fig. 71-9). As resolution improves, MRI and CT angiographies have the potential to replace standard more invasive angiography (Fig. 71-10). Magnetic resonance spectroscopy, perfusion MRI, positron emission tomography scans, and single-photon emission computed tomography (SPECT) are helpful adjunctive diagnostic tools. Positron emission tomography has been used to differentiate tumor recurrence or progression from radiation necrosis. Unfortunately, both of these commonly occur simultaneously rather than in an isolated fashion.

EEG, although a functional diagnostic tool, provides limited confirmation of the presence or absence of a mass lesion. Its primary use is in assessment of the level of consciousness and the presence of epileptogenic activity. Evoked potentials, both visual and auditory, provide information regarding functional assessment. These techniques are valuable in following the course of a patient with a mass lesion but add little to the diagnostic evaluation. Visual evoked responses are most useful in assessing patients with intraorbital or chiasmatic tumors. Auditory short-latency evoked responses are useful for the evaluation of a child with a brainstem mass or acoustic neuroma (Fig. 71-11).

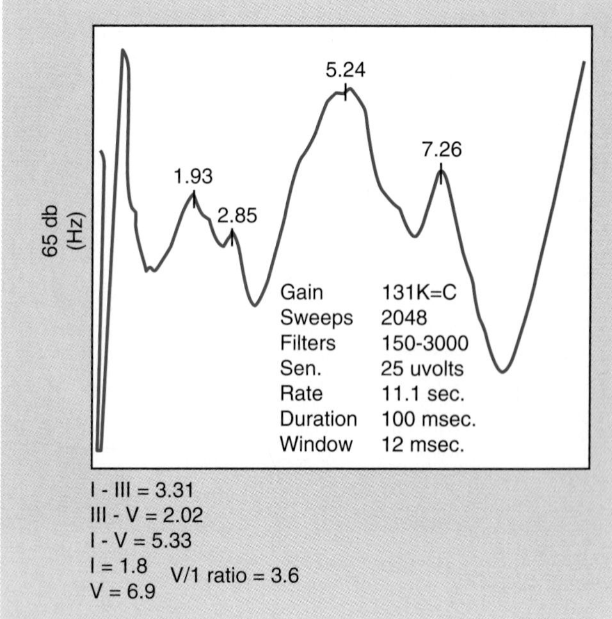

FIGURE 71-11. Brainstem auditory-evoked response in a 16-year-old female with a brainstem glioma. V Jewett wave is prolonged on the left side of the brainstem.

GENERAL PRINCIPLES OF MANAGEMENT

Treatment modalities of CNS cancer are primarily those developed in the middle part of this century. Debulking surgery, in combination with radiation or chemotherapy, are the mainstays of treatment.

At diagnosis, most children with brain tumors have a mass of 0.5 cm or greater, a tumor burden of greater than than 10^9 cells and will have gone through approximately 27 doublings (Fig. 71-12).

All treatment modalities destroy tumor by a log-kill hypothesis. For any treatment, a specific percentage of the cells will be destroyed rather than an absolute number. In a tumor burden of 10^9 cells, 90% surgical removal may reduce the tumor bulk from 10^9 to 10^8. Radiation is believed to add two more log kills, reducing the tumor burden from 10^8 to 10^6, and chemotherapy, in the best of circumstances, will add another one to two log kills or reduce the tumor burden from 10^6 to 10^4. If a treatment is to be effective, the remainder of the cancerous cells must be removed by the body's own immune mechanisms [Silver et al., 1977]. Biologic response modifiers are increasingly used by themselves or in combination with chemotherapy to augment the tumoricidal response.

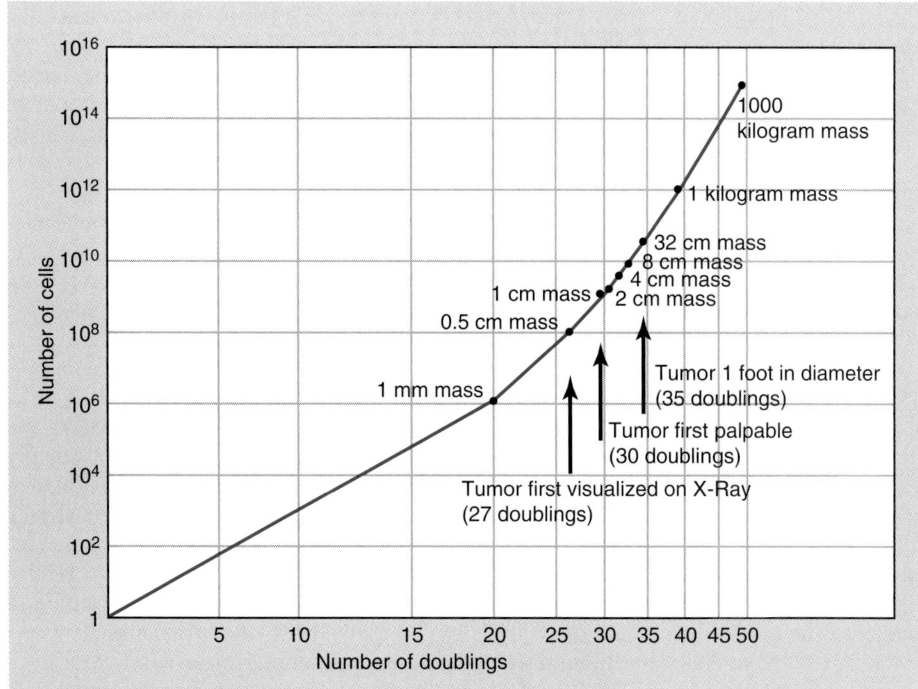

FIGURE 71-12. Tumor size related to number of doublings. (From Silver RT, Young RC, Holland JF. Some new aspects of modern cancer therapy. Am J Med 1977;639:722.)

Surgery

Therapy begins with surgical attempts at bulk removal. Cushing's romantic words describing the surgical approach remain a clarion call for the surgeon today much as they did in 1931:

> "When to take great risks; when to withdraw in the face of unexpected difficulty; whether to force an attempted enucleation of a pathologically favorable tumor to its completion with the prospect of an operative fatality, or to abandon the procedure short of completeness with a certainty that after months or years even greater risks may have to be faced at subsequent session; all this takes surgical judgment which is a matter of long experience and which can scarcely be transmitted by the written word" [Cushing, 1931].

In 1930, Cushing cited a surgical mortality for medulloblastomas of 32% [Cushing, 1930]. With advances in surgery, pediatric anesthesia, the use of the dissecting microscope, laser surgery, and the introduction of the cavitron and stereotactic surgery, operative mortality has declined to less than 2% to 5%. Surgery is not without its risks and needs to be approached with a full knowledge of the possible consequences of treatment. The neurosurgeon should perform a gross total resection when possible, alleviate increased intracranial pressure, relieve local compression of tumor on functional areas, reestablish circulation if obstructed, and provide a tissue diagnosis. Surgical cure can be expected in the treatment of cystic cerebellar astrocytomas, a percentage of craniopharyngiomas, holocord astrocytomas, and extra-axial tumors, such as meningiomas. Although not associated with a definitive cure, it is recognized that gross total resection measurably increases survival in infants younger than 3 years of age with a variety of brain tumors, including medulloblastomas and ependymomas [Duffner et al., 1993].

Surgical techniques continue to evolve. Ultrasonography during surgery permits localization of deep tumors not readily apparent at surgery and provides a means of assessing the extent of tumor resection. For tumors located in eloquent areas such as speech areas, the motor strip, or the brainstem, neuroimaging-guided stereotactic methods are increasingly helpful. Targets can be mapped that encompass tumor volumes and avoid these sensitive areas. Deep-seated tumors can be approached using stereotactic technology coupled with sophisticated imaging.

After surgery, most tumors require some form of radiation or chemotherapy, either independently or in combination. These treatments are not without risk and need to be approached with a full awareness of their possible consequences. With refinement of therapeutic techniques, surgeons are now asked to consider repeat operations in an effort to resect recurrent or residual tumor. This philosophy is recommended in an effort to establish the changing pathology of the tumor, to differentiate radiation necrosis from recurrent tumor and, based on the log-kill hypothesis, to reduce the tumor burden available for adjuvant therapies. Although they can provide irrefutable evidence of a mass, MRI/CT does not reliably differentiate radiation necrosis from recurrent tumor. Increasingly, positron emission tomography, by defining active metabolism of a tumor, is used to differentiate tumor necrosis from recurrent tumor [Valk et al., 1988].

In select cases, specifically in tumors of the posterior fossa, shunting procedures may be necessary to decompress a ventricular system that has expanded secondary to obstruction of cerebrospinal fluid pathways. Shunting provides gradual reduction of ventricular size and reduces the risk associated with sudden decompression as a consequence of tumor removal. As many as 30% of patients require cerebrospinal fluid diversion in the presence of a posterior fossa mass [Raimondi and Tomita, 1979b]. The temporary use of extraventricular drainage may obviate the need for a permanent shunt. Shunts should not be considered routine because they may provide a route for metastasis outside the nervous system. In addition to increasing the potential for metastasis, the presence of a foreign body increases the possibility of postoperative shunt infection, particularly if coupled with subsequent use of immunosuppressive agents. If an aggressive approach to treatment is to be undertaken, the pediatric neurosurgeon must be a strong advocate of the art of the possible and committed to debulk as much tumor as feasible without damaging normal tissue.

Radiation

Radiation may contribute substantially to the patient's progression-free and overall survival. The total dose of radiation necessary to destroy tumor and the amount tolerated by the developing brain are continually reexamined. The goal of therapeutic radiation must be the selective death of tumor cells. Ionizing radiation produces damage either by indirect or direct effects on the cell nucleus. The transfer of energy induced by radiation results in damage to the nucleic acid of the cell. The end result of this process is cell death or sublethal damage to the cell. Sublethal damage may result in either death or subsequent cell repair. Most brain tumors do not undergo active mitosis; therefore large doses of radiation are necessary.

Other concerns are the volume of radiation and the dose per fraction. Volume of radiation refers to the total amount of brain and spinal cord to be irradiated and depends on the tendency of the tumor to seed the neuraxis. Because patients with medulloblastomas and primitive neuroectodermal tumors are prone to develop leptomeningeal disease, craniospinal radiation therapy coupled with a boost to the tumor bed is recommended. Low-grade supratentorial astrocytomas and brainstem gliomas usually do not seed the cerebrospinal fluid. As such, radiation can be limited to the tumor bed alone. Patients with ependymomas (unless they have leptomeningeal disease at diagnosis) are treated with local radiation, as the first site of failure is usually the primary site [Merchant, 2002]. Radiation doses for most CNS tumors, regardless of histology, range from 5500 to 6000 cGy to the tumor bed and 3000 to 3500 cGy to the craniospinal axis, usually given over 6 to 8 weeks.

Most radiation protocols have been determined empirically. Although a great deal is known about radiation biology, the precise dose and schedule needed to destroy tumor and preserve normal tissue are not known. Young children are more susceptible to radiation toxicity than adults. Consequently, the total dose of radiation given to children younger than 2 years of age is generally reduced to a level 10% to 20% of the adult dose. Because the limits of tolerable radiation may have been reached, alternative ways of delivering high-dose radiation are being sought.

Hyperfractionated radiation is an attempt to increase the total dose of radiation given over a defined period without increasing side effects. It is well recognized that radiation side effects can be reduced by decreasing the radiation dose per fraction. In most centers, 150 to 180 cGy of radiation are given as a single dose in a 24-hour period. With hyperfractionation, radiation dose is reduced to 110 to 120 cGy per fraction but given every 12 hours. In this manner the total dose of radiation can theoretically be increased by 10% to 20% without increasing adverse effects on normal tissue.

Hypoxic cells require two to three times the amount of radiation necessary to achieve the same degree of destruction as normally oxygenated tissue. As such, a reduction in oxygen tension below that normally present in tissue may lead to a substantial reduction in cell kill. The use of radiation sensitizers, treatment under increased oxygen tension, and different radiation modalities, such as neutrons or pi-mesons, are attempts to increase the radiation effect on hypoxic cells [Kun, 1994].

Brachytherapy (interstitial brain implants) is a technique used to deliver high-dose radiation to the tumor bed in an effort to improve local tumor control. Radioactive iridium or iodine is loaded into catheters that are stereotactically directed into the tumor bed. These implants are designed to achieve doses of 5000 to 6000 cGy within the radiated tissue over 5 to 6 days. Techniques have been developed to deliver doses as high as 10,000 cGy for intervals up to 7 or 8 weeks. Similarly, instillation of radionuclide colloids within a tumor cavity is used to deliver high-dose radiation.

Radiosurgery (i.e., gamma knife, linear accelerator, proton beam) is the use of collimated radiation from multiple sources focused on a single volume in space. Radiosurgery typically delivers large doses (in excess of 2000 cGy) to tissue within the targeted volume. Although intralesional necrosis can be anticipated, marked injury to surrounding tissue is minimized because of the sharp falloff of the radiation dose from the center [Loeffler and Alexander, 1990]. Both radiosurgery and brachytherapy are limited to tumors less than 5 cm.

In three-dimensional conformal radiation, stereotactic techniques are used to more precisely define a targeted volume, thereby decreasing radiation exposure to surrounding tissue. This technique is currently used in national studies for ependymomas and infants with medulloblastoma.

Chemotherapy

The third arm of the treatment triad consists of chemotherapy. In the late 1950s, drugs became available that theoretically could reach and destroy tumor cells wherever they spread. This development provided a potential treatment not available by either surgery or radiation. In 1955, the Cancer Chemotherapy National Service Center was organized under the auspices of the National Cancer Institute. This plan set in motion a drug development program that included screening, toxicology, pharmacology formulation, clinical trials, and supportive care of patients with cancer. Only since the mid-1970s has interest in the chemotherapy of brain tumors heightened. Reasons for this delay have included the inaccessibility of the CNS to drugs administered systemically, the lack of accrual of large numbers of patients at individual centers, the previous difficulty in quantifying objective responses (before MRI), the fear of drug toxicity, and concerns about quality of life. Since the 1970s, however, there have been increasing numbers of organized efforts to develop chemotherapy protocols applicable for brain tumor trials. Two pediatric cancer cooperative groups (i.e., the Pediatric Oncology Group and the Children's Cancer Study Group) undertook large multicenter trials investigating the use of chemotherapy with and without radiation in children with CNS tumors. These two groups have since combined into the Children's Oncology Group. Enrollment of large numbers of patients into cooperative ventures has permitted questions to be answered regarding the efficacy of new chemotherapeutic agents, delivery systems, immunotherapy, and other modalities of treatment not generally available at a single facility.

All chemotherapeutic agents are first tested in vivo in animal models. Antitumor activity is identified on the basis of increased life span in these animal models. Toxicity is studied in large animals because qualitative and quantitative effects on various organ systems are more parallel to those in humans [Fewer, 1976]. After initial evaluation, chemotherapeutic agents are put through phase I studies in humans. These are essentially studies in which drugs are evaluated for toxic effects. Drugs then enter phase II trials to identify the spectrum of activity against human neoplasms and response of specific cancers to the drug. Phase II studies delineate the optimal dose schedule and establish validity of antitumor activity. Phase III trials are designed to determine whether the agent in question, when used in an adjuvant fashion, offers an advantage over "standard" therapy.

Chemotherapeutic agents, in general, are considered cell cycle specific or cellcycle nonspecific. Knowledge of cell cycle kinetics is basic to the understanding of the mechanisms of action. The cell cycle is divided into four phases: G-1, the phase during which cells synthesize ribonucleic acid, enzymes, and proteins; S phase, the period during which DNA replicates and chromosomal proteins are laid down; G-2, the interval between the completion of DNA synthesis and mitosis; and M phase, mitosis. G-0 consists of those cells, although not actively proliferating, that have the potential to reenter the proliferating pool. Certain chemotherapeutic agents are considered cell cycle specific (i.e., they affect either the proliferating phase of the cell or a specific phase of the cell cycle). Cell cycle–nonspecific agents are effective during any stage of the cell cycle. Because of their broader spectrum of action, these agents have an advantage over cell cycle–specific agents [Valeriote and Vietti, 1977]; however, because the therapeutic index is narrow, significant morbidity often exists.

To enter the CNS, a chemotherapeutic drug must be able to penetrate the blood-brain barrier. Consequently, those properties that allow access into the CNS include low molecular weight, high lipid solubility, nonionizable at physiologic pH, and lack of plasma-protein binding. Compounding the problem of effective drug delivery is the concept of the brain-adjacent tumor (Fig. 71-13). Malignant cells migrating from the center of a necrotic tumor into the periphery of normal brain adjacent to the tumor may be the most viable and have the greatest capacity for proliferation. Because of the intact blood-brain barrier, this region is the least accessible to treatment. Some have suggested that the importance of the blood-brain barrier has been overemphasized and that cellular mechanisms of drug resistance are more likely responsible for failures of chemotherapy than considerations of ability to breach the blood-brain barrier. The inability of a tumor to accumulate and retain drugs, the ability to metabolically degrade drugs, and the ability of a tumor to repair drug-induced damage to cellular constituents may be more important or just as important as drug delivery and the microenvironment of the brain [Phillips, 1991]. Thus location of the tumor, rate of growth, mitotic index, rate of entrance of drugs into the nervous system, and drug resistance all influence the choice of agents [Shapiro, 1975]. The optimum route of administration for chemotherapeutic agents is unknown. Although a great deal is known about mechanism of action, most chemotherapy protocols are developed on an empirical basis. Indications for intrathecal, intravenous, oral, or direct intra-arterial infusions have yet to be established. On theoretical grounds, those tumors that lie near the subarachnoid space should be the most susceptible to intrathecal administration, whereas those tumors occurring in the distribution of a specific arterial channel should be more susceptible to intra-arterial perfusion.

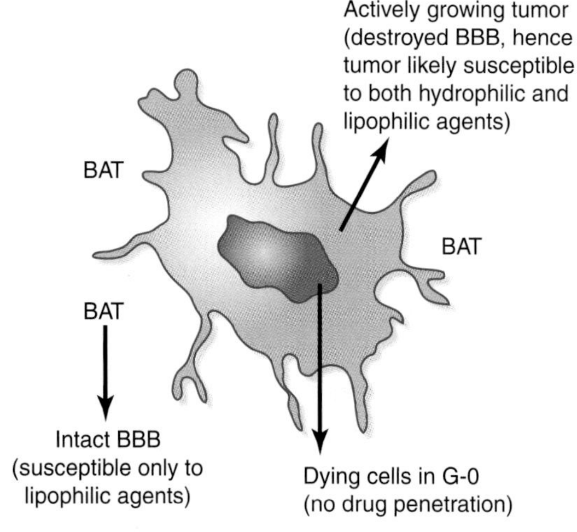

FIGURE 71-13. Diagrammatic representation of the brain-adjacent tumor.

To be effective, the therapeutic approach to patients with brain tumors must address problems inherent in the treatment of any cancer, as well as the added dimensions unique to the brain. These problems include (1) the ability to achieve a gross total resection of the tumor without serious neurologic residual, (2) the problem of pharmacologic sanctuary, and (3) the long-term and irreversible toxicity associated with treatment. The challenge for the future is the development of novel forms of therapy, targeted approaches for delivering current agents, and the development of agents that preserve normal tissue while destroying malignant cells.

MIDLINE TUMORS

Midline tumors are those above the tentorium and that involve the hypothalamus, thalamus, optic pathways, pineal region, or arise in the ventricles. Tumors found in the region of the optic pathways, hypothalamus, and thalamic areas are most likely astrocytomas. Craniopharyngiomas occur in the parasellar area, whereas germ cell tumors are predominantly found in the pineal or suprasellar region. Tumors presenting in the ventricles are generally either choroid plexus papillomas or ependymomas. Less frequently, they may be

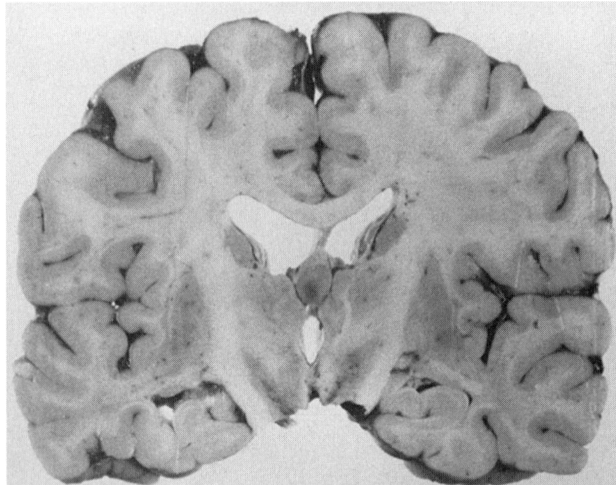

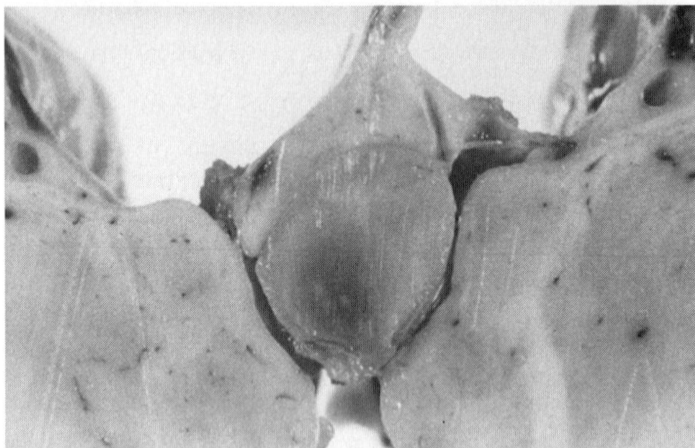

FIGURE 71-14. Colloid cyst of the third ventricle.

meningiomas. Infrequently, a colloid cyst of the third ventricle is identified (Fig. 71-14).

THALAMIC TUMORS

Thalamic tumors are rare, more aggressive, and have a more truncated course than tumors found in the area of the hypothalamus or optic pathways. They are usually of the astrocytic series and vary in malignancy from relatively benign to highly aggressive. Long-term survival without treatment is well documented for low-grade astrocytomas, whereas the more malignant astrocytomas have a poor prognosis despite therapy [Arseni, 1958; Cheek and Taveras, 1966; McKissock and Paine, 1958; Tovi et al., 1961]. Less common tumors occurring in the lateral midline are ganglioneuromas, oligodendrogliomas, and ependymomas.

Patients with thalamic tumors may present with headache, papilledema, confusion, memory loss, and emotional lability. Mental symptoms have been attributed to involvement of the medial thalamic nucleus or anterior thalamic projections. Abnormalities of speech occur with involvement of the ventrolateral nucleus [Ojemann and Ward, 1971]. Involvement of the cerebellar and rubrothalamic tracts may cause unilateral dysmetria, tremor, incoordination, or unsteady gait [Bendhein and Berg, 1981]. Dystonic movements and unilateral chorea implicate abnormalities of the subthalamus or basal ganglia. Visual loss may be secondary to involvement of visual pathways or associated with increased intracranial pressure. Despite location in the thalamus, sensory findings in this region are not common. The thalamic syndrome is virtually never encountered. Behavioral changes may be associated with thalamic masses, suggesting that functional derangement not specifically related to the anatomic site of involvement may occur with tumors of the thalamus.

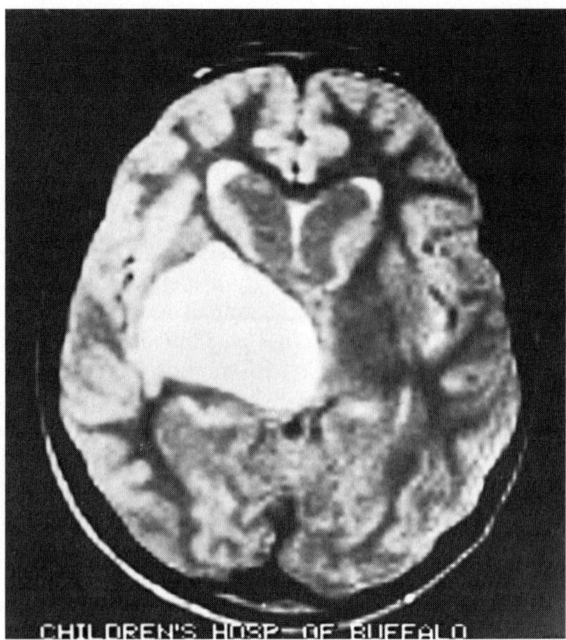

FIGURE 71-15. CT demonstrating large thalamic glioma and obstructive hydrocephalus.

Clinical suspicion of a mass in the thalamus or basal ganglia is confirmed by neuroimaging. Some degree of contrast enhancement on CT (Fig. 71-15) is common. MRI confirms the diagnosis and the anatomic definition of the tumor. EEG findings may consist of bursts of symmetric high-voltage slow waves, delta or theta, occurring in the waking state. EEG may lateralize findings to one hemisphere and consist of ipsilateral depression, normal background, or lateralized polymorphic delta slowing. Sleep spindles may be observed in the waking state.

Hypothalamic Tumors

Astrocytomas occurring in the hypothalamus generally have a different pathology and biology than those occurring in the thalamus. Anterior hypothalamic tumors may blend imperceptibly into the area of the optic chiasm or tracts, thus making the distinction between optic gliomas and hypothalamic tumors arbitrary. Grossly, they are described as avascular, gelatinous masses. Histologically, the tumors are usually pilocytic, characterized by compact and spongy regions consisting of elongated cells surrounding spongy loose areas in which stellate astrocytes are observed. Necrosis, hemorrhage, and Rosenthal fibers may be manifest. An exophytic component is common.

Signs and symptoms are commensurate with the location of the tumor. Hypothalamic tumors may invade the optic chiasm or extend inferior and posterior to invade the intrapeduncular fossa and basal cisterns. Depending on location,

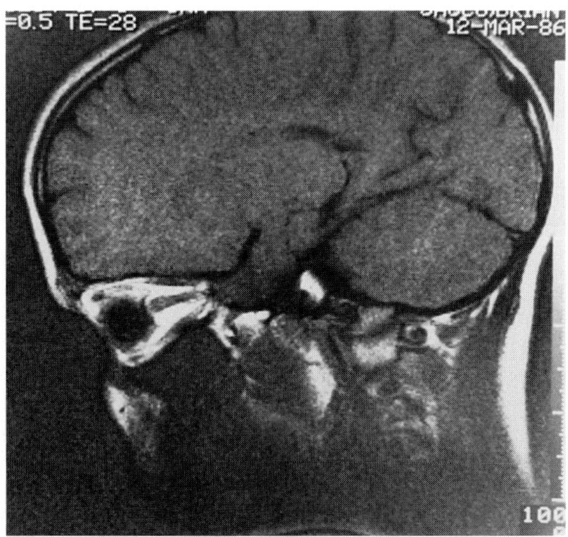

FIGURE 71-16. A 5-year-old male with neurofibromatosis and precocious puberty. MRI demonstrates hypothalamic mass.

presenting signs may be autonomic, endocrinologic, or visual.

Endocrinopathies may be associated with hypothalamic tumors and include failure to thrive, emaciation, loss of subcutaneous fat, sodium loss, hypoglycemia, and accelerated long bone growth [White and Ross, 1963]. Children with tumors in this region, such as hamartomas of the tuber cinereum, may also present with precocious puberty. Astrocytomas, ependymomas, ectopic pinealomas, suprasellar germinomas, suprasellar cysts, and craniopharyngiomas have all been associated with precocious puberty. Non-neoplastic causes of precocious puberty are postinfectious states, neurofibromatosis, and hydrocephalus (Figs. 71-16 and 71-17). Tumors of this region are initially suspected because of the clusters of clinical signs pointing to the hypothalamus. The presence of a tumor is confirmed by the appropriate neuroimaging technique. Searching nystagmus, sometimes erroneously considered to be congenital nystagmus, should suggest a tumor in the region of the optic chiasm with posterior extension into the anterior hypothalamus.

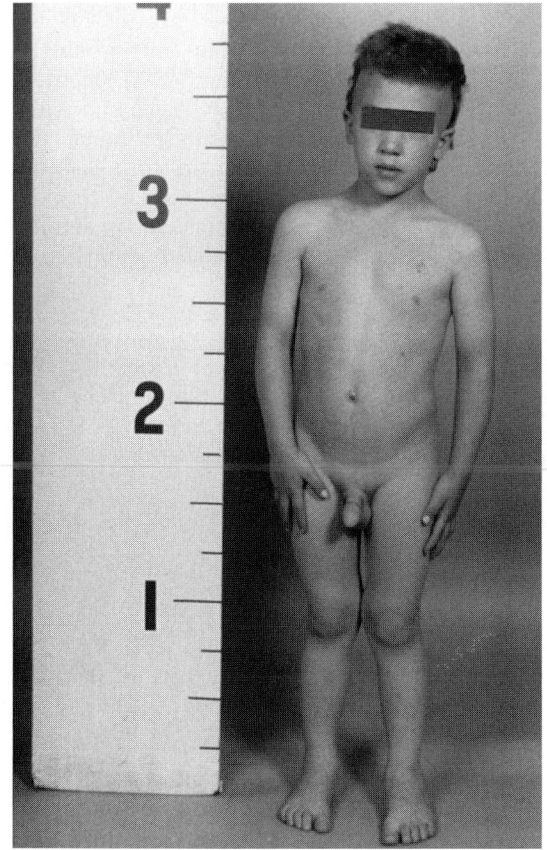

FIGURE 71-17. Patient exhibits precocious puberty.

Although uncommon, the diencephalic syndrome, described by Russell in 1951, has been associated with astrocytomas (typically juvenile pilocytic astrocytomas) of the hypothalamus and optic chiasm [Perilongo et al., 1997; Russell, 1951]. This syndrome manifests in young children between 18 months and 3 years of age and is uncommon in the older child. The child develops normally followed by a period of profound inanition. Hypoglycemia may be present. Excessive appetite, without weight gain, and accelerated long bone growth may be the prominent features. Profound loss of subcutaneous tissue in a happy, normally developing child should raise the possibility of this syndrome. More common symptoms of hypothalamic tumors are obesity, diabetes insipidus, and hypogonadism. Lethargy rather than euphoria is regularly described. With extension into the region of the foramen of Monro, obstructive hydrocephalus may develop with subsequent signs of acute increased intracranial pressure. Leptomeningeal seeding has been increasingly reported in children with the diencephalic syndrome secondary to juvenile pilocytic astrocytomas [Gajjar et al., 1995; Perilongo et al., 1997a] (Fig. 71-18). As such, neuroimaging at diagnosis should include the brain and neuraxis.

Management

"Watchful waiting" is often the approach to tumors of the hypothalamus, particularly for those identified on

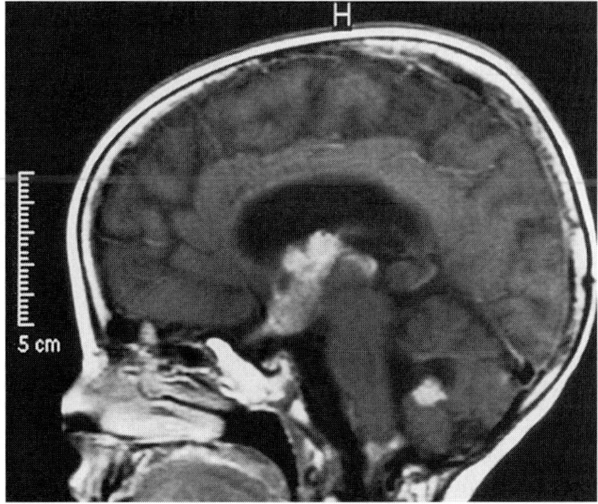

FIGURE 71-18. A 10-month-old child presented with large head, emaciation, and alert appearance. MRI revealed hypothalamic mass with enhancing metastatic lesions in the cerebellum, brainstem, and spinal cord.

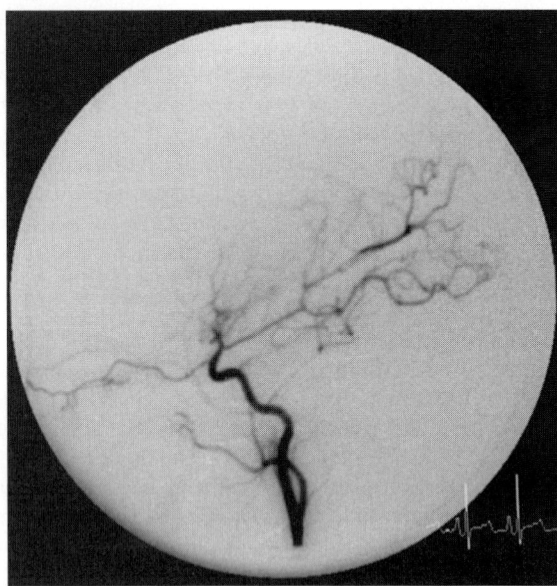

FIGURE 71-19. A 3-year-old child with widely disseminated juvenile pilocytic astrocytomas who developed progressive disease on chemotherapy and therefore received craniospinal radiation. The child developed moyamoya disease as a consequence of her radiation therapy.

"screening" MRIs in children with neurofibromatosis. However, in symptomatic cases, biopsy and, when feasible, debulking surgery is performed followed by consideration of radiation to the tumor bed. Radiation doses between 5000 and 6000 cGy have been associated with reversal of symptoms and even long-term cures. Five-year survival rates of 71% and 10-year survival rates of 56% for children with hypothalamic tumors are well known. In very young children with hypothalamic tumors, in whom there are concerns about radiation-induced vasculopathy, chemotherapy has been used with variable success [McCowage et al., 1996] (Fig. 71-19).

Survival for patients with thalamic tumors is much worse. Treatment generally is limited to high-dose radiation to the tumor bed except in those tumors that seed the cerebrospinal fluid pathways. In such situations, craniospinal radiation therapy is indicated [Bernstein et al., 1984; Bloom et al., 1990; DeSousa et al., 1979]. On recurrence, chemotherapy should be considered.

Optic Pathway Tumors

Optic gliomas comprise approximately 3% to 5% of all childhood tumors. Their association with neurofibromatosis is well recognized [Dutton 1994; Listernick et al., 1997; North, 1998]. The incidence of optic gliomas in children 2 to 9 years of age with neurofibromatosis may approach 3% to 10%. Conversely, of all children with optic gliomas, approximately 50% have neurofibromatosis [Rubinstein et al., 1981; Stern et al., 1979]. As with hypothalamic astrocytomas, most tumors of the anterior visual pathways are generally classified as juvenile pilocytic astrocytomas. Anaplastic astrocytomas and glioblastomas in this area are less common. Gliomas of the optic nerve can be quite variable and may be limited to a single optic nerve, occur bilaterally, involve the optic chiasm, or extend throughout the entire visual pathway [Cohen and Duffner, 1991].

In the absence of neurofibromatosis, diminished visual acuity is the most common presenting sign. Because children as well as adults are generally unaware of gradual decrements in visual acuity, visual loss may not be detected until late in the course of the disease. A nonpulsatile proptosis suggests the presence of an intraorbital mass, whereas nystagmus suggests chiasmatic involvement. The nystagmus usually consists of a series of short arcs and rapid oscillations with scanning or searching slow, wide arc movements [Chutorian et al., 1964]. Spasmus nutans and congenital nystagmus have been confused with the nystagmus occurring in patients with tumors involving the optic chiasm or visual pathways [Anthony et al., 1980]. An afferent pupillary light defect suggests pathology of the optic nerve, whereas a field defect is more apt to be associated with pathology involving the posterior portions of the optic nerve, chiasm, or tract. Field defects in these situations may be congruous or incongruous. Signs of papilledema suggest involvement of the anterior hypothalamus with extension posteriorly to involve the foramen of Monro. Conversely, blurring of the disk and loss of central vision should suggest an intraorbital mass. The presence of optic atrophy may preclude the development of papilledema despite evidence of increased intracranial pressure.

CT and MRI have all but eliminated the need for other neurodiagnostic imaging. Both methods allow direct visualization of the optic nerve in both the axial and coronal projections. Sections cut oblique to the horizontal and longtudinal axis provide greater appreciation of the anatomy. MRI with gadolinium, because of the multiple paradigms of imaging and the ability to image in the coronal, sagittal, and axial planes, has essentially replaced CT. The midsagittal view is valuable in establishing the extent of a chiasmatic lesion but is limited in evaluating intraorbital tumors (Fig. 71-20). Unlike CT, MRI may also identify those T2-weighted lesions associated with neurofibromatosis believed to be non-neoplastic (Fig. 71-21). In patients with neurofibromatosis, streaking along the optic pathway and involving the optic radiations is not unusual and may not represent tumor. Similarly, T2-weighted signals on MRI involving the optic tract and geniculate bodies (Fig. 71-22)

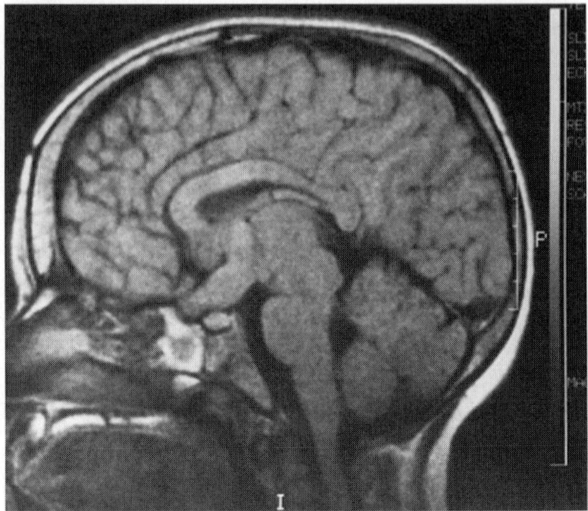

FIGURE 71-20. Chiasmatic glioma in child with neurofibromatosis. T1-weighted MRI demonstrates thickened chiasm.

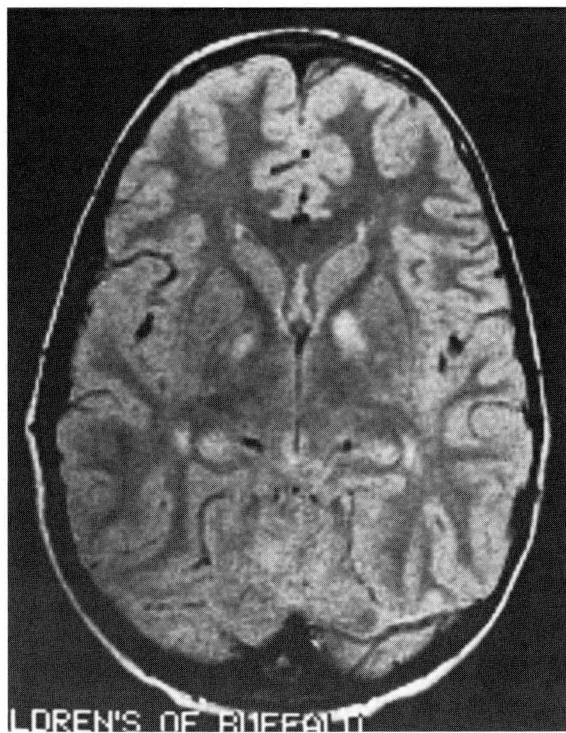

FIGURE 71-21. Increased T2-weighted signals demonstrate unidentified bright objects in the basal ganglia in patient with neurofibromatosis.

have been associated with compression of white matter by an extrinsic lesion; therefore, these findings need to be viewed circumspectly.

Despite knowledge of the existence of optic pathway tumors for more than 150 years, no universally accepted approach to treatment exists [Glaser et al., 1971], although this issue has recently been reevaluated [Listernick et al., 1997]. Many of these tumors are benign and have a long natural history. A consensus is now developing that on recognition of optic pathway tumors, patients should be monitored and not treated until there is evidence of progression either by neuroimaging or by ophthalmologic assessment. Continual evaluation of the patient should include serial MRIs, visual acuity, and visual field testing. MRI is the most sensitive procedure to evaluate progressive disease and, in the presence of known pathology, should be obtained every 3 to 6 months (Fig. 71-23).

Treatment is initiated on evidence of progression as manifested by either continued visual loss or progression on neuroimaging. For patients whose tumors are intraorbital and in whom there is no useful vision, surgical removal of the nerve to the level of the chiasm is warranted. For children younger than 5 years in whom the tumor extends intracranially, the treatment of choice is chemotherapy. As surgical debulking or even biopsy may be associated with visual compromise, this approach remains somewhat controversial. Several reports have advocated the effectiveness of actinomycin D and vincristine [Packer et al., 1988b]. A Pediatric Oncology Group study evaluating 50 patients with progressive optic pathway tumors has shown that carboplatin used as a single agent may be effective [Mahoney and Cohen et al., 2000]. Others have advocated carboplatin in combination with vincristine [Packer et al., 1993]. These two drugs have become the standard chemotherapy for tumors of this region and are the combination that all other agents are measured against. For children older than 5 years of age, radiation with or without chemotherapy continues to be the treatment of choice.

Pineal Region Tumors

Tumors arising in the pineal region are rare. Incidence rates are variable because of imprecise histology, tumor location, and different rates of occurrence in Asian as opposed to Western countries. For example, the incidence of germ cell tumors and pineal region tumors varies from 2.6% to 6.5% in several Japanese articles versus 0.4% to 0.7% in the

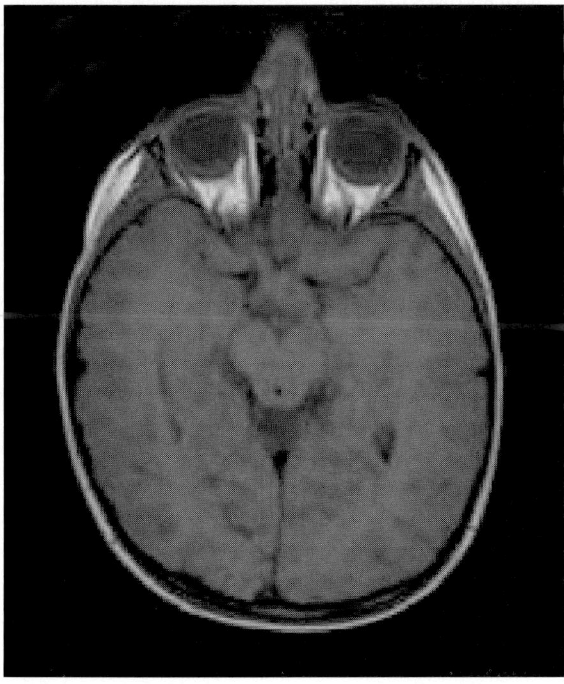

A

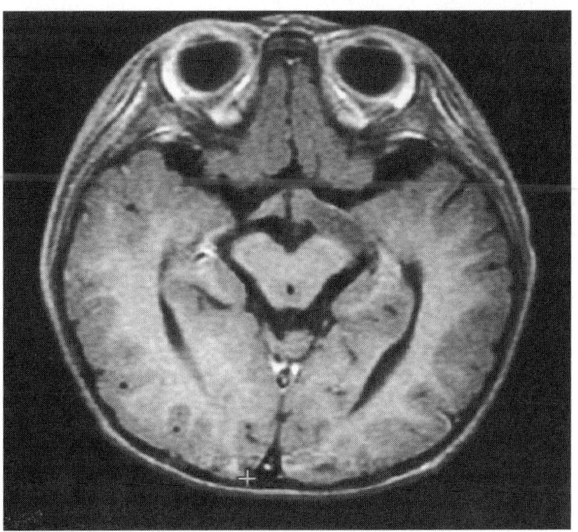

B

FIGURE 71-22. **A**, T1 axial MRI of a 3-year-old with a chiasmatic mass. **B**, T1 axial MRI of an optic pathway tumor involving the left optic tract.

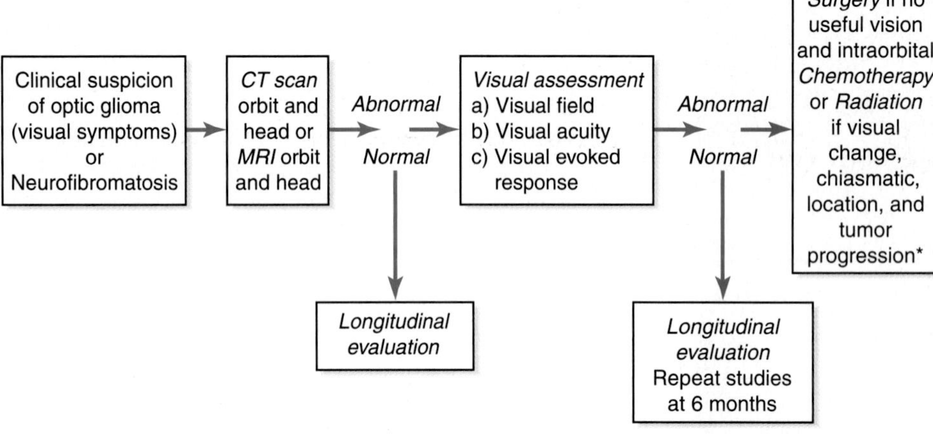

FIGURE 71-23. Suggested approach to the evaluation of an optic pathway tumor. * For children less than 5 years of age, chemotherapy is preferred over radiation therapy. (From Cohen and Duffner, 1994a.)

Western literature [Cohen and Duffner, 1994e; Packer et al., 2000]. Further complicating understanding of the incidence rates is the confusion in the literature in distinguishing parenchymatous tumors of the pineal region from teratomas and germinomas.

Germ cell tumors have been classified into three distinct groups: germ cell tumors that respond to radiation; nongerminomatous germ cell tumors that do not respond to radiation (i.e., embryonal carcinomas, yolk sac or endodermal sinus tumors, choriocarcinomas, and immature teratomas); and mature teratomas. The most common variant is the mixed germ cell tumor.

Tumors that derive from the neuroepithelium of the pineal gland itself (i.e., pineal parenchymal tumors) are divided into pineoblastomas, pineocytomas with and without ganglion cells, and astrocytomas.

Germ cell tumors most commonly occur either in the pineal or suprasellar regions but are also recognized in other areas of the brain including the basal ganglia, thalamus, and fourth ventricle. Germinomas tend to extend into neighboring structures and seed along cerebrospinal fluid pathways. The germinoma consists of large primitive spheroid cells indistinguishable from those of testicular or ovarian germinomas. Lymphoid cells are prominent in their stroma. The embryonal component of these neoplasms is more likely to be associated with elevation of either α-fetoprotein or β-human chorionic gonadotropin (β-HCG) and if so, are not true germinomas. Carcinoembryonic antigen has also been associated with immature and mature teratomas [Allen, 1991; Edwards et al., 1985] (Table 71-2). Nongerminomatous germ cell tumors are more heterogeneous, tend to calcify, and for the most part are limited to the pineal region.

Pineal area tumors peak in the latter half of the second decade of life and are more common in boys than in girls. Suprasellar germinomas, unlike those occurring in the region of the pineal, are more apt to affect the sexes equally or have a female preponderance.

Clinical presentation is variable and may be associated with increased intracranial pressure and Parinaud's phenomena (i.e., lack of convergence, upward gaze, and accommodation). Visual loss, diabetes insipidus, precocious puberty, and emaciation imply an anterior hypothalamic location or are the result of metastasis from the pineal region anteriorly into the third ventricle. The triad of visual loss, hypopituitarism, and diabetes insipidus should suggest a suprasellar location.

CT and MRI demonstrate a vast radiologic heterogeneity in pineal region tumors. They are associated with isodense to variable enhancement with contrast, with or without calcification. Enhancement along the walls of the ventricles suggests cerebrospinal fluid seeding. On MRI, teratomas are characterized by hyperdense, lobulated masses with areas of decreased signal suggesting calcification or multiple cysts (Fig. 71-24). CT more readily identifies calcification.

TABLE 71-2

Tumor Markers and Survival

		TUMOR MARKERS			
HISTOLOGY	INCIDENCE* (% OF GCT)	AFP	HCG	CEA	5-YEAR SURVIVAL* (%)
Pure (56%)					
Germinoma	24	–	+	–	80
Embryonal carcinoma	2	+++	+++	–	<10
Endodermal sinus tumor	2	+++	—	–	<10
Choriocarcinoma	3	–	+++	–	<10
Immature teratoma	10	–	–	+	40
Mature teratoma	15	–	–	+	75
Mixed (44%)	–	–	–	–	–

AFP, alpha-fetoprotein; HCG, human choroids gonadotropin; CEA, carcinoembryonic antigen; GCT, germ cell tumor; –, absent; +, weakly positive; +++, strongly positive.
*Data from Allen, 1991.

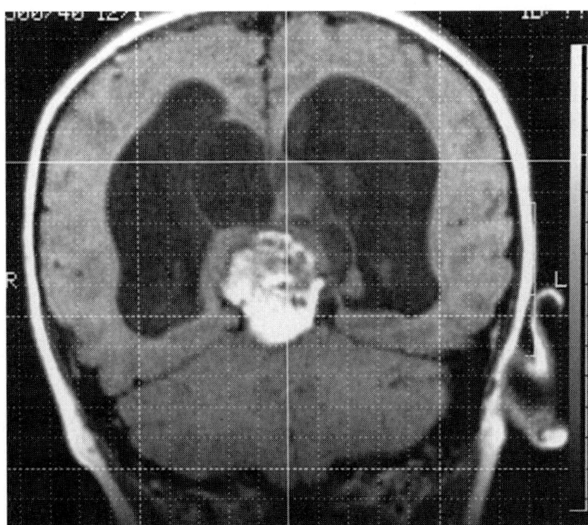

FIGURE 71-24. MRI of 15-year-old male with teratoma who presented with hydrocephalus and visual compromise.

Management

The treatment of children with pineal region tumors is determined by pathology. As such, biopsy (or resection if possible) should be performed on all patients. Although operative mortality of 30% to 60% was previously reported for direct approaches [Davidoff, 1967; DeGirolami and Schmidek, 1973], this rate has dropped dramatically in recent years. Ventricular cisternostomy is the most common diverting procedure for tumors that occupy the cavity of the third ventricle. Direct approaches to the tumor bed are complicated because of the presence of large venous channels in the pineal region. Increasingly, direct approaches to the tumor are being undertaken stereotactically. Nongerminomatous germ cell tumors are not radiosensitive but may respond to chemotherapy, especially platinum-based multiagent chemotherapy [Herrmann et al., 1994]. Conversely, germinomas are radiosensitive and, like their extracranial counterparts, are also chemosensitive. Administration of postoperative chemotherapy has successfully allowed reduction in the dose and volume of radiation in children with germinomas [Allen, 1991]. The 5-year survival rate, after standard radiation, may be as high as 50% to 80% [Brady, 1977; Jenkin et al., 1978; Rao et al., 1981]. Most chemotherapy regimens are platinum based in combination with a variety of other agents (i.e., cyclophosphamide, vinblastine, etoposide, bleomycin, ifosfamide [Allen, 1994; Buckner et al., 1999; Chang et al., 1995].

Overall, the survival for patients with true germinomas treated with 4000 cGy or greater is 90% or higher. The need for craniospinal radiation in the absence of cerebrospinal fluid dissemination remains controversial. There is growing evidence that reduced dose and volume radiation coupled with chemotherapy may provide equivalent survivals with fewer cognitive and endocrine side effects [Packer et al., 2000].

Although the need for prophylactic spinal irradiation in germinomas remains controversial, full neuraxis radiation should be given when the cerebrospinal fluid is positive for cells or MRI of the spine demonstrates seeding. If the tumor is resistant to radiotherapy or in situations in which tumor has regrown, chemotherapy should be considered. Platinum, carboplatin, vincristine, doxorubicin (Adriamycin), cyclophosphamide, and procarbazine all have been associated with responses.

Because pineoblastomas are likely to seed the neuraxis, all patients require craniospinal radiation. Radiation doses of 50 Gy or higher were associated in one study with better control than lower doses [Schild et al., 1996]. Unfortunately, responses and overall survival rate are extremely poor. In a review of 75 children with pineoblastomas, 76% either had died or had progressive disease [Duffner and Cohen, 1997]. Survival rate appears to vary with age because the prognosis is particularly grim in very young children in whom widespread metastases and early death can be anticipated [Duffner et al., 1995a]. In contrast, Jackacki and colleagues [1995] reported that older children treated with craniospinal radiation and either "8 in 1" or vincristine, CCNU, and prednisone had a 3-year progression-free survival of 70%. For patients with benign teratomas, dermoids, gliomas, or arachnoid or pineal cysts, surgery can be curative.

Craniopharyngiomas

Craniopharyngiomas account for approximately 6% to 10% of all tumors in childhood [Rubinstein, 1972]. Diagnosis peaks in the latter half of the first decade and in the early part of the second decade (5 to 14 years). A second peak occurs in late adulthood (50 to 75 years). Survival rates are highest for those diagnosed at a young age. There is no obvious sex predominance. Tumors may be quite variable in location, although most are suprasellar. Occasionally the tumor presents as an intrasellar mass. These tumors usually fill the cavity of the third ventricle or extend inferiorly and posteriorly along the dorsum sella and clivus, displacing structures at the base of the brain (Fig. 71-25).

Craniopharyngiomas putatively arise from embryonic squamous cell rests occurring in the pathway of the involuted tract of the hypophyseal pharyngeal duct. In 1838, Rathke reported the presence of an irregular globular depression at the base of the skull in the roof of the primitive stomatodeum of animals. This depression forms the analog of the anterior portion of the pituitary. Cells along the craniopharyngeal duct are considered to be the site of origin of the craniopharyngioma.

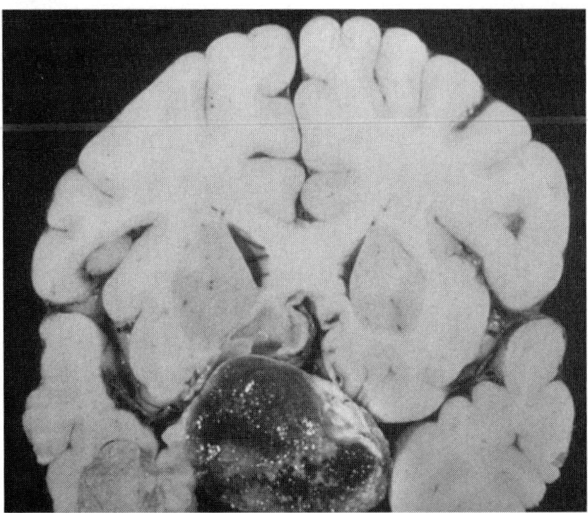

FIGURE 71-25. Gross picture of a craniopharyngioma.

Craniopharyngiomas are largely cystic or partially solid with a firm capsule, usually at the superior end, blending in a finger-like fashion into the surrounding hypothalamus. Cyst contents tend to be thick, brownish yellow, or green, with machine oil-like fluid rich in cholesterol crystals. The cyst content may be gelatinous rather than fluid. Chemical arachnoiditis may result from spillage of cyst contents at surgery. Solid areas contain foci of calcification and early bone formation. Microscopically the tumor represents an epithelial, microcystic tumor. Keratin pearls may be observed among areas of squamous epithelium. Palisading or columnar cells similar to those seen in embryonic dental and oral mucosa have been described and account for the association of this tumor with the adamantinoma found in the jaw. Tumors found in childhood are more likely to resemble the adamantinoma or ameloblastoma of the jaw. Adult tumors are thought to arise from squamous epithelial rest cells rather than the involuted hypophyseal pharyngeal duct and are therefore less likely to resemble dental tissue [Bunin et al., 1998].

As is the case with most intracranial masses, children with craniopharyngiomas complain of headache and vomiting and have nonspecific signs of increased intracranial pressure. Various visual defects may be present, depending on whether the tumor occurs above, below, or behind the visual axis. Endocrine abnormalities include short stature and hypothyroidism. Diabetes insipidus, if not present on presentation, often occurs postoperatively. Less commonly, vegetative states, abnormalities of autonomic function, or disturbances of fluid or electrolyte balance may be recognized [Sotos and Romshe, 1975]. Lateralized neurologic abnormalities are distinctly uncommon.

Diagnosis is made primarily by CT or MRI (Fig. 71-26). Calcification that is patchy, diffuse, or linear may be observed in up to 80% of children with craniopharyngiomas. CT features consist of calcification, areas of low density, cyst formation, and contrast enhancement. Because of the tumor's location in the third ventricle, obstruction of cerebrospinal fluid outflow with resultant hydrocephalus is a common finding. Differentiation of a craniopharyngioma from a chiasmatic or hypothalamic tumor by CT may be quite difficult. MRI is superior to CT in delineating parasellar anatomic structures, such as blood vessels, the optic chiasm, the foramen of Monro, and the pituitary. However, the presence of calcium, a common feature in children with craniopharyngiomas, is best identified by CT.

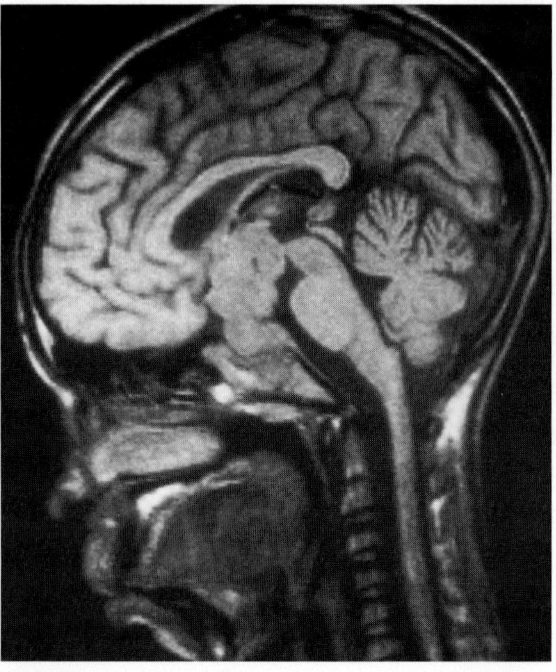

FIGURE 71-26. T1-weighted MRI in a child with craniopharyngioma.

Management

Skilled endocrine management has eliminated fears of intraoperative and postoperative hypopituitarism and has led to more aggressive surgical management. The introduction of steroids has essentially eliminated intraoperative adrenal insufficiency. Currently there are two widely differing surgical approaches. Because the tumor may be densely adherent to the hypothalamus with finger-like projections into its floor, some have suggested that aggressive surgery results in trauma to the hypothalamus with postoperative endocrine and psychologic abnormalities. In these situations, surgical extirpation is not warranted and palliative surgery followed by radiation is the procedure of choice. In tumors in which there is no attachment to the hypothalamus, total surgical removal is contemplated, thereby eliminating the tendency for recurrence and the subsequent need for radiotherapy [Hoffman, 1982; Matson and Crigler, 1969; Yasargil et al., 1990].

Radiation for craniopharyngiomas was initially introduced in 1937. However, only since the 1960s has there been increasing acceptance of the use of radiation in combination with subtotal excision for the treatment of this tumor. The literature suggests that patients with subtotal surgical removal followed by radiotherapy are less apt to experience recurrence and have a better survival rate than patients treated by biopsy and cyst aspiration followed by radiotherapy. Results of total excision alone, compared with subtotal excision and postoperative radiotherapy, are more difficult to analyze. In general, most neurosurgeons and radiotherapists accept the recommendation of radiation once there is evidence of recurrence [Cavazzuti et al., 1983; Danoff et al., 1983; Fischer et al., 1990; Shillito, 1980].

The major morbidity, regardless of treatment, is significant endocrinopathy [Andler et al., 1979]. If not present before treatment, these conditions occur after treatment and consist of delayed or decreased growth hormone production, decreased adrenocorticotropic hormone, thyroid-stimulating hormone, luteinizing hormone/follicle-stimulating hormone, antidiuretic hormone production, and decreased prolactin after thyrotropin-releasing factor stimulation. Normal growth may occur after surgery and radiation despite growth hormone deficiency. The mechanism by which patients with documented low growth hormone levels exhibit catch-up growth after successful treatment of craniopharyngiomas has never been determined. Suggested answers are the levels of somatomedin, insulin, and thyroid and the effects these hormones have in promoting normal growth despite the absence of growth hormone.

Perhaps the major untoward complication of treatment, other than diabetes insipidus, is hyperphagia with morbid obesity. This complication responds only in a limited way to dietary restriction and can be an overwhelming problem for patients and their families.

The decision to irradiate must be tempered by the possibility of radiation necrosis of the brain, damage to the visual axis, and long-term effects on intelligence. Only if total excision is not possible should subtotal excision followed by radiation to the tumor bed be considered. Unfortunately, approximately 50% of patients with a gross surgical resection will have a recurrence and require radiotherapy [Merchant et al., 2002c].

Pituitary Adenomas

Pituitary adenomas causing Cushing's disease are rare in children [Devoe et al., 1997]. Cushing's disease manifests with excessive weight gain and delayed growth due to increased adrenocoticotropic hormone production that results in increased adrenal cortisol production. Diagnosis is established by a positive dexamethasone suppression test, provocative metapyrone and corticotropin-releasing hormone tests, as well as demonstration of the tumor with MRI. The mean age of presentation in one study was 15.7 years [Bickler et al., 1994]. Transsphenoidal surgery is the treatment of choice in children and adolescents. Long-term follow-up studies in 42 children have shown an initial remission rate of 83%. Seven children experienced a relapse of Cushing's disease an average of 4.2 years postoperatively and required repeat transsphenoidal surgery [Devoe et al., 1997].

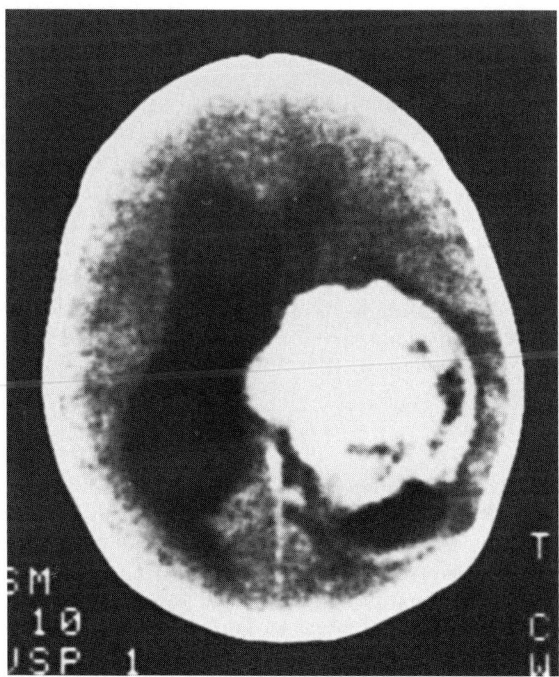

FIGURE 71-27. CT of a 7-month-old female showing a large choroid plexus carcinoma.

VENTRICULAR TUMORS

Choroid Plexus Tumors

Although rare, choroid plexus papillomas are an important tumor of childhood. Davis and Cushing [1925] reported six patients with choroid plexus papillomas and distinguished them from papillary ependymomas. Some continue to consider these tumors an unusual manifestation of ependymoma [Russell and Rubinstein, 1989]. Fourth ventricular choroid plexus papillomas are most commonly found in adults, whereas the lateral ventricles are the usual site in children. The third ventricle is rarely involved. Papillomas arising in the lateral ventricles tend to occur in the atrium of the ventricle. Unlike benign choroid plexus papillomas, the malignant variety is characterized by cellular pleomorphism, mitosis, multinucleated cells, necrosis, and hemorrhage. Spinal fluid seeding may occur with both the benign and malignant varieties. In at least one patient, a choroid plexus papilloma metastasized extraneurally [Valladares et al., 1980]. Malignant transformation has also been reported [Chow et al., 1999]. Presentation usually consists of signs of increased intracranial pressure, vomiting, clumsiness, headache, and seizures. Unilateral calcification in the trigone should suggest a choroid plexus papilloma. Although CT and MRI are the diagnostic methods of choice, angiography is required to define the vascular supply of the tumor (Fig. 71-27).

Management

Treatment of choroid plexus papillomas is primarily surgical but, because of the vascular supply of the tumor, operative mortality remains high. As such, preoperative embolization has become increasingly popular [Pencalet et al., 1998]. Despite the risks, total removal is associated with cure. [Chow et al., 1999; McEvoy et al., 2000]. The use of radiotherapy and chemotherapy is restricted to tumors having malignant features or those that recur after surgery.

The treatment of choroid plexus carcinomas also begins with attempts at gross total resection. In those cases in which a gross total resection is not possible because of the highly vascular nature of the tumor, administration of several courses of chemotherapy has been associated with reduction in tumor vascularity, allowing removal of the tumor in toto at "second look surgery" [St. Clair et al., 1991]. Because most choroid plexus carcinomas occur in infants, surgery is typically followed by chemotherapy for 1 to 2 years. If residual tumor remains or if the tumor grows during chemotherapy, radiation to the tumor bed and neuraxis is required [Chow et al., 1999; Duffner et al., 1995b].

PROGNOSTIC FACTORS

A review of the literature from 1966 to 1998 identified 566 choroid plexus tumors. Prognostic factors included histology, degree of surgical resection, and radiotherapy. Choroid plexus papillomas had 1-, 5-, and 10-year overall survivals of 90%, 81%, and 77% in comparison with 71%, 41%, and 35% for these with choroid plexus carcinomas. Degree of surgical resection was a significant prognostic factor in both choroid plexus papillomas and choroid plexus carcinomas.

Radiotherapy, in this metanalysis, was found to be associated with significantly better survivals for children with choroid plexus carcinomas [Wolff et al., 2002].

In general, the primary treatment of choroid plexus tumors is surgery, ideally a gross total resection. Chemotherapy, followed by "second look" surgery, is helpful in reducing vascularity and allowing complete surgical removal of tumors that were initially incompletely resected. Children with nonmetastatic choroid plexus carcinomas, treated with gross total resection, chemotherapy plus or minus radiation may enjoy long-term survivals. Those that progress on chemotherapy may be "salvaged" with radiation.

Giant Cell Astrocytomas

Another tumor occurring in the region of the ventricles is the subependymal giant cell astrocytoma, found in 6% to 18% of patients with tuberous sclerosis [Franz, 1998]. Giant cells are characteristic. Although considered an astrocytoma, they are of mixed glioneuronal lineage [Goh et al., 2004]. These calcified tumors are commonly found in the region of the foramen of Monro (Fig. 71-28). Presenting signs are usually those of obstructive hydrocephalus.

Management

If the patient is asymptomatic, "watchful waiting" is appropriate. Otherwise, shunting to relieve hydrocephalus may be all that is necessary. Others recommend attempts at surgical resection [Goh et al., 2004]. Long-term prognosis for persons with these tumors is excellent.

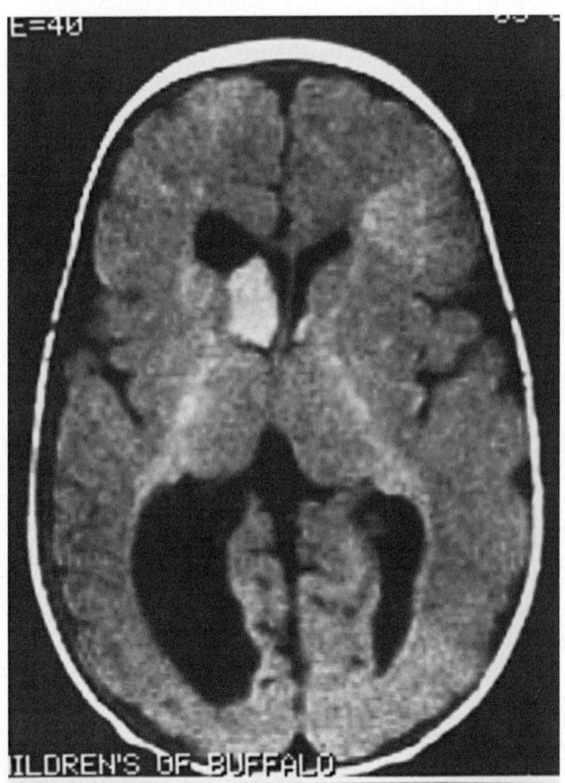

FIGURE 71-28. Subependymal giant cell astrocytoma in a 6-month-old infant with tuberous sclerosis. T1-weighted MRI demonstrates mass in the right lateral ventricle at the level of the foramen of Monro.

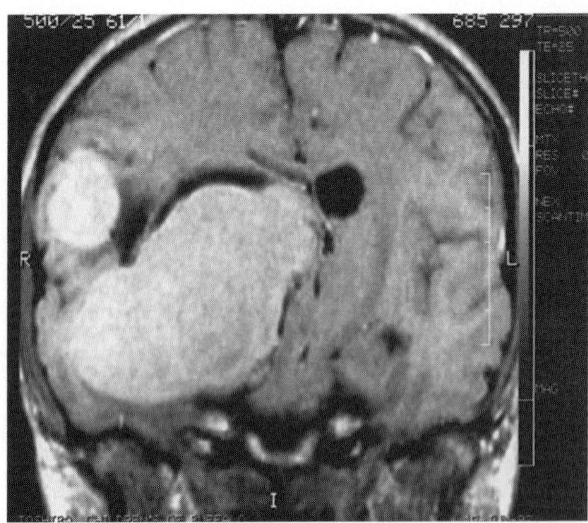

FIGURE 71-29. A 16-year-old male received a scan because he injured his head during a football game. He had a completely normal neurologic examination and no history of neurologic symptoms. The MRI revealed a large enhancing mass extending across the midline. The tumor was a meningioma.

Meningiomas

Meningiomas are uncommon tumors of childhood and, when observed, are more apt to be found in the ventricle or in the posterior fossa [Cohen and Duffner, 1994d]. As with other ventricular tumors, intraventricular meningiomas present with signs of obstructive hydrocephalus, headache, vomiting, visual impairment, and papilledema. CT features are relatively typical, consisting of well-circumscribed or somewhat lobulated, irregular, high-density lesions that enhance with contrast.

Management

Treatment of meningiomas is primarily surgical and when total removal is accomplished, complete cure can be expected; however, because of their bulky size and tendency to be sarcomatous, total surgical removal is difficult. Recurrence rate is high. As with other tumors, lack of total removal or evidence of recurrence are indications for radiation. Factors influencing response to radiation are the tumor's vascularity, location, and growth rate. Specific histology of the tumor may be the least important factor in determining prognosis (Fig. 71-29).

Colloid Cyst

Although benign, the colloid cyst may manifest in a precipitous manner. This tumor originates from ependymal cysts attached to the choroid plexus in the roof of the third ventricle (see Fig. 71-14). The intermittent symptoms and signs of increased intracranial pressure are produced by the ball-valve effect of the tumor related to head position. Intermittent obstruction of the foramen of Monro has been associated with precipitous herniation and sudden death.

Management

Total surgical removal is the treatment of choice.

POSTERIOR FOSSA TUMORS

Tumors of the posterior fossa account for approximately 50% to 55% of all tumors in childhood. Although they are less common in children younger than 1 year of age, the posterior fossa is the most common site for brain tumors in the first decade. Tumors occurring in this area are usually neuronal or glial in origin. Less frequently, hemangioblastomas, dermoids, or arachnoid cysts are encountered. Even rarer in the United States is the tuberculoma. This entity must still be considered in the differential diagnosis of any child living in an endemic area for tuberculosis.

The posterior fossa is the area of the nervous system located beneath the tentorium of the cerebellum. Because the anterior reflection of the tentorium extends to the posterior clinoid process, some authors include tumors of the diencephalon under the rubric of posterior fossa tumors. In this section, we consider neoplasms of the brainstem (i.e., midbrain, pons, and medulla) and cerebellum as posterior fossa tumors. Diencephalic tumors (tumors of the hypothalamus and thalamus) are considered under the classification of midline tumors. The most commonly occurring posterior fossa tumors are medulloblastomas, cerebellar astrocytomas, ependymomas, and brainstem tumors.

Medulloblastomas

Of all childhood brain tumors, the most dramatic change in survival has occurred with medulloblastomas. In Cushing's series of medulloblastomas published in 1930, only 1 of 61 children (1.6%) was alive at the end of 3 years. In the 1980s, the survival rate for medulloblastoma in the SEER Registry data approached 40% [Duffner et al., 1986]. In select series, survival rates of greater than 70% have been reported [Brown et al., 1977; Packer et al., 1988a]. This increase in survival has occurred as a result of more aggressive neurosurgery and the administration of high-dose radiation to the tumor bed coupled with craniospinal irradiation. The best results have been reported in patients older than 3 years of age who have no evidence of tumor after surgery and no evidence of metastasis throughout the subarachnoid space.

The suggested congenital nature of medulloblastoma has led several investigators to apply Collins' rule in predicting the course of the tumor: The period of recurrence risk for an embryonic tumor is 9 months plus the patient's age at diagnosis. Thus, a 1-year-old child with a gross total resection would be considered cured if there was no recurrence in 21 months [Collins, 1955]. Although this concept has some validity in determining the prognosis of patients with medulloblastoma, there have been several reports of late recurrence.

Medulloblastoma is believed to derive from remnants of the fetal external granular layer of the cerebellum or from cell rests found in the posterior medullary velum and possibly the anterior medullary velum of the cerebellum. Although pathologists have more than 50 years of experience with this tumor, there is no consensus as to the nature or origin of the medulloblastoma.

The tumor was termed *medulloblastoma* by Bailey because he believed that the neoplasm consisted of embryonal stem cells with a pluripotential nature [Bailey and Cushing, 1925]. However, the medulloblast, as a normally occurring cell capable of differentiating along multiple cell lines, has never been satisfactorily identified. As such, present day pathologists believe that the medulloblastoma is a primitive neuroectodermal tumor with nonspecific differentiation. Detailed histologic analysis reveals that these tumors may differentiate along ependymal, astroglial, or neuroblastic cell lines. These observations support the concept that the medulloblastoma may represent a tumor of stem cell origin.

As a result of the histologic similarity of medulloblastomas to primitive neuroectodermal tumors these two entities previously were grouped together as primitive neuroectodermal tumors/medulloblastoma. What primarily differentiates the two are location, either above (primitive neuroectodermal tumor) or below the tentorium, response to therapy and presence or absence of molecular markers. Since location and prognosis of these entities are so different despite the histologic similarities, primitive neuroectodermal tumors are currently classified as embryonal/primitive neuroectodermal tumors rather than primitive neuroectodermal tumors/medulloblastoma.

Despite a growing body of literature detailing the existence of biologic markers, their prognostic value has been confusing. TRkC expression and low N-myc expression have been associated with increased survival. Conversely, c-*myc*, deletion of chromosome 1p, increased mitotic index, and alteration of ploidy have been associated with poor prognoses. The most frequent cytogenetic abnormality, found in about 50% of those with medulloblastoma has been the presence of isochromosome 17q [Eberhart et al., 2004].

More recently the atypical teratoid/rhabdoid tumor has been identified. Atypical teratoid/rhabdoid tumors have their highest incidence in children older than 36 months Although superficially similar to primitive neuroectodermal tumors histologically, these tumors have a much more aggressive clinical course and differentiating histologic and cytogenetic features. The term derives from the observation that the tumor has putative epithelial elements (teratoid) or resembles the malignant rhabdoid tumor seen in the kidney, soft tissues, and other organs. An abundance of spindle cells is suggestive of a sarcoma. This entity is associated with either monosomy or deletion of chromosome 22. The specific gene involved has been identified as hSNF5/IN11. This gene maps to chromosome 22q11.2

Atypical teratoid/rhabdoid tumors, like primitive neuroectodermal tumors, are found in the posterior fossa as well as above the tentorium. Rather than the cavity of the fourth ventricle, the tumor has a predilection for the cerebellar hemisphere and cerebellar/pontine angle [MacDonald et al., 2003].

Medulloblastomas occurring in the midline tend to be soft, fleshy, and well demarcated. Hemorrhage, cyst formation, and calcification are uncommon (Fig. 71-30). There is a great deal of heterogeneity in their cytologic features, mitotic activity, and differentiation. Many medulloblastomas have a high mitotic index with potential for local aggressiveness and spread throughout the neural axis. Histo-

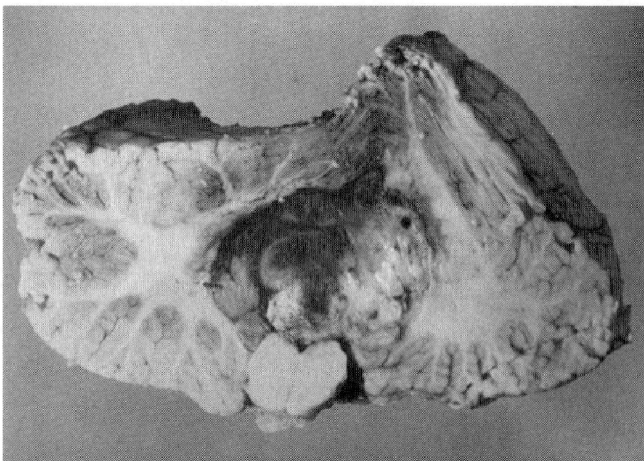

FIGURE 71-30. Gross pathology of a medulloblastoma occurring in the cerebellar vermis.

logically, the tumor is characterized by small round to oval undifferentiated cells with hyperchromatic nuclei in a matrix surrounded by little or poorly defined cytoplasm. Mitosis is variable and has led some pathologists to suggest that a paucity of mitosis, nuclear uniformity and desmoplastic features may be associated with less malignant behavior. Tumors characterized by large cells and anaplasia are considered to have a poor prognosis [Eberhart and Burger, 2003]. However, because there is a limited consensus over the prognostic effect of these pathologic variables, current staging regimens are based solely on clinical and imaging criteria. As with other primitive tumors, medulloblastomas tend to seed the subarachnoid space, both locally and distally. Approximately 70% to 80% recur initially in the posterior fossa. Recurrence in the area of the cribriform plate has been related to the failure to adequately irradiate this region. Extraneural metastases are well documented and, in some series, approach 5% to 30% [Banna et al., 1970; Cohen and Duffner, 1994a; Kleinman et al., 1981].

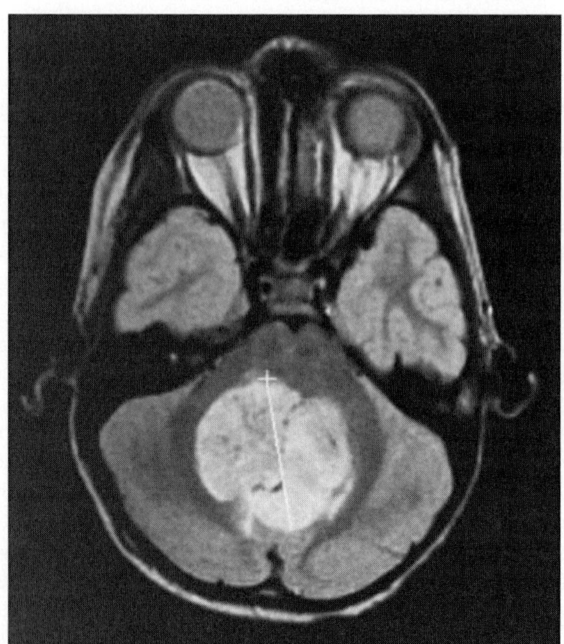

FIGURE 71-31. MRI (T2-weighted image) of 5-year-old child with medulloblastoma.

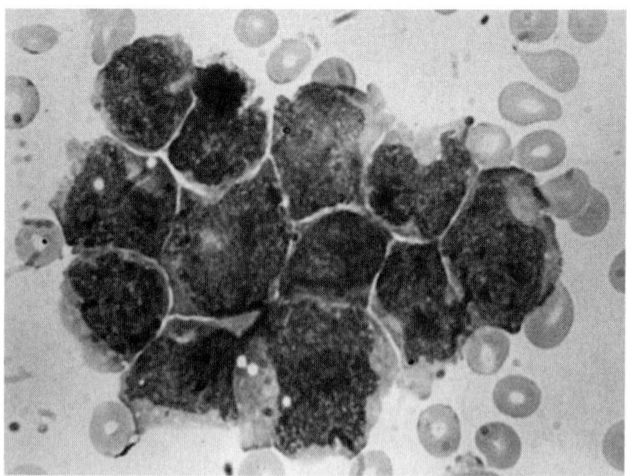

FIGURE 71-32. Cerebrospinal fluid cytology in a patient with medulloblastoma. Note clumped cells containing prominent nuclei and limited cytoplasm.

The primary sites of extraneural metastases are bone and bone marrow.

Clinical Characteristics

Children with medulloblastomas have either nonspecific signs of increased intracranial pressure or a midline cerebellar syndrome. These signs are similar to those present with other posterior fossa tumors. Vomiting, titubation, and headache may reflect increased pressure or invasion of the floor of the fourth ventricle. Head tilt may occur secondary to either ophthalmoparesis or incipient cerebellar herniation. This finding may accompany or precede other signs and may be associated with neck stiffness. Nystagmus is conspicuously absent or mild. As with other cerebellar tumors, hypotonicity, decreased or absent reflexes, and ataxia characterize the motor symptoms.

MRI reveals a gadolinium-enhancing heterogeneous mass presenting in the midline of the cerebellum. The tumor often occupies the cavity of the fourth ventricle, resulting in obstructive hydrocephalus (Fig. 71-31). Presentation in a cerebellar hemisphere is uncommon and is more likely to be associated with an atypical histology. Before treatment, extent of disease should be staged by MRI of the spine, cerebrospinal fluid cytology (Fig. 71-32), bone scan, and bone marrow aspiration.

Management

Treatment of medulloblastomas begins with the attempt to achieve a gross total resection. Aggressive surgery, without compromising neurologic function, provides definitive pathologic diagnosis and reestablishes cerebrospinal fluid integrity. When possible, intraoperative shunting should be avoided in an effort to close a possible portal for extraneural metastasis. In 1930, Cushing recognized the value of bulk removal. In that year he stated: "Radical surgery has greatly augmented the operative mortality rate, which in survivors has notably prolonged the subsequent symptom-free period." Others have concurred that the smaller the amount of tumor left after surgery, the more likely adjuvant therapy will be helpful, and the better the prognosis [Raimondi and Tomita, 1979a; Tait et al.,

1990]. In very young children (<3 years of age), the ability to achieve a gross total resection strongly correlates with improved survival [Duffner et al., 1993].

Many factors have influenced the changing prognosis of medulloblastoma. At the time of diagnosis patients are classified into either a high- or standard-risk group. The standard-risk group are children older than 3 years with less than 1.5 cm^3 postoperative tumor residual who have no evidence of subarachnoid seeding. Parenchymal spread outside the primary tumor site is less of a risk factor. High-risk patients are those with greater than 1.5 cm^3 postoperative residual, subarachnoid seeding, and/or evidence of brainstem involvement. Whereas 5-year survival rates for those with standard-risk disease is more than 80%, those with high-risk disease have a worse prognosis.

There is overwhelming consensus that radiotherapy has been the major reason for improved survival. The use of neuraxis radiation with a boost to the tumor bed has accounted for a major change in survival rates since the early 1950s [Paterson and Farr, 1953]. The reason that medulloblastomas are radiosensitive is not known. Radiosensitivity may relate to in vivo factors, such as tissue oxygenation and growth kinetics, rather than inherent radiosensitivity.

Radiation doses and schedules have changed over the past several decades. In the late 1960s, administration of 40 Gy was considered adequate to the posterior fossa, and 30 Gy was considered adequate for the spinal axis. Current recommended doses are 50 to 60 Gy to the posterior fossa and 24 to 36 Gy to the craniospinal axis. Changes in technology and radiation doses mirror increasing 5-year survival rates. The 5-year survival rates of 20% reported in the 1960s are in marked contrast with the 5-year survival rates of 50% to 70% reported in the 1970s, 1980s, and 1990s [Evans et al., 1990; Hope-Stone, 1970; Hughes et al., 1988; Tarbell et al., 1991].

Recurrence of medulloblastoma, as might be expected, carries a very poor prognosis. However, repeat surgery at the time of recurrence appears to significantly improve prognosis [Balter-Seri et al., 1997]. Chemotherapy, initially single agent but more recently multiagent, has been the most common approach to children with high-risk and recurrent disease [Packer et al., 1999a]. Medulloblastomas are theoretically well suited for treatment with chemotherapy because of their rapid growth rate, high mitotic index, and location in proximity to the ventricular cavity and subarachnoid space.

Although the role of chemotherapy has yet to be fully established, evidence is mounting that supports the benefits of chemotherapy and warrants the continued search for appropriate combinations and routes of administration. The medulloblastoma treatment trials of the International Society of Pediatric Oncology [Bloom et al., 1990], the Children's Cancer Study Group, and the Radiation Therapy Oncology Group have all reached similar conclusions [Evans et al., 1996]. These were two-arm studies. In one arm the children received surgery and radiation, whereas in the other arm the children received surgery, radiation, and chemotherapy. In the Children's Cancer Study Group/Radiation Therapy Oncology Group study, vincristine, prednisone, and CCNU were used, whereas in the International Society of Pediatric Oncology only CCNU and vincristine were used. Initially, the International Society of Pediatric Oncology trial suggested an advantage to the chemotherapy arm; however, long-term differences did not persist ($P = 0.07$). Although an advantage to chemotherapy was not universal, it did persist in certain subgroups, that is, those children who had subtotal or partial excision ($P = 0.007$), those with brainstem involvement ($P = 0.001$), and those with stage T3 and T4 diseases ($P = 0.002$) [Tait et al., 1990]. In the Children's Cancer Study Group trial, the 5-year event-free survival was 59% for children treated with radiation and chemotherapy compared with 50% for patients treated with radiation alone. Both the International Society of Pediatric Oncology and Children's Cancer Study Group studies demonstrated that children with adverse risk factors appeared to benefit from the addition of chemotherapy. Even more impressive have been the results from the Children's Hospital of Philadelphia, where 25 of 26 patients entered in a radiation and chemotherapy pilot were alive and free of disease a median of 24 months from diagnosis [Packer et al., 1988a].

As the number of long-term survivors has increased, concern over the adverse effects of standard dose radiation on intellect and endocrine function has led to trials in which the dose of radiation to the head and neuraxis has been reduced. Studies have been restricted to children considered to be standard risk (i.e., >3 years of age with gross totally resected tumors and no metastases).

In the first multi-institutional trial in which reduced neuraxis radiation (2340 cGy) was compared with standard dose (3600 cGy), children treated on the reduced radiation arm had a significantly higher failure rate overall, as well as in the number of isolated neuraxis relapses [Deutsch et al., 1996]. In the hope that survivals would be improved if chemotherapy were added to reduced neuraxis radiation, the International Society of Pediatric Oncology and the German Society of Pediatric Oncology mounted a study of children with medulloblastoma, which in part asked whether "sandwich therapy" (i.e., up-front postoperative chemotherapy) would allow a reduction in the dose of neuraxis radiation. As in the Pediatric Oncology Group/Children's Cancer Study Group study, the results revealed a worse outcome for children treated with reduced neuraxis radiation, despite the addition of postoperative chemotherapy [Bailey et al., 1995; Kortman et al., 2000]. These studies concluded that the disappointing results were attributed to the delay in giving radiotherapy.

In contrast, other reports have suggested that the addition of chemotherapy to 24 Gy neuraxis radiation (with 50 Gy to the posterior fossa) enhanced rather than decreased survival [Packer et al., 1999b]. There are now multiple reports supporting the view that chemotherapy in conjunction either with reduced neuraxis radiation therapy (2400 cGy) or standard dose radiation therapy (3600 cGy) have consistently shown 5-year survival rates greater than 80% [Evans et al., 1990; Fukunaga-Johnson et al., 1998; Goldwein et al., 1996; Packer et al., 1994; 1999b]. Most of these studies have been in children with standard-risk disease. As a result of the above considerations, adjuvant chemotherapy with reduced dose neuraxis radiation has now become the recommended treatment of choice for both high- and low-risk disease. The choice and degree of intensity of the chemotherapy depend on whether the patient is low risk, high risk, or has recurrent disease.

In summary, treatment of medulloblastomas has been the most successful and serves as the premier example of the value of cooperative trials taking place in the United States as well as internationally. Despite the success of these trials, concern continues about the potential for secondary oncogenesis and endocrine, growth, and intellectual compromise. The search continues for a treatment that provides a cure without the considerable complications associated with current therapies.

Cerebellar Astrocytomas

Cerebellar astrocytomas represent 12% of brain tumors in children younger than 15 years [Duffner et al., 1986]. They are the second most common cerebellar tumor, comprising approximately one third of tumors found in the posterior fossa. Their peak incidence is in the latter half of the first decade, with a second peak in the first half of the second decade [Matson, 1956]. There is no clear-cut gender preference [Pollack and Campbell, 1996].

Astrocytomas may occur anywhere in the cerebellum and may involve the hemispheres, the vermis, or both regions simultaneously. Occasionally, a vermal mass may present largely within the cavity of the fourth ventricle [Ringertz and Nordenstam, 1951]. Invasion of the cerebellar peduncles or brainstem occurs more commonly with tumors of the vermis.

Approximately 80% of cerebellar astrocytomas are cystic [Gol and McKissock, 1959]. Some have suggested that tumors located in the hemisphere are typically cystic, whereas solid tumors are more commonly located in the vermis [Ringertz and Nordenstam, 1951]. The tumors are generally well circumscribed, demarcated from surrounding tissue, and noninvasive. They either consist of a large cyst with a solid mural nodule or they may be largely solid with smaller cysts throughout the substance of the tumor. The wall of the cyst may contain reactive non-neoplastic tissue or occasionally may be fringed by tumor growth. Approximately 20% of cerebellar astrocytomas are solid and similar to those in the cerebral hemispheres (Fig. 71-33).

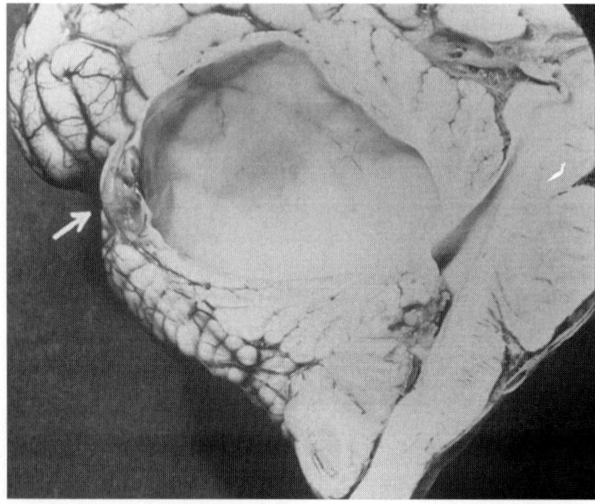

FIGURE 71-33. Gross pathology of cystic hemispheric cerebellar astrocytoma. The *arrow* points to the mural nodule. (From Cohen and Duffner, 1994a.)

The histopathology of most (70% to 85%) cerebellar astrocytomas is that of the typical pilocytic astrocytoma and consists of compact, strongly fibrillated cells that alternate with loose, spongy areas composed of microcysts. Compact areas are generally devoid of microcysts but contain an abundance of Rosenthal fibers. Calcification may be found in 25% of patients. Oligodendroglial cells may be identified. Leptomeningeal dissemination is uncommon but has been reported with spread throughout the neuraxis [Figueiredo et al., 2003]. Dissemination occurs both at diagnosis and years later [Tamura et al., 1998]. Multinucleated giant cells, nuclear hyperchromasia, and endothelial proliferation in the cystic varieties of cerebellar astrocytoma are not necessarily associated with malignant potential. When mitoses are present, however, aggressive tumor behavior should be suspected [Rubinstein, 1972]. Diffuse or fibrillary astrocytomas occur in 15% to 30% of cases.

Attempts to correlate the microscopic appearance of cerebellar astrocytomas with prognosis have been made. Gjerris and Klinken [1978] divided children with astrocytomas into two types: those with the classic juvenile cerebellar astrocytoma and those with diffuse astrocytoma. A total of 70% of the patients had juvenile astrocytomas, whereas 30% had diffuse tumors. The diffuse form was found primarily in the older age group (i.e., 10 to 14 years of age), whereas the juvenile form was found in 88% of children who were younger than 10 years. The 25-year survival rates were 94% for the juvenile and only 38% for the diffuse types. Unlike the cystic cerebellar astrocytoma, the diffuse form of astrocytoma behaved more like the fibrillary astrocytomas of the brainstem or cerebral hemispheres and was associated with recurrence according to the authors. Other more recent studies, however, have not found the marked differences in survival as reported by Gjerris and Klinken [Pollack and Campbell, 1996] (see "Prognostic Factors").

Gilles and associates [1977] also reviewed the histopathology of cerebellar astrocytomas in an attempt to redefine the prognostic meaning of microscopic features. They defined two groups of tumor: glioma A and B. Glioma A, the group defined as having microcysts, Rosenthal fibers, leptomeningeal deposits, and foci of oligodendroglia, is associated with a good prognosis and a 10-year survival rate of 94%. In contrast, the glioma B group has a far worse prognosis with a 10-year survival rate of 29%. Another later study confirmed the prognostic value of the Gilles classification, as patients with glioma B had a higher degree of disease progression and accounted for all deaths in that study [Conway et al., 1991].

Glioblastoma multiforme of the cerebellum is unusual in any age group, particularly in children. Prognosis is invariably poor and, as such, this tumor should be considered a different pathologic entity from the benign cerebellar astrocytoma [Bristot et al., 1999]. Leptomeningeal dissemination, even in the absence of local recurrence, may occur and is associated with a very poor outcome.

Clinical Characteristics

Cerebellar astrocytomas in children typically manifest with signs of increased intracranial pressure. Cerebellar symptoms vary depending on tumor location. Thus, children who have tumors located primarily in the midline will have truncal ataxia, whereas those with primarily hemispheric tumors will have appendicular dysmetria of the ipsilateral limbs. In general, children with cerebellar astrocytomas appear to tolerate increased intracranial pressure far better than children with similar-sized medulloblastomas. Duration of symptoms may vary from days to years. There is generally a longer duration of symptoms before diagnosis in young adults and adolescents compared with younger children. The median duration of symptoms in one study was 3 months [Pollack and Campbell, 1996].

Diagnosis

In the case of cystic cerebellar astrocytomas, a large cystic mass is identified on CT with an enhancing mural nodule. At times, the walls of the cyst may also enhance after intravenous contrast material, which may represent neoplastic lining of the cyst wall. A recent study, however, reported that at least some cases of cysts with enhancement represent reactive tissue rather than neoplasia [Beni-Adani et al., 2000]. Calcification is present in 10% to 20% of cases. Diffuse astrocytomas have slightly decreased density and uniform enhancement. On MRI, cerebellar pilocytic astrocytomas are hypointense or isointense on T1 and hyperintense on T2. Enhancement may be ringlike, nodular or uniform [Pollack and Campbell, 1996]. The mural nodule adjacent to a cyst typically enhances, but most cyst walls do not (64% versus 21%) [Pencalet et al., 1999].

Early postoperative MRI is not accurate in differentiating residual juvenile pilocytic astrocytomas from postoperative changes [Rollins et al., 1998]. CT may help to identify recurrent tumors from postoperative defects because cyst fluid has relatively higher density than cerebrospinal fluid. In addition, compression or alteration in anatomy of the fourth ventricle, cerebellopontine angle, and perimesencephalic cisterns point to recurrent disease [Kingsley and Kendall, 1979; Zimmerman et al., 1978]. In diffuse tumors, MRIs are more valuable in helping to identify recurrence and invasion of the brainstem.

Management

Cushing's surgical experience with cerebellar astrocytomas before 1931 was invariably associated with failure despite removal of the entire cystic mass. Once he recognized that the mural nodule was neoplastic and had to be removed to prevent regrowth of the cyst, survivals improved dramatically [Cushing, 1931]. Today the goal of surgery is complete resection of the tumor. When successful, this approach is associated with more than 90% survival at 10 years [Pollack and Campbell, 1996]. Complete resection may not be possible, however, in the 10% of those with brainstem invasion. Local recurrence is much more common after partial removal of the tumor. Recurrent tumor usually has pathology identical to that of the original tumor; therefore, repeat surgical resection after recurrence may provide a cure [Pollack and Campbell, 1996; Ringertz and Nordenstam, 1951]. Even partial resection has been associated with prolonged survival, although progression-free survivals are significantly less than with gross total resection. As such, there has been controversy about the appropriate postoperative management of those patients with incompletely excised tumor. At least one study reported that children who received radiation therapy after partial resection had better survival rates. Relapse-free survival in those children with partial resection alone was 36%, compared with a relapse-free survival of 83% in those who had irradiation after partial resection [Griffin et al., 1979]. Confirmatory studies have not been reported to date. With the advent of CT and MRI, close, noninvasive follow-up is now possible. When the residual tumor grows, repeat surgery or radiation should be considered.

Surveillance neuroimaging has been recommended at 12, 18, 30, 42, and 66 months with one additional image if definite residual tumor on imaging is identified postoperatively. However, if a gross total resection has been achieved, some authors have not recommended surveillance imaging [Sutton et al., 1996].

The treatment of children with incompletely resected diffuse cerebellar astrocytomas remains controversial. Some investigators would irradiate partially resected diffuse cerebellar astrocytomas because of the putative 38% 25-year survival rate [Leibel et al., 1975]. The validity of this approach has yet to be confirmed. Natural history studies detailing the time interval before recurrence in children with diffuse cerebellar astrocytomas should provide this information.

Children with anaplastic astrocytomas or glioblastomas of the cerebellum are at far greater risk than children with low-grade astrocytomas. Consequently, the recommended treatment is radiation therapy after surgical removal. The volume of radiation is debatable; some authors recommend full craniospinal radiation, whereas others believe radiation to the posterior fossa with wide ports is sufficient [Kopelson, 1982; Salazar and Rubin, 1976]. In view of the risk of leptomeningeal dissemination, even in the absence of local recurrence, craniospinal radiation may be more appropriate than local radiation [Bristot et al., 1999].

There has been little experience in the treatment of cerebellar astrocytomas with chemotherapy, although etoposide [Chamberlain, 1997] and cyclophosphamide have both been used in those with leptomeningeal disease [McCowage et al., 1996]. The tumors generally have such a good prognosis, even at recurrence, that repeat surgery or radiation has been considered to be preferable to chemotherapy.

Quality of life studies of children treated for cerebellar astrocytomas have shown that by adulthood most have done fairly well, that is, they worked and had families but did not fare as well as control groups, especially in terms of depression, socialization, and self-reported life experiences [Pompili et al., 2002]. In another study in which children operated for cerebellar astrocytomas received neuropsychologic evaluations more than 1 year after surgery, poor attention span, poor memory, behavioral issues, and visuospatial deficits were identified in 40% to 70% of children [Aarsen et al., 2004].

PROGNOSTIC FACTORS

Although some authors have attempted to correlate cell proliferation, apoptosis rate and p53 with survival in children with cerebellar pilocytic astrocytomas, they are not prognostic [Haapasalo et al., 1999]. Of interest, although MIB-1 may be high (0.6% to 12%; mean, 4.4%), there is no correlation with clinical behavior, histologic appearance, or neovascularization. Although those cerebellar astrocytomas that appear solid on imaging have significantly higher MIB-1 activity than radiologically cystic tumors with mural nodules, there has been no correlation with progression-free survival [Roessler et al., 2002].

Gross total resection is generally considered a strong prognostic factor [Desai et al., 2001; Bernhardtsen et al., 2003; Morreale et al., 1997], although in at least one study incomplete resection correlated with a worse progression-free survival but not overall survival [Pencalet et al., 1999]. Another important prognostic factor for survival is brainstem involvement [Pencalet et al., 1999; Due-Tønnessen et al., 2002], although, in at least one study, brainstem infiltration was not found to be predictive [Smoots et al., 1998]. Analyses of duration of symptoms before diagnosis have also produced contradictory results, with a short duration of symptoms carrying a good prognosis in one study [Pencalet et al., 1999], whereas others have reported the opposite [Desai et al., 2001].

The previously reported prognostic advantage of cystic over solid tumors has not been supported in recent studies [Pencalet et al., 1999; Smoots et al., 1998] nor has location in the cerebellar hemispheres versus vermis or fourth ventricle been found to be consistently prognostic for survival [Bernhardtsen et al, 2003; Desai et al., 2001]. Even the role of histopathology has not been uniformly accepted. Despite the earlier study by Gjerris and Klinken, pilocytic versus nonpilocytic low-grade histopathology has not had a significant influence on prognosis [Pencalet et al., 1999]. In contrast, it is clear that children with high-grade fibrillary astrocytomas fare worse [Desai et al., 2001].

The literature is decidedly mixed on clearly defined prognostic factors for recurrence and survival. Most studies agree that a gross total resection carries a good prognosis, whereas brainstem infiltration is associated with a worse outcome. Although the earlier studies by Gjerris and Klinken strongly suggested that histopathology was highly prognostic, recent studies have found conflicting results (except for juvenile pilocytic astrocytomas and low-grade fibrillary astrocytomas versus high-grade fibrillary astrocytomas).

Summary

Overall, cerebellar astrocytomas have the best prognosis of any intracranial tumor in childhood. The SEER Registry data reported a 5-year survival rate for cerebellar astrocytomas (excluding glioblastomas of the cerebellum) of 91% that has been confirmed in recent reviews [Duffner et al., 1986b; Pollack and Campbell, 1996]. Preferred treatment is complete surgical removal. In patients with recurrence, repeat surgery is recommended while radiation is reserved for those with progressive disease following a second complete resection or for those with unresectable residual disease who progress [Pollack and Campbell, 1996].

Ependymomas

Ependymomas constitute approximately 8% of brain tumors in children younger than 15 years of age [Duffner et al., 1986]. Most occur in young children, with a mean age at diagnosis of 5 to 6 years. Sixty percent of children with ependymomas are younger than 5 years of age, with only 4% older than 15 years of age at diagnosis [Dohrmann et al., 1976]. In fact, ependymomas represent the second most common malignant brain tumor in children younger than 3 years [Duffner et al., 1993]. Posterior fossa location is more common in younger children (less than 3 years), whereas a supratentorial location is more common in older patients (older than 3 years) [Smyth et al., 2000].

Ependymomas arise in relation to any part of the ventricular system. In general, two thirds of tumors are infratentorial, and one third are supratentorial. Infratentorial tumors arise from the roof, floor, or lateral recesses of the fourth ventricle. The tumor can occlude the ventricle and extend cephalad to the aqueduct. At times, tumor spreads laterally into the cerebellar pontine angle or lateral recesses or extends caudad through the foramina of Lushka and Magendie into the upper cervical canal. Supratentorial ependymomas may be entirely within the lateral or third ventricles or partly intraventricular and partly extraventricular. It is interesting, however, that they may be found anywhere within the cerebral hemispheres and may be entirely extraventricular [Cohen and Duffner, 1994c].

Ependymomas are well-defined, homogeneous, partially encapsulated mass lesions. They may be extensively cystic. Low-grade ependymomas are cellular with a regular histologic pattern. Ependymal rosettes are diagnostic and consist of tumor cells lining a small, central lumen. Pseudorosettes are observed even more commonly. Areas resembling oligodendrogliomas and astrocytomas are also frequently present [Russell and Rubinstein, 1989]. It has been extremely difficult to determine the degree of malignancy of ependymomas based on histologic features. Much of this confusion results from the lack of large numbers and the need to consider histologic characteristics of supratentorial and infratentorial ependymomas separately. The presence of mitotic figures and vascular proliferation has been associated with aggressive lesions, as have the findings of hypercellularity and necrosis. Foci of pleomorphism and hypercellularity may be identified in otherwise benign-appearing ependymomas.

Cytogenetics and Molecular Markers

The most frequent alteration is loss of heterozygosity of chromosome 22q (30% of ependymomas). Other abnormalities of chromosome 22 have also been reported [Debiec-Rychter et al., 2003]. Another common chromosomal abnormality is monosomy 17 (50% of pediatric ependymomas). Loss of heterozygosity was found in one study in the long arms of chromosomes 6 and 9 (30% and 27%, respectively), suggesting that tumor suppressor genes may be found on these chromosomes [Huang et al., 2003]. Although a variety of chromosomal alterations have been identified, no finding is consistent at this time [Teo et al., 2003].

Clinical Characteristics

The symptoms and signs of children with ependymomas vary with tumor location. Children with tumors located in the posterior fossa have signs and symptoms of increased intracranial pressure and cerebellar signs. Supratentorial tumors are more likely associated with focal headaches, seizures, and focal motor signs. Signs vary with tumor location so that nystagmus, meningismus, papilledema, and dysmetria are frequently observed with posterior fossa lesions, whereas hemiparesis, hyperreflexia, and visual field abnormalities are more common with supratentorial tumors [Cohen and Duffner, 1994c; Dohrmann et al., 1976].

Diagnosis

The appearance of ependymomas on precontrast CT scans is that of a usually isodense to gray matter mass, often cystic and typically calcified (50%). At times tumors may be hyperdense. The tumors typically enhance with intravenous contrast. On MRI T1 scans, the tumors may be hypointense or isointense, whereas on T2 scans, tumors are usually isointense to hyperintense [Comi et al., 1998]. Heterogeneous gadolinium enhancement can be quite intense at times. The heterogeneous signals are due to necrosis, hemosiderin, or vascularity [Chen et al., 2004]. Obstructive hydrocephalus is common, especially with infratentorial tumors. The infratentorial tumors tend to "flow" out of the foramen of Lushka and Magendie into the upper cervical canal and pontine cisterns in a manner sometimes called "plasticity." This finding is observed best on MRI scans.

The evaluation of the child with an ependymoma must include examination of the neuraxis (MRI) and cerebrospinal fluid cytology. Although ependymomas do not seed the neuraxis frequently (7%), failure to diagnose leptomeningeal spread will lead to inadequate therapy. As such, surveillance imaging is strongly recommended [Good et al., 2001]. Some authors have suggested that head scans should be obtained every 3 to 6 months for those who have had a gross total resection, whereas those with a subtotal resection should be scanned every 3 months for the first postoperative year. In the second to fifth year, scans of the head are obtained every 6 months. Spine imaging is limited to those with perioperative leptomeningeal disease or those with local recurrence. These recommendations are based on the fact that most children with ependymomas will fail first in the primary site [Goldwein et al., 1990]. However, with the newer approach of three-dimensional conformal radiation to the tumor bed, it might be prudent to perform spinal imaging on all children on a regular basis until long-term follow-up of patterns of failure has been established.

Management

The ability to achieve a gross total resection significantly improves survival rates [Figarella-Branger et al., 2000; Good et al., 2001; Merchant et al., 2002a; Perilongo et al., 1997b; Pollack et al., 1995; VanVeelen-Vincent et al., 2002]. Some have even suggested that in these cases (particularly supratentorial lesions) no further therapy is warranted, but this view is not uniformly accepted [Paulino, 2000]. The importance of radical surgery has led to the increasingly accepted approach of delivering postoperative chemotherapy to children with subtotally resected tumors to improve the likelihood of a complete resection at "second look" surgery [Foreman et al., 1997].

Postoperative radiation is considered standard therapy for older children with ependymomas. As noted above, the only exception is the totally resected supratentorial low-grade ependymoma. A Children's Oncology Group study has a postoperative observation arm for this group. Supratentorial ependymomas, however, are known to recur even after a gross total resection. The approach of withholding radiation to children with gross totally resected supratentorial ependymomas is not universally accepted and should be viewed as experimental only. For children older than 3 years, standard radiation treatment is 5400 cGy in 30 fractions (local) over 6 weeks. Some radiation therapists increase the dose to 5940 cGy in 33 fractions (local) over 6.5 weeks for high-grade tumors. It is of interest that in at least one study, duration of radiation therapy for more than 50 days was a poor prognostic factor [Paulino, 2000]. Previously, there was controversy regarding the volume of radiation (i.e., local versus neuraxis). In response, the Pediatric Oncology Group among others demonstrated that the first site of failure in most patients was the primary location of the tumor [Kovnar et al., 1991]. As such, routine neuraxis radiation is not recommended unless leptomeningeal disease is demonstrated at diagnosis [Chiu et al., 1992; Merchant et al., 1997; Rousseau et al., 1994]. In the presence of widespread disease, there is unanimity that children should receive craniospinal radiation.

New trends in the radiation treatment of children with ependymomas include hyperfractionation (with and without chemotherapy), three-dimensional conformal radiation, and stereotactic radiation. Hyperfractionation given with and without vincristine, cyclophosphamide, and etoposide was not shown to improve survivals compared to historical controls in a large prospective Italian study [Massimino et al., 2004]. In contrast, preliminary data from a Pediatric Oncology Group study of hyperfractionation were promising in children with subtotally resected ependymomas compared with historical controls (3-year event-free survival, 52% versus 27%) [Kovnar, 1996]. Three-dimensional conformal radiation to the tumor bed has had very promising early results in children with ependymomas and has led to an ongoing group-wide Children's Oncology Group study [Merchant et al., 2002c; Paulino, 2001]. If effective, this approach will measurably reduce neurotoxicity. Reports of postoperative stereotactic radiosurgery in children and adults with ependymoma either at diagnosis or recurrence are limited. Preliminary data suggest that this technique may be useful in patients with local recurrence following surgery and external beam radiation, and potentially helpful at diagnosis. Further trials are needed [Mansur et al., 2004; Stafford et al., 2000]. All patients require long-term follow-up because late failures are not uncommon.

The role of chemotherapy at diagnosis and recurrence has been debated. Transient responses to chemotherapy, particularly cisplatinum, have been shown in recurrent tumors [Sexauer et al., 1985]. Various other chemotherapeutic agents have also been used with variable success [Chamberlain, 2001]. A postoperative chemotherapy regimen consisting of cyclophosphamide and vincristine for newly diagnosed children less than 3 years of age with ependymomas was associated with a 48% response rate [Duffner et al., 1993]. Even higher response rates have been observed on other "baby" studies, using dose intensification of the same agents. The role of adjuvant chemotherapy, however, is still unclear. The Children's Cancer Study Group trial of surgery and craniospinal radiation with or without CCNU, vincristine, or prednisone found no difference in outcome between the two arms (10-year progression-free survival of 36% and overall survival of 39%). Bloom and co-workers [1990] reported similarly negative results using CCNU and vincristine. Although the 5-year survival was 70% compared with historical control subjects (40%), the curves converged after 6 to 7 years, and no statistical difference was identified. In contrast, a chemotherapy regimen of carboplatin, vincristine, ifosfamide, and etoposide after surgery and radiation was associated with a 5-year progression-free survival of 74% in one study [Needle et al., 1997]. The French trial of postoperative chemotherapy in children younger than 5 years of age using agents that included procarbazine, carboplatin, etoposide, cisplatin, vincristine, and cyclophosphamide without irradiation was associated with a 4-year survival of 74% in those children who had a gross total resection but only 35% for those with incomplete resection. It is of interest that in contrast to the U.S. baby studies, radiologic responses were limited [Grill et al., 2001]. The German HIT trials combined postoperative radiation with chemotherapy, which included ifosfamide, etoposide, methotrexate, cisplatinum, and cyclophosphamide. The overall survival was 75% at 3 years and the progression-free survival was 59.7%. As with the French study, children with incomplete resection had 3-year progression-free survivals of only 38.5% [Timmermann et al., 2000]. Because several of these studies used both postoperative radiation and chemotherapy, the role and efficacy of the chemotherapy cannot be determined. It appears in general that ependymomas may be chemosensitive but are not chemocurative. As such, it is unlikely that more intense chemotherapy such as bone marrow transplantation will provide improved cure rates. In all of these studies it must be recognized that ependymomas tend to recur late. As such, promising early results must be viewed with caution.

PROGNOSTIC FACTORS

Survival varies with prognostic factors. There is no dispute that a gross total resection is the most significant prognostic factor. In recent years, several authors have reported 5-year progression-free survival of 70% to 80% in children with ependymomas who have had a gross total resection [Korshunov et al., 2004] but 5-year survival has been significantly worse in those who have had a subtotal resection, that is, 20% to 40% [Duffner et al., 1998b; Merchant, 2002a]. This has led to the concept of "second look" surgery, often following two courses of chemotherapy, in children whose tumors have been incompletely resected. Surprisingly, the presence of leptomeningeal seeding has not been consistently identified as a risk factor [Duffner et al., 1998b]. The role of tumor location is also debated as a prognostic factor. Whereas some series have found supratentorial location to be better than infratentorial, others have found conflicting results. Patients with infratentorial tumors located in the lateral recesses appear to have a worse prognosis than those that are more medial, possibly because of the difficulty in achieving a gross total resection in these children [Figarella-Branger et al., 2000; VanVeelen-Vincent et al., 2002].

Very young age (less than 2 years versus 2 to 3 years) was found to be a significant prognostic factor in the first "Baby POG" (Pediatric Oncology Group) study. This may be misleading however, because children younger than 2 years in that study received chemotherapy for 2 years before they were irradiated while those between 2 and 3 years received radiation after only 1 year of chemotherapy. Thus, it may be the delay in radiation beyond 1 year rather than the younger age that led to the worse prognosis [Duffner et al., 1998b]. Young age per se has been considered to be a prognostic factor when children younger than 3 years are compared with older children, however. For example, children younger than 3 years had survivals of 22% versus 75% in those older than 3 [Pollack et al., 1995]. Dose of radiation also has been considered prognostic, that is, a radiation dose of less than 4500 cGy is a negative prognostic factor [Goldwein et al., 1990]. Perhaps the most controversial factor is histologic grade. Results from the first Baby POG study revealed no difference in progression-free or overall survival according to degree of malignancy, that is anaplastic versus low grade [Duffner et al., 1998b]. Recent studies, however, found that high-grade pathology had a significant effect on prognosis [Korshunov et al., 2004; Merchant et al., 2002a]. This area needs clarification because it may affect the type of treatment recommended.

Summary

In summary, gross total resection plus local (possibly conformal) radiation appears to be the most effective treatment regimen at this time. Further studies of adjuvant chemotherapy, particularly to improve the likelihood of achieving a gross total resection at second look surgery, are in progress.

Brainstem Tumors

Approximately 13% to 20% of brain tumors in the pediatric age group are found in the brainstem [CBTRUS, 2004; Duffner et al., 1986; Halperin, 1985]. These tumors occupy the region of the brain traversed by the fourth ventricle and aqueduct of Sylvius. Neoplasms found proximal to the mesencephalon or caudal to the medulla in the cervical spinal cord are not considered under the rubric of brainstem tumors.

Pathologic diagnosis is hampered by the limited amount of tissue that can be obtained at surgery. Stereotactic biopsy is the procedure of choice because of fear of damaging vital brainstem structures and the possibility of brainstem swelling. Small biopsies cannot be viewed as definitive because sampling error and potential for malignant dedifferentiation may complicate interpretation. These considerations led many authors to reject the need for pathologic confirmation. Conversely, others have thought that because most patients have pilocytic tumors that are uniform with little regional variation, sampling error may not be a problem and biopsy is worthwhile [Cohen and Duffner, 1994b].

As with most other tumors, there is a growing tendency to stage these tumors according to location, histology, and clinical behavior. Tumors characteristically associated with the poorest prognosis are those in which symptoms are less than 6 months before diagnosis, have a pontine location, present with an abducens palsy, and engulf the basilar artery.

This group of children has been found to have fibrillary astrocytomas. Those with a better prognosis are those children with tumors either outside the ventral pons, with an exophytic component, a cervical medullary location or a pilocytic histology without the clinical features mentioned above (Fisher et al., 2000). Unlike intrinsic parenchymatous masses, fungating portions of exophytic tumors are surgically accessible. Evacuation of the tumor cysts found in low-grade astrocytomas may be associated with long-term cures and relief of symptoms [Epstein and Wisoff, 1988].

Clinical Characteristics

The triad of long tract signs, cranial neuropathies, and ataxia localizes a suspected lesion to the brainstem. Cranial nerves arising in bulbar and pontine areas are most commonly involved. Vertical nystagmus on upward gaze, bilateral nystagmus on lateral gaze, positional nystagmus on horizontal gaze, and nonfatigable positional nystagmus suggest intrinsic abnormalities of the brainstem. Downbeating, small amplitude, positional nystagmus, with or without ocular myoclonus, suggests a medullary location, whereas localization to the midbrain is suggested by conversion retraction nystagmus. In addition, various oculomotor gaze disturbances have been described. Lower motor neuron facial nerve involvement may suggest a pontine lesion. Bulbar signs, swallowing and feeding difficulties, asymmetry of the palate, absent gag reflex, atrophy of the tongue, and nasal regurgitation imply involvement of the medulla. Appendicular ataxia suggests either involvement of the cerebellum or, more likely, compromise of the pathways passing through any of the three cerebellar peduncles to and from the cerebellum. Motor difficulties may also relate to abnormalities of the descending motor systems [Cohen and Duffner, 1994b].

Neuroimaging confirms the clinical suspicion of a pontine mass. Tumors found in the region of the brainstem on CT may be isodense, cystic, necrotic, or calcified. Low-density lesions with and without contrast enhancement are more likely to behave in a malignant fashion [Segall et al., 1985]. MRI more readily delineates the location and extent of tumor, and may more accurately provide information regarding an exophytic component (Fig. 71-34).

Management

Brainstem tumors are usually considered to be relentlessly progressive, with an inexorable course to death. Duration of symptoms until diagnosis may vary from weeks to several years. In most series, 5-year survival rates range from 5% to 30%. Examination of actuarial survival curves suggests there may be two populations of patients: (1) the majority are short-term survivors who die within the first 1 to 2 years of diagnosis, and (2) a small group of long-term survivors who have a relatively plateaued course [Cohen et al., 1986]. Prognosis depends on location and duration of symptoms before diagnosis, neuroimaging characteristics, and to some extent, histologic diagnosis. Children with signs and symptoms of less than 6 months' duration, tumors that infiltrate the pons, and those that have evidence of two or three brainstem signs have the poorest prognosis. Conversely, lesions that are focal or exophytic or that originate in adjacent anatomic structures, such as the cerebellar peduncle or cervical medullary junction, tend to have a better prognosis and may be amenable to surgery [Robertson et al., 1994]. There is also some suggestion, but not conclusive evidence, that patients with brainstem gliomas who have neurofibromatosis also have a better prognosis. Brainstem tumors occurring in these patients may have a different biology and there are reports of long, progression-free survivals, even in the absence of treatment [Milstein et al., 1989; Pollack et al., 1996; Raffel et al., 1989]. As such, it has been suggested that in patients with neurofibromatosis, intervention should be limited to those with lesions that are relentlessly progressive or cause clinical dysfunction.

Tumors located in the midbrain (tectal, pretectal, or tegmental) regions are another group of brainstem tumors that, other than producing obstructive hydrocephalus, may have a benign course [Robertson et al., 1995]. Periaqueductal location, uniform appearance on MRI with rare enhancement, and long periods of stability without change on clinical examination or neuroimaging are the usual features. Management consists of watchful waiting, periodic imaging studies, and shunting if appropriate [Bowers et al., 2000; Grant et al., 1999].

It has been standard teaching that after clinical evaluation and radiologic confirmation, surgery for typical diffuse pontine gliomas is not indicated and may lead to significant

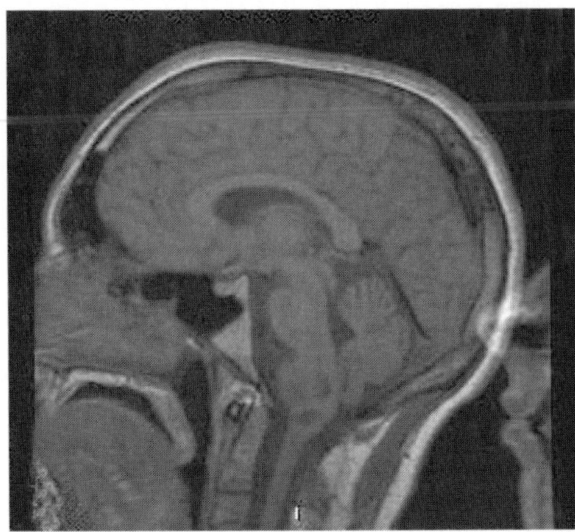
A

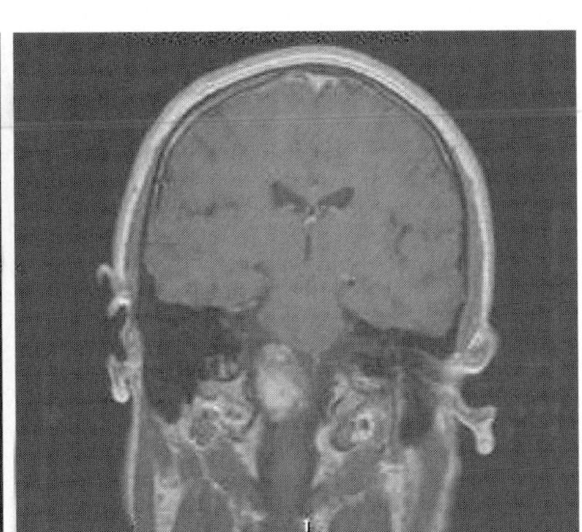
B

FIGURE 71-34. T1 sagittal (**A**) and postcontrast coronal (**B**) views in a 19-year-old male with a large exophytic pilocytic astrocytoma. Following biopsy the patient has been followed for more than 10 years with little evidence of progression.

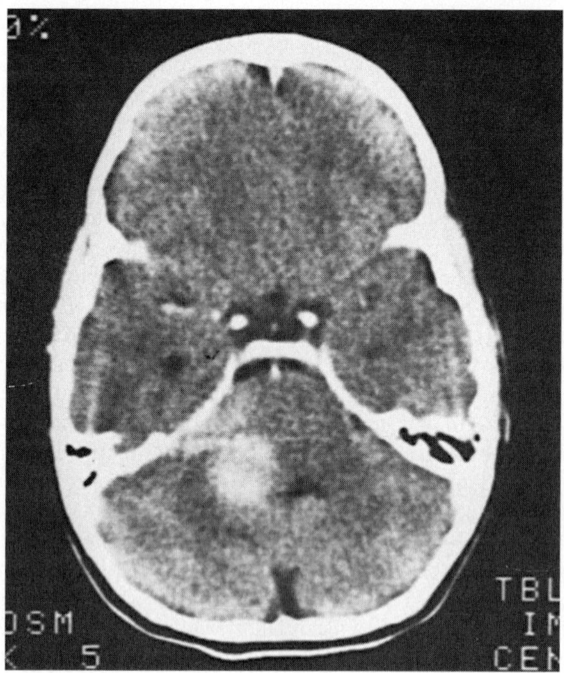

FIGURE 71-35. Axial enhancing CT suggesting a brainstem tumor. After surgery a histopathologic diagnosis of an ependymoma was confirmed. Rather than treat as a brainstem glioma, this child was placed on a Pediatric Oncology Group treatment protocol for ependymoma.

neurologic compromise. This approach prevents pathologic confirmation of the tumor and hampers, to some degree, the ability to develop protocols based on predicted pathologic behavior. Further, imaging cannot effectively exclude the infrequent hemangioma, arachnoid cysts, telangiectasia of the pons, cavernous hemangioma, or hamartoma [Frank et al., 1988]. Using stereotactic biopsy, surgical morbidity can be minimized. With the advent of better anesthesia, agents to control edema, and microsurgery, there is a growing tendency toward surgical exploration and biopsy [Fisher et al., 2000]. Surgical confirmation avoids the pitfalls of wrong diagnosis, allows the removal of an extra-axial mass, and permits evacuation of cyst contents (Fig. 71-35).

Epstein and others [Epstein and Wisoff, 1988; Robertson et al., 1994] have also suggested that prognosis and treatment decisions can be made based on anatomic localization. They defined four categories of brainstem tumors (i.e., diffuse, focal, cystic, cervical medullary). Those that present in a dorsal exophytic manner or at the cervical medullary junction are the most amenable to surgery and are the most likely to benefit from this approach. In this small subset of patients, radical surgery offers the possibility of long-term remission and even cure.

For the majority of patients, the primary treatment of patients with brainstem tumors is radiotherapy. Although survival rates as high as 40% to 50% have been reported, most researchers report 5-year survival rates of less than 30% [Littman et al., 1980]. For children with diffuse pontine gliomas, survival rates are less than 10%. Radiation in doses of 5500 cGy over 5 to 6 weeks is recommended [Kim et al., 1980].

Hyperfractionated radiation has been used as an alternative to standard radiation. Hyperfractionated protocols using treatment schedules from 6400 cGy to as high as 7200 cGy, and even 7800 cGy initially demonstrated trends of increasing time to progression and survival when compared with lower dose levels [Freeman et al., 1991]. Unfortunately, these results have not been sustained. For the most part, a dose-effect relationship regarding toxicity has been observed. Acute toxicity has been minimal, although in a few cases intralesional necrosis has been identified. Because almost all those children have died of progressive disease, long-term toxicity has not been assessed. Overall, although toxicity has been tolerable, survival of children with brainstem gliomas using escalating doses of hyperfractionation have failed to show improvement over that associated with conventional radiation [Mandell et al., 1999].

The margin for error in the treatment of brainstem tumors is extremely limited. Compactness of vital structures and limited room for expansion continue to dampen the enthusiasm for surgery other than biopsy. Poor treatment results using either standard radiation or hyperfractionated radiation have influenced the decision to treat aggressively with chemotherapy. Chemotherapy, that is, multiagent, myeloablative or dose escalating, however, has shown no advantage over radiation alone [Freeman and Perilongo, 1999].

Summary

Despite many innovative attempts at treatment, overall results in this group of tumors have been poor. Even with the poor overall prognosis, there remains a subgroup of patients who have favorable outcomes: those with focal, cystic, or cervical medullary lesions and those associated with neurofibromatosis. These children should be stratified to less aggressive treatment arms. Conversely, the child with diffuse pontine abnormalities on MRI or CT and a short duration of symptoms and signs carries a poor prognosis and merits aggressive therapy (Freeman and Perilongo, 1999).

SUPRATENTORIAL TUMORS

Astrocytomas

Approximately 50% to 60% of primary brain tumors in children are supratentorial in location, most of which are of an astrocytic lineage [CBTRUS, 2004]. CBTRUS coding includes cranial nerves and spinal cord in this assessment. A variety of differing histologies, such as primitive neuroectodermal tumors, oligodendrogliomas, ependymomas, central neurocytomas, and dysembryoplastic neuroepithelial tumors are supratentorial in location. Gliomas account for 46% of the total.

The pathologic nosology of cerebral astrocytomas is complex. Some pathologists have subdivided the tumors according to cytologic architecture, whereas others have graded them according to malignant potential [Bailey and Cushing, 1926; Kernohan et al., 1949]. Unfortunately, because of the multiple classifications, it is often difficult to accurately interpret survival rate and treatment responses from the literature. The classification currently in use is that recognized by the World Health Organization [Kleihues and Cavenee, 2000]. In the World Health Organization classification grade I is benign, grade II is low grade, grade III is anaplastic or intermediately malignant, and grade IV is highly malignant.

TABLE 71-3

Selected Childhood Primary (Malignant and Nonmalignant) Brain and Central Nervous System Tumor Age-Specific Incidence Rates* (Ages 0-19), by Age at Diagnosis, CBTRUS 1995-1999†

	AGE AT DIAGNOSIS											
	0-4		5-9		10-14		15-19		0-19		0-14	
HISTOLOGY	***N***	**Rate**	***N***	**Rate**	***N***	**Rate**	***N***	**Rate**	***N***	**Rate**	***N***	**Rate**
Tumors of Neuroepithelial Tissue	**719**	**3.73**	**665**	**3.37**	**529**	**2.77**	**447**	**2.38**	**2360**	**3.07**	**1913**	**3.29**
Pilocytic astrocytoma	142	0.74	171	0.87	139	0.73	89	0.47	541	0.70	452	0.76
Anaplastic astrocytoma	8	—	27	0.14	19	0.10	21	0.11	75	0.10	54	0.09
Astrocytoma, NOS	59	0.31	60	0.30	55	0.29	50	0.27	224	0.29	174	0.30
Ependymoma/anaplastic ependymoma	90	0.47	35	0.18	25	0.13	30	0.16	180	0.23	150	0.26
Glioma, malignant, NOS	90	0.47	87	0.44	52	0.27	40	0.21	269	0.35	229	0.39
Benign and malignant neuronal/glial, neuronal, and mixed	55	0.29	23	0.12	40	0.21	48	0.26	166	0.22	118	0.20
Embryonal/primitive medulloblastoma	178	0.92	167	0.85	86	0.45	53	0.28	484	0.63	431	0.74
Tumors of Cranial and Spinal Nerves	**—**	**—**	**8**	**—**	**23**	**0.12**	**30**	**0.16**	**65**	**0.08**	**35**	**0.06**
Tumors of the Meninges	**18**	**0.09**	**17**	**0.09**	**35**	**0.18**	**63**	**0.34**	**133**	**0.17**	**70**	**0.12**
Lymphomas and Hematopoietic Neoplasms	**—**	**—**	**—**	**—**	**—**	**—**	**6**	**—**	**16**	**0.02**	**10**	**0.02**
Germ Cell Tumors	**15**	**0.08**	**24**	**0.12**	**42**	**0.22**	**50**	**0.27**	**131**	**0.17**	**81**	**0.14**
Germ cell	15	0.08	24	0.12	42	0.22	50	0.27	131	0.17	81	0.14
Tumors of the Sellar Region	**13**	**0.07**	**39**	**0.20**	**43**	**0.23**	**100**	**0.53**	**195**	**0.25**	**95**	**0.16**
Craniopharyngioma	12	0.068	39	0.20	28	0.15	24	0.13	103	0.13	79	0.14
Local Extensions from Regional Tumors	**—**	**—**	**—**	**—**	**—**	**—**	**6**	**—**	**15**	**0.02**	**9**	**—**
Unclassified Tumors	**41**	**0.21**	**17**	**0.09**	**31**	**0.16**	**29**	**0.15**	**118**	**0.15**	**89**	**0.15**
TOTAL‡	**816**	**4.23**	**774**	**3.92**	**712**	**3.73**	**731**	**3.89**	**3033**	**3.94**	**2302**	**3.96**

*Rates are per 100,000 person-years.
†Includes data from 12 of the 16 registries listed in Table 71-1; New Mexico, North Dakota, Rhode Island, and Texas are excluded.
‡Refers to all childhood brain tumors, including histologies not presented in this table.
CBTRUS, Central Brain Tumor Registry of the United Statess; NOS, not otherwise specified; —, counts are not presented when fewer than 6 cases were reported for the specific histology category, and rates are not presented when fewer than 10 cases were reported for the specifichistology category. The suppressed cases are included in the counts and rates for totals.

The most common astrocytomas seen in children are pilocytic astrocytomas (World Health Organization grade I and grade II astrocytomas). Glioblastoma multiforme is less common but there is the concern that a grade II astrocytoma may dedifferentiate into more malignant pathology.

Composite CBTRUS SEER data reflecting the years 1973 through 1999 indicated that 5- and 10-year survivals for children 0 through 19 years of age with "astrocytomas, not otherwise specified" was 78% and 74.4%: the data for anaplastic astrocytomas were 51.6% and 46.9%; for glioblastomas, 17% and 15%; and for pilocytic astrocytomas, 93.8% and 92%. The survival figures for adults with the same histologies are worse [CBTRUS, 2004] (Table 71-3).

The fibrillary pattern (diffuse astrocytoma) is the most common microscopic pathology. Meningeal fibrils impart a firm consistency to the tumor. Mitoses are absent, and there is no endothelial proliferation. Pilocytic astrocytomas of the cerebrum are often microcystic or may have a single large cyst with a tumor nodule, resembling the cystic cerebellar astrocytoma. Gemistocytic astrocytomas are unusual and have a tendency to evolve into glioblastoma multiforme. Microscopically, the cytoplasm is homogeneous and lightly eosinophilic. Anaplastic astrocytomas have increased cellularity, cellular pleomorphism, and mitoses, as well as features typical of astrocytomas. Glioblastoma multiforme is characterized by pleomorphism, endothelial proliferation, necrosis, and multinucleated giant cells. Mitoses are present in 70% and hemorrhage in 60% [Frankel and German, 1958; Rubinstein, 1972; Russell and Rubinstein, 1989].

Abnormalities of ploidy, loss of heterozygosity, and genetic mutations are increasingly recognized in these tumors. The most common chromosomal abnormalities are deletions of 17p and 22, p53 mutations, and overexpression of platelet-derived growth factor. Chromosomal abnormalities shared by anaplastic gliomas and glioblastomas probably represent the earliest changes in the transformation process from low-grade to high-grade tumor.

Glioblastomas in adults, unlike those arising in children, may not undergo molecular transformation. These so-called de novo tumors are associated with overexpression of epi-

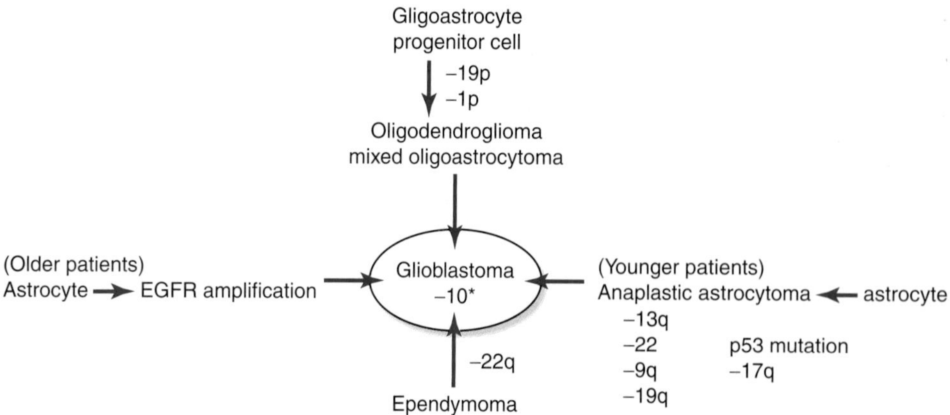

FIGURE 71-36. Graphic showing chromosome deletions associated with astrocytoma progression from benign to more malignant. The progression involves a broad region of chromosome 10. EGFR, epithelial growth factor receptor. (From Furnari FB, Huang HJ, Cavenee WK. Genetics and malignant progression of human brain tumours. Cancer Surv 1996;25:233-275.)

thelial growth factor and chromosome losses on chromosome 10 [Furnari et al., 1996, see illustration; Louis et al., 2001] (Fig. 71-36).

Clinical Characteristics

The signs and symptoms of hemispheric astrocytomas, regardless of grade, relate to the area of cortex involved [Low et al., 1965]. Headaches, visual field abnormalities, seizures, focal motor weakness, and papilledema are common presenting symptoms. Headaches may be focal or nonfocal, but persistently focal headaches correlate with true localization in more than 90% of patients [Jelsma and Bucy, 1967]. Seizures are more common with slower growing tumors. The seizures are usually generalized, partial simple seizures or partial complex seizures with complex symptomatology either with or without secondary generalization. Although brain tumors are an unusual cause of seizures in young children, certain clues to their presence should be recognized. Tumor should be suspected in the child who has had a long-standing seizure disorder and develops (1) change in school performance, (2) increasing frequency of seizures, (3) change in quality of seizures, (4) focal slowing on EEG, (5) change in personality, or (6) change in neurologic examination [Page et al., 1969] (Fig. 71-37).

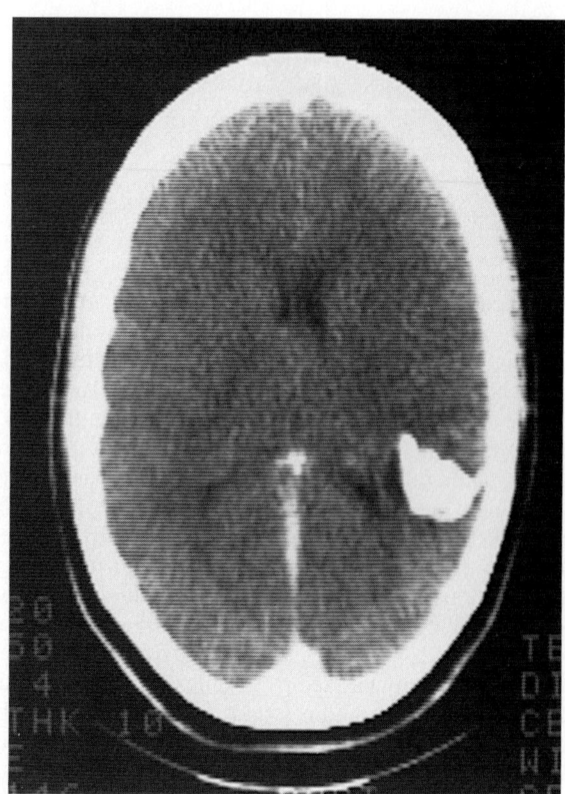

FIGURE 71-37. CT scan of 16-year-old female with long history of seizures. Pathology revealed a low-grade astrocytoma. After surgery and radiation, patient is doing well, with only an occasional seizure.

The duration of symptoms before diagnosis is longer with supratentorial gliomas than with tumors of the posterior fossa, which relates, in part, to the early onset of obstructive hydrocephalus associated with infratentorial tumors. There is an inverse relationship between grade of tumor and duration of symptoms. A longer duration of symptoms before diagnosis tends to carry a better prognosis [Walker et al., 1980].

Diagnosis

CT and more recently MRI have increasingly identified children previously diagnosed as having idiopathic seizure disorders who actually harbor low-grade malignancies. Areas of decreased density on CT or increased signal on T2 MRI images may represent tumor, although mesial temporal sclerosis, trauma, and previous infarct complicate the differential diagnosis. High-grade tumors tend to be associated with alterations in the blood-brain barrier, and consequently enhancement with intravenous contrast occurs in more than 90%. However, not all high-grade tumors enhance on MRI or CT [Barker et al., 1997]. In addition, some low-grade astrocytomas may be associated with contrast enhancement. Thus the presence or absence of contrast enhancement is only suggestive of the degree of malignancy [Barker et al., 1997; Silverman and Marks, 1981; Steinhoff et al., 1978; Tchang et al., 1977].

Management

Although traditional treatment of low-grade astrocytomas has been surgery followed by local irradiation, there are differing approaches to the treatment of low-grade astrocytomas in children older than 5 years. Some neuro-oncologists believe that children with low-grade astrocytomas can be followed longitudinally by CT or MRI before committing the child to either surgery or radiation. Others recommend surgical intervention at diagnosis, followed by "watchful waiting" before committing the child to radiation. In the literature, event-free survival following gross total resection ranges from 50% to 90% [Gajjar et al., 1997]. A third group believes that identification of tumor should be followed by surgery and immediate postoperative local radiation.

Although there may be a question as to whether radiation is indicated at diagnosis, there is universal agreement that when the patient undergoes operation, total removal should be attempted unless the location involves eloquent areas of the nervous system that might be damaged at surgery. As in the cerebellum, surgery is curative for children with cystic pilocytic astrocytomas of the cerebrum if the mural nodule is removed completely. Failures occur in those patients in whom the mural nodule is only partially excised [Palma and Guidetti, 1985]. Total resection is usually possible with tumors occupying the poles of the frontal or temporal lobes. In more deep-seated tumors, such as those involving the thalamus or in high-risk areas, total surgical extirpation may not be possible. The degree of resection can be maximized using stereotactic technology. On evidence of recurrence, attempts at gross total resection are again recommended [Gajjar et al., 1997].

The radiation oncologist's approach to low-grade tumors is usually local volume radiation (the area of the primary tumor with a margin of approximately 2 cm). The dose of radiation is generally 54 Gy. The addition of postoperative radiation for partially resected grade I astrocytomas in adults reportedly increased the 5-year survival rate in one study from 25% to 58% [Sheline, 1977]. Increasingly radiation protocols involve conformal radiation. The margins included in the radiation port usually extend 1 cm beyond the margin of gross tumor [Merchant et al., 2002d]. Unfortunately, the data on children with grade I and II astrocytomas treated with surgery and radiation are difficult to interpret because many of these studies have included cerebellar astrocytomas. Although radiation appears to influence 5-year survival rates, it does not influence 10-year survival rates. Some investigators reported an increase in 5-year survival rates from 13% to 41% with radiation, but by 10 years after diagnosis, irradiated patients had a 26% survival rate compared with a 32% survival rate for patients treated with surgery alone [Fazekas, 1977]. This view has not changed in the past 20 years. At present there are no large, well-documented, prospective studies assessing quality of life or long-term effects in children with low-grade gliomas.

For progressive low-grade tumors, radiation with and without chemotherapy is routinely recommended. There are ongoing phase II chemotherapy trials for efficacy of chemotherapy without radiation in children younger than 10 years of age [Freeman et al.,1998; Gajjar et al., 1997].

An interesting approach to low-grade astrocytomas is a study opened in 1991 by the Pediatric Oncology Group and the Children's Cancer Study Group, which addressed the question of whether radiation improves progression-free survival rate after subtotal surgical resection. Children with totally resected low-grade supratentorial astrocytomas are being followed longitudinally and not committed to radiation; however, children older than 5 years with incomplete resection are randomized to either supportive care, local radiation, or investigators' choice. It is hoped that at publication this study will provide answers regarding the need for radiation as well as the long-term effects of local radiation. In addition, information regarding dedifferentiation of low-grade astrocytomas in children will be clarified.

There is little controversy regarding the need for postoperative radiation treatment of patients with anaplastic astrocytomas and glioblastoma multiforme. Unfortunately, despite postoperative radiation, survival rates are poor. Studies of adults with anaplastic astrocytomas have yielded significantly better survival rates when treatment included radiation: 0% to 3% 5-year survival rates in patients treated with surgery alone compared with 15% to 20% 5-year survival rates in patients treated with surgery and radiation. In contrast, response to treatment of glioblastomas is universally poor. Although radiation does offer a significant advantage over surgery alone, survival is measured in months rather than years [Bloom et al., 1990; Heideman et al., 1997].

Although the literature on glioblastomas and anaplastic astrocytomas in childhood has been limited, children with these tumors appear to have better prognoses than do adults. Survival relates, in part, to the dose of cranial radiation. Children with hemispheric malignant astrocytomas receiving 54 to 60 Gy had a 60% 5-year survival rate in one study compared with 14% for doses of 35 to 50 Gy. In the same study, children with glioblastoma multiforme had a 9% 5-year survival when treated with 54 to 60 Gy versus 0% with 35 to 50 Gy [Marchese and Chang, 1990]. The generally poor outcome of childhood malignant astrocytomas was reconfirmed in 27 patients treated with surgery or radiation, in which the 5-year survival was 25% and 13%, respectively, at 10 years [Hoppe-Hirsch et al., 1993].

Chemotherapy may offer an advantage over radiation alone in pediatric patients with high-grade astrocytomas. The Children's Cancer Study Group reported a trial in which children with high-grade astrocytomas were treated with postoperative radiation alone or radiation plus chemotherapy, including vincristine, CCNU, and prednisone [Sposto et al., 1989]. The 5-year event-free survival was 46% for patients who received radiation and chemotherapy compared with 18% for those who received radiation therapy alone. The presence of mitosis or necrosis was associated with a worse outcome, as was the group who received a biopsy. The study found no difference between gross total resection and partial resection. These results suggest a possible role for chemotherapy in children with high-grade astrocytomas and are of particular interest because similar treatment regimens in adults have not been successful.

Another approach to malignant gliomas of childhood is high-dose chemotherapy followed by autologous bone marrow transplantation [Finlay, 1992]. Although objective responses have been reported, the complications of these regimens, including pulmonary fibrosis (carmustine [BCNU]), leukoencephalopathy (methotrexate), and death from infection or thromboembolic events, currently limit this approach.

Debate continues over the influence of risk factors on prognosis. In one study, deep white matter location carried a worse prognosis than location in the cerebral hemispheres, whereas other authors have not found location to be of prognostic value [Dropcho et al., 1987; Marchese and Chang, 1990]. Controversy also exists over the influence of age on survival. Although children with malignant gliomas and glioblastoma multiforme have better survival rates than adults, the influence of very young age is unclear. In at least one study of children ages 2 to 20 years, children younger than 5 years, and those older than 10 years had significantly better survival rates than any other age group [Al-Mefty et al., 1987]. In contrast, children older than 5 years of age had a better prognosis than children younger than 5 years in another study. In a third study of children 15 months to 18 years of age, a trend toward longer survival was found in children 12 years of age or younger [Dropcho et al., 1987]. The most intriguing group was the 18 infants on Baby POG with high-grade astrocytomas, in whom responses to a chemotherapy regimen of cyclophosphamide and vincristine revealed a 60% response rate and 5-year survival rates of 50% plus or minus 14% [Duffner et al., 1996b]. Reasons for the better survival rates in children compared with adults with similar tumor pathology are not clear but may suggest different tumor biology in different age groups.

Dysembryoplastic Neuroepithelial Tumor

Dysembryoplastic tumors are benign cortical neoplasms usually identified in older children or young adults. They tend to be long standing and may be associated with intractable seizures. Grossly the tumor is nodular and intracortical. Histologically the tumor resembles the oligodendroglioma. Dysembryoplastic tumors are characterized by pleomorphism, glial-neuronal elements, and limited nuclear atypia, cellularity, mitosis, and endothelial proliferation. They initially were thought to be a form of cortical dysplasia without the potential of recurrence following complete surgical excision. However, recent literature has suggested that there are a small group of individuals who despite adequate surgery have recurrence of tumor. Hence, these children require continued surveillance following initial diagnosis and surgery [Nolan, 2004; Pomeroy, 2004].

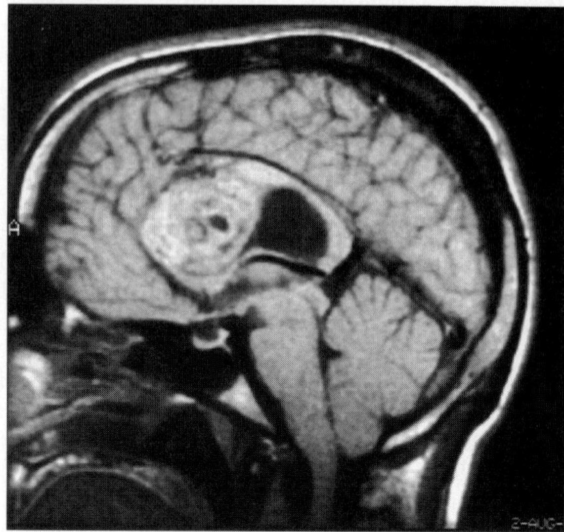

FIGURE 71-38. Neurocytoma manifested in a teenager. The tumor extended to, but did not obstruct, the foramen of Monro.

Central Neurocytoma

This tumor occurs in teenagers and young adults. It manifests as a midline intraventricular calcified mass that rarely obstructs the ventricular system (Fig. 71-38). The tumor is very cellular but has none of the other features of malignancy. Long survivals are the rule with or without surgery or adjuvant therapy [Nishio et al., 1988].

Primitive Neuroectodermal Tumors

Cerebral primitive neuroectodermal tumors were first described in 1973 by Hart and Earle, who reported a group of tumors found in the cerebrum of children and young adults [1973]. The tumors had similar pathologic and clinical features with a rapid course from diagnosis until death. The reported incidence of cerebral primitive neuroectodermal tumors ranges from 2.5% to 7%. They most commonly occur in very young children [Ashwal et al., 1984]. Primitive neuroectodermal tumors are usually supratentorial in location, although occasionally they may be found elsewhere in the CNS, including the spinal cord. As a pathologic entity, the concept of primitive neuroectodermal tumors has not had universal acceptance, in part because Rubinstein [1972] classified neoplasms with similar features as cerebral neuroblastomas. In addition, other primitive neuroepithelial tumors, such as medulloepitheliomas, ependymoblastomas, and pineoblastomas, have been considered separate entities. The most confusing aspect of the primitive neuroectodermal tumor classification is whether to "lump" medulloblastomas with cerebral primitive neuroectodermal tumors. Their similar histopathologic appearance prompted this approach, but their differences in location and especially prognosis have made this approach less useful [Duffner and Cohen, 1997].

Pathology

Grossly, the tumor is sharply delineated from surrounding brain tissue. Necrotic areas, cyst formation, calcification, and hemorrhage are frequently present. On microscopic examination, the tumors are characterized by small, undifferentiated cells with little observable cytoplasm and dark oval to irregular nuclei. The tumors are highly malignant, with numerous mitotic figures, areas of vascular endothelial hyperplasia, and necrosis. The tumor is 90% to 95% undifferentiated, although focal areas of differentiation may be present. On ultrastructural examination, this differentiation along ependymal, neuronal, and astrocytic cell lines can be confirmed [Markesbery and Challa, 1979].

Immunohistochemistry further permits neuropathologists to identify differentiation along various cell lines. Cerebral primitive neuroectodermal tumors in infancy have been found to have a particularly wide range of differentiation [Grieshammer et al., 1991].

Clinical Characteristics

The duration of symptoms prior to diagnosis is brief, usually less than 3 months. The most common presenting symptoms in the literature have been headache, followed by nausea, vomiting, and seizures. Infants and young children typically present with large head circumferences, seizures, and focal motor deficits [Dai et al., 2003]. One of the striking clinical findings has been the patient's ability to accommodate the large tumor mass [Duffner et al., 1981]. This likely reflects the fact that cerebral primitive neuroectodermal tumors are not typically associated with peritumoral edema.

Diagnosis

The diagnosis of primitive neuroectodermal tumors is based on clinical signs and symptoms, abnormal radiologic studies, and pathology. CT demonstrates large, partially calcified hyperdense masses with well-defined margins but without peritumoral edema. There may be cyst formation. Enhancement has ranged from minimal to dense in a heterogeneous or ringlike pattern [Dai et al., 2003; Pigott et al., 1990]. As with CT, MRI reveals well-defined tumor margins and a relative lack of peritumoral edema [Figuerora et al., 1989]. Solid areas range from low- to high-signal intensity [Dai et al., 2003].

Primitive neuroectodermal tumors may seed the cerebrospinal fluid, producing spinal cord metastases in 20% to 40% of patients [Parker et al., 1975; Tomita et al., 1988]. As such, routine MRI of the spine and assessment of cerebrospinal fluid cytology should be performed at diagnosis and follow-up. Extraneural metastases to lung, lymph nodes, pericardium, diaphragm, and liver have been reported [Ashwal et al., 1984; Duffner et al., 1981].

Management

Treatment of primitive neuroectodermal tumors begins with attempts at bulk resection of the tumor. Unlike medulloblastomas, the survival advantage of a gross total resection is not universally accepted [Duffner and Cohen, 1997; Tomita et al., 1988; Zeltzer et al., 1993]. A report from the Children's Cancer Study Group found that less or greater than 1.5 cm^3 postoperative residual tumor did not correlate with significant differences in survival, although a trend toward better survival was identified in children who had minimal residual disease [Albright et al., 1995]. In view of the tumor's tendency to seed the subarachnoid space, craniospinal radiation is recommended [Paulino et al., 2004]. Despite radiotherapy, survivals have been poor [Tomita et al., 1988]. The dose of radiation to the primary site is 5000 to 6000 cGy with 3600 cGy to the neuraxis. Chemotherapy has been considered, in part, because of the chemosensitivity of medulloblastomas. Several authors have reported responses to a variety of chemotherapeutic agents, including carmustine (BCNU), vincristine, methotrexate, procarbazine, and platinum (Fig. 71-39). Despite this, Tomita and associates [1988] were unable to identify a clear survival advantage to chemotherapy versus nonchemotherapy-treated patients. The most successful regimen so far (in a limited number of patients) included surgery, hyperfractionated craniospinal radiation, and an adjuvant chemotherapy regimen of vincristine, cisplatin, and cyclophosphamide [Halperin et al., 1993]. For children with recurrent disease, high-dose chemotherapy with autologous stem cell rescue, usually with radiation, may salvage some patients [Broniscer et al., 2004].

Unfortunately, despite the pathologic resemblance of primitive neuroectodermal tumors to classic medulloblastomas, patients with primitive neuroectodermal tumors have very poor survival rates. A comparison of 5-year survival rates in children with cerebral primitive neuroectodermal tumors and medulloblastoma were 46.9% and 86.3%, respectively [Paulino and Melian, 1999]. Although they may

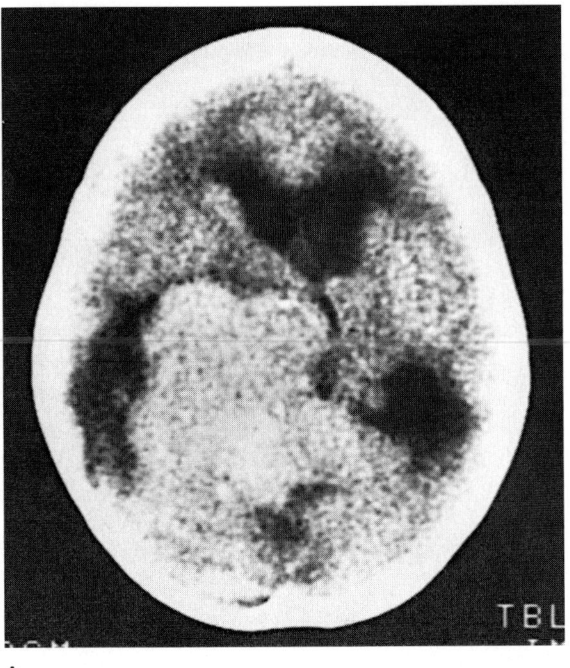

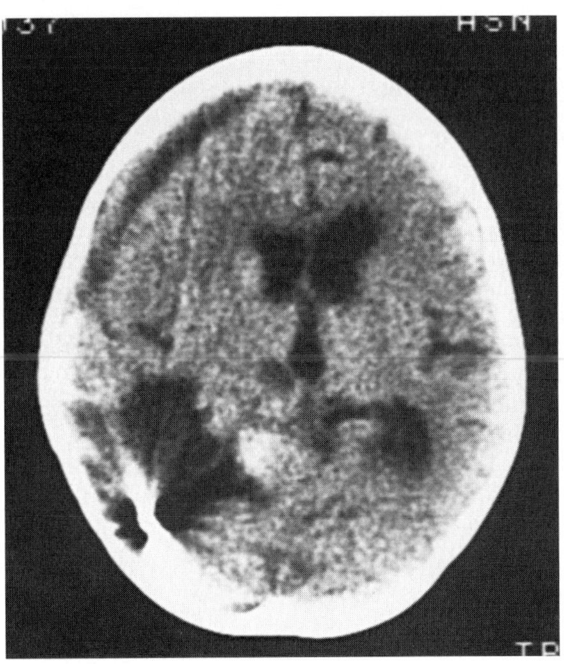

FIGURE 71-39. **A**, CT demonstrating biopsy-confirmed primitive neuroectodermal tumor. **B**, Same patient demonstrating marked reduction in tumor size after chemotherapy. Unfortunately, the response was transient and tumor subsequently recurred.

respond transiently to drugs and radiation, few patients are long-term survivors. The vast majority of children die within 1 to 3 years after diagnosis. Prognostic factors that affect survival adversely include young age (<3 years) and metastatic disease at diagnosis [Albright et al., 1995]. As noted, the benefits of obtaining a gross total resection have been debated [Mikaeloff et al., 1998; Zeltzer et al., 1993].

In summary, primitive neuroectodermal tumors are highly malignant tumors found in childhood that appear to predominate in the very young. Because they tend to seed the cerebrospinal fluid, treatment must be directed to the entire cerebrospinal axis. General treatment recommendations include maximum debulking surgery, craniospinal irradiation, and chemotherapy. In cases of recurrence, there have been reports of transient responses to treatment with chemotherapy, high-dose chemotherapy with bone marrow transplantation, or repeat irradiation.

Oligodendrogliomas

Oligodendrogliomas are rare tumors, accounting for less than 1% of childhood neoplasms [Farwell et al., 1977]. Most oligodendrogliomas are found in the cerebral hemispheres. Occasionally, an intramedullary tumor is encountered. The tumor is rarely found as a pure oligodendroglioma but usually represents the predominant cell type of a mixed glioma. Calcification, as well as cystic and mucoid degeneration, may be present. The tumor may be friable, calcific, or necrotic. Histologically, the tumor is characterized by a honeycomb appearance consisting of a monotonous collection of uniform cells with a rounded appearance and clear cytoplasm. The perinuclear halo gives the honeycomb appearance to the tumor. Compact areas of the tumor may lack such an appearance, suggesting that the finding of oligodendrogliocytes in a mixed glioma, regardless of predominance of cell types, imparts a favorable prognosis to the tumor. Although considered benign, dissemination of oligodendrogliomas in the cerebrospinal fluid pathways is well recognized. Leptomeningeal metastasis with resultant hydrocephalus, as well as remote extracranial metastasis, is occasionally identified.

Seizures are by far the most common presenting symptom. Most oligodendrogliomas are in the cerebral hemispheres; therefore, clinical signs and symptoms relate, in large measure, to the area of involved brain. Many patients with this tumor may have a long, protracted clinical course characterized by seizures, with or without long tract signs. CT usually confirms the presence of a mass. Calcification is commonly present and may appear nodular, shell-like, or winglike. Factors associated with improved survival are age less than 20 years, calcification, low-grade tumor, frontal or parietal location, and lack of contrast enhancement [Shaw et al., 1992]. Of interest, the prognostic value of gross total resection is debated [Razack et al., 1998].

Treatment

Treatment should initially consist of surgery alone because the tumor is slow growing [Hirsch et al., 1989]. With evidence of dissemination of tumor or on recurrence, radiation or combined modality chemotherapy should be considered. In one of the few large-scale retrospective analyses of children with oligodendrogliomas and mixed gliomas, tumor progression was diagnosed in 68% of patients. Of most interest, the median time to progression and overall survival were not affected by postoperative treatment, suggesting that radiation or chemotherapy can be deferred until clinically necessary [Walter et al., 2000]. The 5-year survival in one group of 19 children with oligodendrogliomas and mixed oligodendrogliomas was 65% [Razack et al., 1998].

In the adult population, radiation doses of 60 Gy are required to improve prognosis [Allison et al., 1997]. There has been a great deal of interest in adults with anaplastic oligodendrogliomas because of reports of sensitivity to procarbazine, CCNU, and vincristine with good results as preirradiation therapy and adjuvant therapy or for post-radiation progressive disease [Bouffet et al., 1998; Streffer et al., 2000]. Temozolimide has also had promising results with anaplastic oligodendrogliomas. At least one study found that treatment with postoperative radiation and procarbazine, CCNU, and vincristine in nonanaplastic oligodendrogliomas also produced excellent results, with no local failure in 28 to 240 months. The authors found that radiation alone (60 Gy) was effective but that procarbazine, CCNU, and vincristine without radiation therapy delayed time to progression, and as such may "buy time" for young children until definitive therapy with radiation can be administered [Allison et al., 1997]. Allelic loss of the 1p19q loci may predict the response to chemotherapy and duration of survival in adults with anaplastic oligodendrogliomas [Bauman, 2000].

With the advent of CT and MRI, the incidence of oligodendrogliomas as a cause of long-standing seizures may increase. Any child who has refractory seizures or who has a changing seizure pattern should be evaluated for the possibility of an underlying, slow-growing neoplasm, such as an oligodendroglioma (Fig. 71-40).

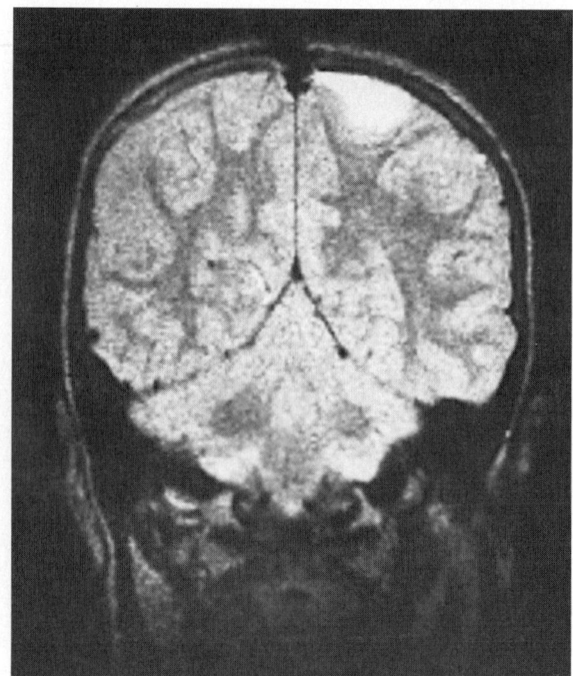

FIGURE 71-40. A 5-year-old female with long-standing seizures. MRI demonstrates an increased T2-weighted signal. An oligodendroglioma was removed at surgery. Patient is doing well with infrequent seizures.

BRAIN TUMORS IN INFANTS AND VERY YOUNG CHILDREN

Approximately 13% of brain tumors in children ranging in age from newborn to 15 years of age are found in those younger than 2 years [Duffner et al., 1986]. The male-to-female ratio is approximately equal, although medulloblastomas in infants, as in older children, tend to be more common in males. Brain tumors in infancy differ in location from those in older children. In the first 6 months of life, most series report a supratentorial predominance. By 7 to 12 months of age, there is a relatively equal distribution between the supratentorial and infratentorial compartments, but after 1 year of age the more typical location is in the posterior fossa. There are approximately equal numbers of supratentorial hemispheric and midline tumors, although there has been some suggestion that midline tumors predominate in the very young infant [Fessard, 1968; Tomita and McLone, 1985].

The types of tumors also tend to vary with age at diagnosis. Whereas most series report astrocytomas as the most common brain tumor in young children, teratomas are prominent in neonates younger than 3 months of age, particularly in Japan. In some Japanese series, teratomas account for 33% to 37% of neonatal brain tumors [Oi et al., 1990]. The most common malignant tumors in children from birth to 3 years of age are medulloblastomas, ependymomas, and primitive neuroectodermal tumors. The last group encompasses ependymoblastomas, pineoblastomas, cerebral neuroblastomas, medulloepitheliomas, and cerebral primitive neuroectodermal tumors (Fig. 71-41). In addition, this grouping encompasses a number of tumors of high-grade malignancy previously designated as "malignant neoplasms not otherwise specified." In contrast with older children, brainstem gliomas and cerebellar astrocytomas are relatively unusual [Duffner et al., 1986]. In several series, high-grade gliomas, such as glioblastomas and anaplastic astrocytomas, have been considered rare [Matson, 1964]; however, wide variability occurs in the various series, depending on the number of patients and referral patterns. Certain tumors characteristically occur in infants. The majority of choroid plexus tumors, discussed earlier in this chapter, are diagnosed before 2 years of age. They tend to occur primarily in the lateral ventricles and less frequently in the third or fourth ventricles in this age group [Matson, 1964]. Approximately 17% are carcinomatous and are associated with a poor prognosis. Meningeal sarcomas also tend to predominate [Raimondi and Tomita, 1983]. Optic gliomas are prominent in all series, representing approximately 2% of patients. These rates will likely change as more children with neurofibromatosis undergo screening neuroimaging.

Clinical Characteristics

Infants with brain tumors are often diagnosed quite late in the disease course. This delay in diagnosis may be one of the reasons that infants have a significantly poorer prognosis than older children. Diagnostic delays occur because the presenting signs and symptoms of brain tumors in infants and very young children are relatively nonspecific and are more often believed to represent common pediatric illnesses than structural CNS disease. Moreover, in young children the early symptoms of increased intracranial pressure may be masked by skull expansion with sutural diastasis. The classical signs and symptoms of increased intracranial pressure may not be present until the tumor bulk is considerable.

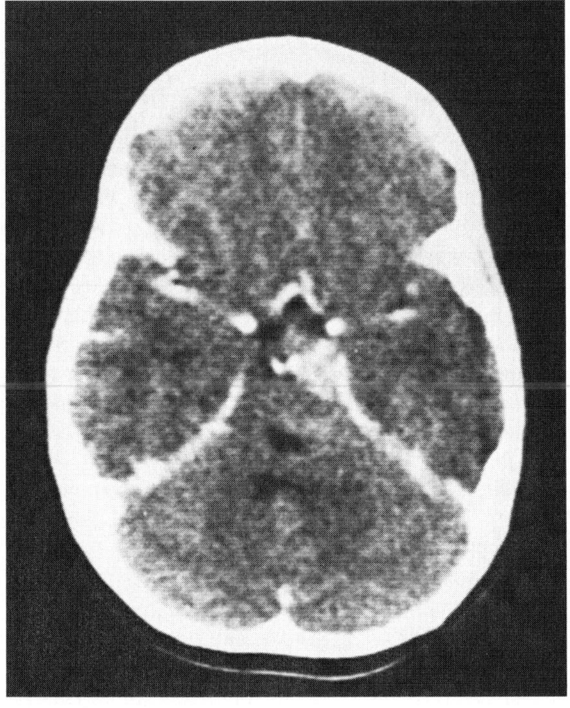

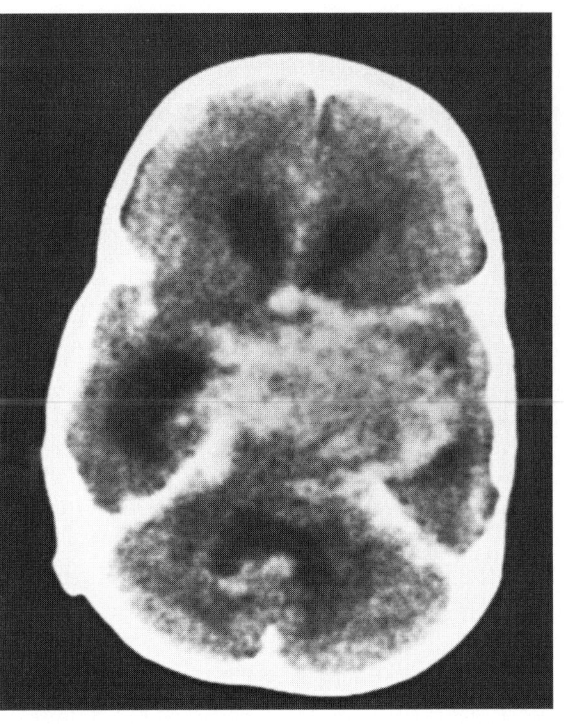

FIGURE 71-41. CT scans of infant with biopsy-confirmed poorly differentiated embryonal tumor. **A**, Initial appearance. **B**, Note rapid increase in size after 3 months despite aggressive therapy.

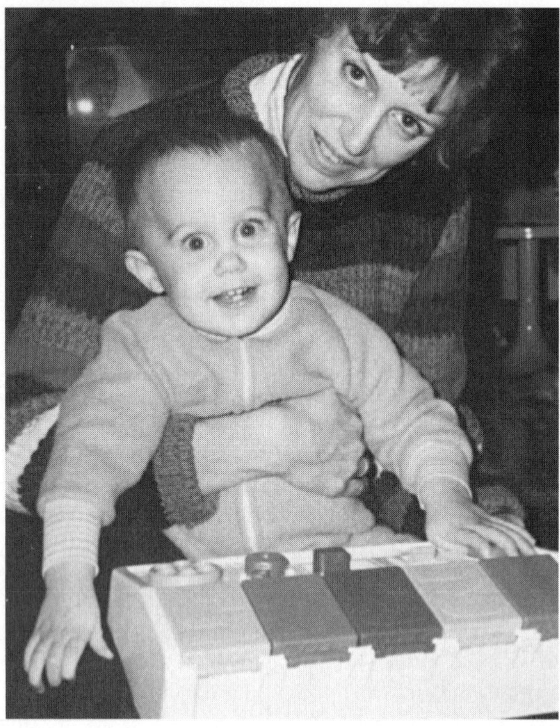

A

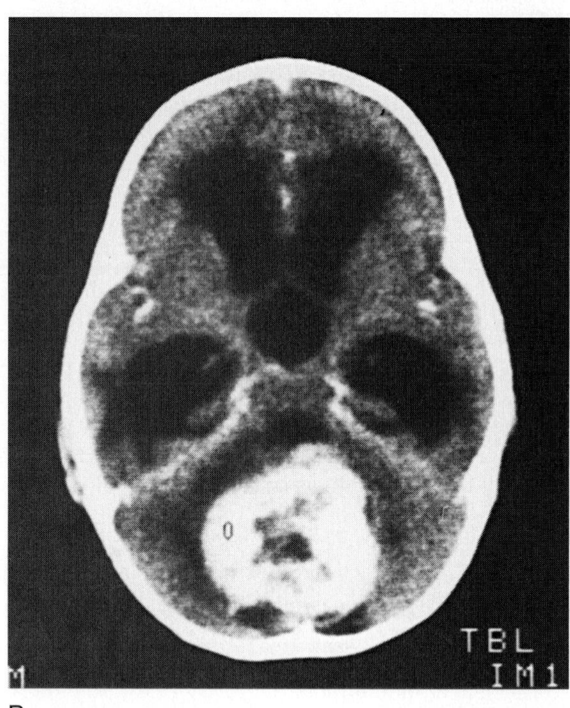

B

FIGURE 71-42. A 14-month-old male with medulloblastoma. **A**, Note prominent forehead secondary to enlarging head circumference. **B**, Axial CT reveals large posterior fossa mass with hydrocephalus.

When the child does present for evaluation, the head may be markedly misshapen because of differential intracranial pressure effects [Jooma et al., 1984] (Fig. 71-42).

One of the most common presenting symptoms is vomiting [Farwell et al., 1978]. Often vomiting is misdiagnosed as gastrointestinal disease, such as gastroesophageal reflux, pyloric stenosis, or intolerance to formula before vomiting secondary to either increased intracranial pressure or direct involvement of the floor of the fourth ventricle is considered [Papadakis et al., 1971].

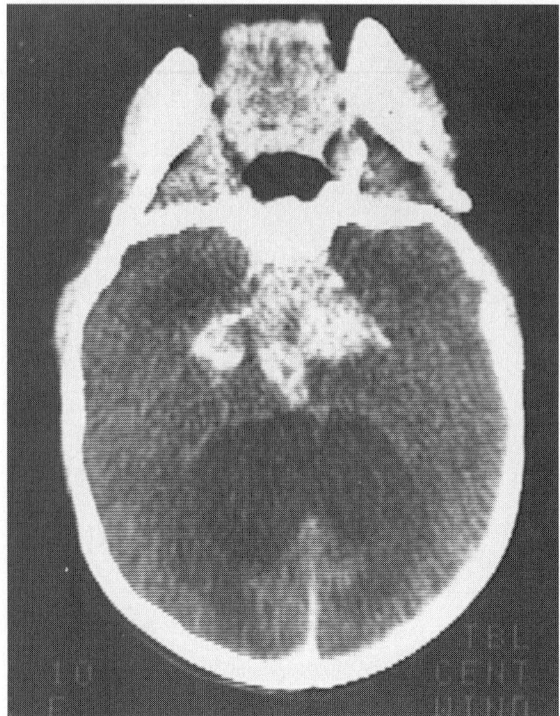

FIGURE 71-43. Axial CT demonstrating a large chiasmatic glioma in a patient erroneously believed to have congenital nystagmus.

Another common symptom in infants with brain tumors is irritability or behavioral changes, sensitive indicators of CNS disease at any age. Because the causes of irritability and behavioral change in infants are diverse, CNS disease is often low in the differential diagnosis.

Seizures are a prominent symptom in most series. As expected, seizures are more common with hemispheric supratentorial tumors and are often partial with or without secondary generalization. Although seizures described as tonic extensor attacks are reported in association with posterior fossa masses, these usually are episodes of opisthotonos related to irritation of the brainstem rather than frank convulsive episodes. There have also been reports of infantile spasms in infants with brain tumors. In two such cases, the infants responded clinically and electroencephalographically to adrenocorticotropic hormone before the tumor was diagnosed [Ruggieri et al., 1989].

Visual loss is difficult to diagnose in the young child and is rarely a presenting symptom in the literature. Moreover, the physical signs of nystagmus or bizarre eye movements are frequently misdiagnosed as spasmus nutans or congenital nystagmus rather than nystagmus resulting from lesions of the chiasm [Baram and Tang, 1986] (Fig. 71-43). Children in the first decade of life with neurofibromatosis are at high risk for the development of visual pathway tumors. Because these children are generally not symptomatic until later in the disease course, routine neuroimaging of the optic nerves and chiasm should be considered.

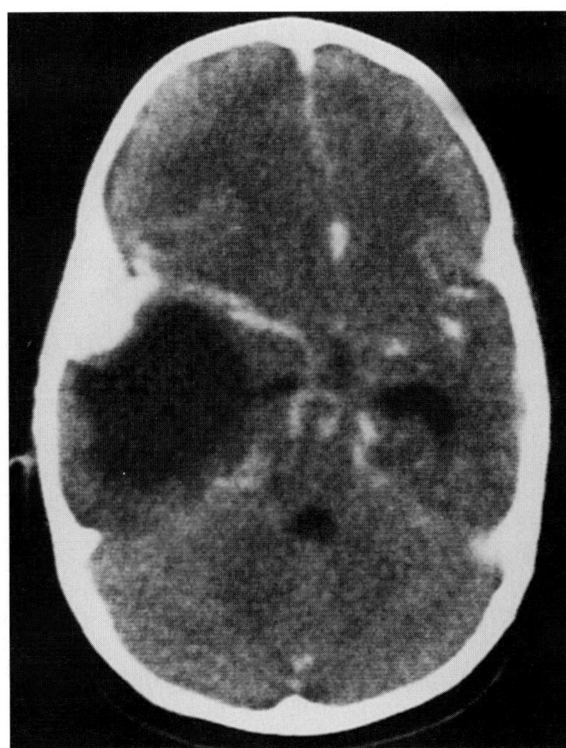

FIGURE 71-44. Contrast-enhanced CT of a 15-month-old child with progressive hemiparesis. Diagnosis was low-grade astrocytoma.

When focal motor signs are present, they are often attributed to static encephalopathy (i.e., hemiparetic cerebral palsy) rather than to progressive intracranial disease. A potentially important differentiating historical point is the presence of early hand preference. In general, children with hemiparetic cerebral palsy have a strong hand preference even from infancy. In contrast, with an expanding mass lesion, the child will be ambidextrous early in life and then develop a hand preference before 12 to 18 months of age. In cases of congenital brain tumors, handedness may be present from birth and strongly mimics static encephalopathy. The association of a focal motor deficit and an expanding head circumference, however, should suggest progressive intracranial pathology rather than the static, nonprogressive encephalopathy characteristic of cerebral palsy (Fig. 71-44).

The presence of meningismus in a child with a large head may reflect incipient herniation rather than meningitis. In many series the constellation of irritability, vomiting, and bulging fontanel has suggested meningitis to the pediatrician, leading to a potentially dangerous lumbar puncture. Although this misdiagnosis inevitably occurs in some patients, careful review of previous head circumferences and the presence of split sutures will suggest a more chronic process and should prompt obtaining a CT scan before considering lumbar puncture [Gordon et al., 1995].

A relatively uncommon but classic presentation of brain tumors in infancy is the diencephalic syndrome, a condition that occurs with tumors involving the hypothalamus. Infants present with a progressive wasting syndrome, especially with loss of subcutaneous tissue in the presence of normal linear growth. The children vomit but not in sufficient amounts to explain the cachexia. They typically appear alert despite their notable emaciation. At times, the diencephalic syndrome may be accompanied by nystagmus, suggesting chiasmatic involvement [Russell, 1951; Simpson et al., 1968].

Diagnosis

The diagnosis of brain tumors in infancy begins with clinical suspicion and then is confirmed by either CT or MRI. Although skull films may demonstrate split sutures and occasionally intracranial calcifications, their usefulness has been replaced by more modern imaging techniques [Jooma et al., 1984]. Cerebrospinal fluid examinations can be misleading because elevation in protein content or pleocytosis may represent a normal finding in infancy. Alternatively, these cerebrospinal fluid findings may suggest infection rather than tumor. Furthermore, the presence of blood in the cerebrospinal fluid may mislead the examiner into believing the child had a subarachnoid or intraventricular hemorrhage rather than bleeding into a necrotic tumor [Fessard, 1968].

The literature on the CT findings of infantile brain tumors is limited. The most striking abnormality on CT and MRI is the extremely large size of the tumor at diagnosis and the severity of hydrocephalus. In their series of children with brain tumors in the first year of life, Asai and colleagues [1989] reported diameters of tumors ranging from 4.6 to 16 cm (Fig. 71-45). MRI is very useful and is replacing CT as the procedure of choice, despite the need for anesthesia.

Once the diagnosis of a brain tumor in an infant is made, a search for neuraxis dissemination is axiomatic. Infants are much more likely to have cerebrospinal fluid metastases than older children with similar tumors [Allen and Epstein, 1982]. Therefore, MRI of the spine and cerebrospinal fluid cytology should be performed in children with medulloblastomas, ependymomas, primitive neuroectodermal tumors (including pineoblastomas), high-grade gliomas, and choroid plexus carcinomas. There have even been reports of infants with juvenile pilocytic astrocytomas with widespread cerebrospinal fluid dissemination [Perilongo et al., 1997a]. Extraneural metastases have also been reported with malignant brain tumors. Therefore, bone marrow biopsy and

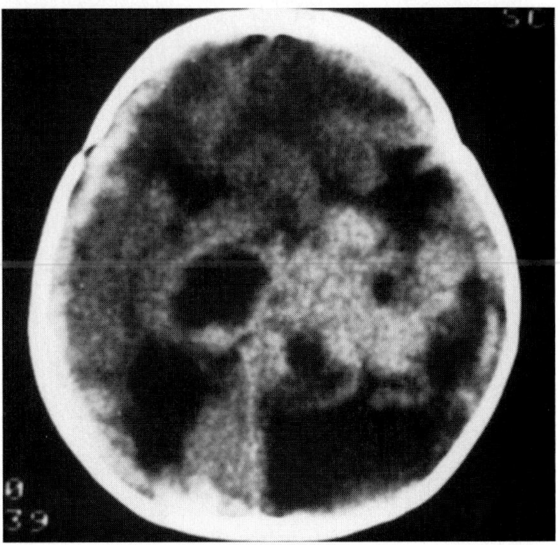

FIGURE 71-45. Contrast-enhanced CT of a 2-month-old child with a glioblastoma multiforme.

bone scan are indicated as part of the metastatic evaluation of children with medulloblastomas and primitive neuroectodermal tumors.

Management

Results of treatment of infants with brain tumors have been disappointing. Successful surgery in the infant with a brain tumor requires an experienced pediatric neurosurgeon, pediatric anesthesiologist, and pediatric intensive care support staff. Surgery of the very young infant is fraught with difficulties. Infants are sensitive to blood loss and hypothermia, and in the older series operative mortality ranged from 19% to 33% [Albright, 1985; Jooma et al., 1984; Raimondi and Tomita, 1983]. Most infants with brain tumors have hydrocephalus. Precraniotomy shunting will improve the infant's condition, but unfortunately provides an entry for malignant cells into the peritoneal cavity [Raimondi and Tomita, 1983]. Although in recent years the mortality associated with surgery has been reduced because of advances in surgery and anesthesia, the morbidity in this age group remains high [DiRocco et al., 1993]. Despite these caveats, surgery is curative in some patients. Choroid plexus papillomas, teratomas, and cerebellar astrocytomas that can be completely excised are associated with a high cure rate. Even in patients in whom the tumor cannot be removed entirely, repeated surgery may be useful at recurrence. Thus the child with a low-grade supratentorial astrocytoma may have surgery and then be followed longitudinally by CT or MRI. In many situations, these children may be monitored for several years before evidence of recurrence. If the child's tumor does recur before 3 years of age, repeated surgery, rather than radiation, may still be the treatment of choice. Thus radiation may be delayed until the child's brain is better able to tolerate this therapy (Fig. 71-46). Even in cases of malignant tumors such as medulloblastomas and ependymomas, the ability to achieve a gross total resection is the single most important indicator of survival [Duffner et al., 1993; 1996a].

In infants with malignant brain tumors, postoperative therapy must be provided. Standard radiation is poorly tolerated by the developing brain and consequently the total dose of radiation is usually decreased by 10% to 20%. This reduction in radiation may be inadequate for tumor control [Deutsch, 1982]. Unfortunately, despite this reduction in radiation dose, young children may still develop treatment-induced mental retardation, vasculopathy, leukoencephalopathy, endocrinopathies, and second malignancies (Fig. 71-47).

Several investigators have explored the concept of treating infants with brain tumors with postoperative chemotherapy in an effort to delay or eliminate radiation [Van Eys et al., 1985]. The largest published study of this approach, Baby POG, opened in 1986 [Duffner et al., 1993]. By closure in 1990, 198 children had been entered. Subsequent group-wide studies, Children's Cancer Group 9921 and Baby POG 2, had 299 and 330 children enrolled, respectively. European investigators have also been using postoperative chemotherapy with or without delayed radiation in children less than 3 years of age with brain tumors. Unfortunately, much of these data are not yet in press. Results vary depending on tumor type.

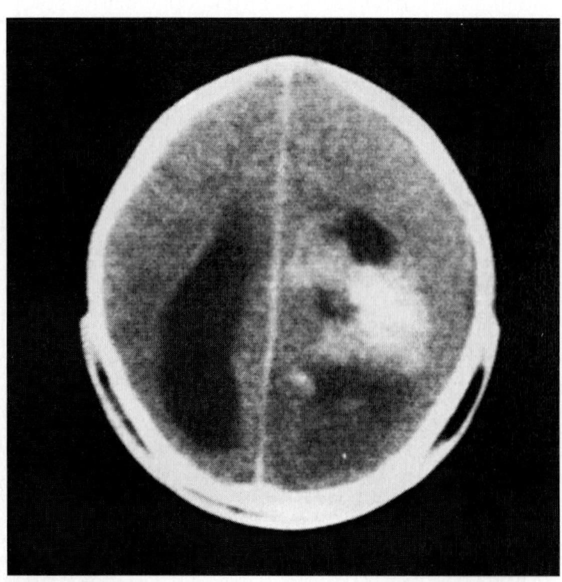

A

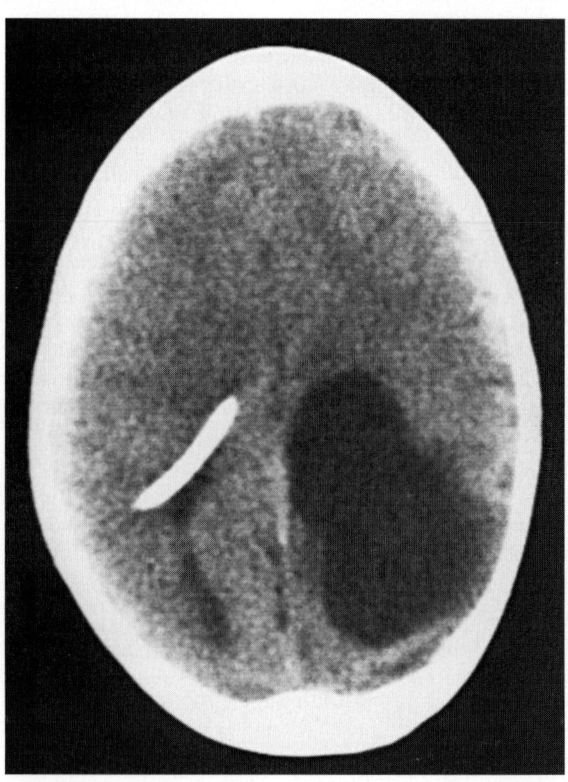

B

FIGURE 71-46. **A**, CT of a male neonate demonstrating a large low-grade astrocytoma. **B**, Same patient at 2 years of age. There has been no progression of the tumor since surgery. No other treatment was given.

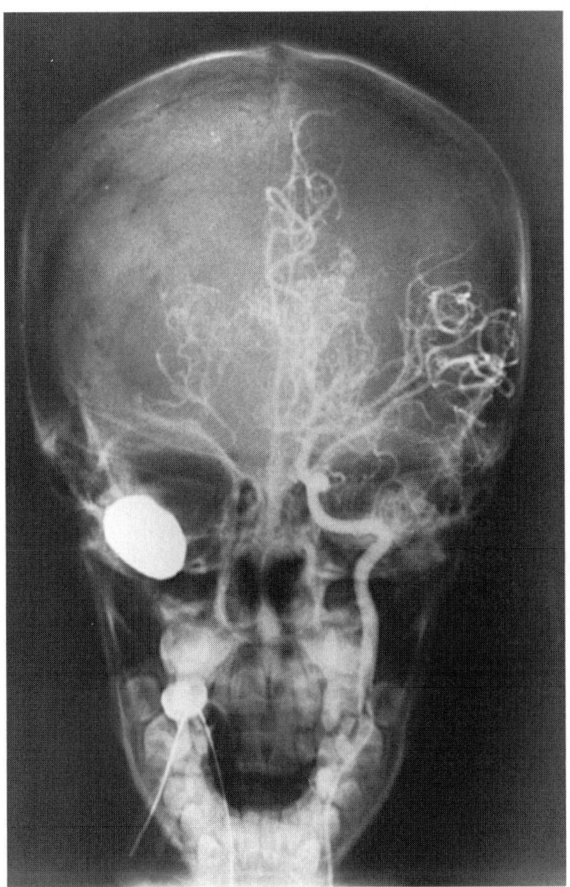

FIGURE 71-47. A 4-year-old patient who developed a severe radiation vasculopathy after radiation for a chiasmatic glioma at 15 months of age. Patient developed bilateral carotid occlusions with subsequent development of moyamoya pattern on serial angiograms.

MEDULLOBLASTOMAS

Sixty-two children younger than 3 years of age with medulloblastomas were treated on Baby POG [Duffner et al., 1993]. Response rates to two cycles of cyclophosphamide and vincristine were high, that is, 48%. Five-year overall survivals were 42%. In those children with a gross total resection, however, survivals were 62%, and in the best prognostic group, that is, gross total resection and no metastases at diagnosis, survival was 69%. Moreover, those children with a gross total resection and no metastases at diagnosis were treated with reduced neuraxis radiation, that is, 2400 cGy with 5000 cGy to the tumor bed and still had excellent survivals, affirming the chemosensitivity of these tumors. Whether eliminating radiation entirely in a subset of children will provide equivalent results, awaits the results of the second Baby POG and Children's Cancer Group infant studies.

EPENDYMOMAS

Forty-eight children younger than 3 years with ependymomas were treated on Baby POG, [Duffner et al., 1998b]. Response rates to two cycles of cyclophosphamide and vincristine were 48%. The overall survival was 40.5%, but in those children with gross total resection, survival was 61%. There was a significant difference in survival according to age less than 2 years versus 2 to 3 years, that is, 30% versus 58.8%, and in those with a gross total resection 37.5% versus 87.5%. The difference between the two groups, other than age, was that children younger than 2 years received chemotherapy for 2 years and then were irradiated, whereas older children received chemotherapy for 1 year and were irradiated. The results of this study strongly suggest that although radiation can be delayed safely for 1 year, it cannot be delayed for 2 years.

In contrast, the French Society of Pediatric Oncology treated 73 children younger than 5 years with ependymomas with postoperative chemotherapy including cycles of procarbazine plus carboplatin, cisplatin plus etoposide, and vincristine plus cyclophosphamide. Radiation was planned only for relapse. Of interest, no complete or partial responses were identified. The 4-year progression-free survival was 22%, whereas the overall survival was 59%. Forty percent of patients were alive without receiving radiation. Prognostic factors included gross total resection and supratentorial location [Grill et al., 2001].

CEREBRAL PRIMITIVE NEUROECTODERMAL TUMORS

Infants and young children with cerebral primitive neuroectodermal tumors have not done well compared with their older counterparts. In the first Baby POG study, the 5-year event-free survival was only 25% and 5-year survival was 27%. Among children with pineoblastomas, all died with widespread dissemination [Duffner et al., 1993; 1995a]. The French SFOP study of 25 children younger than 5 years with supratentorial embryonal tumors had similarly disappointing results. Twenty-four of 25 children relapsed with a median time of 5.5 months, and the 2-year disease-free survival was 4%. This group had been treated with postoperative chemotherapy consisting of cycles of carboplatin, procarbazine, cisplatin plus etoposide, and vincristine plus cyclophosphamide. A better prognosis was found in those with gross total resection (50% versus 8% 1-year event-free survival) and in those with hemispheric location [Marec-Berard et al., 2002].

MALIGNANT GLIOMAS

Whereas most infants and very young children have a significantly worse prognosis than older children with the same tumor pathology, malignant gliomas may be the exception. The first Baby POG study had 18 children younger than 3 years of age with malignant gliomas, including glioblastoma multiforme, anaplastic astrocytoma, and "malignant glioma." Of the 10 children evaluable for neuroradiologic response following two cycles of cyclophosphamide and vincristine, there were six partial responses, that is, more than 60%.

Survivals at 5 years were 50% and have remained stable. Of most interest, four children were not irradiated after 24 months of chemotherapy and none have developed recurrent disease [Duffner et al., 1996b]. Although the data from Baby POG 2 have not yet been published, infants with malignant gliomas also fared well.

RHABDOID TUMORS

One of the most challenging brain tumors in infancy are the atypical teratoid/rhabdoid tumors. These tumors were not diagnosed as separate entities on Baby POG 1, and were likely included in the medulloblastoma grouping. Thirty-six patients younger than 3 years with atypical teratoid/rhabdoid were treated on Baby POG 2 with a postoperative chemotherapy regimen composed of the Baby POG 1 chemotherapy regimen with dose intensification. Results were extremely poor, with all children dying, 31 of disease and 5 of complications from treatment [Strother et al., 2004]. Similarly poor results were reported in 9 children treated with a different postoperative intensive chemotherapy regimen with and without radiation. All died, with a mean survival of 10 months [Reinhardt et al., 2000].

Summary

When reviewing responses to treatment protocols, Collins' rule should be remembered. Tomita and McLone [1985] in a large review of children with malignant tumors during the first 24 months of life found that recurrence did not occur beyond the period of risk indicated by Collins's rule (see earlier) among patients with medulloblastomas, ependymomas, and primitive neuro-ectodermal tumors. However, among patients with astrocytomas, 50% of deaths occurred after the period of risk.

Although there have been advances in survival rates of older children with certain forms of brain tumors in the past 20 years, this improvement has not occurred to the same extent in very young children. Even within specific tumor types, children younger than 3 years of age have fared worse than older children. Not only do they respond poorly to standard therapy, but they are also at greater risk for treatment-induced neurotoxicity. The ultimate goal of prolonged postoperative chemotherapy is to eliminate radiation in those children who have no evidence of residual disease after completion of chemotherapy. Whether this is possible is currently unknown. It has become increasingly clear that although some tumors, such as ependymomas, may respond transiently to chemotherapy, radiation is necessary in most individuals for tumor control.

SPINAL CORD TUMORS

Neoplasms of the spinal cord are less common than those found intracranially. The accepted ratio of intracranial/intraspinal neoplasms for adults is 5:1, whereas for children, depending on the histology of the tumor, the ratio varies from 20:1 to 5:1 [Reimer and Onofrio, 1985]. The literature sugests a 10:1 ratio of adults to children for astrocytomas and 20:1 to 3:1 for ependymomas of the spinal cord [Kopelson et al., 1980].

Because of their relative rarity, there are few series of pediatric spinal cord tumors reported in the literature [Pascual-Castroviejo, 1990]. The large reported series in children are those of Hamby [1944], Matson [1969], and a report from the People's Republic of China [Cheng, 1982]. The Chinese report a much higher incidence of dysembryoplastic neoplasia (i.e., dermoids, epidermoids, teratomas, and chordomas) than is reported in the Western series.

Box 71-2 Common Mistaken Diagnoses in Children with Spinal Cord Tumors

Discitis	Scoliosis
Functional incontinence	Spondylitis
"Growing pains"	Torticollis
Guillain-Barré syndrome	Transverse myelitis
Muscular dystrophy	Trauma
Peripheral neuropathy	

Spinal cord tumors are most commonly found in the thoracic spinal cord followed by location in the cervical, thoracolumbar, and lumbosacral areas. Thus the divisions having the largest number of segments are areas associated with the highest incidence of tumor.

Clinical Characteristics

Signs and symptoms of spinal cord neoplasms can be insidious and misleading. History is often vague, and early in the course of the disease there may be a paucity of clinical signs. Consequently, a high incidence of erroneous diagnoses occurs, as well as a long delay from onset of symptoms until a definitive diagnosis is made (Box 71-2). Complaints may be nonspecific or so nondirected that the physician does not consider spinal cord disease. Common complaints are extremity weakness, abnormalities of gait, or pain in the extremities, back, or even periumbilical region [Baysefer et al., 2004; Murovic and Sundaresan, 1992; Robertson, 1992]. Unfortunately, consideration of a spinal cord mass may not enter the differential diagnosis until there is considerable progression or a spinal cord sensory level becomes obvious. In young children, because enuresis is common, a history of changing patterns of continence may not be elicited. In the very young, who are not bowel or bladder trained, sphincter abnormalities may be over-looked. A clue to the presence of a neurogenic bladder is incontinence of urine associated with crying or straining at stool. Loss of rectal tone is a common finding in pa-tients with spinal cord tumors. An abnormality suggesting a neoplasm of the cervical cord is torticollis [Kiwak et al., 1983].

Changes in posture, nonspecific complaints of back pain, or even unexplained abdominal pain may be associated with disease of the spinal cord. Pain may be classified as root, spinal, or tract in origin. Pain is more often dull, aching, burning, and diffuse, rather than sharp. Sharp pain is uncommon and results from either infiltration of the root entry zone or from swelling of the spinal cord with distortion of the root. Spinal pain refers to epidural or bony involvement adjacent to the tumor. This form of pain is usually dull and aching. Tract pain is vague and burning, whereas paresthesias suggest involvement of the dorsal columns [Epstein and Epstein, 1982]. Classic signs of a sensory level with or without a Brown-Séquard syndrome (i.e., symptoms associated with hemisection of the cord) are rarely encountered.

Any pain accentuated by either Valsalva's maneuvers, such as sneezing, coughing, or straining at stool, or by straight leg raising should be evaluated. These maneuvers, by stretching the meninges, may cause root irritation in a patient with compressive disease of the spinal canal.

Subtle physical findings may be mild scoliosis, discrepancy in foot or leg length, or vasomotor changes in the lower extremities. Findings of hyperreflexia, clonus, and Babinski's responses suggest disease of the corticospinal tracts. Proprioceptive, vibratory loss, or a sensory level, no matter how subtle, should raise suspicion of intraspinal pathology.

Diagnostic Studies

Unlike plain films of the skull, x-rays films of the vertebral column may yield considerable diagnostic information. Radiographs should be obtained in the anteroposterior, lateral, and, for the cervical spine, oblique projections. An increase in the interpedicular distance may suggest a long-standing intramedullary process (Fig. 71-48). Destructive changes of bone are more frequently associated with metastatic disease. Distortion or widening of the neuroforamina may be observed with extramedullary tumors, such as neurofibromas or metastatic disease to the spinal canal (Fig. 71-49). With slowly growing intraspinal tumors, the changing forces of an asymmetrical spinal lesion may alter vertebral growth in such a manner as to cause scoliosis. Bony abnormalities may be associated with a paravertebral soft tissue mass.

Diagnosis is confirmed by neuroimaging. MRI with gadolinium is the procedure of choice. MRI can visualize the entire length of the cord in the sagittal diameter. By this method, intramedullary masses can be readily separated from extramedullary lesions. Further, unlike myelography, MRI readily identifies intramedullary cysts (Fig. 71-50) [Berger et al., 1986; Norman et al., 1983].

Other diagnostic considerations include the use of cystometrograms and cystourethrograms. These techniques help to evaluate bladder function and may confirm the presence of a neurogenic bladder. Electromyography is rarely of much diagnostic use, although it helps to separate lower motor neuron unit disease from upper motor neuron unit disease and may help to establish the level of the lesion.

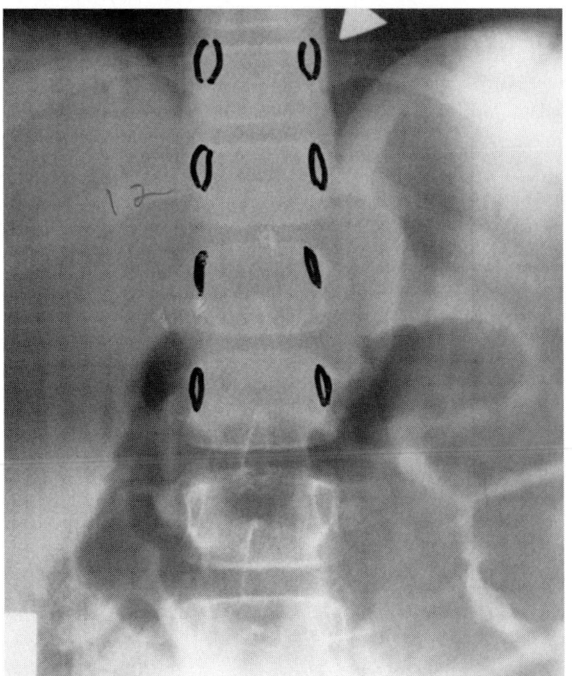

FIGURE 71-48. A 6-year-old male with myxopapillary ependymoma of the cauda equina. L5 spine demonstrates thinning of the pedicle and widening of the interpedicular distance.

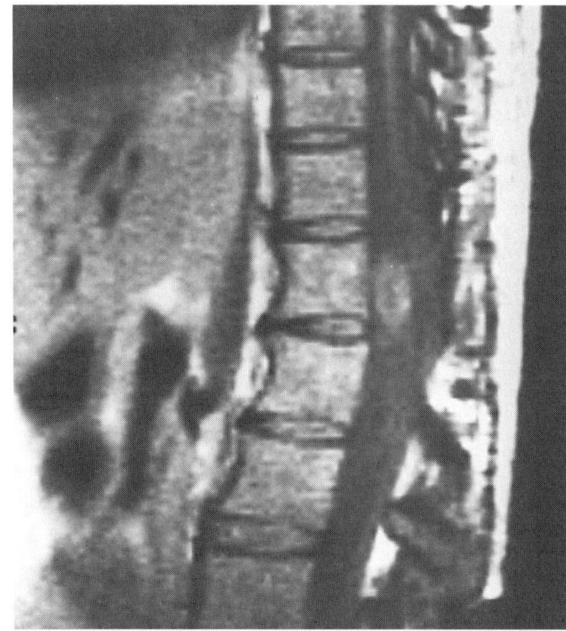

FIGURE 71-49. MRI in the sagittal plane demonstrating an extramedullary neurofibroma displacing the spinal cord posteriorly.

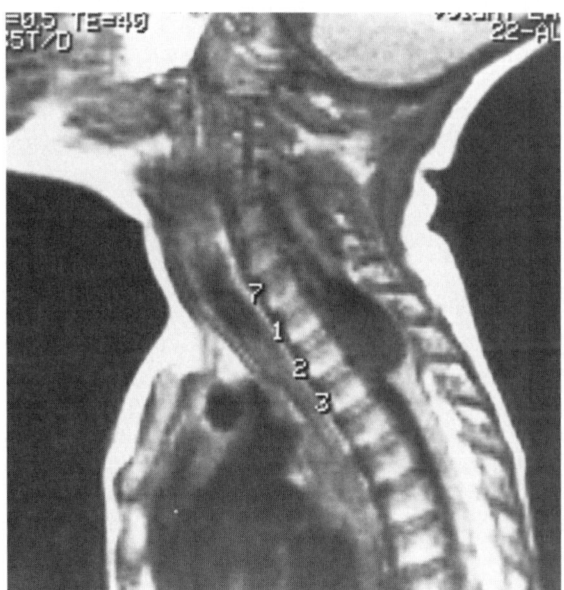

FIGURE 71-50. A 6-month-old patient with a large hydromyelic cavity. The cyst, which was not demonstrated by CT, is easily visualized by MRI.

In the presence of a suspected compressive lesion of the spinal cord, lumbar puncture must be performed judiciously. Protein content is invariably elevated. Froin's syndrome, clotting of cerebrospinal fluid after its removal, is attributed to marked elevation of cerebrospinal fluid protein. This syndrome usually signifies a complete block of the cerebrospinal fluid pathways between the lumbar thecal sac and the subarachnoid space above the area of the block. Cerebrospinal fluid pressure may be variable—either unobtainable or elevated. In an effort to prevent precipitous paraplegia, cerebrospinal fluid examination should be undertaken only

TABLE 71-4

Tumors of the Spinal Cord

INTRAMEDULLARY	EXTRAMEDULLARY
Astrocytomas	Neurofibromas
Cystic	Dysembryoblastic
Noncystic	Dermoids
Ependymomas	Epidermoids
Myxopapillary	Teratomas
Well-differeniated	Lipomas
Oligodendrogliomas	Meningiomas
	Arachnoid cysts
	Metastatic
	Neuroblastoma
	Sarcoma
	Lymphoma

when preparations are made for a subsequent, immediate decompressive laminectomy. In these situations, time is very important.

A rare observation has been the association of spinal cord tumors with increased intracranial pressure and papilledema [Celli et al., 1993]. The etiology for the papilledema has never been fully elucidated [Schijman et al., 1981]. In all likelihood, this association reflects a combination of decreased absorption of cerebrospinal fluid either secondary to hemorrhage within the tumor or as a result of a marked increase in cerebrospinal fluid protein. It is speculated that elevated protein may obstruct the arachnoid villi and axillary sleeves of the spinal roots, thereby limiting reabsorption of cerebrospinal fluid [Ucar et al., 1976].

Types of Tumors

Extramedullary Tumors

Traditionally, tumors of the spinal canal are divided into extramedullary and intramedullary masses (Table 71-4). Extramedullary masses erode the bony vertebral column, present asymmetrically, and involve those sensory and motor tracts placed laterally within the substance of the spinal cord parenchyma. These lesions are likely to represent metastases from sarcomatous or soft tissue masses, such as neuroblastoma, or may represent a more benign neurofibroma.

Patients with neurofibromatosis may have scalloping of the posterior aspects of the bodies of the vertebrae. If scalloping of the vertebrae is found over one or two segments rather than multiple segments, an intraspinal tumor should be considered. Extensive scalloping is more likely associated with dural ectasia. Dumbbell lesions, consisting of neurofibromas presenting both inside and outside the neuroforamina, are occasionally encountered. These tumors can be cured surgically.

Reticulum cell sarcomas, lymphomas, neuroblastomas, and other sarcomatous lesions usually present in the context of neoplasms found elsewhere in the body [Lewis et al., 1986]. In the spinal cord, they occur epidurally and present as compressive lesions. In some cases, metastatic lesions to the spinal canal can be treated with either radiation or chemotherapy without the need for decompressive laminectomy [Young et al., 1980]. Sarcomas may be quite radiosensitive, whereas neuroblastomas are less responsive. Meningiomas are rare in children, except in cases of neurofibromatosis 2 [MacCollin and Mautner, 1998].

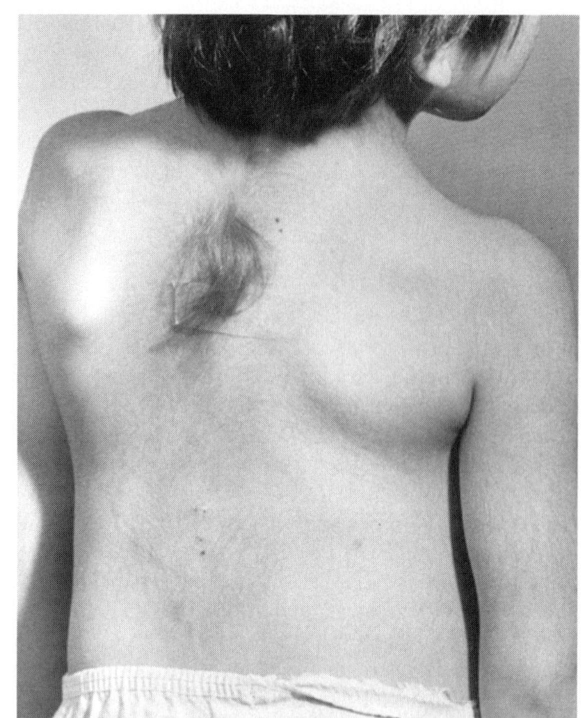

FIGURE 71-51. Hairy patch overlying the spinal cord of a child with spinal dysraphism.

Dysembryoplastic lesions are observed in the younger child. The findings of teeth, bones, or calcification on x-ray film should suggest a dermoid. These findings may be associated with a sinus tract leading from the surface and extending intraspinally. The presence of sinus tracts has been associated with recurrent meningitis. As with dermoids, tumors usually occur in the lumbosacral midline region, although they may occur anywhere in the spinal column, and may be associated with spina bifida, sacral dimple, port-wine nevus, or excessive clumps of coarse hair (Fig. 71-51). At surgery, the tract extends to the conus. Nerve roots of the cauda equina are often enmeshed in the fatty tumor with varying degrees of neurologic abnormalities. The serpiginous nature of these fatty tumors may make surgery difficult. Despite this problem, with or without surgery, patients often remain relatively stable with little progression of symptoms.

Intramedullary Tumors

Thirty-five percent of pediatric intraspinal tumors are intramedullary. Most intramedullary tumors in children are either astrocytomas or ependymomas. Astrocytomas are more common in younger children, whereas ependymomas are seen more often in adults [Houten and Weiner, 2000]. The mean duration of symptoms may vary from 1 day to 4 years [Reimer and Onofrio, 1985].

Astrocytomas present as a mass extending over multiple segments of the cord or the entire length of the spinal cord. They may be partially cystic [Epstein and Farmer, 1991]. Cysts are more common at the caudal end of the lesion and

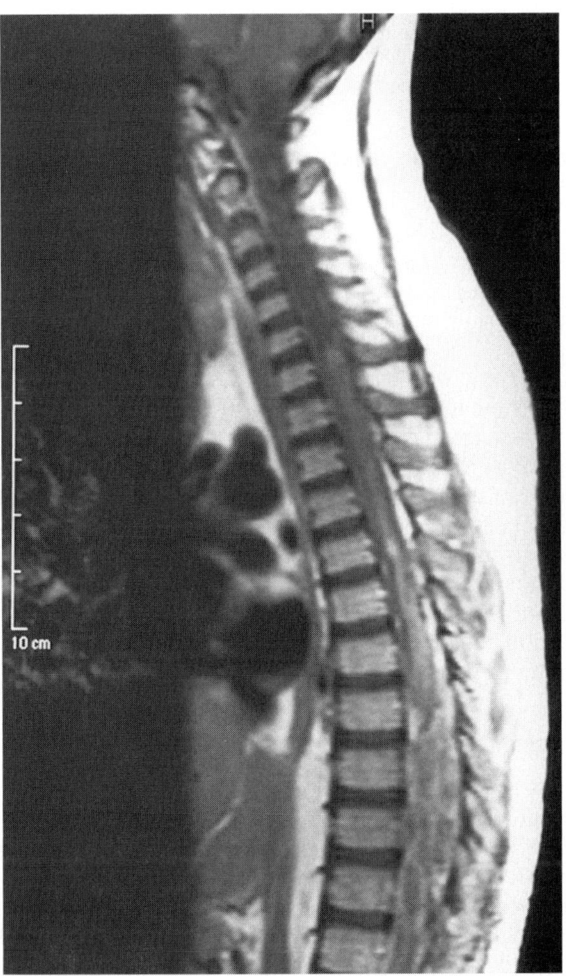

FIGURE 71-52. A 12-year-old child with glioblastoma of the spinal cord. Parents refused postoperative therapy. He developed extensive leptomeningeal dissemination throughout the brain and spinal cord.

may occur in 40% of intramedullary astrocytomas. The cystic component is readily identified by MRI. Because these tumors expand and compress normal tissue, they are more likely to produce slowly progressive signs rather than sudden interruption of neurologic function.

Astrocytomas of the spinal cord have hamartomatous features, consequently their natural history may be quite prolonged. Thus some have recommended a wide decompression with aspiration of cystic contents and bulk removal of the tumor [Epstein and Farmer, 1991; Matson, 1969]. In the presence of a gross total resection, no further therapy is needed [Nadkarni and Rekate, 1999]. Long-term survival of 90% with limited morbidity has been reported. Even in the face of dissemination, radiation can provide long-term survivals [Merchant et al., 2000). In contrast, high-grade astrocytomas of the spinal cord have a poor prognosis, often disseminating widely throughout the neuraxis (Fig. 71-52) [Epstein and Farmer, 1990]. The median survival of these tumors, despite therapy, is up to 12 months. They require, at a minimum, radiation.

Ependymomas are less common than astrocytomas. Ependymomas of the spinal cord are classified into two types: well-differentiated cellular or well-differentiated myxopapillary tumors. The myxopapillary tumor is more likely to involve the conus and cauda equina, whereas the more cellular tumors are found in the substance of the spinal cord. As with astrocytomas, treatment consists of laminectomy with decompression and attempt at total removal. Complete removal is the treatment of choice, resulting in cure [Nadkarni and Rekate, 1999]. In some cases a gross total resection is impossible due to the risks of severe morbidity. The response and need for radiation in both forms of this tumor are controversial. Some favor radiation for patients with subtotally resected cellular ependymomas of the spinal cord [Gilhuis et al., 2003]. The myxopapillary ependymoma is difficult to remove without causing neurologic deficits. As a result, limited resection followed by radiation has been recommended [Merchant et al., 2000] (Fig. 71-53). If a gross total resection can be achieved, however, no further therapy is needed [Gilhuis et al., 2003]. In general, the prognosis for ependymomas of the spinal cord is better than for astrocytoma, with 5-year survival rates of 72% to 100% [Epstein and Farmer, 1990].

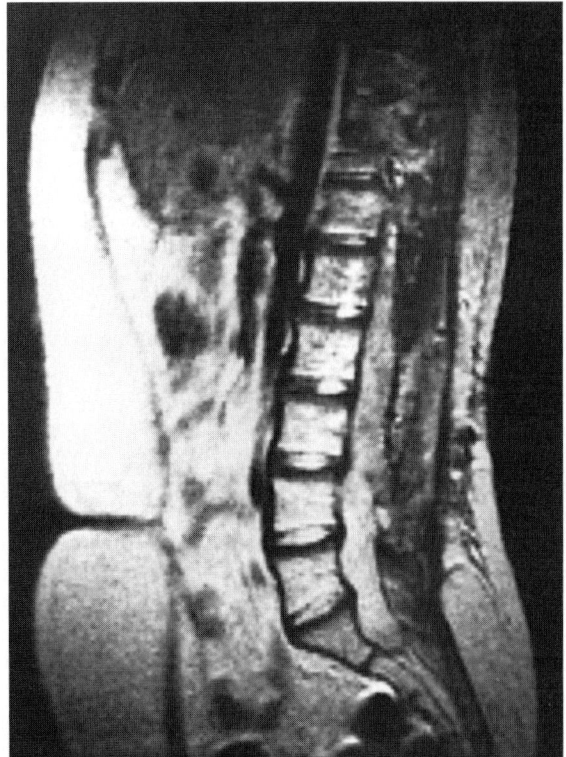

FIGURE 71-53. T2-weighted MRI signal revealing the extent of a myxopapillary ependymoma in a 12-year-old female.

Management

Surgery

After clinical suspicion and confirmation by neurodiagnostic procedures, surgical exploration and removal of tumor should be considered. In all cases, regardless of etiology and the extent of defect, surgical decompression is recommended. The spinal cord is resilient. In general, recovery depends on the length and duration of symptoms. Any evidence of compression of long tract motor or sensory function through the spinal cord limits hope for recovery.

The first report of a patient successfully treated with surgery for a neoplasm involving the spinal cord was by Gowers and Horsley [1888]. In the intervening 100 years there have been marked advances in neurodiagnosis and neurosurgical technology. These changes have resulted in improvements in survival rates. The bipolar coagulating forceps, first used in 1940, permits the surgeon to effectively remove intrinsic tumor without blood loss [Greenwood, 1963]. In 1976 the introduction of the dissecting microscope further enhanced the surgeon's ability to preserve small spinal cord vessels around a tumor [Yasargil et al., 1976]. More recently, the introduction of the ultrasonic surgical aspirator (CUSA system) and laser surgery has helped to minimize intraoperative trauma caused by traction and blunt dissection. The use of intraoperative ultrasonography has aided in defining solid neoplasm from associated intratumoral or extratumoral cysts. Cystic non-neoplastic lesions tend to occur at the rostral or caudal ends of a tumor, are smooth walled, and expand the cord symmetrically. Conversely, tumor cysts are asymmetrical, not smooth walled, and tend to be small. It has also been suggested that ultrasound is useful in planning myelotomies. Ultrasound allows exposure of the tumor at its most voluminous portion, thereby helping to minimize damage to functional neural tissue. Ultrasonography has also been helpful in differentiating astrocytomas from ependymomas of the spinal cord [Raghavendra et al., 1984]. Astrocytomas are relatively isodense and asymmetrical and exhibit heterogeneous signals presumably as a result of calcification or tumor cysts. Conversely, ependymomas are uniformly echogenic and expand symmetrically in a rostral caudal fashion. A tissue plane can be readily identified in ependymomas, whereas in astrocytomas tissue planes tend to blend into normal tissue. Furthermore, Epstein and Farmer [1991] suggested that a persistent abnormal signal will encourage tumor removal at a point at which direct inspection is unclear, which permits more radical resection of tumors previously viewed as inoperable.

In the past, surgical cautery and its associated transmitted heat and movement through tumor adjacent to normal spinal cord led to the destruction of functional tissue and significant morbidity and, as such, prevented significant debulking. In skilled hands the use of the laser and the ultrasonic surgical aspirator (CUSA system) coupled with the operating microscope allow destruction of tumor while preserving normal tissue [Epstein and Farmer, 1991]. Ultrasonic dissection using the CUSA system limits tissue fragmentation to 1 mm from the vibrating tip. Successful myelotomies from the upper cervical segment to the lumbar region with and without associated cysts have been associated with complete cure without reliance on other adjuvant forms of therapy.

At surgery, avoidance of damage to normal tissue can be aided by continuous monitoring of somatosensory evoked potentials. Changes may suggest reversible trauma or traction to the cord at surgery [Grundy, 1983]; however, the use of intraoperative evoked responses continues to remain controversial. During surgery, a loss of temporary signal without clinical correlation or neurologic deficit is frequently reported. The surgeon is often faced with a decision to either terminate the procedure for fear of inflicting irreversible neurologic deficit or continue in an effort to obtain maximum debulking [Epstein and Farmer, 1991]. Several studies, however, have suggested that monitoring somatosensory evoked potentials is beneficial [Kearse et al., 1993; Nadkarni and Rekate, 1999; Stechison et al., 1995].

Adjuvant Management

Radiation is recommended for subtotally resected spinal cord tumors; however, even this approach is not without controversy. Some have suggested that the cystic astrocytomas that occur over multiple segments in the spinal cord may be hamartomatous rather than neoplastic. As such, long-term survival can be expected with or without radiation. Conversely, the long-term survival of most patients with astrocytomas is worse than for patients with ependymomas. Many suggest radiation of all subtotally resected intramedullary tumors, regardless of histology. Recommended radiation doses to the lesion range between 2500 and 5000 cGy in 180 to 200 cGy fractions with a margin of 2 to 3 cm [Kopelson et al., 1980]. The volume to be irradiated should be local, with a margin of one or two vertebral bodies [O'Sullivan et al., 1994]. Furthermore, some suggest that radiation may improve preoperative deficits and lead to improved functional results.

Chemotherapy

There are only limited reports of the use of chemotherapy in low-grade astrocytomas of the spinal cord [Balmaceda, 2000]. Most commonly, varying combinations of carboplatin and vincristine have been used. Two of three such studies reported complete responses with durable remissions (although one patient was 30 years old) [Bouffet et al., 1997; Foreman et al., 1998; Lowis et al., 1998].

There is more experience with high-grade astrocytomas. "Eight in one" was not found to be better than CCNU and vincristine [Allen et al., 1998]. However, several reports of more intensive chemotherapy including one of high-dose chemotherapy followed by autologous bone marrow transplantation with and without radiation produced either complete responses or stable disease [Finlay, 1996; Lowis et al., 1998; Weiss et al., 1997].

The experience with chemotherapy in ependymomas of the spinal cord is exceedingly limited. More research needs to be done in this area, particularly for very young children with intramedullary tumors that have not been completely resected.

Complications

The main complications after treatment of spinal cord tumors are orthopedic. Depending on the extent of the laminectomy and the degree of instability that results from removal of the posterior elements of the vertebral column, significant orthopedic abnormalities may occur. Radiation-associated arachnoiditis or myelopathy also contributes to orthopedic abnormalities. Location of the tumor, age, dose, volume of radiation, and extent of surgery influence the degree of deficit [Fraser et al., 1977; Marks and Adler, 1982; Peschel et al., 1983]. Non-neurologic complications are kyphoscoliosis and, after radiation, limited growth of the vertebral column (Fig. 71-54). The recognition of the dynamic forces that occur in the growing spine has led many to seek a more conservative approach to treatment. The use

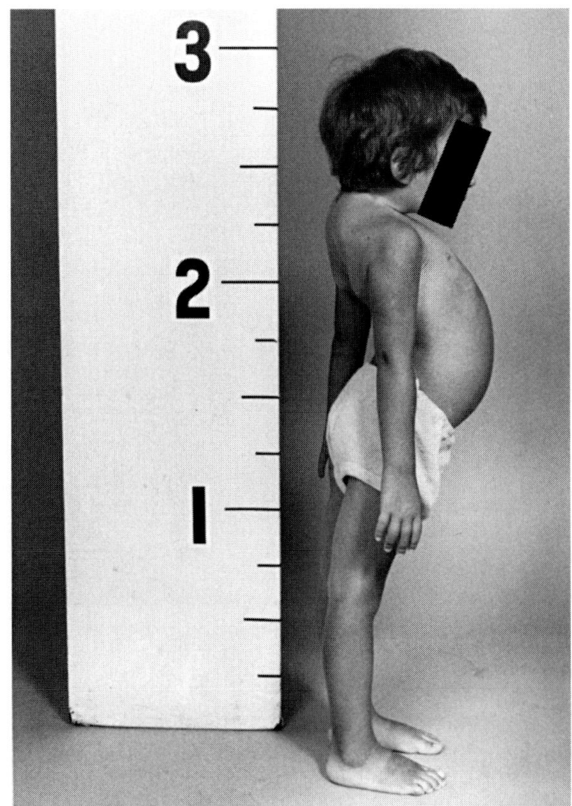

FIGURE 71-54. Severe kyphoscoliosis secondary to spinal surgery and radiation for a cervical cord astrocytoma.

of microsurgical techniques has, to some extent, limited extensive laminectomies. Postoperative bracing and physical therapy can help retard but not prevent the development of significant orthopedic abnormalities [Raimondi et al., 1976; Reimer and Onofrio, 1985].

Neurologic complications after surgical treatment may be flaccid or spastic paraplegia or quadriplegia and bowel or bladder incontinence. Decubitus ulcers, pathologic fractures, and dislocated hips may occur because of loss of trophic neurologic input. Although treatment may be curative, morbidity can be significant. Skilled and continuous rehabilitative care is necessary to maximize the quality of life in such patients.

In conclusion, the prognosis for patients with spinal cord tumors is much better than that for the child with an intracranial tumor. Surgical intervention may delay the growth and progression of these tumors. In the more aggressive tumors, surgery, coupled with judicious use of radiotherapy, has been associated with long-term survival or cure. Unfortunately, morbidity is quite significant. The insidious nature of spinal cord tumors, their relative rarity, and their lack of clinical specificity continue to challenge the most astute neurologic clinicians.

NEUROLOGIC COMPLICATIONS OF LEUKEMIA

Leukemia

Leukemia is the most common malignancy in childhood. In the 1960s, the use of systemic chemotherapy in the treatment of children with acute lymphoblastic leukemia dramatically increased the incidence of bone marrow remission, but approximately 50% of patients developed CNS relapse [Evans et al., 1970]. The introduction of CNS prophylaxis using intrathecal methotrexate reduced this complication to 25% of patients; later the use of cranial radiation therapy in addition to intrathecal methotrexate decreased CNS leukemia to 10% [Holland, 1976]. CNS complications of leukemia relate either to failure of therapy or to adverse effects of this therapy. If CNS leukemia were not prevented, multiple sites in the CNS might become directly involved, including the meninges, brain parenchyma, dural sinuses, and nerve roots. Complications of the disease and treatment include cerebrovascular accidents, infection, and leukoencephalopathy.

Meningeal Leukemia

Infiltration of the superficial arachnoid membrane is the first stage of meningeal leukemia. Leukemic cells are found in the trabeculae of the arachnoid and walls of veins at a time when cells are not commonly identified in the cerebrospinal fluid. In grade II meningeal leukemia, the superficial arachnoid becomes more extensively involved, and the deep arachnoid membrane is infiltrated by tumor cells. The cerebrospinal fluid is consistently contaminated by leukemic cells. Malignant cells penetrate deeply into the Virchow-Robin spaces, but the parenchyma is protected by the pial-glial membrane. In grade III meningeal leukemia, the pial-glial membrane is destroyed and leukemic cells enter the parenchyma. At this stage, there is extensive leukemic involvement of both superficial and deep arachnoid, as well as invasion of the cerebrospinal fluid [Price and Johnson, 1973].

Patients with meningeal leukemia may develop communicating hydrocephalus, presumably secondary to collections of leukemic cells in the subarachnoid space over the surface of the cortex and in the basal cisterns. These cells, by prohibiting or delaying the resorption of cerebrospinal fluid through the arachnoid villi back into the venous system, cause hydrocephalus and increased intracranial pressure [Pierce, 1962]. The child with leptomeningeal disease consequently develops signs and symptoms of increased intracranial pressure, such as headache, early morning vomiting, irritability, papilledema, and nuchal rigidity [Pinkerton and Chessells, 1984]. The association of fever with meningismus may mimic bacterial meningitis. Lumbar puncture reveals increased pressure, pleocytosis, increased protein, and decreased glucose. Blast cells may be identified on cytocentrifugation but in some cases, morphology may be atypical or cell numbers low. In general, high cerebrospinal fluid pressure correlates with high cell counts. Protein elevation is seen in approximately 50% of patients, although values rarely exceed 100 mg/dL. Cerebrospinal fluid glucose has been reported to be less than half the blood glucose level in 60% of patients, but of interest, there is no correlation with cellular response [Pierce, 1962].

Leukemic infiltration of cranial nerves is another typical presenting sign of leptomeningeal disease. Cranial nerves II, VI, VII, and VIII are most commonly involved. Ophthalmic complications of leukemia are found in approximately 9% of children. Involvement of the optic nerve by leukemic infiltration is but one cause of visual problems in patients with leukemia [Ridgway et al., 1976; Weaver et al., 1986].

Although loss of vision is usually due to infiltration of the optic nerve, retinal bleeding and infiltration of the retina, iris, and orbit are also found. Rarely, leukemic infiltration in the subarachnoid space bathing the visual cortex may lead to cortical blindness [Ha et al., 1980].

Cranial nerve VI paresis is usually a nonlocalizing sign of increased intracranial pressure. However, leukemic infiltration of the nerve may also occur.

Facial paresis may occur from infiltration of cranial nerve VII anywhere along its course. Disease may be found intracranially, in the internal auditory meatus, in the middle ear, or at the stylomastoid foramen. At times, facial paresis secondary to leukemic infiltration may be misdiagnosed as a Bell's palsy [Murthy et al., 2002].

Vestibular dysfunction may relate to involvement of the membranous labyrinth by tumor or blood. Sensorineural deafness results from damage either to the intracranial portion of cranial nerve VIII as it enters the pons or from involvement of the end organ. Hearing loss may occur from either mechanism or as a complication of therapy. In addition, conductive deafness occurs when the middle ear is affected by the leukemic process.

The complaint of a numb chin, even with no other findings, suggests infiltration of the mentalis nerve.

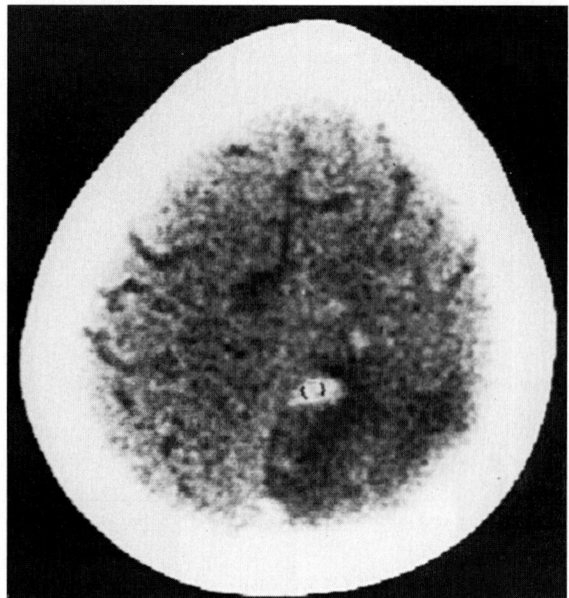

FIGURE 71-55. Axial CT demonstrating an intracerebral hemorrhage secondary to L-asparaginase.

Dural Sinus Thrombosis

Dural sinus thrombosis is a rare complication of CNS leukemia. It may occur while the child is in remission. Sagittal sinus thrombosis may be the cause of increased intracranial pressure in children with acute lymphoblastic leukemia in the absence of cerebrospinal fluid pleocytosis. The etiology is obscure but may be related to leukemic infiltration of the dural sinus or secondary to chemotherapy, such as L-asparaginase [David et al., 1975; Ganick et al., 1978].

Stroke

Hemorrhagic and ischemic strokes occur in 4% of children with acute lymphoblastic leukemia [Packer et al., 1985]. The majority occur within the first year after diagnosis or when the child is no longer responsive to therapy. Hemorrhage commonly develops secondary to thrombocytopenia, disseminated intravascular coagulation, or hematologic toxicity associated with chemotherapy. Patients with low platelet counts and minor head trauma are also at risk for epidural and subdural hematomas, which are readily identified by CT. Patients may occasionally have CNS hemorrhage at diagnosis. Hemorrhage may occur in patients who have a rapid increase of leukocytes to levels of more than 100,000/mm^3. Tendency to hemorrhage appears to be related to the increased viscosity of the blood. Disproportionately high hemoglobin and platelet counts are identified in some patients. With the increased packed cell volume and increased viscosity, cerebroleukostasis and massive hemorrhage follow. Hemorrhage can also develop secondary to expanding leukemic collections within the arachnoid that compress blood vessels. Vascular perfusion of surrounding brain is consequently reduced, leading to ischemic damage, necrosis, and intracerebral hemorrhage [Price and Johnson, 1973]. Patients with elevated white blood cell count levels may also develop thrombotic stroke. More commonly, the cerebrovascular accident is a complication of therapy. The major causative chemotherapeutic agent is L-asparaginase (Fig. 71-55) [Priest et al., 1980]. Typically, thrombotic stroke occurs at the end of induction and presents either as an acute venous sinus thrombosis with seizures and coma or as focal arterial thrombosis. The latter is associated with focal seizures and focal neurologic deficit. L-Asparaginase produces either thrombotic or hemorrhagic stroke, in part because of its tendency to prolong plasma clotting time, lower concentrations of factors IX and XI, depress levels of antithrombin 3, protein C, plasminogen, and produce hypofibrinogenemia [Priest et al., 1980]. Pretreatment with fresh frozen plasma is recommended by some authors [Feinberg and Swenson, 1988].

Other predisposing conditions for stroke in children with acute lymphoblastic leukemia are dehydration and CNS infection. Bacterial or viral sepsis may produce disseminated intravascular coagulation and thrombotic stroke. This condition may mimic a diffuse metabolic encephalopathy, albeit with focal features. The diagnosis may be obscure because the initial area of thrombosis may be in the brain, whereas the systemic manifestations of disseminated intravascular coagulation may not appear for 24 to 48 hours. Fungal meningitis, especially aspergillosis, has been associated with secondary arterial strokes [Packer et al., 1985].

Hypothalamic Syndrome

Hypothalamic infiltration by leukemic cells leads to a syndrome characterized by hyperphagia, headache, vomiting, and increased intracranial pressure. This syndrome was first reported in 1954. Patients with acute lymphoblastic leukemia developed sudden weight gain and voracious appetite. Before CNS prophylaxis, this complication occurred in 15% to 25% of patients with CNS recurrence. Evidence of hypothalamic infiltration dramatically decreased after CNS prophylaxis became routine. Presumably, infiltration of leukemic cells into the ventromedian nucleus of the hypothalamus (satiety center) and the lateral hypothalamus (feeding center) leads to uncontrolled increase in appetite and obesity. Patients with this complication are frequently in bone marrow remission [Greydanus et al., 1978]. Recognition that an increase in appetite and weight gain may represent CNS disease rather than a side effect of steroid therapy may lead to earlier intervention.

Seizures

The incidence of seizures in a population of children with acute lymphoblastic leukemia ranges from 4% to 13%. Approximately two thirds do not have an obvious etiology. Identified etiologies are leukemic infiltration, venous or arterial thrombosis, rapid cell lysis, hemorrhage due to thrombocytopenia, infection, drug complications, or leukoencephalopathy [Ochs et al., 1984]. The majority of seizures are partial simple seizures with or without secondary generalization. Absence seizures and partial complex seizures are rare. Patients often have seizures during therapy but approximately half the children are in remission; the others have a history of prior meningeal leukemia with or without bone marrow relapse.

Seizures have been reported in children within a week following intrathecal methotrexate, of which 50% in one study had prior meningeal leukemia [Maytal et al., 1995]. Seizures may also occur acutely in the presence of intrathecal methotrexate (<2%). Seizures may occur as isolated events or in the face of methotrexate chemical meningitis, a syndrome characterized by fever, headache, dizziness, back pain, nausea, and vomiting. Because methotrexate interferes with dihydrofolate reductase and the reduction of tetrahydrobiopterin, this reaction may secondarily decrease the availability of γ-aminobutyric acid, an inhibitory neurotransmitter, leading to increased seizure susceptibility. Methotrexate is known to be associated with the development of leukoencephalopathy and seizures, especially in patients who have previously received cranial irradiation or in those who have CNS leukemia. CT scans in these patients may reveal evidence of leukoencephalopathy (i.e., ventriculomegaly, calcification, hypodense areas) [Peylan-Ramu et al., 1978]. More recently, intravenous methotrexate, when given frequently and in high doses, has caused leukoencephalopathy in nonirradiated children without CNS disease. In addition to methotrexate-induced complications, seizures may occur with administration of cisplatin due to the development of syndrome of inappropriate antidiuretic hormone, resulting in hyponatremia [Mead et al., 1982]. Another agent, vincristine, may cause the syndrome of inappropriate antidiuretic hormone release with resulting seizures, but seizures have also been reported 5 to 6 days following vincristine when there were no metabolic derangements [Johnson et al., 1973]. L-Asparaginase increases the risk of seizures as well, especially in the presence of hemorrhagic stroke. Metabolic causes of seizures include hyponatremia, hypoglycemia, hypocalcemia, and hypomagnesemia. Narcotics and antiemetics, used commonly in this population, can also lower the seizure threshold.

The evaluation of the child with leukemia and seizures should include assessment of electrolytes, glucose, coagulation studies, and lumbar puncture for cytology, protein, glucose, and bacterial, fungal, and viral cultures. MRI, magnetic resonance venography, and arteriography should also be performed.

The choice of anticonvulsants is problematic for those children still on chemotherapy. Drug-drug interactions may affect the levels of chemotherapy agents as well as anticonvulsants. For example, both phenobarbital and phenytoin displace methotrexate from plasma proteins that then increases the risk of methotrexate neurotoxicity. In addition, because anticonvulsants are given on a daily basis and chemotherapy is given in cycles, dose adjustments can be very difficult.

Another issue with anticonvulsants is their effect on white blood counts, platelets, and liver function. Carbamazepine, for example, commonly causes leukopenia and valproic acid may cause thrombocytopenia, especially in the face of viral infections. Valproic acid, phenytoin, and carbamazepine all have been reported to cause hepatotoxicity. For those children receiving cranial irradiation, phenytoin should be avoided because of the association with erythema multiforme and Stevens-Johnson syndrome [Delattre et al., 1988]. Treating a child with leukemia and seizures may be problematic, making it difficult to know whether hematologic or hepatic abnormalities reflect the leukemia, the chemotherapy, or the anticonvulsants. The newer anticonvulsants such as gabapentin and levetiracetam are not metabolized in the liver and have limited hematologic and hepatic toxicity. As such, they are better choices for these children.

Chemotherapy-Associated Myelopathy

Myelopathy has been reported following intrathecal methotrexate, particularly in children with meningeal disease. It has also been reported, however, in children without CNS leukemia. Cytosine arabinoside has also been implicated in causing myelopathy, even in the absence of methotrexate. Prior radiation to the spinal cord as well as total dose and frequency of drug administration are risk factors [Dunton et al., 1986].

Patients present with weakness or paralysis, a sensory level and loss of bowel and bladder function occurring either immediately or within a short time following chemotherapy. The thoracic cord is primarily affected. There have also been reports of ascending paralysis and death that have occurred as late as 5 weeks following therapy. Just as concerning are cases of progressive paraplegia occurring months after completion of intrathecal therapy [Hahn et al., 1983; McLean et al., 1994; Watterson et al., 1994].

The pathology associated with cytosine arabinoside myelopathy is microvacuolization without inflammation while methotrexate-associated myelopathy has been associated with white matter necrosis and sparing of gray matter [Watterson et al., 1994]. A syndrome that resembles poliomyelitis has also been reported, with destruction of anterior horn cells [Reznik, 1979].

Evaluation includes MRI of the spine and cerebrospinal fluid examination. There is an increase in cerebrospinal fluid protein in approximately half the patients. Elevation in myelin basic protein has been reported to be predictive of future myelopathy [Bates et al., 1985].

The prognosis is poor, with most children dying or remaining permanently paraplegic. There is no effective treatment.

Spinal Cord Compression

Spinal cord compression, an unusual complication of acute lymphoblastic leukemia, occurs in less than 1% of patients [Pui et al., 1985]. It is three times more common in myelogenous than lymphoid leukemia [Lo et al., 1985]. Compression may develop secondary to tumor infiltration. As in other causes of spinal cord compression, patients may have back pain, progressive weakness of lower extremities, and urinary and fecal incontinence. Sensation is generally affected. Diagnosis is often delayed or not recognized in patients treated for acute lymphoblastic leukemia because these symptoms are erroneously believed to be due to neuropathy from chemotherapy rather than secondary to spinal cord disease. Vincristine may cause weakness of the lower extremities and reflex changes, and prednisone may cause proximal muscle weakness and polyuria [Allen, 1978]. Furthermore, complaints of leg pain may be presumed secondary to bone involvement rather than root infiltration [Sullivan, 1963].

The conus medullaris syndrome, characterized by fecal and urinary incontinence with loss of sensation over S2, S3, and S4 dermatomes in the absence of motor weakness, has rarely been reported in acute lymphoblastic leukemia. This syndrome relates to leukemic infiltration of the sacral cord, although it may also be secondary to hemorrhage. Infiltration of the cauda equina by leukemic cells produces a syndrome similar to that of the conus medullaris but distinguished clinically by the presence of asymmetrical weakness or paralysis before sphincter involvement [Peturrson and Boggs, 1981].

The usual site of cord compression is in the thoracic or lumbar region. The lesion is generally epidural and should be readily demonstrated by MRI. Cerebrospinal fluid protein is usually elevated, at times reaching levels of 1000 mg/dL [Peturrson and Boggs, 1981].

Intramedullary lesions, characterized by perivascular cuffing and diffuse myelitis, are much less common. In these cases the picture may be confused with transverse myelitis.

Treatment must be instituted as soon as possible. Local radiation in a dose of 3000 cGy and high-dose dexamethasone are recommended. Laminectomy is rarely necessary because of the sensitivity of the leukemic cells to radiation [Pui et al., 1985]. Results of treatment are generally good, with rapid response to therapy.

Another cause of spinal cord compression is epidural or subdural hematoma in patients who receive lumbar punctures in the presence of thrombocytopenia. In suspected cases, CT or MRI of the affected area will demonstrate blood in the epidural or subdural space. Early evacuation is necessary to prevent permanent neurologic residual.

Infection

Bacterial meningitis is surprisingly uncommon in children with leukemia, which in part relates to the early administration of antibiotics in children with suspected infections. Symptoms such as headache, meningismus, and disorientation should suggest the possibility of bacterial meningitis. Cerebrospinal fluid must be evaluated for the different bacterial, viral, and fungal agents. Meningitis secondary to *Listeria monocytogenes* is suggested by the presence of gram-positive rods in the cerebrospinal fluid. Appropriate therapy includes intravenous ampicillin and gentamicin.

Cryptococcal meningitis is seen in patients with leukemia and other forms of cancer. India ink preparations are positive in 50% of patients. Culture and examination for cryptococcal antigen confirm the diagnosis. Therapy includes systemic amphotericin B in combination with 5-flucytosine.

Brain abscess is suggested by the presence of focal neurologic findings and low-grade fevers. Diagnosis of a bacterial brain abscess is made by MRI or CT with a characteristic ring-enhancing lesion. Cultures may reveal bacterial involvement with either aerobic or anaerobic bacteria. In the presence of pulmonary lesions, *Aspergillus, Mucor, Candida,* and *Nocardia* brain abscesses are more likely (Fig. 71-56). The CT appearance of abscess in fungal disease is usually a poorly circumscribed, low-density area without a capsule [Hara et al., 1984]. Treatment is sulfamethoxazole (Bactrim) for *Nocardia* and amphotericin for fungi (see Chapter 70) [Pizzo, 1981].

Viral encephalitis in patients with leukemia is usually caused by herpes simplex, varicella-zoster, and rubeola. *Toxoplasma gondii* also has a predilection for the CNS. In addition to evidence of CNS involvement characterized by seizures, focal motor deficits, and cranial neuropathies, patients may have more widespread involvement affecting lung, heart, liver, and spleen. There have been several reports of an atypical form of measles encephalitis in children with acute lymphoblastic leukemia who are in remission. Mortality is high, and the diagnosis may be difficult to establish [Campbell et al., 1977].

Previously children with leukemia commonly had cerebrospinal fluid reservoirs placed in an effort to facilitate drug administration. Unfortunately, these reservoirs were foreign bodies and were a nidus for infection [Machado et al., 1985].

LONG-TERM EFFECTS OF CENTRAL NERVOUS SYSTEM THERAPY

As more children with CNS neoplasia survive their disease, the long-term effects of therapy become increasingly

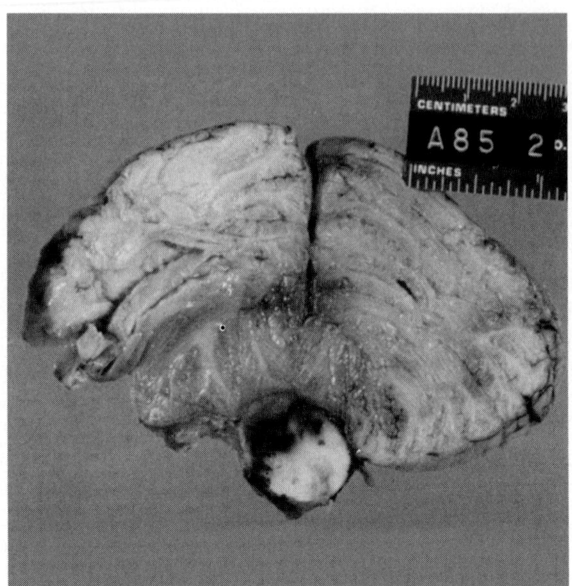

FIGURE 71-56. Gross pathologic section of a patient with acute lymphoblastic leukemia who developed CNS aspergillosis.

relevant. Most studies concerning the late effects of treatment have centered on cranial irradiation in children with leukemia and brain tumors. Chemotherapy is associated with more severe acute toxicity, and the long-term effects have been less well studied than those of radiation [Duffner, 2004a; 2004b].

Radiation

The most common of the early delayed effects of radiation therapy on the cerebrum is the somnolence syndrome. Somnolence associated with anorexia, apathy, and headache occurs 6 to 8 weeks after radiation, with symptoms lasting from 4 to 14 days. Symptoms generally resolve without mental or physical sequelae. First recognized by Druckman in 1929, this syndrome was then reported again in 1973 by Freeman and co-workers, who described the somnolence syndrome in children irradiated for acute lymphoblastic leukemia [Freeman et al., 1973].

A severe form of the early delayed effect of radiation was reported by Lampert and Davis in 1964. This condition is a rapidly progressive syndrome of ataxia, cranial neuropathies, focal motor signs, nystagmus, and death developing over days to weeks after the termination of radiation therapy. Pathology reveals demyelination within the field of radiation therapy, as well as pronounced microglial and astrocytic proliferation [Lampert and Davis, 1964].

Radiation Necrosis

One of the late delayed effects of radiation therapy is radiation necrosis. Radiation necrosis is estimated to occur in 5% of patients between 6 months and 2 years after completion of treatment. Risk increases with total dose and fraction size. Symptoms range from memory loss, dementia, personality change, and agitation to those of recurrent tumor, especially increased intracranial pressure. The pathology is primarily vascular, affecting the endothelium of small arteries and arterioles and leading to thrombosis and ischemia. White matter is also selectively involved with loss of myelin. Differentiating radiation necrosis from recurrent brain tumors is sometimes difficult because both may be associated with elevation in cerebrospinal fluid protein, focal EEG slow wave activity, an avascular mass on angiography, and presence of a mass lesion with a decreased attenuation coefficient and variable enhancement on CT [Marks et al., 1981; Martins et al., 1977]. MRI patterns vary, including a single lesion at or near the site of the original tumor, multiple lesions, subependymal lesions, or lesions remote from the original tumor. Single-photon emission CT and, more reliably, positron emission tomography now offer the potential of distinguishing radiation necrosis from recurrent tumors. However, the ability of positron emission tomography to distinguish these is only 43% [Thompson et al., 1999]. Magnetic resonance spectroscopy may also be useful in differentiating tumor recurrence from radiation necrosis. Patients with postradiation necrosis are more likely to have reduced *N*-acetylaspartate but preserved choline peaks compared with patients with tumor recurrence in which choline is increased [Usenius et al., 1995]. The incidence of radionecrosis has increased with the use of stereotactic radiosurgery, gamma knife, and brachytherapy.

The course of radiation necrosis varies, ranging from spontaneous resolution to stabilization to progression. Steroids are used to decrease acute edema. Others have suggested anticoagulation. Additional agents being studied include pentobarbital, desferoxamine, and pentoxifylline. Surgery is indicated in those with significant mass effect [Glass et al., 1984].

Moyamoya Syndrome

Moyamoya syndrome, a form of late-onset radiation vasculopathy, is a syndrome of basilar stenotic and occlusive disease occurring in the large arteries of the circle of Willis, the terminal parts of the internal carotid artery, and the proximal portions of the middle cerebral and anterior cerebral arteries. Symptoms include transient ischemic attacks, seizures, motor weakness, dementia, and frank strokes. The stenosis is gradual, leading to the development of an extensive collateral circulation. The patient at greatest risk of developing moyamoya syndrome is the child with neurofibromatosis 1 who is younger than 5 years of age and who has been irradiated to the hypothalamic-chiasmatic region with doses greater than 50 Gy. The treatment for this condition is encephaloduroarteriosynangiosis. A segment of the scalp artery is placed on the surface of the brain in order to improve collateral flow. If successful, no further deterioration will occur [Bitzer and Topka, 1995; Kestle et al, 1993; Omura et al, 1997].

Radiation Myelopathy

Radiation myelopathy may occur as a transient phenomenon 6 weeks to 6 months following radiation. This is a temporary condition characterized by L'Hermitte's sign (i.e., electrical buzzing sensations in the limbs and body brought on by movement of the neck) with transient demyelination of the posterior columns and lateral spinothalamic tracts. A much more serious form of radiation myelopathy is the delayed form that occurs months to years following radiation therapy. Patients develop acute or progressive paraplegia or quadriplegia, a sensory level, and loss of bowel and bladder function [Liu et al., 2001]. Radiation myelopathy correlates with total dose (>6000 cGy) and fraction size (>200 cGy). Pathology reflects demyelination and vascular changes including endothelial thickening, vasculitis, telangiectasia, and fibrinoid necrosis. MRI initially reveals spinal cord edema with ring enhancement, but over time spinal cord atrophy develops. Treatment includes steroids for acute edema. Anticoagulation has also been proposed to prevent further damage to the endothelium of small blood vessels [Liu et al., 2001]. Prognosis is poor.

Disturbances in Intellectual Function in Children with Leukemia

The long-term effects of cranial radiation therapy on intellectual function were initially studied in children with acute lymphocytic leukemia who had previously received cranial irradiation as part of CNS prophylaxis. Although cranial radiation therapy is not routinely given to standard-risk children today, there is a large population of long-term survivors who are experiencing significant sequelae. The emphasis on children with leukemia, rather than children with brain tumors, reflects their better overall prognosis, as well as the larger numbers of children with acute lymphocytic leukemia available for study. In addition, because children with CNS leukemia were excluded from many of these studies, effects of treatment could be readily differentiated from the effects of primary CNS disease.

A large, retrospective study of children with acute lymphocytic leukemia found that children who had been irradiated for CNS prophylaxis had significantly lower mean full-scale intelligence quotients than children treated with either intrathecal methotrexate alone or intravenous plus intrathecal methotrexate. Less than 15% of the irradiated patients exceeded the average intelligence quotients, whereas more than 55% from the other two groups had intelligence quotients higher than 100. Furthermore, irradiated children did worse on both wide-range achievement tests and on tests of neuropsychologic function [Rowland et al., 1984] (Fig. 71-57). In other studies, specific deficits in math, visuomotor function, and spatial processing have been recognized. In addition many children have distractibility and attention deficit disorder. Of interest, reading and language abilities are typically preserved [Copeland et al., 1985].

Risk factors include young age at radiation, feminine gender, and CNS relapse. Prospective longitudinal studies have revealed progressive deterioration, with intelligence quotients scores still falling a decade following treatment [Cousens et al., 1988; Fletcher and Copeland, 1988; Kato et al., 1993; Longeway et al., 1990; Mulhern et al., 1987].

The role of chemotherapy in treatment-induced cognitive decline is being reevaluated. Whereas earlier studies suggested that intravenous and/or intrathecal methotrexate was not associated with leukoencephalopathy (unless the child had been irradiated and/or had CNS disease), it is now increasingly accepted that even in the absence of these risk factors, high-dose frequently administered methotrexate may produce leukoencephalopathy and cognitive disorders [Mahoney et al., 1998].

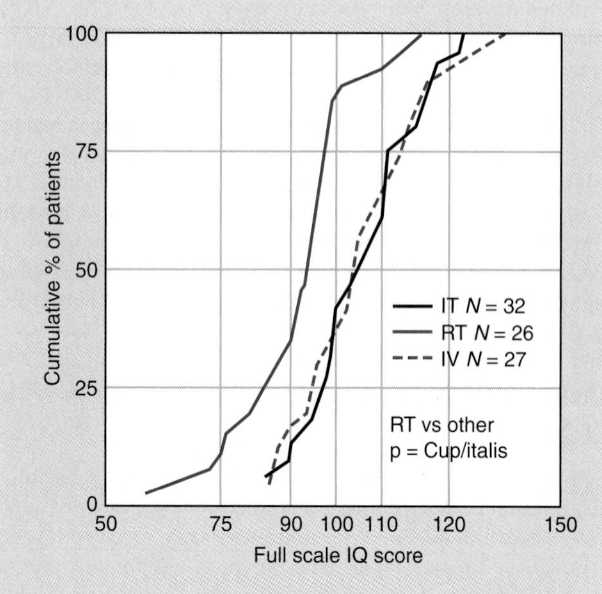

FIGURE 71-57. Full-scale intelligence quotient related to CNS treatment. IT, intrathecal; IV, intravenous; RT, radiation. (From Rowland et al., 1984.)

Disturbances in Intellectual Function in Children with Brain Tumors

Concerns over the potential long-term effects of CNS radiation on children with brain tumors began to surface in the 1980s, as the number of survivors began to increase. Retrospective studies from that decade documented significant intellectual difficulties in children irradiated for brain tumors [Bamford et al., 1976; Broadbent et al., 1981; Duffner et al., 1983b; Raimondi and Tomita, 1979c]. Speculation centered on whether the poor intelligence quotients scores were due to the presence of hydrocephalus, the tumor, or the treatment. In an effort to assess the role of hydrocephalus, intelligence quotients of children with cerebellar astrocytomas treated with surgery alone were compared with children with medulloblastoma treated with surgery and postoperative radiation and chemotherapy. Medulloblastomas and cerebellar astrocytomas, because of their location in the posterior fossa, are both associated with obstructive hydrocephalus secondary to ventricular outflow obstruction. Thus the major difference between the two groups of patients was the postoperative radiation and chemotherapy. Results of this study revealed that only 11% of children with medulloblastomas had intelligence quotients higher than 90, whereas 62% of the patients with cerebellar astrocytomas had intelligence quotients above 90. This study implicated postoperative radiation and chemotherapy as the cause of the intellectual impairment; hydrocephalus was not believed to be a factor [Hirsch et al., 1979]. Subsequent reports confirmed these results [Kun et al, 1983; Mulhern and Kun, 1985].

Although hydrocephalus is not considered a risk factor, several others have been identified as increasing the likelihood of postradiation cognitive disorders. The most important risk factor is age at cranial irradiation. Children irradiated before 3 to 5 years of age have significantly greater intellectual impairment than older children, whereas children irradiated after the age of 8 years are likely spared the most severe deterioration [Packer et al., 1989; Spunberg et al., 1981]. Learning disabilities are almost universal regardless of age. Of great interest was a prospective study performed by Mulhern and colleagues [1989] in which very young children with brain tumors were treated with postoperative chemotherapy and delayed radiation. Only 25% of children had scores in the normal range before any treatment. Thus although radiation damages intellectual function in the very young child, many children may be abnormal before therapy.

Another important risk factor is the volume of radiation. Ellenberg and associates [1987] prospectively studied the intelligence of patients treated for brain tumors and compared those who had received no radiation, local radiation, or whole brain radiation. Children who received whole-brain radiation had a significant decline in intelligence quotients following cranial radiation therapy, whereas children who received local or no cranial radiation therapy remained stable. Others have also found that intellectual dysfunction is more likely in children treated with whole-brain radiation rather than radiation to the posterior fossa alone [Kun et al., 1983].

The dose of radiation is also an important risk factor. Although a safe dose of cranial irradiation has not been defined, children who were irradiated for acute lymphoblastic leukemia in doses of 1800 to 2400 cGy did not demonstrate the severe intellectual sequelae seen in children treated with more than 3600 cGy to the brain. It is important to note, however, that in three different studies reducing the dose of cranial radiation therapy in children with acute lymphocytic leukemia from 2400 to 1800 cGy did not improve intelligence quotient scores [Jankovic et al., 1994; MacLean et al., 1995; Rodgers et al., 1991]. In contrast, studies in which the dose of radiation to the neuraxis in children with brain tumors was reduced have generally found improved scores, for example, full-scale intelligence quotient equal to 76.9 with 25 Gy compared with 63.7 with 35 Gy [Grill et al., 1999]. A Children's Oncology Group study, however, in which children were treated with 2400 cGy craniospinal radiation and chemotherapy found declines in intelligence quotient of 15 to 20 points [Packer et al., 2002].

The site of tumor is also important. Children who have tumors located primarily in the posterior fossa are less likely to be intellectually impaired before treatment than children whose tumors are located either in the supratentorial region or the midline of the brain. After radiation treatment, deterioration may occur regardless of site, but because patients with supratentorial tumors have significantly lower intelligence quotients at baseline than children with posterior fossa tumors, their decline may place them in the frankly abnormal range [Ellenberg et al., 1987]. Several reports have cited hypothalamic and thalamic involvement as being associated with cognitive abnormalities, especially those tumors involving the anterior third ventricle. Patients with pineal region tumors have also been reported to have disorders of memory, visuomotor problem-solving and visuospatial attention [Giglio et al., 2000].

The only chemotherapeutic agent that has been clearly identified as a risk factor for treatment-induced dementia has been methotrexate. Children treated with radiation and intrathecal methotrexate for medulloblastoma in one study, for example, had mean intelligence quotients of only 74.6 2 years after radiation compared with studies by Packer and colleagues [1989] and Jannoun and Bloom [1990], in which irradiated children not treated with methotrexate had scores of 91 and 92, respectively [Riva et al., 1989].

Finally, perioperative morbidity is increasingly recognized as a poor prognostic factor [Chapman et al., 1995; Kao et al., 1994]. Perioperative complications including neurologic deficits, meningitis, shunt infections, and the need for repeat surgery have been correlated with cognitive deficits. The "posterior fossa syndrome" (cerebellar mutism), in particular, has been associated with long-term cognitive decline. A recent report from the Children's Oncology Group found a 24% incidence of posterior fossa syndrome in a group of children with medulloblastomas. As such, long-term cognitive problems for a large group of survivors can be anticipated [Robertson et al., 2002]. This may become more important as attempts at achieving gross total resections are likely to increase in the future.

Prospective studies of children with brain tumors have revealed that intellect may continue to decline over several years. During the first year after radiotherapy, results are inconsistent. However, when follow-up extends to 4 years, progressive deterioration in intellectual functioning is found. Cognition has continued to decline progressively over a 10-year period [Hoppe-Hirsch et al., 1990]. In addition, even children with normal intelligence quotients may have significant learning problems, including attentional difficulties and visual perception problems [Duffner et al., 1985a; Packer et al., 1989].

Disturbances In Endocrine Function

Several groups of investigators have studied the endocrine status of children treated for acute lymphocytic leukemia. These studies demonstrated that levels of growth hormone obtained within 1 to 3 days after a 3-week course of cranial radiation therapy are lower than levels before cranial radiation therapy and, as such, an immediate suppressive effect on the hypothalamic-pituitary axis has been suggested [Dacou-Voutetakis et al., 1977]. The total dose of radiation appears to influence hypothalamic-pituitary function. Doses of less than 2400 cGy may be associated with normal growth hormone response to arginine stimulation, but not to insulin stimulation. In contrast, patients who receive more than 2400 cGy of radiotherapy may have abnormalities of growth hormone release after arginine and insulin stimulation. The theoretical basis for this disparity is that insulin-induced hypoglycemia may produce effects directly on the hypothalamus, whereas arginine stimulation may directly stimulate the pituitary gland. Because the pituitary gland itself is relatively radiation resistant, radiation in low doses may produce growth hormone deficiency resulting primarily from hypothalamic damage. Higher doses of radiation may affect both pituitary and hypothalamic function [Dickinson et al., 1978].

The incidence of biochemical growth hormone deficiency increases if the total dose of radiation is given in larger fractions over a shorter time. Children who receive 2400 cGy of radiation over 2 weeks in 10 fractions experience greater toxicity than children receiving the same dose given in 20 fractions over 4 weeks [Shalet et al., 1976; 1977]. Growth hormone deficiency is not related solely to cranial radiation therapy because it may also be found in children with acute lymphocytic leukemia treated with chemotherapy alone. Children with acute lymphocytic leukemia who were identified as being growth hormone deficient following cranial radiation therapy were initially thought to grow normally. When these children were reassessed after puberty, the irradiated children had shorter adult heights than nonrradiated children, presumably due to their inability to undergo a pubertal growth spurt [Brecher et al, 1992; Uruena et al, 1991; Voorhess et al., 1986]. Risk factors for growth failure in children with acute lymphocytic leukemia are radiation treatment at a young age, feminine gender, and early development of puberty. The effects of chemotherapy are less severe than those caused by radiation.

Because of the much larger doses of cranial radiation therapy administered to children with brain tumors, the risk for endocrine dysfunction is greater than in children with leukemia. Retrospective studies have demonstrated that children with brain tumors treated with cranial radiation therapy are at high risk for the development of growth hormone deficiency. It has been suggested that a minimum dose of 2500 to 2900 cGy delivered to the hypothalamic-pituitary axis may produce growth hormone deficiency in children with brain tumors. Most studies have documented that approximately 80% to 90% of children who have received cranial radiation therapy for brain tumors will develop growth hormone deficiency [Duffner et al., 1985b; Shalet et al., 1978; Wara et al., 1977]. Most growth hormone–deficient children with brain tumors do not grow normally. The reasons for growth failure are multifactorial. Although growth hormone deficiency is a major consideration, another factor is the effect of radiation on the epiphyseal centers in the vertebrae. Shalet and co-workers [1987] reported that radiation of the spine of a child 1 year of age will lead to an absolute loss of height of 9 cm, whereas children irradiated at age 10 years will lose 5 cm. In addition to poor spinal growth, many children develop precocious puberty. Although they have an early growth spurt, they ultimately have short stature. Shalet and co-workers have shown a correlation between age at radiation and onset of puberty, with the earliest onset in those irradiated between 3 and 6 years [Shalet et al., 1988]. The presence of hypothyroidism also adversely affects growth. Finally, the poor nutrition of some children on long-term chemotherapy may contribute to growth failure.

Prospective studies have demonstrated that biochemical growth hormone deficiency begins in some patients as early as 3 months after completion of radiation therapy. Furthermore, the number of patients with growth hormone deficiency increases during the first year after treatment [Duffner et al., 1985b]. Growth hormone deficiency does not appear to be reversible because children have been reported to be growth hormone deficient as long as 8 years after radiation therapy [Duffner et al., 1983a]. Growth deceleration may begin 6 months after completion of radiation and may closely parallel the onset of biochemical growth hormone deficiency. Unless growth deceleration is recognized and treated, clinical growth failure may be permanent (Fig. 71-58). Of interest, some children with brain tumors are growth hormone deficient but continue to grow normally. Explanation for the continued growth in these children is unknown.

Growth hormone deficiency in irradiated patients may be a result of reduced production of growth hormone (pituitary) or deficiencies in growth hormone–releasing factor (ventromedian nucleus of the hypothalamus). Even children who receive radiation to the posterior fossa alone may become growth hormone deficient. Because the anterior limit of the radiation port to the posterior fossa does not include the pituitary gland but does include the ventromedian nucleus of the hypothalamus, it has been suggested that the etiology for some cases of radiation-induced growth hormone deficiency is hypothalamic in origin. Administration of growth hormone–releasing factor produces an elevation in growth hormone levels in some children whose growth hormone deficiency is secondary to cranial radiation therapy. Thus cranial radiation therapy appears to affect growth hormone levels, in part, by damaging hypothalamic growth hormone–releasing factor–secreting neurons [Lustig et al., 1985].

Several investigators have successfully treated radiation-induced growth hormone–deficient children with exogenous growth hormone [Romshe et al., 1984; Shalet et al., 1981]. Unfortunately, although children with brain tumors may respond well for the first year of treatment, others have suggested that a normal growth rate cannot be maintained over a 3-year treatment period [Winter and Green, 1985]. These results are in contrast to other reports in which growth acceleration has been maintained with growth hormone treatment. Growth hormone–releasing factor may also have potential therapeutic value because it causes an increase in growth hormone levels [Lustig et al., 1985]. The long-term efficacy of treatment with both growth hormone and growth hormone–releasing factor needs to be established in larger numbers of patients. Even if growth hormone treatment were effective, normal growth would be unobtainable in children who have abnormal vertebral body growth or in those with precocious puberty. As a result, some investigators have tried to reduce the dose of radiation to the spine, and others have attempted to delay puberty with gonadotropin-releasing hormone analogs [Adan et al., 2000].

Thyroid dysfunction is the next most common endocrinopathy after growth hormone deficiency in children following craniospinal radiation [Hirsch et al., 1979; Larkins and Martin, 1973]. Because the radiation port to the cervical spine includes the thyroid gland, primary hypothyroidism

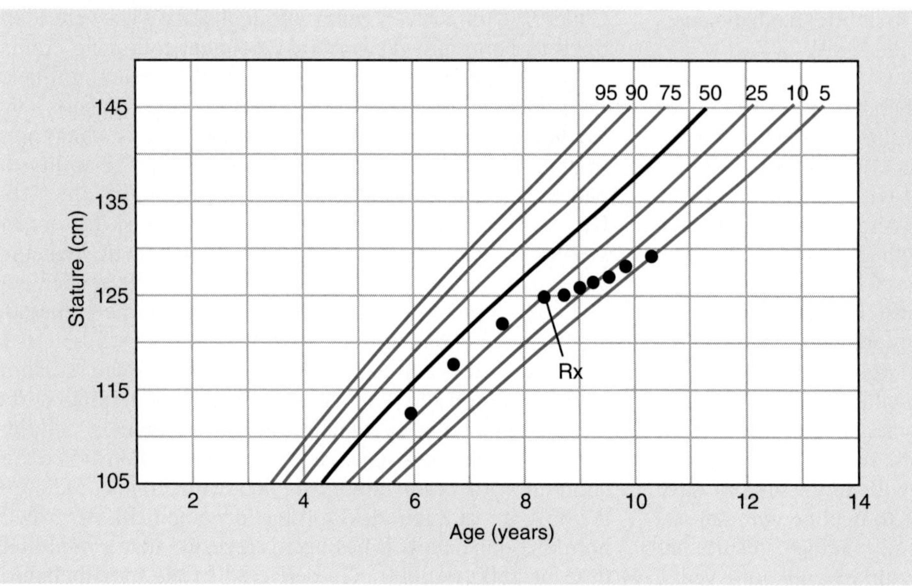

FIGURE 71-58. Abnormal growth in a patient with medulloblastoma treated with radiation and surgery. Patient had documented growth hormone deficiency. The patient's height fell from the 30th percentile to the 5th.

may develop after spinal radiation. The addition of chemotherapy raises the incidence of hypothyroidism from 20% to 69% [Livesey and Brook, 1989]. Giving hyperfractionation rather than standard radiation therapy reduced the incidence of hypothyroidism from 62% to 14% in a group of children with medulloblastoma, despite the fact that adjuvant chemotherapy was given to both groups [Chin et al., 1997; Ricardi et al., 2001]. Children who receive large doses of radiation to the hypothalamic-pituitary axis may also develop secondary or tertiary hypothyroidism, that is, low thyroid-stimulating hormone level in the presence of a low thyroxine level. Children who have a low normal thyroxine level in the presence of elevated thyroid-stimulating hormone (compensated hypothyroidism) should be placed on thyroid replacement even when they are clinically euthyroid because of an increased incidence of thyroid cancer in these patients. Because hypothyroidism may contribute to the child's learning difficulty and may also adversely affect linear growth, prompt recognition and treatment are necessary.

Gonadal function in children with brain tumors has not been studied nearly as well as other endocrinopathies. Radiation to the spine may affect the ovaries. In one study, 35% of girls treated with spinal radiation had evidence of ovarian dysfunction. This problem is compounded when adjuvant chemotherapy is used. Although spinal irradiation does not adversely affect male gonadal function, certain chemotherapeutic agents may be extremely toxic. In particular, cyclophosphamide has a primary effect on the Leydig cells. Although most men do not require androgen replacement, they may develop oligozoospermia or even azoospermia. Gynecomastia and gonadal dysfunction have been reported in adolescent boys treated with combination chemotherapy for Hodgkin's disease [Sherins et al., 1978]. In general, prepubertal patients tend to be more resistant to adverse effects of radiation and chemotherapy on gonadal function, whereas 70% of postpubertal girls may develop oligomenorrhea and 30% of males may have low testosterone levels [Constine et al., 1993; Moshang and Grimberg, 1996]. These findings suggest that gonadal dysfunction in long-term survivors will need to be studied in much greater detail before definitive statements can be made [Clayton et al., 1988].

Leukoencephalopathy

Leukoencephalopathy was first described in children with leukemia and was attributed primarily to treatment with intrathecal methotrexate. Recently, MRI evaluations of children treated only with cranial irradiation for brain tumors have identified leukoencephalopathy in these patients as well. CT scans of affected children are characterized by enlarged ventricles, hypodense areas, and areas of calcification (Fig. 71-59) [Peylan-Ramu et al., 1978]. Typical MRI abnormalities include increased ventricular and sulcal size, with hyperintensity in the periventricular region that stops abruptly at the gray matter–white matter junction. Periventricular hyperintensity is symmetrical and scalloped in appearance (Fig. 71-60). The abnormalities have been graded by Zimmerman and co-workers as ranging from 0, in which there is no evidence of periventricular hyperintensity, to 4, in which there are diffuse white matter abnormalities with increased T2-weighted signals extending from the ventricular lining to the cortical medullary junctions. Intermediate grades range from a pencil-thin continuous line of hyperintensity surrounding the ventricles to a periventricular halo [Zimmerman et al., 1986]. The clinical correlates of CT and MRI leukoencephalopathy are dementia, seizures, and focal motor signs.

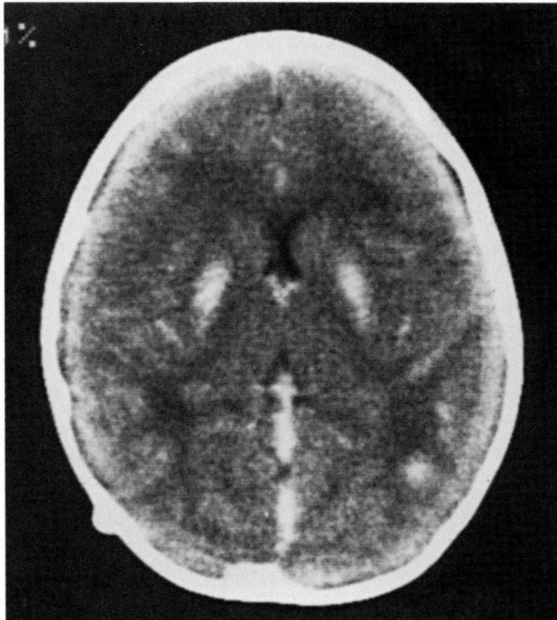

FIGURE 71-59. CT features of leukoencephalopathy (i.e., calcification, hypodense areas, increased sulci).

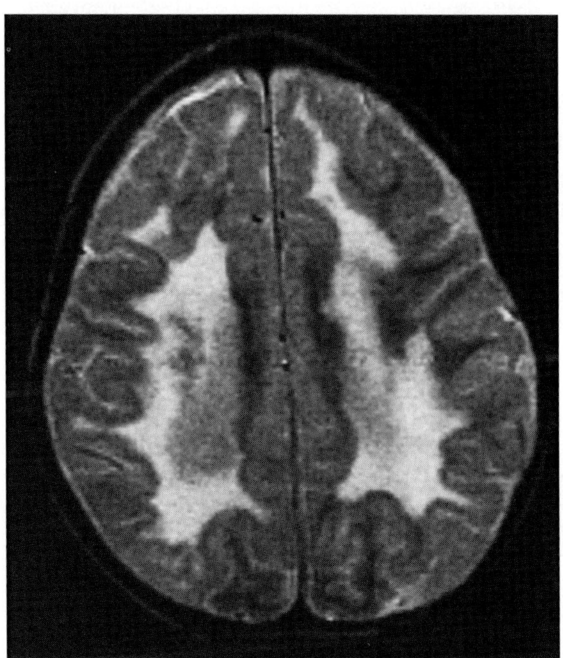

FIGURE 71-60. MRI of leukoencephalopathy characterized by periventricular hyperintensity extending to the gray matter–white matter junction.

Leukoencephalopathy is characterized by diffuse, reactive astrocytosis with multiple noninflammatory necrotic foci [Price and Jamieson, 1975]. Mineralized cellular debris is commonly found. Necrotic areas are found in more severe cases and are typically located in the subcortical white matter of the frontoparietal cortex. In addition to white matter changes, mineralizing microangiopathy and dystrophic calcification have been found, presumably an effect of radiation and chemotherapy [Price and Birdwell, 1978]. The lesion usually involves the lenticular nucleus with or without additional involvement of the cerebral cortex. Calcification and necrosis are present in adjacent neural tissue. Unlike subacute leukoencephalopathy, mineralizing microangiopathy preferentially affects gray matter, especially the putamen and cerebral cortex. It is presumed to be due to small vessel injury secondary to cranial irradiation. The typical distribution is in the border zones of the anterior, middle, and posterior cerebral arteries. Microangiopathy generally begins in the lenticular nuclei, spreading to the cerebral cortex and finally the cerebellar cortex [Price and Birdwell, 1978].

In 1978, methotrexate was implicated as causing leukoencephalopathy in children with leukemia [Peylan-Ramu et al., 1978]. Leukoencephalopathy is particularly likely to develop in children with CNS leukemia and increases with the number of CNS relapses. The addition of radiation further compounds the problem, raising the incidence of leukoencephalopathy to almost 100% [Duffner et al., 1984]. Recently leukoencephalopathy has also been identified in nonirradiated children with acute lymphoblastic leukemia who did not have CNS leukemia. As the dose and frequency of methotrexate administration have increased, so has the likelihood of methotrexate-induced leukoencephalopathy.

Intrathecal and intraventricular routes of methotrexate have been most commonly associated with leukoencephalopathy. Patients with CNS leukemia and patients with brain tumors commonly have alterations in cerebrospinal fluid dynamics secondary to either communicating or obstructive hydrocephalus. When methotrexate is administered either intraventricularly or via the lumbar route to these patients, clearance of methotrexate is slowed or blocked, producing elevated levels of methotrexate for prolonged periods causing subependymal spread of drug into surrounding brain [Shapiro et al., 1973]. Because the toxicity of methotrexate is related not only to its peak level but also to prolonged duration of exposure, children with abnormal cerebrospinal fluid dynamics are more likely to develop leukoencephalopathy. The intraventricular and intrathecal routes of administration of methotrexate should be used only in patients with leptomeningeal disease after cerebrospinal fluid flow studies have demonstrated no abnormalities [Duffner et al., 1984].

Second Malignancies

The oncogenic potential of radiation is increasingly significant as more patients survive their primary tumors. Even low doses of radiation are known to produce secondary malignancies. Children who received low-dose cranial irradiation for tinea capitis had an increased risk of malignant and benign neoplasms of the head and neck compared with control subjects. The most striking increase was in brain tumors, particularly meningiomas, as well as parotid and thyroid tumors [Albert et al., 1966].

Moderate- and high-dose radiation may also be associated with second malignancies. There are several reports of children with acute lymphoblastic leukemia treated with moderate-dose cranial radiation therapy who later developed brain tumors [Chung et al., 1981] (Fig. 71-61). Similarly, a variety of brain tumors have been reported after high-dose radiation treatment for primary brain tumors in children. The interval between treatment of the first tumor and development of the second tumor has ranged from 5 to 26 years. Second tumors include meningiomas, glioblastomas, and astrocytomas. Second malignancies tend to be biologically aggressive, are poorly responsive to treatment, and tend to occur at the site of the original tumor or in locations remote from the original tumor but within the radiation port [Bachman and Ostrow, 1978; Pearl et al., 1980].

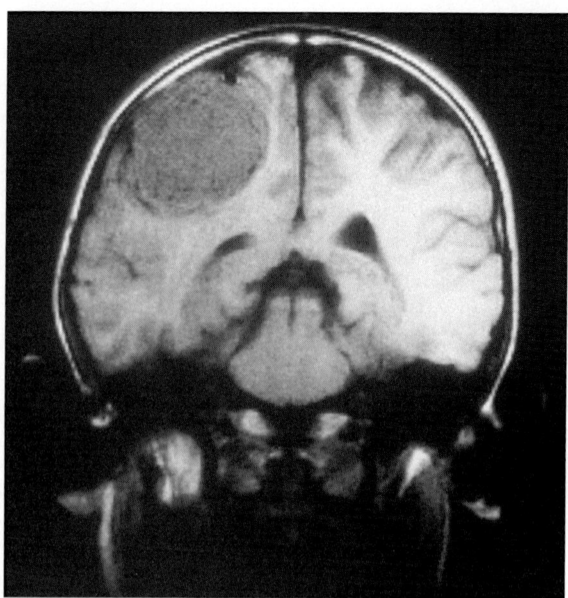

FIGURE 71-61. T1-weighted MRI in a 16 year old with a right frontal parietal meningioma. Fourteen years previously, the patient had been treated with cranial radiation therapy and chemotherapy for acute lymphocytic leukemia.

Chemotherapy can also cause second malignancies. The alkylating agents as well as topoisomerase inhibitors are carcinogenic. There have been reports of infants treated with postoperative chemotherapy for CNS neoplasms who have developed leukemia and myelodysplastic syndrome [Duffner et al., 1998a]. Because these agents are among the most effective chemotherapeutic agents for brain tumors, more such patients are likely to be reported. Non-CNS malignancies may also develop after treatment for brain tumors. Because children with medulloblastomas, primitive neuroectodermal tumors, and some spinal cord tumors receive radiation to the cervical cord, the thyroid gland is irradiated. Cases of thyroid carcinoma have occurred in such children 7 to 18 years after initial irradiation [Roggli et al., 1979]. Because survival time is increasing for all of these brain tumors, the incidence of thyroid carcinoma will likely increase.

Recommendations

Recognition of the risk factors of young age, dose, and volume of radiation has led to changes in the treatment approach to children with brain tumors. As noted throughout this chapter, therapy is being modified to reduce neurotoxicity. For example, very young infants with malignant brain tumors are now treated with prolonged postoperative chemotherapy in an attempt to delay radiation treatment and limit radiation damage to the developing brain. Volume of radiation has been reduced, where possible, by using adjuvant chemotherapy in tumors such as germinomas. Three-dimensional conformal radiation to the tumor bed is now being studied in babies with medulloblastomas and children with ependymomas. Radiation to the craniospinal axis has been eliminated in children with nonmetastatic ependymomas and reduced in dose for some children with medulloblastoma. These studies have as their primary objective the reduction of neurotoxicity while maintaining survival.

Until such time as less toxic therapies are available, certain procedures should be part of the routine follow-up of children treated for brain tumors. Those treated with cranial radiation therapy, with or without accompanying chemotherapy, should have baseline intelligence quotients and achievement tests (when age appropriate). When the child is of school age, reports from the school on academic performance should be obtained. Follow-up intellectual assessments are recommended 1 year after completion of cranial radiation therapy and then yearly for at least 5 years. Audiograms should be obtained routinely because children may have hearing loss resulting from previous radiation or chemotherapy. Communication among the family, psychologist, school, and physician is essential to provide the best possible learning experience for the child. Because many of these children will be long-term survivors, an appropriate program of remedial education is important to maximize quality of life.

Endocrinopathies, which develop as a consequence of treatment, are potentially treatable. Therefore testing of endocrine function should be part of the follow-up of all children with brain tumors. Previous measurements of growth should be reviewed and routine assessments of longitudinal growth with sitting and standing heights made at frequent intervals. Current recommendations are to begin growth hormone therapy 2 years following diagnosis in children who have had growth deceleration. Most authors no longer recommend growth hormone stimulation tests in this population [Albertsson-Wikland et al., 1987; Clarson and Del Maestro, 1999; Romshe et al., 1984]. In those children with precocious puberty or those in whom puberty is advancing rapidly, gonadotropin-releasing hormone analogs are recommended. Failure to diagnose and treat growth hormone deficiency before the patient has epiphyseal fusion will lead to irreversible growth failure. Baseline thyroid testing, including thyroxine and thyroid-stimulating hormone, should be performed and repeated every 6 months for at least 5 years after completion of treatment. Assessment of gonadotropin function is indicated if the child does not exhibit signs of pubertal development by the appropriate age. In children with midline brain tumors, including those involving the diencephalon and pineal region, endocrine evaluations including levels of plasma cortisol, prolactin, and gonadotropins should be performed at 6-month intervals.

Secondary oncogenesis is a serious potential complication of treatment. The physician must be aware that second primary tumors may develop intracranially or extracranially. Children who have received spinal radiation must be closely monitored for the possible development of thyroid carcinoma. If a neoplasm occurs in an unusual location, a second primary tumor rather than tumor recurrence should be considered. Because the second tumor may have a different pathology and respond to surgical excision, repeat explorative surgery and aggressive debulking should be considered.

Recognition of the long-term complications of CNS therapy is important because some are amenable to treatment and others may be prevented by judicious monitoring of administration of drugs and radiation. Careful monitoring can occur only if the physician is aware of the potential adverse effects of treatment. Until newer methods of treatment with fewer long-term side effects are found, awareness of possible consequences of treatment and early intervention, when possible, can help maximize the quality of life of children with brain tumors.

NEW THERAPEUTIC APPROACHES

Historically, the traditional approaches of surgery, radiation, and chemotherapy have yielded notable but limited results. Success has not been without its cost because morbidity to long-term survivors has become increasingly more apparent. Better methods of chemotherapy, improved methods of drug delivery, and imaginative treatment modalities currently available in the laboratory are awaiting clinical studies. Monoclonal antibodies directed against tumor-associated antigens should be available in the future. These antibodies can be used as homing devices and, when attached to a specific chemotherapeutic payload, deliver drug agents directly to the tumor. Monoclonal antibodies targeted with a radioactive label, by attaching to specific tumor antigens, may recognize tumor in unrecognized sanctuaries. This recognition provides the potential for diagnosis of recurrence at a time when the tumor burden is small. In theory, monoclonal antibodies should have considerable clinical application; however, there are several problems yet to be resolved, including antigenic modulation (i.e., a reverse loss of antigenic expression on the surface of cells), multiple antigenic sites, immunoselection, and the development of blocking factors in the presence of natural killer cells or macrophages [Ross et al., 2004; Vulfovich and Saba, 2004]. An increasing understanding in the mechanisms of cell signaling over the past decade has led to development of a new class of drugs. Agents that interfere with cell signaling have the potential of limiting cell proliferation, angioinvasion, and stromal invasion, and in promoting apoptosis. Increasing interest in protein kinase inhibitors has raised the hope that effective molecular options of treatment may soon be available. Several of these agents have shown success in the treatment of non-CNS tumors [Noble et al., 2004].

Two such agents are getfitinib (Irressa) and imatinib (Gleevec): both alter tyrosine kinase signaling activity. Getfitinib alters epidermal growth factor tyrosine kinase signaling. Imatinib inhibits platelet-derived growth factor signaling. Getfitinib has shown limited success in trials involving CNS metastasis. This agent is also being studied as a potential radiation sensitizer. The effect of imatinib to date has been most profound in chronic myelogenous leukemia. A host of other agents involved in inhibiting the tyrosine kinase family of proteins are currently under investigation [Dancey and Freidlin, 2003; Stea et al., 2003; Wong and Witte, 2004].

Other molecular approaches involve phase I and II trials using farnesyl transferase inhibitors. Farnesylation is prominently involved in the activation of *ras* oncogenes. The proteins encoded by these oncogenes are involved in signaling cellular growth, differentiation, and apoptosis. *RAS* genes encode G-proteins responsible for initiating the reproductive events characterizing the cell cycle. Of interest is the observation that neurofibromin; the gene product mutated or altered in neurofibromatosis type 1 is prominently involved in the upstream regulation of *RAS* proteins.

Transferrin receptors have been found to be preferentially expressed in proliferating tissues as opposed to normal brain and may represent a potentially useful target site for transferrin toxic conjugates. Transferrin is a naturally occurring protein and, unlike monoclonal antibodies, is not subject to immune reaction. Anti-transferrin receptor ricin immunotoxins have been used in vitro against glioblastomas in an attempt to obviate the immune responses identified with monoclonal antibodies [Zovickian et al., 1987]. Carrier systems using ricin, abrin, diphtheria toxin, and *Pseudomonas* organisms have been studied in experimental systems but have not been reported in large phase I trials [Weaver and Laske, 2003].

Liposomes and polymers are lipophilic compounds that can carry drugs, radionuclides, toxins, or other materials readily into the CNS. Liposomes are lipid vesicles that can be made from naturally occurring synthetic phospholipids, which are biodegradable and relatively nontoxic. They can be manufactured in sizes ranging from 0.3 to 10 mg and require no chemical binding. Small size offers the advantage of prolonged circulation time and greater likelihood of reaching interstitial spaces.

Biodegradable wafers are being developed that release tumoricidal agents at a predicted rate [DiMeco et al. 2002]. For instance, drugs can be incorporated into albumin microspheres that can be implanted into a tumor. The drug is then released via diffusion. The rate of release can be achieved by modifying the structure of the wafer.

Intra-arterial delivery of drugs is used in an effort to overcome the problems of the blood-brain barrier and to reduce systemic effects. These techniques allow large amounts of drug to be infused directly into the tumor. The basic assumption of regional perfusion is that higher drug concentration leads to greater cell kill, which, in turn, leads to improved tumor response. The advantage of intra-arterial over intravenous administration depends on the fraction of cardiac output flowing through the infused artery and the fraction of drug cleared from the systemic circulation during a single pass. The greater the amount of drug removed during the first pass, the greater the benefit of regional perfusion [Chen and Gross, 1980; Eckman et al., 1974]. If most of a drug such as BCNU or cisplatin administered intra-arterially is extracted during the first pass, large amounts of drug can be delivered with limited concern about systemic, hematologic, or hepatic effects. Techniques are being developed to circumvent the limited ability of chemotherapeutic agents to penetrate the blood-brain barrier. The blood-brain barrier, although disrupted in many tumors, may be intact in the brain-adjacent tumor. This is the region of the brain where the microenvironment of the nervous system is the most inaccessible. Systemic chemotherapy in the absence of an intact blood-brain barrier readily enters the center of a tumor but is excluded from the margins of the tumor and the brain-adjacent tumor because of an intact blood-brain barrier. Seizure, hypertension, hypercapnia, and hyperosmotic agents all have a transient ability to transiently alter the blood-brain barrier. Bradykinin is a nonapeptide that plays a central role in inflammation and host defense against injury. Receptors for these agents are upregulated in regions of tissue damage or injury. The result is increased vascular permeability in cerebral vasculature as well as other areas of the body. In phase I trials bradykinins and their receptor agonists have been found to enhance permeability of selective agents in the region of the brain-adjacent tumor [Elliott et al., 1996, Inamura et al., 1994].

Pro-drugs are substances that must be transformed in vivo to exert their pharmacologic effects. For example, cytosine arabinoside must be phosphorylated in vivo in the target cell to the triphosphate that is the active moiety. Direct administration of the active moiety is of no clinical use because of poor intercellular transport. Attachment of a prodrug to a carrier has the potential to bypass inactivating sites of the agent in question [Bodor, 1984]. Temozolomide is an example of a pro-drug used in treatment trials. This alkylating agent is an analog of dacarbazine, an antimelanoma drug used in the 1970s. The drug is metabolized to a triazene, its active ingredient. The drug's action is to form DNA adducts by methylation in the O^6 position of guanine, thereby hindering DNA replication [Friedman et al., 1995].

Techniques are being developed to enhance chemosensitivity by decreasing the development of drug resistance. Understanding drug resistance depends on knowledge of pharmacokinetics, ability of neoplastic cells to incorporate and retain cytotoxic agents, the ability to attain effective drug concentration by preventing metabolic degradation, and the ability to prevent drug-induced damage to DNA or other parts of the cytosol. Tumors may acquire resistance to drugs by activation of transporter enzymes, such as the multiple-drug–resistant transporter protein. The multiple-drug–resistant gene encodes for the P170 glycoprotein. This gene has been found in both normal and tumor tissues and is believed to encode for a normally protective protein that acts to eliminate natural toxins found in food; therefore, one would expect that the multiple-drug–resistant gene would be operant in transporting those agents that are isolated from naturally occurring sources such as plants, microorganisms, and fungi. This group includes antibiotic agents, such as actinomycin D; doxorubicin; daunorubicin; the mitotic inhibitors, such as vincristine and vinblastine; and epidophyllotoxin. All of these agents are heterocyclic, have large molecular size, and are lipophilic. Calcium channel blockers (e.g., nifedipine, verapamil, calmodulin inhibitors) have been used to circumvent multiple-drug resistance. Metallothionein, another transporter gene, codes for a protein that facilitates the clearance of heavy metals from the cell, such as platinum, copper, and zinc.

Resistance to nitrosoureas is believed to be the result of the attempt of an affected cell to repair damaged DNA. The cytotoxicity of alkylating agents develops through the formulation of covalent bonds between reactive alkyl groups and cellular molecules. Formation of DNA-DNA cross-lengths results in inactivation of DNA with subsequent inhibition of DNA synthesis and ultimately death of the cell. O^6-alkylguanine-DNA alkyltransferase is believed to mediate repair of DNA damage. Saturation of the enzyme by O^6-methylguanine is one mechanism being explored to potentiate alkylating toxicity. Another mechanism of drug resistance is the presence of increased cellular levels of glutathione or glutathione *S*-transferase, which act to decrease the alkylating effect. Depletion of intracellular reduced glutathione by enzyme inhibitors and saturation of the glutathione *S*-transferases by nontoxic substrates have the therapeutic potential of modifying the reparative effect of these enzymes. Butathionine sulfoximine acts by inhibiting the synthesis of glutathione and therefore results in depletion of this agent in brain and extraneural tissues. The diuretic ethacrynic acid has a high substrate affinity for glutathione *S*-transferase and may act as a transferase inhibitor [Phillips, 1991].

Topoisomerase-2 is another enzyme that is believed to confer resistance to alkylators by enhancing the repair of DNA interstrand crosslengths. This enzyme is a nuclear one that may act to facilitate access of enzymes and other proteins involved in the repair of DNA interstrand breaks. As with the glutathione system, understanding the mechanism of action of topoisomerase may lead to ways of inhibiting the activity of this enzyme, thus potentiating drug activity [D'Arpa and Liu, 1989].

FUTURE DIRECTIONS

Since the mid-1990s, despite the increasing interest of neurologists, radiation oncologists, and hematologists/oncologists in the treatment of children with cancer of the nervous system, there has been limited overall change in prognosis. In fact this view extends, unfortunately, to all cancers. A report from the National Center for Health Statistics covering the years 1970 to 1994 indicates that all deaths from cancer have remained the same or have slightly decreased. Despite decades of basic science and clinical efforts focused on improving treatment, the overall results of the war on cancer must be judged a qualified failure. Fortunately, in a select group of cancers, such as leukemia, Hodgkin's disease, Wilms' tumor, and certain CNS tumors, improvements in survival have been noted. Reflecting on the overall state of cancer treatment, Bailar and Gornik [1997] have suggested that a more promising approach to cancer control may be a national commitment to prevention in addition to a focus on funding for research and treatment.

The preceding rather pessimistic view is tempered by the development of new approaches that emphasize chemotherapy screening, virology, immunology, and more recently, molecular genetics. The increased interest in cancer prevention is the result of more attention being placed on the role of the environment and nutrition in initiating oncogenesis. There is now acceptance that genetic damage is central to oncogenesis. As pointed out in the preceding section the knowledge that has been accumulating since 2000 concerning the events occurring at the genomic level that lead to proliferation and differentiation is rapidly being applied to the clinic.

Two different groups of genes, one group that is dominant and the other recessive, are implicated in the development of cancer. These groups have provided hints about specific molecular function and in turn the mechanisms that initiate and promote neoplasia. Dominant oncogenes imply that inheritance of a single mutant allele is sufficient to overcome the effects of the corresponding normal allele, thereby allowing the expression of a malignant phenotype. Recessive oncogenes or tumor suppressor genes, when present on one allele, are associated with orderly regulation of the cell cycle. However, these genes, when deleted or mutated, may be associated with the development of malignancy. Both copies of the gene from a chromosome pair must be absent to cause malignancy. Consistent with the recessive nature of this process, a single mutation may be ineffective. It is only with the second mutation in a given gene's malignant allele partner that malignancy emerges. Thus, a heterozygous cell may function perfectly normally, whereas a cell that has a double mutation of an allelic pair may lose the ability to suppress the development of a tumor. This is called *loss of heterozygosity.*

The types of experiments that enable identification of these two classes of oncogenes [Bishop, 1991; Marshall, 1991] include the analysis of chromosomal translocations, site-directed mutagenesis, and introduction of amplified DNA into transgenic animals with subsequent characterization of inherited kinships. These techniques have resulted in the identification of more than 60 dominant oncogenes. Recessive oncogenes were hinted at by cell fusion studies that indicated that fusion of a normal cell with a transformed cell suppressed malignancy [Bishop, 1991]. More recently, analysis of restriction fragment length polymorphisms in multiple tumors has identified several homozygous gene defects that are candidates for tumor suppressor genes [Marshall, 1991; Pihan and Doxsey, 1999].

It seems likely that malignancies occur as the result of interaction between dominant and recessive genes. Although many oncogenes have been identified, only a few have been sporadically associated with CNS neoplasia. The epidermal growth factor receptor gene has been recognized in up to 40% of malignant gliomas, and c-*myc* amplification has been found in medulloblastomas [Eberhart et al., 2004]. Tumor suppressor genes have been identified on the long arm of chromosome 17 in neurofibromatosis and on the long arm of chromosome 13 in retinoblastoma. Loss of markers that contain the site of the p53 gene on the short arm of chromosome 17 has been found in medulloblastomas and astrocytomas. Mutations in tumor suppressor genes responsible for retinoblastoma and type I neurofibromatosis are more likely to occur on the paternal than on the maternal chromosome, suggesting that germ cell mutations in the paternal line are a reflection of the increasing risk of mutation for spermatocytes.

Identification of the retinoblastoma gene has provided the most information regarding the inherited tendency of cancer. In retinoblastoma, a defect in tumor suppressor genes is inherited on one allele of chromosome 13. The normal remaining allele is inactivated by an epigenetic event, with resultant loss of both tumor suppressor genes. The recessive loss of both alleles, one through the germline and the other autosomally, results in the dominant expression of the tumor. A dominant pattern of inheritance arises from the likelihood that the uninherited normal allele containing the retinoblastoma gene will be lost or inactivated in at least one cell, which subsequently will grow into a tumor. Thus the loss of heterozygosity for the retinoblastoma gene provides for a dominant phenotypic expression [Knudson, 1971; Marshall, 1991].

Oncogenes code for relatively small peptides that are involved in the cellular mechanisms that govern cell growth and proliferation. These proteins may act at the surface of the cell, convey signals from receptors to the cytosol, or code for proteins that orchestrate nuclear functions.

Proto-oncogenes are considered normal components of the cell that act to regulate orderly cell division. When activated by viruses, ionizing radiation, gene amplification, deletion, or loss of tumor suppressors, these genes may induce unregulated cell growth. For the most part, three biologic mechanisms have been described for proto-oncogenes. The first mechanism involves phosphorylation of proteins, primarily at serine, threonine, and tyrosine residues. Protein tyrosine kinases have been the most widely studied and implicated in oncogenesis. Abnormal phosphorylation directed by oncogenes may cause malignant or premalignant transformation. For example, excessive phosphorylation of tyrosine may disrupt the binding of components of the cytoskeleton to the inner surface of the plasma membrane. This disruption may lead to changes that transform cells. It is unknown how this change relates to normal versus malignant, uncontrolled mitosis.

Other oncogenes produce groups of protein that bind to guanosine triphosphate. These proteins transduce exogenous signals at the cell surface into cytoplasmic effects. Disruption of orderly guanosine triphosphate activity is thought to disrupt the regulation of cell division in response to exogenous signals [Tanabe et al., 1985]. A number of proto-oncogenes have been identified that encode nuclear proteins involved in genomic transcription. Oncogenes that affect DNA binding have gene products that relate directly to DNA or DNA-associated nuclear proteins [Donner et al., 1982]. The protein products of these oncogenes are believed to deregulate nuclear mitosis, the activity of which excites excessive mitosis. The result of excessive deregulation may be malignant transformation.

The preceding functions, for the most part, are autocrine. Paracrine functions involve growth factors and growth factor receptors. For instance, platelet-derived growth factors are stored in platelets and released when blood vessels are damaged, stimulating the proliferation of fibroblasts. These factors, as well as other cytokines, play a role in tissue repair, in the phosphorylation of intracellular proteins, and in tyrosine-specific protein kinase activity. It is believed that the mitogenic effect of exogenous growth factor, such as platelet-derived growth factor, activates intercellular growth factor receptors and elicits a cytoplasmic signal protein. The activated signal protein influences nuclear oncogenes, which produce DNA protein. These proteins then act to enhance or suppress one or more of the nuclear regulators of mitosis. This cascade of events leading to cell growth and neoplasia may begin in a paracrine fashion in which the cell of interest is stimulated by one cytokine or another. Growth factor receptors acting on the surfaces of the cell, when stimulated by cytokines, activate intracellular components, which in turn initiate processes that may either upregulate or downregulate mitosis.

The foregoing suggests that in their natural state, oncogenes are relatively quiescent and control mitosis in an orderly manner. When regulation of an oncogene is disturbed, cell division becomes disorderly and derepressed. By directing the activity of protein products that act on the plasma membrane, the cytoplasm, and the nucleus, oncogenes may play a major role in the promotion and orderly control of cell division. The process of cell division is complicated. Its timing must be carefully controlled and coordinated. This mechanism depends on rapid synthesis of many cellular structures. Presumably, many different kinds of oncogenes exist to regulate this ongoing process of cell division and replication [Pihan and Doxsey, 1999].

Identification of oncogenes associated with various neoplasms suggests that in the future determining the malignant potential of the specific neoplasm may be possible. This capability may allow classification of neoplasms based on pathogenesis rather than on morphology alone. Further knowledge of an oncogene may allow development of inhibitors of that gene product. For instance, if a malignant tumor were associated with the production of a growth factor such as the epidermal growth factor receptor on the surface of the cells, a monoclonal antibody directed toward the cell surface receptor might be considered.

The current wisdom is that the malignant phenotype, rather than resulting from one genetic event, is the by-product of the cumulative effects of multiple genetic insults. This model of progressive clonal evolution in tumor cells has been most studied in colorectal cancer [Vogelstein et al., 1988]. Similar approaches in the adult help to define an order for the progressive dedifferentiation of astrocytomas into glioblastomas. Astrocytomas, characterized primarily by hypercellularity, are associated with an allelic loss on the short arm of chromosome 17 in the area of the p53 mutation. Astrocytomas have also been associated with over-expression of the platelet-derived growth factor receptors. The anaplastic astrocytoma, in addition to hypercellularity, is characterized by cellular pleomorphism, mitosis, and vascular proliferation. These changes have been associated with allelic loss on the long arm of chromosome 13 in the region of the retinoblastoma mutation, allelic loss on the short arm of chromosome 9 in the area of genes that code for interferon, and an allelic loss on the long arm of chromosome 19 in the region of DNA repair genes. Necrosis, in addition to the aforementioned histologic features, characterizes the glioblastoma. About 60% to 90% of glioblastomas are associated with allelic losses on both the long and short arms of chromosome 10, suggesting that multiple genes within this chromosome may be responsible for the invasive features of glioblastoma. In addition, in glioblastomas that occur de novo rather than dedifferentiating from astrocytomas, there has been identified a high incidence of amplification of the epidermal growth factor receptor [Furnari et al., 1996].

Biologic response modifiers are being explored as an alternative to chemotherapy. These agents are being considered in conjunction with or as independent modalities to augment the host immune response to evoke an anti-neoplastic effect. Adoptive immunotherapy is that technique in which T cells have been stimulated in vitro with host tumor cells to augment suppressed immune surveillance activity. Tumor infiltrating lymphocytes are an extension of this approach in which lymphocytes at the margin of the tumor are enhanced and reinjected into the patient. Theoretically those cells that are present at the edge of the tumor may be the most immunogenic and therefore the most cytotoxic. These cells have a 100-fold greater anaplastic activity than lymphocytic activated killer cells [Rosenberg et al., 1986]. Other techniques using cytokines such as interleukin-1 and interleukin-2, tumor necrosis factor, and interferon have been used nonspecifically to heighten and augment the immune responsiveness of neoplastic cells. Unfortunately, clinical trials reporting the effectiveness of this approach have yet to be reported [Antonia et al., 2004; Martindale, 2003].

Attenuated retroviruses containing the herpes simplex thymidine kinase gene have been used to infect rapidly growing cells. These cells when exposed to antiviral agents such as ganciclovir have the potential to destroy replicating cells while preserving normal tissues. This approach is undergoing phase II trials in systemic cancers and to a limited extent in CNS tumors. There is also the potential for using antisense technologies to downregulate the expression of specific oncogenes and chemorepair genes. Other techniques available in tissue culture and animal models have suggested that the normal genetic makeup of a cell can be reconstituted using transfection techniques to replace absent tumor suppressor genes.

Although much of the foregoing has yet to make a clinical impact, these techniques offer the hope of providing cures at the cellular level while maintaining the integrity of normal tissue, thereby preserving a good quality of life. Current research suggests that the treatments of tomorrow will be increasingly molecular, with the potential of reducing the need for mutilating surgery, radiation, or highly toxic chemotherapy.

REFERENCES

Aarsen FK, Van Dongen HR, Paquier PF, et al. Long-term sequelae in children after cerebellar astrocytoma surgery. Neurology 2004;62;1311.

Adan L, Sainte-Rose C, Souberbielle JC, et al. Adult height after growth hormone (GH) treatment for GH deficiency due to cranial irradiation. Med Pediatr Oncol 2000;34:14.

Al-Mefty O, Al-Rodhan NR, Phillips RL, et al. Factors affecting survival of children with malignant gliomas. Neurosurgery 1987;20:416.

Albert RE, Omran AR, Brauer EW, et al. Follow-up study of patients treated by x-ray for tinea capitis. Am J Pub Health 1966;56:2114.

Albertsson-Wikland K, Lannering B, Marky I, et al. A longitudinal study on growth and spontaneous growth hormone (GH) secretion in children with irradiated brain tumors. Acta Paediatr Scand 1987;76:966.

Albright AL. Brain tumors in neonates, infants, and toddlers. Contemp Neurosurg 1985;7:1.

Albright AL, Wisoff JH, Zeltzer P, et al. Prognostic factors in children with supratentorial (nonpineal) primitive neuroectodermal tumors. Pediatr Neurosurg 1995;22:1.

Allen JC. The effects of cancer therapy on the nervous system. J Pediatr 1978;93:903.

Allen JC. Controversies in the management of intracranial germ cell tumors. Brain tumors in children. Neurol Clin 1991;9:441.

Allen JC, DaRosso RC, Donahue B, et al. A phase II trial of preirradiation carboplatin in newly diagnosed germinoma of the central nervous system. Cancer 1994;74:940.

Allen JC, Epstein F. Medulloblastoma and other primary malignant neuroectodermal tumors of the CNS: The effect of age and extent of disease on prognosis. J Neurosurg 1982;57:446.

Allen JV, Avivner S, Yates AJ, et al. Treatment of high-grade spinal cord astrocytoma of childhood with "8-in-1" chemotherapy and radiotherapy: A pilot study of CCG-945. J Neurosurg 1998;88:215.

Allison RR, Schulsinger A, Vongtama V, et al. Radiation and chemotherapy improve outcome in oligodendroglioma. Int J Radiat Oncol Biol Phys 1997;37:399.

Andler W, Roosen K, Clar HE. Pre- and post-operative evaluation of hypothalamo-pituitary function in children with craniopharyngiomas. Acta Neurochir 1979;45:287.

Anthony JH, Ouvrier RA, Wise G. Spasmus nutans: A mistaken identity. Arch Neurol 1980;37:373.

Antonia S, Mule JJ, Weber JS. Current developments of immunotherapy in the clinic. Curr Opin Immunol 2004;16:130.

Arseni C. Tumors of the basal ganglia: Their surgical treatment. Arch Neurol Psychiatry 1958;80:18.

Asai A, Hoffman HJ, Hendrick EB, et al. Primary intracranial neoplasms in the first year of life. Childs Nerv Syst 1989;5:230.

Ashwal S, Hinshaw DB Jr, Bedros A. CNS primitive neuroectodermal tumors of childhood. Med Pediatr Oncol 1984;12:180.

Bachman DS, Ostrow PT. Fatal long-term sequelae following radiation cure for ependymoma. Ann Neurol 1978;4:319.

Bailar JC III, Gornik HL. Cancer undefeated. N Engl J Med 1997;336:1569.

Bailey CC, Gnekow A, Wellek S, et al. Prospective randomised trial of chemotherapy given before radiotherapy in childhood medulloblastoma. International Society of Paediatric Oncology (SIOP) and the (German) Society of Paediatric Oncology (GPO): SIOP II. Med Pediatr Oncol 1995;25:166.

Bailey P, Buchanan DN, Bucy PC. Intracranial tumors of infancy and childhood. Chicago: University of Chicago Press, 1939.

Bailey P, Cushing H. Medulloblastoma cerebelli. A common type of mid-cerebellar glioma of childhood. Arch Neurol Psychiatry 1925;14:192.

Bailey P, Cushing H. A classification of the tumors of the glioma group on a histogenetic basis with a correlated study of prognosis. Philadelphia: JB Lippincott, 1926.

Balmaceda C. Chemotherapy for intramedullary spinal cord tumors. J Neurooncol 2000;47:293.

Balter-Seri J, Mor C, Shuper A, et al. Cure of recurrent medulloblastoma. The contribution of surgical resection at relapse. Cancer 1997;79:1241.

Bamford FN, Morris Jones P, Pearson D, et al. Residual disabilities in children treated for intracranial space-occupying lesions. Cancer 1976;37:1149.

Banna M, Lassman LP, Pearce GW. Radiological study of skeletal metastases from cerebellar medulloblastoma. Br J Radiol 1970;43:173.

Baram TZ, Tang R. Atypical spasmus nutans as an initial sign of thalamic neoplasm. Pediatr Neurol 1986;2:375.

Barker FG, Chang SM, Huhn SL, et al. Age and the risk of anaplasia in magnetic resonance—Nonenhancing supratentorial cerebral tumors. Cancer 1997;80:936.

Bates SE, Raphaelson MI, Price RA, et al. Ascending myelopathy after chemotherapy for central nervous system acute lymphoblastic leukemia: Correlation with cerebrospinal fluid myelin basic protein. Med Pediatr Oncol 1985;13:4.

Bauman GS, Ino Y, Ueki K, et al. Allelic loss of chromosome 1p and radiotherapy plus chemotherapy in patients with oligodendrogliomas. Int J Radiat Oncol Biol Phys 2000;48:825.

Baysefer A, Akay KM, Izci Y, et al. The clinical and surgical aspects of spinal tumors in children. Pediatr Neurol 2004;31;261.

Bendhein PE, Berg BO. Ataxic hemiparesis from a midbrain mass. Ann Neurol 1981;9:405.

Beni-Adani L, Gomori M, Spektor S, et al. Cyst wall enhancement in pilocytic astrocytoma: Neoplastic or reactive phenomena. Pediatr Neurosurg 2000;32:234.

Berger PE, Atkinson D, Wilson WJ, et al. High resolution surface coil magnetic resonance imaging of the spine: Normal and pathologic anatomy. Radiographics 1986;6:573.

Bernhardtsen T, Laursen H, Bojsen-Møller, et al. Sub-classification of low-grade cerebellar astrocytoma: Is it clinically meaningful? Childs Nerv Syst 2003;19:729.

Bernstein M, Hoffman HJ, Halliday WC, et al. Thalamic tumors in children. J Neurosurg 1984;61:649.

Bickler SW, McMahon TJ, Campbell JR, et al. Preoperative diagnostic evaluation of children with Cushing's syndrome. J Pediatr Surg 1994;29:671.

Bishop JM. Molecular themes in oncogenesis. Cell 1991;64:235.

Bitzer M, Topka H. Progressive cerebral occlusive disease after radiation therapy. Stroke 1995;26:131.

Bloom HJG, Glees J, Bell J. The treatment and long-term prognosis of children with intracranial tumors: A study of 610 cases, 1950-1981. Intl J Radiat Oncol Biol Phys 1990;18:733.

Bodor N. Soft drugs: Principles and methods for the design of safe drugs. Med Res Rev 1984;4:449.

Bouffet E, Jouvet A, Thiesse P, et al. Chemotherapy for aggressive or anaplastic high-grade oligodendrogliomas and oligoastrocytomas: Better than a salvage treatment. Br J Neurosurg 1998;12:217.
Bouffet F, Amat D, Deveaux Y, et al. Chemotherapy for spinal cord astrocytoma. Med Pediatr Oncol 1997;29:560.
Bowers DC, Georgiades C, Aronson LJ, et al. Tectal gliomas: Natural history of an indolent lesion in pediatric patients. Pediatr Neurosurg 2000;32:24.
Brady LW. The role of radiation therapy. In: Schmidek HH, ed. Pineal tumors. New York: Masson Press, 1977.
Brecher ML, Voorhees MM, Ritchey AK, et al. Adult heights achieved by long-term survivors of childhood acute lymphocytic leukemia (ALL) prophylaxis [Abstract]. Proc Soc Pediatr Res 1992;812:138.
Bristot R, Santoro A, Raco A, et al. Malignant cerebellar astrocytomas. Clinico-pathological remarks on 10 cases. J Neurosurg Sci 1999;43:271.
Broadbent VA, Barnes ND, Wheeler TK. Medulloblastoma in childhood: Long-term results of treatment. Cancer 1981;1:3.
Broniscer A, Nicolaides TP, Dunkel IJ, et al. High-dose chemotherapy with autologous stem-cell rescue in the treatment of patients with recurrent non-cerebellar primitive neuroectodermal tumors. Pediatr Blood Cancer 2004;42:261.
Brown RC, Gunderson L, Plenk HP. Medulloblastoma: A review of the LDS hospital experience. Cancer 1977;40:56.
Buchberg AM, Cleveland LS, Jenkins NA, et al. Sequence homology shared by neurofibromatosis type-I gene and IRA-I, and IRA-2 negative regulators of the RAS cyclic AMP pathway. Nature 1990;347:291.
Buckner JC, Peethambaram PP, Smithson WA, et al. Phase II trial of primary chemotherapy followed by reduced-dose radiation for CNS germ cell tumors. J Clin Oncol 1999;17:933.
Bunin GR, Surawicz TS, Witman PA, et al. The descriptive epidemiology of craniopharyngioma. J Neurosurg 1998;89:547.
Burger PC, Fuller GN. Pathology trends and pitfalls in histologic diagnosis, immunopathology, and applications of oncogene research. Brain tumors in children. Neurol Clin 1991;9:249.
Campbell RHA, Marshall WC, Chessells JM. Neurological complications of childhood leukaemia. Arch Dis Child 1977;52:850.
Cavazzuti V, Fischer EG, Welch K, et al. Neurological and psychological sequelae following different treatments of craniopharyngioma in children. J Neurosurg 1983;59:409.
CBTRUS. Statistical Report: Primary brain tumors in the United States, 1997-2001. Published by the Central Brain Tumor Registry of the United States, 2004-2005. www.CBTRUS.org.
Celli P, Cervoni L, Morselli E, et al. Spinal ependymomas and papilledema: Report of 4 cases and review of the literature. J Neurosurg Sci 1993;37:97.
Chamberlain MC. Recurrent cerebellar gliomas: Salvage therapy with oral etoposide. J Child Neurol 1997;12:200.
Chamberlain MC. Recurrent intracranial ependymoma in children: Salvage therapy with oral etoposide. Pediatrics 2001;24:117.
Chang T, Wong TT, Hwang B. Combination chemotherapy with vinblastine, bleomycin, cisplatin, and etoposide (VBPE) in children with primary intracranial germ cell tumors. Med Ped Oncol 1995;24:368.
Chapman CA, Waber DP, Bernstein JH, et al. Neurobehavioral and neurologic outcome in long-term survivors of posterior fossa brain tumors: Role of age and perioperative factors. J Child Neurol 1995;10:209.
Cheek WR, Taveras JM. Thalamic tumors. J Neurosurg 1966;24:505.
Chen CJ, Tseng YC, Hsu HL, et al. Imaging predictors of intracranial ependymomas. J Comput Assist Tomogr 2004;28:407.
Chen HSG, Gross JF. Intraarterial infusion of anticancer drugs: Theoretic aspects of drug delivery and review of responses. Cancer Treat Rep 1980;64:31.
Cheng MK. Spinal cord tumors in the People's Republic of China: A statistical review. Neurosurgery 1982;10:22.
Chin B, Sklar C, Donahue B, et al. Thyroid function as a late effect in survivors of pediatric medulloblastoma/primitive neuroectodermal tumors: A comparison of hyperfractionated versus conventional radiotherapy. Cancer 1997;80:798.
Chiu JK, Woo SY, Ater J, et al. Intracranial ependymoma in children: Analysis of prognostic factors. J Neurooncol 1992;13:283.
Chow E, Reardon DA, Shah AB, et al. Pediatric choroid plexus neoplasms. Int J Radiat Oncol Biol Phys 1999;44:249.
Chung CK, Stryker JA, Cruse R, et al. Glioblastoma multiforme following prophylactic cranial irradiation and intrathecal methotrexate in a child with acute lymphocytic leukemia. Cancer 1981;47:2563.
Chutorian AM, Schwartz JF, Evans RA, et al. Optic glioma in children. Neurology 1964;14:83.
Clarson CL, Del Maestro RF. Growth failure after treatment of pediatric brain tumors. Pediatrics 1999;103:E37.
Clayton PE, Shalet SM, Price DA. Gonadal function after chemotherapy and irradiation for childhood malignancies. Horm Res 1988;30:104.
Cohen ME, Duffner PK. Optic pathway tumors. Neurol Clin 1991;9:467.
Cohen ME, Duffner PK. Brain tumors in children: Principles of diagnosis and treatment. New York: Raven Press, 1994a.
Cohen ME, Duffner PK. Brainstem tumors. In: Cohen ME, Duffner PK, eds. Brain tumors in children: Principles of diagnosis and treatment, 2nd ed. New York: Raven Press, 1994b.
Cohen ME, Duffner PK. Ependymomas. In: Cohen ME, Duffner PK, eds. Brain tumors in children: Principles of diagnosis and treatment, 2nd ed. New York: Raven Press, 1994c.
Cohen ME, Duffner PK. Meningiomas. In: Cohen ME, Duffner PK, eds. Brain tumors in children: Principles of diagnosis and treatment, 2nd ed. New York: Raven Press, 1994d.
Cohen ME, Duffner PK. Pineal region tumors. In: Cohen ME, Duffner PK, eds. Brain tumors in children: Principles of diagnosis and treatment, 2nd ed. New York: Raven Press, 1994e.
Cohen ME, Duffner PK, Heffner RR, et al. Prognostic factors in brainstem gliomas. Neurology 1986;36:602.
Collins VP. Wilms' tumor: Its behavior and prognosis. J La State Med Soc 1955;197:474.
Comi AM, Backstrom JW, Burger PC, et al. Clinical and neuroradiologic findings in infants with intracranial ependymomas. Pediatr Neurol 1998;18:23.
Constine LS, Woolf PD, Cann D, et al. Hypothalamic-pituitary dysfunction after radiation for brain tumors. N Engl J Med 1993;328:87.
Conway PD, Oechler HW, Kun LE, et al. Importance of histologic condition and treatment of pediatric cerebellar astrocytoma. Cancer 1991;67:2772.
Coon JS, Landay AL, Weinstein RS. Advances in flow cytometry for diagnostic pathology. Lab Invest 1987;57:453.
Copeland DR, Fletcher JM, Pfefferbaum-Levine B, et al. Neuropsychological sequelae of childhood cancer in long-term survivors. Pediatrics 1985;75:745.
Cousens P, Waters B, Said J, et al. Cognitive effects of cranial irradiation in leukaemia: A survey and meta-analysis. J Child Psychol Psychiatry 1988;29:839.
Cushing H. Experiences with cerebellar medulloblastoma: A critical review. Acta Pathol Microbiol Scand 1930;7:1.
Cushing H. Experiences with the cerebellar astrocytomas: A critical review of seventy-six cases. Surg Gynecol Obstet 1931;52:129.
Dacou-Voutetakis C, Xypolyta A, Haidas SK Sr, et al. Irradiation of the head: Immediate effect on growth hormone secretion in children. J Clin Endocrinol Metab 1977;44:791.
Dai AI, Backstrom JW, Burger PC, et al. Supratentorial primitive neuroectodermal tumors of infancy: Clinical and radiologic findings. Pediatr Neurol 2003;29:430.
Dancey JE, Freidlin B. Targeting epidermal growth factor receptor—Are we missing the mark? Lancet 2003;36:62.
Danoff BF, Cowchock FS, Kramer S. Child craniopharyngioma: Survival, local control, endocrine and neurologic function following radiotherapy. Int J Radiat Oncol Biol Phys 1983;9:171.
D'Arpa P, Liu LF. Topoisomerase targeting anti tumor drugs. Biochem Biophys Acta 1989;989:163.
David RB, Hadfield MG, Vines FS, et al. Dural sinus occlusion in leukemia. Pediatrics 1975;56:793.
Davidoff LM. Some considerations in the therapy of pineal tumors: Rudolf Virchow lecture. Bull N Y Acad Med 1967;43:537.
Davis FG, Kupelian V, Freels S, et al. Prevalence estimates for primary brain tumors in the United States by behavior and major histology groups. Neuro-oncol 2001;3:152.
Davis FG, McCarthy BJ, Freels S, et al. The conditional probability of survival of patients with primary malignant brain tumor, surveillance, epidemiology and end results (SEER) data. Cancer 1999;85:485.
Davis LE, Cushing H. Papillomas of the choroid plexus. Arch Neurol Psychiatry 1925;13:681.
Debiec-Rychter M, Biernat W, Zakrzewski K, et al. Loss of chromosome 22 and proliferative potential in ependymomas. Folia Neuropathol 2003;41:191.

DeGirolami U, Schmidek H. Clinicopathological study of 53 tumors of the pineal region. J Neurosurg 1973;39:455.
Delattre JY, Safai B, Posner JB. Erythemia multiforme and Stevens-Johnson syndrome in patients receiving cranial irradiation and phenytoin. Neurology 1988;38:194.
Desai KI, Nadkarni TD, Mazumdar DP, et al. Prognostic factors for cerebellar astrocytomas in children: A study of 102 cases. Pediatr Neurosurg 2001;35:311.
DeSousa AL, Kalsbeck JE, Mealey J, et al. Diencephalic syndrome and its relation to opticochiasmatic glioma: Review of twelve cases. Neurosurgery 1979;4:207.
Deutsch M. Radiotherapy for primary brain tumors in very young children. Cancer 1982;50:2785.
Deutsch M, Thomas PRM, Krischer J, et al. Results of a prospective randomized trial comparing standard dose neuraxis irradiation (3,600 cGy/20) with reduced neuraxis irradiation (2,340 cGy/13) in patients with low-stage medulloblastoma. Pediatr Neurosurg 1996;24:167.
Devoe DJ, Miller WL, Conte FA, et al. Long-term outcome in children and adolescents after transsphenoidal surgery for Cushing's disease. J Clin Endocrinol Metab 1997;82:3196.
Dickinson WP, Berry DH, Dickson L, et al. Differential effects of cranial radiation on growth hormone response to arginine and insulin infusion. J Pediatr 1978;92:754.
DiMeco F, Li KW, Byler BM, et al. Local delivery of mitoxantrone for the treatment of malignant brain tumors in rats. J Neurosurg 2002;97:1173.
DiRocco C, Ceddia A, Iannelli A. Intracranial tumours in the first year of life. A report on 51 cases. Acta Neurochir (Wein) 1993;123:14.
Dohrmann GJ, Farwell JR, Flannery JT. Ependymomas and ependymoblastomas in children. J Neurosurg 1976;45:273.
Donner P, Greiser-Wilke I, Moelling K. Nuclear localization and DNA binding of the transforming gene product of avian myelocytomatosis virus. Nature 1982;296:262.
Dropcho EJ, Wisoff JH, Walker RW, et al. Supratentorial malignant gliomas in childhood: A review of fifty cases. Ann Neurol 1987;22:355.
Due-Tønnessen BJ, Helseth E, Scheie D, et al. Long-term outcome after resection of benign cerebellar astrocytomas in children and young adults (0-19 years): Report of 110 consecutive cases. Pediatr Neurosurg 2002;37:71.
Duffner PK. Long term consequences of CNS therapy. In: Wallace H, Green D, eds. Late effects of childhood cancer. London: Edward Arnold Publishers, 2004a.
Duffner PK. Long-term effects of radiation therapy on cognitive and endocrine function in children with leukemia and brain tumors. Neurologist 2004b;10:293.
Duffner PK, Cohen ME. Primitive neuroectodermal tumors. In: Vecht CJ, ed. Handbook of clinical neurology, 1997;24:68. Neuro-Oncology, Part II, Elsevier Science.
Duffner PK, Cohen ME, Anderson SW, et al. Long-term effects of treatment on endocrine function in children with brain tumors. Ann Neurol 1983a;14:528.
Duffner PK, Cohen ME, Brecher ML, et al. Abnormalities of CT scans and altered methotrexate clearance in children with CNS leukemia. Neurology 1984;34:229.
Duffner PK, Cohen ME, Heffner RR, et al. Primitive neuroectodermal tumors of childhood: An approach to therapy. J Neurosurg 1981;55:376.
Duffner PK, Cohen ME, Kun L, et al. Prognostic factors in infants with ependymomas. Ann Neurol 1996a;38:546.
Duffner PK, Cohen ME, Myers MH, et al. Survival of children with brain tumors: SEER Program, 1973-1980. Neurology 1986;36:597.
Duffner PK, Cohen ME, Parker MS. Prospective intellectual testing in children with brain tumors. Ann Neurol 1985a;18:405.
Duffner PK, Cohen ME, Sanford RA, et al. Lack of efficacy of postoperative chemotherapy and delayed radiation in very young children with pineoblastoma. Med Pediatr Oncol 1995a;25:38.
Duffner PK, Cohen ME, Thomas PRM. Late effects of treatment on the intelligence of children with posterior fossa tumors. Cancer 1983b;51:233
Duffner PK, Horowitz ME, Krischer JP, et al. Postoperative chemotherapy and delayed radiation in children less than three years of age with malignant brain tumors. N Engl J Med 1993;328:1725.
Duffner PK, Krischer JP, Burger PC, et al. Treatment of infants with malignant gliomas: The Pediatric Oncology Group Experience. J Neuro-oncol 1996b;28:245.
Duffner PK, Krischer JP, Horowitz ME, et al. Second malignancies in young children with primary brain tumors following treatment with prolonged postoperative chemotherapy and delayed irradiation: A Pediatric Oncology Group Study. Ann Neurol 1998a;44:313.
Duffner PK, Krischer JP, Sanford RA, et al. Prognostic factors in infants and very young children with intracranial ependymomas. Pediatr Neurosurg 1998b;28:215.
Duffner PK, Kun LE, Burger PC, et al. Postoperative chemotherapy and delayed radiation in infants and very young children with choroid plexus carcinomas. Pediatr Neurosurg 1995b;22:189.
Duffner PK, Voorhess ML, MacGillivray MH, et al. Long-term effects of cranial irradiation on endocrine function in children with brain tumors: A prospective study. Cancer 1985b;56:2189.
Dunton SF, Nitschke R, Spruce WE, et al. Progressive ascending paralysis following administration of intrathecal and intravenous cytosine arabinoside. A Pediatric Oncology Group study. Cancer 1986;57:1083.
Dutton JJ. Gliomas of the anterior visual pathway. Surv Ophthalmol 1994;38:427.
Eberhart CG, Burger PC. Anaplasia and grading in medulloblastomas. Brain Pathol 2003;13:376.
Eberhart CG, Kratz J, Wang Y, et al. Histopathologic and molecular prognostic markers in medulloblastoma: c-myc, N-myc, TrkC, and anaplasia. J Neuropathol Exp Neurol 2004;63:441.
Eckman WW, Patlak CS, Fenstermacher JD. A critical evaluation of the principles governing the advantages of intraarterial infusions. J Pharmacokinet Biopharm 1974;2:257.
Edwards MSB, Davis RL, Laurent JP. Tumor markers and cytologic features of cerebrospinal fluid. Cancer 1985;56:1773.
Ellenberg L, McComb JG, Siegel SE, et al. Factors affecting intellectual outcome in pediatric brain tumor patients. Neurosurgery 1987;21:638.
Elliott PJ, Hayward NJ, Huff MR, et al. Unlocking the blood brain barrier: A role for Cereport in brain tumor therapy. Exp Neurol 1996;141:214.
Epstein F, Epstein N. Intramedullary tumors of the spinal cord. In: Shillito J Jr, Matson DD, eds. Pediatric neurosurgery: Surgery of the developing nervous system. New York: Grune & Stratton, 1982.
Epstein FJ, Farmer JP. Pediatric spinal cord tumor surgery. Neurosurg Clin N Am 1990;1:569.
Epstein FJ, Farmer JP. Trend in surgery: Laser surgery, use of the Cavitron, and debulking surgery. Neurol Clin 1991;9:307.
Epstein F, Wisoff JF. Intrinsic brainstem tumors in childhood: Surgical indications. J Neurooncol 1988;6:304.
Evans AE, Anderson JR, Lefkowitz-Boudreaux IB, et al. Adjuvant chemotherapy of childhood posterior fossa ependymoma: Craniospinal irradiation with or without adjuvant CCNU, vincristine and prednisone: A Children's Cancer Group study. Med Pediatr Oncol 1996;27:8.
Evans AE, Gilbert ES, Zandstra R. The increasing incidence of central nervous system leukemia in children (Children's Cancer Study Group A). Cancer 1970;26:404.
Evans A, Jenkin RDT, Sposto R, et al. The treatment of medulloblastoma: Results of a prospective randomized trial of radiation therapy with and without CCNU, vincristine and prednisone. J Neurosurg 1990;72:572.
Farwell JR, Dohrmann GJ, Flannery JT. Central nervous system tumors in children. Cancer 1977;40:3123.
Farwell JR, Dorhmann GJ, Flannery JT. Intracranial neoplasms in infants. Arch Neurol 1978;35:533.
Fazekas JT. Treatment of grades I & II brain astrocytomas. The role of radiotherapy. Int J Radiat Oncol Biol Phys 1977;2:661.
Feinberg WM, Swenson MR. Cerebrovascular complications of L-asparaginase therapy. Neurology 1988;38:127.
Fessard C. Cerebral tumors in infancy. Am J Dis Child 1968;115:302.
Fewer D. History and general considerations. In: Fewer D, Wilson CB, Levin VA, eds. Brain tumor chemotherapy. Springfield, IL: Charles C Thomas, 1976.
Figarella-Branger D, Civatte M, Bouvier-Labit C, et al. Prognostic factors in intracranial ependymomas in children. J Neurosurg 2000;93:605.
Figueiredo EG, Matushita H, Machado AGG, et al. Leptomeningeal dissemination of pilocytic astrocytoma at diagnosis in childhood. Ara Neuropsiquiatr 2003;61(3-B):842.
Figuerora RE, Gammal TE, Brooks BS, et al. MR findings on primitive neuroectodermal tumors. J Comp Assist Tomogr 1989;13:773.
Finlay JL. High-dose chemotherapy followed by bone marrow rescue for recurrent brain tumors. In: Packer RJ, Bleyer WA, Pochedly C, eds. Pediatric neurooncology. Philadelphia: Hardwood Academic Publishers, 1992.

Finlay JL, Goldman S, Wong MC, et al. Pilot study of high-dose thiotepa and etoposide with autologous bone marrow rescue in children and young adults with recurrent CNS tumors. J Clin Oncol 1996;14:2495.
Fischer EG, Welch K, Shillito J Jr, et al. Craniopharyngiomas in children. Long-term effects of conservative surgical procedures combined with radiation therapy. J Neurosurg 1990;73:534.
Fisher PG, Breiter SN, Carson BS, et al. A clinicopathologic reappraisal of brain stem tumor classification. Identification of pilocystic astrocytoma and fibrillary astrocytoma as distinct entities. Cancer 2000;89:1569.
Fletcher JM, Copeland DR. Neurobehavioral effects of central nervous system prophylactic treatment of cancer in children. J Clin Exp Neuropsychol 1988;10:495.
Foreman NK, Hay TC, Handler M. Chemotherapy for spinal cord astrocytoma. Med Pediatr Oncol 1998;30:311.
Foreman NK, Love S, Gill SS, et al. Second-look surgery for incompletely resected fourth ventricle ependymomas: Technical case report. Neurosurgery 1997;40:856.
Frank F, Fabrizi AP, Frank-Ricci R, et al. Stereotactic biopsy and treatment of brainstem lesions: Combined study of 33 cases (Bologna-Marseille). Acta Neurochir Suppl 1988;42:177.
Frankel SA, German WJ. Glioblastoma multiforme: Review of 219 cases with regard to natural history, pathology, diagnostic methods, and treatment. J Neurosurg 1958;15:489.
Franz DN. Diagnosis and management of tuberous sclerosis complex. Semin Pediatr Neurol 1998;5:253.
Fraser RD, Paterson DC, Simpson DA. Orthopaedic aspects of spinal tumors in children. J Bone Joint Surg 1977;59B:143.
Freeman CR, Farmer JP, Montes J. Low grade astrocytomas in children: Evolving management strategies. Int J Radiat Oncol Biol Phys 1998;41:979.
Freeman CR, Krischer J, Sanford RA, et al. Hyperfractionated radiotherapy in brain tumors: Results of treatment at the 7020 cGy dose level: Pediatric Oncology Group Study #8495. Cancer 1991;68:474.
Freeman CR, Perilongo G. Chemotherapy for brain stem gliomas. Childs Nerv Sys 1999;15:545.
Freeman JE, Johnston PGB, Voke JM. Somnolence after prophylactic cranial irradiation in children with acute lymphoblastic leukemia. BMJ 1973;4:523.
Friedman HS, Dolan ME, Pegg AE, et al. Activity of temozolomide in the treatment of central nervous system xenografts. Cancer Res 1995;55:2853.
Fukunaga-Johnson N, Lee JH, Sandler HM. Patterns of failure following treatment for medulloblastoma: Is it necessary to treat the posterior fossa? Int J Radiat Oncol Biol Phys 1998;42:143.
Furnari FB, Huang HJ, Cavenee WK. Molecular biology of malignant degeneration of astrocytoma. Pediatr Neurosurg 1996;24:41.
Gajjar A, Bhargava R, Jenkins JJ, et al. Low-grade astrocytoma with neuraxis dissemination at diagnosis. J Neurosurg 1995;83:67.
Gajjar A, Sanford RA, Heideman R, et al. Low-grade astrocytoma: A decade of experience at St. Jude Children's Research Hospital. J Clin Oncol 1997;15:2792.
Ganick DJ, Robertson WC Jr, Viseskul C, et al. Dural sinus thrombosis in leukemia. Am J Dis Child 1978;132:1040.
Giglio P, Benedict R, Duffner PK, et al. Cognitive defects in children treated for tumors of the pineal region. Ann Neurol 2000;48:541.
Gilhuis HJ, Kappelle AC, Beute G, et al. Radiotherapy for partially resected spinal ependymomas: A retrospective study of 60 cases. Oncol Rep 2003;10:2079.
Gilles FH, Winston K, Fulchiero A, et al. Histologic features and observational variation in cerebellar gliomas in children. J Natl Cancer Inst 1977;58:175.
Gjerris F, Klinken L. Long-term prognosis in children with benign cerebellar astrocytoma. J Neurosurg 1978;49:179.
Glaser JS, Hoyt WF, Corbett J. Visual morbidity with chiasmal glioma. Arch Ophthalmol 1971;85:3.
Glass JP, Hwang TL, Leavens ME, et al. Cerebral radiation necrosis following treatment of extracranial malignancies. Cancer 1984;54:1966.
Goh S, Butler W, Thiele EA. Subependymal giant cell tumors in tuberous sclerosis complex. Neurology 2004;63:1457.
Gol A, McKissock W. The cerebellar astrocytomas: A report on 98 verified cases. J Neurosurg 1959;16:287.
Goldwein J, Radcliffe J, Johnson J, et al. Updated results of a pilot study of low dose craniospinal irradiation plus chemotherapy for children under five with cerebellar primitive neuroectodermal tumors (medulloblastoma). Int J Radiat Oncol 1996;34:899.
Goldwein JW, Leary JM, Packer RJ, et al. Intracranial ependymomas in children. Int J Radiat Biol Phys 1990;9:1497.
Good CD, Wade AM, Hayward RD, et al. Surveillance neuroimaging in childhood intracranial ependymoma: How effective, how often, and for how long? J Neurosurg 2001;94:27.
Gordon GS, Wallace SJ, Neal JW. Intracranial tumours during the first two years of life: Presenting features. Arch Dis Child 1995;73:345.
Gowers W, Horsley V. A case of tumor of the spinal cord: Removal; recovery. Med Chir Trans Lond 1888;71:377.
Grant GA, Avellino AM, Loeser JD, et al. Management of intrinsic gliomas of the tectal plate in children. A ten year review. Pediatr Neurosurg 1999;31:170.
Greenwood J. Intramedullary tumors of spinal cord: A follow-up study after total surgical removal. J Neurosurg 1963;20:665.
Greydanus DE, Burgert EO, Gilchrist GS. Hypothalamic syndrome in children with acute lymphocytic leukemia. Mayo Clin Proc 1978;53:217.
Grieshammer T, Zimmer C, Vogeley KT. Immunohistochemistry of primitive neuroectodermal tumors in infants with special emphasis on cytokeratin expression. Acta Neuropathol 1991;82:494.
Griffin TW, Beaufait D, Blasko JC. Cystic cerebellar astrocytomas in childhood. Cancer 1979;44:276.
Grill J, Kieffer RV, Bulteau C, et al. Long-term intellectual outcome in children with posterior fossa tumors according to radiation doses and volumes. Int J Radiat Oncol Biol Phys 1999;45:137.
Grill J, Le Deley MC, Gambarelli D, et al. Postoperative chemotherapy without irradiation for ependymoma in children under 5 years of age: A multicenter trial of the French Society of Pediatric Oncology. J Clin Oncol 2001;19:1288.
Grundy BL. Intraoperative monitoring of sensory evoked potentials. Anesthesiology 1983;58:72.
Gurney JG, Davis S, Severson RK, et al. Trends in cancer incidence among children in the U.S. Cancer 1996;78:532.
Ha K, Kanaya S, Ikeda T, et al. Cortical blindness in a child with acute leukemia. Acta Paediatr Scand 1980;69:781.
Haapasalo H, Sallinin S, Sallinen P, et al. Clinicopathological correlation of cell proliferation, apoptosis and p53 cerebellar pilocytic astrocytomas. Neuropathol Appl Neurobiol 1999;25:134.
Hahn AF, Feasby TE, Gilbert JJ. Paraparesis following intrathecal chemotherapy. Neurology 1983;33:1032.
Halperin EC. Pediatric brainstem tumors: Patterns of treatment failure and their implications for radiotherapy. Int J Radiat Oncol Biol Phys 1985;11:1293.
Halperin EC, Friedman HS, Schold SC Jr, et al. Surgery, hyperfractionated craniospinal irradiation, and adjuvant chemotherapy in the management of supratentorial embryonal neuroepithelial neoplasms in children. Surg Neurol 1993;40:278.
Hamby WB. Tumors in the spinal cord in childhood. II. Analysis of the literature of a subsequent decade (1933-1942): Report of a case of meningitis due to an intramedullary epidermoid communicating with a dermoid sinus. J Neuropathol Exp Neurol 1944;3:397.
Hara T, Kishikawa T, Miyazaki S, et al. Central nervous system complications in childhood leukemia: Correlation between clinical and computed tomographic findings. Am J Pediatr Hematol Oncol 1984;6:129.
Hart MN, Earle KM. Primitive neuroectodermal tumors of the brain in children. Cancer 1973;32:890.
Heideman RL, Kuttesch J Jr, Gajjar A, et al. Supratentorial malignant gliomas in childhood: A single institution perspective. Cancer 1997;80:497.
Herrmann, HD, Westphal M, Winkler K, et al. Treatment of nongerminomatous germ-cell tumors of the pineal region. Neurosurgery 1994;34:524.
Hirsch J, Rose CS, Pierre-Kahn A, et al. Benign astrocytic and oligodendrocytic tumors of the cerebral hemispheres in children. J Neurosurg 1989;70:568.
Hirsch JF, Reiner D, Czernichow P, et al. Medulloblastoma in childhood. Survival and functional results. Acta Neurochir 1979;48:1.
Hoffman HJ. Craniopharyngioma: The continuing controversy of management. Concepts Pediatr Neurosurg 1982;2:14.
Holland JF. Oncologist's reply. N Engl J Med 1976;294:440.
Honig PJ, Charney EB. Children with brain tumor headaches. Am J Dis Child 1982;136:121.
Hope-Stone HF. Results of treatment of medulloblastomas. J Neurosurg 1970;32:83.

Hoppe-Hirsch E, Hirsch JF, Lellouch-Tubiana A, et al. Malignant hemispheric tumors in childhood. Childs Nerv Syst 1993;9:131.

Hoppe-Hirsch E, Renier D, LeBouch-Tubiana A, et al. Medulloblastoma in childhood: Progressive intellectual deterioration. Childs Nerv Syst 1990;6:60.

Houten JK, Weiner HL. Pediatric intramedullary spinal cord tumors: Special considerations. J Neurooncol 2000;47:225.

Huang B, Starostik P, Schraut H, et al. Human ependymomas reveal frequent deletions on chromosomes 6 and 9. Acta Neuropathol 2003;106:357.

Hughes EN, Shillito J, Sallan SE, et al. Medulloblastoma at the Joint Center for Radiation Therapy between 1968 and 1984. Cancer 1988;61:1992.

Inamura T, Nomura T, Bartus RT, et al. Intracarotid infusion of Cereport, a bradykinin analog: A method for selective drug delivery to brain tumors. J Neurosurg 1994;81:752.

Jackacki RI, Zeltzer PM, Boyett JM, et al. Survival and prognostic factors following radiation and/or chemotherapy for primitive neuroectodermal tumors of the pineal region in infants and children: A report of the Children's Cancer Group. J Clin Oncol 1995; 131377.

Jankovic M, Brouwers P, Valsecchi MG, et al. Association of 1800 cGy cranial irradiation with intellectual function in children with acute lymphoblastic leukaemia. Lancet 1994;344:224.

Jannoun L, Bloom HJG. Long-term psychological effects in children treated for intracranial tumors. Int J Radiat Oncol Biol Phys 1990;18:747.

Jelsma R, Bucy PC. The treatment of glioblastoma multiforme of the brain. J Neurosurg 1967;27:388.

Jenkin RD, Simpson WJ, Keen CW. Pineal and suprasellar germinomas. J Neurosurg 1978;48:99.

Johnson FL, Bernstein ID, Hartmann Jr, et al. Seizures associated with vincristine sulfate therapy. J Pediatr 1973;82:699.

Jooma R, Hayward RD, Grant DN. Intracranial neoplasms during the first year of life: Analysis of one hundred consecutive cases. Neurosurgery 1984;14:31.

Jukich PJ, McCarthy BJ, Surawicz TS, et al. Trends in incidence of primary brain tumors in the United States, 1984-1994. Neuro-oncol 2001;3:141.

Kao GD, Goldwein JW, Schultz DJ, et al. The impact of perioperative factors on subsequent intelligence quotient deficits in children treated for medulloblastoma/posterior fossa primitive neuroectodermal tumors. Cancer 1994;74:965.

Kato M, Azuma E, Ido M, et al. Ten-year survey of the intellectual deficits in children with acute lymphoblastic leukemia receiving chemoimmunotherapy. Med Pediatr Oncol 1993;21:435.

Kearse LA Jr, Lopez-Bresnahan M, McPeck K, et al. Loss of somatosensory evoked potentials during intramedullary spinal cord surgery predicts postoperative neurologic deficits in motor function. J Clin Anesth 1993;5:392.

Kernohan JW, Mabon RF, Svien H, et al. A simplified classification of the gliomas. Mayo Clin Proc 1949;24:71.

Kestle JRW, Hoffman HJ, Mock AR. Moyamoya phenomenon after radiation for optic glioma. J Neurosurg 1993;79:32.

Kim TH, Chin HW, Pollan S, et al. Radiotherapy of primary brainstem tumors. Int J Radiat Oncol Biol Phys 1980;6:51.

Kingsley DPE, Kendall BE. The CT scanner in posterior fossa tumors of childhood. Br J Radiol 1979;52:769.

Kiwak KJ, Deray MJ, Shields WD. Torticollis in three children with syringomyelia and spinal cord tumor. Neurology 1983;33:946.

Kleihues P, Cavenee WK, eds. World Health Organization Classification of Tumors, Pathology and Genetics of the Nervous System. Lyon, France: International Agency for Research on Cancer Press, 2000.

Kleinman GM, Hochberg FH, Richardson EP. Systemic metastasis from medulloblastoma: Report of two cases and review of the literature. Cancer 1981;48:2296.

Knudson AG. Mutation and cancer: Statistical study of retinoblastoma. Proc Natl Acad Sci U S A 1971;68:820.

Kopelson G. Cerebellar glioblastoma. Cancer 1982;50:308.

Kopelson G, Linggood RM, Kleinman GM, et al. Management of intramedullary spinal cord tumors. Radiology 1980;135:473.

Korshunov A, Golanov A, Sycheva R, et al. The histologic grade is a main prognostic factor for patients with intracranial ependymomas treated in the microneurosurgical era: An analysis of 258 patients. Cancer 2004;100:1230.

Kortman RD, Kuhl J, Timmerman B, et al. Postoperative neoadjuvant chemotherapy before radiotherapy as compared to immediate radiotherapy followed by maintenance chemotherapy in the treatment of medulloblastoma in childhood: Results of the German prospective randomized trial HIT'91;2000. Int J Radiat Oncol Biol Phys 2000;46:269.

Kovnar EH. Hyperfractionated irradiation for childhood ependymoma: Early results of a phase III Pediatric Oncology Group Study. Presented at the Seventh International Symposium of Pediatric Neuro-oncology. Washington, DC, May 15-18, 1996 (abstract).

Kovnar E, Kun L, Krischer. Patterns of dissemination and recurrence in childhood ependymoma: Preliminary results of Pediatric Oncology Group protocol #8532. Ann Neurol 1991;30:457.

Kun L. Principles of radiation therapy. In: Cohen ME, Duffner PK, eds. Brain tumors in children: Principles of diagnosis and treatment. New York: Raven Press, 1994.

Kun LE, Mulhern RK, Crisco JJ. Quality of life in children treated for brain tumors; Intellectual, emotional and academic function. J Neurosurg 1983;58:1.

Lampert PW, Davis RL. Delayed effects of radiation on the human central nervous system early and late delayed reactions. Neurology 1964;14:912.

Larkins RG, Martin FIR. Hypopituitarism after extracranial irradiation: Evidence for hypothalamic origin. BMJ 1973;1:152.

Leibel SA, Sheline GE, Wara WM, et al. The role of radiation therapy in the treatment of astrocytomas. Cancer 1975;35:1551.

Leviton A. Principles of epidemiology. In: Cohen ME, Duffner PK, eds. Brain tumors in children: Principles of diagnosis and treatment, 2nd ed. New York: Raven Press, 1994.

Lewis DW, Packer RJ, Raney B, et al. Incidence, presentation, and outcome of spinal cord disease in children with systemic cancer. Pediatrics 1986;78:438.

Listernick R, Louis DN, Packer RJ, et al. Optic pathway gliomas in children with neurofibromatosis. 1. Consensus statement from the NF1 Optic Pathway Glioma Task Force. Ann Neurol 1997;41:143.

Littman P, Jarrett P, Bilaniuk LT, et al. Pediatric brainstem gliomas. Cancer 1980;45:2787.

Liu CY, Yim BT, Wozniak AJ. Anticoagulation therapy for radiation-induced myelopathy. Ann Pharmacother 2001;35:188.

Livesey SA, Brook CGD. Thyroid dysfunction after radiotherapy and chemotherapy of brain tumours. Arch Dis Child 1989;64:593.

Lo WD, Matthay KK, Kushner J. Spinal cord compression in a child with acute lymphoblastic leukemia. Am J Pediatr Hematol Oncol 1985;7:373.

Loeffler JS, Alexander E. The role of stereotactic radiosurgery in the management of intracranial tumors. Oncology 1990;4:21.

Longeway K, Mulhern R, Crisco J, et al. Treatment of meningeal relapse in childhood acute lymphoblastic leukemia, II: A prospective study of intellectual loss specific to CNS relapse and therapy. Am J Pediatr Hematol Oncol 1990;12:45.

Louis DN, Holland EC, Cairncross JG. Glioma classification: A molecular reappraisal. Am J Pathol 2001;159:779.

Low NL, Correll JW, Hammill JF. Tumors of the cerebral hemispheres in children. Arch Neurol 1965;13:547.

Lowis SP, Pizer BL, Coakham H, et al. Chemotherapy for spinal cord astrocytoma: Can natural history be modified? Childs Nerv Syst 1998;14:317.

Lustig RH, Schriock EA, Kaplan SL, et al. Effect of growth hormone-releasing factor on growth hormone release in children with radiation-induced growth hormone deficiency. Pediatrics 1985;76:274.

MacCollin M, Mautner VF. The diagnosis and management of neurofibromatosis 2 in childhood. Semin Pediatr Neurol 1998;5:243.

MacDonald TJ, Rood BR, Santi MR, et al. Advances on the diagnosis, molecular genetics, and treatment of pediatric embryonal CNS tumors. Oncologist 2003;8:174.

Machado M, Salcman M, Kaplan RS, et al. Expanded role of the cerebrospinal fluid reservoir in neurooncology: indications, causes of revisions, and complications. Neurosurgery 1985;17:600.

MacLean WE, Noll RB, Stehbens JA, et al. Neuropsychological effects of cranial irradiation in young children with acute lymphoblastic leukemia 9 months after diagnosis. Arch Neurol 1995;52:156.

Mahoney DH, Cohen ME, Friedman HS, et al. Carboplatin is effective therapy for young children with progressive optic pathway tumors: A Pediatric Oncology Group Phase II study. Neuro-oncology 2000;2:213.

Mahoney DH Jr, Shuster JJ, Nitschke R, et al. Acute neurotoxicity in children with B-precursor acute lymphoid leukemia: An association

with intermediate-dose intravenous methotrexate and intrathecal triple therapy: A Pediatric Oncology Group study. J Clin Oncol 1998;16:1712.
Mandell LR, Kadota R, Freeman C. There is no role for hyperfractionated radiotherapy in the management of children with newly diagnosed diffuse intrinsic brainstem tumors: Results of a Pediatric Oncology Group phase III trial comparing conventional vs. hyperfractionated radiotherapy. Int J Radiat Oncol Biol Phys 1999;43:959.
Mansur DB, Drzymala RE, Rich KM, et al. The efficacy of stereotactic radiosurgery in the management of intracranial ependymoma. J Neurooncol 2004;66:187.
Marchese MJ, Chang CH. Malignant astrocytic gliomas in children. Cancer 1990;65:2771.
Marec-Berard P, Jouvet A, Thiesse P, et al. Supratentorial embryonal tumors in children under 5 years of age: An SFOP study of treatment with postoperative chemotherapy alone. Med Pediatr Oncol 2002;38:83.
Markesbery WR, Challa VR. Electron microscopic findings in primitive neuroectodermal tumors of the cerebrum. Cancer 1979;44:141.
Marks JE, Adler SJ. A comparative study of ependymomas by site or origin. Int J Radiat Oncol Biol Phys 1982;8:37.
Marks JE, Baglan RJ, Prassad SC, et al. Cerebral radionecrosis: Incidence and risk in relation to dose, time, fractionation, and volume. Int J Radiat Oncol Biol Phys 1981;7:243.
Marshall CJ. Tumor suppressor genes. Cell 1991;64:313.
Martindale D. T cell triumph. Immunotherapy may have finally turned a corner. Sci Am 2003;288:12.
Martins AN, Johnston JS, Henry JM, et al. Delayed radiation necrosis of the brain. J Neurosurg 1977;47:336.
Massimino M, Gandola L, Giangaspero F, et al. Hyperfractionated radiotherapy and chemotherapy for childhood ependymoma: Final results of the first prospective AIEOP (Associazione Italiana di Ematologia-Oncologia Pediatrica) study. Int J Radiat Oncol Biol Phys 2004;58:1336.
Matson DD. Cerebellar astrocytoma in childhood. Pediatrics 1956;18:150.
Matson DD. Intracranial tumors of the first two years of life. West J Surg Obstet Gynecol 1964;72:117.
Matson DD. Neurosurgery of infancy and childhood. Springfield, IL: Charles C Thomas, 1969.
Matson DD, Crigler JF. Management of craniopharyngioma in childhood. J Neurosurg 1969; 30:377.
Maytal J, Grossman R, Yusuf FH, et al. Prognosis and treatment of seizures in children with acute lymphoblastic leukemia. Epilepsia 1995;36:831.
McCowage G, Tien R, McLendon R, et al. Successful treatment of childhood pilocytic astrocytomas metastatic to the leptomeninges with high-dose cyclophosphamide. Med Pediatr Oncol 1996;27:32.
McEvoy AW, Harding BN, Phipps KP, et al. Management of choroids plexus tumours in children: 20 years experience at a single neurosurgical centre. Pediatr Neurosurg 2000;32:192.
McKissock W, Paine KWE. Primary tumours of the thalamus. Brain 1958;81:41.
McLean DR, Clink HM, Ernst P, et al. Myelopathy after intrathecal chemotherapy. Cancer 1994;73:3037.
Mead GM, Arnold AM, Green JA, et al. Epileptic seizures associated with Cisplatin administration. Cancer Treat Rep 1982;66:1719.
Merchant TE. Current management of childhood ependymoma. Oncology 2002;16:629.
Merchant TE, Haida T, Wang MH, et al. Anaplastic ependymoma: Treatment of pediatric patients with or without craniospinal radiation therapy. J Neurosurg 1997;86:943.
Merchant TE, Jenkins JJ, Burger PC, et al. Influence of tumor grade on time to progression after irradiation for localized ependymoma in children. Int J Radiat Oncol Biol Phys 2002a;53:52.
Merchant TE, Kiehna EN, Sanford RA, et al. Craniopharyngioma: The St. Jude Children's Research Hospital experience 1984-2001. Int J Radiat Oncol Biol Phys 2002b;53:533.
Merchant TE, Kiehna EN, Thompson SJ, et al. Pediatric low-grade and ependymal spinal cord tumors. Pediatr Neurosurg 2000;32:30.
Merchant TE, Zhu Y, Thompson SJ, et al. Preliminary results from a phase II trial of conformal radiation therapy for pediatric patients with localized low grade astrocytoma and ependymoma. Int J Radiat Oncol Biol Phys 2002c;52:325.
Mikaeloff Y, Raquin MA, Lellouch-Tubiana A, et al. Primitive cerebral neuroectodermal tumors excluding medulloblastomas: A retrospective study of 30 cases. Pediatr Neurosurg 1998;29:170.
Milstein JM, Geyer JR, Berger MS, et al. Favorable prognosis for brainstem gliomas in neurofibromatosis. J Neurooncol 1989;7:367.
Modan G, Mart H, Baidatz D, et al. Radiation induced head and neck tumors. Lancet 1974;23:277.
Morreale VM, Ebersold MJ, Quast LM, et al. Cerebellar astrocytoma: Experience with 54 cases surgically treated at the Mayo Clinic, Rochester, Minnesota, from 1978 to 1990. J Neurosurg 1997;87:257.
Moshang T Jr, Grimberg A. The effects of irradiation and chemotherapy on growth. Endocrinol Metab Clin North Am 1996;25:731.
Mulhern RK, Horowitz ME, Kovnar EH, et al. Neurodevelopmental status of infants and young children treated for brain tumors with preradiation chemotherapy. J Clin Oncol 1989;7:1660.
Mulhern RK, Kun LE. Neuropsychologic function in children with brain tumors, III: Interval changes in the six months following treatment. Med Pediatr Oncol 1985;13:318.
Mulhern RK, Ochs J, Fairclough D, et al. Intellectual and academic achievement status after CNS relapse: A retrospective analysis of 40 children treated for acute lymphoblastic leukemia. J Clin Oncol 1987;5:933.
Murovic J, Sundaresan N. Pediatric spinal axis tumors. Neurosurg Clin N Am 1992;3:947.
Murthy K, Smith S, Weinstock A, et al. Facial palsy, an unusual presented feature of childhood leukemia. Pediatr Neurol 2002;27:68.
Nadkarni TD, Rekate HL. Pediatric intramedullary spinal cord tumors. Critical review of the literature. Childs Nerv Syst 1999;15:17.
National Radiological Protection Board. Radiol Protection Bull 1981;39:3.
Needle MN, Goldwein JW, Grass J, et al. Adjuvant chemotherapy for the treatment of intracranial ependymoma of childhood. Cancer 1997;80:341.
Nishio S, Tashima T, Takeshita I, et al. Intraventricular neurocytoma: Clinicopathological features of six cases. J Neurosurg 1988;68:665.
Noble ME, Endcott JA, Johnson LN. Protein kinase inhibitors: Insights into drug design from structure. Science 2004;303:1800.
Nolan MA, Sakuta R, Chuang N, et al. Dysembryoplastic neuroepithelial tumors in childhood. Neurology 2004;62:2270.
Norman D, Mills CM, Brant-Zawadzki M, et al. Magnetic resonance imaging of the spinal cord and canal: Potentials and limitations. Am J Roentgenol 1983;141:1147.
North KN. Neurofibromatosis 1 in childhood. Semin Pediatr Neurol 1998;5:231.
Ochs JJ, Bowman WP, Pui CH, et al. Seizures in childhood lymphoblastic leukaemia patients. Lancet 1984;2:1422.
Oi S, Kokumai T, Matsumoto S. Congenital brain tumors in Japan (ISPN Cooperative Study): Special clinical features in neonates. Childs Nerv Syst 1990;6:86.
Ojemann GA, Ward AA. Speech representation in ventrolateral thalamus. Brain 1971;94:669.
Omura M, Aida N, Sekido K. Large intracranial vessel occlusive vasculopathy after radiation therapy in children: Clinical features and usefulness of magnetic resonance imaging. Int J Radiat Oncol Biol Phys 1997;38:241.
O'Sullivan C, Jenkin RD, Doherty MA, et al. Spinal cord tumors in children: Long-term results of combined surgical and radiation treatment. J Neurosurg 1994;81:507.
Packer R, Cogan P, Vezina G, et al. Medulloblastoma: Clinical and biologic aspects. Neuro-oncology 1999a;1:232.
Packer RJ, Cohen BH, Cooney K. Intracranial germ cell tumors. Oncologist 2000;5:312.
Packer RJ, Goldwein J, Nicholson HS, et al. Treatment of children with medulloblastomas with reduced-dose craniospinal radiation therapy and adjuvant chemotherapy: A Children's Cancer Group study. J Clin Oncol 1999b;17:2127.
Packer RJ, Lange B, Ater J, et al. Carboplatin and vincristine for recurrent and newly diagnosed low-grade gliomas of childhood. J Clin Oncol 1993;11:850.
Packer RJ, Rorke LB, Lange BJ, et al. Cerebrovascular accidents in children with cancer. Pediatrics 1985;76:194.
Packer RJ, Siegel KR, Sutton LN, et al. Efficacy of adjuvant chemotherapy for patients with poor risk medulloblastoma: A preliminary report. Ann Neurol 1988a;24:503.
Packer RJ, Sutton LN, Atkins TE, et al. A prospective study of cognitive function in children receiving whole-brain radiotherapy and chemotherapy: 2-year results. J Neurosurg 1989;70:707.
Packer RJ, Sutton LN, Bilaniuk LT, et al. Treatment of chiasmatic/hypothalamic gliomas of childhood with chemotherapy: An update. Ann Neurol 1988b;23:79.

Packer RJ, Sutton LN, Elterman R, et al. Outcome for children with medulloblastoma treated with radiation and cisplatin, CCNU, and vincristine chemotherapy. J Neurosurg 1994;18:690.

Packer RJ, Tarbell N, Jakacki R, et al. Medulloblastoma: Therapeutic progress and treatment strategies of the Children's Oncology Group. Ann Neurol 2002;52 (Suppl 1):S160.

Page LK, Lombrosco CT, Matson DD. Childhood epilepsy with late detection of cerebral glioma. J Neurosurg 1969;31:253.

Palma L, Guidetti B. Cystic pilocytic astrocytomas of the cerebral hemispheres. J Neurosurg 1985;62:811.

Papadakis N, Millan J, Grady DF, et al. Medulloblastoma of the neonatal period and early infancy. J Neurosurg 1971;34:88.

Parker JC, Mortara RH, McCloskey JJ. Biological behavior of the primitive neuroectodermal tumors: Significant supratentorial childhood gliomas. Surg Neurol 1975;4:383.

Pascual-Castroviejo I. Spinal tumors in children and adolescents. Raven Press: New York, 1990.

Paterson R, Farr RF. Cerebellar medulloblastoma: Treatment by irradiation of the whole central nervous system. Acta Radiol 1953;39:323.

Paulino AC. The local field in infratentorial ependymoma: Does the entire posterior fossa need to be treated? Int J Radiat Oncol Biol Phys 2001;49:757.

Paulino AC, Cha DT, Barker JL Jr, et al. Patterns of failure in relation to radiotherapy fields in supratentorial primitive neuroectodermal tumor. Int J Radiat Oncol Biol Phys 2004;58:1171.

Paulino AC, Melian E. Medulloblastoma and supratentorial primitive neuroectodermal tumors: An institutional experience. Cancer 1999;86:142.

Paulino AC, Wen BC. The significance of radiotherapy treatment duration in intracranial ependymoma. Int J Radiat Oncol Biol Phys 2000;47:585.

Pearl GS, Mirra SS, Miles ML. Glioblastoma multiforme occurring 13 years after treatment of a medulloblastoma. Neurosurgery 1980;6:546.

Pencalet P, Maixner W, Sainte-Rose C, et al. Benign cerebellar astrocytomas in children. J Neurosurg 1999;90:265.

Pencalet P, Sainte-Rose C, Lellouch-Tubiana A, et al. Papillomas and carcinomas of the choroid plexus in children. J Neurosurg 1998;88:521.

Perilongo G, Carollo C, Salviati L, et al. Diencephalic syndrome and disseminated juvenile pilocytic astrocytomas of the hypothalamic-optic chiasm region. Cancer 1997a;80:142.

Perilongo G, Massimino M, Sotti G, et al. Analyses of prognostic factors in a retrospective review of 92 children with ependymoma: Italian Pediatric Neuro-Oncology Group. Med Pediatr Oncol 1997b;29:79.

Peschel RE, Kapp DS, Cardinale F, et al. Ependymomas of the spinal cord. Int J Radiat Oncol Biol Phys 1983;9:1093.

Peturrson SR, Boggs DR. Spinal cord involvement in leukemia: A review of the literature and a case of Ph1+ acute myeloid leukemia presenting with a conus medullaris syndrome. Cancer 1981;47:346.

Peylan-Ramu N, Poplack DG, Pizzo PA, et al. Abnormal CT scans of the brain in asymptomatic children with acute lymphocytic leukemia after prophylactic intrathecal chemotherapy. N Engl J Med 1978;298:815.

Phillips PC. Antineoplastic drug resistance. Neurol Clin 1991;9:383.

Pierce MI. Neurologic complications in acute leukemia in children. Pediatr Clin North Am 1962;9:425.

Pigott TJD, Punt JAG, Lowe JS, et al. The clinical, radiological and histopathological features of cerebral primitive neuroectodermal tumours. Br J Neurosurg 1990;4:287.

Pihan GA, Doxsey SJ. The mitotic machinery as a source of genetic instability in cancer. Semin Cancer Biol 1999;9:289.

Pinkerton CR, Chessells JM. Failed central nervous system prophylaxis in children with acute lymphoblastic leukemia: Treatment and outcome. Br J Haematol 1984;57:553.

Pizzo PA. Infectious complications in the child with cancer. III. Management of specific infectious organisms. J Pediatr 1981;98:513.

Plum F, Posner JB. The diagnosis of stupor and coma, 3rd ed, rev. Philadelphia: FA Davis Company, 1982.

Pollack IF, Campbell JW. Cerebellar astrocytomas in children. J Neurooncol 1996a;28:223.

Pollack IF, Gerszten PC, Martinez AJ, et al. Intracranial ependymomas in childhood: Long-term outcome and prognostic factors. Neurosurgery 1995;37:655.

Pollack IF, Shultz B, Mulvihill JJ. The management of brainstem gliomas in patients with neurofibromatosis 1. Neurology 1996;46:1652.

Pomeroy S. Dysembryoplastic neuroepithelial tumor (DNT) in childhood. Neurology 2004;62:2147.

Pompili A, Caperle M, Pace A, et al. Quality-of-life assessment in patients who had been surgically treated for cerebellar pilocytic astrocytoma in childhood. J Neurosurg 2002;96:229.

Price RA, Birdwell DA. The central nervous system in childhood leukemia. III. Mineralizing microangiopathy and dystrophic calcification. Cancer 1978;42:717.

Price RA, Jamieson PA. The central nervous system in childhood leukemia. II. Subacute leukoencephalopathy. Cancer 1975;35:306.

Price RA, Johnson WW. The central nervous system in childhood leukemia. I. The arachnoid. Cancer 1973;31:520.

Priest JR, Ramsay NKC, Latchaw RE, et al. Thrombotic and hemorrhagic strokes complicating early therapy for childhood acute lymphoblastic leukemia. Cancer 1980;46:1548.

Pui CH, Dahl GV, Hustu HO, et al. Epidural spinal cord compression as the initial finding in childhood acute leukemia and non-Hodgkin lymphoma. J Pediatr 1985;106:788.

Raffel C, McComb JG, Bodner S, et al. Benign brainstem lesions in pediatric patients with neurofibromatosis: Case reports. Neurosurgery 1989;25:959.

Raghavendra BN, Epstein FJ, McCleary L. Intramedullary spinal cord tumors in children: localization by intraoperative sonography. AJNR Am J Neuroradiol 1984;5:395.

Raimondi AJ, Gutierrez FA, DiRocco C. Laminotomy and total reconstruction of the posterior spinal arch for spinal canal surgery in childhood. J Neurosurg 1976;45:555.

Raimondi AJ, Tomita T. Brain tumors during the first year of life. Childs Brain 1983;10:193.

Raimondi AJ, Tomita T. Advantages of total resection of medulloblastoma and disadvantages of full head post-operative radiation therapy. Childs Brain 1979a;5:550.

Raimondi AJ, Tomita T. Hydrocephalus and infratentorial tumors. J Neurosurg 1979b;55:174.

Raimondi AJ, Tomita T. Medulloblastoma in childhood. Acta Neurochir 1979c;50:127.

Rao YTR, Medini E, Haselow RE, et al. Pineal and ectopic pineal tumors: The role of radiation therapy. Cancer 1981;48:708.

Razack N, Baumgartner J, Bruner J. Pediatric oligodendrogliomas. Pediatr Neurosurg 1998;28:121.

Reimer R, Onofrio BM. Astrocytomas of the spinal cord in children and adolescents. J Neurosurg 1985;63:669.

Reinhardt D, Benke-Mursch J, Weiss E, et al. Rhabdoid tumors of the central nervous system. Childs Nerv Syst 2000;16:228.

Reznik M. Acute ascending poliomyelomalacia after treatment of acute lymphocytic leukemia. Acta Neuropathol (Berl) 1979;45:153.

Ricardi U, Corrias A, Einaudi S, et al. Thyroid dysfunction as a late effect in childhood medulloblastoma: A comparison of hyperfractionated versus voncentionally fractionated craniospinal radiotherapy. Int J Radiat Oncol Biol Phys 2001;50:1287.

Ridgway EW, Jaffe N, Walton DS. Leukemic ophthalmopathy in children. Cancer 1976;38:1744.

Ringertz N, Nordenstam H. Cerebellar astrocytoma. J Neuropathol Exp Neurol 1951;10:343.

Riva D, Pantaleoni C, Milani N, et al. Impairment of neuropsychological functions in children with medulloblastomas and astrocytomas in the posterior fossa. Childs Nerv Syst 1989;5:107.

Robertson PL. Atypical presentations of spinal cord tumors in children. J Child Neurol 1992;7:360.

Robertson PL, Allen JC, Abbott IR, et al. Cervicomedullary tumors in children: A distinct subset of brainstem gliomas. Neurology 1994;44:1798.

Robertson PL, Muraszko KM, Brunberg JA, et al. Pediatric midbrain tumors: A benign subgroup of brainstem gliomas. Pediatr Neurosurg 1995;22:65.

Robertson PL, Muraszko K, Gajjar A, et al. Cerebellar mutism syndrome (CMS) after posterior fossa surgery: A prospective study of two large cohorts of medulloblastoma. Abstract presented at International Society of Pediatric Neuro-oncology, June 2002.

Rodgers J, Britton PG, Kernahan J, et al. Cognitive function after two doses of cranial irradiation for acute lymphoblastic leukaemia. Arch Dis Child 1991;66:1245.

Roessler K, Bertalanffy A, Jezan H, et al. Proliferative activity as measured by MIB-1 labeling index and long-term outcome of cerebellar juvenile pilocytic astrocytomas. J Neurooncol 2002;58:141.

Roggli VL, Estrada R, Fechner RE. Thyroid neoplasia following irradiation for medulloblastoma. Cancer 1979;43:2232.

Rollins NK, Nisen P, Shapiro KN. The use of early postoperative MR in detecting residual juvenile cerebellar pilocytic astrocytoma. AJNR Am J Neuroradiol 1998;19:151.
Romshe CA, Zipf WB, Miser A, et al. Evaluation of growth hormone release and human growth hormone treatment in children with cranial irradiation-associated short stature. J Pediatr 1984;104;177.
Rosenberg A, Spiess P, Lafreniere R. A new approach to the adoptive immunotherapy of cancer with tumor infiltrating-lymphocytes. Science 1986;233:118.
Ross JS, Schenkein DP, Pietrusko R, et al. Targeted therapies for cancer. Am J Clin Pathol 2004;122:598.
Rousseau P, Habrand JL, Sarrazin D, et al. Treatment of intracranial ependymomas of children: Review of a 15-year experience. Int J Radiat Oncol Biol Phys 1994;28:382.
Rowland JH, Glidewell OJ, Sibley RF, et al. Effects of different forms of central nervous system prophylaxis on neuropsychologic function in childhood leukemia. J Clin Oncol 1984;2:1327.
Rubenstein AE, Mytilineoau C, Yahr MD, et al. Neurological aspects of neurofibromatosis. In: Riccardi VM, Mulvihill JJ, eds. Advances in neurology, vol 29. Neurofibromatosis. New York: Raven, 1981;11.
Rubinstein LJ. Tumors of the central nervous system. Washington, DC: Armed Forces Institute of Pathology, 1972.
Ruggieri V, Caraballo R, Fejerman N. Intracranial tumors and West syndrome. Pediatr Neurol 1989;5:327.
Russell A. A diencephalic syndrome of emaciation in infancy and childhood. Arch Dis Child 1951;26:274.
Russell DS, Rubinstein LF. Pathology of tumors of the nervous system, 4th ed. London: Edward Arnold, 1989.
Salazar OM, Rubin P. The spread of glioblastoma multiforme as a determining factor in the radiation treated volume. Int J Radiat Oncol Biol Phys 1976;1:627.
Schijman E, Zuccaro G, Monges JA. Spinal tumors and hydrocephalus. Childs Brain 1981;8:401.
Schild SE, Scheithauer BW, Haddock MG, et al. Histologically confirmed pineal tumors and other germ cell tumors of the brain. Cancer 1996;78:2564.
Schneck SA, Penn I. De novo brain tumors in renal transplant recipients. Lancet 1971;1:983.
Schoenberg BS, Glista GG, Reagan TJ. The familial occurrence of glioma. Surg Neurol 1975;3:139.
Segall HD, Batnizky S, Zee CS, et al. Computed tomography in the diagnosis of intracranial neoplasms in children. Cancer 1985;56:1748.
Sexauer CL, Khan A, Burger PC, et al. Cis-platinum in recurrent pediatric brain tumors: A POG phase II study. Pediatr Oncol Study Group 1985;56:1497.
Shalet SM, Beardwell C, Aarons BM, et al. Growth impairment in children treated for brain tumours. Arch Dis Child 1978;53:491.
Shalet SM, Beardwell CG, MacFarlane IA, et al. Endocrine morbidity in adults treated with cerebral irradiation for brain tumors during childhood. Acta Endocrinol 1977;84:673.
Shalet SM, Beardwell CG, Morris-Jones PH, et al. Growth hormone deficiency after treatment of acute leukemia in children. Arch Dis Child 1976;51:489.
Shalet SM, Clayton PE, Price DA. Growth and pituitary function in children treated for brain tumours or acute lymphoblastic leukaemia. Horm Res 1988;30:53.
Shalet SM, Gibson B, Swindell R, et al. Effect of spinal irradiation on growth. Arch Dis Child 1987;62:461.
Shalet SM, Whitehead E, Chapman AJ, et al. The effects of growth hormone therapy in children with radiation-induced growth hormone deficiencies. Acta Paediatr Scand 1981;70:81.
Shapiro WR. Chemotherapy of primary malignant brain tumors in children. Cancer 1975;35:965.
Shapiro WR, Chernik NL, Posner VB. Necrotizing encephalopathy following intraventricular installation of methotrexate. Arch Neurol 1973;28:96.
Shaw EG, Scheithauer BW, O'Fallon JR, et al. Oligodendrogliomas: The Mayo Clinic experience. J Neurosurg 1992;76:428.
Sheline GE. Radiation therapy of brain tumors. Cancer 1977;39:873.
Sherins RJ, Oliveny CL, Ziegler JL. Gynecomastia and gonadal dysfunction in adolescent boys treated with combination chemotherapy for Hodgkin's disease. N Engl J Med 1978;299:12.
Shillito J. Craniopharyngiomas: The subfrontal approach or none at all? Clin Neurosurg 1980;27:188.
Silver RT, Young RC, Holland JF. Some new aspects of modern cancer therapy. Am J Med 1977;639:772.
Silverman C, Marks JE. Prognostic significance of contrast enhancement in low-grade astrocytomas of the adult cerebrum. Radiology 1981;139:211.
Simpson DA, Carter RF, Ducrou W. Intracranial tumors in infancy. Dev Med Child Neurol 1968;10:190.
Smith MA, Freidlin B, Ries LA. Trends in reported incidence of primary malignant brain tumors in children in the United States. J Natl Cancer Inst 1998;90:1269.
Smoots DW, Geyer JR, Lieberman DM, et al. Predicting disease progression in childhood cerebellar astrocytoma. Childs Nerv Syst 1998;14:636.
Smyth MD, Horn BN, Russo C, et al. Intracranial ependymomas of childhood: Current management strategies. Pediatr Neurosurg 2000;33:138.
Sotos JF, Romshe CA. Pituitary tumors. In: Gardner LI, ed. Endocrine and genetic disease of childhood and adolescence. Philadelphia: WB Saunders, 1975.
Sposto R, Ertal IA, Jenkin RDT, et al. The effectiveness of chemotherapy for treatment of high grade astrocytoma in children: Results of a randomized trial. J Neurooncol 1989;7:165.
Spunberg JJ, Chang CH, Goldman M, et al. Quality of long-term survival following irradiation for intracranial tumors in children under the age of two. Int J Radiat Oncol Biol Phys 1981;7:727.
St. Clair SK, Humphreys RP, Pillay PK, et al. Current management of choroid plexus carcinoma in children. Pediatr Neurosurg 1991-92;17:225.
Stafford SL, Pollock BE, Foote RL, et al. Stereotactic radiosurgery for recurrent ependymoma. Cancer 2000;88:870.
Stea B, Falsey R, Kislin K, et al. Time and dose-dependent radiosensitization of the glioblastoma U251 cells by the EGF receptor tyrosine kinase inhibitor ZD1839 (Irressa). Cancer Lett 2003;202:43.
Stechison MT, Panagis SG, Reinhart SS. Somatosensory evoked potential. Monitoring during spinal surgery. Acta Neurochir (Wien) 1995;135:56.
Steinhoff H, Grumme TH, Kazner E, et al. Axial transverse computerized tomography in 73 glioblastomas. Acta Neurochir 1978;42:45.
Stern J, DiGiacinto GV, Housepian EM. Neurofibromatosis and optic gliomas: Clinical and morphologic correlations. Neurosurgery 1979;4:524.
Streffer J, Schabet M, Bamberg M, et al. A role for preirradiation PCV chemotherapy for oligodendroglial brain tumors. J Neurol 2000;247:297.
Strother D, Linda S, Burger P, et al. Outcome of therapy for atypical teratoid/rhabdoid tumors (ATRT) on Pediatric Oncology Group study (POG) 9233/34. Presented at ISPNO, Boston, June 2004.
Sullivan MP. Leukemic infiltration of meninges and spinal nerve roots. Pediatrics 1963;32:63.
Sutton LN, Cnaan A, Klatt L, et al. Postoperative surveillance imaging in children with cerebellar astrocytomas. J Neurosurg 1996;84:721.
Swift M, Shulman L, Perry M, et al. Malignant neoplasms in the families of patients with ataxia-telangiectasia. Cancer Res 1976;36:209.
Tait DM, Thornton-Jones H, Bloom HJG, et al. Adjuvant chemotherapy for medulloblastoma: The first multi-centre control trial of the International Society of Paediatric Oncology (SIOP I). Eur J Cancer 1990;26:464.
Tamura M, Zama A, Kurihara H, et al. Management of recurrent pilocytic astrocytoma with leptomeningeal dissemination in childhood. Childs Nerv Syst 1998;14:617.
Tanabe T, Nukada T, Nishikawa Y, et al. Primary structure of the α-subunit of transducin and its relationship to ras proteins. Nature 1985;315:242.
Tarbell NJ, Loeffler JS, Silver B, et al. The change in patterns of relapse in medulloblastoma. Cancer 1991;68:1600.
Tchang S, Scotti G, Terbrugge K, et al. Computerized tomography as a possible aid to histological grading of supratentorial gliomas. J Neurosurg 1977;46:735.
Teo C, Nakaji P, Symons P, et al. Ependymoma. Childs Nerv Syst 2003;19:270.
Thompson TP, Lunsford LD, Kondziolka D. Distinguishing recurrent tumor and radiation necrosis with positron emission tomography versus stereotactic biopsy. Stereotact Funct Neurosurg 1999;73:9.
Timmermann B, Kortmann RD, Kühl J, et al. Combined postoperative irradiation and chemotherapy for anaplastic ependymomas in childhood: Results of the German prospective trials HIT 88/89 and HIT 91. Int J Radiat Oncol Biol Phys 2000;46;287.
Tomita T, McLone DG. Brain tumors during the first twenty-four months of life. Neurosurgery 1985;17:913.

Tomita T, McLone DG, Yasue M. Cerebral primitive neuroectodermal tumors in childhood. J Neurooncol 1988;6:233.

Tovi D, Schisano G, Liljeqvist B. Primary tumors of the region of the thalamus. J Neurosurg 1961;18:730.

Ucar S, Florez G, Garcia J. Increased intracranial pressure associated with spinal cord tumours. Neurochirurgie 1976;19:265.

Ureuna M, Stanhope R, Chessells M, et al. Impaired pubertal growth in acute lymphoblastic leukaemia. Arch Dis Child 1991;66:1403.

Usenius T, Usenius JP, Tenhunen M, et al. Radiation-induced changes in human brain metabolites as studied by ^{1}H nuclear magnetic resonance spectroscopy in vivo. Int J Radiat Oncol Biol Phys 1995;33:719.

Valeriote F, Vietti T. Cellular kinetics and conceptual basis of chemotherapy. In: Sutow W, Vietti T, eds. Clinical pediatric oncology. St. Louis: Mosby, 1977.

Valk PE, Budinger TF, Levin VA, et al. PET of malignant cerebral tumors after interstitial brachytherapy: Demonstration of metabolic activity and correlation with clinical outcome. J Neurosurg 1988;69:830.

Valladares JB, Pery RH, Kalbag RM. Malignant choroid plexus papilloma with extraneural metastasis. J Neurosurg 1980;52:251.

Van Eys J, Cangir A, Coody D, et al. MOPP regimen as primary chemotherapy for brain tumors in infants. J Neurooncol 1985;3:237.

Van Veelen-Vincent ML, Pierre-Kahn A, Kalifa C, et al. Ependymoma in childhood: Prognostic factors, extent of surgery, and adjuvant therapy. J Neurosurg 2002;97:827.

Vogelstein B, Fearon ER, Hamilton SR, et al. Genetic alterations during colorectal-tumor development. N Engl J Med 1988;319:525.

Voorhess M, Brecher ML, Glicksman AS, et al. Hypothalamic-pituitary function in children with acute lymphocytic leukemia following CNS prophylaxis: A retrospective study. Cancer 1986;57:1287.

Vulfovich M, Saba N. Molecular biological design of novel antineoplastic therapies. Expert Opin Investig Drugs 2004;13:577.

Walker MD, Green SB, Byar DD, et al. Randomized comparisons of radiotherapy and nitrosoureas for the treatment of malignant glioma after surgery. N Engl J Med 1980;303:1323.

Walter AW, Gajjar A, Reardon DA, et al. Tamoxifen and carboplatin for children with low-grade gliomas: A pilot study at St. Jude Children's Research Hospital. J Pediatr Hematol Oncol 2000;22:247.

Wara WM, Richards GE, Grumbach MM, et al. Hypopituitarism after irradiation in children. Int J Radiat Oncol Biol Phys 1977;2:549.

Watterson J, Toogood I, Nieder M, et al. Excessive spinal cord toxicity from intensive central nervous system-directed therapies. Cancer 1994;74:3034.

Weaver M, Laske DW. Transferrin receptor ligand-targeted toxin conjugate (Tf-CRM107) for therapy of malignant gliomas. J Neurooncol 2003;65:3.

Weaver RG Jr, Chauvenet AR, Smith TJ, et al. Ophthalmic evaluation of long-term survivors of childhood: acute lymphoblastic leukemia. Cancer 1986;58:963.

Weiss E, Klingbiel T, Kortmann RD, et al. Intraspinal high-grade astrocytoma in a child—Rationale for chemotherapy and more intensive radiotherapy? Childs Nerv Syst 1997;13:108.

White PT, Ross AT. Inanition syndrome in infants with anterior hypothalamic neoplasms. Neurology 1963;13:974.

Winter RJ, Green OC. Irradiation-induced growth hormone deficiency: Blunted growth response and accelerated skeletal maturation to growth hormone therapy. J Pediatr 1985;106:609.

Wolff JE, Sajedi M, Brant R, et al. Choroid plexus tumours. Br J Cancer 2002;87:1086.

Wong S, Witte ON. The BCR-ABL story: Bench to bedside and back. Ann Rev Immunol 2004;22:247.

Yasargil MG, Antic J, Laciga R, et al. The microsurgical removal of intramedullary spinal hemangioblastomas: Report of twelve cases and a review of the literature. Surg Neurol 1976;6:141.

Yasargil MG, Curcic M, Kis M, et al. Total removal of craniopharyngiomas: Approaches and long-term results in 144 patients. J Neurosurg 1990;73:3.

Young JL, Miller RW. Incidence of malignant tumors in U.S. children. J Pediatr 1975;86:254.

Young RF, Post EM, King GA. Treatment of spinal epidural metastases: Randomized prospective comparison of laminectomy and radiotherapy. J Neurosurg 1980;53:741.

Zeller WJ, Ivankovic S, Habs M, et al. Experimental chemical production of brain tumors. Ann N Y Acad Sci 1982;381:250.

Zeltzer PJ, Boyett J, Finlay L, et al. Prognostic factors for survival in high risk primitive neuroectodermal tumors (PNETs) in children: Report from the Children's Cancer Group CCG-921. Proc ASCO 1993;12:415.

Zimmerman RA, Bilaniuk LT, Bruno L, et al. Computed tomography of cerebellar astrocytoma. Am J Roentgenol 1978;130:929.

Zimmerman RD, Fleming CA, Lee BCP, et al. Periventricular hyperintensity as seen by magnetic resonance: Prevalence and significance. AJNR Am J Neuroradiol 1986;7:13.

Zovickian J, Johnson VG, Youle RJ. Potent and specific killing of human malignant brain tumor cells by an anti-transferrin receptor-ricin immunotoxin. J Neurosurg 1987;68:850.

CHAPTER 72

Cerebrovascular Disease

Gabrielle Aline deVeber

PEDIATRIC STROKE—OVERVIEW

Stroke is defined as the sudden occlusion or rupture of cerebral arteries or veins resulting in focal cerebral damage and clinical neurologic deficits. Forms of stroke due to vascular occlusion are arterial ischemic stroke and cerebral sinovenous thrombosis. In arterial ischemic stroke, arterial occlusion is usually due to thromboembolism and results in an arterial infarct. In cerebral sinovenous thrombosis, occlusion of the cerebral veins or venous sinuses may result in a venous infarct or in no parenchymal damage. In either arterial or venous infarction, if the infarct does not contain visible hemorrhage it is called a *bland infarct*. A bland infarct can become a hemorrhagic infarct, occurring when there is bleeding into the area of infarction. Forms of stroke due to vascular rupture are called *hemorrhagic stroke* and are primarily intracerebral and subarachnoid hemorrhage.

Fundamental developmental differences in children and adults make the recognition and treatment of children with stroke challenging. First, stroke in children is relatively rare, frequently resulting in a lack of recognition and delay in diagnosis. Second, the etiologies of stroke in children are legion, and no single risk factor predominates. Multiple risk factors are often present in individual patients. As a result, complex etiologic investigations are often necessary. Third, there have been only limited research studies of medical therapy for childhood stroke. Current treatments for children are therefore necessarily based on therapies used in adult stroke patients; biologic plausibility and safety data in pediatric patients are very limited. There are important maturational differences in the coagulation, cerebrovascular, and neurologic systems of infants and children compared with adults that limit the applicability of research performed in adult stroke patients to pediatric patients with stroke.

During the past several years, a number of clinical and basic research studies have increased our understanding of childhood stroke. Population-based clinical studies have resulted in an increased awareness of the frequencies and outcomes of various types of stroke. Prospective cohort studies have demonstrated the feasibility and safety of several antithrombotic therapies in children with stroke. Advances in neuroimaging and in genetic and other laboratory testing techniques have led to an appreciation of a wider spectrum of stroke subtypes and risk factors.

The purpose of this chapter is, first, to provide a basic understanding of the processes involved in childhood stroke; second, to provide an overview of the epidemiology, investigation, and treatment of pediatric stroke; and, third, to provide a practical clinical approach to the child with stroke. Several comprehensive reviews on the topic of childhood stroke have been published in the form of review articles [Ball, Jr., 1994; Broderick et al., 1993; deVeber, 2002; Kirkham, 1994; Lynch et al., 2002; Nagaraja et al., 1994; Nelson and Lynch, 2004; Rivkin and Volpe, 1996; Trescher, 1992] and reference texts [Andrew et al., 2000; Lasjaunias and Terbrugge, 1997; Roach and Riela, 1995].

For this chapter, a comprehensive review of the literature was conducted searching Medline from 1966 to 2004 using combinations of the key words *child*, *infant*, and *neonate* combined with the terms *stroke*, *cerebrovascular disease*, *cerebral thrombosis* or *embolism*, *cerebral ischemia*, and *sinus thrombosis*. Basic references were supplemented with additional references located through the bibliographies of listed articles. All articles were graded by quality of evidence related to study design as levels I to V, according to previously described criteria [Cook et al., 1995]. Very few clinical treatment trials of childhood stroke were identified that qualified for the classification of levels I to III. Prospective cohort studies were classified as level IV. Retrospective case series were classified as level V. Complete reference lists of the level V studies, which constitute the overwhelming majority, are available on request. Chapter 17 in this book covers neonatal stroke.

Incidence of Pediatric Stroke

Nearly one fourth of strokes in the "young" (i.e., <40 years of age) [Kerr et al., 1993] occur in children. Cerebrovascular disorders are among the top ten causes of death in children, with rates highest in the first year of life. The 1998 U.S. mortality rate for stroke was 7.8/100,000 in children 0 to 1 year of age and was increased in males compared with females and in blacks compared with whites [Murphy, 2000]. Stroke-related mortality in children younger than 1 year of age may have decreased in the past 2 decades [Fullerton et al., 2003].

In the past three decades, the reported incidence rates for pediatric stroke have increased. Previously, reported rates for combined ischemic and hemorrhagic pediatric stroke in the U.S. were 2.5 to 2.7 per 100,000 children per year (0.63 to 1.2 for ischemic stroke and 1.5 to 1.9 for hemorrhagic stroke) [Broderick et al., 1993; Schoenberg et al., 1978]. More recently, an analysis of stroke diagnostic codes in the National Hospital Discharge Survey (NHDS) estimated the incidence of pediatric stroke as 10.7 per 100,000 children per year (2.9 for ischemic stroke and 7.8 for hemorrhagic stroke) [Lynch et al., 2002]. In the city of Dijon, France, the incidence of pediatric stroke was reported as 13 per 100,000 children per year (7.91 for ischemic stroke and 5.11 for hemorrhagic stroke). In Canada, in a prospective population-based registry the estimated incidence of ischemic stroke was at least 1.8 per 100,000 (1.2 for arterial ischemic stroke and 0.67 for cerebral sinovenous thrombosis); hemorrhagic strokes were not assessed [deVeber and Canadian Paediatric Ischemic Stroke Study Group, 2000; deVeber et al., 2001]. In Victoria, Australia, the incidence of cerebral sinovenous thrombosis in children excluding neonates was estimated at 0.34 per 100,000 children per year [Barnes et al., 2004]. The proportion of hemorrhagic versus ischemic stroke in childhood remains to be clarified; two of the above studies reported that hemorrhagic stroke is more frequent [Broderick et al., 1993; Schoenberg et al., 1978] whereas three studies reported that ischemic stroke is more frequent [Giroud et al., 1995; Lanthier et al., 2000; Lynch et al., 2002].

At least two factors likely are responsible for the increased incidence rates. The widespread availability of more sensitive diagnostic tests including computed tomography (CT) and magnetic resonance imaging (MRI) scanning has increased the detection rate for pediatric stroke [Venkataraman et al., 2004; Warach and Baron, 2004; Wiznitzer and Masaryk, 1991]. These tests have also resulted in the identification of a milder spectrum of stroke than previously identified. Second, more effective treatments have increased survival of patients with certain previously lethal primary pediatric diseases that predispose to stroke. Infants and children with a history of prematurity, congenital heart disease, sickle cell disease, and leukemia, for example, now have longer life expectancies, during which time they remain at risk for stroke from the primary disease and its treatments. Ischemic strokes are likely still underdiagnosed in infancy and childhood, particularly cerebral sinovenous thrombosis, because of a lack of clinical suspicion and failure to use appropriate diagnostic tests.

The socioeconomic impact of stroke is considerable. In adults, the lifetime cost of a first stroke per person is estimated to be $228,030 for subarachnoid hemorrhage, $123,565 for intracerebral hemorrhage, $90,981 for ischemic stroke, and $103,576 averaged across all stroke subtypes [Taylor et al., 1996]. On average, developed countries spend 3% of health-care dollars on stroke [Evers et al., 2004]. The economic impact of childhood stroke has not been reported, but because many more decades of disability frequently result, the burden of illness per individual will inevitably be great.

ARTERIAL ISCHEMIC STROKE

Pathophysiology

Arterial Circulation: Anatomy and Physiology

The brain receives its arterial supply via two principal systems: the *anterior circulation*, consisting of the paired carotid arteries and the *posterior circulation*, consisting of the paired vertebral arteries, which join to form the basilar artery (Figs. 72-1 to 72-3). The anterior and posterior communicating arteries link these two systems to form the circle of Willis. The major cerebral arteries arising from the circle of Willis are the paired anterior, middle, and posterior cerebral arteries. The anterior and middle cerebral arteries are the major branches of the internal carotid artery, and the posterior cerebral arteries are the major branches of the vertebrobasilar system. Small *perforator* branches arise from the stem of the anterior, middle, and posterior cerebral

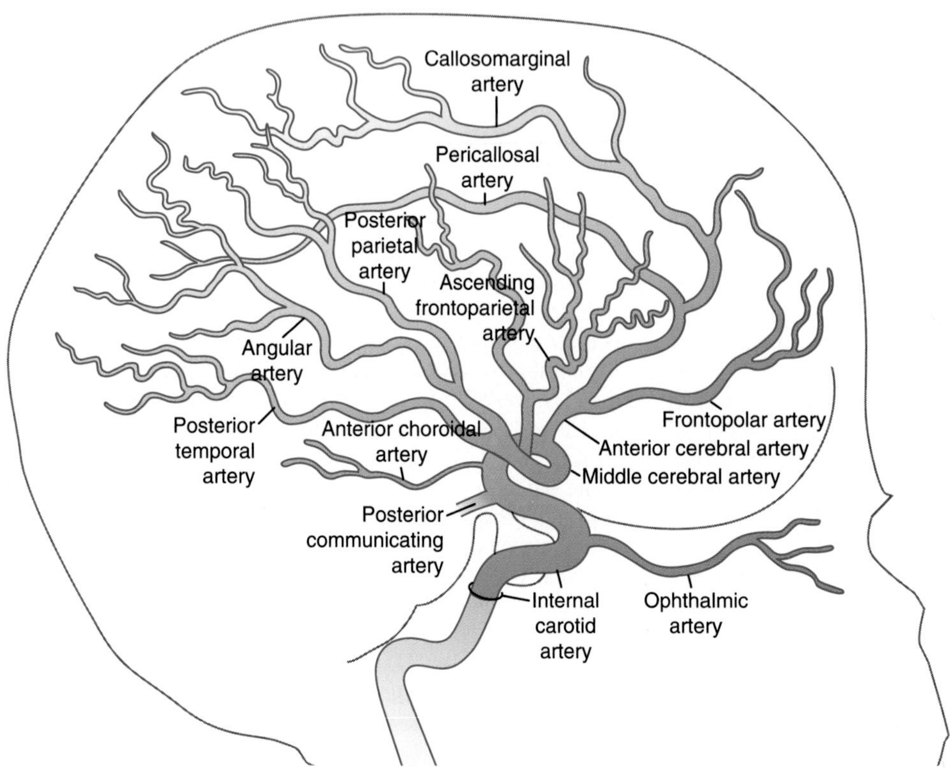

FIGURE 72-1. Lateral view of the cerebral arteries detailing the branches of the anterior and middle cerebral arteries.

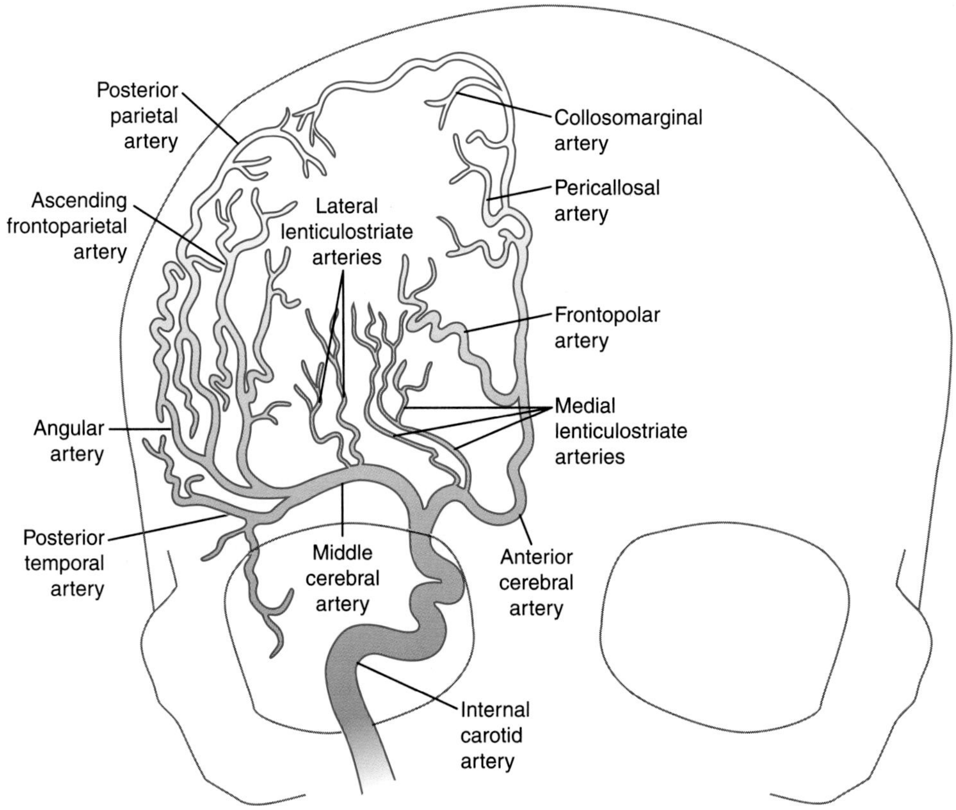

FIGURE 72-2. Anteroposterior view of the cerebral arteries.

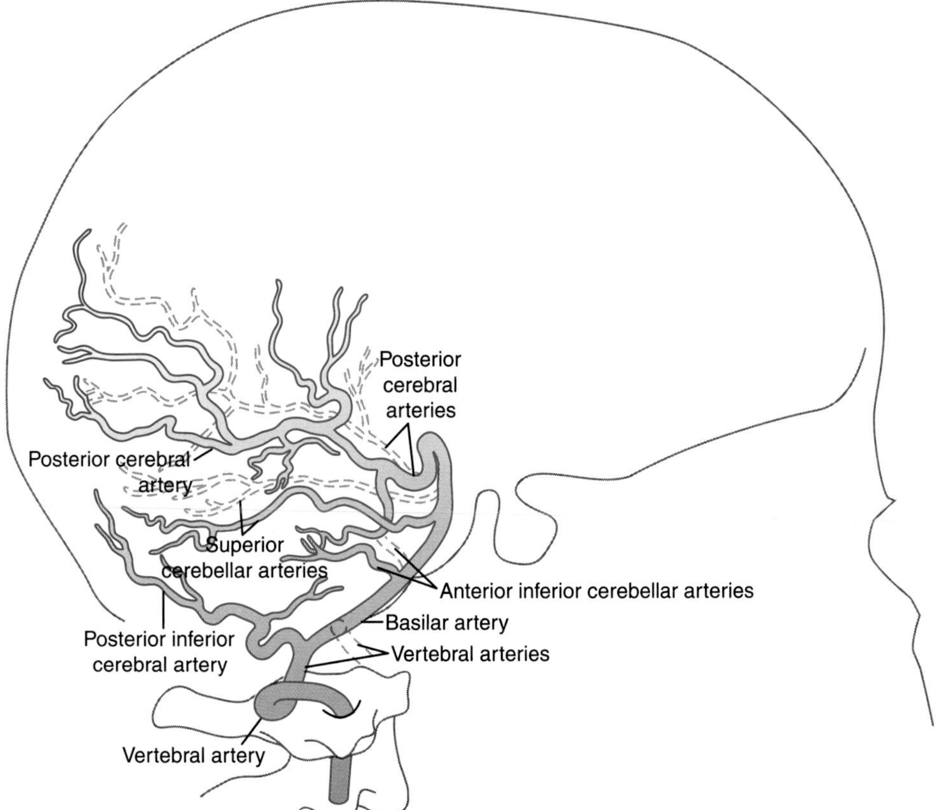

FIGURE 72-3. The vertebral-basilar artery system.

arteries to supply the deep central brain structures, in particular the basal ganglia, thalami, and internal capsules.

Mechanisms of Thromboembolism

Thrombosis arising within cerebral arteries can result from primary disorders of the cerebral arteries or from acquired or congenital prothrombotic states. Under physiologic circumstances, the endothelial lining of the arteries provides an anticoagulant surface that helps to maintain blood in a fluid phase. In situations of low flow, including the normal venous system, the coagulation system plays an increased role in thrombosis, resulting in a predominance of fibrin-rich thrombi. However, in arterial systems including arterial thrombotic stroke, the relative predominance of coagulation activation (fibrin-rich thrombi) or platelet activation (platelet-rich thrombi) is more variable and depends on flow rates, shear stresses, and other factors. When the arterial wall is damaged, as a result of the presence of inflammation or a breach in the endothelial lining, the arterial wall becomes thrombogenic, and thrombosis develops through several mechanisms. The exposure of flowing blood to arterial wall inflammation (as with vasculitis) or to exposed collagen and tissue factors (as with dissection) activates platelets and fibrin clot formation via the coagulation system. The coagulation system is also active in the formation of thrombosis in situations of blood stasis or slow blood flow—for example, arterial occlusion or severe stenosis, In situations of rapid arterial blood flow with "shear" forces, the platelet system becomes activated and promotes formation of platelet-rich thrombi. Age-related differences in both platelet and coagulation activity exist in neonates compared with older children [Carcao et al., 1998; Israels et al., 2001; Roschitz et al., 2001].

Embolic sources for arterial thrombotic stroke in childhood include structural disorders of the heart, aorta, and cerebral arteries. These abnormalities result in cardiogenic embolism or artery-to-artery embolism. A further mechanism is the presence of right-to-left intracardiac shunting that results from ventricular or atrial septal defects, patent foramen ovale, and postoperative residual right-to-left shunts following Fontan and other cardiac surgical procedures. The shunt may be predominantly left to right, but intermittently with Valsalva or other maneuvers may become right to left, during which time a conduit for paradoxical embolism exists. This right-to-left shunting allows systemic venous thrombi to reach the cerebral circulation. Clots of venous origin or intracardiac clots tend to be primarily fibrin-rich thrombi as a result of activation of the coagulation system.

Mechanisms of Infarction

In arterial thrombotic stroke, the severity of cerebral tissue damage and the resultant neurologic impairments are a function of many factors. These include (1) the duration of ischemia, related to the timing and adequacy of restoration of perfusion; (2) the volume and functional components of the brain structures supplied by the involved cerebral artery; (3) the maturational status of the brain; (4) the availability of collateral arterial blood supply; and (5) the concurrent metabolic demands of the ischemic brain tissue. Additional cerebral damage results from early recurrent infarcts. The extent of impairment in the delivery of substrates is directly related to the duration of vascular occlusion and the adequacy of collateral blood flow supplying the ischemic area.

Neuronal damage following arterial occlusion can be reversible or irreversible depending on the severity of ischemia and the rate of neuronal metabolic activity. In transient ischemic attacks, the clinical deficit is usually extremely brief, typically lasting less then 1 hour. In more recent definitions of transient ischemic attacks, no permanent parenchymal lesion is seen by MRI, confirming that the damage is fully reversible [Albers et al., 2002]. In an arterial infarct, the clinical deficit lasts longer, frequently persisting for more than 24 hours, and results in a radiographically confirmed infarct conforming to a vascular territory and appropriate to the neurologic syndrome. In arterial ischemic stroke, there is a central core zone, which represents irreversibly damaged brain, and a surrounding penumbral zone, which represents partially ischemic and potentially viable brain tissue [Schlaug et al., 1999]. The eventual volume of the ischemic infarct is the result of the balance between the rate of delivery of oxygen and glucose and the metabolic activity of the brain, particularly in the penumbra. Cell death in the core or the penumbra occurs with a combination of two major mechanisms, acute necrosis and apoptosis (delayed cell death). In the penumbra, clinical factors that increase the discrepancy between cerebral metabolic rate and the delivery of oxygen and glucose result in additional tissue injury and cell death. Although the core of an infarct is considered irreversibly damaged within several hours of onset, there is the real potential to salvage tissue within the penumbra. Cells in the penumbra are selectively vulnerable to secondary insults, leading to further cell death and enlargement of the stroke.

Aggressive and early specialized care of the child during the first 48 hours after initiation of the ischemic infarct can salvage cerebral tissue, resulting in a smaller volume of infarction. Optimization of cerebral perfusion, tissue oxygenation, and metabolic balance requires careful attention to clinical parameters including blood pressure, abnormal blood glucose levels, and the presence of seizures and fever. Because autoregulation is disturbed in the damaged tissue within an evolving infarct, the peri-infarct area remains extremely vulnerable to decreased cerebral blood flow in the presence of decreased blood pressure.

Cerebral perfusion is a direct function of the mean arterial pressure, intracranial pressure, and vascular resistance and is age-related [Volpe, 2001a]. In adults, the cerebral blood flow is 50 mL per 100 grams of brain tissue per minute. In term neonates, cerebral blood flow is estimated to be approximately 40% of the adult value [Altman et al., 1988]. In children younger than 3 years of age, the cerebral blood flow is around 30 to 50 mL per 100 gm, whereas in children from 3 to 10 years of age these rates significantly increase to about 100 mL per 100 gm of brain tissue per minute. During the late teen years, cerebral blood flow rates again diminish to adult levels. Studies utilizing CT quantitative perfusion have found that the global cerebral blood flow represents 10% to 20% of the global cardiac output for the first 6 months of life, peaks at approximately 55% by 2 to 4 years of age, and stabilizes at approximately 15% by 7 to 8 years of age [Wintermark et al., 2004]. Blood pressure and oxygen and carbon dioxide concentrations alter the degree of vasodilation and vasoconstriction of the cerebral arteries, and hence cerebral perfusion through autoregulation. The extent of autoregulation has not been well studied in the pediatric population; however, in the newborn, autoregulation is normally present between mean arterial blood pressures of 25 and 50 mm Hg [Volpe, 2001a]. The metabolic effects of focal brain ischemia are regional hypoxia and depletion of the high-energy compound adenosine triphosphate, as well as carbohydrate stores. The baseline metabolic rate of cerebral tissue is increased relative to that of other body tissues, and there is a relative paucity of energy stores in the brain [Trescher, 1992]. The cerebral metabolic rate for oxygen is 3.5 mL per 100 grams of brain per minute. Since virtually no oxygen reserve is available, rapid loss of neuronal function results if the oxygen supply is interrupted. Brain glucose reserve is slightly greater, allowing survival of brain tissue for up to 90 minutes if adequate oxygen is supplied. In the newborn, lactate can be used as a substrate for the production of energy, but this capability is lost quickly. When regional hypoxia develops during ischemia, there is a shift from oxidative metabolism to glycolysis. Glucose is metabolized to lactate, which accumulates and results in acidosis, which in turn exacerbates hypoxic injury. Seizures, by increasing the neuronal metabolic rate, dramatically increase the extent of neuronal damage occurring during ischemia. Important functional and anatomic differences between the cerebral arterial and the sinovenous systems result in differing features of thrombotic occlusion. In arterial ischemic stroke, for example, the infarcted brain is a zone of reduced arterial and venous pressure, and delayed recanalization with reperfusion does not relieve the ischemic damage, in contrast to the situation in cerebral sinovenous thrombosis.

Through basic research studies utilizing animal models of stroke, including ischemia-reperfusion injury, exciting information has recently become available about the chain of events that occur in ischemic stroke [Hou and MacManus, 2002]. Additional insights into the timing of mechanisms of stroke have been gained from the application of advanced neuroimaging techniques, including diffusion-weighted MRI. The concept of a neurotoxic cascade of events initiated by acute hypoxia or ischemia has evolved. This neurotoxic biochemical cascade produces permanent cell death over a period of hours (necrosis) to days (apoptosis) following the insult. Accumulation of extracellular glutamate and activation of glutamate receptors play major initiating roles in this cascade, which then involves the accumulation of cytosolic calcium and the activation of multiple calcium-mediated deleterious intracellular events. This neurotoxic cascade, which evolves over many hours, potentially can be arrested by interventions even if instituted after termination of the initial insult. The mechanisms of acute and programmed cell death including apoptosis are further discussed in Chapter 64 of this text.

Neuronal salvage medications aim to minimize neuronal damage at a cellular level by blocking these auto-destructive processes and thereby increasing the viability of the penumbral area. In rodent models, new agents have been found to block excitotoxicity of *N*-methyl-D-aspartate (NMDA) receptors, reduce stroke size, and improve neurologic outcome following middle cerebral arterial occlusion [Aarts et al., 2002], although clinical trials have not shown similar neuroprotection. Among the potential neuroprotective interventions for the immature brain, leading candidates include mild hypothermia, the inhibition of free radical production, and free radical scavengers. Promising clinical data are now available in human infants about the safety of the use of mild hypothermia, and efficacy data are being pursued [Battin et al., 2001]. Immature animal stroke models involving temporary vascular occlusion simulate human ischemia-reperfusion in arterial ischemic stroke and provide a potential means for the development of treatment directed at the inflammatory cascade and apoptosis, events associated with reperfusion injury. These and additional, more recent areas of research, including inhibition of nitric oxide and free-radical formation, the use of iron chelating agents, and the potential role of hypoxia-inducible factors and mediators of caspase activity, growth factors, hypothermia, and administration of magnesium sulfate, have been reviewed [Ashwal and Pearce, 2001].

Other models of vaso-occlusive stroke have been developed, particularly neonatal rodent models. Combined with the use of recent neuroimaging techniques, these can study the events associated with ischemic injury in immature and developing juvenile brains [Qiao et al., 2004]. However, animal models relevant to arterial ischemic stroke in children beyond the neonatal period would need to combine features of cerebral vasculopathies, disordered coagulation, and triggering factors, which underlie most strokes in childhood. Further work and the development of more mature pediatric animal models are necessary to help us understand the effect of stroke on the developing brain.

It has long been held that increased plasticity of neurons and of neuronal pathways in the developing brain could provide increased resistance to damage and increased recovery in the young infant and child with arterial ischemic stroke. However, there has been little data from human studies to address this theory. Some animal studies have documented that the neonatal rodent brain has a decreased tolerance to the effects of ischemia compared with the adult brain [Yager and Thornhill, 1997]. Studies of neonatal, juvenile, and adult rat models have found that brain damage from hypoxic ischemic insult is most severe in 1- and 3-week-old animals, followed by those that were 6 months old. The 6- and 9-week-old groups had significantly less injury than the other three age groups, indicating that the neonatal brain may be more susceptible and that the younger juvenile brain may be relatively protected compared with the adult brain. Similar findings were reported in studies of temporal lobe cortical injury in neonatal, juvenile, and adult rats [Kolb and Cioe, 2003; Kolb et al., 2000]. However, studies of intellectual outcome following stroke in humans have reported conflicting results. Some studies suggest that intellectual outcomes following stroke are best when the stroke occurs either in early infancy or late childhood compared with the occurrence of stroke in early childhood [Bates et al., 1999; Goodman and Yude, 1996]. Recent studies reported that neuropsychologic recovery was better in children older than 1 year of age and worse in infants younger than 1 year age at the time of stroke [Lansing et al., 2004; Max, 2004].

Vascular Patterns

Vascular patterns of arterial ischemic stroke can be classified as large- or small-vessel territory infarcts. Occlusion of large-caliber cerebral arteries results in classic peripheral,

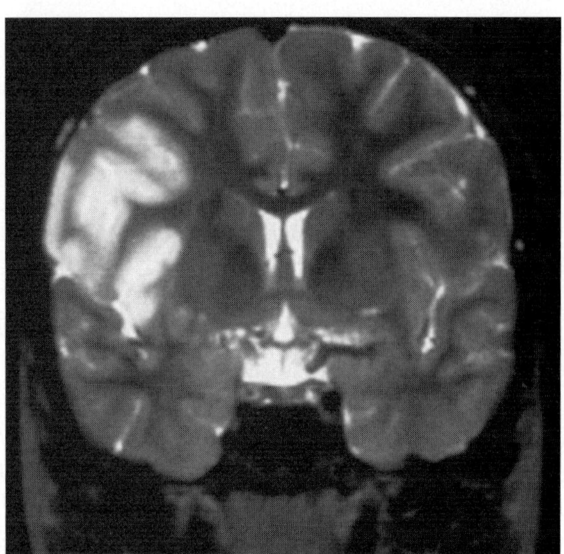

A

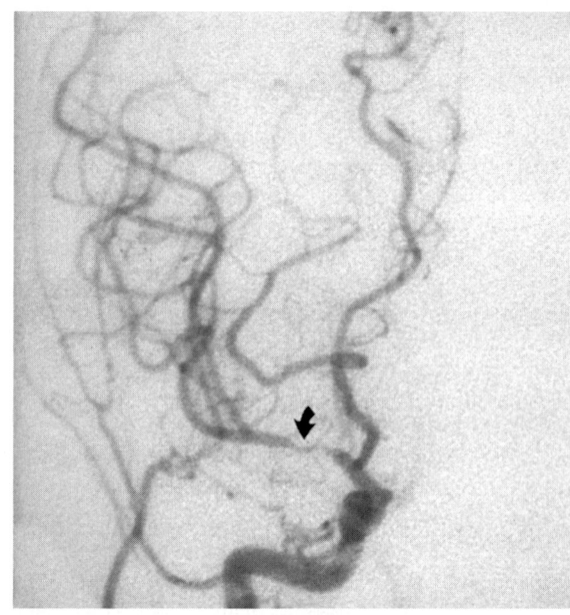

B

FIGURE 72-4. Large-vessel arterial infarct in the right middle cerebral artery (MCA) territory associated with "transient cerebral arteriopathy" of childhood in an 11-year-old female presenting with hemiparesis. **A,** T2-weighted MRI shows right middle cerebral artery (MCA) infarct maximally involving the cortex. **B,** Conventional angiogram shows irregular stenosis in the proximal right MCA. (**B**, Courtesy of Division of Neuroradiology, Hospital for Sick Children, Toronto, Ontario, Canada.)

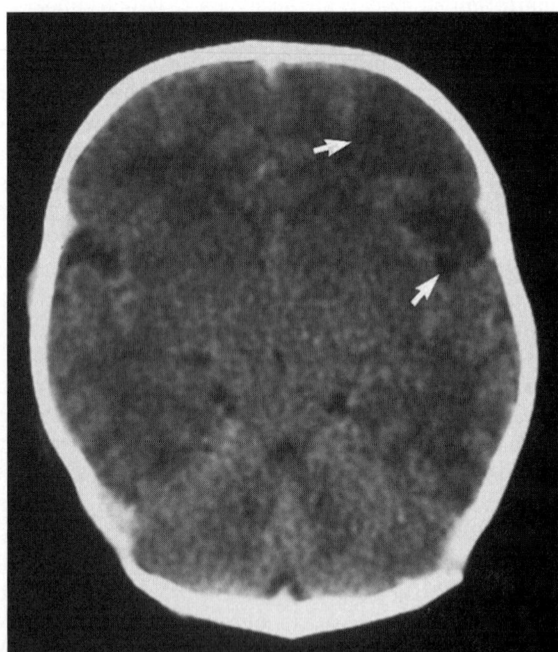

FIGURE 72-5. CT scan shows large-vessel arterial infarct of unknown etiology in the left middle cerebral artery territory in a newborn female presenting with seizures on day 2 of life. (Courtesy of Dr. Laurence Friedman, Children's Hospital at Chedoke McMaster, Ontario, Canada.)

wedge-shaped infarcts involving the cerebral cortex and subjacent white matter in characteristic vascular distributions (Figs. 72-4A and 72-5). Anastamoses at the level of the circle of Willis and through smaller vessels in the leptomeninges can provide collateral blood flow following occlusion of large arteries. In peripheral areas of the brain, at the junction of the areas supplied by the anterior, middle, and posterior cerebral arteries, are so-called watershed zones. Watershed infarctions result when these areas are maximally damaged during global hypoperfusion and to a lesser extent during hypoxia. In the presence of fixed vascular stenosis of the cerebral arteries, global hypoperfusion causes focal infarction. An unusual form of multiple small, "deep" watershed infarcts involving hemispheric white matter has been observed in children with moyamoya disease and occlusion of the distal internal carotid artery. These infarcts appear at the border-zones between penetrating cerebral arterial branches and the perforator arteries arising from the stem of the major cerebral arteries. Occlusion of small-caliber perforator arteries produces infarcts several millimeters to several centimeters in diameter, similar to lacunar infarcts described in adults (Figs. 72-6A and B and 72-7). Such infarcts are concentrated in deep central brain structures, including the basal ganglia and brainstem, that are in the territory of the perforator arteries that arise from the most proximal portions of the anterior, middle, and posterior cerebral arteries. Perforator arteries are functionally classified as end-arteries because they lack vascular anastomoses and collateral supply does not exist. As a result, occlusion of these arteries is more likely to result in permanent infarction. Small-vessel territory infarcts, although small in size, can result in severe clinical manifestations because of the densely concentrated functional pathways located in deep central areas, including the internal capsule. In children with perforator artery territory infarcts, the infarcts tend to be larger "macro-lacunar" infarcts, compared with those in adults, and are probably related to differing mechanisms of occlusion. In adults, lipohyalinosis of the small arteries results in occlusion of individual and distal small artery branches. In childhood, perforator arteries become occluded at their origin off of the stem of the proximal middle, anterior, or posterior cerebral artery, due either to thrombotic occlusion or to inflammation of the wall of

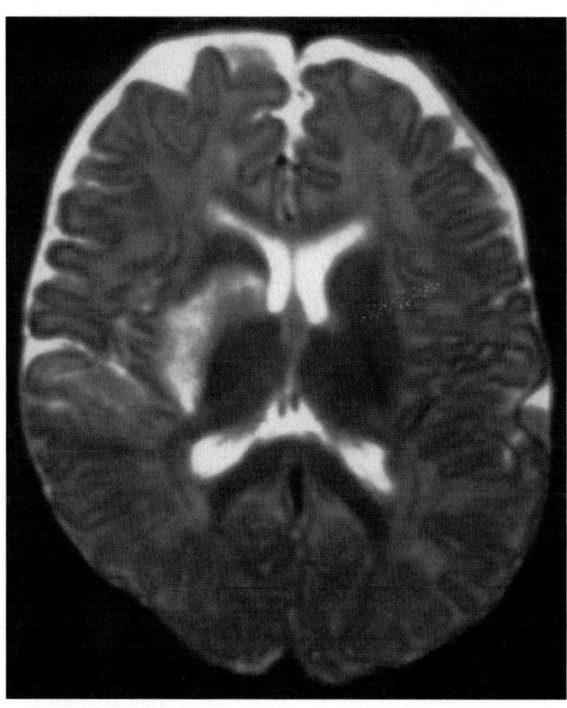

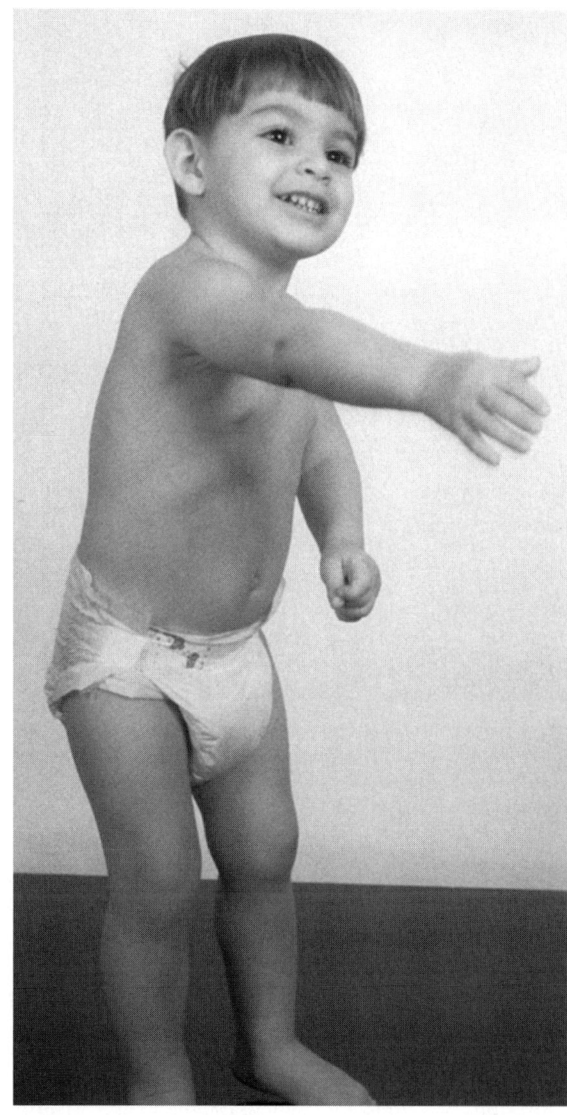

A B

FIGURE 72-6. Small-vessel arterial infarct of unknown etiology in a 10-month-old male. **A,** T2-weighted MRI shows right caudate and putamen infarct. **B,** Same patient 4 months after stroke, residual left hemiparesis with left hand fisting is seen. (Courtesy of Division of Neuroradiology, Hospital for Sick Children, Toronto, Ontario, Canada.)

the large arteries, as in post-varicella angiopathy and transient cerebral arteriopathy of childhood [Askalan et al., 2001; Chabrier et al., 1998]. In population-based studies, arterial infarcts are in the small-vessel distribution in approximately 20% of neonates and in 50% of older infants and children. In both populations, the strokes occur more frequently in the left than in the right hemisphere [deVeber and Canadian Paediatric Ischemic Stroke Study Group, 2000].

Clinical Features

In children with acute arterial ischemic stroke, the recognition of cerebral infarction often is delayed beyond 24 hours because of the lack of public and physician awareness, which is related to the low incidence of arterial ischemic stroke. In one study, the time from clinical onset to first medical contact averaged 28.5 hours, and the time to diagnosis of stroke averaged 35.7 hours [deVeber, 2002]. In children, hemiparesis may be erroneously attributed to migraine, focal seizure, focal encephalitis, or demyelination because of their similar presentations and the increased familiarity of physicians with these conditions in childhood. More subtle symptoms or signs are even less likely to be attributed to stroke, particularly in young infants and children who are unable to verbalize these complaints. To further confuse the issue, seizures at the onset of stroke are relatively frequent in children [Delsing et al., 2001], compared with adults [Trescher, 1992; Yang et al., 1995], and stroke may be incorrectly diagnosed as a postictal Todd's paresis. Children with hypoglycemia also can present with focal neurologic deficits mimicking stroke [Kossoff et al., 2001].

The presenting clinical features of arterial ischemic stroke are age-related. The clinical presentation of stroke occurring in later infancy or childhood is typically an acute neurologic event heralded by hemiparesis with or without seizures. Seizures, fever, headache, and lethargy occur more com-

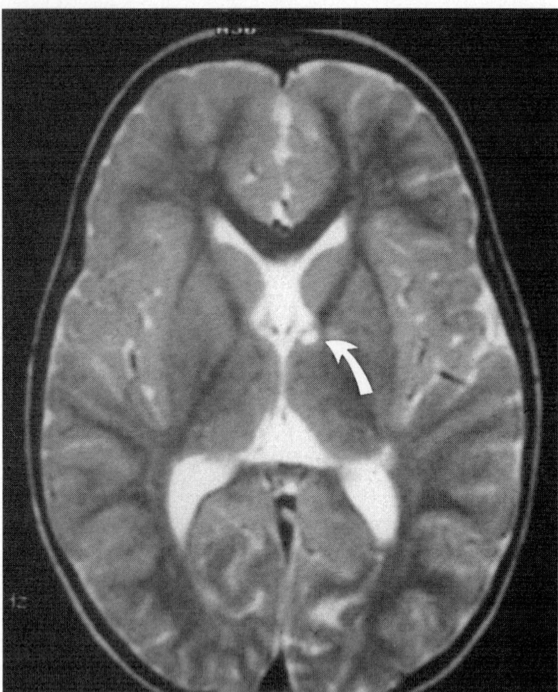

FIGURE 72-7. MRI (T2-weighted) shows left small-vessel arterial infarct not seen on CT in a 5-year-old male who had recurrent episodes of right hemiparesis 6 months after chickenpox and was diagnosed with plasminogen deficiency. (Courtesy of Dr. Laurence Friedman.)

monly in younger children than in older children [Trescher, 1992]. Dystonia is more common in children with basal ganglia infarction than in adults [Demierre and Rondot, 1983]. Although the majority of children with arterial ischemic stroke present with a single episode of focal neurologic deficit, transient ischemic attacks, frequently followed by a stroke, are increasingly recognized in children and infants. The definitions of transient ischemic attack and arterial ischemic stroke are undergoing revision. In the past, these entities were defined solely by the duration of deficit (less than 24 hours for transient ischemic attack and 24 hours or more for arterial ischemic stroke). In reality, a neurologic deficit lasting less than 24 hrs is associated with CT or MRI evidence of an infarct in 2% to 50% of adults. Thus, transient ischemic attack has been recently re-defined as "a brief episode of neurologic dysfunction caused by focal brain or retinal ischemia, with clinical symptoms typically lasting less than one hour, and without evidence of acute infarction." The presence of persistent clinical signs, regardless of duration, or characteristic imaging abnormalities then defines infarction—that is, stroke [Albers et al., 2002].

In children, the differentiation of transient ischemic attack from other causes of brief neurologic deficits can be challenging. However, the development of a clinical deficit that is sudden and maximal at onset, or the presence of cerebral artery stenosis on conventional angiography or magnetic resonance angiography (MRA) suggests a probable thromboembolic etiology. The importance of identifying transient ischemic attacks is that they are frequently followed by stroke, and urgent antithrombotic treatment is advisable.

Risk Factors

Risk factors for arterial ischemic stroke in children differ significantly from those in adults, in whom arteriosclerosis is the leading cause of stroke [deVeber, 2003]. Children are less likely than adult stroke patients to have identifiable risk factors and more likely to have infectious or inflammatory disorders underlying the stroke [Kerr et al., 1993]. In children with stroke, approximately half are previously well [Ganesan et al., 2003]. The reported frequency of identifiable risk factors in children with arterial ischemic stroke beyond the newborn period varies widely across studies, depending on the population of children, criteria for risk factors, and extensiveness of etiologic investigations. In single center tertiary care studies, risk factors are definable in 78% to 90% of children [Chabrier et al., 2000; Ganesan et al., 2003; Lanthier et al., 2000]. In a prospective population-based study, a primary risk factor for cerebral infarction was definable in 72% of children with arterial ischemic stroke [deVeber and Canadian Paediatric Ischemic Stroke Study Group, 2000]. One important risk factor was cardiac disease in 24%. Stroke accompanied cardiac surgery in 20% and catheterization in 17% of these children and occurred spontaneously in 63%. Other risk factors in older children included prothrombotic or hematologic disorders (12%), dissection (7%), moyamoya disease (8%), post-varicella angiopathy (7%), and other vasculopathies (5%). Multiple risk factors frequently were present in individual patients. Another institutional study of risk factors for childhood arterial ischemic stroke reported anemia in 40%, and elevated homocysteine levels or homozygosity for the t-MTHFR mutation in 21% of children [Ganesan et al., 2003]. Trauma and previous varicella zoster infection also were frequently seen. Mechanisms of stroke in another institutional study of 59 children were arteriopathy in 53%, cardioembolic in 12%, and systemic disease in 14% [Chabrier et al., 2000]. In this study, dissection (20%) and transient cerebral arteriopathy (25%) were frequently noted, likely due to the consistent use of and referral for angiography. In 22% of children, no mechanism was identified.

The cause of stroke in some children is obvious—for example, those children with a known structural cardiac disorder or sickle cell disease. Clinical features obtained from the history and physical examination can suggest less obvious etiologies. A recent head or neck injury suggests dissection. A varicella infection in the previous 12 months should lead to consideration of post-varicella angiopathy. A history of head or neck irradiation, especially when focused on the optic chiasm predisposes to postradiation vasculopathy. Migraine, oral contraceptive use, and amphetamine or cocaine use all predispose to infarction. The risk of ischemic stroke is increased in young women using oral contraceptives, including low-estrogen preparations [Gillum et al., 2000]. A family history of stroke, heart attack, lipid problems, leg clots, or lung clots at young ages suggests a hereditary coagulation or lipid disorder. Physical examination may provide additional clues, including head or neck bruits, cardiac murmurs, and skin lesions of tuberous sclerosis, neurofibromatosis, or Fabry's disease.

The interaction of genes with other known risk factors in childhood stroke is being explored [Kirkham, 2004]. Single gene disorders with a significant predisposition to stroke include sickle cell disease, homocystinuria, Menkes' disease, and neurofibromatosis. In children with sickle cell disease, additional gene polymorphisms are associated with different patterns of infarction (small vessel only, large vessel territory with or without small vessel, no strokes) [Hoppe et al., 2004].

The probability of identifying the cause of arterial ischemic stroke depends on the thoroughness of investigation. An underlying predisposing condition should be sought, because children may remain at risk for recurrent thromboembolic events and adverse outcomes are linked to the type and number of risk factors [Chabrier et al., 2000; Lanthier et al., 2000]. Stroke may be the initial manifestation of serious undiagnosed diseases, including heart disease, systemic lupus erythematosus, diabetes, and cancer. Of particular importance is the identification of children with inherited coagulation abnormalities, because treatment for secondary prevention and genetic counseling are available. Additional risk factors for childhood arterial ischemic stroke will undoubtedly be identified over time. Box 72-1 lists the most common causes of arterial ischemic stroke. In the following section, the most important disorders causing arterial ischemic stroke in the pediatric age group are briefly reviewed.

Cardiac Disorders

The most common identifiable cause of childhood ischemic stroke is complex congenital heart disease. Congenital and acquired (endocarditis, cardiomyopathy) cardiac disorders are present in 12% to 28% of older infants and children with arterial ischemic stroke [Chabrier et al., 2000; Ganesan et al., 2003; deVeber and Canadian Paediatric Ischemic Stroke Study Group, 2000]. Thrombi formed in the heart can embolize to the cerebral circulation. Prosthetic heart valves are an important source of emboli. In the presence of an atrial or ventricular septal defect, intermittent right-to-left intracardiac shunting allows systemic venous clots to reach the cerebral circulation. In approximately half of the children with congenital heart disease and stroke, the stroke occurred in relation to the time when cardiac surgery or catheterization procedures were performed. The frequency of stroke following cardiac surgery in children has been recently estimated as 1 in 250 to 1 in 400 procedures [Domi et al., 2002; Menache et al., 2002]. However, following the Fontan procedure, the frequency of immediate or delayed stroke ranged from 3% to 19% [Monagle and Karl, 2002]. Stroke following cardiac catheterization in children is reported to occur in 1 in 600 to 700 procedures [Liu et al., 2001].

Small insignificant intracardiac septal defects, including patent foramen ovale, have been established as risk factors for paradoxical embolism and stroke in young adults [DiTullio et al., 1992]. The Patent Foramen Ovale in Cryptogenic Stroke Study (PICSS), confirmed that patent foramen ovale is more prevalent among patients with cryptogenic stroke and that treatment with aspirin (acetylsalicylic acid) is associated with a low risk of recurrent stroke in the absence of an associated atrial septal aneurysm [Mas et al., 2001]. Prothrombotic disorders apparently combine with patent foramen ovale in the genesis of stroke in such patients [Pezzini et al., 2003; Rodriguez and Homma, 2003]. Echocardiography should be performed in all children with arterial ischemic stroke of undetermined cause. Agitated saline to establish the presence of patent foramen ovale and transesophageal echocardiography increase the sensitivity of testing. These additional echocardiographic techniques should be considered in children with arterial ischemic stroke, especially in children older than 7 years in whom transthoracic echocardiography may have insufficient resolution.

Infection

Fever and nonspecific or nasopharyngeal viral infections frequently are present in children presenting with cerebral infarction. In one recent study, fever was present in nearly 50% and leukocytosis in 26% of children, although specific infectious agents were infrequently identified [Ganesan et al., 2003]. Arterial or venous stroke has been identified in 5% to 12% of children with bacterial meningitis; however, strokes occur in as many as 75% of infants with meningitis in the first year of life [Chang et al., 2003; Chiu et al., 1995; Silverstein and Brunberg, 1995]. Local inflammation of the meninges with thrombophlebitis of cerebral vessels is the primary mechanism. Meningitis should be considered in children with arterial ischemic stroke and fever, and selected cerebrospinal and serum studies assessing for bacterial, tuberculous, and viral meningitis may be indicated. Pediatric stroke has been reported in the following specific infectious disorders: mycoplasma, cat scratch fever, Rocky Mountain spotted fever, Lyme disease, cryptococcus, Japanese encephalitis, coxsackievirus B4 and A9, influenza A, enterovirus, varicella, HIV (human immunodeficiency virus), parvovirus B19 and X, and chlamydia [Guidi et al., 2003]. HIV infection is increasingly recognized as a risk factor for multiple infarcts and cerebral aneurysms. In a recent series, these lesions were found on screening MRI scans in 2.6% of children with HIV and were frequently asymptomatic [Kleinschmidt-DeMasters and Gilden, 2001; Patsalides et al., 2002; Visudtibhan et al., 1999].

Prothrombotic Disorders

Prothrombotic disorders are abnormalities of the coagulation system, fibrinolytic system, endothelial cells, or platelets, which lead to a reduced threshold for pathologic thrombus formation. Inherited or acquired coagulation system disorders have been identified in 50% to 68% of newborns and 20% to 50% of children presenting with arterial ischemic stroke [Barnes and deVeber, 2004; Bonduel et al., 1999; deVeber et al., 1998; Golomb et al., 2001; Gunther et al., 2000]. Acquired prothrombotic states are more frequent than congenital prothrombotic states in children with arterial ischemic stroke [Bonduel et al., 1999; deVeber et al., 1998]. The most frequently reported abnormalities include factor V Leiden deficiency, prothrombin G20210A mutation, elevated lipoprotein(a) and homocysteine levels, protein C deficiency, and antiphospholipid antibodies. In contrast to most prothrombotic states, which primarily promote venous thrombosis, the prothrombin G20210A mutation is more frequently associated with arterial thrombosis, including arterial ischemic stroke, than with venous thrombosis in children [Young et al., 2003]. Recently, anticardiolipin antibodies at modestly increased levels (less than 45 GPL [immunoglobulin G phospholipid] units) have been found not to predict recurrent stroke or transient ischemic attack in

Box 72-1 Disorders Causing Ischemic Stroke

Intravascular

Hematologic Disorders

Hemoglobinopathies (sickle cell anemia)
Immune thrombocytopenic purpura
Thrombotic thrombocytopenic purpura
Thrombocytosis
Polycythemia
Leukemia or other neoplasm

Acquired Prothrombotic States

Prothrombotic medications (oral contraceptives and L-asparaginase)
Pregnancy and the postpartum period
Lupus anticoagulant
Anticardiolipin antibodies
Lipoprotein abnormalities

Congenital or Acquired Prothrombotic States

Antithrombin III deficiency
Protein S deficiency
Protein C deficiency
Plasminogen deficiency

Congenital Prothrombotic States

Factor V Leiden gene defect
Methyltetrahydrofolate reductase
Prothrombin gene defect

Metabolic Disorders

Hyperhomocysteinemia
Hyperlipidemia
Lipoprotein-a elevation

Vascular

Vasculitis

Primary angiitis of the CNS
Meningitis
Systemic lupus erythematosus
Polyarteritis nodosa
Takayasu's arteritis
Rheumatoid arthritis
Dermatomyositis
Inflammatory bowel disease
Drug abuse (cocaine, amphetamines)

Systemic Vascular Disease

Early atherosclerosis
Diabetes
Ehlers-Danlos syndrome
Pseudoxanthoma elasticum
Homocystinuria
Fabry's disease

Vasculopathies

Post-varicella angiopathy*
Transient cerebral arteriopathy*
Arterial fibromuscular dysplasia
Moyamoya disease
Post-radiation vasculopathy

Vasospastic Disorders

Migraine
Ergot poisoning
Vasospasm with subarachnoid hemorrhage

Trauma

Brain herniation and arterial compression
Post-traumatic arterial dissection
Intra-oral trauma
Carotid ligation (e.g., ECMO)
Arteriography

Embolic

Congenital Heart Disease

Complex congenital heart defect
Ventricular/atrial septal defect
Aortic or mitral stenosis
Coarctation
Patent foramen ovale
Patent ductus arteriosus

Acquired Heart Disease

Rheumatic heart disease
Prosthetic heart valve
Bacterial endocarditis
Cardiomyopathy and myocarditis
Atrial myxoma
Cardiac rhabdomyoma
Dysrhythmia

Trauma

Amniotic fluid/placental embolism
Fat or air embolism
Foreign body embolism
Cardiac catheterization

*Likely inflammatory and can be classified as focal vasculitis.
CNS, central nervous system; ECMO, extracorporeal membrane oxygenation.

children, at least with current antithrombotic treatment [Lanthier et al., 2004].

The presence of some prothrombotic states does increase the risk of stroke recurrence in older children, although not in neonates. In a German collaborative study of Caucasian children, stroke recurrence risk was significantly increased in children with familial protein C deficiency or increased lipoprotein (a) levels [Strater et al., 2002]. Children with prothrombotic disorders usually have additional "triggering" risk factors at the time of arterial ischemic stroke [Barreirinho et al., 2003; Strater et al., 2002]. Coagulation testing should be performed in any child with arterial ischemic stroke, including children with other identified risk factors. Children should be tested off anticoagulants if possible. Transient abnormalities in coagulation testing occur for several weeks or longer after the formation of a clot. Testing parents, if the abnormality is a hereditary coagulation abnormality, or retesting the child several months later or both, should confirm abnormal results on samples taken within several weeks of the stroke.

Hematologic Disorders

Sickle cell disease is the most common hematologic disorder associated with cerebrovascular disease. About 25% of patients with sickle cell disease develop cerebrovascular complications that include overt arterial ischemic stroke, subclinical small-vessel occlusive arterial ischemic stroke, and subarachnoid or intracranial hemorrhage [Pegelow, 2001]. Stroke is the cause of death in 10% of children with sickle cell disease [Manci et al., 2003]. Thrombotic stroke occurs as part of the thrombotic crisis or as the result of a progressive cerebral vasculopathy resembling moyamoya disease. Strokes are ischemic in 75% and hemorrhagic in 25% of cases; prior to the mid-teen years hemorrhage is rare. Aneurysms are rare in children with moyamoya disease associated with sickle cell disease with an incidence of only 1.5% [Satoh et al., 1988]. Transcranial Doppler studies are a noninvasive means of following the large-vessel vasculopathy and determining stroke risk in these patients [Adams et al., 1992, 1998]. A randomized, controlled trial has documented that long-term transfusion therapy to reduce the levels of hemoglobin S to less than 20% to 30% reduces the risk of primary stroke in high-risk individuals [Adams et al., 1998]. Since publication of the STOP study in 1998, annual rates of admissions for first stroke for Californian children with sickle cell disease have declined from 0.88 per 100 person-years during 1991 through 1998 to 0.50 in 1999 and 0.17 in 2000 [Fullerton et al., 2004]. In children with sickle cell disease and moyamoya disease, EDAS (encephaloduroarteriosynangiosis) surgery has been used with promising results [Fryer et al., 2003]. Recently, nocturnal hypoxemia has been identified as a significant predictor of stroke in children with sickle cell disease [Kirkham et al., 2001]. Other therapies are under investigation, and hydroxyurea has shown efficacy in the prevention of recurrent stroke in a recent randomized, controlled trial [Ware et al., 2004]. The role of anticoagulant and antiplatelet agents remain unclear but should be considered, especially when large-vessel vasculopathy or prothrombotic abnormalities and recurrent stroke co-exist [Wolters et al., 1995].

Non-sickle cell anemias may be associated more frequently with arterial ischemic stroke than previously recognized and were observed in more than 25% of children with arterial ischemic stroke in one series [Ganesan et al., 2003]. Iron-deficiency anemia also is frequently associated with stroke, particularly in older infants [Hartfield et al., 1997]. The underlying pathophysiology explaining this relation has not been established. Platelet disorders including thrombocytosis can be associated with arterial ischemic stroke.

Arteriopathies

In older infants and children with arterial ischemic stroke, vascular imaging reveals specific arteriopathic disorders in 53% to 59% [Chabrier et al., 2000; Ganesan et al., 2003]. A classification system for arteriopathies associated with arterial ischemic stroke in childhood has been developed recently [Sébire et al., 2004]. Because the presence of vasculopathy increases the risk for arterial ischemic stroke recurrence nearly threefold, cerebrovascular imaging to detect arterial disorders is important [Askalan et al., 2001; Lanthier et al., 2004; Strater et al., 2002].

DISSECTION AND OTHER PHYSICAL INJURIES

Dissection of the carotid or vertebral arteries occurs in 8% to 20% of children with arterial ischemic stroke [Chabrier et al., 2003; Fullerton et al., 2001; Rafay et al., 2002]. In children, dissection can result from intra-oral trauma, mechanical injuries to the neck including external manipulation, or physical exertion, or can occur spontaneously [Chabrier et al., 2003; Rafay et al., 2002]. Headache is a prominent presenting feature in 50% to 75% of children. With current medical therapy, recurrent transient ischemic attacks or strokes are documented in 8% to 19% of children with large-vessel dissection, and recurrent dissection in other arteries occurs in up to 20% of children with dissections involving the anterior circulation [Chabrier et al., 2003; Fullerton et al., 2001; Rafay et al., 2002]. As in adults, initial treatment usually consists of anticoagulation using unfractionated heparin or low-molecular-weight heparins, followed by 3 to 6 months of Coumadin therapy. However, even in adults uncertainty regarding optimal treatment exists, and a randomized, controlled trial assessing aspirin or anticoagulants is needed [Beletsky et al., 2003]. The risk of recurrence and period of endothelial disruption are maximal in the first several weeks from onset. Therefore, a switch from anticoagulant to aspirin therapy may be feasible earlier than is the current practice, especially in patients in whom follow-up vascular imaging indicates rapid resolution of arterial wall abnormalities.

Post-radiation vasculopathy manifests with progressive large-vessel stenosis and transient ischemic attacks or strokes beginning several years after irradiation of optic chiasm gliomas or other sellar or suprasellar region tumors in children (Fig. 72-8). Younger children with increased doses of radiation are particularly susceptible [Omura et al., 1997]. MRI findings of arterial wall thickening and contrast enhancement have been described in this condition [Aoki et al., 2002]. No specific therapy halts the progression of postradiation vasculopathy, although disease progression may spontaneously diminish over time. Cerebral arteries at the base of the brain, particularly the posterior cerebral artery, are susceptible to extrinsic mechanical compression and occlusion. In childhood, this mechanism is observed when intracranial pressure is markedly increased by impending herniation, such as with head trauma, severe diffuse hypoxic ischemic injury, and hydrocephalus.

POSTVARICELLA ANGIOPATHY

Postvaricella angiopathy occurring weeks or months after uncomplicated varicella is probably underdiagnosed. In school-aged children with arterial ischemic stroke, there is a

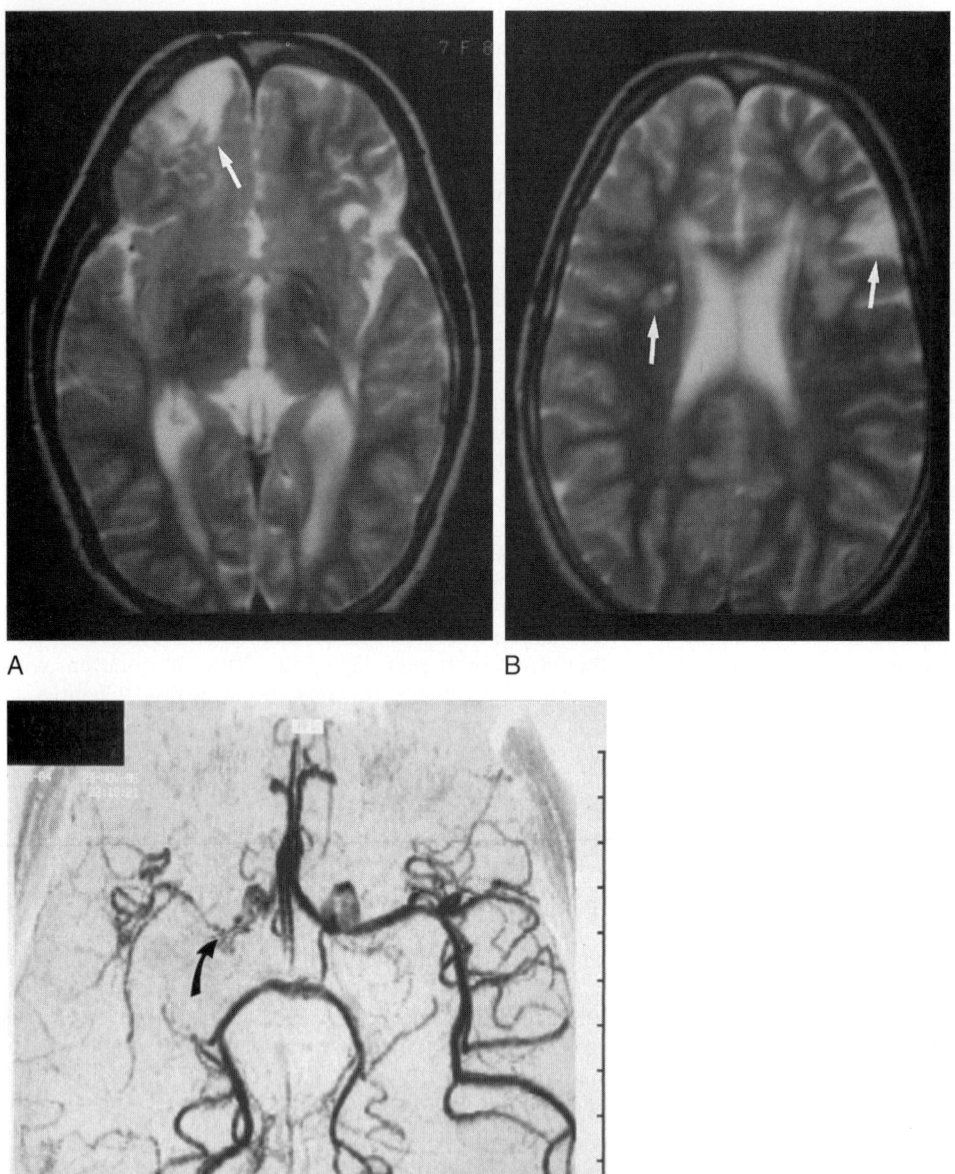

FIGURE 72-8. Nine-year-old female with optic glioma irradiated 3 years earlier and post-radiation vasculopathy with recurrent bilateral artery-to-artery embolic arterial infarcts. **A** and **B,** T2-weighted MRI shows multiple bilateral infarcts. **C,** MR angiogram shows obvious right and subtle left middle cerebral artery stenosis. (Courtesy of Dr. Laurence Friedman.)

threefold increase in preceding varicella infection compared with published population rates, and varicella-associated arterial ischemic stroke accounts for nearly one third of childhood arterial ischemic strokes [Askalan et al., 2001]. Varicella-associated arterial ischemic stroke has characteristic features, including basal ganglia infarction and self-resolving unilateral stenosis of the distal internal carotid or proximal anterior, middle, or (less frequently) posterior cerebral arteries (Fig. 72-9; also see Fig. 72-7) [Askalan et al., 2001]. Elevated cerebrospinal fluid antibody titers to varicella-zoster virus rarely are found [Ueno et al., 2002]. In adults, viral particles or antigens have been detected in the cytoplasm and nuclei of smooth muscle cells from the wall of affected cerebral arteries [Eidelberg et al., 1986; Linnemann and Alvira, 1980; Reshef et al., 1985]. In a 4-year-old female who died of progressive stroke secondary to postvaricella angiopathy, postmortem examination revealed a zoster antigen-positive giant cell arteritis involving the left middle cerebral artery [Berger et al., 2000]. A second case of clinical postvaricella stroke showed lymphocytic arteritis, without evidence of varicella virus, affecting cerebral small vessels in a surgical specimen after decompressive surgery in a 4-year-old male [Hayman et al., 2001]. The most likely mechanism is that the virus is activated in the trigeminal ganglion and spreads along the trigeminal nerve fibers innervating the internal carotid artery and proximal cerebral arteries [Kleinschmidt-DeMasters and Gilden, 2001].

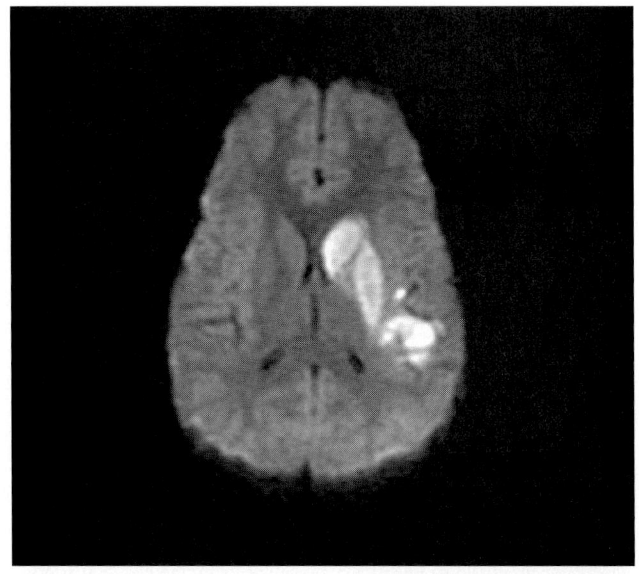

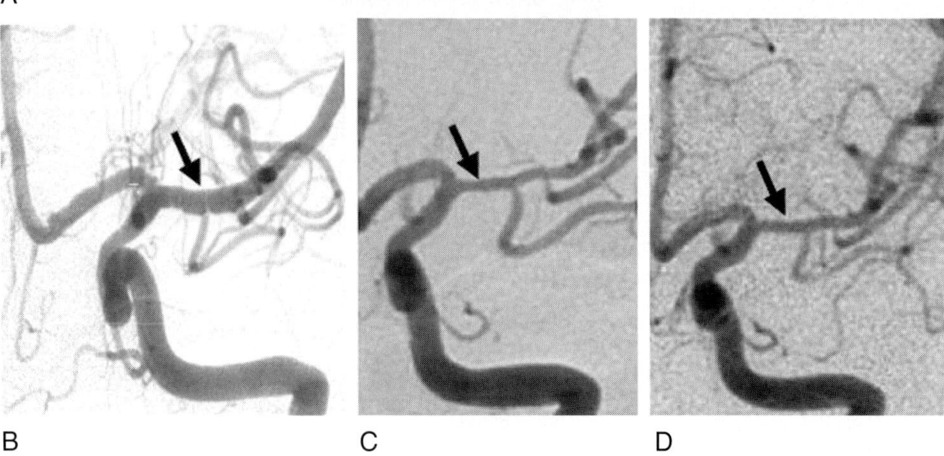

FIGURE 72-9. Postvaricella angiopathy in a 4-year-old male presenting with hemiparesis and speech loss 3 months following chickenpox. **A,** Initial MRI shows a "macro-lacune" involving left basal ganglia. **B,** Initial angiogram shows normal lumen diameter with abnormal striae in the stem (*arrow*) of the left middle cerebral artery (MCA). **C,** Follow-up angiogram 8 weeks later shows stenosis in MCA stem (*arrow*) at the site of the prior abnormality. **D,** Repeat angiogram after another 10 months shows persistence without progression of MCA stem (*arrow*) stenosis. (Courtesy of Derek Armstrong, Division of Neuroradiology, Hospital for Sick Children, Toronto, Ontario, Canada.)

VASCULITIS

Central nervous system vasculitis in childhood may be primary, termed *isolated* or *primary* angiitis of the central nervous system, or secondary to a variety of conditions, including infections, collagen vascular diseases, systemic vasculitides, and malignancies [Benseler and Schneider, 2004]. Systemic vasculitides that can affect the cerebral arteries include Kawasaki's disease, Henoch-Schohnlein purpura, Polyarteritis nodosa, Wegener's granulomatosis, and Takayasu's arteritis [Belostotsky et al., 2002; Berman et al., 1990; Morales et al., 1991; Morfin-Maciel et al., 2002; von Scheven et al., 1998]. Connective tissue diseases, including systemic lupus erythematosus, Behçet's syndrome, dermatomyositis, mixed connective tissue disease, Sjögren's syndrome, and inflammatory bowel disorders, can also cause central nervous system vasculitis in childhood [Benseler and Schneider, 2004; Graf et al., 1993]. Takayasu's arteritis in childhood is rare and presents with progressive stenosis and occlusion of extracranial arteries near their origin from the aorta [Morales et al., 1991]. Although systemic lupus erythematosus is often associated with arterial ischemic stroke, vasculitis as the etiology for stroke is rare [Devinsky et al., 1988]. Isolated angiitis of the central nervous system (IACNS) in childhood has been recently reviewed and classified [Lanthier et al., 2001]. In children, the large, medium-sized, and small vessels can be involved, at times overlapping in individual cases. Histopathologic findings range from a granulomatous to nongranulomatous, primarily lymphocytic process. The aggressive form of IACNS as seen in adults is rare in children. The diagnosis is suspected when progressive, irregular arterial narrowing occurs in the absence of other etiologies (Fig. 72-10). Brain or leptomeningeal biopsy is usually required for confirmation.

Transient cerebral arteriopathy is a unilateral monophasic vasculitis that is frequently recognized in children with arterial ischemic stroke. Transient cerebral arteriopathy is presumed but not proven to represent a form of focal self-limited vasculitis and may well be the most common type of arteriopathy in children with arterial ischemic stroke [Chabrier et al., 1998; Shirane et al., 1992]. The angiographic appearance includes unilateral irregular stenosis involving the distal part of the internal carotid and proximal segments of the anterior cerebral artery (A1 segment), the

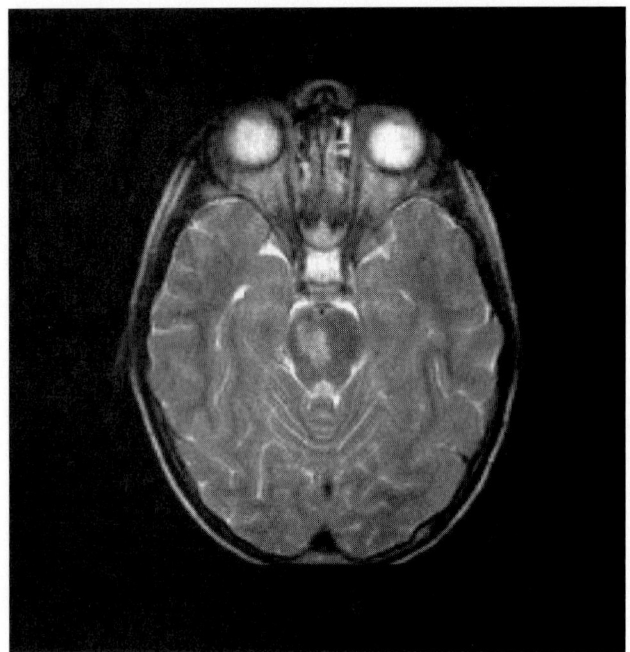

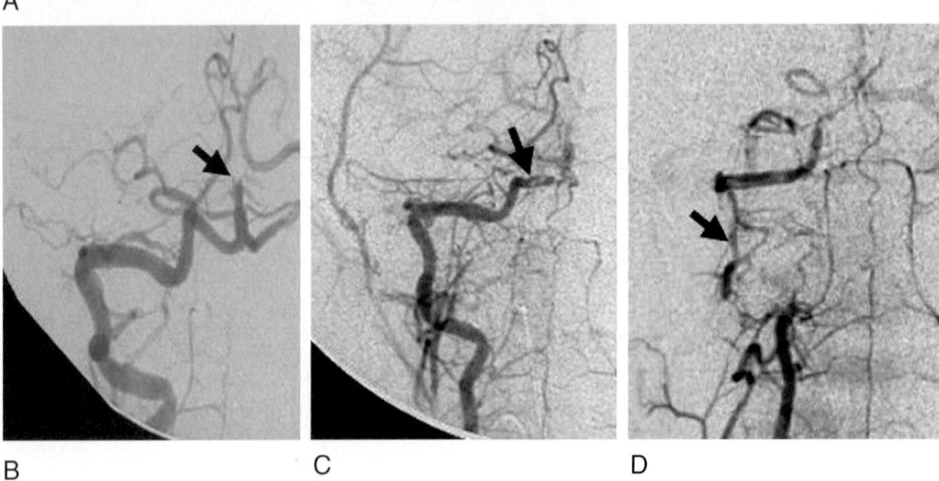

FIGURE 72-10. Progressive, presumed vasculitis of the vertebrovascular system in a 4-year-old male with pontine infarction. **A,** Initial MRI shows pontine infarct. **B,** Initial angiogram demonstrates basilar artery occlusion (*arrow*) with normal vertebral arteries. **C.** Although the clinical course had not changed, follow-up angiogram 4 months later shows presumed vasculitis involving the distal right vertebral artery (*arrow*). **D,** Again, although the clinical course had not changed, a repeat angiogram after the child was on steroid therapy for 5 months shows progression of the presumed vasculitis involving the cervical portion of the vertebral artery (*arrow*). Biopsy was not performed. (Courtesy of Derek Armstrong, Division of Neuroradiology, Hospital for Sick Children, Toronto, Ontario, Canada.)

middle cerebral artery (M1 segment), or the posterior cerebral artery (P1 segment) (see Fig. 72-4B) [Chabrier et al., 1998; Shirane et al., 1992]. Unilateral infarcts located in the basal ganglia and internal capsule are typical features. The average age at onset is 5 years. The natural history includes stabilization or regression of the lesions on angiographic follow-up, with progression of stenosis limited to the initial 3 to 6 months after presentation with arterial ischemic stroke. Serologic markers of vasculitis are rarely seen.

The most plausible pathophysiologic mechanism underlying transient cerebral arteriopathy is a transient acute vasculitis induced by viral infection. When varicella infection precedes the onset of arterial ischemic stroke by less than 12 months, transient cerebral arteriopathy is termed *post-varicella angiopathy*. A worsening of arterial lesions detected on MRA at 6 to 12 months, compared to detection at 3 to 6 months, argues in favor of a chronic cerebral vasculitis [Sébire et al., 2004]. Transient cerebral arteriopathy has been included in the spectrum of IACNS, although this is controversial, and predictors distinguishing this condition from progressive IACNS have been defined [Benseler et al., 2003]. Enteroviral infection also has been associated with transient cerebral arteriopathy [Ribai et al., 2003].

Because vasculitis can involve medium-sized and small vessels that are not well visualized with current MRA techniques, conventional angiography is usually indicated in children with arterial ischemic stroke of unclear etiology. Laboratory tests for vasculitis include the erythrocyte sedimentation rate, complement studies (C3 and C4), rheumatoid factor, antinuclear antibodies, and cerebrospinal examination for pleocytosis. In children with bilateral or distal arterial lesions considered to be possible IACNS, a leptomeningeal and cortical biopsy should be considered to confirm the diagnosis prior to committing to long-term immunosuppressant therapy.

Moyamoya Disease and Moyamoya Syndrome

Moyamoya disease should be distinguished from moyamoya syndrome. Moyamoya disease refers to a specific disease described primarily in the Asian population and characterized

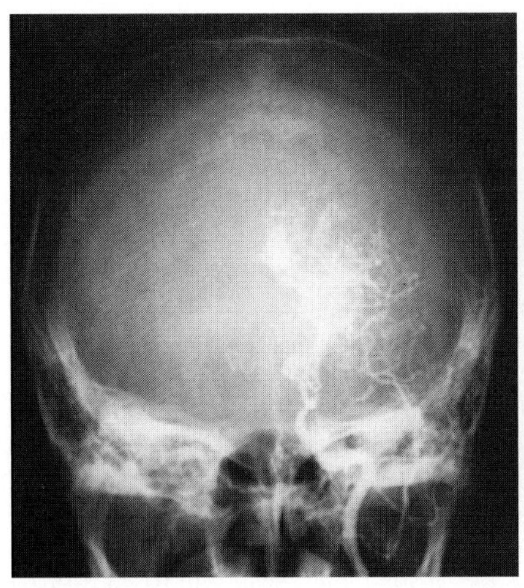
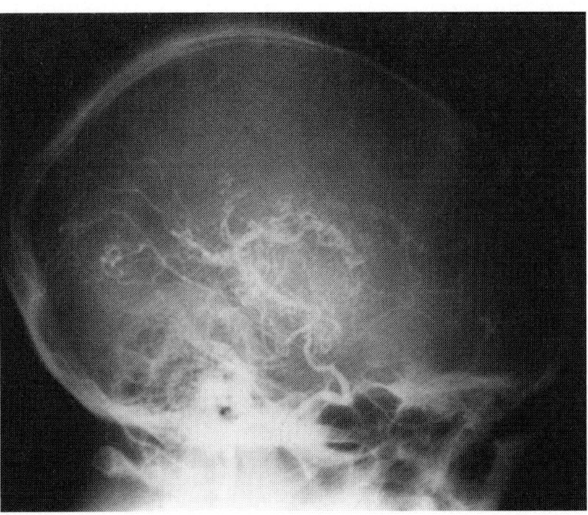

A B

FIGURE 72-11. Moyamoya disease in a developmentally delayed 13-year-old male with left hemiparesis and chorea on the right. **A,** Anterior and middle cerebral arteries are occluded, and a prominent vascular pattern is evident in the basal ganglia. **B,** Lateral projection of same patient.

by progressive idiopathic stenosis and eventual occlusion of the large cerebral arteries involving the circle of Willis. In response to the stenosis, an abnormal network of small collateral vessels develops creating the "puff of smoke" appearance on the angiogram (Fig. 72-11). Moyamoya syndrome includes the angiographic pattern typical of moyamoya disease but occurs secondary to a variety of slowly progressive, occlusive cerebral vasculopathies, such as sickle cell disease and postradiation vasculopathy. A variety of genetic syndromes are associated with moyamoya syndrome, including Down syndrome, neurofibromatosis, and Williams' syndrome. Conventional angiography is the definitive method of diagnosis.

The clinical course consists of recurrent transient ischemic attacks and strokes and progressive cognitive decline. Recurrent infarcts and rapid disease progression are more frequently seen in moyamoya disease presenting prior to age 6 years [Kim et al., 2004]. In contrast to other forms of childhood arterial ischemic stroke, the neurologic events in children with moyamoya disease are frequently related to hyperventilation and breath-holding and appear to have a vasoreactive mechanism responsive to acid-base balance, not simply thromboembolic mechanisms [Mikulis et al., 2004]. Over time, moyamoya disease can remain stable but more typically follows a progressive course with severe motor impairment and intellectual deterioration [Suzuki and Kodama, 1983]. The natural history of moyamoya disease may be less devastating than previously suggested. Hemorrhage is relatively rare in children with moyamoya disease compared with adults [Yoshida et al., 1993].

No specific medical therapy has been found to halt the progression of this disorder, although calcium channel blockers and acetazolamide have been used. Antithrombotic therapy for the prevention of recurrent thromboemboli has not been evaluated but should be considered, as for any other cerebral vasculopathy. Three surgical revascularization procedures have been used to manage this disease: anastamosis of the superficial temporal artery to the cerebral artery ("direct" revascularization), encephalomyosynangiosis, and encephaloduroarteriosynangiosis ("indirect" revascularization). In pial synangiosis, the superficial temporal artery is sutured to the pia mater under microscopic visualization [Ueki et al., 1994]. No clinical trials comparing surgical to nonsurgical management have been conducted. The goal of surgical intervention is to promote development of collateral circulation to the brain, thereby decreasing the risk of stroke, transient ischemic attacks, seizures, and progressive cognitive decline. These surgical techniques are increasingly utilized in the early stages of moyamoya disease with apparently minimal morbidity, and follow-up angiography and perfusion studies demonstrate excellent postoperative establishment of collateral circulation and increased perfusion of ischemic areas of the brain in the majority of patients. In a single center study, 271 pial synangiosis procedures were performed in 143 children, of whom 16 were Asian. In follow-ups ranging from 1 to 17 years, recurrent strokes or transient ischemic attacks were seen in 11 children more than 30 days following surgery and in only 9 children less than 30 days following surgery [Scott et al., 2004].

Migraine

Children with stroke due to migraine have been rarely reported [Feucht et al., 1995; Nezu et al., 1997; Santiago et al., 2001]. The distribution of arterial ischemic stroke is predominantly in the posterior circulation in children with migrainous stroke. When there is an established history of migraine prior to the stroke and a clear migraine headache at the time of the stroke, the causative association is relatively clear. Migraine with aura is a predictor of stroke risk, and in adults migrainous stroke recurs in as many as 15% per year [Rothrock, 1993]. Children frequently develop migraine headache following brain injury, including stroke, and in such cases migraine is likely a result of rather than a cause of the stroke.

Metabolic Vasculopathies

Homozygous homocystinuria predisposes to arterial and venous thrombosis, including cerebral infarcts. Thromboembolic manifestations can precede the ocular and other physical features of the disease [Bodensteiner et al., 1992]. For homozygous homocystinuria, plasma amino acid assays are an adequate diagnostic screen. More subtle forms of hyperhomocysteinemia have been found in up to one fifth of children with arterial ischemic stroke and may play an important pathogenic role [Cardo et al., 2000; Ganesan et al., 2003]. Because hyperhomocysteinemia has a prothrombotic effect, it should be considered even in the absence of a vasculopathy as a possible risk factor for arterial ischemic stroke. Measurement of plasma homocysteine using pediatric normal values is necessary for this diagnosis [Vilaseca et al., 1997]. An oral methionine loading test with pre- and post-methionine plasma homocysteine levels increases the sensitivity of plasma homocysteine testing. In Fabry's disease, caused by alpha-galactosidase deficiency, multiple lacunar cerebral infarcts occur in affected males during the teenage and early adult years. Diagnostic tests for Fabry's disease include examination of the skin for angiokeratoma and testing for increased levels of urinary ceramide trihexoside and decreased levels of leukocyte alpha-galactosidase activity. Children with MELAS syndrome (mitochondrial myopathy, encephalopathy, lactic acidosis and strokelike episodes) present with episodes of nausea, vomiting, headaches, seizures, hemiparesis and cortical blindness. Areas of infarction not conforming to typical vascular distributions are found, usually in the occipital regions [Mudd et al., 1985]. Whether the mechanism for these infarcts includes vascular occlusion has not been established [Michelson and Ashwal, 2005]. However, because focal cortical hyperperfusion is seen in single photon emission computed tomography (SPECT) studies during the strokelike episodes, a more likely explanation is that regional neuronal hyperexcitability results in marked depletion of energy compounds with resultant metabolic infarction [Iizuka et al., 2002]. Elevated serum and cerebrospinal fluid levels of lactate and pyruvate are suggestive of MELAS syndrome, and testing for specific genetic mutations is now available. Children with hyperlipidemia can suffer from stroke [Glueck et al., 1982]. Hypercholesterolemia has been found in up to 9% of children with stroke [Ganesan et al., 2003]. Fasting serum cholesterol, triglycerides, and high-density and low-density lipoprotein fractions should be obtained in any child with idiopathic arterial ischemic stroke. Normal age-related values for these tests are available [Muhonen and Lauer, 1996].

Transient viral or bacterial infections, which involve vasculitis and vascular occlusion in the brain, can trigger idiopathic childhood ischemic stroke on the basis of genetic predisposition [Zou et al., 2002].

Radiographic Features

Computed Tomography

CT of the brain is often normal within the first 12 hours after ischemic stroke [Ball, Jr., 1994]. In children, CT findings of arterial ischemic stroke are similar to those in adults (see Fig. 72-5). Bland infarcts appear as low-density lesions in a vascular territory distribution; hemorrhagic infarcts have additional high-density components. Contrast enhanced CT spiral angiography is a new technique that shows great promise for noninvasive vascular imaging.

Magnetic Resonance Imaging

MRI is more sensitive than CT for detecting early, small, and multiple infarcts [Ameri and Bousser, 1992; Fiebach et al., 2002] (see Fig. 72-7). In the brainstem and cerebellum, MRI is far superior to CT because it avoids bone artifact. MRI is also more sensitive than CT in detecting hemorrhagic conversion of infarcts [Kidwell et al., 2004]. Modifications of MRI that have improved early detection and specificity of the diagnosis of infarct include diffusion-weighted imaging, perfusion-weighted imaging, and proton spectroscopic imaging [Groenendaal et al., 1995; Warach and Baron, 2004]. Recent MRI studies suggest that MRI can predict the volume of ischemic tissue that will progress to infarction and can detect cerebral microbleeds—a risk factor for intracranial hemorrhage [Schlaug et al., 1999; Warach and Baron, 2004]. In children, in whom the differential diagnosis for acute focal deficits is more extensive than in adults, the improved sensitivity of MRI compared to CT in the first 24 hours after arterial ischemic stroke suggests that if a single radiographic study is to be done in suspected acute arterial ischemic stroke, the initial study should be MRI when it is available.

Magnetic Resonance Angiography

MRA can be performed at the same time as MRI and adds valuable information regarding the status of the cerebral arteries. Because time-of-flight MRA visualizes the flow of blood within vessels rather than the structure of the vessels, it is prone to certain artifacts, which must be considered when interpreting the findings. MRA is able to adequately visualize flow in the major cerebral arteries at the level of the circle of Willis (see Fig. 72-8C). When specifically planned, MRA can also image flow in the extracranial carotid and vertebral arteries at sites prone to dissection [Koelfen et al., 1993, 1995; Wiznitzer and Masaryk, 1991]. With continued improvement and refinement, MRA is becoming a realistic noninvasive alternative to conventional angiography, particularly in the pediatric population [Husson and Lasjaunias, 2004]. Recently MRA has been found to correlate well with conventional angiography in children with ischemic stroke [Ganesan et al., 1999; Husson et al., 2002]. However, MRA is less sensitive to the flow effects of diseases involving the medium-sized or small vessels in children, and it also overestimates the degree of vascular stenosis [Ganesan et al., 1999; Husson et al., 2002]. Gadolinium-enhanced MRA and MRA on high-field (3 Tesla) MRI machines reduce the risk of flow-related artifacts and "pseudo-occlusion" seen with regular time-of-flight MRA techniques [Nederkoorn et al., 2003].

Conventional Angiography

Conventional angiography is still considered to be the definitive method of visualizing the extra and intracranial vasculature (see Figs. 72-4B, 72-9, 72-10, and 72-11), despite the increasing availability and value of MRA. With current time-of-flight technique, MRA does not visualize small or medium-sized cerebral arteries reliably, compared with conventional angiography. Specific signs of cerebrovascular disease may be well defined only with conventional angiography, including the "string" and "double lumen" signs of dissection and the "string of beads" seen in vasculitis. Because different management strategies may result from these specific diagnoses, if expertise in pediatric angiography is available, conventional angiography should be performed in children with arterial ischemic stroke in whom a specific etiology has not been determined. In recent studies comparing MRA to conventional angiography in 72 children with arterial ischemic stroke, MRA detected all large-artery lesions but overestimated stenosis and missed small-artery abnormalities in 34% of children [Ganesan et al., 1999; Husson et al., 2002; Husson and Lasjaunias, 2004]. Conventional angiography showed abnormalities in four of nine (44%) patients with normal MRA results.

There are no data assessing the rate of major complications following angiography in children with arterial ischemic stroke; however, clinical experience suggests that they are extremely rare. In adults, since the advent of digital subtraction angiography, the use of conventional angiography in routine clinical practice settings is associated with a 0.5% rate of major complications [Johnston et al., 2001].

Other Neuroimaging Modalities

MR perfusion and single photon emission computed tomography (SPECT) scanning are methods that can detect areas of hypoperfusion that may be present prior to tissue infarction [Shahar et al., 1990]. These techniques provide perfusion information that can be helpful in assessing cerebrovascular reserve in children with severe arterial vasculopathy. Doppler imaging of the carotid arteries and transcranial Doppler imaging provide valuable dynamic information regarding flow patterns through cerebral arteries and can assist in the detection of large-vessel vasculopathy. The value of transcranial Doppler imaging in children with sickle cell disease in predicting the risk of future stroke has been established [Abboud et al., 2004]. Doppler studies, including transcranial Doppler imaging, require expert interpretation because normal values in children differ from those in adults.

Treatment

The treatment of stroke in children has been directed towards stabilizing systemic factors, management of the underlying causes, and prevention of extension or recurrence of thrombotic occlusion of cerebral arteries.

Antithrombotic Therapies

Antithrombotic therapeutic options for arterial ischemic stroke include unfractionated heparin, low-molecular-weight heparin, aspirin, Coumadin, and thrombolytic therapy [Andrew and deVeber, 1999; Monagle et al., 2004]. No randomized, controlled trials have assessed antithrombotic treatments in children with arterial ischemic stroke. Many of the antithrombotic treatment approaches increasingly used in children with cerebrovascular disease have been adapted from studies in adults. Evidence from randomized, controlled trials in children with arterial ischemic stroke is needed. The optimal treatment of children with arterial ischemic stroke using antithrombotic agents can be expected to differ from that of adults, because there are important differences in etiology as well as profound age-dependent differences in the hemostatic system [Andrew et al., 1992], the cerebral vasculature, and the brain [Altman et al., 1988; Roach and Riela, 1995]. These features influence both the pathophysiology of the thrombotic processes and the response to anticoagulant therapy.

In neonates with arterial ischemic stroke, the risk of recurrent arterial ischemic stroke appears to be less than 5%, suggesting that no antithrombotic treatment is required in the majority of cases [deVeber and Canadian Paediatric Ischemic Stroke Study Group, 2000; Kurnik et al., 2003]. However, data now clearly indicate that "no treatment" is not an acceptable option for older children with arterial ischemic stroke, in whom the risk of recurrence is up to 51% when no aspirin or antiplatelet agents are given, nearly double the risk for children treated with these agents [Lanthier et al., 2004].

The use of antithrombotic therapy appears to be increasing for pediatric arterial ischemic stroke beyond the newborn period. In a recent population-based study, 55% of children with arterial ischemic stroke received one or more treatments including unfractionated heparin, low-molecular-weight heparin, aspirin and/or Coumadin [deVeber and Canadian Paediatric Ischemic Stroke Study Group, 2000]. There was a wide variability in indications for and choice of anticoagulants. Accumulating experience with antithrombotic and anticoagulant treatment in children suggests that these agents can be safely used in children with arterial ischemic stroke [Burak et al., 2003; deVeber and Canadian Paediatric Ischemic Stroke Study Group, 2000; Ng W et al., 2002; Strater et al., 2001], although their efficacy and proper dose still need to be established by controlled trials. The use of thrombolytic agents in children with arterial ischemic stroke, however, has been rare, and the risks are as yet unknown.

Antithrombotic treatment guidelines for childhood stroke have been published [Andrew and deVeber, 1999; Monagle et al., 2004; Nowak-Gottl et al., 2003; Paediatric Stroke Working Group, 2004] and reviewed [deVeber, 2005]. The choice of antithrombotic agents in subgroups of children with arterial ischemic stroke is related to the perceived relative roles of platelets and the coagulation system in the initial and future recurrent thrombus formation, that are in turn dependent on the underlying mechanism of stroke. Damage to the arterial intima in dissection, cardiac embolism, venous thrombosis with paradoxical embolism, the presence of prothrombotic abnormalities, and the presence of extremely severe stenosis with slow flow likely promote thrombosis via activation of the coagulation system proportionately more than platelets, and these conditions are frequently treated with anticoagulation, at least for the first days or weeks after initial arterial ischemic stroke. However, idiopathic stroke or the presence of a moderate vascular stenosis that occurs with most vasculopathies is likely to involve platelets in the formation of thrombus, in which case antiplatelet agents are more appropriate.

In individual children, the risks of recurrence or progression of cerebral thromboembolism should be balanced against the risks of treatment, particularly bleeding. If arterial ischemic stroke is associated with initial hemorrhage, hypertension, or other risks to anticoagulants, for example, antithrombotic therapy may not be feasible.

HEPARIN

Heparin, a large heterogeneous polysaccharide complex, functions as an anticoagulant by inhibiting specific enzymes in the coagulation pathway, which in turn prevents clot extension or new clot formation. The major effect of heparin is to potentiate the antithrombin activities of the natural inhibitor antithrombin (AT) by catalyzing its ability to inactivate specific coagulation enzymes, in particular thrombin [Hirsh et al., 1998]. Lower amounts of heparin anticoagulation are needed in children to produce the same anticoagulant effect as in adults [Andrew et al., 1994].

In adults, heparin has been the standard therapy for acute anticoagulation following stroke in situations in which there is a high risk of extension or recurrence of thromboembolic stroke, including acute cardioembolic stroke due to nonvalvular atrial fibrillation, and arterial dissection [Albers et al., 2001; Sandercock et al., 1993]. The results of the International Stroke Trial, in which over 19,000 adults with stroke were randomized to aspirin or heparin or both or neither showed that adults with stroke treated with heparin have significantly fewer recurrent strokes compared with aspirin; however, this benefit is offset by increased risk of cerebral hemorrhage [International Stroke Trial Collaborative Group, 1997].

There have been no large-scale trials of heparin in children with arterial ischemic stroke, but increasing clinical experience suggests that children can be treated along the same lines as adult patients with reasonable safety [deVeber and Canadian Paediatric Ischemic Stroke Study Group, 2000; Monagle et al., 2004]. A decision to use acute anticoagulation in a child with arterial ischemic stroke rests on two questions: What is the likelihood of extension of an infarction or of a second infarction from an embolus that might be prevented by treatment? What is the risk of inducing a hemorrhage because of anticoagulation? Much like the situation in adults, heparin should be considered in children thought to have a high risk of recurrence and a low risk of secondary hemorrhage.

Heparin is commonly used in children for deep vein thrombosis and pulmonary embolism [Monagle et al., 2004]. For anticoagulation for acute or recurrent arterial ischemic stroke, a heparin bolus is usually not given in order to limit the risk of converting a bland infarct to a hemorrhagic infarct. Instead, heparin is given at maintenance doses of 28 units/kg/hour in infants and 20 units/kg/hour in children older than 1 year of age. For older children, the adult dose of 18 units/kg/hour is used. During the maintenance treatment, the dose must be carefully monitored and adjusted according to the activated partial thromboplastin time. The target activated partial thromboplastin time is 60 to 85 seconds or 1.5 to 2 times the baseline value [Andrew et al., 1994]. A nomogram for dose adjustment of standard heparin in children is presented in Box 72-2 [Monagle et al., 2004]. The activated partial thromboplastin time does not reflect the anticoagulant effect of heparin in certain circumstances, such as the presence of a nonspecific inhibitor, which prolongs the activated partial thromboplastin time, or the presence of elevated Factor VIII levels, which shortens the activated partial thromboplastin time. Heparin levels are more accurate but more difficult to obtain. Therapy is usually given for 5 to 7 days, depending on the clinically assessed risk of clot extension or recurrence [Andrew and deVeber, 1999].

Adverse effects of heparin include the risk of hemorrhage, the risk of osteoporosis after long-term courses of therapy, and thrombocytopenia. Children rarely bleed when treated with heparin for deep vein thrombosis or pulmonary embolism [Andrew et al., 1994]. Heparin-induced thrombocytopenia occurs in less than 4% of children [Newall et al., 2003]. When heparin-induced thrombocytopenia occurs, heparinoid or danaproid are alternative anticoagulants.

Box 72-2 Protocol for Systemic Heparin Administration and Dosage Adjustment for Pediatric Patients

I. Loading dose: No loading dose is usually given for stroke.

II. Initial maintenance dose: 28 U/kg/hr for infants younger than 1 year.

III. Initial maintenance dose: 20 U/kg/hr for children older than 1 year.

IV. Adjust heparin dose to maintain activated partial thromboplastin time for 60 to 85 seconds (assuming that this reflects an anti-factor Xa level of 0.30 to 0.70):

APTT (seconds)	BOLUS (U/kg)	HOLD (min)	% RATE CHANGE	REPEAT APTT
<50	50	0	+10%	4 hr
50-59	0	0	+10%	4 hr
60-85	0	0	0	next day
86-95	0	0	−10%	4 hr
96-120	0	30	−10%	4 hr
>120	0	60	−15%	4 hr

V. Obtain blood for APTT 4 hours after initial administration and 4 hours after every change in the infusion rate.

VI. When APTT values are therapeutic, check CBC and APTT levels daily.

APPT, activated partial thromboplastin time; CBC, complete blood count.
From Michelson AD, Bovill E, Andrew M. Antithrombotic therapy in children. Chest 1995;108:506S. Reproduced with permission.

Low-Molecular-Weight Heparins

Low-molecular-weight heparins are molecular subcomponents of the larger compound, unfractionated heparin. They offer several advantages over unfractionated heparin, including reproducible pharmacokinetics [Massicotte et al., 1996], subcutaneous injection, minimal monitoring, and increased safety, with similar efficacy compared with unfractionated heparin in studies of adults. Adults with arterial infarcts who are treated with low-molecular-weight heparin within 48 hours of onset may have a better outcome [Kay et al., 1995]. More recent clinical trials in adults with arterial ischemic stroke have found that survival and disability rates are nearly identical for low-molecular-weight heparin and aspirin [Bath et al., 2001], and the former was therefore not recommended for the routine management of adults with ischemic stroke [Bath et al., 2001].

Low-molecular-weight heparin has become established as the first choice for acute anticoagulant therapy in children. Advantages over standard heparin include a better safety profile, ease of administration (twice-daily subcutaneous injections), and simplicity of monitoring (once weekly or monthly anti-factor Xa levels are usually adequate). In studies of pediatric patients treated for systemic clots with low-molecular-weight heparin, no significant hemorrhagic complications occurred in 100 children [Massicotte et al.,

1996]. Data supporting the safety of low-molecular-weight heparin for acute pediatric arterial ischemic stroke has been published [Burak et al., 2003; deVeber and Canadian Paediatric Ischemic Stroke Study Group, 2000; Ng et al., 2002a; Strater et al., 2001] and treatment of children with cerebral sinovenous thrombosis with low-molecular-weight heparin also appears to be safe [deVeber et al., 2001]. Indications for either standard or low-molecular-weight heparin in children with arterial ischemic stroke include arterial dissection, coagulation disorders, and a high risk of embolism, such as from the heart in the presence of some congenital and acquired disorders [Andrew and deVeber, 1999; Roach and Riela, 1995]. Acute anticoagulation also seems reasonable for treatment of a child with progressing neurologic deficit not due to cerebral hemorrhage during the initial evaluation of a new cerebral infarction [Roach and Riela, 1995]. The recent recommendations of the American Academy of Chest Physicians (AACP) include the use of initial low-molecular-weight or unfractionated heparin at full treatment doses for 5 to 7 days in children with nonhemorrhagic arterial ischemic stroke until dissection or cardiac clot have been excluded [Monagle et al., 2004]. Pediatric stroke guidelines published in the United Kingdom suggest initial aspirin therapy followed by anticoagulation if dissection or cardiac clot are found on investigations [Paediatric Stroke Working Group, 2004].

Box 72-3 Protocol for Subcutaneous Enoxaparin Therapy to Maintain an Anti-Xa Level 4 to 6 Hours Post-dose of 0.5 to 1.0 U/mL for Pediatric Patients

I. Initial maintenance dose: 1.5 mg/kg/dose q12h for infants younger than 2 months of age.

II. Initial maintenance dose: 1.0 mg/kg/dose q12h for infants 2 months of age or older and children.

III. Adjust low-molecular-weight heparin dose to maintain an anti-Xa level of 0.5 to1.0 U/mL.

Anti-Factor Xa Level*	Hold Next Dose?	Dose Change	Repeat Anti-Factor Xa
< 0.35	No	Increase by 25%	4 h after next dose
0.35-0.49	No	Increase by 10%	4 h after next dose
0.5-1.0	No	No	Next day, then 1 wk later, then monthly
1.1-1.5	No	Decrease by 20%	Before next dose
1.6-2.0	3 h	Decrease by 30%	Before next dose, then 4 h after next dose
> 2.0	Until anti-factor Xa = 0.5 U/mL	Decrease by 40%	Before next dose; if not <0.5 U/mL, repeat q12h

Note: Enoxaparin has an anti-factor Xa level of 110 U/mg.

Adapted from Monagle P, Michelson AD, Bovill E, Andrew M. Antithrombotic therapy in children. Chest 2001;119(1 Suppl):344S–370S.

Low-molecular-weight heparins used in children include Lovenox, (Rhone-Poulenc) and Reviparin. Lovenox is given to children subcutaneously at doses of 1 mg/kg every 12 hours (or in infants 2 months of age or younger, 1.5 mg/kg every 12 hours) [Massicotte et al., 1996]. Reviparin dosing for infants and children weighing more than 5 kg is 100 units/kg every 12 hours. Anti-factor Xa levels are used for monitoring low-molecular-weight heparins because the activated partial thromboplastin time does not reflect their activity. The therapeutic range for anti-factor Xa levels is 0.5 to 1.0 units/mL in a sample drawn 4 to 6 hours after the subcutaneous dose. Once therapeutic levels are attained, a weekly check on the anti-factor Xa level is usually sufficient. The initial dosage and nomogram for adjusting the dosage of enoxaparin, the most commonly used low-molecular-weight heparin, are presented in Box 72-3. Low-molecular-weight heparin can be administered using a subcutaneous catheter, which is replaced weekly, further reducing the number of needles required. Because this compound is cleared via the kidneys, its use in patients with renal failure requires close monitoring.

ASPIRIN AND OTHER ANTIPLATELET AGENTS

Aspirin inhibits platelet aggregation by inhibiting the production of thromboxane A2 within platelets. Thromboxane A2 is the principal determinant of the aggregating activity of platelets. The traditional role of aspirin in arterial ischemic stroke has been as an agent for the secondary prevention of recurrent stroke following transient ischemic attack or stroke. In adults, aspirin reduces recurrent stroke by approximately 25% [Albers et al., 2001; Sandercock et al., 1993]. There appears to be a modest benefit from immediate aspirin therapy in acute ischemic stroke [Bousser, 1997; International Stroke Trial Collaborative Group, 1997;]; for longer-term stroke prevention, aspirin is equivalent to warfarin [Mohr et al., 2001].

No clinical trials assessing the efficacy of aspirin for stroke in childhood have been performed. However, aspirin at doses of 1 to 5 mg/kg/day has been found to be safe in children following arterial ischemic stroke [Strater et al., 2001]. The recommended dosage is 1 to 5 mg/ kg/day. Grouping the dosage into every-other-day scheduling is feasible because of the prolonged effect of the medication on platelet function.

Side effects of aspirin are usually mild and include gastric upset, easy bruising and, extremely rare at this dose, hemorrhagic complications. Because of the previous association of Reye's syndrome and aspirin at antipyretic dosages (40 to 60 mg/kg/day) [Hall, 1990], there has been a reluctance to prescribe aspirin for small children. The antiplatelet dosage of 3 to 5 mg/kg/day is less than 10% of the antipyretic doses at which Reye's syndrome occurred, and to date no case of Reye's syndrome has been reported at these doses. Because of the concern about Reye's syndrome, however, precautions such as annual influenza vaccination and reduction of aspirin dosage during febrile illnesses should be observed.

Other antiplatelet drugs used in adults for stroke prevention include ticlopidine and clopidogrel (Plavix), both of which are thienopyridines. Both drugs selectively inhibit ADP-induced platelet aggregation via inhibition of the $P2Y_{12}$ receptor [Ito et al., 1992; Savi et al., 1996]. These agents may offer additional benefit over aspirin alone

[CAPRIE Steering Committee, 1996]. Use of these medications has been limited in children; however, clopidogrel, at doses of approximately 1 mg/kg/day, is currently being used for stroke in children unable to take aspirin [Hune et al., 2004].

WARFARIN

Warfarin and other coumarin anticoagulants reduce the activity of vitamin K–dependent coagulation factors in a dose-dependent manner. Although they may not reduce established clot, they do help prevent further clot formation. The anticoagulant effect occurs in 36 to 72 hours after beginning daily administration.

Warfarin is used in adults for the secondary prevention of stroke in situations in which aspirin therapy has failed or is predicted to be insufficient, including nonvalvular atrial fibrillation. The Warfarin Aspirin Recurrent Stroke Study (WARSS) recently reported that warfarin and aspirin are equivalent for the prevention of recurrent stroke in adults [Mohr et al., 2001]. However, a 30% risk reduction (P = 0.02) was found for warfarin compared with aspirin in nonhypertensive patients with cryptogenic stroke and with infarcts located in the cerebral convexity, or in the convexity plus a deep ispilateral infarct, and in those patients whose infarct was "large and deep," beyond the size boundaries usually considered examples of lacunar infarction (macro-lacunes) [Mohr, 2004]. The latter subtypes of stroke most closely correspond to childhood arterial ischemic stroke, and the implication of this finding is that warfarin may be superior to aspirin for preventing recurrent arterial ischemic stroke in children. The risk of hemorrhage in children appears to be low [Ng et al., 2002b]. The risk of hemorrhage in adults with stroke is increased in the presence of persistent hypertension and advanced age, factors that are rarely or not applicable to children with stroke. A randomized, controlled trial assessing aspirin compared with anticoagulants in pediatric stroke is under development.

In children with cerebrovascular disorders, the major uses of warfarin treatment include long-term treatment for congenital or acquired heart disease, severe hypercoaguable states, arterial dissection, and recurrent arterial ischemic stroke or transient ischemic attack while the patient is taking aspirin. An international normalized ratio of 2.0 to 3.0 is appropriate for most children on warfarin; for children with mechanical heart valves, the international normalized ratio should be 2.5 to 3.5. A nomogram for dose adjustment is shown in Box 72-4 [Monagle et al., 2004]. Because of low levels of Vitamin K in breast milk, safe dosing of warfarin is very difficult in breast-fed infants. Older children may be resistant to oral anticoagulants because of impaired absorption or an excessive amount of Vitamin K in total parenteral nutrition formulas. Experience with long-term anticoagulation to prevent cerebral infarction in children is limited, and there is an additional concern about giving anticoagulants to an active child who may be prone to minor injuries through normal activities. The concern that active children may have an increased risk of hemorrhage due to trauma seems to be largely unfounded, although it is recommended that these children avoid activities that carry an especially high risk of injury (e.g., contact sports). Nevertheless, warfarin is the most effective means of prolonged anticoagulation in children, and clinical experience suggests that warfarin can be used with reasonable safety.

Box 72-4 Protocol for Oral Anticoagulation Therapy to Maintain an INR between 2 and 3 for Pediatric Patients

I. Dose 1: If the baseline INR is 1.0 to 1.3:
Dose = 0.2 mg/kg orally
II. Guidelines for loading doses 2-4:

INR	Action
1.1-1.4	Repeat loading dose
1.5-1.9	50% of loading dose
2.0-3.0	50% of loading dose
3.0-3.5	25% of loading dose
>3.5	Hold until INR <3.5; then restart at 50% less than the previous dose

III. Long-term oral anticoagulation dose guidelines:

INR	ACTION
1.1-1.4	Increase by 20% of dose
1.5-1.9	Increase by 10% of dose
2.0-3.0	No change
3.1-3.5	Decrease by 20% of dose
>3.5	Check INR daily until INR <3.5; then restart at 20% less than the previous dose

INR, international normalized ratio.
From Michelson AD, Bovill E, Andrew M. Antithrombotic therapy in children. Chest 1995;108:506S. Reproduced with permission.

THROMBOLYTIC AGENTS

Thrombolytic agents include recombinant tissue-type plasminogen activator (t-PA), urokinase, prourokinase, and streptokinase. These agents act by converting endogenous plasminogen to plasmin, with the goal of dissolving existing thrombus and recanalizing the occluded blood vessel. A high rate of hemorrhagic complications has limited their use in the past.The use of intravenous t-PA in adults with arterial ischemic stroke has been approved by the U.S. Food and Drug Administration for treating acute ischemic stroke within 3 hours of onset of symptoms, based on the randomized, controlled trial reporting a 30% reduction in death and disability with this therapy [The National Institute of Neurologic Disorders and Stroke rt-PA Stroke Study Group, 1995]. In subsequent trials involving more than 5000 adults with stroke, similar outcome rates have been achieved by following the strict NINDS protocol; however, mortality rates are increased when protocol violations occur, including tPA administration after the 3-hour window [Meschia et al., 2002].

Intra-arterial prourokinase (proUK) given 3 to 6 hours after stroke symptom onset has been assessed in clinical trials in adults. This approach, which delivers an increased concentration of thrombolytic drug to the occlusive thrombus, has been associated with a recanalization rate of 66% for the proUK group compared with 18% for the control group in a randomized, controlled trial ($P < 0.001$). The clinical outcome was also improved at 90 days with recombinant proUK despite an increased frequency of early symptomatic intracranial hemorrhage [Furlan et al., 1999]. The risk of symptomatic intracranial hemorrhage was increased in the presence of acute hyperglycemia [Kase et al., 2001].

Literature reviews and prospective cohort studies of children with extracranial thrombosis treated with thrombolytic agents have shown that although thrombus resolution was achieved in 80% of patients, minor bleeding (not requiring transfusion therapy) was found in over 50% in a pooled literature analysis [Leaker et al., 1996] and in approximately 25% in cohort studies [Leaker et al., 1996]. These bleeding rates suggest that thrombolytic agents should be used with caution in children, particularly because the presence of cerebral infarction would be predicted to increase the risk of intracranial hemorrhage. Recently a low-dose tPA regimen (10% of the standard tPA dose) was assessed in 17 children with systemic thrombosis [Wang et al., 2003]. This regimen was associated with thrombus resolution in approximately 70% of children with "acute" thromboses but required longer duration of therapy than standard tPA dosing.

Thrombolytic agents have not been evaluated in children with arterial ischemic stroke, although several case reports have now been published [Carlson et al., 2001; Cognard et al., 2000; Gruber et al., 2000; Noser et al., 2001]. Theoretically, thrombolytic agents have the potential to be effective as an acute therapy for children with arterial ischemic stroke. However, there are significant concerns about their safety because of unique features of children and childhood arterial ischemic stroke, in particular, the lack of confidence in the diagnosis of arterial ischemic stroke very early in the course. There is a much wider differential diagnosis for acute-onset neurologic deficit in a child with a normal early CT scan than in an adult. Given the risks of intracranial hemorrhage observed in adults who receive thrombolysis when CT shows early signs of the infarct, the risk for bleeding complications of treatment is likely to be unacceptably high in infants and children with CT signs of established arterial ischemic stroke.

Clinical trials evaluating the efficacy of thrombolytic agents in pediatric arterial ischemic stroke are not feasible as yet because of the frequent delay in diagnosis of arterial ischemic stroke in children and the lack of safety data. As the availability of urgent MRI and clinical awareness of pediatric arterial ischemic stroke increase, early diagnosis of this disorder is becoming feasible. Safety studies of tPA in children who arrive at the hospital within the time window for thrombolysis are currently enrolling patients. However, until safety data are available, thombolytic agents as initial stroke therapy in young children with arterial ischemic stroke should be considered potentially dangerous.

Nonantithrombotic Therapies

ACUTE SUPPORTIVE AND NEUROPROTECTIVE CARE

Children with suspected acute stroke should be stabilized promptly and transferred for further management to an institution that can offer specialized pediatric neurovascular care [Hutchison et al., 2004; Paediatric Stroke Working Group, 2004]. Because autoregulation of the cerebral vasculature is impaired during acute stroke, careful supportive therapy, including blood pressure and fluid management, is mandatory. Serum glucose should be carefully monitored because hyperglycemia is known to exacerbate the size of the infarct whereas hypoglycemia will also worsen the effects of stroke [Baird et al., 2003; Yager and Thornhill, 1997]. Maintenance of low-to-normal body temperature is important because hyperthermia exacerbates ischemic brain damage, whereas hypothermia is known to protect against brain damage, including in neonates with hypoxic ischemic encephalopathy [Gluckman et al., 2005; Krieger and Yenari, 2004; Rutherford et al., 2005; Volpe, 2001b]. In adults with stroke, induced hypothermia is feasible but is associated with serious side effects including hypotension, cardiac arrhythmia, and pneumonia [Olsen et al., 2003]. The early use of antiepileptic drugs in children with seizures associated with arterial ischemic stroke is important in order to prevent recurrent seizures that may increase the eventual infarct volume [Wirrell et al., 2001].

Development of malignant cerebral edema within the infarct zone and intracranial hypertension in the first week after acute arterial ischemic stroke may require treatment with intravenous mannitol and hypertonic saline. No beneficial effects of steroids have been demonstrated in adults or children with stroke.

NEUROPROTECTIVE AGENTS

The chain of events occurring at a cellular level in ischemic injury and leading to neuronal death after stroke suggests several potential neuroprotective treatment strategies. In animal studies, several neuroprotective agents given within 6 to 12 hours after stroke onset have been associated with a reduction in infarct volume [Ginsberg and Pulsinelli 1997]. A combination of fibrinolytic and neuroprotective treatments also has been shown to reduce infarct size in animals [Lapchak and Zivin, 2003]. Despite the completion of many human trials, neuroprotective agents have yet to show convincing benefits in adults with arterial ischemic stroke. Whether such agents can be applied to the pediatric stroke population in the future remains to be determined. Unfortunately, irreversible neuronal changes will likely occur before treatment can be initiated in most children with arterial ischemic stroke unless early diagnosis is made. In addition, the effect of such medications on normal maturation and learning processes will require evaluation prior to treatment trials in pediatric patients.

IMMUNOSUPPRESSANT THERAPY

In patients with proven vasculitis or suspected IACNS and, in consultation with rheumatology colleagues, immunosuppressive agents such as prednisone or cyclophosphamide may be indicated (see Chapter 73).

TRANSFUSION THERAPY

For children with sickle cell disease and stroke, long-term transfusion is effective for primary stroke prevention in patients with large-vessel vasculopathy [Adams et al., 1998]. During exchange transfusion it is important to guard against large fluid shifts, as this may increase infarct size.

NEUROSURGICAL PROCEDURES

The use of intracranial pressure monitoring in patients with large-arterial ischemic strokes who have significant cerebral edema is controversial. In patients with large strokes, a decreasing level of consciousness and midline shift are indicators of impending herniation. In the latter situation, emergency decompressive hemicraniectomy can be a life-saving procedure and is associated with good outcomes in young stroke patients [Gupta et al., 2004]. Hemicraniectomy is currently being assessed in adults in a multicenter randomized, controlled trial [Hofmeijer et al., 2003; Schwab et al., 1998]. Early experience with hemicraniectomy in children with progressive edema has been promising.

Additional neurosurgical procedures in children with arterial ischemic stroke include revascularization techniques for moyamoya disease; in some patients. Evacuation of hematomas associated with infarction may be necessary to reduce local, compressive mass effects.

INTERVENTIONAL NEURORADIOLOGIC TECHNIQUES

Intra-arterial thrombolysis has been discussed in a previous section. More aggressive interventional angiographic techniques, including angioplasty, clot retrieval, and stenting of cerebral arteries, are now available for adults with arterial ischemic stroke, and these remain largely unproven and carry significant risks. Their extension to the management of children with arterial ischemic stroke may not be feasible or safe. The smaller caliber and thinner walls of cerebral arteries in children may place them at increased risk for complications from these techniques, such as thrombosis, rupture, and dissection. In addition, long-term complications following these maneuvers, as the cerebral vasculature develops over many decades, are unknown and present additional concerns. Consecutive cohort safety studies are not yet available for pediatric arterial ischemic stroke but are a necessary precursor to the use of these techniques in children.

REHABILITATION THERAPY

Rehabilitation therapies for adults with stroke are gaining an increasing base of evidence. For motor deficits, evidence now supports task-specific approaches and constraint-induced therapy as being more effective than traditional approaches that focus on impairment [Teasell and Kalra, 2004]. Constraint-induced therapy has been shown in a randomized, controlled trial to be effective in children with congenital hemiplegia [Taub et al., 2004]. Botulinum A (botox) injection is an option that is increasingly used for temporary relief of limb hypertonia associated with dystonia or spasticity in children with arterial ischemic stroke. Evidence for this approach is available in populations of children with cerebral palsy and adults with stroke [Bhakta et al., 2000; Fehlings et al., 2000]. Systematic studies assessing speech, occupational, physical, and psychologic therapies in pediatric arterial ischemic stroke are urgently needed. Given the frequency of potentially modifiable neurologic impairments and the known risk of increasing clinical deficits as the child matures, early and aggressive rehabilitation therapy initiated during acute hospitalization for children with persistent deficits is recommended [Paediatric Stroke Working Group, 2004].

Compared with adult stroke victims, infants and young children have additional rehabilitation considerations, including greater complexity of feeding dysfunction and speech therapy, ongoing modification of rehabilitation as the child grows and develops age-related skills, and the potential for ongoing recovery over longer periods of time. Hemiatrophy of affected limbs can create orthopedic problems such as leg length discrepancy and scoliosis. In addition, learning and behavioral deficits unique to this population are common and require intervention by specialized pediatric rehabilitation and education teams. Parents may need encouragement to avoid "overprotection" and to treat the affected child as normally as possible.

SPECIALIZED STROKE CARE

Given the lack of clinical trials and evidence-based treatments of pediatric arterial ischemic stroke, its relative infrequency, and the proven benefit of specialized stroke care in adults, referral to tertiary care centers with expertise in the management of childhood arterial ischemic stroke should be made when feasible. In the care of the child with arterial ischemic stroke, a team approach including pediatric neurol-

Box 72-5 Literature Summary of Outcome in Children with Arterial Ischemic Stroke

Author, Year	Study N (Mean FU)	Death	Normal	Neurologic Deficits	Seizures	Recurrent Stroke	Predictors of Poor Outcome
Isler et al., 1984	87 (30 y)	—	10%	90%	50%	20%	—
Dusser, 1986	44	—	18%	>82%	29%	—	"Symptomatic" stroke
Lanska, 1991	—	—	17%	83%	19%	—	—
Broderick et al., 1993	7	14%	—	—	—	—	—
Ganesan et al., 1999	39	5%	32%	63%	—	—	Large infarct volume
de Schryver et al., 2000	37 (7 y)	11%	41%	59%	24%	27%	—
deVeber, 2000b	126	NA	33%	66%	13%	11%	
deVeber, 2000	660	10%	34%	56%	10%	19%	
Lanthier et al., 2000	51	16%	35%	49%	4%	16%	Multiple RFs
Delsing et al., 2001	31 (3.5 y)	13%	29%	58%		22%	↓LOC, Sz, large MCA infarct
Steinlin et al., 2004	18 (7 y)	2	2	78% handicap 72% handicap		3	Combined cortical and subcortical infarcts

N, number of patients in study; FU, follow-up period; LOC, level of conciousness; Sz, seizures; MCA, middle cerebral artery; neuropsych, neuropsychologic deficits; Rf, risk factors.

ogists, pediatric hematologists, and other subspecialists is important in order to appropriately individualize investigations and therapy [Paediatric Stroke Working Group, 2004].

Outcome

In general, children are observed to recover a greater degree of function and for longer periods of time than adults with the same type of arterial ischemic stroke. The published literature on outcome following pediatric arterial ischemic stroke is summarized in Box 72-5. Following childhood arterial ischemic stroke, the most frequently reported neurologic impairment is hemiparesis (see Fig. 72-6B). However, less obvious residual deficits, including speech and other cortical deficits and subtle problems in learning, socialization, and behavior, also occur and contribute to a reduced quality of life in children with stroke [De Schryver et al., 2000; Friefeld et al., 2004; Steinlin et al., 2004]. Recently, verbal learning and memory have been found to be significantly decreased in children following stroke [Lansing et al., 2004; Max, 2004; Nass and Trauner, 2004]. Younger age at stroke (less than 12 months) was associated with worse outcomes than older age at stroke (more than 12 months) and, in contrast to adults, verbal learning and memory deficits were similar for right and left hemisphere lesions. Movement disorders such as dystonia after basal ganglia infarction have been documented to develop more frequently in children compared with adults, and these can become disabling [Kwak and Jankovic, 2002; Nardocci et al., 1996].

Older studies reported residual neurologic deficits in over 75% of infants and children. [Eeg-Olofsson and Ringheim, 1983; Higgins et al., 1991; Satoh et al., 1988, 1991; Schoenberg et al., 1978]. In more recent population-based studies following neonatal arterial ischemic stroke, a normal outcome was reported in 50% of patients at 9 months' average follow-up interval. The remaining patients had a seizure disorder or neurologic deficit [deVeber and Canadian Paediatric Ischemic Stroke Study Group, 2000]. In children in whom arterial ischemic stroke occurred beyond the neonatal period, outcomes include death in 5% to 13%, neurologic deficits in 56% to 63% of survivors (which are severe in about half), and no neurologic deficit in 29% to 34% [Delsing et al., 2001; deVeber et al., 2000]. Death is related to the underlying infarct in approximately half of the children. Mechanisms of death in adults with arterial ischemic stroke are time-related [Derouesne et al., 1993]. Transtentorial herniation, the main cerebral cause of death, occurs mainly in the first week and is related to large infarcts.

The improved outcome reported in more recent studies of childhood arterial ischemic stroke may reflect the detection of milder forms of stroke enabled by MRI, an increasing trend to use of antithrombotic therapy for this condition, and sources of bias inherent in retrospective study design, which may overestimate abnormal outcome. Another important study design factor is the duration of follow-up interval. The emergence of later neurologic deficits, including subtle learning problems, as the child develops emphasizes the need for longer-term studies over many years in order to accurately define outcome.

Factors predicting poor outcome in childhood arterial ischemic stroke include age younger than 12 months, presentation with an altered level of consciousness or seizures, and infarcts occupying more than 10% of intracranial volume [Delsing et al., 2001; Ganesan et al., 2000; Lansing et al., 2004; Max, 2004]. For both neonates and older children with arterial ischemic stroke, the worst outcome is predicted by the presence of bilateral infarction or of infarction involving both the internal capsule and the cortical middle cerebral artery territory [Golomb et al., 2003; Mercuri et al., 2004]. Neonates having an abnormal background EEG also have worse outcomes [Mercuri et al., 1999].

The likelihood of adverse outcomes following arterial ischemic stroke in neonates and children appears to be increased when prothrombotic abnormalities are defined. Elevated factor VIII (greater than 150 IU per dL and D-dimer levels (greater than 500 ng per mL) at diagnosis have been associated with worse outcomes in neonates and children with thrombotic disorders including stroke [Goldenberg et al., 2004]. In neonates with arterial ischemic stroke the presence of prothrombotic abnormalities, especially factor V Leiden, has been associated with worse outcome [Mercuri et al., 2001].

The reported risk of recurrent stroke or transient ischemic attack in older infants and children ranges from 7% to 35% [deVeber et al., 2000; De Schryver et al., 2000; Chabrier et al., 2000; Isler, 1984; Lanthier et al., 2000, 2004]. In children not treated with antithrombotic therapies, recurrence approaches 50% [Lanthier et al., 2004]. Recurrence is highly correlated with certain etiologies of arterial ischemic stroke, including the presence of an underlying vasculopathy and multiple risk factors [Chabrier et al., 2000; Lanthier et al., 2004].

SINOVENOUS THROMBOSIS

Pathophysiology

Sinovenous Circulation: Anatomy and Physiology

The venous drainage of the brain is achieved by a network of cerebral veins and sinuses (Fig. 72-12). Cerebral sinuses are external to the brain and are enclosed between two layers of fibrous dura mater, the outermost layer being attached to bone along bony suture lines. Because of their rigid attachments, sinuses tend to have a fixed open lumen, and cerebral venous drainage is passive [Capra and Anderson, 1984]. The caliber of sinuses is unresponsive to changes in systemic blood pressure. These factors, combined with the lack of valves in the cerebral veins and sinuses, result in slow flow and the potential for flow reversal. This is in contrast to venous flow in limb veins, in which mechanical pumping action exerted on limb veins by muscle activity, combined with the presence of valves, encourages forward venous flow. Compensating in part for these factors is the effect of gravity when the head is in the upright position.

The superior sagittal sinus is the principal site of the absorption of cerebrospinal fluid. This process occurs as the cerebrospinal fluid is absorbed into "arachnoid granulations," highly vascular structures that protrude across the walls of the sagittal sinus into the subarachnoid space and that drain into the venous system. In sagittal sinus thrombosis or sinus hypertension, the arachnoid granulations become nonfunctional, resulting in communicating hydrocephalus [Bousser and Russell, 1997].

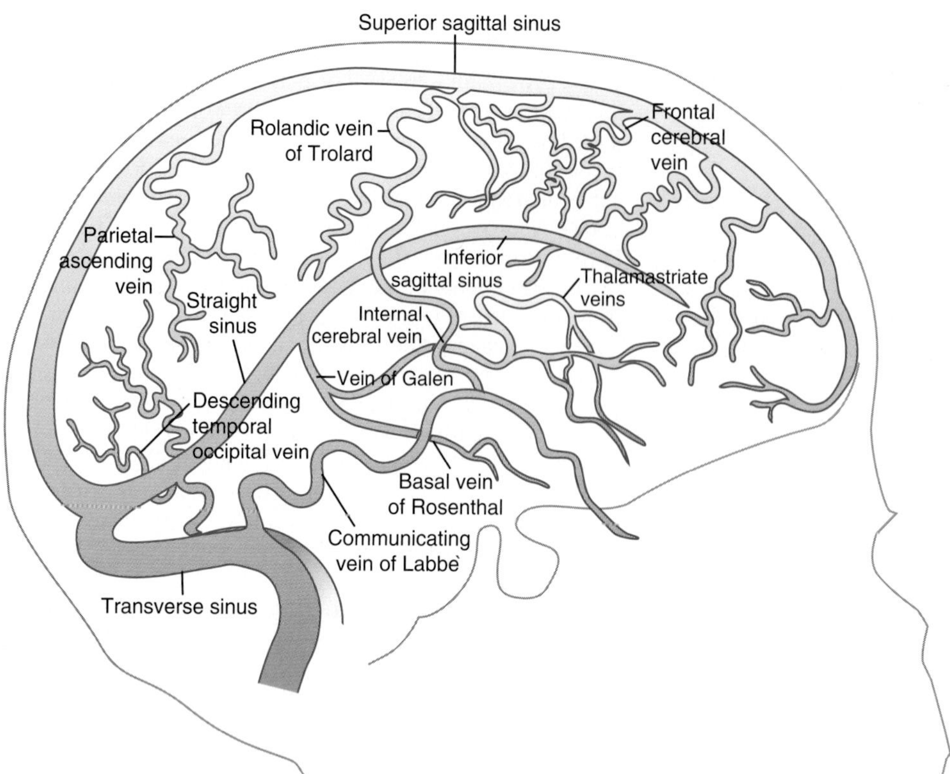

FIGURE 72-12. Lateral view of the cerebral veins.

The principal "superficial venous system" of the brain is provided by cortical veins that drain into the superior sagittal sinus. In most individuals, the superior sagittal sinus empties predominantly into the right lateral sinus (with transverse and sigmoid sinus portions) and the jugular vein. The "deep venous system" includes the inferior sagittal sinus and the paired internal cerebral veins, which join to form the vein of Galen and the straight sinus. This deep system drains predominantly into the smaller-caliber left lateral sinus and jugular vein system [Woodhall, 1936] (see Fig. 72-12). Anteriorly, the paired cavernous sinuses communicate with the jugular system via the petrosal sinuses.

Mechanisms of Thromboembolism

Different factors mediate thrombosis in cerebral sinovenous thrombosis compared with arterial ischemic stroke. In septic cerebral sinovenous thrombosis, a bacterial infection adjacent to the sinuses spreads directly into the sinus, provoking thrombophlebitis. In nonseptic cerebral sinovenous thrombosis, the exact mechanism that initiates thrombosis is not always evident. Platelets appear to play a minimal role in venous thromboembolism, in contrast to the situation in arterial ischemic stroke. There is a relative absence of thrombomodulin in the lining of cerebral sinuses, which may further increase the tendency to thrombosis [Lin et al., 1994]. Because of relatively slower blood flow, the initial formation and subsequent propagation of thrombus may be more likely to occur in cerebral venous channels than in cerebral arteries. Dehydration is a potent risk factor for cerebral sinovenous thrombosis because of hemoconcentration and impaired laminar flow. Inherited or acquired specific coagulation abnormalities including prothrombotic medications (e.g., L-asparaginase) clearly increase clotting risk (Fig. 72-13). Prothrombotic abnormalities play a relatively more important role in promoting venous thrombosis than arterial thrombosis. Mechanical distortion of the major dural sinuses along the bony suture lines occurs during calvarial molding during the birth process [Newton and Gooding, 1975].

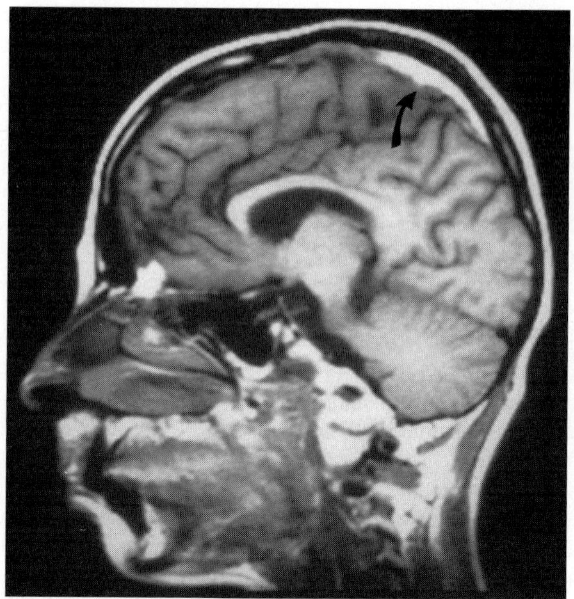

FIGURE 72-13. Sagittal T1-weighted MRI shows superior sagittal sinus thrombosis in an 11-year-old male with non-Hodgkins lymphoma following L-asparaginase chemotherapy. (Courtesy of Division of Neuroradiology, Hospital for Sick Children, Toronto, Ontario, Canada.)

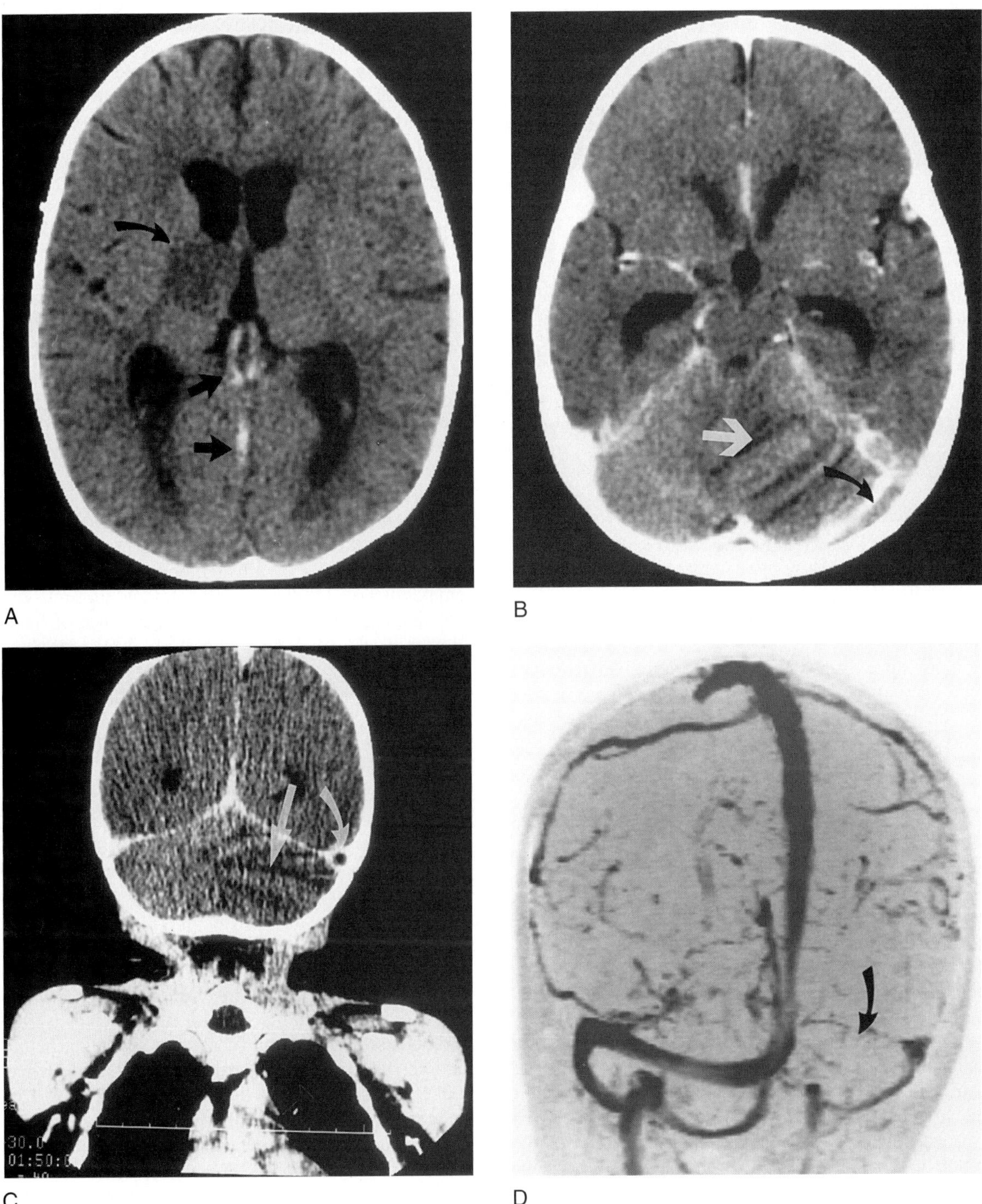

FIGURE 72-14. Nine-month-old female with sinovenous thrombosis after dehydration with iron deficiency anemia. **A,** CT scan without contrast enhancement shows high-density clot within the internal cerebral veins and straight sinus and right thalamic venous infarct (bland). **B** and **C,** Axial and coronal CT scans with contrast enhancement show left cerebellar venous infarct and left lateral sinus thrombus with dural enhancement ("empty triangle"sign). **D,** MR venography scan (coronal) confirms left transverse sinus thrombosis and nonvisualization of the internal sinovenous system (internal cerebral veins and straight sinus). (Courtesy of Manohar Shroff, Division of Neuroradiology, Hospital for Sick Children, Toronto, Ontario, Canada.)

Mechanisms of Infarction

Occlusion of cerebral venous structures initiates a rise in cerebral venous pressure, which, when sudden and severe, results in increased intracranial pressure either diffusely or regionally in the cerebral territory drained by the thrombosed veins. Local tissue pressure elevation results in marked edema as a result of transudation of fluid across venous or capillary channels. Parenchymal lesions can be transient and reversible, likely representing acute focal edema, or permanent, representing tissue infarction (Fig. 72-14A). The increased pressure across capillary channels also accounts for an increased rate of hemorrhagic conversion of infarcts compared with that found in arterial ischemic stroke (Fig. 72-15). Tissue infarction results when the regional increased tissue pressure exceeds the regional arterial

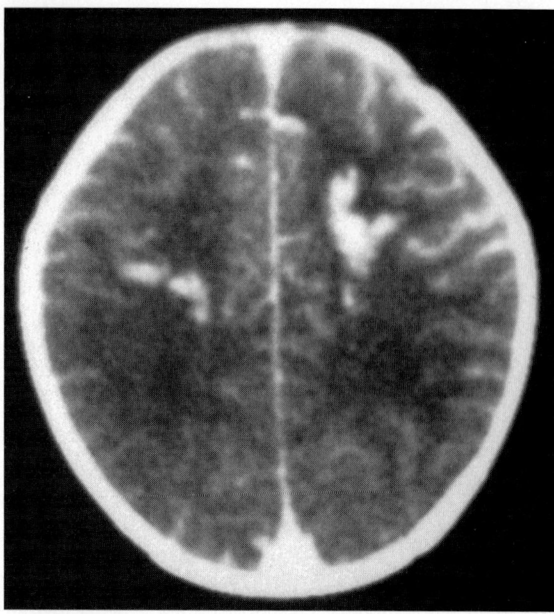

FIGURE 72-15. CT scan without contrast enhancement shows bilateral hemorrhagic venous infarcts due to cerebral sinovenous thrombosis in a 5-week-old infant male with gastroenteritis and dehydration. (Courtesy of Dr. Laurence Friedman, Children's Hospital at Chedoke-McMaster, Ontario, Canada.)

perfusion pressure. Venous infarction is more likely to occur with total occlusion of the sinus or venous lumen, in particular if the entry point of cerebral veins is occluded, and with more rapid rates of occlusion when pial venous collaterals cannot rapidly compensate for the obstruction of venous flow (see Fig. 72-14B and C) [Bousser and Russell, 1997]. Diffusion-weighted imaging studiesof evolving venous infarction demonstrate that initially areas of restricted diffusion (cytotoxic edema) appear to correlate with evolving venous infarction [Carvalho et al., 2001; Forbes et al., 2001]. Unlike the situation in arterial ischemic stroke, early increased diffusion changes are potentially reversible [Ducreux et al., 2001]. When the superior sagittal sinus is occluded, diffusely increased intracranial pressure results from venous congestion as well as from impaired cerebrospinal fluid absorption and a superimposed communicating hydrocephalus.

In contrast to cerebral arterial ischemia, in venous occlusion the affected brain is a zone of prolonged increased venous pressure. As a result, delayed recanalization of the obstruction to venous drainage days and possibly weeks after the initial occlusion can potentially relieve circulatory congestion. At the same time, the low pressure and slower blood flow in the sinovenous system compared with the arterial circulation increases the potential for thrombus propagation throughout the sinovenous system. Accordingly, the role of antithrombotic treatment for cerebral sinovenous thrombosis can be expected to differ from that used for arterial ischemic stroke [Tsao et al., 1999].

Vascular Patterns of Cerebral Sinovenous Thrombosis

Bilateral cortical infarcts, often hemorrhagic, are typical of sagittal sinus thrombosis. Deep venous thrombosis involving the internal cerebral veins, straight sinus or vein of Galen or both may produce thalamic infarction, at times bilateral (see Fig. 72-14A) or intraventricular hemorrhage. However, the site of cerebral sinovenous thrombosis, location of cerebral venous infarction, and type of clinical deficit do not follow the highly correlated patterns seen in arterial ischemic stroke.

Clinical Features

The clinical features of cerebral sinovenous thrombosis may be subtle or overshadowed by concomitant diffuse neurologic syndromes—for example, in a critically ill child with hypoxia or meningitis. Clinical features are age-related. In general, diffuse neurologic signs and seizures at presentation are frequent and focal signs are rare. Typically, the clinical features of cerebral sinovenous thrombosis are subtle and develop gradually over many hours, days, or occasionally, over many weeks.

Neonates and infants less than 1 year of age constitute approximately half of pediatric patients with cerebral sinovenous thrombosis [deVeber et al., 2001; Carvalho et al., 2001]. Males are affected up to twice as frequently as females [Carvalho et al., 2001]. Infants present with seizures, lethargy or jitteriness, with an absence of focal signs [Barron et al., 1992; Carvalho et al., 2001; deVeber et al., 2001; Rivkin et al., 1992]. Seizures occur in over three fourths of neonates compared to nearly half of older infants and children. Hemiparesis is present in only 6% of neonates and 20% of older infants and children [deVeber et al., 2001]. External signs including dilated scalp veins, prominent anterior fontanel, and eyelid swelling have been reported in infants with severe cerebral sinovenous thrombosis [Hartmann et al., 1987] but are rare.

Older infants and preschool-age children frequently present with fever, vomiting, and seizures and, occasionally, focal signs. Older children can present with signs and symptoms suggestive of "idiopathic intracranial hypertension," including headache, papilledema, abducens palsy, and altered levels of consciousness. This clinical presentation is especially frequent when the superior sagittal sinus is the site of thrombosis. Seizures and focal signs including hemiparesis may be superimposed [Barron et al., 1992; deVeber et al., 2001]. Children beyond the neonatal period with cerebral sinovenous thrombosis in the Canadian Registry presented with seizures in 48%, headache in 54%, papilledema in 22%, altered consciousness in 49% and focal neurologic signs in 53% [deVeber et al., 2001]. Recently, a series of 11 children with idiopathic intracranial hypertension were found to have underlying cerebral sinovenous thrombosis, and this study included four children with only lateral sinus thrombosis [Reul et al., 1997]. Clinically unsuspected cerebral sinovenous thrombosis has been found in 25% of children with idiopathic intracranial hypertension undergoing angiography [Ameri and Bousser, 1992], emphasizing the need for a high degree of clinical suspicion. In adults with idiopathic intracranial hypertension, stenosis of the lateral sinuses has been documented in over 90% of patients; however, whether these sinus abnormalities represent the cause of intracranial hypertension or are secondary compression of sinus channels by mass effect is not known [Farb et al., 2003a].

Risk Factors

Traditionally, cerebral sinovenous thrombosis was classified into "septic" and "non-septic" etiologies. Septic cerebral sinovenous thrombosis is defined as thrombosis of venous sinuses associated with head and neck infections such as otitis media, mastoiditis, and sinusitis, has dramatically decreased in incidence but still accounts for 18% of cases of pediatric cerebral sinovenous thrombosis [deVeber et al., 2001].

Risk factors are definable in most children and are frequently multiple. In a prospective population-based study (n = 160), risk factors consisted of prothrombotic disorders in 41% of children, dehydration in 25%, systemic infection in 9%, head and neck infection in 18%, other head and neck disorders in 12%, hematologic disorders in 12%, malignancy in 8%, and cardiac disease in 5%. The majority of cancer patients had had L-asparaginase treatment. Multiple risk factors were present in 65% of patients, with 40% having more than three [deVeber et al., 2001].

Risk factors are age-related. Dehydration is especially common in neonates with cerebral sinovenous thrombosis (see Fig. 72-15). Hematologic disorders, including anemia and structural cardiac disease, predominate in older infants. Iron deficiency anemia has been increasingly reported in older infants with cerebral sinovenous thrombosis and may be an important risk factor [Belman et al., 1990; Hartfield et al., 1997; Meena et al., 2000; Sébire et al., 2005]. Head and neck infections are present in nearly one third of preschool-age children with cerebral sinovenous thrombosis. Chronic systemic diseases are an underlying risk factor in approximately 60% and are clustered in the older age groups. These include systemic lupus erythematosus, nephrotic syndrome, inflammatory bowel disease, hematologic disorders, underlying cardiac disease, and malignancy [deVeber et al., 2001]. The mechanism for sinovenous thrombosis in most chronic diseases is that of an acquired prothrombotic state. For example, nephrotic syndrome causes renal loss of antithrombin, resulting in an acquired antithrombin deficiency, and systemic lupus erythematosus may be associated with a lupus anticoagulant. Acute illnesses, including sepsis and dehydration, are present in nearly one third of children with cerebral sinovenous thrombosis. In older children, head trauma or cranial surgery may damage the dural sinuses, leading to cerebral sinovenous thrombosis [Muthukumar, 2004; Sousa et al., 2004]. In one study of 131 children with head injury requiring a cranial CT scan, cerebral sinovenous thrombosis was found in 8 patients (6.1%) [Stiefel et al., 2000]. In another study, head trauma was the etiology in 9 of 19 children with cerebral sinovenous thrombosis [Huisman et al., 2001].

Prothrombotic disorders have been reported in 20% to 80% of pediatric patients with cerebral sinovenous thrombosis [deVeber et al., 1998, 2001; Ganesan et al., 1996; Riikonen et al., 1996; Vielhaber et al., 1998]. These figures exceed estimates in adults, in whom the incidence is 15% to 21% [Deschiens et al., 1996; Zuber et al., 1996]. In children with cerebral sinovenous thrombosis, acquired prothrombotic states are more frequent than congenital prothrombotic disorders. In the largest study to date, 56% of 149 pediatric patients with cerebral sinovenous thrombosis who underwent systematic coagulation testing had prothrombotic abnormalities, compared with only 21% of controls [Heller et al., 2003]. However, another smaller case-control study showed that there was no increase in thrombophilic markers in children with cerebral sinovenous thrombosis compared with controls, except in children with otherwise idiopathic cerebral sinovenous thrombosis [Kenet et al., 2004]. Factor V Leiden, anticardiolipin antibody, elevated lipoprotein (a), activated protein C resistance, and protein C, protein S, and antithrombin deficiencies are the most frequent abnormalities [deVeber et al., 2001; Ganesan et al., 1996; Gouault-Heilman et al., 1994; Heller et al., 2003; Martinelli et al., 1996; Riikonen et al., 1996; Vielhaber et al., 1998]. Both hyperhomocystinemia and an excess of homozygotes for the thermolabile variant of the methylene tetrahydrofolate reductase (MTFHR) gene compared to control populations have been reported in children and adults with cerebral sinovenous thrombosis [Bonduel et al., 1999; Buoni et al., 2001; Carhuapoma et al., 1997; Vielhaber et al., 1998]. In children, the prothrombotic abnormality acts as a predisposing risk factor, with additional triggering factors usually present [Heller et al., 2003].

Radiographic Features

The radiographic features and diagnostic pitfalls of pediatric cerebral sinovenous thrombosis have been reviewed [Shroff and deVeber, 2003]. The radiographic diagnosis of cerebral sinovenous thrombosis in infants and children is challenging. The location of cerebral sinovenous thrombosis can include any combination of sinuses or veins. However, thrombosis in the superficial system, including the superior sagittal sinus and lateral sinus, predominate (see Fig. 72-13). In the Canadian Registry, thrombosis was located in the superficial system in 86% of infants and children and in the deep system in 38%; nearly half of infants and children (49%) had multiple sinuses or veins involved [deVeber et al., 2001]. Parenchymal lesions such as bland or hemorrhagic venous infarcts are present in nearly half of children with cerebral sinovenous thrombosis (see Figs. 72-14 and 72-15). In the Canadian Registry, 41% had venous infarcts, which were bland in one third and hemorrhagic in two thirds of patients. A small number of patients had transient low-density parenchymal lesions [deVeber et al., 2001].

Radiographic diagnosis has significantly improved in recent years with refinements in CT venography, MRI and MR venography (see Fig. 72-14D) [Casey et al., 1996; Dormont et al., 1994; Lewin et al., 1994; Yuh et al., 1994]. However, cerebral angiography may still be required to confirm the diagnosis when CT and MRI findings are inconclusive.

COMPUTED TOMOGRAPHY

CT performed with and without contrast administration can occasionally suggest the diagnosis of cerebral sinovenous thrombosis. However, CT misses the diagnosis in 10% to 40% of patients and underestimates the extent of sinus involvement and the presence of infarcts [Ameri and Bousser, 1992; Barron et al., 1992; Bousser and Russell, 1997; Jacewicz and Plum, 1990]. In the Canadian Registry, the diagnosis was missed in 16% of CT scans [deVeber et al., 2001]. CT can also yield false positive results [Hamburger et al., 1990] particularly in neonates in whom the increased hematocrit, lower density of unmyelinated brain, and slower venous flow combine to produce a high-density triangle in the torcular area mimicking the "dense triangle" sign [Davies and Slavotinek, 1994; Kriss, 1998; Ludwig et al., 1980]. In addition, subdural hemorrhage layering along the dural walls of the sinuses can be difficult to distinguish from intraluminal thrombus unless high quality coronal images are obtained. Signs of cerebral sinovenous thrombosis on a noncontrast CT include the "filled triangle" or dense triangle signs and the "cord" sign, which represent hyperdense thrombus in sinovenous channels (see Fig. 72-14A). On contrast-enhanced CT, an empty triangle or "delta" sign represents bright contrast enhancement of the dura surrounding a sinovenous clot (see Fig. 72-14C). Multislice contrast-enhanced CT with the capability of submillimeter slices and excellent multiplanar reformations (CT venography) have significantly improved the ability to diagnose cerebral sinovenous thrombosis; however, the increased radiation dose required for CT venography is a concern.

MAGNETIC RESONANCE IMAGING

The absence of radiation and the ability to visualize both absent flow and the presence of thrombus, clot progression and resolution over time, and associated parenchymal lesions have made MRI the diagnostic study of choice in cerebral sinovenous thrombosis [Ameri and Bousser, 1992; Jacewicz and Plum, 1990; Macchi et al., 1986; Medlock et al., 1992; Zimmerman et al., 1992]. On parenchymal MRI, thrombus appears as an increased signal on T1-weighted and T2-weighted images in a cerebral vein or dural sinus. However, slow flow, turbulent flow, angled flow, or flow-related enhancement may produce an increased signal that can mimic intraluminal thrombus. Determining the age of the thrombus may be possible, according to the signal characteristics of the clot [Macchi et al., 1986]. In the subacute phase, a thrombus typically appears as increased signal on T1- and T2-weighted images.

MR venography is frequently used to evaluate the cerebral sinovenous system. The 2-dimensional time-of-flight technique has provided increased diagnostic sensitivity compared with parenchymal MRI techniques. However time-of-flight venography depends on flow signal characteristics and is therefore subject to artifacts. It is associated with "flow gap" artifacts in the transverse sinus in up to 30% of normal adults [Ayanzen et al., 2000]. These artifacts are particularly problematic in the smaller, nondominant transverse sinus. In these situations, particularly common in neonates, confirmatory CT venography may be required. A gadolinium-enhanced MR venography technique is now available [Liang et al., 2001; Takano et al., 1999]. This technique involves the injection of a gadolinium bolus, followed by the acquisition of MR images triggered by the arrival of the gadolinium bolus at the vessel of interest. Gadolinium-enhanced MR venography has proved to be superior to conventional time-of-flight venography [Farb et al., 2003b].

ULTRASOUND

In unstable, ventilated neonates and young infants, MR venography can be difficult to perform. In the presence of an open fontanel, ultrasound provides an inexpensive noninvasive means of screening for and monitoring the course of cerebral sinovenous thrombosis, but its use has not been systematically assessed. Recent ultrasound techniques, including "power Doppler," are specifically designed to determine blood flow and have improved the ability of ultrasound to diagnose cerebral sinovenous thrombosis [Bezinque et al., 1995; Dean and Taylor, 1995]. The power Doppler technique measures the energy of moving red blood cells instead of the velocity and direction of flow and is more sensitive for identifying flow in slow-flow states [Tsao et al., 1999]. The major limitation of Doppler ultrasound is in the evaluation of lateral venous sinuses when there is incomplete occlusion, because residual flow may be mistaken for normal flow [Bezinque et al., 1995; Govaert et al., 1992]. In infants, regular cranial ultrasound can be useful to monitor the presence and severity of centrally located intracranial hemorrhage associated with cerebral sinovenous thrombosis.

CONVENTIONAL ANGIOGRAPHY

Angiography is used in the diagnosis of cerebral sinovenous thrombosis when other techniques cannot confirm the diagnosis, or before intravascular intervention. Classic angiographic findings are similar to those in adults. Partial or complete lack of filling of cerebral veins or sinuses is diagnostic [Ameri and Bousser, 1992]. Angiographic signs that suggest cerebral sinovenous thrombosis include the presence of enlarged collateral veins, delayed venous emptying, reversal of normal venous flow direction, abnormal (broken or corkscrew-like) cortical veins, and regionally or globally delayed venous emptying [Ameri and Bousser, 1992]. Even with angiography, failure to scrutinize the venous phase can result in missing the diagnosis [Scotti et al., 1974], and the distinction between normal left lateral sinus hypoplasia and cerebral sinovenous thrombosis can be difficult [Ameri and Bousser, 1992]. Angiography may cause local thrombosis at the site of catheter insertion, particularly in small infants; however, it is an important alternative to consider when other techniques fail to clarify the diagnosis. In the Canadian Registry, conventional angiography was performed in fewer than 10% of children [deVeber et al., 2001].

Treatment

Antithrombotic Therapies

The treatment of cerebral sinovenous thrombosis in childhood has been strongly influenced by the results of clinical trials in adults because atherosclerosis is not a factor in either age group. Four randomized, controlled trials in adults with cerebral sinovenous thrombosis have reported variable findings. Three of these trials reported a statistically and clinically significant increase in survival and improved neurologic outcome in patients treated with anticoagulants [Einhaupl et al., 1991; Maiti and Chakrabarti, 1997; Nagaraja D et al., 1995]. The fourth trial failed to demonstrate a difference in outcome with anticoagulant treatment; however, this study was underpowered, given the high proportion of patients with good outcomes on placebo [de Bruijn and Stam, 1999]. A meta-analysis of these four trials showed that heparin reduces death and disability with a "number needed to treat" of 7 patients to prevent death. However the published meta-analysis excluded a trial published only in abstract form (Maiti and Chakrabarti, 1997) and a trial that used only CT for the diagnosis (Nagaraja et al., 1995). The combined results from the remaining two randomized, controlled trials showed only a strong trend toward efficacy [Stam et al., 2003]. All of the above trials showed that heparin was safe in adults with cerebral sinovenous thrombosis, including those with initial cerebral hemorrhage [Nagaraja et al., 1995]. These results are supported by large cohort studies that reported an improved outcome in adults with cerebral sinovenous thrombosis, including those with initial hemorrhage, who were treated with heparin therapy with no increase in hemorrhagic complications [Ameri and Bousser, 1992; Milandre et al., 1989; Preter et al., 1996].

The safety of anticoagulation therapy in children with cerebral sinovenous thrombosis has been established in several studies [deVeber et al., 1998, 2001; Dix et al., 2000; Nagaraja et al., 2002; Streif et al., 1999]. Currently anticoagulants are being used in the majority of childhood cerebral sinovenous thrombosis patients without significant hemorrhagic complications [deVeber et al., 1998]. Recent guidelines recommend anticoagulation for neonates without major hemorrhage and for children with cerebral sinovenous thrombosis [Monagle et al., 2004; Paediatric Stroke Working Group, 2004]. For neonates with cerebral sinovenous thrombosis, unfractionated heparin or low-molecular-weight heparin given for 7 days, followed by low-molecular-weight heparin alone for 6 to 12 weeks, should be considered. For older infants and children, unfractioned heparin or low-molecular-weight heparin given for 7 days, followed by Coumadin for 3 to 6 months, is a treatment option based on the practice in adults. If significant intracerebral hemorrhage is associated with initial cerebral sinovenous thrombosis, the use of anticoagulants in children is controversial because of scant pediatric safety data in this situation. The clinical trials data in adults with cerebral sinovenous thrombosis indicating the safety of anticoagulants for hemorrhagic cerebral sinovenous thrombosis are reassuring. If anticoagulants are not used because of hemorrhage or other risks, early (e.g., 5 days) repeated venous imaging is indicated to assess for propagation of the initial thrombus, in which case anticoagulants are usually indicated. In children with cerebral sinovenous thrombosis in whom there is progression of thrombosis in spite of maximal systemic anticoagulation, systemic or intra-clot thrombolytic therapy may be an option and has been used with apparent success in many adults and in several children with cerebral sinovenous thrombosis [Griesemer et al., 1994; Higashida et al., 1989; Roach and Riela, 1995; Wong et al., 1987]. However, a recent Cochrane review found no randomized, controlled trials of thrombolytic treatment in adults with cerebral sinovenous thrombosis and recommended a controlled trial including patients with predictors of poor outcome [Ciccone et al., 2004]. Until more is known about the risk/benefit ratio, thrombolytic therapy should be used only in exceptional circumstances in children with cerebral sinovenous thrombosis.

Nonantithrombotic Therapies

Septic cerebral sinovenous thrombosis requires antibiotics and, in certain cases, surgical removal and drainage of the infection, such as mastoidectomy. Treatment of prolonged, increased intracranial pressure following cerebral sinovenous thrombosis consists of repeat lumbar punctures for removal of excess cerebrospinal fluid, acetazolamide, and, in resistant cases, lumboperitoneal shunting. During prolonged periods of increased intracranial pressure, careful monitoring of the visual fields, in particular the central scotoma, is necessary in order to avoid permanent visual loss. Optic nerve fenestration may be required in situations in which visual field deficits are increasing.

Outcome

In adults with cerebral sinovenous thrombosis, the long-term outcome appears to be favorable. A retrospective study of 77 adults with cerebral sinovenous thrombosis (80% of whom had received anticoagulant therapy after diagnosis) reported neurologic sequelae in only 15% [Preter et al., 1996]. A recent international study of 624 adults with cerebral sinovenous thrombosis with a median follow-up of 16 months reported a normal outcome in 57%, minor or mild impairments in 30%, moderate impairments in 3%, severe handicap in 2%, and death in 8.3% [Ferro et al., 2004]. Overall, the mortality rate is reported to be 6% to 30% and predictors of death or disability include presentation with stupor, coma and intracranial hemorrhage, and thrombosis of the deep cerebral venous system [Ferro et al., 2004; Mehraein et al., 2003]. Symptomatic recurrence of cerebral sinovenous thrombosis (12%), usually in the first year, and pulmonary embolism (11%) occurred in adult patients with cerebral sinovenous thrombosis [Bousser and Russell, 1997; Preter et al., 1996].

The outcome of pediatric cerebral sinovenous thrombosis has been assessed in several cohort studies. In one study utilizing standardized outcome assessments, 63% of 38 consecutive infants and children surviving cerebral sinovenous thrombosis were normal at a mean follow-up of 1.7 years, and the remainder had a mild or moderate neurologic deficit [deVeber et al., 2000]. In a recent study of 17 children with cerebral sinovenous thrombosis, neurologic death occurred in 5 children. The 12 surviving children were followed for a mean of 2.5 years; normal outcomes were demonstrated in 8 children, motor disability in 1, cognitive loss in 2, and reduced quality of life in 3 [De Schryver et al., 2004]. In another study of 27 neonates and children, only 11 of 31 patients had a normal outcome, 17 had residual deficits, and 2 patients died [Carvalho et al., 2001]. In a population-based prospective study of 160 infants and children from the Canadian Pediatric Ischemic Stroke Registry (mean follow-up, 1.6 years) 65% were normal, 35% had a neurologic deficit, 20% had seizures and 9% died [deVeber et al., 2001]. Six of the 7 children who died did not receive anticoagulant therapy. Predictors of death or abnormal neurologic outcome included presentation with venous infarcts or seizures. In the Registry, nearly 25% of children showed an increased severity of neurologic deficits developing over time, reinforcing the need for long-term follow-up. In addition, 13% of children developed recurrent cerebral or systemic thrombosis [deVeber et al., 2001]. In these studies, because one third to one half of the children were treated with anticoagulants, the natural history cannot be extrapolated. In older infants and children with cerebral sinovenous thrombosis, persistent intracranial hypertension is well recognized and may not be influenced by the use of anticoagulants [Higgins et al., 2003].

In adults, recanalization rates on serial neuroimaging have been shown to be maximal 4 months after diagnosis during anticoagulation therapy [Baumgartner et al., 2003]. Recanalization has also been correlated with improved outcome [Strupp et al., 2002]. The rate and extent of recanalization following cerebral sinovenous thrombosis in children has not been established. Recanalization of cerebral sinovenous thrombosis as early as 2 weeks after the onset of clinical symptoms has been reported [Macchi et al., 1986].

HEMORRHAGIC STROKE

Hemorrhagic stroke involves the rupture of normal cerebral blood vessels, as seen in a bleeding diathesis or the rupture of abnormal blood vessels, (e.g., aneurysm or vascular malformation). The result is the extravasation of blood into the brain's parenchyma or the subarachnoid space. Two major types of hemorrhagic stroke reflect the anatomic site of bleeding and are classified as *intracerebral hemorrhage* and *subarachnoid hemorrhage*. Both conditions can occur together—for example, as the result of rupture of an arteriovenous malformation or aneurysm. The most common underlying causes of hemorrhagic stroke are listed in Box 72-6.

Box 72-6 Disorders Causing Hemorrhagic Stroke

Vascular

Congenital Vascular Anomalies

- Arteriovenous malformation
- Venous angioma
- Cavernous malformation
- Hereditary hemorrhagic telangiectasia
- Intracranial aneurysm
- Coarctation with intracranial aneurysm

Vasculopathies

- Ehlers-Danlos syndrome type IV
- Moyamoya
- Pseudoxanthoma elasticum
- Sickle cell disease

Intravascular

Hematologic Disorders

- Immune thrombocytopenic purpura
- Thrombotic thrombocytopenic purpura

Hemophilic states

- Congenital serum C2 deficiency
- Liver dysfunction with coagulation defect
- Vitamin K deficiency
- Factor deficiencies

Systemic Disease

- Systemic hypertension

Vasculitis

- Drug abuse (cocaine, amphetamines)
- Hemolytic-uremic syndrome

Trauma

- Child abuse
- Angioplasty
- Penetrating intracranial trauma

General Features

Important differences exist between pediatric ischemic stroke and pediatric hemorrhagic stroke. A specific cause is more likely to be found for hemorrhagic stroke than for ischemic stroke, and the causes are entirely different in the two conditions [Schoenberg et al., 1978]. In contrast to ischemic stroke, definitive treatment for hemorrhagic stroke frequently requires neurosurgical intervention. Compared with arterial ischemic stroke, hemorrhagic stroke is associated with an increased mortality but improved neurologic recovery in survivors.

Among children with hemorrhagic stroke, subarachnoid hemorrhage is infrequent compared with intracerebral hemorrhage [Giroud et al., 1995; Lanthier et al., 2000]. In one study of 56 children with hemorrhagic stroke, 68% had intracerebral hemorrhage, 25% had subarachnoid hemorrhage and 8% had intraventricular hemorrhage [Blom et al., 2003]. In these children, underlying causes for hemorrhagic stroke included arteriovenous malformations (23); aneurysms (5); hematologic disorders (9); hematologic malignancies, vasculitis, and meningitis (2 each); and Menkes' disease and pinealoma (1 each). In this study, the outcome from hemorrhagic stroke was systematically assessed; 25% had no physical or cognitive deficits at a mean follow-up of 10 years. Death directly related to the hemorrhage occurred in 13 children. In survivors, recurrent hemorrhage was noted in 9 children and was fatal in 3 children. Six children developed long-term seizures. Of 31 survivors, 15 had no physical impairment, 11 had hemiparesis, and 3 had ataxia. Cognitive deficits were found in 15 (50%), despite normal mean IQ scores, and included aphasia in 2 patients. Reduced self-esteem and emotional, behavioral, and other health problems were present in the majority and were increased, compared with normative data on quality of life from American and Dutch populations. Children and their parents reported these latter problems at similar rates [Blom et al., 2003]. Additional studies of hemorrhagic stroke in childhood have found a similar distribution of etiologies and outcomes [Lanthier et al., 2000].

Intraventricular hemorrhage, which should be considered separately from intracerebral hemorrhage, is rare beyond the newborn period and is associated with rupture of vascular malformations and aneurysms as well as with sinus thrombosis and bleeding diatheses. The surgical treatment of hemorrhagic stroke in children has been summarized in two excellent reviews [Punt, 2004; Smith et al., 2002].

The remainder of this chapter is divided into four sections. The sections deal separately with the principal clinical subtypes of hemorrhagic stroke in children—intracerebral (intraparenchymal) hemorrhage, subarachnoid hemorrhage, and traumatic intracranial hemorrhage. In the fourth section, specific vascular disorders underlying hemorrhagic stroke, including vascular malformations, aneurysms, and other vascular disorders, are reviewed.

Intracerebral Hemorrhage

Pathophysiology

Hemorrhage into intracerebral compartments occurs when cerebral arteries or veins rupture. Usually the site of rupture is the medium-sized or smaller branches of the major cerebral arteries distal to their entry point into the brain, where vascular malformations tend to exist. The resulting hematoma mechanically disrupts neuronal structures, causing focal damage. The presence of blood products and damage to the blood-brain barrier promotes cerebral edema, resulting in relatively severe initial neurologic deficits and seizures. When large, a hematoma and the associated cerebral edema can act as a mass lesion, resulting in increased intracranial pressure and focal brain herniation. In particular, in the posterior fossa, hemorrhage may require urgent neurosurgical evacuation in order to prevent fatal brainstem compression. In one series, the location of intracerebral hemorrhage was left hemisphere in 11 cases, right hemisphere in 14, basal ganglia in 5, and cerebellar in 8 [Blom et al., 2003].

Clinical Features

In older children, intracerebral hemorrhage typically presents with a severe headache, focal signs, rapid decrease in consciousness, and seizures. Smaller bleeds may have a more subtle presentation—for example, sudden onset of minor focal neurologic signs. If the posterior fossa is the site of hemorrhage, dysconjugate gaze, ataxia, and rapid deterioration to coma are typical. In a large series in Texas of 68 children with nontraumatic cerebral hemorrhage, clinical presentations included seizures in 37%, hemiparesis in 16%, irritability in 9%, and coma in only 2 children [Al Jarallah et al., 2000].

Risk Factors

In children with nontraumatic intracerebral hemorrhage, risk factors are evident in 85% to 90% and include congenital vascular anomalies in 43% to 62% [Al Jarallah et al., 2000; Lanthier et al., 2000]. Compared with adults, children are less likely to have a generalized cerebral vasculopathy such as congophilic angiopathy or hypertensive vasculopathy underlying parenchymal hemorrhage. However, hemorrhage does occur in the setting of acquired vasculopathies including moyamoya disease, cerebral vasculitis, and metabolic or genetic vasculopathies and in adolescents abusing sympathomimetic drugs [Forman et al., 1989; Levine et al., 1990]. Compared with adults, intracerebral hemorrhage in children is more likely to result from a bleeding diathesis due to inherited hemophilic or thrombocytopenic disorders [Eyster et al., 1978; Roach and Riela, 1995]. These disorders have been found in 32% of children with intracerebral hemorrhage [Al Jarallah et al., 2000] and include hemophilia, thrombocytopenia, liver failure, leukemia, and warfarin therapy. Bleeding from cerebral lesions, including brain tumors and arterial or venous infarcts (see Fig. 72-15), are an important cause of pediatric intracerebral hemorrhage. In one series, 13% of children with intracerebral hemorrhage had brain tumors as the source of their bleeding [Al Jarallah et al., 2000]. In some children, intracerebral hemorrhage is of unclear origin. Conventional angiography should be performed in all older infants and children with intracerebral hemorrhage of unclear origin, because more than 50% will have a definable etiology [Al Jarallah et al., 2000; Zhu et al., 1997].

Outcome

Following cerebral hemorrhage, normal neurologic outcome was present in 50% of the 68 children reported in the Texas series, with death in 9% and neurologic sequelae in the remainder [Al Jarallah et al., 2000]. These sequelae included hemiparesis (25%), aphasia (7%), seizures (10%), and hydrocephalus (5%).

Subarachnoid Hemorrhage

Pathophysiology

The subarachnoid space exists between the pial lining of the brain and the next external layer of leptomeninges, the arachnoid. Normally this space is filled with cerebrospinal fluid. The cerebral arteries forming the circle of Willis and the major branches of these arteries reside in the subarachnoid space, with medium-sized and smaller branches leaving this space as they enter the brain's parenchyma. If the site of cerebral artery rupture is the proximal major arteries at the circle of Willis, as is the case in most aneurysms, or from arteriovenous malformations over the surface of the cerebral hemisphere, the majority of bleeding occurs into the subarachnoid space surrounding the brain. Following subarachnoid hemorrhage, the presence of blood and breakdown products of erythrocytes in the subarachnoid space frequently results in vasospasm in the cerebral arteries, which can be severe enough to cause secondary ischemic infarction. A communicating or noncommunicating hydrocephalus can result from adhesions at the outflow foramina of the fourth ventricle at the base of the brain, or in the arachnoid granulations where cerebrospinal fluid is absorbed.

Clinical Features

In children with subarachnoid hemorrhage, a severe headache with meningeal signs and signs of increased intracranial pressure are typical. Low-grade fever and leukocytosis occasionally are present. Children with vein of Galen malformations may present with abrupt subarachnoid hemorrhage and focal signs. In patients with subarachnoid hemorrhage, retinal examination may reveal subhyaloid retinal hemorrhages. CT detects subarachnoid hemorrhage in most patients acutely, but over the first few days becomes less likely to detect blood. Nonradiographic means of diagnosis of subarachnoid hemorrhage include lumbar puncture, with immediate detection of xanthochromia, and bloody cerebrospinal fluid without reduction or clearing of blood over the duration of the spinal fluid collection. Cerebrospinal fluid glucose may be reduced in subarachnoid hemorrhage. Definitive treatment for subarachnoid hemorrhage depends on finding the source of the hemorrhage and varies according to the type of lesion as discussed later in the fourth section "Specific Vascular Disorders Underlying Hemorrhagic Stroke."

Risk Factors

The principal causes of subarachnoid hemorrhage are the rupture of vascular malformations and aneurysms. In children, subarachnoid hemorrhage is more frequently attributable to aneurysms (mycotic or congenital) than to arteriovenous malformations [Blom et al., 2003; Sedzimir and Robinson, 1973]. In the setting of acute or subacute subarachnoid hemorrhage, if the initial angiogram does not reveal the cause, repeat angiography is usually indicated several weeks or months later because vasospasm, thrombosis, or hemorrhage impinging on the vascular anomaly can result in the lesion's being missed. The diagnostic ability of MR angiography was recently compared with conventional angiography in 19 children with subarachnoid hemorrhage and underlying arteriovenous malformations or aneurysms [Fasulakis and Andronikou, 2003]. There was excellent correlation in the detection of arteriovenous malformations; conventional angiography was superior to MR angiography in demonstrating arterial anatomy, except in identification of lesions in the anterior and posterior communicating arteries, when MRA was superior.

Outcome

The outcome in children with subarachnoid hemorrhage is not well established. In general, children with a depressed level of consciousness or coma at presentation have a poorer outcome than those with retention of normal consciousness [Higgins et al., 1991].

Traumatic Intracranial Hemorrhage

Head trauma, accidental or nonaccidental, is the commonest overall cause of intracranial hemorrhage (as distinct from hemorrhagic stroke) in childhood and, with the exception of inflicted trauma due to child abuse, is usually obvious as a risk factor. Traumatic hemorrhage can occupy any of the classic intracranial compartments: epidural, subdural, subarachnoid, intracerebral, and intraventricular. Intracerebral hemorrhage due to trauma may be associated with a single or several large focal contusions at the site of blunt trauma or may consist of multiple small hemorrhagic foci throughout the white matter, as in diffuse axonal injury. Traumatic subarachnoid hemorrhage can result from the direct rupture of small subarachnoid vessels or can occur as a complication of post-traumatic dissection of cerebral arteries.

In infants, unexplained subdural and other intracranial hemorrhage, particularly when bilateral, should raise suspicion of inflicted trauma. The "shaken baby syndrome" has been assessed in a large cohort study [Morad et al., 2002]. In 75 infants aged 2 to 48 months with shaken baby syndrome, neuroimaging findings included subdural hemorrhage in 94%, cerebral edema in 44%, subarachnoid hemorrhage in 16%, vascular infarction in 12%, intracerebral hemorrhage in 8%, contusion in 8%, and epidural hemorrhage in one child. In 75% of these children, retinal hemorrhages were present and were correlated in severity with the intracranial hemorrhages. Extreme vigilance when treating any infant with intracranial hemorrhage consistent with trauma is necessary because of the frequent absence of external signs of trauma and the difficulty in making a diagnosis of shaken baby syndrome [Committee on Child Abuse and Neglect, 1997]. Head trauma is covered in greater detail in Chapter 63.

Specific Vascular Disorders Underlying Hemorrhagic Stroke

The most important types of vascular disorders, including vascular malformations and aneurysms, and their unique clinical and radiographic features, treatments, and outcomes are briefly reviewed here. Several excellent comprehensive reference texts and reviews covering this topic have been published [Humphreys et al., 1996; Lasjaunias and Terbrugge, 2006; Roach and Riela, 1995].

Vascular Malformations

Vascular malformations are classically divided into four types, based on the caliber and histologic structure of component blood vessels: arteriovenous malformations, cavernous malformations, venous angiomas, and capillary telangiectasias [Russell and Rubenstein, 1989]. Capillary telangiectasias are an infrequent cause of hemorrhagic stroke and are usually associated with neurocutaneous disorders, which are described in Chapter 31.

ARTERIOVENOUS MALFORMATIONS

True arteriovenous malformations consist of an admixture of arteries and veins and can range from several millimeters to several centimeters in size. Development of an arteriovenous malformation results from failure of the formation of the capillary bed between primitive arteries and veins in the brain during the first trimester of fetal life. The incidence of arteriovenous malformations in children is 1 in100,000, and approximately 10% to 20% of all arteriovenous malformations become symptomatic during childhood [Menovsky and van Overbeeke, 1997].

The initial signs of an unruptured arteriovenous malformation include seizures, headaches, and, with large hemispheric arteriovenous malformations, gradually progressive neurologic deficit. In approximately 80% of patients, the initial manifestation is hemorrhage, in the form of either a warning leak or a catastrophic acute intracerebral or subarachnoid hemorrhage [Humphreys et al., 1996]. The probability of a first hemorrhage is 2% to 4% per year, with a recurrence risk as high as 25% by 5 years [Fults and Kelly, 1984]. Familial occurrence has been reported [Yokoyama et al., 1991]. CT with contrast enhancement or MRI can demonstrate an arteriovenous malformation (Fig. 72-16). However, conventional angiography is required in the planning stages of therapy.

Definitive treatment of arteriovenous malformations consists of surgical resection or interventional neuroradiologic techniques employing balloon or coil occlusion of the larger feeding vessels [Burrows et al., 1987]. Successful surgical resection confers immediate protection against recurrent hemorrhage. However, in a recent study, among 36 children with arteriovenous malformations treated with surgical resection, the recurrence rate of bleeding from an arteriovenous malformation was 5.5% at follow-up (mean, 9 years) as a result of an undetected residual nidus [Andaluz et al., 2004]. Radiosurgery is an increasingly available option.

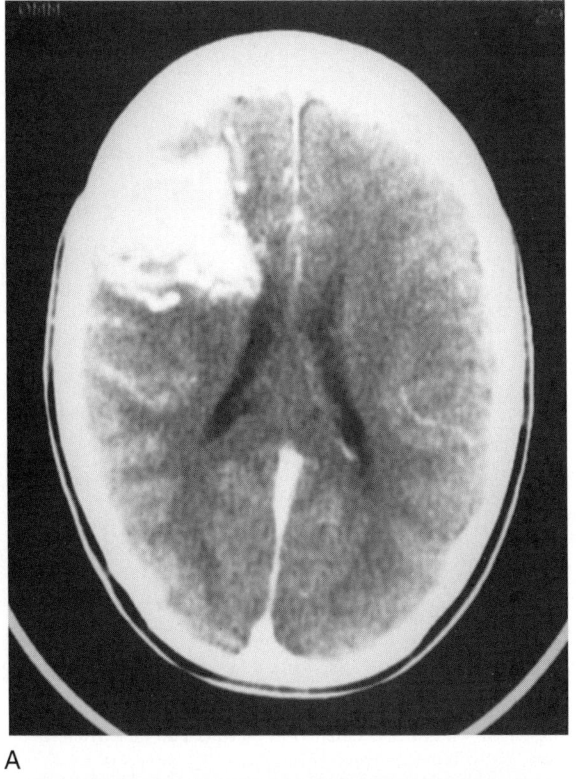

A

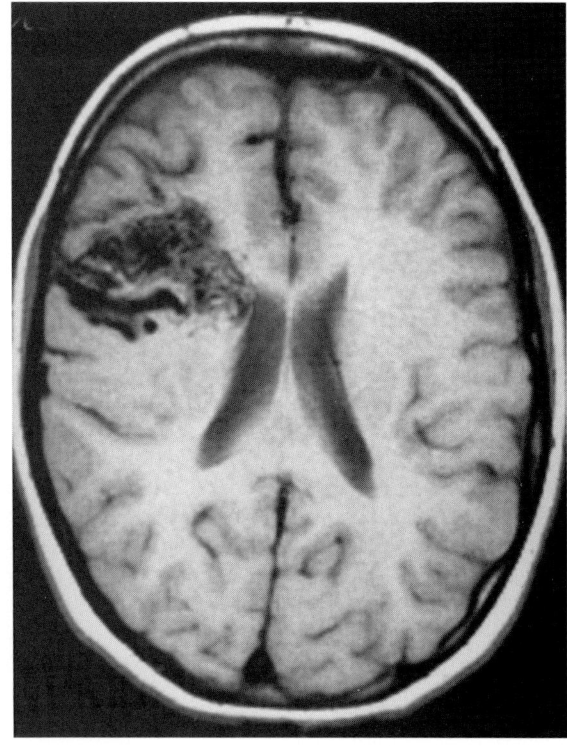

B

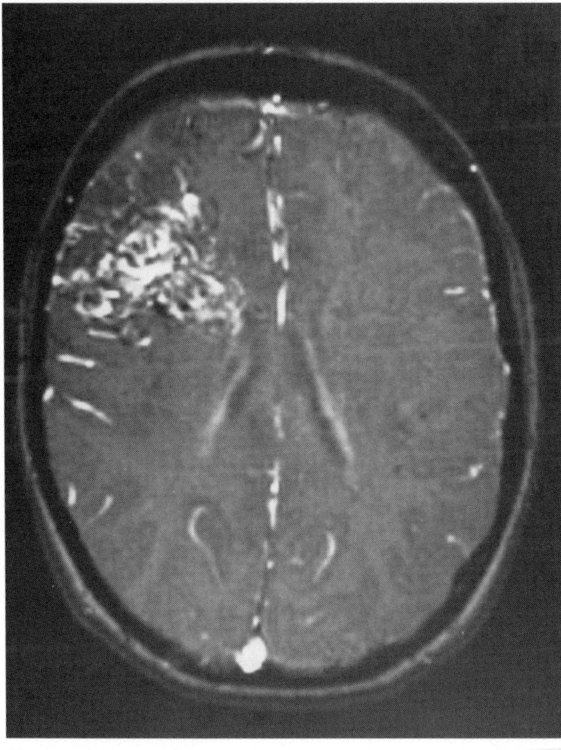

C

FIGURE 72-16. Large hemispheric arteriovenous malformation (AVM) in an 8-year-old child presenting with seizures. **A,** CT scan with contrast enhancement of right frontal mass. **B,** MRI (T1-weighted) shows multiple flow voids in the AVM. **C,** MRI (flow-sensitive sequence) shows flow in abnormal blood vessels within the AVM. (Courtesy of Karel Ter Brugge and Division of Neuroradiology, Hospital for Sick Children, Toronto, Ontario, Canada.)

In smaller lesions, focused gamma knife or proton beam irradiation can obliterate the lesion. A recent study of 31 children treated with this modality reported that in arteriovenous malformations that received at least 18 Gy there was a 10-fold increase in the obliteration rate (63%) compared with arteriovenous malformations that received a lower dose. Lesions smaller than 3 cm^3 were associated with a sixfold increased obliteration rate (53%) compared with lesions larger than 3 cm^3 (8%), but arteriovenous malformation volume was not a statistically significant predictor of response ($P = 0.09$) [Smyth et al., 2002]. The resolution of vascular lesions with radiosurgery is delayed by 1 to 2 years, during which time the patient remains at risk for rupture of the malformation [Loeffler et al., 1990]. In one study, 4 of 53 patients treated with radiosurgery for arteriovenous malformations had subsequent hemorrhages; it is interesting that all occurred more than 2 years after treatment [Levy et al., 2000]. In one study, the cumulative post-treatment hemorrhage rate after stereotactic radiation treatment after stereotactic radiation treatment was reported as 3.2% per patient per year in the first year and 4.3% per patient per year over the first 3 years [Smyth et al., 2002]. However, in another study the annual bleeding rate was 1.5% [Shin et al., 2002].

VEIN OF GALEN MALFORMATION

Vein of Galen aneurysmal malformation is an important form of arteriovenous malformation in infancy. It consists of a high-pressure vascular communication between branches of the major cerebral arteries and the vein of Galen (Fig. 72-17) and results from fistulous connections that develop near the embryonic choroidal plexuses of the 20- to 40-mm embryo. In early infancy, patients typically present with progressive high-output congestive heart failure or failure to thrive, or both, due to the large circulatory shunt into the arteriovenous malformation. In later infancy hydrocephalus can occur. Bleeding is a relatively rare presentation. In recent studies, a more favorable outcome has been reported than was previously observed and was related to an improved understanding of the pathophysiology and improved methods of endovascular therapy. In one study, 52% of 27 children undergoing endovascular treatment had no or only minor developmental delay [Fullerton et al., 2003]. In another large series of 120 infants, 83% were carefully selected for endovascular embolization treatment [Lasjaunias et al., 1996]. Death occurred in all infants in whom the treatment was conservative (i.e., no embolization therapy), and in 9% of those undergoing embolization treatment, giving an overall case mortality rate of 26%. Of the 65% with complete obliteration of the lesion, only 8.5% had severe permanent sequelae. (In this series the treatment consisted of transarterial embolization via the femoral artery with intralesional injection of *N*-butyl cyanoacrylate.)

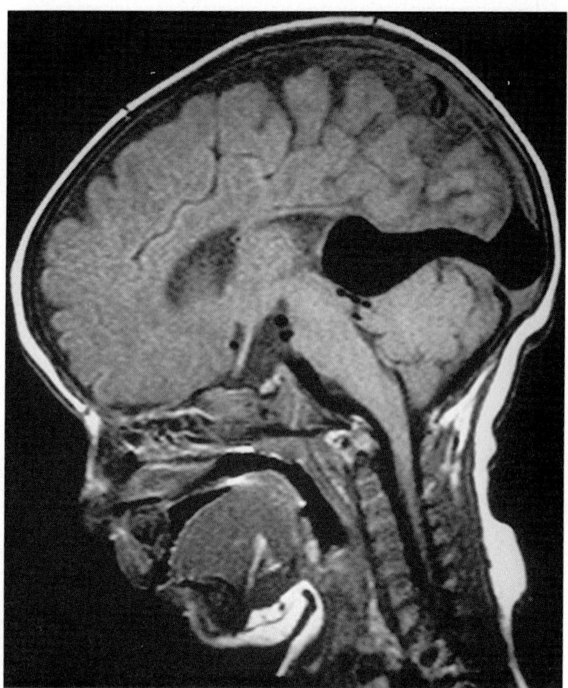

FIGURE 72-17. Vein of Galen malformation in a 3-month old infant presenting with cardiac failure. MRI scan (T1-weighted) shows low-signal flow void within the dilated vein of Galen. (Courtesy of Karel Ter Brugge and Division of Neuroradiology, Hospital for Sick Children, Toronto, Ontario, Canada.)

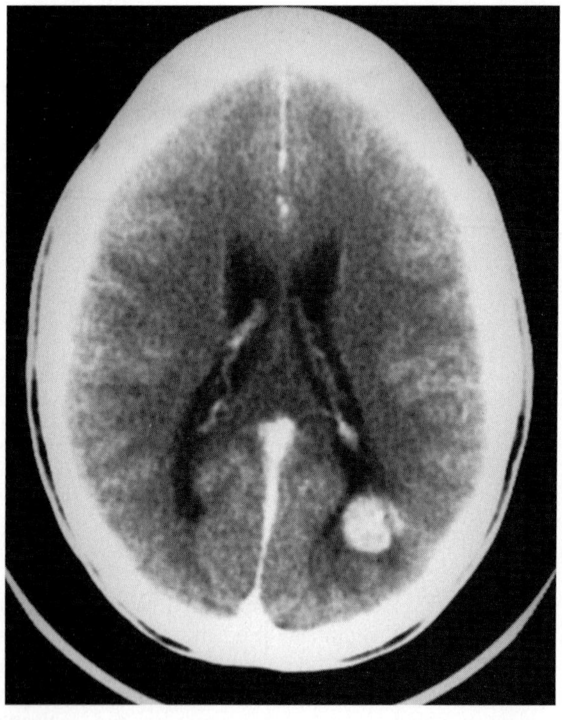

A

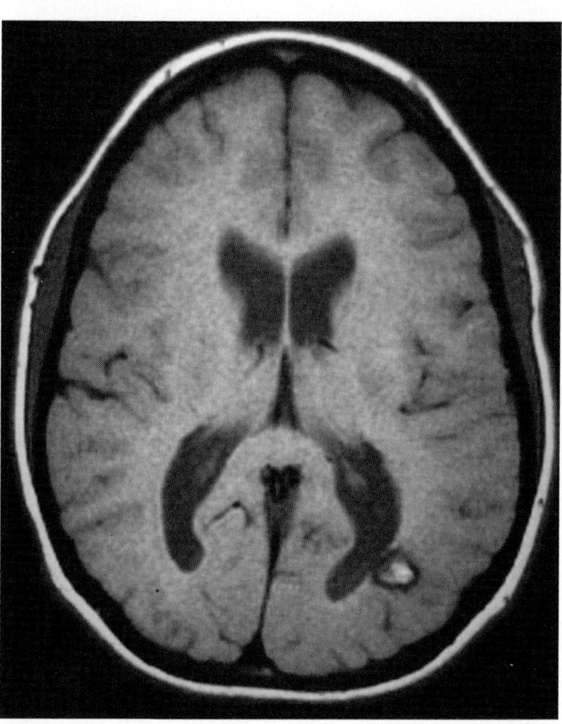

B

FIGURE 72-18. Cavernous malformation in an 18-year-old male presenting with seizures. **A,** CT scan with contrast enhancement of "mulberry" type lesion. **B,** MRI scan (T1-weighted) shows characteristic dark signal rim. (Courtesy of Karel Ter Brugge and Division of Neuroradiology, Hospital for Sick Children, Toronto, Canada.)

Microsurgical techniques utilizing staged surgical procedures have been utilized [Moodie et al., 1983]. However, large, more recent studies assessing surgical treatment are not available. Ventricular shunting is no longer recommended because it is associated with complications and poor neurologic outcome and exacerbates the complex hydrodynamic problems that exist in infants with vein of Galen malformations [Zerah et al., 1992].

CAVERNOUS MALFORMATIONS

Cavernous malformations are dense collections of thin-walled blood vessels distinct from the surrounding brain parenchyma *(*Fig. 72-18*)*. Since the advent of MRI scanning, cavernous malformations are more frequently diagnosed, and they are often asymptomatic. When they are symptomatic, the initial clinical presentation in pediatric patients is approximately one third each with seizures, focal neurologic signs, and intracerebral hemorrhage [Simard et al., 1986]. The risk of hemorrhage is less than 0.25% per person per year [Del Curling et al., 1991]. Unlike hemorrhage resulting from arteriovenous malformations or aneurysms, life-threatening hemorrhage is rare. Familial occurrence of cavernous malformations [Malik et al., 1992] has been frequently reported. In the familial form, lesions tend to be multiple and may have a greater propensity to hemorrhage than nonfamilial cavernous malformations. Retinal cavernous malformations are seen in the familial form. Cavernous malformations have recently been linked to abnormalities in the long arm of chromosome 7 [Sahoo et al., 1999].

Conventional angiography results in cavernous malformations are typically normal. However, cavernous malformation may be associated with other vascular malformations, particularly venous angiomas [Rogner, 1976]. Because of the low risk for bleeding, unruptured cavernous malformations are often managed expectantly, with surgical resection reserved for those patients who have seizure disorders refractory to medical management [Roach and Riela, 1995; Punt, 2004].

VENOUS ANGIOMAS

Venous angiomas are one of the most common types of vascular anomalies but rarely become symptomatic unless they are combined with other vascular malformations [Sarwar and McCormick, 1978]. In isolated venous angioma, hemorrhage is rare, and seizures without hemorrhage are more frequently the presenting clinical sign [Roach and Riela, 1995]. MRI and MR angiography can best demonstrate venous angiomas [Awad et al., 1993] and detect associated parenchymal or vascular lesions. Angiography indicates a caput medusae pattern consisting of a main venous trunk with a cluster of tributary veins (Fig. 72-19) [Agnoli and Hildebrandt, 1985]. Conservative management of isolated venous angiomas is usually recommended, because removal can increase neurologic deficits, presumably due to residual venous congestion in the brain drained by the angioma.

Aneurysms

Approximately 1% to 2% of aneurysms become symptomatic during childhood. Aneurysms in children are frequently associated with other vascular lesions or chronic disorders.

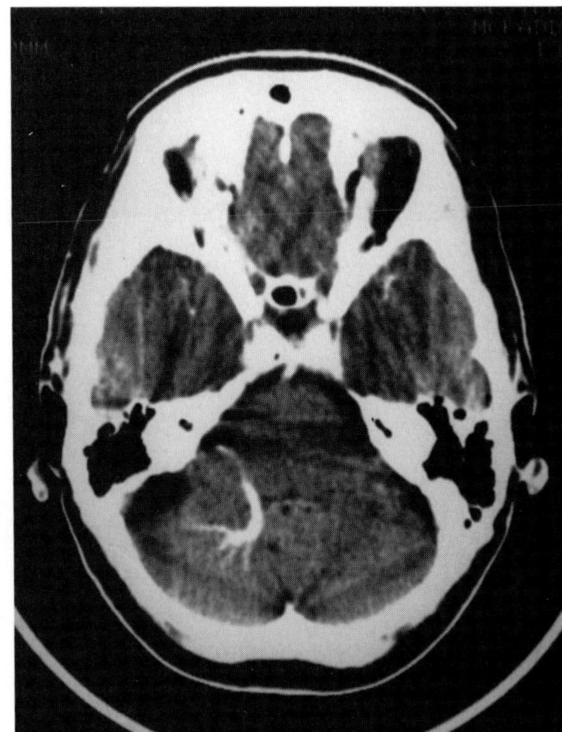

FIGURE 72-19. Venous angioma of the cerebellum of a 6-year-old male presenting with migraine headache. CT scan with contrast enhancement shows characteristic "caput medusae" feeding the draining vein. (Courtesy of Karel Ter Brugge and Divisionof Neuroradiology, Hospital for Sick Children, Toronto, Ontario, Canada.)

Most aneurysms in childhood are saccular and are believed to arise from a focal congenital weakness of the elastic and muscular layers in the cerebral arteries (Fig. 72-20) [Ahlsten et al., 1985; Khoo and Levy, 1999; Rogner, 1976]. Aneurysms tend to rupture in infants younger than 2 years of age and children older than 10 years [Adner et al., 1969] and are twice as common in males as in females [Ostergaard, 1991], in contrast to the preponderance of females in adults with aneurysms. Aneurysms occurring in children younger than 2 years of age are located predominately in the anterior and middle cerebral arteries and internal carotid artery and are larger than 1 centimeter [Crisostomo et al., 1986]. Older children and adolescents have a high proportion of aneurysms at the internal carotid artery bifurcation, with an incidence of around 16%, compared to 4% seen in adults [Khoo and Levy, 1999]. Giant (larger than 10 centimeters) aneurysms are found in 20% to 50% of pediatric cases, and are particularly common in infants [Kasahara et al., 1996]. In children, aneurysms involve the posterior circulation in 20%, nearly three times more frequently than in adults [Khoo and Levy, 1999].

Clinical presentation is usually with acute subarachnoid hemorrhage, frequently associated with intracerebral or intraventricular hemorrhage. Early warning signs are often missed in children and include previous headache or local compressive syndromes such as cranial nerve palsies. Giant aneurysms may manifest clinically with compressive features related to their location. Many systemic and vascular diseases are associated with aneurysms, including systemic arteriovenous malformation, coarctation of the aorta, Ehlers-Danlos syndrome, polycystic kidney disease, and moyamoya disease. Familial occurrence of aneurysms is well described

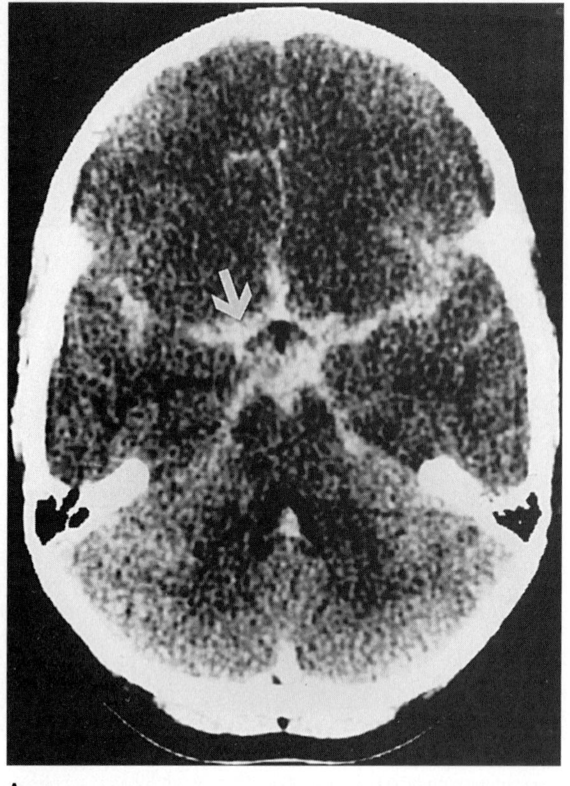

A

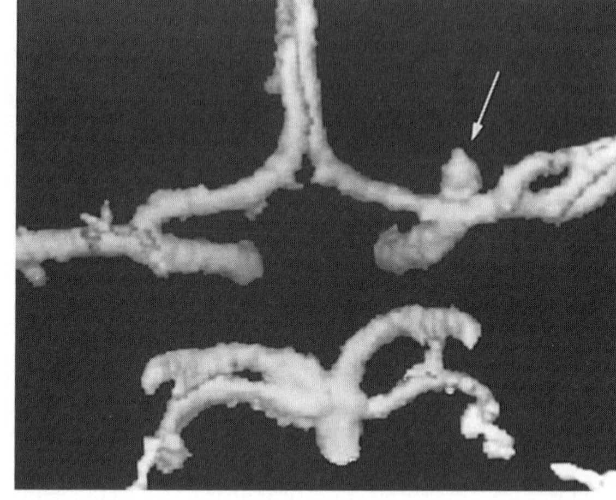

B

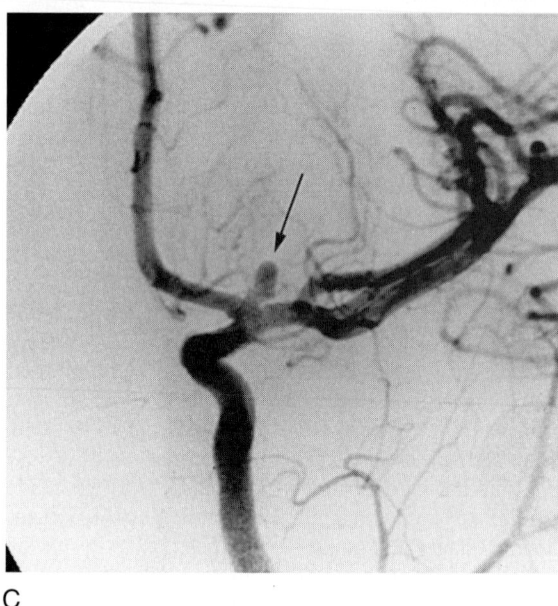

C

FIGURE 72-20. Saccular aneurysm of the left anterior cerebral artery manifesting with subarachnoid hemorrhage. **A,** CT without contrast enhancement shows high-density blood throughout the subarachnoid spaces. **B,** CT spiral angiogram shows left anterior cerebral artery aneurysm. **C,** Conventional angiogram confirms aneurysm. (Courtesy of Karel Ter Brugge and Division of Neuroradiology, Hospital for Sick Children, Toronto, Ontario, Canada.)

and is frequently associated with multiple aneurysms in each family member. MRI and MR angiography can provide good visualization of aneurysms, but angiography is more sensitive and more specific [Ross et al., 1990].

Children with aneurysms may have an increased rebleeding rate compared with adults [Wojtacha et al., 2001]. Because of the risk of early recurrent hemorrhage, surgery the first week after subarachnoid hemorrhage is considered the treatment of choice but may need to be delayed in patients with severe subarachnoid hemorrhage and unstable clinical status [Kassell et al., 1990]. Conservative measures before surgery aimed to decrease the risk of recurrent hemorrhage include sedation, adequate analgesia, prophylaxis against seizures, and prevention of hypertension. The risk of early vasospasm and ischemic infarction, particularly frequent in large subarachnoid hemorrhages, mitigates maintenance of adequate blood pressure, including volume loading. Nimodipine prevents vasospasm in adults but has not been evaluated in children.

Acquired aneurysms are most frequently the result of bacterial endocarditis. In this condition, there is embolization of infected material into cerebral arteries, which results in mycotic aneurysm formation. These aneurysms may be detected on MR or conventional angiography or may manifest with subarachnoid or intracerebral hemorrhage.

Bleeding is the first sign of a mycotic aneurysm in one fourth of cases [Brust et al., 1990]. Surgical resection of such aneurysms, although technically difficult, may be necessary to prevent this complication. Post-traumatic aneurysms may be an under-recognized condition in children [Ventureyra and Higgins, 1994]. In children with cerebral artery dissection, pseudoaneurysms also may be rarely associated with subarachnoid or intracerebral hemorrhage.

Other, Rare Causes of Hemorrhagic Stroke

Rare causes of hemorrhagic stroke due to congenital or acquired disorders of cerebral blood vessels include vasculitis, moyamoya syndrome or moyamoya disease, dissection, Ehlers-Danlos syndrome, and other connective tissue disorders. These disorders present primarily with arterial ischemic stroke and are further discussed in the section on arterial ischemic stroke in this chapter.

REFERENCES

Aarts M, Liu Y, Liu L, et al. Treatment of ischemic brain damage by perturbing NMDA receptor–PSD-95 protein interactions. Science 2002;298:846.

Abboud MR, Cure J, Granger S, et al. Magnetic resonance angiography in children with sickle cell disease and abnormal transcranial Doppler ultrasonography findings enrolled in the STOP study. Blood 2004;103:2822.

Adams R, McKie V, Nichols F, et al. The use of transcranial ultrasonography to predict stroke in sickle cell disease. N Engl J Med 1992;326:605.

Adams RJ, McKie VC, Hsu L, et al. Prevention of a first stroke by transfusions in children with sickle cell anemia and abnormal results on transcranial Doppler ultrasonography. N Engl J Med 1998;339:5.

Adner MM, Fisch GR, Starobin SG, et al. Use of "compatible" platelet transfusions in treatment of congenital isoimmune thrombocytopenic purpura. N Engl J Med 1969;280:244.

Agnoli AL, Hildebrandt G. Cerebral venous angiomas. Acta Neurochir (Wien) 1985;78:4.

Ahlsten G, Ewald U, Tuvemo T. Arachidonic acid–induced aggregation of platelets from human cord blood compared with platelets from adults. Biol Neonate 1985;47:199.

Al Jarallah A, Al Rifai MT, Riela AR, et al. Nontraumatic brain hemorrhage in children: Etiology and presentation. J Child Neurol 2000;15:284.

Albers GW, Amarenco P, Easton JD, et al. Antithrombotic and thrombolytic therapy for ischemic stroke. Chest 2001;119(1 Suppl):300S.

Albers GW, Caplan LR, Easton JD, et al. Transient ischemic attack—proposal for a new definition. N Engl J Med 2002;347:1713.

Altman DI, Powers WJ, Perlman JM. Cerebral blood flow requirements for brain viability in newborn infants is lower than in adults. Ann Neurol 1988;24:218.

Ameri A, Bousser MG. Cerebral venous thrombosis. Neurol Clin 1992;10:87.

Andaluz N, Myseros JS, Sathi S, et al. Recurrence of cerebral arteriovenous malformations in children: Report of two cases and review of the literature. Surg Neurol 2004;62:324.

Andrew M, deVeber G. Pediatric Thromboembolism and stroke protocols, 2nd ed. Hamilton, Ontario, Canada: BC Decker, 1999.

Andrew M, Marzinotto V, Massicotte, P, et al. Heparin therapy in pediatric patients: A prospective cohort study. Pediatr Res 1994;35:78.

Andrew M, Monagle P, Brooker L. Thromboembolic Complications During Infancy and Childhood. Ontario, Canada: BC Decker, 2000.

Andrew M, Vegh P, Johnston M, et al. Maturation of the hemostatic system during childhood. Blood 1992;80:1998.

Aoki S, Hayashi N, Abe O, et al. Radiation-induced arteritis: Thickened wall with prominent enhancement on cranial MR images. Report of five cases and comparison with 18 cases of moyamoya disease. Radiology 2002;223:683.

Ashwal S, Pearce WJ. Animal models of neonatal stroke. Curr Opin Pediatr 2001;13:506.

Askalan R, Laughlin S, Mayank S, et al. Chickenpox and stroke in childhood: A study of frequency and causation. Stroke 2001;32:1257.

Awad IA, Robinson JR Jr, Mohanty S, et al. Mixed vascular malformations of the brain: Clinical and pathogenetic considerations. Neurosurgery 1993;33:179.

Ayanzen RH, Bird CR, Keller PJ, et al. Cerebral MR venography: Normal anatomy and potential diagnostic pitfalls. Am J Neuroradiol 2000;21:74.

Baird TA, Parsons MW, Phanh T, et al. Persistent poststroke hyperglycemia is independently associated with infarct expansion and worse clinical outcome. Stroke 2003;34:2208.

Ball WS Jr. Cerebrovascular occlusive disease in childhood. Neuroimaging Clin N Am 1994;4:393.

Barnes C, deVeber G. Prothrombotic abnormalities in childhood ischaemic stroke. Submitted to Thromb Res 2005; July 20.

Barnes C, Newall F, Furmedge J, et al. Cerebral sinus venous thrombosis in children. J Paediatr Child Health 2004;40:53.

Barreirinho S, Ferro A, Santos M, et al. Inherited and acquired risk factors and their combined effects in pediatric stroke. Pediatr Neurol 2003;28:134.

Barron TF, Gusnard DA, Zimmerman RA, et al. Cerebral venous thrombosis in neonates and children. Pediatr Neurol 1992;8:112.

Bates E, Vicari S, Trauner D. Neural mediation of language development: Perspectives from lesion studies of infants and children. In: Tager-Flausberg H, ed. Neurodevelopmental disorders. Cambridge, MA: MIT Press, 1999;533-582.

Bath PM, Lindenstrom E, Boysen G, et al. Tinzaparin in acute ischaemic stroke (TAIST): A randomised aspirin-controlled trial. Lancet 2001;358:702.

Battin MR, Dezoete JA, Gunn TR, et al. Neurodevelopmental outcome of infants treated with head cooling and mild hypothermia after perinatal asphyxia. Pediatrics 2001;107:480.

Baumgartner RW, Studer A, Arnold M, et al. Recanalisation of cerebral venous thrombosis. J Neurol Neurosurg Psychiatry 2003;74:459.

Beletsky V, Nadareishvili Z, Lynch J, et al. Cervical arterial dissection: Time for a therapeutic trial? Stroke 2003;34:2856.

Belman AL, Roque CT, Ancona R, et al. Cerebral venous thrombosis in a child with iron deficiency anemia and thrombocytosis. Stroke 1990;21:488.

Belostotsky VM, Shah V, Dillon MJ. Clinical features in 17 paediatric patients with Wegener granulomatosis. Pediatr Nephrol 2002;17:754.

Benseler S, Schneider R. Central nervous system vasculitis in children. Curr Opin Rheumatol 2004;16:43.

Benseler S, Silverman E, Tsang L, et al. Transient cerebral arteriopathy and primary angiitis of CNS in children: A spectrum of cerebral arterial disease [Abstract]. Ann Neurol 2003;54(Suppl 7):5.

Berger TM, Caduff JH, Gebbers JO. Fatal varicella-zoster virus antigen-positive giant cell arteritis of the central nervous system. Pediatr Infect Dis J 2000;19:653.

Berman JL, Kashii S, Trachtman MS, et al. Optic neuropathy and central nervous system disease secondary to Sjögren's syndrome in a child. Ophthalmology 1990;97:1606.

Bezinque SL, Slovis TL, Touchette AS, et al. Characterization of superior sagittal sinus blood flow velocity using color flow Doppler in neonates and infants. Pediatr Radiol 1995;25:175.

Bhakta BB, Cozens JA, Chamberlain MA, et al. Impact of botulinum toxin type A on disability and care burden due to arm spasticity after stroke: A randomised double blind placebo controlled trial. J Neurol Neurosurg Psychiatry 2000;69:217.

Blom I, De Schryver EL, Kappelle LJ, et al. Prognosis of haemorrhagic stroke in childhood: A long-term follow-up study. Dev Med Child Neurol 2003;45:233.

Bodensteiner JB, Hille MR, Riggs JE. Clinical features of vascular thrombosis following varicella. Am J Dis Child 1992;146:100.

Bonduel M, Sciuccati G, Hepner M, et al. Prethrombotic disorders in children with arterial ischemic stroke and sinovenous thrombosis. Arch Neurol 1999;56:967.

Bousser MG. Aspirin or heparin immediately after a stroke? Lancet 1997;349:1564.

Bousser MG, Russell RR. Cerebral Venous Thrombosis. Toronto: WB Saunders, 1997.

Broderick J, Talbot GT, Prenger E, et al. Stroke in children within a major metropolitan area: The surprising importance of intracerebral hemorrhage. J Child Neurol 1993;8:250.

Brust JC, Dickinson PC, Hughes JE, et al. The diagnosis and treatment of cerebral mycotic aneurysms. Ann Neurol 1990;27:238.

Buoni S, Molinelli M, Mariottini A, et al. Homocystinuria with transverse sinus thrombosis. J Child Neurol 2001;16:688.

Burak CR, Bowen MD, Barron TF. The use of enoxaparin in children with acute, nonhemorrhagic ischemic stroke. Pediatr Neurol 2003;29:295.

Burrows PE, Lasjaunias PL, Ter Brugge KG, et al. Urgent and emergent embolization of lesions of the head and neck in children: Indications and results. Pediatrics 1987;80:386.

Capra N, Anderson K. Anatomy of the cerebral venous system. In: Knapp JP, Schmidek HH, eds. The Cerebral Venous System and Its Disorders. Orlando, FL: Grune and Stratton, 1984.

CAPRIE Steering Committee. A randomised, blinded, trial of clopidogrel versus aspirin in patients at risk of ischaemic events (CAPRIE). Lancet 1996;348:1329.

Carcao MD, Blanchette VS, Dean JA, et al. The Platelet Function Analyzer (PFA-100): A novel in-vitro system for evaluation of primary haemostasis in children. Br J Haematol 1998;101:70.

Cardo E, Monros E, Colome C, et al. Children with stroke: Polymorphism of the MTHFR gene, mild hyperhomocysteinemia, and vitamin status. J Child Neurol 2000;15:295.

Carhuapoma JR, Mitsias P, Levine SR. Cerebral venous thrombosis and anticardiolipin antibodies. Stroke 1997;28:2363.

Carlson MD, Leber S, Deveikis J, et al. Successful use of rt-PA in pediatric stroke. Neurology 2001;57:157.

Carvalho KS, Bodensteiner JB, Connolly PJ, et al. Cerebral venous thrombosis in children. J Child Neurol 2001;16:574.

Casey SO, Alberico RA, Patel M, et al. Cerebral CT venography. Radiology 1996;198:163.

Chabrier S, Husson B, Lasjaunias P, et al. Stroke in childhood: Outcome and recurrence risk by mechanism in 59 patients. J Child Neurol 2000;15:290.

Chabrier S, Lasjaunias P, Husson B, et al. Ischaemic stroke from dissection of the craniocervical arteries in childhood: Report of 12 patients. Eur J Paediatr Neurol 2003;7:39.

Chabrier S, Rodesch G, Lasjaunias P, et al. Transient cerebral arteriopathy: A disorder recognized by serial angiograms in children with stroke. J Child Neurol 1998;13:27.

Chang CJ, Chang WN, Huang LT, et al. Cerebral infarction in perinatal and childhood bacterial meningitis. QJM 2003;96:755.

Chiu CH, Lin TY, Huang YC. Cranial nerve palsies and cerebral infarction in a young infant with meningococcal meningitis. Scand J Infect Dis 1995;27:75.

Ciccone A, Canhao P, Falcao F, et al. Thrombolysis for cerebral vein and dural sinus thrombosis. Cochrane Database Syst Rev 2004;(1):CD003693. Stroke 2004;35:228.

Cognard C, Weill A, Lindgren S, et al. Basilar artery occlusion in a child: "Clot angioplasty" followed by thrombolysis. Childs Nerv Syst 2000;16:496.

Committee on Child Abuse and Neglect, 1993-1994. Shaken baby syndrome: Inflicted cerebral trauma. Del Med J 1997;69:365.

Cook DJ, Guyatt GH, Laupacis A, et al. Clinical recommendations using levels of evidence for antithrombotic agents. Chest 1995;108(4 Suppl):227S.

Crisostomo EA, Leaton E, Rosenblum EL. Features of intracranial aneurysms in infants and report of a case. Dev Med Child Neurol 1986;28:68.

Davies RP, Slavotinek JP. Incidence of the empty delta sign in computed tomography in the paediatric age group. Australas Radiol 1994;38:17.

Dean LM, Taylor GA. The intracranial venous system in infants: Normal and abnormal findings on duplex and color Doppler sonography. AJR Am J Roentgenol 1995;164:151.

de Bruijn SF, Stam J. Randomized, placebo-controlled trial of anticoagulant treatment with low molecular weight heparin for cerebral sinus thrombosis. Stroke 1999;30:484.

Del Curling O Jr, Kelly DL Jr, Elster AD, et al. An analysis of the natural history of cavernous angiomas. J Neurosurg 1991;75:702.

Delsing BJ, Catsman-Berrevoets CE, Appel IM. Early prognostic indicators of outcome in ischemic childhood stroke. Pediatr Neurol 2001;24:283.

Demierre B, Rondot P. Dystonia caused by putamino-capsulo-caudate vascular lesions. J Neurol Neurosurg Psychiatry 1983;46:404.

Derouesne C, Cambon H, Yelnik A, et al. Infarcts in the middle cerebral artery territory. Pathological study of the mechanisms of death. Acta Neurol Scand 1993;87:361.

Deschiens MA, Conard J, Horellou MH, et al. Coagulation studies, factor V Leiden, and anticardiolipin antibodies in 40 cases of cerebral venous thrombosis. Stroke 1996;27:1724.

De Schryver EL, Blom I, Braun KP, et al. Long-term prognosis of cerebral venous sinus thrombosis in childhood. Dev Med Child Neurol 2004;46:514.

De Schryver EL, Kappelle LJ, Jennekens-Schinkel A, et al. Prognosis of ischemic stroke in childhood: A long-term follow-up study. Dev Med Child Neurol 2000;42:313.

deVeber G, Canadian Pediatric Ischemic Stroke Study Group. Canadian Paediatric Ischemic Stroke Registry: Analysis of children with arterial ischemic stroke [Abstract 12]. Ann Neurol 2000;48:514.

deVeber G. Stroke and the child's brain: An overview of epidemiology, syndromes and risk factors. Curr Opin Neurol 2002;15:133.

deVeber G. Risk factors for childhood stroke: Little folks have different strokes! Ann Neurol 2003;53:149.

deVeber G. In pursuit of evidence-based treatments for paediatric stroke: The UK and Chest guidelines. Lancet Neurol 2005;4:432.

deVeber G, Andrew M, Canadian Pediatric Ischemic Stroke Study Group. Cerebral sinovenous thrombosis in children. N Engl J Med 2001;345:417.

deVeber G, Canadian Paediatric Ischemic Stroke Study Group. Canadian Paediatric Ischemic Stroke Registry: Analysis of children with arterial ischemic stroke. Ann Neurol 2000;48:526.

deVeber G, Chan A, Monagle P, et al. Anticoagulation therapy in pediatric patients with sinovenous thrombosis: A cohort study. Arch Neurol 1998;55:1533.

deVeber G, MacGregor D, Curtis R, et al. Neurologic outcome in survivors of childhood arterial ischemic stroke and sinovenous thrombosis. J Child Neurol 2000;15:316.

deVeber G, Monagle P, Chan A, et al. Prothrombotic disorders in infants and children with cerebral thromboembolism. Arch Neurol 1998;55:1539.

Devinsky O, Petito CK, Alonso DR. Clinical and neuropathological findings in systemic lupus erythematosus: The role of vasculitis, heart emboli, and thrombotic thrombocytopenic purpura. Ann Neurol 1988;23:380.

DiTullio M, Sacco RL, Gopal AS. Patent foramen ovale as a risk factor for cryptogenic stroke. Ann Intern Med 1992;117:461.

Dix D, Andrew M, Marzinotto V, et al. The use of low molecular weight heparin in pediatric patients: A prospective cohort study. J Pediatr 2000;136:439.

Domi T, Edgell D, McCrindle B, et al. Frequency and predictors of vasoocclusive strokes associated with congenital heart disease [Abstract]. Suppl J of Thrombosis & Haemostasis Neurology Society; Washington, DC, Oct. 9–12; Ann Neurol Sept. 2002 (52)(3S): S129–S133.

Dormont D, Anxionnat R, Evrard, S, et al. MRI in cerebral venous thrombosis. J Neuroradiol 1994;21:81.

Ducreux D, Oppenheim C, Vandamme X, et al. Diffusion-weighted imaging patterns of brain damage associated with cerebral venous thrombosis. Am J Neuroradiol 2001;22:261.

Dusser A, Goutieres F, Aicardi J. Ischemic strokes in children. J Child Neurol 1986;1:131.

Eeg-Olofsson O, Ringheim Y. Stroke in children. Clinical characteristics and prognosis. Acta Paediatr Scand 1983;72:391.

Eidelberg D, Sotrel A, Horoupian DS, et al. Thrombotic cerebral vasculopathy associated with herpes zoster. Ann Neurol 1986;19:7.

Einhaupl KM, Villringer A, Meister W, et al. Heparin treatment in sinus venous thrombosis. Lancet 1991;338:597.

Evers SM, Struijs JN, Ament AJ, et al. International comparison of stroke cost studies. Stroke 2004;35:1209.

Eyster ME, Gill FM, Blatt PM, et al. Central nervous system bleeding in hemophiliacs. Blood 1978;51:1179.

Farb RI, Vanek I, Scott JN, et al. Idiopathic intracranial hypertension: The prevalence and morphology of sinovenous stenosis. Neurology 2003a;60:1418.

Farb RI, Scott JN, Willinsky RA, et al. Intracranial venous system: Gadolinium-enhanced three-dimensional MR venography with auto-triggered elliptic centric-ordered sequence—initial experience. Radiology 2003b;226:203.

Fasulakis S, Andronikou S. Comparison of MR angiography and conventional angiography in the investigation of intracranial arteriovenous malformations and aneurysms in children. Pediatr Radiol 2003;33:378.

Fehlings D, Rang M, Glazier J, et al. An evaluation of botulinum-A toxin injections to improve upper extremity function in children with hemiplegic cerebral palsy. J Pediatr 2000;137:331.

Ferro JM, Canhao P, Stam J, et al. Prognosis of cerebral vein and dural sinus thrombosis: Results of the International Study on Cerebral Vein and Dural Sinus Thrombosis (ISCVT). Stroke 2004;35:664.

Feucht M, Brantner S, Scheidinger H. Migraine and stroke in childhood and adolescence. Cephalagia 1995;15:26.

Fiebach JB, Schellinger PD, Jansen O, et al. CT and diffusion-weighted MR imaging in randomized order: Diffusion-weighted imaging results in higher accuracy and lower interrater variability in the diagnosis of hyperacute ischemic stroke. Stroke 2002;33:2206.

Forbes KP, Pipe JG, Heiserman JE. Evidence for cytotoxic edema in the pathogenesis of cerebral venous infarction. Am J Neuroradiol 2001;22:450.

Forman HP, Levin S, Stewart B, et al. Cerebral vasculitis and hemorrhage in an adolescent taking diet pills containing phenylpropanolamine: Case report and review of literature. Pediatrics 1989;83:737.

Friefeld S, Yeboah O, Jones JE, et al. Health-related quality of life and its relationship to neurologic outcome in child survivors of stroke. CNS Spectr 2004;9:465.

Fryer RH, Anderson RC, Chiriboga CA, et al. Sickle cell anemia with moyamoya disease: Outcomes after EDAS procedure. Pediatr Neurol 2003;29:124.

Fullerton HJ, Adams RJ, Zhao S, et al. Declining stroke rates in Californian children with sickle cell disease. Blood 2004;104:336.

Fullerton HJ, Aminoff AR, Ferriero DM, et al. Neurodevelopmental outcome after endovascular treatment of vein of Galen malformations. Neurology 2003;61:1386.

Fullerton HJ, Johnston SC, Smith WS. Arterial dissection and stroke in children. Neurology 2001;57:1155.

Fullerton HJ, Wu YW, Zhao S, et al. Risk of stroke in children: Ethnic and gender disparities. Neurology 2003;61:189.

Fults D, Kelly DL. Natural history of arteriovenous malformations of the brain: A clinical study. Neurosurgery 1984;15:658.

Furlan A, Higashida R, Wechsler L, et al. Intra-arterial prourokinase for acute ischemic stroke. The PROACT II study: A randomized controlled trial. Prolyse in acute cerebral thromboembolism. JAMA 1999;282:2003.

Ganesan V, Hogan A, Shack N, et al. Outcome after ischaemic stroke in childhood. Dev Med Child Neurol 2000;42:455.

Ganesan V, Kelsey H, Cookson J, et al. Activated protein C resistance in childhood stroke. Lancet 1996;96:260.

Ganesan V, Prengler M, McShane MA, et al. Investigation of risk factors in children with arterial ischemic stroke. Ann Neurol 2003;53:167.

Ganesan V, Savvy L, Chong WK, et al. Conventional cerebral angiography in children with ischemic stroke. Pediatr Neurol 1999;20:38.

Gillum LA, Mamidipudi SK, Johnston SC. Ischemic stroke risk with oral contraceptives: A meta-analysis. JAMA 2000;284:72.

Ginsberg MD, Pulsinelli WA. The ischemic penumbra, injury thresholds, and the therapeutic window for acute stroke. Ann Neurol 1997;36:553.

Giroud M, Lemesle M, Gouyon JB. et al. Cerebrovascular disease in children under 16 years of age in the city of Dijon, France: A study of incidence and clinical features from 1985 to 1993. J Clin Epidemiol 1995;48:1343.

Gluckman PD, Wyatt JS, Azzopardi D, et al. Selective head cooling with mild systemic hypothermia after neonatal encephalopathy: Multicentre randomised trial. Lancet 2005;365(9460):663.

Glueck CJ, Daniels SR, Bates S, et al. Pediatric victims of unexplained stroke and their families: Familial lipid and lipoprotein abnormalities. Pediatrics 1982;69:308.

Goldenberg NA, Knapp-Clevenger R, Manco-Johnson MJ. Elevated plasma factor VIII and D-dimer levels as predictors of poor outcomes of thrombosis in children. N Engl J Med 2004;351:1081.

Golomb MR, deVeber GA, MacGregor DL, et al. Independent walking after neonatal arterial ischemic stroke and sinovenous thrombosis. J Child Neurol 2003;18:530.

Golomb MR, MacGregor DL, Domi T, et al. Presumed pre- or perinatal arterial ischemic stroke: Risk factors and outcomes. Ann Neurol 2001;50:163.

Goodman R, Yude C. IQ and its predictors in childhood hemiplegia. Dev Med Child Neurol 1996;38:881.

Gouault-Heilman M, Quentin P, Dreyfus M, et al. Massive thrombosis of venous cerebral sinuses in a 2-year-old boy with a combined inherited deficiency of antithrombin III and protein C. Thromb Haemost 1994;72:782.

Govaert P, Voet D, Achten E. et al. Noninvasive diagnosis of superior sagittal sinus thrombosis in a neonate. Am J Perinatol 1992;9:201.

Graf WK, Milstein JM, Sherry DD. Stroke and mixed connective tissue disease. J Child Neurol 1993;8:256.

Griesemer DA, Theodorou AA, Berg RA, et al. Local fibrinolysis in cerebral venous thrombosis. Pediatr Neurol 1994;10:78.

Groenendaal F, van der Ground J, Witkamp TD, et al. Proton magnetic resonance spectroscopic imaging in neonatal stroke. Neuropediatrics 1995;26:243.

Gruber A, Nasel C, Lang W, et al. Intra-arterial thrombolysis for the treatment of perioperative childhood cardioembolic stroke. Neurology 2000;54:1684.

Guidi B, Bergonzini P, Crisi G, et al. Case of stroke in a 7-year-old male after parvovirus B19 infection. Pediatr Neurol 2003;28:69.

Gunther G, Junker R, Strater R, et al. Symptomatic ischemic stroke in full-term neonates: Role of acquired and genetic prothrombotic risk factors. Stroke 2000;31:2437.

Gupta R, Connolly ES, Mayer S, et al. Hemicraniectomy for massive middle cerebral artery territory infarction: A systematic review. Stroke 2004;35:539.

Hall SM. Reye's syndrome and aspirin: A review. Br J Clin Pract Suppl 1990;70:4.

Hamburger C, Villringer A, Bauer M, et al. Delta (empty triangle) sign in patients without thrombosis of the superior sagittal sinus. In: Einhaupl K, Kempski O, Baethmann A, eds. Cerebral Sinus Thrombosis: Experimental and Clinical Aspects. New York: Plenum Press, 1990.

Hartfield DS, Lowry NJ, Keene DL. et al. Iron deficiency: A cause of stroke in infants and children. Pediatr Neurol 1997;16:50.

Hartmann A, Wappenschmidt J, Solymosi L. Clinical findings and differential diagnosis of cerebral vein thrombosis. In: Einhaupl K, ed. Cerebral Sinus Thrombosis. Experimental and Clinical Aspects. New York: Plenum Press, 1987.

Hayman M, Hendson G, Poskitt KJ. et al. Postvaricella angiopathy: Report of a case with pathologic correlation. Pediatr Neurol 2001;24:387.

Heller C, Heinecke A, Junker R, et al. Cerebral venous thrombosis in children: A multifactorial origin. Circulation 2003;108:1362.

Higashida RT, Helmer E, Halbach VV, et al. Direct thrombolytic therapy for superior sagittal sinus thrombosis. AJNR An J Neuroradiol 1989;10:S4.

Higashida RT, Helmer E, Halbach VV, et al. Inherited prothrombotic risk factors and cerebral venous thrombosis. QJM 1998;91:677.

Higgins JJ, Kammerman LA, Fitz CR. Predictors of survival and characteristics of childhood stroke. Neuropediatrics 1991;22:190.

Higgins JN, Cousins C, Owler BK, et al. Idiopathic intracranial hypertension: 12 cases treated by venous sinus stenting. J Neurol Neurosurg Psychiatry 2003;74:1662.

Hirsh J, Warkentin TE, Raschke R, et al. Heparin and low-molecular-weight heparin: Mechanisms of action, pharmacokinetics, dosing considerations, monitoring, efficacy, and safety. Chest 1998;114(5 Suppl):489S.

Hofmeijer J, van der Worp HB, Amelink GJ, et al. Surgical decompression in space-occupying cerebral infarct: Notification of a randomized trial. Ned Tijdschr Geneeskd 2003;147:2594.

Hoppe C, Klitz W, Cheng S, et al. Gene interactions and stroke risk in children with sickle cell anemia. Blood 2004;103:2391.

Hou ST, MacManus JP. Molecular mechanisms of cerebral ischemia-induced neuronal death. Int Rev Cytol 2002;221:93.

Huisman TA, Holzmann D, Martin E, et al. Cerebral venous thrombosis in childhood. Eur Radiol 2001;11:1760.

Humphreys RP, Hoffman HJ, Drake JM, et al. Choices in the 1990s for the management of pediatric cerebral arteriovenous malformations. Pediatr Neurosurg 1996;25:277.

Hune S, Rafay MF, Domi T, et al. Plavix (clopidogrel) in pediatric stroke: Monitoring of side effects and patient education strategies [Abstract]. Stroke 2004;35:284.

Husson B, Lasjaunias P. Radiological approach to disorders of arterial brain vessels associated with childhood arterial stroke—a comparison between MRA and contrast angiography. Pediatr Radiol 2004;34:10.

Husson B, Rodesch G, Lasjaunias P, et al. Magnetic resonance angiography in childhood arterial brain infarcts: A comparative study with contrast angiography. Stroke 2002;33:1280.

Hutchison JS, Ichord R, Guerguerian AM, et al. Cerebrovascular disorders. Semin Pediatr Neurol 2004;11:139.

Iizuka T, Sakai F, Suzuki N, et al. Neuronal hyperexcitability in stroke-like episodes of MELAS syndrome. Neurology 2002;59:816.

International Stroke Trial Collaborative Group. The International Stroke Trial (IST): A randomised trial of aspirin, subcutaneous heparin, both, or neither among 19,435 patients with acute ischaemic stroke. Lancet 1997;349:1569.

Isler W. Stroke in childhood and adolescence. Eur Neurol 1984;23:421.

Israels SJ, Cheang T, McMillan-Ward EM, et al. Evaluation of primary hemostasis in neonates with a new in vitro platelet function analyzer. J Pediatr 2001;138:116.

Ito MK, Smith AR, Lee ML. Ticlopidine: A new platelet aggregation inhibitor. Clin Pharm 1992;11:603.

Jacewicz M, Plum F. Aseptic cerebral venous thrombosis. In: Einhaupl K, ed. Cerebral Sinus Thrombosis. New York: Plenum Press, 1990.

Johnston DC, Chapman KM, Goldstein LB. Low rate of complications of cerebral angiography in routine clinical practice. Neurology 2001;57:2012.

Kasahara E, Murayama T, Yamane C. Giant cerebral arterial aneurysm in an infant: Report of a case and review of 42 previous cases in infants with cerebral arterial aneurysm. Acta Paediatr Jpn 1996;38:684.

Kase CS, Furlan AJ, Wechsler LR, et al. Cerebral hemorrhage after intra-arterial thrombolysis for ischemic stroke: The PROACT II trial. Neurology 2001;57:1603.

Kassell NF, Torner JC, Haley EC Jr, et al. The International Cooperative Study on the Timing of Aneurysm Surgery. Part 1: Overall management results. J Neurosurg 1990;73:18.

Kay R, Wong KS, Yu YL, et al. Low-molecular-weight heparin for the treatment of acute ischemic stroke. N Engl J Med 1995;333:1588.

Kenet G, Waldman D, Lubetsky A, et al. Paediatric cerebral sinus vein thrombosis. A multi-center, case-controlled study. Thromb Haemost 2004;92:713.

Kerr LM, Anderson DM, Thompson JA, et al. Ischemic stroke in the young: Evaluation and age comparison of patients six months to thirty-nine years. J Child Neurol 1993;8:266.

Khoo L, Levy M. Intracerebral aneurysms. In: Albright A, Pollack I, Adelson PD, eds. Principles and Practice of Pediatric Neurosurgery. New York: Thieme Medical Publishers, 1999.

Kidwell CS, Chalela JA, Saver JL, et al. Comparison of MRI and CT for detection of acute intracerebral hemorrhage. JAMA 2004;292:1823.

Kim SK, Seol HJ, Cho BK, et al. Moyamoya disease among young patients: Its aggressive clinical course and the role of active surgical treatment. Neurosurgery 2004;54:840.

Kirkham F. Stroke in childhood. Curr Pediatr 1994;4:208.

Kirkham F. Paediatric neurology: Genes and the environment. Lancet Neurol 2004;3:18.

Kirkham FJ, Hewes DK, Prengler M, et al. Nocturnal hypoxaemia and central-nervous-system events in sickle-cell disease. Lancet 2001;357:1656.

Kleinschmidt-DeMasters BK, Gilden DH. Varicella-zoster virus infections of the nervous system: Clinical and pathologic correlates. Arch Pathol Lab Med 2001;125:770.

Koelfen W, Freund M, Konig S, et al. Results of parenchymal and angiographic magnetic resonance imaging and neuropsychological testing of children after stroke as neonates. Eur J Pediatr 1993;152:1030.

Koelfen W, Wentz U, Freund M, et al. Magnetic resonance angiography in 140 neuropediatric patients. Pediatr Neurol 1995;12:31.

Kolb B, Cioe J. Recovery from early cortical damage in rats. IX. Differential behavioral and anatomical effects of temporal cortex lesions at different ages of neural maturation. Behav Brain Res 2003;144:67.

Kolb B, Cioe J, Whishaw IQ. Is there an optimal age for recovery from motor cortex lesions? I. Behavioral and anatomical sequelae of bilateral motor cortex lesions in rats on postnatal days 1, 10, and in adulthood. Brain Res 2000;882:62.

Kossoff EH, Ichord RN, Bergin AM. Recurrent hypoglycemic hemiparesis and aphasia in an adolescent patient. Pediatr Neurol 2001;24:385.

Krieger DW, Yenari MA. Therapeutic hypothermia for acute ischemic stroke: What do laboratory studies teach us? Stroke 2004;35:1482.

Kriss VM. Hyperdense posterior falx in the neonate. Pediatr Radiol 1998;28:817.

Kurnik K, Kosch A, Strater R, et al. Recurrent thromboembolism in infants and children suffering from symptomatic neonatal arterial stroke: A prospective follow-up study. Stroke 2003;34:2887.

Kwak CH, Jankovic J. Tourettism and dystonia after subcortical stroke. Mov Disord 2002;17:821.

Lansing AE, Max JE, Delis DC, et al. Verbal learning and memory after childhood stroke. J Int Neuropsychol Soc 2004;10:742.

Lanska MJ, Lanska DJ, Horwitz SJ, Aram DM. Presentation, clinical course, and outcome of childhood stroke. Pediatr Neurol 1991;7:333.

Lanthier S, Carmant L, David M, et al. Stroke in children: The coexistence of multiple risk factors predicts poor outcome. Neurology 2000;54:371.

Lanthier S, Kirkham FJ, Mitchell LG, et al. Increased anticardiolipin antibody IgG titers do not predict recurrent stroke or transient ischemic attack in children. Neurology 2004;62:194.

Lanthier S, Lortie A, Michaud J, et al. Isolated angiitis of the CNS in children. Neurology 2001;56:837.

Lapchak PA, Zivin JA. Ebselen, a seleno-organic antioxidant, is neuroprotective after embolic strokes in rabbits: Synergism with low-dose tissue plasminogen activator. Stroke 2003;34:2013.

Lasjaunias P, Alvarez H, Rodesch G, et al. Aneurysmal malformation of the vein of Galen; Follow-up of 120 children treated between 1984 and 1994. Intervent Neuroradiol 1996;2:15.

Lasjaunias P, Terbrugge K. Vascular Diseases in Neonates, Infants, and Children: Interventional Neuroradiology Management. Heidelberg: Springer-Verlag, 2006.

Leaker M, Massicotte MP, Brooker LA, et al. Thrombolytic therapy in pediatric patients: A comprehensive review of the literature. Thromb Haemost 1996;76:132.

Levine SR, Brust JC, Futrell N, et al. Cerebrovascular complications of the use of the "crack" form of alkaloidal cocaine. N Engl J Med 1990;323:699.

Levy EI, Niranjan A, Thompson TP, et al. Radiosurgery for childhood intracranial arteriovenous malformations. Neurosurgery 2000;47:834.

Lewin JS, Masaryk TJ, Smith AS, et al. Time-of-flight intracranial MR venography: Evaluation of the sequential oblique section technique. AJNR Am J Neuroradiol 1994;15:1657.

Liang L, Korogi Y, Sugahara T, et al. Evaluation of the intracranial dural sinuses with a 3D contrast- enhanced MP-RAGE sequence: Prospective comparison with 2D-TOF MR venography and digital subtraction angiography. AJNR Am J Neuroradiol 2001;22:481.

Lin JH, McLean K, Morser J, et al. Modulation of glycosaminoglycan addition in naturally expressed and recombinant human thrombomodulin. J Biol Chem 1994;269:25021.

Linnemann CC Jr, Alvira MM. Pathogenesis of varicella-zoster angiitis in the CNS. Arch Neurol 1980;37:239.

Liu XY, Wong V, Leung M. Neurologic complications due to catheterization. Pediatr Neurol 2001;24:270.

Loeffler JS, Rossitch E Jr, Siddon R, et al. Role of stereotactic radiosurgery with a linear accelerator in treatment of intracranial arteriovenous malformations and tumors in children. Pediatrics 1990;85:774.

Ludwig B, Brand M, Brockerhoff P. Postpartum CT examination of the heads of full term infants. Neuroradiology 1980;20:145.

Lynch JK, Hirtz DG, deVeber G, et al. Report of the National Institute of Neurologic Disorders and Stroke workshop on perinatal and childhood stroke. Pediatrics 2002;109:116.

Macchi PJ, Grossman RI, Gomori JM, et al. High field MR imaging of cerebral venous thrombosis. J Comp Assisted Tomography 1986;10:10.

Maiti B, Chakrabarti S. Study in cerebral venous thrombosis with specific reference to efficacy of heparin [abstract]. J Neurol Sci 1997;150:S147.

Malik S, Cohen BH, Robinson J, et al. Progressive vision loss. A rare manifestation of familial cavernous angiomas. Arch Neurol 1992;49:170.

Manci EA, Culberson DE, Yang YM, et al. Causes of death in sickle cell disease: An autopsy study. Br J Haematol 2003;123:359.

Martinelli I, Landi G, Merati G, et al. Factor V gene mutation is a risk for cerebral venous thrombosis. Thromb Haemost 1996;75:393.

Mas JL, Arquizan C, Lamy C, et al. Recurrent cerebrovascular events associated with patent foramen ovale, atrial septal aneurysm, or both. N Engl J Med 2001;345:1740.

Massicotte P, Adams M, Marzinotto V, et al. Low-molecular-weight heparin in pediatric patients with thrombotic disease: A dose finding study. J Pediatr 1996;128:313.

Max JE. Effect of side of lesion on neuropsychological performance in childhood stroke. J Int Neuropsychol Soc 2004;10:698.

Medlock MD, Olivero WC, Hanigan WC, et al. Children with cerebral venous thrombosis diagnosed with magnetic resonance imaging and magnetic resonance angiography. Neurosurgery 1992;31:870.

Meena AK, Naidu KS, Murthy JM. Cortical sinovenous thrombosis in a child with nephrotic syndrome and iron deficiency anaemia. Neurol India 2000;48:292.

Mehraein S, Schmidtke K, Villringer A, et al. Heparin treatment in cerebral sinus and venous thrombosis: Patients at risk of fatal outcome. Cerebrovasc Dis 2003;15:17.

Menache CC, du Plessis AJ, Wessel DL, et al. Current incidence of acute neurologic complications after open-heart operations in children. Ann Thorac Surg 2002;73:1752.

Menovsky T, van Overbeeke JJ. Cerebral arteriovenous malformations in childhood: State of the art with special reference to treatment. Eur J Pediatr 1997;156:741.

Mercuri E, Barnett A, Rutherford M, et al. Neonatal cerebral infarction and neuromotor outcome at school age. Pediatrics 2004;113:95.

Mercuri E, Cowan F, Gupte G, et al. Prothrombotic disorders and abnormal neurodevelopmental outcome in infants with neonatal cerebral infarction. Pediatrics 2001;107:1400.

Mercuri E, Rutherford M, Cowan F, et al. Early prognostic indicators of outcome in infants with neonatal cerebral infarction: A clinical, electroencephalogram, and magnetic resonance imaging study. Pediatrics 1999;103:39.

Meschia JF, Miller DA, Brott TG. Thrombolytic treatment of acute ischemic stroke. Mayo Clin Proc 2002;77:542.

Michelson DJ, Ashwal, S. The pathophysiology of stroke in mitochondrial disorders. Mitochondrion 2004;4:665.

Mikulis DJ, Krolczyk G, Desal H, et al. Preoperative and postoperative mapping of cerebrovascular reactivity in moyamoya disease by using blood oxygen level-dependent magnetic resonance imaging. J Neurosurg 2005;103:347.

Milandre L, Gueriot C, Girard N, et al. Cerebral venous thrombosis in adults. Diagnostic and therapeutic aspects in 20 cases. Ann Med Interne (Paris) 1989;139:544.

Mohr JP. Anticoagulation for stroke prevention: Yes, no, maybe. Cleve Clin J Med 2004;71(Suppl 1);S52.

Mohr JP, Thompson JL, Lazar RM, et al. A comparison of warfarin and aspirin for the prevention of recurrent ischemic stroke. N Engl J Med 2001;345:1444.

Monagle P, Chan A, Massicotte P, et al. Antithrombotic therapy in children: The Seventh ACCP Conference on Antithrombotic and Thrombolytic Therapy. Chest 2004;126(3 Suppl):645S.

Monagle P, Karl TR. Thromboembolic problems after the Fontan operation. Semin Thorac Cardiovasc Surg Pediatr Card Surg Annu 2002;5:36.

Moodie DS, Sterba R, Rothner AD, et al. Great vein of Galen malformations in infancy. Cleve Clin Q 1983;50:295.

Morad Y, Kim YM, Armstrong DC, et al. Correlation between retinal abnormalities and intracranial abnormalities in the shaken baby syndrome. Am J Ophthalmol 2002;134:354.

Morales E, Pineda C, Martinez-Lavin M. Takayasu's arteritis in children. J Rheumatol 1991;18:1081.

Morfin-Maciel B, Medina A, Espinosa Rosales F, et al. Central nervous system involvement in a child with polyarteritis nodosa and severe atopic dermatitis. Rev Alerg Mex 2002;49:189.

Mudd SH, Skovby F, Levy, HL, et al. The natural history of homocystinuria due to cystathionine beta-synthase deficiency. Am J Hum Genet 1985;37:1.

Muhonen LA, Lauer RM. Hyperlipidemia in childhood: The United States approach. Bailliere's Clin Pediatr 1996;4:17.

Murphy SL. Deaths: Final data for 1998. Natl Vital Stat Rep 2000;48:1.

Muthukumar N. Uncommon cause of sinus thrombosis following closed mild head injury in a child. Childs Nerv Syst 2004;May 27 (Epub ahead of print).

Nagaraja D, Rao BS, Taly AB, et al. Randomized controlled trial of heparin in puerperal venous sinus thrombosis. Nat Inst Mental Health Neurosci J 1995;13:111.

Nagaraja D, Rao BSS, Taly AB, et al. Safety of low molecular weight heparin at treatment doses in children with arterial ischemic stroke: a consecutive cohort study. Ann Neurol 2002;52: 3S:132.

Nagaraja D, Verma A, Taly AB, et al. Cerebrovascular disease in children. Acta Neurol Scand 1994;90:251.

Nardocci N, Zorzi G, Grisoli M, et al. Acquired hemidystonia in childhood: A clinical and neuroradiological study of thirteen patients. Pediatr Neurol 1996;15:108.

Nass RD, Trauner D. Social and affective impairments are important recovery after acquired stroke in childhood. CNS Spectr 2004;9:420.

National Institute of Neurologic Disorders and Stroke rt-PA Stroke Study Group. Tissue plasminogen activator for acute ischemic stroke. N Engl J Med 1995;333:1580.

Nederkoorn PJ, Elgersma OE, van der Graaf Y, et al. Carotid artery stenosis: Accuracy of contrast-enhanced MR angiography for diagnosis. Radiology 2003;228:677.

Nelson KB, Lynch JK. Stroke in newborn infants. Lancet Neurol 2004;3:150.

Newall F, Barnes C, Ignjatovic V, et al. Heparin-induced thrombocytopenia in children. J Paediatr Child Health 2003;39:289.

Newton TH, Gooding CA. Compression of superior sagittal sinus by neonatal calvarial molding. Neuroradiology 1975;115:635.

Nezu A, Kimura S, Ohtsuki N, et al. Acute confusional migraine and migrainous infarction in childhood. Brain Dev 1997;19:148.

Ng W, Chan AK, Curtis RM. Safety of low molecular weight heparin at treatment of doses in children with arterial ischemic stroke: A consecutive cohort study [Abstract]. Ann Neurol 2002;52(3S):132.

Ng W, Chan AK, Massicotte PM, et al. Safety and feasibility of warfarin in pediatric patients with arterial ischemic stroke: A consecutive cohort study [Abstract]. Ann Neurol 2002;52(3S):S131.

Noser EA, Felberg RA, Alexandrov AV. Thrombolytic therapy in an adolescent ischemic stroke. J Child Neurol 2001;16:286.

Nowak-Gottl U, Straeter R, Sebire G, et al. Antithrombotic drug treatment of pediatric patients with ischemic stroke. Paediatr Drugs 2003;5:167.

Olsen TS, Weber UJ, Kammersgaard LP. Therapeutic hypothermia for acute stroke. Lancet Neurol 2003;2:410.

Omura M, Aida N, Sekido K, et al. Large intracranial vessel occlusive vasculopathy after radiation therapy in children: Clinical features and usefulness of magnetic resonance imaging. Int J Radiat Oncol Biol Phys 1997;38:241.

Ostergaard JR. Aetiology of intracranial saccular aneurysms in childhood. Br.J Neurosurg 1991;5:575.

Paediatric Stroke Working Group. Stroke in Childhood: Clinical Guidelines for Diagnosis, Management and Rehabilitation. London: Royal College of Physicians of London, 2004.

Patsalides AD, Wood LV, Atac GK, et al. Cerebrovascular disease in HIV-infected pediatric patients: Neuroimaging findings. A J R Am J Roentgenol 2002;179:999.

Pegelow CH. Stroke in children with sickle cell anaemia: Aetiology and treatment. Paediatr Drugs 2001;3:421.

Pezzini A, Del Zotto E, Magoni M, et al. Inherited thrombophilic disorders in young adults with ischemic stroke and patent foramen ovale. Stroke 2003;34:28.

Preter M, Tzourio C, Amen A, et al. Long term prognosis in cerebral venous thrombosis: Followup of 77 patients. Stroke 1996;27:243.

Punt J. Surgical management of paediatric stroke. Pediatr Radiol 2004;34:16.

Qiao M, Latta P, Meng S, et al. Development of acute edema following cerebral hypoxia-ischemia in neonatal compared with juvenile rats using magnetic resonance imaging. Pediatr Res 2004;55:101.

Rafay M, MacGregor D, deVeber G. Craniocervical arterial dissection—children are different [Abstract]. Ann Neurol 2002;52(3S):129.

Reshef E, Greenberg SB, Jankovic J. Herpes zoster ophthalmicus followed by contralateral hemiparesis: Report of two cases and review of literature. J Neurol Neurosurg Psychiatry 1985;48:122.

Reul J, Weber U, Kotlarek F, et al. Cerebral vein and sinus thrombosis—an important cause of benign intracranial pressure increase in childhood. Klin Padiatr 1997;209:116.

Ribai P, Liesnard C, Rodesch G, et al. Transient cerebral arteriopathy in infancy associated with enteroviral infection. Eur J Paediatr Neurol 2003;7:73.

Riikonen RS, Vahtera EM, Kekomaki RM. Physiological anticoagulants and activated protein C resistance in childhood stroke. Acta Paediatr 1996;85:242.

Rivkin MJ, Volpe JJ. Strokes in children. Pediatr Rev 1996;17:265.

Rivkin MJ, Anderson ML, Kaye EM. Neonatal idiopathic cerebral venous thrombosis: An unrecognized cause of transient seizures or lethargy. Ann Neurol 1992;32:51.

Roach ES, Riela AR. Pediatric Cerebrovascular Disorders. New York: Futura Publishing, 1995.

Rodriguez CJ, Homma S. Hypercoagulable states in patients with patent foramen ovale. Curr Hematol Rep 2003;2:435.

Rogner G. Heparin level during anticoagulant therapy in mature and premature newborn infants. Kinderarztl Prax 1976;44:193.

Roschitz B, Sudi K, Kostenberger M, et al. Shorter PFA-100 closure times in neonates than in adults: Role of red cells, white cells, platelets and von Willebrand factor. Acta Paediatr 2001;90:664.
Ross JS, Masaryk TJ, Modic MT, et al. Intracranial aneurysms: Evaluation by MR angiography. A J R Am J Roentgenol 1990;155:159.
Rothrock JF. Migrainous stroke. Cephalalgia 1993;13:231.
Russell DS, Rubenstein LJ. Pathology of Tumors of The Nervous System. Baltimore: Williams & Wilkins, 1989.
Rutherford MA, Azzopardi D, Whitelaw A, et al. Mild hypothermia and the distribution of cerebral lesions in neonates with hypoxic-ischemic encephalopathy. Pediatrics 2005;116:1001.
Sahoo T, Johnson EW, Thomas JW, et al. Mutations in the gene encoding KRIT1, a Krev-1/rap1a binding protein, cause cerebral cavernous malformations (CCM1). Hum Mol Genet 1999;8:2325.
Sandercock PA, van den Belt AG, Lindley RI, et al. Antithrombotic therapy in acute ischaemic stroke: An overview of the completed randomised trials [see comments]. J Neurol Neurosurg Psychiatry 1993;56:17.
Santiago R, Dominguez M, Campos J. Cerebral infarct in childhood as a complication of migraine with aura. A case report. Rev Neurol 2001;33:1143.
Sarwar M, McCormick WF. Intracerebral venous angioma. Case report and review. Arch Neurol 1978;35:323.
Satoh S, Shibuya H, Matsushima Y, et al. Analysis of the angiographic findings in cases of childhood moyamoya disease. Neuroradiology 1988;30:111.
Satoh S, Shirane R, Yoshimoto T. Clinical survey of ischemic cerebrovascular disease in children in a district of Japan. Stroke 1991;22:586.
Savi P, Heilmann E, Nurden P. Clopidogrel: An antithrombotic drug acting on the ADP-dependent activation pathway of human platelets. Clin Appl Thromb Haemost 1996;2:35.
Schlaug G, Benfield A, Baird AE, et al. The ischemic penumbra: Operationally defined by diffusion and perfusion MRI. Neurology 1999;53:1528.
Schoenberg BS, Mellinger JF, Schoenberg DG. Cerebrovascular disease in infants and children: A study of incidence, clinical features, and survival. Neurology 1978;28:763.
Schwab S, Steiner T, Aschoff A, et al. Early hemicraniectomy in patients with complete middle cerebral artery infarction. Stroke 1998;29:1888.
Scott RM, Smith JL, Robertson RL, et al. Long-term outcome in children with moyamoya syndrome after cranial revascularization by pial synangiosis. J Neurosurg 2004;100(2 Suppl):142.
Scotti LN, Goldman RL, Hardman DR, et al. Venous thrombosis in infants and children. Radiology 1974;112:393.
Sébire G, Fullerton H, Riou E, et al. Toward the definition of cerebral arteriopathies of childhood. Curr Opin Pediatr 2004;16:617.
Sébire G, Tabarki B, Saunders DE, et al. Cerebral venous sinus thrombosis in children. Brain 2005;128:477.
Sedzimir CB, Robinson J. Intracranial hemorrhage in children and adolescents. J Neurosurg 1973;38:269.
Shahar E, Gilday DL, Hwang PA, et al. Pediatric cerebrovascular disease. Alterations of regional cerebral blood flow detected by TC 99m-HMPAO SPECT. Arch Neurol 1990;47:578.
Shin M, Kawamoto S, Kurita H, et al. Retrospective analysis of a 10-year experience of stereotactic radio surgery for arteriovenous malformations in children and adolescents. J Neurosurg 2002;97:779.
Shirane R, Sato S, Yoshimoto T. Angiographic findings of ischemic stroke in children. Childs Nerv Sys 1992 8:432.
Shroff M, deVeber G. Sinovenous thrombosis in children. Neuroimaging Clin N Am 2003;13:115.
Silverstein FS, Brunberg JA. Postvaricella basal ganglia infarction in children. AJNR Am J Neuroradiol 1995;16:449.
Simard JM, Garcia-Bengochea F, Ballinger WE Jr, et al. Cavernous angioma: A review of 126 collected and 12 new clinical cases. Neurosurgery 1986;18:162.
Smith ER, Butler WE, Ogilvy CS. Surgical approaches to vascular anomalies of the child's brain. Curr Opin Neurol 2002;15:165.
Smyth MD, Sneed PK, Ciricillo SF, et al. Stereotactic radiosurgery for pediatric intracranial arteriovenous malformations: The University of California at San Francisco experience. J Neurosurg 2002;97:48.
Sousa J, O'Brien D, Bartlett R, et al. Sigmoid sinus thrombosis in a child after closed head injury. Br J Neurosurg 2004;18:187.
Stam J, de Bruijn S, deVeber G. Anticoagulation for cerebral sinus thrombosis. Stroke 2003;34:1054.
Steinlin M, Roellin K, Schroth G. Long-term follow-up after stroke in childhood. Eur J Pediatr 2004;163:245.
Stiefel D, Eich G, Sacher P. Posttraumatic dural sinus thrombosis in children. Eur J Pediatr Surg 2000;10:41.
Strater R, Becker S, von Eckardstein A, et al. Prospective assessment of risk factors for recurrent stroke during childhood—a 5-year follow-up study. Lancet 2002;360:1540.
Strater R, Kurnik K, Heller C, et al. Aspirin versus low-dose low-molecular-weight heparin: Antithrombotic therapy in pediatric ischemic stroke patients: A prospective follow-up study. Stroke 2001;32:2554.
Streif W, Andrew M, Marzinotto V, et al. Analysis of warfarin therapy in pediatric patients: A prospective cohort study of 319 patients. Blood 1999;94:3007.
Strupp M, Covi M, Seelos K, et al. Cerebral venous thrombosis: Correlation between recanalization and clinical outcome—long-term follow-up of 40 patients. J Neurol 2002;249:1123.
Suzuki, J, Kodama N. Moyamoya disease—a review. Stroke 1983;14:104.
Takano K, Utsunomiya H, Ono H, et al. Dynamic contrast-enhanced subtraction MR angiography in intracranial vascular abnormalities. Eur Radiol 1999;9:1909.
Taub E, Ramey SL, DeLuca S, et al. Efficacy of constraint-induced movement therapy for children with cerebral palsy with asymmetric motor impairment. Pediatrics 2004;113:305.
Taylor TN, Davis PH, Torner JC, et al. Lifetime cost of stroke in the United States. Stroke 1996;27:1459.
Teasell RW, Kalra L. What's new in stroke rehabilitation. Stroke 2004;35:383.
Trescher WH. Ischemic stroke syndromes in childhood. Pediatr Ann 1992;21:374.
Tsao PN, Lee, WT, Peng SF, et al. Power Doppler ultrasound imaging in neonatal cerebral venous sinus thrombosis. Pediatr Neurol 1999;21:652.
Ueki K, Meyer FB, Mellinger JF. Moyamoya disease: The disorder and surgical treatment. Mayo Clin Proc 1994;69:749.
Ueno M, Oka A, Koeda T, et al. Unilateral occlusion of the middle cerebral artery after varicella-zoster virus infection. Brain Dev 2002;24:106.
Venkataraman A, Kingsley PB, Kalina P, et al. Newborn brain infarction: Clinical aspects and magnetic resonance imaging. CNS Spectr 2004; 9:436.
Ventureyra EC, Higgins MJ. Traumatic intracranial aneurysms in childhood and adolescence. Case reports and review of the literature. Childs Nerv Syst 1994;10:361.
Vielhaber H, Ehrenforth S, Koch HG, et al. Cerebral venous sinus thrombosis in infancy and childhood: Role of genetic and acquired risk factors of thrombophilia. Eur J Pediatr 1998;157:555.
Vilaseca MA, Moyano D, Ferrer I, et al. Total homocysteine in pediatric patients. Clin Chem 1997;43:690.
Visudtibhan A, Visudhiphan P, Chiemchanya S. Stroke and seizures as the presenting signs of pediatric HIV infection. Pediatr Neurol 1999;20:53.
Volpe JJ. Neurology of the Newborn. Philadelphia: WB Saunders, 2001a.
Volpe JJ. Perinatal brain injury: From pathogenesis to neuroprotection. Ment Retard Dev Disabil Res Rev 2001b;7:56.
von Scheven E, Lee C, Berg BO. Pediatric Wegener's granulomatosis complicated by central nervous system vasculitis. Pediatr Neurol 1998;19:317.
Wang M, Hays T, Balasa V, et al. Low-dose tissue plasminogen activator thrombolysis in children. J Pediatr Hematol Oncol 2003;25:379.
Warach S, Baron JC. Neuroimaging. Stroke 2004;35:351.
Ware RE, Zimmerman SA, Sylvestre PB, et al. Prevention of secondary stroke and resolution of transfusional iron overload in children with sickle cell anemia using hydroxyurea and phlebotomy. J Pediatr 2004;145:346.
Wintermark M, Lepori D, Cotting J, et al. Brain perfusion in children: Evolution with age assessed by quantitative perfusion computed tomography. Pediatrics 2004;113:1642.
Wirrell EC, Armstrong EA, Osman LD, et al. Prolonged seizures exacerbate perinatal hypoxic-ischemic brain damage. Pediatr Res 2001;50:445.
Wiznitzer M, Masaryk TJ. Cerebrovascular abnormalities in pediatric stroke: Assessment using parenchymal and angiographic magnetic resonance imaging. Ann Neurol 1991;29:585.
Wojtacha M, Bazowski P, Mandera M, et al. Cerebral aneurysms in childhood. Childs Nerv Syst 2001;17:37.

Wolters HJ, ten Cate H, Thomas LL, et al. Low-intensity oral anticoagulation in sickle-cell disease reverses the prethrombotic state: Promises for treatment? Br J Haematol 1995;90:715.

Wong VK, LeMesurier J, Franceschini R, et al. Cerebral venous thrombosis as a cause of neonatal seizures. Pediatr Neurol 1987;3:235.

Woodhall B. Variations of the cranial venous sinuses in the region of the torcular heterophili. Arch Surg 1936;33:297.

Yager JY, Thornhill JA. The effect of age on susceptibility to hypoxic-ischemic brain damage. Neurosci Biobehav Rev 1997;21:167.

Yang JS, Yong DP, Hartlage P. Seizures associated with stroke in childhood. Pediatr Neurol 1995;12:136.

Yoshida S, Yamamoto T, Yoshioka M, et al. Ischemic stroke in childhood. No Shinkei Geka 1993;21:611.

Young G, Manco-Johnson M, Gill JC, et al. Clinical manifestations of the prothrombin G20210A mutation in children: A pediatric coagulation consortium study. J Thromb Haemost 2003;1:958.

Yuh WT, Simonson TM, Wang AM, et al. Venous sinus occlusive disease: MR findings. AJNR Am J Neuroradiol 1994;15:309.

Zerah M, Garcia-Monaco R, Rodesch G, et al. Hydrodynamics in vein of Galen malformations. Childs Nerv Syst 1992;8:111.

Zhu XL, Chan MS, Poon WS. Spontaneous intracranial hemorrhage: Which patients need diagnostic cerebral angiography? A prospective study of 206 cases and review of the literature. Stroke 1997;28:1406.

Zimmerman RA, Bogdan AR, Gusnard DA. Pediatric magnetic resonance angiography: Assessment of stroke. Cardiovasc Intervent Radiol 1992;15:60.

Zou LP, Guo YH, Fang F, et al. Evidence for human leukocyte antigen-related susceptibility in idiopathic childhood ischemic stroke. Eur Neurol 2002;48:153.

Zuber M, Toulon P, Marnet L, et al. Factor V Leiden mutation in cerebral venous thrombosis. Stroke 1996;27:1721.

CHAPTER 73

Neurologic Manifestations of Rheumatic Disorders of Childhood

Nina Felice Schor, Robert Sheets, Ilona S. Szer, and Stephen Ashwal

The rheumatic disorders of childhood are composed of a wide variety of conditions ranging from simple arthritis to complex multisystem autoimmune diseases. The presence and the degree of nervous system impairment vary widely depending on the diagnosis and course of the disorder. Manifestations of neurologic disease may precede the onset of any other symptoms or occur much later. Classification of the chronic rheumatic disorders has changed, as shown in Box 73-1 [Petty et al., 2004]. The types of autoantibodies found in rheumatic diseases are outlined in Table 73-1.

Neurologic manifestations of rheumatic disorders can arise in both primary and secondary fashion [Benseler and Schneider, 2004]. That is, the antibodies or cellular immune elements responsible for the underlying disease can directly attack and injure or can cause the malfunction of nerves, muscle, brain, spinal cord, and sensory organs. On the other hand, innocent bystander effects of such rheumatic disease accompaniments as the hypercoagulable state, inflammation of the blood vessel wall, and immune complex deposition and side effects of medications used in the treatment of rheumatic disease also take their toll on the nervous system. These neurologic signs and symptoms are often multifactorial in origin, and their treatment may involve approaches to the proximate underlying disease and the more distal symptomatic manifestations.

Rheumatic disease underlies a small but tangible fraction of neurologic syndromes of childhood. For example, vasculitis of infectious or rheumatic origin accounts for approximately 4% of childhood stroke [Williams et al., 1997]. Rheumatic disease should be considered as a possible etiologic factor in neurologic syndromes of childhood when these syndromes are accompanied by persistent fever, weight loss, myalgias, arthralgias, meningeal signs, or multiple nonanatomically contiguous neurologic deficits [Carvalho and Garg, 2002].

CHRONIC ARTHROPATHIES

The key neurologic and laboratory findings in chronic arthropathies are summarized in Table 73-2 [Tan, 1986].

Juvenile Idiopathic Arthritis

The neurologic manifestations and sequelae of juvenile idiopathic arthritis (previously described as juvenile rheumatoid arthritis) and its treatment vary greatly with the subtype of arthritis. Children with pauciarticular or polyarticular disease have only rarely been diagnosed with central nervous system disease, but approximately 20% of those with pauciarticular and 5% of those with polyarticular disease develop uveitis [Rosenberg, 2002]. In contrast, only 1% of children with systemic onset disease develop uveitis [Rosenberg, 2002]. Approximately 6% of children with systemic arthritis develop nervous system symptoms that most often involve the central nervous system.

Neurologic Manifestations of Systemic Juvenile Idiopathic Arthritis

ACUTE ENCEPHALOPATHY WITH OR WITHOUT SEIZURES

The most common form of acute encephalopathy in children with systemic juvenile idiopathic arthritis is macrophage activation syndrome. Symptoms include unremitting fever, rheumatoid rash, seizures, encephalopathy, hepatosplenomegaly, and lymphadenopathy, as well as cardiac, pulmonary and renal failure. Laboratory studies indicate varying degrees of cytopenia, low albumin, elevated D-dimer, and elevated ferritin and lactate dehydrogenase. Elevated liver enzymes as well as triglycerides are common. The sedimentation rate may fall [Ravelli, 2002]. Initial reports of this catastrophic complication implicated the use of acetylsalicylic acid, indomethacin, and gold, but the macrophage activation syndrome has occurred after ingestion of many nonsteroidal anti-inflammatory drugs including sulfasalazine and in the context of no drug intake [Bray and Singleton, 1994]. Immediate treatment with steroids is associated with resolution in most cases. In steroid-resistant cases, cyclosporin A has been effective [Mouy et al., 1996].

In one series of patients, acute hepatic dysfunction, metabolic alterations (including hyponatremia), intracranial hemorrhage, and acute encephalopathy have been described with and without disseminated intravascular coagulation [Hadchouel et al., 1985]. Clinical features are suggestive of a Reye-like syndrome, although cerebral edema, hyperammonemia, and hepatic microvascular fatty infiltration have not been observed. Elevated cerebrospinal fluid protein and cell count were common. These patients demonstrated generalized electroencephalographic slowing, and the neurologic symptoms in five of seven children were attributable to a metabolic encephalopathy associated with hyponatremia. These five children responded well to high-dose corticosteroids. The remaining two children died from disseminated intravascular coagulation [Hadchouel et al., 1985]. In another series of children with systemic juvenile idiopathic arthritis without disseminated intravascular coagulation, an acute encephalopathy associated with generalized and focal seizures, altered states of consciousness, abnormal ictal and interictal electroencephalogram, and moderate elevation of cerebrospinal fluid protein and cells has been reported [Lang

Box 73-1 Classification of the Rheumatic Disorders of Childhood

Juvenile Idiopathic Arthritis (Chronic Arthropathies)

Systemic arthritis (systemic-onset JRA)
Oligoarthritis, persistent or extended (pauciarticular-onset JRA)
Polyarthritis, rheumatoid factor–negative (polyarticular-onset JRA)
Psoriatic arthritis (not previously classified as JRA)
Enthesitis-related arthritis (previously classified as spondyloarthritis)
Undifferentiated arthritis

Arthritis Associated with Infectious Agents

Acute rheumatic fever
Lyme disease
Reiter's syndrome

Connective Tissue Disorders

Systemic lupus erythematosus
Juvenile dermatomyositis
Scleroderma
Mixed connective tissue disease
Sjögren's syndrome

Primary Vasculitic Disorders

Necrotizing Vasculitis

Polyarteritis nodosa
Kawasaki disease
Microscopic polyangiitis
Cogan's syndrome

Leukocytoclastic Vasculitis

Henoch-Schönlein purpura
Hypersensitivity vasculitis

Granulomatous Vasculitis

Churg-Strauss syndrome
Wegener's granulomatosis
Primary angiitis of the central nervous system
Necrotizing sarcoid granulomatosis
Sarcoidosis

Giant Cell Arteritis

Temporal arteritis
Takayasu's arteritis

Miscellaneous Vasculitic Disorders

Behçet's disease

Miscellaneous Disorders

Thrombotic thrombocytopenic purpura
Erythromelalgia

JRA, juvenile rheumatoid arthritis.
Modified from Cassidy JT, Petty RE. Textbook of pediatric rheumatology, 4th ed. Philadelphia: WB Saunders, 2001.

et al., 1974]. Perivascular infiltrates of inflammatory cells within the brain parenchyma have been documented in several children with acute encephalopathy. In one patient, cerebrospinal fluid immune complexes were associated with parenchymal perivascular mononuclear cell infiltrates, suggesting an autoimmune basis of this complication [O'Connor et al., 1980].

Two reports have been published in which there was an association of true Reye syndrome with chronic administration of acetylsalicylic acid in several patients with juvenile idiopathic arthritis when acetylsalicylic acid was the drug of choice for the treatment of chronic childhood arthritis [Silverman et al., 1983; Young et al., 1984]. No reports of Reye syndrome in children with juvenile idiopathic arthritis have emerged since the use of acetylsalicylic acid in children has declined in the United States; furthermore, this complication has not been reported with the use of newer nonsteroidal anti-inflammatory drugs such as naproxen.

NEUROPATHIES

Motor and sensory neuropathies have been reported in children but are far more common in adults. As such, mononeuritis multiplex, the most common neuropathy in adults with rheumatoid arthritis, is seldom if ever present in children. Neuropathologic studies of adult rheumatoid arthritis patients with peripheral neuropathy have demonstrated vasculitis involving both the leptomeninges and the underlying parenchyma with infarction of adjacent neuronal tissue. The

TABLE 73-1

Autoantibodies in Pediatric Rheumatic Diseases

ANTIBODY	CLINICAL FINDING
ANA	97% SLE, but also positive in MCTD, SSc, 10-85% JDMS, 20-88% JRA, SS, and 2-5% of controls
Anti-ds-DNA	30-70% SLE, rarely in other CTDs
Anti-Sm	30% SLE
Anti-RNP	MCTD, also in SLE
Anti-SSA/Ro	25% SLE, 75% SS
Anti-SSB/La	10% SLE, 40% SS
Anti-histone	50% SLE, >90% DILS
Anti-centromere	44-98% CREST syndrome
Anti-Scl-70	27% SSc
Anti-c-ANCA	>90% Wegener's granulomatosis
Anti-p-ANCA	10% Wegener's granulomatosis, 70% CSS, 75% UC, 20% Crohn's disease, 30% SLE
RF A	20% polyarticular JRA, 50% SS; 10-30% SLE, MCTD
LAC	Correlates with thromboembolic risk in SLE
aCL	Correlates with thromboembolic risk in SLE, malignancy; variable in many other diseases

aCL, anticardiolipin antibody; ANA, antinuclear antibody; c-ANCA, cytoplasmic staining antineutrophil cytoplasmic antibody; CREST, calcinosis, *R*aynaud's, *e*sophageal dysmotility, *s*clerodactyly, *t*elangiectasia; CSS, Churg-Strauss syndrome; CTD, connective tissue disease; DILS, drug-induced lupus syndrome; ds-DNA, double-stranded (native) DNA; JDMS, juvenile dermatomyositis, JRA, juvenile rheumatoid arthritis; LAC, lupus anticoagulant; MCTD, mixed connective tissue disease; p-ANCA, perinuclear staining antineutrophil cytoplasmic antibody; RF A, rheumatoid factor A; RNP, ribonucleoprotein; SLE, systemic lupus erythematosus; Sm, Smith; SS, Sjögren's syndrome; SSc, systemic scleroderma; UC, ulcerative colitis.

Adapted from Okano Y. Rheum Dis Clin North Am 1996;22:709; Moder KG. Mayo Clin Proc 1996;71:391; and Bylund DJ, McCallum RM. Vasculitis. In: Henry JB, ed. Clinical diagnosis and management by laboratory methods. Philadelphia: WB Saunders, 1996.

TABLE 73-2

Key Neurologic and Laboratory Findings in the Chronic and Reactive Arthropathies

DISEASE	NEUROLOGIC FINDINGS	LABORATORY FINDINGS
Systemic juvenile idiopathic arthritis	Encephalopathy, seizures, macrophage activation syndrome (Reye-like syndrome), neuropathies	Elevated WBC and ESR, anemia, DIC, elevated CSF protein and cell count, marked increase in ferritin and LDH
Inflammatory bowel disease	Myasthenia gravis, myopathy, neuropathy, seizures, cognitive changes	Elevated ESR, microcytic anemia, melena
Acute rheumatic fever	Chorea, personality changes, seizures	Positive ASO titers, elevated ESR and CRP, abnormal ECG
Lyme disease	Early infection: aseptic meningitis, headache, chorea, cranial nerve palsies, late neuroborreliosis myelitis, MS-like symptoms, subtle encephalopathy, radiculopathy, mononeuritis multiplex	Positive IgG Lyme titer by ELISA, protein by Western blot in serum, positive PCR in CSF

ASO, antistreptolysin O; CRP, c-reactive protein; CSF, cerebrospinal fluid; DIC, disseminated intravascular coagulation; ECG, electrocardiogram; ELISA, enzyme-linked immunosorbent assay; ESR, erythrocyte sedimentation rate; IgG, immunoglobulin G; LDH, lactate dehydrogenase; MS, multiple sclerosis; PCR, polymerase chain reaction; WBC, white blood cell count.

resulting axonal neuropathy may be associated with demyelination caused by vascular occlusion of the vasa nervorum [Peyronnard et al., 1982].

MOOD DISTURBANCES

Reports of psychologic studies of children with juvenile idiopathic arthritis remain uncertain about both the relative frequency of psychologic disorders and the relation of age and severity of arthritis to psychologic symptoms [Baildam et al., 1995; Ungerer et al., 1988]. Premorbid family dynamics, specifically maternal personality, may contribute to subsequent psychologic disorders in the child with juvenile idiopathic arthritis [Vandvik and Eckblad, 1991]. Depression and difficulty with concentration may be secondary to drug interventions, including nonsteroidal anti-inflammatory drugs and sulfasalazine.

MYOSITIS

Approximately 33% of children with juvenile idiopathic arthritis have mild elevations of creatine kinase without weakness [Rachelefsky et al., 1976]. Proximal muscle weakness and biopsy-confirmed myositis are extremely rare, although intermittent myalgias are common, especially in systemic juvenile idiopathic arthritis. Myositis has been localized with magnetic resonance imaging (MRI) in a patient with myalgias and elevated muscle enzymes in systemic juvenile idiopathic arthritis [Miller et al., 1995]. Of note, children with Duchenne's muscular dystrophy, paraplegia, poliomyelitis, and cerebral palsy may have skeletal changes, such as apparent overgrowth of the epiphysis, periarticular osteoporosis, and joint-space narrowing, similar to juvenile idiopathic arthritis [Richardson et al., 1984].

Neurologic Manifestations of Polyarticular Juvenile Rheumatoid Arthritis

MYELOPATHY

Many children with polyarticular or systemic onset juvenile rheumatoid arthritis develop neck stiffness secondary to cervical arthritis. Lateral cervical flexion radiographs may document fusion of the posterior vertebral processes of C2 and C3 followed by fusion of the entire cervical spine. The child with cervical spine fusion is usually able to flex the neck but has severe limitation of cervical extension and rotation. Unlike classic rheumatoid arthritis of adulthood, cervical myelopathy associated with atlantoaxial dislocation is highly unusual.

NEUROPATHOLOGIC ABNORMALITIES OF THE CENTRAL NERVOUS SYSTEM

Neuropathologic studies of children with systemic onset juvenile idiopathic arthritis who have had neurologic complications are rare. Investigations of adults with classic rheumatoid arthritis complicated by central nervous system disease document the presence of rheumatoid nodules in the cranial and spinal dura, falces, leptomeninges, parenchyma, and choroid plexus [Kim, 1980]. Because adult-type (i.e., polyarticular) rheumatoid arthritis is relatively uncommon in children, these manifestations have not been reported but may occur in older children with seropositive (rheumatoid factor–positive) juvenile idiopathic arthritis who have the same disease as their adult counterparts.

Management of Juvenile Idiopathic Arthritis

The treatment of juvenile idiopathic arthritis is dictated by the subtype of the disease. Pauciarticular juvenile idiopathic arthritis is usually managed with either nonsteroidal anti-inflammatory drugs, such as naproxen and tolmetin sodium, or steroid intra-articular joint injection. Iridocyclitis usually responds successfully to topical ophthalmic corticosteroids. Polyarticular juvenile idiopathic arthritis is initially treated with nonsteroidal anti-inflammatory drugs; however, the risk of chronic inflammation of multiple joints may require the use of second-line agents such as methotrexate. If methotrexate fails, a tumor necrosis factor-alpha blocking drug, such as etanercept or infliximab is used. Systemic juvenile idiopathic arthritis may be managed with nonsteroidal anti-inflammatory drugs alone but often requires steroids for control of systemic symptoms. Second-line drugs such as methotrexate are often needed to control arthritis [Cassidy and Petty, 2001]. Once again, etanercept or infliximab are used for disease poorly responsive to prednisone and methotrexate [Quartier et al., 2003]. High-dose methylprednisolone, intravenous immunoglobulin, and cyclophosphamide have been used in recalcitrant disease [Shaikov et al., 1992; Silverman et al., 1994; Uziel et al., 1996]. Antitumor necrosis factor-alpha therapies paradoxically have been associated with worsening of or even emergence of new cases of multiple sclerosis [Sicotte and Voskuhl, 2001].

Because of the chronic nature of juvenile idiopathic arthritis, some children have psychological problems, including depression, anger, adjustment disorders, and troubles with peer and family relations. Counseling of the patient and family is beneficial [Baildam et al., 1995; Quirk and Young, 1990]. In addition, the importance of physical and occupational therapy cannot be overemphasized [Rhodes, 1991].

Neonatal-Onset Multisystem Inflammatory Disease (NOMID) or Chronic Infantile Neurologic Cutaneous and Articular (CINCA) Syndrome

This unusual disorder, which mimics systemic juvenile idiopathic arthritis, has its onset during the first year of life, whereas systemic onset juvenile idiopathic arthritis is a disease of toddlers and children. Clinical manifestations include hectic fever, intermittent rash, lymphadenopathy, hepatosplenomegaly, uveitis, cognitive and developmental delay, chronic meningitis, hydrocephalus, seizures, papilledema, and deforming arthropathy with periosteal changes and bony overgrowth [De Cunto et al., 1997]. In addition, children with this disorder may develop hearing loss, seizures, transient hemiplegia, cerebral atrophy, and an open fontanel, and the electroencephagram results may be abnormal. Long-term prognosis is poor [Prieur, 2000].

Enthesitis-Related and Undifferentiated Syndromes

Although primarily an intestinal disorder, inflammatory bowel disease may present with arthritis and neurologic symptoms. Published studies indicate that approximately 3% of children with inflammatory bowel disease had neurologic involvement during the course of the disease, including one child with myasthenia gravis and others with myopathy, peripheral neuropathy, venous sinus thrombosis, recurrent strokes, myelopathy, cranial neuropathy, seizures, headache, confusional states, meningitis, and syncope [Bridger et al., 1997; del Rosario et al., 1994; Lossos et al., 1995]. A syndrome has been described that includes ileocolonic lymphoid nodular hyperplasia, mild enterocolitis, and developmental delay with autistic features [Wakefield et al., 1998]. Recent reports and reviews have suggested that this disorder is associated with detection of measles virus in the intestinal mucosa of these children [Martin et al., 2002]. Causality has not been demonstrated [Murch et al., 2004]. Other than inflammatory bowel disease, the enthesitis-related syndromes have not been described with neurologic findings.

Patients with inflammatory bowel disease, psoriatic arthritis, and other enthesitis-related arthritides may develop inflammation of the uveal tract. These patients may experience acute episodes of uveitis with eye redness, pain, photophobia, and blurred vision. Prompt attention is required, and treatment with topical ophthalmic corticosteroids usually clears the inflammation. More recent studies and speculation have focused on the inverse situation; that is, the modulation of gastrointestinal inflammation by the nervous system and its chemical messengers [Anton and Shanahan, 1998; Murch, 1998]. It has become clear that both macrophages and lymphocytes bear receptors for various neuropeptides and central nervous system–relevant cytokines, growth factors, and hormone-regulating factors. Furthermore, substance P has emerged as an important mediator, not only of sensory signaling but also of mucosal inflammation. Finally, the absence of significant pain in patients with severe inflammatory bowel disease and consequent mucosal erosion has been linked to altered cortical localization of pain perception as determined by positron emission tomography [Anton and Shanahan, 1998].

ARTHRITIS ASSOCIATED WITH INFECTIOUS AGENTS

Acute Rheumatic Fever

Acute rheumatic fever is an inflammatory illness that follows group A beta-hemolytic streptococcal pharyngitis. The syndrome affects the heart valves, joints, central nervous system, skin, and subcutaneous tissues. Common clinical manifestations include migratory polyarthritis, fever, carditis, and, less frequently, Sydenham's chorea, subcutaneous nodules, and erythema marginatum. The modified Jones criteria, which were last revised in 1992, are used to confirm the diagnosis of acute rheumatic fever and call for the presence of a combination of two major and one minor criteria or one major and two minor criteria, as well as antibody evidence of preceding streptococcal infection (Box 73-2). In the case of isolated Sydenham's chorea, demonstration of preceding streptococcal infection may not always be possible, and in these cases is not a requirement for the diagnosis of acute rheumatic fever [Dajani et al., 1992].

Clinical Characteristics of Sydenham's Chorea

Involuntary, distal, purposeless rapid movements; hypotonia; weakness; and emotional lability characterize Sydenham's chorea. It may be associated with other manifestations of rheumatic fever, or "pure" chorea may appear as the sole manifestations of the disease. Isolated chorea represents 20% to 30% of acute rheumatic fever cases and occurs long after the pharyngitis has resolved, which makes the association with streptococcal infection difficult to demonstrate. Indeed, laboratory evidence of preceding streptococcal infection could not be demonstrated in 35% of children with Sydenham's chorea [Ayoub and Wannamaker, 1966]. Although the onset may be explosive, Sydenham's chorea may develop slowly and insidiously. Chorea may be misdiagnosed as an emotional disorder or as tics with irritability and decreased attention span. Chorea may also be confused with a central nervous system degenerative process, but this is more common in adults than in young children.

In adolescents, chorea occurs almost exclusively in females and may, on rare occasions, be associated with hemichorea or hemiparesis. The hemiparesis, which may be the initial manifestation of the disorder, has an unusual form

Box 73-2 Jones Criteria for Diagnosis of Acute Rheumatic Fever (Revised 1992)

Major*

Carditis: Murmur consistent with aortic regurgitation or mitral insufficiency; echocardiogram findings without significant auscultatory findings are not adequate
Chorea: May be the only manifestation; proof of prior streptococcal infection in only 80%
Erythema marginatum: Rare manifestation; never on the face; transient and migratory
Migratory polyarthritis: Almost always migratory, involving larger joints, responds within 48 hours to aspirin and usually resolves in 1 month
Subcutaneous nodules: Rare manifestation; nontender, on extensor surfaces, usually over elbows, wrists, knees, occipital region, or spinous processes

Minor

Fever: Usually greater than 39° C
Arthralgia: Consider if arthritis not present
Prolonged PR interval: Does not correlate with the development of carditis
Elevated erythrocyte sedimentation rate or C-reactive protein

Adapted from Dajani et al. and The Special Writing Group. Guidelines for the diagnosis of rheumatic fever. Jones Criteria, 1992 update. JAMA 1992; 268:2069.
*Prior episodes of acute rheumatic fever are not criteria; if a patient has had a prior attack of acute rheumatic fever, a new attack may be difficult to diagnose on the basis of changing carditis. In this setting, proof of recent streptococcal infection and either one major or one minor criterion may allow a presumptive diagnosis. Proof of recent streptococcal infection is necessary, except for isolated chorea.

of flaccidity combined with hypotonia and slow relaxation of deep tendon reflexes. Choreiform movements are abrupt and erratic without being rhythmic or repetitive, and usually subside during sleep. Face, hands, and feet are most commonly affected; facial movements include grimacing, frowning, grinning, and pouting. Children commonly are unable to sustain prolonged hand contraction, resulting in the "milkmaid" sign. In other patients, emotional lability, personality changes, restlessness, hyperactivity, irritability, and episodes of anger and tearfulness may herald the onset of chorea. Occasionally, typical "spooning" is observed with hyperextension of the hands [Stollerman, 1985]. Choreiform movements usually subside in 2 to 4 months but may persist for 1 year or more. Chorea and arthritis do not usually accompany each other in acute rheumatic fever; however, carditis frequently develops as the chorea is improving.

Rarely, acute rheumatic fever may be accompanied by other neurologic problems such as meningoencephalitis, encephalitis [Benda, 1948], seizures [Goldenberg et al., 1992], pseudotumor cerebri [Mitkov, 1961], papilledema [Chun et al., 1961], diplopia [Schieken et al., 1973], central retinal occlusion [Ling et al., 1969], transient intellectual loss [Gatti and Rosenheim, 1969], and acute psychosis [Wertheimer, 1961]. Combined, these complications occur in 3% to 5% of all patients.

Chorea, obsessive-compulsive disorder, tic disorder, and Tourette syndrome may all have a common autoimmune pathway. It has been reported that some children with chorea have obsessive-compulsive disorder, and that the obsessive-compulsive disorder resolves before or simultaneously with the resolution of the chorea [Swedo et al., 1993, 1998]. Additionally, an increased prevalence of obsessive-compulsive disorder has been noted in children with tics and Tourette syndrome. An increased prevalence of antineuronal antibodies, as well as increased levels of antistreptococcal antibodies, has been reported in all four of these diseases. It has been shown that in patients with chorea, obsessive-compulsive disorder, or tic disorder, there is an increased incidence of the histocompatability locus antigen marker D8/17, which has been reported more frequently in rheumatic fever patients [Allen et al., 1995; Murphy et al., 1997; Swedo, 1994; Swedo et al., 1997]. The acronym *PANDAS* (*p*ediatric *a*utoimmune *n*europsychiatric *d*isorders *a*ssociated with *s*treptococcal infections) has been suggested for some of these conditions in which there is a combination of behavioral problems, obsessive-compulsive behavior, and tics when associated with an antecedent group A beta-hemolytic streptococcal infection [Garvey et al., 1998]. Some studies refute the connection between group A beta-hemolytic streptococcal infection and obsessive-compulsive disorder with tics, citing evidence that although children with Sydenham's chorea have behavioral difficulties, they do not have an increased incidence of obsessive-compulsive disorder [Faustino et al., 2003]. Inattention was the most common behavioral disturbance found during the acute episodes in children with Sydenham's chorea.

Laboratory Findings in Sydenham's Chorea

Laboratory studies include serologic documentation of antecedent streptococcal infection with an antistreptolysin-O titer, demonstration of a prolonged PR interval on electrocardiogram, elevated C-reactive protein or erythrocyte sedimentation rate, and leukocytosis. Although throat culture may show group A beta-hemolytic streptococci, an elevated or increasing antistreptolysin-O titer is required. An elevated anti-DNase-B increases the sensitivity of an antistreptolysin-O titer alone from 80% to 95% and may be necessary, especially in isolated chorea, in which sensitivity may only be 65%. To exclude other conditions manifesting with chorea, patients may need additional diagnostic studies, including serum ceruloplasmin, thyroxine, calcium, and antinuclear antibody titers. In patients with Sydenham's chorea, electroencephalograms may demonstrate diffuse paroxysmal features and generalized or posterior slowing [Ganji et al., 1988]. Cerebrospinal fluid examinations and neuroimaging are rarely necessary. Of interest is the finding of antineuronal antibodies in the cerebrospinal fluid of patients with chorea [Swedo, 1994]. The specificity of these antibodies is not well known, and they are frequently documented in patients with central nervous system lupus [Bluestein, 1997].

A 3-year-old child with chorea was reported as having the first example of a persistently abnormal MRI, showing a cystic abnormality in the caudate and putamen [Emery and Vieco, 1997]. Subsequent longitudinal radiologic studies of patients with Sydenham's chorea demonstrated that although the majority of patients with this disorder have a normal brain MRI, those with abnormalities during the symptomatic period often continue to demonstrate these same abnormalities when the disease is clinically quiescent or resolved [Faustino et al., 2003]. Most patients with MRI abnormalities demonstrate abnormal signal intensity or cystic changes in the caudate nuclei; subcortical foci and multiple peripheral white matter foci of abnormal signal have also been reported [Emery and Vieco, 1997; Faustino et al., 2003; Robertson and Smith, 2002].

Pathology of Central Nervous System Involvement

Neuropathologic findings in acute rheumatic fever are rare. Rheumatic proliferative endarteritis is limited to the small cortical and meningeal vessels with spotty patches of gray matter degeneration [Halbreich et al., 1976].

Treatment of Sydenham's Chorea

All patients with acute rheumatic fever, including those whose only manifestation is chorea, should receive a 10-day course of penicillin or erythromycin. Prophylaxis with penicillin or sulfadiazine should be started immediately and continued at least until adulthood because of frequent reinfection and the risk of rheumatic heart disease with subsequent streptococcal pharyngitis. More specifically, when residual valvular disease exists, prophylaxis should continue for at least 10 years after the last episode and at least until age 40. If there is no residual valvular disease, the duration of treatment beyond 10 years or into adulthood is not clearly defined. When Sydenham's chorea is diagnosed and there is no valvular disease, the duration of prophylaxis should be at least 5 years or until age 21, whichever is longer [Dajani et al., 1995].

Children who develop chorea as the sole manifestation of acute rheumatic fever during the initial episode of illness have an approximate 50% risk of developing rheumatic heart disease with subsequent infection [Aron et al., 1965]. In addition, studies have suggested that in certain chorea-prone patients, recurrence of Sydenham's chorea may follow either undetectable streptococcal infection or another infectious trigger [Berrios et al., 1985].

Sydenham's chorea has been treated successfully with chlorpromazine, haloperidol [Shenker et al., 1973], phenobarbital, diazepam, valproic acid [Daoud et al., 1990], and corticosteroids [Green, 1978]. In mild cases, cyproheptadine may be effective. Other agents, such as clonidine, pimozide [Shannon and Fenichel, 1990], and corticosteroids [Faustino et al., 2002] may be beneficial in refractory cases. Complete recovery can be expected within 2 to 6 months, although some children may have residual motor, visuomotor, or cognitive dysfunction and a variety of neuropsychiatric manifestations [Bird et al., 1976; Faustino et al., 2002; Leonard et al., 1993; Stehbens and MacQueen, 1972; Swedo et al., 1989].

In some children with Sydenham's chorea, atlantoaxial subluxation may occur during the acute episode of chorea, with symptoms of neck stiffness, decreased mobility, and pain [Coster and Cole, 1990]. In such patients, differentiating this complication from juvenile rheumatoid arthritis may require further clinical and laboratory evaluation and specific orthopedic intervention. In rare instances, recurrences of chorea may occur in patients without evidence of rheumatic cardiac involvement decades after the childhood onset of symptoms [Gibb and Lees, 1989].

Lyme Disease

Lyme disease is an important cause of neurologic symptoms in children. The illness follows a tick bite and occurs in endemic areas during the summer months. The clinical course of Lyme disease is marked by stages similar to the course of syphilis, another spirochetal infection. The early stage begins with the tick bite and includes a flulike illness and the appearance of an oval, expanding rash at the site of the tick bite. At this stage, systemic infection with *Borrelia burgdorferi* may be documented by culture. Within several weeks, the patient may develop early neurologic manifestations, which most commonly include facial nerve palsy and aseptic meningitis but can also include other cranial neuropathies or transverse myelitis and can represent direct invasion of the organism into cerebrospinal fluid [Huisman et al., 1999]. Acute sinovenous thrombosis with consequent pseudotumor cerebri has been reported as well [Ansari et al., 2002]. The illness resolves spontaneously, but the resolution may be hastened by antibiotic treatment (amoxicillin or erythromycin in children younger than 9 years old and tetracycline in children age 9 years or older for 10 to 30 days).

Weeks to months later, the patient who was not treated with antibiotics may develop episodic arthritis of the large joints, primarily the knee. Characteristically, the knee becomes acutely effused, but not particularly tender or hot. The often dramatic joint swelling lasts for several days and resolves but returns multiple times if treatment with antibiotics is not started. The diagnosis may be confirmed after the first few weeks with a positive serum IgG titer against *B. burgdorferi.* Western blotting may be used to confirm the diagnosis if the titer is equivocal [Steere, 1989]. Polymerase chain reaction amplification of the *B. burgdorferi* genome in the cerebrospinal fluid is available as well [Ansari et al., 2002].

Years after the acute infection, some patients develop late neuroborreliosis. In children, this rare complication may manifest as a subtle encephalopathy with stuttering and memory disturbances. Adults may develop a multiple sclerosis–like illness, optic neuritis, seizures, and chronic meningitis. The diagnosis of late neuroborreliosis is confirmed by the demonstration of an elevated intrathecal IgG titer compared with serum titer. Treatment with intravenous ceftriaxone for 1 month to penetrate the blood-brain barrier is indicated, but the response is variable. There is no evidence that treatment lasting longer than 4 weeks is of additional benefit [Bingham et al., 1995; Logigian et al., 1990; Szer et al., 1991].

CONNECTIVE TISSUE DISORDERS

The key neurologic and laboratory findings in connective tissue disorders are summarized in Table 73-3 [Tan, 1986].

Systemic Lupus Erythematosus

Systemic lupus erythematosus is the second most common chronic rheumatic illness of children after juvenile idio-

TABLE 73-3

Key Neurologic and Laboratory Findings in Connective Tissue Diseases

DISEASE	NEUROLOGIC FINDINGS	LABORATORY FINDINGS
SLE	Encephalopathy, chorea, seizures, aseptic meningitis, psychosis, behavioral or cognitive dysfunction, headaches, strokes, neuropathy, myelitis	Elevated ANA, low C3 and C4, pancytopenia, hematuria, proteinuria, autoantibodies, LAC, elevated aCL
Scleroderma: coup-de-sabre deformity	Seizures, blurred vision, bulbar palsy, optic neuritis, trigeminal neuropathy	Elevated ANA and rheumatoid factor
Mixed connective tissue disease	Same as SLE	Same as SLE plus elevated anti-RNP, elevated CK
Sjögren's syndrome	Encephalopathy, optic neuritis, aseptic meningitis, recurrent paresis, myelopathy, neuropathy, autonomic dysfunction	Positive ANA, rheumatoid factor, antibodies to SSA/Ro and SSB/La

aCL, anticardiolipin antibody; ANA, antinuclear antibody; C3, third component of complement; C4, fourth component of complement; CK, creatine kinase; LAC, lupus anticoagulant; RNP, ribonucleoprotein; SLE, systemic lupus erythematosus.

pathic arthritis. At the time of initial presentation, approximately 3.5% of patients with systemic lupus erythematosus are younger than 10 years of age, and 28% are younger than 19 years of age. Approximately 80% of patients are female.

Revised criteria for the classification of systemic lupus erythematosus, developed by the American College of Rheumatology (Box 73-3), call for the presence of at least 4 of 11 specific criteria, including a positive test for antinuclear antibody. The antinuclear antibody alone is not sufficient to establish the diagnosis. It must be associated with multiorgan involvement. Arthritis, arthralgia, fever, and photosensitive rash are the most common initial complaints, with renal, cardiac, and neurologic involvement responsible for chronic disability. Lymphadenopathy, hepatosplenomegaly, pleural and pericardial effusions, pulmonary infiltrates, pericarditis, abdominal pain, and even peritonitis may be present at the time of initial evaluation [Cassidy and Petty, 2001; Szer and Jacobs, 1992].

Box 73-3 Revised Criteria for the Classification of Systemic Lupus Erythematosus (1982)

Seizures or psychosis
Serositis: Pleuritic pain, friction rub, effusion, or pericarditis
Arthritis: Two or more peripheral joints
Nephritis: Proteinuria > 500 mg/day or cellular casts
Malar rash
Oral or nasal ulcers
Discoid lupus rash
Photosensitive rash
Antinuclear antibody: In the absence of a drug known to be associated with drug-induced lupus syndrome
Hematologic disorder: Leukopenia <4000/mm on two or more occasions, or hemolytic anemia with reticulocytosis, or thrombocytopenia <100,000/mm in the absence of offending drugs, or lymphopenia <1500/mm on two or more occasions
Autoantibody: Anti-ds-DNA, anti-Sm, false-positive serologic test for syphilis, positive LAC, elevated aCL

aCL, anticardiolipin antibody; ds-DNA, double-stranded DNA; LAC, lupus anticoagulant; Sm, Smith.
Adapted from Tan EM, et al. Arthritis Rheum 1982;25:1271; and Hochberg MC. Arthritis Rheum 1997;40:1725.

Renal disease occurs in 60% to 80% of children. It may range from an active urinary sediment to clinical renal disease with varying degrees of involvement, including nephrotic syndrome and acute or chronic glomerulonephritis. In addition to an abnormal urinalysis, low serum complement levels, and high antibodies to double-stranded DNA, patients have a decreased glomerular filtration rate and abnormal renal biopsy.

Management of systemic lupus erythematosus is highly individual. Patients with minor organ disease are treated with relatively benign interventions, and children with major organ involvement who are at risk for organ failure are treated aggressively. A thorough evaluation of the extent and intensity of internal organ inflammation and injury dictates the subsequent choice of therapy. In general, acute worsening of organ-specific symptoms should be prevented, because each exacerbation may result in cumulative damage.

The prognosis for children with systemic lupus erythematosus has improved dramatically, with an estimated 10-year survival of 85% [Cassidy and Petty, 2001; Szer and Jacobs, 1992; Takei et al., 1997].

Neurologic Manifestations

Estimates of nervous system involvement in childhood systemic lupus erythematosus range from 20% to 45% [Parikh, 1995; Quintero-Del-Rio and Van Miller, 2000; Sibbitt, 2002; Steinlin et al., 1995]. Early reports in children with systemic lupus erythematosus suggested that central nervous system involvement was the second most common cause of death. More recently, the outcome of children with central nervous system lupus appears favorable, with most showing recovery [Parikh et al., 1995; Steinlin et al., 1995].

SEIZURES

Approximately 10% of children with systemic lupus erythematosus develop generalized and occasionally focal motor seizures [Parikh et al., 1995; Steinlin et al., 1995]. Seizures usually occur during the first year of illness and may be the initial manifestation of systemic lupus erythematosus, but they may occur at any stage. In patients with advanced renal disease, seizures may be secondary to hypertension, uremia, and electrolyte disturbances. Hypertensive encephalopathy may be the presenting symptom of systemic lupus erythematosus in children. After immunosuppressive treatment has begun, opportunistic infections of the central nervous system and cerebral edema may cause seizures. Electroencephalography may show multifocal paroxysmal sharp-wave or slow-wave activity or, in rare instances, focal abnormalities. Quantitative electroencephalograms may show relatively specific changes [Ritchlin et al., 1992].

NEUROPSYCHIATRIC LUPUS

Neuropsychiatric symptoms associated with childhood systemic lupus erythematosus include depression, emotional lability, confusion, headache, anxiety, personality changes, acute psychosis, and progressive dementia. It is estimated that approximately 25% of children with lupus will develop such symptoms; of these patients, approximately 20% to 30% will manifest them as the first symptom of the disease [Parikh et al., 1995; Steinlin et al., 1995]. Depression generally occurs early in the illness, whereas psychosis is observed in later stages. Depression typically is associated with reaction to the serious nature of the disease, to the stress of repeated hospitalizations, and to adolescent concerns about body image and peer rejection. Memory loss, disorientation, impaired cognitive function, and symptoms suggestive of an affective disorder with unusual elation or irritability have also been observed [Silber et al., 1984]. Preexisting psychiatric disorders may be exacerbated during the course of systemic lupus erythematosus [Sergent et al., 1975]. Although they may prove beneficial, antidepressant or antianxiety agents have unpredictable side effects. Acute emotional disturbances may be severe, but the ultimate prognosis may be excellent [Parikh et al., 1995; Steinlin et al., 1995].

In patients who are receiving chronic, intensive therapy for systemic lupus erythematosus, neuropsychiatric lupus can be difficult to distinguish from steroid psychosis. Serum and cerebrospinal fluid studies may be helpful in making this distinction, but in some cases, only close observation of the response to an increase in corticosteroid dose or substitution with cyclophosphamide may crystallize the differential diagnosis [Schor, 2000].

HEADACHE

Headaches are common in children and adolescents with systemic lupus erythematosus [Parikh et al., 1995; Steinlin et al., 1995]. Headache usually occurs during exacerbation of systemic symptoms and frequently is associated with other neurologic symptoms. Unless objective neurologic symptoms are present, the diagnostic workup may yield few abnormalities, although evaluation for a hypertensive encephalopathy should be considered [Parikh et al., 1995; Steinlin et al., 1995]. Most patients will respond to increased dosages of corticosteroids.

In a prospective study of adult patients with systemic lupus erythematosus, it was found that vascular headache developed in 26% of adult patients, and muscle contraction headache in 40% [Vazquez-Cruz et al., 1990].

CHOREA

Chorea occurs in perhaps 5% of children with systemic lupus erythematosus and is the initial symptom in 25% to 30% of patients who present with neurologic symptoms [Herd et al., 1978]. Systemic lupus manifestations often occur within 1 year of onset; rarely, a prolonged latent interval may ensue after the onset of chorea [Parikh et al., 1995; Steinlin et al., 1995]. Approximately 50% of children with lupus chorea develop other central nervous system manifestations, including seizures and neuropsychiatric disturbances. Chorea has also been associated with thromboembolic disease and elevated anticardiolipin antibody [Besbas et al., 1994].

REYE-LIKE SYNDROME

A Reye-like syndrome associated with acetylsalicylic acid treatment of systemic lupus erythematosus has been recognized [Hansen et al., 1985]. Salicylate hepatocellular injury appears to be relatively common in patients with rheumatic disorders, but its relation to Reye's syndrome has raised the possibility of some other etiologic relation between salicylate therapy, various rheumatic disorders, and idiopathic Reye's syndrome. This syndrome has not been seen with other nonsteroidal anti-inflammatory agents.

CEREBROVASCULAR DISEASE

Although it is unusual for a cerebrovascular syndrome to be the initial manifestation of systemic lupus erythematosus, approximately 3% of children develop cerebrovascular occlusive disease that results in hemiplegia, aphasia, or sensory and visual impairments [Parikh et al., 1995; Steinlin et al., 1995]. Most of these patients have serious renal, cardiac, pulmonary, or hematologic disease with hypertension or thrombocytopenia. Even if there is recurrent hemiplegia, significant recovery may occur. Antiphospholipid antibody has been associated with thrombosis in systemic lupus erythematosus, especially when lupus anticoagulant is present [Levy et al., 2003]. Alternatively, thrombotic or thromboembolic disease may be due to a vasculopathy with or without autoimmunity, atheromatous disease, valvular disease, or vasculitis [Bruyn, 1995; West, 1994]. Additionally, in adults it has been reported that elevated homocysteine levels increase the risk of atherothrombotic events [Petri et al., 1996].

A recent case report indicates that perivenous inflammation with secondary calcification may occur in systemic lupus erythematosus. This postmortem finding was preceded by computed tomography (CT) and MRI evidence of foci of breakdown of the blood-brain barrier, calcifications, and a clinical picture consistent with focal vascular dysfunction and diffuse encephalopathy [Matsumoto et al., 1998].

Multifocal cerebral dysfunction with patchy areas of altered signal intensity on MRI have been interpreted as acute vascular lesions associated with pulse steroid therapy in patients with systemic lupus erythematosus. This syndrome responds well to substitution of cyclophosphamide for pulse methylprednisolone, and, as such, it is imperative that it be promptly recognized [Tabata et al., 2002].

HYPERTENSIVE ENCEPHALOPATHY

Headache, seizures, coma, and focal ischemic central nervous system injury have been reported as manifestations of hypertensive encephalopathy associated with lupus nephritis [Cassidy et al., 1977]. Although the mechanism of this encephalopathy is unknown, controlling blood pressure and treatment with corticosteroids frequently result in substantial neurologic improvement.

CRANIAL NERVE, BRAINSTEM, AND SPINAL CORD DYSFUNCTION

Ophthalmoplegia, ptosis, diplopia, facial numbness, vertigo, sensorineural hearing loss [Hisashi et al., 1993], vocal cord paralysis [Teitel et al., 1992], and ataxia have been described in children with systemic lupus erythematosus. Brainstem involvement is usually observed in conjunction with other nervous system symptoms such as chorea and seizures [Gold and Yahr, 1960].

Approximately 6% of children with systemic lupus erythematosus manifest visual symptoms, which include blurred vision, sudden blindness, and field loss [Brandt et al., 1975]. Retinal hemorrhages, cotton wool exudates, papilledema, optic neuritis, and cytoid bodies have all been reported [Cassidy et al., 1977; Hackett et al., 1974]. Retinal artery occlusion may also occur, with resulting transient or permanent visual loss. Papilledema associated with pseudotumor cerebri caused by either the disease or corticosteroid therapy has also been reported [Green et al., 1995]. If papilledema is present, the possible presence of increased pressure or a mass lesion should be assessed before lumbar puncture is performed [Brandt et al., 1975; Carlow and Glaser, 1974]. Patients with either retinal artery occlusion or papilledema should be treated with high doses of corticosteroids after elimination of structural or occlusive cerebrovascular disease.

Transverse myelopathy that causes both paraplegia and sensory loss as the initial or late neurologic manifestations of systemic lupus erythematosus has been reported [Andrianakos et al., 1975; Meislin and Rothfield, 1968]. Other studies in adults have shown an association with antiphospholipid antibodies [Kovacs et al., 1993]. Early treatment with high doses of corticosteroids alone or in combination with cyclophosphamide has been used, but improvement was variable [Berlanga et al., 1992; Boumpas et al., 1990; Chan and Boey, 1996; Propper and Bucknall, 1989].

CENTRAL NERVOUS SYSTEM INFECTIONS

Infection of the central nervous system in children with systemic lupus erythematosus is relatively rare [Cassidy and Petty, 2001; Fish et al., 1977; Walravens and Chase, 1976]. Bacterial meningitis, opportunistic bacterial infection, and fungal meningitis (aspergillosis, nocardiosis, and cryptococcosis) have been reported. Brain abscess may be difficult to differentiate from a multifocal vasculitis, but differentiation may be facilitated by using serial CT scans and angiography. Multiple abscesses of the central nervous system may be relatively silent; if suspected, broad-spectrum antimicrobial or antifungal therapy should be instituted after appropriate cultures are obtained.

LUPUS ASEPTIC MENINGITIS

The syndrome of lupus aseptic meningitis, accompanied by a sterile cerebrospinal fluid lymphocytic pleocytosis, may be manifested by nuchal rigidity, fever, and headache and may occur early in childhood lupus. This syndrome has been reported in association with nonsteroidal anti-inflammatory drugs and trimethoprim-sulfamethoxazole use [Escalante and Stimmler, 1992]. Clinical manifestations and cerebrospinal fluid abnormalities may persist for several weeks before resolving spontaneously. Therapy with corticosteroids may improve this condition, but the data are inconclusive because of the self-limited course [Canoso and Cohen, 1975; Keefe et al., 1974].

PERIPHERAL NERVOUS SYSTEM INVOLVEMENT

Involvement of the peripheral nervous system occurs in approximately 5% of children with systemic lupus erythematosus. Peripheral neuropathies with symptoms consisting of paresthesias, numbness, and distal weakness are usually relatively mild in severity and course, although severe forms of acute lumbosacral plexopathies have been reported [Bailey et al., 1956; Jacob, 1963]. Neuropathy manifesting as either mononeuritis multiplex or acute demyelinating polyneuropathy may occur at any time during systemic lupus erythematosus, may recur, and generally worsens when central nervous system involvement is greater. Polyradiculoneuropathy may mimic Guillain-Barré syndrome in children; however, this pattern is extremely rare [Norris et al., 1977; Robson et al., 1994].

MYOPATHY

Myositis is rare in systemic lupus erythematosus, although myalgias and generalized weakness are common. Myositis can be distinguished from corticosteroid-related myopathy by demonstrating elevated levels of muscle enzymes, electromyography consistent with myopathic and fibrillation activity, and lack of vacuolization in muscle biopsies. One case report demonstrated pyridostigmine-responsive myasthenia gravis complicating childhood systemic lupus erythematosus [Nishimura et al., 1997]. Although children with myasthenia gravis may have circulating serum antinuclear antibodies, clinical systemic lupus erythematosus is highly unusual.

DRUG-INDUCED LUPUS SYNDROME.

Many drugs have been reported to induce a lupus-like syndrome in children and adults [Rubin, 1997]. In general, this disorder is milder than spontaneous systemic lupus erythematosus and occurs with equal frequency in males and females [Totoritis and Rubin, 1985]. Arthritis, pneumonitis, and pericarditis are common, whereas rashes and alopecia are less frequent. Hepatosplenomegaly, lymphadenopathy, and acute pancreatitis may occur in some patients; renal disease appears less often [Rubin, 1997]. Procainamide, hydralazine, and isoniazid are the three drugs that have most commonly induced this syndrome. These drugs share a primary amine or hydrazine portion that is acetylated by the *N*-acetyl transferase system of the liver in two different phenotypic expressions [Rubin, 1997]. The risk of a drug-induced syndrome appears to be much greater in the "slow" acetylators than in the "fast" acetylators.

Antiepileptic drugs and phenothiazines have also been associated with a drug-induced lupus syndrome. Antiepileptic drugs reported to cause this disorder in children include phenytoin, ethosuximide, carbamazepine, and trimethadione [Rubin, 1997; Singsen et al., 1976]. Although children receiving these drugs are usually asymptomatic, approximately 20% of them produce antinuclear antibodies; these children commonly have normal immunoglobulin and serum complement levels and remain free of a clinical lupus-like syndrome. Antiepileptic medication therefore may be continued [Singsen et al., 1976]. Among patients in whom antiepileptic drugs have been discontinued, the presence of antinuclear antibodies may remain for several years.

Recurrent seizures in patients whose initial seizures were well controlled suggest a drug-induced lupus-like syndrome. Moreover, when increasingly higher drug doses produce increased seizure activity, an antinuclear antibody study is appropriate. Although the antinuclear antibody is positive in both systemic and drug-induced systemic lupus erythematosus, specific antihistone antibodies are associated with drug-induced disease, whereas anti-double-stranded DNA tends to be elevated in systemic lupus erythematosus. Discontinuing or substituting other antiepileptic drugs dramatically reduces seizure activity in some patients. Only rarely will corticosteroids be necessary for seizure control.

Drug-induced systemic lupus erythematosus has been associated with etanercept therapy in a child with juvenile idiopathic arthritis [Lepore et al., 2003].

Laboratory Findings

Laboratory features of systemic lupus erythematosus commonly include a positive antinuclear antibody titer, low C3 and C4 levels, leukopenia, direct Coombs-positive hemolytic anemia, hematuria, and proteinuria. Abnormal autoantibodies may include antibody to double-stranded DNA, Sm (Smith), RNP (ribonucleoprotein), Ro (or SSA), La (or SSB), and anticardiolipin. In addition, there may be a paradoxical prolongation of the partial thromboplastin time because of antiphospholipid antibodies. Antibodies to antiphospholipid may also produce a biological false-positive rapid plasma reagin (RPR) or VDRL (Venereal Disease Research Laboratories). In adults a strong correlation between MRI changes and the presence of a positive lupus anticoagulant or anticardiolipin antibody exists, but there is no clear correlation with neuropsychiatric disease [Ishikawa et al., 1994; Manco-Johnson and Nuss, 1995; Molad et al., 1992; Toubi et al., 1995]. Pediatric case reports have also been published showing some correlation between disease and antiphospholipid antibodies as demonstrated by one of these tests [Steinlin et al., 1995; von Scheven et al., 1996]. Elevated lupus anticoagulant (LAC) appears to confer a significant increased risk of arterial or venous thrombotic events [Galli et al., 2003]. Anticardiolipin IgG fraction and anti-β_2-glycoprotein I antibodies may also correlate, but their association is less certain [Galli et al., 2003].

Several mechanisms explaining the pathogenesis of central nervous system lupus have been reported [Bruyn, 1995]. In most patients with documented central nervous system lupus, evidence of immune-mediated abnormalities cannot be found, suggesting multifactorial causes of central nervous system disease. Interestingly, one study found that approximately 75% of observed neurologic events were attributed to metabolic, hematologic, or infectious factors rather than to the primary disease process [Kaell et al., 1986]. Serum complement and autoantibody levels may remain normal. The cerebrospinal fluid is often benign, and imaging modalities are of little value unless there is an ischemic event [Hirohata et al., 1985; Szer and Jacobs, 1992]. However, cerebrospinal fluid examination is often necessary to rule out infectious causes.

In support of a diagnosis of immune disease, studies of cerebrospinal fluid immunoglobulin production have documented elevations of IgG, IgG/albumin ratio, and the cerebrospinal fluid IgG index and the presence of oligoclonal IgG, suggesting accelerated central nervous system IgG synthesis. Further support for immune-mediated disease may be found in the relatively high incidence of antineuronal and antiribosomal P antibody in some children with systemic lupus erythematosus [Reichlin, 2003; Silverman, 1996; West et al., 1995]; however, antiribosomal P was not found to be sensitive for neuropsychiatric manifestations of systemic lupus erythematosus in another series [Press et al., 1996]. In addition, endothelial or vascular injury may be a complement-mediated immunologic insult, because the choroid plexus has been reported as the deposition site of complement and immune complexes; cerebrospinal fluid C4 also appears to be reduced [Hadler et al., 1973; Sher and Pertschuk, 1974]. In addition, cerebrospinal fluid anti-double-stranded DNA complexes and lymphocytotoxic antibodies have been documented in central nervous system lupus [Bluestein, 1997; Carr et al., 1975]. Serial cerebrospinal fluid C4 complement levels may help to distinguish between neuropsychiatric symptoms caused by corticosteroids and those caused by systemic lupus erythematosus. A serial decrease in C4 complement level suggests increased disease activity rather than a drug-induced phenomenon. More recent studies demonstrate moderate levels of interleukin-6 in neuropsychiatric systemic lupus erythematosus. The significance of this finding must be interpreted with caution because significantly high levels of interleukin-6 may be found in central nervous system infection [Tsai et al., 1994]. At present, cerebrospinal fluid findings cannot reliably confirm the diagnosis of neuropsychiatric symptoms associated with central nervous system lupus.

False-positive elevation of antistreptococcal antibody titers can occur in lupus chorea and may incorrectly result in the diagnosis of Sydenham's chorea unless antinuclear antibody titers are obtained. Serum complement is decreased in lupus chorea, but cerebrospinal fluid complement, anti-double-stranded DNA antibody titers, and immunoglobulin synthesis have not been studied [Kukla et al., 1978]. In adults, a significant correlation exists between chorea and the presence of antiphospholipid antibodies [Asherson et al., 1987]. This association has also been reported in children [Besbas et al., 1994].

In patients with transverse myelopathy, cerebrospinal fluid analysis may demonstrate increased protein concentration, decreased glucose, and a monocytic pleocytosis [Al-Husaini and Jamal, 1985].

Neurodiagnostic Testing

Neuroimaging with either CT or MRI scans is essential for evaluating the patient with systemic lupus erythematosus who is suspected of having intracranial disease [Carette

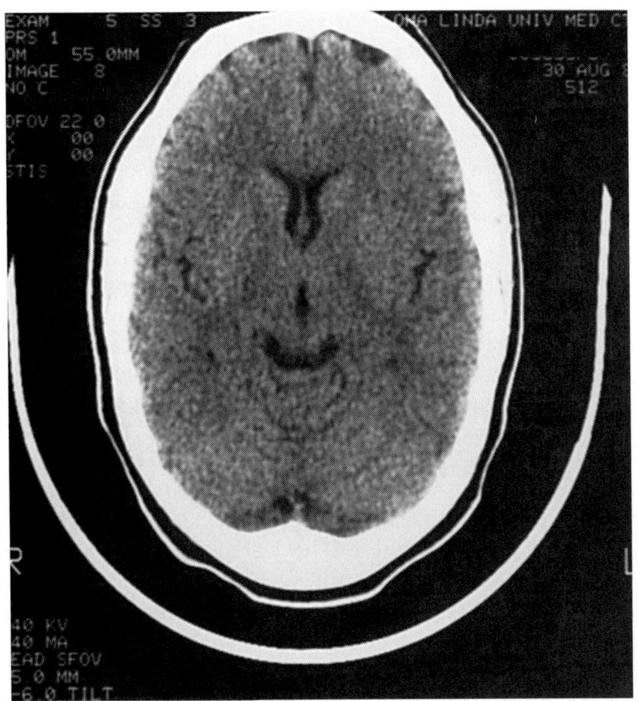
A

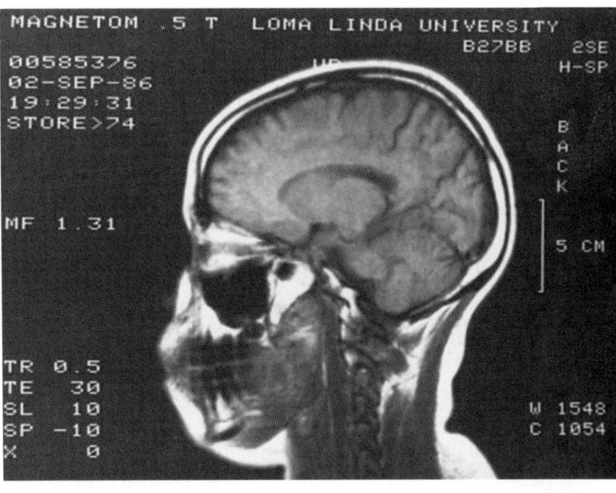

B

FIGURE 73-1. **A,** CT scan of a 14-year-old female with systemic lupus erythematosus, isolated seizures, depressed affect, and intellectual impairment. Cortical atrophy is prominent. **B,** T1-weighted MRI in sagittal plane of same patient, demonstrating mild enlargement of the frontoparietal sulci, indicative of atrophy. (**A,** Courtesy of Dr. Joseph Thompson, and **B,** Courtesy of Dr. David B. Hinshaw, Jr., Department of Neuroradiology, Loma Linda University Children's Hospital.)

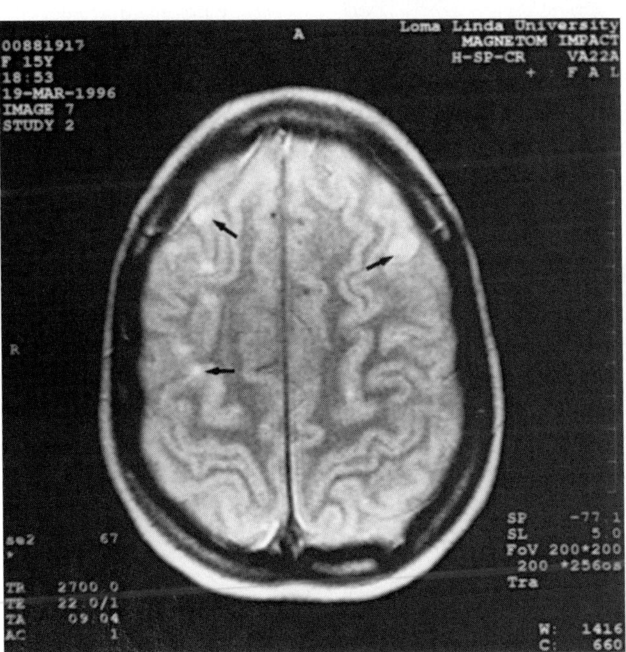

FIGURE 73-2. MRI of a 15-year-old female with systemic lupus erythematosus who developed seizures, depression, generalized weakness, and severe membranous nephritis. Proton density–weighted axial MR image through the high frontal region shows multiple bright cortical lesions (*arrows*; more lesions are visible than those marked). The lesions represent acute microinfarctions that result from small segmental leptomeningeal and parenchymal artery thromboses. With gadolinium, these microinfarctions tend to enhance in the subacute phase. (Courtesy of Dr. Joseph Thompson, Department of Neuroradiology, Loma Linda University Children's Hospital.)

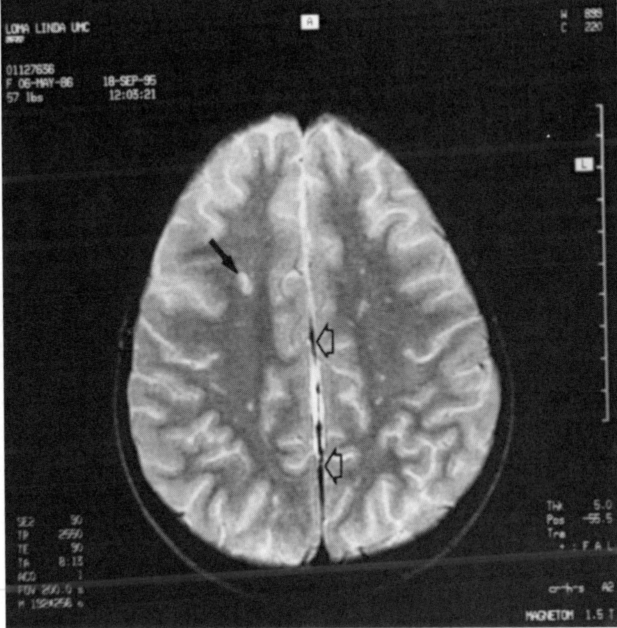

FIGURE 73-3. MRI of a 9-year-old female with systemic lupus erythematosus who had fever, leukopenia, abdominal pain, worsening headache, and cardiomyopathy. A T2-weighted axial image through the centrum semiovale above the lateral ventricles shows multiple bright white matter foci (largest labeled with *arrow*) and intrafalcial hemorrhage *(arrowheads)*. No cortical lesions are discerned. Focal T2 lengthening is somewhat nonspecific as to whether it results from demyelination, microvascular infarction, edema, or more probably a combination of these. Cerebral falx hemorrhage is characterized by a black appearance on T2-weighted images of deoxyhemoglobin and bright adjacent methemoglobin or serum. (Courtesy of Dr. Joseph Thompson, Department of Neuroradiology, Loma Linda University Children's Hospital.)

et al., 1982; Provenzale et al., 1994]. Such studies may show atrophy (Fig. 73-1), infarction (Fig. 73-2), low-density lesions in the cerebral white matter (Fig. 73-3) [Isshi et al., 1994], or hemorrhage [Aisen et al., 1985; Kovacs et al., 1993]. MR angiography or venography may detect sinovenous thrombosis [Steinlin et al., 1995]. Cerebral angiography may be helpful in further differentiating arterial thrombotic from embolic disease but may be normal in children because small vessel arterial changes may not be demonstrable [Jones et al., 1975]. MRI has been used to detect myelopathy in a child as young as 5 years of age [Vieira et al., 2002].

Single-photon emission computed tomography (SPECT) is a sensitive tool for demonstrating diffuse and multiple perfusion abnormalities in children and adults with central nervous system events (Fig. 73-4). Unfortunately, the usefulness of SPECT is limited. It is not specific for central nervous system lupus, and longitudinal assessment with this modality correlates poorly with clinical status [Szer et al., 1993].

Treatment of Neurologic Manifestations

Treatment of the neurologic complications seen in children with systemic lupus erythematosus can be categorized as follows.

Treatment of generalized symptoms requires controlling the underlying inflammatory disorder, correcting metabolic or systemic abnormalities such as hypertension, and administering specific symptom-directed medications such as antiepileptic drugs for the treatment of seizures; analgesic medications for headache; antidepressants, sedatives or tranquilizers, or antipsychotic agents for specific psychiatric symptoms; and dopamine blocking agents for the treatment of chorea. Commonly used antiepileptic drugs in children with seizures associated with systemic lupus erythematosus include phenobarbital, phenytoin, diazepam, lorazepam, valproate, and carbamazepine. Antiepileptic drug use should not be prolonged unnecessarily; discontinuation should be considered when the primary disease is well controlled. In moderate doses, corticosteroids do seem to have beneficial effects in studies of adults with mood or cognitive disorders, suggesting that these are often secondary to neuropsychiatric disease [Carbotte et al., 1995]. However, corticosteroids have also been associated with a variety of behavioral and mood disorders and with psychosis, although the mechanism of this toxic response is unknown. Treatment of lupus chorea with haloperidol, chlorpromazine, valproate, or corticosteroids is usually successful in conjunction with treatment of the underlying disorder.

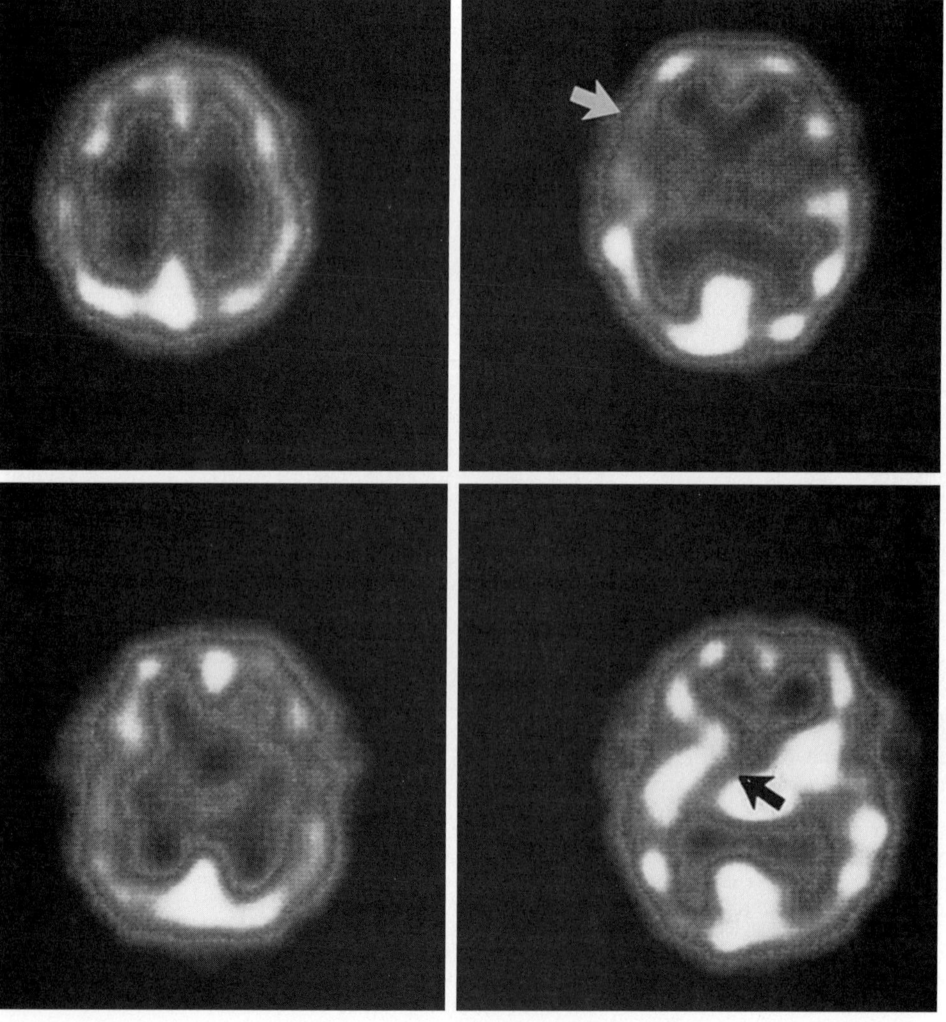

FIGURE 73-4. Representative single-photon emission CT study of a 14-year-old male with systemic lupus erythematosus and acute onset of optic neuritis and transverse myelitis. The study was done immediately after the onset of central nervous system symptoms and shows bilateral cerebral hemisphere decreased perfusion defects in the right frontal region *(white arrow)* and in the right basal ganglia *(black arrow)* compatible with antecedent ischemia. (Courtesy of Dr. M.T. Parisi, Department of Radiology, Children's Hospital of Los Angeles.)

Treatment of central nervous system infection depends on the infectious agent causing the central nervous system disease. The infection will necessitate a diminution of the immunosuppressive therapy until the infection is controlled. Evaluation for central nervous system infection may be indicated in patients in whom the history or clinical examination suggests systemic infection that may have spread to the central nervous system or in patients in whom no definite explanation for their central nervous system symptoms can be determined. A high index of suspicion for fungal infection must be maintained. MRI and cerebrospinal fluid examination provide the most accurate and sensitive methods for such an evaluation.

Anticoagulation may be considered in patients with ischemic cerebrovascular insults who have antiphospholipid antibodies, because there is a significant risk for recurrent thrombotic episodes [Bruyn, 1995; Khamashta et al., 1995]. Agents used in adults have included acetylsalicylic acid, heparin, and warfarin. In adults, prevention of recurrent venous thrombosis may require doses of warfarin with an international normalized ratio of 2 to 3 [Meroni et al., 2003]. It is unclear, even in studies of adults with arterial thromboembolic disease, if anticoagulation is effective, even with a higher international normalized ratio [Brey et al., 2003]. Because of the small number of children with systemic lupus erythematosus with such events, it is unlikely that controlled clinical studies will be completed. Given the nature of children's activities and the reports of hemorrhage in children without systemic lupus erythematosus but with a lupus-type anticoagulant [Becton and Stine, 1997], it might be suspected that the risk of serious or life-threatening hemorrhage would be greater than in adults. Various alternative regimens have been recommended in children [Ravelli and Martini, 1997; Silverman, 1996]. Steroids have not been found to alter the pathology of antiphospholipid manifestations. It is imperative that patients with hypertension and thrombocytopenia do not receive anticoagulants because of the potential risk of central nervous system hemorrhage. Patients on long-term steroid therapy for systemic lupus erythematosus who also require anticoagulation must be monitored for the increased risk of gastrointestinal bleeding.

Immunosuppressive therapy with corticosteroids has proved to be the mainstay of treatment for patients with neuropsychiatric symptoms or symptoms associated with vasculitis [Hammer and Saltissi, 1986; Sanna et al., 2003]. High-dose steroids have also been used for the treatment of coma, seizures, chorea, and transverse myelitis [Chan and Boey, 1996; Eyanson et al., 1980; Harisdangkul et al., 1995; West, 1994]. Adverse neuropsychiatric effects, such as psychosis or vacuolar myopathy, seen with high doses or chronic administration of corticosteroids are unusual [Wysenbeek et al., 1990].

Cytotoxic agents such as mycophenolate [Buratti et al., 2001; Contreras et al., 2004; Kapitsinou et al., 2004] or cyclophosphamide are used in patients with serious renal or neurologic disease. Candidates for such treatment include those who have evidence of diffuse proliferative glomerulonephritis and those with central nervous system lupus or myelopathy who are refractory to corticosteroids. Because there are no prospective controlled trials comparing different immunosuppressive and cytotoxic modalities in the various central nervous system lupus disorders, it is difficult to feel confident about a specific therapeutic regimen [Berlanga et al., 1992; Neuwelt et al., 1995; Propper and Bucknall, 1989]. Whereas mycophenolate is increasingly being used in steroid-resistant major organ disease and diffuse proliferative lupus nephritis, there are no data about the effectiveness of azathioprine or mycophenolate in central nervous system lupus.

Central Nervous System Pathology

Neuropathologic studies of childhood and adult systemic lupus erythematosus are rare, and available reports document a variety of abnormalities. Foci of acute cortical and cerebellar encephalomalacia with neuronal loss and demyelination have been described [Gold and Yahr, 1960; Smith et al., 1994]. Postmortem examination reports of adults who have died from central nervous system lupus have documented diffuse microthrombi and demyelination [Hanly et al., 1992]. Vascular changes have also included vasculitis. Proliferative intimal changes, fibrinoid degeneration, and perivascular inflammation in cerebral arterial vessels have been reported in older studies, but have rarely been observed in recent investigations, suggesting that therapy may have altered the pathologic findings. These vascular changes are less frequent in children than in adults [Walravens and Chase, 1976].

Segmental small artery involvement with leptomeningeal and parenchymal thrombosis may occur, as well as venous sinus thrombosis [Falko et al., 1979; Steinlin et al., 1995]. These individuals have both occlusion and recanalization of vessels without changes in the media and adventitia, suggesting that the cerebrovascular lesions in systemic lupus erythematosus may result from processes acting at the endothelial-blood interface [Smith et al., 1994]. Intravascular coagulation and occlusion may be the primary mechanisms responsible for microinfarction [Falko et al., 1979]. More recent neuropathologic studies in adults implicate platelet thrombi, possibly mediated by antiphospholipid antibodies [Ellison et al., 1993]. Other studies, which do not document vascular involvement, suggest a role for antineuronal antibody-mediated damage in adults with systemic lupus erythematosus [Bluestein, 1997; Kuroe et al., 1994].

A review of the histopathologic studies of lupus patients with chorea rarely indicated abnormalities of the basal ganglia [Kuroe et al., 1994], but there were other central nervous system changes in these patients, such as microinfarction [Kovacs et al., 1993; Penn and Rowan, 1968].

Some neuropathologic studies of patients with peripheral neuropathies have revealed, although rarely, focal areas of necrosis in small arteries supplying nerve bundles, as well as perivascular inflammatory changes, fibrinous exudates, and thrombus formation. Adult patients with myelopathy exhibited large spinal cord infarcts, spinal cord subdural hematoma, and subpial leukomyelopathy [Provenzale and Bouldin, 1992].

Scleroderma

Scleroderma in children occurs in two clinically distinct forms: localized and systemic. Localized scleroderma is further subdivided into morphea, generalized morphea, linear scleroderma, and coup-de-sabre lesions. Coup-de-sabre lesions present as linear sclerodermatous changes of the head or oral cavity. Because there may be underlying central nervous system changes, this form of scleroderma is the most important neurologic finding in children. Systemic scleroderma is subdivided into progressive systemic sclerosis and a generally milder syndrome termed CREST (*c*alcinosis, *R*aynaud's phenomenon, *e*sophageal dysmotility, *s*clerodactyly, and *t*elangiectasia) [Lehman, 1996].

Localized scleroderma is a chronic disorder that generally is not associated with systemic symptoms, except for the coup-de-sabre deformity. Local sequelae of linear scleroderma may include linear growth abnormalities when the process causes joint limitations secondary to local scarring. There have been very rare reports of localized scleroderma progressing to systemic scleroderma [Cassidy and Petty, 2001].

Progressive systemic sclerosis in childhood is a multisystem disease manifesting with progressive hardening of the skin and subcutaneous tissues, with involvement of the gastrointestinal tract, joints, heart, lungs, and kidneys [Uziel et al., 1995]. Children tend to have fewer signs and laboratory parameters of vascular disease compared with adults [Vancheeswaran et al., 1996], but generally the disease is the same [Kornreich et al., 1977; Martinez-Cordero et al., 1993]. Raynaud's phenomenon, severe cardiac and pulmonary disease with congestive heart failure, pulmonary interstitial fibrosis, pulmonary vascular sclerosis, and renal sclerosis with acute renal failure contribute significantly to the mortality associated with this disorder. Although the two disorders may be difficult to differentiate clinically, the CREST syndrome is generally thought to be milder than progressive systemic sclerosis and carries a more favorable prognosis. Systemic sclerosis may have all of the features of the CREST syndrome but is characterized by more severe internal organ involvement [Cassidy and Petty, 2001]. Skin biopsy is diagnostic, demonstrating increased thickness and density of the dermal collagen beneath the epidermis, with scattered foci of perivascular mononuclear cell infiltrate and no evidence of immune complex deposition in any affected organs, including the kidney. Radiographic assessment often demonstrates subcutaneous calcinosis, joint effusions, and diminished esophageal peristalsis. Pulmonary function studies reveal decreased lung diffusion capacity, and echocardiography may document pericardial effusion or pulmonary hypertension.

Neurologic Manifestations

Children with the coup-de-sabre form of localized scleroderma are at risk for central nervous system involvement [Appenzeller et al., 2004]. Progressive facial and scalp lesions may be associated with seizures, blurred vision, diplopia, and contralateral weakness. Vasculitis of small and medium-sized cerebral vessels ipsilateral to the skin lesions has been documented by angiography. A case study with neuropathology has suggested that this may not be a form of central nervous system vasculitis but rather a neurocutaneous syndrome with vascular dysgenesis [Chung et al., 1995].

Periarticular muscle atrophy, common in children with systemic scleroderma, may be attributed to both disuse and subtle myopathic involvement. Muscle biopsy demonstrates findings of a mixed neuromyopathy with group atrophy, suggesting vascular neuropathic involvement as one of the mechanisms associated with the primary disease [Clements et al., 1978]. Despite elevation of creatine kinase activity in 33% of patients with scleroderma, muscle atrophy is rare [Dabich et al., 1974], but clinical weakness is frequent, particularly during the early inflammatory phase of the illness. MRI may be useful in the localization of suspected muscle disease in patients with scleroderma [Olsen et al., 1996].

Children with progressive systemic sclerosis generally do not have primary central nervous system involvement, although cerebral hemorrhage secondary to thrombocytopenia has been reported [Gordon and Silverstein, 1970; Kornreich et al., 1977].

Although neurologic manifestations have been reported rarely in adults with scleroderma, some reviewers [Cerinic et al., 1996; Hietaharju et al., 1993] have argued that these manifestations may be more common than originally believed and include neuropsychiatric symptoms, bulbar palsy, optic neuritis, trigeminal neuropathy, mononeuritis multiplex, and polyneuropathy. There is no consensus regarding treatment of these complications. Of interest is a recent study that demonstrated cerebral hypoperfusion on SPECT scans in half of the neurologically asymptomatic adults with progressive systemic sclerosis [Nobili et al., 2002]. This hypoperfusion is hypothesized to be the result of a noninflammatory microangiopathy that has its origins in endothelial cell damage and dysfunction.

Laboratory Findings

Laboratory evaluation should include determination of antinuclear antibody titers, immunoglobulins, erythrocyte sedimentation rate, rheumatoid factor, and creatine kinase activity. A mild elevation of serum immunoglobulins may be present, and there may be markers of inflammation. Patients with progressive systemic sclerosis may have antibodies to DNA topoisomerase 1 (Scl-70) or RNA polymerase I, II, or III (RNAPs). Patients with the CREST syndrome may have an anticentromere antibody. Approximately 27% of children with progressive systemic sclerosis have Scl-70 antibodies [Vancheeswaran et al., 1996], compared with 14% to 77% of adults, whereas an uncertain number of children with the CREST syndrome have anticentromere antibody, compared with 44% to 98% of adults [Okano, 1996].

Treatment

Treatment of progressive systemic scleroderma is largely supportive, and management of the underlying disease is often not successful. Initial management includes a course of corticosteroids to improve weakness associated with myopathy. D-Penicillamine was initially reported as beneficial for skin fibrosis but generally has not been associated with improvement [Murray and Laxer, 2002]. There has been anecdotal support for the use of steroids and methotrexate in combination for the treatment of linear scleroderma [Uziel et al., 2000]. Raynaud's phenomenon should be treated with calcium channel blockers such as nifedipine or amlodipine. Gastrointestinal symptoms may be relieved by bethanechol chloride, Reglan, or cisapride [Pope, 1996]. Occupational and physical therapy is the mainstay of treatment and is aimed at maintaining and improving joint mobility that is impaired secondary to scarring.

Mixed Connective Tissue Disease

Mixed connective tissue disease is characterized by a combination of signs and symptoms of systemic lupus erythematosus, scleroderma, and dermatomyositis/polymyositis, with specific serologic association of antibodies reactive with the ribonuclease-sensitive component of extractable nuclear antigen (anti-RNP) and speckled pattern antinuclear antibody [Oetgen et al., 1981]. Some children progress to a systemic sclerosis pattern [Kotajima et al., 1996], whereas others follow a course typical of mild systemic lupus erythematosus.

Clinical features include Raynaud's phenomenon as the initial manifestation, followed by polyarthritis, fever, rash, thickening of subcutaneous tissues, hepatosplenomegaly, myositis, and cardiomyopathy. Secondary Sjögren's syndrome may produce parotitis and keratoconjunctivitis sicca (dry eyes). Erythrocyte sedimentation rate and rheumatoid factor are often elevated. Evaluation may demonstrate decreased esophageal motility, diminished tear production, keratoconjunctivitis demonstrated by slit-lamp examination, abnormal parotid sialography, pulmonary effusion demonstrated by chest radiography, and abnormal pulmonary function tests.

Neurologic Characteristics

Proximal muscle weakness, increased creatine kinase activity, myopathic electromyograms, and muscle biopsy are consistent with inflammatory myositis. In one study, asymptomatic children with mixed connective tissue disease had abnormalities detectable on electromyography and biopsy of proximal muscles [Singsen et al., 1980].

Seizures, headache, increased cerebrospinal fluid protein content, and aseptic meningitis have been reported in children with mixed connective tissue disease [Oetgen et al., 1981]. In the original 1972 description of 25 patients, of whom at least 4 were children, none had neurologic symptoms [Sharp et al., 1972]. A follow-up study of 14 of the original cohort indicated myositis as the only neurologic finding in 5 adults. The only surviving child was asymptomatic; the other three died of non-neurologic causes [Nimelstein et al., 1980]. Two additional children have been described with neurologic manifestations [Graf et al., 1993]. The first had an internal carotid artery occlusion and stroke with eventual recovery without evidence of antiphospholipid antibody. The second child had a large intracerebral hematoma and died. Postmortem examination found fibrinoid necrosis of intracerebral capillaries. Trigeminal neuralgia has been observed in adults but has not been reported in children [Sharp, 1975]. Studies of adults have indicated a significant incidence of neuropsychiatric symptoms [Bennet and O'Connell, 1980]. Additionally, an adult with recurrent optic neuropathy and transverse myelopathy has been reported [Flechtner and Baum, 1994], as well as another adult with myelopathy [Mok and Lau, 1995].

Treatment

Treatment of mixed connective tissue disease depends on disease manifestations. For disease with mild organ involvement, hydroxychloroquine may be adequate. For more severe organ system involvement or significant myositis, corticosteroids may be necessary. As there are few long-term studies that clarify the prognosis and best therapy, treatment is empirical [Mier et al., 1996; Tiddens et al., 1993]. Methotrexate, azathioprine, and cyclophosphamide have been used, similar to therapy for systemic lupus erythematosus.

Sjögren's Syndrome

Sjögren's syndrome is a chronic autoimmune disorder in which lymphocytic infiltration of the salivary, lacrimal, and other exocrine glands leads to keratoconjunctivitis sicca, xerostomia, and recurrent inflammation of the salivary glands. Primary Sjögren's syndrome is extremely rare in children, but the secondary form, preceding, accompanying, or following systemic lupus erythematosus, juvenile idiopathic arthritis, mixed connective tissue disease, juvenile dermatomyositis, or scleroderma is more frequent [Nikitakis et al., 2003]. Characteristic laboratory findings include hypergammaglobulinemia, positive antinuclear antibody, anti-SSA, anti-SSB, and classic rheumatoid factor [Anaya et al., 1995]. Confirmation of the diagnosis is obtained by labial salivary gland biopsy, demonstrating periductal lymphocytic infiltration [Cassidy and Petty, 2001]. The Schirmer test, sialogram, and salivary scintiphotography support the diagnosis [Chudwin et al., 1981].

Several children with primary Sjögren's syndrome and neurologic involvement have been reported. A 10-year-old female with optic neuritis and severe central nervous system disease has been described [Berman et al., 1990], as well as an 18-year-old female with aseptic meningitis and small infarctions in both temporal regions and in the right posterior parietal region [Gerraty et al., 1993]. In addition, a 17-year-old female has been described with bilateral carotid and vertebral artery occlusions who was treated with surgical bypass [Nagahiro et al., 1996]. A 9-year-old female who was eventually diagnosed with Sjögren's syndrome developed recurrent paresis with associated nonenhancing lucencies of the left internal capsule and subcortical white matter in the right temporo-occipital regions on CT. MRI confirmed the CT findings and exhibited multiple regions of increased signal intensity on T2-weighted images in the internal capsule and subcortical and periventricular white matter [Ohtsuka et al., 1995]. She developed a rapidly increasing paresis that resulted in quadriplegia but responded fairly well to corticosteroids. T2-weighted images on MRI indicated diffuse swelling of the cervical cord and increased signal intensity from the first cervical to the seventh thoracic vertebra [Ohtsuka et al., 1995]. In adult patients with Sjögren's syndrome and biopsy-documented inflammatory vascular disease, both central nervous system and peripheral nervous system involvement have been reported in 25% to 66% of patients [Alexander, 1992]. Neurologic manifestations in these patients consisted of focal and diffuse brain disease, including seizures, cognitive and behavioral disorders, acute encephalopathy, aseptic meningitis, and forms of progressive myelopathies. Peripheral nervous system involvement included motor and sensory neuropathies and carpal tunnel syndrome [Malinow et al., 1985; Molina et al., 1985]. Further study of these patients revealed one or more cerebrospinal fluid abnormalities in 16 of 21 patients, including increased protein content, pleocytosis, elevated IgG levels, elevated IgG index, increased oligoclonal bands, and abnormal cerebrospinal fluid/serum glucose ratios [Malinow et al., 1985]. Because classification criteria for Sjögren's syndrome vary, it is difficult to interpret the frequency of neurologic symptoms in adults [Alexander, 1992]. MRI may indicate subcortical or periventricular lesions in the white matter in up to 80% of adult patients [Alexander, 1992]. Although the pathogenesis of Sjögren's syndrome is unknown, it has been suggested that the anti-Ro (anti-SSA) antibody may play an immunopathologic role in central nervous system disease [Alexander, 1992].

Treatment

Hydroxychloroquine and supportive care are the mainstays of treatment of non-neurologic manifestations of Sjögren's syndrome [Fox, 1992]. Immunosuppressive management with corticosteroids is needed for significant neurologic manifestations [Anaya et al., 1995; Ostuni et al., 1996]. If there is progressive neurologic disease, cyclophosphamide in addition to corticosteroids has been used successfully [Alexander, 1992]. Long-term prognosis in children with and without neurologic disease is unclear [Anaya et al., 1995; Ostuni et al., 1996].

PRIMARY VASCULITIC DISEASES

Vasculitis may be either primary or secondary to a multisystem disorder. Because the causes of vasculitic disorders remain unknown, classification of the vasculitides is difficult. (In Box 73-1, the vasculitides are organized by pathologic type.) Size and location of the affected vessels may aid in identifying specific disorders. Alternatively, because many of these disorders have distinct clinical patterns of involvement, the diagnosis is often established on clinical grounds with the aid of specific laboratory tests, which help rule out other disorders and confirm the diagnosis.

Although multiple etiologies have been proposed to explain the development of vasculitis, the formation of circulating immune complexes and the production of antiendothelial antibodies are the most commonly accepted theories [Conn, 1990; Kissel, 1989]. In the immune complex model, deposition of circulating antigen-antibody complexes in the vascular wall causes activation of the complement system and release of chemotactic substances that attract circulating polymorphonuclear leukocytes. Leukocytic infiltration of the vascular wall and phagocytosis of immune complexes result in the release of intracellular enzymes that cause localized vascular injury. Activation of the coagulation and kallikrein-kinin systems further contributes to the development of this type of vascular tissue damage. In the antiendothelial cell antibody model, viral infections or the underlying inflammatory disease process may alter the endothelial cell so that a specific antigen site precipitates antibody formation [Cines, 1989; Conn, 1990]. However, the presence of other factors such as tumor necrosis factor, interleukin-1, and interferon gamma appears necessary to sensitize the endothelial cells so that lysis can occur when these cells are exposed to antiendothelial cell antibodies. Once endothelial injury occurs, altered vascular tone causes localized contraction and vasospasm, which presumably happens in conjunction with the release of vasoconstrictor substances such as prostaglandins and calcium, or possibly as the result of inhibition of the release of endothelium-derived relaxing factor [Miller and Burnett, 1990]. The key neurologic findings in the vasculitides are listed in Table 73-4.

Necrotizing Vasculitis

The disorders classified as necrotizing vasculitis include polyarteritis nodosa, microscopic polyangiitis, Kawasaki disease, and Cogan's syndrome. They are characterized by fibrinoid necrosis of small and medium-sized muscular arteries.

TABLE 73-4

Key Neurologic and Laboratory Findings in Childhood Vasculitides

DISEASE	NEUROLOGIC FINDINGS	LABORATORY FINDINGS
Polyarteritis nodosa	Headache, encephalopathy, stroke, seizures, neuropathies	Elevated WBC, ESR, positive HBsAg and c-ANCA
Kawasaki disease	Aseptic meningitis, focal neurologic findings	Coronary aneurysms, thrombocytosis
Cogan's syndrome	Neurosensory hearing loss	None
Henoch-Schönlein purpura	Encephalopathy	Elevated IgA in 50%, hematuria, melena
Churg-Strauss syndrome	Headache, encephalopathy, stroke, seizures, various peripheral neuropathies, coma, intracranial hemorrhage	Eosinophilia, eosinophils on skin biopsy, p-ANCA
Wegener's granulomatosis	Encephalopathy, intracranial hemorrhage, meningitis	c-ANCA
Primary angiitis of the CNS	Headache, encephalopathy, seizures, stroke, myelopathy	Elevated ESR
Sarcoidosis	Obstructive hydrocephalus, seventh nerve palsy, meningitis, seizures, peripheral neuropathies	Noncaseating granuloma
Temporal arteritis	Blindness, encephalopathy, headache	Elevated ESR
Takayasu's arteritis	Headache, stroke, syncope, visual loss	Elevated ESR and factor VIII–related antigen
Behçet's disease	Headache, meningitis, psychiatric disorders, encephalopathy, pseudotumor cerebri, brainstem signs	Elevated ESR

c-ANCA, cytoplasmic staining antineutrophil cytoplasmic antibody; CNS, central nervous system; ESR, erythrocyte sedimentation rate; HBsAg, hepatitis B surface antigen; IgA, immunoglobulin A; p-ANCA, perinuclear staining antineutrophil cytoplasmic antibody; WBC, white blood cell count.

Polyarteritis Nodosa

Polyarteritis nodosa occurs principally in older children and adolescents. Classic polyarteritis nodosa is characterized by unexplained fever, arthralgias, calf discomfort, abdominal pain, recurrent pulmonary infection, renal disease with hypertension, fatigability, weight loss, malar rash, and purpura. Severe kidney impairment and marked hypertension occur early in the course of the disease. Diffuse glomerulonephritis or necrotizing arteritis is found in renal biopsy material. Mesenteric arteritis and resultant bowel wall infarction may lead to gastrointestinal hemorrhage [Bakkaloglu et al., 2001; Maeda et al., 1997].

Laboratory evaluation reveals leukocytosis, anemia, increased sedimentation rate, abnormal urinalysis, and evidence of nephrosis and nephritis, in the absence of complement consumption, antinuclear antibodies, and rheumatoid factor [Ozen et al., 1992]. Patients with polyarteritis nodosa may have circulating antineutrophil cytoplasmic antibodies [Bakkaloglu et al., 2001], elevated factor VIII–related antigen [Ates et al., 1994], and positive serology for hepatitis B surface antigen [Guillevin et al., 1995]. In addition, an association with preceding streptococcal infection has been noted [David et al., 1993; Hoyne and Steiner, 1940]. Angiography may demonstrate aneurysmal dilation of the medium-sized mesenteric, celiac, or renal arteries (Fig. 73-5A). Before corticosteroid therapy, progressive neurologic, renal, and cardiovascular involvement led to a mortality rate of 80% to 90%. Currently, the use of corticosteroids and cytotoxic agents has dramatically reduced the mortality rate to as low as 5% [Bakkaloglu et al., 2001; Maeda et al., 1997]. Unfortunately, polyarteritis nodosa often follows a chronic course characterized by periods of exacerbations despite aggressive immune suppression [Maeda et al., 1997]. Postmortem studies of pediatric patients with arteritis demonstrate necrotizing angiitis accompanied by polymorphonuclear infiltration of small and medium-sized arteries [Ford and Siekert, 1965].

Neurologic Manifestations

Approximately one fourth of patients with polyarteritis nodosa demonstrate neurologic manifestations during their lifetimes [Dillon, 1997]. Seizures frequently accompany polyarteritis nodosa and generally appear early in the illness, become more difficult to control as the disease becomes chronic, and may culminate in episodes of status epilepticus in terminally ill patients. Headache, disturbances of higher cortical function, and affective disorders commonly precede the onset of seizures. This finding suggests central nervous system vasculitis in addition to vasculitis of the internal organs and skin. Cerebrospinal fluid is usually normal, and the presence of blood strongly suggests a ruptured cerebral microaneurysm [Peal et al., 1946]. Commonly reported electroencephalographic abnormalities include diffuse and focal paroxysmal activity and background slowing. Cerebral angiography may indicate segmental narrowing of small and medium-sized vessels and occasional microaneurysmal

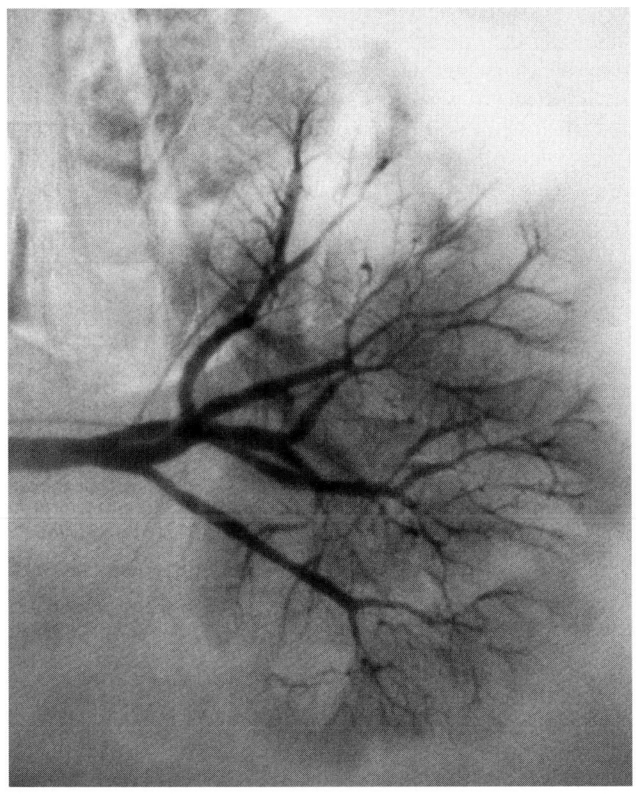
A

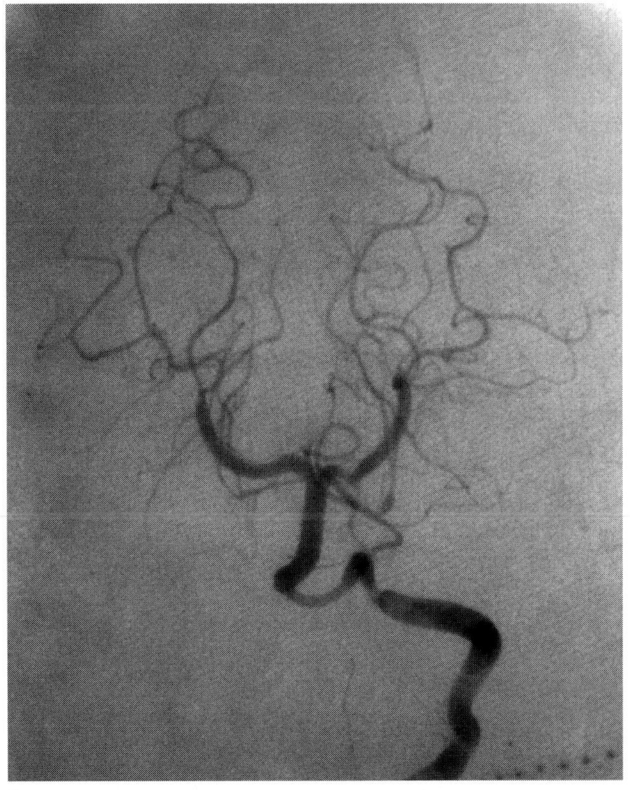
B

FIGURE 73-5. **A,** Renal arteriogram of a child with polyarteritis nodosa demonstrating segmental vasculitis, microaneurysmal dilation, and focal hypoperfusion. **B,** Cerebral angiogram demonstrating segmental narrowing of posterior communicating and posterior cerebral arteries and small branch occlusions in the middle cerebral artery distribution. (Courtesy of Dr. Joseph Thompson, Department of Neuroradiology, Loma Linda University Children's Hospital.)

dilation. Biopsy of the superficial temporal artery is not recommended because only 11% of patients have demonstrable arteritis in the external carotid circulation [Goder, 1956].

Polyarteritis nodosa may manifest with sudden onset of visual field defects, hemiparesis, or increased intracranial pressure. These symptoms tend to occur only in patients with a protracted course. Visual loss associated with proliferative retinitis and fundal hemorrhages may occur independently or accompanying increased intracranial pressure [Fager et al., 1951; Magilavy et al., 1977]. Nystagmus, ophthalmoplegia, diminished corneal reflexes, and ataxia rarely are reported [Ford and Siekert, 1965].

The sudden onset of stroke in a patient with polyarteritis nodosa requires complete assessment of the cerebral circulation initially with MRI and MR angiography, followed by cerebral angiography in selected patients. Although angiography may initially be normal, evidence of segmental arterial narrowing may be demonstrated within several weeks of the central nervous system event (see Fig. 73-5B). Pathology indicates necrotizing angiitis, ruptured microaneurysms of the superficial and deep arteries, subarachnoid hemorrhage, and encephalomalacia caused by ischemia or infarction.

Aseptic meningitis with spinal fluid lymphocytosis and normal protein concentration has also been reported in childhood forms of polyarteritis nodosa. Bacterial meningitis is an uncommon complication in children, despite the use of immunosuppressive agents.

Neuropsychiatric symptoms are uncommon in polyarteritis nodosa despite the diffuse cerebral arteritis [Ford and Siekert, 1965]. Extremely ill patients may develop organic psychosis, a progressive confusional state, and variable states of consciousness that are associated with renal insufficiency. Depression is unusual in the stable patient.

Children with polyarteritis nodosa often experience diffuse myalgia; however, myositis is rarely diagnosed clinically, although it is demonstrated in approximately 11% of postmortem studies. There may be an accompanying increase of creatine kinase activity or evidence of myopathy indicated by electromyography [Blau et al., 1977; Magilavy et al., 1977]. Muscle biopsy may reveal necrotizing arteritis with fibrinoid necrosis and perivascular inflammation. A myopathic pattern is demonstrated in approximately 50% of children with polyarteritis nodosa who undergo electromyography.

Peripheral neuropathy responds well to corticosteroids. Mononeuritis multiplex is the most common and typically early neurologic feature of adult polyarteritis nodosa [Nadeau, 2002]. Sensory and motor nerve conduction velocities are decreased in childhood polyarteritis nodosa. Pathologic studies of the peripheral nervous system reveal fulminant arteritis with thrombotic occlusion of small and medium-sized arteries with accompanying profound nerve infarction and demyelination. Myelopathy occurs rarely and usually only in patients who suffer from chronic disease [Carr and Bryer, 1993].

Microscopic polyangiitis is a subgroup of polyarteritis nodosa and is rarely seen in children [Ozen, 2004]. There is frequent pulmonary hemorrhage, and all patients have glomerulonephritis. They are frequently perinuclear staining antineutrophil cytoplasmic antibody (p-ANCA) positive due to myeloperoxidase antibody. Peripheral neuropathy is less common than in polyarteritis nodosa.

Treatment

Corticosteroids are the mainstay of treatment. Children whose disease follows a chronic course or who develop catastrophic events should be treated with cyclophosphamide both to avoid side effects associated with the use of chronic steroids and to provide greater immune suppression [Lhote and Guillevin, 1995]. Poorer prognosis has been associated with significant central nervous system disease, renal insufficiency, gastrointestinal disease, and cardiomyopathy. Aggressive treatment with high-dose intravenous corticosteroids and cyclophosphamide should be considered for such patients. Plasmapheresis has not been found to be of benefit [Lhote and Guillevin, 1995]. Overall 5-year survival has improved from 10% before corticosteroid use to about 80% in adults, and perhaps even higher in children [Lhote and Guillevin, 1995].

Kawasaki Disease

Kawasaki disease is characterized by aneurysms largely limited to the coronary arteries, although aneurysms have been reported in multiple vessels as well [Burns and Glodé, 2004]. Kawasaki disease is diagnosed by the presence of fever of at least 5 days' duration and four of the following five criteria: (1) bilateral nonpurulent conjunctival injection; (2) changes in the mucosa of the oropharynx, including injected or dry, fissured lips or strawberry tongue; (3) changes in the peripheral extremities, including edema, erythema of hands or feet, and desquamation; (4) rash, which may be polymorphous, but not vesicular; and (5) unilateral cervical lymphadenopathy [Burns and Glodé, 2004].

Prognosis has been excellent since the use of intravenous immunoglobulin and acetylsalicylic acid, with immediate clinical improvement in the majority of children and a decreased rate of coronary artery aneurysmal formation from 20% to 25% to less than 8%. However, myocardial infarction, dysrhythmias, and sudden death were reported in 1% of patients [Melish, 1996].

Neurologic Manifestations

Although pronounced irritability, lethargy, and aseptic meningitis are quite common, other neurologic manifestations are rare [Melish, 1981]. With the exception of a single case report [Engel et al., 1995], cerebral aneurysms have not been demonstrated in infants with Kawasaki disease. This contrasts with polyarteritis nodosa, in which cerebral aneurysms have been reported. In patients who present with an out-of-hospital cardiac arrest secondary to coronary artery involvement, an anoxic encephalopathy may occur.

Postmortem examination of children with Kawasaki disease have failed to reveal prominent cerebrovascular involvement. Major findings have included leptomeningeal thickening, mild endarteritis, and periarteritis.

Treatment

Treatment of Kawasaki disease consists of acetylsalicylic acid, 80 to 100 mg/kg per day in four divided doses, until the patient has been afebrile for about 3 to 7 days, followed by 3 to 5 mg/kg per day in a single dose and continued until inflammatory markers have returned to normal, the thrombocytosis has resolved, and no coronary artery disease exists on follow-up echocardiogram at 4 to 6 weeks. During the acute stage, intravenous immunoglobulin, 2 g/kg as a single dose over 12 hours, is recommended early in the course and preferably before the 10th day [Melish, 1996; Shulman et al., 1995]. The use of corticosteroids in Kawasaki disease is controversial because of one early report of an associated increased frequency of coronary artery aneurysms. This report was not confirmed by others, and children with Kawasaki disease who have failed intravenous immunoglobulin therapy have successfully received corticosteroids [Wright et al., 1996].

Cogan's Syndrome

Cogan's syndrome has been reported rarely in children [Ndiaye et al., 2002]. Although vasculitis may be diffuse, the characteristic features are vertigo, deafness, photophobia, and interstitial keratitis. Eye and ear involvement may precede other systemic symptoms by years. Aortitis and aortic valve insufficiency may also be present [Cassidy and Petty, 2001], along with arthralgia, myalgia, anorexia, episcleritis and/or uveitis, and fever. The noncardiac features generally respond well to corticosteroid therapy, but the aortic valve disease may require surgical replacement of the valve [Olfat and Al-Mayouf, 2001]. Neurologic symptoms have been described in adults [Bicknell and Holland, 1978].

LEUKOCYTOCLASTIC VASCULITIS

Leukocytoclastic vasculitis is a necrotizing vasculitis. Pathologic changes indicate polymorphonuclear leukocytes and necrosis in the walls of small arteries. Nuclear debris is also found in the vessel walls. These changes are seen most commonly in Henoch-Schönlein purpura, systemic lupus erythematosus, and hypersensitivity vasculitis.

Henoch-Schönlein Purpura

Henoch-Schönlein purpura is characterized by palpable purpura, petechiae, or ecchymotic rash, typically found over the buttocks and the lower extremities. It is often associated with large joint arthritis, cramping abdominal pain, fever, peripheral edema, and renal involvement, with a median age of onset of about 6 years [Cassidy and Petty, 2001; Szer, 1996]. Henoch-Schönlein purpura is a common, self-limited illness lasting from about 1 to 3 months. Recurrences may occur over 1 to 2 years. Laboratory tests are usually normal except for microscopic hematuria and guaiac-positive stools. Approximately 50% of patients have elevated IgA levels. Skin, renal, and gastrointestinal biopsies demonstrate leukocytoclastic vasculitis with polymorphonuclear cells within the vessel walls and deposition of IgA, complement, and properdin.

Neurologic Characteristics

Central nervous system complications have been reported in 1% to 8% of children and are secondary to hypertension, renal failure, and vasculitis. Headache, seizures, altered states of consciousness, cerebral vasculitis, intracranial hemorrhage, spastic paralysis, and chorea occur in some patients [Belman et al., 1985; Chen et al., 2000; Østergaard and Storm, 1991; Ritter et al., 1983]. A diffuse encephalopathy in association with or without hypertension has been reported [Belman et al., 1985]. Although the pathogenesis of central nervous system symptoms has not been clearly defined, it has been suggested that IgA immune-complex deposition initiates arteriolar inflammation [Østergaard and Storm, 1991]. Peripheral nervous system complications previously reported include lesions of the femoral, sciatic, and facial nerves; Guillain-Barré syndrome; and isolated mononeuropathies, including mononeuritis multiplex [Bulun et al., 2001; Ritter et al., 1983].

Peripheral nerve dysfunction is believed to result from metabolic disturbances, vasculitis, immune mechanisms, and mechanical compression or entrapment. These peripheral nervous system complications are usually self-limited and resolve with treatment of the underlying disorder and of the specific neurologic symptom (e.g., seizures, chorea, headache).

Management

There is consensus regarding the management of arthritis with nonsteroidal anti-inflammatory drugs and painful cutaneous edema with steroids. Supportive care is required for children who develop massive gastrointestinal bleeding or who become dehydrated or hypertensive [Szer, 1996]. High-dose steroids and plasmapheresis have been used anecdotally for severe central nervous system disease with success [Bulun et al., 2001; Chen et al., 2000; Eun et al., 2003].

Hypersensitivity Angiitis

Hypersensitivity, or allergic, angiitis is an acute necrotizing inflammation of blood vessels similar to Henoch-Schönlein purpura. Unlike the latter, however, recurrent attacks are uncommon. The disorder may be acute and rapidly fatal and may be caused by a hypersensitivity reaction to various drugs, infections, or serums [Cassidy and Petty, 2001; Farooki et al., 1974]. Among adults manifesting similar clinical symptoms, decreased serum complement and cryoglobulinemia have been reported [Cassidy and Petty, 2001]. The occurrence of neurologic complications in the various forms of hypersensitivity angiitis appears to be rare because the cerebral vessels tend to be spared.

GRANULOMATOUS ANGIITIS

Granulomatous angiitis represents a category of systemic necrotizing arteritis manifested by extravascular granulomatous nodules, which consist of a central area of fibrinoid degeneration with surrounding eosinophils and epithelioid and giant cells [Farooki et al., 1974]. Although Churg-Strauss syndrome (allergic granulomatosis), Wegener's granulomatosis, and primary angiitis of the central nervous system are the primary forms of this type of vasculitis, necrotizing sarcoid granulomatosis and sarcoidosis also are discussed in this section because of their granulomatous pathology [Cassidy and Petty, 2001].

Churg-Strauss Syndrome

Churg-Strauss syndrome, also known as allergic granulomatosis, is associated clinically with asthma, fever, eosinophilia, cardiac failure, renal damage, and peripheral neuropathy [Sehgal et al., 1995]. Criteria established by the American College of Rheumatology require the presence of four of the following seven findings: (1) asthma, (2) eosinophilia, (3) history of allergy, (4) mononeuropathy or polyneuropathy, (5) pulmonary infiltrates that are migratory, (6) paranasal sinus abnormality, and (7) extravascular eosinophils on biopsy [Masi et al., 1990]. Approximately 21% of patients are children [Farooki et al., 1974]. The vasculitis is manifested by fibrinoid necrosis of the media of small arteries and veins, with arterial and capillary involvement.

Neurologic involvement appears to be limited to the peripheral nervous system; no reported central nervous system involvement has been observed in children, except for a case report of a 13-year-old female who presented with chorea and associated MRI changes [Kok et al., 1993]. Mononeuritis multiplex or symmetric polyneuropathy is found in 65% to 80% of adult patients. Symptoms are due to a vasculitis of the vasa nervorum. Central nervous system involvement in adults tends to occur late in the course of the disease. Intracranial and subarachnoid hemorrhage, convulsions, and psychosis have been reported. Cranial nerve involvement and optic neuritis also have been described [Acheson et al., 1993; Liou et al., 1994; Sehgal et al., 1995; Tervaert and Kallenberg, 1993].

The treatment of Churg-Strauss syndrome is essentially the same as the therapy for polyarteritis nodosa, and most patients respond well to corticosteroids. Cyclophosphamide has been used for steroid-resistant cases, but usually is not necessary [Lhote and Guillevin, 1995].

Wegener's Granulomatosis

A necrotizing granulomatous vasculitis of the small vessels in the upper and lower respiratory tract and the kidneys characterizes Wegener's granulomatosis. Symptoms frequently include fever, malaise, rhinorrhea, epistaxis, chronic sinusitis, nasal obstruction, pharyngeal ulcers, parenchymal pulmonary lesions, and chronic glomerulonephritis. The most common laboratory abnormality is a cytoplasmic staining antineutrophil cytoplasmic antibody due to anti-PR3 antibodies found in about 90% of patients [Cassidy and Petty, 2001]. Children are rarely affected. The cause of this disorder is unknown.

Of 17 children with Wegener's granulomatosis, 3 had neurologic complications manifested by peripheral neuropathy [Orlowski et al., 1978]. In a more recent review of 23 children, the course was similar to that described in adults except that there was more frequent subglottic stenosis and nasal septal deformity. Central nervous system involvement occurred in 17% of patients and peripheral nervous system involvement in 9% [Rottem et al., 1993]. Two patients had multiple cranial nerve palsies and two had seizures. Cerebral vasculitis has been reported in individual case reports [Haas et al., 2002; von Scheven et al., 1998]. Keratitis, optic nerve granuloma, proptosis, orbital pseudotumor [Wardyn et al., 2003], laryngitis with accompanying aphonia, spasticity, proximal muscle weakness, and diminished deep tendon reflexes have been described [Drachman, 1963; Moorthy et al., 1977]. In contrast to children, approximately 10% of adults with Wegener's granulomatosis had central nervous system involvement, and about 44% had peripheral nervous system involvement [Cruz and Segal, 1997].

Treatment

Prednisone and daily oral cyclophosphamide are often considered the treatments of choice and have lowered the previous mortality rate of up to 100% to the current survival rate of greater than 90% [Langford, 2003]. Pulse cyclophosphamide, intravenous immunoglobulin, trimethoprim-sulfamethoxazole, cyclosporin A, and methotrexate also have been reported to have variable success in inducing remission [Calabrese et al., 1995; Georganas et al., 1996; Jayne and Lockwood, 1996; Reinhold-Keller et al., 1996; Sneller et al., 1995; Stegeman et al., 1996].

Primary Angiitis of the Central Nervous System

Primary angiitis of the central nervous system, also called *granulomatous angiitis*, is characterized by granulomas in 80% of cases. Numerous case reports have been published in the last decade. Clinical criteria require a history or finding of an acquired neurologic deficit associated with angiographic or histopathologic demonstration of vasculitic changes, exclusion of other etiologies, and no evidence of systemic disease [Calabrese, 1995]. It is increasingly recognized as the cause of otherwise unexplained cerebral ischemic episodes in the young [Dillon, 1997] and has been mistaken on occasion for Rasmussen's encephalitis [Derry et al., 2002]. Clinical features include headache, confusion, nausea, altered mental status, focal neurologic deficits, and progressive intellectual deterioration. Primary angiitis of the central nervous system may occur in children as young as 2 years of age and has an equal sex distribution [Barron et al., 1993; Matsell et al., 1990].

Clinical manifestations of primary central nervous system angiitis correlate with the size of the affected vessels. Patients with small vessel disease tend to present with headache, focal seizures, or progressive behavioral or multifocal neurologic impairment. In contrast, patients with medium-sized or large vessel disease tend to present with acute ischemic stroke or transient ischemic attack [Benseler and Schneider, 2004; Lanthier et al., 2001]. In both groups, cranial nerve abnormalities have been described, including diplopia, blurred vision, nystagmus, dysarthria, and pupillary abnormalities. Hemiparesis and language disorders have been observed in approximately 50% of patients. Seizures, spinal cord abnormalities, cerebral hemorrhage, fever, and weight loss also have been reported [Calabrese, 1995].

Laboratory studies reveal elevated erythrocyte sedimentation rate, elevated cerebrospinal fluid protein concentration, and moderately increased monocytosis with increased pressure [Calabrese et al., 1992; Sabharwal et al., 1982]. However, normal acute phase reactants and spinal fluid have been reported in children [Benseler and Schneider, 2004]. Cerebral angiography documents small- and medium-sized vessel occlusion or segmental narrowing with saccular aneurysms and areas of infarction. Neuropathologic studies indicate segmental necrotizing granulomatous vasculitis diffusely affecting the parenchymal and leptomeningeal vessels of the cortex but not the subcortical areas of the brain [Hankey, 1991; Sabharwal et al., 1982]. Patients with small vessel disease are more likely to demonstrate multifocal, hyperintense lesions on T2-weighted MRI with normal cerebrospinal fluid, erythrocyte sedimentation rate, and cerebral angiograms. Those with medium-sized or large vessel disease often demonstrate infarcts on CT and MRI and are more likely than those with small vessel disease to have abnormal cerebrospinal fluid studies, erythrocyte sedimentation rates, and angiograms (Fig. 73-6) [Lanthier et al., 2001].

The course of this disorder fluctuates, and, although initial studies reported that 90% of patients died within a year of onset, it is clear from more recent studies that this disease has a broad spectrum and that the prognosis is much better [Benseler and Schneider, 2004; Calabrese, 1995]. In general, the prognosis for patients with small vessel disease tends to be better than that for patients with stroke due to large vessel disease [Lanthier et al., 2001]. Therapeutic use of corticosteroids, with or without cyclophosphamide, is indicated and should be instituted early in the course of disease [Barron et al., 1993; Lanthier et al., 2001].

The disease in a subgroup of patients seems to follow a benign course termed *benign angiopathy of the central nervous system.* These patients tend to be young women who have a sudden onset of symptoms and near-normal cerebrospinal fluid studies and whose disease often remits after a monophasic course. Unfortunately, some of these patients progress years later to serious and even lethal disease [Calabrese, 1995]. Although most of these patients have been adults, two pediatric patients who experienced complete recovery have been described [Calabrese and Mallek, 1988].

Necrotizing Sarcoid Granulomatosis

Necrotizing sarcoid granulomatosis, first described in 1973, is clinically and pathologically intermediate between sarcoidosis and Wegener's granulomatosis [Kwong et al., 1994]. It consists of a necrotizing granulomatosis and vasculitis similar to that found in Wegener's granulomatosis, with noncaseating granulomas resembling those of sarcoidosis. The condition has been reported in children with multifocal neurologic disease and retinal angiitis. In one child, progressive asymmetric lower limb weakness associated with urinary retention, and diagnosed as an acute myelitis and polyneuritis, responded to treatment with corticosteroids

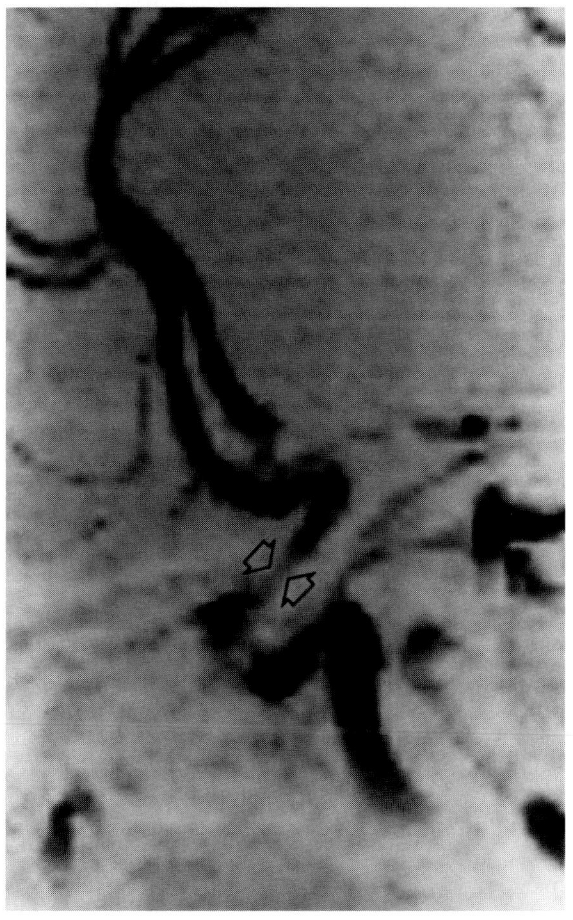

A

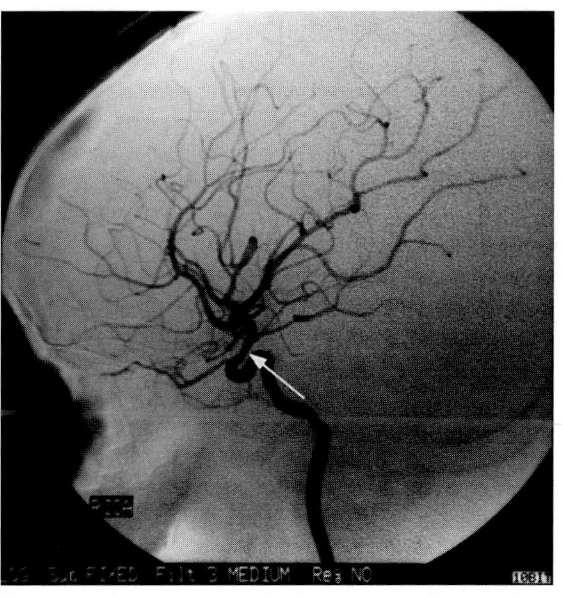

B

FIGURE 73-6. A 4-year-old male with primary angiitis of the central nervous system who had a 2-month history of seizures, chorea, left hemiparesis, and dysarthria; he improved significantly with intravenous immunoglobulin and corticosteroids. **A,** Time-of-flight MR angiogram partitioned for the right distal internal carotid artery shows prominent segmental supraclinoid internal carotid artery narrowing *(arrowheads).* **B,** Lateral right internal carotid digital subtraction arteriogram shows residual segmental narrowing, significantly improved after 2 days of steroid therapy. (Courtesy of Dr. Joseph Thompson, Department of Neuroradiology, Loma Linda University Children's Hospital, Loma Linda, CA.)

[Beach et al., 1980]. A more recent review discussed the previous reported cases, defined the vasculitic features, and differentiated childhood sarcoidosis from familial granulomatous arteritis with arthritis, uveitis, and fever [Kwong et al., 1994]. Findings reported in this disease are similar to those in sarcoidosis and include disc edema and retinal periphlebitis responsive to corticosteroid therapy. Necrotizing sarcoid granulomatosis usually responds to corticosteroids and does not require cytoxic therapy. No significant reports of neurologic involvement have been made [Heinrich et al., 2003]. The extent of this disorder in children and the degree of neurologic involvement are unknown.

Sarcoidosis

Sarcoidosis is a chronic, multisystem granulomatous disease of unknown etiology that is rare in children. Interestingly, sarcoidosis in older children is indistinguishable from adult sarcoidosis, but younger children (younger than 4 years) tend to have different clinical manifestations. In the early onset form, the children tend to present in infancy to preschool years [Fink and Cimaz, 1997]. This form is characterized by relatively painless, boggy polyarthritis with well-preserved range of motion. Uveitis and cutaneous sarcoid lesions are usually present, but pulmonary involvement is rare. Older children tend to present with pulmonary symptoms, hilar adenopathy, fatigue, weight loss, anorexia, headache, fever, and parotid enlargement [Kwong et al., 1994; Pattishall and Kendig, 1996]. This form of sarcoidosis is characterized by hilar and paratracheal adenopathy with interstitial infiltrates, hypercalciuria, leukopenia, and eosinophilia. An elevated erythrocyte sedimentation rate and the presence of elevated serum immunoglobulins further support the diagnosis. Pulmonary function study results are abnormal in most older patients. Noncaseating granulomas obtained from mediastinal or peripheral lymph node biopsies are found in 90% of patients.

Musculoskeletal findings in several children with sarcoidosis have included joint pain with effusions and palpable muscle masses; on biopsy, these muscle masses consist of noncaseating granulomas.

Neurologic findings include obstructive hydrocephalus with noncaseating granulomas throughout the central nervous system, transient cranial nerve VII palsies, and myelopathy. There are reports of optic nerve and orbital involvement, pituitary and hypothalamic lesions, meningitis, and seizures [Cohen-Gadol et al., 2003; Lee et al., 1998; Leiba et al., 1996; Monfort-Gourand et al., 1996; Pattishall and Kendig, 1996].

In adults about 5% of patients with sarcoidosis have neurologic involvement. Central nervous system findings include meningeal, parameningeal, hypothalamic, and pituitary sarcoid infiltration. Adults have presented with symptoms of an apparent intracranial or intramedullary spinal cord tumor. Furthermore, peripheral neuropathies, including postnuclear cranial neuropathies, are associated with sarcoidosis [Scott, 1993]. It appears that the neurologic symptoms are different in children than in adults. Seizures are the most common central nervous system manifestation. Cranial nerve palsy and hypothalamic dysfunction are also frequent. About 25% of patients present with a central nervous system mass lesion [Baumann and Robertson, 2003].

Two reports of intramedullary spinal cord lesions studied by MRI and subsequent biopsy indicate that patchy contrast enhancement and increased T2-weighted signal intensity almost always occurred in sarcoid lesions of the spinal cord. These two relatively small cohorts of patients with non-neoplastic spinal cord lesions differed from one another with regard to the question of whether there was significant expansion of the spinal cord in the region of sarcoid involvement [Cohen-Gadol et al., 2003; Lee et al., 1998].

Treatment of the early-onset form of sarcoidosis has been anecdotal and has consisted of corticosteroids, azathioprine, methotrexate, or, occasionally, cyclophosphamide [Fink and Cimaz, 1997]. Therapy of late-onset or adult-type sarcoidosis depends on whether the arthritis is acute, chronic, or relapsing. Nonsteroidal anti-inflammatory drugs have been used for indolent disease, as well as for acute attacks. More painful episodes have been successfully managed with colchicine. Attacks unresponsive to colchicine have often responded to corticosteroids. Chronic disease unresponsive to nonsteroidal anti-inflammatory drugs has responded to low-dose, alternate-day steroids or methotrexate [Sequeira, 1997].

GIANT CELL ARTERITIS

Temporal Arteritis

Classic giant cell arteritis (temporal arteritis) most often affects men older than 50 years of age [Nordborg et al., 1995]. A recent report of temporal arteritis in a 9-year-old Haitian female with a past medical history remarkable for sensorineural hearing loss; an initial presentation with monocular blindness and a tortuous superficial temporal artery and a temporal artery biopsy study consistent with giant cell arteritis; and a disease course that included a systemic illness with encephalopathy most consistent with polyarteritis nodosa makes it clear that this disorder can occur in childhood [Bert et al., 1999]. Headache, scalp tenderness, visual disturbances, and jaw claudication appearing in association with an elevated sedimentation rate suggest the diagnosis. Biopsy of the superficial temporal artery reveals giant cell perivascular inflammatory infiltrates [Small, 1984]. Hemiparesis, vertigo, hearing loss, brainstem strokes, seizures, oculomotor disorders, and peripheral neuropathies have been reported. Optic neuritis is the most common problem. The superficial temporal, vertebral, ophthalmic, and posterior ciliary arteries are frequently involved. The internal and external carotid and central retinal arteries are less commonly affected, but occlusion of the ophthalmic or central retinal artery can lead to blindness. Intracranial arterial involvement has been documented, although it is rare [Small, 1984]. Myelopathy, transient ischemic attacks, and cerebral infarctions have been reported in adults with temporal arteritis. It is unclear whether the latter two disorders are due to the underlying condition or the patient's age [Caselli and Hunder, 1993].

Before the case report of Bert and colleagues [1999], juvenile temporal arteritis was regarded as a different and even uncommon clinical entity than adult-type temporal arteritis. Two children, 7 and 8 years of age, initially developed unilateral nodules of the temporal arteries without systemic or neurologic symptoms [Lie et al., 1975].

Studies of these lesions failed to demonstrate the classic giant cells but instead revealed perivascular lymphoid hyperplasia with eosinophilia. Occlusion of the temporal artery lumen with thrombus formation and diffuse intimal thickening and focal disruption of the internal elastic lamina and media were observed. This disorder demonstrates a form of non–giant cell granulomatous inflammation of the temporal artery; it is distinct from classic temporal arteritis of adults [Lie et al., 1975]. A more recent review included an additional case report of this syndrome [Lie, 1995].

Takayasu's Arteritis

Takayasu's arteritis, a form of arteritis involving the aorta and its branches, has been reported in children as young as 5 months of age. Onset occurs before 16 years of age in 25% to 30% of patients [Morales et al., 1991], and a recent post-mortem study from India demonstrated a mean age at death of 22.6 ± 10.2 years [Sharma et al., 1998]. In children, the abdominal aorta and its branches are more commonly affected than the aortic arch. The clinical course is variable. Most patients come to medical attention in the prepulseless stage with nonspecific symptoms of fever, fatigue, dyspnea, anorexia, and arthralgia. The obstructive phase of the illness is characterized by aneurysmal dilation and stenosis of the aorta or pulmonary arteries. Because the abdominal aorta is involved in young children, initial symptoms may include abdominal pain or mass, congestive heart failure, and occlusive vascular disease of the abdominal organs or lower extremities [Gronemeyer and Demello, 1982].

Symptoms of claudication, pulselessness, carotid hypersensitivity, and cerebrovascular involvement have been reported in children [Pantell and Goodman, 1981]. Hypertension caused by renal artery stenosis occurs in approximately 70% of patients. Hypertensive encephalopathy has been reported in two children with renal artery stenosis [Millar et al., 1996]. One review noted that neurologic symptoms in childhood are quite rare, but that adults may develop carotid thromboembolic disease, cerebral hypertension, subclavian steal syndrome, or hypersensitivity of the carotid sinus [Tervaert and Kallenberg, 1993]. A review of 26 children emphasized that hypertension, constitutional symptoms, gastrointestinal pain, and heart failure were fairly common. In addition, 50% of patients had significant headache, 12% had convulsions, and 8% developed hemiplegia [Morales et al., 1991]. Another review of 24 patients found similar findings except for a lack of neurologic symptoms [Jain et al., 2000]. In one small study, of patients who succumbed to Takayasu's arteritis, 20% had seizures and 10% had hemiplegia [Sharma et al., 1998]. All of these patients had hypertension as the presenting feature of their disease.

A lymphocytic and plasma cell inflammatory infiltrate in the media and adventitial large vessels occurs in the presence of few giant cells during the active phase of the disease. Subsequently, necrosis and thrombosis occur with accompanying fibrosis, and then narrowing of the arterial lumen.

Treatment with corticosteroids and other immunosuppressive agents improves the long-term prognosis, but most immunosuppressive drugs provide little improvement over corticosteroids [Hoffman, 1996]. Significant improvement has been made with the use of bypass grafts and angioplasty [Hoffman, 1995; Kohrman and Huttenlocher, 1986].

MISCELLANEOUS VASCULITIC DISORDERS

Not all vasculitic disorders can be classified in the previously noted categories of polyarteritis—leukocytoclastic, granulomatous, and giant cell vasculitides. As many as one third of all primary vasculitic diseases of childhood are categorized as idiopathic or "polyangiitis overlap syndrome" [Cassidy and Petty, 2001]. Other diseases, such as Behçet's syndrome, do not fit any of these categories.

Behçet's Disease

Behçet's disease is rare in children [Cassidy and Petty, 2001; Rakover et al., 1989], usually having its onset in the second decade of life. This rarity has led some authors to postulate that juvenile Behçet's disease may differ from adult Behçet's disease in pathogenesis [Koné-Paut et al., 1998]. One study of juvenile Behçet's disease placed the onset of this disorder at or around age 7 [Krause et al., 1999]. The classic clinical triad of Behçet's disease consists of recurrent oral and genital ulcerations and recurrent uveitis [Schor, 2000]. The uveitis tends to be a panuveitis with retinal vasculitis [Tugal-Tutkun and Urgancioglu, 2003]. The following criteria have been proposed for the diagnosis of Behçet's disease: the presence of recurrent aphthous stomatitis and two of the following: (1) recurrent genital ulcers, (2) uveitis or retinal vasculitis, (3) erythema nodosum or pustules, or (4) pathergy (the appearance of a pustular skin lesion after skin puncture) [International Study Group for Behçet's Disease, 1992].

Central nervous system manifestations are reported in as many as 66% of adult patients during the course of the illness. One study found that the prevalence of neurologic manifestations other than headache was much higher in their cohort of patients with childhood Behçet's disease (26.3%) than in their adult counterpart (3.8%) [Krause et al., 1999]. Three forms of central nervous system involvement have been reported in adults and children: (1) diffuse involvement associated with an acute meningoencephalitis, organic psychosis, or dementia; (2) brainstem or spinal cord involvement, with cranial nerve palsies, hemiparesis, and ataxia; and (3) thrombosis of the dural sinuses and intracranial veins manifesting with signs of intracranial hypertension such as headache and papilledema [Davis et al., 1986; Wechsler, 1992]. The central nervous system symptoms occur as isolated recurrent events that evolve slowly [Bahabri et al., 1996; Devlin et al., 1995; Fujikawa and Suemitsu, 1997; Rosenberger et al., 1982]. MRI with or without gadolinium enhancement and SPECT have demonstrated central nervous system involvement in adult patients [Erdem, 1993; Mizukami et al., 1992; Wechsler et al., 1993], although both techniques underestimate the frequency of brain lesions in adults and children. In a study of seven children and one adult with Behçet's disease, all patients demonstrated hypoperfusion, especially in the basal ganglia and frontal and temporal cortex, on ^{99m}Tc-HMPAO SPECT scanning [Nobili et al., 2002].

Neuropathologic studies demonstrate lymphocytic meningitis, vasculitis with perivascular cuffing, and thrombosis of arterioles, venules, veins, and dural venous sinuses. Although the etiopathogenesis of Behçet's disease is unknown, the intraocular fluid of patients with Behçet's disease–associated uveitis, but not that of other uveitis patients, harbors T cells specific for non-peptide prenyl pyrophosphate antigens. This finding suggests that perhaps an autoimmune attack on a specific antigen underlies susceptibility to Behçet's disease [Verjans et al., 2002]. Treatment remains controversial, although early treatment with high doses of corticosteroids appears beneficial [Cassidy and Petty, 2001; O'Duffy and Goldstein, 1976]. Ten children were reviewed recently in whom thalidomide was used successfully in some resistant cases, with good improvement in oral and genital ulcerations [Kari et al., 2001]. In patients with intracranial venous or dural sinus thrombosis, heparinization may be beneficial [Wechsler et al., 1992]. Immunosuppressive agents have been used for the central nervous system manifestations of the disease [Zelenski et al., 1989].

MISCELLANEOUS DISORDERS

Thrombotic Thrombocytopenic Purpura

Rapid onset of thrombocytopenia, severe microangiopathic hemolytic anemia, renal disease, neurologic symptoms, and fever characterizes thrombotic thrombocytopenic purpura [Amorosi and Ultmann, 1966]. Neurologic symptoms in children with thrombotic thrombocytopenic purpura are generally acute and include seizures, confusional states, coma, headache, visual loss, aphasia, and hemiparesis [Lawlor et al., 1997]. Central nervous system symptoms usually persist, unlike the intermittent fluctuating course observed in adults [Thompson et al., 1992]. Retinal hemorrhage is frequent. There have been rare reports of thrombotic thrombocytopenic purpura occurring with systemic lupus erythematosus [Chak et al., 2003]. Thrombotic occlusion may occur in any tissue and may involve the central nervous system, peripheral nervous system, or skeletal muscles. Cerebrospinal fluid examination results are normal in most patients, and electroencephalographic changes are nonspecific. MRI, MR angiography, cerebral angiography [Rinkel et al., 1991; Wijdicks, 1994], and CT scans may reveal evidence of arterial occlusion. A recent study of 12 adult patients with thrombotic thrombocytopenic purpura [Bakshi et al., 1999] demonstrated acute MRI abnormalities in 75%, most commonly reversible posterior leukoencephalopathy and edema associated with hypertension. Ischemic strokes, sometimes multiple in the same patient, were seen in 25% of the patients in this study, and many were complicated by secondary hemorrhage into the area of infarction. Half of the strokes were in the posterior cerebral artery territory, and in general, patients with stroke or primary hematoma (1 patient in this series) had an unfavorable long-term outcome.

Pathologically, amorphous hyaline material occluding small cerebral arteries is usually seen and is indistinguishable from that found in the heart and kidneys. Cerebral gray matter contains many vascular lesions [Silverstein, 1968]. Previously, only 10% of children with thrombotic thrombocytopenic purpura survived for more than 1 year despite aggressive intervention with heparin, intravenous corticosteroids, whole blood transfusion, dextran infusion, and splenectomy. Plasma exchange transfusion has been beneficial for some children, decreasing the mortality to very low levels [Byrnes and Khurana, 1977; Lawlor et al., 1997]. It has been suggested that plasma exchange removes pathogenic substances and supplies other factors that may be deficient in patients with thrombotic thrombocytopenic purpura [Lawlor et al., 1997]. Decreased levels of protease activity with the presence of Von Willebrand factor–protease inhibitors contribute to the bleeding diathesis in this condition [Horton et al., 2003].

Erythromelalgia and Erythermalgia

Erythromelalgia, a rare disorder, consists of intense, asymmetric burning sensations with associated erythema and elevated temperature in the extremities [Mandell et al., 1977]. The transient episodes may last for minutes, hours, or even days. Because of the intense pain and discomfort, patients often do not walk or use their hands. Patients find relief by immersing their hands or feet in ice water. One form of the disorder is associated with thrombocythemia (a fixed increase in the number of platelets). Blood pressure and peripheral pulses are normal during the symptomatic phase. In older patients, this condition has been associated with hypertension, systemic lupus erythematosus, diabetes mellitus, and myeloproliferative diseases. A defect in prostaglandin metabolism was postulated after many patients reported relief of symptoms after using acetylsalicylic acid [Jorgensen and Sondergaard, 1978]. This so-called secondary erythromelalgia has no parallel in childhood [Drenth et al., 1994].

Primary erythromelalgia or "erythermalgia" is a more rare, chronic, symmetric, burning sensation that occurs in children and adults. It is not reliably responsive to medication [Davis et al., 2000], although some patients have responded well to amitriptyline, sodium nitroprusside, regional anesthetic blockade, and gabapentin [Chan et al., 2002; Harrison et al., 2003; McGraw and Kosek, 1997; Rauck et al., 1996]. Regional nerve block has also been used to control pain [Harrison et al., 2003]. Histopathology reveals no consistent vasculitic changes, and erythermalgia is not associated with thrombocythemia [Drenth et al., 1994]. Some studies have demonstrated autonomic and small sensory fiber axonal neuropathy in patients with this disorder [Chan et al., 2002; Davis et al., 2000; Harrison et al., 2003].

The differential for this disorder includes Raynaud's phenomenon and reflex sympathetic dystrophy, but it can usually be distinguished from these conditions by its unique clinical appearance and the relief provided by ice water immersion. In one report, a child with a syndrome resembling erythermalgia was found to have growth hormone deficiency and remission of symptoms with growth hormone replacement therapy; this has raised the question of whether a disorder involving the insulin-like growth factor family of trophic factors and receptors is involved [Cimaz et al., 2001]. Familial instances of erythermalgia have facilitated localization of the gene for susceptibility to this condition to chromosome 2q31-32 [Drenth et al., 2001].

REFERENCES

Acheson JF, Cockerell OC, Bentley CR, et al. Churg-Strauss vasculitis presenting with severe visual loss due to bilateral sequential optic neuropathy. Br J Ophthalmol 1993;77:118.

Aisen AM, Gabrielsen TO, McCune WJ. MR imaging of systemic lupus erythematosus involving the brain. AJR Am J Roentgenol 1985;144:1027.

Alexander E. Central nervous system disease in Sjögren's syndrome. New insights into immunopathogenesis. Rheum Dis Clin North Am 1992;18:637.

Al-Husaini A, Jamal GA. Myelopathy as the main presenting feature of systemic lupus erythematosus. Eur Neurol 1985;24:94.

Allen AJ, Leonard HL, Swedo SE. Case study: A new infection-triggered, autoimmune subtype of pediatric OCD and Tourette's syndrome. J Am Acad Child Adolesc Psychiatry 1995;34:307.

Amorosi EL, Ultmann JE. Thrombotic thrombocytopenic purpura: Report of 16 cases and review of the literature. Medicine 1966;45:139.

Anaya JM, Ogawa N, Talal N. Sjögren's syndrome in childhood. J Rheumatol 1995;22:1152.

Andrianakos AA, Duffy J, Suzuki M, et al. Transverse myelopathy in systemic lupus erythematosus. Ann Intern Med 1975;83:616.

Ansari I, Crichlow B, Gunton KB, et al. A child with venous sinus thrombosis with initial examination findings of pseudotumor syndrome. Arch Ophthalmol 2002;120:867.

Anton PA, Shanahan F. Neuroimmunomodulation in inflammatory bowel disease. How far from "bench" to "bedside"? Ann N Y Acad Sci 1998;840:723.

Appenzeller S, Montenegro MA, Dertkigil SS, et al. Neuroimaging findings in scleroderma en coup de sabre. Neurology 2004;62:1585.

Aron AM, Freeman JM, Carter S. The natural history of Sydenham's chorea. Am J Med 1965;38:83.

Asherson RA, Derksen R, Harris EN, et al. Chorea in systemic lupus erythematosus and "lupus-like"disease: association with antiphospholipid antibodies. Semin Arthritis Rheum 1987;16:253.

Ates E, Bakkaloglu A, Saatci U, et al. Von Willebrand factor antigen compared with other factors in vasculitic syndromes. Arch Dis Child 1994;70:40.

Ayoub EM, Wannamaker LW. Streptococcal antibody titers in Sydenham's chorea. Pediatrics 1966;38:946.

Bahabri SA, al-Mazyed A, al-Balaa S, et al. Juvenile Behçet's disease in Arab children. Clin Exp Rheumatol 1996;14:331.

Baildam EM, Holt PJL, Conway SC, et al. The association between physical function and psychological problems in children with juvenile chronic arthritis. Br J Rheum 1995;34:470.

Bailey AA, Sayre GP, Clark EC. Neuritis associated with systemic lupus erythematosus. AMA Arch Neurol Psychiatry 1956;75:251.

Bakkaloglu A. Ozen S, Baskin E, et al. The significance of antineutrophil cytoplasmic antibody in microscopic polyangiitis and classic polyarteritis nodosa. Arch Dis Child 2001; 85:427.

Bakshi R, Shaikh ZA, Bates VE, et al. Thrombotic thrombocytopenic purpura: Brain CT and MRI findings in 12 patients. Neurology 1999;52:1285.

Barron TF, Ostrov BE, Zimmerman RA, et al. Isolated angiitis of the CNS: Treatment with pulse cyclophosphamide. Pediatr Neurol 1993;9:73.

Baumann RJ, Robertson WC Jr. Neurosarcoid presents differently in children than in adults. Pediatrics 2003;112:e480.

Beach RC, Corrin B, Scopes JW, et al. Necrotizing sarcoid granulomatosis with neurological lesions in a child. J Pediatr 1980;97:950.

Becton DL, Stine KC. Transient lupus anticoagulants associated with hemorrhage rather than thrombosis: The hemorrhagic lupus anticoagulant syndrome. J Pediatr 1997;130:998.

Belman AL, Leicher CR, Moshé SL, et al. Neurologic manifestations of Schönlein-Henoch purpura: Report of three cases and review of the literature. Pediatrics 1985;75:687.

Benda CE. Chronic rheumatic encephalitis. Arch Neurol Psychiatry 1948;59:262.

Bennett RM, O'Connell DJ. Mixed connective tissue disease: A clinicopathologic study of 20 cases. Semin Arthritis Rheum 1980;10:25.

Benseler S, Schneider R. Central nervous system vasculitis in children. Curr Opin Rheumatol 2004;16:43.

Berlanga B, Rubio FR, Moga I, et al. Response to intravenous cyclophosphamide treatment in lupus myelopathy. J Rheumatol 1992;19:829.

Berman JL, Kashii S, Trachtman MS, et al. Optic neuropathy and central nervous system disease secondary to Sjögren's syndrome in a child. Ophthalmology 1990;97:1606.

Berrios X, Quensey S, Morales A, et al. Are all recurrences of "pure" Sydenham chorea true recurrences of acute rheumatic fever? J Pediatr 1985;107:867.

Bert RJ, Antonacci VP, Berman L, et al. Polyarteritis nodosa presenting as temporal arteritis in a 9-year-old child. Am J Neuroradiol 1999;20:167.

Besbas N, Damarguc I, Ozen S, et al. Association of antiphospholipid antibodies with systemic lupus erythematosus in a child presenting with chorea: A case report. Eur J Pediatr 1994;153:891.

Bicknell JM, Holland JV. Neurologic manifestations of Cogan syndrome. Neurology 1978;28:278.

Bingham PM, Galetta SL, Arthreya B, et al. Neurologic manifestation in children with Lyme disease. Pediatrics 1995;96:1053.

Bird MT, Palkes H, Prensky AL. A follow-up study of Sydenham's chorea. Neurology 1976;26:601.

Blau EB, Morris RF, Yunis EJ. Polyarteritis nodosa in older children. Pediatrics 1977;60:227.

Bluestein HG. Antibodies to brain. In: Wallace DJ, Hahn BH, eds. Dubois' Lupus Erythematosus. Baltimore: Williams & Wilkins, 1997.

Boumpas DT, Patronas NJ, Dalakas MR, et al. Acute transverse myelitis in systemic lupus erythematosus: Magnetic resonance imaging and review of the literature. J Rheumatol 1990;17:89.

Brandt KD, Lessell S, Cohen AS. Cerebral disorders of vision in systemic lupus erythematosus. Ann Intern Med 1975;83:163.

Bray VJ, Singleton JD. Disseminated intravascular coagulation in Still's disease. Semin Arthritis Rheum 1994;24:222.

Brey RL, Chapman J, Levine SR, et al. Stroke and the antiphospholipid syndrome: Consensus meeting Taormina 2002. Lupus 2003;12:508.

Bridger S, Evans N, Parker A, et al. Multiple cerebral venous thromboses in a child with inflammatory bowel disease. J Pediatr Gastroenterol Nutr 1997;25:533.

Bruyn GA. Controversies in lupus: Nervous system involvement. Ann Rheum Dis 1995;54:159.

Bulun A, Topaloglu R, Duzova A, et al. Ataxia and peripheral neuropathy: Rare manifestations in Henoch-Schonlein purpura. Pediatr Nephrol 2001;16:1139.

Buratti S, Szer IS, Spencer CH, et al. Mycophenolate mofetil treatment of severe renal disease in pediatric onset systemic lupus erythematosus. J Rheumatol 2001;28:2103.

Burns JC, Glodé MP. Kawasaki syndrome. Lancet 2004;364:533.

Byrnes JJ, Khurana M. Treatment of thrombotic thrombocytopenic purpura with plasma. N Engl J Med 1977;297:1386.

Cabral DA, Petty RE, Malleson PN, et al. Visual prognosis in children with chronic anterior uveitis and arthritis. J Rheumatol 1994;21:2370.

Calabrese LH. Vasculitis of the central nervous system. Rheum Dis Clin North Am 1995;21:1059.

Calabrese LH, Mallek JA. Primary angiitis of the central nervous system: Report of eight new cases, review of the literature and proposal for diagnostic criteria. Medicine 1988;67:20.

Calabrese LH, Furlan AJ, Gragg LA, et al. Primary angiitis of the central nervous system: Diagnostic criteria and clinical approach. Cleve Clin J Med 1992;59:293.

Calabrese LH, Hoffman GS, Guillevin L. Therapy of resistant systemic necrotizing vasculitis. Polyarteritis, Churg-Strauss syndrome, Wegener's granulomatosis, and hypersensitivity vasculitis group disorders. Rheum Dis Clin North Am 1995;21:41.

Canoso JJ, Cohen AS. Aseptic meningitis in systemic lupus erythematosus: Report of three cases. Arthritis Rheum 1975;18:369.

Carbotte RM, Denburg SD, Denburg JA. Cognitive dysfunction in systemic lupus erythematosus is independent of active disease. J Rheumatol 1995;22:863.

Carette S, Urowitz MB, Grosman H, et al. Cranial computerized tomography in systemic lupus erythematosus. J Rheumatol 1982;9:855.

Carlow TJ, Glaser JS. Pseudotumor cerebri syndrome in systemic lupus erythematosus. JAMA 1974;228:197.

Carr J, Bryer A. An isolated myelopathy as a presentation of polyarteritis nodosa. Br J Rheumatol 1993;32:644.

Carr RI, Harbeck RJ, Hoffman AA, et al. Clinical studies on the significance of DNA anti-DNA complexes in the systemic circulation and cerebrospinal fluid (CSF) of patients with systemic lupus erythematosus. J Rheumatol 1975;2:184.

Carvalho KS, Garg BP. Arterial strokes in children. Neurol Clin 2002;20:1079.

Caselli RJ, Hunder GG. Neurologic aspects of giant cell (temporal) arteritis. Rheum Dis Clin North Am 1993;19:941.
Cassidy JT, Petty RE. Textbook of pediatric rheumatology, 4th ed. Philadelphia: WB Saunders, 2001.
Cassidy JT, Sullivan DB, Petty RE, et al. Lupus nephritis and encephalopathy: Prognosis in 58 children. Arthritis Rheum 1977;20(Suppl 2):315.
Cerinic MM, Generini S, Pignone A, et al. The nervous system in systemic sclerosis (scleroderma). Clinical features and pathogenetic mechanisms. Rheum Dis Clin North Am 1996;22:879.
Chak WK, Lam DS, Lo WH, et al. Thrombotic thrombocytopenic purpura as a rare complication in childhood systemic lupus erythematosus: Case report and literature review. Hong Kong Med J 2003;9:363.
Chan KF, Boey ML. Transverse myelopathy in SLE: Clinical features and functional outcomes. Lupus 1996;5:294.
Chan MKH, Tucker AT, Madden S, et al. Erythromelalgia: An endothelial disorder responsive to sodium nitroprusside. Arch Dis Child 2002;87:229.
Chen CL, Chiou YH, Wu CY, et al. Cerebral vasculitis in Henoch-Schonlein purpura: A case report with sequential magnetic resonance imaging changes and treated with plasmapheresis alone. Pediatr Nephrol 2000;15:276.
Chudwin DS, Daniels TE, Wara DW, et al. Spectrum of Sjögren syndrome in children. J Pediatr 1981;98:213.
Chun RWM, Smith NJ, Forster FM. Papilledema in Sydenham's chorea. Am J Dis Child 1961;101:641.
Chung MH, Sum J, Morrell MJ, et al. Intracerebral involvement in scleroderma en coup de sabre: Report of a case with neuropathologic findings. Ann Neurol 1995;37:679.
Cimaz R, Rusconi R, Fossali E, et al. Unexpected healing of cutaneous ulcers in a short child. Lancet 2001;358:211.
Cines DB. Disorders associated with autoantibodies to endothelial cells. Rev Infect Dis 1989;2(Suppl 4):S705.
Clements PJ, Furst DE, Campion DE, et al. Muscle disease in progressive systemic sclerosis. Diagnostic and therapeutic considerations. Arthritis Rheum 1978;21:62.
Cohen-Gadol A, Zikel OM, Miller GM, et al. Spinal cord biopsy: A review of 38 cases. Neurosurgery 2003;52:806.
Conn DL. Polyarteritis. Rheum Dis Clin North Am 1990;16:341.
Contreras G, Pardo V, Leclercq B, et al. Sequential therapies for proliferative lupus nephritis. N Engl J Med 2004;350:971.
Coster TA, Cole HC. Atlanto-axial dislocation in association with rheumatic fever: A case report. Spine 1990;15:591.
Cruz DN, Segal AS. A patient with Wegener's granulomatosis presenting with a subarachnoid hemorrhage: Case report and review of CNS disease associated with Wegener's granulomatosis. Am J Nephrol 1997;17:181.
Dabich L, Sullivan DB, Cassidy JT. Scleroderma in the child. J Pediatr 1974;85:770.
Dajani AS, Ayoub E, Bierman FZ, et al. Guidelines for the diagnosis of rheumatic fever. Jones Criteria, 1992 update. Special Writing Group of the Committee on Rheumatic Fever, Endocarditis, and Kawasaki Disease of the Council on Cardiovascular Disease in the Young of the American Heart Association. JAMA 1992;268:2069.
Dajani A, Taubert K, Ferrieri P, et al. Treatment of acute streptococcal pharyngitis and prevention of rheumatic fever: A statement for health professions. Pediatrics 1995; 96:758.
Daoud AS, Zaki M, Shakir R, et al. Effectiveness of sodium valproate in the treatment of Sydenham's chorea. Neurology 1990;40:1140.
David J, Ansell BM, Woo P. Polyarteritis nodosa associated with streptococcus. Arch Dis Child 1993;69:685.
Davis LE, Hodgin UG, Kornfield M. Recurrent meningoencephalitis with recovery from Behçet's disease. West J Med 1986;145:238.
Davis MDP, O'Fallon WM, Rogers RS, et al. Natural history of erythromelalgia: Presentation and outcome in 168 patients. Arch Dermatol 2000;136:330.
De Cunto CL, Liberatore DI, San Roman JL, et al. Infantile-onset multisystem inflammatory disease: A differential diagnosis of systemic juvenile rheumatoid arthritis. J Pediatr 1997;130:551.
del Rosario JF, Orenstein SR, Bhargava S, et al. Thrombotic complications in pediatric inflammatory bowel disease. Clin Pediatr (Phila) 1994;33:159.
Derry C, Dale RC, Thom M, et al. Unihemispheric cerebral vasculitis mimicking Rasmussen's encephalitis. Neurology 2002;58:327.
Devlin T, Gray L, Allen NB, et al. Neuro-Behçet's disease: Factors hampering proper diagnosis. Neurology 1995;45:1754.
Dillon MJ. Rare vasculitic syndromes. Ann Med 1997;29:175.
Drachman DA. Neurologic complications of Wegener's granulomatosis. Arch Neurol 1963;8:145.
Drenth JP, Finley WH, Breedveld GJ, et al. The primary erythermalgia-susceptibility gene is located on chromosome 2q31-32. Am J Hum Genet 2001;68:1277.
Drenth JP, Michiels JJ, Ozsoylu S. Acute secondary erythermalgia and hypertension in children. Eur J Pediatr 1995;154:882.
Drenth JP, van Genderen PJJ, Michiels JJ. Thrombocythemic erythromelalgia, primary erythermalgia, and secondary erythermalgia: Three distinct clinicopathologic entities. Angiology 1994;45:451.
Ellison D, Gatter K, Heryet A, et al. Intramural platelet deposition in cerebral vasculopathy of systemic lupus erythematosus. J Clin Pathol 1993;46:37.
Emery ES, Vieco PT. Sydenham chorea: Magnetic resonance imaging reveals permanent basal ganglia injury. Neurology 1997;48:531.
Engel DG, Gospe SM Jr, Tracy KA, et al. Fatal infantile polyarteritis nodosa with predominant central nervous system involvement. Stroke 1995;26:699.
Erdem E, Carlier R, Idir AB, et al. Gadolinium-enhanced MRI in central nervous system Behçet's disease. Neuroradiology 1993;35:142.
Escalante A, Stimmler MM. Trimethoprim-sulfamethoxazole induced meningitis in systemic lupus erythematosus. J Rheumatol 1992;19:800.
Eun SH, Kim SJ, Cho DS, et al. Cerebral vasculitis in Henoch-Schonlein purpura: MRI and MRA findings, treated with plasmapheresis alone. Pediatr Int 2003;45:484.
Eyanson S, Passo MH, Aldo-Benson MA, et al. Methylprednisolone pulse therapy for nonrenal lupus erythematosus. Ann Rheum Dis 1980;39:377.
Fager DB, Bigler JA, Simonds JP. Polyarteritis nodosa in infancy and childhood. J Pediatr 1951;39:65.
Falko JM, Williams JC, Harvey DG, et al. Hyperlipoproteinemia and multifocal neurologic dysfunction in systemic lupus erythematosus. J Pediatr 1979;95:523.
Farooki ZQ, Brough AJ, Green EW. Necrotizing arteritis. Am J Dis Child 1974;128:837.
Faustino PC, Terreri MTRA, da Rocha AJ, et al. Clinical, laboratory, psychiatric and magnetic resonance findings in patients with Sydenham chorea. Neuroradiology 2003;45:456.
Fink CW. Polyarteritis and other diseases with necrotizing vasculitis in childhood. Arthritis Rheum 1977;20(Suppl):378.
Fink CW, Cimaz R. Early onset sarcoidosis: Not a benign disease. J Rheumatol 1997;24:174.
Finn R, de M Rudolf N. The electroencephalogram in systemic lupus erythematosus. Lancet 1978;1:1255.
Fish AJ, Blau EB, Westberg NG, et al. Systemic lupus erythematosus within the first two decades of life. Am J Med 1977;62:99.
Flechtner KM, Baum K. Mixed connective tissue disease: Recurrent episodes of optic neuropathy and transverse myelopathy. Successful treatment with plasmapheresis. J Neurol Sci 1994;126:146.
Ford RG, Siekert RG. Central nervous system manifestations of periarteritis nodosa. Neurology 1965;15:114.
Fox RI. Treatment of the patient with Sjögren's syndrome. Rheum Dis Clin North Am 1992;18:699.
Fujikawa S, Suemitsu T. Behçet's disease in children: A nationwide retrospective survey in Japan. Acta Paediatr Jpn 1997;39:285.
Galli M, Luciani D, Bertolini G, Barbui T. Lupus anticoagulants are stronger risk factors for thrombosis than anticardiolipin antibodies in the antiphospholipid syndrome: A systematic review of the literature. Blood 2003;101:1827.
Ganji S, Duncan MC, Frazier E. Sydenham's chorea: Clinical, EEG, CT scan, and evoked potential studies. Clin Electroencephalogr 1988;19:114.
Garvey MA, Giedd J, Swedo SE. PANDAS: The search for environmental triggers of pediatric neuropsychiatric disorders. Lessons from rheumatic fever. J Child Neurol 1998;13:413.
Gatti FM, Rosenheim E. Sydenham's chorea associated with transient intellectual impairment. Am J Dis Child 1969;118:915.
Georganas C, Ioakimidis D, Iatrou C, et al. Relapsing Wegener's granulomatosis: Successful treatment with cyclosporin A. Clin Rheumatol 1996;15:189.
Gerraty RP, McKelvie PA, Byrne E. Aseptic meningoencephalitis in primary Sjögren's syndrome. Response to plasmapheresis and absence of CNS vasculitis at autopsy. Acta Neurol Scand 1993;88:309.
Gibb WR, Lees AJ. Tendency to late recurrence following rheumatic chorea. Neurology 1989;39:999.

Goder G. Periarteritis nodosa in childhood. Z Gesamte Exp Med 1956;11:652.

Gold AP, Yahr MD. Childhood lupus erythematosus: A clinical and pathological study of the neurological manifestations. Trans Am Neurol Assoc 1960;85:96.

Goldenberg J, Ferraz MB, Fonseca AS, et al. Sydenham chorea: Clinical and laboratory findings. Analysis of 187 cases. Rev Paul Med 1992;110:152.

Gordon RM, Silverstein A. Neurologic manifestations in progressive systemic sclerosis. Arch Neurol 1970;22:126.

Graf WD, Milstein JM, Sherry DD. Stroke and mixed connective tissue disease. J Child Neurol 1993;8:256.

Green LN. Corticosteroids in the treatment of Sydenham's chorea. Arch Neurol 1978;35:53.

Green L, Vinker S, Amital H, et al. Pseudotumor cerebri in systemic lupus erythematosus. Semin Arthritis Rheum 1995;25:103.

Gronemeyer PS, Demello DE. Takayasu's disease with aneurysms of right common iliac artery in iliocaval fistula in a young infant. Case report and review of the literature. Pediatrics 1982;69:626.

Guillevin L, Lhote F, Cohen P, et al. Polyarteritis nodosa related to hepatitis B virus. A prospective study with long-term observation of 41 patients. Medicine (Baltimore) 1995;74:238.

Guillevin L, Visser H, Noel LH, et al. Antineutrophil cytoplasm antibodies in systemic polyarteritis nodosa with and without hepatitis B virus infection and Churg-Strauss syndrome—62 patients. J Rheumatol 1993;20:1345.

Haas JP, Metzler M, Ruder H, et al. An unusual manifestation of Wegener's granulomatosis in a 4-year-old girl. Pediatr Neurol 2002;27:71.

Hackett ER, Martinez RD, Larson PF, et al. Optic neuritis in systemic lupus erythematosus. Arch Neurol 1974;31:9.

Hadchouel M, Prieur A, Griscelli C. Acute hemorrhagic, hepatic, and neurologic manifestations in juvenile rheumatoid arthritis. Possible relationship to drugs or infection. J Pediatr 1985;106:561.

Hadler NM, Gerwin RD, Frank MM, et al. The fourth component of complement in the cerebrospinal fluid in systemic lupus erythematosus. Arthritis Rheum 1973;16:507.

Halbreich U, Assael M, Kauly N, et al. Rheumatic brain disease: A disease in its own right. J Nerv Ment Dis 1976;163:24.

Hankey GJ. Isolated angiitis/angiopathy of the central nervous system. Cerebrovasc Dis 1991;1:2.

Hanly JG, Walsh NM, Sangalang V. Brain pathology in systemic lupus erythematosus. J Rheumatol 1992;19:732.

Hanmer O, Saltissi D. Response of acute cerebral lupus in childhood to pulse methylprednisolone in reduced dosage. Ann Rheum Dis 1986;45:606.

Hansen JR, McCray PB, Bale JF, et al. Reye syndrome associated with aspirin therapy for systemic lupus erythematosus. Pediatrics 1985;76:202.

Harisdangkul V, Doorenbos D, Subramony SH. Lupus transverse myelopathy: Better outcome with early recognition and aggressive high-dose intravenous corticosteroid pulse treatment. J Neurol 1995;242:326.

Harrison CM, Goddard JM, Rittey CD. The use of regional anaesthetic blockade in a child with recurrent erythromelalgia. Arch Dis Child 2003;88:65.

Hart RG, Miller VT, Coull BM, et al. Cerebral infarction associated with lupus anticoagulants—preliminary report. Stroke 1984;15:114.

Heinrich D, Gordjani N, Trusen A, et al. Necrotizing sarcoid granulomatosis: A rarity in childhood. Pediatr Pulmonol 2003;35:407.

Herd JK, Medhi M, Uzendoski UM, et al. Chorea associated with SLE: Report of 2 cases and review of literature. Pediatrics 1978;61:308.

Hietaharju A, Jantti V, Korpela M, et al. Central nervous system involvement and psychiatric manifestations in systemic sclerosis (scleroderma): Clinical and neurophysiological evaluation. Acta Neurol Scand 1993;87:382.

Hirohata S, Hirose S, Miyamoto T. Cerebrospinal fluid IgM, IgA, and IgG indexes in systemic lupus erythematosus. Arch Intern Med 1985;145:1843.

Hisashi K, Komune S, Taira T, et al. Anticardiolipin antibody-induced sudden profound sensorineural hearing loss. Am J Otolaryngol 1993;14:275.

Hochberg MC. Updating the American College of Rheumatology. Revised criteria for the classification of systemic lupus erythematosus (letter). Arthritis Rheum 1997;40:1725.

Hoffman GS. Treatment of resistant Takayasu's arteritis. Rheum Dis Clin North Am 1995;21:73.

Hoffman GS. Takayasu arteritis: Lessons from the American National Institutes of Health experience. Int J Cardiol 1996;54:S99.

Horton TM, Stone JD, Yee D, et al. Case series of thrombotic thrombocytopenic purpura in children and adolescents. J Pediatr Hematol Oncol 2003;25:336.

Hoyne AL, Steiner MD. Periarteritis nodosa complicating scarlet fever. Am J Dis Child 1940;59:1271.

Huisman TA, Wohlrab G, Nadal D, et al. Unusual presentations of neuroborreliosis (Lyme disease) in childhood. J Comput Assist Tomog 1999;23:39.

Huttenlocher A, Frieden IF, Emery H. Neonatal onset multisystem inflammatory disease. J Rheumatol 1995;22:1171.

International Study Group for Behçet's Disease. Evaluation of diagnostic ("classification") criteria in Behçet's Disease: Towards internationally agreed criteria. Br J Rheumatol 1992;31:299.

Ishikawa O, Ohnishi K, Miyachi Y, et al. Cerebral lesions in systemic lupus erythematosus detected by magnetic resonance imaging. Relationship to anticardiolipin antibody. J Rheumatol 1994;21:87.

Isshi K, Hirohata S, Hashimoto T, et al. Systemic lupus erythematosus presenting with diffuse low density lesions in the cerebral white matter on computed axial tomography scans: Its implication in the pathogenesis of diffuse central nervous system lupus. J Rheumatol 1994;21:1758.

Jacob JC. Systemic lupus erythematosus in childhood: Report of 35 cases with discussion of 7 apparently induced by anticonvulsant medication, and of prognosis and treatment. Pediatrics 1963;32:257.

Jain S, Sharma N, Singh S, et al. Takayasu arteritis in children and young Indians. Int J Cardiol 2000;75(Suppl 1):S153.

Jayne DR, Lockwood CM. Intravenous immunoglobulin as sole therapy for systemic vasculitis. Br J Rheumatol 1996;35:1150.

Jones JM, Martinez AJ, Joshi VV, et al. Systemic lupus erythematosus. Arch Pathol 1975;99:152.

Jorgensen HP, Sondergaard J. Pathogenesis of erythromelalgia. Arch Dermatol 1978;114:112.

Kaell AT, Shetty M, Lee BC, et al. The diversity of neurologic events in systemic lupus erythematosus. Arch Neurol 1986;43:273.

Kapitsinou PP, Boletis JN, Skopouli FN, et al. Lupus nephritis: Treatment with mycophenolate mofetil. Rheumatol (Oxford) 2004;43:377.

Kari JA, Shah V, Dillon MJ. Behcet's disease in UK children: Clinical features and treatment including thalidomide. Rheumatology 2001;40:933.

Kawasaki T, Kosaki F, Okawa S, et al. A new infantile acute febrile mucocutaneous lymph node syndrome prevailing in Japan. Pediatrics 1974;54:271.

Keeffe EB, Bardana EJ Jr, Harbeck RJ, et al. Lupus meningitis antibody to deoxyribonucleic acid (DNA) and DNA/anti-DNA complexes in cerebrospinal fluid. Ann Intern Med 1974; 80:58.

Khamashta MA, Cuadrado MJ, Mujic F, et al. The management of thrombosis in the antiphospholipid-antibody syndrome. N Engl J Med 1995;332:993.

Kim RC. Rheumatoid disease with encephalopathy. Ann Neurol 1980;7:86.

Kissel JT. Neurologic manifestations of vasculitis. Neurol Clin 1989;7:655.

Kohrman MH, Huttenlocher PR. Takayasu arteritis. A treatable cause of stroke in infancy. Pediatr Neurol 1986;2:154.

Kok J, Bosseray A, Brion JP, et al. Chorea in a child with Churg-Strauss syndrome. Stroke 1993;24:1263.

Koné-Paut I, Yurdakul S, Bahabri SA, et al. Clinical features of Behçet's disease in children: An international collaborative study of 86 cases. J Pediatr 1998;132:721.

Kornreich HK, King KK, Bernstein BH, et al. Scleroderma in childhood. Arthritis Rheum 1977;20:343.

Kotajima L, Aotsuka S, Sumiya M, et al. Clinical features of patients with juvenile onset mixed connective tissue disease: Analysis of data collected in a nationwide collaborative study in Japan. J Rheumatol 1996;23:1088.

Kovacs JA, Urowitz MB, Gladman DD. Dilemmas in neuropsychiatric lupus. Rheum Dis Clin North Am 1993;19:795.

Krause I, Uziel Y, Guedj D, et al. Childhood Behçet's disease: Clinical features and comparison with adult-onset disease. Rheumatology 1999;38:457.

Kukla LF, Reddy C, Silkalns G, et al. Systemic lupus erythematosus presenting as chorea. Arch Dis Child 1978;53:345.

Kuroe K, Kurahashi K, Nakano I, et al. A neuropathological study of a case of lupus erythematosus with chorea. J Neurol Sci 1994;123:59.

Kwong T, Valderrama E, Paley C, et al. Systemic necrotizing vasculitis associated with childhood sarcoidosis. Semin Arthritis Rheum 1994;23:388.
Lang H, Anttila R, Svekus A, et al. EEG findings in juvenile rheumatoid arthritis and other connective tissue diseases in children. Acta Paediatr Scand 1974;63:373.
Langford CA. Wegener's granulomatosis: Current and upcoming therapies. Arthritis Res Ther 2003;5:180.
Lanthier S, Lortie A, Michaud J, et al. Isolated angiitis of the CNS in children. Neurology 2001;56:837.
Lawlor ER, Webb DW, Hill A, et al. Thrombotic thrombocytopenic purpura: A treatable cause of childhood encephalopathy. J Pediatr 1997;130:313.
Laxer RM, Arnold WJD, Petty RE. Juvenile rheumatoid arthritis sparing the lower extremities in a girl with myelodysplasia. Pediatrics 1984a;73:400.
Laxer RM, Dunn HG, Floodmark O. Acute hemiplegia in Kawasaki disease and infantile polyarteritis nodosa. Dev Med Child Neurol 1984b;26:814.
Lee M, Epstein FJ, Rezai A, et al. Nonneoplastic intramedullary spinal cord lesions mimicking tumors. Neurosurgery 1998;43:788.
Lehman TJ. Systemic and localized scleroderma in children. Curr Opin Rheumatol 1996;8:576.
Leiba H, Siatkowski RM, Culbertson WW, et al. Neurosarcoidosis presenting as an intracranial mass in childhood. J Neuroophthalmol 1996;16:269.
Leonard HL, Swedo SE, Lenane MC, et al. A 2- to 7-year follow-up study of 54 obsessive-compulsive children and adolescents. Arch Gen Psychiatry 1993;50:429.
Lepore L, Marchetti F, Facchini S, et al. Drug-induced systemic lupus erythematosus associated with etanercept therapy in a child with juvenile idiopathic arthritis. Clin Exp Rheumatol 2003;21:276.
Levy DM, Massicotte MP, Harvey E, et al. Thromboembolism in paediatric lupus patients. Lupus 2003;12:741.
Lhote F, Guillevin L. Polyarteritis nodosa, microscopic polyangiitis, and Churg-Strauss syndrome. Rheum Dis Clin North Am 1995;21:911.
Lie JT. Bilateral juvenile temporal arteritis. J Rheumatol 1995;22:774.
Lie JT, Gordon LP, Titus JL. Juvenile temporal arteritis: Biopsy study of 4 cases. JAMA 1975;234:496.
Ling W, Oftedal G, Simon T. Central retinal artery occlusion in Sydenham's chorea. Am J Dis Child 1969;118:525.
Liou HH, Yip PK, Chang YC, et al. Allergic granulomatosis and angiitis (Churg-Strauss syndrome) presenting as prominent neurologic lesions and optic neuritis. J Rheumatol 1994;21:2380.
Logigian EL, Kaplan RF, Steere AC. Chronic neurologic manifestations of Lyme disease. N Engl J Med 1990;323:1438.
Lossos A, River Y, Eliakim A, et al. Neurologic aspects of inflammatory bowel disease. Neurology 1995;45:416.
Maeda M, Kobayashi M, Okamoto S, et al. Clinical observation of 14 cases of childhood polyarteritis nodosa in Japan. Acta Paediatr Jpn 1997;39:277.
Magilavy DB, Petty RE, Cassidy JT, et al. A syndrome of childhood polyarteritis. J Pediatr 1977;91:25.
Malinow KL, Molina R, Gordon B, et al. Neuropsychiatric dysfunction in primary Sjögren's syndrome. Ann Intern Med 1985;103:344.
Manco-Johnson MJ, Nuss R. Lupus anticoagulant in children with thrombosis. Am J Hematol 1995;48:240.
Mandell F, Folkman J, Matsumoto S. Erythromelalgia. Pediatrics 1977;59:45.
Martin CM, Uhlmann V, Killalea A, et al. Detection of measles virus in children with ileo-colonic lymphoid nodular hyperplasia, enterocolitis and developmental disorder. Mol Psychiatry 2002;7:S47.
Martinez-Cordero E, Fonseca MC, Aquilar-Leon DE, et al. Juvenile systemic sclerosis. J Rheumatol 1993;20:405.
Masi AT, Hunder GG, Lie JT, et al. The American College of Rheumatology 1990 criteria for the classification of Churg-Strauss syndrome (allergic granulomatosis and angiitis). Arthritis Rheum 1990;33:1094.
Matsell DG, Keene DL, Jimenez C, et al. Isolated angiitis of the central nervous system in childhood. Can J Neurol Sci 1990;17:151.
Matsumoto R, Shintaku M, Suzuki S, et al. Cerebral perivenous calcification in neuropsychiatric lupus erythematosus: A case report. Neuroradiology 1998;40:583.
McGraw T, Kosek P. Erythromelalgia pain managed with gabapentin. Anesthesiology 1997;86:988.
Meislin AG, Rothfield N. Systemic lupus erythematosus in childhood: Analysis of 42 cases, with comparative data on 200 adult cases followed concurrently. Pediatrics 1968;42:37.
Melish ME. Kawasaki syndrome. A new infectious disease? J Infect Dis 1981;143:317.
Melish ME. Kawasaki syndrome. Pediatr Rev 1996;17:153.
Meroni PL, Moia M, Derksen RH, et al. Venous thromboembolism in the antiphospholipid syndrome: Management guidelines for secondary prophylaxis. Lupus 2003;12:504.
Mier R, Ansell B, Hall MA, et al. Long term follow-up of children with mixed connective tissue disease. Lupus 1996;5:221.
Millar AJ, Gilbert RD, Brown RA, et al. Abdominal aortic aneurysms in children. J Pediatr Surg 1996;31:1624.
Miller ML, Levinson L, Pachman LM, et al. Abnormal muscle MRI in a patient with systemic juvenile arthritis. Pediatr Radiol 1995;25(Suppl 1):S107.
Miller WL, Burnett JC Jr. Blood vessel physiology and pathophysiology. Rheum Dis Clin North Am 1990;16:251.
Mitkov V. Cerebral manifestations of rheumatic fever. World Neurol 1961;2:920.
Mizukami K, Shiraishi H, Tanaka Y, et al. CNS changes in neuro-Behçet's disease: CT, MR, and SPECT findings. Comput Med Imaging Graph 1992;16:401.
Moder KG. Use and interpretation of rheumatologic tests: A guide for clinicians. Mayo Clin Proc 1996;71:391.
Mok CC, Lau CS. Transverse myelopathy complicating mixed connective tissue disease. Clin Neurol Neurosurg 1995;97:259.
Molad Y, Sidi Y, Gornish M, et al. Lupus anticoagulant: Correlation with magnetic resonance imaging of brain lesions. J Rheumatol 1992;19:556.
Molina R, Provost TT, Alexander EL. Peripheral inflammatory vascular disease in Sjögren's syndrome: Association with nervous system complications. Arthritis Rheum 1985;28:1341.
Monfort-Gourand M, Chokre R, Dubiez M, et al. Inflammatory pseudotumor of the orbit and suspected sarcoidosis. Arch Pediatr 1996;3:697.
Moorthy AV, Chesney RW, Segar WE, et al. Wegener's granulomatosis in childhood: Prolonged survival following cytotoxic therapy. J Pediatr 1977;91:616.
Morales E, Pineda C, Martínez-Lavín M. Takayasu's arteritis in children. J Rheumatol 1991;18:1081.
Mouy R, Stephan JL, Pillet P, et al. Efficacy of cyclosporine A in the treatment of macrophage activation syndrome in juvenile arthritis: Report of five cases. J Pediatr 1996;129:750.
Murch SH. Local and systemic effects of macrophage cytokines in intestinal inflammation. Nutrition 1998;14:780.
Murch SH, Anthony A, Casson DH, et al. Retraction of an interpretation. Lancet 2004;363:750.
Murphy TK, Goodman WK, Fudge MW, et al. B lymphocyte antigen D8/17: A peripheral marker for childhood-onset obsessive-compulsive disorder and Tourette's syndrome. Am J Psychiatr 1997;154:402.
Murray KJ, Szer W, Grom AA, et al. Antibodies to the 45 kDa DEK nuclear antigen in pauciarticular onset juvenile rheumatoid arthritis and iridocyclitis: Selective association with MHC gene. J Rheumatol 1997;24:560.
Murray KJ, Laxer RM. Scleroderma in children and adolescents. Rheum Dis Clin North Am 2002;28:603.
Nadeau SE. Neurologic manifestations of systemic vasculitis. Neurol Clin 2002;20:123.
Nagahiro S, Mantani A, Yamada K, et al. Multiple cerebral arterial occlusions in a young patient with Sjögren's syndrome: Case report. Neurosurgery 1996;38:592.
Ndiaye IC, Rassi SJ, Wiener-Vacher SR. Cochleovestibular impairment in pediatric Cogan's syndrome. Pediatrics 2002;109:E38.
Neuwelt CM, Lacks S, Kaye BR, et al. Role of intravenous cyclophosphamide in the treatment of severe neuropsychiatric systemic lupus erythematosus. Am J Med 1995;98:32.
Nikitakis NG, Rivera H, Lariccia C, et al. Primary Sjögren syndrome in childhood: Report of a case and review of the literature. Oral Surg Oral Med Oral Pathol Oral Radiol Endod 2003;96:42.
Nimelstein SH, Brody S, McShane D, et al. Mixed connective tissue disease: A subsequent evaluation of the original 25 patients. Medicine 1980;59:239.
Nishimura A, Yamazaki H, Fuchigami T, et al. [A childhood case of systemic lupus erythematosus associated with myasthenia gravis.] No To Hattatsu (in Japanese) 1997;29:390.
Nobili F, Cutolo M, Sulli A, et al. Brain functional involvement by perfusion SPECT in systemic sclerosis and Behçet's disease. N Y Acad Sci 2002;966:409.

Nordborg E, Nordborg C, Malmvall BE, et al. Giant cell arteritis. Rheum Dis Clin North Am 1995;21:1013.

Norris DG, Colon AR, Stickler GB. Systemic lupus erythematosus in children: The complex problems of diagnosis and treatment encountered in 101 such patients at the Mayo Clinic. Clin Pediatr 1977;16:774.

O'Connor D, Bernstein B, Hanson V, et al. Disease of central nervous system in juvenile rheumatoid arthritis. Arthritis Rheum 1980;23:727.

O'Duffy JD, Goldstein NP. Neurologic involvement in seven patients with Behçet's disease. Am J Med 1976;61:170.

Oetgen WJ, Boice JA, Lawless OJ. Mixed connective tissue disease in children and adolescents. Pediatrics 1981;67:333.

Ohtsuka T, Saito Y, Hasegawa M, et al. Central nervous system disease in a child with primary Sjögren syndrome. J Pediatr 1995;127:961.

Okano Y. Antinuclear antibody in systemic sclerosis (scleroderma). Rheum Dis Clin North Am 1996;22:709.

Olfat M, Al-Mayouf SM. Cogan's syndrome in childhood. Rheumatol Int 2001;20:246.

Olsen NJ, King LE Jr, Park JH. Muscle abnormalities in scleroderma. Rheum Dis Clin North Am 1996;22:783.

Orlowski JP, Clough JD, Dyment PG. Wegener's granulomatosis in the pediatric age group. Pediatrics 1978;61:83.

Østergaard JR, Storm K. Neurologic manifestations of Schönlein-Henoch purpura. Acta Paediatr Scand 1991;80:339.

Ostuni PA, Ianniello A, Sfriso P, et al. Juvenile onset of primary Sjögren's syndrome: Report of 10 cases. Clin Exp Rheumatol 1996;14:689.

Ozen S, Besbas N, Saatci U, et al. Diagnostic criteria for polyarteritis nodosa in childhood. J Pediatr 1992;120:206.

Ozen S. Juvenile polyarteritis: Is it a different disease? J Rheumatol 2004;31:831.

Pantell RH, Goodman BW Jr. Takayasu's arteritis. The relationship with tuberculosis. Pediatrics 1981;67:84.

Parikh S, Swaiman KF, Kim Y. Neurologic characteristics of childhood lupus erythematosus. Pediatr Neurol 1995;13:198.

Pattishall EN, Kendig EL Jr. Sarcoidosis in children. Pediatr Pulmonol 1996;22:195.

Peal AR, Gildersleeve N, Lucchesi PF. Periarteritis nodosa complicating scarlet fever. Am J Dis Child 1946;72:310.

Penn AS, Rowan AJ. Myelopathy in systemic lupus erythematosus. Arch Neurol 1968;18:337.

Petri M, Roubenoff R, Dallal GE, et al. Plasma homocysteine as a risk factor for atherothrombotic events in systemic lupus erythematosus. Lancet 1996; 348:1120.

Petty RE, Southwood TR, Manners P, et al. International League of Associations for Theumatology classification of juvenile idiopathic arthritis: Second revision, Edmonton, 2001. J Rheumatol 2004;31:390.

Peyronnard J, Charron L, Beaudet F, et al. Vasculitic neuropathy in rheumatoid disease and Sjögren syndrome. Neurology 1982;32:839.

Pope JE. Treatment of systemic sclerosis. Rheum Dis Clin North Am 1996;22:893.

Prieur AM. A recently recognised chronic inflammatory disease of early onset characterised by the triad of rash, central nervous system involvement and arthropathy. Clin Exp Rheumatol 2000;19:103.

Press J, Palayew K, Laxer RM, et al. Antiribosomal P antibodies in pediatric patients with systemic lupus erythematosus and psychosis. Arthritis Rheum 1996;39:671.

Propper DJ, Bucknall RC. Acute transverse myelopathy complicating systemic lupus erythematosus. Ann Rheum Dis 1989;48:512.

Provenzale J, Bouldin TW. Lupus-related myelopathy: Report of three cases and review of the literature. J Neurol Neurosurg Psychiatry 1992;55:830.

Provenzale JM, Barboriak DP, Gaensler EHL, et al. Lupus-related myelitis: Serial MR findings. Am J Neuroradiol 1994;15:1911.

Quartier P, Taupin P, Bourdeaut F, et al. Efficacy of etanercept for the treatment of juvenile idiopathic arthritis according to the onset type. Arthritis Rheum 2003;48:1093.

Quintero-Del-Rio AI, Van Miller S. Neurologic symptoms in children with systemic lupus erythematousus. J Child Neurol 2000;15:803.

Quirk ME, Young MH. The impact of JRA on children, adolescents, and their families: Current research and implication for future studies. Arthritis Care Res 1990;3:36.

Rachelefsky GS, Kar NC, Coulson A, et al. Serum enzyme abnormalities in juvenile rheumatoid arthritis. Pediatrics 1976;58:730.

Rakover Y, Adar J, Tal I, et al. Behçet disease: Long-term follow-up of three children and review of the literature. Pediatrics 1989;83:986.

Rauck RL, Naveira F, Speight KL, et al. Refractory idiopathic erythromelalgia. Anesth Analg 1996;82:1097.

Ravelli A. Macrophage activation syndrome. Curr Opin Rheumatol 2002;14:548.

Ravelli A, Martini A. Antiphospholipid antibody syndrome in pediatric patients. Rheum Dis Clin North Am 1997;23:657.

Raza A. Anti-TNF therapies in rheumatoid arthritis, Crohn's disease, sepsis, and myelodysplastic syndromes. Microsc Res Tech 2000;50:229.

Reichlin M. Ribosomal P antibodies and CNS lupus. Lupus 2003;12:916.

Reinhold-Keller E, De-Groot K, Rudert H, et al. Response to trimethoprim/sulfamethoxazole in Wegener's granulomatosis depends on the phase of disease. Q J Med 1996;89:15.

Rhodes VJ. Physical therapy management of patients with juvenile rheumatoid arthritis. Phys Ther 1991;71:910.

Richardson ML, Helms CA, Vogler JB, et al. Skeletal changes in neuromuscular disorders mimicking juvenile rheumatoid arthritis and hemophilia. AJR Am J Roentgenol 1984;143:893.

Rinkel GJE, Wijdicks EFM, Hene RJ. Stroke in relapsing thrombotic thrombocytopenic purpura. Stroke 1991;22:1087.

Ritchlin CT, Chabot RJ, Alper K, et al. Quantitative electroencephalography: A new approach to the diagnosis of cerebral dysfunction in systemic lupus erythematosus. Arthritis Rheum 1992;35:1330.

Ritter FJ, Seay AR, Lahey ME. Peripheral mononeuropathy complicating anaphylactoid purpura. J Pediatr 1983;103:77.

Roberts FB, Fetterman GH. Polyarteritis nodosa in infancy. J Pediatr 1963;63:519.

Robertson WC Jr, Smith CD. Sydenham's chorea in the age of MRI: A case report and review. Pediatr Neurol 2002;27:65.

Robson MG, Walport MJ, Davies KA. Systemic lupus erythematosus and acute demyelinating polyneuropathy. Br J Rheumatol 1994;33:1074.

Rosenberg AM. Uveitis associated with childhood rheumatic diseases. Curr Opin Rheumatol 2002;14:542.

Rosenberger A, Adler OB, Haim S. Radiologic aspects of Behçet's disease. Radiology 1982;144:261.

Rothfield N. Clinical features of systemic lupus erythematosus. In: Kelley WN, Harris ED Jr, Ruddy S, et al, eds. Textbook of Rheumatology, 2nd ed. Philadelphia: WB Saunders, 1985.

Rothstein JL, Welt S. Periarteritis nodosa in infancy and in childhood: Report of 2 cases with necropsy observations, abstracts of cases in the literature. Am J Dis Child 1933;45:1277.

Rottem M, Fauci AS, Hallahan CW, et al. Wegener granulomatosis in children and adolescents: Clinical presentation and outcome. J Pediatr 1993;122:26.

Rubin RL. Drug-induced lupus. In: Wallace DJ, Hahn BH, eds. Dubois' lupus erythematosus. Baltimore: Williams & Wilkins, 1997.

Sabharwal UK, Keogh LH, Weisman MH, et al. Granulomatous angiitis of the nervous system. Case report and review of the literature. Arthritis Rheum 1982;25:342.

Sanna G, Bertolaccini ML, Mathieu A. Central nervous system lupus: A clinical approach to therapy. Lupus 2003;12:935.

Schieken R, Anderson WT, Anthony CL. Diplopia: A rare manifestation of chorea. Am J Dis Child 1973;125:586.

Schor NF. Neurology of systemic autoimmune disorders: A pediatric perspective. Semin Pediatr Neurol 2000;7:108.

Scott TF. Neurosarcoidosis: Progress and clinical aspects. Neurology 1993;43:8.

Seaman DE, Londino AV Jr, Kwoh CK, et al. Antiphospholipid antibodies in pediatric systemic lupus erythematosus. Pediatrics 1995;96:1040.

Sehgal M, Swanson JW, DeRemee RA, et al. Neurologic manifestations of Churg-Strauss syndrome. Mayo Clin Proc 1995;70:337.

Sequeira W. Rheumatic manifestations of sarcoidosis. In: Kelley WN, Harris ED Jr, Ruddy S, et al, eds. Textbook of rheumatology, 5th ed. Philadelphia: WB Saunders, 1997.

Sergent JS, Lockshin MD, Klempner MS, et al. Central nervous system disease in systemic lupus erythematosus. Am J Med 1975;58:644.

Shaikov AV, Maximov AA, Speransky AI, et al. Repetitive use of pulse therapy with methylprednisolone and cyclophosphamide in addition to oral methotrexate in children with systemic juvenile rheumatoid arthritis—preliminary results of a long-term study. J Rheumatol 1992;19:612.

Shannon KM, Fenichel GM. Pimozide treatment of Sydenham's chorea. Neurology 1990;40:186.

Sharma BK, Jain S, Radotra BD. An autopsy study of Takayasu arteritis in India. Int J Cardiol 1998;66(Suppl 1):S85.

Sharp GC. Mixed connective tissue disease. Bull Rheum Dis 1975;25:828.

Sharp GC, Irvin WS, Tan EM, et al. Mixed connective tissue disease: An apparently distinct rheumatic disease syndrome associated with a specific antibody to an extractable nuclear antigen (ENA). Am J Med 1972;52:148.

Shenker DM, Grossman HJ, Klawans HL. Treatment of Sydenham's chorea with haloperidol. Dev Med Child Neurol 1973;15:19.

Sher JH, Pertschuk LP. Immunoglobulin G deposits in the choroid plexus of a child with systemic lupus erythematosus. J Pediatr 1974;85:385.

Shulman ST, De lnocencio J, Hirsch R. Kawasaki disease. Pediatr Clin North Am 1995;42:1205.

Sibbitt WL Jr, Brandt JR, Johnson CR, et al. The incidence and prevalence of neuropsychiatric syndromes in pediatric onset systemic lupus erythematosus. J Rheumatol 2002;29:1536.

Sicotte NL, Voskuhl RR. Onset of multiple sclerosis associated with anti-TNF therapy. Neurology 2001;57:1885.

Silber TJ, Chatoor I, White PH. Psychiatric manifestations of systemic lupus erythematosus in children and adolescents. Clin Pediatr 1984;23:331.

Silverman E. What's new in the treatment of pediatric SLE? J Rheumatol 1996;23:1657.

Silverman ED, Cawkwell GD, Lovell DJ, et al. Intravenous immunoglobulin in the treatment of systemic juvenile rheumatoid arthritis: A randomized placebo controlled trial. Pediatric Rheumatology Collaborative Study Group. J Rheumatol 1994;21:2353.

Silverman ED, Miller JJ, Bernstein B, et al. Consumption coagulopathy associated with systemic juvenile rheumatoid arthritis. J Pediatr 1983;103:872.

Silverstein A. Thrombotic thrombocytopenic purpura: The initial neurological manifestations. Arch Neurol 1968;18:358.

Singsen BH, Fishman L, Hanson V. Antinuclear antibodies and lupus-like syndromes in children receiving anticonvulsants. Pediatrics 1976;57:529.

Singsen BH, Swanson VL, Bernstein BH, et al. A histologic evaluation of mixed connective tissue disease in childhood. Am J Med 1980;68:710.

Small P. Giant cell arteritis presenting as a bilateral stroke. Arthritis Rheum 1984;27:819.

Smith RW, Ellison DW, Jenkins EA, et al. Cerebellum and brainstem vasculopathy in systemic lupus erythematosus: Two clinico-pathological cases. Ann Rheum Dis 1994;53:327.

Sneller MC, Hoffman GS, Talar-Williams C, et al. An analysis of forty-two Wegener's granulomatosis patients treated with methotrexate and prednisone. Arthritis Rheum 1995;38:608.

Steere AC. Lyme disease. N Engl J Med 1989;321:586.

Stegeman CA, Tervaert JWC, de Jong PE, et al. Trimethoprim-sulfamethoxazole (co-trimoxazole) for the prevention of relapses of Wegener's granulomatosis. Dutch Co-trimoxazole Wegener Study Group. N Engl J Med 1996;335:16.

Stehbens JA, MacQueen JC. The psychological adjustment of rheumatic fever patients with and without chorea comparisons ten years later. Clin Pediatr 1972;11:638.

Steinlin MI, Blaser SI, Gilday DL, et al. Neurologic manifestations of pediatric systemic lupus erythematosus. Pediatr Neurol 1995;13:191.

Stollerman GH. Rheumatic fever. In: Kelley WN, Harris ED Jr, Ruddy S, et al, eds. Textbook of Rheumatology. Philadelphia: WB Saunders, 1985.

Svantesson H, Marhaug G, Haeffner F. Scoliosis in children with juvenile rheumatoid arthritis. Scand J Rheumatol 1981;10:65.

Swedo SE. Sydenham's chorea. A model for childhood autoimmune neuropsychiatric disorders. JAMA 1994;272:1788.

Swedo SE, Leonard HL, Garvey M, et al. Pediatric autoimmune neuropsychiatric disorders associated with streptococcal infections: Clinical description of the first 50 cases. Am J Psychiatry 1998;155:264.

Swedo SE, Leonard HL, Mittleman BB, et al. Identification of children with pediatric autoimmune neuropsychiatric disorder associated with streptococcal infections by a marker associated with rheumatic fever. Am J Psychiatry 1997;154:110.

Swedo SE, Leonard HL, Schapiro MB, et al. Sydenham's chorea: Physical and psychological symptoms of St. Vitus dance. Pediatrics 1993;91:706.

Swedo SE, Rapoport JL, Cheslow DL, et al. High prevalence of obsessive-compulsive symptoms in patients with Sydenham's chorea. Am J Psychiatry 1989;146:246.

Szer IS. Henoch-Schönlein purpura: When and how to treat. J Rheumatol 1996;23:1661.

Szer IS, Jacobs JC. Pediatric systemic lupus erythematosus. In: Lahita RG, ed. Systemic lupus erythematosus, 2nd ed. New York: Churchill Livingstone, 1992.

Szer IS, Miller JH, Rawlings D, et al. Cerebral perfusion abnormalities in children with central nervous system manifestations of lupus detected by single photon emission computed tomography. J Rheumatol 1993;20:2143.

Szer IS, Sierakowska H, Szer W. A novel autoantibody to the putative oncoprotein DEK in pauciarticular onset juvenile rheumatoid arthritis. J Rheumatol 1994;21:2136.

Szer IS, Taylor E, Steere AC. The long-term course of Lyme arthritis in children. N Engl J Med 1991;325:159.

Tabata Y, Kobayashi I, Kawamura N, et al. Central nervous system manifestations after steroid pulse therapy in systemic lupus erythematosus. Eur J Pediatr 2002;161:503.

Takei S, Maeno N, Shigemori M, et al. Clinical features of Japanese children and adolescents with systemic lupus erythematosus: Results of 1980-1994 survey. Acta Paediatr Jpn 1997;39:250.

Tan EM. Systemic autoimmunity and antinuclear antibodies. Clin Aspects Autoimmunity 1986;1:2.

Tan EM, Cohen AS, Fries JF, et al. The 1982 revised criteria for the classification of systemic lupus erythematosus. Arthritis Rheum 1982;25:1271.

Teitel AD, MacKenzie CR, Stern R, et al. Laryngeal involvement in systemic lupus erythematosus. Semin Arthritis Rheum 1992;22:203.

Tervaert JWC, Kallenberg C. Neurologic manifestations of systemic vasculitides. Rheum Dis Clin North Am 1993;19:913.

Thompson CE, Damon LE, Ries CA, et al. Thrombotic microangiopathies in the 1980's: Clinical features, response to treatment, and the impact of the human immunodeficiency virus epidemic. Blood 1992;80:1890.

Tiddens HA, van der Net JJ, de Graeff-Meeder ER, et al. Juvenile-onset mixed connective tissue disease: Longitudinal follow-up. J Pediatr 1993;122:191.

Totoritis MC, Rubin RL. Drug-induced lupus: Genetic, clinical, and laboratory features. Postgrad Med 1985;78:149.

Toubi E, Khamashta MA, Panarra A, et al. Association of antiphospholipid antibodies with central nervous system disease in systemic lupus erythematosus. Am J Med 1995;99:397.

Tsai CY, Wu TH, Tsai ST, et al. Cerebrospinal fluid interleukin-6, prostaglandin E2 and autoantibodies in patients with neuropsychiatric systemic lupus erythematosus and central nervous system infections. Scand J Rheumatol 1994;23:57.

Tugal-Tutkun I, Urgancioglu M. Childhood-onset uveitis in Behçet's disease: A descriptive study of 36 cases. Am J Ophthalmol 2003;136:1114.

Ungerer JA, Horgan B, Chaitow J, et al. Psychosocial functioning in children and young adults with juvenile arthritis. Pediatrics 1988;81:195.

Uziel Y, Feldman BM, Krafchik BR, et al. Methotrexate and corticosteroid therapy for pediatric localized scleroderma. J Pediatr 2000;136:91.

Uziel Y, Laxer RM, Schneider R, et al. Intravenous immunoglobulin therapy in systemic juvenile rheumatoid arthritis: A follow-up study. J Rheumatol 1996;23:910.

Uziel Y, Miller ML, Laxer RM. Scleroderma in children. Pediatr Clin North Am 1995;42:1171.

Vancheeswaran R, Black CM, David J, et al. Childhood-onset scleroderma. Arthritis Rheum 1996;39:1041.

Vandvik IH, Eckblad G. Mothers of children with recent onset of rheumatic disease: Associations between maternal distress psychosocial variables and the disease of the children. J Dev Behav Pediatr 1991;12:84.

Vazquez-Cruz J, Traboulssi H, Rodriguez-De la Serna A, et al. A prospective study of chronic or recurrent headache in systemic lupus erythematosus. Headache 1990;30:232.

Verjans GM, van Hagen PM, van der Kooi A, et al. Vgamma9Vdelta2 T cells from eyes of patients with Behçet's disease recognize non-peptide prenyl pyrophosphate antigens. J Neuroimmunol 2002;130:46.

Vieira JP, Ortet O, Barata D, et al. Lupus myelopathy in a child. Pediatr Neurol 2002;27:303.

von Scheven E, Athreya BH, Rose CD, et al. Clinical characteristics of antiphospholipid antibody syndrome in children. J Pediatr 1996; 129:339.

von Scheven E, Lee C, Berg BO. Pediatric Wegener's granulomatosis complicated by central nervous system vasculitis. Pediatr Neurol 1998;19:317.

Wada H, Kaneko T, Ohiwa M, et al. Increased levels of vascular endothelial cell markers in thrombotic thrombocytopenic purpura. Am J Hematol 1993;44:101.
Wakefield AJ, Murch SH, Anthony A, et al. Ileal lymphoid-nodular hyperplasia, non-specific colitis, and pervasive developmental disorder in children. Lancet 1998;351:637.
Walravens PA, Chase HP. The prognosis of childhood systemic lupus erythematosus. Am J Dis Child 1976;130:929.
Wardyn KA, Ycinska K, Matuszkiewicz-Rowinska J, Chipczynka, M. Pseudotumour orbitae as the initial manifestation in Wegener's granulomatosis in a 7-year-old girl. Clin Rheumatol 2003;22:472.
Wechsler B, Vidaihet M, Piette JC, et al. Cerebral venous thrombosis in Behçet's disease: Clinical study and long-term follow-up of 25 cases. Neurology 1992;42:614.
Wechsler B, Dell'Isola B, Vidailhet M, et al. MRI in 31 patients with Behçet's disease and neurological involvement: Prospective study with clinical correlation. J Neurol Neurosurg Psychiatry 1993;56:793.
Wertheimer NM. "Rheumatic" schizophrenia. Arch Gen Psychiatry 1961;4:579.
West SG. Neuropsychiatric lupus. Rheum Dis Clin North Am 1994;20:129.
West SG, Emlen W, Wener MH, et al. Neuropsychiatric lupus erythematosus: A 10-year prospective study on the value of diagnostic tests. Am J Med 1995;99:153.
Wijdicks EF. Silent brain infarct in thrombotic thrombocytopenic purpura. Stroke 1994;25:1297.
Williams LS, Garg BP, Cohen M, et al. Subtypes of ischemic stroke in children and young adults. Neurology 1997;49:1541.
Wright DA, Newburger JW, Baker A, et al. Treatment of immune globulin-resistant Kawasaki disease with pulsed doses of corticosteroids. J Pediatr 1996;128:146.
Wysenbeek AJ, Leibovici L, Zoldan J. Acute central nervous system complications after pulse steroid therapy in patients with systemic lupus erythematosus. J Rheumatol 1990;17:1695.
Young RS, Torretti D, Williams RH, et al. Reye's syndrome associated with long-term aspirin therapy. JAMA 1984;251:754.
Zelenski JD, Holden D, Calabrese LH. Central nervous system vasculitis in Behçet's syndrome: Angiographic improvement after therapy with cytotoxic agents. Arthritis Rheum 1989;32:217.

PART XIII

Neuromuscular Disorders

CHAPTER 74

Normal Muscle

V. Venkataraman Vedanarayanan and Owen B. Evans, Jr.

Movement is one of the ultimate expressions of the nervous system and totally depends on the contraction of skeletal muscle. As an organ, skeletal muscle is the largest structure of the body and has other functions besides voluntary movement and the generation of force. This chapter reviews the embryology, anatomy, function, and metabolism of muscle and the common diagnostic procedures used for its study.

EMBRYOLOGY AND DEVELOPMENT

Primitive cells, which are called *premyoblasts,* are the precursors of muscle in the embryonic paraxial mesoderm. The mesoderm gives rise to segmentally arranged somites. Craniofacial muscles arise rostral of the first somite. Discrete condensations of mesenchymal cells, called *dermatomyotomes* and located in the dorsomedial somite, give rise to the axial muscles, and condensations from the lateral somite give rise to the limb muscles (Fig. 74-1) [McLennon, 1994]. Connective tissue and tendons arise from the somatopleural mesoderm, somites, and neural crest. Premyoblasts express the paired box transcription factors *Pax-3* and *Pax-7* and respond to Wnts and sonic hedgehog signals from surrounding embryonic tissues to activate *Myf-5* and *MyoD* myogenic genes [Pownall et al., 2002]. These committed cells, *myoblasts*, migrate to the myotome. The myoblasts divide rapidly within the first several weeks of pregnancy, after a quantal cell cycle under the influence of fetal growth factors. The primordial cells stream ventrally and penetrate between the ectoderm and somatopleura. As the cells migrate, they split and recombine such that individual muscles are formed from several adjacent myotomes. In the limb bud, the cells coalesce into dorsal and ventral masses.

The maturation of premyoblasts to myoblasts begins with the cessation of DNA synthesis. The postmitotic myoblasts elongate and begin attachment and fusion with other myoblasts end to end to form a long and slender primary myotube (Fig. 74-2). The process is facilitated by the appearance of several fetal adhesion molecules on the surface of the myoblast [Schnorrer and Dickson, 2004]. Secondary and tertiary myotubes are formed from side-to-side fusion of myoblasts to existing myotubes and require innervation for the process. Satellite cells provide nuclei to the polar ends of the elongating myotube. Individual muscles begin to form after the initial myotubes appear and the ingrowth of innervation. In the absence of innervation, maturation beyond primary myotubes does not occur, and the muscle develops abnormally.

At about 4 weeks' gestation, the contractile proteins appear and polymerize to form myofilaments, which are produced predominantly in the polar region of the myotube. By the fifth week, the myofilaments aggregate to form the myofibrils, with simultaneous formation of characteristic striations. A microscopic cross-section of the muscle fiber at this stage reveals a tubular structure, with the contractile proteins located around the periphery of the fiber and the center containing the nuclei. The basic shape of an anatomic muscle is apparent by 7 weeks. Movement begins simultaneously with innervation at 8 weeks. In the latter stages of early fetal development, neuron sprouting is intense. Initially, individual mammalian muscle fibers are multiply innervated. Between 16 and 25 weeks' gestation and in association with secondary myotube formation, all but one synapse is eliminated. There is constant denervation and reinnervation as neuromuscular interaction forms physiologic innervations of the motor units. Multiple motor neurons compete for innervation. Competition weakens some synapses and strengthens others, so that ultimately a single input prevails. This process of *synaptic elimination* is stimulated by local factors produced by muscle [Wyatt and Balice-Gordon, 2003]. Several growth factors and receptors appear on the cell surface to facilitate integration of nerve terminals to the muscle cell. The fetal (g) form of the acetylcholine receptor is present until 31 weeks' gestation, after which only the adult type (e) is found. Rhythmic movements that are spinally mediated start shortly after innervation. Most of the fetal membrane proteins that promote growth and differentiation, including the major histocompatibility gene products [Kaparti et al., 1988], are not present on normal mature muscle.

At about 16 weeks' gestation, the nuclei begin migrating to the subsarcolemmal position. Most muscle fibers achieve the histologic features of mature muscle by 25 weeks, although a few continue to have central nuclei. At this stage, the fibers are rounded and loosely arranged within the prominent endomysium. The characteristic polygonal cross-sectional shape becomes apparent after birth.

Distinctive muscle fiber types (see next section) develop after innervation. Primitive fibers, typed as IIc, are undifferentiated and are believed to be precursors of the mature fibers: types I, IIa, and IIb [Landon, 1982]. The myosin in type IIc fibers is immunologically distinct from that of other fiber types [Thornell et al., 1984]. Type I fibers appear at about 18 weeks and are smaller than type II fibers until after birth, when they become somewhat larger. Most muscle fibers in the 20- to 26-week-old fetus are type IIc fibers. Type IIa and IIb fibers appear during the last month of gestation. Only a small percentage of type IIc fibers persist after birth. Differentiation into distinct fiber types is determined by neural influences and causes the biochemical and physiologic diversity of mature fibers. *Calcineurin*, a Ca^{2+}-calmodulin–regulated phosphatase, plays a critical role in

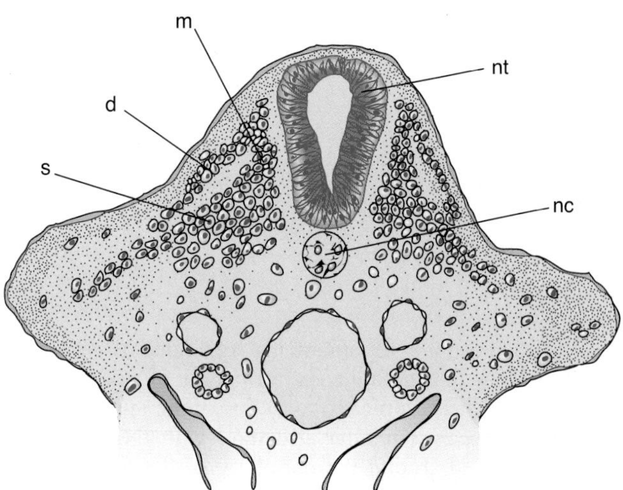

FIGURE 74-1. Cross-section of 28-day fetus at the 21 to 28 somite stage. Early limb buds are apparent. d, Dermatome; m, myotome; nc, notochord; nt, neural tube; s, sclerotome.

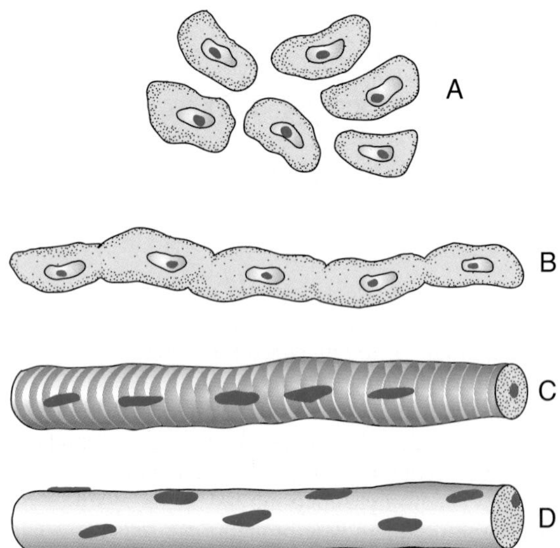

FIGURE 74-2. Development of the muscle fiber. **A,** Premyoblasts. **B,** Myoblast fusion. **C,** Myotube. **D,** Muscle fiber.

the differentiation of physiologic properties in the muscle fiber [Matlin et al., 2001]. Continuous firing of motoneurons causes an increase in intracellular calcium, which activates calcineurin. Activated calcineurin binds and dephosphorylizes nuclear transcription factors, which are translocated to the nucleus and effect gene expression for slow-twitch fiber phenotype. Sporadic motor neuron firing decreases intracellular calcium and deactivates calcineurin. The absence of activated transcription factors in the nucleus results in fast-twitch fibers.

Without innervation, muscle fibers atrophy and undergo cell death. Similarly, spinal motor neurons become nonviable without innervating muscle, so that muscle and neuronal development are ultimately interdependent [McLennon, 1994]. Satellite cells are one of several stem cell types found in muscle and have many features of premyoblasts, although the exact origins are unknown [Chen and Goldhamer, 2003]. These mononuclear muscle cells lie beneath the basement membrane of mature muscle fibers. Subsequent growth and elongation of embryonic muscle fibers depend on fusion of satellite cells for new nuclei. Satellite cells are abundant in fetal muscle, compose 1% to 5% of the total nuclei of mature muscle, and diminish with aging. They are the primary stem cell for regeneration of injured muscle and are capable of forming not only individual muscle fibers but also complete muscle fascicles [Alameddine et al., 1989; Anderson, 2000; Shultz, 1985].

The subsequent growth and strength of muscle after birth depend on functional demand, sex, age, training, and other factors. Enlargement of a muscle results from hypertrophy of muscle fibers rather than from growth of new fibers. Large muscles with a greater workload, such as the quadriceps, have greater cross-sectional diameters of muscle fibers than do other muscles, such as the diaphragm. There is no difference in fiber growth in males and females until puberty, when a noticeable increase appears in males. Training increases the cross-sectional diameter of the muscle fiber, and disuse decreases the diameter. Muscle atrophy associated with aging is caused by loss of muscle fibers, rather than by fiber atrophy, and a decrease in satellite cells to regenerate injured muscle.

Muscle is quite malleable and is under a number of neuronal, hormonal, and usage influences that determine muscle function and contractile properties [Pette, 2001].

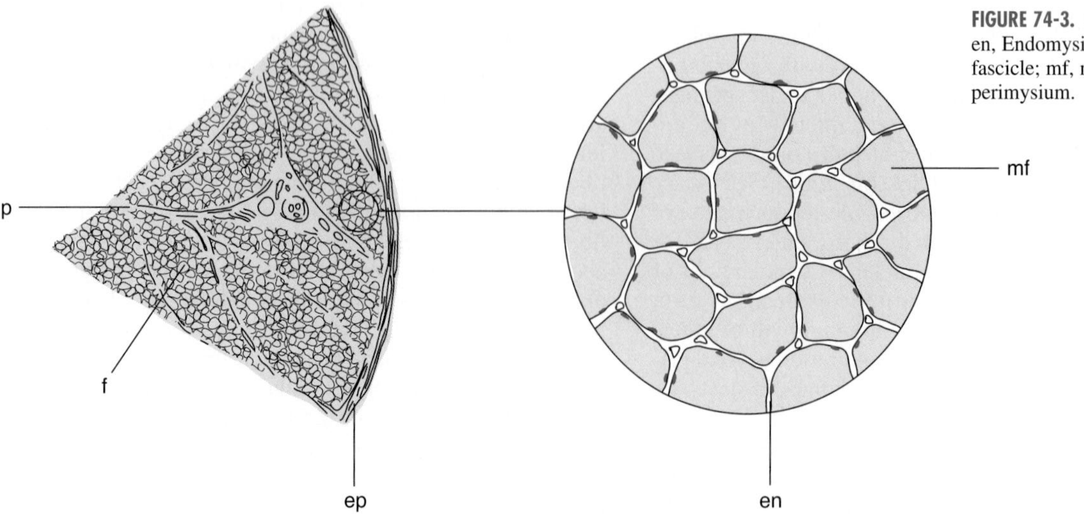

FIGURE 74-3. Morphology of muscle. en, Endomysium; ep, epimysium; f, fascicle; mf, muscle fiber; p, perimysium.

This plasticity of muscle results in changes in fiber type distribution, contractile proteins, calcium uptake of the sarcoplasmic reticulum, and altered energy metabolism.

ANATOMY AND STRUCTURE

Morphology

The muscle as an organ comprises all the individual anatomic muscles. Each anatomic muscle has an origin and an insertion on the skeleton and bridges one or more bony articulations. Contraction of the anatomic muscle thus causes movement across a joint. The anatomic muscle is enclosed within a thick sheet of connective tissue called the *epimysium.* Separating the muscle into individual fascicles is the perimysium, which is contiguous with the epimysium. Within the perimysium are the nutrient blood vessels, intramuscular nerves, and muscle spindles (Fig. 74-3). The confluence of the perimysial and epimysial connective tissue forms the tendons at either end of the muscle belly. The muscle fascicle, which is bounded by perimysial connective tissue, is a wedge-shaped structure comprising several hundred individual muscle fibers. Surrounding each muscle fiber is a network of fine connective tissue, called the *endomysium.* The terminal axons and a rich capillary network reside within the endomysium. Within the muscle fiber are large groups of myofibrils, which contain myofilaments. Myofilaments are made of contractile proteins.

Although a muscle may have almost any shape, all muscles are composed of almost identical muscle fibers. Muscle architecture can be specialized for force production or excursion, depending on the number of muscle fibers arranged in parallel or series, respectively. A muscle fiber, or muscle cell, is a multinucleated, long, tubular structure that varies in diameter from 10 to 20 μm in the infant to about 50 to 70 μm in the adult. Fiber length varies considerably, depending on the size of the muscle and whether the fibers are arranged in series or in parallel orientation, and can be several centimeters in length and can span the entire muscle.

Sarcomere

The most striking feature of skeletal muscle on microscopic examination is the characteristic striations ("striated" muscle), which are especially prominent under polarized light. The striations are caused by the difference in the refractive index of the contractile proteins that are in phase with each other in the myofibrils. A repeating unit is called the *sarcomere,* which comprises interdigitating myofilaments and is bounded by the Z line (Fig. 74-4). The sarcomere has a length of about 2.5 to 3.0 μm and a diameter of 1.0 μm. The Z disk anchors the thin filaments of actin that extend into each adjacent sarcomere and are located in the I band. The M line bisects the sarcomere and also divides the A band, which is formed by an array of thick filaments composed of myosin. The area within the A band in which the thin and thick filaments do not overlap is called the *H band. A* refers to anisotropic and *I* refers to isotropic in reference to the refractile indexes under polarized light.

Contractile and Sarcomeric Proteins

The two major proteins involved in muscle contraction are actin and myosin, which jointly interact with adenosine triphosphate to convert chemical energy to mechanical work. The actin system is complex. The actin molecule has four major domains surrounding a cleft containing adenosine triphosphate or adenosine diphosphate and is tightly bound to a divalent cation [Pollard, 1993]. There are at least 48 classes of actin-binding proteins. The thin filaments are composed of two chains of about 400 polymerized actin molecules arranged in a double helix (Fig. 74-5). The actin molecule has a molecular weight of about 42,000 daltons and is rich in 3-methyl histidine, a unique amino acid found exclusively in muscle. The actin molecule is the same in both fast and slow skeletal muscle fibers. α-Actinin is a major component of the Z disk and plays a role in the binding or cross-linking of actin to other cytoskeletal structures [Critchley, 1993]. Capping proteins anchor the barbed end of actin to the Z line [Cooper et al., 1993]. Mutation in the α-actin gene has been associated with congenital myopathy

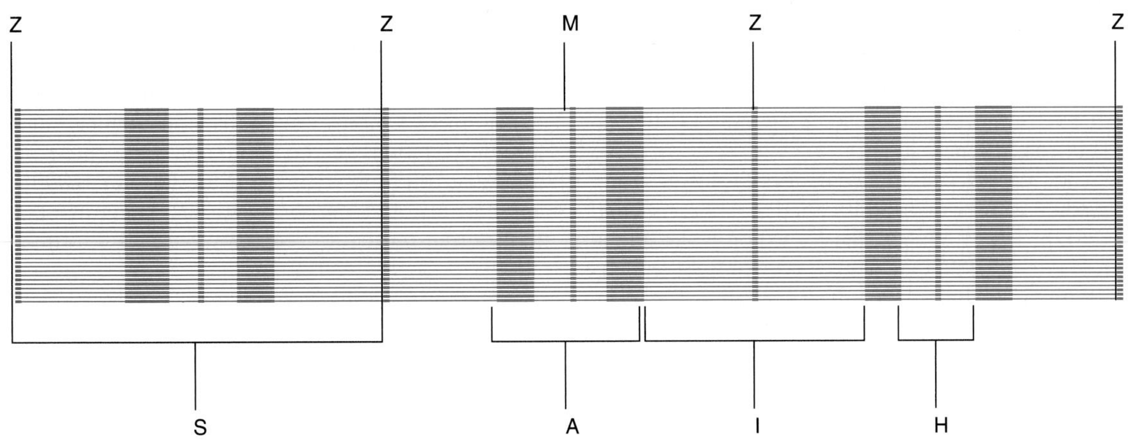

FIGURE 74-4. Sarcomere. A sarcomere extends from Z line to Z line. The thick filaments are made up of myosin and occupy the A band. The thin filaments are made up of actin and make up the I band. The H band is the area in which the thick and thin filaments do not overlap. The M line anchors the thick filaments.

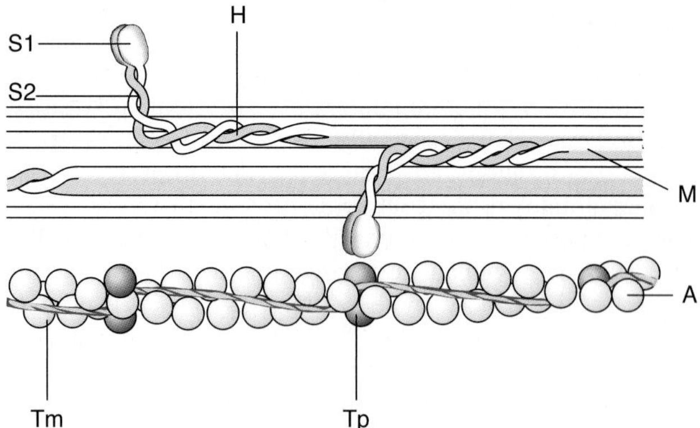

FIGURE 74-5. Contractile proteins. Myosin (M) is located in the thick filaments and is composed of two heavy chains (H) and four light chains located in the head region. The myosin head is divided into two parts: S1 and S2. The thin filaments are composed of actin (A), tropomyosin (Tm), and troponin (Tp).

with excess thin myofilaments and nemaline myopathy [Nowak et al, 1999].

The mechanochemical myosin molecule is a complex protein with a molecular weight of about 500,000 daltons. The myosin molecule consists of at least six polypeptides with two heavy chains and four light chains. The contractile properties of a muscle fiber are related to myosin. Myosin heavy chains are different for type I, IIa, and IIb fibers. The two heavy chains form a double helix that extends along the tail of the molecule. The light chains are of the following three types: two alkali dissociated and one phosphorylated. The light chains are different for type I and II fibers but are the same for IIa and IIb fibers. The structure of myosin is hexameric, composed of two heavy, two alkali dissociated, and two phosphorylated chains. There are nine isoforms of the myosin heavy chain: I, IIA, IIB, IID/X, IIA, α, neonatal, embryonic, and extraocular. The various isoforms of the heavy and light chains create a spectrum of isomyosins that are specific for fast-twitch skeletal muscle, slow-twitch skeletal muscle, cardiac muscle, smooth muscle, brain, and platelets [Whalen, 1985]. Embryonic and neonatal muscle contains distinct sets of isomyosins. Skeletal muscle isomyosins are determined by neural influences (see earlier discussion). "Pure" muscle fibers contain a single myosin heavy chain isoform. "Hybrid" fibers contain more than one myosin isoform, as in muscle fibers transitioning from one fiber type to another during reinnervation. The maximal force, velocity, and power produced by muscle fibers are determined to a large extent by the properties of myosin isoforms [Lutz and Lieber, 2002].

At one end, the myosin molecule evaginates to form globular heads. The myosin head is called the *S2 region* and is attached to the heavy chains. The S2 region is flexible at either end [Huxley, 1982]. One of each type of light chain is associated with the globular heads. The LC1 (light chain 1), or P light chain, somehow modulates the contractile response by specific phosphatase and kinase and exists as P1 and P2 isoforms [Westwood et al., 1984]. The cross-links between actin and myosin occur at the globular heads during excitation. Thus, the myosin molecule is a bipolar structure, with the heavy chains of the tail ordered along the backbone of the thick filament and the heads projected from the side. The heads have a repeating helical arrangement that forms about three cross-bridges per repeating unit [Harrington and Rodgers, 1984]. C proteins exist as several isoforms and can be seen as cross-stripes on the A band on electron microscopy [Fishman, 1993]. The function of C proteins is unknown but is probably regulatory of cross-bridge movements.

Actin and myosin have an inherent affinity, and troponin and tropomyosin are regulatory proteins that enable the actin-myosin interaction to be controlled by the calcium ion [Grabarek et al., 1990]. Tropomyosin is another helical structure, comprising two long filaments that reside within the groove of the actin chains [Smillie, 1993]. There are at least two isoforms of tropomyosin. Fast-twitch skeletal muscle contains both α and β isoforms; slow-twitch muscle contains only β-tropomyosin [Heeley et al., 1985]. Because of the close association with actin, tropomyosin probably also has a structural role.

The troponin molecules are located periodically along tropomyosin and comprise three subunits. Troponin T anchors troponin to tropomyosin. Troponin C binds calcium, which induces a conformational change of the protein and results in activation of actomyosin adenosine triphosphatase, which causes contraction [Gergeley et al., 1993]. Troponin I inhibits actomyosin adenosine triphosphatase. The contraction of striated muscle is regulated by the troponin (Tn) complex, which acts as a Ca^{2+} sensor. Ca^{2+} binding to the regulatory sites of troponin C (TnC) strengthens the interaction of TnC with troponin I (TnI) and weakens the inhibitory activity of TnI for actin and the affinity of troponin T (TnT) for tropomyosin (Tm). Tm then moves toward the groove of the helical actin filament, switching on the myosin active site, which leads to muscle contraction. Tn binds to actin-Tm in the absence of Ca^{2+}, and the changes in interactions among these thin filament components in the presence of Ca^{2+} promote strong binding of myosin to actin [Gomes et al., 2002]. Mutations of sarcomeric genes for troponin T1 and tropomyosin are some of several causes of nemaline myopathy [Wallgren-Pettersson, 2002] and cardiomyopathies [Gomes et al., 2004].

Titin, the largest known protein of about 3 to 3.7 megadaltons constitutes about 10% of myofibrillary proteins and is important for maintaining tension during stretch and re-centering the sarcomere after relaxation [Tskhovrebova and Trinick, 2003]. Opposing molecules of titin span the sarcomere. The NH_2 termini of the titin molecules attach to the Z disk, attaching myosin to the Z disk. The COOH ends extend and overlap in the M band, interconnecting myosin and actin and providing elasticity to the sarcomere. Associated binding proteins with titin in the Z disk include α-actinin, telethonin, and obscurin [Sanger and Sanger, 2001]. Mutations of the telethonin gene cause limb girdle muscular dystrophy type 2G [Moreira et al., 2000]. *Calpain,* another titin-binding protein, has been associated with limb girdle muscular dystrophy type 2A [Sorimachi et al., 2000].

Nebulin is another large filament of the skeletal muscle sarcomere. The COOH terminus is attached to the Z disk, and the NH_2 terminus projects into the I band. Nebulin is closely associated with actin, and although its function is unclear, it may be that of a "ruler" determining the length of the thin filaments [Wang, 1993]. Nebulin is one of several Z-disk proteins that has been associated with nemaline myopathy [Pelin et al., 1999].

Sarcotubular System

A major constituent of muscle fiber is the sarcotubular system (Fig. 74-6). The sarcolemma is the plasma membrane of the muscle cell and is surrounded by the basement membrane and endomysial connective tissue. The sarcolemma is an excitable membrane and shares many properties with the membrane of the neuron. The T tubules are contiguous with the sarcolemma and extend into the interior of the muscle fiber as a tubular system in communication with the sarcolemma. Depolarization of the sarcolemma is propagated throughout the interior of the muscle fiber through this system [Peachey, 1985]. The T tubules project into the interior of the muscle fibers in the area of the junction of the I band and A band, where they come in immediate contact with a second tubular system within the sarcoplasm called the *sarcoplasmic reticulum*. The T tubule bounded on either side by the sarcoplasmic reticulum is a triad. The sarcoplasmic reticulum forms a fine plexus around the myofibrils. Excitation of the sarcolemma and T tubules causes release of calcium from the sarcoplasmic reticulum and initiation of contraction by the myofilaments.

Several important proteins are associated with the junction of the T tubules and the sarcoplasmic reticulum. The voltage sensors of the T-tubule calcium channels are regulated by dihydropyridine receptors. Ryanodine receptors mediate the calcium release of the sarcoplasmic reticulum during muscle activation. Calcium adenosine triphosphatase pumps calcium back into the sarcoplasmic reticulum during relaxation. *Calsequestrin* is a calcium-binding protein that increases the capacity of calcium in the sarcoplasmic reticulum [Franzini-Armstrong, 1999]. Some patients with myasthenia gravis, especially associated with thymoma, have anti–skeletal muscle antibodies to ryanodine receptor antigens, as well as to titin [Skeie et al., 2003; Zhang et al., 1993]. Autosomal-dominant and autosomal-recessive mutations of the ryanodine receptor gene *(RYR)* cause central core disease [Ferreiro et al., 2002] and central core disease with rods [Scacheri et al., 2000].

Other features seen on microscopic examination of muscle are nuclei and the sarcoplasm and its organelles. Normally, nuclei are located beneath the sarcolemma, and each muscle fiber has thousands of nuclei. The sarcoplasm contains many of the elements found in the cytoplasm of other tissues. Most important are the mitochondria, which are located primarily in the intramyofibrillary space near the Z line and adjacent to the A bands. Numerous glycogen granules and fat droplets are located in the same areas.

Cytoskeletal Proteins

The structural integrity of the muscle is maintained against the physical forces of contraction exerted on the sarcolemma membrane by an intricate system of cytoskeletal proteins

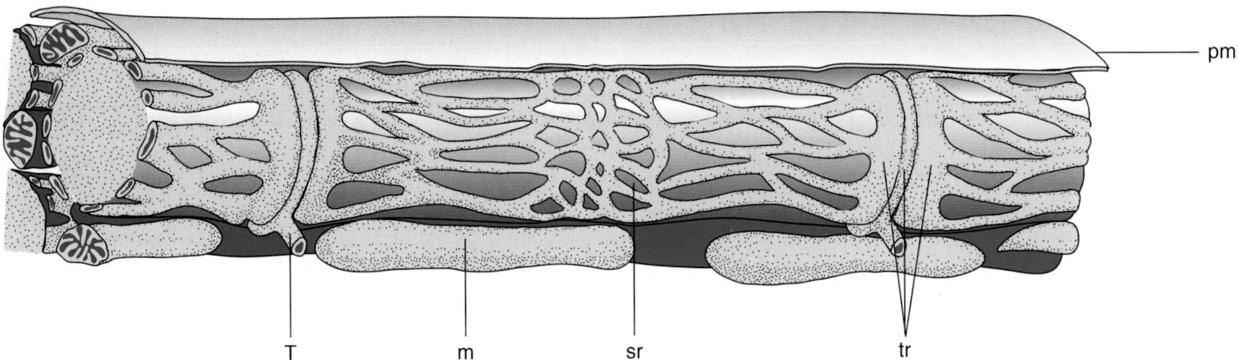

FIGURE 74-6. Sarcotubular system. The drawing illustrates a myofibril of one sarcomere and the associated membrane systems. m, Mitochondrion; pm, plasma membrane; sr, sarcoplasmic reticulum; T, T tubule; tr, triad.

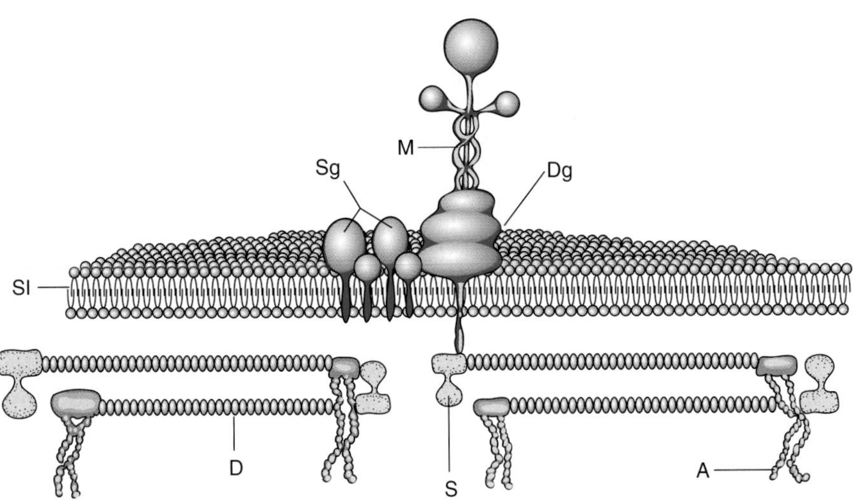

FIGURE 74-7. Sarcolemma-associated cytoskeletal structures. Dystroglycan (Dg) consists of α-Dg associated with merosin (M) and β-Dl, which binds to dystrophin (D). Syntropin (S) is bound to the C-terminal region of dystrophin. The sarcoglycan complex (Sg) consists of four transmembrane subunits: α, β, γ, and δ attached to the sarcolemma (Sl). (Modified from Duggan DJ, Gorospe JR, Fanin M, et al. Mutations in the sarcoglycan genes in patients with myopathy. N Engl J Med 1997;336:618).

TABLE 74-1

Muscle Proteins and Human Genetic Disease

PROTEIN	LOCATION	DISEASE
Plasma Membrane		
Dystrophin	Xp21 DMD	BMD, DMD
α-Sarcoglycan	17q12-q21	LGMD-2D
β-Sarcoglycan	4q12	LGMD-2E
γ-Sarcoglycan	13q12	LGMD-2C
δ-Sarcoglycan	5q33-34	LGMD-2F
Dysferlin	2p13	LGMD-2D, Miyoshi's myopathy
Caveolin-3	3p25	LGMD-1C
Extracellular Matrix		
α_2-Laminin	6q2	Merosin-deficient CMD
Collagen VI	21q22	Ullrich's CMD, Bethlem's myopathy
Sarcoplasmic		
Calpain-3	15q15.1	LGMD-2A
TRIM32	9q31-34	LGMD-2H
Myotubularin	Xq28	Myotubular myopathy
Desmin	11q21-23	Desmin-related myopathy
Plectin	8q24-qter	Epidermolysis bullosa simplex with late-onset muscular dystrophy
Glycosylation Related		
Fukutin	9q31-33	Fukuyama CMD
FKRP	19q1	LGMD-D2, CMD-1C
POMGnT1	1p32-34	Muscle-eye-brain CMD (*O*-mannose β-1,2-*N*-acetylglucosaminyl transferase)
POMT1	9q34	Walker-Warburg CMD (*O*-mannosyltransferase-1)
Sarcomeric Proteins		
Titin	2q	LGMD-2J
Myotilin	5q22-34	LGMD-1A
Telethonin	17q11-12	LGMD-2G
Actin	1q42	Nemaline myopathy
Tropomyosin-3	1q21-23	Nemaline myopathy
Tropomyosin-2	9p13	Nemaline myopathy
Nebulin	2q21-22	Nemaline myopathy
Slow troponin T	19q13	Nemaline myopathy
Ryanodine receptor (RYR1)	19q13.1	Central core disease, central core disease with rods
Nuclear Proteins		
Emerin	Xq28	EDMD
Lamin A/C	1q11-21	LGMD-1B

BMD, Becker muscular dystrophy; CMD, congenital muscular dystrophy; DMD, Duchenne muscular dystrophy; EDMD, Emery-Dreifuss muscular dystrophy; LGMD, limb girdle muscular dystrophy.
Adapted from Vainzof M, Zatz M, 2003.

(Fig. 74-7). These proteins, through a complex pattern of arrangement, anchor the internal structure of the muscle to the basement membrane. Advances in techniques of molecular biology have led to identification and characterization of several of these proteins (Table 74-1).

Dystrophin

The identification and characterization of dystrophin led to understanding the role of cytoskeletal proteins in providing strength and stability to the muscle membrane. Dystrophin is a large protein molecule of about 427 kilodaltons and is composed of 3,685 amino acids. It constitutes 0.01% of total muscle protein and 5% of the sarcolemmal cytoskeletal proteins [Hoffman et al., 1987]. The protein has the shape of a rod, is about 150 nm long, and is arranged as an antiparallel holdimer. It is abundant at the myotendinous junction [Samitt and Bonilla, 1990] and at the postsynaptic membrane of the neuromuscular junction [Byers et al., 1991]. Immunocytochemical studies have localized dystrophin to the cytoplasmic surface of the sarcolemma [Bies et al., 1992]. Dystrophin with two other structural proteins, spectrin and vinculin, are located at the sites of attachment of sarcomeres to the cytoplasmic membrane overlying both the I bands and M lines [Porter et al., 1992]. These findings demonstrate that dystrophin forms an integral part of a muscle's cytoskeleton and links the contractile apparatus to the sarcolemma. There is no difference in the expression of dystrophin in fast- and slow-twitch muscle fibers or in intrafusal muscle fibers [Zubrzycka-Gaarn et al., 1988].

Dystrophin has a binding site for the filamentous form of actin at the 5′ end or domain. The central rod domain contains a number of repeats and demonstrates homology with spectrin and gives the molecule a flexible rod-shaped structure [Pons et al., 1990]. The rod domain is highly conserved in vertebrates, and antibodies against the human dystrophin rod domain cross-react with amphibian and other vertebrate species [Sherratt et al., 1992]. The third domain is rich in cysteine [Suzuki et al., 1992], and the fourth domain, the carboxy terminus, binds with the dystrophin–glycoprotein complex [Ervasti and Campbell, 1991]. The dystrophin-glycoprotein complex consists of dystroglycans (α and β), the sarcoglycans (α, β, γ, δ, ε), sarcospan, the syntrophin, and dystrobrevin [Crawford et al., 2000]. The peripheral members of the complex include neuronal nitric oxide synthase, caveolin, laminin, and merosin [Watkins et al., 2000]. Even though the RNA levels of these proteins are normal in patients with dystrophin deficiency, the protein expression is reduced. The deficiency of these proteins contributes further to the pathologic effects of dystrophin deficiency [Chen et al., 2000].

The gene coding for the protein dystrophin is located on the short arm of the X chromosome near the region Xp21. The dystrophin gene is the largest gene identified so far, covering more than 2.5 megabases (Mb), and contains at least 79 exons [Gutmann and Fischbeck, 1989]. The large size of the gene is responsible for the high rate of mutation in this gene. A 14-kilobase dystrophin messenger RNA is expressed in skeletal, cardiac, and smooth muscle cells. Smaller amounts are expressed in the brain. Isoforms of dystrophin, which are smaller in size, are expressed in nearly all tissues examined. Deficiency of the brain isoform of dystrophin, Dp 140 and Dp 71, is associated with cognitive handicaps. Dystrophin in the brain is important in maintaining synaptic plasticity and participates in cellular signaling pathways involved in modeling synapses [Blake and Kroger, 2000]. Dystrophin isoform Dp 260 is expressed in retina alone [Pillers et al., 1999].

The most important function of dystrophin is to provide mechanical support and structural integrity to the sarcolemma [Lapidos et al., 2004]. Dystrophin is part of the linkage system from the actin cytoskeleton out through the sarcolemmal membrane and basal lamina to the extracellular matrix. Through its linkage to the neuronal nitric oxide synthase, it has a role in regulation of blood flow through muscle during exercise [Sander et al., 2000]. Dystrophin within the dystrophin–glycoprotein complex participates in intracellular signaling. It plays a role in regulation of calcium-dependent kinases in the cell by interacting with calmodulin [Anderson et al., 1996]. Alteration in calcium signaling in dystrophin-deficient muscles plays a major role in altering the normal maturation process of regenerating and developing muscle fibers [Chen et al., 2000].

Deletions or abnormalities of the dystrophin gene cause a deficiency or absence of dystrophin, resulting in the X-linked Duchenne's and Becker's muscular dystrophies.

Dystrophin–Glycoprotein Complex

Biochemical investigation of dystrophin led to the discovery of a large oligomeric complex of glycoprotein localized in the sarcolemma. This dystrophin–glycoprotein complex binds the muscle cytoskeleton to a component of the extracellular matrix, laminin [Campbell and Kahl, 1989; Ervasti et al., 1990]. The dystrophin–glycoprotein complex consists of cytoskeletal, transmembrane, and extracellular components and is composed of two subgroups of protein complexes: the dystroglycans and sarcoglycans. The dystroglycan complex consists of a transmembrane and an extracellular component encoded by a single messenger RNA. The synthesized protein undergoes glycosylation as it passes from endoplasmic reticulum to the sarcolemmal membrane. The α-dystroglycan is a heavily glycosylated protein located on the extracellular side of the sarcolemmal membrane. It plays an active role in basement membrane assembly. It binds to β-dystroglycan (transmembrane component) with its carboxy-terminal region on the intracellular side. The dystroglycan complex plays a pivotal role in linking the cytoskeleton to the extracellular matrix. The dystroglycan complex also plays an important role in normal migration of neurons in the cerebral cortex [Martin and Freeze, 2003; Michele and Campbell, 2003]. The assembly and integration of these proteins occur in the presence of dystrophin; in its absence, these proteins may not be degraded, properly assembled, or integrated into the sarcolemma [Ibraghimov-Beskrovnaya et al., 1992].

No primary mutations in dystroglycans have been identified in human disease. Defective glycosylation of α-dystroglycans causes congenital muscular dystrophies with brain involvement: Fukuyama's congenital muscular dystrophy, muscle-eye-brain disease, Walker-Warburg syndrome, limb girdle muscular dystrophy type 2I [Grewal and Hewitt, 2003].

The sarcoglycan complex consists of α-sarcoglycan (adhalin), β-sarcoglycan, γ-sarcoglycan, and δ-sarcoglycan [Bonnemann et al., 1995]. The sarcoglycan genes *α, β,* and *γ* are located on 17q12-21, 4q12, and 13q12 chromosomes, respectively. Expression of α- and γ-sarcoglycan is limited to skeletal and cardiac muscles [Yamamoto et al., 1994]. The sarcoglycans form a tetrameric complex in the Golgi apparatus and then transition to the sarcolemma as a completely assembled structure. The sarcoglycans consist of a single transmembrane domain, a small intracellular domain, and a large extracellular domain, and their molecular weight ranges from 35 to 50 kilodaltons. The sarcoglycan complex, which is composed of α-, β-, γ-, and δ-sarcoglycan, is part of the dystrophin-associated glycoprotein complex and acts as a link between the extracellular matrix and the cytoskeleton, confers structural stability to the sarcolemma, and protects muscle fibers from mechanical stress during muscle contraction. Mutations in any of the sarcoglycan genes cause destabilization of the complex, produce a decrease in the amount of all sarcoglycan proteins, and cause the different forms of limb girdle muscular dystrophy [Matsumara et al., 1992; Straub and Campbell, 1997].

The diseases associated with sarcoglycan gene mutations (α-sarcoglycan [*SGCA*], limb girdle muscular dystrophy type 2D; β-sarcoglycan [*SGCB*], limb girdle muscular dystropy type 2E; γ-sarcoglycan [*SGSG*], limb girdle muscular dystrophy type 2C; δ-sarcoglycan [*SGCD*], limb girdle muscular dystrophy type 2F) are rare disorders in the general population but represent a sizable proportion of all muscular dystrophies with normal dystrophin (about 10% to 20% of cases). Limb girdle muscular dystrophy type 2D is the most frequent sarcoglycanopathy, followed by types 2C and 2E, whereas the most rare is type 2F [Boito et al., 2003].

The measurement of α-sarcoglycan is a useful screening test to look for sarcoglycan gene mutations in patients with muscular dystrophy [Duggan et al., 1997].

Utrophin

Initially described as dystrophin-related protein or dystrophin-like protein, utrophin is an autosomally encoded protein. It is smaller in size than dystrophin, and it has been localized to the sarcolemmal postsynaptic membrane at the neuromuscular junction and myotendinous junction in the mature muscle fiber [Khurana et al., 1991]. At the neuromuscular junction, it is preferentially concentrated at the acetylcholine receptor–rich crests. Utrophin is present in all tissues tested so far. In the brain, it is localized at the inner plasma face of astrocytic foot processes at the abluminal aspect of the blood-brain barrier [Khurana et al., 1992] Utrophin has a similar amino acid sequence as the carboxy terminus of dystrophin, and it copurifies with α-sarcoglycan. The gene coding for utrophin is localized to the long arm of human chromosome 6, at 6q24. The transcription of utrophin occurs preferentially at the nuclei close to the neuromuscular junctions (subsynaptic nuclei). The transcription of utrophin gene is regulated by growth factors released from neurite, such as heregulin, a neurite-associated growth factor that is a member of the neuregulin family of growth factors. In muscles, growth factors increase the transcription of acetylcholine receptor, sodium channels, and utrophin [Fishbach and Rosen, 1997]. In dystrophin-deficient states, utrophin content is increased and localizes to sarcolemma as well. A number of approaches to upregulate the expression of utrophin in muscles are being explored as treatment for Duchenne's muscular dystrophy.

Dysferlin

Dysferlin is a 237-kilodalton protein composed of 2,080 amino acids. It has a single transmembrane segment at the carboxy terminus. The protein is anchored at the sarcomere by the carboxy terminus, and the rest of the protein is intracytoplasmic. It is distributed at the sarcolemma, similar to dystrophin and the dystrophin–glycoprotein complex. However, the protein is not associated with dystrophin and the dystrophin–glycoprotein complex. The dysferlin protein is coded by a gene located in chromosome 2 p13. The gene is relatively large and spans 150 kilobases. It is composed of 55 exons and is expressed in skeletal and cardiac muscles and placenta. A shorter transcript of 3.5 kilobases is expressed in all regions of the brain. Proteins with homology to dysferlin are seen in other tissues. Fer-1 is present in testes and is required for maturation of spermatozoa. Otoferlin, with 55% homology to dysferlin, is expressed in the inner hair cells. Myoferlin, with 68% homology, is present in the lungs, placenta, heart, and cytoplasm and nuclear membranes of skeletal muscles [Bansal et al., 2003].

The ferlin family of cytoplasmic proteins has motifs that are homologous to so-called C2 domains. The C2 domains are typically found in proteins that function in signal transduction or in membrane trafficking, such as protein kinase C and synaptotamins [Anderson et al., 1999]. These domains interact with multiple targets, including calcium, phospholipids, and other proteins, to mediate signaling events for membrane fusions [De Luna et al., 2004; Rizo and Sudhof, 1998]. The clinical disorders with deficiency, such as distal myopathy of Miyoshi and limb girdle muscular dystrophy type 2B, occur from defects in processes of membrane trafficking or fusion [Bajaoui et al., 1995; Liu et al., 1998; Takahashi et al., 2003].

Caveolin

Caveolae are flask-shaped plasma membrane invaginations that participate in membrane trafficking, sorting, transport, and signal transduction. They are abundant in fibroblasts, adipocytes, endothelial cells, and smooth and striated muscle cells. Caveolin, a family of 21- to 24-kilodalton proteins, is a major constituent of the caveolae. Caveolins form the protein scaffolding upon which the specific proteins and lipids interacting with it are concentrated. Caveolin-3 is expressed in muscles. The human caveolin-3 gene maps to chromosome 3p25, and it codes for a protein of 150 amino acids. The caveolin protein is localized to the sarcolemmal membrane on immunocytochemical studies [Betz et al., 2001].

Mutations in the caveolin-3 gene produce autosomal-dominant limb girdle muscular dystrophy type 1C, hyperC-Kemia, and hereditary rippling muscle disease [Carbone et al., 2000]. The mutant gene produces marked reduction in the caveolin-3 protein, consistent with the dominantly inherited disorder [Cagliani et al., 2003].

Merosin (Laminin-α_2)

Laminin-α_2 is a major component of laminin in the basal lamina of postnatal muscle. It is also expressed in cardiac muscle, pancreas, lung, kidney, adrenal gland, skin, testis, meninges, choroid plexus, and brain. Expression of the laminin-α_2 gene occurs in cells of mesenchymal origin. The gene for laminin-α_2 is localized to chromosome 6q22-23 [Vuolteenaho et al., 1994]. The mature myofiber laminin is a heterodimer composed of laminin-α_2, -β_1, and -γ_1. The laminin interacts with sarcolemma through the dystrophin–glycoprotein and vinculin–integrin complexes. It interacts with basal lamina and extracellular matrix through perlecan, nidogen, and a series of other proteins. Developing and embryonic myofibers express different isoforms of laminin. The laminin isoform expression changes to the α_2 isoform from the α_1 isoform at the time of birth. Mutations of laminin-α_2 in children manifest as congenital muscular dystrophy, complete absence of muscle merosin, and abnormalities of cerebral deep white matter [Jones et al., 2001; Philpot et al., 1995]. Prenatal diagnosis can be made by immunostaining the chorionic villus sample for merosin [Yamamoto et al., 2004].

Intermediate Filaments

Intermediate filaments are cytoskeletal proteins measuring between 10 and 12 nm in thickness [Omary et al., 2004]. Their size is intermediate between actin and the thicker myofilaments such as myosin. Intermediate filaments are seen in cells derived from all three embryonic lineages. Desmin, vimentin, nestin, and lamin are expressed in muscle.

Desmin is the major intermediate filament in skeletal muscle. It is also expressed in cardiac and certain smooth muscles. Desmin is located at the Z band beneath the sarcolemma and is denser at the myotendinous junction [Tidball, 1992]. Desmin is involved with the alignment of sarcomeres with one another and the plasma membrane. It may play a role in the functional and spatial relationship between the nucleus and plasma membrane, and it is presumed to regulate myogenesis because it is more strongly expressed in immature myofibers [Fuchs and Weber, 1994; Gallanti et al., 1992].

Desmin is a 53-kilodalton protein organized in three domains. The highly conserved central α-helical core of 310 amino acids is flanked by a nonhelical amino-terminal head and carboxy-terminal tail. The core is formed of four helical rods: A1, A2, B1, and B2. The desmin polypeptide chains are intertwined in a coiled-coil fashion into a homodimer [Geisler and Weber, 1982]. The desmin filaments interact with other filaments and other proteins to form a cross-linking network, which attaches to membranes. A gene located on chromosome 2q35 encodes the desmin protein [Viegas-Pequignot et al., 1987].

Mutations of the desmin gene result in the desmin-related myopathies, also known as myofibrillar myopathies, and cardiomyopathies [Dalakas et al., 2000, Goldfarb et al., 2004].

Vimentin is an intermediate filament that is also expressed in immature muscle cells during myogenesis. After the postnatal period, its expression in muscle is primarily in regenerating and immature cells [Bornemann and Schmalbruch, 1993]. It is also expressed in tumors of rhabdoid origin.

Nestin is a protein that is expressed with desmin in developing muscle cells [Sjoberg et al., 1994]. Postnatally, the protein is found with desmin in regenerating muscle fibers in patients with dystrophic and inflammatory myopathies.

Plectin, a cytoskeletal linker protein for desmin and keratin organization in muscle and skin, is a large protein (more than 500 kilodaltons) that is expressed in a wide variety of tissues, including muscle and skin. It has a high-affinity binding site for intermediate filaments at its $COOH^-$ terminus. The amino terminus has an actin-binding site, and this site shares similarities with the actin-binding domains of α-actinin, dystrophin, and utrophin. Plectin provides mechanical strength to tolerate the forces of physical stress. Plectin is encoded by a gene localized to 8q24 and has 32 exons [Liu et al., 1996]. Deficiency of plectin has been identified as the cause of recessive epidermolysis bullosa with congenital muscular dystrophy [Whiche, 1998].

Other important cytoskeletal proteins include tubulins and anchor proteins. Microtubules formed from tubulins and other intermediate filaments play an important role in maintaining the cytoplasmic architecture. Anchor proteins link the cytoskeletal proteins to the plasma membrane. Tropomodulin is an integral component of the cytoskeletal structure in the postsynaptic region of the neuromuscular junction [Sussman et al., 1993].

Nuclear Membrane–Related Proteins: Emerin and Lamin A/C

Emerin is a protein associated with the inner nuclear membrane. It is attached to the inner nuclear membrane by its carboxy terminus and extends into the nucleoplasm. Emerin is composed of 254 amino acids and is coded by gene on the X chromosome. Emerin is important in the organization of nuclear membrane during cell division [Fairley et al., 1999]. Mutation of this gene causes X-linked Emery-Dreifuss muscular dystrophy [Haraguchi et al., 2004].

Lamins are major components of the nuclear lamina, which is the major structural framework of nuclei in eukaryotic cells. In humans, two forms of type A (A and C) and B (B1 and B2) are present. Lamins have the helical rod portion and nonhelical portions at the amino and carboxy termini. Lamins differ from other intermediate filaments by the presence of a nuclear localization signal close to their carboxy terminus. The lamins interact with themselves, lamin-associated proteins, and chromatin. The lamins play a role in DNA replication, chromatin organization, spatial arrangement of nuclear pores, nuclear growth, and mechanical stability of the nucleus [Loewinger and McKeon, 1988; Maniotis et al., 1997]. Mutations in the lamin A (A and C) cause autosomal-dominant Emery-Dreifuss muscular dystrophy, dilated cardiomyopathy with conduction defects, and Dunnigan-type familial partial lipodystrophy [Benedetti and Merlini, 2004; van der Kooi et al., 2002].

MUSCLE FIBER TYPES

A single action potential of the neuron causes a transient contraction of the muscle fibers of a motor unit, which is called the *muscle twitch.* The action potential has a duration of about 5 milliseconds, and the onset of contraction occurs about 2 milliseconds after the muscle membrane action potential begins. However, the duration of the muscle fiber contraction varies with the fiber type. Some fibers have rapid twitch times of 5 to 10 milliseconds and are called *fast-twitch* fibers. Other fibers have slow contraction times of 50 to 100 milliseconds and are called *slow-twitch fibers.* Another characteristic of fast-twitch fibers is a relative sensitivity to fatigue and repetitive stimulation. Such fibers often have a grossly pale appearance because they have less myoglobin and mitochondria ("white" muscle). Slow-twitch fibers are resistant to fatigue and have more myoglobin and mitochondria ("red" muscle).

Clinical use commonly divides human muscle fibers into types I and II [Dubowitz and Brook, 1973]. Type I fibers have slow-twitch characteristics and are rich in mitochondria and substrates for aerobic (oxidative) metabolism. They are slightly smaller than type II fibers and have a less well-developed sarcoplasmic reticulum and T-tubule systems. Type II fibers have fast-twitch characteristics and are rich in glycogen and other substrates and enzymes needed for anaerobic (glycolytic) metabolism. Type II fibers can be subdivided into type IIa and IIb fibers. Type IIb fibers are the prototype for the type II fibers, whereas type IIa fibers are intermediate, with both oxidative and glycolytic properties. Type I fibers are generally found in muscles needed for sustained tonic contraction, such as the antigravity muscles of the limbs and trunk. Type I fibers have a more luxurious capillary blood supply. Type II fibers are usually found in muscles concerned with rapid, forceful movement. Table 74-2 summarizes the properties of muscle fiber types. Division of muscle fibers into three basic types is probably an oversimplification. There is a continuum of physiologic properties dependent on the innervation of the motor neuron, which contributes to the plasticity of muscle to adapt to a variety of demands [Buchthal and Schmalbruch, 1980].

The biochemical characteristics of the fiber types can be visualized using histochemical reactions. Type I fibers manifest a strong reaction when stained for the mitochondrial enzymes: succinic dehydrogenase and nicotinamide-adenine dinucleotide (reduced form) transreductase. Nicotinamide-adenine dinucleotide (reduced form) transreductase is also found in abundance in sarcoplasmic reticulum. Myosin adenosine triphosphatase activity can also be used to differentiate fiber types because of the relative abundance of myosin adenosine triphosphatase in type II fibers. Preincubation at various pH levels provides different staining characteristics to various muscle fibers. Type II fibers have an alkali-stable, acid-labile adenosine triphosphatase, whereas type I fibers have the opposite characteristic. Table 74-3 summarizes the histologic and histochemical properties of the muscle fiber types.

All muscle fibers of a motor unit are of a single type. Most of the physiologic, metabolic, and morphologic properties of the muscle fiber depend on innervation from the anterior horn cell. Small α motor neurons innervate type I fibers, and large α motor neurons innervate type II fibers. Reinnervation by the axons of another anterior horn cell alters the muscle fiber properties so that they are identical to the fibers of the donor motor unit [Buller et al., 1960]. The clinical significance of this phenomenon is fiber-type grouping that occurs with reinnervation and can be detected by electromyography and muscle histochemistry. The fibers of a motor unit are normally distributed randomly over several millimeters in the muscle. When a muscle fiber loses its innervation, reinnervation from adjacent, intact axons changes its fiber type. The fiber type can also be altered by changing the characteristics of its innervation [Edgerton et al., 1985], especially its frequency and the quantity of impulses. Prolonged tonic stimulation to a type II fiber can induce type I histochemical characteristics in it [Pette and Vrborá, 1985]. The plasticity of muscle, which alters its characteristics to match changing patterns of innervation, makes the muscle system the most adaptable organ.

FUNCTION

Motor Unit

Contraction of a muscle fiber is initiated by depolarization of its anterior horn cell, which is the final common pathway for all cortical and spinal influences that affect movement. Depolarization of the anterior horn cell membrane is propagated along its axon in the peripheral nerve. At the nerve terminal, axon twigs run parallel within the muscle fascicle to the muscle fibers and innervate the fibers at the neuromuscular junction. Each anterior horn cell innervates about 50 to 200 muscle fibers, depending on the muscle. The anterior horn cell, its peripheral axon, and the innervated muscle fibers compose the motor unit and can be considered a functional unit of the muscle. The muscle fibers within the motor unit are not contiguous but are scattered fairly randomly. In the rat, the motor unit is dispersed over 8% to 76% of the cross-sectional area of the muscle, with some clustering of a few fibers in the motor unit territory [Bodine-Fowler et al., 1990]. When the anterior horn cell discharges, all the muscle fibers innervated by that anterior horn cell contract almost simultaneously. The finer and more coordinated the movement of a muscle, the fewer the fibers in the motor unit. Eye muscles and some hand muscles may have 30 to 50 fibers in the motor unit, whereas some back muscles have hundreds. In general, the larger the muscle, the larger the size of the motor units [McComas, 1991]. For example, there are about 100 fibers per motor unit in the intrinsic muscles of the hand, 200 in the extensor digitorum brevis, and 900 in the larger muscles.

TABLE 74-2

Characteristic Features of Muscle Fiber Types

	I	IIa	IIb
Metabolic Features			
Glycolytic metabolism	Oxidative	Oxidative	Glycolytic
Myoglobin content	High	High	Low
Mitochondria content	High	High	Low
Sarcoplasmic-reticulum-calcium pump capacity	Moderate	High	High myosin isozyme
Adenosine triphosphatase activity	Slow	Fast	Fast
Physiologic Features			
Twitch speed	Slow	Fast	Fast
Twitch duration	Long	Short	Short
Fatigue resistant	Yes	Intermediate	No
Morphologic Features			
Capillary supply	Rich	Intermediate	Poor
Sarcoplasmic reticulum	Intermediate	Rich	Rich
Size	Intermediate	Small	Large
Appearance	Red	Red	White
Other names	Red, slow oxidative	Fast oxidative	White, fast glycolytic

TABLE 74-3

Histochemical Reactions of Human Muscle

	I	IIa	IIb
Myosin ATPase, pH 9.4	Light	Dark	Dark
Myosin ATPase, pH 4.6	Dark	Light	Intermediate
Myosin ATPase, pH 4.3	Dark	Light	Light
Actomyosin ATPase	Light	Dark	Intermediate
NADH-TR	Dark	Intermediate	Light
Succinic dehydrogenase	Dark	Intermediate	Light
α-Glycerophosphate dehydrogenase (menadione linked)	Light	Dark	Dark
Phosphorylase	Light to intermediate	Dark	Dark
Periodic acid–Schiff stain	Light to intermediate	Light	Light
Oil red O stain	Dark	Light	Light

ATPase, adenosine triphosphatase; NADH-TR, nicotinamide-adenine dinucleotide (reduced form) transreductase.

Neuromuscular Transmission

The neuromuscular junction is formed by specialized portions of the nerve and muscle plasma membrane, which are separated by the synaptic cleft (Fig. 74-8). The area on the muscle is the end plate and is located near the center of the muscle at the end-plate zone. The synaptic knob is the terminal dilation of the nerve axon and contains synaptic vesicles of acetylcholine. The motor neuron action potential is propagated down the motor nerve by saltatory conduction. Na^+ channels at the nodes of Ranvier produce current. Within the muscle, the motor nerve fiber branches into terminal fibers that individually innervate muscle fibers within the motor unit. The nerve terminals are unmyelinated, and the membrane excitability is maintained by both K^+ and Na^+. Antibodies to the K^+ antigen cause acquired neuromyotonia, such as Isaac's syndrome [Newsome-Davis et al., 2003].

Depolarization of the nerve terminus opens voltage-gated calcium channels at the synaptic knob. As calcium enters the nerve ending, exocytosis of the synaptic vesicles occurs, releasing acetylcholine. Antibodies directed against the voltage-gated calcium channels causes Lambert-Eaton syndome by reducing the quantal release of acetylcholine [Newsome-Davis, 2004]. Acetylcholine is synthesized from acetyl coenzyme A and choline and exists in a reserve compartment that is not readily available for release and in a mobilization compartment of vesicles. Each synaptic vesicle contains a quantum of about 10,000 acetylcholine molecules. The vesicles are attached to the active zone of the presynaptic membrane. Fifty to 300 vesicles fuse with a nerve terminus depolarization. The process of vesicle formation, fusion, and release is a complex system involving many proteins [Ruff, 2003].

Acetylcholine combines with specific acetylcholine receptors located on the postsynaptic membrane of the muscle sarcolemma. There are about 15,000/μm^2 receptors in the junctional fold concentrated at the tops of the secondary folds. The acetylcholine receptor is a transmembrane glycoprotein with a molecular weight of 250,000 daltons and is composed of four subunits: α, β, δ, and γ [Momoi and Lennon, 1982]. The muscle acetylcholine receptor monomer is constructed with two α subunits and one of each of the other subunits in order: α_1, γ, δ, β_1 [Lindstrom, 2003]. The acetylcholine receptor monomer

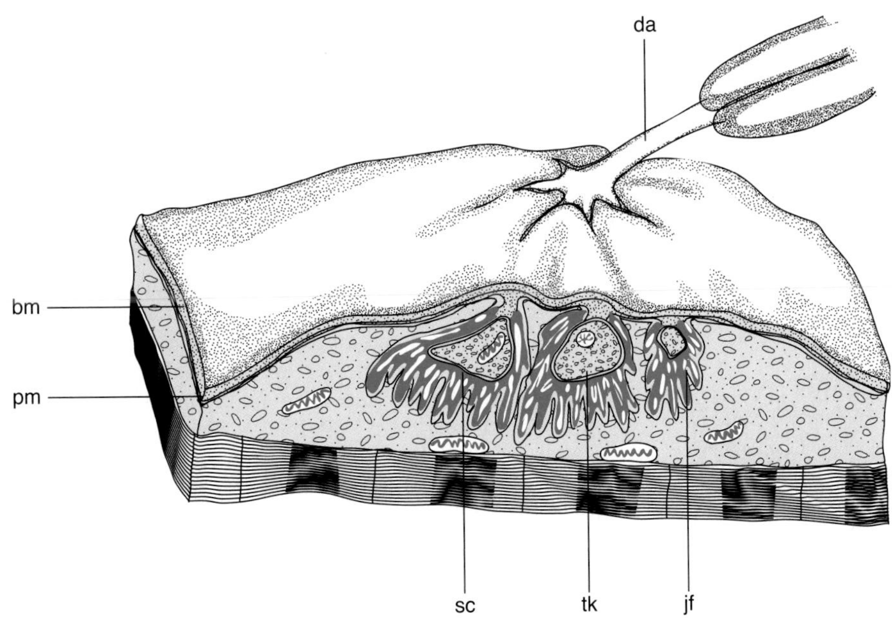

FIGURE 74-8. Neuromuscular junction. bm, Basement membrane; da, distal axon; jf, junctional folds; pm, plasma membrane; sc, synaptic cleft; tk, terminal knob.

contains two acetylcholine-binding sites and the cation-specific channel, whose opening is regulated. The receptor is barrel shaped, traverses the sarcolemma, and projects above its surface. The subunits are arranged around the central channel-like staves (Fig. 74-9) [Kistler et al., 1982]. The acetylcholine receptors are anchored to dystrophin-related protein complexes and connected to the cytoskeleton by dystrophoglycans and sarcoglycan protein complexes. The structure and function of the acetylcholine receptor are remarkably similar in all species studied. Congenital myasthenic syndromes are caused by genetic mutations of the receptor and other synapse structures, whereas myasthenia gravis is caused by antibodies to receptor proteins.

The binding of two acetylcholine molecules with the α subunits of the receptor causes a conformational change in the M2 portion of α-helical structures of each of the five subunits. This change results in a rotational realignment of the helices to open the center of the receptor for a few milliseconds and thereby alter the sodium and potassium permeability by opening ion channels. Increased ion conductance across the sarcolemma causes a localized depolarization of the muscle end plate. A single quantum of acetylcholine interacting with the end plate causes a miniature end-plate potential insufficient to engender a propagated membrane discharge. When depolarization of the terminal axon occurs, 50 to 300 acetylcholine quanta are released. Sufficient interactions between acetylcholine molecules and receptors cause the summation of potentials to reach the threshold potential for the end plate. Thus, an end-plate potential is achieved, and the depolarization is propagated along the sarcolemma and T tubules. Depolarization of the end plate is a statistical phenomenon; given sufficient numbers of acetylcholine molecules and receptors, an interaction will probably occur, followed by depolarization [Katz and Miledi, 1972]. Interference with the release of acetylcholine or a reduction in the number of receptors lessens the likelihood of successful neuromuscular transmission.

Excitation–Contraction Coupling

The major function of muscle is generating movement or force by contraction. This function is accomplished through a series of events called *excitation–contraction coupling,* which is the linkage of the electrical and mechanical properties of muscle. Depolarization of the T tubules at the triad is sensed by dihydropyridine (a calcium-channel blocker) receptors, which are associated with charged molecules within the tubular membrane. Movement of these charged molecules, which can be inhibited by dantrolene [Hui, 1983], causes a conformational change in the "feet," which are structures that bridge the membranes of the T tubules and sarcoplasmic reticulum [Peachey, 1985]. Calsequestrin is a major protein of the sarcoplasmic reticulum that binds calcium and is located close to the sarcoplasmic reticulum calcium efflux channels in register with the "feet" processes [Stadhouders, 1990]. Interaction of these membrane structures at the triad causes the release of calcium from the sarcoplasmic reticulum into the sarcoplasm. During tetany, calcium concentrations decrease in the sarcoplasmic reticulum and increase in the sarcoplasm [Somlyo et al., 1981]. This release of calcium is critical for the mechanics of muscle contractions. Calcium-binding proteins in the sarcoplasm, including calmodulin [Kennelly et al., 1989] and parvalbumin [Heizmann et al., 1990], are essential for regulation of the contractile proteins.

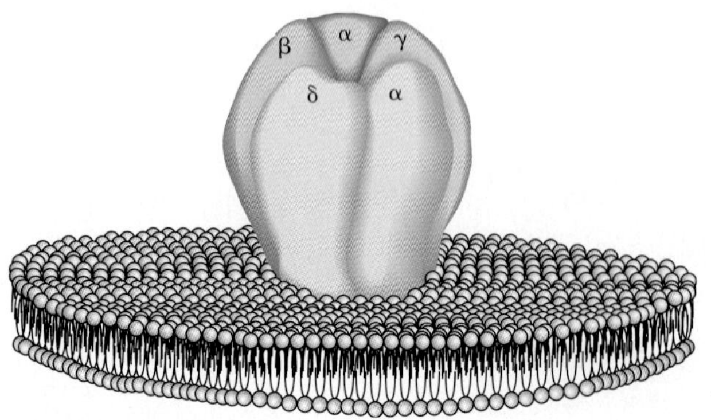

FIGURE 74-9. Acetylcholine receptor. The receptor projects above the plasma membrane and is composed of five subunits arranged around the central ion channel.

Contraction of muscle is brought about by contractile proteins. These proteins have different forms (isoforms), and the presence of a specific isoform within the fiber determines some of the contraction properties of the muscle. The isoforms are similar but have slightly different properties, such as calcium-binding capacity and adenosine triphosphatase activity. Every fiber is capable of synthesizing all isoforms of the contractile proteins, but the precise composition of isoforms within a muscle fiber depends on the many complex mechanisms that coordinate gene expression and the neural influences that ultimately control fiber typing (see earlier discussion).

When it is released by the sarcoplasmic reticulum, calcium binds with calmodulin; the complex acts as a second messenger that activates the myosin light chain troponin C kinase [Kennelly et al., 1989]. This reaction causes an unmasking of a myosin-binding site by displacing troponin I and tropomyosin. The myosin head swings away from the backbone of the thick filament at the hinge area of the S2 region [Horowits et al., 1989]. The myosin head then attaches to actin at an angle, and the hydrolysis of adenosine triphosphate causes the myosin head to swivel to a more acute angle, moving the chains toward one another (Fig. 74-10). Repetition of this event causes shortening of the sarcomere [Vale and Milligan, 2000]. Each attachment, swivel, and reattachment shortens the muscle about 1%, or about 14 nm [Ford et al., 1977]. Myosin hydrolyzes adenosine triphosphate slowly unless combined with actin. Each stroke of the myosin–actin cross-bridge attachment consumes one molecule of adenosine triphosphate: adenosine triphosphate binding to myosin, dissociation of actin and myosin, adenosine triphosphate hydrolysis, reassociation of actin and myosin, and release of hydrolysis products. The rate of stroke cycling and therefore the contraction velocity are dependent on the myosin adenosine triphosphatase isoform [Pollack, 1996]. The exact mechanism of the phase transition that brings about muscle contraction is still not fully known [Brooks, 2003]. The entire process constitutes excitation–contraction coupling.

The tension generated by a muscle is directly proportional to the number of cross-links between the myosin heads of thick filaments and the actin of the thin filaments as

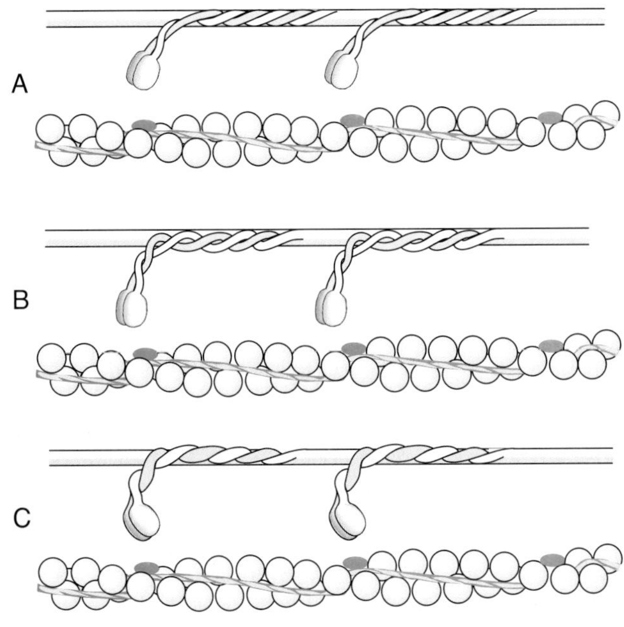

FIGURE 74-10. Myosin head movement. During contraction, the myosin head swivels from its resting position **(A)**, toward actin **(B)**. With hydrolysis of adenosine triphosphate, the orientation of the head closes to a more acute angle, propelling the thin filament to slide **(C)**.

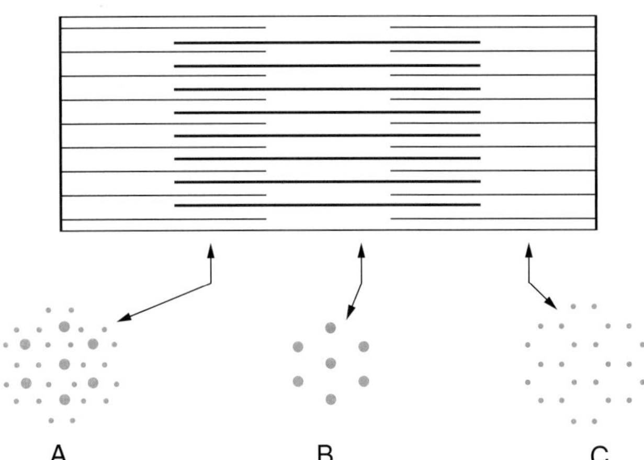

FIGURE 74-11. Schematic diagram of myofilament orientation within the sarcomere. Cross-sections illustrate the relationships of the thick and thin filaments. **A,** A band. **B,** H band. **C,** I band.

determined by length–tension relationships [Pollack and Sugi, 1984]. On cross-section, each myosin heavy chain is surrounded by six actin light chains. This geometric array is found in the area of the sarcomere where there are overlapping myofilaments, as in the A band (Fig. 74-11). The more foreshortened the sarcomere, the more cross-links between the filaments. However, only the thin filaments occur in the I band. Each muscle has a length at which it generates maximum force and at which the greatest interaction between actin and myosin occurs [Hoxley, 1996; Lieber, 1986].

Evidence suggests that contraction of a muscle occurs by heavy and light myofilaments sliding toward one another. When a muscle contracts, the distance between the Z lines decreases at the expense of the I and H bands. The A band remains unchanged (Fig. 74-12). During stretch, the I band increases in length as the actin filament arrays slide in the direction opposite of the myosin filament arrays; thus, the distance between Z lines increases. This sliding is produced by the formation and breakage of the cross-links between actin and myosin.

Neuromuscular transmission is terminated by calcium sequestering within the synaptic knob. Muscle contraction is terminated when the T tubules repolarize; this causes reaccumulation of calcium within the sarcoplasmic reticulum, using a pump that depends on adenosine triphosphate [Peachey, 1985]. Unlike the nerve and muscle plasma membrane, the contraction process has no refractory period. As long as calcium is free in the sarcoplasm and adequate energy stores exist, the muscle will stay contracted. Muscle can stay contracted without excitation of the membrane system, and energy is required for the reuptake of calcium into the sarcoplasmic reticulum. Failure of calcium reuptake from the sarcoplasm when energy stores are depleted inhibits relaxation of the muscle. This mechanism causes rigor mortis and the cramping during exercise found in energy-deficiency disorders, such as McArdle's disease.

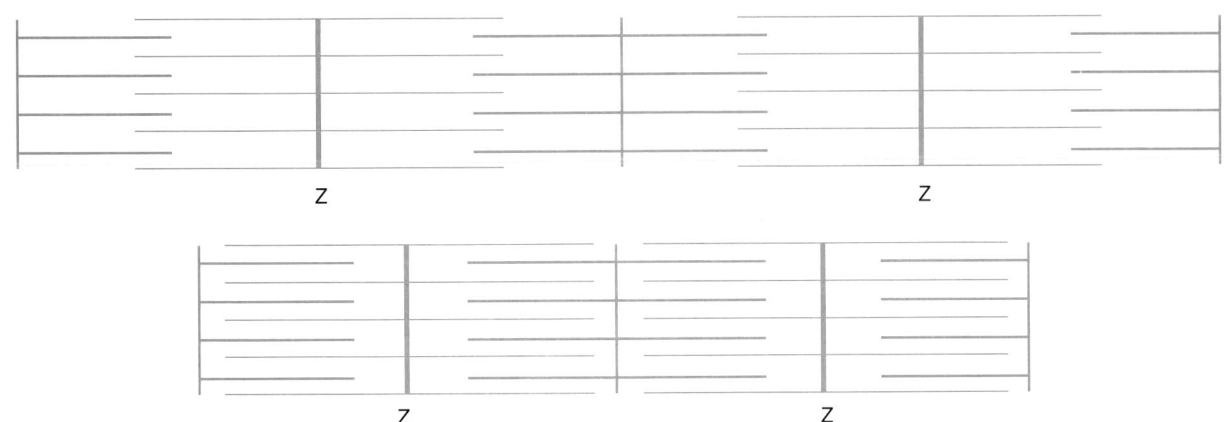

FIGURE 74-12. Sliding filament mechanism of muscle contraction. The thick and thin filaments slide toward one another during contraction, causing the distance between the Z lines to shorten.

NEURAL CONTROL OF MUSCLE CONTRACTION

The sarcomere is the contracting unit of muscle. Whole muscle contraction force is proportional to the number of sarcomeres contracting in parallel, whereas whole muscle contraction velocity is proportional to the number of sarcomeres acting in series [Lieber, 1986]. This interaction generally applies to the muscle fiber and to the architecture of muscle. The more fibers in parallel, the more force is generated by contraction. The longer the muscle fiber, the more sarcomeres are in series and the greater the contraction velocity.

Motor Unit System

The motor unit consists of a single lower motor neuron and the muscle fibers it innervates. The motor unit is the final common pathway of the motor system [Miles, 1994]. The following two control mechanisms are used by the nervous system in generating muscle contraction force: (1) the orderly recruitment of motor units, and (2) the regulation of firing rates of active motor neurons [De Luca, 1985]. There is a rank order of recruitment within a motor neuron pool, so that increasingly larger motor units are recruited for increasing demands of force. Smaller motor units are recruited initially [Henneman, 1985]. Similarly, the rate of discharge of motor units is proportional to the degree of force generated. Current information indicates that the firing rates of motor neurons are not controlled individually, but that the nervous system controls the firing rate of motor neuron pools to modulate force generation. This mechanism has been termed *common drive* [De Luca, 1985]. In general, the recruitment of additional motor units is more important in generating force and power than modulating firing rates [Brooks, 2003].

Motor unit recruitment is the process by which different motor units are activated to produce a specific degree and type of muscle force [Petajan, 1991]. In the graded generation of force, the lower force threshold, slow-twitch motor units are recruited first. Increasing force output increases the firing rate of these first recruited motor neuron pools in fine gradations. Further force generation requires recruitment of large motor neurons with higher force threshold, fast-twitch motor units. This recruitment causes a 5- to 10-fold increase in the graded force. Normally, a motor unit discharges up to rates of 5 to 15 Hz before an additional neuron is recruited. The firing rate of the fastest firing motor unit divided by the number of recruited neurons is normally less than five (e.g., three neurons firing at a rate of 15 Hz). When this recruitment ratio is greater than 10 (e.g., two neurons firing at a rate of 20), it suggests a loss of motor units. At maximal exertion, there is fusion of contractions of the slow-twitch motor units. Because of the short twitch duration of the large motor units, they may not achieve contraction fusion with voluntary effort [De Luca et al., 1982]. During normal activity, slow-twitch motor units discharge more frequently and are active more often than fast-twitch motor units [Hennig and Lomo, 1985].

Changes in the firing rate and the number of motor units recruited for a given muscle contraction are under a variety of controls, including the γ afferents, Golgi tendon organs, and Renshaw cells that facilitate or disfacilitate neurons to produce a graded contraction.

γ Efferent System

The γ efferent system plays a major role in controlling muscle contraction by its effects on the muscle spindle. The muscle spindle is a specialized sensory organ located within the perimysial connective tissue (Fig. 74-13). It is an encapsulated structure containing 2 to 10 small muscle fibers (intrafusal fibers) and special sensory nerve endings. The intrafusal fibers comprise nuclear bag fibers, nuclear chain fibers, and an intermediate type of fiber. Each has distinct ultrastructural and histochemical characteristics [Barker et al., 1972]. The intrafusal fibers of the spindle are arranged in parallel with the extrafusal fibers of the muscle.

The sensory endings are of two types [Scalzi and Price, 1972]. The primary endings (annulospiral) are supplied by large, myelinated, rapidly conducting Ia afferent fibers and end in a spiral or cagelike arrangement around nuclear bag fibers. These endings are sensitive to both stretch of the spindle and the velocity of stretch. Secondary endings of group II sensory nerves terminate in a variety of endings, including cylindrical, flat, and annulospiral or ring-shaped endings, mostly on nuclear chain fibers [Schroder et al., 1989]. Secondary endings are sensitive to the stretch of the spindle.

The fusimotor fibers compose as much as 30% of the total number of ventral root fibers. Most are γ efferents, although a few are β efferents [Barker et al., 1972]. Multiterminal plate endings (i.e., flower-spray) are located on nuclear bag fibers from myelinated γ efferents and probably cause dynamic innervation. Trail endings, however, primarily innervate nuclear chain fibers and arise from smaller myelinated and unmyelinated fibers. Trail fibers supply static innervation.

The afferent fibers of primary endings synapse directly on the anterior horn cells, which supply the extrafusal fibers of the same muscle. The secondary ending afferents probably synapse on motor neurons of other muscles [Scalzi and Price, 1972]. Stretch of a muscle causes distortion of the primary endings and generates a signal to the motor neuron to cause contraction. This signal is the mechanism of the deep tendon reflex. If the muscle were shortened, spindle discharge would decrease, causing muscle relaxation; therefore, spindles serve as a feedback mechanism to maintain muscle length and tone.

The γ efferent system operates in concert with the α motor neuron to effect movement [van der Meulen et al., 1972]. Stimulation of the γ motor neuron causes stretching of the nuclear bag fibers, distortion of the primary endings, and reflex stimulation of the α motor neuron, as discussed previously. The γ motor neurons are regulated by several descending tracts, whose main purpose is to maintain the sensitivity to stretch throughout muscle contraction so that different muscle groups can adjust to the needs of postural control.

The other major sensory innervation of muscle is the Golgi tendon organ [Stuart et al., 1972], which is a netlike structure located around the tendon fascicles supplied by fast-conducting myelinated afferent fibers. The output causes stimulation of inhibitory internuncial neurons, which, in turn, synapse on α motor neurons. The sensory organ is arranged in series with the muscle and thus is more sensitive to changes in muscle force than to changes in

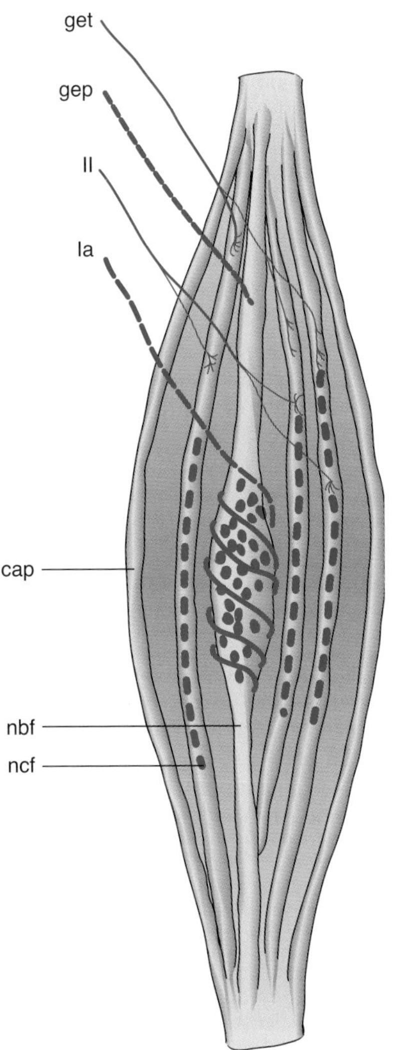

FIGURE 74-13. Muscle spindle. cap, Capsule; get, γ efferent with trail ending; gep, γ efferent with plate ending; II, type II afferent with flower-spray ending; Ia type Ia efferent with annulospiral ending; nbf, nuclear bag fiber; ncf, nuclear chain fiber.

length. Excessive stretch produces an inhibitory influence on the α motor neurons.

MUSCLE METABOLISM

Muscle contraction requires a relatively large amount of energy. The immediate source of this energy is derived from the hydrolysis of adenosine triphosphate, which is synthesized by phosphorylation of adenosine diphosphate. Energy for the formation of adenosine triphosphate is derived from metabolism. At rest, this energy can be stored in the form of phosphocreatine. When needed at the time of exercise, phosphocreatine is hydrolyzed by creatine kinase to form adenosine triphosphate from adenosine diphosphate. After depletion of phosphocreatine stores, muscle metabolism increases to maintain adenosine triphosphate stores.

At rest, high-energy phosphate compounds are produced from the metabolism of available fats and glucose [Hultman, 1995]. Increased lipid supply inhibits glycolysis and carbohydrate use. Excess glucose can be metabolized directly from the circulation or stored as glycogen until needed. With maximal exertion, phosphocreatine and muscle glycogen are the fuels for energy production. Above 60% maximal exertion, type II fibers are preferentially recruited, and carbohydrates are the preferred fuel after a normal meal. Fat utilization is increased with starvation or a high fat intake before exercise. At exercise intensities below 60%, fat is the major fuel corresponding to the recruitment of type I fibers.

In the presence of oxygen, each mole of glucose is converted to 2 mol of pyruvate, which is further oxidized through the citric acid cycle and electron transport chain. For each mole of glucose oxidized, 36 mol of adenosine triphosphate are generated (38 mol from glycogen). In the absence of oxygen, glucose is metabolized to lactic acid. For each mole of glucose consumed, 2 mol of lactic acid are produced, with only 2 mol of adenosine triphosphate. The yield from a glucose unit derived from glycogen under anaerobic conditions is 3 mol of adenosine triphosphate. Tremendous amounts of lactic acid can be generated from breakdown of stored glycogen during brief efforts of anaerobic metabolism, as demonstrated in short sprints and other maximal exertion exercises.

There is a constant relationship among force, phosphate concentrations, and pH [Weiner et al., 1990]. As energy is expended, phosphocreatine concentrations decrease, phosphate increases, and pH decreases. The adenosine triphosphate concentration remains stable [Kushmerick, 1995]. Thus, fatigue is relative to the degree of acidosis and free phosphate concentrations. A lactate–proton cotransport system is important for reducing the accumulation of lactate and H^+ within the muscle [Juel, 1997]. Recovery from fatigue parallels the normalization of these metabolic parameters [Boska et al., 1990].

Lipids can be used, giving a relatively higher yield of adenosine triphosphate per mole of lipid consumed. Mobilizing lipids for energy consumption is a slower process than mobilizing carbohydrates. Activities that require endurance or prolonged effort are associated with higher lipid metabolism. Training increases the vascular perfusion of muscle and oxygen delivery and increases energy production by aerobic metabolism. Training also increases the capacity of the electron transfer system, oxidative phosphorylation, and the lactate–proton cotransport system [Juel, 1997]. Training increases lactate clearance in the muscle by increasing muscle oxidation of lactate and increasing the lactate transporter protein, monocarboxylate transporter [Dubouchaud et al., 2000]. In general, muscle metabolism is quite plastic and adapts relatively rapidly to altered functional requirements.

Muscle has metabolic functions besides energy production. Muscle protein anabolism and catabolism are controlled by many factors in the inverse relationship. The major factors that promote protein synthesis and muscle growth are exercise, amino acid availability, and insulin [Kimball et al., 2002; Wolfe, 2002]. In the adult male, muscle represents about 40% of body weight. It is a vast storehouse for protein, amino acids, fat, and glycogen. Muscle metabolism is intimately involved with metabolism of other tissues, especially the liver. Most lactate in the body is produced from resting muscle. The cell-to-cell lactate shuttle hypothesis suggests that lactate is an intermediate metabolite rather than an end product. It is produced by many tissues, especially muscle, and is used as an energy source in the heart and other highly oxidative tissues and as a precursor of glucose in liver gluconeogenesis (Cori's cycle). Similarly, during fasting or other stresses, muscle releases amino acids, lactate, and other precursors for use by the liver during gluconeogenesis. There is clinical evidence that children with chronic hypoglycemia, as is found in the glycogen storage diseases, have secondary muscle degradation from the chronic muscle catabolism that provides the amino acids necessary for gluconeogenesis [Slonim et al., 1983].

CLINICAL LABORATORY TESTS

Modern investigation of muscle disease includes clinical biochemistry and immunology, electromyography, muscle biopsy pathology, molecular genetics, imaging of muscle, and other modalities [Younger and Gordon, 1996].

Clinical Biochemistry

Several muscle sarcoplasmic enzymes are used in the clinical evaluation of muscle disease. These enzymes are released from the muscle fiber when damaged. Of these enzymes, aldolase and creatine kinase are used most commonly, especially the latter. Creatine kinase exists as several isozymes, including M and B. BB is found almost exclusively in brain tissue, whereas MM is found almost exclusively in muscle and heart tissue. MB is found in several tissues. Determination of creatine kinase isozymes is helpful in differentiating brain from muscle disease but not muscle from heart disease [Vainzof et al., 1985]. Creatine kinase is not found in the liver or erythrocytes.

The normal range of creatine kinase enzyme activity in the blood varies with age, gender, and daily activities. In an inactive male, however, this range may rise to two to three times that of the upper limits. After vigorous extended activity, such as running a marathon or a similar effort, plasma creatine kinase activity may approach 10 times that of normal [Brown et al., 1982]. Elevation of plasma creatine kinase also occurs after trauma, seizures [Wyllie et al., 1985], electroconvulsive therapy [Taylor et al., 1981], and injections. Myopathic disorders cause muscle breakdown and release of creatine kinase and other enzymes into the bloodstream. Increased activities of these enzymes are suggestive, but not diagnostic, of myopathic disease. Creatine kinase can also be mildly elevated in neuropathic diseases. Other enzymes released include transaminases, lactate dehydrogenase, carbonic anhydrase III, and pyruvate kinase. None is as useful as creatine kinase. Serum myoglobin also correlates with muscle breakdown [Norregaard-Hansen and Hein-Sorensen, 1982]. Other biochemical methods that have been used in investigating muscle disease include measuring urinary excretion of creatine and 3-methyl histidine. Their clinical application has not been commonly accepted for various reasons.

Electromyography

Electromyography is the recording of electrical activity by a needle electrode of action potentials of muscle fibers firing singly or in groups near the electrode [Daube, 1991]. Several techniques can be used to study specific features of muscle. The most common is the coaxial needle study. The needle has a central active electrode, which forms the core of the coaxial needle. A surrounding cylinder is insulated from the core and serves as the reference electrode. The needle is inserted into the muscle and records electrical depolarization of the surrounding muscle membranes. The motor unit potential can be visualized on a cathode-ray oscilloscope and is usually amplified through a loudspeaker for auditory analysis. Electromyographic abnormalities are not specific for a given clinical entity but allow for widespread sampling and an indication of the type of neuromuscular disease present [Wilbourn, 1993].

The electromyography study has three aspects. The first aspect is the recording of activity during insertion of the needle electrode. The insertional activity is a reflection of the mechanical damage caused by the needle. Inserting the needle electrode or adjusting the needle usually causes a brief, spontaneous discharge of the surrounding muscle fibers. Abnormal activity on insertion, such as prolonged discharges or activation of spontaneous trains of discharges, indicates disease.

The second part of clinical electromyography is recording the spontaneous resting properties of the muscle. Normally, muscle is electrically silent during rest. End-plate noise can be recorded if the needle is placed near the end-plate zone. End-plate noise is generated by miniature end-plate potentials and single fiber discharges produced by needle irritation [Shahani and Young, 1985]. Spontaneous activities, such as fibrillations, positive sharp waves, fasciculations, or others, usually indicate underlying disease, most commonly neuropathic disorders. Spontaneous repetitive discharges are found in various neuropathic and myopathic disorders, such as the myotonias.

The third part of electromyography is recording motor unit potentials to evaluate the electrical properties of muscle during contraction. The motor unit potential usually has two or three phases and is 5 to 15 milliseconds in duration. The voltage usually does not exceed 5 mV. With a primary muscle disease, a frequent finding is brief, small-amplitude, polyphasic potentials. With chronic neuropathic disease, a common finding is prolonged, large-amplitude, polyphasic potentials. With graded contraction, an increase in the firing rate of individual motor units occurs. Further effort causes an increase in the number of recruited motor units and is proportional to the degree of muscle contractions. Thus, motor units are recruited in response to the degree of effort, and there is a recruitment order of motor units that is relatively fixed [Henneman et al., 1974]. Analysis of the interference pattern can be useful in the diagnosis of neuromuscular disease [Sanders et al., 1996]. At maximal effort, individual motor unit potentials cannot be distinguished (full interference). In primary muscle disease, in which all muscle fibers are similarly affected, a greater number of fibers is needed to perform a given amount of work. Thus, there is an increase in the number of motor units needed to perform the given amount of work. This increase is noticeable with mild effort, and it causes the phenomenon of early recruitment. Conversely, with denervation, in which there is a reduction in the number of motor units, the recruitment pattern is decreased, and thus full interference is not possible.

Single-fiber electromyography is a technique for studying the characteristics of neuromuscular transmission and the localized organization of muscle fibers within a motor unit [Sanders et al., 1996]. A special needle electrode is introduced into the muscle at multiple sites. The number of single muscle fiber action potentials belonging to one motor unit recorded in a given area gives a quantitative measure of the fiber density. Recording from two fibers of the same motor unit enables one to measure "jitter," or the mean consecutive difference in time between the firing of the two fibers, which is usually between 10 and 55 milliseconds. An increase in jitter is commonly observed with defects of neurotransmission. Single-fiber electromyography also detects blocking when the second fiber fails to discharge, which is the basis for the decremental response during repetitive stimulation in patients with myasthenia gravis. Other electrodiagnostic methods are also useful in evaluating myasthenic disorders and peripheral neuropathies. These subjects are discussed in other chapters.

Muscle Biopsy

Muscle biopsy is the definitive test for diagnosing specific muscle diseases and is indicated in the child with suspected neuromuscular disease; however, muscle biopsy is less likely to yield diagnostic findings if creatine kinase and electromyography readings are normal. Muscle biopsy may not be diagnostic early in the course of an illness when the abnormalities are scant and a sampling error can mask the pathologic condition. The pathologic condition may also escape diagnosis late in the course of a disease if the muscle is so altered that no distinguishing features exist ("end-stage" muscle).

The method of muscle biopsy has been reviewed in detail elsewhere [Dubowitz and Brook, 1973]. It can be performed by either an open biopsy or a needle biopsy technique [Heckmatt et al., 1984]. Either method is relatively simple and can be performed on an outpatient basis. The muscle chosen for biopsy should be one affected clinically but not severely.

To obtain optimal results, the material must be handled by experienced technicians and interpreted by those familiar with neuromuscular diseases. Routine histologic stains often used in evaluating a muscle biopsy include the hematoxylin-eosin stain, modified Gomori trichrome stain, periodic acid–Schiff stain for glycogen, and oil red O or Sudan black stain for lipid. The hematoxylin-eosin stain is used most often for evaluating muscle fibers, nuclei, and other cellular constituents. The trichrome stain is used especially for evaluating connective tissue, intramuscular nerves, and certain features of the muscle fiber, such as mitochondria. Other histologic stains are often used for special purposes.

Histochemistry often reveals the most significant information. Adenosine triphosphatase reactions are used to determine fiber typing. The random distribution of the fiber type on the adenosine triphosphatase reaction is a major feature of normal muscle. Normally, there are about equal numbers of type I, IIa, and IIb fibers, although up to 50% of a single type can be found in some muscles [Dubowitz and Brook, 1973]. Oxidative stains and the periodic acid–Schiff stain also reflect fiber typing (see Table 74-3). The oxidative reactions that include succinic dehydrogenase and nicotinamine-adenine dinucleotide transreductase are helpful in identifying mitochondria and the sarcotubular system. Many other histochemical reactions facilitate the study of specific diseases, such as the myophosphorylase reaction that aids in diagnosis of McArdle's disease. Figure 74-14 illustrates the major histologic and histochemical features of muscle.

Immunohistochemistry is becoming increasingly important for the study of normal and diseased muscle. The absence of dystrophin on immunohistochemical staining of muscle tissue is diagnostic of Duchenne's and related muscular dystrophies. Certain congenital myopathies can be classified based on immunohistochemical staining of other cytoskeletal proteins [Duggan et al., 1997; Philpot et al., 1995; Wallgren-Pettersson et al., 1995].

Electron microscopy is rarely needed for accurate diagnosis, but it is often necessary in disorders of the mitochondria and to determine the ultrastructure of central cores, nemaline rods, and other inclusions in congenital myopathy [Younger and Gordon, 1996].

Muscle Imaging

Ultrasonography, computed tomography, and magnetic resonance imaging are used in the diagnosis and management of patients with neuromuscular disease [Clague et al., 1995]. Ultrasonography is a cost-effective method for localization of diseased muscle for biopsy purposes. It is useful for imaging dystrophic muscle [Heckmatt and Dubowitz, 1988]. Magnetic resonance imaging is particularly useful for the diagnosis of inflammatory muscle disease. Inflammation is easily identified and can be distinguished from other causes of weakness [Stonecipher et al., 1994].

Molecular Genetics

Techniques for mapping and sequencing the human genome have brought about an entirely new approach to the diagnosis of human neuromuscular disease [Nawrotzki et al., 1996]. High deletion frequencies, unstable tandem repeat sequences, genomic duplications, and triplet repeat expansions are common abnormalities that enable a molecular genetic diagnosis to be made for such diseases as Duchenne's and Becker's muscular dystrophy, some forms of limb girdle dystrophy, myotonic muscular dystrophy, congenital muscular dystrophy, and many others (see Table 74-1). Often the defective gene product, such as dystrophin in the X-linked dystrophies, can be measured or visualized in muscle samples for diagnostic purposes. Similarly, a number of mitochondrial diseases can be diagnosed from analysis of mitochondrial DNA [Younger and Gordon, 1996].

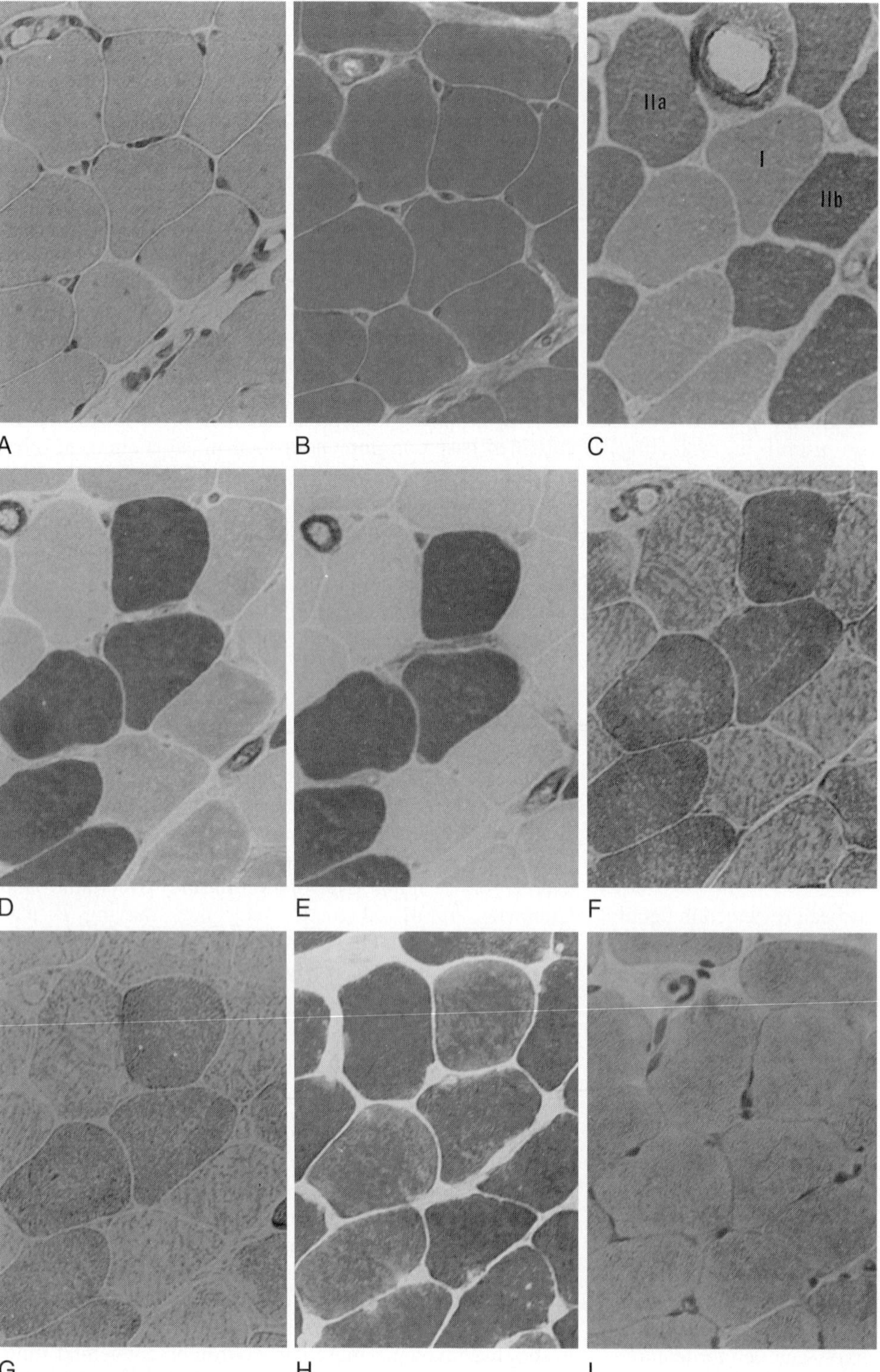

FIGURE 74-14. Muscle histology and histochemistry. Serial sections are stained as follows: **A,** Hematoxylin and eosin. **B,** Modified Gomori trichrome. **C,** Myosin adenosine triphosphate, pH 9.4. **D,** Myosin adenosine triphosphate, pH 4.6. **E,** Myosin adenosine triphosphate, pH 4.3. **F,** Nicotine-adenine dinucleotide transreductase. **G,** Succinic dehydrogenase. **H,** Myophosphorylase. **I,** Periodic acid–Schiff stain.

REFERENCES

Alameddine HS, Dehaupas M, Fardeau M. Regeneration of skeletal muscle fibers from autologous satellite cells multiplied in vitro: An experimental model for testing cultured cell myogenicity. Muscle Nerve 1989;12:544.

Anderson JE. A role for nitric oxide in muscle repair: Nitric oxide-medicated activation of muscle satellite cells. Mol Biol Cell 2000;11:1859.

Anderson JT, Rogers RP, Jarrett HW. Ca2+-calmodulin binds to the carboxyl-terminal domain of dystrophin. J Biol Chem 1996;271:6605.

Anderson LV, Davison K, Moss JA, et al. Dysferlin is a plasma membrane protein and is expressed early in human development. Hum Mol Genet 1999;8:855.

Bajaoui K, Hirabayashi K, Hentati F, et al. Linkage of Miyoshi myopathy (distal autosomal recessive muscular dystrophy) locus to chromosome 2p12-14. Neurology 1995;45:768.

Bansal D, Miyake K, Vogel S, et al. Defective membrane repair in dysferlin-deficient muscular dystrophy. Nature 2003;423(6936):168.

Barker D, Harker D, Stacey MJ, et al. Fusimotor innervation. In: Banker BQ, Przybylski RJ, van der Meulen JP, et al., eds. Research in muscle development and the spindle. Amsterdam: Excerpta Medica, 1972.

Benedetti S, Merlini L. Laminopathies: From the heart of the cell to the clinics. Curr Opin Neurol 2004;17:553.

Betz RC, Schoser BG, Kasper D, et al. Mutations in CAV3 cause mechanical hyperirritability of skeletal muscle in rippling muscle disease. Nat Genet 2001;28:218.

Bies RD, Caskey CT, Fenwick R. An intact cysteine-rich domain is required for dystrophin function. J Clin Invest 1992;90(2):666.

Blake DJ, Kroger S. The neurobiology of Duchenne muscular dystrophy: Learning lessons from muscle? Trends Neurosci 2000;23:92.

Bodine-Fowler S, Garfinkel A, Roy RR, et al. Spatial distribution of muscle fibers within the territory of a motor unit. Muscle Nerve 1990;13:1133.

Boito C, Fanin M, Siciliano G, et al. Novel sarcoglycan gene mutations in a large cohort of Italian patients. J Med Genet 2003;40(5):67.

Bonnemann CG, Modi R, Noguchi S, et al. Beta-sarcoglycan (A3b) mutations cause autosomal recessive muscular dystrophy with loss of the sarcoglycan complex. Nat Genet 1995;11:266.

Bornemann A, Schmalbruch H. Anti-vimentin staining in muscle pathology. Neuropathol Appl Neurobiol 1993;19:414.

Boska MD, Moussavi RS, Carson PJ, et al. The metabolic basis of recovery after fatiguing exercise of human muscle. Neurology 1990;40:240.

Broers JL, Machiels BM, Kuijpers HJ, et al. A- and B-type lamins are differentially expressed in normal human tissues. Histochem Cell Biol 1997;107:505.

Brooks SV. Current topics in skeletal muscle physiology. Adv Physiol Educ 2003;27:171.

Brown LA, McClune JM, Wang HC. Creatine kinase activity following strenuous exercise. JAMA 1982;248:2971.

Buchthal F, Schmalbruch H. Motor unit of mammalian muscle. Physiol Rev 1980;60:90.

Buller AJ, Eccles JC, Eccles RM. Interactions between motor neurons and muscles in respect of the characteristic speeds of their responses. J Physiol 1960;150:417.

Byers TJ, Kunkel LM, Watkins SC. The subcellular distribution of dystrophin in mouse skeletal, cardiac, and smooth muscle. J Cell Biol 1991;115:411.

Cagliani R, Bresolin N, Prelle A, et al. A CAV3 microdeletion differentially affects skeletal muscle and myocardium. Neurology 2003;61(11):1513.

Campbell KP, Kahl SD. Association of dystrophin and an integral membrane glycoprotein. Nature 1989;338:259.

Carbone I, Bruno C, Sotgia F, et al. Mutation in the CAV3 gene causes partial caveolin-3 deficiency and hyperCKemia. Neurology 2000;54:1373.

Chen JC, Goldhamer DJ. Skeletal muscle stem cells. Reprod Biol Endocrinol 2003;13:101.

Chen YW, Zhao P, Borup R, Hoffman EP. Expression profiling in the muscular dystrophies: Identification of novel aspects of molecular pathophysiology. J Cell Biol 2000;151(6):1321.

Clague JE, Roberts N, Gibson H, et al. Muscle imaging in health and disease. Source Neuromusc Disord 1995;5:171.

Cooper JA, Amatruda JF, Hug C, et al. Capping proteins. In: Kreis T, Vale R, eds. Guidebook to the cytoskeletal and motor proteins. New York: Oxford University Press, 1993.

Crawford GE, Gaulkner JA, Crosbie RH, et al. Assembly of the dystrophin-associated protein complex does not require the dystrophin COOH-terminal domain. J Cell Biol 2000;150:1399.

Critchley DR. Alpha-actinins. In: Kreis T, Vale R, eds. Guidebook to the cytoskeletal and motor proteins. New York: Oxford University Press, 1993.

Daube JR. Needle examination in clinical electromyography. Muscle Nerve 1991;14:685.

De Luca C. Control properties of motor units. J Exp Biol 1985;115:125.

De Luca CJ, LeFever RS, McCue MP, et al. Behavior of human motor units in different muscles during linearly varying contractions. J Physiol 1982;329:158.

De Luna N, Gallardo E, Illa I. In vivo and in vitro dysferlin expression in human muscle satellite cells. J Neuropathol Exp Neurol 2004;63(10):1104.

Dubouchaud H, Butterfield GE, Wolfel EE, et al. Endurance training, expression, and physiology of LDH, MCT1 and MCT2 in human skeletal muscle. Am J Physiol Endocrinol Metab 2000;278:E571.

Dubowitz V, Brook MH. Muscle biopsy: A modern approach. Philadelphia: WB Saunders, 1973.

Duggan DJ, Gorospe JR, Fanin M, et al. Mutations in the sarcoglycan genes in patients with myopathy. N Engl J Med 1997;336:618.

Dulakas MC, Park KY, Semino-Mora C, et al. Desmin myopathy, a skeletal myopathy with cardiomyopathy caused by mutations in the desmin gene. N Engl J Med 2003;342:770.

Edgerton VR, Martin TP, Bodine SC, et al. How flexible is the neural control of muscle properties? J Exp Biol 1985;115:393.

Ervasti JM, Campbell KP. Membrane organization of the dystrophin-glycoprotein complex. Cell 1991;66:1121.

Ervasti JM, Ohlendieck K, Kahl SD, et al. Deficiency of a glycoprotein component of the dystrophin complex in dystrophic muscle. Nature 1990;345:315.

Fairley EA, Kendrick-Jones J, Ellis JA. The Emery-Dreifuss muscular dystrophy phenotype arises from aberrant targeting and binding of emerin at the inner nuclear membrane. J Cell Sci 1999;112:2571.

Ferreiro A, Monnier N, Romero NB, et al. A recessive form of central core disease, transiently presenting a multi-minicore disease, is associated with a homozygous mutation in the ryanodine receptor type 1 gene. Ann Neurol 2002;51:750.

Fishbach GD, Rosen KM. ARIA: Neuromuscular junction neuregulin. Annu Rev Neurosci 1997;20:429.

Fishman DA. C-proteins. In: Kreis T, Vale R, eds. Guidebook to the cytoskeletal and motor proteins. New York: Oxford University Press, 1993.

Ford LE, Huxley AF, Simmons EM. Tension responses to sudden length change in stimulated frog muscle fibers near slack length. J Physiol 1977;269:441.

Franzini-Armstrong C. The sarcoplasmic reticulum and the control of muscle contraction. FASEB J 1999;12:S266.

Fuchs E, Weber K. Intermediate filaments: Structure, dynamics, function, and disease. Annu Rev Biochem 1994;63:345.

Galbiati F, Volonte D, Minetti C, et al. Phenotypic behavior of caveolin-3 mutations that cause autosomal dominant limb girdle muscular dystrophy (LGMD-1C). Retention of LGMD-1C caveolin-3 mutants within the Golgi complex. J Biol Chem 1999;274:25632.

Gallanti A, Prelle A, Moggio M, et al. Desmin and vimentin as markers of regeneration in muscle diseases. Acta Neuropathol (Berl) 1992;85:88.

Geisler N, Weber K. The amino acid sequence of chicken muscle desmin provides a common structural model for intermediate filament proteins. EMBO J 1982;1:1649.

Gergeley J, Garbarek Z, Tao T. Troponins. In: Kreis T, Vale R, eds. Guidebook to the cytoskeletal and motor proteins. New York: Oxford University Press, 1993.

Goldfarb LG, Vicart P, Goebel HH, Dalakas MC. Desmin myopathy. Brain 2004;127:723.

Gomes AV, Barnes JA, Harada K, Potter JD. Role of troponin T in disease. Mol Cell Biochem 2004;263(1):115.

Gomes AV, Potter JD, Szczesna-Cordary D. The role of troponins in muscle contraction. IUBMB Life 2002;54:323.

Grabarek Z, Tan RY, Wang T, et al. Inhibition of mutant troponin C activity by an intradomain disulphide bond. Nature 1990;345:132.

Grewal PK, Hewitt JE. Glycosylation defects: A new mechanism for muscular dystrophy? Hum Mol Genet 2003;12:R259.

Gutmann DH, Fischbeck KH. Molecular biology of Duchenne and Becker's muscular dystrophy: Clinical applications. Ann Neurol 1989;26:189.

Haraguchi T, Holaska J, Yamane M, et al. Emerin binding to Btf, a death-promoting transcriptional repressor, is disrupted by a missense mutation that causes Emery-Dreifuss muscular dystrophy. Eur J Biochem 2004;271(5):1035.

Harrington WF, Rodgers ME. Myosin. Annu Rev Biochem 1984;53:35.

Heckmatt J, Dubowitz V. Real time ultrasound imaging of muscle. Muscle Nerve 1988;11:56.

Heckmatt JZ, Moosa A, Hutson C, et al. Diagnostic needle biopsy: A practical and reliable alternative to open biopsy. Arch Dis Child 1984;59:528.

Heeley DH, Dhoot GK, Perry SV. Factors determining the subunit composition of tropomyosin in mammalian skeletal muscle. Biochem J 1985;226:461.

Heizmann C, Rohrenbech J, Kamphuis W. Parvalbumin: Molecular and functional aspects. Adv Exp Med Biol 1990;269:57.

Henneman E. The size-principle: A deterministic output emerges from a set of probabilistic connections. J Exp Biol 1985;115:105.

Henneman E, Clamann JP, Gillies JO, et al. Rank order of motoneurones within a pool: Law of combination. J Neurophysiol 1974;37:1388.

Hennig R, Lomo T. Firing patterns of motor units in normal rats. Nature 1985;314:164.

Hoffman EP, Brown RH, Kunkel LM. Dystrophin: The protein product of the Duchenne muscular dystrophy locus. Cell 1987;51:919.

Horowits R, Maruyama K, Podolsky RJ. Elastic behavior of connecting filaments during thick filament movement in activated skeletal muscle. J Cell Biol 1989;109:2169.

Hui CS. Pharmacological studies of charge movement in frog skeletal muscle. J Physiol 1983;337:509.

Hultman E. Fuel selection of muscle fibre. Proc Nutr Soc 1995;54:107.

Huxley HE. A personal view of muscle and motility mechanisms. Annu Rev Physiol 1996;58:1.

Huxley HE. The mechanism of force production in muscle. In: Schotland DL, ed. Disorders of the motor unit. New York: John Wiley & Sons, 1982.

Ibraghimov-Beskrovnaya O, Ervasti JM, Leveille CJ, et al. Primary structure of dystrophin-associated glycoproteins linking dystrophin to the extracellular matrix. Nature 1992;355:696.

Jones K, Morgan G, Johnston H, et al. The expanding phenotype of laminin alpha 2 (merosin) abnormalities: Case series and review. J Med Genet 2001;38:649.

Juel C. Lactate-proton cotransport in skeletal muscle. Physiol Rev 1997;77:321.

Kaparti G, Pouliot Y, Carpenter S. Expression of immunoreactive major histocompatibility complex products in human skeletal muscles. Ann Neurol 1988;23:64.

Katz B, Miledi R. The statistical nature of the acetylcholine potential and its molecular components. J Physiol 1972;224:665.

Kennelly PJ, Starovasnik M, Krebs EG. Activation of rabbit skeletal light chain kinase by calmodulin. A mechanistic overview. Adv Exp Med Biol 1989;255:155.

Khurana TS, Watkins SC, Chafey P, et al. Immunolocalization and developmental expression of dystrophin related protein in skeletal muscle. Neuromusc Disord 1991;1:185.

Khurana TS, Watkins SC, Kunkel LM. The subcellular distribution of chromosome-6 encoded dystrophin related protein in the brain. J Cell Biol 1992;119:357.

Kimball SR, Farrell PA, Jefferson LS. Invited review: Role of insulin in translational control of protein synthesis in skeletal muscle by amino acids or exercise. J Appl Physiol 2002;93:1168.

Kistler J, Stroud RM, Klymkowsky MW, et al. Structure and function of an acetylcholine receptor. Biophys J 1982;37:371.

Kushmerick MJ. Skeletal muscle: A paradigm for testing principles of bioenergetics. J Bioenerg Biomembr 1995;27:555.

Landon DN. Skeletal muscle: Normal morphology, development, and innervation. In: Mastaglia FL, Walton J, eds. Skeletal muscle pathology. New York: Churchill Livingstone, 1982.

Lapidos KA, Kakkar R, McNally EM, Kass D. The dystrophin glycoprotein complex: Signaling strength and integrity for the sarcolemma. Circ Res 2004;94(8):1023.

Lennmarken C, Bergman T, Larsson J, et al. Skeletal muscle function in man: Force, relation rate, endurance and contraction time-dependence of sex and age. Clin Physiol 1985;5:243.

Lexell J, Henriksson-Larsen K, Winbald B, et al. Distribution of different fiber types in human skeletal muscles: Effects of aging studied in whole muscle cross sections. Muscle Nerve 1983;6:588.

Lieber RC. Skeletal muscle adaptability. I. Review of basic properties. Dev Med Child Neurol 1986;28:390.

Lindstrom JM. Nicotinic acetylcholine receptors of muscles and nerves. Ann N Y Acad Med 2003;998:41.

Liu CG, Maercker C, Castanon MJ, et al. Human plectin: Organization of the gene, sequence analysis, and chromosome localization (8q24). Proc Natl Acad Sci U S A 1996;93:4278.

Liu J, Aoki M, Illa I, et al. Dysferlin, a novel skeletal muscle gene, is mutated in Miyoshi myopathy and limb girdle muscular dystrophy. Nat Genet 1998;20:31.

Loewinger L, McKeon F. Mutations in the nuclear lamin proteins resulting in their aberrant assembly in the cytoplasm. EMBO J 1988;7:2301.

Lutz GJ, Lieber, R. Studies of myosin isoforms in muscle cells: Single cell mechanics and gene transfer. Clin Orthop Relat Res 2002;1(Suppl. 403):S51.

Maniotis AJ, Chen CS, Ingber DE. Demonstration of mechanical connections between integrins, cytoskeletal filaments, and nucleoplasm that stabilize nuclear structure. Proc Natl Acad Sci U S A 1997;94:849.

Martin PT, Freeze H. Glycobiology of neuromuscular disorders. Glycobiology 2003;13(8):67R.

Matlin CA, Delday MI, Siclair DD, et al. Impact of manipulations of myogenesis *in utero* on performance of adult skeletal muscle. Reproduction 2001;122:359.

Matsumura K, Tome FM, Collin H, et al. Deficiency of the 50K dystrophin-associated glycoprotein in severe childhood autosomal recessive muscular dystrophy. Nature 1992;359:320.

McComas AJ. Motor unit estimation: Methods, results and present studies. Muscle Nerve 1991;14:585.

McLennon IS. Neurogenic and myogenic regulation of skeletal muscle formation: A critical re-evaluation. Prog Neurobiol 1994;44:119.

Miles TS. The control of human motor units. Clin Exp Pharmacol Physiol 1994;21:511.

Michele DE, Campbell KP. Dystrophin-glycoprotein complex post-translational processing and dystroglycan function. J Biol Chem 2003;278:15457.

Momoi MY, Lennon VA. Purification and biochemical characterization of nicotinic acetylcholine receptors of human muscle. J Biol Chem 1982;257:12757.

Moreira ES, Wiltshire TJ, Faulkner G, et al. Limb-girdle muscular dystrophy type 2G is caused by mutations in the gene encoding the sarcomeric protein telethonin. Nat Genet 2000;24:163.

Nawrotzki R, Blake DJ, Davies KE. The genetic basis of neuromuscular disorders. Trends Genet 1996;12:294.

Newsome-Davis J. Lambert-Eaton syndrome. Rev Neurol (Paris) 2004;160:177.

Newsome-Davis J, Buckley C, Clover L, et al. Autoimmune disorders of the neuronal potassium channels. Ann N Y Acad Sci 2003;998:2001.

Norregaard-Hansen K, Hein-Sorensen O. Significance of serum myoglobin in neuromuscular diseases and carrier detection of Duchenne muscular dystrophy. Acta Neurol Scand 1982;66:259.

Nowak KJ, Wattanasarichaigoon D, Goebel HH, et al. Mutations in the skeletal muscle alpha-actin gene in patients with actin and nemalin myopathy. Nat Genet 1999;23:208.

Omary MB, Coulombe PA, McLean WHI. Intermediate filament proteins and their associated diseases. N Engl J Med 2004;351:2087.

Peachey LD. Excitation-contraction coupling: The link between the surface and the interior of a muscle cell. J Exp Biol 1985;115:91.

Pelin K, Hilpelä P, Donner K, et al. Mutations in the nebulin gene associated with autosomal recessive nemaline myopathy. Proc Natl Acad Sci U S A 1999;96:2305.

Petajan JH. Motor unit recruitment. Muscle Nerve 1991;14:489.

Pette D. Historical perspectives: Plasticity of mammalian skeletal muscle. J Appl Physiol 2001;90:1119.

Pette D, Heilig A, Klug G, et al. Alterations of phenotype expression of muscle by chronic nerve stimulation. Adv Exp Med Biol 1985;182:169.

Pette D, Vrborá G. Neural control of phenotypic expression in mammalian muscle fibers. Muscle Nerve 1985;8:676.

Philpot J, Sewry C, Pennock J, et al. Clinical phenotype in congenital muscular dystrophy: Correlation with expression of merosin in skeletal muscle. Neuromusc Disord 1995;5:301.

Pillers DAH, Fitzgerald KM, Duncan NM, et al. Duchenne/Becker muscular dystrophy: Correlation of phenotype by electroretinography with sites of dystrophin mutations. Hum Genet 1999;105:2.

Pollack GH. Phase transitions and the molecular mechanism of contraction. Biophys Chem 1996;59:315.

Pollack GH, Sugi H. Contractile mechanisms in muscle. New York: Plenum Press, 1984.

Pollard TD. Actin and actin binding proteins. In: Kreis T, Vale R, eds. Guidebook to the cytoskeletal and motor proteins. New York: Oxford University Press, 1993.

Pons F, Augier N, Heilig R, et al. Isolated dystrophin molecules as seen by electron microscopy. Proc Natl Acad Sci U S A 1990;87:7851.

Porter GA, Dmytrenko GM, Winkelmann JC, et al. Dystrophin colocalizes with beta-spectrin in distinct subsarcolemmal domains in mammalian skeletal muscle. J Cell Biol 1992;117:997.

Pownall ME, Gustafsson MK, Emerson CP, Jr. Myogenic regulatory factors and specific progenitors in vertebrate embryos. Annu Rev Cell Dev Biol 2002;18:747.

Rizo J, Sudhof TC. C2-domains, structure and function of a universal Ca2+-binding domain. J Biol Chem 1998;273:15879.

Ruff RL. Neurophysiology of the neuromuscular junction. Ann N Y Acad Sci 2003;998:1.

Samitt CE, Bonilla E. Immunocytochemical study of dystrophin at the myotendinous junction. Muscle Nerve 1990;13:493.

Sander M, Chavoshan B, Harris SA, et al. Functional muscle ischemia in neuronal nitric oxide synthase-deficient skeletal muscle of children

with Duchenne muscular dystrophy. Proc Natl Acad Sci U S A 2000;97:13818.
Sanders DB, Stalberg EV, Nandedkar SD. Analysis of the electromyographic interference pattern. J Clin Neurophysiol 1996;13:385.
Sanger JW, Sanger JM. Fishing out the proteins that bind to titin. J Cell Biol 2001;154:21.
Scacheri PC, Hoffman EP, Fratkini JD, et al. A novel ryanodine receptor gene mutation causing both cores and rods in congenital myopathy. Neurology 2000;55:1689.
Scalzi HA, Price HM. Electron microscopic observations of the sensory region of the mammalian muscle spindle. In: Banker BQ, Przybylski RJ, van der Meulen JP, et al., eds. Research in muscle development and the spindle. Amsterdam: Excerpta Medica, 1972.
Schnorrer F, Dickson BJ. Muscle building: Mechanisms of myotube guidance and attachment site selection. Dev Cell 2004;7:9.
Schroder JM, Bodden H, Hamacher A, et al. Scanning electron microscopy of teased intrafusal muscle fibers from rat muscle spindle. Muscle Nerve 1989;12:221.
Schultz E. Satellite cells in normal, regenerating and dystrophic muscle. Adv Exp Med Biol 1985;182:73.
Shahani BT, Young RR. Clinical electromyography. In: Baker AB, Joyut RJ, eds. Clinical neurology. Philadelphia: Harper & Row, 1985.
Sherratt TG, Vulliamy T, Strong PN. Evolutionary conservation of the dystrophin central rod domain. Biochem J 1992;287:755.
Sjoberg G, Jiang W-Q, Ringertz NR, et al. Colocalization of nestin and vimentin/desmin in skeletal muscle cells demonstrated by three-dimensional fluorescence digital imaging microscopy. Exp Cell Res 1994;214:447.
Skeie GO, Romi F, Aarli JA, et al. Pathogenesis of myositis and myasthenia associated with titin and ryanodine receptor antibodies. Ann NY Acad Sci 2003;998:343.
Slonim AE, Coleman RA, McElligot MA, et al. Improvement of muscle function in acid maltase deficiency by high protein therapy. Neurology 1983;33:34.
Smillie LB. Tropomyosins. In: Kreis T, Vale R, eds. Guidebook to the cytoskeletal and motor proteins. New York: Oxford University Press, 1993.
Somlyo AV, Gonzalez-Serratos H, Shuman H, et al. Calcium release and ionic changes in the sarcoplasmic reticulum of tetanized muscle: An electron probe study. J Cell Biol 1981;90:577.
Sorimachi H, Ono Y, Suzuki K. Skeletal muscle-specific calpain, p94, and connectin/titin: Their physiologic functions and relationship to limb-girdle muscular dystrophy type 2A. Adv Exp Mol Biol 2000;481:383.
Stadhouders AM. The structural basis of excitation-contraction coupling in muscular contraction. Acta Anaesth Belg 1990;41:65.
Steinbock FA, Wiche G. Role of plectin in cytoskeleton organization and dynamics. J Cell Sci 1999;380:151.
Stonecipher MR, Jorizzo JL, Monu J, et al. Dermatomyositis with normal muscle enzyme concentrations. A single-blind study of the diagnostic value of magnetic resonance imaging and ultrasound. Arch Dermatol 1994;130:1294.
Straub V, Campbell KP. Muscular dystrophies and the dystrophin-glycoprotein complex. Curr Opin Neurol 1997;10:168.
Stuart DG, Mosher CG, Gerlach RL. Properties and central connections of Golgi tendon organs with special reference to locomotion. In: Banker BQ, Przybylski RJ, van der Meulen JP, et al., eds. Research in muscle development and the spindle. Amsterdam: Excerpta Medica, 1972.
Sussman MA, Bilak M, Kedes L, et al. Tropomodulin is highly concentrated at the postsynaptic domain of human and rat neuromuscular junctions. Exp Cell 1993;209:388.
Suzuki A, Yoshida M, Yamamoto H, et al. Glycoprotein-binding site of dystrophin is confined to the cysteine-rich domain and the first half of the carboxy-terminal domain. FEBS Lett 1992;308:154.
Takahashi T, et al. Dysferlin mutations in Japanese Miyoshi myopathy: Relationship to phenotype. Neurology 2003;60(11):1799.
Taylor RJ, Von Witt RJ, Fry AH. Serum creatine phosphokinase activity in psychiatric patients receiving electroconvulsive therapy. J Clin Psychiatr 1981;42:103.
Thornell LE, Billeter R, Butler-Browne GS, et al. Development of fiber types in human fetal muscle. J Neurol Sci 1984;66:107.
Tidball JC. Desmin at myotendinous junctions. Exp Cell Res 1992;199:341.
Tskhovrebova L, Trinick J. Titin: Properties and family relationships. Nat Rev Mol Cell Biol 2003;4:679.
Vainzof M, Zatz M. Protein defects in neuromuscular diseases. Braz J Med Biol Res 2003;36:543:555.
Vale RD, Milligan RA. The way things move: Looking under the hood of molecular motor proteins. Science 2000;288:88.
van der Kooi AJ, Bonne G, Eymard B, et al. Lamin A/C mutations with lipodystrophy, cardiac abnormalities, and muscular dystrophy. Neurology 2002;59:620.
van der Meulen JP, Hellekson CJ, Hinnas RW. The central control of the muscle spindle. In: Banker BQ, Przybylski RJ, van der Meulen JP, et al., eds. Research in muscle development and the spindle. Amsterdam: Excerpta Medica, 1972.
Viegas-Pequignot E, Li ZL, Dutrillaux B, et al. Assignment of human desmin gene to band 2q35 by nonradioactive in site hybridization. Hum Genet 1989;83:33.
Vogler C, Bove KE. Morphology of skeletal muscle in children. Arch Pathol Lab Med 1985;109:238.
Vuolteenaho R, Nissinen M, Sainio K, et al. Human laminin M chain (merosin): Complete primary structure, chromosomal assignment, and expression of the M and A chain in human fetal tissues. J Cell Biol 1994;124:381.
Wallgren-Pettersson C. Nemaline and myotubular myopathies. Semin Pediatr Neurol 2002;9:132.
Wallgren-Pettersson C, Clarke A, Samson F, et al. The myotubular myopathies: Differential diagnosis of the X linked recessive, autosomal dominant, and autosomal recessive forms and present state of DNA studies. J Med Genet 1995;32:673.
Wang K. Nebulin. In: Kreis T, Vale R, eds. Guidebook to the cytoskeletal and motor proteins. New York: Oxford University Press, 1993.
Watkins SC, Cullen MJ, Hoffman EP, Billington L. Plasma membrane cytoskeleton of muscle: A fine structural analysis. Microsc Res Tech 2000;48:131.
Weiner MW, Moussavi RS, Baker AJ, et al. Constant relationship between force phosphate concentration, and pH in muscles with differential fatigability. Neurology 1990;40:1888.
Westwood SA, Hudlicka O, Perry SV. The effect of contractile activity on the phosphorylation of the P light chain of myosin of rabbit skeletal muscle. Biochem J 1984;218:841.
Whalen RG. Myosin isoenzymes as molecular markers for muscle physiology. J Exp Biol 1985;115:43.
Whiche G. Role of plectin in cytoskeletal organization and dynamics. J Cell Sci 1998;111:247.
Wilbourn AJ. The electrodiagnostic examination with myopathies. J Clin Neurophysiol 1993;10:132.
Wolfe RR. Regulation of muscle protein by amino acids. J Nutr 2002;132:3219S.
Worton R. Muscular dystrophies: Diseases of the dystrophin glycoprotein complex. Science 1995;270:755.
Wyatt RM, Balice-Gordon RJ. Activity-dependent elimination of neuromuscular synapses. J Neurocytol 2003;32:777.
Wyllie E, Leuders H, Pippenger C, et al. Postictal serum creatine kinase in the diagnosis of seizure disorders. Arch Neurol 1985;42:123.
Yamamoto H, Mizuno Y, Hayashi K, et al. Expression of dystrophin-associated protein 35DAG (A4) and 50DAG (A2) is confined to striated muscles. J Biochem 1994;115:162.
Yamamoto L, Gollop T, Naccache N, et al. Protein and DNA analysis for the prenatal diagnosis of [alpha]2-laminin-deficient congenital muscular dystrophy. Diagn Mol Pathol 2004;13(3):167.
Yasunaga S, Grati M, Chardenoux S, et al. OTOF encodes multiple long and short isoforms: Genetic evidence that the long ones underlie recessive deafness DFNB9. Am J Hum Genet 2000;67:591.
Younger DS, Gordon PH. Diagnosis in neuromuscular diseases. Neurol Clin 1996;14:135.
Zhang Y, Chen HS, Khanna VK, et al. A mutation in the human ryanodine receptor gene associated with central core disease. Nat Genet 1993;5:46.

CHAPTER 75

Anterior Horn Cell and Cranial Motor Neuron Disease

Anne M. Connolly and Susan T. Iannaccone

Anterior horn cells (a motor neurons), located in the anterior gray masses of the cord, are found at every cord segment and are concentrated in the cervical and lumbosacral enlargements. Morphologic differentiation of the anterior horn cells is most evident from 12 to 14 weeks' gestation [Vassilopoulos and Emery, 1977]. There is a period of normal differentiation followed by programmed cell death [Fidzianska and Rafalowska, 2002; Yachnis et al., 1998] Anterior horn cells are clustered into medial and lateral cell divisions (Fig. 75-1). The medial group is subdivided into ventromedial and dorsomedial components. The ventromedial component innervates the superficial larger muscles, and the dorsomedial component innervates the small, deep muscles adjacent to the spine.

The lateral cell mass is also subdivided into groups. The ventrolateral group innervates extensor muscles, and the centrodorsal group innervates flexor muscles [Romanes, 1951]. Because these groups of neurons are located in a relatively small region, deleterious influences harm cells from more than one group, and weakness may be widespread.

The motor neurons in the nuclei of the cranial nerves are homologous to spinal cord anterior horn cells. Therefore, pathologic mechanisms that compromise the cranial motor neurons may initiate symptoms and signs that mimic anterior horn cell dysfunction. Atrophy, severe weakness, and fasciculations without sensory deficit are signs of anterior horn cell disease. When sensory function is impaired in conjunction with anterior horn cell disease, dysfunction of adjacent tracts of the spinal cord or the peripheral nerves must be present.

CONGENITAL DEFECTS

Diastematomyelia

Diastematomyelia is an abnormal division of the spinal cord, usually almost equally, by a septum of variable caudal-rostral length (Fig. 75-2). The mesodermal septum is composed of fibrous tissue, bone, cartilage, or a mixture of these. The septum traverses the neural canal, thus splitting the spinal cord, and is usually anchored posteriorly on the dura or bony neural arch [Moes and Hendrick, 1963]. The neural tube forms a closed cavity when normal maturation occurs during the first fetal month. The tube becomes distended, the dorsal surface (roof) becomes permeable, and fluid flows into the adjacent space; this space develops into the subarachnoid space. The point of failure of the developmental process that results in diastematomyelia is still not completely understood.

Surgical manipulation of the chick embryo shows it is possible to produce a chick with diastematomyelia by intraspinal grafting of a somite. Transplanted quail cells may form a septum between the dorsal surface (roof) and floor, dividing the neural tube into two parts. However, in some chicks, the same experiment leads to the chick host eliminating quail cells, and in some, spina bifida is produced. This finding suggests that spontaneous diastematomyelia may be the consequence of abnormal gastrulation, the process by which the two early germ layers convert to three distinctive germ layers [Klessinger and Christ, 1996].

When diastematomyelia is present, the mesodermal septum commonly compromises the anterior horn cell column and subsequently causes muscle atrophy, decreased or absent deep tendon reflexes, and moderate-to-severe weakness of the distal muscles of the legs and feet. This weakness is often the patient's first complaint. Involvement is usually bilateral. Deformities of the feet, particularly talipes equinovarus, commonly occur. Atonic bladder with urinary retention or incontinence may occur. Cutaneous lesions over the spine often accompany the condition; these lesions include sacrococcygeal sinus, lipoma, hypertrichosis, soft tissue swelling, myelomeningocele, and pigmented nevi or hemangiomas over the lower spine [James and Lassman, 1964].

Because of its location, the septum transects nerve fibers as they cross from one side of the spinal cord to the other. These fibers transmit pain and temperature sensations. Therefore, pain and temperature perception may be impaired. Superficial sensation (light touch) may also be affected. When the septum is wide enough or laterally placed, corticospinal tract compromise may be evidenced by upper motor unit symptoms and signs.

Radiography, computed tomography (CT), or magnetic resonance imaging (MRI) usually demonstrates the septum; the deposition of calcium, which may be delayed for years, facilitates identification [Bruhl et al., 1990; Harwood-Nash and McHugh, 1990; Thron and Schroth, 1986]. More recently, diastematomyelia has been diagnosed prenatally with ultrasound and MRI (Fig. 75-3), allowing earlier intervention [Allen and Silverman, 2000; Sonigo-Cohen et al., 2003]. The septum is usually located in the lower thoracic and lumbar areas but may be present as high as the cervical vertebra [Balci et al., 2002; Cowie, 1951] One patient with involvement of the basicranium has been described [Pfeifer, 1991]. Spina bifida occulta or tethered cord may be associated [Guthkelch and Hoffmann, 1981]. Kyphoscoliosis or scoliosis may accompany the other characteristic findings. Intersegmental laminar fusion occurring with spina bifida at or adjacent to the level of fusion should suggest the diagnosis of diastematomyelia [Hilal et al., 1974]. Diastematomyelia has been associated with

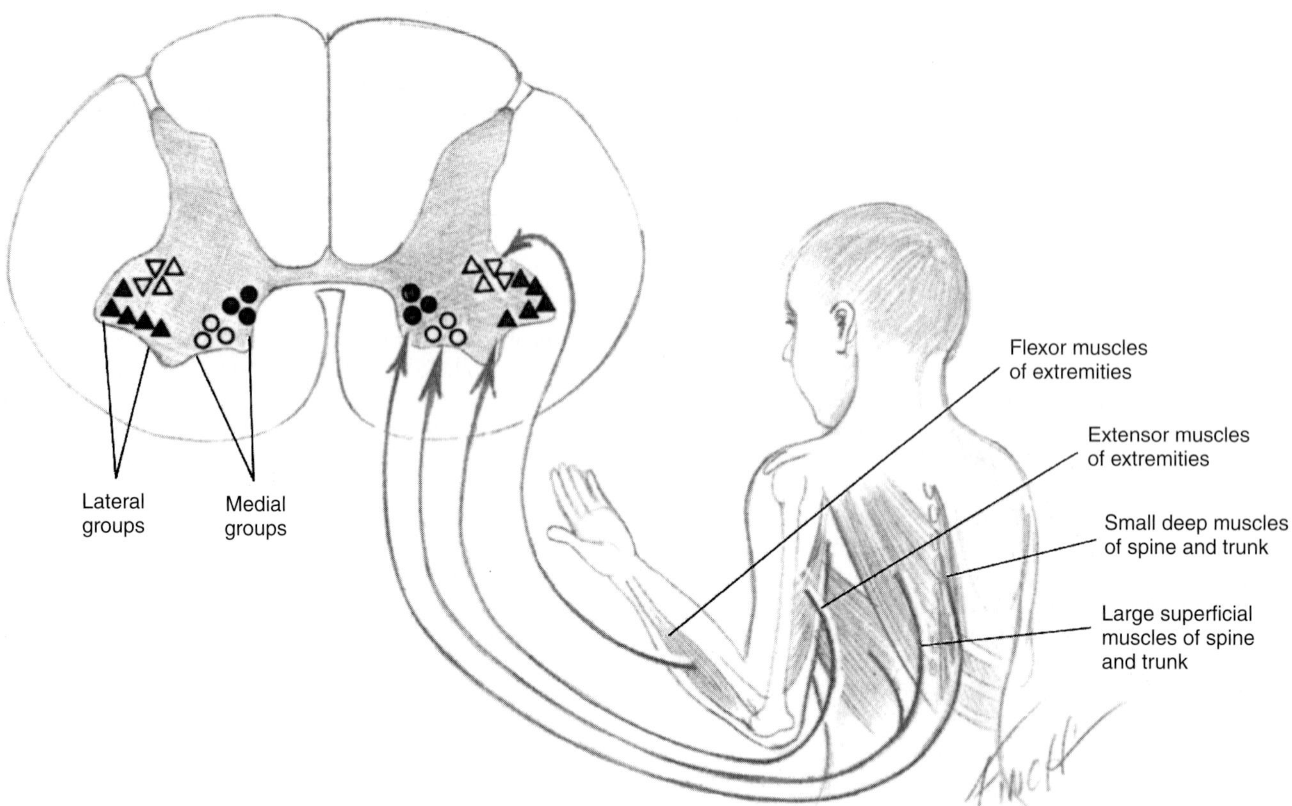

FIGURE 75-1. The a motor neurons located in the anterior horn of the spinal cord (anterior horn cells) are clustered in a specific pattern. The medial cell groups are associated with muscles of the spine and trunk. The lateral cell groups are associated with muscles of the extremities.

epidermoid cysts and syrinx [Sheehan et al., 2002] or teratoma [Hader et al., 1999]. Because these may not occur at the same level, imaging of all levels is indicated.

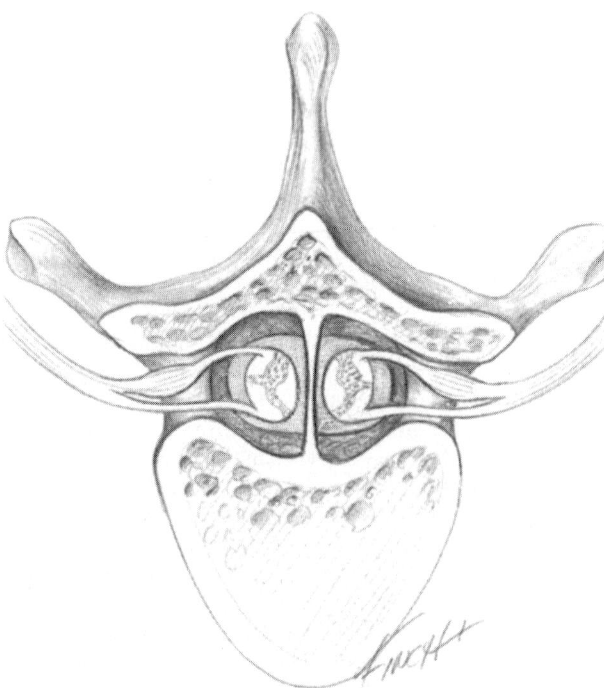

FIGURE 75-2. The spinal cord is cleaved by a central or paracentral mesodermal septum. The cord is usually separated asymmetrically. The mesodermal septum may become calcified and thus readily identifiable with radiographic techniques.

Symptoms, particularly pain, may be prevented or significantly ameliorated by surgery [Kim et al., 1994; Meacham, 1967; Schijman, 2003]. Clinical and radiographic correlations suggest three subsets of patients with diastematomyelia: those with associated tethered cord, those with midline cutaneous stigmata, and those with meningocele or meningomyelocele [Schijman, 2003]. Excision of the mesodermal septum, including all portions attached to the anterior dural surface, and subsequent laminectomy are indicated in all but those with very severe associated meningomyelocele. Neurologic deficits may remain [Kim et al., 1994]. Failure to remove the septum almost always results in scoliosis.

Syringomyelia

Syringomyelia is a slowly progressive cavity formation within the spinal cord, medulla oblongata, or both that is associated with gliosis. When the medulla is involved, the condition is called *syringobulbia.* Cavity formation usually occurs in the cervical and lumbar cord segments. On cross-section, the destruction occurs in the area of the anterior white commissure, interrupting crossing fibers of the lateral spinothalamic tracts, with resultant bilateral loss of temperature and pain sensation (Fig. 75-4). Superficial sensation is normal because fiber tracts associated with this function are located dorsally and do not cross the cord. Dissociation of sensation occurs when there is concurrent preservation of light touch perception and decrease or absence of pain and temperature perception. The anterior horn cells are affected only after the lesion has reached significant proportions.

Although the lesion is virtually always bilateral, involvement is usually asymmetric early in the course of the dis-

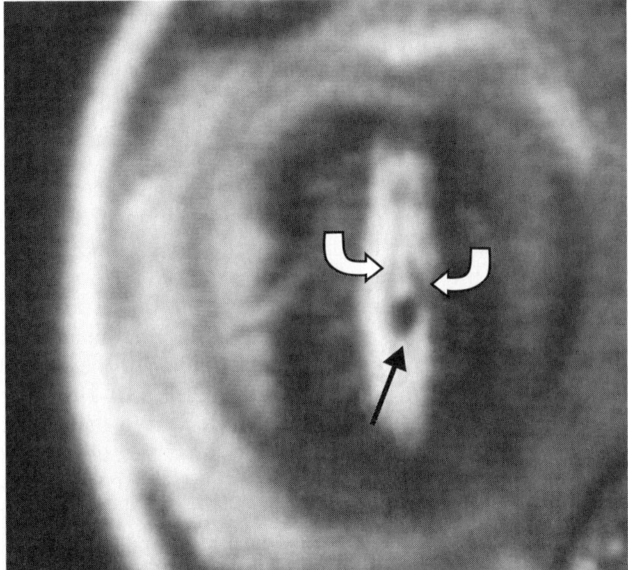

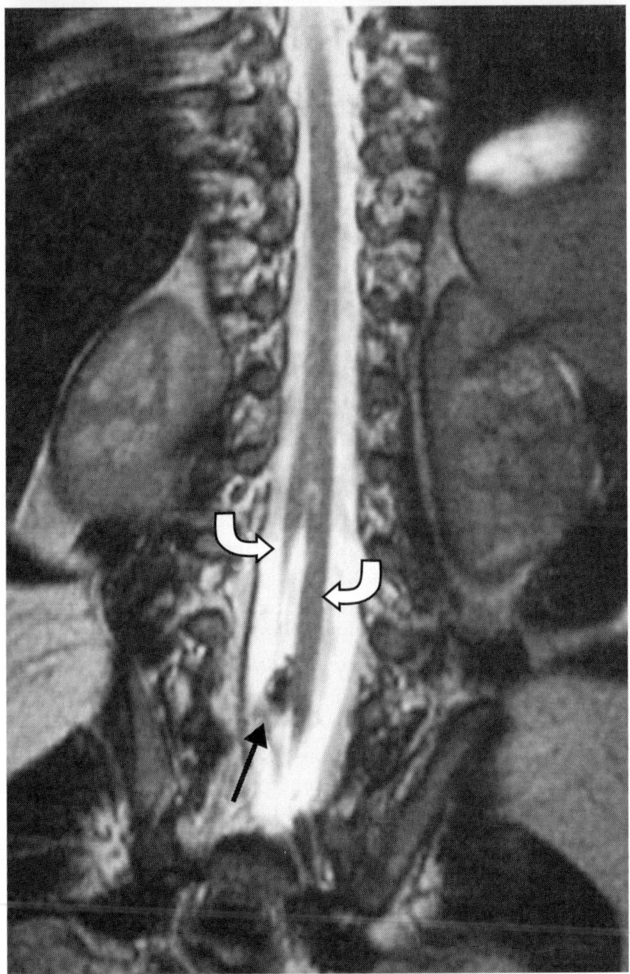

FIGURE 75-3. Coronal T2-weighted fetal magnetic resonance images (**A**) 26 weeks' gestation and (**B**) 3 months of age show the subdivision into two asymmetric cords (*white arrows*) and the hyposignal bony spur (*black arrows*) at the level of the diastematomyelia.

ease. The long tracts, including the corticospinal tracts, are not affected until after the cavitary lesion has become very large. Involvement of the sympathetic nervous system neurons in the cervical cord may cause Horner's syndrome.

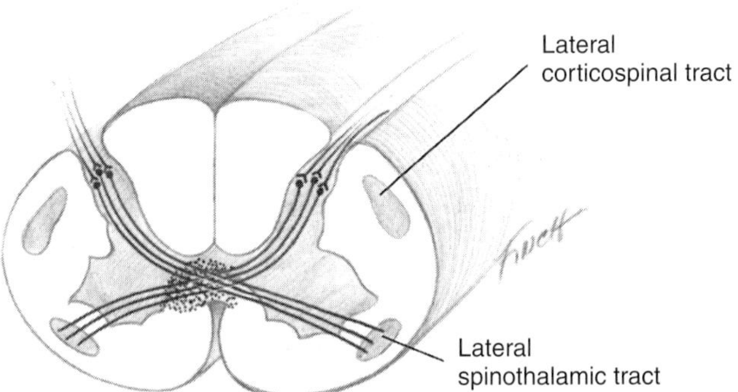

FIGURE 75-4. The anterior white commissure is often compromised in syringomyelia. Severing the crossing fibers from the lateral spinothalamic tracts results in bilateral loss of pain and temperature sensation. Enlargement of the lesion often leads to disruption of the anterior horns.

Chiari I malformations are often accompanied by syringomyelia or hydromyelia [Gillespie et al., 1986; Inoue et al., 2003; Isu et al., 1990, 1992]. The association of Chiari I malformation with syringomyelia is poorly understood [Gillespie et al., 1986; Iqbal et al., 1992]. In one set of monozygotic twins, both had syringomyelia, but they were discordant for Chiari I malformation [Tubbs et al., 2004]. Other congenital structural abnormalities, including basilar impression, Klippel-Feil syndrome, cervical ribs, and scoliosis, may be associated with syringomyelia [Berke and Magee, 1976; Isu et al., 1990, 1992; Jaeger et al., 1997].

The earliest clinical presentation of syringomyelia may be isolated congenital scoliosis or kyphosis. MRI studies of these infants indicate that 31% have spinal cord abnormalities, including syringomyelia (3 of 41), diastematomyelia (5 of 41), and tethered cord (12 of 41) [Suh et al., 2001].

Incomplete closure of the neural tube during the fourth week of gestation is the likely cause of congenital syringomyelia. The normal pattern of cell differentiation causes an inner clustering of spongioblastic cells, which subsequently form glial tissue, and an outer clustering of neuroblastic cells, which subsequently form neurons and their processes. Congenital syringomyelia may result from delayed differentiation of the spongioblastic cells, with ensuing cavitation and gliosis [Leyden, 1876].

Another theory cites a possible congenital structural defect of the hindbrain reminiscent of the one that leads to myelomeningocele and the Chiari deformity. Gardner reported many instances in which the foramen of Magendie was sealed by a membrane [Gardner, 1960]. Clear fluid appeared to accumulate between the syrinx and the fourth ventricle. Failure of the foramen to form an adequate passageway for the fluid during gestation may cause distention of the syrinx and fourth ventricle. Although these findings occasionally may reflect hydromyelia, it is more likely that the pathophysiologic defect is an abnormal intramedullary vascular pattern. The vessels appear to be susceptible to occlusion; thus, infarction or hemorrhage is likely to occur and cause cavitation [Netsky, 1953]. This vascular compromise may come as a result of intermittent compression from increased pressure [Levine, 2004].

Another explanation for syringomyelia evolved from a questionnaire designed to determine whether a high number of mothers of patients with syringomyelia had experienced difficult labor [Williams, 1977]. An unexpectedly high number of patients had undergone forceps delivery. The number of instances in which the patient with syringomyelia was the firstborn was also significantly increased. It was suggested that, as a result of birth injury, the tonsils descend through the foramen magnum and cause arachnoiditis. This mechanism may only be relevant for infants who already have a Chiari malformation [Newman et al., 1981]. The difference in fluid pressure between cranial and spinal compartments may lead to ongoing insidious descent of the tonsils, resulting in communicating syringomyelia.

Recent animal models to study syringomyelia have focused on post-traumatic models. These models have very high syrinx formations when an excitotoxic agent is added to the traumatic injury. In the rat model, fluid enters the syrinx from the subarachnoid space through perivascular spaces. There is more flow in the perivascular spaces at the levels of the syrinx [Brodbelt et al., 2003a, 2003b, 2003c; Yang et al., 2001a].

Patients with syringomyelia have limited abilities to monitor pain and temperature. Trophic ulcers of the fingers are often present. Weakness of the limbs is often profound because the cervical and lumbosacral enlargements bear the brunt of the cavitation and gliosis. Muscle atrophy is often first appreciated in the distal small hand muscles. Deep tendon reflexes are either difficult to elicit or absent. Fasciculations are visible in muscles of the shoulder, elbow, and hip. Cervical syringomyelia has been accompanied by papilledema. Elevated intracranial pressure may be present and results from hydrocephalus, mass lesions, or obstruction of the foramina of Luschka and Magendie [Alpers and Comroe, 1931]. Rarely, syringomyelia may be acquired from tumors or infections of the spinal cord. These acquired types are unusual in infants and young children. Trauma may be a more common cause of acquired syringomyelia in older children and adults [Schurch et al., 1996; Silver, 2001].

Intramedullary cord tumors may cause signs and symptoms similar to those of syringomyelia and prove confounding [Gillespie et al., 1986; Madsen and Scott, 1993; Williams and Timperley, 1977]. Differentiation between syringomyelia and intramedullary tumors should be possible with modern imaging techniques.

Spinal fluid dynamics and constituents are usually normal in syringomyelia, although the fluid may be xanthochromic, and flow may be obstructed. The Valsalva maneuver, which accompanies coughing, straining, and postural changes, may increase pressure and grossly exaggerate findings associated with cysts in the cord. The transient increased pressure may enhance the formation of syringomyelia and syringobulbia [Bertrand, 1973; Levine, 2004].

MRI appears to be the most sensitive method in the detection of syringomyelia [Gillespie et al., 1986; Iqbal et al., 1992]. Management of syringomyelia accompanied by Chiari I malformation consists of posterior fossa decompression, which is beneficial in almost 75% of such patients [Vaquero et al., 1990].

Hydromyelia

Hydromyelia is a congenital deformity resulting from distention of the central canal, which in turn compresses the surrounding cord structures, including the anterior horn cells. The clinical findings are similar to those in syringomyelia. Hydromyelia or syringomyelia is found in more than 50% of patients with Chiari I malformations [Menezes, 1991]. Hydromyelia is found most frequently in the cervical and lumbar cord enlargements. The pathologic distention may involve the cord throughout its entire length. The hydromyelic cavity is lined with ependymal cells, in contrast to the glial cell lining of the syrinx [Levine, 2004].

Although the cause of hydromyelia is unknown, its association with Chiari I malformation is well established [Wisoff, 1988]. The lack of patency in the foramina of the fourth ventricle may underlie the distention of the central canal [Gardner, 1965; Lassman et al., 1968]. However, cerebrospinal fluid protein content differs from that of the hydromyelic segment, and the measured pressure in the syrinx is higher than that of cerebrospinal fluid at rest. As with syringomyelia, erect position, cough, or strain may transiently elevate the cerebrospinal fluid pressure, causing an increase in fluid in the syrinx [Levine, 2004]. Hydromyelia develops in about one fourth of patients with post-traumatic cord injuries and is more likely to develop if there is more than 14 degrees of kyphosis or more than 25% stenosis [Abel et al., 1999]. Current therapeutic approaches in patients with Chiari I malformations are similar to those used in patients with syringomyelia and include posterior fossa decompression with or without duraplasty [Munshi et al., 2000].

SPINAL MUSCULAR ATROPHIES

The history of the spinal muscular atrophies began in the 1890s when Guido Werdnig, a retired battalion physician who was working at the Institute of Anatomy and Physiology of the Central Nervous System at the University of Vienna, gave a lecture entitled "On a Case of Muscular Dystrophy with Positive Spinal Cord Findings" [Groger, 1990]. In 1891, he published the paper entitled "Two Early Infantile Hereditary Cases of Progressive Muscular Atrophy Appearing as Dystrophy, but on a Neurotic Basis." The next year, Professor Johann Hoffmann of Heidelberg University coined the term *spinal muscular atrophy*, in German *spinale muskelatrophie* [Hoffmann, 1892a]. Together, their papers presented a complete picture of the clinical and pathologic aspects of infantile spinal muscular atrophies: onset during the first year of life, occurrence in siblings with normal parents, progressive floppiness and weakness, hand tremor, and death from pneumonia in early childhood. Moreover, Hoffmann talked about "progressive" and chronic ("*chronische*") types of spinal muscular atrophies [Hoffmann, 1892a, 1892b, 1896]. In the tradition of German neurology of the late 19th century, both conducted postmortem examinations on their patients and described the striking atrophy of the ventral roots on gross examination. They correlated this finding with the histologic appearance of the anterior horns, which were lacking in the usual number of motor neurons, and with a pattern of atrophy in muscle fibers [Iannaccone et al., 1990].

For the next 50 years, confusion reigned in the nosology of spinal muscular atrophies. Some of this confusion stemmed from the teaching of Hermann Oppenheim, an influential neurologist at the turn of the 20th century [Iannaccone et al., 1990]. In 1900, he published a paper in German "... und Localisierte Atonie der Muskulatur [Myatonie] ..." that was translated into English unfortunately as "amyotonia" [Oppenheim, 1900]. His patients most likely had spinal muscular atrophies, but he claimed that some of them improved with time, unlike the patients of Hoffmann and Werdnig [Greenfield and Stern, 1928]. During the first part of the 20th century, then, many floppy infants were labeled with *amyotonia congenita* or *Oppenheim's amyotonia,* when specific diagnostic tests, such as electromyography or biopsy, were unavailable for clarification. With the birth of myology as a subspecialty of neurology in the 1950s, muscle biopsy came into widespread use, and it became apparent that not all floppy infants had the same disease. Only then did discussion begin about whether all congenital disease of the anterior horn cell should be called *spinal muscular atrophies*.

Beginning with Byers and Banker, the classification of spinal muscular atrophies according to severity was used to facilitate prognostication [Byers and Banker, 1961]. The relationship between age of onset and severity was supported by Dubowitz's observations [Dubowitz, 1964]. As a result of international collaboration [Dubowitz, 1995; Munsat, 1991b], most pediatric neurologists now use the following nomenclature: *spinal muscular atrophy type I,* for onset of symptoms before age 6 months; *spinal muscular atrophy type II,* for onset between 6 and 18 months; and *spinal muscular atrophy type III,* for onset after age 18 months (Table 75-1). The three types may be subdivided on the basis of mortality or highest motor milestone achieved. For example, patients with type I spinal muscular atrophy are almost never able to sit without support [Iannaccone et al., 1993]. In fact, most patients with spinal muscular atrophy of any type can never pull themselves to sitting position or roll over at any age. Patients with type I spinal muscular atrophy and onset before 3 months of age have the highest mortality rate (90%), whereas those with onset after age 3 months may survive to adulthood, albeit with severe motor handicap. Patients with type III spinal muscular atrophy often are independently ambulatory at least for part of their life and often have a normal life expectancy [Russman et al., 1992]. On the other hand, the distribution of the three types is such that most spinal muscular atrophy patients have type I, with decreasing incidence for types II and III, respectively. In other words, the incidence is highest for type I, followed by type II; type III has the lowest incidence. Considering the relative mortality rates, it is not surprising that the highest prevalence is for spinal muscular atrophies types II and III.

Spinal Muscular Atrophy Type I

Synonyms for spinal muscular atrophy type I are *infantile onset spinal muscular atrophy* and *Werdnig-Hoffmann disease*. Spinal muscular atrophy type I is the most severe form of the disease, beginning at birth or in the first few months of life and frequently resulting in death from respiratory failure before 2 years of age. These infants have severe weakness of the limbs and intercostal muscles. There is a paucity of spontaneous movement at the shoulder and

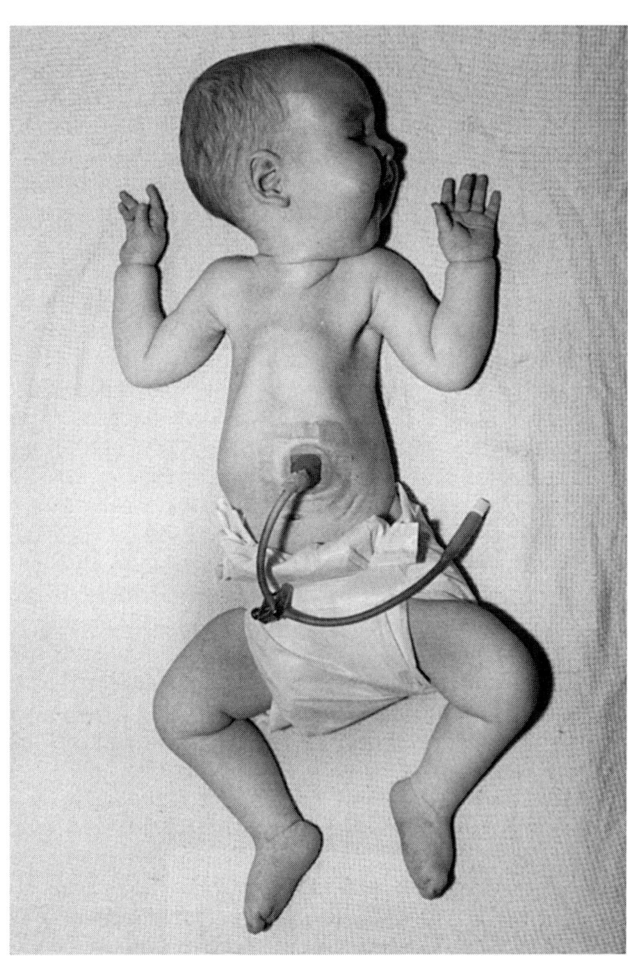

FIGURE 75-5. This patient with spinal muscular atrophy type I, or Werdnig-Hoffmann disease, is severely affected and required a gastric feeding tube. There is little or no movement of the shoulders, whereas the fingers and toes remain active. The typical posture of flexion of the knees and abduction of the legs at the hips is evident. The weakness of the intercostal muscles, coupled with relatively normal diaphragmatic contractions, results in marked chest deformity.

TABLE 75-1

Clinical Features of Spinal Muscular Atrophy (SMA) Linked to the *SMN* Gene

SMA TYPE	ONSET OF WEAKNESS	HIGHEST FUNCTION	MORTALITY
SMA I	<6 mo	Most nonsitters; few sitters	>90%; few survive to second decade
SMA II	6–18 mo	Most sitters; few walkers	Variable; most survive to second or third decade
SMA III	18 mo	Many walkers	Many with normal life expectancy

hip girdle. In contrast, there is some antigravity movement in the hands and feet (Fig. 75-5). The only spontaneous movement of the extremities may be that of the fingers and toes. Frequently, hand movement is characterized by a fine tremor called *polyminimyoclonus.* Often the infant assumes a frog-leg position, with the legs externally rotated, abducted, and flexed at the hips and knees. Typically, slight elbow flexion occurs, and the hands are held at chest level. There is often a narrowed thorax with a pectus excavatum deformity and flaring of the lower ribs (bell-shaped chest). These deformities are caused by weak intercostal muscles countered by diaphragmatic muscle contraction. Affected infants have diaphragmatic or "paradoxical" breathing pattern. Evidence of upper cranial nerve motor dysfunction is rare (i.e., cranial nerves III, IV, V, VI, and VII). Weakness of the tongue and accompanying fasciculations are commonly observed. However, the examiner must carefully distinguish fasciculations from normal movements during crying. The tongue should be examined at rest, in the mouth. Atrophy of the tongue may be manifest as scalloping of the border (see Fig. 2-6). Deep tendon reflexes are usually absent, whereas sphincter tone and sensation remain intact. There is a striking discrepancy between the infant's high level of social interaction and lack of motor skills.

Such infants tire quickly during feeding and, if breast-fed, may begin to lose weight before it is evident that they are not taking in appropriate calories. Their respiratory insufficiency exacerbates this fatigue and makes them susceptible to aspiration. Any minor upper respiratory tract infection may quickly become a life-threatening pneumonia. Bilateral eventration or paralysis of the diaphragm may be a presenting manifestation before the loss of deep tendon reflexes or the detection of muscle weakness [Bove and Iannaccone, 1988; McWilliam et al., 1985; Mellins et al., 1974]. Paralysis of the diaphragm, either unilateral or bilateral, before the age of 3 months is the most common presenting complaint in spinal muscular atrophy with respiratory distress (SMARD1).

At the time of disclosure of diagnosis to the family, it is important to counsel them about the high risk for death from pneumonia [Samaha et al., 1994]. It is also important to review management, considering the possible need for nasogastric feedings and airway clearance. Parents should be taught how to handle a severely floppy infant and be provided with appropriate seating for feeding and for automobile travel. Most specialty clinics teach parents to provide prophylactic chest percussion therapy and advise full immunization against influenza, respiratory syncytial virus, and pneumonia. Intervention with ventilatory support has been provided for some patients on an individual basis. Long-term survival under such circumstances is rare and requires constant monitoring, although new technology makes mobility, even with ventilators, feasible [Wang et al., 1994].

Spinal Muscular Atrophy Type II

Synonyms for spinal muscular atrophy type II include *juvenile spinal muscular atrophy, intermediate spinal muscular atrophy,* and *chronic spinal muscular atrophy* [Dubowitz, 1996; Hausmanowa-Petrusewicz, 1978]. Weakness and hypotonia are the rule, although patients usually achieve normal milestones up to 6 to 8 months of age. The lower extremities tend to be more involved than the upper extremities, so that failure to walk is a typical chief complaint. Patients may be thought to have a paraparesis and occasionally have clubfoot deformity. The pattern of deep tendon reflexes may be variable, with preservation in muscle groups that are fairly strong. Minipolymyoclonus may be prominent in these infants. The movements are intermittent, irregular, and of small amplitude. Distal muscles, particularly of the fingers, are primarily affected. No movements are evident during relaxation or sleep. Fatigue, stress, and self-consciousness increase the amplitude. The pathophysiologic origin of these movements is not known, although fasciculations of the intrinsic hand muscles may participate. These movements do not occur in myopathic processes [Spiro, 1970].

Many patients with type II are able to sit without support if placed in position; rarely, some are able to stand or walk with aid. The age at death is quite variable, from 7 months to 7 years [Byers and Banker, 1961] or in the third decade [Guinter et al., 1977]. The eldest patient in one prospective study died at age 72 years [Russman et al., 1996].

Spinal Muscular Atrophy Type III

The mildest form of spinal muscular atrophy is type III and is also called *Wohlfart-Kugelberg-Welander syndrome* and *mild spinal muscular atrophy* [Kugelberg and Welander, 1954, 1956]. It usually presents in late childhood or adolescence as a proximal neurogenic muscular atrophy that may be confused with limb girdle muscular dystrophy [Furukawa et al., 1968; Lunt et al., 1989; Topaloglu et al., 1989; Zerres and Rudnik-Schoneborn, 1995]. Frequently, patients have elevated serum creatine kinase levels [Kugelberg, 1975]. This syndrome is distinguished from Werdnig-Hoffmann disease by later onset and long survival [Kugelberg and Welander, 1954, 1956]. It is distinguished from amyotrophic lateral sclerosis by the benign course and absence of any involvement of corticospinal tracts.

Spinal muscular atrophy type III patients may have a waddling gait, with lumbar lordosis, genu recurvatum, and a protuberant abdomen. Deep tendon reflexes may or may not be elicited but are never pathologically hyperactive. In one report, six of eight children were able to stand without aid between 1 and 2 years of age; however, only two of the eight were eventually able to walk without assistance [Byers and Banker, 1961]. The prognosis for continued independent ambulation can be correlated with age of onset of weakness [Zerres et al., 1997a]. If onset is before 2 years of age, the patient is likely to stop walking by age 15, whereas if onset occurs later than 2 years, it is highly likely that ambulation will be possible into the fifth decade [Russman et al., 1996]. A large, prospective clinical study found little or no progression of weakness over several years in patients with type II or III [Russman et al., 1992]. The authors suggested that spinal muscular atrophy may not be a neurodegenerative disease, but new information indicates that this conclusion was wrong [Bromberg and Swoboda, 2002]. Scoliosis is the most serious orthopedic problem experienced [Schwentker and Gibson, 1976].

Neuropathologic findings include loss of anterior horn motor neurons [Byers and Banker, 1961; Greenfield and Stern, 1928; Walsh et al., 1987]. Dicarboxylic aciduria was reported in one infant with classic Werdnig-Hoffmann disease [Harpey et al., 1990; Kelley and Sladky, 1986], but the significance of such findings is unclear. Acidosis in some cases may be secondary to chronic malnutrition and loss of glycogen reserves in the context of extremely low muscle bulk. However, there is now concern that a subpopulation of spinal muscular atrophy patients may have a primary metabolic disturbance that must be identified before beginning experimental therapy, such as with histone deacetylase inhibitors [Brichta et al., 2003; Sumner et al., 2003; Tein et al., 1995].

Hexosaminidase A deficiency represents an interesting, albeit rare, variant of late-onset spinal muscular atrophy [Johnson et al., 1982, 1983]. This syndrome is discussed in more detail in the sections on GM_2 gangliosidosis and on hexosaminidase variants and neuromuscular syndromes.

Epidemiologic studies always indicated an autosomal-recessive mode of inheritance [Zellweger et al., 1969] and nearly equal sex distribution, with a slight predominance in males [Hausmanowa-Petrusewicz et al., 1984], but apparent autosomal-dominant transmission is a rare occurrence [Jansen et al., 1986]. Several families have been described in which the co-occurrence of spinal muscular atrophy and amyotrophic lateral sclerosis was documented [Appelbaum et al., 1992; Shaw et al., 1992]. Linkage of autosomal recessive spinal muscular atrophy to chromosome 5q11.2-13.3 was reported by Gilliam and associates [Gilliam et al., 1990]. This international consortium studied families with evidence of recessive transmission only, although they were able to document phenotypic heterogeneity within families [Brzustowicz et al., 1990; Muller et al., 1992; Munsat et al., 1990]. Melki and colleagues reported the occurrence of major deletions at 5q11.2-13.3 in patients with severe spinal muscular atrophy (Werdnig-Hoffmann phenotype), compared with patients with mild spinal muscular atrophy (Wohlfart-Kugelberg-Welander phenotype) who had no deletions or smaller deletions [Melki et al., 1990]. Clinical evidence suggests that early-onset spinal muscular atrophy represents a spectrum of disease, a finding consistent with a single gene locus [Iannaccone et al., 1991; Melki et al., 1994].

Thus, the most common form of spinal muscular atrophy is an autosomal-recessive disorder [Hoffmann, 1900a, 1900b] linked to the 5q11 locus [Brzustowicz et al., 1990; Lefebvre et al., 1995; Melki et al., 1990; Muller et al., 1992; Roy et al., 1995]. Mutations occur in as many as 98% of children with spinal muscular atrophy, and mutation analysis has replaced electrodiagnostic studies and muscle biopsy in primary diagnosis of this disease. Deletions occur with less frequency among patients with mild spinal muscular atrophy than among those with type I [Gilliam et al., 1990; Melki et al., 1994; Rudnik-Schoneborn et al., 1996].

Most spinal muscular atrophy cases are associated with deletions or mutations in exons 7 and 8 of the telomeric copy of the spinal muscular atrophy gene (called *SMN1*), although cases of small deletions or mutations in other parts of the gene have also been reported. The centromeric copy of *SMN* (called *SMN2*) is a disease-modifying gene. The number of copies correlates with the type or severity of disease; mild cases tend to have more copies than severe cases [Burghes, 1997; Campbell et al., 1997; Gilliam et al., 1990].

SMN protein, found in structures called *gems*, was absent from motor neurons of infants with type I disease. Protein was present in type II or III disease but in decreased amounts compared with controls [Lefebvre et al., 1997]. These findings suggest that the severity of disease is proportional to the loss of SMN protein [Zerres et al., 1997b] and that a correlation between the SMN protein level and the disease state has been established [Lefebvre et al., 1997; Zerres et al., 1997b]. Patients with type I or II spinal muscular atrophy have reduced amounts of SMN protein compared with normal controls; this decrease ranges from 5% to 100% [Lefebvre et al., 1997]. Type III patients have normal amounts of intracellular SMN protein. SMN protein level and disease severity are most likely a consequence of *SMN2* gene copy number [Burghes, 1997; Coovert et al., 1997; Lefebvre et al., 1997]. In addition, motor unit counts appear to correspond with *SMN2* copy counts [Swoboda et al., 2005].

All patients have at least one copy of *SMN2* because complete loss of all *SMN* genes appears to be an embryonic lethal lesion [DiDonato et al., 1999; Monani et al., 2000]. *SMN1* produces full-length *SMN* messenger RNA. *SMN2* expresses dramatically reduced full-length and abundant levels of transcript lacking exon 7 (Δ7-*SMN*) [Gavrilov et al., 1998]. The protein product of *SMN2* differs from normal full-length SMN protein in sequence and function [Monani et al., 1999] because the *SMN2* gene has a single base-pair change in exon 7 producing truncated messenger RNA transcript. A single nucleotide difference (C-to-T transition in exon 7) in *SMN2* causes exon 7 skipping and a transcript that encodes for a less stable protein [Monani et al., 1999; Lorson, 1999, 2000]. Several studies demonstrated that the C to T change on the +6 position of exon 7 results in exon skipping of SMN2 during its transcription [Cartegni, 2002; Lemaire, 2002].

The gene product of *SMN1* forms a large complex with other proteins called Gemin2, Gemin4, Gemin5, Gemin6, and Gemin7 [Pellizzoni et al., 2002]; this complex interacts with spliceosomes [Fischer et al., 1997; Liu et al., 1997; Strasswimmer et al., 1999]. There have been only a few studies to date that have investigated SMN protein [Coovert et al., 1997; Lefebvre et al., 1997] and RNA expression [Gavrilov et al., 1998; Gennarelli et al., 1995; Patrizi et al., 1999] in spinal muscular atrophy patients. Patients produced two to three times more Δ7-*SMN* compared with full-length *SMN* messenger RNA expression [Gavrilov et al., 1998; Gennarelli et al., 1995; Patrizi et al., 1999]. A number of studies investigated the relationship between *SMN2* gene copy number and disease severity, suggesting that the number of *SMN2* copies is directly related to a mild spinal muscular atrophy phenotype.

Animal models for spinal muscular atrophy recently became available for therapeutic studies [Schmalbruch and Haase, 2001]. Mice have only one *SMN* gene, and the knockout $Smn^{-/-}$ mouse dies in utero before implantation. Heterozygotes ($Smn^{+/-}$) had an *SMA* phenotype, but it was mild despite a 50% reduction in SMN protein level. Two groups constructed *SMN2* transgenic mice and crossed them with $Smn^{+/-}$ to produce a knockout mouse with the human *SMN2* gene, the $Smn^{-/-}$ *SMN2* mouse [Hsieh-Li et al., 2000; Monani et al., 2000]. Littermates demonstrated a range of phenotypes similar to that seen in humans with spinal muscular atrophy types I, II, and III. Furthermore, the severity of the phenotype was inversely proportional to the number of *SMN2* copies (and therefore the amount of SMN protein), exactly as seen in human subjects. The importance of SMN protein in producing the disease phenotype has been reinforced by the finding that an A2G missense mutation modulates the mouse phenotype [Monani et al., 2003]. In other words, increasing the presence of SMN protein, even abnormal protein, may be a reasonable therapeutic strategy. A concurrent strategy is to examine many compounds for their ability to alter splicing and to produce full-length protein in vitro using cells from patients or from *Smn* mice [Zerres et al., 1997b].

Frugier and associates cross-bred three mice: one with a transgene expressing Cre recombinase controlled by the neuron specific enolase promoter, the *Smn*$^{+/-}$ mouse, and finally one homozygous for *Smn* exon 7 being flanked by loxP recombination sites [Frugier et al., 2000]. This cross-breeding produced the *Smn*$^{F7/-}$ NSE-Cre mouse that expresses *Smn* exon 7 deletion in neurons only [Salah et al., 2002]. Both animal models are being used to test drugs and compounds for their effect on SMN protein production in vivo.

The largest class of compounds to upregulate *SMN* messenger RNA ratios are histone deacetylase inhibitors [Andreassi et al., 2001; Jarecki et al., 2002]. Histone deacetylase inhibitors include the following drugs: valproic acid, commonly used as an antiepileptic in children; hydroxyurea; sodium butyrate; and sodium vanadate. Butyrate, a histone deacetylase inhibitor, can induce transcriptional activation of a number of genes and induce cellular differentiation as histone acetylation levels increase. Butyrate was found to induce γ-globin expression through changes in histone acetylation [McCaffrey et al., 1997; Pace et al., 2002]. Chang and colleagues have treated the *Smn*$^{-/-}$ *SMN2* mouse with sodium butyrate [Chang et al., 2001]. Survival in the treated group was significantly improved. There was elevation of exon 7 containing SMN protein in treated animal tissues including motor neurons. Experiments using sodium butyrate in lymphoid cell lines from spinal muscular atrophy patients showed an increased number of full-length *SMN* transcripts. Sodium butyrate increased the amount of exon 7 containing SMN protein in spinal muscular atrophy lymphoid cell lines. Mercuri and colleagues reported a significant improvement in functional strength in a short pilot trial of phenylbutyrate in children with spinal muscular atrophy [Carducci et al., 2001; Mercuri et al., 2004].

Clinical Laboratory Tests

The diagnostic evaluation for spinal muscular atrophy has changed since the discovery of the survival motor neuron gene. The diagnosis now can begin with blood DNA analysis for mutations in this gene [Parano et al., 1996; Rudnik-Schoneborn et al., 1996]. For infants who have mutations, no further evaluation is necessary. If mutations cannot be identified, a more traditional approach may be necessary for diagnosis.

This approach includes measurement of serum muscle enzymes, electrodiagnosis with nerve conduction velocities and electromyography, and muscle biopsy. As already stated, serum levels of the muscle enzyme creatine kinase may or may not be elevated, although it usually is normal in spinal muscle atrophy types I and II.

The electrodiagnostic characteristics that accompany anterior horn cell impairment are often readily detectable by electromyography. Evidence of acute denervation such as fibrillation potentials is common. Infants may exhibit spontaneous rhythmic firing of motor units, whereas electromyographic patterns of patients with long-standing disease often display pseudomyotonic volleys [Hausmanowa-Petrusewicz et al., 1987; Hausmanowa-Petrusewicz and Jozwik, 1986]. There usually is also evidence of reinnervation in the form of large polyphasic motor units and increased recruitment.

Measurement of motor nerve conduction velocities in infants may be difficult because of the small-sized limbs and short distance between stimulus and recording electrodes. Examination usually documents either normal conduction velocities or, occasionally, faster conduction velocities than expected [Moosa and Dubowitz, 1976]. Normal sensory conduction velocities have been found in the sural or median nerves of patients in all three groups and in patients with juvenile proximal hereditary muscular atrophy [Schwartz and Moosa, 1977]. If there is profound muscle atrophy, it may be difficult to interpret responses to nerve stimulus. Conventional diagnostic criteria mandate that the diagnosis of spinal muscular atrophy (in the absence of an identifiable gene mutation) must be accompanied by normal motor and sensory nerve conduction velocities.

Ultrasonography of the muscles is usually abnormal and has been used as a screening test for neurogenic atrophy in patients with mild clinical disability [Kamala et al., 1985].

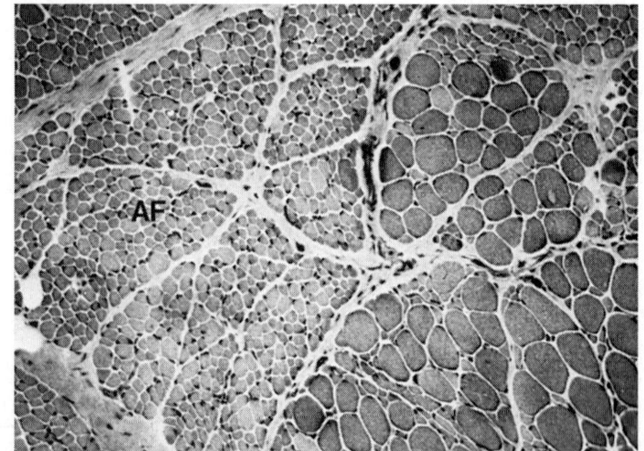

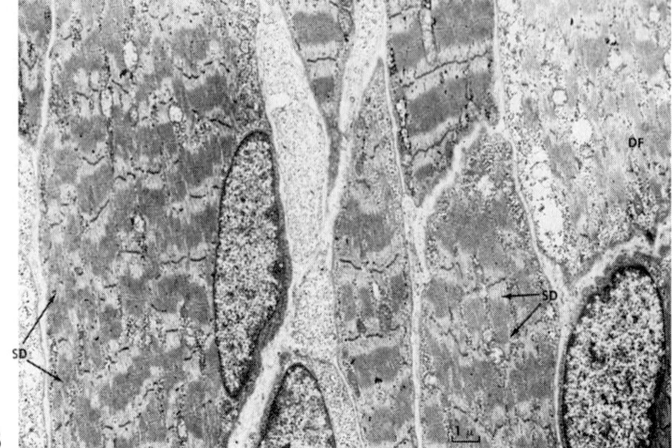

FIGURE 75-6. Infantile spinal muscular atrophy: biceps muscle from a 3-month-old infant. **A,** Fascicles with atrophic muscle fibers (AF) and fascicles with atrophic and normal fibers. (Trichrome stain, ×160.) **B,** Ultrastructural appearance showing small fibers, sarcomere disruption (SD), and degenerating fiber (DF) (×7000). (Courtesy of Dr. Stephen A. Smith.)

However, it is not as reliable or specific as other diagnostic tests.

Muscle biopsy should indicate neurogenic atrophy or evidence of reinnervation (Fig. 75-6). The affected fibers are smaller in diameter than normal, and fat tissue is more abundant between the fiber bundles. Disproportionate preservation of large, rounded fibers in the denervated fasciculi is common [Byers and Banker, 1961]. This is frequently called the *infantile pattern of neurogenic atrophy*. From mid-childhood, one may see angular fibers indicating acute denervation and type grouping indicating reinnervation. Fidzianska described three types of muscle cells found in a study of muscle tissue taken from seven children with spinal muscular atrophy: normal cells, small cells with a large central nucleus appearing as older myoblasts, and cells resembling myotubes containing a common basement membrane [Fidzianska, 1976]. The latter two types were believed to represent arrested maturation rather than atrophy. Nonspecific changes such as fiber size disproportion may occur, possibly as a result of sampling error [Bove and Iannaccone, 1988]. In such a case, repeat biopsy of another muscle or at a later age may suggest more typical evidence of neurogenic atrophy. Many fibers reveal a loss of filaments from their myofibrils, a change typical of denervation atrophy. Other atrophic fibers contain clumps of thin filaments frequently seen in young myoblasts, suggesting either active regeneration or cessation of maturation [Shafiq et al., 1967]. However, no changes in the muscle spindles have been reported.

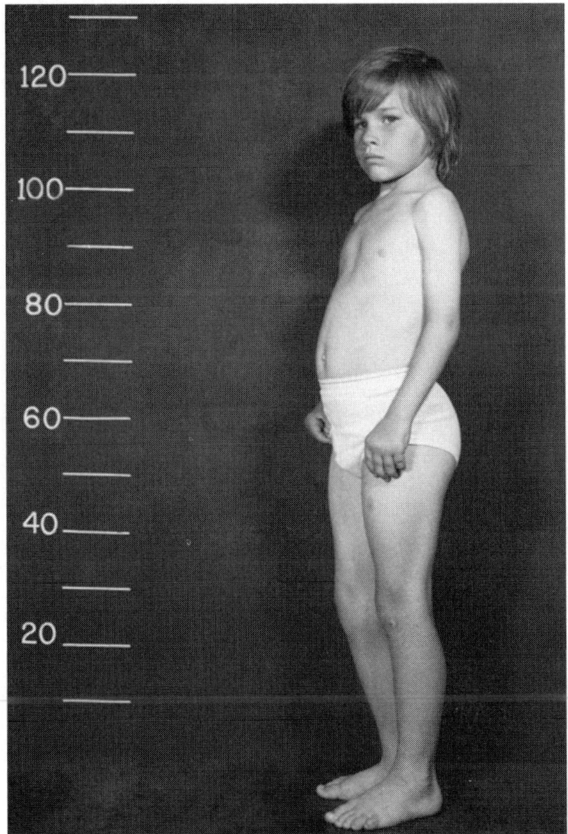

FIGURE 75-7. This patient with juvenile proximal hereditary muscular atrophy (Kugelberg-Welander disease) has generalized weakness. Marked weakness and atrophy of the shoulder girdle are present. Lumbar lordosis, as well as abdominal protuberance related to abnormal weakness, is common.

Imaging of the central nervous system (CNS) is done infrequently. The brain should have normal structure. Anomalies of the CNS may occur with motor neuron disease but not with spinal muscle atrophy that is linked to the 5q locus. Variants of spinal muscle atrophy are discussed in a later section.

Management

Because there is no effective therapy for spinal muscle atrophy [Dubowitz, 1996; Eng et al., 1984], management consists of preventing or treating the complications. Complications of severe weakness include restrictive lung disease, poor nutrition, orthopedic deformities, immobility, and psychosocial problems (Fig. 75-7).

Restrictive lung disease results from weakness of intercostal muscles and diaphragm causing hypoventilation and weak cough. Aggressive prophylaxis against pneumonia may include assisted cough, chest percussion therapy, and intermittent positive-pressure breathing. Patients require assistance to maintain good pulmonary toilet even when not experiencing an acute infection and may require intervention to prevent progressive atelectasis [Bach, 1994; Bach and Alba, 1990, 1991]. Risk for pneumonia increases as forced vital capacity decreases and may occur even without significant change in limb or trunk strength. Oxygen therapy should be contraindicated except in the context of acute infection. Patients with restrictive lung disease develop retention of CO_2 before hypoxia, and administration of oxygen may cause death from apnea secondary to suppression of the respiratory drive. It is helpful to monitor blood gases on a regular basis along with the forced vital capacity. When CO_2 retention occurs, noninvasive ventilation, either positive or negative pressure, during sleep may be helpful and restorative.

Recent studies indicate that noninvasive ventilation can improve quality of life, prolong survival, and decrease morbidity in patients with restrictive lung disease, including spinal muscular atrophy patients [Birnkrant et al., 1998; Wallgren-Pettersson et al., 2004]. Other technology is also available to improve airway clearance, including insufflators-exsufflators and intermittent P ventilation [Finder et al., 2004; Miske et al., 2004; Toussaint et al., 2003].

Poor nutrition often occurs as a result of a weak suck, unprotected airway, or easy fatigability. A feeding evaluation can be done by a team of occupational therapists and dietitians. Recommendations may include adjusting the feeding schedule, positioning, or food textures to maximize caloric intake. The child should be examined during a modified barium swallow using several food textures, including liquid, semiliquid, soft, and solid food. If aspiration occurs, a gastrostomy may be recommended. In some cases, supplemental gastrostomy feedings may be indicated in the absence of aspiration because the child cannot take in enough by mouth before fatiguing.

Scoliosis is the most serious orthopedic problem among patients with spinal muscular atrophy. Nonwalkers tend to develop spinal deformities earlier than walkers. Most curves are thoracolumbar in location. Spinal orthoses usually do not prevent or retard scoliosis; however, they may help patients sit. Surgical correction should be undertaken only after careful consideration because patients should be in good health at the time, and they will experience no further linear growth after spine surgery [Schwentker and Gibson, 1976]. Vigorous preoperative and postoperative physical therapy is required to prevent loss of strength or function after spinal fusion, as well as respiratory complications. Marked improvement in the degree of scoliosis is often possible after fusion or instrumentation, with associated improvement in vital capacity, sitting, balance, and comfort [Aprin et al., 1982; Daher et al., 1985a; Piasecki et al., 1986]. Patients who do not undergo correction of scoliosis typically experience progressive deformity with discomfort, inability to position, and further decompensation of pulmonary functions.

Walking may occasionally be facilitated by lightweight orthoses for the legs, although for spinal muscle atrophy type I or II patients, it may be a temporary skill [Russman et al., 1996; Wilkins and Gibson, 1976]. Power chairs should be prescribed as close to the second birthday as possible to provide some independent mobility at an appropriate developmental age [Siegel and Silverman, 1984]. Because children with spinal muscle atrophy often have high cognitive function [Whelan, 1987], they easily learn how to maneuver a joystick. The motor speed can be adjusted as needed, and the parents should be encouraged to set consistent limits for behavior. As the child grows, pneumatic lifts, special mattresses, and bath accessories are beneficial for many patients. An in-home occupational therapy consult will ensure that the patient receives appropriate equipment.

School-aged children may benefit from a full-time aide who can help with toileting and feeding and maintain the respiratory and physical therapy regimens during the school day. Parents can be encouraged to seek resources for such help and to communicate freely with school district officials to provide their child with an education that will maximize academic abilities.

KENNEDY'S DISEASE

Kennedy's disease, or spinal and bulbar muscular atrophy, was first described in 1968 [Kennedy et al., 1968]. It is a rare motor neuron disease that causes proximal weakness, bulbar weakness with dysphagia and aspiration, asymmetric or symmetric facial weakness, and gynecomastia. Age of onset is variable, and clinical diagnosis may not be possible until gynecomastia develops after the fourth decade. Inheritance is X-linked. Fischbeck and colleagues localized the gene in 7 families to Xq12-22 [Fischbeck et al., 1986]. Subsequently, the human androgenic receptor gene (*hAR*) was localized to Xq11-12, and examination of *hAR* in spinal and bulbar muscular atrophy patients demonstrated that there was an abnormal expansion of exon 1 to more than twice normal size [Choi et al., 1993]. The expansion was found to be caused by CAG repeats, normally numbering 15 to 31 in *hAR*, but numbering more than 40 in the spinal and bulbar muscular atrophy mutation [Belsham et al., 1992; La Spada et al., 1991, 1994].

Although clinical and genetic diagnosis is usually established in the fourth of fifth decade of life when weakness is present, the earliest symptoms may be present in the second decade of life and include gynecomastia, muscle cramps, and fatigue [Sperfeld et al., 2002]. This weakness is slowly progressive and involves bulbar musculature, including a weak, atrophic tongue. There are no signs of spinal cortical tract dysfunction; deep tendon reflexes are diminished or normal. Fasciculations and cramps in limb muscles are common. Hypesthesia and decreased vibratory sense are present in about half of patients. There may be mild elevation of muscle enzymes, but electrodiagnostic study and muscle biopsy are indicative of motor neuron disease. Once the clinical phenotype is recognized in a patient, diagnosis may be confirmed by mutation analysis in a blood sample.

TABLE 75-2

Rare and Atypical Forms of Spinal Muscular Atrophy (SMA) Not Linked to the *SMN* Gene

NAME	GENE/INHERITANCE	CLINICAL	REFERENCES
Scapuloperoneal SMA	AD; 12q24.1-q24.31	Congenital absence of muscles; progressive weakness of scapuloperoneal, distal, and laryngeal muscles	DeLong and Siddique, 1992; Isozumi et al., 1996
Spinal SMA 2	AR or X-linked	Onset 1 year; proximal more than distal	Nevo et al., 1998
Pontocerebellar hypoplasia with SMA (PCH I)	AR	Onset 0–6 mo; progressive CNS hypotrophic cerebellum and brainstem; absent dentate nucleus; neuronal loss in basal ganglia; cortical atrophy	Barth, 1993; Chou, 1993; Chou et al., 1990; Gorgen-Pauly et al., 1999; Rudnik-Schoneborn et al., 2003; Ryan et al., 2000
Distal infantile SMA with diaphragm paralysis (SMARD1)	AR; 11q13.2-q13.4 Immunoglobulin-γ–binding protein-2 (IGHMBP2)	Onset 1–2 mo; diaphragmatic paralysis; death <3 mo	Grohmann et al., 2003; Mellins et al., 1974; Rudnik-Schoneborn et al., 2004
Distal hereditary motor neuropathy, Jerash type	AR; 9p21.1-p12	Onset 6–10 yr; legs involved first then hands	Christodoulou et al., 2000; Middleton et al., 1999
X-linked infantile SMA with arthrogryposis	Xp11.3-q11.2	Onset birth or infant; contractures; death <2 yr	Greenberg et al., 1988; Kobayashi et al., 1995
SMA, congenital nonprogressive, of lower limbs	AD; 12q23-24	Late walking proximal and distal weakness; mild knee contractures; pes equinovarus	Fleury and Hageman, 1985

AD, autosomal dominant; AR, autosomal recessive; CNS, central nervous system.

TABLE 75-3

Distal Hereditary Motor Neuropathy (HMN) or Distal Spinal Muscular Atrophy (SMN)

NAME	GENE/INHERITANCE	CLINICAL	INVESTIGATORS
HMN 1	AD	Onset 2–40 yr; symmetric weakness; no upper motor neuron signs	
HMN 2	AD; HSPB8 (HSP22); 12q24 (same gene mutated in Charcot-Marie-Tooth disease 2L)	Onset 14–35 yr; weak toe extensors with progression to complete paralysis of distal leg muscles in 5 years	(Irobi et al., 2004b; Timmerman et al., 1992)
HMN 5	AD; 7p14; glycyl transfer RNA synthetase (allelic with Charcot-Marie-Tooth disease 2D); GARS protein (aminoacyl transfer RNA synthetase)	Onset of weakness is in hands with mean age 17 yr; lower extremity involved in 50% after 2 yr; slowly progressive	(Christodoulou et al., 1995; Ellsworth et al., 1999)
HMN 5B	AD; 11q13; BSCL2 protein; seipin (allelic to Beradinelli-Seip congenital lipodystrophy, type 2, and SPG-17—Silver's syndrome)	Onset in hands with mean onset age 15 yr (range, 2–40 yr); slow progression over decades with lower extremity involvement in 95%	(Irobi et al., 2004a; Windpassinger et al., 2004)
HMN 7	AD; 2q14	Onset second decade with voice or gait disorder; slow progression but vocal cord paralysis can lead to respiratory failure	(Boltshauser et al., 1989; Young and Harper, 1980)
HMN + vocal cord (2)	AD: 2p13; dynactin 1	Early adult onset with respiratory failure with vocal cord paralysis; progressive; hands and then feet	(Puls et al., 2003)
Distal SMA, X-linked	X-linked; Xq13.1-q21	Onset 1–10 yr; very slow	(Takata et al., 2004)

AD, autosomal dominant; SPG, spastic paraplegia.

RARE AND ATYPICAL FORMS OF SPINAL MUSCULAR ATROPHY

Molecular genetics have allowed specific identification of several atypical forms of spinal muscular atrophy that may occur distally or proximally (Tables 75-2 and 75-3). Scapuloperoneal spinal muscular atrophy was first described clinically by Emery and co-workers before the identification of the *SMN* gene, and Mawatari recognized sporadic and X-linked cases [Emery et al., 1968; Mawatari and Katayama, 1973]. More recently, a clinically similar syndrome with onset in the first decade of life and slow progression has been linked to chromo-some 12 with autosomal-dominant inheritance [DeLong and Siddique, 1992; Isozumi et al., 1996].

In progressive bulbar paralysis of childhood, or Fazio-Londe disease, motor neurons in cranial nerve nuclei may be progressively impaired and decreased in number, with resultant progressive bulbar paralysis and little or no accompanying anterior spinal cord involvement [Gomez et al., 1962]. Although the condition may be genetically transmitted [Fazio, 1892; Londe, 1893, 1894], sporadic cases are more common [McShane et al., 1992; Suresh and Deepa, 2004]. Age of onset varies and may be as early as 3 years. Bulbar paralysis is only one facet of progressive motor neuron disease in many of these patients, and pathologic study confirms widespread degenerative changes in the brainstem. Morphologic involvement of anterior horn cells has been demonstrated despite the absence of clinical signs [Alexander et al., 1976]. Involvement of the anterior horn cells in the cervical and upper thoracic cord segments is often associated with demonstrable loss of neurons in other locations, including decreased neuronal population in the dentate nucleus. Of the cranial nerves, cranial nerve VII is almost always affected. Cranial nerve XII is usually affected pathologically, and clinical manifestations are apparent in the early-onset patients. The nuclei of cranial nerves III, IV, VI, and X may also be involved. Clinical impairment of extraocular movement is rare.

Juvenile-onset bulbospinal muscular atrophy associated with deafness [Brown-Vialetto-Van Laere syndrome) manifests late in the first decade or in the second decade [Brown, 1894; Van Laere, 1966; Vialetto, 1936]. Bulbar impairment is indicated by dysarthria, dysphagia, and facial diplegia [Gallai et al., 1981; Summers et al., 1987]

MÖBIUS' SYNDROME

First described in 1898 by Thomas, Möbius' syndrome is a congenital, static condition manifested by facial palsy (often bilateral) and involvement (usually bilateral) of cranial nerve VI [Thomas, 1898]. The lower face is usually less involved than the upper face. Impaired lateral rectus muscle contraction results in unopposed medial rectus muscle action, with resultant convergence (Fig. 75-8). Conjugate eye movements in the vertical plane are usually present, although ptosis may also be present. Dysfunction of other cranial nerves, including cranial nerves V, X, XI, and XII, often accompanies the abnormalities of cranial nerves VI and VII. Associated absence of the pectoral muscles may occur. The clinical findings are correlated with failure of

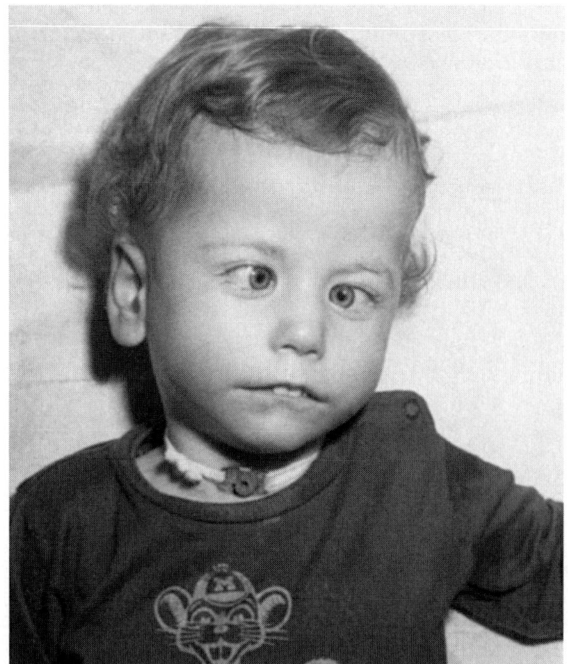

FIGURE 75-8. Patient with Möbius' syndrome who has bilateral weakness of cranial nerves VI and VII. Recurrent swallowing impairment resulted in multiple episodes of pneumonitis, which necessitated tracheostomy.

development or degeneration of the involved cranial nerve motor cells. Several gene loci have been identified, and the nomenclature now refers to Möbius' syndromes 1, 2, and 3 (Table 75-4). Möbius' syndrome has also been associated with exposure to cocaine or misoprostol in utero [de Muelenaere, 1999; Goldberg et al., 2001; Kankirawatana et al., 1993; Leong and Ashwell, 1997; Marques-Dias et al., 2003; Pastuszak et al., 1998; Shepard, 1995; Vargas et al., 2000].

Although the differential diagnosis includes non–motor neuron involvement, including supranuclear or myopathic conditions such as facial scapulohumeral dystrophy, myotubular myopathy, or myotonic dystrophy, other clinical features usually distinguish Möbius' syndrome from these.

AMYOTROPHIC LATERAL SCLEROSIS

Amyotrophic lateral sclerosis represents a spectrum of motor system degeneration involving the corticospinal and corticobulbar pathways and motor neurons associated with the cranial nerves and anterior horn cells of the spinal cord. Onset may be as early as adolescence, although most cases present after the fourth decade of life. Dysfunction of upper and lower motor neurons produces clinical manifestations of both spasticity and muscular atrophy.

Amyotrophic lateral sclerosis is inherited in about 10% of cases as an autosomal-dominant disorder with increasing penetrance after 50 years of age [Emery, 1991]. Sporadic and familial amyotrophic lateral sclerosis are clinically indistinguishable. Familial amyotrophic lateral sclerosis has been studied to understand pathogenesis. Multiple genes or gene loci have now been identified in familial amyotrophic lateral sclerosis (Table 75-5). The most common, superoxide dismutase (*SOD*), a gene that encodes a cytosolic Cu/Zn-binding superoxide dismutase, is causative in amyotrophic lateral sclerosis type 1 [Deng et al., 1993; Rosen et al., 1993]. The role of superoxide dismutase in controlling free radical tissue levels made it a logical choice as a candidate gene in familial amyotrophic lateral sclerosis. Superoxide is known to be cytotoxic, but the accumulation of superoxide by an inhibition of superoxide dismutase may be exacerbated by activation of excitatory neurotransmitters, such as glutamate [Coyle and Puttfarcken, 1993]. However, this initial concept of pathogenesis has not been confirmed because humans studies show that amyotrophic lateral sclerosis severity is independent of enzyme activity, and neither the *SOD1* knockout nor the *SOD1*-overexpressing wild-type mice develop weakness [Shibata, 2001]. Instead, severity of weakness in *SOD1* mutant mice is related to transgene copy number. Mice with high copy numbers develop progressive weakness and motor neuron loss resulting in death [Borchelt et al., 1998; Shibata, 2001]. This toxic gain of function may be caused by either a gain of oxidative function or gain of abnormal protein-protein interactions [Liochev and Fridovich, 2003].

There are three well-recognized amyotrophic lateral sclerosis syndromes with onset in the first two decades of life (see Table 75-5). Amyotrophic lateral sclerosis type 2 is due to mutations in the Alsin gene (*ALS2*) [Hadano et al., 2001; Yang et al., 2001b]. This gene, which has sequence homology to guanosine triphosphatase regulatory proteins, bears mutations that predict truncation of the protein and loss of function. Children present in the first decade of life with spasticity involving face and limbs and may develop a pseudobulbar affect. Symptoms are very slowly progressive with difficulty walking after 40 years of age. An allelic condition, progressive lateral sclerosis with onset in infancy, has also been associated with mutations in this gene [Eymard-Pierre et al., 2002; Gros-Louis et al., 2003].

The second juvenile-onset form of amyotrophic lateral sclerosis is type 4, an autosomal-dominant inherited distal motor neuronopathy with pyramidal symptoms [Chance et al., 1998]. Symptoms begin in the second decade of life

TABLE 75–4

Genetic Forms of Möbius' Syndrome

NAME	GENE LOCI	INHERITANCE /OMIM	ASSOCIATED FEATURES	INVESTIGATORS
MBS 1	13q12.2-q13	AD; 157900	CN IV; arthrogryposis; mental retardation	(Parkes, 1999; Slee et al., 1991)
MBS 2	3q21-q22	AD; 601471	Asymmetric CN VII; no ophthalmoplegia; incomplete penetrance	(Kremer et al., 1996)
MBS 3		AD; 604185	Asymmetric, bifacial weakness; variable hearing loss; reduced penetrance	(Verzijl et al., 1999)

AD, autosomal dominant; CN, cranial nerve.

TABLE 75–5

Genetic Forms of Amyotrophic Lateral Sclerosis (ALS)

NAME	GENE/LOCI/PROTEIN	INHERITANCE	ONSET	INVESTIGATORS
ALS 1	*SOD1*/21q22.1/Cu/Zn-binding superoxide dismutase	AD	Adult	(Rosen, 1993)
ALS 2	*ALS2*/2q33/alsin	AR	Child	(Hadano et al., 2001; Yang et al., 2001b)
ALS 3	18q21	AD	Adult	(Hand et al., 2002)
ALS 4	9q34/senataxin	AD	Child	(Blair et al., 2000; Chen et al., 2004)
ALS 5	15q15	AR	Child	(Hentati et al., 1998)
ALS 6	16q12	AD	Adult	(Ruddy et al., 2003; Sapp et al., 2003)
ALS 7	20p13	AD	Adult	(Sapp et al., 2003)
ALS 8	*VAPB*/20q13	AD	Adult	(Nishimura et al., 2004)
ALS-FTD*	9q21-22	AD	Adult	(Hosler et al., 2000)
	22q12/neurofilament heavy chain	Unknown	Adult	(Al-Chalabi et al., 1999)
	12q12/peripherin	Unknown	Adult	(Gros-Louis et al., 2004)

*ALS with frontotemporal dementia.
AD, autosomal dominant; AR, autosomal recessive; SOD, superoxide dismutase.

with difficulty walking, and examination shows both upper and lower motor neuron involvement. Electrophysiology confirms localization to the level of the anterior horn cell [Rabin et al., 1999]. The clinical course has a slow progression with a normal life span. Recently causative mutations in the senataxin gene (*SETX*) have been demonstrated. Although the precise function is unknown, the Senataxin gene has homology to genes involved in RNA processing [Chen et al., 2004].

The third form of amyotrophic lateral sclerosis with childhood onset is type 5, localized to chromosome 15q15.1-q21.1, and is recessively inherited. No specific gene has been identified. This form of juvenile amyotrophic lateral sclerosis has been described in multiple ethnic groups from North Africa, South Asia, and Europe. There are two clinical subtypes. Onset for both is in the second decade of life. Type 1 affects arms more than legs, and bulbar symptoms develop late. Type 2 has much more spasticity and much more prominent involvement in legs and may be a form of familial spastic paraparesis [Hentati et al., 1998].

BENIGN CONGENITAL HYPOTONIA

When examining tone in infants and young children, both axillary and appendicular tones are assessed. Infants with CNS injury often demonstrate decreased axial tone but increased appendicular tone after the first months of life. However, in the first months, tone in both areas may be decreased in these infants. In contrast, children with hypotonia secondary to disorders of spinal cord (spinal muscular atrophy), nerve, neuromuscular junction, or myopathy usually maintain low axial and appendicular tone and have clear weakness throughout infancy and childhood.

The initial reports of children with "benign congenital hypotonia" cited 17 infants with hypotonia with no apparent weakness at birth or in first months of life. Eight improved completely by 10 years, and the other nine improved but had definite muscle weakness or marked ligamentous laxity at follow-up. All eight children who recovered had deep tendon reflexes when initially examined, although three had reflexes that were difficult to elicit [Walton, 1957]. Although there was no clinical evidence of muscular dystrophy, infantile spinal muscular atrophy, mental deficiency, or upper motor neuron disease clinically in these children, diagnostic studies at that time were limited. Only two had muscle biopsies, with hematoxylin and eosin staining only [Walton, 1957].

Children with "benign hypotonia" may have various conditions, including nonprogressive congenital myopathies identified with more detailed testing [Spagnoli et al., 1985; Thompson, 2002]. Because some of these disorders have clinical or hereditary implications, making these specific diagnoses is important. Other children with hypotonia in infancy without weakness may have cognitive difficulties later [Dubowitz, 1968; Shuper et al., 1987; Zellweger, 1983]. Thus, some suggest that this diagnosis be eliminated or replaced with the term *central hypotonia* because the prognosis is not necessarily benign. The cause in those children without a neuromuscular diagnosis is likely related to improper modulatory influences on the gamma loop from the CNS. As the brain matures, typical motor deficits may develop that are consistent with a diagnosis of cerebral palsy. The condition may be accompanied by cognitive deficit [Dubowitz, 1968]. In short-term follow-up to age 3 years, 44% of 36 children still had hypotonia and gross motor delay, and a small number had speech delay [Shuper et al., 1987]. One follow-up of 25 children with a clinical diagnosis of benign congenial hypotonia demonstrated that by age 6 to 8 years, these children still had inferior gross motor performance for coordination and strength compared with 26 healthy controls [Parush et al., 1998].

Thus, the clinician must be wary of making the diagnosis of benign congenital hypotonia because of the large differential diagnosis, which includes infantile spinal muscular atrophy and congenital myopathies [Thompson, 2002; Zellweger, 1983]. Follow-up examination to determine whether the appendicular tone increases or stays low and whether weakness becomes apparent is critical to deciding which children should have more detailed diagnostic studies [Thompson, 2002; Zellweger, 1983]. It is also possible that some children with congenital hypotonia without persistent weakness have variable degrees of ligament laxity [Carboni et al., 2002; McGrory et al., 1997].

ARTHROGRYPOSIS MULTIPLEX CONGENITA

Arthrogryposis multiplex congenita, a syndrome manifesting at birth, is characterized by multiple, fixed contractures of large joints. The pathologic features of arthrogryposis cover a broad spectrum [Banker, 1985, 1986, 1994]. General and genetic classifications have been proposed [Hall, 1997].

Fetal hypokinesia or restricted movement in utero of any cause will result in congenital contractures. Congenital anomalies of the brain are common (e.g., hydrocephalus, hydranencephaly, microcephaly) [Hageman et al., 1987; Hennekam et al., 1991] and may be accompanied by anomalies of other organs [Vlaanderen et al., 1991]. Inheritance of anterior horn cell arthrogryposis, when determinable, is most often autosomal recessive. However, autosomal-dominant transmission has been reported [Fleury and Hageman, 1985].

Anterior horn cell arthrogryposis results from a marked decrease of the anterior horn cell population in the cervical and lumbar spinal cord enlargements. More than 90% of patients with arthrogryposis have anterior horn cell–related disease [Adams et al., 1988; Banker, 1985]. Most affected infants hold their arms rotated inwardly; elbow position varies. The forearms are held pronated, with ulnar deviation at the wrists. The hands are flexed, and the fingers are curled tightly. The thighs are usually externally rotated and flexed at the hips. There is either flexion or extension of the knees, but the feet are almost always positioned in an equinovarus deformity (Fig. 75-9). The limbs are slender (Fig. 75-10); conversely, the joints appear greatly enlarged (Fig. 75-11).

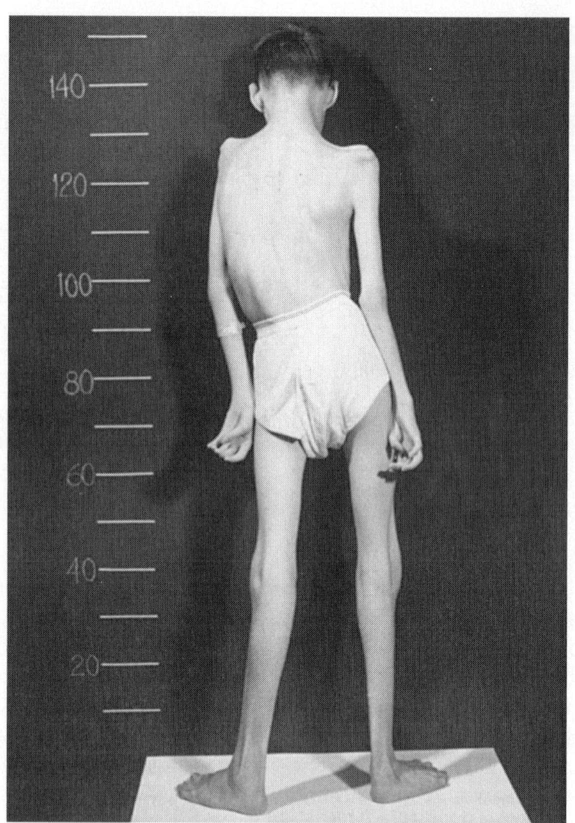

FIGURE 75-10. This patient with anterior cell arthrogryposis has had a number of orthopedic procedures. Marked scoliosis and generalized muscle wasting, particularly of the shoulder girdle, are clearly demonstrated.

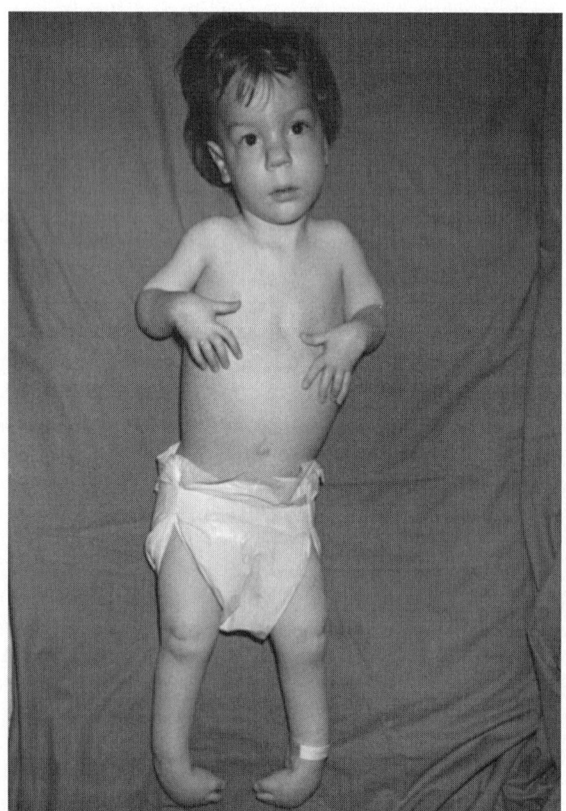

FIGURE 75-9. This 6-month-old male has the neurogenic form of arthrogryposis. The marked deformities of the ankles and feet are evident. There are flexion contractures of the wrists, elbows, and knees.

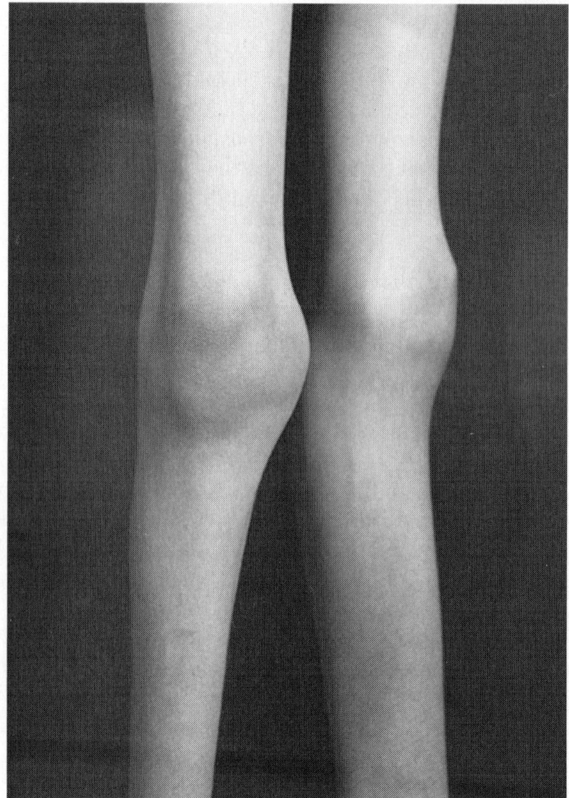

FIGURE 75-11. Close-up view of the knees of the patient in Figure 75-10. The knee joints, although of normal size, appear relatively enlarged because of the marked muscle wasting.

The patella may be very small or absent. Other abnormalities may include inguinal hernias, cleft palate, scoliosis, ankylosis of the temporomandibular joint, and cardiac malformations [Drachman and Banker, 1961].

Passive movement of the affected joints is possible, but only a small range is present. Deep tendon reflexes are not elicitable, and electromyographic examination confirms electrical abnormalities consistent with anterior horn cell impairment. The few available pathologic studies of the involved muscles revealed markedly decreased bulk [Drachman and Banker, 1961] or even absence [Adams et al., 1988]. Hip contractures develop from unopposed contraction of the iliopsoas muscles. Muscle spindles are normal. Few pathologic alterations are evident in endomysial connective tissue, but perimysial connective tissue may be decidedly increased. One affected member each in two sets of identical twins has been reported [Drachman and Banker, 1961].

Children with arthrogryposis associated with anterior horn cell disease present in infancy and may demonstrate autosomal recessive, sporadic, or X-linked inheritance. The genetically defined syndromes are described in Table 75-2. Pathologic features of arthrogryposis multiplex congenita associated with anterior horn cell dysfunction were studied in infants from two families. These infants had flexed elbows, extended wrists, acute flexion of the knee and hip joints, and bilateral talipes equinovarus [Hooshmand et al., 1971; Pena et al., 1968]. Postmortem examination documented nodular fibrosis of the anterior spinal roots along the entire length of the spinal cord and absence of myelin and axis cylinders. Central chromatolysis was evident in a few anterior cells; the morphologic changes were believed to be secondary to the anterior root lesions. The voluntary muscle exhibited neurogenic muscular atrophy. Identification of muscle tissue in some areas was impossible because of extensive replacement by fat [Pena et al., 1968].

A rare form of lethal arthrogryposis multiplex congenita related to abnormal Schwann cell development was reported [Charnas et al., 1988]. Contractures have accompanied neonatal myasthenia gravis, although anticholinesterase therapy does not improve them [Holmes et al., 1980; Smit and Barth, 1980].

Prenatal diagnosis has been done using ultrasound [Bonilla-Musoles et al., 2002; Stoll et al., 1991]. Newborns with arthrogryposis may have myotonic dystrophy [Sarnat et al., 1976]. The lower extremities are predominantly involved. These infants often have loose, wrinkled skin and a paucity of subcutaneous tissue. Neck muscle weakness precludes normal neck flexion. Serum creatine kinase activity may be elevated. Diagnosis can be confirmed by blood DNA analysis, which reveals an expansion of the triplet repeat in the myotonic dystrophy gene.

Considering the differential diagnosis, it is not surprising that muscle pathology varies greatly in arthrogryposis patients. All of the congenital myopathies have been associated with arthrogryposis, including central core disease, nemaline myopathy, and centronuclear myopathy, as well as congenital muscular dystrophy [Moerman et al., 1985; Quinn et al., 1991; Schmalbruch et al., 1987]. Selective distal arthrogryposis is more likely to be caused by specific muscle mutations [Sung et al., 2003a, 2003b]. Administration of anesthesia during surgical intervention may be complicated by malignant hyperthermia, especially in children with muscular dystrophy or central core disease [Baines et al., 1986].

Kuskokwim disease, named for the river delta on which the original cases were diagnosed, is a form of arthrogryposis in Alaskan Eskimos [Petajan et al., 1969]. Multiple contractures of the joints, commonly of the knees and ankles, characterize the disease. The primary pathologic process is associated with the connective tissue. There is no indication of myopathy, neuropathy, or motor cell disease. The disease manifests in the first decade of life and is transmitted as an autosomal-recessive trait. Contractures at the elbows and knees may be seen during the first few months of life. Accompanying internal tibial torsion and profound planovalgus occur. Flexion hip contractures are also present. The deep tendon reflexes are usually elicitable in the biceps and Achilles tendons but are frequently absent in the triceps and quadriceps tendons. Although one infant had a small cataract at 3 years of age, cataracts are uncommon in adults. Radiographic examinations have revealed cysts in the proximal long bones of several patients. Other patients have had pigmented nevi and diminished corneal reflexes. This form of arthrogryposis may be associated with webbed-neck or Klippel-Feil deformity and with anomalies of the genitourinary system [Beckerman and Buchino, 1978].

New information describing genes that control development of limb buds suggests that abnormalities in transcription factors may be theoretically responsible for some cases of arthrogryposis [Nelson et al., 1996; Roberts and Tabin, 1994]. In such cases, there would be no evidence of muscle or nerve disease, but muscle development in the limbs may be severely defective or absent (amyoplasia) [Sells et al., 1996]. To date, no such mutations have been found. On the other hand, mutations in contractile proteins, such as tropomyosin 2 and troponin I, have been shown to cause amyoplasia or distal arthrogryposis [Sung et al., 2003a, 2003b].

Orthopedic procedures performed on patients with arthrogryposis often provided sufficient alignment and stability of the legs to allow independent ambulation [Bennett et al., 1985; Fisher et al., 1970; Guidera and Drennan, 1985]. Nonsurgical casting and manipulation methods introduced by Penseti have replaced early surgical approaches in children with clubfoot deformity [Ponseti, 1998] but require careful follow-up and compliance to be successful [Dobbs et al., 2004]. Talectomy before walking ability is acquired is rarely done currently but may prove beneficial in severe clubfoot deformity [Joseph and Myerson, 2004]. Scoliosis may be a prominent problem and may require surgical correction [Daher et al., 1985b]. Some improvement in arm and hand function is usually possible with physical therapy and exercise. Anesthesia for these patients requires special consideration [Baines et al., 1986; Oberoi et al., 1987; Oda et al., 1990]. Otolaryngologic management may be necessary for poor suck reflex, omega-shaped epiglottis, airway compromise, achalasia, and micrognathia [Laureano and Rybak, 1990].

INFECTIOUS DISEASES

Poliomyelitis

Poliomyelitis is a viral disease of motor neurons caused by poliovirus. Nonparalytic poliomyelitis is the most common form of the disease. From a clinical standpoint, it is largely indistinguishable from other meningoencephalitides. About 25% of patients reported in one series had nonparalytic poliomyelitis, 50% had spinal poliomyelitis, about 12% had bulbar poliomyelitis, and 10% had bulbospinal involvement [Auld et al., 1960; Lepow and Spence, 1965].

Three immunologically different types of virus that do not produce cross-immunity have been isolated as causing poliomyelitis; infection with a specific type results in permanent immunity to that type. In many countries, immunization with killed-virus and attenuated live-virus vaccines has effectively ended the large-scale epidemics of the disease that previously occurred in the summer and early fall. Transmission of the virus is from human to human, primarily through secretions of the upper respiratory tract or through fecal contamination. In the United States, a few cases have occurred in adults whose immune status had diminished with time or in siblings not yet immunized; transmission could be traced to a child recently immunized with live vaccine.

Onset is indicated by signs of malaise, which are usually accompanied by muscular pains or stiffness. Headaches occur frequently, and symptoms of upper respiratory tract infection are common in children. The patient may experience some degree of nuchal rigidity and a low-grade fever as the disease progresses. Muscular tightness then becomes noticeable, primarily in the hamstring, thigh, and neck. Poliomyelitis characterized by a triad of fever, nuchal rigidity, and spasm of the back muscles may affect infants who are younger than 1 year of age [Abramson and Greenberg, 1955]. Spinal involvement is more common than bulbar involvement in infants. The course of the disease may range from slowly progressive to fulminating; the more rapid the progression, the more severe the eventual involvement.

The anterior horn cells are the prime target of the virus, and motor weakness is the hallmark of the clinical pattern. In most cases, the weakness is asymmetric. The incidence of quadriplegia and trunk muscle compromise is greater after the first year of life. Bulbar involvement is life threatening, resulting in embarrassment of the respiratory, autonomic, and circulatory centers of the brainstem and in profound weakness of the muscles of respiration and swallowing [Auld et al., 1960; Baker et al., 1950]. Poliomyelitis has occurred in utero on numerous occasions and can result in death during the neonatal period [Pugh and Dudgeon, 1954].

Clinical Laboratory Tests

Evidence of pleocytosis with mononuclear cells and a normal or slightly elevated protein concentration can usually be obtained through spinal fluid examination. Polymorphonuclear cells may become prevalent early in the course of the disease. The spinal fluid glucose content is usually normal. Direct analysis of cerebrospinal fluid for virus DNA makes diagnosis rapid and accurate.

Management

Treatment is supportive. Mechanical ventilation and support of circulation may be required in the presence of bulbar symptoms. Prolonged rehabilitation is generally the rule after patients have recovered from the acute stage of polio, and permanent motor deficits are common. Postpolio syndrome may begin two or more decades after the illness and is associated with progressive loss of strength and atrophy of an already affected limb. Its cause is unknown [Munsat, 1991a].

Other Viruses Causing Polio-like Paralysis

Although poliovirus immunization has led to marked reduction of this form of anterior horn cell disease, it is clear that many other viruses, including Epstein-Barr virus [Wong et al., 1999], enterovirus 71 [Hayward et al., 1989], ECHO (enteric cytopathogene human orphan) virus type 4 [Kopel et al., 1965], and coxsackievirus [Grist, 1962; Jarcho et al., 1963] are capable of causing a "polio-like syndrome." Most recently, West Nile virus has also been demonstrated to cause producing flaccid paralysis that localizes by examination, imaging, and electrophysiologically to the anterior horn cell [Solomon and Willison, 2003].

West Nile Poliomyelitis

West Nile virus is a single-strand RNA flavivirus that is transmitted between Culex mosquitoes and birds, with incidental infections developing in humans. It is endemic to Africa, the Middle East, and Southwest Asia. An epidemic in New York City in 1999 has led to the virus spreading across North America [Asnis et al., 2000, 2001]. There is a 5- to 15-day incubation period, and infection through blood productions has been documented [Pealer et al., 2003]. Most infections are asymptomatic, with 20% of affected patients developing a mild febrile illness.

Symptomatic infections are more common in adults older than 50 years but have been described in children. Systemic features include fever, nausea, vomiting, and headache, and meningoencephalitis is present in 63%. Cerebrospinal fluid studies find elevated protein, normal glucose, and pleocytosis [Petersen and Marfin, 2002]. Children with West Nile virus infection have less severe illnesses [Hayes and O'Leary, 2004].

Neurologic involvement develops in between 1 in 140 and 1 in 320 infections [Horga and Fine, 2001]. Weakness over days may be associated with encephalopathy. The weakness may involve the face and may be asymmetric involving a single limb. Sensory examination is normal, and electrophysiologic studies indicate normal conduction velocities but small compound muscle action potentials and asymmetric denervation changes [Al-Shekhlee and Katirji, 2004; Flaherty et al., 2003; Leis et al., 2002]. MRI changes are not uniformly present but may include cauda equina enhancement, spinal cord parenchymal signal abnormalities, and parenchymal or leptomeningeal signal changes in the brain [Heresi et al., 2004; Jeha et al., 2003]. Although most patients well studied electrophysiologically have localization to the anterior horn cells, a demyelinating, Guillain-Barré–like picture has also been described [Ahmed et al., 2000].

Although neurologic manifestations are less common in children, encephalitis and aseptic meningitis developed in two hospitalized children in the original outbreak [Horga and Fine, 2001]. The polio-like illness has been described in a single child [Heresi et al., 2004].

Pathologic features include perivascular and leptomeningeal inflammation, microglial nodules, and neuronophagia, involving the temporal lobes and brainstem in patients with meningoencephalitis [Kelley et al., 2003]. In patients with polio-like illness, similar findings are present in the spinal cord [Kelley et al., 2003; Sampson et al., 2003].

Diagnosis is confirmed by demonstrating rising immunoglobulin M titer to the virus. Although this test is sensitive, antibodies to West Nile virus may cross-react with dengue or St. Louis encephalitis, so that positive results should be confirmed using reverse-transcriptase polymerase chain reaction [Horga and Fine, 2001].

Transverse Myelitis Associated with Immune-Mediated Processes, Infection, or Both

Transverse myelitis associated with infection or associated immune-mediated processes is usually viral in origin, although other microorganisms may be involved. Many of the clinical characteristics of the infectious myelitides are similar, thus allowing for a general discussion.

The thoracic area of the cord is most often affected. The illness begins acutely and progresses quickly for 1 to 2 days. Early manifestations of spinal cord dysfunction may follow

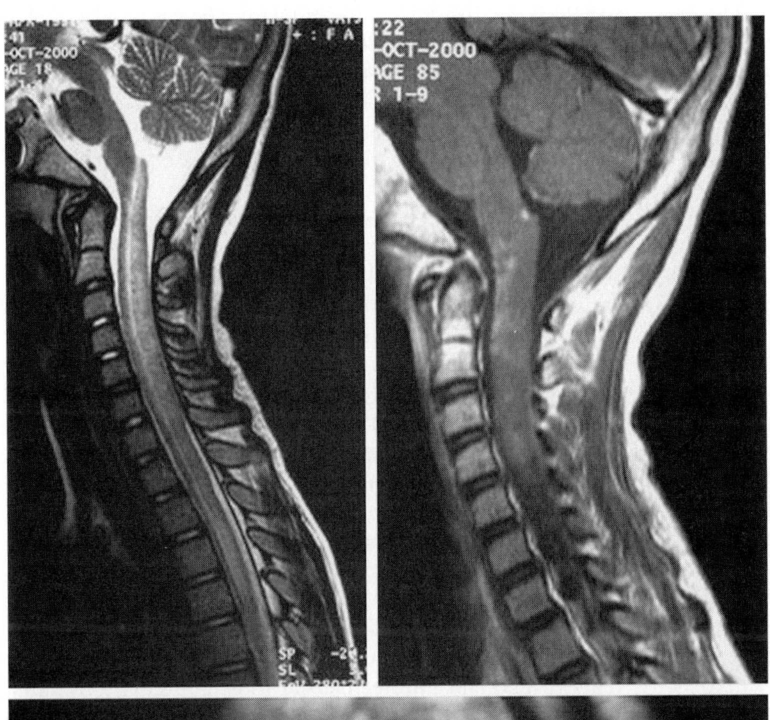

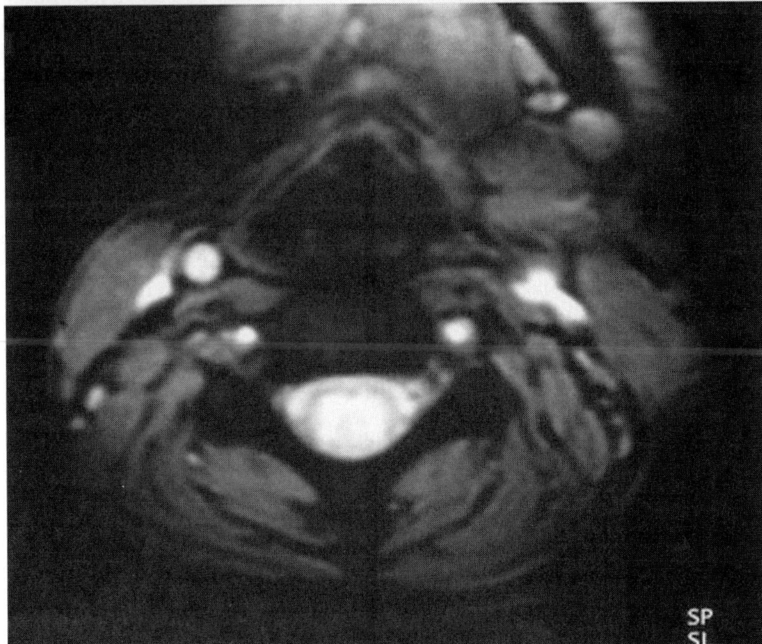

FIGURE 75-12. Magnetic resonance imaging findings in a child with transverse myelitis. Sagittal (**A**) and axial (**B**) T2-weighted images of the cervical cord demonstrate diffuse hyperintense signal from the obex to T4. **C,** Gadolinium-enhanced sagittal T1-weighted image demonstrates patchy enhancement of the cord over the same area.(From Andronikou S, Albuquerque-Jonathan G, Wilmshurst J, et al. MRI findings in acute idiopathic transverse myelopathy in children. Pediatr Radiol 2003;33:624.)

or be accompanied by fever, lethargy, malaise, and myalgia. Paresthesias of the legs are common. Back pain at the segmental level of the involved cord frequently occurs. Anterior horn cell disruption in the cervical or lumbar enlargements causes symptoms and signs of lower motor unit dysfunction in the arms and legs. The permanency of the weakness is not predictable from its characteristics. The sequence of involvement most often exhibited is weakness and even flaccidity of the legs with subsequent loss of rectal and bladder sphincter control. Sensory impairment usually extends to the segmental level of motor impairment. The transitional zone between the involved and uninvolved areas may be the site of dysesthesias and hyperalgesia. Deprivation of autonomic innervation below the cord lesion causes loss of sweating.

Recovery may be evident within a week of onset; more commonly, improvement may not occur for several weeks or months, if it occurs at all. Unfortunately, flaccidity in limbs innervated caudal to the spinal segment interruption may slowly transform into spasticity after several weeks. Consonant with the appearance of spasticity, hyperreflexia associated with ankle clonus and extensor toe signs may occur. Aggressive corticosteroid therapy may be beneficial.

Examination of cerebrospinal fluid usually reveals pleocytosis with a high percentage of lymphocytes. Protein content is usually normal, but a slight increase may occur when the rootlets or peripheral nerves are compromised. Glucose concentration is usually normal. Electromyographic examination may be normal or may demonstrate anterior horn cell dysfunction in the involved cord segments. MRI may depict the degree and extent of the lesion, with T2-weighted images indicating hyperintensity and patchy enhancement with gadolinium (Fig. 75-12) [Andronikou et al., 2003; Awerbuch et al., 1987]. Importantly, the severity of MRI involvement does not correlate with the severity of presentation or outcome [Andronikou et al., 2003].

Numerous viral and other infections, as well as other agents and processes, including immune-mediated phenomena that are associated with inflammation, have been implicated in transverse myelitis and accompanying anterior horn cell involvement. They include acquired multiple sclerosis [Rust, 2000], immune deficiency syndrome [Barakos et al., 1990], infectious mononucleosis [Clevenbergh et al., 1997; Grose and Feorino, 1973; Grose et al., 1975; Junker et al., 1991; Tsutsumi et al., 1994], mumps [Benady et al., 1973; Caksen and Ustunbas, 2003; Nussinovitch et al., 1992; Venketasubramanian, 1997], *Mycoplasma pneumoniae* infection [Candler and Dale, 2004; Francis et al., 1988; Parisi and Filice, 2001], rabies vaccination [Harrington and Olin, 1971; Label and Batts, 1982], smallpox vaccination [Shyamalan et al., 1964], rubella, rubeola, small pox [Booss and Davis, 2003], and varicella.

TRAUMA-RELATED ANTERIOR HORN CELL DISEASE

Incomplete or total transection of the spinal cord may follow birth trauma, falls, motor vehicle crashes, or blows to the spinal column. Neurologic dysfunction, reflected in diverse functional impairment, may result. Fractures or dislocations of the vertebrae are often present. The pattern of clinical involvement is determined by the areas of anatomic disruption. Therefore, signs and symptoms of corticospinal tract, posterior column, and lateral spinothalamic tract interruption may be present. Limb weakness, consonant with the segmental level of injury, and loss of deep and superficial sensations below that level are seen. Compromise of bladder function is common.

Findings characteristic of anterior horn cell dysfunction are evident in the limbs as a sequel to spinal cord trauma in the cervical or lumbosacral enlargements. Neurologic impairment resulting from trauma localized to the anterior horn cell column is unlikely unless the anterior spinal artery is the primary site of injury.

Trauma accompanying delivery, particularly in a breech presentation, usually affects the middle and lower cervical segments of the spinal cord [Abroms et al., 1973]. Radiographic documentation of dislocation or fracture of the spinal column is rare. Although flaccidity is present at birth, spasticity of the legs may gradually develop. The distribution of weakness in the arms and hands is variable. The pattern may be such that bilateral Erb's paralysis is erroneously diagnosed. The combination of compromise of the small muscles of the hands and paresis of the legs should suggest spinal cord involvement rather than brachial plexus injury.

Development of pectus excavatum in these patients results from unopposed diaphragmatic respiration by the intercostal muscles. The abdominal muscles are frequently weak, and protrusion of the abdomen occurs. Impairment of bladder function with resultant urinary retention followed by infection may become a major problem. Depending on the level of involvement, Horner's syndrome may be present. Decreased or absent perspiration below the segmental levels innervated by the upper thoracic nerves may alter temperature homeostasis, resulting in hyperthermia that may prove life threatening if the ambient temperature is high. Providing an air-conditioned environment may be obligatory for these infants.

Although motor vehicle crashes are the most common cause of traumatic spinal cord injury in infants and children, etiologies vary by age [Cirak et al., 2004]. Children 2 to 9 years of age had injuries caused most commonly by falls, and children 10 to 14 years of age had sports injuries as the most common cause [Cirak et al., 2004]. In neonates, many reports corroborate the relatively high risk for middle or lower cervical cord trauma during breech delivery when there is hyperextension of the head. In one report, complete transection of the cervical cord occurred in 21% of the 88 patients reviewed. None of the infants delivered by cesarean section sustained spinal cord injury [Abroms et al., 1973]. Other causes of spinal cord injury in the neonatal period, including ischemia, are common associated problems [Ruggieri et al., 1999]. Unfortunately, no specific treatment exists, although physical and occupational therapy may be helpful.

VASCULAR CONDITIONS

Anterior Spinal Artery Occlusion

The anterior spinal artery originates where the vertebral arteries meet and traverses the anterior median sulcus over the entire course of the spinal cord. The radicular arteries are divided into anterior and posterior radicular arteries. Blood from the anterior radicular arteries that enter with the nerve roots between the third cervical and third lumbar segments flows into the anterior spinal artery (Fig. 75-13). The anterior spinal artery is then further separated into several sulcal branches that pierce the central gray matter, perfuse the anterior horn cells, and then form numerous small penetrating vessels that supply the white matter of the anterior and lateral columns. Because the penetrating branches of the anterior spinal artery are end arteries, their occlusion results in infarction of the anterior half of the spinal cord. The anatomic relationship between the two posterior spinal arteries provides a much different vascular pattern for the posterior cord than the anterior spinal arteries do for the anterior cord. The posterior circulation has a more extensive collateral system. Therefore, occlusion of the posterior spinal arteries usually does not cause severe clinical dysfunction.

Steegman reported the clinical effects of obstruction of anterior spinal artery circulation [Steegman, 1952]. Occlusion of the anterior spinal artery often results from arteriosclerotic vascular disease in adults, a condition uncommon in children. However, certain childhood pathologic conditions may lead to similar obstruction of blood flow. Trauma and infectious conditions are among the most common causes of anterior spinal artery insufficiency in children [Blennow and Starck, 1987; Goebel and Muller, 1977]. Other causes include embolism from cardiac disease and thrombosis from hypercoagulable states [Oller-Navarro et al., 1979].

Compromise of blood circulation in rhesus monkeys occurring inferior to the first lumbar vertebra causes the development of a lesion that expands from the central gray matter toward the periphery [Fried and Aparicio, 1973]. The most devastated areas of infarction are found in the third and sixth lumbar segments. The region superior to the experimental ligation is relatively unaffected. The central gray matter is entirely infarcted. In the lesions that are associated with the greatest degree of destruction, only a thin rim of the peripheral white matter is preserved. In lesions that are less extensive, the neighboring circumferential white matter is disrupted. This occasional survival of the peripheral white matter and the lateral area of the anterior horn may result from perfusion from pial plexus vessels and vasa corona, both receiving blood supplies from the posterior spinal arteries. As much as 50% of the outer rim of white matter may receive its circulation from these sources [Fried and Aparicio, 1973].

Clinical findings associated with anterior spinal artery occlusion depend on the level at which the artery is occluded [Steegman, 1952]. Obstruction of the anterior spinal artery near its inception from the two vertebral arteries initiates brainstem compromise. Clinical findings may be unilateral but are usually bilateral. Loss of pain and temperature sensation and spastic quadriplegia occur and are commonly associated with some loss of superficial sensation inferior to the involved segmental level. Ischemia or infarction of the cervical spinal cord causes flaccid paralysis of the arms because of disruption of the anterior horn cells in the cervical enlargement. Weakness, muscle atrophy, and absence of deep tendon reflexes in the legs follow occlusion of the anterior spinal artery in the region of the lumbar enlargement.

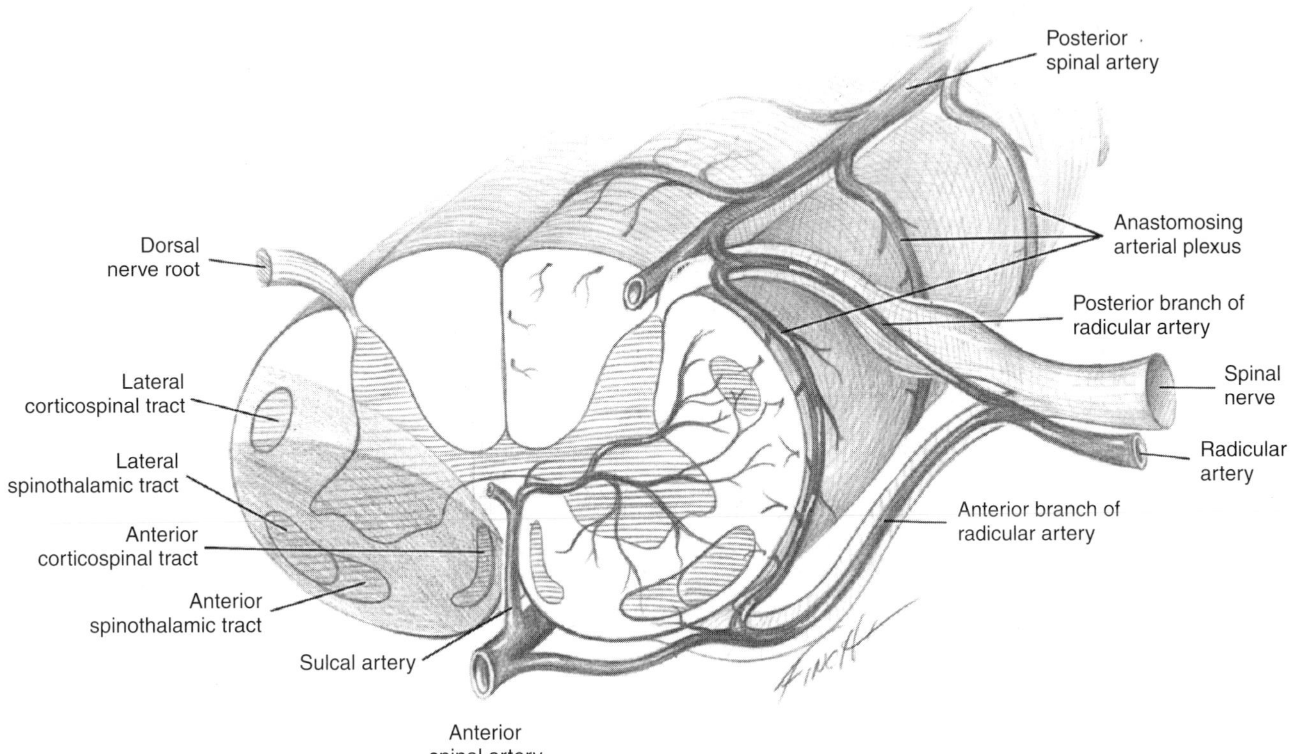

FIGURE 75-13. The anterior spinal artery supplies most of the anterior spinal cord as well as the lateral column area of the cord *(darkly shaded area)*. Some areas of the cord are supplied by both the anterior and posterior circulation *(light-gray shaded area)*; there is variation among individuals. The anterior horn cells and lateral spinothalamic tracts rely on the anterior spinal artery for blood supply.

Temperature and pain perception are often affected in the legs.

Pain and temperature perception can be lost while superficial sensation remains intact (dissociation of sensation) in the presence of certain lesions below the medulla because of the anatomic arrangement. The myelinated tracts subserving temperature and pain sensations cross in the anterior white commissure of the spinal cord; in this area of intersection, they are subject to damage when anterior spinal artery obstruction occurs. However, the tracts responsible for superficial sensation ascend in the cord without crossing and thus are not at risk when the anterior spinal artery is occluded.

Bladder function is impaired with occlusion of the anterior spinal artery, and dysfunction may become the most difficult treatment problem. Return of automatic and occasionally voluntary bladder function may occur after several weeks.

Tumors and congenital vascular malformations are among the conditions that must be considered in the differential diagnosis of anterior spinal artery interruption in children. Vascular syndromes of the spinal cord may be seen in association with coarctation of the aorta [Darwish et al., 1979; Owens and Swan, 1963; Servais et al., 2001]. During corrective surgery, blood flow must be maintained from the proximal to the distal portions of the aorta. Surgical anastomosis requires removal of the stenotic section of the aorta and establishment of an adequate anastomosis. One and occasionally two radicular arteries in the thoracic region originate in the aorta; they in turn provide blood flow for the anterior spinal artery through radicular branches. If the radicular artery is cut or clamped for a significant period during surgery, clinical findings of anterior spinal artery compromise may develop [Weenink and Smilde, 1964].

Sensory impairment may initially be severe after ischemia induced during surgery but tends to relent in the first few postoperative weeks; unfortunately, the motor deficits often remain. The deficits appear to mirror anterior horn cell dysfunction. This pattern may reflect the fact that the anterior horn cells are in the region of greatest oxidative metabolic dependency in the spinal cord [Dodson and Landau, 1973]. The anterior spinal artery syndrome has been reported with coarctation of the aorta in children who have not had surgical correction [Weenink and Smilde, 1964].

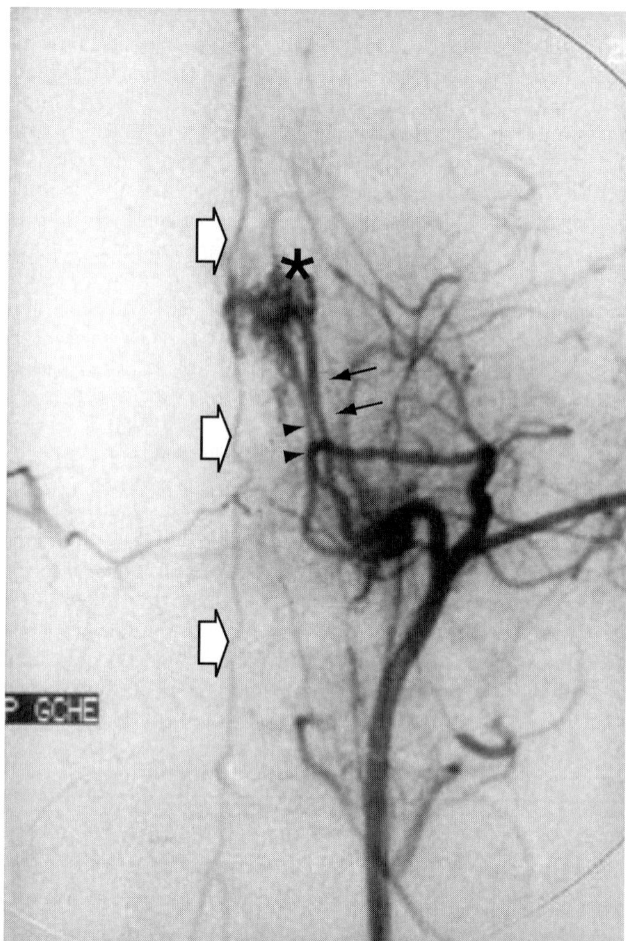

FIGURE 75-14. Angiogram of 11-year-old child with nidus-type arteriovenous malformation located at thoracic level 4. The lesion (*asterisk*) is supplied by a radiculomedullary artery (*arrowheads*), participating in the continuity of the anterior spinal axis (*open arrows*). The nidus drains through a radicular vein (*arrows*) toward the upper thoracic epidural plexuses. (From Rodesch G, Hurth M, Alvarez H, et al. Angio-architecture of spinal cord arteriovenous shunts at presentation. Clinical correlations in adults and children. The Bicetre experience on 155 consecutive patients seen between 1981–1999. Acta Neurochir [Wien] 2004;146:217.)

Spinal Cord Vascular Anomalies

Although arteriovenous malformations of the spinal cord are rare, symptoms during the first two decades of life develop in 20% of patients [Rodesch et al., 2004]. Of the 30 children in one large series, 21 presented with hemorrhage. In 11 of these, hematomyelia developed, and in 10, the hemorrhage was subarachnoid. Twenty of the 30 children had nidus-type arteriovenous malformations, and 10 had fistulous type (Fig. 75-14). The fistulous-type shunts were divided into microarteriovenous and macroarteriovenous fistulas. Five of the six with macroarteriovenous fistulas had hereditary hemorrhagic telengiectasia [Rodesch et al., 2004]. Infarction is accompanied by pain in the back or abdomen; the loss of strength and sensation in the legs may develop gradually or suddenly. The lower extremities become flaccid over the next 12 to 24 hours, and bladder control ceases [Buchanan and Walker, 1941]. During the next few weeks, the leg flaccidity gradually relents, only to be replaced by spasticity. Priapism, which may be intractable, may occur. Imaging studies and surgical exploration demonstrate a large mass of pulsating vessels in the spinal canal.

Despite anterior horn cell compromise, concurrent impairment of the corticospinal and spinothalamic tracts results in a clinical picture primarily of loss of temperature and pain perception and of upper motor unit dysfunction manifested by acute flaccidity that evolves into spasticity after several weeks. Lumbar puncture reveals normal cerebrospinal fluid pressure. The cerebrospinal fluid may be xanthochromic. Normal cerebrospinal fluid flow is often obstructed, with resultant marked elevation of protein content. Myelography may not faithfully depict the extent of the lesion. Angiography or magnetic resonance angiogram may be necessary for adequate visualization of the arteriovenous malformation [Pattany et al., 2003; Tobin and Layton, 1976]. Based on angiography, three types of lesions have been described: single coiled vessel, glomus, and juvenile. CT and MRI may be most useful in delineating the vascular lesions. The relative benefit of surgery is determined by such factors as residual damage, number of feeding vessels, and extent and pattern of the abnormal vessels within the mass.

ACKNOWLEDGMENT

We would like to thank Dr. Alan Pestronk of the Neuromuscular Disease Center, Washington University School of Medicine, St. Louis, MO. (World Wide Web URL: http://www.neuro.wustl.edu/neuromuscular/.)

REFERENCES

Abel R, Gerner HJ, Smit C, et al. Residual deformity of the spinal canal in patients with traumatic paraplegia and secondary changes of the spinal cord. Spinal Cord 1999;37:14.

Abramson H, Greenberg M. Acute poliomyelitis in infants under one year of age: Epidemiological and clinical features. Pediatrics 1955;16:478.

Abroms IF, Bresnan MJ, Zuckerman JE, et al. Cervical cord injuries secondary to hyperextension of the head in breech presentations. Obstet Gynecol 1973;41:369.

Adams C, Becker LE, Murphy EG. Neurogenic arthrogryposis multiplex congenita: Clinical and muscle biopsy findings. Pediatr Neurosci 1988;14:97.

Ahmed S, Libman R, Wesson K, et al. Guillain-Barre syndrome: An unusual presentation of West Nile virus infection. Neurology 2000;55:144.

Al-Chalabi A, Andersen PM, Nilsson P, et al. Deletions of the heavy neurofilament subunit tail in amyotrophic lateral sclerosis. Hum Mol Genet 1999;8:157.

Al-Shekhlee A, Katirji B. Electrodiagnostic features of acute paralytic poliomyelitis associated with West Nile virus infection. Muscle Nerve 2004;29:376.

Alexander MP, Emery ES 3rd, Koerner FC. Progressive bulbar paresis in childhood. Arch Neurol 1976;33:66.

Allen LM, Silverman RK. Prenatal ultrasound evaluation of fetal diastematomyelia: Two cases of type I split cord malformation. Ultrasound Obstet Gynecol 2000;15:78.

Alpers B, Comroe B. Syringomyelia with choked disk. J Nerv Ment Dis 1931;73:577.

Andreassi C, Jarecki J, Zhou J, et al. Aclarubicin treatment restores SMN levels to cells derived from type I spinal muscular atrophy patients. Hum Mol Genet 2001;10:2841.

Andronikou S, Albuquerque-Jonathan G, Wilmshurst J, et al. MRI findings in acute idiopathic transverse myelopathy in children. Pediatr Radiol 2003;33:624.

Appelbaum JS, Roos RP, Salazar-Grueso EF, et al. Intrafamilial heterogeneity in hereditary motor neuron disease. Neurology 1992;42:1488.

Aprin H, Bowen JR, MacEwen GD, et al. Spine fusion in patients with spinal muscular atrophy. J Bone Joint Surg Am 1982;64:1179.

Asnis DS, Conetta R, Teixeira AA, et al. The West Nile Virus outbreak of 1999 in New York: The Flushing Hospital experience. Clin Infect Dis 2000;30:413.

Asnis DS, Conetta R, Waldman G, et al. The West Nile virus encephalitis outbreak in the United States (1999–2000): From Flushing, New York, to beyond its borders. Ann N Y Acad Sci 2001;951:161.

Auld PA, Kevy SV, Eley RC. Poliomyelitis in children. Experience with 956 cases in the 1955 Massachusetts epidemic. N Engl J Med 1960;263:1093.

Awerbuch G, Feinberg WM, Ferry P, et al. Demonstration of acute post-viral myelitis with magnetic resonance imaging. Pediatr Neurol 1987;3:367.

Bach JR. Update and perspective on noninvasive respiratory muscle aids. Part 2: The expiratory aids. Chest 1994;105:1538.

Bach JR, Alba AS. Management of chronic alveolar hypoventilation by nasal ventilation. Chest 1990;97:52.

Bach JR, Alba AS. Intermittent abdominal pressure ventilator in a regimen of noninvasive ventilatory support. Chest 1991;99:630.

Baines DB, Douglas ID, Overton JH. Anaesthesia for patients with arthrogryposis multiplex congenita: What is the risk of malignant hyperthermia? Anaesth Intensive Care 1986;14:370.

Baker AB, Matzke HA, Brown JR. Bulbar poliomyelitis: A study of medullary function. Arch Neurol Psychiatry 1950;63:257.

Balci S, Oguz KK, Firat MM, et al. Cervical diastematomyelia in cervico-oculo-acoustic (Wildervanck) syndrome: MRI findings. Clin Dysmorphol 2002;11:125.

Banker BQ. Neuropathologic aspects of arthrogryposis multiplex congenita. Clin Orthop 1985;194:30.

Banker BQ. Arthrogryposis multiplex congenita: Spectrum of pathologic changes. Hum Pathol 1986;17:656.

Banker BQ. The congenital muscular dystrophies. In: Engel AG, Franzini-Armstrong C, eds. Myology, Vol. 2. New York: McGraw-Hill, 1994;1275.

Barakos JA, Mark AS, Dillon WP, et al. MR imaging of acute transverse myelitis and AIDS myelopathy. J Comput Assist Tomogr 1990;14:45.

Barth PG. Pontocerebellar hypoplasias. An overview of a group of inherited neurodegenerative disorders with fetal onset. Brain Dev 1993;15:411.

Beckerman RC, Buchino JJ. Arthrogryposis multiplex congenita as part of an inherited symptom complex: Two case reports and a review of the literature. Pediatrics 1978;61:417.

Belsham DD, Yee WC, Greenberg CR, et al. Analysis of the CAG repeat region of the androgen receptor gene in a kindred with X-linked spinal and bulbar muscular atrophy. J Neurol Sci 1992;112:133.

Benady S, Zvi AB, Szabo G. Transverse myelitis following mumps. Acta Paediatr Scand 1973;62:205.

Bennett JB, Hansen PE, Granberry WM, et al. Surgical management of arthrogryposis in the upper extremity. J Pediatr Orthop 1985;5:281.

Berke JP, Magee KR. Craniofacial dysostosis with syringomyelia and associated anomalies. Arch Neurol 1976;33:63.

Bertrand G. Dynamic factors in the evolution of syringomyelia and syringobulbia. Clin Neurosurg 1973;20:322.

Birnkrant DJ, Pope JF, Martin JE, et al. Treatment of type I spinal muscular atrophy with noninvasive ventilation and gastrostomy feeding. Pediatr Neurol 1998;18:407.

Blair IP, Bennett CL, Abel A, et al. A gene for autosomal dominant juvenile amyotrophic lateral sclerosis (ALS4) localizes to a 500-kb interval on chromosome 9q34. Neurogenetics 2000;3:1.

Blennow G, Starck L. Anterior spinal artery syndrome. Report of seven cases in childhood. Pediatr Neurosci 1987;13:32.

Boltshauser E, Lang W, Spillmann T, et al. Hereditary distal muscular atrophy with vocal cord paralysis and sensorineural hearing loss: A dominant form of spinal muscular atrophy? J Med Genet 1989;26:105.

Bonilla-Musoles F, Machado LE, Osborne NG. Multiple congenital contractures (congenital multiple arthrogryposis). J Perinat Med 2002;30:99.

Booss J, Davis LE. Smallpox and smallpox vaccination: Neurological implications. Neurology 2003;60:1241.

Borchelt DR, Wong PC, Sisodia SS, et al. Transgenic mouse models of Alzheimer's disease and amyotrophic lateral sclerosis. Brain Pathol 1998;8:735.

Bove KE, Iannaccone ST. Atypical infantile spinomuscular atrophy presenting as acute diaphragmatic paralysis. Pediatr Pathol 1988;8:95.

Brichta L, Hofmann Y, Hahnen E, et al. Valproic acid increases the SMN2 protein level: A well-known drug as a potential therapy for spinal muscular atrophy. Hum Mol Genet 2003:12:2481.

Brodbelt AR, Stoodley MA, Watling A, et al. The role of excitotoxic injury in post-traumatic syringomyelia. J Neurotrauma 2003a;20:883.

Brodbelt AR, Stoodley MA, Watling AM, et al. Altered subarachnoid space compliance and fluid flow in an animal model of posttraumatic syringomyelia. Spine 2003b;28:E413.

Brodbelt AR, Stoodley MA, Watling AM, et al. Fluid flow in an animal model of post-traumatic syringomyelia. Eur Spine J 2003c;12:300.

Bromberg MB, Swoboda KJ. Motor unit number estimation in infants and children with spinal muscular atrophy. Muscle Nerve 2002;25:445.

Brown CH. Infantile amyotrophic lateral sclerosis of the family type. J Nerv Ment Dis 1894;21:707.

Bruhl K, Schwarz M, Schumacher R, et al. Congenital diastematomyelia in the upper thoracic spine. Diagnostic comparison of CT, CT-myelography, MRI, and US. Neurosurg Rev 1990;13:77.

Brzustowicz LM, Lehner T, Castilla LH, et al. Genetic mapping of chronic childhood-onset spinal muscular atrophy to chromosome 5q11.2-13.3. Nature 1990;344:540.

Buchanan DN, Walker AE. Vascular anomalies of the spinal cord in children. Am J Dis Child 1941;61:928.

Burghes AH. When is a deletion not a deletion? When it is converted. Am J Hum Genet 1997;61:9.

Byers RK, Banker BQ. Infantile muscular atrophy. Arch Neurol 1961;5:140.
Caksen H, Ustunbas HB. A fatal case of acute transverse myelitis associated with mumps. J Emerg Med 2003;24:341.
Campbell L, Potter A, Ignatius J, et al. Genomic variation and gene conversion in spinal muscular atrophy: Implications for disease process and clinical phenotype. Am J Hum Genet 1997:61:40.
Candler PM, Dale RC. Three cases of central nervous system complications associated with Mycoplasma pneumoniae. Pediatr Neurol 2004;31:133.
Carboni P, Pisani F, Crescenzi A, et al. Congenital hypotonia with favorable outcome. Pediatr Neurol 2002;26:383.
Carducci MA, Gilbert J, Bowling MK, et al. A phase I clinical and pharmacological evaluation of sodium phenylbutyrate on an 120-h infusion schedule. Clin Cancer Res 2001;7:3047.
Cartegni L, Krainer AR. Disruption of an SF2/ASF-dependent exonic splicing enhancer in SMN2 causes spinal muscular atrophy in the absence of SMN1. Nat Genet 2002;30:377.
Chance PF, Rabin BA, Ryan SG, et al. Linkage of the gene for an autosomal dominant form of juvenile amyotrophic lateral sclerosis to chromosome 9q34. Am J Hum Genet 1998;62:633.
Chang JG, Hsieh-Li HM, Jong YJ, et al. Treatment of spinal muscular atrophy by sodium butyrate. Proc Natl Acad Sci U S A 2001;98:9808.
Charnas L, Trapp B, Griffin J. Congenital absence of peripheral myelin: Abnormal Schwann cell development causes lethal arthrogryposis multiplex congenita. Neurology 1988;38:966.
Chen YZ, Bennett CL, Huynh HM, et al. DNA/RNA helicase gene mutations in a form of juvenile amyotrophic lateral sclerosis (ALS4). Am J Hum Genet 2004;74:1128.
Choi WT, MacLean HE, Chu S, et al. Kennedy's disease: Genetic diagnosis of an inherited form of motor neuron disease. Aust N Z J Med 1993;23:187.
Chou SM. Controversy over Werdnig-Hoffmann disease and multiple system atrophy. Curr Opin Neurol 1993;6:861.
Chou SM, Gilbert EF, Chun RW, et al. Infantile olivopontocerebellar atrophy with spinal muscular atrophy (infantile OPCA + SMA). Clin Neuropathol 1990;9:21.
Christodoulou K, Kyriakides T, Hristova AH, et al. Mapping of a distal form of spinal muscular atrophy with upper limb predominance to chromosome 7p. Hum Mol Genet 1995;4:1629.
Christodoulou K, Zamba E, Tsingis M, et al. A novel form of distal hereditary motor neuronopathy maps to chromosome 9p21.1-p12. Ann Neurol 2000;48:877.
Cirak B, Ziegfeld S, Knight VM, et al. Spinal injuries in children. J Pediatr Surg 2004;39:607.
Clevenbergh P, Brohee P, Velu T, et al. Infectious mononucleosis complicated by transverse myelitis: Detection of the viral genome by polymerase chain reaction in the cerebrospinal fluid. J Neurol 1997;244:592.
Coovert DD, Le TT, McAndrew PE, et al. The survival motor neuron protein in spinal muscular atrophy. Hum Mol Genet 1997;6:1205.
Cowie TN. Diastematomyelia with vertebral column defects:observations on its radiological diagnosis. Br J Radiol 1951;24:156.
Coyle JT, Puttfarcken P. Oxidative stress, glutamate, and neurodegenerative disorders. Science 1993;262:689.
Daher YH, Lonstein JE, Winter RB, et al. Spinal surgery in spinal muscular atrophy. J Pediatr Orthop 1985a;5:391.
Daher YH, Lonstein JE, Winter RB, et al. Spinal deformities in patients with arthrogryposis. A review of 16 patients. Spine 1985b;10:609.
Darwish H, Archer C, Modin J. The anterior spinal artery collateral in coarctation of the aorta. A clinical angiographic correlation. Arch Neurol 1979;36:240.
de Muelenaere C. Misoprostol and Möbius syndrome. S Afr Med J 1999;89:12.
DeLong R, Siddique T. A large New England kindred with autosomal dominant neurogenic scapuloperoneal amyotrophy with unique features. Arch Neurol 1992;49:905.
Deng HX, Hentati A, Tainer JA, et al. Amyotrophic lateral sclerosis and structural defects in Cu,Zn superoxide dismutase. Science 1993;261:1047.
DiDonato CJ, Brun T, Simard LR. Complete nucleotide sequence, genomic organization, and promoter analysis of the murine survival motor neuron gene (Smn). Mamm Genome 1999;10:638.
Dobbs MB, Rudzki JR, Purcell DB, et al. Factors predictive of outcome after use of the Ponseti method for the treatment of idiopathic clubfeet. J Bone Joint Surg Am 2004;86:22.
Dodson WE, Landau WM. Motor neuron loss due to aortic clamping in repair of coarctation. Neurology 1973;23:539.
Drachman DB, Banker BQ. Arthrogryposis multiplex congenita. Case due to disease of the anterior horn cells. Arch Neurol 1961;5:77.
Dubowitz V. Infantile muscular strophy. A prospective study with particular reference to a slowly progressive variety. Brain 1964;87:707.
Dubowitz V. The floppy infant: A practical approach to classification. Dev Med Child Neurol 1968;10:706.
Dubowitz V. Disorders of the lower motor neurone: The spinal muscular atrophies. In: Dubowitz V, ed. Muscular disorders in childhood. London: WB Saunders, 1995.
Dubowitz V. 38th ENMC International Workshop. Spinal muscular atrophy trial group 10–12 December 1995, Naarden, The Netherlands. Neuromuscul Disord 1996;6:293.
Ellsworth RE, Ionasescu V, Searby C, et al. The CMT2D locus: Refined genetic position and construction of a bacterial clone-based physical map. Genome Res 1999;9:568.
Emery AE. Population frequencies of neuromuscular diseases. II. Amyotrophic lateral sclerosis (motor neurone disease). Neuromuscul Disord 1991;1:323.
Emery ES, Fenichel GM, Eng G. A spinal muscular atrophy with scapuloperoneal distribution. Arch Neurol 1968;18:129.
Eng GD, Binder H, Koch B. Spinal muscular atrophy: Experience in diagnosis and rehabilitation management of 60 patients. Arch Phys Med Rehabil 1984;65:549.
Eymard-Pierre E, Lesca G, Dollet S, et al. Infantile-onset ascending hereditary spastic paralysis is associated with mutations in the alsin gene. Am J Hum Genet 2002;71:518.
Fazio M. Ereditarieta della paralisi bulbare progressiva. Riforma Med 1892;8:327.
Fidzianska A. Morphological differences between the atrophied small muscle fibres in amyotrophic lateral sclerosis and Werdnig-Hoffmann disease. Acta Neuropathol (Berl) 1976;34:321.
Fidzianska A, Rafalowska J. Motoneuron death in normal and spinal muscular atrophy-affected human fetuses. Acta Neuropathol (Berl) 2002;104:363.
Finder JD, Birnkrant D, Carl J, et al. Respiratory care of the patient with Duchenne muscular dystrophy: ATS consensus statement. Am J Respir Crit Care Med 2004;170:456.
Fischbeck KH, Ionasescu V, Ritter AW, et al. Localization of the gene for X-linked spinal muscular atrophy. Neurology 1986;36:1595.
Fischer U, Liu Q, Dreyfuss G. The SMN-SIP1 complex has an essential role in spliceosomal snRNP biogenesis. Cell 1997;90:1023.
Fisher RL, Johnstone WT, Fisher WH Jr, et al. Arthrogryposis multiplex congenita: A clinical investigation. J Pediatr 1970;76:255.
Flaherty ML, Wijdicks EF, Stevens JC, et al. Clinical and electrophysiologic patterns of flaccid paralysis due to West Nile virus. Mayo Clin Proc 2003;78:1245.
Fleury P, Hageman G. A dominantly inherited lower motor neuron disorder presenting at birth with associated arthrogryposis. J Neurol Neurosurg Psychiatry 1985;48:1037.
Francis DA, Brown A, Miller DH, et al. MRI appearances of the CNS manifestations of Mycoplasma pneumoniae: A report of two cases. J Neurol 1988;235:441.
Fried LC, Aparicio O. Experimental ischemia of the spinal cord. Histologic studies after anterior spinal artery occlusion. Neurology 1973;23:289.
Frugier T, Tiziano FD, Cifuentes-Diaz C, et al. Nuclear targeting defect of SMN lacking the C-terminus in a mouse model of spinal muscular atrophy. Hum Mol Genet 2000;9:849.
Furukawa T, Nakao K, Sugita H, et al. Kugelberg-Welander disease with particular reference to sex-influenced manifestations. Arch Neurol 1968;19:156.
Gallai V, Hockaday JM, Hughes JT, et al. Ponto-bulbar Palsy with deafness (Brown-Vialetto-Van Laer syndrome): A report on three cases. J Neurol Sci 1981;50:259.
Gardner WJ. Myelomeningocele, the result of rupture of the embryonic neural tube. Cleve Clin Q 1960;27:88.
Gardner WJ. Hydrodynamic mechanism of syringomyelia: Its relationship to myelocele. J Neurol Neurosurg Psychiatry 1965;28:247.
Gavrilov DK, Shi X, Das K, et al. Differential SMN2 expression associated with SMA severity. Nat Genet 1998;20:230.
Gennarelli M, Lucarelli M, Capon F, et al. Survival motor neuron gene transcript analysis in muscles from spinal muscular atrophy patients. Biochem Biophys Res Commun 1995;213:342.

Gillespie JE, Jenkins JP, Metcalfe RA, et al. Magnetic resonance imaging in syringomyelia. Acta Radiol Suppl 1986;369:239.

Gilliam TC, Brzustowicz LM, Castilla LH, et al. Genetic homogeneity between acute and chronic forms of spinal muscular atrophy. Nature 1990;345:823.

Goebel HH, Muller J. The unusual features of traumatic neurogenic muscular atrophy in the infant: an anatomic study. Neuropadiatrie 1977;8:274.

Goldberg AB, Greenberg MB, Darney PD. Misoprostol and pregnancy. N Engl J Med 2001;344:38.

Gomez MR, Clermont V, Bernstein J. Progressive bulbar paralysis in childhood (Fazio-Londe's disease). Report of a case with pathologic evidence of nuclear atrophy. Arch Neurol 1962;6:317.

Gorgen-Pauly U, Sperner J, Reiss I, et al. Familial pontocerebellar hypoplasia type I with anterior horn cell disease. Eur J Paediatr Neurol 1999;3:33.

Greenberg F, Fenolio KR, Hejtmancik JF, et al. X-linked infantile spinal muscular atrophy. Am J Dis Child 1988;142:217.

Greenfield JG, Stern RO. The anatomical identity of the Werdnig-Hoffmann and Oppenheim forms of infantile muscular atrophy. Brain 1927;(652).

Grist NR. Type A7 Coxsackie (type 4 poliomyelitis) virus infection in Scotland. J Hyg (Lond) 1962;60:323.

Groger H. The founders of child neurology. San Francisco: Norman Publishing, 1990.

Grohmann K, Varon R, Stolz P, et al. Infantile spinal muscular atrophy with respiratory distress type 1 (SMARD1). Ann Neurol 2003;54:719.

Gros-Louis F, Lariviere R, Gowing G, et al. A frameshift deletion in peripherin gene associated with amyotrophic lateral sclerosis. J Biol Chem 2004;279:45951.

Gros-Louis F, Meijer IA, Hand CK, et al. An ALS2 gene mutation causes hereditary spastic paraplegia in a Pakistani kindred. Ann Neurol 2003;53:144.

Grose C, Feorino PM. Epstein-Barr virus and transverse myelitis. Lancet 1973;1:892.

Grose C, Henle W, Henle G, et al. Primary Epstein-Barr-virus infections in acute neurologic diseases. N Engl J Med 1975;292:392.

Guidera KJ, Drennan JC. Foot and ankle deformities in arthrogryposis multiplex congenita. Clin Orthop 1985;194:93.

Guinter RH, Hernried LS, Kaplan AM. Infantile neurogenic muscular atrophy with prolonged survival. J Pediatr 1977;90:95.

Guthkelch AN, Hoffmann GT. Tethered spinal cord in association with diastematomyelia. Surg Neurol 1981;15:352.

Hadano S, Hand CK, Osuga H, et al. A gene encoding a putative GTPase regulator is mutated in familial amyotrophic lateral sclerosis 2. Nat Genet 2001;29:166.

Hader WJ, Steinbok P, Poskitt K, et al. Intramedullary spinal teratoma and diastematomyelia. Case report and review of the literature. Pediatr Neurosurg 1999;30:140.

Hageman G, Willemse J, van Ketel BA, et al. The pathogenesis of fetal hypokinesia. A neurological study of 75 cases of congenital contractures with emphasis on cerebral lesions. Neuropediatrics 1987;18:22.

Hall JG. Arthrogryposis multiplex congenita: Etiology, genetics, classification, diagnostic approach, and general aspects. J Pediatr Orthop B 1997;6:159.

Hand CK, Khoris J, Salachas F, et al. A novel locus for familial amyotrophic lateral sclerosis, on chromosome 18q. Am J Hum Genet 2002;70:251.

Harpey JP, Charpentier C, Paturneau-Jouas M, et al. Secondary metabolic defects in spinal muscular atrophy type II. Lancet 1990;336:629.

Harrington RB, Olin R. Incomplete transverse myelitis following rabies duck embryo vaccination. JAMA 1971;216:2137.

Harwood-Nash DC, McHugh K. Diastematomyelia in 172 children: The impact of modern neuroradiology. Pediatr Neurosurg 1990;16:247.

Hausmanowa-Petrusewicz I, Askanas W, Badurska B, et al. Infantile and juvenile spinal muscular atrophy. J Neurol Sci 1968;6:269.

Hausmanowa-Petrusewicz I, Friedman A, Kowalski J, et al. Spontaneous motor unit firing in spinal muscular atrophy of childhood. Electromyogr Clin Neurophysiol 1987;27:259.

Hausmanowa-Petrusewicz I, Jozwik A. The application of the nearest neighbor decision rule in the evaluation of electromyogram in spinal muscular atrophy (SMA) of childhood. Electromyogr Clin Neurophysiol 1986;26:689.

Hausmanowa-Petrusewicz I, Zaremba J, Borkowska J, et al. Chronic proximal spinal muscular atrophy of childhood and adolescence: Sex influence. J Med Genet 1984;21:447.

Hayes EB, O'Leary DR. West Nile virus infection: A pediatric perspective. Pediatrics 2004;113:1375.

Hayward JC, Gillespie SM, Kaplan KM, et al. Outbreak of poliomyelitis-like paralysis associated with enterovirus 71. Pediatr Infect Dis J 1989;8:611.

Hennekam RC, Barth PG, Van Lookeren Campagne W, et al. A family with severe X-linked arthrogryposis. Eur J Pediatr 1991;150:656.

Hentati A, Ouahchi K, Pericak-Vance MA, et al. Linkage of a commoner form of recessive amyotrophic lateral sclerosis to chromosome 15q15-q22 markers. Neurogenetics 1998;2:55.

Heresi GP, Mancias P, Mazur LJ, et al. Poliomyelitis-like syndrome in a child with West Nile virus infection. Pediatr Infect Dis J 2004;23:788.

Hilal SK, Marton D, Pollack E. Diastematomyelia in children. Radiographic study of 34 cases. Radiology 1974;112:609.

Hoffmann J. Ueber familiare progressive spinale muskelatrophie. Arch Psych (Berlin) 1892a;24:644.

Hoffmann J. Ueber chronische spinale muskelatrophieim kindesalter auf familiare basis. Dtsch Zeit Nervenheilk 1892b;3.

Hoffmann J. Weiterer beitrag zur lehre von der hereditaren progressiven spinalen muskelatrophie im kindesalter nebst bemerkungen (ber den fortschreitenden muskelschwund im Allgemeinen. Dtsch Zeit Nervenheilk 1896;10:292.

Hoffmann J. Dritter beitrag zur lehre bon der hereditaren progressiven spinalen muskelatrophie im kindesalter. Dtsch Zeit Nervenheilk 1900a;18:217.

Hoffmann J. Uber die hereditare progressive spinal muskelatrophie im kindesalter. Munch Med Wschr 1900b;47:1649.

Holmes LB, Driscoll SG, Bradley WG. Contractures in a newborn infant of a mother with myasthenia gravis. J Pediatr 1980;96:1067.

Hooshmand H, Martinez AJ, Rosenblum WI. Arthrogryposis multiplex congenita. Simultaneous involvement of peripheral nerve and skeletal muscle. Arch Neurol 1971;24:561.

Horga MA, Fine A. West Nile virus. Pediatr Infect Dis J 2001;20:801.

Hosler BA, Siddique T, Sapp PC, et al. Linkage of familial amyotrophic lateral sclerosis with frontotemporal dementia to chromosome 9q21-q22. JAMA 2000;284:1664.

Hsieh-Li HM, Chang JG, Jong YJ, et al. A mouse model for spinal muscular atrophy. Nat Genet 2000;24:66.

Iannaccone ST, Browne RH, Samaha FJ, et al. Prospective study of spinal muscular atrophy before age 6 years. DCN/SMA Group. Pediatr Neurol 1993;9:187.

Iannaccone ST, Caneris O, Hoffman J. Founders of child neurology. San Francisco: Norman Publishing, 1990.

Iannaccone ST, Russman BS, Samaha F. Spinal muscular atrophy: Functional testing before age five. Ann Neurol 1991;30:502.

Inoue M, Nakata Y, Minami S, et al. Idiopathic scoliosis as a presenting sign of familial neurologic abnormalities. Spine 2003;28:40.

Iqbal JB, Bradey N, Macfaul R, et al. Syringomyelia in children: Six case reports and review of the literature. Br J Neurosurg 1992;6:13.

Irobi J, Van den Bergh P, Merlini L, et al. The phenotype of motor neuropathies associated with BSCL2 mutations is broader than Silver syndrome and distal HMN type V. Brain 2004a;127:2124.

Irobi J, Van Impe K, Seeman P, et al. Hot-spot residue in small heat-shock protein 22 causes distal motor neuropathy. Nat Genet 2004b;36:597.

Isozumi K, DeLong R, Kaplan J, et al. Linkage of scapuloperoneal spinal muscular atrophy to chromosome 12q24.1-q24.31. Hum Mol Genet 1996;5:1377.

Isu T, Chono Y, Iwasaki Y, et al. Scoliosis associated with syringomyelia presenting in children. Childs Nerv Syst 1992;8:97.

Isu T, Iwasaki Y, Akino M, et al. Hydrosyringomyelia associated with a Chiari I malformation in children and adolescents. Neurosurgery 1990;26:591; discussion, 596.

Jaeger HJ, Schmitz-Stolbrink A, Mathias KD. Cervical diastematomyelia and syringohydromyelia in a myelomeningocele patient. Eur Radiol 1997;7:477.

James CC, Lassman LP. Diastematomyelia. A critical survey of 24 cases submitted to laminectomy. Arch Dis Child 1964;39:125.

Jansen PH, Joosten EM, Jaspar HH, et al. A rapidly progressive autosomal dominant scapulohumeral form of spinal muscular atrophy. Ann Neurol 1986;20:538.

Jarcho LW, Fred HL, Castle CH. Encephalitis and polio-myelitis in the adult due to Coxsackie virus group B, type 5. N Engl J Med 1963;268:235.

Jarecki J, Chen J, Whitney M, et al. Identification and profiling of compounds that increase full-length SMN mRNA levels, Vol. 6. Sixth Annual International Spinal Muscular Atrophy Research Group Meeting. 2002:34.

Jeha LE, Sila CA, Lederman RJ, et al. West Nile virus infection: A new acute paralytic illness. Neurology 2003:61:55.

Johnson WG, Hogan E, Hanson PA, et al. Prognosis of late-onset hexosaminidase deficiency with spinal muscular atrophy. Neurology 1983;33[Suppl 2]:155.

Johnson WG, Wigger HJ, Karp HR, et al. Juvenile spinal muscular atrophy: A new hexosaminidase deficiency phenotype. Ann Neurol 1982;11:11.

Joseph TN, Myerson MS. Use of talectomy in modern foot and ankle surgery. Foot Ankle Clin 2004;9:775.

Junker AK, Roland EH, Hahn G. Transverse myelitis and Epstein-Barr virus infection with delayed antibody responses. Neurology 1991;41:1523.

Kamala D, Suresh S, Githa K. Real-time ultrasonography in neuromuscular problems in children. J Clin Ultrasound 1985;13:465.

Kankirawatana P, Tennison MB, D'Cruz O, et al. Möbius syndrome in infant exposed to cocaine in utero. Pediatr Neurol 1993;9:71.

Kelley RI, Sladky JT. Dicarboxylic aciduria in an infant with spinal muscular atrophy. Ann Neurol 1986;20:734.

Kelley TW, Prayson RA, Ruiz AI, et al. The neuropathology of West Nile virus meningoencephalitis. A report of two cases and review of the literature. Am J Clin Pathol 2003;119:749.

Kennedy WR, Alter M, Sung JH. Progressive proximal spinal and bulbar muscular atrophy of late onset. A sex-linked recessive trait. Neurology 1968;18:671.

Kim SK, Chung YS, Wang KC, et al. Diastematomyelia: Clinical manifestation and treatment outcome. J Korean Med Sci 1994;9:135.

Klessinger S, Christ B. Diastematomyelia and spina bifida can be caused by the intraspinal grafting of somites in early avian embryos. Neurosurgery 1996;39:1215.

Kobayashi H, Baumbach L, Matise TC, et al. A gene for a severe lethal form of X-linked arthrogryposis (X-linked infantile spinal muscular atrophy) maps to human chromosome Xp11.3-q11.2. Hum Mol Genet 1995;4:1213.

Kopel FB, Shore B, Hodes HL. Nonfatal bulbospinal paralysis due to ECHO 4 virus. J Pediatr 1965;67:588.

Kremer H, Kuyt LP, van den Helm B, et al. Localization of a gene for Möbius syndrome to chromosome 3q by linkage analysis in a Dutch family. Hum Mol Genet 1996;5:1367.

Kugelberg E. Chronic proximal (pseudomyopathic) spinal muscular atrophy. In: Vinkyn B, ed. Handbook of clinical neurology. Amsterdam: North-Holland Publishing, 1975.

Kugelberg E, Welander L. Familial neurogenic (spinal?) muscular atrophy simulating ordinary proximal dystrophy. Acta Psychiatr Scand 1954;29:42.

Kugelberg E, Welander L. Heredofamilial juvenile muscular atrophy simulating muscular dystrophy. AMA Arch Neurol Psychiatry 1956;75:500.

Label LS, Batts DH. Transverse myelitis caused by duck embryo rabies vaccine. Arch Neurol 1982;39:426.

La Spada AR, Paulson HL, Fischbeck KH. Trinucleotide repeat expansion in neurological disease. Ann Neurol 1994:36;814.

La Spada AR, Wilson EM, Lubahn DB, et al. Androgen receptor gene mutations in X-linked spinal and bulbar muscular atrophy. Nature 1991;352:77.

Lassman LP, James CC, Foster JB. Hydromyelia. J Neurol Sci 1968;7:149.

Laureano AN, Rybak LP. Severe otolaryngologic manifestations of arthrogryposis multiplex congenita. Ann Otol Rhinol Laryngol 1990;99:94.

Lefebvre S, Burglen L, Reboullet S, et al. Identification and characterization of a spinal muscular atrophy-determining gene. Cell 1995;80:155.

Lefebvre S, Burlet P, Liu Q, et al. Correlation between severity and SMN protein level in spinal muscular atrophy. Nat Genet 1997;16:265.

Leis AA, Stokic DS, Polk JL, et al. A poliomyelitis-like syndrome from West Nile virus infection. N Engl J Med 2002;347:1279.

Lemaire R, Prasad J, Kashima T, et al. Stability of a PKCl-1–related mRNA is controlled by the splicing factor ASF/SF2: A novel function for SR proteins. Genes Dev 2002;16:594.

Leong S, Ashwell KW. Is there a zone of vascular vulnerability in the fetal brain stem? Neurotoxicol Teratol 1997;19:265.

Lepow ML, Spence DA. Effect of trivalent oral poliovirus vaccine in an institutionalized population with varying natural and acquired immunity to poliomyelitis. Pediatrics 1965;35:236.

Levine DN. The pathogenesis of syringomyelia associated with lesions at the foramen magnum: A critical review of existing theories and proposal of a new hypothesis. J Neurol Sci 2004;220:3.

Leyden E. Ueber hydromyelus und Syringomyelie. Virchows Arch A Pathol Anat Histopathol 1876;68:1.

Liochev SI, Fridovich I. Mutant Cu,Zn superoxide dismutases and familial amyotrophic lateral sclerosis: evaluation of oxidative hypotheses. Free Radic Biol Med 2003;34:1383.

Liu Q, Fischer U, Wang F, et al. The spinal muscular atrophy disease gene product, SMN, and its associated protein SIP1 are in a complex with spliceosomal snRNP proteins. Cell 1997;90:1013.

Londe P. Paralysie bulbaire progressive infantile et familiale. Rev Med 1893;13:1020.

Londe P. Paralysie bulbaire progressive infantile et familiale. Rev Med 1894;14:212.

Lorson CL, Androphy EJ. An exonic enhancer is required for inclusion of an essential exon in the SMA determining gene SMN. Hum Mol Genet 2000;9:259.

Lorson CL, Hahmen E, Androphy EJ, Wirth B. A single nucleotide in the SMN gene regulates splicing and is responsible for spinal muscular atrophy. Proc Natl Acad Sci U S A 1999;96:6307.

Lunt PW, Cumming WJ, Kingston H, et al. DNA probes in differential diagnosis of Becker muscular dystrophy and spinal muscular atrophy. Lancet 1989;1:46.

Madsen JR, Scott RM. Chiari malformations, syringomyelia, and intramedullary spinal cord tumors. Curr Opin Neurol Neurosurg 1993;6:559.

Marques-Dias MJ, Gonzalez CH, Rosemberg S. Möbius sequence in children exposed in utero to misoprostol: Neuropathological study of three cases. Birth Defects Res A Clin Mol Teratol 2003;67:1002.

Mawatari S, Katayama K. Scapuloperoneal muscular atrophy with cardiopathy. An X-linked recessive trait. Arch Neurol 1973;28:55.

McCaffrey PG, Newsome DA, Fibach E, et al. Induction of gamma-globin by histone deacetylase inhibitors. Blood 1997;90:2075.

McGrory BJ, Burke DW, Moran SJ. Posterior instability of the hip in an adult. A case report. Clin Orthop 1997;341:151.

McShane MA, Boyd S, Harding B, et al. Progressive bulbar paralysis of childhood. A reappraisal of Fazio-Londe disease. Brain 1992;115(Pt 6):1889.

McWilliam RC, Gardner-Medwin D, Doyle D, et al. Diaphragmatic paralysis due to spinal muscular atrophy. An unrecognised cause of respiratory failure in infancy? Arch Dis Child 1985;60:145.

Meacham WF. Surgical treatment of diastematomyelia. J Neurosurg 1967;27:78.

Melki J. Gene for chronic proximal spinal muscular atrophies maps to chromosome 5q. Nature 1990;344:767.

Melki J, Lefebvre S, Burglen L, et al. De novo and inherited deletions of the 5q13 region in spinal muscular atrophies. Science 1994;264:1474.

Mellins RB, Hays AP, Gold AP, et al. Respiratory distress as the initial manifestation of Werdnig-Hoffmann disease. Pediatrics 1974;53:33.

Menezes AH. Chiari I malformations and hydromyelia: Complications. Pediatr Neurosurg 1991;17:146.

Mercuri E, Bertini E, Messina S, et al. Pilot trial of phenylbutyrate in spinal muscular atrophy. Neuromuscul Disord 2004;14:130.

Middleton LT, Christodoulou K, Mubaidin A, et al. Distal hereditary motor neuronopathy of the Jerash type. Ann N Y Acad Sci 1999;883:65.

Miske LJ, Hickey EM, Kolb SM, et al. Use of the mechanical in-exsufflator in pediatric patients with neuromuscular disease and impaired cough. Chest 2004;125:1406.

Moerman P, Fryns JP, Van Dijck H, et al. Congenital muscular dystrophy associated with lethal arthrogryposis multiplex congenita. Virchows Arch A Pathol Anat Histopathol 1985;408:43.

Moes CA, Hendrick EB. Diastematomyelia. J Pediatr 1963;63:238.

Monani UR, Coovert DD, Burghes AH. Animal models of spinal muscular atrophy. Hum Mol Genet 2000;9:2451.

Monani UR, Lorson CL, Parsons DW, et al. A single nucleotide difference that alters splicing patterns distinguishes the SMA gene SMN1 from the copy gene SMN2. Hum Mol Genet 1999;8:1177.

Monani UR, Pastore MT, Gavrilina TO, et al. A transgene carrying an A2G missense mutation in the SMN gene modulates phenotypic severity in mice with severe (type I) spinal muscular atrophy. J Cell Biol 2003;160:41.

Moosa A, Dubowitz V. Motor nerve conduction velocity in spinal muscular atrophy of childhood. Arch Dis Child 1976;51:974.

Muller B, Melki J, Burlet P, et al. Proximal spinal muscular atrophy (SMA) types II and III in the same sibship are not caused by different alleles at the SMA locus on 5q [see Comments]. Am J Hum Genet 1992;50:892.

Munsat TL. Poliomyelitis: New problems with an old disease. N Engl J Med 1991a;324:1206.

Munsat TL. Workshop report: International SMA collaboration. Neuromusc Disord 1991b;1:81.

Munsat TL, Skerry L, Korf B, et al. Phenotypic heterogeneity of spinal muscular atrophy mapping to chromosome 5q11.2-13.3 (SMA 5q). Neurology 1990;40:1831.

Munshi I, Frim D, Stine-Reyes R, et al. Effects of posterior fossa decompression with and without duraplasty on Chiari malformation-associated hydromyelia. Neurosurgery 2000;46:1384; discussion, 1389.

Nelson CE, Morgan BA, Burke AC, et al. Analysis of Hox gene expression in the chick limb bud. Development 1996;122:1449.

Netsky MG. Syringomyelia: A clinicopathologic study. AMA Arch Neurol Psychiatry 1953;70:741.

Nevo Y, Kramer U, Legum C, et al. SMA type 2 unrelated to chromosome 5q13. Am J Med Genet 1998;75:193.

Newman PK, Terenty TR, Foster JB. Some observations on the pathogenesis of syringomyelia. J Neurol Neurosurg Psychiatry 1981;44:964.

Nishimura AL, Mitne-Neto M, Silva HC, et al. A mutation in the vesicle-trafficking protein VAPB causes late-onset spinal muscular atrophy and amyotrophic lateral sclerosis. Am J Hum Genet 2004;75:822.

Nussinovitch M, Brand N, Frydman M, et al. Transverse myelitis following mumps in children. Acta Paediatr 1992;81:183.

Oberoi GS, Kaul HL, Gill IS, et al. Anaesthesia in arthrogryposis multiplex congenita: Case report. Can J Anaesth 1987;34:288.

Oda Y, Yukioka H, Fujimori M. Anesthesia for arthrogryposis multiplex congenita: Report of 12 cases. J Anesth 1990;4:275.

Oller-Navarro JL, Rivera-Reyes L, Rodriguez-Rivera AA. Juvenile diabetic myelopathy. A 14-year-old girl with juvenile diabetes mellitus complicated by acute transverse myelopathy. Clin Pediatr (Phila) 1979;18:60.

Oppenheim H. Ber allgemeine und localisierte atonie der muskulatur (myatonie) im fruhen kindesalter. Mschr Psych Neur 1900;8:232.

Owens JC, Swan H. Complications in the repair of coarctation of the aorta. J Cardiovasc Surg (Torino) 1963;117:816.

Pace BS, White GL, Dover GJ, et al. Short-chain fatty acid derivatives induce fetal globin expression and erythropoiesis in vivo. Blood 2002;100:4640.

Parano E, Pavone L, Falsaperla R, et al. Molecular basis of phenotypic heterogeneity in siblings with spinal muscular atrophy. Ann Neurol 1996;40:247.

Parisi A, Filice G. Transverse myelitis associated with Mycoplasma pneumoniae pneumonitis: A report of two cases. Infez Med 2001;9:39.

Parkes JD. Genetic factors in human sleep disorders with special reference to Norrie disease, Prader-Willi syndrome and Moebius syndrome. J Sleep Res 1999;8(Suppl 1):14.

Parush S, Yehezkehel I, Tenenbaum A, et al. Developmental correlates of school-age children with a history of benign congenital hypotonia. Dev Med Child Neurol 1998;40:448.

Pastuszak AL, Schuler L, Speck-Martins CE, et al. Use of misoprostol during pregnancy and Möbius' syndrome in infants. N Engl J Med 1998;338:1881.

Patrizi AL, Tiziano F, Zappata S, et al. SMN protein analysis in fibroblast, amniocyte and CVS cultures from spinal muscular atrophy patients and its relevance for diagnosis. Eur J Hum Genet 1999;7:301.

Pattany PM, Saraf-Lavi E, Bowen BC. MR angiography of the spine and spinal cord. Top Magn Reson Imaging 2003;14:444.

Pealer LN, Marfin AA, Petersen LR, et al. Transmission of West Nile virus through blood transfusion in the United States in 2002. N Engl J Med 2003;349:1236.

Pellizzoni L, Baccon J, Rappsilber J, et al. Purification of native survival of motor neurons complexes and identification of Gemin6 as a novel component. J Biol Chem 2002;277:7540.

Pena CE, Miller F, Budzilovich GN, et al. Arthrogryposis multiplex congenita. Report of two cases of a radicular type with familial incidence. Neurology 1968;18:926.

Petajan JH, Momberger GL, Aase J, et al. Arthrogryposis syndrome (Kuskokwim disease) in the Eskimo. JAMA 1969;209:1481.

Petersen LR, Marfin AA. West Nile virus: A primer for the clinician. Ann Intern Med 2002:137;173.

Pfeifer JD. Basicranial diastematomyelia: A case report. Clin Neuropathol 1991;10:232.

Piasecki JO, Mahinpour S, Levine DB. Long-term follow-up of spinal fusion in spinal muscular atrophy. Clin Orthop 1986;207:44.

Ponseti IV. Correction of the talar neck angle in congenital clubfoot with sequential manipulation and casting. Iowa Orthop J 1998;18:74.

Pugh RC, Dudgeon JA. Fatal neonatal poliomyelitis. Arch Dis Child 1954;29:381.

Puls I, Jonnakuty C, LaMonte BH, et al. Mutant dynactin in motor neuron disease. Nat Genet 2003;33:455.

Quinn CM, Wigglesworth JS, Heckmatt J. Lethal arthrogryposis multiplex congenita: A pathological study of 21 cases. Histopathology 1991;19:155.

Rabin BA, Griffin JW, Crain BJ, et al. Autosomal dominant juvenile amyotrophic lateral sclerosis. Brain 1999;122(Pt 8):1539.

Roberts DJ, Tabin C. The genetics of human limb development. Am J Hum Genet 1994;55:1.

Rodesch G, Hurth M, Alvarez H, et al. Angio-architecture of spinal cord arteriovenous shunts at presentation. Clinical correlations in adults and children. The Bicetre experience on 155 consecutive patients seen between 1981–1999. Acta Neurochir (Wien) 2004;146:217; discussion, 226.

Romanes GJ. The motor cell columns of the lumbo-sacral spinal cord of the cat. J Comp Neurol 1951;94:313.

Rosen DR. Mutations in Cu/Zn superoxide dismutase gene are associated with familial amyotrophic lateral sclerosis. Nature 1993;364:362.

Rosen DR, et al. Mutations in Cu/Zn superoxide dismutase gene are associated with familial amyotrophic lateral sclerosis. Nature 1993;362:59.

Roy N, Mahadevan MS, McLean M, et al. The gene for neuronal apoptosis inhibitory protein is partially deleted in individuals with spinal muscular atrophy [see Comments]. Cell 1995;80:167.

Ruddy DM, Parton MJ, Al-Chalabi A, et al. Two families with familial amyotrophic lateral sclerosis are linked to a novel locus on chromosome 16q. Am J Hum Genet 2003;73:390.

Rudnik-Schoneborn S, Forkert R, Hahnen E, et al. Clinical spectrum and diagnostic criteria of infantile spinal muscular atrophy: further delineation on the basis of SMN gene deletion findings. Neuropediatrics 1996;27:8.

Rudnik-Schoneborn S, Stolz P, Varon R, et al. Long-term observations of patients with infantile spinal muscular atrophy with respiratory distress type 1 (SMARD1). Neuropediatrics 2004;35:174.

Rudnik-Schoneborn S, Sztriha L, Aithala GR, et al. Extended phenotype of pontocerebellar hypoplasia with infantile spinal muscular atrophy. Am J Med Genet A 2003;117:10.

Ruggieri M, Smarason AK, Pike M. Spinal cord insults in the prenatal, perinatal, and neonatal periods. Dev Med Child Neurol 1999;41:311.

Russman BS, Buncher CR, White M, et al. Function changes in spinal muscular atrophy II and III. The DCN/SMA Group. Neurology 1996;47:973.

Russman BS, Iannacone ST, Buncher CR, et al. Spinal muscular atrophy: New thoughts on the pathogenesis and classification schema. J Child Neurol 1992;7:347.

Rust RS. Multiple sclerosis, acute disseminated encephalomyelitis, and related conditions. Semin Pediatr Neurol 2000;7:66.

Ryan MM, Cooke-Yarborough CM, Procopis PG, et al. Anterior horn cell disease and olivopontocerebellar hypoplasia. Pediatr Neurol 2000;23:180.

Salah N, Desforges G, Cifuentes-Diaz C, et al. Therapeutic strategies in SMA mouse models, Vol. 6. Sixth Annual International Spinal Muscular Atrophy Research Group Meeting, Schaumburg, IL, June 21-22, 2002.

Samaha FJ, Buncher CR, Russman BS, et al. Pulmonary function in spinal muscular atrophy. J Child Neurol 1994;9:326.

Sampson BA, Nields H, Armbrustmacher V, et al. Muscle weakness in West Nile encephalitis is due to destruction of motor neurons. Hum Pathol 2003;34:628.

Sapp PC, Hosler BA, McKenna-Yasek D, et al. Identification of two novel loci for dominantly inherited familial amyotrophic lateral sclerosis. Am J Hum Genet 2003;73:397.

Sarnat HB, O'Connor T, Byrne PA. Clinical effects of myotonic dystrophy on pregnancy and the neonate. Arch Neurol 1976;33:459.

Schijman E. Split spinal cord malformations: Report of 22 cases and review of the literature. Childs Nerv Syst 2003;19:96.

Schmalbruch H, Haase G. Spinal muscular atrophy: present state. Brain Pathol 2001;11:231.

Schmalbruch H, Kamieniecka Z, Arroe M. Early fatal nemaline myopathy: Case report and review. Dev Med Child Neurol 1987;29:800.

Schurch B, Wichmann W, Rossier AB. Post-traumatic syringomyelia (cystic myelopathy): A prospective study of 449 patients with spinal cord injury. J Neurol Neurosurg Psychiatry 1996;60:61.

Schwartz MS, Moosa A. Sensory nerve conduction in the spinal muscular atrophies. Dev Med Child Neurol 1977;19:50.

Schwentker EP, Gibson DA. The orthopaedic aspects of spinal muscular atrophy. J Bone Joint Surg Am 1976;58:32.

Sells JM, Jaffe KM, Hall JG. Amyoplasia, the most common type of arthrogryposis: the potential for good outcome. Pediatrics 1996;97:225.

Servais LJ, Rivelli SK, Dachy BA, et al. Anterior spinal artery syndrome after aortic surgery in a child. Pediatr Neurol 2001;24:310.

Shafiq SA, Milhorat AT, Gorycki MA. Fine structure of human muscle in neurogenic atrophy. Neurology 1967;17:934.

Shaw PJ, Ince PG, Goodship J, et al. Adult-onset motor neuron disease and infantile Werdnig-Hoffmann disease (spinal muscular atrophy type 1) in the same family. Neurology 1992;42:1477.

Sheehan JP, Sheehan JM, Lopes MB, et al. Thoracic diastematomyelia with concurrent intradural epidermoid spinal cord tumor and cervical syrinx in an adult. Case report. J Neurosurg Spine 2002;97:231.

Shepard TH. Möbius syndrome after misoprostol: A possible teratogenic mechanism. Lancet 1995;346:780.

Shibata N. Transgenic mouse model for familial amyotrophic lateral sclerosis with superoxide dismutase-1 mutation. Neuropathology 2001;21:82.

Shuper A, Weitz R, Varsano I, et al. Benign congenital hypotonia. A clinical study in 43 children. Eur J Pediatr 1987;146:360.

Shyamalan NC, Singh SS, Bisht DB. Transverse myelitis after vaccination. BMJ 1964;5380: 434.

Siegel IM, Silverman M. Upright mobility system for spinal muscular atrophy patients. Arch Phys Med Rehabil 1984;65:418.

Silver JR. History of post-traumatic syringomyelia: post traumatic syringomyelia prior to 1920. Spinal Cord 2001;39:176.

Slee JJ, Smart RD, Viljoen DL. Deletion of chromosome 13 in Moebius syndrome. J Med Genet 1991;28:413.

Smit LM, Barth PG. Arthrogryposis multiplex congenita due to congenital myasthenia. Dev Med Child Neurol 1980;22:371.

Solomon T, Willison H. Infectious causes of acute flaccid paralysis. Curr Opin Infect Dis 2003;16:375.

Sonigo-Cohen P, Schmit P, Zerah M, et al. Prenatal diagnosis of diastematomyelia. Childs Nerv Syst 2003;19:555.

Spagnoli LG, Palmieri G, Bertini E. Benign congenital hypotonia with uniform type 1 fibers and aspecific ultrastructural changes in the muscle: a case with esophagus involvement. Ital J Neurol Sci 1985;6:317.

Sperfeld AD, Karitzky J, Brummer D, et al. X-linked bulbospinal neuronopathy: Kennedy disease. Arch Neurol 2002;59:1921.

Spiro A. Minpolymyoclonus. A neglected sign in childhood spinal muscular atrophy. Neurology 1970;20:1124.

Steegman AT. Syndrome of the anterior spinal artery. Neurology 1952;2:15.

Stoll C, Ehret-Mentre MC, Treisser A, et al. Prenatal diagnosis of congenital myasthenia with arthrogryposis in a myasthenic mother. Prenat Diagn 1991;11:17.

Strasswimmer J, Lorson CL, Breiding DE, et al. Identification of survival motor neuron as a transcriptional activator-binding protein. Hum Mol Genet 1999:8:1219.

Suh SW, Sarwark JF, Vora A, et al. Evaluating congenital spine deformities for intraspinal anomalies with magnetic resonance imaging. J Pediatr Orthop 2001;21:525.

Summers BA, Swash M, Schwartz MS, et al. Juvenile-onset bulbospinal muscular atrophy with deafness: Vialetta-van Laere syndrome or Madras-type motor neuron disease? J Neurol 1987;234:440.

Sumner CJ, Huynh TN, Markowitz JA, et al. Valproic acid increases SMN levels in spinal muscular atrophy patient cells. Ann Neurol 2003;54:647.

Sung SS, Brassington AM, Grannatt K, et al. Mutations in genes encoding fast-twitch contractile proteins cause distal arthrogryposis syndromes. Am J Hum Genet 2003a;72:681.

Sung SS, Brassington AM, Krakowiak PA, et al. Mutations in TNNT3 cause multiple congenital contractures: A second locus for distal arthrogryposis type 2B. Am J Hum Genet 2003b;73:212.

Suresh PA, Deepa C. Congenital suprabulbar palsy: A distinct clinical syndrome of heterogeneous aetiology. Dev Med Child Neurol 2004;46:617.

Swoboda KJ, Prior TW, Scott CB, et al. Natural history of denervation in SMA: Relation to age, SMN2 copy number, and function. Ann Neurol 2005;57:704.

Takata RI, Speck Martins CE, Passosbueno MR, et al. A new locus for recessive distal spinal muscular atrophy at Xq13.1-q21. J Med Genet 2004;41:224.

Tein I, Sloane AE, Donner EJ, et al. Fatty acid oxidation abnormalities in childhood-onset spinal muscular atrophy: Primary or secondary defect(s)? Pediatr Neurol 1995;12:21.

Thomas HM. Congenital facial paralysis. J Nerv Ment Dis 1898;25:571.

Thompson CE. Benign congenital hypotonia is not a diagnosis. Dev Med Child Neurol 2002;44:283.

Thron A, Schroth G. Magnetic resonance imaging (MRI) of diastematomyelia. Neuroradiology 1986;28:371.

Timmerman V, Raeymaekers P, Nelis E, et al. Linkage analysis of distal hereditary motor neuropathy type II (distal HMN II) in a single pedigree. J Neurol Sci 1992;109:41.

Tobin WD, Layton DD. The diagnosis and natural history of spinal cord arteriovenous malformations. Mayo Clin Proc 1976;51:637.

Topaloglu H, Renda Y, Kale G, et al. Muscular dystrophy or spinal muscular atrophy? Lancet 1989;1:960.

Toussaint M, De Win H, Steens M, et al. Effect of intrapulmonary percussive ventilation on mucus clearance in Duchenne muscular dystrophy patients: a preliminary report. Respir Care 2003;48:940.

Tsutsumi H, Kamazaki H, Nakata S, et al. Sequential development of acute meningoencephalitis and transverse myelitis caused by Epstein-Barr virus during infectious mononucleosis. Pediatr Infect Dis J 1994;13:665.

Tubbs RS, Wellons JC 3rd, Blount JP, et al. Syringomyelia in twin brothers discordant for Chiari I malformation: Case report. J Child Neurol 2004;19:459.

Van Laere J. Paralysie bulbo-pontine chronique frogressive familial avec surdite: Un cas de syndrome de Klippel-Trénaunay das la meme fratrie (problems diagnostiques et gentiques). Rev Neurol 1966;115:289.

Vaquero J, Martinez R, Arias A. Syringomyelia-Chiari complex: Magnetic resonance imaging and clinical evaluation of surgical treatment. J Neurosurg 1990;73:64.

Vargas FR, Schuler-Faccini L, Brunoni D, et al. Prenatal exposure to misoprostol and vascular disruption defects: a case-control study. Am J Med Genet 2000;95:302.

Vassilopoulos D, Emery AE. Quantitative histochemistry of the spinal motor neurone nucleus during human fetal development. J Neurol Sci 1977;32:275.

Venketasubramanian N. Transverse myelitis following mumps in an adult: A case report with MRI correlation. Acta Neurol Scand 1997;96:328.

Verzijl HT, van den Helm B, Veldman B, et al. A second gene for autosomal dominant Möbius syndrome is localized to chromosome 10q, in a Dutch family. Am J Hum Genet 1999;65:752.

Vialetto E. Contibuto alla forma ereditaria della paralisi bulbare progressiva. Riv Sper Frenait 1936;40:1.

Vlaanderen W, Manschot TA, Vermeulen-Meiners C. A dominant-hereditary variation of the Pena-Shokeir syndrome: A case report. Eur J Obstet Gynecol Reprod Biol 1991;40:163.

Wallgren-Pettersson C, Bushby K, Mellies U, et al. 117th ENMC workshop: Ventilatory support in congenital neuromuscular disorders—congenital myopathies, congenital muscular dystrophies, congenital myotonic dystrophy and SMA (II) 4-6 April 2003, Naarden, The Netherlands. Neuromuscul Disord 2004;14:56.

Walsh FS, Moore SE, Lake BD. Cell adhesion molecule N-CAM is expressed by denervated myofibres in Werdnig-Hoffman and Kugelberg-Welander type spinal muscular atrophies. J Neurol Neurosurg Psychiatry 1987;50:439.

Walton JN. The limp child. J Neurol Neurosurg Psychiatry 1957;20:144.

Wang TG, Bach JR, Avilla C, et al. Survival of individuals with spinal muscular atrophy on ventilatory support. Am J Phys Med Rehabil 1994;73:207.

Weenink HR, Smilde J. Spinal cord lesions due to coarctatio aortae. Psychiatr Neurol Neurochir 1964;67:259.

Whelan TB. Neuropsychological performance of children with Duchenne muscular dystrophy and spinal muscle atrophy. Dev Med Child Neurol 1987;29:212.

Wilkins KE, Gibson DA. The patterns of spinal deformity in Duchenne muscular dystrophy. J Bone Joint Surg Am 1976;58:24.

Williams B. Difficult labour as a cause of communicating syringomyelia. Lancet 1977;2:51.

Williams B, Timperley WR. Three cases of communication syringomyelia secondary to midbrain gliomas. J Neurol Neurosurg Psychiatry 1977;40:80.

Windpassinger C, Auer-Grumbach M, Irobi J, et al. Heterozygous missense mutations in BSCL2 are associated with distal hereditary motor neuropathy and Silver syndrome. Nat Genet 2004;36:271.

Wisoff JH. Hydromyelia: A critical review. Childs Nerv Syst 1988;4:1.

Wong M, Connolly AM, Noetzel MJ. Poliomyelitis-like syndrome associated with Epstein-Barr virus infection. Pediatr Neurol 1999;20:235.

Yachnis AT, Giovanini MA, Eskin TA, et al. Developmental patterns of BCL-2 and BCL-X polypeptide expression in the human spinal cord. Exp Neurol 1998;150:82.

Yang L, Jones NR, Stoodley MA, et al. Excitotoxic model of post-traumatic syringomyelia in the rat. Spine 2001a;26:1842.

Yang Y, Hentati A, Deng HX, et al. The gene encoding alsin, a protein with three guanine-nucleotide exchange factor domains, is mutated in a form of recessive amyotrophic lateral sclerosis. Nat Genet 2001b;29:160.

Young ID, Harper PS. Hereditary distal spinal muscular atrophy with vocal cord paralysis. J Neurol Neurosurg Psychiatry 1980;43:413.

Zellweger H. The floppy infant: A practical approach. Helv Paediatr Acta 1983;38:301.

Zellweger H, Schneider H, Schuldt DR. A new genetic variant of spinal muscular atrophy. Neurology 1969;19:865.

Zerres K, Rudnik-Schoneborn S. Natural history in proximal spinal muscular atrophy. Clinical analysis of 445 patients and suggestions for a modification of existing classifications. Arch Neurol 1995;52:518.

Zerres K, Rudnik-Schoneborn S, Forrest E, et al. A collaborative study on the natural history of childhood and juvenile onset proximal spinal muscular atrophy (type II and III SMA): 569 patients. J Neurol Sci 1997;146:67.

Zerres K, Wirth B, Rudnik-Schoneborn S. Spinal muscular atrophy: Clinical and genetic correlations. Neuromuscul Disord 1997;7:202.

CHAPTER 76

Peripheral Neuropathies

Stephen A. Smith and Robert Ouvrier

Disorders of peripheral nerves may be considered acute or chronic, divided by the type of peripheral nerve involved (primarily motor, sensory, or autonomic), or classified as acquired or hereditary. Some neuropathies are radicular in distribution. Pathologically, neuropathies are demyelinating or axonal, depending on whether the main disruption involves the axon or the myelin supported by the Schwann cell. This chapter discusses neuropathies occurring in children, and categorization is by disease.

ANATOMY

The peripheral nervous system is made up of cranial nerves III through XII, the spinal roots, the nerve plexuses, the peripheral nerves, and the autonomic ganglia. (The autonomic nervous system is addressed separately and is not discussed in this chapter.) Neuronal cell bodies subserving the nerves in the peripheral nervous system reside in the brainstem, anterior horn cells of the spinal cord, intermediolateral cell column where the autonomic system originates, and the dorsal root ganglia for afferent sensory function. Peripheral nerves innervate all skeletal muscles through large myelinated nerve fibers. Sensory input from skin, joints, and muscles is transmitted through a combination of unmyelinated and myelinated nerve fibers from the periphery to the central nervous system (CNS). The outer connective tissue sheath of a peripheral nerve, the epineurium, encases bundles of nerves in fascicles. Each fascicle has a sheath termed the *perineurium.* Myelinated and unmyelinated nerve fibers surrounded by collagenous fibers, the endoneurium, are present in fascicles (Fig. 76-1). Peripheral nerves are very vascular, with arteries and arterioles in the epineurium, arterioles in the perineurium, and primarily capillaries in the endoneurium. The venous system is similarly represented.

Fetal nerve is initially unmyelinated, with multiple nerve fibers contained within single Schwann cell investments. By 20 weeks of gestation, there are many more Schwann cells, and myelin is beginning to form [Davison et al., 1973]. The biochemical composition of the peripheral nerve becomes more complicated after 20 weeks. Myelination continues after birth. The perineurium creates a diffusion barrier responsible for the maintenance of endoneurial homeostasis. The perineurium matures relatively late during human peripheral nerve development [Pummi et al., 2004].

Evaluation of peripheral nerve diseases includes obtaining a clear history of the distribution and rate of progression of the condition; conducting an appropriate examination; obtaining an electromyogram with nerve conduction velocities, amplitudes, and latencies plus indicated muscle needle electrode study; and often performing a sural nerve biopsy. Many peripheral neuropathies are familial, and other family members may need to be studied.

Facial Nerve Paralysis (Bell's Palsy)

Acute dysfunction of cranial nerve VII caused by lesions of the facial nerve nucleus in the pons or axial or extra-axial facial nerve is called *Bell's palsy.* The result is partial or complete paralysis of the upper and lower face muscles. Bell's palsy most often results from edema and inflammation of the nerve as it traverses the facial canal within the temporal bone.

Cranial nerve VII is a complex nerve that has motor, sensory, and autonomic components (Fig. 76-2). The nonmotor functions of the facial nerve are mediated by parasympathetic afferent fibers, which innervate lacrimal and salivary glands; efferent fibers, which subserve taste; and other fibers that mediate the auditory reflex. Motor functions are subserved by somatic afferent fibers innervating muscle fibers of facial movement.

Lesions of the facial nerve nucleus and nerve distal to the nucleus result in paralysis of upper (forehead) and lower facial muscles. Because bihemispheral pathways from the motor cortex extend to the facial nerve nuclei subserving frontalis and orbicularis oculi muscles, a lesion in one cerebral hemisphere causes facial weakness confined strictly to the lower face and spares forehead muscles. This condition is termed *central facial nerve palsy*. It is important to ascertain whether facial paralysis is due to upper or lower motor unit involvement before the diagnosis of Bell's palsy is considered. When forehead muscles are involved, a lower motor lesion of the facial nerve or peripheral facial nerve palsy is present.

Clinical Features

The incidence of Bell's palsy is 2.7 per 100,000 below the age of 10 years and 10.1 per 100,000 during the second decade of life [Katusik et al., 1986]. Female and male incidence is equal. Ear pain near the mastoid process is the first manifestation of impending facial nerve involvement half of the time. Unilateral inability to close the eyelid and maintain normal facial movement is the initial indication of motor involvement. Facial weakness develops rapidly over several hours to 3 days, resulting in paresis to complete paralysis. Bell's palsy commonly follows an upper respiratory tract infection, indicating possible postinfectious demyelination. Drinking and eating are impaired because of the inability to close the mouth on the involved side. Depending on the site of facial nerve involvement (Table 76-1; see Fig. 76-2), lacrimation may be decreased and taste distorted.

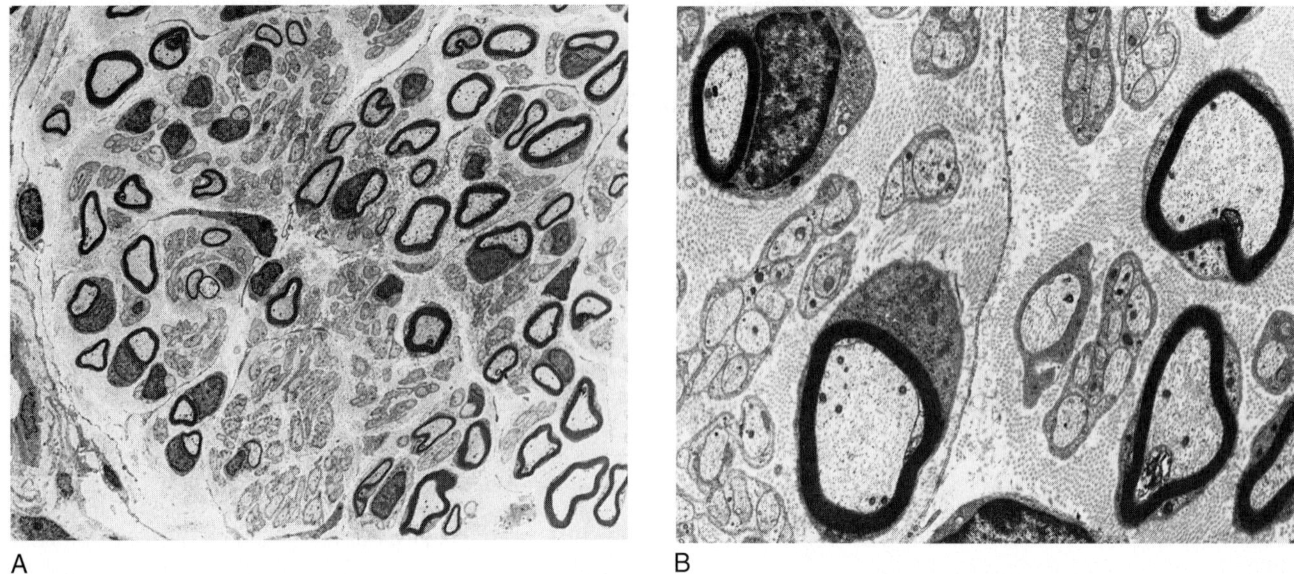

FIGURE 76-1. Normal sural nerve in an infant. **A**, Low-power view showing part of the perineurium surrounding a nerve fascicle and unmyelinated and myelinated nerve fibers (×1980). **B**, Higher-power view showing multiple unmyelinated nerve fibers invested by Schwann cells and individual myelinated fibers with Schwann cell investment (×10,800).

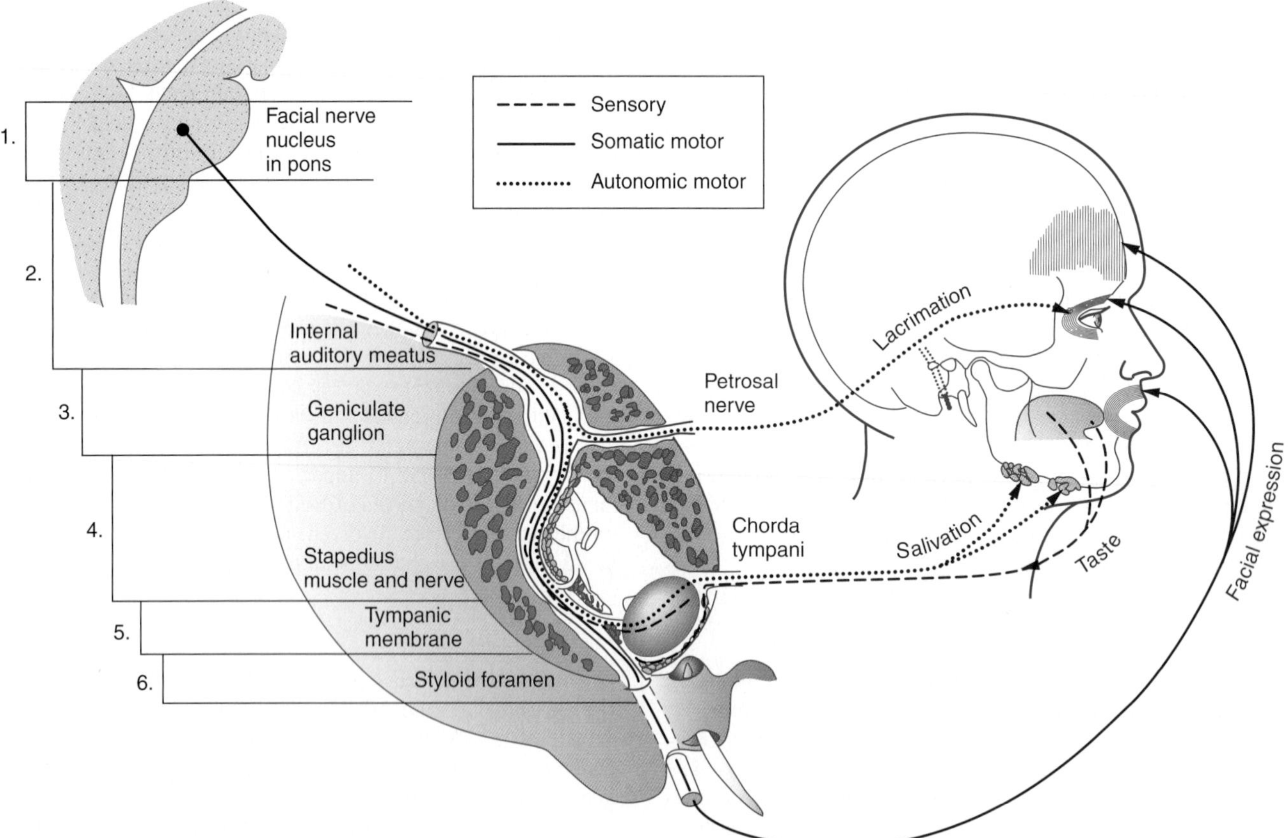

FIGURE 76-2 Schematic pathway of the facial nerve (cranial nerve VII). (Modified from Haymaker W. Bing's local diagnosis in neurological diseases, 15th ed. St Louis: Mosby, 1969; Rasmussen AT. The principal nervous pathways. New York: Macmillan, 1951; and Swaiman KF, Wright FS. Pediatric neuromuscular diseases. St Louis: Mosby, 1979.)

Taste sensation is evaluated by alternately applying solutions of sugar and salt to the anterior edge of the tongue on the involved side while holding the tongue with a piece of gauze. The tongue should not be retracted during the examination because the solutions will intermix. Lacrimation may be reduced on the ipsilateral side. However, if the parasympathetic pathways of lacrimation are intact, excessive tearing can occur from corneal irritation. Diminished lacri-

TABLE 76-1

Clinical Localization of Facial Nerve Lesions

ANATOMIC SITE*	FACIAL MOVEMENT	LACRIMATION	TASTE	SALIVATION	HYPERACUSIS
Nucleus (1)	Defective	Normal	Normal	Normal	Present
Pons to internal auditory meatus (2)	Defective	Defective	Normal	Defective	Present
Geniculate ganglion (3)	Defective	Defective	Defective	Defective	Present
Ganglion to stapedius nerve (4)	Defective	Normal	Defective	Defective	Present
Stapedius nerve to chorda tympani (5)	Defective	Normal	Defective	Defective	Absent
Below chorda tympani (6)	Defective	Normal	Normal	Normal	Absent

*Numbers refer to Figure 76-2.

mation may be determined by hooking filter paper over both lower eyelid margins and observing decreased wetting of the paper on the involved side over 5 minutes (Schirmer test). Stapedius nerve function is evaluated by audiologic study.

The differential diagnosis of facial paralysis includes trauma, acute and chronic infections of the inner ear, herpes simplex infection, herpes zoster infection, *Mycoplasma pneumoniae* infection [Klar et al., 1985], Epstein-Barr virus infection [Andersson and Sterner, 1985], and Lyme disease (*Borrelia* species infection) (Box 76-1). Hypertension may be responsible for an acute facial paresis resembling Bell's palsy [Lloyd et al., 1966]. Melkersson-Rosenthal and Möbius' syndromes have facial paralysis. Guillain-Barré syndrome, motor neuron disorders, myasthenia gravis, various myopathies, leprosy, and Tangier disease may cause facial paresis.

In rare circumstances, Bell's palsy can present bilaterally in children, although one side is usually more involved than the other. The more-affected side usually is paralyzed first, and the less-involved side by the next day. Bilateral facial nerve palsy is often associated with Guillain-Barré syndrome.

Bilateral, congenital facial paralysis, usually in conjunction with ophthalmoplegia involving cranial nerve VI, presents in the newborn as Möbius' syndrome. The condition is the result of aplasia or hypoplasia of cranial nerves and nuclei VI and VII [Jaradeh et al., 1996]. Muscles innervated by other cranial nerves may be involved. Arthrogryposis may be present. Mental retardation may be diagnosed later. Möbius' syndrome may be sporadic or inherited as a dominant condition linked to chromosomes 13q12.2-13 or 3q [Kremer et al., 1996; Nishikawa et al., 1997]. Differential diagnosis includes traumatic delivery with skull fracture and injury to the nerve in the facial canal, sacral pressure on the facial nerve during delivery, or pressure over the parotid area from forceps application with nerve compression. Möbius' syndrome may be related in some instances to maternal ingestion of ergotamine in early pregnancy [Smets et al., 2004].

Simple asymmetry of facial expression when infants and children cry is common. A rare syndrome, the cardiofacial syndrome, referred to as *Cayler's syndrome,* is due to congenital hypoplasia of the depressor anguli oris causing the asymmetric crying facies syndrome. Unilateral partial lower facial weakness is noted in infants when smiling or crying. The syndrome is associated with congenital heart disease [Caksen et al., 1996; Cayler et al., 1971; Nelson and Eng, 1972; Punal et al., 2001]. Anomalies of the head and neck, heart, skeleton, genitourinary tract, and CNS accompany the syndrome [Lin et al., 1997]. Cardiofacial syndrome links to chromosome 22q11.2, including in one infant without cardiac involvement and in another with hypoparathyroidism [Giannotti and Mingarelli, 1994; Lindsay et al., 1995; Stewart and Smith, 1997]. Frameshift mutation of the *EYA1* gene has been described [Shimasaki et al., 2004]. Most children with asymmetric crying facies are otherwise normal.

Laboratory Findings

Uncomplicated facial palsy that resolves relatively quickly does not need detailed evaluation. Palsy that persists or seems atypical requires study. Evaluation for infection is appropriate, but peripheral leukocyte and differential counts and erythrocyte sedimentation rate are usually normal. Cerebrospinal fluid studies may show pleocytosis and blood-brain barrier alterations in Lyme disease (*Borrelia* species infection) [Roberg et al., 1991]. Imaging of the cranium is performed to exclude skull fracture, osteomyelitis, mastoiditis, increased intracranial pressure, calcification, and osteopetrosis. Magnetic resonance imaging (MRI) has been used in adults to predict the outcome of acute facial nerve palsy during the first few days after onset of symptoms [Kress et al., 2004]. The time to recovery from onset may increase from 6 to 14 weeks if enhancement on post-contrast images is present [Yetiser et al., 2003]. MRI can be used in children to find rare tumors invading the facial nerve [Koerbel el al., 2003]. Small lesions inside the temporal bone and at the cerebellopontine angle can be detected using gadolinium-enhanced MRI [Becelli et al., 2003]. Electrodiagnostic techniques may be useful in assessing the severity of facial nerve involvement and predicting the outcome. These studies include determination of nerve conduction velocity [Langworth and Taverner, 1963], detection of the level or threshold of response to stimulation [Campbell et al., 1962; Devi et al., 1978], nerve conduction latencies, and electrical stimulation of the tongue [Peiris and Miles, 1965]. Serial studies may be helpful [Fisch, 1984]. Nerve degeneration can be detected electrically by 72 hours after onset of paralysis.

Because Bell's palsy may be a component of a more widespread disease affecting other cranial and peripheral nerves, obtaining a complete electromyographic evaluation and extremity nerve conduction velocities is sometimes helpful [Bueri et al., 1984].

Treatment and Prognosis

The prognosis for recovery in children is good [Singhi and Jain, 2003]. Most children do not need drug therapy

Box 76-1 Facial Weakness in Childhood

Congenital, Structural
Chiari malformation
Depressor anguli oris muscle absence (cardiofacial syndrome)
Inner ear or facial nerve malformations
Möbius' syndrome
Syringobulbia

Genetic
Facioscapulohumeral dystrophy
Familial cranial neuropathy (recurrent)
Fazio-Londe disease
Myasthenia gravis (non–immune mediated)
Myotonic dystrophy
Nemaline myopathy

Infectious, Inflammatory
Basilar meningitis
Bell's palsy
Epstein-Barr infection (infectious mononucleosis)
Guillain-Barré syndrome
Miller-Fisher syndrome
Mycoplasma pneumoniae infection
Lyme disease (*Borrelia* species infection)
Otitis media and mastoiditis
Parotitis
Poliomyelitis
Ramsay Hunt syndrome (herpes zoster)
Sarcoidosis
Trichinosis
Tuberculosis

Trauma, Nerve Compression
Forceps pressure during delivery
Cleidocranial dysostosis
Histiocytosis X
Hyperostosis cranialis interna
Increased intracranial pressure
Petrous bone fracture
Pressure from maternal sacrum

Metabolic Conditions
Hyperparathyroidism
Hypothyroidism
Idiopathic infantile hypercalcemia
Osteopetrosis

Neoplasms
Brainstem glioma
Parotid gland tumors

Vascular
Arterial hypertension
Vascular syndromes of the cranial nerves

Other
Idiopathic cranial neuropathy
Melkersson-Rosenthal syndrome
Multiple sclerosis
Myasthenia gravis (immune mediated)
Myasthenia gravis (transient neonatal)

[Salman and MacGregor, 2001]. A number of drugs have been used, particularly steroids. Surgical decompression has been recommended in some patients when progressive paralysis and thus nerve degeneration occur [Jenkins et al., 1985]. Prednisone is the most widely used drug; it is given in high dosage for 1 week, followed by tapering the second week. It should be started within 1 week of disease onset. The degree to which steroid therapy can alter the natural history of Bell's palsy is unknown, although it appears to be more helpful in completely paralyzed than paretic individuals [Wolf et al., 1978]. Most children recover completely without treatment. Recovery usually begins within 2 to 4 weeks, reaching its maximum within 6 to 12 months. Wetting solutions to maintain corneal moisture and an eye patch for protection may be needed when the child cannot close the eye.

Recurrent Facial Paralysis

Recurrent unilateral facial paralysis indicates the need to exclude a neoplasm or vascular malformation. The Melkersson-Rosenthal syndrome is a rare cause of recurrent facial nerve paralysis [Graham and Kemink, 1986; Rogers, 1996]. It is a dominant syndrome with incomplete penetrance linked to chromosome 9p11. Onset is usually before 16 years of age. This syndrome consists of recurrent unilateral or bilateral facial paralysis accompanied by orofacial edema manifested as a fissured, reddish-brown appearance of swollen lips or facial edema. Fissured tongue (lingua plicata) is present in up to half of patients. Facial nerve decompression may be recommended.

BRACHIAL PLEXUS

Nerve roots from the fifth cervical through the first thoracic nerves form the three primary trunks of the brachial plexus. Once formed, they divide promptly into anterior and posterior divisions (Fig. 76-3). The posterior divisions join to form the posterior cord, which gives rise to the upper and lower subscapular, thoracodorsal, axillary, and radial nerves. The anterior divisions of the fifth, sixth, and seventh nerves form the lateral cord, and the anterior divisions of the eighth cervical and first thoracic nerves form the medial cord. The lateral cord subsequently gives rise to the musculocutaneous nerve and a branch to the coracobrachialis. The medial cord gives rise to the ulnar, medial antebrachial cutaneous, and medial brachial cutaneous nerves. Additional branches from the lateral and medial cords unite to form the median nerve.

Injury

Birth-related brachial plexus injuries occur in 0.5 to 1 of 1000 live births. Although traditionally thought to be associated with excessive traction to the affected extremity during breech delivery or traction to the head and neck during vertex delivery [Adler and Patterson, 1967], brachial plexus injuries can occur in the absence of fetal trauma [Ouzounian et al., 1997]. A recent study found that half of cases of Erb's palsy occur in normal-sized infants without trauma at delivery [Graham et al., 1997]. Brachial plexus injury is observed often in infants with shoulder dystocia [Greenwald et al.,

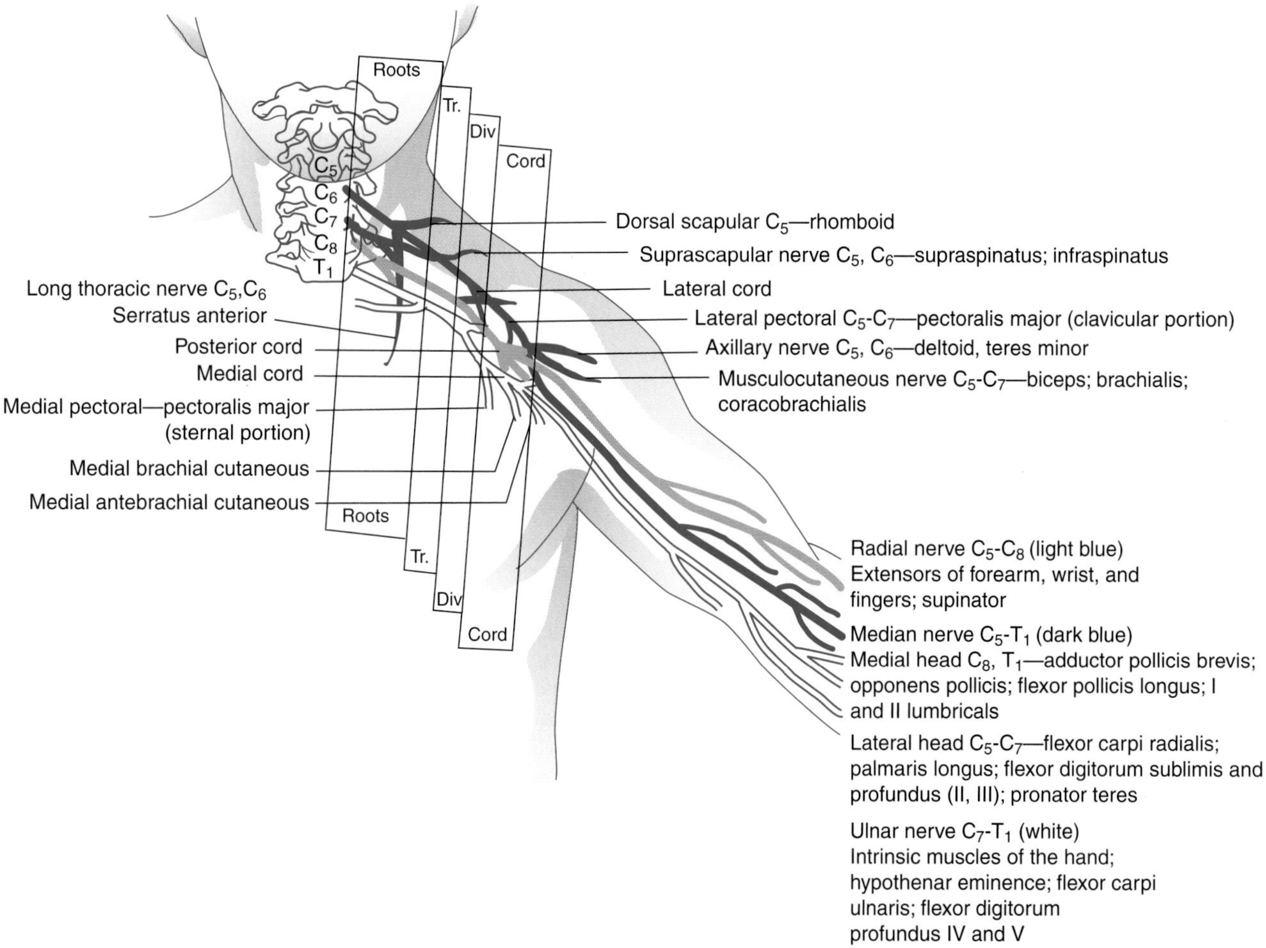

FIGURE 76-3. Relationship of the brachial plexus to peripheral nerves of the shoulder and arm. Note the formation of the brachial plexus from nerve roots of spinal segments C5 to T1. The brachial plexus is divided into roots, trunks, divisions, and cords. The origin of the peripheral nerves and their muscle innervations are listed. The median nerve has a lateral head from the lateral cord (C5, C6, C7) and a medial head from the medial cord (C8, T1). The ulnar nerve also arises from the medial cord, whereas the radial nerve comes directly from the posterior cord.

1984; Rossi et al., 1982; Tada et al., 1984], although other studies question this assumption [Ecker et al., 1997; Graham et al., 1997]. Birth-related brachial plexus injury is associated with clavicle fracture in 10% of cases and humerus fracture in 10%.

The most common brachial plexus injury is Erb's palsy, which composes 80% to 90% of newborn brachial plexus injuries. Damage to the fifth and sixth cervical nerves or the upper trunk of the brachial plexus results in paralysis of the upper arm. The infant with this condition typically lies with the humerus adducted and internally rotated with the elbow extended, forearm pronated, and wrist flexed. The deltoid, biceps, brachialis, supinator, and extensors of the wrist and finger muscles are paralyzed (Fig. 76-4). The biceps and radioperiosteal reflexes are absent. Unless there has been avulsion of nerve roots, recovery occurs in part, if not completely. It is important to protect the arm and brachial plexus from further injury by pinning the forearm in a sleeve sling in front of the chest. Two to three weeks later, passive range of motion is appropriate to prevent contracture of the shoulder. Although quick recovery may be observed, complete recovery may take many months. Good return of hand and arm function by 6 months is a good prognostic sign [DiTaranto et al., 2004].

Surgery for newborn brachial nerve lesions is becoming more popular, especially when electrophysiologic and neuroimaging data indicate primary injury to the plexus and no nerve root evulsion. Primary nerve reconstruction followed by appropriate tendon transfers provides return of function in select patients [Piatt, 2004; Tonkin et al., 1996].

Injury to the lower trunk of the plexus, involving the eighth cervical nerve and first thoracic nerve, is known as *Klumpke's paralysis.* This condition is rare, composing less than 1% of newborn brachial plexus injuries [al-Qattan et al., 1995]. Weakness of the forearm extensors, flexors of the wrist and fingers, and intrinsic muscles of the hand occurs. Horner's syndrome is often present as a result of involvement of the sympathetic fibers accompanying the first thoracic nerve. The elbow is typically flexed, the forearm is supinated, the wrist is extended, and a clawlike deformity of the hand with hyperextension of the wrist and fingers is present. The triceps reflex may be diminished, and the grasp reflex is usually absent. As with Erb's palsy, protection of the plexus initially, followed by passive range-of-motion therapy, in this instance to the wrist and fingers, is appropriate during recovery.

The most severe newborn brachial plexus injury occurs when all three trunks of the brachial plexus are involved.

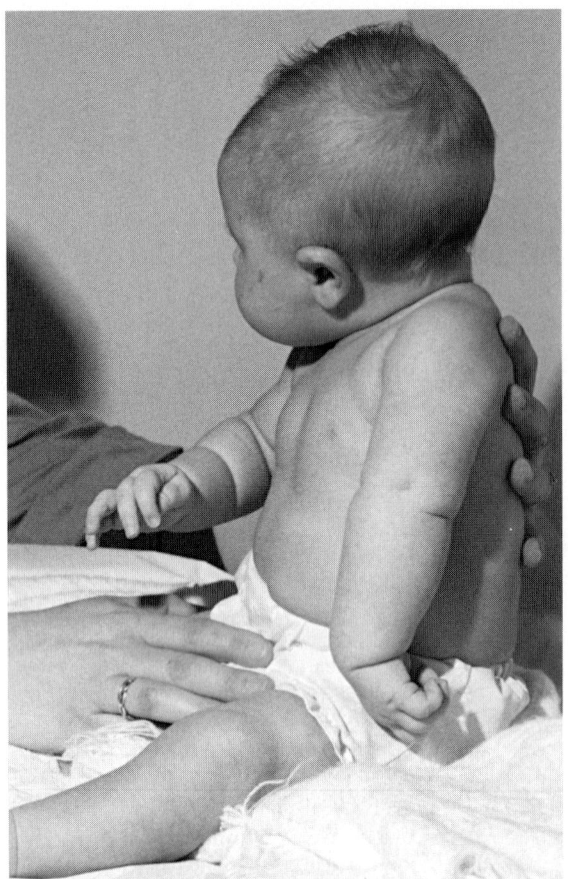

FIGURE 76-4. Erb's palsy caused by birth injury. The arm position is characteristic. The arm is adducted, with the humerus internally rotated, elbow extended, forearm pronated, and wrist flexed. The fingers are not involved. (Courtesy of the Division of Pediatric Neurology, University of Minnesota Medical School, Minneapolis, MN.)

Total brachial plexus involvement is present 10% of the time in newborn injuries. The arm hangs limply from the shoulder with no muscle movement. This is associated with tendon areflexia and decreased sensation over the arm and hand. The outlook for recovery after complete brachial plexus injury is poorer than with isolated upper or lower trunk injury because of the larger distribution of involvement and the usually greater severity of nerve injury. In this circumstance, nerve roots have often been avulsed or nerves in the plexus divided by severe stretching. In up to 10% to 20% of newborn brachial plexus injuries, bilateral involvement is present. Rare instances of brachial neuritis have been reported in children and may be associated with diphtheria-pertussis-tetanus vaccinations [Martin and Weintraub, 1973].

Inherited Conditions

Recurrent inherited brachial plexus neuritis, referred to as *hereditary neuralgic amyotrophy* and carried on chromosome 17q24-q25 as a dominantly inherited condition [Guillozet and Mercer, 1973; Wiederholt, 1974], is typically diagnosed in childhood. This recurrent syndrome manifests with pain and is followed by brachial plexus innervated muscle weakness, often including facial paresis. The long thoracic nerve is involved, with scapular winging present. Lumbar plexus involvement may be noted. Tendon reflexes are reduced. Residual weakness may develop after exacerbations. Autonomic nerves are affected [Dunn et al., 1978]. Short stature, hypotelorism, small face and palpebral fissures, prominent epicanthal folds, and syndactyly are part of the syndrome. Axonal loss is demonstrated by electrophysiologic testing. The condition is believed to be an immune complex disease that causes damage to blood vessel walls. In most instances, recovery occurs spontaneously, and there is no specific treatment [Rubin, 2001].

Hereditary neuropathy with liability to pressure palsies may present in children. This autosomal dominantly inherited condition due to a deletion involving the *PMP22* gene carried on chromosome 17p11.2-p12 may cause recurrent brachial neuropathy. The condition is painless, demyelination is corroborated electrophysiologically, and recovery is common [Windebank et al., 1995].

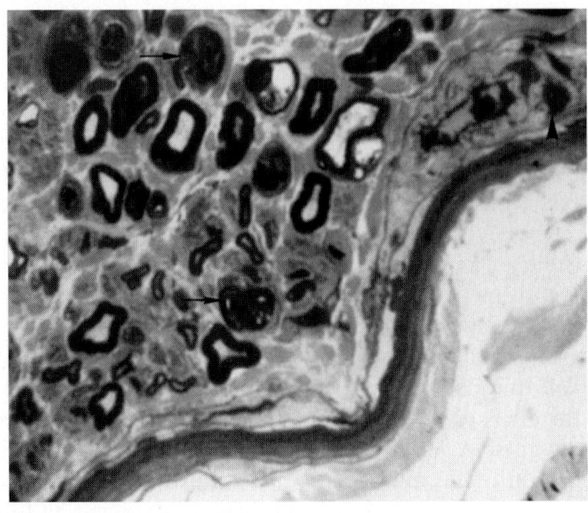

A

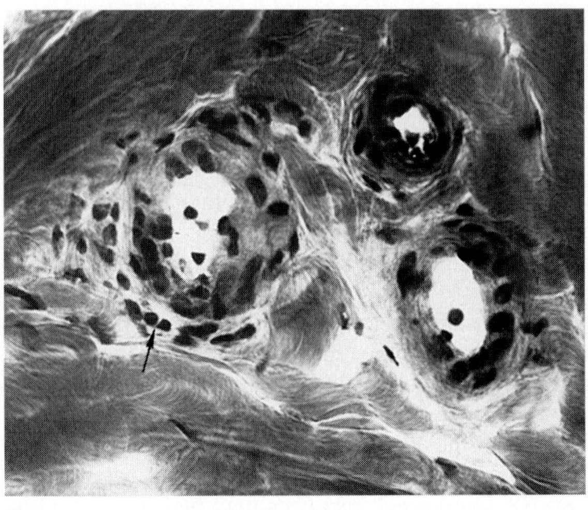

B

FIGURE 76-5. Sural nerve biopsy from a 14-year-old male with acute inflammatory demyelinating polyradiculoneuropathy. **A**, Part of a nerve fascicle demonstrating demyelinating nerve fibers *(arrows)* and perivascular infiltration *(arrowhead)* (×1180). **B**, Perivenular lymphocytic infiltrate *(arrow)* (×1560).

INFLAMMATORY NEUROPATHIES

Acute Inflammatory Demyelinating Polyradiculoneuropathy (Guillain-Barré Syndrome)

Acute inflammatory demyelinating polyradiculoneuropathy is commonly known as *Guillain-Barré syndrome* (see Chapter 72). It is an inflammatory, demyelinating disorder of spinal nerve roots and peripheral nerves of acute to subacute onset. Activated cellular and humoral immune mechanisms, induced by an antecedent, presumably viral infection, trigger inflammation and demyelination [Arnason and Soliven, 1993; Asbury et al., 1969; Brechenmacher et al., 1987; Cook and Dowling, 1981; Hartung et al., 1995a; Honavar et al., 1991; Prineas, 1981]. Cytomegalovirus, Epstein-Barr virus, *M. pneumoniae* infection, vaccinia virus, and *Campylobacter jejuni* bacterial diarrhea are recognized causes of prodromal illness preceding acute inflammatory demyelinating polyradiculoneuropathy [Hartung et al., 1995b; Kuwabara, 2004; Winer et al., 1988]. An antecedent infectious disease is recognized in 65% of cases 3 days to 6 weeks before the onset of symptoms caused by demyelination [Beghi et al., 1985; Hartung et al., 1995b]. The resultant neuropathy is predominantly motor [Guillain et al., 1916] and is typically accompanied by mild sensory loss and sensory ataxia. Severe sensory deficit is rare [Dawson et al., 1988]. Autonomic involvement occurs in children and may be quite severe for some [Hodson et al., 1984].

Pathology

Demyelination and mononuclear cell infiltration of peripheral nerve may be found on nerve biopsy [Honavar et al., 1991; Prineas, 1981]. Varying degrees of edema, endoneurial lymphocytic cell infiltration, and segmental demyelination occur (Fig. 76-5). Macrophage invasion of Schwann cells can be seen ultrastructurally [Brechenmacher et al., 1987]. Spinal roots and proximal and distal nerves display focal and perivenular lymphocytes and macrophages [Hall et al., 1992]. In addition to demyelination, axonal degeneration may be found [Feasby et al., 1993] or may even predominate (acute motor axonal neuropathy) [Hafer-Macko et al., 1996]. Complement-fixing antibodies to peripheral nerve myelin may be demonstrated in some cases [Koski et al., 1987], but not all patients with acute inflammatory demyelinating polyradiculoneuropathy have immunoglobulin deposits on myelin sheaths [Honavar et al., 1991]. Cerebrospinal fluid protein is elevated within the first week, accompanied by a lack of inflammatory cellular response, with usually less than 10 lymphocytes/mm^3.

Clinical Characteristics

The overall incidence of acute inflammatory demyelinating polyradiculoneuropathy is 1 to 2 per 100,000 each year; in the population younger than 18 years, the incidence is 0.8 per 100,000 each year [Beghi et al., 1985]. The incidence rate for males is 1.5 times that for females [Koobatian et al., 1992]. Muscle pain may be the initial manifestation of the disease in children, involving the anterior and posterior thighs, buttocks, and lower back [Ropper and Shahani, 1984]. Pain and paresthesias after infection are quickly followed by symmetric, progressive weakness of extremity and facial muscles. Bladder dysfunction, mental alterations, headache, ataxia, and meningismus may be accompanying features. Tendon reflexes are diminished or lost. The disease may progress for days to several weeks before plateauing, and then improves over a period of months. Weakness may proceed rapidly with complete paralysis, including bulbar paralysis developing within 24 hours of onset. Ventilatory support may be necessary even early in the course of the illness. Eighty percent of patients make an excellent recovery.

Autonomic involvement may produce blurred vision, cramping abdominal pain, postural hypotension, cardiac dysrhythmia, and bladder and bowel incontinence. These symptoms may occur transiently in the course of predominantly motor and sensory involvement.

Electrophysiologic evaluation usually provides evidence for peripheral nerve demyelination often accompanied by changes indicative of axonal involvement. Distal motor and F wave latencies are prolonged to more than 150% of normal. Nerve conduction velocities are reduced to 70% below normal. Compound motor action potentials are reduced with prolonged terminal dispersions, these being the most common electrophysiologic findings in children [Bradshaw and Jones, 1992]. Children younger than 10 years of age have greater slowing of motor nerve conduction velocities than children older than 10. More profound slowing corresponds to high antibody levels against peripheral nerve myelin during the first week of illness [Rudnicki et al., 1992]. In cases in which the pathologic change is one of mainly axonal degeneration, nerve conduction studies reveal normal or mildly slow conduction with diminished amplitude of compound muscle action potentials.

The youngest reported patients are neonates. A 4-month-old child presented with advancing hypotonia [Carroll et al., 1977]. Several other children younger than 6 months of age have been reported. The rate of progression, degree of impairment, and time for improvement vary greatly; however, recovery does not continue after 2 years from onset [Ropper, 1986]. Poor prognosis is related to the need for ventilation and failure to improve after 3 weeks of reaching peak deficit [Winer et al., 1985]. The mortality rate approaches 5% in adults but should be negligible in children; 10% to 15% of adults remain permanently disabled [Arnason, 1984].

Management

Because prognosis is usually excellent for spontaneous recovery, the mainstay of treatment is supportive. Mechanical ventilation may be needed, and careful attention to nutritional, fluid, and electrolyte balance is necessary. When paralyzed and ventilated, children are still mentally alert. They need psychologic support from parents and caregivers. The ordeal may be very frightening.

Plasmapheresis may be effective if started within 7 days of illness onset [French Cooperative Group, 1987; Greenwood et al., 1984; Guillain-Barré Syndrome Study Group, 1985; Osterman et al., 1984; Smith and Hughes, 1992]. If patients lose the ability to walk unaided, have significant reduction in respiratory capacity, or have bulbar insufficiency, plasmapheresis or intravenous immune globulin therapy is indicated. Although most plasmapheresis studies have been performed on adults, a study on children demonstrated shortened recovery time in 5 of 6 children aged 5 to 15 years [Lamont et al., 1991]. A retrospective study documented faster recovery of independent ambulation in 9 children who received plasmapheresis, compared with 14 who did not receive plasmapheresis [Epstein and Sladky, 1990]. Intravenous immune globulin is more convenient in small children and shortens the course of illness [Kleyweg et al., 1988; Sladky, 2004]. In adults, intravenous immune globulin given during the first week is at least as effective as plasmapheresis and may be of greater efficacy [van der Meché et al., 1992]. There is no documented benefit to using both therapies [Bril et al., 1996; Hughes et al., 1996]. Corticosteroids, thought to be of little value, may improve outcome in combination with intravenous immune globulin.

Chronic Inflammatory Demyelinating Polyradiculoneuropathy

Chronic inflammatory demyelinating polyradiculopathy was the cause of polyneuropathy in 8.8% to 11.6% of children in two series of childhood polyneuropathy [Ouvrier and McLeod, 1988; Sladky et al., 1986]. A low frequency of antecedent events is described. Precipitous onset of weakness accompanied by sensory loss and diminished tendon reflexes is typical [Nevo et al., 1996; Simmons et al., 1997]. Pain and cranial neuropathies are uncommon. Progressive weakness for 2 months is required for the diagnosis of chronic inflammatory demyelinating polyradiculoneuropathy, although one of five affected children reach their nadir by this time [Simmons et al., 1993]. For some children, a monophasic disease progresses beyond 2 months, and for others, relapses are common.

Pathology

Cerebrospinal protein is elevated with a normal cell count. Slowed conduction velocities, prolonged distal latencies, and temporal dispersion are present electrophysiologically. Sural nerve biopsy, if performed, shows demyelination, remyelination, and usually a lymphocytic inflammatory infiltrate. Onion bulb formation indicates chronicity of the condition (Fig. 76-6).

Management

Patients, including children, improve with therapy [Colan et al., 1980; Gorson et al., 1997; Nevo et al., 1996; Sladky et al., 1986; Uncini et al., 1991], which most often begins with intravenous immune globulin or, less commonly, plasmapheresis. Plasmapheresis combined with prednisone or prednisone alone has also been used. Sustained recovery is expected with treatment [Simmons et al., 1997], and even without treatment, most children eventually improve.

HEREDITARY NEUROPATHIES

About 70% of chronic neuropathies seen in children are hereditary. In Dyck's classification of these conditions [Dyck, 1984], the broad categories of hereditary motor, hereditary sensory and autonomic, and hereditary motor and sensory neuropathies are subdivided on the basis of clinical, genetic, and (rarely) biochemical characteristics. The main basis for inclusion in one of these three groups is whether the peripheral motor, peripheral sensory, or both are mainly affected. The peripheral motor neuropathies are called the *spinal muscular atrophies* in other classifications and are described in Chapter 75. The original Dyck classification of the hereditary motor and sensory neuropathies did not allow for the inclusion of autosomal and X-linked recessive forms of hereditary motor and sensory neuropathy types I and II. Nor could it have included the striking recent advances in the understanding of the molecular biology of these disorders. Because the question of classification is in flux, a modified version of Dyck's classification is included in Tables 76-2 and 76-3.

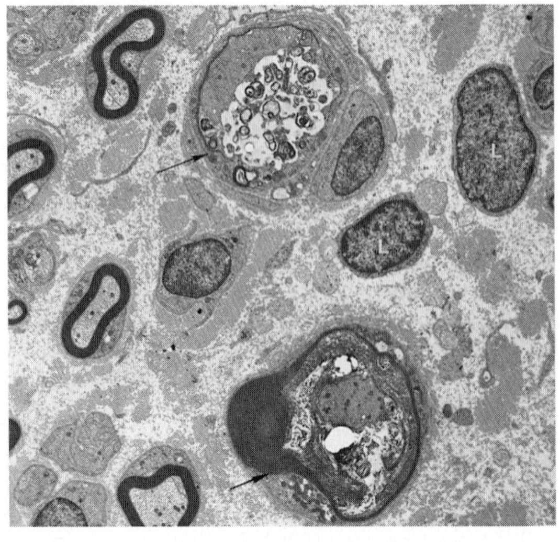

A

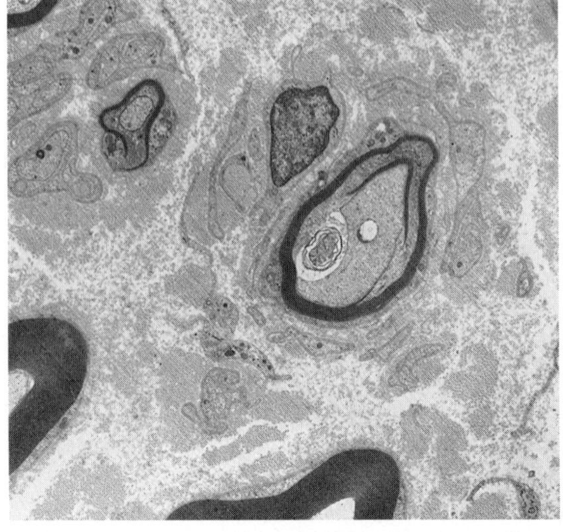

B

FIGURE 76-6. Sural nerve biopsy from a 5-year-old female with chronic inflammatory demyelinating polyradiculoneuropathy. **A**, Demyelination of two nerve fibers *(arrows)* with lymphocytes (L) located nearby (×6100). **B**, Partial demyelination of a nerve fiber surrounded by redundant Schwann cell elements, including excessive basement membrane. This process represents early onion bulb formation, which develops as the disease progresses (×8400).

TABLE 76-2

Subclassifications of Charcot-Marie-Tooth (CMT) Syndrome

DISORDER (OMIM NO.)	INHERITANCE	CHROMOSOMAL LOCUS	PATHOLOGIC MECHANISM	HISTOPATHOLOGIC FEATURES	CLINICAL FEATURES
CMT 1A (118220)	AD	Chromosome 17, 1.5-Mb duplication at 17p11.2-12	DNA duplication, PMP 22 protein	Sheath hypertrophy, onion bulb formation	Distal weakness; mild functional impairment; slowing of NCVs
CMT 1B (118200)	AD	1q21-23	Duffy linked, myelin protein P0 mutation	Similar to CMT 1A or more severe	Similar to CMT 1A or more severe (see Dejerine-Sottas syndrome)
CMT 1C	AD	16p13.1-p12.1	LITAF missense		
CMT 1D	AR	10q21.1-q22.1	EGR2/KROX20 mutation		
CMT 1E (118300)	AD	17p11.2	*PMP22* mutation		Associated with sensorineural deafness
CMT 1F	AR, AD	8p21	*NEFL* mutation		Early onset, severe; is confused with Dejerine-Sottas syndrome
CMT 1	AR	Unknown		Fewer classic onion bulbs; basal lamina bulbs more frequent; tomacula present	Early onset, similar to CMT 1A but more complex
CMT X1 (302800)	X-linked AD	Xq13.1	Connexin 32 (gap junction protein [GJB1] mutation); NB GJB1 and P0 mutations have also been found in CMT 2 patients.	Demyelination and axonal degeneration; minimal hypertrophy; MNCVs lower than normal but faster than CMT 1A	X-linked: absence of male-to-male transmission; females mildly affected; males more severely affected than in CMT 1A
CMT X2 (302801)	X-linked AR	Xp22.2	Unknown		Rare X-linked: only 1 family affected; females very mildly affected
CMT X3 (302802)	X-linked AR	Xq26	Unknown		As for CMT X2 but 2 families studied
CMT 2A (118210)	AD	1p35-36	Kinesin family member gene 1B (*KIF1B*) mutation; mitofusin 2 (MFN2)	Axonal degeneration	Normal NCVs; later onset than CMT 1A
CMT 2B	AD	3q13-q22	RAB7 missense	Large and small fiber loss	Single kindred; sensory features
CMT 2B1 (605588)	AR	1q21.2-3	LMNA missense		Confined to a small Moroccan pedigree
CMT 2B2 (605589)	AR	19q13.3	Unknown		Confined to a small inbred Costa Rican pedigree
CMT 2C (606071)		Linked to chromosome 12	Unknown		Severe, including respiratory failure and vocal weakness
CMT 2D (601472)	AD	7p15	*GARS* mutation		Clinically similar to CMT 2A; spinal atrophy
CMT 2E (607684)	AD	8p21	*NEFL* gene mutation		Few kindreds
CMT 2F (606595)	AD	7q11-q21	HSPB1/ HSP27; small heat-shock protein		
CMT 2G (607706)	AR	8q13-q21.1	GDAP1 missense		Several kindreds, some severe with vocal weakness
CMT 2H (607731)	AR	8q21.3	GDAP1 missense		Pyramidal features; single Tunisian kindred
CMT 2I (607677)	AD	1q22, 8q21.3	*MPZ* (P0) mutation GDAP1 missense		Late onset
CMT 2J (607736)	AR	1q22	*MPZ* (P0) mutation		Sensory and pupillary abnormalities

continued

TABLE 76-2, *cont'd*

Subclassifications of Charcot-Marie-Tooth (CMT) Syndrome

DISORDER (OMIM NO.)	INHERITANCE	CHROMOSOMAL LOCUS	PATHOLOGIC MECHANISM	HISTOPATHOLOGIC FEATURES	CLINICAL FEATURES
CMT 2K (607831)	AR	8q13-q21.1	*GDAP1* missense		Single Moroccan kindred
CMT 3 (145900) (Dejerine-Sottas syndrome)	AR, AD	19q13.1, 17p11.2, 1q22 (a number of specific allelic variants have been reported)	Periaxin (*PRX*), *PMP22, MPZ* (P0), *EGR2*	Hypomyelination; basal lamina onion bulb formation; MNCVs < 10 m/sec	Clinically severe; infantile onset; global delay; cranial and spinal nerve involvement (shares features with severe CMT 1A, especially in the tetrasomic homozygous variants)
CMT 4A (214400)	AR, occasionally AD	8q13-q21.1	*GDAP1* mutation	Axonal degeneration	Early and severe onset; complete distal (to elbows and knees) paralysis by teens; often nonambulatory
CMT 4B1 (601382)	AR	11q22	*MTMR2* gene mutation	Congenital hypomyelination; excessive myelin out-folding; onion bulbs; slow NCVs	Clinically mild to severe; early distal weakness and pes cavus; cranial nerve signs; confined to small pedigrees; glaucoma in CMT 4B2
CMT 4B2 (604563)	AR	11p15	*MTMR* 13 (SBF2) mutation		
CMT 4C (601596)	AR	5q32	*KIAA*1985 mutation		
CMT 4D (601455) Lom type	AR	8q24.3	*NDRG1* mutation		Closed gypsy pedigree; associated with deafness
CMT 4E (605253)	AR	10q21-22	*EGR2* (Krox20 mouse homolog) mutation		
CMT 4F (145900)	AR	19q13	Periaxin (PRX)		See CMT 3 (Dejerine-Sottas syndrome)
CMT 5 (600631)	AD	Not known; linkages excluded at chromosomes 1, 3, 7, 10, 17	Unknown	Axonal degeneration	Two families; pyramidal features; marked leg cramps; late onset
CMT intermediate A (608340)	AR	8q13-q21.1	*GDAP1* mutation	Intermediate NCVs	Two Turkish families; mixed axonal and demyelinating features; fairly mild
CMT intermediate B (606482)	AD	19p13.2-p12	Unknown		
CMT intermediate C (608323)	AD	1p35	Unknown		Two unrelated families
CMT intermediate D (607791)	AD	1q22-q23	*MPZ* (P0) mutation		
Hereditary neuropathy with liability to pressure palsies (HNPP) (162500)		Chromosome 17, 1.5-Mb deletion at 17p11.2-12	DNA deletion (or missense mutation) affecting PMP 22 protein synthesis	Presence of tomaculous changes on biopsy with uncompacted myelin; mild slowing of MNCVs, but conduction block may be present	Acute onset of weakness and sensory loss following nerve trauma; often the functional deficit is temporary, returning to baseline levels over time; may be episodic
Roussy-Lévy syndrome (180800)		Chromosome 17, 500-Kb partial duplication at 17p11.2; 1q22-q23	*PMP22* or *MPZ* (P0) mutation		Similar features to CMT 1A but with associated gait ataxia and tremor; in later life may suffer neuropathic foot ulcers

AD, autosomal dominant; AR, autosomal recessive; MNCV, motor nerve conduction velocity; NCV, nerve conduction velocity.
Data from Auer-Grumbach and Strasser-Fuchs, 1998; Chance, 2001; Murakami et al., 1996; Ouvrier, 1996; Vance et al., 2000; and the National Institutes of Health On-line Mendelian Inheritance in Man database.

TABLE 76-3

Hereditary Sensory and Autonomic Neuropathies

TYPE	INHERITANCE	COMMENTS
I	Autosomal dominant	Linked to 9q22.1-22.3
II	Autosomal recessive	—
III	Autosomal recessive	Riley-Day syndrome
IV	Autosomal recessive	Possibly due to TRKA receptor defect
V	Possibly autosomal recessive	—
Other	—	—

Note: The term *CMT 3* should be reserved for hereditary neuropathies in which hypomyelination is the dominant feature. This would include congenital hypomyelinating neuropathy, Dejerine-Sottas syndrome, and congenital amyelinating neuropathy.

Hereditary Motor and Sensory Neuropathy

Hereditary motor and sensory neuropathy types I and II are often referred to as *Charcot-Marie-Tooth disease.* Charcot-Marie-Tooth disease is characterized by weakness of the extremities and foot deformities, including pes cavus and permanently flexed "hammer" toes. Variable loss of sensation is present. This condition is also referred to as *peroneal muscular atrophy* because of characteristic muscle wasting and weakness in legs early in the course of the illness. The distinction between types I and II is discussed later. Charcot-Marie-Tooth disease is present throughout the world, with an estimated prevalence of up to 40 per 100,000. In most countries, hereditary motor and sensory neuropathy type I is three or four times more common than type II disease.

Type I

Hereditary motor and sensory neuropathy type I is a heterogeneous disorder causing a progressive motor and sensory demyelinating neuropathy. It is a dominantly inherited disorder with onset in the first or second decade of life. In certain families, the defective gene maps to chromosome 1 [Chance et al., 1990; Lebo et al., 1990], where it has been found to cause mutations of myelin protein zero (P0), the most abundant protein in peripheral myelin [Hayasaka et al., 1993]. Much more commonly, the defective gene links to the short arm of chromosome 17 in the region 17p11.2 [Middleton-Price et al., 1990; Raeymakers et al., 1989; Vance et al., 1989]. In most type I families, affected members have a 1.5 million base-pair tandem DNA duplication at that site [Hallam et al., 1992; Lupski et al., 1991; Raeymakers et al., 1991]. This region contains the gene for the myelin protein PMP22, increased amounts of which may lead to excessive or faulty production of myelin. Rare cases of hereditary motor and sensory neuropathy type I have been due to point mutations of the *PMP22* gene. The disease carried on chromosome 17 is designated *type Ia,* and the condition carried on chromosome 1 is called *type Ib.* Although cases of hereditary motor and sensory neuropathy types Ia and Ib caused by point mutations tend to be more severely affected than cases caused by the duplication on chromosome 17, the frequent exceptions to the rule make it difficult to separate these subtypes on clinical or neurophysiologic grounds. Cases of autosomal-dominant hereditary motor and sensory neuropathy type I exist in which no abnormalities of the *PMP22* or *MPZ* gene can be demonstrated. Hereditary motor and sensory neuropathy *type Ic* is due to mutations of the *LITAF* gene, whereas *type Id* is due to *EGR2* mutation and *type If* is due to mutation in the neurofilament light-chain gene.

There is also a "spinal" form of Charcot-Marie-Tooth disease, known as *distal spinal muscular atrophy,* in which degeneration of specific anterior horn cells leads to a clinical picture similar to hereditary motor and sensory neuropathy type I or II but without any sensory nerve involvement.

PATHOLOGY

The peripheral nerves in hereditary motor and sensory neuropathy type I are often easily palpated because they are hypertrophied as a result of excessive Schwann cell and

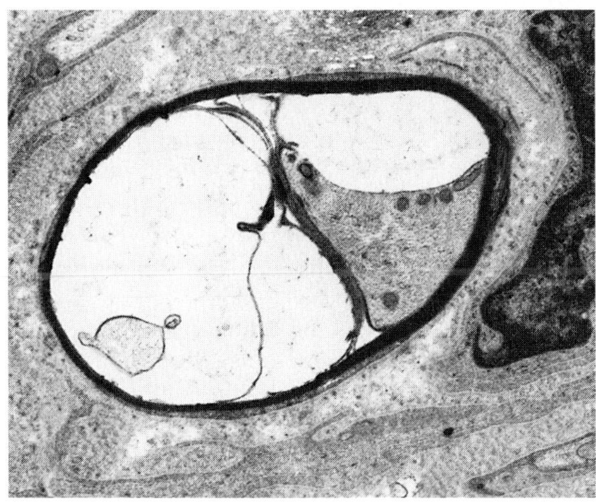
A

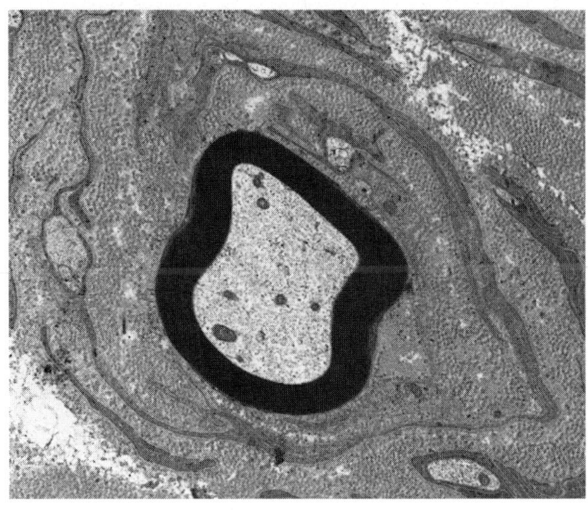
B

FIGURE 76-7. Sural nerve biopsy from a 15-year-old female with hereditary motor and sensory neuropathy type I, the hypertrophic form of Charcot-Marie-Tooth disease. **A**, Demyelination and axonal disruption are noted (×17,400). **B**, Typical onion bulb formation with a myelinated nerve fiber surrounded by redundant Schwann cell investments, basement laminae, and collagen (×10,100).

fibroblast activity. This situation creates redundant wrappings of Schwann cell investments around nerve fibers accompanied by excessive collagen deposition, known as *onion bulbs* [Thomas et al., 1974]. Sural nerve biopsies disclose a loss of myelinated fibers, especially the large myelinated fibers. With advancing age, there is progressive reduction in the myelinated fiber density, an increased number of fibers undergoing demyelination, and increased frequency of onion bulb formations [Low et al., 1978]. In this setting, onion bulb formations are the result of repeated episodes of demyelination and remyelination (Fig. 76-7). Some loss of axonal neurotubules and filaments may eventually be observed, indicating that, although demyelination is predominant, some axonal degeneration is part of the disease process and is responsible for the progression of the weakness and wasting [Nordborg et al., 1984].

CLINICAL CHARACTERISTICS

The disease is typically recognized during the first decade of life or in early adolescence, but it may be evident even at birth. A large variation in the age of onset and severity of disease among individuals in the same family has sometimes been observed [Birouk et al., 1997; Hagberg and Lyon, 1981]. Early onset, although uncommon, usually results in greater disability later in life than that seen in individuals with later onset, who are often able to ambulate and work until old age.

The disease presents with distal lower extremity muscle wasting and weakness, accompanied by development of pes cavus. Progressive weakness of the tibialis anterior and peroneal muscles, which are more involved clinically than the tibialis posterior muscle, is associated with the development of the high arch of the foot or pes cavus. The hammer toe deformities occur as the long toe extensors attempt to make up for the foot dorsiflexor (tibialis anterior) atrophy and weakness. Gradual loss of sensation is noted, especially loss of proprioception, which causes unsteady gait in darkness and a positive Romberg sign. Vibration and big toe position sense are both diminished. Tendon reflexes are usually lost early at the ankle and later at the knee. Muscle wasting and weakness slowly spread proximally, so that atrophy of the medial rectus muscle and distal rectus femoris in the quadriceps group becomes apparent. Classically, the leg assumes a storklike appearance, with little motor function remaining, but this is rare in children with hereditary motor and sensory neuropathy type I. As the lower extremities become more involved, atrophy of the hand intrinsic muscles with accompanying weakness is recognized, which leads to difficulty with fine motor skills, including writing. Distal sensory loss soon becomes evident in the upper extremities. Kyphosis and scoliosis develop in about 10% of cases. Variability of expression among families makes it difficult to describe a uniform rate of change. Typically, younger age of clinical recognition and more rapid progression in a parent are associated with similar expression in affected children. Some individuals require wheelchair assistance because of severe muscle weakness. Much more commonly, patients remain ambulatory, often assisted by leg braces or corrective foot surgery at the end of the second decade or in the third decade. The condition is compatible with normal longevity.

CLINICAL NEUROPHYSIOLOGY

Motor and sensory conduction velocity is within the "demyelinating" range and is thus less than 60% of normal values in infants; in patients older than 3 years, it is less than 38 m/second in all peripheral nerves. Conduction velocity changes little with increasing age, but there is a progressive reduction in the amplitude of the evoked muscle action potential, indicating axonal loss [Roy et al., 1989].

GENETICS

Hereditary motor and sensory neuropathy types Ia through If are dominantly inherited. In addition, autosomal recessive [Gabreels-Festen et al., 1992; Harding and Thomas, 1980] and X-linked forms of a similar disorder exist [Hahn et al., 1990; Rozear et al., 1987]. Autosomal-recessive forms, which are designated Charcot-Marie-Tooth disease type 4, tend to have an earlier onset and a higher incidence of ataxia, complete areflexia, and kyphoscoliosis than dominant types. Several recessive varieties have been cloned or linked to specific chromosomal regions, such as in inbred Tunisian (chromosome 8q13-21) [Ben Othmane et al., 1993], Bulgarian (chromosome 8q24) [Kalaydjieva et al., 1996], and Algerian (chromosome 5q23-33) [Kessali et al., 1997] families. Another form with florid myelin sheath changes, known as *hereditary motor and sensory neuropathy with focally folded myelin* or *congenital dysmyelinating neuropathy,* has been linked to chromosome 11q23. Even this latter condition, however, is heterogeneous. Charcot-Marie-Tooth disease type 4B1 is due to mutations of the myotubularin gene, whereas type 4B2 is due to a mutation of the *SBF2* gene.

The classification of Charcot-Marie-Tooth disease and related disorders has become complex and confused and is likely to remain so because of the ever-expanding list of gene mutations that are continuing to be discovered. A recent classification is shown in Table 76-2.

MANAGEMENT

Treatment is supportive. Early in the course of the disease, strengthening exercises for the feet and legs with active stretching of the feet may be beneficial, although there is no objective evidence for this. Typically, the hind foot can be dorsiflexed well beyond 90 degrees, but tightness in the plantar fascia may inhibit normal forefoot dorsiflexion as the pes cavus deformity becomes more pronounced. Special attention to stretching of the forefoot in late childhood and early adolescence may be of considerable benefit in helping maintain gait without footdrop. Using polypropylene ankle-foot orthoses to stabilize the feet and correct the footdrop reduces the likelihood of falling. The lightweight polypropylene orthoses slip conveniently into supportive shoes and can be covered by socks. In adolescence, orthopedic surgery on the foot to reduce the pes cavus deformity and eliminate footdrop by fusing the ankle bones together may be helpful. After such stabilizing surgery, some adolescents have been able to resume strenuous activities, such as water skiing and tennis.

Involvement of the wrist and hand may call for the use of special adaptive devices for the hands, such as cock-up splints or specially adapted writing instruments, communicators, and utensils.

It is hoped that as the genes causing the various forms of Charcot-Marie-Tooth disease are isolated and their gene products identified, more specific therapies will become available.

Type II

Hereditary motor and sensory neuropathy (Charcot-Marie-Tooth disease) type II is heterogeneous and is usually dominantly inherited. Autosomal recessive and X-linked forms of the disorder are known and will be discussed further [Hahn et al., 1990; Harding and Thomas, 1980; Rozear et al., 1987]. Hereditary motor and sensory neuropathy type II does not link to chromosome 17 [Loprest et al., 1992]. The known gene mutations and linkages for type II are shown in Table 76-2. In general, onset of clinical manifestations tends to be later in dominantly inherited hereditary motor and sensory neuropathy type II than in type I. Muscle atrophy and weakness are milder and more prominent than sensory deficits compared with the type I disorder. Otherwise, the clinical course of type II disease is similar to that found in type I.

The pathology is marked by axonal degeneration. Nerve hypertrophy and palpable nerve enlargement are not present. The onion bulb formation typical of type I disease is rarely seen. In one variant, focally enlarged myelinated axons with aggregations of neurofilaments have been described [Goebel et al., 1986]. In addition to the focal accumulation of intra-axonal neurofilaments in the myelinated fibers, similar structures have been seen without axonal enlargement in the nonmyelinated axons. Similar structures have been noted in fibroblasts and endothelial cells in muscle and skin. Whether these intra-axonal filaments describe a different disease process is unknown. Nerve conduction velocities are low normal to slightly reduced.

A rather severe form of hereditary motor and sensory neuropathy type II, which is usually of autosomal-recessive inheritance, was designated *hereditary motor and sensory neuropathy of neuronal type with onset in early childhood.* Two large series of such patients were reported [Gabreels-Festen et al., 1991; Ouvrier et al., 1981]. The disorder accounts for up to 5% of childhood chronic neuropathies. The features of the disorder include sporadic occurrence or evidence of autosomal-recessive or, less commonly, autosomal-dominant inheritance. In addition, onset of weakness within the first 5 years of life, rapid progression of weakness to almost complete paralysis below the elbows and knees by the second decade, moderate sensory changes in most cases, clinical electrophysiologic studies consistent with an axonal degenerative polyneuropathy, and histologic studies indicating neuronal (axonal) atrophy and degeneration of peripheral motor and sensory neurons are noted. Cerebrospinal fluid is usually normal. The condition advances rather rapidly, so that most patients are nonambulatory by the middle to late teens. The chromosomal localization of this group of disorders is not yet known.

Congenital Axonal Types

Some infants are born with arthrogryposis secondary to an axonal neuropathy. This condition is often a nonprogressive disorder, presumably secondary to some intrauterine insult. It is not clear whether these disorders are hereditary. Cases have been described in which infants a few weeks old have presented with rapidly progressive respiratory distress leading to death or permanent ventilatory support within the first year of life [Appleton et al., 1994; Vanasse and Michaud, 1992]. In these cases, clinical electrophysiologic and histopathologic examinations have been consistent with a form of spinal muscular atrophy affecting the diaphragm and distal muscles preferentially. In others, investigations have suggested the presence of an axonal neuropathy. Mutations of the gene encoding the immunoglobulin mu binding protein (*IGHMBP2*) cause these disorders.

Type III (Dejerine-Sottas Disease) and Hypomyelinating Neuropathies

Hypomyelinating neuropathies are disorders in which Schwann cells are, to a variable extent, incapable of forming normal myelin. Histopathologically, they are characterized by the presence of thin myelin sheaths, often with few or poorly compacted myelin lamellae, and by the presence of onion bulbs, which are often large and made up of thin lamellae and basal lamina remnants.

The most extreme form of hypomyelinating neuropathy, in which the patient is severely affected at birth by a condition resembling congenital spinal muscular atrophy, is sometimes termed *congenital amyelinating neuropathy* [Charnas et al., 1988; Karch and Urich, 1975; Kasman et al., 1976; Palix and Coignet, 1978; Seitz et al., 1986]. In this group, arthrogryposis is common, presumably because of lack of limb movements in utero. Because of respiratory problems and swallowing difficulties, these infants usually die when very young. Nerve conduction velocity is either unrecordable or extremely low. Peripheral nerve histopathologic examination reveals no (amyelination) or very little myelin and virtually absent onion bulbs. Such cases probably represent examples of the extreme end of the spectrum of clinical and pathologic severity resulting from myelin protein mutations.

Dejerine-Sottas disease (hereditary motor and sensory neuropathy type III) pathologically is associated with hypomyelination. In most cases, hypotonia, delay in developmental milestones, or both are noted within the first year of life. The onset of walking is often delayed beyond the second year, but most hereditary motor and sensory neuropathy type III toddlers eventually do walk, although coordination is never fully normal. Ataxia is present in all patients and is probably due to a proprioceptive deficit. Distal weakness, more marked in the lower limbs, is present early. Proximal weakness and deformity of the hands and feet are not common in early childhood. Both become increasingly more obvious with advancing age, so that by the second decade, proximal weakness is the rule. Deep tendon reflexes are usually absent. Clinical enlargement of nerves, with the median and other peripheral nerves feeling thicker than a pencil, is present in most hereditary motor and sensory neuropathy type III patients by the end of the first decade or earlier. By the time adequate testing can be performed, moderate-to-severe sensory loss is present in most patients. By comparison, such sensory loss is rarely seen in hereditary motor and sensory neuropathy type I cases. Scoliosis often occurs early and tends to progress. Nerve conduction velocities are typically lower than 10 m/second, probably because of loss of saltatory conduction. Prognosis is variable [Guzzetta et al., 1982]. Some patients clearly deteriorate over the first two decades [Tyson et al., 1997], but most patients whom we have been able to follow have experienced little change over many years, except for the progression of limb deformities and scoliosis [Ouvrier et al., 1987].

Many, perhaps most, cases of congenital hypomyelinating neuropathy and Dejerine-Sottas syndrome are the result of myelin protein mutations. The (dominant) heterozygous PMP22 and myelin P0, as well as homozygous myelin P0, mutations have been reported to cause the Dejerine-Sottas phenotype [Tyson et al., 1997; Valentijn et al., 1995; Warner et al., 1996]. In addition, homozygous inheritance of the chromosome 17p11.2 -12 duplication (in which the patient has four copies of the *PMP22* gene), compound heterozygous states involving a deletion and a point mutation of the *PMP22* gene [Gonnaud et al., 1995], and a case of apparent homozygosity for hereditary motor and sensory neuropathy type II [Sghirlanzoni et al., 1992] caused by a myelin P0 mutation [Taroni et al., 1996] have all been associated with the Dejerine-Sottas phenotype. There is probably also a rare autosomal-recessive form. The complexity of the genetics of the Dejerine-Sottas syndrome makes it important to study such cases and their families before genetic counseling is given. In addition to the preceding studies, two remarkable cases of recovery from a congenital hypomyelinating neuropathy were reported [Ghamdi et al., 1997; Levy et al., 1997].

Types IV to VII

The term *hereditary motor and sensory neuropathy type IV* was applied by Dyck to Refsum's disease but is not widely used. Dyck designated patients with spastic paraplegia, who had abnormalities in quantitative testing of sensation, of sensory nerve conduction, and of histometric evaluation of sural nerve, as well as a pattern of autosomal-dominant inheritance, as cases of *hereditary motor and sensory neuropathy type V*. Harding and Thomas [1984] reported 25 cases of peroneal muscular atrophy with pyramidal features. In contrast to Dyck and colleagues [1975], these authors believed that peroneal muscular atrophy with pyramidal features is a separate disorder from hereditary spastic paraplegia but that it also demonstrates heterogeneity. The combination of hereditary motor and sensory neuropathy with optic atrophy was designated *hereditary motor and sensory neuropathy type VI* by Dyck and colleagues [1975]. First described by Vizioli [1879], this rare condition may be transmitted by autosomal-dominant or autosomal-recessive inheritance [Ippel et al., 1995]. The combination of a neuropathy with familial retinitis pigmentosa, first reported by Massion-Verniory and associates [1946] from Belgium, was designated *hereditary motor and sensory neuropathy type VII* by Dyck and colleagues [1975]. In the original family, a 34-year-old male rather abruptly developed visual and gait difficulties that worsened over the next 9 years. Two of his sisters had pigmentary retinopathy without evidence of neuropathy. Cerebrospinal fluid protein was elevated. A nerve biopsy was unhelpful. Cases of this combination are rare and, to the authors' knowledge, have not been reported in childhood.

X-Linked Forms

X-LINKED DOMINANT FORMS (X-LINKED DOMINANT CHARCOT-MARIE-TOOTH DISEASE)

About 10% of hereditary motor and sensory neuropathies are transmitted by X-linked inheritance. The cardinal features of X-linked dominant hereditary motor and sensory neuropathy are as follows:

1. A pattern of inheritance consistent with X-linked transmission, as indicated by absence of male-to-male transmission, a tendency for females to be less severely affected than males, or demonstration of genetic linkage with X chromosome markers, as well as absence of the DNA duplication seen on chromosome 17 in hereditary motor and sensory neuropathy type Ia patients
2. Onset of symptoms within the first or second decade
3. Progressive wasting and weakness of distal limb musculature, more marked in affected males than females, and with more severe involvement, especially of the hands, in males with X-linked hereditary motor and sensory neuropathy than males with hereditary motor and sensory neuropathy type Ia
4. Median nerve motor conduction velocity usually between 30 and 40 m/second
5. Presence of some obligate carrier females with nerve conduction velocities varying in a range from 25 m/second to normal
6. Histopathologic features predominantly of axonal degeneration and regeneration but with some evidence of segmental demyelination in sural nerve biopsies

Clinical Manifestations

The clinical features of X-linked hereditary motor and sensory neuropathy are broadly similar to those of hereditary motor and sensory neuropathy type Ia, but the disease is more severe in X-linked hereditary motor and sensory neuropathy males and less severe in females than in hereditary motor and sensory neuropathy type Ia. Gait difficulties are usually the first manifestation. Wasting of leg muscles and subsequently of the intrinsic muscles of the hands is more marked in X-linked hereditary motor and sensory neuropathy males than females and more obvious than in males with hereditary motor and sensory neuropathy type Ia. The patellar reflexes are retained in about 50% of affected females but only in 10% of males. The ankle jerks are absent in most cases [Nicholson and Nash, 1993]. Sensory loss is present in more than 75% of affected adult men and women. Clinical hypertrophy of nerves is not a feature. Despite the presence of the condition, few adults with the disorder are sufficiently disabled to interfere with work until age 50 or 60 years. Affected males often require canes to stabilize their gait when elderly, but they are not often wheelchair bound.

Clinical Neurophysiology

Motor nerve conduction velocities in X-linked hereditary motor and sensory neuropathy males tend to be lower than normal but faster than those in typical hereditary motor and sensory neuropathy type I cases. Nicholson and Nash [1993] found a mean median motor nerve velocity of 31 m/second in a group of 20 X-linked hereditary motor and sensory neuropathy males from two kindreds, compared with a mean median motor nerve conduction velocity of 45 m/second in 32 affected females.

The histopathologic findings on sural nerve biopsy have been variable. Biopsies in patients with proven connexin mutations demonstrate a mixture of demyelination and axonal degeneration. Fiber loss and regenerative cluster formation are evident in transverse sections but with some onion bulb formation. Rarely there are marked changes of chronic demyelination.

Genetics

As an X-linked dominant condition, expression is more severe in affected males than affected females. Fathers transmit the gene to all of their daughters but none of their sons. Affected females transmit the gene to half their sons and half their daughters. Thus, fewer males are affected than females.

The gene is localized to the DXYS1 region at Xq13.1 on the proximal long arm of the X chromosome near the centromere [Bergoffen et al., 1993b; Fischbeck et al., 1986]. More recently, it was recognized that the gene for the gap junction protein (connexin 32) was located in the same chromosomal segment. Direct sequencing of the connexin 32 gene has revealed mutations in individuals with X-linked Charcot-Marie-Tooth disease [Bergoffen et al., 1993a]. There is remarkable variability in the connexin 32 mutations, with mostly different mutations in tested patients with X-linked hereditary motor and sensory neuropathy [Scherer et al., 1995]. Connexin 32 is normally expressed in myelinated peripheral nerve and appears to be localized mainly at the nodes of Ranvier and Schmidt-Lanterman incisures. It is postulated that connexin 32 may form intracellular gap junctions that connect the folds of Schwann cell cytoplasm, allowing transfer of ions, nutrients, and other small molecules around and across the compact myelin to the innermost myelin layers, perhaps also providing indirect sustenance to the axon as well [Bergoffen et al., 1993a].

X-LINKED RECESSIVE FORMS

X-linked recessive inheritance of a condition resembling hereditary motor and sensory neuropathy type II has also been reported. The specific characteristics of these disorders are poorly defined.

Hereditary Sensory and Autonomic Neuropathies

Type I

Hereditary sensory and autonomic neuropathy type I is a dominantly inherited disorder, usually evident in the second or third decade of life [Dyck, 1984]. The condition is mapped to 9q22.1-22.3 [Nicholson et al., 1996]. The disorder is caused by mutations of the *SPTLC1* gene encoding serine palmitoyl transferase [Dawkins et al., 2001]. In some instances, genetic analysis has indicated that a similar disease may be inherited as an autosomal-recessive condition rather than as the typical dominantly inherited condition with variable expression [Kondo et al., 1974]. Characteristically, the patient experiences lightning-like pains and develops perforating ulcers of the feet.

Cutaneous sensation and tendon reflexes are lost in the lower extremities [Berginer et al., 1984]. Pes cavus, hammer toes, and peroneal muscular weakness develop. Variability of disease expression is so great that some affected relatives may be asymptomatic, but 100% penetrance is evident by the age of 30 years, as reported in the large kindred by Nicholson and colleagues [1996]. Spontaneous amputations of the distal limbs have occurred. Pathologic studies from such individuals have demonstrated nerve degeneration and bone necrosis [Teot et al., 1985]. As individuals advance into adulthood, the loss of all peripheral sensory modalities, except those of the face, has been reported [Nance and Kirby, 1985]. Hereditary deafness is an associated feature [Fitzpatrick et al., 1976; Nicholson et al., 1996]. Increased immunoglobulin A levels were found in members of three unrelated families [Whitaker et al., 1974]. In a separate family, both immunoglobulin A and G levels rose as the disease progressed [Iwabuchi et al., 1976]. Sural nerve biopsy reveals marked loss of myelinated nerve fibers, especially large myelinated fibers, and loss of unmyelinated nerve fibers [Danon and Carpenter, 1985]. Treatment is limited and is generally preventive. Protection of the feet from injury by wearing appropriate shoes and avoiding jumping and falling is important. Meticulous attention to proper toenail trimming and treatment of plantar ulcers are other important measures. If conservative efforts fail, amputation of affected extremities is necessary [Gwathmey and House, 1984].

Type II

Hereditary sensory and autonomic neuropathy type II occurs as a congenital sensory neuropathy that seems to be recessively inherited [Ohta et al., 1973]. In addition to loss of pain and temperature sensation, affected children have great difficulty recognizing objects by touch. Recurrent infections are common in the digits, and fractures may occur. As the disease progresses, mutilation of fingers and toes occurs. Nerve biopsies reveal a marked decrease in myelinated fibers of all calibers, as well as of unmyelinated fibers. There are possibly several subtypes of this disorder, one of which is thought to be nonprogressive [Ferrière et al., 1992].

Type III

Hereditary sensory and autonomic neuropathy type III is otherwise known as *familial dysautonomia* or the *Riley-Day syndrome* (see Chapter 85).

Type IV

Hereditary sensory and autonomic neuropathy type IV is a congenital recessively inherited sensory neuropathy usually associated with mental retardation [Dyck, 1984]. Anhidrosis is a feature of the condition [Gillespie and Perucca, 1960; Pinsky and DiGeorge, 1966; Swanson, 1963; Vassalla et al., 1968]. Rosemberg and associates [1994] summarized the findings in 32 cases, 16 sporadic and 16 from seven kindreds. Of the 16 sporadic cases, parental consanguinity was present in four. The condition is similar to hereditary sensory and autonomic neuropathy type II except for the sweating deficit and possibly the preservation of fungiform papillae on the tongue. Oral lacerations and self-mutilation are particularly prominent, leading to infection and scarring of the tongue, lips, and gums and sometimes to osteomyelitis of the jaw. The condition differs from hereditary sensory and autonomic neuropathy type III in that overflow tears are preserved in type IV and excessive sweating is a feature of dysautonomia. The anhidrosis leads to episodes of apparently unexplained fevers and hyperthermia, particularly in infancy, which are often associated with febrile convulsions.

The incidence and degree of mental retardation are apparently higher than in hereditary sensory and autonomic neuropathy type II, although normal intellect has been reported. Although often attributed to episodes of hyperthermia, mental disability occurs in the absence of overt episodes of the latter. When measured, intelligence quotients have varied from 41 to 78, the majority being in the 60 to 92 range. Microcephaly is sometimes described [Rosemberg et al., 1994]. Decreased cerebrospinal fluid levels of substance P were found in four patients with hereditary sensory and autonomic neuropathy type IV. This reduction may be a secondary effect of the loss of primary sensory neurons, which might in turn be the result of a prenatal deficiency of nerve growth factor [Iwanaga et al., 1996]. The long-term prognosis is poorly defined but, in the authors' experience, rather unsatisfactory. Chronic infections, particularly of the bones and joints, cause multiple hospitalizations and deformities. Death before the age of 4 years occurs in about 20% of cases [Rosemberg et al., 1994], usually secondary to hyperthermia or sepsis.

This disorder is of autosomal recessive inheritance. Indo and associates [1996] reported four unrelated patients with consanguineous parents who had deletion, splice, and missense mutations of TRKA, a receptor tyrosine kinase for nerve growth factor. Mouse models lacking TRKA indicate diminished responses to painful stimuli and develop skin ulcerations, missing digits, and corneal opacities. They also demonstrate deficits in cholinergic basal forebrain projections to the hippocampus and cortex [Smeyne et al., 1994]. The striking similarity of these mouse models to human hereditary sensory and autonomic neuropathy type IV suggests that a deficit in TRKA is responsible for this disorder, which also explains the cognitive difficulties.

Type V

Individuals with hereditary sensory and autonomic neuropathy type V do not perceive pain or temperature normally, but other sensory modalities are relatively well preserved [Dyck et al., 1983; Low et al., 1978]. Strength and deep tendon reflexes are normal, as are conventional nerve conduction studies. Nerve biopsy discloses absence of small myelinated fibers but preservation of the large ones. These findings explain the preservation of tendon reflexes and the normal nerve conduction studies.

Other Inherited Sensory Neuropathies

Several entities have been described that do not fit into the preceding categories. These include sensory neuropathy in association with spasticity [Cavanagh et al., 1979], skeletal dysplasia [Axelrod et al., 1983], keratitis [Donaghy et al., 1987], growth hormone deficiency [Liberfarb et al., 1993], ichthyosis and anterior chamber syndrome [Quinlivan et al., 1993], deafness, and ovarian agenesis [Linssen et al., 1994]. In addition, two different types of sensory neuropathy have been described in Navajo children [Appenzeller et al., 1976; Johnsen et al., 1993]. Most of these conditions appear to be of autosomal-recessive inheritance, but an X-linked sensory neuropathy was described by Jestico and colleagues [1985].

Acquired Sensory Neuropathy

Acquired sensory neuropathies are rare in childhood. Roach and colleagues [1985] reported self-injurious behavior in a 2-year-old child with a sensory neuropathy after organophosphate ingestion. A delayed sensory neuropathy resulting from chlorpyriphos (another organophosphate) was reported in 14- and 15-year-old siblings by Kaplan and colleagues [1993]. Sensory neuropathy of acute or subacute onset has been reported after administration of excessive doses of pyridoxine [Albin et al., 1987; Schaumburg et al., 1983]. Acute sensory neuropathy is a monophasic disorder characterized by the rapid onset of generalized paresthesia, ataxia, and areflexia associated with a severe, mainly proprioceptive sensory defect. The site of the lesion is thought to be at the dorsal root ganglion and is probably mediated by an autoimmune response. Fernandez and colleagues [1994] described such a case in a 9-year-old male. Leprosy may be associated with sensory neuropathy, which presents even in childhood, but the neuropathy is usually patchy or thermally distributed. Associated clinical features, coupled with family history, usually make diagnosis easy once suspicion is aroused [Sabin and Thomas, 1984]. It is exceptional for amyloidosis to present before the age of 15 years. Diagnosis is readily apparent on sural nerve biopsy [O'Connor et al., 1984].

FRIEDREICH'S ATAXIA

Friedreich's ataxia is an autosomal-recessive disease characterized by slowly progressive ataxia commencing in childhood. The ataxia affects all motor functions, and the gait disturbance eventually requires use of a wheelchair, usually in the second decade of life. Intellect is preserved. Skeletal deformities of pes cavus, hammer toes, and kyphoscoliosis are typical. Cardiomyopathy is often present. A sensory neuropathy resulting from progressive degeneration of dorsal ganglion cells with "dying back" of their central and peripheral axons is the principal cause of disease progression [Lamarche et al., 1984]. This process results in an alteration in sensory nerve potentials and conduction [Dunn, 1973; Oh and Halsey, 1973]. Motor nerve conduction velocities remain typically in the low-normal range at the time when sensory conduction velocities are markedly impaired. These findings are in addition to those of the spinal cord posterior column and corticospinal tract degeneration. A loss of myelinated nerve fibers, particularly of large caliber, is seen in peripheral sensory nerves. Axonal degeneration, with some secondary demyelination in the later stages, is the predominant finding in nerve biopsies.

When strict diagnostic criteria are applied, all cases of Friedreich's ataxia are inherited by autosomal-recessive transmission [Barbeau, 1976]. The Friedreich's ataxia locus was linked to chromosome 9 in typical families [Chamberlain et al., 1988]. Subsequent testing of late-onset and Acadian cases, as well as of families with early-onset ataxia with retained tendon reflexes, also indicated linkage homogeneity [Chamberlain et al., 1989; De Michele et al., 1994; Keats et al., 1990; Klockgether et al., 1993; Palau et al., 1995]. In 1996, Campuzano and colleagues identified the responsible gene *X25* in the critical region on chromosome 9q13 [Campuzano et al, 1996]. The gene encodes a 210–amino acid protein, frataxin, the function of which is currently unknown. Most Friedreich's ataxia patients (98%) are homozygous for an unstable GAA trinucleotide in the first intron of *X25*, but a few (about 1%) have point mutations of the frataxin gene. It is thought that the triplet GAA expansion causes disease by suppressing frataxin gene expression, which, in some way, causes spinal cord, heart, and pancreatic degeneration. This is the first autosomal-recessive disease in which a triplet repeat expansion has been demonstrated.

Further studies have shown that virtually all patients with typical Friedreich's disease, Acadian Friedreich's disease, late-onset Friedreich's disease, and early-onset ataxia with retained tendon reflexes carry two copies of the GAA triplet expansion. Cases with larger GAA expansions tend to have earlier onset and are more likely to demonstrate additional manifestations of the disease, such as optic atrophy, hearing loss, and possibly cardiomyopathy (see Chapter 57) [Montermini et al., 1997].

GIANT AXONAL NEUROPATHY

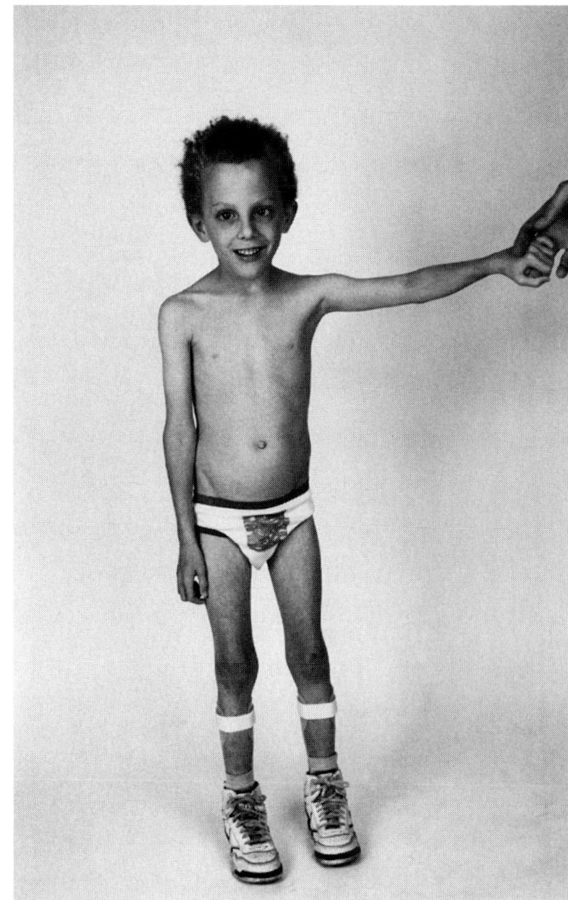

FIGURE 76-8. A 6-year-old male with giant axonal neuropathy. Note his kinky hair and need to grasp a finger for support because of gait unsteadiness. Ankle-foot orthoses counteract footdrop.

Giant axonal neuropathy was first described in 1972 by Berg and colleagues in a 6-year-old female as a slowly progressive peripheral neuropathy resembling Friedreich's ataxia [Berg et al., 1972]. With reports of four more children, it became clear that this disorder is a generalized one of increased, abnormal cytoplasmic microfilaments involving a number of body tissues, including Schwann cells, fibroblasts, and vascular endothelium [Carpenter et al., 1974; Igisu et al., 1975; Koch et al., 1977; Ouvrier et al., 1974]. Axons are swollen with densely packed neurofilaments. The initial descriptions of children younger than 9 years of age noted the presence of unusually kinky hair (Fig. 76-8). Parental consanguinity was recorded for six involved children, suggesting autosomal-recessive inheritance [Donaghy et al., 1988; Gambarelli et al., 1977; Igisu et al., 1975; Ouvrier et al., 1974]. Reports of siblings with the disease further suggested recessive inheritance [Jones et al., 1979; Takebe et al., 1981]. The responsible gene, gigaxonin, located on chromosome 16q24 [Bomont et al., 2000], is a cytoskeletal protein that may play a role in neurofilament architecture. Progressive gait disturbance, kinky hair, long curly eyelashes, a prominently high forehead, and variable CNS involvement, including optic atrophy, abnormal ocular motility, mental retardation, and spasticity, are hallmarks of the condition [Dooley et al., 1981; Fois et al., 1985; Kirkham et al., 1980]. Leukoencephalopathy on brain imaging studies may be accompanied clinically by deterioration of cognitive function [Stollhoff et al., 1991].

As the disease advances, motor function declines. Not all systems are equally affected; for example, some wheelchair-bound children retain normal mental capacity [Boltshauser et al., 1977; Pfeiffer et al., 1977]. Rapid progression of the sensory motor neuropathy leads to early death. Abnormal electroencephalograms and visual, auditory, and somatosensory-evoked potentials have been recorded [Majnemer et al., 1986]. Nerve conduction studies provide evidence of axonal neuropathy.

Thickened, distal axons distended by an increased number of neurofilaments accompanied by axonal loss constitute the peripheral nerve pathologic findings [Asbury et al., 1972; Carpenter et al., 1974]. Other pathologic descriptions note the presence of cytoplasmic microfilaments in Schwann cells, endothelial cells, perineurial cells, endoneurial fibroblasts, and melanocytes (Fig. 76-9) [Bonerandi et al., 1981; Klymkowsky and Plummer, 1985; Prineas et al., 1976]. Skin biopsy may demonstrate accumulation of microfilaments in endothelial cells, melanocytes, and fibroblasts [Takebe and Koide, 1981]. Neurofilaments that accumulate in sural nerve have the same protein composition as normal neurofilaments [Ionasescu et al., 1983; Pena, 1982]. One newborn with hypotonia had axonal swelling in peripheral nerves and distal degeneration of long spinal cord tracts without involvement of the cerebral cortex or brainstem [Kinney et al., 1985]. Severe cerebellar degeneration and optic atrophy clinically were demonstrated at postmortem examination to be caused by degeneration and gliosis of the optic nerves and tracts [Thomas et al., 1987]. Ultrastructurally, the hair has characteristic longitudinal grooves [Treiber-Held et al., 1994].

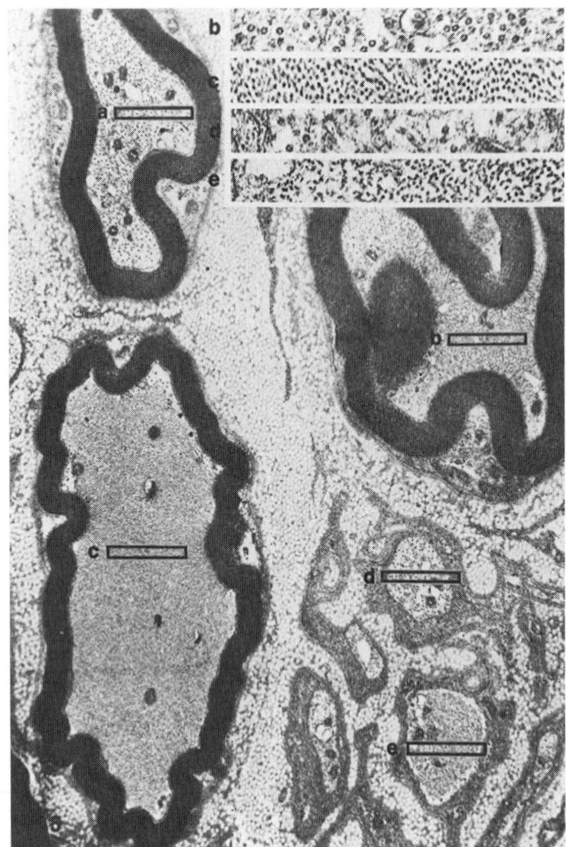

FIGURE 76-9. Nerve biopsy from a child with giant axonal neuropathy displaying one myelinated and one unmyelinated fiber (b and d, respectively) with excessive tubules. Fibers c and e show axons composed largely of tightly packed neurofilaments (×12,000). **Inset**, ×22,000. (From Prineas JW, Ouvrier RA, Wright RG, et al. Giant axonal neuropathy: A generalized disorder of cytoplasmic microfilament formation. J Neuropathol Exp Neurol 1976;35:458.)

In summary, giant axonal neuropathy presents in early infancy or early childhood with hypotonia, distal weakness, diminished tendon reflexes, gait disturbance if the child is already walking, and kinky hair. Electromyographic findings demonstrate an axonal, motor sensory neuropathy; sural nerve examination reveals numerous large, swollen axons distended by neurofilaments. Numerous other body cells, including Schwann cells and fibroblasts, also contain the filamentous inclusions, indicating that this is a disease associated with abnormal cytoskeleton proteins. The defective gene is gigaxonin. This disorder is recessively inherited.

INFANTILE NEUROAXONAL DYSTROPHY (SEITELBERGER'S DISEASE)

Infantile neuroaxonal dystrophy is a progressive central and peripheral nervous system disorder characterized pathologically by the presence of axonal spheroids. Onset of symptoms is recognized between ages 1 and 2 years. Loss of mental and motor milestones denotes the regressive nature of the condition. Seizures typically develop. Progressive motor sensory neuropathy causes loss of sensation in particular with subsequent limb mutilation. Hypotonia associated with diminished tendon reflexes in an infant exhibiting regression of milestones is a clear sign of the disorder. Urinary retention may become a problem as the disease advances. Hypothalamic failure results in diabetes insipidus and hypothyroidism. The autonomic nervous system is affected, with decreased tearing and poor temperature regulation clinically apparent. One infant presented unusually early in the neonatal period with hypertonia, axonal spheroids on biopsy, and mineralization of the basal ganglia observed by imaging studies and at postmortem examination [Venkatesh et al., 1994]. MRI indicates cerebellar atrophy and cerebellar hyperintensity on T2-weighted images [Tanabe et al., 1993], corresponding to marked loss of cerebellar neurons and astrogliosis found at postmorterm examination. The MRI changes are characteristic early in the course of the disease and may aid in diagnosis. Children with infantile neuroaxonal dystrophy do not survive beyond their preschool years. Later-onset forms of neuroaxonal dystrophy have been reported.

Central, peripheral, and autonomic neurons and nerve fibers contain spheroids of varying sizes with a predilection for involvement of sensory nerves [Itoh et al., 1993]. Sural nerve biopsy displays periodic acid–Schiff stain–positive, ballooned axons, the spheroids that contain mitochondria, glycogen-like granules, dense bodies, vesicles, and electron lucent material (Fig. 76-10) [Shimono et al., 1976]. Membranotubular and granulovesicular profiles are found ultrastructurally in spheroids [Malandrini et al., 1995]. Peripheral nerve lesions mimic those found in the CNS [Duncan et al., 1970; Martin and Martin, 1972]. Biceps muscle biopsy may

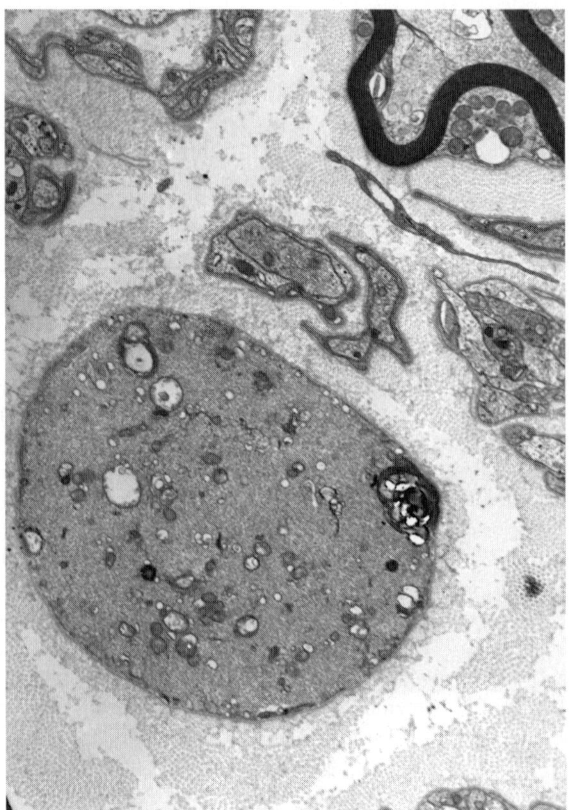

FIGURE 76-10. Sural nerve biopsy from a child with neuroaxonal dystrophy ultrastructurally displaying a spheroid containing mitochondria, membranotubular profiles, granulovesicular inclusions, dense bodies, and vesicles (×15,000).

be useful for diagnostic purposes, revealing axonal spheroid bodies in intermuscular nerve fibers, neuromuscular junctions, and motor nerve endings [Miike et al., 1986]. Early muscle biopsy may require an intense ultrastructural investigation of presynaptic neurons at the neuromuscular junction to demonstrate dystrophic axons [Wakai et al., 1993]. Immunohistochemistry of spheroids is positive for ubiquitin and negative for β-tubulin and β-amyloid. Lack of reactivity to tubulin in spheroids suggests that loss of microtubules may be part of the mechanism in the formation of axonal spheroids [Moretto et al., 1993]. Activation of the ubiquitin system is an attempt of the neuron to remove abnormal proteins. The morphologic findings of infantile neuroaxonal dystrophy are remarkably similar to those reported in α-*N*-acetylgalactosaminidase deficiency [Wolfe et al., 1995].

METABOLIC NEUROPATHIES

Diabetes Mellitus

It has been known for a long time that 10% of children with insulin-dependent diabetes mellitus have symptoms and signs caused by peripheral neuropathy associated with diabetes [Gamstorp et al., 1966]. These bilaterally symmetric changes, especially in the lower extremities, include mild distal weakness, loss of touch and pain sensation, and decreased ankle tendon reflexes. Despite good management of diabetes, impaired nerve function occurs.

In a large prospective study of nerve conductions and autonomic nervous system function in diabetic children, slowed sensory nerve conduction velocities and impaired autonomic function were present in 25% of children at the time of diagnosis [Solders et al., 1997]. Follow-up measurements of nerve conduction velocities and parasympathetic function (R-R variations) 2 years later indicated deterioration from baseline of sensory and motor nerve conductions and autonomic nerve function. The degree of deterioration correlated with blood sugar control. After 3 years of diabetes, all motor and sensory nerve conduction times were slowed [Hyllienmark et al., 1995]. By contrast to the electrophysiologic changes, only 4% of children at onset of diabetes have symptoms or signs suggestive of neuropathy despite early nerve conduction slowing. In another approach to peripheral nerve function, vibration perception threshold was measured in diabetic males. Compared with age-matched control subjects, impaired vibration perception was present in diabetic males in the absence of clinical symptoms of peripheral or autonomic neuropathy [Olsen et al., 1994].

Mildly impaired autonomic nervous system function is found in 30% to 50% of children with diabetes when measured soon after diagnosis [Donaghue et al., 1996; Verrotti et al., 1995]. The percentage involved does not change over 3 years [Donaghue et al., 1996]; abnormalities are not related to age, duration of diabetes, or degree of blood sugar control. Heart rate variation during Valsalva maneuver and a maximum-to-minimum ratio of 30:15 are the most sensitive indexes to detect autonomic abnormalities in children [Verrotti et al., 1995]. Further, asymptomatic diabetic children have diminished sensation of bladder filling [Barkai and Szabó, 1993]. If cardiovascular autonomic dysfunction is present in addition, loss of bladder filling sensation is even more striking. Loss of bladder filling sensation correlates with duration of diabetes and poor blood sugar control.

It is clear that careful clinical and electrophysiologic follow-up is required to monitor altered peripheral and autonomic nerve function in childhood-onset diabetes mellitus. In another study comparing diabetic and nondiabetic children, both motor and sensory peripheral nerve abnormalities were related to poor blood sugar control as measured by hemoglobin A1c and duration of diabetes [Fiçicioglu et al., 1994]. These results emphasize the importance of metabolic control and duration of diabetes in the pathogenesis of diabetic neuropathy. The findings suggest that peripheral neuropathy is common in young, insulin-dependent diabetic patients. Because nerve function tests are easy to conduct and are sensitive, they may help to achieve better metabolic control and prevent diabetic complications.

Uremic Neuropathy

Uremic neuropathy is rarely diagnosed in children. When recognized, it is characterized by burning sensations in the feet and a symmetric motor sensory neuropathy with progressive muscle weakness. Motor nerve and sensory nerve conduction velocities are decreased early in the course of the disease, often before clinical symptoms appear [Di Paolo et al., 1982]. In particular, the proximal 1a sensory and motor nerve conduction velocities are significantly slowed early, compared with distal values in uremic neuropathy [Panayiotopoulos and Lagos, 1980]. The H-reflex response latency can be used to detect early changes in some patients [Knoll and Dierker, 1980]. Parathyroid hormone levels have been correlated with early peripheral nerve conduction delays in some instances [Di Paolo et al., 1982], but not in others [Aiello et al., 1982]. The facial nerve is a sensitive indicator of uremic neuropathy [Mitz et al., 1984]. In vitro inhibition of tubulin 6s polymerization by uremic toxins suggests a mechanism for initiating uremic neuropathy [Braguer et al., 1986]. The plasma of uremic patients contains high concentrations of middle molecules in the 300 to 1500 dalton range, which cause toxic effects [Babb et al., 1981]. A b4-2 peak correlates with the neuropathy [Faguer et al., 1983].

The predominant change in the peripheral nerve is a demyelinating neuropathy, but some individuals experience a progressive axonal neuropathy with secondary segmental demyelination. An acute axonal neuropathy is rarely observed [Said et al., 1983]. In the more rapidly progressive neuropathies, ischemic changes related to accelerated hypertension and possibly to septicemia may be etiologically related to rapid progression [McGonigle et al., 1985]. Biotin therapy has been recommended for patients with advanced renal failure before the neuropathy becomes manifest [Yatzidis et al., 1984].

Acute Intermittent Porphyria

Acute intermittent porphyria, a rare inborn error of metabolism inherited on an autosomal-dominant basis, is caused by defects in the gene encoding hydroxymethylbilane synthase on the long arm of chromosome 11. There is a marked increase of δ-aminolevulinic acid, porphobilinogen, uroporphyrin, and coproporphyrin in the urine. δ-Aminolevulinic acid synthetase activity is typically increased in body tissues. Although the disease has occurred within the first decade of life, it typically presents after puberty. Gene carriers are at risk for developing potentially fatal neurogenic attacks if exposed to precipitating factors [Wassif et al., 1994]. Axonal damage observed both on sural nerve biopsy [Defanti et al., 1985] and postmortem examination suggests that the neuropathy is primarily axonal [Yamada et al., 1984].

Acute, severe, colicky abdominal pain is a typical manifestation of an acute episode accompanied by CNS and peripheral nervous system impairment. Peripherally, motor weakness is most striking, but sensory impairment may also occur. A flaccid paralysis resembling Guillain-Barré syndrome has been observed. The proximal muscles may be more involved than distal muscles when weakness occurs. Reflexes are often diminished or absent. The motor cranial nerves, particularly cranial nerves III, VII, and X, may be involved. Urinary retention or incontinence occurs. Centrally, mental changes consisting of confusion, delirium, and hallucinations may develop. Autonomic function involving the sympathetic and parasympathetic nervous systems may be affected. Typically the symptoms remit with resolution of the episode, but parasympathetic dysfunction has been detected during remission and when the patient is otherwise asymptomatic [Laiwah et al., 1985]. Barbiturates and other antiepileptic drugs may trigger attacks. No successful treatment has been described. Lead poisoning and Guillain-Barré syndrome must be considered in the differential diagnosis.

Vitamin Deficiency

Thiamine, or vitamin B_1, is a water-soluble vitamin that serves as a coenzyme in carbohydrate metabolism. Classic thiamine deficiency in children causes peripheral neuropathy, encephalopathy, and high-output cardiac failure [Debuse, 1992]. Infantile beriberi disease has been described in infants born to mothers with thiamine deficiency. Symptoms consist of anorexia, vomiting, and lethargy occurring within the first 3 months of life as a result of vasoconstriction, hypotension, and severe metabolic acidosis. The infant may be pale, puffy, and listless on examination. Cranial nerve dysfunction has been noted, with ptosis, optic atrophy, and laryngeal paralysis causing a hoarse cry. Cardiac enlargement with heart failure has also been found. A thiamine-dependent state has also been described [Mandel et al., 1984]. Treatment allows for reversal of symptoms with or without sequelae [Román, 1994].

Congenital Pernicious Anemia

Two forms of pernicious anemia in children are associated with peripheral neuropathy. One occurs as a congenital disease or an early-onset disease in children [Heisel et al., 1984]. Congenital pernicious anemia occurs before age 5 years as a result of a vitamin B_{12} deficiency caused by isolated absence of gastric intrinsic factor. There is adequate gastric-free acid and a normal gastric mucosa. The patient has a macrocytic anemia, a decreased serum vitamin B_{12} level, a lack of intrinsic factor in the gastric juice, but an otherwise normal gastric acid content and gastric mucosa. There is an absence of the antibodies to the parietal cell and intrinsic factor. Select infants with this form of pernicious anemia have been reported to have neuropathies. There may be a delay in acquiring motor milestones and growth failure. Treatment is with parenteral vitamin B_{12} and results in recovery to normal hemoglobin levels in 4 to 6 weeks.

A later-onset form of pernicious anemia resembles that seen in adults. This form is histamine-fast achlorhydria associated with gastric mucosal atrophy and the presence of antibodies to parietal cells and intrinsic factor in the serum. These children may experience a variety of endocrinologic disorders. Pathologic changes develop in the spinal cord and less commonly in the peripheral nerve and brain.

Infants who are breast-fed by strictly vegetarian mothers or who have undiagnosed pernicious anemia are at risk for developing a megaloblastic anemia because of a deficiency of vitamin B_{12}. A loss of acquired milestones with seeming neurologic regression occurs [Higginbottom et al., 1978]. Cystathioninuria, glycinuria, methylmalonic aciduria, 3-hydroxy propionic aciduria, and formic aciduria may develop. Inadequate tissue availability of vitamin B_{12} results in increased concentrations of methylmalonic acid and homocysteine caused by inhibition of methylmalonyl-coenzyme A mutase and methionine synthase, respectively. It can be prevented by supplementing the vegetarian mother's diet with vitamin B_{12} (cobalamin).

Abetalipoproteinemia

Abetalipoproteinemia, known as *Bassen-Kornzweig syndrome,* is characterized by progressive ataxic neuropathy, retinitis pigmentosa, steatorrhea, hypolipidemia, deficiency of fat-soluble vitamins, and acanthocytosis [Bassen and Kornzweig, 1950; Selimoglu et al., 2001]. The onset of symptoms in this autosomal-recessive disorder occurs between early childhood and the late teen years. Apoprotein B, required for synthesis and structural integrity of chylomicrons and low-density and very-low-density lipoproteins, is missing in plasma because of lack of synthesis [Salt et al., 1960]. The result is absence of lipoproteins. Intestinal fat absorption is absent from birth and results in a progressive deficiency of fat-soluble vitamins A, D, E, and K. Many of the clinical problems of the syndrome are due to vitamin E deficiency, and treatment with vitamin E is recommended [Miller and Lloyd, 1982]. Sensory neuropathy exists with reduced amplitude responses [Lowry et al., 1984].

Pathology

Degeneration of posterior columns, spinal cerebellar pathways, and cerebellum caused by vitamin E deficiency [Mino, 1993] is the major pathologic change. Loss of anterior horn cells is found in the spinal cord. Posterior column degeneration leads to abnormal somatosensory-evoked potentials [Brin et al., 1986]. Sural nerve biopsy indicates decreased numbers of large myelinated fibers and clusters of regenerating fibers [Wichman et al., 1985]. The posterior fundus of the eye exhibits a loss of photoreceptors, loss or attenuation of pigment epithelium, and preservation of submacular pigment epithelium, with an excessive accumulation of lipofuscin [Cogan et al., 1984]. Macrophage-like pigmented cells invade the retina.

Clinical Characteristics

The most significant neurologic finding is a progressive ataxia that may be present as early as 2 years of age but certainly by age 6 years. Generalized weakness, ptosis, and extraocular muscle weakness develop. The lower cranial nerves may be involved, with facial and tongue weakness plus twitching movements. A progressive peripheral sensory neuropathy causing hypesthesia, hypalgesia, and proprioceptive loss is associated with absent tendon reflexes. Generalized muscle weakness and wasting may be severe. Intestinal malabsorption produces bulky, foul stools and leads to a delay in normal growth.

Clinical Laboratory Tests

The most significant finding is the inborn absence of the major apoprotein of low-density plasma lipoproteins [Lange and Steck, 1984], leading to an abnormal serum and red-cell lipid profile, along with spiny erythrocytes or acanthocytosis. Fat-soluble vitamin deficiency is typically present. The electroretinogram may be nonrecordable because of the pigmentary retinopathy [Judisch et al., 1984]. There are wide variations in the appearance of the acanthocytes. Erythrocyte membrane phospholipids and cholesterol are increased [Iida et al., 1984].

Management

High doses of vitamin E provide clinical amelioration and electrophysiologic improvement with increased evoked motor unit potentials and improved nerve conduction velocities [Brin et al., 1986; Hegele and Angel, 1985; Runge et al., 1986]. In addition to large doses of oral vitamin E therapy, a low-fat diet and supplements of the other fat-soluble vitamins are recommended. If these dietary changes are started early enough, the progressive retinopathy can most likely be prevented.

α-Lipoprotein Deficiency (Tangier Disease)

Tangier disease is an uncommon familial disorder of lipoprotein metabolism notable for the absence of normal high-density lipoprotein from plasma and the accumulation of cholesterol esters in multiple organs. Extremely low plasma cholesterol levels are present. Physical examination indicates patches of yellow-orange lymphoid tissue in the tonsils and pharynx and hepatosplenomegaly. Yellow patches are present on the surface of the liver, and liver biopsy specimens contain cholesterol esters. Fiberscopic rectal examination documents orange-brown spots present throughout the rectum. Foam cells are present in the lymphoid tissue of both the pharynx and rectal mucosa, and rectal mucosal biopsy is recommended for diagnostic purposes [Tarao et al., 1984]. Widespread storage of lipid material by the reticuloendothelial system is present, and foamy histiocytes can be easily found [Dechelotte et al., 1985]. Onset is between 2 and 67 years of age [Pietrini et al., 1985].

Clinical Characteristics

Recurrent neuropathy occurs in children with fluctuating asymmetric sensory involvement mostly in the lower extremities, sometimes accompanied by progressive development of weakness of both distal and proximal muscles. Complaints of numbness and tingling in the distal extremities are early symptoms, followed by signs of the neuropathy and weakness. A dissociated loss of pain and temperature sensation may occur. More severe forms of neuropathy have been described in older individuals, suggesting more than one type of neuropathic involvement [Marbini et al., 1985; Pietrini et al., 1985]. Facial diplegia may develop. Hand atrophy occurs. Sural nerve biopsy in more severely affected individuals indicates a reduction of smaller myelinated and unmyelinated fibers, with an abundance of abnormal non–membrane-bound vacuoles in the Schwann cells, fibroblasts, macrophages, and perineurial cells [Gibbels et al., 1985].

Biochemistry

Tangier disease is characterized by low levels of apo-A-1 and high-density lipoproteins. A higher than normal amount of pro-apo-A-1 lipoprotein is present in Tangier disease, but there is no deficiency of the converting enzyme activity to mature apo-A-1 [Bojanovski et al., 1984]. The turnover rate from pro-apo-lipoprotein to mature apo-lipoprotein may be abnormal [Edelstein et al., 1984]. In normal circumstances, high-density lipoproteins bind to monocytes at the cell surface, and the lipoprotein is internalized and subsequently resecreted without significant degradation. Conversely, high-density lipoproteins bind to Tangier monocytes more actively, and when internalized, they are found in secondary lysosomes; that is, when they are resecreted, most of the high-density lipoprotein is degraded. At least one of the abnormal mechanisms in this disease is apparently the abnormal cellular metabolism of high-density lipoproteins in Tangier monocytes [Schmitz et al., 1985]. Another biochemical abnormality demonstrated in Tangier disease is a significant reduction of endoneurial sodium, potassium adenosine triphosphatase, and magnesium adenosine triphosphatase activities demonstrated in six sural nerve biopsies from patients with the condition [Sutherland and Pollock, 1984]. All these patients had either mononeuropathy multiplex or a progressive axonal neuropathy. The reduced level of the adenosine triphosphatase activity may relate to altered endoneurial lipid metabolism and impaired axoplasmic flow.

Management

Treatment by restriction of dietary fat may be one way to reduce the accumulation of the cholesterol esters in the reticuloendothelial system [Herbert et al., 1978], possibly resulting in clinical improvement.

Krabbe's Disease (Globoid Cell Leukodystrophy)

Galactosylceramide lipidosis, known as *Krabbe's disease* or *globoid cell leukodystrophy,* is an autosomal-recessive neurodegenerative disorder that presents most often in infants 3 to 5 months of age (see Chapter 27). Deficiency of galactosylceramide β-galactosidase results from mutations and heterogeneous deletions in the galactocerebrosidase gene on chromosome 14q31 [Luzi et al., 1995; Rafi et al., 1995; Tatsumi et al., 1995]. The clinical profile is a highly irritable infant with spasticity, optic atrophy, intellectual delay, and polyneuropathy. The disease leads to a loss of milestones, microcephaly, severe failure to thrive, and progressive demyelinating peripheral neuropathy with slowed conduction velocities with prolonged latencies. Hyperacusis is part of the irritability. Cerebrospinal fluid protein is elevated. Average age of death is 13 months. An earlier, neonatal onset is associated with failure to thrive, infantile spasms, and hemiplegia [Hagberg, 1984]. A small number of patients have later-onset forms of the condition, up to age 50 years [Rafi et al., 1995], causing spasticity, motor polyneuropathy, dysarthria, and optic atrophy [Loonen et al., 1985].

The central and peripheral manifestations are due to abnormalities in the metabolism of myelin with accumulation of galactosylceramide, which causes an infiltration of macrophages that subsequently transform into globoid cells in the brain [Suzuki, 1984]. The peripheral neuropathy is characterized by uniform marked slowing of conduction velocities [Miller et al., 1985]. Hypomyelination is noted pathologically in infantile Krabbe's disease. Segmental demyelination is more important in later-onset globoid cell leukodystrophy and can be demonstrated on sural nerve biopsy. Ultrastructurally, curvilinear lamellar cytoplasmic inclusions are present in Schwann cells and histiocytes creating the globoid cell.

Krabbe's disease may present initially as a peripheral neuropathy. A 13-year-old with scoliosis and pes cavus displayed distal leg weakness and sensory loss. Electrophysiologic nerve study indicated demyelinating neuropathy. Four years later, spasticity developed, and the diagnosis was established [Marks et al., 1997].

Metachromatic Leukodystrophy

Metachromatic leukodystrophy is a recessively inherited disease affecting children and adults (see Chapter 27). The basic disorder is a failure of the catabolism of sulfatide, the sulfate ester of galactose cerebroside. This lipid is a component of the myelin membrane and is probably also a component of neuronal membranes [McKhann, 1984]. The storage of metachromatic material in Schwann cell lysosomes and macrophages associated with segmental demyelination is well recognized in the late infantile, juvenile, and adult forms (Fig. 76-11) [Luijten et al., 1978]. Given the abnormal storage of lipid in the central and peripheral nervous system, a combination of upper and lower motor neuron disease is recognized clinically. Nerve conduction velocities are slowed, and the latencies of evoked potentials are prolonged. Sensory nerve conduction velocities are generally delayed earlier and more severely than are motor nerve conduction velocities [Takakura et al., 1985].

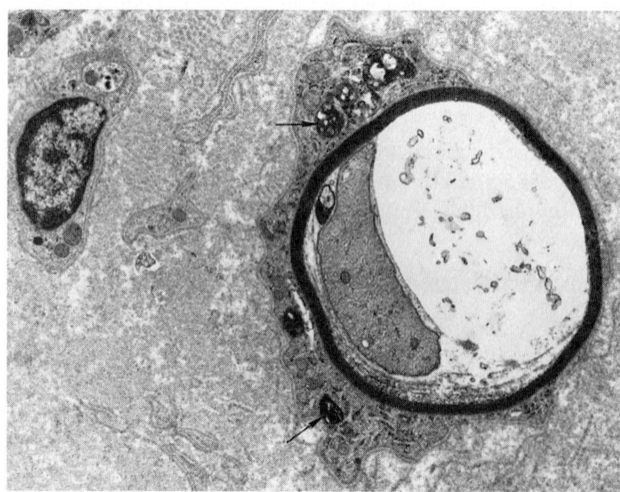

FIGURE 76-11. Sural nerve biopsy from a child with metachromatic leukodystrophy demonstrating sulfatide storage *(arrows)* in a Schwann cell and degeneration of the axon in myelinated nerve fiber (×17,400).

Clinically, in the infantile form of metachromatic leukodystrophy, the infant acquires normal milestones until 1 to 2 years of age and then begins to exhibit signs of the disease. An unsteady gait is an early sign, accompanied by loss of language, intellectual deterioration, and later, spasticity. The juvenile form of the disease occurs after several years of age, again with gait disturbance followed by intellectual deterioration. Given the greater variability of presentation in the adult form, dementia may be the initial presentation without other obvious neurologic deficits. The disease can be suspected when evoked potentials are delayed and peripheral nerve conduction velocities are slowed [Wulff and Trojaborg, 1985].

Bone marrow transplantation has shown some promise for at least delaying the progression of the late infantile and juvenile forms of metachromatic leukodystrophy [Bayever et al., 1985; Krivit et al., 1990; Lipton et al., 1986]. Follow-up studies indicate arrest of CNS disease but not of peripheral neuropathy.

Refsum's Disease (Heredopathia Atactica Polyneuritiformis)

Refsum's disease is a recessively inherited condition caused by a deficiency in phytanic acid oxidase activity, allowing the accumulation of phytanic acid in body tissues. Anorexia, ataxia, ichthyosis, and sensorineural hearing loss were originally described [Refsum, 1946; Refsum et al., 1949] (see Chapter 29). Malabsorption and steatorrhea may be present early [Mandel et al., 1992]. In the classic form of the disease, clinical characteristics can be divided into three groups. Congenital abnormalities, such as skeletal deformities unrelated to the level of phytanic acid, constitute one group. Retinitis pigmentosa, which develops slowly, is another clinical group, unrelated to the plasma phytanic acid level. A third group of lesions includes the neuropathy, rash, and cardiac dysrhythmias, which can deteriorate or improve according to plasma phytanic acid level [Gibberd et al., 1985]. The sensorimotor neuropathy is of the chronic hypertrophic demyelinating type with very reduced nerve conduction velocity and raised cerebrospinal fluid protein levels. Exacerbations of the neuropathy and rash can be precipitated by a low calorie intake, with mobilization of phytanic acid from adipose tissue.

Patients with Refsum's disease lack the ability to degrade phytanic acid to pristanic acid and carbon dioxide. This defect can be analyzed in fibroblasts [Skjeldal et al., 1986]. The gene responsible for the metabolic defect codes for phytanoyl–coenzyme A hydroxylase. Serial plasma exchanges to reduce the level of phytanic acid have been correlated with significant clinical improvement, in particular of the neuropathy and cerebellar ataxia [Hungerbeuhler et al., 1985].

When this is combined with a diet low in phytanic acid, clinical improvement, which correlates with a lowered serum phytanic acid level, can be sustained.

An infantile form of Refsum's disease is recognized as a result of excessive phytanic acid storage. Pigmentary retinopathy is again observed, along with hypotonia, severe hearing impairment, and severe developmental delay [Weleber et al., 1984]. Facial dysmorphism and hepatomegaly have also been described [Budden et al., 1986]. Two patients had intracranial hemorrhage secondary to a vitamin K–responsive clotting defect, and both had steatorrhea. The affected infant may have protracted diarrhea and low serum cholesterol level. There is an absence of the normal hepatic peroxisomes [Van den Branden et al., 1986] compared with the adult form of Refsum's disease in which peroxisomes and fibroblasts are not diminished [Beard et al., 1985]. The plasma of patients with the infantile, but not adult, form of Refsum's disease contains increased amounts of pipecolic acid and at least two abnormal bioacids [Poulos et al., 1984]. Cultured skin fibroblasts demonstrate a marked increase in the concentration of the long-chain fatty acid hexacosanoic acid [Poulos and Sharp, 1984]. Infantile Refsum's disease appears to share several biochemical features with the cerebrohepatorenal syndrome (Zellweger's disease) and adrenoleukodystrophy. Both the patients with infantile Refsum's disease and patients with Zellweger's disease have a deficiency in phytanic acid oxidase activity, and all three are considered neonatal peroxisomal disorders [Aubourg et al., 1986; Poulos et al., 1985].

Chédiak-Higashi Syndrome

Chédiak-Higashi syndrome produces albinism with abnormal pigmentation of the hair and skin, pancytopenia, susceptibility to infection, and an increased risk for lymphoreticular malignancy. Psychomotor retardation, seizures, and muscular weakness have been described. Leukocytes contain characteristic peroxidase-positive granules.

Axonal sensory neuropathy with loss of myelinated nerve fibers in sural nerve biopsy is associated with the syndrome [Misra et al., 1991]. In more advanced neuropathy, abnormal granules are present in Schwann cells [Lockman et al., 1967]. Spinocerebellar degeneration has been observed and is often associated with features of parkinsonism [Pettit and Berdal, 1984]. Muscle biopsy in advanced disease indicates neurogenic muscular atrophy secondary to the peripheral neuropathy. In addition, acid phosphatase–positive granules, indicating abnormal lysosomes, are found in normal-appearing muscle fibers. These correspond ultrastructurally to autophagic vacuoles containing glycogen particles and membranous structures [Uchino et al., 1993]. These findings indicate that Chédiak-Higashi syndrome is a generalized lysosomal disorder. The defective gene has been localized to chromosome 1q42-44 [Barbosa et al., 1997].

TOXIC NEUROPATHIES

Diphtheria

Diphtheria is an uncommon disease in the Western hemisphere because most individuals are immunized with diphtheria-pertussis-tetanus vaccine. The disease occurs in unimmunized children and in adults who have lost immunity. An exotoxin produced by the *Corynebacterium diphtheriae* infection in the throat produces cardiomyopathy and neuropathy. A systemic radiculoneuropathy with onset 1 to 16 weeks after infection marked by sensory loss may develop [Gaskill and Korb, 1946]. Clinically, blurred vision and swallowing difficulties mark the onset of diphtheric neuropathy. A generalized motor sensory demyelinating polyneuropathy with distal, symmetric involvement is recognized [Créange et al., 1995]. Lower cranial nerves are affected. Proximal and distal muscle weakness and muscle tenderness are present. Proprioceptive modalities are altered in the lower extremities. Spinal fluid protein may be elevated with or without pleocytosis. Recovery is usually complete within several months [Buzzi, 1982]. The exotoxin may produce a localized effect on pharyngeal and palatal muscles secondary to nerve involvement adjacent to the infection. Complete recovery is anticipated.

Neuropathy of Serum Sickness

Serum sickness is a systemic illness resulting from hypersensitivity to an injected foreign protein, such as tetanus or diphtheria antisera, producing encephalomyelitis, neuropathy, or brachial plexus neuropathies [Igbal and Arnason, 1984; McCombe and Pender, 1991]. Fever, joint swelling, abdominal pain, diarrhea, and cutaneous eruptions develop within days of receiving foreign protein. Deposition of antigen–antibody complexes is associated with disease.

Botulism

See Chapter 78.

Antibiotic-Induced Neuropathy

A number of antibiotic, antifungal, and antituberculous drugs have been known to cause peripheral neuropathy in a small percentage of cases. For example, chloramphenicol can cause mild, primarily sensory peripheral neuropathy after long-term use at relatively high doses. Nitrofurantoin may produce a polyneuropathy of sudden onset on rare occasion. Isoniazid causes an axonal neuropathy responsive to pyridoxine therapy in 1% to 2% of patients. The primarily sensory neuropathy begins with paresthesias. Ethambutol, an antituberculous drug, occasionally causes a sensory neuropathy associated with optic neuritis.

Pyridoxine-Induced Polyneuropathy

Pyridoxine taken in large doses can cause a sensory neuropathy with paresthesias, diffuse sensory loss, sensory ataxia, and autonomic dysfunction [Albin et al., 1987; Schaumburg et al., 1983]. Strength is intact. Sural nerve biopsy documents marked loss of large myelinated nerve fibers [Santoro et al., 1991]. Recovery may be incomplete. A chronic neuropathy from lower-dose ingestion has similar and milder symptoms and a better prognosis [Dordain and Deffond, 1994]. There is a dose-dependent relationship to the development of neuropathy [Berger et al., 1992]. Most reports in the literature concern adults; however, a report of an 18-year-old with pyridoxine-dependent seizures describes onset of sensory neuropathy by 2 years of age as a result of 2 g/day of pyridoxine therapy for seizure control. The neuropathy did not progress from age 2 to 18 years. Electrophysiologic studies indicate a pure sensory neuronopathy [McLachlan and Brown, 1995].

Nitrous Oxide–Induced Polyneuropathy

Severe myeloneuropathy and macrocytic anemia associated with a low vitamin B_{12} level are reported after prolonged exposure to nitrous oxide [Stacy et al., 1992]. Vitamin B_{12} supplementation alone does not result in improvement, but the addition of methionine does arrest the progression of neuropathy. Chronic nitrous oxide exposure inhibits methionine synthetase activity, which remains suppressed after nitrous oxide exposure has ended, underscoring the need for treatment with methionine. Continuous exposure to nitrous oxide for longer than 3 hours causes neuropathy, especially in vitamin B_{12}–deficient individuals [Louis-Ferdinand, 1994].

Chemotherapeutic Agent–Induced Neuropathy

Peripheral neuropathy may develop after the use of chemotherapeutic agents to treat neoplasms. Sensorimotor peripheral neuropathy may develop after high-dose cytosine arabinoside therapy manifested pathologically by axonal degeneration and scattered destruction of myelin sheaths [Borgeat et al., 1986]. The neuropathy is marked by dysesthesias, muscle aching, and progressive weakness. Cytosine arabinoside neuropathic pain may respond to carbamazepine [Malapert and Degos, 1989]. In 1% of patients treated with high-dose cytosine arabinoside, demyelinating polyneuropathy develops, resulting in quadriparesis and need for ventilatory support [Openshaw et al., 1996]. In addition to peripheral neuropathy, brachial plexus neuropathy has been observed with high-dose cytosine arabinoside [Scherokman et al., 1985].

Adenine arabinoside has also been reported to cause a sensory neuropathy with pain and tingling in the feet [Lok et al., 1984]. Combination therapy with cancer chemotherapeutic agents may induce peripheral neuropathy.

Vincristine is perhaps the best known chemotherapeutic agent, causing peripheral neuropathy and, less commonly, autonomic and cranial nerve neuropathy [Shapiro and Young, 1984]. Tingling sensations, absent reflexes (particularly at the heels), distal weakness, and impaired vibration and superficial sensation develop secondary to vincristine use. Vincristine neuropathy is most profound in children with hereditary motor and sensory neuropathy type I and is associated with incomplete recovery after discontinuation of the drug. Neuropathy is less severe in hereditary motor and sensory neuropathy type II with better recovery of nerve function after drug use is discontinued [Igarashi et al., 1995]. Vincristine should be avoided in hereditary motor and sensory neuropathy type I [Graf et al., 1996].

Cisplatin may cause profound axonal loss in peripheral nerves, producing a sensory neuropathy. Paresthesias and numbness occur months after initiating cancer therapy with this agent. Proprioception is also impaired, with diminished vibration and joint position sensation. Occasionally, mild distal muscle weakness is noted. In select protocols treating germ cell tumors in children and using cisplatin as one therapeutic agent, the incidence of neuropathy was very low [Göbel et al., 1989; Hartmann et al., 1988]. High-tone hearing loss was noted, which may be due to the combination of cisplatin and etoposide.

Vaccine-Induced Polyneuropathy

The diphtheria-pertussis-tetanus vaccine may produce a peripheral neuropathy, probably because of the tetanus toxoid component. The influenza, or 1976 swine flu, vaccine allegedly caused Guillain-Barré syndrome, but this has been questioned by reevaluation of the statistical evidence on which the initial allegation rested.

Heavy-Metal Neuropathy

Lead toxicity may cause a motor and to a lesser extent sensory neuropathy. Lower extremities are particularly affected in children. Axonal neuropathy is demonstrated electrophysiologically and pathologically. Chelation therapy with penicillamine or ethylenediaminetetra-acetic acid may be indicated, and slow recovery is anticipated with elimination of lead exposure. Lead levels can be measured. Coproporphyrin is elevated. Other presentations include colic and pallor. Encephalopathy may be present with or without neuropathy, and weakness is typical of lead poisoning, which can be caused by both organic and inorganic forms of the heavy metal. Organic tetra-alkyl derivatives are fat soluble and easily cross the blood-brain barrier. They produce an encephalopathy without neuropathy in both adults and children. The inorganic salts produce alterations that are age dependent. In infants and children, inorganic lead poisoning usually causes an encephalopathy, whereas in adults, a neuropathy is produced. Abdominal pain, constipation, anemia, and neuropathy are the typical clinical features. The anemia is usually microcytic and hypochromic, with basophilic stippling of the red cells. Children may also have an iron-deficiency anemia.

Slowing of nerve conduction occurs in children environmentally exposed to lead, who are otherwise asymptomatic [Schwartz et al., 1988]. Current concern is raised for developmental problems in children exposed to continuous, low-level lead in the environment.

In lead poisoning, inhibition of erythrocyte aminolevulinic acid occurs, leading to an increase in aminolevulinic acid, which is detectable in the urine when the blood lead level reaches 40 to 50 mg/dL. In adults, the most common exposure is industrial, but in children, the ingestion of old, lead-based paint or chewing on paint chips causes the intoxication. Obviously, removing the source of the lead is most important, and a chelating agent may be of value.

Rare instances of arsenic poisoning, usually purposely perpetrated against an individual, have been reported, producing an axonal, primarily sensory neuropathy. Exposure may be by overdose, producing a subacute neuropathy, or may be more chronic, causing a slowly progressing neuropathy. Environmental exposure from industrial waste is associated with skin pigmentation, palmar and plantar keratosis, gastrointestinal symptoms, liver disease, and peripheral neuropathy [Mazumder et al., 1992].

Mercury poisoning was described in Minamata Bay in Japan. The poisoning resulted from industrial discharge of short-chain alkyl mercury compounds, which were picked up by microorganisms and subsequently entered the food chain, concentrated in fish and shellfish.

Organic mercury poisoning in children produces acrodynia, or pink disease, consisting of generalized erythema, especially of the hands, feet, and face, with swelling of the hands and feet. Stomatitis, loss of teeth, increased perspiration, and irritability are present. Elemental mercury is absorbed from a saturated atmosphere of mercury vapor, leading to subacute exposure. Several patients with predominantly axonal motor neuropathy resulting from vapor exposure have been recorded [Ross, 1964; Swaiman and Flagler, 1971]. Chronic exposure results in sensory and motor neuropathy, encephalopathy, and autonomic dysfunction. Chronic exposure may produce a subclinical neuropathy detected electrophysiologically [Zampollo et al., 1987]. Removing the source of mercury is important, and chelation therapy may be of value.

Accidental ingestion of rat poison or insecticides containing thallium causes an acute or subacute syndrome of gastrointestinal disturbance and neuropathy. A sensory and motor axonal severe peripheral neuropathy with abdominal pain, nausea, vomiting, and alopecia is typical. One transplacental case is known. If death does not ensue, recovery is usually complete [Desenclos et al., 1992; Rangel-Guerra et al., 1990]. Thallium was banned in the United States as a rodenticide in 1972.

Critical Illness Polyneuropathy

Critical illness polyneuropathy occurs in patients with sepsis and multiple organ failure. Initially reported in adults with severe systemic illnesses in intensive care units [Bolton et al., 1986], it is often first recognized when it proves difficult to wean the patient from mechanical ventilation. The accompanying signs of generalized weakness, muscle wasting, and depressed reflexes may be difficult to detect or may be misinterpreted in the intensive care setting. The differential diagnosis includes paraparesis or tetraparesis secondary to spinal cord lesions, prolonged neuromuscular blockade, steroid- or relaxant-induced myopathy, acute necrotizing myopathy, hypophosphatemia, toxic (including nitrous oxide) and thiamine deficiency neuropathies, the asthma-amyotrophy (Hopkins) syndrome, and Guillain-Barré syndrome. These can be eliminated by systematic investigation by imaging, serum creatine kinase and phosphate levels, clinical neurophysiologic studies, and, if doubt persists, nerve and muscle biopsies. In typical cases of critical illness polyneuropathy, nerve conduction and histopathologic studies confirm widespread axonal degeneration with extensive muscle denervation.

The condition has been reported in childhood secondary to sepsis associated with severe asthma [Sheth and Bolton, 1995], sepsis accompanying brain contusion or craniectomy [Petersen et al., 1999], status epilepticus, cardiac surgical complications, and hemorrhagic shock encephalopathy syndrome. It has occurred with complications of bone marrow transplantation [Banwell et al., 2003]. A similar condition may follow severe burns.

Treatment is mainly supportive, but therapy with intravenous immune globulins, given within 24 hours of the onset of the sepsis, has been encouraging [Mohr et al., 1997].

REFERENCES

Adler JB, Patterson RL. Erb's palsy: Long term results of treatment in eighty-eight cases. J Bone Joint Surg Am 1967;49:1052.

Aiello I, Serra G, Gilli P, et al. Uremic neuropathy: Correlations between electroneurographic parameters and serum levels of parathyroid hormone and aluminum. Eur Neurol 1982;21:396.

Albin RL, Albers JW, Greenberg HS, et al. Acute sensory neuropathy-neuronopathy from pyridoxine overdose. Neurology 1987;37:1729.

al-Qattan MM, Clarke HM, Curtis CG. Klumpke's birth palsy. Does it really exist? J Hand Surg 1995;20:19.

Andersson J, Sterner G. A 16-month-old boy with infectious mononucleosis, parotitis and Bell's palsy, Acta Paediatr Scand 1985;74:629.

Appenzeller O, Kornfeld M, Snyder R. Acromutilating, paralyzing neuropathy with corneal ulceration in Navajo children. Arch Neurol 1976;33:733.

Appleton R, Riordan A, Tedman B, et al. Congenital peripheral neuropathy presenting as apnoea and respiratory insufficiency. Dev Med Child Neurol 1994;36:545.

Arnason BGW. Acute inflammatory demyelinating polyneuropathies. In: Dyck PJ, Thomas PK, Lambert EH, Bunge R, eds. Peripheral neuropathy, 2nd ed., vol. 2. Philadelphia: WB Saunders, 1984.

Arnason BGW, Soliven B. Acute inflammatory demyelinating polyradiculoneuropathy. In: Dyck PJ, Thomas PK, Griffin JW, et al., eds. Peripheral neuropathy, 3rd ed., vol. 2. Philadelphia: WB Saunders, 1993.

Asbury AK, Arnason BG, Adams RD. The inflammatory lesion in idiopathic polyneuritis. Medicine 1969;48:173.

Asbury AK, Gary MK, Cox SC, et al. Giant axonal neuropathy: A unique case with segmental neurofilamentous masses. Acta Neuropathol 1972;20:237.

Aubourg P, Scotta J, Rocchicciolo F, et al. Neonatal adrenoleukodystrophy. J Neurol Neurosurg Psychiatry 1986;49:77.

Auer-Grumbach M, Strasser-Fuchs S, Wagner K, et al. Roussy-Levy syndrome is a phenotypic variant of Charcot-Marie-Tooth syndrome IA associated with a duplication on chromosome 17p11.2. J Neurol Sci 1998;154:72.

Axelrod FB, Pearson J, Tepperberg J, Ackerman BD. Congenital sensory neuropathy with skeletal dysplasia. J Pediatr 1983;102:727.

Babb AL, Ahmad S, Bergstrom J, et al. The middle molecule hypothesis in perspective. Am J Kidney Dis 1981;1:46.

Banwell BL, Mildner MD, Hassall AC, et al. Muscle weakness in critically ill children. Neurology 2003;61:1779.

Barbeau A. Friedreich's ataxia 1976: An overview. Can J Neurol Sci 1976;3:389.

Barbosa MD, Barratt FJ, Tchernev VT, et al. Identification of mutations in two major mRNA isoforms of the Chediak-Higashi syndrome gene in human and mouse. Hum Mol Genet 1997;6:1091.

Barkai L, Szabó L. Urinary bladder dysfunction in diabetic children with and without subclinical cardiovascular autonomic neuropathy. Eur J Pediatr 1993;152:190.

Bassen FA, Kornzweig AL. Malformation of the erythrocytes in a case of atypical retinitis pigmentosa. Blood 1950;5:381.

Bayever E, Ladisch S, Philippart M, et al. Bone-marrow transplantation for metachromatic leukodystrophy. Lancet 1985;2:471.

Beard ME, Sapirstein V, Kolodny EH, et al. Peroxisomes in fibroblasts from skin of Refsum's disease patients. J Histochem Cytochem 1985;33:480.

Becelli R, Perugini M, Carboni A, Renzi G. Diagnosis of Bell palsy with gadolinium magnetic resonance imaging. J Craniofac Surg 2003;14:51.

Beghi E, Kurland LT, Mulder DW, et al. Guillain-Barré syndrome: Clinicoepidemiologic features and effect of influenza vaccine. Arch Neurol 1985;42:1053.

Ben Othmane K, Hentati F, Lennon F, et al. Linkage of a locus (CMT4A) for autosomal recessive Charcot-Marie-Tooth disease to chromosome 8q. Hum Mol Genet 1993;10:1625.

Berg BO, Rosenberg S, Asbury AK. Giant axonal neuropathy. Pediatrics 1972;49:894.

Berger AR, Schaumburg HH, Schroeder C, et al. Dose response, coasting, and differential fiber vulnerability in human toxic neuropathy:

A prospective study of pyridoxine neurotoxicity. Neurology 1992;42:1367.

Berginer V, Baruchin A, Ben-Yakar Y, et al. Plantar ulcers in hereditary sensory neuropathy: A plea for conservative treatment. Int J Dermatol 1984;23:664.

Bergoffen J, Scherer SS, Wang S, et al. Connexin mutations in X-linked Charcot-Marie-Tooth disease. Science 1993a;262:2039.

Bergoffen J, Trofatter J, Pericek-Vance MA, et al. Linkage localisation of X-linked Charcot-Marie-Tooth disease. Am J Hum Genet 1993b;52:312.

Birouk N, Gouider R, Le Guern E, et al. Charcot-Marie-Tooth disease type Ia with 17p11.2 duplication. Clinical and electrophysiological phenotype study and factors influencing disease severity in 119 cases. Brain 1997;120:813.

Bojanovski D, Gregg RE, Brewer HB Jr. Tangier disease: In vitro conversion of proapo-A-I Tangier to mature apo-A-I Tangier. J Biol Chem 1984;259:6049.

Bolton CF, Laverty DA, Brown JD, et al. Critically ill polyneuropathy: Electrophysiological studies and differentiation from Guillain-Barré syndrome. J Neurol Neurosurg Psychiatry 1986;49:563.

Boltshauser E, Bischoff A, Isler W. Giant axonal neuropathy. J Neurol Sci 1977;31:269.

Bomont P, Cavalier L, Blondeau F, et al. The gene encoding gigaxonin, a new member of the cytoskeletal BTB/kelch repeat family, is mutated in giant axonal neuropathy. Nat Genet 2000;26:370.

Bonerandi JJ, Gambarelli D, Livet MO, et al. Melanocytic involvement in giant axonal neuropathy. J Cutan Pathol 1981;8:313.

Borgeat A, De Muralt B, Stalder M. Peripheral neuropathy associated with high-dose ara-C therapy. Cancer 1986;58:852.

Bradshaw DY, Jones HR. Guillain-Barré syndrome in children: Clinical course, electrodiagnosis, and prognosis. Muscle Nerve 1992;15:500.

Braguer D, Gallice P, Monti JP, et al. Inhibition of microtubule formation by uremic toxins: Action mechanism and hypothesis about the active component. Clin Nephrol 1986;25:212.

Brechenmacher C, Vital C, Deminiere C, et al. Guillain-Barré syndrome: An ultrastructural study of peripheral nerve in 65 patients. Clin Neuropathol 1987;6:19.

Bril V, Ilse WK, Pearce R, et al. Pilot trial of immunoglobulin versus plasma exchange in patients with Guillain-Barré syndrome. Neurology 1996;46:100.

Brin MF, Pedley TA, Lovelace RE, et al. Electrophysiologic features of abetalipoproteinemia: Functional consequences of vitamin E deficiency. Neurology 1986;36:669.

Budden SS, Kennaway NG, Buist NR, et al. Dysmorphic syndrome with phytanic acid oxidase deficiency, abnormal very long chain fatty acids, and pipecolic acidemia: Studies in four children. J Pediatr 1986;108:33.

Bueri JA, Cohen LG, Panizza ME, et al. Peripheral nerve involvement in Bell's palsy. Arq Neuropsiquiatr 1984;42:341.

Buzzi S. Diphtheria toxin treatment of human advanced cancer. Cancer Res 1982;42:2054.

Caksen H, Kurtoglu S, Ustünbau HB, et al. A case of the cardiofacial syndrome (Cayler's syndrome). Acta Paediatr Jpn 1996;38:3256.

Campbell EDR, Hickey RP, Nixon KH, et al. Value of nerve-excitability measurements in prognosis of facial palsy. BMJ 1962;2:7.

Campuzano V, Montermini L, Moltò MD, et al. Friedreich's ataxia: Autosomal recessive disease caused by an intronic GAA triplet repeat expansion. Science 1996;271:1423.

Carpenter S, Karpati G, Andermann F, et al. Giant axonal neuropathy: A clinically and morphologically distinct neurological disease. Arch Neurol 1974;31:312.

Carroll JE, Jedziniak M, Guggenheim MA. Guillain-Barré syndrome: Another cause of the "floppy infant." Am J Dis Child 1977;131:699.

Cavanagh NP, Eames RA, Galvin RJ, et al. Hereditary sensory neuropathy with spastic paraplegia. Brain 1979;102:79.

Cayler G, Blumenfeld CM, Anderson RL. Further studies of patients with the cardiofacial syndrome. Chest 1971;60:161.

Chamberlain S, Shaw J, Rowland A, et al. Mapping of mutation causing Friedreich's ataxia to human chromosome 9. Nature 1988;334:248.

Chamberlain S, Shaw J, Wallis J, et al. Genetic homogeneity at the Friedreich ataxia locus on chromosome 9. Am J Hum Genet 1989;44:518.

Chance PF. Molecular basis of hereditary neuropathies. Phys Med Rehabil Clin North Am 2001;12:277.

Chance PF, Bird TD, O'Connel P, et al. Genetic linkage and heterogeneity in type I Charcot-Marie-Tooth disease (hereditary motor and sensory neuropathy type I). Am J Hum Genet 1990;47:915.

Charnas L, Trapp B, Griffin J. Congenital absence of peripheral myelin: Abnormal Schwann cell development causes lethal arthrogryposis multiplex congenita. Neurology 1988;38:966.

Cogan DG, Rodrigues M, Chu FC, et al. Ocular abnormalities in abetalipoproteinemia: A clinicopathologic correlation. Ophthalmology 1984;91:991.

Colan RV, Snead OC, Oh SJ, Benton JW. Steroid-responsive polyneuropathy with subacute onset in childhood. J Pediatr 1980;97:374.

Cook SD, Dowling PC. The role of autoantibody and immune complexes in the pathogenesis of Guillain-Barré syndrome. Ann Neurol 1981;9(Suppl):70.

Créange A, Meyrignac C, Roualdes B, et al. Diphtheric neuropathy. Muscle Nerve 1995;18:1460.

Danon MJ, Carpenter S. Hereditary sensory neuropathy: Biopsy study of an autosomal dominant variety. Neurology 1985;35:1226.

Davison AN, Duckett S, Oxberry JM. Correlative morphological and biochemical studies of the human fetal sciatic nerve. Brain Res 1973;58:327.

Dawkins JL, Hulme DJ, Brahmbhatt SB, et al. Mutations in SPTLC1, encoding serine palmitoyltransferase, long chain base subunit-1, cause hereditary sensory neuropathy type I. Nat Genet 2001;27:309.

Dawson DM, Samuels MA, Morris J. Sensory form of acute polyneuritis. Neurology 1988;38:1728.

Debuse PJ. Shoshin beriberi in an infant of a thiamine-deficient mother. Acta Paediatr 1992;81:723.

Dechelotte P, Kantelip B, de Laguillaumie BV, et al. Tangier disease: A histological and ultrastructural study. Pathol Res Pract 1985;180:424.

Defanti CA, Sghirlanzoni A, Bottacchi E, et al. Porphyric neuropathy: A clinical, neurophysiological and morphological study. Ital J Neurol Sci 1985;6:521.

De Michele G, Filla A, Cavalcanti F, et al. Late onset Friedreich's disease: Clinical features and mapping of mutation to the FRDA locus. J Neurol Neurosurg Psychiatry 1994;57:977.

Desenclos JC, Wilder MH, Coppenger GW, et al. Thallium poisoning: An outbreak in Florida, 1988. South Med J 1992;85:1203.

Devi S, Challenor Y, Duarte N, et al. Prognostic value of minimal excitability of facial nerve in Bell's palsy. J Neurol Neurosurg Psychiatry 1978;41:649.

Di Paolo B, Cappelli P, Spisni C, et al. New electrophysiological assessments for the early diagnosis of encephalopathy and peripheral neuropathy in chronic uremia. Int J Tissue React 1982;4:301.

DiTaranto P, Campagna L, Price AE, Grossman JA. Outcome following nonoperative treatment of brachial plexus birth injuries. J Child Neurol 2004;19:87.

Donaghue KC, Fung AT, Fairchild JM, et al. Prospective assessment of autonomic and peripheral nerve function in adolescents with diabetes. Diabet Med 1996;13:65.

Donaghy M, Brett EM, Ormerod IEC, et al. Giant axonal neuropathy, observations on a further patient. J Neurol Neurosurg Psychiatry 1988;51:991.

Donaghy M, Hakin RN, Bamford JM, et al. Hereditary sensory neuropathy with neurotrophic keratitis. Description of an autosomal recessive disorder with a selective reduction of small myelinated nerve fibres and a discussion of the classification of the hereditary sensory neuropathies. Brain 1987;110:563.

Dooley JM, Oshima Y, Becker LE, et al. Clinical progression of giant-axonal neuropathy over a twelve year period. Can J Neurol Sci 1981;8:321.

Dordain G, Deffond D. Pyridoxine neuropathies. Review of the literature. Therapie 1994;49:333.

Duncan C, Strub R, McGarry P, et al. Peripheral nerve biopsy as an aid to diagnosis in infantile neuroaxonal dystrophy. Neurology 1970;20:1024.

Dunn HG. Nerve conduction studies in children with Friedreich's ataxia and ataxia-telangiectasia. Dev Med Child Neurol 1973;15:324.

Dunn HG, Daube JR, Gomez MR. Heredofamilial brachial plexus neuropathy (hereditary neuralgic amyotrophy with brachial predilection) in childhood. Dev Med Child Neurol 1978;20:28.

Dyck PJ. Neuronal atrophy and degeneration predominantly affecting peripheral sensory and autonomic neurons. In: Dyck PJ, Thomas PK, Lambert EH, Bunge R, eds. Peripheral neuropathy, Vol. 2, 2nd ed. Philadelphia: WB Saunders, 1984.

Dyck PJ, Mellinger JF, Reagan TJ, et al. Not "indifference to pain" but varieties of hereditary sensory and autonomic neuropathy. Brain 1983;106:373.

Dyck PJ, Thomas PK, Lambert EH, eds. Peripheral neuropathy, Vol. 2. Philadelphia: WB Saunders, 1975.

Ecker JL, Greenberg JA, Norwitz ER, et al. Birth weight as a predictor of brachial plexus injury. Obstet Gynecol 1997;89:643.

Edelstein C, Gordon JI, Vergani CA, et al. Comparative in vitro study of the pro-apolipoprotein A-I to apolipoprotein A-I converting activity between normal and Tangier plasma. J Clin Invest 1984;74:1098.

Epstein MA, Sladky JT. The role of plasmapheresis in childhood Guillain-Barré syndrome. Ann Neurol 1990;28:65.

Faguer P, Man NK, Cueille G, et al. Improved separation and quantification of the "middle molecule": B4-2 in uremia. Clin Chem 1983;29:703.

Feasby TE, Hahn AF, Brown WF, et al. Severe axonal degeneration in acute Guillain-Barré syndrome: Evidence of two different mechanisms? J Neurol Sci 1993;116:185.

Fernandez JM, Dávalos A, Ferrer I, et al. Acute sensory neuronopathy: Report of a child with remarkable clinical recovery. Neurology 1994;44:762.

Ferrière G, Guzzetta F, Kulakowski S, Evrard P. Nonprogressive type II hereditary sensory autonomic neuropathy: A homogeneous clinicopathologic entity. J Child Neurol 1992;7:364.

Fiçicioglu C, Aydin A, Haktan M, Kiziltan M. Peripheral neuropathy in children with insulin-dependent diabetes mellitus. Turk J Pediatr 1994;36:97.

Fisch U. Progressive value of electrical tests in acute facial paralysis. Am J Otolaryngol 1984;5:494.

Fischbeck KH, Ar-Rushdi HN, Pericek-Vance MA, et al. X-linked neuropathy: Gene localisation with DNA probes. Ann Neurol 1986;20:527.

Fitzpatrick DB, Hooper RE, Seife B. Hereditary deafness and sensory radicular neuropathy. Arch Otolaryngol 1976;102:552.

Fois A, Balestri P, Farnetani MA, et al. Giant axonal neuropathy: Endocrinological and histological studies. Eur J Pediatr 1985;144:274.

French Cooperative Group on Plasma Exchange in Guillain-Barré syndrome. Efficiency of plasma exchange in Guillain-Barré syndrome: Role of replacement fluids. Ann Neurol 1987;22:753.

Gabreels-Festen AAWM, Gabreels FJM, Jennekens FGI, et al. Autosomal recessive form of hereditary motor and sensory neuropathy type I. Neurology 1992;42:1755.

Gabreels-Festen AAWM, Joosten EMG, Gabreels F, et al. Hereditary motor and sensory neuropathy of neuronal type with onset in early childhood. Brain 1991;114:1855.

Gambarelli D, Hassoun J, Pellissier JF, et al. Giant axonal neuropathy: Involvement of peripheral nerve, myenteric plexus and extra-neuronal area. Acta Neuropathol 1977;39:261.

Gamstorp I, Shelburne SA Jr, Engleson G, et al. Peripheral neuropathy in juvenile diabetes. Diabetes 1966;15:411.

Gaskill HS, Korb M. Occurrence of multiple neuritis in cases of cutaneous diphtheria. Arch Neurol Psychiatry 1946;55:559.

Ghamdi M, Armstrong D, Miller G. Congenital hypomyelinating neuropathy: A reversible case. Pediatr Neurol 1997;16:71.

Giannotti A, Mingarelli R. Cayler cardiofacial syndrome and del 22q11: Part of the CATCH22 phenotype [Letter]. Am J Med Genet 1994;53:303.

Gibbels E, Schaefer HE, Runne U, et al. Severe polyneuropathy in Tangier disease mimicking syringomyelia or leprosy: Clinical, biochemical, electrophysiological, and morphological evaluation, including electron microscopy of nerve, muscle, and skin biopsies. J Neurol 1985;232:283.

Gibberd FB, Billimoria JD, Goldman JM, et al. Heredopathia atactica polyneuritiformis: Refsum's disease. Acta Neurol Scand 1985;72:1.

Gillespie JB, Perucca LG. Congenital generalized indifference to pain (congenital analgia). Am J Dis Child 1960;100:124.

Göbel U, Bamberg M, Haas RJ, et al. Non-testicular germ cell tumors: Analysis of the therapy study MAKEI$^{83}/_{86}$ and changes in the protocol for the follow-up study. Klin Padiatr 1989;201:247.

Goebel HH, Vogel P, Gabriel M. Neuropathologic and morphometric studies in hereditary motor and sensory neuropathy type II with neurofilament accumulation. Ital J Neurol Sci 1986;7:325.

Gonnaud PM, Sturtz F, Fourbil Y, et al. DNA analysis as a tool to confirm the diagnosis of asymptomatic hereditary neuropathy with liability to pressure palsies (HNPP) with further evidence for the occurrence of de novo mutations. Acta Neurol Scan 1995;92:313.

Gorson KC, Allam G, Simovic D, Ropper AH. Improvement following interferon-alpha 2A in chronic inflammatory demyelinating polyneuropathy. Neurology 1997;48:777.

Graf WD, Chance PF, Lensch MW, et al. Severe vincristine neuropathy in Charcot-Marie-Tooth disease type 1A. Cancer 1996;77:1356.

Graham EM, Forouzan I, Morgan MA. A retrospective analysis of Erb's palsy cases and their relation to birth weight and trauma at delivery. J Matern Fetal Med 1997;6:1.

Graham MD, Kemink JL. Total facial nerve decompression in recurrent facial paralysis and the Melkersson-Rosenthal syndrome: A preliminary report. Am J Otol 1986;7:34.

Greenwald AG, Schute PC, Shiveley JL. Brachial plexus birth palsy: A 10-year report on the incidence and prognosis. J Pediatr Orthop 1984;4:689.

Greenwood RJ, Newsom-Davis J, Hughes RA, et al. Controlled trial of plasma exchange in acute inflammatory polyradiculoneuropathy. Lancet 1984;1:877.

Guillain G, Barré JA, Strohl A. Sur un syndrome de radiculo-nevrite avec hyperalbuminose de liquide cephalo-rachidien sans réaction cellulaire: Remarques sur les caractères cliniques et graphiques des reflexes tendineux. Bull Soc Med Hop Paris 1916;40:1462.

Guillain-Barré Syndrome Study Group. Plasmapheresis and acute Guillain-Barré syndrome. Neurology 1985;35:1096.

Guillozet N, Mercer RD. Hereditary recurrent brachial neuropathy. Am J Dis Child 1973;125:884.

Guzzetta F, Ferrière G, Lyon G. Congenital hypomyelination polyneuropathy: Pathological findings compared with polyneuropathies starting later in life. Brain 1982;105:395.

Gwathmey FW, House JH. Clinical manifestations of congenital insensitivity of the head and classification of syndromes. J Hand Surg 1984;9A:863.

Hafer-Macko C, Hsieh ST, Li CY, et al. Acute motor axonal neuropathy: An antibody-mediated attack on axolemma. Ann Neurol 1996;40:635.

Hagberg B. Krabbe's disease: Clinical presentation of neurological variants. Neuropediatrics 1984;15:11.

Hagberg B, Lyon G. Pooled European series of hereditary peripheral neuropathies in infancy and childhood: A "correspondence work shop" report of the European Federation of Child Neurology Societies (EFCNS). Neuropediatrics 1981;12:9.

Hahn AF, Brown WF, Koopman WJ, et al. X-linked dominant hereditary motor and sensory neuropathy. Brain 1990;113:1511.

Hall SM, Hughes RAC, Atkinson PF, et al. Motor nerve biopsy in severe Guillain-Barré syndrome. Ann Neurol 1992;31:441.

Hallam PJ, Harding AE, Berciano J, et al. Duplication of part of chromosome 17 is commonly associated with hereditary motor and sensory neuropathy type I (Charcot-Marie-Tooth disease type I). Ann Neurol 1992;31:570.

Harding AE, Thomas PK. The clinical features of hereditary motor and sensory neuropathy types I and II. Brain 1980;103:259.

Harding AE, Thomas PK. Peroneal muscular atrophy with pyramidal features. J Neurol Neurosurg Psychiatry 1984;47:168.

Hartmann O, Pinkerton CR, Philip T, et al. Very-high-dose cisplatin and etoposide in children with untreated advanced neuroblastoma. J Clin Oncol 1988;6:44.

Hartung HP, Pollard JD, Harvey GK, Toyka KV. Immunopathogenesis and treatment of the Guillain-Barré syndrome: Part I. Muscle Nerve 1995a;18:137.

Hartung HP, Pollard JD, Harvey GK, Toyka KV. Immunopathogenesis and treatment of the Guillain-Barré syndrome: Part II. Muscle Nerve 1995b;18:154.

Hayasaka K, Takada G, Ionasescu VV, et al. Mutation of the myelin Po gene in Charcot-Marie-Tooth neuropathy type IB. Hum Mol Genet 1993;2:1369.

Hegele RA, Angel A. Arrest of neuropathy and myopathy in abetalipoproteinemia with high-dose vitamin E therapy. Can Med Assoc J 1985;132:41.

Heisel MA, Siegel SE, Falk RE, et al. Congenital pernicious anemia: Report of seven patients, with studies of the extended family. J Pediatr 1984;105:564.

Herbert PN, Forte T, Heinen RJ, et al. Tangier disease: One explanation of lipid storage. N Engl J Med 1978;299:519.

Higginbottom MC, Sweetman L, Nyhan WL. A syndrome of methylmalonic aciduria, homocystinuria, megaloblastic anemia and neurologic abnormalities in a vitamin B-12 deficient breast-fed infant of a strict vegetarian. N Engl J Med 1978;299:317.

Hodson AK, Hurwitz BJ, Albrecht R. Dysautonomia in Guillain-Barré syndrome with dorsal root ganglioneuropathy, wallerian degeneration, and fatal myocarditis. Ann Neurol 1984;15:88.

Honavar M, Tharakan JK, Hughes RAC, et al. A clinicopathological study of the Guillain-Barré syndrome. Nine cases and literature review. Brain 1991;114:1245.

Hughes RAC, for the Plasma Exchange/Sandoglobin Guillain Barré Syndrome Trial Group. Comparison of plasma exchange, intravenous immunoglobulin, and plasma exchange followed by intravenous immunoglobulin in the treatment of the Guillain Barré syndrome. Ann Neurol 1996;3:551(abstr).

Hungerbeuhler JP, Meier C, Rousselle L, et al. Refsum's disease: Management by diet and plasmapheresis. Eur Neurol 1985;24:153.

Hyllienmark L, Brismar T, Ludvigsson J. Subclinical nerve dysfunction in children and adolescents with IDDM. Diabetologia 1995;38:685.

Igarashi M, Thompson EI, Rivera GK. Vincristine neuropathy in type I and type II Charcot-Marie-Tooth disease (hereditary motor sensory neuropathy). Med Pediatr Oncol 1995;25:113.

Igbal A, Arnason BG. Neuropathy of serum sickness. In: Dyck PJ, Thomas PK, Lambert EH, Bunge R, eds. Peripheral neuropathy, 2nd ed, vol. 2. Philadelphia: WB Saunders, 1984.

Igisu H, Ohta M, Tabira T, et al. Giant axonal neuropathy: A clinical entity affecting the central as well as peripheral nervous system. Neurology (Minneapolis) 1975;25:717.

Iida H, Takashima Y, Maeda S, et al. Alterations in erythrocyte membrane lipids in abetalipoproteinemia: Phospholipid and fatty acyl composition. Biochem Med 1984;32:79.

Indo Y, Tsuruta M, Hayashida Y, et al. Mutations in the TRKA/NGF receptor gene in patients with congenital insensitivity to pain with anhidrosis. Nat Genet 1996;13:485.

Ionasescu V, Searby C, Rubenstein P, et al. Giant axonal neuropathy: Normal protein composition of neurofilaments. J Neurol Neurosurg Psychiatry 1983;46:551.

Ippel E, Wittebol-Post D, Jennekens FGI, Bijlsma JB. Genetic heterogeneity of hereditary motor and sensory neuropathy type VI. J Child Neurol 1995;10:459.

Itoh K, Negishi H, Obayashi C, et al. Infantile neuroaxonal dystrophy: Immunohistochemical and ultrastructural studies on the central and peripheral nervous systems in infantile neuroaxonal dystrophy. Kobe J Med Sci 1993;39:133.

Iwabuchi S, Yoshino Y, Goto H, et al. Analysis of serum immunoglobulins in hereditary sensory radicular neuropathy. J Neurol Sci 1976;30:29.

Iwanaga R, Matsuishi T, Ohnishi A, et al. Serial magnetic resonance images in a patient with congenital sensory neuropathy with anhidrosis and complications resembling heat stroke. J Neurol Sci 1996;142:79.

Jaradeh S, D'Cruz O, Howard JF Jr, et al. Mobius syndrome: Electrophysiologic studies in seven cases. Muscle Nerve 1996;19:1148.

Jenkins HA, Herzog JA, Coker NJ. Bell's palsy in children: Cases of progressive facial nerve degeneration. Ann Otol Rhinol Laryngol 1985;94:331.

Jestico JV, Urry PA, Efphimiou J. An hereditary sensory and autonomic neuropathy transmitted as an X-linked recessive trait. J Neurol Neurosurg Psychiatry 1985;48:1259.

Johnsen SD, Johnson PC, Stein SR. Familial sensory autonomic neuropathy with arthropathy in Navajo children. Neurology 1993;43:1120.

Jones MZ, Nigro MA, Barre PS. Familial "giant axonal neuropathy." J Neuropathol Exp Neurol 1979;38:324(abstr).

Judisch GF, Rhead WJ, Miller DK. Abetalipoproteinemia: Report of an unusual patient. Ophthalmologica 1984;189:73.

Kalaydjieva L, Hallmayer J, Chandler D, et al. Gene mapping in gypsies identifies a novel demyelinating neuropathy on chromosome 8q24. Nat Genet 1996;14:214.

Kaplan JG, Kessler J, Rosenberg N, et al. Sensory neuropathy associated with Dursban (chlorpyrifos) exposure. Neurology 1993;43:2193.

Karch SB, Urich H. Infantile polyneuropathy with defective myelination: An autopsy study. Dev Med Child Neurol 1975;17:504.

Kasman M, Bernstein L, Schulman S. Chronic polyradiculoneuropathy of infancy: A report of three cases with familial incidence. Neurology 1976;26:565.

Katusik S, Beard CM, Wiederholt WC, et al. Incidence, clinical features and prognosis in Bell's palsy, Rochester, Minnesota 1968–1982. Ann Neurol 1986;20:622.

Keats BJB, Ward LJ, Shaw J, et al. "Acadian" and "classical" forms of Friedreich ataxia are most probably caused by mutations at the same locus. Am J Med Genet 1990;33:266.

Kessali M, Zemmouri R, Guilbot A, et al. A clinical, electrophysiological, neuropathologic and genetic study of two large Algerian families with an autosomal recessive demyelinating form of Charcot-Marie-Tooth disease. Neurology 1997;48:867.

Kinney RB, Gottfried MR, Hodson AK, et al. Congenital giant axonal neuropathy. Arch Pathol Lab Med 1985;109:639.

Kirkham TH, Guitton D, Coupland SG. Giant axonal neuropathy: Visual and oculomotor deficits. Can J Neurol Sci 1980;7:177.

Klar A, Gross-Kieselstein E, Hurvitz H, et al. Bilateral Bell's palsy due to *Mycoplasma pneumoniae* infection. Isr J Med Sci 1985;21:692.

Kleyweg RP, van der Meché FGA, Meulstee J. Treatment of Guillain-Barré syndrome with high-dose gammaglobulin. Neurology 1988;38:1639.

Klockgether T, Chamberlain S, Wullner U, et al. Late onset Friedreich's ataxia. Molecular genetics, clinical neurophysiology, and magnetic resonance imaging. Arch Neurol 1993;50:803.

Klymkowsky MW, Plummer DJ. Giant axonal neuropathy: A conditional mutation affecting cytoskeletal organization. J Cell Biol 1985;100:245.

Knoll O, Dierker E. Detection of uremic neuropathy by reflex response latency. J Neurol Sci 1980;47:305.

Koch T, Schultz P, Williams R, et al. Giant axonal neuropathy: A childhood disorder of microfilaments. Ann Neurol 1977;1:438.

Kondo K, Horikawa Y, Japan N. Genetic heterogeneity of hereditary sensory neuropathy. Arch Neurol 1974;30:336.

Koobatian TJ, Birkhead GS, Schramm MM, et al. The use of hospital discharge data for public health surveillance of Guillain-Barré syndrome. Ann Neurol 1992;30:618.

Koerbel A, Prevedello DM, Tatsui CE, et al. Posterior fossa gangliocytoma with facial nerve invasion: Case report. Arq Neuropsiquiatr 2003;61:274.

Koski CL, Sanders ME, Swoveland PT, et al. Activation of terminal components of complement in patients with Guillain-Barré syndrome and other demyelinating neuropathies. J Clin Invest 1987;80:1492.

Kremer H, Kuyt LP, van den Helm B, et al. Localization of a gene for Möbius syndrome to chromosome 3q by linkage analysis in a Dutch family. Hum Mol Genet 1996;5:1367.

Kress B, Griesbeck F, Stippich C, et al. Bell palsy: Quantitative analysis of MR imaging data as a method of predicting outcome. Radiology 2004;230:504.

Krivit W, Shapiro E, Kennedy W, et al. Treatment of late infantile metachromatic leukodystrophy by bone marrow transplantation. N Engl J Med 1990;322:28.

Kuwabara S. Guillain-Barré syndrome: Epidemiology, pathophysiology and management. Drugs 2004;64:597.

Laiwah AC, Macphee GJ, Boyle P, et al. Autonomic neuropathy in acute intermittent porphyria. J Neurol Neurosurg Psychiatry 1985;48:1025.

Lamarche JB, Lemieux B, Lieu HB. The neuropathology of "typical" Friedreich's ataxia in Quebec. Can J Neurol Sci 1984;11:592.

Lamont PJ, Johnston HM, Berdoukas VA. Plasmapheresis in children with Guillain-Barré syndrome. Neurology 1991;41:1928.

Lange Y, Steck TL. Mechanism of red blood cell acanthocytosis and echinocytosis in vivo. J Membr Biol 1984;77:153.

Langworth EP, Taverner D. The prognosis in facial palsy. Brain 1963;86:465.

Lebo R, Lynch E, Wiegant J, et al. Multicolor fluorescence in situ hybridization dissects demyelinating Charcot-Marie-Tooth disease gene region. J Neurol Sci 1990;98(Suppl):106.

Lee EL, Oh GC, Lam K, et al. Experience and reason briefly recorded: Congenital sensory neuropathy with anhidrosis. A case report. Pediatrics 1976;57:259.

Levy BK, Fenton GA, Loaiza S, Hayat GR. Unexpected recovery in a newborn with severe hypomyelinating neuropathy. Pediatr Neurol 1997;16:245.

Liberfarb RM, Jackson AH, Eavey RD, Robb RM. Unique hereditary sensory and autonomic neuropathy with growth hormone deficiency. J Child Neurol 1993;8:271.

Lin AE, Ardinger HH, Ardinger RH Jr, et al. Cardiovascular malformations in Smith-Lemli-Opitz syndrome. Am J Med Genet 1997;68:270.

Lindsay EA, Greenberg F, Shaffer LG, et al. Submicroscopic deletions at 22q11.2: Variability of the clinical picture and delineation of a commonly deleted region. Am J Med Genet 1995;56:191.

Linssen WHJP, Van den Bent MJ, Brunner HG, Poels PJE. Deafness, sensory neuropathy, and ovarian dysgenesis: A new syndrome or a broader spectrum Perrault syndrome. Am J Med Genet 1994;51:81.

Lipton M, Lockman LA, Ramsay NK, et al. Bone marrow transplantation in metachromatic leukodystrophy. Birth Defects 1986;22:57.

Lloyd AV, Jewitt DE, Still JD. Facial paralysis in children with hypertension. Arch Dis Child 1966;41:292.

Lockman LA, Kennedy WR, White JG. Chédiak-Higashi syndrome: Electrophysiological and electron microscopic observation on the peripheral neuropathy. J Pediatr 1967;70:942.

Lok AS, Wilson LA, Thomas HC. Neurotoxicity associated with adenine arabinoside monophosphate in the treatment of chronic hepatitis B virus infection. J Antimicrob Chemother 1984;14:93.

Loonen MC, Van Diggelen OP, Janse HC, et al. Late-onset globoid cell leucodystrophy (Krabbe's disease): Clinical and genetic delineation of two forms and their relation to the early-infantile form. Neuropediatrics 1985;16:137.

Loprest LJ, Pericek-Vance MA, Stajich J, et al. Linkage studies in Charcot-Marie-Tooth disease type 2: Evidence that CMT types 1 and 2 are distinct genetic entities. Neurology 1992;42:597.

Louis-Ferdinand RT. Myelotoxic, neurotoxic and reproductive adverse effects of nitrous oxide. Adverse Drug React Toxicol Rev 1994;13:193.

Low PA, McLeod JG, Prineas JW. Hypertrophic Charcot-Marie-Tooth disease: Light and electron microscope studies of the sural nerve. J Neurol Sci 1978;35:93.

Lowry NJ, Taylor MJ, Belknapp W, et al. Electrophysiological studies in five cases of abetalipoproteinemia. Can J Neurol Sci 1984;11:60.

Luijten JA, Straks W, Blikkendaal-Lieftinck LF, et al. Metachromatic leukodystrophy: A comparative study of the ultrastructural findings in the peripheral nervous system of three cases, one of the later infantile, one of the juvenile and one of the adult form of the disease. Neuropaediatrie 1978;9:338.

Lupski JR, Montes de Oca-Luna R, Slaugenhaupt S, et al. DNA duplication associated with Charcot-Marie-Tooth disease type 1A. Cell 1991;66:219.

Luzi P, Rafi MA, Wenger DA. Characterization of the large deletion in the GALC gene found in patients with Krabbe's disease. Hum Mol Genet 1995;4:2335.

Majnemer A, Rosenblatt B, Watters G, et al. Giant axonal neuropathy: Central abnormalities demonstrated by evoked potentials. Ann Neurol 1986;19:394.

Malandrini A, Cavallaro T, Fabrizi GM, et al. Ultrastructure and immunoreactivity of dystrophic axons indicate a different pathogenesis of Hallervorden-Spatz disease and infantile neuroaxonal dystrophy. Virchows Arch 1995;427:415.

Malapert D, Degos JD. Painful legs and moving toes. Neuropathy caused by cytarabine. Rev Neurol (Paris) 1989;145:869.

Mandel H, Berant M, Hazani A, et al. Thiamine-responsive anemia syndrome. N Engl J Med 1984;311:836.

Mandel H, Meiron D, Schutgens RB, et al. Infantile Refsum's disease: Gastrointestinal presentation of a peroxisomal disorder. J Pediatr Gastroenterol Nutr 1992;14:83.

Marbini A, Gemignani F, Ferrarini G, et al. Tangier disease: A case with sensorimotor distal polyneuropathy and lipid accumulation in striated muscle and vasa nervorum. Acta Neuropathol (Berl) 1985;67:121.

Marks HG, Scavina MT, Kolodny EH, et al. Krabbe's disease presenting as a peripheral neuropathy. Muscle Nerve 1997;20:1024.

Martin GI, Weintraub MI. Brachial neuritis and seventh nerve palsy: A rare hazard of DPT vaccination. Clin Pediatr 1973;12:506.

Martin JJ, Martin L. Infantile neuroaxonal dystrophy: Ultrastructural study of the peripheral nerves and of the motor end plates. Eur Neurol 1972;8:239.

Massion-Verniory L, Dumont E, Potvin AM. Amyotrophie neurogene avec la retinite pigmentaire. Rev Neurol (Paris) 1946;78:561.

Mazumder DN, Das Gupta J, Chakraborty AK, et al. Environmental pollution and chronic arsenicosis in south Calcutta. Bull World Health Organ 1992;70:481.

McCombe PA, Pender MP. Lack of neurological abnormalities in Lewis rats with experimental chronic serum sickness. Clin Exp Neurol 1991;28:139.

McGonigle RJ, Bewick M, Weston MJ, et al. Progressive, predominantly motor uraemic neuropathy. Acta Neurol Scand 1985;71:379.

McKhann GM. Metachromatic leukodystrophy: Clinical and enzymatic parameters. Neuropediatrics 1984;15:4.

McLachlan RS, Brown WF. Pyridoxine dependent epilepsy with iatrogenic sensory neuronopathy. Can J Neurol Sci 1995;22:50.

Middleton-Price HR, Harding AE, Monteiro C, et al. Linkage of hereditary motor and sensory neuropathy type I to the pericentromeric region of chromosome 17. Am J Hum Genet 1990;46:92.

Miike T, Ohtani Y, Nishiyama S, et al. Pathology of skeletal muscle and intramuscular nerves in infantile neuroaxonal dystrophy. Acta Neuropathol 1986;69:117.

Miller DPR, Lloyd JK. Effect of large oral doses of vitamin E on the neurological sequelae of patients with abetalipoproteinemia. Ann NY Acad Sci 1982;393:133.

Miller RG, Gutmann L, Lewis RA, et al. Acquired versus familial demyelinative neuropathies in children. Muscle Nerve 1985;8:205.

Mino M. Vitamin A and E deficiency in children, including the marginal deficiency. Nippon Rinsho 1993;51:972.

Misra VP, King RH, Harding AE, et al. Peripheral neuropathy in the Chediak-Higaski syndrome. Acta Neuropathol (Berl) 1991;81:354.

Mitz M, Di Benedetto M, Klingbeil GE, et al. Neuropathy in end-stage renal disease secondary to primary renal disease and diabetes. Arch Phys Med Rehabil 1984;65:235.

Mohr M, Englisch L, Roth A, et al. Effects of early treatment with immunoglobulin on critical illness polyneuropathy following multiple organ failure and gram-negative sepsis. Intensive Care Medicine 1997;23:1144.

Montermini L, Richter A, Morgan K, et al. Phenotypic variability in Friedreich ataxia: Role of the associated GAA triplet repeat expansion. Ann Neurol 1997;41:675.

Moretto G, Sparaco M, Monaco S, et al. Cytoskeletal changes and ubiquitin expression in dystrophic axons of Seitelberger's disease. Clin Neuropathol 1993;12:34.

Murakami T, Garcia CA, Reiter LT, et al. Charcot-Marie-Tooth disease and related inherited neuropathies. Medicine (Baltimore) 1966;75:233.

Nance PW, Kirby RL. Rehabilitation of an adult with disabilities due to congenital sensory neuropathy. Arch Phys Med Rehabil 1985;66:123.

Nelson KB, Eng GD. Congenital hypoplasia of the depressor anguli oris muscle: Differentiation from congenital facial palsy. J Pediatr 1972;81:16.

Nevo Y, Pestronk A, Kornberg AJ, et al. Childhood chronic inflammatory demyelinating neuropathies: Clinical course and long-term follow-up. Neurology 1996;47:98.

Nicholson GA, Dawkins JL, Blair IP, et al. The gene for hereditary sensory neuropathy type I (HSN-I) maps to chromosome 9q22.1-q22.3. Nat Genet 1996;13:101.

Nicholson G, Nash J. Intermediate nerve conduction velocities define X-linked Charcot-Marie-Tooth neuropathy families. Neurology 1993;43:2558.

Nishikawa M, Ichiyama T, Hayashi T, Furukawa S. Möbius-like syndrome associated with a 1;2 chromosome translocation. Clin Genet 1997;51:122.

Nordborg C, Conradi N, Sourander P, et al. Hereditary motor and sensory neuropathy of demyelinating and remyelinating type in children: Ultrastructural and morphometric studies on sural nerve biopsy specimens from ten sporadic cases. Acta Neuropathol (Berl) 1984;64:1.

O'Connor CR, Rubinow A, Brandwein S, Cohen AS. Familial amyloid polyneuropathy: A new kinship of German ancestry. Neurology 1984;34:1096.

Oh SJ, Halsey JH. Abnormality in nerve potentials in Friedreich's ataxia. Neurology 1973;23:52.

Ohta M, Ellefson RD, Lambert EH, et al. Hereditary sensory neuropathy, type II: Clinical, electrophysiologic, histologic and biochemical studies of a Quebec kinship. Arch Neurol 1973;29:23.

Olsen BS, Nir M, Kjaer I, et al. Elevated vibration perception threshold in young patients with type 1 diabetes in comparison to non-diabetic children and adolescents. Diabetes Med 1994;11:888.

Openshaw H, Slatkin NE, Stein AS, et al. Acute polyneuropathy after high dose cytosine arabinoside in patients with leukemia. Cancer 1996;78:1899.

Osterman PG, Lundemo G, Pirskanem R, et al. Beneficial effects of plasma exchange in acute inflammatory polyradiculoneuropathy. Lancet 1984;2:1296.

Ouvrier RA. Hereditary neuropathies in children: The contribution of the new genetics. Semin Pediatr Neurol 1996;3:140.

Ouvrier RA, McLeod JG. Chronic peripheral neuropathy in childhood: An overview. Aust Paediatr J 1988;24(Suppl 1):80.

Ouvrier RA, McLeod JG, Conchin TE. The hypertrophic forms of hereditary motor and sensory neuropathy: A study of hypertrophic Charcot-Marie-Tooth disease (HMSN Type I) and Dejerine-Sottas disease (HMSN Type III) in childhood. Brain 1987;110:121.

Ouvrier RA, McLeod JG, Morgan GJ, et al. Hereditary motor and sensory neuropathy of neuronal type with onset in early childhood. J Neurol Sci 1981;51:181.

Ouvrier RA, Prineas J, Walsh JC, et al. Giant axonal neuropathy: A third case. Proc Aust Assoc Neurol 1974;11:137.

Ouzounian JG, Korst LM, Phelan JP. Permanent Erb palsy: A traction-related injury? Obstet Gynecol 1997;89:139.

Palau F, De Michele G, Vilchez JJ, et al. Early-onset ataxia with cardiomyopathy and retained tendon reflexes maps to Friedreich's ataxia locus on chromosome 9q. Ann Neurol 1995;37:359.

Palix C, Coignet J. Un cas de polyneuropathie périphérique neo-natale par amyélinisation. Pédiatrie 1978;33:201.

Panayiotopoulos CP, Lagos G. Tibial nerve H-reflex and F-wave studies in patients with uremic neuropathy. Muscle Nerve 1980;3:423.

Peiris OA, Miles DW. Galvanic stimulation of the tongue as a prognostic index in Bell's palsy. BMJ 1965;2:1162.

Pena SD. Giant axonal neuropathy: An inborn error of organization of intermediate filaments. Muscle Nerve 1982;5:166.

Petersen B, Schneider C, Strassburg HM, Schrod L. Critical illness neuropathy in pediatric intensive care patients. J Paediatr Neurol 1999;21:749.

Pettit RE, Berdal KG. Chédiak-Higashi syndrome: Neurologic appearance. Arch Neurol 1984;41:1001.

Pfeiffer J, Schlote W, Bischoff AS, et al. General giant axonal neuropathy. Acta Neuropathol 1977;40:213.

Piatt JH Jr. Birth injuries of the brachial plexus. Pediatr Clin North Am. 2004;51(2):421.

Pietrini V, Rizzuto N, Vergani C, et al. Neuropathy in Tangier disease: A clinicopathologic study and a review of the literature. Acta Neurol Scand 1985;72:495.

Pinsky L, DiGeorge AM. Congenital familial sensory neuropathy with anhidrosis. J Pediatr 1966;68:1.

Poulos A, Sharp P. Plasma and skin fibroblast C26 fatty acids in infantile Refsum's disease. Neurology 1984;34:1606.

Poulos A, Sharp P, Fellenberg AJ, et al. Cerebro-hepato-renal (Zellweger) syndrome, adrenoleukodystrophy, and Refsum's disease: Plasma changes and skin fibroblast phytanic acid oxidase. Hum Genet 1985;70:172.

Poulos A, Sharp P, Whiting M. Infantile Refsum's disease (phytanic acid storage disease): A variant of Zellweger's syndrome. Clin Genet 1984;26:579.

Prineas JW. Pathology of the Guillain-Barré syndrome. Ann Neurol 1981;9(Suppl):6.

Prineas JW, Ouvrier RA, Wright RG, et al. Giant axonal neuropathy: A generalized disorder of cytoplasmic microfilament formation. J Neuropathol Exp Neurol 1976;35:458.

Pummi KP, Heape AM, Grenman RA, et al. Tight junction proteins ZO-1, occludin, and claudins in developing and adult human perineurium. J Histochem Cytochem 2004;52:1037.

Punal JE, Siebert MF, Angueira FB, et al. Three new patients with congenital unilateral facial nerve palsy due to chromosome 22q11 deletion. J Child Neurol 2001;16:450.

Quinlivan R, Robb S, Hughes RA, et al. Congenital sensory neuropathy in association with ichthyosis and anterior chamber cleavage syndrome. Neuromusc Disord 1993;3:217.

Raeymakers P, Timmerman V, DeJonghe P, et al. Localization of the mutation in an extended family with Charcot-Marie-Tooth neuropathy (HMSNI). Am J Hum Genet 1989;45:953.

Raeymakers P, Timmerman V, Nelis E, et al. Duplication in chromosome 17p11.2-12 in Charcot-Marie-Tooth neuropathy type 1a (CMT1a). Neuromusc Disord 1991;1:93.

Rafi MA, Luzi P, Chen YQ, Wenger DA. A large deletion together with a point mutation in the GALC gene is a common mutant allele in patients with infantile Krabbe's disease. Hum Mol Genet 1995;4:1285.

Rangel-Guerra R, Martínez HR, Villarreal HJ. Thallium poisoning: Experience with 50 patients. Gac Med Mex 1990;126:487.

Refsum S. Heredopathia atactica polyneuritiformis: A familial syndrome not hitherto described. A contribution to the clinical study of the hereditary diseases of the nervous system. Acta Psychiatr Scand 1946;(Suppl 38):1.

Refsum S, Salomonsen L, Skatvedt M. Heredopathia atactica polyneuritiformis in children. J Pediatr 1949;35:335.

Roach ES, Abramson JS, Lawless MR. Self-injurious behavior in acquired sensory neuropathy. Neuropediatrics 1985;16:159.

Roberg M, Ernerudh J, Fosberg P, et al. Acute peripheral facial palsy: CSF findings and etiology. Acta Neurol Scand 1991;83:55.

Rogers RS 3rd. Melkersson-Rosenthal syndrome and orofacial granulomatosis. Dermatol Clin 1996;14:371.

Román GC. An epidemic in Cuba of optic neuropathy, sensorineural deafness, peripheral sensory neuropathy and dorsolateral myeloneuropathy. J Neurol Sci 1994;127:11.

Ropper AH. Severe acute Guillain-Barré syndrome. Neurology 1986;36:429.

Ropper AH, Shahani BT. Pain in Guillain-Barré syndrome. Arch Neurol 1984;41:511.

Rosemberg S, Marie SK, Kliemann S. Congenital insensitivity to pain with anhidrosis (hereditary sensory and autonomic neuropathy type IV). Pediatric Neurol 1994;11:50.

Ross AT. Mercuric polyneuropathy with albumino-cytologic dissociation and eosinophilia. JAMA 1964;188:830.

Rossi LN, Vassella F, Mumenthaler M. Obstetrical lesions of the brachial plexus. Eur Neurol 1982;21:1.

Roy EP 3d, Gutmann L, Riggs JE. Longitudinal conduction studies in hereditary motor and sensory neuropathy type 1. Muscle Nerve 1989;12:52.

Rozear MP, Pericek-Vance MA, Fischbeck K, et al. Hereditary motor and sensory neuropathy, X-linked: A half century follow-up. Neurology 1987;37:1460.

Rubin DI. Neuralgic amyotrophy: Clinical features and diagnostic evaluation. Neurologist 2001;7(6):350.

Rudnicki S, Vriesendorp F, Koski CL, et al. Electrophysiologic studies in the Guillain-Barré syndrome: Effects of plasma exchange and antibody rebound. Muscle Nerve 1992;15:57.

Runge P, Muller DP, McAllister J, et al. Oral vitamin E supplements can prevent the retinopathy of abetalipoproteinaemia. Br J Ophthalmol 1986;70:166.

Sabin TD, Thomas TR. Leprosy. In: Dyck PJ, Thomas PK, Lambert EH, Bunge R, eds. Peripheral neuropathy, 2nd ed., Vol. 2. Philadelphia: WB Saunders, 1984.

Said G, Boudier L, Selva J, et al. Different patterns of uremic polyneuropathy: Clinicopathologic study. Neurology 1983;33:567.

Salman MS, MacGregor DL. Should children with Bell's palsy be treated with corticosteroids? A systematic review. J Child Neurol 2001;16(8):565.

Salt HB, Wolff OH, Lloyd JK, et al. On having no beta-lipoprotein: A syndrome comprising abetalipoproteinaemia, acanthocytosis and steatorrhoea. Lancet 1960;IIL:325.

Santoro L, Ragno M, Nucciotti R, et al. Pyridoxine neuropathy. A four-year electrophysiological and clinical follow-up of a severe case. Acta Neurol 1991;13:13.

Schaumburg H, Kaplan J, Windebank A, et al. Sensory neuropathy from pyridoxine abuse: A new megavitamin syndrome. N Engl J Med 1983;309:445.

Scherer SS, Deschennes S, Xu YT, et al. Connexin 32 is a myelin-related protein in the PNS and CNS. J Neurosci 1995;15:8281.

Scherokman B, Filling-Katz MR, Tell D. Brachial plexus neuropathy following high-dose cytarabine in acute monoblastic leukemia. Cancer Treat Rep 1985;69:1005.

Schmitz G, Assmann G, Robenek H, et al. Tangier disease: A disorder of intracellular membrane traffic. Proc Natl Acad Sci U S A 1985;82:6305.

Schwartz J, Landrigan PJ, Feldman RG, et al. Threshold effect in lead-induced peripheral neuropathy. J Pediatr 1988;112:12.

Seitz RJ, Wechsler W, Mosny DS, Lenard HG. Hypomyelination neuropathy in a female newborn presenting as arthrogryposis multiplex congenita. Neuropediatrics 1986;17:1326.

Selimoglu MA, Esrefoglu M, Gundoglu C, Kilic A. Abetalipoproteinemia: A case report. Turk J Pediatr 2001;43:243.

Sghirlanzoni A, Pareyson D, Balestrini MR, et al. HMSN III phenotype due to homozygous expression of a dominant HMSN-II gene. Neurology 1992;42:2201.

Shapiro WR, Young DF. Neurological complications of antineoplastic therapy. Acta Neurol Scand 1984;100:125.

Sheth RD, Bolton CF. Neuromuscular complications of sepsis in children. J Child Neurol 1995;10:346.

Shimasaki N, Watanabe K, Hara M, Kosaki K. EYA1 mutation in a newborn female presenting with cardiofacial syndrome. Pediatr Cardiol 2004;25(4):411.

Shimono M, Ohta M, Asada M, et al. Infantile neuroaxonal dystrophy: Ultrastructural study of peripheral nerve. Acta Neuropathol (Berl) 1976;36:71.

Simmons Z, Albers JW, Bromberg MB, Feldman EL. Presentation and initial clinical course in patients with chronic inflammatory demyelinating polyradiculoneuropathy: Comparison of patients without and with monoclonal gammopathy. Neurology 1993;43:2202.

Simmons Z, Wald JJ, Albers JW. Chronic inflammatory demyelinating polyradiculoneuropathy in children. I. Presentation, electrodiagnostic studies, and initial clinical course, with comparison to adults. Muscle Nerve 1997;20:1008.

Singhi P, Jain V. Bell's palsy in children. Semin Pediatr Neurol 2003;10:289.

Skjeldal OH, Stokke O, Norseth J, et al. Phytanic acid oxidase activity in cultured skin fibroblasts: Diagnostic usefulness and limitations. Scand J Clin Lab Invest 1986;46:283.

Sladky JT. Guillain-Barré syndrome in children. J Child Neurol 2004;19:191.

Sladky JT, Brown MJ, Berman PH. Chronic inflammatory demyelinating polyneuropathy of infancy: A corticosteroid-responsive disorder. Ann Neurol 1986;20:76.

Smets K, Zecic A, Willems J. Ergotamine as a possible cause of Möbius sequence: Additional clinical observation. J Child Neurol 2004;19:398.

Smeyne RJ, Klein R, Schnapp A, et al. Severe sensory and sympathetic neuropathies in mice carrying a disrupted Trk/NGF receptor gene. Nature 1994;368:246.

Smith GD, Hughes RAC. Plasma exchange treatment and prognosis of Guillain-Barré syndrome. Q J Med 1992;85:751.

Solders G, Thalme B, Aguirre-Aquino M, et al. Nerve conduction and autonomic nerve function in diabetic children. A 10-year follow-up study. Acta Paediatr 1997;86:361.

Stacy CB, Di Roco A, Gould RJ. Methionine in the treatment of nitrous-oxide-induced neuropathy and myeloneuropathy. J Neurol 1992;239:401.

Stewart HS, Smith JC. Two patients with asymmetric crying facies, normal cardiovascular systems and deletion of chromosome 22q11. Clin Dysmorphol 1997;6:165.

Stollhoff K, Albani M, Goebel HH. Giant axonal neuropathy and leukodystrophy. Pediatr Neurol 1991;7:69.

Sutherland WH, Pollock M. Endoneurial adenosine triphosphatase activity in Tangier disease and other peripheral neuropathies. Muscle Nerve 1984;7:447.

Suzuki K. Biochemical pathogenesis of genetic leukodystrophies: Comparison of metachromatic leukodystrophy and globoid cell leukodystrophy (Krabbe's disease). Neuropediatrics 1984;15:32.

Swaiman KF, Flagler DG. Penicillamine therapy of the Guillain-Barré syndrome caused by mercury poisoning. Neurology 1971;21:456.

Swanson AG. Congenital insensitivity to pain with anhidrosis. Arch Neurol 1963;8:299.

Tada K, Tsuyuguchi Y, Kawai H. Birth palsy: Natural recovery course and combined root avulsion. J Pediatr Orthop 1984;4:279.

Takakura H, Nakano C, Kasagi S, et al. Multimodality evoked potentials in progression of metachromatic leukodystrophy. Brain Dev 1985;7:424.

Takebe Y, Koide N. Giant axonal neuropathy report of two siblings with endocrinological and histological studies. Neuropediatrics 1981;12:392.

Takebe Y, Koide N, Takahashi G. Giant axonal neuropathy: Report of two siblings with endocrinological and histological studies. Neuropediatrics 1981;12:392.

Tanabe Y, Iai M, Ishii M, et al. The use of magnetic resonance imaging in diagnosing infantile neuroaxonal dystrophy. Neurology 1993;43:110.

Tarao K, Iwamura K, Fujii K, et al. Japanese adult siblings with Tangier disease and statistical analysis of reported cases. Tokai J Exp Clin Med 1984;9:379.

Taroni F, Botti S, Sghirlanzoni A, Pareyson D. PMP22 and MPZ point mutations in Italian families with hereditary neuropathy with liability to pressure palsies (HNPP) and Dejerine-Sottas disease (DSD). Am J Hum Genet 1996;59:A288(abstr 1688).

Tatsumi N, Inui K, Sakai N, et al. Molecular defects in Krabbe's disease. Hum Mol Genet 1995;4:1865.

Teot L, Arnal F, Humeau C, et al. Ultrastructural aspects of nerves, bones, and vessels in hereditary sensory neuropathy. J Orthop Res 1985;3:226.

Thomas C, Love S, Powell HC, et al. Giant axonal neuropathy: Correlation of clinical findings with postmortem neuropathology. Ann Neurol 1987;22:79.

Thomas PK, Calne DB, Stewart G. Hereditary motor and sensory polyneuropathy (peroneal muscular atrophy). Ann Hum Genet 1974;38:111.

Tonkin MA, Eckersley JR, Gschwind CR. The surgical treatment of brachial plexus injuries. Aust N Z J Surg 1996;66:29.

Treiber-Held S, Budjarjo-Welim H, Riemann D, et al. Giant axonal neuropathy: A generalized disorder of intermediate filaments with longitudinal grooves in the hair. Neuropediatrics 1994;25:89.

Tyson J, Ellis D, Fairbrother U, et al. Hereditary demyelinating neuropathy of infancy. A genetically complex syndrome. Brain 1997;120:47.

Uchino M, Uyama E, Hirano T, et al. A histochemical and electron microscopic study of skeletal muscle in an adult case of Chédiak-Higashi syndrome. Acta Neuropathol (Berl) 1993;86:521.

Uncini A, Parano E, Lange DJ, et al. Chronic inflammatory demyelinating polyneuropathy in childhood: Clinical and electrophysiological features. Childs Nerv Syst 1991;7:191.

Valentijn LJ, Ouvrier RA, van den Bosch NH, et al. Dejerine-Sottas neuropathy is associated with a de novo PMP22 mutation. Hum Mutat 1995;5:76.

Vanasse M, Michaud J. Congenital axonal neuropathy. Pediatr Neurol 1992;8:404(abstr).

Van den Branden C, Vamacq J, Wybo I, et al. Phytol and peroxisome proliferation. Pediatr Res 1986;20:411.

van der Meché FGA, Schmitz PIM, Dutch Guillain-Barré Study Group. A randomized trial comparing intravenous immune globulin and plasma exchange in Guillain-Barré syndrome. N Engl J Med 1992;326:1123.

Vance JM. The many faces of Charcot-Marie-Tooth disease. Arch Neurol 2000;57:638.

Vance JM, Nicholson GA, Yamaoka LH, et al. Linkage of Charcot-Marie-Tooth neuropathy type 1a to chromosome 17. Exp Neurol 1989;104:186.

Vassalla F, Emrich HM, Kraus-Ruppert R, et al. Congenital sensory neuropathy with anhidrosis. Arch Dis Child 1968;43:124.

Venkatesh S, Coulter DL, Kemper TD. Neuroaxonal dystrophy at birth with hypertonicity and basal ganglia mineralization. J Child Neurol 1994;9:74.

Verrotti A, Chiarelli F, Blasetti A, Morgese G. Autonomic neuropathy in diabetic children. J Paediatr Child Health 1995;31:545.

Wakai S, Asanuma H, Tachi N, et al. Infantile neuroaxonal dystrophy: Axonal changes in biopsied muscle tissue. Pediatr Neurol 1993;9:309.

Warner LE, Hilz MJ, Appel SH, et al. Clinical phenotypes of different MPZ (Po) mutations may include Charcot-Marie-Tooth type IB, Dejerine-Sottas, and congenital hypomyelination. Neuron 1996;17:451.

Wassif WS, Deacon AC, Floderus Y, et al. Acute intermittent porphyria: Diagnostic conundrums. Eur J Clin Chem Clin Biochem 1994;32:915.

Weleber RG, Tongue AC, Kennaway NG, et al. Ophthalmic manifestations of infantile phytanic acid storage disease. Arch Ophthalmol 1984;102:1317.

Whitaker JN, Falchuck ZM, Engel WK, et al. Hereditary sensory neuropathy: Association with increased synthesis of immunoglobulin A. Arch Neurol 1974;30:359.

Wichman A, Buchthal F, Pezeshkpour GH, et al. Peripheral neuropathy in abetalipoproteinemia. Neurology 1985;35:1279.

Wiederholt WC. Hereditary brachial neuropathy: Report of two families. Arch Neurol 1974;30:252.

Williams LL, O'Dougherty MM, Wright FS, et al. Dietary essential fatty acids, vitamin E, and Charcot-Marie-Tooth disease. Neurology 1986;36:1200.

Windebank AJ, Schenone A, Dewald GW. Hereditary neuropathy with liability to pressure palsies and inherited brachial plexus neuropathy: Two genetically distinct disorders. Mayo Clin Proc 1995;70:743.

Winer JB, Hughes RAC, Anderson MJ, et al. A prospective study of acute idiopathic neuropathy. II. Antecedent events. J Neurol Neurosurg Psychiatry 1988;51:613.

Winer JB, Hughes RA, Greenwood RJ, et al. Prognosis in Guillain-Barré syndrome. Lancet 1985;1:1202.

Wolf SM, Wagner JH Jr, Davidson S, et al. Treatment of Bell palsy with prednisone: A prospective randomized study. Neurology 1978;28:158.

Wolfe DE, Schindler D, Desnick RJ. Neuroaxonal dystrophy in infantile alpha-*N*-acetylgalactosaminidase deficiency. J Neurol Sci 1995;132:44.

Wulff CH, Trojaborg W. Adult metachromatic leukodystrophy: Neurophysiologic findings. Neurology 1985;35:1776.

Yamada M, Konodo M, Tanaka M, et al. An autopsy case of acute porphyria with a decrease of both uroporphyrinogen I synthetase and ferrochelatase activities. Acta Neuropathol (Berl) 1984;64:6.

Yatzidis H, Koutsicos D, Agroyannis B, et al. Biotin in the management of uremic neurologic disorders. Nephron 1984;36:183.

Yetiser S, Kazkayas M, Altinok D, Karadeniz Y. Magnetic resonance imaging of the intratemporal facial nerve in idiopathic peripheral facial palsy. Clin Imaging 2003;27(2):77.

Zampollo A, Baruffini A, Cirla AM, et al. Subclinical inorganic mercury neuropathy: Neurophysiological investigations in 17 occupationally exposed subjects. Ital J Neurol Sci 1987;8:249.

CHAPTER 77

Inflammatory Neuropathies

John T. Sladky and Stephen Ashwal

Although children and adults with peripheral neuropathies exhibit similar clinical and electrophysiologic features, the incidence and nature of the underlying disorders responsible for peripheral nerve diseases in children and adults are widely divergent. Perhaps the most salient difference is that most peripheral nerve diseases in children are immune mediated and potentially treatable. Table 77-1 shows a broad categorical breakdown of the etiologies for neuropathy in a group of 249 children evaluated over 12 years at a tertiary pediatric referral center. Acquired inflammatory neuropathies were the most frequently occurring peripheral nerve diseases in this group of patients, followed by the genetically determined neuropathies. Table 77-2 illustrates a more specific classification of the acquired immune-mediated neuropathies seen in this group. Acute and chronic inflammatory demyelinating neuropathies were the most common cause of neuropathy in the inflammatory subgroup. Some children with collagen vascular diseases developed neuropathy as a complication of rheumatoid arthritis, systemic lupus erythematosus, or mixed connective tissue disease. Necrotizing vasculitis selectively affecting the peripheral nervous system was also seen. The category of "other immune/infectious disorders" included children with graft-versus-host disease after bone marrow transplantation [Adams et al., 1995; Perry et al., 1994] and children who developed a chronic immune demyelinating polyneuropathy-like presentation in the course of primary Lyme disease. Although children with human immunodeficiency virus infection and acquired immune deficiency syndrome were frequently evaluated for neurologic complications, only one adolescent developed an associated peripheral neuropathy [Leger, 1992], presumably as a complication of treatment.

Inflammatory neuropathies, by virtue of their frequency and potential to respond to therapeutic intervention, are important to consider when evaluating children with peripheral nerve disease. As noted earlier, Guillain-Barré syndrome constitutes the most common variety of acquired immune-mediated neuropathy in childhood. The pathologic manifestations of Guillain-Barré syndrome are protean, with immunologic-targeted antigens resulting primarily in segmental demyelination or axonal degeneration. The clinical manifestations of the disease are determined by the nature of the pathology and the populations of axons that come under immunologic attack. Although the salient clinical feature of Guillain-Barré syndrome is weakness, any organ system that relies on peripheral nerve for reporter or executive functions may be affected by the illness. It is reasonable to conceptualize this syndrome as an inhomogeneous spectrum of clinical features with specific constellations of clinical characteristics clustering in distinct patterns, permitting definitions of subcategories of Guillain-Barré syndrome.

ACUTE INFLAMMATORY DEMYELINATING POLYNEUROPATHY

Epidemiology

Acute inflammatory demyelinating polyneuropathy, one of several discrete varieties of Guillain-Barré syndrome, accounts for about 90% of the disease in North America and Western Europe. It is the most common paralytic illness affecting children in countries with established immunization programs. The incidence of Guillain-Barré syndrome has been estimated in population-based studies to be between 0.25 and 1.5 cases per 100,000 children younger than 16 years [Rantala et al., 1994]. Based on these estimates, about 400 to 600 children per year would be diagnosed with Guillain-Barré syndrome in the United States [Prevots et al., 1997]. Similar data have been reported from Canada [McLean et al., 1994], England, Europe, and the Scandinavian countries [Farkkila et al., 1991; Korinthenberg et al., 1996]; Latin America [Asbury and Cornblath, 1990; Hart et al., 1994; Korinthenberg and Monting, 1996; Molinero et al., 2003; Olive et al., 1997]; and Taiwan [Hung et al., 1994]. Both sexes are affected, although most pediatric series have noted a slight male preponderance.

Diagnostic Criteria

As part of a nationwide program to evaluate the possible relation of swine-flu immunization to Guillain-Barré syndrome, diagnostic criteria were developed under the sponsorship of the National Institute of Neurological Disorders and Stroke and were later modified after analysis of data from several multicenter treatment trials [Asbury and Cornblath, 1990]. Boxes 77-1 and 77-2 provide summaries of the consensus statement describing the clinical characteristics necessary to diagnose Guillain-Barré syndrome along with those features, including electrophysiologic testing and laboratory measurements, that mitigate for or against the diagnosis.

Clinical Features

The clinical presentation of Guillain-Barré syndrome is similar in children and adults [Bradshaw and Jones, 1992; Kleyweg et al., 1989; Korinthenberg and Monting, 1996; Rantala et al., 1991; Sakakihara et al., 1991; Sarada et al., 1994; Sladky, 2004] Although there is considerable variability in the nature of the initial symptoms, the overall pattern of the evolution of the clinical syndrome and the ultimate severity of disability usually conform to a triphasic model: (1) onset and progression of symptoms and signs that reach a nadir, followed by (2) a plateau phase and

TABLE 77-1

Etiologies of Neuropathy in 249 Children (1980–1992)

CATEGORY	PATIENTS (%)
Immune and inflammatory disorders	45
Genetically determined disorders	42
Other causes of neuropathy	13

Data from unpublished observations of John T. Sladky, MD.

TABLE 77-2

Causes of Inflammatory and Immune Neuropathy in 112 Children

DIAGNOSIS	PATIENTS (%)
Guillain-Barré syndrome	58
Chronic inflammatory demyelinating polyneuropathy	31
Cases associated with collagen vascular disease	7
Other immune and infectious disorders	4

Data from unpublished observations of John T. Sladky, MD.

Box 77-1 Clinical and Laboratory Features in the Diagnosis of Guillain-Barré Syndrome

I. Required for diagnosis
- Progressive motor weakness of more than one limb
- Areflexia—loss of ankle-jerk reflex and diminished knee and biceps reflexes suffice if other features are consistent with the diagnosis

II. Strongly supportive of the diagnosis
- Progression—weakness may develop rapidly but cease to progress after 4 weeks; roughly 50% will plateau within 2 weeks, 80% by 3 weeks, and 90% after 4 weeks
- Relative symmetry
- Mild sensory symptoms or signs
- Cranial nerve involvement; facial weakness develops in about half of patients
- Autonomic dysfunction
- Absence of fever at the onset of neurologic symptoms
- Recovery—usually recovery begins 2 to 4 weeks after progression ceases; it may be delayed for months
- Variants
  Fever at onset of symptoms
  Severe sensory loss with pain
  Progressive phase longer than 4 weeks
  Lack of recovery or major permanent residual deficit
- Sphincter dysfunction—sphincters are usually spared, although transient bladder paralysis may occur
- CNS involvement

III. Features casting doubt on diagnosis
- Marked persistent asymmetry in motor function
- Persistent bowel or bladder dysfunction
- Bowel or bladder dysfunction at onset of symptoms
- Discrete sensory level

IV. Features that exclude the diagnosis
- History of recent Hexa carbon abuse
- Evidence of porphyria
- Recent diphtheria
- Features consistent with lead neuropathy and evidence of lead intoxication
- A pure sensory syndrome
- Definite diagnosis of an alternate paralytic disorder

From Asbury AK, Cornblath DR. Assessment of current diagnostic criteria for Guillain-Barré syndrome. Ann Neurol 1990;27:S21.

Box 77-2 Consensus Electrophysiologic Features Supportive of a Diagnosis of Multifocal Demyelinating Neuropathy of Guillain-Barré Syndrome

Must demonstrate three of the following four features:

1. Reduction in conduction velocity in two or more motor nerves
   a. <80% of LLN if CMAP amplitude >80% LLN
   b. <70% of LLN if CMAP amplitude <80% LLN
2. Conduction block or excessive temporal dispersion of proximally evoked CMAP in one or more motor nerves (peroneal, between ankle and below fibular head; median, between wrist and elbow; ulnar, between wrist and below elbow)
   a. Criteria for partial conduction block: <15% change in CMAP duration between proximal and distal sites and 20% drop in negative-peak area of peak-to-peak amplitude between proximal and distal sites
   b. Criteria for abnormal temporal dispersion and possible conduction block: >15% increase in CMAP duration between distal and proximal stimulation sites and >20% decrease in negative-peak CMAP area or peak-to-peak amplitude between distal and proximal stimulation sites
3. Prolonged distal latencies in two or more nerves
   a. >125% of ULN if amplitude >80% of LLN
   b. >150% of ULN if amplitude <80% LLN
4. Absent F waves or prolonged minimum F-wave latencies (10 to 15 trials) in two or more motor nerves
   a. >120% of ULN if amplitude >80% of LLN
   b. >150% of ULN if amplitude <80% of LLN

CMAP, compound motor unit action potential; LLN, lower limit of normal; ULN, upper limit of normal.

From Asbury AK, Cornblath DR. Assessment of current diagnostic criteria for Guillain-Barré syndrome. Ann Neurol 1990;27:S21.

finally (3) recovery that takes place over weeks or months. The initial phase is generally relentless and rapid. Between 50% and 75% of patients develop maximal weakness within 2 weeks, and 90% to 98% by 4 weeks [Asbury and Cornblath, 1990; Korinthenberg and Monting, 1996; Italian Guillain-Barré Study Group, 1996]. In several series describing the natural history of the disorder, in both adults and children, the mean duration of the progressive phase was in the range of 10 to 12 days. A small number of patients continue to progress for longer than 4 weeks. This latter group overlaps to some degree with patients diagnosed with chronic inflammatory demyelinating polyneuropathy. The duration of the plateau phase is similar to that of the progressive phase, averaging 10 to 12 days but ranging from several days to 4 weeks [Italian Guillain-Barré Study Group, 1996]. Patients who develop severe axonal degeneration have a prolonged plateau phase and tend to have more severe residual weakness [Cornblath, 1990]. In a series primarily of adult patients, about half recovered within 6 months, and more than 80% by 24 months [Italian Guillain-Barré Study Group, 1996].

A multicenter study of 175 children with Guillain-Barré syndrome has reported similar findings [Korinthenberg and Monting, 1996]. At the height of the disease, 26% of patients remained able to walk, but 16% required artificial ventilation. The median time from onset of symptoms to first recovery was 17 days, to walk unaided 37 days, and to be free of symptoms 66 days. The population in this study was heterogeneous, with many children receiving some form of treatment including plasmapheresis, intravenous immune globulin, and corticosteroids. A large number of children have a relatively benign course, and a smaller group a more severe and protracted course of their disease. At 6 months' follow-up evaluation, 98 of 106 children were free of symptoms, and the others were able to walk unaided. As in series of adult patients, the maximum degree of disability at clinical nadir appears to be the most powerful predictive factor for incomplete recovery.

In the past, there has been debate about whether the natural history of Guillain-Barré syndrome in children is more benign or comparable to that among adults. Advocates have positioned themselves on both sides of the question. The argument may ultimately be unresolvable because of the absence of large prospective controlled treatment trials in children compared with adults with Guillain-Barré syndrome. There are only a few case series that include descriptions of the natural course of this syndrome in untreated children with consistent end-point measures. Two benchmark studies in adults are the North American Treatment Trial and the French Plasmapheresis Treatment Trial.

Table 77-3 summarizes some of the presenting complaints seen in a series of 49 children hospitalized with

TABLE 77-3

Clinical Features in 49 Children Younger than 18 Years with Guillain-Barré Syndrome

FEATURE	PREVALENCE
Age	7.1 years (mean)
Male-to-female ratio	1.2:1
Weakness	73%
Pain	55%
Ataxia	44%
Paresthesias	18%
Shortness of breath	4%

Data from unpublished observations of John T. Sladky, MD. Two patients had findings consistent with Miller Fisher syndrome.

TABLE 77-4

Clinical Grading Scale from the U.S. Guillain-Barré Syndrome Plasmapheresis Trial

SCORE	CLINICAL CRITERIA
0	Health
1	Minor signs or symptoms
2	Able to walk 5 m without a walker or equivalent support
3	Able to walk 5 m with a walker or support
4	Bed or chair bound (unable to walk 5 m with a walker or support)
5	Requires assisted ventilation (for at least part of the day)
6	Dead

From the Guillain-Barré Syndrome Study Group. Neurology 1985;35:1096.

Guillain-Barré syndrome. Not surprisingly, weakness was the most common initial complaint. Pain, particularly in the back and lower extremities, was also a prominent feature. A history of difficulty with balance early in the course of the illness was elicited in almost half of the children. The classic triad, characteristic of the Miller Fisher variant of Guillain-Barré syndrome (ataxia, ophthalmoparesis, and areflexia), was present in only two children. All children had evidence of progression. Maximal disability was quantitated according to the 1985 Guillain-Barré Syndrome Study Group grading scale (Table 77-4). At the time of maximal neurologic deficit, 25% of children were able to ambulate 5 meters without assistance (grade 2). Another 11 children (22%) reached a nadir of grade 3 (unable to walk 5 meters without assistance). The largest group of children (39%) were bed or wheelchair confined (grade 4), and 7 children (14%) required mechanical ventilatory assistance (grade 5). There were no fatalities. Autonomic dysfunction was present in 14 children (28%) and included labile hypertension in 9 children and urinary or bowel incontinence in 6 children.

The duration of symptoms in children with Guillain-Barré syndrome requiring hospitalization varies in the reported studies. The incidence of admission to pediatric intensive care units for treatment of respiratory failure or other serious medical problems (e.g., infection) or for plasmapheresis ranges between 17% and 68%, with the average length of stay about 11 days [Jansen et al., 1993]. The average duration for mechanical ventilation ranges from 17 to 22 days. The mean duration of hospitalization is also quite variable, ranging from 12 to 84 days [Jansen et al., 1993; Jones, 1996]. Time to independent walking reported in a multicenter study in Western Europe [Korinthenberg and Monting, 1996] was somewhat shorter than in other pediatric series, which reported durations of 43 days [Lamont et al., 1991] or 52 days [Epstein and Sladky, 1990]. The European study was a questionnaire-based survey that included children from community hospitals along with tertiary referral centers, which the authors thought may represent a less severely affected population. In addition, many of these children received therapies, including corticosteroids, intravenous immune globulin, and plasmapheresis.

Autonomic dysfunction has been reported in 12.5% to 25% of children with Guillain-Barré syndrome [Bradshaw and Jones, 1992; Hung et al., 1994] and is similar to that in adults [Ropper, 1994; Zochodne, 1994]. Symptoms are usually intermittent and include postural hypotension, supraventricular tachycardia, bradycardia, and fluctuating blood pressure. Gastrointestinal complaints are numerous and related to impaired swallowing, gastroesophageal dysmotility, pseudo-obstruction, and constipation. Urinary retention also occurs, and the potential need for catheterization and bladder decompression should be considered in children with more severe symptoms during the acute phase of the illness. On rare occasions, cardiac arrest secondary to autonomic dysfunction has been observed in children with Guillain-Barré syndrome [Bos et al., 1987; Briscoe et al., 1987].

Although acute inflammatory demyelinating polyneuropathy is often regarded as an entity in which motor symptoms predominate, pain is a common symptom, occurring in up to 79% of children [Bradshaw and Jones, 1992; Nguyen et al., 1999; Sladky, 2004] and 72% of adult patients [Pentland and Donald, 1994]. Pain is among the initial manifestations of Guillain-Barré syndrome in roughly 60% of children. The types of pain are protean and include paresthesias, dysesthesias, axial and radicular pain, meningismus, myalgia, joint pain, and visceral discomfort. Pain intensity on admission appears to correlate poorly with the degree of initial neurologic disability and is not predictive of prognosis [Moulin et al., 1997]. Patients may also present with or develop pain in a variety of clinical settings, such as the intensive care unit or pediatric ward, or during the more chronic phase of the disease when in rehabilitation or at home. Back and leg pain usually resolves over the first 8 weeks, but dysesthetic extremity pain may persist longer in 5% to 10% of patients despite motor recovery.

Moderate-to-severe pain requires aggressive treatment. In a recent study of adult patients with Guillain-Barré syndrome, 75% required oral opioid analgesics, and 29% received parenteral morphine to provide adequate pain relief [Hahn, 1996]. Despite aggressive therapy, most adults with

TABLE 77-5

Variants of Immune-Mediated Acute and Chronic Demyelinating and Axonal Disorders Seen in Children

GUILLAIN-BARRÉ SYNDROME SUBTYPE	DESCRIPTION	REFERENCES*
Acute inflammatory demyelinating polyneuropathy (AIDP)	Acute onset of ascending weakness and hyporeflexia with elevated CSF protein and EMG showing demyelinating neuropathy; triphasic course usually with good recovery	Hung et al., 1994; Jones, 1996, 2000; Korinthenberg and Monting, 1996
Acute motor and sensory axonal neuropathy (AMSAN)	Acute onset of ascending weakness and hyporeflexia with elevated CSF protein and EMG showing axonal involvement with reduction of CMAP; triphasic course usually with poor or limited recovery	Alma, 1998; Chowdhury, 2001; Currie et al., 1990; Reisin et al., 1993
Acute motor axonal neuropathy (AMAN)	Clinical syndrome similar to AIDP or AMSAN; elevated CSF protein; electrophysiologic and histopathologic evidence of degeneration strictly limited to sensory axons	Griffin et al., 1995; Ho et al., 1995, 1997b; Lu et al., 2000; Paradiso et al., 1999
Miller Fisher syndrome	Acute onset of ophthalmoplegia, hyporeflexia, and ataxia with elevated CSF protein and subsequent recovery	Hughes et al., 1999; Jones, 2000; Sladky, 2004; Willison and O'Hanlon, 1999
Polyneuritis cranialis	Acute onset of multiple cranial nerve palsies (usually bilateral VII and sparing of II) with elevated CSF protein, slowing of motor conduction velocities and recovery	McFarland, 1976; Morosini et al., 2003; Polo et al., 1992
Acute sensory neuropathy	Acute onset of sensory loss, areflexia, elevated CSF protein, slowing of motor conduction velocities and recovery	Sahashi et al., 1985; Seneviratne et al., 2002; Wilmshurst et al., 1999
Acute pandysautonomia	Acute onset of multiple dysautonomic symptoms with limited or no motor involvement, CSF protein elevation, and good recovery	Chistiansen and Brodersen, 2003; Fagius et al., 1983; Low, 1994; Nass and Chutorian, 1982; Zochodne, 1994
Chronic inflammatory demyelinating polyneuropathy	Subacute or indolent onset of weakness and hyporeflexia with elevated CSF protein and EMG showing demyelinating neuropathy; symptoms persist for > 8 weeks and may remain chronic or become progressive	Connolly, 2001; Korinthenberg, 1999; Nevo, 1998; Ryan et al., 2000
Chronic inflammatory relapsing demyelinating polyneuropathy	Acute or subacute onset of weakness and hyporeflexia with elevated CSF protein and EMG showing demyelinating neuropathy; symptoms persist for > 8 weeks and follow a chronic relapsing course	Connolly, 2001; Gorson and Chaudhry, 1999; Hahn, 1998; Hahn et al., 1996a; Hughes, 1994; Nevo, 1998; Ryan et al., 2000; Said, 2002; Sladky et al., 1986
Chronic inflammatory axonal polyneuropathy	Subacute or indolent onset of weakness and hyporeflexia with elevated CSF protein and EMG consistent with an axonal neuropathy; symptoms follow a chronic course; sural nerve biopsy is normal	Chin et al., 2004; Feasby, 1990; Hughes, 1994; Uncini et al., 1991
Guillain-Barré syndrome with encephalopathic features	Acute onset of weakness and hyporeflexia with elevated CSF protein and EMG showing demyelinating neuropathy accompanied by encephalopathic and brainstem symptoms that may have a protracted course	Bradshaw and Jones, 2001; Brashear et al., 1985; Feasby et al., 1990; Gamstorp, 1974; Maier et al., 1997; Nadkarni and Lisak, 1993; Uncini et al., 1991

*References listed are for pediatric case series if available.

CMAP, compound motor unit action potentials; CSF, cerebrospinal fluid; EMG, electromyography;

grade 4 or 5 disease severity reported that their pain was inadequately treated. Few data regarding pain symptoms in children with this syndrome have been published. The principles of pain management for Guillain-Barré syndrome patients have been well described [Moulin et al., 1997; Pentland and Donald, 1994].

Clinical Variants of Guillain-Barré Syndrome

Several clinical forms of Guillain-Barré syndrome have been characterized (Table 77-5). Some of the more clearly defined entities are discussed in this section.

Acute Motor and Sensory Axonal Neuropathy

Whether acute motor and sensory axonal neuropathy is distinct from the more common acute inflammatory demyelinating polyneuropathy or part of a continuum of disease remains a topic for ongoing discussion. The initial clinical presentations in these disorders are virtually identical; however, children and adults with acute motor and sensory axonal neuropathy with a severe extent of axonal degeneration are more likely to have incomplete recovery. The electrophysiologic hallmark of this syndrome is the decrement or absence of sensory and motor action potential amplitudes with only minimal slowing of nerve conduction velocities commensurate with the degree of axonal loss. In most instances, pathologic evaluation of the peripheral nervous system from patients within the spectrum of Guillain-Barré syndrome illnesses reveals evidence of endoneurial inflammation with both primary demyelination and axonal degeneration [Berciano et al., 1993]. Either process can predominate in an individual patient, within a particular peripheral nerve, or in a nerve segment [Berciano et al., 1997]. The mechanism through which the immune system targets specific constituents of the peripheral nervous system remains poorly understood. It is clear that the immune response can be remarkably specific in isolating predominantly myelin-related epitopes, those associated with axolemma, or an admixture of both [Griffin et al., 1996a, 1996b; Hughes et al., 1999]. There have been a number of studies attempting to associate the presence of circulating immunoglobulin directed against specific ganglioside moieties with specific Guillain-Barré syndrome–related entities. For the most part, there has been only limited correlation between the targeted antigens and the syndrome phenotype. The strongest associations have been reported in Miller Fisher syndrome with an immune response to GQ1B [Hughes et al., 1999; Saida, 1996].

Reisin and colleagues [1993, 1996] reported a series of 44 children with an acute axonal form of Guillain-Barré syndrome. These patients initially had severe reduction in the amplitude of compound motor action potentials (<10% of lower limit of normal) and after 2 weeks of illness had diffuse, severe denervation on needle electrode examination. Compared with patients with compound motor action potentials that were greater than 10% of normal, they were more likely to require assisted ventilation (60% versus 6.2%), were more frequently quadriplegic at the peak of their disability (80% versus 18.7%), and required longer periods to improve one functional grade (mean, 63.6 days versus 16.6 days) and to become ambulatory (mean, 156 versus 17.6 days).

Acute Motor Axonal Neuropathy

Although there may have been earlier recognition of this unique form of Guillain-Barré syndrome, the first clear and detailed description of acute motor axonal neuropathy resulted from studies of clustered outbreaks of the disease in rural regions of northern China. The clinical presentation of the disease is similar to that of acute inflammatory demyelinating polyneuropathy or acute motor and sensory axonal neuropathy but is distinguished by the discrete involvement of motor axons with sparing of sensory axons [Lu et al., 2000]. Electrophysiologic hallmarks of the disease are normal sensory nerve conduction studies and diminished compound motor action potential amplitudes, with normal, or nearly so, motor conduction velocities [McKhann et al., 1991]. Diffuse denervation is present during needle electromyography. Histopathologic examination reveals normal-appearing sensory nerves with degeneration of motor axons within motor nerve roots and motor fibers in the peripheral nervous system [Griffin et al., 1995, 1996a, 1996b; Ho et al., 1995, 1997a; Lu et al., 2000; McKhann et al., 1993]. Just as acute inflammatory demyelinating polyneuropathy and acute motor and sensory axonal neuropathy have been found to occur after gastrointestinal infection with *Campylobacter jejuni*, the association in acute motor axonal neuropathy is even stronger. Patients who develop acute motor axonal neuropathy in northern China typically come from rural areas where the ability to purify communal drinking water is often limited or nonexistent. Paradiso and colleagues made similar observations in a series of children with Guillain-Barré syndrome who were treated in Buenas Aires [Paradiso et al., 1999]. The patients with acute motor axonal neuropathy constituted 30% of children with Guillain-Barré syndrome with a high incidence of evidence of prior infection with *C. jejuni*.

Miller Fisher Syndrome

Ophthalmoplegia, ataxia, and areflexia characterize this Guillain-Barré syndrome variant described originally in adults in 1956 [Arakawa et al., 1993; Bradshaw and Jones, 1992; Eggenberger et al., 1993; Jones 2000; Sladky, 2004; Wong, 1997]. The incidence of Miller Fisher syndrome is probably 2% to 4% in children with Guillain-Barré syndrome-like illnesses (see Table 77-5) [Bradshaw and Jones, 1992; Jones 2000; Sladky, 2004]. Cerebrospinal fluid protein elevation is seen in virtually all patients, and in most patients, complete recovery occurs. Brainstem auditory-evoked potentials have demonstrated peripheral and central auditory conduction defects in children [Wong, 1997] Of interest are recent investigations demonstrating antibodies against the ganglioside GQ1b that recognize similar epitopes from specific *C. jejuni* strains [Jacobs et al., 1997a]. Cross-reactivity with the GQ1b ganglioside, which is present in cranial and other peripheral nerves, may in part account for the restricted involvement seen in patients with Miller Fisher syndrome [Willison et al., 1993, 1999]. This is in contrast to the classic form of Guillain-Barré syndrome in which molecular mimicry has been described between anti-GM1 antibodies and *C. jejuni* [Ang et al., 2001; Carpo et al., 1998; Kuroki et al., 2001]. Successful treatment with intravenous immune globulin has been reported in a 3-year-old boy with Miller Fisher syndrome [Arakawa et al., 1993].

Polyneuritis Cranialis

Polyneuritis cranialis can occur in children, and it manifests with the acute onset of multiple cranial nerve palsies (usually bilateral VII and sparing of II) with elevated cerebrospinal fluid protein, slowing of motor conduction velocities, and good recovery [Lyu et al., 2004; Polo et al., 1992, 2002]. Bilateral facial weakness, dysphonia, and dysphagia are typical symptoms. Evidence suggests some association with cytomegalovirus infection. Visser studied 20 cytomegalovirus-associated Guillain-Barré syndrome patients, comparing the findings with earlier established data of *C. jejuni*-related Guillain-Barré syndrome patients, and found that they were significantly younger, initially had a severe course indicated by a high frequency of respiratory insufficiency, and often developed cranial nerve involvement and severe sensory loss [Visser et al., 1996]. This finding was in contrast to patients with *C. jejuni* infection, which was more commonly associated with an acute inflammatory demyelinating polyneuropathy phenotype. Enhancement of multiple cranial nerves seen with postcontrast magnetic resonance imaging (MRI) has also been documented, but clinical symptoms and electrodiagnostic studies reflected abnormalities caused by some, but not all, of the enhancing cranial nerves [Fulbright et al., 1995; Morosini et al., 2003].

Guillain-Barré Syndrome with Central Nervous System Manifestations

Although rare, Guillain-Barré syndrome with central nervous system (CNS) manifestations is reasonably well described in both adults and children [Bradshaw and Jones, 2001; Gamstorp 1974; Maier et al., 1997; Nadkarni and Lisak, 1993; Okumura et al., 2002]; however, the incidence, severity, neuroimaging, and pathologic characterization of Guillain-Barré syndrome immune-mediated or toxic encephalopathy in children remains elusive. Maier and colleagues reported on 13 postmortem examinations of adult patients with Guillain-Barré syndrome whose death ranged from 1 day to 12 months from the onset of neurologic symptoms. CNS pathologic findings were predominantly secondary to injury to spinal nerve roots and cranial nerves. Evidence of primary inflammation was present, especially within the spinal cord, medulla, and pons, with clusters of mononuclear cells around small vessels. Although features of primary demyelination were identified in the peripheral nervous system in 12 of 13 patients, it was not detected in the CNS in any patients. Nadkarni and Lisak [1993] reported a 28-year-old patient with acute Guillain-Barré syndrome who developed bilateral optic neuritis and extensive CNS white matter lesions on MRI. This illness was associated with *Mycoplasma pneumoniae* infection and suggested some degree of overlap with acute disseminated encephalomyelitis. It was hypothesized that certain infections might have a shared epitope that targets both the peripheral nervous system and CNS. The finding of abnormal central conduction using somatosensory evoked potentials in children with Guillain-Barré syndrome and Miller Fisher syndrome supports the possibility that CNS involvement may also occur in children. It is likely that such involvement in young children, particularly if there is severe generalized weakness with or without respiratory failure, may be clinically difficult to detect.

Differential Diagnosis

A variety of other peripheral and occasionally CNS disorders can be confused with Guillain-Barré syndrome. These are outlined in Box 77-3, and the reader is referred to the specific chapters that discuss these conditions.

Clinical Laboratory Evaluation

The diagnosis of Guillain-Barré syndrome is based on clinical features. Confirmatory laboratory studies include cerebrospinal fluid examination, electrophysiologic testing, and occasionally MRI to look for enhancement in spinal roots after contrast administration.

Box 77-3 Differential Diagnosis of Guillain-Barré Syndrome

Cerebral
- Bilateral strokes
- Hysteria

Cerebellar
- Acute cerebellar ataxia syndrome (multiple etiologies)
- Posterior fossa structural lesion

Spinal
- Compressive myelopathy
- Transverse myelitis
- Anterior spinal artery syndrome

Peripheral nerve
- Toxic neuropathy
- Drugs: amitriptyline, dapsone, glutethimide, hydralazine, isoniazid, nitrofurantoin, nitrous oxide, incrusting
- Toxins: acrylamide, glue sniffing, fish toxins, heavy metals (lead, arsenic, mercury, thallium), insecticides, *N*-hexane and other solvents, organophosphates
- Critical illness neuropathy
- Diphtheria
- Tick paralysis
- Porphyria

Neuromuscular Junction
- Botulism
- Myasthenia gravis
- Neuromuscular-blocking agents

Muscle Diseases
- Acute viral myositis
- Acute inflammatory myopathies (polymyositis, dermatomyositis)
- Metabolic myopathies (multiple types)
- Periodic paralysis

Modified from Evans OB. Guillain-Barré syndrome in children. Pediatr Rev 1986;8:69; and Jones HR. Childhood Guillain-Barré syndrome: Clinical presentation, diagnosis, and therapy. J Child Neurol 1996;11:4.

Cerebrospinal Fluid

A characteristic laboratory finding supporting the diagnosis of Guillain-Barré syndrome is albuminocytologic dissociation or a disproportionate elevation of cerebrospinal fluid protein in the absence of significant evidence of inflammation (i.e., >10 mononuclear cells/mm^3 of cerebrospinal fluid) after the first week of symptoms of the disease. The presence of significant cerebrospinal fluid pleocytosis (>50 mononuclear cells/mm^3) or the presence of polymorphonuclear leukocytes in the cerebrospinal fluid should raise doubt about the diagnosis of Guillain-Barré syndrome [Asbury and Cornblath, 1990; Jones 1996]. Elevation of cerebrospinal fluid protein includes both albumin and immunoglobulin moieties. This feature of the illness is due to breakdown of the blood-nerve barrier within the subarachnoid space surrounding spinal nerve roots. Cerebrospinal fluid protein elevation may not be detectable early in the course of Guillain-Barré syndrome in about 20% of children. If sites of inflammation within the course of the peripheral nervous system are distal to the intraspinal roots, protein elevation within cerebrospinal fluid may be minimal. In most reported pediatric series, the increase in cerebrospinal fluid protein has been in the range of 80 to 200 mg/dL (normal being less than 40 mg/dL) [Briscoe et al., 1987; Epstein and Sladky, 1990; Jones, 1996, 2000; Rantala et al., 1991].

Electrophysiologic Testing

The pathologic hallmark of Guillain-Barré syndrome is multifocal, immune-mediated demyelination within spinal roots and peripheral nerves [Asbury et al., 1969]. The electrophysiologic correlate is the presence of multifocal slowing of nerve conduction or conduction block [Alma et al., 1998; Cros et al., 1996; Hadden et al., 1998; Vriesendorp et al., 1995]. In the case of acute inflammatory demyelinating polyneuropathy, the task of the clinical electrophysiologist is to demonstrate electrophysiologic evidence of multifocal demyelination in sensory and motor peripheral nerves indicative of an acquired, inflammatory disorder. This task requires demonstrating asymmetric slowing of nerve conduction along the course of peripheral nerves, disparate conduction velocities among comparable nerve segments, or the presence of conduction block. Asymmetric slowing along the course of a peripheral nerve might be manifest as disproportionate prolongation of the distal motor latency compared with the degree of conduction slowing in a more proximal nerve segment. Alternatively, markedly prolonged F-wave or H-reflex latencies in the face of reasonably normal distal motor latency and nerve conduction velocity in the limb are indicative of slowing of conduction in proximal nerve segments or spinal roots. Conduction block and temporal dispersion of proximally evoked compound motor action potentials are also features of multifocal segmental demyelination in peripheral nerves and are indicative of an acquired inflammatory demyelinating neuropathy. Box 77-2 includes the revised consensus criteria of electrodiagnostic features considered supportive of the diagnosis of Guillain-Barré syndrome [Asbury and Cornblath, 1990]. Application of a form of these criteria in recent studies resulted in 60% of adult patients with Guillain-Barré syndrome fulfilling the criteria for polyneuropathy at the first examination (mean time interval, 6 days since disease onset) [Meulstee and van der Meche, 1995].

Magnetic Resonance Imaging

Because the differential diagnosis includes transverse myelitis, a possibility that is underscored when weakness is confined to the lower extremities and the child is complaining of back pain, spinal MRI studies may occasionally need to be performed as part of the diagnostic evaluation. Several observers have noted marked gadolinium enhancement of the cauda equina and lumbar nerves that is indicative of an inflammatory process confined to dorsal and ventral spinal nerve roots [Baran et al., 1993; Bertorini et al., 1995; Crino et al., 1994].

Conspicuous nerve root enhancement in some studies appeared to correlate with pain, Guillain-Barré syndrome disability grade, and duration of recovery [Gorson et al., 1996]. Nerve root enhancement was also 83% sensitive in the diagnosis of acute Guillain-Barré syndrome and was present in 95% of typical cases; it is potentially useful in patients in whom the electrophysiologic abnormalities are equivocal.

Pathologic Findings

The pathologic findings of Guillain-Barré syndrome are confined predominantly to spinal nerve roots and peripheral nerves [Asbury et al., 1969]. The pathogenesis of the disorder is immune orchestrated with macrophage-mediated demyelination of sensory and motor axons within the peripheral nervous system [Hafer-Macko et al., 1996b; Hartung et al., 1996; Hughes et al., 1999]. There is also evidence that epitopes expressed on axolemma may also be a target for immune attack and result in concomitant axonal degeneration that commonly accompanies the demyelinating process [Hafer-Macko et al., 1996b; Hartung et al., 1999; Hughes et al., 1999]. It is likely that both myelin–Schwann cell and axonal surface epitopes are immunologically targeted to variable degrees during the active phase of Guillain-Barré syndrome, resulting in the spectrum of clinical manifestations of the disease. The typical pathogenic mechanism in Guillain-Barré syndrome involves macrophages insinuating themselves under the myelin sheath at the node of Ranvier or between myelin lamellae and stripping myelin from the underlying axon [Hafer-Macko et al., 1996b; Hartung et al., 1996, 2002; Hughes et al., 1992, 1999; Kiefer et al., 2001; Steck et al., 1998]. Documenting the early events in the immune-mediated attack on the peripheral nervous system is, for obvious reasons, difficult in humans. The early pathologic changes have been characterized in a laboratory model, experimental allergic neuritis, a nearly homologous disorder to Guillain-Barré syndrome. Experimental allergic neuritis can be induced in laboratory rodents immunized with constituents of peripheral nerve myelin or with transfer of activated T cells from animals with the disease (Fig. 77-1) [Rostami, 1997]. A different pattern of injury has been described (Fig. 77-2) in acute motor axonal neuropathy related to *Campylobacter* species infection. In these patients, macrophages have again been found to interrupt axoglial tight junctions at nodes of Ranvier and attack and

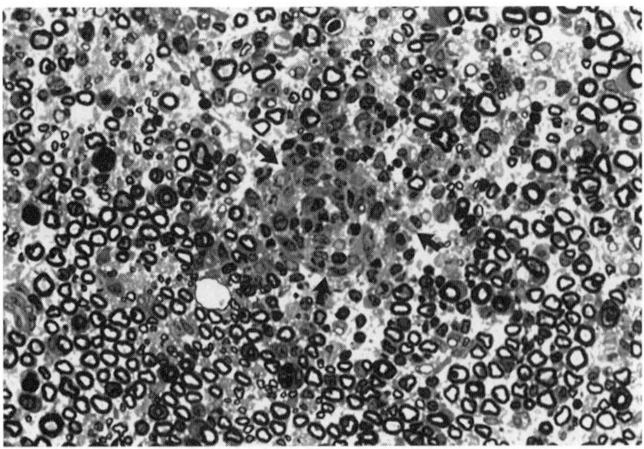

FIGURE 77-1. Cross-section through a sciatic nerve from a Lewis rat during the acute phase of experimental allergic neuritis. There is a large collection of mononuclear cells within the endoneurium during this acute phase of the illness (bounded by *arrows*) (×250). (Courtesy of John Sladky, MD.)

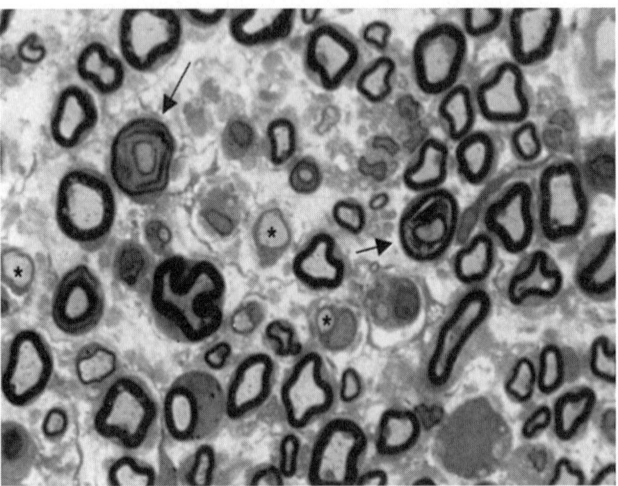

FIGURE 77-2. Cross-section through a sciatic nerve from a Lewis rat during the acute phase of experimental allergic neuritis. Note that there are several demyelinated axons (some indicated with *asterisks*) and thinly myelinated axons in the early stages of remyelination. Large-caliber myelinated axons demonstrating splitting and fragmentation of myelin lamellae in the early stage of macrophage-mediated demyelination are present *(arrows)* (×650). (Courtesy of John Sladky, MD.)

destroy the motor axon, sparing the circumferential myelin, which then secondarily breaks down [Griffin et al., 1995, 1996a, 1996b; Hafer-Macko et al., 1996a; McKhann et al., 1993]. This process results in a relatively pure motor syndrome without evidence of primary demyelination on histopathologic examination or electrophysiologic testing [Griffin et al., 1995, 1996a, 1996b; Hafer-Macko et al., 1996a; McKhann et al., 1993].

The sequence of events that engenders autoimmune neuromuscular disorders such as Guillain-Barré syndrome is incompletely understood. Dalakas [1995] emphasized that several sequential steps are required to orchestrate autoimmune-mediated tissue injury. The first is breaking of tolerance in which molecular mimicry, cytokine stimulation, or superantigens, individually or in concert, activate T cells to recognize autoantigens. The second requires antigen recognition by T-cell receptors and antigen processing through the class I or II major histocompatibility complexes. This second step is modulated by costimulatory factors, such as B7 and B7-binding proteins, and intercellular adhesion molecule-1. The activated T cells must then gain access to their targeted autoantigens. In the peripheral nervous system, they must traverse the blood-nerve barrier, usually through a pathway of adhesion molecules including selectins and leukocyte integrins and their counter-receptors on endoneurial vascular endothelial cells. Finally, activated T cells and autoantibodies enter the endoneurium along with macrophages and bind targeted epitopes on Schwann cells, axons, or both, resulting in tissue injury and phagocytosis [Dalakas, 1995, 1999a, 1999b; Hartung et al., 2001, 2002; Hughes et al., 1999]. The presence of proinflammatory and anti-inflammatory cytokines acts to modulate the intensity of the autoimmune attack on endoneurial contents.

Nerve fibers in peripheral nerves are relatively protected from systemic immune responses and inflammatory reactions by the specialized endoneurial, endothelial, and perineural barriers [Dalakas, 1995; Hartung et al., 2001, 2002; Hughes et al., 1999]. Compared with peripheral nerve trunks, there are more macrophage-like cells and more permeable blood vessels in the dorsal root ganglia and spinal roots that are preferred sites for the inflammatory response in experimental allergic neuritis. As noted earlier, experimental allergic neuritis can be induced by immunization with either myelin proteins or fragments of the proteins. P0 and P2 proteins have been most consistently used to induce this Guillain-Barré syndrome model; a similar but less inflammatory, more chronic demyelinating neuropathy can be induced in rabbits with the glycolipid galactocerebroside [Harvey et al., 1987]. In myelin protein–induced experimental allergic neuritis, $CD4^+$ helper T-cell responses are sufficient to transfer full-blown disease, but antibodies of undefined specificity may also play a part. In rabbit galactocerebroside neuritis, antibodies are probably more important and are directed predominantly against a haptenic group including galactose. A small proportion of patients with Guillain-Barré syndrome and chronic immune demyelinating polyneuropathy show T-cell responses to P0 or P2, which may mark important pathogenetic reactions. In addition, some patients with Guillain-Barré syndrome and chronic immune demyelinating polyneuropathy have antibodies to gangliosides, including for instance the most abundant peripheral nerve ganglioside, GM1, which may also be important. In particular, patients with acute severe Guillain-Barré syndrome and marked axonal degeneration often have immunoglobin G antibodies to GM1 and GD1b, whereas patients with Miller Fisher syndrome are characterized by antibodies to GQ1b. Autoimmune responses to neural antigens have become useful diagnostically in some diseases and probably indicate important pathogenetic mechanisms. In inflammatory demyelinating neuropathy, macrophage-mediated demyelination is probably targeted by both antibody and T-cell-mediated autoimmune responses. The nature of the autoantigen and the relative importance of T-versus B-cell responses are likely to vary depending on the nature of the initial immunologic stimulus.

Antecedent events associated with the subsequent development of Guillain-Barré syndrome have been infection, immunization, drugs [Awong et al., 1996], trauma, or parturition. It is likely that many of the reported associations

TABLE 77-6

Infectious Agents Associated with Guillain-Barré Syndrome

INFECTIOUS AGENT	REFERENCES
Borrelia burgdorferi	Bouma et al., 1989; Horneff et al., 1993; Lopez de Munain et al., 1990; Mancardi et al., 1989; Shapiro, 1998
Brucellosis	Al-Eissa et al., 1996; Berciano et al., 2003; Garcia et al., 1989; Namiduru et al., 2003
Campylobacter species	Griffin et al., 1993; Hadden and Gregson, 2001; Hughes, 2004; Rees et al., 1995b
Cytomegalovirus	Jacobs et al., 1997c, 1998; Yuki, 2001
Epstein-Barr virus	Hadden et al., 2001; Hughes et al., 1999; Jacobs et al., 1998
Enteroviral infections	Alexander et al., 1994; McMinn et al., 2001; Mori et al., 2000; Usui et al., 1974
Hantavirus	Esselink et al., 1994; Rabaud et al., 1995
Hepatitis virus	Murthy, 1994; Ono et al., 1994; Tabor, 1987; Tsukada et al., 1987
Herpes virus	Dowling and Cook, 1981; Jacobs et al., 1997c; Merelli et al., 1992; Ormerod and Cockerell, 1993
Measles	Coe, 1989; Lidin-Janson et al., 1972; Murthy, 1994; Phillips, 1972
Mumps	Duncan et al., 1990; Ghosh, 1967; Murthy, 1994
Mycoplasma	Ang et al., 2002; Jacobs et al., 1998; Kusunoki et al., 2001; Meseguer et al., 1998
Rocky Mountain spotted fever	Toerner et al., 1996
Typhoid fever	Aldrey et al., 1999; Berger et al., 1986; Chanmugam and Waniganetti, 1969; Donoso, 1988; Ozen et al., 1993

are purely coincidental. The relations between several common infections and immunizations and Guillain-Barré syndrome that seem relatively solid are summarized in Table 77-6. Some of the more well-established infections include cytomegalovirus [Jacobs et al., 1997c], Epstein-Barr virus [Grose et al., 1972; Jacobs et al., 1998] and other herpes viruses [Dowling et al., 1981], hepatitis [Tabor, 1987], and *Mycoplasma* species infections [Susuki et al., 2004; Thomas et al., 1993]. Of the acute viral infections that have been implicated as possible antecedent events, only cytomegalovirus and Epstein-Barr virus have been found, using serologic markers, to be statistically related to subsequent Guillain-Barré syndrome illnesses [Jacobs et al., 1998; Winer et al., 1988]. The subgroups of Guillain-Barré syndrome—acute inflammatory demyelinating polyneuropathy, acute motor and sensory axonal neuropathy, and acute motor axonal neuropathy—have all been associated with antecedent or coincident systemic infection with *Campylobacter* species [Hadden and Gregson, 2001; Hughes, 2004; Jacobs et al., 1997b; McCarthy et al., 2001; Melendez-Vasquez et al., 1997; Rees et al., 1995a; Toyka, 1999]. Controversy exists concerning the oral polio vaccine and its relation to Guillain-Barré syndrome. In 1993, the Institute of Medicine found that the evidence favored acceptance of a causal relationship between oral polio vaccine and Guillain-Barré syndrome [Ismail et al., 1998; Stratton et al., 1994], although other epidemiologic studies have found no such correlation [Rantala et al., 1994]. This issue is discussed further in Chapter 91.

Treatment

Immunomodulating strategies for the treatment of Guillain-Barré syndrome can include agents to interrupt the autoimmune process at several stages from T-cell activation to macrophage-mediated tissue injury [Hahn, 1997; Hughes et al., 1999; Saida, 1996]. There is reasonable evidence that it is possible to blunt the severity of tissue injury by interfering with the autoimmune process at multiple levels, including interventions that (1) block or interfere with antigen recognition or T-cell activation, (2) blunt costimulatory pathways and cytokine activity, (3) impair access of activated cells and autoantibodies to target tissues, (4) selectively eliminate activated lymphocyte subpopulations through cytotoxic T-cell receptor ligands, (5) interrupt macrophage targeting or lysosomal activity at antigen recognition sites in the endoneurium, and (6) interfere with effector proteases that mediate cytoskeletal injury [Deretzi et al., 1999; Gabriel et al., 1997; Hartung et al., 2000; Hughes et al., 1998; Jung et al., 1995; Kiefer et al., 2001; Laura et al., 2002; Redford et al., 1997; Stoll, 2002; Yu et al., 2002; Zou et al., 1999, 2000, 2002].

The mechanisms by which plasmapheresis and intravenous immune globulin administration act in Guillain-Barré syndrome or chronic inflammatory demyelinating polyneuropathy are not entirely understood. It is likely that the primary effect of plasmapheresis is to remove circulating antibody directed toward peripheral nerve antigens. The predominant effect of intravenous immune globulin is speculative. High-dose intravenous immune globulin administration may act by binding anti-idiotypic antibodies, absorbing complement, or down-regulating B-cell–mediated antibody production. Other actions that may also play a role include blockade of activated receptors, enhancement of suppressor cell activity, and interference with lymphocyte proliferation (Thornton and Griggs, 1994). Both of these therapies also down-regulate production of proinflammatory cytokines, which play an important role in enhancing the severity of the immune-mediated injury [Aarli, 2003; Creange et al., 1996; Jander et al., 2001; Lisak et al., 1997; Sharief et al., 1999; Stoll, 2002].

There are no definitive, prospectively derived data to indicate that treatment of children with Guillain-Barré syndrome with plasmapheresis or intravenous immune globulin is efficacious. Nevertheless, several limited studies indicate that both treatments may be effective for this disorder [Abd-Allah et al., 1997; Baskin et al., 1996; Epstein and Sladky, 1990; Gurses et al., 1995; Jansen et al., 1993; Kanra et al., 1997; Khatri et al., 1990; Lamont et al., 1991; McKhann, 1990; Shahar and Leiderman, 2003; Singhi et al., 1999; Sladky, 2004; Vajsar et al., 1994]. Evidence in large prospective trials of plasmapheresis and intravenous immune globulin involving predominantly adults has confirmed that both treatment modalities reduce morbidity associated with Guillain-Barré syndrome and that they are comparable in efficacy [French Cooperative Group on Plasma

Exchange in Guillain-Barré Syndrome, 1987; Plasma Exchange/Sandoglobulin Guillain-Barré Syndrome Trial Group, 1997]. Both modalities appear to reduce the duration of the disease and improve the neurologic outcome [Plasma Exchange/Sandoglobulin Guillain-Barré Syndrome Trial Group, 1997]. In addition, the Guillain-Barré Syndrome Study Group documented that treatment with high-dose intravenous corticosteroids was not only ineffective but also likely to be harmful in adults with Guillain-Barré syndrome [Guillain-Barré Syndrome Steroid Trial Group, 1993]. In a subsequent study by these same investigators, plasmapheresis and intravenous immune globulin were found to be comparable in efficacy, and these two treatments in combination were not superior to either treatment alone in adults with Guillain-Barré syndrome [Plasma Exchange/Sandoglobulin Guillain-Barré Syndrome Trial Group, 1997)]. Subsequent studies have examined the benefit of performing two, four, or six plasmaphereses in patients with varying degrees of severity of Guillain-Barré syndrome [French Cooperative Group on Plasma Exchange in Guillain-Barré Syndrome, 1987]. The conclusions of this study recommended that patients with mild Guillain-Barré syndrome on admission receive two cycles of plasmapheresis, whereas patients with moderate or severe forms would benefit from two additional exchanges. More than four exchanges did not enhance the pace or completeness of recovery.

Plasmapheresis

Available data on treatment of children with Guillain-Barré syndrome are derived from small, nonrandomized series using, for the most part, historical controls (Table 77-7). One of these studies looking at treatment and control groups that were reasonably well matched in terms of demographic characteristics and disease severity indicated that plasmapheresis significantly shortened the time required for nonambulatory patients to regain independent ambulation from 60 to 24 days [Epstein and Sladky, 1990]. This observation has been confirmed by other studies in at least 50 pediatric patients [Jansen et al., 1993; Khatri et al., 1990; Lamont et al., 1991]. In adult studies, plasmapheresis was particularly effective when started within 7 days of the onset of symptoms. Similar observations have been noted in several of the studies of children with severe Guillain-Barré syndrome [Jansen et al., 1993]. Rantala and colleagues [1995] have suggested that certain factors increase the risk for respiratory failure in children with Guillain-Barré syndrome and that, if present, early treatment with plasmapheresis or intravenous immune globulin is warranted. In this study, signs and symptoms predictive of respiratory failure included (1) onset of symptoms of Guillain-Barré syndrome within 8 days after a preceding infection, (2) presence of cranial nerve involvement, and (3) cerebrospinal fluid protein level greater than 800 mg/L during the first week of illness [Rantala et al., 1995].

Plasmapheresis appears to be safe in children but is limited to some degree by size constraints of the patient and the availability of a technically trained staff and appropriately sized equipment. Children as young as 8 months of age have been treated [Delgado, 1996], and the reported morbidity associated with plasmapheresis in children is minimal [Epstein and Sladky, 1990; Jansen et al., 1993]. Potential

TABLE 77-7

Results of Treatment with Plasmapheresis or Intravenous Immune Globulin in Children with Guillain-Barré Syndrome*

REFERENCE	NO. OF PATIENTS IMPROVED/ TREATED	TIME TO WALKING: TREATMENT GROUP (DAYS)	TIME TO WALKING: CONTROL GROUP (DAYS)	OTHER COMMENTS
Plasmapheresis				
Niparko et al., 1989	Not stated/15	NA	NA	All patients were in ICU with ventilatory assistance
Epstein and Sladky, 1990	9/9	24	60	14 control GBS patients
Khatri et al., 1990	10/11	NA	NA	At 6 months, 9 of 11 were normal
Lamont et al., 1991	5/6	17	43	18 control GBS patients
Jansen et al., 1993	8/8	NA	NA	Lower GBS scores in treatment group
Hernandez Gonzalez et al., 1993	3/5	NA	NA	Cardiac arrest in 1 patient
Hammersjö, 1995	0/11	—	—	—
Intravenous Immune Globulin				
Shahar et al., 1997	25/26	NA	NA	20 patients able to walk within 1 week of IVIG
Reisin et al., 1996	0/13	NA	NA	Not improved, particularly those with low CMAP
Vallee et al., 1993	12/13	12	51	8 control GBS patients
Vajsar et al., 1994	9/10	NA	NA	Time to improve 2 GBS scores was 17 days in IVIG group and 48 days in plasmapheresis group
Goodhew et al., 1996 Abd-Allah et al., 1997	7/7	NA	NA	IVIG treatment similar to plasmapheresis
Kanra et al., 1997	Not stated/75	NA	NA	Mean time to improve 1 clinical grade 20.8 days in IVIG group, 64.2 days in controls

*Only reports with at least five pediatric patients are included in this table.
CMAP, compound motor unit action potential; GBS, Guillain-Barré syndrome; ICU, intensive care unit; IVIG, intravenous gamma globulin; NA, not available.

complications include hemorrhage, hypotension, transfusion reactions, transmitted infections, septicemia, hypocalcemia, arrhythmias, cardiac arrest, and local tissue injury. There have been no reported deaths caused by plasmapheresis in children.

Intravenous Immunoglobulin

Similar results have also been reported in trials of intravenous immune globulin in children with Guillain-Barré syndrome [Abd-Allah et al., 1997; al-Qudah, 1994; Kanra et al., 1997; Reisin et al., 1996; Shahar et al., 1997] and are summarized in Table 77-7. Shahar and colleagues, in an open prospective multicenter study of 26 children with severe Guillain-Barré syndrome, concluded that intravenous immune globulin was effective and safe in severe childhood-onset disease and considered it the initial treatment of choice [Shahar et al., 1997]. They administered a total dose of 2 g/kg on 2 consecutive days and found marked and rapid improvement in 25 children (improvement by 1 to 2 disability grade scales within 2 weeks of treatment). Twenty were able to walk independently by 1 week, and one could be weaned off ventilatory support. Eighteen children recovered by 2 weeks. The rest recuperated in 4 months, including a child who was artificially ventilated for 4 weeks. Abd-Allah and colleagues compared a group of seven children treated with intravenous immune globulin with another cohort of eight children treated with plasmapheresis and found that intravenous immune globulin was equally effective [Abd-Allah et al., 1997]. They reviewed data on 74 previously treated pediatric patients and also concluded that intravenous immune globulin should be considered the initial choice of treatment.

Critical Care Management

Despite the dramatic therapeutic advances made during the past two decades, Guillain-Barré syndrome remains a serious disorder that requires careful management, particularly for patients who develop respiratory failure or lose the ability to swallow and maintain nutrition. The mortality rate for adults with Guillain-Barré syndrome remains at 5% to 8% [Hahn, 1996]. Within industrialized countries, the mortality from Guillain-Barré syndrome in children is virtually zero. For reasons incompletely understood, the mortality in countries with more limited resources remains in the range of 10% [Molinero et al., 2003]. Several articles, predominantly focusing on adult patients with Guillain-Barré syndrome, have reviewed selected aspects of care in the critical-care setting [Fulgham and Wijdicks, 1997; Hahn, 1996; Henderson et al., 2003; Hughes, 1992, 1998; Hughes et al., 2003b; Kieseier et al., 2004; Ng et al., 1995; Ropper, 1994; Zochodne et al., 1996].

By definition, children with Guillain-Barré syndrome who require intensive care unit care admission are the most severely affected. In addition to paralysis and respiratory failure, which is the usual reason for admission to the intensive care unit, attendant concerns include secondary infection, gastrointestinal dysfunction, urinary obstruction, and the risk for pulmonary embolism. Other dysautonomic symptoms, including hypertension and hypotension, volume loss caused by excessive perspiration, and cardiac dysrhythmias, may also complicate the course [Ropper, 1994; Zochodne, 1994]. Additional care must be taken with children concerning their fragile nutrition and hydration status. Intravenous hyperalimentation frequently is required, and occasionally, in long-term severely compromised patients, percutaneous gastrostomy is necessary. Many of these severely affected children also have marked dysesthetic symptoms, and adequate pain control is essential. Attention to the stress of illness on the family and awareness of the problems attendant with the loss of verbal and nonverbal forms of communication, particularly in children, are critical in the successful management of these patients [Khatri and Pearlstein, 1997; Manners and Murray, 1992; McDouall and Tasker, 2004; Mikati and DeLong, 1985; Moulin et al., 1997; Nguyen et al., 1999; Pentland and Donald, 1994; Roca et al., 1998; Ropper and Shahani, 1984]. In Guillain-Barré syndrome, as in other acute debilitating disorders, the early implementation of a comprehensive rehabilitation program, preferably within the intensive care unit for severely affected patients, will prevent many secondary complications of the disease.

Prognosis

Most series indicate that the prognosis for children who develop Guillain-Barré syndrome is generally excellent and probably better than that for older age groups [Briscoe et al., 1987; Cole and Matthew, 1987; Kleyweg et al., 1989; Korinthenberg and Monting 1996; Ortiz Corredor et al., 2003; Rantala et al., 1991; Sladky, 2004; Vajsar et al., 2003]. Opinion in the literature is not unanimous, and dissenting viewpoints argue that the clinical course and prognosis are similar in children and adults [Kleyweg et al., 1989]. In the group of 49 children listed in Table 77-3, 80% achieved complete functional recovery within 6 months of the onset of illness. About 20% had mild residual neurologic deficits, including mild weakness in the facial or lower extremity muscles and decreased deep tendon reflexes [Barbara Martin, M.D., personal communication]. Similar findings, as reviewed earlier in this chapter, were reported from a retrospective international multicenter study of 175 children with Guillain-Barré syndrome [Korinthenberg and Monting 1996].

A limitation in our ability to draw definitive conclusions regarding the prognosis of Guillain-Barré syndrome in children is the absence of prospectively defined, systematically collected clinical data. The numbers of children included in individual published studies are small, which contributes to the variable fashion in which these limited observations are interpreted. The consensus in the literature is that children will do at least as well if not better than older patients with Guillain-Barré syndrome [Jones, 2000; Korinthenberg and Monting, 1996; Sladky, 2004]. This opinion is reinforced by several nonprospective studies looking at treatment in which children recover faster after plasmapheresis or intravenous immune globulin administration than published recovery rates in adults [Epstein and Sladky, 1990; Jansen et al., 1993; Jones 2000; Korinthenberg and Monting 1996; Lamont et al., 1991; Reisin et al., 1996; Sladky, 2004]. These studies are not directly comparable and need to be interpreted with caution; however, there is emerging consensus that prognosis in childhood

Box 77-4 Research Criteria for the Diagnosis of Chronic Inflammatory Demyelinating Polyneuropathy

I. Clinical
  A. Mandatory—progressive or relapsing motor and sensory, rarely only motor or sensory, dysfunction of more than one limb of a peripheral nerve nature, developing over at least 2 months
  B. Supportive—large-fiber sensory loss predominates over small-fiber sensory loss
  C. Exclusion
    1. Mutilation of hands or feet, retinitis pigmentosa, ichthyosis, appropriate history of drug or toxic exposure known to cause a similar peripheral neuropathy, or family history of a genetically based peripheral neuropathy
    2. Sensory level
    3. Unequivocal sphincter disturbance

II. Physiologic studies
  A. Mandatory—nerve conduction studies including studies of proximal nerve segments in which the predominant process is demyelination; must have three of the following four:
    1. Reduction in CV in two or more motor nerves:
      a. <80% of LLN if amplitude >80% of LLN
      b. <70% of LLN if amplitude <80% of LLN
    2. Partial conduction block or abnormal temporal dispersion in one or more motor nerves (either peroneal nerve between ankle and below fibular head, median nerve between wrist and elbow, or ulnar nerve between wrist and below elbow)
      a. Criteria suggestive of partial conduction block: <15% change in duration between proximal and distal sites and >20% drop in -p area or p-p amplitude between proximal and distal sites
      b. Criteria for abnormal temporal dispersion and possible conduction block: >15% change in duration between proximal and distal sites and >20% drop in –p area or p-p amplitude between proximal and distal sites

These criteria are only suggestive of partial conduction block because they are derived from studies of normal individuals. Additional studies, such as stimulation across short segments or recording of individual motor unit potentials, are required for confirmation.

    3. Prolonged distal latencies in two or more nerves:
      a. >125% of ULN if amplitude >80% of LLN
      b. >150% of ULN if amplitude <80% of LLN
    4. Absent F waves or prolonged minimum F-wave latencies (10 to 15 trials) in two or more motor nerves:
      a. >120% of ULN if amplitude >80% of LLN
      b. >150% of ULN if amplitude <80% of LLN
  B. Supportive
    1. Reduction in sensory CV <80% of LLN
    2. Absent H reflexes

I. Pathologic features
  A. Mandatory—nerve biopsy demonstrating unequivocal evidence of demyelination and remyelination
    1. Demyelination by either electron microscopy (>5 fibers) or teased fiber studies (>12% of 50 teased fibers, minimum of four internodes each, demonstrating demyelination/remyelination)
  B. Supportive
    1. Subperineurial or endoneurial edema
    2. Mononuclear cell infiltration
    3. Onion bulb formation
    4. Prominent variation in the degree of demyelination between fascicles
  C. Exclusion
    1. Vasculitis, neurofilamentous swollen axons, amyloid deposits, or intracytoplasmic inclusions in Schwann cells or macrophages indicating adrenoleukodystrophy, metachromatic leukodystrophy, globoid cell leukodystrophy, or other evidence of specific pathologic conditions

IV. Cerebrospinal fluid studies
  A. Mandatory
    1. Cell count $<10/mm^3$ if HIV seronegative or $<50/mm^3$ if seropositive
    2. Negative VDRL

IV. Diagnostic categories for research purposes
  A. Definite: clinical A and C, physiology A, pathology A and C, and cerebrospinal fluid A
  B. Probable: clinical A and C, physiology A, and cerebrospinal fluid A
  C. Possible: Clinical A and C, and physiology A

VI. Laboratory studies—depending on the results of the laboratory tests, those patients meeting the aforementioned criteria are classified into the groups listed below. The following studies are suggested: complete blood count, erythrocyte sedimentation rate, Sequential Multiple Analyzer–6/12, creatine kinase, antinuclear antibodies, thyroid function, serum and urine immunoglobulin studies (to include either immunofixation electrophoresis or immunoelectrophoresis), and HIV and hepatitis serology. The list of laboratory studies is not comprehensive. For instance, in certain clinical circumstances, other studies may be indicated, such as phytanic acid, long-chain fatty acids, porphyrins, urine heavy metals, α-lipoprotein, β-lipoprotein, glucose tolerance test, imaging studies of the central nervous system, and lymph node or bone marrow biopsy.
  A. Idiopathic CIDP—no concurrent disease
  B. Concurrent diseases with CIDP (depending on laboratory studies or other clinical features):
    1. Systemic lupus erythematosus
    2. HIV infection

Box 77-4 Research Criteria for the Diagnosis of Chronic Inflammatory Demyelinating Polyneuropathy cont'd

3. Monoclonal or biclonal gammopathy (macroglobulinemia, POEMS [polyneuropathy, organomegaly, endocrinopathy, M protein, skin changes] syndrome, osteosclerotic myeloma)
4. Castleman's disease
5. Monoclonal gammopathies of undetermined significance
6. Diabetes
7. Central nervous system demyelinating disease

CV, conduction velocity; HIV, human immunodeficiency virus; LLN, lower limit of normal; –p, negative peak; p-p, peak-to-peak; ULN, upper limit of normal.

From the Ad Hoc Subcommittee of the American Academy of Neurology AIDS Task Force. Research criteria for the diagnosis of chronic inflammatory demyelinating polyneuropathy (CIDP). Neurology 1991;41:617.

Guillain-Barré syndrome is good and may be enhanced with developing treatment modalities.

CHRONIC INFLAMMATORY DEMYELINATING POLYNEUROPATHY

Chronic inflammatory demyelinating polyneuropathy is an immune-mediated polyneuropathy of more than 2 months' duration. Criteria for the diagnosis of this condition were developed in 1991 by an ad hoc subcommittee of the American Academy of Neurology and are listed in Box 77-4. These criteria were developed for research purposes and may be somewhat restrictive for general clinical practice. They provide, however, helpful benchmarks for evaluating patients with suspected chronic inflammatory demyelinating polyneuropathy. Chronic progressive and relapsing subtypes have been described.

Epidemiology

The true incidence of this disorder in children is unknown and probably unlikely to come to light. Although it represents the most common acquired, potentially treatable chronic neuropathy in childhood, it is nonetheless rare. Ascertaining the incidence of this disease in the pediatric population is further complicated by its propensity for mimicking genetically determined neuropathies, except that the often anticipated history of dominant transmission in the kinship is lacking. Because many children affected with this disorder respond well to immunosuppressive therapy, it is critical to consider this disease in the differential diagnosis of any child with chronic neuropathy, particularly when there are features of demyelination and when evidence for a hereditary pattern cannot be elicited [Connolly, 2001; Korinthenberg, 1999; McLeod et al., 1999; Nevo, 1998; Rodriguez-Casero et al., 2003; Ryan et al., 2000; Sladky, 1996].

Clinical Features

The clinical features of chronic inflammatory demyelinating polyneuropathy are protean, and diagnosis can be difficult. It can present as an indolently progressive, predominantly motor neuropathy and closely resemble hereditary motor and sensory neuropathy type I, including several genotypic variants [Carter et al., 2004]. Active demyelination may be confined to proximal nerve segments, and electrophysiologic testing may be most compatible with an axonal neuropathy, with the disease masquerading as hereditary motor and sensory neuropathy type II. It has been reported to present in infancy with extremely slow nerve conduction velocity measurements resembling hereditary motor and sensory neuropathy type III disease [Sladky, 1996]. It may also present with features of sensory ataxia and can mimic Friedreich's ataxia. Alternatively, the clinical manifestations may include any combination of these presentations. In some children, the disease presentation is more typical, with the distinct onset of neuropathic symptoms in a previously healthy child, a negative family history with normal examination of both parents, and confirmatory laboratory studies. This scenario is usually the exception, and the likelihood of diagnosing children with more subtle presentations of chronic inflammatory demyelinating polyneuropathy is directly related to the persistence and expertise of the neurologist evaluating such patients. In summary, the disease may present in any age group, the rate of progression may be subacute to indolent, and it may affect selective populations of peripheral nerve axons and interrupt function of any organ system that relies on peripheral nerve function for feedback or regulatory input.

There have been several series reporting the clinical, electrophysiologic, histopathologic, and prognostic features in children with chronic inflammatory demyelinating polyneuropathy [Connolly, 2001; Hattori et al., 1998; Korinthenberg, 1999; Nevo et al., 1996; Simmons et al., 1997a, 1997b; Sladky, 1996]. As one might predict, there are divergent observations among individual reports, presumably as a consequence of relatively small numbers in each series. Looking at the papers in aggregate, several common themes emerge. First, like adults with chronic inflammatory demyelinating polyneuropathy, the clinical course and response to treatment are variable. Similarly, children may present with a subacute course or a more subtle indolent progression of symptoms. Lower extremity weakness is the most common presenting complaint, whereas sensory symptoms are relatively uncommon. Areflexia is the rule. Second, the pace of progression of the initial symptoms may be subacute, over 2 to 3 months, or may exhibit a more protracted course. On some occasions, the initial temporal progression of the disease may be so indolent as to mimic genetically determined neuropathies. Those with a more rapid pace of onset of their chronic inflammatory demyelinating polyneuropathy may have a better likelihood of responding to treatment and a more benign outcome. Third, electrophysiologic testing is a useful diagnostic tool and will, in most cases, confirm the acquired nature of the neuropathy. These tests, however, have only limited predictive value regarding prognosis. Fourth, chronic inflammatory demyelinating polyneuropathy is an eminently treatable disease in children. Therapeutic outcomes fall roughly into three categories. Most children initially improve in response to treatment with corticosteroids. About half the children with chronic inflammatory demyelinating polyneuropathy have a monophasic course and are able to be weaned from steroids, albeit, in many cases, over a protracted period of time. The balance become refractory to steroid treatment and require alternative immunosuppressants or suffer one or more relapses. Most of this group will respond to immunosuppressant therapies, and many achieve remission. A small fraction of children with chronic inflammatory demyelinating polyneuropathy may become refractory to aggressive immunotherapy and become dependent on chronic immunosuppression or sustain severe, widespread peripheral nerve injury with substantial residual neurologic disability. Like the situation in Guillain-Barré syndrome, the prognosis for children with chronic inflammatory demyelinating polyneuropathy is more favorable than among adults.

Laboratory Evaluation

Although there are persuasive arguments to the contrary, it is sometimes useful to look at Guillain-Barré syndrome and chronic inflammatory demyelinating polyneuropathy as different ends of the spectrum of the same disease. In that context, the similarities between the disorders are more striking than the differences. Like the children with the more fulminant Guillain-Barré syndrome, children with chronic inflammatory demyelinating polyneuropathy may evidence pathognomonic features of multifocal demyelination on electrophysiologic testing. These features have been reviewed extensively [Albers et al., 1989; Connolly 2001; Hattori et al., 1998; McCombe et al., 1987; Simmons et al., 1997b].

Sensory and motor nerve conduction studies are the most useful and practical way to assess the physiologic properties of saltatory conduction in large-caliber myelinated fibers. Such data may be useful in distinguishing inherited from acquired disorders. However, none of the electrophysiologic measures are, in themselves, absolute discriminators. Excluding those rare kinships with steroid-responsive inherited demyelinating neuropathy [Bird et al., 1991; Dyck et al., 1982c], some children with typical hereditary motor and sensory neuropathy type I may demonstrate dispersion of proximal evoked compound motor action potentials and conduction block. Conversely, some children with chronic inflammatory demyelinating polyneuropathy may have electrophysiologic characteristics that suggest a genetically determined disease. When the clinical history is suggestive of an acquired disorder and electrophysiologic testing is compatible with an axonal neuropathy, cerebrospinal fluid examination may be helpful in demonstrating an elevated protein concentration typical of demyelinating neuropathies. Measurement of circulating antibodies to myelin protein constituents is rarely useful in children. Contrast-enhanced MRI may indicate blood-nerve barrier breakdown caused by spinal nerve root inflammation [Bertorini et al., 1995; Crino et al., 1993; Kuwabara et al., 1997]. Nerve biopsy may be necessary to assist in discriminating acquired from sporadic or recessively transmitted genetic disorders [Gabreels-Festen et al., 1993]. Because de novo mutations can result in the appearance of a sporadic disorder, testing for an abnormality in the more common gene mutations associated with hereditary motor and sensory neuropathy type I phenotype may establish a diagnosis and define implications for prognosis and genetic counseling. Finally, when the clinical and laboratory data remain inconclusive, including clinical and electrophysiologic examination of family members, a therapeutic trial of immunosuppressive therapy may be warranted.

Pathologic Findings

The most characteristic histopathologic features on nerve biopsy of patients with chronic inflammatory demyelinating polyneuropathy are loss of myelinated axons, particularly larger-caliber axons; evidence of segmental demyelination and remyelination; and regional variability in the severity of fiber loss and inflammation [Baba et al., 1993; Gabreels-Festen et al., 1993; Matsumuro et al., 1994; Sladky et al., 1986]. The presence of inflammatory cells and selective fascicular variability in the expression of pathologic abnormalities are the only characteristics helpful in distinguishing an acquired from a genetically determined disorder [Gabreels-Festen et al., 1993]. The presence of thinly remyelinated internodes, segmental demyelination and remyelination, and onion bulb formations (indicative of chronicity) may be seen in any chronic demyelinating neuropathy. Specific features of inflammation (i.e., mononuclear cellular infiltrates) are present in a minority of biopsies from children and infants with chronic inflammatory demyelinating polyneuropathy. Most children with chronic inflammatory demyelinating polyneuropathy demonstrate evidence of subperineurial and endoneurial edema and an increased number of inflammatory cells dispersed within the endoneurium [Sladky et al., 1986]. Discrete perivascular collections of inflammatory cells around epineurial or endoneurial vessels are relatively rare. Teased fiber preparations demonstrating isolated demyelinated internodes or random variability in internodal length and myelin thickness are also highly suggestive of a multifocal inflammatory demyelinating process (Fig. 77-3). Electron microscopy may confirm these features and demonstrate fragmentation of myelin sheaths with splitting of myelin lamellae and intralamellar insinuation of macrophages ingesting internodal myelin. Immunocytochemical testing may be helpful to confirm activated lymphocytic subpopulations within the endoneurium and demonstrate expression of class I and II major histocompatibility complex markers on Schwann cell surfaces in areas of active demyelination. Similar findings have been reported in Guillain-Barré syndrome as well [Asbury et al., 1969; Hughes et al., 1992]. More recently, circulating antibodies to myelin-related gangliosides have been reported and associated, for the most part loosely, with specific Guillain-Barré syndrome subtypes. However, antibodies to any of these candidate myelin autoantigens were not significantly more frequent in patients with chronic inflammatory demyelinating polyneuropathy than in controls or other groups studied. In addition, serologic evidence of *C. jejuni* or cytomegalovirus infection was not detected.

The ability to make a conclusive diagnosis from a biopsy specimen in a multifocal process such as chronic inflammatory demyelinating polyneuropathy is limited by the problem of sampling error. Because only a finite amount of tissue is removed, pathognomonic histopathologic features may not be

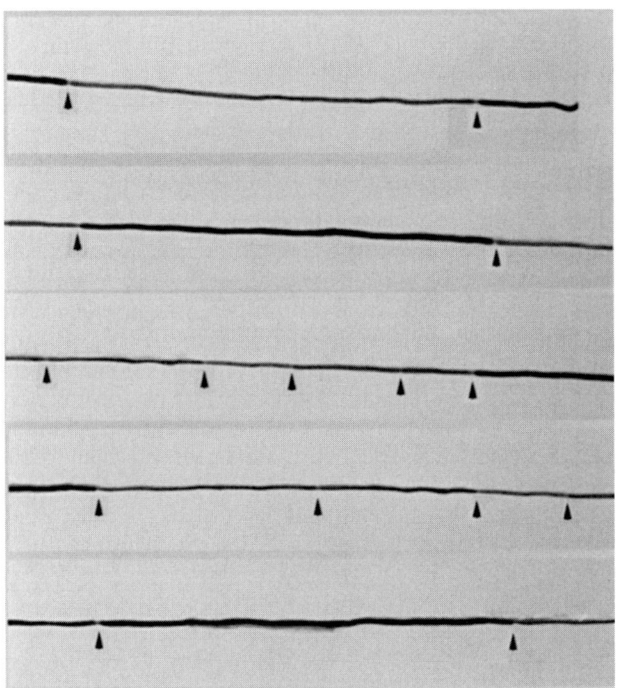

FIGURE 77-3. Teased fiber preparation of osmicated axons from a patient with chronic immune demyelinating polyneuropathy. Sequential internodes along the course of an individual myelinated axon are shown. (Individual nodes of Ranvier are indicated with *arrowheads.*) The random variability in internodal length and myelin thickness is pathognomonic for a multifocal demyelinating process and could be seen in chronic immune demyelinating polyneuropathy or during the recovery stage in Guillain-Barré syndrome (×75). (Courtesy of John Sladky, MD.)

present in the sample obtained for pathologic inspection. This situation is of particular concern in chronic inflammatory demyelinating polyneuropathy, in which inflammation with secondary axonal injury may be confined to proximal nerve segments. A biopsy specimen from a sural nerve site well "downstream" from the area of active inflammation may indicate only evidence of wallerian degeneration of distal axons below the level of primary injury.

Treatment

Several therapeutic modalities have been found to be effective in the management of chronic inflammatory demyelinating polyneuropathy, including corticosteroids, plasmapheresis, intravenous immune globulin, and other immunosuppressive agents [Baba et al., 1993, 1996; Barnett et al., 1998; Berger et al., 2003; Brannagan, 2002; Brannagan et al., 2002; Choudhary and Hughes, 1995; Comi et al., 2003; Connolly, 2001; Dalakas, 2002, 2004a, 2004b; Dyck et al., 1982a, 1982b, 1985a, 1985b, 1986, 1994; Good et al., 1998; Gorson et al., 2004; Gorson et al., 1998; Hahn et al., 1996a, 1996b; Hodgkinson et al., 1990; Hughes et al., 2003a; Kissel, 2003; Mahattanakul et al., 1996; Mendell et al., 2001; Meriggioli and Rowin, 2000; Molenaar et al., 1997; Mowzoon et al., 2001; Vallat et al., 2003; van Doorn and Ruts, 2004]. However, there are few data comparing the relative efficacy of these treatments [Choudhary and Hughes, 1995; Choudhary et al., 1995b]. It remains unclear which treatment should be a first-line regimen in the treatment of chronic inflammatory demyelinating polyneuropathy.

In patients with suspected or definite chronic inflammatory demyelinating polyneuropathy, initial treatment with prednisone at a dose of 2 mg/kg/day for 6 to 8 weeks has been successful. Most previously untreated children with the disease demonstrate substantial functional improvement within that time frame [Baba et al., 1996; Connolly, 2001; Korinthenberg, 1999; Nevo, 1998; Sladky, 1996]. Lack of significant clinical improvement in this setting implies that (1) the child cannot metabolize prednisone to an active form, (2) the child will not respond well enough to corticosteroids to justify potential long-term side effects, or (3) the child does not have chronic inflammatory demyelinating polyneuropathy. A small number of individuals are unable to metabolize prednisone to an active form. In prednisone nonresponders who also are not demonstrating other clinical signs of steroid effects after 6 to 8 weeks of treatment (i.e., cushingoid facies and weight gain), this possibility should be entertained and methyl prednisolone substituted before discarding corticosteroid therapy. Patients nonresponsive to corticosteroids can be tapered off medication over several weeks. In steroid-responsive individuals, it is desirable to gradually reduce the dosage schedule over 6 months to an alternate-day dose of about 1 mg/kg/day or a dose of 30 mg on alternate days in children weighing more than 30 kg. A cumulative daily dose of 0.5 mg/kg is considered to pose little significant risk for opportunistic infection, osteopenia, or cataract formation. This regimen can be slowly reduced over the next 4 to 6 months. About half the children will remain in remission after treatment is discontinued. In a pilot study involving a small group of patients, pulsed high-dose dexamethasone (six cycles at 40 mg/day for 4 days every 28 days) has been reported in adults to be an alternative effective treatment [Molenaar et al., 1997].

Although most children with chronic inflammatory demyelinating polyneuropathy initially respond to corticosteroids, some become refractory or require unacceptably high doses to maintain stable function. Human intravenous immune globulin or plasmapheresis is the next alternate therapeutic option to consider in such patients [Barnett et al., 1998; Gay et al., 1986; Hahn, 2000; Hahn et al., 1996a, 1996b; Kiprov et al., 2003; Tanaka, 1998; Vedanarayanan et al., 1991; Walk et al., 2004]. Intravenous immune globulin has the advantage of permitting treatment at home using visiting nursing teams if the child has exhibited no untoward reactions to an initial course of treatment in the hospital. In older children who are large enough to establish adequate peripheral venous access for plasmapheresis, the procedure can be initiated on an outpatient basis. The choice between therapies depends more on logistical and technical factors than on the inherent superiority of one or the other modality. A small number of children become refractory to these treatments as well and will require more potent immunosuppressive agents to maintain remission. Again, there are no data to guide the clinician as to which immunosuppressant will be best for an individual patient. It is probably wisest to begin with an agent with which the treating physician has the most experience. Clinicians have been inclined to avoid cyclophosphamide and azathioprine in the past because of the potential risk for developing future malignancies. However, there are probably only small differences in the risk for this late complication among different chemotherapeutic agents. Methotrexate is not commonly helpful in chronic inflammatory demyelinating polyneuropathy, but it is worth consideration because it can be given orally on a weekly basis and is associated with few complications when serum levels are carefully monitored. Cyclosporine can be useful in treating selected refractory cases of chronic inflammatory demyelinating polyneuropathy [Barnett et al., 1998; Jongen et al., 1988; Mahattanakul et al., 1996; Ryan et al., 2000]. This agent is given orally at an initial dose of 3 to 5 mg/kg twice a day. It is generally a safe drug if renal function and serum levels are carefully followed.

Prognosis

The prognosis in children is generally favorable [Ryan et al., 2000; Simmons et al., 1997b; Sladky, 1996; Sladky et al., 1986]. About 50% respond well to corticosteroids and remain in remission after treatment is discontinued. Another 25% to 30% respond to additional treatment modalities and require a prolonged course of treatment. The long-term prognosis in this group of patients remains uncertain. A small number of children respond poorly to all treatment strategies or, more typically, become refractory to treatment or develop significant side effects to protracted immunosuppression and suffer substantial neurologic disability [Connolly, 2001; Nevo, 1998; Nevo et al., 1996; Pollard, 1994, 2002; Ryan et al., 2000; Simmons et al., 1997a, 1997b].

OTHER IMMUNE-MEDIATED NEUROPATHIES IN CHILDREN

Table 77-8 summarizes some of the other types of immune-mediated peripheral neuropathies that have been observed in children. These occur relatively infrequently and are usually associated with evidence of other systemic symptoms [Tan et al., 2003]. Although peripheral nerve disorders are described as being relatively frequent in patients with human immunodeficiency virus infection, many of the affected children have been identified based on electrodiagnostic criteria and often have little clinical evidence of peripheral nerve involvement [Floeter et al., 1997]. Many of these children are also receiving multiple drugs, and it is likely that peripheral neuropathy in this population is, in some cases, a side effect of treatment rather than a complication of infection. Inflammatory neuropathy, often with electrophysiologic evidence of demyelination, can occur in the course of graft-versus-host disease after bone marrow transplantation [Adams et al., 1995; Amato et al., 1993; Imrie et al., 1994; Openshaw, 1997; Sladky, 1996]. There are a number of reports associating *Borrelia burgdorferi* infection with peripheral neuropathy, especially chronic inflammatory demyelinating polyneuropathy. Most of these reports have involved older individuals. Chronic peripheral neuropathy including chronic inflammatory demyelinating polyneuropathy developing in the course of active Lyme disease is rare in childhood [Belman et al., 1993]. As in the case of many associations, a causal relationship between chronic inflammatory demyelinating polyneuropathy and neuropathy may be inferred, but not proved. Finally, vasculitis confined to peripheral nerves and presenting as mononeuritis multiplex is extremely uncommon [Mok et al., 2001] but can occur in children and may respond well to corticosteroids or other immunosuppressant modalities [Bulun et al., 2001].

TABLE 77-8

Immune-Mediated Neuropathies Other than Guillain-Barré Syndrome and Chronic Immune Demyelinating Polyneuropathy in Children

IMMUNE DISORDER	NO. OF PATIENTS (TOTAL OF 10)
Bone marrow transplantation	4
Collagen vascular diseases (juvenile rheumatoid arthritis, lupus erythematosus, mixed connective tissue disease)	3
Human immunodeficiency virus infection	1
Lyme disease	1
Peripheral nerve vasculitis	1

Data from unpublished observations of John T. Sladky, MD.

REFERENCES

Aarli JA. Role of cytokines in neurological disorders. Curr Med Chem 2003;10:1931.

Abd-Allah SA, Jansen PW, Ashwal S, et al. Intravenous immunoglobulin as therapy for pediatric Guillain-Barré syndrome. J Child Neurol 1997;12:376.

Adams C, August CS, Maguire H, et al. Neuromuscular complications of bone marrow transplantation. Pediatr Neurol 1995;12:58.

Albers JW, Kelly JJ Jr. Acquired inflammatory demyelinating polyneuropathies: Clinical and electrodiagnostic features. Muscle Nerve 1989;12:435.

Aldrey JM, Fernandez-Rial A, Lopez-Gonzalez FJ, et al. Guillain-Barré syndrome as first manifestation of typhoid fever. Clin Infect Dis 1999;28:1171.

Al-Eissa YA, Al-Herbish AS. Severe hypertension: An unusual presentation of Guillain-Barré syndrome in a child with brucellosis. Eur J Pediatr 1996;155:53.

Alexander JP Jr, Baden L, Pallansch MA, et al. Enterovirus 71 infections and neurologic disease—United States, 1977-1991. J Infect Dis 1994;169:905.

al-Qudah AA. Immunoglobulins in the treatment of Guillain-Barré syndrome in early childhood. J Child Neurol 1994;9:178.

Alma TA, Chaudhry V, Cornblath DR. Electrophysiological studies in the Guillain-Barré syndrome: Distinguishing subtypes by published criteria. Muscle Nerve 1998;21:1275.

Amato AA, Barohn RJ, Sahenk Z, et al. Polyneuropathy complicating bone marrow and solid organ transplantation. Neurology 1993;43:1513.

Ang CW, De Klerk MA, Endtz HP, et al. Guillain-Barré syndrome– and Miller Fisher syndrome–associated Campylobacter jejuni lipopolysaccharides induce anti-GM1 and anti-GQ1b antibodies in rabbits. Infect Immun 2001;69:2462.

Ang CW, Tio-Gillen AP, Groen J, et al. Cross-reactive anti-galactocerebroside antibodies and Mycoplasma pneumoniae infections in Guillain-Barré syndrome. J Neuroimmunol 2002;130:179.

Arakawa Y, Yoshimura M, Kobayashi S, et al. The use of intravenous immunoglobulin in Miller Fisher syndrome. Brain Dev 1993;15:231.

Asbury AK, Arnason BG, Adams RD. The inflammatory lesion in idiopathic polyneuritis. Its role in pathogenesis. Medicine 1969;48:173.

Asbury AK, Cornblath DR. Assessment of current diagnostic criteria for Guillain-Barré syndrome. Ann Neurol 1990;27:S21.

Awong IE, Dandurand KR, Keeys CA, et al. Drug-associated Guillain-Barré syndrome: A literature review. Ann Pharmacother 1996;30:173.

Baba M, Ogawa M, Matsunaga M. Treatment of chronic inflammatory demyelinating polyneuropathy (CIDP). Rinsho Shinkeigaku 1996;36:1336.

Baba M, Takada H, Tomiyama M, et al. Chronic inflammatory demyelinating polyneuropathy in childhood. No To Shinkei 1993;45:233.

Baran GA, Sowell MK, Sharp GB, et al. MR findings in a child with Guillain-Barré syndrome. AJR Am J Roentgenol 1993;161:161.

Barnett MH, Pollard JD, Davies L, et al. Cyclosporin A in resistant chronic inflammatory demyelinating polyradiculoneuropathy. Muscle Nerve 1998;21:454.

Baskin E, Turkay S, Icagasioglu D, et al. High-dose intravenous immune globulin in the management of severe Guillain-Barré syndrome. Turk J Pediatr 1996;38:119.

Belman AL, Iyer M, Coyle PK, et al. Neurologic manifestations in children with North American Lyme disease. Neurology 1993;43:2609.

Berciano J, Coria F, Monton F, et al. Axonal form of Guillain-Barré syndrome: Evidence for macrophage-associated demyelination. Muscle Nerve 1993;16:744.

Berciano J, Figols J, Garcia A, et al. Fulminant Guillain-Barré syndrome with universal inexcitability of peripheral nerves: A clinicopathological study. Muscle Nerve 1997;20:846.

Berciano J, Pascual J. Selective contrast enhancement of anterior spinal nerve roots on magnetic resonance imaging: A suggestive sign of Guillain-Barré syndrome and neurobrucellosis. J Peripher Nerv Syst 2003;8:135.

Berger AR, Bradley WG, Brannagan TH, et al. Guidelines for the diagnosis and treatment of chronic inflammatory demyelinating polyneuropathy. J Peripher Nerv Syst 2003;8:282.

Berger JR, Ayyar DR, Kaszovitz B. Guillain-Barré syndrome complicating typhoid fever. Ann Neurol 1986;20:649.

Bertorini T, Halford H, Lawrence J, et al. Contrast-enhanced magnetic resonance imaging of the lumbosacral roots in the dysimmune inflammatory polyneuropathies. J Neuroimaging 1995;5:9.

Bird SJ, Sladky JT. Corticosteroid-responsive dominantly inherited neuropathy in childhood. Neurology 1991;41:437.

Bos AP, van der Meche FG, Witsenburg M, et al. Experiences with Guillain-Barré syndrome in a pediatric intensive care unit. Intensive Care Med 1987;13:328.

Bouma PA, Carpay HA, Rijpkema SG. Antibodies to Borrelia burgdorferi in Guillain-Barré syndrome. Lancet 1989;2:739.

Bradshaw DY, Jones HR. Pseudomeningoencephalitic presentation of pediatric Guillain-Barré syndrome. J Child Neurol 2001;16:505.

Bradshaw DY, Jones HR Jr. Guillain-Barré syndrome in children: Clinical course, electrodiagnosis, and prognosis. Muscle Nerve 1992;15:500.

Brannagan TH 3rd. Intravenous gammaglobulin (IVIg) for treatment of CIDP and related immune-mediated neuropathies. Neurology 2002;59(12 Suppl 6):S33.

Brannagan TH 3rd, Pradhan A, Heiman-Patterson T, et al. High-dose cyclophosphamide without stem-cell rescue for refractory CIDP. Neurology 2002;58:1856.

Brashear HR, Bonnin JM, Login IS. Encephalomyeloneuritis simulating Guillain-Barré syndrome. Neurology 1985;35:1146.

Briscoe DM, McMenamin JB, O'Donohoe NV. Prognosis in Guillain-Barré syndrome. Arch Dis Child 1987;62:733.

Bulun A, Topaloglu R, Duzova A, et al. Ataxia and peripheral neuropathy: Rare manifestations in Henoch-Schönlein purpura. Pediatr Nephrol 2001;16:1139.

Carpo M, Pedotti R, Lolli F, et al. Clinical correlate and fine specificity of anti-GQ1b antibodies in peripheral neuropathy. J Neurol Sci 1998;155:186.

Carter GT, England JD, Chance PF. Charcot-Marie-Tooth disease: Electrophysiology, molecular genetics and clinical management. IDrugs 2004;7:151.

Chanmugam D, Waniganetti A. Guillain-Barré syndrome associated with typhoid fever. BMJ 1969;1:95.

Chin RL, Latov N, Sander HW, et al. Sensory CIDP presenting as cryptogenic sensory polyneuropathy. J Peripher Nerv Syst 2004;9:132.

Choudhary PP, Hughes RA. Long-term treatment of chronic inflammatory demyelinating polyradiculoneuropathy with plasma exchange or intravenous immunoglobulin. QJM 1995;88:493.

Choudhary PP, Thompson N, Hughes RA. Improvement following interferon beta in chronic inflammatory demyelinating polyradiculoneuropathy. J Neurol 1995;242:252.

Christiansen I, Brodersen P. Pandysautonomia. Severe autonomic dysfunction accompanying polyneuropathy. Ugeskr Laeger 2003;165:1366.

Coe CJ. Guillain-Barré syndrome in Korean children. Yonsei Med J 1989;30:81.

Cole GF, Matthew DJ. Prognosis in severe Guillain-Barré syndrome. Arch Dis Child 1987;62:288.

Comi G, Quattrini A, Fazio R, et al. Immunoglobulins in chronic inflammatory demyelinating polyneuropathy. Neurol Sci 2003;24(Suppl 4):S246.

Connolly AM. Chronic inflammatory demyelinating polyneuropathy in childhood. Pediatr Neurol 2001;24:177.

Cornblath DR. Electrophysiology in Guillain-Barré syndrome. Ann Neurol 1990;27:S17.

Creange A, Belec L, Clair B, et al. Circulating tumor necrosis factor (TNF)-alpha and soluble TNF-alpha receptors in patients with Guillain-Barré syndrome. J Neuroimmunol 1996;68:95.

Crino PB, Grossman RI, Rostami A. Magnetic resonance imaging of the cauda equina in chronic inflammatory demyelinating polyneuropathy. Ann Neurol 1993;33:311.

Crino PB, Zimmerman R, Laskowitz D, et al. Magnetic resonance imaging of the cauda equina in Guillain-Barré syndrome. Neurology 1994;44:1334.

Cros D, Triggs WJ. Guillain-Barré syndrome: Clinical neurophysiologic studies. Rev Neurol (Paris) 1996;152:339.

Currie DM, Nelson MR, Buck BC. Guillain-Barré syndrome in children: Evidence of axonal degeneration and long-term follow-up. Arch Phys Med Rehabil 1990;71:244.

Dalakas MC. Basic aspects of neuroimmunology as they relate to immunotherapeutic targets: Present and future prospects. Ann Neurol 1995;37(Suppl 1):S2.

Dalakas MC. Advances in chronic inflammatory demyelinating polyneuropathy: Disease variants and inflammatory response mediators and modifiers. Curr Opin Neurol 1999a;12:403.

Dalakas MC. Intravenous immunoglobulin in the treatment of autoimmune neuromuscular diseases: Present status and practical therapeutic guidelines. Muscle Nerve 1999b;22:1479.

Dalakas MC. Mechanisms of action of IVIg and therapeutic considerations in the treatment of acute and chronic demyelinating neuropathies. Neurology 2002;59(12 Suppl 6):S13.

Dalakas MC. Intravenous immunoglobulin in autoimmune neuromuscular diseases. JAMA 2004a;291:2367.

Dalakas MC. The use of intravenous immunoglobulin in the treatment of autoimmune neuromuscular diseases: evidence-based indications and safety profile. Pharmacol Ther 2004b;102:177.

Delgado MR. Guillain-Barré syndrome: A pediatric challenge. J Child Neurol 1996;11:1.

Deretzi G, Pelidou S, Zou L, et al. Suppression of chronic experimental autoimmune neuritis by nasally administered recombinant rat interleukin-6. Immunology 1999;97:69.

Donoso R. Guillain-Barré syndrome following typhoid fever [letter]. Ann Neurol 1988;23:627.

Dowling PC, Cook SD. Role of infection in Guillain-Barré syndrome: Laboratory confirmation of herpes viruses in 41 cases. Ann Neurol 1981;9(Suppl):44.

Duncan S, Will RG, Catnach J. Mumps and Guillain-Barré syndrome. J Neurol Neurosurg Psychiatry 1990;53:709.

Dyck PJ, Daube J, O'Brien P, et al. Plasma exchange in chronic inflammatory demyelinating polyradiculoneuropathy. N Engl J Med 1986;314:461.

Dyck PJ, Kurtzke JF. Plasmapheresis in Guillain-Barré syndrome. Neurology 1985a;35:1105.

Dyck PJ, Litchy WJ, Kratz KM, et al. A plasma exchange versus immune globulin infusion trial in chronic inflammatory demyelinating polyradiculoneuropathy. Ann Neurol 1994;36:838.

Dyck PJ, O'Brien P, Swanson C, et al. Combined azathioprine and prednisone in chronic inflammatory-demyelinating polyneuropathy. Neurology 1985b;35:1173.

Dyck PJ, O'Brien PC, Oviatt KF, et al. Prednisone improves chronic inflammatory demyelinating polyradiculoneuropathy more than no treatment. Ann Neurol 1982a;11:136.

Dyck PJ, Pineda A, Swanson C, et al. The Mayo Clinic experience with plasma exchange in chronic inflammatory-demyelinating polyneuropathy (CIDP). Prog Clin Biol Res 1982b;106:197.

Dyck PJ, Swanson CJ, Low PA, et al. Prednisone-responsive hereditary motor and sensory neuropathy. Mayo Clin Proc 1982c;57:239.

Eggenberger ER, Coker S, Menezes M. Pediatric Miller Fisher syndrome requiring intubation: A case report. Clin Pediatr (Phila) 1993;32:372.

Epstein MA, Sladky JT. The role of plasmapheresis in childhood Guillain-Barré syndrome. Ann Neurol 1990;28:65.

Esselink RA, Gerding MN, Brouwers PJ, et al. Guillain-Barré syndrome associated with hantavirus infection. Lancet 1994;343:180.

Fagius J, Westerberg CE, Olsson Y. Acute pandysautonomia and severe sensory deficit with poor recovery. A clinical, neurophysiological and pathological case study. J Neurol Neurosurg Psychiatry 1983;46:725.

Farkkila M, Kinnunen E, Weckstrom P. Survey of Guillain-Barré syndrome in southern Finland. Neuroepidemiology 1991;10:236.

Feasby TE, Hahn AF, Koopman WJ, et al. Central lesions in chronic inflammatory demyelinating polyneuropathy: An MRI study. Neurology 1990;40:476.

Floeter MK, Civitello LA, Everett CR, et al. Peripheral neuropathy in children with HIV infection. Neurology 1997;49:207.

French Cooperative Group on Plasma Exchange in Guillain-Barré Syndrome. Efficiency of plasma exchange in Guillain-Barré syndrome: Role of replacement fluids. Ann Neurol 1987;22:753.

Fulbright RK, Erdum E, Sze G, et al. Cranial nerve enhancement in the Guillain-Barré syndrome. AJNR Am J Neuroradiol 1995;16(4 Suppl):923.

Fulgham JR, Wijdicks EF. Guillain-Barré syndrome. Crit Care Clin 1997;13:1.

Gabreels-Festen AA, Gabreels FJ, Hoogendijk JE, et al. Chronic inflammatory demyelinating polyneuropathy or hereditary motor and sensory neuropathy? Diagnostic value of morphological criteria. Acta Neuropathol (Berl) 1993;86:630.

Gabriel CM, Gregson NA, Redford EJ, et al. Human immunoglobulin ameliorates rat experimental autoimmune neuritis. Brain 1997;120:1533.

Gamstorp I. Encephalo-myelo-radiculo-neuropathy: Involvement of the CNS in children with Guillain-Barré-Strohl syndrome. Dev Med Child Neurol 1974;16:654.

Garcia T, Sanchez JC, Maestre JF, et al. Brucellosis and acute inflammatory polyradiculoneuropathy. Neurologia 1989;4:145.

Gay T, Katz B. Plasma exchange as sole treatment for chronic inflammatory demyelinating polyneuropathy. Med J Aust 1986;144:503.

Ghosh S. Guillain-Barré syndrome complicating mumps. Lancet 1967;1:895.

Good JL, Chehrenama M, Mayer RF, et al. Pulse cyclophosphamide therapy in chronic inflammatory demyelinating polyneuropathy. Neurology 1998;51:1735.

Goodhew PM, Johnston HM. Immune globulin therapy in children with Guillain-Barré syndrome. Muscle Nerve 1996;19:1490.

Gorson KC, Amato AA, Ropper AH. Efficacy of mycophenolate mofetil in patients with chronic immune demyelinating polyneuropathy. Neurology 2004;63:715.

Gorson KC, Chaudhry VV. Chronic inflammatory demyelinating polyneuropathy. Curr Treat Options Neurol 1999;1:251.

Gorson KC, Ropper AH, Clark BD, et al. Treatment of chronic inflammatory demyelinating polyneuropathy with interferon-alpha 2a. Neurology 1998;50:84.

Gorson KC, Ropper AH, Muriello MA, et al. Prospective evaluation of MRI lumbosacral nerve root enhancement in acute Guillain-Barré syndrome. Neurology 1996;47:813.

Griffin JW, Ho TW. The Guillain-Barré syndrome at 75: The Campylobacter connection. Ann Neurol 1993;34:125.

Griffin JW, Li CY, Ho TW, et al. Pathology of the motor-sensory axonal Guillain-Barré syndrome. Ann Neurol 1996a;39:17.

Griffin JW, Li CY, Ho TW, et al. Guillain-Barré syndrome in northern China. The spectrum of neuropathological changes in clinically defined cases. Brain 1995;118:577.

Griffin JW, Li CY, Macko C, et al. Early nodal changes in the acute motor axonal neuropathy pattern of the Guillain-Barré syndrome. J Neurocytol 1996b;25:33.

Grose C, Feorino PM. Epstein-Barr virus and Guillain-Barré syndrome. Lancet 1972;2:1285.

Guillain-Barré Syndrome Steroid Trial Group. Double-blind trial of intravenous methylprednisolone in Guillain-Barré syndrome. Lancet 1993;341:586.

Guillain-Barré Syndrome Study Group. Plasmapheresis and acute Guillain-Barré syndrome. Neurology 1985;35:1096.

Gurses N, Uysal S, Cetinkaya F, et al. Intravenous immunoglobulin treatment in children with Guillain-Barré syndrome. Scand J Infect Dis 1995;27:241.

Hadden RD, Cornblath DR, Hughes RA, et al. Electrophysiological classification of Guillain-Barré syndrome: Clinical associations and outcome. Plasma Exchange/Sandoglobulin Guillain-Barré Syndrome Trial Group. Ann Neurol 1998;44:780.

Hadden RD, Gregson NA. Guillain-Barré syndrome and Campylobacter jejuni infection. Symp Ser Soc Appl Microbiol 2001;30:145S.

Hadden RD, Karch H, Hartung HP, et al. Preceding infections, immune factors, and outcome in Guillain-Barré syndrome. Neurology 2001;56:758.

Hafer-Macko C, Hsieh ST, Li CY, et al. Acute motor axonal neuropathy: An antibody-mediated attack on axolemma. Ann Neurol 1996a;40:635.

Hafer-Macko CE, Sheikh KA, Li CY, et al. Immune attack on the Schwann cell surface in acute inflammatory demyelinating polyneuropathy. Ann Neurol 1996b;39:625.

Hahn AF. Management of Guillain-Barré syndrome (GBS). Baillieres Clin Neurol 1996;5:627.

Hahn AF. Guillain-Barré syndrome: An evolving concept. Curr Opin Neurol 1997;10:363.

Hahn AF. Treatment of chronic inflammatory demyelinating polyneuropathy with intravenous immunoglobulin. Neurology 1998;51(6 Suppl 5):S16.

Hahn AF. Intravenous immunoglobulin treatment in peripheral nerve disorders—indications, mechanisms of action and side-effects. Curr Opin Neurol 2000;13:575.

Hahn AF, Bolton CF, Pillay N, et al. Plasma-exchange therapy in chronic inflammatory demyelinating polyneuropathy. A double-blind, sham-controlled, cross-over study. Brain 1996a;119:1055.

Hahn AF, Bolton CF, Zochodne D, et al. Intravenous immunoglobulin treatment in chronic inflammatory demyelinating polyneuropathy. A double-blind, placebo-controlled, cross-over study. Brain 1996b;119:1067.

Hammersjö JA. Plasma exchange in childhood Guillain-Barré syndrome. Acta Paediatr 1995;84:355.

Hart DE, Rojas LA, Rosario JA, et al. Childhood Guillain-Barré syndrome in Paraguay, 1990 to 1991. Ann Neurol 1994;36:859.

Hartung HP, Kieseier BC. Antibody responses in the Guillain-Barré syndrome. J Neurol Sci 1999;168:75.

Hartung HP, Kieseier BC. The role of matrix metalloproteinases in autoimmune damage to the central and peripheral nervous system. J Neuroimmunol 2000;107:140.

Hartung HP, Kieseier BC, Kiefer R. Progress in Guillain-Barré syndrome. Curr Opin Neurol 2001;14:597.

Hartung HP, Willison HJ, Kieseier BC. Acute immunoinflammatory neuropathy: Update on Guillain-Barré syndrome. Curr Opin Neurol 2002;15:571.

Hartung HP, Zielasek J, Jung S, et al. Effector mechanisms in demyelinating neuropathies. Rev Neurol (Paris) 1996;152:320.

Harvey GK, Pollard JD, Schindhelm K, et al. Chronic experimental allergic neuritis. An electrophysiological and histological study in the rabbit. J Neurol Sci 1987;81:215.

Hattori N, Ichimura M, Aoki S, et al. Clinicopathological features of chronic inflammatory demyelinating polyradiculoneuropathy in childhood. J Neurol Sci 1998;154:66.

Henderson RD, Lawn ND, Fletcher DD, et al. The morbidity of Guillain-Barré syndrome admitted to the intensive care unit. Neurology 2003;60:17.

Hernandez Gonzalez A, Rubio Quinones F, Quintero Otero S, et al. The treatment of the Guillain-Barré syndrome in childhood by plasmapheresis. An Esp Pediatr 1993;39:240.

Ho TW, Hsieh ST, Nachamkin I, et al. Motor nerve terminal degeneration provides a potential mechanism for rapid recovery in acute motor axonal neuropathy after Campylobacter infection. Neurology 1997a;48:717.

Ho TW, Li CY, Cornblath DR, et al. Patterns of recovery in the Guillain-Barré syndromes. Neurology 1997b;48:695.

Ho TW, Mishu B, Li CY, et al. Guillain-Barré syndrome in northern China. Relationship to Campylobacter jejuni infection and anti-glycolipid antibodies. Brain 1995;118:597.

Hodgkinson SJ, Pollard JD, McLeod JG. Cyclosporin A in the treatment of chronic demyelinating polyradiculoneuropathy. J Neurol Neurosurg Psychiatry 1990;53:327.

Horneff G, Huppertz HI, Muller K, et al. Demonstration of Borrelia burgdorferi infection in a child with Guillain-Barré syndrome. Eur J Pediatr 1993;152:810.

Hughes PM, Wells GM, Clements JM, et al. Matrix metalloproteinase expression during experimental autoimmune neuritis. Brain 1998;121:481.

Hughes RA. The management of Guillain-Barré syndrome. Hosp Pract (Off Ed) 1992;27:107.

Hughes RA. The spectrum of acquired demyelinating polyradiculoneuropathy. Acta Neurol Belg 1994;94:128.

Hughes RA. Management of acute neuromuscular paralysis. J R Coll Physicians Lond 1998;32:254.

Hughes R. Campylobacter jejuni in Guillain-Barré syndrome. Lancet Neurol 2004;3:644.

Hughes R, Atkinson P, Coates P, et al. Sural nerve biopsies in Guillain-Barré syndrome: Axonal degeneration and macrophage-associated demyelination and absence of cytomegalovirus genome. Muscle Nerve 1992;15:568.

Hughes RA, Hadden RD, Gregson NA, et al. Pathogenesis of Guillain-Barré syndrome. J Neuroimmunol 1999;100:74.

Hughes RA, Swan AV, van Doorn PA. Cytotoxic drugs and interferons for chronic inflammatory demyelinating polyradiculoneuropathy. Cochrane Database Syst Rev 2003a;1:CD003280.

Hughes RA, Wijdicks EF, Barohn R, et al. Practice parameter: Immunotherapy for Guillain-Barré syndrome. Report of the Quality Standards Subcommittee of the American Academy of Neurology. Neurology 2003b;61:736.

Hung KL, Wang HS, Liou WY, et al. Guillain-Barré syndrome in children: A cooperative study in Taiwan. Brain Dev 1994;16:204.

Imrie KR, Couture F, Turner CC, et al. Peripheral neuropathy following high-dose etoposide and autologous bone marrow transplantation. Bone Marrow Transplant 1994;13:77.

Ismail EA, Shabani IS, Badawi M, et al. An epidemiologic, clinical, and therapeutic study of childhood Guillain-Barré syndrome in Kuwait: Is it related to the oral polio vaccine? J Child Neurol 1998;13:488.

Italian Guillain-Barré Study Group. The prognosis and main prognostic indicators of Guillain-Barré syndrome. A multicentre prospective study of 297 patients. Brain 1996;119:2053.

Jacobs BC, Endtz HP, van der Meche FG, et al. Humoral immune response against Campylobacter jejuni lipopolysaccharides in Guillain-Barré and Miller Fisher syndrome. J Neuroimmunol 1997a;79:62.

Jacobs BC, Hazenberg MP, van Doorn PA, et al. Cross-reactive antibodies against gangliosides and Campylobacter jejuni lipopolysaccharides in patients with Guillain-Barré or Miller Fisher syndrome. J Infect Dis 1997b;175:729.

Jacobs BC, Rothbarth PH, van der Meche FG, et al. The spectrum of antecedent infections in Guillain-Barré syndrome: A case-control study. Neurology 1998;51:1110.

Jacobs BC, van Doorn PA, Groeneveld JH, et al. Cytomegalovirus infections and anti-GM2 antibodies in Guillain-Barré syndrome. J Neurol Neurosurg Psychiatry 1997c;62:641.

Jander S, Stoll G. Interleukin-18 is induced in acute inflammatory demyelinating polyneuropathy. J Neuroimmunol 2001;114:253.

Jansen PW, Perkin RM, Ashwal S. Guillain-Barré syndrome in childhood: Natural course and efficacy of plasmapheresis. Pediatr Neurol 1993;9:16.

Jones HR Jr. Childhood Guillain-Barré syndrome: Clinical presentation, diagnosis, and therapy. J Child Neurol 1996;11:4.

Jones HR Jr. Guillain-Barré syndrome: Perspectives with infants and children. Semin Pediatr Neurol 2000;7:91.

Jongen PJ, Joosten EM, Berden JH, et al. Cyclosporine therapy in chronic inflammatory demyelinating polyradiculoneuropathy: A preliminary report of clinical results in two patients. Transplant Proc 1988;20(3 Suppl 4):329.

Jung S, Toyka KV, Hartung HP. Soluble complement receptor type 1 inhibits experimental autoimmune neuritis in Lewis rats. Neurosci Lett 1995;200:167.

Kanra G, Ozon A, Vajsar J, et al. Intravenous immunoglobulin treatment in children with Guillain-Barré syndrome. Eur J Paediatr Neurol 1997;1:7.

Khatri A, Pearlstein L. Pain in Guillain-Barré syndrome. Neurology 1997;49:1474.

Khatri BO, Flamini JR, Baruah JK, et al. Plasmapheresis with acute inflammatory polyneuropathy. Pediatr Neurol 1990;6:17.

Kiefer R, Kieseier BC, Stoll G, et al. The role of macrophages in immune-mediated damage to the peripheral nervous system. Prog Neurobiol 2001;64:109.

Kieseier BC, Kiefer R, Gold R, et al. Advances in understanding and treatment of immune-mediated disorders of the peripheral nervous system. Muscle Nerve 2004;30:131.

Kiprov DD, Hofmann JC. Plasmapheresis in immunologically mediated polyneuropathies. Ther Apher Dial 2003;7:189.

Kissel JT. The treatment of chronic inflammatory demyelinating polyradiculoneuropathy. Semin Neurol 2003;23:169.

Kleyweg RP, van der Meche FG, Loonen MC, et al. The natural history of the Guillain-Barré syndrome in 18 children and 50 adults. J Neurol Neurosurg Psychiatry 1989;52:853.

Korinthenberg R. Chronic inflammatory demyelinating polyradiculoneuropathy in children and their response to treatment. Neuropediatrics 1999;30:190.

Korinthenberg R, Monting JS. Natural history and treatment effects in Guillain-Barré syndrome: A multicentre study. Arch Dis Child 1996;74:281.

Kuroki S, Saida T, Nukina M, et al. Three patients with ophthalmoplegia associated with Campylobacter jejuni. Pediatr Neurol 2001;25:71.

Kusunoki S, Shiina M, Kanazawa I. Anti-Gal-C antibodies in GBS subsequent to mycoplasma infection: Evidence of molecular mimicry. Neurology 2001;57:736.

Kuwabara S, Nakajima M, Matsuda S, et al. Magnetic resonance imaging at the demyelinative foci in chronic inflammatory demyelinating polyneuropathy. Neurology 1997;48:874.

Lamont PJ, Johnston HM, Berdoukas VA. Plasmapheresis in children with Guillain-Barré syndrome. Neurology 1991;41:1928.

Laura M, Gregson NA, Curmi Y, et al. Efficacy of leukemia inhibitory factor in experimental autoimmune neuritis. J Neuroimmunol 2002;133:56.

Leger JM. Involvement of the peripheral nervous system in HIV infection: Electromyographic study and nerve conduction velocity. Neurophysiol Clin 1992;22:403.

Lidin-Janson G, Strannegard O. Guillain-Barré syndrome after measles. BMJ 1972;4:553.

Lisak RP, Skundric D, Bealmear B, et al. The role of cytokines in Schwann cell damage, protection, and repair. J Infect Dis 1997;176(Suppl 2):S173.

Lopez de Munain A, Espinal Valencia JB, Marti-Masso JF, et al. Antibodies to Borrelia burgdorferi in Guillain-Barré syndrome. Lancet 1990;335:1168.

Low PA. Autonomic neuropathies. Curr Opin Neurol 1994;7:402.

Lu JL, Sheikh KA, Wu HS, et al. Physiologic-pathologic correlation in Guillain-Barré syndrome in children. Neurology 2000;54:33.

Lyu RK, Chen ST. Acute multiple cranial neuropathy: A variant of Guillain-Barré syndrome? Muscle Nerve 2004;30:433.

Mahattanakul W, Crawford TO, Griffin JW, et al. Treatment of chronic inflammatory demyelinating polyneuropathy with cyclosporin-A. J Neurol Neurosurg Psychiatry 1996;60:185.

Maier H, Schmidbauer M, Pfausler B, et al. Central nervous system pathology in patients with the Guillain-Barré syndrome. Brain 1997;120:451.

Mancardi GL, Del Sette M, Primavera A, et al. Borrelia burgdorferi infection and Guillain-Barré syndrome. Lancet 1989;2:985.

Manners PJ, Murray KJ. Guillain-Barré syndrome presenting with severe musculoskeletal pain. Acta Paediatr 1992;81:1049.

Matsumuro K, Izumo S, Umehara F, et al. Chronic inflammatory demyelinating polyneuropathy: Histological and immunopathological studies on biopsied sural nerves. J Neurol Sci 1994;127:170.

McCarthy N, Giesecke J. Incidence of Guillain-Barré syndrome following infection with Campylobacter jejuni. Am J Epidemiol 2001;153:610.

McCombe PA, Pollard JD, McLeod JG. Chronic inflammatory demyelinating polyradiculoneuropathy. A clinical and electrophysiological study of 92 cases. Brain 1987;110:1617.

McDouall SF, Tasker RC. Are anticonvulsants a satisfactory alternative to opiate analgesia in patients experiencing pain with Guillain-Barré syndrome? Arch Dis Child 2004;89:686.

McFarland HR. Polyneuritis cranialis as the sole manifestation of the Guillain-Barré syndrome. Mo Med 1976;73:227.

McKhann GM. Guillain-Barré syndrome: Clinical and therapeutic observations. Ann Neurol 1990;27:S13.

McKhann GM, Cornblath DR, Griffin JW, et al. Acute motor axonal neuropathy: A frequent cause of acute flaccid paralysis in China. Ann Neurol 1993;33:333.

McKhann GM, Cornblath DR, Ho T, et al. Clinical and electrophysiological aspects of acute paralytic disease of children and young adults in northern China. Lancet 1991;338:593.

McLean M, Duclos P, Jacob P, et al. Incidence of Guillain-Barré syndrome in Ontario and Quebec, 1983-1989, using hospital service databases. Epidemiology 1994;5:443.

McLeod JG, Pollard JD, Macaskill P, et al. Prevalence of chronic inflammatory demyelinating polyneuropathy in New South Wales, Australia. Ann Neurol 1999;46:910.

McMinn P, Stratov I, Nagarajan L, et al. Neurological manifestations of enterovirus 71 infection in children during an outbreak of hand, foot, and mouth disease in Western Australia. Clin Infect Dis 2001;32:236.

Melendez-Vasquez C, Redford J, Choudhary PP, et al. Immunological investigation of chronic inflammatory demyelinating polyradiculoneuropathy. J Neuroimmunol 1997;73:124.

Mendell JR, Barohn RJ, Freimer ML, et al. Randomized controlled trial of IVIg in untreated chronic inflammatory demyelinating polyradiculoneuropathy. Neurology 2001;56:445.

Merelli E, Sola P, Faglioni P, et al. Newest human herpesvirus (HHV-6) in the Guillain-Barré syndrome and other neurological diseases. Acta Neurol Scand 1992;85:334.

Mericle RA, Triggs WJ. Treatment of acute pandysautonomia with intravenous immunoglobulin. J Neurol Neurosurg Psychiatry 1997;62:529.

Meriggioli MN, Rowin J. Chronic inflammatory demyelinating polyneuropathy after treatment with interferon-alpha. Muscle Nerve 2000;23:433.

Meseguer MA, Aparicio M, Calvo A, et al. Mycoplasma pneumoniae antigen detection in Guillain-Barré syndrome. Eur J Pediatr 1998;157:1034.

Meulstee J, van der Meche FG. Electrodiagnostic criteria for polyneuropathy and demyelination: Application in 135 patients with Guillain-Barré syndrome. Dutch Guillain-Barré Study Group. J Neurol Neurosurg Psychiatry 1995;59:482.

Mikati MA, DeLong GR. Childhood Guillain-Barré syndrome masquerading as a protracted pain syndrome. Arch Neurol 1985;42:839.

Mok CC, Lau CS, Wong RW. Neuropsychiatric manifestations and their clinical associations in southern Chinese patients with systemic lupus erythematosus. J Rheumatol 2001;28:766.

Molenaar DS, van Doorn PA, Vermeulen M. Pulsed high dose dexamethasone treatment in chronic inflammatory demyelinating polyneuropathy: A pilot study. J Neurol Neurosurg Psychiatry 1997;62:388.

Molinero MR, Varon D, Holden KR, et al. Epidemiology of childhood Guillain-Barré syndrome as a cause of acute flaccid paralysis in Honduras: 1989–1999. J Child Neurol 2003;18:741.

Mori M, Takagi K, Kuwabara S, et al. Guillain-Barré syndrome following hand-foot-and-mouth disease. Intern Med 2000;39:503.

Morosini A, Burke C, Emechete B. Polyneuritis cranialis with contrast enhancement of cranial nerves on magnetic resonance imaging. J Paediatr Child Health 2003;39:69.

Moulin DE, Hagen N, Feasby TE, et al. Pain in Guillain-Barré syndrome. Neurology 1997;48:328.

Mowzoon N, Sussman A, Bradley WG. Mycophenolate (CellCept) treatment of myasthenia gravis, chronic inflammatory polyneuropathy and inclusion body myositis. J Neurol Sci 2001;185:119.

Murthy JM. Guillain-Barré syndrome following specific viral infections: An appraisal. J Assoc Physicians India 1994;42:27.

Nadkarni N, Lisak RP. Guillain-Barré syndrome (GBS) with bilateral optic neuritis and central white matter disease. Neurology 1993;43:842.

Namiduru M, Karaoglan I, Yilmaz M. Guillain-Barré syndrome associated with acute neurobrucellosis. Int J Clin Pract 2003;57:919.

Nass R, Chutorian A. Dysaesthesias and dysautonomia: A self-limited syndrome of painful dysaesthesias and autonomic dysfunction in childhood. J Neurol Neurosurg Psychiatry 1982;45:162.

Nevo Y. Childhood chronic inflammatory demyelinating polyneuropathy. Eur J Paediatr Neurol 1998;2:169.

Nevo Y, Pestronk A, Kornberg AJ, et al. Childhood chronic inflammatory demyelinating neuropathies: Clinical course and long-term follow-up. Neurology 1996;47:98.

Ng KK, Howard RS, Fish DR, et al. Management and outcome of severe Guillain-Barré syndrome. Q J Med 1995;88:243.

Nguyen DK, Agenarioti-Belanger S, Vanasse M. Pain and the Guillain-Barré syndrome in children under 6 years old. J Pediatr 1999;134:773.

Niparko N, Goldie WD, Mitchell W, et al. The use of plasmapheresis in the management of Guillain-Barré syndrome in pediatric patients. Ann Neurol 1989;26:448.

Okumura A, Ushida H, Maruyama K, et al. Guillain-Barré syndrome associated with central nervous system lesions. Arch Dis Child 2002;86:304.

Olive JM, Castillo C, Castro RG, et al. Epidemiologic study of Guillain-Barré syndrome in children <15 years of age in Latin America. J Infect Dis 1997;175(Suppl 1):S160.

Ono S, Chida K, Takasu T. Guillain-Barré syndrome following fulminant viral hepatitis A. Intern Med 1994;33:799.

Openshaw H. Peripheral neuropathy after bone marrow transplantation. Biol Blood Marrow Transplant 1997;3:202.

Ormerod IE, Cockerell OC. Guillain-Barré syndrome after herpes zoster infection: A report of 2 cases. Eur Neurol 1993;33:156.

Ortiz Corredor F, Mieth Alviar KW. Prognostic factors for walking in childhood Guillain-Barré syndrome. Rev Neurol 2003;36:1113.

Ozen H, Cemeroglu P, Ecevit Z, et al. Unusual neurologic complications of typhoid fever (aphasia, mononeuritis multiplex, and Guillain-Barré syndrome): A report of two cases. Turk J Pediatr 1993;35:141.

Paradiso G, Tripoli J, Galicchio S, et al. Epidemiological, clinical, and electrodiagnostic findings in childhood Guillain-Barré syndrome: A reappraisal. Ann Neurol 1999;46:701.

Pentland B, Donald SM. Pain in the Guillain-Barré syndrome: A clinical review. Pain 1994;59:159.

Perry A, Mehta J, Iveson T, et al. Guillain-Barré syndrome after bone marrow transplantation. Bone Marrow Transplant 1994;14:165.

Phillips PE. Guillain-Barré syndrome after measles. BMJ 1972;4:50.

Plasma Exchange/Sandoglobulin Guillain-Barré Syndrome Trial Group. Randomised trial of plasma exchange, intravenous immunoglobulin, and combined treatments in Guillain-Barré syndrome. Lancet 1997;349:225.

Pollard JD. Chronic inflammatory demyelinating polyradiculoneuropathy. Baillieres Clin Neurol 1994;3:107.

Pollard JD. Chronic inflammatory demyelinating polyradiculoneuropathy. Curr Opin Neurol 2002;15:279.

Polo A, Manganotti P, Zanette G, et al. Polyneuritis cranialis: Clinical and electrophysiological findings. J Neurol Neurosurg Psychiatry 1992;55:398.

Polo JM, Alana-Garcia M, Cacabelos-Perez P, et al. Atypical Guillain-Barré syndrome: Multiple cranial neuropathy. Rev Neurol 2002;34:835.

Prevots DR, Sutter RW. Assessment of Guillain-Barré syndrome mortality and morbidity in the United States: Implications for acute flaccid paralysis surveillance. J Infect Dis 1997;175(Suppl 1):S151.

Rabaud C, May T, Hoen B, et al. Guillain-Barré syndrome associated with hantavirus infection. Clin Infect Dis 1995;20:477.

Rantala H, Cherry JD, Shields WD, et al. Epidemiology of Guillain-Barré syndrome in children: Relationship of oral polio vaccine administration to occurrence. J Pediatr 1994;124:220.

Rantala H, Uhari M, Cherry JD, et al. Risk factors of respiratory failure in children with Guillain-Barré syndrome. Pediatr Neurol 1995;13:289.

Rantala H, Uhari M, Niemela M. Occurrence, clinical manifestations, and prognosis of Guillain-Barré syndrome. Arch Dis Child 1991;66:706; discussion, 708.

Redford EJ, Smith KJ, Gregson NA, et al. A combined inhibitor of matrix metalloproteinase activity and tumour necrosis factor-alpha processing attenuates experimental autoimmune neuritis. Brain 1997;120:1895.

Rees JH, Gregson NA, Hughes RA. Anti-ganglioside antibodies in patients with Guillain-Barré syndrome and Campylobacter jejuni infection. J Infect Dis 1995a;172:605.

Rees JH, Soudain SE, Gregson NA, et al. Campylobacter jejuni infection and Guillain-Barré syndrome. N Engl J Med 1995b;333:1374.

Reisin RC, Cersosimo R, Garcia Alvarez M, et al. Acute "axonal" Guillain-Barré syndrome in childhood. Muscle Nerve 1993;16:1310.

Reisin RC, Pociecha J, Rodriguez E, et al. Severe Guillain-Barré syndrome in childhood treated with human immune globulin. Pediatr Neurol 1996;14:308.

Roca B, Mentero A, Simon E. Pain and opioid analgesics in Guillain-Barré syndrome. Neurology 1998;51:924.

Rodriguez-Casero MV, Shield LK, Coleman LT, et al. Childhood chronic inflammatory demyelinating polyneuropathy with central nervous system demyelination resembling multiple sclerosis. Neuromuscul Disord 2003;13:158.

Ropper AH. Intensive care of acute Guillain-Barré syndrome. Can J Neurol Sci 1994;21:S23.

Ropper AH, Shahani BT. Pain in Guillain-Barré syndrome. Arch Neurol 1984;41:511.

Rostami AM. P2-reactive T cells in inflammatory demyelination of the peripheral nerve. J Infect Dis 1997;176(Suppl 2):S160.

Ryan MM, Grattan-Smith PJ, Procopis PG, et al. Childhood chronic inflammatory demyelinating polyneuropathy: Clinical course and long-term outcome. Neuromuscul Disord 2000;10:398.

Sahashi K, Takahashi A, Ibi T, et al. Acute predominantly sensory neuropathy. Klin Wochenschr 1985;63:319.

Said G. Chronic inflammatory demyelinative polyneuropathy. J Neurol 2002;249:245.

Saida K. The immunopathology of Guillain-Barré syndrome. Curr Opin Neurol 1996;9:329.

Sakakihara Y, Kamoshita S. Age-associated changes in the symptomatology of Guillain-Barré syndrome in children. Dev Med Child Neurol 1991;33:611.

Sarada C, Tharakan JK, Nair M. Guillain-Barré syndrome. A prospective clinical study in 25 children and comparison with adults. Ann Trop Paediatr 1994;14:281.

Seneviratne U, Gunasekera S. Acute small fibre sensory neuropathy: Another variant of Guillain-Barré syndrome? J Neurol Neurosurg Psychiatry 2002;72:540.

Shahar E, Leiderman M. Outcome of severe Guillain-Barré syndrome in children: Comparison between untreated cases versus gamma-globulin therapy. Clin Neuropharmacol 2003;26:84.

Shahar E, Shorer Z, Roifman CM, et al. Immune globulins are effective in severe pediatric Guillain-Barré syndrome. Pediatr Neurol 1997;16:32.

Shapiro EE. Guillain-Barré syndrome in a child with serologic evidence of Borrelia burgdorferi infection. Pediatr Infect Dis J 1998;17:264.

Sharief MK, Ingram DA, Swash M, et al. I.V. immunoglobulin reduces circulating proinflammatory cytokines in Guillain-Barré syndrome. Neurology 1999;52:1833.

Simmons Z, Wald JJ, Albers JW. Chronic inflammatory demyelinating polyradiculoneuropathy in children: I. Presentation, electrodiagnostic studies, and initial clinical course, with comparison to adults. Muscle Nerve 1997a;20:1008.

Simmons Z, Wald JJ, Albers JW. Chronic inflammatory demyelinating polyradiculoneuropathy in children: II. Long-term follow-up, with comparison to adults. Muscle Nerve 1997b;20:1569.

Singhi SC, Jayshree M, Singhi P, et al. Intravenous immunoglobulin in very severe childhood Guillain-Barré syndrome. Ann Trop Paediatr 1999;19:167.

Sladky JT. Guillain-Barré syndrome in children. J Child Neurol 2004;19:191.

Sladky JT. Immune neuropathies in childhood. Baillieres Clin Neurol 1996;5:233.

Sladky JT, Brown MJ, Berman PH. Chronic inflammatory demyelinating polyneuropathy of infancy: A corticosteroid-responsive disorder. Ann Neurol 1986;20:76.

Steck AJ, Schaeren-Wiemers N, Hartung HP. Demyelinating inflammatory neuropathies, including Guillain-Barré syndrome. Curr Opin Neurol 1998;11:311.

Stoll G. Inflammatory cytokines in the nervous system: Multifunctional mediators in autoimmunity and cerebral ischemia. Rev Neurol (Paris) 2002;158:887.

Stratton KR, Howe CJ, Johnston RB Jr. Adverse events associated with childhood vaccines other than pertussis and rubella. Summary of a report from the Institute of Medicine. JAMA 1994;271:1602.

Susuki K, Okada M, Mori M, et al. Acute motor axonal neuropathy after mycoplasma infection: Evidence of molecular mimicry. Neurology 2004;62:949.

Tabor E. Guillain-Barré syndrome and other neurologic syndromes in hepatitis A, B, and non-A, non-B. J Med Virol 1987;21:207.

Tan MJ, Kandler R, Baxter PS. Focal neuropathy in children with critical illness. Neuropediatrics 2003;34:149.

Tanaka M. Plasmapheresis in chronic inflammatory demyelinating polyradiculoneuropathy. Rinsho Shinkeigaku 1998;38:853; author reply, 4.

Thomas NH, Collins JE, Robb SA, et al. Mycoplasma pneumoniae infection and neurological disease. Arch Dis Child 1993;69:573.

Thornton CA, Griggs RC. Plasma exchange and intravenous immunoglobulin treatment of neuromuscular disease. Ann Neurol 1994;35:260.

Toerner JG, Kumar PN, Garagusi VF. Guillain-Barré syndrome associated with Rocky Mountain spotted fever: Case report and review. Clin Infect Dis 1996;22:1090.

Toyka KV. Eighty three years of the Guillain-Barré syndrome: Clinical and immunopathologic aspects, current and future treatments. Rev Neurol (Paris) 1999;155:849.

Tsukada N, Koh CS, Inoue A, et al. Demyelinating neuropathy associated with hepatitis B virus infection. Detection of immune complexes composed of hepatitis B virus surface antigen. J Neurol Sci 1987;77:203.

Uncini A, Gallucci M, Lugaresi A, et al. CNS involvement in chronic inflammatory demyelinating polyneuropathy: an electrophysiological and MRI study. Electromyogr Clin Neurophysiol 1991;31:365.

Usui T, Hamada Y, Arita M. A case of Guillain-Barré syndrome associated with Coxsackie b-5 virus infection. Tokushima J Exp Med 1974;21:17.

Vajsar J, Fehlings D, Stephens D. Long-term outcome in children with Guillain-Barré syndrome. J Pediatr 2003;142:305.

Vajsar J, Sloane A, Wood E, et al. Plasmapheresis vs intravenous immunoglobulin treatment in childhood Guillain-Barré syndrome. Arch Pediatr Adolesc Med 1994;148:1210.

Vallat JM, Hahn AF, Leger JM, et al. Interferon beta-1a as an investigational treatment for CIDP. Neurology 2003;60(8 Suppl 3):S23.

Vallee L, Dulac O, Nuyts JP, et al. Intravenous immune globulin is also an efficient therapy of acute Guillain-Barré syndrome in affected children. Neuropediatrics 1993;24:235.

van Doorn PA, Ruts L. Treatment of chronic inflammatory demyelinating polyneuropathy. Curr Opin Neurol 2004;17:607.

Vedanarayanan VV, Kandt RS, Lewis DV Jr, et al. Chronic inflammatory demyelinating polyradiculoneuropathy of childhood: treatment with high-dose intravenous immunoglobulin. Neurology 1991;41:828.

Visser LH, van der Meche FG, Meulstee J, et al. Cytomegalovirus infection and Guillain-Barré syndrome: the clinical, electrophysiologic, and prognostic features. Dutch Guillain-Barré Study Group. Neurology 1996;47:668.

Vriesendorp FJ, Triggs WJ, Mayer RF, et al. Electrophysiological studies in Guillain-Barré syndrome: Correlation with antibodies to GM1, GD1B and Campylobacter jejuni. J Neurol 1995;242:460.

Walk D, Li LY, Parry GJ, et al. Rapid resolution of quadriplegic CIDP by combined plasmapheresis and IVIg. Neurology 2004;62:155.

Willison HJ, O'Hanlon GM. The immunopathogenesis of Miller Fisher syndrome. J Neuroimmunol 1999;100:3.

Willison HJ, Veitch J, Paterson G, et al. Miller Fisher syndrome is associated with serum antibodies to GQ1b ganglioside. J Neurol Neurosurg Psychiatry 1993;56:204.

Wilmshurst JM, Macleod MJ, Hughes E, et al. Acute sensory neuropathy in an adolescent girl following BCG vaccination. Eur J Paediatr Neurol 1999;3:277.

Winer JB, Hughes RA, Anderson MJ, et al. A prospective study of acute idiopathic neuropathy. II. Antecedent events. J Neurol Neurosurg Psychiatry 1988;51:613.

Wong V. A neurophysiological study in children with Miller Fisher syndrome and Guillain-Barré syndrome. Brain Dev 1997;19:197.

Yu S, Chen Z, Mix E, et al. Neutralizing antibodies to IL-18 ameliorate experimental autoimmune neuritis by counter-regulation of autoreactive Th1 responses to peripheral myelin antigen. J Neuropathol Exp Neurol 2002;61:614.

Yuki N. Infectious origins of, and molecular mimicry in, Guillain-Barré and Fisher syndromes. Lancet Infect Dis 2001;1:29.

Zochodne DW. Autonomic involvement in Guillain-Barré syndrome: A review. Muscle Nerve 1994;17:1145.

Zochodne DW, Bolton CF. Neuromuscular disorders in critical illness. Baillieres Clin Neurol 1996;5:645.

Zou LP, Abbas N, Volkmann I, et al. Suppression of experimental autoimmune neuritis by ABR-215062 is associated with altered Th1/Th2 balance and inhibited migration of inflammatory cells into the peripheral nerve tissue. Neuropharmacology 2002;42:731.

Zou LP, Deretzi G, Pelidou SH, et al. Rolipram suppresses experimental autoimmune neuritis and prevents relapses in Lewis rats. Neuropharmacology 2000;39:324.

Zou LP, Ma MH, Wei L, et al. IFN-beta suppresses experimental autoimmune neuritis in Lewis rats by inhibiting the migration of inflammatory cells into peripheral nervous tissue. J Neurosci Res 1999;56:123.

CHAPTER 78

Diseases of the Neuromuscular Junction

Gil I. Wolfe and Richard J. Barohn

Both acquired and inherited disorders of the neuromuscular junction occur in childhood. As with adults, the most common neuromuscular junction disorders are autoimmune and respond to immunosuppressive therapy. These include myasthenia gravis and the rarer Lambert-Eaton myasthenic syndrome. A number of genetically determined disorders of neuromuscular transmission, the congenital myasthenic syndromes, are unique to childhood and are discussed later in this chapter. Botulism, a toxin-mediated disorder of the neuromuscular junction, most commonly occurs in infancy. All neuromuscular junction disorders have the ability to produce generalized weakness and fatigability with a propensity for oculobulbar involvement. Electrophysiologic studies detect an impairment of neuromuscular transmission in most of these disorders [Harper, 1996]. Before the various neuromuscular junction disorders are described, normal relevant physiology is reviewed.

THE NEUROMUSCULAR JUNCTION

Familiarity with the pathophysiology, diagnosis, and treatment of neuromuscular junction disorders requires a fundamental understanding of normal neuromuscular transmission (Fig. 78-1). Acetylcholine is the natural neurotransmitter of the neuromuscular junction. It is synthesized and stored in vesicles in the motor nerve terminal [Drachman, 1978; Miller, 1985]. Each vesicle contains a quantum (about 10,000 molecules) of neurotransmitter. At rest, individual vesicles spontaneously release their quantum of acetylcholine at special release sites on the presynaptic membrane. The released neurotransmitter migrates and binds to acetylcholine receptors (AchRs) located on the postsynaptic membrane, producing a transient increase in the permeability of sodium and potassium ions. The local endplate depolarization that results is known as a *miniature endplate potential.* It has been hypothesized that miniature endplate potentials help to maintain resting muscle tone by producing a perpetual background of cholinergic stimulation [Liu and Erickson, 1994].

Miniature endplate potentials are dwarfed by the larger depolarizations that occur when nerve action potentials arrive at the presynaptic terminal. The nerve action potentials rapidly depolarize the presynaptic membrane. Depolarization produces an influx of calcium ions into the motor terminal, leading to exocytosis of a large number of acetylcholine vesicles (150 to 200 quanta). The resulting postsynaptic depolarization is termed an *endplate potential.* Because of a physiologic safety factor, the endplate potential is normally sufficient to generate an action potential along the muscle membrane. Propagation of this muscle action potential leads to a cascade of events that drives muscle contraction.

The amplitude of the endplate potential is directly related to the number of acetylcholine molecules that bind to their receptors. Normally an adequate number of neurotransmitter-receptor interactions occurs to produce a muscle action potential [Miller, 1985]. As discussed later, the immunologic defect in myasthenia gravis directly reduces this safety margin, and muscle weakness ensues.

Neuromuscular transmission is rapid, taking only milliseconds to complete the entire sequence. The process is terminated by diffusion of acetylcholine from the synapse and its rapid hydrolysis by acetylcholinesterase [Liu and Erickson, 1994].

By 20 weeks of gestation, the structure of the neuromuscular junction is well established, with further refinement of the postsynaptic membrane continuing until term [Sanes and Jessell, 2000]. Clustering of AchR in utero depends on muscle-specific receptor tyrosine kinase (MuSK) and rapsyn. Both the AchR and MuSK have been implicated as postsynaptic targets of the immune system in myasthenia gravis [Hoch et al., 2001]. Other neuromuscular junction antigens targeted by plasma factors are likely to be discovered in the future (Plested et al., 2002).

AUTOIMMUNE MYASTHENIA GRAVIS

Myasthenia gravis is the best understood autoimmune disease of the nervous system [Vincent et al., 2001]. The immune-mediated nature of myasthenia gravis was suspected as early as 1960 when Simpson speculated that it was an autoimmune disease with antibodies directed against the skeletal muscle AchR. A series of breakthroughs in the 1970s confirmed Simpson's hypothesis. Lindstrom and colleagues [1976a; Patrick and Lindstrom, 1973] developed the animal model of experimental autoimmune myasthenia gravis by immunizing rabbits and rats with highly purified AchR from the electric organ of the eel. Not only did the animals develop weakness and respiratory insufficiency in about 3 weeks, but they also responded to anticholinesterase medications and demonstrated typical decremental responses on repetitive nerve stimulation [Seybold et al., 1976]. These animals also had high anti-AchR antibody titers in serum. Subsequently, these titers were found in the serum of myasthenia gravis patients [Lindstrom et al., 1976b]. Engel and co-workers [Engel and Arahata, 1987; Engel et al., 1977b] localized both the immunoglobulin G (IgG) antibody and complement to the myasthenia motor endplate. This finding implied that circulating IgG antibody directed against the AchR became bound to the postsynaptic

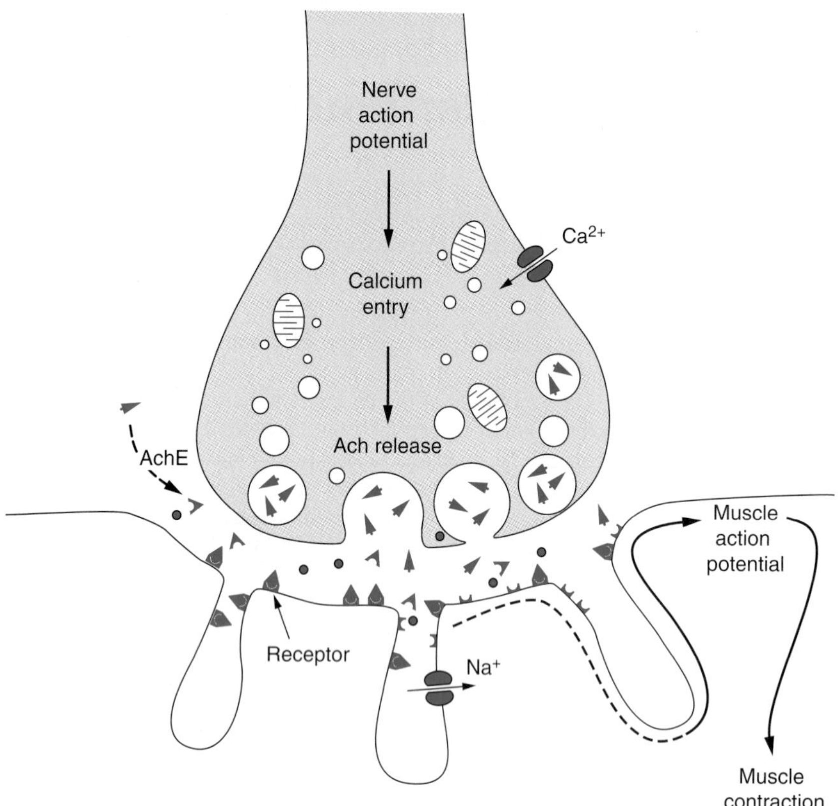

FIGURE 78-1. Diagram of the neuromuscular junction. At top, a nerve action potential arrives at the motor terminal and produces rapid depolarization. The depolarization initiates an influx of calcium ions into the motor axon, which leads to synchronized fusion of vesicles containing acetylcholine (Ach) with the presynaptic membrane. Released Ach molecules diffuse across the synapse, bind to their postsynaptic receptors, and generate a localized endplate potential (EPP). If the EPP reaches threshold, the muscle membrane undergoes an increase in sodium conductance, with subsequent generation of a muscle action potential. Propagation of the muscle action potential through the muscle fiber culminates in a cascade of events that drive contraction. Neuromuscular transmission is terminated by diffusion of Ach from the synapse and its rapid cleavage by acetylcholinesterase (AchE).

membrane and activated the terminal complement sequence (C5b-9), or membrane attack complex, which resulted in lysis of the AchR with subsequent degeneration.

Elevated membrane attack complex levels have been demonstrated in the plasma of patients with myasthenia gravis [Barohn and Brey, 1993]. Anti-AchR antibody has also been found to block neuromuscular transmission and accelerate turnover of AchR crosslinked by IgG [Drachman, 1978]. As a result of this process, the postsynaptic membrane becomes simplified, with decreased junctional folds [Engel et al., 1976]. In addition, the neuromuscular blockade is passively transferred by injecting animals with IgG from myasthenia gravis patients [Toyka et al., 1977]. The same phenomenon occurs when an infant born to a mother with myasthenia gravis exhibits symptoms at birth, so-called neonatal myasthenia gravis [Papazian, 1992].

The AchR is a large protein consisting of five subunits, and the antibody response in myasthenia gravis and experimental autoimmune myasthenia gravis is polyclonal. The portion of the protein primarily responsible for inducing antibodies that produce the disease is debated. Although the existence of a main immunogenic region in the alpha subunit has been promoted [Tzartos and Lindstrom, 1980], other investigators have challenged this evidence [Lennon and Greismann, 1989]. It is possible that if the most pathogenic determinants of the AchR can be identified, a more rational and specific immune therapy can be designed [Krolick et al., 1994].

The process that initiates the immune-mediated neuromuscular junction dysfunction is still unknown. The thymus gland may play a role, inasmuch as 75% of myasthenia gravis patients who undergo thymectomy have thymic pathologic findings; 15% are tumors of the thymus, and the remainder consist of lymphoid hyperplasia [Castleman, 1966]. Lymphocytes in the thymus and peripheral blood appear to be sensitized to muscle in myasthenia gravis patients [Sommer et al., 1990, 1991]. Muscle-like myoid cells are found in the thymus gland, and thymus tissue from myasthenia gravis patients with and without thymoma is enriched in AchR-reactive T cells [Kao and Drachman, 1977; Wekerle et al., 1975]. The close association of lymphocytes and myoid cells in the thymus, along with some stimulus causing the disruption of immune tolerance, may lead to the autoimmune response. There may be a hereditary predisposition to develop myasthenia gravis because there is an increased incidence of certain human leukocyte antigens in various myasthenia gravis populations [Behan, 1980; Compston et al., 1980].

Clinical Features

Myasthenia gravis has a prevalence of approximately 125 cases per million population [Drachman, 1994]. Approximately 11% to 24% of all patients with myasthenia gravis experience disease onset in childhood or adolescence [Millichap and Dodge, 1960; Simpson, 1958]. There is a slight female predominance of 3:2 at those ages but a male predominance in older age groups. The disease can arise at any age, but peaks are observed in the third and sixth decades.

Myasthenia gravis is characterized by weakness and fatigability of ocular, bulbar, and extremity striated muscles. The ocular manifestations are ptosis and diplopia, whereas the bulbar manifestations are dysarthria, dysphagia, and dyspnea. Proximal muscles tend to be weaker than distal extremity muscles. Symptoms of myasthenia gravis tend to worsen with stress, with exertion, and as the day progresses. These temporal symptoms, however, may be difficult to elicit in many patients. Myasthenic crisis, characterized by respiratory weakness and the inability to handle secretions or swallow, may punctuate a more stable clinical course in some children.

The best data on the natural history of myasthenia gravis are from Grob and co-workers [1987], who carefully studied more than 1400 patients between 1940 and 1985. Some of the key points from their work are as follows:

- Most patients present with ocular symptoms. Initial symptoms were ocular in 53% (ptosis in 25%, diplopia in 25%, blurred vision in 3%); leg, arm, face, neck, or trunk weakness in 20%; bulbar symptoms in 16% (difficulty swallowing in 6%, slurred or nasal speech in 5%, difficulty chewing in 4%, dyspnea in 1%); and generalized fatigue in 9%.
- Most patients exhibit progression of the disease. One year after onset, the disease was purely ocular in 40%, generalized in 35%, confined to the extremities in 10%, and bulbar or oculobulbar in 15%. However, myasthenia gravis remained purely ocular in only 14% over the entire follow-up period. Therefore, 86% of patients eventually progress to generalized involvement.
- If a patient with ocular myasthenia gravis is going to develop general symptoms, this occurs relatively early. Of the patients who presented with purely ocular disease, 56% progressed to generalized disease by 6 months, 78% by the first year, 85% by the second year, and 92% by the third year.
- Mortality statistics for myasthenia gravis have fallen dramatically over time. Between 1940 and 1957, the mortality rate was 31%, whereas between 1966 and 1985, the mortality rate was 7%. The two primary reasons for this reduced mortality rate were the improvement in intensive respiratory care and the introduction of corticosteroids. Death from myasthenia gravis is an uncommon event in current practice.

Clinical Classification

Osserman [1958] classified myasthenia gravis patients according to disease severity. The most commonly used modification of the original classification is as follows:

- Group I: ocular
- Group IIA: mild generalized
- Group IIB: moderate-to-severe generalized
- Group III: acute, severe, developing over weeks to months
- Group IV: late, severe with marked bulbar involvement

The Osserman classification has several shortcomings, including the vague descriptive terminology and lack of distinctions between some of the groups. For instance, differentiating between mild and moderate generalized disease may be difficult. The scheme also fails to include a category for patients in remission. Other myasthenia gravis classifications have been developed to more clearly differentiate between mild, moderate, and severe disease states and to include remission as a separate category [Barohn and Jackson, 1994; Mohan et al., 1994]. A task force of the Myasthenia Gravis Foundation of America developed a new classification system (Box 78-1) that is more descriptive and provides better distinction between classes [Barohn, 2003; Jaretzki et al., 2000].

Box 78-1 Myasthenia Gravis Foundation of America (MGFA) Classification System

Class I: Any ocular muscle weakness; there may be weakness of eye closure. All other muscle strength is normal.

Class II: Mild weakness affecting muscles other than ocular muscles; there may also be ocular muscle weakness of any severity.

IIa. Predominantly affecting limb, axial muscles, or both. There may also be lesser involvement of oropharyngeal muscles.

IIb. Predominantly affecting oropharyngeal, respiratory muscles, or both. There may also be lesser or equal involvement of limb, axial muscles, or both.

Class III: Moderate weakness affecting muscles other than ocular muscles; there may also be ocular muscle weakness of any severity.

IIIa. Predominantly affecting limb, axial muscles, or both. There may also be lesser involvement of oropharyngeal muscles.

IIIb. Predominantly affecting oropharyngeal, respiratory muscles, or both. There may also be lesser or equal involvement of limb, axial muscles, or both.

Class IV: Severe weakness affecting muscles other than ocular muscles; there may also be ocular muscle weakness of any severity.

IVa. Predominantly affecting limb, axial muscles, or both. There may also be lesser involvement of oropharyngeal muscles.

IVb. Predominantly affecting oropharyngeal, respiratory muscles, or both. There may also be lesser or equal involvement of limb, axial muscles, or both.

Class V: Defined as intubation, with or without mechanical ventilation, except when used during routine postoperative management. The use of a feeding tube without intubation places the patient in class IVb.

Categories of Myasthenia Gravis in Childhood

Autoimmune myasthenia gravis in children is most commonly divided into neonatal transient and juvenile types.

Neonatal transient myasthenia gravis occurs in infants of myasthenic mothers. Placental transfer of anti-AchR antibody or immunocytes results in transient impairment of neuromuscular transmission in the neonate [Barlow, 1981; Donaldson et al., 1981]. Findings such as a weak suck or cry, ptosis, dysphagia, generalized weakness, decreased spontaneous movement, and respiratory distress are usually present in the first few hours of life but may not be evident until the third day [Millichap and Dodge, 1960]. Hypotonia may be the primary manifestation. The disorder usually resolves in the first 4 weeks but may persist for months [Branch et al., 1978; Desmedt and Borenstein, 1977]. The severity of the disorder in the infant is not correlated with the degree of maternal involvement. A prior history of neonatal myasthenia gravis in a sibling is the only predictive factor. Fortunately, only 10% to 15% of infants born to myasthenic mothers develop the disorder [Ahlsten et al., 1992; Fraser and Turner, 1953; Namba et al., 1970]. Prior thymectomy or remission of disease in the mother does not prevent development of neonatal transient myasthenia gravis [Elias et al., 1979; Geddes and Kidd, 1951]. Careful monitoring of pregnant women with myasthenia gravis is critical because there is a 40% chance of disease exacerbation during pregnancy and a 30% risk in the puerperium. The perinatal mortality rate is approximately 68 per 1000 births, five times the risk in uncomplicated pregnancies [Plauche, 1991].

Juvenile myasthenia gravis represents the childhood onset of autoimmune myasthenia gravis seen in adults. The onset is usually after 10 years of age, and disease manifestations appear before puberty in half the cases. Onset before 1 year of age is exceptional [Andrews et al., 1993; Fenichel, 1978; Geh and Bradbury, 1998]. Juvenile myasthenia gravis is more common in girls, but a large proportion of cases in boys is prepubertal [Anlar et al., 1996; Batocchi et al., 1990; Rodriguez et al., 1983]. In one study, predominance was in girls at a rate of 1.3:1 in prepubertal cases, in comparison with 1.8:1 in peripubertal and 14:1 in postpubertal cases [Andrews et al., 1993]. As with adults, ptosis is the most common clinical finding, frequently accompanied by ophthalmoparesis (Fig. 78-2). Ptosis was unilateral at onset in one third of patients with juvenile myasthenia gravis but subsequently spread to the other eye in nearly 90% of cases [Afifi and Bell, 1993]. Facial and oropharyngeal weakness, other common findings, lead to dysarthria, dysphagia, and difficulty chewing. Facial weakness without ocular involvement is an unusual but recognized presentation of juvenile myasthenia gravis [Kini, 1995]. Extremity weakness can occur and is usually most prominent proximally. Bulbar weakness, characterized by slow chewing, dysphagia, nasal dysarthria, and weak cough, develops in up to 75% of patients [Rodriguez et al., 1983]. Respiratory failure from either diaphragmatic or intercostal muscle weakness or airway compromise related to bulbar dysfunction produces myasthenic crisis, an exacerbation severe enough to endanger the patient's life. As in adults, the disease may be generalized at onset, but isolated ocular involvement is a more common presentation, followed by generalization at a later time. However, children with ocular myasthenia gravis appear more likely than adults to remain with purely ocular involvement and not progress to generalized disease. As many as 85% of adults with ocular myasthenia gravis later develop generalized disease [Evoli et al., 1988; Weinberg et al., 1994]. In children, this percentage is closer to 50% to 75% [Afifi and Bell, 1993; Andrews, 2004]. In children of Chinese descent, pure ocular myasthenia gravis is the predominant disease type and has been linked to certain human leukocyte antigen types [Chan-Lui et al., 1984; Hawkins et al., 1989].

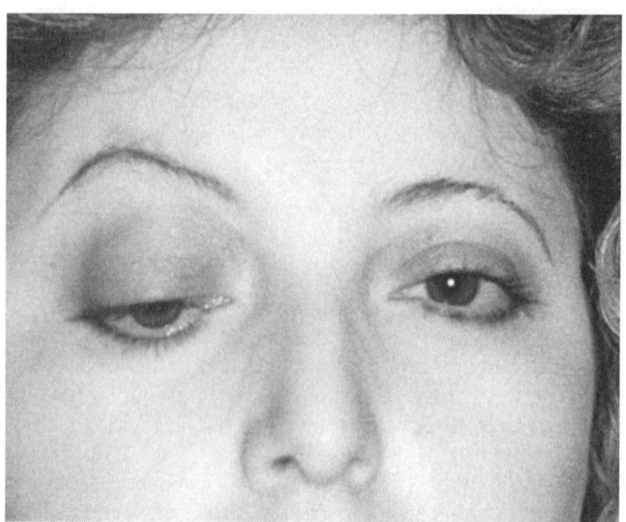

FIGURE 78-2. Ptosis of the right eyelid in a young woman with juvenile myasthenia gravis. A hypertropia of the left eye is also present.

Myasthenia gravis is frequently associated with other diseases, specifically those with an immune etiology. The most common associations are with rheumatoid arthritis, thyroid disease, systemic lupus erythematosus, and diabetes mellitus [Afifi and Bell, 1993; Millichap and Dodge, 1960; Rodriguez et al., 1983]. Nonimmune disorders associated with juvenile myasthenia gravis include epilepsy in 3% to 13% [Rodriguez et al., 1983; Snead et al., 1980] and various forms of neoplasia, particularly thymoma and, later in life, breast carcinoma. Thymoma cases in juvenile myasthenia gravis, present in fewer than 5% of children with myasthenia gravis [Rodriguez et al., 1983], are rare in comparison with adult cases and are found mainly in children with onset of myasthenia gravis in adolescence [Andrews, 2004].

Neurologic Examination

On examination, it is important to determine whether ptosis is present. Normally the upper eyelid should be positioned at least 1 mm above the pupil. Observing for upper eyelid fatigue in sustained upward gaze can be helpful, but this phenomenon is often not present and may be difficult to assess in children. Any restriction of ocular motility is documented, as is whether the patient has diplopia in primary position, on horizontal gaze to the right or left, or on vertical gaze.

Testing for weakness in the orbicularis oculi muscle is crucial but often overlooked. Many patients with symptomatic myasthenia gravis have bilateral weakness of this muscle group. Strength should also be tested in the lower facial muscles (blowing out cheeks against resistance) and in the tongue. Attention to speech patterns may disclose a nasal dysarthria. It is important to check for neck flexion and extension weakness because those muscle groups are frequently involved. Testing of extremity strength should include proximal and distal muscle groups in the arms and legs. Proximal limb muscles tend to be more affected than distal muscles. In rare cases, however, patients with myasthenia gravis may demonstrate a tendency for weakness in distal muscle groups, especially finger extensors [Nations et al., 1997].

Symptoms and signs can be quantified by using a validated myasthenia gravis scoring system and activities of

TABLE 78-1

Quantitative Myasthenia Gravis Scale

TEST ITEM	GRADE 0	1	2	3
Double vision on lateral gaze **right** or **left** (circle one)	61 seconds	11-60 seconds	1-10 seconds	Spontaneous
Ptosis (upward gaze)	61 seconds	11-60 seconds	1-10 seconds	Spontaneous
Facial muscles	Normal lid	Complete, weak, some resistance	Complete, without resistance	Incomplete
Swallowing 4 oz. of water (1/2 cup)	Normal	Minimal coughing or throat clearing	Severe coughing/choking or nasal regurgitation	Cannot swallow (test not attempted)
Speech following counting aloud from 1-50 (onset of dysarthria)	None at #50	Dysarthria at #30-49	Dysarthria at #10-29	Dysarthria at #9
Right arm outstretched (90 degrees sitting)	240 seconds	90-239 seconds	10-89 seconds	0-9 seconds
Left arm outstretched (90 degrees sitting)	240 seconds	90-239 seconds	10-89 seconds	0-9 seconds
Vital capacity (% predicted)	≥80%	65%-79%	50%-64%	<50%
Right hand grip				
Male (kg-force)	≥45	15-44	5-14	0-4
Female	≥30	10-29	5-9	0-4
Left hand grip				
Male (kg-force)	≥35	15-34	5-14	0-4
Female	≥5	10-24	5-9	0-4
Head, lifted (45 degrees supine)	120 seconds	30-119 seconds	1-29 seconds	0 seconds
Right leg outstretched (45 degrees supine)	100 seconds	31-99 seconds	1-30 seconds	0 seconds
Left leg outstretched (45 degrees supine)	100 seconds	31-99 seconds	1-30 seconds	0 seconds
Total QMG Score ______				

From Barohn RJ, McIntire D, Herbelin L, et al. Reliability testing of the quantitative myasthenia gravis score. Ann N Y Acad Sci 1998;841:769.

TABLE 78-2

Myasthenia Gravis Activities of Daily Living Scale

TEST ITEM	GRADE 0	1	2	3
Talking	Normal	Intermittent slurring or nasal speech	Constant slurring or nasal, but can be understood	Difficult to understand speech
Chewing	Normal	Fatigue with solid food	Fatigue with soft food	Gastric tube
Swallowing	Normal	Rare episode of choking	Frequent choking, necessitating changes in diet	Gastric tube
Breathing	Normal	Shortness of breath with exertion	Shortness of breath at rest	Ventilator dependence
Impairment of ability to brush teeth or comb hair	None	Extra effort, but no rest periods needed	Rest periods needed	Cannot do one of these functions
Impairment of ability to arise from a chair	None	Mild, sometimes uses arms	Moderate, always uses arms	Severe, requires assistance
Double vision	None	Occurs, but not daily	Daily, but not constant	Constant
Eyelid droop	None	Occurs, but not daily	Daily, but not constant	Constant
Total MG-ADL Score ______				

From Wolfe GI, Herbelin L, Nations SP, et al. Myasthenia gravis activities of daily living profile. Neurology 1999;52:1487.

daily living scale (Tables 78-1 and 78-2). The activities of daily living score is correlated with the objective quantitative myasthenia gravis score [Wolfe et al., 1999]. A Myasthenia Gravis Foundation of America task force has recommended that the quantitative myasthenia gravis score be used as an outcome measure for therapy trials in myasthenia gravis [Barohn, 2003; Jaretzki et al., 2000]. The scales are readily administered to adolescents as young as 15 years of age [Barohn et al., 1998].

Clinical and Laboratory Tests

In most instances, the clinician can be confident about the diagnosis of myasthenia gravis on the basis of abnormalities revealed through the neurologic history and examination. However, one or more tests are usually performed to confirm the clinical diagnosis.

Edrophonium (Tensilon) Test

The intravenous administration of up to 10 mg of edrophonium is often the first diagnostic test performed in the evaluation of a potential myasthenia gravis patient. However, the edrophonium test has a number of pitfalls. The most common mistake is that the physician performing the test does not have an objective parameter to measure before and after edrophonium administration. The most useful parameter is the degree of ptosis in each eye. The best indication of a positive test result is a significant increase in the palpebral fissure aperture or the opening of a completely ptotic eye. If no ptosis is present, the edrophonium test result may be difficult to interpret even in clear-cut cases of myasthenia gravis. If the patient has a severe restriction of extraocular movement and edrophonium dramatically improves the motility, the test result is considered positive. However, subjective diplopia may not resolve unless edrophonium corrects alignment for both eyes, which is rare. Significant improvement in dysarthria or in swallowing is another indication of a positive edrophonium test result. A mild improvement in limb strength or in subjective well-being is not sufficient for claiming a positive result. In addition, a positive edrophonium test result is not specific because transient subjective improvement is reported in other neurologic disorders, such as motor neuron disease and peripheral neuropathy [Oh and Cho, 1990].

The edrophonium test is performed in a straightforward manner. First, 1 mL (10 mg) of edrophonium is drawn up into a 1-mL tuberculin syringe. The edrophonium is often injected directly into a vein (usually antecubital), but in smaller children, a "butterfly" intravenous line can be started, connecting the tuberculin syringe directly to the intravenous catheter. In children weighing less than 30 kg, the total delivered dose should not exceed 0.1 mg/kg. For children weighing more than 30 kg, a total dose up to 0.2 mg/kg may be given, not to exceed 10 mg. Initially, a test dose of 0.01 mg/kg is injected. If after 30 to 60 seconds the patient experiences no side effects from the drug (fasciculations, sweating, nausea), further aliquots of 0.01 to 0.02 mg/kg are injected, not exceeding the total dose suggested. When the drug is injected into an intravenous catheter, catheter flushes with saline are needed with each aliquot. Children are more likely than adults to experience nausea, and so an emesis basin should be available. More serious side effects, such as bronchospasm or lightheadedness caused by bradycardia, are quite uncommon, but atropine should be readily available. When either side effects or a positive response is obtained, no further edrophonium need be given. The mean dose of edrophonium needed to produce a positive response was 3.3 mg (±1.6 mg standard deviation) for ptosis and 2.6 mg (±1.1 mg standard deviation) for oculomotor dysfunction in a survey of 83 adult patients [Kupersmith et al., 2003].

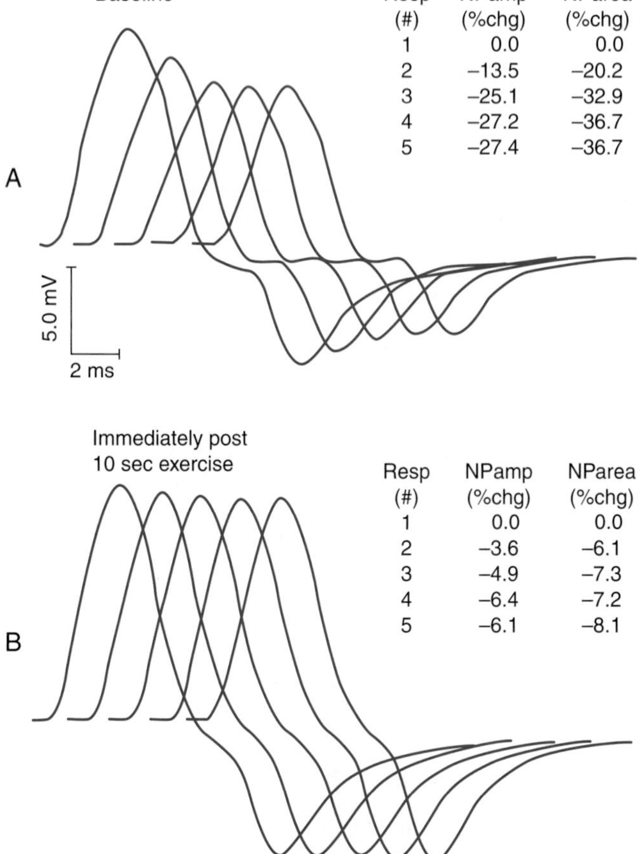

FIGURE 78-3. Repetitive stimulation of the ulnar nerve at 3 Hz, recorded in the adductor digiti minimi. **A,** Baseline; there is an abnormal amplitude decrement of 27%. **B,** Immediately after 10 seconds of exercise, the decrement has resolved, demonstrating postexercise facilitation. NPamp, negative peak amplitude; NParea, negative peak area; Resp, response.

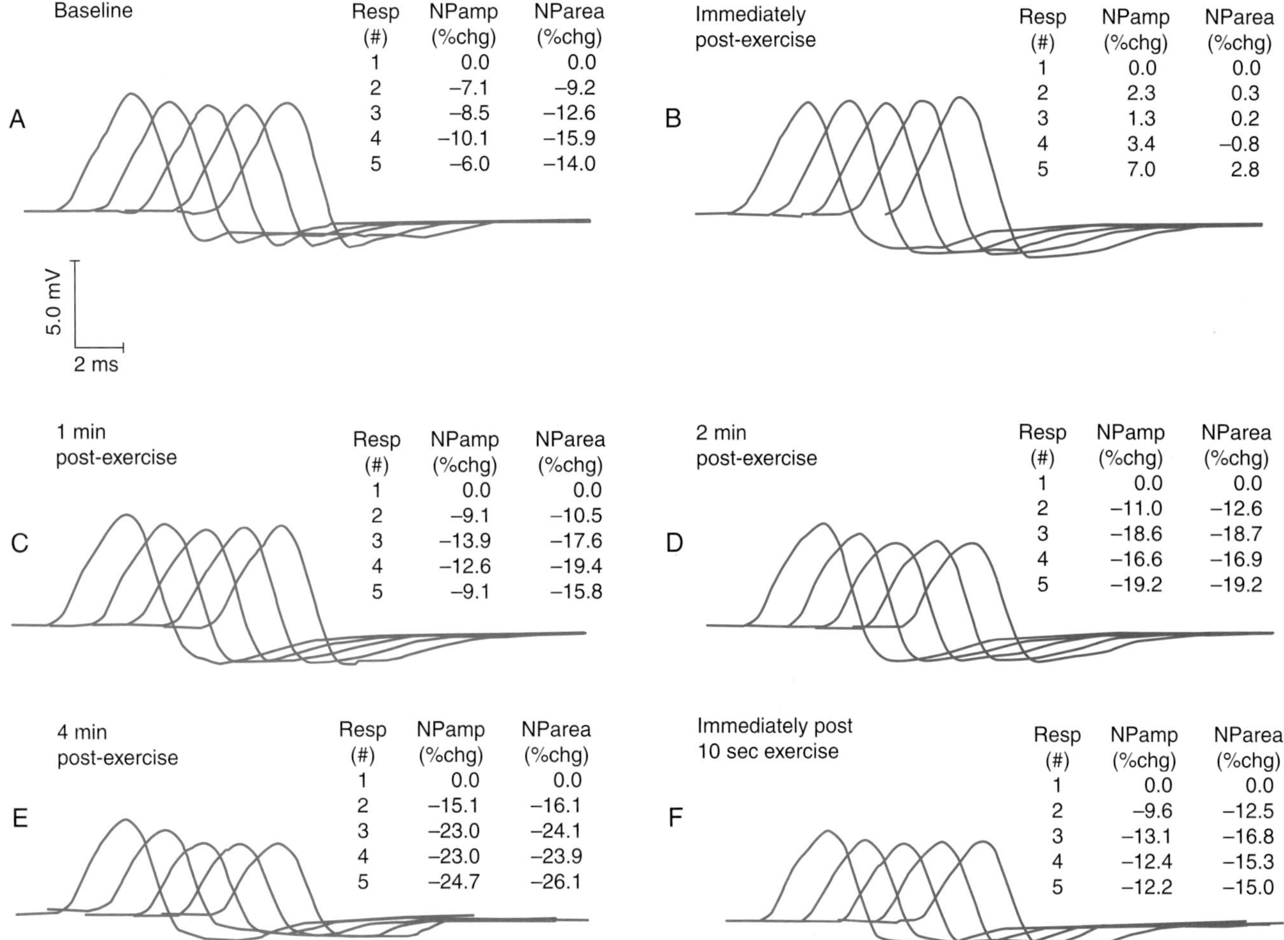

FIGURE 78-4. Repetitive stimulation (RS) of the ulnar nerve at 3 Hz, recorded in the adductor digiti minimi. At baseline (**A**), there is only a borderline decrement at response 4. Immediately after exercise (**B**), there is no decrement, but a 12% to 14% decrement develops 1 minute (**C**) after exercise, and this worsens at 2 and 4 minutes (**D** and **E**), demonstrating postexercise exhaustion. After 10 seconds of brief exercise (**F**), the decrement improves. NPamp, negative peak amplitude; NParea, negative peak area; Resp, response.

If a patient has ptosis, it is crucial that the palpebral fissure aperture be measured and its size recorded before and after edrophonium administration. In most children a placebo injection before edrophonium is likely unnecessary. In patients with less objective findings that do not enable easy measurement, edrophonium should likely not be given in the first place. Thus a placebo injection is rarely useful.

In infants and younger children who are too uncooperative to monitor for a brief time, longer acting neostigmine may be favored over edrophonium. The intramuscular dose is 0.15 mg/kg and intravenous dose 0.05 mg/kg [Andrews, 2004]. Intravenous use can be hazardous because of severe muscarinic side effects [Wolfe et al., 1997]. A positive response is generally evident by 15 minutes and is most obvious after 30 minutes. Positive results on edrophonium or neostigmine testing are seen in up to 90% of juvenile myasthenia gravis cases [Afifi and Bell, 1993]. It is a good idea to have injectable atropine available in the case of severe side effects whenever neostigmine is used.

Electrophysiologic Testing

REPETITIVE STIMULATION

The classic electrophysiologic demonstration of a neuromuscular junction transmission defect is the documentation of a decremental response of the compound muscle action potential to repetitive stimulation of a motor nerve [Oh, 1988]. The decrement results from failure of some muscle fibers to reach threshold and contract when successive volleys of acetylcholine vesicles are released at the neuromuscular junction. Failure to reach the threshold endplate potential to achieve muscle contraction is called *blocking.* The percentage decreases in amplitude and area are calculated between the first compound muscle action potential produced by a train of stimuli and each successive potential. In most laboratories, five or six responses are obtained at 2 or 3 Hz, and the maximal percentage decrement can be measured at the fourth or fifth response. A decrement exceeding 10% is considered a positive result of a repetitive stimulation study (Fig. 78-3).

In some patients a decremental response can be demonstrated at baseline. However, often a brief period of exercise (usually 1 minute) is necessary to elicit fatigue in the neuromuscular junction so that the decrement can be observed. This phenomenon of postexercise exhaustion usually occurs at 2 to 4 minutes after exercise (Fig. 78-4). In addition, postexercise facilitation, or an improvement in the decrement, can sometimes be observed immediately (within seconds) after brief exercise (see Fig. 78-3).

Repetitive stimulation is typically first recorded in a distal thenar or hypothenar muscle after the median or ulnar nerve, respectively, is stimulated. If no decrement is observed, repetitive stimulation can be performed on a proximal limb muscle (i.e., trapezius, deltoid, or biceps) or on a facial muscle (orbicularis oculi). An arm board is used to immobilize the hand muscles. False-positive results are more of a problem in proximal limb muscles because of motion artifact.

Because repetitive stimulation is a reflection of the integrity of neuromuscular junction transmission, a decrement is more often observed in clinically weak muscles. Thus, even if a patient has generalized myasthenia gravis and if there is only facial and proximal limb weakness, a decrement in a hand muscle is unlikely. In a patient with pure ocular myasthenia gravis a decrement may not be present in the orbicularis oculi unless that muscle is found to be weak on examination.

As with the edrophonium test, repetitive stimulation does not have to be performed on every patient with myasthenia gravis if the diagnosis is certain according to the clinical findings and a positive finding of anti-AchR antibody.

A protocol for repetitive stimulation of the ulnar nerve recording over the adductor digiti minimi is as follows:

- Apply electrodes and immobilize the patient's hand.
- Obtain a normal baseline compound muscle action potential and increase to supramaximal intensity.
- If there is a small compound muscle action potential amplitude at baseline, screen for Lambert-Eaton myasthenic syndrome before doing repetitive stimulation (see later discussion).
- After establishing a stable baseline compound muscle action potential, give five shocks at 3 Hz.
- If there is no decrement, exercise the hand by having the patient spread the fingers for 1 minute. Repeat repetitive stimulation immediately after exercise and 1, 2, 3, 4, and 6 minutes after exercise.
- If there is a decrement after exercise (postexercise exhaustion), briefly exercise the muscle again for 10 seconds and repeat repetitive stimulation at 3 Hz. If the decrement improves, this indicates postexercise facilitation.
- If there is a marked decrement at baseline to 3-Hz repetitive stimulation (>20%), exercise for only 10 seconds and repeat repetitive stimulation immediately. If the decrement improves, this is also postexercise facilitation. In this case, the protocol for demonstrating postexercise exhaustion described previously is optional.

A decremental response is more likely present in a proximal muscle than in a distal muscle. In the series by Stalberg and Sanders [1981], a decrement in a distal muscle was

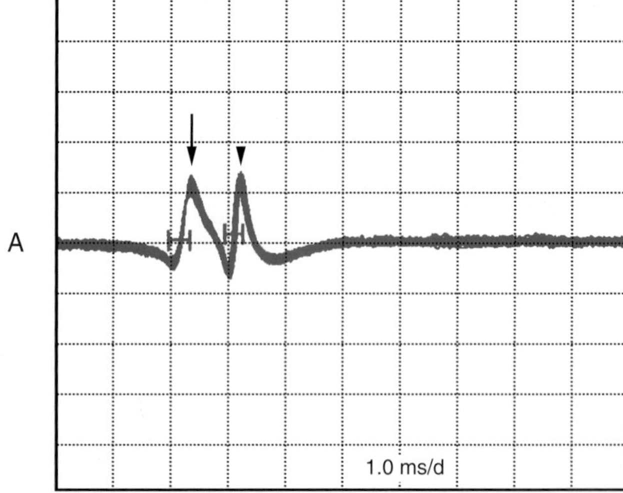

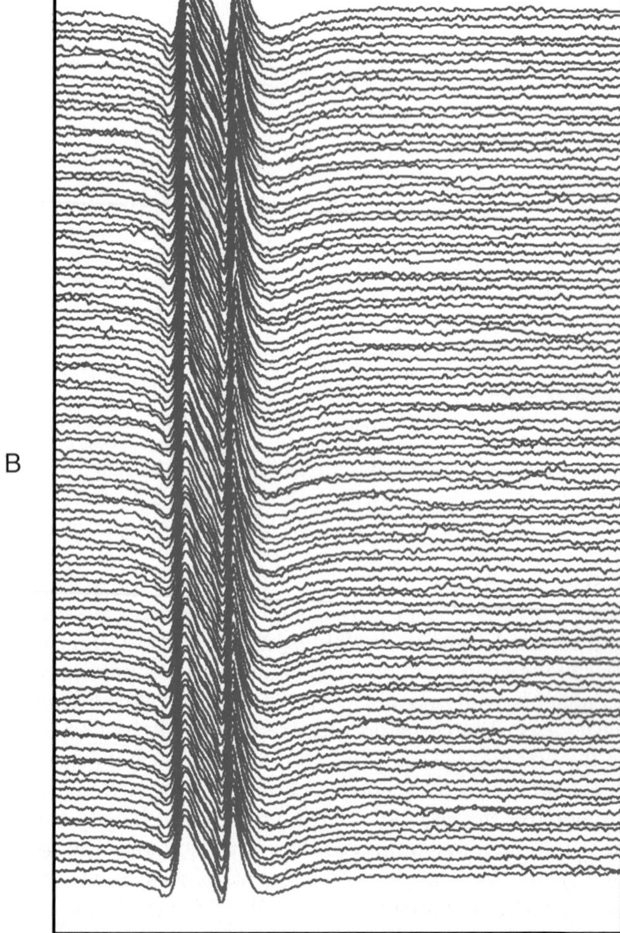

FIGURE 78-5. Recruited single-fiber electromyogram of the extensor digitorum communis muscle. The single-fiber needle is inserted in the muscle with the patient extending the digit so that action potentials from at least two muscle fibers from the same motor unit are recorded (**A**). A trigger is placed on the initial potential under the *arrow*. Because both potentials are from the same motor unit, the second potential (under the *arrowhead*) appears at approximately the same time in relation to the triggered potential. One hundred successive acquisitions are obtained (**B**). The degree of variability in the time that the second potential occurs in the successive pairs is the jitter, measured as the mean consecutive difference. In this normal pair, the mean consecutive difference is 14.3 microseconds (normal <35 microseconds).

reported in 38% of patients, whereas a decrement in proximal muscles occurred in 64%. Similar findings have been described by other authors [Oh et al., 1992; Vial et al., 1991]. In a study of 27 juvenile myasthenic patients, Afifi and Bell [1993] found that the chance of finding a decrement was doubled to 66% by including proximal muscles. In children with generalized disease at onset, 80% demonstrated a decrement when proximal muscles were studied. In ocular myasthenia gravis, decrements are less common, occurring in 20% to 50% of patients [Evoli et al., 1988; Stalberg and Sanders, 1981]. Repetitive stimulation at faster rates (i.e., 20 or 50 Hz) is usually not performed unless there is con-cern about Lambert-Eaton myasthenic syndrome, a rare condition in children.

SINGLE-FIBER ELECTROMYOGRAPHY

Conventional electromyography is rarely helpful in the diagnosis of myasthenia gravis in children. Single-fiber electromyography, however, is a more sensitive measure of neuromuscular transmission than is repetitive stimulation and can be considered in selected children. In myasthenia gravis, the time required for the endplate potential at the neuromuscular junction to reach threshold is extremely variable. The measurement of this variability in the endplate potential rise time is known as *jitter.* The jitter value, calculated in microseconds, is the most important piece of data obtained from single-fiber electromyographic study. Everyone, including healthy individuals, has some degree of jitter (Fig. 78-5). Myasthenic patients have increased jitter values (Fig. 78-6). In addition, blocking occurs in myasthenic patients if a muscle fiber's endplate potential never reaches threshold and depolarization does not occur. The frequency of blocking, expressed as a percentage, is also determined with single-fiber electromyography. In healthy individuals, the percentage of blocking is zero (see Fig. 78-6).

Single-fiber electromyography is undoubtedly the most sensitive test for myasthenia gravis in adults. It is abnormal in 94% of patients with generalized myasthenia gravis and 80% of those with ocular myasthenia gravis [Oh et al., 1992]. However, single-fiber electromyography has several disadvantages. It is a tedious and lengthy study that requires considerable patient cooperation and is poorly tolerated by many children. Stimulated single-fiber electromyography can be performed with the patient under sedation, requires less patient cooperation, and may be preferred for children, although it is still a lengthy procedure [Jabre et al., 1989]. An abnormal result of a single-fiber electromyographic study is not specific for myasthenia gravis because increased jitter commonly occurs as a result of other neuromuscular diseases, such as motor neuron disease, peripheral neuropathy, and many myopathies [Oh, 1988]. Fortunately, it is seldom necessary to perform single-fiber electromyography to diagnose myasthenia gravis in children. It is likely most useful in children who present difficult diagnostic dilemmas and who otherwise have normal results of laboratory studies for myasthenia gravis. Single-fiber electromyographic abnormalities may be seen in 12% to 33% of first-degree relatives of patients with juvenile myasthenia gravis [Anlar et al., 1995; Stalberg et al., 1976].

A

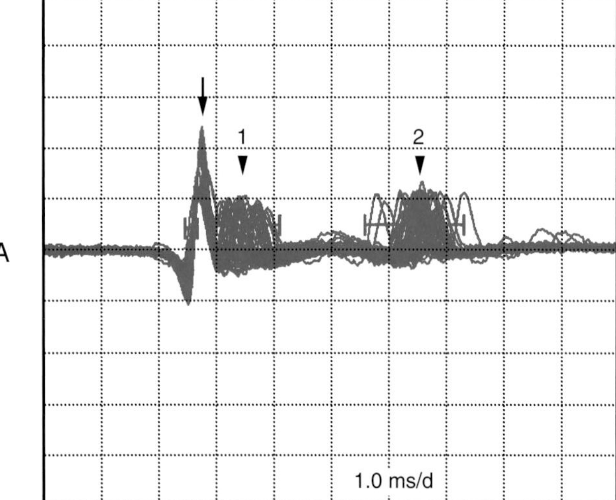

B

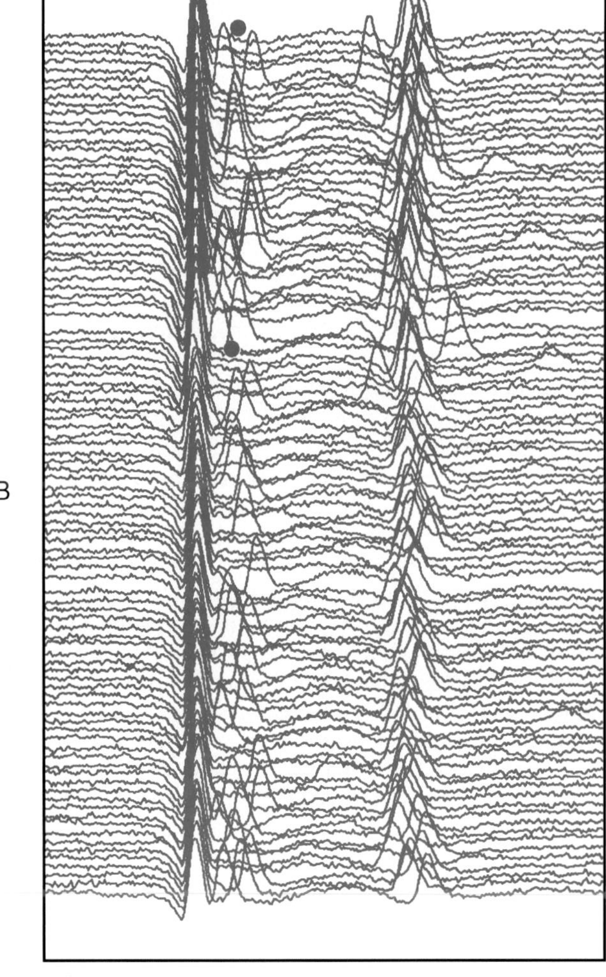

FIGURE 78-6. Recruited single-fiber electromyogram from the extensor digitorum communis in a patient with myasthenia gravis. Three muscle fiber potentials from the same motor unit are recorded (**A**), and 100 successive recordings are captured (**B**). The *arrow* identifies the triggered potential. The degree of jitter for potential 1 is 270 microseconds and for potential 2 it is 187 microseconds (normal <35 microseconds). In addition, potential 1 demonstrates blocking in 50% of the acquisitions (two of these instances are indicated by the *closed circles* in **B**).

Antibody Testing

ANTI-AchR ANTIBODIES

Finding anti-AchR antibody in the serum of a suspected myasthenia gravis patient is the most specific and definitive finding for supporting the diagnosis. When the anti-AchR antibody assay yields positive results, it can be argued that no other diagnostic studies for myasthenia gravis are needed. Most hospitals and medical centers do not run the assay in-house, but the test is commercially available through a number of reference laboratories. It generally takes 1 week to receive the results from the reference laboratory. Thus, the clinician who is initially making the diagnosis is often in the position of performing the edrophonium and electrophysiologic tests while awaiting the results of the study.

Anti-AchR antibody levels are not elevated in all patients with myasthenia gravis. The assay is most informative in adults with generalized myasthenia gravis; it is positive in 85% of such patients [Drachman, 1994; Lindstrom et al., 1976b; Oh et al., 1992; Vincent and Newsom-Davis, 1985]. Only 50% of patients with ocular myasthenia gravis, however, have a measurable anti-AchR antibody. Children represent another group of myasthenia gravis patients whose results are often antibody negative. In one study, only 56% of prepubertal children with autoimmune juvenile myasthenia gravis were seropositive [Andrews et al., 1993], in comparison with 82% who had peripubertal onset of the disease. All 15 children with onset after puberty were seropositive. Similarly, seropositivity was more common in females with onset of juvenile myasthenia gravis after 11 years of age [Anlar et al., 1996]. Seronegativity was more common in pure ocular forms, mild disease, and remission [Afifi and Bell, 1993; Andrews et al., 1993; Anlar et al., 1996]. Only 13% of patients with generalized myasthenia gravis at the time of antibody testing were seronegative [Andrews et al., 1993]. These serologic data support the view that sex and hormonal status influence disease frequency and anti-AchR antibody levels in juvenile myasthenia gravis [Andrews et al., 1993]. Because congenital myasthenic syndromes and seronegative autoimmune myasthenia gravis manifest in early childhood, it is often difficult to differentiate these disorders when the family history is negative [Andrews et al., 1993]. Fluctuating weakness or disease severity and good responses to pharmacologic therapy favor an autoimmune basis [Anlar et al., 1996].

The most common anti-AchR antibody test is the binding radioimmunoassay with bungarotoxin, measured in nanomoles per liter. The upper limit of normal level varies among reference laboratories (usually between 0.03 and 0.5 nmol/liter) [Lennon, 1982]. Other assays that block bungarotoxin binding to AchR ("blocking" assay) or that reduce the density of AchR on cultured human myotubes (modulating antibody assay) are also commercially available [Howard et al., 1987]. These additional assays may be useful in patients with suspected myasthenia gravis whose tests yielded negative results with the standard binding assay [Howard et al., 1987]. Anti-AchR antibodies can also be detected using human rhabdomyosarcoma cell lines [Tami et al., 1994; Voltz et al., 1991], but these are still primarily research laboratory assays.

Anti-AchR antibody titers are poorly correlated with myasthenia gravis severity [Roses et al., 1981]. Although the titer may fall in some patients as the clinical condition improves, antibody titers in general do not guide therapeutic decisions. Indeed, myasthenia gravis patients in clinical remission may still have elevated titers, but this is not an indication to continue immunosuppressive therapy.

ANTI-MuSK ANTIBODIES

Since 2001, IgG from 40% to 70% of seronegative patients with generalized myasthenia gravis has been found to bind to the extracellular domain of MuSK [Hoch et al., 2001; McConville et al., 2004; Sanders et al., 2003]. Marked female predominance with mean age at onset in the fourth decade has been a typical finding [Evoli et al., 2003; Sanders et al., 2003], although Evoli and associates encountered a child with disease onset at age 6 years, and two patients from the initial series presented before age 10 [Hoch et al., 2001]. A child with severe bulbar involvement beginning at age 9 years has also been encountered with this antibody. Patients with anti-MuSK myasthenia gravis often have prominent oculobulbar involvement [Scuderi et al., 2002] or neck, shoulder, and respiratory involvement [Sanders et al., 2003] that is more refractory to conventional treatment. Anti-MuSK antibodies appear to be rare in pure ocular myasthenia gravis and only as recently as 2004 were identified in patients who also were seropositive for anti-AchR antibody [Ohta et al., 2004]. It has been hypothesized that anti-MuSK antibodies impede agrin-mediated clustering of AchR and disrupt normal postsynaptic architecture, but this hypothesis has been placed into question by initial studies on human intercostal muscle; therefore, the pathogenesis remains unclear [Selcen et al., 2004]. Testing for anti-MuSK antibodies is commercially available.

STRIATED MUSCLE ANTIBODIES

Antibodies to striated muscle in patients with myasthenia gravis were discovered before anti-AchR antibodies. These antibodies can be directed against a number of striated muscle proteins, including myosin, actin, α-actinin, titin, and tropomyosin. It is generally believed that if anti–striated muscle antibodies are present in a myasthenia gravis patient, they should raise suspicion for thymoma, because they are reported in up to 84% of patients with thymoma [Limburg et al., 1983]. However, this high a frequency has not been duplicated in all series [Mohan et al., 1994], and the antibody has limited specificity, being present in one third of patients without thymoma [Limburg et al., 1983]. The absence of anti–striated muscle antibodies also does not exclude a thymoma. Thus, the predictive value of this assay may be overemphasized [Lanska, 1991]. From an adult perspective, anti-titin antibodies have been suggested as a marker for more severe disease in patients with myasthenia gravis onset after age 40 and demonstrated a better correlation with disease severity than did anti-AchR antibodies [Romi et al., 2000].

Treatment

Most patients with juvenile myasthenia gravis who require maintenance therapy are treated with anticholinesterase agents with or without a variety of immunosuppressive medications. Pyridostigmine is recommended as an initial intervention [Snead et al., 1980]. As with the adult form of the disease, corticosteroids and other immunosuppressive medications have been useful [Engel, 1984], although few randomized, controlled clinical trials have been conducted for any myasthenia gravis population. Thymectomy plays an important role in treating older children at most centers. Plasmapheresis [Pinching et al., 1976] and intravenous gamma globulin [Arsura, 1989] are generally reserved for patients with more refractory disease or for those in myasthenic crisis. Plasmapheresis is also used to maximize function before thymectomy. Short-term supportive care and anticholinesterase agents are usually adequate for neonatal transient myasthenia gravis. Management for the different types of childhood myasthenia gravis is reviewed in the following sections.

Neonatal Myasthenia Gravis

Neonates with transient myasthenia gravis are at risk of respiratory and bulbar dysfunction. If there is no significant respiratory or swallowing impairment, medications are not necessary. In more severe cases, oral pyridostigmine is given in syrup form (60 mg/5 mL) at a recommended daily dose of 7 mg/kg. The dose should be divided during the day and given 30 minutes before feedings. For neonates unable to swallow, intramuscular injections of pyridostigmine should be given. To convert from oral doses, 1 mg of intramuscular pyridostigmine is equivalent to 30 mg orally. Intramuscular neostigmine is an alternative but has more muscarinic side effects. Treatment for 4 to 6 weeks is usually all that is required.

Juvenile Myasthenia Gravis

ACETYLCHOLINESTERASE INHIBITORS

In juvenile myasthenia gravis, the aggressiveness of management should be in accordance with disease severity. In general, management attempts should first focus on pyridostigmine. A total daily dose up to 7 mg/kg a day is delivered in five to six divided doses [Wolfe et al., 1997]. Older children can use 60-mg tablets that can be split in half as needed. Typical doses in older children and adults are 60 mg three to five times a day. If symptoms are poorly controlled on a pyridostigmine dose exceeding 300 mg/day, it is likely necessary to add immunomodulating therapy. Prolonged-release pyridostigmine is also available (Mestinon TS, 180 mg). However, because of variable absorption, difficulty adjusting doses, and increased side effects, many clinicians discourage use of this preparation.

Although weakness, which is a nicotinic receptor side effect that results from pyridostigmine use, is relatively uncommon, muscarinic side effects occur frequently. The most common of these are gastrointestinal cramps and diarrhea. These symptoms can limit the amount of pyridostigmine that a patient can tolerate. Oral hyoscyamine sulfate, glycopyrrolate, atropine, and over-the-counter loperamide can be prescribed on an as-needed basis or prophylactically with selected pyridostigmine doses to minimize these side effects.

If a child with juvenile myasthenia gravis is hospitalized and cannot take oral pyridostigmine, intravenous pyridostigmine can be substituted. This situation arises most often if a myasthenic patient is admitted for surgery unrelated to the myasthenia gravis and is not permitted to take oral fluids or medications. The general rule is that intravenous pyridostigmine is given at one thirtieth the dose of oral pyridostigmine. Thus, 60 mg of oral pyridostigmine is equivalent to 2 mg given intravenously. The frequency of administration can remain the same. A second scenario is the critically ill myasthenic patient who is unable to swallow or requires mechanical ventilation for crisis. However, it is accepted practice in this setting to withhold all pyridostigmine, simplifying airway management by avoiding cholinergic overstimulation. Once the patient has improved with other therapeutic interventions and bed rest, oral pyridostigmine can be resumed. Pyridostigmine is usually not the deciding factor in withdrawing patients from the ventilator and resolving myasthenic crisis.

THYMECTOMY

When a child's symptoms can no longer be controlled by anticholinesterase agents alone, a decision must be made regarding whether to pursue thymectomy or immunosuppressive therapy. In 1939, Blalock and co-workers reported the remission of generalized myasthenia gravis in a 21-year-old woman after removal of the cystic remains of a necrotic thymic tumor. Since then, thymectomy, with or without the presence of thymoma, has gained widespread acceptance as a treatment for myasthenia gravis. Thus, thymectomy was the first attempt at "immunotherapy" for myasthenia gravis and continues to be one of the most common treatments for the disease.

There is a general consensus that patients between puberty and 60 years of age with generalized myasthenia gravis benefit from thymectomy [Lanska, 1990; Rowland, 1987]. However, randomized studies of thymectomy that control for medical therapy have never been conducted. A critical review of the largely retrospective literature continues to raise questions about the ability of the procedure to induce remission or produce clinical improvement [Lanska, 1991; McQuillen and Leone, 1977]. The use of thymectomy in very young children, in itself, is controversial because of concerns for a subsequent impairment in immune protection or an enhanced risk of cancer. A review of incidental thymectomy and thymectomy as treatment for myasthenia gravis in young children, however, did not reveal a consistent association between thymectomy and these proposed risks in children older than 1 year [Seybold, 1998]. In a survey that included 56 neurologists with expertise in myasthenia gravis, lower age limits for thymectomy ranged from 1 year to puberty, the median being 7.5 years [Lanska, 1990].

In an evidence-based practice parameter from the American Academy of Neurology, Gronseth and Barohn [2000] analyzed retrospective, controlled, nonrandomized studies of thymectomy in myasthenia gravis. A total of 28 studies published between 1953 and 1998 were identified. The effect of surgery was broadly favorable in most series. However, the benefit of surgery was generally small. For example, the median relative rate favoring surgery over nonoperative treatment for achieving remission was 2.1 (a modest gain in view of the fact that the median remission rate in the nonthymectomized groups was 10%). Other median relative rates were 1.6 for asymptomatic status, 1.7 for improvement, and 1.1 for survival. Patient subgroup analysis indicated that only patients with myasthenia gravis who had moderate weakness or greater (Osserman group IIB) exhibited a significant improvement after thymectomy in comparison with control subjects. Of importance was that the modest benefits ascribed to thymectomy were confounded by baseline differences between the operative and nonoperative groups as well as by limited thymic resections performed in a significant percentage of the patients. No study included blinded assessments. As a result, the authors expressed uncertainty as to whether claims of improved myasthenia gravis outcomes were a result of thymectomy or related to differences in baseline characteristics between operative and nonoperative groups. The authors concluded that thymectomy be considered a treatment *option* in patients without thymoma [Gronseth and Barohn, 2000]. To address this uncertainty, an international prospective, single-blinded, randomized trial controlling for medical therapy is being organized for nonthymomatous myasthenia gravis [Wolfe et al., 2003].

Thymectomy has been widely used for the treatment of juvenile myasthenia gravis, resulting in a higher likelihood of remission when performed early in the disease course than did no operative treatment [Seybold, 1998]. In the largest study, 85 (57%) of 149 patients with juvenile myasthenia gravis underwent thymectomy. Of the thymectomized patients, 42 (49%) entered remission and another 25 (29%) improved clinically [Rodriguez et al., 1983]. In contrast, only 34% of patients who did not undergo thymectomy entered remission. Remission rates were 260 per 1000 person-years in the first year after thymectomy, falling to 95 per 1000 person-years over the next year after surgery [Rodriguez et al., 1983]. After 3 years, the remission rate decreased to 20 per 1000 person-years, similar to the spontaneous remission rate. Favorable predictors for postoperative remission included surgery during the first year after disease onset, bulbar symptoms, absence of ocular or generalized involvement, onset of symptoms between ages 12 and 16 years, and the presence of other autoimmune disorders [Rodriguez et al., 1983]. Sex of the child or thymic pathologic findings did not appear to influence remission rates. Histologic findings of the thymus were normal in 16%, hyperplastic in 78%, and neoplastic in 3%.

Other series suggest that the clinical benefit from thymectomy may not be realized for as long as 7 to 10 years [Mulder et al., 1989]. Adams and co-workers [1990] reported that, of 24 patients with juvenile myasthenia gravis who underwent thymectomy, 16 entered complete remission and 7 experienced improvement. Of 12 black children with juvenile myasthenia gravis who underwent thymectomy, 6 entered remission and 4 experienced much improvement in follow-up periods ranging from 1 to 10 years [Lakhoo et al., 1997]. These favorable clinical responses and the low rates of morbidity and mortality from thymectomy in childhood cases bolster its widespread use [Batocchi et al., 1990; Ryniewicz and Badurska, 1977; Youssef, 1983], prompting some investigators to consider the procedure at the onset of generalized symptoms [Adams et al., 1990]. Clinical improvement after thymectomy has been observed regardless of whether there is a reduction in circulating anti-AchR antibody levels [Oosterhuis et al., 1985].

Transsternal thymectomy remains the preferred surgical technique [Younger et al., 1987], although transcervical and infra-axillary video-assisted approaches have been used [Cooper et al., 1988; Mack et al., 1996; Papatestas et al., 1975]. There is some evidence to support the view that the more extensive the resection, the better the long-term results [Jaretzki, 1997]. After a "maximal" thymectomy approach that included both transcervical and transsternal incisions, life-table analyses demonstrated an 81% remission rate at 7.5 years [Jaretzki and Wolff, 1988]. Comparative remission rates for transcervical approaches have been in the range of 30% to 45% at 7 years [Jaretzki et al., 2003], and approximately 50% at 6 years after either an extended transsternal or a video-assisted thoracoscopic procedure that includes a transverse cervical incision [Mantegazza et al., 2003]. It should be noted that remission rates in surgical series are often unexpectedly high. Definitions of remission, as well as its duration, vary between studies, and the retrospective determination of these outcomes is certainly open to bias [Gronseth and Barohn, 2000; Jaretzki, 1997]. Transcervical and video-assisted thoracoscopic procedures offer advantages from a cosmetic and postoperative recovery standpoint. Thoracoscopic procedures have been found to reduce the length of hospital stay and patient care costs in comparison with open thoracic surgery [Hazelrigg et al., 1993].

The presence of a thymoma is, of course, the one absolute indication for thymectomy. All newly diagnosed myasthenia gravis patients must undergo computed tomography or magnetic resonance imaging of the chest with contrast medium to look for evidence of a thymoma. Up to 25% of thymic tumors may not be detected on routine chest radiographs [Batra et al., 1987]. Although there is a consensus among neurologists that thymectomy should be considered in all but the youngest children with generalized myasthenia gravis whose disease is not controlled by anticholinesterase agents alone, there is less enthusiasm for the procedure in isolated ocular myasthenia gravis. Response to thymectomy was lacking in a report of 12 patients with anti-MuSK antibodies, 5 with typical myasthenia gravis findings and 7 with proximal neck/shoulder or respiratory muscle weakness but without ocular involvement [Sanders et al., 2003]. Further studies of patients with anti-MuSK antibodies are needed to better guide treatment decisions. Nevertheless, work to date suggests that thymic tissue in the population with anti-MuSK antibodies does not demonstrate morphologic abnormalities and that thymectomy does not produce significant clinical improvement for these patients [Lauriola et al., 2004].

In several reviews, authors have discussed the preoperative management of patients with myasthenia gravis who undergo thymectomy, including the use of intravenous immune globulin or plasmapheresis to reduce the risk of perioperative complications [Dillon, 2004; Huang et al., 2003; Juel, 2004].

CORTICOSTEROIDS

Despite its many potential side effects, prednisone is considered by many physicians to be the most effective oral immunosuppressive agent for the treatment of myasthenia gravis. Although corticosteroids can potentially suppress the immune system in a variety of ways, the exact explanation for the beneficial response in myasthenia gravis is unknown. However, prednisone can reduce anti-AchR antibody titers, and this may be correlated with clinical improvement [Tindall, 1980].

Typically, oral prednisone is initiated at 1.5 to 2 mg/kg daily. If clinical improvement occurs in the first 4 weeks, the patient can be switched immediately to an alternate-day dose of 1.5 to 2 mg/kg [Warmolts and Engel, 1972]. Longer daily regimens must be followed by a slower alternate-day gradual withdrawal. If corticosteroid therapy is initiated at moderate to high doses, an improvement is usually apparent in 2 to 3 weeks [Johns, 1984; Pascuzzi et al., 1984]. However, in some patients, daily dosing may be necessary for 2 to 3 months before there is clinical improvement. The main concern when initiating prednisone therapy at these doses is the transient worsening that occurs in one third to one half of patients [Badurska et al., 1992; Johns, 1984; Miller et al., 1986; Pascuzzi et al., 1984]. The mechanism may involve a direct effect of corticosteroids to impair neuromuscular junction function [Miller et al., 1986]. In one study, 8.6% of patients who experienced transient worsening required intubation [Pascuzzi et al., 1984]. In another report, 3 of 20 children started on corticosteroids developed respiratory failure [Badurska et al., 1992]. Thus, an advised practice is to admit patients with myasthenia gravis to the hospital for 5 to 7 days when high-dose prednisone therapy is initiated. During this time, bulbar function and forced vital capacity are monitored daily. If the patient remains stable over this interval, he or she can be safely discharged with a prescription for oral prednisone.

The therapeutic efficacy of prednisone in adult myasthenia gravis has been clearly demonstrated [Johns, 1984; Pascuzzi et al., 1984]. In a study of 116 patients, prednisone produced pharmacologic remission (asymptomatic on medication) in 28%, marked improvement in 53% (minor symptoms and return to activities of daily living), moderate improvement in 15% (functional limitations), and no improvement in only 5% [Pascuzzi et al., 1984]. The mean time needed to achieve maximum prednisone benefit was 5.5 months (range, 2 weeks to 6 years). This study also made clear the disappointing fact that only 14% of patients were able to discontinue prednisone treatment and maintain improvement. Similar response rates have been reported in children [Andrews, 2004].

It is noteworthy that a retrospective analysis suggested that prednisone reduces the incidence of disease generalization at 2 years in patients presenting with pure ocular myasthenia gravis [Kupersmith et al., 2003]. Only 7% of such patients receiving prednisone developed generalized disease, in comparison with 36% receiving only pyridostigmine or no medication. Similar observations were made from two smaller retrospective series [Mee et al., 2003; Monsul et al., 2004].

After significant improvement is observed, there should not be a rush to withdraw the prednisone. Most patients remain on alternate-day doses of prednisone for at least 6 to 8 months. Premature withdrawal of prednisone is a common management error. When the withdrawal is begun, it is best to proceed slowly by reducing the dose no faster than 5 mg every 2 weeks. When the patient's dose has been reduced to 20 mg every other day, withdrawing at an even slower rate is advisable. Although an attempt should be made for the patient to withdraw fully from prednisone, it is not uncommon for patients to require low-dose therapy (5 to 10 mg every other day) for many years or indefinitely. Prior thymectomy does not appear to influence the outcome of steroid withdrawal [Miano et al., 1991].

The side effects of corticosteroids are well appreciated and significant. Children should be closely monitored for cataracts, hypertension, diabetes mellitus, weight gain, growth retardation, and cognitive or affective disturbance [Drachman, 1994; Massey, 1997; Pascuzzi et al., 1984; Andrews, 2004]. Adverse effects of corticosteroids on early stages of bone mineralization and development are also of concern, emphasizing the need for "steroid-sparing" strategies in children whose disease is refractory to gradual withdrawal.

AZATHIOPRINE

Azathioprine (Imuran), an antimetabolite that blocks cell proliferation and inhibits T lymphocytes, has been used more frequently because of the side effects associated with corticosteroids. Most reports describe its use in adults. It is used most often in patients who have a relapse while taking prednisone or who have been taking prednisone for lengthy periods in the hope that the steroid dose can be decreased or eliminated. Azathioprine is commonly used as a first-line immunosuppressive agent instead of prednisone in Europe [Hohlfeld et al., 1988; Mantegazza et al., 1988; Matell, 1987; Myasthenia Gravis Clinical Study Group, 1993].

Retrospective studies of azathioprine therapy have demonstrated that 70% to 90% of patients with myasthenia gravis experience improvement [Hohlfeld et al., 1988; Mantegazza et al., 1988; Matell, 1987; Mertens et al., 1981; Myasthenia Gravis Clinical Study Group, 1993], regardless of whether it is used as a first- or second-line immunosuppressive drug. However, the response is slow, ranging up to 12 months or more. In a double-blind study, the use of oral prednisolone was compared with prednisolone plus azathioprine. Patients receiving azathioprine had fewer relapses, longer remissions, and fewer side effects with less weight gain [Palace et al., 1998]. At 3 years, 63% of patients receiving azathioprine had completely withdrawn from prednisolone, in comparison with 20% who had received prednisolone alone. However, the beneficial effect of azathioprine was not statistically documented until month 18 of the study. Thus, if a patient already taking pyridostigmine is quite weak and a rapid response is required, azathioprine is not a practical choice. Azathioprine may be used in combination with plasmapheresis in children whose disease is refractory to other management modalities [Carter et al., 1980]. Azathioprine is reported to lower anti-AchR antibody levels [Mantegazza et al., 1988].

Azathioprine is supplied as a 50-mg, dumbbell-shaped tablet that can be easily broken in half. The initial dose of azathioprine in children should be no more than 25 to 50 mg daily for 1 week. If there are no systemic side effects, the dose is increased to a target level of 2 to 3 mg/kg/day. Although azathioprine is generally well tolerated, there are three important and limiting side effects [Kissel et al.,

1986]: (1) Approximately 10% of patients have an idiosyncratic systemic reaction within the first several weeks of therapy that consists of fever, abdominal pain, nausea, vomiting, and anorexia. Such patients feel as if they have the flu. When the drug is stopped, the symptoms resolve quickly. If such a patient is rechallenged, the symptoms invariably recur. (2) In addition, patients can develop leukopenia and hepatotoxicity. Blood counts and hepatic enzymes need to be monitored monthly. If the white blood cell count falls below 4000 cells/mm^3, it is advisable to decrease the dose. If it falls below 3000 cells/mm^3, medication should be temporarily withheld until the cell count returns to normal. Similarly, medication should be temporarily withheld if there is evidence of hepatocellular dysfunction. Although the patient can be rechallenged after the laboratory values return to normal, toxicity often recurs, requiring discontinuation of the drug. (3) Late development of malignancy after long-term use of azathioprine is of theoretical concern [Andrews, 2004].

CYCLOSPORINE

Cyclosporine (Sandimmune, Neoral) is an accepted option for immunosuppressive therapy in adult myasthenia gravis. Data on its use in juvenile myasthenia gravis are not available, although it is frequently used in pediatric transplant recipients. Cyclosporine inhibits helper T lymphocytes and allows the expression of suppressor T lymphocytes. It blocks the production and secretion of interleukin-2 by helper T cells. Cyclosporine was subjected to randomized, double-blinded, placebo-controlled trials in myasthenia gravis [Tindall et al., 1987, 1993]. These studies demonstrated that cyclosporine was more effective than placebo in improving myasthenia gravis when a quantitative myasthenia gravis scale was used as the primary efficacy measure. In addition, cyclosporine lowered anti-AchR antibody levels. Corticosteroid doses could be reduced after cyclosporine was initiated [Tindall et al., 1993].

The onset of clinical benefit for cyclosporine is 1 to 2 months. This is somewhat faster than azathioprine and slower than prednisone. Doses for cyclosporine range between 3 and 6 mg/kg/day. The drug is usually given in two divided doses rather than as a single dose, to reduce potential nephrotoxicity. Cyclosporine is available as 25- or 100-mg capsules or as an oral solution (100 mg/mL). Side effects include hirsutism, tremor, gum hyperplasia, paresthesias, and hepatotoxicity. Hypertension and nephrotoxicity are the main limitations to therapy. More than one fourth of adult patients taking cyclosporine experience increases in serum creatinine levels between 30% and 70% above baseline levels [Ciafaloni et al., 2000]. Blood pressure, renal function, and trough plasma cyclosporine levels are monitored monthly.

MYCOPHENOLATE MOFETIL

Mycophenolate mofetil (MM, CellCept) is the latest immunosuppressive agent to enter common practice at myasthenia gravis centers, having exhibited initial promise in several uncontrolled, open-label series demonstrating favorable responses in two thirds of adult patients [Chaudhry et al., 2001; Ciafaloni et al., 2001]. Benefits have included improved functional status and a corticosteroid-sparing effect. According to a retrospective analysis of 85 patients in which Myasthenia Gravis Foundation of America postintervention classifications were used, 73% achieved pharmacologic remission, minimal manifestation status, or improvement with mycophenolate mofetil [Meriggioli et al., 2003]. Patients with severe weakness (Myasthenia Gravis Foundation of America class IV) were less likely to respond. Mycophenolate mofetil had a relatively rapid onset of action, with improvement observed at a mean of 9 to 11 weeks and maximal improvement by approximately 6 months. In some subjects, however, the initial response was delayed up to 40 weeks. The most common adult dosing regimen is 1 gram by mouth twice daily, although doses up to 3 grams a day have been used. It is used in the pediatric transplant population at doses 600 mg/m^2 twice daily. Children with body surface areas greater than 1.5 m^2 are dosed at 1 gram twice daily.

Mycophenolate mofetil blocks inosine monophosphate dehydrogenase, which results in selective inhibition of B and T lymphocyte proliferation by blocking purine synthesis. It is routinely used in allogeneic transplant recipients and has been well tolerated in the population with myasthenia gravis. Main side effects are diarrhea, vomiting, increased risk for infection, and leukopenia, which is relatively uncommon. Complete blood counts are checked weekly for the first month and then less frequently. Long-term safety for mycophenolate mofetil is still in question, but malignancy rates do not appear higher in the transplant population. With its more rapid onset of action and favorable side-effects profile, mycophenolate mofetil is replacing azathioprine as the first-line "steroid sparer" in many myasthenia gravis centers and is being studied in two multicenter, randomized, controlled trials.

CYCLOPHOSPHAMIDE

The use of cyclophosphamide (Cytoxan), a nitrogen mustard alkylating agent that blocks cell proliferation, is mainly reserved for patients with refractory myasthenia gravis. Reported use is limited. In one study, 42 adults had been treated with cyclophosphamide; 23 were also taking prednisone [Perez et al., 1981]. At the time of the retrospective data analysis, 25 of the 42 patients had become asymptomatic, and 12 were in complete remission and had discontinued all medications. Of 10 children with juvenile myasthenia gravis, 8 improved when cyclophosphamide was added to regimens that included azathioprine and corticosteroids [Badurska et al., 1992].

In a randomized, placebo-controlled, double-blinded study, monthly intravenous pulses of cyclophosphamide, 500 mg/m^2, were given to 23 adult myasthenia gravis patients with severe, refractory disease or steroid-related side effects [De Feo et al., 2002]. At month 12, the group receiving cyclophosphamide had significantly improved muscle strength on the Quantitative Myasthenia Gravis Scale. At both 6 and 12 months, steroid doses were significantly lower for the patients receiving cyclophosphamide. Similarly, impressive therapy responses were seen in three adult patients with refractory disease who received high-dose (50 mg/kg) intravenous cyclophosphamide for 4 days, followed by "rescue" with granulocyte colony-stimulating factor [Drachman et al., 2003]. Marked improvement in strength without disease recurrence over several years was observed.

The high rate and severity of toxicity are the drawbacks for cyclophosphamide. In one study, alopecia occurred in 75%, leukopenia in 35%, and nausea and vomiting in 25% [Perez et al., 1981]. The increased risk of bladder and lymphoreticular malignancy with prolonged administration of cyclophosphamide should be of particular concern. As a result, cyclophosphamide should be considered only in the most refractory cases of juvenile myasthenia gravis.

PLASMAPHERESIS

Plasma exchange was first used for myasthenia gravis in 1976 [Pinching et al., 1976] and is employed primarily in the short-term, acute management of severe disease, including crisis, and in readying weak patients for thymectomy [Behan et al., 1979; Campbell et al., 1980; Dau et al., 1977; Rowland, 1980]. Plasmapheresis removes anti-AchR antibodies from the circulation of patients with myasthenia gravis, and improvement is measured in several days, rather than weeks for corticosteroids and months for immunosuppressive agents. Two other circumstances in which plasmapheresis is considered include the treatment of severely weak patients admitted for initiation of prednisone therapy and a chronic intermittent therapy in patients with refratory disease. Plasmapheresis has been lifesaving in some children [Snead et al., 1980].

In general, a course of plasmapheresis consists of four to six exchanges in which approximately 50 mL of plasma per kilogram of the patient's weight are removed at each treatment. Decisions regarding the number of exchanges and total amount removed are largely driven by the status of the patient, including clinical response and tolerability of the hemodynamic shifts from the procedure. Improvement is often seen within 48 hours after the first or second exchange. Treatments are usually administered every other day or on no more than 2 of 3 consecutive days, so that a full course is completed in 7 to 10 days [Andrews, 2004].

The main limitations of plasmapheresis are (1) intravenous access, because a double-lumen catheter is required in younger children; (2) complications, including pneumothorax, hypotension, sepsis, and pulmonary embolism; (3) expense of the procedure; and (4) the relatively brief clinical benefit, which persists for only a few weeks.

INTRAVENOUS IMMUNE GLOBULIN

Intravenous immune globulin is increasingly used by neurologists for various immune-mediated neuromuscular diseases, including myasthenia gravis. In an analysis of eight published retrospective studies, a response rate to intravenous immune globulin of 73% was derived, with clinical responses seen in 4 to 5 days [Arsura, 1989]. The effect can persist for several weeks to several months. A randomized, double-blinded, placebo-controlled trial of intravenous immune globulin in generalized myasthenia gravis was initiated but was terminated before an adequate number of subjects could be enrolled, and the trial was underpowered [Wolfe et al., 2002]. In the open-label intravenous immune globulin extension, favorable trends in quantitative strength and electrophysiologic outcome measures were seen in patients who had initially received placebo, which was consistent with qualitative improvement seen in prior reports. In a Cochrane Database review, data from four randomized controlled trials of intravenous immune globulin that enrolled 147 subjects were analyzed [Gajdos et al., 2003]. No significant efficacy difference was observed between intravenous immune globulin and either plasma exchange or methylprednisolone in disease exacerbations [Gajdos et al., 1997]. Although no studies have focused on the pediatric population, children and adolescents have responded favorably to intravenous immune globulin [Andrews, 2004].

The initial dose of intravenous immune globulin is usually 2 grams/kg. This can be given over 2 to 5 days. When given over the shorter interval, the infusion runs nearly continuously. A common practice is to then schedule two or three subsequent infusions of 0.4 to 1 gram/kg at 2- to 4-week intervals. Patients are then reevaluated to determine whether further treatments are needed.

Advantages of intravenous immune globulin over plasma exchange include the relative ease of administration and the favorable side effects profile in both children and adults. Headache, transient flulike symptoms, and hyperactivity are the adverse events most common to the pediatric population [Andrews, 2004]. Patients who suffer migraine are prone to develop a severe headache related to aseptic meningitis. The

Box 78-2 Drugs That May Worsen Myasthenia Gravis or Interfere with Neuromuscular Transmission

- Antibiotic agents
  - Aminoglycosides
  - Erythromycin
  - Tetracycline
  - Penicillins
  - Sulfonamides
  - Fluoroquinolones
  - Clindamycin
  - Lincomycin
- Anesthetic agents
  - Neuromuscular blocking agents
  - Lidocaine
  - Procaine
- Antiepileptic drugs
  - Phenytoin
  - Mephenytoin
  - Trimethadione
- Cardiovascular drugs
  - Beta blockers
  - Procainamide
  - Quinidine
- Rheumatologic drugs
  - Chloroquine
  - D-Penicillamine
- Miscellaneous
  - Iodinated contrast
  - Chlorpromazine
  - Corticosteroids
  - Lithium

outbreak of hepatitis C in relation to some intravenous immune globulin products [Schiff, 1994] has been controlled with improved donor screening and sterilization techniques. Major complications are observed in up to 5% of adults, including cardiovascular, cerebrovascular, and deep venous thrombotic events; congestive heart failure; and acute nephrotoxicity [Brannagan et al., 1996; Go and Call, 2000; Steg and Leflowitz, 1994; Tan et al., 1993].

Drugs to Avoid

Children with myasthenia gravis, like adults with myasthenia gravis, are sensitive to nondepolarizing neuromuscular blocking agents. Intermediate-acting nondepolarizing blockers such as atracurium and vecuronium should be used with care [Baraka, 1992]. It is advisable to administer small increments of these agents, with neuromuscular monitoring as a guide [Brown et al., 1990]. Other commonly used drugs known to exacerbate myasthenia gravis or interfere with neuromuscular transmission are listed in Box 78-2. Of these agents, aminoglycoside antibiotics are perhaps the agents that most commonly affect neuromuscular transmission, and they should be used in patients with myasthenia gravis only when there are no reasonable alternatives.

LAMBERT-EATON MYASTHENIC SYNDROME

Lambert-Eaton myasthenic syndrome is an acquired autoimmune disorder of neuromuscular junction transmission in which the defect is in the presynaptic nerve terminal. Lambert and co-workers [1956] and Eaton and Lambert [1957] are credited for defining the syndrome, including the electrophysiologic abnormalities seen on routine electromyography. Elmqvist and Lambert [1968] then found that the neuromuscular junction defect resulted from inadequate presynaptic release of acetylcholine.

An immune-mediated basis for Lambert-Eaton myasthenic syndrome was suspected when the disease was passively transferred from the purified IgG of patients to mice [Lang et al., 1981]. At about the same time, it was found that the number of voltage-gated calcium channels is reduced in the motor nerve terminal [Fukunga et al., 1982]. A number of investigators have subsequently provided data as evidence that the Lambert-Eaton syndrome IgG is directed at voltage-gated calcium channels [Kim and Neher, 1988; Lang et al., 1989; Sher et al., 1989]. This action inhibits the influx of calcium into the motor nerve terminal. As a result, the number of quanta of acetylcholine vesicles released with each action potential that reaches the nerve terminal is decreased.

Clinical Features

Lambert-Eaton myasthenic syndrome is characterized by fatigability and weakness in a limb-girdle distribution [Mareska and Gutmann, 2004; O'Neill et al., 1988]. Unlike patients with myasthenia gravis, these patients may note that the weakness is worse soon after awakening and lessens later in the day. Although exercise can transiently improve strength, persistent exertion causes fatigue. Cranial nerve and respiratory involvement are less common than in myasthenia gravis. Up to 50% of patients have a mild degree of ptosis, diplopia, dysphagia, and dysarthria. Patients also have autonomic involvement, including dry mouth and eyes, impotence, blurred vision, and orthostasis. On examination, there is a limb-girdle pattern of weakness, and deep tendon reflexes are reduced or absent. In some patients, improvement in strength or the reflex response can be demonstrated after a few seconds of voluntary contraction. This reaction is called *postexercise facilitation of reflexes* and was observed in 44% of 16 patients in one study [Odabasi et al., 2002].

A malignancy is present in approximately 50% of adult patients with Lambert-Eaton myasthenic syndrome. The tumor is usually a small cell carcinoma of the lung; other malignancies include renal cell carcinoma and hematologic tumors. Lambert-Eaton myasthenic syndrome can be the presenting manifestation of a small cell carcinoma and can precede the detection of the tumor by months. Seventy percent of men with Lambert-Eaton myasthenic syndrome and only 25% of women with Lambert-Eaton myasthenic syndrome have a malignancy.

Lambert-Eaton myasthenic syndrome is only rarely described in children. The first report was about a 10-year-old boy with leukemia [Dahl and Sato, 1974]. The literature contains only a handful of cases in which the patient is younger than 15 years [Argov et al., 1995; Chelmicka-Schorr et al., 1979; Shapira et al., 1974; Tsao et al., 2002], often in association with a lymphoproliferative disorder. A congenital case of Lambert-Eaton myasthenic syndrome not diagnosed until age 4 years has been reported [Bady et al., 1987].

Clinical Laboratory Tests

A diagnosis of Lambert-Eaton myasthenic syndrome is often first suggested by findings on nerve conduction studies and repetitive stimulation. Edrophonium may produce mild improvement in strength, but its results do not differentiate Lambert-Eaton myasthenic syndrome from myasthenia gravis. The classic electrophysiologic triad of Lambert-Eaton myasthenic syndrome is (1) low-amplitude compound muscle action potential that increases dramatically after brief exercise, (2) decremental response at low rates of repetitive stimulation (2 to 5 Hz), and (3) incremental response at high rates (20 to 50 Hz) of repetitive stimulation [Oh, 1988]. These electrophysiologic features are illustrated in Figure 78-7.

The diagnosis of Lambert-Eaton myasthenic syndrome often becomes apparent first in the electromyography laboratory when, in the process of performing routine motor nerve conduction studies, diffusely small-amplitude compound muscle action potentials are found. At this point, it is useful to conduct the Lambert-Eaton myasthenic syndrome screen test. After the baseline compound muscle action potential amplitude is obtained (e.g., in the adductor digiti minimi), the patient is asked to spread the fingers apart against resistance for 10 seconds. Then the single nerve stimulation is immediately repeated and the compound muscle action potential recorded. In Lambert-Eaton myasthenic syndrome there is a dramatic, often greater than 100% increase in the compound muscle action potential amplitude and area. The physiologic effect of either brief exercise or tetanic stimulation produces enough influx of

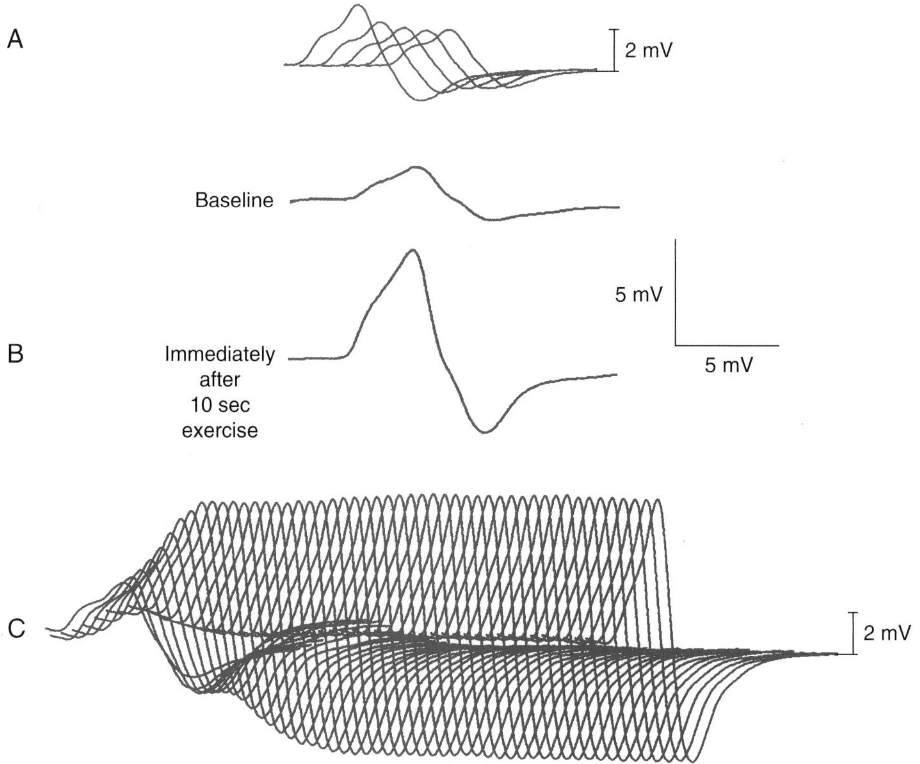

FIGURE 78-7. Repetitive stimulation of the ulnar nerve, recorded in the adductor digiti minimi in a patient with Lambert-Eaton myasthenic syndrome. **A,** Low-frequency (3-Hz) repetitive stimulation elicited a 32% decrement. **B,** After 10 seconds of exercise (brief exercise test), the compound motor action potential demonstrated a 220% increment over baseline. **C,** High-frequency repetitive stimulation elicited a 195% increment. (From Katz J, Wolfe GI, Bryan WW, et al. Acetylcholine receptor antibodies in the Lambert-Eaton myasthenic syndrome. Neurology, 1998;50:470.)

calcium into the presynaptic terminal to overcome the underlying defect in quantal release.

Incremental responses consistent with Lambert-Eaton myasthenic syndrome should be at least 100%. Normal individuals can have incremental responses as great as 40% [Oh, 1989]. Single-fiber electromyography indicates increased jitter in Lambert-Eaton myasthenic syndrome, but this does not differentiate the disease from myasthenia gravis.

Antibody testing for Lambert-Eaton myasthenic syndrome is now available in select laboratories. In a study of 72 patients ranging from 16 to 80 years of age, 92% were seropositive for antibodies to P/Q-type voltage-gated calcium channel [Motomura et al., 1996]. In contrast, only 33% were seropositive for anti-N-type voltage-gated calcium channel antibodies. All patients with anti-N-type voltage-gated calcium channel antibodies were also seropositive for anti-P/Q-type voltage-gated calcium channel antibodies. Lennon and co-workers [1995] found that all patients with Lambert-Eaton myasthenic syndrome who had a diagnosis of cancer had anti-P/Q-type voltage-gated calcium channel antibodies, in comparison with 91% of such patients without cancer [Lennon et al., 1995]. Nakao and colleagues [2002] found that of 110 patients with Lambert-Eaton myasthenic syndrome, 85% had anti-P/Q-type voltage-gated calcium channel antibodies and that seronegative patients were less likely to have small cell carcinoma (12% versus 70% of the seropositive population). Anti-N-type voltage-gated calcium channel antibodies were present in only 49% of patients with Lambert-Eaton myasthenic syndrome. These results support the notion that anti-P/Q-type voltage-gated calcium channel antibodies are primarily responsible for the presynaptic defect in Lambert-Eaton myasthenic syndrome. Children with P/Q-type voltage-gated calcium channel antibodies and typical features of Lambert-Eaton myasthenic syndrome were first reported as recently as 2002 [Tsao et al., 2002]. On occasion, adult patients with Lambert-Eaton myasthenic syndrome also have anti-AchR antibodies in the serum [Katz et al., 1998].

Treatment

As in the adult form of the disorder, clinical improvement in childhood Lambert-Eaton myasthenic syndrome has been observed with anticholinesterase agents [Dahl and Sato, 1974], prednisone [Chelmicka-Schorr et al., 1979], and guanidine hydrochloride [Bady et al., 1987; Chelmicka-Schorr et al., 1979]. As expected, treatment guidelines are mostly drawn from reports of adult patients. In general, a trial of pyridostigmine is the first intervention, although it is often of limited benefit. Ideally, drugs that increase the release of acetylcholine vesicles should be tried. Guanidine hydrochloride is the oldest drug in this group and has been beneficial in some Lambert-Eaton myasthenic syndrome patients [Cherington, 1976]. However, the side effects of guanidine are prohibitive and include bone marrow depression, renal failure, gastrointestinal distress, ataxia, hypotension, paresthesias, confusion, dry skin, and atrial fibrillation. One report suggested that lower doses of guanidine not exceeding 1000 mg daily, combined with pyridostigmine, may be more tolerable [Oh et al., 1997]. 3,4-Diaminopyridine increases the duration of the presynaptic action potential by blocking the outward potassium efflux. This effect indirectly prolongs the activation of voltage-gated calcium channel and increases calcium entry in nerve terminals. In clinical trials, 3,4-diaminopyridine improves strength and compound muscle action potential amplitudes in patients with Lambert-Eaton myasthenic syndrome [McEvoy et al., 1989; Sanders et al., 1993]. Most patients tolerated the drug with only minor side effects. Unfortunately, 3,4-diaminopyridine is available only as an investigational agent in the United States.

There are surprisingly few clinical studies on immunosuppressive therapy in Lambert-Eaton myasthenic syndrome. Newsom-Davis and Murray [1984] reported that plasmapheresis, corticosteroids, and azathioprine can be effective in both neoplastic and nonneoplastic Lambert-Eaton myasthenic syndrome. Other reports describe the effectiveness of intravenous immune globulin in a small number of Lambert-Eaton myasthenic syndrome patients [Bird, 1992; Rich et al., 1997]. Muscle strength improved in a placebo-controlled crossover trial of intravenous immune globulin in nine patients with Lambert-Eaton myasthenic syndrome [Bain et al., 1996]. The improvement peaked 2 to 4 weeks after infusion and was associated with a significant decline in voltage-gated calcium channel antibody titers. A sustained response to cyclosporine was reported in two children who had only limited responses to intravenous immune globulin and plasmapheresis [Tsao et al., 2002]. A Cochrane Database review of Lambert-Eaton myasthenic syndrome treatment concluded that randomized, controlled trials of 3,4-diaminopyridine and intravenous immune globulin demonstrated improved muscle strength scores and compound muscle action potential amplitudes [Maddison and Newsom-Davis, 2003]. In general, the regimens and doses for the immunotherapies outlined for myasthenia gravis can be applied to Lambert-Eaton myasthenic syndrome.

CONGENITAL MYASTHENIC SYNDROMES

Congenital myasthenic syndromes compose a heterogeneous group of relatively uncommon childhood diseases that present a diagnostic challenge to the clinician. The estimated prevalence is 1 to 2 per million. Some forms are life threatening, whereas others produce only mild weakness and are treatable [Engel, 1990; Shillito et al., 1993]. Therefore, an accurate diagnosis is necessary for rational therapy. Unlike myasthenia gravis and Lambert-Eaton myasthenic syndrome, the congenital myasthenic syndromes are not autoimmune; antibody determinations are negative, and immunosuppressive therapy is not effective. Although clinical and electrophysiologic data may suggest congenital myasthenic syndrome, specialized microelectrode analysis of neuromuscular transmission, ultrastructural studies of the neuromuscular junction, biochemical skeletal muscle assays, and molecular analysis are necessary to make a precise diagnosis [Engel, 1993; Engel et al., 1998; Harper, 2004]. These genetically determined disorders all compromise in some way the safety factor that normally preserves the integrity of neuromuscular transmission, either directly or through secondary alterations at the neuromuscular junction [Engel, 1994].

The earliest report of a congenital myasthenic syndrome was in 1937 by Rothbart, who described four brothers who developed a myasthenic condition before the age of 2 years. Bowman [1948] coined the term *congenital myasthenia* to describe the condition of an infant who had normal parents and whose myasthenic symptoms persisted into childhood.

Box 78-3 Classification of the Congenital Myasthenic Syndromes

- Presynaptic defects
  - Paucity of synaptic vesicles and decreased quantal release
  - Congenital myasthenic syndromes with episodic apnea (choline acetyltransferase deficiency)
  - Lambert-Eaton syndrome–like form
- Synaptic defects
  - Endplate acetylcholinesterase deficiency
- Postsynaptic defects
  - Primary acetylcholine receptor deficiency
  - Reduced receptor expression as a result of acetylcholine receptor mutations
  - Reduced receptor expression as a result of rapsyn mutations
  - Reduced receptor expression with plectin deficiency
  - Primary acetylcholine receptor kinetic abnormality with or without acetylcholine receptor deficiency
  - Slow-channel syndrome
  - Fast-channel syndrome
  - Sodium-channel mutations

By 1972, 97 familial cases of early-onset myasthenia had been documented [Bundey, 1972]. Forty-one had presented before 2 years of age. Using refined techniques, Engel and co-workers [1977a] subsequently described three forms of congenital myasthenic syndrome: endplate acetylcholinesterase deficiency [Engel et al., 1977a], slow-channel syndrome [Engel et al., 1982], and impaired resynthesis or vesicular packaging of acetylcholine [Mora et al., 1987], also known as *familial infantile myasthenia* [Greer and Schotland, 1960; Robertson et al., 1980]. Work by Engel's group has identified other forms of congenital myasthenic syndrome related to kinetically abnormal or deficient AchRs [Engel et al., 1997]. Box 78-3 summarizes the syndromes that have been characterized to this point [Harper, 2004].

Clinical Features

Most patients with congenital myasthenic syndrome present in the first 2 years of life, with many becoming symptomatic in the neonatal period or in early infancy [Misulis and Fenichel, 1989; Shillito et al., 1993]. However, clinical involvement may not occur until adolescence or adulthood, particularly in the slow-channel syndrome. Symptoms in familial infantile myasthenia can be episodic or worsen with fever and emotional stimuli. There is considerable variation between families and even siblings sharing the same type of congenital myasthenic syndrome, which confounds the clinical definition and classification of these disorders [Misulis and Fenichel, 1989; Vincent et al., 1981].

Typical clinical findings in congenital myasthenic syndrome include feeding difficulty, respiratory dysfunction, ophthalmoparesis, ptosis, hypotonia, and limb fatigability. Symptoms may worsen with crying or physical activity in the neonatal period [Engel, 1994]. The attainment of developmental milestones, as well as progression and regression of symptoms, should be carefully documented.

Response to various pharmacologic challenges may assist in defining the syndrome. A positive family history is obviously suggestive of congenital myasthenic syndrome, but a negative family history does not exclude autosomal-recessive inheritance, incomplete penetration, or a new mutation.

Clinical Laboratory Tests

Preliminary testing should include nerve conduction studies and needle electromyography. These studies often yield normal results, but repetitive motor action potential discharges to a single electrical stimulus suggest acetylcholinesterase deficiency or slow-channel syndrome [Engel, 1993]. Low-frequency repetitive nerve stimulation usually reveals a decrement in weak muscles and should be performed at baseline and after exercise. To exclude autoimmune myasthenia or myasthenic syndrome, antibodies against AchR, skeletal muscle, and calcium channels should be assayed. Routine muscle biopsy for light microscopy and electron microscopy may yield normal results or reveal nonspecific abnormalities such as type 1 fiber predominance or type 2 fiber atrophy. Small groups of atrophic fibers and vacuolar changes near the endplate are seen in slow-channel syndrome.

Although the specialized, intensive testing required for definitive diagnosis is available in only a handful of tertiary centers, routine clinical data can be very helpful in classifying patients. Table 78-3 summarizes distinctive clinical and electrodiagnostic features of the various forms of congenital myasthenic syndrome.

Specialized studies include microscopic and ultrastructural examination of muscle specimens to assess synaptic vesicle content, acetylcholinesterase assay, AchR abundance, and destructive postsynaptic changes that may reflect cholinergic overactivity [Engel and Ohno, 2002]. Microelectrode electrophysiologic studies on intercostal or anconeus muscle biopsies can localize the process to a presynaptic, synaptic, or postsynaptic defect and can define factors responsible for the impairment in neuromuscular transmission. Miniature endplate potential amplitude and frequency, endplate potential amplitude, the number and probability of quanta released by nerve impulses, and quantal content are determined. Patch clamp recording of individual AchRs defines the amplitude and duration of single currents to determine kinetic abnormalities of the receptor. A number of developments since the mid-1990s have accelerated the molecular characterization of these disorders. These include the identification of the complementary DNA sequence for the various subunits of the AchR and acetylcholinesterase, improved resolution of patch clamping techniques in human intercostal muscle to allow recording of single-channel currents, and the ability to study mutant neuromuscular junction proteins in engineered mammalian systems [Engel and Ohno, 2002].

If the evaluation demonstrates features consistent with a defect in a candidate gene or protein, molecular analysis follows. If a mutation is found, genetically engineered models of the mutant molecule can be used to confirm the pathogenicity and further define the properties of the mutation. This approach has led to the discovery of more than 100 mutations combined in various subunits of the AchR, acetylcholinesterase, and choline acetyltransferase [Ohno and Engel, 2000].

Presynaptic Defects

Three major types of presynaptic defects have been identified: congenital myasthenic syndrome with episodic apnea related to disturbances in acetylcholine resynthesis, paucity of synaptic vesicles with reduced quantal release, and a Lambert-Eaton myasthenic syndrome–like form of congenital myasthenic syndrome.

Disturbances in Acetylcholine Resynthesis

Patients with defective acetylcholine resynthesis have distinctive, sudden episodes of generalized and bulbar weakness with apnea precipitated by infections, fever, vomiting episodes, or emotional stimuli. Some infants present at birth with hypotonia and bulbar and respiratory weakness necessitating mechanical ventilation; others are normal at birth and do not experience apneic episodes until childhood. Ptosis, poor suck, feeble cry, and generalized weakness may be present early, but there is little or no extraocular involvement. Affected infants often demonstrate spontaneous improvement after several weeks and by adolescence may appear normal except for easy fatigability with exercise [Engel, 1990; Shillito et al., 1993]. Episodic crises may occur at any age, however, potentially leading to respiratory failure and death in infancy and early childhood [Conomy et al., 1975; Gay and Bodensteiner, 1990]. A family history of "sudden infant death syndrome" in older siblings is not uncommon [Ohno et al., 2001]. Apneic episodes become less frequent and severe as the child grows older. Decremental responses are typical on low-rate repetitive stimulation in presynaptic congenital myasthenic syndromes [Albers et al., 1984; Lecky et al., 1986; Vincent et al., 1981], at times occurring only after exercise [Engel, 1980; Hart et al., 1979]. In milder cases, prolonged repetitive stimulation at rates of 10 to 15 Hz may be necessary to demonstrate neuromuscular transmission failure [Harper, 2004]. The progressive decrement seen with prolonged stimulation is more severe and recovers more slowly (over 10 to 15 minutes) than in autoimmune myasthenia gravis or congenital myasthenic syndrome related to AchR deficiency and sodium channel defects.

These patients closely resemble those described in earlier reports of "familial infantile myasthenia" [Greer and Schotland, 1960; Misulis and Fenichel, 1989], but this term should be avoided because all congenital myasthenic syndromes are familial and most manifest in the neonatal period. On microelectrode studies, miniature endplate potentials are normal at rest but decrease abnormally on repetitive stimulation over several minutes, which is consistent with a defect in acetylcholine resynthesis. Later studies established that mutations in the *CHAT* gene encoding endplate choline acetyltransferase, the rate-limiting enzyme in resynthesis of acetylcholine from choline and acetyl coenzyme A, are responsible [Ohno et al., 2001].

Low doses of anticholinesterases improve muscle strength in these patients and should be available in intramuscular form (neostigmine) for episodic crises [Engel, 1994]. Installation of apnea monitors is advised, as is training of family members in hand-assisted ventilatory devices. Nutritional support and aggressive treatment of underlying infections are important during crises [Harper, 2004]. 3,4-Diaminopyridine may produce transient benefit but over time can exacerbate symptoms when

TABLE 78-3

Distinctive Clinical and Electrodiagnostic Features of Congenital Myasthenic Syndromes

CMS Syndrome	Autosomal dominant inheritance	Episodic apnea triggered by stressors	Neonatal hypotonia and respiratory insufficiency	Skeletal deformities	Delayed pupillary light responses	Prominent neck, wrist and finger extensor weakness	Repetitive CMAPs after single stimulus	Progressive decrement with prolonged exercise or repetitive stimulation	Marked increment (>200%) with high-frequency repetitive stimulation	Decrement repairs with AchE inhibitors	Clinical improvement with AchE inhibitors	Clinical worsening with AchE inhibitors
Presynaptic												
Choline acetyl-transferase deficiency		x	x					x				
LEMS-like form			x						x			
Synaptic												
AchE deficiency			x (in severe cases)	x	x		x					x
Postsynaptic												
Primary AchR deficiency			x (in severe cases)	x				x		x		
Slow-channel CMS	x (most mutations)					x	x					x
Fast-channel CMS				x (in severe cases)						x	x	

AchE, acetylcholinesterase; AchR, acetylcholine receptor; CMAPs, compound muscle action potentials; CMS, congenital myasthenic syndrome; LEMS, Lambert-Eaton myasthenic syndrome.

acetylcholine stores are depleted [Harper, 2004; Palace et al., 1991].

Paucity of Synaptic Vesicles

Paucity of synaptic vesicles with reduced quantal release clinically resembles autoimmune myasthenia gravis with symptoms beginning in infancy in the one documented case [Walls et al., 1993]. Slow-rate repetitive stimulation revealed a decrement that repaired after exercise. There was a marked reduction in quantal release in response to nerve impulses, and morphologic studies documented a reduction in density of synaptic vesicles. The molecular basis for this disorder is unknown, and whether it relates to defective axonal transport of vesicle constituents or impaired recycling is unclear. Anticholinesterase medications produced modest benefit.

Lambert-Eaton Myasthenic Syndrome-like Form

The Lambert-Eaton myasthenic syndrome–like syndrome shares the electrophysiologic signature of autoimmune Lambert-Eaton myasthenic syndrome discussed previously, with greater than 100% facilitation on high-frequency stimulation [Albers et al., 1984; Maselli et al., 2001]. Infants present with severe hypotonia and respiratory insufficiency [Harper, 2004]. There are no significant morphologic alterations, and synaptic vesicle density appears normal. Defective P/Q-type voltage-gated calcium channels or impaired vesicle release mechanisms may be responsible. Anticholinesterase agents, guanidine, and 3,4-diaminopyridine may provide some benefit.

Synaptic Defects

Endplate Acetylcholinesterase Deficiency

The initial description of acetylcholinesterase deficiency was in 1977 [Engel et al., 1977a] and was followed by several reports of either sporadic cases or autosomal-recessive pedigrees [Engel et al., 1981; Hutchinson et al., 1993; Walls et al., 1989]. Symptoms begin in the neonatal period with ptosis, poor suck, feeble cry, and generalized moderate to severe weakness. Motor milestones are delayed. Lordosis and scoliosis are prominent features. Ophthalmoparesis is variable, seen in about half of patients [Engel, 1990, 1994]. Pupillary light responses may also be abnormally sluggish. Decremental responses are seen on repetitive stimulation. Multiple motor action potential discharges may follow a single stimulus on routine nerve conduction studies, a characteristic but nonspecific finding that is also seen in slow-channel syndrome and in the setting of excessive anticholinesterase use [Shillito et al., 1993]. Acetylcholinesterase deficiency can be differentiated from slow-channel syndrome by a test in which cholinesterase inhibitors are administered: The number and size of the repetitive discharges after a single stimulus increases in slow-channel syndrome but does not change in the setting of acetylcholinesterase deficiency [Harper, 2004].

The primary abnormality is deficient acetylcholinesterase activity at the endplate on cytochemical and immunocytochemical studies, resulting in prolonged miniature endplate potential and endplate potential durations [Engel et al., 1977a; Hutchinson et al., 1993]. Recessive mutations in the *COLQ* gene, which encodes the triple-stranded collagenic tail of acetylcholinesterase, have been identified in affected patients [Ohno et al., 2000]. The ColQ tail is responsible for anchoring catalytic subunits of acetylcholinesterase to the basal lamina of the postsynaptic membrane. Neuromuscular transmission appears to be impaired by the small size of nerve terminals, an endplate myopathy resulting from cholinergic overstimulation, and by densensitization/ depolarization block of AchRs [Engel and Ohno, 2002]. Treatment is difficult, inasmuch as the condition is refractory or worsens with anticholinesterase agents [Harper, 2004]. Medications that enhance neurotransmitter release from the nerve terminal, such as 3,4-diaminopyridine, would likely have a similar effect. Ephedrine may produce subjective improvement [Milone and Engel, 1996].

Postsynaptic Defects

Postsynaptic defects represent the most common forms of congenital myasthenic syndrome (Box 78-4). These disorders arise predominantly from a variety of AchR subunit mutations that either enhance or reduce their response to neurotransmitter. Although phenotypes vary, postsynaptic defects tend to be less severe than other forms of congenital myasthenic syndrome and, at times, respond more favorably to pharmacologic therapy. Muscle AchR is a transmembrane structure composed of five homologous subunits: two alpha, one beta, one delta, and one gamma subunit in the fetal form that is replaced by an epsilon subunit in the adult AchR. On the basis of extensive studies, two major kinetic abnormalities of the AchR have been described: slow-channel and fast-channel syndromes [Engel and Ohno, 2002]. Primary AchR deficiency, which may be accompanied by kinetic abnormalities, and congenital myasthenic syndrome related to perijunctional sodium channel mutations round out the postsynaptic defects.

Slow-Channel Congenital Myasthenic Syndrome

The slow channel syndrome was first described by Engel and co-workers in 1982. Whereas most forms of congenital myasthenic syndrome demonstrate recessive inheritance, the majority of slow-channel syndromes result from dominant gain-of-function mutations [Harper, 2004]. These mutations prolong channel opening events and slow the decay of endplate currents, which result in cationic overload in muscle fibers and an endplate myopathy with fixed weakness [Gomez et al., 1997; Milone et al., 1997]. Onset of symptoms varies considerably, ranging from infancy to adulthood [Shillito

Box 78-4 Localization of Defect in 134 Patients with Congenital Myasthenic Syndromes [Engel and Ohno, 2002]

Type of Congenital Myasthenic Syndromes	Number of Cases
Presynaptic	1 (8%)
Synaptic	23 (17%)
Postsynaptic	96 (72%)
No identified defect	4 (3%)

et al., 1993], although late onset is more typical of this syndrome than for other forms of congenital myasthenic syndrome. Clinical findings also vary, although there is a propensity for early cervical, scapular, wrist, and finger extensor weakness that helps to distinguish the syndrome. Ptosis and ophthalmoplegia are less prominent. Lower extremities may be less involved than upper extremities [Engel, 1990]. Weakness in most patients is slowly progressive.

Decremental responses up to 40% and increased jitter are seen on electrophysiologic testing. Repetitive potentials to single stimuli are characteristic of both weak and strong muscles and are best seen at rates below 0.2 Hz, inasmuch as at higher stimulation rates, the second potential is often of very small amplitude [Oosterhuis et al., 1987]. Cholinesterase inhibitors increase the number and amplitude of the repetitive responses in slow-channel syndrome but not in endplate acetylcholinesterase deficiency; this difference helps distinguish these two forms of congenital myasthenic syndrome. Specialized electrophysiologic studies on intercostal muscle have shown normal or slightly reduced miniature endplate potential amplitudes and normal quantal content of the endplate potential but prolonged decay time of the miniature endplate potential and endplate potential. Although it was suspected earlier, it was not until 1992 that prolonged open time of the AchR was clearly demonstrated to account for the slowed decay of endplate currents [Engel et al., 1993]. On exposure to acetylcholine, the abnormal AchRs have prolonged activation, resulting in abnormally slowed decay of endplate potential. Spontaneous openings of the AchR are also observed. This change in kinetic activity produces cationic overloading and an endplate myopathy with loss of junctional folds and AchRs, widening of synaptic space, and other morphologic alterations [Engel and Ohno, 2002]. These changes, in addition to the depolarization block that occurs when prolonged endplate potentials extend beyond the refractory period of muscle fibers, compromise neuromuscular transmission.

A number of dominant mutations in the alpha, beta, and epsilon subunits of AchR have been described in slow-channel syndrome. Autosomal recessive mutations in the epsilon subunit have also been described [Croxen et al., 2002]. Not surprisingly, acetylcholinesterase inhibitors and 3,4-diaminopyridine worsen the condition. The worsening with acetylcholinesterase inhibitors can help distinguish slow-channel syndrome from autoimmune myasthenia gravis and all other forms of congenital myasthenic syndrome except for endplate acetylcholinesterase deficiency. Quinidine at doses of 200 mg two to three times a day and fluoxetine at doses of 80 to 160 mg per day have improved clinical and electrophysiologic measures in a small number of patients [Harper and Engel, 1998; Harper et al., 2003]. These two agents partially correct for prolonged AchR activation episodes in cell cultures expressing mutated receptors and clinically have demonstrated both short-term and long-term improvement of weakness. Quinidine may be problematic because of drug allergies, and fluoxetine is often better tolerated.

Fast-Channel Congenital Myasthenic Syndrome

More recently described are the less common fast-channel syndromes. These are related to recessive loss-of-function mutations of the AchR. Common features of these postsynaptic syndromes are rapid decay of endplate currents, brief channel activation episodes, and reduced probability of channel opening in response to acetylcholine, which result in reduced miniature endplate potential amplitudes [Engel and Ohno, 2002]. A variety of kinetic abnormalities have been described in the fast-channel syndromes in relation to mutations in the alpha and epsilon subunits of the AchR. The syndromes result from a mutant subunit allele that dominates the clinical phenotype combined with a null or missense mutation on the second allele. Phenotypic severity varies from a disabling congenital myasthenic syndrome related to low-affinity channels [Uchitel et al., 1993] to a mild syndrome associated with gating abnormalities. Typical patients present in infancy to early childhood with ptosis, opthalmoparesis, bulbar symptoms, and exertional limb weakness [Harper, 2004]. Decrements are present at slow rates of repetitive stimulation that can repair with exercise, high-frequency stimulation, and anticholinesterases. A static or slowly progressive course is usually observed. As would be predicted, fast-channel syndromes respond favorably to 3,4-diaminopyridine combined with anticholinesterases, because these agents enhance AchR activation by either increasing quantal release or reducing acetylcholine degradation in the synapse [Engel and Ohno, 2002].

Primary Acetylcholine Receptor Deficiency

AchR deficiency states have most commonly been linked to homozygous or heterozygous recessive mutations of AchR subunits. Most mutations have involved the epsilon subunit [Engel et al., 1996]. This propensity may arise because null mutations of other subunits are lethal, whereas the fetal gamma subunit can partially compensate for the absence of the epsilon subunit. In addition, the epsilon subunit gene may be more susceptible to DNA rearrangements. The mutations reduce AchR density; in addition, some mutations produce minor kinetic abnormalities. Recessive mutations in the gene that encodes rapsyn, a protein synthesized by muscle that, through agrin and muscle-specific kinases, mediates the clustering of AchRs on the postsynaptic membrane, have also been associated with congenital myasthenic syndrome [Burke et al., 2003; Maselli et al., 2003; Ohno et al., 2002]. A single case report of reduced AchR counts associated with myopathy has been described with plectin deficiency [Banwell et al., 1999].

Disease severity in AchR deficiency states, whether from receptor subunit or rapsyn mutations, is variable, with onset occurring between the neonatal period and childhood [Harper, 2004]. Ptosis, ophthalmoplegia, and generalized hypotonia and weakness are typical. Epsilon subunit mutations generally produce milder manifestations [Engel et al., 2003]. Fixed weakness and skeletal anomalies, including high-arched palate and facial dysmorphism, are observed. In most cases, there is a nonprogressive course or even improvement with age. Repetitive stimulation at slow rates demonstrates a decrement in most but not all patients that repairs with anticholinesterases. In more severe cases, the decrement may worsen with stimulation frequencies above 10 Hz. Ultrastructural studies demonstrate increased numbers of endplate regions over an increased span of muscle fibers [Engel and Ohno, 2002]. Junctional folds appear to be preserved, although some endplates are small and simplified. There is a notable reduction in the density and numbers of AchRs. As with fast-channel forms of congenital myasthenic syndrome, anticholinesterases and 3,4-diaminopyridine may provide benefit [Harper, 2004].

Sodium-Channel Congenital Myasthenic Syndrome

Sodium-channel congenital myasthenic syndrome was described in a single patient who harbored two recessive mutations in the skeletal muscle-sodium channel gene *SCN4A* [Tsujino et al., 2003]. Expression of the mutation in a human cell line exhibited enhanced fast inactivation of the sodium channel, thereby decreasing the safety margin of neuromuscular transmission by increasing the size of the endplate potential needed to generate a muscle action potential.

Weakness began at birth with ptosis and bulbar and skeletal involvement. Brief exacerbations of bulbar and respiratory symptoms lasting no longer than 30 minutes persisted into early adulthood. Routine repetitive stimulation studies were normal. Decrements were seen only after stimulation for periods longer than 1 minute at rates of 10 to 50 Hz. The drop in compound motor action potential amplitude repaired rapidly within several minutes, a faster repair than that seen in choline acetyltransferase deficiency [Harper, 2004].

BOTULISM

Botulism is caused by a toxin produced by *Clostridium botulinum,* a gram-positive anaerobic organism found commonly in soil and agricultural products [Cherington, 1990, 2004; Glatman-Freedman, 1996]. Eight immunologically distinct toxins have been identified; most human cases are caused by type A, B, or E. After binding irreversibly to receptors on presynaptic nerve terminals, the botulinum toxin is translocated across the membrane and blocks the calcium-dependent release of acetylcholine [Gutierrez et al., 1994]. The action of the toxin appears independent of calcium entry. Impaired release of acetylcholine results in failed neuromuscular transmission. Damage to nerve terminals may be permanent, resulting in a prolonged clinical recovery believed to be dependent on the formation of new neuromuscular junctions. Three forms of botulism exist, the most common being the form that occurs in infants.

Classic Botulism

The classic form of botulism almost always follows ingestion of food contaminated by previously formed toxin [Cherington, 1998]. The stereotypical presentation features the development of bulbar symptoms, including blurred vision, diplopia, ptosis, dysarthria, and dysphagia, within 12 to 36 hours after ingestion of the contaminated food. A descending pattern of weakness and, in some cases, respiratory paralysis follows. Antitoxins have not clearly improved outcome, but supportive care measures have improved survival rates, and nearly full recovery is expected for surviving patients.

Infantile Botulism

Infantile botulism was first described in 1976 [Pickett et al., 1976] and has since become the most frequently reported form of botulism. It is also a common cause of hypotonia in this age group [Gay and Bodensteiner, 1990]. An interesting observation is that most reported cases in the United States occur in California, Pennsylvania, and Utah, states with high counts of *C. botulinum* spores in the soil [Cherington, 1990]. In infantile botulism, spores of *C. botulinum* are ingested and then germinate and propagate in the gastrointestinal tract, producing toxin in vivo. Consumption of honey and corn syrup has been associated with infantile botulism, but in most cases, the source of infection is not evident [Glatman-Freedman, 1996; Spika et al., 1989]. Infantile botulism typically manifests in infants between 6 weeks and 9 months of age and is heralded by the onset of severe constipation [Cherington, 1990; Gay and Bodensteiner, 1990]. A descending paralysis with cranial nerve paralysis, poor suck, feeble cry, and reduced facial expressions ensues and is followed by limb weakness [Wilson et al., 1982]. The child appears hypotonic, with ptosis, decreased extraocular motility, sluggish pupillary light responses, facial diplegia, weak suck, and a reduced gag response. Deep tendon reflexes and spontaneous bowel sounds are reduced. There is usually no associated fever. Both respiratory and autonomic compromise may occur, with the disease progressing over several days to a week.

Although the presentation is often quite typical, the diagnostic approach should be tailored to exclude other possible etiologies, including systemic infection, tick paralysis, organophosphate poisoning, Guillain-Barré syndrome, congenital myopathies, and autoimmune and congenital myasthenic conditions. Electrophysiologic studies support a presumptive diagnosis of botulism while results of the bacteriologic studies are awaited. Sensory nerve conduction studies are normal. Compound muscle action potential amplitudes are normal to reduced, and motor conduction velocities are preserved. Repetitive stimulation study results confirm a presynaptic defect in neuromuscular transmission. Decremental responses are variably seen on slow rates of repetitive stimulation, but increments are present at rapid rates (20 to 50 Hz). An incremental response at rapid rates was the most distinctive finding in one study, observed in 92% of cases [Cornblath et al., 1983]. The increment averaged 73%. Post-tetanic facilitation is also seen in Lambert-Eaton myasthenic syndrome, but the facilitation is particularly prolonged in botulism, persisting up to 20 minutes [Gutierrez et al., 1994]. On needle electromyography, fibrillation potentials are seen in approximately 50% of affected infants, and short-duration, low-amplitude motor units in more than 90% [Cornblath et al., 1983]. Diagnosis is confirmed by isolation of the organism or toxin in stool samples. Toxin isolation is accomplished by the mouse neutralization test, usually performed at state health departments [Cherington, 1990]. Polymerase chain reaction assays have been developed but are not routinely available. In infantile botulism, the toxin is only rarely found in the serum [Cherington, 1990].

Treatment of infantile botulism is supportive; complete recovery requires several weeks to months. Case fatality rates of hospitalized patients in the United States are below

5% [Glatman-Freedman, 1996; Wilson et al., 1982]. Nasogastric or parenteral nutrition is needed if the child is unable to drink or eat. Mechanical ventilation may also be required. Aminoglycosides and other agents that impair neuromuscular transmission should be used with extreme caution. The length of hospitalization averages 4 weeks, but some infants may require supportive care for as long as 5 months [Wilson et al., 1982].

Wound Botulism

Wound contamination with *C. botulinum* leads to production of botulinum toxin after bacterial incubation, producing clinical symptoms 4 to 14 days after the wound has been infected. The condition has been described in a small number of individuals from age groups ranging from adolescents to older adults [Burningham et al., 1994; Mechem and Walter, 1994]. The disease may be severe, producing diffuse muscle weakness, including bulbar dysfunction, that necessitates ventilatory support. Prompt recognition and support are important for preventing respiratory failure.

REFERENCES

Adams C, Theodorescu D, Murphy EG, et al. Thymectomy in juvenile MG. J Child Neurol 1990;5:215.

Afifi AK, Bell WE. Tests for juvenile myasthenia gravis: Comparative diagnostic yield and prediction of outcome. J Child Neurol 1993;8:403.

Ahlsten G, Lefvert AK, Osterman PO, et al. Follow-up study of muscle function in children of mothers with myasthenia gravis. J Child Neurol 1992;7:264.

Albers JW, Faulkner JA, Dorovini-Zis K, et al. Abnormal neuromuscular transmission in an infantile myasthenic syndrome. Ann Neurol 1984;16:28.

Andrews PI. Autoimmune myasthenia gravis in childhood. Sem Neurol 2004;24:101.

Andrews PI, Massey JM, Sanders DB. Acetylcholine receptor antibodies in juvenile myasthenia gravis. Neurology 1993;43:977.

Anlar B, Kuruoglu R, Varli K, et al. Acetylcholine receptor antibodies and single-fiber EMG in first-degree relatives of children with myasthenia gravis. Neuropediatrics 1995;26:335.

Anlar B, Ozdirim E, Renda Y, et al. Myasthenia gravis in childhood. Acta Paediatr 1996;85:838.

Argov Z, Shapira Y, Averbuch-Heller L, et al. Lambert-Eaton myasthenic syndrome (LEMS) in association with lymphoproliferative disorders. Muscle Nerve 1995;18:715.

Arsura E. Experience with intravenous immunoglobulin in myasthenia gravis. Clin Immunol Immunopathol 1989;53:S170.

Badurska B, Ryniewicz B, Strugalska H. Immunosuppressive treatment for juvenile myasthenia gravis. Eur J Pediatr 1992;151:215.

Bady B, Chauplannaz G, Carrier H. Congenital Lambert-Eaton myasthenic syndrome. J Neurol Neurosurg Psychiatry 1987;50:476.

Bain PG, Motomura M, Newsom-Davis J, et al. Effects of intravenous immunoglobulin on muscle weakness and calcium-channel autoantibodies in the Lambert-Eaton myasthenic syndrome. Neurology 1996;47:678.

Banwell BL, Russel J, Fukudome T, et al. Myopathy, myasthenic syndrome, and epidermolysis bullosa simplex due to plectin deficiency. J Neuropathol Exp Neurol 1999;58:832.

Baraka A. Anaesthesia and myasthenia gravis. Can J Anaesth 1992;39:476.

Barlow CF. Neonatal myasthenia gravis. Am J Dis Child 1981;135:209.

Barohn R. Standards of measurements in myasthenia gravis. Ann N Y Acad Sci 2003;998:432.

Barohn RJ, Brey RC. Soluble terminal complement components in human myasthenia gravis. Clin Neurol Neurosurg 1993;95:285.

Barohn RJ, Jackson CE. New classification system for myasthenia gravis [Abstract]. J Child Neurol 1994;9:205.

Barohn RJ, McIntire D, Herbelin L, et al. Reliability testing of the quantitative myasthenia gravis score. Ann N Y Acad Sci 1998;841:769.

Batocchi AP, Evoli A, Palmisani MT, et al. Early-onset myasthenia gravis: Clinical characteristics and response to therapy. Eur J Pediatr 1990;150:66.

Batra P, Herrmann C Jr, Mulder D. Mediational imaging in myasthenia gravis: Correlation of chest radiography, CT, MR, and surgical findings. AJR Am J Roentgenol 1987;148:515.

Behan PO. Immune disease and HLA associations with myasthenia gravis. J Neurol Neurosurg Psychiatry 1980;43:611.

Behan PO, Shakir AA, Simpson JA, et al. Plasma exchange combined with immunosuppressive therapy in myasthenia gravis. Lancet 1979;2:438.

Bird SJ. Clinical and electrophysiologic improvement in Lambert-Eaton syndrome with intravenous immunoglobulin therapy. Neurology 1992;42:1422.

Blalock A, Mason MF, Morgan HJ, et al. Myasthenia gravis and tumors of the thymic region. Report of a case in which the tumor was removed. Ann Surg 1939;505:607.

Bowman JR. Myasthenia gravis in young children: Report of three cases: One congenital. Pediatrics 1948;1:472.

Branch CE, Swift TR, Dyken PR. Prolonged neonatal myasthenia gravis: Electrophysiological studies. Ann Neurol 1978;3:416.

Brannagan TH, Nagle KJ, Lange DJ et al. Complications of intravenous immune globulin treatment in neurologic disease. Neurology 1996;47:674.

Brown TC, Gebert R, Meretoja OA, et al. Myasthenia gravis in children and its anaesthetic implications. Anaesth Intensive Care 1990;18:466.

Bundey S. A genetic study of infantile and juvenile myasthenia gravis. J Neurol Neurosurg Psychiatry 1972;35:41.

Burke G, Cossins J, Maxell S, et al. Rapsyn mutations in hereditary myasthenia: Distinct early- and late-onset phenotypes. Neurology 2003;61:826.

Burningham MD, Walter FG, Mechem C, et al. Wound botulism. Ann Emerg Med 1994;24:1184.

Campbell WW, Leshner RT, Swift TR. Plasma exchange in myasthenia gravis: Electrophysiologic studies. Ann Neurol 1980;8:584.

Carter B, Harrison R, Lunt GG, et al. Anti-acetylcholine receptor antibody titres in the sera of myasthenia patients treated with plasma exchange combined with immunosuppressive therapy. J Neurol Neurosurg Psychiatry 1980;43:397.

Castleman B. The pathology of the thymus gland in myasthenia gravis. Ann N Y Acad Sci 1966;135:496.

Chan-Lui WY, Leung NK, Lau TT. Myasthenia gravis in Chinese children. Dev Med Child Neurol 1984;26:717.

Chaudhry V, Cornblath DR, Griffin JW, et al. Mycophenolate mofetil: A safe and promising immunosuppressant in neuromuscular diseases. Neurology 2001;56:94.

Chelmicka-Schorr E, Bernstein LP, Zurbrugg E, et al. Eaton-Lambert syndrome in a 9-year-old girl. Arch Neurol 1979;36:572.

Cherington M. Guanidine and germine in Eaton-Lambert syndrome. Neurology 1976;26:944.

Cherington M. Botulism. Semin Neurol 1990;10:27.

Cherington M. Clinical spectrum of botulism. Muscle Nerve 1998;21:701.

Cherington M. Botulism: update and review. Semin Neurol 2004;2:153.

Ciafaloni E, Massey JM, Tucker-Lipscomb B, et al. Mycophenolate mofetil for myasthenia gravis: An open-label study. Neurology 2001;56:97.

Ciafaloni E, Nikhar NK, Massey JM, et al. Retrospective analysis of the use of cyclosporine in myasthenia gravis. Neurology 2000;55:448.

Compston DAS, Vincent A, Newsom-Davis J, et al. Clinical, pathological, HLA antigen and immunological evidence for disease heterogeneity in myasthenia gravis. Brain 1980;103:579.

Conomy JP, Levinsohn M, Fanaroff A. Familial infantile myasthenia gravis: A cause of sudden death in young children. J Pediatr 1975;87:428.

Cooper JD, Al-Jilaihawa AN, Pearson FG, et al. An improved technique to facilitate transcervical thymectomy for myasthenia gravis. Ann Thorac Surg 1988;45:242.

Cornblath DR, Sladky JT, Sumner AJ. Clinical electrophysiology of infantile botulism. Muscle Nerve 1983;6:448.

Croxen R, Hatton C, Shelley C, et al. Recessive inheritance and variable penetrance of slow-channel congenital myasthenic syndromes. Neurology 2002;59:162.

Dahl DS, Sato S. Unusual myasthenic state in a teen-age boy. Neurology 1974;24:897.

Dau PC, Lindstrom JM, Cassel CK, et al. Plasmapheresis and immunosuppressive drug therapy in myasthenia gravis. N Engl J Med 1977;297:1134.

De Feo LG, Schottlender J, Martelli NA, et al. Use of intravenous pulsed cyclophosphamide in severe, generalized myasthenia gravis. Muscle Nerve 2002;26:31.

Desmedt JE, Borenstein S. Time course of neonatal myasthenia gravis and unsuspectedly long duration of neuromuscular block in distal muscles. N Engl J Med 1977;296:633.

Dillon FX. Anesthesia issues in the perioperative management of myasthenia gravis. Semin Neurol 2004;24:83.

Donaldson JO, Penn AS, Lisak RP, et al. Antiacetylcholine receptor antibody in neonatal myasthenia gravis. Am J Dis Child 1981;135:222.

Drachman DB. Myasthenia gravis: Part I. N Engl J Med 1978;298:136.

Drachman DB. Myasthenia gravis. N Engl J Med 1994;330:1797.

Drachman DB, Jones RJ, Brodsky RA. Treatment of refractory myasthenia: "Rebooting" with high-dose cyclophosphamide. Ann Neurol 2003;53:29

Eaton LM, Lambert EH. Electromyography and electric stimulation of nerve in diseases with motor units. Observations on myasthenic syndrome associated with malignant tumors. JAMA 1957;163:1117.

Elias SB, Butler I, Appel SH. Neonatal myasthenia gravis in the infant of a myasthenic mother in remission. Ann Neurol 1979;6:72.

Elmqvist D, Lambert EH. Detailed analysis of neuromuscular transmission in a patient with the myasthenic syndrome sometimes associated with bronchogenic carcinoma. Mayo Clin Proc 1968;43:689.

Engel AG. Morphologic and immunopathologic findings in myasthenia gravis and in congenital myasthenic syndromes. J Neurol Neurosurg Psychiatry 1980;43:577.

Engel AG. Myasthenia gravis and myasthenic syndromes. Ann Neurol 1984;16:519.

Engel AG. Congenital disorders of neuromuscular transmission. Semin Neurol 1990;10:12.

Engel AG. The investigation of congenital myasthenic syndromes. Ann N Y Acad Sci 1993;681:425.

Engel AG. Congenital myasthenic syndromes. Neurol Clin 1994;12:401.

Engel AG, Arahata K. The membrane attack complex of complement at the end-plate in myasthenia gravis. Ann N Y Acad Sci 1987;505:326.

Engel AG, Hutchinson DO, Nakano S, et al. Myasthenic syndromes attributed to mutations affecting the epsilon subunit of the acetylcholine receptor. Ann N Y Acad Sci 1993;681:496.

Engel AG, Lambert EH, Gomez MR. A new myasthenic syndrome with end-plate acetylcholinesterase deficiency, small nerve terminals, and reduced acetylcholine release. Ann Neurol 1977a;1:315.

Engel AG, Lambert EH, Howard FM. Immune complexes (IgG and C3) at the motor end-plate in myasthenia gravis: Ultrastructural and light microscopic localization and electrophysiologic correlations. Mayo Clin Proc 1977b;52:267.

Engel AG, Lambert EH, Mulder DM, et al. Recently recognized congenital myasthenic syndromes: (A) End-plate acetylcholine (Ach) esterase deficiency. (B) Putative abnormality of the Ach induced ion channel. (C) Putative defect of Ach resynthesis or mobilization: Clinical features, ultrastructure and cytochemistry. Ann N Y Acad Sci 1981;377:614.

Engel AG, Lambert EH, Mulder DM, et al. A newly recognized congenital myasthenic syndrome attributed to a prolonged open time of the acetylcholine-induced ion channel. Ann Neurol 1982;11:553.

Engel AG, Ohno K. Congenital myasthenic syndromes. In: Pourmand R, Harati Y, eds. Advances in neurology: Neuromuscular disorders. Philadelphia: Lippincott Williams & Wilkins, 2002;203.

Engel AG, Ohno K, Bouzat C, et al. End-plate acetylcholine receptor deficiency due to nonsense mutations in the epsilon subunit. Ann Neurol 1996;40:810.

Engel AG, Ohno K, Milone M, et al. Congenital myasthenic syndromes caused by mutations in acetylcholine receptor genes. Neurology 1997;48 (Suppl 5):S28.

Engel AG, Ohno K, Milone M, et al. Congenital myasthenic syndromes: New insights from molecular genetic and patch-clamp studies. Ann NY Acad Sci 1998;841:140.

Engel AG, Ohno K, Shen XM, et al. Congenital myasthenic syndromes: Multiple molecular targets at the neuromuscular junction. Ann N Y Acad Sci 2003;998:138.

Engel AG, Tsujihata M, Lindstrom JM, et al. The motor end-plate in myasthenia gravis and in experimental autoimmune myasthenia gravis: A quantitative ultrastructural study. Ann N Y Acad Sci 1976;274:60.

Evoli A, Tonali P, Bartoccioni E, et al. Ocular myasthenia: Diagnostic and therapeutic problems. Acta Neurol Scand 1988;77:31.

Evoli A, Tonali PA, Padua L, et al. Clinical correlates with anti-MuSK antibodies in generalized seronegative myasthenia gravis. Brain 2003;126:2304.

Fenichel GM. Clinical syndrome of myasthenia in infancy and childhood. Arch Neurol 1978;35:97.

Fraser D, Turner JW. Myasthenia gravis and pregnancy. Lancet 1953;2:417.

Fukunga H, Engel AG, Osame M, et al. Paucity and disorganization of presynaptic membrane active zones in the Lambert-Eaton myasthenic syndrome. Muscle Nerve 1982;5:686.

Gajdos P, Chevret S, Clair B, et al. Clinical trial of plasma exchange and high-dose intravenous immunoglobulin in myasthenia gravis. Ann Neurol 1997;41:789.

Gajdos P, Chevret S, Toyka K. Intravenous immunoglobulin for myasthenia gravis. Cochrane Database Syst Rev 2003;(2):CD002277.

Gay CT, Bodensteiner JB. The floppy infant: Recent advances in the understanding of disorders affecting the neuromuscular junction. Neurol Clin 1990;8:715.

Geddes AK, Kidd HM. Myasthenia gravis of the newborn. Can Med Assoc J 1951;64:152.

Geh VS, Bradbury JA. Ocular myasthenia presenting in an 11-month-old boy. Eye 1998;12:319.

Glatman-Freedman A. Infant botulism. Pediatr Rev 1996;17:185.

Go RS, Call TG. Deep venous thrombosis of the arm after intravenous immunoglobulin infusion: Case report and literature review of intravenous immunoglobulin–related thrombotic complications. Mayo Clin Proc 2000;75:83.

Gomez CM, Maselli R, Gundeck JE, et al. Slow-channel transgenic mice: A model of postsynaptic organellar degeneration at the neuromuscular junction. J Neurosci 1997;17:4170.

Greer M, Schotland M. Myasthenia gravis in the newborn. Pediatrics 1960;26:101.

Grob D, Asura EL, Brunner NG, et al. The course of myasthenia gravis and therapies affecting outcome. Ann N Y Acad Sci 1987;505:472.

Gronseth GS, Barohn RJ. Thymectomy for non-thymomatous autoimmune myasthenia gravis (an evidence-based review). Neurology 2000;55:7.

Gutierrez AR, Bodensteiner J, Gutmann L. Electrodiagnosis of infantile botulism. J Child Neurol 1994;9:362.

Harper CM. Neuromuscular transmission disorders in childhood. In: Jones HR Jr., Bolton CF, Harper CM, eds. Pediatric clinical electromyography. Philadelphia: Lippincott-Raven, 1996;353.

Harper CM. Congenital myathenic syndromes. Sem Neurol 2004;24:111.

Harper CM, Engel AG. Quinidine sulfate therapy for the slow-channel congenital myasthenic syndrome. Neurology 1998;43:480

Harper CM, Fukodome T, Engel AG. Treatment of slow-channel congenital myasthenic syndrome with fluoxetine. Neurology 2003;60:1710.

Hart ZH, Sahasashi K, Lambert EH, et al. A congenital, familial myasthenic syndrome caused by a presynaptic defect of transmitter resynthesis or mobilization [Abstract]. Neurology 1979;29:556.

Hawkins BR, Yu YL, Wong V, et al. Possible evidence for a variant of myasthenia gravis based on HLA and acetylcholine receptor antibody in Chinese patients. Q J Med 1989;70:235.

Hazelrigg SR, Nunchuck SK, Landrenau RJ, et al. Cost analysis for thoracoscopy: Thoracoscopic wedge resection. Ann Thorac Surg 1993;56:633.

Hoch W, McConville J, Helms S, et al. Auto-antibodies to the receptor tyrosine kinase MuSK in patients with myasthenia gravis without acetylcholine receptor antibodies. Nat Med 2001;7:365.

Hohlfeld R, Michels M, Heininger K, et al. Azathioprine toxicity during long-term immunosuppression of generalized myasthenia gravis. Neurology 1988;8:258.

Howard FM, Lennon VA, Finley J, et al. Clinical correlations of antibodies that bind, block, or modulate human acetylcholine receptors in myasthenia gravis. Ann N Y Acad Sci 1987;505:526.

Huang CS, Hsu HS, Kao KP, et al. Intravenous immunoglobulin in the preparation of thymectomy for myasthenia gravis. Acta Neurol Scand 2003;108:136.

Hutchinson DO, Walls TJ, Nakano S, et al. Congenital endplate acetylcholinesterase deficiency. Brain 1993;116:633.

Jabre JF, Chirico-Post J, Weiner M. Stimulation SFEMG in myasthenia gravis. Muscle Nerve 1989;12:38.

Jaretzki A 3rd. Thymectomy for myasthenia gravis: Analysis of the controversies regarding technique and results. Neurology 1997;48 (Suppl 5):S52.

Jaretzki A 3rd, Aarli JA, Kaminski HJ, et al. Thymectomy for myasthenia gravis: Evaluation requires controlled prospective studies. Ann Thorac Surg 2003;76:1.

Jaretzki A 3rd, Barohn RJ, Ernstoff RM, et al. Myasthenia gravis: Recommendations for clinical research standards. Neurology 2000;55:16.

Jaretzki A 3rd, Wolff M. Maximal thymectomy for myasthenia gravis: Surgical anatomy and operative technique. J Thorac Cardiovasc Surg 1988;96:711.

Johns TR. Long-term corticosteroid treatment of myasthenia gravis. Ann N Y Acad Sci 1984;505:568.

Juel VC. Myasthenia gravis: Management of myasthenic crisis and perioperative care. Semin Neurol 2004;24:75.

Kao I, Drachman DB. Thymic muscle cells bear acetylcholine receptors: Possible relation to myasthenia gravis. Science 1977;195:74.

Katz J, Wolfe GI, Bryan WW, et al. Acetylcholine receptor antibodies in the Lambert-Eaton myasthenic syndrome. Neurology, 1998;50:470.

Kim YI, Neher E. IgG from patients with Lambert-Eaton syndrome blocks voltage-dependent calcium channels. Science 1988;239:405.

Kini PG. Juvenile myasthenia gravis with predominant facial weakness in a 7 year-old boy. Int J Pediatr Otorhinolaryngol 1995;32:167.

Kissel JT, Levy RJ, Mendell JR, et al. Azathioprine toxicity in neuromuscular disease. Neurology 1986;36:35.

Krolick KA, Thompson PA, Zoda TE, et al. Immunological factors that influence disease severity in experimental autoimmune myasthenia gravis. In: Hohlfeld R, ed. Immunology of neuromuscular disease. Dordrecht, the Netherlands: Kluwer, 1994;209.

Kupersmith MJ, Latkany R, Homel P. Development of generalized disease at 2 years in patients with ocular myasthenia gravis. Arch Neurol 2003;60:243.

Lakhoo K, De Fonseca J, Rodda J, et al. Thymectomy in black children with juvenile myasthenia gravis. Pediatr Surg Int 1997;12:113.

Lambert EH, Eaton LM, Rooke ED. Defect of neuromuscular conduction associated with malignant neoplasms. Am J Physiol 1956;187:612.

Lang B, Newsom-Davis J, Wray D, et al. Autoimmune etiology for myasthenic (Eaton-Lambert) syndrome. Lancet 1981;2:224.

Lang B, Vincent A, Murray NMF, et al. Lambert-Eaton myasthenic syndrome: Immunoglobulin G inhibition of Ca^{2+} flux in tumor cells correlates with disease severity. Ann Neurol 1989;25:265.

Lanska DJ. Indications for thymectomy in myasthenia gravis. Neurology 1990;40:1828.

Lanska DJ. Diagnosis of thymoma in myasthenics using anti-striated muscle antibodies: Predictive value and gain in diagnostic certainty. Neurology 1991;41:520.

Lauriola L, Guerriero M, Bartoccioni E, et al. Thymus changes in anti-MuSK-positive and -negative myasthenia gravis [Abstract]. Neurology 2004;62:A183

Lecky BRF, Morgan-Hughes JA, Murray NMF, et al. Congenital myasthenia: Further evidence of disease heterogeneity. Muscle Nerve 1986;9:233.

Lennon VA. Myasthenia gravis. Diagnosis by assay of serum antibodies. Mayo Clin Proc 1982;57:723.

Lennon VA, Greismann GE. Evidence against acetylcholine receptor having a main immunogenic region and detection of similarities between subunits. Proc Natl Acad Sci U S A 1989;77:755.

Lennon VA, Kryzer TJ, Griesmann GE, et al. Calcium-channel antibodies in Lambert-Eaton syndrome and other paraneoplastic syndromes. N Engl J Med 1995;332:1467.

Limburg PC, The TH, Hummel-Tapel E, et al. Anti-acetylcholine receptor antibodies in myasthenia gravis. Part 1. Relation to clinical parameters in 250 patients. J Neurol Sci 1983;58:357.

Lindstrom J, Lennon V, Seybold ME, et al. Experimental autoimmune myasthenia gravis and myasthenia gravis: Biochemical and immunochemical aspects. Ann N Y Acad Sci 1976a;274:254.

Lindstrom JM, Seybold ME, Lennon VA, et al. Antibody to acetylcholine receptor in myasthenia gravis. Prevalence, clinical correlates, and diagnostic value. Neurology 1976b;26:1054.

Liu JHK, Erickson K. Cholinergic agents. In: Albert DM, Jakobiec FA, eds. Principles and practice of ophthalmology: Basic sciences. Philadelphia: WB Saunders, 1994;985.

Mack MJ, Landreneau RJ, Yim AP, et al. Results of video-assisted thymectomy in patients with myasthenia gravis. J Thorac Cardiovasc Surg 1996;112:1352.

Maddison P, Newsom-Davis J. Treatment for Lambert-Eaton myasthenic syndrome. Cochrane Database Syst Rev 2003;(2):CD003279.

Mantegazza R, Antozzi C, Peluchitte D, et al. Azathioprine as a single drug or in combination with steroids in the treatment of myasthenia gravis. J Neurol 1988;235:449.

Mantegazza R, Baggi F, Bernasconi P, et al. Video-assisted thoracoscopic extended thymectomy and extended thymectomy (T-3b) in non-thymomatous myasthenia gravis patients: Remission after 6 years of follow-up. J Neurol Sci 2003;212:31.

Mareska M, Gutmann L. Lambert-Eaton myasthenic syndrome. Semin Neurol 2004;24:149.

Maselli RA, Dunne V, Pascual-Pascual SI, et al. Rapsyn mutations in myasthenic syndrome due to impaired receptor clustering. Muscle Nerve 2003;28:293.

Maselli RA, Kong DZ, Bowe CM, et al. Presynaptic congenital myasthenic syndrome due to quantal release deficiency. Neurology 2001;57:279.

Massey JM. Treatment of acquired myasthenia gravis. Neurology 1997;48 (Suppl):S46.

Matell G. Immunosuppressive drugs: Azathioprine in the treatment of myasthenia gravis. Ann N Y Acad Sci 1987;505:588.

McConville J, Farrugia ME, Beeson D, et al. Detection and characterization of MuSK antibodies in seronegative myasthenia gravis. Ann Neurol 2004;55:580.

McEvoy KM, Windebank AJ, Daube JR, et al. 3,4-Diaminopyridine in the treatment of Lambert-Eaton myasthenic syndrome. N Engl J Med 1989;321:1567.

McQuillen MP, Leone MG. A treatment carol: Thymectomy revisited. Neurology 1977;27:1103.

Mechem CC, Walter FG. Wound botulism. Vet Hum Toxicol 1994;36:233.

Mee J, Paine M, Byrne E, et al. Immunotherapy of ocular myasthenia gravis reduces conversion to generalized myasthenia gravis. J Neuroophthalmol 2003;23:251.

Meriggioli MN, Ciafaloni E, Al-Hayk KA, et al. Mycophenolate mofetil for myasthenia gravis: An analysis of efficacy, safety, and tolerability. Neurology 2003;61:1438.

Mertens HG, Hertel P, Reuter P, et al. Effect of immunosuppressive drugs (azathioprine). Ann N Y Acad Sci 1981;337:691.

Miano MA, Bosley TM, Heiman-Patterson TD, et al. Factors influencing outcome of prednisone dose reduction in myasthenia gravis. Neurology 1991;41:919.

Miller NR: Myopathies and disorders of neuromuscular transmission. In: Walsh TJ, Hoyt WF, eds. Clinical Neuro-Ophthalmology, 4th ed. Baltimore: Williams & Wilkins, 1982;785.

Miller RG, Milner-Brown S, Mirka A. Prednisone-induced worsening of neuromuscular function in myasthenia gravis. Neurology 1986;36:729.

Millichap JG, Dodge PR. Diagnosis and treatment of myasthenia gravis in infancy, childhood, and adolescence. Neurology 1960;10:1007.

Milone M, Engel AG. Block of the endplate acetylcholine receptor channel by the sympathomimetic agents ephedrine, pseudoephedrine, and albuterol. Brain Res 1996;740:346.

Milone M, Wang HL, Ohno K, et al. Slow-channel myasthenic syndrome caused by enhanced activation enhanced activation, desensitization, and agonist binding affinity attributable to mutation in the M2 domain of the acetylcholine receptor alpha subunit. J Neurosci 1997;17:5651.

Misulis KE, Fenichel GM. Genetic forms of myasthenia gravis. Pediatr Neurol 1989;5:205.

Mohan S, Barohn RJ, Jackson CE, et al. Evaluation of myosin-reactive antibodies from a panel of myasthenia gravis patients. Clin Immunol Immunopathol 1994;70:266.

Monsul NT, Patwa HS, Knorr AM, et al. The effect of prednisone on the progression from ocular to generalized myasthenia gravis. J Neurol Sci 2004;217:131.

Mora M, Lambert EH, Engel AG. Synaptic vesicle abnormality in familial infantile myasthenia. Neurology 1987;37:206.

Motomura M, Lang B, Johnston I, et al. Incidence of serum anti–P/Q-type and anti–N-type calcium channel autoantibodies in the Lambert-Eaton myasthenic syndrome. J Neurol Sci 1996;147:35.

Mulder DG, Graves M, Hermann C. Thymectomy for myasthenia gravis: Recent observation and comparisons with past experience. Ann Thorac Surg 1989;48:551.

Myasthenia Gravis Clinical Study Group. A randomized clinical trial comparing prednisone and azathioprine in myasthenia gravis. Results of the second interim analysis. J Neurol Neurosurg Psychiatry 1993;53:1157.

Nakao YK, Motomura M, Fukudome T, et al. Seronegative Lambert-Eaton myasthenic syndrome. Study of 110 Japanese patients. Neurology 2002;59:1773

Namba T, Brown SB, Grob D. Neonatal myasthenia gravis: Report of two cases and review of the literature. Pediatrics 1970;45:488.

Nations SP, Wolfe GI, Amato AA, et al. Clinical features of patients with distal myasthenia gravis. Neurology 1997;48:A64.

Newsom-Davis J, Murray NMF. Plasma exchange and immunosuppressive drug treatment in the Lambert-Eaton myasthenic syndrome. Neurology 1984;34:480.

Odabasi Z, Demirci M, Kim DS, et al. Postexercise facilitation of reflexes is not common in Lambert-Eaton myasthenic syndrome. Neurology 2002;59:1085.

Oh SJ. Electromyography: Neuromuscular transmission studies. Baltimore: Williams & Wilkins, 1988.

Oh SJ. Diverse electrophysiological spectrum of the Lambert-Eaton myasthenic syndrome. Muscle Nerve 1989;12:464.

Oh SJ, Cho HK. Edrophonium responsiveness not necessarily diagnostic of myasthenia gravis. Muscle Nerve 1990;13:187.

Oh SJ, Kim DS, Head TC, et al. Low-dose quinidine and pyridostigmine: Relatively safe and effective long-term symptomatic therapy in Lambert-Eaton myasthenic syndrome. Muscle Nerve 1997;20:1146.

Oh SJ, Kim DS, Kuruoglu R, et al. Diagnostic sensitivity of the laboratory tests in myasthenia gravis. Muscle Nerve 1992;15:720.

Ohno K, Engel AG. Congenital myasthenic syndromes: Gene mutations. Neuromusc Disord 2000;10:534

Ohno K, Engel AG, Brengman JM, et al. The spectrum of mutations causing end-plate acetylcholinesterase deficiency. Ann Neurol 2000;47:162.

Ohno K, Engel AG, Shen XM, et al. Rapsyn mutations in humans cause endplate acetylcholine-receptor deficiency and myasthenic syndrome. Am J Hum Genet 2002;70:875.

Ohno K, Tsujino A, Brengman JM, et al. Choline acetyltransferase mutations cause myasthenic syndrome associated with episodic apnea in humans. Proc Natl Acad Sci U S A 2001;98:2017.

Ohta K, Shigemoto K, Kubo S, et al. MuSK antibodies in AchR Ab-seropositive MG vs AchR Ab-seronegative MG. Neurology 2004;62:2132.

O'Neill JH, Murrah NMF, Newsom-Davis J. The Lambert-Eaton myasthenic syndrome: A review of 50 cases. Brain 1988;111:577.

Oosterhuis HJ, Limburg PC, Hummel-Tappel E, et al. Antiacetylcholine receptor antibodies in myasthenia gravis. Part 3. The effect of thymectomy. J Neurol Sci 1985;69:335.

Oosterhuis HJ, Newsom-Davis J, Wokke JHJ, et al. The slow channel syndrome. Two new cases. Brain 1987;110:1061.

Osserman KE. Myasthenia gravis. New York: Grune & Stratton, 1958.

Palace J, Newsom-Davis J, Lecky B, et al. A randomized double-blind trial of prednisolone alone or with azathioprine in myasthenia gravis. Neurology 1998;50:1778.

Palace J, Wiles CM, Newsom-Davis J. 3,4-Diaminopyridine in the treatment of congenital (hereditary) myasthenia. J Neurol Neurosurg Psychiatry 1991;54:1069.

Papatestas AE, Genkins G, Kornfeld P, et al. Transcervical thymectomy in myasthenia gravis. Surg Gynecol Obstet 1975;140:535.

Papazian O. Transient neonatal myasthenia gravis. J Child Neurol 1992;7:135.

Pascuzzi RM, Coslett HB, Johns TR. Long-term corticosteroid treatment of myasthenia gravis: Report of 116 patients. Ann Neurol 1984;5:291.

Patrick J, Lindstrom J. Autoimmune response to Ach receptor. Science 1973;180:871.

Perez MC, Buot WL, Mercado-Danguilan C, et al. Stable remissions in myasthenia gravis. Neurology 1981;31:32.

Pickett JB, Berg B, Chaplin E, et al. Syndrome of botulism in infancy: Clinical and electrophysiologic study. N Engl J Med 1976;295:770.

Pinching A, Peters DK, Newsom-Davis J. Remission of myasthenia gravis following plasma exchange. Lancet 1976;2:1373.

Plauche WC. Myasthenia gravis in mothers and their newborns. Clin Obstet Gynecol 1991;34:82.

Plested CP, Tang T, Spreadbury I, et al. AchR phosphorylation and indirect inhibition of AchR function in seronegative MG. Neurology 2002;59:1682.

Rich MM, Teener JW, Bird SJ. Treatment of Lambert-Eaton syndrome with intravenous immunoglobulin. Muscle Nerve 1997;20:614.

Robertson WC, Chun RWM, Kornguth SE. Familial infantile myasthenia. Arch Neurol 1980;37:117.

Rodriguez M, Gomez MR, Howard FM, et al. Myasthenia gravis in children: Long-term follow-up. Ann Neurol 1983;13:504.

Romi R, Skeie GO, Aarli JA, et al. The severity of myasthenia gravis correlates with serum concentration of titin and ryanodine receptor antibodies. Arch Neurol 2000;57:1596.

Roses AD, Olanow W, McAdams MW, et al. No direct correlation between anti-acetylcholine receptor antibody levels and clinical state of individual patients with myasthenia gravis. Neurology 1981;31:220.

Rothbart HB. Myasthenia gravis in children: Its familial incidence. JAMA 1937;108:715.

Rowland LP. Controversies about the treatment of myasthenia gravis. Neurology 1980;43:644.

Rowland LP. General discussion on therapy in myasthenia gravis. Ann N Y Acad Sci 1987;505:607.

Ryniewicz B, Badurska B. Follow-up study of myasthenic children after thymectomy. J Neurol 1977;217:133.

Sanders DB, El-Salem K, Massey JM, et al. Clinical aspects of MuSK antibody positive seronegative MG. Neurology 2003;60:1978.

Sanders DB, Howard JF Jr, Massey JM. 3,4-Diaminopyridine in Lambert-Eaton myasthenic syndrome and myasthenia gravis. Ann N Y Acad Sci 1993;681:588.

Sanes JR, Jessell TM. The formation and generation of synapses. In: Kandel ER, Schwartz JH, Jessell TM, eds. Principles of neuroscience, 4th ed. New York: McGraw-Hill, 2000;1087.

Schiff RI. Transmission of viral infections through intravenous immune globulin. N Engl J Med 1994;331:1607.

Scuderi F, Marino M, Colonna L, et al. Anti-P110 autoantibodies identify a subtype of "seronegative" myasthenia gravis with prominent oculobulbar involvement. Lab Invest 2002;82:1139.

Selcen D, Fukuda T, Shen X-M, et al. Are MuSK antibodies the primary cause of myasthenic symptoms? Neurology 2004;62:1945.

Seybold ME. Thymectomy in childhood myasthenia gravis. Ann N Y Acad Sci 1998;841:731.

Seybold ME, Lambert EH, Lennon VA, et al. Experimental autoimmune myasthenia: Clinical, neurophysiologic, and pharmacologic aspects. Ann N Y Acad Sci 1976;274:275.

Shapira Y, Civdalli G, Szabo G, et al. A myasthenic syndrome in childhood leukemia. Develop Med Child Neurol 1974;16:668.

Sher E, Gotti C, Canal N, et al. Specificity of calcium channel autoantibodies in Lambert-Eaton myasthenic syndrome. Lancet 1989;2:640.

Shillito P, Vincent A, Newsom-Davis J. Congenital myasthenic syndromes. Neuromusc Disord 1993;3:183.

Simpson JA. An evaluation of thymectomy in myasthenia gravis. Brain 1958;81:112.

Simpson JA. Myasthenia gravis: A new hypothesis. Scott Med J 1960;5:419.

Snead OC, Benton JW, Dwyer D, et al. Juvenile myasthenia gravis. Neurology 1980;30:732.

Sommer N, Harcourt GC, Willcox N, et al. Acetylcholine receptor–reactive T lymphocytes from healthy subjects and myasthenia gravis patients. Neurology 1991;41:1270.

Sommer N, Willcox N, Harcourt GC, et al. Myasthenic thymus and thymoma are selectively enriched in acetylcholine receptor–reactive T cells. Ann Neurol 1990;28:312.

Spika JS, Shaffer N, Hargrett-Bean N, et al. Risk factors for infant botulism in the United States. Am J Dis Child 1989;143:828.

Stalberg E, Sanders DB. Electrophysiologic testing of neuromuscular transmission. In: Stalberg E, Young RR, eds. Clinical neurophysiology. London: Butterworth, 1981;88.

Stalberg E, Trontelj JV, Schwartz MS. Single-muscle-fiber recording of the jitter phenomenon in patients with myasthenia gravis and in members of their families. Ann N Y Acad Sci 1976;274:189.

Steg RE, Leflowitz DM. Cerebral infarction following intravenous immunoglobulin therapy for myasthenia gravis. Neurology 1994;44:1180.

Tami JA, Krolick K, Jackson C, et al. Detection of human antibodies to acetylcholine receptor (AchR) in patients with myasthenia gravis (MG) by immunohistochemistry and flow cytometry. Neurology 1994;44:A290.

Tan E, Hajinazarian M, Bay W, et al. Acute renal failure resulting from intravenous immunoglobulin therapy. Arch Neurol 1993;50:137.

Tindall RSA. Humoral immunity in myasthenia gravis: Effect of steroids and thymectomy. Neurology 1980;30:554.

Tindall RSA, Phillips JT, Rollins JA, et al. A clinical therapeutic trial of cyclosporine in myasthenia gravis. Ann N Y Acad Sci 1993;681:539.

Tindall RSA, Rollins JA, Phillips JT, et al. Preliminary results of a double-blind, randomized, placebo-controlled trial of cyclosporine in myasthenia gravis. N Engl J Med 1987;316:719.

Toyka KV, Drachman DB, Griffin DE, et al. Myasthenia gravis: Study of humoral immune mechanisms by passive transfer to mice. N Engl J Med 1977;296:125.

Tsao C-Y, Mendell JR, Friemer ML, et al. Lambert-Eaton myasthenic syndrome in children. J Child Neurol 2002;17:74.

Tsujino A, Maertens C, Ohno K, et al. Myasthenic syndrome caused by mutation of the SCN4A sodium channel. Proc Natl Acad Sci U S A 2003;100:7377.

Tzartos SJ, Lindstrom JM. Monoclonal antibodies used to probe acetylcholine receptor structure: localization of the main immunogenic region and detection of similarities between subunits. Proc Natl Acad Sci U S A 1980;77:755.

Uchitel O, Engel AG, Walls TJ, et al. Congenital myasthenic syndromes: II. Syndrome attributed to abnormal interaction of acetylcholine with its receptor. Muscle Nerve 1993;16:1293.

Vial C, Charles N, Chauplannaz G, et al. Myasthenia gravis in childhood and infancy: Usefulness of electrophysiologic studies. Arch Neurol 1991;48:847.

Vincent A, Cull-Candy SG, Newsom-Davis J, et al. Congenital myasthenia: End-plate acetylcholine receptors and electrophysiology in five cases. Muscle Nerve 1981;4:306.

Vincent A, Newsom-Davis J. Acetylcholine receptor antibody as a diagnostic test for myasthenia gravis: Results in 153 validated cases and 2967 diagnostic assays. J Neurol Neurosurg Psychiatry 1985;48:1246.

Vincent A, Palace J, Hilton-Jones D. Myasthenia gravis. Lancet 2001;357:2122.

Voltz R, Hohlfeld R, Fateh-Moghadam A, et al. Myasthenia gravis: Measurement of AchR autoantibodies using cell line TE671. Neurology 1991;41:1836.

Walls TJ, Engels AG, Harper CM, et al. Congenital neuromuscular junction acetylcholinesterase deficiency. Ann Neurol 1989;26:147.

Walls TJ, Engel AG, Nagel AS, et al. Congenital myasthenic syndrome associated with paucity of synaptic vesicles and reduced quantal release. Ann N Y Acad Sci 1993;681:461.

Warmolts JR, Engel WK. Benefit from alternate-day prednisone in myasthenia gravis. N Engl J Med 1972;286:17.

Weinberg DA, Lesser RL, Vollmer TL. Ocular myasthenia: A protean disorder. Surv Ophthalmol 1994;39:169.

Wekerle H, Paterson B, Ketelsen U-P, et al. Striated muscle fibers differentiate in monolayer cultures of adult thymus reticulum. Nature 1975;256:493.

Wilson R, Morris JG, Snyder JD, et al. Clinical characteristics of infant botulism in the United States: A study of the non-California cases. Pediatr Infect Dis 1982;1:148.

Wolfe GI, Barohn RJ, Foster BM, et al. Randomized, controlled trial of intravenous immunoglobulin in myasthenia gravis. Muscle Nerve 2002;26:549.

Wolfe GI, Barohn RJ, Galetta SL. Drugs for the diagnosis and treatment of myasthenia gravis. In: Zimmerman TJ, Kooner KS, Sharir M, et al., eds. Textbook of ocular pharmacology. Philadelphia: Lippincott-Raven, 1997;837.

Wolfe GI, Herbelin L, Nations SP, et al. Myasthenia gravis activities of daily living profile. Neurology 1999;52:1487.

Wolfe GI, Kaminski HJ, Jaretzki III A, et al. Development of a thymectomy trial in nonthymomatous myasthenia gravis patients receiving immunosuppressive therapy. Ann N Y Acad Sci 2003;998:473.

Younger DS, Jaretzki A III, Penn AS, et al. Maximum thymectomy for myasthenia gravis. Ann N Y Acad Sci 1987;505:832.

Youssef S. Thymectomy for myasthenia gravis in children. J Pediatr Surg 1983;18:537.

CHAPTER 79

Muscular Dystrophies

Diana M. Escolar and Robert T. Leshner

Muscular dystrophies are progressive, inherited skeletal muscle disorders resulting in muscle degeneration and loss of strength. This heterogeneous group of disorders has been further characterized at the clinical and molecular level since the 1980s, giving rise to the many unique forms of muscular dystrophies known today. The time of clinical onset of these disorders ranges from the neonatal period to late adulthood. The distribution of predominant muscle weakness can help identify six major phenotypes [Emery, 2002]:

- Duchenne-like, involving shoulder and pelvic girdle, neck flexors muscle with calf hypertrophy.
- Emery-Dreifuss–type with scapulohumeral peroneal distribution.
- Limb-girdle (pelvic and shoulder).
- Fascioscapulohumeral peroneal involvement.
- Distal muscle involvement (distal myopathy).
- Oculopharyngeal, as seen in oculopharyngeal muscular dystrophy, with involvement of these muscles plus shoulder and limb girdle.

The congenital forms of muscular dystrophies are generalized.

The mode of inheritance in muscular dystrophies can be autosomal dominant, autosomal recessive, or X-linked. The underlying molecular defects responsible for these disorders are very diverse, including extracellular matrix proteins (laminin-2, collagen VI), transmembrane- and sarcolemma-associated proteins (dystrophin, sarcoglycans, caveolin-3, α5 and α7 integrins, dysferlin), cytoplasmatic proteases (calpain-3), cytoplasmatic proteins associated with organelles and sarcomeres (titin, fukutin, telethonin), and nuclear membrane proteins (lamin, emerin). The molecular characterization of the different muscular dystrophies since the 1990s has helped increase the understanding of the sarcolemmal organization and underlying muscle biology responsible for the normal structure and maintenance of the normal sarcolemma. Figure 79-1 depicts an updated version of the muscle membrane. Binding relationships among proteins have turned out to be more complex than once thought, and the specific relation of these proteins, as well as the presence of phosphorylation sites, provides the basis for the pathophysiology that has been associated with these disorders. Disorders caused by mutations of these proteins are listed in the figure.

In view of the widely variable manifestation of the muscular dystrophies, the broad spectrum of other organs that might be involved in addition to muscle (i.e., myotonic dystrophies), and the diverse group of proteins that can cause these disorders, it seems that the only common feature among them is the characteristic pathologic changes in muscle that allows characterization of these disorders as a "dystrophy," although at times these features can be very mild.

An updated molecular-based classification of the muscular dystrophies is presented in Table 79-1. Many of these disorders first manifest clinically in adulthood and are not covered in detail in this chapter. The most common muscular dystrophy in children is Duchenne muscular dystrophy, and it is the main focus of this chapter. Extensive investigations of this disorder have shed light on the pathophysiology of other muscular dystrophies, especially those related to the dystrophin-associated glycoprotein complex (DGC), and so most of these features are discussed only in the Duchenne muscular dystrophy section.

DYSTROPHINOPATHIES

Dystrophinopathies are a group of muscular dystrophies resulting from mutations in the dystrophin gene, located on the short arm of the X chromosome in the Xp21 region [Baumbach et al., 1989]. Of these, Duchenne muscular dystrophy is the most common dystrophinopathy resulting from complete absence of the dystrophin gene product, the subsarcolemmal protein dystrophin. Its allelic variant, Becker muscular dystrophy, is rarer. Becker muscular dystrophy is a consequence of different types of mutations in the same gene (in-frame mutations) that result in decreased quantity or decreased quality of the dystrophin protein, giving rise to a disease with varied severity and time of onset, ranging from childhood to adulthood. Whereas Duchenne muscular dystrophy typically manifests before age 4 years, Becker muscular dystrophy can be asymptomatic for many decades.

Duchenne Muscular Dystrophy

History

In a communication to the Royal Medical and Chirurgical Society of London in December 1851 (published in the Transactions of the Society the following year), Edward Meryon, an English physician, described in considerable detail a disease affecting eight males in three families. He was particularly impressed by the predilection for male members and its familial nature and by the fact that the progressive muscle wasting and weakness resulted from a disease of muscle and not the nervous system. He described meticulous histologic studies that revealed no abnormality of the spinal cord or nerves, but in muscle tissue he observed extensive "granular degeneration" and, in particular, that the sarcolemma was broken down and destroyed. He appears to

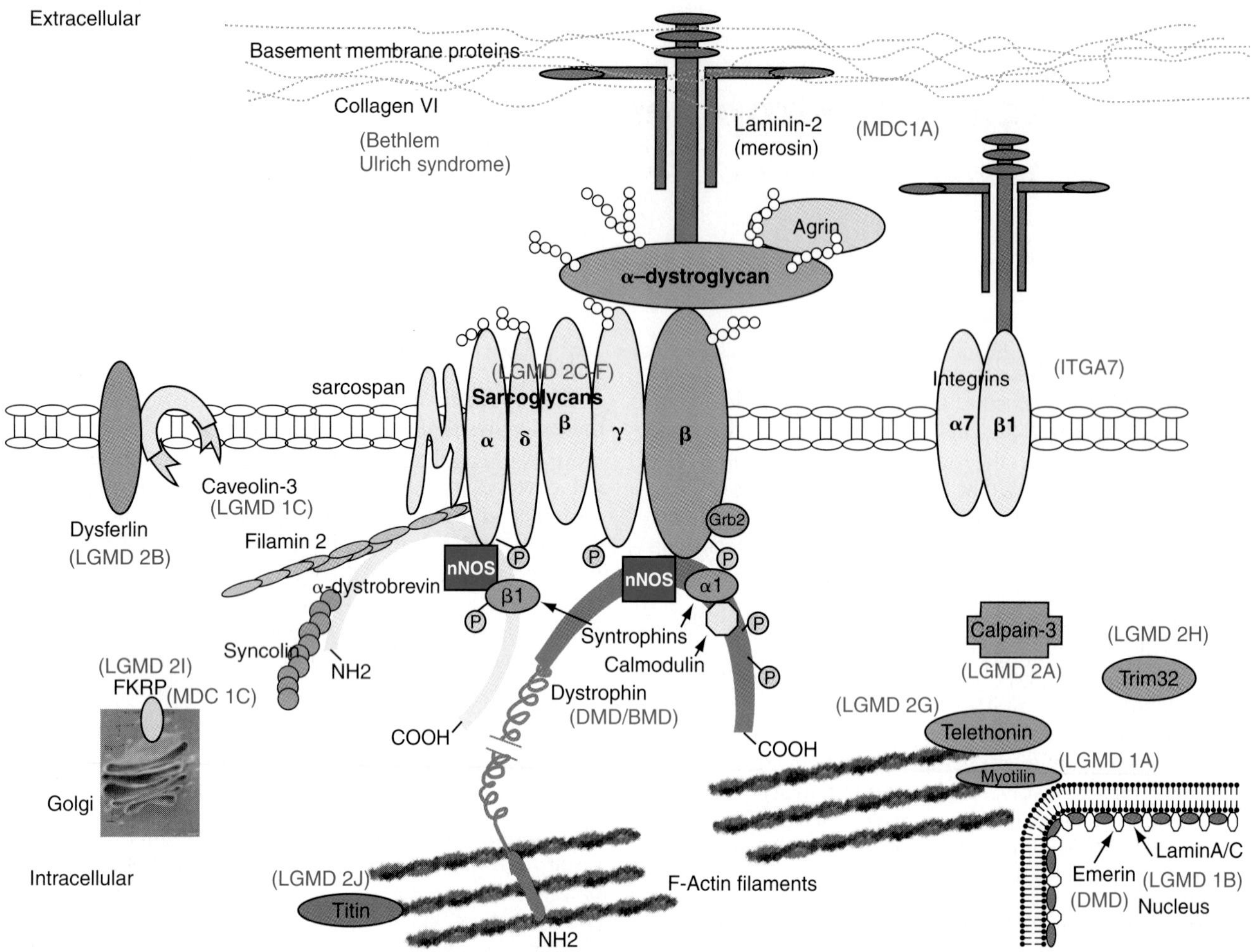

FIGURE 79-1. Diagram of the muscle membrane as known today, illustrating association of dystrophin-glycoprotein complex linkage to contractile proteins, extracellular matrix proteins, and other proteins with signaling properties (syntrophins, Grb2). It also illustrates the multiple phosphorylation sites in the 3′ end of dystrophin, dystrobrevin, and dystroglycans. Diseases associated with defect in individual proteins are also listed in parentheses. BMD, Becker muscular dystrophy; DMD, Duchenne muscular dystrophy; ITGA7, integrin α7; LGMD, limb-girdle muscular dystrophy; MDC1A, merosin-negative congenital muscular dystrophy; MDC1C, merosin-positive congenital muscular dystrophy; nNOS, neuronal nitric oxide synthetase. See also Color Plate.

have been the first physician to make a detailed clinical, genetic, and pathologic study of the disorder several years before Guillaume-Benjamin Duchenne [Emery, 1993]. Later, in 1868, Duchenne, a French neurologist and student of electrical stimulation of muscle, described a syndrome characterized by muscular paralysis associated with muscle hypertrophy that resulted from accumulation of large amounts of fat and connective tissue in muscle. Duchenne described the first instrument capable of procuring muscle for biopsy and analysis, and his description of pseudohypertrophic, X-linked muscular dystrophy bears his name.

The discovery of the molecular defect in this disorder constitutes the first example of reverse cloning. Restriction fragment length polymorphisms were used to track the cosegregation of the disease phenotype with DNA markers within a family. The initial cloning of the Duchenne dystrophy gene occurred in 1985 and 1986 [Kunkel et al., 1985; Monaco et al., 1985; Ray et al., 1985], followed by isolation of the DNA clones complementary to the Duchenne dystrophy gene [Burghes et al., 1987; Cross et al., 1987; Monaco et al., 1986]. These complementary DNA clones, which were made from RNA transcripts from the Duchenne gene, contain the coding sequences or exons in the Duchenne gene. Subsequently, the protein product of the human Duchenne muscular dystrophy locus was identified through the use of polyclonal antibodies directed against fusion proteins containing two distinct regions of the Duchenne muscular dystrophy locus's complementary DNA. This protein was named *dystrophin* [Hoffman et al., 1987a].

Molecular Pathogenesis

Duchenne muscular dystrophy is a relentlessly progressive skeletal muscle disorder caused by a genetic mutation in the X-linked dystrophin gene, resulting in absence of a critical protein, dystrophin [Hoffman et al., 1987a, 1988; Koenig et al., 1987].

The dystrophin gene includes 86 exons (including seven promoters linked to unique first exons), which make up only 0.6% of the gene; the rest consists of introns. The gene spans a genetic distance of more than 2.5 million base pairs and is the largest human gene isolated to date [Burmeister and Lehrach, 1986].

In more than 90% of males with the Duchenne muscular dystrophy genotype, there is an absence of dystrophin corresponding to an "out-of-frame" mutation that disrupts

TABLE 79-1

Classification of the Muscular Dystrophies

DISEASE	GENE LOCUS	GENE PRODUCT	MODE OF INHERITANCE
Limb-Girdle Muscular Dystrophy (LGMD) Caused by Sarcolemma or Cytosolic Protein Defects			
Duchenne/Becker muscular dystrophy	Xp21	Dystrophin	XR
LGMD1A	5q22	Myotilin	AD
LGMD1B	1q11-q21	Lamin A/C	AD
LGMD1C	3p25	Caveolin-3	AD
LGMD1D	6q23	Not identified	AD
LGMD1E	7q	Not identified	AD
LGMD1F	2q	Not identified	AD
LGMD2A	15q15	Calpain-3	AR
LGMD2B/Myoshi's myopathy	2p13	Dysferlin	AR
LGMD2C	13q12	γ-Sarcoglycan	AR
LGMD2D	17q112	α-Sarcoglycan	AR
LGMD2E	4q12	β-Sarcoglycan	AR
LGMD2F	5q23	δ-Sarcoglycan	AR
LGMD2G	17q11	TCAP	AR
LGMD2H	9q31	TRIM32	AR
LGMD2I	13q13	FKRP	AR
LGMD2J/Tibial muscular dystrophy	2q31	Titin	AR/AD
Congenital Muscular Dystrophies (CMDs) Secondary to Glycosylation Disorder			
Fukuyama's muscular dystrophy	9q31-q33	Fukutin	AR
Muscle-eye-brain disease	1p3	POMGnT1 glycosyltransferase	AR
Walker-Warburg syndrome	9q34	POMT1	AR
MDC1A	6q22	Laminin-2 (merosin)	AR
MDC1B	1q42	Not identified	AR
MDC1C	19q13	FKRP	AR
MDC1D	22q12	LARGE	AR
Other Congenital Muscular Dystrophies			
CMD with early rigid spine	1p36	Selenoprotein 1	AR
CMD with ITGA7 mutations	12q	Integrin α7	AR
Ullrich's syndrome/Bethlem's myopathy	21q22.3 (A1, A2) 2q37(A3)	Collagen 6 A1, A2, and A3	AD
Muscular Dystrophies Secondary to Nuclear Envelope Defects ("Nuclear Envelopathies")			
Emery-Dreifuss muscular dystrophy (EDMDX)	Xq28	Emerin	XR
Emery-Dreifuss muscular dystrophy (EDMD1)	1q11-q23	Lamin A/C	AD/sporadic
Muscular Dystrophies Secondary to RNA Metabolism Defect			
Myotonic dystrophy 1 (DM1)	19q13	DM	AD
Myotonic dystrophy 2 (DM2)	3q21	ZFN9	AD
Muscular Dystrophies of Unknown Mechanism			
Facioscapulohumeral muscular dystrophy	4q35	Not identified	AD
Oculopharyngeal muscular dystrophy	14q11.2-q13	PABp2	AD

AD, autosomal dominant; AR, autosomal recessive; MDC, merosin-negative congenital muscular dystrophy; XR, X-linked recessive.

normal dystrophin transcription [Gillard et al., 1989]. These mutations cause a premature stop codon and early termination of messenger RNA transcription. As a result, an unstable RNA is produced, undergoes rapid decay, and eventually leads to the production of nearly undetectable concentrations of truncated proteins. If the mutation maintains translational reading, an "in-frame" deletion, the Becker muscular dystrophy phenotype, with variably decreased amounts of abnormal molecular weight dystrophin, is present [Hoffman et al., 1988]. This reading frame hypothesis holds for over 90% of afflicted individuals and is commonly used both as a diagnostic confirmation of dystrophinopathies and for the differential diagnosis of Duchenne muscular dystrophy and Becker muscular dystrophy.

Exceptions to these two typical situations occur in approximately 10% of patients. Out-of-frame deletions affecting exons 3 to 7, 5 to 7, 3 to 6 or downstream at exons 51, 49 to 50, 47 to 52, 44, or 45 can result in a milder Becker muscular dystrophy phenotype. The most common explanation for the presence of at least some dystrophin in these patients is exon skipping, which occurs through alternative splicing [Nicholson et al., 1992; Patria et al., 1996]. In this form of Becker muscular dystrophy, the carboxy-terminus is always preserved [Arahata et al., 1991]. Exon skipping is also the underlying mechanism for the revertant fibers (muscle fibers exhibiting dystrophin staining in muscle biopsies) evident in about 50% of males with Duchenne muscular dystrophy [Winnard et al., 1995]. The limited expression of dystrophin results in a slower progression of muscle weakness than in the usual Duchenne phenotype [Arahata et al., 1989; Baumbach et al., 1989; Koenig et al., 1989; Malhotra et al., 1988]. A new therapeutic strategy in Duchenne muscular dystrophy is being developed on the basis of this natural finding, attempting to pharmacologically induce "exon-skipping" in Duchenne muscular dystrophy patients to allow for production of some quantity of dystrophin to ameliorate the phenotype (see therapeutic approaches).

Another exception to the reading frame hypothesis might occur with large in-frame deletions in the 5′ end that extend to the middle of the rod domain (i.e., deletions of exons 3 to 31, 3 to 25, 4 to 41, and 4 to 18) [Nevo et al., 2003], as well as with small in-frame deletions of exons 3 to 13 [Muntoni et al., 1994] that cause the severe Duchenne muscular dystrophy phenotype. These small and large mutations affect another actin-binding domain in this N-terminus of dystrophin and therefore may have significant functional consequences, resulting in the worsened phenotype. Other mechanisms, such as unexpected effect of the deletion on splicing behavior, might also be implicated in determining the phenotypic outcome [Muntoni et al., 1994].

After the complete dystrophin complementary DNA was isolated [Koenig et al., 1987], it became evident that about 60% of patients with Duchenne and Becker muscular dystrophies manifest structural rearrangements of the deletion type [Darras et al., 1988; den Dunnen et al., 1987; Forrest et al., 1987; Koenig et al., 1987; Kunkel, 1986]. Deletions and, more rarely, duplications can happen almost anywhere in the dystrophin gene; however, two deletion hot spots are known. The most commonly mutated region includes exons 45 to 55 with genomic breakpoints (i.e., the end points of where the deletions actually occur) lying within intron 44. The second hot spot is located toward the 5′ end and includes exons 2 to 19 with genomic breakpoints commonly found in introns 2 and 7 [Beggs et al., 1990; den Dunnen et al., 1989; Nobile et al., 1995; Oudet et al., 1992]. The other 40% of patients have mutations that result from small mutations (point mutations resulting in frameshift or nonsense mutations) or duplications.

The incidence of Duchenne muscular dystrophy is approximately 1 per 3300 male births [Brooks and Emery, 1977; Jeppesen et al., 2003]. Although the most common mode of inheritance is X-linked recessive (mother is a carrier), this disorder is associated with a high spontaneous mutation rate, which accounts for approximately 30% of cases [Brooks and Emery, 1977; Moser, 1984; Scheuerbrandt et al., 1986; van Essen et al., 1992]. Therefore, almost one third of males with Duchenne muscular dystrophy have no family history of muscular dystrophy. This mutation rate is estimated to be 10 times higher than for any other genetic disorder [Hoffman et al., 1992] because of the extremely large Duchenne gene size [Hoffman and Kunkel, 1989]. The 2.5 million base pairs constituting the gene (a full 1% of the X chromosome) provide a large target for random mutational events. Nonfamilial Duchenne muscular dystrophy patients might be the product of germinal mosaicism on the X chromosome (a mutation occurring before the birth of the mother) [Bakker et al., 1989; Bunyan et al., 1994; Lanman et al., 1987; Smith et al., 1999], in which case the mother is a Duchenne muscular dystrophy carrier, but no other family member is affected with Duchenne muscular dystrophy. Another possibility is that the mother or father has gonadal mosaicism: a new mutation in maternal or paternal germ cells in an unaffected father or mother whose other maternal cells (i.e., muscle, lymphocytes) are normal [Darras et al., 1988; Hurko et al., 1989; Lanman et al., 1987]. This mother neither is an obligate carrier nor has the muscle characteristics of the Duchenne muscular dystrophy carrier. The remaining new mutations are partial gene duplications [Hu et al., 1989, 1990].

Because the genetic defect is an X-linked recessive trait, dystrophinopathies are expressed primarily in boys and young men. However, females may manifest symptoms of Duchenne muscular dystrophy if they also exhibit skewed X-inactivation, wherein the abnormal X chromosome is expressed in an excessively abnormal proportion [Kinoshita et al., 1990; Lesca et al., 2003; Pena et al., 1987; Yoshioka et al., 1986]. Females with both Duchenne muscular dystrophy and Turner's syndrome have been described. This rare combination arises because the single X chromosome contains a mutant gene [Bjerglund Nielsen and Nielsen, 1984; Ferrier et al., 1965; Lescaut et al., 2004].

GENOTYPE/PHENOTYPE CORRELATION

There is no simple relationship between the size of the deletion and the resultant clinical disease. For example, large deletions, which may involve nearly 50% of the gene, have been described in patients with Becker muscular dystrophy [England et al., 1990], whereas deletions of small exons, such as exon 44, typically results in classic Duchenne muscular dystrophy. The central and distal rod domains seem to be almost dispensable functionally; some deletions in this region are associated with a syndrome characterized only by myalgia and muscle cramps or by an isolated increase in creatine kinase [Beggs et al., 1991; Gospe et al., 1989]. This finding has been reported in patients with in-frame deletions in exons 32 to 44, 48 to 51, or 48 to 53, all of whom had normal or near normal dystrophin concentrations [Melis et al., 1998]. The effect of the genetic mutations on the phenotype depends on whether it does or does not disrupt the reading frame (reading frame hypothesis) and on specific essential signaling or binding sites in the dystrophin protein that might be affected by the mutation.

Good correlation is generally found between the severity of the phenotype and the effect of the deletion on the reading frame: Deletions that disrupt the reading frame result in a severe phenotype, whereas in-frame deletions are associated with a milder disease course [Gillard et al., 1989]. These assumptions hold true for about 90% of the cases in which mutations are in the rod domain of the dystrophin protein. Rare exceptions to this rule exist, mainly resulting from frameshift mutations in the 5′ region of the gene (in particular, deletions involving exons 3 to 7) which are associated with a milder phenotype than expected [Malhotra et al., 1988]. When mutations arise in the 5′ region of the gene, especially in the first 13 exons of the dystrophin gene, one third of them have a phenotype different from that theoretically expected [Muntoni et al., 1994]. Affected patients can have a severe clinical phenotype despite the presence of a small in-frame deletion, or they can have a mild phenotype with an out-of-frame deletion. In the first case, a Duchenne phenotype is associated with in-frame deletions of exon 5, of exon 3, and of exons 3 to 13. In the second case, an intermediate Duchenne muscular dystrophy or Becker phenotype is seen with out-of-frame deletions involving not only the usual exons 3 to 7 but also 5 to 7 and 3 to 6 [Muntoni et al., 1994]. Because of this, a high proportion of patients with a deletion in the 5′ end of the gene have a phenotype that is not predictable on the basis of the effect of the deletion on the reading frame.

Very large chromosomal deletions, such as the Xp21 chromosomal microdeletion syndrome, cause multisystem disorders along with the Duchenne muscular dystrophy phenotype [Francke et al., 1985].

The Leiden database (http://www.dmd.nl/) is a useful resource for phenotype/genotype correlation in situations in which genetic testing and phenotype do not appear to be clearly correlated.

Pathophysiology

DYSTROPHIN PROTEIN

The normal dystrophin gene creates a 14-kilobase dystrophin messenger RNA that encodes 3685 amino acids, producing a 427-kD protein called *dystrophin.* Dystrophin localizes to the subsarcolemmal region in skeletal and cardiac muscle and constitutes 0.002% of total muscle protein [Hoffman et al., 1987a, 1987b; Knudson et al., 1988]. Dystrophin binds to the cytoskeletal actin and to the cytoplasmic tail of the transmembrane DGC protein β-dystroglycan and thus forms a link from the cytoskeleton to the extracellular matrix (see Fig. 79-1).

Dystrophin contains 3685 amino acids and is separated into four domains: the N-terminus, the rod domain, a cysteine-rich area, and the C-terminus [Koenig et al., 1987]. The N-terminus consists of the first 240 amino acids and provides an F-actin binding site at three distinct regions with α-actinin homology. The rod region is a succession of 25 triple-helical repeats similar to spectrin and contains about 3000 residues, including four proline-rich regions that may act as hinges. Another F-actin binding site is located near the middle of the dystrophin rod domain but with significantly lower affinity than the N-terminus site [Rybakova et al., 1996]. A cysteine-rich area with amino acids 3080 to 3360 has a WW domain that binds to the protein β-dystroglycan, an essential protein through which dystrophin links to other integral membrane components of the DGC [Ozawa, 1995; Ozawa et al., 1995]. The site at which dystrophin binds to β-dystroglycan extends to the first half of the carboxy-terminal domain (C-terminus) [Watkins et al., 2000]. The C-terminus comprises the last 420 amino acids and has homology to utrophin and dystrobrevin. This area contains many potential phosphorylation sites and also binds to syntrophins at exon 74 and possibly to dystrophin-associated glycoproteins [Rybakova et al., 1996].

Dystrophin is organized in costamers and is present in greater amounts at myotendinous and neuromuscular junctions than in other muscle areas. In the heart, it is also associated with T tubules. In smooth muscle, it is discontinuous along membranes, alternating with vinculin.

Besides the full dystrophin protein just described, seven different dystrophin transcripts can be identified. These transcripts have different promoter regions and initial exons. The N-terminus region is excluded in smaller dystrophins, but the C-terminus region is found in all seven dystrophin transcripts. The transcripts are specific to cell types. Three full-length isoforms have the same number of exons but are derived from three independent promoters in brain, muscle, and Purkinje cerebellar neurons. The best characterized of these transcripts is the previously described muscle protein, expressed not only in skeletal muscle but also in cardiac muscle, smooth muscle, and retina. A cortical 427-kDa transcript is found in cortical postsynaptic densities, retina, and skeletal muscle [Boyce et al., 1991]. A Purkinje cell 427-kDa transcript is found in the cerebellum [Gorecki et al., 1992]. There is also a retinal 260-kDa transcript, a brain and kidney 140-kDa transcript, and a Schwann cell 116-ka protein resulting from transcription beginning on exon 56 [Byers et al., 1993]. A glial 71-kDa transcript resulting from transcription beginning at exon 63 can be found in glia, viscera, and cardiac muscle [Rapaport et al., 1992]. The presence or absence of these seven dystrophin transcripts in Duchenne muscular dystrophy depends on the location and size of deletion in the dystrophin gene, which determines phenotypic expression.

PRIMARY AND SECONDARY (DOWNSTREAM) EVENTS

An important concept that has evolved is that muscle cell death in the muscular dystrophies (by apoptosis and necrosis) is conditional and reflects a propensity that varies between muscles and changes with age [Rando, 2001b]. The fact that adjacent muscle groups in Duchenne muscular dystrophy can be completely normal and others are undergoing active necrosis not only supports this concept but also argues against the concept of inevitability. If endogenous biochemical mechanisms alter the ability of a muscle cell to live or die while the genetic and biochemical defects remain constant, then pharmacologic modulation of these pathways should result in successful therapies for Duchenne muscular dystrophy and other muscular dystrophies [Rando, 2001b]. Whereas dystrophin deficiency is the primary cause of Duchenne muscular dystrophy, multiple secondary pathways are responsible for the progression of muscle necrosis, abnormal fibrosis, and failure of regeneration that results in a progressively worsening clinical status. Since the mid-1990s, hypothesis-driven research has dissected several abnormal pathways involved in muscular dystrophy progression. There is ample literature establishing evidence of oxidative radical damage to myofibers [Baker and Austin, 1989; Haycock et al., 1996a, 1996b; Murphy and Kehrer, 1986; Rando et al., 1998], inflammation [Cai et al., 2000; Kissel et al., 1993; Lagrota-Candido et al., 2002; McDouall et al., 1990; Nahirney et al., 1997; Porter et al., 2002; Shaw et al., 1996; Spencer et al., 2000; Spencer and Tidball, 2001], abnormal calcium homeostasis [Baker and Austin, 1989; De Luca et al., 2002; Leijendekker et al., 1996; Murphy and Kehrer, 1986; Pulido et al., 1998; Ruegg et al., 2002; Wrogemann and Pena, 1976], myonuclear apoptosis [Adams et al., 2001; Rando, 2001b; Sandri et al., 1995, 1997, 1998a, 1998b, 2001; Smith et al., 2000; Spencer et al., 1997; Tews, 2002; Tews and Goebel, 1997; Tindall et al., 1987], and abnormal fibrosis and failure of regeneration [Bernasconi et al., 1995, 1999; D'Amore et al., 1994; Iannaccone et al., 1995; Luz et al., 2002; Melone et al., 2000; Morrison et al., 2000; Murakami et al., 1999; Passerini et al., 2002; Rando, 2001b; Yamazaki et al., 1994]. This evidence has been validated by cross-sectional genome-wide approaches that allow an overall analysis of multiple defective mechanisms in Duchenne muscular dystrophy

[Chen et al., 2000; Porter et al., 2002]. The increasing understanding of these events has led to the discovery of potential pharmacologic targets designed to reverse, stop, or slow down muscle damage and progression of disease, even if the primary genetic defect cannot at present be repaired. Thus, it is important to understand these mechanisms as the basis of present and future therapies for this otherwise fatal disease.

Mechanical Membrane Fragility

Dystrophin is a link between the intracellular cytoskeleton and the extracellular matrix. The carboxy-terminal of dystrophin is attached to the sarcolemma, the surface membrane of striated muscle cells [Arahata et al., 1988; Bonilla et al., 1988; Watkins et al., 1988; Zubrzycka-Gaarn et al., 1988], binding to β-dystroglycan [Jung et al., 1995] and, through this, to other dystrophin-associated glycoproteins [Ervasti and Campbell, 1991]. When dystrophin is lost, disconnection of the link between contractile proteins to β-dystroglycan results in loss of β-dystroglycan and DGC from sarcolemma, expressed as reduced α-sarcoglycan immunoreactivity.

The location of dystrophin supported the original idea of fragile membranes in Duchenne muscular dystrophy and Becker muscular dystrophy, with membrane gaps that allow leakage of cytoplasmic components, such as creatine kinase, and the influx of excessive Ca^{2+}. Initially, it was thought that the main function of dystrophin was to provide mechanical reinforcement to the sarcolemma and thereby protect it from the mechanical stress of muscle contraction [Petrof et al., 1993]. Indeed, dystrophin is a load-bearing element, and deficiency in dystrophin leads to muscle membrane fragility and aberrant mechanotransduction [Kumar et al., 2004]. In the absence of dystrophin, there is disruption to normal force transmission and greater stress placed on myofibrillar and membrane proteins, leading to muscle damage [Lynch, 2004], especially during lengthening (eccentric) contractions, during which a muscle contracts against a mechanical force pulling in the opposite direction [Lynch et al., 2000]. The consequent muscle membrane fragility and abnormal permeability characteristics allow increased Ca^{2+} influx intracellularly [Mallouk and Allard, 2000; Mallouk et al., 2000] and initiate some aspects of the pathologic cascade of events that result in muscle necrosis and fibrosis [Ruegg and Gillis, 1999; Ruegg et al., 2002]. However, it does not appear that Ca^{2+} enters the cell through a "broken" membrane.

Abnormal Permeability to Calcium and Chronic Increase of Intracellular Calcium

Although the theory of increased membrane microdisruptions with subsequent increased Ca^{2+} permeability cannot be refuted, there is accumulating evidence that abnormal Ca^{2+} handling may be related to direct dystrophin regulation of mechanosensitive transient receptor potential channels [Vandebrouck et al., 2002b; Yeung and Allen, 2004], as well as abnormal Ca^{2+} intracellular cycling [Doran et al., 2004; Dowling et al., 2004; Woods et al., 2004]. Several nifedipine-insensitive, voltage-independent Ca^{2+} channels might be involved in the initial abnormal Ca^{2+} entry. This new evidence is extremely important, because modulation of these channels could be new therapeutic targets. Although there is concordant evidence of increased Ca^{2+} influx to the cell, there is no consensus on an overall increase in resting intracellular Ca^{2+} concentration [Gillis, 1996]. As explained later, not only are Ca^{2+} currents increased, but release of Ca^{2+} from the sarcoplasmic reticulum appears to be decreased, and many Ca^{2+} buffering proteins are abnormal, so that the overall intracellular Ca^{2+} concentration at rest might be difficult to measure.

One line of evidence involves abnormal function of "stretch-activated" and "stretch-inactivated" Ca^{2+} channels, a subfamily of the transient receptor potential channels [Clapham, 2003]. These stretch-activated channels are abnormally active under mechanical stimulation in mdx (murine model of Duchenne muscular dystrophy) myotubes and result in an increase in intracellular Ca^{2+} [Mallouk and Allard, 2000; Vandebrouck et al., 2002a, 2002b]. In addition, there is evidence that a large number of these channels, when subjected to mild mechanical stress, irreversibly shift to a stretch-inactivated channel form [Franco and Lansman, 1990] that remains open at rest and allows a chronic increase of calcium currents [Franco-Obregon and Lansman, 2002]. Accumulation of abnormally active Ca^{2+} leak channels over time results in a gradual loss of Ca^{2+} homeostasis and eventual cell death [Alderton and Steinhardt, 2000]. This increase of Ca^{2+} current might also be initiated by other types of Ca^{2+} permeable, growth factor–activated channels. The latter are normally localized in the cytoplasm of skeletal muscle, and translocate to the plasma membrane only under insulin-like growth factor 1 and possibly other growth factor stimuli [Iwata et al., 2003]. In dystrophic muscle, these channels are abnormally increased in the sarcolemma and seem to be directly involved with the increased in intracellular Ca^{2+} and abnormal creatine kinase efflux seen during mechanical stress of dystrophic muscle membrane [Iwata et al., 2003]. The increase in intracellular Ca^{2+} further increases the translocation of cytoplasmic growth factor–activated channels to the membrane, with subsequent increase of intracellular Ca^{2+} in a vicious cycle.

Of practical importance is that blockade of these stretch-activated channels has been achieved by the nonselective transient receptor potential blockers gadolinium and mycin, as well as by the selective cationic transient receptor potential blocker GsMTx4 (spider venom toxin) and has resulted in normalization of intracellular calcium and muscle force generation ex vivo in mdx mouse muscle [Yeung et al., 2003, 2005]. Furthermore, treatment of mdx mice with oral streptomycin resulted in decreased muscle necrosis, which is suggestive of its possible use in clinical trials [Yeung et al., 2005]. Forced expression of the full length and mini-dystrophin protein in dystrophin-deficient So18 skeletal myotubes also rectified steady-state levels of subcellular concentrations of Ca^{2+} and of Ca^{2+} transients [Marchand et al., 2001, 2004].

The L-type, voltage gated Ca^{2+} channels appear to be abnormal in the absence of dystrophin, as it was demonstrated that the Ca^{2+} currents in response to an action potential were much smaller in mdx mice than in normal control subjects. A disrupted direct or indirect linkage of dystrophin with these channels may be crucial for proper excitation-contraction coupling to initiate Ca^{2+} release from the sarcoplasmic reticulum. This linkage seems to be fully restored in the presence of mini-dystrophin [Friedrich et al., 2004].

Calcium cycling within the dystrophic muscle cell is also altered in mdx mice. Although the subsarcolemmal Ca^{2+}

concentration might be elevated [Mallouk et al., 2000], release of Ca^{2+} by the sarcoplasmic reticulum in response to an action potential is much decreased in this model [Plant and Lynch, 2003; Woods et al., 2004] and might contribute to abnormal activation-contraction coupling and subsequent muscle weakness. The Ca^{2+} buffering system in dystrophin myotubes is equally affected. A key luminal Ca^{2+}-binding protein, sarcalumenin, is affected in mdx skeletal muscle, which results in an abnormal shuttling of Ca^{2+} between the Ca^{2+}-uptake sarco-endoplasmic reticulum Ca^{2+}-adenosine triphosphatase and calsequestrin and might indirectly amplify the Ca^{2+} leak channel-induced increase in cytosolic Ca^{2+} levels [Dowling et al., 2004].

Abnormal intracellular Ca^{2+} levels result in abnormal activation of Ca^{2+}-activated proteases (e.g., calpain) with subsequent abnormal degradation of intracellular proteins that likely contribute to the abnormal functioning of the leak channels [Turner et al., 1993]. There is evidence that exercise worsens the abnormalities in calcium homeostasis in mdx [Fraysse et al., 2004]. This finding is not surprising because it is well known that excessive exercise by individuals with Duchenne muscular dystrophy may be deleterious and exacerbate muscle weakness [Allen, 2004; Ansved, 2003].

Abnormal Immunologic Response

In normal skeletal muscle, contraction-induced damage is followed by an inflammatory response involving multiple cell types that subsides over several days. This transient inflammatory response is a normal homeostatic reaction to muscle damage. In contrast, a persistent inflammatory response is observed in dystrophic skeletal muscle that leads to an altered extracellular environment that includes an increased presence of inflammatory cells (i.e., macrophages) and elevated levels of various inflammatory cytokines (i.e., tumor necrosis factor α, transforming growth factor β). Therefore, the signals that lead to successful muscle repair in healthy muscle may promote muscle wasting and fibrosis in dystrophic muscle.

Evidence supporting the role of the immune system in promoting muscle pathology in Duchenne muscular dystrophy, as well as the active role of cytotoxic T cells and myeloid cells in the pathophysiology of progressive muscle necrosis and fibrosis in Duchenne muscular dystrophy and mdx mice, has accumulated since the mid-1990s [Spencer and Tidball, 2001]. More recently, genome-wide approaches investigating the gene expression profile of Duchenne muscular dystrophy and mdx mouse muscles have revealed that an abnormal immunologic response is induced very early and is maintained at a low level in Duchenne muscular dystrophy patients and mdx mice from early in the neonatal period [Chen et al., 2000; Porter et al., 2003a]. Microarray experiments conducted longitudinally in mdx mice have allowed identification of abnormally increased cytokines and their receptors within the muscle cells, which implies that the dystrophic muscle might contribute to abnormal chemotaxis [Porter et al., 2002, 2003a]. These cytokine pathways could be new therapeutic targets.

Several pathways are involved in abnormal immune response in Duchenne muscular dystrophy. First, invasion of antigen-presenting cells activate cytotoxic and helper T cells [Banchereau and Steinman, 1998; Hart, 1997]. These release interleukin-2 that initiates polyclonal expansion of cytotoxic T cells [Gussoni et al., 1994; Spencer et al., 1997, 2001], which in turn mediates muscle necrosis by perforin-mediated [Cai et al., 2000; Spencer et al., 1997, 2001] and cytokine-mediated (tumor necrosis factor α and transforming growth factor β) killing mechanisms [Isenberg et al., 1986; Lundberg et al., 1995; Morrison et al., 2000; Spencer et al., 2000; Tews and Goebel, 1996]. Another pathway is through circulating dermal dendritic cells, which are abundant in Duchenne muscular dystrophy muscle [Chen et al., 2000] and through $CD4^+$ cells, which in turn activate (through interleukin-2) $CD8^+$ cells. Finally, another immune pathway starts by the invasion of muscle by myeloid cells, including macrophages, neutrophils, eosinophils, and mast cells [Arahata and Engel, 1988; Cai et al., 2000; Gorospe et al., 1994b; McDouall et al., 1990]. Most of these can kill target cells by liberating cytokines (tumor necrosis factor α; macrophage inflammatory protein 1αβ, RANTES), and by generating high concentrations of oxidative radicals. Mast cells can also promote muscle fibrosis [Gorospe et al., 1994a; Granchelli et al., 1996]. Muscle cells might become autoreactive as they liberate tumor necrosis factor α and could be an additional source of antigen-presenting cells [Behrens et al., 1998]. Many of these specific pathways are known to be blocked by prednisone, including induction of the transcription of I B (inhibitor), which keeps nuclear factor κβ in the inactive state; decreased production of proinflammatory cytokines; and induction of genes that inhibit cyclooxygenase-2, adhesion molecules, and other inflammatory mediators.

Abnormal Signaling Functions

Although the mechanical theory remains an important one and is well documented [Kumar et al., 2004], there is accumulating evidence that the DGC complex has important muscle cell–signaling functions, and its integrity is essential for muscle cell viability [Rando, 2001a]. These functions include transmembrane signaling (through β-dystroglycan), docking of signal transduction molecules (e.g., caveolin-3) and interaction with or regulation of other transmembrane complexes (e.g., integrins). A review of this line of evidence is beyond the scope of this chapter; the interested reader is referred to an excellent published summary [Rando, 2001a]. The absence of dystrophin causes extensive abnormalities and disruption of the DGC, in which sarcoglycans, neuronal nitric oxide synthetase [Rando, 2001b], and other members of the DGC lose their association with the sarcolemma. Many of the putative signaling cascades and molecules associated with this complex are known to regulate the balance between pro- and anti-apoptotic pathways [Rando, 2001a]. In addition to direct regulation of apoptosis, the defective DGC signaling might alter the metabolic pathways necessary to modulate cell susceptibility to injury. Of these important pathways that are clearly involved in Duchenne muscular dystrophy pathogenesis and that lead to cell death when disrupted, those involving oxidative radical metabolism [Baker and Austin, 1989; Haycock et al., 1996b; Kumar and Boriek, 2003; Ragusa et al., 1997; Rando, 2002; Spencer et al., 2001] and intracellular Ca^{2+} regulation are of particular interest because they could be targets of pharmacologic modulation. In addition, mechanical stretch has been demonstrated to abnormally activate the classic nuclear factor κβ pathway (in a Ca^{2+}- independent manner) in the mdx mouse, resulting in increased expression of inflammatory cytokines interleukin-1β and tumor necrosis factor α, which precedes the onset of muscular dystrophy [Kumar and Boriek, 2003].

The "vascular" theory of Duchenne muscular dystrophy pathogenesis was supported in the past by morphologic evidence in Duchenne muscular dystrophy and mdx mouse muscle fiber group necrosis, which occurred very early in the disease, presumably secondary to ischemia. Indeed, more recent findings indicate that the mislocalization and reduction of neuronal nitric oxide synthetase in dystrophic muscle affects smooth vessel vasodilation in response to alpha-adrenergic stimuli during exercise [Thomas et al., 2003], and results in muscle ischemia [Sander et al., 2000]. Dystrophin-associated α-syntrophin appears to be essential for the membrane localization of neuronal nitric oxide synthetase [Thomas et al., 2003].

Abnormal Fibrosis and Muscle Regeneration

Fibrosis (excessive deposition of endomysial and perimysial extracellular matrix) is a phenomenon known to be secondary to chronic muscle inflammation and fiber degeneration in Duchenne muscular dystrophy [Porter et al., 2002]. However, the amount of fibrosis in Duchenne muscular dystrophy seems disproportionate in relation to the clinical severity in the earlier stages of the disease, which raises the hypothesis that an abnormal fibrotic process might be directly related to the absence of dystrophin and might occur in parallel to (as well as after) muscle necrosis and degeneration. In fact, there is enough evidence that both enhanced fibrinogenesis and decreased fibrinolysis [von Moers et al., 2005] are implicated in the development of muscle fibrosis in Duchenne muscular dystrophy. There is a clear increase in expression of the fibrogenic cytokine transforming growth factor β1 in muscle of Duchenne muscular dystrophy patients [Bernasconi et al., 1995] and in serum samples of individuals with Duchenne muscular dystrophy [Bernasconi et al., 1999]. Moreover, preclinical studies in mdx mice have revealed that transforming growth factor β1 levels are also significantly elevated in the diaphragm, the muscle in this model that better mimics human skeletal muscle pathology [Hartel et al., 2001; Iannaccone et al., 1995; Morrison et al., 2000; Passerini et al., 2002; Porter et al., 2002]. Similar findings of abnormal cytokine levels and fibrosis early in the disease process are found in the golden retriever model of Duchenne muscular dystrophy [Passerini et al., 2002]. The level of messenger RNA transcript for transforming growth factor β1 was found to be increased in mononucleated cells around areas of fiber necrosis in 6- and 9-week-old mdx mice but not in 12-week-old mdx mice [Gosselin et al., 2004]. These findings indicate a role of transforming growth factor β1 during the early stages of fibrogenesis in dystrophic diaphragmatic muscle. Transforming growth factor β1 induces organ fibrosis by increasing extracellular matrix synthesis [Gosselin et al., 2004] and by simultaneously inhibiting matrix-degradation proteases such as matrix metalloproteases, especially matrix metalloprotease 1 [Herbst et al., 1997; von Moers et al., 2005]. Another abnormal fibrotic pathway in Duchenne muscular dystrophy relates to an increase in levels of platelet-derived growth factor and its receptors, which have an important modulating role in the active stage of tissue destruction, as well as initiation and promotion of muscle fibrosis [Zhao et al., 2003]. Of concern is that fibroblasts in Duchenne muscular dystrophy appear to have a paracrine function inhibiting satellite cell growth [Melone et al., 2000], in which case abnormal fibrosis would directly decrease muscle regeneration.

Temporal gene expression profiling studies in Duchenne muscular dystrophy have demonstrated that inflammatory and profibrinogenic pathways predominate in the presymptomatic stages of the disease, whereas the acute activation of transforming growth factor β and failure of metabolic pathways occur later in the disease [Chen, 2005]. In hind limb mdx muscle, inflammation, proteolysis, and extracellular matrix upregulation and fibrosis are initiated very early in the course of the disease, represent a substantial component of the transcriptional response at that early age, and are tightly coordinated [Porter et al., 2003b]. Pharmacologic blockade of these pathways may have promising therapeutic implications, especially in symptomatic subjects [De Luca et al., 2005; Porter et al., 2002].

Clinical Characteristics

The natural history of untreated Duchenne muscular dystrophy follows a predictable course. However, the disease course can be modified with aggressive pharmacologic (corticosteroids) and rehabilitation treatments. The following sequence of events occurs in treated and untreated patients with Duchenne muscular dystrophy but at a much later age in the former.

The disease is present in infancy, with muscle fiber necrosis and a high serum creatine kinase enzyme level; however, clinical manifestations are typically not recognized until the child is 3 years of age or older. This "therapeutic window" has been previously underemphasized; however, it lends itself to the development of early therapeutic interventions to prevent or delay the onset of symptoms secondary to advanced muscle degeneration. Walking often begins later than in normal children, and affected children experience more falling than expected. Gait abnormality often becomes apparent at 3 to 4 years of age, prompting clinical evaluation. Muscle weakness is present initially in neck flexor muscles, with power being less than antigravity. As a result, the child needs to turn on his side when getting up from a supine position on the floor, which is the initial sign of the Gowers maneuver (Fig. 79-2). Hypertrophy of calf muscles typically occurs, often being very prominent by age 3 or 4 years (Fig. 79-3). Hypertrophy of other muscles may also develop, especially involving the vastus lateralis; infraspinous; deltoid; and, less frequently, the gluteus maximus, triceps, and masseter muscles. Muscle mass is usually decreased in later stages in the pectoral, peroneal, and anterior tibial muscles.

Hip girdle muscles are affected earlier than shoulder girdle muscles. Because of weakness of the hip extensor muscles that act as "shock absorbers" when weight is placed on one leg, these patients tend to rock from side to side when walking, which produces a waddling gait. Anterior hip rotation caused by muscle weakness results in increased lumbar lordosis, which is necessary to keep the center of balance stable, with shoulders lined up over hips, knees, and ankles. The preschooler has difficulty rising from the floor, turning 45, then 90, and finally 180 degrees (depending on the

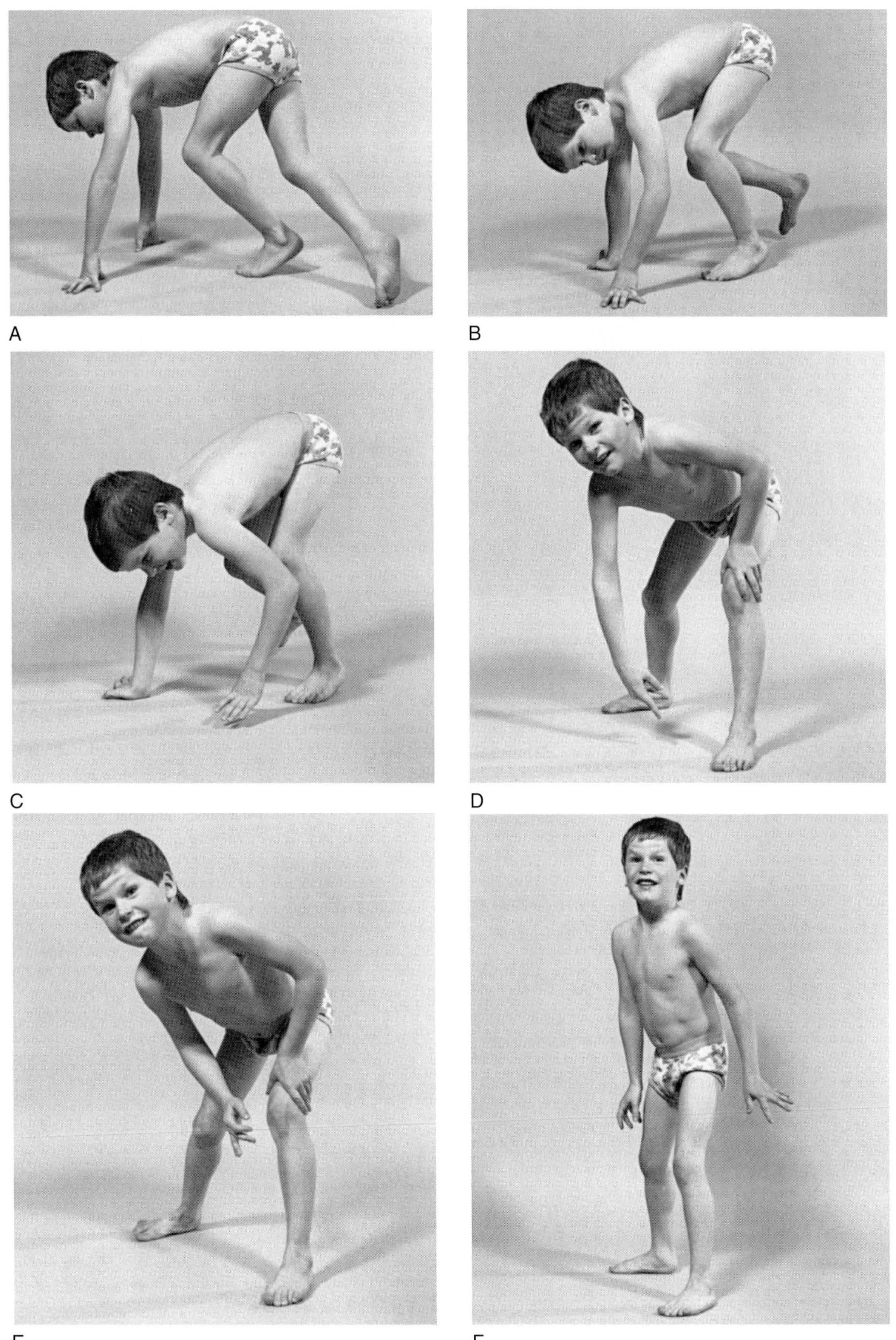

FIGURE 79-2. Boy with Duchenne muscular dystrophy demonstrates the sequence of maneuvers that constitute Gowers' sign. The child pushes off the floor with all four extremities, then prepares to push up by moving his hands along the floor closer to the feet, and finally places the hands on the thighs and pushes up to the erect position. The maneuver is necessary primarily because of marked weakness of the hip extensors.

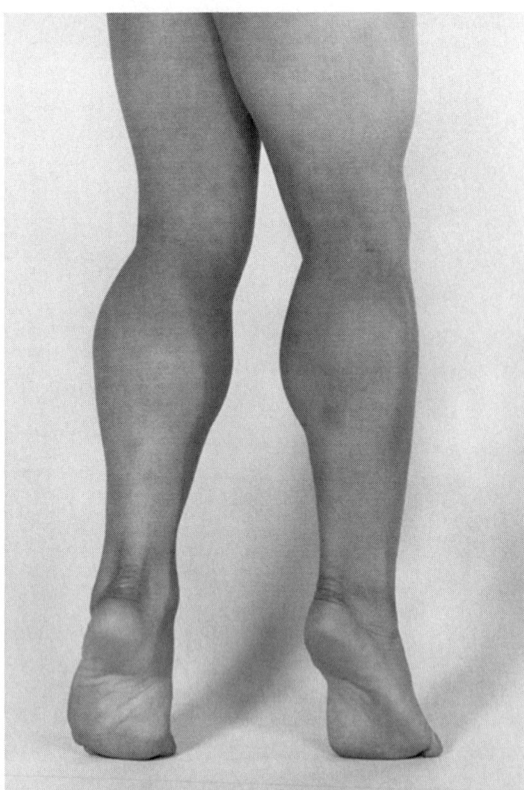

FIGURE 79-3. Pseudohypertrophy of the gastrocnemius muscles is usually profound. The large muscle mass is secondary to replacement of normal muscle with adipose and collagen tissue.

degree of neck flexor weakness), and placing the hands on the floor to get up. Later, the complete Gowers sign (see Fig. 79-2) is exhibited. The patient assumes a locked-leg, buttocks-first position, followed by pushing off the floor with the hands, literally pushing the trunk erect by bracing the arms against the anterior thighs. The maneuver is necessary because of pronounced weakness of the hip muscles, predominantly the gluteus maximus, and is present by age 5 or 6 years. As muscle deterioration proceeds, climbing stairs becomes difficult, necessitating use of both hands on a railing or crawling on all four extremities. Distal muscles of the arms and legs exhibit weakness as the disease progresses.

The patellar tendon reflex is often diminished early in the course of Duchenne muscular dystrophy. In contrast, the Achilles tendon reflex can usually be elicited for many years. Contractures of heel cords, necessitating vigorous, daily stretching, may be a major problem as early as 4 to 5 years of age in males with untreated Duchenne muscular dystrophy. Iliotibial bands and hip flexors also may become contracted because of the alteration in gait that results from the distribution of muscle weakness. If contractures are allowed to advance to a fixed equinovarus position, the patient walks on his toes and often falls. Locking of the knees to compensate for less-than-antigravity quadriceps strength with resultant genu recurvatum posture is common as the gastrocnemius muscles attempt to compensate for the quadriceps deficiency.

Accelerated deterioration in strength and balance often results from intercurrent disease or surgically induced immobilization. If tendon release surgery is performed, immediate mobilization in a walking splint or cast is necessary to prevent deterioration in muscle strength from disuse. When ambulation is no longer possible—usually near the end of the first decade in untreated Duchenne muscular dystrophy and about 3 to 10 years later in steroid-treated Duchenne muscular dystrophy—a wheelchair is required. Contractures become more pronounced in the lower extremities and soon involve the shoulders. Kyphoscoliosis may develop after ambulation is lost. Maintaining an erect posture with long leg braces or a stander after ambulation is lost may help prevent scoliosis. Proper wheelchair sizing, solid seating, and solid back support are important. Both manual and power wheelchairs are useful. Cardiac and respiratory involvement often occurs in this later disease stage.

Adolescent patients manifest increasing weakness and are unable to perform routine tasks with their arms, hands, and fingers. The head may progressively flex forward as extensor neck muscles lose strength. Lower facial muscles may be involved in the advanced phase.

PULMONARY INVOLVEMENT

Pulmonary function becomes compromised because of weakness of intercostal and diaphragmatic muscles and severe scoliosis, occurs later in the disease in nonambulatory patients, and is the primary cause of mortality in Duchenne muscular dystrophy. Delaying the time to reach nonambulatory status can have a significant impact on the development of scoliosis and respiratory function. This postponement can be achieved by the use of steroids [Moxley et al., 2005] (which prolongs ambulation) and the use of standers to keep children upright even when they are not walking [Galasko et al., 1995]. Use of mechanical ventilation and good pulmonary and cardiac care have increased survival [Gomez-Merino and Bach, 2002] to about 58% at age 25 years even in patients in some countries who have not been treated with steroids [Eagle et al., 2002].

Muscle weakness affects all aspects of lung function, including mucociliary clearance, gas exchange at rest and during exercise, and respiratory control during wakefulness and sleep [Gozal, 2000]. It is important to recognize that Duchenne muscular dystrophy is often associated with sleep-disordered breathing, which could be asymptomatic or only mildly symptomatic. Patients can have normal waking oxygen saturation and capillary blood gas levels and normal or near-normal forced vital capacity. Overnight polysomnography is useful for detecting abnormalities [Kirk et al., 2000].

CARDIAC INVOLVEMENT

Children with Duchenne muscular dystrophy are at risk for cardiomyopathy, especially if they have deletion of exons 48 to 53 [Nigro et al., 1994]. Early screening for cardiomyopathy at ages 5 to 6 years and then again at 10 to 12 years with an electrocardiogram and echocardiogram allows detection of cardiomyopathy with impaired cardiac output, often before signs of heart failure are apparent. If heart failure occurs, rigorous intervention to improve cardiac function and output is necessary to prevent terminal cardiac failure. Mild degrees of cardiac compromise in Duchenne muscular dystrophy may occur in up to 95% of affected males [Melacini et al., 1996]. Chronic heart failure may affect up to 50% [Melacini et al., 1996; Wahi et al., 1971]. Sudden cardiac failure can occur, especially during adolescence. In one series of 19 patients, postmortem studies revealed that 84% had demonstrable cardiac involvement [Leth and Wulff, 1976]. Characteristic electrocardiographic changes include sinus tachycardia; tall R1 wave in lead V_1; prominent Q wave in leads I, aVL, and V_6 or in leads II, III, and aVF; increased QT dispersion; and possibly autonomic dysfunction [Danzig et al., 2003; Finsterer and Stollberger, 2003]. Initially, routine echocardiography yields normal findings. However, very early abnormalities in cardiac function can be detected with newer ultrasound techniques in children between the ages of 4 and 10 years [Giglio et al., 2003]. Some young children with Duchenne muscular dystrophy might exhibit regional wall motion abnormalities in areas of fibrosis [Melacini et al., 1996]. With spreading of fibrosis, left ventricular dysfunction and ventricular dysrhythmias can occur. In the final stages of the disease, systolic function may lead to heart failure and sudden death. Subclinical or clinical cardiac insufficiency is present in about 90% of patients with Duchenne muscular dystrophy or Becker muscular dystrophy but is the cause of death in only 20% of those with Duchenne muscular dystrophy and 50% of those with Becker muscular dystrophy [Finsterer and Stollberger, 2003; Melacini et al., 1996].

NEUROPSYCHOLOGIC INVOLVEMENT

Males with Duchenne muscular dystrophy, overall, have an intelligence quotient (IQ) curve shifted to the left [Ogasawara, 1989]. The mean IQ score in one study was 83 (range, 46 to 134). However, other investigators have not been able to demonstrate a difference in overall IQ [Bushby et al., 1995; Felisari et al., 2000; Hinton et al., 2000; Roccella et al., 2003]. It has become evident that certain cognitive areas are more affected than others in patients with Duchenne muscular dystrophy: namely, verbal memory [Hinton et al., 2000]. Genotype/phenotype studies have revealed that deletions localized in central and 3′ parts of the gene are preferentially associated with mental impairment, some of these directly affecting the regulatory and coding sequences for the three central nervous system-specific carboxy-terminal isoforms [Giliberto et al., 2004]. Another study of 137 males with Duchenne muscular dystrophy/Becker muscular dystrophy confirmed these findings, demonstrating that all patients with deletions upstream of the 5′ end of the gene were mentally normal, whereas all patients with mental retardation or autism had deletions containing the 3′ end of the gene. Some researchers have found average intelligence [Sollee et al., 1985] but difficulties with immediate memory [Wicksell et al., 2004]. Specifically, children with Duchenne muscular dystrophy have poor performance on measures of story recall, digit span, and auditory comprehension. This profile indicates that verbal working memory skills are selectively impaired in Duchenne muscular dystrophy, and this could contribute to poor academic achievement [Hinton et al., 2001]. Morphologic changes in the central nervous system have been reported; however, the results of brain postmortem examination and, more recently, brain imaging studies have been inconsistent. Although many investigators have found no pathologic or radiologic brain abnormalities in Duchenne muscular dystrophy, others, using positron emission tomographic scanning, have reported hypometabolism in the cerebral and cerebellar hemispheres [Bresolin et al., 1994; Rae et al., 1998]. Pathologic studies have revealed mild-to-striking abnormalities, including neuronal loss, heterotopias, gliosis, neurofibrillary tangles, Purkinje cell loss, dendritic abnormalities (length, branching, and intersections), disordered architecture, astrocytosis, and perinuclear vacuolation [Anderson et al., 2002]. There is some evidence that patients with Duchenne muscular dystrophy who have identifiable brain abnormalities, especially mild brain atrophy, also have cognitive impairment [Septien et al., 1991], but these findings have not been confirmed by other investigators [al-Qudah et al., 1990]. Overall, there is no firm evidence that an abnormality of the brain, either gross or histologic, is common in patients with Duchenne muscular dystrophy, and a correlation between abnormality and intellectual impairment has yet to be clearly established [Anderson et al., 2002].

OTHER ORGAN INVOLVEMENT

Males with Duchenne muscular dystrophy can have an early abnormality in gastric motility caused by deranged regulatory mechanisms and later the result of smooth muscle involvement. Symptoms can include megacolon, volvulus, abdominal cramping, and malabsorption [Borrelli et al., 2005]. In the era before steroids and ventilation, death usually occurred late in the second decade of life (median age of 18 years), and only 25% of males with Duchenne muscular dystrophy lived beyond 21 years of age [Gardner-Medwin, 1970]. This natural history has changed [Eagle et al., 2002], and in current studies, researchers are trying to characterize the impact of steroid treatment, age at start of treatment, noninvasive ventilation, rehabilitation, scoliosis surgery, and pulmonary care on the quality of life and survival of patients with Duchenne muscular dystrophy.

FEMALE DUCHENNE MUSCULAR DYSTROPHY CARRIERS AND MANIFESTING CARRIERS

Female carriers are heterozygous with a normal dystrophin gene on one X chromosome and a mutant gene on the other. More than 90% of female carriers are asymptomatic. However, female carriers may manifest various degrees of muscle weakness because random inactivation of one X chromosome, according to the Lyon hypothesis, may leave more than half of mutant X chromosomes operant in muscle cells (skewed X-inactivation). When more than half the X chromosomes in a given muscle fiber express a mutant gene for Duchenne muscular dystrophy, the muscle fiber is prone to degeneration. The number of potentially abnormal muscle fibers in a given muscle determines whether that muscle displays weakness. The degree of strength from one muscle to another may vary from normal strength to significant weakness.

In the presence of muscle fiber degeneration resulting from a burden of more than half mutant X chromosomes in muscle nuclei, muscle fiber degeneration is followed by regeneration. The new fiber, formed from fused myoblasts, may have less than half or more than half mutant X chromosomes and be susceptible to degeneration. Overall, individual muscle groups may express less than normal strength but with time either become stronger or weaker or stay the same. Each muscle responds separately. The tendency in muscles with a high percentage of mutant X chromosomes is that with remodeling of the muscle through cycles of degeneration and regeneration, there is an increase in the number of normal X chromosomes but not necessarily a parallel increase in dystrophin content [Pegoraro et al., 1995]. Immunohistochemical and immunoblot analysis of muscle biopsies in these female carriers reveals a mosaic of dystrophin-normal and dystrophin-abnormal muscle fibers [Minetti et al., 1991].

Signs and symptoms of female dystrophinopathy include muscle weakness, myopathic muscle biopsy specimens, elevated levels of creatine kinase enzymes, and partial absence of dystrophin in the muscle [Hoffman et al., 1992]. This absence is seen in about one fifth of Duchenne muscular dystrophy carriers [Hoogerwaard et al., 1999a]. Search for female dystrophinopathy should be initiated in women with elevated creatine kinase enzyme levels and muscle weakness, even in the absence of a Duchenne muscular dystrophy-positive family history [Hoffman, 1996].

Female patients with Duchenne muscular dystrophy and severe weakness and absence of muscle dystrophin are affected when chromosomal translocation has taken place, allowing expression of an abnormal Duchenne muscular dystrophy gene. The female Duchenne muscular dystrophy phenotype resembling the male Duchenne muscular dystrophy phenotype is occasionally present with Turner's syndrome.

Duchenne muscular dystrophy carriers appear to have an increased incidence of cardiomyopathy. Different studies have revealed an incidence of asymptomatic cardiomyopathy in 8% to 48% among adult Duchenne muscular dystrophy carriers [Grain et al., 2001; Hoogerwaard et al., 1999a, 1999b] and in 0% to 15% among Duchenne muscular dystrophy carrier girls younger than 16 years [Nolan et al., 2003].

Diagnosis

CLINICAL LABORATORY TESTS

The serum creatine kinase level is the most valuable and universally used diagnostic enzyme indicator of Duchenne dystrophinopathy. Levels of creatine kinase, the muscle isoenzyme, are greatly elevated, typically from 10,000 to 30,000 times normal, early in the disease. Gaps in the sarcolemma allow efflux of the enzyme into the circulation. Serum creatine kinase levels can vary greatly with activity and decrease as muscle mass is lost with disease progression. There is no correlation between the serum creatine kinase level and clinical severity in Duchenne muscular dystrophy, and the use of creatine kinase levels as a surrogate marker of treatment response is not well supported. Because of the leakage of intracellular muscle proteins, other muscle isoenzyme levels also increase in the circulation. These include lactate dehydrogenase, alanine aminotransferase, and, to a lesser degree, aspartate aminotransferase, all usually tested routinely as markers of liver function in normal children. It is not unusual that pediatricians embark in extensive unnecessary liver studies before it is realized that these are muscle isoenzymes and their abnormal levels parallel that of creatine kinase. This occurrence is more common in Becker muscular dystrophy because these patients might not have any muscle symptoms for decades [Korones et al., 2001; Lin et al., 1999; Tay et al., 2000; Zamora et al., 1996].

GENETIC TESTING

Genetic test for Duchenne muscular dystrophy and Becker muscular dystrophy is widely available, especially for the deletions in the two hot spots of the gene. The screening of only 19 exons by multiplex polymerase chain reaction identifies about 98% of all deletions [Beggs et al., 1990]. Southern blot analysis of these samples can frequently predict whether the deletion, when in the rod domain, will shift the reading frame, and thus is conclusive for Duchenne muscular dystrophy or Becker muscular dystrophy. This technique is very effective for the molecular diagnosis of common deletions (60% of patients); however, it cannot be used to identify duplications or to establish genotype in female carriers. Other diagnostic approaches, such as quantitative polymerase chain reaction [Abbs and Bobrow, 1992; Yau et al., 1996] or multiplex amplifiable probe hybridization [White et al., 2002] might be used for carrier diagnosis. With more recent technology, it is possible to screen the entire dystrophin gene for the specific molecular defects responsible in the other 40% of patients with Duchenne muscular dystrophy and Becker muscular dystrophy in whom a genetic abnormality has not been detected. These techniques include a protein truncation test [Tuffery-Giraud et al., 1999a, 1999b], single-condition amplification/internal primer sequencing [Mendell et al., 2001] and denaturing high-performance liquid chromatography followed by sequencing, which enables the detection of small mutations in nearly all the 79 exons [Bennett et al., 2001]. In a large series with single-condition amplification/internal primer sequencing, deletions of one or more exons were found in 66% of probands, which was consistent with the frequency of deletions in the previously reported literature. Point mutations were found in 18%, including premature stop codons in 13% and missense mutations in 4% of the total mutations. Frameshift mutations were found in 3% of patients. Fourteen subexonic mutations were also found, and these included nonsense mutations in 9 (64%); missense mutations in 3 (21%), and frameshift mutations in 2 (14%). This testing modality might be more sensitive for detecting deletions than is multiplex polymerase chain reaction. Of the 45 deletions detected, 3 (7%) either were undetected or would have been undetected by that technique [Dent et al., 2005]. Duplications were detected in 6% of patients, and no disease-causing mutation was identified in 7% of the evaluated patients [Dent et al., 2005].

There are few commercial laboratories offering gene sequencing at present, but these methods will become routinely available for diagnosis of suspected dystrophinopathy patients, as well as for carrier detection and prenatal diagnosis.

MUSCLE BIOPSY

Histologic study reveals fiber size variation, degenerating and regenerating fibers, clusters of smaller fibers, endo-

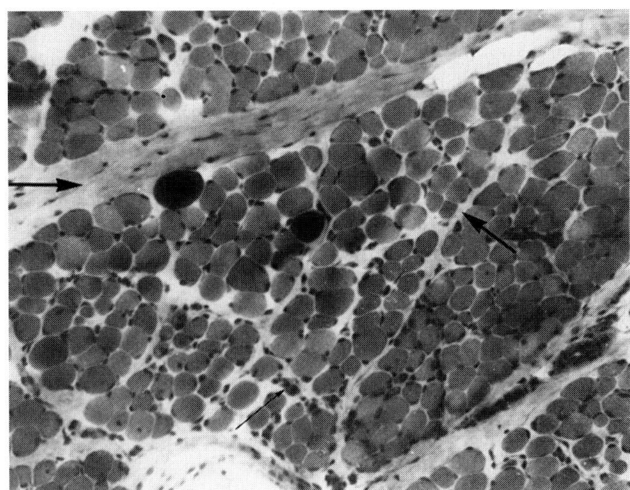

FIGURE 79-4. Biceps muscle biopsy sample from a 2-year-old child with Duchenne muscular dystrophy, revealing dark, opaque fibers, variable fiber size, and excessive connective tissue (*large arrows*). A basophilic, regenerating fiber is identified by the *small arrow.* (Hematoxylin and eosin staining; ×390.)

mysial fibrosis, and a few scattered lymphocytes. Large, opaque fibers distinguished by intense staining with the modified Gomori trichrome are prominent (Fig. 79-4). As the disease progresses and degeneration exceeds regeneration, a decrease in the number of muscle fibers is apparent, with replacement of muscle with fat and connective tissue. Fiber typing with adenosine triphosphatase histochemistry is less distinct than expected. Oxidative histochemistry is maintained. Absence of immunoreactivity for dystrophin with monoclonal antibodies against the C-terminal, rod domain, and N-terminal are necessary for accurate diagnosis of Duchenne muscular dystrophy (Fig. 79-5). Quantitative dystrophin analysis by immunoblot is more accurate for diagnosis than is immunostaining, with levels of dystrophin being less than 5% of normal in Duchenne muscular dystrophy patients. On electron microscopic study, gaps in the sarcolemma with preservation of the basement lamina are seen in non-necrotic fibers (Figs. 79-6 and 79-7).

Management

Children with Duchenne muscular dystrophy and Becker muscular dystrophy are best cared for in a multidisciplinary setting, in which physicians (neurologists, psychiatrists, orthopedic surgeons, cardiologists, and pulmonary medicine), physical and occupational therapists, nutritionists, exercise physiologists, and social workers can work together for the overall well-being of the child and the family.

Parents of the patient with Duchenne dystrophinopathy should be kept informed on a timely basis about the expected clinical course, the need for regular evaluations, and available treatment programs, including clinical trials, for their participation. Initial counseling is with parents, but as the patient becomes older, he or she should be involved directly with team members. For example, an explanation of how muscles function and the concept of weakness are im-

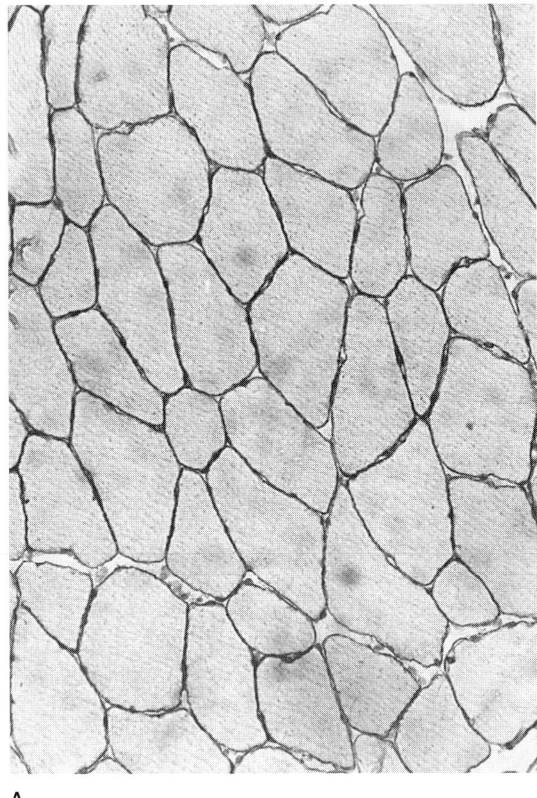

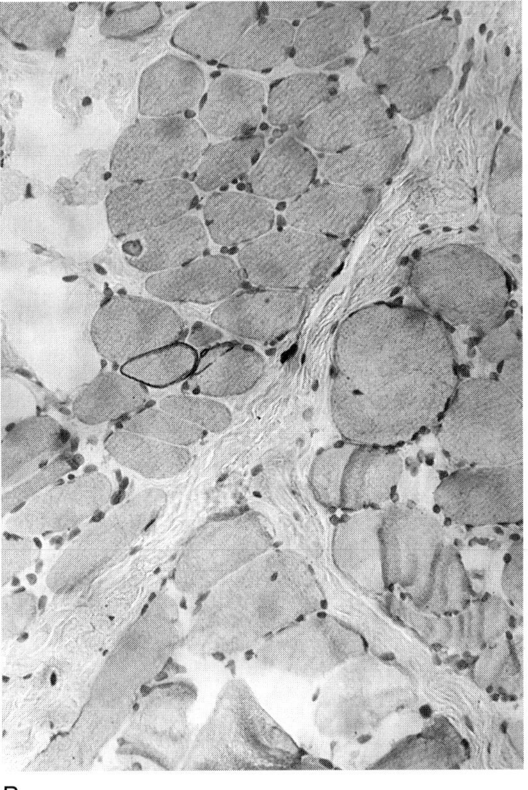

A B

FIGURE 79-5. Immunocytochemical staining for dystrophin with a monoclonal antibody (DYS 2) reacting to muscle protein dystrophin. This antibody recognizes a distal portion of the dystrophin molecule that represents the last 17 amino acids of the carboxy-terminus on the dystrophin gene. **A,** Control muscle exhibiting normal dystrophin localization to the sarcolemma, demonstrated with peroxidase staining (×230). **B,** Muscle from a 5-year-old male with Duchenne muscular dystrophy, devoid of sarcolemmal staining for dystrophin except for one recombinant fiber in the center of the field (×260).

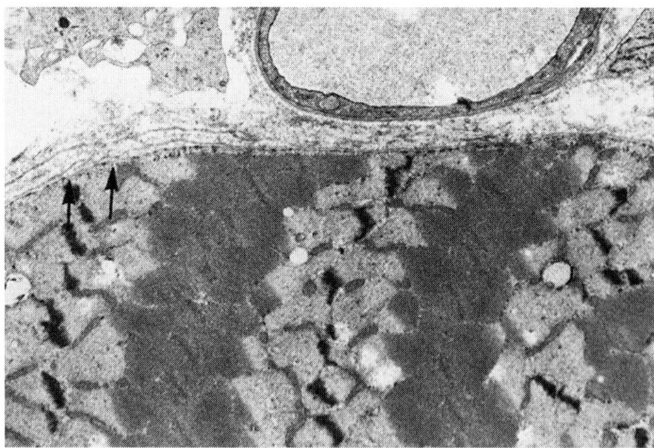

FIGURE 79-6. Electron micrograph of a speciment from a 6-year-old child with Duchenne muscular dystrophy, revealing sarcolemmal (plasma cell wall) disruption (*arrows*) with redundant basement membranes (×10,800).

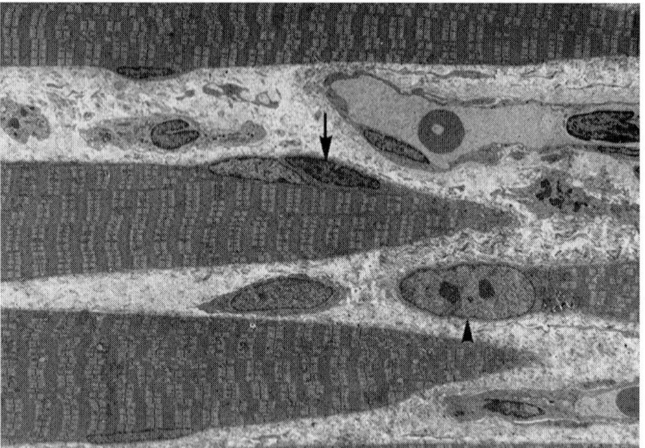

FIGURE 79-7. Longitudinally oriented, plastic-embedded resin section from a 2-year-old child with Duchenne muscular dystrophy. Note the vesicular muscle nucleus with prominent nucleoli (*arrowhead*) and satellite cell (*arrow*) adjacent to a mildly vesicular muscle nucleus. A capillary, fibroblasts, and prominent endomysial connective tissue are present. (Toluidine blue staining; ×2400.)

portant. Many children with Duchenne muscular dystrophy have known for a long time before they are told about their disease that they "were different" and not as athletic as their peers, which frequently causes serious self-esteem issues. Interacting with playmates and school peers and adjusting to a nonambulatory life are key adjustments that must be made. It may be necessary for appropriate team members to contact school authorities or even participate in school team meetings to educate teachers and peers on how to support the child with Duchenne muscular dystrophy and yet let the child be as independent as possible. Support groups for the family, siblings, and patient and special camps should be made available, and participation in them should be encouraged.

PHARMACOLOGIC TREATMENT

Daily prednisone stabilizes or improves the strength of children with Duchenne muscular dystrophy and it is the only demonstrated treatment for this disease [Moxley et al., 2005]. Drachman and associates [1974] first reported a beneficial effect of prednisone in an open trial of 2 mg/kg/day. This finding was duplicated in other open-design trials [Brooke et al., 1987; DeSilva et al., 1987] and subsequently, through the collaboration of the Clinical Investigation of Duchenne Dystrophy investigators, in double-blinded placebo-controlled trials [Fenichel et al., 1991; Griggs et al., 1993; Mendell et al., 1989]. The most effective dose is 0.75 mg/kg/day. There is a dose-response effect, the lower effective dose being 0.3 mg/kg/day [Mendell et al., 1989]. Effects on strength are seen as soon as 10 days after treatment starts, with a peak at 3 months and then a stabilization period [Griggs et al., 1991]. In a 3-year follow-up study, improvement was maintained in children who were kept on doses of at least 0.5 and 0.6 mg/kg/day [Fenichel et al., 1991]. It is hoped that long-term monitoring of these patients will confirm continuous benefit in muscle strength and respiratory function. Children with Duchenne muscular dystrophy treated with prednisone from an early age usually remain ambulatory into their teens, have a lower incidence of scoliosis [Alman et al., 2004; Biggar et al., 2004] and of contractures [Yilmaz et al., 2004], and maintain normal or near-normal respiratory function [Angelini et al., 1994; Biggar et al., 2004; Campbell and Jacob, 2003; Merlini et al., 2003]. Daily deflazacort yields a similar benefit in strength with decreased incidence of weight gain, but it carries an increased rate of asymptomatic cataract formation [Angelini et al., 1994; Biggar et al., 2001; Bonifati et al., 2000; Campbell and Jacob, 2003; Mesa et al., 1991; Moxley et al., 2005]. Weight gain and cushingoid features, two common side effects of prednisone, although somewhat less, also occur more frequently in children treated with deflazacort in comparison with placebo. The suggested dosage is 0.9 to 1.2 mg/kg/day. However, this drug is not available in the United States; therefore, U.S. patients must import the drug from other countries. This medication should be recommended only for patients with Duchenne muscular dystrophy who are already overweight before treatment and in a more advanced stage of the disease. Lower dosage regimens, including alternate-day corticosteroids and treatment for the first 10 days of the month, have not demonstrated sustained efficacy [Fenichel et al., 1991; Sansome et al., 1993]. Other immunosuppressive medications have produced mixed results. Whereas azathioprine yields no benefit [Griggs et al., 1993], there is uncontrolled evidence that cyclosporine is efficacious in managing Duchenne muscular dystrophy [Mendell et al., 1995; Sharma et al., 1993].

In spite of the fact that prednisone remains the only drug that has been proved effective in 80% of children with Duchenne muscular dystrophy, this therapy has not become the standard of care for treatment of this disease because of its feared significant side effects. An American Academy of Neurology Practice Parameter paper on the use of steroids in treating Duchenne muscular dystrophy [Moxley et al., 2005] and a Cochrane Database review of all trials [Manzur et al., 2004] support the use of corticosteroids for Duchenne muscular dystrophy. Clearly, the benefits of steroids outweigh the risks. There is accumulating evidence that treatment should start as soon as the diagnosis is made [Dubowitz et al., 2002; Kinali et al., 2002; Merlini et al., 2003]. However, early steroid treatment is associated with significant decrease in linear growth. A pilot study of 10 mg/kg given over 2 consecutive days of the week (Friday and Saturday) demonstrated that males with Duchenne muscular dystrophy had improved muscle strength and function while maintaining linear growth and did not have an increase in their basal metabolic index in comparison with males with untreated Duchenne muscular dystrophy [Connolly et al., 2002]. A larger trial is ongoing. Such a dosage regimen, if proven equally effective, could encourage physicians and parents to start treatment earlier.

With the standard treatment of daily prednisone, the most common side effects are increased appetite with weight gain, irritability, hirsutism, cushingoid facies, and decreased linear growth [Moxley et al., 2005]. The most serious side effects of prednisone (e.g., diabetes, hypertension, ulcers, and infections) are extremely rare in this population. The effect of steroids on bone metabolism and subsequent osteoporosis is difficult to discern, because baseline osteoporosis might be present secondary to decreased activity [Aparicio et al., 2002; Bianchi et al., 2003; Larson and Henderson, 2000]. A study of deflazacort in children with Duchenne muscular dystrophy revealed that treated patients had better bone density than did untreated patients [Biggar et al., 2004]. However, other studies have yielded opposite results [Bianchi et al., 2003], leaving this an area for further research [Biggar et al., 2005]. Children with Duchenne muscular dystrophy who are treated with prednisone or deflazacort should be supplemented orally with calcium and vitamin D. There is no consensus regarding the need for monitoring bone density with dual-energy x-ray absorptiometric scans, inasmuch as the relationship of decreased Z scores and the incidence of fractures in this population (and the general population) has not been established. There is no indication for treatment of asymptomatic children with Duchenne muscular dystrophy who have osteoporosis. However, in the setting of spontaneous pathologic fractures and osteoporosis, treatment with alendronate or similar drugs could be offered, although the safety of these drugs has not been proven in children [Biggar et al., 2005].

Obesity is often a major problem in patients with Duchenne muscular dystrophy, even if steroids are not used. For uncertain reasons, children with Duchenne muscular dystrophy may gain excessive weight, which often becomes apparent before ambulation is lost. The obesity becomes more prominent after the patient can no longer walk. Boredom, diminished physical activity, and depression may lead to inappropriate food intake [Zanardi et al., 2003], and rigorous measures are required to forestall weight gain. Obesity reduces the period of walking capability, hastens scoliosis, and fosters respiratory and cardiac insufficiency. Therefore, if steroid treatment is prescribed, these patients need to follow a strict dietary caloric intake to prevent excessive weight gain. A diet high in proteins, fresh fruits, and vegetables and low in fat and carbohydrates is ideal. A nutritionist should be part of the medical team of a patient with Duchenne muscular dystrophy who receives continuous steroid treatment. Experience suggests that the patient and the entire family must embrace these healthier eating habits to avoid excessive weight gain. Obesity in the parents is a bad prognostic factor for the child's compliance with diet.

The mechanism of action of prednisone in Duchenne muscular dystrophy is not entirely known and likely involves immunosuppressive actions, gene transcription regulation, and modulation of intracellular calcium [Kissel et al., 1993; Liu and Sun, 1996; Passaquin et al., 1998; Ruegg et al., 1998, 2002; St-Pierre et al., 2004; Wershil et al., 1995] and might prevent exercise-induced apoptosis [Lim et al., 2004] and thus prevent some muscle damage related to exercise.

Other immunosuppressive and other pharmacologic treatments have undergone limited investigation. Cyclosporine (5 mg/kg/day) produced improvement in strength tested on an isolated muscle [Sharma et al., 1993]. The anabolic steroid oxandrolone was tried in a randomized trial, and there was a trend toward improvement of muscle strength as a secondary, but not primary, outcome measure (quantitative isometric muscle force) [Fenichel et al., 2001]. A randomized, controlled, blinded trial of creatine monohydrate and glutamine supplementation in ambulant Duchenne muscular dystrophy patients (aged 5 to 11) also yielded negative findings based on manual muscle testing (primary outcome). However, there were consistent and clear trends toward improvement in isometric muscle strength in the older patients with creatine and increase in function in the younger children with creatine and glutamine [Escolar et al., 2005]. Other studies have demonstrated increases in muscle strength and body mass index with creatine in Duchenne muscular dystrophy [Tarnopolsky et al., 2004; Walter et al., 2000]. No significant side effects were seen with doses of 5 grams/day for at least 6 months [Escolar et al., 2005].

In an attempt to repair mutant dystrophin genes in vivo, gentamicin, an aminoglycoside antibiotic that binds the ribosome and causes "read-through" of premature stop codon (nonsense) mutations, was tried first in the mdx murine model of Duchenne muscular dystrophy [Barton-Davis et al., 1999] and then in a clinical trial on four patients with Duchenne muscular dystrophy or Becker muscular dystrophy [Wagner et al., 2001]. Although the mdx experiments revealed positive dystrophin measurements in about 15% of previously dystrophin-negative muscle fibers, the investigators were unable to duplicate this finding in humans. Efforts with similar but more potent drugs are ongoing. Other approaches involving gene repair mechanisms are being evaluated in experimental models. These include delivery to dystrophin-deficient cells of RNA-DNA oligonucleotides that target the specific mutation and cause it to revert to the normal sequence (chimeraplasts) [Rando et al., 2000] and the delivery of antisense RNA molecules to dystrophin-deficient cells so that semifunctional dystrophin can be produced [Errington et al., 2003; Gebski et al., 2003; Lu et al., 2003; Mann et al., 2001; Wells et al., 2003]. This method forces the cell-splicing machinery to skip the dystrophin gene exon that contains the gene mutation, which results in the full translation of dystrophin messenger RNA (minus the mutant exon) into an "in-frame" semifunctional dystrophin protein. These antisense oligonucleotides are small molecules and could be systemically delivered, which makes them an exciting prospect for effective therapy. Preclinical studies involving delivery of functional mini-dystrophin genes to replace the missing dystrophin, through adeno-associated viral vectors, are also in progress. In this model, dystrophin can be produced, the immune response can be prevented, and there is evidence of improved function and amelioration of pathology [Wang et al., 2000] in young and older animals [DelloRusso et al., 2002; Hartigan-

O'Connor et al., 2001; Scott et al., 2002]. A last hurdle was crossed when systemic delivery of an adeno-associated virus type 6 vector with a mini-dystrophin gene was achieved in the older mdx mouse [Gregorevic et al., 2004]. This approach is expected to move toward the clinical phase by 2010.

Results of myoblast transfer and other stem cell approaches are not encouraging [Partridge, 2002]. Myoblast transplantation was attempted in children with Duchenne muscular dystrophy with no success [Miller et al., 1997; Munsat, 1990; Neumeyer et al., 1998], although they were effective in mdx mice [Huard et al., 1994].

RESPIRATORY CARE

With the progression of muscle weakness, loss of respiratory muscle strength, with ensuing ineffective cough and decreased ventilation, leads to pneumonia, atelectasis, and respiratory insufficiency in sleep and during wakefulness [Gozal, 2000]. These complications are generally preventable with careful monitoring and assessments of respiratory function. Patients with Duchenne muscular dystrophy should have routine immunizations by a primary care physician, as recommended for well children by the American Academy of Pediatrics. In addition, these patients should receive the pneumococcal vaccine and an annual influenza vaccine.

The older ambulatory patients with Duchenne muscular dystrophy should undergo annual spirometry. Once the child can no longer walk and if either the forced vital capacity falls below 80% of predicted or the child is 12 years of age, or both, the child should be seen twice a year by a physician specializing in pediatric respiratory care [Finder et al., 2004]. Patients in more advanced stages of the disease who require mechanically assisted airway clearance therapy or mechanically assisted ventilation should see a pulmonologist every 3 to 6 months. Routine evaluations at these visits should include oxyhemoglobin saturation by pulse oxymetry, spirometry, and measures of inspiratory and expiratory pressures and peak cough flow [Bach et al., 1997].

Maintaining good pulmonary toilet is essential; hence, these patients should be taught strategies to improve airway clearance and how to employ these techniques early and aggressively. The use of assisted cough technologies should be recommended when peak cough flow is less than 270 liters/minute or when the maximal expiratory pressures are less than 60 cm H_2O, or both [Finder et al., 2004].

Patients with Duchenne muscular dystrophy have an increased risk for sleep apnea, nocturnal hypopnea, and hypoxemia. Treatment of these problems with noninvasive nocturnal ventilation can significantly increase the quality of life [Baydur et al., 2000; Vianello et al., 1994].

A polysomnographic study with continuous CO_2 monitoring is the best way to assess the need for ventilatory support. Pulse oximetry, especially during the waking state, is suboptimal. Decisions regarding long-term ventilation, either invasive or noninvasive, should involve the patient, caregivers, and medical teams. Physicians have a legal and ethical responsibility to disclose treatment options and must avoid using their own perceptions of quality of life as the main factor in deciding whether to offer this type of information [Gibson, 2001]. End-of-life decision-making should be discussed earlier, with all possible information available to the patient [Hilton et al., 1993].

REHABILITATION

Unfortunately, no large prospective studies have been conducted to evaluate the role of physical therapy, stretching exercises, use of braces, and types of physical activity in Duchenne muscular dystrophy, and so the scientific evidence to support solid recommendations is poor.

Exercise

On the basis of the preclinical data in the mdx murine model of Duchenne muscular dystrophy, there is a general consensus that high-resistance exercises, especially those involving eccentric contractions (e.g., weight lifting), are damaging to the muscle cell membrane and should be avoided [Ansved, 2003; Petrof, 1998]. However, a sedentary life is equally damaging [McDonald, 2002]. Furthermore, another line of evidence in mdx mice indicates that sustained, nonresistive activity might produce a histochemical shift of the muscle cells toward fatigue resistance with benefits in activity and fatigability measures [Carter et al., 1995; Hayes et al., 1993; Petrof, 1998]. Therefore, active nonresistive exercises are encouraged. Swimming is perhaps the best sport for these children and is usually recommended. Keeping an active life style will also prevent excessive weight gain, especially if the child is taking steroids. Regular periods of daily walking for several hours enhance maintenance of strength and retard contracture formation. Swivel walkers may be used to provide low-energy ambulation and improve the quality of life [Sibert et al., 1987]. Both the nature and degree of activity should be modified so that fatigue does not remain after a night's sleep. Wheelchair games can be played when ambulation is lost. Children confined to bed because of intercurrent disease, injury, or surgery require physical therapy, including range-of-motion exercises, with return to more active exercise, including walking, as soon as possible; if such exercise is not resumed, patients may lose the capacity to ambulate. In the event of leg fractures, walking casts should be used as soon as possible [Siegel, 1977].

Contractures

Contractures of the Achilles tendons and, later, of other joints is common. With early hip girdle weakness, anterior rotation of the hips and posterior displacement of the shoulders to keep the center of gravity perpendicular to the ground through the shoulders, hips, and ankles occur. When this happens, there is excessive force in the gastrocnemius musculature that ultimately shortens the heel cord tendons. Active range-of-motion exercises supplemented by passive stretching are important for preventing contractures. Nighttime stretching orthoses (similar to the static ankle-foot orthoses but with a hinge at the ankle and adjustable straps) are useful and should be recommended at age 5 to 6. A standing board tilted up 20 degrees may be used for 20 minutes twice per day to provide constant stretching of the Achilles tendons. Keeping the heel cords stretched through vigorous passive stretching by parents and physical therapists helps the patient maintain better gait mechanics. This program requires stretching of the tensor fascia lata, hamstrings, knee flexors, and ankle plantar flexors. If strenuous stretching is not effective, surgical release of tight heel cords may be beneficial [Do, 2002], even if both the quadriceps and gastrocnemius muscle groups have

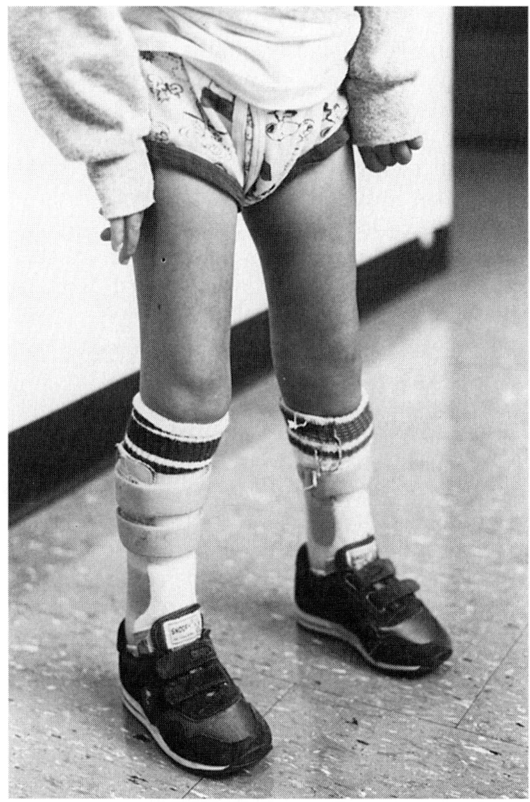

FIGURE 79-8. Orthotic devices stabilize the position of the feet in relation to the ankles after Achilles tenotomy and are temporally helpful and necessary to help maintain position.

less-than-antigravity in strength. In the latter case, long leg bracing can be offered to keep some ambulation after contractures are corrected. Mobilization in a walking cast immediately after surgery is essential for preventing loss of strength. Temporary bracing after surgery is necessary for optimal results after tenotomy procedures (Fig. 79-8).

The iliotibial bands may also tighten because of the broad-based gait used to maintain stability. Hip flexors may become contracted when ambulation is still present as a result of the anterior rotation of the hips or, later, because of sitting for prolonged periods in a wheelchair. Hip flexion contractures may benefit from surgical release, followed by application of long leg braces. Resection of the tensor fascia lata (Rideau procedure) may be beneficial for some patients [Do, 2002].

Scoliosis

Nearly all patients with Duchenne muscular dystrophy develop scoliosis after losing independent ambulation. The use of solid seat and back inserts in properly fitted wheelchairs is helpful in preventing scoliosis by keeping truncal posture erect. For some patients, long leg braces can be fitted to allow braced upright daily standing to prevent curvature. Baseline back radiographs to document the degree of curvature if scoliosis begins to develop should be obtained for comparison with future films. The use of steroids—perhaps because it prolongs ambulation beyond the growth spurt of early teenage years—delays or prevents scoliosis, even if the child is eventually unable to walk [Alman et al., 2004; Yilmaz et al., 2004].

Once the scoliotic curve reaches 30 degrees, it progresses with age and growth [Yamashita et al., 2001a]. Failure to repair scoliosis in Duchenne muscular dystrophy can result in increased hospitalization rates, worsening of pulmonary function, and poor quality of life [Finder et al., 2004; Yamashita et al., 2001b]. In fact, monitoring vital capacity may help determine the relative need for surgical stabilization of the spine [Rideau et al., 1984]. Surgical intervention should be undertaken when lung and cardiac function are satisfactory (with best recovery when the forced vital capacity exceeds 40%). However, there are no absolute contraindications to scoliosis surgery that are based on pulmonary function [Finder et al., 2004]. Surgery is usually scheduled once the Cobb angle measured on scoliosis films is between 30 and 50 degrees [Brook et al., 1996]. Immobilization attendant to surgical intervention for scoliosis may adversely affect the patient's residual strength if proper physical therapy is not provided.

CARDIAC MANAGEMENT

The mechanism of muscle damage discussed previously appears to be the same for cardiac muscle degeneration. In Duchenne muscular dystrophy and Becker muscular dystrophy, the left posterobasal and lateral walls are more extensively affected, with sparing of the left and right atria and the right ventricle [Finsterer and Stollberger, 2003]. The conduction system does not appear to be involved until there is advanced fibrosis; however, most cardiac deaths occur secondary to left ventricular cardiac failure [Corrado et al., 2002]. Two families with promoter and exon 1 involvement presenting with X-linked dilated cardiomyopathy enabled the discovery of a novel regulatory element, DEM2, which appears to be involved with the expression of dystrophin in the heart [Bastianutto et al., 2002].

Although electrocardiographic abnormalities are common in Duchenne muscular dystrophy, the best correlation of cardiac involvement with prognosis is measuring left ventricular dysfunction with echocardiography [Corrado et al., 2002]. Guidelines for the study of cardiac involvement in Duchenne muscular dystrophy [Bushby et al., 2003; Finsterer and Stollberger, 2003] recommend that Duchenne muscular dystrophy patients undergo electrocardiography and echocardiography at the time of diagnosis and then be screened every 2 years up to age 10 and subsequently every year. Early, preventive use of angiotensin-converting enzyme inhibitors and, later, β blockers may be needed and should be considered [Bushby et al., 2003; Finsterer and Stollberger, 2003].

GENETIC COUNSELING

Duchenne muscular dystrophy and Becker muscular dystrophy are inherited in an X-linked recessive manner, and the risk to siblings of a patient depends on the carrier status of the mother. Female carriers have a 50% chance of transmitting the Duchenne muscular dystrophy mutation in each pregnancy. Sons who inherit the abnormal gene are affected, whereas daughters who inherit it are carriers. Male patients with Duchenne muscular dystrophy do not reproduce. However, male patients with Becker muscular dystrophy and X-linked dilated cardiomyopathy may reproduce. All their daughters are carriers, but none of the sons inherits his father's dystrophin mutation. Prenatal testing for fetuses at risk is possible. Until the molecular genetics of Duchenne muscular dystrophy and Becker muscular dystrophy were understood, diagnosis of maternal and female sibling carriers was based on pedigree analysis and indirect assays. These included serum creatine kinase determinations [Griggs et al., 1985; Milhorat and Goldstone, 1965], the occasional finding of histologic abnormalities in muscle obtained from carriers [Maunder-Sewry and Dubowitz, 1981], and in vitro muscle ribosomal protein synthesis [Ionasescu et al., 1971a, 1971b, 1980]. Today, the specific molecular characterization of a patient makes genetic counseling easier. If a specific mutation is found in a child with Duchenne muscular dystrophy or Becker muscular dystrophy, genetic testing of the mother or sister for the exact mutation determines whether she is or is not a carrier; appropriate counseling for future pregnancies can be performed. When DNA analysis in the patient is not informative, muscle biopsy of a fetus can be used for diagnosis [Kuller et al., 1992]. Study of muscle from male fetuses with Duchenne muscular dystrophy reveals morphologic changes by the second trimester, especially greater muscle nuclear size in comparison with fetuses of the same gestational age [Vassilopoulos and Emery, 1977]. Immunoreaction for dystrophin is absent. When a deletion or specific mutation in the Duchenne muscular dystrophy/Becker muscular dystrophy gene has been demonstrated in another family member, the deletion may be detected in fetal tissue or earlier by chorionic villus sampling. This means that intrauterine diagnosis is possible by the seventh week of gestation in male embryos suspected of being affected. A genetic counselor is an essential part of the multidisciplinary team that diagnoses and monitors patients with Duchenne muscular dystrophy. The genetic counselor should give the family a full explanation of the X-linked recessive inheritance pattern of Duchenne muscular dystrophy, and molecular genetic testing should be made available to the patient and other family members as necessary.

DRUG PRECAUTIONS

Use of anticholinergic drugs and ganglionic blocking agents should be avoided because of their tendency to decrease muscle tone. Patients with Duchenne muscular dystrophy may be susceptible to malignant hyperthermia, and proper evaluation and preparation before administration of general anesthesia are recommended [Heiman-Patterson et al., 1986]. Cardiotoxic drugs, such as halothane, should not be used, and caution is advised in inducing general anesthesia [Smith and Bush, 1985].

EMOTIONAL AND BEHAVIORAL ABNORMALITIES

Dysthymic disorder and major depressive disorder can occur in children with Duchenne muscular dystrophy, especially during adolescence [Fitzpatrick et al., 1986; Witte, 1985]. An affected child's preoccupation with self and subsequent withdrawal may lead many families to seek counseling. Depression may develop in a patient who has lost an older sibling or close friend with Duchenne muscular dystrophy. Depression is often associated with intellectual limitation, which may induce low tolerance for frustration. Psychologic evaluation and counseling may be necessary. Neuropsychologic screening for intellectual deficits and behavioral problems is ideally conducted at time of school entry and should be repeated in preadolescence. Appropriate follow-up with the family and school officials is important. Mothers identified as carriers of Duchenne muscular dystrophy may suffer from feelings of guilt and require psychologic support [Nereo et al., 2003]. Depression is also common among parents and should be recognized [Abi Daoud et al., 2004]. End-of-life care, including home mechanical ventilation, may be appropriate [Hilton et al., 1993].

Becker Muscular Dystrophy

A "late-onset X-linked muscular dystrophy" was reported by Becker and Kiener in 1955. Like Duchenne muscular dystrophy, Becker muscular dystrophy is an X-linked recessive condition with mutation at Xp21. When the dystrophin reading frame is not shifted, there is no stop codon, and dystrophin is present but in reduced amounts. Distal rod deletions involving exons 45 to 48 result in a relatively high level of dystrophin, whereas N-terminus deletions are associated with low levels of dystrophin, perhaps as low as 10% of normal. The distal rod in-frame deletions result in a moderate Becker phenotype. A more severe Becker phenotype is associated with N-terminus deletions. The most severe phenotype, resembling Duchenne muscular dystrophy with the presence of minimal dystrophin, results from carboxy-terminus deletions. Further discussion of molecular genetics is found under Duchenne Muscular Dystrophy. At times, routine immunohistochemistry studies might demonstrate normal dystrophin in patients with increased creatine kinase and only mild or no muscle weakness. In these patients, immunostaining for neuronal nitric oxide synthetase has been found useful, revealing complete absence in 3 patients who were later found to have in-frame deletions in the common rod domain exons (in these cases 48, 45 to 51, and 47 to 53) that were consistent with Becker muscular dystrophy [Torelli et al., 2004]. In one family, deletion of exon 48 was demonstrated in five members (a 4-year-old female and four male relatives, aged 8 to 58), all of whom had normal muscle strength. These individuals by definition have Becker muscular dystrophy but represent one end of the clinical spectrum. This finding means that molecular genetic studies alone cannot be used for counseling purposes [Morrone et al., 1997]. With in-frame deletions in the proximal third of the rod domain involving exons 13 to 17, the clinical manifestation is cramps and myalgia. In this particular Becker phenotype, immunoreactivity over the sarcolemma for dystrophin often appears normal.

Creatine kinase levels in Becker muscular dystrophy are usually between 2000 and 20,000 U/liter but may be in the normal range for mildly affected male patients. Because these patients can be asymptomatic for decades, it is not uncommon that they receive misdiagnoses of a liver disorder when routine laboratory testing indicates elevated transaminase levels (aspartate aminotransferase and alanine aminotransferase), which are, in reality, muscle isoenzymes, abnormally elevated in parallel with the creatine kinase serum levels. These children might undergo several liver biopsies, with repeated normal results, before a creatine kinase level is measured and a diagnosis of Becker muscular dystrophy is established after further testing is performed [Tay et al., 2000; Zamora et al., 1996].

Muscle biopsy histologic findings are similar to those in Duchenne muscular dystrophy, but findings are less pronounced. The sarcolemmal gaps displayed ultrastructurally in Duchenne muscular dystrophy are not as readily seen in Becker muscular dystrophy. When monoclonal antibodies are directed to separate regions of dystrophin, immunoreactivity over the sarcolemma has a variety of staining patterns, ranging from intact to absent with one or more antibodies [Jay et al., 1993]. Becker muscular dystrophy is present in 3 to 6 per 100,000 male births [Gardner-Medwin, 1970].

The onset of Becker muscular dystrophy usually occurs after age 7 years and often in the second decade. Ambulation is typically maintained beyond age 30. Pseudohypertrophy, proximal hip weakness resulting in Gowers' sign, and electrocardiographic abnormalities associated with Duchenne muscular dystrophy are also common in Becker muscular dystrophy (Fig. 79-9). A few patients with earlier onset Becker muscular dystrophy have the same phenotype as patients with Duchenne muscular dystrophy but prove later, with muscle dystrophin and molecular genetic testing, to have Becker muscular dystrophy [Hoffman, 1991]. A number of children and adolescents with Becker muscular dystrophy experience calf pain or muscle cramps after exercise, which may be the initial symptom [Samaha and Quinlan, 1996]. In other individuals, strength may be nearly normal, but vigorous exercise produces severe cramps and occasionally rhabdomyolysis [Figarella-Branger et al., 1997]. A few teenagers with Becker muscular dystrophy initially have heart failure caused by a dilated cardiomyopathy before weakness is recognized. Sudden cardiac failure caused by heart block may occur in Becker muscular dystrophy. Early-onset

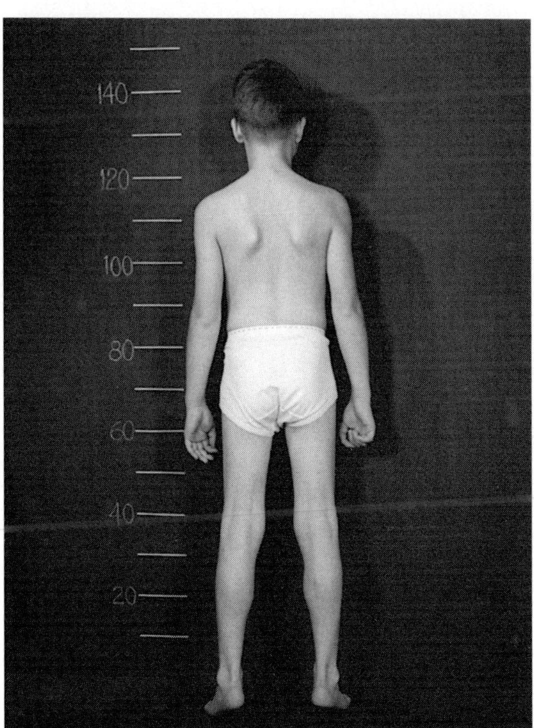

FIGURE 79-9. This 14-year-old male with Becker muscular dystrophy manifests moderate pseudohypertrophy of the calf muscles and wasting of the muscles of the shoulder girdle.

cardiomyopathy with mild muscle weakness is associated with muscle promoter and exon 1 deletion.

The likelihood of intellectual retardation, although greater than that in the general population, is less than that in Duchenne muscular dystrophy. However, mental retardation (IQ range, 60 to 68) and psychiatric disturbance in the absence of muscle weakness have been reported in Becker muscular dystrophy [North et al., 1996].

Therapeutic suggestions and measures appropriate for Duchenne muscular dystrophy are applicable at some point for Becker muscular dystrophy. This approach includes the use of prednisone in the more severely affected patients. Patients with Becker muscular dystrophy may be predisposed to malignant hyperthermia, and appropriate precautions should be taken when general anesthesia is necessary [Breucking et al., 2000; Kleopa et al., 2000].

Chromosome Xp21 Microdeletion Syndromes

The Xp21 microdeletion syndromes are a series of syndromes that include Duchenne muscular dystrophy, Aland's eye disease, adrenal hypoplasia, glycerol kinase deficiency, retinitis pigmentosa (RP3), mental retardation (MRX1), and ornithine transcarbamylase deficiency. The combination of these conditions led to the discovery of the Duchenne muscular dystrophy gene on Xp21 [Francke et al., 1985].

LIMB-GIRDLE MUSCULAR DYSTROPHIES

The limb-girdle muscular dystrophies (LGMDs) are a diverse group of disorders characterized by progressive muscle weakness, usually affecting the large muscles around the shoulder and pelvic girdles. However, as specific phenotypes corresponding to individual causative mutations have been characterized, the distribution of weakness around the limb-girdles has been found not universal, and some forms of LGMD affect distal muscles and can be confused with the most common phenotype of a neuropathy. These disorders are caused by a multiplicity of genes encoding proteins involved in all aspects of muscle cell biology. Initial classification of these disorders were based on the mode of inheritance, and were divided into autosomal-dominant (type 1: LGMD1), autosomal-recessive (type 2: LGMD2), and X-linked. With the discovery of causative genes in these three categories, each new entity was given a nominal letter, which resulted in the confusing and unpractical denomination of LGMD1A to 1F and LGMD2A to 2K. To date, there are 6 autosomal-dominant forms and 11 autosomal-recessive forms. Most loci defined by linkage have been identified, with the exception of LGMD1D to 1F, which are not included in the classification table. The majority of cases of LGMD are autosomal-recessive. Autosomal-dominant forms are found only in a few families, except for LGMD1B, which is the autosomal-dominant form of Emery-Dreifuss muscular dystrophy. An integrated classification taking into account the type and localization of the proteins has been proposed [Emery, 2002]. The age at onset and the key clinical findings are added to this classification scheme in this chapter to provide a clinical-biochemical classification more useful to the practitioner evaluating these disorders. This classification is presented in Table 79-2. Many of these syndromes are

TABLE 79-2

Clinical and Biochemical Classification of the Limb-Girdle Muscular Dystrophies (LGMDs)

PROTEINS	PROPOSED PROTEIN FUNCTION	NOMENCLATURE	AGE AT ONSET	KEY CLINICAL FINDINGS	MODE OF INHERITANCE	FREQUENCY
Sarcolemma Associated						
γ-Sarcoglycan α-Sarcoglycan β-Sarcoglycan δ-Sarcoglycan	Stabilize DGC at the sarcolemma δ and γ bind γ-filamin Signaling	LGMD2C LGMD2D LGMD2E LGMD2F	Infancy to young adult	Variable in severity from DMD to BMD phenotype Dilated cardiomyopathy in δ-sarcoglycan	AR	Variable proportion in different countries worldwide
Caveolin-3	Concentration of signaling molecules/biogenesis of T tubules	LGMD1C	Childhood (age 5)	Calf hypertrophy, increased CK, rippling muscle disease	AD	Uncommon, but worldwide
Dysferlin	Membrane repair	LGMD2B	Teens to early 20s	May manifest with distal or proximal weakness Biopsy reveals inflammation Worsens with steroids	AR	Relatively common Worldwide
Extracellular Matrix						
Collagen 6A1, A2, and A3	Anchors basal lamina in extracellular matrix Bridges cells with extracellular matrix through integrins	Bethlem's myopathy	Neonatal to adulthood	Proximal weakness, atrophy, distal contractures	AD	Rare
Proteins with Enzymatic Activity						
Calpain-3 (cytosolic)	Regulates nuclear factor κβ/Iκβα in protection from apoptosis Binds titin Cleaves γ-filamin	LGMD 2A	Infancy to young adult	Atrophic disease, early Achilles contractures, and trunk muscle involvement	AR	Relatively common in many countries
Fukutin-related protein (Golgi apparatus)	Glycosylation of α-dystroglycan	LGMD 2I	Birth to adulthood	Calf hypertrophy, common cardiac and respiratory involvement	AR	Commonest LGMD in many countries
Protein *O*-mannosyl-transferase (POMT) 1 (endoplasmic reticulum)	Glycosylation of α-dystroglycan	LGMD2K	Infancy	Mild muscle hypertrophy, microcephaly, mental retardation, normal brain MRI	AR	Rare: described in Turkish and British families
Sarcomeric Proteins						
Myotilin (z-line)	Binds α-actinin, γ-filamin and bundles α-actin	LGMD 1A	Teens to young adult. Anticipation?	Dysarthria, tight Achilles tendons, 50% cardiomyopathy	AD	Rare
Telethonin (Z line)	Substrate for titin kinase	LGMD 2G	9 to 15 years	Proximal weakness and footdrop Calf hypertrophy or atrophy, cardiomyopathy	AR	Rare: described only in Brazil
Titin	Specifies sarcomeric structure Has intrinsic kinase activity	LGMD 2J	Childhood	Allelic with Finnish tibial myopathy, more severe, high CK level	AR	Rare: described only in Finland

AD, autosomal dominant; AR, autosomal recessive; BMD, Becker muscular dystrophy; CK, creatine kinase; DGC, dystrophin-associated glyprotein complex; DMD, Duchenne muscular dystrophy.

extremely rare; only a few affected families have been described in the literature, and so these rarer forms are not reviewed in detail in this chapter [see Laval and Bushby, 2004, for a recent review]. In this classification, proteins causing solely a congenital muscular dystrophy phenotype have been purposefully excluded because those are better classified as listed later in Table 79-4 and described in the later section on congenital muscular dystrophies.

The pathophysiology of the syndromes caused by defects of sarcolemmal proteins, as part of the DGC, is similar to that described for dystrophinopathies. In contrast, other LGMDs have distinct pathophysiologic mechanisms. For example, dysferlin deficiency causes abnormal muscle membrane repair, whereas calpain-3 deficiency involves abnormal regulation of anti-apoptotic pathways and likely abnormal cytoskeletal remodeling.

Limb-Girdle Muscular Dystrophy 1C: Caveolinopathy

Caveolins are small transmembrane proteins with intracellular domains that undergo extensive oligomerization to form membrane complexes known as *caveolae.* Skeletal muscle disorders result from mutations on chromosome 3p25 in the gene that encodes caveolin-3, which interacts with neuronal nitric oxide synthase and the dystrophin-associated protein complex via the intracellular portion of β-dystroglycan [Song et al., 1996; Tang et al., 1996]. During muscle differentiation, caveolin-3 is associated with developing T tubules [Parton et al., 1997]. In the original reports of caveolinopathy, the disorders resulted from heterozygous changes in the membrane-spanning domain, which produced an autosomal-dominant LGMD phenotype [Minetti et al., 1998]. The clinical features of subsequently reported cases have been heterogeneous, and too few cases have been reported to define a predominant phenotype. Symptoms can begin in childhood with slowly progressive weakness. Calf hypertrophy is present, and creatine kinase levels are elevated 4- to 20-fold. Other families may manifest only elevated serum creatine kinase levels (hypercreatine kinase-emia) and postexertional myalgia and cramping, which may also begin in the first decade [Herrmann et al., 2000; Merlini et al., 2002]. Caveolin-3 mutations have been defined in autosomal-dominant rippling muscle disease [Betz et al., 2001], and severe rippling muscle symptoms have been reported in two unrelated patients with homozygous caveolin-3 mutations [Kubisch et al., 2003]. A single case of distal myopathy has been described [Tateyama et al., 2002]. The broad spectrum of clinical symptoms and the possibility that spontaneous or germline mutations produce simplex cases frequently raise the possibility of caveolinopathy. The postulated dominant negative effect of a number of caveolin-3 mutations leads to a substantial or complete loss of caveolin-3 immunoreactivity, allowing for screening with immunohistochemical techniques [Carbone et al., 2000; Herrmann et al., 2000].

Limb-Girdle Muscular Dystrophy 2A: Calpainopathy

Calpainopathy is a relatively frequent, childhood-onset LGMD that was fully characterized, and the molecular and biochemical abnormalities were described, in 1995 [Chiannilkulchai et al., 1995; Richard et al., 1995]. This type has been reported as the most frequent autosomal-recessive LGMD in several series [Chae et al., 2001; Dincer et al., 1997; Richard et al., 1997; Topaloglu et al., 1997]. The abnormal protein, calpain-3, is a nonlysosomal intracellular, muscle-specific, Ca^{2+}-activated neutral protease [Johnson, 1990]. Before recogition of this new LGMD, the focus on calpain-3 was in relation to its abnormal activation in Duchenne muscular dystrophy secondary to increased levels of intracellular Ca^{2+}. Type 2A was the first form of LGMD identified that is caused by deficiency of a nonstructural protein; this deficiency emphasizes the role of abnormal molecular signaling as the basis for muscle cell degeneration that has been discussed before for Duchenne muscular dystrophy.

Molecular Pathogenesis

The gene responsible for LGMD2A (CAPN3) is located at chromosome region 15q15.1-q21.1 [Chiannilkulchai et al., 1995] and consists of 24 exons extending over a genomic region of 50 kilobases [Richard et al., 1995]. It is expressed as a 3.5-kilobase transcript, a 94-kDa translated protein. More than 140 different mutations have been reported, including different nonsense, splice site, frameshift, or missense calpain-3 mutations, most of which are "unique" mutations [Saenz et al., 2005]. In addition, several ethnic groups have unique mutations that co-segregate with the disease [Canki-Klain et al., 2004; Chae et al., 2001; Chrobakova et al., 2004; Cobo et al., 2004; Fanin et al., 2004; Jia et al., 2001; Kramerova et al., 2004; Passos-Bueno et al., 1999]. In a large series, it was found that 87% of mutant alleles are concentrated in seven exons (exons 1, 4, 5, 8, 10, 11, and 21) and 61% correspond to only eight mutations, which indicates the regions to which future molecular analysis could be restricted [Fanin et al., 2004]. In patients in Brazil, most mutations are found in exons 1, 2, 4, 5, 11, and 22 [Zatz et al., 2003]. However, other investigators have not found the same deletion pattern [Saenz et al., 2005], which suggests that these hot spots could be related to confounder mutations in the area. Mutations can be homozygous or compound heterozygous. Homozygous null-null mutations appear to confer the most severe phenotype, in terms of earlier wheelchair need, whereas a heterozygous missense mutation confers a milder phenotype [Saenz et al., 2005].

Calpain-3 is a muscle specific protein that belongs to the calpain family of proteins. This protein has many unique features and is considered a "modulator protease." Several lines of evidence suggest that calpain-3 is mostly in an inactive state in muscle and needs a signal to be activated. Activated calpain-3 has several relationships with important cytoskeleton proteins. Some of its substrates include titin and filamin C [Taveau et al., 2003]. The interaction of calpain-3 with these cytoskeletal proteins may modulate remodeling during myofibrillogenesis by affecting scaffolding of titin for sarcomere assembling [Kramerova et al., 2004], and by cleaving filamin C and inhibiting its regulation of sarcoglycan assembly [Guyon et al., 2003]. There is also evidence that when calpain-3 is activated, its proteolytic activity leads to disruption of the actin cytoskeleton. Thus, calpain-3 appears to be a cytoskeleton modulator with an important role in muscle maturation [Spencer et al., 2002]. Other pathogenic hypotheses are proposed to explain why mutations in this gene might cause muscular dystrophy. Calpain-3 could have a protective effect and be involved in muscle detoxification preventing degradation of the muscle fiber [Zatz et al., 2003]. It may also play a role in intracellular signaling pathways and its deficiency might be associated with myonuclear apoptosis by deregulation of the Iκβα/nuclear factor κβ pathway [Baghdiguian et al., 1999].

The majority of the LGMD2A mutations appear to affect domain-domain interaction, which may be critical in the assembly and activation of the multidomain calpain-3 [Jia et al., 2001]. Under normal circumstances, calpain-3 undergoes rapid autocatalytic activity after translation, [Taveau et al., 2003]. During the short time (less than 5 minutes in muscle cultures) that the protein is present, it is in a resting state, unless it is activated by signaling mechanisms [Rey and Davies, 2002]. The autocatalytic activity resides in a Ca^{2+}-sensitive region between domains II and III of the protein. In the 20% to 40% [Fanin et al., 2003; Saenz et al., 2005] of patients with genetically proven LGMD2A, in which Western blots fail to reveal any protein abnormality, the mutations are in these autocatalytic regions (R490Q, R489Q, R490W missense mutations), resulting in a reduced autocatalytic activity by lowering the Ca^{2+} sensitivity [Fanin et al., 2003].

Clinical Manifestations

LGMD2A has a characteristic phenotype in about 64% of the genetically confirmed patients. Interfamilial and intrafamilial variability is not uncommon [Zatz et al., 2003]. The age at onset of symptoms is between 2 and 49 years; the mean age at presentation is 14 (±8) years [Saenz et al., 2005]. The disease causes symmetric weakness of the pelvic and shoulder girdle muscles. There is preferential involvement of the posterior compartment of the thighs and posterior superficial calves that can be seen clinically and by computed tomographic or magnetic resonance imaging (MRI) studies. Facial, oculomotor, and cardiac muscles are not affected. Scapular winging can be observed early [Beckmann and Bushby, 1996]. Contractures, if present, occur late in the disease and do not extend into the spine [Beckmann and Bushby, 1996]. Most patients become unable to walk about 25 years after symptom onset. The creatine kinase level is 5- to 20-fold elevated. However, occasional patients (reported in Brazil) have normal creatine kinase levels, and so this should not be an exclusion criterion. Cognition is not impaired. The clinical phenotype can be confused with that of LGMD2I (fukutin-related protein gene [FKRP]) or facioscapulohumeral muscular dystrophy because of the presence of scapular winging. However, the distribution of weakness and the muscle MRI findings are very characteristic and distinct from those of these two disorders [Mercuri et al., 2005].

Diagnosis

Diagnosis of a calpainopathy is based on a typical phenotype, a muscle biopsy sample revealing Western blot abnormalities, and genetic testing indicating two mutations on two alleles. The combination of a typical phenotype with an abnormal Western blot result in muscle biopsy samples (at least two abnormal bands) increases the probability that an affected patient has a calpainopathy to 90% [Saenz et al., 2005]. However, if one of these variables is missing, the probability is reduced to about 75% [Saenz et al., 2005]. False-negative reports with Western blots in 20% to 40% of these patients indicates that genetic sequencing has to be pursued when a calpainopathy is clinically suspected on the basis of the typical phenotype [Fanin et al., 2003; Saenz et al., 2005].

Muscle pathologic findings are positive for necrosis, regeneration, altered myofibrillar architecture, increased numbers of centrally placed nuclei, fibrosis, fiber type I predominance, and normal immunoreactivity for dystrophin and α-sarcoglycan. Muscle biopsy samples in preclinical cases have exhibited an unusual pattern of isolated fascicles of degenerating fibers in an almost normal muscle. This pattern has not been seen in patients early in the disease course who are affected by other forms of LGMD, which suggests that a peculiar pattern of focal degeneration occurs early in calpainopathy, independently of the type of mutation or the amount of calpain-3 in the muscle [Vainzof et al., 2003].

Western blot analysis of muscle calpain-3 can reveal total, partial, or no deficiency, with no relation between protein expression and severity of phenotype [Saenz et al., 2005; Zatz et al., 2003]. Secondary reduction of calpain-3 can be seen in other conditions, specifically dysferlinopathies and LGMD2I secondary to FKRP deficiency [Vainzof et al., 2000a].

Limb-Girdle Muscular Dystrophy 2B: Dysferlinopathy

Mutations in the dysferlin gene on chromosome 2p13 cause distinct phenotypes of muscular dystrophy: LGMD type 2B (LGMD2B), Miyoshi's myopathy, and distal anterior compartment myopathy, which are known by the term *dysferlinopathies.* This form represents 1% of recessive LGMD and about 33% of distal LGMD. Although the distributions of weakness in Miyoshi's myopathy and LGMD2B are different (distal and proximal, respectively), both syndromes manifest in the late teens, progress slowly, and are associated with high serum creatine kinase levels. Moreover, identical mutations can give rise to both phenotypes in the same family; therefore, environmental or other factors might contribute to the differential expression of muscle weakness [Kawabe et al., 2004].

Molecular Pathogenesis

Molecular pathogenesis is an autosomal-recessive LGMD that is caused by mutations in the dysferlin gene on chromosome 2p13 [Bashir et al., 1996; Passos-Bueno et al., 1996a, 1996b]. In humans, the dysferlin gene encompasses 55 exons spanning more than 150 kilobases of genomic DNA [Aoki et al., 2001]. The dysferlin gene encodes a 230-kDa protein with widespread expression in tissues such as skeletal muscle, cardiac muscle, the kidneys, the placenta, the lungs, and the brain. Although dysferlin is expressed most abundantly in skeletal and cardiac muscles, there is no evidence for cardiac muscle dysfunction in dysferlin-deficient patients. Immunohistochemical studies revealed that in skeletal muscle, dysferlin is located at the plasma membrane, as well as in cytoplasmic vesicles [Bansal et al., 2003].

The pathogenesis of this class of muscular dystrophy is distinct in that the defect lies in the maintenance, not the structure, of the plasma membrane. Histopathologic and immunohistochemical studies in these patients reveal absence of dysferlin [Matsuda et al., 1999]. In addition, a very active inflammatory and degenerative process is characteristic in this disease and can lead to a misdiagnosis of polymyositis. However, the immune response is different, with macrophages being more common than T cells; the presence of perivascular and interstitial infiltrate consisting of $CD8^+$ and $CD4^+$ cells, but no B cells; and overexpression of major histocompatibility complex class I on muscle fibers [Gallardo et al., 2001]. These findings differ from polymyositis but are closely similar to those in SJL/J mice (murine model of dysferlin deficiency); this emphasizes a direct relationship between absence of dysferlin and immune system abnormalities in muscle [Confalonieri et al., 2003], perhaps in response to an inefficient muscle membrane repair and regenerative system [Cenacchi et al., 2005].

Ultrastructural studies provide evidence for the abnormal membrane repair mechanism when dysferlin is absent. Electron microscopy studies demonstrate prominent aggregations of small vacuoles, likely derived from the Golgi apparatus in the subsarcolemmal region, consisting of empty, swollen cisternae. The sarcolemma has multiple small gaps and microvillus-like projections. The basal lamina is thick and has focal duplications, thus having a multilayered appearance [Cenacchi et al., 2005; Selcen et al., 2001]. These alterations are seen mostly over plasmalemmal defects. Characteristic of this disorder is the presence of one to several layers of small vesicles just beneath the sarcolemma as proof of a defective resealing mechanism that fails to repair the sarcolemma [Cenacchi et al., 2005].

Clinical Presentation

There are two common phenotypes, LGMD2B and Miyoshi's myopathy, both manifesting in the second decade of life [Takahashi et al., 2003]. Two other phenotypes, distal anterior compartment type and scapuloperoneal type, also exist and are seen especially early in the clinical course [Ueyama et al., 2002]. Patients undergo normal early developmental milestones without weakness in childhood and development of slowly progressive muscle weakness and wasting starting in adolescence [Mahjneh et al., 2001]. The LGMD2B phenotype is a predominantly proximal muscular dystrophy. Affected individuals have onset of pelvic girdle muscle weakness, with lower limbs abducted and externally rotated and hyperlordosis as a result of hip muscle weakness. The anterior muscles of the distal legs and distal arms are relatively normal in these patients, even at the later stages of the disease. In contrast, the Miyoshi myopathy phenotype is a predominantly distal muscular dystrophy with early involvement of the posterior compartments of the lower limb; a common early symptom is the inability to stand on tiptoes. These patients manifest hyperextension of the lower limbs caused by weakness of the quadriceps and gastrocnemius muscle. As a result, physical examination reveals extensive wasting of the distal posterior muscles of the leg and, later, of the thigh [Ueyama et al., 2002]. Although previously described mainly in Japan, Miyoshi's myopathy has been increasingly recognized in Western countries. Ten years after the onset of the disease, pronounced gait abnormalities are present in both the LGMD2B and the Miyoshi myopathy phenotypes: The foot leaves the ground with a double flexion of the knee and the hip. At this stage, upper extremity weakness is also evident and at times has a distal pattern. Laboratory evaluation demonstrates markedly increased serum creatine kinase levels.

There is no specific treatment for this disorder, and the management is in the realm of rehabilitation medicine. Ankle-foot orthosis can improve gait when footdrop is pronounced. Despite the pronounced inflammatory response in muscle biopsy samples, steroids are not beneficial and might worsen the disorder.

Diagnosis

Diagnosis of dysferlinopathy is based on the absence of dysferlin expression on immunoblots or cryostat sections and on exclusion of dystrophinopathy, sarcoglycanopathy, calpainopathy, and calveolinopathy, because dysferlin deficiency is rarely secondary in other myopathies. However, severe reduction of dysferlin expression is seen only in Miyoshi's myopathy or LGMD2A [Anderson et al., 2000]. The diagnosis of dysferlinopathy can also be made by measuring dysferlin expression in peripheral blood mononuclear cells by immunoblot analysis, which has excellent correlation with muscle biopsy findings [Ho et al., 2002]. This test is available commercially.

Limb-Girdle Muscular Dystrophies 2C, 2D, 2E, 2F: Sarcoglycanopathies

The sarcoglycanopathies are a family of autosomal recessive disorders that often manifest with an early and severe phenotype. The four sarcoglycans constitute a tetrameric complex of membrane proteins that contributes to the stability of the plasma membrane cytoskeleton and facilitates the association of dystrophin with the dystroglycans. The four sarcoglycan genes (α, β, γ, and δ) are related to each other structurally and functionally, but each has a discrete chromosomal location. Mutations in each gene may produce partial or complete loss of the entire complex [Nigro et al., 1996b]. Patients with sarcoglycanopathies were initially distinguished from children with a severe Duchenne-like presentation who proved dystrophin positive and in whom autosomal-recessive inheritance was likely [Zatz et al., 1989]. The term *severe childhood autosomal recessive muscular dystrophy* was used to describe the condition of these children; some of them were later found to have a deficiency of a 50-kDa dystrophin-associated protein, the gene for which was localized to chromosome 13q12, the locus for γ-sarcoglycan [Azibi et al., 1993; Matsumura et al., 1992]. Sister proteins were identified [Mizuno et al., 1994], and the phenotypes associated with sarcoglycanopathies broadened to include less severely involved children.

Mutations in each of the four sarcoglycans are found worldwide. In outbred populations such as those in Europe, North America, and Brazil, the relative frequencies of symptomatic mutations of the four genes are, from highest to lowest, α, β, γ, and δ in an 8:4:2:1 ratio [Duggan et al., 1997]. In other populations, this ratio may vary. A founder mutation *Thr151Arg* in β-sarcoglycan has been identified in the Indiana Amish community [Duclos et al., 1998]. Specific mutations of γ-sarcoglycan cause the majority of cases of LGMD among Gypsies and persons in northern Africa [Merlini et al., 2000; Noguchi et al., 1995], and a specific mutation of δ-sarcoglycan is seen in a relatively higher frequency in African-Brazilians [Nigro et al., 1996a; Vainzof et al., 1999]. Although the worldwide epidemiology of sarcoglycanopathies has not been extensively studied, data obtained in northern Italy suggest an incidence of 5.6 per million [Fanin et al., 1997].

Before a child is evaluated for sarcoglycanopathy, a primary dystrophinopathy must be excluded. Fewer than 5% of males with a Duchenne/Becker phenotype have a sarcoglycanopathy or other limb girdle muscular dystrophy. Young females with a Duchenne/Becker phenotype are nearly as likely to be carriers of a dystrophinopathy as to have an alternative diagnosis [Hoffman and Clemens, 1996]. The majority of dystrophin-positive children presenting with an early-onset Duchenne-like phenotype have a sarcoglycanopathy [Duggan et al., 1996; Vainzof et al., 1999]. In contrast, only about 10% of patients with a more benign phenotype evolving in adolescence or young adulthood manifest a sarcoglycanopathy.

Immunostaining of muscle with antisarcoglycan antibodies is the standard screening for new cases of sarcoglycanopathy. Muscle biopsy samples from patients with primary dystrophinopathy reveal reduced sarcoglycan immunoreactivity. Therefore, both dystrophin and sarcoglycan immunostaining must be performed on the same muscle tissue. The finding of normal dystrophin staining and deficiency in immunostaining of any of the sarcoglycans suggests that a sarcoglycan mutation is present. Many laboratories perform immunostaining only for α-sarcoglycan, relying on a reduction or absence of immunoreactivity to reflect a mutation in any of the four sarcoglycans. Because the entire sarcoglycan complex tends to be affected as a unit in response to mutations in any of the four components, this is usually adequate. However, staining with antibodies to all four sarcoglycans can provide clues regarding the protein that reflects the primary mutation. This information helps direct DNA testing for definitive diagnosis of the specific sarcoglycan mutation. On occasion, immunoreactivity of components within the sarcoglycan complex appears normal in the presence of a documented reduction in immunostaining of another component [Higuchi et al., 1998; Vainzof et al., 2000b]. γ-Sarcoglycanopathy in particular may produce a marked reduction in γ-sarcoglycan immunoreactivity with relatively good preservation of α- and δ-sarcoglycan staining [Nowak et al., 2000; Vainzof et al., 1996]. The pathophysiology of sarcoglycanopathies relates to that of dystrophinopathies, discussed in detail in the preceding section and is not covered here.

γ-Sarcoglycanopathy (Limb-Girdle Muscular Dystrophy 2C)

The gene for γ-sarcoglycan is found on chromosome 13q12. It codes for a 35-kDa protein expressed predominantly in skeletal muscle. In addition to its role as a stabilizer of the dystrophin-associated complex, γ-sarcoglycan binds γ-filamin/filamin C [Noguchi et al., 1995]. Minor expression in smooth muscle occurs as well [Barresi et al., 2000]. The most common γ-sarcoglycan mutation is the deletion of a single thymidine residue, *del521T* [Noguchi et al., 1995], that originated in northern Africa as a founder mutation. This mutation produces a truncated protein. However, the clinical severity is variable even within families, ranging from a Duchenne-like to a mild Becker phenotype [McNally et al., 1996a, 1996b]. The mean age at symptom onset is 5 years. The distribution of weakness is most notable in the glutei and thigh adductors. Upper extremity weakness usually begins in the periscapular muscle and later involves the deltoid and biceps muscles. In contrast to Duchenne muscular dystrophy, the quadriceps tends to be spared and is usually as powerful as the hamstrings. Calf and tongue muscle hypertrophy is common. Cardiac problems occur late in the disease, with evidence of right ventricular hypertrophy on electrocardiograms and asymptomatic ventricular dysfunction [Melacini et al., 1999]. Cognition is normal. Mild sensorineural hearing loss may evolve. Loss of independent ambulation occurs at mean age of 16 years (range, 10 to 37 years). Orthopedic problems include progressive lordosis. Surgical stabilization of the spine is rarely needed.

Laboratory studies reveal gross elevations of creatine kinase level, usually more than 10-fold normal. Muscle biopsy samples yield dystrophic findings of degeneration and regeneration and occasional foci of inflammation. Immunostaining of sarcoglycans with a dystrophin-immunostaining control sample is the diagnostic procedure of choice. Patients with γ-sarcoglycan can have near-normal α-sarcoglycan immunostaining, which yields a false-negative muscle biopsy result [Nowak et al., 2000].

α-Sarcoglycanopathy (Limb-Girdle Muscular Dystrophy 2D)

α-Sarcoglycan is encoded on chromosome 17q21. The 50-kDa protein originally called *adhalin* is expressed only in skeletal and cardiac muscle. Most mutations are missense in the extracellular domain [Piccolo et al., 1995]. Worldwide, α-sarcoglycanopathy is the most common of the sarcolycan disorders, accounting for over 50% of patients [Hayashi and Arahata, 1997]. The *Arg787Cys* missense mutation is the most common, accounting for a third of all cases of α-sarcoglycanopathy [Carrie et al., 1997]. Null mutations are associated with total absence of α-sarcoglycan and often confer a severe phenotype with onset of symptoms in the first 3 years of life [Duggan et al., 1997].

Onset of motor problems occurs between 2 and 15 years; earlier onset is predictive of more rapid deterioration and low or absent α-sarcoglycan. In patients with late onset, ambulation may be preserved for decades. Occasional patients manifest a high creatine kinase level in the absence of weakness. The distribution of weakness, atrophy, and hypertrophy is similar to that described for γ-sarcoglycan, but the quadriceps tends to be involved in patients with severe, early-onset disease. The phenotype varies from a severe Duchenne phenotype to a mild Becker phenotype. Early scapular weakness is common. Symptomatic cardiomyopathy is rare, although evidence of cardiac dysfunction is present in about 30% of patients [Melacini et al., 1999]. Cognition is normal. Serum creatine kinase levels are high, usually over 5000 IU.

Small therapeutic trials of corticosteroids have been conducted, with reports of benefits similar to those seen in steroid-treated Duchenne muscular dystrophy patients [Connolly et al., 1998].

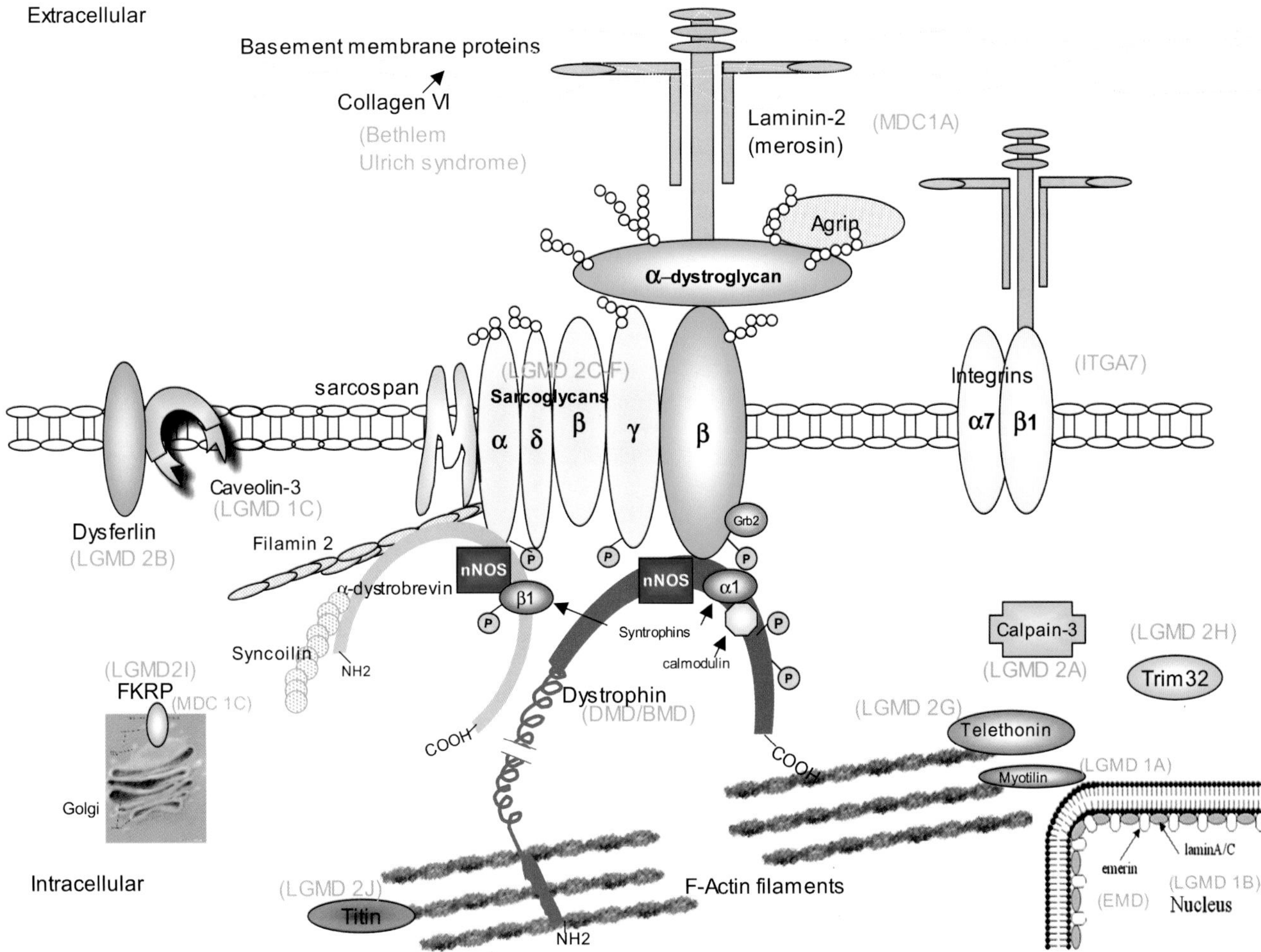

FIGURE 79-1. Diagram of the muscle membrane as known today, illustrating association of dystrophin-glycoprotein complex linkage to contractile proteins, extracellular matrix proteins, and other proteins with signaling properties (syntrophins, Grb2). It also illustrates the multiple phosphorylation sites in the 3′ end of dystrophin, dystrobrevin, and dystroglycans. Diseases associated with defect in individual proteins are also listed in parenthesis. BMD, Becker muscular dystrophy; DMD, Duchenne muscular dystrophy; ITGA7, integrin α7; LGMD, limb-girdle muscular dystrophy; MDC1A, merosin-negative congenital muscular dystrophy; MDC1C, merosin-positive congenital muscular dystrophy; nNOS, neuronal nitric oxide synthetase.

β-Sarcoglycanopathy (Limb-Girdle Muscular Dystrophy 2E)

β-Sarcoglycan is coded on chromosome 4q12. It is a 43-kDa protein that is expressed not only in skeletal and cardiac muscle but also in brain and kidney tissue. Worldwide, it accounts for about 25% of reported cases of sarcoglycanopathy. However, certain populations have a much higher incidence of β-sarcoglycan mutations, including the Indiana Amish.

The clinical spectrum is similar to that described for the γ- and α-sarcoglycanopathies, with onset occurring between age 3 years and the mid-teens and faster progression with earlier onset. Independent walking is often lost between the ages of 10 and 15 and nearly always by age 25. Muscle hypertrophy is prominent in the calves. Symptomatic cardiomyopathy is rarely seen.

Creatine kinase levels are approximately 5000 IU. Muscle biopsy specimens usually reveal absence of all sarcoglycan immunostaining, and there is occasional reduction of dystrophin immunostaining as well. A knockout mouse model of β-sarcoglycanopathy has been developed, and attempts at gene transfer have been initiated [Dressman et al., 2002].

δ-Sarcoglycanopathy (Limb-Girdle Dystrophy 2F)

The gene for δ-sarcoglycanopathy in chromosome region 5q33-q34 codes for a 35-kDa protein localized to the subsarcolemmal region of skeletal and cardiac muscle. It is the rarest of the sarcoglycanopathies. Missense and nonsense mutations are reported, as is a frameshift mutation that produces a premature truncation of protein found in affected Brazilian families [Nigro et al., 1996a]. The clinical phenotype is universally severe, with onset of symptoms occurring between 2 and 10 years of age and progression to full-time wheelchair use by the mid-teens. Most patients do not survive their second decade. A dilated cardiomyopathy may occur with or without skeletal myopathy [Politano et al., 2001; Tsubata et al., 2000].

Limb-Girdle Muscular Dystrophy 2I: Fukutin-Related Protein Gene Deficiency

LGMD2I is a newly characterized LGMD, whose causative gene was discovered in 2001 [Brockington et al., 2001b]. Since then, it has become apparent that this is one of the most common forms of LGMD, representing from 11% [Zatz et al., 2003] to 19% [Krasnianski et al., 2004; Walter et al., 2004] of all cases of LGMD in different series.

Molecular Pathogenesis

The disease is caused by a mutation in the fukutin-related protein gene in chromosome 19q13.3 [Brockington et al., 2001a]. The most common mutation is a single point (826C>A) missense mutation in one allele (>90%) causing a Leu276Ileu (C826A) [Brockington et al., 2001b]. Disease severity correlates with a mutation on the second allele; consequently, patients with homozygous mutations causing a Leu276Ileu exhibit a less severe phenotype [Brockington et al., 2002; Mercuri et al., 2003]. Patients heterozygous for this mutation usually have a second heteroallelic mutation on the other allele [Walter et al., 2004]. This disorder is allelic to congenital muscular dystrophy with muscle hypertrophy and a normal central nervous system (merosin-positive congenital muscular dystrophy type [MDC1C]) [Brockington et al., 2001a].

FKRP is a ubiquitous protein with highest levels in skeletal muscle, heart, and placenta tissue. FKRP localizes to rough endoplasmic reticulum and has glycosyltransferase activity [Matsumoto et al., 2004]. FKRP and fukutin are targeted to the medial Golgi apparatus through their N-termini and transmembrane domains [Esapa et al., 2002]. Together with fukutin, FKRP appears to be involved in the initial steps of *O*-mannosylglycan synthesis of α-dystroglycan [Matsumoto et al., 2004].

Clinical Manifestations

Age at onset ranges from 0.5 to 27 years; 61% of patients present before age 5 years. Patients present with either a Duchenne muscular dystrophy phenotype (heterozygous mutations) or, with a later onset, milder limb-girdle syndrome (homozygous mutations). The clinical course varies, usually involving weakness and wasting of the shoulder girdle muscles and proximal extremities, with significant calf hypertrophy, and elevated serum creatine kinase levels, ranging from 5- to 70-fold increases. There is a characteristic predilection for muscles of the lower extremities, with weakness of hip flexion and adduction, knee flexion, and ankle dorsiflexion being more predominant [Fischer et al., 2005]. Other clinical manifestations have been described, including exercise-induced myalgia in addition to weakness and isolated myalgia, cramps, elevated serum creatine kinase levels, and dilated cardiomyopathy without muscle weakness [Krasnianski et al., 2004]. In some series, most patients presented with muscle pain and myoglobinuria as the earliest symptoms [Walter et al., 2004]. Cardiac and respiratory involvement are relatively common in the heterozygous, earlier presentation cases, occurring in about 30% of patients, and at times while they are still ambulatory [Mercuri et al., 2003; Poppe et al., 2003].

Diagnosis

Methods for genetic sequencing of the FKRP gene from peripheral blood are commercially available, and so diagnosis can be confirmed.

Muscle biopsy samples reveal characteristic dystrophin changes, with muscle fiber size variation, muscle fiber necrosis and regeneration, and mild increase in connective tissue. The most consistent abnormality is secondary abnormal laminin-2 immunostaining. Most patients also have a marked decrease in immunostaining of muscle α-dystroglycan and a reduction in its molecular weight on Western blot analysis [Brockington et al., 2001a, 2001b].

MRI of muscle demonstrates a distinct and consistent pattern of muscular involvement in LGMD2I that is correlated with the pattern of muscle weakness in these patients. Predominant weakness of shoulder adduction and internal rotation, elbow flexion, hip flexion and adduction, knee flexion, and ankle dorsiflexion, independent of the individual disease duration and the level of clinical severity, are corroborated by the findings on muscle MRI analysis

[Fischer et al., 2005]. This pattern is very similar to that of LGMD2A (calpain-3 deficiency) but distinct from dysferlinopathies, sarcoglycanopathies, and dystrophinopathies. In LGMD2I, marked hyperintense signal changes on T1-weighted images can be seen in the adductor and posterior thigh muscles that clearly exceed the changes in the abductor and anterior thigh muscles. Hypertrophy of the gracilis and sartorius muscle seems to be a frequent finding. Furthermore, the degree of signal abnormalities in affected muscles mirrors the degree of muscle weakness in individual patients [Fischer et al., 2005].

Management

There is no specific treatment for this disorder, and its management does not differ from other muscular dystrophies. There is no evidence of a response to steroids or other pharmacologic treatments. Cardiac and respiratory function need to be evaluated at diagnosis, with follow-up frequency determined from the baseline measurements and clinical evolution.

Limb-Girdle Muscular Dystrophy 1A, 2G, and 2J: Sarcomeric Protein Deficiencies

Limb-Girdle Muscular Dystrophy 1A (Myotilinopathy)

LGMD1A was the first autosomal-dominant limb-girdle dystrophy to be linked to a specific gene locus. Initial clinical observations of the co-segregating of two rare diseases, muscular dystrophy and Pelger-Huët syndrome [Schneiderman et al., 1969], in a kindred were followed years later by linkage studies localizing the gene to chromosome region 5q31-q33 [Yamaoka et al., 1994] and the discovery of the first of several missense mutations in the gene coding for the sarcomeric protein myotilin [Hauser et al., 2002].

Myotilin localizes to the Z-disk and interacts with α-actinin and F-actin, efficiently cross-linking thin filaments. This protein also interacts with other filaments, including filamin C. In vitro studies suggest that the expression of myotilin in muscle cells is tightly regulated to become active in the later stages of in vitro myofibrillogenesis, when preassembled myofibrils begin to align. Thus, myotilin appears to have an indispensable role in stabilization and anchorage of the thin filaments that may be needed for correct Z-disk orientation [Salmikangas et al., 2003]. The mutations observed in LGMD1A do not disrupt binding of myotilin to α-actinin but result in Z-disk streaming.

Myotilin has been implicated in other diseases, including a causal role in some cases of myofibrillar myopathy [Selcen and Engel, 2004; Selcen et al., 2004] and a secondary role in central core disease and nemaline myopathy [Schroder et al., 2003].

Missense mutations underlie the pathophysiology in the initially reported family and the seven additional families expressing this disorder. Patients in the initial kindred had symptoms of proximal weakness in young adulthood, with a mean age at onset of 27 [Hauser et al., 2000]. A suggestion of anticipation has been reported with a reduction in age at onset by 13 years from one generation to the next, an observation uncommon in diseases not caused by nucleotide repeat expansions. About half of patients with LGMD1A develop nasal dysarthria. Ankle contractures are common. Progression of the disease is slow, and ambulation is maintained for decades. Creatine kinase level elevations from 2- to 10-fold are common. Electrodiagnostic study findings are consistent with a myonecrotic myopathy. Cardiac involvement occurs in about half of the patients but is rarely debilitating. Muscle biopsies reveal Z-line streaming, muscle fiber degeneration, fiber splitting, and central nucleation. Rimmed autophagic vacuoles are reported [Hauser et al., 2002].

Establishing the diagnosis in new patients is challenging. Immunostaining of myotilin is normal. A history of slowly progressive limb-girdle weakness with a family history consistent with autosomal-dominant transmission may be obtained, but the incidence of spontaneous mutation is unknown. The findings of heel cord contracture, nasal dysarthria, mild-to-moderate elevation of creatine kinase level, and muscle biopsy findings of Z-line streaming and autophagic vacuoles should increase clinical suspicion. Mutation analysis of the myotilin gene is needed for a definitive diagnosis.

Limb-Girdle Muscular Dystrophy 2G (Telethonin)

Telethonin is a small 19-kDa sarcomeric protein expressed in skeletal and cardiac muscle [Valle et al., 1997]. Its gene maps to chromosome region 17q11-q12, the candidate site to which samples from members of a Brazilian family with an early-onset LGMD phenotype had mapped [Moreira et al., 1997]. Subsequent studies of this and three other Brazilian families confirmed mutations of the telethonin gene [Moreira et al., 2000]. Telethonin has been implicated in myofibrillar assembly [Mason et al., 1999]. It is phosphorylated by the serine kinase domain of titin and may serve to cap titin in the Z-disk [Knoll et al., 2002]; telethonin is also known as T-CAP.

Patients with telethonin mutations have not been recognized outside Brazil. The onset of symptoms has occurred between 9 and 15 years of age. Weakness is mainly proximal, but of the 13 patients described, 7 had prominent distal weakness with lower extremity atrophy and footdrop. Paradoxically, six patients evidenced calf hypertrophy. Only one patient has remained independently ambulatory after age 43. Five of 9 of these original 13 patients studied for cardiac abnormality had mild cardiomyopathy. Creatine kinase levels were elevated 3- to 30-fold in all patients early in their disease. Muscle biopsy revealed degenerating and regenerating muscle fibers and rimmed vacuoles (an unusual finding for LGMD but not for distal myopathy syndromes) [Moreira et al., 1997]. Patients can be screened with immunohistochemical techniques through the use of antitelethonin antibodies. Mutation analysis is simplified because the telethonin gene contains only two exons.

Limb-Girdle Muscular Dystrophy 2J (Titin)

Titin is a giant structural protein of the sarcomere with a molecular weight of over 3800 kDa. It is the largest human protein and forms the third filament system in striated muscle along with actin and myosin. Single titin molecules span half sarcomeres from Z-disks to M-lines in skeletal and cardiac muscle. Titin contributes to sarcomere assembly and passive tension of myofibrils and serves sensor and signaling functions [Granzier and Labeit, 2004; McElhinny et al., 2004]. Titin serine kinase phosphorylates telethonin, another sarcomeric protein that is implicated in LGMD2G.

Mutations in the titin gene on chromosome 2q31 most often produce autosomal-dominant tibial muscular dystrophy, a distal muscular dystrophy of mid-adult life with prominent involvement of the tibialis anterior and toe extensor muscles [Hackman et al., 2002]. This disorder is most commonly seen in persons of Finnish descent. Patients with mutations causing truncated titins have autosomal-dominant familial dilated cardiomyopathy without skeletal muscle disease [Gerull et al., 2002]. Homozygous mutations have produced an adult-onset limb-girdle disorder, LGMD2J [Hackman et al., 2003]. Severe calpain-3 deficiency is seen in patients with LGMD2J and may be an important downstream pathway [Haravuori et al., 2001]. A review of 207 patients heterozygous for the specific C-terminal M-line titin mutation illustrated variability of clinical expression, including one child with infantile-onset generalized weakness and one with onset of a LGMD phenotype at age 6 [Udd et al., 2005].

X-LINKED SYNDROMES

McLeod's cardiomyopathy is a dilated cardiomyopathy with limited findings for myopathy linked to chromosome Xp21.1 as a recessive condition involving Kx membrane transport protein. Muscle weakness is mild. Central nervous system involvement includes chorea, seizures, and cerebral and caudate nucleus atrophy [Malandrini et al., 1994]. Acanthocytosis is present, and erythrocytes have abnormal expression of Kell blood group and Kx surface antigens. Creatine kinase levels tend to be high.

Another X-linked dilated cardiomyopathy, known as *Barth's syndrome,* is linked to chromosome Xp28. Tafazzin protein, which belongs to a superfamily with acyl transferases involved in phospholipid synthesis, is abnormal. Onset occurs in infancy. Motor development is delayed. Recurrent neutropenia and early infections, including pyodermia, are present. Ventricular hypertrophy with endocardial fibroelastosis is present. The creatine kinase level is normal. Muscle is mildly myopathic. In the endocardium, abnormal mitochondria are found with concentric cristae. Urinary organic acids 3-methylglutaconic acid, 3-methylglutarate, and 2-ethylacrylic acid are excreted. Early death in childhood from cardiac failure or sepsis may happen. Other patients exhibit gradual improvement in cardiac funcion, motor development, and resolving infections.

X-linked vacuolar myopathy is expressed pathologically with excessive autophagic vacuoles and granular material in the basement membrane. It is located on chromosome Xq28 near the Emery-Dreifuss locus as a recessive condition. Onset occurs in early childhood with weakness proximally and at the ankles. Progression of the disease is slow. The creatine kinase level is elevated 2 to 10 times normal.

EMERY-DREIFUSS MUSCULAR DYSTROPHY

Overview

Emery-Dreifuss muscular dystrophy was recognized as a distinct phenotype in the mid-1960s [Emery and Dreifuss, 1966]. Emery-Dreifuss muscular dystrophy is characterized by a clinical triad of early contractures, muscle wasting and weakness in a humeroperoneal distribution, and cardiomyopathy. Considerable phenotypic variability exists regarding age at onset and rate of progression. X-linked transmission and autosomal-dominant transmission are recognized.

Molecular Biology

Both X-linked and autosomal-dominant Emery-Dreifuss muscular dystrophy result from mutations in genes coding for nuclear envelop proteins. The X-linked form of Emery-Dreifuss muscular dystrophy is caused by mutations of the STA gene located at Xq28 which encodes a 34-kDa ubiquitously expressed nuclear envelop protein, emerin [Bione et al., 1994]. Of mutations producing X-linked Emery-Dreifuss muscular dystrophy, 95% are null mutations associated with a complete absence of emerin in skeletal muscle, as well as in smooth muscle, skin fibroblasts, leukocytes, and exfoliative buccal cells. A mosaic pattern is seen in female carriers, and the diagnosis of X-linked Emery-Dreifuss muscular dystrophy in males and identification of female heterozygotes is therefore possible with immunohistochemical studies of muscle and more easily accessed tissue [Emery, 2000; Manilal et al., 1997].

Autosomal-dominant Emery-Dreifuss muscular dystrophy and autosomal-recessive Emery-Dreifuss muscular dystrophy (a single reported case [Raffaele Di Barletta et al., 2000]) result from mutations of the LMNA gene located on 1q21, which encodes two nuclear envelope proteins, lamins A and C [Bonne et al., 1999]. Lamins A and C are alternatively spliced products of the same gene and constitute part of the nuclear lamina; they interact with chromatin and other proteins of the inner nuclear membrane, including emerin [Gruenbaum et al., 2003]. Mutations of the lamins A and C genes that produce the autosomal-dominant Emery-Dreifuss muscular dystrophy phenotype are missense mutations that allow translation of full-length lamins A and C. Immunostaining of lamins A and C is therefore not reliable for confirmation of the diagnosis of autosomal-dominant Emery-Dreifuss muscular dystrophy [Emery, 2000]. The diagnosis of lamin A or C disorders requires DNA sequencing or mutation scanning [Bonne et al., 2000, 2003; Brown et al., 2001]. The Emery-Dreifuss muscular dystrophy phenotype and its variants have focused attention on the importance of nuclear envelope proteins [Nagano and Arahata, 2000], but the pathophysiologic mechanisms of the diseases remain conjectural.

Clinical Features

Although X-linked Emery-Dreifuss muscular dystrophy and autosomal-dominant Emery-Dreifuss muscular dystrophy usually share a similar phenotype, wide clinical variation with poor genotype-phenotype correlation has been documented in both X-linked Emery-Dreifuss muscular dystrophy and autosomal-dominant Emery-Dreifuss muscular dystrophy [Bonne et al., 2000; Fujimoto et al., 1999; Muntoni et al., 1998]. Inter- and intrafamilial phenotypic variability may exist in patients sharing identical mutations.

The onset of contractures occurs early in the disease, in the first or second decade, and often precedes clinically significant weakness. Contractures are most prominent at the elbows, Achilles tendons, and posterior cervical muscles [Emery, 1989] (Figs. 79-10 and 79-11). Upper extremity contractures often precede axial and lower extremity deformities. The arms are held in a semiflexed position (Fig. 79-12). The feet are set in talipes equinus, often in association with toe walking. Posterior cervical contractures preclude full neck flexion (Fig. 79-13; see also Fig. 79-11). Contractures usually remain disproportionate to the degree of weakness [Emery, 2000] and may be the major factor in functional impairment. Muscle weakness is relatively mild and slowly progressive. The distribution of motor deficits is humeroperoneal with upper extremity weakness (in biceps, triceps, and spinatus muscles) occurring earlier than leg weakness (in tibialis anterior and peroneal muscles). Pseudohypertrophy is not seen, and its absence helps clinically differentiate X-linked Emery-Dreifuss muscular dystrophy from dystrophinopathy (Becker muscular dystrophy).

Cardiac symptoms may include palpitations, syncope, and diminished exercise tolerance. Supraventricular dysrhyth-

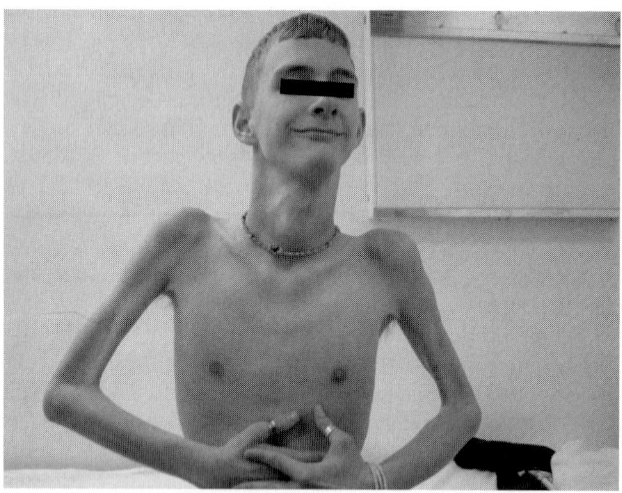

FIGURE 79-10. Sixteen-year-old male with X-linked Emery-Dreifuss muscular dystrophy. This male exhibits significant humeral atrophy, elbow flexion contractures, and neck hyperextension secondary to neck extensor contractures. Facial muscles are spared.

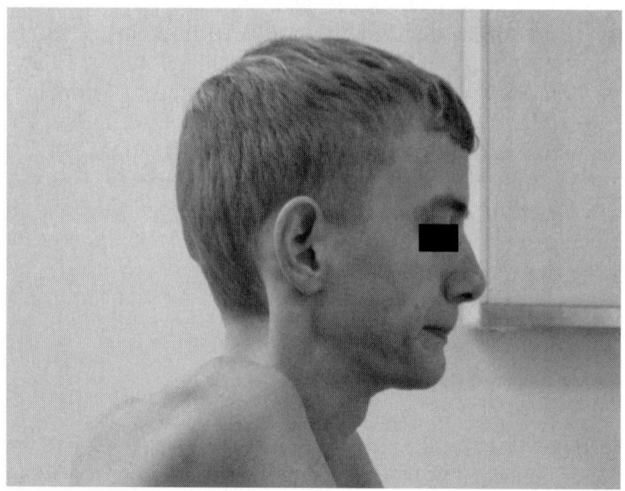

FIGURE 79-11. Same male with X-linked Emery-Dreifuss muscular dystrophy. Significant neck extensor contractures severely limit neck flexion.

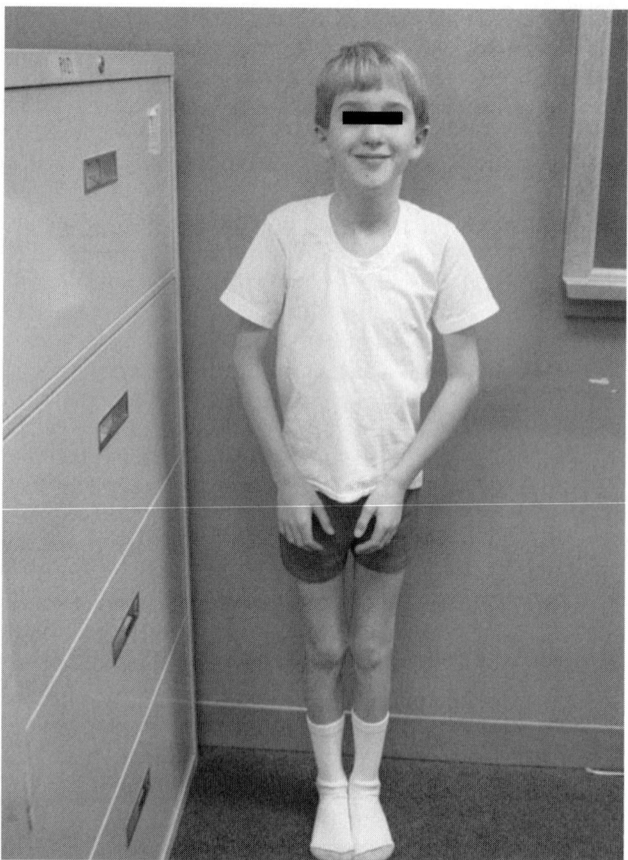

A

B

FIGURE 79-12. Seven-year-old male with autosomal-dominant Emery-Dreifuss muscular dystrophy. The presenting symptom was mild weakness; however, elbow flexor contractures (**A**) and mild neck extension contractures (**B**) were obvious on examination, as depicted in this photograph.

mias, atrioventricular conduction block, ventricular dysrhythmias, and restrictive or dilated cardiomyopathy may evolve. The risk of ventricular dysfunction and dysrhythmias is greater in autosomal-dominant than in X-linked Emery-Dreifuss muscular dystrophy [Becane et al., 2000; Bonne et al., 2003], but symptomatic cardiomyopathy may occur in women heterozygous for null emerin mutations. Cardiac symptoms usually evolve after the second decade.

Phenotypic variability in emerin deficiency relates to the age at onset and disease progression in X-linked Emery-Dreifuss muscular dystrophy. A broad spectrum of phenotypes has been discovered for mutations of the lamin A or C gene. Skeletal and cardiac myopathy without early contracures characterizes autosomal-dominant LGMD1B (see Fig. 79-13). Disorders of peripheral nerve, including an autosomal-recessive axonal form of Charcot-Marie-Tooth syndrome (type 2B1) and an autosomal-dominant peripheral neuropathy, are seen in other lamin A or C mutations [De Sandre-Giovannoli et al., 2002]. Dunnigan-type familial partial lipodystrophy [Shackleton et al., 2000] and generalized lipoatrophy with insulin resistance [Caux et al., 2003] have been reported. Autosomal-dominant Hutchinson-Gilford progeria [De Sandre-Giovannoli et al., 2003] and atypical Werner's syndrome [Chen et al., 2003] are more recent additions to the spectrum of laminopathies.

Management

Treatment is largely based on symptoms. The high incidence of cardiac dysfunction mandates early and regular cardiology evaluations. Mothers and sisters of males with X-linked Emery-Dreifuss muscular dystrophy should also receive cardiology consultation. Orthopedic interventions may be helpful in addressing limb contractures. In the late stage of Emery-Dreifuss muscular dystrophy, respiratory aids, including cough-assistive devices and noninvasive nocturnal respiratory support, may be helpful.

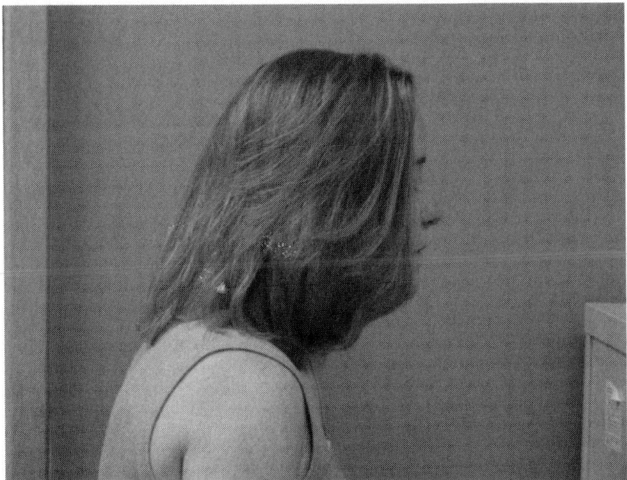

FIGURE 79-13. Mother of the male in Figure 79-12. She was asymptomatic, and her condition was undiagnosed; however, her neck extensor contractures are obvious, as depicted in this picture of her attempting to flex her neck.

FACIOSCAPULOHUMERAL MUSCULAR DYSTROPHY

Overview

Facioscapulohumeral muscular dystrophy was described by Landouzy and Dejerine in 1885. This disease is inherited as an autosomal-dominant disorder with high penetrance and variable expression. Ten percent to 30% of cases represent new mutations [Zatz et al., 1995]. Prevalence is estimated at 1 per 20,000. Clinical signs and symptoms are usually present before age 20 years and are manifested by weakness of the facial muscles, fixators of the scapula, and dorsiflexors of the ankle. Severity is highly variable. Although skeletal muscle symptoms dominate the clinical picture, other systems are often involved, which implies a more widespread developmental/degenerative process.

Molecular Genetics

Facioscapulohumeral muscular dystrophy maps to chromosome 4q35 [Wijmenga et al., 1993]. More than 95% of patients with facioscapulohumeral muscular dystrophy have a reduced number of 3.3-kilobase tandem repeat sequences termed D4Z4. The D4Z4 repeat region lies within a region of telomeric heterochromatin. There is no known gene within or telomeric to the D4Z4 repeat region, and the molecular biology underlining skeletal muscle and systemic abnormalities remains conjectural. An inverse correlation exists between the D4Z4 size and disease severity [Zatz et al., 1995]. Abnormal restriction enzyme EcoRI fragments are 34 kilobases or smaller (i.e., fewer than 10 repeats) [Upadhyaya et al., 1997]. The largest deletions have been associated with severe, congenital-onset facioscapulohumeral muscular dystrophy [Brouwer et al., 1994, 1995]. A large deletion with a 10- to 13-kilobase remaining DNA fragment usually produces symptoms by 16 years of age, and these may be severe. In some instances, this may be a new mutation. An intermediate deletion with a remaining DNA fragment greater than 16 kilobases is associated with large families expressing the dominantly inherited condition beginning between ages 8 and 22 years. Small deletions are usually found in kindreds with disease of later onset, usually from 15 to 23 years. In these families, a few individuals carrying the small deletion phenotypically appear normal, which is suggestive of nonpenetrance.

Possible mechanisms by which truncation of the D4Z4 repeat sequences produces facioscapulohumeral muscular dystrophy include altered interactions with transcription factors or chromatin modifiers at the nuclear envelope. Shortening of the D4Z4 repeat sequence may also allow position effect variegation (a change in the expression of a gene adjacent to heterochromatin) [Winokur et al., 1994]. The possibility of de-repression of silent genes or pathologic maintenance of genes in a transcriptionally active state after expression should have been downregulated is supported by studies demonstrating upregulation of the expression of genes that lie immediately upstream of the D4Z4 repeats [Tsien et al., 2001].

Commercially available testing of chromosome 4q35 is the most specific and sensitive diagnostic test for facioscapulohumeral muscular dystrophy. Subtelomeric translocations between chromosomes 4q35 and 10q26 occur relatively frequently in the general population and may complicate molecular diagnosis. A D4Z4 deletion results in disease if the deletion occurs on chromosome 4, but deletions on chromosome 10 have no clinical significance. Detection of a deletion in an individual with a 4;10 translocation must be interpreted with caution [van der Maarel et al., 1999; van Deutekom et al., 1996]. In 5% of facioscapulohumeral muscular dystrophy patients a 4q35 deletion is not identified, which suggests that at least one additional genetic disorder, designated facioscapulohumeral muscular dystrophy 1B, produces the facioscapulohumeral muscular dystrophy phenotype [Yamanaka et al., 2004].

Clinical Features

Clinical diagnostic criteria have been established by the facioscapulohumeral muscular dystrophy consortium [Tawil et al., 1998]. They specify autosomal-dominant inheritance; bifacial weakness; and weakness of the scapular stabilizer muscles, ankle dorsiflexor muscles, or both. Supporting criteria include asymmetry of motor deficits (a finding far more common in facioscapulohumeral muscular dystrophy than any other muscular dystrophy); sparing of deltoid, neck flexor, and calf muscles; and involvement of wrist extensors and abdominal muscles. Hearing loss involving high frequencies and retinal vasculopathy (Coats' disease) are additional supportive findings. Exclusion criteria include eyelid ptosis, extraocular muscle weakness, skin rash, elbow contractures, cardiomyopathy, sensory loss, neurogenic changes documented in muscle biopsy, and myotonia or neurogenic motor unit potentials documented on needle electromyography.

Weakness is usually first appreciated in the facial muscles. Patients have difficulty with puckering the lips, whistling, sipping through a straw, or blowing up balloons because of weakness of the orbicularis oris muscle. Most patients have a transverse smile and limited facial expression. Weakness of the orbicularis oculi is usually asymptomatic, but the examiner can appreciate it by observing incomplete burying of the eyelashes with forced eyelid closure and the ease with which the closed eyelids can be pried apart. A history of sleeping with the eyes open may be offered by a parent or spouse. Facial weakness may not be symmetric (Figs. 79-14 and 79-15).

Weakness of scapular fixation is evidenced by scapular winging accentuated by arm elevation in a forward plane (Fig. 79-16). The scapulae ride high on the back, producing the illusion of hypertrophied trapezius muscles (Fig. 79-17). Arm abduction is impaired in the presence of normal power and bulk of the deltoid muscles. Wasting of the biceps and triceps with preservation of deltoid and forearm muscles yields a "Popeye" configuration to the arms. Wasting of the clavicular head of the pectoral muscles produces a reversal of the axillary folds with a deep upward slope. Weakness of lower abdominal muscles may result in a "potbelly" when standing and a positive Beevor sign (cephalad movement of the umbilicus with neck flexion) when the patient lies supine.

Lower extremity weakness is usually first evident in the ankle dorsiflexors, with compromised heel walking or overt footdrop. Atrophy is most prominent in the tibialis anterior muscle. Preservation or hypertrophy of the extensor digitorum brevis muscle clinically excludes a neurogenic etiology of the footdrop. Axial paraspinal muscle weakness may result in marked lumbar lordosis, especially in patients with childhood-onset facioscapulohumeral muscular dystrophy.

Motor deficits are slowly progressive. Some patients report long periods of clinical stability punctuated by abrupt stepwise loss of power in restricted muscle groups. Asymmetry of weakness and muscle atrophy is the rule and may be striking. Most patients remain functionally independent throughout life. About 20% of facioscapulohumeral mus-

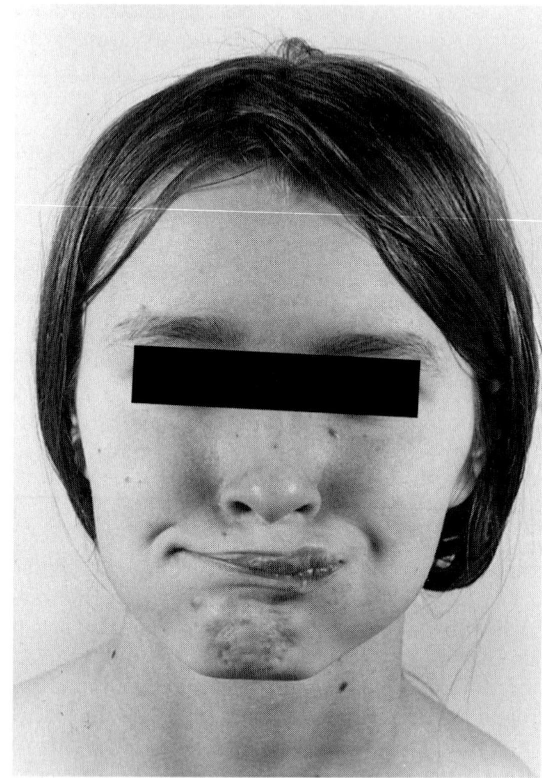

FIGURE 79-14. Marked facial weakness of this patient with facioscapulohumeral muscular dystrophy leads to a smooth, unlined, relatively inanimate face. The patient is attempting to blow her cheeks outward without success.

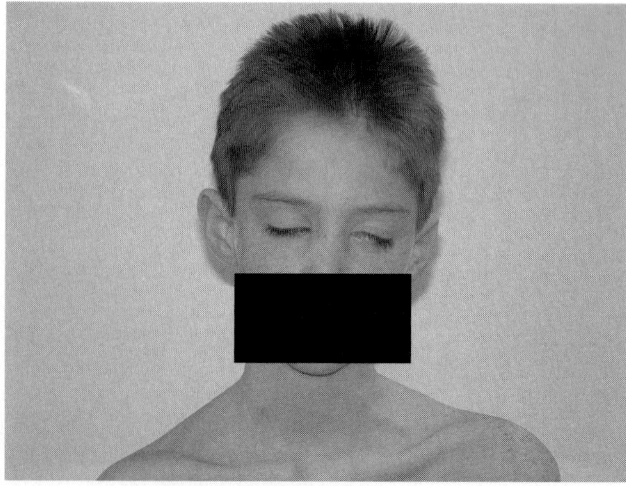

FIGURE 79-15. Marked facial weakness in patient with facioscapulohumeral muscular dystrophy, manifesting with asymmetric orbicularis oculi weakness and incomplete eyelid closure (inability to bury the eyelashes).

cular dystrophy patients (usually those with early disease onset) eventually require a wheelchair. Life expectancy is normal. Men appear to be more severely affected than women, and greater penetrance of the disorder has been documented in male patients [Zatz et al., 1998]. Sensorineural hearing loss is frequently documented, especially in children presenting before 10 years of age [Takeya et al., 1990; Voit et al., 1986] but can often be asymptomatic.

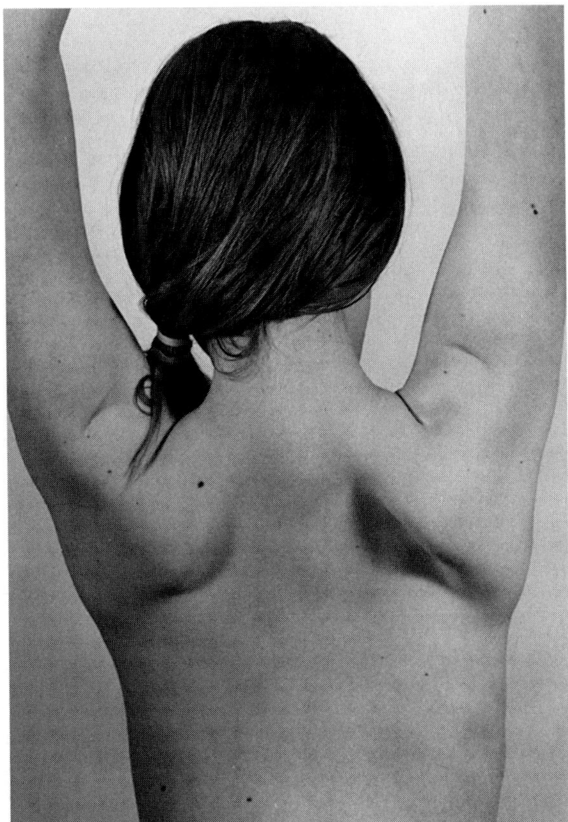

FIGURE 79-16. Patient with facioscapulohumeral muscular dystrophy exhibits extreme wasting of the muscles responsible for scapular stabilization.

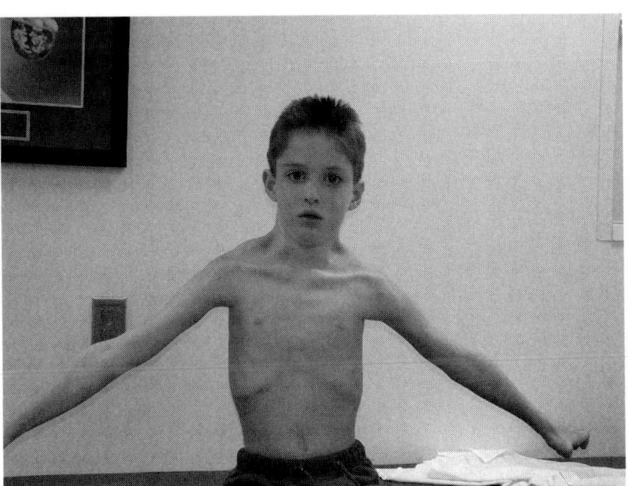

FIGURE 79-17. Patient with facioscapulohumeral muscular dystrophy exhibits scapular high-riding on the back as a consequence of abnormal scapular fixation, giving the appearance of hypertrophied trapezius muscles.

Retinal vasculopathy with telangiectasia and retinal detachment (Coats' disease) may develop [Fitzsimons et al., 1987; Gurwin et al., 1985; Padberg et al., 1995]; regular ophthalmology evaluations are warranted.

Congenital onset of facioscapulohumeral muscular dystrophy has been associated with mental retardation and epilepsy in children with the largest D4Z4 deletions (EcoRI fragment size of 10 kilobases; i.e., fewer than 10 repeats). The congenital-onset, or infantile, phenotype is severe and rapidly progressive, accompanied by sensorineural hearing loss and Coats' disease [Fitzsimons et al., 1987; Small, 1968; Taylor et al., 1982]. Marked shoulder and pelvic girdle weakness is present before 6 years of age, with loss of ambulation by 15 years. The condition may be mistaken for Möbius' syndrome. Profound weakness of facial, including extraocular, muscles is typical (Fig. 79-18).

Laboratory Findings

Creatine kinase determinations are either normal or slightly elevated; creatine kinase levels exceeding five times the laboratory norms are suggestive of an alternative diagnosis. Genetic testing has largely replaced electrodiagnostic and muscle biopsy evaluations in persons with suspected facioscapulohumeral muscular dystrophy. Electromyographic studies of moderately weak muscles reveal brief, low-amplitude motor unit potentials consistent with myopathy; sparse fibrillations reflecting muscle fiber necrosis are also present. However, the needle electromyographic examination may be normal in clinically powerful muscles. Neurogenic motor units are virtually never seen and, if present, should raise the possibility of another disorder, such as

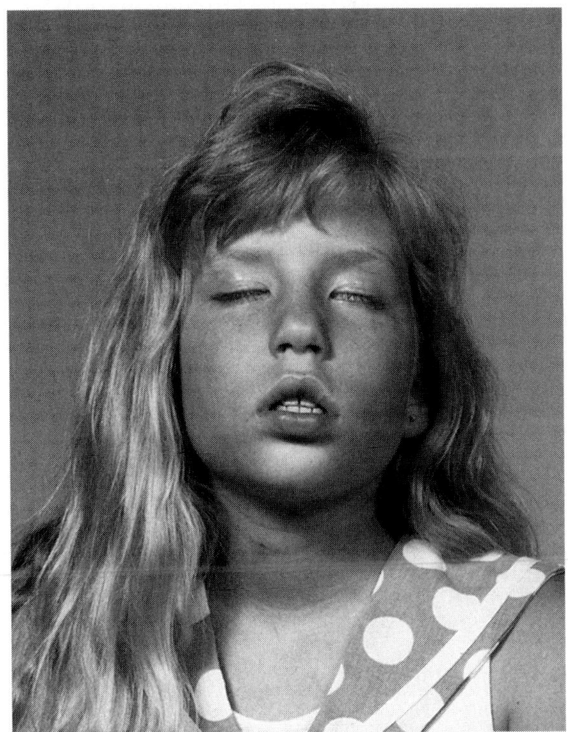

FIGURE 79-18. The early-onset or infantile form of facioscapulohumeral muscular dystrophy, manifesting with incomplete eyelid closure and lack of facial expression.

X-linked spinal and bulbar muscular atrophy. Muscle biopsy findings are often nonspecific, with occasional small angular fibers, necrotic fibers, and regenerating fibers. A modest increase in the percentage of hypertrophy type II muscle fibers may be seen. Foci of inflammatory cells in a perivascular or endomysial distribution are commonly encountered and on occasion may lead to a pathologic misdiagnosis of polymyositis [Rothstein et al., 1971].

Treatment

There is no definitive treatment for facioscapulohumeral muscular dystrophy. Results of therapeutic trials of corticosteroids [Rose and Tawil, 2004] and the β-adrenergic agonist albuterol [Kissel et al., 2001] have been disappointing. A larger trial of albuterol is currently in progress. Footdrop is best managed with ankle-foot orthoses. Orthopedic scapular fixation may improve upper extremity function [Bunch and Siegel, 1993; Twyman et al., 1996] but the gain may be short-lived. Muscle strengthening exercises may be of some benefit for preserving power in relatively unaffected muscle groups. Severe weakness of the orbicularis oculi may predispose to corneal injury; artificial tears can be helpful.

OCULOPHARYNGEAL MUSCULAR DYSTROPHY

The earliest description of oculopharyngeal muscular dystrophy is credited to Taylor [1915], who described the combination of ptosis and pharyngeal palsy, key findings of the disorder, in related family members. Oculopharyngeal muscular dystrophy typically manifests after 50 years of age [Brais et al., 1995]. Many affected individuals of French-Canadian descent are traced to a single ancestor from France [Barbeau, 1966].

Oculopharyngeal muscular dystrophy is recognized in the fourth to sixth decades by onset of ptosis, partial extraocular muscle paresis, dysphagia, and tongue weakness. Weakness of the proximal upper and lower extremity muscles slowly develops. The creatine kinase level may be normal or mildly elevated.

Progressive oculopharyngeal dysfunction is described in Greek siblings, aged 11 and 14 years, both of whom had rimmed vacuoles; one was found to have cytoplasmic and intranuclear tubulofilamentous inclusions 25 nm in diameter on muscle biopsy [Rose et al., 1997]. Another childhood-onset oculopharyngeal syndrome manifested with intestinal pseudo-obstruction [Amato et al., 1995]. These may be examples of recessively inherited conditions similar to dominantly inherited oculopharyngeal muscular dystrophy. Progressive ophthalmoplegia in a child should be interpreted with caution. Most likely, this is secondary to a mitochondrial disorder, rather than a muscular dystrophy [Rowland et al., 1997].

CONGENITAL MUSCULAR DYSTROPHY

The congenital muscular dystrophies are a heterogeneous group of autosomal-recessive disorders characterized by hypotonia, weakness, and variable degrees of muscle contractures. Signs and symptoms are evident in the neonatal period or the first few months of life. Serum creatine kinase levels are usually elevated. Muscle biopsy abnormalities suggestive of a myopathic or dystrophic process, including variation in muscle fiber size, necrotic and regenerating fibers, and an increase in endomysial connective tissue, establish a working diagnosis of congenital muscular dystrophy (Fig. 79-19).

Delineation of a precise diagnosis requires integration of muscle and systemic findings, immunostaining or Western blot of extracellular proteins, and DNA testing when available. The congenital muscular dystrophy syndromes are divided into those associated with brain and eye malformations (syndromic congenital muscular dystrophy) and those without (nonsyndromic or "classic" congenital muscular dystrophy). Within this broad classification, considerable phenotypic variation exists, and clinical differences may be more quantitative than qualitative. However, evidence supports genetically distinct bases for the different congenital muscular dystrophy subgroups. The summed incidence of all forms of congenital muscular dystrophy is approximately 1 per 21,500 [Mostacciuolo et al., 1996].

Nonsyndromic (Classic) Congenital Muscular Dystrophy

Merosin-Negative Congenital Muscular Dystrophy

Merosin-negative congenital muscular dystrophy (MDC1A) is the most common of the congenital muscular dystrophy disorders and accounts for about 50% of cases of nonsyndromic congenital muscular dystrophy (Table 79-3). Patients with complete absence of merosin present as hypotonic infants. Limb weakness is usually more prominent than bulbar or respiratory impairment, but feeding difficulties including aspiration [Philpot et al., 1999], and ventilatory insufficiency necessitating respiratory support may occur [Fardeau et al., 1996]. Most patients achieve independent sitting, but few stand or walk unassisted. Multiple

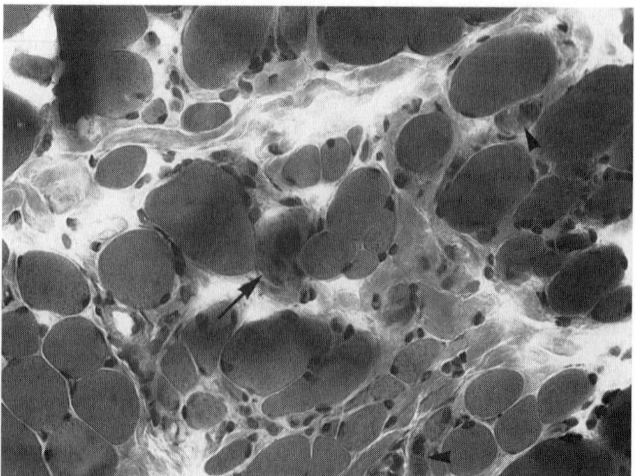

FIGURE 79-19. Muscle biopsy from an infant with congenital muscular dystrophy. Note the fiber size variation, muscle necrosis (*arrow*), and regenerating fibers (*arrowheads*) surrounded by increased endomysial connective tissue. (Hematoxylin and eosin staining; ×300.)

TABLE 79-3

Nonsyndromic (Classic) Congenital Muscular Dystrophies (CMDs)

DISEASE	GENE LOCUS	PROTEIN PRODUCT	TESTING
CMD with complete merosin deficiency (MDC1A)	6q22-q23 LAMA2 (merosin gene)	Laminin α_2 chain (merosin)	Immunostaining
CMD with secondary merosin deficiency (MDC1B)	1q42	Unknown	—
CMD type 1C (MCD1C)	19q13.3	Fukutin-related protein	DNA testing available
CMD with integrin α7 mutations	12q13	Integrin α7	Research
CMD with early rigid spine	1p36-p35	SEPN1 (Selenoprotein)	Research
Ullrich's CMD with collagen 6 mutations	21q22.3 2q37	COL6A1, COL6A2, COL6A3	Research

joint contractures may be present at birth or develop in infancy or early childhood. Weakness tends to be stable or slowly progressive (Fig. 79-20). Most patients exhibit normal brain structure and cognitive development. Focal cortical dysplasia of the occipital lobes occurs in some cases with concurrent intellectual impairment [Taratuto et al., 1999], but the extensive neuronal migration abnormalities characteristic of patients with syndromic congenital muscular dystrophy is not seen. Epilepsy occurs frequently even in patients with normal intellect [Pegoraro et al., 1998].

Virtually all merosin-negative congenital muscular dystrophy patients have characteristic white matter lesions on MRI scans most prominent on T2-weighted images. These findings may not be evident at birth but invariably develop by age 6 months. White matter abnormalities involve the centrum semiovale and spare the corpus callosum, internal capsule, cerebellum, and brainstem [Caro et al., 1999]. The MRI findings are consistent with abnormal water distribution in the white matter that results from disruption of the blood-brain barrier secondary to merosin deficiency in cerebral vasculature [Villanova et al., 1997].

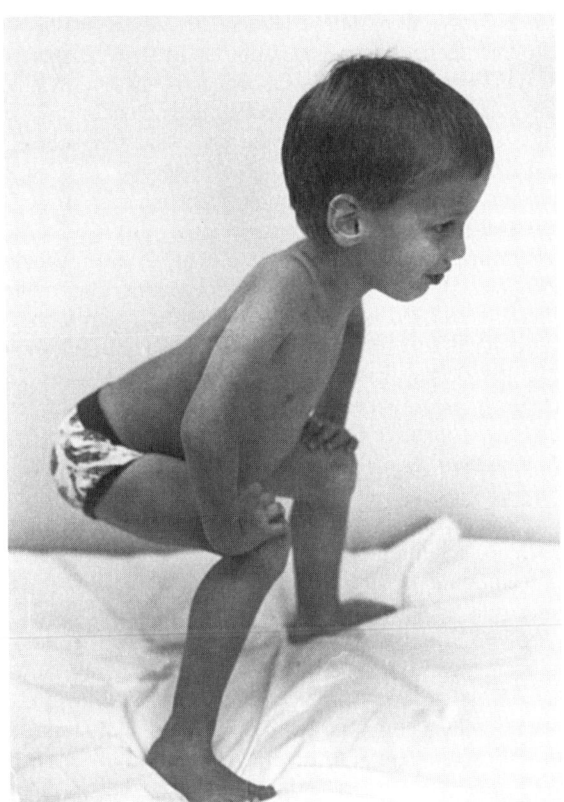

FIGURE 79-20. A 3-year-old male with congenital muscular dystrophy getting up from a sitting position by using a modified Gowers maneuver. Note the generalized, proximal weakness, which is greater than distal weakness.

Serum creatine kinase levels are usually elevated in the neonatal period in excess of 1000 U/liter but tend to decrease over years. Electrodiagnostic studies yield nonspecific myopathic findings on needle electromyography. Nerve conduction studies reveal slowing of conduction velocity, which is consistent with demyelinating polyneuropathy [Gilhuis et al., 2002]. Muscle biopsy samples demonstrate changes consistent with a dystrophic process, including adipose tissue replacement and connective tissue proliferation. In addition, inflammatory changes may be striking enough to suggest a diagnosis of infantile polymyositis [Pegoraro et al., 1996].

Merosin is the heavy α_2 chain of laminin 2 (LAMA2). The laminins are heterotrimeric proteins that influence cell adhesion, growth, and migration. LAMA2 is expressed in the basement membrane of muscle fibers, Schwann cells of intramuscular nerves and at neuromuscular junctions. LAMA2 promotes myotube stability and inhibits apoptosis [Vachon et al., 1996]. Absence of immunohistochemical staining for the laminin α_2 chain on snap frozen muscle biopsy tissue provides confirmation of the diagnosis of merosin deficiency. The merosin (LAMA2) gene located on chromosome 6q22 contains 64 exons with mutations distributed through a large coding sequence of 9.5 kilobases, which makes routine mutation screening impractical at present. Partial merosin deficiency has been reported in rare patients with a benign childhood- or adult-onset LGMD phenotype [Allamand et al., 1997]; routine immunohistochemical staining for LAMA2 is therefore suggested in evaluating patients with both congenital muscular dystrophy and LGMD phenotypes. Prenatal diagnosis of merosin-deficient congenital muscular dystrophy is possible by direct mutation analysis of chorionic villus biopsy material, but because of the lack of predictable hot spots of mutation, linkage analysis is a more commonly used approach. Direct immunostaining of trophoblasts from chorionic villus samples with laminin α_2 chain antibodies provides an additional method for prenatal diagnosis.

Merosin-Positive, Nonsyndromic Congenital Muscular Dystrophies

Patients with nonsyndromic congenital muscular dystrophy who express merosin are a heterogeneous group. A small percentage of patients have mutations of the LAMA2 gene and may present with an LGMD or mild congenital muscular dystrophy phenotype. The majority of patients with normal merosin expression or partial merosin deficiency presenting with a congenital muscular dystrophy phenotype have other genetic disorders that do not link to the region of chromosome 6q; their clinical course is similar to but usually milder than that of merosin-negative children. The distribution of weakness and contractures is comparable. Patients lack the cerebral white matter MRI abnormalities seen in merosin-negative patients.

Congenital Muscular Dystrophy Type 1C Caused by Fukutin-Related Protein Deficiency

MDC1C usually manifests at birth or in the first few weeks of life with hypotonia and leg muscle hypertrophy. Creatine kinase values are greatly increased (1000 to 10,000 IU/liter). Children follow a regressive course that may include cardiomyopathy. Routine histochemical analysis of muscle biopsy specimens does not differentiate these patients from children with merosin-negative congenital muscular dystrophy.

Immunohistochemical staining reveals partial merosin deficiency and severely reduced α-dystroglycan. In addition, reduced molecular weight of α-dystroglycan on Western blot indicates defective glycosylation, which is important in the pathophysiology of MDC1C. The genetic defect maps to chromosome 19q13.3 and the gene coding for fukutin-related protein. The spectrum of this protein deficiency therefore includes the milder limb-girdle phenotype LGMD2I and a congenital muscular dystrophy phenotype [Brockington et al., 2001a, 2002]. DNA testing is commercially available.

Congenital Muscular Dystrophy with Integrin α7 Deficiency

This rare disorder was discovered during analysis of muscle biopsy specimens from 117 patients with unclassified congenital myopathy and congenital muscular dystrophy phenotypes. Three patients evidenced integrin α7 deficiency on muscle immunohistochemistry profiles, which was correlated with three different mutations in the integrin α7 deficiency gene on chromosome 12q13 [Hayashi et al., 1998]. Another study of 210 patients with undefined myopathy indicates that secondary deficiencies of this type of congenital muscular dystrophy also occur, complicating the diagnostic significance of this protein [Pegoraro et al., 2002].

Congenital Muscular Dystrophy with Early Rigid Spine Syndrome

Development of axial paraspinal muscle contractures produces the rigid spine syndrome in a number of congenital myopathies and muscular dystrophies including Emery-Dreifuss muscular dystrophy. A distinct phenotype-genotype correlation was defined in consanguineous families of Moroccan, Turkish, and Iranian descent [Moghadaszadeh et al., 2001]. The gene for rigid spine syndrome in these patients mapped to chromosome region 1p35-p46, coding for a selenoprotein (SEPN1) known to be expressed in skeletal muscle.

In another American family presenting a phenotype of infantile hypotonia, prominent cervical muscle weakness, and early spinal rigidity and scoliosis, linkage to the chromosome 1p rigid spine syndrome locus was proved [Flanigan et al., 2000]. Restrictive lung disease often complicates rigid spine syndrome and mandates close observation for nocturnal hypoventilation and early institution of noninvasive respiratory support.

Ullrich's Congenital Muscular Dystrophy and Bethlem's Myopathy

Ullrich's congenital muscular dystrophy is characterized by infantile onset of weakness, hypotonia, and early findings of severe proximal joint contractures in the face of striking hyperlaxity of distal joints [Furukawa and Toyokura, 1977]. Other orthopedic findings may include congenital hip dislocation, prominent calcanei, and transient kyphosis. Progressive flexion contractures of the wrists, fingers, and ankles may replace distal limb laxity. The disease is slowly progressive. Although some youngsters acquire independent ambulation, weakness and orthopedic deformities lead to full-time wheelchair use. Involvement of chest wall and diaphragm muscles often necessitates nocturnal ventilatory assistance, but cardiac function is usually unaffected. Serum creatine kinase levels are usually normal or slightly elevated. Muscle biopsy samples demonstrate nonspecific myopathic or dystrophic changes of degenerating and regenerating muscle cells with increased endomysial connective tissue. Collagen 6 immunostaining of muscle basal lamina and endomysial connective tissue is severely reduced or absent [Higuchi et al., 2003].

Ullrich's congenital muscular dystrophy is caused by autosomal-recessive mutations in any of three collagen genes [Vanegas et al., 2002; Zhang et al., 2002]. Collagen 6 is composed of three different α peptide chains. The α_1 and α_2 chains are encoded by two genes (COL6A1 and COL6A2) located head to tail at chromosome 21q22.3 [Heiskanen et al., 1995]. The gene for COL6A3 maps to locus 2q37. Collagen 6 is an extracellular matrix protein expressed in nearly all connective tissues.

The phenotype of Ullrich's congenital muscular dystrophy merges with that of Bethlem's myopathy, originally described as a benign myopathy with autosomal dominant inheritance [Bethlem and Wijngaarden, 1976]. The clinical manifestation is far more variable than that of Ullrich's congenital muscular dystrophy. The onset of signs and symptoms of proximal weakness is usually in early childhood, manifesting by difficulty climbing stairs and running. Gowers' sign is often present. In more severe cases, findings may be present in the neonatal period with mild hypotonia, foot deformities, congenital torticollis, or arthrogryposis. Unlike the progressive contractures in Ullrich's syndrome, the neonatal arthrogryposis seen in patients with Bethlem's myopathy tends to improve spontaneously. Weakness is usually nonprogressive. However, contractures may develop late in the first decade, often localized to the ankles, elbow flexors and finger flexors. In other patients, the clinical presentation is delayed until the fourth decade. Dominant mutations in any of the collagen 6 genes may produce the Bethlem's myopathy phenotype or a clinical picture of Ullrich's congenital muscular dystrophy [Jobsis et al., 1999]. The family history is helpful in determining whether the disorder has been transmitted as an autosomal-dominant or -recessive trait, but de novo mutations and parental germline mosaicism may complicate this assessment. Immunostaining for collagen 6 is usually normal in Bethlem's myopathy; therefore, DNA studies of the COL6A genes are necessary for definitive diagnosis [Lampe et al., 2005].

Management of Ullrich's congenital muscular dystrophy and Bethlem's myopathy is symptomatic. Aggressive physical therapy and surgical intervention address contractures. Severely affected children need active mobilization, and standing frames are often helpful. Nocturnal ventilatory support is often required [Wallgren-Pettersson et al., 2004]. The combination of restrictive lung disease and progressive orthopedic deformity in severely affected children make the timing of surgical interventions critical.

Syndromic Congenital Muscular Dystrophy

There are three clinically defined congenital muscular dystrophies (Table 79-4) with associated brain malformations. The genes and protein products of these disorders are involved in glycosylation of extracellular muscle and brain protein. All three diseases arise from mutations in known or putative glycosyltransferase enzymes and share a common feature of a hypoglycosylated form of α-dystroglycan in skeletal muscle. Brain pathology is characterized by neuronal migration past a defective glial limiting membrane into the subpial space, which produces a developmental anomaly termed the *cobblestone complex.* It is appreciated that deficiency of fukutin-related protein seen in MDC1C and LGMD2I does not result in pathologic neuronal migration.

Fukuyama's Congenital Muscular Dystrophy

Fukuyama's congenital muscular dystrophy is one of the most common autosomal-recessive diseases and the second most common form of muscular dystrophy in Japan, where the carrier frequency is estimated at 1 per 90 [Toda et al., 2000]. The disease is uncommon outside of Japan. Hypotonia and generalized muscle weakness are usually present before 9 months of age, and 50% of affected infants manifest a poor suck and weak cry. Facial weakness and a tented upper lip are frequent findings. Calf hypertrophy is present in 50% of patients. Gross motor milestones are severely delayed. Affected children often achieve independent sitting but never gain independent ambulation. Contractures are not marked at birth but develop by 1 year of age and involve the hips, knees, ankles, and elbows.

Mental retardation is often severe, with IQ scores ranging from 30 to 50. Seizures occur in 40% of affected children. Ocular abnormalities are common but not universal and include myopia, cataracts, optic disc pallor, and retinal detachment. Most children have a rapid deterioration in motor abilities after the age of 6 years, and death occurs in early adolescence.

Laboratory studies reveal consistent elevations of creatine kinase levels. Electrodiagnostic studies reveal myopathic potentials on needle electromyography; nerve conduction velocities are normal. Brain imaging studies and postmortem studies reveal brain malformations, including polymicrogyria, pachygyria, and agyria of the cerebrum and cerebellum (type II cobblestone lissencephaly), with a lack of the normal lamination of the cerebral cortex. There is a paucity of cortical gyrations in the temporal and occipital regions.

Fukuyama's congenital muscular dystrophy is caused by mutations of chromosome 9q31 on the gene coding for fukutin, a protein localized to the basement membrane of muscle. The protein is also found in fetal but not in postnatal neurons. The most common mutation is a 3-kilobase retrotransposon, which is suggestive of a founder effect [Kobayashi et al., 1998]. Fukutin deficiency is associated with decreased immunostaining for α-dystroglycan and merosin with preservation of the dystrophin-related complex [Hayashi et al., 2001]

Muscle-Eye-Brain Disease

Approximately 30 patients have been reported with this disorder, the majority from Finland. The clinical picture is dominated by neonatal hypotonia, profound developmental delay with psychomotor retardation, and ocular abnormalities. Affected children may attain independent ambulation by age 4 years. Some acquire limited language skills. Motor abilities decline late in the first decade in association with the development of contractures and spasticity. Visual failure is in the form of severe myopia, followed by retinal degeneration and cataracts. Seizures are common. Central nervous system dysgenesis includes cobblestone lissencephaly type II, frontal pachygyria, and occipital micropolygyria. There is severe disorganization of the cerebral and cerebellar cortices [Haltia et al., 1997]. The associated myopathy may be overshadowed by central nervous system and ocular abnormalities. However, creatine kinase levels are increased, especially after the first year of life, and electromyography studies indicate myopathic abnormalities.

The muscle-eye-brain disease gene localizes to chromosome region 1p32-p34 [Cormand et al., 2001] and codes for loss of function mutations in *O*-mannose β1,2-*N*-acetylglucosaminyltransferase. DNA testing for at-risk families is available.

TABLE 79-4

Syndromic Congenital Muscular Dystrophies (CMDs)

DISEASE	GENE LOCUS	PROTEIN PRODUCT	TESTING
Fukuyama's CMD	9q31	Fukutin	DNA testing available
Muscle-eye-brain disease (POMGnT1)	1q32-34	*O*-mannoside β1,2-*N*-acetylglucosaminyl-transferase	DNA testing available
Walker-Warburg syndrome (POMT1)	9q34.1	*O*-mannosyltransferase 1	DNA testing available

Walker-Warburg Syndrome

Unlike Fukuyama's congenital muscular dystrophy and muscle-eye-brain disease, Walker-Warburg syndrome does not have an ethnic predominance. The clinical stigmata are dominated by the most severe brain malformations seen in any congenital muscular dystrophy syndrome, including lissencephaly type II, hydrocephalus, occipital encephalocele, fusion of the cerebral hemispheres, absence of the corpus callosum, and hypoplasia of the cerebellum and brainstem. Ocular findings have included congenital cataracts, microphthalmia, buphthalmus, and Peter's anomaly. At birth, affected children are blind, markedly hypotonic, and poor feeders. Myopathy is manifest by mild elevations of creatine kinase level and variable abnormalities on muscle biopsy samples. All affected infants manifest profound psychomotor retardation, and the median length of survival is only 4 months. Clinical similarities in muscle-eye-brain disease and Walker-Warburg syndrome cause debate as to whether they are separate entities or a spectrum of a single autosomal recessive disorder. Detection of a distinct gene locus on chromosome 9q34.1 coding for protein *O*-mannosyltransferase 1 in 6 of 30 patients with Walker-Warburg syndrome favors classifying this condition as a separate disease. Only limited DNA testing is available for at-risk families.

REFERENCES

Abbs S, Bobrow M. Analysis of quantitative PCR for the diagnosis of deletion and duplication carriers in the dystrophin gene. J Med Genet 1992;29:191.

Abi Daoud MS, Dooley JM, Gordon KE. Depression in parents of children with Duchenne muscular dystrophy. Pediatr Neurol 2004;31:16.

Adams V, Gielen S, Hambrecht R, et al. Apoptosis in skeletal muscle. Front Biosci 2001;6:D1.

al-Qudah AA, Kobayashi J, Chuang S, et al. Etiology of intellectual impairment in Duchenne muscular dystrophy. Pediatr Neurol 1990;6:57.

Alderton JM, Steinhardt RA. How calcium influx through calcium leak channels is responsible for the elevated levels of calcium-dependent proteolysis in dystrophic myotubes. Trends Cardiovasc Med 2000;10:268.

Allamand V, Sunada Y, Salih MA, et al. Mild congenital muscular dystrophy in two patients with an internally deleted laminin alpha2-chain. Hum Mol Genet 1997;6:747.

Allen DG. Skeletal muscle function: Role of ionic changes in fatigue, damage and disease. Clin Exp Pharmacol Physiol 2004;31:485.

Alman BA, Raza SN, Biggar WD. Steroid treatment and the development of scoliosis in males with Duchenne muscular dystrophy. J Bone Joint Surg Am 2004;86:519.

Amato AA, Jackson CE, Ridings LW, et al. Childhood-onset oculopharyngodistal myopathy with chronic intestinal pseudo-obstruction. Muscle Nerve 1995;18:842.

Anderson JL, Head SI, Rae C, et al. Brain function in Duchenne muscular dystrophy. Brain 2002;125 (Pt 1):4.

Anderson LV, Harrison RM, Pogue R, et al. Secondary reduction in calpain 3 expression in patients with limb girdle muscular dystrophy type 2B and Miyoshi myopathy (primary dysferlinopathies). Neuromuscul Disord 2000;10:553.

Angelini C, Pegoraro E, Turella E, et al. Deflazacort in Duchenne dystrophy: Study of long-term effect. Muscle Nerve 1994;17:386. [Published erratum appears in Muscle Nerve 1994;17:833.]

Ansved T. Muscular dystrophies: Influence of physical conditioning on the disease evolution. Curr Opin Clin Nutr Metab Care 2003;6:435.

Aoki M, Liu J, Richard I, et al. Genomic organization of the dysferlin gene and novel mutations in Miyoshi myopathy. Neurology 2001;57:271.

Aparicio LF, Jurkovic M, DeLullo J. Decreased bone density in ambulatory patients with Duchenne muscular dystrophy. J Pediatr Orthop 2002;22:179.

Arahata K, Beggs AH, Honda H, et al. Preservation of the C-terminus of dystrophin molecule in the skeletal muscle from Becker muscular dystrophy. J Neurol Sci 1991;101:148.

Arahata K, Engel AG. Monoclonal antibody analysis of mononuclear cells in myopathies. IV: Cell-mediated cytotoxicity and muscle fiber necrosis. Ann Neurol 1988;23:168.

Arahata K, Hoffman EP, Kunkel LM, et al. Dystrophin diagnosis: Comparison of dystrophin abnormalities by immunofluorescence and immunoblot analyses. Proc Natl Acad Sci U S A 1989;86:7154.

Arahata K, Ishiura S, Ishiguro T, et al. Immunostaining of skeletal and cardiac muscle surface membrane with antibody against Duchenne muscular dystrophy peptide. Nature 1988;333:861.

Azibi K, Bachner L, Beckmann JS, et al. Severe childhood autosomal recessive muscular dystrophy with the deficiency of the 50 kDa dystrophin-associated glycoprotein maps to chromosome 13q12. Hum Mol Genet 1993;2:1423.

Bach JR, Ishikawa Y, Kim H. Prevention of pulmonary morbidity for patients with Duchenne muscular dystrophy. Chest 1997;112:1024.

Baghdiguian S, Martin M, Richard I, et al. Calpain 3 deficiency is associated with myonuclear apoptosis and profound perturbation of the IkappaB alpha/NF-kappaB pathway in limb-girdle muscular dystrophy type 2A. Nat Med 1999;5:503.

Baker MS, Austin L. The pathological damage in Duchenne muscular dystrophy may be due to increased intracellular OXY-radical generation caused by the absence of dystrophin and subsequent alterations in Ca^{2+} metabolism. Med Hypotheses 1989;29:187.

Bakker E, Veenema H, Den Dunnen JT, et al. Germinal mosaicism increases the recurrence risk for "new" Duchenne muscular dystrophy mutations. J Med Genet 1989;26:553.

Banchereau J, Steinman RM. Dendritic cells and the control of immunity. Nature 1998;392:245.

Bansal D, Miyake K, Vogel SS, et al. Defective membrane repair in dysferlin-deficient muscular dystrophy. Nature 2003;423:168.

Barbeau A. [Ocular myopathy in French Canada. A preliminary study.] J Genet Hum (in French) 1966;15 (Suppl):49.

Barresi R, Moore SA, Stolle CA, et al. Expression of gamma-sarcoglycan in smooth muscle and its interaction with the smooth muscle sarcoglycan-sarcospan complex. J Biol Chem 2000;275:38554.

Barton-Davis ER, Cordier L, Shoturma DI, et al. Aminoglycoside antibiotics restore dystrophin function to skeletal muscles of mdx mice. J Clin Invest 1999;104:375.

Bashir R, Keers S, Strachan T, et al. Genetic and physical mapping at the limb-girdle muscular dystrophy locus (LGMD2B) on chromosome 2p. Genomics 1996;33:46.

Bastianutto C, De Visser M, Muntoni F, et al. A novel muscle-specific enhancer identified within the deletion overlap region of two XLDC patients lacking muscle exon 1 of the human dystrophin gene. Genomics 2002;80:614.

Baumbach LL, Chamberlain JS, Ward PA, et al. Molecular and clinical correlations of deletions leading to Duchenne and Becker muscular dystrophies. Neurology 1989;39:465.

Baydur A, Layne E, Aral H, et al. Long term non-invasive ventilation in the community for patients with musculoskeletal disorders: 46 year experience and review. Thorax 2000;55:4.

Becane HM, Bonne G, Varnous S, et al. High incidence of sudden death with conduction system and myocardial disease due to lamins A and C gene mutation. Pacing Clin Electrophysiol 2000;23 (11 Pt 1):1661.

Becker PE, Kiener F. [A new x-chromosomal muscular dystrophy] [in German]. Arch Psychiatr Nervenkr Z Gesamte Neurol Psychiatr 1955;193:427.

Beckmann JS, Bushby KM. Advances in the molecular genetics of the limb-girdle type of autosomal recessive progressive muscular dystrophy. Curr Opin Neurol 1996;9:389.

Beggs AH, Hoffman EP, Snyder JR, et al. Exploring the molecular basis for variability among patients with Becker muscular dystrophy: Dystrophin gene and protein studies. Am J Hum Genet 1991;49:54.

Beggs AH, Koenig M, Boyce FM, et al. Detection of 98% of DMD/BMD gene deletions by polymerase chain reaction. Hum Genet 1990;86:45.

Behrens L, Kerschensteiner M, Misgeld T, et al. Human muscle cells express a functional costimulatory molecule distinct from B7.1 (CD80) and B7.2 (CD86) in vitro and in inflammatory lesions. J Immunol 1998;161:5943.

Bennett RR, den Dunnen J, O'Brien KF, et al. Detection of mutations in the dystrophin gene via automated DHPLC screening and direct sequencing. BMC Genet 2001;2:17.

Bernasconi P, Di Blasi C, Mora M, et al. Transforming growth factor-beta1 and fibrosis in congenital muscular dystrophies. Neuromuscul Disord 1999;9:28.

Bernasconi P, Torchiana E, Confalonieri P, et al. Expression of transforming growth factor-beta 1 in dystrophic patient muscles correlates with fibrosis. Pathogenetic role of a fibrogenic cytokine. J Clin Invest 1995;96:1137.

Bethlem J, Wijngaarden GK. Benign myopathy, with autosomal dominant inheritance. A report on three pedigrees. Brain 1976;99:91.

Betz RC, Schoser BG, Kasper D, et al. Mutations in CAV3 cause mechanical hyperirritability of skeletal muscle in rippling muscle disease. Nat Genet 2001;28:218.

Bianchi ML, Mazzanti A, Galbiati E, et al. Bone mineral density and bone metabolism in Duchenne muscular dystrophy. Osteoporos Int 2003;14:761.

Biggar WD, Bachrach LK, Henderson RC, et al. Bone health in Duchenne muscular dystrophy: A workshop report from the meeting in Cincinnati, Ohio, July 8, 2004. Neuromuscul Disord 2005;15:80.

Biggar WD, Gingras M, Fehlings DL, et al. Deflazacort treatment of Duchenne muscular dystrophy. J Pediatr 2001;138:45.

Biggar WD, Politano L, Harris VA, et al. Deflazacort in Duchenne muscular dystrophy: A comparison of two different protocols. Neuromuscul Disord 2004;14:476.

Bione S, Maestrini E, Rivella S, et al. Identification of a novel X-linked gene responsible for Emery-Dreifuss muscular dystrophy. Nat Genet 1994;8:323.

Bjerglund Nielsen L, Nielsen IM. Turner's syndrome and Duchenne muscular dystrophy in a girl with an X;autosome translocation. Ann Genet 1984;27:173.

Bonifati MD, Ruzza G, Bonometto P, et al. A multicenter, double-blind, randomized trial of deflazacort versus prednisone in Duchenne muscular dystrophy. Muscle Nerve 2000;23:1344.

Bonilla E, Samitt CE, Miranda AF, et al. Duchenne muscular dystrophy: Deficiency of dystrophin at the muscle cell surface. Cell 1988;54:447.

Bonne G. [The laminopathy saga.] Rev Neurol (in Spanish) 2003;37:772.

Bonne G, Di Barletta MR, Varnous S, et al. Mutations in the gene encoding lamin A/C cause autosomal dominant Emery-Dreifuss muscular dystrophy. Nat Genet 1999;21:285.

Bonne G, Mercuri E, Muchir A, et al. Clinical and molecular genetic spectrum of autosomal dominant Emery-Dreifuss muscular dystrophy due to mutations of the lamin A/C gene. Ann Neurol 2000;48:170.

Bonne G, Yaou RB, Beroud C, et al. 108th ENMC International Workshop, 3rd Workshop of the MYO-CLUSTER project: EUROMEN, 7th International Emery-Dreifuss Muscular Dystrophy (Emery-Dreifuss muscular dystrophy) Workshop, 13-15 September 2002, Naarden, The Netherlands. Neuromuscul Disord 2003;13:508.

Borrelli O, Salvia G, Mancini V, et al. Evolution of gastric electrical features and gastric emptying in children with Duchenne and Becker muscular dystrophy. Am J Gastroenterol 2005;10:695.

Boyce FM, Beggs AH, Feener C, et al. Dystrophin is transcribed in brain from a distant upstream promoter. Proc Natl Acad Sci U S A 1991;88:1276.

Brais B, Xie YG, Sanson M, et al. The oculopharyngeal muscular dystrophy locus maps to the region of the cardiac alpha and beta myosin heavy chain genes on chromosome 14q11.2-q13. Hum Mol Genet 1995;4:429.

Bresolin N, Castelli E, Comi GP, et al. Cognitive impairment in Duchenne muscular dystrophy. Neuromuscul Disord 1994;4:359.

Breucking E, Reimnitz P, Schara U, et al. [Anesthetic complications. The incidence of severe anesthetic complications in patients and families with progressive muscular dystrophy of the Duchenne and Becker types.] Anaesthesist (in German) 2000;49:187.

Brockington M, Blake DJ, Brown SC, et al. The gene for a novel glycosyltransferase is mutated in congenital muscular dystrophy MDC1C and limb girdle muscular dystrophy 2I. Neuromuscul Disord 2002;12:233.

Brockington M, Blake DJ, Prandini P, et al. Mutations in the fukutin-related protein gene (FKRP) cause a form of congenital muscular dystrophy with secondary laminin alpha2 deficiency and abnormal glycosylation of alpha-dystroglycan. Am J Hum Genet 2001a;69:1198.

Brockington M, Yuva Y, Prandini P, et al. Mutations in the fukutin-related protein gene (FKRP) identify limb girdle muscular dystrophy 2I as a milder allelic variant of congenital muscular dystrophy MDC1C. Hum Mol Genet 2001b;10:2851.

Brook PD, Kennedy JD, Stern LM, et al. Spinal fusion in Duchenne's muscular dystrophy. J Pediatr Orthop 1996;16:324.

Brooke MH, Fenichel GM, Griggs RC, et al. Clinical investigation of Duchenne muscular dystrophy. Interesting results in a trial of prednisone. Arch Neurol 1987;44:812.

Brooks AP, Emery AE. The incidence of Duchenne muscular dystrophy in the South East of Scotland. Clin Genet 1977;11:290.

Brouwer OF, Padberg GW, Bakker E, et al. Early onset facioscapulohumeral muscular dystrophy. Muscle Nerve 1995;2:S67.

Brouwer OF, Padberg GW, Wijmenga C, et al. Facioscapulohumeral muscular dystrophy in early childhood. Arch Neurol 1994;51:387.

Brown CA, Lanning RW, McKinney KQ, et al. Novel and recurrent mutations in lamin A/C in patients with Emery-Dreifuss muscular dystrophy. Am J Med Genet 2001;102:359.

Bunch WH, Siegel IM. Scapulothoracic arthrodesis in facioscapulohumeral muscular dystrophy. Review of seventeen procedures with three to twenty-one-year follow-up. J Bone Joint Surg Am 1993;75:372.

Bunyan DJ, Robinson DO, Collins AL, et al. Germline and somatic mosaicism in a female carrier of Duchenne muscular dystrophy. Hum Genet 1994;93:541.

Burghes AH, Logan C, Hu X, et al. A cDNA clone from the Duchenne/Becker muscular dystrophy gene. Nature 1987;328:434.

Burmeister M, Lehrach H. Long-range restriction map around the Duchenne muscular dystrophy gene. Nature 1986;324:582.

Bushby K, Muntoni F, Bourke JP. 107th ENMC international workshop: The management of cardiac involvement in muscular dystrophy and myotonic dystrophy. 7th-9th June 2002, Naarden, the Netherlands. Neuromuscul Disord 2003;13:166.

Bushby KM, Appleton R, Anderson LV, et al. Deletion status and intellectual impairment in Duchenne muscular dystrophy. Dev Med Child Neurol 1995;37:260.

Byers TJ, Lidov HG, Kunkel LM. An alternative dystrophin transcript specific to peripheral nerve. Nat Genet 1993;4:77.

Cai B, Spencer MJ, Nakamura G, et al. Eosinophilia of dystrophin-deficient muscle is promoted by perforin-mediated cytotoxicity by T cell effectors. Am J Pathol 2000;156:1789.

Campbell C, Jacob P. Deflazacort for the treatment of Duchenne dystrophy: A systematic review. BMC Neurol 2003;3:7.

Canki-Klain N, Milic A, Kovac B, et al. Prevalence of the 550delA mutation in calpainopathy (LGMD 2A) in Croatia. Am J Med Genet A 2004;125:152.

Carbone I, Bruno C, Sotgia F, et al. Mutation in the CAV3 gene causes partial caveolin-3 deficiency and hyperCKemia. Neurology 2000;54:1373.

Caro PA, Scavina M, Hoffman E, et al. MR imaging findings in children with merosin-deficient congenital muscular dystrophy. AJNR Am J Neuroradiol 1999;20:324.

Carrie A, Piccolo F, Leturcq F, et al. Mutational diversity and hot spots in the alpha-sarcoglycan gene in autosomal recessive muscular dystrophy (LGMD2D). J Med Genet 1997;34:470.

Carter GT, Wineinger MA, Walsh SA, et al. Effect of voluntary wheel-running exercise on muscles of the mdx mouse. Neuromuscul Disord 1995;5:323.

Caux F, Dubosclard E, Lascols O, et al. A new clinical condition linked to a novel mutation in lamins A and C with generalized lipoatrophy, insulin-resistant diabetes, disseminated leukomelanodermic papules, liver steatosis, and cardiomyopathy. J Clin Endocrinol Metab 2003;88:1006.

Cenacchi G, Fanin M, De Giorgi LB, et al. Ultrastructural changes in dysferlinopathy support defective membrane repair mechanism. J Clin Pathol 2005;58:190.

Chae J, Minami N, Jin Y, et al. Calpain 3 gene mutations: Genetic and clinico-pathologic findings in limb-girdle muscular dystrophy. Neuromuscul Disord 2001;11:547.

Chen L, Lee L, Kudlow BA, et al. LMNA mutations in atypical Werner's syndrome. Lancet 2003;362:440.

Chen YW, Zhao P, Borup R, et al. Expression profiling in the muscular dystrophies: Identification of novel aspects of molecular pathophysiology. J Cell Biol 2000;151:1321.

Chiannilkulchai N, Pasturaud P, Richard I, et al. A primary expression map of the chromosome 15q15 region containing the recessive form of limb-girdle muscular dystrophy (LGMD2A) gene. Hum Mol Genet 1995;4:717.

Chrobakova T, Hermanova M, Kroupova I, et al. Mutations in Czech LGMD2A patients revealed by analysis of calpain3 mRNA and their phenotypic outcome. Neuromuscul Disord 2004;14:659.

Clapham DE. TRP channels as cellular sensors. Nature 2003;426:517.
Cobo AM, Saenz A, Poza JJ, et al. A common haplotype associated with the basque 2362AG Æ TCATCT mutation in the muscular calpain-3 gene. Hum Biol 2004;76:731.
Confalonieri P, Oliva L, Andreetta F, et al. Muscle inflammation and MHC class I up-regulation in muscular dystrophy with lack of dysferlin: An immunopathological study. J Neuroimmunol 2003;142:130.
Connolly A, Schierbecker J, Renna R, et al. High dose weekly oral prednisone improves strength in boys with Duchenne muscular dystrophy. Neuromuscul Disord 2002;12:917.
Connolly AM, Pestronk A, Mehta S, et al. Primary alpha-sarcoglycan deficiency responsive to immunosuppression over three years. Muscle Nerve 1998;21:1549.
Cormand B, Pihko H, Bayes M, et al. Clinical and genetic distinction between Walker-Warburg syndrome and muscle-eye-brain disease. Neurology 2001;56:1059.
Corrado G, Lissoni A, Beretta S, et al. Prognostic value of electrocardiograms, ventricular late potentials, ventricular arrhythmias, and left ventricular systolic dysfunction in patients with Duchenne muscular dystrophy. Am J Cardiol 2002;89:838.
Cross GS, Speer A, Rosenthal A, et al. Deletions of fetal and adult muscle cDNA in Duchenne and Becker muscular dystrophy patients. EMBO J 1987;6:3277.
D'Amore PA, Brown RH Jr, Ku PT, et al. Elevated basic fibroblast growth factor in the serum of patients with Duchenne muscular dystrophy. Ann Neurol 1994;35:362.
Danzig V, Fiksa J, Hani AB, et al. [Cardiac problems in patients with progressive muscular dystrophy.] Sb Lek (in Czech) 2003;104:273.
Darras BT, Blattner P, Harper JF, et al. Intragenic deletions in 21 Duchenne muscular dystrophy (DMD)/Becker muscular dystrophy (BMD) families studied with the dystrophin cDNA: Location of breakpoints on HindIII and BglII exon-containing fragment maps, meiotic and mitotic origin of the mutations. Am J Hum Genet 1988;43:620.
De Luca A, Nico B, Liantonio A, et al. A multidisciplinary evaluation of the effectiveness of cyclosporine a in dystrophic mdx mice. Am J Pathol 2005;166:477.
De Luca A, Pierno S, Liantonio A, et al. Pre-clinical trials in Duchenne dystrophy: What animal models can tell us about potential drug effectiveness. Neuromuscul Disord 2002;12 (Suppl 1):S142.
De Sandre-Giovannoli A, Bernard R, Cau P, et al. Lamin a truncation in Hutchinson-Gilford progeria. Science 2003;300:2055.
De Sandre-Giovannoli A, Chaouch M, Kozlov S, et al. Homozygous defects in LMNA, encoding lamin A/C nuclear-envelope proteins, cause autosomal recessive axonal neuropathy in human (Charcot-Marie-Tooth disorder type 2) and mouse. Am J Hum Genet 2002;70:726.
DelloRusso C, Scott JM, Hartigan-O'Connor D, et al. Functional correction of adult mdx mouse muscle using gutted adenoviral vectors expressing full-length dystrophin. Proc Natl Acad Sci U S A 2002;99:12979.
den Dunnen JT, Bakker E, Breteler EG, et al. Direct detection of more than 50% of the Duchenne muscular dystrophy mutations by field inversion gels. Nature 1987;329:640.
den Dunnen JT, Grootscholten PM, Bakker E, et al. Topography of the Duchenne muscular dystrophy (DMD) gene: FIGE and cDNA analysis of 194 cases reveals 115 deletions and 13 duplications. Am J Hum Genet 1989;45:835.
Dent KM, Dunn DM, von Niederhausern AC, et al. Improved molecular diagnosis of dystrophinopathies in an unselected clinical cohort. Am J Med Genet A 2005;134:295.
DeSilva S, Drachman DB, Mellits D, et al. Prednisone treatment in Duchenne muscular dystrophy. Long-term benefit. Arch Neurol 1987;44:818.
Dincer P, Leturcq F, Richard I, et al. A biochemical, genetic, and clinical survey of autosomal recessive limb girdle muscular dystrophies in Turkey. Ann Neurol 1997;42:222.
Do T. Orthopedic management of the muscular dystrophies. Curr Opin Pediatr 2002;14:50.
Doran P, Dowling P, Lohan J, et al. Subproteomics analysis of Ca^{2+}-binding proteins demonstrates decreased calsequestrin expression in dystrophic mouse skeletal muscle. Eur J Biochem 2004;271:3943.
Dowling P, Doran P, Ohlendieck K. Drastic reduction of sarcalumenin in Dp427 (dystrophin of 427 kDa)–deficient fibres indicates that abnormal calcium handling plays a key role in muscular dystrophy. Biochem J 2004;379 (Pt 2):479.
Drachman DB, Toyka KV, Myer E. Prednisone in Duchenne muscular dystrophy. Lancet 1974;2:1409.
Dressman D, Araishi K, Imamura M, et al. Delivery of alpha- and beta-sarcoglycan by recombinant adeno-associated virus: Efficient rescue of muscle, but differential toxicity. Hum Gene Ther 2002;13:1631.
Dubowitz V, Kinali M, Main M, et al. Remission of clinical signs in early Duchenne muscular dystrophy on intermittent low-dosage prednisolone therapy. Eur J Paediatr Neurol 2002;6:153.
Duclos F, Broux O, Bourg N, et al. Beta-sarcoglycan: Genomic analysis and identification of a novel missense mutation in the LGMD2E Amish isolate. Neuromuscul Disord 1998;8:30.
Duggan DJ, Fanin M, Pegoraro E, et al. Alpha-sarcoglycan (adhalin) deficiency: Complete deficiency patients are 5% of childhood-onset dystrophin-normal muscular dystrophy and most partial deficiency patients do not have gene mutations. J Neurol Sci 1996;140:30.
Duggan DJ, Gorospe JR, Fanin M, et al. Mutations in the sarcoglycan genes in patients with myopathy. N Engl J Med 1997;336:618.
Eagle M, Baudouin SV, Chandler C, et al. Survival in Duchenne muscular dystrophy: Improvements in life expectancy since 1967 and the impact of home nocturnal ventilation. Neuromuscul Disord 2002;12:926.
Emery AE. Emery-Dreifuss syndrome. J Med Genet 1989;26:637.
Emery AE. Duchenne muscular dystrophy—Meryon's disease. Neuromuscul Disord 1993;3:263.
Emery AE. Emery-Dreifuss muscular dystrophy—A 40 year retrospective. Neuromuscul Disord 2000;10:228.
Emery AE. The muscular dystrophies. Lancet 2002;359:687.
Emery AE, Dreifuss FE. Unusual type of benign X-linked muscular dystrophy. J Neurol Neurosurg Psychiatry 1966;29:338.
England SB, Nicholson LV, Johnson MA, et al. Very mild muscular dystrophy associated with the deletion of 46% of dystrophin. Nature 1990;343:180.
Errington SJ, Mann CJ, Fletcher S, et al. Target selection for antisense oligonucleotide induced exon skipping in the dystrophin gene. J Gene Med 2003;5:518.
Ervasti JM, Campbell KP. Membrane organization of the dystrophin-glycoprotein complex. Cell 1991;66:1121.
Esapa CT, Benson MA, Schroder JE, et al. Functional requirements for fukutin-related protein in the Golgi apparatus. Hum Mol Genet 2002;11:3319.
Escolar DM, Buyse G, Henricson E, et al. CINRG randomized controlled trial of creatine and glutamine in Duchenne muscular dystrophy. Ann Neurol 2005;58:151.
Fanin M, Duggan DJ, Mostacciuolo ML, et al. Genetic epidemiology of muscular dystrophies resulting from sarcoglycan gene mutations. J Med Genet 1997;34:973.
Fanin M, Fulizio L, Nascimbeni AC, et al. Molecular diagnosis in LGMD2A: Mutation analysis or protein testing? Hum Mutat 2004;24:52.
Fanin M, Nascimbeni AC, Fulizio L, et al. Loss of calpain-3 autocatalytic activity in LGMD2A patients with normal protein expression. Am J Pathol 2003;163:1929.
Fardeau M, Tome FM, Helbling-Leclerc A, et al. [Congenital muscular dystrophy with merosin deficiency: Clinical, histopathological, immunocytochemical and genetic analysis.] Rev Neurol (Paris) (in French) 1996;152:11.
Felisari G, Martinelli Boneschi F, Bardoni A, et al. Loss of Dp140 dystrophin isoform and intellectual impairment in Duchenne dystrophy. Neurology 2000;55:559.
Fenichel GM, Florence JM, Pestronk A, et al. Long-term benefit from prednisone therapy in Duchenne muscular dystrophy. Neurology 1991;41:1874.
Fenichel GM, Griggs RC, Kissel J, et al. A randomized efficacy and safety trial of oxandrolone in the treatment of Duchenne dystrophy. Neurology 2001;56:1075.
Ferrier P, Bamatter F, Klein D. Muscular dystrophy (Duchenne) in a girl with Turner's syndrome. J Med Genet 1965;42:38.
Figarella-Branger D, Baeta Machado AM, Putzu GA, et al. Exertional rhabdomyolysis and exercise intolerance revealing dystrophinopathies. Acta Neuropathol (Berl) 1997;94:48.
Finder JD, Birnkrant D, Carl J, et al. Respiratory care of the patient with Duchenne muscular dystrophy: ATS consensus statement. Am J Respir Crit Care Med 2004;170:456.
Finsterer J, Stollberger C. The heart in human dystrophinopathies. Cardiology 2003;99:1.
Fischer D, Walter MC, Kesper K, et al. Diagnostic value of muscle MRI in differentiating LGMD2I from other LGMDs. J Neurol 2005;252:538.

Fitzpatrick C, Barry C, Garvey C. Psychiatric disorder among boys with Duchenne muscular dystrophy. Dev Med Child Neurol 1986;28:589.

Fitzsimons RB, Gurwin EB, Bird AC. Retinal vascular abnormalities in facioscapulohumeral muscular dystrophy. A general association with genetic and therapeutic implications. Brain 1987;110 (Pt 3):631.

Flanigan KM, Kerr L, Bromberg MB, et al. Congenital muscular dystrophy with rigid spine syndrome: A clinical, pathological, radiological, and genetic study. Ann Neurol 2000;47:152.

Forrest SM, Cross GS, Speer A, et al. Preferential deletion of exons in Duchenne and Becker muscular dystrophies. Nature 1987;329:638.

Francke U, Ochs HD, de Martinville B, et al. Minor Xp21 chromosome deletion in a male associated with expression of Duchenne muscular dystrophy, chronic granulomatous disease, retinitis pigmentosa, and McLeod syndrome. Am J Hum Genet 1985;37:250.

Franco A Jr, Lansman JB. Calcium entry through stretch-inactivated ion channels in mdx myotubes. Nature 1990;344:670.

Franco-Obregon A, Lansman JB. Changes in mechanosensitive channel gating following mechanical stimulation in skeletal muscle myotubes from the mdx mouse. J Physiol 2002;539 (Pt 2):391.

Fraysse B, Liantonio A, Cetrone M, et al. The alteration of calcium homeostasis in adult dystrophic mdx muscle fibers is worsened by a chronic exercise in vivo. Neurobiol Dis 2004;17:144.

Friedrich O, Both M, Gillis JM, et al. Mini-dystrophin restores L-type calcium currents in skeletal muscle of transgenic mdx mice. J Physiol 2004;555 (Pt 1):251.

Fujimoto S, Ishikawa T, Saito M, et al. Early onset of X-linked Emery-Dreifuss muscular dystrophy in a boy with emerin gene deletion. Neuropediatrics 1999;30:161.

Furukawa T, Toyokura Y. Congenital, hypotonic-sclerotic muscular dystrophy. J Med Genet 1977;14:426.

Galasko CS, Williamson JB, Delaney CM. Lung function in Duchenne muscular dystrophy. Eur Spine J 1995;4:263.

Gallardo E, Rojas-Garcia R, de Luna N, et al. Inflammation in dysferlin myopathy: Immunohistochemical characterization of 13 patients. Neurology 2001;57:2136.

Gardner-Medwin D. Mutation rate in Duchenne type of muscular dystrophy. J Med Genet 1970;7:334.

Gebski BL, Mann CJ, Fletcher S, et al. Morpholino antisense oligonucleotide induced dystrophin exon 23 skipping in mdx mouse muscle. Hum Mol Genet 2003;12:1801.

Gerull B, Gramlich M, Atherton J, et al. Mutations of TTN, encoding the giant muscle filament titin, cause familial dilated cardiomyopathy. Nat Genet 2002;30:201.

Gibson B. Long-term ventilation for patients with Duchenne muscular dystrophy: Physicians' beliefs and practices. Chest 2001;119:940.

Giglio V, Pasceri V, Messano L, et al. Ultrasound tissue characterization detects preclinical myocardial structural changes in children affected by Duchenne muscular dystrophy. J Am Coll Cardiol 2003;42:309.

Gilhuis HJ, ten Donkelaar HJ, Tanke RB, et al. Nonmuscular involvement in merosin-negative congenital muscular dystrophy. Pediatr Neurol 2002;26:30.

Giliberto F, Ferreiro V, Dalamon V, et al. Dystrophin deletions and cognitive impairment in Duchenne/Becker muscular dystrophy. Neurol Res 2004;26:83.

Gillard EF, Chamberlain JS, Murphy EG, et al. Molecular and phenotypic analysis of patients with deletions within the deletion-rich region of the Duchenne muscular dystrophy (DMD) gene. Am J Hum Genet 1989;45:507.

Gillis JM. Membrane abnormalities and Ca homeostasis in muscles of the mdx mouse, an animal model of the Duchenne muscular dystrophy: A review. Acta Physiol Scand 1996;156:397.

Gomez-Merino E, Bach JR. Duchenne muscular dystrophy: Prolongation of life by noninvasive ventilation and mechanically assisted coughing. Am J Phys Med Rehabil 2002;81:411.

Gorecki DC, Monaco AP, Derry JM, et al. Expression of four alternative dystrophin transcripts in brain regions regulated by different promoters. Hum Mol Genet 1992;1:505.

Gorospe JR, Tharp M, Demitsu T, et al. Dystrophin-deficient myofibers are vulnerable to mast cell granule–induced necrosis. Neuromuscul Disord 1994a;4:325.

Gorospe JR, Tharp MD, Hinckley J, et al. A role for mast cells in the progression of Duchenne muscular dystrophy? Correlations in dystrophin-deficient humans, dogs, and mice. J Neurol Sci 1994b;122:44.

Gospe SM Jr, Lazaro RP, Lava NS, et al. Familial X-linked myalgia and cramps: A nonprogressive myopathy associated with a deletion in the dystrophin gene. Neurology 1989;39:1277.

Gosselin LE, Williams JE, Deering M, et al. Localization and early time course of TGF-beta 1 mRNA expression in dystrophic muscle. Muscle Nerve 2004;30:645.

Gozal D. Pulmonary manifestations of neuromuscular disease with special reference to Duchenne muscular dystrophy and spinal muscular atrophy. Pediatr Pulmonol 2000;29:141.

Grain L, Cortina-Borja M, Forfar C, et al. Cardiac abnormalities and skeletal muscle weakness in carriers of Duchenne and Becker muscular dystrophies and controls. Neuromuscul Disord 2001;11:186.

Granchelli JA, Avosso DL, Hudecki MS, et al. Cromolyn increases strength in exercised mdx mice. Res Commun Mol Pathol Pharmacol 1996;91:287.

Granzier HL, Labeit S. The giant protein titin: A major player in myocardial mechanics, signaling, and disease. Circ Res 2004;94:284.

Gregorevic P, Blankinship MJ, Allen JM, et al. Systemic delivery of genes to striated muscles using adeno-associated viral vectors. Nat Med 2004;10:828.

Griggs RC, Mendell JR, Brooke MH, et al. Clinical investigation in Duchenne dystrophy: V. Use of creatine kinase and pyruvate kinase in carrier detection. Muscle Nerve 1985;8:60.

Griggs RC, Moxley RT 3rd, Mendell JR, et al. Prednisone in Duchenne dystrophy. A randomized, controlled trial defining the time course and dose response. Clinical Investigation of Duchenne Dystrophy Group. Arch Neurol 1991;48:383.

Griggs RC, Moxley RT 3rd, Mendell JR, et al. Duchenne dystrophy: Randomized, controlled trial of prednisone (18 months) and azathioprine (12 months). Neurology 1993;43 (3 Pt 1):520.

Gruenbaum Y, Goldman RD, Meyuhas R, et al. The nuclear lamina and its functions in the nucleus. Int Rev Cytol 2003;226:1.

Gurwin EB, Fitzsimons RB, Sehmi KS, et al. Retinal telangiectasis in facioscapulohumeral muscular dystrophy with deafness. Arch Ophthalmol 1985;103:1695.

Gussoni E, Pavlath GK, Miller RG, et al. Specific T cell receptor gene rearrangements at the site of muscle degeneration in Duchenne muscular dystrophy. J Immunol 1994;153:4798.

Guyon JR, Kudryashova E, Potts A, et al. Calpain 3 cleaves filamin C and regulates its ability to interact with gamma- and delta-sarcoglycans. Muscle Nerve 2003;28:472.

Hackman JP, Vihola AK, Udd AB. The role of titin in muscular disorders. Ann Med 2003;35:434.

Hackman P, Vihola A, Haravuori H, et al. Tibial muscular dystrophy is a titinopathy caused by mutations in TTN, the gene encoding the giant skeletal-muscle protein titin. Am J Hum Genet 2002;71:492.

Haltia M, Leivo I, Somer H, et al. Muscle-eye-brain disease: A neuropathological study. Ann Neurol 1997;41:173.

Haravuori H, Vihola A, Straub V, et al. Secondary calpain3 deficiency in 2q-linked muscular dystrophy: Titin is the candidate gene. Neurology 2001;56:869.

Hart DN. Dendritic cells: Unique leukocyte populations which control the primary immune response. Blood 1997;90:3245.

Hartel JV, Granchelli JA, Hudecki MS, et al. Impact of prednisone on TGF-beta1 and collagen in diaphragm muscle from mdx mice. Muscle Nerve 2001;24:428.

Hartigan-O'Connor D, Kirk CJ, Crawford R, et al. Immune evasion by muscle-specific gene expression in dystrophic muscle. Mol Ther 2001;4:525.

Hauser MA, Conde CB, Kowaljow V, et al. Myotilin mutation found in second pedigree with LGMD1A. Am J Hum Genet 2002;71:1428.

Hauser MA, Horrigan SK, Salmikangas P, et al. Myotilin is mutated in limb girdle muscular dystrophy 1A. Hum Mol Genet 2000;9:2141.

Hayashi YK, Arahata K. [The frequency of patients with adhalin deficiency in a muscular dystrophy patient population.] Nippon Rinsho (in Japanese) 1997;55:3165.

Hayashi YK, Chou FL, Engvall E, et al. Mutations in the integrin alpha7 gene cause congenital myopathy. Nat Genet 1998;19:94.

Hayashi YK, Ogawa M, Tagawa K, et al. Selective deficiency of alpha-dystroglycan in Fukuyama-type congenital muscular dystrophy. Neurology 2001;57:115.

Haycock JW, Jones P, Harris JB, et al. Differential susceptibility of human skeletal muscle proteins to free radical induced oxidative damage: A histochemical, immunocytochemical and electron microscopical study in vitro. Acta Neuropathol (Berl) 1996a;92:331.

Haycock JW, MacNeil S, Jones P, et al. Oxidative damage to muscle protein in Duchenne muscular dystrophy. Neuroreport 1996b;8:357.

Hayes A, Lynch GS, Williams DA. The effects of endurance exercise on dystrophic mdx mice. I. Contractile and histochemical properties of intact muscles. Proc R Soc Lond B Biol Sci 1993;253:19.

Heiman-Patterson TD, Natter HM, Rosenberg HR, et al. Malignant hyperthermia susceptibility in X-linked muscle dystrophies. Pediatr Neurol 1986;2:356.

Heiskanen M, Saitta B, Palotie A, et al. Head to tail organization of the human COL6A1 and COL6A2 genes by fiber-FISH. Genomics 1995;29:801.

Herbst H, Wege T, Milani S, et al. Tissue inhibitor of metalloproteinase-1 and -2 RNA expression in rat and human liver fibrosis. Am J Pathol 1997;150:1647.

Herrmann R, Straub V, Blank M, et al. Dissociation of the dystroglycan complex in caveolin-3–deficient limb girdle muscular dystrophy. Hum Mol Genet 2000;9:2335.

Higuchi I, Horikiri T, Niiyama T, et al. Pathological characteristics of skeletal muscle in Ullrich's disease with collagen VI deficiency. Neuromuscul Disord 2003;13:310.

Higuchi I, Kawai H, Umaki Y, et al. Different manners of sarcoglycan expression in genetically proven alpha-sarcoglycan deficiency and gamma-sarcoglycan deficiency. Acta Neuropathol (Berl) 1998;96:202.

Hilton T, Orr RD, Perkin RM, et al. End of life care in Duchenne muscular dystrophy. Pediatr Neurol 1993;9:165.

Hinton VJ, De Vivo DC, Nereo NE, et al. Poor verbal working memory across intellectual level in boys with Duchenne dystrophy. Neurology 2000;54:2127.

Hinton VJ, De Vivo DC, Nereo NE, et al. Selective deficits in verbal working memory associated with a known genetic etiology: The neuropsychological profile of Duchenne muscular dystrophy. J Int Neuropsychol Soc 2001;7:45.

Ho M, Gallardo E, McKenna-Yasek D, et al. A novel, blood-based diagnostic assay for limb girdle muscular dystrophy 2B and Miyoshi myopathy. Ann Neurol 2002;51:129.

Hoffman EP. Molecular diagnostics of Duchenne/Becker dystrophy: New additions to a rapidly expanding literature [Editorial]. J Neurol Sci 1991;101:129.

Hoffman EP. Clinical and histopathological features of abnormalities of the dystrophin-based membrane cytoskeleton. Brain Pathol 1996;6:49.

Hoffman EP, Arahata K, Minetti C, et al. Dystrophinopathy in isolated cases of myopathy in females. Neurology 1992;42:967.

Hoffman EP, Brown RH Jr, Kunkel LM. Dystrophin: The protein product of the Duchenne muscular dystrophy locus. Cell 1987a;51:919.

Hoffman EP, Clemens PR. HyperCKemic, proximal muscular dystrophies and the dystrophin membrane cytoskeleton, including dystrophinopathies, sarcoglycanopathies, and merosinopathies. Curr Opin Rheumatol 1996;8:528.

Hoffman EP, Fischbeck KH, Brown RH, et al. Characterization of dystrophin in muscle-biopsy specimens from patients with Duchenne's or Becker's muscular dystrophy. N Engl J Med 1988;318:1363.

Hoffman EP, Knudson CM, Campbell KP, et al. Subcellular fractionation of dystrophin to the triads of skeletal muscle. Nature 1987b;330:754.

Hoffman EP, Kunkel LM. Dystrophin abnormalities in Duchenne/Becker muscular dystrophy. Neuron 1989;2:1019.

Hoogerwaard EM, Bakker E, Ippel PF, et al. Signs and symptoms of Duchenne muscular dystrophy and Becker muscular dystrophy among carriers in The Netherlands: A cohort study. Lancet 1999a;353:2116.

Hoogerwaard EM, van der Wouw PA, Wilde AA, et al. Cardiac involvement in carriers of Duchenne and Becker muscular dystrophy. Neuromuscul Disord 1999b;9:347.

Hu X, Burghes A, Bulman D. Evidence for mutation by unequal sister chromatid exchange in the Duchenne muscular dystrophy gene. Am J Hum Genet 1989;44:855.

Hu X, Ray P, Murphy E, et al. Duplicational mutation at the Duchenne muscular dystrophy locus: Its frequency, distribution, origin, and phenotypegenotype correlation. Am J Hum Genet 1990;46:682.

Huard J, Acsadi G, Jani A, et al. Gene transfer into skeletal muscles by isogenic myoblasts. Hum Gene Ther 1994;5:949.

Hurko O, Hoffman EP, McKee L, et al. Dystrophin analysis in clonal myoblasts derived from a Duchenne muscular dystrophy carrier. Am J Hum Genet 1989;44:820.

Iannaccone S, Quattrini A, Smirne S, et al. Connective tissue proliferation and growth factors in animal models of Duchenne muscular dystrophy. J Neurol Sci 1995;128:36.

Ionasescu V, Burmeister L, Hanson J. Discriminant analysis of ribosomal protein synthesis findings in carrier detection of Duchenne muscular dystrophy. Am J Med Genet 1980;5:5.

Ionasescu V, Zellweger H, Conway TW. A new approach for carrier detection in Duchenne muscular dystrophy. Protein synthesis of muscle polyribosomes in vitro. Neurology 1971a;21:703.

Ionasescu V, Zellweger H, Conway TW. Ribosomal protein synthesis in Duchenne muscular dystrophy. Arch Biochem Biophys 1971b;144:51.

Isenberg DA, Rowe D, Shearer M, et al. Localization of interferons and interleukin 2 in polymyositis and muscular dystrophy. Clin Exp Immunol 1986;63:450.

Iwata Y, Katanosaka Y, Arai Y, et al. A novel mechanism of myocyte degeneration involving the Ca^{2+}-permeable growth factor–regulated channel. J Cell Biol 2003;161:957.

Jay V, Becker LE, Ackerley C, et al. Dystrophin analysis in the diagnosis of childhood muscular dystrophy: An immunohistochemical study of 75 cases. Pediatr Pathol 1993;13:635.

Jeppesen J, Green A, Steffensen BF, et al. The Duchenne muscular dystrophy population in Denmark, 1977-2001: Prevalence, incidence and survival in relation to the introduction of ventilator use. Neuromuscul Disord 2003;13:804.

Jia Z, Petrounevitch V, Wong A, et al. Mutations in calpain 3 associated with limb girdle muscular dystrophy: Analysis by molecular modeling and by mutation in m-calpain. Biophys J 2001;80:2590.

Jobsis GJ, Boers JM, Barth PG, et al. Bethlem myopathy: A slowly progressive congenital muscular dystrophy with contractures. Brain 1999;122 (Pt 4):649.

Johnson P. Calpains (intracellular calcium-activated cysteine proteinases): Structure-activity relationships and involvement in normal and abnormal cellular metabolism. Int J Biochem 1990;22:811.

Jung D, Yang B, Meyer J, et al. Identification and characterization of the dystrophin anchoring site on beta-dystroglycan. J Biol Chem 1995;270:27305.

Kawabe K, Goto K, Nishino I, et al. Dysferlin mutation analysis in a group of Italian patients with limb-girdle muscular dystrophy and Miyoshi myopathy. Eur J Neurol 2004;11:657.

Kinali M, Mercuri E, Main M, et al. An effective, low-dosage, intermittent schedule of prednisolone in the long-term treatment of early cases of Duchenne dystrophy. Neuromuscul Disord 2002;12 (Suppl 1):S169.

Kinoshita M, Ikeda K, Yoshimura M, et al. [Duchenne muscular dystrophy carrier presenting with mosaic X chromosome constitution and muscular symptoms—With analysis of the Barr bodies in the muscle.] Rinsho Shinkeigaku (in Japanese) 1990;30:643.

Kirk VG, Flemons WW, Adams C, et al. Sleep-disordered breathing in Duchenne muscular dystrophy: A preliminary study of the role of portable monitoring. Pediatr Pulmonol 2000;29:135.

Kissel JT, Lynn DJ, Rammohan KW, et al. Mononuclear cell analysis of muscle biopsies in prednisone- and azathioprine-treated Duchenne muscular dystrophy. Neurology 1993;43 (3 Pt 1):532.

Kissel JT, McDermott MP, Mendell JR, et al. Randomized, double-blind, placebo-controlled trial of albuterol in facioscapulohumeral dystrophy. Neurology 2001;57:1434.

Kleopa KA, Rosenberg H, Heiman-Patterson T. Malignant hyperthermia-like episode in Becker muscular dystrophy. Anesthesiology 2000;93:1535.

Knoll R, Hoshijima M, Hoffman HM, et al. The cardiac mechanical stretch sensor machinery involves a Z disc complex that is defective in a subset of human dilated cardiomyopathy. Cell 2002;111:943.

Knudson CM, Hoffman EP, Kahl SD, et al. Evidence for the association of dystrophin with the transverse tubular system in skeletal muscle. J Biol Chem 1988;263:8480.

Kobayashi K, Nakahori Y, Miyake M, et al. An ancient retrotransposal insertion causes Fukuyama-type congenital muscular dystrophy. Nature 1998;394:388.

Koenig M, Beggs AH, Moyer M, et al. The molecular basis for Duchenne versus Becker muscular dystrophy: Correlation of severity with type of deletion. Am J Hum Genet 1989;45:498.

Koenig M, Hoffman EP, Bertelson CJ, et al. Complete cloning of the Duchenne muscular dystrophy (DMD) cDNA and preliminary genomic organization of the DMD gene in normal and affected individuals. Cell 1987;50:509.

Korones DN, Brown MR, Palis J. "Liver function tests" are not always tests of liver function. Am J Hematol 2001;66:46.

Kramerova I, Kudryashova E, Tidball JG, et al. Null mutation of calpain 3 (p94) in mice causes abnormal sarcomere formation in vivo and in vitro. Hum Mol Genet 2004;13:1373.

Krasnianski M, Neudecker S, Deschauer M, et al. [The clinical spectrum of limb-girdle muscular dystrophies type 2I in cases of a mutation in the "fukutin-related-protein"-gene.] Nervenarzt (in German) 2004;75:770.

Kubisch C, Schoser BG, von During M, et al. Homozygous mutations in caveolin-3 cause a severe form of rippling muscle disease. Ann Neurol 2003;53:512.

Kuller JA, Hoffman EP, Fries MH, et al. Prenatal diagnosis of Duchenne muscular dystrophy by fetal muscle biopsy. Hum Genet 1992;90:34.

Kumar A, Boriek AM. Mechanical stress activates the nuclear factor-kappaB pathway in skeletal muscle fibers: A possible role in Duchenne muscular dystrophy. FASEB J 2003;17:386.

Kumar A, Khandelwal N, Malya R, et al. Loss of dystrophin causes aberrant mechanotransduction in skeletal muscle fibers. FASEB J 2004;18:102.

Kunkel LM. Analysis of deletions in DNA from patients with Becker and Duchenne muscular dystrophy. Nature 1986;322:73.

Kunkel LM, Monaco AP, Middlesworth W, et al. Specific cloning of DNA fragments absent from the DNA of a male patient with an X chromosome deletion. Proc Natl Acad Sci U S A 1985;82:4778.

Lagrota-Candido J, Vasconcellos R, Cavalcanti M, et al. Resolution of skeletal muscle inflammation in mdx dystrophic mouse is accompanied by increased immunoglobulin and interferon-gamma production. Int J Exp Pathol 2002;83:121.

Lampe AK, Dunn DM, von Niederhausern AC, et al. Automated genomic sequence analysis of the three collagen VI genes: Applications to Ullrich congenital muscular dystrophy and Bethlem myopathy. J Med Genet 2005;42:108.

Lanman JT Jr, Pericak-Vance MA, Bartlett RJ, et al. Familial inheritance of a DXS164 deletion mutation from a heterozygous female. Am J Hum Genet 1987;41:138.

Larson CM, Henderson RC. Bone mineral density and fractures in boys with Duchenne muscular dystrophy. J Pediatr Orthop 2000;20:71.

Laval SH, Bushby KM. Limb girdle muscular dystrophies—from genetics to molecular pathology. Neuropathol Appl Neurobiol 2004;30:91.

Leijendekker WJ, Passaquin AC, Metzinger L, et al. Regulation of cytosolic calcium in skeletal muscle cells of the mdx mouse under conditions of stress. Br J Pharmacol 1996;118:611.

Lesca G, Demarquay G, Llense S, et al. [Symptomatic carriers of dystrophinopathy with chromosome X inactivation bias.] Rev Neurol (Paris) (in French) 2003;159:775.

Lescaut W, Butori C, Soriani MH, et al. [Report of four women with Duchenne or Becker muscular dystrophy.] Rev Med Interne (in French) 2004;25:464.

Leth A, Wulff K. Myocardiopathy in Duchenne progressive muscular dystrophy. Acta Paediatr Scand 1976;65:28.

Lim JH, Kim DY, Bang MS. Effects of exercise and steroid on skeletal muscle apoptosis in the mdx mouse. Muscle Nerve 2004;30:456.

Lin YC, Lee WT, Huang SF, et al. Persistent hypertransaminasemia as the presenting findings of muscular dystrophy in childhood. Acta Paediatr Taiwan 1999;40:424.

Liu X, Sun B. [Suppressive effect of corticosteroids on the gene expression of interleukin-5 and eosinophil activation in asthmatics.] Zhonghua Nei Ke Za Zhi (in Chinese) 1996;35:231.

Lu QL, Mann CJ, Lou F, et al. Functional amounts of dystrophin produced by skipping the mutated exon in the mdx dystrophic mouse. Nat Med 2003;9:1009.

Lundberg I, Brengman JM, Engel AG. Analysis of cytokine expression in muscle in inflammatory myopathies, Duchenne dystrophy, and non-weak controls. J Neuroimmunol 1995;63:9.

Luz MA, Marques MJ, Santo Neto H. Impaired regeneration of dystrophin-deficient muscle fibers is caused by exhaustion of myogenic cells. Braz J Med Biol Res 2002;35:691.

Lynch GS. Role of contraction-induced injury in the mechanisms of muscle damage in muscular dystrophy. Clin Exp Pharmacol Physiol 2004;31:557.

Lynch GS, Rafael JA, Chamberlain JS, et al. Contraction-induced injury to single permeabilized muscle fibers from mdx, transgenic mdx, and control mice. Am J Physiol Cell Physiol 2000;279:C1290.

Mahjneh I, Marconi G, Bushby K, et al. Dysferlinopathy (LGMD2B): A 23-year follow-up study of 10 patients homozygous for the same frameshifting dysferlin mutations. Neuromuscul Disord 2001;11:20.

Malandrini A, Fabrizi GM, Truschi F, et al. Atypical McLeod syndrome manifested as X-linked chorea-acanthocytosis, neuromyopathy and dilated cardiomyopathy: Report of a family. J Neurol Sci 1994;124:89.

Malhotra SB, Hart KA, Klamut HJ, et al. Frame-shift deletions in patients with Duchenne and Becker muscular dystrophy. Science 1988;242:755.

Mallouk N, Allard B. Stretch-induced activation of Ca(2+)-activated K(+) channels in mouse skeletal muscle fibers. Am J Physiol Cell Physiol 2000;278:C473.

Mallouk N, Jacquemond V, Allard B. Elevated subsarcolemmal Ca^{2+} in mdx mouse skeletal muscle fibers detected with Ca^{2+}-activated K^+ channels. Proc Natl Acad Sci U S A 2000;97:4950.

Manilal S, Sewry CA, Man N, et al. Diagnosis of X-linked Emery-Dreifuss muscular dystrophy by protein analysis of leucocytes and skin with monoclonal antibodies. Neuromuscul Disord 1997;7:63.

Mann CJ, Honeyman K, Cheng AJ, et al. Antisense-induced exon skipping and synthesis of dystrophin in the mdx mouse. Proc Natl Acad Sci U S A 2001;98:42.

Manzur AY, Kuntzer T, Pike M, et al. Glucocorticoid corticosteroids for Duchenne muscular dystrophy. Cochrane Database Syst Rev 2004;(2):CD003725.

Marchand E, Constantin B, Balghi H, et al. Improvement of calcium handling and changes in calcium-release properties after mini- or full-length dystrophin forced expression in cultured skeletal myotubes. Exp Cell Res 2004;297:363.

Marchand E, Constantin B, Vandebrouck C, et al. Calcium homeostasis and cell death in Sol8 dystrophin-deficient cell line in culture. Cell Calcium 2001;29:85.

Mason P, Bayol S, Loughna PT. The novel sarcomeric protein telethonin exhibits developmental and functional regulation. Biochem Biophys Res Commun 1999;257:699.

Matsuda C, Aoki M, Hayashi YK, et al. Dysferlin is a surface membrane-associated protein that is absent in Miyoshi myopathy. Neurology 1999;53:1119.

Matsumoto H, Noguchi S, Sugie K, et al. Subcellular localization of fukutin and fukutin-related protein in muscle cells. J Biochem (Tokyo) 2004;135:709.

Matsumura K, Tome FM, Collin H, et al. Deficiency of the 50K dystrophin-associated glycoprotein in severe childhood autosomal recessive muscular dystrophy. Nature 1992;359:320.

Maunder-Sewry CA, Dubowitz V. Needle muscle biopsy for carrier detection in Duchenne muscular dystrophy. Part 1. Light microscopy—Histology, histochemistry and quantitation. J Neurol Sci 1981;49:305.

McDonald CM. Physical activity, health impairments, and disability in neuromuscular disease. Am J Phys Med Rehabil 2002;81 (11 Suppl):S108.

McDouall RM, Dunn MJ, Dubowitz V. Nature of the mononuclear infiltrate and the mechanism of muscle damage in juvenile dermatomyositis and Duchenne muscular dystrophy. J Neurol Sci 1990;99:199.

McElhinny AS, Perry CN, Witt CC, et al. Muscle-specific RING finger-2 (MURF-2) is important for microtubule, intermediate filament and sarcomeric M-line maintenance in striated muscle development. J Cell Sci 2004;117 (Pt 15):3175.

McNally EM, Duggan D, Gorospe JR, et al. Mutations that disrupt the carboxyl-terminus of gamma-sarcoglycan cause muscular dystrophy. Hum Mol Genet 1996a;5:1841.

McNally EM, Passos-Bueno MR, Bonnemann CG, et al. Mild and severe muscular dystrophy caused by a single gamma-sarcoglycan mutation. Am J Hum Genet 1996b;59:1040.

Melacini P, Fanin M, Duggan DJ, et al. Heart involvement in muscular dystrophies due to sarcoglycan gene mutations. Muscle Nerve 1999;22:473.

Melacini P, Vianello A, Villanova C, et al. Cardiac and respiratory involvement in advanced stage Duchenne muscular dystrophy. Neuromuscul Disord 1996;6:367.

Melis MA, Cau M, Muntoni F, et al. Elevation of serum creatine kinase as the only manifestation of an intragenic deletion of the dystrophin gene in three unrelated families. Eur J Paediatr Neurol 1998;2:255.

Melone MA, Peluso G, Galderisi U, et al. Increased expression of IGF-binding protein-5 in Duchenne muscular dystrophy (DMD) fibroblasts correlates with the fibroblast-induced downregulation of DMD myoblast growth: An in vitro analysis. J Cell Physiol 2000;185:143.

Mendell JR, Buzin CH, Feng J, et al. Diagnosis of Duchenne dystrophy by enhanced detection of small mutations. Neurology 2001;57:645.

Mendell JR, Kissel JT, Amato AA, et al. Myoblast transfer in the treatment of Duchenne's muscular dystrophy. N Engl J Med 1995;333:832.

Mendell JR, Moxley RT, Griggs RC, et al. Randomized, double-blind six-month trial of prednisone in Duchenne's muscular dystrophy [see comments]. N Engl J Med 1989;320:1592.

Mercuri E, Brockington M, Straub V, et al. Phenotypic spectrum associated with mutations in the fukutin-related protein gene. Ann Neurol 2003;53:537.

Mercuri E, Bushby K, Ricci E, et al. Muscle MRI findings in patients with limb girdle muscular dystrophy with calpain 3 deficiency (LGMD2A) and early contractures. Neuromuscul Disord 2005;15:164.

Merlini L, Carbone I, Capanni C, et al. Familial isolated hyperCKaemia associated with a new mutation in the caveolin-3 (CAV-3) gene. J Neurol Neurosurg Psychiatry 2002;73:65.

Merlini L, Cicognani A, Malaspina E, et al. Early prednisone treatment in Duchenne muscular dystrophy. Muscle Nerve 2003;27:222.

Merlini L, Kaplan JC, Navarro C, et al. Homogeneous phenotype of the gypsy limb-girdle MD with the gamma-sarcoglycan C283Y mutation. Neurology 2000;54:1075.

Mesa LE, Dubrovsky AL, Corderi J, et al. Steroids in Duchenne muscular dystrophy—Deflazacort trial. Neuromuscul Disord 1991;1:261.

Milhorat AT, Goldstone L. The carrier state in muscular dystrophy of the Duchenne type. JAMA 1965;194:130.

Miller RG, Sharma KR, Pavlath GK, et al. Myoblast implantation in Duchenne muscular dystrophy: The San Francisco study. Muscle Nerve 1997;20:469.

Minetti C, Chang HW, Medori R, et al. Dystrophin deficiency in young girls with sporadic myopathy and normal karyotype. Neurology 1991;41:1288.

Minetti C, Sotgia F, Bruno C, et al. Mutations in the caveolin-3 gene cause autosomal dominant limb-girdle muscular dystrophy. Nat Genet 1998;18:365.

Mizuno Y, Noguchi S, Yamamoto H, et al. Selective defect of sarcoglycan complex in severe childhood autosomal recessive muscular dystrophy muscle. Biochem Biophys Res Commun 1994;203:979.

Moghadaszadeh B, Petit N, Jaillard C, et al. Mutations in SEPN1 cause congenital muscular dystrophy with spinal rigidity and restrictive respiratory syndrome. Nat Genet 2001;29:17.

Monaco AP, Bertelson CJ, Middlesworth W, et al. Detection of deletions spanning the Duchenne muscular dystrophy locus using a tightly linked DNA segment. Nature 1985;316:842.

Monaco AP, Neve RL, Colletti-Feener C, et al. Isolation of candidate cDNAs for portions of the Duchenne muscular dystrophy gene. Nature 1986;323:646.

Moreira ES, Vainzof M, Marie SK, et al. The seventh form of autosomal recessive limb-girdle muscular dystrophy is mapped to 17q11-12. Am J Hum Genet 1997;61:151.

Moreira ES, Wiltshire TJ, Faulkner G, et al. Limb-girdle muscular dystrophy type 2G is caused by mutations in the gene encoding the sarcomeric protein telethonin. Nat Genet 2000;24:163.

Morrison J, Lu QL, Pastoret C, et al. T-cell–dependent fibrosis in the mdx dystrophic mouse. Lab Invest 2000;80:881.

Morrone A, Zammarchi E, Scacheri PC, et al. Asymptomatic dystrophinopathy. Am J Med Genet 1997;69:261.

Moser H. Duchenne muscular dystrophy: Pathogenetic aspects and genetic prevention. Hum Genet 1984;66:17.

Mostacciuolo ML, Miorin M, Martinello F, et al. Genetic epidemiology of congenital muscular dystrophy in a sample from north-east Italy. Hum Genet 1996;97:277.

Moxley RT, 3rd, Ashwal S, Pandya S, et al. Practice parameter: Corticosteroid treatment of Duchenne dystrophy: Report of the Quality Standards Subcommittee of the American Academy of Neurology and the Practice Committee of the Child Neurology Society. Neurology 2005;64:13.

Munsat TL. Clinical trials in neuromuscular disease. Muscle Nerve 1990;13 (Suppl):S3.

Muntoni F, Gobbi P, Sewry C, et al. Deletions in the 5′ region of dystrophin and resulting phenotypes. J Med Genet 1994;31:843.

Muntoni F, Lichtarowicz-Krynska EJ, Sewry CA, et al. Early presentation of X-linked Emery-Dreifuss muscular dystrophy resembling limb-girdle muscular dystrophy. Neuromuscul Disord 1998;8:72.

Murakami N, McLennan IS, Nonaka I, et al. Transforming growth factor-beta2 is elevated in skeletal muscle disorders. Muscle Nerve 1999;22:889.

Murphy ME, Kehrer JP. Free radicals: A potential pathogenic mechanism in inherited muscular dystrophy. Life Sci 1986;39:2271.

Nagano A, Arahata K. Nuclear envelope proteins and associated diseases. Curr Opin Neurol 2000;13:533.

Nahirney PC, Dow PR, Ovalle WK. Quantitative morphology of mast cells in skeletal muscle of normal and genetically dystrophic mice. Anat Rec 1997;247:341.

Nereo NE, Fee RJ, Hinton VJ. Parental stress in mothers of boys with Duchenne muscular dystrophy. J Pediatr Psychol 2003;28:473.

Neumeyer AM, Cros D, McKenna-Yasek D, et al. Pilot study of myoblast transfer in the treatment of Becker muscular dystrophy. Neurology 1998;51:589.

Nevo Y, Muntoni F, Sewry C, et al. Large in-frame deletions of the rod-shaped domain of the dystrophin gene resulting in severe phenotype. Isr Med Assoc J 2003;5:94.

Nicholson LV, Bushby KM, Johnson MA, et al. Predicted and observed sizes of dystrophin in some patients with gene deletions that disrupt the open reading frame. J Med Genet 1992;29:892.

Nigro G, Politano L, Nigro V, et al. Mutation of dystrophin gene and cardiomyopathy. Neuromuscul Disord 1994;4:371.

Nigro V, de Sa Moreira E, Piluso G, et al. Autosomal recessive limb-girdle muscular dystrophy, LGMD2F, is caused by a mutation in the delta-sarcoglycan gene. Nat Genet 1996a;14:195.

Nigro V, Piluso G, Belsito A, et al. Identification of a novel sarcoglycan gene at 5q33 encoding a sarcolemmal 35 kDa glycoprotein. Hum Mol Genet 1996b;5:1179.

Nobile C, Galvagni F, Marchi J, et al. Genomic organization of the human dystrophin gene across the major deletion hot spot and the 3′ region. Genomics 1995;28:97.

Noguchi S, McNally EM, Ben Othmane K, et al. Mutations in the dystrophin-associated protein gamma-sarcoglycan in chromosome 13 muscular dystrophy. Science 1995;270:819.

Nolan MA, Jones OD, Pedersen RL, et al. Cardiac assessment in childhood carriers of Duchenne and Becker muscular dystrophies. Neuromuscul Disord 2003;13:129.

North KN, Miller G, Iannaccone ST, et al. Cognitive dysfunction as the major presenting feature of Becker's muscular dystrophy. Neurology 1996;46:461.

Nowak KJ, Walsh P, Jacob RL, et al. Severe gamma-sarcoglycanopathy caused by a novel missense mutation and a large deletion. Neuromuscul Disord 2000;10:100.

Ogasawara A. Downward shift in IQ in persons with Duchenne muscular dystrophy compared to those with spinal muscular atrophy. Am J Ment Retard 1989;93:544.

Oudet C, Hanauer A, Clemens P, et al. Two hot spots of recombination in the DMD gene correlate with the deletion prone regions. Hum Mol Genet 1992;1:599.

Ozawa E. [Dystrophin, dystrophin-associated protein and dystrophinopathy.] Nihon Shinkei Seishin Yakurigaku Zasshi (in Japanese) 1995;15:289.

Ozawa E, Yoshida M, Suzuki A, et al. Dystrophin-associated proteins in muscular dystrophy. Hum Mol Genet 1995;4 (Spec No):1711.

Padberg GW, Brouwer OF, de Keizer RJ, et al. On the significance of retinal vascular disease and hearing loss in facioscapulohumeral muscular dystrophy. Muscle Nerve 1995;2:S73.

Parton RG, Way M, Zorzi N, et al. Caveolin-3 associates with developing T-tubules during muscle differentiation. J Cell Biol 1997;136:137.

Partridge T. Myoblast transplantation. Neuromuscul Disord 2002;12 (Suppl 1):S3.

Passaquin AC, Lhote P, Ruegg UT. Calcium influx inhibition by steroids and analogs in C2C12 skeletal muscle cells. Br J Pharmacol 1998;124:1751.

Passerini L, Bernasconi P, Baggi F, et al. Fibrogenic cytokines and extent of fibrosis in muscle of dogs with X-linked golden retriever muscular dystrophy. Neuromuscul Disord 2002;12:828.

Passos-Bueno MR, Moreira ES, Marie SK, et al. Main clinical features of the three mapped autosomal recessive limb-girdle muscular dystrophies and estimated proportion of each form in 13 Brazilian families. J Med Genet 1996a;33:97.

Passos-Bueno MR, Moreira ES, Vainzof M, et al. Linkage analysis in autosomal recessive limb-girdle muscular dystrophy (AR LGMD) maps a sixth form to 5q33-34 (LGMD2F) and indicates that there is at least one more subtype of AR LGMD. Hum Mol Genet 1996b;5:815.

Passos-Bueno MR, Vainzof M, Moreira ES, et al. Seven autosomal recessive limb-girdle muscular dystrophies in the Brazilian population: From LGMD2A to LGMD2G. Am J Med Genet 1999;82:392.

Patria SY, Alimsardjono H, Nishio H, et al. A case of Becker muscular dystrophy resulting from the skipping of four contiguous exons (71-74) of the dystrophin gene during mRNA maturation. Proc Assoc Am Physicians 1996;108:308.

Pegoraro E, Cepollaro F, Prandini P, et al. Integrin alpha 7 beta 1 in muscular dystrophy/myopathy of unknown etiology. Am J Pathol 2002;160:2135.

Pegoraro E, Mancias P, Swerdlow SH, et al. Congenital muscular dystrophy with primary laminin alpha2 (merosin) deficiency presenting as inflammatory myopathy. Ann Neurol 1996;40:782.

Pegoraro E, Marks H, Garcia CA, et al. Laminin alpha2 muscular dystrophy: Genotype/phenotype studies of 22 patients. Neurology 1998;51:101.

Pegoraro E, Schimke RN, Garcia C, et al. Genetic and biochemical normalization in female carriers of Duchenne muscular dystrophy: Evidence for failure of dystrophin production in dystrophin-competent myonuclei. Neurology 1995;45:677.

Pena SD, Karpati G, Carpenter S, et al. The clinical consequences of X-chromosome inactivation: Duchenne muscular dystrophy in one of monozygotic twins. J Neurol Sci 1987;79:337.

Petrof BJ. The molecular basis of activity-induced muscle injury in Duchenne muscular dystrophy. Mol Cell Biochem 1998;179:111.

Petrof BJ, Shrager JB, Stedman HH, et al. Dystrophin protects the sarcolemma from stresses developed during muscle contraction. Proc Natl Acad Sci U S A 1993;90:3710.

Philpot J, Cowan F, Pennock J, et al. Merosin-deficient congenital muscular dystrophy: The spectrum of brain involvement on magnetic resonance imaging. Neuromuscul Disord 1999;9:81.

Piccolo F, Roberds SL, Jeanpierre M, et al. Primary adhalinopathy: A common cause of autosomal recessive muscular dystrophy of variable severity. Nat Genet 1995;10:243.

Plant DR, Lynch GS. Depolarization-induced contraction and SR function in mechanically skinned muscle fibers from dystrophic mdx mice. Am J Physiol Cell Physiol 2003;285:C522.

Politano L, Nigro V, Passamano L, et al. Evaluation of cardiac and respiratory involvement in sarcoglycanopathies. Neuromuscul Disord 2001;11:178.

Poppe M, Cree L, Bourke J, et al. The phenotype of limb-girdle muscular dystrophy type 2I. Neurology 2003;60:1246.

Porter JD, Guo W, Merriam AP, et al. Persistent over-expression of specific CC class chemokines correlates with macrophage and T-cell recruitment in mdx skeletal muscle. Neuromuscul Disord 2003a;13:223.

Porter JD, Khanna S, Kaminski HJ, et al. A chronic inflammatory response dominates the skeletal muscle molecular signature in dystrophin-deficient mdx mice. Hum Mol Genet 2002;11:263.

Porter JD, Merriam AP, Leahy P, et al. Dissection of temporal gene expression signatures of affected and spared muscle groups in dystrophin-deficient (mdx) mice. Hum Mol Genet 2003b;12:1813.

Pulido SM, Passaquin AC, Leijendekker WJ, et al. Creatine supplementation improves intracellular Ca^{2+} handling and survival in mdx skeletal muscle cells. FEBS Lett 1998;439:357.

Rae C, Scott RB, Thompson CH, et al. Brain biochemistry in Duchenne muscular dystrophy: A 1H magnetic resonance and neuropsychological study. J Neurol Sci 1998;160:148.

Raffaele Di Barletta M, Ricci E. Galluzzi G, et al. Different mutations in the LMNA gene cause autosomal dominant and autosomal recessive Emery-Dreifuss muscular dystrophy. Am J Hum Genet 2000;66:1407.

Ragusa RJ, Chow CK, Porter JD. Oxidative stress as a potential pathogenic mechanism in an animal model of Duchenne muscular dystrophy. Neuromuscul Disord 1997;7:379.

Rando TA. The dystrophin-glycoprotein complex, cellular signaling, and the regulation of cell survival in the muscular dystrophies. Muscle Nerve 2001a;24:1575.

Rando TA. Role of nitric oxide in the pathogenesis of muscular dystrophies: A "two hit" hypothesis of the cause of muscle necrosis. Microsc Res Tech 2001b;55:223.

Rando TA. Oxidative stress and the pathogenesis of muscular dystrophies. Am J Phys Med Rehabil 2002;81 (11 Suppl):S175.

Rando TA, Disatnik MH, Yu Y, et al. Muscle cells from mdx mice have an increased susceptibility to oxidative stress. Neuromuscul Disord 1998;8:14.

Rando TA, Disatnik MH, Zhou LZ. Rescue of dystrophin expression in mdx mouse muscle by RNA/DNA oligonucleotides. Proc Natl Acad Sci U S A 2000;97:5363.

Rapaport D, Lederfein D, den Dunnen JT, et al. Characterization and cell type distribution of a novel, major transcript of the Duchenne muscular dystrophy gene. Differentiation 1992;49:187.

Ray PN, Belfall B, Duff C, et al. Cloning of the breakpoint of an X;21 translocation associated with Duchenne muscular dystrophy. Nature 1985;318:672.

Rey MA, Davies PL. The protease core of the muscle-specific calpain, p94, undergoes Ca^{2+}-dependent intramolecular autolysis. FEBS Lett 2002;532:401.

Richard I, Brenguier L, Dincer P, et al. Multiple independent molecular etiology for limb-girdle muscular dystrophy type 2A patients from various geographical origins. Am J Hum Genet 1997;60:1128.

Richard I, Broux O, Allamand V, et al. Mutations in the proteolytic enzyme calpain 3 cause limb-girdle muscular dystrophy type 2A. Cell 1995;81:27.

Rideau Y, Glorion B, Delaubier A, et al. The treatment of scoliosis in Duchenne muscular dystrophy. Muscle Nerve 1984;7:281.

Roccella M, Pace R, De Gregorio MT. Psychopathological assessment in children affected by Duchenne de Boulogne muscular dystrophy. Minerva Pediatr 2003;55:267.

Rose MR, Landon DN, Papadimitriou A, et al. A rapidly progressive adolescent-onset oculopharyngeal somatic syndrome with rimmed vacuoles in two siblings. Ann Neurol 1997;41:25.

Rose MR, Tawil R. Drug treatment for facioscapulohumeral muscular dystrophy. Cochrane Database Syst Rev 2004;(2):CD002276.

Rothstein TL, Carlson CB, Sumi SM. Polymyositis with facioscapulohumeral distribution. Arch Neurol 1971;25:313.

Rowland LP, Hirano M, DiMauro S, et al. Oculopharyngeal muscular dystrophy, other ocular myopathies, and progressive external ophthalmoplegia. Neuromuscul Disord 1997;7 (Suppl 1):S15.

Ruegg U, Passaquin A, Lhote P. Calcium influx inhibition by steroids and analogs in C2C12 skeletal muscle cells. Br J Pharmacol 1998;124:1751.

Ruegg UT, Gillis JM. Calcium homeostasis in dystrophic muscle. Trends Pharmacol Sci 1999;20:351.

Ruegg UT, Nicolas-Metral V, Challet C, et al. Pharmacological control of cellular calcium handling in dystrophic skeletal muscle. Neuromuscul Disord 2002;12 (Suppl 1):S155.

Rybakova IN, Amann KJ, Ervasti JM. A new model for the interaction of dystrophin with F-actin. J Cell Biol 1996;135:661.

Saenz A, Leturcq F, Cobo AM, et al. LGMD2A: Genotype-phenotype correlations based on a large mutational survey on the calpain 3 gene. Brain 2005;128:732.

Salmikangas P, van der Ven PF, Lalowski M, et al. Myotilin, the limb-girdle muscular dystrophy 1A (LGMD1A) protein, cross-links actin filaments and controls sarcomere assembly. Hum Mol Genet 2003;12:189.

Samaha FJ, Quinlan JG. Dystrophinopathies: Clarification and complication. J Child Neurol 1996;11:13.

Sander M, Chavoshan B, Harris SA, et al. Functional muscle ischemia in neuronal nitric oxide synthase-deficient skeletal muscle of children with Duchenne muscular dystrophy. Proc Natl Acad Sci U S A 2000;97:13464.

Sandri M, Carraro U, Podhorska-Okolov M, et al. Apoptosis, DNA damage and ubiquitin expression in normal and mdx muscle fibers after exercise. FEBS Lett 1995;373:291.

Sandri M, El Meslemani AH, Sandri C, et al. Caspase 3 expression correlates with skeletal muscle apoptosis in Duchenne and facioscapulo human muscular dystrophy. A potential target for pharmacological treatment? J Neuropathol Exp Neurol 2001;60:302.

Sandri M, Massimino ML, Cantini M, et al. Dystrophin deficient myotubes undergo apoptosis in mouse primary muscle cell culture after DNA damage. Neurosci Lett 1998a;252:123.

Sandri M, Minetti C, Pedemonte M, et al. Apoptotic myonuclei in human Duchenne muscular dystrophy. Lab Invest 1998b;78:1005.

Sandri M, Podhorska-Okolow M, Geromel V, et al. Exercise induces myonuclear ubiquitination and apoptosis in dystrophin-deficient muscle of mice. J Neuropathol Exp Neurol 1997;56:45.

Sansome A, Royston P, Dubowitz V. Steroids in Duchenne muscular dystrophy; pilot study of a new low-dosage schedule. Neuromuscul Disord 1993;3:567.

Scheuerbrandt G, Lundin A, Lovgren T, et al. Screening for Duchenne muscular dystrophy: An improved screening test for creatine kinase and its application in an infant screening program. Muscle Nerve 1986;9:11.

Schneiderman LJ, Sampson WI, Schoene WC, et al. Genetic studies of a family with two unusual autosomal dominant conditions: Muscular dystrophy and Pelger-Huët anomaly. Clinical, pathologic and linkage considerations. Am J Med 1969;46:380.

Schroder R, Reimann J, Salmikangas P, et al. Beyond LGMD1A: Myotilin is a component of central core lesions and nemaline rods. Neuromuscul Disord 2003;13:451.

Scott JM, Li S, Harper SQ, et al. Viral vectors for gene transfer of micro-, mini-, or full-length dystrophin. Neuromuscul Disord 2002;12 (Suppl 1):S23.

Selcen D, Engel AG. Mutations in myotilin cause myofibrillar myopathy. Neurology 2004;62:1363.

Selcen D, Ohno K, Engel AG. Myofibrillar myopathy: Clinical, morphological and genetic studies in 63 patients. Brain 2004;127 (Pt 2):439.

Selcen D, Stilling G, Engel AG. The earliest pathologic alterations in dysferlinopathy. Neurology 2001;56:1472.

Septien L, Gras P, Borsotti JP, et al. [Mental development in Duchenne muscular dystrophy. Correlation of data of the brain scanner.] Pediatrie (in French) 1991;46:817.

Shackleton S, Lloyd DJ, Jackson SN, et al. LMNA, encoding lamin A/C, is mutated in partial lipodystrophy. Nat Genet 2000;24:153.

Sharma KR, Mynhier MA, Miller RG. Cyclosporine increases muscular force generation in Duchenne muscular dystrophy. Neurology 1993;43 (3 Pt 1):527.

Shaw RA, Mantsch HH, Anderson JE. Infrared spectroscopy of dystrophic mdx mouse muscle tissue distinguishes among treatment groups. J Appl Physiol 1996;81:2328.

Sibert JR, Williams V, Burkinshaw R, et al. Swivel walkers in Duchenne muscular dystrophy. Arch Dis Child 1987;62:741.

Siegel IM. Fractures of long bones in Duchenne muscular dystrophy. J Trauma 1977;17:219.

Small RG. Coats' disease and muscular dystrophy. Trans Am Acad Ophthalmol Otolaryngol 1968;72:225.

Smith CL, Bush GH. Anaesthesia and progressive muscular dystrophy. Br J Anaesth 1985;57:1113.

Smith J, Goldsmith C, Ward A, et al. IGF-II ameliorates the dystrophic phenotype and coordinately down-regulates programmed cell death. Cell Death Differ 2000;7:1109.

Smith TA, Yau SC, Bobrow M, et al. Identification and quantification of somatic mosaicism for a point mutation in a Duchenne muscular dystrophy family. J Med Genet 1999;36:313.

Sollee ND, Latham EE, Kindlon DJ, et al. Neuropsychological impairment in Duchenne muscular dystrophy. J Clin Exp Neuropsychol 1985;7:486.

Song KS, Scherer PE, Tang Z, et al. Expression of caveolin-3 in skeletal, cardiac, and smooth muscle cells. Caveolin-3 is a component of the sarcolemma and co-fractionates with dystrophin and dystrophin-associated glycoproteins. J Biol Chem 1996;271:15160.

Spencer MJ, Guyon JR, Sorimachi H, et al. Stable expression of calpain 3 from a muscle transgene in vivo: Immature muscle in transgenic mice suggests a role for calpain 3 in muscle maturation. Proc Natl Acad Sci U S A 2002;99:8874.

Spencer MJ, Marino MW, Winckler WM. Altered pathological progression of diaphragm and quadriceps muscle in TNF-deficient, dystrophin-deficient mice. Neuromuscul Disord 2000;10:612.

Spencer MJ, Montecino-Rodriguez E, Dorshkind K, et al. Helper (CD4(+)) and cytotoxic (CD8(+)) T cells promote the pathology of dystrophin-deficient muscle. Clin Immunol 2001;98:235.

Spencer MJ, Tidball JG. Do immune cells promote the pathology of dystrophin-deficient myopathies? Neuromuscul Disord 2001;11:556.

Spencer MJ, Walsh CM, Dorshkind KA, et al. Myonuclear apoptosis in dystrophic mdx muscle occurs by perforin-mediated cytotoxicity. J Clin Invest 1997;99:2745.

St-Pierre SJ, Chakkalakal JV, Kolodziejczyk SM, et al. Glucocorticoid treatment alleviates dystrophic myofiber pathology by activation of the calcineurin/NF-AT pathway. FASEB J 2004;18:1937.

Takahashi T, Aoki M, Tateyama M, et al. Dysferlin mutations in Japanese Miyoshi myopathy: Relationship to phenotype. Neurology 2003;60:1799.

Takeya T, Hamano K, Kawashima K, et al. [Facioscapulohumeral muscular dystrophy (FSH) and hearing loss.] No To Hattatsu (in Japanese) 1990;22:24.

Tang Z, Scherer PE, Okamoto T, et al. Molecular cloning of caveolin-3, a novel member of the caveolin gene family expressed predominantly in muscle. J Biol Chem 1996;271:2255.

Taratuto AL, Lubieniecki F, Diaz D, et al. Merosin-deficient congenital muscular dystrophy associated with abnormal cerebral cortical gyration: An autopsy study. Neuromuscul Disord 1999;9:86.

Tarnopolsky MA, Mahoney DJ, Vajsar J, et al. Creatine monohydrate enhances strength and body composition in Duchenne muscular dystrophy. Neurology 2004;62:1771.

Tateyama M, Aoki M, Nishino I, et al. Mutation in the caveolin-3 gene causes a peculiar form of distal myopathy. Neurology 2002;58:323.

Taveau M, Bourg N, Sillon G, et al. Calpain 3 is activated through autolysis within the active site and lyses sarcomeric and sarcolemmal components. Mol Cell Biol 2003;23:9127.

Tawil R, Figlewicz DA, Griggs RC, et al. Facioscapulohumeral dystrophy: A distinct regional myopathy with a novel molecular pathogenesis. FSH Consortium. Ann Neurol 1998;43:279.

Tay SK, Ong HT, Low PS. Transaminitis in Duchenne's muscular dystrophy. Ann Acad Med Singapore 2000;29:719.

Taylor DA, Carroll JE, Smith ME, et al. Facioscapulohumeral dystrophy associated with hearing loss and Coats syndrome. Ann Neurol 1982;12:395.

Taylor EW. Progressive vagus-glossopharyngeal paralysis with ptosis. Contribution to group of family diseases. J Nerv Ment Dis 1915;42:129.

Tews DS. Apoptosis and muscle fibre loss in neuromuscular disorders. Neuromuscul Disord 2002;12:613.

Tews DS, Goebel HH. Cytokine expression profile in idiopathic inflammatory myopathies. J Neuropathol Exp Neurol 1996;55:342.

Tews DS, Goebel HH. DNA-fragmentation and expression of apoptosis-related proteins in muscular dystrophies. Neuropathol Appl Neurobiol 1997;23:331.

Thomas GD, Shaul PW, Yuhanna IS, et al. Vasomodulation by skeletal muscle-derived nitric oxide requires alpha-syntrophin–mediated sarcolemmal localization of neuronal nitric oxide synthase. Circ Res 2003;92:554.

Tindall RS, Rollins JA, Phillips JT, et al. Preliminary results of a double-blind, randomized, placebo-controlled trial of cyclosporine in myasthenia gravis. N Engl J Med 1987;316:719.

Toda T, Kobayashi K, Kondo-Iida E, et al. The Fukuyama congenital muscular dystrophy story. Neuromuscul Disord 2000;10:153.

Topaloglu H, Dincer P, Richard I, et al. Calpain-3 deficiency causes a mild muscular dystrophy in childhood. Neuropediatrics 1997;28:212.

Torelli S, Brown SC, Jimenez-Mallebrera C, et al. Absence of neuronal nitric oxide synthase (nNOS) as a pathological marker for the diagnosis of Becker muscular dystrophy with rod domain deletions. Neuropathol Appl Neurobiol 2004;30:540.

Tsien F, Sun B, Hopkins NE, et al. Methylation of the FSHD syndrome–linked subtelomeric repeat in normal and FSHD cell cultures and tissues. Mol Genet Metab 2001;74:322.

Tsubata S, Bowles KR, Vatta M, et al. Mutations in the human delta-sarcoglycan gene in familial and sporadic dilated cardiomyopathy. J Clin Invest 2000;106:655.

Tuffery-Giraud S, Chambert S, Demaille J, et al. [Genotypic diagnosis of Duchenne and Becker muscular dystrophies.] Ann Biol Clin (Paris) (in French) 1999a;57:417.

Tuffery-Giraud S, Chambert S, Demaille J, et al. Point mutations in the dystrophin gene: Evidence for frequent use of cryptic splice sites as a result of splicing defects. Hum Mutat 1999b;14:359.

Turner PR, Schultz R, Ganguly B, et al. Proteolysis results in altered leak channel kinetics and elevated free calcium in mdx muscle. J Membr Biol 1993;133:243.

Twyman RS, Harper GD, Edgar MA. Thoracoscapular fusion in facioscapulohumeral dystrophy: Clinical review of a new surgical method. J Shoulder Elbow Surg 1996;5:201.

Udd B, Vihola A, Sarparanta J, et al. Titinopathies and extension of the M-line mutation phenotype beyond distal myopathy and LGMD2J. Neurology 2005;64:636.

Ueyama H, Kumamoto T, Horinouchi H, et al. Clinical heterogeneity in dysferlinopathy. Intern Med 2002;41:532.

Upadhyaya M, Maynard J, Rogers MT, et al. Improved molecular diagnosis of facioscapulohumeral muscular dystrophy (FSHD): Validation of the differential double digestion for FSHD. J Med Genet 1997;34:476.

Vachon PH, Loechel F, Xu H, et al. Merosin and laminin in myogenesis; Specific requirement for merosin in myotube stability and survival. J Cell Biol 1996;134:1483.

Vainzof M, Anderson LVB, Moreira ES. Characterization of the primary defect in LGMD 2A and analysis of its secondary effect in other LGMDs. Neurology 2000a;54(A):436.

Vainzof M, de Paula F, Tsanaclis AM, et al. The effect of calpain 3 deficiency on the pattern of muscle degeneration in the earliest stages of LGMD2A. J Clin Pathol 2003;56:624.

Vainzof M, Moreira ES, Canovas M, et al. Partial alpha-sarcoglycan deficiency with retention of the dystrophin-glycoprotein complex in a LGMD2D family. Muscle Nerve 2000b;23:984.

Vainzof M, Passos-Bueno MR, Canovas M, et al. The sarcoglycan complex in the six autosomal recessive limb-girdle muscular dystrophies. Hum Mol Genet 1996;5:1963.

Vainzof M, Passos-Bueno MR, Pavanello RC, et al. Sarcoglycanopathies are responsible for 68% of severe autosomal recessive limb-girdle muscular dystrophy in the Brazilian population. J Neurol Sci 1999;164:44.

Valle G, Faulkner G, De Antoni A, et al. Telethonin, a novel sarcomeric protein of heart and skeletal muscle. FEBS Lett 1997;415:163.

van der Maarel SM, Deidda G, Lemmers RJ, et al. A new dosage test for subtelomeric 4;10 translocations improves conventional diagnosis of facioscapulohumeral muscular dystrophy (FSHD). J Med Genet 1999;36:823.

van Deutekom JC, Bakker E, Lemmers RJ, et al. Evidence for subtelomeric exchange of 3.3 kb tandemly repeated units between chromosomes 4q35 and 10q26: Implications for genetic counselling and etiology of FSHD1. Hum Mol Genet 1996;5:1997.

van Essen AJ, Busch HF, te Meerman GJ, et al. Birth and population prevalence of Duchenne muscular dystrophy in The Netherlands. Hum Genet 1992;88:258.

Vandebrouck C, Duport G, Raymond G, et al. Hypotonic medium increases calcium permeant channels activity in human normal and dystrophic myotubes. Neurosci Lett 2002a;323:239.

Vandebrouck C, Martin D, Colson-Van Schoor M, et al. Involvement of TRPC in the abnormal calcium influx observed in dystrophic (mdx) mouse skeletal muscle fibers. J Cell Biol 2002b;158:1089.

Vanegas OC, Zhang RZ, Sabatelli P, et al. Novel COL6A1 splicing mutation in a family affected by mild Bethlem myopathy. Muscle Nerve 2002;25:513.

Vassilopoulos D, Emery AE. Muscle nuclear changes in fetuses at risk for Duchenne muscular dystrophy. J Med Genet 1977;14:13.

Vianello A, Bevilacqua M, Salvador V, et al. Long-term nasal intermittent positive pressure ventilation in advanced Duchenne's muscular dystrophy. Chest 1994;105:445.

Villanova M, Sewry C, Malandrini A, et al. Immunolocalization of several laminin chains in the normal human central and peripheral nervous system. J Submicrosc Cytol Pathol 1997;29:409.

Voit T, Lamprecht A, Lenard HG, et al. Hearing loss in facioscapulohumeral dystrophy. Eur J Pediatr 1986;145:280.

von Moers A, Zwirner A, Reinhold A, et al. Increased mRNA expression of tissue inhibitors of metalloproteinase-1 and -2 in Duchenne muscular dystrophy. Acta Neuropathol (Berl) 2005;109:285.

Wagner KR, Hamed S, Hadley DW, et al. Gentamicin treatment of Duchenne and Becker muscular dystrophy due to nonsense mutations. Ann Neurol 2001;49:706.

Wahi PL, Bhargava KC, Mohindra S. Cardiorespiratory changes in progressive muscular dystrophy. Br Heart J 1971;33:533.

Wallgren-Pettersson C, Bushby K, Mellies U, et al. 117th ENMC workshop: Ventilatory support in congenital neuromuscular disorders—Congenital myopathies, congenital muscular dystrophies, congenital myotonic dystrophy and SMA (II) 4-6 April 2003, Naarden, The Netherlands. Neuromuscul Disord 2004;14:56.

Walter MC, Lochmuller H, Reilich P, et al. Creatine monohydrate in muscular dystrophies: A double-blind, placebo-controlled clinical study. Neurology 2000;54:1848.

Walter MC, Petersen JA, Stucka R, et al. FKRP (826C>A) frequently causes limb-girdle muscular dystrophy in German patients. J Med Genet 2004;41:e50.

Wang B, Li J, Xiao X. Adeno-associated virus vector carrying human minidystrophin genes effectively ameliorates muscular dystrophy in mdx mouse model. Proc Natl Acad Sci U S A 2000;97:13714.

Watkins SC, Cullen MJ, Hoffman EP, et al. Plasma membrane cytoskeleton of muscle: A fine structural analysis. Microsc Res Tech 2000;48:131.

Watkins SC, Hoffman EP, Slayter HS, et al. Immunoelectron microscopic localization of dystrophin in myofibres. Nature 1988;333:863.

Wells KE, Fletcher S, Mann CJ, et al. Enhanced in vivo delivery of antisense oligonucleotides to restore dystrophin expression in adult mdx mouse muscle. FEBS Lett 2003;552:145.

Wershil BK, Furuta GT, Lavigne JA, et al. Dexamethasone and cyclosporin A suppress mast cell–leukocyte cytokine cascades by multiple mechanisms. Int Arch Allergy Immunol 1995;107:323.

White S, Kalf M, Liu Q, et al. Comprehensive detection of genomic duplications and deletions in the DMD gene, by use of multiplex amplifiable probe hybridization. Am J Hum Genet 2002;71:365.

Wicksell RK, Kihlgren M, Melin L, et al. Specific cognitive deficits are common in children with Duchenne muscular dystrophy. Dev Med Child Neurol 2004;46:154.

Wijmenga C, Frants RR, Hewitt JE, et al. Molecular genetics of facioscapulohumeral muscular dystrophy. Neuromuscul Disord 1993;3:487.

Winnard AV, Mendell JR, Prior TW, et al. Frameshift deletions of exons 3-7 and revertant fibers in Duchenne muscular dystrophy: Mechanisms of dystrophin production. Am J Hum Genet 1995;56:158.

Winokur ST, Bengtsson U, Feddersen J, et al. The DNA rearrangement associated with facioscapulohumeral muscular dystrophy involves a heterochromatin-associated repetitive element: Implications for a role of chromatin structure in the pathogenesis of the disease. Chromosome Res 1994;2:225.

Witte RA. The psychosocial impact of a progressive physical handicap and terminal illness (Duchenne muscular dystrophy) on adolescents and their families. Br J Med Psychol 1985;58 (Pt 2):179.

Woods CE, Novo D, DiFranco M, et al. The action potential-evoked sarcoplasmic reticulum calcium release is impaired in mdx mouse muscle fibres. J Physiol 2004;557 (Pt 1):59.

Wrogemann K, Pena SD. Mitochondrial calcium overload: A general mechanism for cell-necrosis in muscle diseases. Lancet 1976;1:672.

Yamanaka G, Goto K, Ishihara T, et al. FSHD-like patients without 4q35 deletion. J Neurol Sci 2004;219:89.

Yamaoka LH, Westbrook CA, Speer MC, et al. Development of a microsatellite genetic map spanning 5q31-q33 and subsequent placement of the LGMD1A locus between D5S178 and IL9. Neuromuscul Disord 1994;4:471.

Yamashita T, Kanaya K, Kawaguchi S, et al. Prediction of progression of spinal deformity in Duchenne muscular dystrophy: A preliminary report. Spine 2001a;26:E223.

Yamashita T, Kanaya K, Yokogushi K, et al. Correlation between progression of spinal deformity and pulmonary function in Duchenne muscular dystrophy. J Pediatr Orthop 2001b;21:113.

Yamazaki M, Minota S, Sakurai H, et al. Expression of transforming growth factor-beta 1 and its relation to endomysial fibrosis in progressive muscular dystrophy. Am J Pathol 1994;144:221.

Yau SC, Bobrow M, Mathew CG, et al. Accurate diagnosis of carriers of deletions and duplications in Duchenne/Becker muscular dystrophy by fluorescent dosage analysis. J Med Genet 1996;33:550.

Yeung EW, Allen DG. Stretch-activated channels in stretch-induced muscle damage: Role in muscular dystrophy. Clin Exp Pharmacol Physiol 2004;31:551.

Yeung EW, Head SI, Allen DG. Gadolinium reduces short-term stretch-induced muscle damage in isolated mdx mouse muscle fibres. J Physiol 2003;552 (Pt 2):449.

Yeung EW, Whitehead NP, Suchyna TM, et al. Effects of stretch-activated channel blockers on [Ca^{2+}]i and muscle damage in the mdx mouse. J Physiol 2005;562 (Pt 2):367.

Yilmaz O, Karaduman A, Topaloglu H. Prednisolone therapy in Duchenne muscular dystrophy prolongs ambulation and prevents scoliosis. Eur J Neurol 2004;11:541.

Yoshioka M, Itagaki Y, Saida K, et al. Clinical and genetic studies of muscular dystrophy in young girls. Clin Genet 1986;29:137.

Zamora S, Adams C, Butzner JD, et al. Elevated aminotransferase activity as an indication of muscular dystrophy: Case reports and review of the literature. Can J Gastroenterol 1996;10:389.

Zanardi MC, Tagliabue A, Orcesi S, et al. Body composition and energy expenditure in Duchenne muscular dystrophy. Eur J Clin Nutr 2003;57:273.

Zatz M, de Paula F, Starling A, et al. The 10 autosomal recessive limb-girdle muscular dystrophies. Neuromuscul Disord 2003;13:532.

Zatz M, Marie SK, Cerqueira A, et al. The facioscapulohumeral muscular dystrophy (FSHD1) gene affects males more severely and more frequently than females. Am J Med Genet 1998;77:155.

Zatz M, Marie SK, Passos-Bueno MR, et al. High proportion of new mutations and possible anticipation in Brazilian facioscapulohumeral muscular dystrophy families. Am J Hum Genet 1995;56:99.

Zatz M, Passos-Bueno MR, Rapaport D. Estimate of the proportion of Duchenne muscular dystrophy with autosomal recessive inheritance. Am J Med Genet 1989;32:407.

Zhang RZ, Sabatelli P, Pan TC, et al. Effects on collagen VI mRNA stability and microfibrillar assembly of three COL6A2 mutations in two families with Ullrich congenital muscular dystrophy. J Biol Chem 2002;277:43557.

Zhao Y, Haginoya K, Sun G, et al. Platelet-derived growth factor and its receptors are related to the progression of human muscular dystrophy: An immunohistochemical study. J Pathol 2003;201:149.

Zubrzycka-Gaarn EE, Bulman DE, Karpati G, et al. The Duchenne muscular dystrophy gene product is localized in sarcolemma of human skeletal muscle. Nature 1988;333:466.

CHAPTER 80

Congenital Myopathies

Jonathan B. Strober

The congenital myopathies are a group of disorders characterized by their histopathologic findings on muscle biopsy. The discovery of this heterogeneous group grew out of the ability to investigate abnormal muscle by histochemical techniques introduced in the 1950s and 1960s [Jungbluth et al., 2003]. Since then, electron microscopy, proteomics, and genomics have expanded the understanding of these conditions, as well as complicated physicians' ability to create a simple classification schema.

The majority of these conditions manifest at or shortly after birth with hypotonia, static or nonprogressive muscle weakness, normal to decreased deep tendon reflexes, and delays in reaching milestones [Riggs et al., 2003; Taratuto, 2002]. They can also become manifest in late childhood or adulthood. Patients may have a mildly progressive course or may even be asymptomatic when presenting later in life [Riggs et al., 2003]. The serum creatine kinase level is typically normal or mildly elevated, and electromyography often reveals a myopathic pattern: namely, short, small-action potentials with rapid recruitment. A muscle biopsy is usually necessary to classify the condition and improve the clinician's ability to prognosticate for the patient and family. The findings commonly seen in the biopsy include type I fiber predominance or hypotrophy, or both, with the absence of fiber necrosis and other evidence of chronic degeneration, such as endomysial fibrosis and fatty infiltration, findings typically seen in muscular dystrophies. Protein aggregation, often of defective proteins, then allows for final classification. Overall, there are no cures for these conditions, but supportive care is important for quality of life and longevity.

The more common and better known congenital myopathies are central core disease, nemaline myopathy, and myotubular myopathy. These are discussed in this chapter, along with some of the rarer disorders that have been described.

CENTRAL CORE DISEASE

Central core disease was the first congenital myopathy described by Magee and Shy [1956]. It was named from the round delineated areas, typically within type I muscle fibers, that are devoid of oxidative enzyme activity [Jungbluth et al., 2003; Quinlivan et al., 2003; Taratuto, 2002].

Clinical Features

In addition to the hypotonia, muscle weakness (which typically affects the pelvic girdle), and developmental delay, children often present with skeletal deformities such as scoliosis, congenital hip dislocation, and pes cavus [Jungbluth et al., 2003; Quinlivan et al., 2003; Taratuto, 2002]. Facial weakness can also be present, is usually mild, and may be seen only in the inability to bury the eyelashes completely [De Cauwer et al., 2002; Jungbluth et al., 2003]. It mainly manifests in infancy or early childhood, although it can appear later in life or even never. The weakness tends to be static or slowly progressive. Many patients are eventually able to walk, and some families may report muscle cramping [Jungbluth et al., 2003]. It is allelic with malignant hyperthermia [Quinlivan et al., 2003]. The serum creatine kinase level tends to be normal to mildly elevated.

Pathology

Muscle biopsy specimens from patients with central core disease demonstrate type I fiber predominance, with cores seen in the center of many type 1 fibers that extend throughout a large part of the fiber's length [Jungbluth et al., 2003; Taratuto, 2002]. The cores are most easily seen when stained with the nicotinamide adenine dinucleotide–tetrazolium reductase technique [Riggs et al., 2003].

The 1995 diagnostic criteria created by the European Neuromuscular Centre include the presence of cores, which are central, although they may be eccentric or multiple, and well demarcated, visible with oxidative stains and affecting only type 1 fibers [De Cauwer et al., 2002]. Histologic diagnosis also requires distinctive electron microscopy and a type 1 fiber predominance. Corelike lesions can also be seen with denervation and are called targetoid lesions or targets if they are trilayered [Goebel, 2003]. Various proteins have been found to accumulate within cores (Table 80-1), and this often helps differentiate central core disease from mini-core disease, which is discussed later.

Genetics

Central core disease is most commonly an autosomal-dominant condition with variable penetrance; however, sporadic cases have been reported [Jungbluth et al., 2003; Riggs et al., 2003; Taratuto, 2002]. It has been mapped to chromosome region 19q12-p13.1 [Fananapazir et al., 1993; Haan et al., 1990; Monnier et al., 2000; Tilgen, et al., 2001], which is also associated with malignant hyperthermia. This locus is linked to a ryanodine receptor (RYR1), which is a ligand-gated release channel for calcium [McCarthy et al., 2000], mediating calcium release after sarcolemma depolarization [Taratuto, 2002]. Mutations in this gene can give rise to malignant hyperthermia, central core disease, or both and account for almost 80% of cases of central core disease [Taratuto, 2002]. There are three regions on the RYR1 gene where mutations have been found. The majority of lesions are found in regions 1 and 2, which reside in the myoplasmic foot domain [Tilgen et al., 2001]. Mutations have more recently been reported in region 3, which is located in the highly conserved transmembrane C-terminal region. A mutation in this region has been found in a French family with a severe form of the disease with malignant hyperthermia and cores and rods in muscle fibers on biopsy [Monnier et al., 2000]. Central core disease has also been reported with hypertrophic cardiomyopathy, but not malignant hyperthermia, and found to result from a mutation in β-myosin heavy gene [Fananapazir et al., 1993].

MULTI-MINI-CORE DISEASE

Multi-mini-core disease is histologically similar to central core disease; however, there are many significant differences. It was first described by Engel and associates in 1971 and is characterized by multiple small areas of sarcomeric disorganization lacking oxidative activity [Ferreiro and Fardeau, 2002].

Clinical Features

There are four phenotypic groups identified, all of which are characterized by approximately normal creatine kinase levels, myopathic findings on electromyography, and no cardiac involvement [Ferreiro and Fardeau, 2002]. Patients typically present at birth or within the first 18 months of life. The classic form, or first group, manifests with severe neonatal hypotonia; predominant axial muscle weakness, especially in neck flexors; delayed motor development; severe scoliosis; and significant respiratory involvement. Its characteristics are similar to those of congenital muscular dystrophy with early rigidity of the spine (RSMD1) [Jungbluth et al., 2003]. Limb joint hyperlaxity and myopia have been found in many of the patients [Ferreiro and Fardeau, 2002; Taratuto, 2002]. The second group, or ophthalmoplegia form, consists of the typical findings plus variable ophthalmoplegia and often severe facial weakness. The third group manifests with early onset and arthrogryposis, and the fourth group is characterized by slow progression and hand amyotrophy.

Pathology

There are several pathologic differences between central core and mini-core disease. In multi-mini-core disease, the lesions tend to have poorly defined boundaries and are short; thus, longitudinal muscle sections must be evaluated to help differentiate the two conditions. Mini-cores are found in both fiber types, as opposed to just type 1 fibers in central core disease [Ferreiro and Fardeau, 2002], and contain different proteins (see Table 80-1) [Goebel, 2003].

Genetics

These disorders are mostly autosomal recessive, but many sporadic cases have been reported [Jungbluth et al., 2003]. Recessive mutations have been found in the *RYR1* gene in patients with group 3 disease [Jungbluth et al., 2002] and in one family with distal weakness and amyotrophy [Ferreiro et al., 2002a]. Patients with the classic form have been found to have recessive mutations in the selenoprotein N gene [Ferreiro et al., 2002b] and in the RSMD1 gene [Moghadaszadeh et al., 2001]. Selenoprotein N is a glycoprotein found in the endoplasmic reticulum, expressed mostly in fetal tissues and in dividing cells [Petit et al., 2003].

TABLE 80-1

Protein Accumulation in Core Disease

Central Core Disease	
Actin	Gelsolin
α-Actin	Myosin (slow)
α_1-antichymotrypsin	Neural cell adhesion molecule
β-Amyloid precursor protein	Nebulin
β_2-Microglobulin	Tau
Caveolin	Tubulin
Desmin	Ubiquitin
Dysferlin	Utrophin
Dystrophin	Vimentin
Mini-Core Disease	
αB-crystallin	
Desmin	
γ-Filamin/filamin 2C	
Myozenin/calsarcin	
Telethonin	

Adapted from Goebel HH. Congenital myopathies at their molecular dawning. Muscle Nerve 2003;27:527.

NEMALINE MYOPATHY

Nemaline myopathy was the second congenital myopathy to be reported. Its classification system has undergone a dramatic change as a result of advances in molecular genetics, and six different clinical forms can be identified [Goebel, 2003].

Clinical Features

The severe congenital form manifests with no spontaneous movements or respirations at birth and may be associated with contractures and congenital fractures [Wallgren-Pettersson and Laing, 2000]. The fetal akinesia sequence has been reported to be associated with intrauterine onset [Lammens et al., 1997]. High-arched palate [Taratuto, 2002], cardiomyopathy, and ophthalmoplegia have also been associated with this form [Wallgren-Pettersson and Laing, 2000]. Children affected with the intermediate congenital type are able to breathe and move at birth, but during early childhood they become unable to breathe independently and typically cannot sit or walk [Wallgren-Pettersson and Laing, 2000]. Contractures tend to develop early. The typical form manifests in early childhood with proximal weakness, especially in neck flexors, in association with facial, bulbar, and respiratory weakness [Wallgren-Pettersson and Laing, 2000]. Distal involvement can occur later, but affected children are able to reach their milestones, albeit delayed, and have a slowly progressive or even nonprogressive course [Wallgren-Pettersson and Laing, 2000]. The mild childhood or juvenile form is similar to the classic form without facial weakness [Goebel, 2003]. There is also an adult-onset form and other, less common forms that may manifest with an unusual distribution of weakness [Wallgren-Pettersson and Laing, 2000].

Pathology

Nemaline myopathy is histopathologically characterized through the use of the Gomori trichrome technique by red staining "rods" that are predominantly subsarcolemmal [Jungbluth et al., 2003], although they can be intermyofibrillar or intranuclear and are reactive to α-actin [Taratuto, 2002]. They are associated with the Z-disk and often are in continuity with the Z-lines [Jungbluth et al., 2003; Riggs et al., 2003]. They have a similar lattice structure and are composed of filaments. There is no correlation between the amount of rods seen and the severity of the condition [Jungbluth et al., 2003; Taratuto, 2002]. The rods can be seen solely in type I fibers or in both fiber types and measure 2 to 7 mm in length [Riggs et al., 2003]. These findings are typically in conjunction with type 1 fiber predominance or type 1 fiber hypotrophy, or both.

Genetics

Currently, five filament encoding genes have been found to carry mutations. The rods have been found to be morphologically the same among all types [Goebel, 2003]. The most common mutations have been found in the α-actin and nebulin genes. α-Actin gene mutations, which account for 10% to 20% of cases [Taratuto, 2002], are frequently reported in the severe cases [Wallgren-Pettersson and Laing, 2001], although the presentation in patients with these mutations is heterogeneous [Agrawal et al., 2004]. Autosomal-dominant and -recessive forms have also been described [Nowak et al., 1999]. The α-actin gene is at chromosome 1q42.1 [Goebel, 2003; Taratuto, 2002], and most cases are sporadic [Agrawal et al., 2004]. Nebulin gene mutations have also been reported in the severe congenital form [Wallgren-Pettersson et al., 2002]. The nebulin gene is located on chromosome region 2q21.2-q22 [Pelin et al., 1999]. Mutations are usually recessive and are associated with the typical form [Jungbluth et al., 2003; Wallgren-Pettersson and Laing, 2003].

The first genetic locus to be reported in nemaline myopathy is in the slow α-tropomyosin gene, found on chromosome region 1q21-q23 [Laing et al., 1992, 1995]. It, along with β-tropomyosin, are actin-related skeletal muscle fiber proteins [Goebel, 2003]. α-Tropomyosin gene mutations [Laing et al., 1995] and, less frequently, β-tropomyosin gene mutations are located on 9p13.2-p13.1 [Donner et al., 2002] and have been reported in the mild form. The often fatal infantile autosomal-recessive type has been associated with a mutation in the troponin T1 gene on chromosome 19q13.4 in an Amish population [Johnston et al., 2000]. Troponins are a component of the actin filaments [Goebel, 2003]. Finally, an autosomal-dominant phenotype consisting of muscle slowness and proximal muscle weakness with associated corelike lesions on muscle biopsy was found in a Dutch family [Gommans et al., 2002] and has been linked to chromosome region 15q21-q23 [Gommans et al., 2003]. However, no disease-associated mutations in the α-tropomyosin-1 gene, which is located within the critical region, could be found.

Management

Nemaline myopathy is the only myopathy in this group with a possible treatment apart from supportive care. L-Tyrosine has been reported to improve certain clinical aspects of patients with this condition [Wallgren-Pettersson and Laing, 2003]. Tyrosine treatment appears to diminish drooling and increase appetite and physical activity level. These symptoms returned on cessation of the supplement and were again controlled with reinstituting the treatment. Tyrosine is a nonessential amino acid required in the synthesis of catecholamines, which possibly helps explain the benefits seen from supplementation. Several trials evaluating the benefits of tyrosine in patients with nemaline myopathy are currently in progress.

CENTRONUCLEAR/MYOTUBULAR MYOPATHY

Myotubular (centronuclear) myopathy is likely the most severe of all the congenital myopathies, and the majority of cases are X-linked autosomal-recessive [Taratuto, 2002]. Pathologically, there are numerous centrally located nuclei in muscle fibers, which appear similar to the myotube, the immature stage of the muscle fiber [Goebel, 2003]. It is this appearance that led to the name *myotubular myopathy* [Spiro et al., 1966], and later *centronuclear myopathy* [Sher et al., 1967].

Clinical Features

Respiratory failure typically leads to death within the first year of life [Taratuto, 2002] and often necessitates ventilatory dependence [Bertini et al., 2004]. Milder forms with the development of spontaneous breathing have been reported [Barth and Dubowitz, 1998]. Associated conditions include polyhydramnios, reduced to absent fetal movements, severe hypotonia, and limited extraocular movements [Jungbluth et al., 2003; Taratuto, 2002]. It appears to be a nonprogressive condition; however, affected infants do not exhibit progress in motor developmental milestones [Jungbluth et al., 2003]. Female carriers are usually asymptomatic [Taratuto, 2002], although they can develop early limb-girdle weakness with secondary kyphoscoliosis. Facial weakness and dysarthria can develop. These findings are more likely caused by an abnormal expression or distribution of myotubularin, the abnormal protein leading to this condition, rather than by X-inactivation [Sutton et al., 2001]. Other clinical courses have been described. Patients with onset during late infancy or childhood present with weakness that includes the extraocular muscles, hypotonia, and delayed achievement of milestones [Riggs et al., 2003]. Other patients present in adulthood with mild-to-moderate lower extremity weakness.

Pathology

Muscle nuclei, which normally are peripherally placed, are found displaced centrally in a large number of muscle fibers in patients with this disorder. Perinuclear halos—areas with absence of myofilaments—often surround these central nuclei [Jungbluth et al., 2003]. As with the other myopathies in this category, type 1 fiber predominance is usually seen with type 1 fiber hypotrophy. Central nuclei can be seen in just type 1 fibers or in both fiber types [Riggs et al., 2003]. Although the disorder has been named after the similar appearance that muscle fibers seen on biopsy samples have to fetal myotubes, studies have demonstrated the presence of mature myofibrillar proteins [Jungbluth et al., 2003].

Genetics

The severe form of this disorder tends to arise from mutations in the myotubularin gene on chromosome Xq28 [Laporte et al., 1996] and likely accounts for up to 80% of X-linked cases [Laporte et al., 2000]. Myotubularin is a tyrosine phosphatase [Laporte et al., 1996] that dephosphorylates phosphatidylinositol-3-phosphate, a second messenger, and exerts its effects during myogenesis by regulating cellular levels of this lipid [Taylor et al., 2000]. Most mutations lead to absence or inactivation of myotubularin [Bertini et al., 2004]. Eight other forms of myotubularin have been reported [Goebel, 2003], and mutations in one have been found in patients with one of the demyelinating forms of Charcot-Marie-Tooth disease [Bolino et al., 2000; Houlden et al., 2001]. Autosomal-dominant forms, which tend to be milder and manifest later in life, and autosomal-recessive forms, with variable manifestation from mild generalized weakness with external ophthalmoplegia to early onset with severe proximal muscle weakness, have also been reported in myotubular myopathy [Jungbluth et al., 2003].

FIBER TYPE DISPROPORTION MYOPATHY

Case reports of patients with presentations similar to the congenital myopathies and the finding of type 1 fibers being at least 12% smaller than type 2 fibers were published in the 1960s and 1970s [Clarke and North, 2003]. The term *congenital fiber type disproportion* was then coined by Brooke [1973]. However, since then, these pathologic findings have been reported in the other congenital myopathies and in myotonic dystrophy, other myopathies, neuropathies, and central nervous system disorders [Clarke and North, 2003; Imoto and Nonaka, 2001; Taratuto, 2002] (Table 80-2). This condition should therefore be diagnosed only through exclusion, if at all.

Clinical Features

Overall, children with a diagnosis of this condition tend to have proximal and limb-girdle static weakness in association with myopathic facies and high-arched palate [Clarke and North, 2003]. Most cases have a mild-to-moderate course, although severe cases have been reported. There is often a positive family history of this condition, but the disease can also be sporadic.

TABLE 80-2

More Common Causes of Fiber Size Disproportion

Congenital myopathies	Spinal muscular atrophy
Muscular dystrophies	Cerebral malformations
Mitochondrial myopathies	Spinocerebellar degeneration
Arthrogryposis multiplex congenita	Perinatal asphyxia
Peripheral neuropathies	Globoid cell leukodystrophy

Adapted from Clarke NF, North KN. Congenital fiber type disproportion—30 years on. J Neuropathol Exp Neurol 2003;62:977.

OTHER STRUCTURAL CONGENITAL MYOPATHIES

Many other forms of congenital myopathy have been reported over the years as resulting from abnormal structural arrangements seen on biopsy (Table 80-3). Some have emerged as a result of the presence of intracytoplasmic inclusions or aggregates of filaments, whereas others have been characterized by vacuolated areas. As knowledge of the proteins involved in muscle structure and function increases, investigators have been able to determine the underlying etiology for some of these conditions. Cases of congenital myopathy with unusual inclusions previously reported include zebra bodies, which are a nonspecific finding in muscle at the myotendinous junction and in extraocular muscles; cylindric spirals; caps; and reducing bodies, which have also been observed in a congenital myopathy with rigid spine [Taratuto, 2002]. Several other myopathies that contain inclusions are described as follows.

Desminopathies

Desmin is a 52-kDa chief intermediate filament of skeletal and cardiac muscle [Dalakas et al., 2000] that has been found to accumulate in a group of myopathies known as myofibrillar myopathies [Taratuto, 2002]. These aggregates appear as cytoplasmic, sarcoplasmic, and spheroid bodies and can also be seen as granulofilamentous material [Goebel, 2003; Taratuto, 2002]. Several structural desmin-related myopathies have also been discovered and include αB-crystallinopathy, hereditary inclusion body myopathies, and possibly hyaline body myopathy [Goebel and Fardeau, 2002].

TABLE 80-3

Congenital Myopathy Genetics

CONGENITAL MYOPATHY	INHERITANCE	LOCUS	PROTEIN
Myotubular myopathy	XR	Xq28	Myotubularin
Central core	AD	19q13.1	Skeletal muscle ryanodine receptor
Nemaline myopathy	AD (NEM1)	1q21-q23	α-Tropomyosin
	AR (NEM2)	2q21.2-q22	Nebulin
	AR	19q13.4	Troponin T1
	AD	9p13.2-p13.1	β-Tropomyosin
(Actinopathy)	AD and AR	1q42.1	α-Actin, skeletal muscle

AD, autosomal dominant; AR, autosomal recessive; XR, X-linked recessive.

Clinical Features

Desminopathies typically manifest with distal muscle weakness. Cardiac conduction defects may be present, as may a cardiomyopathy [Taratuto, 2002]. When a cardiomyopathy was present, granulofilamentous material was seen on muscle biopsy [Goebel, 2003]. Peripheral neuropathy can accompany these features as well, and giant axons resulting from neurofilament accumulation are seen on nerve biopsy [Goebel, 2003]. The protein aggregates of desmin, which have been found to be hyperphosphorylated [Goebel, 2003], are typically surrounded by areas lacking oxidative enzymes [Taratuto, 2002]. Autosomal-dominant and -recessive types have been reported [Goebel and Fardeau, 2002; Taratuto, 2002]. The desmin gene maps to chromosome 2q35 [Viegas-Pequignot et al., 1989]. A desmin knockout mouse develops normally but becomes afflicted with an early skeletal and cardiac myopathy accompanied by vascular disease [Goebel, 2003].

αB-Crystallinopathy

A French family with a clinical picture suggestive of a desminopathy and accompanied by small lens opacities was found to have a mutation on chromosome 11 in a gene encoding αB-crystallin [Goebel and Fardeau, 2002], a protein that co-aggregates with desmin [Goebel, 2003]. αB-crystallin is a small heat shock protein the acts as a chaperone protein that participates in the breakdown of intracellular proteins outside of the lysosome [Goebel, 2003]. Therefore, mutated αB-crystallin would naturally lead to protein accumulation. αB-crystallin has been found in many tissues, including skeletal muscle, and lens tissue and in cardiocytes [Goebel, 2003].

Hyaline Body Myopathy

Hyaline body myopathy, which was known as myofibrillar lysis myopathy [Goebel and Fardeau, 2002], is characterized by non–membrane-bound subsarcolemmal aggregation of dense, disorganized filaments in continuity with myosin staining, also known as hyaline bodies [Goebel and Anderson, 1999; Taratuto, 2002]. These bodies are usually seen in 10% to 30 % of type 1 fibers, exhibit myosin immunoreactivity, and stain intensely with acid myosin adenosine triphosphatase [Goebel and Anderson, 1999]. Children affected with this disorder typically present with mild, nonprogressive scapuloperoneal weakness and atrophy early in life [Goebel and Anderson, 1999; Taratuto, 2002]. Most cases are sporadic, but autosomal-dominant and -recessive forms have been described [Goebel and Fardeau, 2002; Taratuto, 2002].

Myosin-Related Myopathy

Two disorders have so far been linked to mutations in the genes encoding myosin heavy chains. The first is in a Swedish family with a progressive myopathy and rimmed vacuoles, tubulofilamentous aggregates, and mini-core–like lesions. This condition was once called *hereditary inclusion body myopathy type 3* and now is known as *type 1c* [Goebel, 2003]. The gene is on chromosome 17 and encodes for myosin heavy chain IIa. Hereditary cardiomyopathies have also been associated with mutations in cardiac myosin heavy chains.

Fingerprint Body Myopathy

Fingerprint body myopathy was first described by Engel and colleagues in 1972 and manifests with early onset, limb and trunk weakness, and delayed motor development [Riggs et al., 2003]. Fingerprint bodies are identified on electron microscopy as subsarcolemmal inclusions of osmiophilic lamellae that resemble fingerprints [Goebel and Anderson, 1999; Riggs et al., 2003]. There is one case report of a pair of siblings with proximal muscle weakness and susceptibility to malignant hyperthermia who were found to have central cores in conjunction with fingerprint bodies [Stojkovic et al., 2001]. No mutations in the RYR1 gene were found. Fingerprint bodies have been reported in other muscle disorders, such as myotonic dystrophy [Tomé and Fardeau, 1973], a patient with Marfan's syndrome and slowly progressive weakness [Jadro-Santel et al., 1980], and oculopharyngeal muscular dystrophy, as well as other myopathies and neurodegenerative disorders [Riggs et al., 2003; Stojkovic et al., 2001]. They have also been found in fetal muscle, which suggests that these bodies may be transient structures of developmental significance, which could account for their infrequent occurrence in these conditions [Ambler et al., 1987].

Tubular Aggregate Myopathies

Tubular aggregates are basophilic deposits made up of fascicles of parallel tubules possibly derived from the sarcoplasmic reticulum [Riggs et al., 2003]. They have been reported to be seen in up to 98% of muscle fibers on biopsy in a family with slowly progressive weakness of the iliopsoas, deltoid, triceps, and sternocleidomastoid muscles. This condition is inherited in an autosomal-dominant fashion [Goebel and Anderson, 1999]. However, like fingerprint bodies, tubular aggregates have been reported in many other neurologic conditions, such as periodic paralyses; myalgic syndromes, in which the aggregates were in type 2 fibers; and familial myopathies, in which they were seen in both fiber types [Riggs et al., 2003].

Vacuolar Myopathy

Families have been reported with what appears to be X-linked mental retardation, cardiomyopathy, and a vacuolar myopathy [Goebel and Anderson, 1999; Muntoni et al., 1994]. Affected males developed proximal and axial muscle weakness in their teens and a cardiomyopathy in their 20s. They all had moderate-to-severe cognitive impairment. Creatine kinase values were moderately elevated, and muscle biopsy specimens revealed severe vacuolar changes in association with many fibers' having internal nuclei.

REFERENCES

Agrawal PB, Strickland CD, Midgett C, et al. Heterogeneity of nemaline myopathy cases with skeletal muscle alpha-actin gene mutations. Ann Neurol 2004;56:86.

Ambler MW, Neave C, Entwistle R. Fingerprint inclusions in normal fetal muscle. Acta Neuropathol (Berl) 1987;73:185.

Barth PG, Dubowitz V. X-linked myotubular myopathy—A long-term follow-up study. Eur J Paediatr Neurol 1998;2:49.

Bertini E, Biancalana V, Bolino A, et al. 118th ENMC International Workshop on Advances in Myotubular Myopathy. 26-28 September 2003, Naarden, The Netherlands. (5th Workshop of the International Consortium on Myotubular Myopathy). Neuromuscul Disord 2004;14:387.

Bolino A, Muglia M, Conforti FL, et al. Charcot-Marie-Tooth type 4B is caused by mutations in the gene encoding myotubularin-related protein-2. Nat Genet 2000;25:17.

Brooke MH. Congenital fiber type disproportion. In: Kakulas BA, ed. 2nd International Congress on Muscle Disease, November 22-29, 1971. Perth, Australia: Excerpta Medica, 1973;147.

Clarke NF, North KN. Congenital fiber type disproportion—30 years on. J Neuropathol Exp Neurol 2003;62:977.

Dalakas MC, Park KY, Semino-Mora C, et al. Desmin myopathy, a skeletal myopathy with cardiomyopathy caused by mutations in the desmin gene. N Engl J Med 2000;342:770.

De Cauwer H, Heytens L, Martin JJ. Workshop report of the 89th ENMC International Workshop: Central Core Disease, 19th-20th January 2001, Hilversum, The Netherlands. Neuromuscul Disord 2002;12:588.

Donner K, Ollikainen M, Ridanpaa M, et al. Mutations in the beta-tropomyosin (TPM2) gene—A rare cause of nemaline myopathy. Neuromuscul Disord 2002;12:151.

Engel AG, Angelini C, Gomez MR. Fingerprint body myopathy, a newly recognized congenital muscle disease. Mayo Clin Proc 1972;47:377.

Engel AG, Gomez MR, Groover RV. Multicore disease. A recently recognized congenital myopathy associated with multifocal degeneration of muscle fibers. Mayo Clin Proc 1971;46:666.

Fananapazir L, Dalakas MC, Cyran F, Cohn G, Epstein ND. Missense mutations in the beta-myosin heavy-chain gene cause central core disease in hypertrophic cardiomyopathy. Proc Natl Acad Sci U S A 1993;90:3993.

Ferreiro A, Fardeau M. 80th ENMC International Workshop on Multi-Minicore Disease: 1st International MmD Workshop. 12-13th May, 2000, Soestduinen, The Netherlands. Neuromuscul Disord 2002;12:60.

Ferreiro A, Monnier N, Romero NB, et al. A recessive form of central core disease, transiently presenting as multi-minicore disease, is associated with a homozygous mutation in the ryanodine receptor type 1 gene. Ann Neurol 2002a;51:750.

Ferreiro A, Quijano-Roy S, Pichereau C, et al. Mutations of the selenoprotein N gene, which is implicated in rigid spine muscular dystrophy, cause the classical phenotype of multiminicore disease: Reassessing the nosology of early-onset myopathies. Am J Hum Genet 2002b;71:739.

Goebel HH. Congenital myopathies at their molecular dawning. Muscle Nerve 2003;27:527.

Goebel HH, Anderson JR. Structural congenital myopathies (excluding nemaline myopathy, myotubular myopathy and desminopathies): 56th European Neuromuscular Centre (ENMC) sponsored International Workshop. December 12-14, 1997, Naarden, The Netherlands. Neuromuscul Disord 1999;9:50.

Goebel HH, Fardeau M. Desmin—Protein surplus myopathies, 96th European Neuromuscular Centre (ENMC)–sponsored International Workshop held 14-16 September 2001, Naarden, The Netherlands. Neuromuscul Disord 2002;12:687.

Gommans IM, Davis M, Saar K, et al. A locus on chromosome 15q for a dominantly inherited nemaline myopathy with core-like lesions. Brain 2003;126(Pt 7):1545.

Gommans IM, van Engelen BG, ter Laak HJ, et al. A new phenotype of autosomal dominant nemaline myopathy. Neuromuscul Disord 2002;12:13.

Haan EA, Freemantle CJ, McCure JA, et al. Assignment of the gene for central core disease to chromosome 19. Hum Genet 1990;86:187.

Houlden H, King RH, Wood NW, et al. Mutations in the 5 region of the myotubularin-related protein 2 (MTMR2) gene in autosomal recessive hereditary neuropathy with focally folded myelin. Brain 2001;124(Pt 5):907.

Imoto C, Nonaka I. The significance of type 1 fiber atrophy (hypotrophy) in childhood neuromuscular disorders. Brain Dev 2001;23:298.

Jadro-Santel D, Grcevic N, Dogan S, et al. Centronuclear myopathy with type I fibre hypotrophy and "fingerprint" inclusions associated with Marfan's syndrome. J Neurol Sci 1980;45:43.

Johnston JJ, Kelley RI, Crawford TO, et al. A novel nemaline myopathy in the Amish caused by a mutation in troponin T1. Am J Hum Genet 2000;67:814.

Jungbluth H, Muller CR, Halliger-Keller B, et al. Autosomal recessive inheritance of RYR1 mutations in a congenital myopathy with cores. Neurology 2002;59:284.

Jungbluth H, Sewry CA, Muntoni F. What's new in neuromuscular disorders? The congenital myopathies. Eur J Paediatr Neurol 2003;7:23.

Laing NG, Majda BT, Akkari PA, et al. Assignment of a gene (NEMI) for autosomal dominant nemaline myopathy to chromosome I. Am J Hum Genet 1992;50:576.

Laing NG, Wilton SD, Akkari PA, et al. A mutation in the alpha tropomyosin gene TPM3 associated with autosomal dominant nemaline myopathy NEM1. Nat Genet 1995;10:249.

Lammens M, Moerman P, Fryns JP, et al. Fetal akinesia sequence caused by nemaline myopathy. Neuropediatrics 1997;28:116.

Laporte J, Biancalana V, Tanner SM, et al. MTM1 mutations in X-linked myotubular myopathy. Hum Mutat 2000;15:393.

Laporte J, Hu LJ, Kretz C, et al. A gene mutated in X-linked myotubular myopathy defines a new putative tyrosine phosphatase family conserved in yeast. Nat Genet 1996;13:175.

Magee KR, Shy GM. A new congenital non-progressive myopathy. Brain 1956;79:610.

McCarthy TV, Quane KA, Lynch PJ. Ryanodine receptor mutations in malignant hyperthermia and central core disease. Hum Mutat 2000;15:410.

Moghadaszadeh B, Petit N, Jaillard C, et al. Mutations in SEPN1 cause congenital muscular dystrophy with spinal rigidity and restrictive respiratory syndrome. Nat Genet 2001;29:17.

Monnier N, Romero NB, Lerale J, et al. An autosomal dominant congenital myopathy with cores and rods is associated with a neomutation in the RYR1 gene encoding the skeletal muscle ryanodine receptor. Hum Mol Genet 2000;9:2599.

Muntoni F, Catani G, Mateddu A, et al. Familial cardiomyopathy, mental retardation and myopathy associated with desmin-type intermediate filaments. Neuromuscul Disord 1994;4:233.

Nowak KJ, Wattanasirichaigoon D, Goebel HH, et al. Mutations in the skeletal muscle alpha-actin gene in patients with actin myopathy and nemaline myopathy. Nat Genet 1999;23:208.

Pelin K, Hilpela P, Donner K, et al. Mutations in the nebulin gene associated with autosomal recessive nemaline myopathy. Proc Natl Acad Sci U S A 1999;96:2305.

Petit N, Lescure A, Rederstorff M, et al. Selenoprotein N: An endoplasmic reticulum glycoprotein with an early developmental expression pattern. Hum Mol Genet 2003;12:1045.

Quinlivan RM, Muller CR, Davis M, et al. Central core disease: Clinical, pathological, and genetic features. Arch Dis Child 2003;88:1051.

Riggs JE, Bodensteiner JB, Schochet SS Jr. Congenital myopathies/dystrophies. Neurol Clin 2003;21:779.

Sher JH, Rimalovski AB, Athanassiades TJ, Aronson SM. Familial centronuclear myopathy: A clinical and pathological study. Neurology 1967;17(8 Pt 1):727.

Spiro AJ, Shy GM, Gonatas NK. Myotubular myopathy. Persistence of fetal muscle in an adolescent boy. Arch Neurol 1966;14:1.

Stojkovic T, Maurage CA, Moerman A, et al. Congenital myopathy with central cores and fingerprint bodies in association with malignant hyperthermia susceptibility. Neuromuscul Disord 2001;11:538.

Sutton IJ, Winer JB, Norman AN, et al. Limb girdle and facial weakness in female carriers of X-linked myotubular myopathy mutations. Neurology 2001;57:900.

Taratuto AL. Congenital myopathies and related disorders. Curr Opin Neurol 2002;15:553.

Taylor GS, Maehama T, Dixon JE. Inaugural article: Myotubularin, a protein tyrosine phosphatase mutated in myotubular myopathy, dephosphorylates the lipid second messenger, phosphatidylinositol 3-phosphate. Proc Natl Acad Sci U S A 2000;97:8910.

Tilgen N, Zorzato F, Halliger-Keller B, et al. Identification of four novel mutations in the C-terminal membrane spanning domain of the ryanodine receptor 1: Association with central core disease and alteration of calcium homeostasis. Hum Mol Genet 2001;10:2879.

Tomé FM, Fardeau M. "Fingerprint inclusions" in muscle fibres in dystrophia myotonica. Acta Neuropathol (Berl) 1973;24:62.

Viegas-Pequignot E, Li ZL, Dutrillaux B, et al. Assignment of human desmin gene to band 2q35 by nonradioactive in situ hybridization. Hum Genet 1989;83:33.

Wallgren-Pettersson C, Donner K, Sewry C, et al. Mutations in the nebulin gene can cause severe congenital nemaline myopathy. Neuromuscul Disord 2002;12:674.

Wallgren-Pettersson C, Laing NG. Report of the 70th ENMC International Workshop: Nemaline myopathy, 11–13 June 1999, Naarden, The Netherlands. Neuromuscul Disord 2000;10:299.
Wallgren-Pettersson C, Laing NG. Report of the 83rd ENMC International Workshop: 4th Workshop on Nemaline Myopathy, 22–24 September 2000, Naarden, The Netherlands. Neuromuscul Disord 2001;11:589.
Wallgren-Pettersson C, Laing NG. 109th ENMC International Workshop: 5th workshop on nemaline myopathy, 11th-13th October 2002, Naarden, The Netherlands. Neuromuscul Disord 2003;13:501.

CHAPTER 81

Metabolic Myopathies

Ingrid Tein

UTILIZATION OF BIOENERGETIC SUBSTRATES IN EXERCISE

Defects of energy metabolism may profoundly disrupt the function of muscle and other highly energy-dependent tissues, such as those of the brain, nerves, heart, kidneys, liver, and bowel. The limits of energy utilization in skeletal muscle are set by the adenosine triphosphatases (ATPases), which couple muscle contraction (myosin ATPase) and ion transport (calcium and sodium, potassium ATPases) to the hydrolysis of adenosine triphosphate (ATP) to adenosine diphosphate (ADP) and inorganic phosphate [Kushmerick, 1995]. ADP and inorganic phosphate, in turn, activate energy-producing reactions that regenerate ATP. Without this, ATP stores would be exhausted in seconds. The substrates that are used to replenish ATP are determined by the intrinsic properties of these fuels and by the intensity and duration of exercise that modulates fuel selection [Astrand and Rodahl, 1986; Gollnick, 1985]. The creatine kinase reaction and anaerobic glycogenolysis are the major anaerobic sources of ADP phosphorylation. Increases in ADP and adenosine monophosphate (AMP) that occur in strenuous exercise are buffered primarily by the coupled adenylate kinase (myokinase), adenylate deaminase (myoadenylate deaminase) reactions. Anaerobic glycogenolysis and phosphocreatine hydrolysis support rates of muscle energy production that are twofold to fourfold higher than those supported by oxidative metabolism [Sahlin, 1986]. Anaerobic energy is crucial for rapid bursts of exercise and for fueling the transition from rest to exercise. The acceleration to high rates of energy production occurs instantly for ATP, in less than a second for phosphocreatine, and within seconds for anaerobic glycogenolysis. In contrast, maximal oxidative power requires from 3 minutes (with glycogen as the oxidative substrate) to 30 minutes (for peak fatty acid oxidation). Anaerobic fuels are rapidly depleted and lead to the accumulation of metabolic end products such as protons and inorganic phosphates that promote fatigue.

If exercise needs to be sustained for more than a few minutes, then oxidative phosphorylation is necessary and provides the most abundant source of ATP synthesis. Glycogen is the major endogenous oxidative fuel of skeletal muscle, whereas blood glucose and free fatty acids are the major exogenous fuels. A small percentage of muscle energy needs are supplied by amino acids, predominantly branched-chain amino acids, which are oxidized to a limited extent. Oxidative metabolism provides higher yields of ATP per mole of substrate, rising from 2 to 36 for glucose and from 3 to 37 per glycosyl unit of glycogen metabolized anaerobically rather than oxidatively. Furthermore, the metabolic end products of oxidative metabolism, namely, carbon dioxide and water, are easily removed from working muscle and do not promote fatigue. The most abundant and critical fuel for the support of prolonged, moderate exercise is lipid. Carbohydrate stores in the form of muscle and hepatic glycogen and blood glucose (derived mainly from hepatic glycogenolyis) are limited and can support high-intensity exercise for only 1 to 2 hours. However, carbohydrate, particularly muscle glycogen, is critical for normal oxidative metabolism. Glycogen supports a peak rate of oxidative phosphorylation that is about twofold greater than that for fat. Although this process is incompletely understood, it may be based on a requirement for glycogen-derived pyruvate to support optimal function of the tricarboxylic acid cycle [Gibala et al., 1997; Sahlin et al., 1990, 1995]. The proportion of carbohydrate in relation to lipid oxidation increases progressively as the intensity of the aerobic exercise increases until carbohydrate is the exclusive fuel of maximum oxidative metabolism [Sahlin, 1986; van Loon et al., 2001]. Glycogen is also able to accelerate to maximal oxidative power output more rapidly than are other fuels [Haller and Vissing, 2002; Sahlin, 1986]. Third, the molar ratio of ATP produced to oxygen consumed is higher for glycogen (6.17) and glucose (5.98) than for fatty acids (5.61) [Rennie and Edwards, 1981]. The importance of this point lies in the fact that peak oxygen utilization in healthy humans is limited by oxygen delivery [Saltin, 1988].

The combustion of fuels in oxidative metabolism involves the generation of reducing equivalents in β-oxidation, glycolysis, and the tricarboxylic acid cycle that are oxidized through the respiratory chain, in which the phosphorylation of ADP is coupled to the reduction of molecular oxygen to water. Normal oxidative metabolism requires a highly integrated physiologic support system to regulate the flow of oxygen from the lungs to the respiring muscle mitochondria, as well as to functional mitochondria, that can efficiently extract the available oxygen from blood. Muscle oxygen utilization in oxidative phosphorylation may increase 50-fold or greater from rest to peak exercise. This increase is achieved by increases in the level of oxygen extraction from oxyhemoglobin in red blood cells and in the rate of delivery of oxygenated blood to working muscle by the circulation.

The primary source of energy for resting muscle is derived from fatty acid oxidation [Felig and Wahren, 1975]. At rest, glucose utilization accounts for 10% to 15% of total oxygen consumption [Wahren, 1977]. Both slow- and fast-twitch fibers have similar levels of glycogen content at rest [Essen, 1978]. The choice of the bioenergetic pathway in working muscle depends on the type, intensity, and duration of exercise [Essen, 1977; Gollnick et al., 1974] but also on diet and physical conditioning [DiMauro and Haller, 1999]. In the first 5 to 10 minutes of moderate exercise, high-energy phosphates are used first to regenerate ATP. This period is followed by muscle glycogen breakdown, which is indicated by a sharp rise in lactate during the first 10 minutes. Blood lactate levels then drop as muscle triglycerides and blood-borne fuels are used [Felig and Wahren, 1975; Lithell et al., 1979]. After 90 minutes, the major fuels are glucose and free fatty acids. During 1 to 4 hours of mild-to-moderate prolonged exercise, muscle uptake of free fatty acids increases approximately 70%, and after 4 hours, free fatty acids are used twice as much as carbohydrates.

Symptoms in muscle energy defects are directly related to a mismatch between the rate of ATP utililization (energy demand) and the capacity of the muscle metabolic pathways to regenerate ATP (energy supply). This energy supply/demand mismatch impairs energy-dependent processes that power muscle contraction (resulting in weakness and exertional fatigue), mediate muscle relaxation (muscle cramping, tightness), and/or maintain membrane ion gradients necessary for normal membrane excitability (fatigue, weakness) and muscle cell integrity (muscle pain, injury, myoglobinuria). In metabolic myopathies, the specific metabolic mediators of premature fatigue, cramping, pain, and muscle injury are complex and vary among the different metabolic disorders. Disorders of glycogen, lipid, or mitochondrial metabolism may cause two main clinical syndromes in muscle: (1) acute, recurrent, reversible muscle dysfunction with exercise intolerance and acute muscle breakdown or myoglobinuria (with or without cramps), such as phosphorylase, phosphorylase b kinase, phosphofructokinase, phosphoglycerate kinase, phosphoglycerate mutase, and lactate dehydrogenase among the glycogenoses, and carnitine palmitoyltransferase II, very-long-chain acyl-coenzyme A (CoA) dehydrogenase (VLCAD), trifunctional protein, short-chain *L*-3-hydroxyacyl-CoA dehydrogenase (SCHAD) deficiency among the disorders of fatty acid oxidation, and complex II and coenzyme Q10 deficiencies among the mitochondrial disorders; and (2) progressive weakness, such as acid maltase, debrancher enzyme, brancher enzyme, and aldolase enzyme deficiencies among the glycogenoses; long-chain acyl-CoA dehydrogenase (LCAD), VLCAD, trifunctional protein, glutaric aciduria type II, and short-chain acyl-CoA

Box 81-1 Heritable Causes of Myoglobinuria

- I. Biochemical abnormality known
  - A. Glycolysis/glycogenolysis
    1. Phosphorylase deficiency [McArdle, 1951]*
    2. Phosphofructokinase deficiency [Layzer et al., 1967; Tarui et al., 1965]
    3. Phosphoglycerate kinase deficiency [DiMauro et al., 1981a]*
    4. Phosphoglycerate mutase deficiency [DiMauro et al., 1981b]*
    5. Lactate dehydrogenase deficiency [Kanno et al., 1980]*
    6. Phosphorylase b kinase deficiency [Abarbanel et al., 1986]
    7. Debrancher deficiency [Brown, 1986]
    8. Aldolase A deficiency [Kreuder et al., 1996]*
  - B. Fatty acid oxidation
    1. Carnitine palmitoyltransferase II deficiency [DiMauro and DiMauro, 1973]*
    2. Long-chain acyl-CoA dehydrogenase deficiency [Roe, cited in Stanley, 1987]
    3. Very long-chain acyl-CoA dehydrogenase deficiency [Ogilvie et al., 1994]
    4. Medium-chain acyl-CoA dehydrogenase deficiency [Ruitenbeek et al., 1995]
    5. Short-chain L-3-hydroxyacyl CoA dehydrogenase deficiency [Tein et al., 1991]*
    6. Trifunctional enzyme deficiency [Dionisi-Vici et al., 1991]*
    7. Medium-chain 3-ketoacyl CoA thiolase deficiency [Kamijo et al., 1997]*
  - C. Pentose phosphate pathway
    1. Glucose-6-phosphate dehydrogenase deficiency [Bresolin et al., 1989]*
  - D. Purine nucleotide cycle
    1. Myoadenylate deaminase deficiency [Hyser et al., 1989]
  - E. Respiratory chain
    1. Complex I deficiency [de Lonlay-Debeney et al., 1999]*
    2. Coenzyme Q10 deficiency [Ogasahara et al., 1989]
    3. Complex II and aconitase deficiencies [Haller et al., 1991]*
    4. Complex III deficiency (cytochrome b deficiency) [Andreu et al., 1999]
    5. Complex IV deficiency (cytochrome oxidase deficiency) (Keightley et al., 1996]*
    6. Multiple mitochondrial DNA deletions [Ohno et al., 1991]*
- II. Biochemical abnormality incompletely characterized
  - A. Impaired long-chain fatty acid oxidation [Engel et al., 1970]*
  - B. Impaired function of the sarcoplasmic reticulum (?) in familial malignant hyperthermia (predisposition in central core disease, Duchenne muscular dystrophy, Becker muscular dystrophy, myotonic dystrophy, myotonia congenita, Schwartz-Jampel syndrome, King-Denborough syndrome)*
  - C. Abnormal composition of the sarcolemma in Duchenne and Becker muscular dystrophies [Bonilla et al., 1989; Hoffman et al., 1989; Medori et al., 1989]*
- III. Biochemical abnormality unknown
  - A. Familial recurrent myoglobinuria*
  - B. Repeated attacks in sporadic cases*

Modified from Tein I, DiMauro S, Rowland LP. In: Rowland LP, DiMauro S, eds. Handbook of clinical neurology, vol 18 (62). Myopathies. Amsterdam: Elsevier Science, 1992;553.

*Etiologies that have been documented to cause recurrent myoglobinuria beginning in childhood.

dehydrogenase (SCAD) deficiencies and plasmalemmal carnitine transporter (OCTN2) defect among the fatty acid oxidation defects; and mitochondrial enzyme deficiencies such as complex I, cytochrome oxidase deficiency, multiple mitochondrial DNA (mtDNA) deletions, and mtDNA depletion syndrome (Box 81-1). Progressive weakness and recurrent myoglobinuria can also occur together in a given disorder (e.g., LCAD, VLCAD, SCHAD, trifunctional protein, and severe carnitine palmitoyltransferase II deficiencies among the fatty acid oxidation defects, as well as multiple mtDNA deletions and coenzyme Q10 deficiency).

MYOGLOBINURIA

Myoglobinuria is a clinical syndrome, not just a biochemical state [Rowland, 1984]. In the alert patient, myalgia and limb weakness are the most common presenting symptoms. Urine color is usually brownish rather than red, and the urine tests positive for both albumin and heme (a concentration of at least 4 μg/mL). There are few or no red blood cells. Myoglobin can be identified by immunochemical methods. Concentrations of the sarcoplasmic enzymes, including serum creatine kinase, are usually elevated to more than 100 times normal. Less frequent features include hyperphosphatemia, hyperuricemia, hypocalcemia, or hypercalcemia. If renal failure occurs, serum potassium and calcium levels may rise. If the patient is comatose or if the presenting disorder is one of acute renal failure, there may be no muscle symptoms or signs. Under these conditions, the diagnosis can be made if (1) there is renal failure and (2) the serum content of sarcoplasmic enzymes is 100 times normal. The potentially life-threatening hazards of an attack of myoglobinuria include renal or respiratory failure and cardiac dysrhythmias. The etiologies of heritable myoglobinuria in adults differ from those in children. In a study of 77 adult patients aged 15 to 65 years, Tonin and associates [1990] identified the enzyme abnormality in 36 patients (47%) as follows: carnitine palmitoyltransferase deficiency in 17 patients; glycolytic defects in 15 patients (including phosphorylase in 10, phosphorylase b kinase in 4, and phosphoglycerate kinase in 1); myoadenylate deaminase in 3; and combined carnitine palmitoyltransferase and myoadenylate deaminase deficiencies in 1. In contrast, in 100 cases of recurrent childhood-onset myoglobinuria, cases have been diagnosed biochemically in a lower percentage of affected children (24%): 16 had carnitine palmitoyltransferase deficiency, 1 had SCHAD deficiency, and 7 had various glycolytic defects (2 had phosphorylase deficiency, 1 had phosphoglycerate kinase deficiency, 3 had phosphoglycerate mutase deficiency, and 1 had lactate dehydrogenase deficiency) [Tein et al., 1990b]. These children could be divided into two groups: a type I exertional group, in which exertion was the primary precipitating factor (56 cases), and a type II toxic group, in which leukocytosis and infection and/or fever were the primary precipitants (37 cases). The type II toxic childhood-onset group was distinguished from the type I exertional childhood-onset and adult-onset groups by the etiologies, which were limited to fatty acid oxidation defects, as well as its slight female predominance, which was in contrast to the marked male predominance in the latter two groups. The type II toxic group was further distinguished by the earlier age at onset of myoglobinuria, the presence of a more generalized disease (e.g., ictal bulbar signs, seizures, encephalopathy, developmental delay), and a higher mortality rate. Currently, the most common etiology for recurrent myoglobinuria in both adults and in children is carnitine palmitoyltransferase II deficiency [Tein et al., 1992].

GLYCOGENOSES

Only glycogenoses affecting skeletal muscle, alone or in association with other tissues, are discussed in this section (Fig. 81-1) [DiMauro and Bresolin, 1986]. Molecular genetic analysis has led to the cloning of genes encoding the

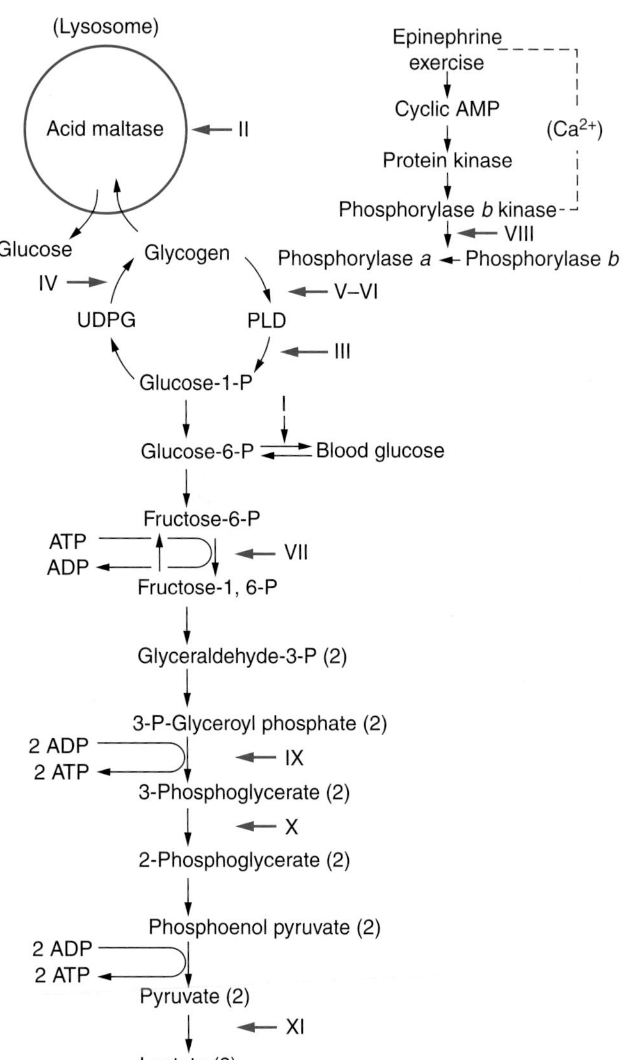

FIGURE 81-1. Scheme of glycogen metabolism and glycolysis. Roman numerals refer to glycogenoses resulting from defects of the following enzymes: I, glucose-6-phosphatase; II, acid maltase; III, debrancher; IV, brancher; V, muscle phosphorylase; VI, liver phosphorylase; VII, phosphofructokinase; VIII, phosphorylase b kinase; IX, phosphoglycerate kinase; X, phosphoglycerate mutase; XI, lactate dehydrogenase. ADP, adenosine diphosphate; AMP, adenosine monophosphate; ATP, adenosine triphosphate; P, phosphate; PLD, phosphorylase-limit-dextrin, D; UDPG, uridine diphosphate glucose. (From DiMauro S, Miranda AF, Sakoda S, et al. Metabolic myopathies. Am J Med Genet 1986;25:635-651.)

TABLE 81-1

Chromosomal Assignment of Human Genes Encoding Glycogenolytic and Glycolytic Enzymes

ENZYME	SUBUNIT OR ISOZYME	CHROMOSOME	REFERENCE
Acid maltase	—	17q23→q25	Engel and Hirschhorn, 1994
Phosphorylase b kinase	α (M)	Xq12→q13	Francke et al., 1989
	α (L)	Xp22.2→p22.1	Davidson et al., 1992
	β	16q12→q13	Francke et al., 1989
	γ	7p12-q21	Jones et al., 1990
Phosphorylase	M	11q13	Lebo et al., 1984
	L	14q21→q22	Newgard et al., 1986; Billingsley et al., 1994
	B	10, 20p11.2	Newgard et al., 1988; Rao et al., 1992
Debrancher	—	1p21	Yang-Feng et al., 1992
Phosphofructokinase	M	1(cen→q32)	Vora et al., 1982
	P	10p	Vora et al., 1983b
	L	21q22.3	Van Keuren et al., 1986
Aldolase A	M	16q22-q24	Kukita et al., 1987
Phosphoglycerate kinase	A	Xq13	Meera Khan et al., 1971
Phosphoglycerate mutase	M	7	Edwards et al., 1989
	B	10	Junien et al., 1982
Lactate dehydrogenase	M	11	Boone et al., 1972
	H	12	Chen et al., 1973

Modified from DiMauro S, Tsujino S. Nonlysosomal glycogenoses. In: Engel AG, Franzini-Armstrong C, eds. Myology, vol 2. New York: McGraw-Hill, 1994;1554.
A, the isoform of phosphoglycerate kinase present in all tissues except spermatogenic cells; B, brain; H, heart; L, liver; M, muscle; P, platelets.

enzymes involved in most glycogenoses, as well as their chromosomal localization (Table 81-1). All are autosomal recessive in inheritance with the exception of phosphoglycerate kinase, which is X-linked recessive, and phosphorylase b kinase, which may be either. In the glycogenoses, fixed weakness is the primary manifestation in deficiencies of acid maltase, debrancher, aldolase, and brancher enzymes, whereas exercise intolerance with cramps, myalgia, and recurrent myoglobinuria are the primary manifestations in deficiencies of phosphorylase kinase, phosphorylase, phosphofructokinase, phosphoglycerate kinase, phosphoglycerate mutase, β-enolase, and lactate dehydrogenase [DiMauro and Lamperti, 2001].

Pathophysiology

The immediate source of energy for contraction and relaxation is provided by the hydrolysis of ATP. Oxidative phosphorylation provides the largest contribution of energy overall, whereas anaerobic glycolysis plays a relatively minor role, limited primarily to conditions of sustained isometric contraction when blood flow and oxygen delivery to exercising muscles are drastically reduced. The dynamic form of exercise, such as walking or running, depends primarily on aerobic glycolysis. Therefore, the pathophysiology of glycogenoses relates more to the impairment of aerobic than anaerobic glycolysis [Lewis and Haller, 1986; Lewis et al., 1991].

Which energy substrates are used by muscle for aerobic metabolism depends on the type, intensity, and duration of exercise, as well as on physical conditioning and diet. During intense exercise (close to maximal oxygen uptake [Vo_{2max}], in dynamic exercise or maximal force generation in isometric exercise), energy is derived from anaerobic glycolysis, particularly when there is a burst of activity with rapid acceleration to maximal exercise [DiMauro and Tsujino, 1994]. During low-intensity exercise (below 50% Vo_{2max}), the primary sources of energy are blood glucose and free fatty acids. At higher intensities, the proportion of energy derived from carbohydrate oxidation increases, and glycogen becomes an important fuel. At 70% to 80% of Vo_{2max}, the critical energy source is provided by the aerobic metabolism of glycogen, and fatigue occurs when glycogen stores are exhausted [DiMauro and Tsujino, 1994]. Individuals with defective glycolysis/glycogenolysis are most vulnerable during the initial stages of intense exercise, and they must rest soon after beginning exercise because of muscle cramps. However, if they continue to exercise at low intensity, they are able to continue for a longer time. This is known as the *second-wind phenomenon* and has been attributed to a metabolic switch from carbohydrate to fatty acid utilization [Felig and Wahren, 1975] and to increased circulation with increased availability of blood glucose from hepatic glycogenolysis [Haller et al., 1985]. A decrease in ATP levels could first cause muscle contracture. In theory, a more severe depletion could lead to myoglobinuria [Rowland, 1984], although this has not been proved.

The forearm ischemic exercise test developed by McArdle [1951] is a useful test for the detection of enzymatic defects in the nonlysosomal glycogenolytic and glycolytic pathways. This test can be performed in cooperative children as young as 6 years of age. A catheter is placed in a superficial antecubital vein, and basal lactate and ammonia levels are obtained without stasis. A sphygmomanometer cuff is then placed above the elbow and inflated above arterial pressure. The patient is asked to rhythmically squeeze another rolled-up cuff to well above 120 mm Hg for 1 minute of exercise. This test requires constant encouragement from the observer because significant discomfort can occur even in healthy control subjects. The test should be discontinued if the patient develops an acute cramp, because myonecrosis or a compartment syndrome or both may occur in an individual with a glycolytic disorder [Lindner et al., 2001; Meinck et al., 1982). After 1 minute of exercise, the cuff around the arm is deflated, and blood samples are sequentially obtained 1, 3, 5, 7, 10, and 15 minutes afterward. In healthy subjects, there is a fourfold to sixfold increase of lactate concentrations over baseline, with the peak occurring 1 to 2 minutes after the exercise, and then a decline to baseline values by 15 minutes. This pattern is paralleled by a similar fivefold or more increase in ammonia concentrations, which generally peak 2 to 5 minutes after the exercise in individuals with normal myoadenylate deaminase activity. In healthy subjects, venous ammonia and lactate concentrations are linearly related [Sinkeler et al., 1985]. In individuals with a defect in glycolysis/glycogenolysis, there is an insufficient rise in lactate (less than twofold), with a compensatory and exaggerated increase in ammonia, which also indicates sufficient effort on the part of the individual. This exaggerated rise in ammonia is attributable to high cellular levels of ADP, which result from a combination of blocked glycogenolysis/glycolysis and absence of cellular acidosis. An insufficient lactate rise has been demonstrated in deficiencies of phosphorylase, debrancher enzyme, phosphofructokinase, phosphoglycerate kinase, phosphoglycerate mutase, and lactate dehydrogenase but not in acid maltase or phosphorylase b kinase deficiency. The major limitation of this test is that the rise of venous lactate in individuals who do not have a defect in this pathway is highly dependent on the patient's ability and willingness to exercise. Therefore, patients in whom lactate levels are low, because of either poor effort or placement of the venous catheter in other than the median cubital vein, exhibit proportionally blunted ammonia responses.

In view of the potential risk of myoglobinuria, alternatives to the traditional ischemic forearm test have been described. One of these uses sustained, intense (70% of maximal voluntary contraction) isometric handgrip exercise [Hogrel et al., 2001]. However, this form of testing is as ischemic as the use of a blood pressure cuff, inasmuch as the intramuscular pressure in isometric contractions of more than 50% of maximal voluntary contraction completely occludes muscle blood flow. Therefore, any reduction in the incidence of muscle contractures depends on shortening the duration of the test, which is also effective in minimizing contractures in the traditional ischemic forearm test. An alternative nonischemic forearm test involves 30 maximal handgrip contractions in 1 minute without a blood pressure cuff [Kazemi-Esfarjani et al., 2002]. The degree of increases in lactate and ammonia concentrations in control subjects and the diagnostic sensitivity in patients were similar to those in the ischemic exercise test. However, in contrast to the ischemic tests, the retained oxidative capacity helps protect individuals from contractures or significant pain [Kazemi-Esfarjani et al., 2002].

Glycolytic/Glycogenolytic Defects

Acid Maltase Deficiency

CLINICAL FEATURES

Acid maltase deficiency (glycogenosis type II) results in three very different clinical presentations [DiMauro and Lamperti, 2001]: (1) A severe generalized disease of infancy described by Pompe [1932] that is invariably fatal before 2 years of age as a result of respiratory weakness and cardiac failure. This infantile form (Pompe's disease) manifests with diffuse hypotonia and weakness in the first weeks or months of life and is associated with macroglossia, massive cardiomegaly, and moderate hepatomegaly. (2) A juvenile variant that affects exclusively muscle, with onset in childhood. It causes severe proximal, truncal, and respiratory muscle weakness, usually leading to death in the second or third decade. (3) A milder, adult-onset variant simulating limb-girdle dystrophy or polymyositis. In adult acid maltase deficiency a slowly progressive myopathy begins in the third or fourth decade with early ventilatory insufficiency. Affected adults often complain of headache upon waking, caused by sleep hypercapnia. Slonim and co-workers [2000] described a subgoup of patients who have the neonatal onset and the muscle morphologic features of the infantile form, but their condition differs from typical Pompe's disease in that the heart is not involved and survival is longer.

LABORATORY TESTS

In all forms of acid maltase deficiency, there is an increase in serum creatine kinase concentration. Electromyographic studies reveal myopathic abnormalities and may also demonstrate fibrillation potentials, positive waves, complex repetitive discharges, and myotonic discharges [DiMauro and Lamperti, 2001]. These are more frequently demonstrated in the paraspinal muscles. The electrocardiogram demonstrates characteristic, although not specific, changes, including a short PR interval, giant QRS complexes, and signs of biventricular hypertrophy in infantile acid maltase deficiency. In adults, there is markedly reduced vital capacity.

PATHOLOGY

In infantile acid maltase deficiency, glycogen accumulation is evident in all tissues, most notably the heart. There is significant involvement of the anterior horn cells of the spinal cord, leading to severe weakness and fasciculations, and of brainstem nuclei. Glycogen accumulation in Schwann cells is seen in peripheral nerve biopsy specimens. There is vacuolar myopathy on muscle biopsy samples in all three forms of acid maltase deficiency [DiMauro et al., 1992]. In the infantile form, all muscle fibers contain many vacuoles, which often coalesce into a lacework pattern and contain periodic acid–Schiff stain–positive, diastase-digestible material and stain positively for acid phosphatase. Electron microscopic study reveals excess glycogen within lysosomal vacuoles and free in the cytoplasm.

INHERITANCE

The three forms of acid maltase deficiency are allelic disorders that are transmitted as autosomal recessive traits. The gene encoding acid maltase is located on chromosome 17. Acid maltase activity can be measured in cultured amniocytes for the purposes of prenatal diagnosis.

BIOCHEMISTRY AND MOLECULAR GENETICS

Although the enzyme defect is generalized and can be documented in lymphocytes [Shanske and DiMauro, 1981] or in cultured skin fibroblasts, biochemical measurement of acid maltase in muscle establishes the diagnosis. It is not entirely clear why symptoms are confined mainly to muscle in the childhood and adult forms. However, differences in clinical expression may in part relate to the amounts of residual activity [Mehler and DiMauro, 1977; Reuser et al., 1987; Van Der Ploeg et al., 1988]. Also, genetic heterogeneity has been demonstrated. In a study of 14 patients, Martiniuk and colleagues [1990a, 1990b] found that messenger RNA was lacking in 5 of 10 cases of infantile acid maltase deficiency and was present in all four adult cases, although it was shorter in two cases. The defective lysosomal enzyme, α-glucosidase, is encoded by a gene on chromosome 17 [D'Ancona et al., 1979; Solomon et al., 1979; Weil et al., 1979], and more than 55 mutations have been identified in patients with the three variants [DiMauro and Lamperti, 2001]. The correlation between genotype and phenotype is hard to establish because of the frequent compound heterozygosity. However, there is good correlation between the severity of the mutation and the severity of the clinical phenotype. Therefore, deletions and nonsense mutations are usually associated with the infantile variant, whereas "leaky" mutations, such as the IVS1 (–13T>G) splice site mutations, are associated with the adult-onset variant [Hirschhorn, 1995]. Childhood acid maltase deficiency is often the result of compound heterozygosity [Huie et al., 1998], but it has also been associated with at least one homozygous, apparently specific mutation [Adams et al., 1997].

TREATMENT

Trials with lysosome-labilizing agents and activators of glycogenolysis have been unsuccessful in Pompe's disease [DiMauro et al., 1992]. The use of an acid maltase precursor containing phosphorylated, *N*-linked, high-mannose carbohydrate chains, which is efficiently taken up by cultured muscle cells from patients, may be more promising [Van Der Ploeg et al., 1988]. Enzyme replacement also looks promising, particularly for patients with childhood- and adult-onset acid maltase deficiency. Recombinant human α-glucosidase obtained from the milk of transgenic rabbits and injected into knockout mice lacking acid maltase fully corrected the enzyme defect in all tissues except brain tissue [Bijvoet et al., 1999]. Amalfitano and associates [2001] reported the results of a phase I/II open-label study of recombinant human α-glucosidase administered intravenously twice weekly in three infants with infantile acid maltase deficiency. The results of more than 250 administrations revealed that recombinant human α-glucosidase was generally well tolerated. Steady decreases in heart size and maintenance of normal cardiac function for more than 1 year were observed in all three infants. These infants lived past the critical first birthday and also exhibited improvements in skeletal muscle function. In another study of late-onset acid maltase deficiency, three patients (aged 11, 16, and 32 years)—all wheelchair dependent and two ventilator dependent with a history of deteriorating pulmonary function—received 3 years of treatment with weekly intravenous infusions of recombinant α-glucosidase from rabbit milk; they exhibited stabilized pulmonary function and reported less fatigue [Winkel et al., 2004]. The youngest and least affected patient demonstrated significant improvement of skeletal muscle strength and function and, after 72 weeks of treatment, could walk without support. There have also been promising gene therapy results both in vitro and in vivo using E1-deleted recombinant adenovirus encoding human α-glucosidase. Transduction of the viral construct into enzyme-deficient human fibroblasts in culture resulted in a dose-dependent return of acid maltase activity, which was localized within lysosomes [Pauly et al., 1998]. Equally encouraging results were obtained by injecting a similar viral construct into the pectoral muscle of acid maltase-deficient Japanese quails, which are an avian model of acid maltase deficiency [Tsujino et al., 1998]. Individuals with childhood or adult acid maltase deficiency may require ventilatory assistance. A high-protein diet has improved strength and respiratory function in some but not all patients [DiMauro et al., 1992; Slonim et al., 1983].

Phosphorylase b Kinase Deficiency

CLINICAL FEATURES

Phosphorylase b kinase deficiency (glycogenosis type VIII) may be divided into four clinical syndromes [DiMauro and Tsujino, 1994]. These can be differentiated by inheritance and tissue distribution as follows:

- Liver disease that is usually benign, begins in infancy or childhood, and is characterized by hepatomegaly, abnormal liver function tests, gross motor delay, failure to thrive, and fasting hypoglycemia [Willems et al., 1990]. Inheritance is X-linked recessive, encoded by a gene in chromosome region Xp22.2-p22.1, or, on occasion, autosomal recessive. The defect is expressed in liver and erythrocytes [Van der Berg and Berger, 1990]. Burwinkel and co-workers [1998] described eight new mutations in the gene encoding the liver isoform of the phosphorylase b kinase alpha subunit and the phenotypic consequence in patients with X-linked liver glycogenosis.
- Liver and muscle disease characterized by childhood-onset hepatomegaly, fasting hypoglycemia, and nonprogressive myopathy. This disease is autosomal recessive and caused by mutations in the beta subunit encoded by a gene in chromosome region 16q12-q13.
- Myopathy that appears to be X-linked recessive [DiMauro and Lamperti, 2001]. Most patients have childhood- or adolescent-onset exercise intolerance with cramps and weakness in exercising muscles; six patients have been reported with exercise-induced pigmenturia [Abarbanel et al., 1986; Carrier et al., 1990]. Two molecular defects have been identified in the muscle isoform of the alpha subunit, including a nonsense mutation [Wehner et al., 1994] and a splice-junction mutation that causes skipping of one exon [Bruno et al., 1998].
- Fatal infantile cardiomyopathy, which may be autosomal recessive [Mizuta et al., 1984; Servidei et al., 1988a].

LABORATORY FEATURES

The resting serum creatine kinase level is variably increased in most patients. The electromyogram may appear normal or may reveal nonspecific myopathic changes. Muscle biopsy specimens may be normal or contain subsarcolemmal accumulations of glycogen, located primarily in type 2B fibers. The phosphorylase stain is normal. There are pools of free, normal-looking glycogen particles on electron microscopic studies [DiMauro and Tsujino, 1994].

BIOCHEMISTRY AND MOLECULAR GENETICS

Phosphorylase b kinase participates in glycogen metabolism regulation by acting on the two main enzymes involved in glycogen synthesis and degradation: glycogen synthetase and phosphorylase [Heilmeyer, 1991]. Phosphorylase b kinase converts phosphorylase from the less active "b" form to the more active "a" form and simultaneously converts glycogen synthetase from a more active, dephosphorylated form to a less active, phosphorylated form. Thus, when glycogen synthesis is turned on, glycogen degradation is turned off, and vice versa. Phosphorylase b kinase is a multimeric enzyme composed of four different subunits (alpha, beta, gamma, and delta) [DiMauro and Tsujino, 1994]. The alpha and beta subunits are regulatory, the gamma subunit is catalytic, and the delta subunit is identical to calmodulin and confers calcium sensitivity to the enzyme [DiMauro and Lamperti, 2001]. In addition, there are two isoforms for the alpha subunit (muscle and liver) that are encoded by genes on the X chromosome. The two isoforms for the gamma subunit (muscle and testis) and the beta subunit are encoded by autosomal genes. Glycogen is normal or moderately increased in patients with myopathy, and the phosphorylase b kinase activity is absent or markedly decreased [DiMauro and Tsujino, 1994].

It is not easy to account for the tissue specificity in the different clinical variants. Two distinct genes have been identified. One gene (*PHKA1*) is on the proximal long arm at chromosome Xq13, which encodes a muscle isozyme; the other gene (*PHKA2*) is on the distal short arm of the X chromosome at Xp22.2-p22.1, which encodes a nonmuscle isozyme, and is in the same region to which the gene for X-linked liver glycogenosis resulting from phosphorylase b kinase deficiency has been mapped [Willems et al., 1991]. Tissue-specific isozymes may be the result of alternative RNA splicing. DiMauro and Tsujino [1994] suggested that mutations in tissue that specifically expressed exons of the beta subunit [Harmann et al., 1991] could explain the apparently autosomal-recessive forms of myopathy and fatal infantile cardiomyopathy.

TREATMENT

Although there is no specific therapy for phosphorylase b kinase deficiency, a high-protein diet may be helpful.

Phosphorylase Deficiency

CLINICAL FEATURES

Myophosphorylase deficiency (type V glycogenosis, or McArdle's disease) is a rare disease but an important cause of recurrent myoglobinuria. Exercise intolerance generally starts in childhood, but overt episodes of muscle cramping and myoglobinuria develop later in adolescence. Brief isometric contraction (e.g., as in lifting heavy objects) and less intense but sustained dynamic exercise (e.g., as in climbing stairs) are the two primary precipitants. Approximately 50% of affected patients experience episodes of muscle necrosis and myoglobinuria after exercise, 27% of whom develop acute renal failure. Although there is usually complete functional recovery after the episode of myoglobinuria, about one third of patients have fixed mild proximal weakness greater than distal weakness, which is more commonly seen in older patients [DiMauro and Bresolin, 1986]. The diagnosis is usually made in the second or third decade of life. There may be a marked variation in the severity of symptoms. In some, progressive weakness may begin late in life (the sixth decade) with no history of cramps or pigmenturia [DiMauro and Bresolin, 1986; Pourmand et al., 1983]. The cumulative effect of recurrent muscle damage over the years may explain the appearance of fixed weakness in older individuals. In contrast, there have been four unique childhood cases with severe generalized muscle and respiratory weakness documented at or soon after birth with death in infancy [DiMauro and Hartlage, 1978; DiMauro and Tsujino, 1994; Milstein et al., 1989]. One hypotonic 1-year-old infant has been described with repeated episodes of hyper–creatine kinase–emia during febrile episodes [Ito et al., 2003].

LABORATORY DATA

Between episodes of myoglobinuria, the serum creatine kinase is variably increased in 93% of cases. This serves as a feature differentiating phosphorylase b kinase deficiency from carnitine palmitoyltransferase deficiency, in which the resting creatine kinase is generally normal. Electromyography between episodes of myoglobinuria demonstrates fibrillations, myotonic discharges, and positive waves in up to 50% of patients, which are suggestive of mild myopathy [DiMauro and Tsujino, 1994]. There is a lack of cytoplasmic acidification on phosphorus 31 nuclear magnetic resonance (^{31}P-NMR) spectroscopy during aerobic or ischemic exercise, as well as an abnormally steep drop in the phosphocreatine/inorganic phosphate ratio [Argov and Bank, 1991; Ross et al., 1981].

INHERITANCE

There is an unexplained, marked male predominance despite the autosomal-recessive pattern of inheritance. The muscle isoform gene has been localized to chromosome 11 [Lebo et al., 1984]. The appearance of the disease in two families with apparent autosomal-dominant transmission [Chui and Munsat, 1976; Schimrigk et al., 1967] may be explained on the basis of subsequent generations of homozygotes and manifesting heterozygotes, in whom the residual activity was below a critical threshold [Papadimitriou et al., 1990; Schmidt et al., 1987]. In a third family, Tsujino and associates [1993a] demonstrated that the affected mother was a compound heterozygote carrying two different point mutations in the phosphorylase gene, the unaffected father was heterozygous for a third point mutation, and the three affected children were compound heterozygotes.

MUSCLE BIOPSY

There may or may not be focal accumulations of glycogen between myofibrils and in the subsarcolemmal regions on periodic acid-Schiff stain. The phosphorylase stain [Takeuchi and Kuriaki, 1955] reveals no staining in muscle fibers, in contrast to normal staining of the smooth muscle in the walls of intramuscular vessels. DiMauro and Tsujino [1994] pointed out that a positive histochemical reaction may be seen in McArdle's disease under the following two conditions: (1) when there are regenerating fibers and (2) when there is residual enzyme activity. A false-positive reaction in regenerating fibers results from expression of a different isozyme in immature muscle cells [DiMauro et al., 1978; Sato et al., 1977]. Accumulation of normal-looking glycogen beta particles under the sarcolemma and between myofibrils and myofilaments may be seen on electron microscopy [DiMauro and Tsujino, 1994].

BIOCHEMICAL CONSIDERATIONS

Phosphorylase (α-1,4-glucan orthophosphate glycosyl transferase) initiates glycogen breakdown by removing 1,4-glucosyl residues phosphorolytically from the outer branches of the glycogen molecule with liberation of glucose-1-phosphate until the peripheral chains have been shortened to approximately four glucosyl units. The debranching enzyme catalyzes the further breakdown. The combined action of these two enzymes degrades glycogen to glucose-1-phosphate (approximately 93%) and glucose (approximately 7%). Muscle phosphorylase exists as an active phosphorylated alpha form and a less active dephosphorylated beta form. The muscle phosphorylase activity is undetectable in most or up to 10% of normal residual activity in affected patients [DiMauro and Tsujino, 1994]. Glycogen accumulation is moderate (about twofold) or normal. The glycogen structure is normal. There is no immunologically detectable enzyme protein in muscle by sodium dodecylsulfate polyacrylamide gel electrophoresis, immunoblot, and enzyme-linked immunosorbent assay in the majority of patients [McConchie et al., 1991; Servidei et al., 1988b]. Normal mature human muscle has a single phosphorylase isozyme, whereas cardiac muscle and brain have three different isozymes on polyacrylamide gel electrophoresis: (1) a minor, slow-migrating isozyme identical to muscle phosphorylase and representing about 13% of total activity in the heart and 8% in the brain; (2) a major, fast-migrating brain isozyme representing 58% of total activity in the heart and 64% in the brain; and (3) an intermediate band (29% of total activity in the heart and 28% in the brain), which is a hybrid of the muscle and brain isozymes [Bresolin et al., 1983]. Lack of the muscle isozyme should therefore cause partial defects in the heart and brain. A defect of the brain isozyme would be expected to cause heart and brain involvement [DiMauro and Tsujino, 1994].

PATHOPHYSIOLOGY

The pathophysiology of exercise intolerance in McArdle's disease involves a combination of interconnected factors related to impaired ATP production from both aerobic and anaerobic glycolysis. The decrease of ATP generated during anaerobic glycolysis may selectively affect muscle ATPases [James et al., 1996], including Na^+/K^+-ATPase. This inhibition, together with a decrease in Na^+/K^+ pump numbers, may lead to excessive increases in levels of blood and extracellular potassium, which are typically seen during exercise in McArdle's disease [Haller et al., 1998a]. These changes can, in turn, explain the sarcolemmal inexcitability during repetitive neural stimulation [Dyken et al., 1967]. Furthermore, the lack of lactic acid production and intracellular acidification during exercise alters the equilibrium of the creatine kinase reaction, resulting in an exaggerated rise of ADP during exercise. The excessive intracellular ADP is converted to AMP, inosine monophosphate, ammonia, and adenine nucleotide degradation products, including inosine, hypoxanthine, and uric acid [Mineo et al., 1987]. Premature fatigue may result from impaired excitation-contraction coupling, mediated by excessive accumulation of ADP [Lewis and Haller, 1991a]. Oxidative metabolism is also affected in McArdle's disease, because the block in glycogenolysis impairs production of pyruvate, which is a major anaplerotic substrate for the Krebs cycle [Sahlin et al., 1995]. In patients with McArdle's disease, oxygen extraction and maximal oxygen uptake are decreased; these can be partially restored by administration of intravenous glucose [Haller et al., 1985].

MOLECULAR GENETICS

The three phosphorylase isozyme genes have been cloned, sequenced, and localized to different chromosomes [Billingsley et al., 1994; Lebo et al., 1984; Newgard et al., 1986, 1988; Rao et al., 1992] (see Table 81-1). Tsujino and associates [1993a] identified three different point mutations in the muscle isozyme gene: a C-to-G mutation in codon 49 of exon 1 (converting an arginine molecule to a stop codon), a G-to-A mutation in codon 204 of exon 5 (converting a glycine molecule to a serine molecule), and an A-to-C mutation in codon 542 of exon 14 (converting a lysine molecule to a threonine molecule). In an analysis of 32 patients, 15 were homozygous for the first mutation, and 12 were compound heterozygotes [Tsujino et al., 1993a]. More than 30 mutations have been identified in the muscle isozyme gene, which will facilitate carrier identification [DiMauro and Lamperti, 2001; DiMauro and Tsujino, 1994; Tsujino et al., 1993a, 1994a, 1994b, 1994c]. These include missense, nonsense, and splice-junction mutations. The most common mutation in Europe and North America is the Arg49Stop, which accounts for 81% of the alleles in British patients [Bartram et al., 1993] and 63% of alleles in a survey of U.S. patients [El-Schahawi et al., 1996]. The high frequency of this mutation, on at least one allele, has facilitated molecular diagnosis in blood samples from patients with suspected McArdle's disease. However, it is important to realize that the frequency of different mutations varies in different ethnic groups. The frequency of the Arg49Stop mutation appears to decrease from north to south in Europe from 81% of alleles in the United Kingdom [Bartram et al., 1993] to 56% in Germany [Vorgerd et al., 1998] and 32% in Italy [Martinuzzi et al., 1996].

To date, there has been no clear genotype:phenotype correlation in McArdle's disease. For example, the common homozygous Arg49Stop mutation was also present in an infant with the fatal myopathic variant [Tsujino et al., 1993a] and in a child who died of sudden infant death syndrome [El-Schahawi et al., 1997]. This lack of clear correlation between genotype and phenotype was also documented in a study of 54 Spanish patients with McArdle's disease from

40 unrelated families [Martin et al., 2001]. One possible explanation for increased severity of clinical manifestation would be the presence of additional gene defects, such as myoadenylate deaminase deficiency [Rubio et al., 1997; Tsujino et al., 1995a].

TREATMENT

A key therapeutic strategy has been the attempt to bypass the metabolic block by providing the muscle with glycolytic substrates [DiMauro and Tsujino, 1994]. The oral administration of glucose or fructose to raise the blood glucose concentration has been helpful but has resulted in weight gain. Glucagon injections were impractical and yielded inconsistent results. Although exercise tolerance was increased by raising the serum free fatty acid concentration through the use of fat emulsions, fasting, and the administration of norepinephrine or heparin, more practical regimens such as a high-fat, low-carbohydrate diet have not been effective [DiMauro and Bresolin, 1986]. An alternative strategy was to supply branched-chain amino acids, which are taken up, rather than released, by tissue of patients with McArdle's disease during exercise [Wahren et al., 1973]. Slonim and Goans [1985] demonstrated an improvement of muscle endurance and strength in a patient with weakness after institution of a high-protein diet. Direct administration of branched-chain amino acids to six patients, however, resulted in an impairment rather than an improvement of bicycle exercise capacity in five of the six patients, possibly because of a lowering of free fatty acid levels by the amino acids [MacLean et al., 1998]. In contrast, aerobic training in four McArdle's patients improved peak cycle exercise capacity, circulatory capacity, and oxygen uptake [Haller et al., 1998b].

Vitamin B_6 is another potential therapeutic aid, inasmuch as overall body stores of pyridoxal phosphate are depleted in McArdle's disease because of the lack of enzyme protein to which pyridoxal phosphate is bound [Haller et al., 1983]. One patient experienced a beneficial effect with vitamin B_6 supplementation [Phoenix et al., 1998] but further studies need to be done. In addition, oral creatine monohydrate supplementation in a placebo-controlled crossover trial involving nine patients was demonstrated to alleviate symptoms and increase patients' capacity for ischemic, isometric forearm exercise [Vorgerd et al., 2000]. Another strategy has been the ingestion of sucrose before exercise to increase the availability of glucose [Vissing and Haller, 2003]. In a single-blind, randomized, placebo-controlled crossover study, 12 patients were studied. Ingestion of sucrose before exercise improved exercise tolerance and sense of well-being.

Finally, a first-generation adenoviral recombinant containing the full-length human myophosphorylase complementary DNA has been efficiently transduced into phosphorylase-deficient sheep myoblasts and human myoblasts, resulting in restoration of phosphorylase activity [Pari et al., 1999].

Debrancher Deficiency

CLINICAL FEATURES

Debrancher deficiency (glycogenosis type III) is characterized by childhood-onset liver dysfunction with hepatomegaly, growth failure, fasting hypoglycemia, and infrequently hypoglycemic seizures. Spontaneous resolution may occur around puberty with normal adult liver function [Smit et al., 1990], although cirrhosis and liver failure may develop later [Fellows et al., 1983]. The myopathy tends to appear late in the third or fourth decade in 70% of cases and involves primarily distal leg and intrinsic hand muscles. It is slowly progressive and rarely incapacitating. Childhood onset was documented in 7 of 22 patients. Two patients had exercise intolerance, cramps, and premature fatigue [Murase et al., 1973; Ozand et al., 1967], and five others had diffuse weakness and wasting, growth failure, and gross motor delay [Badurska et al., 1970; Slonim et al., 1982]. Myoglobinuria was reported in one case [Brown, 1986]. Enzymatic deficiency was documented in the muscle of 16 patients, 11 of whom had no weakness [Moses et al., 1986]. However, in view of the young ages of these patients (2 to 27 years), it is possible that clinical myopathy developed later. Peripheral neuropathy has also been documented [Moses et al., 1986]. Although clinical cardiomyopathy is infrequent, cardiac involvement has been demonstrated in most patients with myopathy [Brunberg et al., 1971; Miller et al., 1972; Moses et al., 1989]. Of interest, Cleary and associates [2002] reported consistent facial features in seven patients with glycogenosis type III, which included midfacial hypoplasia with a depressed nasal bridge and a broad upturned nasal tip, indistinct philtral pillars, and blow-shaped lips with a thin vermillion border. In addition, younger patients had deep-set eyes. Several children had clinical problems such as persistent otitis media or recurrent sinusitis.

LABORATORY DATA

Administration of glucagon or epinephrine in the fasting state does not increase blood glucose levels, which indicates liver involvement [DiMauro and Tsujino, 1994]. All patients with myopathy have an increase in serum creatine kinase levels. The electromyogram has characteristics of myopathy but may also demonstrate fibrillation activity, and the nerve conduction velocities are frequently decreased [Brunberg et al., 1971; Moses et al., 1986]. Evidence of left ventricular or biventricular hypertrophy may be seen on the electrocardiogram and echocardiogram [Brunberg et al., 1971; Moses et al., 1989; Smit et al., 1990].

INHERITANCE

There is a male predominance. The gene has been assigned to chromosome 1p21 [Yang-Feng et al., 1992]. Prenatal diagnosis can be made by a qualitative assay on the basis of persistence of the abnormal polysaccharide in cultured amniocytes exposed to a glucose-free medium [Yang et al., 1990].

PATHOLOGY

A severe vacuolar myopathy, which contains periodic acid-Schiff stain–positive material that is digested by diastase, is seen on muscle biopsy. This myopathy corresponds to large pools of free and apparently normal glycogen particles seen on electron microscopic studies [DiMauro and Tsujino, 1994]. Excessive glycogen is also seen in skin biopsy specimens [Sancho et al., 1990], cultured muscle [Miranda et al., 1981], endomyocardial biopsy specimens [Olson et al.,

1984], intramuscular nerves [Powell et al., 1985], and Schwann cells and axons of sural nerve [Ugawa et al., 1986], and brain tissue [Hug and Schubert, 1966].

BIOCHEMISTRY

The debrancher enzyme is a single 160-kDa polypeptide with two distinct catalytic functions. After digestion of glycogen to four glucosyl units by phosphorylase, the residual stubs are removed by the debrancher enzyme in two steps, a transferase and a glucosidase, which are located in different domains of the polypeptide [Bates et al., 1975]. On the basis of enzymatic and immunologic assays, debrancher deficiency has been classified into three groups [Chen et al., 1987; Ding et al., 1990]: (1) common type IIIA, characterized by lack of both transferase and glucosidase activity and lack of cross-reacting material in both muscle and liver; (2) less frequent type IIIB, characterized both by lack of enzymatic activities and by a lack of or marked decrease in cross-reacting material in liver, with sparing of the muscle and heart; and (3) type IIIC, characterized by the selective loss of transferase activity in both liver and muscle and the presence of cross-reacting material.

MOLECULAR GENETICS

Human debrancher complementary DNA has been isolated and sequenced [Yang et al., 1992]. A number of mutations have been described in glycogenosis type IIIa [Okubo et al., 1996, 1999, 2000; Parvari et al., 1998; Shaiu et al., 2000; Shen et al., 1996, 1997] and in glycogenosis type IIIb [Shen et al., 1996]. It is interesting to note that most patients with the type IIIb variant have mutations in exon 3 of the debrancher gene, which are expected to result in truncated proteins [Shen et al., 1996]. Whereas the overall incidence of type III glycogenosis in the U.S. is about 1 in 100,000 live births, it is unusually frequent among Jews of north African descent in Israel (prevalence, 1 per 5400; carrier prevalence, 1 per 35) [Parvari et al., 1997]. Another ethnic group with a high prevalence of glycogenosis type III—1 per 3600, with a carrier frequency of 1 per 30—are individuals from the Faroe Islands [Santer et al., 2001].

TREATMENT

Fasting hypoglycemia should be avoided in infants and young children with debrancher deficiency through the implementation of frequent feedings and nocturnal gastric glucose infusions and uncooked cornstarch [Fernandes, 1990]. A marked improvement after institution of a high-protein diet overnight for 6 months was documented in a 7-year-old child with severe weakness and wasting [Slonim et al., 1982]. However, a 6-month high-protein diet had no significant effect on an adult with myopathy and distal wasting [DiMauro and Tsujino, 1994].

Phosphofructokinase Deficiency

CLINICAL FEATURES

Muscle phosphofructokinase deficiency (glycogenosis type VII) has been reported in fewer than 40 patients [Rowland et al., 1986]. Exercise intolerance with cramps and compensated hemolysis are the main clinical features. Fixed weakness of late adult onset was prominent in three patients. Myoglobinuria has been documented in 10 of 25 patients. Six children have been reported with early severe myopathy, with or without contractures [Amit et al., 1992; DiMauro and Tsujino, 1994]. One male also had a cardiomyopathy and died at 21 months of age [Amit et al., 1992]. None of the infantile cases had hemolysis, which is suggestive of different molecular etiologies. Other associated multisystem signs in infants or very young children have included seizures, cortical blindness, corneal opacifications, and cardiomyopathy [DiMauro and Lamperti, 2001]. Four patients had hemolysis without myopathy; two of these patients had normal or only mildly decreased muscle activity and about half-normal erythrocyte phosphofructokinase activity. This finding was attributed to instability of the muscle-specific subunit of phosphofructokinase [Etiemble and Kahn, 1976; Kahn et al., 1975]. Minor clinical differences from McArdle's disease include more common reports of nausea and vomiting during exercise-induced crises of myalgia, cramps, and weakness and lesser frequency of attacks of myoglobinuria [DiMauro and Lamperti, 2001]. Considering that phosphofructokinase deficiency blocks both the metabolism of muscle glycogen and blood glucose, Haller and Vissing [2004] studied five individuals with muscle phosphofructokinase deficiency and 29 patients with McArdle's disease during continuous cycle exercise. They found that no phosphofructokinase-deficient patient developed a spontaneous second-wind phenomenon under conditions that consistently produced one in patients with McArdle's disease and concluded that the ability to metabolize blood glucose was critical to the development of a typical spontaneous second-wind phenomenon.

LABORATORY DATA

The serum creatine kinase concentration is usually increased in patients with muscle disease. Hemolysis is indicated by an increased serum bilirubin level and moderate reticulocytosis [DiMauro and Tsujino, 1994]. Most patients have an increase in uric acid. The electromyogram may appear normal or myopathic. ^{31}P-NMR spectroscopy reveals a pattern different from that obtained in McArdle's disease, because in phosphofructokinase deficiency, as well as in other defects of distal glycolysis, glycolytic intermediates accumulate in muscle as phosphorylated monoesters and can be detected as a distinct spectral peak [Argov and Bank, 1991].

INHERITANCE

The gene encoding the muscle (M) subunit is located on chromosome 1 [Vora et al., 1982].

MUSCLE BIOPSY

Diagnosis can be made from a negative histochemical phosphofructokinase stain [Bonilla and Schotland, 1970]. The definitive diagnosis comes from the biochemical analysis but only if the muscle specimen is snap-frozen at the time of biopsy, because phosphofructokinase is highly labile and its activity declines rapidly in specimens kept at room temperature or on wet ice, which is why partial phosphofructoinase deficiencies with residual activities above 10% or 20% of normal should be considered skeptically [DiMauro and Lamperti, 2001]. An important feature differentiating this condition from McArdle's disease is the presence of an abnormal polysaccharide in some cases, particularly older patients [Hays et al., 1981]. This abnormal polysaccharide has the characteristics of polyglucosan and stains intensely with the periodic acid-Schiff reaction but is resistant to diastase digestion, and, ultrastructurally, it is composed of finely granular and filamentous material, similar to the storage material seen in branching enzyme deficiency and in Lafora's disease [DiMauro and Lamperti, 2001].

BIOCHEMISTRY

Phosphofructokinase (ATP:D-fructose-1-phosphotransferase) is a tetrameric enzyme under the control of three structural loci that encode three distinct subunits: M (muscle), L (liver), and P (platelet) [Vora, 1983; Vora et al., 1983a]. The three subunits have variable expression in different tissues. Mature human muscle expresses only the M subunit, whereas erythrocytes express both the M and L subunits, thereby containing five isozymes. In the typical form of phosphofructokinase deficiency, genetic defects of the M subunit cause total lack of activity in muscle and partial enzyme deficiency in erythrocytes, in which the homotetramer L4 is responsible for the residual activity. Other tissues, such as liver, that express predominantly the L subunit are not affected.

PATHOPHYSIOLOGY

The functional consequences of phosphofructokinase deficiency are similar to those observed in McArdle's disease and are related to the inability of muscle to generate pyruvate [DiMauro and Tsujino, 1994]. With the ischemic exercise test, the venous lactate levels fails to rise [Tarui et al., 1965). However, phosphofructokinase deficiency differs signific-antly from phosphorylase deficiency by the inability of phosphofructokinase-deficient muscle to use glucose. Because of this inability, maximal oxygen uptake has been increased by increasing free fatty acid availability [Haller and Lewis, 1991]. Exercise intolerance is not decreased by glucose administration, which is potentially harmful because it reduces the concentration of free fatty acids and ketones. This problem explains why high-carbohydrate meals exacerbate exercise intolerance in patients with phosphofructokinase deficiency, a situation referred to as the *out-of-wind phenomenon* [Haller and Lewis, 1991]. The excessive exercise-induced degradation of muscle purine nucleotides likely accounts for the hyperuricemia present in phosphofructokinase-, phosphorylase-, and debrancher-deficient patients [Mineo et al., 1987]. Finally, in phosphofructokinase deficiency, as in McArdle's disease, exercise triggers increases in heart rate, cardiac output, and blood flow, which are exaggerated in relation to the muscle's capacity to use oxygen [Lewis et al., 1991].

MOLECULAR GENETICS

The genes encoding the M, P, and L subunits have been assigned to chromosomes 1, 10, and 21 (see Table 81-1) [Van Keuren et al., 1986; Vora et al., 1982, 1983b]. The M subunit complementary DNA has been isolated and sequenced [Nakajima et al., 1987], and evidence for tissue-specific alternative messenger RNA splicing has been documented [Nakajima et al., 1990]. At least 20 mutations responsible for muscle phosphofructokinase deficiency have been identified [DiMauro and Lamperti, 2001; DiMauro et al., 1995; Sherman et al., 1994; Tsujino et al., 1994d]. Raben and Sherman [1995] tabulated 15 disease-inducing mutations of the muscle phosphofructokinase gene and several polymorphisms. These included splicing defects, frameshifts, and missense mutations in patients from six different ethnic backgrounds, supporting of genetic heterogeneity of the disease. This disorder appeared to be particularly prevalent among individuals of Ashkenazi Jewish descent. The most frequent mutation in these patients was an exon 5 splicing defect, which accounted for approximately 68% of the mutant alleles. Patients in whom muscle phosphofructokinase deficiency is diagnosed in the United States have been of Ashkenazi Jewish origin, and the several mutations identified in them differ from those described in the non-Ashkenazi Italian and Japanese patients [DiMauro et al., 1995].

TREATMENT

Glucose is not an alternative substrate in phosphofructokinase deficiency. A high-protein diet may be beneficial, although this has not been tried [DiMauro and Tsujino, 1994]. A 2-year-old male with the severe infantile form of phosphofructokinase deficiency, including arthrogryposis multiplex congenita, respiratory insufficiency, slowed motor nerve conduction velocities, and abnormal electroencephalographic patterns had a significant improvement in strength, electromyographic features, and electroencephalographic patterns on the ketogenic diet [Swoboda et al., 1997]. Unfortunately, the child died of complications of pneumonia at 35 months.

Phosphoglycerate Kinase Deficiency

CLINICAL FEATURES

Phosphoglycerate kinase deficiency (glycogenosis type IX) manifests with nonspherocytic hemolytic anemia and dysfunction of the central nervous system [Boivin et al., 1974; Valentine et al., 1960]. Neurologic problems have included behavioral abnormalities, mental retardation, seizures, and strokes. In hemizygous male patients, the severe hemolytic anemia manifests soon after birth with jaundice, splenomegaly, and hemoglobinuria. Childhood mortality has been reported in four members of one family [Valentine et al., 1960]. Heterozygous females may be normal or may have mild chronic hemolytic anemia. Myopathic features have included myopathy in males [DiMauro et al., 1981a, 1983a; Morimoto et al., 2003; Rosa et al., 1982; Tonin et al., 1993] with exercise intolerance, cramps, and myoglobinuria. Twenty phosphoglycerate kinase variants with reduced phosphoglycerate kinase activity have been identified; myopathy was present in eight of these variants [Tsujino et al., 1995b].

LABORATORY DATA

Myopathic patients demonstrate an inconsistent increase in resting serum creatine kinase level.

INHERITANCE

Phosphoglycerate kinase is located on the long arm of the X chromosome (see Table 81-1). The defect is expressed in fibroblasts, and prenatal diagnosis is possible [DiMauro and Tsujino, 1994].

MUSCLE BIOPSY

Periodic acid–Schiff stain for glycogen illustrated mildly increased levels in one patient. Electron microscopic studies demonstrated glycogen accumulation in all patients [DiMauro and Tsujino, 1994].

BIOCHEMISTRY

Human phosphoglycerate kinase is a single polypeptide encoded on the X chromosome for all tissues except spermatogenic cells [DiMauro and Tsujino, 1994]. The complete amino acid sequence of normal human phosphoglycerate kinase has been determined [Huang et al., 1980a, 1980b], and mutations have been identified. Patients with hemoglobinuria and those with myopathy demonstrate genetic heterogeneity in enzyme activities. Phosphoglycerate kinase mutant genes associated with myopathy have been named *Creteil* [Rosa et al., 1982], *New Jersey* [DiMauro et al., 1983a], *Alberta* [Tonin et al., 1993], *Hamamatsu* [Sugie et al., 1989], *Shizuoka* [Fujii et al., 1992], and *North Carolina* [Tsujino et al., 1994e]. Because phosphoglycerate kinase is a monomer, there are no tissue-specific isoforms with the exception of phosphoglycerate kinase 2, which is confined to spermatogenic cells; therefore the defect should be expressed in all tissues. In three patients with myopathy, phosphoglycerate kinase was documented to be significantly decreased in erythrocytes, leukocytes, platelets, fibroblasts, and muscle culture [DiMauro et al., 1983a; Rosa et al., 1982; Tonin et al., 1993].

PATHOPHYSIOLOGY

It is difficult to explain the lack of clinical myopathy in many patients with hemolytic anemia and conversely, the selective involvement of muscle in other patients [DiMauro and Tsujino, 1994]. However, one patient with phosphoglycerate kinase Shizuoka has been described with chronic hemolysis and myoglobinuria [Fujii et al., 1992], and a second patient has been described with hemolytic anemia, central nervous system dysfunction, and myopathy [Sugie et al., 1994]. Systematic correlation of molecular genetic, biochemical, and clinical data in future patients may provide insight into the explanation for the striking clinical heterogeneity of phosphoglycerate kinase deficiency [Tsujino et al., 1995b].

MOLECULAR GENETICS

A full-length complementary DNA for the normal phosphoglycerate kinase gene on the X chromosome has been isolated [Michelson et al., 1983], and genetic heterogeneity has been documented [Tonin et al., 1993]. Seven missense mutations and one splice-junction mutation have been identified in eight patients, three of whom had myopathy [Fujii et al., 1992; Morimoto et al., 2003; Tsujino et al., 1994e, 1995b]. The testicular isozyme, phosphoglycerate kinase 2, is encoded by a gene on chromosome 19 [DiMauro and Lamperti, 2001].

Phosphoglycerate Mutase Deficiency

CLINICAL FEATURES

Phosphoglycerate mutase deficiency (glycogenosis type X) has been reported in four men and two women [DiMauro et al., 1981b; DiMauro and Tsujino, 1994]. Exercise intolerance, cramps, and myoglobinuria are the main clinical features.

LABORATORY DATA

Four patients demonstrated an increase in serum creatine kinase concentration between attacks. Results of electromyographic and nerve-conduction studies were normal.

MUSCLE BIOPSY

A variable increase in the periodic acid–Schiff stain reaction has been demonstrated on histochemical examination, and electron microscopic studies have confirmed mild glycogen accumulation in most cases [DiMauro and Tsujino, 1994].

BIOCHEMISTRY

Phosphoglycerate mutase catalyzes the conversion of 3-phosphoglycerate to 2-phosphoglycerate and is very active in normal human muscle [DiMauro et al., 1981b, 1982]. The glycogen concentration in muscle was normal in four patients and moderately increased in two [DiMauro and Tsujino, 1994]. Insufficient in vitro lactate production has been demonstrated in three patients during anaerobic glycolysis [DiMauro et al., 1981b; Servidei and DiMauro, 1989]. The residual phosphoglycerate mutase activity varied from 2.1% to 6% of normal. Human phosphoglycerate mutase is a dimeric enzyme that consists of different proportions of a slow-migrating muscle (MM) isozyme, a fast-migrating brain (BB) isozyme, and an intermediate hybrid (MB) form in different tissues [Omenn and Cheung, 1974; Omenn and Hermodson, 1975]. The electrophoretic pattern of normal adult human muscle phosphoglycerate mutase reveals a marked predominance of the MM band, with only faint BB and MB bands [DiMauro et al., 1981b, 1982; Omenn and Cheung, 1974; Omenn and Hermodson, 1975]. The only other tissues containing substantial amounts of the M subunit are heart and sperm, although there is no evidence of cardiomyopathy or male infertility in phosphoglycerate mutase deficiency [DiMauro and Lamperti, 2001]. In cardiac muscle, the MM isozyme predominates, although all three bands are seen [DiMauro et al., 1981b; Omenn and Hermodson, 1975]. In most other tissues, such as those of the brain, liver, leukocytes, and erythrocytes, BB is the only isozyme present on electrophoresis of PGAM-BB [Omenn and Cheung, 1974; Omenn and Hermodson, 1975].

PATHOPHYSIOLOGY

Normal lactate production was demonstrated in one patient during maximal aerobic exercise [Kissel et al., 1985]. ^{31}P-NMR studies revealed exercise-induced accumulation of phosphorylated monoesters and mild intracellular acidosis [Argov et al., 1987].

MOLECULAR GENETICS

A full-length ccomplementary DNA [Shanske et al., 1987] and the genomic clone for phosphoglycerate mutase-M [Tsujino et al., 1989] have been isolated and sequenced, and the gene has been localized to chromosome 7 [Edwards et al., 1989]. Tsujino and associates [1993b] identified three distinct point mutations in five patients with phosphoglycerate mutase-M deficiency. A full-length complementary DNA has been identified for phosphoglycerate mutase-B [Sakoda et al., 1988]. The gene has been localized to chromosome 10 [Junien et al., 1982].

Lactate Dehydrogenase Deficiency

CLINICAL FEATURES

Lactate dehydrogenase deficiency (glycogenosis type XI) has been reported in two young men with exercise intolerance and recurrent myoglobinuria [Bryan et al., 1990; Kanno et al., 1980]. It has also been reported in an asymptomatic woman through blood screening [Maekawa et al., 1984]. In addition to muscle symptoms, three affected Japanese women suffered from dystocia, which necessitated cesarean sections, and a few patients had dermatologic problems [Kanno et al., 1995]. Takayasu and colleagues [1991] reported a 16-year-old Japanese female who had desquamating erythematosquamous lesions primarily on the extensor surface of the extremities. The epidermis of the diseased skin and scalp hair follicles were virtually devoid of lactate dehydrogenase activity.

LABORATORY DATA

The forearm ischemic exercise test demonstrated an abnormally low increase in venous lactate, in contrast to an excessive increase in pyruvate, in all three patients studied. The muscle biopsy specimen was normal in one patient [Bryan et al., 1990].

BIOCHEMISTRY

Lactate dehydrogenase is a tetrameric enzyme composed of two subunits, M (or A) and H (or B), which result in five isozymes, the two homotetramers, M4 and H4, and the three hybrid forms. The M subunit-containing isozymes predominate in skeletal muscle. The H subunit-containing isozymes predominate in heart and other tissues [DiMauro and Tsujino, 1994].

MOLECULAR GENETICS

The gene encoding lactate dehydrogenase-M has been assigned to chromosome 11 [Boone et al., 1972]. The gene encoding lactate dehydrogenase-H has been assigned to chromosome 12 [Chen et al., 1973]. Five mutations have been described that lead to muscle lactate dehydrogenase deficiency [DiMauro et al., 1995; Maekawa et al., 1990, 1991, 1994].

Branching Enzyme Deficiency

CLINICAL FEATURES

Branching enzyme (brancher) deficiency (glycogenosis type IV) manifests in infancy as a rapidly progressive disease dominated by liver dysfunction with hepatosplenomegaly and cirrhosis, with death from hepatic failure or gastrointestinal bleeding by 4 years of age [DiMauro and Tsujino, 1994]. Other clinical features include hypotonia, muscle wasting, and contractures [Fernandes and Huijing, 1968; Zellweger et al., 1972]. Cardiomyopathy has also been documented in several affected children [Farrans et al., 1966; Servidei et al., 1987]. Isolated myopathy has been reported in six patients, three siblings with delayed motor development and chronic proximal weakness [Reusche et al., 1992], a child with myopathy and hepatic involvement [Bruno et al., 1999], and two adults in whom proximal weakness had started at 26 and 49 years of age [Bornemann et al., 1996; Ferguson et al., 1983]. Schroder and co-workers [1993] reported a case of juvenile type IV glycogenosis with total brancher deficiency in skeletal muscle and liver in a male patient who presented with severe myopathy, dilated cardiomyopathy, heart failure, dysmorphic features, and subclinical neuropathy and who died at age 19 of sudden cardiac death. Alegria and associates [1999] reported hydrops fetalis as a presenting manifestation of glycogenosis type IV. The infant was delivered by cesarean section at 34 weeks and had generalized edema, severe hypotonia, and arthrogryposis of the lower limbs at birth and died at 4 days of age. Cox and colleagues [1999] reported three sibling fetuses who were documented to have type IV glycogenosis by pathologic and biochemical studies and who had onset of hydrops, limb contractures, and akinesia early in the second trimester. This disease has considerable clinical heterogeneity. Brancher deficiency has been identified in the leukocytes of two Israeli patients with adult polyglucosan body disease [Lossos et al., 1991]. Adult polyglucosan body disease has been described in approximately 15 patients and is characterized by progressive upper and lower motor neuron involvement, sensory loss, sphincter problems, neurogenic bladder, and, in some cases, dementia [Bruno et al., 1993; Cafferty et al., 1991].

LABORATORY DATA

Carbohydrate tolerance tests and the response of blood glucose to glucagon or epinephrine are normal in affected patients with liver disease [DiMauro and Tsujino, 1994]. The serum creatine kinase concentration is inconsistently increased. Echocardiography revealed cardiac dilatation and impaired shortening of the left ventricular ejection fraction in one patient [Servidei et al., 1987]. Sensorimotor axonopathy has been demonstrated in patients with adult polyglucosan body disease [Bruno et al., 1993; Cafferty et al., 1991].

INHERITANCE

Prenatal diagnosis is possible in fibroblasts and amniocytes [Brown and Brown, 1989].

MUSCLE BIOPSY

Muscle biopsy demonstrates deposits of basophilic, intensely periodic acid–Schiff stain–positive material, which is only partially sensitive to diastase digestion. Electron microscopy reveals storage material consisting of filamentous and finely granular material often associated with normal-looking glycogen beta particles [DiMauro and Tsujino, 1994]. The abnormal polysaccharide is found in skin, liver, muscle, heart, and the central nervous system. In adult polyglucosan body disease, polyglucosan bodies have been found in both gray and white matter in the processes of neurons and astrocytes. In sural nerve biopsies, the bodies are in the axoplasm primarily of myelinated fibers and in Schwann cells [Cafferty et al., 1991].

BIOCHEMISTRY

Branching enzyme catalyzes the last step in glycogen biosynthesis by attaching a short glucosyl chain in an α-1,6-glucosidic link to a naked peripheral chain of nascent glycogen [DiMauro and Tsujino, 1994]. The polysaccharide that accumulates has peripheral chains that are longer than normal and fewer branching points than does normal glycogen.

MOLECULAR GENETICS

Several mutations have been identified in patients with different clinical presentations [Bao et al., 1996; Bruno et al., 1999]. One of these, Tyr329Ser, was present in seven patients with adult polyglucosan body disease [Lossos et al., 1998].

TREATMENT

A number of strategies have been used, including administration of glucagon; long-term use of steroids; a high-protein, low-carbohydrate diet; and administration of fungal α-1,4-glucosidase and α-1,6-glucosidase. These strategies have been ineffective [DiMauro and Tsujino, 1994]. Liver transplantation was thought to be beneficial in 10 children [Selby et al., 1991], although one child developed intractable cardiomyopathy 2 years after transplantation [Sokal et al., 1992].

Aldolase A Deficiency (Glycogenosis Type XII)

CLINICAL FEATURES

This disorder was discovered in 1996 in a 4-year-old male who presented with episodic exercise intolerance and weakness after febrile illnesses [Kreuder et al., 1996]. This boy was considered to have myoglobinuria even though his highest serum creatine kinase concentration was 6480 U/liter (normal, <60 U/liter). He also had proximal muscle wasting with weakness and episodes of nonspherocytic hemolytic anemia and jaundice.

BIOCHEMISTRY

Biochemical assays revealed a profound reduction in muscle and red blood cell aldolase levels and a decrease in the thermostability of the residual enzyme [Kreuder et al., 1996]. The enzyme is a tetramer of identical 40,000-Da subunits. Vertebrates have three aldolase isozymes that are distinguished by their electrophoretic and catalytic properties [Charlesworth, 1972].

MOLECULAR GENETICS

The aldolase A gene has been mapped to chromosome region 16q22-q24, and two pseudogenes were found on chromosomes 3 and 10 [Kukita et al., 1987; Serero et al., 1988]. The patient described by Kreuder and colleagues [1996] was found to be homozygous for a germline mutation in which a negatively charged glutamic acid is changed to a positively charged lysine at residue 206, a residue that is highly conserved within the subunit interface region.

FATTY ACID OXIDATION DISORDERS

Historical Background

Fatty acid oxidation disorders are an important group of diseases because they potentially are rapidly fatal and are a source of major morbidity. They manifest with a spectrum of clinical disorders, including recurrent myoglobinuria; progressive lipid storage myopathy; neuropathy, progressive cardiomyopathy; recurrent hypoglycemic hypoketotic encephalopathy, or Reye-like syndrome; seizures; and mental retardation. All of the currently known conditions are inherited as autosomal-recessive traits. Thus, there is frequently a family history of sudden infant death syndrome in siblings. Early recognition and prompt institution of therapy, appropriate preventive measures, and, in certain cases, specific therapy may be lifesaving and may significantly decrease long-term morbidity, particularly with regard to central nervous system sequelae. There are at least 20 recognized defects in fatty acid oxidation, most of which have been diagnosed since 1990. With the significant advances in bioedical technology, there has been a rapid increase in the number of subsequently diagnosed cases. For example, in a study of 410 consecutive neonatal blood-spot cards in a northern English population for the most common mutation for MCAD deficiency (substitution of a guanine for an adenine at base pair 985 in the MCAD gene), the data suggested a heterozygote carrier state of 1 per 68 for this particular mutation, with a projected homozygote frequency of approximately 1 per 18,500 births [Blakemore et al., 1991; Gregersen et al., 1991]. The incidence for MCAD deficiency was even higher, at 1 per 8930 live births, in a more recent survey from the Pennsylvania neonatal screening program, in which diagnosis by tandem mass spectrometry was followed by confirmation through molecular analysis for several common mutations [Ziadeh et al., 1995].

The delay in recognition of these disorders can be attriuted to three major factors. First, fatty acid oxidation does not play a major role in energy production until relatively late in fasting. Thus, affected individuals may remain clinically asymptomatic until they experience periods of fasting beyond 12 hours or prolonged exercise. In a number of cases, the acute decompensation may be precipitated by an intercurrent infection with fasting, vomiting, and shivering thermogenesis. Second, results of routine laboratory tests, such as that for urinary ketones, may not demonstrate the defect in fatty acid oxidation, unless the blood and urine samples are obtained at the time of the acute episode. If they are obtained after the child has received intravenous glucose therapy or has recovered from the acute illness, the defect may be missed. Thirdly, there has been a rapid expansion in the methods for identifying defects in fatty acid oxidation. For example, methods to identify abnormal fatty acid metabolites in the urine through gas chromatography/mass spectrometry have been available only since the mid-1970s. The identification of certain characteristic organic acid profiles in urine specimens taken during the acute episode has been seminal in the diagnosis of the probable site of defect.

Fasting Adaptation

Fats constitute the most important and efficient fuel for oxidative metabolism and are the largest reserve of fuel in the body. Because liver glycogen stores are depleted within a few hours of a meal, and because there are no reserve stores of protein in the body, fatty acids become the predominant substrate for oxidation quite early in fasting [Stanley, 1987]. In adults, fatty acids provide approximately 80% of caloric requirements after a 24-hour period of fasting; this proportion increases to 94% during more prolonged fasting. Fatty acids serve three major functions. First, the partial oxidation of fatty acids by the liver produces ketones, which are an important auxiliary fuel for almost all tissues and particularly for the brain. Because the blood-brain barrier prevents the direct use of long-chain fatty acids by the brain, ketones provide an important mechanism with which to spare glucose oxidation and proteolysis during prolonged fasting [Cahill, 1970]. Second, fatty acids serve as a major fuel for cardiac and skeletal muscle. During mild-to-moderate prolonged exercise and during rest, muscle depends primarily on fatty acid oxidation [Essen, 1978; Felig and Wahren, 1975; Gollnick et al., 1974]. Third, the high rates of hepatic gluconeogenesis and ureagenesis needed for maintaining fasting homeostasis are sustained by the production of energy (ATP), reducing equivalents, and metabolic intermediates derived from fatty acid oxidation [Hale and Bennett, 1992].

Increased Susceptibility of the Child

There are several reasons for an increased risk of problems with fasting adaptation in infants and young children [Aynsley-Green, 1982; Bier et al., 1977; Pildes et al., 1973]. First, because of the large ratio of surface area to body mass, basal energy needs in the infant are high so as to maintain body temperature. Shivering thermogenesis, which maintains body temperature, is highly dependent on efficient fatty acid oxidation. Second, infants have a larger brain in comparison with body size. The developing brain is highly dependent on glucose and has a high rate of metabolism [Hale and Bennett, 1992]; therefore, infants and children exhibit even earlier activation of fatty acid oxidation with hyperketonemia within 12 to 24 hours of fasting. Third, there is a lower activity of several key enzymes involved in energy production in the infant than in the older child and

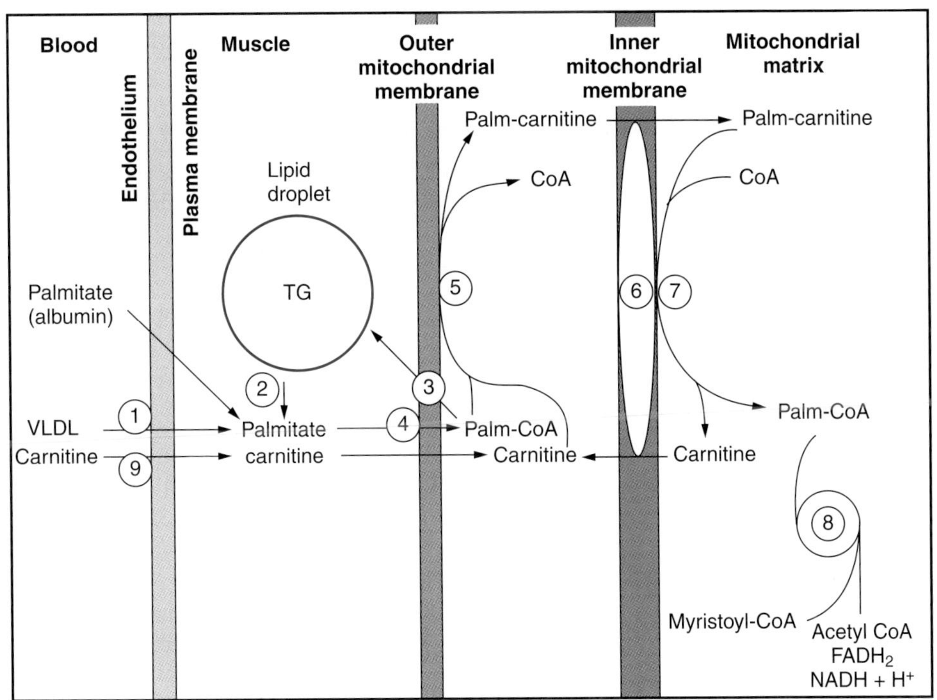

FIGURE 81-2. Schematic representation of long-chain fatty acid metabolism in muscle. Blood-borne substrates are represented by fatty acids bound to albumin and by triglycerides in the form of very-low-density lipoproteins (VLDL). Endogenous lipid stores are triglycerides (TG) in lipid droplets. Enzymes or enzyme complexes are indicated by circled numbers adjacent to or within the membrane to which they are bound: 1, lipoprotein lipase; 2, intracellular neutral triglyceride, diglyceride, and monoglyceride lipase; 3, triglyceride synthetic pathway; 4, palmitoyl (Palm)-coenzyme A (CoA) synthetase; 5, CPT I; 6, carnitine-acylcarnitine translocase; 7, carnitine palmitoyltransferase II; 8, beta oxidation pathway; 9, active transport system for carnitine. $FADH_2$, flavin adenine dinucleotide, reduced form; H^+, hydrogen ion; Mit, mitochondrial; NADH, nicotinamide adenine dinucleotide, reduced form. (From DiMauro S, Tonin P, Servidei S. In: Rowland LP, DiMauro S, eds. Handbook of clinical neurology, vol 18, Myopathies. Amsterdam: Elsevier Science, 1992;479–526.)

adult, which leads to further impairment of the infant's ability to maintain glucose homeostasis [Pagliara et al., 1973].

Normal Pathway of Fatty Acid Oxidation

The pathway of mitochondrial fatty acid oxidation is outlined in Figure 81-2 [DiMauro et al., 1992]. Free fatty acids are liberated from adipocytes during fasting and are transported to other tissues either as triglyceride-rich lipoproteins or bound to serum albumin [Stremmel et al., 1986]. Once across the plasma membrane, short-chain (e.g., four-carbon) and medium-chain (e.g., eight-carbon) fatty acids of fewer than 10 carbon atoms are able to cross the outer and inner mitochondrial membranes as free acids to enter the mitochondrial matrix. They are then activated into their CoA esters for ensuant intramitochondrial beta oxidation. The mitochondrial membrane is impermeable to long-chain (e.g., 16-carbon) fatty acids. Therefore, long-chain fatty acids diffuse or are transported to the outer mitochondrial membrane and to the endoplasmic reticulum, where they are activated by conversion to their CoA thioesters by long-chain acyl-CoA synthetase [Schulz, 1985]. The inner mitochondrial membrane is impermeable to CoA and its derivatives. Therefore, the long-chain acyl-CoA must first be converted into its acylcarnitine form (e.g., palmitoylcarnitine), with release of free CoA by carnitine palmitoyltransferase I, which is located on the inner side of the outer mitochondrial membrane [Murthy and Pande, 1987]. The palmitoylcarnitine is then translocated across the inner mitochondrial membrane by carnitine-acylcarnitine translocase [Pande, 1975]. In the mitochondrial matrix, palmitoylcarnitine in the presence of free CoA is then converted back to palmitoyl-CoA and carnitine by carnitine palmitoyltransferase II on the inner side of the inner mitochondrial membrane.

There are four sequential steps in mitochondrial beta oxidation, which is composed of chain length–specific enzymes. Until recently, it was held that the complete intramitochondrial oxidation of long-chain fatty acids required a minimum of nine enzymes, including the three genetically distinct acyl-CoA dehydrogenases (short-, medium-, and long-chain) [Ikeda et al., 1983], at least two enoyl-CoA hydratases (crotonase and long-chain enoyl-CoA hydratase) [Fong and Schulz, 1981], two *L*-3-hydroxyacyl-CoA dehydrogenases (short- and long-chain) [El-Fakhri and Middleton, 1982], and two 3-ketoacyl-CoA thiolases (acetoacetyl-CoA thiolase and generalized 3-ketoacyl-CoA thiolase) [Middleton, 1975]. Further characterization has revealed the presence of an additional VLCAD enzyme [Izai et al., 1992; Kelley, 1992] and of a trifunctional enzyme, which combines the activities of the long-chain enoyl-CoA hydratase, long-chain *L*-3-hydroxyacyl-CoA dehydrogenase (LCHAD), and the long-chain thiolase enzymes [Carpenter et al., 1992; Hashimoto, 1992; Luo et al., 1993]. The trifunctional protein is a heterocomplex of four alpha and four beta subunits, which are encoded by two nuclear genes. The alpha subunit contains the long-chain enoyl-CoA hydratase and LCHAD activities, and the beta subunit contains the long-chain 3-ketoacyl-CoA thiolase activity [Kamijo et al., 1993]. There are two different biochemical phenotypes of trifunctional protein deficiency [Jackson et al., 1992; Kamijo et al., 1994]. The first includes deficiency of all three enzyme activities of the trifunctional protein, with loss of both alpha and beta subunits documented by immunoblotting studies. The second has isolated LCHAD deficiency with preservation of the long-chain enoyl-CoA hydratase and 3-ketoacyl-CoA thiolase activities and normal amounts of alpha and beta subunit proteins.

With each complete cycle of intramitochondrial beta oxidation, a two-carbon fragment is cleaved, and an acetyl-CoA moiety is released. Most tissues, such as those of muscle and the heart, oxidize acetyl-CoA for energy production through the tricarboxylic acid cycle. In liver, approximately 90% of the hepatic acetyl-CoA is converted into ketones via the coordinated action of acetyl-CoA acetyltransferase, β-hydroxy-β-methylglutaryl-CoA lyase, and β-hydroxybutyrate dehydrogenase [Reed and Lane, 1975]. The ketones are then exported for final oxidation by other tissues, such as brain.

Alternative Pathways for Fatty Acid Metabolism

Mitochondrial beta oxidation accounts for the majority of fatty acid oxidation under normal circumstances. The peroxisome may contribute up to 20% of total cellular fatty acid oxidation, under conditions of prolonged fasting, through omega oxidation, which leads to the formation of dicarboxylic acids [Krahling et al., 1978]. The specific pattern of dicarboxylic acids in serum or urine may be useful in the identification of specific inborn errors of fatty acid oxidation. When there is an impairment in mitochondrial beta oxidation, three additional mechanisms may be important. These include the deacylation of CoA by thioesterases and the conjugation of acyl groups to glycine and to carnitine [Kolvraa and Gregersen, 1986; Roe et al., 1985]. Measurement of acylcarnitines and acylglycines is also diagnostically useful in the identification of genetic defects in fatty acid oxidation [Baretz et al., 1976; Millington, 1986; Rinaldo et al., 1988].

Clinical and Biochemical Features of Identified Defects

Common Features of Fatty Acid Oxidation Disorders

Hale and Bennett [1992] suggested that there are at least four clinical and laboratory features that should lead the clinician to suspect a genetic defect in fatty acid oxidation: (1) acute metabolic decompensation in association with fasting, (2) chronic involvement of tissues highly dependent on efficient fatty acid oxidation (e.g., heart, muscle, and liver), (3) recurrent episodes of hypoketotic hypoglycemia, and (4) alterations in the quantity of total carnitine or in the percentage of esterified carnitine in plasma and tissue.

METABOLIC DECOMPENSATION IN ASSOCIATION WITH FASTING

Children with fatty acid oxidation defects are most prone to decompensation, within the context of depleted glycogen and glucose reserves, during conditions that place stress on the fatty acid oxidation pathway for fuel generation. These conditions include prolonged exercise (particularly after 1 hour of mild-to-moderate aerobic exercise), fasting, infection with vomiting, and cold-induced shivering thermogenesis.

In cold exposure, ketogenesis is stimulated in normal individuals [Johnson et al., 1961], and shivering, which is an involuntary form of muscle activity, also depends on long-chain fatty acid oxidation [Bell and Thompson, 1979]. After an overnight fast, affected children are most likely to be found comatose in the early morning hours. During infection, there may be an added problem with vomiting and decreased oral intake. Children may also present with a Reye-like syndrome. Infants and younger children are at greater risk during fasting because of their decreased abilities to adapt to fasting. Prolonged fasting for an infant younger than 1 year is 6 to 10 hours, in comparison with 12 hours for a child between 1 and 4 years of age [Hale and Bennett, 1992].

INVOLVEMENT OF FATTY ACID OXIDATION–DEPENDENT TISSUES

Tissues such as skeletal muscle, heart, and liver have high energy demands and are therefore dependent on efficient fatty acid oxidation. When there is a defect in hepatic ketogenesis, glucose becomes the only available fuel and thus becomes rate limiting under conditions of fatty acid oxidation stress when glycogen and glucose stores have been depleted. As a result, free fatty acids, which are liberated during fasting and cannot be metabolized because of the block, may be stored in the cytosol as triglycerides. This situation produces a progressive lipid storage myopathy with weakness; hypertrophic or dilatative cardiomyopathy, or both; and a fatty liver. Increased content of short- or medium-chain fatty acids and, in particular, their dicarboxylic metabolites, from compensatory omega oxidation, may cause a variety of secondary biochemical abnormalities, including an impairment of gluconeogenesis, beta oxidation, and the citric acid cycle [Corkey et al., 1988; Tonsgard, 1986; Tonsgard and Getz, 1985], leading to a further decrease in cellular ATP production. In addition, in the long-chain fatty acid oxidation disorders, which may have recurrent episodes of acute muscle breakdown or myoglobinuria (e.g., carnitine palmitoyltransferase II, VLCAD, and trifunctional enzyme deficiencies), the accumulation of long-chain fatty acids and long-chain acylcarnitines may have detergent-like actions on muscle membranes. Excessive amounts of palmitoyl-CoA and palmitoylcarnitine have detergent properties on isolated canine myocytic sarcolemmal membranes and potentiate free radical–induced lipid membrane peroxidative injury in ischemia [Mak et al., 1986]. Long-chain acylcarnitines also activate calcium channels in cardiac [Inoue and Pappano, 1983; Spedding, 1985] and smooth muscle myocytes [Spedding, 1985; Spedding and Mir, 1987]. They may thus potentiate the increase in cytosolic calcium associated with arrhythmogenesis, as seen in ischemic myocardium [Lee et al., 1987].

HYPOKETOTIC HYPOGLYCEMIA

The pattern of hypoketotic hypoglycemia reflects the accelerated rate of glucose utilization that occurs when fatty acids cannot be used as fuels and ketone bodies are not generated to spare glucose/glycogen stores. An increase in the ratio of serum free fatty acids to ketones from the normal 1:1 to greater than 2:1 therefore suggests a block in beta oxidation.

ALTERATIONS IN PLASMA AND TISSUE CONCENTRATIONS OF CARNITINE

In most cases of intramitochondrial beta oxidation defects, the total carnitine concentration is decreased (<50% or normal), and the acylcarnitine fraction is increased (>50% esterified; normal is 10% to 25% in the fed state and 30% to 50% in the fasting state) [Hale and Bennett, 1992]. In the intramitochondrial beta oxidation disorders, the excessive acyl-CoAs that accumulate proximal to the metabolic block may be converted into acylcarnitines by chain length–specific carnitine acyltransferases [Bremer, 1983]. These acylcarnitines, when filtered through the kidneys, compete with free carnitine at the renal tubular reabsorptive site. Because the longer chain–length acylcarnitines have an increasingly higher affinity for the carnitine transporter than does free carnitine [Stanley et al., 1991], the free carnitine is excreted, which leads to a decrease in free carnitine in the serum. In the case of the high-affinity plasmalemmal carnitine transporter OCTN2 defect, the total carnitine is markedly reduced (e.g., <5% of normal) and the esterified fraction is normal [Tein et al., 1990a] because the transport defect, which is also expressed in kidney, leads to a decreased renal threshold for carnitine reabsorption.

Additional Laboratory Findings

During acute catabolic crises, other biochemical derangements may be present. A modest hyperammonemia (100 to 200 μmol/liter) accompanied by threefold to fivefold elevations of liver transaminases may be documented during the Reye-like syndrome manifestation [Hale and Bennett, 1992]. In acute myoglobinuria, there are marked increases in the concentrations of sarcoplasmic enzymes, including that of serum creatine kinase, which may rise higher than 100,000 IU/liter (normal, <250 IU/liter). The serum concentrations of amino acids (especially taurine), creatinine, potassium, phosphate, and urate may also be increased [Tein et al., 1990b]. These changes may have deleterious renal and cardiac effects, thereby further exaggerating the damage [Knochel, 1976]. Lactic acidosis may also be present during the acute catabolic episodes. This presence may reflect either poor tissue perfusion or inhibition of critical enzymes, such as pyruvate carboxylase, by accumulated metabolites [Corkey et al., 1988]. Urine organic acid screening may demonstrate unusual or excessive amounts of organic acids, which may be diagnostic of a specific block in beta oxidation.

Specific Features of Individual Genetic Defects

For most of the defects in fatty acid oxidation—with the exeption of MCAD, carnitine uptake (OCTN2) defect, classic late-onset carnitine palmitoyltransferase II, VLCAD, LCHAD, α-electron transfer flavoprotein (α-ETF) and ETF-coenzyme Q deficiencies, and 3-hydroxy-3-methylglutaryl (HMG)-CoA lyase deficiency—fewer than 25 cases have been reported in the literature, although more cases may have been diagnosed. Thus, the clinical and laboratory characteristics presented here are based on a review of these cases and are summarized in Table 81-2 [Rinaldo et al., 2002; Tein, 1995, 2000a].

There are several differentiating features. In the defects involving the transport of fatty acids into the mitochondria (carnitine uptake defect, carnitine palmitoyltransferase I,

TABLE 81-2

Clinical Features Associated with Specific Genetic Defects of Fatty Acid Oxidation

DEFICIENCY	FASTING DISORDER	TISSUE INVOLVED	HYPOKETOTIC HYPOGLYCEMIA	ALTERED CARNITINE	DICARBOXYLIC ACIDS	REYE-LIKE SYNDROME	SUDDEN INFANT DEATH SYNDROME
LCFAUD	+	Liver	+	+	NR	NR	NR
CUD	+	Heart, muscle	+	+	NR	+	NR
CPT I	+	Kidney	+	+	NR	+	NR
TRANS	+	Heart, muscle, (myoglobinuria)	+	+	NR	+	+
CPT II (mild)	+/–	Muscle, myoglobinuria, pancreatitis	NR	+	NR	NR	NR
CPT II (severe)	+	Heart, muscle, myoglobinuria, liver	+	+	NR	+	+
VLCAD/LCAD	+	Heart, muscle, myoglobinuria, liver	+	+	+	+	+
Trifunctional/ LCHAD	+	Heart, muscle, myoglobinuria, liver, neuropathy, pancreatitis, retinopathy	+	+	+	+	+
Dienoyl-CoA reductase	NR	Muscle, dysmorphic features, brain, (heart)	NR	+	NR	NR	NR
MCAD	+	(Myoglobinuria)	+	+	+	+	+
SCAD	+	Muscle, brain, dysmorphic features, heart	+/–	+	+	NR	+
SCHAD	+	Heart, muscle, myoglobinuria liver	+	+	+	NR	+
ETF and ETF-Qo	+	Muscle, heart, kidney, brain, dysmorphic features	+	+	+	NR	+
HMG-CoA lyase	+	Brain, pancreatitis	+	+	+	+	+ ?

CoA, coenzyme A; CPT, carnitine palmitoyltransferase; CUD, carnitine uptake defect; ETF, electron transfer flavoprotein; HMG, β-hydroxy-β-methylglutaryl; LCAD, long-chain acyl-CoA dehydrogenase; LCHAD, long-chain L-3-hydroxyacyl-CoA dehydrogenase; LCFAUD, long-chain fatty acid uptake defect; MCAD, medium-chain acyl-CoA dehydrogenase; NR, no case yet reported; Qo, coenzyme Q oxidoreductase; SCAD, short-chain acyl-CoA dehydrogenase; SCHAD, short-chain *L*-3-hydroxyacyl-CoA dehydrogenase; TRANS, carnitine acylcarnitine translocase; trifunctional, long-chain enoyl-CoA hydratase + long-chain *L*-3-hydroxyacyl-CoA dehydrogenase + long-chain 3-ketoacyl-CoA thiolase; VLCAD, very-long-chain acyl-CoA dehydrogenase.

Modified from Tein I. Fatty acid oxidation and associated defects. In American Academy of Neurology Proceedings, 1995. Madison, WI: Omnipress, 1995, 269:9–38.

carnitine-acylcarnitine translocase, carnitine palmitoyltransferase II), there is generally not an associated abnormal dicarboxylicaciduria. However, this has been reported in one case of severe infantile carnitine palmitoyltransferase II deficiency [Elpeleg et al., 1993] and, on one occasion, during an acute metabolic decompensation in an individual with infantile carnitine palmitoyltransferase I deficiency who presented with recurrent Reye-like syndrome [Poll-The et al., 1992]. The carnitine uptake (high-affinity carnitine transporter OCTN2) defect, carnitine palmitoyltransferase I, and carnitine acylcarnitine translocase defects involve both skeletal and cardiac muscle and manifest in infancy or early childhood. The carnitine uptake defect is characterized by a progressive hypertrophic or dilatative cardiomyopathy, or both, which pathologically resembles endocardial fibroelastosis [Tripp et al., 1981]. Of importance is that this defect is exquisitely responsive to high-dose oral carnitine supplementation, which reverses the cardiomyopathy [Stanley et al., 1991; Tein et al., 1990a]. Renal tubular acidosis has been documented in one case of carnitine palmitoyltransferase I deficiency [Falik-Borenstein et al., 1992]. Classic adult carnitine palmitoyltransferase II deficiency is characterized by adolescent-onset recurrent episodes of acute myoglobinuria precipitated by prolonged exercise or fasting, in which power between episodes is normal and in which lipid accumulation in muscle is present only under conditions of fasting and prolonged exercise [DiMauro and Papadimitriou, 1986]. Fasting ketogenesis is generally normal in this condition, although it may be delayed, and there is no fixed cardiomyopathy, although dysrhythmias secondary to hyperkalemia and hypocalcemia may occur during the acute myoglobinuric crises. Statistically speaking, classic carnitine palmitoyltransferase II deficiency is the most common cause for recurrent myoglobinuria in children and in adults [Tein et al., 1990b; Tonin et al., 1990]. Several cases of severe infantile carnitine palmitoyltransferase II deficiency have been described as manifesting with recurrent Reye-like syndrome; hepatomegaly with hypoketotic hypoglycemia and elevated liver aminotransferase concentration; cardiomegaly with cardiac dysrhythmias and elevated serum creatine kinase concentration; and evidence of lipid storage in the heart, skeletal muscle, liver, and kidney [Demaugre et al., 1991; Elpeleg et al., 1993; Hug et al., 1991]. In these cases, the activity of carnitine palmitoyltransferase II in cultured skin fibroblasts was less than 10% of control values, in contrast to the 25% residual activity documented in classic carnitine palmitoyltransferase II deficiency [Demaugre et al., 1991], which may explain the differences in severity of the clinical phenotype.

In addition to the high-affinity plasmalemmal carnitine transporter OCTN2 defect, there is another plasma membrane fatty acid oxidation disorder: long-chain fatty acid transport/binding defect [Al-Odaib et al., 1998]. This defect in the active transport of long-chain free fatty acids across the plasma membrane has been described in two young males who presented with acute liver failure accompanied by hyperammonemia, hyperbilirubinemia, coagulopathy, and mild encephalopathy, with no evidence of cardiac or skeletal myopathy, and who required liver transplantation. One boy had documented hypoketotic hypoglycemia. The uptake of oleic acid (C18:1) in skin fibroblasts from the patients was lower than in control subjects. The features that were atypical for a fatty acid oxidation defect included the absence of fatty liver with low concentrations of long-chain free fatty acids and elevated carnitine concentrations in liver homogenate, caused by defective transport of long-chain free fatty acids.

The intramitochondrial beta-oxidation defects (SCAD, MCAD, LCAD, VLCAD, ETF, ETF-coenzyme Q, SCHAD, medium-and short-chain *L*-3-hydroxyacyl-CoA dehydrogenase (M/SCHAD), trifunctional/LCHAD, medium-chain 3-ketoacyl-CoA thiolase, 2,4-dienoyl-CoA reductase, HMG-CoA synthase, HMG-CoA lyase deficiencies) share many features, although there are differentiating characteristics. Those cases previously attributed to LCHAD deficiency are known to be related to a defect in the trifunctional enzyme that combines the activities of the long-chain enoyl-CoA hydratase, LCHAD, and long-chain 3-ketoacyl-CoA thiolase enzymes [Hashimoto, 1992; Sims et al., 1995], although isolated LCHAD deficiency appears to be more common than trifunctional protein deficiency [Rinaldo et al., 2002]. A number of previously diagnosed cases of LCAD deficiency are believed to be attributable instead to VLCAD deficiency [Aoyama et al., 1995b; Ogilvie et al., 1994; Yamaguchi et al., 1993]. Cardiac involvement (cardiomegaly, cardiomyopathy) is more commonly found in the long-chain defects (e.g., LCAD, VLCAD, trifunctional) [Glasgow et al., 1983; Hale et al., 1985, 1990a, 1990b; Strauss et al., 1995; Tein et al., 1995], although it has also been documented in one case of SCHAD deficiency [Tein et al., 1991] and one case of SCAD deficiency [Tein et al., 1999a]. Cardiomyopathy has been documented in 17 of 24 reported cases of trifunctional enzyme deficiency with presumed or proved marked deficiency of the LCHAD component [Tein et al., 1995].

Chronic skeletal muscle weakness is seen in all of the intramitochondrial beta oxidation defects but less commonly in MCAD [Stanley et al., 1990] and HMG-CoA lyase deficiency [Gibson et al., 1988]. A unique case of SCAD deficiency has been reported in a 13-year-old-female with progressive external ophthalmoplegia, ptosis, cardiomyopathy, and multi-core myopathy [Tein et al., 1999a]. Additional cases of SCAD deficiency with multi-core myopathy have since been identified. Recurrent myoglobinuria has been reported with LCAD [Hale et al., 1990a], VLCAD [Ogilvie et al., 1994], trifunctional [Dionisi-Vici et al., 1991; Tein et al., 1995], and SCHAD deficiencies [Tein et al., 1991]. A first episode of myoglobinuria has also been described in an adult with MCAD deficiency [Ruitenbeek et al., 1995].

All intramitochondrial enzyme defects demonstrate hepatic dysfunction at the time of catabolic decompensation. Persistent dysfunction has been documented in trifunctional enzyme [Hagenfeldt et al., 1990], severe carnitine palmitoyltransferase II [Elpeleg et al., 1993], and LCAD/VLCAD [Hale et al., 1985] deficiencies. Of importance is that isolated LCHAD deficiency in children may also be associated with severe illness in the heterozygous mother during pregnancies with affected fetuses who have a common mutation (G1528C, E474Q) in one or both alleles [Ibdah et al., 1998b; Sims et al., 1995; Tein, 2000b; Treem et al., 1996; Wilcken et al., 1993]. The maternal illnesses include the acute fatty liver of pregnancy syndrome; the syndrome of hypertension or hemolysis, elevated liver enzymes, and low platelets (HELLP); and hyperemesis gravidarum. In acute fatty liver of pregnancy syndrome, the mother may suffer fulminant liver failure and die. In both syndromes, there is microvesicular fatty infiltration of the maternal liver. In addition to the recurrent episodes of myoglobinuria, trifunctional protein/LCHAD deficiency may manifest with progressive pigmentary retinopathy [Tyni et al., 1998, 2004] and motor-sensory neuropathy [Spiekerkoetter et al., 2004]. Thus, the myoneuropathic variant of trifunctional protein/LCHAD deficiency may mimic the spinal muscular atrophy phenotype. There appear to be three major phenotypes of trifunctional protein/LCHAD deficiency with variable overlap: a hepatic form with Reye-like syndrome that is associated with acute fatty liver of pregnancy syndrome; a neonatal cardiomyopathic form; and a less common, milder, myoneuropathic form. These phenotypes appear to be correlated with specific genotypes [Ibdah et al., 1998a, 1999; Isaacs et al., 1996; Sims et al., 1995].

Maternal complications in pregnancy are not limited to carriers of LCHAD mutations. Patients with deficiencies of carnitine palmitoyltransferase I, MCAD, and SCAD were also born to mothers who developed liver disease during their pregnancies [Innes et al., 2000; Matern et al., 2001; Nelson et al., 2000; Walter, 2000]. Therefore, all infants born after pregnancies that are complicated by acute fatty liver of pregnancy or HELLP syndrome should be considered at risk for having a defect in beta oxidation.

SCAD deficiency is a clinically heterogeneous disorder in which the clinical phenotype varies from fatal metabolic decompensation, including intermittent metabolic acidosis and neonatal hyperammonemia, to infantile-onset lipid storage myopathy with failure to thrive, developmental delay, hypotonia, seizures, and hyperreflexia [Bhala et al., 1995] to more subtle later onset progressive myopathy, including multi-core myopathy [Tein et al., 1999a], to asymptomatic states [Ribes et al., 1998]. The characteristic metabolites of ethylmalonic and methlysuccinic acids in SCAD deficiency may also result from the presence of one of two relatively common variants of SCAD (625G>A and 511C>T) that predispose to excessive ethylmalonic acid production. These variants may represent disease susceptibility variations when occurring in combination with other genetic or environmental factors or both, especially fever [Corydon et al., 2001; Gregersen et al., 1998].

Multiple acyl-CoA dehydrogenase deficiency or glutaric acidemia type II is caused by defects of the ETF or ETF-ubiquinone oxidoreductase, which are nuclear encoded proteins through which electrons from flavoprotein acyl-CoA dehydrogenases, dimethylglycine dehydrogenase, and sarcosine dehydrogenase enter the respiratory chain [Frerman and Goodman, 1989]. These cases can be divided into three groups, each consistent within a family, and have been designated as (1) neonatal onset with congenital anomalies, (2) neonatal onset without anomalies, and (3) mild or later onset. Patients in the first two groups are sometimes said to have severe multiple acyl-CoA dehydrogenase deficiency and the third group to have a mild form of this deficiency. Patients with the neonatal onset form and congenital anomalies are often premature, presenting within the first 24 to 48 hours after birth with severe hypoglycemia, hypotonia, hepatomegaly, metabolic acidosis, and an odor similar to that of sweaty feet. Affected infants may have enlarged kidneys and facial dysmorphism (e.g., high forehead, low-set ears, hypertelorism, hypoplastic midface), rocker-bottom feet, muscular defects of the anterior abdominal wall, and anomalies of the external genitalia (hypospadius, chordee). Most of these patients die within the first week after birth. In others, congenital anomalies are not documented, but renal cysts are found at postmortem examination. Affected infants without congenital anomalies usually develop hypotonia, tachypnea, hepatomegaly, hypoglycemia, metabolic acidosis, and a "sweaty foot" odor within the first few days after birth, many in the first 24 hours. The few infants with this form who have survived beyond the first week of life, as a result of prompt diagnosis and treatment, have died within a few months, usually of severe cardiomyopathy. A few other infants have been hypoglycemic in the neonatal period, have later developed typical Reye-like episodes, and have survived longer. The late-onset glutaric acidemia type II is extremely variable in age at manifestation and course of the disease. One infant presented at 7 weeks of age with intermittent episodes of vomiting, hypoglycemia, and acidosis, whereas another patient was asymptomatic during childhood and presented in adulthood with episodic vomiting, hypoglycemia, hepatomegaly, and proximal myopathy. Some individuals have had progressive lipid storage myopathy with carnitine deficiency.

SCHAD deficiency has been only rarely reported. It is also now known as M/SCHAD deficiency, given its broader chain length specificity [Kobayashi et al., 1996]. Three distinct clinical and biochemical phenotypes have been described. One female presented with recurrent myoglobinuria, myopathy, cardiomyopathy, and hypoketotic hypoglycemic encephalopathy and died at 16 years of age [Tein et al., 1991]. SCHAD activity was deficient in muscle but not in cultured skin fibroblasts, although these fibroblasts demonstrated marked microvesicular steatosis when cultured in a glucose-free medium to simulate fasting stress [Renaud et al., 2002]. Other tissues were not examined enzymatically. A second phenotype manifesting with ketotic hypoglycemia and SCHAD deficiency was described in isolated mitochondria from cultured skin fibroblasts, but no other tissues were studied [Bennett et al., 1996]. A third group of patients presented with hepatic involvement and steatosis; SCHAD activity was deficient in liver but normal in muscle and fibroblasts [Bennett et al., 1999]. Mutation analysis of the SCHAD gene in these patients has been inconclusive, which suggests that other proteins in addition to M/SCHAD may be necessary for enzymatic activity and that these proteins may have a tissue-specific distribution. Apparent disease-causing mutations have been described in a patient with fulminant hepatic failure who required transplantation [O'Brien et al., 2000].

Only one patient with 2,4-dienoyl-CoA reductase deficiency in muscle and liver has been reported; that patient presented with neonatal hypotonia, microcephaly, a small ventricular septal defect, and dysmorphism and died at 4 months of age of respiratory acidosis; biventricular hypertrophy was evident at postmortem examination [Roe et al., 1990]. The clinical significance of the biochemical abnormalities therefore cannot be confirmed until additional patients have been identified. In addition, one patient with medium-chain 3-ketoacyl-CoA thiolase deficiency has been described in a Japanese male neonate who died at 13 days of age after presenting at 2 days of age with vomiting, dehydration, metabolic acidosis, liver dysfunction, and myoglobinuria [Kamijo et al., 1997].

There are several disorders of ketone body production. Deficiency of HMG-CoA lyase, which is also active in the metabolism of leucine, manifests with hypoketotic hypoglycemia, hyperammonemia, and acidosis [Mitchell and Fukao, 2001]. Succinyl-CoA:3-keto-acid CoA transferase (SCOT) functions in conjunction with mitochondrial acetoacetyl-CoA thiolase to generate ketones in extrahepatic tissues. SCOT deficiency manifests as persistent ketonuria in the first 1 to 2 years of life, whereas acetoacetyl-CoA thiolase deficiency manifests with variable clinical symptoms and exaggerated ketoacidosis in response to minor physiologic stresses [Fukao et al., 1995, 1997; Kassovska-bratinova et al., 1996; Pretorius et al., 1996]. HMG-CoA synthetase deficiency has been reported in a child who presented with fasting hypoketotic hypoglycemia [Thompson et al., 1997].

Differentiating Laboratory Features

Analysis of the fatty acid intermediates in the serum or urine of affected children may suggest the site of defect, depending on the chain-length specificity and the species type of the intermediates. Identification of these intermediates often requires specialized biomedical technology, which may necessitate referral to specialized metabolic laboratories. Particularly useful are the assessment of plasma total and free carnitine, serum acylcarnitines, urine acylcarnitines and urine acylglycines, and organic acids. These intermediates may be absent at times when the child is metabolically stable and receiving adequate supplies of glucose, because this state would reduce the stress on the fatty acid oxidation pathway. They are best detected in the serum and urine of children during acute catabolic crises or during times of fasting. Specific intermediates characteristic for individual defects are listed in Table 81-3 [Tein, 1995].

Carnitine

Fatty acid oxidation disorders are associated with a decrease in plasma total carnitine concentration (<30 μmol/liter; normal, 40 to 60 μmol/liter). The carnitine uptake defect has

TABLE 81-3

Laboratory Features Associated with Genetic Defects of Fatty Acid Oxidation

DEFICIENCY	LEVELS OF CARNITINE Total	Free	UNIQUE OR SPECIFIC METABOLITES Acyl-Carnitine	Acyl-Glycine	Organic Acids
LCFAUD	Low	Low	NR	NR	NR
CUD	Very low	Low	NR	NR	NR
CPT I	Normal/high	High	NR	NR	NR(+)
TRANS	Low	Very low	Long-chain	NR	NR
CPT II (mild)	Low	Very low	Long-chain	NR	NR
CPT II (severe)	Low	Very low	Long-chain	NR	+
VLCAD/LCAD	Low	Low	Long-chain	NR	Adipic, suberic, sebacic
Trifunctional	Low	Low	Long-chain	NR	Adipic, suberic, sebacic; 3-hydroxy intermediates
Dienoyl-CoA reductase	Low	Low	Decadienoyl	NR	NR
MCAD	Low	Low	Octanoyl	Suberyl, hexanoyl, phenylpropionyl	Adipic, suberic, sebacic
SCAD	Low	Low	Butyryl	Butyryl	Adipic, suberic, sebacic; ethylmalonic; methylsuccinate
SCHAD	Low	Low	NR	NR	Adipic, suberic, sebacic; 3-hydroxy intermediates
ETF and ETF-Qo	Low	Low	Octanoyl, glutaryl, butyryl, isovaleryl	Suberyl, hexanoyl, butyryl, isovaleryl	Adipic, suberic, sebacic; glutaric; ethylmalonic
HMG-CoA lyase	Low	Low	3-Methylglutaryl	?	3-Hydroxy-3-methylglutaric; 3-methyl-glutaconic; 3-methyl-glutaric, adipic; 3-hydroxy- isovaleric

CoA, coenzyme A; CPT, carnitine palmitoyltransferase; CUD, Carnitine uptake defect; ETF, electron transfer flavoprotein; HMG, β-hydroxy-β-methylglutaryl; LCAD , long-chain acyl-CoA dehydrogenase; LCFAUD, long-chain fatty acid uptake defect; MCAD, medium-chain acyl-CoA dehydrogenase; NR, no case yet reported; Qo, coenzyme Q oxidoreductase; SCAD, short-chain acyl-CoA dehydrogenase; SCHAD, short-chain *L*-3-hydroxyacyl-CoA dehydrogenase; TRANS, carnitine acylcarnitine translocase; trifunctional, long-chain enoyl-CoA hydratase + long-chain *L*-3-hydroxyacyl-CoA dehydrogenase + long-chain 3-ketoacyl-CoA thiolase; VLCAD, very long-chain acyl-CoA dehydrogenase.

Modified from Tein I. Fatty acid oxidation and associated defects. In American Academy of Neurology Proceedings, Seattle, 1995. Madison, WI: Omnipress, 1995;269;9–38.

the lowest concentrations, which are usually less than 5% of control values [Stanley et al., 1991]. In the intramitochondrial beta oxidation defects, the plasma total carnitine concentrations vary between 10% and 50% of normal. In carnitine palmitoyltransferase I deficiency, in contrast, the total plasma carnitine concentration may be normal or increased because the esterification of palmitate to carnitine is defective [Stanley et al., 1992].

In most fatty acid oxidation defects, with the exception of the carnitine uptake and carnitine palmitoyltransferase I defects, there is an increase in the ratio of esterified carnitine to total carnitine. This increase reflects the esterification to carnitine of the excessive acyl-CoAs that accumulate proximal to the block in beta oxidation. Estimates of the amount of acylcarnitines are based on the difference between the free and total carnitine measurements. Under normal conditions, the esterified carnitine is 10% to 25% of total in the fed state and 30% to 50% of total in the fasting state [Hale and Bennett, 1992]. The carnitine esters can be further separated on the basis of the acid insolubility of long-chain acylcarnitine esters [Hale and Bennett, 1992]. Increased amounts of long-chain acylcarnitines are found in defects of long-chain fatty acid oxidation [Glasgow et al., 1983]. Further separation and identification of the individual acylcarnitine esters have been facilitated by fast atom bombardment-tandem mass spectrometry and isotopic exchange high-performance liquid chromatography [Kerner and Bieber, 1983; Millington et al., 1992]. Profiles of specific serum acylcarnitines have been useful in the diagnosis of certain defects (e.g., octanoyl-carnitine in MCAD deficiency) [Millington, 1986]. They are particularly helpful in the diagnosis of long-chain fatty acid oxidation disorders because they overcome the problem of the renal threshold effect, whereby long-chain acylcarnitines are selectively reabsorbed at the renal carnitine transporter site at the expense of free carnitine. This limits the urinary excretion and detection of long-chain acylcarnitines. Serum acylcarnitine measurements also overcome the problem of the poor solubility of long-chain fatty acids in urine. A novel approach that has been successfully applied to skin fibroblasts for the diagnosis of various fatty acid oxidation defects involves probing the beta oxidation pathway by incubating the cells in the presence of a stable, isotopically labeled long-chain fatty acid and then analyzing the produced acylcarnitine intermediates by tandem mass spectrometry [Nada et al., 1995a, 1995b]. This method has also been used for the successful prenatal diagnosis of MCAD and VLCAD deficiencies in cultured amniocytes [Nada et al., 1996].

Dicarboxylic Acids

Dicarboxylic acids (adipic, suberic, and sebacic acids) are found in all identified intramitochondrial beta oxidation defects [Gregersen et al., 1982a]. Hale and Bennett [1992] pointed out that there are several limitations to the value of these compounds in the recognition of fatty acid oxidation defects:

- These dicarboxylic acids may be found in children receiving certain formulas containing medium-chain triglycerides or in children who are seriously ill (e.g., with diabetic ketoacidosis) [Mortensen and Gregersen, 1982]. They are also found in children who are receiving certain medications that interfere with fatty acid oxidation, such as valproic acid [Mortensen, 1981]. In each of these cases, however, the amount of ketones exceeds the amount of dicarboxylic acids, whereas in the intramitochondrial fatty acid oxidation defects, the amount of dicarboxylic acids equals or exceeds the amount of ketones when the children are fasting.
- These dicarboxylic acids are not present when children are not catabolic, are well and eating regularly, or are receiving intravenous glucose at rates in excess of normal hepatic glucose production rates. Under these conditions, there is a reduction in dependence on fatty acid oxidation and the production of fatty acid metabolites.
- Increased concentrations of dicarboxylic acids in the urine are generally not seen in the disorders involving the transport of fats into the mitochondria. Therefore, a fatty acid oxidation defect can be suspected in the presence of an excess of dicarboxylic acids relative to ketones, but the absence of dicarboxylic acids does not necessarily exclude a defect.

The site of defect may be suggested by the organic acid pattern. For example, children with LCAD/VLCAD deficiency excrete primarily medium- and long-chain saturated dicarboxylic acids, in contrast to children with trifunctional enzyme deficiency, who excrete almost equimolar amounts of the saturated and the 3-hydroxydicarboxylic acids [Hale et al., 1990a, 1990b]. However, toxic reactions with acetaminophen and intrinsic liver disease may also manifest with urinary excretion of 3-hydroxy compounds [Pollitt, 1990]. Further advances in stable-isotope dilution mass spectrometry have improved the ability to quantify metabolites in very small amounts [Gregersen et al., 1986] in plasma or urine. Acylglycines that are consistently excreted in small quantities in the urine do not appear to have the same limitations of dicarboxylic acids. Useful glycine metabolites therefore have been identified for several defects, including MCAD, SCAD, ETF, and ETF-coenzyme Q oxidoreductase deficiencies [Rinaldo et al., 1988].

Diagnostic Approaches and Screening Methods

History and Physical Examination

The key to investigation of these patients is a thorough history and a careful clinical examination. The presentation may be either acute and recurrent or more chronic and slowly progressive. The more typical presentation is the acute one in which the child has a history of decreased oral intake during the preceding 24 to 36 hours, followed by increasing lethargy and progressive obtundation or coma. The important initial investigations in a comatose child should include serum glucose and urine ketone measurements. Determination of urine ketones may be complicated because ill children are often dehydrated and have concentrated urine that may demonstrate a relatively spurious elevation in ketones. A blood glucose level above 3.3 mmol/ liter (60 mg/dL) and accompanied by large amounts of urinary ketones tends to rule out a fatty acid oxidation disorder. However, a blood glucose level lower than 3.3 mmol/ liter with trace or small amounts of urine ketones suggests the possibility of a fatty acid oxidation disorder and warrants further investigation. Most important, samples from the acute presentation, particularly before intravenous glucose therapy, should be saved for the determination of total and free serum carnitine, serum acylcarnitines, serum free fatty acids and ketones, urine organic acids, acylglycines, and acylcarnitines. With normal fatty acid oxidation, the ratio of serum free fatty acids to ketones is 1:1. In the event of a block in fatty acid oxidation, this ratio increases to greater than 2:1 and is therefore useful as an initial screen. The serum and urine specimens during the acute episode can also be used to assess the integrity and hormonal regulation of the biochemical pathways involved in glucose homeostasis.

Total Carnitine Measurement

The differentiation among the carnitine uptake defect, carnitine palmitoyltransferase I, and the intramitochondrial defects on the basis of total and free plasma carnitine concentrations has been previously discussed.

Urinary Organic Acids

It is crucial to obtain urine specimens during the acute catabolic episode, before intravenous glucose is administered, because production of fatty acid metabolites ceases quickly during normoglycemia. The chain length and species type of the organic acids help identify the specific site of fatty acid oxidation block.

Fasting Studies

If the important samples have not been taken during an acute catabolic event, a fasting study may be considered in order to distinguish a fatty acid oxidation defect from the other etiologies of hypoglycemia. However, if a fasting study is to be undertaken, it must be done under carefully controlled hospital conditions with continuous monitoring and by physicians who are knowledgeable with regard to hypoglycemia, hypopituitarism, hyperinsulinism, and fatty acid oxidation disorders. It is thought by some authorities that fasting studies should not be performed in children with fatty acid oxidation disorders, because diagnostic fasting may precipitate an acute metabolic crisis, leading to further morbidity or death. It has been suggested instead that loading tests with carnitine or phenylpropionate can be used to aid in diagnosis. Hale and Bennett [1992] outlined advantages and disadvantages of each method. The specific advantages of a fasting study are the following:

- The duration of fasting tolerance can be determined under carefully controlled conditions. This control may provide useful information regarding the long-term management of the affected patient and provide guidelines for the prevention of hypoglycemia.

- The full spectrum of abnormal fasting adaptation can be studied through the assessment of a number of laboratory parameters, including hormonal measurements.
- The time to precipitation of acute clinical decompensation can be documented. As previously emphasized, the cardinal risk is the precipitation of an acute catabolic crisis that leads to morbidity and death. It is preferable instead to collect the appropriate samples during an acute catabolic event that the child has suffered.

The primary advantage of loading tests and the measurement of specific metabolites is their safety. The disadvantages are that (1) they are useful only in certain fatty acid oxidation defects (e.g., MCAD deficiency) and thus a negative test result does not exclude all fatty acid oxidation defects, and (2) they do not evaluate the spectrum of fasting adaptation.

The purpose of the fasting study is to identify the defective metabolic pathway through an analysis of temporal changes in substrates (glucose, free fatty acids, lactate, ketones), metabolites (carnitine, dicarboxylic acids), and relevant hormones (growth hormone, cortisol, insulin). The fast should be promptly terminated when the child demonstrates the first symptoms or has a blood glucose level of less than 3.3 mmol/liter (60 mg/dL). If at this point there is a deficient ketogenic response in the presence of a significant dicarboxylic aciduria, and if the ratio of serum free fatty acids to ketones is greater than 2:1, there is strong presumptive evidence of a defect in the fatty acid oxidation pathway.

Other Studies

Once presumptive evidence of a defect in fatty acid oxidation has been established, the clinical picture in combination with an analysis of serum acylcarnitines, urinary organic acid profiles, and urinary acylglycines may suggest a specific site of defect and the chain-length specificity of the defect (e.g., short-, medium-, or long-chain). Further investigations to identify the specific site of defect are discussed next.

TABLE 81-4

Enzymatic and Molecular Characterization of Fatty Acid Oxidation Disorders

DEFICIENCY	ASSAY	GENE	CHROMOSOME LOCATION	PROTEIN AND MOLECULAR CHARACTERIZATION; REFERENCES
CUD (OCTN2 transporter)	Carnitine uptake in cultured skin fibroblasts, lymphoblasts, myoblasts	*SLC22A5*	5q33.1	Wu et al., 1998; Tamai et al., 1998; Lamhonwah and Tein, 1998
CPT I, liver	Fibroblasts, muscle, liver	*CPTIA*	11q13	Esser et al., 1993; Britton et al., 1995; Yamazaki et al., 1996
TRANS	Fibroblasts	*SLC25A20*	3p21.31	Indiveri et al., 1990, 1991; Palmieri et al., 1996
CPT II	Fibroblasts, muscle, liver	*CPT2*	1p32	Woeltje et al., 1990; Finocchiaro et al., 1991; Taroni et al., 1993; Gellera et al., 1994; Verderio et al., 1995
VLCAD	Fibroblasts, muscle	*ACADVL*	17p11.2-p.11.1	Kelley, 1992; Izai et al., 1992; Strauss et al., 1995; Aoyama et al., 1995a, 1995b; Andresen et al., 1996a, 1996b
LCAD	Fibroblasts, muscle, liver	*ACADL*	2q34-q35	Indo et al., 1991b
Trifunctional/LCHAD	Fibroblasts, muscle, liver	*HADHB/HADHA*	2p23	Carpenter et al., 1992; Luo et al., 1993; Uchida et al., 1992; Jackson et al., 1992; Kamijo et al., 1993, 1994; Sims et al., 1995; Strauss, 1997
Dienoyl-CoA reductase	Muscle, liver	*DECR1*	8q21.3	Helander et al., 1997
MCAD	Fibroblasts, liver, leukocytes	*ACADM*	1p31	Kelly et al., 1987; Strauss et al., 1990; Gregersen et al., 1991; Blakemore et al., 1991
SCAD	Fibroblasts, muscle, liver	*ACADS*	12q22-qter	Finocchiaro et al., 1987; Naito et al., 1989; Corydon et al., 1996; Gregersen et al., 1996
SCHAD	Fibroblasts, muscle, (liver)	*HADHSC*	4q22-q26	Vredendaal et al., 1996
ETF	Fibroblasts			
	α-Subunit	*ETFA*	15q23-q25	Finocchiaro et al., 1988; Indo et al., 1991a
	β-Subunit	*ETFB*	19q13.3	Finocchiaro et al., 1993
ETF/Qo	Fibroblasts	*ETFDH*	4q32.qter	Goodman et al., 1992
HMG-CoA lyase	Fibroblasts, liver, leukocytes	*HMGCL*	1pter-p33	Mitchell et al., 1993; Roberts et al., 1994
HMG-CoA synthase	Liver	*HMGCS2*	1p13-p12	Bouchard et al., 2001; Mascaro et al., 1995

CoA, coenzyme A; CPT, carnitine palmitoyltransferase; CUD, Carnitine uptake defect; ETF, electron transfer flavoprotein; HMG, β-hydroxy-β-methylglutaryl; LCAD, long-chain acyl-CoA dehydrogenase; LCFAUD, long-chain fatty acid uptake defect; LCHAD, long-chain *L*-3-hydroxyacyl-CoA dehydrogenase; MCAD, medium-chain acyl-CoA dehydrogenase; OCTN2, an organic cation/carnitine transporter; Qo, coenzyme Q oxidoreductase; SCAD, short-chain acyl-CoA dehydrogenase; SCHAD, short-chain L-3-hydroxyacyl-CoA dehydrogenase; TRANS, carnitine acylcarnitine translocase; trifunctional, long-chain enoyl-CoA hydratase + long-chain L-3-hydroxyacyl-CoA dehydrogenase + long-chain 3-ketoacyl-CoA thiolase; VLCAD, very long-chain acyl-CoA dehydrogenase.

Modified from Tein I. Fatty acid oxidation and associated defects. In American Academy of Neurology Proceedings, Seattle, 1995. Madison, WI: Omnipress, 1995;269:9–38.

FATTY ACID OXIDATION STUDIES

Provided the defect is expressed in cultured skin fibroblasts, a useful screening tool is the measurement of the oxidation rates of [1–carbon 14]–labeled palmitate (C16), octanoate (C8), and butyrate (C4) in the fibroblasts to establish the chain-length specificity of the defect [Rhead, 1990]. Another screening test useful for suggesting an underlying defect in fatty acid oxidation is to culture skin fibroblasts in a glucose-free medium, which will simulate fasting and exacerbate microvesicular steatosis in the fibroblasts expressing a genetic defect in fatty acid oxidation [Renaud et al., 2002]. Another method for quantitative acylcarnitine profiling by electrospray ionization–tandem mass spectrometry in human skin fibroblasts with unlabeled palmitic acid as substrate has revealed pathognomonic acylcarnitine profiles in a variety of short-, medium- and long-chain fatty acid oxidation defects [Okun et al., 2002]. In addition, this method delineates different variants of MCAD deficiency, such as mild and classic. A rapid method for acylcarnitine profiling with stable isotopically labeled palmitate and intact mitochondria prepared from homogenates of fresh muscle biopsy specimens, which reduces the delay in diagnosis related to tissue culture, has also been described [Tyni et al., 2002].

ENZYMATIC ASSAYS

Depending on the suspected site of defect, a direct enzymatic assay may then be performed for the specific enzyme (Table 81-4) [Tein, 1995]. These assays can be performed in cultured skin fibroblasts or in muscle biopsy specimens for carnitine palmitoyltransferase I, carnitine palmitoyltransferase II, SCAD, LCAD, SCHAD, and trifunctional enzyme deficiencies, among others. However, certain of these defects may be tissue specific, such as muscle SCHAD deficiency [Tein et al., 1991], in which case the defect is expressed in muscle biopsy specimens and not in fibroblasts and therefore may be missed unless the affected tissue is examined. Carnitine acylcarnitine translocase deficiency [Pande et al., 1993] and MCAD deficiency can be measured in cultured skin fibroblasts. Evidence for a defect in ETF or ETF-coenzyme Q relies on demonstration of a combined deficiency in the activities of the SCAD, MCAD, and LCAD enzymes. Carnitine palmitoyltransferase II deficiency has been rapidly diagnosed prenatally by enzyme assay in 10 mg of chorionic villus sampling at the 11th week of gestation in combination with haplotyping with polymorphic markers linked to the carnitine palmitoyltransferase II gene [Vekemans et al., 2003].

CARNITINE UPTAKE STUDIES

For the carnitine uptake defect, diagnosis is confirmed by in vitro studies of carnitine uptake in cultured skin fibroblasts. This study demonstrates negligible uptake of carnitine in the homozygous patients, thereby precluding the calculation of K_m and V_{max} values [Tein et al., 1990a; Treem et al., 1988]. This finding supports the concept that primary carnitine deficiency is caused by a defect in the specific high-affinity, low-concentration, carrier-mediated OCTN2. Heterozygotes demonstrate normal K_m values but reduced V_{max} values, ranging from 13% to 44% of control values [Stanley et al., 1991; Tein et al., 1990a]. This suggests that heterozygotes have a reduced number of normally functioning transporters. This is the most sensitive study for detection of the carrier state because serum carnitine concentrations in the heterozygotes may be normal. Negligible carnitine uptake has also been demonstrated in the cultured lymphoblasts [Tein and Xie, 1996] and myoblasts [Pons et al., 1997] of affected children.

MOLECULAR STUDIES

Molecular characterization of the specific defects include Western blotting to determine whether the defects are positive for cross-reacting material, suggestive of a kinetic deficiency, or whether they are negative for cross-reacting material, suggestive of a decrease in the production of the affected enzyme. Western blotting has also been used in the determination of the amounts of the alpha and beta subunits of ETF [Finocchiaro et al., 1990]. A number of the enzymes (e.g., carnitine palmitoyltransferase I, carnitine palmitoyltransferase II, VLCAD, LCAD, SCAD, MCAD, trifunctional enzymes) and transporters (e.g., high-affinity OCTN2) have been cloned (see Table 81-4). This cloning has led to the discovery of specific mutations resulting in the defective activity, which has given rise to the development of specific molecular probes. These probes can be used for the precise and rapid detection of certain specific defects. Specific mutations have been documented for carnitine palmitoyltransferase II [Taroni et al., 1993; Verderio et al., 1995], VLCAD [Andresen et al., 1996a, 1996b; Souri et al., 1996; Strauss et al., 1995], MCAD [Blakemore et al., 1991; Gregersen et al., 1991], SCAD [Corydon et al., 1996; Gregersen et al., 1996; Naito et al., 1990], trifunctional enzyme [Sims et al., 1995; Strauss, 1997], and OCTN2 defects [Lamhonwah et al., 2002], among others. The types of mutations may include missense mutations, small amino acid deletions and insertions, truncating mutations, nonsense mutations, out-of-frame deletions and insertions, and splice-site mutations [Gregersen et al., 2001]. The most straightforward application of mutation analysis is to confirm the diagnosis in suspected patients, particularly in the context of family studies and for prenatal/preimplantation analysis.

Treatment

Because of the small number of patients in any given institution, it is difficult to systematically evaluate any single treatment regimen. However, the mainstay of therapy is the avoidance of precipitating factors, particularly prolonged fasting. General treatment strategies are discussed next.

Avoidance of Precipitating Factors

Avoidance of precipitating factors, such as prolonged fasting, prolonged aerobic exercise (>30 minutes), and cold exposure leading to shivering thermogenesis, is key. Prolonged fasting is 6 to 10 hours for the infant younger than 1 year and 12 hours for the child between 1 and 4 years of age. In the event of progressive lethargy, obtundation, or an inability to take oral feedings because of vomiting, the child should be taken immediately to the emergency room for intravenous glucose therapy. Intravenous glucose should be provided at rates sufficient to prevent fatty acid mobilization (8 to 10 mg/kg/minute of glucose) [Hale and Bennett, 1992]. This regimen should be continued until the catabolic cascade has been reversed and the child is able to take oral feedings again. It is wise to avoid prolonged exercise (i.e., >30 minutes) because during this time there is increased fat mobilization. A high-carbohydrate load before exercise is advisable with a rest period and a repeat carbohydrate load at 15 minutes. Avoidance of cold exposure is essential.

High-Carbohydrate, Low-Fat Diet

In general, it is advisable to institute a high-carbohydrate, low-fat diet with frequent feedings throughout the day that would be commensurate with the nutritional needs at the child's age. This goal is best achieved with the aid of a dietitian, aiming toward approximately 70% to 75% of calories from carbohydrate sources, 15% from protein, and approximately 10% to 15% from fat. Monitoring of essential fatty acid levels is important to ensure that the child is receiving adequate essential fatty acids, which may necessitate supplementation. Augmentation of the diet with essential fatty acids (at 1% to 2% of total energy intake) is often used to reduce the risk of essential fatty acid deficiency [Gillingham et al., 1999; Solis and Singh, 2002; Uauy et al., 1989]. Flaxseed, canola, walnut, or safflower oil can be used for this purpose.

An older child should have three regular meals per day with three equidistantly scheduled intermeal snacks, including a bedtime snack. In younger children, oral or nasogastric tube administration of an appropriate formula is indicated. In HMG-CoA lyase deficiency, a high-carbohydrate, low-fat, low-protein diet with leucine restriction should be implemented [Gibson et al., 1988].

Uncooked Cornstarch

To delay the onset of fasting overnight, the nightly institution of uncooked cornstarch, in doses similar to those used in the treatment of glycogen storage disease (1 to 2 grams per kilogram of body weight per day as a single nighttime dose), will prolong the postabsorptive state and delay fasting [Dionisi-Vici et al., 1991]. Cornstarch provides a sustained-release source of glucose, thereby preventing hypoglycemia and lipolysis [Fernandes and Smit, 2001]. Cornstarch is usually initiated at 8 months of age, when pancreatic enzymes are first able to function at full capacity for appropriate absorption [Hayde and Widhalm, 1990]. The initial recommended dose is generally 1.0 gram/kg/day, which can be gradually increased to 1.5 to 2.0 grams/kg/day by age 2 years as needed [Fernandes and Smit, 2001].

Specific measures for individual fatty acid oxidation disorders include the following:

- *Medium-chain triglyceride oil:* Medium-chain triglyceride oil as a nutritional source could be useful in long-chain fatty acid oxidation disorders because the medium-chain fatty acids would circumvent the block in long-chain fatty acid oxidation and thereby facilitate ATP production from the remainder of the patent fatty acid oxidation pathway. The medium-chain triglyceride oil could be started at a dosage of 0.5 gram/kg/day divided in three daily doses and could be increased up to 1 or 1.5 grams/kg/day as tolerated. The major side effect is diarrhea. The usefulness of this approach, however, may be limited because excess medium-chain triglyceride would ultimately be stored as long-chain fats in adipocytes. The success of medium-chain triglyceride oil supplementation in LCHAD deficiency has been variable [Tein et al., 1995]. When a high percentage of energy from fat is provided by medium-chain triglyceride oil, patients are at risk for essential fatty acid deficiency, and their diet should therefore be supplemented with essential fatty acids (1% to 2% of total energy intake) [Solis and Singh, 2002].
- *Riboflavin:* Certain cases of the multiple acyl-CoA dehydrogenase deficiencies (e.g., ETF or ETF-coenzyme Q–linked deficiencies) are responsive to riboflavin supplementation [Gregersen et al., 1982b]. The dosage is approximately 50 mg three times a day for infants and young children and 100 mg three times a day for older children.
- *Carnitine:* The essential indication for carnitine therapy is the OCTN2 defect, which is characterized by carnitine-responsive cardiomyopathy and very low plasma and tissue concentrations of carnitine (generally <5% of normal) [Stanley et al., 1991; Tein et al., 1990a]. There was a dramatic improvement in the cardiomyopathy and myopathy in all 22 patients treated with high-dose oral carnitine supplementation within the first few weeks, as well as a reduction of heart size toward normal within a few months of therapy. In addition, three children with significant failure to thrive before therapy demonstrated a marked improvement in growth after therapy [Tein et al., 1990a]. Of 19 patients treated with carnitine therapy for 5 to 20 years, 18 continue to be healthy [Cederbaum et al., 2002; Stanley et al., 1991]. Thus, in the OCTN2 defect, high-dose oral L-carnitine supplementation at 100 mg/kg/day in four divided daily doses is critical and lifesaving, significantly reversing the pathology in this otherwise progressive and lethal disease. Furthermore, in children in whom the condition is prospectively diagnosed at birth, early carnitine therapy from birth has been demonstrated to prevent the development of the clinical phenotype [Lamhonwah et al., 2002].

In the intramitochondrial beta oxidation defects with secondary carnitine deficiency, the results of carnitine therapy have been highly variable and insufficiently evaluated. Theoretically, carnitine has been given to limit the intracellular concentrations of potentially toxic acyl-CoA intermediates within the cell through transesterification and to thereby liberate CoA, which is a critical intracellular cofactor [Hale and Bennett, 1992]. However, there has been no objective prospective study to prove that carnitine administration has had a beneficial effect. In one study of a patient with MCAD deficiency, Stanley and colleagues [1990] demonstrated that the associated carnitine deficiency was not the cause of the defect in fatty acid oxidation, as indicated by the lack of effect of carnitine replacement on fasting ketogenesis. After 3 months of oral carnitine therapy, this patient had no increase in plasma ketones and continued to become ill and hypoglycemic after 14 hours of fasting. Furthermore, there is increasing evidence to suggest that carnitine administration may have deleterious effects in the long-chain fatty acid oxidation disorders. In these disorders, there is an accumulation of long-chain acyl-CoAs proximal to the metabolic block, which on esterification become long-chain acylcarnitines. Excessive palmitoylcarnitine may have detergent effects on membranes and arrhythmogenic effects as previously discussed [Inoue and Pappano, 1983; Lee et al., 1987; Mak et al., 1986; Spedding, 1985; Spedding and Mir, 1987]. This field warrants further investigation.

SPECIFIC THERAPIES FOR LCHAD/TRIFUNCTIONAL PROTEIN DEFICIENCY

Oral prednisone has led to a dramatic reversal of the limb-girdle myopathy and marked reduction in the episodic myoglobinuria in one male with the myoneuropathic form of LCHAD deficiency [Tein et al., 1995]. Several children with LCHAD deficiency who had asssociated pigmentary retinopathy were documented to have a deficiency of the n-3-polyunsaturated fatty acid docosahexaenoic acid, and subsequent supplementation with docosahexaenoic acid led to some improvement in visual function [Gillingham et al., 1997; Harding et al., 1999]. Furthermore, the daily oral administration of a cod liver oil extract containing high amounts of docosahexaenoic acid led to a marked clinical and electrophysiologic recovery of the progressive peripheral sensorimotor axonopathy in one male with the myoneuropathic form of LCHAD deficiency [Tein et al., 1999b].

TRIHEPTANOIN

Use of the anaplerotic odd-chain triglyceride triheptanoic acid has been reported to be of value in the therapy for long-chain fatty acid oxidation defects [Roe et al., 2002]. In three patients with VLCAD deficiency fed controlled diets in which the fat component was switched from medium-length even-chain triglycerides to triheptanoin, this treatment led rapidly to clinical improvement that included the resolution of chronic cardiomyopathy, myoglobinuria, and muscle weakness for more than 2 years in one child and of myoglobinuria and weakness in the others. This finding warrants further investigation.

Genetics and Presymptomatic Recognition

All known fatty acid oxidation disorders are inherited as autosomal-recessive conditions. Therefore, screening for other affected siblings is important because institution of preventive measures is relatively simple, and without treatment, morbidity and mortality are significant. Although screening of family members after identification of an affected individual is of benefit to the family, this approach fails to identify individuals who do not belong to this high-risk group.

One approach to screening would be to evaluate populations that are considered at risk for a fatty acid oxidation defect, such as those manifesting with sudden infant death syndrome, "near-miss" sudden infant death syndrome, and Reye's syndrome. Bennett and co-workers [1987] demonstrated that the incidence of dicarboxylic aciduria in an acutely ill pediatric population is approximately 1 per 12,000 and that in most cases the organic acid pattern was consistent with a defect in fatty acid oxidation. In another study of 7058 dried filter-paper blood spot specimens obtained at postmortem examination by electrospray tandem mass spectrometric analysis of acylcarnitine profiles from infants with unexplained causes of death, there were 23 cases of MCAD deficiency, 9 cases of VLCAD deficiency, 8 cases of glutaric acidemia type II, 6 cases of carnitine palmitoyltransferase II/translocase deficiencies, 4 cases of severe carnitine deficiency, and 4 cases of LCHAD/trifunctional protein deficiency [Chace et al., 2001].

More recently, specific molecular probes have been used to screen for one of the more common defects, MCAD deficiency. In one study, through use of the specific molecular probe for the gene mutation found in more than approximately 60% of children in the United Kingdom with MCAD deficiency (A985G point mutation), Blakemore and associates [1991] examined 410 consecutive neonatal blood-spot cards in a northern English population. The data suggested that the carrier state for this mutation is 1 in 68, which would correspond to a frequency of approximately 1 in 18,500 births for the homozygous MCAD-deficient state in this particular population group.

Tandem mass spectrometry has made screening possible for most fatty acid oxidation defects on the basis of the profiling of acylcarnitines in blood spots [Rinaldo and Matern, 2000]. The inclusion of fatty acid oxidation disorders in screening programs is highly desirable to prevent morbidity and mortality, implement preventive measures and treatment strategies, and to contain the cost of care of affected patients. For example, the incidence for MCAD deficiency was 1 per 8930 live births in a survey from the Pennsylvania neonatal screening program, obtained through tandem mass spectrometry, followed by confirmation through molecular analysis for several common mutations [Ziadeh et al., 1995].

MITOCHONDRIAL ENCEPHALOMYOPATHIES

Although all of the mitochondrial myopathies that are expressed in muscle are at potential risk for the development of myopathy and exercise intolerance, the specific defects in which acute episodes of myoglobinuria have been documented to date include defects of complexes I, II, III, and IV activities, as well as multiple mtDNA deletions and coenzyme Q10 deficiency. Chapter 28 is dedicated to the detailed discussion of the individual mitochondrial disorders; therefore, the following sections serve to summarize and highlight the key clinical, morphologic, biochemical, genetic, and physiologic features of this group of disorders.

Historical Considerations

In 1962 the concept of mitochondrial disease was first introduced when Luft and colleagues [1962] reported a young Swedish woman who suffered from severe hypermetabolism that was not caused by thyroid dysfunction. Muscle biopsy revealed abnormal mitochondria, and biochemical investigation revealed loose coupling of oxidation and phosphorylation in isolated muscle mitochondria. In the 1960s and

1970s, investigation of muscle biopsy specimens led to the recognition of different patterns of mitochondrial changes [Shy and Gonatas, 1964; Shy et al., 1966]. In 1963 the modification of the Gomori trichrome stain by Engel and Cunningham [1963] allowed identification of abnormal deposits of mitochondria as ragged-red fibers. In the 1970s and 1980s, systematic biochemical investigation led to a rational biochemical classification of mitochondrial diseases into five main groups. With advances in mitochondrial genetics, which contain their own DNA (mtDNA), a genetic classification has subsequently been proposed on the basis of nuclear or mitochondrial inheritance or both.

Morphologic Considerations

Although the finding of ragged-red fibers or ultrastructural alterations of mitochondria in muscle biopsy specimens suggests the possibility of a mitochondrial disorder, there are important limitations, as pointed out by DiMauro [1993]:

- In nonmitochondrial disorders, such as muscular dystrophies, polymyositis, and some glycogenoses, ragged-red fibers, or ultrastructural mitochondrial abnormalities in which they likely represent secondary changes, may be present.
- Conversely, in many primary mitochondrial diseases, such as enzyme defects in metabolic pathways other than the respiratory chain (e.g., the pyruvate dehydrogenase complex, carnitine palmitoyltransferase, beta oxidation, and fumarase deficiencies), ragged-red fibers are not present.

In addition, there are defects of the respiratory chain, such as the form of Leigh's syndrome secondary to cytochrome c oxidase (COX) deficiency, in which ragged-red fibers tend not to be present. Although ragged-red fibers are most often present in transfer RNA encoding mtDNA defects (which affect the respiratory chain), protein coding defects, such as the syndrome of neurogenic muscle weakness, ataxia, and retinitis pigmentosa (NARP) and Leber's hereditary optic neuropathy, have only subtle mitochondrial changes, without ragged-red fibers [Uemura et al., 1987]. Furthermore, the appearance of ragged-red fibers may also depend on the stage of the disease and on the threshold effect (the percentage of mutant mtDNA). Succinate dehydrogenase and COX stains are two other useful histochemical stains. Ragged-red fibers are often COX-negative, although not all COX-negative fibers are ragged-red fibers [DiMauro, 1993]. COX-negative ragged-red fibers are seen in patients with progressive external ophthalmoplegia and mtDNA deletions and in the syndrome of myoclonus and epilepsy with ragged-red fibers (MERRF). They are not seen in the syndrome of mitochondrial encephalomyopathy, lactic acidosis, and strokelike episodes (MELAS), in which COX-positive ragged-red fibers are usually present. There may be increased numbers of mitochondria (pleoconial myopathy), increased size (megaconial myopathy), disoriented or rarefied cristae, or osmiophilic or paracrystalline inclusions [DiMauro, 1993] on electron microscopic samples. The paracrystalline inclusions are deposits of mitochondrial creatine kinase [Stadhouders et al., 1990]. Lipid or glycogen storage may also be documented on muscle biopsy, signifying a defect of terminal oxidation [Jerusalem et al., 1973].

Clinical Considerations

The prevalence of mtDNA-related disorders has only been estimated. In northeastern England, mtDNA defects were the cause of disease in 6.57 per 100,000 adults of working age [Chinnery et al., 2000]. Overall, it was estimated that 12.48 per 100,000 individuals in the adult and child population either had mtDNA disease or were at risk of developing mtDNA disease. In western Sweden, the incidence of mitochondrial diseases overall was 1 per 11,000 preschool children [Darin et al., 2001]. Certain mtDNA mutations are relatively common, such as the A3243G MELAS mutation in northern Finland, which was estimated to occur in 16.3 per 100,000 in the adult population [Majamaa et al., 1998]. These prevalence rates support the conclusion that mitochondrial diseases are among the most common metabolic disorders, at least in northern Europe [Vu et al., 2002].

Mitochondrial diseases are clinically heterogeneous. There may be variation in the age at onset, course, and distribution of weakness in pure myopathies [DiMauro, 1993]. Additional features may include exercise intolerance and premature fatigue. In clinical classification, there has been controversy between the "lumpers" and the "splitters." Originally, three specific clinical syndromes were described: Kearns-Sayre, MERRF, and MELAS syndromes, each resulting from three distinct mutations in mtDNA. All three share the features of short stature, dementia, sensorineural hearing loss, lactic acidosis, and ragged-red fibers [DiMauro, 1993]. Mitochondria and mtDNA are ubiquitous, which explains why every tissue in the body can be affected by mtDNA mutations. The most common presenting clinical features include short stature, sensorineural hearing loss, migraine headaches, ophthalmoparesis, myopathy, axonal neuropathy, diabetes mellitus, hypertrophic cardiomyopathy, and renal tubular acidosis. Additional features may include strokelike episodes, seizures, myoclonus, retinitis pigmentosa, optic atrophy, ataxia, and gastrointestinal pseuo-obstruction. In the case of mtDNA mutations, there may be a diverse spectrum of associated syndromes, even in a single pedigree, because of heteroplasmy and the threshold effect, whereby different tissues harboring the same mtDNA muttion may be affected to different degrees or not at all. Furthermore, the same mutation can cause different syndromes (e.g., the T8993G mutation can cause either NARP or maternally inherited Leigh's syndrome), and different mutations can cause the same phenotype (e.g., A3243G mutation, single deletion, and multiple deletions of the mtDNA can all cause progressive external opththalmoplegia) [Moraes et al., 1993; Vu et al., 2002]. Thus, the diagnosis of mtDNA-related disorders often requires a careful synthesis of the clinical history, signs, mode of inheritance, laboratory data, neuroradiologic findings, exercise physiology, muscle biopsy findings, biochemistry profile, and molecular genetics.

Biochemical Classification

Mitochondrial encephalomyopathies can be classified into five groups [DiMauro, 1993] according to the area of mitochondrial metabolism specifically affected: (1) defects of transport, (2) defects of substrate utilization, (3) defects of

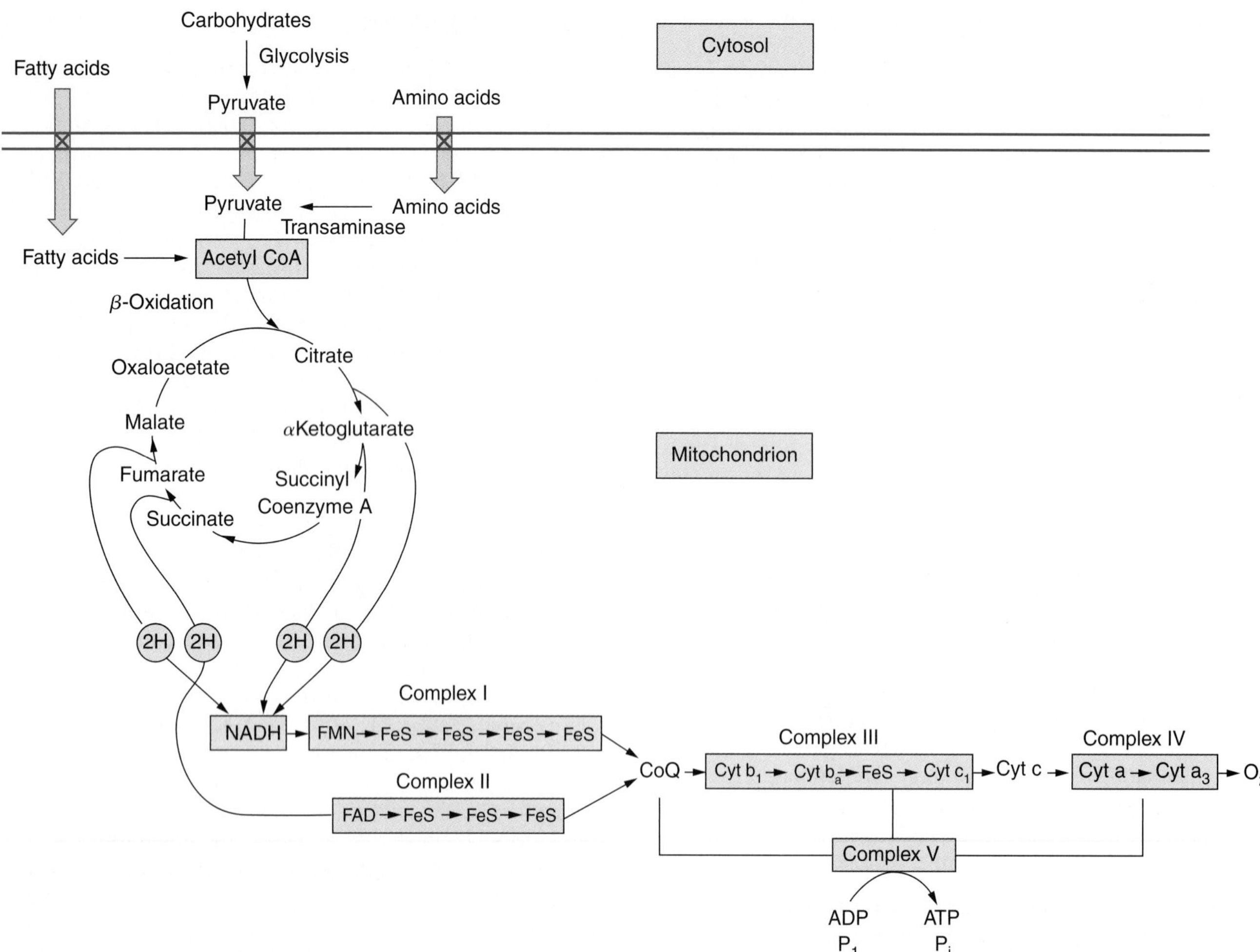

FIGURE 81-3. Scheme of mitochondrial metabolism. ADP, adenosine diphosphate; ATP, adenosine triphosphate; CoA, coenzyme A; CoQ, coenzyme Q; Cyt, cytochrome; FAD, flavin adenine dinucleotide; FeS, nonheme iron-sulfur protein; FMN, flavin mononucleotide; NADH, nicotinamide adenine nucleotide, reduced; Pi, inorganic phosphate. (From DiMauro S, DeVivo DC. Diseases of carbohydrate, fatty acid, and mitochondrial metabolism. In: Siegel GJ, Agranoff BW, Albers W, et al., eds. Basic neurochemistry: Molecular, cellular, and medical aspects, 4th ed. New York: Raven Press, 1989;647.)

the Krebs cycle, (4) defects of the respiratory chain, and (5) defects of oxidation/phosphorylation coupling (Fig. 81-3) [DiMauro and De Vivo, 1989]. Limitations of this classification scheme relate to the respiratory chain defects that can result from genetic defects of mtDNA, which are usually heteroplasmic, and to deletions of mtDNA or point mutations in transfer RNA, which affect mtDNA translation as a whole and may lead to multiple respiratory chain defects.

Genetic Classification

Mitochondria are the only subcellular organelles with their own DNA (mtDNA) [Nass and Nass, 1963] that are capable of synthesizing a vital set of proteins. Human mtDNA is a small (16.5-kilobase), circular, double-stranded molecule that has been completely sequenced [Anderson et al., 1981]. It encodes 13 structural proteins, all of which are subunits of respiratory chain complexes, as well as two ribosomal RNAs and 22 transfer RNAs needed for translation.

Human mtDNA has a number of unique features [DiMauro, 1993]:

- Its genetic code differs from that of nuclear DNA.
- It is subject to spontaneous mutations at a higher rate than is nuclear DNA.
- It contains no introns and is therefore tightly packed with information.
- It is transmitted by maternal inheritance.
- Its repair mechanisms are less efficient than those of nuclear DNA.
- It is present in hundreds or thousands of copies per cell.

In the formation of the zygote, mtDNA is contributed only by the oocyte [Giles et al., 1980]. Therefore, a mother carrying an mtDNA mutation passes it on to all her children, but only her daughters will transmit it to their progeny. If there is a mutation in some mtDNA in the ovum or zygote, this may be passed on randomly to subsequent generations of cells, some of which will receive primarily or exclusively mutant genomes (mutant homoplasmy); others will receive few or no mutant genomes (normal or wild type of homoplasmy); and still others will receive a mixed population of mutant and wild-type mtDNAs (heteroplasmy).

Maternal inheritance and heteroplasmy have several important implications [DiMauro, 1993]:

- Inheritance of disease is maternal, as in X-linked traits, but both sexes are equally affected.
- Phenotypic expression of an mtDNA mutation will depend on relative proportions of mutant and wild-type genomes; a minimum critical number of mutant genomes is necessary for expression (threshold effect). The threshold for disease is lower in tissues that are highly dependent on oxidative metabolism, such as brain, heart, skeletal muscle, retina, renal tubule, and endocrine gland tissue. Therefore, these tissues are especially vulnerable to the effects of pathogenic mutations in mtDNA.
- At cell division, the proportion may shift in daughter cells (mitotic segregation), leading to a corresponding phenotypic change. This shift explains the age-related, and even tissue-related, variability of clinical features frequently observed in mtDNA-related disorders.
- Subsequent generations will be affected at a higher rate than in autosomal-dominant diseases.

The critical number of mutant mtDNA needed for the threshold effect may vary, depending on the specific vulnerability of the tissue to impairments of oxidative metabolism. It may also vary according to the vulnerability of the same tissue over time, which may increase with age [Moraes et al., 1991a; Ozawa, 1995; Wallace et al., 1988b]. A current

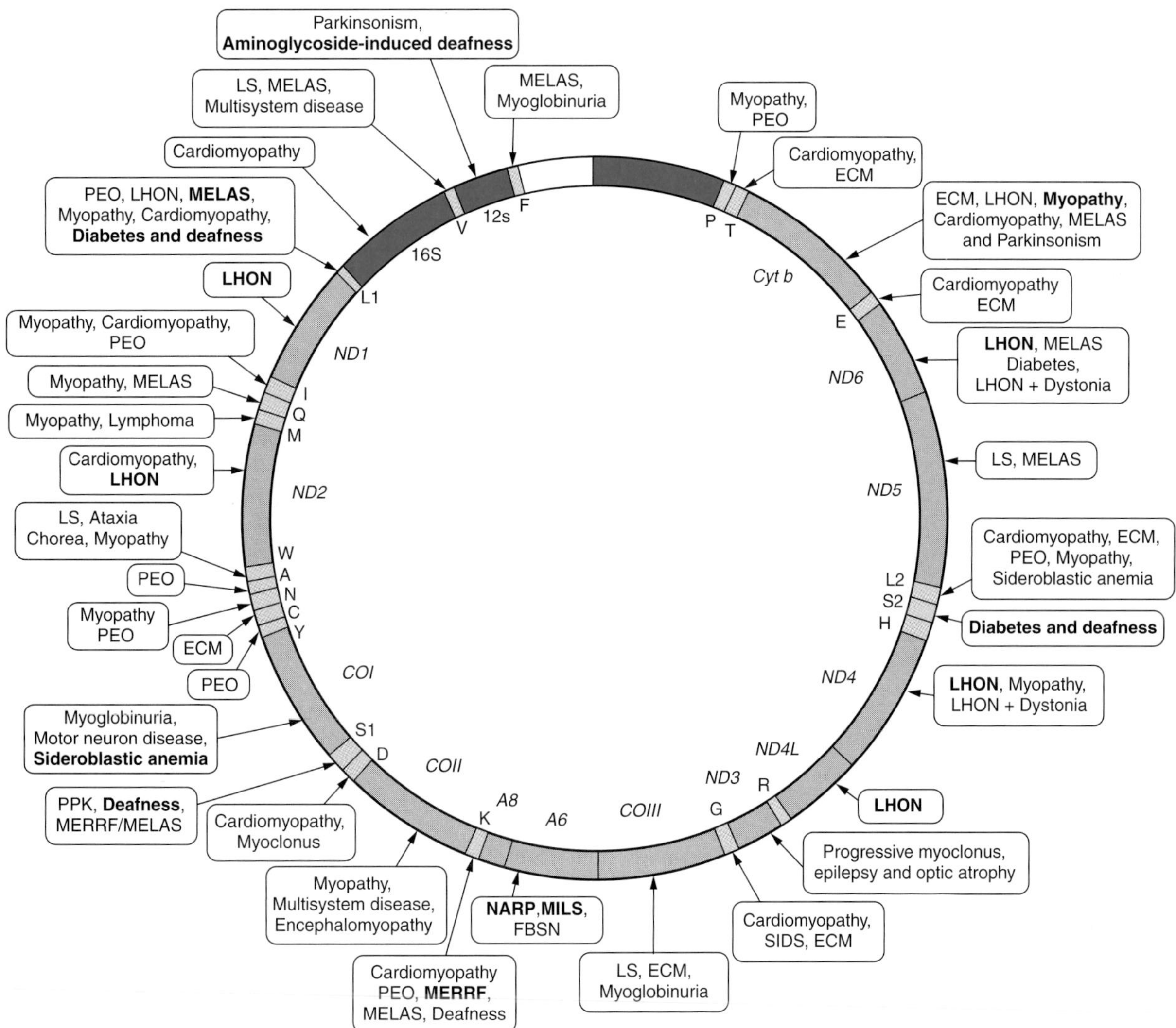

FIGURE 81-4. Morbidity map of the human mitochondrial genome as of January 1, 2004. See also Color Plate. In the map of the 16,569-kilobase mitochondrial DNA, differently shaded areas represent the protein-coding genes for the seven subunits of complex 1 (ND1 to ND4, ND4L, ND5, ND6), the three subunits of cytochrome oxidase (COX), cytochrome b (Cyt b), and the two subunits of adenosine triphosphate synthetase (A8, A6) (*red*); the 12S and 16S ribosomal RNAs (12S, 16S) (*dark blue*), and the 22 transfer RNAs identified by one-letter codes and by L1, L2, S1, and S2 for the corresponding amino acids (*light blue*). Diseases caused by mutations that impair mitochondrial protein synthesis are named in *blue;* diseases caused by mutations in protein-coding genes are named in *red.* ECM, encephalomyopathy; FBSN, familial bilateral striatal necrosis; KSS, Kearns-Sayre syndrome; LHON, Leber's hereditary optic neuropathy; LS, Leigh's syndrome; MELAS, mitochondrial encephalomyopathy, lactic acidosis, and strokelike episodes; MERRF, myoclonus, epilepsy with ragged-red fibers; MILS, maternally inherited Leigh's syndrome; NARP, neuropathy, ataxia, retinitis pigmentosis; PEO, progressive external opththalmoplegia; PPK, palmoplantar keratoderma; SIDS, sudden infant death syndrome. (From DiMauro S. Mitochondrial diseases. Biochim Biophys Acta 2004;1658:83, Fig. 3; modified from DiMauro S, Schon EA. Mitochondrial respiratory-chain diseases. New Engl J Med 2003;348:2660, Fig. 3. Copyright " 2003 Massachusetts Medical Society. All rights reserved.)

morbidity map of the human mitochondrial genome is shown in Figure 81-4 [DiMauro, 2004].

Although the mtDNA-encoded peptides are functionally important, they represent only a small proportion of the total mitochondrial protein. Of the approximately 80 proteins that make up the respiratory chain, only 13 are encoded by mtDNA. Complexes I, III, IV, and V contain some subunits encoded by mtDNA: seven for complex 1 (ND1-ND4, ND4L, ND5, and ND6), one for complex III (cytochrome b), three for complex IV (COX I to COX III), and two for complex V (ATPase 6 and ATPase 8) [DiMauro, 2004]. In contrast, complex II, coenzyme Q, and cytochrome c are encoded exclusively by nuclear DNA. Thus, the majority of mitochondrial proteins are encoded by nuclear DNA. The nuclear DNA-encoded proteins are synthesized in the cytoplasm and then imported into mitochondria. This transport of proteins requires a complex series of post-translational events and translocation machinery. This series involves synthesis of larger precursors in the cytosol, amino terminal leader peptides, which function as address signals and recognize specific mitochondrial membrane receptors. This synthesis is followed by translocation across the mitochondrial membrane and cleavage of the

TABLE 81-5

Genetic Classification of Mitochondrial Diseases

Defects of mtDNA
Single-deletions (usually sporadic)
Duplications or duplications/deletions (maternal transmission)
Point mutations (maternal transmission)
Structural genes
Transfer RNA genes
Defects of Nuclear DNA (Mendelian Transmission)
Mutations in genes encoding enzymes or translocases
Defects of substrate transport
Defects of substrate utilization
Defects of the respiratory chain
Defects of oxidation/phosphorylation coupling
Defects of mitochondrial protein importation
Defects of intergenomic dialogue
Multiple deletions of mtDNA
Depletion of mtDNA

From Vu TH, Hirano M, DiMauro S. Mitochondrial diseases. Neurol Clin North Am 2002;20:810.
mtDNA, mitochondrial DNA.

TABLE 81-6

Genetic and Biochemical Classification of the Mitochondrial Diseases

GENOME	GENE	[mtDNA]	BIOCHEMISTRY	CLINICAL PHENOTYPE
mtDNA		Single deletion	Decreased protein synthesis	Kearns-Sayre syndrome; ocular myopathy; Pearson's syndrome
	$tRNA^{Leu(UUR)}$		Decreased protein synthesis	MELAS syndrome
	$tRNA^{Lys}$		Decreased protein synthesis	MERRF syndrome
	Other tRNAs		Decreased protein synthesis	Multiple phenotypes
	ATPase 6		Decreased ATP synthesis	Neurogenic muscle weakness, ataxia, retinitis pigmentosa (NARP)/maternally inherited Leigh's syndrome
	ND1, ND4, ND6		Decreased complex I	Leber's hereditary optic neuropathy
	ND1, ND4		Decreased complex I	Myopathy†
	Cytochrome b		Decreased complex III	Myopathy†
	COX III		Decreased complex IV	Myopathy†
Nuclear DNA				
	NDUF		Decreased complex I	Leigh's syndrome
	SDHA		Decreased complex II	Leigh's syndrome
	BCSIL		Decreased complex III	GRACILE
	SURF1		Decreased complex IV	Leigh's syndrome
	SCO1		Decreased complex IV	Hepatoencephalomyopathy
	SCO2		Decreased complex IV	Cardioencephalomyopathy
	COX 10		Decreased complex IV	Nephroencephalomyopathy
	COX 15		Decreased complex IV	Cardioencephalomyopathy
	ATP 12		Decreased complex V	Fatal infantile multisystemic disease
	TP	Multiple deletions*	Decreased _	Mitochondrial neurogastrointestinal encephalomyopathy
	ANT1	Multiple deletions*	Decreased protein synthesis	Autosomal-dominant PEO-plus‡
	Twinkle	Multiple deletions*	Decreased protein synthesis	Autosomal-dominant PEO-plus‡
	POLG	Multiple deletions*	Decreased protein synthesis	Autosomal-dominant/recessive PEO-plus‡
	dGK	Depletion*	Decreased protein synthesis	Hepatocerebral syndrome
	TK2	Depletion*	Decreased protein synthesis	Myopathy; spinal muscular atrophy
	TAZ		Decreased cardiolipin	Barth's syndrome
	OPA1		Decreased mitochondrial motility	Autosomal-dominant optic atrophy

*[mtDNA] indicates changes of mtDNA secondary to nuclear DNA mutations (defects of intergenomic signaling).

†Mutations in cytochrome b and *COX* genes can also cause multisystemic diseases.

‡"Plus" refers to proximal weakness, neuropathy, psychiatric disorders, and parkinsonism.

ATP, adenosine triphosphate; ATPase, adenosine triphosphatase; COX, cytochrome c oxidase; GRACILE, growth retardation, aminoaciduria, cholestasis, lactic acidosis, and early death; MELAS, mitochondrial encephalomyopathy, lactic acidosis, and strokelike episodes; MERRF, myoclonus, epilepsy associated with ragged-red fibers; mtDNA, mitochondrial DNA; PEO, progressive external ophthalmoplegia; tRNA, transfer RNA.

From DiMauro S. Mitochondrial diseases. Biochim Biophys Acta 2004;1658:81.

leader peptides with assembly of mature peptides at their final intramitochondrial location [Schatz, 1991].

Therefore, the genetic classification of mitochondrial diseases must take into account defects of nuclear DNA or mtDNA and defects of communication between the two genomes (Table 81-5) [Vu et al., 2002]. The corresponding biochemical defects and the disease phenotypes arising from mutations in the currently recognized nuclear and mitochondrial genes are summarized in Table 81-6 [DiMauro, 2004].

Physiologic Considerations

Standard exercise physiology tests, such as cycle ergometers or treadmills, can be used to detect alterations of oxidative metabolism [Haller et al., 1989; Lewis and Haller, 1991b]. Maximal oxygen uptake is the most useful indicator of a patient's capacity for oxidative metabolism [DiMauro, 1993]. Typical physiologic responses in patients with defects in oxidative metabolism are as follows [Haller et al., 1989, 1991; Taivassalo et al., 2003]:

- The increase of cardiac output during exercise is greater than normal in relation to the rate of oxidative metabolism. In a study of 40 patients with mitochondrial myopathies who engaged in maximal cycle exercise, the increase in cardiac output relative to oxygen uptake (Vo_2) (15.0 ± 13.6; range, 3.3 to 73) was found to be exaggerated in comparison with control subjects (5.1 ± 0.7).
- Oxygen extraction per unit of blood remains almost unchanged from rest to maximal exercise. In patients during maximal cycle exercise, the mean peak systemic arteriovenous oxygen difference was 7.7 ± 3.5 mL/dL (range, 2.7 to 17.6), in comparison with control subjects, whose values were 15.2 ± 2.1 mL/dL. This problem leads to a gross mismatch between oxygen transport and utilization.
- Ventilation is normal at rest but increases excessively in relation to oxygen uptake. In patients during maximal cycle exercise, the increase in ventilation in relation to Vo_2 (mean peak ventilation/Vo_2 = 65 ± 24; range, 21 to 104) was exaggerated in comparison with control subjects (ventilation/Vo_2 = 41.2 ± 7.4).
- The level of venous lactate, which is usually elevated at rest, increases excessively in relation to workload and oxygen uptake. Furthermore, during maximal cycle exercise in 40 patients with mitochondrial myopathies, the mean peak work capacity (0.88 ± 0.6 [watts]/kg) and oxygen uptake (Vo_2 = 16 ± 8 mL/kg/minute) were significantly lower ($P < 0.01$) than in control subjects (mean work capacity, 2.2 ± 0.7 W/kg; Vo_2 = 32 ± 7 mL/kg/minute), but the patient range was broad (mean work capacity, 0.17 to 3.2 W/kg; Vo_2 = 6 to 47 mL/kg/minute) [Taivassalo et al., 2003]. The investigators concluded that the degree of exercise intolerance in mitochondrial myopathies was correlated directly with the severity of impaired muscle oxidative phosphorylation, as indicated by the peak capacity for muscle oxygen extraction. The exaggerated circulatory and ventilatory responses to exercise were a direct consequence of the level of impaired muscle oxidative phosphorylation and increased exponentially in relation to increasing severity of oxidative impairment.

Aerobic forearm exercise provides an easily performed screening test that sensitively detects impaired oxygen use and accurately assesses the severity of oxidative impairment in patients with mitochondrial myopathy and exercise intolerance. In a study of 13 patients with mitochondrial myopathy and exercise intolerance, the exercise venous oxygen tension (Po_2) paradoxically rose from 27.2 ± 4.0 mm Hg to 38.2 ± 13.3 mm Hg, whereas the oxygen tension fell from 27.2 ± 4.2 mm Hg to 24.2 ± 2.7 mm Hg in healthy subjects [Taivassalo et al., 2002]. The range of elevated venous oxygen tension during forearm exercise in the patients (32 to 82 mm Hg) was correlated closely with the severity of oxidative impairment as assessed during cycle exercise. Impaired oxygen extraction by exercising muscles can also be detected by near-infrared spectroscopy, which measures the degree of deoxygenation of hemoglobin [Bank et al., 1998].

Mitochondrial function in muscle in vivo can be evaluated quantitatively with ^{31}P-NMR [Radda et al., 1995]. The ratio of phosphocreatine to inorganic phosphate can be measured in muscle at rest, during exercise, and during recovery. In patients with mitochondrial dysfunction, ratios of phosphocreatine to inorganic phosphate are lower than normal at rest, decrease excessively during exercise, and return to baseline values more slowly than normal [Argov and Bank, 1991].

Defects of Mitochondrial DNA

Defects in Mitochondrial Protein Synthesis

MITOCHONDRIAL DNA REARRANGEMENTS: SINGLE DELETIONS AND DUPLICATIONS

Single deletions of mtDNA have been associated with three conditions that are usually sporadic [DiMauro and Hirano, 2003a]: (1) Kearns-Sayre syndrome, a multisytem disorder; (2) progressive external ophthalmoplegia, with or without proximal limb weakness, which is often compatible with a normal life span; and (3) Pearson syndrome, a rapidly fatal disorder of infancy characterized by sideroblastic anemia and exocrine pancreas dysfunction.

Duplications of mtDNA can occur in isolation or together with single deletions and have been documented in patients with Kearns-Sayre syndrome or with diabetes mellitus and deafness [DiMauro, 2004]. Duplications and duplications/deletions are rare and are usually transmitted by maternal inheritance.

Kearns-Sayre Syndrome

The clinical criteria for diagnosing Kearns-Sayre syndrome are (1) onset before age 20; (2) progressive external ophthalmoplegia; (3) pigmentary retinopathy; and (4) at least one of the following: heart block, cerebellar ataxia, or a cerebrospinal fluid protein level above 100 mg/dL. Other relatively common but nonspecific features include dementia, sensorineural hearing loss, and multiple endocrine abnormalities (short stature, diabetes, hypoparathyroidism) [DiMauro, 1993]. Ragged-red fibers and variable COX-negative fibers are seen on muscle biopsy. The prognosis is poor despite pacemaker placement. The course is progressively downhill, with death by the third or fourth decade. Renal tubular acidosis [Eviatar et al., 1990; Goto et al., 1990a] and Lowe's syndrome [Moraes et al., 1991b] are unusual clinical variants. A few overlapping cases, such as two children with Kearns-Sayre syndrome and strokelike episodes [Zupanc et al., 1991], have been described. The genetic basis of Kearns-Sayre syndrome is attributable to mtDNA deletions in the great majority of cases [Holt et al., 1989; Moraes et al., 1989].

Sporadic Progressive External Opththalmoplegia with Ragged-Red Fibers

Sporadic progressive external opththalmoplegia with ragged-red fibers is a clinically benign condition characterized by adolescent- or young adult–onset ophthalmoplegia, ptosis, and proximal limb weakness, which is slowly progressive and compatible with a relatively normal life span. The muscle biopsy reveals ragged-red fibers and COX-negative fibers. Approximately 50% of patients with progressive external opththalmoplegia have mtDNA deletions [Moraes et al., 1989]. The family history is negative.

In terms of therapy, one woman with adult-onset chronic progressive external ophthalmoplegia, ptosis, mild proximal weakness, and muscle mtDNA deletion was treated with 7 months of oral lipoic acid; she demonstrated an increase in brain energy availability and skeletal muscle performance, as illustrated by in vivo ^{31}P-NMR spectroscopy [Barbiroli et al., 1995].

DELETIONS OF MITOCHONDRIAL DNA: MOLECULAR BIOLOGY

Deletions of mtDNA range from approximately 2 to 8.5 kilobases and are confined primarily to an 11-kilobase region [DiMauro, 1993]. Regardless of clinical presentation, 30% to 40% of all deletions are identical. They span 4977 base pairs from the ATPase 8 gene to the ND5 gene [Holt et al., 1989; Shoffner et al., 1989; Tanaka et al., 1989]. These deletions can be divided into two main classes [Mita et al., 1990]. The distribution and relative abundance of mtDNA deletions in different tissues appear to determine the clinical phenotype [DiMauro, 1993].

MITOCHONDRIAL DNA POINT MUTATIONS

Point mutations have been identified in mtDNA from a variety of disorders, most of which are maternally inherited and multisystemic, although some are sporadic and tissue specific. Two of the more common syndromes among the maternally inherited encephalomyopathies are the MERRF and MELAS syndromes. Syndromes associated with transfer RNA mutations may be multisystemic, affecting vision (optic atrophy, retinitis pigmentosa, cataracts), hearing (sensorineural hearing loss), the endocrine system (short stature, diabetes mellitus, hypoparathyroidism), the heart (hypertrophic cardiomyopathies, cardiac conduction blocks), the gastrointestinal tract (exocrine pancreatic dysfunction, intestinal pseudo-obstruction, gastroesophageal reflux), and the kidneys (renal tubular acidosis).

MERRF Syndrome

MERRF syndrome is characterized by myoclonus, seizures, mitochondrial myopathy, and cerebellar ataxia. Less common signs include dementia, optic atrophy, spasticity, hearing loss, and peripheral neuropathy. Inheritance is maternal; however, expression depends on the percentage of mutant mtDNA. The highly specific, although not exclusive, point mutation is an A8344G in the transfer RNA^{Lys} gene of mtDNA [Shoffner et al., 1990]. This facilitates identification of patients independent of the severity of their clinical phenotype. Genetic heterogeneity is suggested by the absence of the mutation in four patients with typical MERRF syndrome [Hammans et al., 1991; Zeviani et al., 1991]. Other identified mutations in the transfer RNA^{Lys} gene that have been associated with MERRF syndrome are the T8356C and G8363A point mutations [DiMauro, 2004]. In one patient with MERRF syndrome, a mutation has been identified in a different transfer RNA: G611A in the transfer RNA^{Phe} gene [Mancuso et al., 2004a].

Onset may occur in childhood or in adulthood, and the course may be slowly progressive or rapidly downhill. Wallace and associates [1988b] suggested that there may be a hierarchy of vulnerability of different organs in which the brain suffers first, followed by muscle and heart. However, there may be variations among patients in the sequence of organ involvement [Lombes et al., 1989; Tsairis et al., 1973]. Muscle biopsy reveals ragged-red fibers, although exceptions occur [Hammans et al., 1991]. There are two populations of mitochondria: those that have normal COX activity and immunoreactivity for subunit II and those with decreased COX activity and COX II immunoreactivity [Lombes et al., 1989]. Neuropathologic findings include neuronal loss and gliosis, affecting in particular the dentate nucleus and inferior olivary complex, with some dropout of Purkinje cells and neurons of the red nucleus. There is pallor of the posterior columns of the spinal cord [DiMauro, 1993]. Muscle biochemistry profiles have revealed variable defects of complex III [Berkovic et al., 1989; Morgan-Hughes et al., 1982], complexes II and IV [Berkovic et al., 1989], complexes I and IV [Wallace et al., 1988b], or complex IV alone [Lombes et al., 1989]. Combined partial defects of all complexes with subunits encoded by mtDNA have been suggested by studies in which investigators used human cell lines completely devoid of mtDNA (rho0 cells) [Chomyn et al., 1991; King and Attardi, 1989]. There is no specific therapy, although coenzyme Q10 appeared to benefit a mother and daughter with the MERRF mutation [Wallace et al., 1991].

MELAS Syndrome

MELAS is a clinical syndrome that is characterized by (1) strokelike episodes (computed tomography or magnetic resonance imaging provides evidence of focal brain abnormalities); (2) lactic acidosis, ragged-red fibers, or both; and (3) at least two of the following: dementia, focal or generalized seizures, recurrent headache, or vomiting [Ciafaloni et al., 1992; Pavlakis et al., 1984]. In one series, onset was before 15 years of age in 62% of patients, and hemianopia or cortical blindness was the most common manifestation [Ciafaloni et al., 1992]. Inheritance is maternal, and there is a highly specific, although not exclusive, point mutation at nucleotide 3243 in the transfer RNA$^{Leu(UUR)}$ gene of mtDNA [Goto et al., 1990b; Kobayashi et al., 1990]. Other point mutations have also been described. Cerebrospinal fluid protein levels were abnormally increased in approximately

50% of patients [Ciafaloni et al., 1992]. Basal ganglia calcifications were demonstrated in 6 of 22 patients and dilatative or hypertrophic cardiomyopathy in 4 [Ciafaloni et al., 1992]. Ragged-red fibers are usually but not always seen on muscle biopsy specimens [Ciafaloni et al., 1992]. Mitochondrial accumulations have been demonstrated in smooth muscle cells of intramuscular vessels [Sakuta and Nonaka, 1989] and of brain arterioles [Ohama et al., 1987] and in epithelial cells and blood vessels of the choroid plexus [Ohama and Ikuta, 1987]. Muscle complex I deficiency has been demonstrated in many cases [Kobayashi et al., 1987; Koga et al., 1988]; however, multiple defects involving complexes I, III, and IV have also been demonstrated [Ciafaloni et al., 1992]. Because the number of mutant genomes is lower in blood than in muscle [Ciafaloni et al., 1992], the mutation may not be detectable in blood cells from some patients in whom it is detectable in muscle. The prognosis in patients with the full syndrome is poor. Therapeutic trials have included corticosteroids [Shapira et al., 1975] and coenzyme Q10 [Yamamoto et al., 1987]. In some patients with severe lactic acidosis, the use of dichloroacetate to lower serum lactate levels has led to significant biochemical [De Stefano et al., 1995] or clinical improvement [D. C. De Vivo, personal communication, 1992] [Saijo et al., 1991]; however, this has not occurred in all cases. Furthermore, peripheral neuropathy is an important complication of chronic dichloroacetate therapy [Spruijt et al., 2001].

Defects of Protein-Coding Genes

In this category, two syndromes are more common. The first syndrome has two phenotypic manifestations, NARP and maternally inherited Leigh's syndrome, and the second syndrome is Leber's hereditary optic neuropathy.

ATPASE 6 MUTATION

ATPase 6 mutation is a maternally inherited disorder that manifests with either Leigh's syndrome or developmental delay, retinitis pigmentosa, dementia, seizures, ataxia, proximal weakness, and sensory neuropathy and is caused by a point mutation at nucleotide 8993 within the ATPase 6 gene [Holt et al., 1990]. The severity of disease manifestation appears to correlate with the percentage of mutant mtDNA. When the degree of heteroplasmy is moderate (around 70%), the clinical expression is NARP, a subacute or chronic disease of young adults, but when the degree of heteroplasmy is very high (about 90%), the clinical expression is a rapidly progressive encephalopathy of infancy or childhood, Leigh's syndrome [Tatuch et al., 1992]. Maternally inherited Leigh's syndrome is a more severe infantile encephalopathy with characteristic symmetric lesions in the basal ganglia and the brainstem. There are two recognized mutations, namely, T8993G and T8993C, with the T-to-G mutation being both clinically and biochemically more deleterious than the T-to-C change [Vazquez-Memije et al., 1998].

LEBER'S HEREDITARY OPTIC NEURORETINOPATHY

Leber's hereditary optic neuropathy is characterized by onset, usually between 18 and 30 years of age, of acute or subacute loss of vision resulting from severe bilateral optic atrophy. There is a marked male predominance [Newman and Wallace, 1990]. The classic ophthalmologic features include circumpapillary telangiectatic microangiopathy and pseudoedema of the optic disc. Associated features may include cardiac conduction abnormalities (pre-excitation syndrome), cerebellar ataxia, hyperreflexia, and peripheral neuropathy. About a dozen different mtDNA point mutations in structural genes have been associated with Leber's hereditary optic neuropathy, but only three appear to be pathogenic even when present in isolation. A homoplasmic G-to-A transition at nucleotide 11778, which causes the replacement of a highly conserved arginine residue by histidine at position 340 of the ND4 protein of complex 1, was first described in 11 American pedigrees [Wallace et al., 1988a]. Another point mutation was found in which a G-to-A transition at nucleotide 3460 in the ND1 gene was identified in three Finnish families [Huoponen et al., 1991]. A third pathogenic mutation, namely, T14484C in ND6 has been identified [Carelli, 2002]. All three mutations affect genes of complex I. Predominance of affected men (approximately 50% of male patients but only approximately 20% of female patients have optic atrophy) has been attributed to the influence of the nuclear gene on the X chromosome [DiMauro, 1993]. Complex I deficiency was demonstrated in platelets from four affected members of an Australian family in which the molecular genetic defect was not documented [Parker et al., 1989].

Interestingly, point mutations in mtDNA protein-coding genes often escape the rules of mitochondrial genetics in that they affect single individuals and single tissues and most commonly involve skeletal muscle [DiMauro et al., 2003]. For example, patients with exercise intolerance, myalgia, and occasionally recurrent myoglobinuria may have isolated defects of complex I, complex III or complex IV, caused by pathogenic mutations in genes encoding ND subunits, COX subunits, and, in particular, cytochrome b [Andreu et al., 1999]. The lack of maternal inheritance and the involvement of muscle alone would suggest that the mutations arose de novo in myogenic stem cells after germ layer differentiation ("somatic mutations") [DiMauro, 2004].

Diseases Caused by Mutations in Nuclear DNA

There are numerous disorders caused by mutations in nuclear DNA, not only because most respiratory chain subunits are nucleus-encoded but also because the correct structure and functioning of the respiratory chain requires a series of steps, all of which are under the control of nuclear DNA. These steps include the following [DiMauro, 2004]:

- Nuclear factors are needed for the proper assembly of respiratory chain complexes. Mutations in these ancillary proteins have been associated with numerous disorders, particularly Leigh's syndrome.
- The integrity and replication of mtDNA require nuclear DNA–encoded factors, and there has been rapid progress in the understanding of the molecular basis of disorders of intergenomic signaling, such as syndromes associated with multiple mtDNA deletions and mtDNA depletion.

- Hereditary defects in the complex machinery involved in the transport of nuclear DNA–encoded proteins from the cytoplasm into the mitochondria have been documented.
- The respiratory chain is embedded in the lipid bilayer of the inner mitochondrial membrane. Alterations of this lipid milieu can lead to disease, as seen in Barth's syndrome, in which there is altered synthesis of cardiolipin.
- Mitochondria move around the cell, divide by fission, and fuse with one another. Disorders of motility can cause disease, as seen in autosomal dominant optic neuropathy.

Defects of Substrate Transport

The carnitine uptake defect and carnitine palmitoyltransferase deficiency were discussed earlier.

Defects of Substrate Oxidation

Defects in beta oxidation have already been discussed. Within pyruvate metabolism, pyruvate may be converted to acetyl-CoA by the pyruvate dehydrogenase complex. Defects of the pyruvate dehydrogenase complex can affect each of three catalytic components—E1 (pyruvate decarboxylase), E2 (dihydrolipoyl transacetylase), or E3 (dihydrolipoyl dehydrogenase)—as well as the regulatory component, pyruvate dehydrogenase–phosphatase, which activates it and the protein X–lipoate component. The most common enzyme defect, E1 (pyruvate decarboxylase), is composed of two subunits that are encoded by a gene on the X chromosome at Xp22.1-p22.2 [Brown et al., 1989] and two beta subunits that are encoded by a gene on chromosome 3 [Ho et al., 1988]. The E1 defects are caused by mutations in the E1-alpha gene, which is X-linked. This particular E1 defect can manifest in three ways, with a graded spectrum from most to least severe [Robinson, 1995] as follows:

- A neonatal form with onset in the first days or weeks of life and death usually before 6 months of age. This is characterized by hypotonia, seizures, episodic apnea and lethargy, failure to thrive, and severe lactic acidosis, with frequent agenesis of the corpus callosum.
- An infantile form with onset before 6 months of age, which is characterized by psychomotor delay, hypotonia, seizures, episodic apnea and lethargy, ophthalmoplegia, optic atrophy, ataxia, and mild to moderate lactic acidosis, with death usually by 3 years of age. The neuropathologic findings are characteristic of Leigh's syndrome.
- A benign form with mild developmental delay and with episodes of intermittent ataxia or exercise intolerance, which is found only in male patients and appears to respond to thiamine administration.

Because of the central importance of the pyruvate dehydrogenase complex in central nervous system metabolism, the E1-alpha mutations can manifest in both male and female patients. Most defects in the E1-alpha gene are de novo mutations. In male patients, the defects are either missense mutations or mutations that affect only the 3′ end of the coding sequence. In female patients, deletions and insertions that completely nullify one allele are more common. The remaining defects of the pyruvate dehydrogenase complex are extremely rare [Robinson, 1995]. The E2 and protein X-lipoate defects result in severe psychomotor retardation. The E3 lipoamide deydrogenase defect leads to deficient activity in the pyruvate dehydrogenase complex and in the alpha-ketoglutarate and branched-chain keto-acid dehydrogenase complexes. Pyruvate dehydrogenase phosphatase deficiency has been documented in three patients with Leigh's disease and a fourth with unremitting lactic acidemia.

Alternatively, pyruvate may be converted to oxaloacetate by pyruvate carboxylase. Pyruvate carboxylase deficiency has three major manifestations [Robinson, 1995]. In the simple (A) form, which has been documented in the Algonkian-speaking American Indian population, onset occurs in the first few months of life with a mild to moderate lactic acidemia and delayed development, leading to severe mental retardation and often death in childhood. In the more complex (B) form, which occurs in patients in France and the United Kingdom, the onset is soon after birth with a severe lactic acidemia accompanied by hyperammonemia, citrullinemia, and hyperlysinemia. Death usually occurs before 3 months of age. In a single case (C), the manifestation was mild and consisted only of episodic acidosis with no pyschomotor retardation. There is good evidence to suggest that patients in group A have some residual pyruvate carboxylase activity, whereas those in group B have no activity at all.

Defects of the Krebs Cycle

Defects in the Krebs cycle include alpha-ketoglutarate dehydrogenase, fumarase, and aconitase deficiency. Aconitase deficiency has been described in an individual who had exercise intolerance and myoglobinuria, as well as complex II deficiency [Haller et al., 1991].

Defects of the Respiratory Chain: Mutations in Genes Encoding Subunits or Ancillary Proteins of the Respiratory Chain

Defects of the respiratory chain may be caused by defects of nuclear DNA or mitochondrial DNA. As previously mentioned, mtDNA encodes only 13 subunits of the respiratory chain, whereas nuclear DNA encodes all subunits of complex II, most subunits of the other four complexes, as well as coenzyme Q10 and cytochrome c. The following syndromes are presumed to be caused by nuclear DNA defects.

Direct "hits" are mutations in genes encoding respiratory chain subunits, which includes subunits of complex I [Triepels et al., 2001] and of complex II [Bourgeron et al., 1995]. Most of these have been associated with autosomal recessive forms of Leigh's syndrome. Indirect "hits" are mutations in genes encoding proteins that are not themselves components of the respiratory chain but are required for the proper assembly and function of the respiratory chain complexes. Examples of such ancillary proteins are best demonstrated by mendelian defects of COX (complex IV). Mutations in five ancillary proteins, SURF1, SCO2, SCO1, pathy) and those with tissue-specific defects, thy or cardiomyopathy. Among the multi- fatal infantile form was described in a child lactic acidosis; hypotonia; complex III defi- e, heart, kidney, and liver tissue; and a 75% ochrome b in muscle [Birch-Machin et al., set encephalomyopathies (childhood to adult fested with a variable spectrum of weakness, ementia, sensorineural deafness, pigmentary xia, sensory neuropathy, and pyramidal signs 88; Morgan-Hughes et al., 1985]. The myo- tation is characterized by exercise intolerance e fatigue and hyperpnea and is often asso- xed weakness [Kennaway, 1988; Morgan- 1985]. Tissue specificity is suggested by the ormal complex III activity in fibroblasts and s of one patient with pure myopathy [Darley- 1986]. Menadione (vitamin K_3) and ascorbate ave been used as treatment strategies [Eleff In one young woman with myopathy [Darley- ., 1983], this treatment resulted in prompt ovement [Argov et al., 1986; Eleff et al., 1984]. nt, however, proved ineffective in two other pa- ding an infant with encephalomyopathy 1987] and an adult with myopathy [Reich- , 1986]. Another phenotype of complex III s been described in one patient with an unusual ioscapulohumeral muscular dystrophy [Slipetz]. The cardiomyopathic symptoms caused by and reducible cytochrome b deficiency in the n were documented in one infant with a rare fatal cardiomyopathy [Papadimitriou et al., 1984]. proved to be tissue-specific to heart tissue.

DEFICIENCY

yzes the transfer of reducing equivalents from c to molecular oxygen. The generated energy ransmembrane proton-pumping activity. The COX ontains two copper atoms and two unique heme A yrins as redox centers, which are bound to a nit protein frame that is embedded in the inner drial membrane [DiMauro, 1993]. The apoprotein ed of 13 polypeptides. The three largest subunits III) perform both catalytic and proton-pumping and are encoded by mtDNA. The 10 smaller IV, Va, Vb, VIa, VIb, VIc, VIIa, VIIb, VIIc, and encoded by nuclear DNA [Kadenbach et al., 1983]. length cDNAs of all the subunits of human COX n elucidated [DiMauro et al., 1990; Koga et al., he clinical manifestations can be divided into a ic form and a multisystemic form, which is d by encephalopathy [DiMauro et al., 1990]. There forms of myopathy. Both manifest soon after birth ere diffuse weakness, respiratory distress, and lactic although they have different outcomes. The fatal myopathy is often accompanied by associated renal with DeToni-Fanconi syndrome and results in death year of age. Autosomal recessive inheritance is sug- y pedigree analysis, and immunocytochemical studies cumented a selective defect of COX subunit VIIa in tients [Tritschler et al., 1991]. In addition, an infantile myopathy with associated cardiomyopathy is not thought to be genetically related to the fatal infantile myopathy [Hart and Chang, 1988; Zeviani et al., 1986]. The benign infantile myopathy manifests with severe weakness and, frequently, a need for ventilator assistance and gavage feedings in early life. Subsequently, there is spontaneous improvement and a return to normal by 2 or 3 years of age [DiMauro et al., 1983b]. There is a lack of both subunit VIIa and subunit II on muscle immunocytochemistry profiles in the benign form, with a spontaneous recovery toward normal COX activity both histochemically and biochemically [DiMauro et al., 1983b]. It is postulated that the defect most likely involves a nuclear DNA–encoded COX subunit that is tissue specific and developmentally regulated and that corrects as the mature isozyme is expressed [DiMauro, 1993].

COX deficiency is the most common biochemical cause of Leigh's syndrome (subacute necrotizing encephalomyelopathy) [Van Coster et al., 1991]. Leigh's syndrome is a devastating encephalopathy of infancy or childhood (rarely of adulthood). It is characterized by psychomotor regression, usually beginning at 1 year of age, with ataxia, optic atrophy, ophthalmoplegia, nystagmus, tremor, dystonia, pyramidal signs, and respiratory abnormalities. The classic pathologic findings consist of focal, symmetric areas of necrosis in the thalamus, brainstem, and posterior columns of the spinal cord, which are spongiform lesions characterized by cystic cavitation, vascular proliferation, neuronal loss, and demyelination [DiMauro, 1993]. There may be increased numbers of mitochondria in muscle on electron microscopic study. Involvement of nuclear DNA has been confirmed by fusion experiments [Miranda et al., 1989]. Inheritance is autosomal recessive. Patients with Leigh's syndrome have a generalized but partial defect of COX activity [DiMauro, 1993]. This defect is expressed in fibroblasts in most patients, making possible prenatal diagnosis from chorionic villi sampling [Ruitenbeek et al., 1988].

COX deficiency has also been documented in the muscle biopsy specimens of two unrelated cases of Alpers' disease [Prick et al., 1983].

COMPLEX V DEFICIENCY

Complex V or ATP synthase converts the transmembrane proton gradient generated in the respiratory chain into chemical energy by synthesizing ATP from ADP and inorganic phosphate. The complex consists of a membrane portion, F0, and a catalytic portion, F1, which are joined by a stalk. It is composed of 12 to 14 subunits, two of which (subunits 6 and 8) are encoded by mtDNA [Hatefi, 1985]. Two phenotypes have been described. One was in a 17-year-old male with a multisystem syndrome of weakness, ataxia, retinopathy, dementia, and peripheral neuropathy [Clark et al., 1983]. The other was a 37-year-old female with congenital, slowly progressive myopathy, ragged-red fibers, and intramitochondrial paracrystalline inclusions [Schotland et al., 1976].

COMBINED DEFECTS OF THE RESPIRATORY CHAIN

Combined defects of the respiratory chain are often caused by defects in mtDNA but can also be caused by defects of nuclear DNA. Potential mechanisms include (1) mutations of regulatory genes controlling more than one complex,

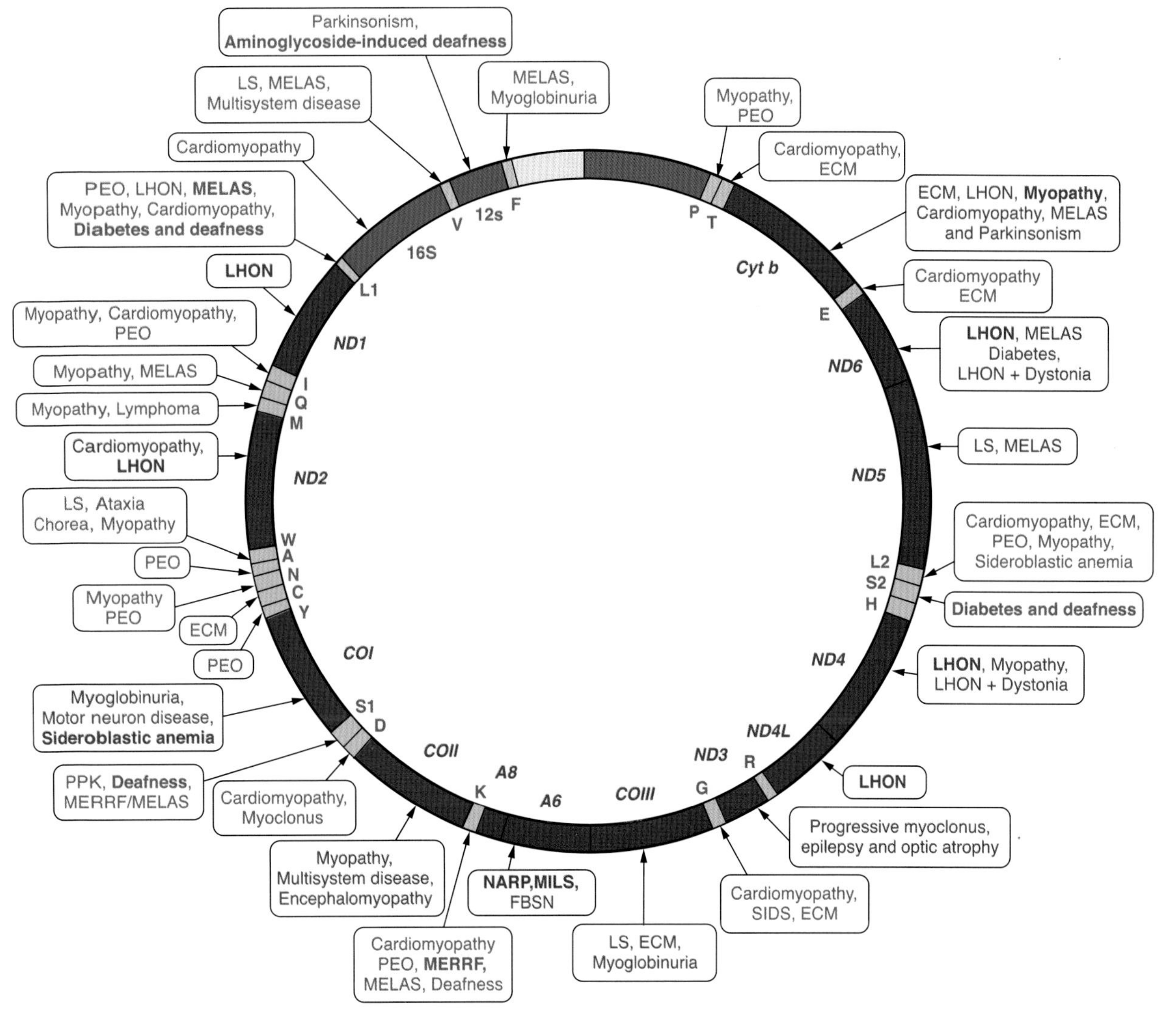

FIGURE 81-4. Morbidity map of the human mitochondrial genome as of January 1, 2004. In the map of the 16,569-kilobase mitochondrial DNA, differently shaded areas represent the protein-coding genes for the seven subunits of complex 1 (ND1 to ND4, ND4L, ND5, ND6), the three subunits of cytochrome oxidase (COX), cytochrome b (Cyt b), and the two subunits of adenosine triphosphate synthetase (A8, A6) (*red*); the 12S and 16S ribosomal RNAs (12S, 16S) (*dark blue*), and the 22 transfer RNAs identified by one-letter codes and by L1, L2, S1, and S2 for the corresponding amino acids (*light blue*). Diseases caused by mutations that impair mitochondrial protein synthesis are named in *blue;* diseases caused by mutations in protein-coding genes are named in *red.* ECM, encephalomyopathy; FBSN, familial bilateral striatal necrosis; LHON, Leber's hereditary optic neuropathy; LS, Leigh's syndrome; MELAS, mitochondrial encephalomyopathy, lactic acidosis, and strokelike episodes; MERRF, myoclonus, epilepsy with ragged-red fibers; MILS, maternally inherited Leigh's syndrome; NARP, neuropathy, ataxia, retinitis pigmentosis; PEO, progressive external opththalmoplegia; PPK, palmoplantar keratoderma; SIDS, sudden infant death syndrome. (From DiMauro S. Mitochondrial diseases. Biochim Biophys Acta 2004;1658:83, Fig. 3; modified from DiMauro S, Schon EA. Mitochondrial respiratory-chain diseases. New Engl J Med 2003;348:2660, Fig. 3. Copyright " 2003 Massachusetts Medical Society. All rights reserved.)

COX10, and COX15, have been associated with COX-deficient Leigh's syndrome [Sacconi et al., 2003; Tiranti et al., 1998; Zhu et al., 1998] or other multisystemic fatal infantile disorders, in which encephalopathy is associated with cardiomyopathy [Antonicka et al., 2003; Papadopoulou et al., 1999] (SCO2, COX15), nephropathy [Valnot et al., 2000] (COX10), or hepatopathy [Valnot et al., 1999] (SCO1). Mutations in a complex III assembly protein, BCSIL, have been associated with Leigh-like syndromes [de Lonlay et al., 2001] and with the lethal infantile disorder of growth retardation, aminoaciduria, cholestasis, iron overload, lacticacidosis, and early death (GRACILE) [Fellman, 1992; Visapaa et al., 2002]. There is also a newly recognized defect of complex V, caused by mutations in the assembly protein ATP12, that is associated with congenital lactic acidosis and a fatal infantile multisystemic disease involving the brain, liver, heart, and muscle [De Meirleir et al., 2004].

This is an important field of research from both theoretic and practical points of view as identification of mutations allows prenatal diagnosis. Furthermore, in certain cases there are potentially novel approaches to future therapy, such as copper administration to infants with mutations in SCO2, a protein involved in copper homeostasis in complex IV, as suggested by studies in cultured human cells [Jaksch et al., 2001; Salviati et al., 2002a].

COMPLEX I DEFICIENCY

Reduced nicotinamide adenine dinucleotide (NADH)-coenzyme Q reductase is the largest complex of the respiratory chain. It contains 46 different polypeptides (7 encoded by mtDNA) and several nonprotein components, including flavin mononucleotides, eight nonheme iron-sulfur clusters, and phospholipid [Hatefi, 1985; DiMauro, 2004]. Three main clinical syndromes have been characterized:

- A fatal infantile multisystem disorder characterized by severe congenital lactic acidosis, psychomotor delay, diffuse hypotonia and weakness, cardiomyopathy, and cardiorespiratory failure, which leads to death in the neonatal period [Moreadith et al., 1984; Robinson et al., 1986]. The enzymatic defect is multisystemic. Therapeutic trials with biotin, thiamine, carnitine, and the ketogenic diet have proved unsuccessful [Moreadith et al., 1984]. Some subunits may be encoded by genes on the X chromosome [Day and Scheffler, 1982].
- Myopathy with exercise intolerance, followed by fixed weakness. This form can start in childhood or adulthood and is usually accompanied by lactic acidosis at rest, which may be exaggerated by exercise [Morgan-Hughes et al., 1988]. In view of the tissue specificity of this disorder, it is possible that one or more of the nuclear DNA-encoded complex I subunits may exist as tissue-specific isoforms. Therapy with riboflavin was of benefit to one patient with weakness [Arts et al., 1983].
- Mitochondrial encephalomyopathy (excluding MELAS syndrome) with onset in childhood or adulthood. This form can have multiple combinations of ophthalmoplegia, seizures, dementia, ataxia, sensorineural hearing loss, pigmentary retinopathy,

sensory r
[Morgan-
were repo
this heter
nuclear D
[DiMauro,

Pitkanen and
plex I deficiency
oxide radicals a
superoxide dism
Hydrogen peroxi
would generate
that could then ca
and would be lik
morbidity, and mo

COMPLEX II DEFICIENC

The clinical spectr
five patients [DiMa
vaglia et al., 1990; H
cise intolerance, ex
succinate dehydroge
et al., 1991]. Anothe
ciency [Haller et al.,

COENZYME Q10 DEFICIEN

Exercise intolerance
axial and proximal lim
extraocular muscles, w
hara et al., 1989]. Autos
gested by the family hi
myoglobinuria in assoc
infections. Excessive lip
were documented on mu
suggested a muscle- (5%
isozyme defect of coen
improved both brain and

It is now apparent that
can cause three major sy
pathic disorder with recur
antly encephalopathic dis
atrophy, and a generalized
possible that the different m
different biosynthetic enzyr
mented [DiMauro, 2004].
of the significant clinical r
supplementation.

COMPLEX III DEFICIENCY

Complex III is composed of
high-molecular weight core p
chrome b (encoded by mtD
chrome c1, and a nonheme iro
Rieske protein [Hatefi, 1985].
use of both nicotinamide ade
adenine dinucleotide-linked su
neity in the clinical manifestati
into two major groups: those

(2) mutations of subunits shared by two or more complexes, (3) mutations affecting the milieu of the complexes, and (4) defects of mitochondrial protein importation affecting subunits of multiple complexes [DiMauro, 1993].

DEFECTS OF OXIDATION/PHOSPHORYLATION COUPLING

Luft's disease (nonthyroidal hypermetabolism) or loose coupling of oxidation/phosphorylation has been reported in two patients with sporadic cases: a Swedish woman [Luft et al., 1962] and a Jordanian woman [DiMauro et al., 1976; Haydar et al., 1971]. The clinical manifestation was that of onset in adolescence with fever, heat intolerance, profuse perspiration, polyphagia, polydipsia, and resting tachycardia with exercise intolerance and mild-to-moderate weakness. Myopathic changes were documented on electromyography, and muscle biopsy demonstrated numerous ragged-red fibers with greatly enlarged mitochondria, many of which contained osmiophilic inclusions. The possibility that Luft's disease may be the result of a nuclear DNA defect is suggested by the lack of evidence for maternal inheritance, apparent muscle specificity of the disease, and lack of mtDNA deletions [Moraes et al., 1989].

Defects of Mitochondrial Protein Importation

Mitochondrial proteins that are synthesized in the cytoplasm are given mitochondrial targeting signals that direct their entry into mitochondria. Transport across outer and inner membranes requires a series of factors, including docking protein, chaperonins, and proteases. In addition, it involves unfolding and refolding of the protein to be translocated [Okamoto et al., 2002]. Several mutations in targeting sequences that prevent individual proteins from reaching their destination have been documented. At least two disorders have been associated with mutations in components of the transport machinery. One is an X-linked disease, the deafness-dystonia syndrome (Mohr-Tranebjaerg syndrome), which is characterized by neurosensory hearing loss, dystonia, cortical blindness and psychiatric symptoms. It is caused by mutations in the *TIMM8A* gene, which encodes the deafness-dystonia protein (DDP1), an intermembrane space component of the transport machinery [Roesch et al., 2002]. The second is an autosomal-dominant form of hereditary spastic paraplegia caused by mutations in the chaperonin HSP60 [Hansen et al., 2002].

Defects of Intergenomic Signaling

For its function and replication, mtDNA is highly dependent on numerous factors encoded by nuclear genes. Mutations in these genes cause mendelian disorders that are characterized by qualitative or quantitative alterations of mtDNA [Hirano et al., 2001; Suomalainen and Kaukonen, 2001]. Qualitative alterations of mtDNA include autosomal-dominant or autosomal-recessive multiple deletions of mtDNA, which are usually accompanied clinically by progressive external ophthalmoplegia plus a variety of other signs and symptoms [Hirano and DiMauro, 2001]. Quantitative alterations of mtDNA include severe or partial expression of mtDNA depletion, which is usually characterized clinically by congenital or childhood forms of autosomal-recessively inherited myopathy or hepatopathy [Moraes et al., 1991a; Vu et al., 1998].

MULTIPLE MITOCHONDRIAL DNA DELETIONS

Multiple deletions of mtDNA were documented in an Italian family with an autosomal-dominant disease characterized by progressive external opththalmoplegia, cataracts, hearing loss, exercise intolerance, proximal and respiratory muscle weakness, and early death with lactic acidosis and ragged-red fibers documented on muscle biopsy [Servidei et al., 1991; Zeviani et al., 1989]. Other families with autosomal dominantly inherited progressive external opththalmoplegia have also been described [Cormier et al., 1991; Zeviani et al., 1990]. Associated multisystemic features have included mental retardation, tremor, ataxia, and peripheral neuropathy [Zeviani et al., 1990]. Other abnormalities have included hypoparathyroidism and hypodensities of the basal ganglia, centrum ovale, and brain peduncle documented by computed tomographic scan [Cormier et al., 1991]; nystagmus; and abnormal electroencephalographic findings [Iannaccone et al., 1974]. There were different clinical and family histories in two sets of Japanese brothers [Ohno et al., 1991; Yuzaki et al., 1989] whose parents were apparently asymptomatic. In one family, the brothers had ptosis but no ophthalmoplegia, myopathy, optic atrophy, or peripheral neuropathy [Yuzaki et al., 1989]. In the other family, the brothers suffered from recurrent myoglobinuria precipitated by exercise, fasting, or alcohol intake but had no ptosis or ophthalmoplegia [Ohno et al., 1991]. Muscle biochemistry demonstrated combined defects of the respiratory chain in one family [Servidei et al., 1991], complex I deficiency in another [Cormier et al., 1991], and normal respiratory chain enzymes in the patients with myoglobinuria [Ohno et al., 1991].

Four of these conditions have been characterized at a molecular level. Mutations in the gene encoding one isoform of adenine nucleotide translocator (*ANT1*) have been documented in some, but not all, patients with autosomal-dominant progressive external opththalmoplegia [Kaukonen et al., 2000]. Mutations in the gene for thymidine phosphorylase (*TP*) lead to an autosomal-recessive multisystemic syndrome, named MNGIE (mitochondrial neurogastrointestinal encephalomyopathy) [Nishino et al., 1999, 2000]. Both types of mutations affect the mitochondrial nucleotide pools and may have similar pathogenic mechanisms. Mutations in the *Twinkle* gene, which is a helicase, are associated with autosomal dominant progressive external opththalmoplegia [Spellbrink et al., 2001]. Finally, mutations in the gene encoding polymerase γ (*POLG*) may lead to either autosomal-dominant or autosomal recessive progressive external opththalmoplegia, which is occasionally associated with psychiatric symptoms or parkinsonism [Mancuso et al., 2004b; VanGoethem et al., 2001].

DEPLETION OF MITOCHONDRIAL DNA

Depletion of mtDNA has been described in a number of patients and can be divided into those with severe depletion and those with partial depletion [Boustany et al., 1983; Moraes et al., 1991a; Tritschler et al., 1992]. Clinical manifestation has been variable in severe mtDNA depletion. The spectrum has included different combinations of diffuse myopathy in the first weeks of life, necessitating ventilator support; liver disease; renal dysfunction with glycosuria, phosphaturia, and generalized amino aciduria (DeToni-Fanconi-Debre syndrome); seizures with evidence of hypsarrhythmia; and, in rare cases, progressive external opththalmoplegia, with death between 3 and 9 months of age. All patients had severe lactic acidosis and ragged-red fibers in muscle. One family history was suggestive of autosomal-recessive inheritance [Boustany et al., 1983]. In each case, mtDNA depletion was observed only in the affected tissues. In children with partial mtDNA depletion, the primary feature was myopathy, with onset between 5 and 12 months of age and death between 11 months and 3 years of age. Serum lactate levels were normal. Muscle biochemistry demonstrated combined defects of respiratory chain complexes containing mtDNA-encoded subunits, such as complexes I, III, and IV, which were more severe in patients with severe depletion. A male with normal early growth and development until 1 year of age, followed by a severe progressive neuromuscular disorder resembling spinal muscular atrophy, lost his ability to walk at 3 years of age and subsequently received a diagnosis of mtDNA depletion syndrome. An initial muscle biopsy at $2^1/_2$ years of age was consistent with denervation, but there were no deletions in exons 7 and 8 of the survival motor neuron gene on DNA analysis [Pons et al., 1996].

Thus, mtDNA depletion is usually characterized clinically by congenital or childhood forms of autosomal recessively inherited myopathy or hepatopathy [Moraes et al., 1991a; Vu et al., 1998]. Although skeletal muscle and liver seem to be the main target tissues, other tissues are often affected in both conditions, including kidney (renal tubular acidosis) and the central nervous system. Central nervous system involvement often simulates spinal muscular atrophy, and mtDNA depletion should be considered in children with the spinal muscular atrophy phenotype but without mutations in the *SMN* gene [Mancuso et al., 2002, 2003].

The decrease in mtDNA is documented by densitometry of Southern blot analysis and confirmed by immunocytochemistry with anti-DNA antibodies and by in situ hybridization [Andreeta et al., 1991; Moraes et al., 1991a; Tritschler et al., 1992]. In severe cases, depletion of muscle mtDNA varies between 83% and 98%, and in less severe cases, it varies between 66% and 92%. Mutations in two genes, both of which are involved in mitochondrial nucleotide homeostasis, have been associated with mtDNA depletion syndromes, even though they do not explain all cases. Mutations in the gene encoding thymidine kinase 2 (*TK2*) are frequently documented in patients with the myopathic mtDNA depletion syndrome [Mancuso et al., 2002; Saada et al., 2001]. Mutations in the gene encoding deoxyguano--sine kinase (*dGK*) predominate in patients with hepatic or multisystemic mtDNA depletion syndromes [Mandel et al., 2001; Salviati et al., 2002b].

Alterations of the Lipid Milieu of the Inner Mitochondrial Membrane

An example of this etiology is provided by Barth's syndrome, an X-linked recessive disorder characterized by mitochondrial myopathy, cardiomyopathy, growth retardation, and neutropenia [Barth et al., 1999]. This disorder is caused by mutations in the tafazzin (*TAZ*) gene, which encodes a family of proteins ("tafazzins") that are homologous to phospholipid acyltransferases [Bione et al., 1996]. Analysis of phospholipids in target tissues from patients with Barth's syndrome and *TAZ* mutations revealed decreased cardiolipin in all tissues from patients with genetically proven Barth's syndrome [Schlame et al., 2002, 2003]. The cardiolipin was selectively affected, whereas the other phospholipid levels were normal.

Alterations of Mitochondrial Motility or Fission

Mitochondria are dynamic organelles that are propelled within the cell by energy-requiring dynamins along cytoskeletal microtubular rails [Boldogh et al., 2001]. Mutations in a gene (*OPA1*) that encodes a dynamin-related guanosine triphosphatase have been associated with an autosomal-dominant form of optic atrophy resulting in early-onset blindness [Alexander et al., 2000; Delettre et al., 2000]. Morphologically, mitochondria were clumped together rather than uniformly distributed in the cytoplasm of monocytes from these patients.

Differential Diagnosis of Lactic Acidemia

The ratio of lactate to pyruvate in the blood is a helpful indicator of the underlying problem and may help to direct further investigations. A ratio of lactate to pyruvate below 25, which is considered to be in the normal range, suggests a defect of either pyruvate dehydrogenase or one of the gluconeogenic enzymes, whereas a consistently elevated ratio of lactate to pyruvate, particularly one of 35 or greater, suggests a pyruvate carboxylase (type A) deficiency or a respiratory chain defect [Robinson et al., 1987, 1989].

MYOADENYLATE DEAMINASE DEFICIENCY

Clinical Presentation

Myoadenylate deaminase deficiency is detected in 1% to 3% of all muscle biopsy samples and may be characterized by exercise-related myalgia and cramps [Sabina, 1993]. However, the pathogenetic significance of this defect is controversial because (1) in patients with unexplained myopathy, symptoms are generally mild, ill-defined, and often subjective and (2) more than 50% of patients had either well-defined myopathies, such as Duchenne or Becker muscular dystrophy, McArdle's disease, spinal muscular atrophy, or amyotrophic lateral sclerosis. Therefore, Fishbein [1985] divided myoadenylate deaminase into the following two forms: (1) a primary (hereditary) myoadenylate deaminase deficiency characterized by myopathy alone with exercise intolerance, myalgia, and cramps; very low residual activity (<1% of normal); and lack of cross-reacting material in muscle and (2) a secondary (acquired) myoadenylate deaminase deficiency associated with well-defined myopathies or neuromuscular disorders in which there is higher residual activity and detectable cross-reacting material. Isolated myoadenylate deaminase deficiency may manifest with recurrent myoglobinuria [Baumeister et al., 1993; Tonin et al., 1990].

Laboratory Tests

The resting serum creatine kinase level is usually normal but may increase after exercise. The forearm ischemic exercise test demonstrates a normal rise in venous lactate but no rise in ammonia or inosine monophosphate. The electromyogram may appear normal or may demonstrate nonspecific myopathic features.

Pathology

Muscle biopsy specimens are usually normal; however, decreased myoadenylate deaminase activity can be detected by histochemical staining [Fishbein et al., 1980].

Biochemistry and Molecular Genetics

There are three tissue-specific subunits: M (muscle), L (liver), and E (erythrocyte), which are under separate genetic control. Adult human muscle contains almost exclusively the M homotetramer. AMP deaminase converts AMP to inosine monophosphate and ammonia. The complementary DNA and gene of muscle AMP deaminase have been cloned, sequenced, and localized to chromosome 1p13-p21 [Gross, 1994; Sabina et al., 1990], and a C34T mutation leading to recurrent myoglobinuria has been identified [Baumeister et al., 1993]. The AMP deaminase-1 gene maps to chromosome 1p21-p13 [Morton et al., 1989].

ACKNOWLEDGMENTS

Part of the work described here was supported by an operating grant from the Heart and Stroke Foundation of Ontario (T-5424) and the physicians of Ontario, Canada, through the Physicians' Services Incorporated Foundation. Ingrid Tein is a recipient of a Detweiler Travelling Fellowship from the Royal College of Physicians and Surgeons of Canada.

REFERENCES

Abarbanel JM, Bashan N, Potashnik R, et al. Adult muscle phosphorylase "b" kinase deficiency. Neurology 1986;36:560.

Adams EM, Becker JA, Griffith L, et al. Glycogenosis type II: A juvenile-specific mutation with an unusual splicing pattern and a shared mutation in African Americans. Hum Mutat 1997;10:128.

Al-Odaib A, Shneider BL, Bennett MJ, et al. A defect in the transport of long-chain fatty acids associated with acute liver failure. N Engl J Med 1998;339:1752.

Alegria A, Martins E, Dias M, et al. Glycogen storage disease type IV presenting as hydrops fetalis. J Inherit Metab Dis 1999;22:330.

Alexander C, Votruba M, Pesch UEA, et al. OPA1, encoding a dynamin-related GTPase, is mutated in autosomal dominant optic atrophy linked to chromosome 3q28. Nat Genet 2000;26:211.

Amalfitano A, Bengur AR, Morse RP, et al. Recombinant human acid alpha-glucosidase enzyme therapy for infantile glycogen storage disease type II: Results of a phase I/II clinical trial. Genet Med 2001;3:132.

Amit R, Bashan N, Abarbanel JM, et al. Fatal familial infantile glycogen storage disease: Multisystem phosphofructokinase deficiency. Muscle Nerve 1992;15:455.

Anderson S, Bankier AT, Barrell BG, et al. Sequence and organization of the human mitochondrial genome. Nature 1981;290:457.

Andreeta F, Tritschler HJ, Schon EA, et al. Localization of mitochondrial DNA in normal and pathological muscle using immunological probes: A new approach to the study of mitochondrial myopathies. J Neurol Sci 1991;105:88.

Andresen BS, Bross P, Vianey-Saban C, et al. Cloning and characterization of human very-long-chain acyl-CoA dehydrogenase cDNA, chromosomal assignment of the gene and identification in four patients of nine different mutations within the VLCAD gene. Hum Mol Genet 1996a;5:461.

Andresen BS, Vianey-Saban C, Bross P, et al. The mutational spectrum in very long-chain acyl-CoA dehydrogenase deficiency. J Inherit Metab Dis 1996b;19:169.

Andreu AL, Hanna MG, Reichmann H, et al. Exercise intolerance due to mutations in the cytochrome b gene of mitochondrial DNA. N Engl J Med 1999;341:1037.

Antonicka H, Mattman A, Carlson CG, et al. Mutations in COX15 produce a defect in the mitochondrial heme biosynthetic pathway, causing early-onset fatal hypertrophic cardiomyopathy. Am J Hum Genet 2003;72:101.

Aoyama T, Souri M, Ueno I, et al. Cloning of human very-long-chain acyl-coenzyme A dehydrogenase and molecular characterization of its deficiency in two patients. Am J Hum Genet 1995a;57:273.

Aoyama T, Souri M, Ushikubo S, et al. Purification of human very-long-chain acyl-coenzyme A dehydrogenase and characterization of its deficiency in seven patients. J Clin Invest 1995b;95:2465.

Argov Z, Bank WJ, Boden B, et al. Phosphorus magnetic resonance spectroscopy of partially blocked muscle glycolysis. Arch Neurol 1987;44:614.

Argov Z, Bank WJ, Maris J, et al. Treatment of mitochondrial myopathy due to complex III deficiency with vitamins K_3 and C: A ^{31}P-NMR follow-up study. Ann Neurol 1986;19:598.

Argov Z, Bank WJ. Phosphorus magnetic resonance spectroscopy (^{31}P MRS) in neuromuscular disorders. Ann Neurol 1991;30:90.

Astrand PO, Rodahl K. Textbook of work physiology: Physiological basis of exercise. New York: McGraw-Hill, 1986.

Arts WFM, Scholte HR, Bogaard JM, et al. NADH-CoQ reductase deficiency myopathy: Successful treatment with riboflavin. Lancet 1983;2:581.

Aynsley-Green A. Hypoglycemia in infants and children. Clin Endocrinol Metab 1982;11:159.

Badurska B, Fidzianska A, Kwiatkowska Z. Muscular glycogenosis (type 3) in a 15-year-old boy. Neuropatol Pol 1970;8:265.

Bank W, Park J, Lech G, et al. Near-infrared spectroscopy in the diagnosis of mitochondrial disorders. Biofactors 1998;7:243.

Bao Y, Kishnani P, Tang TT, et al. Hepatic and neuromuscular forms of glycogen storage disease type IV caused by mutations in the same glycogen-branching enzyme. J Clin Invest 1996;97:941.

Barbiroli B, Medori R, Tritschler HJ, et al. Lipoic (thioctic) acid increases brain energy availability and skeletal muscle performance as shown by in vivo ^{31}P-MRS in a patient with mitochondrial cytopathy. J Neurol 1995;242:472.

Baretz BH, Ramsdell HS, Tanaka K. Identification of *N*-hexanoylglycine in urines from two patients with Jamaican vomiting sickness. Clin Chim Acta 1976;73:199.

Barth PG, Wanders RJA, Vreken P, et al. X-linked cardioskeletal myopathy and neutropenia (Barth syndrome). J Inherit Metabol Dis 1999;22:555.

Bartram C, Edwards R, Clague J, et al. McArdle's disease: A nonsense mutation in exon 1 of the muscle glycogen phosphorylase gene explains some but not all cases. Hum Mol Genet 1993;2:1291.

Bates EJ, Heaton GM, Taylor C, et al. Debranching enzyme from rabbit skeletal muscle: Evidence for the location of two active centers on a single polypeptide chain. FEBS Lett 1975;58:181.

Baumeister FA, Gross M, Wagner DR, et al. Myoadenylate deaminase deficiency with severe rhabdomyolysis. Eur J Pediatr 1993;152:513.

Bell AW, Thompson GE. Free fatty acid oxidation in bovine muscle in vivo: Effects of cold exposure and feeding. Am J Physiol 1979;237:E309.

Bennett MJ, Spotswood SD, Ross KF, et al. Fatal hepatic short-chain *L*-3-hydroxyacyl-coenzyme A dehydrogenase deficiency: Clinical, biochemical, and pathological studies on three subjects with this recently identified disorder of mitochondrial beta-oxidation. Pediatr Dev Pathol 1999;2:337.

Bennett MJ, Weinberger MJ, Kobori JA, et al. Mitochondrial short-chain *L*-3-hydroxybutyryl-CoA dehydrogenase deficiency: A new defect of fatty acid oxidation. Pediatr Res 1996;39:185.

Bennett MJ, Worthy E, Pollitt RJ. The incidence and presentation of dicarboxylic aciduria. J Inherit Metab Dis 1987;10:241.

Berkovic SF, Carpenter S, Evans A, et al. Myoclonus epilepsy and ragged-red fibers (MERRF). 1. A clinical, pathological, biochemical, magnetic resonance spectrographic and positron emission tomographic study. Brain 1989;112:1231.

Bhala A, Willi SM, Rinaldo P, et al. Clinical and biochemical characterization of short-chain acyl-coenzyme A dehydrogenase deficiency. J Pediatr 1995;126:910.

Bier DM, Leake RD, Haymond MW, et al. Measurement of "true" glucose production rates in infancy and childhood with 6,6-dideuteroglucose. Diabetes 1977;26:1016.

Bijvoet AG, Van Hirtum H, Kroos MA, et al. Human acid alpha-glucosidase from rabbit milk has therapeutic effect in mice with glycogen storage disease type II. Hum Mol Genet 1999;8:2145.

Billingsley GD, Cox DW, Duncan AM, et al. Regional localization of loci on chromosome 14 using somatic cell hybrids. Cytogenet Cell Genet 1994;66:33.

Bione S, D'Adamo P, Maestrini E, et al. A novel X-linked gene, G4.5, is responsible for Barth syndrome. Nat Genet 1996;12:385.

Birch-Machin MA, Shepherd IM, Watmaugh NJ, et al. Fatal lactic acidosis in infancy with a defect of complex III of the respiratory chain. Pediatr Res 1989;25:553.

Blakemore AIF, Singleton H, Pollitt RJ, et al. Frequency of the G985 MCAD mutation in the general population. Lancet 1991;337:298.

Boivin P, Hakim J, Manderau J, et al. [Erythrocyte and leucocyte 3-phosphoglycerate kinase deficiency. Studies of properties of the enzyme, phagocytic activity of the polymorphonuclear leucoytes and a review of the literature]. Nouv Rev Fr Hematol (in French) 1974;14:495.

Boldogh IR, Yang HC, Nowakowski WD, et al. Arp 2/3 complex and actin dynamics are required for actin-based mitochondrial motility in yeast. Proc Natl Acad Sci U S A 2001;98:3162.

Bonilla E, Chang HW, Miranda AF, et al. Duchenne muscular dystrophy: The disease, the protein. In: Benzi G, ed. Advances in myochemistry II. Toronto-Paris: John Libbey Eurotext, 1989;173.

Bonilla E, Schotland DL. Histochemical diagnosis of muscle phosphofructokinase deficiency. Arch Neurol 1970;22:8.

Boone CM, Chen TR, Ruddle FH. Assignment of three human genes to chromosomes (LDH-A to 11, TK to 17, and IDH to 20) and evidence for translocation between human and mouse chromosomes in somatic cell hybrids. Proc Natl Acad Sci U S A 1972;69:510.

Bornemann A, Besser R, Shin YS, et al. A mild adult myopathic variant of type IV glycogenosis. Neuromuscul Disord 1996;6:95.

Bouchard L, Robert MF, Vinarov D, et al. Mitochondrial 3-hydroxy-3-methylglutaryl-CoA synthase deficiency: Clinical course and description of causal mutations in two patients. Pediatr Res 2001;49:326.

Bourgeron T, Rustin P, Chretien D, et al. Mutation of a nuclear succinate dehydrogenase gene results in mitochondrial respiratory chain deficiency. Nat Genet 1995;11:144.

Boustany RN, Aprille JR, Halperin J, et al. Mitochondrial cytochrome deficiency presenting as a myopathy with hypotonia, external ophthalmoplegia, and lactic acidosis in an infant and as fatal hepatopathy in a second cousin. Ann Neurol 1983;14:462.

Bremer J. Carnitine-metabolism and functions. Physiol Rev 1983;63:1420.

Bresolin N, Bet L, Moggio M, et al. Muscle glucose-6-phosphate dehydrogenase deficiency. J Neurol 1989;236:193.

Bresolin N, Miranda AF, Jacobsen MP, et al. Phosphorylase isoenzymes of human brain. Neurochem Pathol 1983;1:171.

Britton CH, Schultz RA, Zhang B, et al. Human liver mitochondrial carnitine palmitoyltransferase I: Characterization of its cDNA and chromosomal localization and partial analysis of the gene. Proc Natl Acad Sci U S A 1995;92:1984.

Brown BI. Debranching and branching enzyme deficiencies. In: Engel AG, Banker B, eds. Myology. New York: McGraw-Hill, 1986;1653.

Brown BI, Brown DH. Branching enzyme activity of cultured amniocytes and chorionic villi: Prenatal testing for type IV glycogen storage disease. Am J Hum Genet 1989;44:378.

Brown RM, Dahl H-HM, Brown GK. X-chromosome localization of the functional gene for the E1 subunit of the human pyruvate dehydrogenase complex. Genomics 1989;4:174.

Brunberg JA, McCormick WF, Schochet SS. Type III glycogenosis: An adult with diffuse weakness and muscle wasting. Arch Neurol 1971;25:171.

Bruno C, DiRocco M, Doria Lama L, et al. A novel missense mutation in the glycogen branching enzyme gene in a child with myopathy and hepatopathy. Neuromuscul Disord 1999;9:403.

Bruno C, Manfredi G, Andreu AL, et al. A splice junction mutation in the alpha-M gene of phosphorylase kinase in a patient with myopathy. Biochem Biophys Res Comm 1998;249:648.

Bruno C, Servidei S, Shanske S, et al. Glycogen branching enzyme deficiency in adult polyglucosan body disease. Ann Neurol 1993;33:88.

Bryan W, Lewis SF, Bertocci L, et al. Muscle lactate dehydrogenase deficiency: A disorder of anaerobic glycogenolysis associated with exertional myoglobinuria [Abstract]. Neurology 1990;40:203.

Burwinkel B, Amat L, Gray RG, et al. Variability of biochemical and clinical phenotype in X-linked liver glycogenosis with mutations in the phosphorylase kinase PHKA2 gene. Hum Genet 1998;102:423.

Cafferty MS, Lovelace RE, Hays AP. Polyglucosan body disease. Muscle Nerve 1991;14:102.

Cahill GF Jr. Starvation in man. N Engl J Med 1970;282:668.

Carelli V. Leber's hereditary optic neuropathy. In: Schapira AHV, DiMauro S, eds. Mitochondrial Disorders in Neurology, vol. 2. Boston: Butterworth-Heinemann, 2002;115.

Carpenter K, Pollitt RJ, Middleton B. Human liver long-chain 3-hydroxyacyl-coenzyme A dehydrogenase is a multifunctional membrane-bound beta-oxidation enzyme of mitochondria. Biochem Biophys Res Commun 1992;183:443.

Carrier H, Maire I, Vial C, et al. Myopathic evolution of an exertional muscle pain syndrome with phosphorylase b kinase deficiency. Acta Neuropathol 1990;81:84.

Cederbaum SD, Koo-McCoy S, Tein I, et al. Carnitine membrane transporter deficiency: A long-term follow up and OCTN2 mutation in the first documented case of primary carnitine deficiency. Mol Genet Metab 2002;77:195.

Chace DH, DiPerna JC, Mitchell BL, et al. Electrospray tandem mass spectrometry for analysis of acylcarnitines in dried postmortem blood specimens collected at autopsy from infants with unexplained cause of death. Clin Chem 2001;47:1166.

Charlesworth D. Starch-gel electrophoresis of four enzymes from human red blood cells: Glyceraldehyde-3-phosphate dehydrogenase, fructoaldolase, glyoxalase II and sorbital dehydrogenase. Ann Hum Genet 1972;35:477.

Chen TR, McMorris FA, Creagan R, et al. Assignment of the genes for malate oxidoreductase to chromosome 6 and peptidase B and lactate dehydrogenase B to chromosome 12 in man. Am J Hum Genet 1973;25:200.

Chen YT, He JK, Ding JH, et al. Glycogen debranching enzyme: Purification, antibody characterization, and immunoblot analysis of type III glycogen storage disease. Am J Hum Genet 1987;41:1002.

Chinnery PF, Johnson MA, Wardell TM, et al. Epidemiology of pathogenic mitochondrial DNA mutations. Ann Neurol 2000;48:188.

Chomyn A, Meola G, Bresolin N, et al. In vitro genetic transfer of protein synthesis and respiration defects to mitochondrial DNA–less cells with myopathy-patient mitochondria. Mol Cell Biol 1991;11:2236.

Chui LA, Munsat TL. Dominant inheritance of McArdle syndrome. Arch Neurol 1976;33:636.

Ciafaloni E, Ricci E, Shanske S, et al. MELAS: Clinical features, biochemistry, and molecular genetics. Ann Neurol 1992;31:391.

Clark JB, Hayes DJ, Byrne E, et al. Mitochondrial myopathies: Defects in mitochondrial metabolism in human skeletal muscle. Biochem Soc Trans 1983;11:626.

Cleary MA, Walter JH, Kerr BA, et al. Facial appearance in glycogen storage disease type III. Clin Dysmorphol 2002;11:117.

Corkey BE, Hale DE, Glennon MC, et al. Relationship between unusual hepatic acyl coenzyme A profiles and the pathogenesis of Reye syndrome. J Clin Invest 1988;82:782.

Cormier V, Rotig A, Tardieu M, et al. Autosomal dominant deletions of the mitochondrial genome in a case of progressive encephalomyopathy. Am J Hum Genet 1991;48:643.

Corydon MJ, Gregersen N, Lehnert W, et al. Ethylmalonic aciduria is associated with an amino acid variant of short chain acyl-coenzyme A dehydrogenase. Pediatr Res 1996;39:1059.

Corydon MJ, Vockley J, Rinaldo P, et al. Role of common gene variations in the molecular pathogenesis of short-chain acyl-CoA dehydrogenase deficiency. Pediatr Res 2001;49:18.

Cox PM, Brueton LA, Murphy KW, et al. Early-onset fetal hydrops and muscle degeneration in siblings due to a novel variant of type IV glycogenosis. Am J Med Genet 1999;86:187.

D'Ancona GG, Wurm J, Croce C. Genetics of type II glycogenosis: Assignment of the human gene for acid glucosidase to chromosome 17. Proc Nat Acad Sci U S A 1979;76:4526.

Darin N, Oldfors A, Moslemi AR, et al. The incidence of mitochondrial encephalomyopathies in childhood: Clinical features and morphological, biochemical, and DNA abnormalities. Ann Neurol 2001;49:377.

Darley-Usmar VM, Kennaway NG, Buist NR, et al. Deficiency in ubiquinone cytochrome c reductase in a patient with mitochondrial myopathy and lactic acidosis. Proc Natl Acad Sci U S A 1983;80:5103.
Darley-Usmar VM, Watanabe M, Uchiyama Y, et al. Mitochondrial myopathy: Tissue-specific expression of a defect in ubiquinol-cytochrome c reductase. Clin Chim Acta 1986;158:253.
Davidson JJ, Özçelik T, Hamacher C, et al. cDNA cloning of a liver isoform of the phosphorylase kinase a subunit and mapping of the gene to Xp22.2-p22.1, the region of human X-linked liver glycogenosis. Proc Natl Acad Sci U S A 1992;89:2096.
Day CE, Scheffler IE. Mapping of the genes of some components of the electron transport chain (complex I) on the X chromosome of mammals. Somat Cell Mol Genet 1982;8:691.
de Lonlay-Debeney P, Edery P, Cormeir-Daire V, et al. Respiratory chain deficiency presenting as recurrent myoglobinuria in childhood. Neuropediatrics. 1999;30:42.
de Lonlay P, Valnot I, Barrientos A, et al. A mutant mitochondrial respiratory chain assembly protein causes complex III deficiency in patients with tubulopathy, encephalopathy, and liver failure. Nat Genet 2001;29:57.
De Meirleir L, Seneca S, Lissens W, et al. Respiratory chain complex V deficiency due to a mutation in the assembly gene ATP12. J Med Genet 2004;41:120.
De Stefano N, Matthews PM, Ford B, et al. Short-term dichloroacetate treatment improves indices of cerebral metabolism in patients with mitochondrial disorders. Neurology 1995;45:1193.
Delettre C, Lenaers G, Griffoin JM, et al. Nucelar gene OPA1, encoding a mitochondrial dynamin-related protein, is mutated in dominant optic atrophy. Nat Genet 2000;26:207.
Demaugre F, Bonnefont JP, Mitchell G, et al. Hepatic and muscular presentations of carnitine palmitoyltransferase deficiency: Two distinct entities. Pediatr Res 1988;24:308.
DiMauro S. Mitochondrial encephalomyopathies. In: Rosenberg RN, Prusiner SB, DiMauro S, et al., eds. The molecular and genetic basis of neurological disease. Boston: Butterworth-Heinemann, 1993;665.
DiMauro S. Mitochondrial diseases. Biochim Biophys Acta 2004;1658: 80.
DiMauro S, Arnold S, Miranda AF, et al. The mystery of reappearing phosphorylase activity in muscle culture. A fetal isoenzyme. Ann Neurol 1978;3:60.
DiMauro S, Bonilla E, Lee CP, et al. Luft's disease. Further biochemical and ultrastructural studies of skeletal muscle in the second case. J Neurol Sci 1976;27:217.
DiMauro S, Bonilla E, Mancuso M, et al. Mitochondrial myopathies. Basic Appl Myol 2003;13:145.
DiMauro S, Bresolin N. Phosphorylase deficiency. In: Engel AG, Banker BQ, eds. Myology. New York: McGraw-Hill, 1986;1585.
DiMauro S, Dalakas M, Miranda AF. Phosphoglycerate kinase (PGK) deficiency: A new cause of recurrent myoglobinuria [Abstract]. Ann Neurol 1981a;10:90.
DiMauro S, Dalakas M, Miranda AF. Phosphoglycerate kinase deficiency: Another cause of recurrent myoglobinuria. Ann Neurol 1983a;13:11.
DiMauro S, De Vivo DC. Diseases of carbohydrate, fatty acid, and mitochondrial metabolism. In: Siegel GJ, Agranoff BW, Albers W, et al., eds. Basic neurochemistry: Molecular, cellular, and medical aspects, 4th ed. New York: Raven Press, 1989;647.
DiMauro S, DiMauro PMM. Muscle carnitine palmitoyltransferase deficiency and myoglobinuria. Science 1973;182:929.
DiMauro S, Haller RG. Metabolic myopathies: Substrate use defects. In: Schapira AHV, Griggs RC, eds. Muscle Diseases. Boston: Butterworth-Heinemann, 1999;225.
DiMauro S, Hartlage PL. Fatal infantile form of muscle phosphorylase deficiency. Neurology 1978;28:1124.
DiMauro S, Hirano M. Mitochondrial DNA deletion syndromes, GeneReviews at Gene Tests: Medical Genetics Information Resource [database online]. Available at: ed/.http://www.genetest.org, University of Washington, Seattle, 2003a.
DiMauro S, Hirano M. MELAS, Gene Reviews at Gene Tests: Medical Genetics Information Resource [database online] ed. University of Washington, Seattle, 2003b.
DiMauro S, Hirano M, Kaufmann P, et al. Clinical features and genetics of myoclonic epilepsy with ragged red fibres. In: Fahn S, Frucht SJ, Hallett M, et al., eds. Myoclonus and paroxysmal dyskinesia. Philadelphia: Lipppincott Williams & Wilkins, 2002;217.
DiMauro S, Lamperti C. Muscle glycogenoses. Muscle and Nerve 2001;24:984.
DiMauro S, Lombes A, Nakase H, et al. Cytochrome c oxidase deficiency. Pediatr Res 1990;28:536.
DiMauro S, Miranda AF, Khan S, et al. Human muscle phosphoglycerate mutase deficiency: A newly discovered metabolic myopathy. Science 1981b;212:1277.
DiMauro S, Miranda AF, Olarte M, et al. Muscle phosphoglycerate mutase deficiency. Neurology 1982;32:584.
DiMauro S, Miranda AF, Sakoda S, et al. Metabolic myopathies. Am J Med Genet 1986;25:635.
DiMauro S, Nicholson JF, Hays AP, et al. Benign infantile mitochondrial myopathy due to reversible cytochrome c oxidase deficiency. Ann Neurol 1983b;14:226.
DiMauro S, Papadimitriou A. Carnitine palmitoyltransferase deficiency. In: Engel AG, Banker BQ, eds. Myology, vol 2. New York: McGraw-Hill, 1986;1697.
DiMauro S, Tonin P, Servidei S. Metabolic myopathies. In: Rowland LP, DiMauro S, eds. Handbook of clinical neurology, vol 18(62). Myopathies. Amsterdam, The Netherlands: Elsevier Science, 1992;479.
DiMauro S, Tsujino S. Nonlysosomal glycogenoses. In: Engel AG, Banker BQ, eds. Myology, vol 2. New York: McGraw-Hill, 1994.
DiMauro S, Tsujino S, Shanske S, et al. Biochemistry and molecular genetics of human glycogenoses: An overview. Muscle Nerve 1995;3:S10.
Ding JH, DeBarsy TH, Brown BI, et al. Immunoblot analysis of glycogen debranching enzyme in different subtypes of glycogen storage disease type III. J Pediatr 1990;116:95.
Dionisi-Vici C, Burlina AB, Bertini E, et al. Progressive neuropathy and recurrent myoglobinuria in a child with long-chain 3-hydroxyacyl-coenzyme A dehydrogenase deficiency. J Pediatr 1991;118:744.
Dyken M, Smith D, Peake R. An electromyographic diagnostic screening test in McArdle's disease and a case report. Neurology 1967;17:45.
Edwards YH, Sakoda S, Schon EA, et al. The gene for human muscle-specific phosphoglycerate mutase, PGAMM, mapped to chromosome 7 by polymerase chain reaction. Genomics 1989;5:948.
El-Fakhri M, Middleton B. The existence of an inner-membrane-bound, long acyl-chain–specific 3-hydroxyacyl-CoA dehydrogenase in mammalian mitochondria. Biochem Biophys Acta 1982;713:270.
El-Schahawi M, Bruno C, Tsujino S, et al. Sudden infant death syndrome (SIDS) in a family with myophosphorylase deficiency. Neuromuscul Disord 1997;7:81.
El-Schahawi M, Tsujino S, Shanske S, et al. Diagnosis of McArdle's disease by molecular genetic analysis of blood. Neurology 1996;47:579.
Eleff S, Kennaway NG, Buist NR, et al. ^{31}P NMR study of improvement in oxidative phosphorylation by vitamins K_3 and C in a patient with a defect in electron transport at complex III in skeletal muscle. Proc Natl Acad Sci U S A 1984;81:3529.
Elpeleg ON, Joseph A, Branski D, et al. Recurrent metabolic decompensation in profound carnitine palmitoyltransferase II deficiency. J Pediatr 1993;122:917.
Engel AG, Hirschhorn R. Acid maltase deficiency. In: Engel AG, Banker BQ, eds: Myology, vol 2. New York: McGraw-Hill, 1994;1533.
Engel WK, Cunningham CG. Rapid examination of muscle tissue: An improved trichrome stain method for fresh-frozen biopsy sections. Neurology 1963;13:919.
Engel WK, Vick NA, Glueck CJ, et al. A skeletal-muscle disorder associated with intermittent symptoms and a possible defect of lipid metabolism. N Engl J Med 1970;282:697.
Essen B. Glycogen depletion of different types in human skeletal muscle during intermittent and continuous exercise. Acta Physiol Scand 1978;103:446.
Essen B. Intramuscular substrate utilization during prolonged exercise. Ann N Y Acad Sci 1977;301:30.
Esser V, Britton CH, Weis BC, et al. Cloning, sequencing, and expression of a cDNA encoding rat liver carnitine palmitoyltransferase I. J Biol Chem 1993;268:5817.
Etiemble J, Kahn APB. Hereditary hemolytic anemia with erythrocyte phosphofructokinase deficiency. Hum Genet 1976;31:83.
Eviatar L, Shanske S, Gauthier B, et al. Kearns-Sayre syndrome presenting as renal tubular acidosis. Neurology 1990;40:1761.
Falik-Borenstein ZC, Jordan SC, Saudubray JM, et al. Brief report: Renal tubular acidosis in carnitine palmitoyltransferase type 1 deficiency. N Engl J Med 1992;327:24.

Farrans VJ, Hibbs RG, Walsh JJ, et al. Cardiomyopathy, cirrhosis of the liver and deposits of a fibrillar polysaccharide. Am J Cardiol 1966;17:457.

Felig P, Wahren J. Fuel homeostasis in exercise. N Engl J Med 1975;293:1078.

Fellman V. The GRACILE syndrome, a neonatal lethal metabolic disorder with iron overload. Blood Cells Mol Diseases 1992;29:444.

Fellows IW, Lowe JS, Ogilvie AL, et al. Type III glycogenosis presenting as liver disease in adults with atypical histological features. J Clin Pathol 1983;36:431.

Ferguson IT, Mahon M, Cumming WJ. An adult case of Andersen's disease—Type IV glycogenosis. A clinical, histochemical, ultrastructural and biochemical study. J Neurol Sci 1983;60:337.

Fernandes J. The glycogen storage diseases. In: Fernandes J, Saudubray JM, Tada K, eds. Inborn metabolic diseases. Berlin: Springer-Verlag, 1990;69.

Fernandes J, Huijing F. Branching enzyme-deficiency glycogenosis: Studies in therapy. Arch Dis Child 1968;43:347.

Fernandes J, Smit G. The glycogen storage diseases. In: Fernandes J, Saudubray J, Van den Berghe C, eds. Inborn error of metabolic diseases, diagnosis and treatment, 3rd ed. New York: Springer, 2001;88.

Finocchiaro G, Colombo I, Garavaglia B, et al. cDNA cloning and mitochondrial import of the beta subunit of the human electron-transfer flavoprotein. Eur J Biochem 1993;213:1003.

Finocchiaro G, Ikeda Y, Ito M, et al. Biosynthesis, molecular cloning and sequencing of electron transfer flavoprotein. In: Tanaka K, Coates PM, eds. Progress in clinical and biological research, vol 321. Fatty acid oxidation: Clinical, biochemical and molecular aspects. New York: Alan R. Liss, 1990;637.

Finocchiaro G, Ito M, Ikeda Y, et al. Molecular cloning and nucleotide sequence of cDNAs encoding the a-subunit of human electron transfer flavoprotein. J Biol Chem 1988;265:15773.

Finocchiaro G, Ito M, Tanaka K. Purification and properties of short chain acyl-CoA, medium chain acyl-CoA, and isovaleryl-CoA dehydrogenases from human liver. J Biol Chem 1987;262:7982.

Finocchiaro G, Taroni F, Rocchi M, et al. cDNA cloning, sequence analysis, and chromosomal localization of the gene for human carnitine palmitoyltransferase. Proc Natl Acad Sci USA 1991;88:661.

Fishbein WN. Myoadenylate deaminase deficiency: Inherited and acquired forms. Biochem Med 1985;33:158.

Fishbein WN, Griffin JL, Armbrustmacher VW. Stain for skeletal muscle adenylate deaminase: An effective tetrazolium stain for frozen biopsy specimens. Arch Pathol Lab Med 1980;104:462.

Fong JC, Schulz H. Short-chain and long-chain enoyl-CoA hydratases from pig heart muscle. Methods Enzymol 1981;71:390.

Francke U, Darras BT, Zander NF, et al. Assignment of human genes for phosphorylase kinase subunits alpha (PHKA) to Xq12-q13 and beta (PHKB) to 16q12-q13. Am J Hum Genet 1989;45:276.

Frerman FE, Goodman SI. Glutaric aciduria type II and defects of the mitochondrial respiratory chain. In: Scriver CR, Beaudet AL, Sly WS, et al., eds. The metabolic basis of inherited disease. New York: McGraw-Hill, 1989;915.

Fujii H, Kanno H, Hirono A, et al. A single amino acid substitution (157 Gly to Val) in a phosphoglycerate kinase variant (PGK Shizuoka) associated with chronic hemolysis and myoglobinuria. Blood 1992;79:1582.

Fukao T, Song XQ, Yamaguchi S, et al. Identification of three novel frameshift mutations (83delAT, 754insCT, and 435 + 1G to A) of mitochondrial acetoacetyl-coenzyme A thiolase gene in two Swiss patients with CRM-negative beta-ketothiolase deficiency. Hum Mutat 1995;9:277.

Fukao T, Yamaguchi S, Orii T, et al. Molecular basis of beta-ketothiolase deficiency: Mutations and polymorphisms in the human mitochondrial acetoacetyl-coenzyme A thiolase gene. Hum Mutat 1995;5:113

Garavaglia B, Antozzi C, Girotti F, et al. A mitochondrial myopathy with complex II deficiency [Abstract]. Neurology 1990;40 (Suppl 1):294.

Gellera C, Verderio E, Floridia G, et al. Assignment of the human carnitine palmitoyltransferase II gene (CPT II) to chromosome 1p32. Genomics 1994;24:195.

Gibala MJ, MacLean DA, Graham TE, et al. Anaplerotic processes in human skeletal muscle during brief dynamic exercise. J Physiol 1997;502:703

Gibson EM, Breuer J, Nyhan WL. 3-Hydroxy-3-methylglutaryl-coenzyme A lyase deficiency: Review of 18 reported patients. Eur J Pediatr 1988;148:180.

Giles RE, Blanc H, Cann RM, et al. Maternal inheritance of human mitochondrial DNA. Proc Natl Acad Sci U S A 1980;83:9611.

Gillingham M, Van Calcar S, Ney D, et al. Dietary management of long-chain 3-hydroxyacyl-CoA dehydrogenase deficiency (LCHADD): a case report and survey. J Inherit Metab Dis 1999;22:123.

Gillingham MB, Mills MD, Vancalcar SC, et al. DHA supplementation in children with long-chain 3-hydroxyacyl-CoA dehydrogenase deficiency. 7th International Congress of Inborn Errors of Metabolism, Vienna, Austria, May 21-25, 1997.

Glasgow AM, Engel AG, Bier DM, et al. Hypoglycemia, hepatic dysfunction, muscle weakness, cardiomyopathy, free carnitine deficiency and long-chain acylcarnitine excess responsive to medium-chain triglyceride diet. Pediatr Res 1983;17:319.

Gollnick PD. Metabolism of substrates: Energy substrate metabolism during exercise and as modified by training. Fed Proc 1985;44:353.

Gollnick PD, Piehl K, Saltin B. Selective glycogen depletion pattern in human muscle fibers after exercise of varying intensity and at varying pedalling rates. J Physiol 1974;241:45.

Goodman SI, Bemelen KF, Frerman FE. Human cDNA encoding ETF dehydrogenase (ETF; ubiquinone oxidoreductase), and mutations in glutaric acidemia type II. In: Coates PM, Tanaka K, eds. Progress in clinical and biological research, vol 375. New developments in fatty acid oxidation. New York: Wiley-Liss Inc, 1992;567.

Goto Y, Itami N, Kajii N, et al. Renal tubular involvement mimicking Bartter syndrome in a patient with Kearns-Sayre syndrome. J Pediatr 1990a;116:904.

Goto YI, Nonaka I, Horai S. A mutation in the tRNALeu(UUR) gene associated with the MELAS subgroup of mitochondrial encephalomyopathies. Nature 1990b;348:651.

Gregersen N, Andresen BS, Bross P, et al. Characterization of a disease-causing Lys329 to Glu mutation in 16 patients with medium-chain acyl-CoA dehydrogenase deficiency. J Inherit Metab Dis 1991;14:314.

Gregersen N, Andresen BS, Corydon MJ, et al. Mutation analysis in mitochondrial fatty acid oxidation defects: Exemplified by acyl-CoA dehydrogenase deficiencies, with special focus on genotype-phenotype relationship. Hum Mutat 2001;18:169.

Gregersen N, Kølvraa S, Mortensen PB, et al. C6-C10-dicarboxylic aciduria: Biochemical considerations in relation to diagnosis of β-oxidation defects. Scand J Clin Lab Invest 1982a;42 (Suppl 161):15.

Gregersen N, Kølvraa S, Mortensen PB. Acyl-CoA: glycine N-acyltransferase: In vitro studies on the glycine conjugation of straight- and branched-chained acyl-CoA esters in human liver. Biochem Med Metab Biol 1986;35:210.

Gregersen N, Winter VS, Corydon MJ, et al. Characterization of four new mutations in the short-chain acyl-CoA dehydrogenase (SCAD) gene in two patients with SCAD deficiency [Abstract]. J Inherit Metab Dis 1996; (Suppl 1):19.

Gregersen N, Winter VS, Corydon MJ, et al. Identification of four new mutations in the short-chain acyl-CoA dehydrogenase (SCAD) gene in two patients: One of the variant alleles, 511CÆT, is present at an unexpectedly high frequency in the general population, as was the case for 625GÆA, together conferring susceptibility to ethylmalonic aciduria. Hum Mol Genet 1998;7:619.

Gregersen N, Wintzensen H, Kølvraa S, et al. C6-C10-dicarboxylic aciduria: Investigations of a patient with riboflavin responsive multiple acyl-CoA dehydrogenation defects. Pediatr Res 1982b;16:861.

Gross M. Molecular biology of AMP deaminase deficiency. Pharm World Sci 1994;16:55.

Hagenfeldt L, von Döbein U, Holme E, et al. 3-Hydroxydicarboxylic aciduria: A fatty acid oxidation defect with severe prognosis. J Pediatr 1990;116:387.

Hale DE, Batshaw ML, Coates PM, et al. Long-chain acyl coenzyme A dehydrogenase deficiency: An inherited cause of nonketotic hypoglycemia. Pediatr Res 1985;19:666.

Hale DE, Bennett MJ. Fatty acid oxidation disorders: A new class of metabolic diseases. J Pediatr 1992;121:1.

Hale DE, Stanley CA, Coates PM. The long-chain acyl-CoA dehydrogenase deficiency. In: Tanaka K, Coates PM, eds. Progress in clinical and biological research, vol 321. Fatty acid oxidation: Clinical, biochemical and molecular aspects. New York: Alan R. Liss, 1990a;303.

Hale DE, Thorpe C. Short-chain 3-OH acyl-CoA dehydrogenase deficiency. Pediatr Res 1989;25:199A.

Hale DE, Thorpe C, Braat K, et al. The *L*-3-hydroxyacyl-CoA dehydrogenase deficiency. In: Tanaka K, Coates PM, eds. Progress in clinical and biological research, vol 321. Fatty acid oxidation: Clinical, biochemical and molecular aspects. New York: Alan R. Liss, 1990b;503.

Haller RG, Clausen T, Vissing J. Reduced levels of skeletal muscle $Na^{+}K^{+}$-ATPase in McArdle disease. Neurology 1998a;50:37.

Haller RG, Dempsey W, Feit H, et al. Low muscle levels of pyridixone in McArdle's syndrome. Am J Med 1983;74:217.

Haller RG, Henriksson KG, Jorfeldt L, et al. Deficiency of skeletal muscle succinate dehydrogenase and aconitase. Pathophysiology of exercise in a novel human muscle oxidative defect. J Clin Invest 1991;88:1197.

Haller RG, Lewis SF. Glucose-induced exertional fatigue in muscle phosphofructokinase deficiency. N Engl J Med 1991;324:364.

Haller RG, Lewis SF, Cook JD, et al. Myophosphorylase deficiency impairs muscle oxidative metabolism. Ann Neurol 1985;17:196.

Haller RG, Lewis SF, Eastabrook RW, et al. Exercise intolerance, lactic acidosis, and abnormal cardiopulmonary regulation in exercise associated with adult skeletal muscle cytochrome c oxidase deficiency. J Clin Invest 1989;84:155.

Haller RG, Vissing J. Spontaneous second wind and glucose-induced second, second wind in McArdle disease: Oxidative mechanisms. Arch Neurol 2002;59:1395.

Haller RG, Vissing J. No spontaneous second wind in muscle phosphofructokinase deficiency. Neurology 2004;62:82.

Haller RG, Wyrick P, Cavender D, et al. Aerobic conditioning: An effective therapy in McArdle's disease. Neurology 1998b;50:A369.

Hammans SR, Sweeney MG, Brockington M, et al. Mitochondrial encephalomyopathies: Molecular genetic diagnosis from blood samples. Lancet 1991;337:1311.

Hansen JJ, Durr A, Couruu-Reibex C, et al. Hereditary spastic paraplegia SPG13 is associated with a mutation in the gene encoding the mitochondrial chaperonin HP60. Am J Hum Genet 2002;70:1328.

Harding CO, Gillingham MB, Van Calcar SC, et al. Docosahexaenoic acid and retinal function in children with long-chain 3-hydroxyacyl-CoA dehydrogenase deficiency. J Inherit Metab Dis 1999;22:276.

Harmann B, Zander NF, Kilimann MW. Isoform diversity of phosphorylase kinase α and β subunits generated by alternative RNA splicing. J Biol Chem 1991;266:15631.

Hart Z, Chang CH. A newborn infant with respiratory distress and stridulous breathing. J Pediatr 1988;113:150.

Hashimoto T. Peroxisomal and mitochondrial enzymes. In: Coates PM, Tanaka K, eds. Progress in clinical and biological research, vol 375. New developments in fatty acid oxidation. New York: Wiley-Liss, 1992;19.

Hatefi Y. The mitochondrial electron transport and oxidative phosphorylation system. Annu Rev Biochem 1985;54:1015.

Haydar NA, Conn HL, Afifi A, et al. Severe hypermetabolism with primary abnormality of skeletal muscle mitochondria. Ann Intern Med 1971;74:548.

Hayde M, Widhalm K. Effects of cornstarch treatment in very young children with type I glycogen storage diseases. Eur Pediatr 1990;149:630.

Hays AP, Hallett M, Delfs J, et al. Muscle phosphofructokinase deficiency: Abnormal polysaccharide in a case of late-onset myopathy. Neurology 1981;31:1077.

Heilmeyer LMG. Molecular basis of signal integration in phosphorylase kinase. Biochim Biophys Acta 1991;1094:168.

Helander HM, Koivuranta KT, Horelli-Kuitunen N, et al. Molecular cloning and characterization of the human mitochondrial 2,4-dienoyl-CoA reductase gene (DECR). Genomics 1997;46:112.

Hirano M, DiMauro S. ANT1, Twinkle, POLG, and TP: New genes open our eyes to ophthalmoplegia. Neurology 2001;57:2163.

Hirano M, Marti R, Ferreira-Barros C, et al. Defects of intergenomic communication: Autosomal disorders that cause multiple deletions and depletion of mitochondrial DNA. Cell Dev Biol 2001;12:417.

Hirschhorn R. Glycogen storage disease type II: Acid alpha-glucosidase (acid maltase) deficiency. In: Scriver CR, Beaudet AL, Sly WS, et al., eds. The metabolic and molecular bases of inherited diseases. New York: McGraw-Hill, 1995;2443.

Ho L, Javed AA, Pepin RA, et al. Identification of a cDNA clone for the beta-subunit of the pyruvate dehydrogenase component of human pyruvate dehydrogenase complex. Biochem Biophys Res Commun 1988;150:904.

Hoffman EP, Kunkel LM, Angelini C, et al. Improved diagnosis of Becker muscular dystrophy by dystrophin testing. Neurology 1989;39:1011.

Hogrel JY, Laforet P, Yaou RB, et al., A non-ischemic forearm exercise test for the screening of patients with exercise intolerance. Neurology 2001;56:1733

Holt IJ, Harding AE, Cooper JM, et al. Mitochondrial myopathies: Clinical and biochemical features of 30 patients with major deletions of muscle mitochondrial DNA. Ann Neurol 1989;26:699.

Holt IJ, Harding AE, Petty RKH, et al. A new mitochondrial disease associated with mitochondrial DNA heteroplasmy. Am J Hum Genet 1990;46:428.

Huang I-Y, Rubinfien E, Yoshida A. Complete amino acid sequence of human phosphoglycerate kinase: Isolation and amino acid sequence of tryptic peptides. J Biol Chem 1980a;255:6408.

Huang IY, Welch CD, Yoshida A. Complete amino acid sequence of human phosphoglycerate kinase: Cyanogen bromide peptides and complete amino acid sequence. J Biol Chem 1980b;255:6412.

Huie ML, Tsujino S, Sklower Brooks S, et al. Glycogen storage disease type II: Identification of four novel missense mutations (D645N, G648S, R672W, R672Q) and two insertions/deletions in the acid alpha-glucosidase locus of patients of differing phenotype. Biochem Biophys Res Comm 1998;244:921.

Hug G, Bove KE, Soukup S. Lethal neonatal multiorgan deficiency of carnitine palmitoyltransferase II. N Engl J Med 1991;325:1862.

Hug G, Schubert WK. Glycogenosis associated with degenerative disease of the brain: Biochemical and electron microscopic findings. Clin Res 1966;14:441

Huoponen K, Vilkki J, Aula P, et al. A new mtDNA mutation associated with Leber hereditary optic neuroretinopathy. Am J Hum Genet 1991;48:1147.

Hyser CL, Clarke PRH, DiMauro S, et al. Myoadenylate deaminase deficiency and exertional myoglobinuria [Abstract]. Neurology 1989;39:335.

Iannaccone ST, Griggs RC, Markesbery WR, et al. Familial progressive external ophthalmoplegia and ragged-red fibers. Neurology 1974;24:1033.

Ibdah JA, Bennett MJ, Rinaldo P, et al. A fetal fatty acid oxidation disorder as a cause of liver disease in pregnant women. N Engl J Med 1999;340:1723.

Ibdah JA, Tein I, Dionisi-Vici C, et al. Mild trifunctional protein deficiency is associated with progressive neuropathy and myopathy and suggests a novel genotype-phenotype correlation. J Clin Invest 1998a;102:1193.

Ibdah JA, Zhao M, Hill I, et al. The association between maternal liver disease and the common mutation in mitochondrial trifunctional protein is significant. Hepatology 1998b;28:316.

Ikeda Y, Dabrowski C, Tanaka K. Separation and properties of five distinct acyl-CoA dehydrogenases from rat liver mitochondria. Identification of a new 2-methyl-branched-chain acyl-CoA dehydrogenase. J Biol Chem 1983;258:1066.

Indiveri C, Tonazzi A, Palmieri F. Identification and purification of the carnitine carrier from rat liver mitochondria. Biochim Biophys Acta 1990;1020:81.

Indiveri C, Tonazzi A, Prezioso G, et al. Kinetic characterization of the reconstituted carnitine carrier from rat liver mitochondria. Biochim Biophys Acta 1991;1065:231.

Indo Y, Glassberg R, Yokota I, et al. Molecular characterization of variant α-subunit of electron transfer flavoprotein in three patients with glutaric acidemia type II and identification of glycine substitution for valine-157 in the sequence of the precursor, producing an unstable mature protein in a patient. Am J Hum Genet 1991a;49:575.

Indo Y, Tang-Feng T, Glassberg R, et al. Molecular cloning and nucleotide sequence of cDNAs encoding human long chain acyl-CoA dehydrogenase and assignment of the location of its gene (ACADL) to chromosome 2. Genomics 1991b;11:609.

Innes AM, Seargeant LE, Balachandra K, et al. Hepatic carnitine palmitoyltransferase I deficiency presenting as maternal illness in pregnancy. Pediatr Res 2000;47:43.

Inoue D, Pappano AJ. L-palmitoylcarnitine and calcium ions act similarly on excitatory ionic currents in avian ventricular muscle. Circ Res 1983;52:625.

Isaacs JD Jr, Sims HF, Powell CK, et al. Maternal acute fatty liver of pregnancy associated with fetal trifunctional protein deficiency: Molecular characterization of a novel mutant allele. Pediatr Res 1996;40:393.

Ito Y, Saito K, Shishikura K, et al. A 1-year-old infant with McArdle disease associated with hyper–creatine kinase–emia during febrile episodes. Brain Dev 2003;25:438.

Izai K, Uchida Y, Orii T, et al. Novel fatty acid β-oxidation enzymes in rat liver mitochondria. I. Purification and properties of very long-chain acyl-coenzyme A dehydrogenase. J Biol Chem 1992;267:1027.

Jackson S, Kler RS, Bartlett K, et al. Combined enzyme defect of mitochondrial fatty acid oxidation. J Clin Invest 1992;90:1219.

Jaksch M, Paret C, Stucka R, et al. Cytochrome c oxidase deficiency due to mutations in SCO2, a copper-binding protein, is rescued by copper in human myoblasts. Hum Mol Genet 2001;10:3025.

James JH, Fang CH, Schrantz SJ, et al. Linkage of anaerobic glycolysis to sodium-potassium transport in rat skeletal muscle. J Clin Invest 1996;98:2388.

Jerusalem F, Angelini C, Engel AG, et al. Mitochondria-lipid-glycogen (MLG) disease of muscle. Arch Neurol 1973;29:162.

Johnson RE, Possmore R, Sargent F. Multiple factors in experimental human ketosis. Arch Intern Med 1961;107:43.

Jones TA, da Cruz e Silva EF, Spurr NK, et al. Localization of the gene encoding the catalytic gamma subunit of phosphorylase kinase to human chromosome bands 7p12-q21. Biochim Biophys Acta 1990;1048:24.

Junien C, Despoisse S, Turleau C, et al. Assignment of phosphoglycerate mutase (PGAMA) to human chromosome 10: Regional mapping of GOT1 and PGAMA subbands 10q26.1 (or q25.3). Ann Genet 1982;25:25.

Kadenbach B, Ungibauer BM, Jarausch J, et al. The complexity of respiratory complexes. Trends Biochem Sci 1983;8:398.

Kahn A, Etiemble J, Meienhofer MC, et al. Erythrocyte phosphofructokinase deficiency associated with an unstable variant of muscle phosphofructokinase. Clin Chim Acta 1975;61:415.

Kamijo T, Aoyama T, Miyazaki J, et al. Molecular cloning of the cDNAs for the subunits of rat mitochondrial fatty acid β-oxidation multienzyme complex. J Biol Chem 1993;268:26452.

Kamijo T, Indo Y, Souri M, et al. Medium-chain 3-ketoacyl-coenzyme A thiolase deficiency: A new disorder of mitochondrial fatty acid β-oxidation. Pediatr Res 1997;42:569.

Kamijo T, Wanders RJA, Saudubray JM, et al. Mitochondrial trifunctional protein deficiency. Catalytic heterogeneity of the mutant enzyme in two patients. J Clin Invest 1994;93:1740.

Kanno T, Maekawa M. Lactate dehydrogenase M-subunit deficiency: Clinical features, metabolic background, and genetic heterogeneities. Muscle Nerve 1995;3:S54.

Kanno T, Sudo K, Takeuchi I, et al. Hereditary deficiency of lactate dehydrogenase M-subunit. Clin Chim Acta 1980;108:267.

Kassovskabratinova S, Fukao T, Song XQ, et al. Succinyl CoA-3-oxoacid CoA transferase (SCOT): Human cDNA cloning, human chromosomal mapping to 5p13, and mutation detection in a SCOT-deficient patient. Am J Hum Genet 1996;59:519.

Kaukonen J, Juselius JK, Tiranti V, et al. Role of adenine nucleotide translocator 1 in mtDNA maintenance. Science 2000;289:782.

Kazemi-Esfarjani P, Skomorowoska E, Dysgaard TD, et al. A nonischemic forearm exercise test for McArdle disease. Ann Neurol 2002;52:153.

Keightley JA, Hoffbuhr KC, Burton MD, et al. A microdeletion in cytochrome c oxidase (COX) subunit III associated with COX deficiency and recurrent myoglobinuria. Nat Genet 1996;12:410.

Kelley RI. Beta-oxidation of long-chain fatty acids by human fibroblasts: Evidence for a novel long-chain acyl-coenzyme A dehydrogenase. Biochem Biophys Res Commun 1992;182:1002.

Kelly DP, Kim JJ, Billadello JJ, et al. Nucleotide sequence of MCAD mRNA. Proc Natl Acad Sci U S A 1987;84:4068.

Kennaway NG. Defects in the cytochrome bc1 complex in mitochondrial diseases. J Bioenerg Biomembr 1988;20:325.

Kerner J, Bieber LL. A radioisotopic exchange method for quantitation of short-chain (acid soluble) acylcarnitines. Anal Biochem 1983;134:459.

King MP, Attardi G. Human cells lacking mtDNA: Repopulation with exogenous mitochondria by complementation. Science 1989;246:500.

Kissel JT, Beam W, Bresolin N, et al. Physiologic assessment of phosphoglycerate mutase deficiency: Incremental exercise tests. Neurology 1985;35:828.

Knochel JP. Renal injury in muscle disease. In: Suki WN, Eknoyan G, eds. The kidney in systemic disease. New York: John Wiley & Sons, 1976;129.

Kobayashi A, Jiang LL, Hashimoto T. Two mitochondrial 3-hydroxyacyl-CoA dehydrogenases in bovine liver. J Biochem 1996;119:775.

Kobayashi M, Morishita H, Sugiyama N, et al. Two cases of NADH-coenzyme Q reductase deficiency: Relationship to MELAS syndrome. J Pediatr 1987;110:223.

Kobayashi Y, Momo MY, Tominaga K, et al. A point mutation in the mitochondrial $tRNA^{Leu(UUR)}$ gene in MELAS. Biochem Biophys Res Commun 1990;173:816.

Koga Y, Fabrizi GM, Mita S, et al. Sequence of a cDNA specifying subunit VIIc of human cytochrome c oxidase. Nucleic Acid Res 1990;18:684.

Koga Y, Nonaka I, Kobayashi M, et al. Findings in muscle in complex I (NADH coenzyme Q reductase) deficiency. Ann Neurol 1988;24:749.

Kølvraa S, Gregersen N. Acyl-CoA:glycine *N*-acyltransferase: Organelle localization and affinity toward straight-and branched-chained acyl-CoA esters in rat liver. Biochem Med Metab Biol 1986;36:98.

Krahling JB, Gee R, Murphy PA, et al. Comparison of fatty acid oxidation in mitochondria and peroxisomes from rat liver. Biochem Biophys Res Commun 1978;82:136.

Kreuder J, Borkhardt A, Repp R, et al. Brief report: Inherited metabolic myopathy and hemolysis due to a mutation in aldolase A. New Eng J Med 1996;334:1100.

Kukita A, Yoshida MC, Fukushige S, et al. Molecular gene mapping of human aldolase A (ALDOA) gene to chromosome 16. Hum Genet 1987;76:20.

Kushmerick MJ. Skeletal muscle: A paradigm for testing principles of bioenergetics. J Bioenerg Biomembr 1995;27:555.

Lamhonwah AM, Olpin SE, Pollitt RJ, et al. Novel OCTN2 mutations: No genotype-phenotype correlations: Early carnitine therapy prevents cardiomyopathy. Am J Med Genet 2002;111:271.

Lamhonwah AM, Tein I. Carnitine uptake defect: Frameshift mutations in the human plasmalemmal carnitine transporter gene. Biochem Biophys Res Commun 1998;252:396.

Lamperti C, Naini A, Hirano M, et al. Cerebellar ataxia and coenzyme Q10 deficiency. Neurology 2003;60:1206.

Layzer RB, Rowland LP, Ranney HM. Muscle phosphofructokinase deficiency. Arch Neurol 1967;17:512.

Lebo RV, Gorin F, Fletterick RJ, et al. High-resolution chromosome sorting and DNA spot-blot analysis assign McArdle's syndrome in chromosome 11. Science 1984;225:57.

Lee HC, Smith N, Mohabir R, et al. Cytosolic calcium transients from the beating mammalian heart. Proc Natl Acad Sci U S A 1987;84:7793.

Lewis SF, Haller RG. The pathophysiology of McArdle's disease: Clues to regulation in exercise and fatigue. J Appl Physiol 1986;61:391.

Lewis SF, Haller RG. Fatigue in skeletal muscle disorders. In: Atlan G, Belivau L, Bouissou P, eds. Muscle fatigue: Biochemical and physiological aspects. Paris: Masson, 1991a;119.

Lewis SF, Haller RG. Physiologic measurement of exercise and fatigue with special reference to chronic fatigue syndrome. Rev Infect Dis 1991b;13 (Suppl 1):S98.

Lewis SF, Vora S, Haller RG. Abnormal oxidative metabolism and O_2 transport in muscle phosphofructokinase deficiency. J Appl Physiol 1991;70:391.

Lindner N, Reichert M, Eichorn M, et al. Acute compartment syndrome after forearm ischemic work test in a patient with McArdle's disease. Neurology 2001;56:1779.

Lithell H, Orlander J, Schele R, et al. Changes in lipoprotein-lipase activity and lipid stores in human skeletal muscle with prolonged heavy exercise. Acta Physiol Scand 1979;107:257.

Lombes A, Mendell JR, Nakase H, et al. Myoclonic epilepsy and ragged-red fibers with cytochrome c oxidase deficiency: Neuropathology, biochemistry, and molecular genetics. Ann Neurol 1989;26:20.

Lossos A, Barash V, Soffer D, et al. Hereditary branching enzyme dysfunction in adult polyglucosan body disease: A possible metabolic cause in two patients. Ann Neurol 1991;30:655.

Lossos A, Meiner Z, Barash V, et al. Adult polyglucosan body disease in Ashkenazi Jewish patients carrying the Tyr329Ser mutation in the glycogen-branching enzyme gene. Ann Neurol 1998;44:867.

Luft R, Ikkos D, Palmieri G, et al. A case of severe hypermetabolism of nonthyroid origin with a defect in the maintenance of mitochondrial respiratory control: A correlated clinical, biochemical, and morphological study. J Clin Invest 1962;41:1176.

Luo MJ, He XY, Sprecher H, et al. Purification and characterization of the trifunctional β-oxidation complex from pig heart mitochondria. Arch Biochem Biophys 1993;304:266.

MacLean D, Vissing J, Vissing SF, et al. Oral branched-chain amino acids do not improve exercise capacity in McArdle disease. Neurology 1998;51:1456.

Maekawa M, Kanda S, Sudo K, et al. Estimation of the gene frequency of lactate dehydrogenase subunit deficiencies. Am J Hum Genet 1984;36:1204.

Maekawa M, Sudo K, Kanno T, et al. Molecular characterization of genetic mutation in human lactate dehydrogenase-A (M) deficiency. Biochem Biophys Res Comm 1990;168:677.

Maekawa M, Sudo K, Kanno T, et al. A novel deletion mutation of lactate dehydrogenase A (M) gene in the fifth family with the enzyme deficiency. Hum Mol Genet 1994;3:825.

Maekawa M, Sudo K, Li SS, et al. Analysis of genetic mutations in human lactate dehydrogenase (LDH-A) deficiency using DNA conformation polymorphism in combination with polyacrylamide gel and silver staining. Biochem Biophys Res Comm 1991;180:1083.

Majamaa K, Moilanen JS, Uimonen S, et al. Epidemiology of A3243G, the mutation for mitochondrial encephalomyopathy, lactic acidosis, and strokelike episodes: Prevalence of the mutation in an adult population. Am J Hum Genet 1998;63:447.

Mak IT, Kramer JH, Weglicki WB. Potentiation of free radical-induced lipid peroxidative injury to sarcolemmal membranes by lipid amphiphiles. J Biol Chem 1986;26:1153.

Mancuso M, Filosto M, Hirano M, et al. Spinal muscular atrophy and mitochondrial DNA depletion. Acta Neuropathol 2003;105:621.

Mancuso M, Filosto M, Mootha VK, et al. A novel mitochondrial $tRNA^{Phe}$ mutation causes MERRF syndrome. Neurology 2004a;62:2119.

Mancuso M, Filostos M, Oh SJ, et al. A novel polymerase gamma mutation in a family with ophthalmoplegia, neuropathy, and Parkinsonism. Arch Neurol 2004b;61:1777.

Mancuso M, Salviati L, Sacconi S, et al. Mitochondrial DNA depletion: Mutations in thymidine kinase gene with myopathy and SMA. Neurology 2002;59:1197.

Mandel H, Szargel R, Labay V, et al. The deoxyguanosine kinase gene is mutated in individuals with depleted hepatocerebral mitochondrial DNA. Nat Genet 2001;29:337.

Martin MA, Rubio JC, Buchbinder J, et al. Molecular heterogeneity of myophosphorylase deficiency (McArdle's disease): A genotype-phenotype correlation study. Ann Neurol 2001;50:574.

Martiniuk F, Mehler M, Tzall S, et al. Extensive genetic heterogeneity in patients with alpha glucosidase deficiency as detected by abnormalities of DNA and mRNA. Am J Hum Genet 1990a;47:73.

Martiniuk F, Mehler M, Tzall S, et al. Sequence of the cDNA and 5′-flanking region for human acid alpha-glucosidase, detection of an intron in the 5′ untranslated leader sequence, definition of 18-bp polymorphisms, and differences with previous cDNA and amino acid sequence. DNA Cell Biol 1990b;9:85.

Martinuzzi A, Tsujino S, Vergani L, et al. Molecular characterization of myophosphorylase deficiency in a group of patients from Northern Italy. J Neurol Sci 1996;137:14.

Mascaro C, Buesa C, Ortiz JA, et al. Molecular cloning and tissue expression of human mitochondrial 3-hydroxy-3-methylglutaryl-CoA synthase. Arch Biochem Biophys 1995;317:385.

Matern D, Hart P, Murtha A, et al. Acute fatty liver of pregnancy assoicated with short-chain acyl-coenzyme A dehydrogenase deficiency. J Pediatr 2001;138:585.

McArdle B. Myopathy due to a defect in muscle glycogen breakdown. Clin Sci 1951;10:13.

McConchie SM, Coakley J, Edwards RHT, et al. Molecular heterogeneity in McArdle's disease. Biochim Biophys Acta 1991;1096:26.

Medori R, Brooke MH, Waterston R. Two dissimilar brothers with Becker's dystrophy have an identical genetic defect. Neurology 1989;39:1493.

Meera Khan P, Westerveld A, Grzeschik KH, et al. X-linkage of human phosphoglycerate kinase confirmed in man-mouse and man-Chinese hamster somatic cell hybrids. Am J Hum Genet 1971;23:614.

Mehler M, DiMauro S. Residual acid maltase activity in late-onset acid maltase deficiency. Neurology 1977;27:178.

Meinck H, Goebel H, Rumpf K, et al. The forearm ischaemic work test—hazardous to McArdle patients. J Neurol 1982;45:1144.

Michelson AM, Markham AF, Orkin SH. Isolation and DNA sequence of a full-length cDNA clone for human X chromosome encoded phosphoglycerate kinase. Proc Natl Acad Sci U SA 1983;80:472.

Middleton B. 3-Ketoacyl-CoA thiolases of mammalian tissues. In: Lowenstein JM, ed. Methods in enzymology. Part B, vol 35, Lipids. New York: Academic Press, 1975;128.

Miller CG, Alleyne GA, Brooks SEH. Gross cardiac involvement in glycogen storage disease type III. Br Heart J 1972;34:862.

Millington DS. New methods for the analysis of acylcarnitines and acyl-coenzyme A compounds. In: Gaskell SJ, ed. Mass spectrometry in biomedical research. New York: John Wiley & Sons, 1986;Chapter 7.

Millington DS, Terada N, Chace DH, et al. The role of tandem mass spectrometry in the diagnosis of fatty acid oxidation disorders. In: Coates PM, Tanaka K, eds. Progress in clinical and biological research, vol 375. New developments in fatty acid oxidation. New York: Wiley-Liss, 1992;339.

Milstein JM, Herron TM, Haas JE. Fatal infantile muscle phosphorylase deficiency. J Child Neurol 1989;4:186.

Mineo I, Kono N, Hara N, et al. Myogenic hyperuricemia. A common pathophysiologic feature of glycogenosis types III, V, and VII. N Engl J Med 1987;317:75.

Miranda AF, DiMauro S, Antler A, et al. Glycogen debrancher deficiency is reproduced in muscle culture. Ann Neurol 1981;9:283.

Miranda AF, Ishii S, DiMauro S, et al. Cytochrome c oxidase deficiency in Leigh's deficiency: Genetic evidence for a nuclear DNA-encoded mutation. Neurology 1989;39:697.

Mita S, Rizzuto R, Moraes CT, et al. Recombination via flanking direct repeats is a major cause of large-scale deletions of human mitochondrial DNA. Nucleic Acid Res 1990;18:561.

Mitchell GA, Fukao T. Inborn errors of ketone body metabolism. In: Scriver C, Beaudet AL, Sly W, et al., eds. The metabolic and molecular basis of inherited disease, 8th ed. New York: McGraw-Hill, 2001;2327.

Mitchell GA, Robert MF, Hruz PW, et al. 3-Hydroxy-3-methylglutaryl coenzyme A lyase (HL). Cloning of human and chicken liver HL cDNAs and characterization of a mutation causing human HL deficiency. J Biol Chem 1993;25:4376.

Mizuta K, Hashimoto E, Tsutou A, et al. A new type of glycogen storage disease caused by deficiency of cardiac phosphorylase kinase. Biochem Biophys Res Commun 1984;119:582.

Moraes CT, Ciacci F, Silvestri G, et al. Atypical clinical presentations associated with the MELAS mutation at position 3243 of human mitochondrial DNA. Neuromuscul Disord 1993;3:43.

Moraes CT, DiMauro S, Zeviani M, et al. Mitochondrial DNA deletions in progressive external ophthalmoplegia and Kearns-Sayre syndrome. N Engl J Med 1989;320:1293.

Moraes CT, Shanske S, Tritschler HJ, et al. MtDNA depletion with variable tissue expression: A novel genetic abnormality in mitochondrial diseases. Am J Hum Genet 1991a;48:492.

Moraes CT, Zeviani M, Schon EA, et al. Mitochondrial DNA deletion in a girl with manifestations of Kearns-Sayre and Lowe syndromes: An example of phenotypic mimicry? Am J Hum Genet 1991b;41:301.

Moreadith RW, Batshaw ML, Ohnishi T, et al. Deficiency of the iron-sulfur clusters of mitochondrial reduced nicotinamide-adenine dinucleotide–ubiquinone oxidoreductase (complex I) in an infant with congenital lactic acidosis. J Clin Invest 1984;74:685.

Morgan-Hughes JA, Hayes D, Clark J, et al. Mitochondrial encephalomyopathies. Biochemical studies in two cases revealing defects in the respiratory chain. Brain 1982;105:553.

Morgan-Hughes JA, Hayes DJ, Cooper M, et al. Mitochondrial myopathies: Deficiencies localized to complex I and complex III of the mitochondrial respiratory chain. Biochem Soc Trans 1985;13:648.

Morgan-Hughes JA, Schapira AHV, Cooper JM, et al. Molecular defects of NADH–ubiquinone oxidoreductase (complex I) in mitochondrial diseases. J Bioenerg Biomembr 1988;20:365.

Morimoto A, Ueda I, Hirashima Y, et al. A novel missense mutation (1060G>C) in the phosphoglycerate kinase gene in a Japanese boy with chronic hemolytic anemia, developmental delay and rhabdomyolysis. Br J Hemat 2003;122:1009.

Mortensen PB. Inhibition of fatty acid oxidation by valproate. Lancet 1981;2:856.

Mortensen PB, Gregersen N. The biological origin of ketotic dicarboxylic aciduria. II. In vivo and in vitro investigations of the β-oxidation of C8-C16-dicarboxylic acids in unstarved, starved and diabetic rats. Biochim Biophys Acta 1982;710:477.

Morton CC, Eddy RL, Shows TB, et al. Human AMP deaminase-1 gene (AMPD1) is mapped to chromosome 1. Cytogenet Cell Genet 1989;51:1048.

Moses SW, Gadoth N, Bashan N, et al. Neuromuscular involvement in glycogen storage disease type III. Acta Paediatr Scand 1986;75:289.

Moses SW, Wanderman KL, Myroz A, et al. Cardiac involvement in glycogen storage disease type III. Eur J Pediatr 1989;148:764.

Murase T, Ikeda H, Muro T, et al. Myopathy associated with type III glycogenosis. J Neurol Sci 1973;20:287.

Murthy MSR, Pande SV. Malonyl-CoA binding site and the overt carnitine palmitoyltransferase activity reside on the opposite sides of the outer mitochondrial membrane. Proc Natl Acad Sci USA 1987;84:378.

Nada MA, Chace DH, Sprecher H, et al. Investigation of β-oxidation intermediates in normal and MCAD deficient human fibroblasts using tandem mass spectrometry. Biochem Mol Med 1995a;54:59.

Nada MA, Rhead JW, Sprecher H, et al. Evidence for intermediate channelling in mitochondrial beta-oxidation. J Biol Chem 1995b;270:530.

Nada MA, Vianey-Saban C, Roe CR, et al. Prenatal diagnosis of mitochondrial fatty acid oxidation defects. Prenat Diagn 1996;16:117.

Naito E, Indo Y, Tanaka K. Identification of two variant short chain acyl-coenzyme A dehydrogenase alleles, each containing a different point mutation in a patient with short chain acyl-coenzyme A dehydrogenase deficiency. J Clin Invest 1990;85:1575.

Naito E, Ozasa H, Ikeda Y, et al. Molecular cloning and nucleotide sequence of complementary DNAs encoding human short chain acyl-coenzyme A dehydrogenase and the study of the molecular basis of human short chain acyl-coenzyme A dehydrogenase deficiency. J Clin Invest 1989;83:1605.

Nakajima H, Kono N, Yamasaki T, et al. Tissue specificity in expression and alternative RNA splicing of human phosphofructokinase-M and -L genes. Biochem Biophys Res Commun 1990;173:1317.

Nakajima H, Noguchi T, Yamasaki T, et al. Cloning of human muscle phosphofructokinase cDNA. FEBS Lett 1987;223:113.

Nass S, Nass MMK. Intramitochondrial fibers with DNA characteristics. J Cell Biol 1963;19:593.

Nelson J, Lewis B, Walters B. The HELLP syndrome associated with fetal medium-chain acyl-CoA dehydrogenase deficiency. J Inherit Metab Dis 2000;23:18.

Newgard CB, Littman DR, van Genderen C, et al. Human brain glycogen phosphorylase: Cloning, sequence analysis, chromosomal mapping, tissue expression and comparison with the human liver and muscle isozymes. J Biol Chem 1988;263:3850.

Newgard CB, Nakano K, Hwang PK, et al. Sequence analysis of the cDNA encoding human liver glycogen phosphorylase reveals tissue-specific codon usage. Proc Natl Acad Sci U S A 1986;83:8132.

Newman NJ, Wallace DC. Mitochondria and Leber's hereditary optic neuropathy. Am J Ophthalmol 1990;109:726.

Nishino L, Spinazzola A, Hirano M. Thymidine phosphorylase gene mutations in MNGIE, a human mitochondrial disorder. Science 1999;283:689.

Nishino L, Spinazzola A, Papadimitrious A, et al. Mitochondrial neurogastrointestinal encephalomyoapthy: An autosomal recessive disorder due to thymidine phosphorylase mutations. Ann Neurol 2000;47:792.

O'Brien LK, Rinaldo P, Sims HF, et al. Fulminant hepatic failure associated with mutations in the medium and short chain *L*-3-hydroxyacyl-CoA dehydrogeanse gene. J Inher Metab Dis 2000;23 (Suppl):127.

Ogasahara S, Engel AG, Frens D, et al. Muscle coenzyme Q deficiency in familial mitochondrial encephalomyopathy. Proc Natl Acad Sci USA 1989;86:2379.

Ogilvie I, Pourfarzam M, Jackson S, et al. Very long-chain acyl coenzyme A dehydrogenase deficiency presenting with exercise-induced myoglobinuria. Neurology 1994;44:467.

Ohama E, Ikuta F. Involvement of choroid plexus in mitochondrial encephalomyopathy (MELAS). Acta Neuropathol 1987;76:1.

Ohama E, Ohara S, Ikuta F, et al. Mitochondrial angiopathy in cerebral blood vessels of mitochondrial encephalomyopathy. Acta Neuropathol 1987;74:226.

Ohno KM, Tanaka K, Sahashi T, et al. Mitochondrial DNA deletions in inherited recurrent myoglobinuria. Ann Neurol 1991;29:364.

Okamoto K, Brinker A, Paschen SA, et al. The protein import motor of mitochondria: A targeted molecular ratchet driving unfolding and translocation. EMBO J 2002;21:3659.

Okubo M, Aoyama Y, Murase T. A novel donor splice site mutation in the glycogen debranching enzyme gene is associated with glycogen storage disease type III. Biochem Biophys Res Comm 1996;224:493.

Okubo M, Horinishi A, Takeuchi M, et al. Heterogeneous mutations in the glycogen-debranching enzyme gene are responsible for glycogen storage disease type IIIa in Japan. Hum Genet 2000;106:108.

Okubo M, Kanda F, Horinishi A, et al. Glycogen storage disease type IIIa: First report of a causative missense mutation (G1448R) of the glycogen debranching enzyme gene found in a homozygous patient. Hum Mutat 1999;14:542.

Okun JG, Kolker S, Schulze A, et al. A method for quantitative acylcarnitine profiling in human skin fibroblasts using unlabelled palmitic acid: Diagnosis of fatty acid oxidation disorders and differentiation between biochemical phenotypes of MCAD deficiency. Biochim Biophys Acta 2002;1584:91.

Olson LJ, Reeder GS, Edwards WD, et al. Cardiac involvement in glycogen storage disease III: Morphologic and biochemical characterization with endomyocardial biopsy. Am J Cardiol 1984;53:980.

Omenn GS, Cheung CY. Phosphoglycerate mutase isozyme marker for tissue differentiation in man. Am J Hum Genet 1974;26:393.

Omenn GS, Hermodson MA. Human phosphoglycerate mutase: Isozyme marker for muscle differentiation and neoplasia. In: Markert CM, ed. Isozymes: III. Developmental biology. New York: Academic Press, 1975;1005.

Ozand P, Tokatli M, Amiri S. Biochemical investigation of an unusual case of glycogenosis. J Pediatr 1967;71:225.

Ozawa T. Mitochondrial DNA mutations associated with aging and degenerative diseases. Exp Gerontol 1995;30:269.

Pagliara AS, Karl IE, Haymond M, et al. Hypoglycemia in infancy and childhood, part I. J Pediatr 1973;82:365.

Palmieri F, Bisaccia F, Capobianco L, et al. Mitochondrial metabolite transporters. Biochim Biophys Acta 1996;1275:127.

Pande SV. A mitochondrial carnitine acylcarnitine translocase system. Proc Natl Acad Sci U S A 1975;72:883.

Pande SV, Brivet M, Slama A, et al. Carnitine-acylcarnitine translocase deficiency with severe hypoglycemia and auriculoventricular block. J Clin Invest 1993;91:1247.

Papadimitriou A, Manta P, Divari R, et al. McArdle's disease: Two clinical expressions in the same pedigree. J Neurol 1990;237:267.

Papadimitriou A, Neustein HB, DiMauro S, et al. Histiocytoid cardiomyopathy of infancy: Deficiency of reducible cytochrome b in heart mitochondria. Pediatr Res 1984;18:1023.

Papadopoulou LC, Sue CM, Davidson MM, et al. Fatal infantile cardioencephalomyopathy with COX deficiency and mutations in SCO2, a COX assembly gene. Nat Genet 1999;23:333.

Pari G, Crerar MM, Nalbantoglu J, et al. Myophosphorylase gene transfer in McArdle's disease myoblasts in vitro. Neurology 1999;53:1352.

Parker WD, Oley CA, Parks JK. A defect in mitochondrial electron-transport activity (NADH-coenzyme Q oxidoreductase) in Leber's hereditary optic neuropathy. N Engl J Med 1989;320:1331.

Parvari R, Moses S, Shen J, et al., A single-base deletion in the 3-prime coding region of glycogen-debranching enzyme is prevalent in glycogen storage disease type IIIA in a population of North African Jewish patients. Europ J Hum Genet 1997;5:266.

Parvari R, Shen J, Hershkovitz E, et al. Two new mutations in the 3′ coding region of the glycogen debranching enzyme in a glycogen storage disease type IIIa Ashkenazi Jewish patient. J Inher Metab Dis 1998;21:141.

Pauly DF, Johns DC, Matelis LA, et al. Complete correction of acid alpha-glucosidase deficiency in Pompe disease fibroblasts in vitro, and lysosomally targeted expression in neonatal rat cardiac and skeletal muscle. Gene Ther 1998;5:473.

Pavlakis SG, Phillips PC, DiMauro S, et al. Mitochondrial myopathy, encephalopathy, lactic acidosis, and stroke-like episodes: A distinctive clinical syndrome. Ann Neurol 1984;16:481.

Phoenix J, Hopkins P, Bartram C, et al. Effect of vitamin B_6 supplementation in McArdle's disease: A strategic case study. Neuromuscul Disord 1998;8:210.

Pildes RS, Patel DA, Nitzan M. Glucose disappearance rate in symptomatic neonatal hypoglycemia. Pediatrics 1973;52:75.

Pitkanen S, Robinson BH. Mitochondrial complex I deficiency leads to increased production of superoxide radicals and induction of superoxide dismutase. J Clin Invest 1996;98:345.

Poll-The BT, Duran M, Mousson B, et al. Carnitine palmitoyl transferase I deficiency: Is there a diagnostic dicarboxylic aciduria? Proceedings of the 30th Annual Symposium of the Society for the Study of Inborn Errors of Metabolism, Leuven, Belgium, September 8-11, 1992 (Abstract p. 128).

Pollitt RJ. Clinical and biochemical presentations in twenty cases of hydroxydicarboxylic aciduria. In: Tanaka K, Coates PM, eds. Progress in clinical and biological research, vol 321. Fatty acid oxidation: Clinical, biochemical, and molecular aspects. New York: Alan R. Liss, 1990;495.

Pompe JC. Over idiopatische hypertrophie van het hart. Ned Tijdschr Geneeskd 1932;76:304.

Pons R, Andreetta F, Wang CH, et al. Mitochondrial myopathy simulating spinal muscular atrophy. Pediatr Neurol 1996;15:153.

Pons R, Carrozzo R, Tein I, et al. Deficient muscle carnitine transport in primary carnitine deficiency. Pediatr Res 1997;42:583.

Pourmand R, Sanders DB, Corwin HM. Late-onset McArdle's disease with unusual electromyographic findings. Arch Neurol 1983;40:374.

Powell HC, Haas R, Hall CL, et al. Peripheral nerve in type III glycogenosis: Selective involvement of unmyelinated fiber Schwann cells. Muscle Nerve 1985;8:667.

Pretorius CJ, Son GGL, Bonnici F, et al. Two siblings with episodic ketoacidosis and decreased activity of succinyl-CoA:3-ketoacid CoA-transferase in cultured fibroblasts. J Inherit Metab Dis 1996;19:296.

Prick MJJ, Gabreels FJM, Trijbels JMF, et al. Progressive poliodystrophy (Alpers' disease) with a defect in cytochrome aa_3 in muscle: A report of two unrelated patients. Clin Neurol Neurosurg 1983;85:57.

Przyrembel H. Therapy of mitochondrial disorders. J Inherit Metab Dis 1987;10 (Suppl 2):129.

Raben N, Sherman JB. Mutations in muscle phosphofructokinase gene. Hum Mutat 1995;6:1.

Radda GK, Odoom J, Kemp G, et al. Assessment of mitochondrial function and control in normal and diseased states. Biochim Biophys Acta 1995;1271:15.

Rao PN, Hayworth R, Akots G, et al. Physical localization of chromosome 20 markers using somatic cell hybrid cell lines and fluorescence in situ hybridization. Genomics 1992;14:532.

Reed WD, Lane MD. Mitochondrial 3-hydroxy-3-methylglutaryl-CoA synthetase from chicken liver. In: Lowenstein JM, ed. Methods in enzymology. Part B, vol 35, Lipids. New York: Academic Press, 1975;155.

Reichmann H, Rohkamm R, Zeviani M, et al. Mitochondrial myopathy due to complex III deficiency with normal reducible cytochrome b concentration. Arch Neurol 1986;43:957.

Renaud DL, Edwards V, Wilson GJ, et al. Glucose-free medium exacerbates microvesicular steatosis in cultured skin fibroblasts of genetic defects in fatty acid oxidation. A novel screening test. J Inherit Metab Dis 2002;25:547.

Rennie MJ, Edwards RHT. Carbohydrate metabolism of skeletal muscle and its disorders. In: Randle P, ed. Carbohydrate metabolism and its disorders. New York: Academic Press, 1981;1.

Reusche E, Aksu F, Goebel HH, et al. A mild juvenile variant of type IV glycogenosis. Brain Dev 1992;14:36.

Reuser AJJ, Kroos M, Willemsen R, et al. Clinical diversity in glycogenosis type II. J Clin Invest 1987;79:1689.

Rhead WJ. Screening for inborn errors of fatty acid oxidation in cultured fibroblasts: An overview. In: Tanaka K, Coates PM, eds. Progress in clinical and biological research, vol 321. Fatty acid oxidation: Clinical, biochemical and molecular aspects. New York: Alan R. Liss, 1990;365.

Ribes A, Riudor E, Garavaglia B, et al. Mild or absent clinical signs in twin sisters with short-chain acyl-CoA dehydrogenase deficiency. Eur J Pediatr 1998;157:317.

Rinaldo P, Matern D. Disorders of fatty acid transport and mitochondrial oxidation: Challenges and dilemmas of metabolic evaluation. Genet Med 2000;2:338.

Rinaldo P, Matern D, Bennett MJ. Fatty acid oxidation disorders. Annu Rev Physiol 2002;64:477.

Rinaldo P, O'Shea JJ, Coates PM, et al. Medium-chain acyl-CoA dehdyrogenase deficiency. Diagnosis by stable isotope dilution measurement of urinary *N*-hexanoylglycine and 3-phenylpropionylglycine. N Engl J Med 1988;319:1308.

Roberts JR, Narasimhan C, Hruz PW, et al. 3-Hydroxy-3-methylglutaryl-CoA lyase: Expression and isolation of the recombinant human enzyme and investigation of a mechanism for regulation of enzyme activity. J Biol Chem 1994;269:17841.

Robinson BH. Lactic acidemia. In: Scriver CR, Beaudet AL, Sly WS, et al., eds. The metabolic basis of inherited disease, 6th ed. New York: McGraw-Hill, 1989;869.

Robinson BH. Lactic acidemia (disorders of pyruvate carboxylase, pyruvate dehydrogenase). In: Scriver CR, Beaudet AL, Sly WS, et al., eds. The metabolic and molecular bases of inherited disease, 7th ed. New York: McGraw-Hill, 1995;1479.

Robinson BH, De Meirleir LJ, Glerum M, et al. Clinical presentation of patients with mitochondrial respiratory chain defects in NADH-coenzyme Q reductase and cytochrome oxidase: Clues to the pathogenesis of Leigh disease. J Pediatr 1987;110:216.

Robinson BH, Ward J, Goodyer P, et al. Respiratory chain defects in the mitochondria of cultured skin fibroblasts from three patients with lactic acidemia. J Clin Invest 1986;77:1422.

Roe CR as cited by Stanley, CA. New genetic defects in mitochondrial fatty acid oxidation and carnitine deficiency. Adv Pediatr 1987;34:59.

Roe CR, Millington DS, Maltby DA, et al. Diagnostic and therapeutic implications of medium-chain acylcarnitines in the medium-chain acyl-CoA dehydrogenase deficiency. Pediatr Res 1985;19:459.

Roe CR, Millington DS, Norwood DL, et al. 2,4-Dienoyl-coenzyme A reductase deficiency: A possible new disorder of fatty acid oxidation. J Clin Invest 1990;85:1703.

Roe CR, Sweetman L, Roe DS, et al. Treatment of cardiomyopathy and rhabodmyolysis in long-chain fat oxidation disorders using an anaplerotic odd-chain triglyceride. J Clin Invest 2002;110:259.

Roesch K, Curran SP, Tranebjaerg L, et al. Human deafness, dystonia syndrome is caused by a defect in assembly of the DDP1/TIMM8-TIMM13 complex. Hum Mol Genet 2002;11:477.

Rosa R, George C, Fardeau M, et al. A new case of phosphoglycerate kinase deficiency: PGK Creteil associated with rhabdomyolysis and lacking hemolytic anemia. Blood 1982;60:84.

Ross BD, Radda GK, Gadian DG, et al. Examination of a case of suspected McArdle's syndrome by ^{31}P nuclear magnetic resonance. N Engl J Med 1981;304:1338.

Rowland LP. Myoglobinuria. Can J Neurol Sci 1984;11:1.

Rowland LP, DiMauro S, Layzer RB. Phosphofructokinase deficiency. In: Engel AG, Banker BQ, eds. Myology. New York: McGraw-Hill, 1986;1603.

Rubio JC, Martin MA, Bautista J, et al. Association of genetically proven deficiencies of myophosphorylase and AMP deaminase: A second case of "double trouble." Neuromuscul Disord 1997;7:387.

Ruitenbeek W, Poels PJE, Turnbull DM, et al. Rhabdomyolysis and acute encephalopathy in late onset medium chain acyl-CoA dehydrogenase deficiency. J Neurol Neurosurg Psychiatry 1995;58:209.

Ruitenbeek W, Sengers R, Albani M, et al. Prenatal diagnosis of cytochrome c oxidase deficiency by biopsy of chorionic villi [Letter]. N Engl J Med 1988;319:1095.

Saada A, Shaag A, Mandel H, et al. Mutant mitochondrial thymidine kinase in mitochondrial DNA depletion myopathy. Nat Genet 2001;29:337.

Sabina RL. Myoadenylate deaminase deficiency. In: Rosenberg RN, Prusiner SB, DiMauro S, et al., eds. The molecular and genetic basis of neurological disease. Boston: Butterworth-Heinemann, 1993;261.

Sabina RL, Morisaki T, Clarke P, et al. Characterization of the human and rat myoadenylate deaminase genes. J Biol Chem 1990;265:9423.

Sacconi S, Salviati L, Sue CM, et al. Mutation screening in patients with isolated cytochrome c oxidase deficiency. Pediatr Res 2003;53:224.

Sahlin K. Metabolic changes limiting muscle performance. In: Saltin B, ed. Biochemistry of exercise VI. Champaign, IL: Human Kinetics, 1986;323.

Sahlin K, Jorfeldt L, Henriksson K, et al. Tricarboxylic acid cycle intermediates during incremental exercise: Attenuated increase in McArdle's disease. Clin Sci 1995;88:687.

Sahlin K, Katz A, Broberg S. Tricarboxylic acid cycle intermediates in human muscle during prolonged exercise. Am J Physiol 1990;259:C834.

Saijo T, Naito E, Ito M, et al. Therapeutic effect of sodium dichloroacetate on visual and auditory hallucinations in a patient with MELAS. Neuropediatrics 1991;22:166.

Sakoda S, Shanske S, DiMauro S, et al. Isolation of a cDNA encoding the B isozyme of human phosphoglycerate mutase (PGAM) and characterization of the PGAM gene family. J Biol Chem 1988;263:16899.

Sakuta R, Nonaka I. Vascular involvement in mitochondrial myopathy. Ann Neurol 1989;25:594.

Saltin B. Capacity of blood flow delivery to exercising skeletal muscle in humans. Am J Cardiol 1988;62:30E.

Salviati L, Hernandez-Rosa E, Walker WF, et al. Copper supplementation restores cytochrome c oxidase activity in cultured cells from patients with SCO2 mutations. Biochem J 2002a;363:321.

Salviati L, Sacconi S, Mancuso M, et al. Mitochondrial DNA depletion and dGK gene mutations. Ann Neurol 2002b;52:311.

Sancho S, Navarro C, Fernández J, et al. Skin biopsy findings in glycogenosis III: Clinical, biochemical, and electrophysiological correlations. Ann Neurol 1990;27:480.

Santer R, Kinner M, Steuerwald U, et al. Molecular genetic basis and prevalence of glycogen storage disease type IIIA in the Faroe Islands. Eur J Hum Genet 2001;9:388.

Sato K, Imai F, Hatayama I, et al. Characterization of glycogen phosphorylase isoenzymes present in cultured skeletal muscle from patients with McArdle's disease. Biochem Biophys Res Commun 1977;78:663.

Schatz G. The mitochondrial protein import machinery. In: Sato T, DiMauro S, eds. Mitochondrial encephalomyopathies. New York: Raven Press, 1991;57.

Schimrigk K, Mertens HG, Ricker K, et al. [McArdle's syndrome (myopathy in muscle phosphorylase deficiency)]. Klin Wochenschr (in German) 1967;45:1.

Schlame M, Kelley RI, Feigenbaum A, et al. Phospholipid abnormalities in children with Barth syndrome. J Am Coll Cardiol 2003;42:1994.

Schlame M, Towbin JA, Heerdt PM, et al. Deficiency of tetralinoleoyl-cardiolipin in Barth syndrome. Ann Neurol 2002;51:634.

Schmidt B, Servidei S, Gabbai AA, et al. McArdle's disease in two generations: Autosomal recessive transmission with manifesting heterozygote. Neurology 1987;37:1558.

Schotland DL, DiMauro S, Bonilla E, et al. Neuromuscular disorder associated with a defect in mitochondrial energy supply. Arch Neurol 1976;33:475.

Schroder JM, May R, Shin YS, et al. Juvenile hereditary polyglucosan body disease with complete branching enzyme deficiency (type IV glycogenosis). Acta Neuropathol 1993;85:419.

Schulz H. Oxidation of fatty acids. In: Vance DE, Vance JE, eds. Biochemistry of lipids and membranes. Menlo Park, CA: Benjamin Cummings, 1985;116.

Selby R, Starzl TE, Yunis E, et al. Liver transplantation for type IV glycogen storage disease. N Engl J Med 1991;324:39.

Serero S, Maire P, Van Cong N, et al. Localization of the active gene of aldolase on chromosome 16, and two aldolase A pseudogenes on chromosomes 3 and 10. Hum Genet 1988;78:167.

Servidei S, DiMauro S. Disorders of glycogen metabolism of muscle. Neurol Clin 1989;7:159.

Servidei S, Metlay LA, Chodosh J, et al. Fatal infantile cardiopathy caused by phosphorylase b kinase deficiency. J Pediatr 1988a;113:82.

Servidei S, Riepe RE, Langston C, et al. Severe cardiopathy in branching enzyme deficiency. J Pediatr 1987;111:51.

Servidei S, Shanske S, Zeviani M, et al. McArdle disease. Biochemical and molecular genetic studies. Ann Neurol 1988b;24:774.

Servidei S, Zeviani M, Manfredi G, et al. Dominantly inherited mitochondrial myopathy with multiple deletions of mitochondrial DNA: Clinical, morphologic, and biochemical studies. Neurology 1991;41:1053.

Shaiu WL, Kishnani PS, Shen J, et al. Genotype-phenotype correlation in two frequent mutations and mutation update in type III glycogen storage disease. Mol Genet Metab 2000;69:16.

Shanske S, DiMauro S. Late-onset acid maltase deficiency. Biochemical studies of leukocytes. J Neurol Sci 1981;50:57.

Shanske S, Sakoda S, Hermodson MA, et al. Isolation of a cDNA encoding the muscle-specific subunit of human phosphoglycerate mutase. J Biol Chem 1987;262:14612.

Shapira Y, Cederbaum SD, Cancilla PA, et al. Familial poliodystrophy, mitochondrial myopathy, and lactate acidemia. Neurology 1975;25:614.

Shen JJ, Bao Y, Chen YT. A nonsense mutation due to a single base insertion in the 3′-coding region of glycogen debranching enzyme gene is associated with a severe phenotype in a patient with glycogen storage diseases type IIIa. Hum Mutat 1997;9:37.

Shen JJ, Bao Y, Liu HM, et al. Mutations in exon 3 of the glycogen debranching enzyme gene are associated with glycogen storage disease type III that is differentially expressed in liver and muscle. J Clin Invest 1996;98:352.

Sherman JB, Raben N, Nicastri C, et al. Common mutations in the phosphofructokinase-M gene in Ashkenazi Jewish patients with glycogenosis VII—and their population frequency. Am J Hum Genet 1994;55:305.

Shoffner JM, Lott MT, Lezza AMS, et al. Myoclonic epilepsy and ragged-red fiber disease (MERRF) is associated with a mitochondrial DNA $tRNA^{Lys}$ mutation. Cell 1990;61:931.

Shoffner JM, Lott MT, Voljavec AS, et al. Spontaneous Kearns-Sayre/chronic external ophthalmoplegia plus syndrome associated with mitochondrial DNA deletion: A slip-replication model and metabolic therapy. Proc Natl Acad Sci U S A 1989;86:7952.

Shy GM, Gonatas NK. Human myopathy with giant abnormal mitochondria. Science 1964;145:493.

Shy GM, Gonatas NK, Perez M. Two childhood myopathies with abnormal mitochondria. I. Megaconial myopathy. II. Pleoconial myopathy. Brain 1966;89:133.

Sims HF, Brackett JC, Powell CK, et al. The molecular basis of pediatric long chain 3-hydroxyacyl-CoA dehydrogenase deficiency associated with maternal acute fatty liver of pregnancy. Proc Natl Acad Sci USA 1995;92:841.

Sinkeler STP, Daanen HAM, Wevers RA, et al. The relation between blood lactate and ammonia in ischemic handgrip exercise. Muscle Nerve 1985;8:523.

Slipetz DM, Aprille JR, Goodyer PR, et al. Deficiency of complex III of the mitochondrial respiratory chain in a patient with facioscapulohumeral disease. Am J Hum Genet 1991;48:502.

Slonim AE, Balone L, Ritz S, et al. Identification of two subtypes of infantile acid maltase deficiency. J Pediatr 2000;137:283.

Slonim AE, Coleman RA, McElligot MA, et al. Improvement of muscle function in acid maltase deficiency by high-protein therapy. Neurology 1983;33:34.

Slonim AE, Goans PJ. Myopathy in McArdle's syndrome. Improvement with a high protein diet. N Engl J Med 1985;312:355.

Slonim AE, Weisberg C, Benke P, et al. Reversal of debrancher deficiency myopathy by the use of high-protein nutrition. Ann Neurol 1982;11:420.

Smit GPA, Fernandes J, Leonard JV, et al. The long-term outcome of patients with glycogen storage diseases. J Inherit Metab Dis 1990;13:411.

Sokal EM, Van Hoof F, Alberti D, et al. Progressive cardiac failure following orthotopic liver transplantation for type IV glycogenosis. Eur J Pediatr 1992;151:200.

Solis JO, Singh RH. Management of fatty acid oxdation disorders : A survery of current treatment strategies. J Am Diet Assoc 2002;102:1800.

Solomon E, Swallow D, Burgess S, et al. Assignment of human acid alpha glucosidase (aGLU) to chromosome 17 using somatic cell hybirds. Ann Hum Genet 1979;42:273.

Souri M, Aoyama T, Orii K, et al. Mutation analysis of very-long-chain acyl-coenzyme A dehydrogenase (VLCAD) deficiency: Identification and characterization of mutant VLCAD cDNAs from four patients. Am J Hum Genet 1996;58:97.

Spedding M. Activators and inactivators of Ca^{++} channels: New perspectives. J Pharmacol (Paris) 1985;16:319.

Spedding M, Mir AK. Direct activation of Ca^{++} channels by almitoyl carnitine, a putative endogenous ligand. Br J Pharmacol 1987;92:457.

Spellbrink JN, Li FY, Tiranti V, et al. Human mitochondrial DNA deletions associated with mutations in the gene encoding *Twinkle*, a phage T7 gene 4-like protein localized in mitochondria. Nat Genet 2001;28:223.

Spiekerkoetter U, Bennett MJ, Ben-Zeev B, et al. Peripheral neuropathy, episodic myoglobinuria, and respiratory failure in deficiency of the mitochondrial trifunctional protein. Muscle Nerve 2004;29:66.

Spruijt L, Naviaux RK, McGown KA, et al. Nerve conduction changes in patients with mitochondrial diseases treated with dichloroacetate. Muscle Nerve 2001;24:916.

Stadhouders A, Jap P, Walliman TH. Biochemical nature of mitochondrial crystals. J Neurol Sci 1990;98 (Suppl):304.

Stanley CA. New genetic defects in mitochondrial fatty acid oxidation and carnitine deficiency. Adv Pediatr 1987;34:59.

Stanley CA, Deleeuw S, Coates PM, et al. Chronic cardiomyopathy and weakness or acute coma in children with a defect in carnitine uptake. Ann Neurol 1991;30:709.

Stanley CA, Hale DE, Coates PM. Medium-chain acyl-CoA dehydrogenase deficiency. In: Tanaka K, Coates PM, eds. Progress in clinical and biological research, vol 321. Fatty acid oxidation: Clinical, biochemical, and molecular aspects. New York: Alan R. Liss, 1990;291.

Stanley CA, Sunaryo F, Hale DE, et al. Elevated plasma carnitine in the hepatic form of carnitine palmitoyltransferase-1 deficiency. J Inherit Metab Dis 1992;15:785.

Strauss AW. Genotype-phenotype correlations in mitochondrial trifunctional protein deficiency. Proceedings of the 7th International Congress of Inborn Errors of Metabolism, Vienna, Austria, May 21-25, 1997.

Strauss AW, Duran M, Zhang Z, et al. Molecular analysis of medium chain acyl-CoA dehydrogenase deficiency. In: Tanaka K, Coates PM, eds. Progress in clinical and biological research, vol 321. Fatty acid oxidation: Clinical, biochemical and molecular aspects. New York: Alan R. Liss, 1990;609.

Strauss AW, Powell CK, Hale DE et al. Molecular basis of human mitochondrial very-long-chain acyl-CoA dehydrogenase deficiency causing cardiomyopathy and sudden death in childhood. Proc Natl Acad Sci U S A 1995;92:10496.

Stremmel W, Strohmeyer G, Berk PD. Hepatocellular uptake of oleate is energy dependent, sodium linked, and inhibited by an antibody to a hepatocyte plasma membrane fatty acid binding protein. Proc Natl Acad Sci U S A 1986;83:3584.

Sugie H, Sugie Y, Nishida M, et al. Recurrent myoglobinuria in a child with mental retardation: Phosphoglycerate kinase deficiency. J Child Neurol 1989;4:95.

Sugie H, Sugie Y, Tsurui S, et al. Phosphoglycerate kinase deficiency [Comment]. Neurology 1994;44:1364.

Suomalainen A, Kaukonen J. Diseases caused by nuclear genes affecting mtDNA stability. Am J Med Genet 2001;106:53.

Swoboda KJ, Specht L, Jones HR, et al. Infantile phosphofructokinase deficiency with arthrogryposis: Clinical benefit of a ketogenic diet. J Pediatr 1997;131:932.

Taivassalo T, Abbott A, Wyrick P, et al. Venous oxygen levels during aerobic forearm exercise: An index of impaired oxidative metabolism in mitochondrial myopathy. Ann Neurol 2002;51:38.

Taivassalo T, Dysgaard Jensen T, Kennaway N, et al. The spectrum of exercise tolerance in mitochondrial myopathies: A study of 40 patients. Brain 2003;126:413.

Takayasu S, Fujiwara S, Waki T. Hereditary lactate dehydrogenase M-subunit deficiency: Lactate dehydrogenase activity in skin lesions and in hair follicles. J Am Acad Dermatol 1991;24:339.

Takeuchi T, Kuriaki H. Histochemical detection of phosphorylase in animal tissues. J Histochem Cytochem 1955;3:153.

Tamai I, Ohashi R, Nezu J, et al. Molecular and functional identification of sodium ion-dependent, high affinity human carnitine transporter OCTN2. J Biol Chem 1998;273:293.

Tanaka M, Sato W, Ohno K, et al. Direct sequencing of deleted mitochondrial DNA in myopathic patients. Biochem Biophys Res Commun 1989;164:156.

Taroni F, Verderio E, Dworzak F, et al. Identification of a common mutation in the carnitine palmitoyltransferase II gene in familial recurrent myoglobinuria patients. Nat Genet 1993;4:314.

Tarui S, Okuno G, Ikura Y, et al. Phosphofructokinase deficiency in skeletal muscle: A new type of glycogenosis. Biochem Biophys Res Commun 1965;19:517.

Tatuch Y, Christodoulou J, Feigenbaum A, et al. Heteroplasmic mtDNA mutation (T>G) at 8993 can cause Leigh disease when the percentage of abnormal mtDNA is high. Am J Hum Genet 1992;50:852.

Tein I. Fatty acid oxidation and associated defects. In: Proceedings of the 47th Annual Meeting of the American Academy of Neurology, Seattle, Washington. Madison, WI: Omnipress, 1995;269:9.

Tein I. Fatty acid oxidation and associated defects. In: Proceedings of the 52nd Annual Meeting of the American Academy of Neurology, San Diego, CA. Evaluation of Metabolic Myopathies. Madison, WI: Omnipress, 2000a;3AS.008.

Tein I. Metabolic disease in the fetus predisposes to maternal hepatic complications of pregnancy. Pediatr Res 2000b;47:6.

Tein I, De Vivo DC, Bierman F, et al. Impaired skin fibroblast carnitine uptake in primary systemic carnitine deficiency manifested by childhood carnitine-responsive cardiomyopathy. Pediatr Res 1990a;28:247.

Tein I, De Vivo DC, Hale DE, et al. Short-chain *L*-3-hydroxyacyl-CoA dehydrogenase deficiency in muscle: A new cause for recurrent myoglobinuria and encephalopathy. Ann Neurol 1991;30:415.

Tein I, DiMauro S, De Vivo DC. Recurrent childhood myoglobinuria. Adv Pediatr 1990b;37:77.

Tein I, DiMauro S, Rowland LP. Myoglobinuria. In: Rowland LP, DiMauro S, eds. Handbook of clinical neurology, vol 18(62). Myopathies. Amsterdam: Elsevier Science Publishers BV, 1992;553.

Tein I, Donner EJ, Hale DE, et al. Clinical and neurophysiologic response of myopathy and neuropathy in long-chain *L*-3-hydroxyacyl-CoA dehydrogenase deficiency to oral prednisone. Pediatr Neurol 1995;12:68.

Tein I, Halsam RH, Rhead WJ, et al. Short-chain acyl-CoA dehydrogenase deficiency: A cause of ophthalmoplegia and multicore myopathy. Neurology 1999a;52:366.

Tein I, Vasjar J, MacMillan L, et al. Long-chain L-3-hydroxyacyl-coenzyme A dehydrogenase deficiency neuropathy: response to cod liver oil. Neurology 1999b;52:640.

Tein I, Xie ZW. The human plasmalemmal carnitine transporter defect is expressed in cultured lymphoblasts: A new non-invasive method for diagnosis. Clin Chim Acta 1996;252:201.

Thompson GN, Hsu BYL, Pitt JJ, et al. Fasting hypoketotic coma in a child with deficiency of mitochondrial 3-hydroxy-3-methylglutaryl-CoA synthase. N Engl J Med 1997;337:1203.

Tiranti V, Hoertnagel K, Carrozzo R, et al. Mutations of SURF-1 in Leigh disease associated with cytochrome c oxidase deficiency. Am J Hum Genet 1998;63:1609.

Tonin P, Lewis P, Servidei S, et al. Metabolic causes of myoglobinuria. Ann Neurol 1990;27:181.

Tonin P, Shanske S, Miranda AF, et al. Phosphoglycerate kinase deficiency: Biochemical and molecular genetic studies in a new myopathic variant (PGK Alberta). Neurology 1993;43:387.

Tonsgard JH. Serum dicarboxylic acids in patients with Reye syndrome. J Pediatr 1986;109:440.

Tonsgard JH, Getz GS. Effect of Reye's syndrome serum on isolated chinchilla liver mitochondria. J Clin Invest 1985;76:816.

Treem WR, Shoup ME, Hale DE, et al. Acute fatty liver of pregnancy, hemolysis, elevated liver enzymes and low platelets syndrome and long-chain 3-hydroxyacyl-coenzyme A dehydrogenase deficiency. Am J Gastroenterol 1996;91:2293.

Treem WR, Stanley CA, Finegold DN, et al. Primary carnitine deficiency due to a failure of carnitine transport in kidney, muscle and fibroblasts. N Engl J Med 1988;319:1331.

Triepels RH, Van Den Heuvel LP, Trijbels JM, et al. Respiratory chain complex I deficicncy. Am J Med Genet 2001;106:37.

Tripp ME, Katcher ML, Peters HA, et al. Systemic carnitine deficiency presenting as familial endocardial fibroelastosis. A treatable cardiomyopathy. N Engl J Med 1981;305:385.

Tritschler HJ, Andreetta F, Moraes CT, et al. Mitochondrial myopathy of childhood associated with depletion of mitochondrial DNA. Neurology 1992;42:209.

Tritschler HJ, Bonilla E, Lombes A, et al. Differential diagnosis of fatal and benign cytochrome c oxidase-deficient myopathies of infancy: An immunohistochemical approach. Neurology 1991;41:300.

Tsairis P, Engel WK, Kark P. Familial myoclonic epilepsy syndrome associated with skeletal muscle mitochondrial abnormalities. Neurology 1973;23:408.

Tsujino S, Kinoshita N, Tashiro T, et al. Adenovirus-mediated transfer of human acid maltase gene reduces glycogen accumulation in skeletal muscle of Japanese quail with acid maltase deficiency. Hum Gene Ther 1998;9:1609.

Tsujino S, Rubin LA, Shanske S, et al. An A-to-C substitution involving the translation initiation codon in myophosphorylase deficiency (McArdle's disease). Hum Mutat 1994a;4:73.

Tsujino S, Sakoda S, Mizuno R, et al. Structure of the gene encoding the muscle-specific subunit of human phosphoglycerate mutase. J Biol Chem 1989;264:15334.

Tsujino S, Servidei S, Tonin P, et al. Identification of three novel mutations in non-Ashkenazi Italian patients with muscle phosphofructokinase deficiency. Am J Hum Genet 1994d;54:812.

Tsujino S, Shanske S, Carroll JE, et al. Double trouble: Combined myophosphorylase and AMP deaminase deficiency in a child homozygous for nonsense mutations at both loci. Neuromuscul Disord 1995a;5:263.

Tsujino S, Shanske S, DiMauro S. Molecular genetic heterogeneity of myophosphorylase deficiency (McArdle's disease). N Engl J Med 1993a;329:241.

Tsujino S, Shanske S, DiMauro S. Molecular genetic heterogeneity of phosphoglycerate kinase (PGK) deficiency. Muscle Nerve 1995b;3:S45.

Tsujino S, Shanske S, Goto Y, et al. Two mutations, one novel and one frequently observed, in Japanese patients with McArdle's disease. Hum Mol Genet 1994b;3:1005.

Tsujino S, Shanske S, Nonaka I, et al. Three new mutations in patients with myophosphorylase deficiency (McArdle's disease). Am J Hum Genet 1994c;54:44.

Tsujino S, Shanske S, Sakoda S, et al. The molecular genetic basis of muscle phosphoglycerate mutase (PGAM) deficiency. Am J Hum Genet 1993b;52:472.

Tsujino S, Tonin P, Shanske S, et al. A splice junction mutation in a new myopathic variant of phosphoglycerate kinase deficiency (PGK North Carolina). Ann Neurol 1994e;35:349.

Tyni T, Paetau A, Strauss A, et al. Mitohcondrial fatty acid (beta) oxidation in the human eye and brain: Implications for retinopathy of long-chain-3-hydroxyacyl-CoA dehydrogenase deficiency. Pediatr Res 2004;56:744.

Tyni T, Pihko H, Kivela T. Ophthalmic pathology in long-chain 3-hydroxyacyl-CoA dehydrogenase deficiency caused by the G1528C mutation. Curr Eye Res 1998;17:551.

Tyni T, Pourfarzam M, Turnbull DM. Analysis of mitochondrial fatty acid oxdation intermediates by tandem mass spectrometry from intact mitochondria prepared from homogenates of cultured fibroblasts, skeletal muscle cells, and fresh muscle. Pediatr Res 2002;52:64.

Uauy R, Treen M, Hoffman DR. Essential fatty acid metabolism and requirements during development. Semin Perinatol 1989;13:118.

Uchida Y, Izai K, Orii T, et al. Novel fatty acid β-oxidation enzymes in rat liver mitochondria. II. Purification and properties of enoyl-coenzyme A (CoA) hydratase/3-hydroxyacyl-CoA dehydrogenase/3-ketoacyl-CoA thiolase trifunctional protein. J Biol Chem 1992;267:1034.

Uemura A, Osame M, Nakagawa M, et al. Leber's hereditary optic neuropathy: Mitochondrial and biochemical studies on muscle biopsies. Br J Ophthalmol 1987;71:531.

Ugawa Y, Inoue K, Takemura T, et al. Accumulation of glycogen in sural nerve axons in adult-onset type III glycogenosis. Ann Neurol 1986;19:294.

Valentine WM, Hsieh H, Paglia DE, et al. Hereditary hemolytic anemia associated with phosphoglycerate kinase deficiency in erythrocytes and leukocytes. N Engl J Med 1960;280:528.

Valnot I, Osmond S, Gigarel N, et al. Mutations in the SCO1 gene in mitochondrial cytochrome c oxidase deficiency with neonatal onset hepatic failure and encephalopathy. Am J Hum Genet 1999;67:1104.

Valnot J, von Kleist-Retzow JC, Barrientos A, et al. A mutation in the human heme-A:farnesyltransferase gene (COX 10) causes cytochrome c oxidase deficiency. Hum Mol Genet 2000;9:1245.

Van Coster R, Lombes A, De Vivo DC, et al. Cytochrome c oxidase–associated Leigh syndrome: Phenotypic features and pathogenetic speculations. J Neurol Sci 1991;104:97.

Van der Berg IET, Berger R. Phosphorylase b kinase deficiency in man: A review. J Inherit Metab Dis 1990;13:442.

Van Der Ploeg AT, Bolhuis PA, Wolterman, RA, et al. Prospect for enzyme therapy in glycogenosis type II variants: A study on cultured muscle cells. J Neurol 1988;235:392.

Van Keuren M, Drabkin H, Hart I, et al. Regional assignment of human liver-type 6-phosphofructokinase to chromosome 21q22.3 by using somatic cell hybrids and a monoclonal anti-L antibody. Hum Genet 1986;74:34.

Van Loon LJ, Greenhaff PL, Constantin-Teodosiu D, et al. The effects of increasing exercise intensity on muscle fuel utilization in humans. J Physiol 2001: 536:295.

VanGoethem G, Dermaut B, Lofgren A, et al. Mutation of POLG is assoicated with progressive external ophthalmoplegia characterized by mtDNA deletions. Nat Genet 2001;28:211.

Vazquez-Memije ME, Shanske S, Santorelli FM, et al. Comparative biochemical studies of ATPases in cells from patients with the T8993G or the T8993C mitochondrial DNA mutations. J Inherit Metab Dis 1998;21:829.

Vekemans BC, Bonnefont JP, Aupetit J, et al. Prenatal diangosis of carnitine palmitoyltransferase 2 deficiency in chorionic villi: A novel approach. Prenatal Diagn 2003;23:884.

Verderio E, Cavadini P, Montermini L, et al. Carnitine palmitoyltransferase II deficiency: Structure of the gene and characterization of two novel disease-causing mutations. Hum Mol Genet 1995;4:19.

Visapaa L, Fellman V, Vesa J, et al. GRACILE syndrome, a lethal metabolic disorder with iron overload, is caused by a point mutation in BCSIL. Am J Hum Genet 2002;71:863.

Vissing J, Haller RG. The effect of oral sucrose on exercise tolerance in patients with McArdle's disease. N Engl J Med 2003;349:2503.

Vora S. Isozymes of human phosphofructokinase: Biochemical and genetic aspects. Isozymes 1983;11:3.

Vora S, Davidson M, Seaman C, et al. Heterogeneity of the molecular lesions in inherited phosphofructokinase deficiency. J Clin Invest 1983a;72:1995.

Vora S, Durham S, de Martinville B, et al. Assignment of the human gene for muscle-type phosphofructokinase (PFKM) to chromosome 1 (region cen-q32) using somatic cell hybrids and monoclonal anti-M antibody. Somatic Cell Genet 1982;8:95.

Vora S, Miranda AF, Hernandez E, et al. Regional assignment of the human gene for platelet-type phosphofructokinase (PFKP) to chromosome 10p: Novel use of polyspecific rodent antisera to localize human enzyme genes. Hum Genet 1983b;63:374.

Vorgerd M, Grehl T, Jager M, et al. Creatine therapy in myophosphorylase deficiency (McArdle disease). Arch Neurol 2000;57:956.

Vorgerd M, Kubisch C, Burwinkel B, et al. Mutation analysis in myophosphorylase deficiency (McArdle's disease). Ann Neurol 1998;43:326.

Vredendaal PCJM, van den Berg IET, Malingre HEM, et al. Human short-chain *L*-3-hydroxyacyl-CoA dehydrogenase: Cloning and characterization of the coding sequence. Biochem Biophys Res Commun 1996;223:718.

Vu TH, Hirano M, DiMauro S. Mitochondrial diseases. Neurol Clin North Am 2002;20:809.

Vu TH, Sciacco M, Tanji K, et al. Clinical manifestations of mitochondrial DNA depletion. Neurology 1998;50:1783.

Wahren J. Glucose turnover during exercise in man. Ann N Y Acad Sci 1977;301:45.

Wahren J, Felig P, Havel RJ, et al. Amino acid metabolism in McArdle's syndrome. N Engl J Med 1973;288:774.

Wallace DC, Shoffner JM, Lott MT, et al. Myoclonic epilepsy and ragged-red fiber disease (MERRF): A mitochondrial $tRNA^{Lys}$ mutation responsive to coenzyme Q10 (CoQ) therapy [Abstract]. Neurology 1991;41 (Suppl 1):280.

Wallace DC, Singh G, Lott MT, et al. Mitochondrial DNA mutation associated with Leber's hereditary optic neuropathy. Science 1988a;242:1427.

Wallace DC, Zheng X, Lott MT, et al. Familial mitochondrial encephalomyopathy (MERRF): Genetic, pathophysiological and biochemical characterization of a mitochondrial DNA disease. Cell 1988b;55:601.

Wanders RJA, Duran M, Ijlst L, et al. Sudden infant death and long-chain 3-hydroxyacyl-CoA dehydrogenase. Lancet 1989;2:52.

Walter JH. Inborn errors of metabolism and pregnancy. J Inherit Metab Dis 2000;23:229.

Wehner M, Clemens PR, Engel AG, et al. Human muscle glycogenosis due to phosphorylase kinase deficiency associated with a nonsense mutation in the muscle isoform of the alpha subunit. Hum Mol Genet 1994;3:1983.

Weil D, Cong N, Gross MS, et al. [Localization of the gene for human acid alpha-glucosidase (alpha-GLUa) on the 17q21→17qter by interspecific hybridization]. Hum Genet (in French) 1979;52:249.

Wilcken B, Leung KC, Hammond J, et al. Pregnancy and fetal long-chain 3-hydroxyacyl coenzyme A dehydrogenase deficiency. Lancet 1993;341:407.

Willems PJ, Gerver WJ, Berger R, et al. The natural history of liver glycogenosis due to phosphorylase kinase deficiency: A longitudinal study of 41 patients. Eur J Pediatr 1990;149:268.

Willems PJ, Hendrickx J, Van der Auwera BJ, et al. Mapping of the gene for X-linked liver glycogenosis due to phosphorylase kinase deficiency to human chromosome region Xp22. Genomics 1991;9:565.

Winkel LP, Van den Hout JM, Kamphoven JH, et al. Enzyme replacement therapy in late-onset Pompe's disease: A three-year follow-up. Ann Neurol 2004;55:495.

Woeltje KF, Esser V, Weist BC, et al. Cloning, sequencing, and expression of a cDNA encoding rat liver mitochondrial carnitine palmitoyltransferase II. J Biol Chem 1990;265:10720.

Wu Z, Prasad PD, Leibach FH, et al. cDNA sequence, transport function, and genomic organization of human OCTN2, a new member of the organic cation transporter family. Biochem Biophys Res Commun 1998;246:589.

Yamaguchi S, Indo Y, Coates PM, et al. Identification of very-long-chain acyl-CoA dehydrogenase deficiency in three patients previously diagnosed with long-chain acyl-CoA dehydrogenase deficiency. Pediatr Res 1993;34:111.

Yamamoto M, Sato T, Anno M, et al. Mitochondrial myopathy, encephalopathy, lactic acidosis, and stroke-like episodes with recurrent abdominal symptoms and coenzyme Q10 administration. J Neurol Neurosurg Psychiatry 1987;50:1475.

Yamazaki N, Shinohara Y, Shima A, et al. Isolation and characterization of cDNA and genomic clones encoding human muscle type carnitine palmitoyltransferase I. Biochem Biophys Acta 1996;1307:157.

Yang BZ, Ding JH, Brown BI, et al. Definitive prenatal diagnosis for type III glycogen storage disease. Am J Hum Genet 1990;47:735.

Yang BZ, Ding JH, Enghild JJ, et al. Molecular cloning and nucleotide sequence of cDNA encoding human muscle glycogen debranching enzyme. J Biol Chem 1992;267:9294.

Yang-Feng TL, Zheng K, Yu J, et al. Assignment of the human glycogen debrancher gene to chromosome 1p21. Genomics 1992;13:931.

Yuzaki M, Ohkoshi N, Kanazawa I, et al. Multiple deletions in mitochondrial DNA at direct repeats of non–D-loop regions in cases of familial mitochondrial myopathy. Biochem Biophys Res Commun 1989;164:1352.

Zellweger H, Mueller S, Ionasescu V, et al. Glycogenosis: IV. A new cause of infantile hypotonia. J Pediatr 1972;80:842.

Zeviani M, Amati P, Bresolin N, et al. Rapid detection of the A-to-G(8344) mutation of mtDNA in Italian families with myoclonus epilepsy and ragged-red fibers (MERRF). Am J Hum Genet 1991;48:203.

Zeviani M, Bresolin N, Gellera C, et al. Nucleus-driven multiple large-scale deletions of the human mitochondrial genome: A new autosomal dominant disease. Am J Hum Genet 1990;47:904.

Zeviani M, Servidei S, Gellera C, et al. An autosomal dominant disorder with multiple deletions of mitochondrial DNA starting at the D-loop region. Nature 1989;339:309.

Zeviani M, Van Dyke DH, Servidei S, et al. Myopathy and fatal cardiopathy due to cytochrome c oxidase deficiency. Arch Neurol 1986;43:1198.

Zhu Z, Yao J, Johns T, et al. SURF1, encoding a factor involved in the biogenesis of cytochrome c oxidase, is mutated in Leigh syndrome. Nat Genet 1998;20:337.

Ziadeh R, Hoffman EP, Finegold DN, et al. Medium chain acyl-CoA dehydrogenase deficiency in Pennsylvania: Neonatal screening shows high incidence and unexpected mutation frequencies. Pediatr Res 1995;37:675.

Zupanc ML, Moraes CT, Shanske S, et al. Deletion of mitochondrial DNA in patients with combined features of Kearns-Sayre and MELAS syndromes. Ann Neurol 1991;29:680.

CHAPTER 82

Inflammatory Myopathies

Anthony A. Amato and John T. Kissel

The inflammatory myopathies are a heterogeneous group of disorders all characterized pathologically by inflammation in skeletal muscle with resulting muscle fiber damage and subsequent clinical weakness. There are two major categories of inflammatory myopathy—idiopathic and infectious (Box 82-1). Although several types of muscular dystrophy may be associated with inflammation (e.g., facioscapulohumeral dystrophy), these disorders are traditionally excluded from classifications of inflammatory myopathy because they result from a fundamental genetic defect. The classic idiopathic inflammatory myopathies are usually considered autoimmune diseases, although a genetic predisposition may exist for many of these diseases based on inherited human leukocyte antigen haplotypes.

As a group, the inflammatory myopathies are the most common acquired myopathies of childhood. The infectious myositides are the most prevalent conditions worldwide, with acute viral myositis clearly the most common variety in North America and Europe. The idiopathic varieties are relatively uncommon, with a combined incidence (including adult cases) of approximately 1 in 100,000 [Dalakas, 1991; Medsger et al., 1970]. There are three major forms of idiopathic inflammatory myopathy—dermatomyositis, polymyositis, and inclusion body myositis, with dermatomyositis by far the most common form in childhood [Pachman, 1994]. Polymyositis is relatively uncommon in children and is usually seen as an overlap syndrome with other connective tissue disorders. Inclusion body myositis is exclusively a disease of adulthood and therefore is not discussed here.

IDIOPATHIC INFLAMMATORY MYOPATHIES

Although clinicians frequently conceptualize the idiopathic inflammatory myopathies as a single entity (e.g., polymyositis is dermatomyositis without the rash), the disorders are clinically, histologically, and pathogenetically distinct. Banker and Victor [1966] first reported the unique vascular changes of juvenile dermatomyositis and highlighted the involvement of organs other than muscle and skin. Subsequent immunologic and pathologic observations have confirmed a differing pathophysiology for these disorders. Although there have been occasional reports of siblings or parent/child cases of both dermatomyositis and polymyositis, most cases are sporadic.

Dermatomyositis

Clinical Features

Juvenile dermatomyositis can present at any age, including infancy, although most cases occur between ages 5 and 14 years [Medsger et al., 1970]. Females are affected more commonly than males. Onset of weakness is typically over weeks to a few months, although fatigue, muscle aches and stiffness, decreased activity, and fever can precede the onset of weakness by months. More acute, fulminate onset (over days) or an indolent, slowly progressive course (sometimes lasting a year) also has been described [Kissel et al., 1991; Pachman, 1994, 1995; Tymms and Webb, 1985]. Weakness typically affects the neck flexors and shoulder and pelvic girdle muscles first, so that the child may have difficulty getting up from the floor, riding a bicycle, running, climbing steps, or raising the arms above the head. Distal weakness is usually present, although not as severe as in proximal muscles. Complete sparing of distal strength should always lead the clinician to suspect another diagnosis, particularly one of the dystrophies. Dysphagia occurs in approximately one third of patients, and rarely individuals will also have chewing

Box 82-1 THE INFLAMMATORY MYOPATHIES

I. Idiopathic
   A. Juvenile dermatomyositis
   B. Polymyositis
   C. Inclusion body myositis
   D. Myositis as overlap syndrome
      1. Mixed connective tissue disease
      2. Scleroderma
      3. Systemic lupus erythematosus
      4. Rheumatoid arthritis
      5. Sjögren's syndrome
   E. Other inflammatory myopathies
      1. Eosinophilic myositis
      2. Focal nodular myositis
      3. Sarcoid myopathy
II. Infectious
   A. Viral myositides
      1. Influenza
      2. Human immunodeficiency virus
      3. Others (coxsackievirus, parainfluenza, mumps, measles, adenovirus, herpes simplex, cytomegalovirus, hepatitis B, Epstein-Barr virus, respiratory syncytial virus, echovirus, and possibly arboviruses)
   B. Parasitic myositis
      1. Trichinosis
      2. Toxoplasmosis
      3. Cysticercosis
   C. Bacterial myositis
   D. Fungal myositis

difficulties, dysarthria, and speech delay because of oropharyngeal involvement.

The rash frequently precedes the muscle symptoms and often provides the most important clue to diagnosis [Bowyer et al., 1986; Crowe et al., 1982; Sontheimer, 1999]. Skin changes typically involve the fingers and periorbital regions first, although any area may be involved. A purplish discoloration of the eyelids (heliotrope rash) with periorbital edema and extension onto the cheeks and forehead is typical (Fig. 82-1). On the hands, the periungual regions become erythematous and scaly, with dilated capillary loops in the nailbeds (Fig. 82-2). Papular, erythematous, scaly lesions over the knuckles (Gottron's sign) are characteristic, with similar lesions occurring on the elbows, knees, and malleoli. A more macular, erythematous rash may appear on the face, neck, and anterior chest (V sign) or on the shoulders and upper back (shawl sign). Subcutaneous calcifications, which do not occur in adult cases, occur in 30% to 70% of childhood cases. The calcinosis tends to develop over pressure points (e.g., buttocks, knees, elbows) and occurs more commonly when the diagnosis has been delayed or the treatment inadequate [Bowyer et al., 1983; Pachman, 1995]. The lesions typically appear as painful, hard nodules that erupt through the skin in severe cases. Occasional patients have the characteristic rash but never develop weakness [Euwer and Sontheimer, 1993; Stonecipher, 1993].

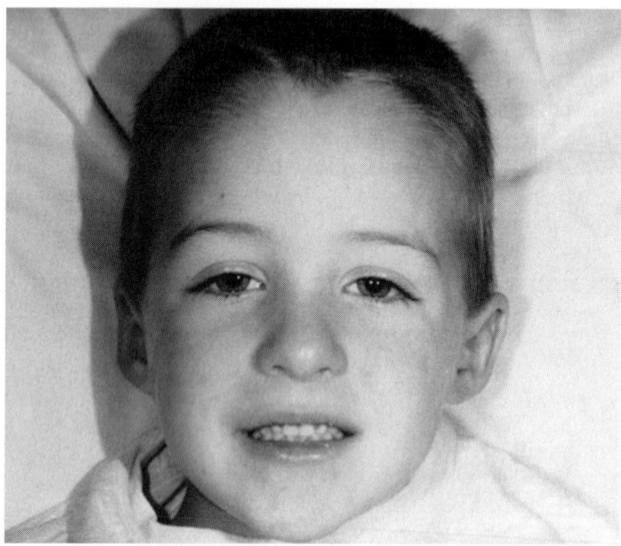

FIGURE 82-1. An 8-year-old male with juvenile dermatomyositis has a mild, erythematous rash over the cheeks, nasal bridge, and eyelids with mild periorbital edema. (Photo courtesy Albert Tsao, MD.)

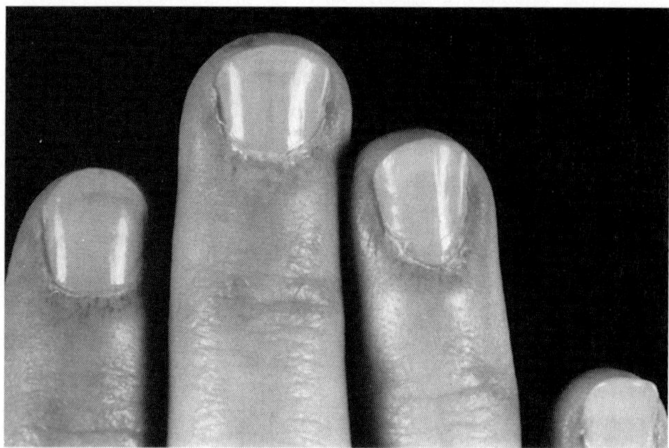

FIGURE 82-2. Close-up view of the fingers of a 17-year-old female with juvenile dermatomyositis. The cuticles are thickened, cracked, and irregular; there are dilated capillary loops at the nail base, especially in the first finger.

ASSOCIATED MANIFESTATIONS

Although involvement of organs other than muscle and skin has become less common with the advent of effective immunosuppressive therapies, some children will develop clinical manifestations in addition to weakness and rash on the basis of the underlying vasculopathy. About 50% will have electrocardiographic abnormalities, including conduction defects and dysrhythmias, and pericarditis, myocarditis, and congestive heart failure can occur [Askari, 1984; Haupt and Hutchins, 1982; Tymms and Webb, 1985]. Pulmonary function tests may demonstrate restrictive defects and reduced diffusion capacity even in patients with no pulmonary symptoms [Pachman, 1994]. Approximately 10% of patients, particularly those with antibodies to histidyl transfer ribonucleic acid synthetase (Jo-1), develop frank interstitial lung disease or bronchiolitis obliterans and organizing pneumonia [Love et al., 1991; Targoff, 1994]. Vasculopathic involvement of the gastrointestinal tract can result in malabsorption, mucosal ulceration, perforation, and hemorrhage. Dysphagia and delayed gastric emptying caused by inflammatory involvement of the alimentary skeletal and smooth muscles are more common.

Arthralgias are common, but true arthritis occurs mainly in children with an "overlap" connective tissue disorder (see later). Ophthalmic involvement on the basis of vascular changes in the retina and conjunctiva can occur [Pachman, 1995]. Renal compromise is rare and results from acute tubular necrosis in the setting of myoglobinuria after fulminant muscle necrosis [Rose et al., 1996]. In contrast to adult dermatomyositis patients, no definitive increased incidence of malignancy has been demonstrated in children [Callen, 1994; Sigugeirsson et al., 1992].

Laboratory Features

The laboratory evaluation of patients with inflammatory myopathy should include muscle enzyme analysis, electrodiagnostic studies, and muscle biopsy. Muscle imaging studies can indicate areas of inflammation in affected muscles but are seldom useful in making a diagnosis [Fraser et al., 1991; Hernandez et al., 1993].

Serologic Studies

Creatine kinase is the most reliable, sensitive, and specific marker for muscle destruction. The creatine kinase level is elevated in more than 90% of patients sometime during the course of the disease, with levels up to 50 times normal [Amato et al., 1996; Dalakas, 1994a; Tymms and Webb, 1985]. Creatine kinase levels often do not correlate with weakness and can be normal even in children with significant weakness. Rarely, serum aldolase can be elevated when the serum creatine kinase is normal. Serum myoglobin, lactate dehydrogenase, aspartate aminotransferase, and alanine aminotransferase can also be elevated but provide no additional information to the creatine kinase. Erythrocyte sedimentation rate is normal or mildly elevated and does not correlate with severity. Antinuclear antibodies occur in 25% to 50% of patients, most commonly in those with overlap syndromes.

Myositis-specific antibodies are associated with specific human leukocyte antigen haplotypes and can be demonstrated in a minority of patients (usually adults) with inflammatory myopathy. There have been few reports of these antibodies in childhood dermatomyositis, and their role in the pathogenesis of the inflammatory myopathies is unclear [Love et al., 1991; Plotz et al., 1995]. Although these antibodies provide some information about prognosis [Joffe et al., 1993; Miller, 1993; Targoff, 1994], their value in managing patients is limited. The only exception is the Jo-1 antibody, which is commonly present in patients with interstitial lung disease. In these Jo-1–positive patients, the interstitial lung disease is often more refractory to treatment, and may require the initiation of therapy with prednisone and a second-line immunosuppressive agent (see "Treatment" later). The presence of interstitial lung disease is also a contraindication to the use of methotrexate, which can itself cause interstitial pulmonary fibrosis.

ELECTROMYOGRAPHY

Electromyography is indispensable in demonstrating that the patient's weakness is myopathic in origin and in determining which muscle to biopsy in patients with mild weakness [Mastaglia and Laing, 1996]. Typical electromyographic features include increased spontaneous activity with fibrillation potentials, positive sharp waves, and occasionally pseudomyotonic and complex repetitive discharges, as well as small-duration, low-amplitude, polyphasic motor unit potentials, which recruit early but at normal frequencies. The amount of spontaneous activity generally reflects the ongoing disease activity.

MUSCLE BIOPSY

Every child suspected of having dermatomyositis should undergo muscle biopsy before therapy is instituted. A characteristic histologic feature is perifascicular atrophy, which occurs in 90% of childhood cases and is relatively specific for dermatomyositis (Fig. 82-3). Traditional teaching has been that the perifascicular small fibers represent the residuals of ischemic damage [Carpenter et al., 1976], but recent evidence suggests that other factors may be involved [Greenberg and Amato, 2004]. Dermatomyositis is clearly associated with a microvasculopathy with capillary loss, and the earliest demonstrable histologic abnormality is deposition of C5b-9 complement membrane attack complex around small blood vessels (as well as immunoglobulin M and other complement components, including C3 and C9) [Emslie-Smith and Engel, 1990; Kissel et al., 1986]. These findings have led to the hypothesis that complement-mediated necrosis of small blood vessels leads to reduced capillary density and ischemic damage of muscle fibers. Supporting this view is the finding that inflammatory cells in dermatomyositis biopsies are predominantly perivascular and perimysial in location (Fig. 82-4). Electron microscopy reveals small intramuscular arterioles and capillaries with endothelial hyperplasia, microvacuoles, and cytoplasmic inclusions.

Pathogenesis

Dermatomyositis is believed to be an autoimmune, humorally mediated microangiopathic disorder. The vascular deposits of immunoglobulin M, C3, and membrane attack complex suggest that the primary immunologic event in dermatomyositis is generation of an antibody directed against antigens located within the walls of intramuscular blood vessels. According to this traditional hypothesis, the microangiopathy then leads to ischemic damage to muscle fibers. The triggers that initiate the immunologic events are uncertain, however, and the putative vascular antigens are unknown. It is also not known whether the complement deposition results from activation of the direct or indirect complement

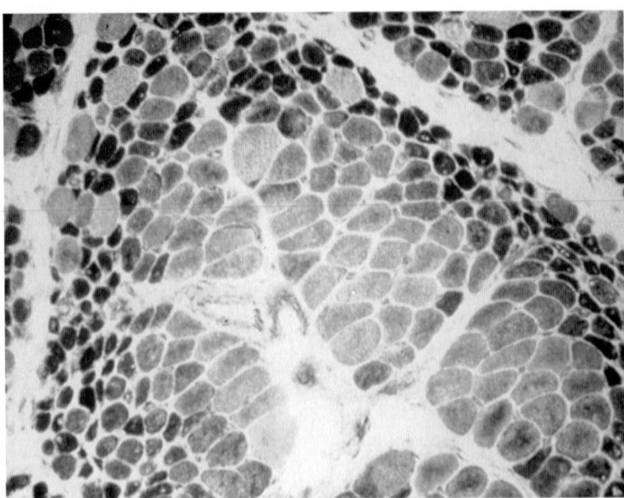

FIGURE 82-3. Bicep biopsy from a patient with dermatomyositis showing characteristic perifascicular atrophy with relative sparing of the central fascicle (ATPase stain, pH 4.6, ×200).

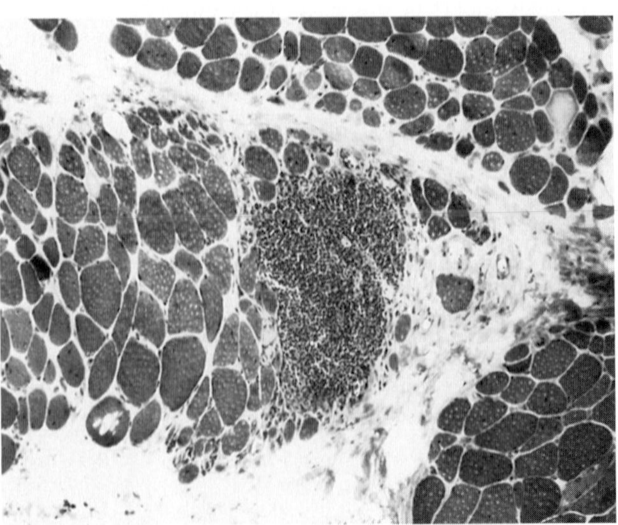

FIGURE 82-4. Muscle biopsy from a patient with juvenile dermatomyositis showing striking focus of perivascular inflammation in a perimysial blood vessel (modified Gomori trichrome, ×400).

cascade or if it is an epiphenomenon, unrelated to the main cause of the capillary destruction [Greenberg and Amato, 2004]. Gene expression studies on muscle biopsies have suggested increased expression of type 1 interferons in patients with dermatomyositis as well as perivascular, perimysial, and endomysial plasmacytoid dendritic cells (primary producers of type 1 interferons) [Greenberg et al., 2005]. This finding suggests that the innate immune system may also be involved in the pathogenesis of dermatomyositis.

Treatment

Although corticosteroids are generally regarded as the most effective therapy for dermatomyositis, there is controversy surrounding the best route of administration, dosing regimen, duration of therapy, and parameters to monitor during therapy [Amato and Griggs, 2003a]. There have been no controlled trials to examine these issues, although retrospective studies have demonstrated that prednisone reduces morbidity and improves strength and function [Adams and Plotz, 1995; Chwalinska-Sadowska and Madykowa, 1990; Dalakas, 1994a; Joffe et al., 1993; Oddis, 1994].

CORTICOSTEROIDS

Prednisone is the usual first line of treatment for dermatomyositis. Short courses of intravenous methylprednisolone (Solu-Medrol) (20 to 30 mg/kg/day or every other day for 3 to 5 days) may be the best way to initiate therapy in severely affected individuals, especially because this therapy may prevent calcinosis [Callen et al., 1994; Laxer et al., 1987]. A more traditional regimen involves oral therapy (1 to 2 mg/kg/day) given as a single morning dose. After 3 to 6 weeks of daily prednisone, the dosage can usually be switched directly to an alternate-day regimen at the same dose, although occasional patients will require persistent daily therapy. The high dose is maintained while strength is carefully monitored. Although the creatine kinase level can sometimes be useful in monitoring response, it should *never* be the primary determinant when therapeutic decisions are made.

Patients should be evaluated at least monthly during this phase of treatment. When the child's strength has returned to normal or improvement has reached a plateau (usually within 4 to 6 months), the prednisone can be tapered at a rate no faster than 5 mg every 2 to 4 weeks. If an exacerbation occurs during the tapering, the prednisone dose is increased back to its original level and again given daily. When strength has recovered, the prednisone taper can be resumed. Although occasional patients will require daily dosing, or even split daily doses to maintain adequate disease control, alternate-day dosing is preferred because it is associated with fewer side effects. Most patients (approximately 80%) improve with therapy, with approximately two thirds having a complete response [Amato et al., 1996; Pachman, 1995].

Because most patients require therapy for 1 to 2 years to achieve remission, limiting the side effects of prednisone is an important part of management [Boumpas et al., 1993]. Patients should be started on a low-sodium, low-carbohydrate, high-protein, low-calorie diet to limit weight gain and reduce the risk of hypertension. Calcium supplementation (1000 to 1500 mg/day) and vitamin D reduce the risk of osteoporosis, as does physical therapy with axial exercise as tolerated by the patient's weakness. Baseline determination of bone density through dual-energy x-ray absorptiometry scanning is indispensable in diagnosing and following osteoporosis in this population. Exercise also reduces the risk of steroid myopathy [Escalante et al., 1993]. Blood pressure, serum glucose and potassium levels, and ocular status (for cataracts and glaucoma) should be assessed periodically. Hip pain in a child on prednisone must be investigated aggressively because avascular necrosis is an uncommon but devastating development in these individuals. Growth retardation and delayed puberty can occur with prolonged therapy.

Although the rash usually responds along with the muscle response, occasional patients require separate treatment for their skin changes. Hydroxychloroquine, chloroquine, topical steroids, topical tacrolimus, and sunscreen have been used to treat the rash when weakness is mild or not apparent [Euwer and Sontheimer, 1993; Sontheimer, 1999; Stonecipher, 1993]. Treatment of calcinosis is more difficult. Colchicine, probenecid, warfarin, and phosphate buffers have been used with only limited success [Pachman, 1994]. Surgery may be indicated, but the lesions may recur or worsen despite surgery.

OTHER AGENTS

Patients who respond poorly to steroids, relapse repeatedly as prednisone is tapered, or develop intolerable side effects are candidates for alternative therapy (Table 82-1). Methotrexate is probably the drug of choice in children, although there are no prospective, controlled studies to guide its use.

TABLE 82-1

Steroid-Sparing Immunosuppressive Therapy for Inflammatory Myopathies

AGENT	ROUTE	DOSE	SIDE EFFECTS	MONITOR
Methotrexate	PO	10-20 mg/m^2/wk	Hepatotoxicity, leukopenia, alopecia, stomatitis, neoplasia	LFTs, CBC
	IV	1-3 mg	Same	Same
Cyclophosphamide	PO	1-2 mg/kg/day	Leukopenia, cystitis, alopecia, infections, neoplasia	CBC, urinalysis
	IV	50-75 mg/m^2	Same, nausea and vomiting	Same
Cyclosporine	PO	0.5-7.5 mg/kg/day	Renal toxicity, hypertension, hirsutism, hepatotoxicity, infection, gum hyperplasia	BP, BUN, Cr, LFTs, drug levels
IVIG	IV	2 g/kg over 2 days	Fevers, chills, diaphoresis, aseptic meningitis, headache, hypotension, leukopenia	BP, BUN, Cr

BP, blood pressure; BUN, blood urea nitrogen; CBC, complete blood count; Cr, creatinine; IV, intravenous; LFTs, liver function tests; PO, orally; IVIG, intravenous immunoglobulin.

In a retrospective series, approximately 75% of children refractory to prednisone improved with methotrexate therapy [Cagnoli et al., 1991; Joffe et al., 1993; Miller et al., 1992b]. Methotrexate must be used with caution because of side effects, including alopecia, stomatitis, oncogenicity, infection, interstitial lung disease, and bone marrow, renal, and liver toxicity. Pulmonary function tests, blood counts, and liver functions must be monitored. Azathioprine, mycophenolate mofetil, cyclophosphamide, and cyclosporine have also been used in refractory patients (see Table 82-1) [Amato and Barohn, 1997; Amato and Griggs, 2003a].

On the basis of a double-blind, placebo-controlled study suggesting benefits in 15 adult dermatomyositis patients, intravenous immunoglobulin has become an important component of the treatment of dermatomyositis [Dalakas et al., 1993]. Although originally used only for refractory cases, it is finding increasing use as both a steroid-sparing agent and a primary agent because of its low incidence of long-term side effects. Treatment is usually initiated at a dose of 2 g/kg given slowly over 2 to 5 days with repeat infusions at variable intervals (usually every 2 to 6 weeks) for at least 3 months [Thornton and Griggs, 1994]. Patients should have an immunoglobulin A level checked before therapy because patients with low immunoglobulin A levels may have anti-immunoglobulin A antibodies, which can cause anaphylactic reactions. Flulike symptoms (i.e., headaches, myalgias, fever, chills, and nausea) may occur in as many as 50% of patients during the infusions but are usually mild. Rash, aseptic meningitis, transient leukopenia, renal failure, and stroke have been described rarely. A controlled trial of plasmapheresis and leukopheresis demonstrated no improvement with either modality in dermatomyositis [Miller et al., 1992a].

Polymyositis

Polymyositis, although common in adults, is relatively rare in children as an isolated entity [Amato and Griggs, 2003b; Dalakas and Hohlfeld, 2003, Hoogendijk et al., 2004; Van der Meulen et al., 2003]. In one epidemiologic study, juvenile dermatomyositis was 10 to 20 times more common than polymyositis [Hanissian et al., 1982]. When polymyositis does occur in children, it is often in the setting of an "overlap" condition with features of another connective tissue disorder [Pachman, 1994; Rider and Miller, 1994]. Because of the absence of the rash, the diagnosis is often delayed compared with dermatomyositis.

Clinical Features

As in dermatomyositis, patients typically present after weeks to months of neck flexor and symmetric proximal greater than distal arm and leg weakness. Muscle pain and tenderness are common. Dysphagia occurs in approximately one third of patients secondary to oropharyngeal and esophageal involvement. Mild facial weakness occasionally may be demonstrated. Sensation and tendon reflexes are usually preserved. As in adults, in children, other organs, most notably the heart and lungs, can be involved, although the incidence appears to be less than in adults. Congestive heart failure or conduction abnormalities and interstitial lung disease are found in rare patients, the latter more commonly in patients

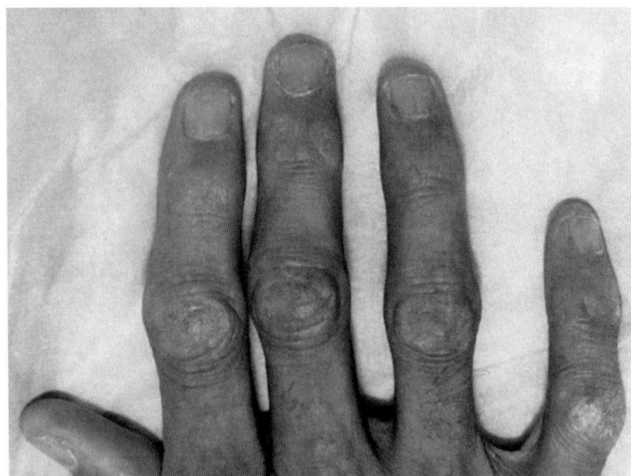

FIGURE 82-5. Scleroderma/dermatomyositis overlap syndrome in a 16-year-old male. There is tapering of the digits with a scaly, erythematous rash over the interphalangeal joints and tightness and thinning of the skin.

with serum anti–Jo-1 antibodies [Love et al., 1991]. Polyarthritis has been reported in as many as 45% of polymyositis patients at the time of diagnosis.

OVERLAP SYNDROMES

In children, polymyositis more frequently occurs as part of an overlap syndrome, where the myositis is associated with another connective tissue disorder, than as an isolated entity. The common overlap syndromes associated with polymyositis (and often dermatomyositis) include scleroderma, mixed connective tissue disease, Sjögren's syndrome, systemic lupus erythematosus, polyarteritis nodosa, and rheumatoid arthritis [Rider and Miller, 1994]. Involvement of the skin, joints, kidneys, eyes, and salivary glands is identical to that seen for each disorder in isolation (Fig. 82-5), and the serologic abnormalities are also similar. Weakness in these patients is not always due to myositis because disuse and type 2 fiber atrophy from chronic steroid treatment of the underlying condition can also result in muscle weakness. In these individuals, it is crucial to document the nature of the muscle involvement with serologic and electromyographic studies and often muscle biopsy. The prognosis is often related to the underlying disorder, and treatment may have to be modified based on the associated condition.

Laboratory Features

Laboratory evaluation in polymyositis is similar to that in dermatomyositis. Unlike dermatomyositis, the serum creatine kinase is essentially always elevated in polymyositis. The serum creatine kinase level can be helpful in monitoring response to therapy but only in conjunction with the physical examination. Positive antinuclear antibodies are present in approximately 30%. Muscle-specific antibodies have been reported to be more common in polymyositis than dermatomyositis [Love et al., 1991; Plotz et al., 1995; Targoff, 1994]. Close analysis of these reports, however, indicates that the muscle histopathology in many of the antibody-positive cases does not demonstrate the typical pathologic features of polymyositis (e.g., there is usually no invasion of non-necrotic muscle fibers by $CD8^+$ T-lympho-

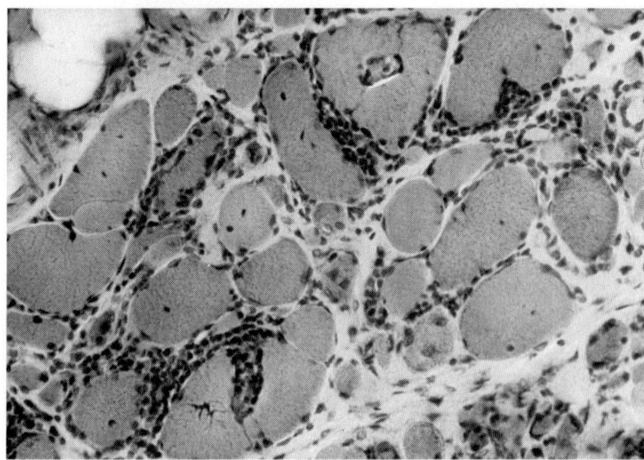

FIGURE 82-6. Muscle biopsy from a patient with polymyositis revealing endomysial inflammation surrounding and occasionally invading *(top right)* individual non-necrotic muscle fibers (hematoxylin and eosin stain, ×500).

cytes). [Greenberg et al., 2002; Miller et al., 2002; Mozaffar et al., 2000]. In some cases, the biopsies are more suggestive of a microangiopathic disorder similar to that seen in dermatomyositis. Electromyography is similar to that in dermatomyositis, with a myopathic picture of increased spontaneous activity, small polyphasic motor units, and early recruitment.

MUSCLE BIOPSY

The pathologic findings of polymyositis are distinct from dermatomyositis and reflect basic differences in the underlying pathophysiology [Amato and Griggs, 2003b; Dalakas and Hohlfeld, 2003; Van der Meulen et al., 2003]. Biopsies are characterized by variability in fiber size, with scattered necrotic and regenerating fibers, and endomysial inflammation, with invasion of non-necrotic muscle fibers by $CD8^+$ cytotoxic/suppressor T cells and macrophages (Fig. 82-6) [Arahata and Engel, 1984; Engel and Arahata, 1984]. The invaded (and some noninvaded) fibers express major histocompatibility complex class 1 antigen, which is not present on normal fibers [Emslie-Smith et al., 1989]. The vascular changes of dermatomyositis are not seen.

Pathogenesis

Polymyositis results from a human leukocyte antigen-restricted, antigen-specific, cell-mediated immune response against muscle fibers. The T-cell receptors of the muscle-invading T cells have an oligoclonal pattern of gene rearrangement, suggesting that the immune response is antigen specific [Mantegazza et al., 1993]. The antigen against which the immune response is generated and the trigger for the autoimmune attack are not known. Although speculation has centered around a viral infection triggering the immune response, viral antigens and genomes have not been identified in the muscle fibers of patients with polymyositis [Leff et al., 1992; Plotz et al., 1995].

Treatment

The treatment of children with polymyositis does not differ in any substantive way from that of dermatomyositis. Corticosteroids are the mainstay of treatment, with secondary agents used as indicated by the response [Amato and Griggs, 2003a]. The role of intravenous immunoglobulin in polymyositis is less clear than in dermatomyositis and should probably be reserved for refractory cases. Treatment of patients with an overlap syndrome is occasionally dictated more by the degree of joint, kidney, or skin involvement than by the muscle disease. Although the majority of patients with polymyositis respond to therapy, the response is often less robust and less sustained than in dermatomyositis. Fewer patients (approximately 20%) attain a complete remission, so that more long-term therapy, along with its associated side effects from medications, is frequently required. Unfortunately, no prospective studies have examined in detail the long-term prognosis of these patients.

Congenital Inflammatory Myopathy

Over the past three decades, there have been scattered reports of infants with "congenital inflammatory myopathy" or "infantile myositis" [Kinoshita et al., 1980, 1986; Nagai et al., 1992; Roddy et al., 1986; Shevell et al., 1990; Thompson, 1982]. The disorder is characterized by perinatal hypotonia and generalized weakness with elevated serum creatine kinase levels, myopathic electromyography, and striking inflammation on muscle biopsy. In one case of well-documented congenital myositis [Roddy et al., 1986], the child was later diagnosed as having Prader-Willi syndrome. Most of the other patients did not improve with corticosteroid therapy, and it is likely that many of these cases had a form of muscular dystrophy with secondary inflammation. Inflammation on biopsy is not specific for a primary inflammatory myopathy and can be demonstrated in Duchenne, facioscapulohumeral, dysferlin-related, and Fukuyama-type muscular dystrophies; Walker-Warburg syndrome; and the Occidental type of congenital dystrophy with hypomyelination and laminin alpha-2 deficiency [Olney and Miller, 1983; Pegoraro et al., 1996]. The diagnosis of inflammatory muscle disease should be made with extreme caution in infants and only after the various dystrophies have been carefully considered.

Other Idiopathic Inflammatory Myopathies

Several other extremely rare inflammatory myositides have been described in children. Eosinophilic myositis has been described in several children with peripheral eosinophilia and focal eosinophilic infiltration in isolated muscles [Agrawal and Giesen, 1981; Kaufman et al., 1993; Nagar and Bar-Ziv, 1993]. The reported cases in children may differ from those in adults in occasionally being a focal rather than diffuse myositis, occurring without a drug or toxin exposure, and sometimes resolving without treatment. The condition usually occurs as a part of the hypereosinophilic syndrome.

Focal nodular myositis, as the name implies, is also a focal disorder associated with mononuclear infiltration in individual muscles causing the subacute onset of focal pain, swelling, and weakness [Flaisler et al., 1993]. Some patients go on to develop generalized polymyositis. Improvement has been reported after surgical excision of the mass but can also occur spontaneously.

A myositis with noncaseating granulomas can occur in sarcoid myopathy, a condition that may respond partially to prednisone [Banker, 1994].

INFLAMMATORY MYOPATHY ASSOCIATED WITH INFECTIONS

Although myositis can occur after a wide variety of bacterial, parasitic, fungal, or viral infections, the viral myositides (especially those caused by influenza), toxoplasmosis, and trichinosis are the disorders most likely to be encountered by the clinician.

Influenza Myositis

Influenza A, B, and rarely C are common upper respiratory tract pathogens. Acute infection is commonly associated with myalgias when fever and other constitutional symptoms are present. The myalgias are presumably caused by the systemic release of cytokines, although a true myositis can develop [Hays and Gamboa, 1994].

Clinical Features

As respiratory symptoms subside, pain, swelling, and muscle tenderness herald the onset of myositis [Hays and Gamboa, 1994; Mejlszenkier et al., 1973; Ruff and Secrist, 1982]. The pain can be so severe as to interfere with the child's ability to walk or perform routine activities, and muscle swelling and induration may be present. Weakness can be profound and myoglobinuria has been reported [Christianson et al., 1990]. The symptoms are self-limited, lasting less than 1 week, although rare patients have recurrent symptoms associated with different influenza types [Ruff and Secrist, 1982].

Laboratory Features

The creatine kinase level is usually elevated, often markedly so, whereas it is typically normal in uncomplicated influenza infection. Electromyography reveals features of an active necrotizing myopathy. Muscle biopsy is rarely indicated but indicates scattered necrotic and regenerating fibers, with occasional interstitial inflammatory cells. Influenza virus has only occasionally been isolated on culture of the muscle specimen [Hays and Gamboa, 1994].

PATHOGENESIS

The mechanism of muscle injury in these patients is unclear. Although muscle damage may result from direct attack of the virus on muscle, electron microscopy has not revealed viral particles in the muscle biopsies, and viral cultures are rarely positive for influenza [Farrell et al., 1980]. An immune-mediated attack on muscle triggered by the virus is another possible mechanism for muscle injury.

TREATMENT

The disorder is usually self-limited, and treatment is supportive, with bed rest, hydration, and acetaminophen or nonsteroidal anti-inflammatory drugs.

OTHER VIRAL MYOSITIDES

Acute viral myositis is not specific for influenza infection, and similar syndromes can complicate infections with coxsackievirus, parainfluenza, mumps, measles, adenovirus, herpes simplex, cytomegalovirus, hepatitis B, Epstein-Barr virus, respiratory syncytial virus, echovirus, and possibly arboviruses [Hays and Gamboa, 1994]. Like influenza, the myositis associated with these viruses is usually self-limited and requires only supportive therapy. Acute and convalescent viral titers (3 or 4 weeks after infection), as well as blood, stool, urine, and throat cultures, can be useful in identifying the responsible virus but seldom add to the management of the muscle symptoms.

An inflammatory myopathy has also been described with infection by human immunodeficiency virus. This disorder usually develops in patients with acquired immune deficiency syndrome but can also occur in early human immunodeficiency virus infection. It has been reported exclusively in adults, although human immunodeficiency virus-infected children are also at risk. The presentation is similar to that of polymyositis with subacute progressive, symmetric proximal weakness, an elevated creatine kinase level, and myopathic electromyography. The disorder must be distinguished from zidovudine (AZT) myotoxicity, human immunodeficiency virus–wasting syndrome, and other disorders that can complicate human immunodeficiency virus infection [Dalakas, 1994b; Illa et al., 1991].

Trichinosis

Trichinosis, the most common parasitic disease of skeletal muscle, is caused by the nematode *Trichinella spiralis,* which is ingested in inadequately cooked meat (usually pork). Most infected patients are asymptomatic.

Clinical Features

Two to 12 days after ingestion, the larval form of the nematode disseminates through the bloodstream and invades the muscles [Davis et al., 1976]. Patients develop fever, headache, abdominal pain, diarrhea, generalized myalgias, and weakness during the acute systemic reaction. Periorbital edema, ptosis, subconjunctival hemorrhage, and an erythematous urticarial or petechial rash are also often present. Myalgias and weakness peak in the third week of the infection but can last for months. Severe disease can be complicated by myocarditis, pneumonitis, and central nervous system infection.

Laboratory Features

Most patients have a marked eosinophilic leukocytosis and elevated serum creatine kinase level. Serum antibodies against *T. spiralis* can be demonstrated 3 to 4 weeks after infection. Electromyography demonstrates the typical features of an inflammatory myopathy. In the early stage of infection, muscle biopsy reveals infiltration of the muscle by eosinophils and polymorphonuclear leukocytes. With more chronic infection, mononuclear inflammatory cells are more common [Gross and Ochoa, 1979]. Larvae, cysts with focal calcification, fibrosis, and granulomas may be observed months after the initial infection (Fig. 82-7).

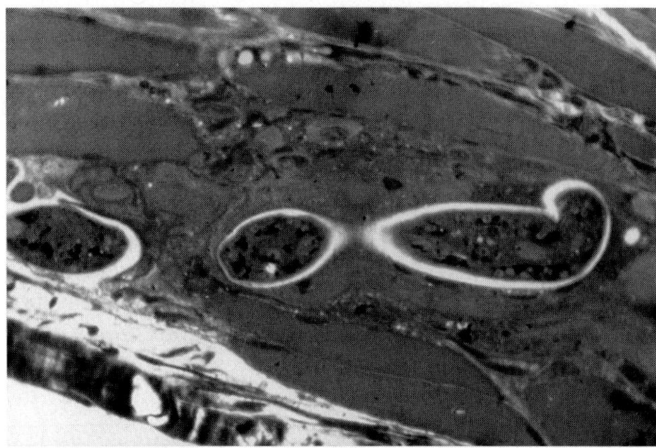

FIGURE 82-7. Muscle biopsy from a patient with trichinosis documenting encysted larvae of the *Trichinella* organism (modified Gomori trichrome, ×550). (Photo courtesy Jerry Mendell, MD.)

Treatment

Thiabendazole (25 mg/kg twice daily to a maximum dose of 3 g/day) is the drug of choice for killing the larvae and adult nematode, with 7 days usually an adequate course of therapy. Thiabendazole is not effective against the encysted larvae, and mebendazole may be a better agent in this regard. Because a Herxheimer-like reaction can develop after degeneration of the larvae, concurrent prednisone administration is beneficial (2 mg/kg/day for several weeks). The majority of patients respond quickly to treatment.

Toxoplasmosis

Toxoplasmosis is caused by the protozoon *Toxoplasma gondii*. The common mode of infection is through the ingestion of food, usually undercooked meat, contaminated with oocysts or cysts containing bradyzoites of the organism. The cysts mature and enter the bloodstream and lymphatics to invade other organs. Exposure to the organism is common worldwide, although symptomatic infection usually occurs in immunocompromised patients. Skeletal muscle involvement can occur in isolation or as part of more generalized infection [Banker, 1994].

Clinical and Laboratory Features

In most patients, symptoms are mild and nonspecific, including fever, malaise, fatigue, and myalgias. Patients with more severe disease have lymphadenopathy, hepatosplenomegaly, uveitis, pneumonia, myocarditis, rash, or meningoencephalopathy. Weakness develops in those with significant muscle involvement [Gherardi et al., 1992; Pollock, 1979]. The serum creatine kinase level is elevated, and the typical myopathic picture is evident on electromyography. Muscle biopsy may reveal cysts containing the organism, along with inflammation and giant cells. The diagnosis is confirmed through serologic studies indicating immunoglobulin M reactivity to the organism.

Treatment

A combination of pyrimethamine and sulfadiazine or trisulfapyrimidines is the treatment of choice for the primary infection, although once the organisms have become encysted in muscle no medication is effective. Clindamycin is also an effective agent and can be used in place of sulfadiazine. The duration of therapy is variable and depends on the severity of the illness.

Cysticercosis

Cysticercosis is caused by the tapeworm *Taenia solium*, another organism usually transmitted through eating undercooked meat. Although central nervous system infection usually dominates the clinical picture, with focal neurologic deficits, seizures, and encephalopathy, skeletal muscles can also be involved. Weakness, myalgias, muscle tenderness, and muscle pseudohypertrophy are accompanied by an elevated creatine kinase level and eosinophilia [Banker, 1994; Sawney et al., 1976]. The biopsy is characterized by fibrosis, inflammation with eosinophils, giant cells, and encysted organisms. Praziquantel (50 mg/kg/day in three divided doses for 2 weeks) is effective against central nervous system infection, but its efficacy in muscle is less clear. Albendazole (15 mg/kg/day in divided doses for 8 days) also has been used. Niclosamide and paromomycin are useful for treating the adult worms, and corticosteroids suppress the inflammatory reaction against degenerating parasites.

Bacterial Infections

Pyomyositis refers to the multifocal abscesses associated with bacterial infection of the muscle. Although bacterial infections are more common in developing countries, they are being seen with increasing frequency in developed countries as a result of human immunodeficiency virus infection and intravenous drug abuse [Antony and Kerodle, 1996; Hsueh et al., 1996; Rodgers et al., 1993].

Muscle pain, tenderness, and fever are the initial symptoms, most commonly affecting the quadriceps, glutei, and deltoids. Most patients have a neutrophilic pleocytosis, elevated erythrocyte sedimentation rate, and normal or elevated serum creatine kinase level. Blood cultures are usually negative early in the infection until the patient becomes septic. Ultrasound, computed tomography, and magnetic resonance imaging of muscle can be useful in localizing abscesses for diagnostic needle aspiration. The most common organisms are *Staphylococcus aureus*, streptococci, *Escherichia coli, Yersinia* organisms, and *Legionella* organisms [Akman et al., 1996; Collazos et al., 1996; O'Neill et al., 1996]. Pyomyositis usually arises as an extension of infection from adjacent tissues or via hematologic spread of the organisms. Early in the illness, the infection may respond to appropriate antibiotics, although more severe infections require incision and drainage.

Fungal Myositides

Fungal infection of the muscles is very uncommon and usually occurs in an immunosuppressed adult patient. Candidiasis is the most common fungal myositis and almost always is associated with disseminated disease [Arena et al., 1981; Jarowski et al., 1978]. Diffuse muscle pain, tenderness, weakness, fever, and a papular erythematous rash are evident but may be obscured by other systemic involvement.

Muscle biopsy demonstrates infiltration of the muscle by hyphal and yeast forms of the organism, inflammation, and hemorrhagic necrosis. Myositis has also been reported complicating cryptococcal infection, sporotrichosis, actinomycosis, and histoplasmosis [Halverson et al., 1985; Heffner, 1993; Wrzolek et al., 1990].

REFERENCES

Adams EM, Plotz PH. The treatment of myositis. How to approach resistant disease. Rheum Clin North Am 1995;21:179.

Agrawal BL, Giesen PC. Eosinophilic myositis: An unusual cause of pseudotumor and eosinophilia. JAMA 1981;246:70.

Akman I, Ostrov B, Varma BK, et al. Pyomyositis: Report of three patients and review of the literature. Clin Pediatr 1996;35:397.

Amato AA, Barohn RJ. Idiopathic inflammatory myopathies. Neurol Clin 1997;15:615.

Amato AA, Gronseth GS, Jackson CE, et al. Inclusion body myositis: Clinical and pathological boundaries. Ann Neurol 1996;40:581.

Amato AA, Griggs RC. Inflammatory myopathies. Curr Opin Neurol 2003a;16:569.

Amato AA, Griggs RC. Unicorns, dragons, polymyositis and other mythical beasts. Neurology 2003b;61:316.

Antony SJ, Kerodle DS. Nontropical pyomyositis in patients with AIDS. J Natl Med Assoc 1996;88:865.

Arahata K, Engel AG. Monoclonal antibody analysis of mononuclear cells in myopathies. I. Quantitative of subsets according to diagnosis and sites of accumulation and demonstration and counts of muscle fibers invaded by T cells. Ann Neurol 1984;16:193.

Arena AP, Perlin M, Brahman H, et al. Fever, rash, and myalgias of disseminated candidiasis during antifungal therapy. Arch Intern Med 1981;141:1233.

Askari AD. Inflammatory disorders of muscle: Cardiac abnormalities. Clin Rheum Dis 1984;10:131.

Banker BQ. Other inflammatory myopathies. In: Engel AG, Franzini-Armstrong C, eds. Myology, 2nd ed. New York: McGraw-Hill, 1994.

Banker BQ, Victor M. Dermatomyositis (systemic angiopathy) of childhood. Medicine (Baltimore) 1966;45:261.

Boumpas DT, Chrousos GP, Wilder RL, et al. Glucocorticoid therapy for immune-mediated diseases: Basic and clinical correlates. Ann Intern Med 1993;119:1198.

Bowyer SL, Blane CE, Sullivan DB. Childhood dermatomyositis: Factors predicting functional outcome and development of dystrophic calcification. J Pediatr 1983;103:882.

Bowyer SL, Clark RAF, Ragsdale CG, et al. Juvenile dermatomyositis: Histologic findings and pathogenic hypothesis for the associated skin changes. J Rheumatol 1986;13:753.

Cagnoli M, Marchesoni A, Tosi S. Combined steroid, methotrexate, and chlorambucil therapy for steroid resistant dermatomyositis. Clin Exp Rheumatol 1991;9:658.

Callen JP. Relationship of cancer to inflammatory muscle diseases: Dermatomyositis, polymyositis, and inclusion body myositis. Rheum Dis Clin North Am 1994;20:943.

Carpenter S, Karpati G, Rothman S, et al. The childhood type of dermatomyositis. Neurology 1976;26:952.

Christianson JC, San Joaquin VH. Influenza-associated rhabdomyolysis in a child. Pediatr Infect Dis J 1990;9:60.

Chwalinska-Sadowska H, Madykowa H. Polymyositis-dermatomyositis: 25 year follow-up of 50 patients—Disease course, treatment, prognostic factors. Mater Med Pol 1990;22:213.

Collazos J, Fernandez A, Martinez E, et al. Pneumococcal pyomyositis. Case report, review of the literature, and comparison with classic pyomyositis caused by other bacteria. Arch Intern Med 1996;156:1470.

Crowe WE, Love KE, Levinson JE, et al. Clinical and pathogenetic implications of histopathology in childhood polydermatomyositis. Arthritis Rheum 1982;25:126.

Dalakas MC. Polymyositis, dermatomyositis, and inclusion body myositis. N Engl J Med 1991;325:1487.

Dalakas MC. How to diagnose and treat the inflammatory myopathies. Semin Neurol 1994a;14:137.

Dalakas MC. Retrovirus-related muscle disease. In: Engel AG, Franzini-Armstrong C, eds. Myology, 2nd ed. New York: McGraw-Hill, 1994b.

Dalakas MC, Illa I, Dambrosia JM, et al. A controlled trial of high dose intravenous immunoglobulin infusions as treatment for dermatomyositis. N Engl J Med 1993;329:1993.

Dalakas MC, Holhfeld R. Polymyositis and dermatomyositis. Lancet 2003;362:971.

Davis MJ, Cilo M, Platitakis A, et al. Trichinosis. Severe myopathic involvement with recovery. Neurology 1976;26:37.

Emslie-Smith AM, Arahata K, Engel AG. Major histocompatibility complex 1 antigen expression, immunolocalization of interferon subtypes, and T cell–mediated cytotoxicity in myopathies. Hum Pathol 1989;20:224.

Emslie-Smith AM, Engel AG. Microvascular changes in early and advanced dermatomyositis: A quantitative study. Ann Neurol 1990;27:343.

Engel AG, Arahata K. Monoclonal antibody analysis of mononuclear cells in myopathies. II: Phenotypes of autoinvasive cells in polymyositis and inclusion body myositis. Ann Neurol 1984;16:209.

Escalante A, Miller L, Beardmore TD. Resistive exercise in the rehabilitation of polymyositis/dermatomyositis. J Rheumatol 1993;20:1340.

Euwer RL, Sontheimer RD. Amyopathic dermatomyositis: A review. J Invest Dermatol 1993;100:124S.

Farrell MK, Partin JC, Bove KE, et al. Epidemic influenza myopathy in Cincinnati in 1977. J Pediatr 1980; 96:545.

Flaisler F, Blin D, Asencio G, et al. Focal myositis: A localized form of polymyositis? J Rheumatol 1993;20:1414.

Fraser DD, Frank JA, Dalakas M, et al. Magnetic resonance imaging in idiopathic inflammatory myopathies. J Rheumatol 1991;18:1693.

Gherardi R, Baidrimont M, Lionnet F, et al. Skeletal muscle toxoplasmosis in patients with acquired immunodeficiency syndrome. Ann Neurol 1992;32:535.

Greenberg SA, Bradshaw EM, Pinkus GS, et al. Interferon α/β-mediated innate mechanisms in dermatomyositis. Ann Neurol 2005;57:664.

Greenberg SA, Sanoudou D, Haslett JN, et al. Molecular profiles of the inflammatory myopathies. Neurology 2002;59:1170.

Greenberg SA, Amato AA. Uncertainties in the pathogenesis of DM. Curr Opin Neurol 2004;13:356.

Gross B, Ochoa J. Trichinosis: Clinical report and histochemistry of muscle. Muscle Nerve 1979;2:394

Halverson PB, Lahiri S, Wojno WC, et al. Sporotrichal arthritis presenting as granulomatous myositis. Arthritis Rheum 1985;28:1425.

Hanissian AS, Masi AT, Pitner SE, et al. Polymyositis and dermatomyositis in children: An epidemiologic and clinical comparative analysis. J Rheumatol 1982;9:390

Haupt HM, Hutchins GM. The heart and conduction system in polymyositis-dermatomyositis. Am J Cardiol 1982;50:998.

Hays AP, Gamboa ET. Acute viral myositis. In: Engel AG, Franzini-Armstrong C, eds. Myology, 2nd ed. New York: McGraw-Hill, 1994.

Heffner RR. Inflammatory myopathies. A review. J Neuropathol Exp Neurol 1993;52:339.

Hernandez RJ, Sullivan DB, Chenevert TL, et al. MR imaging in children with dermatomyositis: Findings and correlations with clinical and laboratory findings. Am J Roentgenol 1993;161:359.

Hoogendijk JE, Amato AA, Lecky BR, et al. Workshop report. 119th ENMC international workshop: Trial design in adult idiopathic inflammatory myopathies, with the exception of inclusion body myositis. Naarden, The Netherlands, October 10-12, 2003. Neuromusc Disord 2004;14:337.

Hsueh PR, Hsiue TR, Hsieh WC. Pyomyositis in intravenous drug abusers: Report of a unique case and review or the literature. Clin Infect Dis 1996;22:858.

Illa I, Nath A, Dalakas MC. Immunocytochemical and virological characteristics of HIV-associated inflammatory myopathies: Similarities with seronegative polymyositis. Ann Neurol 1991;29:474.

Jarowski CI, Fialk MA, Murray HW, et al. Fever, rash, and muscle tenderness. A distinctive clinical presentation of disseminated candidiasis. Arch Intern Med 1978;138:544.

Joffe MM, Love LA, Leff RL. Drug therapy of idiopathic inflammatory myopathies: Predictors of response to prednisone, azathioprine, and methotrexate and a comparison of their efficacy. Am J Med 1993;94:379.

Kaufman LD, Kephart GM, Seidman RJ, et al. The spectrum of eosinophilic myositis: Clinical and immunopathologic studies of three patients, and a review of the literature. Arthritis Rheum 1993;36:1014.

Kinoshita M, Nishina M, Koya N. Ten years follow-up study of steroid therapy for congenital encephalomyopathy. Brain Dev 1986;8:281.
Kinoshita M, Iwasaki Y, Wada F, et al. A case of congenital polymyositis—A possible pathogenesis of "Fukuyama type congenital muscular dystrophy." Clin Neurol 1980;20:911.
Kissel JT, Halterman RK, Rammohan KW, et al. The relationship of complement-mediated microvasculopathy to the histologic features and clinical duration of disease in dermatomyositis. Arch Neurol 1991;48:26.
Kissel JT, Mendell JR, Rammohan KW. Microvascular deposition of complement membrane attack complex in dermatomyositis. N Engl J Med 1986;314:331.
Laxer RM, Stein LD, Petty RE. Intravenous pulse methylprednisolone treatment of juvenile dermatomyositis. Arthritis Rheum 1987;30:328.
Leff RL, Love LA, Miller FW, et al. Viruses in idiopathic inflammatory myopathies. Absence of viral candidate genomes in muscle. Lancet 1992;339:1192.
Love LA, Leff RL, Fraser DD, et al. A new approach to the classification of idiopathic inflammatory myopathy: Myositis-specific autoantibodies define useful homogeneous patient groups. Medicine 1991;70:360.
Mantegazza R, Andreetta F, Bernasconi P, et al. Analysis of T cell receptor of muscle-infiltrating T lymphocytes in polymyositis: Restricted V alpha/beta rearrangements may indicate antigen-driven selection. J Clin Invest 1993;91:2880.
Mastaglia FL, Laing NG. Investigation of muscle disease. J Neurol Neurosurg Psychiatry 1996;60:256.
Medsger TA Jr, Dawson WN, Masi AT. The epidemiology of polymyositis. Am J Med 1970;48:715.
Mejlszenkier JD, Safran AP, Healy JJ, et al. The myositis of influenza. Arch Neurol 1973;29:441.
Miller FW. Myositis-specific antibodies. Touchstones for understanding the inflammatory myopathies. JAMA 1993;270:1846.
Miller FW, Leitman SF, Cronin ME, et al. Controlled trial of plasma exchange and leukopheresis in polymyositis and dermatomyositis. N Engl J Med 1992a;326:1380.
Miller LC, Sisson BA, Tucker LB, et al. Methotrexate treatment of recalcitrant childhood dermatomyositis. Arthritis Rheum 1992b;35:1143.
Miller T, Al-Lozi MT, Lopate G, et al. Myopathy with antibodies to the signal recognition particle: Clinical and pathological features. J Neurol Neurosurg Psychiatry 2002;73:420.
Mozaffar T, Pestronk A. Myopathy with anti-Jo-1 antibodies: Pathology in perimysium and neighbouring muscle fibres. J Neurol Neurosurg Psychiatry 2000;68:472.
Nagai T, Hasgawa T, Saito M, et al. Infantile polymyositis: A case report. Brain Dev 1992;14:167.
Nagar H, Bar-Ziv Y. Focal eosinophilic myositis: Unusual cause of a tumour on the chest wall. Eur J Surg 1993;159:187.
Oddis CV. Therapy of inflammatory myopathy. Rheum Dis Clin North Am 1994; 20:899.
Olney RK, Miller RG. Inflammatory infiltration in Fukayama type congenital muscular dystrophy. Muscle Nerve 1983;6:75.
O'Neill DS, Baquis G, Moral L. Infectious myositis. A tropical disease steals out of its zone. Postgrad Med 1996;100:193.
Pachman LM. Inflammatory myopathy in children. Rheum Dis Clin North Am 1994;20:919.
Pachman LM. Juvenile dermatomyositis. Pathophysiology and disease expression: Pediatr Rheumatol 1995;42:1071.
Pegoraro E, Mancias P, Swerdlow SH, et al. Congenital muscular dystrophy with primary laminin 2 (merosin) deficiency presenting as inflammatory myopathy. Ann Neurol 1996;40:782.
Plotz PH, Rider LG, Targoff IN, et al. Myositis: Immunologic contributions to understanding cause, pathogenesis, and therapy. Ann Intern Med 1995;122:715.
Pollock JL. Toxoplasmosis appearing to be dermatomyositis. Arch Dermatol 1979;115:736.
Rider LG, Miller FW. New perspectives on the idiopathic inflammatory myopathies of childhood. Curr Opin Rheumatol 1994;6:575.
Roddy SM, Ashwal S, Peckham N, et al. Infantile myositis: A case diagnosed in the neonatal period. Pediatr Neurol 1986;2:241.
Rodgers WB, Yodlowski ML, Mintzer CM. Pyomyositis in patients who have the human immunodeficiency virus. Case report and review of the literature. J Bone Joint Surg 1993;75:588.
Rose MR, Kissel JT, Bickley LS, et al. Sustained myoglobinuria: The presenting manifestation of dermatomyositis. Neurology 1996;47:119.
Ruff RL, Secrist D. Viral studies in benign acute childhood myositis. Arch Neurol 1982;39:261.
Sawney BB, Chopra JS, Banerji AK, et al. Pseudohypertrophic myopathy in cysticercosis. Neurology 1976;26:270
Shevell M, Rosenblatt B, Silver K, et al. Congenital inflammatory myopathy. Neurology 1990;40:1111.
Sigugeirsson B, Lindelöf B, Edhag, et al. Risk of cancer in patient with dermatomyositis or polymyositis. N Engl J Med 1992;326:363.
Sontheimer RD. Cutaneous features of classic dermatomyositis and amyopathic dermatomyositis. Curr Opin Rheum 1999;11:475.
Stonecipher MR. Cutaneous changes of dermatomyositis in patients with normal muscle enzymes: Dermatomyositis sine myositis? J Am Acad Dermatol 1993;28:951.
Targoff IN. Immune manifestations of inflammatory disease. Rheum Dis Clin North Am 1994;20:857.
Thompson CE. Infantile myositis. Dev Med Child Neurol 1982;24:307.
Thornton CA, Griggs RC. Plasma exchange and intravenous immunoglobulin treatment of neuromuscular disease. Ann Neurol 1994;35:260.
Tymms KE, Webb J. Dermatomyositis and other connective tissue diseases: A review of 105 cases. J Rheumatol 1985;12:1140.
Van der Meulen MFG, Bronner M, Hoogendijk JE, et al. Polymyositis: A diagnostic entity reconsidered. Neurology 2003;61:316.
Wrzolek MA, Sher JH, Kozlowski PB, et al. Skeletal muscle pathology in AIDS: An autopsy study. Muscle Nerve 1990;13:508.

CHAPTER 83

Channelopathies: Myotonic Disorders and Periodic Paralysis

Richard T. Moxley III and Rabi Tawil

The term *channelopathies* has been extended to include disorders affecting all organ systems, but this chapter focuses on *channelopathies of skeletal muscle.* The initial identification of channelopathies of skeletal muscle began with a number of diseases associated with mutations in the genes for specific channels, including the channels for chloride [Davies and Hanna, 2003; Fahlke et al., 1997a, 1997b; George et al., 1993; Jurkat-Rott and Lehmann-Horn, 2004; Koch et al., 1992; Meyer-Kleine et al., 1995; Zhang et al., 1996], sodium [Cannon, 1996, 2001; Fournier et al., 2004; Lehmann-Horn and Rudel, 1996; Ptacek, 1997; Ptacek et al., 1993], calcium [Greenberg, 1997; McCarthy and Mackrill, 2004], and potassium [Cannon, 2002; Choi et al., 2004; Donaldson et al., 2004; Sanguinetti and Spector, 1997] ions. Periodic symptoms are typical for most channelopathies and occur in disorders other than muscle diseases. For example, familial migraine and hereditary episodic ataxia result from mutations in the calcium channel. These two diseases have joined a growing list of disorders, including familial hypokalemic periodic paralysis, malignant hyperthermia, central core disease, and Lambert-Eaton myasthenic syndrome, that are also calcium channelopathies [Greenberg, 1997]. This chapter limits its discussion to the disorders listed in Box 83-1 and refers the reader to the preceding references for discussion of other channelopathies.

Box 83-1 General Classification of the Channelopathies Seen in Children: Myotonias and Periodic Paralyses

Myotonic disorders of unknown mechanism
- Myotonic dystrophy type 1 (DM1)
- Myotonic dystrophy type 2 (DM2)

Chloride channel myotonias
- Autosomal-dominant myotonia congenita (Thomsen's disease)
- Autosomal-recessive myotonia congenita (Becker's disease)

Sodium channel myotonias
- ***Without periodic paralysis***
- Acetazolamide-responsive myotonia
- Myotonia fluctuans
- ***With periodic paralysis***
- Paramyotonia congenita
- Paramyotonia congenita with hyperkalemic periodic paralysis
- Hyperkalemic periodic paralysis with myotonia
- **Possible sodium or potassium channel abnormality with periodic paralysis**
- **Calcium channel abnormality with periodic paralysis**
- **Possible calcium channel abnormality with periodic paralysis**

THE MYOTONIC DYSTROPHIES: MYOTONIC DYSTROPHY TYPE 1 OF STEINERT AND MYOTONIC DYSTROPHY TYPE 2 (PREVIOUSLY TERMED PROXIMAL MYOTONIC MYOPATHY)

The myotonic dystrophies represent a group of dominantly inherited, multisystem (eye, heart, brain, endocrine, gastrointestinal tract, uterus, skin) diseases that share the core features of myotonia, weakness, and early-onset cataracts (younger than 50 years). Table 83-1 summarizes myotonic dystrophy types 1 and 2. Clinicians considered myotonic dystrophy to be a single disease up until the later part of the 1990s. Steinert and colleagues described the disorder clearly in the early 1900s, and that description is still valid [Harper, 2001]. After the discovery of the gene defect responsible for myotonic dystrophy of Steinert in 1992 [Brook et al., 1992; Fu et al., 1992; Mahadevan et al., 1992] DNA testing revealed a group of patients with dominantly inherited myotonia, proximal greater than distal weakness, and cataracts who were previously diagnosed as having myotonic dystrophy but who after testing lacked the gene defect responsible for myotonic dystrophy of Steinert. Subsequent clinical studies of kindreds with patients having these characteristics led to the use of new diagnostic labels for these patients, myotonic dystrophy type 2 [Thornton et al., 1994] and proximal myotonic myopathy (PROMM) [Ricker et al., 1994a]. Later studies demonstrated that many of the families identified as having myotonic dystrophy type 2 or PROMM had the same disease, a disorder that results from an unstable four nucleotide repeat expansion [CCTG] on chromosome 3 [Liquori et al., 2001]. This disease is similar to, but distinct from, classic myotonic dystrophy of Steinert. It is referred to as myotonic dystrophy type 2 [Day et al., 1999, 2003; Thornton et al., 1994].

The existence of different types of myotonic dystrophy has created a need to develop a diagnostic classification. To address this need, the International Myotonic Dystrophy Consortium developed a new nomenclature and guidelines for deoxyribonucleic acid (DNA) testing [IDMC, 2000].

Myotonic dystrophy of Steinert, the classic form of myotonic dystrophy that results from an unstable trinucleotide repeat expansion on chromosome 19, is now termed myotonic dystrophy type 1 (DM1). Patients with the clinical picture of myotonic dystrophy type 2/proximal myotonic

TABLE 83-1

Myotonias Due to Unstable Nucleotide Repeat Expansion

CLINICAL FEATURES	MYOTONIC DYSTROPHY OF STEINERT (MYOTONIC DYSTROPHY TYPE 1, [DM1])	MYOTONIC DYSTROPHY TYPE 2 (PROXIMAL MYOTONIC MYOPATHY—DM2)
Inheritance	Dominant	Dominant
Gene defect	Chromosome 19; CTG expansion affecting a protein kinase; repeat size ranges from 50 to >2000; normal 5-37 repeats	Chromosome 3; CCTG expansion affecting the zinc finger 9 protein gene; repeat sizes vary from 78 >11,000; normal <78 repeats
Age of onset	Broad range of ages (infancy to adulthood), with infant onset in most severe cases	Broad range of ages (late childhood to late adulthood)
Myopathy	Face, eyes, forearm, hands, and legs, with generalized weakness and hypotonia in affected infants	Mild; thighs, hips, neck flexors, occasional calf muscle hypertrophy
Myotonia	Primarily affects hand and forearm muscles and tongue; occasionally affects respiratory muscles and smooth muscle, such as intestine or uterus; myotonia improves with heat and exercise; myotonia results from a decrease in chloride channel protein	Mainly in hands and thighs; varies; frequently hard to detect; pain occurs sometimes with and without myotonia; myotonia improves with repeated contractions; myotonia results from a decrease in chloride protein
Provocative stimuli	Myotonia worsened by rest and cold; myotonia is relatively constant in severity and muscles affected	Myotonia worsened by rest but varies in severity, occasionally being absent on clinical examination; hand grip and thigh stiffness are usual sites
Therapy for symptoms	Bracing; cataract removal; monitoring dysrhythmias and respiratory insufficiency; pacemaker; antimyotonia therapy (mexiletine); avoid depolarizing muscle relaxants, opiates, and barbiturates with surgery for all of these myotonic disorders	Cataract removal; occasional need for pacemaker; antimyotonia therapy often not necessary (mexiletine); monitor carefully during and after surgery for muscle rigidity and rhabdomyolysis

myopathy (DM2), who have positive DNA testing for the unstable four nucleotide repeat expansion on chromosome 3, are now classified as having DM2. Patients with myotonia, proximal greater than distal weakness, and early onset cataracts with negative DNA testing for DM1 and DM2 are classified as having the "PROMM syndrome" or as having possible DM3 or as having an unclassified form of myotonic dystrophy [Meola and Moxley, 2004]. Reliability of DNA testing to establish the diagnosis of or to exclude DM1 is close to 100% [Harper, 2001]. However, caution is necessary in excluding the diagnosis of DM2. DNA testing methodology used in the recent past to screen for DM2 may have failed to detect as many as 20% of affected individuals [Day et al., 2003]. It will be necessary to use the more sensitive DNA testing methodologies for DM2 [Bachinski et al., 2003; Day et al., 2003] to rule out this disorder. Patients need to undergo this more sensitive DNA testing before a care provider raises the possibility that the individual has another form of myotonic dystrophy, such as DM3 and so on.

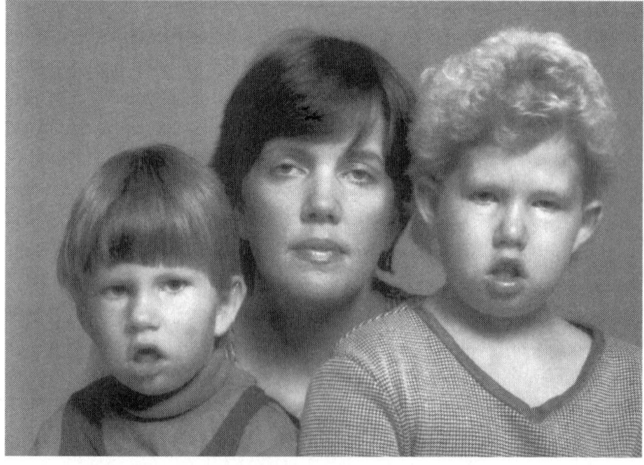

A

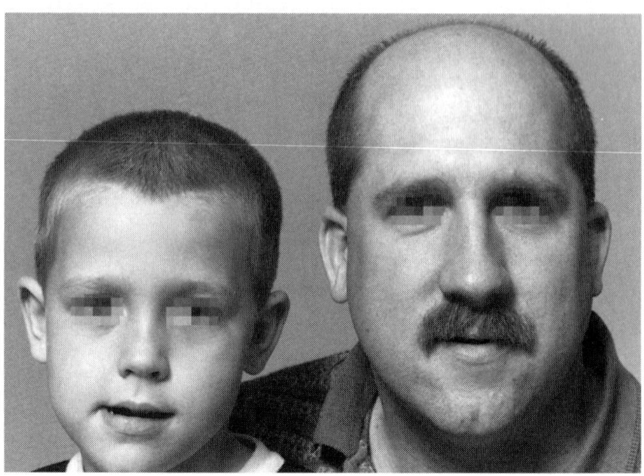

B

FIGURE 83-1. Mother with mild-to-moderate myotonic dystrophy with her two children, both of whom have the congenital form of myotonic dystrophy *(upper panel)*. Father and son both have mutations in the gene for the skeletal muscle sodium channel and have the acetazolamide-responsive form of sodium channel myotonia *(lower panel)*.

Myotonic Dystrophy Type 1

Clinical Features and Subclassification

DM1 is a multisystem, autosomal dominantly inherited, highly variable muscle disease with an incidence of 1 in 8000 individuals (see Table 83-1) [Harper, 2001; Moxley, 2003]. In childhood it presents as a severe congenital form or in a milder form in early school years. The congenital form presents at birth with respiratory failure, poor feeding, generalized hypotonia, clubfoot deformity, and an increased risk of intracerebral hemorrhage and eventration of the diaphragm [Harper, 2001]. During gestation there are often reduced fetal movements and a history of polyhydramnios. There is an increased frequency of placenta previa and miscarriage [Harper, 2001; Rudnik-Schoneborn and Zerres,

2004], and not uncommonly a failed labor may require urgent cesarean section. During the perinatal period, infants with congenital myotonic dystrophy may require continuous ventilator support, and those remaining ventilator dependent beyond 4 weeks of age have a poor prognosis for survival [Campbell et al., 2004; Harper 2001]. During the first 2 years of life, children with congenital myotonic dystrophy are at increased risk for aspiration pneumonitis and difficulties with feeding. Mental retardation and learning disabilities are common in congenital myotonic dystrophy. Determining the degree of cognitive deficit requires careful evaluation because these patients have marked facial weakness and are unable to speak and communicate well until mid to late childhood. There is also an increased incidence of hearing loss [Harper, 2001]. These problems complicate results of neuropsychologic testing. The upper panel of Figure 83-1 shows a mother with two daughters, both of whom have congenital myotonic dystrophy. Both children have delayed ability to speak and cognitive impairment. Their mother has mild ptosis, minimal grip myotonia, and minimal distal weakness. She is fully employed and has no cognitive impairment. This mother has the classic adult-onset form of myotonic dystrophy [Harper, 2001; Moxley, 2003].

The later childhood-onset form usually is evident from nonmuscular manifestations of the disease, such as intellectual deficiency, difficulty with speech or hearing, clumsiness, or rarely with a cardiac dysrhythmia or postoperative apnea [Harper, 2001; Moxley, 2003; Sabovic et al., 2003]. An increased sensitivity to sedative medications, especially barbiturates and opiates, occurs in DM1 and occasionally muscle stiffness/myotonia worsens during general anesthesia [Harper et al., 2004; Moxley, 2003]. Cardiac arrhythmias are more common complications for the adult-onset forms of DM1 [Bhakta et al., 2004; Harper, 2001]. However, other nonmuscular manifestations, such as gastrointestinal hypomotility with chronic constipation, and intermittent urinary tract symptoms, such as urgency or frequent urination, are common in childhood myotonic dystrophy [Harper, 2001; Harper et al., 2004].

Genetics

DM1 results from an unstable trinucleotide expansion in the 3′ untranslated region of a gene on chromosome 19 that codes for a serine/threonine protein kinase, DMPK [Brook et al., 1992; Fu et al., 1992; Mahadevan et al., 1992]. The function of this kinase, DMPK, remains unclear. The cause of the unstable CTG repeat expansion is also unknown. Recent research suggests that premutations arise from the upper normal range of CTG sizes and become pathologically enlarged within a few generations [Abbruzzese et al., 2002; Martorell et al., 2001]. More recent investigation demonstrates that mitomycin C can enhance enlargement of pathologically expanded repeats and promote enlargement of normal repeats [Pineiro et al., 2003]. Inhibitors of replication also modulate instability of the CTG repeat in the DM1 gene in cultured cells [Yang et al., 2003]. These observations raise the possibility that environmental/external factors may influence the development of pathologic enlargement of CTG repeats at the DM1 locus. The normal size of the [CTG]n repeats ranges from 5 to 37 repeats. Children with the congenital form of DM1 have expansions typically greater than 1500 repeats [Harley et al., 1993; Lavedan et al., 1993; Redman et al., 1993; Tsilfidis et al., 1992]. Moderately affected adults with DM1 have [CTG]n sizes ranging from 300 to 1000 repeats, and mildly affected individuals have expansions from 50 to 200 repeats.

The unstable expansion of the DM1 gene provides an explanation for the well-described phenomenon of anticipation, that is, the earlier onset of more severe manifestations of disease in successive generations. Figure 83-1 emphasizes the phenomenon of anticipation in that the mother who has mild-to-moderate DM1 has had two children with severe congenital DM1.

Pathophysiology

There are no examples of point mutations in the DMPK gene locus that have caused the clinical picture of DM1. There is evidence in a recently described mouse model of DM1 that certain disease manifestations may result largely from the CTG repeat expansion alone [Mankodi et al., 2000] without requiring either the presence of or disturbance of the DMPK gene or flanking genes. The molecular pathomechanism of DM1 appears in large part to result from a toxic effect of the abnormally expanded mRNA that accumulates in the nuclei of target tissues [Mankodi and Thornton, 2002; Mankodi et al., 2003; Ranum and Day, 2002; Timchenko et al., 2002]. The abnormal mutant transcripts contain expansions of CUG repeats that interfere with the normal regulation of splicing of specific premessenger ribonucleic acids. Accumulation in muscle nuclei of this expanded mRNA interrupts the production of important proteins, such as the insulin receptor and the skeletal muscle chloride channel. Investigations of muscle biopsies from DM1 patients have discovered abnormal splicing of the insulin receptor [Savkur et al., 2001] and the skeletal muscle chloride channel [Charlet et al., 2002; Mankodi et al., 2002]. The previously mentioned transgenic mouse model of DM1 also demonstrates a defect in splicing and offers a means to examine the pathophysiologic alterations that occur [Mankodi et al., 2000, 2002]. Studies of the transgenic DM1 mouse model demonstrate that the myotonia results from a severe decrease in chloride conductance that is associated with a marked deficiency of normal chloride channel protein. The severity of the defect in production of the chloride channel relates directly to the size of the CUG repeat in the transgene and to its level of expression [Mankodi et al., 2002].

Clues as to how the accumulations of expanded ribonucleic acid lead to the defect in splicing of specific pre-mRNAs have come from studies of muscleblind knockout mouse models of DM1 [Kanadia et al., 2003] and from studies of muscleblind staining in muscle biopsies from DM1 patients [Mankodi et al., 2003]. Disruption of the muscleblind 1 gene in mice leads to muscle, eye, and RNA splicing abnormalities that are characteristic of DM1 [Kanadia et al., 2003]. The double-stranded RNA binding nuclear regulatory factor, muscleblind, binds to CUG repeats in the intranuclear accumulations containing the abnormally expanded DM1 mRNA, and only proteins in the muscleblind family are recruited to these foci [Mankodi et al., 2003]. A deficiency of muscleblind or at least an improper distribution of this nuclear regulatory protein occurs in DM1 and appears to be an important contributor to the defect in splicing and the disease manifestations.

The cause of the muscle wasting and weakness remains a mystery. In the DM1 mouse model the mice do not develop muscle wasting or significant weakness. In patients there are hormonal abnormalities, including testosterone deficiency, insulin resistance, hyperinsulinemia, and altered release of growth hormone, which may contribute to muscle wasting due to deficient anabolism; but, to date, therapeutic trials restoring or exceeding physiologic levels of these hormones have failed to reverse the weakness and wasting [Harper, 2001; Moxley et al., 2004].

Clinical Laboratory Tests

Identification of the abnormal expansion of [CTG]n repeats in the DMPK gene on chromosome 19 establishes the diagnosis of DM1. Electromyography to detect myotonia is helpful in older children, but myotonia may be absent in infancy or in early childhood. Slit-lamp examination to identify the typical iridescent, spokelike posterior capsular cataracts is helpful. Muscle biopsy is not necessary to diagnose DM1 but may be useful to exclude other disorders. Careful examination of the mothers of patients with suspected congenital DM1 is more useful than a muscle biopsy. The biopsy in adults indicates prominent central nuclei, scattered angular fibers, pyknotic nuclear clumps, and type 1 fiber atrophy. Creatine kinase levels may be normal or elevated and are not of primary value in the diagnosis.

Treatment

With the discovery of the gene defect in DM1, it is possible to perform both prenatal and perinatal genetic counseling. Analysis of the DNA isolated from amniocytes or chorionic villus samples can predict the delivery of affected infants and the severity of illness [Harley et al., 1993; Harper, 2001; Redman et al., 1993].

Treating patients with congenital myotonic dystrophy involves ventilatory support, use of a feeding tube, and bracing for clubfoot deformities when present (Fig. 83-2) [Harper, 2001; Harper et al., 2004]. Figure 83-2 shows the molded plastic orthosis that helps treat foot deformity later in childhood. Speech problems and abdominal pain may improve with antimyotonia treatment. Mexiletine is sometimes helpful in alleviating some of the symptoms, especially in later childhood or adolescence when patients may have recurrent dislocation of the mandible and pain and muscle spasm in the masseter muscles. Electrocardiographic monitoring is necessary on a regular basis, particularly during treatment with mexiletine to search for covert dysrhythmias. Treatment should be coordinated with the child's school to ensure that cognitive deficiencies and hearing deficits are monitored. The increased risk for cardiac dysrhythmia and apnea after administration of general anesthesia for surgery

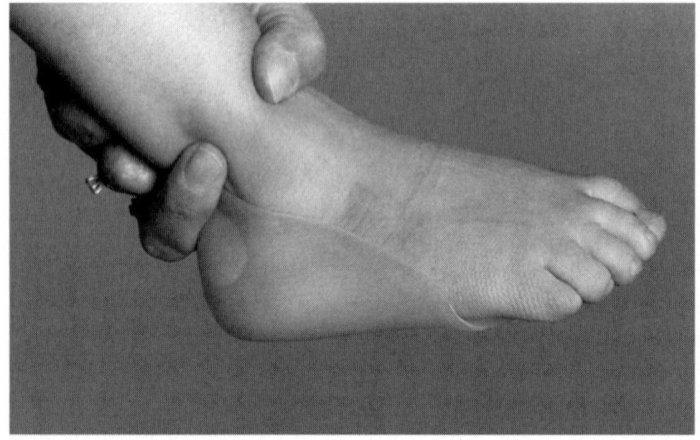
A

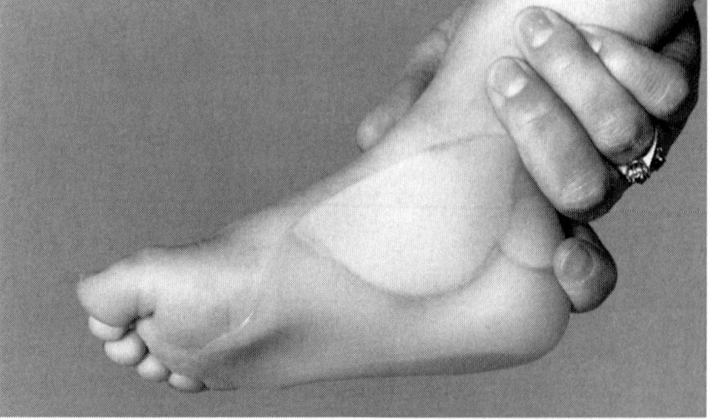
B

C

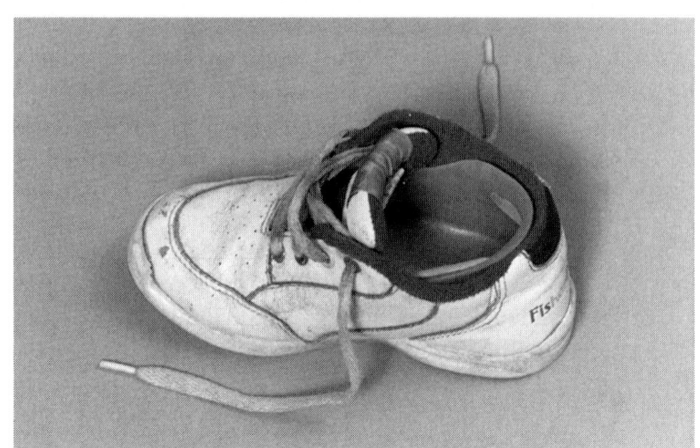
D

FIGURE 83-2. An example of the plastic, molded foot orthosis that is useful in the treatment of clubfoot deformity in congenital myotonic dystrophy.

requires overnight hospitalization with monitoring. Apnea can develop several hours after a patient has been extubated [Harper et al., 2004; Moxley, 2003]. No specific limitation on physical activity is necessary during childhood provided the child has gained sufficient strength and coordination to carry out activities requested in the school environment.

Myotonic Dystrophy Type 2 (Formerly Proximal Myotonic Myopathy)

Clinical Features

DM2/PROMM typically appears in adult life and has variable manifestations, such as early-onset cataracts (younger than 50 years), varying grip myotonia, thigh muscle stiffness, and muscle pain, as well as weakness (hip flexors, hip extensors, or long flexors of the fingers) [Day et al., 1999, 2003; Meola, 2000; Moxley et al., 2002; Ricker et al., 1994a, 1995; Schoser et al., 2004; Thornton et al., 1994]. These complaints often appear between 20 and 50 years of age, and patients as well as their care providers ascribe them to overuse of muscles, "pinched nerves," "sciatica," arthritis, or fibromyalgia. Younger patients may complain of stiffness or weakness when running up steps. The muscle pain has no consistent relationship to exercise or to the severity of myotonia found on clinical examination. The pain, which tends to come and go without obvious cause, usually fluctuates in intensity and distribution over the limbs. It can last for days to weeks. This pain seems qualitatively different from the muscle and musculoskeletal pain that occurs in patients with DM1.

Early in the presentation of DM2 there is only mild weakness of hip extension, thigh flexion, and finger flexion. Myotonia of grip and thigh muscle stiffness vary from minimal to moderate severity over days to weeks. Direct percussion of forearm extensor and thenar muscles is the most sensitive clinical test for myotonia in DM2. Myotonia of grip is sometimes prominent and often has a jerky quality that seems to differ from that in DM1 and the nondystrophic myotonias. Myotonia is often less apparent in DM2 compared with patients with DM1. In cases of late-onset DM2, myotonia may only appear on electromyographic testing after examination of several muscles [Day et al., 2003; Ricker et al., 1995]. Facial weakness is mild in DM2 as is muscle wasting in the face and limbs. Weakness of neck flexors is frequent. Trouble arising from a squat is common, especially as the disease progresses. Calf muscle hypertrophy occasionally is prominent [Ricker et al., 1994a, 1995; Thornton et al., 1994]. Other manifestations, such as excessive sweating, hypogonadism, glucose intolerance, cardiac conduction disturbances, and cognitive/neuropsychologic alterations may also occur and worsen over time [Day et al., 1999, 2003; Meola et al., 1999, 2003].

At present there is no evidence of a congenital form of DM2 [Day et al., 2003]. However, there is evidence of anticipation, with earlier onset of more prominent symptoms, in studies of parent-child pairs [Schneider et al., 2000]. When symptoms occur in childhood, they typically are transient and relate to grip myotonia in the hands and thighs. Proximal weakness, muscle pain, cataracts, and occasional cardiac dysrhythmias usually do not develop until mid or late adult life [Ricker et al., 1995; Thornton et al., 1994].

Genetics

DM2 results from an unstable four nucleotide repeat expansion, CCTG, in intron 1 of the zinc finger protein 9 gene on chromosome 3q21 [Bachinski et al., 2003; Liquori et al, 2001, 2003; Ranum et al., 1998]. The cause for the unstable expansion is unknown. The size of the CCTG repeat appears to increase over time in the same individual, and, like DM1, it is a dynamic gene defect [Day et al., 2003]. The size of the CCTG repeat in normal leukocyte DNA is less than 75 repeats [Day et al., 2003; Liquori et al., 2001]. The size in DM2 ranges from 75 to over 11,000 repeats [Day et al., 2003; Liquori et al., 2001]. The gene mutation responsible for DM2 appears to have arisen from a northern European founder [Bachinski et al., 2003; Liquori et al., 2003].

Pathophysiology

The molecular pathomechanism leading to the manifestations of DM2 is believed to be similar to that in DM1 and relates to a toxic effect of the abnormally expanded RNA that accumulates in the muscle nuclei [Mankodi and Thornton 2002; Mankodi et al., 2003; Ranum and Day, 2002; Timchenko et al., 2002]. There is no apparent relationship between the putative functions of the zinc finger protein 9 gene at 3q21 and the DM1 gene at 19q13.3 or their gene products [Liquori et al., 2001]. Flanking genes are not similar for the DM2 and DM1 loci. A toxic effect of the ribonucleic acid made from the unstable, abnormally expanded, nucleotide repeats in the DM2 and DM1 genes is likely to serve as the common mechanism for their disease manifestations. Both DM2 and DM1 have intranuclear accumulations of abnormally expanded ribonucleic acid, and both have ribonuclear foci that bind the nuclear regulatory protein, muscleblind [Mankodi et al., 2003]. Muscleblind is necessary for the muscle cell to produce the proper type of chloride channel. Abnormal splicing of the skeletal muscle chloride channel [Mankodi et al., 2002] and insulin receptor [Savkur et al., 2001, 2004] occurs in both DM2 and DM1, and DM2 and DM1 produce a severe deficiency of chloride channel protein on immunostaining of muscle biopsies from the patients [Mankodi et al., 2002]. Sequestering of muscleblind and thwarting of its normal function appears responsible for the abnormal splicing.

The cause for the weakness in DM2 is unclear. Patients with DM2, in contrast to patients with classic DM1, usually have only mild muscle wasting. However, there is an uncommon, adult-onset variant of DM2, termed proximal myotonic dystrophy [Udd et al., 1997] that causes severe wasting of proximal arm and thigh muscles as the illness progresses. Patients with the proximal myotonic dystrophy variant of DM2 have the identical CCTG repeat expansion at 3q21 that occurs in patients with DM2 [Bachinski et al., 2003]. The reason for the severe muscle wasting in this variant compared with DM2 patients is unknown. Whether individuals with proximal myotonic dystrophy [Udd et al., 1997] share an underlying mechanism responsible for muscle wasting that is similar to the mechanism in DM1 remains to be established. If the pathomechanism of muscle wasting in this variant of DM2 is the same as DM1, what cellular mechanism limits the loss of muscle in DM2?

Clinical Laboratory Tests

Leukocyte DNA testing is available for DM2. DNA testing methodology used in the recent past to screen for DM2 may have failed to detect as many as 20% of affected individuals [Day et al., 2003]. It is necessary to use the more sensitive DNA testing methodologies for DM2 [Bachinski et al., 2003; Day et al., 2003; Jakubiczka et al., 2004; Sallinen et al., 2004] to rule out this disorder. Patients need to undergo this more sensitive DNA testing before considering the possibility that the individual has another form of myotonic dystrophy.

Slit-lamp examination to detect early cataract formation and electromyography, especially of the first dorsal interosseous, anterior tibialis, and anterior thigh muscles, are useful. Grip myotonia varies in severity and may be absent. Some patients have an elevation (twofold to fourfold) in creatine kinase and gamma glutamyltransferase levels. Patients with elevated creatine kinase values may have greater postoperative complications [Ricker et al., 1995]. A recent comparison of muscle biopsy findings in DM2 with those in classic DM1 indicates that there is less severe atrophy of fibers in DM2, and that in DM2 there are subgroups of very small type 2 fibers and nuclear clumps [Vihola et al., 2003]. Both DM2 and DM1 display abundant central nuclei on their biopsies [Day et al., 2003; Harper, 2001; Vihola et al., 2003], but it appears that DM2 is predisposed to type 2 fiber atrophy and DM1 to type 1 fiber atrophy [Schoser et al., 2004b; Vihola et al., 2003].

Treatment

In general the management of DM2 is similar to that of DM1, but there is less need for supportive care, such as bracing, scooters, or wheelchairs. Cataracts require monitoring, and serial monitoring with an electrocardiogram (ECG) is necessary to check for covert dysrhythmia. Disturbances in cardiac rhythm are less frequent in DM2, but abnormalities do occur [Day et al., 2003; Moxley et al., 2002]. Hypogonadism and insulin resistance need monitoring as in DM1. Myotonia tends to be less marked and less troublesome in DM2, but in specific circumstances antimyotonia therapy is helpful, especially if muscle stiffness is frequent and persistent. Cognitive difficulties also occur in DM2 as in DM1 but become manifest in adult life and appear to be associated with decreased cerebral blood flow to frontal and anterior temporal lobes [Meola et al., 1999] and decreased brain volume [Akiguchi et al., 1999; Chang et al., 1998; Flachenecker et al., 2003]. The changes are less severe than in DM1. Their etiology is unknown but may relate to the toxic effect of intranuclear accumulations of abnormally expanded RNA. Management of these brain symptoms is similar to that for DM1.

A frequent and difficult problem in DM2 is the peculiar muscle pain described earlier. The exact mechanism underlying the pain is unknown, and there is no well-established, effective treatment. Carbamazepine or mexiletine along with nonsteroidal anti-inflammatory medications ameliorate this pain in some patients.

Autosomal-Dominant and Autosomal-Recessive Myotonia Congenita

Thomsen's disease (autosomal-dominant myotonia congenita) and Becker's disease (autosomal-recessive myotonia congenita) represent two forms of chloride channelopathies (Table 83-2).

The chloride channelopathies that produce myotonia as their primary symptom resemble the sodium channel disorders without periodic paralysis and may resemble mild forms of DM1 and DM2. Other causes of muscle stiffness or poor coordination, including central nervous system diseases affecting the frontal lobes, brainstem, and cerebellum, require initial consideration but are rarely confused with these channelopathies.

Clinical Features

Generalized painless myotonia is the major clinical symptom in dominant and recessive forms of chloride channel

TABLE 83-2

Chloride Channel Myotonias

CLINICAL FEATURES	AUTOSOMAL-DOMINANT MYOTONIA CONGENITA OF THOMSEN	AUTOSOMAL-RECESSIVE GENERALIZED A MYOTONIA OF BECKER
Inheritance	Dominant	Recessive
Gene defect	Chromosome 7; mutation in skeletal muscle chloride channel	Chromosome 7; mutation in skeletal muscle chloride channel
Age of onset	Infancy to early childhood	Late childhood, occasionally starts earlier or begins in teens
Myopathy	Muscle hypertrophy frequent; no myopathy, although variants uncommonly develop weakness	Occasional muscle wasting and weakness can occur late; hypertrophy of muscles frequently occurs in legs
Myotonia	Generalized stiffness, especially after rest; improves with exercise; prominent myotonia of eye closure, but not paradoxical myotonia	Generalized stiffness, especially after rest; transient weakness is prominent after complete relaxation for several minutes; myotonia occurs in eyes; no paradoxical myotonia
Provocative stimuli	Prolonged rest or maintenance of the posture	Prolonged rest or maintenance of the same posture
Therapy for symptoms	Exercise; antimyotonia therapy (e.g., mexiletine); Achilles' tendon stretching helps prevent need for heel cord–lengthening surgery	Exercise; especially avoiding prolonged rest; antimyotonia therapy (e.g., mexiletine); transient weakness does not improve after mexiletine

myotonia congenita. Symptoms develop in the first or second decade of life. Myotonic stiffness occurs with sudden physical exertion after a period of rest. Repeated muscle contractions ameliorate the stiffness. This response is the "warm-up phenomenon," which helps distinguish chloride channel myotonia congenita from certain forms of sodium channel myotonia that display increasing muscle stiffness with repeated contractions, a paramyotonic response. DM1 and DM2, like chloride channel myotonia, demonstrate the typical warm-up response.

In contrast to Thomsen's disease, patients with autosomal-recessive myotonia congenita have transient muscle weakness. The transient weakness appears for a few seconds during the initial attempt at a specific movement after a period of inactivity [Zwarts and VanWeerden, 1989]. Muscle strength improves to normal after several strong contractions [Baumann et al., 1996; Zwarts and VanWeerden, 1989].

Patients have prominent muscle hypertrophy, especially in the legs in both the autosomal-dominant and autosomal-recessive forms of myotonia congenita. Tendon reflexes, cerebellar function, sensation, and strength are normal. Myotonia is present in the grip on eye closure, and there is a lid lag. If patients lie supine for 5 to 10 minutes and suddenly arise, generalized myotonic stiffness in the proximal and paraspinous muscles becomes apparent.

Genetics

Point mutations in the gene for the skeletal muscle chloride channel cause both autosomal-dominant [Fahlke et al., 1997a; Grunnet et al., 2003; Koch et al., 1992; Pusch, 2002; Pusch et al., 1995] and autosomal-recessive [Koch et al., 1992; Pusch, 2002; Zhang et al., 1996] forms of myotonia congenita. Autosomal-dominant myotonia congenita (Thomsen's disease) may vary considerably in age of onset and severity of myotonia [Duno et al., 2004; Koty et al., 1996]. It is possible to screen for known point mutations in the chloride channel gene on chromosome 7 [Abdalla et al., 1992], but this genetic testing for the more than 60 mutations is not routinely available.

Pathophysiology

Electrophysiologic studies in myotonic goats [Lipicky and Bryant, 1993] and human muscle tissue from patients with autosomal-dominant and autosomal-recessive [Koch et al., 1992; Rudel et al., 1994] myotonia congenita demonstrate a decreased chloride conductance. The decreased chloride conductance across the transverse tubular system renders the muscle membrane hyperexcitable, which leads to after-depolarization and repetitive firing, creating clinical myotonia. Both autosomal-dominant myotonia congenita (Thomsen's disease) and generalized autosomal-recessive myotonia congenita (Becker's disease) involve mutations at the same locus [George et al., 1993; Koch et al., 1992]. Current models for the chloride channel indicate that two subunits combine to form a double-barreled entry gate for chloride ions and a single outflow channel [Duffield et al., 2003; Fahlke et al., 1997a, 1997b; Jentsch et al., 2002; Pusch, 2002; Saviane et al., 1999]. Dominant mutations affect the common outflow channel (slow flow channel) and recessive mutations require involvement of the two faster flow entry gates [Duffield et al., 2003]. The model proposes that involvement of only one entry gate does not cause clinical disease. Recessive mutations cause a pathologic reduction in chloride current because both fast gates undergo blockade, and dominant mutations cause pathologically reduced current because they affect the slower, common exit channel for chloride ions. The variations in the clinical severity of certain very rare dominantly inherited forms chloride channel myotonia, such as "myotonia levior" [Ryan et al., 2002; Wu et al., 2002], and "fluctuating myotonia" [Wagner et al., 1998], are interesting, and point to limitations in our current version of the model as explanation for the clinical spectrum of findings. A more recent report further emphasizes the limitation of the model. This report describes two unrelated families with the Becker recessive form and two unrelated families with the Thomsen dominant form of myotonia congenita, all of whom have a common R894X mutation [Duno et al., 2004]. The dominant family with the most severe phenotype expressed twice the expected amount of the R894X mRNA allele. These findings suggest that allelic variation may be an important modifier of disease progression in myotonia congenita.

The model for the chloride channel also does not provide an explanation for the transient weakness that is a prominent clinical feature in generalized autosomal recessive (Becker's myotonia) myotonia congenita. Its cause remains to be discovered.

Clinical Laboratory Tests

Evaluation of patients with suspected myotonia congenita should include consideration of other myotonic disorders, such as DM1, DM2, paramyotonia congenita, sodium channel myotonias of other types, and chondrodystrophic myotonia (Schwartz-Jampel syndrome) (see Table 83-2). DM1 patients typically have facial and distal muscle weakness. DNA analysis reveals an abnormal expansion of [CTG]n repeats in the DMPK gene on chromosome 19. Patients with DM2 have an abnormal expansion of [CCTG]n repeats in the zinc finger 9 protein gene on chromosome 3. Patients with chondrodystrophic myotonia (Schwartz-Jampel syndrome) have typical dysmorphic features, dwarfism, and distinctive myotonic discharges on electromyography, which are neurogenic in origin.

Distinguishing patients with chloride channel myotonia, either autosomal-dominant or autosomal-recessive forms, from those with sodium channel myotonic disorders is difficult. Both cause myotonic stiffness and muscle hypertrophy, especially in the legs. One distinguishing feature of sodium channel myotonia is the paradoxical myotonia of the eyelids that develops with repeated forceful eye closure. Figure 83-3 shows the response to looking up and down and to eye closure in a patient with DM1. The patient in Figure 83-4 has sodium channel myotonia, exhibiting lid lag and persisting myotonia after forceful closure of the eyes. If this patient repeats the forceful closure of his eyes, his myotonia worsens. Persistent myotonia of the eyelids also occurred in this patient's son. In contrast, patients with autosomal-dominant and autosomal-recessive forms of chloride channel myotonia exhibit warm-up after repeated contractions. Patients with chloride channel myotonia do not have a

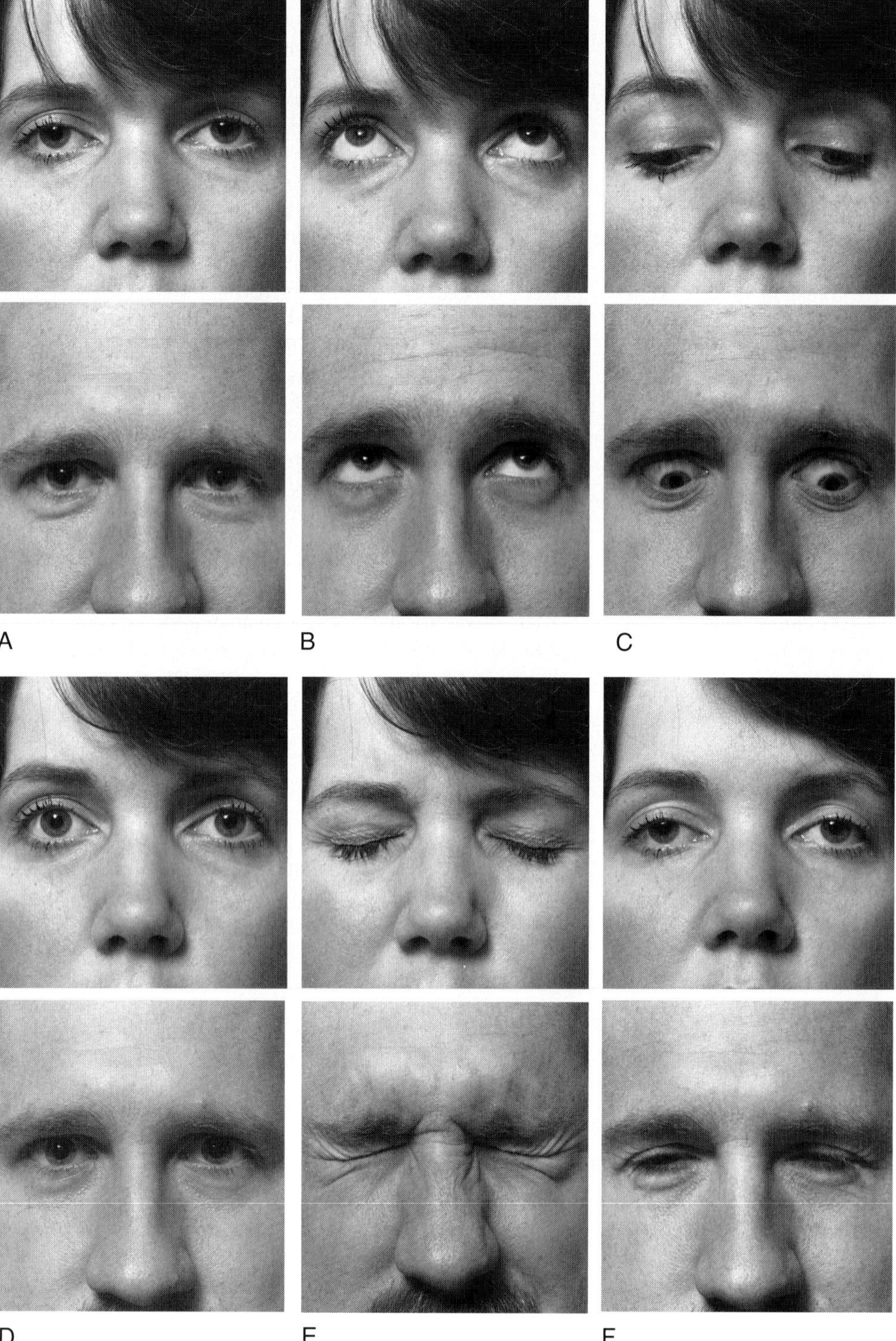

FIGURE 83-3. Sequential photographs of the mother with myotonic dystrophy in Figure 83-1 looking up, looking down, and closing her eyes *(upper panel)*. Sequential photographs of the father with acetazolamide-responsive sodium channel myotonia in Figure 83-1 looking up, looking down, and closing his eyes *(lower panel)*.

worsening of myotonic stiffness or paralysis after prolonged exposure of muscle to cold. To search for cold-induced paralysis, it is necessary to soak the hand or forearm muscles in cold water (15° C) for 15 to 20 minutes. If there is weakness with exercise after this cold exposure, this strongly favors sodium channel myotonia rather than chloride channel disease. The subsequent section on sodium channel myotonia briefly describes the laboratory evaluation of the sodium channelopathy disorder, hyperkalemic periodic paralysis. In that section the use of provocative testing using potassium loading as a diagnostic test is discussed. Sodium channel myotonic disorders are typically "potassium sensitive." An elevation in extracellular potassium markedly worsens myotonia in sodium channelopathies but not in chloride channel myotonia.

Treatment

Antimyotonia treatment with mexiletine is often helpful [Ceccarelli et al., 1992]. Before initiating treatment with mexiletine, a baseline ECG is necessary to identify patients with unsuspected cardiac conduction abnormalities. Side effects of mexiletine, which are usually mild and dose related, include dysgeusia, light-headedness, and diarrhea. Tocainide, another lidocaine derivative similar to mexiletine, was another useful alternative [Kwiecinski et al., 1992], but it is no longer available. Isolated reports suggest that carbamazepine may be a readily available alternative antimyotonia medication for myotonia congenita [Berardinelli et al., 2000; Sheela, 2000]. Children with moderately severe myotonia develop heel cord shortening and contractures at their elbows. If these contractures do not respond to stretching and other physical therapy exercises, it is appropriate to initiate antimyotonia treatment even when patients do not complain of stiffness.

Acetazolamide-Responsive Sodium Channel Myotonia and Myotonia Fluctuans

Two disorders that mimic myotonia congenita and are forms of sodium channel myotonia without periodic paralysis include acetazolamide-responsive sodium channel myotonia and myotonia fluctuans (Table 83-3).

The discovery that hyperkalemic periodic paralysis and paramyotonia congenita result from mutations in the gene for the skeletal muscle sodium channel [Cannon, 2002; Lehmann-Horn and Jurkat-Rott, 1999; Ptacek and Bendahhou, 2001] has led to further investigations that have identified a group of patients with myotonia without episodic weakness, whose myotonia is worsened by potassium intake and who have mutations in the gene for the skeletal muscle sodium channel [Lerche et al., 1993; Ptacek et al., 1992, 1994b; Ricker et al., 1990, 1994b; Trudell et al., 1987]. This section reviews two of these disorders, acetazolamide-responsive myotonia [Ptacek et al., 1994b; Trudell et al., 1987] and myotonia fluctuans [Ricker et al., 1990, 1994b], which resembles chloride channel myotonia. A review of two other rare nondystrophic myotonic disorders caused by mutations in the sodium channel, myotonia permanens and chronic myotonia [Lerche et al., 1993], is not included. The reader is referred to the reports describing these uncommon disorders.

Clinical Features

Acetazolamide-responsive sodium channel myotonia often initially presents to the pediatrician rather than the neurologist with common complaints, such as clumsiness causing frequent falls, a lazy eye, growing pains, back muscle spasm, or stridor. Parents may observe that after prolonged crying an infant or young child will have "their eyes stuck." This is a manifestation of paradoxical eyelid myotonia that develops with repeated bouts of forceful closure of the eyes during crying. Myotonia is most apparent in the face, eyes, and larynx in very young patients. Stiffness in the hands, proximal limb muscles, and paraspinous muscles is more apparent in middle childhood. Muscle hypertrophy, especially in the legs, is frequent. Cerebellar function, sensory testing, tendon reflexes, and muscle strength are normal. Grip and percussion myotonia, as well as lid lag, are present. The severity of these complaints varies both in affected individuals within the same kindred and between kindreds. Episodes of painful muscle spasm occur in some patients, usually during or immediately after exercise. Pain is not common in most myotonic disorders. Acetazolamide-responsive sodium channel myotonia and DM2 are exceptions.

The clinical findings in myotonia fluctuans are similar to those described previously for acetazolamide-responsive sodium channel myotonia, with one important additional finding. The severity of the muscle stiffness fluctuates to a greater degree in this illness. On "good days" the myotonia can vanish. The fluctuating myotonia also has an interesting relationship to prolonged exercise. A phenomenon termed *exercise-induced delayed-onset myotonia* occurs [Ricker et al., 1990]. Patients report that after a period of rest following vigorous exercise, if they resume exercise "at the wrong time," severe muscle stiffness may develop. The time interval between the period of rest and the resumption of exercise is critical. If it is only a few minutes or an hour or more, stiffness does not occur. During the intermediate time interval, the fluctuation and provocation of severe myotonia happen.

The myotonic symptoms in both acetazolamide-responsive sodium channel myotonia and myotonia fluctuans tend to persist throughout a patient's lifetime. Some individuals note a lessening in severity in mid to late adulthood. This finding may represent only an adjustment to the illness and a decrease in physical activity.

Genetics

Acetazolamide-responsive sodium channel myotonia results from a mutation in the gene for the skeletal muscle sodium

TABLE 83-3

Sodium Channel Myotonias without Periodic Paralysis

CLINICAL FEATURES	ACETAZOLAMIDE-RESPONSIVE SODIUM CHANNEL MYOTONIA	MYOTONIA FLUCTUANS
Inheritance	Dominant	Dominant
Gene defect	Chromosome 17; mutation in skeletal muscle sodium channel	Chromosome 17; mutation in skeletal muscle sodium channel
Age of onset	First decade	First or second decade
Myopathy	Rare	Rare; muscle hypertrophy common
Myotonia	Face, paraspinal muscles, paradoxical myotonia of eyelids, grip limbs; varies in severity and often there is pain with myotonia	Face, limbs, eyelids; frequently fluctuates in severity, especially after exercise
Provocative stimuli	Fasting, cold, oral potassium, infection	Exercise-rest-exercise, oral potassium
Therapy for symptoms	Acetazolamide, mexiletine; avoid high-potassium diet; monitor during and after surgery for rigidity and rhabdomyolysis	Mexiletine; avoid high-potassium diet; monitor during and after surgery for rigidity and rhabdomyolysis

channel [Ptacek et al., 1994b] as does myotonia fluctuans [Ricker et al., 1994b]. The mutations in these two disorders of the sodium channel are not identical. Two separate mutations produce myotonia fluctuans [Ricker et al., 1994b]. Both disorders are autosomal dominant.

Pathophysiology

Both of these nondystrophic sodium channel myotonic disorders worsen with an elevation in extracellular potassium. The myotonic stiffness can totally disable a patient under these circumstances. The specific mechanism by which the fluctuation in severity of myotonia occurs remains unclear, but it may relate in part to hormonal fluctuations. The levels of insulin, corticosteroids, and other hormones may exert an important influence on extracellular potassium levels [Lehmann-Horn et al., 1994; Ricker et al., 1994b].

Clinical Laboratory Tests

Routine DNA testing is not available; however, several research laboratories screen for known mutations in the gene for the sodium channel in selected patients. The remainder of the laboratory evaluation is as described previously for chloride channel myotonia.

Treatment

Acetazolamide often controls myotonic stiffness and pain in acetazolamide-responsive sodium channel myotonia [Ptacek et al., 1994b]. This treatment usually ameliorates the muscle pain. Annual ultrasound of the abdomen is useful to detect early formation of kidney stones, which are the major complication of acetazolamide [Tawil et al., 1993]. Dysesthesia and dysgeusia are common side effects. Attacks of severe muscle spasm and pain often improve with cyclobenzaprine. Patients undergoing surgery require monitoring during and after the procedure for signs of worsening muscle stiffness. Maintaining plasma potassium levels between 3.8 and 4.2 mEq/L helps to decrease perioperative muscle stiffness. Stress, muscle tissue damage, and bleeding all elevate plasma potassium levels and worsen myotonia. Postoperatively, intravenous diazepam or lorazepam may be necessary to decrease myotonic stiffness, especially if patients are unable to take medications by mouth. Mexiletine is an effective alternative to acetazolamide, and, if necessary, these drugs can be used in combination.

The management of myotonia fluctuans is similar to that of acetazolamide-responsive sodium channel myotonia. Careful attention to the pattern and timing of exercise helps to decrease episodes of severe muscle stiffness. Intraoperative and postoperative monitoring is important, as noted previously.

PERIODIC PARALYSES

This section focuses on those disorders listed in Tables 83-4 and 83-5, which are associated with periodic paralyses, including channelopathies affecting the sodium, potassium, and calcium channels in skeletal muscle. The general classification of the periodic paralyses is as primary (inherited) or secondary (acquired) forms and as to the change in serum potassium level, such as hyperkalemic or hypokalemic. Paralytic attacks may last from less than 1 hour to several days. Weakness can be localized or generalized. Tendon reflexes decrease or disappear during attacks. Muscle fibers become unresponsive to either direct or indirect electrical stimulation. The generalized attacks of weakness usually begin in proximal muscles and spread to distal ones. Respiratory and cranial muscles tend to be spared but occasionally may become paralyzed. Rest after exercise tends to provoke weakness in the muscles that have undergone the exercise, but continued mild exercise may abort attacks. Exposure to cold may provoke weakness in certain sodium channel-related forms of periodic paralysis. Complete recovery usually occurs after attacks. Permanent weakness and irreversible pathologic changes sometimes occur.

Disorders that cause periodic weakness in otherwise normal individuals are uncommon. In patients with a clear autosomal-dominant family history and in whom the serum potassium level indicates a clear increase or decrease during the paralytic attack, the diagnosis of a specific type of periodic paralysis is obvious. However, on many occasions a patient has an episode of weakness at home or arrives late in the attack or after recovery. Some patients have relatively

TABLE 83-4

Sodium Channel Myotonias with Periodic Paralysis

CLINICAL FEATURES	PARAMYOTONIA CONGENITA	PARAMYOTONIA CONGENITA WITH HYPERKALEMIC PERIODIC PARALYSIS	HYPERKALEMIC PERIODIC PARALYSIS WITH MYOTONIA
Inheritance	Dominant	Dominant	Dominant
Gene defect	Chromosome 17; mutation in skeletal muscle sodium channel	Chromosome 17; mutation in skeletal muscle sodium channel	Chromosome 17; mutation in skeletal muscle sodium channel
Age of onset	First decade	First decade	First decade
Myopathy	Very rare	Rare	Infrequent
Myotonia	Especially paradoxical myotonia of the eyelids, and grip	Especially paradoxical myotonia of the eyelids, and grip	Especially paradoxical myotonia of the eyelids
Provocative stimuli	Cold exposure followed by exercise leads to focal paralysis; occasionally exercise provokes stiffness, but cold does not cause weakness	Oral potassium load, rest after exercise mainly in morning (hyperkalemic weakness), cold exposure followed by exercise (focal paralysis)	Rest after exercise, cold, oral potassium
Therapy for symptoms	Mexiletine, mild exercise, keep patient warm	Mild exercise, thiazides, mexiletine	Thiazides, acetazolamide, sodium restriction

TABLE 83-5

Channelopathies with Hypokalemic Periodic Paralysis

CLINICAL FEATURES	ANDERSEN'S SYNDROME: PERIODIC PARALYSIS WITH CARDIAC DYSRHYTHMIA	CALCIUM CHANNEL PERIODIC PARALYSIS	SODIUM CHANNEL PERIODIC PARALYSIS	POTASSIUM CHANNEL PERIODIC PARALYSIS	PERIODIC PARALYSIS WITH THYROID DISEASE
Inheritance	Dominant	Dominant	Dominant	Dominant	Sporadic—occasionally dominant
Gene defect	Chromosome 17; affects Kir2.1 potassium channel	Chromosome 1; affects skeletal muscle calcium channel	Chromosome 17; affects skeletal muscle sodium channel	Chromosome 11; affects MiRP2 subunit of potassium channel	Unknown
Age of onset	First or second decade	First to third decade	First to third decade	Second to third decade	Third decade (males 20:1)
Myopathy	Typical; also short stature; dysmorphic features; prolonged QT interval on electrocardiogram; ventricular dysrhythmias	Moderately common late; vacuoles frequently seen on biopsy	Not yet determined	Not yet determined	Infrequent
Myotonia	No	No	No	No	No
Provocative stimuli	Rest after exercise, oral glucose	High-carbohydrate meals, rest after exercise, cold, emotional stress/ excitement	High-carbohydrate meals, rest after exercise, cold, emotional stress/ excitement	Usually by strenuous exercise followed by rest. Less consistent provocation after high carbohydrate intake	High-carbohydrate meals, rest after exercise, acetazolamide
Therapy for symptoms	Mild exercise, glucose, high sodium intake, acetazolamide, dichlorphenamide	Acetazolamide, dichlorphenamide, potassium, spirolactone	Acetazolamide, dichlorphenamide, potassium, spirolactone	Acetazolamide	Propranolol, restoration of euthyroid state, oral potassium, spironolactone

mild attacks, and diagnostic laboratory findings or clues from physical examination are not present. Some patients with inherited forms of periodic paralysis have other medical problems, and these coexisting problems may complicate the history and findings as the care provider attempts to develop a differential diagnosis. Certain general guidelines are useful to consider.

The hereditary forms of periodic paralysis manifest symptoms within the first two decades of life, and on initial evaluation there is usually no difficulty distinguishing the cause of the weakness from the cause of weakness in patients with cerebral dysfunction, spinal cord disease, nerve root damage, or neuromuscular transmission failure. Muscle weakness, fatigue, or gait instability caused by illnesses involving the central nervous system, nerve roots, or neuromuscular junction become manifest during exercise. This contrasts with symptoms of periodic paralysis, which virtually never develop during exercise. Occasionally there is a lack of clear-cut family history or clinical findings to identify autosomal dominant inheritance. If other family members have symptoms, molecular genetic testing can assist in confirming the diagnosis. Ultimately, however, some children need to undergo provocative testing with potassium loading, cold exposure, and glucose loading to establish a diagnosis.

Hyperkalemic Periodic Paralysis

Clinical Features

Table 83-4 outlines the major clinical and diagnostic features of hyperkalemic periodic paralysis, as well as important issues in management. All three forms are transmitted as autosomal dominant with high penetrance in both sexes [Cannon, 2002; Lehmann-Horn and Jurkat-Rott, 1999; Moxley, 2000; Ptacek, 1998]. Attacks begin in childhood and are usually brief, being shorter and more frequent than attacks in hypokalemic periodic paralysis. The attacks can occur with or without myotonia and in certain families hyperkalemic paralysis occurs in combination with coexisting paramyotonia congenita [Cannon, 2002; Lehman-Horn and Jurkat-Rott, 1999; Moxley 2000; Ptacek, 1998]. At the onset of an attack, myalgia may develop. Patients with hyperkalemic periodic paralysis plus myotonia frequently develop muscle stiffness and prominent paradoxical myotonia of the eyelids during attacks. Similar symptoms occur in patients with hyperkalemic periodic paralysis in association with paramyotonia congenita. Most patients with hyperkalemic attacks manifest signs of myotonia and notice increasing muscle tension, especially in the paraspinous muscles.

Genetics

All clinical variants of hyperkalemic periodic paralysis result from mutations in the gene for the skeletal muscle sodium channel [Barchi, 1995; Cannon, 1997, 2002; Lehmann-Horn and Jurkat-Rott, 1999; Lehmann-Horn et al., 1994; Miller et al., 2004; Ptacek et al., 1993, 1994a], but the exact mutation can differ despite the fact that clinical symptoms are indistinguishable.

Pathophysiology

In hereditary primary hyperkalemic periodic paralyses with and without myotonia, the net movement of potassium is opposite of that which occurs in hereditary hypokalemic periodic paralysis. There is an enhanced urinary excretion of potassium, a decrease in serum sodium concentration and in urinary excretion of sodium, and a decrease or unaltered serum chloride level [Moxley, 1994]. These findings are consistent with the egress of potassium and entry of sodium into muscle cells during attacks. During attacks of weakness in both hyperkalemic periodic paralysis and in paramyotonia congenita, there is an abnormally increased sodium conductance leading to depolarization of the muscle [Lehmann-Horn et al., 1994]. Patients with hyperkalemic periodic paralysis have a strong diurnal sensitivity to attacks of weakness, which occur primarily in the morning [Ricker et al., 1989]. This sensitivity may relate to circulating factors, such as glucocorticoids and beta-adrenergic hormones. Interestingly, salbutamol and metaproterenol, both beta-adrenergic drugs, are capable of increasing muscle strength during attacks [Lehmann-Horn et al., 1994; Ricker et al., 1989].

Clinical Laboratory Tests

The primary laboratory evaluation involves monitoring of serum electrolytes during attacks to identify hyperkalemia or hypokalemia and monitoring the ECG to search for any evidence of dysrhythmia or other conduction disturbance, such as the ECG changes that occur in Andersen-Tawil syndrome. A dominant family history helps to limit additional laboratory testing to search for secondary forms of hyperkalemia, which might lead to muscle weakness. Laboratory evaluation for secondary hyperkalemic weakness should include a search for hormonal disturbances, such as insulin deficiency or adrenal insufficiency, or toxic effects of medications, such as beta-adrenergic antagonists, alpha-adrenergic agonists, digitalis intoxication, or the use of succinylcholine. In patients not observed during a spontaneous attack of weakness, it may be necessary to perform provocative testing with oral potassium loading or exercise followed by potassium challenge [Moxley, 2000].

Treatment

Attacks of weakness in hyperkalemic periodic paralysis are seldom severe enough to require emergency room evaluation. Oral glucose hastens recovery. Severe attacks usually respond to 2 g/kg of glucose by mouth and 15 to 20 units of crystalline insulin subcutaneously. Occasionally, severe attacks may fail to respond to these treatments. Calcium gluconate, 0.5 to 2 g intravenously, is sometimes effective, as is the inhalation of beta-adrenergic agents, such as metaproterenol, every 15 minutes for three doses.

Preventive treatment includes avoidance of fasting, exposure to cold, and overexertion. A prudent consumption of frequent meals high in carbohydrate content is helpful. Diuretics that promote kaluresis, such as hydrochlorothiazide and carbonic anhydrase inhibitors, are the primary therapies.

Paramyotonia Congenita

Clinical Features

Symptoms develop usually during the first decade of life and have a predilection for facial, lingual, neck, and hand muscles (see Table 83-4) [Lehmann-Horn and Jurkat-Rott, 1999; Moxley, 2000]. Attacks of increased muscle stiffness followed by paralysis occur on exposure to cold followed by exercise. The hallmark clinical sign is paradoxical myotonia or paramyotonia, that is, stiffness that worsens with repeated muscle contraction. This sign is most prominent in the muscles of eye closure. Clinical myotonia may be restricted to the eye muscles and not be apparent in grip or after percussion.

Genetics

Mutations in the gene for the skeletal muscle sodium channel in several locations cause paramyotonia congenita [Cannon, 2002; Lehmann-Horn and Jurkat-Rott, 1999; Miller et al., 2004; Ptacek, 1998], but they tend to fall into the following two general groups: (1) those in the S3-S4 segments in domain 4 near the extracellular surface of the membrane; and, (2) those in the cytoplasmic loop between domains 3 and 4. Patients with paramyotonia congenita associated with hyperkalemic periodic paralysis have mutations in the cytoplasmic loop between domains 3 and 4 [Bouhours et al., 2004; Lehmann-Horn and Jurkat-Rott, 1999; Ptacek, 1998]. There is considerable variation in the severity of symptoms both within and between kindreds, and this variation does not correlate closely with the exact mutation [Lehmann-Horn and Jurkat-Rott, 1999; Mohammadi et al., 2003]. One recent report indicates that the combined form of hyperkalemic periodic paralysis and paramyotonia congenita, with the severe phenotype beginning in infancy, involves a specific mutation, methionine substitution at codon 704 (T704M) [Brancati et al., 2003]. More studies are necessary to establish this phenotype-genotype correlation.

Clinical Laboratory Tests

Standardized testing using immersion of the hand and forearm in cold water for 15 minutes followed by exercise is effective in provoking paramyotonic stiffness and paralysis in most patients [Moxley, 2000; Ricker et al., 1990]. Most cooperative children can tolerate this testing. If no clear evidence of cold-induced muscle stiffness and weakness is apparent, further laboratory testing as indicated previously under hyperkalemic periodic paralysis and as noted under laboratory tests for chloride channel myotonia may be necessary. DNA analysis to search for known mutations in the gene for the sodium channel is available in selected research laboratories and in the future may become routinely available.

Pathophysiology

As in hyperkalemic periodic paralysis caused by sodium channel dysfunction, paramyotonia congenita also has increased sodium conductance and excessive depolarization of the muscle membrane [Cannon, 2002; Bouhours et al., 2004; Lehmann-Horn and Jurat-Rott, 1999]. The electrophysiologic defect in hyperkalemic periodic paralysis and paramyotonia congenita differs. This difference is apparent in the response of forearm muscle to cooling and exercise. In hyperkalemic periodic paralysis, cooling of forearm muscle followed by forceful contractions leads to mild

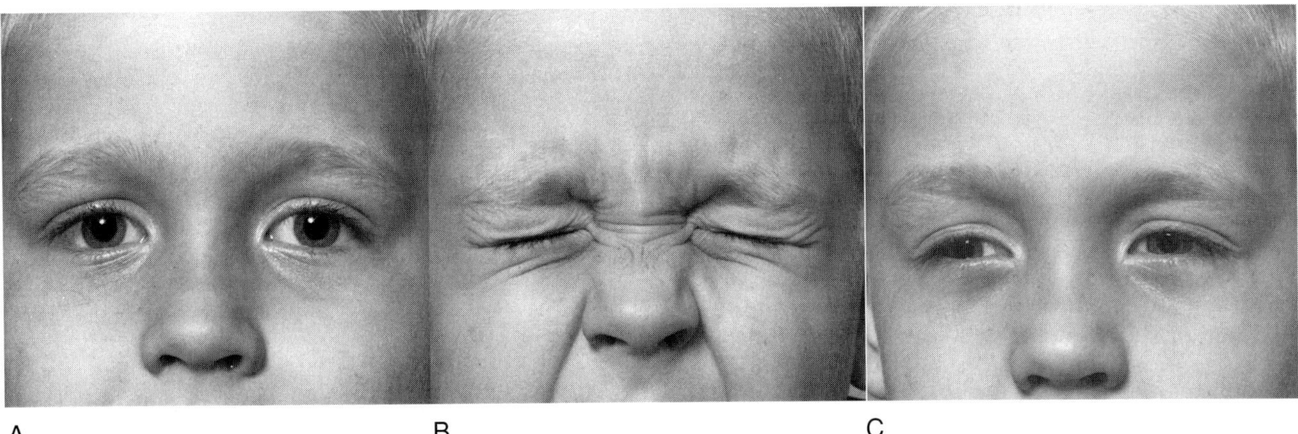

FIGURE 83-4. Patient has acetazolamide-responsive sodium channel myotonia. The patient appears in Figure 83-1 with his father, who is also shown in Figure 83-3. Sequential photographs of the patient before and after forced closure of the eyes. Myotonia appears and worsens after repeated eye closure (e.g., paramyotonia).

weakness, but muscle fibers do not display the marked depolarization observed in the muscle of patients with paramyotonia congenita. Treatment with tocainide, which is effective in paramyotonia congenita, does not reduce the mild weakness provoked by cooling and exercise in hyperkalemic periodic paralysis, in contrast to its beneficial protective effect on forearm muscle strength in paramyotonia congenita [Rudel et al., 1994]. In paramyotonia congenita, exercise after exposure to cold provokes muscle stiffness and occasionally prolonged paralysis. More research is necessary to clarify the mechanism of cold-induced weakness in paramyotonia and its variation within individuals in the same and different kindreds.

Treatment

Mexiletine is usually effective in preventing attacks of cold-induced weakness. Tocainide is also effective, but is no longer available. Patients having the combination of paramyotonia congenita plus hyperkalemic periodic paralysis require additional treatment with either a thiazide diuretic or acetazolamide.

Hypokalemic Periodic Paralysis

Hypokalemic periodic paralysis is an autosomal-dominant disorder caused most commonly by mutations in a skeletal muscle calcium channel gene [Fouad et al., 1997; Jurkat-Rott et al., 1994, 1998; Ptacek et al., 1994a]. A clinically identical form of hypokalemic periodic paralysis can also result from specific mutations of the same skeletal muscle sodium channel associated with hyperkalemic periodic paralysis [Bulman et al., 1999; Jurkat-Rott et al., 2000; Struyk et al., 2000].

Clinical Features

Attacks of hypokalemic periodic paralysis usually have their onset in the first or second decade, and about 60% of patients are affected before the age of 16 years [Engel et al., 1965; Lapie et al., 1997; Lehmann-Horn et al., 1994; Moxley, 1994; Shy et al., 1961]. Initially, attacks tend to be infrequent but eventually may recur daily. Diurnal fluctuations in strength may develop so that patients demonstrate greatest weakness during the night or early morning hours and gradually gain strength as the day passes. During major attacks, the serum potassium level decreases but not always to below normal. There is urinary retention of sodium, potassium, chloride, and water [Lehmann-Horn et al., 1994; Moxley, 1994]. Oliguria or anuria develops during such attacks, and patients tend to be constipated. Sinus bradycardia and ECG signs of hypokalemia appear when the serum potassium falls below normal. Usually during the fourth and fifth decades of life, attacks become less frequent and may cease. However, repeated attacks may leave the patient with permanent residual weakness [Dalakas and Engel, 1983; Dyken et al., 1969; Griggs et al., 1970; Odor et al., 1967].

Genetics

Familial hypokalemic periodic paralysis results from mutations in the gene for the skeletal muscle voltage-gated calcium channel on chromosome 1 and typically affects the dihydropyridine receptor [Jurkat-Rott et al., 1994; Lapie et al., 1997; Ptacek et al., 1994a; Sillen et al., 1997]. The mutations affect segment S4 of domains 3 and 4 [Lapie et al., 1997]. The prevalence of familial hypokalemic periodic paralysis is approximately 1 in 100,000 [Lapie et al., 1997; Lehmann-Horn et al., 1994]. The symptoms are more severe in males, as is the case in hyperkalemic periodic paralysis.

About 10% of hypokalemic periodic paralysis results from specific mutations of the skeletal muscle sodium channel gene [Miller et al., 2004].

Pathophysiology

In hereditary hypokalemic periodic paralysis, the muscle fiber develops reduced excitability and an increased sodium conductance that, unlike sodium channel forms of periodic paralysis, cannot be prevented by application of the sodium channel blocker tetrodotoxin [Lehmann-Horn et al., 1994; Moxley, 1994]. The in vitro electrophysiologic behavior of muscle fibers with sodium channel mutations associated with hypokalemic periodic paralysis appears to be similar to those with mutated calcium channels [Cannon, 2002].

The precise mechanism by which the skeletal muscle calcium channel permits this inexcitability of the muscle fiber remains unknown.

Clinical Laboratory Tests

Evaluation of serum electrolytes and ECG during attacks of weakness is essential to diagnosis and treatment. Muscle biopsy is usually not necessary but may reveal vacuoles, especially in patients with fixed weakness [Lehmann-Horn et al., 1994]. In patients not observed during attacks of weakness, it may be necessary to undertake careful provocative testing. This testing requires hospitalization and continuous monitoring of the ECG as indicated in previously published protocols [Moxley, 1994, 2000]. Occasionally, hypokalemic paralysis develops from acquired, secondary causes. Causes for secondary hypokalemic weakness include hypokalemia in association with hyperthyroidism, beta-adrenergic stimulation, excessive insulin, alkalemia, barium poisoning, poor potassium intake (e.g., alcoholics, anorexia nervosa), excessive potassium excretion (e.g., diarrhea, laxative abuse, profuse sweating during athletic training), and renal loss of potassium (e.g., renal tubular acidosis, osmotic diuresis, and medication use, such as large doses of penicillin antibiotics) [Moxley, 1994].

Treatment

Acute attacks may respond to oral potassium chloride (0.2 to 0.4 mmol/kg) repeated at 15- to 30-minute intervals [Moxley, 1994]. Monitoring ECG and serum potassium levels and muscle strength helps determine the frequency of these doses. Milder attacks resolve spontaneously, and mild exercise of the weakened muscles speeds recovery. If a patient has a severe attack and is unable to swallow or is vomiting, cautious intravenous infusion of potassium may be necessary. Treating physicians should keep in mind that a patient's serum potassium levels do not represent a total body deficit of potassium but rather a temporary intracellular shift. Therefore potassium replacement formulas tend to overestimate the replacement needs and result in potentially dangerous hyperkalemia.

Preventive therapy for attacks of hypokalemic weakness is usually needed. A low-sodium (2 to 3 g/day) and low-carbohydrate (60 to 80 g/day) diet, avoidance of exposure to cold and overexertion, and supplemental doses of potassium chloride (2.5 to 7.5 g as a 10% solution) taken two to four times daily are preventive measures that may help [Moxley, 1994]. However, no convincing data are available to indicate that oral potassium chloride prevents attacks.

Acetazolamide in divided doses usually abolishes attacks of weakness in most patients when taken daily [Griggs et al., 1970; Lehmann-Horn et al., 1994; Moxley, 1994]. Dichlorphenamide is another carbonic anhydrase inhibitor that is useful as preventive treatment if acetazolamide proves ineffective [Dalakas and Engel, 1983; Lehmann-Horn et al., 1994; Moxley, 1994; Tawil et al., 2000]. Both of these carbonic anhydrase inhibitors produce a metabolic acidosis, and despite their kaluretic action and their tendency to lower serum potassium levels, they appear to act on skeletal muscle to stabilize potassium flux, especially during insulin stimulation [Corbett et al., 1984]. Side effects are as described in the section on hyperkalemic periodic paralysis.

There are rare familial cases of hypokalemic periodic paralysis in which acetazolamide exacerbates attacks of weakness [Torres et al., 1981]. This weakness appears to be a consistent but not universal feature of hypokalemic periodic paralysis families carrying sodium channel mutations [Cannon, 2002; Venance et al., 2004]. In these families, triamterene or spironolactone may control the attacks.

Myotonic Chondrodystrophy: Schwartz-Jampel Syndrome

The Schwartz-Jampel syndrome is diagnosed in early childhood by the presence of myotonia, short stature, mask-like facies, muscle pseudohypertrophy, skeletal dysplasia with bone and joint abnormalities, and growth retardation [Aberfeld et al., 1965; Cao et al., 1978; Schwartz and Jampel, 1962]. This classic form of Schwartz-Jampel syndrome is proposed as type 1A [Giedion et al., 1997] and is linked to chromosome 1p34-p35 [Fontaine et al., 1996; Nicole et al., 1995]. The perlecan, a large heparin sulfate proteoglycan, is involved in Schwartz-Jampel syndrome causation. Mutations in the perlecan gene (HSPG2) are associated with Schwartz-Jampel syndrome [Arikawa-Hirasawa et al., 2002]. The defective protein that is encoded leads to abnormal cartilage development and anomalous neuromuscular activity [Ho et al., 2003].

A similar Schwartz-Jampel syndrome, type 1B, is recognizable at birth with more pronounced bone dysplasia. A more severe form of the syndrome, designated type 2, manifests at birth with increased mortality and bone dysplasia. More severe skeletal abnormalities and feeding difficulties are present [Al Gazali et al., 1996]. The presence in neonates of chondrodysplasia; congenital bowing of shortened femora and tibiae; and facial manifestations consisting of a small mouth, micrognathia, and pursed lips should suggest the diagnosis of Schwartz-Jampel syndrome [Spranger et al., 2000].

Death resulting from respiratory complications may occur in type 2. A second locus appears to be responsible for this severe neonatal type of Schwartz-Jampel syndrome [Brown et al., 1997].

In typical Schwartz-Jampel syndrome, range of motion at joints becomes progressively restricted, which may be due to unchecked myotonia. Although carpal tunnel syndrome is rare in childhood, it does occur with some frequency in Schwartz-Jampel syndrome [Van Meir and De Smet, 2003]. Malignant hyperpyrexia may occur, complicating orthopedic surgical procedures [Seay and Ziter, 1978]. Mental retardation is present in 25% of affected children, and developmental language disorder and attention-deficit disorder may be present [Paradis et al., 1997]. Severe microcephaly has been reported [Pinto-Escalante et al., 1997].

Serum creatine kinase activity is mildly increased. Striking high-frequency potentials associated with myotonia are demonstrated electrophysiologically. Electrical silence does not occur during rest, during general anesthesia, or after curarization [Taylor et al., 1972]. Muscle biopsy demonstrates myopathic findings [Brown et al., 1975; Huttenlocher et al., 1969]. Computed tomography of muscles reveals diffuse high attenuation in sternocleidomastoid muscles and low attenuation in the paraspinal, quadriceps, sartorius, soleus, and gastrocnemius muscles [Iwata et al., 2000]. Somatosensory-evoked potentials are delayed [Singh et al., 1997], although visual and brainstem auditory-evoked potentials and nerve conduction velocities are normal.

Phenytoin administration increases range of motion through relaxation of myotonia. Carbamazepine treatment also reduces myotonia [Topaloglu et al., 1993]. Early initiation of treatment tends to lessen skeletal malformations [Squires and Prangley, 1996].

Periodic Paralysis with Cardiac Arrhythmia: Andersen-Tawil Syndrome

Clinical Features

Andersen syndrome [Bendahhou et al., 2003; Donaldson et al., 2003; Miller et al., 2004; Tristani-Firouzi et al., 2002] or, as recently recognized, Andersen-Tawil Syndrome [Bendahhou et al., 2003], is a rare inherited disorder characterized by periodic paralysis, long QT syndrome, ventricular dysrhythmias, and skeletal developmental abnormalities. The early reports of this disorder raised the possibility of hyperkalemia during attacks of weakness, but as more specific identification of kindreds with Andersen-Tawil syndrome has occurred, it is apparent that the disorder is a variant of hypokalemic periodic paralysis [Bendahhou et al., 2003; Donaldson et al., 2003; Miller et al., 2004; Tristani-Firouzi et al., 2002]. Patients with this type of hypokalemic weakness have dysmorphic features, such as short stature, clinodactyly, and microcephaly, as well as ventricular dysrhythmias (Fig. 83-5). Attacks of weakness develop during the first or second decade [Andersen et al., 1971; Fukuda et al., 1988; Gould et al., 1985; Klein et al., 1963; Kramer et al., 1979; Levitt et al., 1972; Lisak et al., 1972; Sansone et al., 1997; Stubbs, 1976; Tawil et al., 1994; Yoshimura et al., 1983]. The attacks of limb weakness can vary from mild, resembling those in the sodium channel form of hyperkalemic periodic paralysis, to severe, resembling the typical calcium channel form of hypokalemic periodic paralysis. The major difference is that occasionally the episodes of weakness are associated with syncopal attacks and rarely sudden death. The cardiac arrhythmias and extrasystoles improve with an elevation in extracellular potassium, while hypokalemia tends to aggravate the cardiac dysrhythmias. In carriers of the potassium channel mutation, Kir2.1, associated with Andersen-Tawil syndrome, 64% had attacks of weakness, 71% had long QT intervals, and 78% had dysmorphic features [Tristani-Firouzi et al., 2002]. Cardiac symptoms can be provoked by digitalis; are refractory to disopyramide phosphate, propranolol, and phenytoin; and may respond to imipramine [Sansone et al., 1997; Tawil et al., 1994].

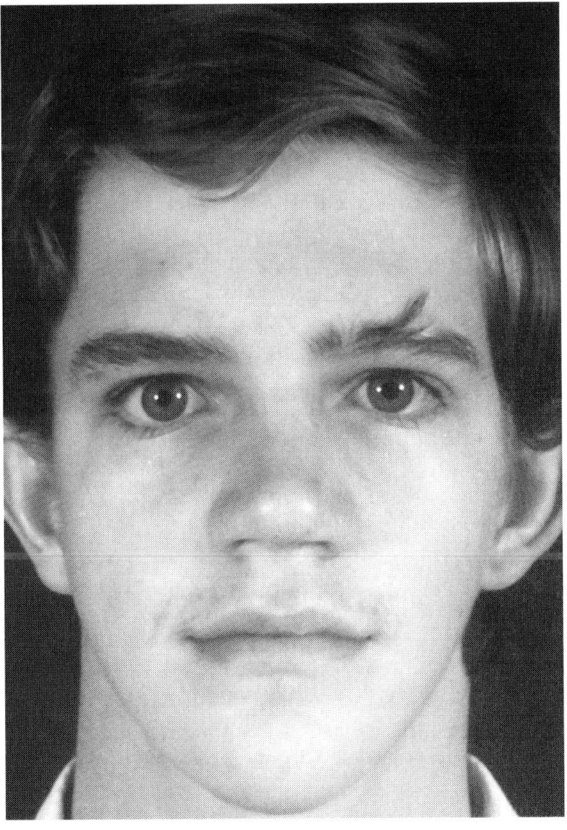

A

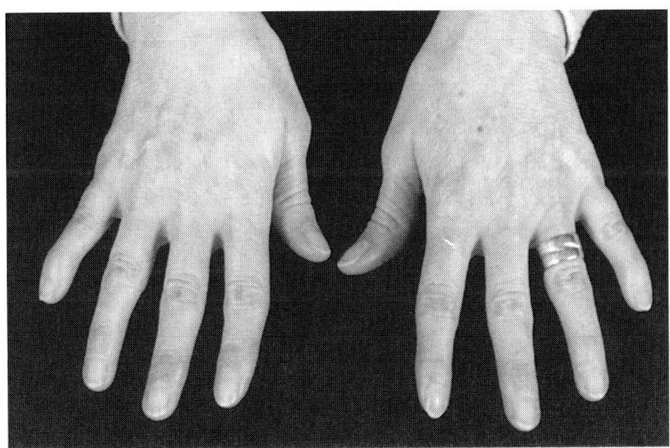

B

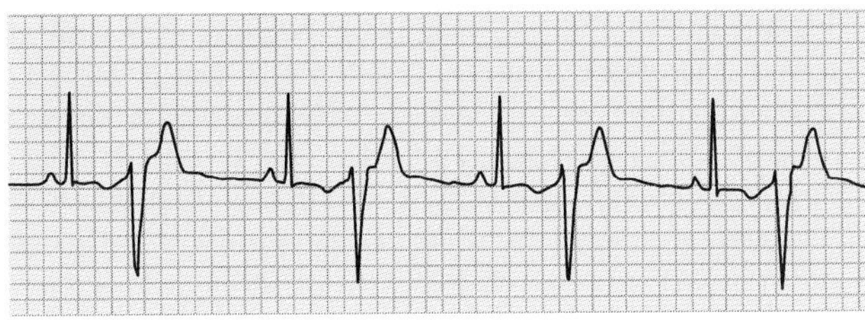

C

FIGURE 83-5. Facial appearance of a teenager with Andersen's syndrome (hyperkalemic periodic paralysis with cardiac dysrhythmias), the hands of his mother, who also has mild dysmorphic features of Andersen's syndrome, and the electrocardiograph (ECG) in this teenage patient demonstrating the typical dysrhythmia. During attacks of generalized weakness in which the serum potassium level rises above 5 mEq/L, the ECG in this patient typically returns to normal. (From Sansone V et al., 1997; and Tawil R et al., 1994. Copyright 1994 Wiley-Liss, Inc., a Wiley Company. Reproduced with permission of John Wiley & Sons, Inc.)

Genetics

One of the responsible mutations involves the gene encoding the inward-rectifying potassium channel Kir2.1 [Ai et al., 2002; Andelfinger et al., 2002; Plaster et al., 2001]. Autosomal-dominant inheritance occurs with variable severity within families [Bendahhou et al., 2003; Donaldson et al., 2003; Miller et al., 2004; Tristani-Firouzi et al., 2002]. Aside from the individuals with known mutations in the Kir2.1 gene, approximately 40% of cases with the clinical features of Andersen-Tawil syndrome have unknown mutations [Donaldson et al., 2004].

Pathophysiology

The 21 different mutations thus far identified in 30 kindreds with Andersen-Tawil syndrome appear to affect channel function through heterogeneous mechanisms [Donaldson et al., 2004]. These include (a) reduced activation of the channel due to altered binding of membrane-associated phosphatidylinositol 4,5 bisphosphate [Donaldson et al., 2003] and (b) mutated channels co-assembled and co-localized to the muscle membrane, with normal channels causing a dominant negative effect on their function [Bendahhou et al., 2003]. Other gene mutations that cause Andersen-Tawil syndrome likely share a common pathway or function with Kir2.1 or facilitate the activity of this ion channel.

Clinical Laboratory Tests

Periodic monitoring of the ECG is important to identify covert dysrhythmias. DNA testing as it becomes available will also be very helpful in establishing the diagnosis [Donaldson et al., 2004]. Muscle biopsy may help to distinguish patients with Andersen-Tawil syndrome from those with other myopathic disorders, especially various congenital myopathies. Provocative testing with potassium may be necessary. Patients with Andersen's syndrome are potassium sensitive [Sansone et al., 1997; Tawil et al., 1994], and occasionally more detailed provocative testing may be necessary [Moxley, 1994].

Treatment

Acetazolamide in doses used to treat sodium channel forms of hyperkalemic periodic paralysis is sometimes effective in preventing attacks of weakness. Dichlorphenamide may provide an effective alternative if acetazolamide fails [Tawil et al., 2000]. Cardiac dysrhythmias are less frequent if serum potassium is permitted to range from 4 to 4.4 mEq/L. However, this elevation in potassium may be difficult to achieve because it is typically not feasible with the use of carbonic anhydrase inhibitors. Occasionally, patients require the use of a spironolactone diuretic in combination with a carbonic anhydrase inhibitor to achieve a slightly higher serum potassium. Management of the cardiac dysrhythmia is best handled by a cardiologist. It is typically difficult to control.

Thyrotoxic Periodic Paralysis

Clinical Features

Attacks of thyrotoxic periodic paralysis are unusual in the first decade or early in the second decade of life but tend to develop in the late teens and during the 20s. It is much more frequent in Asians and males; 95% of cases are sporadic [Moxley, 1994; Ober, 1992; Resnick et al., 1969]. Cardiac problems, including sinus tachycardia, atrial fibrillation, supraventricular tachycardia, and ventricular fibrillation, can occur [Moxley, 1994; Ober, 1992; Resnick et al., 1969].

Pathophysiology

Pathophysiology of thyrotoxic periodic paralysis remains a mystery, but it is clear that the hyperthyroid state is an essential factor in mediating the hypokalemia and attacks of weakness [Moxley, 1994]. Patients have attacks only when they are hyperthyroid, and attacks cannot be precipitated by insulin and carbohydrate administration once patients become euthyroid in contrast with patients with hereditary hypokalemic periodic paralysis [Moxley, 1994; Ober, 1992]. Even after patients have become euthyroid and symptom free, paralytic attacks recur if the patient experiences a relapse into a thyrotoxic state or if hyperthyroidism is produced again with exogenous thyroid hormone [Moxley, 1994; Ober, 1992; Okihiro and Nordyke, 1966]. Hyperthyroidism alters plasma membrane permeability to sodium and potassium and increases responsiveness to catecholamines, probably through an increase in the sodium potassium adenosine triphosphatase in skeletal muscle [Ewart and Klip, 1995; Norgaard and Kjeldsen, 1991]. However, hypokalemia does not appear to be the primary regulator of weakness in thyrotoxic periodic paralysis because some patients regain their strength in the presence of persistent hypokalemia [Shayne and Hart, 1994; Yeung and Tse, 1974]. Moreover, a degree of hypokalemia sufficient to provoke a paralytic attack in a hyperthyroid patient may have no effect when that same patient is euthyroid [Ober, 1992], emphasizing that the relationship between hypokalemia and thyrotoxic periodic paralysis is complex. The fact that propranolol can prevent paralytic attacks at a level of hypokalemia, which in the same individual typically precipitates weakness [Ober, 1992; Yeung and Tse, 1974], raises additional questions about the specific role of changes in serum potassium in the etiology of thyrotoxic periodic paralysis.

Genetics

The gene defect responsible for thyrotoxic hypokalemic periodic paralysis remains unclear. One recent report described an R83H mutation in the potassium channel gene, KCNE3 [Dias da Silva et al., 2002] in a man who developed symptoms with the onset of Graves' disease. The mutation was found in two of three descendants. Three more recent reports have failed to confirm this observation. One study of 97 Chinese men with thyrotoxic periodic paralysis compared the genetic findings in this group to those in 77 Graves' disease patients without periodic paralysis and to 100 normal males [Kung et al., 2004]. None of the men with known thyrotoxic periodic paralysis had mutations in the calcium channel, sodium channel, or potassium channel genes previously reported to be associated with periodic paralysis. Another study describes an analysis of the entire coding sequence of KCNE3 gene in 79 Chinese patients with thyrotoxic periodic paralysis and compared their findings with those from 111 men with thyrotoxicosis without periodic paralysis [Tang et al., 2004]. No mutations were found in the

KCNE3 gene. A third report describes genetic studies in 19 Chinese men with thyrotoxic periodic paralysis and compared them to evaluations in 48 thyrotoxic patients and 32 normal individuals [Ng et al., 2004]. No mutations were found in the calcium or sodium channel genes previously reported to cause hypokalemic periodic paralysis. Despite the close similarity between familial autosomal-dominant hypokalemic periodic paralysis and thyrotoxic periodic paralysis, there does not appear to be a common genetic basis for these disorders.

Clinical Laboratory Tests

Measurement of thyroid function tests and the ECG are essential in establishing the diagnosis and in directing treatment. Other aspects of clinical laboratory evaluation are as described for familial hypokalemic periodic paralysis.

Treatment

Treatment consists of antithyroid therapy until the patient achieves the euthyroid state. Preventive measures should be undertaken after treatment of the acute attack as described for primary familial hypokalemic periodic paralysis. Propranolol is often effective in preventing attacks in thyrotoxic periodic paralysis [Ober, 1992; Yeung and Tse, 1974]. One recent report has emphasized the importance of propranolol as an initial treatment and has suggested caution about the use of potassium replacement [Tassone et al., 2004]. Acetazolamide is ineffective and may worsen or precipitate symptoms in thyrotoxic hypokalemic periodic paralysis and should be avoided [Moxley, 1994]. In general, beta-blocking drugs are helpful to use throughout the early stages of management until the patient becomes euthyroid.

MYOTONIC-LIKE DISORDERS AFFECTING PERIPHERAL AND CENTRAL NERVOUS SYSTEM OR THE BASEMENT MEMBRANE OF NEUROMUSCULAR JUNCTION AND CARTILAGE

This section briefly considers those disorders that have myotonic-like skeletal muscle manifestations but have their primary defect in nonmuscle tissues. These disorders include Schwartz-Jampel syndrome [Aberfeld et al., 1965; Ho et al., 2003; Pascuzzi, 1991; Schwartz and Jampel, 1962], hereditary familial episodic ataxia type 1 [Brunt and

TABLE 83-6

Disorders of Central and Peripheral Nervous System Causing Myotonic-like Muscle Contractions

CLINICAL FEATURES	STIFF PERSON SYNDROME	ACQUIRED GENERALIZED PERIPHERAL NERVE HYPEREXCITABILITY	HEREDITARY FAMILIAL EPISODIC ATAXIA TYPE 1
Inheritance	Acquired	Acquired	Autosomal dominant
Gene defect	Associated with elevated titers of antibodies against glutamic acid decarboxylase, the rate limiting enzyme for synthesis of γ-aminobutyric acid, the major inhibitory neurotransmitter in the brain. A subgroup of patients have antiamphiphysin autoantibodies of paraneoplastic origin	Associated with autoantibody-mediated or autoimmune-associated disorders that have antibodies against voltage-gated potassium channels; also associated with certain toxins, e.g., timber rattlesnake venom	Chromosome 12p13; mutations identified in voltage-gated potassium channel gene, KCNA1
Age of onset	Early to late adulthood	Childhood to late adulthood	Infancy or childhood
Main findings	Emotional stress and startle provoke sudden episodic muscle spasms; predominantly affects spinal and lower extremity muscles; females more than males 2:1; paraneoplastic variant occurs with breast cancer	Muscle twitching, cramps, stiffness, delayed muscle relaxation after contraction, spontaneous carpal or pedal spasm occurs; hyperhydrosis common; one third have distal paresthesias	Episodic brief attacks (seconds to minutes) of ataxia, dysarthria, and rippling muscles (myokymia) occur; muscle hypertrophy, joint contractures, skeletal deformity, and postural abnormalities may develop
Myotonia	Electromyography during the muscle spasms indicates normal motor units that discharge in a pattern of spasmodic reflex myoclonus; affects agonist and antagonist muscles simultaneously; transcranial magnetic stimulation demonstrates enhanced motor cortex excitability	Delayed muscle contractions and spontaneous snakelike muscle movements occur in association with myokymic and/or neuromyotonic discharges on electromyography; these discharges persist during sleep and general anesthesia but disappear following curare blockade	Electromyography usually reveals ongoing myokymic discharges even in the absence of clinical signs of myokymia or delayed muscle contraction; neuromyotonic discharges also occur
Provocative stimuli	Emotional stimuli; sudden noise; gentle skin stimulation	Exercise or muscle contraction (voluntary or electrically evoked)	Strenuous exercise, emotional stress, sudden limb movement, startle, and elevated body temperature or local elevation of temperature (hot bath, hair dryer)
Therapy for symptoms	Symptomatic treatment with γ-aminobutyric acid-enhancing agents (benzodiazepines, valproate, vigabatrin, tigabine, gabapentin, baclofen; immunotherapy (corticosteroids, other); plasmapheresis, periodic intravenous immunoglobulin infusions	Symptomatic treatment with carbamazepine and phenytoin; plasma exchange or intravenous immunoglobulin infusions as short-term treatment; long-term immunotherapy (corticosteroids, other); treat specific toxins or other associated diseases	Symptomatic treatment with carbamazepine and phenytoin

van Weerden, 1990; Gancher and Nutt, 1986], acquired generalized peripheral nerve hyperexcitability [Gamstorp and Wohlfart, 1959; Hart, 2000; Hart et al., 2002; Isaacs, 1961], and stiff person syndrome [Dalakas et al., 2000; Koerner et al., 2004; Moersch and Woltman, 1956; Murinson et al., 2004]. Table 83-6 summarizes their characteristics and treatments. Schwartz-Jampel syndrome and episodic ataxia type 1 occur early in childhood, whereas acquired generalized peripheral nerve hyperexcitability, which usually presents in adults, occasionally has an onset in childhood or adolescence. Stiff person syndrome presents almost exclusively in adults, but in principle the underlying pathophysiologic process can occur in children. Clinical features, especially the characteristics of the muscle contractions and the associated electromyographic findings, distinguish the myotonic-like disorders from the primary myotonic diseases and the periodic paralyses. Below are highlights of the clinical findings and comments about treatment that complement the information provided in Table 83-6.

Schwartz-Jampel Syndrome

Clinical Features

The phenotype of Schwartz-Jampel syndrome has considerable variability. Severe forms appear in infancy and milder forms usually develop manifestations between 2 and 3 years of age [Ho et al., 2003; Pascuzzi, 1991]. Patients have a short neck, protuberant abdomen, and sparse subcutaneous tissue. Joint contractures develop, along with a typical facial appearance (small palpebral fissures, pursed lips, low hairline, and low-set ears). The abnormal facies becomes increasingly prominent with age. The bony abnormalities, such as pectus carinatum, kyphoscoliosis, pes planus, hip dysplasia, platybasia, and flattened small vertebrae often are apparent early in the disease. Patients have a stooped posture with their shoulders flexed forward. Muscle hypertrophy and hirsutism are common. Orthopedic consultation may precede neurologic evaluation, and comments by a radiologist about the spinal x-ray appearance may point to the diagnosis of Schwartz-Jampel syndrome. On neurologic examination the combination of action and percussion myotonia, hyporeflexia, typical facies and body appearance, and electromyographic evidence of continuous muscle fiber activity (high frequency discharges occurring both at rest and exacerbated by muscle contraction) is diagnostic for Schwartz-Jampel syndrome. The electromyographic findings differ from classic myotonic discharges that disappear at rest, have a lower frequency, and wax and wane [Huttenlocher et al., 1969; Taylor et al., 1972]. Local infusion of curare abolishes continuous discharges in some patients [Cadilhac et al., 1975; Edwards and Root, 1982; Taylor et al., 1972]. This finding supports the hypothesis that the electrical discharges are neural or neuromuscular junction mediated [Arikawa-Hirasawa et al., 2002].

Genetics

Genetic heterogeneity accompanies the phenotypic variability in Schwartz-Jampel syndrome [Arikawa-Hirasawa et al., 2002; Brown et al., 1997; Fontaine et al., 1996; Giedion et al., 1997; Nicole et al., 2000] as indicated in Table 83-6. One type of Schwartz-Jampel syndrome (type 1A and type 1B) is linked to chromosome 1p34-36 [Al Gazali et al., 1996; Arikawa-Hirasawa et al., 2002; Fontaine et al., 1996; Giedion et al., 1997; Brown et al., 1997; Nicole et al., 2000] and the other (Schwartz-Jampel syndrome type 2) is not linked to this locus [Brown et al., 1997].

Mutations in the perlecan gene (HSPG2) are responsible for most cases of Schwartz-Jampel syndrome [Arikawa-Hirasawa et al., 2002; Nicole et al., 2000]. Perlecan is a large heparan sulfate proteoglycan and is a component of the basement membrane [Brown et al., 1997; Costell et al., 1999; Friedrich et al., 1999; Iozzo et al., 1994]. Evidence supports the hypothesis that a deficiency of perlecan causes Schwartz-Jampel syndrome and that complete absence of perlecan causes a severe neolethal condition, Silverman-Handmaker disorder [Arikawa-Hirasawa et al., 2001, 2002].

Pathophysiology

The electrophysiologic evidence noted earlier that suggests that the hyperexcitability of nerve-muscle transmission in Schwartz-Jampel syndrome relates to alterations at the neuromuscular junction secondary to a deficiency of perlecan. Recent evidence indicates that perlecan is a key molecule for localizing acetylcholine esterase at the synapse of the neuromuscular junction [Arikawa-Hirasawa et al., 2002; Peng et al., 1999]. Studies of muscle biopsies of Schwartz-Jampel syndrome patients demonstrate nonspecific alterations in muscle fibers on typical histochemical staining but have weak immunostaining of perlecan with domain-specific antiperlecan antibodies [Arikawa-Hirasawa et al., 2002]. It seems likely that a deficiency of perlecan at the neuromuscular junction in Schwartz-Jampel syndrome allows sufficient but altered regulation of neuromuscular transmission. This alteration in turn leads to continuous muscle fiber activity and myotonic-like muscle contractions. Absence of perlecan in contrast may not permit sufficient neuromuscular transmission and in turn accounts for the rapid demise of the patient and the lack of clinical signs of myotonic-like muscle contractions.

Treatment

Therapy in Schwartz-Jampel syndrome is supportive and focuses on specific symptoms and potential complications. Orthopedic consultation and physical and occupational therapy are necessary to treat the bony deformities and contractures. Carbamazepine (20 mg/kg/day in infants [Squires and Prangley, 1996; Topaloglu et al., 1993] and 600 mg of extended release twice daily in older children [Ho et al, 2003]) is effective in controlling the myotonia and continuous muscle fiber activity. Procainamide is another potential antimyotonia treatment [Huttenlocher et al., 1969] and phenytoin may provide a modest benefit [Edwards and Root, 1982; Taylor et al., 1972]. Response to other antimyotonia drugs, such as mexiletine, has not been reported. Some patients require nasal bilevel positive airway pressure for obstructive sleep apnea [Cook and Borkowski, 1997] and some benefit from levator aponeurosis surgery [Cruz et al., 1998]. Anesthesiology consultation before surgery is prudent, since difficulty with intubation [Cook and Borkowski, 1997] and malignant hyperthermia [Ho et al., 2003; Seay and Ziter, 1978] are potential complications.

Hereditary Familial Episodic Ataxia Type 1

Clinical Features

The classic description of episodic ataxia type 1 includes the appearance of sudden episodes of cerebellar ataxia, lasting a few minutes, often provoked by startle, and beginning in childhood [Brunt and van Weerden, 1990; Gancher and Nutt, 1986]. Some patients display prominent myokymia [Hanson et al., 1977; Vaamonde et al., 1991; Van Dyke et al., 1975]. However, recent clinical studies demonstrate that there is considerable phenotypic variation in episodic ataxia type 1 [Eunson et al., 2000; Kinali et al., 2004; Klein et al., 2004]. Some patients have grip myotonia, muscle stiffness, limited jaw opening, contractures (elbows and ankles), muscle hypertrophy, and kyphoscoliosis [Kinali et al., 2004], a clinical picture that resembles the childhood form of Schwartz-Jampel syndrome. Some individuals within a kindred only display seizures and have no episodes of ataxia or muscle stiffness [Eunson et al., 2000]. In contrast, one report describes a patient with prolonged episodes (10 to 12 hours in duration) of painful muscle stiffness triggered by fever and exertion associated with wrist flexion, thumb adduction, and myokymia in the periorbital muscles [Klein et al., 2004]. Ataxia was not a feature of these episodes. Dysarthria and double vision along with swelling of the feet occurred at the onset of attacks in this patient [Klein et al., 2004]. Tendon reflexes may be diminished, normal, or hyperactive. Electromyographic studies reveal continuous myokymic discharges and occasional neuromyotonic discharges [Gutmann and Gutmann, 2004]. Nerve conduction is normal. Usually the clinical picture and the family history of a dominantly inherited episodic disorder confirm the diagnosis.

Genetics and Pathophysiology

Episodic ataxia type 1 links to mutations in the KCNA1 gene on chromosome 12p13 that encodes the Shaker-type potassium channel subunit hKv1.1 [Litt et al., 1994]. There are at least five mutations associated with episodic ataxia type 1 [Eunson et al., 2000; Kinali et al., 2004; Klein et al., 2004; Rea et al., 2002]. Recent evidence suggests that the specific molecular defect and the phenotype vary with the location of the mutation [Imbrici et al., 2003; Klein et al., 2004; Rea et al., 2002]. Mutations that cause typical episodic ataxia type 1 (V4041, I177N) or neuromyotonia (P244H) alone are associated with altered kinetics of the potassium channel [Imbrici et al., 2003; Rea et al., 2002]. A mutation (R417stop) that causes a severe medication-resistant form of episodic ataxia type 1 impairs both tetramerization of the R417stop with the wild type of hKv1.1 subunits and the membrane targeting of the heterotetramers. Two other mutations (T226R, A242P) that lead to a severe phenotype of episodic ataxia type 1, including seizures, produce a combination of defects in channel assembly, membrane trafficking, and abnormal channel kinetics [Rea et al., 2002]. Another mutation, which involves a single nucleotide change at position 785 T>C, causes prolonged (10 to 12 hours), painful episodes of stiffness triggered by fever and exertion. These clinical findings [Klein et al., 2004] are similar to those in patients with antibody-mediated acquired generalized peripheral nerve hyperexcitability [Hart et al., 2002], and have led the investigators to hypothesize that the 785 T>C mutation causes channel dysfunction similar to that in the autoimmune disorder [Klein et al., 2004]. Further research is necessary to establish phenotype-genotype relationships.

Treatment

Therapy is symptomatic. Reducing opportunities for stress, startle, and overexertion lessen the frequency of episodes. Physical therapy and orthopedic consultation are helpful in patients with contractures. Acetazolamide may reduce episodes of ataxia, but carbamazepine is necessary to control muscle stiffness and myokymia [Klein et al., 2004]. Phenytoin can also ameliorate myokymia and stiffness [Kinali et al., 2004].

Acquired Generalized Peripheral Nerve Hyperexcitability

Clinical Findings

Acquired generalized peripheral nerve hyperexcitability represents a heterogeneous group of disorders that have included diagnoses such as Isaacs' syndrome, cramp-fasciculation syndrome, and neuromyotonia [Gutmann and Gutmann, 2004; Hart, 2000; Hart et al., 2002; Newsom-Davis et al., 2003]. Autoimmune, toxic, degenerative, and hereditary forms are included in the classification [Hart et al, 2002]. The core clinical symptoms are muscle twitching, exercise triggered muscle cramps, and muscle stiffness [Hart et al., 2002]. Delayed relaxation after muscle contraction (pseudomyotonia) occurs less commonly (36%) [Hart et al., 2002]. Acquired generalized peripheral nerve hyperexcitability is very uncommon in childhood. In a recent series of 42 patients, only 3 patients were younger than 20 years of age (5, 10, and 15 years of age) [Hart et al., 2002]. One of these patients developed symptoms in early childhood and went untreated for many years. He had growth retardation and presented for evaluation in a wheelchair with severe muscle stiffness and cramps that had been mistaken for spasticity. Patients typically have normoactive or diminished tendon reflexes, and approximately one third have sensory complaints. Excessive sweating is common (50%), but specific alterations of the autonomic nervous system are not. At the time of presentation most patients have muscle overactivity affecting the legs alone or legs and trunk combined [Hart et al., 2002]. Electromyography reveals spontaneous firing of motor units as doublet, triplet, or multiple discharges that have a high burst frequency (40 to 400 Hz) and in more than 90% of cases, the discharges occur at irregular intervals of 1 to 30 seconds [Hart, 2000]. Voluntary contractions or electrically evoked contractions often provoke prolonged after-discharges. Abnormal spontaneous activity can occur without visible myokymia. These discharges disappear after blockade of neuromuscular transmission and lessen or disappear in some patients after epidural anesthesia or proximal nerve block [Hart, 2000]. These findings support the hypothesis that the spontaneous discharges result from peripheral nerve hyperactivity [Hart, 2000; Hart et al., 2002].

Pathophysiology

Immune-related diseases, such as myasthenia gravis, diabetes mellitus, and rheumatoid arthritis, are more frequent in acquired generalized peripheral nerve hyperexcitability as is lung cancer. Approximately 40% of patients have antibodies to the voltage-gated potassium channel [Hart et al., 2002], and these antibodies appear to have a central role in the pathophysiology [Arimura et al., 2002; Hart et al., 2002; Tomimitsu et al., 2004]. Studies of cultured cell lines incubated with patient sera indicate there is antibody-mediated suppression of outward-gated potassium current [Arimura et al., 2002; Tomimitsu et al, 2004]. Recent in vitro investigations using neuronal cell lines indicate that the reduction in potassium currents by antibodies to the voltage-gated potassium channel is independent of added complement; however, F(ab′)2 fragments isolated from patient sera significantly reduce potassium currents. These findings make it likely that cross-linking of the voltage-gated potassium channels by divalent antibodies is an important mechanism in reducing the potassium current [Tomimitsu et al., 2004].

Other circulating factors cause acquired generalized peripheral nerve hyperexcitability, such as timber rattlesnake envenomation [Gutmann and Gutmann, 2004]. The venom enters the circulation, causing generalized myokymia involving the face and extremities. Symptoms abate within hours of administering antivenin therapy [Gutmann and Gutmann, 2004].

Treatment

Carbamazepine and phenytoin are the primary symptomatic medications for the neuromyotonia and usually control symptoms of muscle overactivity [Hart, 2000]. In refractory cases or in the initial management of severe cases, plasma exchange [Hart, 2000; Hayat et al., 2000; Newsom-Davis et al., 2003] or immune globulin infusion [Alessi et al., 2000; Hart, 2000; Newsome-Davis et al., 2003] may produce rapid resolution of symptoms. Prednisone and azathioprine may prove useful for long-term treatment, as well as other immunosuppressive agents [Hart, 2000; Newsom-Davis et al., 2003], but long-term controlled trials are necessary to confirm this clinical impression.

Stiff Person Syndrome

Clinical Findings

Stiff person syndrome is a rare neurologic disorder with autoimmune features. Its primary manifestation is progressive, severe muscle rigidity or stiffness, most prominently affecting the spine and lower extremities [Dalakas et al., 2000; Murinson et al., 2004; Rakocevic et al., 2004]. Occasionally the muscle stiffness may resemble myotonia with a delay in relaxation, but the typical manifestations in skeletal muscle are readily distinguished from true myotonia. In stiff person syndrome there is an insidious onset of muscular rigidity in limb and axial musculature [Dalakas et al., 2000]. The stiffness is most prominent in the abdominal and thoracolumbar muscles and causes difficulty in turning and bending. Electromyographic recordings demonstrate that there is continuous co-contraction of agonist and antagonist muscles, and the patient is unable to relax. Episodic muscle spasms that may occasionally resemble myotonic-like contractions are superimposed on this rigidity and are precipitated by unexpected noises, tactile stimuli, or emotional stress. These manifestations occur in the absence of any other neurologic disease or underlying chronic pain syndrome that might produce prolonged muscle rigidity and spasms. Many patients have an elevated titer of antibodies to glutamic acid decarboxylase antibodies, and they often have diabetes or other autoimmune diseases [Dalakas et al., 2000; Koerner et al., 2004; Lohmann et al., 2003; Murinson et al., 2004; Rakocevic et al., 2004]. Uncommonly, in perhaps 5% of stiff person syndrome patients there is a paraneoplastic origin for the illness associated with antibodies against amphiphysin [Petzold et al., 2004].

Stiff person syndrome is rare in children. One recent study of 116 stiff person syndrome patients with elevated levels of glutamic acid decarboxylase antibodies included only 1 teenage patient; the remaining 115 patients were older than 30 years of age [Murinson et al., 2004]. In an earlier study of 20 selected patients the average age was 41.2 years [Dalakas et al., 2000], and in another recent report of 16 patients with stiff person syndrome the ages ranged from 37 to 62 years, with a median age of 52 years [Rakocevic et al., 2004].

Pathophysiology

Electromyographic investigations in patients with stiff person syndrome disclose the presence of low-frequency firing of normal motor units, especially in the muscles of the trunk, which increases for seconds or minutes to a dense pattern during a spontaneous or provoked muscle spasm [Koerner et al., 2004; Martinelli et al., 1996; Meinck et al., 1995]. These bursts of electrical activity are highly variable in location, duration, and intensity. Investigators have described a stereotyped motor response to stimulation of peripheral nerves in stiff person syndrome patients that consists of a sequence of one to three synchronous myoclonic bursts, 60 to 70 milliseconds after median nerve stimulation, followed by tonic decrescendo activity over a number of seconds [Meinck et al., 1995]. They call this response spasmodic reflex myoclonus, and have used it to explain certain aspects of the pathophysiology of stiff person syndrome. They speculate that the stiffness is a fragment of spasms and that both are due to a common neuronal mechanism of abnormal regulation of interneurons in the spinal gray matter [Meinck et al., 1995]. Other studies support this mechanism and suggest an important role for motor cortex hyperexcitability in stiff person syndrome [Koerner et al., 2004; Martinelli et al., 1996]. The most recent study using transcranial magnetic stimulation methodology points out that the elevation of glutamic acid decarboxylase antibodies directly correlates with the enhanced cortical excitability and that γ-aminobutyric acid–mimetic medications reduce intracortical facilitation [Koerner et al., 2004]. These observations suggest a clear role for glutamic acid decarboxylase antibodies in mediating the stiffness and muscle spasms. However, the precise pathophysiologic role of glutamic acid decarboxylase antibodies in stiff person syndrome requires further investigation [Dalakas et al., 2001b].

One recent study of 16 adults with stiff person syndrome notes that there is no correlation between the glutamic acid decarboxylase antibody titers in serum or cerebrospinal fluid and the severity of disease [Rakocevic et al., 2004]. The authors emphasize that an elevation of glutamic acid decarboxylase antibodies serve as an excellent marker for stiff person syndrome, but monitoring their titers during the course of the disease may not have practical value. Another recent study stresses the importance of establishing an appropriate threshold elevation of glutamic acid decarboxylase antibodies before making a diagnosis of stiff person syndrome [Murinson et al., 2004] because nonaffected individuals, such as some diabetic people, may have modest elevations of glutamic acid decarboxylase antibodies. This study also notes that elevation of glutamic acid decarboxylase antibodies do not correlate with the age or duration of stiff person syndrome [Murinson et al., 2004]. It is interesting to note that two children born to two different mothers with stiff person syndrome had high titers of glutamic acid decarboxylase antibodies for the first 24 months of life, and having reached the ages of 6 and 8 years have not had any manifestations of stiff person syndrome [Nemni et al., 2004]. Clinical criteria remain the benchmark for the diagnosis of stiff person syndrome [Chang and Lang, 2004].

Treatment

Diazepam is an effective medication to control muscle spasms and the dose needs to be titrated to each patient. Its beneficial effect is likely mediated by its actions on the γ-aminobutyric acid ($GABA_A$) receptor. Baclofen, gabapentin, clonazepam, Dantrium, and vigabatrin have provided lesser benefit. Plasma exchange and intravenous immune globulin infusions have proved effective, especially in times of acute worsening or in patients who develop refractoriness to symptomatic therapy with these medications [Dalakas et al., 2000, 2001a]. Controlled trials are needed to establish the role of long-term treatment with immunosuppressive medications such as corticosteroids and mycophenolate, and are also needed to determine the comparative effectiveness of plasmapheresis and immune globulin therapy.

REFERENCES

Abbruzzese C, Costanzi PS, Mariani B, et al. Instability of a premutation allele in homozygous patients with myotonic dystrophy type 1. Ann Neurol 2002;52(4):435.

Abdalla JA, Casley WL, Cousin HK, et al. Linkage of Thomsen disease to the T-cell-receptor beta (Tcrb) locus on chromosome-7Q35. Am J Hum Genet 1992;51(3):579.

Aberfeld DC, Hinterbuchner LP, Schneider M. Myotonia, dwarfism, diffuse bone disease and unusual ocular and facial abnormalities (a new syndrome). Brain 1965;88:313.

Ai T, Fujiwara Y, Tsuji K, et al. Novel KCNJ2 mutation in familial periodic paralysis with ventricular dysrhythmia. Circulation 2002;105:2592.

Akiguchi I, Nakano S, Shiino A, et al. Brain proton magnetic resonance spectroscopy and brain atrophy in myotonic dystrophy. Arch Neurol 1999;56(3):325.

Al Gazali LI, Varghese M, Varady E, et al. Neonatal Schwartz-Jampel syndrome: A common autosomal recessive syndrome in the United Arab Emirates. J Med Genet 1996;33:203.

Alessi G, De Reuck J, De Bleecker J, Vancayzeele S. Successful immunoglobulin treatment in a patient with neuromyotonia. Clin Neurol Neurosurg 2000;102(3):173.

Andelfinger G, Tapper AR, Welch RC, et al. KCNJ2 mutation results in Andersen syndrome with sex-specific cardiac and skeletal muscle phenotypes. Am J Hum Genet 2002;71(3):663.

Andersen ED, Krasilnikoff PA, Overvad H. Intermittent muscular weakness, extrasystoles, and multiple developmental anomalies. A new syndrome? Acta Paediatr Scand 1971;60(5):559

Arikawa-Hirasawa E, Le AH, Nishino I, et al. Structural and functional mutations of the perlecan gene cause Schwartz-Jampel syndrome, with myotonic myopathy and chondrodysplasia. Am J Hum Genet 2002;70:1368.

Arikawa-Hirasawa E, Wilcox WR, Le AH Jr, et al. Dyssegmental dysplasia, Silverman-Handmaker type, is caused by functional null mutations of the perlecan gene. Nat Genet 2001;27:431.

Arimura K, Sonoda Y, Watanabe O, et al. Isaacs' syndrome as a potassium channelopathy of the nerve. Muscle Nerve 2002(Suppl 11):S55.

Bachinski LL, Udd B, Meola G, et al. Confirmation of the type 2 myotonic dystrophy (CCTG)n expansion mutation in patients with proximal myotonic myopathy/proximal myotonic dystrophy of different European origins: A single shared haplotype indicates an ancestral founder effect. Am J Hum Genet 2003;73(4):835.

Barchi RL. Molecular pathology of skeletal-muscle sodium-channel. Ann Rev Physiol 1995;57:355.

Baumann P, Siira P, Vanharanta H, et al. Quantification of muscle strength in recessive myotonia congenita. Eur Neurol 1996;36(5):284.

Bendahhou S, Donaldson MR, Plaster NM, et al. Defective potassium channel Kir2.1 trafficking underlies Andersen-Tawil syndrome. J Biol Chem 2003;278(51):51779.

Berardinelli A, Gorni K, Orcesi S. Response to carbamazepine of recessive-type myotonia congenita. Muscle Nerve 2000;23(1):138.

Bhakta D, Lowe MR, Groh WJ. Prevalence of structural cardiac abnormalities in patients with myotonic dystrophy type I. Am Heart J 2004;147(2):224.

Bouhours M, Sternberg D, Davoine CS, et al. Functional characterization and cold sensitivity of T1313A, a new mutation of the skeletal muscle sodium channel causing paramyotonia congenita in humans. J Physiol 2004;554(Pt 3):635.

Brancati F, Valente EM, Davies NP, et al. Severe infantile hyperkalaemic periodic paralysis and paramyotonia congenita: Broadening the clinical spectrum associated with the T704M mutation in SCN4A. J Neurol Neurosurg Psychiatry 2003;74(9):1339.

Brook JD, McCurrach ME, Harley HG, et al. Molecular basis of myotonic dystrophy: Expansion of a trinucleotide (CTG) repeat at the 3′ end of a transcript encoding a protein kinase family member. Cell 1992;(68):799.

Brown KA, al-Gazali LI, Moynihan LM, et al. Genetic heterogeneity in Schwartz-Jampel syndrome: Two families with neonatal Schwartz-Jampel syndrome do not map to human chromosome 1p34-p36.1. J Med Genet 1997;34:685.

Brown S, Garcia-Mullin R, Murai Y. The Schwartz-Jampel syndrome (myotonic chondrodystrophy) in the adult. Neurology 1975;25:365.

Brunt ER, van Weerden TW. Familial paroxysmal kinesigenic ataxia and continuous myokymia. Brain 1990;113(Pt 5):1361.

Bulman DE, Scoggan KA, van Oene MD, et al. A novel sodium channel mutation in a family with hypokalemic periodic paralysis. Neurology 1999;53(9):1932.

Cadilhac J, Baldet P, Greze J, et al. Studies of two family cases of the Schwartz and Jampel syndrome (osteo-chondro-muscular dystrophy with myotonia). Electromyogr Clin Neurophysiol 1975;15:5.

Campbell C, Sherlock R, Jacob P, et al. Congenital myotonic dystrophy: Assisted ventilation duration and outcome. Pediatrics 2004;113(4):811.

Cannon SC. Sodium channel defects in myotonia and periodic paralysis. Annu Rev Neurosci 1996;19:141.

Cannon SC. From mutation to myotonia in sodium channel disorders. Neuromuscul Disord 1997;7(4):241.

Cannon SC. Voltage-gated ion channelopathies of the nervous system. Clin Neurosci Res 2001;1:104.

Cannon SC. An expanding view for the molecular basis of familial periodic paralysis. Neuromuscul Disord 2002;12(6):533.

Cao A, Cianchetti C, Culisti L, et al. Schwartz-Jampel syndrome: Clinical, electrophysiological, and histopathological study of a severe variant. J Neurol Sci 1978;35:175.

Ceccarelli M, Rossi B, Siciliano G, et al. Clinical and electrophysiological reports in a case of early onset myotonia congenita (Thomsen's disease) successfully treated with mexiletine. Acta Paediatr 1992;81(5):453.

Chang L, Ernst T, Osborn D, et al. Proton spectroscopy in myotonic dystrophy: Correlations with CTG repeats. Arch Neurol 1998;55(3):305.

Chang T, Lang B. GAD antibodies in stiff-person syndrome. Neurology 2004;63:1999.

Charlet B, Savkur RS, Singh G, et al. Loss of the muscle-specific chloride channel in type 1 myotonic dystrophy due to misregulated alternative splicing. Mol Cell 2002;10(1):45.

Choi GR, Porter CB, Ackerman MJ. Sudden cardiac death and channelopathies: A review of implantable defibrillator therapy. Pediatr Clin North Am 2004;51(5):1289.

Cook SP, Borkowski WJ. Obstructive sleep apnea in Schwartz-Jampel syndrome. Arch Otolaryngol Head Neck Surg 1997;123:1348.

Costell M, Gustafsson E, Aszodi A, et al. Perlecan maintains the integrity of cartilage and some basement membranes. J Cell Biol 1999;147:1109.

Cruz AA, Souza CA, Plastino LS, Jr. Levator aponeurosis surgery in Schwartz-Jampel syndrome. Ophthal Plast Reconstr Surg 1998;14:271.

Corbett A, Kingston W, Griggs RC, et al. Effect of acetazolamide on insulin sensitivity in myotonic disorders. Arch Neurol 1984;41(7):740.

Dalakas MC, Engel WK. Treatment of "permanent" muscle weakness in familial hypokalemic periodic paralysis. Muscle Nerve 1983;6(3):182.

Dalakas MC, Fujii M, Li M, et al. The clinical spectrum of anti-GAD antibody-positive patients with stiff-person syndrome. Neurology 2000;55:1531.

Dalakas MC, Fujii M, Li M, et al. High-dose intravenous immune globulin for stiff-person syndrome. N Engl J Med 2001a;345:1870.

Dalakas MC, Li M, Fujii M, et al. Stiff person syndrome: Quantification, specificity, and intrathecal synthesis of GAD65 antibodies. Neurology 2001b;57:780.

Davies NP, Hanna MG. The skeletal muscle channelopathies: Distinct entities and overlapping syndromes. Curr Opin Neurol 2003;16(5):559.

Day JW, Ricker K, Jacobsen JF, et al. Myotonic dystrophy type 2: Molecular, diagnostic and clinical spectrum. Neurology 2003;60(4):657.

Day JW, Roelofs R, Leroy B, et al. Clinical and genetic characteristics of a five-generation family with a novel form of myotonic dystrophy (DM2). Neuromuscul Disord 1999;9(1):19.

Dias da Silva MR, Cerutti JM, Arnaldi LA, et al. A mutation in the KCNE3 potassium channel gene is associated with susceptibility to thyrotoxic hypokalemic periodic paralysis. J Clin Endocrinol Metab 2002;87(11):4881.

Donaldson MR, Jensen JL, Tristani-Firouzi M, et al. PIP2 binding residues of Kir2.1 are common targets of mutations causing Andersen syndrome. Neurology 2003;60(11):1811.

Donaldson MR, Yoon G, Fu YH, et al. Andersen-Tawil syndrome: a model of clinical variability, pleiotropy, and genetic heterogeneity. Ann Med 2004;36(Suppl 1):92.

Duffield M, Rychkov G, Bretag A, et al. Involvement of helices at the dimer interface in ClC-1 common gating. J Gen Physiol 2003;121(2):149.

Duno M, Colding-Jorgensen E, Grunnet M, et al. Difference in allelic expression of the CLCN1 gene and the possible influence on the myotonia congenita phenotype. Eur J Hum Genet 2004;12(9):738.

Dyken M, Zeman W, Rusche T. Hypokalemic periodic paralysis. Children with permanent myopathic weakness. Neurology 1969;19(7):691.

Edwards WC, Root AW. Chondrodystrophic myotonia (Schwartz-Jampel syndrome): Report of a new case and follow-up of patients initially reported in 1969. Am J Med Genet 1982;13:51.

Engel AG, Lambert EH, Rosevear JW, et al. Clinical and electromyographic studies in a patient with primary hypokalemic periodic paralysis. Am J Med 1965;38:626.

Eunson LH, Rea R, Zuberi SM, et al. Clinical, genetic, and expression studies of mutations in the potassium channel gene KCNA1 reveal new phenotypic variability. Ann Neurol 2000;48:647.

Ewart HS, Klip A. Hormonal regulation of the Na(+)-K(+)-ATPase: Mechanisms underlying rapid and sustained changes in pump activity. Am J Physiol 1995;269(2 Pt 1):C295.

Fahlke C, Beck CL, George AL, Jr. A mutation in autosomal dominant myotonia congenita affects pore properties of the muscle chloride channel. Proc Natl Acad Sci U S A 1997a;94(6):2729.

Fahlke C, Knittle T, Gurnett CA, et al. Subunit stoichiometry of human muscle chloride channels. J Gen Physiol 1997b;109(1):93.

Flachenecker P, Schneider C, Cursiefen S, et al. Assessment of cardiovascular autonomic function in myotonic dystrophy type 2 (DM2/PROMM). Neuromuscul Disord 2003;13(4):289.

Fontaine B, Nicole S, Topaloglu H, et al. Recessive Schwartz-Jampel syndrome (SJS): Confirmation of linkage to chromosome 1p, evidence of genetic homogeneity and reduction of the SJS locus to a 3-cM interval. Hum Genet 1996;98:380.

Fouad G, Dalakas M, Servidei S, et al. Genotype-phenotype correlations of DHP receptor alpha 1-subunit gene mutations causing hypokalemic periodic paralysis. Neuromuscul Disord 1997;7(1):33.

Fournier E, Arzel M, Sternberg D, et al. Electromyography guides toward subgroups of mutations in muscle channelopathies. Ann Neurol 2004;56(5):650.

Friedrich MV, Gohring W, Morgelin M, et al. Structural basis of glycosaminoglycan modification and of heterotypic interactions of perlecan domain. J Mol Biol 1999;294:259.

Fu YH, Pizzuti A, Fenwick RG, et al. An unstable triplet repeat in a gene related to myotonic muscular dystrophy. Science 1992;(255):1256.

Fukuda K, Ogawa S, Yokozuka H, et al. Long-standing bidirectional tachycardia in a patient with hypokalemic periodic paralysis. J Electrocardiol 1988;21(1):71.

Gamstorp I, Wohlfart G. A syndrome characterized by myokymia, myotonia, muscular wasting and increased perspiration. Acta Psychiatr Neurol Scand 1959;34:181.

Gancher ST, Nutt JG. Autosomal dominant episodic ataxia: A heterogeneous syndrome. Mov Disord 1986;1:239.

George AL, Jr., Crackower MA, Abdalla JA, et al. Molecular basis of Thomsen's disease (autosomal dominant myotonia congenita). Nat Genet 1993;3:305.

Giedion A, Boltshauser E, Briner J, et al. Heterogeneity in Schwartz-Jampel chondrodystrophic myotonia. Eur J Pediatr 1997;156:214.

Gould RJ, Steeg CN, Eastwood AB, et al. Potentially fatal cardiac dysrhythmia and hyperkalemic periodic paralysis. Neurology 1985;35(8):1208.

Greenberg DA. Calcium channels in neurological disease. Ann Neurol 1997;42(3):275.

Griggs RC, Engel WK, Resnick JS. Acetazolamide treatment of hypokalemic periodic paralysis. Prevention of attacks and improvement of persistent weakness. Ann Intern Med 1970;73(1):39.

Grunnet M, Jespersen T, Colding-Jorgensen E, et al. Characterization of two new dominant ClC-1 channel mutations associated with myotonia. Muscle Nerve 2003;28(6):722.

Gutmann L, Gutmann L. Myokymia and neuromyotonia 2004. J Neurol 2004;251:138.

Hanson PA, Martinez LB, Cassidy R. Contractures, continuous muscle discharges, and titubation. Ann Neurol 1977;1:120.

Harley HG, Rundle SA, MacMillan JC, et al. Size of the unstable CTG repeat sequence in relation to phenotype and parental transmission in myotonic dystrophy. Am J Hum Genet 1993;52(6):1164.

Harper PS. Myotonic dystrophy, 3rd ed. London: W.B. Saunders Company, 2001.

Harper PS, van Engelen B, Eymard et al. Myotonic dystrophy: Present management, future therapy. Oxford: Oxford University Press, 2004.

Hart IK. Acquired neuromyotonia: A new autoantibody-mediated neuronal potassium channelopathy. Am J Med Sci 2000;319:209.

Hart IK, Maddison P, Newsom-Davis J, Vincent A, Mills KR. Phenotypic variants of autoimmune peripheral nerve hyperexcitability. Brain 2002;125:1887.

Hayat GR, Kulkantrakorn K, Campbell WW, Giuliani MJ. Neuromyotonia: Autoimmune pathogenesis and response to immune modulating therapy. J Neurol Sci 2000;181(1-2):38.

Ho NC, Sandusky S, Madike V, et al. Clinico-pathogenetic findings and management of chondrodystrophic myotonia (Schwartz-Jampel syndrome): A case report. BMC Neurol 2003;3:3.

Huttenlocher PR, Landwirth J, Hanson V, et al. Osteo-chondro-muscular dystrophy. A disorder manifested by multiple skeletal deformities, myotonia, and dystrophic changes in muscle. Pediatrics 1969;44:945.

Imbrici P, Cusimano A, D'Adamo MC, et al. Functional characterization of an episodic ataxia type-1 mutation occurring in the S1 segment of hKv1.1 channels. Pflugers Arch 2003;446:373.

The International Myotonic Dystrophy Consortium (IDMC). New nomenclature and DNA testing guidelines for myotonic dystrophy type 1 (DM1). The International Myotonic Dystrophy Consortium (IDMC). Neurology 2000;54(6):1218.

Iozzo RV, Cohen IR, Grassel S, et al. The biology of perlecan: The multifaceted heparan sulphate proteoglycan of basement membranes and pericellular matrices. Biochem J 1994;302:625.

Isaacs H. A syndrome of continuous muscle-fiber activity. J Neurol Neurosurg Psychiat 1961;24:319.

Iwata H, Ozawa H, Kamei A, et al: Siblings of Schwartz-Jampel syndrome with abnormal muscle computed tomographic findings. Brain Dev 22;494: 2000.

Jakubiczka S, Vielhaber S, Kress W, et al. Improvement of the diagnostic procedure in proximal myotonic myopathy/myotonic dystrophy type 2. Neurogenetics 2004;5(1):55.

Jentsch TJ, Stein V, Weinreich F, et al. Molecular structure and physiological function of chloride channels. Physiol Rev 2002;82(2):503.

Jurkat-Rott K, Lehmann-Horn F. Electrophysiology and molecular pharmacology of muscle channelopathies. Rev Neurol (Paris) 2004;160:S43.

Jurkat-Rott K, Lehmann-Horn F, Elbaz A, et al. A calcium channel mutation causing hypokalemic periodic paralysis. Hum Mol Genet 1994;3(8):1415.

Jurkat-Rott K, Mitrovic N, Hang C, et al. Voltage-sensor sodium channel mutations cause hypokalemic periodic paralysis type 2 by enhanced inactivation and reduced current. Proc Natl Acad Sci U S A 2000;97(17):9549.

Jurkat-Rott K, Uetz U, Pika-Hartlaub U, et al. Calcium currents and transients of native and heterologously expressed mutant skeletal muscle DHP receptor alpha1 subunits (R528H). FEBS Lett 1998;423(2):198.

Kanadia RN, Johnstone KA, Mankodi A, et al. A muscleblind knockout model for myotonic dystrophy. Science 2003;302(5652):1978.

Kinali M, Jungbluth H, Eunson LH, et al. Expanding the phenotype of potassium channelopathy: Severe neuromyotonia and skeletal deformities without prominent episodic ataxia. Neuromuscul Disord 2004;14:689.

Klein A, Boltshauser E, Jen J, Baloh RW. Episodic ataxia type 1 with distal weakness: A novel manifestation of a potassium channelopathy. Neuropediatrics 2004;35(2):147.

Klein R, Ganelin R, Marks JF, et al. Periodic paralysis with cardiac arrhythmia. J Pediatr 1963;62:371.

Koch MC, Steinmeyer K, Lorenz C, et al. The skeletal muscle chloride channel in dominant and recessive human myotonia. Science 1992;257(5071):797.

Koerner C, Wieland B, Richter W, et al. Stiff-person syndromes: Motor cortex hyperexcitability correlates with anti-GAD autoimmunity. Neurology 2004;62(8):1357.

Koty PP, Pegoraro E, Hobson G, et al. Myotonia and the muscle chloride channel: Dominant mutations show variable penetrance and founder effect. Neurology 1996;47(4):963.

Kramer LD, Cole JP, Messenger JC, et al. Cardiac dysfunction in a patient with familial hypokalemic periodic paralysis. Chest 1979;75(2):189.

Kung AW, Lau KS, Fong GC, et al. Association of novel single nucleotide polymorphisms in the calcium channel alpha 1 subunit gene (Ca(v)1.1) and thyrotoxic periodic paralysis. J Clin Endocrinol Metab 2004;89(3):1340.

Kwiecinski H, Ryniewicz B, Ostrzycki A. Treatment of myotonia with antiarrhythmic drugs. Acta Neurol Scand 1992;86(4):371.

Lapie P, Lory P, Fontaine B. Hypokalemic periodic paralysis: An autosomal dominant muscle disorder caused by mutations in a voltage-gated calcium channel. Neuromuscul Disord 1997;7(4):234.

Lavedan C, Hofmann-Radvanyi H, Shelbourne P, et al. Myotonic dystrophy: Size- and sex-dependent dynamics of CTG meiotic instability, and somatic mosaicism. Am J Hum Genet 1993;52(5):875

Lehmann-Horn F, Engel AG, Ricker K, et al. The periodic paralysis and paramyotonia congenita. In: Engel AG, Franzini-Armstrong C, eds. Myology. New York: McGraw-Hill, 1994;1303.

Lehmann-Horn F, Jurkat-Rott K. Voltage-gated ion channels and hereditary disease. Physiol Rev 1999;79(4):1317.

Lehmann-Horn F, Rudel R. Channelopathies: The nondystrophic myotonias and periodic paralyses. Semin Pediatr Neurol 1996;3(2):122.

Lerche H, Heine R, Pika U, et al. Human sodium channel myotonia: Slowed channel inactivation due to substitutions for a glycine within the III-IV linker. J Physiol 1993;470:13.

Levitt LP, Rose LI, Dawson DM. Hypokalemic periodic paralysis with arrhythmia. N Engl J Med 1972;286(5):253.

Lipicky RJ, Bryant SH. A biophysical study of the human myotonias. In: Desmedt JE, ed. New developments in electromyography and clinical neurophysiology. Basel: S. Karger, 1993.

Liquori CL, Ikeda Y, Weatherspoon M, et al. Myotonic dystrophy type 2: Human founder haplotype and evolutionary conservation of the repeat tract. Am J Hum Genet 2003;73(4):849.

Liquori CL, Ricker K, Moseley ML, et al. Myotonic dystrophy type 2 caused by a CCTG expansion in intron 1 of ZNF9. Science 2001;293(5531):864.

Lisak RP, Lebeau J, Tucker SH, et al. Hyperkalemic periodic paralysis and cardiac arrhythmia. Neurology 1972;22(8):810.

Litt M, Kramer P, Browne D, et al. A gene for episodic ataxia/myokymia maps to chromosome 12p13. Am J Hum Genet 1994;55:702.

Lohmann T, Londei M, Hawa M, et al. Humoral and cellular autoimmune responses in stiff person syndrome. Ann N Y Acad Sci 2003;998:215.

Lubbers WJ, Brunt ER, Scheffer H, et al. Hereditary myokymia and paroxysmal ataxia linked to chromosome 12 is responsive to acetazolamide. J Neurol Neurosurg Psychiatry 1995;59(4):400.

Mahadevan M, Tsilfidis C, Sabourin L, et al. Myotonic dystrophy mutation: An unstable CTG repeat in the 3′ untranslated region of the gene. Science 1992;(255):1253.

Mankodi A, Logigian E, Callahan L, et al. Myotonic dystrophy in transgenic mice expressing an expanded CUG repeat. Science 2000;289(5485):1769.

Mankodi A, Takahashi MP, Jiang H, et al. Expanded CUG repeats trigger aberrant splicing of ClC-1 chloride channel pre-mRNA and hyperexcitability of skeletal muscle in myotonic dystrophy. Mol Cell 2002;10(1):35.

Mankodi A, Teng-Umnuay P, Krym M, et al. Ribonuclear inclusions in skeletal muscle in myotonic dystrophy types 1 and 2. Ann Neurol 2003;54(6):760.

Mankodi A, Thornton CA. Myotonic syndromes. Curr Opin Neurol 2002;15(5):545.

Martinelli P, Nassetti S, Minardi C, et al. Electrophysiological evaluation of the stiff-man syndrome: Further data. J Neurol 1996;243(7):551.

Martorell L, Monckton DG, Sanchez A, et al. Frequency and stability of the myotonic dystrophy type 1 premutation. Neurology 2001;56(3):328.

McCarthy TV, Mackrill JJ. Unravelling calcium-release channel gating: Clues from a 'hot' disease. Biochem J 2004;380(Pt 2):e1.

Meinck HM, Ricker K, Hulser PJ, et al. Stiff man syndrome: Neurophysiological findings in eight patients. J Neurol 1995;242(3):134.

Meola G. Clinical and genetic heterogeneity in myotonic dystrophies. Muscle Nerve 2000;23(12):1789.

Meola G, Moxley RT, III. Myotonic dystrophy type 2 and related myotonic disorders. J Neurol 2004;251(10):1173.

Meola G, Sansone V, Perani D, et al. Reduced cerebral blood flow and impaired visual-spatial function in proximal myotonic myopathy. Neurology 1999;(5):1042.

Meola G, Sansone V, Perani D, et al. Executive dysfunction and avoidant personality trait in myotonic dystrophy type 1 (DM-1) and in proximal myotonic myopathy (PROMM/DM-2). Neuromuscul Disord 2003;13(10):813.

Meyer-Kleine C, Steinmeyer K, Ricker K, et al. Spectrum of mutations in the major human skeletal muscle chloride channel gene (CLCN1) leading to myotonia. Am J Hum Genet 1995;57(6):1325.

Miller TM, Dias da Silva MR, Miller HA, et al. Correlating phenotype and genotype in the periodic paralyses. Neurology 2004;63(9):1647.

Moersch FP, Woltman HW. Progressive fluctuating muscular rigidity and spasm ("stiff-man" syndrome); report of a case and some observations in 13 other cases. Mayo Clin Proc 1956;31:421.

Mohammadi B, Mitrovic N, Lehmann-Horn F, et al. Mechanisms of cold sensitivity of paramyotonia congenita mutation R1448H and overlap syndrome mutation M1360V. J Physiol 2003;547(Pt 3):691.

Moxley RT III. Metabolic and endocrine myopathies. In: Walton J, Karpati G, Hilton-Jones D, eds. Disorders of voluntary muscle. Edinburgh: Churchhill Livingstone, 1994;647.

Moxley RT III. Channelopathies. Curr Treat Options Neurol 2000;2(1):31.

Moxley RT III. Myotonic dystrophy. Medlink neurology 2003. Available at: www.medlink.com.

Moxley RT III, Meola G, Udd B, et al. Report of the 84th ENMC workshop: PROMM (proximal myotonic myopathy) and other myotonic dystrophy-like syndromes: 2nd workshop, Loosdrecht, The Netherlands, October, 13-15, 2000. Neuromuscul Disord 2002;12(3):306.

Moxley RT III, Pandya S, Thornton CA, et al. Therapeutic trials and future advances. In: Harper PS, van Engelen BGM, Eymard B, Wilcox DE, eds. Myotonic dystrophy: Present management, future therapy. Oxford: Oxford University Press, 2004;219.

Murinson BB, Butler M, Marfurt K, et al. Markedly elevated GAD antibodies in SPS: Effects of age and illness duration. Neurology 2004;63(11):2146.
Nemni R, Caniatti LM, Gironi M, et al. Stiff person syndrome does not always occur with maternal passive transfer of GAD65 antibodies. Neurology 2004;62(11):2101.
Newsom-Davis J, Buckley C, Clover L, et al. Autoimmune disorders of neuronal potassium channels. Ann N Y Acad Sci 2003;998:202.
Ng WY, Lui KF, Thai AC, et al. Absence of ion channels CACN1AS and SCN4A mutations in thyrotoxic hypokalemic periodic paralysis. Thyroid 2004;14(3):187.
Nicole S, Ben Hamida C, Beighton P, et al. Localization of the Schwartz-Jampel syndrome (SJS) locus to chromosome 1p34-p36.1 by homozygosity mapping. Hum Mol Genet 1995;4:1633.
Nicole S, Davoine CS, Topaloglu H, et al. Perlecan, the major proteoglycan of basement membranes, is altered in patients with Schwartz-Jampel syndrome (chondrodystrophic myotonia). Nat Genet 2000;26(4):480.
Norgaard A, Kjeldsen K. Interrelation of hypokalaemia and potassium depletion and its implications: A re-evaluation based on studies of the skeletal muscle sodium, potassium-pump [editorial]. [Review] [53 refs]. Clin Sci 1991;81(4):449.
Ober KP. Thyrotoxic periodic paralysis in the United States. Report of 7 cases and review of the literature. [Review] [121 refs]. Medicine 1992;71(3):109.
Odor DL, Patel AN, Pearce LA. Familial hypokalemic periodic paralysis with permanent myopathy. A clinical and ultrastructural study. J Neuropathol Exper Neurol 1967;26(1):98.
Okihiro MM, Nordyke RA. Hypokalemic periodic paralysis. Experimental precipitation with sodium liothyronine. JAMA 1966;198(8):949.
Paradis CM, Gironda F, Bennett M. Cognitive impairment in Schwartz-Jampel syndrome: A case study. Brain Lang 1997;56:301.
Pascuzzi RM. Schwartz-Jampel syndrome. Semin Neurol 1991;11(3):267.
Peng HB, Xie H, Rossi SG, Rotundo RL. Acetylcholinesterase clustering at the neuromuscular junction involves perlecan and dystroglycan. J Cell Biol 1999;145(4):911.
Petzold GC, Marcucci M, Butler MH, et al. Rhabdomyolysis and paraneoplastic stiff-man syndrome with amphiphysin autoimmunity. Ann Neurol 2004;55(2):286.
Pineiro E, Fernandez-Lopez L, Gamez J, et al. Mutagenic stress modulates the dynamics of CTG repeat instability associated with myotonic dystrophy type 1. Nucleic Acids Res 2003;31(23):6733.
Pinto-Escalante D, Ceballos-Quintal JM, Canto-Herrera J. Identical twins with the classical form of Schwartz-Jampel syndrome. Clin Dysmorphol 1997;6:45.
Plaster NM, Tawil R, Tristani-Firouzi M, et al. Mutations in Kir2.1 cause the developmental and episodic electrical phenotypes of Andersen's syndrome. Cell 2001;105(4):511.
Ptacek L. The familial periodic paralyses and nondystrophic myotonias. Am J Med 1998;105(1):58.
Ptacek L, Bendahhou S. Ion channel disorders of muscle. In: Karpati G, Hilton-Jones D, Griggs RC, eds. Disorders of voluntary muscle. Cambridge: Cambridge University Press, 2001;604.
Ptacek LJ. Channelopathies: Ion channel disorders of muscle as a paradigm for paroxysmal disorders of the nervous system. Neuromuscul Disord 1997;7(4):250.
Ptacek LJ, Johnson KJ, Griggs RC. Genetics and physiology of the myotonic muscle disorders. N Engl J Med 1993;328(7):482.
Ptacek LJ, Tawil R, Griggs RC, et al. Linkage of atypical myotonia congenita to a sodium channel locus. Neurology 1992;42(2):431.
Ptacek LJ, Tawil R, Griggs RC, et al. Dihydropyridine receptor mutations cause hypokalemic periodic paralysis. Cell 1994a;77(6):863.
Ptacek LJ, Tawil R, Griggs RC, et al. Sodium channel mutations in acetazolamide-responsive myotonia congenita, paramyotonia congenita, and hyperkalemic periodic paralysis. Neurology 1994b;44(8):1500.
Pusch M, Steinmeyer K, Koch MC, et al. Mutations in dominant human myotonia congenita drastically alter the voltage dependence of the CIC-1 chloride channel. Neuron 1995;15(6):1455.
Pusch M. Myotonia caused by mutations in the muscle chloride channel gene CLCN1. Hum Mutat 2002;19(4):423.
Rakocevic G, Raju R, Dalakas MC. Anti-glutamic acid decarboxylase antibodies in the serum and cerebrospinal fluid of patients with stiff-person syndrome: Correlation with clinical severity. Arch Neurol 2004;61(6):902.
Ranum LP, Day JW. Myotonic dystrophy: Clinical and molecular parallels between myotonic dystrophy type 1 and type 2. Curr Neurol Neurosci Rep 2002;2(5):465.
Ranum LP, Rasmussen PF, Benzow KA, et al. Genetic mapping of a second myotonic dystrophy locus. Nat Genet 1998;19(2):196.
Rea R, Spauschus A, Eunson LH, et al. Variable K(+) channel subunit dysfunction in inherited mutations of KCNA1. J Physiol 2002;538(Pt 1):5.
Redman JB, Fenwick RJ, Fu YH, et al. Relationship between parental trinucleotide GCT repeat length and severity of myotonic dystrophy in offspring. JAMA 1993;269(15):1960.
Resnick JS, Dorman JD, Engel WK. Thyrotoxic periodic paralysis. Am J Med 1969;47(5):831.
Ricker K, Camacho LM, Grafe P, et al. Adynamia episodica hereditaria: What causes the weakness? Muscle Nerve 1989;12(11):883.
Ricker K, Koch MC, Lehmann-Horn F, et al. Proximal myotonic myopathy: A new dominant disorder with myotonia, muscle weakness, and cataracts. Neurology 1994a;44(8):1448.
Ricker K, Koch MC, Lehmann-Horn F, et al. Proximal myotonic myopathy. Clinical features of a multisystem disorder similar to myotonic dystrophy. Arch Neurol 1995;52(1):25.
Ricker K, Lehmann-Horn F, Moxley RT. Myotonia fluctuans [see comments]. Arch Neurol 1990;47(3):268.
Ricker K, Moxley RT, Heine R, et al. Myotonia fluctuans. A third type of muscle sodium channel disease. Archives of Neurology 1994b;51(11):1095.
Rudel R, Lehmann-Horn F, Ricker K. The nondystrophic myotonias. In: Engel AG, Franzini-Armstrong C, eds. Myology. New York: McGraw-Hill, 1994;1291.
Rudnik-Schoneborn S, Zerres K. Outcome in pregnancies complicated by myotonic dystrophy: A study of 31 patients and review of the literature. Eur J Obstet Gynecol Reprod Biol 2004;114(1):44.
Ryan A, Rudel R, Kuchenbecker M, et al. A novel alteration of muscle chloride channel gating in myotonia levior. J Physiol 2002;545(Pt 2):345.
Sabovic M, Medica I, Logar N, et al. Relation of CTG expansion and clinical variables to electrocardiogram conduction abnormalities and sudden death in patients with myotonic dystrophy. Neuromuscul Disord 2003;13(10):822.
Sallinen R, Vihola A, Bachinski LL, et al. New methods for molecular diagnosis and demonstration of the (CCTG)n mutation in myotonic dystrophy type 2 (DM2). Neuromuscul Disord 2004;14(4):274.
Sanguinetti MC, Spector PS. Potassium channelopathies. Neuropharmacology 1997;36(6):755.
Sansone V, Griggs RC, Meola G, et al. Andersen's syndrome: A distinct periodic paralysis. Ann Neurol 1997;42(3):305.
Saviane C, Conti F, Pusch M. The muscle chloride channel ClC-1 has a double-barreled appearance that is differentially affected in dominant and recessive myotonia. J Gen Physiol 1999;113(3):457.
Savkur RS, Philips AV, Cooper TA. Aberrant regulation of insulin receptor alternative splicing is associated with insulin resistance in myotonic dystrophy. Nat Genet 2001;29(1):40.
Savkur RS, Philips AV, Cooper TA, et al. Insulin receptor splicing alteration in myotonic dystrophy type 2. Am J Hum Genet 2004;74(6):1309.
Schoser BG, Kress W, Walter MC, et al. Homozygosity for CCTG mutation in myotonic dystrophy type 2. Brain 2004a;127(Pt 8):1868.
Schneider C, Ziegler A, Ricker K, et al. Proximal myotonic myopathy: Evidence for anticipation in families with linkage to chromosome 3q. Neurology 2000;55(3):383.
Schwartz O, Jampel R. Congenital blepharophimosis associated with a unique generalized myopathy. Arch Ophthal 1962;68:52.
Seay AR, Ziter FA. Malignant hyperpyrexia in a patient with Schwartz-Jampel syndrome. J Pediatr 1978;93(1):83.
Shayne P, Hart A. Thyrotoxic periodic paralysis terminated with intravenous propranolol. Ann Emerg Med 1994;24(4):736.
Sheela SR. Myotonia congenita: Response to carbamazepine. Indian Pediatr 2000;37(10):1122.
Shy G, Wanko T, Rowley P, et al. Familial periodic paralysis. Exper Neurol 1961;3:53.
Sillen A, Sorensen T, Kantola I, et al. Identification of mutations in the CACNL1A3 gene in 13 families of Scandinavian origin having hypokalemic periodic paralysis and evidence of a founder effect in Danish families. Am J Med Genet 1997;69(1):102.
Singh B, Biary N, Jamil AA, al-Shahwan SA. Schwartz-Jampel syndrome: Evidence of central nervous system dysfunction. J Child Neurol 1997;12:214.
Spranger J, Hall BD, Hane B, et al: Spectrum of Schwartz-Jampel syndrome includes micromelic chondrodysplasia, kyphomelic dysplasia, and Burton disease. Am J Med Genet 94:287-95, 2000.

Squires LA, Prangley J. Neonatal diagnosis of Schwartz-Jampel syndrome with dramatic response to carbamazepine. Pediatr Neurol 1996;15:172.

Struyk AF, Scoggan KA, Bulman DE, et al. The human skeletal muscle Na channel mutation R669H associated with hypokalemic periodic paralysis enhances slow inactivation. J Neurosci 2000;20(23):8610.

Stubbs WA. Bidirectional ventricular tachycardia in familial hypokalaemic periodic paralysis. Proc R Soc Med 1976;69(3):223.

Tang NL, Chow CC, Ko GT, et al. No mutation in the KCNE3 potassium channel gene in Chinese thyrotoxic hypokalaemic periodic paralysis patients. Clin Endocrinol (Oxf) 2004;61(1):109.

Tassone H, Moulin A, Henderson SO. The pitfalls of potassium replacement in thyrotoxic periodic paralysis: A case report and review of the literature. J Emerg Med 2004;26(2):157.

Tawil R, Moxley RT, Griggs RC. Acetazolamide-induced nephrolithiasis: Implications for treatment of neuromuscular disorders. Neurology 1993;43(6):1105.

Tawil R, Ptacek LJ, Pavlakis SG, et al. Andersen's syndrome: Potassium-sensitive periodic paralysis, ventricular ectopy, and dysmorphic features [see comments]. Ann Neurol 1994;35(3):326.

Tawil R, McDermott MP, Brown R, Jr., et al. Randomized trials of dichlorphenamide in the periodic paralyses. Working Group on Periodic Paralysis. Ann Neurol 2000;47(1):46.

Taylor RG, Layzer RB, Davis HS, et al. Continuous muscle fiber activity in the Schwartz-Jampel syndrome. Electroencephalogr Clin Neurophysiol 1972;33(5):497.

Thornton CA, Griggs RC, Moxley RT. Myotonic dystrophy with no trinucleotide repeat expansion [see comments]. Ann Neurol 1994;35(3):269.

Timchenko LT, Tapscott SJ, Cooper TA, et al. Myotonic dystrophy: Discussion of molecular basis. Adv Exp Med Biol 2002;516:27.

Tomimitsu H, Arimura K, Nagado T, et al. Mechanism of action of voltage-gated K+ channel antibodies in acquired neuromyotonia. Ann Neurol 2004;56:440.

Topaloglu H, Serdaroglu A, Okan M, et al. Improvement of myotonia with carbamazepine in three cases with the Schwartz-Jampel syndrome. Neuropediatrics 1993;24:232.

Torres CF, Griggs RC, Moxley RT, et al. Hypokalemic periodic paralysis exacerbated by acetazolamide. Neurology 1981;31(11):1423.

Tristani-Firouzi M, Jensen JL, Donaldson MR, et al. Functional and clinical characterization of KCNJ2 mutations associated with LQT7 (Andersen syndrome). J Clin Invest 2002;110(3):381.

Trudell RG, Kaiser KK, Griggs RC. Acetazolamide-responsive myotonia congenita. Neurology 1987;37(3):488.

Tsilfidis C, MacKenzie AE, Mettler G, et al. Correlation between CTG trinucleotide repeat length and frequency of severe congenital myotonic dystrophy. Nature Genetics 1992;1(3):192.

Udd B, Krahe R, Wallgren-Pettersson C, et al. Proximal myotonic dystrophy—A family with autosomal dominant muscular dystrophy, cataracts, hearing loss and hypogonadism: Heterogeneity of proximal myotonic syndromes? Neuromuscul Disord 1997;7(4):217.

Vaamonde J, Artieda J, Obeso JA. Hereditary paroxysmal ataxia with neuromyotonia. Mov Disord 1991;6:180.

VanDyke DH, Griggs RC, Murphy MJ, Goldstein MN. Hereditary myokymia and periodic ataxia. J Neurol Sci 1975;25(1):109.

Van Meir N, De Smet L: Carpal tunnel syndrome in children. Acta Orthop Belg 2003;69:38.

Venance SL, Jurkat-Rott K, Lehmann-Horn F, et al. SCN4A-associated hypokalemic periodic paralysis merits a trial of acetazolamide. Neurology 2004;63(10):1977.

Vihola A, Bassez G, Meola G, et al. Histopathological differences of myotonic dystrophy type 1 (DM1) and PROMM/DM2. Neurology 2003;60(11):1854.

Wagner S, Deymeer F, Kurz LL, et al. The dominant chloride channel mutant G200R causing fluctuating myotonia: Clinical findings, electrophysiology, and channel pathology. Muscle Nerve 1998;21(9):1122.

Wu FF, Ryan A, Devaney J, et al. Novel CLCN1 mutations with unique clinical and electrophysiological consequences. Brain 2002;125(Pt 11):2392.

Yang Z, Lau R, Marcadier JL, et al. Replication inhibitors modulate instability of an expanded trinucleotide repeat at the myotonic dystrophy type 1 disease locus in human cells. Am J Hum Genet 2003;73(5):1092.

Yeung RT, Tse TF. Thyrotoxic periodic paralysis. Effect of propranolol. Am J Med 1974;57(4):584.

Yoshimura T, Kaneuji M, Okuno T, et al. Periodic paralysis with cardiac arrhythmia. Eur J Pediatr 1983;140(4):338.

Zhang J, George ALJ, Griggs RC, et al. Mutations in the human skeletal muscle chloride channel gene (CLCN1) associated with dominant and recessive myotonia congenita. Neurology 1996;47(4):993.

Zwarts MJ, van Weerden TW. Transient paresis in myotonic syndromes. A surface EMG study. Brain 1989;112(Pt 3):665.

PART XIV

Neuroendocrine and Autonomic Nervous System Disorders

CHAPTER 84

Endocrine Disorders of the Hypothalamus and Pituitary

Qing Dong and Stephen M. Rosenthal

Through integrated neural and hormonal signaling, the hypothalamus and pituitary regulate a broad range of physiologic processes, including statural growth, sexual maturation, lactation, metabolic actions ascribed to adrenal (glucocorticoid) and thyroid hormones, appetite, and water balance. Each of these physiologic processes involves hypothalamic/pituitary regulation of a variety of target tissues, which in turn, regulate hypothalamic/pituitary function through feedback loops. Although a comprehensive endocrine approach to abnormalities of any of these physiologic loops or axes requires consideration of disorders intrinsic to the hypothalamus/pituitary or intrinsic to the target tissues, this chapter will focus on those disorders specifically caused by endocrine abnormalities of the hypothalamus and pituitary. An overview of hypothalamic/pituitary anatomy and physiology is followed by a review of endocrine disorders of these structures grouped by principal signs and symptoms.

ANATOMIC AND PHYSIOLOGIC ASPECTS

The hypothalamus, the ventral part of the diencephalon, is an evolutionarily conserved region of the mammalian brain. The hypothalamus is separated by the third ventricle and connected to the pituitary by the hypophysial stalk. The hypothalamus functions as the primary control center for a variety of physiologic processes, integrating neural and hormonal signaling. Hypothalamic nuclei are not well-demarcated regions; however, these cell groups in the walls of the third ventricle possess specific physiologic functions [Pansky et al., 1988]. The supraoptic and paraventricular nuclei produce arginine vasopressin (also known as *antidiuretic hormone*) and oxytocin. Paraventricular nuclei and arcuate nuclei release thyrotropin-releasing hormone, corticotropin-releasing hormone, somatostatin, growth hormone-releasing hormone, gonadotropin-releasing hormone, and dopamine into the hypophysial portal circulation to regulate the synthesis and release of anterior pituitary hormones. In addition, hypothalamic neurons that regulate appetite and energy balance are also located in the paraventricular and arcuate nuclei of the hypothalamus, such as pro-opiomelanocortin and neuropeptide Y and agouti-related protein–expressing neurons [Cone et al., 2003].

The pituitary (hypophysis) is housed in the sella turcica, and, as noted, is attached to the hypothalamus by the hypophysial stalk. The stalk, also called the *infundibulum*, is a collective term for the median eminence (the most inferior extension of the tuber cinereum), and the infundibular stalk (a hollow process extending from the tuber cinereum to the posterior hypophysis). The stalk serves as an anatomic and functional link between the hypothalamus and the pituitary. The optic chiasm is situated directly anterior to the pituitary stalk (Fig. 84-1). The pituitary itself is small, weighing an average of about half a gram, and is divided into the anterior lobe (adenohypophysis), the posterior lobe (neurohypophysis), and a vestigial intermediate lobe. Six hormones—growth hormone, thyroid-stimulating hormone, adrenocorticotropin hormone, follicle-stimulating hormone, luteinizing hormone, and prolactin—are synthesized and stored in the anterior lobe from well-differentiated distinct cell types (somatotrophs, thyrotrophs, corticotrophs, gonadotrophs, and lactotrophs). However, some cell types, such as mammosomatotrophs, can express multiple hormones (prolactin and growth hormone). The neurohypophysis synthesizes, stores, and secretes arginine vasopressin and oxytocin [Cone et al., 2003].

The blood supply in the hypothalamic-pituitary-portal system allows bidirectional hypothalamic-pituitary hormonal interaction. The superior hypophysial arteries from the internal carotid arteries form a primary plexus in the median eminence. These vessels travel down to the anterior pituitary as the major blood supply. The hypothalamic-pituitary-portal circulation carries the hypothalamic-releasing and hypothalamic-inhibiting hormones to the adenohypophysis. Retrograde blood flow within the internal capillary plexus (gomitoli) derived from the stalk branches of the superior hypophysial arteries provides local hormonal feedback to the hypothalamus. The blood supply for the posterior pituitary gland is derived from the inferior hypophysial arteries, in turn, derived from the internal carotid arteries [Bergland and Page, 1979; Stanfield, 1960].

Organogenesis of the hypothalamus and the pituitary is a complex process. The alar plates from the myelencephalon form the lateral walls of the diencephalon. During brain development the hypothalamic sulcus divides the alar plates into dorsal and ventral regions. The hypothalamus, as part of the lower and ventral portion of the alar plates, differentiates into hypothalamic nuclei that serve as control centers for life-sustaining physiologic processes. The pituitary, however, develops from two distinct areas. The adenohypophysis derives from the oral ectoderm (Rathke's pouch), and the neurohypophysis is a downward extension of the diencephalon [Sadler, 1990]. Since the mid 1990s, significant progress has been made in our understanding of the molecular events that regulate embryogenesis of the adenohypophysis. Bone morphogenic protein-4 and fibroblast growth factor-8 are critical for anterior pituitary gland development. In addition, differentiation of anterior pituitary cell types requires a spatiotemporally regulated cascade of homeodomain transcription factors. Several

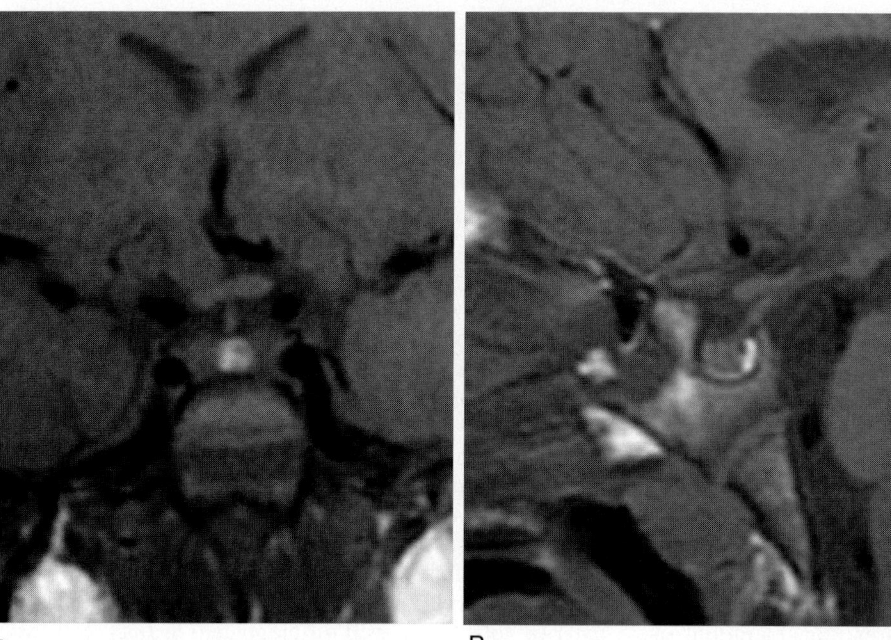

FIGURE 84-1. Coronal (**A**) and sagittal (**B**) T1-weighted images of normal hypothalamus/pituitary in an 8-year-old female by MRI. Note the location of the pituitary stalk, and the intense bright signal from the posterior pituitary (bright spot) in the sagittal view.

pituitary-specific transcription factors, such as Lhx3/Lhx4 (LIM homeobox-3 and -4), Rpx (Rathke's pouch homeobox, also known as Hesx1), Pitx (pituitary homeobox), Prop-1, Pit-1, and Sox3, are important determinants of pituitary cell lineages. Mutations in these transcription factors can lead to either isolated or combined pituitary hormone deficiencies with or without detectable anatomic abnormalities [Cohen and Radovick, 2002; Dattani et al., 1998, 2000; Rizzoti et al., 2004].

HYPOTHALAMIC/PITUITARY DISORDERS OF PUBERTAL DEVELOPMENT

Normal Physiology of Puberty and Adrenarche

Puberty is the transitional period between the juvenile state and adulthood, characterized by attainment of secondary sex characteristics and reproductive capability. The control center of puberty is composed of hypothalamic gonadotropin-releasing hormone neurosecretory neurons (pulse generator) located in the medial basal hypothalamus [King et al., 1985]. Puberty is not a sudden event but rather reflects a milestone on a continuum that begins before birth. The gonadotropin-releasing hormone pulse generator becomes pulsatile by midgestation, and remains active in early infancy until about 6 months of age in males and 12 to 24 months in females [Grumbach, 2002]. Between late infancy and the onset of puberty, the gonadotropin-releasing hormone pulse generator becomes relatively quiescent as a consequence of an as yet poorly defined central nervous system (CNS) inhibitory mechanism. After a quiescent period of approximately 10 years, the gonadotropin-releasing hormone pulse generator is disinhibited, leading to increased amplitude and frequency of luteinizing hormone and follicle-stimulating hormone secretion resulting in increased sex steroid production (principally estradiol and testosterone) and attainment of physical puberty [Grumbach, 2002].

Adrenarche refers to the prepubertal rise of adrenal androgen precursors, in particular dehydroepiandrosterone and its sulfated form, as a consequence of maturation of the zona reticularis of the adrenal cortex. Dehydroepiandrosterone can be peripherally converted to testosterone, thus adrenarche is clinically typified by mild androgenic effects, such as a change in body odor and the appearance of axillary and pubic hair and acne. The mechanisms that regulate adrenarche are not well understood. Adrenache is independent of the maturation of the hypothalamic-pituitary-gonadal axis, preceding the onset of puberty by about 2 years [Miller, 1999].

The normal age of onset of secondary sexual characteristics (defined as 2.5 standard deviations on either side of the mean, or where approximately 99% of the population falls) is 6 to 13 years in females and 9 to 14 years in males. The appearance of secondary sexual characteristics, acceleration of growth, and the capacity of reproduction are hallmarks of puberty. The development of puberty is characterized by sequential events that are specific for each sex. In females, secondary sexual characteristics include breast development, the appearance of pubic and axillary hair, maturation of the labia, and estrogenization of the vaginal mucosa. The development of pubic and axillary hair is influenced by androgens produced in both the adrenal cortex (adrenarche) and the ovary. Menarche usually occurs 2 to 3 years after initiation of breast development. The pubertal growth spurt, which normally occurs in the early stages of puberty for females, can result in a gain in height of 25 cm or more. In males, puberty begins with testicular enlargement (≥2.5 cm in longest dimension) followed by the appearance of sexual hair and phallic enlargement. The growth spurt occurs during midpuberty, which results in an average 28 cm gain in height [Grumbach and Styne, 2003].

General abnormalities of puberty include sexual precocity and delayed or arrested puberty, each with a broad differential diagnosis. Although pubertal disorders can arise from defects at the level of the hypothalamus, pituitary, or gonads, the focus of this discussion is on hypothalamic and pituitary causes of sexual precocity and delayed puberty.

Sexual Precocity

Sexual precocity is usually defined as the development of secondary sexual characteristics before 7 years of age in females [Herman-Giddens et al., 1997], and before 9 years of age in males. In all cases thus far described, sexual precocity results from an increase in circulating sex steroids. An endocrine approach to the differential diagnosis of sexual precocity would include consideration of exogenous and endogenous sources of these steroids. Endogenous causes include the gonads and adrenal cortex, either of which may inappropriately secrete sex steroids as the result of a primary process intrinsic to these tissues, or secondary to a circulating stimulatory factor. As previously noted, this chapter focuses only on hypothalamic/pituitary causes of sexual precocity.

Precocious puberty (sometimes referred to as *true* or *central precocious puberty*) is defined as early puberty specifically resulting from premature reactivation of the gonadotropin-releasing hormone pulse generator. Precocious puberty is most commonly idiopathic but can result from a broad range of abnormalities, including CNS tumors, hamartoma of the tuber cinereum, congenital malformations, subarachnoid cysts, CNS infection, irradiation, and trauma. The incidence of precocious puberty is significantly higher in females. In studies of females with precocious puberty, idiopathic precocious puberty ranges from 63% to 74% [Cisternino et al., 2000; Pescovitz et al., 1986]. In contrast, precocious puberty is idiopathic in only 6% of males with this condition [Pescovitz et al., 1986]. Idiopathic precocious puberty is a diagnosis of exclusion and it is thus essential to search for underlying neurologic causes. Tumors involving in the posterior hypothalamus, such as glioma, germinoma, and teratoma can cause precocious puberty. Most of these tumors are thought to trigger early puberty by interfering with mechanisms that normally inhibit the gonadotropin-releasing hormone pulse generator. Few luteinizing hormone/ follicle-stimulating hormone–secreting adenomas have been reported in adults, [Demura et al., 1977; Sassolas et al., 1988]; however, they are extremely rare in children [Tashiro et al., 1999]. Hamartoma of the tuber cinereum, a congenital malformation, can cause central precocious puberty. Hamartomas are small lesions (4 to 25 mm), may be sessile or pedunculated, and usually do not enlarge with time (Fig. 84-2). Histologically, they appear to be composed of normal brain tissue and contain gonadotropin-releasing hormone secretory neurons, which may serve as an "ectopic pulse generator" [Mahachoklertwattana et al., 1993]. In some hypothalamic hamartomas, the production of transforming growth factor α can initiate early puberty by activating the normal gonadotropin-releasing hormone pulse generator [Jung et al., 1999]. Hamartomas of the tuber cinereum are often associated with gelastic (laughing) seizures.

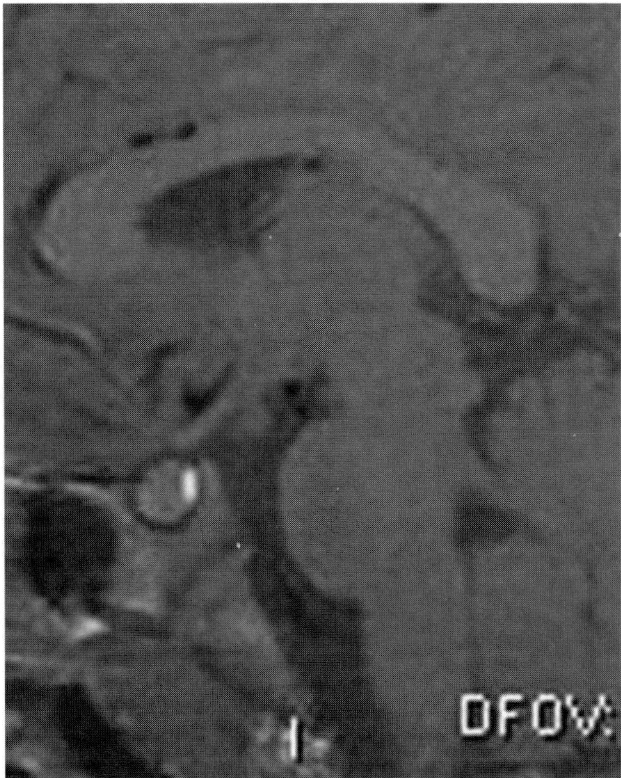

FIGURE 84-2. Hamartoma of the tuber cinereum in a 3-year-old female by MRI. Note a small (6 × 6 mm), pedunculated and isointense hypothalamic mass in the sagittal view. The patient had midpubertal breast development, and an advanced bone age of 6 years at a chronologic age of 3 years.

Ectopic human chorionic gonadotropin–secreting tumors in the CNS (and elsewhere), for example, hypothalamic germinomas, can cause sexual precocity in males [Sklar et al., 1981]. Such patients do not have pituitary gonadotropin-dependent precocious puberty in that they do not have premature reactivation of the hypothalamic gonadotropin-releasing hormone pulse generator. Rather, the ectopic human chorionic gonadotropin interacts with the luteinizing hormone/human chorionic gonadotropin receptor on testicular Leydig cells, resulting in increased testosterone secretion and virilization. In females, ovarian estrogen secretion requires both luteinizing hormone and follicle-stimulating hormone. Thus, ectopic secretion of human chorionic gonadotropin alone causes sexual precocity almost exclusively in boys [Grumbach and Styne, 2003].

The accurate diagnosis of precocious puberty and its cause requires detailed history, physical examination, hormonal testing, and imaging studies of the CNS. Idiopathic precocious puberty is often familial. The occurrence of early breast and pubic hair development is often seen in females with precocious puberty, and testicular enlargement and other signs of virilization are seen in males with precocious puberty. Hormonal analysis demonstrates increased amplitude and frequency of luteinizing hormone and follicle-stimulating hormone pulsatile secretion, resulting from increased pulsatile secretion of gonadotropin-releasing hormone. This finding can be demonstrated either by serial sampling of luteinizing hormone and follicle-stimulating hormone or by single luteinizing hormone/ follicle-stimulating hormone measurements using highly sensitive immunochemiluminescent assays. Dynamic testing using gonadotropin-releasing hormone or a gonadotropin-releasing hormone agonist is also routinely used to diagnose precocious puberty. Magnetic resonance imaging (MRI) with particular attention to the hypothalamic-pituitary area should be carried out in any child diagnosed with precocious puberty.

Management

If a CNS lesion that causes precocious puberty is identified, an appropriate treatment plan for that lesion should be developed. Previously, treatment of hamartomas of the tuber cinereum was principally surgical. However, such treatment carried a significant risk of morbidity and mortality [Rosenfeld et al., 2001; Valdueza et al., 1994]. A long-term follow-up study demonstrated an excellent response to gonadotropin-releasing hormone agonist without surgical resection [Mahachoklertwattana et al., 1993]. Rarely, after treatment of CNS disorders causing precocious puberty, the rapid progression of pubertal development is reversed or arrested. More commonly, once puberty has been initiated, it will often continue despite intervention to address a primary CNS disorder. Such patients require treatment to suppress the hypothalamic-pituitary-gonadal axis. State-of-the-art treatment consists of administration of a gonadotropin-releasing hormone agonist, which desensitizes pituitary gonadotropin-releasing hormone receptors, leading to suppression of the hypothalamic-pituitary-gonadal axis [Breyer et al., 1993]. This treatment is commonly given by a monthly depot intramuscular injection. Long-term studies demonstrate resumption of normal puberty after discontinuation of gonadotropin-releasing hormone agonist [Feuillan et al., 2001].

Delayed or Arrested Puberty

Delayed puberty may be defined in males by the absence of testicular enlargement by 14 years of age, and in females by the absence of breast development by 13 years of age. The differential diagnosis of delayed puberty can be divided into three major categories: constitutional delay in growth and development, hypogonadotropic hypogonadism, and hypergonadotropic hypogonadism. Constitutional delay in growth, the most common cause of delayed puberty, is a normal variant, and is thought to result from a prolonged quiescent period of the gonadotropin-releasing hormone pulse generator. Such patients often have a family history of delayed puberty and have delayed skeletal maturation without evidence of endocrinopathy or other organic diseases. Hypergonadotropic hypogonadism, which indicates a defect at the level of the gonads, is not reviewed in this section. Hypogonadotropic hypogonadism indicates a defect at the level of the hypothalamus or pituitary, and may result from a variety of CNS disorders that can lead to delayed or absent puberty. Hypogonadotropic hypogonadism can be congenital or acquired, can occur alone or in association with multiple hypothalamic and pituitary hormone deficiencies, and may be organic or functional in etiology.

Isolated Congenital Hypogonadotropic Hypogonadism

The most common form of isolated gonadotropin deficiency is Kallmann's syndrome (olfactory-genital-dysplasia), which occurs in 1 in 10,000 males and 1 in 50,000 females [Rugarli and Ballabio, 1993]. Considerable genetic heterogeneity exists for Kallmann's syndrome. Classic Kallmann's syndrome is transmitted in an X-linked or autosomal-dominant fashion with variable penetrance, characterized by hypogonadotropic hypogonadism and anosmia/hyposmia. Some patients may also have unilateral renal agenesis, synkinesia (mirror movements), and pes cavus. Mirror movements occur in 85% of patients with classic Kallmann's syndrome, associated with bilateral hypertrophy of the corticospinal tract [Krams et al., 1999]. Mutations in the *KAL1* gene account for half of males with X-linked hypogonadotropic hypogonadism [Hardelin et al., 1993] and 5% of sporadic cases [Georgopoulos et al., 1997]. The *KAL1* gene resides close to the pseudoautosomal region of the X-chromosome. The cause in females is unknown. The concurrence of anosmia/hyposmia and hypogonadism may reflect disruption of comigration of gonadotropin-releasing hormone and olfactory neurons from the olfactory placode into the hypothalamus during early embryonic development [Wray et al., 1989]. Lack of correlation between genotype and phenotype has been described in Kallmann's syndrome. For instance, within the same family, one patient may have normal gonadal function and anosmia, whereas another may have hypogonadism and a normal sense of smell. However, isolated gonadotropin deficiency with normal sense of smell is rare.

Another form of X-linked hypogonadotropic hypogonadism is associated with adrenal hypoplasia congenita due to defects of *DAX1* (dose-sensitive sex reversal adrenal hypoplasia congenita–associated gene on the X chromosome). *DAX1* encodes a transcription factor that appears to play key developmental roles in the hypothalamus, pituitary, gonad, and adrenal cortex. Males with *DAX1* mutations who survive adrenal failure in infancy and early childhood can present with hypogonadotropic hypogonadism. Rarely, a mild mutation may present in adulthood with mild adrenal insufficiency and incomplete pubertal development. Females homozygous for a *DAX1* nonsense mutation can present with isolated hypogonadotropic hypogonadism [Kalantaridou and Chrousos, 2002]. In addition, mutations in the ß subunits of follicle-stimulating hormone and luteinizing hormone have been reported in association with primary amenorrhea and hypogonadism [Kalantaridou and Chrousos, 2002].

Isolated hypogonadotropic hypogonadism on an autosomal basis is also found in patients with mutations in genes encoding the gonadotropin-releasing hormone receptor [Kalantaridou and Chrousos, 2002] and GPR54, a G protein–coupled receptor [Colledge, 2004; de Roux et al., 2003; Seminara et al., 2003]. Isolated gonadotropin deficiency also occurs in association with Prader-Willi syndrome and Laurence-Moon-Biedl syndrome [Crino et al., 2003; Hashimoto and Kumahara, 1979].

Hypogonadotropic Hypogonadism Associated with Multiple Hypothalamic/Pituitary Hormone Deficiencies

Hypogonadotropic hypogonadism can also present in combination with other hypothalamic/pituitary hormone deficiencies. Human mutations of pituitary transcription factors known to cause delayed puberty include Prop-1 and Lhx3. Prop-1 (prophet of Pit-1) is a paired-like homeodomain transcription factor expressed only in the anterior pituitary. Combined pituitary hormone deficiencies caused by mutations in Prop-1 occur with an incidence of about 1 in 8000 births. Patients with mutations in Prop-1 have combined pituitary hormone deficiencies, which may include deficiencies of growth hormone, prolactin, thyroid-stimulating hormone, and gonadotropins. Such patients have hypogonadotropic hypogonadism in association with short stature and hypothyroidism [Wu et al., 1998]. Lhx3 is a LIM-type homeodomain protein. Mutations in Lhx3 have been associated with anterior pituitary hypoplasia and complete deficits of growth hormone, prolactin, thyroid-stimulating hormone, and gonadotropins. Lhx3 mutations are also associated with decreased range of motion in the cervical spine [Netchine et al., 2000].

Other genetic factors that lead to delayed puberty include mutations of prohormone convertase-1, leptin, and leptin receptor genes. A defect in prohormone convertase-1 has been found to disrupt gonadotropin-releasing hormone processing and results in hypogonadotropic hypogonadism and obesity associated with impaired processing of insulin and proopiomelanocortin. Mutations in leptin and the leptin receptor are associated with a similar clinical picture of hypogonadotropic hypogonadism, hyperinsulinemia, and obesity [Beier and Dluhy, 2003; Kalantaridou and Chrousos, 2002]. Congenital midline defects of the CNS, such as septo-optic dysplasia, empty sella syndrome, and Rathke's cyst are often associated with hypothalamic/pituitary dysfunction, which may include hypogonadotropic hypogonadism. The genetics of septo-optic dysplasia and its related pituitary hormone deficiencies are reviewed in detail in the section on hypothalamic/pituitary disorders of statural growth.

Numerous CNS lesions can lead to hypogonadotropic hypogonadism, including CNS tumors (primarily third ventricular), CNS infection, invasive diseases, cranial irradiation, and trauma. These CNS disorders often present with combined anterior and posterior pituitary hormone deficiencies. CNS tumors of the sella and parasellar region associated with multiple hypothalamic/pituitary hormone deficiencies include craniopharyngioma, pituitary adenomas, optic and hypothalamic gliomas, and germ cell tumors. Delayed or arrested puberty is the second most common presenting symptom of CNS tumors after headache. Craniopharyngiomas, the most common tumor of the sella and parasellar region in children, are slow-growing, space-occupying tumors (Fig. 84-3). Most patients present before their teenage years with headache, visual loss, and multiple hypothalamic/pituitary hormone deficits. Pituitary adenomas in children usually present as microadenomas with pituitary hormone hypersecretion. Nonsecreting adenomas in children are rare and are usually macroadenomas. Prolactinoma is the most common pituitary adenoma in the pediatric population and is frequently associated with delayed or arrested puberty. Nonsecreting macroadenomas also can cause delayed puberty, at least in part, through elevation of prolactin as a consequence of stalk compression [Kunwar and Wilson, 2001]. Cranial irradiation to the third ventricular area may also be associated with hypogonadotropic hypogonadism.

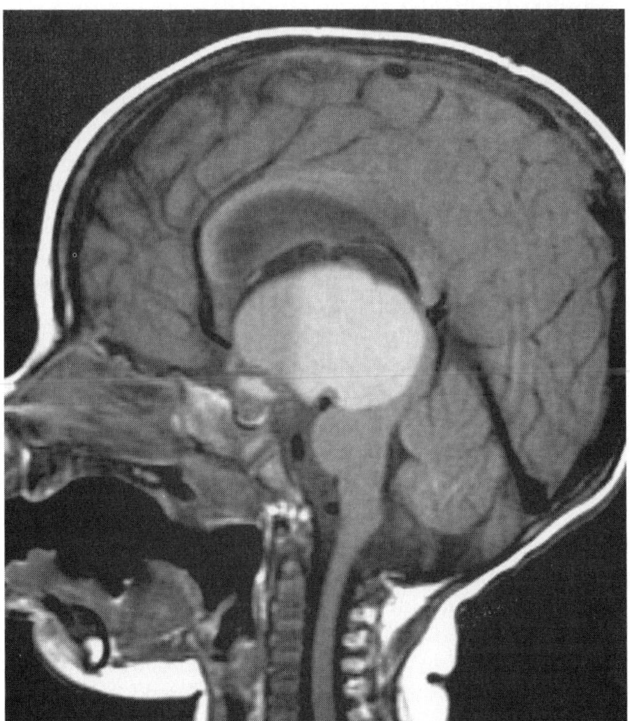

FIGURE 84-3. Craniopharyngioma in a child by MRI. Note a large suprasellar mass elevating the floor of the third ventricle.

Functional Hypogonadotropic Hypogonadism

Reproductive capability is intimately linked to nutritional and metabolic homeostasis. Chronic systemic disease, malnutrition, hypothyroidism, hypercortisolism, poorly controlled diabetes mellitus, and anorexia nervosa are known to cause delayed or arrested pubertal development as a consequence of hypogonadotropic hypogonadism. Functional gonadotropin deficiency may be associated with marijuana use and may occur in some female athletes and ballet dancers. In general, weight loss to less than 80% of ideal weight may result in functional gonadotropin deficiency.

Evaluation of Delayed or Arrested Puberty

As part of an initial evaluation, basal gonadotropin levels (luteinizing hormone, follicle-stimulating hormone) should be measured. Elevated gonadotropins indicate primary ovarian or testicular failure, whereas low or normal gonadotropins indicate either constitutional delay or hypogonadotropic hypogonadism. A gonadotropin-releasing hormone stimulation test is often useful in distinguishing patients with constitutional delay from those with hypogonadotropic hypogonadism. If hypogonadotropic hypogonadism is strongly suspected, further evaluation to identify a specific etiology should be undertaken. An important aspect of the physical examination is evaluation of the sense of smell. Any patient with proven hypogonadotropic hypogonadism should have a thorough evaluation of all hypothalamic/pituitary hormones and should undergo an MRI with particular focus on the third ventricular area.

Management

Once the etiology of delayed or arrested puberty has been established, an appropriate treatment plan can be designed.

For constitutionally delayed pubertal development, short-term (3 to 6 months) sex steroid replacement may be useful to induce maturation of the gonadotropin-releasing hormone pulse generator. Permanent hypogonadotropic hypogonadism requires long-term sex hormone replacement. Testosterone for males can be administrated either by intramuscular injection or topically. Long-term hormonal therapy for females includes the use of estrogen and progestin cycling.

DISORDERS OF PROLACTIN SECRETION

Normal Biochemistry and Physiology of Prolactin

Prolactin was identified in humans in the early 1970s after the lactogenic acitivity of growth hormone was blocked by growth hormone antiserum. Prolactin is a 199–amino acid peptide synthesized in lactotroph cells, which constitute 15% to 25% of functioning anterior pituitary cells. Prolactin has homology to growth hormone and placental lactogen in its structure and function. Regulation of prolactin secretion is distinct from that of other anterior pituitary hormones. Prolactin is the only pituitary hormone that is predominantly regulated by the hypothalamus through an inhibitory mechanism mediated by dopamine via the hypothalamic-pituitary portal circulation. Other inhibitory factors include transforming growth factor β and endothelin-1, thought to act via paracrine mechanisms. Stimulatory factors include thyrotropin-releasing hormone, oxytocin, and vasoactive intestinal polypeptide. The principal physiologic functions of prolactin are enhanced mammary gland development during pregnancy and lactation. Prolactin may be increased through physiologic and pathologic mechanisms. Physiologic stimuli include pregnancy, lactation, stress, sleep, and exercise. Pathologic causes of hyperprolactinemia include prolactinomas, injury to the hypothalamic-pituitary stalk secondary to tumors or other CNS disease (infiltration, granuloma, irradiation, infection, trauma), a variety of systemic disorders, including chronic renal failure and cirrhosis, and a variety of drugs ranging from dopamine receptor blockers and dopamine synthesis inhibitors to oral contraceptives.

Clinical Features and Management of Hyperprolactinemia

The principal clinical feature of hyperprolactinemia, regardless of the cause, is galactorrhea, which may be unilateral or bilateral. Other clinical features may include delayed or arrested puberty, amenorrhea in females, and gynecomastia in males. Prolactinoma is the most common tumor of the pituitary, comprising about 50% of anterior pituitary adenomas. Most prolactinomas are less than 1 cm in diameter, such as microprolactinomas, and normally do not cause significant mass effects. However, with macroprolactinoma, headache and visual disturbance can be the first presenting symptoms. Rarely, patients with macroprolactinoma present with hydrocephalus, cranial nerve palsies, and seizures [Colao et al., 1998].

If a prolactinoma is diagnosed, therapeutic options include medical management with dopamine agonists, surgery, and adjunctive radiotherapy. Although medical management is often considered the principal intervention, numerous reports indicate that microprolactinomas can be removed surgically, though with variable recurrence rates. Macroprolactinomas are less likely to be cured surgically and often require chronic dopamine agonist treatment. Adjunctive radiotherapy has been considered beneficial in some patients with macroprolactinoma. The skill and experience of the surgeon clearly play a role in determining the optimal treatment and outcome.

HYPOTHALAMIC/PITUITARY DISORDERS OF GLUCOCORTICOID PRODUCTION

The hypothalamic-pituitary-adrenal axis is responsible for glucocorticoid production by the zona fasciculata of the adrenal cortex. Adrenocorticotropic hormone is produced by pituitary corticotrophs in response to stimulation by hypothalamic corticotropin-releasing hormone. Adrenocorticotropic hormone increases adrenal production of cortisol, the principal glucocorticoid, by a cyclic adenosine monophosphate-dependent mechanism. Cortisol, in turn, regulates the production of both corticotropin-releasing hormone and adrenocorticotropic hormone through negative-feedback loops. An intact hypothalamic-pituitary-adrenal axis is essential for general homeostasis, including regulation of blood pressure and glucose, and for response to stress. Hypersecretion of pituitary adrenocorticotropic hormone leads to Cushing's disease, whereas inadequate production of corticotropin-releasing hormone/adrenocorticotropic hormone causes adrenal glucocorticoid insufficiency.

Adrenocorticotropic Hormone Excess

Excessive production of adrenocorticotropic hormone from the pituitary arises either from corticotrophin-releasing hormone overproduction or from a primary adrenocorticotropic hormone–producing adenoma (Cushing's disease). The first sign of Cushing's disease in a growing child is often impaired linear growth [Mindermann and Wilson, 1995]. Other classic signs and symptoms of Cushing's disease include excessive weight gain (central obesity), buffalo hump, plethora, "moon facies," acne, striae, hypertension, hirsutism, fatigue, pubertal delay or arrest, bruising, and headache [Devoe et al., 1997; Magiakou et al., 1994, 2002]. Usually, at the time of diagnosis, adrenocorticotropic hormone–producing adenomas are significantly smaller than other pituitary adenomas (Fig. 84-4). These tumors are usually not well demarcated and are often less than 10 mm in diameter (microadenoma).

The diagnosis of Cushing's disease can pose significant challenges. Endogenous hypercortisolism is either adrenocorticotropic hormone dependent or adrenocorticotropic hormone independent. Of the adrenocorticotropic hormone–dependent causes, a pituitary adenoma (Cushing's disease) is most common. A less common adrenocorticotropic hormone–dependent cause is ectopic adrenocorticotropic hormone production associated with a variety of extrapituitary neoplasms. Adrenocorticotropic hormone–independent causes of hypercortisolism are rare in the pediatric

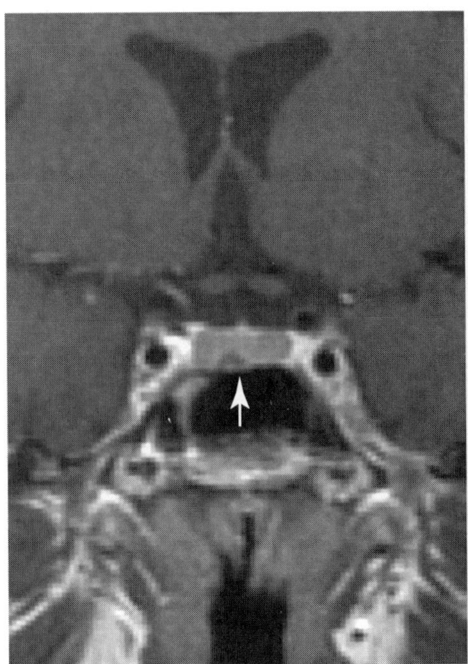

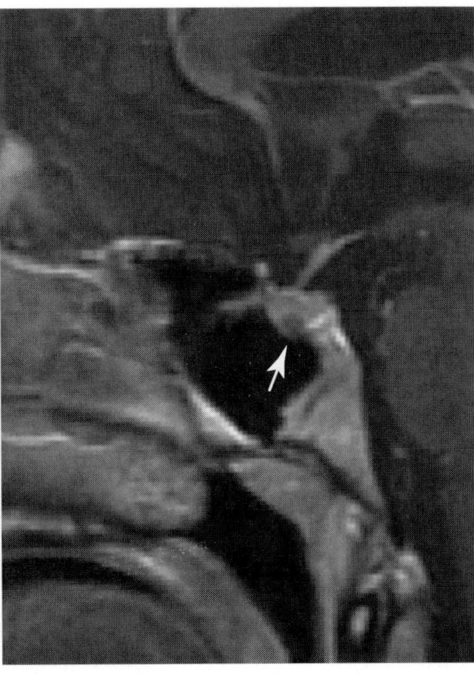

FIGURE 84-4. Adrenocorticotropic hormone–secreting pituitary adenoma in a 15-year-old female by MRI. A crescent-shaped hypodense area is indicated in the coronal view (**A**). A 3 × 2-mm hypodense nodule in the inferior aspect of the pituitary is indicated by the arrow in the sagittal view (**B**).

population. Biochemical evidence of hypercortisolism can be demonstrated by 24-hour urine collections for free cortisol. Patients with hypercortisolism will demonstrate loss of normal diurnal variation in plasma cortisol and adrenocorticotropic hormone. A single midnight serum cortisol value has been reported to effectively distinguish Cushing's syndrome from a pseudo-Cushing condition (e.g., exogenous obesity, depression, stress) [Papanicolaou et al., 1998]. The main challenge in the differential diagnosis of Cushing's syndrome is distinguishing Cushing's disease from ectopic adrenocorticotropic hormone production. In general, patients with Cushing's disease experience suppression of cortisol and adrenocorticotropic hormone with dexamethasone administration (20 μg/kg every 6 hours for 2 days). However, up to 20% of patients with Cushing's disease do not suppress under these conditions. An MRI of the hypothalamic/pituitary area should be obtained if Cushing's disease is suspected, although small adenomas may not be visualized [Devoe et al., 1997; Magiakou et al., 1994].

Transsphenoidal resection of pituitary adenomas has emerged as the treatment of choice for Cushing's disease [Devoe et al., 1997]. Due to small size, some of these tumors are difficult to identify intraoperatively. The recurrence rate after surgery is about 15% to 25% even in the hands of skilled neurosurgeons. Radiotherapy can be effective for unsuccessful transsphenoidal surgery [Estrada et al., 1997]. Other therapeutic options for recurrent Cushing's disease include repeated pituitary exploration, bilateral adrenalectomy, and the use of pharmacologic agents that directly impair cortisol synthesis and secretion.

Adrenocorticotropic Hormone Deficiency

Secondary adrenal insufficiency is defined as hypocortisolism as a consequence of adrenocorticotropic hormone deficiency. Secondary adrenal insufficiency can be isolated or occur as part of multiple hypothalamic/pituitary deficiencies; such deficiencies can be idiopathic or associated with structural malformations or various CNS diseases as previously discussed in the section on gonadotropin deficiency. Chronic suppression of corticotropin-releasing hormone and adrenocorticotropic hormone by long-term glucocorticoid therapy can also result in secondary adrenal insufficiency.

Isolated adrenocorticotropic hormone deficiency is a rare cause of secondary adrenal insufficiency, due to either corticotropin-releasing hormone deficiency or a primary decrease in adrenocorticotropic hormone production by corticotrophs. Clinical presentation is highly variable. Neonatal onset of isolated adrenocorticotropic hormone deficiency usually presents with sudden, severe episodes of hypoglycemia, sometimes with seizure and coma. Neonates may also present with prolonged cholestatic jaundice. Death may occur if treatment is not initiated promptly. More than 70% of these patients have a loss of function mutation in the TPIT gene, which encodes a transcription factor that is specifically expressed in corticotrophs and is required for expression of pro-opiomelanocortin, the precursor of adrenocorticotropic hormone. Other genetic factors leading to isolated adrenocorticotropic hormone deficiency remain to be elucidated. As noted, adrenocorticotropic hormone deficiency can be associated with multiple hypothalamic/pituitary hormone deficiencies. The genetic basis of some forms of combined pituitary hormone deficiencies has been elucidated. As previously noted, mutations in Prop-1 can present with growth hormone, prolactin, thyroid-stimulating hormone, gonadotropin, and adrenocorticotropic hormone deficiencies [Agarwal et al., 2000]. Adrenocorticotropic hormone deficiency is also found in patients who have mutations in the Lhx4 gene, which is closely related to Lhx3 as described in the section on delayed puberty. Mutations in either Lhx3 or Lhx4 can also lead to deficiencies in both growth hormone and thyroid-stimulating hormone [Machinis et al., 2001]. CNS tumors involving the third ventricular area, such as craniopharyngioma, germinoma, and astrocytoma can cause multiple pituitary deficiencies, including adrenocorticotropic hormone deficiency. In addition, adrenocorticotropic hormone deficiency with other pituitary hormone deficiencies can be seen in a variety of CNS disorders, including infection, invasive disease, irradiation, congenital malformation, and trauma. Long-term glucocorticoid therapy, for example, in patients with chronic inflammatory and autoimmune diseases, will often suppress the hypothalamic-pituitary-adrenal axis.

Cortisol (hydrocortisone) replacement is based on studies of the cortisol secretory rate in the pediatric population [Kerrigan et al., 1993; Linder et al., 1990; Metzger et al., 1993]. During periods of significant stress, such as febrile illness and surgery, such patients are routinely managed with a temporary increase in glucocorticoids (given orally or parenterally) at doses up to 50 mg/m^2/day of hydrocortisone.

HYPOTHALAMIC/PITUITARY DISORDERS OF STATURAL GROWTH

Statural growth is a complex process influenced by multiple factors. Endocrine regulation of growth postnatally stems from hormones produced in the hypothalamus and the pituitary, including growth hormone–releasing hormone, somatostatin, growth hormone, thyrotropin-releasing hormone, thyroid-stimulating hormone, corticotropin-releasing hormone, and adrenocorticotropic hormone. Inadequate thyrotropin-releasing hormone/thyroid-stimulating hormone and excessive corticotropin-releasing hormone/adrenocorticotropic hormone/cortisol lead to suboptimal linear growth, as discussed in other sections of this chapter. Abnormal statural growth related to either growth hormone deficiency or growth hormone excess (gigantism) is discussed in this section.

Human growth hormone is synthesized, stored, and secreted by somatotrophs in the lateral regions of the adenohypophysis. Human growth hormone is a single-chain peptide hormone composed of 191 amino acids. Pulsatile growth hormone secretion is regulated by two hypothalamic regulatory peptides: growth hormone–releasing hormone and somatostatin, which in turn are regulated by multiple neurotransmitters and neuropeptides. For instance, ghrelin, a 28–amino acid peptide secreted from oxyntic cells in the stomach fundus and duodenum, increases growth hormone secretion by either increasing growth hormone–releasing hormone in the hypothalamus, or by directly stimulating growth hormone in the pituitary. Other hormones that affect growth hormone secretion include glucocorticoids, thyroid hormones, and sex steroids. Although acute glucocorticoid administration stimulates growth hormone secretion, chronically elevated glucocorticoids inhibit growth hormone, as seen in Cushing's disease and during chronic administration of glucocorticoids. Sex steroids (estradiol and testosterone) stimulate growth hormone secretion, contributing to a pubertal rise in growth hormone. In addition, growth hormone levels are decreased in hypothyroidism. The growth-promoting effects of growth hormone are mediated principally through endocrine, autocrine, and paracrine production of insulin-like growth factors. Growth hormone also has direct effects on lipid metabolism and glucose regulation [Rosenfeld and Cohen, 2002].

Growth Hormone Deficiency

The incidence of growth hormone deficiency is estimated to be as high as 1:3480 in the United States [Lindsay et al., 1994]. Children with congenital growth hormone deficiency are of normal size at birth. However, after approximately 6 months of life, growth failure becomes apparent when linear growth becomes growth hormone dependent. Usually, children with growth hormone deficiency are short and cherubic with a doll-like appearance. Approximately 10% to 20% of growth hormone–deficient patients present with severe hypoglycemia in addition to short stature. In the neonatal period, hypoglycemia and microphallus strongly suggest growth hormone deficiency.

Abnormalities can occur at any level of the growth hormone-releasing hormone/growth hormone–insulin-like growth factor-I axis, but the majority of these abnormalities occur at the hypothalamic/pituitary level. In fact, most patients with growth hormone deficiency (80% to 90%) are growth hormone–releasing hormone deficient, and are capable of secreting growth hormone in response to exogenous growth hormone–releasing hormone. As with gonadotropins or adrenocorticotropic hormone, a deficiency of growth hormone may be isolated or associated with other hypothalamic/pituitary hormone abnormalities. Growth hormone deficiency may be idiopathic, genetic, associated with a variety of CNS disorders (midline developmental defect syndrome, tumors, infection, irradiation, and trauma) and may occur in association with significant emotional deprivation. Isolated growth hormone deficiency is rarely due to a growth hormone gene deletion. Mutations in the homeobox gene Rpx/Hesx1 are associated with septo-optic dysplasia, also known as *de Morsier's syndrome*, a common midline malformation. This syndrome is characterized by the classical triad of optic nerve hypoplasia, midline malformations (such as agenesis of the corpus callosum and absence of the septum pellucidum), and pituitary hypoplasia with consequent panhypopituitarism. Mutations in Rpx/Hesx1 also can cause isolated growth hormone deficiency. However, more commonly, these mutations found in pituitary transcription factors cause multiple hormonal deficiencies and congenital midline defects. The phenotypes of mutations in Rpx/Hesx1 gene are highly variable, ranging from isolated growth hormone deficiency without any midline defects to the complete spectrum of the disease with panhypopituitarism [Thomas et al., 2001].

Evaluation of a child with suspected growth hormone deficiency includes a thorough history, physical examination, and careful review of growth charts and laboratory studies. Severe neonatal hypoglycemia is suggestive of growth hormone deficiency. Most children with growth hormone deficiency will have not only short stature but also a subnormal height velocity with relative preservation of weight and head circumference. The diagnosis of growth hormone deficiency is often difficult to make with a single blood test in view of the pulsatile nature of growth hormone secretion. Growth hormone–dependent insulin-like growth factor-I and insulin-like growth factor–binding protein-3 levels and provocative tests of growth hormone secretion have been widely used to evaluate growth hormone status. If a diagnosis of growth hormone deficiency is made, it is essential to evaluate all anterior and posterior pituitary hormones and to obtain a cranial MRI with particular attention to the third ventricular area.

The primary treatment of children with growth hormone deficiency is recombinant synthetic growth hormone. Typically, growth hormone is administered as a daily subcutaneous injection. Some children with growth hormone deficiency on the basis of growth hormone–releasing hormone deficiency have been successfully treated with growth hormone–releasing hormone. Adequacy of treatment is determined by assessment of growth velocity and serum insulin-like growth factor-I and insulin-like growth factor–binding protein-3 levels. Recent studies demonstrate beneficial effects of continued growth hormone treatment (at lower doses) after final height is reached in adolescents with permanent growth hormone deficiency. Growth hormone treatment is occasionally associated with side effects, such as increased intracranial pressure, hyperglycemia, and slipped femoral capital epiphysis.

Growth Hormone Excess

Growth hormone excess can lead to tall stature (gigantism) in children who have open epiphyses and acromegaly in adolescents who have closed epiphyses. Gigantism is a rare condition caused by growth hormone oversecretion primarily due to increased growth hormone production from the pituitary [Abe and Ludecke, 1999; Kunwar and Wilson, 1999]. Growth hormone–producing adenomas constitute up to 10% of pituitary adenomas [Kunwar and Wilson, 2001]. Ectopic growth hormone–releasing hormone overproduction is a rare cause of growth hormone excess [Thorner et al., 1982]. In addition, McCune-Albright syndrome can present with gigantism. The constitutively active G proteins in somatotrophs can result in a rise in cyclic adenosine monophosphate, leading to increased growth hormone secretion in patients with McCune-Albright syndrome [Cuttler et al., 1989; Geffner et al., 1987].

Accelerated longitudinal growth and acromegalic features (enlarged head, large hands and feet, big tongue, and broad nose) are the most prominent signs of growth hormone excess. In girls, menstrual irregularity is common. Mass effect of the tumor can cause impaired vision and headache due to increased intracranial pressure. Some patients may also have hyperprolactinemia as a result of an adenoma from somatolactotrophs. A diagnosis of pituitary gigantism is made by demonstrating nonsuppressible growth hormone in response to glucose infusion in association with elevated insulin-like growth factor-I and insulin-like growth factor–binding protein-3 levels. Usually, cranial MRI will reveal a pituitary mass.

The goal of treatment in growth hormone–secreting adenomas is normalization of growth hormone and insulin-like growth factor-I levels. Transsphenonoidal surgery has resulted in a greater than 80% cure rate. If surgery is unsuccessful, somatostatin analogs, growth hormone antgonists, and dopamine agonists can be used; radiotherapy may be beneficial.

HYPOTHALAMIC/PITUITARY DISORDERS OF THYROID FUNCTION

Normal Thyroid Physiology

Under regulation by the hypothalamus and pituitary, the thyroid gland produces thyroxine and triiodothyronine, which have broad effects on metabolism, general growth, and central nervous system development [Anderson et al., 2000]. Embryonic development of the hypothalamic-pituitary-thyroid axis begins during the first trimester, marked by significant concentrations of thyrotropin-releasing hormone in the hypothalamus, the median eminence, and the supraoptic tract. The thyroid gland forms as an invagination of endoderm at the base of the tongue and descends along the midline to its final position anterior to the second to fourth tracheal cartilage rings [Fisher and Brown, 2000]. Maturation of the human hypothalamic-pituitary-thyroid axis is a complex process involving ontogenesis of hypothalamic thyrotropin-releasing hormone, pituitary thyroid–stimulating hormone, and thyroid hormone secretory processes, as well as maturation of their respective receptors, and of pituitary iodothyronine monodeiodinase enzyme activities [Fisher and Brown, 2000]. Thyroid-stimulating hormone is a heterodimeric glycoprotein consisting of α and β subunits. The α subunit is common to thyroid-stimulating hormone, luteinizing hormone, follicle-stimulating hormone, and human chorionic gonadotropin, whereas the β subunit confers specificity. Thyroid-stimulating hormone acts on the thyroid gland to stimulate thyroid hormone synthesis and secretion. Thyroid-stimulating hormone is negatively regulated by thyroid hormones and positively regulated by thyrotropin-releasing hormone. Thyroid hormone signaling is mediated by specific nuclear receptors that regulate the expression of target genes at the levels of transcription and protein synthesis [Anderson et al., 2000]. More than 90% of circulating thyroxine and triiodothyronine are bound to thyroid-binding proteins (thyroid-binding globulin, transthyretin, and albumin) [Refetoff, 1989]. Thyroxine serves largely as a prohormone that is peripherally converted to the more potent triiodothyronine [Anderson, et al., 2000].

Central Hypothyroidism

Central (hypothalamic/pituitary) hypothyroidism is rare in comparison with primary hypothyroidism, and may be congenital or acquired. Signs and symptoms associated with hypothyroidism may arise insidiously and are often nonspecific. In the neonatal period, newborns may have lethargy, hypotonia, hypothermia, or prolonged jaundice. Untreated hypothyroidism during infancy and early childhood can result in developmental delay, mental retardation, and poor statural growth. Presenting symptoms in older children include weight gain, subnormal height velocity, constipation, cold intolerance, hoarse voice, dry skin, and lethargy.

Congenital thyroid-stimulating hormone deficiency occurs in 1:50,000 to 1:150,000 newborns [Fisher, 2002]. Underlying etiologies include isolated thyroid-stimulating hormone deficiency, developmental defects of the hypothalamus and pituitary, and familial panhypopituitarism. Patients with congenital thyroid-stimulating hormone deficiency are usually not detected by neonatal screening for hypothyroidism because most programs are designed to screen for hyperthyrotropinemia that accompanies the more primary hypothyroidism.

Isolated thyroid-stimulating hormone deficiency is usually autosomal recessive. Mutations in the thyroid-stimulating hormone β subunit prevent formation of the active thyroid-stimulating hormone heterodimer [Hayashizaki et al., 1989, 1990; Karges et al., 2004; McDermott et al., 2002]. Thyroid-stimulating hormone deficiency in combination with other pituitary hormone deficiencies is frequently seen in patients with *HESX1, PIT1,* and *PROP1* mutations. As described previously in sections on disorders of statural growth and puberty, these genes are pituitary transcription factors critical for pituitary development. In addition, isolated central hypothyroidism can result from a loss-of-function mutation in the thyrotropin-releasing hormone receptor [Collu et al., 1997].

Acquired central hypothyroidism may result from CNS insults including tumors invading the third ventricular area, irradiation, infection, and trauma. Acquired central hypothyroidism is usually associated with multiple hypothalamic/pituitary hormone deficiencies.

With respect to laboratory assessment of thyroid function, it is critical to recognize that normal ranges vary significantly with age [Nelson et al., 1993]. In particular, thyroid-stimulating hormone and free thyroxine are relatively high in newborns in comparison with older infants, children, and adolescents. The principal goals of treating central hypothyroidism are prevention of mental retardation and growth impairment. Thus, thyroxine replacement should be instituted promptly after diagnosis of hypothyroidism, regardless of etiology.

Central Hyperthyroidism

Most cases of hyperthyroidism in the pediatric population are autoimmune and thyroid-stimulating hormone independent. Central hyperthyroidism as a consequence of a pituitary thyroid-stimulating hormone–secreting adenoma is exceedingly rare [Tolis et al., 1978]. Such patients may have a prominent local mass effect of the tumor, such as loss or partial loss of vision from optic atrophy, and may have hydrocephalus. Other signs and symptoms of hyperthyroidism such as agitation, tall stature, goiter, tremor, and palpitation are also manifested in central hyperthyroidism. Biochemically, patients with central hyperthyroidism have elevated concentrations of thyroid-stimulating hormone in the context of elevated thyroxine and triiodothyronine. If a pituitary adenoma is not identifiable on imaging studies, rare selective pituitary triiodothyronine resistance should be considered. Surgical removal of the tumor is the treatment of choice for thyroid-stimulating hormone–secreting pituitary adenoma. However, the treatment of selective pituitary triiodothyronine resistance remains a therapeutic challenge.

HYPOTHALAMIC DISORDERS OF APPETITE REGULATION AND ENERGY BALANCE

Appetite and energy balance are regulated by a complex network in which the hypothalamus serves as the central processing unit for hormonal, nutritional, and neuronal input from both peripheral tissue and higher brain centers. In humans it is well known that hypothalamic damage (e.g., from a tumor, surgery, trauma, or radiation) can lead to hypothalamic obesity [Bray and Gallagher, 1975]. These patients present with excessive weight gain without response to caloric restriction or exercise [Bray et al., 1981]. Traditionally, the ventromedial hypothalamus has been viewed as the "satiety" center because damage to the ventromedial hypothalamus can cause hyperphagic obesity. In contrast, the lateral hypothalamus has been viewed as the "feeding" center because its disruption leads to hypophagia and weight loss [Flier and Maratos-Flier, 1998].

Insights into mechanisms of hypothalamic obesity derive from advances in our understanding of hypothalamic control of appetite regulation and energy balance (Fig. 84-5). Energy storage and appetite are regulated at the hypothalamus through signaling by leptin, an anorexigenic hormone secreted by adipocytes, and by insulin. Both leptin and insulin stimulate anorexigenic and inhibit orexigenic pathways in the hypothalamus. In the anorexigenic pathway, leptin and insulin maintain expression of pro-

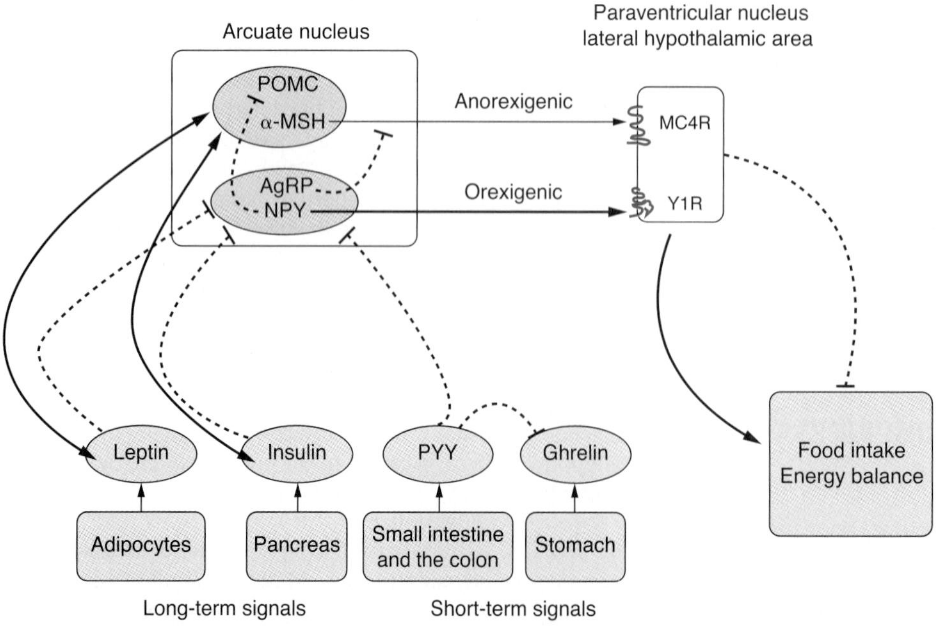

FIGURE 84-5. Hormonal regulation of food intake and energy balance in the hypothalamus. The dashed lines indicate inhibitory effects and the solid lines with arrows indicate stimulatory effects. Long-term signals affecting body fat mass include leptin and insulin, whereas short-term signals determining meal initiation and termination include peptide YY_{3-36} and ghrelin. α-MSH, α-melanocyte–stimulating protein; AgRP, agouti-related protein; MC4R, melanocortin-4 receptor; NPY, neuropeptide Y; POMC, pro-opiomelanocortin; PYY, peptide YY_{3-36}; Y1R, Y1 subtype of the neuropeptide Y receptor.

opiomelanocortin in the arcuate nuclei within the ventromedial hypothalamus, and pro-opiomelanocortin–derived α-melanocyte–stimulating hormone activates the melanocortin-4 receptor in the paraventricular nuclei and the lateral hypothalamic area. This melanocortin signal is appetite suppressing and leads to decreased food intake. In addition, leptin and insulin inhibit neuropeptide Y and agouti-related protein within the arcuate nuclei, both of which are appetite-stimulating peptides [Schwartz et al., 2003]. Neuropeptide Y decreases pro-opiomelanocortin expression through the neuropeptide Y1 receptor. Agouti-related protein is an inverse agonist for melanocortin-4 receptor, thus antagonizing the interaction of α-melanocyte–stimulating hormone and the melanocortin-4 receptor and leading to increased food intake [Korner and Leibel, 2003].

Short-term signals that affect appetite and determine meal initiation and termination are derived from gut hormones, such as ghrelin (secreted by oxyntic cells in the stomach fundus) and peptide $YY_{3\text{-}36}$ secreted by endocrine L cells in the distal small bowel and colon). Ghrelin signals hunger and increases food intake by stimulating ghrelin receptors on hypothalamic neuropeptide Y and agouti-related protein-expressing neurons [Cummings et al., 2002]. In contrast, peptide $YY_{3\text{-}36}$ signals satiety and decreases food intake by inhibiting neuropeptide Y/agouti-related protein–expressing neurons via the neuropeptide Y2 receptor and by decreasing ghrelin levels [Batterham et al., 2002, 2003].

Both long-term and short-term hormonal signals are received in the arcuate nuclei, constituting the afferent system of the feedback loop for appetite and energy balance. Through the paraventricular and lateral nuclei, these signals are transmitted into a complex and less well-understood efferent system that controls appetite and energy balance. The autonomic system plays a critical role in regulating energy expenditure. It is known that the ventromedial hypothalamus has direct neuronal projections to spinal cord that regulate sympathetic outflow. Activation of the sympathetic nervous system results in increased energy expenditure, such as increased local heat production and increased lipolysis. In addition, the ventromedial hypothalamus has projections to the dorsal motor nucleus of the vagus that innervate the gastrointestinal system. Disinhibition of vagal firing by ventromedial hypothalamus lesions is associated with relative insulin hypersecretion and subsequent increased energy storage [Lustig, 2002].

Examples of monogenic obesity are those caused by mutations in either pro-opiomelanocortin or melanocortin-4 receptor. In the former, two patients have been reported with loss-of-function mutations in pro-opiomelanocortin, leading to defective synthesis of adrenocorticotropic hormone and α-melanocyte–stimulating hormone [Krude et al., 1998, 2003]. Both patients have red hair, adrenal insufficiency, hyperphagia, and morbid obesity. In the latter, heterogeneous mutations in melanocortin-4 receptor have been found in 2.5% of obese children, representing the most common genetic defects in human obesity [Farooqi et al., 2000; Vaisse et al., 2000].

Congenital leptin deficiency and leptin receptor abnormalities are extremely rare monogenic forms of morbid obesity. Only two United Kingdom families of Pakistani origin [Farooqi et al., 2002; Montague et al., 1997], one Canadian family of Pakistani origin [Gibson et al., 2004], and one Turkish family [Licinio et al., 2004] with mutations in the leptin gene have been described thus far. The first three children reported were born to two consanguineous Pakistani families [Farooqi et al., 2002]. They had normal birth weight but became hyperphagic in infancy and developed severe obesity with undetectable levels of leptin. Exogenous administration of leptin induced sustained weight loss due to loss of fat mass in these patients. Similar results were observed in three adults who have congenital leptin deficiency [Licinio et al., 2004]. Leptin replacement in these adults resulted in profound weight loss, increased physical activity, and resolution of insulin resistance and hypogonadism. Homozygous mutation of the leptin receptor is also associated with severe childhood obesity. These patients have early onset of morbid obesity associated with high levels of leptin. In addition, they have absent pubertal development and reduced levels of both thyrotropin and growth hormone [Clement et al., 1998].

As previously noted, hypothalamic obesity is frequently seen in children with hypothalamic insults such as brain tumor, surgery, irradiation, or trauma. Approximately 50% of children with craniopharyngioma develop hypothalamic obesity. Other tumors, such as germinoma, optic glioma, prolactinoma, hypothalamic astrocytoma, also are associated with hypothalamic obesity. These patients usually have unrelenting weight gain after tumor removal or radiotherapy without documented excessive food intake [Harz et al., 2003]. Other risk factors associated with hypothalamic obesity include dose of hypothalamic irradiation (>51 Gy), and associated hypothalamic endocrinopathy (growth hormone deficiency, hypothyroidism, adrenocorticotropic hormone deficiency, precocious or delayed puberty, and diabetes insipidus) [Lustig et al., 2003]. A recent report indicates that reduced physical activity rather than increased energy intake is primarily responsible for obesity in patients with craniopharyngioma [Harz et al., 2003]. In patients with hypothalamic obesity and apparent insulin hypersecretion, the somatostatin agonist octreotide has been found to decrease or stabilize body weight [Lustig et al., 1999].

HYPOTHALAMIC/PITUITARY DISORDERS OF WATER BALANCE

Under normal circumstances plasma osmolality is maintained within a relatively narrow range (280 to 295 mOsm/kg). This homeostasis requires adequate water intake regulated by an intact thirst mechanism and appropriate free water excretion by the kidneys, mediated by appropriate secretion of vasopressin (arginine vasopressin), that is, antidiuretic hormone [Robertson, 2001]. Arginine vasopressin is produced in the magnocellular neurons in the paraventricular and supraoptic nuclei of the hypothalamus. Axons from these neurons project through the pituitary stalk and terminate in the posterior pituitary gland [Robertson, 2001]. A gene on chromosome 20p13 encodes both arginine vasopressin and its carrier protein, neurophysin II. Arginine vasopressin and neurophysin II are synthesized as a single polypeptide, cleaved within neurosecretory granules, reassembled into an arginine vasopressin/neurophysin II complex, and secreted [Rutishauser et al., 2002]. Arginine vasopressin exerts its antidiuretic action by binding to the X chromosome–encoded V2 vasopressin receptor (V2R), a G protein–coupled receptor on the basolateral membrane of renal collecting duct epithelial cells. After V2 vasopressin receptor activation, increased intracellular cyclic adenosine monophosphate mediates shuttling of the water channel aquaporin-2 to the apical membrane of collecting duct epithelial cells, resulting in increased water permeability and antidiuresis [Schrier and Cadnapaphornchai, 2003].

Arginine vasopressin secretion is regulated mainly by changes in plasma osmolality and in effective circulating volume [Robertson, 2001]. Osmoreceptors in the hypothalamus stimulate secretion of arginine vasopressin when plasma osmolality increases by as little as 1% in healthy individuals. Arginine vasopressin levels are normally low and do not increase until plasma osmolality exceeds 280 mOsm/kg [Robinson and Verbalis, 2003]. Arginine vasopressin secretion is also regulated by changes in blood volume. Baroreceptors in the systemic venous circulation, right side of the heart, and left atrium ("low pressure" areas), as well as in the systemic arterial systems of the carotid sinus and aortic arch ("high pressure" areas) signal the hypothalamus via the vagus and glossopharyngeal nerves, respectively. These baroreceptors become activated when stretched by increases in intravascular volume, leading to inhibition of arginine vasopressin secretion. In addition, a variety of other factors affect arginine vasopressin secretion. Arginine vasopressin is stimulated by pain, stress, and a variety of drugs and is inhibited by multiple factors [Robinson and Verbalis, 2003]. Adequate water intake, governed by an intact thirst mechanism, is regulated by hypothalamic osmoreceptors located near vasopressinergic neurons.

Clinical disorders of water balance are common, and abnormalities in many steps involving arginine vasopressin secretion and responsiveness have been described [Robertson, 2001]. The focus of this section is on the principal hypothalamic/pituitary disorders of water balance, diabetes insipidus, and the syndrome of inappropriate antidiuretic hormone (SIADH) secretion.

Diabetes Insipidus

Diabetes insipidus may result from a deficiency of arginine vasopressin or from nephrogenic causes [Baylis and Cheetham, 1998; Robinson and Verbalis, 2003; Verbalis, 2003]. Nephrogenic diabetes insipidus may be congenital, resulting from inactivating mutations in the V2 vasopressin receptor gene or from autosomal-recessive or autosomal-dominant lesions in the aquaporin-2 gene, or acquired, resulting from a variety of conditions including some forms of primary renal disease, obstructive uropathy, hypokalemia, hypercalcemia, sickle cell disease, and a variety of drugs including lithium and demeclocycline [Baylis and Cheetham, 1998; Morello and Bichet, 2001; Robinson and Verbalis, 2003; Verbalis, 2003]. Prolonged polyuria of any cause can result in some degree of nephrogenic diabetes insipidus secondary to a reduction of tonicity in the renal medullary interstitium and a subsequent decrease in the gradient necessary to concentrate the urine.

Central diabetes insipidus is rarely congenital and more frequently acquired. Congenital central diabetes insipidus may be caused by hypothalamic structural malformations and through both autosomal-dominant and autosomal-recessive mutations in the arginine vasopressin/neurophysin II gene. Of the latter, the autosomal-dominant causes are more common and are thought to be a consequence of heterozygous mutations in the arginine vasopressin/neurophysin II gene, which lead to misfolding of the precursor arginine vasopressin/neurophysin II protein [Rutishauser et al., 2002]. The dominant negative effect is thought to occur as a consequence of the misfolded precursor protein that accumulates in the endoplasmic reticulum of vasopressinergic neurons, ultimately resulting in death of these neurons and gliosis [Robinson and Verbalis, 2003; Rutishauser et al., 2002]. In such patients, clinical diabetes insipidus usually develops several months to years after birth. A rare autosomal-recessive form of central diabetes insipidus has been reported in association with a mutation in the arginine vasopressin/neurophysin II gene, resulting in a biologically inactive arginine vasopressin [Willcutts et al., 1999].

Acquired forms of diabetes insipidus occur in association with a variety of disorders in which there is destruction or degeneration of vasopressinergic neurons. Etiologies include primary tumors (e.g., craniopharyngioma germinoma) or metastases, infection (meningitis, encephalitis), histiocytosis, granuloma, vascular disorders, and autoimmune disorders (lymphocytic infundibuloneurohypophysitis) [Baylis and Cheetham, 1998; Robinson and Verbalis, 2003; Verbalis, 2003]. Acquired diabetes insipidus may occur in association with trauma and surgery. Idiopathic diabetes insipidus is a diagnosis of exclusion, and one that is made with decreasing frequency concurrent with improved sensitivity of CNS MRI imaging and of cerebrospinal fluid and serum tumor markers [Maghnie et al., 2000; Mootha et al., 1997].

The principal presenting sign of diabetes insipidus is polyuria, which in addition to deficiency or impaired responsiveness to arginine vasopressin, may result from an osmotic agent (e.g., hyperglycemia in diabetes mellitus) or from excessive water intake (primary polydipsia). Hypernatremia usually does not occur if patients have an intact thirst mechanism, adequate access to fluids, and no additional ongoing fluid losses (e.g., diarrhea). Infants with diabetes insipidus, in addition to polyuria and polydipsia, may be irritable and have fever of unknown origin, growth failure secondary to inadequate caloric intake, and hydronephrosis. Older children may also have nocturia and enuresis. Diabetes insipidus may not be apparent in patients with coexisting untreated anterior pituitary-mediated adrenal glucocorticoid insufficiency, because cortisol is required to generate a normal free water loss [Robinson and Verbalis, 2003].

A diagnosis of diabetes insipidus can be made if screening laboratory studies reveal serum hyperosmolality concurrent with urine that is inappropriately dilute. However, because most patients with diabetes insipidus do not have hyperosmolality and hypernatremia, as noted above, a standardized water deprivation test is useful to distinguish diabetes insipidus from primary polydipsia. Urine osmolality of greater than 750 mOsm/kg after 7 to 8 hours of water deprivation is thought to exclude diabetes insipidus [Baylis and Cheetham, 1998]. Urine osmolality in the 300-

to 750-mOsm/kg range may indicate partial diabetes insipidus [Baylis and Cheetham, 1998]. If diabetes insipidus is suspected, a plasma sample should be obtained for arginine vasopressin radioimmunoassay. Arginine vasopressin or a synthetic analog (desmopressin) should then be administered to distinguish arginine vasopressin deficiency from arginine vasopressin unresponsiveness.

Once a diagnosis of central diabetes insipidus is made, a brain MRI with particular attention to the third ventricular area should be obtained. An absent posterior pituitary "bright spot" is seen in virtually all patients with central diabetes insipidus. Under normal circumstances a posterior pituitary bright spot is seen on T1-weighted images due to stored arginine vasopressin in neurosecretory granules (see Fig. 84-1). In patients with diabetes insipidus as a consequence of an autosomal-dominant mutation in the arginine vasopressin/neurophysin II gene, a posterior pituitary bright spot may be seen in the early stages of the disease [Robinson and Verbalis, 2003]. In central diabetes insipidus patients with an absent posterior pituitary bright spot, an otherwise normal MRI warrants close follow-up with cerebrospinal fluid tumor markers and cytology, serum tumor markers, and serial contrast-enhanced brain MRIs for early detection of an evolving occult hypothalamic-stalk lesion [Mootha et al., 1997].

In addition to treating a primary disease causing central diabetes insipidus, the drug of choice for most patients with arginine vasopressin deficiency is desmopressin. This arginine vasopressin analog has markedly reduced pressor activity in comparison with native arginine vasopressin, has a prolonged half-life, and can be administered orally, intranasally, or by subcutaneous injection.

Syndrome of Inappropriate Antidiuretic Hormone Secretion

SIADH is characterized by the inability to excrete a free water load, with inappropriately concentrated urine, and resultant hyponatremia, hypo-osmolality, and natriuresis [Bartter and Schwartz, 1967; Baylis, 2003; Robinson and Verbalis, 2003]. Following from the original criteria established by Bartter and Schwartz [1967], a diagnosis of SIADH is made when the following occur: (1) plasma hypo-osmolality (<275 mOsm/kg); (2) less than maximally dilute urine (urine osmolality >100 mOsm/kg); (3) euvolemia (secondary to regulatory adaptations); (4) natriuresis; (5) normal renal function; and (6) no evidence of thyroxine or cortisol deficiency. Whereas most patients with SIADH have inappropriately measurable or elevated levels of plasma arginine vasopressin relative to plasma osmolality, 10% to 20% of patients with SIADH do not have measurable arginine vasopressin levels. This finding may reflect issues of assay sensitivity or may indicate a syndrome resembling SIADH, such as the recently described nephrogenic syndrome of inappropriate antidiuresis associated with an activating mutation in the X-linked G protein–coupled V2 vasopressin receptor and unmeasurable circulating levels of arginine vasopressin [Feldman et al., 2004].

Euvolemia in chronic SIADH is an important distinguishing factor in the evaluation of a patient with serum hypo-osmolality and has a bearing on treatment issues, as is discussed subsequently. Euvolemia in chronic SIADH is thought to represent an adaptation to water overload. This adaptation is mediated, in part, at the cellular level through depletion of intracellular electrolytes (potassium) and organic osmolytes [Robinson and Verbalis, 2003]. The loss of brain solutes is thought to allow effective regulation of brain volume during chronic hyponatremia and SIADH. Natriuresis, thought to be mediated in part through secretion of atrial natriuretic peptide, also contributes to volume regulation in chronic SIADH [Cogan et al., 1988]. Cerebral salt wasting, associated with some intracranial diseases (e.g., subarachnoid hemorrhage), is often considered in the differential diagnosis of SIADH. However, the hypo-osmolality, hyponatremia, and natriuresis in cerebral salt wasting are associated with volume contraction, which distinguishes this disorder from the euvolemic condition of SIADH [Robinson and Verbalis, 2003].

A large number of disorders and conditions are associated with SIADH, and can be grouped into five categories: (1) disorders of the CNS, including infection, trauma, cerebrovascular accident, tumors (nonarginine vasopressin producing), hydrocephalus, neonatal hypoxia; (2) a variety of pulmonary disorders (e.g., pneumonia, asthma); (3) non-CNS tumors with ectopic production of arginine vasopressin (e.g., bronchogenic carcinoma, lymphoma; (4) a large variety of drugs (e.g., phenothiozines, tricylic antidepressants); and (5) general surgery (mechanism not well understood) [Baylis, 2003; Robinson and Verbalis, 2003].

Therapy for SIADH includes treatment of the underlying disorder (or discontinuation of an offending drug) and fluid restriction. Replacement of lost body sodium may also be necessary but usually can be achieved through normal dietary salt intake. Severe hyponatremia (serum sodium <120 mEq/L) may be associated with CNS abnormalities, including seizures, and may require treatment with hypertonic (3%) intravenous sodium chloride solution. Concurrent use of a diuretic, such as furosemide, may be indicated when volume expansion is severe. Other therapeutic approaches include the use of agents that induce nephrogenic diabetes insipidus, such as demeclocycline and lithium, although both are contraindicated, particularly in younger pediatric patients, because of untoward side effects. Urea has been used as an osmotic diuretic in pediatric SIADH [Huang et al., 2004]. A variety of nonpeptide V2 vasopressin receptor antagonists are currently in clinical trials [Verbalis, 2002].

If SIADH and hyponatremia are acute (<48 hours), it is thought that hyponatremia can be corrected quickly. However, if SIADH and hyponatremia are chronic (>48 hours), overzealous treatment can result in CNS damage, including central pontine myelinolysis [Robinson and Verbalis, 2003]. Brain solute loss, although an important regulatory mechanism in chronic SIADH, may predispose to the development of central pontine myelinolysis with rapid correction of serum osmolality. It is generally recommended that plasma sodium be corrected to a "safe" level of approximately 120 to 125 mEq/L at a rate of no greater than 0.5 mEq/L per hour with an overall correction that does not exceed 12 mEq/L in the initial 24 hours and 18 mEq/L in the initial 48 hours of treatment [Robinson and Verbalis, 2003].

REFERENCES

Abe T, Ludecke DK. Recent primary transnasal surgical outcomes associated with intraoperative growth hormone measurement in acromegaly. Clin Endocrinol (Oxf) 1999;50:27.

Agarwal G, Bhatia V, Cook S, et al. Adrenocorticotropin deficiency in combined pituitary hormone deficiency patients homozygous for a novel PROP1 deletion. J Clin Endocrinol Metab 2000;85:4556.

Anderson GW, Mariash CN, Oppenheimer JH. Molecular actions of thyroid hormone, 8th ed. Philadelphia: Lippincott Williams & Wilkins, 2000.

Bartter FC, Schwartz WB. The syndrome of inappropriate secretion of antidiuretic hormone. Am J Med 1967;42:790.

Batterham RL, Cohen MA, Ellis SM, et al. Inhibition of food intake in obese subjects by peptide YY3-36. N Engl J Med 2003;349:941.

Batterham RL, Cowley MA, Small CJ, et al. Gut hormone PYY(3-36) physiologically inhibits food intake. Nature 2002;418:650.

Baylis PH. The syndrome of inappropriate antidiuretic hormone secretion. Int J Biochem Cell Biol 2003;35:1495.

Baylis PH, Cheetham T. Diabetes insipidus. Arch Dis Child 1998;79:84.

Beier DR, Dluhy RG. Bench and bedside—The G protein–coupled receptor GPR54 and puberty. N Engl J Med 2003;349:1589.

Bergland RM, Page RB. Pituitary-brain vascular relations: A new paradigm. Science 1979;204:18.

Bray GA, Gallagher TF, Jr. Manifestations of hypothalamic obesity in man: A comprehensive investigation of eight patients and a review of the literature. Medicine (Baltimore) 1975;54:301.

Bray GA, Inoue S, Nishizawa Y. Hypothalamic obesity. The autonomic hypothesis and the lateral hypothalamus. Diabetologia 1981;20 (Suppl):366.

Breyer P, Haider A, Pescovitz OH. Gonadotropin-releasing hormone agonists in the treatment of girls with central precocious puberty. Clin Obstet Gynecol 1993;36:764.

Cisternino M, Arrigo T, Pasquino AM, et al. Etiology and age incidence of precocious puberty in girls: A multicentric study. J Pediatr Endocrinol Metab 2000;13 (Suppl 1):695.

Clement K, Vaisse C, Lahlou N, et al. A mutation in the human leptin receptor gene causes obesity and pituitary dysfunction. Nature 1998;392:398.

Cogan E, Debieve MF, Pepersack T, et al. Natriuresis and atrial natriuretic factor secretion during inappropriate antidiuresis. Am J Med 1988;84:409.

Cohen LE, Radovick S. Molecular basis of combined pituitary hormone deficiencies. Endocr Rev 2002;23:431.

Colao A, Loche S, Cappa M, et al. Prolactinomas in children and adolescents. Clinical presentation and long-term follow-up. J Clin Endocrinol Metab 1998;83:2777.

Colledge WH. GPR54 and puberty. Trends Endocrinol Metab 2004;15:448.

Collu R, Tang J, Castagne J, et al. A novel mechanism for isolated central hypothyroidism: inactivating mutations in the thyrotropin-releasing hormone receptor gene. J Clin Endocrinol Metab 1997;82:1561.

Cone RD, Low MJ, Elmquist JK, et al. Neuroendocrinology, 10th ed. Philadelphia: Saunders, 2003.

Crino A, Schiaffini R, Ciampalini P, et al. Hypogonadism and pubertal development in Prader-Willi syndrome. Eur J Pediatr 2003;162:327.

Cummings DE, Weigle DS, Frayo RS, et al. Plasma ghrelin levels after diet-induced weight loss or gastric bypass surgery. N Engl J Med 2002;346:1623.

Cuttler L, Jackson JA, Saeed uz-Zafar M, et al. Hypersecretion of growth hormone and prolactin in McCune-Albright syndrome. J Clin Endocrinol Metab 1989;68:1148.

Dattani ML, Martinez-Barbera J, Thomas PQ, et al. Molecular genetics of septo-optic dysplasia. Horm Res 2000;53 (Suppl 1):26.

Dattani MT, Martinez-Barbera JP, Thomas PQ, et al. Mutations in the homeobox gene HESX1/Hesx1 associated with septo-optic dysplasia in human and mouse. Nat Genet 1998;19:125.

de Roux N, Genin E, Carel JC, et al. Hypogonadotropic hypogonadism due to loss of function of the KiSS1-derived peptide receptor GPR54. Proc Natl Acad Sci U S A 2003;100:10972.

Demura R, Kubo O, Demura H, et al. FSH and LH secreting pituitary adenoma. J Clin Endocrinol Metab 1977;45:653.

Devoe DJ, Miller WL, Conte FA, et al. Long-term outcome in children and adolescents after transsphenoidal surgery for Cushing's disease. J Clin Endocrinol Metab 1997;82:3196.

Estrada J, Boronat M, Mielgo M, et al. The long-term outcome of pituitary irradiation after unsuccessful transsphenoidal surgery in Cushing's disease. N Engl J Med 1997;336:172.

Farooqi IS, Matarese G, Lord GM, et al. Beneficial effects of leptin on obesity, T cell hyporesponsiveness, and neuroendocrine/metabolic dysfunction of human congenital leptin deficiency. J Clin Invest 2002;110:1093.

Farooqi IS, Yeo GS, Keogh JM, et al. Dominant and recessive inheritance of morbid obesity associated with melanocortin 4 receptor deficiency. J Clin Invest 2000;106:271.

Feldman BJ, Rosenthal SM, Vargas GA, et al. Nephrogenic syndrome of inappropriate antidiuresis. N Engl J Med, 2005;352:1884.

Feuillan PP, Jones JV, Barnes K, et al. Follow-up of children and young adults after GnRH-agonist therapy or central precocious puberty. J Endocrinol Invest 2001;24:734.

Fisher DA. Disorders of the thyroid in the new born and infant, 2nd ed. Philadelphia: WB Saunders, 2002.

Fisher DA, Brown RS. Thyroid physiology in the perinatal period and during childhood, 8th ed. Philadelphia: Lippincott Williams & Wilkins, 2000.

Flier JS, Maratos-Flier E. Obesity and the hypothalamus: Novel peptides for new pathways. Cell 1998;92:437.

Geffner ME, Nagel RA, Dietrich RB, et al. Treatment of acromegaly with a somatostatin analog in a patient with McCune-Albright syndrome. J Pediatr 1987;111:740.

Georgopoulos NA, Pralong FP, Seidman CE, et al. Genetic heterogeneity evidenced by low incidence of KAL-1 gene mutations in sporadic cases of gonadotropin-releasing hormone deficiency. J Clin Endocrinol Metab 1997;82:213.

Gibson WT, Farooqi IS, Moreau M, et al. Congenital leptin deficiency due to homozygosity for the delta133G mutation: Report of another case and evaluation of response to four years of leptin therapy. J Clin Endocrinol Metab 2004;89:4821.

Grumbach MM. The neuroendocrinology of human puberty revisited. Horm Res 2002;57 (Suppl 2):2.

Grumbach MM, Styne DM. Puberty: Ontogeny, neuroendocrinology, physiology, and disorders, 10th ed. Philadelphia: WB Saunders, 2003.

Hardelin JP, Levilliers J, Blanchard S, et al. Heterogeneity in the mutations responsible for X chromosome-linked Kallmann syndrome. Hum Mol Genet 1993;2:373.

Harz KJ, Muller HL, Waldeck E, et al. Obesity in patients with craniopharyngioma: Assessment of food intake and movement counts indicating physical activity. J Clin Endocrinol Metab 2003;88:5227.

Hashimoto T, Kumahara Y. Concerning hypogonadism of Laurence-Moon-Biedl syndrome. Metabolism 1979;28:370.

Hayashizaki Y, Hiraoka Y, Endo Y, et al. Thyroid-stimulating hormone (TSH) deficiency caused by a single base substitution in the CAGYC region of the beta-subunit. EMBO J 1989;8:2291.

Hayashizaki Y, Hiraoka Y, Tatsumi K, et al. Deoxyribonucleic acid analyses of five families with familial inherited thyroid stimulating hormone deficiency. J Clin Endocrinol Metab 1990;71:792.

Herman-Giddens ME, Slora EJ, Wasserman RC, et al. Secondary sexual characteristics and menses in young girls seen in office practice: A study from the Pediatric Research in Office Settings network. Pediatrics 1997;99:505.

Huang EA, Geller DH, Gitelman SE. The use of oral urea in the treatment of chronic syndrome of inappropriate antidiuretic hormone secretion (SIADH) in children. In: Pediatric research. San Francisco: 2004; 161A.

Jung H, Carmel P, Schwartz MS, et al. Some hypothalamic hamartomas contain transforming growth factor alpha, a puberty-inducing growth factor, but not luteinizing hormone-releasing hormone neurons. J Clin Endocrinol Metab 1999;84:4695.

Kalantaridou SN, Chrousos GP. Clinical review 148: Monogenic disorders of puberty. J Clin Endocrinol Metab 2002;87:2481.

Karges B, LeHeup B, Schoenle E, et al. Compound heterozygous and homozygous mutations of the TSHbeta gene as a cause of congenital central hypothyroidism in Europe. Horm Res 2004;62:149.

Kerrigan JR, Veldhuis JD, Leyo SA, et al. Estimation of daily cortisol production and clearance rates in normal pubertal males by deconvolution analysis. J Clin Endocrinol Metab 1993;76:1505.

King JC, Anthony EL, Fitzgerald DM, et al. Luteinizing hormone-releasing hormone neurons in human preoptic/hypothalamus: Differential intraneuronal localization of immunoreactive forms. J Clin Endocrinol Metab 1985;60:88.

Korner J, Leibel RL. To eat or not to eat—How the gut talks to the brain. N Engl J Med 2003;349:926.

Krams M, Quinton R, Ashburner J, et al. Kallmann's syndrome: Mirror movements associated with bilateral corticospinal tract hypertrophy. Neurology 1999;52:816.

Krude H, Biebermann H, Gruters A. Mutations in the human proopiomelanocortin gene. Ann N Y Acad Sci 2003;994:233.

Krude H, Biebermann H, Luck W, et al. Severe early-onset obesity, adrenal insufficiency and red hair pigmentation caused by POMC mutations in humans. Nat Genet 1998;19:155.

Kunwar S, Wilson CB. Pediatric pituitary adenomas. J Clin Endocrinol Metab 1999;84:4385.

Kunwar S, Wilson CB. Sellar and parasellar tumors in children, 4th ed. Philadelphia: WB Saunders, 2001.

Licinio J, Caglayan S, Ozata M, et al. Phenotypic effects of leptin replacement on morbid obesity, diabetes mellitus, hypogonadism, and behavior in leptin-deficient adults. Proc Natl Acad Sci U S A 2004;101:4531.

Linder BL, Esteban NV, Yergey AL, et al. Cortisol production rate in childhood and adolescence. J Pediatr 1990;117:892.

Lindsay R, Feldkamp M, Harris D, et al. Utah Growth Study: Growth standards and the prevalence of growth hormone deficiency. J Pediatr 1994;125:29.

Lustig RH. Hypothalamic obesity: The sixth cranial endocrinopathy. Endocrinologist 2002;12:210.

Lustig RH, Post SR, Srivannaboon K, et al. Risk factors for the development of obesity in children surviving brain tumors. J Clin Endocrinol Metab 2003;88:611.

Lustig RH, Rose SR, Burghen GA, et al. Hypothalamic obesity caused by cranial insult in children: altered glucose and insulin dynamics and reversal by a somatostatin agonist. J Pediatr 1999;135:162.

Machinis K, Pantel J, Netchine I, et al. Syndromic short stature in patients with a germline mutation in the LIM homeobox LHX4. Am J Hum Genet 2001;69:961.

Maghnie M, Cosi G, Genovese E, et al. Central diabetes insipidus in children and young adults. N Engl J Med 2000;343:998.

Magiakou MA, Chrousos GP. Cushing's syndrome in children and adolescents: Current diagnostic and therapeutic strategies. J Endocrinol Invest 2002;25:181.

Magiakou MA, Mastorakos G, Chrousos GP. Final stature in patients with endogenous Cushing's syndrome. J Clin Endocrinol Metab 1994;79:1082.

Mahachoklertwattana P, Kaplan SL, Grumbach MM. The luteinizing hormone–releasing hormone-secreting hypothalamic hamartoma is a congenital malformation: natural history. J Clin Endocrinol Metab 1993;77:118.

McDermott MT, Haugen BR, Black JN, et al. Congenital isolated central hypothyroidism caused by a "hot spot" mutation in the thyrotropin-beta gene. Thyroid 2002;12:1141.

Metzger DL, Wright NM, Veldhuis JD, et al. Characterization of pulsatile secretion and clearance of plasma cortisol in premature and term neonates using deconvolution analysis. J Clin Endocrinol Metab 1993;77:458.

Miller WL. The molecular basis of premature adrenarche: A hypothesis. Acta Paediatr Suppl 1999;88:60.

Mindermann T, Wilson CB. Pituitary adenomas in childhood and adolescence. J Pediatr Endocrinol Metab 1995;8:79.

Montague CT, Farooqi IS, Whitehead JP, et al. Congenital leptin deficiency is associated with severe early-onset obesity in humans. Nature 1997;387:903.

Mootha SL, Barkovich AJ, Grumbach MM, et al. Idiopathic hypothalamic diabetes insipidus, pituitary stalk thickening, and the occult intracranial germinoma in children and adolescents. J Clin Endocrinol Metab 1997;82:1362.

Morello JP, Bichet DG. Nephrogenic diabetes insipidus. Annu Rev Physiol 2001;63:607.

Nelson JC, Clark SJ, Borut DL, et al. Age-related changes in serum free thyroxine during childhood and adolescence. J Pediatr 1993;123:899.

Netchine I, Sobrier ML, Krude H, et al. Mutations in LHX3 result in a new syndrome revealed by combined pituitary hormone deficiency. Nat Genet 2000;25:182.

Pansky B, Allen DJ, Budd CC. Hypothalamic fiber connections and nuclear summary, 2nd ed. New York: Macmillan Publishing Company, 1988.

Papanicolaou DA, Yanovski JA, Cutler GB Jr, et al. A single midnight serum cortisol measurement distinguishes Cushing's syndrome from pseudo-Cushing states. J Clin Endocrinol Metab 1998;83:1163.

Pescovitz OH, Comite F, Hench K, et al. The NIH experience with precocious puberty: Diagnostic subgroups and response to short-term luteinizing hormone releasing hormone analogue therapy. J Pediatr 1986;108:47.

Refetoff S. Inherited thyroxine-binding globulin abnormalities in man. Endocr Rev 1989;10:275.

Rizzoti K, Brunelli S, Carmignac D, et al. SOX3 is required during the formation of the hypothalamo-pituitary axis. Nat Genet 2004;36:247.

Robertson GL. Antidiuretic hormone. Normal and disordered function. Endocrinol Metab Clin North Am 2001;30:671.

Robinson AG, Verbalis JG. Posterior pituitary gland, 10th ed. Philadelphia: WB Saunders, 2003.

Rosenfeld JV, Harvey AS, Wrennall J, et al. Transcallosal resection of hypothalamic hamartomas, with control of seizures, in children with gelastic epilepsy. Neurosurgery 2001;48:108.

Rosenfeld RG, Cohen P. Disorders of growth hormone/insulin-like growth factor secretion and action, 2nd ed. Philadelphia: WB Saunders, 2002.

Rugarli EI, Ballabio A. Kallmann syndrome. From genetics to neurobiology. JAMA 1993;270:2713.

Rutishauser J, Kopp P, Gaskill MB, et al. Clinical and molecular analysis of three families with autosomal dominant neurohypophyseal diabetes insipidus associated with a novel and recurrent mutations in the vasopressin-neurophysin II gene. Eur J Endocrinol 2002;146:649.

Sadler TW. Central nervous system, 6th ed. Baltimore: Williams & Wilkins, 1990.

Sassolas G, Lejeune H, Trouillas J, et al. Gonadotropin-releasing hormone agonists are unsuccessful in reducing tumoral gonadotropin secretion in two patients with gonadotropin-secreting pituitary adenomas. J Clin Endocrinol Metab 1988;67:180.

Schrier RW, Cadnapaphornchai MA. Renal aquaporin water channels: From molecules to human disease. Prog Biophys Mol Biol 2003;81:117.

Schwartz MW, Woods SC, Seeley RJ, et al. Is the energy homeostasis system inherently biased toward weight gain? Diabetes 2003;52:232.

Seminara SB, Messager S, Chatzidaki EE, et al. The GPR54 gene as a regulator of puberty. N Engl J Med 2003;349:1614.

Sklar CA, Grumbach MM, Kaplan SL, et al. Hormonal and metabolic abnormalities associated with central nervous system germinoma in children and adolescents and the effect of therapy: Report of 10 patients. J Clin Endocrinol Metab 1981;52:9.

Stanfield JP. The blood supply of the human pituitary gland. J Anat 1960;94:257.

Tashiro H, Katabuchi H, Ohtake H, et al. A follicle-stimulating hormone-secreting gonadotroph adenoma with ovarian enlargement in a 10-year-old girl. Fertil Steril 1999, 72:158.

Thomas PQ, Dattani MT, Brickman JM, et al. Heterozygous HESX1 mutations associated with isolated congenital pituitary hypoplasia and septo-optic dysplasia. Hum Mol Genet 2001;10:39.

Thorner MO, Perryman RL, Cronin MJ, et al. Somatotroph hyperplasia. Successful treatment of acromegaly by removal of a pancreatic islet tumor secreting a growth hormone-releasing factor. J Clin Invest 1982;70:965.

Tolis G, Bird C, Bertrand G, et al. Pituitary hyperthyroidism. Case report and review of the literature. Am J Med 1978;64:177.

Vaisse C, Clement K, Durand E, et al. Melanocortin-4 receptor mutations are a frequent and heterogeneous cause of morbid obesity. J Clin Invest 2000;106:253.

Valdueza JM, Cristante L, Dammann O, et al. Hypothalamic hamartomas: With special reference to gelastic epilepsy and surgery. Neurosurgery 1994;34:949.

Verbalis JG. Vasopressin V2 receptor antagonists. J Mol Endocrinol 2002;29:1.

Verbalis JG. Diabetes insipidus. Rev Endocr Metab Disord 2003;4:177.

Willcutts MD, Felner E, White PC. Autosomal recessive familial neurohypophyseal diabetes insipidus with continued secretion of mutant weakly active vasopressin. Hum Mol Genet 1999;8:1303.

Wray S, Grant P, Gainer H. Evidence that cells expressing luteinizing hormone–releasing hormone mRNA in the mouse are derived from progenitor cells in the olfactory placode. Proc Natl Acad Sci U S A 1989;86:8132.

Wu W, Cogan JD, Pfaffle RW, et al. Mutations in PROP1 cause familial combined pituitary hormone deficiency. Nat Genet 1998;18:147.

CHAPTER 85

Disorders of the Autonomic Nervous System: Autonomic Dysfunction in Pediatric Practice

Christopher J. Mathias

The autonomic nervous system supplies and influences every organ in the body with a network of efferent pathways whose activities depend on a number of factors (Fig. 85-1). These include afferent information from various sources, cerebral and spinal cord integration, and local factors in target organs. The peripheral effector pathways consist of the sympathetic and parasympathetic nervous systems, in addition to the enteric nervous system. Dysfunction of the autonomic nervous system in childhood may occur for a variety of reasons; these include developmental abnormalities in the neonate that result in clinical presentation at birth, genetic disorders that manifest later in childhood, and the many causes of generalized or localized dysfunction as observed in adults.

Autonomic disorders in children, as in adults, cover many disciplines; dysfunction may be a complication of various diseases and thus can pose particular challenges. At different stages in children, specific aspects linked to developmental changes may need to be considered. This chapter, based predominantly on adult clinical practice, provides an emphasis on disorders occurring in childhood. There are brief descriptions also of adult autonomic disorders, which are of relevance because this information may have implications for genetic advice and for screening of children.

ANATOMIC, PHYSIOLOGIC, AND BIOCHEMICAL BASIS OF AUTONOMIC NERVOUS SYSTEM FUNCTION

The development of the autonomic nervous system has been well described in recent reviews [Ashwal, 1999; Hammil and La Gamma, 2002]. The effector components of the autonomic nervous system develop in the basal plate of the spinal cord and in the neural crest. In the third week of gestation, the neural plate begins to fuse and the neural tube is closed by the fourth week. Neural crest cells migrate as the neural tube fuse; crest cells in cephalic regions detach and migrate before the neural tube has closed. These cells undergo modification and differentiate to form the sympathetic and parasympathetic nervous systems. The sympathetic nervous system, in the thoracolumbar portion of the spinal cord, is formed from neural crest cells from the sixth somite to the posterior end of the neural crest. By the fifth week of gestation, primitive sympathetic ganglia appear, and later other preganglionic fibers pass through the paravertebral ganglia without synapsing, forming the splanchnic nerves that innervate the viscera.

Preganglionic parasympathetic fibers arise from neural crest cells in the diencephalon and cranial part of the mesencephalon (III cranial nerve), rhombencephalon (migrating cranially to form cranial nerves VII, IX, and X), and the second to fourth sacral segments of the developing spinal cord (parasympathetic supply to the pelvic viscera). Pupils, salivary glands, heart, gastrointestinal tract, and lungs become innervated from the fifth to the seventh week. In the 10th week, cardiac conducting fibers have appeared. Development of the enteric nervous system is from three different regions—the neural crest, vagal trunk, and sacrum—with neuroblasts first detected in the 24th week.

A variety of intrinsic and extrinsic factors affect the development of the autonomic nervous system, and these are both intrinsic and extrinsic. Genes, growth factors, and neurotrophins control various stages, and each may be critical at different development phases. These factors may in part be responsible for genetic and familial disorders, which include Hirschsprung's disease; Riley-Day syndrome; dopamine beta hydroxylase deficiency; hereditary, sensory, and autonomic neuropathies; and tumors affecting sympathoadrenal tissue.

The autonomic nervous system is essentially an effector (efferent) system that often operates in the form of a reflex arc. The sympathetic outflow is connected with major nuclei in the hypothalamus, midbrain, and brainstem and descends through the cervical spinal cord, where axons synapse in the intermediolateral cell mass. From the thoracic and upper lumbar spinal segments, myelinated axons emerge in white rami and synapse in paravertebral ganglia, which are some distance from target organs. The major ganglionic neurotransmitter is acetylcholine. Postganglionic fibers, which are unmyelinated, rejoin the mixed nerve through the gray rami and innervate target organs, except for the adrenal medulla, which has only a preganglionic supply. The neurotransmitter at postganglionic sites is predominantly noradrenaline, although sympathetic cholinergic fibers (with acetylcholine as the transmitter) supply sweat glands. There are complex pathways in neurotransmitter formation, release, and function, as illustrated with the catecholamines (Fig. 85-2). Many neurons have multiple neurotransmitters, which may be nonadrenergic and noncholinergic (Fig. 85-3). Vasoactive intestinal polypeptide is co-secreted with acetylcholine, which explains the inability of atropine to block all the effects of parasympathetic stimulation. Neuropeptide Y may be co-released with noradrenaline, accounting for why alpha-adrenoceptor blockers may not completely prevent the effects of sympathetic neural stimulation. The autonomic nervous system, despite the multiplicity of neurotransmitters and neuromodulators, however, selectively controls responses in specific regional vascular territories and organs, making it a highly complex but precisely regulated and integrated system.

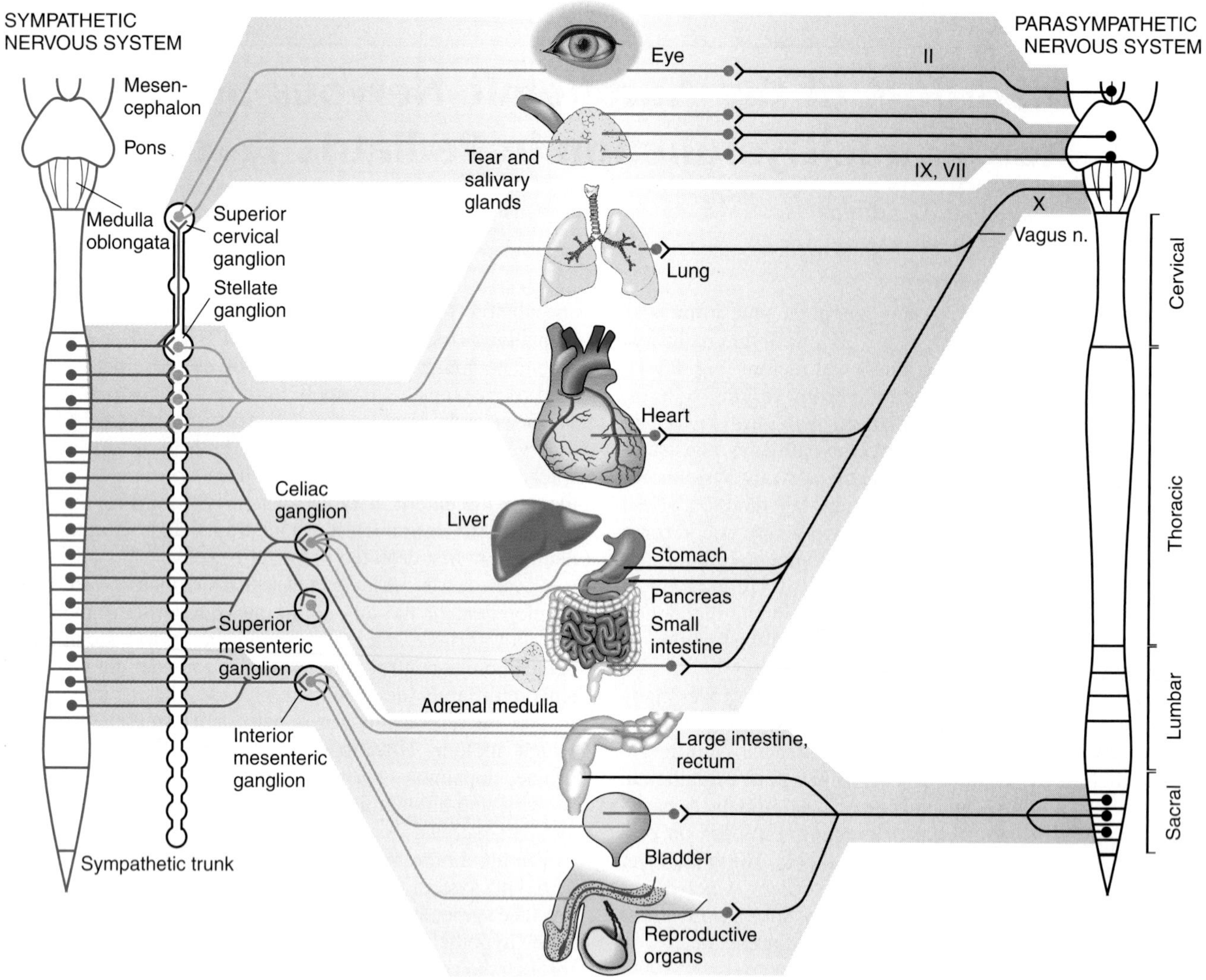

FIGURE 85-1. Parasympathetic and sympathetic innervation of major organs. (From Janig, 1989.)

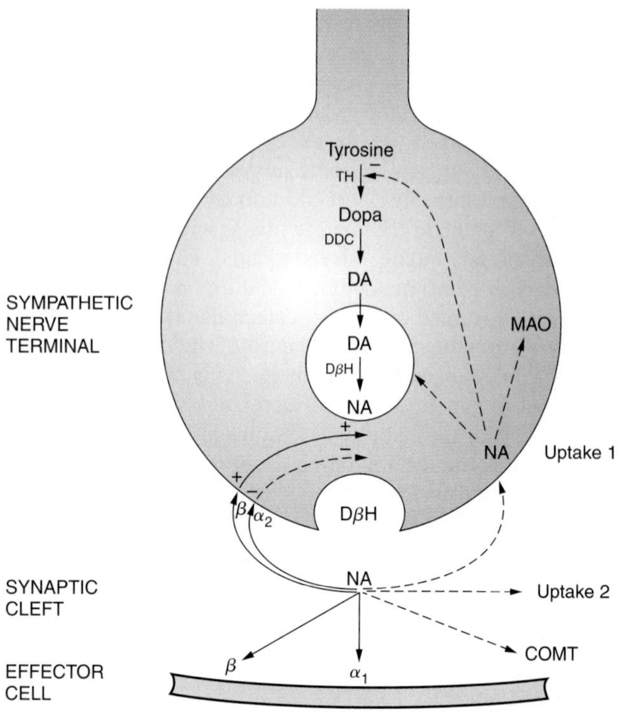

FIGURE 85-2. Schema of some pathways in the formation, release, and metabolism of noradrenaline from sympathetic nerve terminals. Tyrosine is converted into dihydroxyphenylalanine (dopa) by tyrosine hydroxylase (TH). Dopa is converted into dopamine (DA) by dopa decarboxylase (DDC). In the vesicles DA is converted into noradrenaline (NA) by dopamine β-hydroxylase (DβH). Nerve impulses release both DβH and NA into the synaptic cleft by exocytosis. NA acts predominantly on alpha$_1$-adrenoceptors (α_1) but has actions on beta-adrenoceptors (β) on the effector cell of target organs. It also has presynaptic adrenoceptor effects. Those acting on alpha$_2$ adrenoceptors inhibit NA release; those on beta-adrenoceptors stimulate NA release. NA may be taken up by a neuronal (uptake 1) process into the cytosol, where it may inhibit further formation of dopa through the rate-limiting enzyme TH. NA may be taken into vesicles or metabolized by monoamine oxidase (MAO) in the mitochondria. NA may be taken up by a higher capacity but lower affinity extraneuronal process (uptake 2) into peripheral tissues, such as vascular and cardiac muscle and certain glands. NA is also metabolized by catechol-*O*-methyltransferase (COMT). NA measured in plasma is the overspill not affected by these numerous processes. (Adapted from Mathias, 2004.)

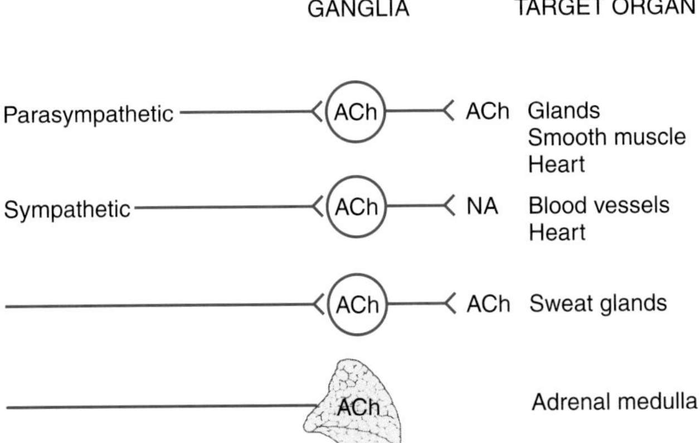

FIGURE 85-3. Outline of the major transmitters at autonomic ganglia and postganglionic sites on target organs supplied by the sympathetic and parasympathetic efferent pathways. The acetylcholine receptor at all ganglia is of the nicotinic subtype. Ganglionic blockers such as hexamethonium thus prevent both parasympathetic and sympathetic activation. Atropine, however, acts only on the muscarinic (ACH-m) receptor at postganglionic parasympathetic and sympathetic cholinergic sites. The co-transmitter is also indicated. NA, noradrenaline. (Adapted from Mathias, 1998.)

The parasympathetic outflow consists of cranial and sacral efferents. Cranial efferents accompany cranial nerves III, VII, IX, and X and supply the eye, lacrimal and salivary glands, heart and lungs, and gastrointestinal tract with associated structures, down to the level of the colon. The sacral outflow supplies the urinary tract and bladder, the large bowel, and reproductive system. Cerebral and spinal parasympathetic nuclei have specific control, for example, the Edinger-Westphal nucleus in pupillary control and Onuf's nucleus in the second and third sacral segments in urinary sphincter function. Most parasympathetic ganglia are close to target organs, and acetylcholine is the major transmitter at ganglia and at postganglionic sites.

Each sensory pathway has the capability to influence autonomic activity, as has been described in relation to autonomic control of blood pressure. The major baroreceptor afferents in the carotid sinus and aortic arch relay information to the brain through cranial nerves IX (glossopharyngeal) and X (vagal). Receptors in the heart and lungs (cardiopulmonary baroreceptors), skin, muscle, and viscera also influence blood pressure. Their role may be unmasked in tetraplegic subjects with cervical cord lesions above the spinal sympathetic outflow, where the peripheral sympathetic and cranial parasympathetic nervous systems function independently of the brain.

The major cerebral centers concerned with autonomic regulation include the insula, amygdyla, hypothalamus, midbrain (Edinger-Westphal nucleus and locus ceruleus), and brainstem (nucleus tractus solitarius and vagal nuclei). A combination of neuroimaging and physiologic studies indicates that a variety of cerebral areas, in different situations and in response to different stimuli, influence autonomic function (Benarroch, 2002; Critchley et al., 2001a, 2001b; Spyer, 2002).

CLASSIFICATION OF AUTONOMIC DISORDERS IN CHILDREN

Autonomic disorders may be primary, in which no cause has been determined, or secondary to specific diseases, such as diabetes mellitus (Table 85-1). Drugs are a major cause of autonomic dysfunction (Table 85-2). An intermittent autonomic abnormality occurs in neurally mediated syncope and the postural tachycardia syndrome. Table 85-3 provides examples of autonomic disorders in which localized deficits affect specific organs.

CLINICAL FEATURES OF AUTONOMIC DYSFUNCTION

Disorders of the autonomic nervous system can result in a wide spectrum of clinical manifestations (Table 85-4). Sympathetic adrenergic failure results in orthostatic (postural) hypotension and ejaculatory failure (in the postpubertal male), whereas sympathetic cholinergic failure causes anhidrosis. The reverse, sympathetic overactivity may result in hypertension, tachycardia, and hyperhidrosis. Parasympathetic failure causes a fixed heart rate, an atonic urinary bladder, a sluggish large bowel, and erectile failure; overactivity can result in bradycardia and even cardiac arrest. The clinical features depend on the extent of the lesion, the associated disease, and the ensuing functional deficit.

Some disorders are recognized at birth, such as the Riley-Day syndrome (familial dysautonomia), in which there usu-

TABLE 85-1

Outline Classification of Autonomic Failure

PRIMARY
Acute/Subacute Dysautonomias
Pure pandysautonomia
Pandysautonomia with neurologic features
Pure cholinergic dysautonomia
Chronic Autonomic Failure Syndromes
Pure autonomic failure
Multiple system atrophy (Shy-Drager syndrome)
Autonomic failure with Parkinson's disease
SECONDARY
Congenital
Nerve growth factor deficiency
Hereditary
Hereditary sensory and autonomic neuropathies
Riley-Day syndrome (familial dysautonomia)
Congenital insensitivity to pain with anhidrosis
Familial amyloid neuropathy
Dopamine β-hydroxylase deficiency
Metabolic
Diabetes mellitus
Chronic renal failure
Chronic liver disease
Alcohol-induced
Inflammatory
Guillain-Barré syndrome
Transverse myelitis
Infections
Bacterial tetanus
Viral human immunodeficiency infection
Neoplasia
Brain tumors, especially of third ventricle or posterior fossa
Paraneoplastic, to include adenocarcinomas of lung and pancreas
Trauma
Spinal cord lesions
DRUGS, CHEMICALS, POISONS, TOXINS (also see Table 85-2)
By their direct effects
By causing a neuropathy

Adapted from Mathias, 2003.

TABLE 85-2

Drugs, Chemicals, Poisons, and Toxins Causing Autonomic Dysfunction

Decreasing Sympathetic Activity

Centrally Acting
Clonidine
Methyldopa
Moxonidine
Reserpine
Barbiturates
Anesthetics
Peripherally acting
Sympathetic nerve endings (guanethidine, bethanidine)
Alpha-adrenoceptor blockade (phenoxybenzamine)
Beta-adrenoceptor blockade (propranolol)

Increasing Sympathetic Activity

Amphetamines
Releasing noradrenaline (tyramine)
Uptake blockers (imipramine)
Monoamine oxidase inhibitors (tranylcypromine)
Beta-adrenoceptor stimulants (isoprenaline)

Decreasing Parasympathetic Activity

Antidepressants (imipramine)
Tranquilizers (phenothiazines)
Antidysrhythmics (disopyramide)
Anticholinergics (atropine, probanthine, benztropine)
Toxins (botulinum)

Increasing Parasympathetic Activity

Cholinomimetics (carbachol, bethanechol, pilocarpine, mushroom poisoning)
Anticholinesterases
Reversible carbamate inhibitors (pyridostigmine, neostigmine)
Organophosphorous inhibitors (parathion, sarin)

Miscellaneous

Alcohol, thiamine (vitamin B_1) deficiency
Vincristine, perhexiline maleate
Thallium, arsenic, mercury
Mercury poisoning (pink disease)
Ciguatera toxicity
Jellyfish and marine animal venoms
First dose of certain drugs (prazosin, captopril)
Withdrawal of chronically used drugs (clonidine, opiates, alcohol)

Adapted from Mathias CJ. Disorders of the autonomic nervous system. In: Bradley WG, Daroff RB, Fenichel GM, Jankovic J, eds. Neurology in clinical practice, 4th ed. Philadelphia: Butterworth-Heinemann, 2004;2406.

TABLE 85-3

Examples of Localized Autonomic Disorders

Horner's syndrome
Holmes-Adie pupil
Crocodile tears (Bogorad's syndrome)
Gustatory sweating (Frey's syndrome)
Reflex sympathetic dystrophy
Idiopathic palmar or axillary hyperhidrosis
Chagas' disease *(Trypanosoma cruzi)**
Surgical procedures[†]
Sympathectomy (regional)
Vagotomy and gastric drainage procedures in "dumping" syndrome
Organ transplantation (heart, lungs)

*Listed here because it specifically targets intrinsic cholinergic plexuses in the heart and gut.
[†]Surgery also may cause other localized disorders, such as Frey's syndrome after parotid surgery.

TABLE 85-4

Some Clinical Manifestations of Autonomic Dysfunction

Cardiovascular	
Postural hypotension	Supine hypertension
Lability of blood pressure	Paroxysmal hypertension
Tachycardia	Bradycardia
Sudomotor	
Hypohidrosis or anhidrosis	Hyperhidrosis
Gustatory sweating	Hyperpyrexia
Heat intolerance	
Alimentary	
Xerostomia	Dysphagia
Gastric stasis	Dumping syndromes
Constipation	Diarrhea
Urinary	
Nocturia	Frequency
Urgency; retention	Incontinence
Sexual	
Erectile failure	Ejaculatory failure
Retrograde ejaculation	
Eye	
Pupillary abnormalities	Ptosis
Alacrima	Abnormal lacrimation with food ingestion

ally is a history of consanguinity in parents of Ashkenazi Jewish origin. Vasovagal syncope frequently presents in teenage years. In familial amyloid polyneuropathy, symptoms often occur in adulthood. In later years, after the age of 50, a number of neurodegenerative disorders such as multiple system atrophy present; in this particular disorder, there is no familial or known genetic link, which is important to the family of such patients. There may be sex preponderance; vasovagal syncope and the postural tachycardia syndrome are more common in females. A detailed history is essential and must include drug medication and previous exposure to chemical substances. The history should include gestational details, including the use of drugs taken during pregnancy.

In secondary autonomic disorders the features of the underlying or associated disorder need consideration because they may exacerbate autonomic manifestations. Individual assessments are necessary, especially of their psychologic state, in certain forms of vasovagal syncope, also known as *emotional syncope*.

The clinical findings may be confined to an area or an organ or may involve an entire system or systems. Impairment of the parasympathetic supply to the iris musculature occurs in the Holmes-Adie pupil; in essential hyperhidrosis, only the palms and soles may be affected. In generalized disorders a cardinal feature often is orthostatic (postural) hypotension (Fig. 85-4). This feature is defined as a decrease in systolic blood pressure of more than 20 mm Hg, or a fall in diastolic blood pressure of more than 10 mm Hg, while standing or during head-up tilt to 60 degrees for at least 3 minutes (Schatz et al., 1996). A variety of symptoms accompany the fall in blood pressure (Bleasdale-Barr and Mathias, 1998, Mathias et al., 1999) (Table 85-5). These depend on the rapidity and degree of fall in blood pressure, the extent to which compensatory factors come into play,

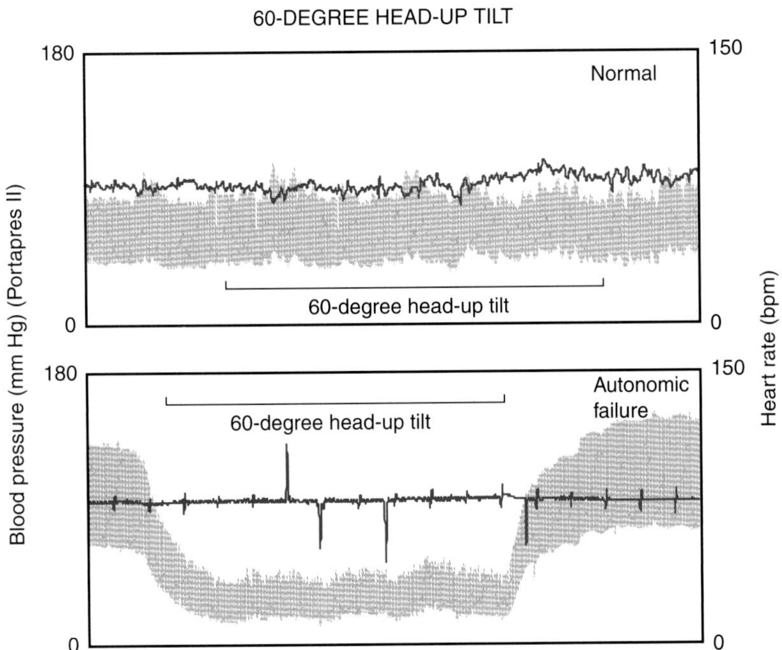

FIGURE 85-4. Blood pressure and heart rate before, during, and after head-up tilt in a normal subject *(upper panel),* and in a patient with autonomic failure *(lower panel).* In the normal subject, there is no fall in blood pressure during head-up tilt, unlike a subject with autonomic failure in whom blood pressure falls promptly and remains low with a blood pressure overshoot on return to the horizontal. In this subject, there is only a minimal change in heart rate despite the marked blood pressure fall. In each subject, continuous blood pressure and heart rate was recorded with the Portapres II monitor. (Adapted from Mathias, 2005.)

and the underlying disorder. Many factors influence orthostatic hypotension (Table 85-6). Stimuli in daily life such as food ingestion and mild exercise (Figs. 85-5 and 85-6) can lower supine blood pressure and unmask or exaggerate orthostatic hypotension (Mathias et al., 1991; Smith et al., 1993). The effect of drugs should be considered. Determination of the mechanisms contributing to orthostatic hypotension is of importance in management.

TABLE 85-5

Some of the Symptoms Resulting from Orthostatic Hypotension and Impaired Perfusion of Various Organs

Cerebral Hypoperfusion
- Dizziness
- Visual disturbances
  - Blurred—tunnel
  - Scotoma
  - Graying out—blacking out
  - Color defects
- Loss of consciousness
- Cognitive deficits

Muscle Hypoperfusion
- Paracervical and suboccipital ("coat hanger") ache
- Lower back/buttock ache

Subclavian Steal-like Syndrome

Renal Hypoperfusion
- Oliguria

Spinal Cord Hypoperfusion

Nonspecific
- Weakness, lethargy, fatigue
- Falls

Adapted from Mathias, 2003.

INVESTIGATION OF AUTONOMIC DYSFUNCTION

Autonomic activity may be measured directly or indirectly. Sympathetic nerve activity can be recorded using the electrophysiologic technique of microneurography or biochemically by measuring plasma noradrenaline and adrenaline levels using spillover techniques (Esler et al., 2003; Wallin, 2002). Each has its limitations. Some are invasive and measurements in a particular territory may not reflect activity in the whole body or other regions than from where the measurements are made. In clinical practice, functional effects are measured with systems- and organ-directed investigations (Mathias and Bannister, 2002a) (Table 85-7). Testing always should be in combination with the clinical history and examination. The main objectives of investigation are:

TABLE 85-6

Factors That May Influence Orthostatic Hypotension

- Speed of positional change
- Time of day (worse in the morning)
- Prolonged recumbency
- Warm environment (hot weather, hot bath)
- Raising intrathoracic pressure—micturition, defecation, or coughing
- Water ingestion*
- Food and alcohol ingestion
- Physical exertion
- Physical maneuvers and positions (bending forward, abdominal compression, leg crossing, squatting, activating calf muscle pump)**
- Drugs with vasoactive properties

*This raises blood pressure in autonomic failure.
†These maneuvers usually reduce the postural fall in blood pressure in neurogenic causes of orthostatic hypotension, unlike the others.
Adapted from Mathias, 2003.

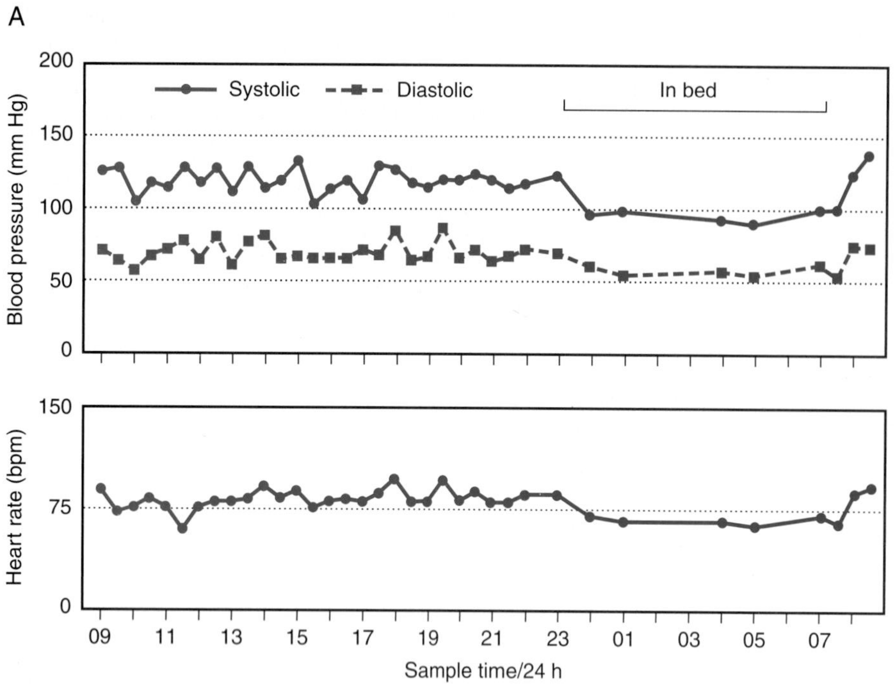

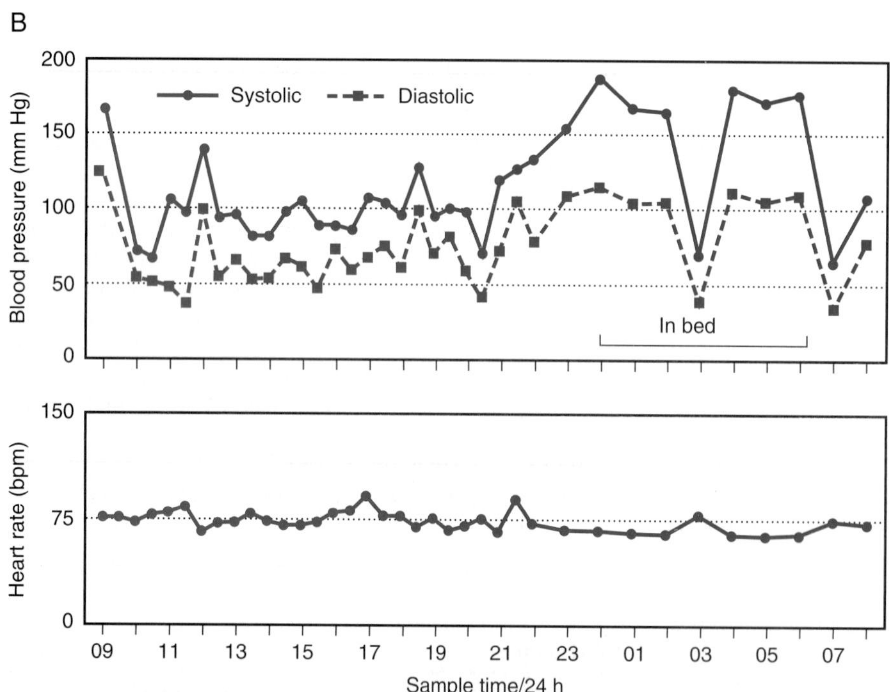

FIGURE 85-5. Twenty-four-hour noninvasive ambulatory blood pressure profile, showing systolic *(dark circles)* and diastolic *(dark squares)* blood pressure and heart rate at intervals through the day and night. **A,** Normal. The changes in a normal subject with no postural fall in blood pressure; there was a fall in blood pressure at night while asleep, with a rise in blood pressure on waking. **B,** Patient with autonomic failure. The marked falls in blood pressure usually are the result of postural changes, either sitting or standing. Supine blood pressure, particularly at night, is elevated. Getting up to micturate causes a marked fall in blood pressure (at 0300 hours). There is a reversal of the diurnal changes in blood pressure. There are relatively small changes in heart rate, considering the marked changes in blood pressure. (From Mathias and Bannister, 2002b. Reprinted with permission of Oxford University Press.)

1. To assess if autonomic function is normal or abnormal.
2. If the latter, to ascertain the degree of autonomic dysfunction with an emphasis on the site of lesion and functional deficit.
3. To determine the underlying or associated disease because this disease will need concurrent treatment with management of autonomic dysfunction.

Investigation of the autonomic nervous system ideally should utilize noninvasive techniques that are safe, reproducible, and patient friendly so that they can be used for initial screening and if needed for repeat testing to determine disease progression and the effects of therapy. This comforting approach is of importance in young children. Different autonomic laboratories are unlikely to have similar equipment and an identical set of procedures, despite attempts to standardize such approaches. High specificity and sensitivity, although desirable, may not be achievable or practical, and the findings must be considered in the context of a wide variety of factors, including the patient's ability to cooperate while being tested. The effect of drugs is another confounding factor, because some have effects directly or indirectly on autonomic function. Finally, the results must be linked with the relevant clinical symptoms and signs. Difficulties mainly arise in mild or moderate cases with

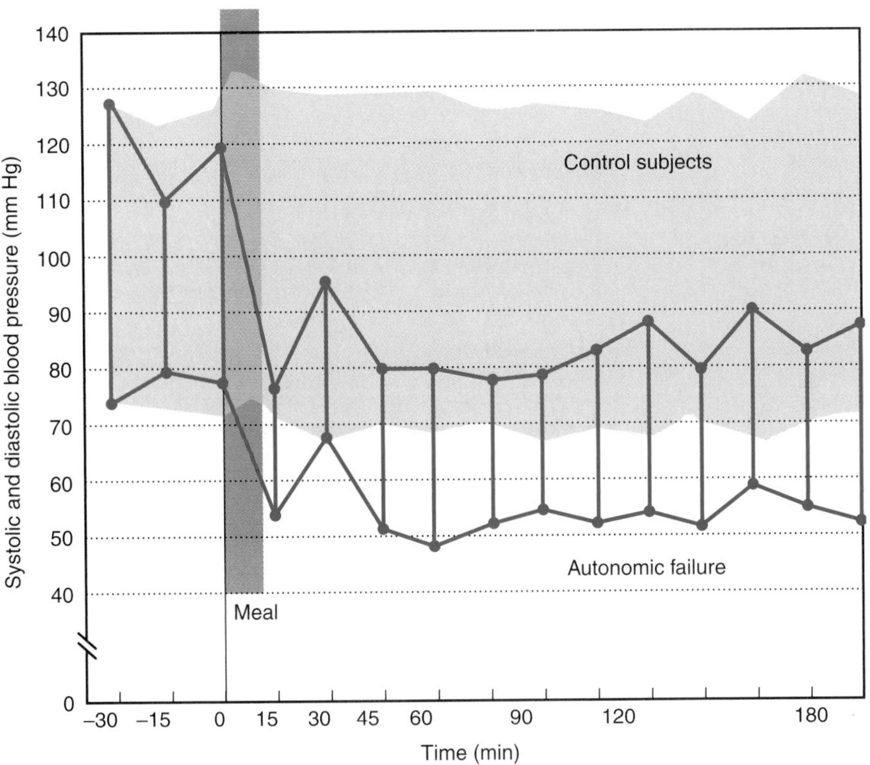

FIGURE 85-6. Supine systolic and diastolic blood pressure before and after a standard meal in a group of normal subjects *(stippled area)* and in a patient with autonomic failure. Blood pressure does not change in the normal subjects after a meal taken while lying flat. In the patient, there is a rapid fall in blood pressure to levels around 80/50 mm Hg, which remains low while in the supine position over the 3-hour observational period. (From Mathias and Bannister, 2002b. Reprinted with permission of Oxford Univeristy Press.)

questionable autonomic involvement, unlike patients with definite abnormalities.

Cardiovascular System

A postural fall in blood pressure, especially if consistently more than 20 mm Hg systolic, or less in the presence of symptoms, warrants further investigation. Head-up tilt often is used as the postural stimulus, especially when the neurologic deficit or severe hypotension makes it difficult for the patient to stand (see Fig. 85-3). In some, orthostatic hypotension may be unmasked by exercise (Smith and Mathias, 1995) because vasodilatation in skeletal muscle is not appropriately counteracted by autonomic reflexes. Food ingestion also may be a provoking factor (Mathias et al., 1989), presumably because of splanchnic vasodilatation not compensated for by vasoconstriction in other regions. Non-neurogenic causes of orthostatic hypotension also must be considered (Table 85-8). The same may occur with drugs that cause vasodilatation, even if this usually is only a minor side effect.

Both blood pressure and heart rate can be accurately measured using noninvasive techniques, many of which are automated and provide a printout at preset intervals. Intermittent ambulatory recordings over a 24-hour period using small computerized devices are of particular value, especially at home to determine the effects of various stimuli in daily life (see Fig. 85-5). They may be of value in determining the beneficial effects of therapy in different situations. Beat-by-beat measurement of blood pressure and heart rate is essential in neurally mediated syncope when the changes in blood pressure often are rapid and would be missed because of the slow response time of most noninvasive sphygmomanometers; furthermore they may be independent of changes in heart rate. The Finometer, Portapres, and CNS Taskforce machines enable noninvasive and beat-by-beat blood pressure and heart rate recordings with a finger cuff and provide a reliable measure of change in blood pressure (Wieling and Karemaker, 2002).

Screening investigations help determine the site and extent of the cardiovascular autonomic abnormality. With these tests, cooperation is an essential component, which may be difficult to ensure, especially in younger children. The responses to the Valsalva maneuver during which intrathoracic pressure is raised depend on the integrity of the entire baroreflex pathway. Changes in heart rate alone, even in the absence of blood pressure recordings, provide a useful guide. Some patients may, however, raise mouth pressure without necessarily raising intrathoracic pressure, resulting in a falsely abnormal response. Stimuli that raise blood pressure, such as isometric exercise (by sustained hand grip for 3 minutes), the cold pressor test (immersing the hand in ice slush for 90 seconds), and mental arithmetic (using serial-7 or serial-17 subtraction), activate different afferent or central pathways, which then stimulate the sympathetic outflow. The heart rate responses to postural change, deep breathing (sinus dysrhythmia; see Fig. 85-5), and hyperventilation assess cardiac vagal efferent pathways.

Additional investigations may be needed to determine factors causing or contributing to orthostatic hypotension and syncope. These include determining the responses to food ingestion and exercise. To assess postprandial hypotension, the cardiovascular responses to a balanced liquid meal containing carbohydrate, protein, and fat are determined while supine, with comparisons of the blood pressure response to head-up tilt before the meal and 45 minutes later (Mathias et al., 1991) (see Fig. 85-6). To evaluate exercise-induced hypotension, responses are obtained during graded

TABLE 85-7

Outline of Investigations in Autonomic Dysfunction

Cardiovascular	
Physiologic	Head-up tilt (60 degrees)*; standing*; Valsalva's maneuver*
	Pressor stimuli* (isometric exercise, cold pressor, mental arithmetic)
	Heart rate responses—deep breathing,* hyperventilation,* standing,* head-up tilt,* 30:15 R-R interval ratio
	Liquid meal challenge
	Exercise testing
	Carotid sinus massage
Biochemical	Plasma noradrenaline: supine and head-up tilt or standing; urinary catecholamines; plasma renin activity and aldosterone
Pharmacologic	Noradrenaline: alpha-adrenoceptors, vascular
	Isoprenaline: beta-adrenoceptors, vascular and cardiac
	Tyramine: pressor and noradrenaline response
	Edrophonium: noradrenaline response
	Atropine: parasympathetic cardiac blockade
Endocrine	Clonidine—$alpha_2$-adrenoceptor agonist: noradrenaline suppression; growth hormone stimulation
Sudomotor	Central regulation thermoregulatory sweat test
	Sweat gland response to intradermal acetylcholine, quantitative sudomotor axon reflex test, localized sweat test
	Sympathetic skin response
Gastrointestinal	Videocine fluoroscopy, barium studies, endoscopy, gastric emptying studies, lower gut studies
Renal Function and Urinary Tract	Day and night urine volumes and sodium/potassium excretion
	Urodynamic studies, intravenous urography, ultrasound examination, sphincter electromyography
Sexual Function	Penile plethysmography
	Intracavernosal papaverine
Respiratory	Laryngoscopy
	Sleep studies to assess apnea and oxygen desaturation
Eye and Lachrymal Function	Pupil function, pharmacologic and physiologic
	Schirmer's test

*Indicates screening autonomic tests used in the author's London unit.
Adapted from Mathias and Bannister, 2002b. Reprinted with permission of Oxford University Press.

TABLE 85-8

Examples of Non-neurogenic Causes of Orthostatic Hypotension

Low Intravascular Volume	
Blood/plasma loss	Hemorrhage, burns, hemodialysis
Fluid/electrolyte deficiency	
Diminished intake	Anorexia nervosa
Loss from gut	Vomiting, ileostomy losses, diarrhea
Loss from kidney	Salt-losing nephropathy, diuretics
Endocrine deficiency	Adrenal insufficiency (Addison's disease)
Cardiac Insufficiency	
Myocardial	Myocarditis
Impaired ventricular filling	Atrial myxoma, constrictive pericarditis
Impaired output	Aortic stenosis
Vasodilatation	
Endogenous	Hyperpyrexia
	Hyperbradykininism
	Systemic mastocytosis
	Varicose veins
Exogenous	Drugs that are vasodilators
	Alcohol
	Excessive heat

Adapted from Mathias, 2003.

incremental supine exercise using a bicycle ergometer with measurement of postural responses before and after exercise (Smith and Mathias, 1995) (Fig. 85-7).

Measurement of plasma catecholamine levels may provide valuable information about the site of lesion. Thus in postganglionic lesions, as observed in acute sympathetic failure and adults with pure autonomic failure, the supine basal level of plasma noradrenaline is low, indicating a distal lesion. This finding differs from that in patients with central lesion (as in the adult with multiple system atrophy), in whom supine levels often are within the normal range (Fig. 85-8). In both groups, however, there is an attenuation or lack of rise in plasma noradrenaline levels during head-up tilt, indicating impairment of sympathetic neural activity. However, in patients with high spinal cord lesions who also have preganglionic lesions, basal plasma noradrenaline and adrenaline levels are low and do not rise with postural change (Mathias et al., 1975). There is a rise (but only moderately above the basal levels of normal subjects) during severe hypertension accompanying autonomic dysreflexia (Mathias et al., 1976) that differentiates these patients from pheochromocytoma in which paroxysmal hypertension often is associated with elevated plasma noradrenaline or adrenaline levels.

Extremely low or undetectable levels of plasma noradrenaline and adrenaline with elevated plasma dopamine levels occur in sympathetic failure caused by deficiency of the enzyme dopamine β-hydroxylase, which converts dopamine into noradrenaline (Mathias and Bannister, 2002b). Plasma levels of this enzyme are undetectable, but this situation may occur in 10% of normal individuals and is not diagnostic of the disorder. Immunohistochemical studies confirm the absence of the enzyme in tissues such as skin.

Many techniques capitalize on applying the advances of modern technology, as demonstrated with the study of cardiovascular autonomic function. These include techniques for the noninvasive measurement of cardiac function and blood flow in various regions (Chandler and Mathias, 2002; Puvi-Rajasingham et al., 1997), a variety of computer and spectral analytic techniques that assess heart rate (Parati et al., 2002), and methods (some invasive) that measure total body and regional noradrenaline spillover in the heart, splanchnic, renal, and brain circulation (Esler et al., 2003; Lambert et al., 1997). Techniques to visualize sympathetic innervation of cardiac tissue include radionuclide 123-metaiodobenzylguanidine (Hakusui et al,. 1994, Mantysaari et al., 1996), and positron emission tomography scanning with 6-[^{18}F]fluorodopamine (Goldstein et al,. 1997). These

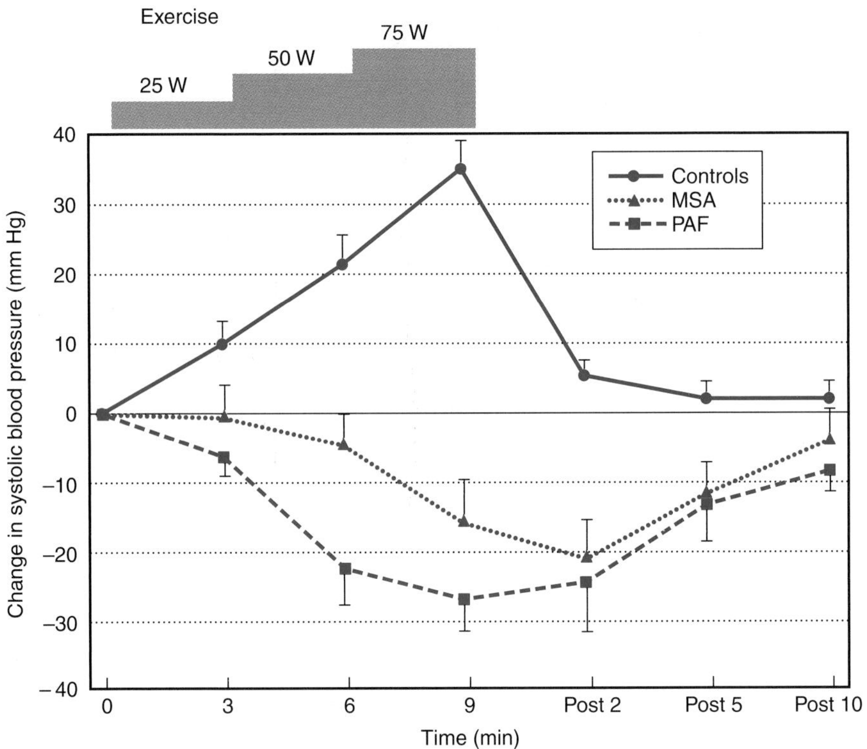

FIGURE 85-7. Changes in systolic blood pressure during supine bicycle exercise at three incremental levels (25, 50, and 75 watts) in normal subjects (controls) and patients with multiple system atrophy (MSA) and pure autonomic failure (PAF). The bars indicate standard error of the mean. Unlike controls in whom there is a rise, there is a fall in blood pressure in both MSA and PAF. Blood pressure returns rapidly to the baseline in controls, unlike in the two patient groups in whom it takes almost 10 minutes. All remained horizontal during and for 10 minutes postexercise. (From Smith et al., 1995b.)

techniques have a role in the clinical research setting, mainly in adults, and some are applied to the clinical investigation of cardiovascular autonomic function.

In the majority of autonomic disorders affecting the circulation, physiologic testing using head-up postural challenge, a series of pressor tests, Valsalva's maneuver, deep breathing, and hyperventilation is often adequate for screening purposes. Depending on the disorder, additional tests may be needed, such as food and exercise challenge, ocular massage, and appropriate biochemical and pharmacologic studies.

Sweating

The thermoregulatory sweating response is tested by elevating body temperature by 10° C, with either a heat cradle or hot water bottles and a space blanket. This process tests the integrity of central pathways, from the hypothalamus to the sweat glands. Sweating is assessed using powders such as Ponceau red, which turns from a pale pink to vivid red on exposure to moisture. In autonomic failure, the thermoregulatory sweating response is lost, and additional tests are needed to distinguish between central and peripheral lesions. In postganglionic lesions, the sudomotor and pilomotor response to intradermal acetylcholine is lost. Various measures can be used, including the quantitative sudomotor axon reflex test. Intradermal pilocarpine assesses the function of sweat glands directly. In dopamine β-hydroxylase deficiency syndrome, sympathetic cholinergic function and sweating is preserved, providing a clue to selective impairment of sympathetic noradrenergic function. In gustatory sweating, spicy foods, cheese, or substances containing tyramine are ingested to provoke sweating (Fig. 85-9).

The sympathetic skin response measures electrical potentials from electrodes on the foot and hand and provides a measure of sympathetic cholinergic activity to sweat glands. The sympathetic skin response can be induced by stimuli that are physiologic (inspiratory gasps, loud noise, or touch) or electrical (median nerve stimulation) (Cariga et al., 2001a, 2001b; Nicotra et al., 2004). In peripheral autonomic disorders, such as pure autonomic failure and pure cholinergic dysautonomia (Fig. 85-10), the sympathetic skin response is a reliable marker of sympathetic cholinergic function. However, this reliability depends on the presence or absence of the response, rather than latency and amplitude, which are highly variable (Magnifico et al., 1998).

Gastrointestinal Tract

Video or cinefluoroscopy is of value in assessing swallowing and the presence of oropharyngeal dysphagia. A barium swallow, meal, and follow-through are helpful in suspected upper gastrointestinal disorders, although alternative investigation by endoscopy provides the opportunity for biopsy. Caution should be exercised when there is suspected widespread cholinergic involvement and colonic stasis. Esophageal manometry is of value in disorders of motility and esophagogastric function. Several methods (radioisotope methods and scintigraphic scanning) are available to determine gastric motility noninvasively. When bacterial overgrowth is a suspected cause of diarrhea, a therapeutic trial with broad-spectrum antibiotics, such as neomycin or tetracycline, may be used along with investigations such as jejunal aspiration and the C14 glycocholate test. In the adult with chronic primary autonomic failure, such as multiple system atrophy and pure autonomic failure (Maule et al.,

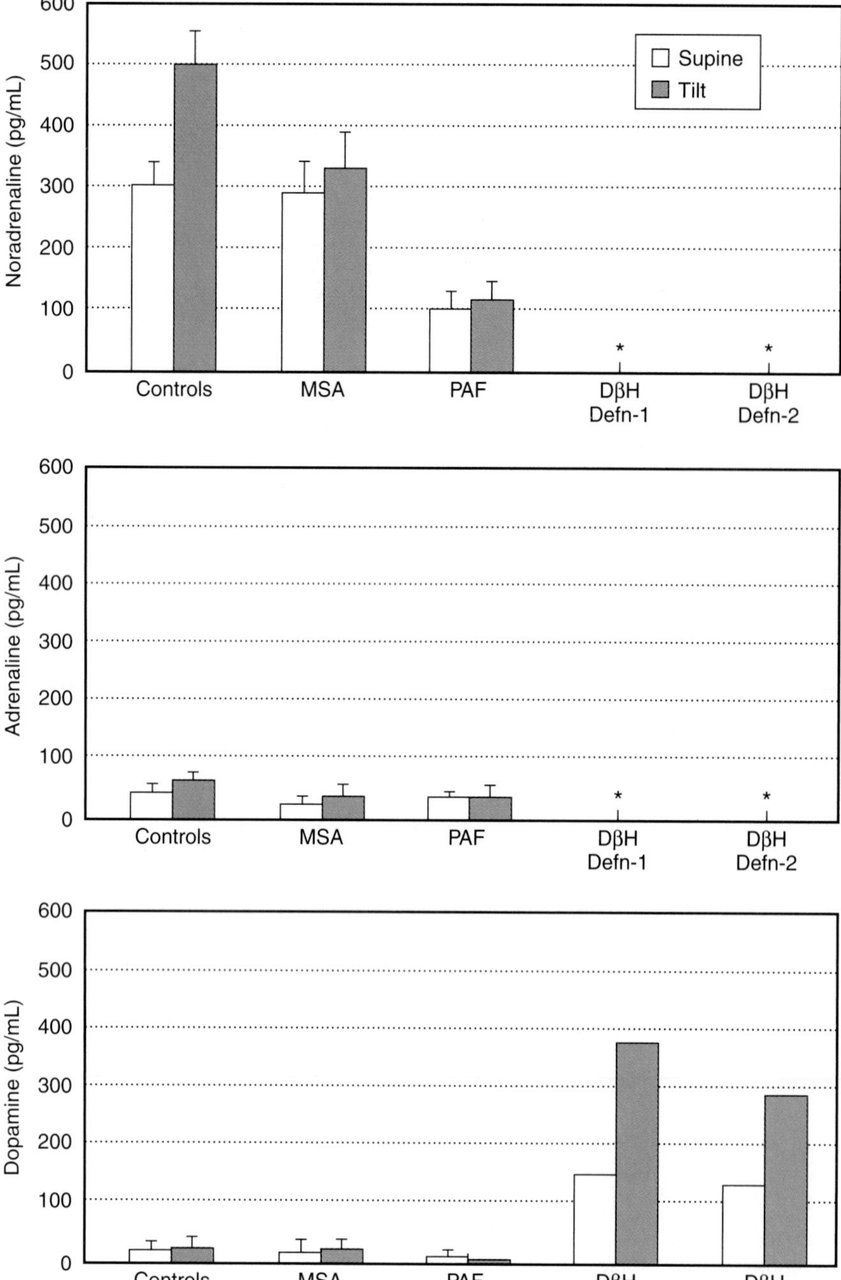

FIGURE 85-8. Plasma noradrenaline, adrenaline, and dopamine levels (measured by high-pressure liquid chromatography) in normal subjects (controls), patients with multiple system atrophy (MSA) or pure autonomic failure (PAF), and two individual patients with dopamine β-hydroxylase (DβH) while supine and after head-up tilt to 45 degrees for 10 minutes. The asterisk indicates levels below the detection limits for the assay, which are less than 5 pg/mL for noradrenaline and adrenaline and less than 20 pg/L for dopamine. Bars indicate ± SEM. (From Mathias and Bannister, 2002b. Reprinted with permission of Oxford University Press.)

2002), *Helicobacter pylori* infection is common and may contribute to gastric dysfunction; whether this occurs in children is unclear. Small bowel manometry and telemetric devices are of value in separating myopathic from neuropathic disorders of the gut. The measurement of transit time and proctologic function are used to investigate lower bowel disorders causing diarrhea, constipation, and fecal incontinence.

Urinary Tract

Nocturnal polyuria can be assessed by separate day and night measurement of urine volume. Measurements of urine osmolarity and the concentration of sodium and potassium may be helpful. When the urinary bladder is involved, an intravenous pyelogram and micturating cystometrogram may be needed. Urodynamic measurements are valuable in defining the function of the bladder musculature and sphincter mechanisms. Measurement of postmicturition residual volume (e.g., by ultrasound) is of particular importance. It may be high when the urinary bladder is involved; this residual may cause urinary infection, which should be detected early and promptly treated. In some, such as patients with spinal cord lesions, particular care must be provided because recurrent infections, along with calculi, may cause chronic renal failure.

Respiratory System

Respiratory rate and arterial blood gases should be measured to determine the degree of hypoxia, especially during

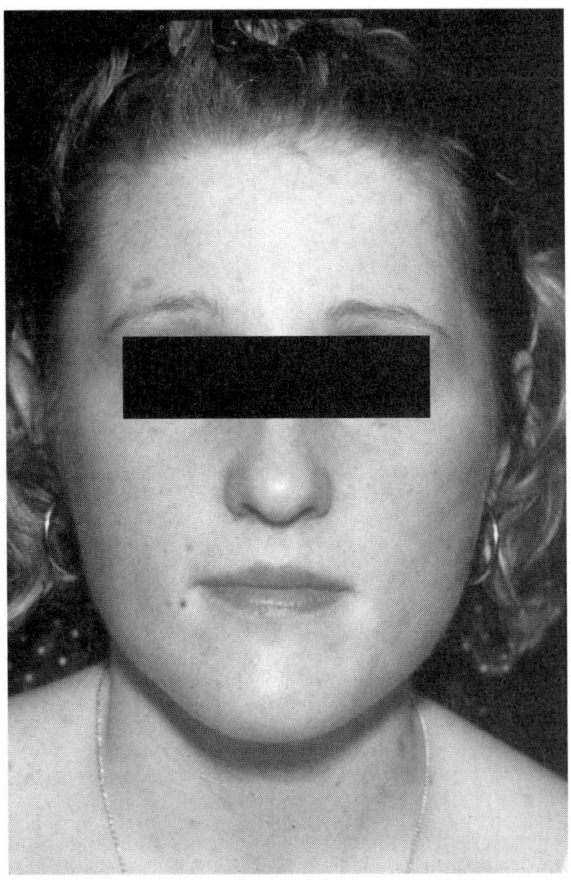

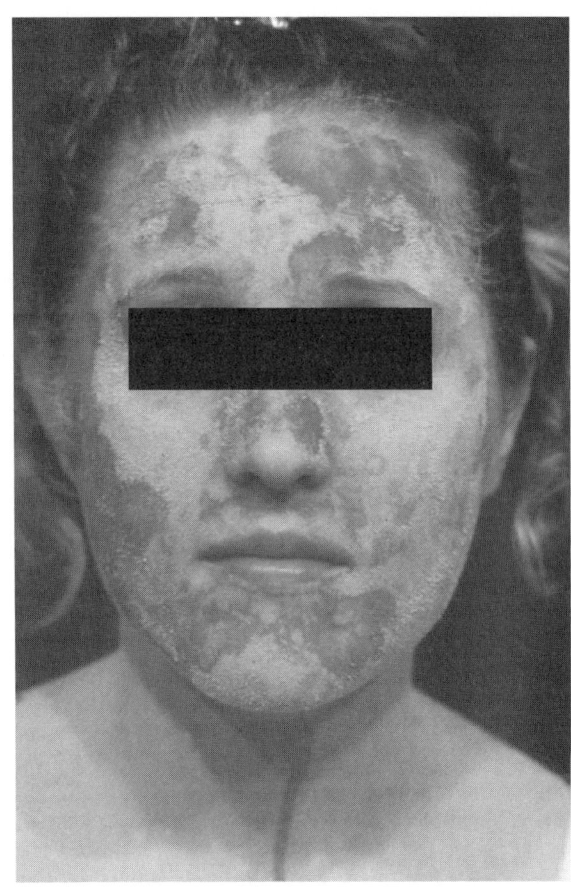

FIGURE 85-9. Gustatory sweating induced by food in a subject recovering from an acute pandysautonomia. On contact with moisture, the pale powder, hardly visible in **A**, turns a vivid red, with sweat dripping down the neck (as observed in **B**). (From Mathias, 1996. ©1996. Reproduced with permission from The McGraw-Hill Companies.)

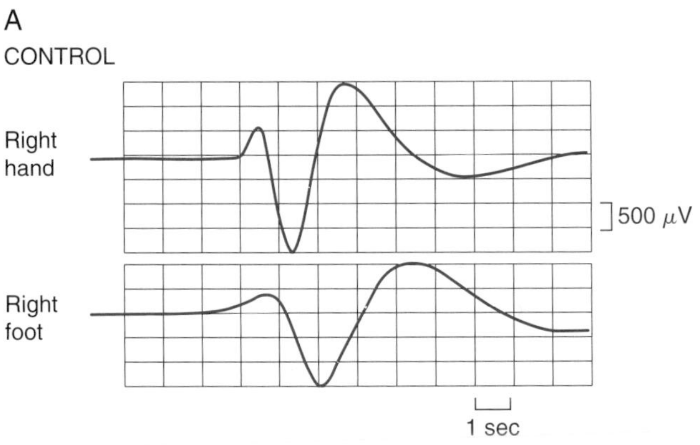

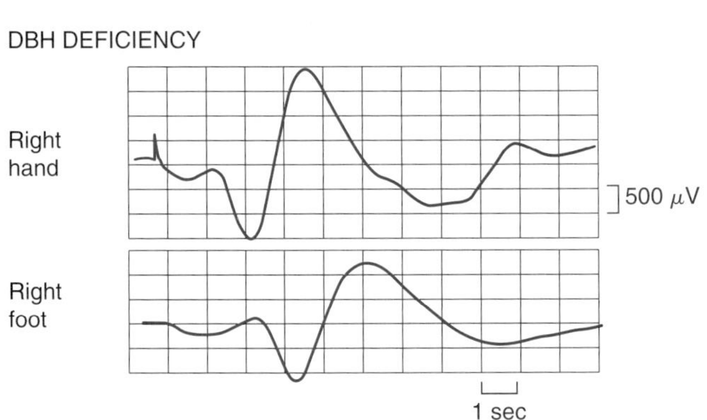

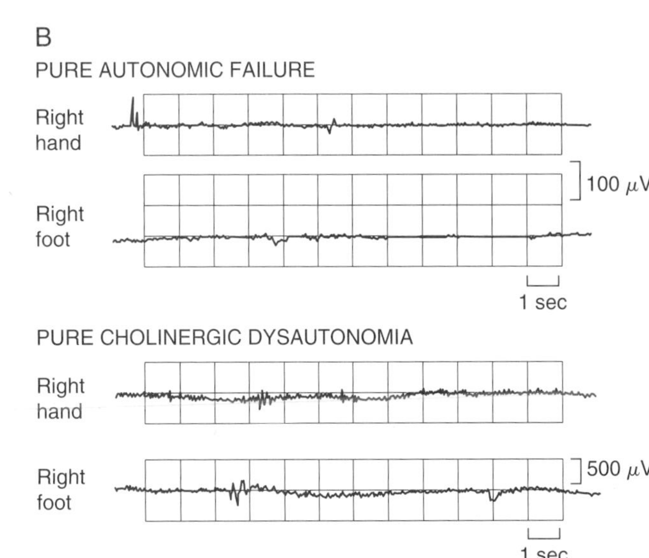

FIGURE 85-10. A, The sympathetic skin response (in microvolts) from the right hand and right foot of a normal subject (control) and a patient with dopamine β-hydroxylase (DβH) deficiency. **B**, The sympathetic skin response could not be recorded in two patients, one with pure autonomic failure and the other with pure cholinergic dysautonomia. (From Magnifico et al., 1998. Reprinted with kind permission of Springer Science and Business Media.)

sleep in patients with apneic episodes. Indirect and direct laryngoscopy detects laryngeal abductor paresis.

Eye

Various pharmacologic preparations administered locally help determine the degree of sympathetic or parasympathetic involvement of pupils. Lacrimal secretion can be tested by Schirmer's test, and damage from deficient secretion can be assessed using rose bengal instillation followed by slit-lamp examination.

Skin

The flare response is elicited by intradermal injection of histamine. A positive response is indicated by local swelling and redness. Absence of pain, piloerection, and flare are typical in autonomic dysfunction.

Miscellaneous

Additional nonautonomic investigations may be needed to determine the cause of the disorder or associated complications. Computed tomographic scans and magnetic resonance imaging (MRI) of the brain help in assessing basal ganglia, cerebellar, and brainstem involvement. Positron emission tomography scanning has provided valuable information in adults with central autonomic disorders, such as multiple system atrophy (Brooks, 2002). In suspected peripheral nerve involvement, electrophysiologic studies together with sural nerve biopsy are indicated. In amyloidosis, a rectal or renal biopsy may be diagnostic; the latter is indicated if there is renal involvement. Genetic testing is helpful in familial amyloid polyneuropathy. To exclude adrenal insufficiency, a short or long Synacthen test should be performed.

In patients with localized lesions, specific investigations to determine the cause may be warranted. In Horner's syndrome, for example, investigations may include brain neuroimaging to exclude a midbrain or medullary hemorrhage, bronchoscopy, and radiography to exclude an apical bronchial neoplasm, and carotid artery angiography to assess lesions of the internal carotid artery.

Measurement of plasma cortisol, plasma renin activity, and plasma aldosterone levels is useful in certain cases. In Addison's disease and adrenocortical failure, basal plasma renin levels are markedly elevated, whereas plasma aldosterone is low or absent. In diabetic autonomic neuropathy, there may be low levels of both plasma renin and aldosterone, which contribute to hyperkalemia.

MANAGEMENT OF ORTHOSTATIC HYPOTENSION

Orthostatic hypotension may cause considerable disability. In some children, as in dopamine β-hydroxylase deficiency, it may be the reason for inability to exercise. In others there is the potential risk of serious injury. In non-neurogenic orthostatic hypotension, the underlying problem may need to be resolved rapidly because it may be an indicator of substantial blood or fluid loss or of a serious underlying disorder, such as adrenal insufficiency (Table 85-9).

TABLE 85-9

Some of the Approaches Used in the Management of Orthostatic Hypotension Caused by Autonomic Failure

NONPHARMACOLOGIC MEASURES
To be avoided
Sudden head-up postural change (especially on waking)
Prolonged recumbency
Straining during micturition and defecation
High environmental temperature (including hot baths)
"Severe" exertion
Large meals (especially with refined carbohydrate)
Alcohol
Drugs with vasodepressor properties
To be introduced
Head-up tilt during sleep
Small frequent meals
High salt intake
Judicious exercise (including swimming)
Body positions and maneuvers
To be considered
Elastic stockings
Abdominal binders
Water ingestion
PHARMACOLOGIC MEASURES
Starter drug—fludrocortisone
Sympathomimetics—ephedrine, midodrine
Specific targeting—octreotide, desmopressin, erythropoietin

Adapted from Mathias, 2003.

Approaches to therapy may include reducing fluid loss, replacing blood and fluids, correcting the endocrine deficiency, improving cardiac function, and preventing vasodilatation. In some patients with neurogenic orthostatic hypotension, treatment may be highly effective, as in dopamine β-hydroxylase deficiency; in the majority, however, cure is less likely. The management depends on the pathophysiologic processes and primary disease responsible. It should be emphasized that the management of associated non-neurogenic factors (such as those resulting from fluid and blood loss), also is essential because they can considerably exacerbate neurogenic orthostatic hypotension. Nonpharmacologic measures are an essential component of management, even when drugs are used. Because no single drug can effectively mimic the actions of the sympathetic nervous system, a multipronged approach is needed (Table 85-10), which includes factors to avoid, institute, and consider.

Even in young children, increasing awareness of the many factors that lower blood pressure is important. These include simple measures such as avoiding rapid postural change, especially in the morning when getting out of bed, because the supine blood pressure often is lowest at this time, in those in whom nocturnal polyuria reduces extracellular fluid volume. Prolonged bed rest and recumbency, especially postoperatively, should be avoided. Head-up tilt at night is beneficial and may reduce salt and water loss by stimulating the renin-angiotensin-aldosterone system or by activating other hormonal, neural, or local renal hemodynamic mechanisms, which reduce recumbency-induced diuresis. When head-up tilt is impractical or the degree of tilt achieved inadequate, nocturnal polyuria and nocturia can be reduced with the antidiuretic agent desmopressin (Mathias and Young, 2003; Mathias et al., 1986). Straining during micturition and bowel movement should be avoided. In hot weather there

TABLE 85-10

Outline of the Major Actions by Which a Variety of Drugs May Reduce Orthostatic Hypotension.

Reducing salt loss/plasma volume expansion
Mineralocorticoids (fludrocortisone)
Reducing nocturnal polyuria
V_2-receptor agonists (desmopressin)
Vasoconstriction—sympathetic
On resistance vessels (ephedrine, midodrine, phenylephrine, noradrenaline, clonidine, tyramine with monoamine oxidase inhibitors, yohimbine, L-dihydroxyphenylserine)
On capacitance vessels (dihydroergotamine)
Vasoconstriction—nonsympathomimetic
V_1 receptor agents—terlipressin
Ganglionic nicotinic-receptor stimulation
Anticholinesterase inhibitors
Preventing vasodilatation
Prostaglandin synthetase inhibitors (indomethacin, flurbiprofen)
Dopamine receptor blockade (metoclopramide, domperidone)
$Beta_2$-adrenoceptor blockade (propranolol)
Preventing postprandial hypotension
Adrenosine receptor blockade (caffeine)
Peptide release inhibitors (somatostatin analog: octreotide)
Increasing cardiac output
Beta blockers with intrinsic sympathomimetic activity (pindolol, xamoterol)
Dopamine agonists (ibopamine)
Increasing red cell mass
Erythropoietin

Adapted from Mathias, 2003.

may be elevation of body temperature if thermoregulatory mechanisms, such as sweating, are impaired; this elevation may further increase vasodilatation and worsen orthostatic hypotension. Ingestion of alcohol or large meals, especially those containing a high carbohydrate content, may cause postprandial hypotension and aggravate postural hypotension. Various physical maneuvers such as leg crossing, squatting, sitting in the knee-chest position, and abdominal compression, are of value in reducing orthostatic hypotension (Wieling et al., 1993).

Consideration should be given to introducing means to prevent venous pooling during standing. These include lower limb elastic stockings and abdominal binders (Tanaka et al., 1997). Each has its limitations and may increase susceptibility to orthostatic postural hypotension when not in use. Tachypacing with an implanted cardiac pacemaker is of no benefit in the management of neurogenic orthostatic hypotension except in the rare situation when bradycardia also occurs (Bannister et al., 1986, Sahul et al., 2004). This result occurs because raising heart rate without increasing venous return does not elevate cardiac output and therefore does not raise blood pressure.

Recent observations indicate that ingestion of 500 mL of water raises supine blood pressure substantially in older adults (Jordan et al., 2000) and raises supine blood pressure and improves orthostatic hypotension in primary autonomic failure (Cariga et al., 2001a; Young and Mathias, 2004) (Fig. 85-11).

Drugs to raise blood pressure are needed in some patients, in addition to the nonpharmacologic measures described above. They act in various ways (see Table 85-10). In autonomic failure, enhanced blood pressure responses usually occur to pressor and vasodepressor agents; the former may result in severe hypertension, especially when supine, whereas vasodepressor substances may cause marked hypotension.

Although there is no evidence of a mineralocorticoid deficiency in primary autonomic failure, a valuable starter drug is fludrocortisone, in a low dose of 0.1 or 0.2 mg at night. Low-dose fludrocortisone reduces the inability to retain salt and water, especially when recumbent, and increases the sensitivity of blood vessels to pressor substances. In low doses it is less likely to induce side effects such as ankle edema and hypokalemia. If nocturnal polyuria is not reduced by head-up tilt, fludrocortisone can be effectively combined with desmopressin, a vasopressin-2 receptor agonist with potent antidiuretic but minimal direct pressor activity. A dosage of 5 to 40 mg intranasally or 100 to 400 mg orally at night reduces the diuresis but when used without fludrocortisone does not prevent nocturnal natriuresis. These trials have been performed mainly in chronic autonomic failure. Smaller doses (usually 5 to 10 mg only) are used in postganglionic lesions (such as pure autonomic

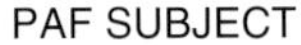

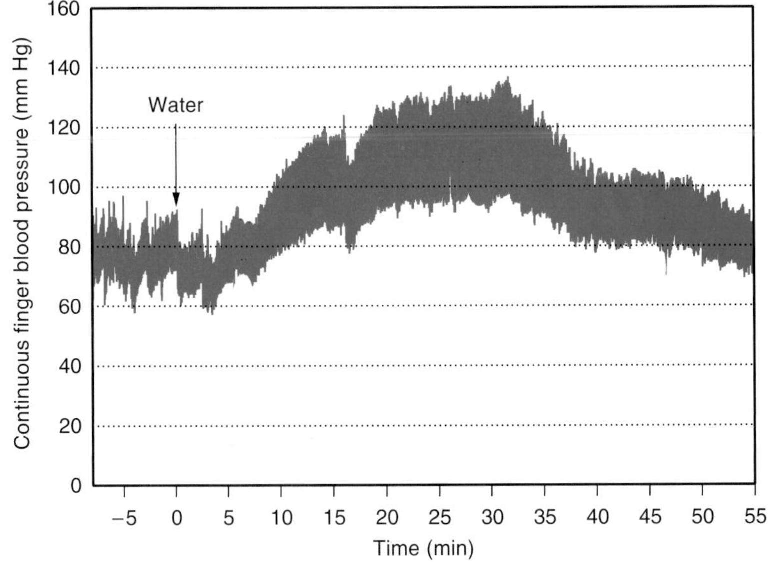

FIGURE 85-11. Changes in blood pressure before and after 500 mL distilled water ingested at time "0" in a patient with pure autonomic failure (PAF). Blood pressure is measured continuously using the Portapres II monitor. (From Cariga and Mathias, 2001. ©The Biochemical Society. Reproduced with permission.)

failure) because they appear to be more sensitive to the drug than in patients with central lesions (such as multiple system atrophy). Plasma sodium must be monitored to exclude hyponatremia and water intoxication. These can be reversed by stopping the drug and withholding water, but a diuresis then ensues, which may enhance orthostatic hypotension.

Sympathetic failure is a feature of neurogenic orthostatic hypotension and sympathomimetics often are used with fludrocortisone. Drugs that mimic the activity of noradrenaline, either directly or indirectly, include ephedrine and midodrine. Ephedrine acts both directly and indirectly, and is of value in central and incomplete autonomic lesions, including multiple system atrophy. A dose of 15 mg three times daily initially can be increased to 30 or 45 mg three times daily, although central side effects (loss of appetite and insomnia) may limit use of the higher doses. In severe peripheral sympathetic lesions (as in pure autonomic failure), it may have minimal or no effects. Drugs that act directly on alpha-adrenoceptors include midodrine, which is converted to the active metabolite, desglymidodrine (Low et al., 1997). The ergot alkaloid dihydroergotamine acts predominantly on venous capacitance vessels, but its effects are limited by its poor absorption; high oral doses (5 to 10 mg three times daily) may be needed.

In individuals with a precise biochemical deficit, such as in dopamine β-hydroxylase deficiency, agents can be given that bypass deficient enzyme systems and result in appropriate neurotransmitter replacement (Fig. 85-12). The amino acid L-threo-3,4-dihydroxyphenylserine is directly converted by dopa-decarboxylase into noradrenaline. Whether this occurs intra- or extraneuronally (or both) is unclear. It may be of value in the management of orthostatic hypotension in primary autonomic failure (Kaufmann et al., 2003; Mathias et al., 2001a).

Some drugs act through pre- and postsynaptic alpha$_2$-adrenoceptor mechanisms although they have limited application in practice. The alpha$_2$-adrenoceptor agonist clonidine, which lowers blood pressure mainly through a central reduction in sympathetic outflow, also acts on peripheral postsynaptic alpha$_2$-adrenoceptors, and may raise blood pressure in the presence of pressor supersensitivity. Yohimbine blocks presynaptic alpha$_2$-adrenoceptors, which normally suppress release of noradrenaline and should theoretically benefit in incomplete sympathetic lesions, as observed in single-dose studies. Recently the acetylcholinesterase inhibitor pyridostigmine has been reported to raise blood pressure when given in single doses (Singer et al., 2003). Their value in long-term management is not known.

In adults the management of orthostatic hypotension, especially with drugs, may cause supine hypertension, may occur in chronic autonomic failure, and may be worsened by treatment. It is unclear if this is a problem in children. It may occasionally result in cerebral hemorrhage, aortic dissection, myocardial ischemia, or cardiac failure. This effect may be a greater problem with certain drug combinations, such as tyramine (which releases noradrenaline) and monoamine oxidase inhibitors (such as tranylcypromine and moclobemide), which prolong its actions. Supine hypertension may increase symptoms of cerebral ischemia during subsequent postural change, probably through an unfavorable resetting of cerebral autoregulatory mechanisms. To prevent these problems, head-up tilt, omission of the evening dose of vasopressor agents, a prebedtime snack to induce postprandial hypotension, and even nocturnal use of short-acting vasodilators have been suggested.

To overcome the problems with lability of blood pressure, a subcutaneous infusion pump (as in the control of hyperglycemia with insulin in diabetes mellitus) has been used in adults, infusing the short-acting vasoconstrictor, noradrenaline. Previous studies with a pilot device had been successful, but with a number of practical problems, including the difficulty of accurate monitoring of blood pressure without an intra-arterial catheter. Some of these problems have been overcome (Oldenberg et al., 2001). This may benefit the severely hypotensive patient refractory to the combination of nonpharmacologic and conventionally administered drug therapy.

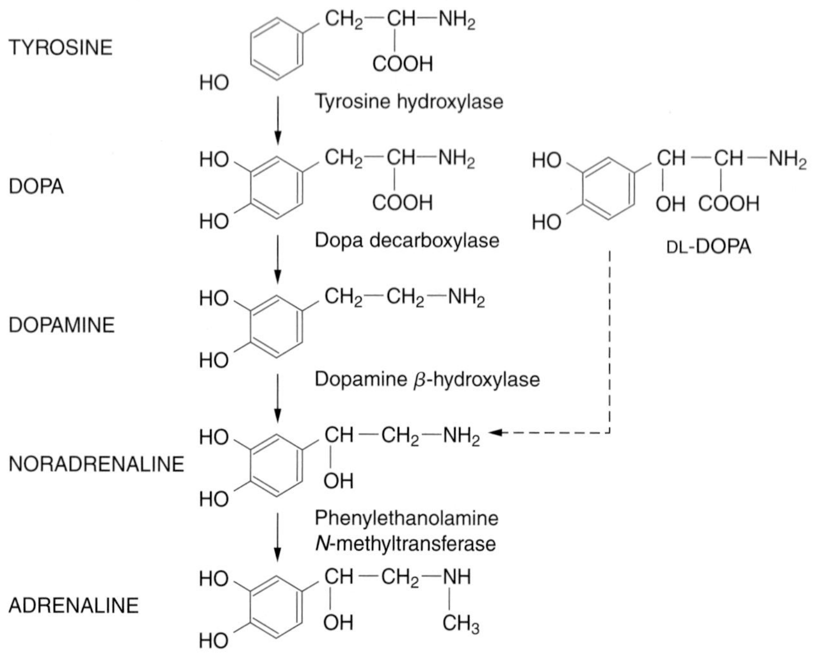

TYROSINE — Tyrosine hydroxylase → DOPA — Dopa decarboxylase → DOPAMINE — Dopamine β-hydroxylase → NORADRENALINE — Phenylethanolamine *N*-methyltransferase → ADRENALINE; DL-DOPA → NORADRENALINE

FIGURE 85-12. Biosynthetic pathway in the formation of adrenaline and noradrenaline. The structure of DL-DOPA is indicated on the right. It is converted directly to noradrenaline by dopa decarboxylase, thus bypassing dopamine β-hydroxylase. (From Mathias et al., 1990. Reprinted with permission of Oxford University Press.)

A variety of drugs have been used in adults, sometimes with success. They include the prostaglandin synthetase inhibitors, indomethacin and flurbiprofen. They may act by blocking vasodilatory prostaglandins, by causing salt and water retention through their renal effects, or both. They have potentially serious side effects, however, such as gastrointestinal ulceration and hemorrhage. The dopamine antagonists metoclopramide and domperidone may be of value when an excess of dopamine is contributory.

Beta-adrenoceptor blockers, such as propranolol, may be successful when orthostatic hypotension is accompanying tachycardia; the combination of blocking beta$_2$-adrenoceptor vasodilatation and beta$_1$-adrenoceptor–induced tachycardia may account for the benefit. Beta-adrenoceptor blockers with high intrinsic sympathomimetic activity, such as pindolol, may raise blood pressure and probably increase cardiac output, but may cause cardiac failure.

Various therapeutic approaches have been used to reduce severe postprandial hypotension. Caffeine, which blocks vasodilatory adenosine receptors, has been used in a dose of 250 mg (the equivalent of two cups of coffee). The prodrug L-dihydroxyphenylserine, presumably through adrenoceptor-induced vasoconstriction, reduces postprandial hypotension in primary autonomic failure (Freeman et al., 1996). The somatostatin analog octreotide, which inhibits release of a variety of gastrointestinal tract peptides, including those with vasodilatory properties, has been successfully used to prevent postprandial hypotension; it also may partly reduce postural and exercise-induced hypotension (Smith et al., 1995b). It does not enhance nocturnal (supine) hypertension (Alam et al., 1995). The need for subcutaneous administration is a drawback. Exercise-induced hypotension may respond to octreotide or midodrine (Schrage et al., 2004). Anemia may occur in some subjects with primary autonomic failure and dopamine β-hydroxylase deficiency; it may be associated with renal impairment in diabetes mellitus and primary amyloidosis. Erythropoietin, which raises red cell mass and hemoglobin concentration, reduces orthostatic hypotension in such circumstances (Hoeldtke and Streeten, 1993).

DESCRIPTION OF AUTONOMIC DISORDERS

Primary Autonomic Failure

In autonomic disorders the etiology is unknown and there is no clear association with either specific lesions or known diseases. The acute-subacute dysautonomias are relatively rare, unlike the chronic forms of primary autonomic failure that occur mainly in adults (Mathias, 2004). The latter consists of pure autonomic failure in which only the autonomic nervous system is affected, unlike multiple system atrophy, in which there are additional neurologic deficits. The latter is a neurodegenerative disorder that mainly occurs older than the age of 55 and is sporadic in nature with no familial or hereditary component.

Acute or Subacute Dysautonomias

There are three forms of dysautonomia: pure cholinergic dysautonomia, pure pandysautonomia (with both sympathetic and parasympathetic failure), and pandysautonomia with other neurologic features, in which the peripheral nerves often are affected. The precise causes are unclear and may include viral infections, with immunologic damage as a contributory factor. The prognosis in the pandysautonomias is variable, with complete recovery in some.

Pure cholinergic dysautonomia mainly affects children and young adults (Hopkins et al., 1974; Inander et al., 1982; Takayama et al., 1987; Tomashevsky et al., 1972). Symptoms of parasympathetic failure include blurred vision, dry eyes, xerostomia, dysphagia involving mainly the lower esophagus, constipation, and urinary retention. Symptoms of sympathetic cholinergic failure are anhidrosis and a tendency to hyperthermia. The signs include dilated pupils, raised heart rate, dry and hot skin, a distended abdomen, and a palpable urinary bladder. Orthostatic hypotension is absent, as sympathetic vasoconstrictor function is not impaired. Only cholinergic muscarinic synapses are affected. There is a response to cholinomimetic agents, such as bethanechol, indicating preservation of postsynaptic cholinergic receptor function and suggesting a presynaptic lesion. A barium meal examination must be avoided because it will be retained in the colon (Fig. 85-13). The prognosis is good if complications are avoided. Recovery of cholinergic function is unlikely.

The differential diagnosis in pure cholinergic dysautonomia includes the effects of anticholinergic drugs, poisons, and toxins. In jimsonweed *(Datura stramonium)* seed poisoning, there are similar autonomic features, along with additional features including hallucinations, hyperreflexia, and clonic jerking movements; recovery usually

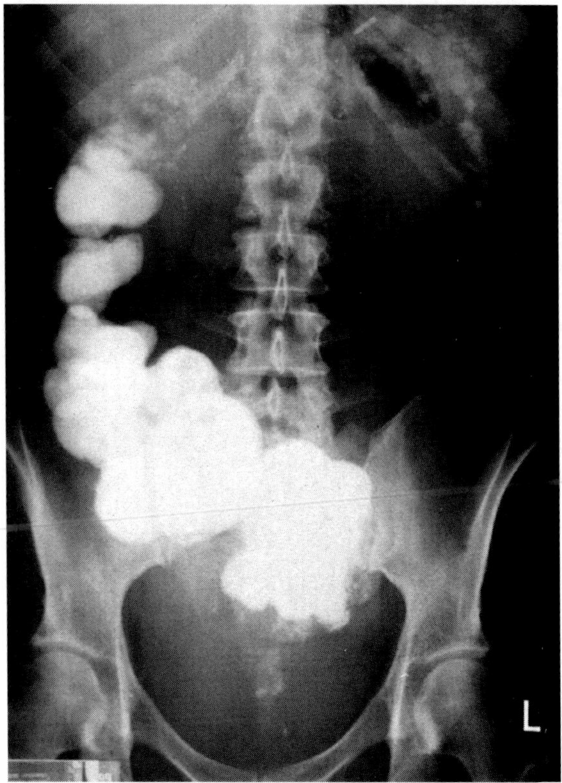

FIGURE 85-13. Retention of barium in the colon of a patient with acute cholinergic dysautonomia 3 months after barium ingestion. Attempts to dislodge the barium failed. She needed a laparotomy, with partial colectomy. (From Mathias, 1996. ©1996. Reproduced with permission from The McGraw-Hill Companies.)

occurs in a few days (Mikolich et al., 1975). A variant of botulism, botulism B, which spares motor pathways and appears to preferentially affect the cholinergic system, has been described; in such cases, however, there is substantial recovery within 3 months (Jenzer et al., 1975; Merz et al., 2003).

In the pandysautonomias there is sympathetic and parasympathetic involvement that may occur with other neurologic features (Kanda et al., 1990; Young et al., 1975). In addition to cholinergic features, as described earlier, there are manifestations of sympathetic failure. Postural hypotension is often a major problem. The symptoms and clinical features, therefore, are more extensive and the investigation additionally indicates postural hypotension, diminished pressor responses, and an abnormal Valsalva maneuver. The degree of autonomic impairment varies from case to case; in those with neurologic deficits, electrophysiologic studies are often suggestive of a peripheral neuropathy and abnormal features are seen on nerve biopsy. The cerebrospinal fluid protein levels may be elevated.

The prognosis in the pandysautonomias is variable; in some patients there may a substantial recovery, whereas in others, as with pure cholinergic dysautonomia, recovery may be minimal. These disorders may have an immunologic basis, and intravenous immunoglobulin has been used with success in some (Heafield et al., 1996; Smit et al., 1997); currently there is no clear evidence in favor of such an approach. The management consists of supportive therapy. Postural hypotension often impedes rehabilitation and usually calls for a combination of nondrug and drug therapy. Hyperthermia should be prevented. Adequate fluid intake and nutrition is important, particularly if there is a paralytic ileus. The investigation of dysphagia must not include the use of barium because this can result in deposition in the large bowel; a recent patient needed, in due course, a hemicolectomy with a colostomy. Blurred vision can be prevented with low-dose pilocarpine eyedrops. Artificial tears, such as hypromellose, are needed to prevent ocular complications. Artificial saliva is helpful. Cholinomimetics such as bethanechol and carbachol, which can be given either orally or parenterally to improve bowel and bladder activity, are helpful. The prognosis in the early stages largely depends on establishing an early diagnosis and on supportive management to prevent complications. As children grow, there may be new problems, as in males when they reach adulthood and experience erectile and ejaculatory dysfunctions.

Secondary Autonomic Failure

Hereditary Sensory and Autonomic Neuropathies

There are a number of hereditary autonomic disorders that are characterized by additional sensory involvement (Hilz, 2002) and have been classified into predominantly five types. Some, such as type III, the Riley-Day syndrome, can be diagnosed at birth. Types II, IV, and V appear in infancy or early childhood and type I in adulthood. There are varying autonomic abnormalities. In types I and IV, anhidrosis is a feature, being severe in the latter (congenital insensitivity to pain with anhidrosis). In type II, there is episodic hyperhidrosis, as in types II and V, but with fever, bladder, and gastrointestinal dysfunctions, tonic pupils, and apnea. A variety of autonomic abnormalities occur in type III, as described later. Autonomic investigation should include the intradermal histamine flare response, with an impaired response common in these disorders.

There are other autonomic disorders with overlapping features, some of which may be related to nerve growth factor deficiency (Anand et al., 1991). Anhidrosis may be an integral component of some of the hereditary sensory and autonomic neuropathies (Houlden et al., 2001) or may be congenital and without other features (Cevoli et al., 2002).

Riley-Day Syndrome (Familial Dysautonomia)

Because there are a number of familial autonomic disorders (including familial amyloid polyneuropathy and dopamine β-hydroxylase deficiency), the Riley-Day syndrome probably is a more appropriate designation. It is an autosomal-recessive disorder predominantly affecting autonomic and sensory neurons (Axelrod, 2002; Mahloud et al., 1970). The parents usually are normal; it occurs mainly in Ashkenazi Jews and there is a strong history of consanguinity. In a newborn infant, absent fungiform papillae, lack of corneal reflexes, decreased deep tendon reflexes, and a diminished response to pain in a child of Ashkenazi Jewish extraction should point to the diagnosis. An abnormal intradermal histamine skin test (with an absent flare response) and pupillary hypersensitivity to cholinomimetics would confirm the diagnosis. The chromosome abnormality is linked to 9Q31 and there is a mutation in the gene *IK-BKAP* in 99% of cases; there is sufficient sensitivity to genetic probe to ascertain whether the fetus is affected (Anderson et al., 2001; Blumenfeld et al., 1993).

A variety of symptoms, resulting from both autonomic underactivity and overactivity may occur. These include a labile blood pressure (with hypertension and postural hypotension), parasympathetic abnormalities (with periodic vomiting, dysphagia, constipation, and diarrhea), and urinary bladder disturbances. Neurologic abnormalities, associated skeletal problems (scoliosis), and renal failure previously contributed to a poor prognosis. The ability to anticipate complications and provide adequate support and therapy has resulted in a number of children reaching adulthood.

The clinical manifestations are variable and are usually present from birth, with additional features appearing with increasing age. These include a labile blood pressure with postural hypotension and impaired responses to pressor stimuli. Hypertension, however, may also occur (Fig. 85-14). There may be episodes of sweating and blotchy erythema, sometimes at mealtimes and when patients are excited. Excretion of homovanillic acid (a metabolite of dopamine) and vanillylmandelic acid (a metabolite of noradrenaline) is reduced. Plasma dopamine β-hydroxylase levels may be low. Parasympathetic abnormalities include periodic vomiting, dysphagia (which may be associated with impaired motility in the lower third of the esophagus), constipation, and diarrhea. Urinary bladder control is often disturbed. The eyes are affected with diminished tear secretion, and there is hypersensitivity of the pupil to cholinomimetics such as dilute methacholine or pilocarpine. There is sensory

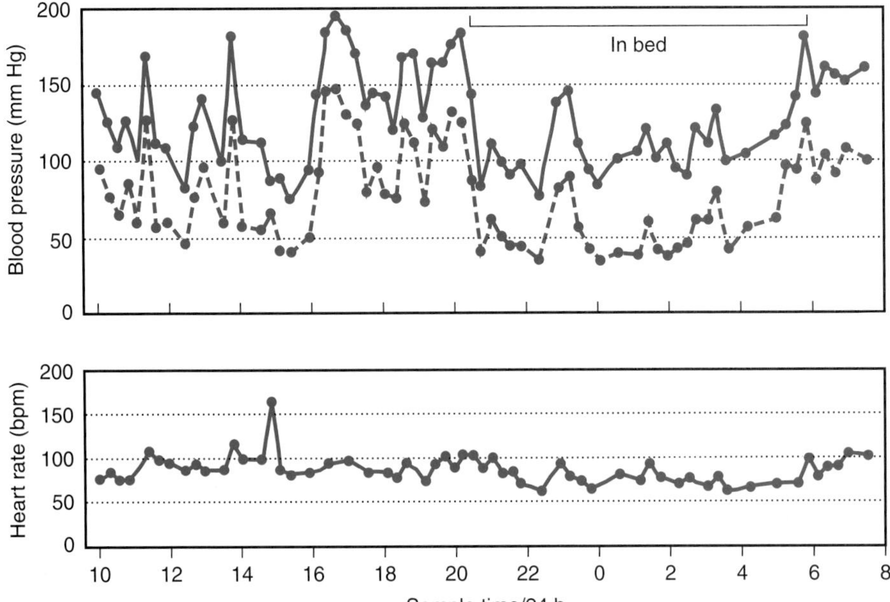

FIGURE 85-14. Twenty-four-hour noninvasive ambulatory blood pressure profile, showing systolic *(dark circles)* and diastolic *(dark squares)* blood pressure and heart rate at intervals through the day and night in a subject with the Riley-Day syndrome (familial dysautonomia). There is considerable lability of blood pressure, with hypotension and hypertensive episodes. (Adapted from Mathias, 1996. ©1996. Reproduced with permission from The McGraw-Hill Companies.)

involvement. Corneal hypesthesia may lead to corneal ulceration and scar formation. Other sensory system abnormalities include an abnormal taste sensation and a pale, smooth tongue because of lack of fungiform papillae.

The prognosis depends on anticipating complication and on supportive therapy. The average life expectancy has been steadily rising; before 1960, some 50% of these patients died before the age of 5 years. Many now reach adulthood, with 50% reaching the age of 30 years. Many lead independent lives and some have married and had normal offspring. In the past, many would have been dead by the early second decade. Death is often sudden and may be the result of a cardiorespiratory arrest. Cardiac pacemakers may be of value. A prolonged Q-T interval in the electrocardiograph is seen in one third of patients; it is unclear if this predisposes them to cardiac dysrhythmias. Renal failure can occur in older children and adults.

The management of patients includes control of blood pressure, which can be difficult because of its lability. Impaired thermoregulation can occur with extremes of temperature and requires appropriate therapy. Reduced food intake because of periodic vomiting and impaired gastroesophageal motility may impair growth and result in anemia; a gastrostomy is often helpful. There are a wide variety of neurologic disturbances, in addition to those affecting impaired sensation. Gait disturbances are common and scoliosis frequently occurs with increasing age. There may be a range of psychometric abnormalities.

Congenital Insensitivity to Pain with Anhidrosis

This is an autosomal-recessive disorder characterized by anhidrosis, recurrent episodic fever, and absence of afferent neurons causing pain insensitivity and self-mutilation (Swanson, 1963). It occurs in Greek, Italian, Arabic, Bedouin, Japanese, Pakistani, and Indian families; there is consanguinity in about 50%. The chromosomal abnormality is linked to 1q21-22 and the abnormal gene is *NTRK1*, with multiple mutations involving the *NTRK1*/tyrosine kinase domain of the nerve growth factor receptor (Indo et al., 1996; Mardy et al., 1999).

Familial Amyloid Polyneuropathy

In familial amyloid polyneuropathy, symptoms occur in the adult. However, the diagnosis has considerable implications for children. Sensory, motor, and autonomic abnormalities result from deposition in peripheral nerves of mutated amyloid protein, mainly produced in the liver. Motor and sensory neuropathy often begins in the lower limbs. Classification of familial amyloid polyneuropathy is based on the chemical and molecular nature of the constituent proteins and not on clinical presentation. There are various forms: transthyretin (TTR30) FAP, FAP Ala 60 (Irish/Appalachian), and FAP Ser 84 and His 58. The cardiovascular system, gut, and urinary bladder can be affected at any stage. The disease relentlessly progresses but at a variable speed. There is increasing evidence of differences in autonomic dysfunction in the various mutations resulting in familial amyloid polyneuropathy. There may be dissociation of autonomic symptoms from functional deficits; this dissociation is of importance because evaluation of cardiovascular autonomic abnormalities may be essential in preventing morbidity and mortality especially during hepatic transplantation. Currently this is the only way to reduce levels of variant transthyretin and its deposition in nerves. Thus it appears to prevent progression and may reverse some neuropathic features. It may be of greater value if performed before substantial nerve damage, or cardiac deposition, occurs.

Genetic testing for familial amyloid polyneuropathy is of value although the potentially damaging aspects of a positive test in children need to be considered.

In the adult, light chain amyloid deposition results in autonomic dysfunction (Reilly and Thomas, 2002). In this form, amyloid is derived from monoclonal light chains, secondary to multiple myeloma, malignant lymphoma, or Waldenström's macroglobulinemia. There appear to be no genetic implications.

Dopamine β-Hydroxylase Deficiency

This disorder has been described in nine patients, two who are siblings (Deinum et al., 2004; Gomes et al., 2003; Mathias and Bannister, 2002a). Presentation often is in childhood, although an autonomic disorder was not considered until they became teenagers, when orthostatic hypotension was first recognized. Whether the symptoms become more prominent, or are easier to detect, at this time is unclear. The clinical features indicate sympathetic adrenergic failure with sparing of sympathetic cholinergic and parasympathetic function (Man in't Veld et al., 1987; Mathias et al., 1990; Robertson et al., 1986). Sweating is preserved and urinary bladder and bowel functions are normal; in one of the males erection was possible but ejaculation was difficult to achieve. The diagnosis may be made from basal levels of plasma catecholamines because noradrenaline and adrenaline levels are undetectable while dopamine levels are elevated. The enzymatic defect is highly specific, with the sympathetic nerve pathways and terminals otherwise intact, as has been demonstrated by both electron microscopy and preservation of muscle sympathetic nerve activity using microneurography. These subjects, therefore, are a unique model of superselective sympathetic adrenergic failure. In six patients, several different mutations of the dopamine β-hydroxylase gene, leading to truncated proteins or an altered sequence in certain regions have been described (Deinum et al., 2004; Kim et al., 2002); one of the mutations, a splice site variant, was common in five. Absence of dopamine β-hydroxylase in plasma, without the functional deficit seen in these patients, also may occur, through a locus in the 5′ flanking region of the dopamine β-hydroxylase gene (Deinum et al., 2004)

Treatment is with the prodrug L-dihydroxyphenylserine (see Fig. 85-12), which has a structure similar to noradrenaline except for a carboxyl group that is acted on by the enzyme dopa decarboxylase, which is widely distributed, thus transforming it into noradrenaline. This transformation reduces orthostatic hypotension and has resulted in remarkable improvements in their ability to lead active lives. In those with anemia, there is a favorable response to erythropoietin (Gomes et al., 2003); the cause of low erythropoietin and anemia is unclear and may be related to noradrenergic failure.

Diabetes Mellitus

Impairment of the autonomic nervous system can result in a variety of abnormalities, especially in older, long-standing adult diabetics on insulin therapy (Watkins, 1998). Whether autonomic neuropathy occurs in children is not entirely clear. However, the early onset of microvascular complications has been reported in single cases (Hamilton et al., 2004) and a recent study reported that nearly a third of young patients had profound neuropathy (Tesfaye et al., 2005) and within a short time frame a fourth developed neuropathy. The probability of autonomic involvement thus remains higher than previously considered (Perkins and Bril, 2005).

In the adult with diabetic autonomic neuropathy, morbidity and mortality are considerably higher than in those without a neuropathy. It initially often involves the vagus, with characteristic features of cardiac vagal denervation (Watkins and Edmonds, 2002). This may occur in conjunction with partial preservation of the cardiac sympathetic and may predispose diabetic patients, many of whom have ischemic heart disease, to sudden death from cardiac dysrhythmias. The type of diabetes may influence the neuropathy; in type 2 diabetes sympathetic neuropathies seem to occur more frequently than parasympathetic impairment (Sundqvist et al., 1998). In those with sympathetic failure, orthostatic hypotension may be enhanced by insulin. Awareness of hypoglycemia, which depends on autonomic activation, is diminished. There may be involvement of the gastrointestinal tract (gastroparesis diabeticorum and diabetic diarrhea), the urinary bladder (diabetic cystopathy), and in the male, impotence. Sudomotor abnormalities include gustatory sweating. Damage to other organs may occur through non-neuropathic factors and compound the problems caused by the neuropathy.

Other than maintaining normoglycemia, there is no known means to prevent and reverse the neuropathy except possibly by pancreatic transplantation.

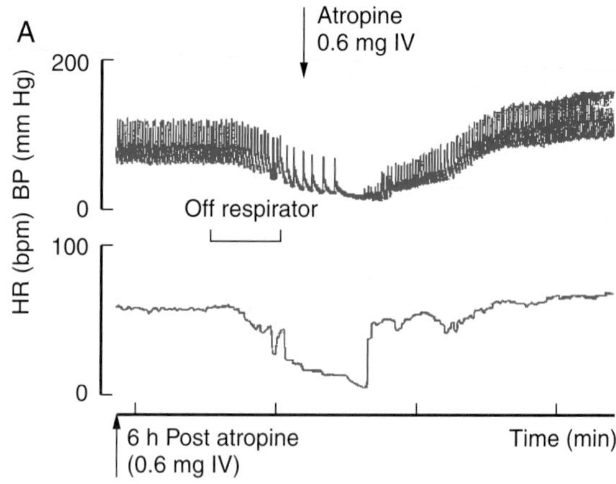

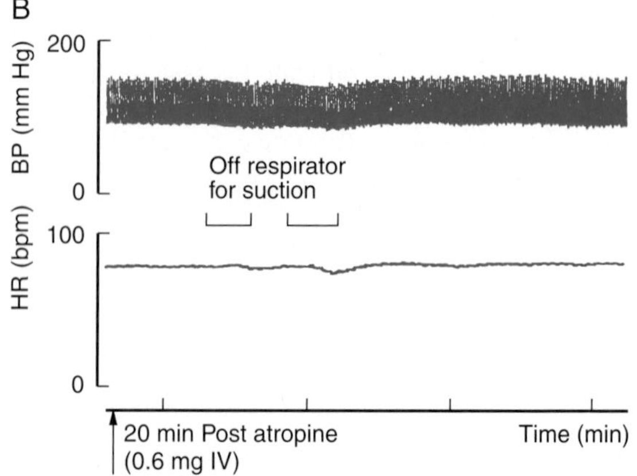

FIGURE 85-15. **A,** The effect of disconnecting the respirator (as required for aspirating the airways) on the blood pressure (BP) and heart rate (HR) of a recently injured tetraplegic patient (C4-5 lesion) in spinal shock, 6 hours after the last dose of intravenous (IV) atropine. Sinus bradycardia and cardiac arrest (also observed on the electrocardiograph) were reversed by reconnection, intravenous atropine and external cardiac massage. **B,** The effect of tracheal suction, 20 minutes after atropine. Disconnection from the respirate and tracheal suction did not lower either heart rate or blood pressure. (**A**, from Frankel et al., 1975; **B,** from Mathias, 1976.)

Spinal Cord Lesions

Autonomic dysfunction affecting various systems occurs in spinal cord lesions and injuries because the entire sympathetic and the sacral sympathetic outflow is from the spinal cord (Mathias and Frankel, 2002). The level of completeness of lesion determines the degree of dysfunction.

In children spinal cord damage can result from a variety of causes—trauma (causing spinal cord transaction), syringomyelia, and transverse myelitis. There can be varying degrees of autonomic involvement, depending on the site and extent of the lesion. The disturbances affect the cardiovascular, thermoregulatory, gastrointestinal, urinary, and reproductive systems (Mathias and Frankel, 2002). In the majority of cases, there may be both autonomic underactivity and at times overactivity, which can pose special problems.

In recently injured tetraplegics, the basal supine level of blood pressure usually is lower than normal (Mathias et al., 1979). This condition depends on a number of factors, including complicating trauma and drug therapy. The lower levels of blood pressure appear secondary to diminution in sympathetic nervous activity, which normally accounts for about 20% of vascular tone. It is unlikely that skeletal muscle paralysis alone is the explanation because tetraplegics, due to poliomyelitis, often have normal or even higher levels of blood pressure. The basal heart rate, especially in high lesions, also can be low, reflecting a relative increase in cardiac vagal activity in the absence of other neural and humoral adrenergic stimuli to the heart. This imbalance is likely to contribute to bradycardia and even cardiac arrest at times, especially in high lesions that depend on artificial respiration (Fig. 85-15). It can be a particular problem during tracheal suction, which stimulates vagal and glossopharyngeal afferents to reflexively increase vagal efferent activity (Mathias, 1976). Normally this is opposed by factors that raise heart rate and that include the pulmonary inflation vagal reflex and sympathoneuronal activity. Bradycardia effectively is prevented by atropine, emphasizing that the efferent limb of the reflex is the cardiac vagus. Knowledge of these mechanisms is important because the prevention of hypoxia, care during tracheal suction, and, if necessary, the use of maintenance atropine or even a temporary demand pacemaker, may be critical in the early phases when high lesions need respiratory support.

The return of isolated spinal cord activity, with skeletal muscle spasms and spinal autonomic reflexes, in cervical and high thoracic lesions, may cause considerable lability in blood pressure. In the early stages of rehabilitation, movement from the horizontal to the upright position can result in pronounced orthostatic hypotension (Fig. 85-16) with symptoms resulting from organ hypoperfusion (see Table 85-5). Symptoms include cervical pain, in the "coat hanger" region (Cariga et al., 2002b). Loss of consciousness may occur, although this is more frequent in the early stages of rehabilitation and in chronic lesions after prolonged recumbency. With frequent postural changes and time, along with drugs such as ephedrine if needed, the blood pressure decrease with head-up change is reduced. Importantly, there is greater tolerance to lower levels of blood pressure; this tolerance may be related to the increasing ability of the cerebral circulation to autoregulate in the face of a low perfusion pressure. In the later stages, additional factors that aid blood pressure recovery during postural change include activation of the renin-angiotensin-aldosterone system and the initiation of spinal sympathetic reflexes.

Spinal sympathetic reflex activity may be induced by stimuli below the level of lesion resulting from visceral, skeletal muscle, or cutaneous stimulation. There may be a widespread increase in autonomic activity, mainly beneath the level of the lesion. In high lesions (above T6), this may result in autonomic dysreflexia. In this syndrome, blood

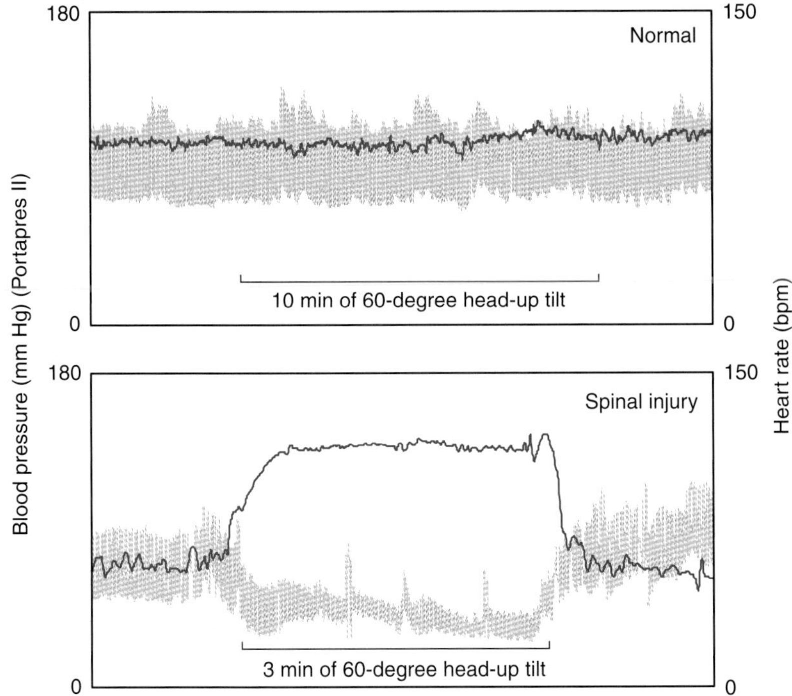

FIGURE 85-16. Blood pressure and heart rate measured continuously with the Portapres II monitor in a patient with a high cervical spinal cord lesion. There is a fall in blood pressure because of impairment of the sympathetic outflow disrupted in the cervical spine. Heart rate rises because of withdrawal of vagal activity in response to the rise in pressure. (From Mathias, 2005.)

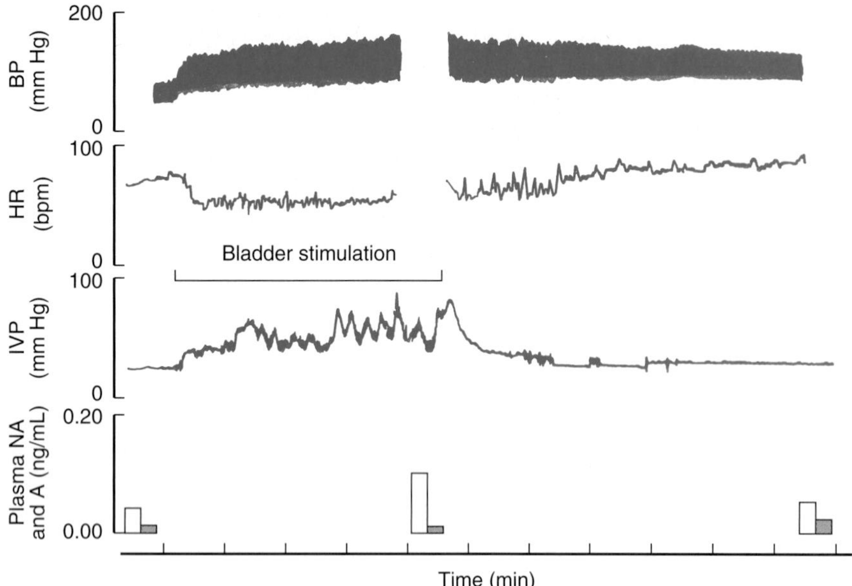

FIGURE 85-17. Blood pressure (BP), heart rate (HR), intravesical pressure (IVP), and plasma noradrenaline (NA) and adrenaline (A) levels in a tetraplegic patient before, during, and after bladder stimulation induced by suprapubic percussion of the anterior abdominal wall. The rise in BP is accompanied by a fall in heart rate as a result of increased vagal activity in response to the rise in blood pressure. Level of plasma NA *(open histograms),* but not A *(filled histograms)* rises, suggesting an increase in sympathetic neural activity independently of adrenomedullary activation. (From Mathias and Frankel, 2002.)

pressure is elevated; there is constriction of blood vessels (arterial and venous) below the level of the lesion, reducing peripheral blood flow and causing cold limbs, and a rise in levels of plasma noradrenaline but not adrenaline (Fig. 85-17). Sometimes evacuation of the urinary bladder and lower bowel, penile erection, and skeletal muscle spasms occur; these are components of the "mass reflex" described by Head and Riddoch (1917). Above the lesion there is usually dilatation of blood vessels with flushing over the face and neck, along with sweating. These episodes may be severe and prolonged, causing a throbbing headache and excessive perspiration above the lesion and, at times, death because of intracerebral hemorrhage. It is important to determine the cause of autonomic dysreflexia and rectify it; sometimes this is not possible and maneuvers and drugs are needed, especially to reduce hypertension (Hickey et al., 2004; McGinnis et al., 2004). These approaches may involve blocking afferent activity to the cord (lignocaine into the bladder), diminishing spinal autonomic activity (a spinal anesthetic), centrally acting drugs (clonidine) or drugs that act on sympathetic ganglia (hexamethonium), adrenoreceptors (phenoxybenzamine, prazosin, and terazosin) (Vaidyanathan et al., 1998). Agents that act indirectly on the target organs, such as glyceryltrinitrate and nifedipine, dilate blood vessels to lower blood pressure. Propantheline bromide, which blocks muscarinic cholinergic receptors, can prevent sweating.

The abnormalities arising from disordered sudomotor function and cutaneous vascular function predispose such patients to abnormal body temperature regulation. Hyperthermia can occur because of the inability to vasodilate and to sweat appropriately, whereas the reverse, hypothermia, may occur especially in high lesions because of the inability to vasoconstrict and to increase heat production because of impaired shivering thermogenesis (Fig. 85-18). Measurement of core temperature, as with a low-reading rectal thermometer, is critical because axillary and oral temperature measurements may be misleading.

Gastrointestinal dysfunction is common. In high lesions, paralytic ileus may occur in the early stages of shock and cause abdominal distention and meteorism, which reduces

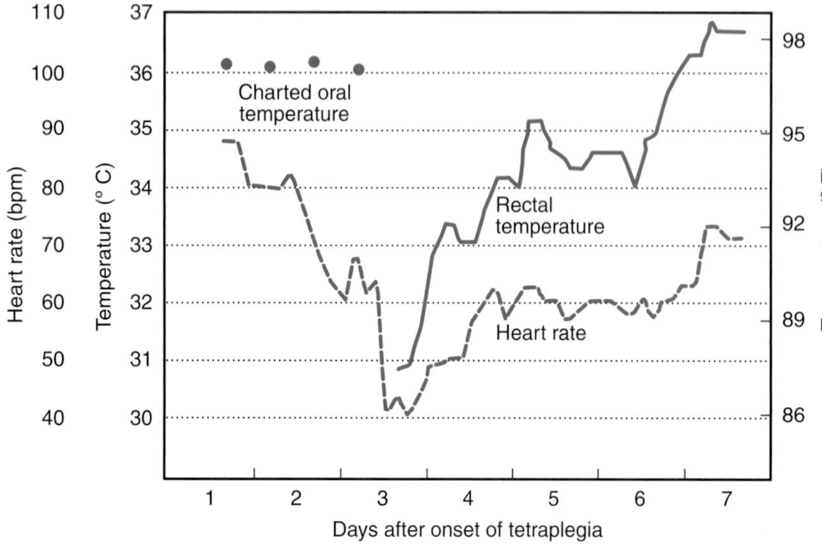

FIGURE 85-18. Fall in central temperature (measured as rectal temperature) and heart rate in a recently injured tetraplegic in a temperate climate. Hypothermia is ideally monitored by a low reading rectal thermometer or tympanic temperature, as a measure of core temperature. It may be missed, as indicated in this case initially, if oral temperature alone is recorded. (From Pledger, 1962. Reproduced with permission and copyright © of the British Editorial Society of Bone and Joint Surgery.)

diaphragmatic improvement; additionally, there are associated problems with nutrition and fluid balance. Bowel atony in the early stages is followed by a return of function with reflex activation by distention of the bowel. This can be used in reconditioning of large bowel function. The same applies to the urinary bladder; in the early stages catheterization is needed, preferably with intermittent catheterization, but with return of reflex function and a neurogenic bladder training is often successful. The sequelae of disturbed urinary bladder function, especially with a discoordinated bladder (detrusor contraction against a contracted sphincter), include autonomic dysreflexia; in some patients this may lead to hydronephrosis, recurrent urinary infections, and ultimately, renal failure.

Abnormalities in sexual function usually are not of relevance to children with high spinal cord lesions. Penile erection may occur reflexively, as part of autonomic dysreflexia, during cutaneous stimulation of the glans penis, such as before urethral catheterization.

Infectious Diseases

A combination of autonomic underactivity and overactivity may occur in disorders associated with bacterial, viral, or parasitic illness. In the Guillain-Barré syndrome, tachycardia and hypotension may alternate with bradycardia and hypertension. There are differences between the axonal and myelinated forms of the Guillain-Barré syndrome (Asahina et al., 2001). Autonomic disturbances contribute to both morbidity and mortality. The precise mechanisms are unclear and the possibilities should be anticipated because appropriate drugs may be needed. Cardiovascular disturbances of a similar nature may occur in tetanus, especially in those who suffer muscle paralysis and are on assisted respiration. In acquired immunodeficiency syndrome, a cardiovascular and gut neuropathy has been reported (Craddock et al., 1987).

Drugs, Chemicals, and Toxins

A variety of drugs, chemicals, heavy metals, and toxins may cause or contribute to autonomic dysfunction through their recognized pharmacologic effects, such as the sympatholytic agents (see Table 85-3), or by other actions (such as causing a neuropathy) (Tonkin and Frewin, 2002). A side effect of a drug may cause clinical problems when used in high dosage or over a prolonged period (such as the anticholinergic effects of antidepressants), or when deficits are unmasked or induced in susceptible individuals. Examples are the ability of pressor agents to cause severe hypertension in autonomic failure because of denervation supersensitivity (Polinsky, 2002). Drugs such as vincristine, by causing an autonomic neuropathy, may induce autonomic dysfunction independently of their pharmacologic properties.

In some cases the relationship may be obvious, although there are situations in which it may be less so. Examples include the beta-adrenoceptor blockers such as atenolol for treatment of gestation hypertension; this drug may cause bradycardia in the fetus and newborn infant (Shifferli and Caldeyro-Barcia, 1973). Certain drugs taken by mothers who are breast-feeding have the potential, through secretion in breast milk, to affect the infant. In children undergoing organ transplantation, cyclosporine can increase sympathetic neural activity (Scherrer et al., 1990); this effect may be a contributory factor to hypertension, which is common in transplantees.

Children are more likely than adults to accidentally ingest toxins and poisonous substances that can impair the autonomic nervous system. Increased parasympathetic activity may result from mushroom poisoning, whereas the reverse, decreased parasympathetic activity, may occur after ingestion of atropine-like substances. These include the shining black berries of deadly nightshade *(Atropa belladonna),* the seed of the thorn apple (jimsonweed or *D. stramonium*) and various parts of henbane *(Hyoscyamus niger)* (Cooper and Johnson, 1984).

Neurally Mediated Syncope

Intermittent dysfunction of the autonomic nervous system is a common cause of syncope and presyncope, once cardiac and nonautonomic neurologic causes have been excluded (Mathias et al., 2001b). In neurally mediated syncope, there may be increased cardiac parasympathetic activity resulting in bradycardia (the cardioinhibitory form), diminished sympathetic vasoconstrictor activity resulting in hypotension (the vasodepressor form), or a combination of the two. Cardiac vagal tone is considerably greater (vagotonia) in children and may be a contributory factor to their death in certain situations. Stimulation of facial receptors triggering an associated vagal response, for instance, may be responsible for apnea and cardiac arrest when a child falls even into a shallow pool of cold water. In those children with near death experiences, there often is an exaggerated cardiac response to ocular compression (Kahn et al., 1983). It is essential in children to exclude disorders with a prolonged Q-T interval, such as the Romano-Ward and Jervell and Lange-Nielsen syndromes.

There are three major causes of neurally mediated syncope. These include vasovagal syncope, in the young, carotid sinus hypersensitivity, especially in patients older than 50 years, and miscellaneous causes, often referred to as *situational syncope.*

Vasovagal Syncope

Vasovagal syncope probably is the most common form of neurally mediated syncope. There are three forms: cardioinhibitory, vasodepressor, and mixed form (Fig. 85-19). The history often provides an important clue. Episodes may begin in the very young; there may be sudden collapse and seizures due to anoxia, hence the use of the abbreviation RAS that may indicate reflex anoxic syncope, reflex anoxic seizures, or even reflex asystolic syncope (Stephenson, 1990). It may be, because of the greater degree of vagotonia in children, that the cardioinhibitory form is more common. A cardiac demand pacemaker often is of value in such cases.

Another cluster occurs around the teenage years, with fainting often associated with a postural component especially while standing still, such as at assembly. There may be a clear provoking factor that includes blood, needles, or pain. Sometimes even the sight of a needle or mention of venipuncture may induce an attack. In those presenting as teenagers, there often is a strong family history, which in some studies also has been associated with friends of the patient (Camfield and Camfield, 1990; Mathias et al., 1998,

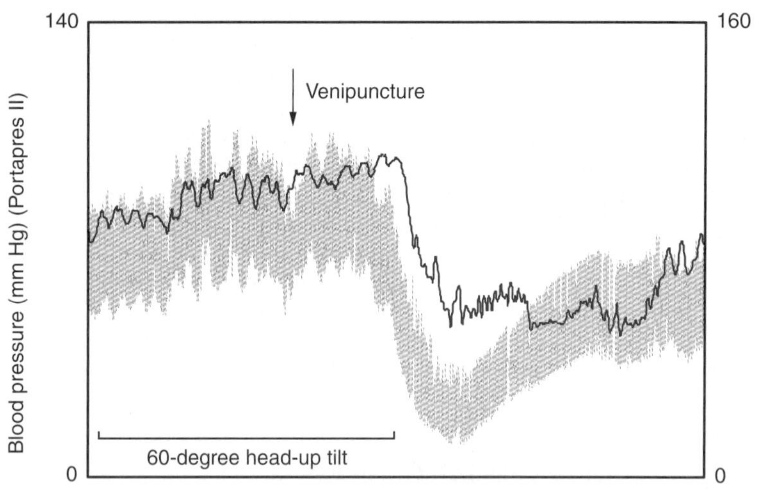

FIGURE 85-19. Blood pressure *(blue shading)* and heart rate *(blue line)* with continuous recordings from the Portapres II monitor in a patient with the mixed (cardioinhibitory and vasodepressor) form of vasovagal syncope. (From Mathias, 2005.)

2001). Whether this indicates an acquired or genetic predisposition or both, is unclear. In some with vasovagal syncope, recurrent attacks may be the result of pseudosyncope, which can cause considerable difficulties in diagnosis and management (Mathias et al., 2001b).

The investigation of vasovagal syncope in older children includes tilt-table testing, often with a provocative stimulus, which in recent studies has included venipuncture and even pseudovenipuncture (Mathias et al., 2001b). In the mixed form, when the role of bradycardia is not clear and a cardiac demand pacemaker is being considered, an atropine test is often useful. Atropine elevates heart rate and if with repeat head-up tilt hypotension is reduced with fewer or no symptoms, this result favors the beneficial effect of cardiac pacing. A lack of effect suggests that vasodepression is the key component and that a pacemaker is unlikely to be of benefit. There is, however, unpredictability in inducing an episode with head-up tilt tests, and this has led to combining additional physiologic and pharmacologic stimuli to induce an attack (El Badawi and Hainsworth, 1994). These include lower body negative pressure, or drugs such as isoprenaline, GTN, and adenosine. Such testing may result in false positives.

The management of vasovagal syncope includes reducing or preventing exposure to precipitating causes, although these may be unclear. In some, especially with phobias, cognitive behavioral psychotherapy is needed. A combination of nonpharmacologic approaches should include a high-salt diet, fluid repletion, exercise especially to strengthen lower limb muscles, measures that activate the sympathetic nervous system such as sustained hand grip, the use of the calf muscle pump to prevent pooling, and various maneuvers that range from leg crossing to simulating the tying of shoelaces (Brignole et al., 2004; Cooper et al., 2002; Mathias and Young, 2004; van Dijk et al., 2000). The ideal in such patients when they have symptoms suggestive of an oncoming attack is to sit and lie, head down, if needed, with legs upright. Drugs are used especially when there is a low supine blood pressure and nonpharmacologic measures alone are not successful. They include low-dose fludrocortisone and sympathomimetics such as ephedrine and midodrine. The 5-hydroxytryptamine uptake release inhibitors have been used with varying success in adults. There appears to be a limited role for beta blockers. In the cardioinhibitory form, a cardiac demand pacemaker may be of value (Benditt, 1999). The long-term prognosis is favorable, and in many young subjects the frequency of attacks is reduced after the third decade.

Carotid Sinus Hypersensitivity

Carotid sinus hypersensitivity is a disease of adults, rarely diagnosed before the age of 50 (McIntosh et al., 1993); the incidence increases with advancing age. It is more common than previously thought and may be the cause of unexplained falls. The provocative stimulus of carotid sinus massage should be performed in the laboratory when upright, which is when there is a greater dependence on autonomic activity (Mathias et al., 1991). In carotid sinus hypersensitivity a cardiac pacemaker often is of benefit. The disorder is not familial and there are no genetic implications.

Miscellaneous Causes

There are a variety of situations, often referred to as *situational syncope*, that can cause bradycardia and hypotension, again by mechanisms similar to those observed in vasovagal syncope. These findings may occur in high spinal cord injuries, especially in tetraplegic patients on artificial respirators, where increased vagal activity not opposed by sympathetic activity may result from tracheal stimulation (see Fig. 85-17). The first-dose hypotensive effect of certain drugs may be neurally mediated via the Bezold-Jarisch reflex. In otherwise normal adults, intermittent syncope has been reported with swallowing (in some associated glossopharyngeal neuralgia) (Deguchi and Mathias, 1999), and during pelvic and rectal examination. In some cases instrumentation, even during anesthesia, may result in cardiac arrest. Micturition- and defecation-induced syncope has been reported mainly in adults, as has laughter-induced and cough syncope. Syncope may occur in trumpet blowers and weight lifters. Changes in intrathoracic pressure may contribute, as in cough- and laughter-induced syncope, trumpet blowing, and voluntary syncope ("fainting lark"). The fainting lark is due to a combination of the Valsalva maneuver and gravity (lowering blood pressure with hyperventilation causing hypocapnea and cerebral vasoconstriction) (Fig. 85-20). Fainting is induced by squatting, overbreathing, standing up suddenly, and blowing

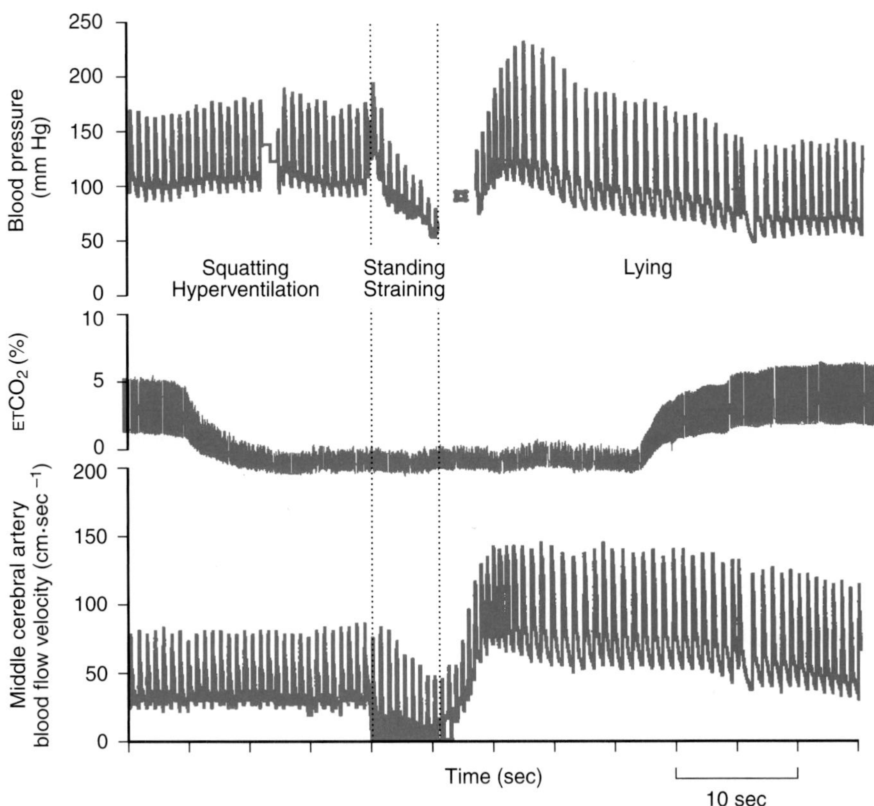

FIGURE 85-20. Finger arterial blood pressure at heart level, end tidal carbon dioxide concentration (ETCO$_2$), and middle cerebral artery blood flow velocity in a normal subject during squatting and hyperventilating, followed by standing and straining. There is a rapid fall in blood pressure and the subject can readily lose consciousness. This phenomenon is the basis of the "fainting lark" as used by children. (From Wieling and van Lieshout, 2002. Reprinted with kind permission of Springer Science and Business Media.)

against a closed glottis (Howard et al., 1951). It may be self-induced and has been reported in mentally retarded children (Gastaut et al., 1982). In children, increased vagal activity and vagotonia may contribute to their being more susceptible to bradycardia. This susceptibility may explain why the young are more prone to cardiac arrest and sudden death during blunt impact to the chest during sports activities; the precise cause of "commotio cordis" is unclear and the possibility of excessive vagal activity in the presence of apnea remains likely (Maron et al., 1995).

Transient Orthostatic Hypotension

Instantaneous or transient orthostatic hypotension has been described in children with normal autonomic function, who have appropriate vasoconstrictor responses to gravitational

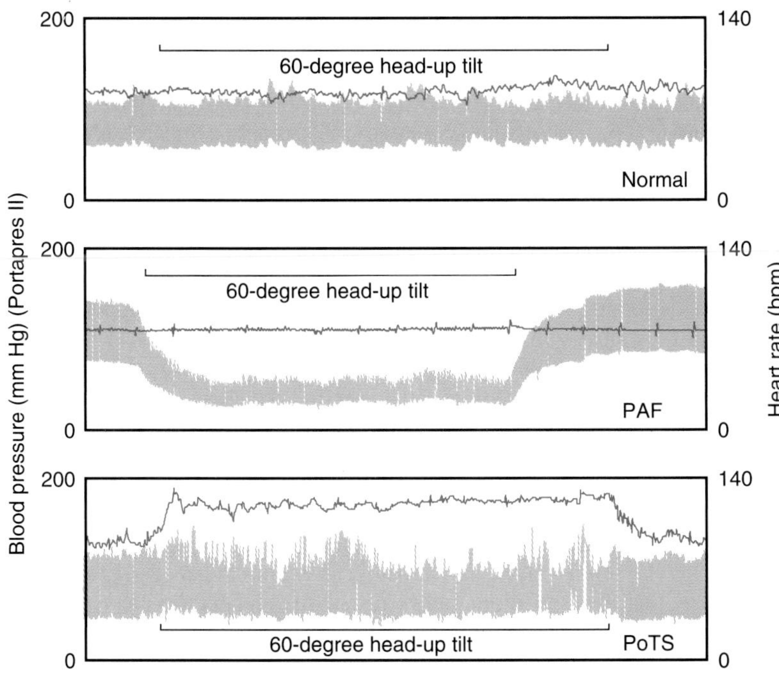

FIGURE 85-21. Blood pressure and heart rate measured (noninvasively) continuously before, during, and after 60-degree head-up tilt (by the Portapres II monitor) in a normal subject and in a subject with two different autonomic disorders: with pure autonomic failure (PAF) and the postural tachycardia syndrome (PoTS). (From Mathias, 2002.)

stimuli (Stewart, 2002; Tanaka et al., 1999). This response may be an exaggeration of the initial transient fall in blood pressure described in normal adults (Wieling and Karemaker, 2002). There may be a greater proportion of young with the chronic fatigue syndrome with this transient change, which may cause dizziness; impaired cerebral hemodynamics may contribute, but does not explain all the findings (Tanaka et al., 2002)

Postural Tachycardia Syndrome

Symptoms of orthostatic intolerance (light-headedness and other manifestations of cerebral hypoperfusion), often with palpitations and without orthostatic hypotension are the hallmark of the postural tachycardia syndrome (Low et al., 2001). The symptoms occur on standing and during even mild exertion. Investigations exclude orthostatic hypotension and autonomic failure; during postural challenge the heart rate increases by more than 30 beats per minute or rises above 120 beats per minute (Fig. 85-21). In the adult it has been predominantly observed in young females between 20 and 50 years of age. Whether the same criterion of heart rate change with head-up posture should apply in children needs consideration (Stewart et al., 1999).

There are similarities between postural tachycardia syndrome and various syndromes, including those initially described by Da Costa and by Lewis (also known as *soldier's heart* or *neurocirculatory asthenia*). There is an association with mitral valve prolapse, chronic fatigue syndrome, and deconditioning after prolonged bed rest and microgravity during space flight. In a family with identical twins, a genetic basis with a defect in the noradrenaline transporter system has been described, which accounted for the raised basal noradrenaline levels; mutation of the gene encoding the noradrenaline transporter was thought to be responsible (Shannon et al., 2000). In some it appears to follow a viral infection, raising the possibility of immunologically mediated autonomic neuropathy. Investigations indicate predominantly lower limb autonomic denervation affecting vascular and sudomotor function (Jacob et al., 2000; Schondorf and Low, 1993; Streeten, 1990). Venous pooling may be a problem (Streeten et al., 1998). Antibodies to autonomic ganglia have been observed in some patients and are related to the autonomic deficits (Vernino et al., 2000). There is a strong association with the joint hypermobility syndrome (Ehler-Danlos type III) (Gazit et al., 2003). Psychogenic components need to be evaluated, especially when hyperventilation is thought to contribute.

In postural tachycardia syndrome, the symptoms may warrant use of drug approaches similar to those used for orthostatic hypotension, and include fludrocortisone and midodrine. Correcting hypovolemia and contributory factors (such as hyperventilation) is important. Beta blockers, especially those that are cardioselective, may reduce tachycardia. As in neurally mediated syncope, use of nonpharmacologic measures should be introduced. With time, some recover spontaneously. The complications of associated disorders, such as the joint hypermobility syndrome, need to be addressed.

"Localized" Autonomic Disorders

There are many autonomic disorders affecting single organs or specific systems. Examples of these are listed in Table 85-4.

The lacrimal glands have a rich autonomic innervation. Alacrima may occur as part of a generalized autonomic disorder. "Crocodile" tears may result from aberrant reinnervation of the lacrimal gland with fibers from the salivary glands. The mechanisms are similar to gustatory sweating, due to aberrant connections between nerves to salivary and facial sweat glands. Triple A (Allgrove) children have alacrima, achalasia, and adrenal failure (Allgrove et al., 1978). The disorder is autosomal recessive, with mutations of the *ALADIN* gene, along with other neurologic and autonomic deficits (Houlden et al., 2002).

The Holmes-Adie pupil is characteristically dilated and sluggishly responsive to light but responds to near vision, hence the descriptive term *near-light dissociation*. It results from parasympathetic denervation, probably of the ciliary ganglia, with supersensitivity of the iris musculature to locally applied cholinomimetics. The term *Holmes-Adie syndrome* is used when associated with absent tendon reflexes; this probably is due to involvement of dorsal root ganglia, accounting for the absent H reflex on electrophysiologic testing. Some patients have areas of anhidrosis, although they often complain of hyperhidrosis that is likely to be compensatory in nature (Ross' syndrome). Others may have cardiovascular autonomic deficits, a chronic dry cough, and diarrhea (Kimber et al., 1998). Although considered benign, in some adults the disorder may be progressive, with baroreceptor reflex dysfunction causing labile hypertension and orthostatic hypotension. The disorder is not familial.

In Horner's syndrome, there is partial ptosis and a small pupil as the sympathetic fibers to the face are affected. It may result from a lesion along the course of the facial sympathetic supply, in the brain, spinal cord, the upper thoracic ganglia, or postganglionic efferents that follow the vasculature. Although it causes few, if any, symptoms, it may be a harbinger of a serious disorder.

In essential (primary) hyperhidrosis there is excessive palmar, plantar, and sometimes whole-body hyperhidrosis. There is no peripheral neural abnormality; whether hypothalamic dysfunction or altered behavioral responses are the mechanisms causing hyperhidrosis is unclear. There is a familial component in some (Kaufmann et al., 2003). The treatment of hyperhidrosis, especially of localized areas (Kaufmann et al., 2003) such as the palms and face, includes percutaneous endoscopic transthoracic sympathectomy, with bilateral ablation of ganglia between T2 and T4; compensatory hyperhidrosis affecting the trunk and lower limbs may occur postoperatively that in some patients may be worse than the original complaint. Injection of botulinum toxin, especially into small areas such as the palm, face, and axillae, has been successful but needs to be repeated and long-term benefits are unknown (Naumann et al., 1997a, 1997b; Tugnoli et al., 2002).

In reflex sympathetic dystrophy (chronic regional pain syndrome type 2), there is debate about whether features such as sweating and vascular changes have an autonomic basis (Schott, 1998); in some these abnormalities are relieved by sympatholytic (guanethidine) blockade.

Localized disorders of the gut include Hirschsprung's disease. In Chagas' disease (after infection with *Trypanosoma cruzi*), the intrinsic autonomic ganglia in the esophagus, colon, and heart are specifically targeted, probably by an immunologic process. Various surgical procedures may be complicated by autonomic dysfunction, an example being the dumping syndrome complicating vagotomy and gastric drainage procedures. Denervation of transplanted organs such as heart or kidneys also may result in dysfunction; reinnervation may occur in due course.

REFERENCES

Alam M, Smith GDP, Bleasdale-Barr K, et al. Effects of the peptide release inhibitor, octreotide, on daytime hypotension and on nocturnal hypertension in primary autonomic failure. J Hypertens 1995;13:1669.

Allgrove J, Clayden GS, Grant DB, Macaulay JC. Familial glucocorticoid deficiency with achalasia of the cardia and deficient tear production. Lancet 1978;1:1284.

Anand P, Rudge P, Mathias CJ, et al. New autonomic and sensory neuropathy with loss of adrenergic sympathetic function and sensory neuropeptides. Lancet 1991;337:1253.

Anderson SL, Coli R, Daly IW et al. Familial dysautonomia is caused by mutation of the IKAP gene. Am J Hum Genet 2001;68:753.

Asahina M, Kuwabara S, Suzuki A, Hattori T. Autonomic function in demyelinating and axonal subtypes of Guillain-Barre syndrome. Acta Neurol Scand 2001;105:1.

Ashwal S. Neonatal and infantile development of the autonomic nervous system: Function and clinical implications. In: Appenzeller O, ed. Handbook of clinical neurology. St. Louis: Elsevier Science, 1999;199.

Axelrod FB. Familial dysautonomia. In: Mathias CJ. Bannister R, eds. Autonomic failure. A textbook of clinical disorders of the autonomic nervous system, 4th ed. Oxford: Oxford University Press, 2002;402.

Bannister R, da Costa DF, Hendry GH, et al. Atrial demand pacing to protect against vagal over-activity in sympathetic autonomic neuropathy. Brain 1986;109:345.

Benarroch EE. Central neurotransmitters and neuromodulators in cardiovascular regulation. In: Mathias CJ, Bannister R, eds. Autonomic failure. A textbook of clinical disorders of the autonomic nervous system, 4th ed. Oxford: Oxford University Press, 2002;37.

Benditt DG. Cardiac pacing for prevention of vasovagal syncope. J Am Coll Cardiol 1999;33:21.

Bleasdale-Barr K, Mathias CJ. Neck and other muscle pains in autonomic failure: Their association with orthostatic hypotension. J Royal Soc Med 1998;91:355.

Blumenfeld A, Slaughenhaupt SA, Axelrod FB, et al. Localisation of the gene for familia dysautonomia on chromosome 9 and definition of DNA markers for genetic diagnosis. Nature Genet 1993;4:160.

Brignole M, Croci F, Menozzi C, et al. Isometric arm contraction at the onset of prodromal symptoms: A new first-line treatment for vasovagal syncope. In: Raviele A, ed. Cardiac arrhythmias. New York: Springer, 2004:641.

Brooks DJ. Neuroimaging and allied studies in autonomic failure syndromes. In: Mathias CJ, Bannister R, eds. Autonomic failure. A textbook of clinical disorders of the autonomic nervous system, 4th ed. Oxford: Oxford University Press, 2002:320.

Camfield PR, Camfield CS: Syncope in children: A case control clinical study of the familial tendency to faint. Can J Neurol Sci 1990;17:306.

Cariga P, Ahmed S, Mathias CJ, Gardner BP. The prevalence and association of neck (coat-hanger) pain and orthostatic (postural) hypotension in human spinal cord injury. Spinal Cord 2002b;40:77.

Cariga P, Catley M, Savic G, et al. Organisation of the sympathetic skin response in spinal cord injury. J Neurol Neurosurg Psychiatry 2002a;72;356.

Cariga P, Mathias CJ. The haemodynamics of the pressor effect of oral water in human sympathetic denervation due to autonomic failure. Clin Sci 2001;101:313.

Cevoli S, Pierangeli F, Magnifico F, et al. The circardian rhythm of body core temperature (CRT) is normal in a patient with congenital generalized anhidrosis. Clin Aut Res 2002;12:170.

Chandler, MP, Mathias CJ. Haemodynamic responses during head-up tilt and tilt reversal in two groups with chronic autonomic failure: Pure autonomic failure and multiple system atrophy. J Neurol 2002;249:542.

Cooper MR, Johnson AV. Poisonous plants in Britain and their effects on animals and man. London: Her Majesty's Stationery Office, 1984.

Cooper VL, Hainsworth R. Effects of dietary salt on orthostatic tolerance, blood pressure and baroreceptor sensitivity in patients with syncope. Clin Auton Res 2002;12:234.

Craddock G, Pasvol G, Bull R, et al. Cardiorespiratory arrest and autonomic neuropathy in AIDS. Lancet 1987;2:16.

Critchley HD, Mathias CJ, Dolan RJ. Neural activity relating to reward anticipation in human brain. Neuron 2001a;29:537.

Critchley HD, Mathias CJ, Dolan RJ. Neuroanatomical basis for first-and second-order representations of bodily states. Nature Neurosci 2001b;4:207.

Deguchi K, Mathias CJ. Continuous haemodynamic monitoring in an unusual case of swallow-induced syncope. J Neurol Neurosurg Psychiatry 1999;67:220.

Deinum J, Steenbergen-Spanjers GCH, Jansen M, et al. DBH gene variants that cause low plasma dopamine β hydroxylase with or without a severe orthostatic syndrome. J Med Genet 2004;41:1.

El Badawi KM, Hainsworth R. Combined head-up tilt and lower body suction: a test of orthostatic intolerance. Clin Auton Res 1994;4:41.

Esler M, Lambert G, Brunner-La Rocca HP, et al. Sympathetic nerve activity and neurotransmitter release in humans: Translation from pathophysiology into clinical practice. Acta Physiol Scand 2003;177:275.

Frankel HL, Mathias CJ, Spalding JMK. Mechanisms of reflex cardiac arrest in tetraplegic patients. Lancet 1975;2:1183.

Freeman R, Young J, Landsbert L, Lipsitz L. The treatment of postprandial hypotension in autonomic failure with 3,4-DL-threo-dihydroxyphenylserine. Neurology 1996;47:1414.

Gastaut H, Broughton R, De Leo G. Syncopal attacks compulsively self-induced by the Valsalva maneouvre in children with mental retardation. Electroencephalogr Clin Neurophysiol (Suppl 35):323.

Gazit Y, Nahir AM, Grahame R, Jacob G. Dysautonomia in the joint hypermobility syndrome. Am J Med 2003;115:33.

Goldstein DS, Holmes C, Cannon RO III, et al. Sympathetic cardioneuropathy in dysautonomias. N Engl J Med 1997;336:696.

Gomes MER, Deinum J, Timmers, HJLM, Lenders JWM. Occam's razor; anaemia and orthostatic hypotension. Lancet 2003;362:1282.

Hakusui S, Yasuda T, Yanagi T, et al. A radiological analysis of heart sympathetic functions with meta-[^{123}I] iodobenzylguanadine in neurological patients with autonomic failure. J Auton Nerv Syst 1994;49:81.

Hamill R, LaGamma EF. Autonomic nervous system development. In: Mathias CJ, Bannister R, eds. Autonomic failure. A textbook of clinical disorders of the autonomic nervous system, 4th ed. Oxford: Oxford University Press, 2002;16.

Hamilton J, Brown M, Silver R, Daneman D. Early onset of severe diabetes mellitus-related microvascular complications. J Pediatr 2004;144:281.

Head H, Riddoch G. The autonomic bladder, excessive sweating and some other reflex conditions in gross injuries of the spinal cord. Brain 1917;40:188.

Heafield MT, Gammage MD, Nightingale S, Williams AC. Idiopathic dysautonomia treated with intravenous gammaglobulin. Lancet 1996;347:28.

Hickey KJ, Vogel LC, Willis KM, Anderson CJ. Prevalence and etiology of autonomic dysreflexia in children with spinal cord injuries. J Spinal Cord Med 2004;27 (Suppl 1):S54.

Hilz M. Assessment and evaluation of hereditary sensory and autonomic neuropathies with autonomic and neurophysiological examinations. Clin Aut Res 2002;12 (Suppl 1):33.

Hoeldtke RD, Streeten DHP. Treatment of orthostatic hypotension with erythropoietin. N Engl J Med 1993;329:611.

Hopkins A, Neville B, Bannister R. Autonomic neuropathy of acute onset. Lancet 1974;1:769.

Houlden H, King RHM, Hashemi-Nejad A, et al. A novel TRK A *(NTRK1)* mutation associated with hereditary sensory and autonomic neuropathy type V. Ann Neurol 2001;49:521.

Houlden H, Smith S, de Carvalho M, et al. Clinical and genetic characterization of families with triple A (Allgrove) syndrome. Brain 2002;125:2681.

Howard HO, Leathart GL, Dornhorst AC, et al. The 'mess trick' and the 'fainting lark.' BMJ 1951;2:382.

Inander S, Easton LB, Lester G. Acquired post-ganglionic cholinergic dysautonomia: Case report and review of the literature. Pediatrics 1982;70:976.

Indo Y, Tsuruta M, Hayashida Y, et al. Mutations in the TRKA/NGF receptor gene in patients with anhidrosis. Nat Genet 1996;13:485.

Jacob G, Costa F, Shannon JR, et al. The neuropathic postural tachycardia syndrome. N Engl J Med 2000;343:1008.

Janig W. Autonomic nervous system. In: Schmidt RF, Thews G, eds. Human physiology, 2nd ed. Berlin: Springer, 1989;333.

Jenzer G, Mumenthaler M, Luden HP, Robert F. Autonomic dysfunction in botulism B: A clinical report. Neurology 1975;25:150.

Jordan J, Shannon JR, Black BK, et al. The pressor response to water drinking in humans: A sympathetic reflex? Circulation 2000;101:504.

Kanda F, Uchida T, Jinnai K, et al. Acute autonomic and sensory neuropathy: A case report. J Neurol 1990;237:42.

Kaufmann H, Saadia D, Polin C, et al. Primary hyperhidrosis—Evidence for autosomal dominant inheritance. Clin Auton Res 2003;13:96.

Kaufmann H, Saadia D, Voustianiouk A, et al. Norepinephrine precursor therapy in neurogenic orthostatic hypotension. Circulation 2003;108:724.

Khan AA, Riazi J, Bloom D. Oculocardiac reflex in near-miss for sudden infant death syndrome infants. Pediatrics 1983;71:49.

Kim CH, Zabetian CP, Cubells JF, et al. Mutations in the dopamine beta-hydroxylase gene are associated with human norepinephrine deficiency. Am J Med Genet 2002;108:140.

Kimber J, Mitchell D, Mathias CJ. Chronic cough in the Holmes-Adie syndrome: Association in five cases with autonomic dysfunction. J Neurol Neurosurg Psychiatry 1998;65:583.

Lambert GW, Thompson JM, Turner AG, et al. Cerebral noradrenaline spillover and its relation to muscle sympathetic nervous activity in healthy human subjects. J Auton Nerv Syst 1997;64:57.

Low PA, Gilden JL, Freeman R, et al. Efficacy of midodrine vs. placebo in neurogenic orthostatic hypotension. A randomized, double-blind multicenter study. JAMA 1997;277:1046.

Low PA, Schondorf R, Rummans TA. Why do patients have orthostatic symptoms in PoTS? Clin Auton Res 2001;11:223.

Magnifico F, Misra VP, Murray NMF, Mathias CJ. The sympathetic skin response in peripheral autonomic failure—Evaluation in pure autonomic failure, pure cholinergic dysautonomia and dopamine beta-hydroxylase deficiency. Clin Auton Res 1998;8:133.

Mahloud JIM, Brunt PW, McKusick VA. Clinical neurological aspects of familial dysautonomia. J Neurol Sci 1970;11:383.

Man in't Veld AJ, Boomsma F, Moleman P, et al. Congenital dopamine beta-hydroxylase deficiency. A novel orthostatic syndrome. Lancet 1987;1:183.

Mantysaari M, Kuikka J, Mustonem J, et al. Measurement of myocardial accumulation of 123-metaiodobenzylguanidine for studying cardiac autonomic neuropathy in diabetes mellitus. Clin Auton Res 1996;6:163.

Mardy S, Miura Y, Endo F, et al. Congenital insensitivity to pain with anhidrosis: Novel mutations in the the TRKA(NTRK1) gene encoding a high-affinity receptor for nerve growth factor. Am J Hum Genet 1999;64:1570.

Maron BJ, Poliac LC, Kaplan JA, Mueller RO. Blunt impact to the chest leading to sudden death from cardiac arrest during sports activities. N Engl J Med 1995;333:337.

Mathias CJ. Bradycardia and cardiac arrest during tracheal suction—Mechanisms in etraplegic patients. Eur J Intensive Care Med 1976;2:147.

Mathias CJ. Disorders of the autonomic nervous system in childhood. In: Berg B, ed. Principles of child neurology. New York: McGraw-Hill, 1996;413.

Mathias CJ. Autonomic disorders. In: Bogousslavsky J, Fisher M, eds. Textbook of neurology. Boston: Butterworth-Heinemann, 1998;519.

Mathias CJ. To stand on one's own legs. Clin Med 2002;2:237.

Mathias CJ. Autonomic diseases—Clinical features and laboratory evaluation. J Neurol Neurosurg Psychiatry 2003a;74:31.

Mathias CJ. Autonomic diseases: Management. J Neurol Neurosurg Psychiatry 2003b;74:iii42.

Mathias CJ. Disorders of the autonomic nervous system. In: Bradley WG, Daroff RB, Fenichel GM, Jancovich J, eds. Neurology in clinical practice, 3rd ed. Boston: Butterworth-Heinemann, 2004;2403.

Mathias CJ. Orthostatic hypotension and orthostatic intolerance. In: De Groot LJ, Jameson JL, eds. Endocrinology, 5th ed. Philadelphia: Elsevier, in press, 2005.

Mathias CJ, Bannister R. Dopamine beta-hydroxylase deficiency and other genetically determined autonomic disorders. In: Mathias CJ, Bannister R, eds. Autonomic failure. A textbook of clinical disorders of the autonomic nervous system, 4th ed. Oxford: Oxford University Press, 2002a;387.

Mathias CJ, Bannister R. Investigation of autonomic disorders. In: Mathias CJ, Bannister R, eds. Autonomic failure. A textbook of clinical disorders of the autonomic nervous system, 4th ed. Oxford: Oxford University Press, 2002b;169.

Mathias CJ, Bannister R, Cortelli P, et al. Clinical autonomic and therapeutic observations in two siblings with postural hypotension and sympathetic failure due to an inability to synthesize noradrenaline from dopamine because of a deficiency of dopamine beta-hydroxylase. Q J Med, New Series 1990;278:617.

Mathias CJ, Christensen NJ, Corbett JL, et al. Plasma catecholamines, plasma renin activity and plasma aldosterone in tetraplegic man, horizontal and tilted. Clin Sci Molec Med 1975;49:291.

Mathias CJ, Christensen NJ, Corbett JL, et al. Plasma catecholamines during paroxysmal neurogenic hypertension in quadriplegic man. Circ Res 1976;39:204.

Mathias CJ, Christensen NJ, Frankel HL, Spalding JMK. Cardiovascular control in recently injured tetraplegics in spinal shock. Q J Med, New Series 1979;48:273.

Mathias CJ, da Costa DF, Fosbraey P, et al. Cardiovascular, biochemical and hormonal changes during food induced hypotension in chronic autonomic failure. J Neurol Sci 1989;94:255.

Mathias CJ, Deguchi K, Bleasdale-Barr K, Kimber JR. Frequency of family history in vasovagal syncope. Lancet 1998;352:33.

Mathias CJ, Deguchi K, Schatz I. Observations on recurrent syncope and presyncope in 641 patients. Lancet 2001b;357:348.

Mathias CJ, Frankel H. Autonomic disturbances in spinal cord lesions. In: Mathias CJ, Bannister R, eds. Autonomic failure. A textbook of clinical disorders of the autonomic nervous system, 4th ed. Oxford: Oxford University Press, 2002;494.

Mathias CJ, Fosbraey P, da Costa DF, et al. The effect of desmopressin on nocturnal polyuria, overnight weight loss and morning postural hypotension in patients with autonomic failure. BMJ 1986;293:353.

Mathias CJ, Holly E, Armstrong E, et al. The influence of food on postural hypotension in three groups with chronic autonomic failure: Clinical and therapeutic implications. J Neurol Neurosurg Psychiatry 1991;54:726.

Mathias CJ, Mallipeddi R, Bleasdale-Barr K. Symptoms associated with orthostatic hypotension in pure autonomic failure and multiple system atrophy. J Neurol 1999;246:893.

Mathias CJ, Senard J, Braune S, et al. L-threo-dihydroxphenylserine (L-threo-DOPS; droxidopa) in the management of neurogenic orthostatic hypotension: A multi-national, multi-centre, dose-ranging study in multiple system atrophy and pure autonomic failure. Clin Auton Res 2001a;11:235.

Mathias CJ, Young TM. Plugging the leak—The benefits of the vasopressin-2 agonist, desmopressin in autonomic failure. Clin Auton Res 2003;13:85.

Mathias CJ, Young TM. Water drinking in the management of orthostatic intolerance orthostatic hypotension, vasovagal syncope and the postural tachycardia syndrome. Eur J Neurol 2004;11:613.

Maule S, Lombardo L, Rossi C, et al. *Helicobacter pylori* and gastric function in primary autonomic neuropathy. Clin Auton Res 2002;12:193.

McGinnis KB, Vogel LC, McDonald CM, et al. Recognition and management of autonomic dysreflexia in pediatric spinal cord injury. J Spinal Cord Med 2004;27 (Suppl 1):S61.

McIntosh SJ, Lawson J, Kenny RA. Clinical characteristics of vasodepressor, cardioinhibitory and mixed carotid sinus syndrome in the elderly. Am J Med 1993;95:203.

Merz B, Bigalke H, Stoll G, Naumann M. Botulism type B presenting as pure autonomic dysfunction. Clin Auton Res 2003;13:337.

Mikolich JR, Paulson GW, Cross CJ. Acute anti-cholinergic syndrome due to Jimson seed ingestion: Clinical and laboratory observation in six cases. Ann Intern Med 1975;83:321.

Naumann M, Flachenecker P, Brocker E-B, et al. Botulinum toxin for palmar hyperhidrosis. Lancet 1997a;349:252.

Naumann M, Zellner M, Toyka KV, Reiners K. Treatment of gustatory sweating with botulinum toxin. Ann Neurol: 1997b;42:973.

Nicotra A, Asahina M, Mathias CJ. Skin vasodilator response to local heating in human chronic spinal cord injury. Eur J Neurol 2004;11:835.

Oldenburg O, Mitchell AN, Nurnberger J, et al. Ambulatory norepinephrine treatment of severe autonomic orthostatic hypotension. J Am Coll Cardiol 2001;37:219.

Perkins BA, Bril V. Early vascular risk factor modification in type 1 diabetes. N Engl J Med 2005;352:408.

Parati G, Di Rienzo M, Omboni S, Mancia G. Computer analysis of blood pressure and heart rate variability in subjects with normal and abnormal autonomic cardiovascular control. In: Mathias CJ, Bannister R, eds. Autonomic failure. A textbook of clinical disorders of the autonomic nervous system, 4th ed. Oxford: Oxford University Press, 2002;211.

Pledger HG. Disorders of temperature regulation in acute traumatic paraplegia. J Bone Joint Surg 1962;44B:110.

Polinsky RJ. Neuropharmacological investigation of autonomic failure. In: Mathias CJ, Bannister R, eds. Autonomic failure. A textbook of clinical disorders of the autonomic nervous system, 4th ed. Oxford: Oxford University Press, 2002;232.

Puvi-Rajasingham S, Smith GDP, Akinola A, Mathias CJ. Abnormal regional blood flow responses during and after exercise in human sympathetic denervation. J Physiol 1997;505:481.

Reilly MM, Thomas PK. Amyloid polyneuropathy. In: Mathias CJ, Bannister R, eds. Autonomic failure. A textbook of clinical disorders of the autonomic nervous system, 4th ed. Oxford: Oxford University Press, 2002;410.

Robertson D, Goldberg MR, Onrot J, et al. Isolated failure of autonomic noradrenergic neurotransmission. Evidence for impaired beta-hydroxylation of dopamine. N Engl J Med 1986;314:494.

Sahul ZH, Trusty JM, Erickson M, et al. Pacing does not improve hypotension in patients with severe orthostatic hypotension—A prospective randomized cross-over pilot study. Clin Auton Res 2004;14:255.

Schatz IJ, Bannister R, Freeman RL, et al. Consensus statement on the definition of orthostatic hypotension, pure autonomic failure and multiple system atrophy. Clin Auton Res 1996;6:125.

Scherrer U, Vissing SF, Morgan BJ, et al. Cyclosporine-induced sympathetic activation and hypertension after heart transplantation. N Engl J Med 1990;323:693.

Schondorf R, Low PA. Idiopathic postural tachycardia syndrome: An attenuated form of acute pandysautonomia? Neurology 1993;3:132.

Schott GD. Interrupting the sympathetic outflow in causalgia and reflex sympathetic dystrophy. A futile procedure for many patients. BMJ 1998;316:792.

Schrage WG, Eisenach JH, Dinenno FA, et al. Effects of midodrine on exercise-induced hypotension and blood pressure recovery in autonomic failure. J Appl Physiol 2004;97:1978.

Shannon JR, Flatten NL, Jordan J, et al. Orthostatic intolerance and tachycardia associated with norepinephrine-transporter deficiency. N Eng J Med 2000;342:541.

Shifferli PY, Caldeyro-Barcia R. Effects of atropine and beta-adrenergic drugs on the heart rate of the human fetus. In: Boreus LO, ed. Fetal pharmacology. New York: Raven Press, 1973;259.

Singer W, Opfer-Gehrking TL, McPhee BR, et al. Acetylcholinesterase inhibition: A novel approach in the treatment of neurogenic orthostatic hypotension. J Neurol Neurosurg Psychiatry 2003;74:1294.

Smit AAJ, Hardjowijono MA, Wieling W. Are portable folding chairs useful to combat orthostatic hypotension? Ann Neurol 1997;42:975.

Smith GDP, Alam M, Watson LP, Mathias CJ. Effects of the somatostatin analogue, octreotide, on exercise induced hypotension in human subjects with chronic sympathetic failure. Clin Sci 1995a;89:367.

Smith GDP, Bannister R, Mathias CJ. Post exercise dizziness as the sole presenting symptom in autonomic failure. Br Heart J 1993;69:359.

Smith GDP, Mathias CJ. Postural hypotension enhanced by exercise in patients with chronic autonomic failure. Q J Med 1995;88:251.

Smith GDP, Watson LP, Pavitt DV, Mathias CJ. Abnormal cardiovascular and catecholamine responses to supine exercise in human subjects with sympathetic dysfunction. J Physiol (Lond) 1995b;484:255.

Spyer KM. Central nervous control of the cardiovascular system. In: Mathias CJ, Bannister R, eds. Autonomic failure. A textbook of clinical disorders of the autonomic nervous system, 4th ed. Oxford: Oxford University Press, 2002;45.

Stephenson JBP. Fits and faints. In: Clinical and Developmental Medicine No 109. Oxford, Mac Keith Press, Blackwell, 1900.

Stewart JM. Transient orthostatic hypotension is common in adolescents. J Pediatr 2002;140:418.

Stewart JM, Gewitz MH, Weldon A, Munoz J. Patterns of orthostatic intolerance: The orthostatic tachycardia syndrome and adolescent chronic fatigue. J Pediatr 1999;135:218.

Streeten DH. Pathogenesis of hyperadrenergic orthostatic hypotension: Evidence of disordered venous innervation exclusively in the lower limbs. J Clin Invest 1990;86:1582.

Streeten DH, Anderson GH Jr, Richardson R, Thomas FD. Abnormal orthostatic changes in blood pressure and heart rate in subjects with intact sympathetic nervous function: Evidence for excessive venous pooling. J Lab Clin Med 1998;111:326.

Sundqvist G, Bornmyr S, Svensson H, et al: Sympathetic neuropathy is more frequent than parasympathetic neuropathy in patients with a short duration of type 2 diabetes. Clin Auton Res 1998;8:281.

Swanson AG. Congenital insensitivity to pain with anhidrosis. Arch Neurol 1963;8:299.

Takayama H, Kazahay Y, Kashihara N, et al. A case of post-ganglionic cholinergic dysautonomia. J Neurol Neurosurg Psychiatry 1987;50:915.

Tanaka H, Matsushima R, Tamai H, Kajimoto Y. Impaired postural cerebral hemodynamics in young patients with chronic fatigue and without orthostatic intolerance. J Pediatr 2002;140:412.

Tanaka H, Yamaguchi H, Matsushima R, et al. Instantaneous orthostatic hypotension in Japanese children and adolescents: A new entity of orthostatic intolerance. Pediatr Res 1999;46:691.

Tanaka H, Yamaguchi H, Tamai H. Treatment of orthostatic intolerance with inflatable abdominal band. Lancet 1997;349:175.

Tesfaye S, Chaturvedi N, Eaton SE, et al. Vascular risk factors and diabetic neuropathy. N Engl J Med 2005;352:341.

Tomashevsky AJ, Horowitz SJ, Finegold MH. Acute autonomic neuropathy. Neurology 1972;22:251.

Tonkin AL, Frewin DB. Drugs, chemicals and toxins that alter autonomic function. In: Mathias CJ, Bannister R, eds. Autonomic failure. A textbook of clinical disorders of the autonomic nervous system, 4th ed. Oxford: Oxford University Press, 2002;527.

Tugnoli V, Marchese Ragona R, Eleopra R, et al. The role of gustatory flushing in Frey's syndrome and its treatment with botulinum toxin type A. Clin Auton Res 2002;12:174.

Vaidyanathan S, Soni BM, Sett P, et al. Pathophysiology of autonomic dysreflexia: Long-term treatment with terazosin in adult and paediatric spinal cord injury patients manifesting recurrent dysreflexic episodes. Spinal Cord 1998;36:761.

van Dijk N, Harms MP, Linzer M, Wieling W. Treatment of vasovagal syncope: Pacemaker or crossing legs? Clin Auton Res 2000;10:347.

Vernino S, Low PA, Fealey RD, et al. Autoantibodies to ganglionic acetylcholine receptors in autoimmune autonomic neuropathies. N Engl J Med 2000;343:847.

Wallin BG. Intraneural recordings of normal and abnormal sympathetic activity in humans. In: Mathias CJ, Bannister R, eds. Autonomic failure. A textbook of clinical disorders of the autonomic nervous system, 4th ed. Oxford: Oxford University Press, 2002;224.

Watkins PJ. The enigma of autonomic failure in diabetes. J R Coll Phys Lond 1998;32:360.

Watkins PJ, Edmonds ME. Diabetic autonomic failure. In: Mathias CJ, Bannister R, eds. Autonomic failure. A textbook of clinical disorders of the autonomic nervous system, 4th ed. Oxford: Oxford University Press, 2002;378.

Wieling W, Karemaker JM. Measurement of heart rate and blood pressure to evaluate disturbances in neurocardiovascular control. In: Mathias CJ, Bannister R, eds. Autonomic failure. A textbook of clinical disorders of the autonomic nervous system, 4th ed. Oxford: Oxford University Press, 2002;196.

Wieling W, van Lieshout JJ. The fainting lark. Clin Auton Res 2002;12:207.

Wieling W, van Lieshout JJ, van Leeuwen AM. Physical manoeuvres that reduce postural hypotension. Clin Auton Res 1993;3:57.

Young RR, Asbury AK, Corbett JL, et al. Pure pandysautonomia with recovery: Description and discussion of diagnostic criteria. Brain 1975;98:613.

Young TM, Mathias CJ. The effects of water ingestion on orthostatic hypotension in two groups with chronic autonomic failure: Multiple system atrophy and pure autonomic failure. J Neurol Neurosurg Psychiatry 2004;75:1737.

CHAPTER 86

Disorders of Micturition and Defecation

Bhuwan P. Garg

DISORDERS OF MICTURITION

Micturition is an intricate function that results from a coordinated activity of the muscles of the urinary bladder and urethral sphincter. Knowledge, particularly of normal mechanisms, is accruing primarily from animal studies. Volitional and automatic functions are integrated [Bradley, 1986]. The automatic activities are controlled by the autonomic nervous system. In infants, autonomic control is primary, and as development proceeds, voluntary control over micturition is exerted. Voiding is frequent and largely uninhibited for the first 16 months of life. However, recent studies have found that there is cortical arousal in response to a full bladder even in newborns [Yeung et al., 1995]. Voiding frequency gradually decreases, and between 1 and 2 years of age, the child becomes aware of the sensation of a full bladder. By 2 years of age, children begin to retain their urine for brief periods, although most children cannot willfully initiate voiding. By 3 years of age, diurnal control is established, and most children acquire nocturnal control by age 4 years. By 5 years of age, 85% of children have achieved complete bladder control [Himsel and Hurwitz, 1991]. Bowel control precedes bladder control with the sequence of control as follows: (1) nocturnal bowel control, (2) diurnal bowel control, (3) diurnal bladder control, and (4) nocturnal bladder control [Perlmutter, 1985].

Toilet training is necessary for achieving continence. As a general rule children are ready for toilet training when they can appreciate the sensation of voiding and recognize a wet or soiled diaper. Similarly, ability to largely remain dry through an afternoon nap is a sign that a child is ready to stop wearing a diaper at night. Toilet training is a complex process and includes not only the recognition of an urge to void but also the ability to undress, void, wipe, dress again, flush, and wash hands [Stadtler et al.,1999]. Isolated day wetting or wetting both day and night is urinary incontinence. Nocturnal enuresis, or more commonly enuresis (derived from the Greek word *enourein,* "to void urine"), is usually used to denote bedwetting only in sleep. In nocturnal enuresis there is a mismatch between the nocturnal bladder capacity and the amount of urine produced during the night, as well as an inability of the child to wake up in response to a full bladder. In one study of micturition habits of healthy children, 12% of boys and 7% of girls at 7 years of age and 0.3% of boys and 0.6% of girls at 17 years of age reported bedwetting [Hellström et al., 1995]. In another study, daytime urinary incontinence (at least once a month) occurred in 6.3% of first graders and 4.3% of fourth graders. Bedwetting (at least once a month) was reported in 7.1% and 2.7%, respectively. In first graders, fecal incontinence was present in 9.8% and in fourth graders in 5.6%. Daytime urinary incontinence was strongly associated with fecal incontinence [Soderstrom et al., 2004].

Micturition is primarily a parasympathetic function; the sympathetic nervous system is involved in determining bladder capacity and urine storage. Voluntary control of the external sphincter, periurethral muscles, and abdominal muscles is effected through conventional pathways of the corticospinal connections. Knowledge of the specific mechanisms of normal micturition remains incomplete, thereby frustrating efforts directed toward precise diagnosis and management.

Anatomy and Embryology

The urinary bladder, a hollow viscus, receives urine from the kidneys through the two ureteral orifices and discharges urine through a solitary urethral orifice [Elbadawi, 1996]. The mucous membrane of the bladder is lined by transitional epithelium, which is supported by an underlying loose submucous coat. A three-layer muscular coat of smooth muscle fibers forms the bulk of the bladder wall. There are inner longitudinal, middle circular, and outer longitudinal layers of muscle fibers (i.e., detrusor muscle). The inner longitudinal layer is the thinnest. The middle circular layer, strongest of the three layers, forms a ring ventrally around the internal urethral orifice. The outer longitudinal layer ventrally forms a collar-like structure called the *collare vesicae;* around the bladder neck this structure is called the *nodus vesicae* [Dorschner et al., 1994]. The detrusor muscle is bilaterally innervated and functions as a syncytium [Zimmern et al., 1996]. Gap-type junctions (electrical synapses) occur frequently; axoaxonal-type synapses are also present. Stretch receptors are arranged in series with the detrusor muscle fibers [Bradley, 1986].

The urinary bladder originates from the enlarged terminal portion of the hindgut (the cloaca), which forms during the early somite stage. Ventrally the entodermal cloacal lining is in direct contact with the surface ectoderm, forming the cloacal membrane. During the fourth to seventh weeks of gestation, the cloaca subdivides into an anterior primitive urogenital sinus and a posterior anorectal canal. This subdivision is accomplished by the caudad growth of the urorectal septum. The entrance of the mesonephric ducts into this primitive urogenital sinus divides the sinus into two portions—the vesicourethral canal above and the definitive urogenital sinus below. The urinary bladder and the upper portion of the urethra are formed from the vesicourethral canal. Therefore the epithelial lining of the bladder is derived from the embryonic entoderm. Some controversy exists regarding the origin of the epithelium of the trigone of the bladder, which may be partially of mesodermal origin. The detrusor muscle arises from the visceral mesoderm.

Nerve Supply

The urinary bladder has two chief sources of nerve supply—the autonomic nervous system, primarily concerned with impulses of involuntary nature, and the cerebrospino-pudendal pathway, which subserves volitional control.

The pathways that provide cerebral control of the detrusor neurons have been delineated with horseradish peroxidase and immunohistochemical techniques. In the rat the urinary bladder appears to be innervated by axons from the caudal portion of the nucleus laterodorsalis tegmenti, which connects with the medial frontal cortex [Sakanaka et al., 1983]. The projections in the rat appear to be ipsilateral and also extend to the ipsilateral septal area; the latter area is involved with emotional and motivational activities [Bradley, 1986]. In humans the cerebrocortical areas concerned with pudendal and detrusor activation are located in the medial aspect of the area immediately anterior to the rolandic fissure [Haldeman et al., 1982a; 1982b].

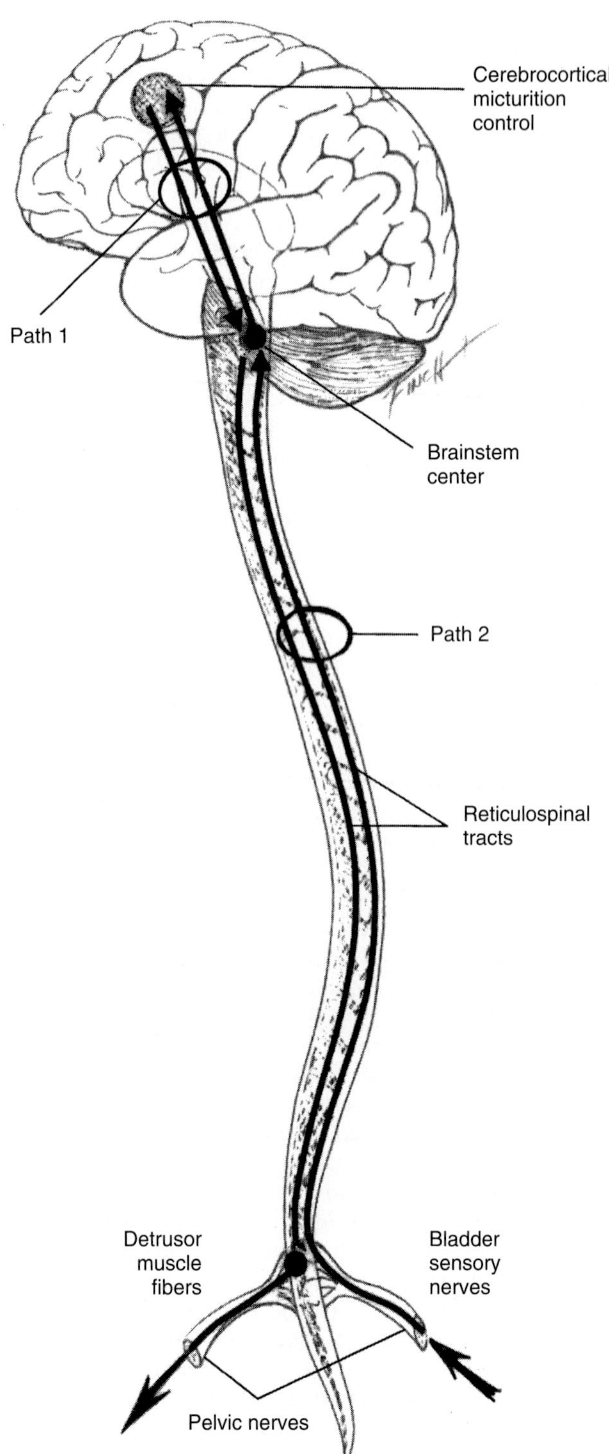

FIGURE 86-1. Paths 1 and 2. (Redrawn from Bradley, 1986.)

Bradley [1986] has divided the various neural interconnections into loops (paths). Path 1 is a bidirectional pathway between brainstem and cerebral cortex that includes connections to subcortical nuclei (e.g., thalamus, basal ganglia, and amygdaloid nucleus) (Fig. 86-1).

Path 2, which is also bidirectional, is traversed by ascending impulses from the detrusor muscle to the brainstem detrusor nucleus and by descending impulses from the brainstem detrusor nucleus to the sacral spinal cord (see Fig. 86-1).

Path 3 comprises the following: (1) afferent axons from the detrusor muscle and periurethral striated muscle that impinge on the sacral pudendal nucleus and (2) efferent motor axons that originate in the sacral pudendal nucleus and terminate in the striated sphincter muscles (Fig. 86-2).

Path 4 consists of supraspinal (path 4a) and segmental (path 4b) portions. Path 4a comprises the following: (1) a sensory pathway that traverses the posterior columns and (2) an efferent motor pathway that originates in the motor cortex and connects with the sacral alpha motor and gamma motor neurons (Fig. 86-3). The afferent portion of path 4b comprises the following: (1) sensory fibers originating in the striated-muscle spindles of the periurethral area and (2) the axons that travel upward to connect with the sensorimotor cortex. The efferent portion of path 4b comprises the following: (1) the alpha motor fibers that issue from the alpha motor neurons in the sacral cord and innervate the periurethral striated muscle and (2) the gamma motor fibers that originate in the gamma motor neurons in the anterior horn of the spinal cord and innervate the muscle spindle fibers in the periurethral striated muscle (Fig. 86-4).

Three other minor pathways have been described, which include proximal urethra to detrusor muscle, periurethral striated muscle to detrusor (which inhibits contraction), and sacral afferents to the lumbar cord that cause excitation of lumbar efferents to the pelvic ganglia, which in turn inhibit synaptic transmission in the pelvic ganglia [Bradley, 1986].

Paths 1 and 4a provide for cortical control or modification of the detrusor and pudendal pathways. Path 2 provides for brainstem control of the detrusor pathways. Path 3 provides for segmental control of pudendal pathways. Path 4b is a conventional pathway that contains alpha motor neuron, gamma motor neuron, and axonal connections with the sensorimotor and motor cortex and striated muscle of the periurethral area.

The spinal cord detrusor nucleus is located in the region of the parasympathetic nerve cells at S3 in the intermediolateral cell column. S2 and S4 also contribute to the nerve supply (Fig. 86-5) [Saper, 1995]. The axons from these cell bodies, after traversing the ventral roots, form the pelvic nerve that innervates the detrusor muscle; both ipsilateral and contralateral innervation occurs.

The sympathetic motor nerve supply to the bladder originates in the cell bodies of the intermediolateral column

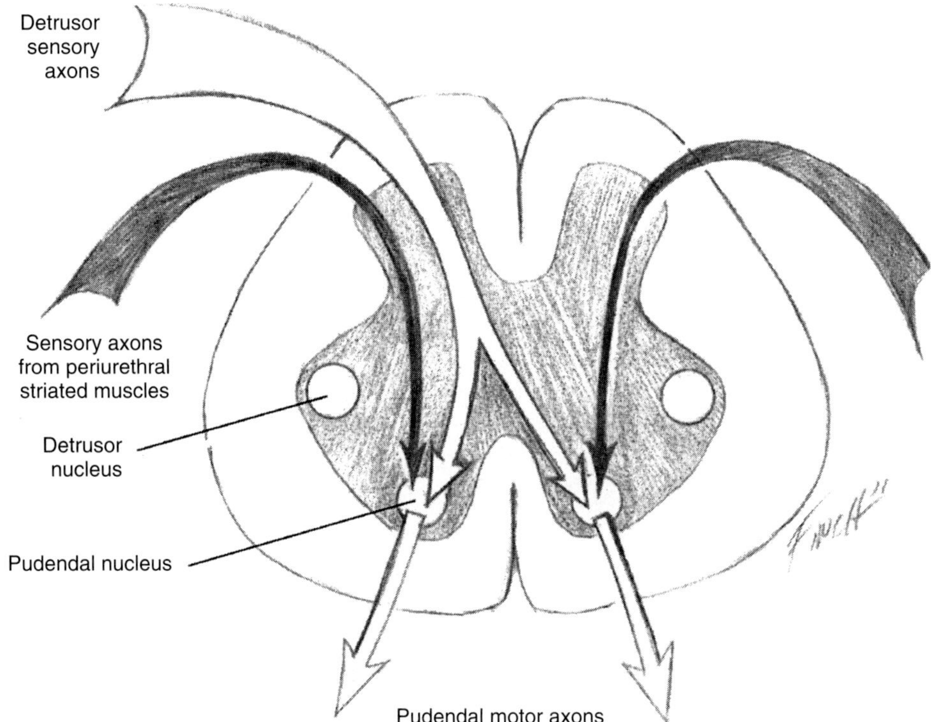

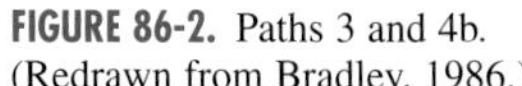

FIGURE 86-2. Paths 3 and 4b. (Redrawn from Bradley, 1986.)

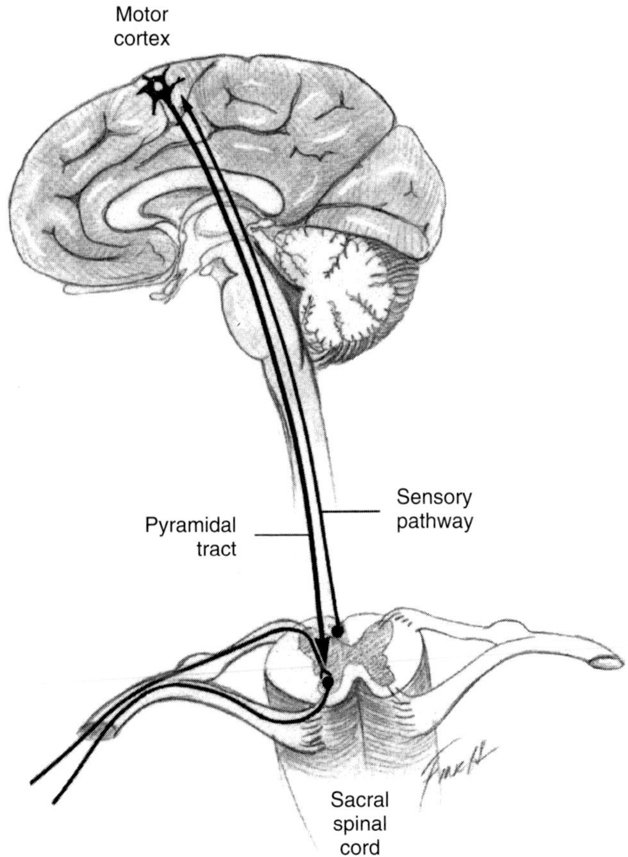

FIGURE 86-3. Paths 4a and 4b. (Redrawn from Bradley, 1986.)

of the spinal cord extending from T11 to L2. The preganglionic nerve fibers from these cell bodies synapse in the sympathetic ganglia of the hypogastric plexus and emerge as postganglionic fibers in the hypogastric nerve. These sympathetic fibers innervate the trigone region of the bladder [Chai and Steers, 1996; Wein and Barrett, 1992].

The cerebrospinopudendal pathway subserves volitional control of micturition. The pudendal nerve arises from the pudendal nucleus (Onuf's nucleus), which is located in the anterior horn cell column of S3 and S4 (see Fig. 86-5). The nerve innervates the external urethral sphincter, as well as the accessory urethral and perineal muscles. The pudendal nucleus is innervated through the pyramidal tract from the upper motor neuron cells situated on the medial surface of the frontal lobe anterior to the rolandic fissure (the paracentral lobule). Somatic afferent impulses, which are transmitted in the pudendal nerve, enter the dorsal roots of S2 to S4.

Pathophysiology

Most children with lower urinary tract dysfunction suffer from neurologic compromise [Fidas et al., 1987; Sensirivatana et al., 1987]. The micturition reflex is primarily a brainstem reflex and requires intact brainstem reticular formation pathways to the spinal cord (reticulospinal tracts), although other portions of the brain exert significant influence on the micturition reflex. Important areas of brain control of micturition include the frontal sensorimotor cortex (medial surface anterior to the rolandic fissure), the midbrain, and the dorsal tegmental area of the pons (brainstem detrusor motor nucleus); they exert either a facilitatory or an inhibitory effect on the micturition reflex [Carpenter and Sutin, 1983; Chai and Steers, 1996; Wein and Barrett, 1992]. The precise role of the thalamus, hypothalamus, limbic system, and basal ganglia remains largely unknown, although the general contributions of these regions have been partially delineated. The activities in the cerebral cortex, basal ganglia, anterior hypothalamus, and anterior midbrain inhibit the reflex detrusor contraction that is induced by

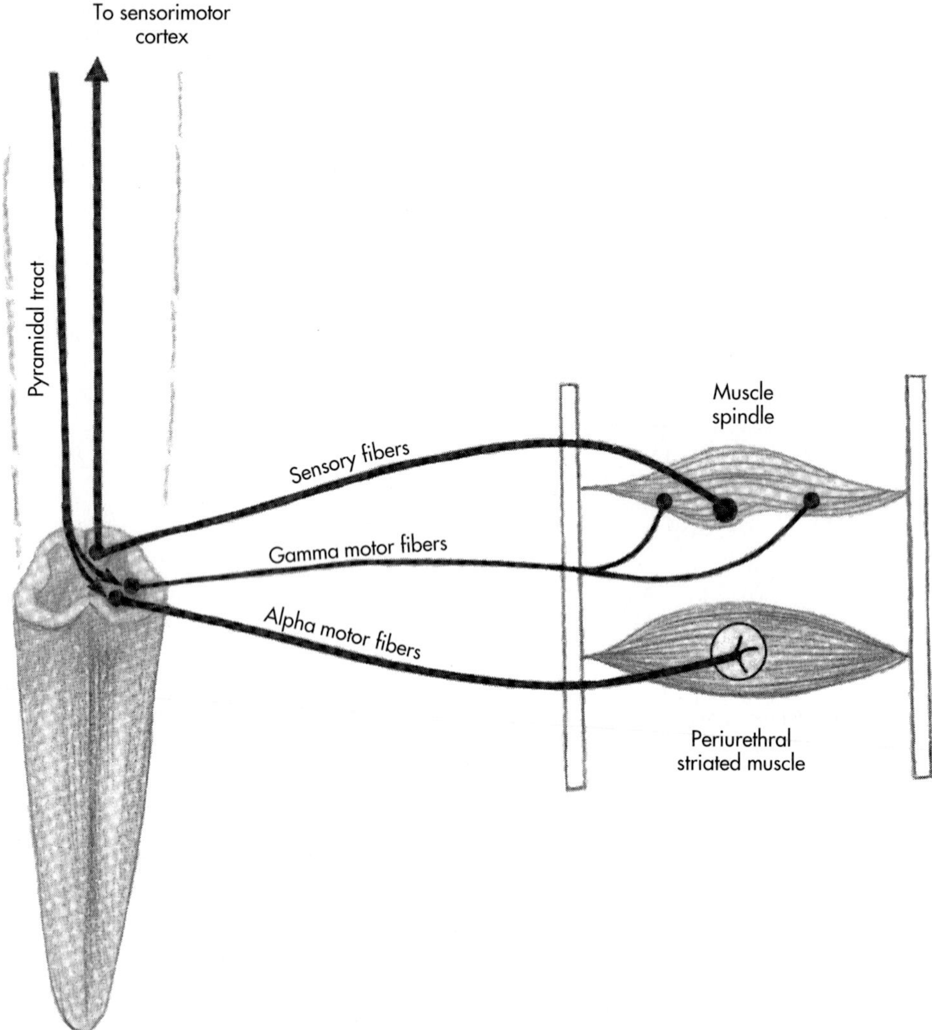

FIGURE 86-4. Path 4b. (The pyramidal tract actually descends on the same side as the ascending tract to the sensorimotor cortex.) (Redrawn from Bradley, 1986.)

bladder filling. Although connections between the cerebellum and urinary bladder have been established and possible cerebellar influence on micturition hypothesized [Bradley, 1986], little specific information is available concerning this relationship.

The brainstem detrusor motor nucleus is located in the caudal portion of the dorsal tegmental area of the pons rostral to the nucleus locus ceruleus [Tohyama et al., 1978]. Two projections emanate from this nucleus—one to the lateral hypothalamic area and one to the sacral spinal cord [Saper, 1995]. Bilateral lesions involving the pontine tegmentum, resulting in an inability to empty the bladder and urinary retention, have been described [Manente et al., 1996].

Detrusor muscle and the striated urethral sphincter muscles act in a complex reciprocal manner during bladder filling and voiding. Concurrent relaxation of the striated muscles of the internal and external urethral sphincters and contraction of detrusor muscle results in voiding. Reverse interaction results in bladder filling.

The stretch receptors in the detrusor muscle are activated by bladder filling and initiate the micturition reflex [Bradley, 1986]. Some of these stretch receptor-initiated impulses travel in the pelvic nerve afferents, which synapse with the pudendal neurons in the sacral cord (path 3; see Fig. 86-2). Impulses inhibit the pudendal neurons, with resultant relaxation of the striated muscles of the internal and external urethral sphincters. Other afferents are directed over a long pathway to the brainstem pudendal nucleus; from there they travel down the reticulospinal tract to terminate on the sacral detrusor neurons, with resultant muscle contraction (path 2).

The voluntary control of the urethral sphincter is mediated through path 4a, which originates in the neurons of the corticospinal tract (pyramidal tract) in the medial anterior frontal cortex. The axons of the pyramidal tract terminate on the pudendal neurons in the sacral cord and by effecting activity in path 4b exert voluntary control over the sphincter muscle (cerebrospinopudendal pathway) [Nakagawa, 1980]. Tonic activity in the pudendal nerves innervating the urethral sphincter maintains closure of the sphincter during both waking and sleeping states. The muscle stretch receptors in the sphincter-striated muscle modulate and maintain this tonic activity. Commanding the patient to contract the sphincter provides a test for evaluating these neural connections. Because the innervation of the urethral and anal sphincter is the same for purposes of analysis, anal sphincter monitoring is useful for assessing urethral sphincter function. An anourethral reflex has also been described [Shafik, 1992]. Urethral sphincter function may also be assessed electromyographically by examination of the pelvic floor muscles [Siroky, 1996].

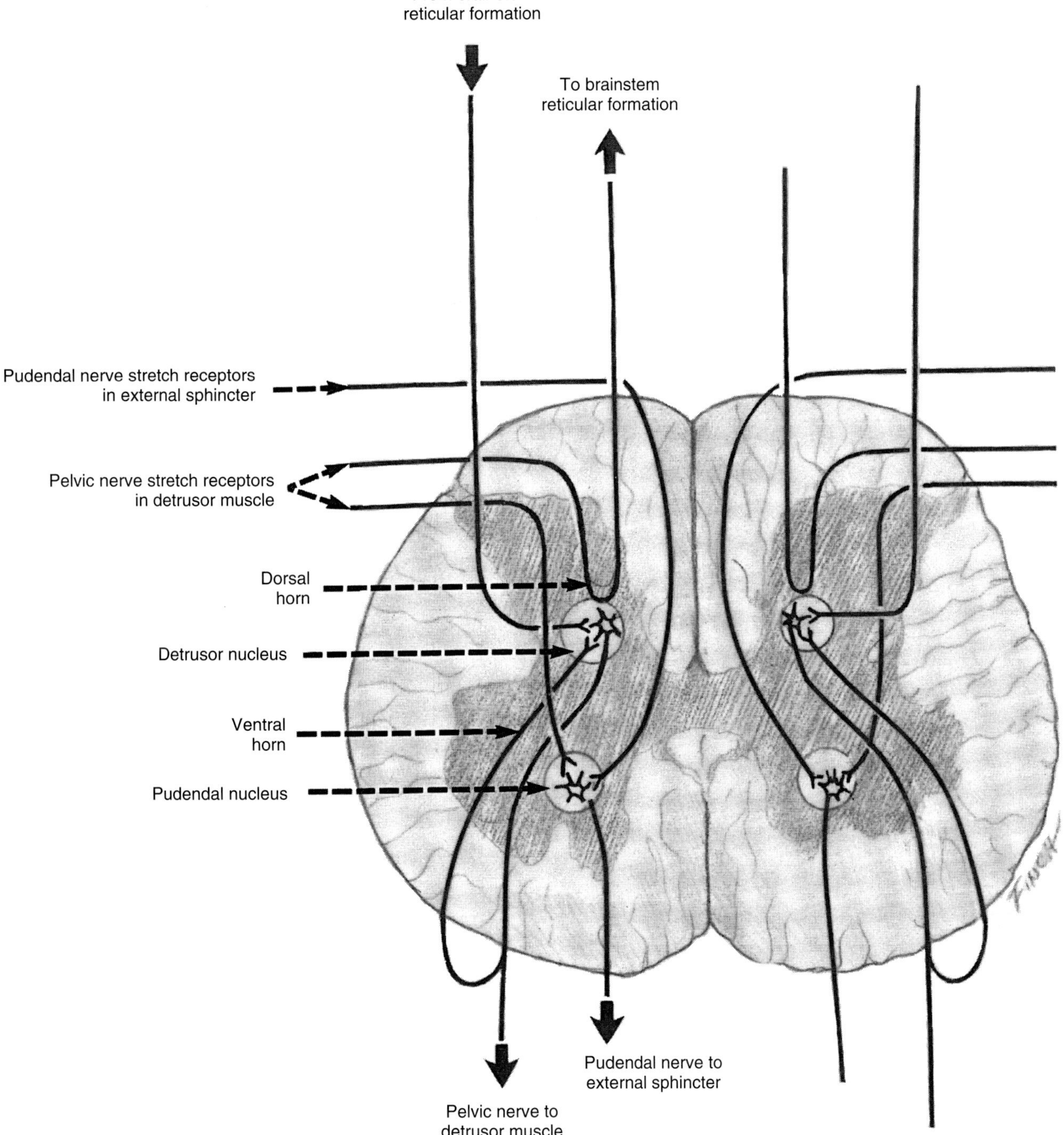

FIGURE 86-5. Input-output relationships of conus medullaris. Recurrent inhibition pathways are observed in the pelvic motor nerves. (Redrawn from Bradley, 1986.)

The frontal lobes exert some voluntary control over the detrusor muscle. The integrity of this pathway can be readily demonstrated by the ability of the patient to suppress the detrusor reflex contraction on command during micturition and cystometric examination. Pathologic compromise of this pathway results in detrusor hyperreflexia, which is characterized during the cystometric examination by the reaction of a detrusor reflex at a low-volume threshold; the reflex cannot be interdicted volitionally by the patient. The impairment may be so subtle that the clinical manifestations may be evident only on postural change or during walking.

Bilateral pathologic involvement of the pyramidal tract, usually in the spinal cord, results in impaired volitional control of the urethral sphincter; therefore the urethral sphincter may undergo inappropriate relaxation, or increased sphincter activity may occur during detrusor contraction. This imbalance is termed *detrusor-urethral sphincter dyssynergia* [Hinman, 1980].

Box 86-1 Micturition Disorders: Sites of Dysfunction

Upper motor neuron unit lesions
- Frontal and parietal lobes
- Limbic system and hypothalamus
- Basal ganglia
- Brainstem
- Cerebellum
- Spinal cord

Lower motor neuron unit lesions
- Afferent (sensory) pathways
- Efferent (motor) pathways
- Preganglionic
- Postganglionic
- Muscle fibers

Detrusor vesicle outlet structural alterations

Box 86-2 Functional Classification of Urinary Incontinence

A. Impaired urine storage
  1. Detrusor dysfunction
    a. Hyperreflexia
    b. Increased tone
    c. Decreased elasticity
  2. Altered outflow resistance
    a. Incompetent sphincter
    b. Structural abnormalities

B. Impaired bladder emptying
  1. Detrusor dysfunction
    a. Hypotonicity
    b. Areflexia
  2. Increased outflow resistance
    a. Sphincter dyssynergia
    b. Structural abnormalities

Anatomic and functional classifications of the disorders of micturition, including incontinence, are provided in Boxes 86-1 and 86-2.

Patient Evaluation

History

A detailed history is essential in eliciting clues regarding onset and the site of pathologic involvement in disorders of micturition. The presence or absence of incontinence or change in urinary habits must be ascertained. Frequency, urgency, force of the urinary stream, urinary volume, pattern of incontinence, and associated discomfort are crucial aspects of the history. Questioning a child concerning these symptoms requires patience and imagination. Allowing the child to describe the urinary dysfunction, with particular emphasis on the sensations associated with urination and the procedures and sensations associated with initiating and terminating micturition, may be crucial to ascertaining the correct diagnosis. One should suspect children who void by the Valsalva or Credé maneuver. In infants, whether the infant has to strain to void, the number of diapers changed, and the interval between changes must be determined. Chronic genital dermatitis despite frequent diaper changes may indicate constant dribbling and a neurogenic bladder.

Intact afferent and efferent connections to the detrusor muscle are prerequisites for instigation of the desire to void. Lesions in the afferent pathways from the bladder result in an absence of the desire to void. Sensations of imminent micturition and of ongoing micturition indicate that the requisite sensory pathways are intact. Lesions of the efferent pathways to the bladder lead to a dysfunction of micturition in the presence of a normal desire to void. In this situation, structural obstruction to the flow of urine must be excluded.

In spinal cord lesions the level of injury determines the symptom complex. In lesions of the spinal cord at or below T10, the sensation of suprapubic fullness is generally preserved [Bauer, 1992]. If the lesion is rostral to T6, autonomic overactivity may be present and manifested by bradycardia, chills and diaphoresis, piloerection, paroxysmal hypertension, headache, and suffusion of the head and neck. This overactive autonomic response is the result of exaggerated reflex sympathetic activity in the isolated spinal cord. Plasma catecholamine concentrations are elevated, and peripheral sympathetic activity is increased.

Circumstances surrounding the initiation and termination of urination provide further evidence of the type of neural lesion involved. The abrupt urge to void, with resultant sudden micturition, signifies an incomplete suprasegmental lesion. When the lesion is complete, the patient has no warning and no sensation associated with reflex micturition. In peripheral motor lesions involving injury of S2 to S4 segments (conus medullaris lesions), bladder pressure must be increased with the use of the abdominal muscles, and/or the bladder must be manually compressed to effect voiding. In this instance, micturition may cease when the patient discontinues straining or applying pressure to the abdominal wall. In suprasegmental lesions a momentary, involuntary interruption of the urinary stream may occur. If the patient can volitionally interrupt and resume urination, the efferent pathway may be presumed to be intact.

Nocturnal enuresis is defined as persistent nighttime bedwetting beyond 5 years of age because 85% of children are urinary bladder continent by this age. Nocturnal enuresis has an uneven age and sex distribution; more boys than girls have this complaint at corresponding ages [Mattsson, 1994; Rushton, 1995]. Sleep polygraphic studies suggest immaturity of the central nervous system (CNS) inhibition of micturition reflex in sleep in enuretic children [Robert et al., 1993]. In a child who never achieved complete bladder control, the enuresis is said to be primary. Secondary enuresis is bedwetting after a dry period, indicating successful urinary bladder control. A few children, more females than males, exhibit daytime giggle micturition (enuresis risoria), which should be distinguished from stress incontinence [Elzinga-Plomp et al., 1995]. Diurnal or nocturnal enuresis occurring beyond the expected age of urinary control requires systematic evaluation. In enuretic children any associated impairment of sensory or motor function, particularly of the legs and perianal areas, should be carefully delineated because of the possibility of cord involvement.

When present, incontinence should be categorized. Frequency of urination, urgency with a need to rush to the bathroom, and urge incontinence (often accompanied by a squatting posture in girls) usually indicate an overactive bladder. The likely mechanism in this instance is uninhibited detrusor contractions during bladder filling. Infrequent voiding may be due to a hypocontractile and distended bladder. Weak urinary stream, difficulty in initiating urination, or necessity to strain during micturition should lead to a suspicion of overactive sphincter, dysfunctional voiding, and structural obstruction. Urge syndrome is the most common voiding dysfunction in children [Saedi and Schulman, 2003]. *Overflow incontinence,* relatively rare in childhood, may accompany involvement of central or peripheral motor mechanisms. Loss of urine when lifting objects, coughing, or walking indicates *stress incontinence,* which may result from a peripheral motor lesion compromising either the detrusor muscle or the muscles of the pelvic floor. Abrupt, uncontrolled voiding is associated with neurologic lesions, such as those involving the cerebral hemispheres or the suprasegmental areas of the spinal cord.

Neurologic Examination

The classic neurologic conceptualization of disease resulting from either upper or lower motor neuron unit involvement is inadequate for evaluating problems of micturition. Effects of CNS lesions vary widely because these lesions, depending on location, have significant inhibitory or facilitatory influences on micturition. Other confounding factors associated with these lesions are chronic infection and bladder distention, which lead to alterations in detrusor muscle contractility and neuronal excitability; these changes must be differentiated from primary neurologic conditions.

Uninhibited neurogenic bladder may occur with bilateral involvement of the medial frontal lobe areas (e.g., superior sagittal sinus thrombosis). Frequency and urgency of urination are increased; bladder sensation is preserved. As the bladder fills, the detrusor contracts and increases intravesical pressure. The bladder may become so contracted that a minute quantity of urine induces micturition. Ultimately, automatic micturition develops [Saper, 1995]. Suprasegmental lesions of the spinal cord above the lumbar segments are accompanied by urgency, incontinence, increased frequency, and nocturia.

The neurologic examination should be directed at excluding focal or progressive spinal cord lesions. The cutaneous area over the spine should be scrutinized for midline abnormalities that may indicate underlying congenital malformations. The spine should be evaluated for tenderness and scoliosis. Skeletal muscle spasticity, hyperreflexia, clonus, and extensor toe signs accompany suprasegmental lesions. Muscle atrophy, muscle weakness, and decreased or absent deep-tendon reflexes accompany lower motor neuron unit lesions originating in the lumbosacral cord; associated sensory changes are often evident. Syndromes of the epiconus, conus medullaris, and cauda equina are distinguishable by clinical findings and are summarized in Table 86-1 [Wright, 1982].

When the epiconus (L4, L5, S1, and S2) is involved, profound motor involvement of the lower legs and feet occurs [Saper, 1995]. External rotation and dorsiflexion of the thigh are most affected. Abduction at the hip, flexion at the knee, and flexion and extension at the ankle are also involved. The Achilles tendon reflex is absent.

When the conus medullaris (S3 to Coc1) is involved (conus syndrome), paralytic bladder incontinence and, usually, bladder distention occur [Bauer, 1992; Saper, 1995]. Bowel incontinence is also present. There is loss of perianal sensation consonant with impairment of the lower sacral (S3 and S4) and coccygeal cord segments. Rectal sphincter reflex (anal wink) is absent, and denervation of the voluntary anal sphincter causes loss of anal sphincter tone. No motor abnormalities of the legs and feet occur. The Achilles tendon reflex is uninvolved. In a study of traumatic conus lesions, the prognosis was somewhat better than has been widely appreciated [Taylor and Coolican, 1988]. In the cauda equina syndrome, there is involvement of nerve roots from spinal segments L3 to Coc1. It may be difficult to distinguish cauda equina from conus lesions. All forms of sensibility are involved. Spontaneous pain, especially in the perineum over the sacrum and bladder, may dominate the clinical pattern [Saper, 1995]. Peroneal weakness, including footdrop, may occur. Fibrillary twitching in affected muscles is common. When preferential interruption of motor innervation occurs, detrusor contraction is greatly compromised, although bladder sensation is preserved (motor paralytic bladder).

Clinical Laboratory Tests

Studies are chosen to clarify the nature of the bladder dysfunction [Borzyskowski, 1996]. Urinalysis and urine

TABLE 86-1

Differentiating Features of Lower Spinal Cord Lesions

	EPICONUS L4-S2	CONUS MEDULLARIS S3-Coc1	CAUDA EQUINA L3-Coc1 ROOTS
Onset	Variable	Usually sudden and bilateral	Usually gradual and unilateral
Motor	Considerable motor dysfunction in the lower extremities (see text for details)	Usually mild, symmetric motor dysfunction; fasciculations may be present	Asymmetric, marked motor dysfunction; fasciculation uncommon
Sensory	Disturbances in L4-S2 segments	Bilateral, symmetric saddle distribution; dissociation of sensory loss may be present	Asymmetric, saddle distribution; may be unilateral; no dissociation of sensation
Reflexes	Achilles tendon reflex absent	Achilles tendon reflex may be diminished	Patellar and Achilles tendon reflexes may be absent
Bladder and rectal symptoms	Small, contracted "spastic" bladder, loss of voluntary control with incontinence	Paralytic, distended bladder and patulous anus, incontinence	Paralytic, distended bladder and patulous anus, incontinence; involvement late and less severe
Pain	Variable	Absent or symmetric bilateral mild pain in perineum or thighs	Radicular pain; asymmetric, unilateral pain that may be severe and prominent

culture, blood urea nitrogen, and serum creatinine are necessary studies. Results of these tests may indicate primary renal or other non-neurologic conditions. Ultrasonography of the kidneys and bladder has been of great value in rapidly assessing structural changes. In one series of children studied with ultrasonography, 32% of 74 children with voiding problems had one or more of the following: thickened detrusor muscle; large bladder capacity with or without residual urine; fecal impaction; suspected bladder neck obstruction, which later required internal urethrotomy; or small bladder capacity [Maizels et al., 1987]. A wide bladder neck anomaly has been recognized as a common cause of incontinence in children [Murray et al., 1987]. Abnormal cystic masses, bladder diverticula, and other structural abnormalities may be recognized; however, interpretation may occasionally be difficult and lead to erroneous diagnoses [Vick et al., 1983].

Urodynamic study of the free-flow curve provides valuable data without invasive instrumentation or an extensive urodynamic study. If the free-flow curve is normal and there is no residual urine, a significant voiding abnormality, whether functional or anatomic in origin, is unlikely [Griffiths and Scholtmeijer, 1984]. Study methods particularly adapted to children and norms for children have been developed [Di Scipio et al., 1986; Pompino and Hoffmann, 1983]. Video urodynamic studies of children with grossly intact neurologic function often reveal detrusor dysfunction and abnormal sphincter activity [Webster et al., 1984]. Computer-monitored voiding studies can provide useful information concerning detrusor muscle function and allow categorization of the dysfunction [van Mastrigt and Griffiths, 1986]. Urodynamic evaluation and follow-up care are important in the diagnosis and optimal management of many children with micturition problems [Churchill et al., 1987].

Plain radiographs of the lumbosacral area, intravenous pyelography, and a voiding cystourethrogram all provide further information. Bladder prolapse, with the bladder neck situated below the upper margin of the pubic symphysis, has been described as a urographic radiologic sign of urethral sphincter denervation in children with myelodysplasia [Zerin et al., 1990]. Conventional invasive urologic examinations, now less commonly required because of modern imaging techniques, should be performed when other examinations have not provided sufficient data [Ewalt and Bauer, 1996; Walther and Kaplan, 1979].

Detrusor muscle function can be evaluated by cystometry if other methods are insufficient. A slow-fill cystometrogram triggers bladder contraction after dilatation with instilled fluid. Detrusor tone, reflex threshold, sensation, and volitional ability to inhibit detrusor contraction can be assessed. Reflex abnormalities of the detrusor (i.e., hyperreflexia, hyporeflexia, or areflexia) may be documented [Bauer, 1992; Rushton, 1995]. Voiding cystourethrography and other radiologic techniques provide useful additional information [Bisset et al., 1987; Lebowitz, 1985].

Although infrequently performed, percutaneous stimulation of the sacral roots can be performed, in conjunction with transducer placement in the bladder, to monitor peripheral reflex pathways. Intact preganglionic pathways to the bladder are necessary for optimal detrusor response after percutaneous stimulation. Currently, sacral-evoked responses are used to evaluate these pathways, typically by determining the latency of the bulbocavernosus reflex [Vodusek, 1996; Wein and Barrett, 1992].

Testing of the postganglionic pathways is more complex. The effect of percutaneous stimulation is assessed, as well as the detrusor contraction in response to direct electrical stimulation applied through a cystoscope and the intravesical pressure response to bethanechol chloride [Chai and Steers, 1996; Ewalt and Bauer, 1996; Wein and Barrett, 1992]. Muted or absent response to percutaneous and direct electrical stimulation and denervation hypersensitivity to bethanechol suggest impaired postganglionic pathways. Lack of a con-

Box 86-3 Selected Differential Diagnosis of Neurologically Induced Disorders of Micturition and Defecation

Congenital malformations
- Caudal regression syndrome
- Diastematomyelia
- Diplomyelia
- Hydromyelia
- Myelodysplasia
- Myelomeningocele
- Sacral agenesis
- Spondylosis
- Syringobulbia
- Syringomyelia
- Tethered cord

Infectious and inflammatory conditions
- Acute disseminated encephalomyelitis (postvaccinal, postinfectious)
- Adhesive arachnoiditis of the spinal cord
- Anterior horn cell infection (e.g., coxsackie, poliomyelitis)
- Guillain-Barré syndrome
- Herpes zoster
- Suppurative infection of the spine with extension to the cord (e.g., tuberculosis)
- Transverse myelitis

Vascular conditions
- Anterior spinal artery occlusion or hemorrhage
- Hematomyelia
- Sagittal sinus thrombosis
- Spinal cord arteriovenous malformation
- Spinal cord epidural hemorrhage

Metabolic conditions
- Diabetes mellitus

Traumatic conditions
- Birth injury (e.g., spinal cord traction)
- Spinal anesthesia complications
- Spinal cord injury (e.g., crush injury, stab injury)
- Vertebral fracture or dislocation with spinal cord disruption

Tumors
- Cauda equina tumor (e.g., teratoma, lipoma)
- Cerebral tumors (e.g., parasagittal meningioma)
- Sacrococcygeal mass (e.g., teratoma, lipoma, dermoid)
- Spinal cord tumor (e.g., ependymoma, lymphoma)

Demyelinating diseases
- Devic's disease
- Multiple sclerosis

tractile response to direct stimulation and lack of denervation hypersensitivity may indicate myopathic detrusor changes, which result from bladder overdistention or infection.

Patient Evaluation

Differential Diagnosis

Nocturnal enuresis is the most common disorder of micturition in childhood. Neurologic disease must be excluded in any child who either does not develop or subsequently loses urinary continence. Box 86-3 presents a list of differential diagnoses in disorders of micturition. Several dysfunctional voiding syndromes without associated neurologic dysfunction (non-neurogenic voiding disorders) have been described and respond to a variety of therapeutic interventions [Homsy, 1994; Jayanthi et al., 1997; Yang and Mayo, 1997]. Chronic constipation may sometimes be associated with urinary incontinence in children [Loening-Baucke, 1997].

Management

Individuals with impaired bladder and bowel control report a low self-concept and low self-esteem with lower perceived quality of life on several domains and have greater difficulty in creating new social relationships [Hicken et al., 2001; Moore et al., 2004]. Precise diagnosis is required for a systematic and effective therapeutic approach. Neurogenic bladder dysfunction must be countermanded so that urinary control and normal renal function are allowed to continue [Chandra, 1995]. The goals of treatment are to preserve renal function, prevent urinary infection, and promote urinary continence in older children [Fernandes et al., 1994]. Optimal neurogenic therapy prevents infections (Table 86-2). Patients require regular monitoring. Medications commonly employed in treating bladder dysfunction are listed in Table 86-2.

Hyperreflexic bladder, the result of impairment of suprasegmental governance of the detrusor muscle, is associated with increased resting bladder tone, uncontrollable bladder contraction with incontinence, frequency and urgency of urination, and diminished bladder volume. Therapeutic measures are directed at these cardinal features [Chua et al., 1996; Sakakibara et al., 1996; Wyndaele, 1995].

Administration of anticholinergic drugs decreases contractility. Therapy with propantheline bromide is often effective. Oxybutynin may be used in some children [Kaplinski et al., 1996; Mizunaga et al., 1994; Palmer et al., 1997]. Trials with new anticholinergic agents demonstrate promise [Hehir and Fitzpatrick, 1985; Mazur et al., 1995; Otto-Unger, 1985]. Unfortunately, anticholinergic therapy may be associated with urinary retention and an increase in residual urine; therefore residual urine volume should be estimated and urinary output monitored. Intermittent catheterization may prove necessary if retention occurs [Cass et al., 1984]. Credé's or Valsalva's maneuver may sometimes be sufficient to completely empty the bladder [Bauer, 1992]. Renal rupture after the Credé maneuver has been described [Reinberg et al., 1994].

Drugs that augment the noradrenergic system appear to facilitate continence; in addition, drugs that depress or block dopamine activity may produce urinary incontinence. Dopamine agonists and specific catecholamine agents may prove valuable in managing urinary incontinence [Ambrosini, 1984].

A sympathomimetic agent is used if detrusor muscle hypertonicity rather than uninhibited detrusor reflex contractions exists. Management is usually initiated with imipramine hydrochloride. The child (and parents) should be instructed concerning the features of urinary retention. Difficulty in initiating micturition; failing to completely empty the bladder, which leads to urinary retention; and dribbling incontinence are characteristic of detrusor hyporeflexia or areflexia. Bladder capacity is usually significantly increased. Management in this instance is directed toward increasing effective intravesicular pressure and decreasing bladder outlet resistance. Credé's or Valsalva's maneuver, as well as intermittent catheterization, may be used to empty the bladder. Cholinergic stimulation (e.g., with bethanechol chloride) should be used with caution because it may aggravate urinary dysfunction in such patients.

Neurogenic bladder outlet obstruction may respond to alpha-adrenergic blocking agents. Alpha-blocker therapy with doxazosin also has been used succesfully to reduce postvoid residual urine volume in children with complex neuropathic and non-neuropathic voiding dysfunction [Cain

TABLE 86-2

Drugs Used in Neurogenic Bladder Dysfunction

BLADDER DYSFUNCTION	DRUG	ACTION	USUAL MINIMUM DOSE PER DAY (mg/kg)	USUAL MAXIMUM DOSE PER DAY (mg/kg)
Impaired Urine Storage				
Decreased bladder capacity	Propantheline	Anticholinergic	1	2
	Oxybutynin	Anticholinergic	0.4	0.8
	Flavoxate	Direct muscle action	6	9
	Dicyclomine	Anticholinergic	1	2
	Terodiline	Calcium antagonist	12.5	25 mg/day
Decreased outflow resistance	Phenylpropranolol	Sympathomimetic	5	7.5
	Ephedrine	Sympathomimetic	1	3
	Imipramine	Complex	1.4	2.4
Impaired Bladder Emptying				
Increased bladder capacity	Bethanechol	Cholinergic	2	3
Increased outflow resistance	Phenoxybenzamine	Sympatholytic	0.6	1.5
	Dantrolene	Direct muscle action	1	8 to 10

Modified from Bauer, 1992.

et al., 2003]. The phentolamine test can be used to predict which patients are likely to benefit from phenoxybenzamine therapy [Smey et al., 1980]. Use of oral baclofen may be of limited benefit in a few patients. It probably relaxes the external sphincter and may be used as an adjunct. Intravesical medications may be used in children who either cannot tolerate or have poor and inadequate response to oral therapy [Greenfield and Fera, 1991; Kato et al., 1991]. Intrathecal baclofen has also been used [Frost et al., 1989]. Botulinum A toxin injection into the external urethral sphincter has been used for the treatment of detrusor-sphincter dyssynergia in patients with spinal cord injury [Schurch et al., 1997]. Newer drugs with both anticholinergic and calcium antagonist properties, such as terodiline, are being used in children [Langtry and McTavish, 1990]. An understanding of the role of serotonin (5-HT_4) receptors in urinary bladder function may also lead to the development of newer drugs [Hegde and Eglen, 1996].

Functional bladder-sphincter dyssynergia may be successfully treated by using electromyographic biofeedback with exercises, which consist of alternate tensing and relaxing lower pelvic muscles [Libo et al., 1983]. Other biofeedback training programs have also been effective in managing children with probable non-neurogenic bladder disturbances [Hellström et al., 1987; Jerkins et al., 1987].

Mechanical compression (Credé's or Valsalva's maneuver), intermittent self-catheterization [Bauer, 1992; Cass et al., 1984; Chai et al., 1995], and various surgical techniques may be of value. Clean, intermittent catheterization has been widely used in children, but its use and effectiveness in infants have only recently been recognized. Early implementation of this method helps preserve renal function, especially in children with myelodysplasia. It may be used in combination with anticholinergic drugs in infants [Baskin et al., 1990; Joseph et al., 1989; Lapides et al., 1972]. Surgical techniques include transurethral incision of the external urethral sphincter, urinary stream diversion operations, implantation of an artificial urinary sphincter [Khoury and Churchill, 1987; Light, 1985; Simeoni et al., 1996], bladder augmentation [Krishna et al., 1995], bladder replacement [Hensle and Burbige, 1985; King et al., 1987], free autogenous muscle transplantation [Hakelius et al., 1984], and differential sacral nerve root rhizotomy and electrical stimulation [Sindou et al., 1994; Tanagho et al., 1989]. Nonsurgical therapies should be exhausted before surgical therapy is undertaken. Early intervention may sometimes be necessary to preserve normal function or avoid progressive dysfunction, especially in children with spinal dysraphism [Bauer, 1992; Keating et al., 1988].

Several incontinent products are available for use in children with urinary incontinence. [Sanders, 2002]

DISORDERS OF DEFECATION

Defecation is the conscious act of emptying the bowel, and continence is the ability to control defecation voluntarily. Fecal soiling is the presence of stool in the underwear independent of whether an organic or anatomic lesion is present. Fecal incontinence is fecal soiling when there is an organic or anatomic lesion such as meningomyelocele or other neuromuscular disorders, anal malformations, anal surgery, or traumatic lesions [Loening-Baucke, 1996]. Reflex neuromuscular mechanisms and the anatomy of the rectum, anus, and sphincters contribute to anal continence in a normal child. Bowel control usually precedes bladder control in children [Perlmutter, 1985]. Conscious bowel control is achieved at 28 months of age on average [Brazelton, 1962]. Toilet training is a complex multistep process as mentioned in the preceding discussion.

Anatomy and Embryology

The rectum and anal canal are derived from the primitive anorectal canal and originate from entoderm and ectoderm, respectively. The muscular anal sphincters are mesodermal in origin. The pelvic diaphragm, formed by the levator ani muscles, demarcates the anal canal from the rectum. The anal canal proceeds dorsocaudally through the levator ani muscles to the anus and is surrounded by the internal and external anal sphincters. The ringlike internal anal sphincter is a thickening of the circular muscle of the rectum. The external anal sphincter, which envelops the internal sphincter, is elliptic in outline and is divided into three portions. The deep division is separated from the internal sphincter by strands of the longitudinal coat, whose fibers also interdigitate partially with those of the levator ani. The superficial division is the principal part. It is attached to the coccyx dorsally and to the central tendon ventrally. The subcutaneous division surrounds the anus and has no bony attachments.

The course of the rectum is aligned at an approximate 90-degree angle to the axis of the anal canal. The sharp angular bend favors anal continence. The pelvic floor is formed from the levator ani muscles, which elevate the anorectal junction and thrust it anteriorly during contraction. The resultant straightening of the path between the anal canal and rectum facilitates defecation. Fecal continence is the result of the interrelationships among the two anal sphincters and the levator ani muscles [Rao, 1996, 1997].

Nerve Supply

In a simplistic sense, the sympathetic nervous system modulates rectal filling, and the parasympathetic system controls bowel emptying. Activation of the parasympathetic system results in contraction of the sigmoid and rectal smooth muscles with concomitant relaxation of the internal sphincter. Activation of the sympathetic system causes the reverse pattern—relaxation of the sigmoid and rectum and contractions of the internal sphincter [Rao, 1996, 1997].

Innervation of the rectum parallels that of the bladder; the previous discussion of bladder neuroanatomy should be reviewed for further information. Pudendal nucleus cells (S2 to S4) are located in the region of parasympathetic nerve cells, give rise to the pudendal nerve, and innervate the external anal sphincter. Sympathetic innervation is derived primarily from L1 and L2 through the hypogastric plexus and innervates the internal anal sphincter.

The anal canal contains numerous sensory nerve endings. Light touch, pain, and temperature sensations are transmitted to the sacral cord through the pudendal nerves, where they are distributed through conventional sensory pathways and also participate in path 3, which was described in the discussion on bladder innervation.

The neural circuitry for defecation is complex. Some afferent impulses travel through the pudendal nerve to the spinal cord and then ascend to the cerebrum, which exerts voluntary control. Motor impulses (efferent) arising in the cerebrum descend by way of the lateral columns and reach the T6 to T12 motor neurons and initiate abdominal muscle contraction. This contraction increases intra-abdominal pressure and secondarily exerts pressure on the rectum.

Distention of the rectal ampulla causes the sensation of fullness in the perineum. Increasing distention causes awareness that defecation is imminent. Sensory information is also provided by the numerous free endings and by the extensive myenteric plexus in the rectum. Pararectal nerve stimulation and stretching of the sensory nerve endings in the levator ani muscles (especially the puborectalis muscle) may also contribute to the urge to defecate.

In the initial (involuntary) phase of defecation, fecal material reaches the rectum as a result of the peristaltic movement originating in the sigmoid colon. The elevation in rectal pressure, which results from fecal matter pushing against the anorectal ring (puborectalis muscle), results in the urge to defecate. The next phase consists of volitional contraction of the abdominal muscles, followed by an increase in abdominal pressure and simultaneous relaxation of rectal sphincters, causing defecation.

Interaction of tone and reflex activity is essential in the physiology of continence. Reflex and voluntary contractions of the puborectalis muscle and internal and external sphincters are important components of continence during sleep and waking. Because of the intricate relationship of the sphincters, determining their contribution to maintenance of resting pressure is difficult; however, the resting pressure appears primarily to be the result of contraction of the internal sphincter [Pemberton and Kelly, 1986].

Incontinence occurs when the pressure induced by the peristaltic movement in the distal rectum overcomes the anorectal pressure. There are three types of incontinence—true incontinence, partial incontinence, and overflow incontinence [Wright, 1982]. Deficient anorectal muscles (e.g., imperforate anus) or impaired neuromuscular function results in true incontinence. There may be insufficient anorectal pressure or impaired sensation of peristaltic movement and bowel distention. Fecal soiling is the result of partial incontinence because the final stage of defecation is inadequate and is followed by continuing passage of small amounts of stool. Overflow incontinence, not a true form of incontinence, results from chronic fecal impaction and leakage of liquid feces through the dilated anorectal ring.

Patient Evaluation

History

Fecal incontinence is the usual complaint of patients seeking help. It is essential to determine whether bowel control was lost after it had been achieved or whether bowel control was never present. The age at onset, frequency, related circumstances (e.g., time of day, association with sleep, behavioral aspects), and alterations in bowel habits, stool mass, stool color, and stool consistency should be established. Overall integrity of afferent and efferent pathways may be evaluated by further questioning. Inquiries should be designed to ascertain whether rectal sensation, including pressure of fecal volume and need to defecate, as well as the ability to differentiate between passage of flatus and feces, is present. Similarly, efferent function can be evaluated by questions related to volitional inhibition of defecation. Fecal incontinence is unlikely to be due to spinal cord disease in the absence of urinary symptoms or neurologic abnormalities in the lower limbs.

Neurologic Examination

Because the neural pathways are similar, neurologic evaluation of bowel incontinence parallels that described for disorders of micturition.

In lesions above the sacral cord (suprasegmental lesions), voluntary control over the sphincter ani is lost. Sphincter tone is increased, and fecal retention occurs, leading to chronic fecal impaction and consequent soiling. During rectal examination the patient should be able to contract and relax the sphincter on request. Sphincter tone is often increased and contracted with suprasegmental lesions [Wright, 1982]. Paralysis of the sphincter ani accompanies sacral cord disturbance. The anus is patulous, the anal sphincter reflex is lacking, and the patient is unable to contract the sphincter on command. In contrast with bladder function, the extent of preservation or return of anal and rectal sensation in conus medullaris lesions is important in achieving bowel control. The involuntary passage of flatus is a distressing symptom in such patients if they cannot distinguish it from feces for which sensory input is essential [Taylor and Coolican, 1988]. Further information on the examination of the patient with lower cord and cauda equina lesions can be found in the section on urinary incontinence.

Clinical Laboratory Tests

Proctoscopy and fiberoptic studies of the lower bowel are efficient methods of excluding the presence of structural abnormalities. Barium enema studies are sometimes necessary as are defecography studies, which visually monitor the functional events during defecation [Mezwa et al., 1993].

Special studies include anal sphincter electromyography [Lewis and Rudolph, 1997; Rao, 1996, 1997; Shafik, 1992]. Denervation potentials indicate a recent lower motor neuron process. Pudendal nerve terminal motor latency is especially useful when neuropathy is suspected. Overall electrodiagnostic studies are helpful in the evaluation of fecal incontinence, although less so in very young children [Cheong et al., 1995]. A manometric study may also be useful [Rao, 1996]. The correlation between the clinical findings and the manometric assessment of sphincters in response to rectal distention has often been thought to be poor; recent re-evaluation suggests otherwise [Rao and Patel, 1997]. Computed tomography allows imaging of the puborectal muscle and external sphincters and identification of associated anomalies [Ikawa et al., 1985; Kohda et al., 1985]. Sacral ratios less than 0.52 correlate well with spinal cord anomalies and with unfavorable prognosis in children with anorectal malformations. Sacral ratio is determined by dividing the distance from the lowest point of the sacrum (or of the coccyx, if present) to the line joining the two posterior iliac spines by the distance from that latter line to the line joining the upper limits of the iliac crests [Torre et al., 2001].

Differential Diagnosis

Bowel dysfunction is produced by the conditions listed in Box 86-3. Lumbosacral defects may be associated with reduced or absent external sphincter function, which is demonstrated by sphincter electromyography. Denervation potentials or reduced large-amplitude potentials may be observed. In Hirschsprung's disease, manometric studies demonstrate an absence of the rectoanal inhibitory reflex; that is, the internal sphincter fails to relax in response to a transient rectal distention. The relaxation wave is absent.

The most common cause of bowel incontinence is encopresis, which is not associated with neurologic dysfunction. Encopresis is fecal incontinence without organic cause for more than a month in children 4 years of age or older. Males outnumber females 3.5 to 1 [Bellman, 1966]. The cardinal feature of encopresis is withholding of stools: This condition is often not recognized by parents. Neurogenic and other organic conditions causing bowel dysfunction must be excluded [Loening-Baucke, 1996; Nolan and Oberklaid, 1993].

Management

Assessment of contributing factors, including psychosocial milieu, anorectal examination, and appropriate neurologic evaluation, is necessary for adequate management. Therapeutic approaches include dietary, behavioral, pharmacologic, and surgical methods [Wald, 1986]. Education is important in achieving good outcome [King et al., 1994].

Dietary measures to harden stools may be attempted for some patients. The stools can then be evacuated by manual pressure over the abdomen and by straining of the abdominal muscles. Some children may perceive the urge to defecate when the stools are bulkier, which can be achieved by using stool-bulking agents (e.g., Metamucil). High-fiber diet may be appropriate in some cases. Rectal suppositories (bisacodyl) or a saline enema may empty the rectum before it fills and cause reflex relaxation of the internal sphincter. This approach may prevent soiling in some children. Excessive flatus and soiling may also be controlled by avoiding certain foods, such as legumes, and by giving attention to strict dietary and bowel habits. Antegrade colonic enemas have been used in children who have failed usual medical treatment [Griffiths and Malone, 1995; Squire et al., 1993].

Biofeedback training [Owen-Smith and Chesterfield, 1986], behavior modification [Whitehead et al., 1986], muscle training, and medications are often beneficial [Scharli, 1987]. New devices to control both fecal and urinary incontinence have shown promise [Numanoglu, 1987]. Surgical intervention may be considered if conservative treatment fails [Bass and Yazbeck, 1987; Chen and Zhang, 1987; Kottmeier et al., 1986; Peña, 1994]. Artificial anal sphincter, gracilis muscle transposition, and dynamic graciloplasty have also been used with good outcome in children who fail medical management [Baeten et al., 1995; Han et al., 1995; Wong et al., 1996].

REFERENCES

Ambrosini PJ. A pharmacological paradigm for urinary incontinence and enuresis. J Clin Psychopharmacol 1984;4:247.

Baeten CGMI, Geerdes BP, Adang EMM, et al. Anal dynamic graciloplasty in the treatment of intractable fecal incontinence. N Engl J Med 1995;332:1600.

Baskin LS, Kogan BA, Benard F. Treatment of infants with neurogenic bladder dysfunction using anticholinergic drugs and intermittent catheterization. Br J Urol 1990;66:532.

Bass J, Yazbeck S. Reoperation by anterior perineal approach for missed puborectalis. J Pediatr Surg 1987;22:761.

Bauer SB. Neuropathology of the lower urinary tract. In: Kelalis PP, King LR, Belman AB, eds. Clinical pediatric urology, 3rd ed. Philadelphia: WB Saunders, 1992.

Bellman M. Studies in encopresis. Acta Paediatr Scand 1966;170 (Suppl):1.

Bisset GS III, Strife JL, Dunbar JS. Urography and voiding cystourethrography. Findings in girls with urinary tract infection. Am J Roentgenol 1987;148:479.

Borzyskowski M. An update on the investigation of the child with a neuropathic bladder. Dev Med Child Neurol 1996;38:744.

Bradley WE. Physiology of the urinary bladder. In: Walsh PC, Gittes BF, Perlmutter AD, et al., eds. Campbell's urology. Philadelphia: WB Saunders, 1986.

Brazelton TB. A child oriented approach to toilet training. Pediatrics 1962;29:121.

Cain MP, Wu SD, Austin PF, et al. Alpha blocker therapy for children with dysfunctional voiding and urinary retention. J Urol 2003;170:1514.

Carpenter MB, Sutin J. Human neuroanatomy. Baltimore: Williams & Wilkins, 1983.

Cass AS, Luxenberg M, Gleich P, et al. Clean intermittent catheterization in the management of the neurogenic bladder in children. J Urol 1984;132:526.

Chai T, Chung AK, Belville WD, et al. Compliance and complications of clean intermittent catheterization in the spinal cord injured patient. Paraplegia 1995;33:161.

Chai TC, Steers WD. Neurophysiology of micturition and continence. Urol Clin North Am 1996;23:221.

Chandra M. Reflux nephropathy, urinary tract infection, and voiding disorders. Curr Opin Pediatr 1995;7:164.

Chen YL, Zhang XH. Reconstruction of rectal sphincter by transposition of gluteus muscle for fecal incontinence. J Pediatr Surg 1987;22:62.

Cheong DMO, Vaccaro CA, Salanga VD, et al. Electrodiagnostic evaluation of fecal incontinence. Muscle Nerve 1995;18:612.

Chua HC, Tow A, Tan ES. The neurogenic bladder in spinal cord injury: Pattern and management. Ann Acad Med Singapore 1996;25:553.

Churchill BM, Gilmour RF, Williot P. Urodynamics. Pediatr Clin North Am 1987;34:1133.

Di Scipio WJ, Smey P, Kogan SJ, et al. Impromptu micturitional flow parameters in normal boys. J Urol 1986;136:1049.

Dorschner W, Stolzenburg JU, Leutert G. A new theory of micturition and urinary continence based on histomorphological studies. Urol Int 1994;52:61.

Elbadawi A. Functional anatomy of the organs of micturition. Urol Clin North Am 1996;23:177.

Elzinga-Plomp A, Boemers TML, Messer AP, et al. Treatment of enuresis risoria in children by self-administered electric and imaginary shock. Br J Urol 1995;76:775.

Ewalt DH, Bauer SB. Pediatric neurourology. Urol Clin North Am 1996;23:501.

Fernandes ET, Reinberg Y, Vernier R, et al. Neurogenic bladder dysfunction in children: Review of pathophysiology and current management. J Pediatr 1994;124:1.

Fidas A, Elton RA, McInnes A, et al. Neurophysiological measurement of the voiding reflex arcs in patients with functional disorders of the lower urinary tract. Br J Urol 1987;60:205.

Frost F, Nanninga J, Penn R, et al. Intrathecal baclofen infusion effect on bladder management programs in patients with myelopathy. Am J Phys Med Rehabil 1989;68:112.

Greenfield SP, Fera M. The use of intravesical oxybutynin chloride in children with neurogenic bladder. J Urol 1991;146:532.

Griffiths DJ, Scholtmeijer RJ. Place of the free flow curve in the urodynamic investigation of children. Br J Urol 1984;56:474.

Griffiths DM, Malone PS. The Malone antegrade continence enema. J Pediatr Surg 1995;30:68.
Hakelius L, Gierup J, Grotte G. Urinary incontinence in children. Treatment with free autogenous muscle transplantation. Prog Pediatr Surg 1984;17:155.
Haldeman S, Bradley WE, Bhatia NN, et al. Pudendal somatosensory evoked potentials. Arch Neurol 1982a;39:280.
Haldeman S, Bradley WE, Bhatia NN, et al. Evoked responses from pudendal nerve. J Urol 1982b;128:974.
Han SJ, Park HJ, Kmi CB, et al. Long-term follow-up of gracilis muscle transposition in children. Yonsei Med J 1995;36:372.
Hegde SS, Eglen RM. Peripheral 5-HT_4 receptors. FASEB J 1996;1398.
Hehir M, Fitzpatrick JM. Oxybutynin and the prevention of urinary incontinence in Spina Bifida. Eur Urol 1985;11:254.
Hellström A, Hanson E, Hansson S, et al. Micturition habits and incontinence at age 17 reinvestigation of a cohort studies at age 7. Br J Urol 1995;76:231.
Hellström AL, Hjalmask K, Jodal U. Rehabilitation of the dysfunctional bladder in children: method and 3-year follow up. J Urol 1987;138:847.
Hensle TW, Burbige KA. Bladder replacement in children and young adults. J Urol 1985;133:1004.
Hicken BL, Putzke JD, Richards JS, Bladder management and quality of life after spinal cord injury. Am J Phys Med Rehabil 2001;80:916.
Himsel KK, Hurwitz RS. Pediatric urinary incontinence. Urol Clin North Am 1991;18:283.
Hinman F. Syndromes of vesical incoordination. Urol Clin North Am 1980;7:311.
Homsy YL. Dysfunctional voiding syndromes and vesicoureteral reflux. Pediatr Nephrol 1994;8:116.
Ikawa H, Yokoyama J, Sanbonmatsu T, et al. The use of computerized tomography to evaluate anorectal anomalies. J Pediatr Surg 1985;20:640.
Jayanthi VR, Khoury AE, McLorie GA, et al. The nonneurogenic neurogenic bladder of early infancy. J Urol 1997;158:1281.
Jerkins GR, Noe HN, Vaughn WR, et al. Biofeedback training for children with bladder sphincter incoordination. J Urol 1987;138:1113.
Joseph DB, Bauer SB, Colodny AH, et al. Clean, intermittent catheterization of infants with neurogenic bladder. Pediatrics 1989;84:78.
Kaplinsky R, Greenfield S, Wan J, et al. Expanded follow-up of intravesical oxybutynin chloride use in children with neurogenic bladder. J Urol 1996;156:753.
Kato K, Kondo A, Saito M, et al. In vitro intravesical instillation of anticholinergic, antispasmodic and calcium blocking agents to decrease bladder contractility. Urol Int 1991;47(Suppl 1):36.
Keating MA, Rink RC, Bauer SB, et al. Neurological implications of the changing approach in management of occult spinal lesions. J Urol 1988;140:1299.
Khoury AE, Churchill BM. The artificial urinary sphincter. Pediatr Clin North Am 1987;34:1175.
King JC, Currie DM, Wright E. Bowel training in spina bifida: Importance of education, patient compliance, age, and anal reflexes. Arch Phys Med Rehabil 1994;5:243.
King LR, Webster GD, Bertram RA. Experiences with bladder reconstruction in children. J Urol 1987;138:1002.
Kohda E, Fujioka M, Ikawa H, et al. Congenital anorectal anomaly. CT evaluation. Radiology 1985;157:349.
Kottmeier PK, Velcek FT, Klotz DH, et al. Results of levatorplasty for anal incontinence. J Pediatr Surg 1986;21:647.
Krishna A, Gough DCS, Fishwick J, et al. Ileocystoplasty in children: Assessing safety and success. Eur Urol 1995;27:62.
Langtry HD, McTavish D. Terodiline. A review of its pharmacological properties and therapeutic use in the treatment of urinary incontinence. Drugs 1990;40:748.
Lapides J, Diokno AC, Silber SJ, et al. Clean, intermittent self catheterization in the treatment of urinary tract disease. J Urol 1972;107:458.
Lebowitz RL. Pediatric uroradiology. Pediatr Clin North Am 1985;32:1353.
Lewis G, Rudolph CD. Practical approach to defecation disorders in children. Pediatr Ann 1997;26:260.
Libo LM, Arnold GE, Woodside JR, et al. EMG biofeedback for functional bladder-sphincter dyssynergia. A case study. Biofeedback Self Regul 1983;8:243.
Light JK. The artificial urinary sphincter in children. Experience with AS800 series and bowel reconstruction. Urol Clin North Am 1985;12:103.
Loening-Baucke V. Encopresis and soiling. Pediatr Clin North Am 1996;43:279.
Loening-Baucke V. Urinary incontinence and urinary tract infection and their resolution with treatment of chronic constipation of childhood. Pediatrics 1997;100:228.
Maizels M, Zaontz MR, Houlihan DL, et al. In-office ultrasonography to image the kidneys and bladder of children. J Urol 1987;138:1031.
Manente G, Melchionda D, Uncini A. Urinary retention in bilateral pontine tumour: Evidence for a pontine micturition center in humans. J Neurol Neurosurg Psychiatry 1996;61:528.
Mattsson S. Urinary incontinence and nocturia in healthy schoolchildren. Acta Paediatr 1994;83:950.
Mazur D, Wehnert J, Dorschner W, et al. Clinical and urodynamic effects of propiverine in patients suffering from urgency and urge incontinence. Scand J Urol Nephrol 1995;29:289.
Mezwa DG, Feczko PJ, Bosanko C. Radiologic evaluation of constipation and anorectal disorders. Radiol Clin North Am 1993;31:1375.
Mizunaga M, Miyata M, Kaneko S, et al. Intravesical instillation of oxybutynin hydrochloride therapy for patients with a neuropathic bladder. Paraplegia 1994;32:25.
Moore C, Kogan BA, Parekh A. Impact of urinary incontinence on self concept in children with spina bifida. J Urol 2004;17:1659.
Murray K, Nurse D, Borzykowski M, et al. The "congenital" wide bladder neck anomaly. A common cause of incontinence in children. Br J Urol 1987;59:533.
Nakagawa S. Onuf's nucleus of the sacral cord in a South American monkey *(Saimiri):* Its location and bilateral cortical input from area 4. Brain Res 1980;191:337.
Nolan T, Oberklaid F. New concepts in the management of encopresis. Pediatr Rev 1993;14:447.
Numanoglu I. Anal and urinary control device. Artif Organs 1987;11:420.
Otto-Unger G. Treatment of the unstable bladder in children with the anticholinergic agent propiverin hydrochloride (mictonorm/mictonets). Z Urol Nephrol 1985;78:145.
Owen-Smith VH, Chesterfield BW. Computerized biofeedback achieving continence in high anal atresia. Arch Dis Child 1986; 1:1033.
Palmer LS, Zebold K, Firlit CF, et al. Complications of intravesical oxybutynin chloride therapy in the pediatric myelomeningocele population. J Urol 1997;157:638.
Pemberton JH, Kelly KA. Achieving enteric continence: Principles and applications. Mayo Clin Proc 1986;61:586.
Peña A. The posterior sagittal approach: Implication in adult colorectal surgery. Dis Colon Rectum 1994;37:1.
Perlmutter AD. Enuresis. In: Kelalis PP, King LR, Belman AB, eds. Clinical pediatric urology. Philadelphia: WB Saunders, 1985.
Pompino HJ, Hoffmann D. Normal urinary flow for girls aged 3-14 years. Z Kinderchir 1983;38:177.
Rao SS. Manometric evaluation of constipation. Part I. Gastroenterologist 1996;4:145.
Rao SS. Manometric evaluation of defecation disorders: Part II. Fecal incontinence. Gastroenterologist 1997;5:99.
Rao SSC, Patel RS. How useful are manometric tests of anorectal function in the management of defecation disorders? Am J Gastroenterol 1997;92:469.
Reinberg Y, Fleming T, Gonzales R. Renal rupture after the Credé maneuver. J Pediatr 1994;124:279.
Robert M, Averous M, Besset A, et al. Sleep polygraphic studies using cystomanometry in twenty patients with enuresis. Eur Urol 1993;24:97.
Rushton HG. Wetting and functional voiding disorders. Urol Clin North Am 1995;22:75.
Saedi NA, Schulman SL. Natural history of voiding dysfunction. Pediatr Nephrol 2003;18:894.
Sakakibara R, Takamichi H, Yasuda K, et al. Micturition disturbance in acute transverse myelitis. Spinal Cord 1996;34:481.
Sakanaka M, Shiosaka S, Takatsuki K, et al. Evidence for the existence of substance P containing pathway from the nucleus laterodorsalis tegmenti (castaldi) to the medial frontal cortex of the rat. Brain Res 1983;259:123.
Sanders C. Choosing incontinence products for children. Nurs Stand 2002;16:39.
Saper CB. Bing and Haymaker's neurological diagnosis. St. Louis: Mosby, 1995.
Scharli AF. Anorectal incontinence: Diagnosis and treatment. J Pediatr Surg 1987;22:693

Schurch B, Hodler J, Rodic B. Botulinum A toxin as a treatment of detrusor-sphincter dyssynergia in patients with spinal cord injury: MRI controlled transperineal injections. J Neurol Neurosurg Psychiatry 1997;63:474.

Sensirivatana R, Watana D, Sornmani W, et al. Diagnostic study of urinary frequency in children. Urology 1987;30:50.

Shafik A. Anourethral reflex. Description of a reflex and its clinical significance: Preliminary study. Paraplegia 1992;30:210.

Simeoni J, Guys JM, Mollard P, et al. Artificial urinary sphincter implantation for neurogenic bladder: A multi-institutional study in 107 children. Br J Urol 1996;78:287.

Sindou M, Turano G, Pantieri R, et al. Intraoperative monitoring of spinal cord SEPs during microsurgical DREZotomy (MDT) for pain, spasticity, and hyperactive bladder. Stereotact Funct Neurosurg 1994;62:164.

Siroky MB. Electromyography of the perineal floor. Urol Clin North Am 1996;23:299.

Smey P, King LR, Firlit CF. Dysfunctional voiding in children secondary to internal sphincter dyssynergia: Treatment with phenoxybenzamine. Urol Clin North Am 1980;7:337.

Soderstrom U, Hoelcke M, Alenius L, et al. Urinary and faecal incontinence: A population-based study. Acta Paediatr 2004;93:386.

Squire R, Kiely EM, Carr B, et al. The clinical application of the Malone antegrade colonic enema. J Pediatr Surg 1993;28:1012.

Stadtler AC, Gorski PA, Brazelton TB, Toilet training methods, clinical interventions, and recommendations. American Academy of Pediatrics. Pediatrics 1999;103:1359.

Tanagho EA, Schmidt RA, Orvis BR. Neural stimulation for control of voiding dysfunction: A preliminary report in 22 patients with serious neuropathic voiding disorders. J Urol 1989;142:340.

Taylor TKF, Coolican MJR. Injuries of the conus medullaris. Paraplegia 1988;26:393.

Tohyama M, Satoh K, Sakaumoto T. Organization and projections of the neurons in the dorsal tegmental area of the rat. J Hirnforsch 1978;19:165.

Torre M, Martucciello G, Jasonni V, Sacral development in anorectal malformations and in normal population. Pediatr Radiol 2001;31:858.

Van Mastrigt R, Griffiths DJ. An evaluation of contractility parameters determined from isometric contractions and micturition studies. Urol Res 1986;14:45.

Vick CW, Viscomi GN, Mannes E, et al. Pitfalls related to the urinary bladder in pelvic sonography: A review. Urol Radiol 1983;5:253.

Vodusek DB. Evoked potential testing. Urol Clin North Am 1996;23:427.

Wald A. Fecal incontinence. Effective nonsurgical treatments. Postgrad Med 1986;80:123.

Walther PC, Kaplan GW. Cystoscopy in children: Indications for its use in common urologic problems. J Urol 1979;122:717.

Webster GD, Koefoot RB Jr, Sihelnik S. Urodynamic abnormalities in neurologically normal children with micturition dysfunction. J Urol 1984;132:74.

Wein AJ, Barrett DM. Physiology of micturition and urodynamics. In: Kelalis PP, King LR, Belman AB, eds. Clinical pediatric urology, 3rd ed. Philadelphia: WB Saunders, 1992.

Whitehead WE, Parker L, Bosmajian L, et al. Treatment of fecal incontinence in children with spina bifida. Comparison of biofeedback and behavior modification. Arch Phys Med Rehabil 1986;67:218.

Wong WD, Jensen LL, Bartolo DCC, et al. Artificial anal sphincter. Dis Colon Rectum 1996;39:1345.

Wright FS. Disorders of micturition and defecation. In: Swaiman KF, Wright FS, eds. The practice of pediatric neurology, 2nd ed. St. Louis: Mosby, 1982.

Wyndaele JJ. Development and evaluation of the management of the neuropathic bladder. Paraplegia 1995;33:305.

Yang CC, Mayo ME. Morbidity of dysfunctional voiding syndrome. Urology 1997;49:445.

Yeung CK, Godley ML, Ho CKW, et al. Some new insights into bladder function in infancy. Br J Urol 1995;76:235.

Zerin MJ, Lebowitz RL, Bauer SB. Descent of the bladder neck: A urographic finding in denervation of the urethral sphincter in children with myelodysplasia. Radiology 1990;174:833.

Zimmern PE, Lin VK, McConnell JD. Smooth-muscle physiology. Urol Clin North Am 1996;23:211.

PART XV

Systemic Diseases and Their Effect on the Nervous System

CHAPTER 87

Poisoning and Drug-Induced Neurologic Diseases

Laurence E. Walsh and Bhuwan P. Garg

Many substances are potential nervous system toxins. Manufactured and naturally occurring agents, including pharmaceutical compounds and recreational drugs, may be ingested, inhaled, injected, or absorbed, with a subsequent deleterious effect on a child's central or peripheral nervous system. Effects may be acute, subacute, or chronic and occur in adolescents, young children, infants, or fetuses. Neurologic dysfunction may be isolated or part of a systemic derangement.

Poisonings are common. In 2003, nearly 2.4 million cases of poisoning were reported to the nation's poison control centers, 93% of which occurred at home [Watson et al., 2004]. Of these, 1.58 million involved persons younger than 20 years of age, and 1.24 million (or 52% of all poisoning victims) were children younger than 5 years [Watson et al., 2004]. Intoxication is the second most common injury (behind falls) in children younger than 48 months [Agran et al., 2003]. Data from other countries suggest similar demographics [Andiran and Sarikayalar, 2004].

Neurotoxins are among the most commonly encountered toxins, although they less commonly are the culprits in children younger than 6 years [Watson et al., 2004]. Poisonings and drug-induced neurologic disease may mimic infection, trauma, neoplasm, psychiatric illness, or metabolic disorders. Intoxications should be considered in the differential diagnosis of a child with an unexplained change in sensorium, seizures, ataxia, involuntary movements, muscle weakness, or autonomic dysfunction. Prompt recognition and management of intoxication reduce both mortality and morbidity in most cases.

Neurotoxins may have more long-term cognitive sequelae. Unfortunately, studies of low-level environmental exposures often suffer from imperfect control of confounding factors [Mink et al., 2004; Weiss et al., 2004]; this situation may limit conclusions that may be drawn from these studies.

Most childhood poisonings are accidental [Nhachi and Kasilo, 1994; Singh et al., 1995; Watson et al., 2004]. The most common agents implicated in children younger than 6 years are cosmetics, personal care products, and household cleaning solutions. Important factors contributing to accidental poisonings include parental factors, such as improper medicinal or chemical storage, lapses in child monitoring, and ignorance of poison control methods. Likewise, children may be noncompliant, may mistake a potential toxin for food, may imitate parental medication-taking behavior, or simply may be curious. One unusual example was that of an 11-year-old male who ingested 35% hydrogen peroxide solution. Although H_2O_2 exposure may result in irreversible cerebral injury, his magnetic resonance imaging (MRI) test demonstrated bilateral posterior reversible diffusion restriction; he later made a full recovery [Cannon et al., 2003]. Failure of "childproof" containers was cited in 18% of poisonings in one study [Brayden et al., 1993].

Adolescents and preadolescents are at risk for recreational drug and solvent abuse. The rate of substance abuse by preteens in the United Kingdom approaches 5% [McArdle, 2004]. Poisoning occurs deliberately in suicide attempts, child abuse, and other attempts to harm a child. In a 2002 Polish study, 14% of poisonings in children younger than 15 years were intentional (including self-inflicted) [Kotwica and Czerczak, 2002]. Two thirds of suicide victims younger than 19 years in the United Kingdom use self-poisoning [Camidge et al., 2003]. In Hong Kong, poisoning is implicated in 15% to 20% of murders and suicides in the general population [Chan et al., 2003]. These high percentages of nonaccidental poisoning deaths compared with the United States may reflect differences in firearm regulation. Among the pediatric population, those at highest risk for abuse are infants and preschoolers; teenagers have the highest risk for suicide [McClure, 1994; McClure et al., 1996]. Abuse of alcohol and other recreational drugs may predict suicide attempts, although the method may involve neither [Hawton and Fagg, 1992, 1993]. Common suicide methods identified recently in teenagers include hanging, exhaust inhalation, and overdose on medications, including paracetamol, benzodiazepines, and tricyclic antidepressants [Andiran and Sarikayalar, 2004; Ghazi-Khansari and Oreizi]. Pesticides, herbicides, and caustic agents may also be used; fatalities caused by ingestion of such agents may be the result of suicidal intent rather than accidental exposure more often in adolescents than in adults [Andiran and Sarikayalar, 2004; Klein-Schwartz and Smith, 1997; Thompson et al., 1995].

Poisoning as a result of child abuse usually occurs in conjunction with a background of other, separate injuries. Still, poisoning may occur in isolation or within a more cryptic history of unexplained illnesses; this is especially evident in Munchausen's syndrome by proxy [Chadwick, 1997]. A diagnosis of Munchausen's syndrome by proxy suggests the secondary gain of medical contact as motive; it is sometimes difficult to differentiate Munchausen's syndrome by proxy from other causes of nonaccidental injury. The incidence of nonaccidental poisoning in the British Isles is more than 2.8 per 100,000 children younger than 1 year each year and more than 0.5 per 100,000 children younger than 16 years each year [McClure et al., 1996]. Methods reported include forced ingestion of antiepileptic drugs, opioids, and caustics, as well as various other agents [Gotschlich and Beltran, 1995; McClure et al., 1996]. Unfortunately, escalation of Munchausen's syndrome by proxy often occurs, with suffocation a frequent terminal event [Chadwick, 1977; McClure et al.,

1996]. One instructive case of Munchausen's syndrome by proxy was that of an 11-year-old female with a history of cyclic vomiting. Investigation eventually revealed arsenic poisoning by her mother [Embry, 1987].

Conversely, some children and adults present with complaints of symptoms that are believed to be the result of a toxic exposure, but for which no toxin is identified. In these cases, symptoms often are vague; litigation is common (30%); and the patients or families do not easily accept refutation of the alleged exposure [Leikin et al., 2004].

Finally, chemical agents have been used as weapons against groups of people. Although their use in battle is not new, recent events have raised concern over covert use of chemical agents to attack civilian populations. In the 1994 Matsumoto nerve agent terrorist attack using sarin, 58 of 600 exposed people required hospital admission, and 7 died. The most common symptom was miosis. Central nervous system (CNS) effects and transient cardiomyopathy also occurred [Okudera, 2002]. The U.S. Department of Health and Human Services has published a brief guide to toxidromes associated with likely covertly used chemical weapons [Patel et al., 2003].

Clinical trials, preclinical studies, anecdotal reports, and epidemiologic data have contributed to our understanding of neurotoxins [Erinoff, 1995; Fray and Robbins, 1996; Indulski and Lutz, 1996; Kurz et al., 1995]. Detailed discussion of antiepileptic drugs and immunization side effects is omitted here; these topics are covered in other chapters.

EMERGENCY EVALUATION AND MANAGEMENT

Management of the poisoned child requires skilled immediate stabilization of the patient and appropriate corrective and supportive therapy. It requires also that the physician review the history and examine the child carefully for clues that may suggest poisoning or drug effects. Discovery of such evidence is not always easy, and a high index of suspicion is necessary. Three fourths of all poisonings are by ingestion. Although cosmetics and household cleaning solutions are ingested, medications account for most deaths [Litovitz et al., 1995; Watson et al., 2004]. Careful physical examination helps to establish the cause of the child's distress and guide therapy. Neurologic findings may result from the drug or toxic agent itself or from CNS hypoxia or ischemia caused by a generalized disturbance of circulation and respiration. Systemic abnormalities that occur after various types of intoxication may include cardiac dysrhythmias, gastrointestinal disturbances, and varying degrees of metabolic acidosis. Dysrhythmias, including marked degrees of bradycardia with cyanide or physostigmine intoxication, may be clues to the identity of the toxic agent and signal the need for emergency treatment. Cardiac conduction abnormalities, such as prolonged QT interval with phenothiazine overdose and widened QRS interval with tricyclic antidepressants, quinine, or quinidine overdose, may be present. Gastrointestinal complications, including severe diarrhea and vomiting, may occur with lithium, mercury, phosphorus, arsenic, mushroom, and organophosphate poisoning. Metabolic acidosis with a large anion gap may result from intoxication with cyanide, methyl alcohol, ethylene glycol, propylene glycol, and salicylates [Gardner et al., 2004].

Box 87-1 Suggested General Management of Suspected Intoxications and Poisoning

1. Establish patent airway, adequate respirations, pulse, and systemic perfusion; monitor level of consciousness and urine output.
2. Establish intravenous access.
3. Administer oxygen, glucose, and naloxone as necessary, especially in patients with acute alteration of mental status.
4. Obtain pertinent history and perform careful physical examination, specifically looking for entry sites for envenomation, needle tracks, or other evidence of agent entry (e.g., nasal mucosa, mouth, genital orifices); examine for systemic signs of intoxication, including fever, abnormal vital signs, excessive tearing or salivation, odor, skin and nailbed color, hyperhydrosis or anhydrosis, trauma, or hemorrhages.
5. Perform age-appropriate neurologic examination, including mental status examination and cranial nerve, speech, motor, cerebellar, muscle stretch reflex, and sensory evaluations. Observe patient for posture and gait.
6. Obtain laboratory studies, such as a chemistry profile, including serum glucose and electrolyte levels, blood pH, complete blood count, urine and serum toxicologic studies (for specific agents when indicated), and drug levels if suggested by history or physical examination.
7. Prevent further absorption or maximize elimination of the toxic agent using gastric lavage or activated charcoal only when indicated [Zimmerman, 2004].
8. Administer specific antidote when indicated.
9. Obtain electrocardiogram and, when indicated, neuroimaging studies (e.g., CT, MRI), electroencephalogram, and cerebrospinal fluid for examination.
10. Monitor closely; reassess the child frequently.

Finally, steps should be taken to protect the child from future exposures. Appropriate general management steps are outlined in Box 87-1; details may be found in several recent references [Arena, 1985; Banner et al., 1994; Chan et al., 1993; Goetz, 1985; Gosselin et al., 1984; Haddad and Winchester, 1983; Leikin and Osterhoudt et al., 2004; Paloucek, 1995; POISINDEX, 2005; Zimmerman, 2003]. Therapy for specific toxidromes is discussed with the individual agents.

Testing

The value of routine toxicologic testing in cases of possible intoxications is debated in the literature. The low sensitivity of specific tests and the inability to test for all possible agents, medicolegal concerns, and cost effectiveness have fueled arguments that routine testing should be limited [Bond, 1995]. Ideally, history and physical examination narrow the list of possible exposures and direct specific toxicologic testing. However, young children may not provide adequate history, and poisoned children sometimes present with unfamiliar or atypical clinical features [Lifshitz et al., 1997]. These situations may require a more extensive search for the toxic agent.

Toxicologic screening methods have other limitations as well. Most are not designed specifically for use in children, although modified panels or pediatric protocols are available [Badcock and Zoanetti, 1996]. Many physicians are unaware of the agents actually identified by the blood and urine panels available at their institutions. A standard screen for drugs of abuse may detect barbiturates, benzodiazepines, opioids, amphetamines, cocaine metabolites (benzoylecgonine), phencyclidine palmitate, and marijuana metabolites (tetrahydrocannabinol) by immunoassay, but other drugs, such as lysergic acid diethylamide, may remain undetected [Bond, 1995]. Other broad drug screens may detect phenothiazines, tricyclic antidepressants, ethanol or other volatile substances, and sympathomimetic amines. Urine screens for drugs of abuse may detect two to nine agents (e.g., tetrahydrocannabinol, cocaine, opioids, amphetamines, barbiturates, benzodiazepines, methamphetamines, phencyclidine palmitate, tricyclic antidepressants in Diagnostix kits). Other commercially available screens include EMIT (Behring Diagnostics, San Jose, California), Abuscreen (Roche Diagnostic Systems, Basel, Switzerland), and others. Thin-layer chromatography and ultraviolet spectroscopy are also popular, but older tests, including crude spot tests, are still available. The sensitivity of the screens and the need for subsequent confirmation (i.e., by high-performance liquid chromatography) depend on the methods used. Likewise, routine urine screens for heavy metals may identify only arsenic, mercury, and lead. Results from some screens may be obtained in less than 1 hour, but broad screens may require 24 hours for results; specific tests may require a week [Pathology and Laboratory Medicine, 1994]. Hair sample–based toxicologic testing has become increasingly popular and overcomes many limitations of other modalities. The test is minimally invasive, does not rely on dilution methods, and gives historical information. Use of a wide variety of substances can be determined from hair samples, including drugs of abuse, haloperidol, antidepressants, sympathomimetics, and heavy metals [Hoffman and Nelson, 2001; Leikin, 1995]. The primary cocaine metabolite, benzoylecgonine, and acidic, polar drugs are difficult to identify reliably in hair samples, and the test is probably not appropriate for acute toxicity testing situations, although in the case of cocaine, qualitative and semiquantitative analysis of more chronic use can be demonstrated [Katikaneni et al., 2002; Stephens et al., 2004].

In a prospective pediatric emergency department study, using urine gas chromatography–mass spectrometry drug screens, the best clinical predictors of poisoning were odor on the child's breath, symptoms and signs consistent with poisoning, and poison actually on the child's clothing [Hwang et al., 2003]. Positive predictive values for these three variables were 100%, 92%, and 86%, respectively.

Other Ancillary Testing

Ancillary testing is directed by specific clinical findings. Electroencephalography is important to exclude subtle or subclinical seizures in intoxicated patients who display altered mental status. Neuroimaging studies have at least three roles. First, in the acutely intoxicated child or teenager, a head computed tomography (CT) scan may be required if there is suspicion of concomitant trauma or hemorrhage. Second, brain MRI findings may explain a patient's neurologic findings when clinical history and other laboratory studies do not. As neuroimaging of an increasing number of poisoned children and adults has occurred, a couple of recurring MRI patterns have become evident. Agents that cause hypoxic injury, including cellular respiratory poisons, may result in an MRI picture of bilateral symmetric cortical and subcortical gray matter injury, although white matter changes occur as well [Halavaara et al., 2002; Kim et al., 2003; Rachinger et al., 2002]. Medications used for immunosuppression and those that cause hypertension or changes in blood-brain barrier permeability may contribute to a characteristic neuroradiographic pattern of bilateral posterior reversible leukoencephalopathy (so-called posterior reversible leukoencephalopathy syndrome) [Renard et al., 2004]. Third, the increasing use of diffusion-weighted MRI sequences and apparent diffusion coefficient calculations (apparent diffusion coefficient mapping) often provides a method to delineate early cerebral injury.

Neurologic Examination

Examination of a poisoned child includes initial and serial assessment of neurologic status; this assessment guides clinical management, predicts prognosis, and often identifies the offending agent. Assessment of mental status is important because several poisons, medications, and recreational drugs may be associated with affective symptoms and may also cause acute changes in sensorium such as irritability, other affective symptoms, delirium, coma, lethargy, and seizures. Although psychotropic or analgesic medications have the greatest potential to cause these effects, antihistamines and other routinely used pediatric medications are common culprits [Bassett et al., 1996]. Environmental and biologic toxins may likewise cause change in sensorium, although more often in younger children. More chronic effects include dementia, subtle learning difficulties, and apparent psychiatric illness. Agents that cause seizures or changes in sensorium are listed in Box 87-2.

Cranial nerve examination may reveal specific toxin-induced syndromes. Decreased visual acuity or changes in color perception may suggest anticholinergic or cardiac glycoside toxicity, respectively. Papilledema reflects increased intracranial pressure and may suggest pseudotumor cerebri, or benign intracranial hypertension, caused by systemically administered steroids, excessive vitamin A intake, or use of outdated tetracyclines. Visual impairment and a macular cherry red spot has been reported in association with dapsone poisoning. The patient had concomitant peripheral neuropathy, and the macular changes were considered secondary to toxic retinal damage [Abhayambika et al., 1990]. Pupillary dysfunction may be caused by medication use, abuse of street drugs, and exposure to various environmental or biologic toxins [Leikin and Paloucek, 1995; Slamovits and Glaser, 1990]. Nystagmus is common in intoxications, especially with antiepileptic agents; bradykinetic extraocular movements follow exposure to antidopaminergic

Box 87-2 Selected Agents That Cause Changes in Sensorium or Seizures

Medications
- Allopurinol
- Antiarrhythmics
- Antibiotics
- Anticholinergic agents
- Antidepressants
- Antiepileptic drugs
- Antifungal agents
- Antihistamines
- Antihypertensives
- Antineoplastics
- Antiparasitic agents
- Antipsychotics
- Antitubercular drugs
- Antiviral agents
- Anxiolytics
- Baclofen [Chen et al., 2003]
- Benzodiazepines
- β-Agonists
- β-Blockers [Gleiter and Deckert, 1996]
- Bismuth subgallate
- Bromides [Frances et al., 2003]
- Bromocriptine
- Camphor
- Carbinols
- Castor oil
- Chloral hydrate
- Cholinergic agents
- Cisapride
- Clomiphene
- Cocaine
- Colchicine [Goldbart et al, 2000]
- Cyclobenzaprine
- Dantrolene
- Dextromethorphan
- Disulfiram
- Diuretics
- Erythropoietin
- Glutethimide, zolpidem
- Granisetron, nabilone
- Guaifenesin
- Hallucinogens
- Hydrogen peroxide [Cannon et al., 2003]
- Immunomodulators
- Isotretinoin
- Ketamine
- Levodopa
- Levothyroxine
- Lithium
- Lovastatin
- Muromonab-CD3 [Thaisetthawatkul et al., 2001]
- Nabilone
- Narcotics
- Niacin (acute)
- Nitrous oxide
- Nonsteroidal anti-inflammatory drugs, salicylates [Easley and Altemeier, 2000; Hesslinger et al., 1996]
- Omeprazole (acute)
- Steroids
- Sucralfate
- Sulfasalazine
- Sumatriptan
- Sympathomimetics, stimulants
- Vitamin A

Industrial Toxins
- Acrylamide
- Alcohols (ethanol, isopropanol, methanol)
- Aluminum compounds
- Ammonium chloride (toilet bowl cleaners)
- Antifreeze components
- Boric acid (antiseptics, insecticides)
- Camphor
- Carbon monoxide
- Cyanide
- Ethylene oxide
- Formaldehyde
- Gasoline
- Heavy metals
- Hexachlorophene
- Metaldehyde (snail bait, fire starters)
- Naphthalene
- Organophosphate insecticides
- Rodenticides
- Solvents
- Zinc, manganese [Mergler et al., 1994]

Biologic Toxins
- Baneberry (*Actaea* species)
- Box jellyfish (sea wasp)
- Box thorn (*Lycium halmifolium*)
- Buckeye (*Aesculus* species)
- Copperhead, cottonmouth, some rattlesnake venom
- Corn lily (*Helleborus* species)
- Daphne
- Death Camus (*Zigadenus* species)
- Foxglove (*Digitalis purpurea*)
- Ginkgo nuts [Miwa et al., 2001]
- *Hyoscyamus niger*
- Jimson weed (*Datura stramonium*)
- Lupine
- Marijuana (*Cannabis sativa*)
- Mayapple (*Podophyllum peltatum*)
- Mescaline, peyote
- Methcathinone
- Morning glory (*Ipomoea purpurea, Rivea corymbosa*)
- Mushrooms (especially *Amanita muscaria, Pantherina, Psilocybe, Panaeolus, Copelandia,* and *Gymnopilus* species)
- Nutmeg
- Oleander
- Peony, *Paeonia* species (high doses in medicinal preparations)
- Potato (leaves, stems, immature tubers)
- Shellfish (domoic acid poisoning)
- *Shigella* toxin [Lahat et al., 1990]
- *Solanum* species (Jerusalem cherry or ornamental pepper, black nightshade)

Box 87-2 Selected Agents That Cause Changes in Sensorium or Seizures, cont'd

Star fruit [Chan et al., 2002]
Star of Bethlehem, Indian tobacco (*Lobelia inflata*)
Strychnine ("slang nut") [Katz et al., 1996]
Tobacco (nicotine, acute)

medications, and extraocular muscle paresis is an important indicator of botulism poisoning [Glaser and Bachynski, 1990]. Loss of the blink reflex and facial paresis may occur as part of a generalized encephalopathy, such as in profound narcotic intoxications, or occur in isolation, such as in botulism or vincristine-induced neuropathy. Acute hearing loss resulting from poisoning is uncommon but may be caused by aminoglycoside use, toxicity, or overdose of nicotine or lithium. Vestibular dysfunction is one of the most common presenting symptoms of drug-induced neurologic syndromes, including those caused by exposure to antiepileptic drugs, antibiotics, and metals [Mount et al., 1995; Wood et al., 1996]. Vestibular dysfunction should be differentiated from vagally mediated "dizziness," although both may result from intoxications. Isolated toxin-induced disorders of the pharyngeal and neck musculature (e.g., loss of ability to swallow in clostridial toxidromes) are rare, but dysgeusia is not; the latter occurs commonly with use of lithium-containing preparations. Table 87-1 lists toxins that cause cranial nerve deficits.

Motor weakness may be due to poisoning of the anterior horn cells, peripheral nerves, neuromuscular junction, or muscles. Proximal myopathies (e.g., caused by steroid use) or distal motor neuropathies (e.g., caused by metal exposure) should be differentiated from infectious, inflammatory, metabolic, and degenerative processes. Profound weakness may occur with use of depolarizing agents and neuromuscular blockers. Rigidity may result from either central or peripheral disinhibition (Boxes 87-3 to 87-5) [Katz et al., 1996; Reeves et al., 1996]. Extrapyramidal disorders may be caused by exposure to environmental toxins but are also well-recognized side effects of many medications (Box 87-6). Drugs implicated most frequently in movement disorders are antipsychotics and related agents, calcium channel antagonists, CNS stimulants, antidepressants, antiepileptic drugs, antiparkinsonian drugs, and lithium [Jimenez-Jimenez et al., 1997; Kerrick et al., 1995]. With severe intoxications, the cardiovascular effects of many of these medications overshadow the acute neurologic symptoms. Antibiotics, antidepressants, and some antineoplastic drugs may cause myoclonus (Box 87-7) [Chow et al., 2003].

Ataxia may be due to cerebellar or peripheral nerve dysfunction (Box 87-8). Cerebellar dysfunction may also manifest as nystagmus, scanning speech, hypotonia with pendular reflexes, dyssynergy, dysmetria, or dysdiadochokinesis [DeJong, 1967; Findley, 1996]. Tremor is common in several intoxications (Box 87-9).

TABLE 87-1

Selected Agents Causing Cranial Nerve Deficits

CRANIAL NERVE DEFICIT	MEDICATIONS	INDUSTRIAL TOXINS	BIOLOGIC TOXINS
General	Methotrexate, vincristine	Organic mercury, ethylene glycol	Cobra venom
Olfactory	Levodopa	—	—
Optic nerve and retina	Antibiotics, phenothiazines [Glaser, 1990], antineoplastics, cyclosporine, disulfiram (retrobulbar neuritis), isoniazid, minoxidil, quinines, valproic acid	Cyanide, methanol, lead, thallium, organic mercury, hexachlorophene	Lathyrus
Extraocular Muscles	Botulinum A toxin, bretylium, antiepileptics, interferon	—	*Clostridium botulinum* toxin
Mydriasis	Antihistamines, anticholinergics, nortriptyline barium, bromides, carbamazepine, cocaine, cyclobenzaprine, glutethimide, sertraline, sympathomimetics	Ethylene glycol, benzene, cyanide	Black nightshade (*Solanum nigrum*), box thorn (*Lycium halmifolium*), lupine, morning glory, potato (leaves, stems, immature tubers), tetrodotoxin (puffer fish, others), water hemlock (*Cicuta* species), mescaline, peyote
Miosis	Buspirone, cholinergics, narcotics	—	—
Dysgeusia	Dipyridamole, disulfiram, selegiline, ethambutol, lithium, nedocromil tocainide	Dimethyl sulfoxide	Ciguatera toxin (red snapper, farm-raised salmon)
Auditory	Antibiotics, especially aminoglycosides, antifungals, antineoplastics, lithium (acute), nonsteroidal anti-inflammatory drugs and salicylates, quinine antiarrhythmics, angiotensin-converting enzyme inhibitors, danazol, dantrolene, dapsone, antidepressants, digoxin, dimenhydrinate, diuretics, vitamin A	Carbon monoxide, cyanide, ` methanol, solvents, mercury (organic)	Tobacco (acute), lathyrus

Box 87-3 Selected Agents Associated with Myopathies

Amphetamine
Amiodarone
Barium
β-Blockers
Caffeine
Chloroquine, hydroxychloroquine
Cimetidine
Clofibrate
Cocaine
Colchicine
Corticosteroids: prednisone
Cromolyn sodium
Cyclosporine
Diltiazem
Doxepin
D-Penicillamine
Ethanol
Etretinate
Heroin
Hydrogen peroxide
Licorice
Lovastatin
Minoxidil
Niacin
Phencyclidine palmitate (PCP)
Procainamide
Propylthiouracil
Pyrithioxine
Quinolones, penicillin, nalidixic acid
Salicylates
Sulfasalazine
Tiopronin
Vincristine, paclitaxel
Zidovudine

Common Toxidromes

The neurologic examination may indicate poisonings and drug intoxications that fit clinically into one of several toxidromes resulting from a predominant neurotransmitter derangement or disruption of one arm of the autonomic nervous system [Babe and Serafin, 1996; Brown and Taylor, 1996; Haddad and Winchester, 1983; Hoffman and Lefkowitz, 1996; Leikin and Paloucek, 1995; Reisine and Pasternak, 1996; Sanders-Bush and Mayer, 1996]. The major toxidromes include the following: anticholinergic, cholinergic, sympathomimetic, serotonergic, antihistaminic, and narcotic/sedative-hypnotic syndromes.

The anticholinergic syndrome is readily recognizable. Features may be divided into peripheral muscarinic signs, including tachycardia, dry skin and mucous membranes, dilated pupils, decreased gastrointestinal motility, urinary retention, and fever, and central anticholinergic signs, including confusion, disorientation, agitation, hallucinations, incoordination, ataxia, and frank psychosis ("mad, hot, dry, and blind"). The anticholinergic toxidrome is caused by atropine, belladonna alkaloids, plants (jimson weed), antihistamines, low-potency phenothiazines, and antidepressants, especially tricyclic antidepressants. The tricyclic antidepressants may also be associated with a depressed level of consciousness, seizures, and cardiac dysrhythmias.

Box 87-4 Selected Agents Causing Peripheral Neuropathy

Medications
- Amiodarone
- Amitriptyline (acute polyradiculopathy)
- Antibiotics: nitrofurantoin, chloramphenicol, quinolones, aminoglycosides, polymyxin B
- Antineoplastic agents: vinca alkaloids, paclitaxel, procarbazine (mixed), cisplatin, cytosine arabinoside
- Antiparasitic agents: metronidazole, chloroquine, hydroxychloroquine [Gupta et al., 2003]
- Antitubercular agents [Lewin and McGreal, 1993]
- Colchicine
- Dapsone (distal motor neuropathy) [Abhayambika et al., 1990]
- Digitoxin
- Disulfiram
- Ethanol
- Ethionamide
- Hydralazine
- Interferons (sensory)
- Nitrous oxide
- Phenytoin, fosphenytoin
- Pyridoxine (sensory) [Parry and Bredesen, 1985]
- Streptokinase (Guillain-Barré syndrome) [Taylor et al., 1995]
- Thalidomide (sensory)

Industrial Toxins
- Acrylamide (sensory)
- Carbon monoxide
- Chlorophenoxy herbicides (sensory)
- Dinitrophenols
- Ethylene oxide (mixed motor, sensory) [Crystal et al., 1988; Schaumburg and Berger, 1993]
- Heavy metals
- Organophosphate pesticides
- Solvents

Biologic Toxins
- Cyanide (cassavism)
- Diphtheria
- Lathyrus
- Podophyllum (ingestion)
- Stonefish (Scorpaenidae)

Additional references: Le Quintrec and Le Quintrec, 1991; Dyck and Thomas, 1993; Leikin and Paloucek, 1995; Patel et al., 2003; REPROTOX, 2005.

Cholinergic toxidromes, which include both muscarinic and nicotinic effects, are produced by organophosphate insecticides, carbamate insecticides, nicotine, physostigmine, and their congeners. Consciousness may be extremely depressed, and the patient may be comatose with respiratory depression; pinpoint pupils; widespread fasciculations; *s*alivation, *l*acrimation, *u*rination, and *d*efecation (SLUD syndrome); bronchoconstriction; pulmonary edema; hypotension or hypertension; and bradycardia.

Box 87-5 Selected Agents Associated with Paralysis and Muscular Rigidity

Paralysis

Medications and Industrial Toxins

- Aminoglycoside antibiotics
- β-Blockers
- Chloroquine (with color vision shift)
- Cholinesterase inhibitors: neostigmine, pyridostigmine
- D-Penicillamine
- Pesticides: organophosphates, carbamates
- Pyrithioxine
- Trimethadione

Biologic Toxins

- Cobra venom
- Poison hemlock *(Conium maculatum)*
- Scorpion fish (Scorpaenidae)
- Snake venom, ticks, botulinum toxin
- Star of Bethlehem *(Hippobroma longiflora)*
- Sweet pea *(Lathyrus odoratus)*
- Tetrodotoxin (puffer fish, blue-ringed octopus, others)

Muscular Rigidity

- Black widow spider venom *(Latrodectus mactans)* [Reeves et al., 1996]
- Strychnine (*Strychnos nux vomica,* "slang nut") [Katz et al., 1996]
- Tetanus toxin

Box 87-7 Selected Agents Associated with Myoclonus

Medications

- Antibiotics (β-lactams)
- Antidepressants [Bak et al., 1995]
- Antineoplastics: busulfan, chlorambucil
- Carbamazepine, vigabatrin [Neufeld and Vishnevska, 1995]
- Clozapine [Bak et al., 1995]
- Levodopa [Bak et al., 1995]
- Lidocaine
- Lithium [Bak et al., 1995]
- Lorazepam (preterm infants) [Reiter and Stiles, 1993]
- Methaqualone
- Morphine [Jacobsen et al., 1995]
- Nitroprusside
- Piperazine [Conners, 1995]

Industrial Toxins

- Camphor
- Chlorophenoxy herbicides
- Gasoline

Biological Toxins

- Buckeye (*Aesculus* species)
- Lupine
- Shellfish (domoic acid poisoning)

Box 87-6 Selected Agents Associated with Parkinsonism and Other Acute Extrapyramidal Reactions

Medications

- Amiodarone
- Anticholinergic agents: benztropine
- Antidepressants (including selective serotonin reuptake inhibitors) [Eisenhauer and Jermain, 1993]
- Antiepileptic drugs
- Antifungal agents
- Antihistamines
- Antipsychotics and related drugs (including "novel" agents) [Buzan, 1996; Lindstrom et al., 1995]
- Bethanechol
- Bupropion (acute)
- Buspirone
- Captopril (acute)
- Clonazepam
- Diazoxide
- Digoxin (chorea)
- Estrogen (chorea)
- Heroin
- Ketamine
- Levodopa
- Lithium (chorea)
- 1-Methyl-4-phenyl-1,2,3,6,-tetrahydropyridine (MPTP)
- Metronidazole (oculogyric crisis)
- Narcotics
- Ofloxacin (Tourette-like syndrome) [Thomas and Reagan, 1996]
- Reserpine
- Stimulants
- Sulfasalazine (chorea)
- Vinblastine

Industrial Toxins

- Carbon monoxide
- Metals: manganese, thallium, aluminum [Normandin et al., 2002]
- Methanol
- Trichloroethylene

Biologic Toxins

- *Arthrinium* mycotoxin [He et al., 1995]

Seizures may occur. Young children, however, may not display typical peripheral cholinergic signs and symptoms [Lifshitz et al., 1997; Patel et al., 2003]. Sympathomimetic, or stimulant, toxidromes occur with ingestion (sometimes at subtherapeutic doses) of amphetamines, methylphenidate, xanthines (caffeine), ephedrine and related agents, nicotine, and cocaine. Signs range from restlessness, anorexia, and insomnia to euphoria and, in severe cases, seizures [Conway et al., 1990; Rivkin and Gilmore, 1989]. Mydriasis is present, and increased motor activity and tremor may also occur.

Although serotonergic side effects have been noted with several drugs (isoniazid, tranylcypromine, and L-tryptophan in combination with monoamine oxidase inhibitors), the proliferation of newer, relatively selective, serotonin re-

Box 87-8 Selected Toxic Causes of Ataxia

Medications
- Acetohexamide
- Amiodarone
- Anticholinergic agents
- Antidepressants, including selective serotonin reuptake inhibitors
- Antiepileptic drugs
- Antihistamines
- Antimicrobials, antifungals
- Antineoplastics
- Antiparasitics [Conners, 1995; Lewin and McGreal, 1993]
- Baclofen
- Buspirone
- Dextromethorphan
- Disulfiram
- Ethanol
- Fenfluramine
- Lithium
- Lysergic acid diethylamide (LSD), phencyclidine palmitate (PCP)
- Mexiletine
- Sedatives, narcotics

Industrial Toxins
- Aluminum compounds
- Butyl alcohol
- Carbon monoxide
- Carbon tetrachloride
- Ethylene glycol
- Formaldehyde
- Gasoline
- Manganese
- Metaldehyde (snail bait, fire starters)
- Paradichlorobenzene (moth repellent, diaper pail deodorant)
- Rodenticides: aluminum phosphide, sodium monofluoroacetate
- Solvents

Biologic Toxins
- Belladonna, hyoscyamine
- Buckeye (*Aesculus* species)
- Mayapple *(Podophyllum peltatum)*
- Mescaline, peyote
- Podophyllum (ingested)
- Poison hemlock (*Conium maculatum*)

Box 87-9 Selected Agents Associated with Tremor

Medications
- Aluminum compounds
- Aminophylline, theophylline
- Amiodarone
- Antiepileptic drugs
- Antihistamines
- Chlorambucil
- Ciprofloxacin
- Cyclosporine, tacrolimus (FK-506)
- Dextromethorphan
- Digitoxin, lidocaine
- Fenfluramine
- Levothyroxine
- Lithium
- Nortriptyline
- Piperazine
- Sympathomimetics, stimulants

Industrial Toxins
- Carbon tetrachloride
- Fluoride
- Metaldehyde (snail bait, fire starters)
- Organic mercury
- Pyrethrins [Miyamoto et al., 1995]
- Rodenticides: aluminum phosphide

Biologic Toxins
- Hyoscyamine
- Mescaline, peyote
- Star of Bethlehem, Indian tobacco *(Lobelia inflata)*
- Tobacco (nicotine)

uptake inhibitors used to treat depression, obsessive-compulsive disorder, and headache has fostered new interest in this toxidrome. Onset is often sudden. Central manifestations of this syndrome include confusion, myoclonus, tremor, ataxia, hyperreflexia, and fever; peripheral findings consist of sweating, facial flushing, trismus, and diarrhea [Sternbach, 1991].

Antihistaminic agents can be divided into histamine$_1$ and histamine$_2$ blockers. Both may cause significant CNS side effects at therapeutic doses, although the degree to which they do so is agent specific. Older histamine$_1$ blockers, such as chlorpheniramine, act at both central and peripheral histamine$_1$ receptors, monoaminergic receptors, and muscarinic receptors. They cause sedation and delirium, the latter especially in children, and subtle cognitive deficits [Gengo, 1996]. They may also have significant toxicity, including movement disorders and autonomic dysfunction related to their antagonism of dopaminergic, β-adrenergic, serotonergic, and muscarinic receptors. With overdose, ataxia and seizures may supervene. Agents such as terfenadine and clemastine are less likely to cause CNS toxicity as a result of more histamine$_1$ selectivity and less CNS penetration [Babe and Serafin, 1996]. However, toxicity may be delayed by several days because of slower CNS penetration. Histamine$_2$ blockers, such as cimetidine, ranitidine, and newer agents, tend not to have significant antihistaminic side effects (except cimetidine) in children at therapeutic doses. At high doses, mental status changes predominate, especially with cimetidine.

The opioid-induced toxidrome, which is readily diagnosable and treatable by administration of naloxone, includes CNS depression with coma, pinpoint pupils, muscle flaccidity, respiratory depression, and bradycardia. All opioid-derived agents may cause this syndrome. Sedative-barbiturate toxidromes are manifested primarily by lethargy or more profound depression and respiratory depression, miotic pupils, and generalized hypotonia with areflexia and ataxia. Signs and symptoms may be progressive, especially in intoxication with longer-acting agents, such as phenobarbital. In the absence of administration of a specific antidote, such as naloxone for opioids or flumazenil for benzodiazepines, differentiation between causative agents may prove difficult on clinical grounds.

Chronic Fatigue Syndrome and Related Disorders

Fatigue is a common complaint in both adult and pediatric medicine. It may take the form of simple "lack of energy" or present as a more pervasive syndrome attended by an "infectious" prodrome and a host of somatic symptoms, including weakness, malaise, and sleep, appetite, and emotional or neuropsychiatric disturbances. This cluster of symptoms has been codified as *chronic fatigue syndrome*. The disorder is marked by extreme, disabling fatigability of longer than 6 months' duration, lasting an average of 2 to 3 years, but usually with eventual full recovery. In a cohort of Chicago primary care adolescent patients the rate of chronic fatigue syndrome was 4.4% [Mears et al., 2004]. Diagnostic criteria have been developed, although the disorder's heterogeneity is recognized [Farrar et al., 1995].

Putative etiologies for chronic fatigue syndrome are numerous. Postinfectious and postviral causes have been explored most thoroughly, although there is little direct evidence of an association between infection and chronic fatigue syndrome. In one study an apparent infection rate of 72% in chronic fatigue syndrome patients yielded a proven infection rate of only 7% [Salit, 1997]. Other contributing factors included trauma, surgery, antecedent stressful events, and allergies. Psychiatric factors are also suggested [Huibers et al., 2004]. Allergies have been implicated as a result of findings of possible but inconsistent immunologic alterations in chronic fatigue syndrome patients, a 65% rate of positive allergy history in chronic fatigue syndrome patients, and anecdotal reports of chronic fatigue syndrome onset after immunizations [Farrar et al., 1995; Salit, 1997]. Rigorous evaluation of the cohort of Salit revealed no correlation between chronic fatigue syndrome and exposure to animals, raw milk, meat, cigarette smoking, or foreign travel [Salit, 1997].

Neurobehavioral abnormalities in children are also ascribed frequently to allergies or "environmental toxins." Some models for testing the causal relationship in adults exist but are applicable only in individual assessments, and the field is in its infancy [Weiss, 1994]. There are no large-scale studies of toxic causes for childhood behavioral disorders. A systematic approach to a child in whom there is concern for such a causal exposure begins with a careful history and physical examination to discern any evidence of exposure to known toxins. Temporal and spatial aspects of the history may be especially important. Other possible causes, including psychosocial factors, should be investigated as well. Results of this evaluation should direct any subsequent testing. Elimination of the putative offending agent (or removal of the child from the environment) should be an option, but disruption of the child's life is a significant consideration in cases in which there is little evidence of environmental toxic exposure. Cognitive behavioral therapy has been associated with improvement in chronic fatigue syndrome symptoms in adolescents and adults. Although relapse of some symptoms is common, functional outcome, including school attendance, improves [Stulemeijer et al., 2005].

SPECIFIC AGENTS

Toxic effects of several specific agents deserve additional discussion. Although there is much overlap in toxicity among various poisons and therapeutically used medications (see preceding discussion of toxidromes), individual classes of toxins, and in some cases individual agents, may have unique effects and specific remedies.

Poisons and Environmental Toxins

Biologic Toxins

Biologic toxins include snake, tick, insect, and fish toxins, botanical toxins, and bacterial toxins (e.g., diphtheria, tetanus, botulism). Botanical poisonings are especially common among children; whereas most are mild and result from ingestion of easily accessible houseplants, other botanical poisonings may have more serious consequences (see Table 87-1 and Boxes 87-2 and 87-4 to 87-9) [Krenzelok et al., 1996]. See also reviews by Hardin and Arena [1974], Kunkel [1983], and Langford and Boor [1996].

Snake venoms, which in the United States are primarily from rattlesnakes and copperheads, are strong neurotoxins. In addition to the local effects of envenomation, there are systemic symptoms of fever, nausea, vomiting, diarrhea, and tachycardia, as well as altered blood coagulation. Neurotoxins affect the neuromuscular junction, causing paralysis of the diaphragm and the intercostal and limb muscles and, more rarely, altered states of consciousness and convulsions. There is controversy concerning the use of local incisions, fasciotomy, application of ice packs, and steroids. Exercise hastens absorption of venom. Intravenous administration of specific antivenoms is recommended [Grant et al., 1997; Hawgood, 1996; Podgorny, 1983]. The occurrence of the various envenomations depends partially on regional fauna. In New South Wales, Australia, the percentage of poisoning from envenomation range from 3.1% (females aged 15 to 19 years) to 84.1% (males aged 5 to 9 years) [Lam, 2003].

Tick paralysis is an infrequent but treatable cause of acute paralysis or ataxia caused by neurotoxins from *Dermacentor andersoni* (wood tick), *Dermacentor variabilis* (dog tick), *Amblyomma americanum* (Lone Star tick), *Amblyomma maculatum*, *Ixodes scapularis* (black-legged tick), and *Ixodes pacificus* (western black-legged tick) [Centers for Disease Control and Prevention, 1996a]. Although most prevalent in states west of the Rocky Mountains, tick paralysis also occurs in the southeastern and northeastern United States. Small children are most likely to be paralyzed. The scalp and neck at the hairline are the most common sites for attachment of the gravid tick, which produces a neurotoxin that prevents liberation of acetylcholine at the neuromuscular junction [Swift and Ignacio, 1975]. Within 5 to 6 days after tick attachment, the child develops restlessness and irritability, followed within 24 hours by progressive ataxia and difficulty walking or by symmetric ascending flaccid paralysis with loss of deep tendon reflexes. Removal of the tick in the early stage of the disease leads to reversal of the clinical manifestations within 24 hours, whereas failure to remove the tick may result in progressive bulbar paralysis and death. Insect repellents, especially permethrin-containing products applied to children's clothing, may be used as a preventive measure.

Botulinum toxin blocks presynaptic release of acetylcholine and causes neuromuscular junction blockade. Infection with *Clostridium botulinum* spores results in three different clinical syndromes. Food-borne botulism occurs after ingestion of food, which is frequently home cooked and canned, that is contaminated with *C. botulinum*. Nonacidic canned vegetable products and soups are frequently implicated, and recent reports also implicate dairy products as a source of botulism poisoning [Aureli et al., 1996; Townes et al., 1996]. There are prominent gastrointestinal symptoms of diarrhea and vomiting, followed by rapidly developing progressive paralytic disease associated with visual blurring and diplopia, dysphagia, dysarthria, and subsequent weakness of extremities and intercostal muscles. Antitoxin is effective only if given early [Cherington, 1974].

Infantile botulism, which occurs almost exclusively in the first months of life, can be a severe paralytic disease affecting the limbs, trunk, bulbar musculature, and cranial nerves. It is preceded almost universally by a history of severe constipation without other gastrointestinal symptoms. This illness has been reported in clusters in both California and Pennsylvania, but it has also been observed in isolated instances throughout the United States and in some instances has been related to the ingestion of honey-containing botulinum spores [Glatman-Freedman, 1996; Johnson et al., 1979; Midura, 1996].

Wound botulism, the rarest form of botulism, is both a local infection of contaminated wounds and a systemic intoxication. It can produce a paralytic illness that may be indistinguishable clinically from the disorder produced by food-borne botulism. The most common cause of wound botulism in the United States is secondary to intravenous drug abuse [Centers for Disease Control and Prevention, 1996b]. Rarely, wound botulism may result from small intranasal or septal abscesses in nasal cocaine abusers. Botulism mimicking Guillain-Barré syndrome has been reported [Griffin et al., 1997].

Insecticides

Organophosphate and carbamate insecticides account for most childhood insecticide exposures. Fortunately, most childhood exposures do not result in poisoning. Fewer than 10% of the 8500 insecticide exposures reported to 16 regional poison control centers in 1983 were symptomatic or associated with more than minor symptoms [Veltri and Litovitz, 1984]. A later nine-state study from 1999 to 2002 confirmed that even with active community spraying programs, symptomatic exposure was rare. In that study, 133 cases were reported among a population of 118 million people. Of these cases, 29 resulted from a single incident in which a mosquito-control truck inadvertently sprayed a malathion-containing product during a softball game. Only one person, who survived, had severe toxicity [Patel et al., 2003]. However, these agents are acetylcholinesterase inhibitors, which may result in serious cholinergic signs. Toxins can be absorbed through the skin and gastrointestinal tract, but most childhood poisonings are the result of ingestion. Signs of acute intoxication occur usually within 12 to 24 hours but can develop in minutes after an acute exposure, indicating severe intoxication and a medical emergency. Salivation, lacrimation, bronchoconstriction, wheezing, and increased pulmonary secretions are all muscarinic manifestations. Peripheral nicotinic signs include muscle weakness, decreased respiratory effort, and muscle fasciculations. CNS signs are anxiety, restlessness, confusion, headache, slurred speech, ataxia, and generalized seizures. Opsoclonus has been reported with diazinon poisoning in an adult [Liang et al., 2003]. With low-dose organophosphate exposure, muscarinic signs predominate, but in more severe acute intoxication, the nicotinic and CNS signs appear. Nicotinic effects appear to mediate delayed peripheral toxicity. With longer-acting agents, such as chlorpyrifos (Dursban), recovery is protracted and possibly incomplete [Sherman, 1995]. Rarely a myopathy may complicate the picture [Marrs, 1993; Rusyniak and Nanagas, 2004].

A scoring system called Acute Physiology and Chronic Health Evaluation II (APACHE II) has been applied to adults with organophosphate poisoning and has indicated high predictive value for intensive care unit admission and subsequent mortality [Lee and Tai, 2001]. Cholinesterase levels may be used to predict subsequent weaning of mechanical ventilation in surviving patients.

Treatment includes decontamination, general supportive therapy, and administration of specific antidote, including atropine and pralidoxime or obidoxime, the oximes being cholinesterase reactivators [Mortensen, 1986]. Prompt decontamination protects both the patient and attendant health-care workers [Stacey et al., 2004]. The dose of atropine for children younger than 12 years is 0.02 to 0.05 mg/kg, followed by maintenance doses of 0.02 to 0.05 mg/kg repeated every 10 to 30 minutes (maximum dose, 1 to 2 mg) until cholinergic signs are reversed. For children older than 12 years, the adult dose of atropine (1 to 2 mg) may be used. Because pralidoxime does not cross the blood-brain barrier, atropine must be continued in addition to pralidoxime to reverse central and muscarinic receptor overstimulation. The response to antidote virtually confirms the diagnosis suggested by the history of exposure and the characteristic acute cholinergic symptoms, although intermediate (1 to 4 days after exposure) and delayed effects are not influenced by atropine or oxime therapy [Marrs, 1993]. These delayed effects are not seen generally in insecticides available in the United States and Europe, and it is thought that the delayed central effects are mediated not by cholinergic mechanisms but rather by direct phosphorylation of neuronal structures [Marrs, 1993]. A newer therapeutic agent, liposome encapsulating organophosphorus hydrolase, has demonstrated promise in the laboratory, raising the median lethal dose of paraoxon beyond that provided by pralidoxime and atropine combined [Petrikovics et al., 2004].

Endosulfan, a chlorinated hydrocarbon, may pose a chronic and endemic threat to children with repeated exposure. Acute intoxication causes respiratory distress, gagging, vomiting, diarrhea, agitation, convulsions, ataxia, and coma in severe cases. Fatal status epilepticus occurs, and endosulfan-related fatalities occurred in Sri Lanka in 1998 before the agent was banned that year [Roberts et al., 2003]. Dewan and associates reported recurrent convulsions and several deaths in a rural area of India due to wheat flour being stored in containers previously used for endosulfan storage [Dewan et al., 2004]. Amitraz, a formamidine pesticide, has side effects similar to clonidine overdose (CNS depression, miosis, bradycardia, hypotension, emesis, and hyperglycemia). With adequate support, death is rare [Aydin et al., 2002].

Nerve Agents

Nerve agents are chemically related to organophosphate insecticides but are far more potent [Newmark, 2004]. A single drop of VX on the skin may kill a person. Childhood exposure would likely be as result of deliberate attack with nerve agents. They are divided into two classes: G agents and V agents. Tabun (GA), Sarin (GB), and Soman (GD), are clear, tasteless, and colorless, and mostly odorless. Tabun and Soman may have a slightly fruity odor, but this property is not clinically useful. VX is amber and oily but also odorless and tasteless. All may exert their effects within seconds to minutes depending on route of exposure. Onset after cutaneous exposure may be delayed up to 18 hours. Management, as with insecticide poisoning, rests on decontamination; airway, breathing, and cardiovascular stabilization; and specific antidotes as described previously [Rotenberg and Newmark, 2003; Smythies and Golomb, 2004]. The Centers for Disease Control and Prevention maintain a web site outlining exposure and management information for these agents (http://www.atsdr.cdc.gov/MHMI/mmg166.html) [Patel et al., 2003].

LINDANE

Lindane (1,2,3,4,5,6-hexachlorocyclohexane) is a topical pediculicide used commonly throughout the world. Its use has been associated with significant neurotoxicity, especially in infants. Lindane passes easily into the CNS; brain levels may greatly exceed blood levels [Fischer, 1994].

Acute lindane neurotoxicity manifests usually as generalized seizures. Mental status changes and extrapyramidal movements may occur as well. Onset of symptoms after topical use occurs within a few hours, with generally complete resolution within 48 hours. Although topical lindane poisoning in young adults is reported, it most commonly results from inappropriate or excessive use of the medication in children [Boffa et al., 1995; Fischer, 1994; Forrester et al., 2004]. Occupational exposure may result in chronic lindane poisoning manifesting as emotional changes, muscle jerking, and alteration of the electroencephalogram [Aks et al., 1995]. Accidental ingestion of lindane is usually reported in toddlers. This situation appears to result from parental misunderstanding of application instructions. High levels may be attained quickly, and vomiting and seizures result, although vomiting and ocular pain are common [Forrester et al., 2004]. Myonecrosis may occur with blood lindane levels exceeding 0.6 g/mL, whereas blood levels in excess of 1.2 g/mL may be fatal [Aks et al., 1995].

Treatment of acute topical exposure is supportive, with control of seizures necessary. Barbiturates or benzodiazepines are the antiepileptic drugs of choice; phenytoin should be avoided because it may exacerbate lindane-induced seizures [Aks et al., 1995]. Gastric lavage may be attempted within 30 to 60 minutes after ingestion; subsequently, activated charcoal or cholestyramine speeds gastrointestinal excretion of lindane. Prevention of lindane poisoning is easier than its treatment. Permethrin 5% preparations may be safer in infants and young toddlers. Repeated exposures within 7 days and increased topical absorption (e.g., with open wounds or after a hot bath) enhance toxicity. Finally, pediculicidal preparations available in the United States contain 1% lindane; lindane 0.3% preparations have been effective in other nations [Surber and Rufli, 1995].

INSECT REPELLENTS

The most effective general insect repellent currently in use is diethyltoluamide (permethrin is more effective against ticks), a compound available in many topical preparations. Although increasing the diethyltoluamide concentration up to 75% increases its efficacy, preparations containing more than 20% diethyltoluamide are likely to cause neurotoxicity, and most products for children contain 8% to 10% diethyltoluamide [Brown and Herbert, 1997]. Children using compounds with as little as 20% diethyltoluamide may suffer seizures (8 to 48 hours after exposure), ataxia, and tremor [Oransky et al., 1989; Sudakin, 2003]. There is some evidence, in fact, that there is no absolutely safe level of diethyltoluamide exposure for children [Briassoulis et al., 2001].

Metals

LEAD

Acute lead poisoning is rare. The syndrome of acute lead encephalopathy in children with pica who ate lead paint chips from peeling paint and plaster in older dwellings consisted of listlessness, drowsiness, and irritability, followed by seizures and signs and symptoms of acutely increased intracranial pressure. Severe cerebral edema resulting from acute lead encephalopathy often resulted in significant neurologic sequelae. Use of lead-based paints for indoor use was banned in the United States in 1978, with a consequent decrease in lead toxicity since.

Chronic lead exposure as a result of ingestion of lead paint, inhalation of automobile exhaust fumes, or inhalation of industrial pollutants may result in high levels of blood lead and is the more common form of intoxication today. Lead poisoning is defined as a blood lead level of greater than 10 µg/dL, although this threshold is undergoing critical reappraisal as perhaps too liberal [Lidsky and Schneider, 2003; Wilken et al., 2004]. Most children with lead poisoning are asymptomatic. A lead concentration of 25 µg/dL or higher in blood is reported to be associated with learning problems and neurobehavioral effects [Bellinger, 1995; Bellinger et al., 1991; Landrigan et al., 1975; LaPorte and Talbott, 1978; Winneke et al., 1990, 1996]. Measurement of full-scale intelligence may be relatively insensitive in detecting the deleterious effects of chronic lead exposure in children; subtests measuring visual motor and reaction performance skills appear to be more sensitive. Some authorities recommend treatment with ethylenediaminetetraacidic acid for children who have even mildly elevated lead levels (i.e., greater than 25 µg/dL) [American Academy of Pediatrics, 1995; Piomelli et al., 1984; Trachtenbarg, 1996]. A newer oral chelation agent, meso 2,3-dimercapto-succinic acid, has been approved recently and used for children with blood lead levels greater than 45 µg/dL [Berlin, 1997]. Acute lead encephalopathy at any blood lead level constitutes a life-threatening emergency and should be managed accordingly [American Academy of Pediatrics Committee on Drugs, 1995].

MERCURY

Mercury poisoning can result from both inorganic and organic mercury exposure. The former can occur acutely after accidental ingestion of an antiseptic solution containing mercury. Chronic poisoning may follow prolonged use of mercury-containing teething powders, repeated applications of ammoniated mercury ointment to the skin, or application of mercury-containing antiseptics to the oral mucosa. Acute inorganic mercury poisoning results primarily in severe gastrointestinal problems without neurologic symptoms, whereas chronic or subacute mercury toxicity is manifested by the development of coarse tremor, irritability, and peripheral neuropathy. Symptoms of acrdynia, now mainly of historical interest, include irritability and signs of profound peripheral neuropathy.

Organic mercury poisoning has occurred as a result of ingestion of fish (contaminated by mercury-polluted water), grain (contaminated by mercurial fungicides), or pork (contaminated by feeding pigs mercury fungicide–treated grain) [Cranmer et al., 1996; Zepp et al., 1974]. Minamata disease occurred in people who ate fish from mercury-contaminated waters and exemplified the danger of organic mercury bioamplification as it ascends the food chain [Bigham and Vandal, 1996]. The symptoms and signs of organic mercury poisoning include ataxia, peripheral neuropathy, choreoathetosis, visual loss, confusion, and coma [Patel et al., 2003]. Subclinical mercury neurotoxicity has been demonstrated as well in occupational exposures, using visual-evoked potentials and electromyography [Urban et al., 1996]. Dimercaprol and 2,3-dimercaptosuccinic acid effectively chelate and remove mercury from the tissues but do not necessarily reverse the clinical manifestations. Heavy-metal poisoning may also cause a peripheral neuropathy, although this is rare in children. Ingestion of elemental mercury, such as from a broken thermometer, does not usually cause mercury poisoning; however, Koyun and colleagues reported serious mercury intoxication in three unrelated teenagers after exposure to a broken manometer [Koyun et al., 2004]. Despite chelation therapy, one patient died. Although other heavy-metal poisoning is usually associated with industrial exposure affecting workers, poisoning may also occur in children. Smelting operations may release large amounts of lead, zinc, cadmium, and arsenic into the surrounding environment [American Academy of Pediatrics Committee on Drugs, 1997].

Perhaps no topic concerning mercury has resulted in as much controversy as an alleged link between thimerosal and autism. In such debates, causal links are difficult to prove, and often even more difficult to disprove once suggested. Most peer-reviewed literature does not support an association beyond coincident timing of vaccines and manifestations of autism. Furthermore, historical evidence (e.g., Minamata disease) reveals a different developmental neuropathology regarding mercury poisoning [Nelson and Bauman, 2003].

THALLIUM

Thallium was once used as treatment for night sweats in tuberculosis and topically for ringworm in children (with mortality rates reported as high as 5%) [Dyck and Thomas, 1993]. The primary modern sources of thallium are rodenticides and insecticides. Ingestion may be accidental or intentional. Thallium poisoning presents with the clinical triad of abdominal pain, alopecia, and mixed peripheral neuropathy. Although there may be gastritis and hepatic injury, abdominal pain is usually secondary to peripheral neuropathy [Burnett, 1990]. Alopecia occurs suddenly after a 2- to 3-week delay and is associated with an acneiform rash over the nose, cheeks, and nasolabial folds [Dyck and Thomas, 1993]. The neuropathy is both demyelinating and axonal. Other neurologic effects of thallium include cranial neuropathies involving optic and oculomotor nerves, CNS depression, dementia, delirium, and seizures. CNS levels of thallium may continue to rise for at least a few days after the initial exposure [Sharma et al., 2004]. Cardiovascular involvement includes hypertension and myocardial damage, with shock and death occurring in massive doses [Sharma et al., 2004]. In adults, acute exposure to as little as 1 g of thallium may be fatal; 5 mg/kg is toxic in children [Burnett, 1990; Patel et al., 2003]. Additional clues to diagnosis of thallium poisoning include the presence of painful distal glossitis, Mees' lines, and black thallium deposits at the base of abnormally tapered hairs [Feldman and Levisohn, 1993]. Cerebrospinal fluid protein may be elevated as well. Thallium crosses the placenta and may affect the fetus.

ARSENIC

Chronic arsenic poisoning is well recognized. Although intentional poisoning captures the imagination, accidental exposure through the workplace or environmental contamination poses a larger public health problem. Because inorganic arsenic poses a greater threat of acute poisoning than does the less toxic organic arsenic, most severe accidental poisonings occur by contamination of water supply [Abernathy et al., 2003]. Acute poisoning manifests with nausea and vomiting, abdominal pain, and diarrhea, together with cutaneous and neurologic findings [Ratnaike, 2003]. Severe inorganic arsenic poisoning also results in encephalopathy in older children [Patel et al., 2003]. Reports describe endemic chronic arsenic intoxication within entire families and towns resulting from contamination of the local water supply or from chronic dust exposure [Gerr et al., 2000]. In these epidemics, children are affected with the typical keratoderma and distal peripheral neuropathy and may also be mentally retarded [Das et al., 1995; Foy et al., 1992–1993; Mazumder et al., 1992]. Other acute cutaneous findings may include facial edema, transient flushing, conjunctival hemorrhage, and maculopapular rash in intertriginous areas. Mees' lines may be found several months after exposure [Uede and Furukawa, 2003]. Unlike thallium, arsenic typically does not cause alopecia [Rusyniak et al., 2002].

Heavy-metal exposure, including cadmium, lead, arsenic, mercury, and thallium, may occur from intake of medicinals. Ernst and Coon provide a review of such metal toxicity in traditional Chinese medicines [Ernst and Coon, 2001].

Solvents

Isopropyl alcohol poisoning most commonly results from the ingestion of common household "rubbing alcohol." Isopropyl alcohol vaporizes readily and is rapidly absorbed through the lungs. Alcohol sponging for fever reduction, especially in a poorly ventilated room, can result in intoxication and coma. Ingestion of as little as 20 mL can produce symptoms [McFadden and Haddow, 1969]. Peak serum levels are reached in about 1 hour, with adverse initial symptoms, primarily gastrointestinal complaints, occurring within 30 minutes after ingestion. CNS effects include headache, confusion, dizziness, ataxia, stupor, and deep coma, which may be caused partially by the formation of acetone during metabolism [Mydler et al., 1993]. Hypotension and hypothermia may occur. The diagnosis is suggested by history, characteristic odor on the patient's breath, and the presence of large amounts of ketones in the urine without significant metabolic acidosis. Urine toxicology may be revealing [Mydler et al., 1993]. Treatment is primarily supportive. Intermittent or continuous gastric lavage has been suggested, but use of syrup of ipecac is contraindicated; charcoal may be beneficial [Leikin and Paloucek, 1995].

Intoxication has also been reported with benzyl alcohol, which was used as an antibacterial agent and a preservative in saline solution. This form of intoxication, called the *gasping syndrome,* was reported after the administration of saline solutions as intravenous flushes in small, preterm infants [American Academy of Pediatrics Committee on Drugs, 1997; Gershanik et al., 1982]. The infusion of small amounts of flush solutions containing 0.9% benzyl alcohol may cause severe metabolic acidosis, encephalopathy, respiratory depression with gasping, and death. Intoxication from other sources of benzyl alcohol (i.e., as a preservative in medications other than saline) is unlikely.

Children may suffer from clinically significant environmental exposure to solvents. This exposure may occur especially in areas with little child labor protection, resulting in occupational exposure [Saddik et al., 2003].

Other Nonpharmacologic Compounds

A patient presented after ingesting matchstick heads, of which potassium chlorate is the major component, in coma; his MRI indicated bilateral symmetric deep gray matter and temporal lobe hyperintensity on T2-weighted images. He recovered after hyperbaric oxygen therapy and supportive care [Mutlu et al., 2003].

Drugs of Abuse

Cocaine

Cocaine abuse has reached epidemic proportions, especially among young adults. Lifetime incidence of cocaine use is 15% among high school seniors and more than 20% among college students. There is a suggestion of a decrease in cocaine use, although the same may not be true of crack cocaine. Almost 1 in 20 high school seniors have tried crack cocaine [O'Malley et al., 1991].

Cocaine, a stimulant alkaloid, is derived from the leaves of the shrub *Erythroxyline cocoa.* Cocaine inhibits reuptake of norepinephrine, dopamine, and serotonin. Acute toxicity, manifested by tremors, diaphoresis, tachycardia, cardiac dysrhythmias, vasoconstriction, and hypertension, is probably the result of cocaine's effect on norepinephrine reuptake. Behavioral effects are most likely caused by its actions on the dopaminergic system. Cocaine use results in an enhanced sense of well-being, increased alertness and excitement, and apparent enhancement of the reward response. These effects are followed by anxiety, depression, exhaustion, and sometimes paranoid psychosis. Addiction follows continued use. Stroke, intracranial hemorrhage, and seizures have been reported [Levine et al., 1990; Mody et al., 1988; Sloan et al., 1991; Walsh and Garg, 1997]. Infants and children passively exposed to cocaine may have similar complications; however, some have disputed these effects [Wurtzel et al., 1988]. Increased cerebral blood flow velocity has been found in infants exposed to cocaine [Van de Bor et al., 1990].

Narcotics

Data regarding numbers of established narcotic users in childhood are scanty; a great percentage of narcotic users never come to the attention of poison control centers. High school students are among the population at risk, as are children younger than 5 years of age who reside with adults who are narcotic abusers. Narcotics such as morphine, heroin, hydromorphone (Dilaudid), levorphanol (Dromoran), meperidine (Demerol), and methadone share the toxic properties of the opiate group, but the onset and duration of toxic signs vary after ingestion. Opiate users may also be simultaneously exposed to multiple other toxic agents, which are either adulterants of the opiates or are taken concurrently. The signs and symptoms of acute opiate poisoning most commonly follow rapid intravenous administration and include apnea, circulatory collapse, convulsions, and cardiopulmonary arrest. The less severely poisoned patient experiences varying degrees of CNS depression, ranging from drowsiness to profound coma, miotic pupils, and respiratory depression.

Narcotic poisoning in younger children more commonly results from ingestion of various analgesics, such as meperidine, codeine, oxycodone (Percodan), and pentazocine (Talwin). Ingestion of a large dose, whether accidental or iatrogenic, of the antidiarrheal medication diphenoxylate (Lomotil), which also contains atropine, may result in signs of opiate toxicity with CNS and respiratory depression, as well as signs of atropine overdose, such as facial flushing, tachycardia, dry mouth, hyperpyrexia, and agitation [Brunton, 1996; POISINDEX, 2005].

Treatment of opiate intoxication includes administration of naloxone, a specific and highly effective opiate antagonist, and maintenance of respiration and circulation. The initial dose of naloxone is 0.01 mg/kg; if there is no response, the dose can be increased up to 10-fold, to 0.1 mg/kg. Naloxone can be given intravenously, intramuscularly, or even through an endotracheal tube, with effects lasting 30 to 45 minutes. Constant monitoring of the patient is required, with repeated doses of naloxone administered as needed in addition to supportive care.

Nanan and associates reported the case of a 14-year-old female with intentional morphine sulfate overdose and leukoencephalopathy involving the corpus callosum, centrum semiovale, and cerebellar white matter [Nanan et al., 2000]. The MRI findings were not explained adequately by hypoxic-ischemic injury, and a drug-induced neurotoxicity was suggested. Other cases of severe neurotoxicity resulting from polypharmacy are reported [Nebelsieck, 2004]. Injected heroin also has been reported to produce a spongiform leukoencephalopathy [Robertson et al., 2001]

Cannabis

Cannabis usually is taken recreationally by inhalation (smoking marijuana cigarettes) or ingestion. The active compound is tetrahydrocannabinol. Tetrahydrocannabinol intoxication produces psychomotor slowing acutely, short-term memory loss, analgesia, and appetite stimulation. Coma has been reported in children ingesting cannabis-laced cookies. Cannabis ingestion should be considered in cases of coma, especially when associated with conjunctival hyperemia, pupillary dilation, and tachycardia and when there is no other obvious cause [Boros et al., 1996].

Tetrahydrocannabinol acts through the CB1 receptor [Iverson, 2003]. Interestingly, anandamide, an endogenous ligand for the CB1 receptor, has been implicated in the "runner's high" [Sparling et al., 2003]. Long-term biologic sequelae of cannabis use are ill defined. Dependency may occur, as may apparently reversible mild cognitive impairment. Psychosocial consequences may be more severe.

γ-Hydroxybutyrate

γ-Hydroxybutyrate is a schedule I sedative-hypnotic drug. Although it is used volitionally as a recreational drug, its most infamous use is when it is given surreptitiously as a "date-rape" drug. There is suggestion in the literature that its sedative effects may be reversed by physostigmine, but no conclusive data exist [Caldicott and Kuhn, 2001; Traub et al., 2002].

Volatile Solvents and Propellants

Hydrocarbon-based solvents are frequently used by adolescents for their euphoria-producing effects. The compounds commonly in use include various glues, rubber and model airplane cements, typewriter correction fluids, gasoline, lighter fluids, and aerosols [Doring et al., 2002]. Neurologic effects develop within minutes and last several hours, with an initial excitatory stage of euphoria, mental confusion, ataxia, and dysarthria, followed by lethargy, sleep, and coma. Cerebellar dysfunction and sensorimotor neuropathy from chronic gasoline sniffing have been reported [Prockop, 1979; Prockop et al., 1974; Young et al., 1977]. Permanent cognitive impairment and CT evidence of diffuse atrophy of the cerebral hemispheres, cerebellum, and brainstem have also been documented [Hormes et al., 1986]. More sequelae occur with abuse of leaded gasoline [Cairney et al., 2004]. One MRI series demonstrated cerebral atrophy, white matter hyperintensity on T2-weighted images, and hypointensity involving the basal ganglia and thalami on T2-weighted images, as well as focal enhancement. Although a correlation was found between the degree of neurologic impairment and extent of white matter disease, no correlation was seen between radiographic evidence of damage to subcortical gray structures and clinical findings [Caldemeyer et al., 1996].

Nitrous Oxide

Nitrous oxide abuse is governed by access and therefore is rare in children. Neurotoxicity is related to nitrous oxide's ability to interfere with the cobalamin cofactor of methionine synthetase. Neurologic toxicity, which occurs after months of daily use, presents as subacute combined degeneration of the spinal cord [Seppelt, 1995].

Hallucinogens

Phencyclidine, also known as *angel dust* or *PCP*, is a readily available drug of abuse that is commonly inhaled or ingested. The clinical syndrome of phencyclidine palmitate toxicity includes euphoria and a "high" appearance, at times with violent behavior associated with extreme muscular rigidity and Herculean displays of muscle strength. Vertical and horizontal nystagmus is common, along with marked pupillary dilation. Instead of excitation, the intoxicated patient may manifest a syndrome of catatonic rigidity, opisthotonus, dystonic posturing, stupor or profound fluctuations in the level of consciousness, seizures, and myoclonus. Extreme elevations of blood pressure are common. Intracranial hemorrhage has been reported [Bessen, 1982; Boyko et al., 1987]. The phencyclidine palmitate–intoxicated patient should be sedated, especially if agitated or seizing, cooled for extreme degrees of hyperthermia, and treated for systolic hypertension with hydralazine or diazoxide [Kulberg, 1986]. Gastric lavage is helpful in removing ingested but unabsorbed drug. Urinary acidification promotes drug excretion.

Lysergic acid diethylamide remains a potent and frequently abused hallucinogen. Lysergic acid diethylamide intoxication results in acute personality changes, hallucinations, and feelings of depersonalization. Acute panic reactions, or "bad trips," may occur with neurologic signs of excitation, including ataxia, tremors, diaphoresis, convulsions, and, with severe toxicity, coma and respiratory arrest. Most of the milder cases resolve spontaneously; there is no specific antidote or treatment for lysergic acid diethylamide poisoning other than general support and sedation.

Finally, coma has been reported in children ingesting cannabis-laced cookies. Cannabis ingestion should be considered in cases of coma, especially when associated with conjunctival hyperemia, pupillary dilation, and tachycardia and when there is no other obvious cause [Boros et al., 1996].

Amphetamines

Amphetamines such as dextroamphetamine, benzedrine, and methamphetamine cause clinically similar effects, including a sense of well-being and decreased fatigue. With increasing doses, acute paranoid psychosis may develop, with mania, hyperactivity, and severe sympathomimetic effects, including mydriasis, flushing, diaphoresis, and tachycardia. Convulsions are rare. Cerebral vasculitis, cerebral infarction, and intracranial hemorrhage have been reported with amphetamine use [Delaney and Estes, 1980; Matick et al., 1983; Rothrock et al., 1988]. Gastric lavage is useful in elimination of the toxin. Severe agitation or seizures may be treated with intravenous benzodiazepines; hallucinations may also be treated with haloperidol. Hyperthermia should be treated aggressively; diazoxide or nitroprusside may be indicated for severe hypertension. Adverse effects of medicinal amphetamine use are discussed later in this chapter.

"Ecstasy"

3,4-Methylenedioxymethamphetamine (commonly known as *ecstasy*) continues to be a popular drug of abuse. Its primary mode of action is to both stimulate and block reuptake of serotonin (5-hydroxytryptamine) [Parrott, 2002]. It also has lesser effect on other monoaminergic neurotransmitters. Taken at dance parties called *raves*, it promotes a feeling of closeness and heightens sensory experience. It also causes euphoria. Acutely, it commonly causes serotonergic symptoms of confusion, hyperkinesis, and increased body temperature. These symptoms may be exacerbated by conditions that may prevail at raves: overcrowding, high ambient temperature, and coincident use of other stimulants. Rarely these symptoms can develop into a full-blown serotonergic syndrome and a medical emergency. Once the acute effects wear off, depressive symptoms resulting from monoaminergic depletion occur. There are both laboratory animal and human data suggesting subsequent serotonergic axonal damage [Parrott, 2002].

Ethanol

Ethanol is abused increasingly often by children; acute alcohol intoxication and even chronic alcoholism have become serious problems in children as young as 10 years of age. The signs of acute alcohol intoxication are familiar, but a pediatrician confronted with a child who exhibits incoordiation, ataxia, wide mood swings, impaired awareness, and gastrointestinal distress may not consider the diagnosis. Profound CNS depression follows ingestion of large amounts of alcohol. Alcohol withdrawal syndromes are rare in children. Alcohol intoxication may occur in mixed substance abuse. Accidental alcohol intoxication has also been reported in young children drinking attractively packaged and flavored mouthwashes. These mouthwashes have a significant ethanol content (14.2% to 26.9%) [Selbst et al., 1985], as do a variety of medicinal preparations, including cough medicines, decongestants, and teething preparations [Pruitt, 1984]. Chronic ethanol exposure in pregnant women causes fetal alcohol syndrome, as well as lesser fetal alcohol effects (see later discussion); some studies have suggested radiographically demonstrable brain injury in infants born to pregnant women consuming large amounts of alcohol [Holzman et al., 1995; Mattson et al., 1994]. Alcohol abuse may have a relationship to teenage suicide [Esposito-Smythers and Spirito, 2004]. Alcohol intoxication may increase the risk for suicidal attempts acutely. Its long-term disruptive influence on the young person's life also may lead to further depressive symptoms and subsequent suicidal behavior.

Barbiturates

Barbiturate poisoning in small children is usually the result of accidental ingestion, whereas barbiturate poisoning in teenagers is often seen in suicide attempts. Barbiturate intoxication produces confusion and varying degrees of sedation and coma; lesser amounts may result in ataxia. Respiratory depression, flaccid areflexia, miotic pupils, and absent brainstem reflexes occur with more severe poisoning. Although barbiturates are absorbed rapidly, gastric lavage should be used within 1 hour of ingestion. Activated charcoal is also indicated in the management of barbiturate poisoning; the half-life of longer-acting barbiturates is shortened by repeated doses of activated charcoal administered over 3 to 4 days. Urine alkalinization and forced diuresis enhance the clearance of barbiturates. Because there are no antidotes to barbiturates and the use of stimulant drugs is contraindicated, the prime consideration in the treatment of the child with barbiturate intoxication is respiratory and circulatory support. Renal function monitoring is necessary because renal failure may be a consequence of hypotension and shock. Hemodialysis is of unproved value but may benefit severely intoxicated patients.

Barbiturates are an uncommon cause of reflex sympathetic dystrophy [Falasca et al., 1994; Botella et al., 1996].

Other Medications

Benzodiazepines

Intoxication with benzodiazepines is common because of their ready availability. These compounds produce depression and sedation at low doses and confusion, somnolence, and coma at higher doses. Respiratory depression and hypotension may occur. The combination of benzodiazepines and other CNS depressants is potentially fatal. Treatment consists of supportive care and administration of flumazenil, a specific benzodiazepine antagonist. An optimal dose is not defined, but an initial dose of 0.01 to 0.02 mg/kg (maximum dose, 0.125 mg) is suggested; repeated doses or continuous infusion may be necessary. Flumazenil-induced convulsions may occur in individuals with chronic benzodiazepine use [Leiken and Paloucek, 1995; Perry and Shannon, 1996].

Other Sedatives

Chloral hydrate, ethchlorvynol (Placidyl), methaqualone, and glutethimide (Doriden) are sedatives that can cause severe intoxication with CNS depression. With mild intoxication, the child may be lethargic, confused, and ataxic; with severe intoxication, profound hypotonia, coma, and ophthalmoplegia may occur. Glutethimide in particular is associated with prolonged periods of unconsciousness. Careful attention must be given to respiratory support, which may be prolonged, and premature weaning must be avoided [Nicholson, 1983]. Glutethimide and its metabolites persist in the blood because they recirculate from fat stores and undergo enterohepatic circulation, resulting in reabsorption from the gastrointestinal tract; however, there is a poor correlation between plasma levels of glutethimide and clinical effects. Activated charcoal and resin hemoperfusion have been used in patients who have not responded to standard supportive measures. There are no specific antidotes for these sedative agents, although methylene blue is used to treat glutethimide-induced methemoglobinemia.

Despite its notoriety as a teratogen, the hypnotic agent thalidomide has been used in many infectious and inflammatory conditions, including human immunodeficiency virus–related complications, leprosy, graft-versus-host disease, and lupus erythematosus. Although it typically causes limb and craniofacial birth defects, fetal thalidomide exposure can also cause congenital cranial neuropathies. Its effects suggest a toxic neural cristopathy. Postnatally, thalidomide acts as a potent neurotoxin, causing a potentially severe and often prolonged, if not permanent, sensory neuropathy [Alexander and Wilcox, 1997; Forsyth et al., 1996; Haslett et al., 1997; LeQuesne, 1993; Rodier et al., 1997].

Antipsychotic Agents (Neuroleptics)

Major tranquilizers include phenothiazines and related compounds, as well as butyrophenones, which are associated with a variety of serious neurologic complications, including sedation, acute dystonic reactions, akathisia, pseudoparkinsonism, withdrawal, emergent dyskinesia, tardive dyskinesia, and neuroleptic malignant syndrome. Newer antipsychotic agents include clozapine, sertindole, olanzapine, and risperidone and reportedly have fewer neurologic side effects [Caroff et al., 2002]. Acute intoxication in a young child usually results in a confusional state or depressed level of consciousness. Acute dystonic reactions, often observed in children after a single dose of phenothiazine or haloperidol, may manifest as an oculogyric crisis or sudden dystonic posturing of the head and neck, including opisthotonus, retrocollis, torticollis, facial grimacing, and tongue thrusting. These acute reactions are not necessarily dose related and are usually readily reversed with the intravenous administration of 25 to 50 mg of diphenhydramine. Miosis, coma, hypothermia or hyperthermia, and hypotension may occur after ingestion of a large dose of either phenothiazines or butyrophenones. Respiratory depression suggests the ingestion of additional agents, such as narcotics [Knight and Roberts, 1986].

Akathisia, an internal feeling of restlessness, is a dose-related neurologic complication of neuroleptic treatment and is thought to be rare in children [Sachdev, 1995]. It is one of the most distressing adverse effects of neuroleptic use but usually responds to treatment with anticholinergic drugs or blockers.

Neuroleptic malignant syndrome is a rare complication of neuroleptic drug therapy and is characterized by fever, muscular rigidity, autonomic dysfunction, and altered sensorium with waxing and waning of consciousness. The patient may be in a catatonic-like stupor and may be mute. In children, neuroleptic malignant syndrome occurs during therapy with neuroleptics, as well as after accidental phenothiazine ingestion [Klein et al., 1985b]. Myoglobinuria and acute renal failure may supervene. Treatment consists of intensive supportive care with monitoring of vital signs, aggressive fluid management, and in selected cases dantrolene administration [Caroff and Mann, 1993; Tueth, 1994]. Although reported more often in association with older antipsychotic medications, neuroleptic malignant syndrome occurs also with newer agents such as clozapine, albeit possibly with less dramatic clinical and laboratory findings [Sachdev et al., 1995]. A clinical presentation of confusion, myoclonus, hyperreflexia, diaphoresis, and diarrhea progressing to fever, coma, and rigidity that improved over 10 days with bromocriptine and aggressive intensive care unit care was seen in a young woman taking risperidone and fluvoxamine [Reeves et al., 2002].It was thought that this may not have been neuroleptic malignant syndrome but rather serotonin syndrome.

Tardive dyskinesia after chronic phenothiazine or haloperidol use is extremely rare in children [Singer, 1986]. The propensity to develop tardive dyskinesia may be related to the patient's underlying neural substrate, as found in a recent study. Juckel and colleagues [1995], using auditory event–related potentials, demonstrated an association between a small P300 evoked potential and subsequent tardive dyskinesia.

The newer "novel" antipsychotics, such as clozapine, risperidone, olanzapine, and sertindole, have clinically significant pharmacologic activity at multiple receptors and fewer typical antidopaminergic side effects such as acute parkinsonism, akathisia, and tardive movement disorders [Baldessarini, 1996; Casey, 1996a; Krebs, 1995; Lindstrom et al., 1995; Schooler, 1996]. Clozapine, in particular, appears to be associated with less bradykinesia and akathisia than haloperidol, although not necessarily less tremor [Kurz et al., 1995]. Acute extrapyramidal effects have been seen in children after an overdose of 100 mg of clozapine [Goetz et al., 1993; POISINDEX, 2005]. Confusion, lethargy, and ataxia have also been reported in children. Although clozapine-associated seizures have been reported at doses of 250 mg/day, the prevalence of seizures is higher (5%) in adults taking 600 to 900 mg/day [Haller and Binder, 1990; Tueth, 1994]. Myoclonus has also been reported at higher doses [Bak et al., 1995]. Extrapyramidal side effects (acutely, dystonia) and tardive dyskinesia are reported infrequently with risperidone [Buzan, 1996; Daniel et al., 1996; Faulk et al., 1996]. Olanzapine appears to have an extrapyramidal side-effect profile intermediate between that of the older antipsychotics and its newer cousins [Casey, 1996b].

Antidepressants

Tricyclic antidepressants, such as amitriptyline, imipramine, and desipramine, have been associated with acute toxicity and significant morbidity and mortality. Acute encephalopathy occurs within 4 hours of ingestion and includes ataxia, hallucinations, and nystagmus. Somnolence occurs subsequently, and tremor or myoclonus may occur. Cardiac conduction abnormalities, including tachycardia, heart block, atrial fibrillation, and ventricular flutter, are the most common and serious non-neurologic results of tricyclic intoxication [Pimentel and Trommer, 1994]. Dry mouth, palpitations, and tachycardia occur as typical anticholinergic effects. Death may occur as a result of progressive coma, seizures, and cardiac conduction defects. In acute poisoning, activated charcoal with a cathartic may be helpful; lavage may be attempted if fewer than 6 hours have passed since ingestion. Up to 2 mg of physostigmine administered intravenously may awaken a comatose patient but should be avoided in patients with bradycardia. Keeping the blood pH slightly alkaline (e.g., 7.5) helps in the treatment of tachyarrhythmias. A prolonged QRS interval is a good predictor of seizures and cardiac dysrhythmias in acute intoxication with tricyclics, but serious CNS depression may occur with relatively normal QRS intervals [Boehnert and Lovejoy, 1985]. Amoxapine, a newer tricyclic antidepressant, also frequently induces seizures when taken in toxic amounts, but unlike the other drugs of this class, it does not seriously alter the electrocardiogram [Rogol et al., 1984].

Selective serotonin reuptake inhibitors are some of the most frequently used medications in the United States at the present time. Such popularity stems from their broad range of efficacy and relatively favorable side-effect profile. Although cases of selective serotonin reuptake inhibitor toxicity have increased as a result of this wide availability, serious neurotoxicity is limited generally to accidental ingestions or intentional overdoses, especially in combination with other medications or drugs of abuse [Klein-Schwartz and Anderson, 1996; Lavin et al., 1993; Litovitz et al., 1995]. Paradoxic behavioral reactions and selective sertonin re-uptake inhibitor–induced hyperkinetic movement disorders are perhaps the most likely adverse neurologic effects. In a review of 469 selective serotonin reuptake inhibitor intoxication cases in adults, a more severe serotonergic syndrome, with coma or convulsions, occurred in 2.4% and 1.9%, respectively [Isbister et al., 2004]. Of note, of the five different selective serotonin reuptake inhibitors involved, citalopram had relative QTc prolongation, although its clinical significance was unclear. In a study of isolated accidental fluoxetine ingestion of 20 mg or more in 120 children younger than 6 years, 96% were asymptomatic. Sedation and vomiting were the only side effects reported in symptomatic children [Baker and Morgan, 2004]. Recently, a neonatal withdrawal syndrome including neonatal convulsions has been described in newborns whose mothers were taking selective serotonin reuptake inhibitors during the pregnancy [Sanz et al, 2005].

Lithium

Lithium carbonate, used for the treatment of bipolar depression in adults, is effective in the treatment of certain behavioral and affective disorders in children [Goetting, 1985]. Most cases of lithium intoxication occur during the course of prolonged therapy. The typical patient has apathy, drowsiness, nystagmus, tinnitus, dysarthria, ataxia, coarse muscle tremors, vomiting, and diarrhea. Choreiform movements, dystonic posturing, and cogwheel rigidity may occur. Severity of symptoms correlates well with the serum lithium concentration. Seizures and coma indicate severe toxicity (i.e., serum lithium level, >3.0 mmol/L). Treatment of acute poisoning should include induction of emesis or gastric lavage. However, because of the slow excretion of lithium, symptoms may progress despite cessation of the medication. There is no specific treatment other than attention to fluid balance and support. Sodium chloride administration enhances urinary excretion, particularly if the patient is hyponatremic. Peritoneal dialysis or hemodialysis is used in cases of clinically severe intoxication with serum lithium levels greater than 3 mmol/L [Tueth, 1994]. Prolonged hemodialysis may be necessary to prevent a rebound in serum lithium concentration [Sansone and Ziegler, 1985].

Salicylates and Acetaminophen

Salicylates are present in a myriad of medicinal preparations ranging from aspirin tablets to oil of wintergreen and long-used Chinese medicinal oils [Chan et al., 1995; Chan, 1996]. Poisoning has been reported with all forms through both oral and topical routes [Abdel-Magid and el-Awad Ahmed, 1994]. Absorption rate depends on the preparation. Neurologic, hepatic, and pulmonary toxicity occurs in concert with other metabolic derangements [Bari, 1995]. Symptom onset in acute intoxications is within a few hours. Salicylates directly affect the CNS and cause central hyperventilation with respiratory alkalosis. Poisoning of the Krebs cycle and increased skeletal muscle metabolism result in increased oxygen consumption, increased carbon dioxide production, and metabolic acidosis. Salicylates also contribute directly to this acidosis. Mortality is related to brain salicylate concentration; respiratory decompensation and subsequent worsening acidosis facilitate salicylic acid passage into the CNS [Yip et al., 1994]. Severe intoxication is more likely in children younger than 4 years.

Chronic toxicity occurs after several days of use and may be more difficult to discern sometimes because of symptoms of the patient's underlying illness. CNS disturbances occur in up to 60% of patients and include lethargy, coma, and convulsions; however, the predominant toxicity with chronic salicylism is pulmonary edema [English et al., 1996; Yip et al., 1994]. Poisoning also may result from chronic excessive use of bismuth subsalicylate (Pepto-Bismol). The combination of typical signs of chronic salicylate toxicity and radiopaque bismuth precipitate seen on radiographs of the abdomen suggests the diagnosis [Hearney et al., 1996; Vernace et al., 1994].

Failure to recognize and aggressively treat salicylate poisoning contributes to morbidity and mortality. Supportive therapy and aggressive measures to speed elimination of salicylates from the body are the mainstays of treatment. Fluid diuresis coupled with urinary alkalinization is used in milder cases; more severe poisonings may require blood alkalinization. This alkalinization and early hemodialysis may be life saving in severe intoxications [Yip et al., 1994]. Activated charcoal is beneficial, but the advantage of multiple-dose over single-dose regimens is not proved [Cienki et al., 1995]. Hypoglycemia may complicate salicylate poisoning. Intravenous fluids should contain at least 5% glucose; 10% glucose solutions should be used in young children with documented hypoglycemia or mental status changes. Aspirin tablets may form bezoars within the stomach; these provide a reservoir for prolonged salicylate absorption and may require dilutional catharsis.

Unlike salicylates, acetaminophen (and paracetamol) appears not to have a recognizable primary toxic effect on the brain. CNS effects result from acetaminophen-induced liver failure. Hepatic coma and life-threatening cerebral edema may be present in severe acute overdoses, although peak symptoms may not occur until 1 to 3 days after ingestion [Leikin and Paloucek, 1995]. Early lack of symptoms does not exclude a potentially fatal ingestion, and need for therapy is directly related to dose and measured acetaminophen blood level. Conservative estimates of the acute pediatric toxic dose are 140 to 150 mg/kg, but many authors use doses of 200 mg/kg, up to an adult toxic dose of about 7.5 g [Anker and Smilkstein, 1994]. Home ipecac administration for this and other suspected poisonings once was considered standard of care; however, the current American Academy of Pediatrics recommendation is to not have ipecac in the home [American Academy of Pediatrics Committee on Injury, Violence, and Poison Prevention, 2003; Bond, 1995; Shannon, 2003;]. Gastric lavage is effective if performed within 1 hour after ingestion. Activated charcoal should be given up to 4 hours after ingestion. If dosage at or above toxic range is suspected, *N*-acetylcysteine should be started; efficacy of oral versus intravenous therapy is debated. A 4-hour postingestion blood acetaminophen level is compared with a standard nomogram to determine the need to continue *N*-acetylcysteine therapy [Brandwene et al., 1996]. *N*-acetylcysteine coupled with a molecular absorbant recirculating system, if started early, may allow hepatic regeneration and obviates the need for liver transplantation [Koivusalo et al., 2003]. After ingestion of extended-release acetaminophen preparations, a second blood acetaminophen level should be obtained 4 to 6 hours after the first (but at least 8 to 12 hours after ingestion) [Cetaruk et al., 1997; Leikin and Paloucek, 1995].

Stimulants

Stimulant medications, such as dextroamphetamine, pemoline, and methylphenidate, used for the treatment of attention-deficit–hyperactivity disorder may produce increased activity and varying dyskinesias, including motor tics and chorea [Jimenez-Jimenez et al., 1997; Nakamura et al., 2002; Stork and Cantor, 1997]. Some children receiving methylphenidate may develop Tourette's syndrome, but a recent study of males with attention-deficit–hyperactivity disorder and Tourette's syndrome demonstrated that tics increased reversibly with stimulant use [Castellanos et al., 1997].

Theophylline

Theophylline and aminophylline, commonly used for treating apnea of prematurity and asthma, may cause neurologic symptoms as a result of either accidental ingestion or therapeutic error. Although theophylline concentrations higher than 20 mg/L are believed to be toxic, and clinical toxicity with nausea, vomiting, tachycardia, and agitation followed by seizures is more common when theophylline levels are greater than 30 to 40 mg/L, some children suffer lesser side effects with levels above 12 to 15 mg/L [Barr et al., 1994]. Gastrointestinal symptoms do not necessarily precede the onset of seizures, and seizures may occur with serum theophylline concentrations as low as 25 mg/L, although they are more common when concentrations exceed 50 mg/L [Gal et al., 1980; Jira et al., 1996]. Treatment of theophylline toxicity is supportive. Although activated charcoal absorbs the drug well within the gastrointestinal tract, hemoperfusion is considered the definitive treatment. Peritoneal dialysis has been used successfully in neonates and infants [Colonna et al., 1996; Jira et al., 1996]. Ipecac should be avoided. Seizures may be difficult to control but should be treated initially with benzodiazepines [Leikin and Paloucek, 1995]. Status epilepticus associated with increased theophylline levels carries a risk for increased morbidity over status epilepticus in general [Dunn and Parekh, 1991]. This risk may be secondary to theophylline-induced decreased cerebral blood flow or to increased risk for hypoxia due to underlying pulmonary disease.

Atropine and Related Alkaloids

Many drugs with anticholinergic properties, such as atropine, may produce an acute anticholinergic syndrome if taken in excess (see previous toxidrome discussion). Examples of drugs with significant anticholinergic properties include atropine, scopolamine, and local mydriatics, such as cyclopentolate (Cyclogyl) and tropicamide (Mydriacyl); a few antihistaminics, such as diphenhydramine and tripelennamine; gastrointestinal antispasmodics, such as dicyclomine (Bentyl) and propantheline (Pro-Banthīne); and older tricyclic antidepressants. The scopolamine-containing transdermal patches used for the prevention of motion sickness are a novel way to administer excessive amounts of scopolamine to children. The transdermal patch was developed primarily for adults and contains 1.5 mg of scopolamine, which can produce toxic psychosis in children and should be used with caution [Klein et al., 1985a; Lewis et al., 1994]. These patches also are used in some developmentally disabled children (e.g., with cerebral palsy) to decrease drooling. Poisoning may also occur after ingestion of plants containing belladonna alkaloids (*Atropa belladonna*, also known as *deadly nightshade*). Recreational abuse of such plants (e.g., tea made with *Brugmansia* [*Angel's trumpet*] and *Datura* species) in teenagers has been reported, although seizures or fatalities resulting from drinking the prepared tea appear unlikely [Isbister et al., 2003; Patel et al., 2003].

Supportive measures are the mainstay of therapy. Physostigmine may be used but may precipitate cholinergic toxicity, including seizures and bradyarrhythmias, and its use requires availability of adequate supportive therapy for these potential complications [Kulig and Rumack, 1983]. Physostigmine (0.5 mg intravenously) is administered slowly in children; it may be repeated every 10 minutes for a maximum total dose of 2 mg.

Drugs Used in Organ Transplantation

Organ transplantation may result in severe neurologic complications. Severe neurologic sequelae may occur in 10% to 15% of children who undergo hematopoietic stem cell transplantation [Faraci et al., 2002]. In a large Italian study, risk factors were allogeneic donor, presence of graft-versus-host disease, and use of total brain irradiation.

Cyclosporine

Cyclosporine, a potent immunosuppressant, is being used increasingly in solid organ transplantation [de Groen et al., 1987; Lee and Vacanti, 1996]. It probably is implicated most in neurologic sequelae of transplantation drugs [Faraci et al., 2002]. Neurotoxicity, nephrotoxicity, and hypertension are complications of cyclosporine therapy. Cyclosporine is lipophilic, a property that allows it relatively easy access to the CNS. The most common side effects of cyclosporine on the nervous system are headache, confusion, and seizures, but cortical blindness, hemiparesis, ataxia, and tremor are also reported [Adams et al., 1987; Boon et al., 1988; Garg et al., 1993; Ghalie et al., 1990; Miller, 1996; Reece, 1991; Soy et al., 1995; Trzepacz et al., 1993]. A syndrome of encephalopathy, seizures, and cerebral white matter changes has also been described. The white matter changes are more prominent in the parieto-occipital areas and resemble posterior reversible encephalopathy syndrome [Miller, 1996; Truwit et al., 1991; Nishie et al., 2003]. Marchiori and associates reported a case of cyclosporine-associated posterior reversible encephalopathy syndrome and reversible opsoclonus in a teenager after orthotopic liver transplantation [Marchiori et al., 2004]. These complications seem to be reversible but may require a decrease in the cyclosporine dose. Side effects are usually associated with high levels of cyclosporine. Other factors that exacerbate cyclosporine toxicity include hypertension, fever, hypomagnesemia, hypocholesterolemia, aluminum overload (especially in patients undergoing renal transplantation), and concurrent methylprednisolone treatment [Bhatt, 1988; de Groen, 1987; Thompson et al., 1984; Trzepacz et al., 1993].

OKT3

OKT3 is a murine monoclonal anti–pan-T-cell antibody of the immunoglobulin G2a isotype. OKT3 has been used extensively as an immunosuppressant agent in acute cellular allograft rejection or graft-versus-host disease [Norman, 1989]. The target of OKT3 is CD3, a 17- to 20-kDa molecule found on mature T cells that is selectively removed during treatment with this monoclonal antibody. OKT3 blocks both the generation and function of cytotoxic T cells. The half-life of injected OKT3 is about 18 hours [Fung, 1991; Norman, 1989]. A picture of aseptic meningitis with fever, photophobia, cephalgia, and cerebrospinal fluid pleocytosis has been described with OKT3 use [Adair et al., 1991; Emmons, 1986; Martin et al., 1988]. Other complications have included cerebral edema, seizures, cerebritis, and tremor [Capone and Cohen, 1991; Garg et al., 1993; Thomas et al., 1987; Trzepacz et al., 1993].

Tacrolimus (FK-506)

Tacrolimus, or FK-506, is used primarily to prevent organ rejection in liver transplant recipients [Diasio and LoBuglio, 1996; Lee and Vacanti, 1996]. Like cyclosporine, it inhibits interleukin-2 and is thought to act by inhibiting T-cell activation. Serum levels of tacrolimus are altered significantly by multiple drugs, including cyclosporine, methylprednisolone, metoclopramide, some antiepileptic drugs, and various antifungal agents.

Tacrolimus has clinical toxicity similar to that of cyclosporine. At serum levels greater than 3 ng/mL, delirium has been reported [Trzepacz et al., 1993]. Other neurologic side effects include dysphasia, seizures, and tremor. The dose relationship of these side effects is unclear, although increased toxicity has been noted with concomitant use of agents that increase tacrolimus delivery to the small intestine (e.g., metoclopramide) [Backman et al., 1994; Trzepacz et al., 1993; Prescott et al., 2004]. MRI may indicate white matter change, but reversibility may be predicted by apparent diffusion coefficient mapping [Shimono et al., 2003; Furukawa et al., 2001].

Antibiotics

Chloramphenicol

Chloramphenicol has been associated with the development of a reversible optic neuritis, demonstrable clinically and by visual-evoked potentials, in patients with cystic fibrosis who undergo long-term treatment with chloramphenicol [Leikin and Paloucek, 1995; Leitman et al., 1964; Spaide et al., 1987].

Nitrofurantoin

Polyneuropathy is a known complication in patients treated over prolonged periods with nitrofurantoin, particularly in the presence of impaired renal function. Patients have ascending sensory and motor polyneuropathy associated with increased spinal fluid protein [Spring et al., 2001].

Aminoglycosides

Aminoglycosides are potentially ototoxic. Recent data suggest that susceptibility to aminoglycoside-induced ototoxicity is associated with a mitochondrial mutation (nucleotide 1555) [Usami et al., 1997]. Symptoms may arise not only from oral or parenteral administration of the drugs but also after wound irrigation. A myasthenic-like syndrome accompanied by generalized muscle weakness, which is partially antagonized by neostigmine, may result from the administration of aminoglycosides such as streptomycin, neomycin, kanamycin, bacitracin, colistin, and gentamicin. This reaction usually occurs in association with the simultaneous administration of a neuromuscular blocking agent (e.g., succinylcholine, D-tubocurarine, decamethonium bromide). This neuromuscular blocking effect is especially pronounced when these antibiotics are placed in the pleural or abdominal cavities, with resultant rapid absorption and high plasma levels. These antibiotics may also cause a transient clinical deterioration in patients with myasthenia gravis [Kaeser, 1984].

β-Lactam Antibiotics

The β-lactam antibiotics are a diverse group of medications with potential for myriad systemic and neurologic side effects. Seizures caused by the penicillins, cephalosporins, and carbapenems result from the inhibition of γ-aminobutyric acid receptors [Asensi et al., 1993; Sunagawa and Nouda, 1996]. Movement disorders and change in sensorium may occur also. Effects may be magnified in a child with an altered blood-brain barrier.

Antiviral Agents

Anti–human immunodeficiency virus drugs have prolonged the lives of many patients with acquired immune deficiency syndrome. They have also been associated with significant neurotoxicity. Use of two older agents, dideoxycytidine and dideoxyinosine, as well as a newer reverse transcriptase inhibitor, stavudine, has been associated with peripheral neuropathy [Brew and Currie, 1993; Mueller, 1997]. So far, therapy with protease inhibitors has not demonstrated significant neurotoxicity, but only preliminary data are available [Mueller, 1997].

Anticytomegalovirus agents (acyclovir, ganciclovir, and foscarnet) have some CNS side effects, such as alteration in consciousness or seizures, but they are usually overshadowed by neurologic sequelae of concomitant systemic toxicity (i.e., myelosuppression and nephrotoxicity).

Antineoplastic Drugs

Use of chemotherapeutic agents has produced striking improvement in the outcome of childhood malignant disease and is associated with a number of neurologic complications in children and adults [Armstrong and Gilbert, 2004].

Vinca Alkaloids

Vincristine and vinblastine are potent antineoplastic agents with variable degrees of neurotoxicity, some of which is reversible. Impaired nutrition appears to increase susceptibility to vincristine toxicity. Greater neurotoxicity is also related to higher concentrations of drug per dose and increased frequency and duration of therapy. Some degree of symmetric peripheral neuropathy, with areflexia involving early and consistent loss of Achilles tendon reflexes, slapping gait, muscle atrophy, and leg weakness, develops frequently, even with customary doses of vincristine. Numbness and tingling paresthesias in hands and feet are common with preserved cutaneous sensation, although the child may complain of hand clumsiness before the onset of footdrop [Tuxen and Hansen, 1994]. Muscle cramps are also a frequent symptom of vincristine-associated motor neuropathies, occurring in both proximal and distal distributions [Haim et al., 1991]. Cranial nerve palsies may also occur with involvement of cranial nerves II to VIII and X. The most common ocular findings are variable degrees of ophthalmoparesis and ptosis. Autonomic dysfunction is another aspect of vincristine neurotoxicity, with colicky abdominal pain, paralytic ileus and constipation (in 33% to 46% of patients), and bladder atony (Christensen et al., 1994; Tuxen and Hansen, 1994). Generalized seizures and inappropriate secretion of antidiuretic hormone are additional but rare complications of vincristine treatment [Sandler et al., 1969; Shurin et al., 1982]. Vincristine's peripheral neurotoxic effects may be potentiated by itraconazole [Ariffin et al., 2003; Kamaluddiin et al., 2001]. Vinorelbine has the potential to cause similar neurotoxic effects but, possibly because of its greater selectivity for mitotic rather than axonal microtubules, does so less often [Tuxen and Hansen, 1994].

Vincristine also causes a necrotizing myopathy [Le Quintrec and Le Quintrec., 1991]. Especially with concomitant steroid therapy, a combined myoneuropathy picture may develop [Bradley et al., 1970; DeAngelis et al, 1991]. Improvement usually ensues with completion of therapy.

Methotrexate

Myelopathy, headache, vomiting, nuchal rigidity with aseptic meningitis, truncal ataxia, tremor, paraplegia, delirium, and somnolence have been described as complications of both intrathecal and systemic therapy with methotrexate. Meningoencephalopathy can occur as late as several months after completion of methotrexate therapy. Scattered subcortical intracerebral calcifications may result from large cumulative doses of intravenous methotrexate, and concurrent administration of cytosine arabinoside may increase the risk for this complication [McIntosh et al., 1977]. The most devastating effect of methotrexate therapy, originally thought to be related to a combination of a high dose of intrathecal methotrexate and CNS irradiation, is a subacute and usually progressive leukoencephalopathy. A characteristic pattern of decreased density of periventricular white matter is evident on CT or as increased periventricular signal on T2-weighted MRI. Clinical manifestations include mental deterioration with dementia, seizures, and focal neurologic deficits. This complication may occur between 3 and 9 months after high-dose methotrexate therapy. An immediate and fatal necrotizing leukoencephalopathy has been reported in association with an inadvertent, more than 50-fold intrathecal overdose of methotrexate [Ettinger, 1982]. Leukoencephalopathy can occur with intravenous methotrexate therapy plus cranial irradiation without intrathecal administration of the methotrexate [McIntoshet al., 1977; Price and Jamieson, 1975; Weiss et al., 1974; Shuper et al., 2002]. Animal studies suggest that concomitant administration of steroids may play a role in this neurotoxicity [Mullenix et al., 1994]. In addition, underlying disease may potentiate methotrexate toxicity. Miller and Wilkinson describe 79% to 93% reduction in local cerebrospinal fluid clearance of intraventricularly administered methotrexate in three individuals with carcinomatous meningitis [Miller and Wilkinson, 1989]. Improvement also has been reported in a single report using a combination of high-dose folinic acid and aminophylline [Jaksic et al., 2004].

L-Asparaginase

L-Asparaginase therapy may produce changes in mentation, somnolence, and electroencephalogram slowing [Moure et al., 1970; Tuxen and Hansen, 1994]. Intracranial thrombosis or hemorrhage and peripheral arterial thrombosis with headache, obtundation, hemiparesis, and seizures have also been recognized as complications in 1% to 2% of children receiving L-asparaginase [Priest et al., 1982]. The associated coagulation disorder is thought to be secondary to L-asparaginase–induced decrease in antithrombin III level [Kieslich et al., 2003]. Despite this, it is not yet clear that L-asparaginase–related cerebrovascular thrombosis responds to replacement of factors, or that it is resistant to low-molecular-weight heparin therapy.

Platinum Agents

Ototoxicity is a common complication of cisplatin therapy; peripheral sensory neuropathy may also occur with dysesthesias and paresthesias, diminished reflexes, decreased vibratory and light touch sensation, and sensory ataxia [Cavaletti et al., 1996; Thompson et al., 1982; Steeghs et al., 2003; Markman, 2003]. Although retinal toxicity is reported in adults, it is rare in children and may be associated with abnormal renal function [Hilliard et al., 1997]. Autonomic neuropathy is rare. Oxaliplatin has similar neurotoxic potential; carboplatin appears somewhat less toxic to the nervous system [Tuxen and Hansen, 1994]. Possible neuroprotectant agents that may minimize this neurotoxicity include calcium channel antagonists, thiol compounds, adrenocorticotropic hormone analogs, and neurotropic factors [Cavaletti et al., 1996].

Cytosine Arabinoside

Cytosine arabinoside has been associated with transient paraplegia after intrathecal administration. In childhood acute myelogenous leukemia, patients given intrathecal and intravenous cytosine arabinoside have exhibited progressive ascending paralytic disease, with onset delayed up to 6 months after treatment, accompanied by spinal cord demyelination [Dunton et al., 1986]. Cytosine arabinoside may also cause cerebellar ataxia, change in sensorium (the latter at high doses), and rarely peripheral neuropathy or brachial plexopathy [Tuxen and Hansen, 1994].

Cyclophosphamide and Ifosfamide

Cyclophosphamide and ifosfamide both may cause CNS toxicity (10% to 30% incidence in the case of the latter) [DiMaggio et al., 1994; Tuxen and Hansen, 1994]. This toxicity is manifest as mental status changes, seizures, and ataxia. Cranial neuropathies are also possible. In the case of ifosfamide, toxicity may be evident within 2 hours after infusion is begun and may continue for 1 to 3 days after a 5-day course of therapy [Pratt et al., 1989; Nicolao and Giometto, 2003; Rieger et al., 2004]. It is more likely to occur in the face of common concomitants of malignancy, including hepatic or renal dysfunction, hypoalbuminemia, acidosis, or prior CNS abnormality. Improvement has been reported with methylene blue administration [Raj et al., 2004; Orbach et al., 2003].

Other Agents Used in Cancer Chemotherapy

Fludarabine, cladribine, and pentostatin are newer purine analogs that are used currently more often in adults than in children. They carry potential for fatal neurotoxicity at higher-than-recommended doses; at the recommended dosage, each carries a 15% risk for (usually reversible) neurotoxicity [Cheson et al., 1994].

Finally, as cytokines find increasing roles in cancer chemotherapy, their neurotoxicity is becoming more evident. Evidence is strongest for interferon and interleukin-2. Interferon therapy has been associated with frontal lobe dysfunction (decreased executive functions, transient aphasia), migraine, parkinsonism and akathisia, and peripheral neuropathy. Conversely, interleukin-2 use has been linked to neurobehavioral changes ranging from lethargy to delirium. The mechanism of neurotoxicity is unclear, although it is postulated that they circumvent the blood-brain barrier through a poorly understood mechanism. Quantification of the degree of toxicity awaits prospective studies [Forman, 1994; Margolin, 1994].

Steroids

Neurologic complications of steroid therapy include delirium, cortical atrophy, pseudotumor cerebri, and steroid myopathy. More subtle neurobehavioral effects of steroids, especially anabolic and androgenic steroids used (and abused) by athletes, are catalogued elsewhere [Lukas, 1996; Pope and Katz, 1994]. Brain atrophy (ascertained by neuroimaging studies) and pseudotumor cerebri related to steroids occur primarily in children receiving prolonged corticosteroid treatment, the latter at times after drug withdrawal. There does not appear to be any relationship between pseudotumor cerebri and the disorder for which steroids were being administered. Autonomic neuropathy has also been reported [Rosener et al., 1996]. Proximal myopathy may be a common complication of steroid therapy. Onset may be insidious, and it may occur after only a short duration (<14 days) of steroid therapy. Although often mild, myopathy may occur in up to 60% of patients treated with steroids [Batchelor et al., 1997].

Radiographic Contrast Agents

Metrizamide, a contrast agent for myelographic procedures, may cause a transient encephalopathy manifested by confusional state, hallucinations, myoclonus, and asterixis.

There is evidence that metrizamide reaches the intracranial subarachnoid space in these patients [Junck and Marshall, 1983]. Headache is common after metrizamide myelography. The incidence of seizures is 0.1%; many of the reported seizures have occurred in patients with a history of seizures [Torvik and Walday, 1995]. Rare transient adverse effects of metrizamide include paraparesis, loss of reflexes, blindness, speech disturbances, and diplopia. Cerebrospinal fluid pleocytosis and clinical evidence of aseptic meningitis may occur after metrizamide myelography [Junck and Marshall, 1983; DiMario, 1985]. Seizures have also been reported with diatrizoate meglumine (Hypaque) [Karl et al., 1994]. Newer nonionic contrast agents, including iohexol and iodixanol, appear to have less risk, although similar side effects have been reported anecdotally [Torvik and Walday, 1995]. Symptoms occur 2 to 12 hours after injection and may last 24 to 72 hours.

Iophendylate (Pantopaque), an oily contrast agent that is used occasionally for myelography, may induce acute and chronic meningeal reactions. The acute reaction consists of headache, fever, meningismus, and cerebrospinal fluid pleocytosis and is usually self-limited. Patients with adhesive arachnoiditis from chronic inflammation may have back pain and signs and symptoms of lumbar and sacral root dysfunction within several months of myelography. Complete removal of any residual iophendylate after myelography is recommended as a preventive measure. Systemic or intrathecal corticosteroid therapy may be beneficial.

ADVERSE DRUG REACTIONS

Adverse drug reactions affecting the nervous system are not necessarily a result of accidental ingestions, inappropriate dosage, or therapeutic error but may occur during the course of therapy. Such reactions may be due to (1) vehicle or method of medication preparation, (2) method of drug administration, (3) pharmacogenetic susceptibility, (4) drug interactions, (5) developmental immaturity, (6) underlying disease, or (7) idiosyncrasy or exaggeration of the normal pharmacologic action of drugs.

Method of Preparation

Propylene glycol has been commonly used as a drug solubilizer for various medications, including vitamins and certain parenteral drug products such as phenytoin and diazepam. CNS and respiratory depression, hypotension, and cardiac dysrhythmias may result from intravenous injection of products containing propylene glycol. Otherwise unexplained CNS depression in small children has occurred after large doses of oral vitamin D–containing propylene glycol for treatment of vitamin D–deficiency rickets [Pruitt et al., 1985].

Technique of Drug Administration

Intramuscular injections of medications, particularly into the buttocks, may result in peripheral nerve injury, especially in infants and small children. Sciatic neuropathy may result from a buttock injection when the needle is directed inadvertently into the sciatic nerve; this injection error may occur more easily in a small, struggling infant. Sciatic neuropathy has occurred after intramuscular administration of penicillin, promethazine, chlorpromazine, and vitamin K [Gilles and Matson, 1970]. The clinical syndrome classically occurs within 12 hours after an injection presumably has been given in the upper outer quadrant of the buttock. The child complains of pain and tingling paresthesia in the buttock and down the back of the leg to the lateral margin of the foot. The pain and dysesthesias may be so severe that the child refuses to walk. Within weeks, footdrop and calf muscle atrophy develop, with decreased sensation over the lateral aspect of the foot and diminished Achilles tendon reflex. Before the institution of aggressive rehabilitation and neurolysis, only 30% to 60% of children had good recovery. This figure now approaches 100%, although lack of electrical activity and muscle strength in innervated muscles portend a less favorable outcome [Villarejo and Pascual, 1993]. Because of this complication, the recommended site for intramuscular injections in infants and children is the lateral or anterolateral aspect of the upper thigh.

Injections into the lateral or anterolateral aspect of the thigh, however, are not entirely free of complications. Repeated intramuscular injections into this area may result in fibrosis and contracture of the quadriceps muscle with loss of knee flexion. In addition, these children have palpable cords of connective tissue in the thighs, with associated atrophy and dimpling of the overlying skin and subcutaneous tissue. Affected patients usually have been given repeated injections of antibiotics for the treatment of serious illnesses in the neonatal period [Norman et al., 1970]. Progressive fibrosis involving the deltoid muscle has been reported in children after repeated injections in the upper arm. Deltoid muscle injury and fibrosis may result in progressive abduction contracture of the arm at the shoulder, with winging of the scapula accompanied by weakness or pain in the shoulder. Neonatal sciatic nerve palsy has resulted from umbilical artery injections with subsequent vasoconstriction of the umbilical artery and vasospasm of the hypogastric and inferior gluteal arteries. The injection of hypertonic sodium bicarbonate or 50% glucose solutions may produce this effect [San Augustin et al., 1962]. Paraplegia has also occurred as a complication of umbilical artery catheterization, with flaccid paralysis of the lower extremities and profound sensory deficit, presumably resulting from ischemic injury to the spinal cord. With the advent of therapeutic botulinum toxin injections to treat myriad neuromuscular problems, there is potential for inadvertent regional effects of neuromuscular blockade. In one report, botulinum toxin injections administered to alleviate adductor spasticity produced prolonged urinary retention [Schnider et al., 1995].

Finally, intramuscular injection of phenytoin may lead to sterile abscess. It is hoped that the introduction of fosphenytoin will eliminate this complication.

Pharmacogenetic Susceptibility

Adverse reactions to some drugs may be related to individual genetic variation rather than to the drug itself. Sex, race, and ethnicity influence drug response and metabolism [Matthews, 1995]. Although isoniazid poisoning is known to occur after excessive doses of the drug, adverse reactions, including toxic psychosis, seizures, and peripheral neuropathy, may also occur in genetically susceptible individuals on conventional therapeutic doses of isoniazid. Such individuals are slow inactivators of isoniazid, a genetically transmitted autosomal recessive trait. These slow isoniazid inactivators are also predisposed to phenytoin intoxication when given both isoniazid and phenytoin simultaneously.

Impaired parahydroxylation of phenytoin, another genetically determined defect in drug metabolism, is another cause of unexplained phenytoin toxicity manifested by nystagmus, ataxia, and mental clouding. This autosomal-dominant trait results in the accumulation of unmetabolized phenytoin, with marked elevation of serum phenytoin concentrations despite the use of conventional dosages of the drug. Idiosyncratic reactions to both phenytoin and carbamazepine were linked previously to defective microsomal epoxide hydrolase, although more recent studies have not confirmed this association [Davis et al., 1995; Gaedigk et al., 1994; Green et al., 1995].

Pseudocholinesterase deficiency, an autosomal recessive trait, results in abnormal reactions to succinylcholine manifested by prolonged muscle relaxation with profound weakness and apnea. The adverse response follows the administration of therapeutic doses of succinylcholine during surgery. Individuals with this disorder have an atypical plasma cholinesterase that hydrolyzes succinylcholine at markedly reduced rates, with resultant persistent elevation of plasma succinylcholine concentrations.

Patients with acute intermittent porphyria and some of the other genetically determined disorders of porphyrin metabolism (e.g., variegate porphyria and hereditary coproporphyria) have recurrent attacks of severe abdominal pain. Presumably these attacks are related to autonomic and peripheral neuropathy that, in addition to delirium, coma, and seizures, may be precipitated by several drugs, including antiepileptic drugs, sulfonamides, griseofulvin, barbiturates, and other sedative hypnotic agents.

Malignant hyperthermia is an inherited disorder precipitated by the administration of halothane, isoflurane, and muscle relaxants such as succinylcholine, decamethonium, gallamine, and D-tubocurarine [Nelson and Flewellen, 1983]. The clinical syndrome is characterized by the rapid development of tachycardia, cardiac dysrhythmias, muscle fasciculations, muscular rigidity, and high fever after agent administration. Myoglobinuria, elevation of blood creatine kinase and potassium levels, and severe metabolic acidosis are prominent laboratory findings. Complications include swelling, pain, necrosis of skeletal muscle, renal failure, disseminated intravascular coagulation, and encephalopathy. Pretreatment with dantrolene is effective in preventing the clinical syndrome. The prophylactic oral dose in children is 4 to 8 mg/kg per day divided into four doses for 1 to 2 days preceding anesthetic administration; the time between the last dose and induction of anesthesia should be 3 to 4 hours for oral dosing and 75 minutes for intravenous administration, the latter at a dose of 2.5 mg/kg [Leikin and Paloucek, 1995]. Emergency administration of dantrolene, discontinuation of the inciting drug, and vigorous supportive care are effective treatment measures for individuals who appear to be developing the clinical disorder. Other potentially at-risk individuals include children with central core disease, those with muscular dystrophies such as Duchenne's muscular dystrophy, and a group of children with a unique constellation of unusual physical features resembling those seen in Noonan's syndrome, including short stature, thoracic kyphosis, lumbar lordosis, hypoplastic mandible, low-set ears, webbed neck, down-slanting palpebral fissures, and cryptorchidism [King and Denborough, 1973; Online Mendelian Inheritance in Man, 1997]. The halothane-caffeine contracture test on muscle biopsy tissue is the most specific test for laboratory confirmation of the disorder; however, it is not always diagnostic in children younger than 5 years.

Drug Interactions

The administration of one drug may alter the pharmacologic activity of another by changing the hepatic metabolism of the second drug or by interfering with its protein binding or renal clearance. For example, addition of felbamate alters the metabolism of phenytoin, carbamazepine, and valproic acid and usually requires reduction in their doses by as much as one third. Other such antiepileptic drug interactions are discussed in Chapter 49. Likewise, concurrent administration of erythromycin in patients taking cimetidine or carbamazepine produces CNS toxicity with confusion, slurred speech, delirium, hallucinations, and coma despite doses of cimetidine that are not usually intoxicating [Caroff and Mann, 1993].

Developmental Immaturity

Sulfisoxazole (Gantrisin) was implicated in the pathogenesis of kernicterus in preterm infants [Silverman et al., 1956]. This finding remains one of the clearest examples of iatrogenic neurologic disease related to the adverse effect of a drug and an immature hepatic enzyme system. The sulfonamide given to these infants competed with bilirubin for albumin binding sites, displacing the bilirubin and allowing free unconjugated bilirubin to diffuse into the brain with subsequent kernicterus. Salicylates, caffeine, sodium benzoate, and oxacillin may similarly displace bilirubin from albumin with increased risk for kernicterus. Another similar form of drug-induced neonatal jaundice and kernicterus was related to the administration of large doses of two synthetic, water-soluble vitamin K analogs (e.g., menadione sodium diphosphate, menadione sodium bisulfate) for the prevention of hemorrhagic disease in the newborn [Lucey and Dolan, 1959].

A variety of analgesic drugs administered to the mother may affect the newborn, causing significant degree of sedation, hypotonia, poor suck, and decreased Moro response. In addition, tranquilizing agents, such as phenothiazines administered during labor to reduce the requirement of maternal analgesic medications, may produce lethargy. Neonatal withdrawal syndromes have been related to chronic maternal use of various sedative-hypnotics, barbiturates, and opiates, including heroin, morphine, hydromorphone, methadone, codeine, pentazocine, propoxyphene (Darvon), ethchlorvynol (Placidyl), hydroxyzine hydrochloride (Atarax), and desmethylimipramine [TERIS, 2005; Webster, 1973]. In the case of heroin-using mothers, 40% to 80% of at-risk infants display withdrawal or abstinence syndromes. These are manifested by irritability, hypertonicity, vomiting, diarrhea, sneezing, poor suck, shrill cry, jitteriness, tremors, and, rarely, seizures [Alroomi, 1988; Lam et al., 1992; Zuckerman et al., 1995]. Onset is most often 24 hours to 7 days postpartum (depending on the narcotic used) and appears to be less evident in preterm infants. The latter observation may be attributed to either decreased fat stores or receptor immaturity in preterm infants [Zuckerman et al., 1995]. The syndrome usually lasts about 3 weeks but may be more prolonged. The treatment of choice is paregoric, using one of a number of titration schedules; alternatively, phenobarbital may be used. Duration of treatment is individualized, but 10 to 30 days' duration is common [Kendall, 1995].

Magnesium sulfate used for the treatment of toxemia may produce neonatal respiratory depression, lethargy, diminished tone, and absent reflexes. Such infants usually have significant elevation of magnesium above the upper normal level of 2.9 mg/dL; the severity of the neurologic disorder correlates well with the serum magnesium level.

Chronic use of tranquilizers and psychotropic agents during pregnancy may have adverse effects on the fetus and newborn. An association between neuroleptic use and neonatal behavioral abnormalities has been noted, often after large maternal doses [Hammond and Toseland, 1970; Levy and Wisniewski, 1974; Tamer et al., 1969; TERIS, 2005]. The abnormalities closely resemble the extrapyramidal signs seen in patients taking these agents, with prominent rigidity, hypertonia, and tremor. The symptoms resolve gradually but may persist for months. This association has been reported for chlorpromazine, haloperidol, and perphenazine, among others [Handal et al., 1995; Sexson and Barak, 1989].

Neonates born to mothers treated during pregnancy with the antidepressant clomipramine may develop significant lethargy, hypotonia, and respiratory irregularity, which only gradually subside within the first weeks of life [Ostergaard and Pedersen, 1982].

There is mounting evidence that maternal selective serotonin re-uptake inhibitor use during pregnancy may result in a withdrawal syndrome in neonates [Lanz et al, 2005]. This syndrome has been reported with paroxetine and may relate to the pharmacokinetics of the various selective serotonin re-uptake inhibitor agents. The clinical picture is one of an encephalopathy, with jitteriness and hyperreflexia starting within the first day of life. Infants are described as hypotonic, but tone may be variable. Seizures and respiratory distress may occur, requiring aggressive intervention. Neonates suspected of selective serotonin re-uptake inhibitor withdrawal should be monitored in a neonatal intensive care unit. Although the symptoms usually resolve over several days, they can last up to a month [Herbst and Gortner, 2003].

Among the risk factors associated with the development of intraventricular hemorrhage is the maternal use of aspirin. The incidence of intraventricular hemorrhage appears significantly higher in preterm infants exposed to aspirin compared with those not exposed [Rumack et al., 1981].

Coagulation defects have been noted in infants born to mothers who had received antiepileptic medications. Intracranial, abdominal, or thoracic hemorrhage may occur, and these infants should be carefully monitored. Although vitamin K administration reverses the clotting abnormalities, critical reappraisal of data in maternal-fetal pairs receiving enzyme-inducing antiepileptic drugs has suggested that the actual number of infants at risk for serious bleeding is smaller than previously suggested [Hey, 1999; Kaaja et al., 2002; Montouris et al., 1979].

Finally, many additional substances find their way into the neonate through breast milk. Assessment of risk is inexact. A rough estimate of level of exposure may be obtained by consideration of the milk-to-plasma ratio of the possible toxin, metabolic alteration of the drug by maternal organs (including the breast), correlation of feeding schedule and agent half-life, and pharmacokinetics of the agent in the infant [Bailey and Ito, 1997]. Although convincing studies are limited, a few agents have demonstrated toxicity when introduced through breast-feeding, although long-term sequelae of these exposures are unknown. The incidence of neonatal hypotonia correlated with polychlorinated biphenyl levels in the breast milk of the infants' mothers [Huisman et al., 1995; Rogan et al., 1986, 1988]. Isolated cases of adverse effects on breast-fed newborns have also been reported with phenobarbital, primidone, carbamazepine, clemastine, and ergots. If the mother is still actively using cocaine postpartum, breast-feeding is contraindicated [Kendall, 1995]. In the absence of reassuring data, a recent review suggested avoidance of drugs of abuse, ethanol, antineoplastic agents, gold, iodine, and lithium [Bailey and Ito, 1997]. Although lead and mercury are both found in breast milk, the prevailing concentrations are much lower than for maternal blood. They probably pose little risk to the breast-fed infant [Dorea, 2004].

Underlying Disease

The pharmacokinetics of a drug may be altered by a child's underlying disease. Impaired renal clearance increases the ototoxic potential of kanamycin, gentamicin, and colistin and the peripheral neurotoxicity of nitrofurantoin (Macrodantin) and related drugs. Similarly, lactam antibiotic-induced myoclonus and generalized tonic-clonic seizures occur more frequently in renal patients and in those who are neurologically abnormal [Asensi et al., 1993; Grondahl and Langmoen, 1993; Keskin and Konkol, 1993].

Severe chronic constipation with functional megacolon or congenital aganglionic megacolon increases the likelihood of water intoxication as a complication of enemas with tap water or hypotonic solutions. Functional megacolon is a recognized complication in psychiatric and neurologic patients, although its causes in this population are heterogeneous [Fehlow et al., 1995]. Patients with colon dilation, associated with severe chronic constipation, have an increased absorptive surface and decreased peristaltic function and thus absorb large amounts of hypotonic fluids after administration of these enemas [Ziskin and Gellis, 1958]. Patients may develop headache, vomiting, decreased awareness, coma, and convulsions. After the administration of hypertonic enemas, especially those containing large amounts of sodium phosphate and biphosphate, patients with megacolon may develop tetany, coma, and convulsions from hypernatremia, hyperphosphatemia, and severe hypocalcemia.

Use of hypertonic contrast media may increase the risk for stroke in patients with sickle cell disease because of increased sickling [Zagoria, 1994]. Alternate strategies, such as use of low-osmolality contrast agents or substitution of MRI or magnetic resonance angiography where appropriate, may be considered [Allison et al., 1994; Hunter et al., 1994].

Neuroteratology

A variety of adverse effects on the fetus may occur as a result of administration of drugs during pregnancy. The effects of these drugs depend on the timing of administration; the dose, distribution, and metabolism in maternal tissues; placental transfer; and subsequent concentration and distribution of the drug in fetal tissues. Brain development, including phases of neuronal proliferation and migration, arborization and synaptogenesis, and myelination, represents a long period of developmental vulnerability [Rodier, 2004].

Assessment of neuroteratogenic effects of a given agent is difficult. Teratogenic risk is frequently underestimated or overestimated. Improved methods of ascertainment are being developed, including mathematic models and models derived from animal studies [Leroux et al., 1996; Slikker, 1994; Zhang et al., 1995]. Sparse data and confounding factors limit conclusive recommendations. Discussion is limited to agents in which a neuroteratogenic effect seems likely based on human data or in which animal data reflect a likely human scenario (i.e., in the case of some antineoplastic agents). Omitted here is discussion of agents in which massive animal exposures to agents are associated with teratogenicity but for which there are no supporting human data, as well as agents described as possible behavioral teratogens without either strong statistical support or corresponding structural anomalies (Table 87–2).

Fetal ethanol exposure is the most common preventable chemical cause of mental retardation in the United States.

TABLE 87-2

Selected Human Neuroteratogens

DRUG/TOXIN	EFFECT ON NERVOUS SYSTEM	REFERENCE
Aminoglycoside antibiotics	Cranial nerve VIII damage (10%–15%)	Hanson, 1996; Warkany, 1979
Antiepileptic drugs: oxazolidinediones (trimethadione), phenytoin, valproic acid, carbamazepine	CNS malformations, mental retardation, developmental delay, microcephaly, neural tube defect; spina bifida (1%-2%)	Adams et al., 1990; Feldman et al., 1977; Gladstone et al., 1992; Hanson, 1986, 1996; Omtzigt et al., 1992; REPROTOX, 2005
Cisplatin	Cranial nerve III	REPROTOX, 2005
Chloroquine, hydroxychloroquine, quinine	Hydrocephalus, optic nerve hypoplasia, cranial nerve VIII damage (10%-15%)	Dannenberg et al., 1983; Hanson, 1996; Nishimura and Tanimura, 1976
Cocaine	CNS hemorrhage, infarction	Heier et al., 1991; REPROTOX, 2005
Coumarin anticoagulants	Mental retardation, microcephaly, optic nerve hypoplasia, midline CNS malformations	Gulba, 1996; Hanson, 1996
Ethanol (dose related)	Mental retardation, developmental and behavioral disabilities, dyscoordination, microcephaly, CNS midline malformations and migrational errors	Hanson, 1996; Swayze et al., 1997
Folic acid antagonists (aminopterin, methotrexate)	Cranial malformations, mental retardation	Hanson, 1996
Hyperthermia	Neural tube defect, migrational errors, Möbius' syndrome	Graham et al., 1988; Hanson, 1996; Layde et al., 1980
Ionizing radiation (>200 Gy)	CNS malformation, microcephaly	Hanson, 1996; Leikin and Paloucek, 1995
Lead	Learning disabilities	Dietrich et al., 1987; Hanson, 1996; Winneke, 1996
Maternal diabetes mellitus	Caudal regression, holoprosencephaly-arhinencephalia	Barr et al., 1981; Hanson, 1996
Organic mercury	CNS malformation, microcephaly	Hanson, 1996; Leikin and Paloucek, 1995; Matusmoto et al., 1965
Solvents: gasoline, xylene, toluene (as substances of abuse)	Caudal regression malformation, CNS malformations, mental retardation	Hanson, 1996; Arnold et al., 1994; Pearson et al., 1994
Retinoids, vitamin A	Holoprosencephaly, neural tube defect, microcephaly, posterior fossa cysts, cranial nerve palsies (II, III, VII)	Hanson, 1996
Thiouracil, propylthiouracil (PTU), iodine-131	Mental retardation (congenital hypothyroidism)	Cheron et al., 1981; Hanson, 1996
Undertreated maternal phenylketonuria	Mental retardation (>90% in untreated mothers)	Hanson, 1996
Vinyl chloride	CNS malformation	Leikin and Paloucek, 1995

The 1985 Household Survey on Drug Abuse sponsored by the National Institute on Drug Abuse suggested that 60.9% of women of childbearing age (between 15 and 44 years of age; 34 million of the about 56 million women in this age group) were current (meaning within the past month) users of alcohol. By 1990, this figure was reduced to 50.8%, or about 30.5 million women [Adams et al., 1989; Khalsa and Gfroerer, 1991]. In a survey of 19,991 pregnant women, 0.8% to 3.1% reported "binge" drinking sometime during pregnancy, most before 6 weeks of gestation [Gladstone et al., 1997]. Alcohol consumed during pregnancy is associated with increased risk for fetal abnormalities. There is an estimated 6% risk that an alcoholic mother will have a child with fetal alcohol syndrome; the risk is 70% for subsequent offspring. This number compares with a risk of 1.9 per 1000 in the general population [Abel and Sokol, 1987]. Although most studies suggest that significant risk to the fetus occurs with maternal ethanol consumption of about two drinks a week or a few "weekend binges" during pregnancy, there is no defined "safe" threshold consumption value. Cardinal features of fetal alcohol syndrome are (1) prenatal and postnatal growth deficiency; (2) CNS anomalies, usually involving microcephaly and mental retardation, with irritability and restlessness in infants; and (3) craniofacial anomalies that include short palpebral fissures, frontonasal alterations, midface hypoplasia with flat midface, thin upper lip, hypoplastic maxilla, and sometimes hypoplastic mandible [Jones, 1996; Swayze et al., 1997; TERIS, 2005]. Partial morphologic expression of alcohol effect is sometimes referred to as *alcohol-related birth defects* or *fetal alcohol effects*. Long-term follow-up suggests that patients with fetal alcohol syndrome continue to have growth retardation, craniofacial anomalies, and cognitive and behavioral problems in school. Children with fetal alcohol syndrome had lower weight, shorter length, and smaller head circumference at 3 years of age [Day et al., 1991]. Decrease in intelligence quotient at 4 and 7 years of age has been reported [Streissguth et al., 1989, 1990].

Antiepileptic medications are also teratogens. Although it is difficult to separate the effects of epilepsy and antiepileptic drugs in the production of fetal abnormalities, phenytoin administered to pregnant women is associated with a specific fetal malformation syndrome of facial and digital anomalies, growth deficiency, and mental deficiency [Hanson and Smith, 1975; Jones, 1996; Online Mendelian Inheritance in Man, 2005; Phelan et al., 1982]. Carbamazepine, trimethadione, and valproic acid are also teratogenic [Feldman et al., 1977; Jones, 1996; TERIS, 2005]. Neural tube defects occur in about 1% to 2% of valproate- or carbamazepine-exposed fetuses [Jones, 1996]. There may also be more subtle effects of valproic acid [Koch et al., 1996]. Maternal folic acid supplementation may reduce the risk for antiepileptic drug–associated neural tube defects.

Isotretinoin (Accutane), a vitamin A analog used to treat acne, is a recently identified teratogen. It produces a characteristic pattern of malformation involving craniofacial, cardiac, thymic, and CNS structures. The CNS malformations include hydrocephalus, posterior fossa defects, and focal cortical abnormalities. The syndrome is thought to relate to isotretinoin's ability to interfere with neural crest cell development [Coberly et al., 1996; Hanson, 1996; Lammer et al., 1985].

Although the evidence is strongest for the agents listed in Table 87-2, suggestive animal or human data support the teratogenicity of other substances. These substances include antineoplastic medications, including azacitidine, carmustine, and etoposide [Rosen et al., 1990; Takahashi et al., 1986; Thompson et al., 1974]; polychlorinated biphenyls [Huisman et al., 1995; Jacobson and Jacobson, 1997; Winneke et al., 2002]; and less conclusively, manganese (in manganese-based contrast agents), ribavirin, and combinations of tobacco and caffeine [Misselwitz et al., 1995; Nehlig and Debry, 1994; TERIS, 2005]. Severe intrauterine methylmercury exposure may result in mental retardation, visual and hearing deficits, and a cerebral palsy–like picture. Stable low-level maternal exposure to mercury also appears to have neuropsychologic consequences at least into early school age [Grandjean et al., 2003; Mendola et al., 2002]. The U.S. National Research Council has concluded that 0.1 g/kg body weight per day probably is a safe level of methylmercury exposure for maternal-fetal pairs [Mahaffey, 2000].

Finally, prenatal exposure to cocaine may have both short- and long-term CNS sequelae. Although the existence of a consistent dysmorphic "syndrome" in cocaine-exposed neonates is debated, congenital urogenital malformations are linked more firmly to prenatal cocaine exposure [Zuckerman et al., 1995]. Infants and children may be exposed to cocaine through transplacental transfer, breast-milk ingestion, and passive inhalation [Bateman and Heagarty, 1989; Chasnoff et al., 1986; Shannon et al., 1989]. The potential public health impact of prenatal cocaine exposure is not trivial. In the 1985 Household Survey on Drug Abuse sponsored by the National Institute on Drug Abuse, 3.5% of women of childbearing age reported cocaine use in the preceding month [Khalsa and Gfroerer, 1991]. Although this figure had dropped to 0.5% by 1990, current data do not support this apparent trend. The percentage of pregnant women testing positive for cocaine metabolites in one inner-city clinic in Atlanta was 5% of those who consented to testing [Khalsa and Gfroerer, 1991; Lindsay et al., 1997]. Another study from Toronto produced a self-reported rate of cocaine use among pregnant women of 1.1% in the control group (11% in an ethanol-binge group) [Gladstone et al., 1997]. Screening based on self-reporting (and possibly on urine testing) underestimates cocaine use [Kline et al., 1997]. Finally, neonatal and meconium cocaine testing yielded positive results in 0.25% to 0.6% in "low-prevalence" rural populations [Little et al., 1996; O'Connor et al., 1997].

Infants exposed to cocaine prenatally have intrauterine growth retardation and reduced head circumference [Little and Snell, 1991; Little et al., 1996; Napiorkowski et al., 1996; Zuckerman et al., 1989]. Sharp waves and spikes may be seen in the neonatal electroencephalogram, and there is maturational delay in the brainstem auditory-evoked response in neonates exposed prenatally to cocaine [Doberczak et al., 1988; Salamy et al., 1990]. Maternal cocaine use has been associated with intracranial hemorrhage and antenatal or perinatal cerebral infarction [Chasnoff et al., 1986; Dusick et al., 1991]. Effects on neurobehavioral performance in 3-week-old infants after intrauterine cocaine exposure have also been reported recently [Tronick et al., 1996]. Infants are frequently irritable and tremulous with a high-pitched cry and sometimes hypertonia and hyperreflexia [Dempsey et al., 2000]. Poor feeding, abnormal sleep patterns, inappropriate response to stimulation, and difficulties with state regulation may also be present [Griffith et al., 1988; Madden et al., 1986]. Long-term follow-up data are limited, but there is a suggestion that cocaine-exposed children at 3 years of age are highly distractible with poorly developed verbal, language, and motor skills despite average test scores; microcephaly persists [Freier et al., 1991; Griffith et al., 1990; Zuckerman et al., 1995]. Two prospective studies addressed this issue further. One revealed dose-dependent abnormalities on standardized neonatal behavioral tests; the other demonstrated deficits in prenatally exposed children's ability to attend to a computer vigilance task but revealed no effect on academic achievement or classroom behavior through age 6 years [Martin et al., 1996; Richardson et al., 1996].

CONCLUDING REMARKS AND ADDITIONAL SOURCES

Fifty years ago, more than 400 children in the United States died each year as a result of poisoning. From a stack of index cards and other informal efforts grew our current system of regional and local poison control centers. The American Association of Poison Control Centers compiles Toxic Exposure Surveillance System data from regional centers in the United States. This effort, combined with educational efforts by the American Academy of Pediatrics and the National Association of Medical Examiners' Pediatric Toxicology (PedTox) Registry and local poison control center public and professional education, has reduced pediatric poison-related deaths in this country to less than 50 children each year [Burda and Burda, 1997; Hanzilck, 1996]. Other nations have similar programs and results.

New information concerning poisoning and drug effects on the nervous system appears rapidly. Because no text chapter can incorporate this burgeoning body of knowledge, the following section lists several other sources for current toxicology information. Internet URLs are current as of early 2005. The sites have links to other sites involving specific subtopics.

Internet Sites

Poison Control Centers (United States)

American Association of Poison Control Centers: http://www.aapcc.org/

Poison Control Centers (International)

Canada: http://www.uoguelph.ca/cntc/
Europe: http://www.eapcct.org/
Asia: http://prn.usm.my/prnnet.html

REFERENCES

Abdel-Magid EH, el-Awad Ahmed FR. Salicylate intoxication in an infant with ichthyosis transmitted through skin ointment. Pediatrics 1994;94:939.

Abel E, Sokol R. Incidence of fetal alcohol syndrome and economic effect of FAS related anomalies. Drug Alcohol Depend 1987;19:51.

Abernathy CO, Thomas DJ, Calderon RL. Health effects and risk assessment of arsenic. J Nutrition 2003;133 (Suppl 1):1536S.

Abhayambika K, Chacko A, Mahadevan K, et al. Peripheral neuropathy and haemolytic anaemia with cherry red spot on macula in dapsone poisoning. J Assoc Physicians India 1990;38:564.

Adair JC, Woodley SL, O'Connell JB, et al. Aseptic meningitis following cardiac transplantation: Clinical characteristics and relationship to immunosuppressive regimen. Neurology 1991;41:249.

Adams DH, Ponsford S, Gunson B, et al. Neurological complications following liver transplantation. Lancet 1987;1:949.

Adams E, Gfroerer JC, Rouse BA. Epidemiology of substance abuse including alcohol and cigarette smoking. Ann N Y Acad Sci 1989;562:1420.

Adams J, Vorhees CV, Middaugh LD. Developmental neurotoxicity of anticonvulsants: Human and animal evidence on phenytoin. Neurotoxicol Teratol 1990;12:203.

Agran PF, Anderson C, Winn D, et al. Rates of pediatric injuries by 3-month intervals for children 0 to 3 years of age. Pediatrics 2003;111:683.

Aks SE, Krantz A, Hryhrczuk DO, et al. Acute accidental lindane ingestion in toddlers. Ann Emerg Med 1995;26:647.

Alexander LN, Wilcox CM. A prospective trial of thalidomide for the treatment of HIV-associated idiopathic esophageal ulcers. AIDS Res Hum Retrovir 1997;13:301.

Allison JW, Glasier CM, Stark JE, et al. Head and neck MR angiography in pediatric patients: A pictorial essay. Radiographics 1994;14:795.

Alroomi LG, Davidson J, Evans TJ, et al. Maternal narcotic abuse and the newborn. Arch Dis Child 1988;63:81.

American Academy of Pediatrics Committee on Drugs. Treatment guidelines for lead exposure in children. Pediatrics 1995;96:155.

American Academy of Pediatrics Committee on Drugs. "Inactive" ingredients in pharmaceutical products: Update. Pediatrics 1997;99:268.

American Academy of Pediatrics Committee on Injury, Violence, and Poison Prevention. Poison treatment in the home. Pediatrics 2003;112:1182.

Andiran N, Sarikayalar F. Pattern of acute poisonings in childhood in Ankara: What has changed in twenty years? Turk J Pediatr 2004;46:147.

Anker AL, Smilkstein MJ. Acetaminophen. Concepts and controversies. Emerg Med Clin North Am 1994;12:335.

Arena JM. Poisoning, toxicology symptoms, treatments, 5th ed. Springfield, IL: Charles C. Thomas, 1985.

Ariffin H, Omar KZ, Ang EL, et al. Severe vincristine neurotoxicity with concomitant use of itraconazole. J Paediatr Child Health 2003;39:638.

Armstrong T, Gilbert MR. Central nervous system toxicity from cancer treatment. Curr Oncol Rep 2004;6:11.

Arnold GL, Kirby RS, Langendoerfer S, et al. Toluene embryopathy: Clinical delineation and developmental follow-up. Pediatrics 1994;93:216.

Asensi F, Otero MC, Perez-Tamarit D, et al. Risk/benefit in the treatment of children with imipenem-cilastatin for meningitis caused by penicillin-resistant pneumococcus. J Chemother 1993;5:133.

Aureli P, Franciosa G, Pourshaban M. Foodborne botulism in Italy [Letter]. Lancet 1996;348:1594.

Aydin K, Hüseyin P, Kurtoglu S, et al. Amitraz poisoning in children. Eur J Pediatr 2002;161:349.

Babe KS Jr, Serafin WE. Histamine, bradykinin, 5-hydroxytryptamine, and their antagonists. In: Hardman JG, Limbird LE, Molinoff PB, et al., eds. Goodman and Gilman's the pharmacologic basis of therapeutics, 9th ed. New York: McGraw-Hill, 1996.

Backman L, Nicar M, Levy M, et al. Whole blood and plasma levels of FK506 after liver transplantation: Correlation with toxicity. Transplant Proc 1994;26:1804.

Badcock NR, Zoanetti GD. Modifications to Toxi-Lab for the routine screening for drugs in paediatric toxicology. Ann Clin Biochem 1996;33:75.

Bailey B, Ito S. Breastfeeding and maternal drug use. Pediatr Clin North Am 1997;44:41.

Bak TH, Bauer M, Schaub RT, et al. Myoclonus in patients treated with clozapine: A case series. J Clin Psychiatry 1995;56:418.

Baker SD, Morgan DL. Fluoxetine exposures: Are they safe for children? Am J Emerg Med 2004;22:211.

Baldessarini RJ. Drugs and the treatment of psychiatric disorders: Psychosis and anxiety. In: Hardman JG, Limbird LE, Molinoff PB, et al., eds. Goodman and Gilman's the pharmacologic basis of therapeutics, 9th ed. New York: McGraw-Hill, 1996.

Banner W Jr, Timmons OD, Vernon DD. Advances in the critical care of poisoned paediatric patients. Drug Saf 1994;10:83.

Bari N. Salicylate poisoning. J Pak Med Assoc 1995;45:160.

Barr JT, Schumacher GE, Luks DB, et al. Mild theophylline-related adverse reactions and serum theophylline concentration. Am J Hosp Pharm 1994;51:2688.

Barr M, Hanson JW, Currey K, et al. Holoprosencephaly in infants of diabetic mothers. J Pediatr 1981;102:565.

Bassett KE, Schunk JE, Crouch BI. Cyclizine abuse by teenagers in Utah. Am J Emerg Med 1996;14:472.

Batchelor TT, Taylor LP, Thaler HT, et al. Steroid myopathy in cancer patients. Neurology 1997;48:1234.

Bateman DA, Heagarty MC. Passive free-base cocaine ("crack") inhalation by infants and toddlers. Am J Dis Child 1989;143:25.

Bellinger DC, Sloman A, Leviton A, et al. Low level lead exposure and children's cognitive function in the preschool years. Pediatrics 1991;87:219.

Bellinger DC. Interpreting the literature on lead and child development: The neglected role of the "experimental system." Neurotoxicol Teratol 1995;17:201.

Berlin CM. Lead poisoning in children. Curr Opinion Pediatr 1997;9:173.

Bessen HA. Intracranial hemorrhage associated with phencyclidine abuse. JAMA 1982;248:585.

Bhatt BD, Meriano FV, Buchwald D. Cyclosporine associated central nervous system toxicity. N Engl J Med 1988;318:788.

Bigham GN, Vandal GM. A drainage basin perspective of mercury transport and bioaccumulation: Onondaga Lake, New York. Neurotoxicology 1996;17:279.

Boehnert MT, Lovejoy FH. Value of the QRS duration versus the serum drug level in predicting seizures and ventricular arrhythmias after an acute overdose of tricyclic antidepressants. N Engl J Med 1985;313:474.

Boffa MJ, Brough PA, Ead RD. Lindane neurotoxicity. Br J Dermatol 1995;133:1013.

Bond GR. The poisoned child. Evolving concepts in care. Emerg Med Clin North Am 1995;13:343.

Boon AP, Adams DH, Carey MP, et al. Cyclosporin-associated cerebral lesions in liver transplantation [Letter]. Lancet 1988;1:1457.

Boros CA, Parsons DW, Zoanetti GD, et al. Cannabis cookies: A cause of coma. J Paediatr Child Health 1996;32:194.

Boyko OB, Burger PC, Heinz ER. Pathological and radiological correlation of subarachnoid hemorrhage in phencyclidine abuse. J Neurosurg 1987;67:446.

Bradley WG, Lassman LP, Pearce GW, et al. The neuromyopathy of vincristine in man. Clinical, electrophysiological, and pathological studies. J Neurol Sci 1970;10:107.

Brandwene EL, Williams SR, Tunget-Johnson C, et al. Refining the level for anticipated hepatotoxicity in acetaminophen poisoning. J Emerg Med 1996;14:691.

Brayden RM, MacLean WE Jr, Bonfiglio JF, et al. Behavioral antecedents of pediatric poisonings. Clin Pediatr (Phila) 1993;32:30.

Brew BJ, Currie JN. HIV-related neurological disease. Med J Austr 1993;158:104.

Brisse H, Doz F. Central neurological manifestations during chemotherapy in children [in French]. Arch de Pediatrie 2003;10:533.

Brown JH, Taylor P. Muscarinic receptor agonists and antagonists. In: Hardman JG, Limbird LE, Molinoff PB, et al., eds. Goodman and Gilman's the pharmacologic basis of therapeutics, 9th ed. New York: McGraw-Hill, 1996.

Brown M, Herbert AA. Insect repellents: An overview. J Am Acad Dermatol 1997;36:243.

Brunton LL. Agents affecting gastrointestinal water flux and motility; emesis and antiemetics; bile acids and pancreatic enzymes. In: Hardman JG, Limbird LE, Molinoff PB, et al., eds. Goodman and Gilman's the pharmacologic basis of therapeutics, 9th ed. New York: McGraw-Hill, 1996.

Burda AM, Burda NM. The nation's first poison control center: Taking a stand against accidental childhood poisoning in Chicago. Vet Hum Toxicol 1997;39:115.

Burnett JW. Thallium poisoning. Cutis 1990;46:112.

Buzan RD. Risperidone-induced tardive dyskinesia [Letter]. Am J Psychiatry 1996;153:734.

Cairney S, Maruff P, Burns CB, et al. Neurological and cognitive impairment associated with leaded gasoline encephalopathy. Drug Alcohol Depend 2004;73:183.

Caldemeyer KS, Armstrong SW, George KK, et al. The spectrum of neuroimaging abnormalities in solvent abuse and their clinical correlation. J Neuroimag 1996;6:167.

Caldicott DG, Kuhn M. Gamma-hydroxybutyrate overdose and physostigmine: Teaching new tricks to an old drug? Ann Emerg Med 2001;37:99.

Camidge DR, Wood RJ, Bateman DN. The epidemiology of self-poisoning in the UK. Br J Clin Pharmacol 2003;56:613.

Cannon G, Caravati EM, Filloux FM. Hydrogen peroxide neurotoxicity in childhood: Case report with unique magnetic resonance imaging features. J Child Neurol 2003;18:805.

Capone PM, Cohen ME. Seizures and cerebritis associated with administration of OKT3. Pediatr Neurol 1991;7:299.

Caroff SN, Mann SC. Neuroleptic malignant syndrome. Med Clin North Am 1993;77:185.

Caroff SN, Mann SC, Campbell EC, et al. Movement disorders associated with atypical antipsychotic drugs. J Clin Psychiatry 2002;63 (Suppl 4):12.

Casey DE. Extrapyramidal symptoms in old and new antipsychotics. In: Kane JM, chairperson. Choosing among old and new antipsychotics. J Clin Psychiatry 1996a;57:427.

Casey DE. Side effect profiles of new antipsychotic agents. J Clin Psychiatry 1996b;57 (Suppl 11):40.

Castellanos FX, Giedd JN, Elia J, et al. Controlled stimulant treatment of ADHD and comorbid Tourette's syndrome: Effects of stimulant and dose. J Am Acad Child Adolesc Psychiatry 1997;36:589.

Cavaletti G, Cascinu S, Venturino P, et al. Neuroprotectant drugs in cisplatin neurotoxicity. Anticancer Res 1996;16:3149.

Centers for Disease Control and Prevention. Tick paralysis—Washington, 1995. JAMA 1996a;275:1470.

Centers for Disease Control and Prevention. Wound botulism—California, 1995. JAMA 1996b;275:95.

Cetaruk EW, Dart RC, Hurlbut KM, et al. Tylenol extended relief overdose. Ann Emerg Med 1997;30:104.

Chadwick DL. The diagnosis of inflicted injury in infants and young children. Del Med J 1997;69:3

Chan B, Gaudry P, Grattan Smith TM, et al. The use of Glasgow Coma Scale in poisoning. J Emerg Med 1993;11:579.

Chan CY, Beh SL, Broadhurst RG. Homicide-suicide in Hong Kong, 1989–1998. Forensic Sci Int 2003;137:165.

Chan TH, Wong KC, Chan JC. Severe salicylate poisoning associated with the intake of Chinese medicinal oil ("red flower oil"). Aust N Z J Med 1995;25:57.

Chan YL, Ng HK, Leung CB, et al. (31) Phosphorous and single voxel proton MR spectroscopy and diffusion-weighted imaging in a case of star fruit poisoning. AJNR Am J Neuroradiol 2002;23:1557.

Chasnoff IJ, Bussey ME, Savich R, et al. Perinatal cerebral infarction and maternal cocaine use. J Pediatr 1986;108:456.

Chen YC, Chang CT, Fang JT, et al. Baclofen neurotoxicity in uremic patients: Is continuous ambulatory peritoneal dialysis less effective than intermittent hemodialysis? Renal Failure 2003;25:297.

Cherington M. Botulism: 10 Year experience. Arch Neurol 1974;30:432.

Cheron RG, Kaplan MM, Larsen PR, et al. Neonatal thyroid function after propylthiouracil therapy for maternal Graves disease. N Engl J Med 1981;304:525.

Cheson BD, Vena DA, Foss FM, et al. Neurotoxicity of purine analogs: A review. J Clin Oncol 1994;12:2216.

Chow KM, Szeto CC, Hui AC, et al. Retrospective review of neurotoxicity induced by cefepime and ceftazidime. Pharmacotherapy 2003;23:369.

Christensen ML, Mahmoud H, Evans WE. Pharmacokinetics of vincristine in children and adolescents with acute lymphoblastic leukemia. J Pediatr 1994;125:642.

Cienki J, Akhtar J, Donovan JW. Activated charcoal and salicylate. Ann Emerg Med 1995;26:569.

Coberly S, Lammer E, Alashari M. Retinoic acid embryopathy: Case report and review of literature. Pediatr Pathol Lab Med 1996;16:823.

Colonna F, Trappan A, de Vonderweid U, et al. Peritoneal dialysis in a 6-weeks old preterm infant with severe theophylline intoxication. Minerva Pediatr 1996;48:383.

Conners GP. Piperazine neurotoxicity: Worm wobble revisited. J Emerg Med 1995;13:341.

Conway EE, Mezey AP, Powers K. Status epilepticus following the oral ingestion of cocaine in an infant. Pediatr Emerg Care 1990;6:189.

Cranmer M, Gilbert S, Cranmer J. Neurotoxicity of mercury: Indicators and effects of low-level exposure. Neurotoxicology 1996;17:9.

Crystal HA, Schaumburg HH, Grober E, et al. Cognitive impairment and sensory loss associated with chronic low-level ethylene oxide exposure. Neurology 1988;38:567.

Daniel DG, Smith K, Hyde T, et al. Neuroleptic-induced tardive dyskinesia [Letter]. Am J Psychiatry 1996;153:734.

Dannenberg AL, Dorfman SF, Johnson J. Use of quinine for self-induced abortion. South Med J 1983;76:846.

Das D, Chatterjee A, Mandal BK, et al. Arsenic in the ground water in six districts of West Bengal, India: The biggest arsenic calamity in the world. Part 2. Arsenic concentration in drinking water, hair, nails, urine, skin-scale and liver tissue (biopsy) of the affected people. Analyst 1995;120:917.

Davis CD, Pirmohamed M, Kitteringham NR, et al. Kinetic parameters of lymphocyte microsomal epoxide hydrolase in carbamazepine hypersensitivity patients. Assessment by radiometric HPLC. Biochem Pharmacol 1995;50:1361.

Day NL, Robles N, Richardson GA, et al. The effects of prenatal alcohol use on the growth of children at three years of age. Alcohol Clin Exp Res 1991;15:67.

de Groen PC, Aksamit AJ, Rakela J, et al. Central nervous system toxicity after liver transplantation. N Engl J Med 1987;14:861.

DeAngelis LM, Gnecco C, Taylor L, et al. Evolution of neuropathy and myopathy during intensive vincristine/corticosteroid chemotherapy for non-Hodgkin's lymphoma. Cancer 1991;67:2241.

DeJong R. The cerebellum. In: DeJong R, ed. The neurologic examination, 3rd ed. New York: Hoeber Medical Division, Harper & Row, 1967.

Delaney P, Estes M. Intracranial hemorrhage with amphetamine abuse. Neurology 1980;30:1125.

Dempsey DA, Hajnal BL, Partridge JC, et al. Tone abnormalities are associated with maternal cigarette smoking during pregnancy in in utero cocaine-exposed infants. Pediatrics 2000;106:79.

Dewan A, Bhatnager VK, Mathur ML, et al. Repeated episodes of endosulfan poisoning. J Toxicol Clin Toxicol 2004;42:363.

Diasio RB, LoBuglio AF. Immunomodulators: Immunosuppressive agents and immunostimulants. In: Hardman JG, Limbird LE, Molinoff PB, et al., eds. Goodman and Gilman's the pharmacologic basis of therapeutics, 9th ed. New York: McGraw-Hill, 1996.

Dietrich KN, Krafft KM, Bornschein RL, et al. Low-level fetal lead exposure effect on neurobehavioral development in early infancy. Pediatrics 1987;80:721.

DiMaggio JR, Brown R, Baile WF, et al. Hallucinations and ifosfamide neurotoxicity. Cancer 1994;73:1509.

DiMario FJ. Aseptic meningitis secondary to metrizamide lumbar myelography in a 4 month old infant. Pediatrics 1985;76:259.

Doberczak TM, Shanzer S, Senie RT, et al. Neonatal neurologic and electroencephalographic effects of intrauterine cocaine exposure. J Pediatr 1988;113:354.

Dorea JG. Mercury and lead during breast-feeding. Br J Nutr 2004;92:21.

Doring G, Baumeister FA, Peters J, et al. Butane abuse associated encephalopathy. Klinische Padiatrie 2002;214:295.

Dunn DW, Parekh HU. Theophylline and status epilepticus. Neuropediatrics 1991;22:24.

Dunton SF, Nitschke R, Spruce WE, et al. Progressive ascending paralysis following administration of intrathecal and intravenous cytosine arabinoside. Cancer 1986;5:1083.

Dusick AM, Covert RF, Tebbett IR, et al. Prenatal cocaine exposure and intracranial hemorrhage in very low birthweight babies. Pediatr Res 1991;29:212.

Dyck PJ, Thomas PK. Peripheral neuropathy, 3rd ed. Philadelphia: WB Saunders, 1993.

Easley RB, Altemeier WA III. Central nervous system manifestations of an ibuprofen overdose reversed by naloxone. Pediatr Emerg Care 2000;16:39.

Eisenhauer G, Jermain DM. Fluoxetine and tics in an adolescent. Ann Pharmacother 1993;27:725.

Embry CK. Toxic cyclic vomiting in an 11-year-old girl. J Am Acad Child Adolesc Psychiatry 1987;26:447.

Emmons C, Smith J, Flanigan M. Cerebrospinal fluid inflammation during OKT3 therapy. Lancet 1986;2:510.

English M, Marsh V, Amukoye E, et al. Chronic salicylate poisoning and severe malaria. Lancet 1996;347:1736.

Erinoff L. General considerations in assessing neurotoxicity using neuroanatomical methods. Neurochem Int 1995;26:111.

Ernst E, Coon JT. Heavy metals in traditional Chinese medicines: A systematic review. Clin Pharmacol Ther 2001;70:497.

Esposito-Smythers C, Spirito A. Adolescent substance use and suicidal behavior: A review with implications for treatment research. Alcoholism Clin Exp Res 2004;28 (Suppl 5):77S.

Ettinger LJ. Pharmacokinetics and biochemical effects of a fatal intrathecal methotrexate overdose. Cancer 1982;50:444.

Falasca GF, Toly TM, Reginato AJ, et al. Reflex sympathetic dystrophy associated with antiepileptic drugs. Epilepsia 1994;35:394.

Faraci M, Lanino E, Dini G, et al. Severe neurologic complications after hematopoietic stem cell transplantation in children [erratum appears in Neurology 2003;60:1055]. Neurology 2002;59:1895.

Farrar DJ, Locke SE, Kantrowitz FG. Chronic fatigue syndrome: 1. Etiology and pathogenesis. Behav Med 1995;21:5.

Faulk RS, Gilmore JH, Jensen EW, et al. Risperidone-induced dystonic reaction [Letter]. Am J Psychiatry 1996;153:577.

Fehlow P, Walther F, Miosge W. An increased incidence of megacolon in psychiatric and neurologic patients. Nervenarzt 1995;66:57.

Feldman GL, Weaver DD, Lovrien EW. The fetal trimethadione syndrome: Report of an additional family and further delineation of this syndrome. Am J Dis Child 1977;131:1389.

Feldman J, Levisohn DR. Acute alopecia: Clue to thallium toxicity. Pediatr Dermatol 1993;10:29.

Findley LJ. Classification of tremors. J Clin Neurophysiol 1996;13:122.

Fischer TF. Lindane toxicity in a 24-year-old woman. Ann Emerg Med 1994;24:972.

Forman AD. Neurologic complications of cytokine therapy. Oncology 1994;8:105.

Forrester MB, Sievert JS, Stanley SK. Epidemiology of lindane exposures for pediculosis reported to Poison Centers in Texas, 1998–2002. J Toxicol Clin Toxicol 2004;42:55.

Forsyth CJ, Cremer PD, Torzillo P, et al. Thalidomide responsive chronic pulmonary GVHD. Bone Marrow Transplant 1996;17:291.

Foy HM, Tarmapai S, Eamchan P, et al. Chronic arsenic poisoning from well water in a mining area in Thailand. Asian Pac J Public Health 1992–1993;6:150.

Frances C, Hoizey G, Lamiable D, et al. Bromism from daily over intake of bromide salt. J Toxicol Clin Toxicol 2003;41:181.

Fray PJ, Robbins TW. CANTAB battery: Proposed utility in neurotoxicology. Neurotoxicol Teratol 1996;18:499.

Freier MC, Griffith DR, Chasnoff IJ. In utero drug exposure: Developmental follow up and maternal-infant interaction. Semin Perinatol 1991;15:310

Fung J. Prophylactic use of OKT3 in liver transplantation: A review. Dig Dis Sci 1991;10:1427.

Furukawa M, Terae S, Chu BC, et al. MRI in seven cases of tacrolimus (FK-506) encephalopathy: Utility of FLAIR and diffusion-weighted imaging. Neuroradiology 2001;43:615.

Gabriel Botella F, Labios Gomez M, Galindo Puerto MJ, et al. Reflex sympathetic dystrophy syndrome associated with phenobarbital [Letter]. Ann Med Interne (Paris) 1996;13:336.

Gaedigk A, Spielberg SP, Grant DM. Characterization of the microsomal epoxide hydrolase gene in patients with anticonvulsant adverse drug reactions. Pharmacogenetics 1994;4:142.

Gal P, Roop C, Robinson H, et al. Theophylline induced seizures in accidentally overdosed neonates. Pediatrics 1980;65:547.

Gardner TB, Manning HL, Beelen AP, et al. Ethylene glycol toxicity associated with ischemia, perforation, and colonic oxaliate crystal deposition. J Clin Gastroenterol 2004;38:435.

Garg BP, Walsh LE, Pescovitz MD, et al. Neurologic complications of pediatric liver transplantation. Pediatr Neurol 1993;9:444.

Gengo FM. Reduction of the central nervous system adverse effects associated with antihistamines in the management of allergic disorders: Strategies and progress. J Allergy Clin Immunol 1996;98:S319.

Gerr F, Letz R, Ryan PB, et al. Neurological effects of environmental exposure to arsenic in dust and soil among humans. Neurotoxicology 2000;21:475.

Gershanik J, Beocler B, Ensley H, et al. The gasping syndrome and benzyl alcohol poisoning. N Engl J Med 1982;307:1384.

Getz R, Siegel E, Scaglione J, et al. Suspected moonflower intoxication—Ohio, 2002. MMWR Morb Mortal Wkly Rep 2003;52:788.

Ghalie R, Fitzsimmons WE, Bennett D, et al. Cortical blindness: A rare complication of cyclosporine therapy. Bone Marrow Transplant 1990;6:147.

Ghazi-Khansari M, Oreizi S. A prospective study of fatal outcomes of poisoning in Tehran. Vet Hum Toxicol 1995;37:449.

Gilles FH, Matson D. Sciatic nerve injury following misplaced gluteal injection. J Pediatr 1970;76:247.

Gladstone DJ, Bologa M, Maguire C, et al. Course of pregnancy and fetal outcome following maternal exposure to carbamazepine and phenytoin: A prospective study. Reprod Toxicol 1992;6:257.

Gladstone J, Levy M, Nulman I, et al. Characteristics of pregnant women who engage in binge alcohol consumption. Can Med Assoc J 1997;156:789.

Glaser JS. Topical diagnosis: Prechiasmal visual pathways. In: Glaser JS, ed. Neuro-ophthalmology, 2nd ed. Philadelphia: JB Lippincott, 1990.

Glaser JS, Bachynski B. Infranuclear disorders of eye movement. In: Glaser JS, ed. Neuro-ophthalmology, 2nd ed. Philadelphia: JB Lippincott, 1990.

Glatman-Freedman A. Infant botulism. Pediatr Rev 1996;17:185.

Gleiter CH, Deckert J. Adverse CNS effects of beta-adrenoceptor blockers. Pharmacopsychiatry 1996;29:201.

Goetting MG. Acute lithium poisoning in a child with dystonia. Pediatrics 1985;76:978.

Goetz CG. Neurotoxins in clinical practice. New York: Spectrum Publications, 1985.

Goetz CM, Love RC, Schuster P. Overdose of clozapine in a child. Vet Hum Toxicol 1993;35:338.

Goldbart A, Press J, Sofer S, et al. Near fatal acute colchicine intoxication in a child. A case report. Eur J Pediatr 2000;159:895.

Gosselin RE, Smith RP, Hodge HC, et al., eds. Clinical toxicology of commercial products, 5th ed. Baltimore: Williams & Wilkins, 1984.

Gotschlich T, Beltran RS. Poisoning of a 21-month-old child by a baby-sitter. Clin Pediatr 1995;34:52.

Graham JM, Edwards MJ, Lipson AH, et al. Gestational hyperthermia as a cause for Moebius syndrome [Abstract]. Teratology 1988;37:461.

Grandjean P, White RF, Weihe P, et al. Neurotoxic risk caused by stable and variable exposure to methylmercury from seafood. Ambul Pediatr 2003;3:18.

Grant GA, Al-Rabiee R, Xu XL, et al. Critical interactions at the dimer interface of kappa-bungarotoxin, a neuronal nicotinic acetylcholine receptor antagonist. Biochemistry 1997;36:3353.

Green VJ, Pirmohamed M, Kitteringham NR, et al. Genetic analysis of microsomal epoxide hydrolase in patients with carbamazepine hypersensitivity. Biochem Pharmacol 1995;50:1353.

Griffin PM, Hatheway CL, Rosenbaum RB, et al. Endogenous antibody production to botulinum toxin in an adult with intestinal colonization botulism and underlying Crohn's disease. J Infect Dis 1997;175:633.

Griffith DR, Chasnoff IJ, Dirkes K, et al. Neurobehavioral development of cocaine-exposed infants in the first month of life. Pediatr Res 1988;23:55.

Griffith DR, Chasnoff IJ, Freier MC. Developmental follow up of cocaine exposed infants through three years. Infant Behav Dev 1990;13:126.

Grondahl TO, Langmoen IA. Epileptogenic effect of antibiotic drugs. J Neurosurg 1993;78:938.

Gulba DC. Anticoagulant drugs. Herz 1996;21:12.

Gupta AK, Agarwal MP, Avasthi R, et al. Metronidazole-induced neurotoxicity. J Assoc Physicians India 2003;51:617.

Haddad LM, Winchester JF. Clinical management of poisoning and drug overdose. Philadelphia: WB Saunders, 1983.

Haim N, Barron SA, Robinson E. Muscle cramps associated with vincristine therapy. Acta Oncol 1991;30:707.

Halavaara J, Valanne L, Setala K. Neuroimaging supports the clinical diagnosis of methanol poisoning. Neuroradiology 2002;44:924.

Haller E, Binder RL. Clozapine and seizures. Am J Psychiatry 1990;147:1069.

Hammond JE, Toseland PA. Placental transfer of chlorpromazine. Arch Dis Child 1970;45:139.
Handal M, Matheson I, Bechensteen AG, et al. Antipsychotic agents and pregnant women. A case report. Tidsskr Nor Laegeforen 1995;115:2537.
Hanson JW. Teratogen update: Fetal hydantoin effects. Teratology 1986;33:349.
Hanson JW. Human teratology. In: Rimoin DL, Connor JM, Pyeritz RE, eds. Emery and Rimoin's principles and practice of medical genetics, 3rd ed. New York: Churchill-Livingstone, 1996.
Hanson JW, Smith DW. Fetal hydantoin syndrome. J Pediatr 1975;87:285.
Hanzilck R. National Association of Medial Examiner's Pediatric Toxicology (PedTox) Registry. Toxicology 1996;107:153.
Hardin JW, Arena JM. Human poisoning from native and cultivated plants. Durham, NC: Duke University Press, 1974.
Haslett P, Tramontana J, Burroughs M, et al. Adverse reactions to thalidomide in patients infected with human immunodeficiency virus. Clin Infect Dis 1997;24:1223.
Hatzis T. Toxic encephalopathy associated with use of DEET insect repellents: A case analysis of its toxicity in children. Hum Exp Toxicol 2001;20:8.
Hawgood BJ. Sir Joseph Fayrer MD FRS (1824–1907) Indian Medical Service: Snakebite and mortality in British India. Toxicon 1996;34:171.
Hawton K, Fagg J. Deliberate self-poisoning and self-injury in adolescents. A study of characteristics and trends in Oxford, 1976–89. Br J Psychiatry 1992;161:816.
Hawton K, Fagg J, Platt S. Factors associated with suicide after parasuicide in young people. BMJ 1993;306:1641.
He F, Zhang S, Qiam F, et al. Delayed dystonia with striatal CT lucencies induced by a mycotoxin. Neurology 1995;45:2178.
Hearney EG, Fuhrer J, Marioz P. Photo quiz. Pepto Bismol poisoning. Clin Infect Dis 1996;23:37, 159.
Heier LA, Carpanzano CR, Mast J, et al. Maternal cocaine abuse: The spectrum of radiologic abnormalities in the neonatal CNS. AJNR Am J Neuroradiol 1991;12:951.
Herbst F, Gortner L. Paroxetine withdrawal syndrome as differential diagnosis of acute neonatal encephalopathy? [in German]. Z Geburtshilfe Neonatol 2003;207:232.
Hesslinger B, Hellwig B, Sester U, et al. An acute psychotic disorder caused by perfloxacin: A case report. Prog Neuropsychopharmacol Biol Psychiatry 1996;20:343.
Hey E. Effect of maternal anticonvulsant treatment on neonatal blood coagulation. Arch Dis Child Fetal Neonatal Ed 1999;81:F208.
Hilliard LM, Berkow RL, Watterson J, et al. Retinal toxicity associated with cisplatin and etoposide in pediatric patients. Med Pediatr Oncol 1997;28:310.
Hoffman BB, Lefkowitz RJ. Catecholamines, sympathomimetic drugs, and adrenergic receptor antagonists. In: Hardman JG, Limbird LE, Molinoff PB, et al., eds. Goodman and Gilman's the pharmacologic basis of therapeutics, 9th ed. New York: McGraw-Hill, 1996.
Hoffman RJ, Nelson L. Rational use of toxicology testing in children. Curr Opin Pediatr 2001;13:183.
Holzman C, Paneth N, Little R, et al. Perinatal brain injury in premature infants born to mothers using alcohol in pregnancy. Neonatal Brain Hemorrhage Study Team. Pediatrics 1995;95:66.
Hormes JT, Filley CM, Rosenberg NL. Neurologic sequelae of chronic solvent vapor abuse. Neurology 1986;36:698.
Huibers MJ, Bultman U, Kasl SV, et al. Predicting the two-year course of unexplained fatigue and the long-term sickness absence in fatigued employees: results from Cohort Study. J Occupat Environ Med 2004;46:1041.
Huisman M, Kooperman-Esseboom C, Fidler B, et al. Perinatal exposure to polychlorinated biphenyls and dioxins and its effect on neonatal neurological development. Early Hum Dev 1995;41:111.
Hunter TB, Dye J, Duval JF. Selective use of low-osmolality contrast agents for IV urography and CT: Safety and effect on cost. AJR Am J Roentgenol 1994;163:965.
Hwang CF, Foot CL, Eddie G, et al. The utility of the history and clinical signs of poisoning in childhood: A prospective study. Ther Drug Monit 2003;25:728.
Indulski JA, Lutz W. Biomarkers of neurotoxic effects induced by environmental chemicals. Med Pr 1996;47:383.
Isbister GK, Bowe SJ, Dawson A, et al. Relative toxicity of selective serotonin reuptake inhibitors (SSRIs) in overdose. J Toxicol Clin Toxicol 2004;42:277.
Isbister GK, Oakley P, Dawson AH, et al. Presumed Angel's trumpet (Brugmansia) poisoning: Clinical effects and epidemiology. Emerg Med 2003;15:376.
Iverson L. Cannabis and the brain. Brain 2003;126 (Pt 6):1252.
Jacobsen LS, Olsen AK, Sjogren P, et al. Morphine-induced hyperalgesia, allodynia and myoclonus: New side effects of morphine? Ugeskr Laeger 1995;57:3307.
Jacobson JL, Jacobson SW. Teratogen update: Polychlorinated biphenyls. Teratology 1997;55:338.
Jaksic W, Veljkovic D, Pozza C, et al. Methotrexate-induced leukoencephalopathy reversed by aminophylline and high-dose folinic acid. Acta Haematol 2004;111:230.
Jessel N, Stiskal JA. Neonatal encephalopathy after antidepressant exposure during pregnancy. Z Geburtshilfe Neonatol 2004;208:75.
Jimenez-Jimenez FJ, Garcia-Ruiz PJ, Molina JA. Drug-induced movement disorders. Drug Saf 1997;16:180.
Jira PE, Semmekrot BA, Vree TB, et al. Theophylline poisoning in children. Nederlands Tijdschrift voor Geneeskunde 1996;140:1608.
Johnson RO, Clay SA, Arnon SS. Diagnosis and management of infant botulism. Am J Dis Child 1979;133:586.
Jones KL. Smith's recognizable patterns of human malformation, 5th ed. Philadelphia: WB Saunders, 1996.
Juckel HU, Muller-Schubert A, Pietzcker A, et al. Schizophrenics with small P300: A subgroup with a neurodevelopmental disturbance and a high risk for tardive dyskinesia. Acta Psychiatr Scand 1995;91:120.
Junck L, Marshall WH. Neurotoxicity of radiological contrast agents. Ann Neurol 1983;13:469.
Kaaja E, et al. Enzyme-inducing antiepileptic drugs in pregnancy and the risk of bleeding in the neonate. Neurology 2002;58:549.
Kaeser HE. Drug induced myasthenic syndromes. Acta Neurol Scand 1984;70 (Suppl 100):39.
Kamaluddiin M, McNally P, Breatnach F, et al. Potentiation of vincristine toxicity by itraconazole in children with lymphoid malignancies. Acta Paediatr 2001;90:1204.
Karl HW, Talbott GA, Roberts TS. Intraoperative administration of radiologic contrast agents: potential neurotoxicity. Anesthesiology 1994;81:1067.
Katz J, Prescott K, Woolf AD. Strychnine poisoning from a Cambodian traditional remedy. Am J Emerg Med 1996;14:475.
Kendall SR. Treatment options for drug-exposed infants. NIDA Res Monogr 1995;149:78.
Kerrick JM, Kelley BJ, Maister BH, et al. Involuntary movement disorders associated with felbamate. Neurology 1995;45:185.
Keskin S, Konkol RJ. Seizure exacerbation related to beta-lactam antibiotics in a child with cerebral dysgenesis. Dev Med Child Neurol 1993;35:267.
Khalsa JH, Gfroerer J. Epidemiology and health consequences of drug abuse among pregnant women. Semin Perinatol 1991;15:265.
Kieslich M, Porto L, Lantermann H, et al., Cerebrovascular complications of L-asparaginase in the therapy of acute lymphoblastic leukemia. J Pediatr Hematol Oncol 2003;25:484.
Kim JH, Chang KH, Song IC, et al. Delayed encephalopathy of acute carbon monoxide intoxication: Diffusivity of cerebral white matter lesions. AJNR Am J Neuroradiol 2003;24:1592.
King JO, Denborough MA. Anesthetic induced malignant hyperpyrexia in children. J Pediatr 1973;83:37.
Klein BL, Ashenburg CA, Reed MD. Transdermal scopolamine intoxication in a child. Pediatr Emerg Care 1985a;1:208.
Klein SK, Levinsohn MW, Blume JL. Accidental chlorpromazine ingestion as a cause of neuroleptic malignant syndrome in children. J Pediatr 1985b;107:970.
Klein-Schwartz W, Anderson B. Analysis of sertraline-only overdoses. Am J Emerg Med 1996;14:456.
Klein-Schwartz W, Smith GS. Agricultural and horticultural chemical poisonings: Mortality and morbidity in the United States. Ann Emerg Med 1997;29:232.
Kline J, Ng SK, Schittini M, et al. Cocaine use during pregnancy: Sensitive detection by hair assay. Am J Public Health 1997;87:352.
Knight MR, Roberts RJ. Phenothiazine and butyrophenone intoxication in children. Pediatr Clin North Am 1986;33:229.
Koch S, Jager-Roman E, Losche G, et al. Antineoplastic drug treatment in pregnancy: Drug side-effects in the neonate and neurologic outcome. Acta Paediatr 1996;85:739.
Koivusalo AM, Yildirim Y, Vakkuri A, et al. Experience with albumin dialysis in five patients with severe overdoses of paracetamol. Acta Anaesthesiol Scand 2003;47:1145.

Kotwica M, Czerczak S. Intentional poisonings in children below 15 years of age in the city of Lodz. Vet Hum Toxicol 2002;44:248.
Koyun M, Akman S, Guven AG. Mercury intoxication resulting from school barometers in three unrelated adolescents. Eur J Pediatr 2004;163:131.
Krebs MO. Current data on neurologic sequelae caused by neuroleptics. Encephale 1995;21:49.
Krenzelok EP, Jacobsen TD, Aronis JM. Plant exposures: A state profile of the most common species. Vet Hum Toxicol 1996;289.
Kulberg A. Substance abuse: Clinical identification and management. Pediatr Clin North Am 1986;33:325.
Kulig K, Rumack BH. Anticholinergic poisoning. In: Haddad LM, Winchester JF, eds. Clinical management of poisoning and drug overdose. Philadelphia: WB Saunders, 1983.
Kunkel DB. Poisonous plants. In: Haddad LM, Winchester JF, eds. Clinical management of poisoning and overdose. Philadelphia: WB Saunders, 1983.
Kurz M, Hummer M, Oberhauer H, et al. Extrapyramidal side effects of clozapine and haloperidol. Psychopharmacology 1995;118:52.
Lahat E, Katz Y, Bistritzer T, et al. Recurrent seizures in children with Shigella-associated convulsions. Ann Neurol 1990;28:393.
Lam LT. Childhood and adolescence poisoning in NSW, Australia: An analysis of age, sex, geographic, and poison types. Inj Prev 2003;9:338.
Lam SK, To WK, Duthie SJ, et al. Narcotic addiction in pregnancy with adverse maternal and perinatal outcome. Aust N Z J Obstet Gynaecol 1992;32:216.
Lammer EJ, Chen DT, Haas RM, et al. Retinoic acid embryopathy. N Engl J Med 1985;313:837.
Landrigan PJ, Gehlbach SH, Rosenblum BF, et al. Neuropsychological dysfunction in children with chronic low level lead absorption. Lancet 1975;1:708.
Langford SD, Boor PJ. Oleander toxicity: An examination of human and animal toxic exposures. Toxicology 1996;109:1.
LaPorte RE, Talbott EE. Effects of low level lead exposure on cognitive function: A review. Arch Environ Health 1978;33:236.
Lavin MR, Mendelowitz A, Block SH. Adverse reaction to high-dose fluoxetine [Letter]. J Clin Psychopharmacol 1993;13:452.
Layde PM, Edmonds LD, Erickson JD. Maternal fever and neural tube defects. Teratology 1980;21:105.
Lee H, Vacanti JP. Liver transplantation and its long-term management in children. Pediatr Clinics North Am 1996;43:99.
Lee P, Tai DY. Clinical features of patients with acute organophosphate poisoning requiring intensive care. Intensive Care Med 2001;27:694.
Leikin JB, Mycyk MB, Bryant S, et al. Characteristics of patients with no underlying toxicologic syndrome evaluated in a toxicology clinic. J Toxicol 2004;42:643.
Leikin JB, Paloucek FP. Poisoning and toxicology handbook 1996–97, 2nd ed. Hudson, OH: Lexi-Comp, 1995.
Leitman PS, diSant Agnese PA, Wong VA. Optic neuritis in cystic fibrosis of the pancreas: Role of chloramphenicol therapy. JAMA 1964;189:924.
LeQuesne PM. Neuropathy due to drugs. In: Dyck PJ, Thomas PK, eds. Peripheral neuropathy, 3rd ed. Philadelphia: WB Saunders, 1993.
Le Quintrec JS, Le Quintrec JL. Drug-induced myopathies. Baillieres Clin Rheumatol 1991;5:21.
Leroux BG, Leisenring WM, Moolgavkar SH. A biologically-based dose-response model for developmental toxicology. Risk Anal 1996;16:449.
Levine SR, Futrelln N, Ho K-L, et al. A comparative study of cerebrovascular complications of cocaine: Alkaloidal versus cocaine hydrochloride. Ann Neurol 1990;28:225.
Levy W, Wisniewski K. Chlorpromazine causing extrapyramidal dysfunction in newborn infant of psychotic mother. N Y State Med J 1974;74:684.
Lewin PK, McGreal D. Isoniazid toxicity with cerebellar ataxia in a child. Can Med Assoc J 1993;48:49.
Lewis DW, Fontana C, Mehallick LK, et al. Transdermal scopolamine for reduction of drooling in developmentally delayed children. Dev Med Child Neurol 1994;36:484.
Li WF, Costa LG, Richter RJ, et al. Catalytic efficiency determines the in-vivo efficacy of PON1 for detoxifying organophosphorus compounds. Pharmacogenetics 2000;10:767.
Liang TW, Balcer LJ, Solomon D, et al. Supranuclear gaze palsy and opsoclonus after Diazinon poisoning. J Neurol Neurosurg Psychiatry 2003;74:677.
Lidsky TI, Schneider JS. Lead neurotoxicity in children: Basic mechanisms and clinical correlates. Brain 2003;126 (Pt 1):5.
Lifshitz M, Shahak E, Bolotin A. Carbamate poisoning in early childhood and adults. J Toxicol 1997;35:25.
Lindsay MK, Carmichael S, Peterson H, et al. Correlation between self-reported cocaine use and urine toxicology in an inner-city prenatal population. J Natl Med Assoc 1997;89:57.
Lindstrom E, Eriksson B, Hellgren A, et al. Efficacy and safety of risperidone in the long-term treatment of patients with schizophrenia. Clin Ther 1995;17:402.
Litovitz TL, Felberg L, Soloway RA, et al. 1994 Annual report of the American Association of Poison Control Centers Toxic Exposure Surveillance System. Am J Emerg Med 1995;13:551.
Litovitz TL, Smilkstein M, Felberg L, et al. 1996 Annual report of the American Association of Poison Control Centers Toxic Exposure Surveillance System. Am J Emerg Med 1997;15:447.
Little BB, Snell LM. Brain growth among fetuses exposed to cocaine in utero: Asymmetrical growth retardation. Obstet Gynecol 1991;77:361.
Little BB, Wilson GN, Jackson G. Is there a cocaine syndrome? Dysmorphic and anthropometric assessment of infants exposed to cocaine. Teratology 1996;54:145.
Lucey JF, Dolan RG. Hyperbilirubinemia of the newborn infants associated with the parenteral administration of vitamin K analogue to the mothers. Pediatrics 1959;23:553.
Luft FC. Thinking about zinc: Clinical implications. J Mol Med 2003;81:597.
Lukas SE. CNS effects and abuse liability of anabolic-androgenic steroids. Annu Rev Pharmacol Toxicol 1996;36:333.
Madden JD, Payne TF, Miller S. Maternal cocaine abuse and effects on the newborn. Pediatrics 1986;77:209.
Mahaffey KR. Recent advances in recognition of low-level methylmercury poisoning. Curr Opin Neurol 2000;13:699.
Marchiori PE, Mies S, Scaff M. Cyclosporine A–induced ocular opsoclonus and reversible leukoencephalopathy after orthotopic liver transplantation: brief report. Clin Neuropharmacol 2004;27:195.
Margolin K. The Forman article reviewed. Oncology 1994;8:116.
Markman M. Toxicities of the platinum antineoplastic agents. Expert Opin Drug Safety 2003;2:597.
Marrs TC. Organophosphate poisoning. Pharmacol Ther 1993;58:51.
Martin JC, Barr HM, Martin DC, et al. Neonatal neurobehavioral outcome following prenatal exposure to cocaine. Neurotoxicol Teratol 1996;18:617.
Martin MA, Massanari M, Dai D, et al. Nosocomial aseptic meningitis associated with administration of OKT 3. JAMA 1988;259:2002.
Matick H, Anderson D, Brumlik J. Cerebrovasculitis associated with oral amphetamine overdose. Arch Neurol 1983;40:253.
Matthews HW. Racial, ethnic, and gender differences in response to medicines. Drug Metab Drug Interact 1995;12:77.
Mattson SN, Riley EP, Jernigan TL, et al. A decrease in the size of the basal ganglia following prenatal alcohol exposure: A preliminary report. Neurotoxicol Teratol 1994;16:283.
Matusmoto HG, Goyo K, Takevchi T. Fetal Minamata disease: A neuropathological study of two cases of intrauterine intoxication by a methylmercury compound. Neuropathol Exp Neurol 1965;24:563.
Mauer MP, Rosales R, Sievert J, et al. Surveillance for acute insecticide-related illness associated with mosquito-control efforts—nine states, 1999–2002. MMWR Morb Mortal Wkly Rep 2003;52:629.
Mazumder DN, Das Gupta J, Chakraborty AK. Environmental pollution and chronic arsenicosis in south Calcutta. Bull World Health Org 1992;70:481.
McArdle P. Substance abuse by children and young people: A contemporary disease. Arch Dis Child 2004;89:701.
McClure GM. Suicide in children and adolescents in England and Wales 1960–1990. Br J Psychiatry 1994;165:510.
McClure RJ, Davis PM, Meadow SR, et al. Epidemiology of Munchausen syndrome by proxy, non-accidental poisoning, and non-accidental suffocation. Arch Dis Child 1996;75:57.
McFadden SW, Haddow JE. Coma produced by topical application of isopropanol. Pediatrics 1969;43:622.
McIntosh S, Fischer DB, Rothman SG, et al. Intracranial calcifications in childhood leukemia. J Pediatr 1977;91:909.
Mears CJ, Taylor RR, Jordan KM, et al. Sociodemographic and symptom correlates of fatigue in an adolescent: Primary care sample. J Adolesc Health 2004;35:528e.21.

Mendola P, Selevan SG, Gutter S, et al. Environmental factors associated with a spectrum of neurodevelopmental deficits. Ment Retard Dev Disabil Res Rev 2002;8:188.

Mergler D, Huel G, Bowler R, et al. Nervous system dysfunction among workers with long-term exposure to manganese. Environ Res 1994;64:151.

Midura TF. Update: Infant botulism. Clin Microbiol Rev 1996;9:119.

Miller KT, Wilkinson DS. Pharmacokinetics of methotrexate in the cerebrospinal fluid after intracerebroventricular administration in patients with meningeal carcinomatosis and altered cerebrospinal fluid flow dynamics. Ther Drug Monit 1989;11:231.

Miller LW. Cyclosporin-associated neurotoxicity. The need for a better guide for immunosuppressive therapy. Circulation 1996;94:1209.

Mink PJ, Goodman M, Barraj LM, et al. Evaluation of uncontrolled confounding in studies of environmental exposures and neurobehavioral testing in children. Epidemiology 2004;15:385.

Misselwitz B, Muhler A, Weinmann HJ. A toxicologic risk for using manganese complexes? A literature survey of existing data through several medical specialties. Invest Radiol 1995;30:611.

Miwa H, Iijima M, Tanaka S, et al. Generalized convulsions after consuming a large amount of ginkgo nuts. Epilepsia 2001;42:280.

Miyamoto J, Kaneko H, Tsuji R, et al. Pyrethroids, nerve poisons: How their risks to human health should be assessed. Toxicol Lett 1995;82–83:933.

Mody CK, Miller BL, McIntyre HB, et al. Neurologic complications of cocaine abuse. Neurology 1988;38:1189.

Montouris GD, Fenichel GM, McLain LW Jr. The pregnant epileptic: A review and recommendations. Arch Neurol 1979;36:601.

Mortensen ML. Management of acute childhood poisonings caused by selected insecticides and herbicides. Pediatr Clin North Am 1986;33:421.

Mount RJ, Takeno S, Wake M, et al. Carboplatin ototoxicity in the chinchilla: Lesions of the vestibular sensory epithelium. Acta Otolaryngol Suppl 1995;519:60.

Moure JMB, Whitecare JP, Bodey GP. Electroencephalogram changes secondary to asparaginase. Arch Neurol 1970;23:365.

Mueller BU. Antiviral chemotherapy. Curr Opin Pediatr 1997;9:178.

Mullenix PJ, Kernan WJ, Schunior A, et al. Interactions of steroid, methotrexate, and radiation determine neurotoxicity in an animal model to study therapy for childhood leukemia. Pediatr Res 1994;35:171.

Mutlu H, Silit E, Pekkafali Z, et al. Cranial MR imaging findings of potassium chlorate intoxication. AJNR Am J Neuroradiol 2003;24:1396.

Mydler TT, Wasserman GS, Watson WA. Two-week-old infant with isopropanol intoxication. Pediatr Emerg Care 1993;9:146.

Nakamura H, Blumer JL, Reed MD. Pemoline ingestion in children: A report of five cases and review of the literature. J Clin Pharmacol 2002;42:275.

Nanan R, von Stockhausen HB, Petersen B, et al. Unusual pattern of leukoencephalopathy after morphine sulphate intoxication. Neuroradiology 2000;42:845.

Napiorkowski B, Lester BM, Freier MC, et al. Effects of in utero substance exposure on infant neurobehavior. Pediatrics 1996;98:71.

Nebelsieck H. Recreational and designer drugs—the risks to heart and brain (in German). MMW Fortschritte Medizin 2004;146:40.

Nehlig A, Debry G. Potential teratogenic and neurodevelopmental consequences of coffee and caffeine exposure: A review of human and animal data. Neurotoxicol Teratol 1994;16:531.

Nelson KB, Bauman ML. Thimerosal and autism? Pediatrics 2003;111:674.

Nelson TE, Flewellen EH. Current concepts: The malignant hyperthermia syndrome. N Engl J Med 1983;309:445.

Neufeld MY, Vishnevska S. Vigabatrin and multifocal myoclonus in adults with partial seizures. Clin Neuropharmacol 1995;18:280.

Newmark J. Nerve agents: Pathophysiology and treatment of poisoning. Semin Neurol 2004;24:185.

Nhachi CF, Kasilo OM. Household chemicals poisoning admissions in Zimbabwe's main urban centres. Hum Exp Toxicol 1994;13:69.

Nicholson DP. The immediate management of overdose. Clin North Am 1983;67:1279.

Nicolao P, Giometto B. Neurological toxicity of ifosfamide. Oncology 2003;65 (Suppl 2):11.

Nishie M, Kurahishi K, Ogawa M, et al. Posterior encephalopathy subsequent to cyclosporin A presenting as irreversible abulia. Intern Med 2003;42:750.

Nishimura H, Tanimura T. Clinical aspects of the teratogenicity of drugs. New York: Excerpta Medica, American Elsevier, 1976.

Norman DJ. The clinical role of OKT3. Immunol Allerg Clin North Am 1989;9:9.

Norman MG, Temple AR, Murphy JV. Infantile quadriceps femoris contracture resulting from intramuscular injection. N Engl J Med 1970;282:964.

Normandin L, Panisset M, Zayed J. Manganese neurotoxicity: Behavioral, pathological, and biochemical effects following various routes of exposure. Rev Environ Health 2002;17:189.

O'Connor TA, Bondurant HH, Siddiqui J. Targeted perinatal drug screening in a rural population. J Matern Fetal Neonatal Med 1997;6:108.

Okudera H. Clinical features on nerve gas terrorism in Matasumoto. J Clin Neurosci 2002;9:17.

O'Malley PM, Johnston LD, Bachman JG. Quantitative and qualitative changes in cocaine use among American high school seniors, college students, and young adults. NIDA Res Monogr 1991;110:19.

Omtzigt JGC, Los FJ, Grobbee DE, et al. The risk of spina bifida aperta after first-trimester exposure to valproate in a prenatal cohort. Neurology 1992;42 (Suppl 5):119.

Online Mendelian Inheritance in Man, OMIM (TM). Center for Medical Genetics, Johns Hopkins University (Baltimore, MD) and National Center for Biotechnology Information, National Library of Medicine (Bethesda, MD), 1997. Available at: http://www3.ncbi.nlm.nih.gov/omim/.

Oransky S, Roseman B, Fish D. Seizures temporally associated with the use of DEET repellent: New York and Connecticut. MMWR Morb Mortal Wkly Rep 1989;38:678.

Ostergaard GZ, Pedersen SE. Neonatal effects of maternal clomipramine treatment. Pediatrics 1982;69:233.

Osterhoudt KC, Durbin D, Alpern ER, et al. Risk factors for emesis after therapeutic use of activated charcoal in acutely poisoned children. Pediatrics 2004;113:806.

Parrott AC. Recreational Ecstasy/MDMA, the serotonin syndrome, and serotonergic neurotoxicity. Pharmacol Biochem Behav 2002;71:837.

Parry GJ, Bredesen DE. Sensory neuropathy with low-dose pyridoxine. Neurology 1985;35:1466.

Patel M, Schier J, Belson M, et al. Recognition of illness associated with exposure to chemical agents—United States, 2003. MMWR Morb Mortal Wkly Rep 2003;52:938.

Pathology and laboratory medicine. Handbook of Services for Indiana University Medical Center, Wishard Memorial Hospital and Clinics, and Veteran's Administration Hospital and Medical Center. Hudson, OH: Lexi-Comp, 1994.

Pearson MA, Hoyme HE, Seaver LH, et al. Toluene embryopathy: Delineation of phenotype and comparison with fetal alcohol syndrome. Pediatrics 1994;93:211.

Perry HE, Shannon MW. Diagnosis and management of opioid- and benzodiazepine-induced comatose overdose in children. Curr Opin Pediatr 1996;8:243.

Petrikovics I, Papahadjopoulos D, Hong K, et al. Comparing therapeutic and prophylactic protection against the lethal effect of paraoxon. Toxicol Sciences 2004;77: 258.

Phelan MP, Pellock JM, Nance WE. Discordant expression of fetal hydantoin syndrome in heteropaternal dizygotic twins. N Engl J Med 1982;307:99.

Pimentel L, Trommer L. Cyclic antidepressant overdoses. A review. Emerg Med Clin North Am 1994;12:533.

Piomelli S, Rosen JF, Chisolm JJ, et al. Management of childhood lead poisoning. Pediatrics 1984;105:523.

Podgorny G. Venomous reptiles and arthropods of the United States and Canada. In: Haddad LM, Winchester JF, eds. Clinical management of poisoning and drug overdose. Philadelphia: WB Saunders, 1983.

POISINDEX/TERIS(Rx) 1974–2005. Micromedex Inc.

Pope HG Jr, Katz DL. Psychiatric and medical effects of anabolic-androgenic steroid use. Arch Psychiatry 1994;51:375.

Pratt CB, Douglass EC, Etcubanas EL, et al. Ifosfamide in pediatric malignant solid tumors. Can Chemother Pharmacol 1989;24 (Suppl 1):S24.

Prescott WA Jr, Callahan BL, Park JM. Tacrolimus toxicity associated with concomitant metoclopramide therapy. Pharmacotherapy 2004;24:532.

Price RA, Jamieson PA. The central nervous system in childhood cancer. Cancer 1975;35:306.

Priest JR, Ramsay NKC, Steinherz PG, et al. A syndrome of thrombosis and hemorrhage complicating L-asparaginase therapy for childhood acute lymphoblastic leukemia. J Pediatr 1982;100:984.
Prockop LD. Neurotoxic volatile substances. Neurology 1979;29:862.
Prockop LD, Alt M, Tison J. Huffner's neuropathy. JAMA 1974;229:1083.
Pruitt AW. Committee on Drugs, American Academy of Pediatrics. Ethanol in liquid preparations intended for children. Pediatrics 1984;73:405.
Pruitt AW, Kauffman RE, Mofenson HC, et al. Committee on Drugs, American Academy of Pediatrics. Inactive ingredients in pharmaceutical products. Pediatrics 1985;76:635.
Raatnaike RN. Acute and chronic arsenic toxicity. Postgrad Med J 2003;79:391.
Rachinger J, Fellner FA, Stieglbauer K, et al. MR changes after acute cyanide intoxication. AJNR Am J Neuroradiol 2002;23:1398.
Raj AB, Bertolone SJ, Jaffe N. Methylene blue reversal of ifosfamide-related encephalopathy. J Pediatr Hematol Oncol 2004;26:116.
Reece DE. Neurologic complications in allogeneic bone marrow transplant patients receiving cyclosporin. Marrow Transplant 1991;8:393.
Reeves JA, Allison J, Goodman PE. Black widow spider bite in a child. Am J Emerg Med 1996;14:469.
Reeves RR, Mack JE, Beddingfield JJ. Neurotoxic syndrome associated with risperidone and fluvoxamine. Ann Pharmacother 2002;36:1293.
Reisine T, Pasternak G. Opioid agonists and antagonists. In: Hardman JG, Limbird LE, Molinoff PB, et al., eds. Goodman and Gilman's the pharmacologic basis of therapeutics, 9th ed. New York: McGraw-Hill, 1996.
Reiter PD, Stiles AD. Lorazepam toxicity in a premature infant. Ann Pharmacother 1993;27:727.
Renard D, Westhovens R, Vandenbussche E, Vandenberghe R. Reversible posterior leucoencephalopathy during oral treatment with methotrex. Neurology 2004;251:226.
REPROTOX (computer database). Micromedex Inc., 1974–2005.
Richardson GA, Conroy ML, Day NL. Prenatal cocaine exposure: Effects on the development of school-age children. Neurotoxicol Teratol 1996;18:627.
Rieger C, Fiegl M, Tischer J, et al. Incidence and severity of ifosfamide-induced encephalopathy. Anticancer Drugs 2004;15:347.
Rivkin M, Gilmore HE. Generalized seizures in an infant due to environmentally acquired cocaine. Pediatrics 1989;84:1100.
Roberts DM, Karunarathna A, Buckley NA, et al. Influence of pesticide regulation on acute poisoning deaths in Sri Lanka. Bull World Health Org 2003;81:789.
Robertson AS, Jain S, O'Neil RA. Spongiform leucoencephalopathy following intravenous heroin abuse: radiological and histopathological findings. Australas Radiol 2001;45:390.
Rodier PM. Environmental causes of central nervous system maldevelopment. Pediatrics 2004;113 (Suppl 4):1076.
Rodier PM, Ingram JL, Tisdale B, et al. Linking etiologies in humans and animal models: Studies of autism. Reprod Toxicol 1997;11:417.
Rogan WJ, Gladen BC, Hung K-L. Congenital poisoning by polychlorinated biphenyls and their contaminants in Taiwan. Science 1988;241:334.
Rogan WJ, Gladen BC, McKinney JD, et al. Neonatal effects of transplacental exposure to PCBs and DDE. J Pediatr 1986;109:335.
Rogol AD, Schoumacher R, Spyker DA. Generalized convulsions as the presenting sign of amoxapine intoxication. Clin Pediatr 1984;23:235.
Rosen MB, House HS, Francis BM, et al. Teratogenicity of 5-azacytidine in the Sprague-Dawley rat. J Toxicol Environ Health 1990;29:201.
Rosener M, Martin E, Zipp F, et al. Neurologic side-effects of pharmacologic corticoid therapy. Nervenarzt 1996;67:983.
Rotenberg JS, Newmark J. Nerve agents attacks on children: Diagnosis and management. Pediatrics 2003;112 (3 Pt 1):648.
Rothrock JF, Rubenstein R, Lyden PD. Ischemic stroke associated with methamphetamine inhalation. Neurology 1988;38:589.
Rumack CM, Guggenheim MA, Rumack BH, et al. Neonatal intracranial hemorrhage and maternal use of aspirin. Obstet Gynecol 1981;58:52S.
Rusyniak DE, Furbee RB, Kirk MA. Thallium and arsenic poisoning in a small Midwestern town., Ann Emerg Med 2002;39:307.
Rusyniak DE, Nanagas KA. Organophosphate poisoning. Semin Neurol 2004;24:197.
Sachdev P. The epidemiology of drug-induced akathisia: Part II. Chronic, tardive, and withdrawal akathisias. Schizophr Bull 1995;21:451.
Sachdev P, Kruk J, Kneebone M, et al. Clozapine-induced neuroleptic malignant syndrome: review and report of new cases. J Clin Psychopharmacol 1995;15:365.
Saddik B, Muwayhid I, Williamson A, et al. Evidence of neurotoxicity in working children in Lebanon. Neurotoxicology 2003;24:733.
Salamy A, Eldredge L, Anderson J, et al. Brain-stem transmission time in infants exposed to cocaine in utero. J Pediatr 1990;117:627.
Salit IE. Precipitating factors for the chronic fatigue syndrome. J Psychiatr Res 1997;31:59.
San Augustin M, Nitowsky HM, Borden JN. Neonatal sciatic palsy after umbilical vessel injection. J Pediatr 1962;60:408.
Sanders-Bush E, Mayer SE. 5-Hydroxytryptamine (serotonin) receptor agonists and antagonists. In: Hardman JG, Limbird LE, Molinoff PB, et al., eds. Goodman and Gilman's the pharmacologic basis of therapeutics, 9th ed. New York: McGraw-Hill, 1996.
Sandler SG, Tobin W, Henderson ES. Vincristine-induced neuropathy. Neurology 1969;19:367.
Sansone MEG, Ziegler DK. Lithium toxicity: A review of neurologic complications. Clin Neuropharmacol 1985;8:242.
Sanz EJ, De-las-Cuevas C, Kiuru A, et al. Selective serotonin reuptake inhibitors in pregnant women and neonatal withdrawal syndrome: A database analysis. Lancet 2005;365:482.
Schaumburg HH, Berger AR. Human toxic neuropathy due to industrial agents. In: Dyck PJ, Thomas PK, eds. Peripheral neuropathy, 3rd ed. Philadelphia: WB Saunders, 1993.
Schnider P, Berger T, Schmied M, et al. Increased residual urine volume after local injection of botulinum A toxin. Nervenarzt 1995;66:465.
Schooler NR. Clozapine and risperidone: Recent findings in two new drugs. In: Kane JM, chairperson. Choosing among old and new antipsychotics. J Clin Psychiatry 1996;57:427.
Selbst SM, DeMaio JG, Boenning D. Mouthwash poisoning. Clin Pediatr 1985;24:162.
Seppelt IM. Neurotoxicity from overuse of nitrous oxide [Letter]. Med J Austr 1995;163:280.
Sexson WR, Barak Y. Withdrawal emergent syndrome in an infant associated with maternal haloperidol therapy. J Perinatol 1989;9:170.
Shannon M. The demise of ipecac. Pediatrics 2003;112:1180.
Shannon M, Lacouture PG, Roe J, et al. Cocaine exposure among children seen at a pediatric hospital. Pediatrics 1989;83:337.
Sharma AN, Nelson LS, Hoffman RS. Cerebrospinal fluid analysis in fatal thallium poisoning: Evidence for delayed distribution into the central nervous system. Am J Forens Med Pathol 2004;25:156.
Sherman JD. Organophosphates pesticides: Neurological and respiratory toxicity. Toxicol Industr Health 1995;11:33.
Shimono T, Miki Y, Toyoda H, et al. MR imaging with quantitative diffusion mapping of Tacrolimus-induced neurotoxicity in organ transplant patients. Eur Radiol 2003;13:986.
Shuper A, Stark B, Kornreich L, et al. Methotrexate-related neurotoxicity in the treatment of childhood acute lymphoblastic leukemia. Israel Med Assoc J 2002;4:1050.
Shurin SB, Rekate HL, Annable W. Optic atrophy induced by vincristine. Pediatrics 1982;70:288.
Silverman WA, Andersen DH, Blanc WA, et al. A difference in mortality rate and incidence of kernicterus among premature infants allotted to two prophylactic antibacterial regimens. Pediatrics 1956;18:614.
Singer HS. Tardive dyskinesia: A concern for the pediatrician. Pediatrics 1986;77:553.
Singh S, Singhi S, Sood NK, et al. Changing pattern of childhood poisoning (1970–1989): Experience of a large north Indian hospital. Indian Pediatr 1995;32:331.
Slamovits TL, Glaser JS. The pupils and accommodation. In: Glaser JS, ed. Neuro-ophthalmology, 2nd ed. Philadelphia: JB Lippincott, 1990.
Slikker W Jr. Principles of developmental neurotoxicology. Neurotoxicology 1994;15:11.
Sloan MA, Kittner SJ, Rigamonti D, et al. Occurrence of stroke associated with use/abuse of drugs. Neurology 1991;41:1358.
Smythies J, Golomb B. Nerve gas antidotes. J Royal Soc Med 2004;97:32.
Soy D, Campistol JM, Brunet M, et al. Role of cyclosporin metabolites and clinical toxicity in organ transplantation. Transplant Proc 1995;27:2415.
Spaide RF, Diamond G, D'Amico RA. Ocular findings in cystic fibrosis. Am J Ophthalmol 1987;103:204.
Sparling PB, Giuffrida A, Piomelli D, et al. Exercise activates the endocannabinoid system. Neuroreport 2003;14:2209

Spring PJ, Sharpe DM, Hayes MW. Nitrofurantoin and peripheral neuropathy: A forgotten problem. Med J Aust 2001;174:153.

Stacey R, Morfey D, Payne S. Secondary contamination in organophosphate poisoning: Analysis of an incident. Q J Med 2004;97:75.

Steeghs N, deJongh PE, Sillevis Smitt PA, et al. Cisplatin-induced encephalopathy and seizures. Anticancer Drugs 2003;14:443.

Sternbach H. The serotonin syndrome. Am J Psychiatry 1991;148:705.

Stork CM, Cantor R. Pemoline induced acute choreoathetosis: Case report and review of the literature. J Toxicol Clin Toxicol 1997;35:105.

Streissguth AP, Barr HM, Sampson PD, et al. IQ at age 4 in relation to maternal alcohol use and smoking during pregnancy. Dev Psychol 1989;25:30.

Streissguth AP, Barr HM, Sampson PD. Moderate prenatal alcohol exposure: Effects on child IQ and learning problems at age 7 years. Alcohol Clin Exp Res 1990;14:662.

Stulemeijer M, de Jong LW, Fiselier TJ, et al. Cognitive behaviour therapy for adolescents with chronic fatigue: Randomised controlled trial. BMJ 2005;330:14.

Sudakin DL. DEET: A review and update of safety and risk in the general population. J Toxicol Clin Toxicol 2003;41:831.

Sunagawa M, Nouda H. Neurotoxicity of carbapenem compounds and other beta-lactam antibiotics. Jpn J Antibiot 1996;49:1.

Surber C, Rufli T. Lindane. Hautarzt 1995;46:528.

Swayze VW 2nd, Johnson VP, Hanson JW, et al. Magnetic resonance imaging of brain anomalies in fetal alcohol syndrome. Pediatrics 1997;99:232.

Swift TR, Ignacio OJ. Tick paralysis, electrophysiologic studies. Neurology 1975;25:1130.

Takahashi N, Kai S, Kohmura H, et al. Reproduction studies of VP 16-213 (II): Oral administration to rats during the period of fetal organogenesis. J Toxicol Sci 1986;11(Suppl 1):195.

Tamer A, McKey R, Arias D, et al. Phenothiazine induced extra-pyramidal dysfunction in the neonate. J Pediatr 1969;75:479.

Taylor BV, Mastaglia FL, Stell R. Guillain-Barré syndrome complicating treatment with streptokinase. Med J Aust 1995;162:214.

Thaisetthawatkul P, Weinstock A, Kerr SL, et al. Muromonab-CD3-induced neurotoxicity: Report of two siblings, one of whom had subsequent cyclosporin-induced neurotoxicity. J Child Neurol 2001;16:825.

Thomas DM, Nicholls AJ, Feest TG, et al. OKT3 and cerebral edema. BMJ 1987;295:1486.

Thomas RJ, Reagan DR. Association of a Tourette-like syndrome with ofloxacin. Ann Pharmacother 1996;30:138.

Thompson CB, June CH, Sullivan KM, et al. Association between cyclosporine neurotoxicity and hypomagnesemia. Lancet 1984;2:1116.

Thompson DJ, Molello JA, Strebing RJ, et al. Reproduction and teratology studies with oncolytic agents in the rat and rabbit. I. 1,3-Bis(2-chloroethyl)-1-nitrosourea (BCNU). Toxicol Appl Pharmacol 1974;30:422.

Thompson JP, Casey PB, Vale JA. Deaths from pesticide poisoning in England and Wales 1990–91. Hum Exp Toxicol 1995;14:437.

Thompson SW, Davis LE, Kornfeld N, et al. Cisplatin neuropathy: Clinical, electrophysiologic, morphologic and toxicologic studies. Neurology 1982;32:A133.

Torvik A, Walday P. Neurotoxicity of water-soluble contrast media. Acta Radiol 1995;399 (Suppl):221.

Townes JM, Cieslak PR, Hatheway CL, et al. An outbreak of type A botulism associated with a commercial cheese sauce. Ann Intern Med 1996;125:558.

Trachtenbarg DE. Getting the lead out: When is treatment necessary? Postgrad Med 1996;99:201.

Traub SJ, Nelson LS, Hoffman RS. Physostigmine as a treatment for gamma-hydroxybutyrate toxicity: A review. J Toxicol Clin Toxicol 2002;40:781.

Tronick EZ, Frank DA, Cabral H, et al. Late dose-response effects of prenatal cocaine exposure on newborn neurobehavioral performance. Pediatrics 1996;98:76.

Truwit CL, Denaro CP, Lake JR, et al. MR imaging of reversible cyclosporin A-induced neurotoxicity. AJNR Am J Neuroradiol 1991;12:651.

Trzepacz PT, DiMartini A, Tringali R. Psychopharmacologic issues in organ failure and psychiatric aspects of immunosuppressants and anti-infectious agents. Psychosomatics 1993;24:199.

Tueth MJ. Emergencies caused by side effects of psychiatric medications. Am J Emerg Med 1994;12:212.

Tuxen MK, Hansen SW. Neurotoxicity secondary to antineoplastic drugs. Cancer Treat Rev 1994;20:171.

Uede K, Furukawa F. Skin manifestations in acute arsenic poisoning from the Wakayama curry-poisoning incident. Br J Dermatol 2003;149:757.

Urban P, Lukas E, Benicky L. Neurological and electrophysiological examination on workers exposed to mercury vapors. Neurotoxicology 1996;17:191.

Usami S, Abe S, Kasai M, et al. Genetic and clinical features of sensorineural hearing loss associated with the 1555 mitochondrial mutation. Laryngoscope 1997;107:483.

Van de Bor M, Walther WF, Lenis ME. Increased cerebral blood flow velocity in infants of mothers who abuse cocaine. Pediatrics 1990;85:733.

Veltri JC, Litovitz TL. Annual report of the American Association of Poison Control Centers national data collection system. Am J Emerg Med 1984;4:420.

Vernace MA, Bellucci AG, Wilkes BM. Chronic salicylate toxicity due to consumption of over-the-counter bismuth subsalicylate. Am J Med 1994;97:308.

Villarejo FJ, Pascual AM. Injection injury of the sciatic nerve (370 cases). Child Nerv Sys 1993;9:229.

Walsh LE, Garg BP. Ischemic stroke in children: A review. Indian J Pediatr 1997;64:613.

Warkany J. Antituberculous drugs. Teratology 1979;20:133.

Watson WA, Litovitz TL, Klein-Schwartz W, et al. 2003 Annual report of the American Association of Poison Control Centers Toxic Exposure Surveillance System. Am J Emerg Med 2004;22:335.

Webster PAC. Withdrawal symptoms in neonates associated with maternal antidepressant therapy [Letter]. Lancet 1973;2:318.

Weiss B. Low-level chemical sensitivity: A perspective from behavioral toxicology. Toxicol Indust Health 1994;10:605

Weiss B, Amler S, Amler RW. Pesticides. Pediatrics 2004;113(Suppl 4):1030.

Weiss HD, Walker MD, Wiernik PH. Neurotoxicity of commonly used antineoplastic drugs. N Engl J Med 1974;291:75.

Wilkin M, Currier S, Abel-Zieg C, et al. A survey of compliance: Medicaid's mandated blood lead screenings for children age 12–18 months in Nebraska. BMC Public Health 2004;4:1471.

Winneke G. Inorganic lead as a developmental neurotoxicant: Some basic issues and the Dusseldorf experience. Neurotoxicology 1996;17:565.

Winneke G, Brockhaus A, Ewers U, et al. Results from the European multicenter study on lead neurotoxicity in children: Implications for risk assessment. Neurotoxicol Teratol 1990;12:553.

Winneke G, Walkowiak J, Lilienthal H. PCB-induced neurodevelopmental toxicity in human infants and its potential medication by endocrine dysfunction. Toxicology 2002;181–182:161.

Wood PJ, Ioannides-Demos LL, Li SC. Minimization of aminoglycoside toxicity in patients with cystic fibrosis. Thorax 1996;51:369.

Wurtzel D, Porat R, Brodsky N. No increased risk for intracranial hemorrhage (ICH) in preterm infants exposed in utero to cocaine. Pediatr Res 1988;23:431.

Yip L, Dart RC, Gabow PA. Concepts and controversies in salicylate toxicity. Emerg Med Clin North Am 1994;12:351.

Young RSK, Grzyb SE, Crimson L. Recurrent cerebellar dysfunction as related to chronic gasoline sniffing in adolescent girls. Clin Pediatr 1977;16:706.

Zagoria RJ. Iodinated contrast agents in neuroradiology. Neuroimag Clin North Am 1994;4:1.

Zepp EA, Thomas JA, Knotts GR. The toxic effects of mercury. Clin Pediatr 1974;13:783.

Zhang LL, Collier PA, Ashwell KW. Mechanisms in the induction of neuronal heterotopiae following prenatal cytotoxic brain damage. Neurotoxicol Teratol 1995;17:297.

Zimmerman JL. Poisonings and overdoses in the intensive care unit: General and specific management issues. Crit Care Med 2003;31:2794.

Ziskin A, Gellis S. Water intoxication following tap water enemas. Am J Dis Child 1958;96:699.

Zuckerman B, Frank D, Brown E. Overview of the effects of abuse and drugs on pregnancy and offspring. NIDA Res Monogr 1995;149:16.

Zuckerman B, Frank DA, Hingson R, et al. Effects of maternal marijuana and cocaine on fetal growth. N Engl J Med 1989;320:762.

CHAPTER 88

Neurologic Disorders Associated with Cardiac Disease

Cecil D. Hahn and Adré J. du Plessis

Congenital heart disease is recognized in approximately 0.5% to 1.25% of live births [Rosenthal, 1998]. Of approximately 40,000 infants born yearly in the United States with some form of congenital heart disease, about one half have critical congenital heart disease that will require surgical intervention in the first year of life [Benson, 1989; Castaneda et al., 1974; Castaneda et al., 1989]. It is therefore not surprising that children with congenital heart disease and its complications constitute one of the largest inpatient populations in most major pediatric centers. Neurologic injury is one of the most common extracardiac complications of congenital heart disease, and the morbidity of this injury tends to be prolonged. Consequently, the child neurologist is increasingly faced with diagnostic and management decisions for affected children.

The predominant cause of acquired neurologic dysfunction in this population is mediated by cerebral hypoxia-ischemia or reperfusion injury. This result occurs primarily because of the nervous system's exquisite dependence on a consistent and responsive supply of oxygen and metabolic substrate. In children with congenital heart disease, cerebral hypoxia-ischemia or reperfusion injury may be mediated by global hypoperfusion (e.g., cardiac arrest) and focal vaso-occlusive insults (e.g., cardiogenic stroke).

The major advances in management of congenital heart disease in recent decades have changed the mechanisms and manifestations of hypoxic-ischemic brain injury in these infants. In earlier years, neurologic complications of congenital heart disease were related in large part to the effects of right-to-left shunting and chronic cyanosis [Berthrong and Sabiston, 1951; Cottrill and Kaplan, 1973; Martelle and Linde, 1961; Phornphutkul et al., 1973; Terplan, 1976; Tyler and Clark, 1957a, 1957b]. With the development in 1953 of cardiopulmonary bypass, the ability to provide extracorporeal circulatory support facilitated the development of open-heart surgery. However, for the ensuing 2 decades, the surgical options for complex lesions were limited by the small size of the infant's heart and the constricted surgical field. Repeated palliative procedures were often necessary until growth of the infant allowed definitive procedures to be performed. During this delay of the final repair, infants remained exposed to cumulative brain injury from chronic hypoxia, polycythemia, and right-to-left shunts, as well as from the effects of repeated cardiopulmonary bypass and surgery [Newburger et al., 1984].

The next major advance in the surgical management of congenital heart disease occurred in the early 1970s with the development of low-flow cardiopulmonary bypass and deep hypothermic circulatory arrest. These techniques allowed the reduction of blood flow or complete circulatory arrest during critical phases of the operation, thereby clearing the surgical field of blood and cannulas and exposing small and complex lesions for repair. A prerequisite for low-flow cardiopulmonary bypass and deep hypothermic circulatory arrest was the development of techniques such as deep hypothermia that effectively suppress cellular metabolism and oxygen requirements and "prepare" vital organs for the marked decrease in oxygen delivery. These developments have been pivotal in allowing definitive anatomic repair in ever-younger infants. As a result, neonatal heart repair has become commonplace in many major centers. These techniques are largely responsible for the dramatic increase in survival of infants with congenital heart disease, particularly those with lesions that are more complex.

The impact of these advances on the incidence of neurologic morbidity in infants undergoing cardiac surgery unfortunately has not paralleled the decrease in mortality. Instead, these surgical advances have heightened concerns about the neurologic outcome of these children [Limperopoulos et al., 1999, 2000]. Although cardiac repair in the newborn has reduced exposure to earlier risk factors such as chronic hypoxia, there has been a paradoxical increase in other forms of neurologic morbidity. First, severe heart lesions may be associated with profound hemodynamic shock and acidosis in the newborn period. These previously lethal conditions have become amenable to early correction, and the long-term neurologic consequences of such early-life hemodynamic disturbances are beginning to emerge in survivors. Second, the techniques responsible for increasing survival (i.e., low-flow cardiopulmonary bypass and deep hypothermic circulatory arrest) have their own inherent risks for neurologic injury. Consequently, the striking increase in survival of infants with severe congenital heart disease has been accompanied by the emergence of a population in whom cardiac morbidity has been replaced by chronic, often lifelong, neurodevelopmental dysfunction.

This chapter reviews the neurologic complications of cardiac surgical interventions and considers inherited and acquired conditions with combined neurologic and cardiac dysfunction unrelated to surgery.

NEUROLOGIC COMPLICATIONS OF CARDIAC SURGERY

The advance of neonatal heart repair into the earliest days of the newborn period has had a significant impact on the neurologic complications in this population. First, the shorter period before cardiac correction has decreased the brain's exposure to the deleterious effects of an uncorrected cardiovascular anatomy (e.g., chronic hypoxia). Second, the marked circulatory and metabolic changes intrinsic to many neonatal cardiac operations now occur more frequently in patients with a structurally and functionally immature cerebral vasculature. The increased vascular fragility and tenuous autoregulatory function of the immature brain have prompted increasing concern about hemorrhagic (e.g., germinal matrix–intraventricular hemorrhage) and ischemic (e.g., periventricular leukomalacia) injury occurring in the perioperative period of neonatal cardiac surgery.

Children undergoing cardiac surgery are at risk for brain injury before, during, and after the operative procedure. The residual neurologic deficits are likely the cumulative result of insults sustained during these periods. Insults that occur during earlier phases may render the cerebral vasculature and parenchyma vulnerable to injury in subsequent phases. Despite this complex interplay of potential injurious mechanisms and the difficulty of delineating the precise role of insults in these different phases, this chapter considers the preoperative, intraoperative, and postoperative mechanisms separately.

Mechanisms of Neurologic Injury in Cardiac Surgical Patients

Intraoperative Mechanisms

The principal cause of perioperative neurologic dysfunction is hypoxic-ischemic or reperfusion injury. The ability to identify imminent hypoxia-ischemia in the individual patient has been limited by a lack of reliable techniques for the intraoperative measurement of cerebral blood flow and oxygenation. Near-infrared spectroscopy is a promising technique that has provided important insights in animal and human studies [du Plessis et al., 1995c; Sakamoto et al., 2001, 2004; Wardle et al., 1998]. The potential mechanisms for the development of hypoxic-ischemic or reperfusion injury are multiple and include global (Box 88-1) and focal insults (Box 88-2). In adults undergoing cardiac surgery, the predominant form of brain injury is embolic, resulting when atheromatous debris dislodged from the aorta enters the arteriosclerotic cerebrovascular bed. Conversely, in the young infant undergoing open-heart surgery, the cerebral hypoxic-ischemic or reperfusion insults are primarily mediated by global hypoperfusion. This notion is supported by the neuropathologic features at postmortem examination, which correspond in topography to other forms of global hypoxic-ischemic or reperfusion injury. Specifically, cortical laminar necrosis, periventricular leukomalacia, and parasagittal injury are seen; focal infarctions occur less commonly [Bozoky et al., 1984; Terplan, 1973, 1976]. The lesions are likely acquired for the most part during periods of low or absent blood flow required for open-heart surgery. A multitude of complex, dynamic, and interrelated phenomena simultaneously may affect cerebral oxygen delivery and demand (see Box 88-1) during the core cooling, low- or no-flow bypass, and rewarming phases of deep hypothermic cardiac surgery. The precise role and contribution of each of these phenomena in the ultimate neurologic outcome in individually affected infants are unclear. In essence, the anesthetist-perfusionist team assumes control of the complex autoregulatory systems that normally maintain the delicate balance between cerebral oxygen supply and use. Guidelines for this external regulation of cerebral oxygen supply and demand are based on theoretical parameters of safety for techniques, such as duration of circulatory arrest and depth of hypothermia.

Box 88-1 Intraoperative Determinants of Global Cerebral Oxygen Delivery and Use

Factors That Decrease Cerebral Oxygen Use
- Hypothermia
- Drugs (e.g., barbiturates)
- After hypoxia or ischemia

Factors That Decrease Cerebral Oxygen Supply

Cerebral perfusion pressure decreases
- Deep hypothermic circulatory arrest or low-flow cardiopulmonary bypass
- Nonpulsatile perfusion
- Disturbed autoregulation
- Increased central venous pressure

Oxygen-carrying capacity decreases
- Hemodilution

Oxygen delivery decreases
- Increased oxyhemoglobin affinity (i.e., hypothermia and alkalosis)

Box 88-2 Potential Mechanisms for Focal Intraoperative Vaso-occlusive Insults

Embolic Insults

From bypass circuit
- Synthetic debris
- Platelet emboli
- Air emboli

From surgical field
- Fat emboli
- Air emboli
- Platelet emboli

From venous system
- Systemic veins after deep hypothermic circulatory arrest
- Pulmonary veins after bypass

Thrombotic Insults
- Arterial: possible inflammatory vascular changes
- Venous: increased central venous pressure

There has been intense research into techniques that reduce the risk of intraoperative hypoxia-ischemia. Clinical trial data have provided important insights into strategies that optimize intraoperative cerebral oxygen delivery. A randomized clinical trial of deep hypothermic circulatory arrest versus low-flow bypass in 171 infants with transposition of the great arteries found that circulatory arrest was associated with higher perioperative morbidity [Newburger et al., 1993] and worse developmental outcome at ages 1, 4, and 8 years [Bellinger et al., 1997, 1999, 2003]. As a result, current bypass strategies favor the maintenance

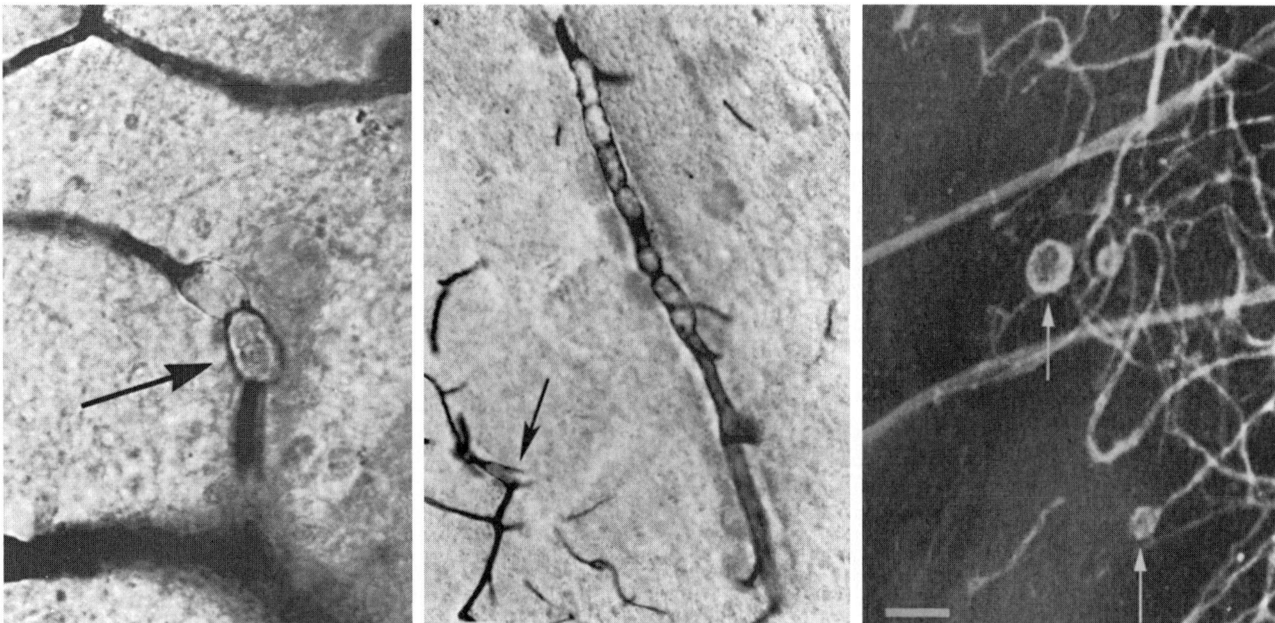

FIGURE 88-1. Aneurysmal dilatations *(arrows)* in the cerebral microvasculature after cardiopulmonary bypass. (From Moody D, Bell M, Challa VR, et al. Brain microemboli during cardiac surgery or aortography. Ann Neurol 1990;28:477-486. Copyright © 1990 Wiley-Liss, Inc., a Wiley Company. Reproduced with permission of John Wiley & Sons, Inc.)

of low blood flow during surgery, and they minimize circulatory arrest times.

Another area of controversy has been the approach to acid-base management. Both the more alkalotic alpha-stat strategy and the more acidotic pH-stat strategy have theoretical advantages. The alpha-stat approach is based on the natural alkaline shift in tissue that accompanies hypothermia, and it is thought to optimize enzyme function at low temperatures. Conversely, the pH-stat technique uses the addition of carbon dioxide to counter this alkaline shift, and it is used to enhance tissue oxygen delivery. The more hypercarbic perfusate increases cerebral perfusion and increases oxygen release in tissues by countering the increased oxygen-hemoglobin affinity associated with hypothermia. A randomized clinical trial comparing these two pH management strategies found that infants managed by the pH-stat strategy had less perioperative morbidity and a shorter time to recovery of electrocortical activity [du Plessis et al., 1997]. In many centers, the pH-stat strategy has become the preferred method of acid-base management in infants undergoing cardiopulmonary bypass.

Another area of investigation has been the management of hematocrit during infant cardiopulmonary bypass. Hemodilution is widely used in adult cardiopulmonary bypass to improve blood flow in the microcirculation. However, the benefits of improved perfusion are countered by the reduced oxygen-carrying capacity of blood. A randomized clinical trial of different hematocrit levels in infants undergoing hypothermic cardiopulmonary bypass found that hemodilution was associated with greater perioperative hemodynamic instability and worse psychomotor development at 1 year of age [Jonas et al., 2003].

Vaso-occlusive insults play a lesser role in intraoperative brain injury during infant cardiac surgery. Cardiopulmonary bypass and the surgical field may generate particulate (e.g., platelet, synthetic, fat) (Fig. 88-1) or gaseous (e.g., air) emboli [Boyajian et al., 1993; Fish, 1988; Moody et al., 1990; Padayachee et al., 1987]. Young infants commonly develop a post-bypass systemic inflammatory syndrome [Kirklin et al., 1983; Westaby, 1987], with systemic vascular injury manifesting with marked edema. This syndrome is related to the relatively large blood volume required for priming bypass pumps and the prolonged exposure of this blood to artificial surfaces. The elevated levels of cytokines (i.e., interleukins-6, -8, and -10; tumor necrosis factor-α; and endothelin-1) measured in bypass blood may mediate vascular and cellular injury [Bando et al., 1998; Elliott, 1999; Elliott and Finn, 1993; Jansen et al., 1992; Journois et al., 1996; Kirklin et al., 1983; Millar et al., 1993; Steinberg et al., 1993]. Ultrafiltration of blood during or after cardiopulmonary bypass reduces cytokine levels and excess free plasma water [Gaynor, 2003]. Ultrafiltration has been associated with improved postoperative hemodynamics [Bando et al., 1998] and improved myocardial function [Chaturvedi et al., 1999; Davies et al., 1998], but a significant long-term benefit has not been demonstrated. It is not known whether the beneficial effects of ultrafiltration result primarily from a reduction in postoperative cytokine levels or from hemoconcentration. The possible contribution of this systemic inflammatory response to intraoperative brain injury has received limited attention, and its importance remains uncertain.

Perioperative Mechanisms

In the preoperative and early postoperative periods, circulatory and oxygenation derangements may be severe. A detailed understanding of this complex cerebrovascular pathophysiology is essential for effective prevention of perioperative brain injury in this population. Infants with complex heart lesions may present with shock, hypoxemia, and acidosis before surgery. After open-heart surgery, significant

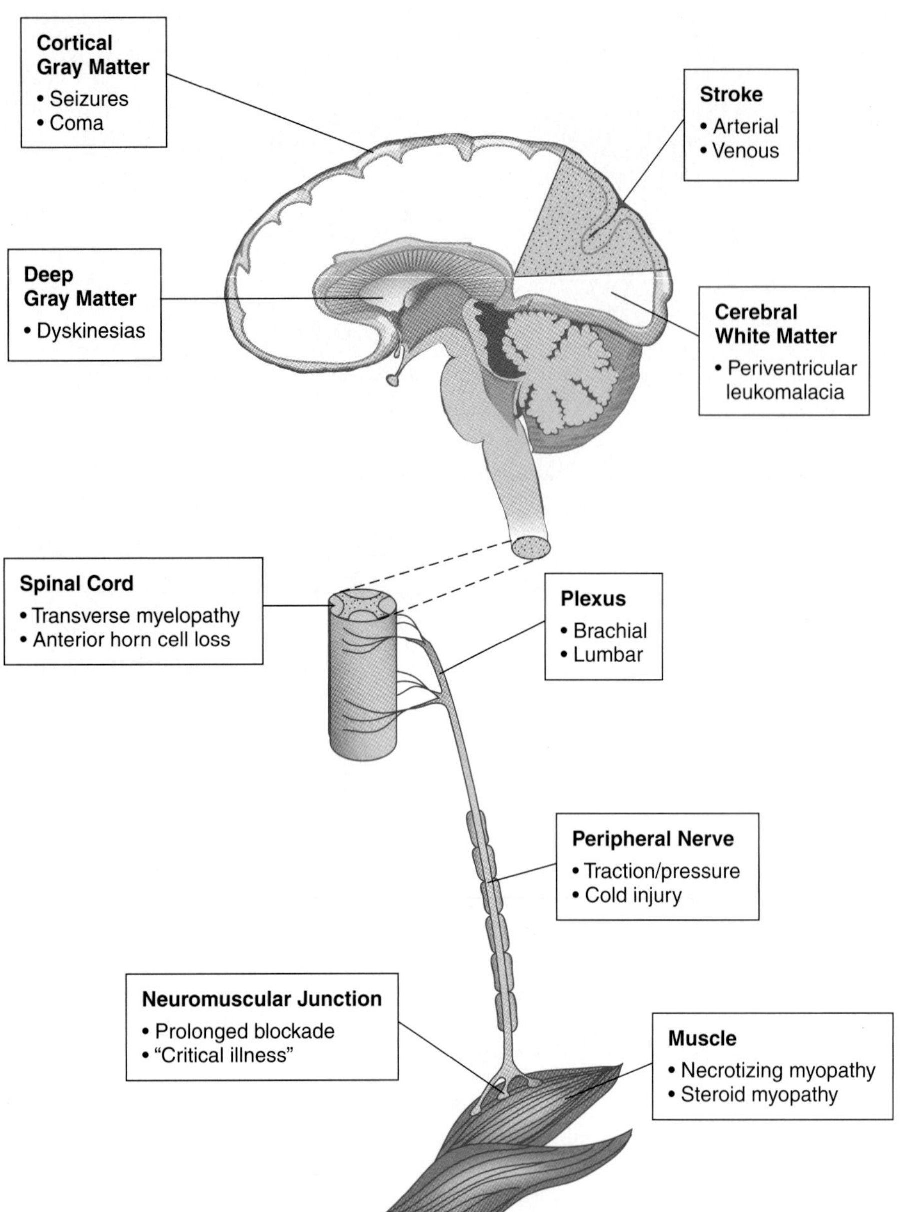

FIGURE 88-2. Diagram of the neuraxis demonstrates the different levels at which neurologic injury may occur during the intraoperative and perioperative periods in children undergoing cardiac surgery.

cardiopulmonary dysfunction can complicate the early postoperative course. The brain's vulnerability to this systemic hemodynamic instability may be further accentuated by postoperative disturbances in cerebral vasoregulation [du Plessis et al., 1995b; O'Hare et al., 1995; Rodriguez et al., 1995].

Perioperative and intraoperative injury to the nervous system may occur at any or multiple levels of the neuraxis (Fig. 88-2). However, the clinical diagnosis of neurologic dysfunction at the bedside of these critically ill infants may be complicated by the subtle manifestations of cerebrovascular injury and further obscured by the widespread use of sedating or paralyzing medications. These confounding factors have delayed the accurate diagnosis of perioperative brain dysfunction and limited the formulation of rational management strategies.

Preoperative Neurologic Complications

Neonatal Cerebrovascular Disease

The leading cause of neurologic injury in the newborn infant is mediated by cerebrovascular disturbances. The most important factors predisposing to this form of brain injury are vascular immaturity (structural and functional) and systemic hemodynamic instability. In the premature infant, this cerebrovascular vulnerability manifests as hemorrhagic or ischemic injury (i.e., intraventricular-periventricular hemorrhage and periventricular leukomalacia). Compared with the newborn population overall, the prevalence of cerebrovascular injury is increased among infants with congenital heart disease [Glauser et al., 1990a; Leviton and Gilles, 1974]. This vulnerability is related to the intrinsic circulatory disturbances associated with congenital heart disease and the increasingly immature infants rescued by modern cardiac surgery.

Congenital heart disease prolongs the risk period for this maturity-dependent injury. The incidence of antenatal cerebrovascular injury is increased [van Houten et al., 1996], and the risk extends into later gestation than for the overall population of newborn infants. In term infants with congenital heart disease, cranial ultrasound studies revealed a 59% incidence of cerebral abnormalities; the most common lesions were cerebral atrophy (41%), linear echodensities of the deep gray matter (20%), intraventricular hemorrhage (16%), and parenchymal echodensities (16%) [van Houten et al., 1996]. Brain lesions of antenatal origin are most common in coarctation of the aorta and ventricular septal defect. Term infants with these cardiac lesions occurring in combination had a 70% incidence of an abnormality at birth identified by cranial ultrasound [van Houten et al., 1996], possibly because of disturbed intrauterine cerebral perfusion because of limited flow through the preductal aorta. Cranial ultrasound studies performed preoperatively and postoperatively in a cohort of infants undergoing cardiac surgery identified a 24% incidence of new lesions after cardiac surgery, with new hemorrhagic lesions in 6% of cases [Krull et al., 1994].

Preoperative and postoperative magnetic resonance imaging (MRI) of 24 term newborns with congenital heart disease undergoing open-heart surgery confirmed the importance of preoperative and intraoperative contributions to neurologic injury. Preoperative elevations in brain lactate were seen in 53% of newborns by magnetic resonance (MR) spectroscopy. Periventricular leukomalacia was present in 16% of newborns before surgery and developed in another 48% of newborns after surgery. New postoperative infarctions were seen in 19%, and new intraparenchymal hemorrhages were seen in 33% of patients. Overall, new postoperative lesions or worsening of preoperative lesions occurred in 67% of patients [Mahle et al., 2002]. Another study using MRI and MR spectroscopy in 10 newborns with transposition of the great arteries revealed preoperative brain injury in 4, and age-adjusted levels of lactate were higher in the patients with heart disease compared with controls, confirming the larger study of Mahle [Miller et al., 2004].

Diagnosis of Preoperative Cerebrovascular Injury

The accurate diagnosis of cerebrovascular lesions before cardiopulmonary bypass and cardiac surgery correlates with the potential for extending or consolidating reversible tissue injury during the procedure. The induced hemodynamic and coagulation changes required during open-heart surgery may extend hemorrhagic and ischemic lesions, as well as cause hemorrhagic transformation of a bland infarct. One MRI study comparing the preoperative and postoperative appearance of asymptomatic intracranial hemorrhage in neonates with congenital heart disease demonstrated increased hemorrhage in 43%, decreased hemorrhage in 26%, and no change in 30% of patients [Tavani et al., 2003]. Other than this study, the overall paucity of prospective data has hampered the formulation of guidelines for the diagnosis and management of preoperative hemorrhagic or ischemic brain lesions. Until such data become available, a reasonable approach is to obtain preoperative brain ultrasound scans for infants with birth weights less than 1500 grams, hemodynamic compromise sufficient to cause metabolic acidosis, neurologic dysfunction, coagulation disturbances, or certain cardiac lesions at particular risk, such as hypoplastic left heart syndrome, with its inherent hemodynamic instability [Glauser et al., 1990a], and coarctation of the aorta, with its increased prevalence of intracranial vascular malformations and hypertension [Volpe, 2001; Young et al., 1982]. Infants with focal neurologic deficits suggestive of stroke (e.g., preoperative focal seizures) are best evaluated by computed tomography (CT) or MRI if their medical conditions allow transport.

Management of Preoperative Cerebrovascular Injury

Recent cerebrovascular injury in infants awaiting cardiac surgery presents a difficult management dilemma. The timing and management of cardiac surgery in children with acute cerebrovascular injury should aim to balance the risks of extending brain injury during cardiac surgery with the hemodynamic instability of uncorrected heart disease. These decisions are influenced by the severity of cardiac dysfunction, the nature of the brain lesion, and the anticipated complexity of the operation. Informed management guidelines are limited by the lack of prospective outcome data.

The optimal timing of surgery in the newborn infant with intraventricular-periventricular hemorrhage presents a dilemma similar to that confronting clinicians using extracorporeal membrane oxygenation [Rudack et al., 1994; von Allmen et al., 1992]. Minor subependymal hemorrhages are at minimal risk for extension and should not delay surgery. Conversely, in infants with intraventricular or intraparenchymal vaso-occlusive stroke (with its tenuous penumbral region), cardiopulmonary bypass should be delayed for a week or longer, provided the cardiovascular status of the child remains stable. Hemorrhagic transformation is a concern, particularly after large, major arterial strokes, venous thrombosis, and infected emboli (discussed later). Prospective studies are needed to better define these issues.

Early Postoperative Neurologic Complications

As many as 25% of children undergoing open-heart operations demonstrate neurologic dysfunction in the early postoperative period [Ferry, 1987, 1990; Newburger et al., 1993]. These early postoperative neurologic complications are often transient, and they were previously considered to be of little long-term consequence. However, some studies have demonstrated that these early complications may be associated with long-term adverse outcomes [Bellinger et al., 1995]. As the long-term significance of these early complications emerges, neurologists will be called on more frequently to evaluate and treat these conditions.

Delayed Recovery of Consciousness

Excessive delay in the recovery of consciousness after cardiac surgery, anesthesia, and sedation is a frequent postoperative complication. The standard diagnostic guidelines [Plum and Posner, 1985] for the evaluation of altered mental status should be applied to these patients. The precise mechanism of this complication remains unclear in most patients. Ultimately, many of these infants demonstrate features compatible with cerebral hypoxic-ischemic or reperfusion injury. However, because intraoperative events specific for hypoxic-ischemic or reperfusion injury are often lacking, other potentially reversible causes should be excluded, including postoperative hepatic or renal impairment with accumulation of toxic metabolites and impaired metabolism or excretion of sedating drugs. Prolonged use of neuromuscular blocking agents for ventilatory management may be associated with delayed recovery of motor function [Gooch et al., 1991; Partridge et al., 1990; Waitling and Dasta, 1994], and in severe cases, the situation may mimic impaired consciousness. Neuromuscular blockade may be excluded with a bedside peripheral nerve stimulator or with nerve conduction studies. A significant minority of infants develops postoperative seizures, which may recur serially and are often clinically silent [Newburger et al., 1993]. In the absence of other causes for persistent loss of consciousness, such occult seizures or a prolonged postictal state should be considered.

Seizures

Seizures are among the most common manifestations of neurologic dysfunction after infant open-heart surgery. Past series have reported clinical seizures in up to 15% of infants in the early postoperative period [Ehyai et al., 1984; Miller et al., 1995; Newburger et al., 1993], whereas clinically silent, electrographic seizures were detected by continuous electroencephalographic (EEG) monitoring in up to 20% of infants [Helmers et al., 1997]. Later studies from large pediatric cardiac surgery centers reported widely disparate postoperative seizure rates of 1.2% to 17.7% [Clancy et al., 2003; Menache et al., 2002]. Risk factors for postoperative seizures include the use of deep hypothermic cardiac arrest (rather than low-flow bypass), prolonged deep hypothermic circulatory arrest times, presence of a ventricular septal defect, and preexisting genetic conditions [Clancy et al., 2003; Helmers et al., 1997]. The recent decline in seizure incidence observed in some centers may be attributable to refinements in extracorporeal perfusion support, such as the minimization of circulatory arrest in favor of low-flow bypass and the adoption of a pH-stat strategy.

Two forms of early postoperative seizures may be distinguished: seizures with a readily identifiable cause and seizures without an identified cause. The usual causes of seizures should be excluded, particularly reversible causes such as hypoglycemia and electrolyte disturbances. Cyclosporin toxicity is a common cause of seizures in heart transplant recipients [Menache et al., 2002].

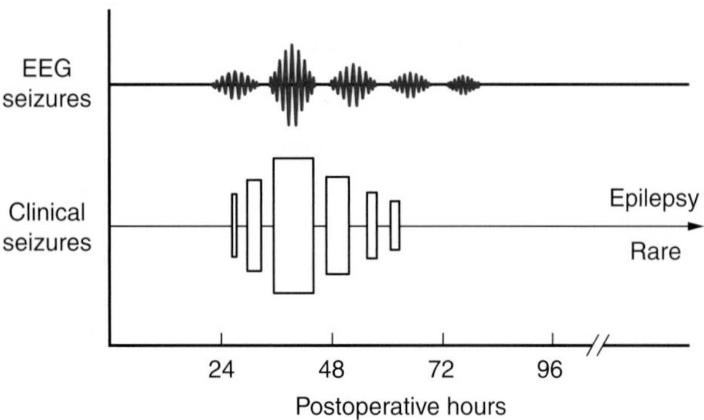

FIGURE 88-3. Diagram of the circumscribed postoperative susceptibility period for electroencephalographic (EEG) and clinical seizures.

POSTPUMP SEIZURES

In previous years, most postoperative seizures did not have a clearly identified cause. The frequency of these cryptogenic postoperative seizures, widely known as *postpump seizures*, appears to be decreasing. Postpump seizures tend to have certain characteristic clinical features, and they are confined almost exclusively to young infants. Conversely, postoperative seizures in older infants and children are usually associated with an identifiable cause. Postpump seizures often are assumed to reflect intraoperative hypoxic-ischemic or reperfusion injury; however, they differ from other hypoxic-ischemic or reperfusion (e.g., birth asphyxia) seizures in several ways. First, the onset of postpump seizures (including EEG seizures) is typically delayed until 24 to 48 hours postoperatively. This delay is significantly later than postasphyxial seizures, which often manifest within the first 12 hours after birth. Second, the long-term outcome after these seizures [Bellinger et al., 1995] is markedly better than the 50% incidence of adverse neurologic outcomes seen after postasphyxial seizures [Andre et al., 1990; Bergman et al., 1983; Volpe, 2001].

The temporal predilection for postpump seizures is relatively circumscribed to a window of several days (Fig. 88-3). During this period, seizures tend to recur, and status epilepticus commonly develops. After several days, the tendency for further seizures decreases rapidly. The clinical manifestations of postpump seizures may be subtle, especially in infants on sedating or paralyzing drugs. Behavioral changes may be confined to paroxysmal changes in autonomic function and pupillary size. Convulsive activity, when evident, is often focal or multifocal. Bedside electroencephalography helps distinguish true epileptic phenomena from other behavioral or autonomic changes [Mizrahi, 1987; Scher and Painter, 1990]. The ability of electroencephalography to detect clinically occult seizure activity helps guide therapy with antiepileptic drugs. Highly focal EEG abnormalities may reflect an underlying stroke, indicating the need for neuroimaging.

The therapeutic approach to postpump seizures is best dictated by their typical clinical course. After reversible causes such as hypoglycemia, hypomagnesemia, and hypocalcemia [Lynch and Rust, 1994; Satur et al., 1993] have been excluded, antiepileptic therapy should commence. In view of the tendency toward repeated seizures and status epilepticus, the initial goal is rapid achievement of therapeutic antiepileptic levels by an intravenous route. Most postoperative seizures are controlled by standard antiepileptic drug regimens used in infants. Careful cardiorespiratory monitoring is essential when using potentially cardiotoxic antiepileptic drugs during the postoperative period, when myocardial dysfunction or dysrhythmias are prevalent. In infants with established myocardial dysfunction, cautious administration of phenobarbital is advisable, whereas preexistent conduction disturbances, particularly bradyarrhythmias, necessitate careful monitoring of phenytoin therapy [Cranford et al., 1978]. The apparently circumscribed window of susceptibility for these postpump seizures and the rarity of subsequent epilepsy allow successful early withdrawal of antiepileptic agents, often before hospital discharge.

PROGNOSIS

The prognosis for postoperative seizures depends on the underlying cause. Postpump seizures without an obvious cause were previously considered benign, transient events. However, a significant association between postoperative seizures and worse neurodevelopmental outcome and MRI abnormalities has been demonstrated in a large, prospective study [Bellinger et al., 1995; Rappaport et al., 1998]. Although epilepsy is a rare sequel to typical postpump seizures [Ehyai et al., 1984], the West syndrome has been described in occasional survivors of intractable postoperative seizures [du Plessis et al., 1994a]. The long-term outcome of infants with an identified cause for their postoperative seizures is related to the specific cause. The prevalence of developmental brain anomalies is increased in infants with congenital heart disease (discussed later). Seizures in infants with brain dysgenesis are associated with an almost universally poor long-term outcome, and epilepsy is a common complication. Stroke in young infants commonly manifests with seizures. The overall risk for subsequent epilepsy in these infants ranges from 20% to 30% [Lanska et al., 1991; Yang et al., 1995], and it is related to the age at stroke and the post-stroke latency to first seizure. Specifically, the risk for later epilepsy is lowest when stroke occurs in the newborn infant [Levy et al., 1985] and when seizures are an early manifestation of stroke [Yang et al., 1995]. These features should be considered when planning maintenance antiepileptic drug therapy.

Movement Disorders

For almost 4 decades, movement disorders have been a dreaded complication of deep hypothermic cardiac surgery [Barrat-Boyes, 1990; Bergouignan et al., 1961; Bjork and Hultquist, 1962; Brunberg et al., 1974; Chaves and Scaltsas-Persson, 1988; Curless et al., 1994; DeLeon et al., 1990; Donaldson et al., 1990; Huntley et al., 1993; Medlock et al., 1993; Robinson et al., 1988; Wical and Tomasi, 1990; Wong et al., 1992]. Choreoathetosis is the most frequently reported dyskinesia after cardiac surgery, but a spectrum of movement disorders, including oculogyric crises [du Plessis et al., 1994b], akathisia, and parkinsonian syndromes [Straussberg et al., 1993] may be encountered. These dyskinesias are likely underdiagnosed and underreported, making the true incidence difficult to ascertain; however, in reported case series, the incidence of postoperative choreoathetosis has ranged from 0.5% [Wessel and du Plessis, 1995] to 19% [Brunberg et al., 1974]. Despite the relative infrequency of this complication, these postoperative movement disorders are often dramatic, frequently intractable, and ultimately debilitating. Severe forms are associated with substantial mortality.

Postoperative choreoathetosis has a fairly stereotypic presentation and clinical course (Fig. 88-4). The involuntary movements are preceded in most cases by a latent period of 2 to 7 days, during which neurologic recovery from surgery is unremarkable. The dyskinesia is almost invariably heralded by subacute changes in mental status, including often severe insomnia and irritability. These mental status changes are soon followed by "restlessness" progressing to frankly abnormal involuntary movements. The dyskinesia usually commences in the distal extremities and orofacial muscles and progresses proximally to involve the girdle muscles and trunk. In severe cases, violent ballismic thrashing may develop. The dyskinesia is present during wakefulness, becomes more noticeable during distress, and resolves during the brief and fitful periods of sleep. An oromotor apraxia may become prominent, disrupting oral feeding and expressive language. Parents and caretakers often develop concerns about "blindness" in these infants, because they appear not to look at or show signs of recognizing familiar faces. This problem rarely is caused by blindness and instead results from a supranuclear ophthalmoplegia or oculomotor apraxia, with loss of voluntary gaze. Reflex extraocular movements and optokinetic nystagmus remain spared. Over the course of days to a week, the involuntary movements intensify and then plateau over 1 to 2 weeks. This period is

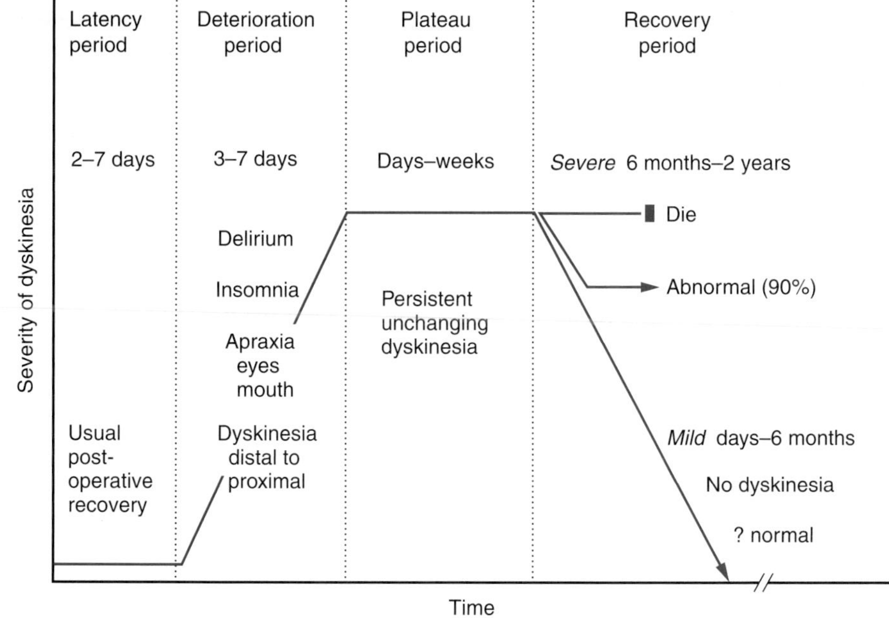

FIGURE 88-4. Diagram of the time course and evolution of postoperative dyskinesia.

followed by a recovery phase that is more variable in duration, depending on the severity of the initial dyskinetic syndrome.

Most cases of mild dyskinesia tend to resolve completely within days to weeks; by 6 months, none of these children exhibits involuntary movements. The quality of their voluntary movements and cognitive abilities has not been studied in detail. In survivors of severe postoperative dyskinesia, the involuntary movements may gradually improve for up to 2 years, after which the chances for further meaningful recovery are unlikely.

Diagnosis of these postoperative hyperkinetic syndromes is essentially clinical. Adjunctive neurodiagnostic techniques have been useful only insofar as they exclude other disorders. Neuroimaging studies, including CT and MRI, have indicated nonspecific and nonfocal changes, the most common picture being one of diffuse cerebral atrophy [Medlock et al., 1993; Robinson et al., 1988; Wong et al., 1992]. Single-photon emission computed tomography (SPECT) functional brain imaging studies have found a high incidence of cortical and subcortical perfusion defects, even in the absence of structural defects detected using CT or MRI [du Plessis et al., 1994b]. The EEG pattern is usually normal or demonstrates diffuse slowing. The involuntary movements are not associated with ictal changes. Postmortem examination studies in these patients are limited and the inconsistent neuropathologic changes have not elucidated the mechanisms of injury [Chaves and Scaltsas-Persson, 1988; Kupsky et al., 1995]. The characteristic features of focal or global hypoxic-ischemic or reperfusion insults are typically absent. The basal ganglia do not exhibit infarction, and the topography of the selective neuronal loss and gliosis (i.e., in the external globus pallidus) is uncharacteristic of hypoxic-ischemic or reperfusion injury occurring at normothermia [Kupsky et al., 1995]. However, an animal model of deep hypothermic circulatory arrest [Johnston et al., 1995; Redmond et al., 1994] has suggested that when hypoxic-ischemic or reperfusion injury occurs at deep hypothermia, the topography and evolution of injury may be modified. In this model, selective neuronal necrosis is prominent in the globus pallidus.

The prognosis of these conditions depends largely on their initial severity. Based on the severity and persistence of the dyskinesias, two forms of postpump choreoathetosis may be distinguished: a mild, transient form and a severe, persistent form [Wong et al., 1992]. In the mild, transient form, involuntary movements are confined to the distal extremities or face, and they tend to resolve over several weeks to months in virtually all cases [du Plessis et al., 2002]. However, a significant minority of these children has persistent disturbances in gait, fine motor function, and language. In contrast, children with severe postpump choreoathetosis invariably have a much less favorable course. Their involuntary movements persist long after the onset, and they have pervasive disturbances in behavior and cognition, frequently meeting the criteria for mental retardation [du Plessis et al., 2002]. These severe cases are associated with a mortality rate approaching 40% because of respiratory complications such as aspiration pneumonia, massive caloric consumption, and infection [Wong et al., 1992].

Dyskinesias have also been associated with the use of fentanyl and midazolam, widely used postoperative analgesics and sedatives. These medication-associated forms of movement disorder have a good prognosis, with less prominent sensorium changes and mild involuntary movements that resolve over days to weeks [Bergman et al., 1991; Lane et al., 1991; Petzinger et al., 1995].

The effective management of postoperative dyskinesias, both preventive and symptomatic, remains a frustrating challenge. Prevention of these disorders is limited by the current lack of a discernible mechanism of injury. However, certain preventable risk factors have been identified in retrospective studies. Children at particular risk tend to be older than 9 months at the time of surgery, have cyanotic congenital heart disease with systemic-to-pulmonary collaterals from the head and neck and, during surgery, have shorter cooling periods before attenuation of intraoperative blood flow [Wong et al., 1992]. These guidelines have been incorporated into the surgical management protocol at Children's Hospital, Boston. In patients with correction of heart lesions at earlier ages, close attention to systemic-to-pulmonary collaterals, more gradual cooling, and decreased use of deep hypothermic circulatory arrest have resulted in a marked decline in the incidence of postoperative dyskinesia [Wessel and du Plessis, 1995].

Acute and long-term management of these postoperative dyskinesias has remained frustrating. No agents reliably control the adventitious movements while preserving alertness. In the acute phase, essential management goals should be amelioration of the agitated delirium, protection of the airway, and anticipation of the skin breakdown and increased nutritional demands. General measures against the profound irritability should include a decrease in the level of external (e.g., noise, light) and internal (e.g., pain) stimuli. Sedation should be used judiciously, and it should aim to restore the fragmented sleep-wake cycle. During the acute phase, mild dyskinesias can be managed by sedating agents alone, such as benzodiazepines and chloral hydrate. Despite the generally refractory nature of severe movement disorders, a cautious trial with more specific antidyskinetic agents is a reasonable approach. If the child's hemodynamic status is stable, a trial of haloperidol may be warranted. This agent should be started at low doses (0.025 mg/kg/day, given in divided doses three times daily) and gradually increased while monitoring closely for cardiodepressant effects of dopamine blockade. If sedation becomes evident without a clear decrease in involuntary movements or if myocardial depression develops, these agents should be replaced by more specific sedating agents, such as clonazepam. The often-prominent oromotor dyskinesia impairs feeding and predisposes to aspiration. Nasogastric or even gastrostomy tube feedings may be necessary to meet the high caloric demands of the constant involuntary movements.

Equally exasperating has been the pursuit of long-term pharmacologic control of residual dyskinesias. A wide spectrum of medications effective against other forms of hyperkinetic movement disorders has been tried, including dopamine receptor antagonists (e.g., phenothiazines, butyrophenones), dopamine-depleting agents (e.g., reserpine, tetrabenazine), dopamine agonists (L-dopa), γ-aminobutyric acid agents (e.g., benzodiazepines, barbiturates, baclofen), and other agents, including valproic acid, carbamazepine, phenytoin, diphenhydramine, and chloral hydrate. The efficacy of these agents for movement control has been modest at best and often occurs at the expense of excessive sedation. The benefit-risk ratio of several of these agents is further compromised by their risks for cardiac dysfunction and the development of secondary dyskinesias (e.g., tardive dyskinesias).

Spinal Cord Injury

Spinal cord injury is a rare complication of cardiac surgery in infants and children, and it is most commonly [Puntis and Green, 1985] seen after aortic coarctation repair, occurring in 0.4% [Brewer et al., 1972] to 1.5% [Lerberg et al., 1982; Pennington et al., 1979] of patients. During aortic surgery, spinal cord injury results from a watershed type of hypoxic-ischemic or reperfusion insult. In the spinal cord, end-zone or watershed territories of arterial supply are located transversely at the lower thoracic level and longitudinally between the supply territories of the anterior and posterior spinal arteries. Transverse ischemia at the thoracic level is the usual form of cord injury seen after coarctation repair. Clamping of the aorta distal to the subclavian arteries renders the distal cord vulnerable to ischemia for several reasons. First, perfusion to the distal cord depends on a highly variable, inconsistent collateral supply. Second, aortic cross-clamping may precipitate hypertension that increases cerebrospinal fluid pressure and further decreases perfusion pressure to the lower cord. Transverse cord ischemia manifests as postoperative paraplegia with pyramidal features, with or without a thoracolumbar sensory level and bladder and bowel dysfunction.

The longitudinal cord syndrome is rare and is mediated by systemic hypotension, as occurs with birth asphyxia [Sladky and Rorke, 1986] or with cardiac defects [Rousseau et al., 1993]. Injury is maximal in the ventral gray matter columns, with selective anterior horn cell loss. Unlike the predominant pyramidal features of transverse cord ischemia, longitudinal cord injury causes a prominent lower motor neuron syndrome, with acute and long-term hypotonia and weakness with decreased or absent reflexes; posterior column sensory function is relatively spared. Some authorities have advocated intraoperative monitoring of spinal cord function during coarctation surgery by using somatosensory-evoked potentials [Guerit et al., 1997; Laschinger et al., 1983, 1988]. However, this technique evaluates posterolateral spinal pathways rather than the more vulnerable anterior horn cells, and consequently, it has not been universally adopted [Laschinger et al., 1988].

Strategies for the prevention of this complication have been investigated in experimental models and adults undergoing aortic aneurysm surgery [Coles et al., 1983; Colon et al., 1987; Lange et al., 1997; Laschinger et al., 1984, 1987; Nylander et al., 1982; Robertson et al., 1986]. In infants and children, the relatively low prevalence of aortic coarctation and the rare occurrence of intraoperative spinal injury have limited the design of prospective clinical trials for prevention.

Peripheral Neuromuscular Injury

The often prolonged periods of immobility during and after cardiac procedures expose the peripheral nervous system to pressure and traction injuries. The child with congenital heart disease also is at risk for toxic metabolic injury to the peripheral nerve, neuromuscular junction, and muscle.

PLEXOPATHIES

Plexopathies, particularly brachial, can occur after cardiac procedures [Kent et al., 1994; Lederman et al., 1982]. The brachial plexus is vulnerable to traction injury during the intraoperative retraction of a sternal thoracotomy incision; this form of plexopathy is more common in older patients. Cardiac catheterization, particularly newer interventional techniques such as radiofrequency ablation of aberrant conduction pathways and the placement of devices to occlude septal defects, may require prolonged shoulder hyperabduction in the sedated patient. This treatment may result in traction injury, usually to the lower brachial plexus. The patient presents in the postcatheterization period with weakness in the wrist and finger extensors and the intrinsic muscles of the hand, occasionally associated with Horner's syndrome. Because the lesion is usually neurapraxic, it usually improves over time [Dawson and Fischer, 1977]. Conversely, upper plexus lesions most commonly result from direct injury or extravasated blood associated with indwelling central venous catheters in the neck vessels. The clinical manifestation of such upper brachial plexus injuries depends on the precise level of injury but most commonly involves the abductors and external rotators of the shoulder. Prognosis for recovery from these direct traumatic lesions is more guarded.

Catheterization by using the femoral vessels in the inguinal region may be complicated by a localized hematoma or false aneurysm formation. The compressive and inflammatory effects of extravasated blood may injure the lumbar plexus (with retroperitoneal hematomas) or the femoral nerve and its branches (with inguinal hematomas). Although these neuropathies may be acutely debilitating, recovery is usually complete [Kent et al., 1994].

MONONEUROPATHIES

Pressure palsies may develop at a variety of dependent sites, most commonly the peroneal and ulnar nerves. Phrenic nerve injury is another relatively common complication of hypothermic cardiac surgery. This form of injury results in diaphragmatic paralysis and should be considered in the evaluation of any child with postoperative ventilator dependence. The precise mechanism of injury is often unclear, but it is thought to reflect direct cold injury from ice packed around the heart or inadvertent transection of the nerve as it courses alongside the heart [Dunne et al., 1991; Mok et al., 1991; Watanabe et al., 1987]. The diagnosis may be established by ultrasound or fluoroscopy of the diaphragm or by bedside phrenic nerve conduction and diaphragmatic electromyography [Bolton, 1993; Swenson and Rubenstein, 1992]. In most cases, the phrenic nerve palsies are transient and presumably neurapraxic in origin. Less commonly, phrenic palsies are permanent and require diaphragmatic plication or rarely require diaphragmatic pacing [Weese-Mayer et al., 1992].

POLYNEUROPATHY AND MYOPATHY

Several reports [Gooch et al., 1991; Waitling and Dasta, 1994] have described a prolonged neuromuscular syndrome emerging after withdrawal of nondepolarizing neuromuscular blocking drugs. Agents such as vecuronium and pancuronium are commonly used to facilitate post-thoracotomy ventilatory management. Patients with renal and hepatic failure appear to be at increased risk for developing this syndrome. Administration of acetylcholinesterase inhibitors may result in improved strength, but this effect is unpredictable and usually transient. The neuropathology of this syndrome is highly variable, ranging from an axonal motor neuropathy to myopathic changes [Danon and Carpenter, 1991; Subramony et al., 1991]. The neuropathy associated with neuromuscular blockers may be difficult to distinguish clinically from "critical illness polyneuropathy" [Sheth and Bolton, 1995]. This syndrome occurs in patients with sepsis and multiorgan failure, conditions that may complicate congenital heart disease and surgery.

Prolonged neuromuscular blockade may be complicated by an often severe myopathy. The risk of this form of myopathic complication is increased when neuromuscular blocking agents and high-dose steroids are used together [Hirano et al., 1992]. This combination of drugs is often used after cardiac transplantation. Unlike the neuropathies described previously, muscle weakness associated with these myopathic syndromes is usually maximal in proximal muscles. Tendon reflexes are reduced or absent, and sensory function is preserved. Two forms of myopathy may complicate neuromuscular blockade: an acute necrotizing myopathy and an acute myosin-deficiency myopathy [Al-Lozi et al., 1994; Hirano et al., 1992]. These myopathies may be distinguished by electromyography, which demonstrates markedly increased spontaneous activity in the necrotizing variety that is not seen in the myosin-deficiency myopathy. Muscle biopsy indicates a severe myofiber necrosis or, in the latter condition, relative preservation of myofibers with deficiency of myosin relative to actin filaments.

Delayed Postoperative Neurologic Complications

The delayed neurologic manifestations of cardiac surgery may be considered in two categories. First, there are the developmental and cognitive deficits that emerge later in children who have suffered transient acute postoperative neurologic complications such as seizures and choreoathetosis. For example, although epilepsy is a rare sequel to postpump seizures, these infants are at higher risk for long-term neurodevelopmental deficits [Bellinger et al., 1995]. The second category of delayed neurologic manifestations includes those that develop ab initio remote from surgical procedures. Two specific manifestations, stroke and headache, are the focus of this section.

Stroke

Stroke in the child with congenital heart disease is predominantly thromboembolic in origin. Less commonly, arteriopathic or stenotic lesions of the intracranial vasculature may be seen in patients with certain congenital heart lesions.

THROMBOEMBOLIC CARDIOGENIC STROKE

Although thromboembolic stroke may complicate congenital heart disease at any time in the preoperative, intraoperative, and early postoperative periods, most cardiogenic strokes occur remote from surgery. The overall annual incidence of childhood stroke ranges from 2.5 [Schoenberg et al., 1978] to 7.9 per 100,000 children [Giroud et al., 1995] each year. Congenital heart disease remains the leading known risk factor for stroke in childhood; it occurs in 25% to 30% of cases [Lanska et al., 1991; Riela and Roach, 1993; Schoenberg et al., 1978]. Risk factors for cardiogenic stroke in earlier years (e.g., polycythemia, right-to-left shunt) have decreased with the surgical correction of heart lesions in early infancy [Berthrong and Sabiston, 1951; Cottrill and Kaplan, 1973; Martelle and Linde, 1961; Phornphutkul et al., 1973; Terplan, 1976; Tyler and Clark, 1957a, 1957b]. Postmortem examination studies from earlier decades described cerebrovascular ischemic lesions in up to 20% of children with congenital heart disease [Berthrong and Sabiston, 1951; Terplan, 1976]. The prevalence of stroke in the modern era of cardiac surgery is unknown because of the lack of neuropathologic studies.

In patients who survive cyanotic congenital heart disease into adulthood, the risk for stroke persists and likely increases. One study found a stroke incidence of 1 case per 100 patient-years for patients with cyanotic congenital heart disease who were older than 18 years [Ammash and Warnes, 1996]. Similar to earlier studies in children [Cottrill and Kaplan, 1973; Linderkamp et al., 1979], the strongest risk factor for stroke in this cyanotic population was microcytosis. The proposed mechanism is a procoagulant shift resulting from an increased blood viscosity caused by the microcytic erythrocytosis.

The major physiologic and anatomic risk factors for stroke, including the three elements of Virchow's triad (i.e., altered vascular surface, stasis [du Plessis et al., 1995a; Rosenthal et al., 1995a, 1995b], and hypercoagulability [Cromme-Dijkhuis et al., 1990; Komp and Sparrow, 1970; Linderkamp et al., 1979], commonly exist in children with

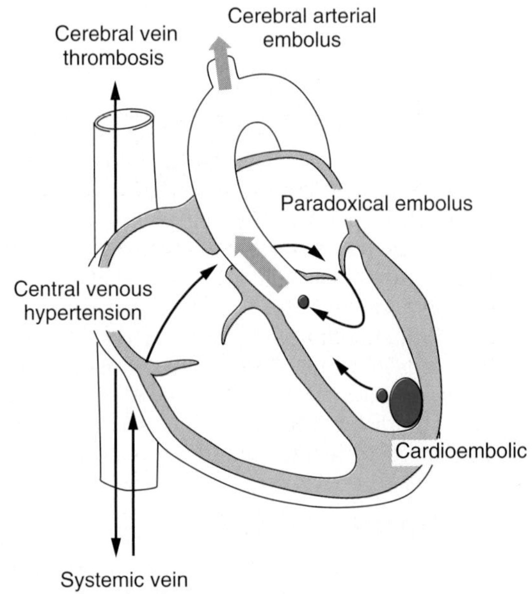

FIGURE 88-5. The three broad mechanisms of cardiogenic stroke: cardioembolic (i.e., intracardiac embolic source), paradoxical (i.e., systemic venous embolic source), and cerebral vein thrombosis.

congenital heart disease. The presence of paradoxical vascular pathways between the systemic venous system and the cerebral arteries constitute a further major risk factor for cardiogenic stroke. In broad terms, cardiogenic stroke may be mediated by three mechanisms (Fig. 88-5). First, arterial emboli may emanate from an intracardiac embolic source (i.e., *cardioembolic stroke*). Second, emboli may arise from a systemic venous or right heart source and bypass the pulmonary circulation through a right-to-left shunt (i.e., *paradoxical embolic stroke*). *Cerebral venous thrombosis* may result from a combination of central venous hypertension, venous stasis, and polycythemia. In earlier postmortem examination reports, venous thrombosis was the most common form of cerebral vaso-occlusive lesion [Cottrill and Kaplan, 1973].

Although most strokes occur beyond the early postoperative period, certain features of open-heart surgery and the immediate postoperative period predispose patients to stroke and warrant brief review. During the intraoperative period, embolic and thrombotic mechanisms may predispose patients to cerebral vaso-occlusive disease. Particulate and gaseous emboli originating from the cardiopulmonary bypass apparatus or surgical field bypass the normal pulmonary filtration system during cardiopulmonary bypass and enter the systemic circulation directly [Boyajian et al., 1993; Moody et al., 1990; Padayachee et al., 1987; Solis et al., 1975]. Improvements in bypass circuits, particularly the replacement of bubble oxygenators by membrane oxygenators, have decreased the incidence of macroembolic injury [Nussmeier and McDermott, 1988]. The impact of these advances on the incidence of microvascular injury [Fish, 1988] is unclear. The often-marked inflammatory response triggered by the extensive and prolonged exposure between bypass blood and artificial surfaces [Kirklin et al., 1983; Millar et al., 1993; Steinberg et al., 1993] is known to trigger complex cascades, including endothelial–leukocyte interactions [del Zoppo, 1994; Elliott and Finn, 1993; Feuerstein et al., 1994; Lucchesi, 1993]. The resulting microvascular dysfunction may predispose to intravascular thrombosis or thromboembolism, manifesting with vaso-occlusive brain injury.

In the early postoperative period, several factors predispose to cardiogenic stroke. First, vascular stasis may result from localized areas of low flow within the heart [du Plessis et al., 1995a; Rosenthal et al., 1995a, 1995b] or global ventricular dysfunction. Prolonged postoperative immobility predisposes to systemic venous stasis and thrombosis. Transient pulmonary hypertension is common after cardiopulmonary bypass, elevating venous pressure and decreasing the rate of blood flow through the right heart chambers and central veins. Injury to native tissue or the presence of prosthetic tissue alters vascular surfaces in contact with the circulation. A number of these stroke risk factors may apply after the Fontan procedure, the most common final operation for congenital heart disease with a single-ventricle physiology [Day et al., 1995; Dobell et al., 1986; du Plessis et al., 1995a; Hutto et al., 1991; Mathews et al., 1986; Rosenthal et al., 1995a, 1995b]. In this procedure, venous blood returning to the right atrium is redirected to the pulmonary arterial system, bypassing the single ventricle, which then serves as the pump for systemic perfusion. Consequently, right atrial pressure is often elevated, slowing flow through this chamber and the central veins supplying it. The procoagulant effect of this slow venous flow is further enhanced by the use of a prosthetic "tunnel" or baffle within the atrium to redirect flow. These factors combine to predispose to thrombus formation within the right atrium and central veins. In

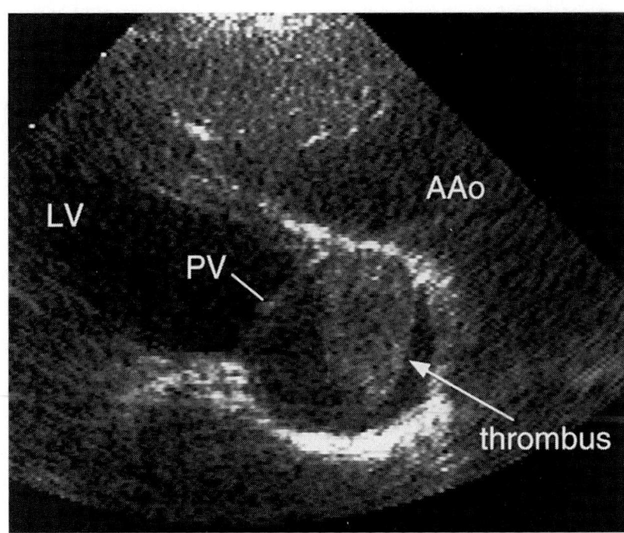

A

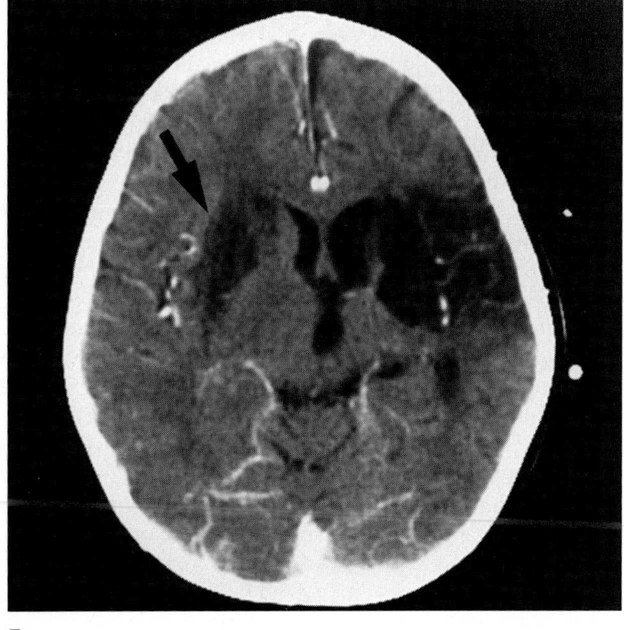

B

FIGURE 88-6. Recurrent strokes after a Fontan procedure for congenital heart disease with single-ventricle physiology with persistent or recurrent thrombus in the pulmonary artery stump. **A**, The echocardiogram shows a thrombus *(arrow)* in the proximal, blind-ending stump of the ligated main pulmonary artery. AAo, arch of aorta; LV, left ventricle; PV, pulmonary valve. **B**, Computed tomographic brain scan with contrast demonstrates a recurrent stroke *(arrow)* in the right middle cerebral artery distribution. This stroke occurred 14 months after an initial large, left-sided stroke despite therapeutic levels of anticoagulation. It was presumably caused by an embolus from the persistent or recurrent pulmonary artery thrombus in **A**.

the fenestrated Fontan modification, a right-to-left interatrial defect is created in the baffle or tunnel. This fenestrated modification, which has markedly reduced the mortality of the Fontan operation, essentially connects the thrombogenic right atrium to the cerebral arterial supply.

Another potential area of thrombus formation after the Fontan procedure results when the main pulmonary artery is ligated, leaving a blind-ending low flow stump. Thrombi in this location (Fig. 88-6A) are capable of generating emboli directly into the aorta and cerebral circulation (see Fig. 88-6B). Retrospective studies of patients after the Fontan procedure confirm the increased stroke risk, with a prevalence ranging from 2.6% [du Plessis et al., 1995a] to 8.8% [Day et al., 1995]. This risk for stroke after the Fontan operation persists for up to 3 [du Plessis et al., 1995a] to 15 years [Rosenthal et al., 1995b] after the procedure.

Stroke therapies may be considered in broad terms as rescue or preventive strategies. Rescue strategies aim to limit the extent of stroke by salvaging injured but potentially viable brain. Rescue therapies include thrombolytic agents [del Zoppo et al., 1988; Mori et al., 1988] or agents directed at limiting the injurious biochemical cascades triggered by hypoxic-ischemic or reperfusion insults [Gerlach et al., 1995; Vannucci, 1990]. Because these rescue therapies are confined to experimental and adult trials, they are not discussed further here. Preventive therapies for stroke may be primary (i.e., treatment of high-risk patients to prevent a first stroke) or secondary (i.e., aimed at preventing stroke recurrence) [Anderson, 1991].

A universally accepted approach for the primary or secondary prevention of cardiogenic stroke in children is lacking. For the most part, the guidelines in current clinical practice are based on the adult stroke experience. However, many aspects of stroke prophylaxis in adults are still in dispute, and the mechanisms and long-term consequences of stroke differ markedly in children compared with adults. These issues emphasize the need for prospective therapeutic trials for the prevention of stroke in congenital heart disease. Widely accepted indications for primary stroke prophylaxis in congenital heart disease include children with prosthetic heart valves, dilated cardiomyopathy, or intracardiac thrombus identified by echocardiogram. Stroke prophylaxis should also be considered in patients with combined risk factors such as elevated right atrial pressure, intracardiac prosthetic material, right-to-left shunt, and prolonged bed rest. Because post-Fontan patients have a number of these risk factors, many centers use prophylactic antithrombotic agents after this operation. Although low-dose aspirin is most commonly used, the optimal agent and duration of treatment are unclear.

Some patients with critical end-stage heart disease have been supported by mechanical circulatory support devices that serve as a bridge to heart transplantation. These devices may be extracorporeal membrane oxygenation or intracardiac devices used to augment ventricular function. The prolonged interface between circulating blood and prosthetic material predisposes the patient to thrombus formation and stroke. The theoretical risk of stroke in children on these support devices has not been studied in any detail; consequently, the optimal prophylactic anticoagulation strategy has not been established.

Secondary stroke prevention with anticoagulant therapy is controversial, particularly in the early period after stroke [Pessin et al., 1993]. The aim of secondary prophylaxis is to balance the risks of recurrent embolism and hemorrhagic transformation of a bland infarction. Unfortunately, the magnitude of these risks is unknown for childhood cardiogenic stroke. In adults with stroke after myocardial infarction, the risk of recurrent cerebral embolism is approximately 1% per day during the first 2 weeks [Anderson et al., 1992; Cerebral Embolism Study Group, 1984, 1987; Cerebral Embolism Task Force, 1989], whereas the risk for spontaneous hemorrhagic transformation of the infarct may be as high as 20% to 40% [Hart and Easton, 1986; Hart et al., 1995]. The risk of significant clinical deterioration is higher when hemorrhagic transformation occurs in the anticoagulated patient [Okada et al., 1989; Sherman et al., 1992]. Certain broad guidelines have emerged for the use of anticoagulation after acute stroke. Overall, 70% of strokes that ultimately undergo hemorrhagic transformation do so within the first 48 hours after the onset of cerebral infarction [Sherman et al., 1992]. Large infarcts are at greater risk for secondary hemorrhage, particularly when an entire cerebral lobe or more than 30% of a hemisphere are involved [Okada et al., 1989; Sherman et al., 1992; Yatsu et al., 1988]. Other risk factors for bleeding into stroke include uncontrolled systemic hypertension, stroke due to septic emboli (see Fig. 88-9), and cerebral venous thrombosis.

The risk of hemorrhagic complications may be decreased by newer low-molecular-weight heparin preparations. Initial experience with these agents in children at risk for thrombosis is encouraging, but full evaluation awaits a randomized clinical trial [Massicotte et al., 1996]. Long-term administration of these agents through a subcutaneous catheter may facilitate home therapy for children at risk for stroke.

Seizures are a common manifestation of childhood stroke, particularly in the young infant [Clancy et al., 1985; Lanska et al., 1991; Levy et al., 1985]. The combination of antiepileptic and antithrombotic therapies may result in important drug interactions. Phenobarbital and carbamazepine tend to decrease the anticoagulant effect of warfarin (Coumadin), necessitating higher warfarin doses, whereas phenytoin may increase or decrease this effect. The coagulation profile should be followed closely, particularly after discontinuation of antiepileptic agents, when excessive anticoagulation may occur.

ARTERIOPATHIC STROKE

Various forms of progressive stenotic or occlusive vasculopathy involving the intracranial circulation have been reported in patients with congenital heart disease. Although these conditions are not usually related to cardiac surgery, they are discussed here because they should be included in the differential diagnosis of stroke in congenital heart disease. Several cardiac lesions have been associated with intracranial arteriopathy, and they may be grouped into two broad categories: conotruncal defects and obstructive lesions of the aorta or pulmonary arteries. In one report, five patients with congenital heart disease who developed repeated strokes and seizures had moyamoya disease [Lutterman et al., 1998]. This slowly obliterative angiopathy involves the supraclinoid internal carotid artery and the anterior and middle (more than the posterior) cerebral arteries. Moyamoya disease results from progressive intimal thickening and the development of extensive collateral vessels [Suzuki and Kodama, 1983]. This syndrome most commonly manifests with repeated transient ischemic attacks and seizures. Over months to years, affected children develop progressive motor deterioration, mental retardation, and epilepsy. Coarctation of the aorta has also been associated with other neurovascular lesions, such as aneurysms [Orsi et al., 1993] of the circle of Willis and spinal arteries [Ling and Bao, 1994], and arteriovenous malformations [LeBlanc et al., 1968; Shearer et al., 1970; Tomlinson et al., 1992; Young et al., 1982]. Children with aortic coarctation who develop hypertension may be particularly vulnerable to intracranial hemorrhage from these intracranial vascular defects. After coarctation repair, patients who develop stroke symptoms (particularly when referable to the posterior circulation) should be evaluated for a subclavian steal syndrome [Saalouke et al., 1978].

The vasculopathy originally described in Williams' syndrome was confined to stenosis of the supravalvar aortic region. The arterial luminal narrowing is more widespread than previously recognized, with reports describing involvement of the carotid, vertebral, and intracranial arteries. There have been several reports of stroke in patients with Williams' syndrome [Ardinger et al., 1994; Kaplan, 1995; Soper et al., 1995]. Histopathologically, this multifocal intracranial arteriopathy is characterized by medial fibroelastic dysplasia, hypertrophied smooth muscle cells, and disorganized elastin fibers. This angiopathy is thought to result from a deficiency of elastin in the vessel media, caused by deletion of the elastin gene [Ewart et al., 1993]. Two older patients (i.e., 18 and 22 years) with Williams' syndrome have been described as having moyamoya disease [Kawai et al., 1993; Soper et al., 1995]. However, the histopathology of moyamoya disease [Graham, 1992] differs from that of Williams' syndrome, exhibiting predominant fibrocellular thickening of the intima rather than the medial changes seen in Williams' syndrome. The relationship between the various angiopathic syndromes seen in patients with congenital heart disease needs further study.

Headache

Intracranial mechanisms of headache are mediated by stimulation of nerve endings in the dura and blood vessels by processes as diverse as inflammation and tension or pressure. Because many of the physiologic changes capable of stimulating these structures (e.g., vasodilation, intracranial hypertension) occur in congenital heart disease, it is not surprising that headaches are a common complication of congenital heart disease. For example, decreased cerebral oxygen delivery and hypercarbia can cause vasodilation. Elevated cerebral venous pressure may cause headaches by venous distention and, if sustained, by causing communicating hydrocephalus due to impaired cerebrospinal fluid absorption [Rosman and Shands, 1978]. Headaches are particularly common in adolescent and adult survivors of earlier palliative procedures, in whom progressive pulmonary hypertension, central venous hypertension, and polycythemia develop over time. Certain surgical procedures (i.e., Fontan and Glenn operations) are prone to central venous hypertension and are commonly complicated by headaches. In patients with venous hypertension and polycythemia, the development of headaches may herald dural vein thrombosis. The intensity and frequency of headaches associated with progressive polycythemia tend to parallel the rising hematocrit and to respond to erythropheresis.

Headache is the most common initial complaint in the often subtle clinical presentation of brain abscess [Aicardi, 1992b]. Consequently, a diagnosis of brain abscess must be excluded before the direct measurement of cerebrospinal fluid pressure when doing a lumbar puncture in congenital heart disease patients with papilledema. Sudden-onset, severe headaches should always raise concern about the

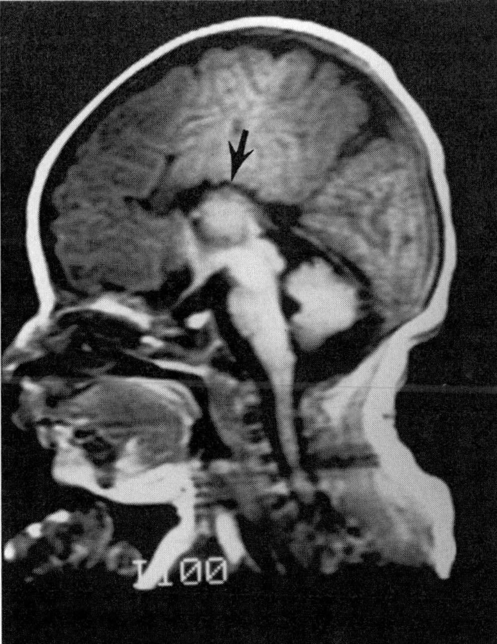

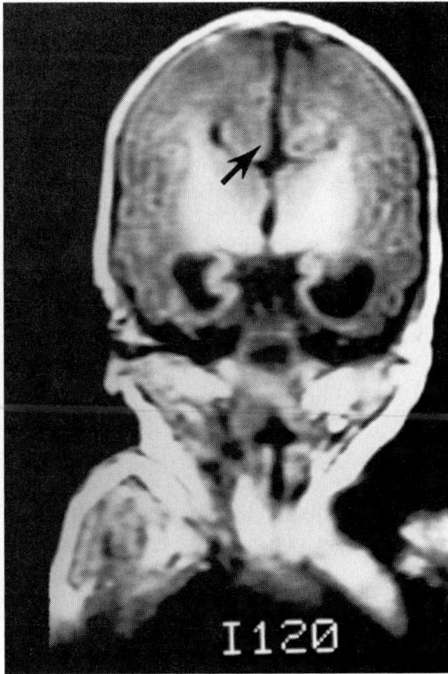

FIGURE 88-7. T1-weighted magnetic resonance imaging of the brain of a 3-week-old infant with transposition of the great arteries who developed postoperative seizures after an arterial switch operation. The scan shows cerebral dysgenesis in the form of agenesis of the corpus callosum *(arrows)* and a small cerebellar vermis.

possibility of subarachnoid hemorrhage, particularly in patients with infective endocarditis [Bohmfalk et al., 1978; Jones and Sieker, 1989] and in hypertensive patients with coarctation of the aorta [LeBlanc et al., 1968; Shearer et al., 1970; Tomlinson et al., 1992; Young et al., 1982].

NEUROLOGIC COMPLICATIONS UNRELATED TO CARDIAC SURGERY

A substantial proportion of the neurologic morbidity complicating childhood heart disease is unrelated to the acute or chronic effects of cardiac surgery. The mechanisms and manifestations of neurologic dysfunction in these cases depend on the associated form of heart disease: structural congenital heart disease; inherited disease of the heart, brain, and muscle; and acquired heart disease. Considerable neurologic morbidity is associated with extracorporeal membrane oxygenation (ECMO).

Structural Congenital Heart Disease

The nonoperative neurologic complications of structural congenital heart disease may be developmental or have an infectious cause. Dysgenetic disorders often manifest in infancy, whereas infectious complications tend to occur later.

Cerebral Dysgenesis

The prevalence of dysgenetic brain lesions is increased among children with congenital heart disease, ranging from 10% to 29% in postmortem examination studies [Glauser et al., 1990b; Jones, 1991; Miller and Vogel, 1999; Terplan, 1976]. Cerebral dysgenesis should be considered in any child with congenital heart disease and unexplained neurologic dysfunction (Fig. 88-7). The prevalence of dysgenetic brain lesions appears to be particularly increased among patients with certain cardiac lesions [Glauser et al., 1990b; Jones, 1991; Terplan, 1976]. For example, a range of cerebral dysgenesis, from microdysgenesis to gross malformations such as holoprosencephaly, has been described at postmortem examination in infants with the hypoplastic left heart syndrome [Glauser et al., 1990b]. Clinically, these dysgenetic lesions may manifest in the newborn period with seizures, alterations in level of consciousness, and abnormalities in motor tone. Conversely, the lesions may remain clinically occult until later infancy and childhood, when they manifest with developmental delay, epilepsy, and cerebral palsy. Diagnosis is best confirmed by MRI of the brain. The increasing availability and resolution of neuroimaging likely will delineate more clearly the association between congenital heart disease and brain dysgenesis.

Infectious and Parainfectious Complications

Congenital heart disease is a known risk factor for infective endocarditis and brain abscess. Although earlier corrective surgery and modern antibiotic therapy have been associated with a marked decline in the incidence of these potentially devastating infectious complications, they continue to occur in children with congenital heart disease.

INFECTIVE ENDOCARDITIS

Neurologic injury complicates infective endocarditis in 20% to 40% of patients [Francioli, 1991; Saiman et al., 1993]. The neurologic manifestations of infective endocarditis are protean and include meningitis, brain abscess, seizures, and most commonly, cerebrovascular injury. Systemic embolization occurs in up to 50% of patients with infective endocarditis [Lutas et al., 1986; Pelletier and Petersdorf, 1977; Roy et al., 1976], with as many as 65% of embolic events targeting the brain, usually the middle cerebral artery territory [Pruitt et al., 1978]. Several factors have been identified that increase the risk for dissemination of septic emboli [Pruitt et al., 1978]: endocarditis caused by *Staphylococcus aureus* or *Candida albicans*; vegetations on the mitral (25%) more than the aortic (10%) valve (Fig. 88-8), particularly the anterior mitral leaflet; vegetations exceeding 10 mm; and the first 2 to 4 weeks after the initiation of antibiotic treatment.

Cerebrovascular complications are the most common form of neurologic injury, and they are the most lethal

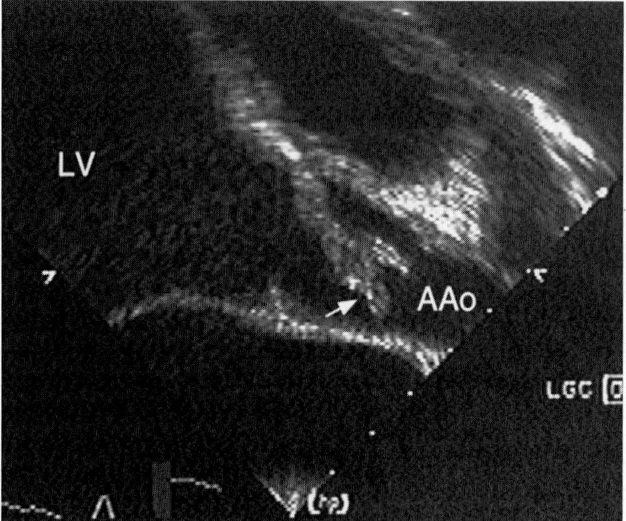

A

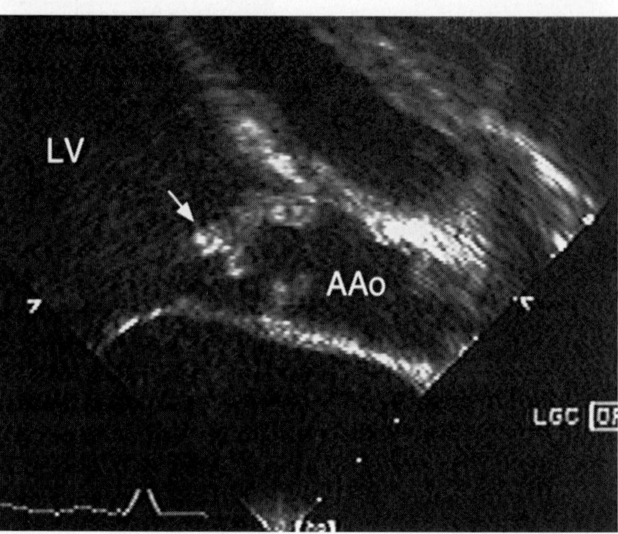

B

FIGURE 88-8. The echocardiogram demonstrates the aortic valve during systole (**A**) and diastole (**B**). Vegetations on the valve leaflets are indicated by *arrows*. AAo, aortic arch; LV, left ventricle.

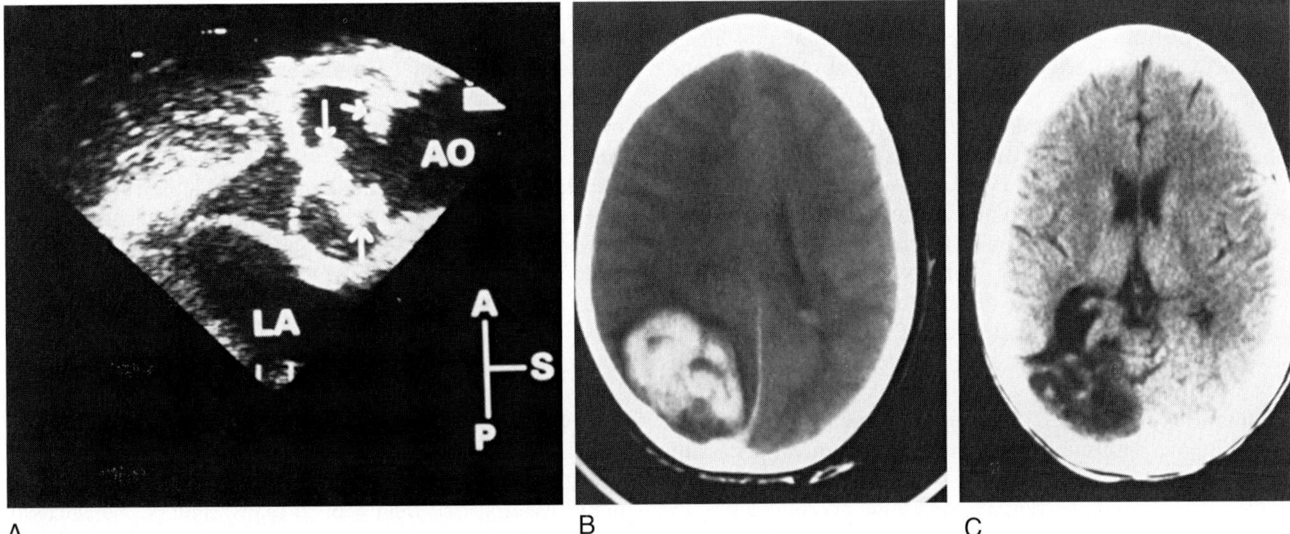

FIGURE 88-9. Cerebral hemorrhagic infarction in a 16-year-old boy with bacterial endocarditis. **A,** Echocardiogram of the aortic (AO) root demonstrates vegetations on the aortic valve leaflets *(arrows)*. LA, left atrium. **B,** Computed tomography (CT) of the brain shows large area of hemorrhage in the right occipitoparietal region several days after the development of seizures. **C,** Follow-up CT of the brain 3 months later shows a large residual area of encephalomalacia in the right occipitoparietal region.

[Pruitt et al., 1978]. Cerebrovascular lesions are at particular risk for bleeding when mediated by infected emboli, whether into an infarct or through a mycotic aneurysm. For these reasons, anticoagulant therapy is contraindicated in children with infective endocarditis who develop neurologic symptoms [Pruitt et al., 1978].

CEREBRAL MYCOTIC ANEURYSMS

Cerebral mycotic aneurysms are an infrequent but often lethal complication of infective endocarditis. Although mycotic aneurysms complicate only 1.2% to 5% of cases of infective endocarditis, the overall mortality of this lesion approaches 60% [Bohmfalk et al., 1978]. Two thirds of cerebral mycotic aneurysms occur at the more distal bifurcations, particularly the middle cerebral artery. The remaining aneurysms are more centrally located at the branches of the circle of Willis [Corr et al., 1995]. Angiographic studies have determined that multiple aneurysms are present in approximately 30% of patients [Corr et al., 1995]. The clinical presentation is highly variable, with features ranging from those of sudden catastrophic hemorrhage (Fig. 88-9), a mass lesion, or an embolic lesion. Presentation and outcome depend primarily on the location and integrity of the aneurysm. The mortality rate for patients with intact aneurysms is about 30%, and it increases to 90% if the aneurysm ruptures [Bohmfalk et al., 1978; Jones and Sieker, 1989]. Aneurysms that leak rather than rupture are associated with a sterile meningeal syndrome with elevations of spinal fluid protein and of red and white blood cell counts.

Mycotic aneurysms should be excluded in all cases of infective endocarditis complicated by severe headaches, "sterile" meningitis, strokelike events, or cranial nerve abnormalities. The screening technique of choice is high-resolution, contrast-enhanced CT, because it is capable of identifying the presence of cerebral hemorrhage and the location of mycotic aneurysms. The definitive diagnostic test remains four-vessel angiography. Current MR angiography techniques remain insensitive to aneurysms smaller than 5 mm [Huston et al., 1994].

Management of mycotic aneurysms is complex and includes medical and surgical approaches [D'Angelo et al., 1995; Elowiz et al., 1995; Utoh et al., 1995]. A 6-week course of antimicrobial therapy directed at the organism responsible for the underlying endocarditis should be completed. Hereafter, follow-up angiography is indicated to assess the response to treatment and to detect enlarging or new aneurysms [Corr et al., 1995]. Subsequent treatment is based on these angiographic findings. When angiograms are repeated after a full course of appropriate antimicrobial therapy, complete resolution of the aneurysms is seen in 33% to 50%, whereas 17% to 30% exhibit a decrease in size [Bingham, 1977; Corr et al., 1995]. In 17%, there is no change in size [Corr et al., 1995]; in 20%, the aneurysms enlarge [Bingham, 1977]. Despite a full course of treatment, new aneurysms may develop in up to 10% of cases [Bingham, 1977]. Up to 50% of patients have full clinical recovery of their neurologic deficits after a 6-week course of treatment [Corr et al., 1995].

Indications for surgical intervention remain controversial [Wilson et al., 1982] but include the presence of single or multiple aneurysms distal to the first middle cerebral artery bifurcation that persist, enlarge, or bleed despite appropriate antibiotic therapy [Corr et al., 1995; Scotti et al., 1996]. The usual surgical approach to these aneurysms is direct excision or clip application, but endovascular procedures [Scotti et al., 1996] have been used to manage selected, severe cases of deep or distal mycotic aneurysms.

BRAIN ABSCESS

Brain abscess is a rare condition in childhood [Ghosh et al., 1988]. However, among children diagnosed with brain abscess, almost one half had congenital heart disease [Aebi et al., 1991]. In children with congenital heart disease, brain abscess is rare before the age of 2 years, with a peak incidence between 4 and 7 years of age [Kagawa et al., 1983]. The risk is highest in cyanotic congenital heart disease; earlier studies reported that brain abscess develops in 2% to 6% of patients [Shu-yuan, 1989]. The risk for brain abscess is highest in children with polycythemia and right-to-left shunts [Tyler and Clark, 1957a], particularly tetralogy of Fallot [Aebi et al., 1991]. The incidence, morbidity, and mortality rates of brain abscess in congenital heart disease are inversely correlated with circulating arterial oxygenation [Shu-yuan, 1989]. Infants with higher oxygen saturations are less likely to develop brain abscess and more likely to recover. During periods of systemic illness and dehydration, polycythemia may critically disturb cerebral microvascular perfusion, with subsequent localized areas of ischemia. A right-to-left shunt allows organisms to bypass the pulmonary filtration system and to gain direct access to the brain. In areas of necrosis, organisms breach the disrupted blood-brain barrier, passing into necrotic areas to form focal septic cerebritis that may evolve to frank cerebral abscess. The recent marked decrease in incidence of brain abscess among children with congenital heart disease likely results from a number of factors, including earlier corrective surgery, decreased exposure to polycythemia and hypoxia, and more aggressive rehydration.

Clinical manifestations of brain abscess are determined by the degree of intracranial hypertension, focal neurologic injury, and sepsis. The location of the abscess influences the neurologic presentation. Seventy-five percent of brain abscesses are supratentorial. Posterior fossa abscesses are less common but more dangerous because they often remain clinically silent until the onset of rapid deterioration from tonsillar herniation and brainstem compression (Fig. 88-10). Cerebral abscesses are multifocal in about 20% of patients.

The manifestation of brain abscess is usually subtle, with the exception of seizures, and the course is slowly progressive. The most common presenting features are headache and vomiting [Aicardi, 1992a]. Up to 75% of patients are afebrile and have minimal peripheral leukocytosis. Diagnosis of brain abscess is best established by contrast-enhanced CT or MRI scan. On CT, brain abscess appears as an area of hypodensity with contrast ring enhancement. The lesion is often surrounded by marked cerebral edema. After brain imaging has excluded significant mass effect, cerebrospinal fluid should be obtained. Typically, results suggest elevated levels of protein but only mild leukocytosis (see Chapter 68).

Optimal management of brain abscess remains controversial [Dodge and Pomeroy, 1992]. Surgery by direct resection or CT-guided aspiration is still considered the definitive first-line treatment in many centers. Advances in antibiotic therapy and neuroimaging surveillance have allowed a more conservative approach [Berg et al., 1978; Rosenblum et al., 1980]. This approach remains controversial, but it may prove effective in early cases of focal cerebritis without rapid progression. Whether combined with surgery or not, high-dose antibiotic therapy should be maintained for at least 6 weeks.

Initial antimicrobial management should be directed at the most common causative organisms (i.e., mixed aerobic and anaerobic streptococci and staphylococci) [Ghosh et al., 1988]. Third-generation cephalosporins used in combination with anti-staphylococcal and anaerobic agents have largely superseded earlier antibiotic regimens. Subsequent

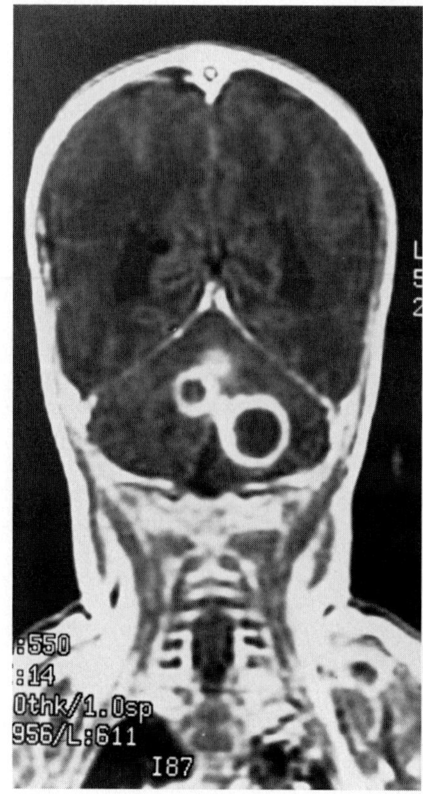

A

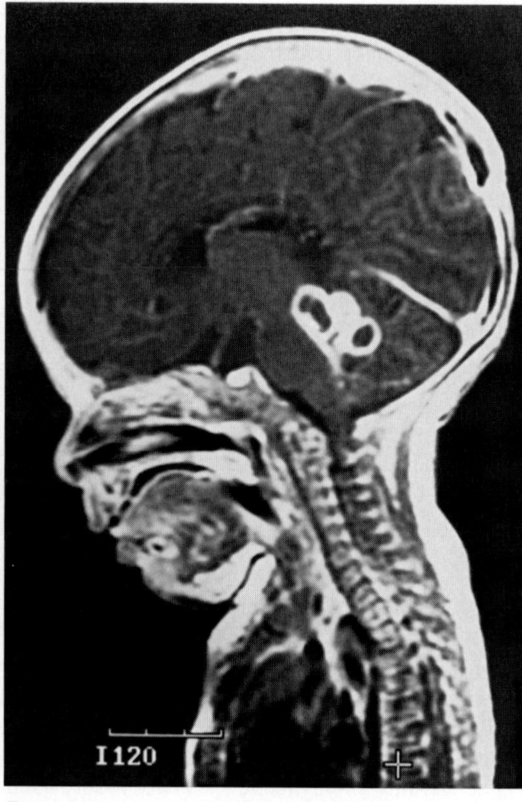

B

FIGURE 88-10. T1-weighted magnetic resonance imaging reveals multiple brain abscesses in the cerebellum and fourth ventricle of an infant with cyanotic congenital heart disease. **A,** Coronal view. **B,** Sagittal view.

antibiotic treatment should be guided by microbial culture results. In immunosuppressed patients (e.g., after cardiac transplantation), other lower-virulence organisms, fungi (e.g., *Aspergillus*), and parasites (e.g., *Toxoplasma*) should be considered. Because the clinical presentation of brain abscess may closely resemble stroke in up to 30% of patients [Kurlan and Griggs, 1983], it has been suggested that children with cyanotic congenital heart disease and a strokelike presentation should be managed with antibiotic therapy until a brain abscess is excluded [Kurlan and Griggs, 1983].

Diagnostic and therapeutic advances have reduced the mortality of brain abscess from 40% [Kagawa et al., 1983] to 10% [Dodge and Pomeroy, 1992]. However, in survivors, the prevalence of neurologic sequelae has remained largely unchanged at about 35% to 45% [Aebi et al., 1991; Dodge and Pomeroy, 1992]. Epilepsy may develop, often years later, in up to 30% of survivors [Aebi et al., 1991].

Inherited Disorders of Heart, Muscle, and Nervous System

Combined cardiac and neurologic dysfunction may develop in certain inherited disorders of metabolism and neuromuscular disorders. Certain chromosomal disorders may have prominent cardiac and nervous system malformations. This discussion is confined to the more common of these rare syndromes. Diagnostic and therapeutic approaches to these conditions are discussed in more detail elsewhere in this textbook.

Inborn Errors of Metabolism

Cardiac dysfunction may be a prominent feature, and it is often the cause of death of patients with several inherited metabolic disorders [Lyon et al., 1996]. The inheritance of these conditions is usually recessive (autosomal, rarely X-linked) or mitochondrial. The cardiac dysfunction results from a hypertrophic or dilated cardiomyopathy resulting from myocardial infiltration or energy failure rather than from a primary structural lesion. The cardiac involvement in these conditions manifests clinically with myocardial failure, valvular insufficiency, dysrhythmias, or coronary insufficiency (in storage disorders) with myocardial ischemia. Neurologic manifestations may be due primarily to the underlying enzyme defect, or it may result from global or focal cerebral hypoperfusion caused by diminished cardiac output.

Disorders of Energy Production

MITOCHONDRIAL FATTY ACID OXIDATION DEFECTS

Conditions caused by mitochondrial fatty acid oxidation defects include a group of autosomal recessive disorders that may manifest with combined cardiac and neurologic dysfunction (see Chapters 23 and 28). These conditions manifest with several clinical syndromes, including recurrent metabolic crises, depressed mental status, and ataxia. Primary systemic carnitine deficiency results from a defect in carnitine transport, and it is the only disorder of carnitine metabolism with prominent cardiomyopathic features. Children with long-chain acyl-CoA dehydrogenase (LCAD) deficiency commonly develop a hypertrophic or dilated cardiomyopathy owing to myocardial fat deposition. Infants with the neonatal-onset form of multiple acyl-CoA dehydrogenase deficiency (glutaric aciduria type II) may present with dysmorphic features, a "sweaty feet" odor, and a severe, often catastrophic illness within the first days of life. Neuronal loss and gliosis lead to caudate and putaminal atrophy [Chow et al., 1989], with a prominent ataxic and dyskinetic syndrome. The cardiomyopathy in this condition is severe and usually lethal within weeks to months.

DISORDERS OF OXIDATIVE PHOSPHORYLATION

Disorders of oxidative phosphorylation result from enzyme defects in pyruvate metabolism and the mitochondrial electron transport chain. Brain and muscle are the most commonly involved systems. Cardiac dysfunction may be prominent, with the presenting features related to the age at onset. In young infants, a rapidly progressive and usually fatal hypertrophic cardiomyopathy develops, whereas older patients with later-onset cardiac involvement are more likely to develop dysrhythmias and conduction defects [Guenthard et al., 1995]. Patients with certain respiratory chain enzyme defects, such as complex I (i.e., NADH CoQ reductase) [Rustin et al., 1994] and complex IV (i.e., cytochrome *c* oxidase) [Zeviani and Van Dyke, 1986] deficiencies (often in combination) [Nagai et al., 1993] are more prone to cardiac dysfunction. Complex III (i.e., reduced CoQ-cytochrome *c* reductase) deficiency may cause an isolated cardiomyopathy. Cytochrome *c* oxidase deficiency may manifest in the newborn or young infant as a severe, rapidly fatal condition or as a benign, reversible form. Initially, the benign form may be indistinguishable from the lethal form; the lactic acidemia may be more severe in the benign form [DiMauro et al., 1990]. Because infants with the benign form may recover fully with supportive management, an aggressive approach is warranted until the clinical distinction becomes evident. Kearns-Sayre syndrome usually is associated with complex I or IV deficiencies, and it causes retinal degeneration and chronic progressive external ophthalmoplegia. Cardiac involvement results in atrioventricular heart block, with syncopal spells or sudden death occurring between late childhood and adulthood.

Storage Disorders of the Heart and Nervous System

GLYCOGEN STORAGE DISEASES

Among the different forms of glycogen storage disease, combined cardiac and neurologic dysfunction is largely confined to the early-infantile form of type II glycogen storage disease caused by acid maltase (acid α-glucosidase) deficiency (see Chapter 25). Later-onset type II glycogen storage disease manifesting after age 2 years is not associated with cardiac dysfunction. Glycogen deposition in the early-infantile form causes macroglossia, a hypertrophic cardiomyopathy, and a rapidly progressive diffuse skeletal myopathy. In the nervous system, glycogen deposition is confined to the anterior horn cells of the spinal cord and brainstem [Martin et al., 1973], sparing cerebral cortical neurons.

The progressive obstructive cardiomyopathy and respiratory weakness caused by myopathy and anterior horn cell involvement usually culminate in cardiorespiratory death before 1 year of age.

LYSOSOMAL STORAGE DISEASES

Lysosomal storage diseases are slowly progressive conditions in which the clinical manifestations of hypertrophic or dilated cardiomyopathy are delayed until well after the typical features (e.g., coarse facial features, hepatomegaly, corneal clouding) and neurodegeneration are established. Patients with the mucopolysaccharidoses may develop myocardial thickening, valvular dysfunction, coronary insufficiency, and pulmonary hypertension. Refsum's disease results from a deficiency of phytanic acid oxidase with abnormal storage of phytanic acid. Cardiac dysfunction is confined to a later-onset form of Refsum's disease and manifests with atrioventricular conduction defects and bundle branch block, progressive cardiac failure, and sudden death. Cardiac complications tend to develop late, after the typical features of retinitis pigmentosa, peripheral polyneuropathy, cerebellar ataxia, and sensorineural deafness are established.

Inherited Neuromuscular Disorders with Cardiac Complications

X-LINKED MUSCULAR DYSTROPHIES

The dystrophinopathies of Duchenne and Becker may be complicated by a dilated cardiomyopathy that usually manifests years after the skeletal muscle syndrome becomes established. Severe and rapidly progressive cardiac deterioration may occur in Duchenne's dystrophy because of papillary muscle dysfunction with subsequent valvular (particularly mitral) incompetence, cardiac (mainly atrial) dysrhythmias, and myocardial fibrosis. Another X-linked condition, Emery-Dreifuss muscular dystrophy, manifests with slowly progressive humeral-peroneal muscle weakness and wasting with prominent, early contractures. Cardiac dysfunction caused by atrial flutter, fibrillation, and permanent atrial inexcitability is a frequent cause of death that may be prevented by cardiac pacing.

MYOTONIC DYSTROPHY

Myotonic dystrophy is an autosomal-dominant condition that involves multiple tissues, including skeletal, smooth, and cardiac muscle. Although myocardial dystrophy is usually mild in this condition, severe cardiac conduction defects may develop, causing dysrhythmias and heart block.

FRIEDREICH'S ATAXIA

Friedreich's ataxia is an autosomal recessive disorder caused by a GAA trinucleotide repeat expansion in the *FXN* gene encoding the protein frataxin, which is involved in mitochondrial iron metabolism [Durr et al., 1996]. The frataxin deficiency seen in Friedreich's ataxia causes mitochondrial iron accumulation, resulting in toxic free radical generation and oxidative cellular injury. Years after their neurologic diagnosis is established, patients with Friedreich's ataxia frequently develop a hypertrophic cardiomyopathy, which may progress to a hypokinetic dilated cardiomyopathy, which carries a particularly poor prognosis. Pathologic Q waves on electrocardiography may identify patients who are more likely to develop the hypokinetic dilated cardiomyopathy [Casazza and Morpurgo, 1996]. Clinical trials of the free radical scavenger idebenone have demonstrated modest improvement in the cardiomyopathy but no improvement in neurologic function [Buyse et al., 2003; Mariotti et al., 2003].

Chromosomal Disorders Involving the Heart and Brain

Combined structural cardiac defects and cerebral dysgenesis may be prominent in certain chromosomal disorders. Approximately 40% of children with trisomy 21 have congenital heart disease, typically endocardial cushion defects. The most common cardiac lesions in trisomies 13 and 18 are ventricular septal defects and patent ductus arteriosus.

A spectrum of chromosome 22 deletion syndromes [Morrow et al., 1995] has been delineated. The phenotypic similarities have led to the acronym CATCH-22 spectrum (i.e., *c*ardiac defect, *a*bnormal facies, *t*hymic hypoplasia, *c*left palate, *h*ypocalcemia, chromosome 22q11 deletions) [Demczuk et al., 1995; Driscoll, 1994; Lindsay et al., 1995; Morrow et al., 1995; Shprintzen et al., 1992]. This spectrum includes the DiGeorge syndrome and velocardiofacial (Shprintzen's) syndrome, both of which may manifest initially with hypocalcemic seizures and subsequently manifest neurologic or cognitive disturbances [Moss et al., 1995]. A second genetic locus for DiGeorge syndrome and velocardiofacial syndrome *(DGS2)* has been identified on chromosome 10p [Bartsch et al., 2003; Daw et al., 1996].

The most common cardiac defects in DiGeorge syndrome are interrupted aortic arch type B, truncus arteriosus, and tetralogy of Fallot. Features typical of the velocardiofacial syndrome include cleft palate or velopharyngeal insufficiency and a typical facial appearance (Fig. 88-11), with a broad, prominent nose and retrognathia. Ventricular septal defects and tetralogy of Fallot are the most common structural defects in the velocardiofacial syndrome, and developmental brain lesions include a small posterior fossa and vermis and small cystic lesions adjacent to the frontal horns of the lateral ventricle. Developmental and learning disabilities are conspicuous features of the velocardiofacial syndrome. The mean IQ is 70, with a marked discrepancy between verbal and performance IQ [Moss et al., 1995]. Hearing and speech impairment is often striking. During childhood, a peculiar and inappropriately blunt affect emerges [Golding-Kushner et al., 1985], and adults with this syndrome appear at increased risk for psychotic illness [Pulver et al., 1994; Shprintzen et al., 1992].

The most common cardiac lesions seen in patients with Williams' syndrome are supravalvar aortic stenosis, peripheral pulmonary stenosis, and ventricular or atrial septal defects. These patients are prone to neurologic dysfunction [Ardinger et al., 1994; Chapman et al., 1995; Kaplan, 1995; Soper et al., 1995] and usually have obvious cognitive impairment; the average IQ is approximately 55. This impairment is further compounded by learning and social disabilities. Gross motor, fine motor, and oromotor dysfunctions are common, as are visuospatial and constructional difficulties [Chapman et al., 1995]. Children with Williams' syndrome may present with stroke because of an intracranial

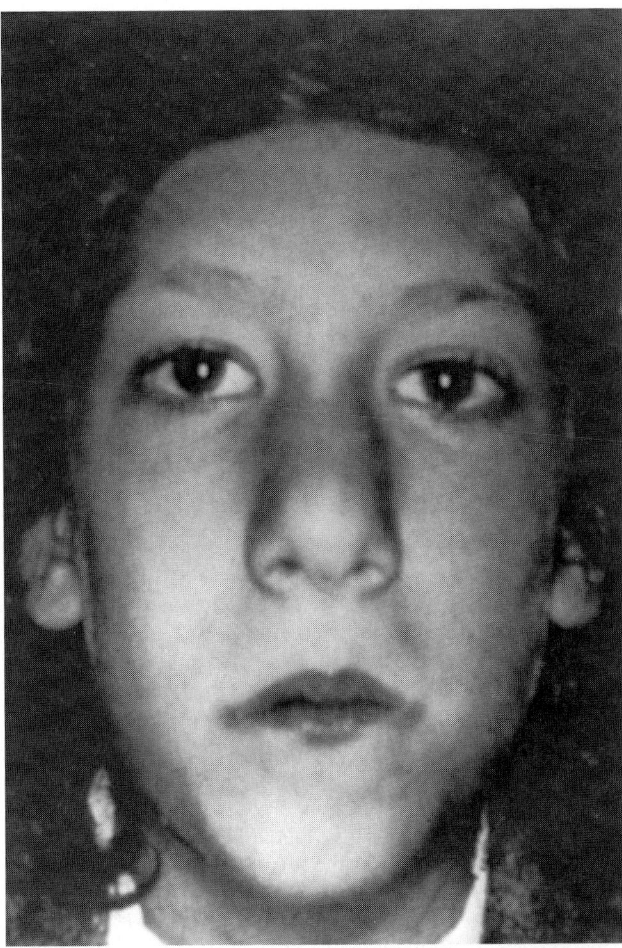

FIGURE 88-11. Facial features of a female with velocardiofacial syndrome include the typical elongated face and broad nasal bridge. (From Jones KL, ed. Smith's recognizable patterns of human malformation, 4th ed. Philadelphia: WB Saunders, 1988:225.)

arteriopathy [Ardinger et al., 1994; Kaplan, 1995; Soper et al., 1995].

Acquired Heart Disease

Acquired heart disease in children for the most part has an infectious or para-infectious origin. Among the more common forms of infectious cardiac disease associated with neurologic dysfunction are viral myocarditis and rheumatic carditis, both of which predispose patients to the generation of emboli and focal cerebral ischemia. In viral myocarditis, ventricular dilation and hypokinesia predispose to thrombus and embolus formation. In rheumatic carditis with valvular disease, bland emboli from vegetations and septic emboli from secondary infective endocarditis may compromise the cerebral circulation. Because these complications were discussed earlier, this section focuses on the other major neurologic complication of rheumatic fever: Sydenham's chorea.

Rheumatic Heart Disease

Sydenham's chorea, the major neurologic complication of acute rheumatic fever [Special Writing Group, 1992], was in earlier years the most common form of acquired chorea in childhood [Eschel et al., 1993]. For several decades, there has been a global decline in the incidence of rheumatic fever and in the incidence of chorea as a complication of rheumatic fever [Eschel et al., 1993]. Possible reasons for this decline are an alteration in the virulence or epitopes of rheumatogenic streptococci and a decrease in antigen cross-reactivity with the basal ganglia. However, outbreaks of rheumatic fever in the United States [Ayoub, 1992] and elsewhere [Karademir et al., 1994] have again focused attention on this condition.

Chorea complicates rheumatic fever in only 10% to 25% of patients [Eschel et al., 1993]. Chorea may emerge 1 week to 8 months after the onset of rheumatic fever and then persist for 1 to 6 months [Eschel et al., 1993]. Sydenham's chorea is rare in children younger than 3 years, and it occurs more commonly in females than in males. In some patients, chorea may be the only clinical manifestation of rheumatic fever. The onset of this disorder is often subtle, and the abnormal movements tend to be preceded by psychologic-emotional symptoms such as anxiety, emotional lability, distractibility, the emergence or exacerbation of attention-deficit–hyperactivity disorder, obsessive-compulsive symptoms, and sleep disturbances [Swedo, 1994; Swedo and Kiessling, 1994]. Occasionally, the onset of psychologic-emotional prodrome and dyskinesia may be explosive. The motor activity that at first is described as "fidgety" soon becomes choreiform, evolving from initial brief, myoclonic-like proximal muscle jerks to more complex and writhing distal movements. The handgrip often has a rippling character due to inconsistently sustained finger pressure (i.e., milkmaid's grip). The chorea may be asymmetric, and in some cases, pure hemichorea develops. Muscle hypotonia and mild-to-moderate weakness are often present. Patients may have difficulty initiating and sustaining spontaneous motor activity. Speech and oral motor activity are often affected; an explosive dysarthria may develop, evolving in severe cases to complete mutism. These symptoms usually begin to subside after about 2 to 6 months, but they may recur in the setting of subsequent illnesses, particularly streptococcal infections, pregnancy (i.e., chorea gravidarum), or oral contraceptive use.

The diagnosis of acute rheumatic fever is based on specific (Jones) criteria [Special Writing Group, 1992], which may be major or minor, depending on their diagnostic importance. A patient with two major criteria or with one major and two minor criteria has a high probability of having rheumatic fever. The major criteria are carditis, polyarthritis, chorea, erythema marginatum, and subcutaneous nodules. The minor criteria are based on clinical features (e.g., fever, arthralgia, previous rheumatic fever) or laboratory features (e.g., acute-phase reaction, elevated erythrocyte sedimentation rate, leukocytosis, C-reactive protein, prolonged PR interval on electrocardiogram). Additional laboratory findings, such as an elevated anti-streptolysin O titer or positive throat cultures for group A β-hemolytic streptococci, may be helpful. The diagnosis of chorea is purely clinical. Despite the causal relationship to streptococcal infection, the onset of chorea is often delayed. Consequently, serologic evidence of streptococcal disease may be absent in 25% of patients. Rheumatogenic strains of group A streptococci contain particular (M-type) proteins that share antigenic determinants with neurons in the basal ganglia, particularly in the caudate and subthalamic nuclei. Autoantibodies against these neurons (i.e., antineuronal antibodies) have been detected in up to 90% of patients in some studies [Swedo, 1994; Swedo et al., 1997].

Because this condition is seldom fatal, neuropathologic data are limited. However, neuronal loss with vascular and perivascular inflammatory changes has been described in the caudate, putamen, and frontoparietal cortex. The topography of these earlier neuropathologic findings has been supported by MRI [Giedd et al., 1995; Heye et al., 1993] and SPECT [Heye et al., 1993]. These techniques have also demonstrated disturbances in the blood-brain barrier with localized edema, presumably resulting from vasculitis [Heye et al., 1993].

Current management of the chorea includes dopamine-blocking agents such as haloperidol, given as 0.5 to 1 mg twice daily for 2 to 6 months and then gradually withdrawn. Other agents used include carbamazepine and valproic acid [Aicardi, 1992b; Swedo et al., 1993]. These drugs often diminish the intensity of the chorea, but they fail to completely control it. In severe cases, prednisone has been used with limited success. Prophylaxis against group A streptococcal infections with penicillin or monthly intramuscular benzathine penicillin is recommended because even asymptomatic future infections may precipitate recurrence of chorea. The high incidence of antineuronal antibodies [Swedo, 1994; Swedo and Kiessling, 1994] and anticardiolipin antibodies [Diniz et al., 1994; Figueroa et al., 1992] in these patients has led to trials of plasmapheresis and intravenous immunoglobulin therapy; results from these studies are not yet available.

Extracorporeal Membrane Oxygenation

Extracorporeal membrane oxygenation has been used for some time in tertiary centers to support children with severe respiratory failure. More recently, extracorporeal membrane oxygenation has been used to support children with severe cardiac failure due to congenital or acquired heart disease. The short-term benefit of extracorporeal membrane oxygenation is well demonstrated, with multicenter reports of 83% survival rates among infants with a predicted mortality rate of greater than 80% [Stolar et al., 1991]. Extracorporeal membrane oxygenation may be performed through a veno-venous or, more commonly, a veno-arterial circuit. Veno-venous extracorporeal membrane oxygenation provides oxygenation for respiratory failure, whereas veno-arterial extracorporeal membrane oxygenation provides oxygenation and circulatory support for cardiac failure. In both veno-venous and veno-arterial circuits, venous blood is drained from the right atrium through a catheter placed in the right internal jugular vein. After oxygenation, removal of carbon dioxide, and rewarming, the blood is pumped by a nonpulsatile flow into the right atrium through the second lumen of a double-lumen catheter (i.e., veno-venous circuit) or to the aortic arch through a catheter in the right common carotid artery (i.e., veno-arterial circuit). Systemic heparinization is required to prevent clotting in the extracorporeal membrane oxygenation circuit. The rostral segments of the cannulated vessels (i.e., jugular vein and, in veno-arterial extracorporeal membrane oxygenation, the right common carotid) are ligated as part of the procedure. The right common carotid artery has been reconstructed after termination of extracorporeal membrane oxygenation.

Indications

Extracorporeal membrane oxygenation is indicated for pulmonary failure that is refractory to treatment but potentially reversible (e.g., meconium aspiration syndrome, congenital diaphragmatic hernia, persistent pulmonary hypertension, sepsis, respiratory distress syndrome), for potentially reversible cardiac disease (e.g., cardiomyopathy), because of an inability to wean off cardiopulmonary bypass after cardiac surgery, and as a bridge to cardiac transplantation.

Contraindications

Absolute contraindications to extracorporeal membrane oxygenation include gestational age of less than 34 weeks (because of excessive morbidity and mortality related to intracranial hemorrhage), birth weight less than 2000 grams (because of limitations of cannula size), any uncontrollable coagulopathy or bleeding, and a preexisting grade III intraventricular hemorrhage or periventricular hemorrhagic infarction. Relative contraindications include preexisting grade I or II intraventricular hemorrhage, other intracranial hemorrhage, cerebral infarction, and sepsis, which increases the risk for intracranial hemorrhage [Cilley et al., 1986; Kim and Stolar, 2000; Sell et al., 1986].

Mechanisms of Neurologic Injury

Extracorporeal membrane oxygenation may injure the brain through multiple mechanisms that promote ischemic or hemorrhagic injury. Carotid ligation causes an immediate reduction in blood flow to the ipsilateral middle cerebral artery, which may be only partially restored by collateral flow from the anterior communicating artery, from the posterior circulation through circle of Willis, and from the external carotid artery. This reduced flow may cause direct ischemia, and it may interfere with cerebral autoregulation, rendering that hemisphere vulnerable to systemic hypotension. Jugular vein ligation can result in cerebral venous hypertension, which may predispose to venous infarction. Systemic heparinization increases the risk of intracranial hemorrhage, which may be primary or result from hemorrhagic transformation of an ischemic lesion. Extracorporeal membrane oxygenation causes elevated levels of inflammatory cytokines, which may contribute to the development of periventricular leukomalacia [Fortenberry et al., 1996; Kinney and Back, 1998].

Neurologic Complications

Intracranial hemorrhage and infarction are the primary neurologic complications of extracorporeal membrane oxygenation. The overall risk of hemorrhage or infarction is between 25% and 50%, whereas 10% to 20% of infants experience severe hemorrhage or infarction [Volpe, 2001]. The most common sites of hemorrhage are intraventricular and posterior fossa. Cerebral ischemia may be global or focal, or it may manifest as periventricular leukomalacia [Jarjour and Ahdab-Barmada, 1994; Kinney and Back, 1998]. Clinical and electrographic seizures are common among neonates treated with extracorporeal membrane oxygenation, with a reported incidence of 20% to 70% [Kim and Stolar, 2000]. However, the risk for subsequent epilepsy is low. Sensorineural hearing impairment is reported in 4% to 15% of neonates after extracorporeal membrane oxygenation, but many of these deficits resolve over time [Desai et al., 1997; Hofkosh et al., 1991; Schumacher et al., 1991]. Reports of neurocognitive outcome after extracorporeal membrane oxygenation indicate that 10% to 29% of extracorporeal membrane oxygenation neonates have developmental quotients less than 70, with smaller infants at the greatest risk for developmental delays [Hamrick et al., 2003; Revenis et al., 1992].

REFERENCES

Aebi C, Kaufmann F, Schaad U. Brain abscess in childhood: Long-term experiences. Eur J Pediatr 1991;150:282.

Aicardi J. Postnatally acquired infectious diseases. In: Aicardi J. Diseases of the nervous system in childhood, Vol. 115/118. London: MacKeith Press, 1992a:590.

Aicardi J. Para-infectious and other inflammatory disorders of immunological origin. In: Aicardi J. Diseases of the nervous system in childhood, Vol. 115/118. London: MacKeith Press, 1992b:697.

Al-Lozi M, Pestronk A, Yee W, et al. Rapidly evolving myopathy with myosin-deficient muscle fibers. Ann Neurol 1994;35:273.

Ammash N, Warnes C. Cerebrovascular events in adult patients with cyanotic congenital heart disease. J Am Coll Cardiol 1996;28:768.

Anderson D. Cardioembolic stroke: Primary and secondary prevention. Postgrad Med 1991;90:67.

Anderson RV, Siegman MG, Balaban RS, et al. Hyperglycemia increases cerebral intracellular acidosis during circulatory arrest. Ann Thorac Surg 1992;54:1126.

Andre M, Matisse N, Vert P. Prognosis of neonatal seizures. In: Wasterlain CG, Vert P, eds. Neonatal seizures. New York: Raven Press, 1990:61.

Ardinger R, Goertz K, Matteoli L. Cerebrovascular stenosis with cerebral infarction in a child with Williams syndrome. Am J Med Genet 1994;51:200.

Ayoub E. Resurgence of rheumatic fever in the United States. Postgrad Med 1992;92:133.

Bando K, Turrentine MW, Vijay P, et al. Effect of modified ultrafiltration in high-risk patients undergoing operations for congenital heart disease. Ann Thorac Surg 1998;66:821.

Barrat-Boyes B. Choreoathetosis as a complication of cardiopulmonary bypass. Ann Thorac Surg 1990;50:693.

Bartsch O, Nemeckova M, Kocarek E, et al. DiGeorge/velocardiofacial syndrome: FISH studies of chromosomes 22q11 and 10p14, and clinical reports on the proximal 22q11 deletion. Am J Med Genet 2003;117A:1.

Bellinger DC, Jonas RA, Rappaport LA, et al. Developmental and neurologic status of children after heart surgery with hypothermic circulatory arrest or low-flow cardiopulmonary bypass. N Engl J Med 1995;332:549.

Bellinger DC, Rappaport LA, Wypij D, et al. Patterns of developmental dysfunction after surgery during infancy to correct transposition of the great arteries. J Dev Behav Pediatr 1997;18:75.

Bellinger DC, Wypij D, du Plessis AJ, et al. Neurodevelopmental status at eight years in children with dextro-transposition of the great arteries: The Boston Circulatory Arrest Trial. J Thorac Cardiovasc Surg 2003;126:1385.

Bellinger DC, Wypij D, Kuban KC, et al. Developmental and neurological status of children at 4 years of age after heart surgery with hypothermic circulatory arrest or low-flow cardiopulmonary bypass. Circulation 1999;100:526.

Benson D. Changing profile of congenital heart disease. Pediatrics 1989;83:790.

Berg B, Franklin G, Cuneo R, et al. Nonsurgical cure of brain abscess: Early diagnosis and follow-up with computerized tomography. Ann Neurol 1978;3:474.

Bergman I, Painter M, Hirsch R, et al. Outcome in neonates with convulsions treated in an intensive care unit. Ann Neurol 1983;14:642.

Bergman I, Steeves M, Burckart G, et al. Reversible neurologic abnormalities associated with prolonged intravenous midazolam and fentanyl administration. J Pediatr 1991;119:644.

Bergouignan M, Fontan F, Trarieux M. Syndromes choreiformes de l'enfant au décours d'interventions cardio-chirurgicales sous hypothermic profounde. Rev Neurol 1961;105:48.

Berthrong M, Sabiston D. Cerebral lesions in congenital heart disease. Bull Johns Hopkins Hosp 1951;89:384.

Bingham W. Treatment of mycotic intracranial aneurysms. J Neurosurg 1977;46:428.

Bjork V, Hultquist G. Contraindications to profound hypothermia in open-heart surgery. J Thorac Cardiovasc Surg 1962;44:1.

Bohmfalk G, Story J, Wissinger J, et al. Bacterial intracranial aneurysm. J Neurosurg 1978;48:369.

Bolton C. Clinical neurophysiology of the respiratory system. Muscle Nerve 1993;16:809.

Boyajian RA, Sobel DF, DeLaria GA, et al. Embolic stroke as a sequela of cardiopulmonary bypass. J Neuroimaging 1993;3:1.

Bozoky B, Bara D, Kertesz E. Autopsy study of cerebral complications of congenital heart disease and cardiac surgery. J Neurol 1984;3:153.

Brewer L, Fosburg R, Mulder G, et al. Spinal cord complications following surgery for coarctation of the aorta. J Thorac Cardiovasc Surg 1972;64:68.

Brunberg J, Doty D, Reilly E. Choreoathetosis in infants following cardiac surgery with deep hypothermia and circulatory arrest. J Pediatr 1974;84:232.

Buyse G, Mertens L, Di Salvo G, et al. Idebenone treatment in Friedreich's ataxia: Neurological, cardiac, and biochemical monitoring. Neurology 2003;60:1679.

Casazza F, Morpurgo M. The varying evolution of Friedreich's ataxia cardiomyopathy. Am J Cardiol 1996;77:895.

Castaneda AR, Lamberti J, Sade RM, et al. Open-heart surgery during the first three months of life. J Thorac Cardiovasc Surg 1974;68:719.

Castaneda AR, Mayer JE, Jonas RA, et al. The neonate with critical congenital heart disease: Repair—a surgical challenge. J Thorac Cardiovasc Surg 1989;98:869.

Cerebral Embolism Study Group. Immediate anticoagulation of embolic stroke: Brain hemorrhage and management options. Stroke 1984;15:779.

Cerebral Embolism Study Group. Cardioembolic stroke, immediate anticoagulation, and brain hemorrhage. Arch Intern Med 1987;147:636.

Cerebral Embolism Task Force. Cardiogenic brain embolism. The second report of the Cerebral Embolism Task Force. Arch Neurol 1989;46:727.

Chapman C, du Plessis A, Pober B. Neurologic findings in children and adults with Williams syndrome. J Child Neurol 1995;10:63.

Chaturvedi RR, Shore DF, White PA, et al. Modified ultrafiltration improves global left ventricular systolic function after open-heart surgery in infants and children. Eur J Cardiothorac Surg 1999;15:742.

Chaves E, Scaltsas-Persson I. Severe choreoathetosis (CA) following congenital heart disease (CHD) surgery [Abstract]. Neurology 1988;38:284.

Chow C, Frerman F, Goodman S, et al. Striatal degeneration in glutaric aciduria type II. Acta Neuropathol 1989;77:554.

Cilley RE, Zwischenberger JB, Andrews AF, et al. Intracranial hemorrhage during extracorporeal membrane oxygenation in neonates. Pediatrics 1986;78:699.

Clancy R, Malin S, Laraque D, et al. Focal motor seizures heralding stroke in full-term neonates. Am J Dis Child 1985;139:601.

Clancy RR, McGaurn SA, Wernovsky G, et al. Risk of seizures in survivors of newborn heart surgery using deep hypothermic circulatory arrest. Pediatrics 2003;111:592.

Coles J, Wilson G, Sima A, et al. Intraoperative management of thoracic aortic aneurysm: Experimental evaluation of perfusion cooling of the spinal cord. J Thorac Cardiovasc Surg 1983;85:292.

Colon R, Frazier O, Cooley D, et al. Hypothermic regional perfusion for protection of the spinal cord during periods of ischemia. Ann Thorac Surg 1987;43:639.

Corr P, Wright M, Handler L. Endocarditis-related cerebral aneurysms: Radiologic changes with treatment. Am J Neuroradiol 1995;16:745.

Cottrill C, Kaplan S. Cerebral vascular accidents in cyanotic congenital heart disease. Am J Dis Child 1973;125:484.

Cranford R, Leppik I, Patrick B, et al. Intravenous phenytoin: Clinical and pharmacological aspects. Neurology 1978;28:874.

Cromme-Dijkhuis A, Henkens C, Bijleveld C, et al. Coagulation factor abnormalities as possible thrombotic risk factors after Fontan operations. Lancet 1990;336:1087.

Curless RG, Katz DA, Perryman RA, et al. Choreoathetosis after surgery for congenital heart disease. J Pediatr 1994;124:737.

D'Angelo V, Fiumara E, Gorgoglione L, et al. Surgical treatment of a cerebral mycotic aneurysm using the stereo-angiographic localizer. Surg Neurol 1995;44:263.

Danon M, Carpenter S. Myopathy with thick filament (myosin) loss following prolonged paralysis with vecuronium during steroid treatment. Muscle Nerve 1991;14:1131.

Davies MJ, Nguyen K, Gaynor JW, et al. Modified ultrafiltration improves left ventricular systolic function in infants after cardiopulmonary bypass. J Thorac Cardiovasc Surg 1998;115:361.

Daw SC, Taylor C, Kraman M, et al. A common region of 10p deleted in DiGeorge and velocardiofacial syndromes. Nat Genet 1996;13:458.

Dawson D, Fischer E. Neurologic complications of cardiac catheterization procedures. Neurology 1977;27:496.

Day R, Boyer R, Tait V, et al. Factors associated with stroke following the Fontan procedure. Pediatr Cardiol 1995;16:270.

del Zoppo G. Microvascular changes during cerebral ischemia and reperfusion. Cerebrovasc Brain Metab Rev 1994;6:47.

del Zoppo G, Ferbert A, Otis S, et al. Local intra-arterial fibrinolytic therapy in acute carotid territory stroke: A pilot study. Stroke 1988;19:307.

DeLeon S, Ilbawi M, Arcilla R, et al. Choreoathetosis after deep hypothermia without circulatory arrest. Ann Thorac Surg 1990;50:714.

Demczuk S, Levy A, Aubry M, et al. Excess of deletions of maternal origin in the DiGeorge/velo-cardio-facial. A study of 22 new patients and review of the literature. Hum Genet 1995;96:9.

Desai S, Kollros PR, Graziani LJ, et al. Sensitivity and specificity of the neonatal brain-stem auditory evoked potential for hearing and language deficits in survivors of extracorporeal membrane oxygenation. J Pediatr 1997;131:233.

DiMauro S, Lombes A, Nakase H, et al. Cytochrome *c* oxidase deficiency. Pediatr Res 1990;28:536.

Diniz R, Goldenberg J, Andrade L, et al. Antiphospholipid antibodies in rheumatic fever chorea. J Rheumatol 1994;21:1367.

Dobell A, Trusler G, Smallhorn J, et al. Atrial thrombi after the Fontan operation. Ann Thorac Surg 1986;42:664.

Dodge P, Pomeroy S. Parameningeal infections (including brain abscess, epidural abscess, subdural empyema). In: Feigin R, Cherry J, eds. Textbook of pediatric infectious diseases, Vol. II. Philadelphia: WB Saunders, 1992:455.

Donaldson D, Fullerton D, Gollub R, et al. Choreoathetosis in children after cardiac surgery. Neurology 1990;40:337.

Driscoll DA. Genetic basis of DiGeorge and velocardiofacial syndromes. Curr Opin Pediatr 1994;6:702.

du Plessis AJ, Bellinger DC, Gauvreau K, et al. Neurologic outcome of choreoathetoid encephalopathy after cardiac surgery. Pediatr Neurol 2002;27:9.

du Plessis A, Chang A, Wessel D, et al. Cerebrovascular accidents following the Fontan procedure. Pediatr Neurol 1995a;12:230.

du Plessis AJ, Jonas RA, Wypij D, et al. Perioperative effects of alpha-stat versus pH-stat strategies for deep hypothermic cardiopulmonary bypass in infants. J Thorac Cardiovasc Surg 1997;114:991.

du Plessis A, Kramer U, Jonas R, et al. West syndrome following deep hypothermic cardiac surgery. Pediatr Neurol 1994a;11:246.

du Plessis AJ, Newburger J, Jonas RA, et al. Cerebral CO_2 vasoreactivity is impaired in the early postoperative period following hypothermic infant cardiac surgery. Eur J Neurol 1995b;2:68A.

du Plessis AJ, Newburger J, Jonas RA, et al. Cerebral oxygen supply and utilization during infant cardiac surgery. Ann Neurol 1995c;37:488.

du Plessis A, Treves S, Hickey P, et al. Regional cerebral perfusion abnormalities after cardiac operations. J Thorac Cardiovasc Surg 1994b;107:1036.

Dunne JW, Reutens DC, Newman M, et al. Phrenic nerve injury in open heart surgery. Muscle Nerve 1991;14:883.

Durr A, Cossee M, Agid Y, et al. Clinical and genetic abnormalities in patients with Friedreich's ataxia. N Engl J Med 1996;335:1169.

Ehyai A, Fenichel G, Bender H. Incidence and prognosis of seizures in infants after cardiac surgery with profound hypothermia and circulatory arrest. JAMA 1984;252:3165.

Elliott M. Modified ultrafiltration and open heart surgery in children. Paediatr Anaesth 1999;9:1.

Elliott M, Finn A. Interaction between neutrophils and endothelium. Ann Thorac Surg 1993;56:1503.

Elowiz E, Johnson W, Milhorat T. Computerized tomography (CT) localized stereotactic craniotomy for excision of a bacterial intracranial aneurysm. Surg Neurol 1995;44:265.

Eschel G, Lahat E, Azizi E, et al. Chorea as a manifestation of rheumatic fever: A 30 year survey (1960-1990). Eur J Pediatr 1993;152:645.

Ewart A, Morris C, Atkinson D, et al. Hemizygosity at the elastin locus in a developmental disorder, Williams syndrome. Nat Genet 1993;5:11.

Ferry PC. Neurologic sequelae of cardiac surgery in children. Am J Dis Child 1987;141:309.

Ferry PC. Neurologic sequelae of open-heart surgery in children. An "irritating question." Am J Dis Child 1990;144:369.

Feuerstein G, Liu T, Barone F. Cytokines, inflammation, and brain injury: Role of tumor necrosis factor-a. Cerebrovasc Brain Metab Rev 1994;6:341.

Figueroa F, Berrios X, Gutierrez M, et al. Anticardiolipin antibodies in acute rheumatic fever. J Rheumatol 1992;19:1175.

Fish KJ. Microembolization: Etiology and prevention. In: Hilberman M, ed. Brain injury and protection during cardiac surgery. Boston: Martinus Nijhoff, 1988:67.

Fortenberry JD, Bhardwaj V, Niemer P, et al. Neutrophil and cytokine activation with neonatal extracorporeal membrane oxygenation. J Pediatr 1996;128:670.

Francioli P. Central nervous complications of infective endocarditis. In: Scheld W, Whiteley R, Durack D, eds. Infections of the central nervous system. New York: Raven Press, 1991:515.

Gaynor JW. The effect of modified ultrafiltration on the postoperative course in patients with congenital heart disease. Semin Thorac Cardiovasc Surg Pediatr Card Surg Annu 2003;6:128.

Gerlach M, Riederer P, Youdim M. Neuroprotective therapeutic strategies: Comparison of experimental and clinical results. Biochem Pharmacol 1995;50:1.

Ghosh S, Chandy M, Abraham J. Brain abscess and congenital heart disease. J Indian Med Assoc 1988;88:312.

Giedd J, Rapoport J, Kruesi M, et al. Sydenham's chorea: Magnetic resonance imaging of the basal ganglia. Neurology 1995;45:2199.

Giroud M, Lemesle M, Gouyon J-B, et al. Cerebrovascular disease in children under 16 years of age in the city of Dijon, France: A study of incidence and clinical features from 1985 to 1993. J Clin Epidemiol 1995;48:1343.

Glauser T, Rorke L, Weinberg P, et al. Acquired neuropathologic lesions associated with the hypoplastic left heart syndrome. Pediatrics 1990a;85:991.

Glauser T, Rorke L, Weinberg P, et al. Congenital brain anomalies associated with the hypoplastic left heart syndrome. Pediatrics 1990b;85:984.

Golding-Kushner K, Weller G, Shprintzen R. Velo-cardio-facial syndrome: Language and psychological profiles. J Craniofac Genet 1985;5:259.

Gooch JL, Suchyta MR, Balbierz JM, et al. Prolonged paralysis after treatment with neuromuscular junction blocking agents. Crit Care Med 1991;19:1125.

Graham DI. Hypoxia and vascular disorders. In: Adams JH, Duchen LW, eds. Greenfield's neuropathology. New York: Oxford University Press, 1992:153.

Guenthard J, Wyler F, Fowler B, et al. Cardiomyopathy in respiratory chain disorders. Arch Dis Child 1995;72:223.

Guerit JM, Witdoeckt C, Rubay J, et al. The usefulness of the spinal and subcortical components of the posterior tibial nerve SEPs for spinal cord monitoring during aortic coarctation repair. Electroencephalogr Clin Neurophysiol 1997;104:115.

Hamrick SE, Gremmels DB, Keet CA, et al. Neurodevelopmental outcome of infants supported with extracorporeal membrane oxygenation after cardiac surgery. Pediatrics 2003;111:e671.

Hart R, Easton J. Hemorrhagic infarcts. Stroke 1986;17:586.

Hart R, Boop B, Anderson D. Oral anticoagulants and intracranial hemorrhage. Facts and hypotheses. Stroke 1995;26:1471.

Helmers SL, Wypij D, Constantinou JE, et al. Perioperative electroencephalographic seizures in infants undergoing repair of complex congenital cardiac defects. Electroencephalogr Clin Neurophysiol 1997;102:27.

Heye N, Jergas M, Hotzinger H, et al. Sydenham chorea: Clinical, EEG, MRI and SPECT findings in the early stages of the disease. J Neurol 1993;240:121.

Hirano M, Ott B, Raps E, et al. Acute quadriplegic myopathy: A complication of treatment with steroids, nondepolarizing blocking agents, or both. Neurology 1992;42:2082.

Hofkosh D, Thompson AE, Nozza RJ, et al. Ten years of extracorporeal membrane oxygenation: Neurodevelopmental outcome. Pediatrics 1991;87:549.

Huntley D, Al-Mateen M, Menkes J. Unusual dyskinesia complicating cardiopulmonary bypass surgery. Dev Med Child Neurol 1993;35:631.

Huston JI, Nichols D, Luetmer P, et al. Blinded retrospective evaluation of the sensitivity of MR angiography to known intracranial aneurysms: Importance of aneurysm size. Am J Neuroradiol 1994;15:1607.

Hutto R, Williams J, Maertens P, et al. Cerebellar infarct: Late complication of the Fontan procedure. Pediatr Neurol 1991;7:293.

Jansen NJ, van Oeveren W, Gu YJ, et al. Endotoxin release and tumor necrosis factor formation during cardiopulmonary bypass. Ann Thorac Surg 1992;54:744.

Jarjour IT, Ahdab-Barmada M. Cerebrovascular lesions in infants and children dying after extracorporeal membrane oxygenation. Pediatr Neurol 1994;10:13.

Johnston MV, Redmond JM, Gillinov AM, et al. Neuroprotective strategies in a model of selective neuronal necrosis from hypothermic circulatory arrest. In: Moskowitz MA, Caplan LR, eds. Cerebrovascular diseases. Boston: Butterworth-Heinemann, 1995:165.

Jonas RA, Wypij D, Roth SJ, et al. The influence of hemodilution on outcome after hypothermic cardiopulmonary bypass: Results of a randomized trial in infants. J Thorac Cardiovasc Surg 2003;126:1765.

Jones H, Sieker R. Neurologic manifestations of infective endocarditis. Brain 1989;122:1295.

Jones KL, ed. Smith's recognizable patterns of human malformation, 4th ed. Philadelphia: WB Saunders, 1988:225.

Jones M. Anomalies of the brain and congenital heart disease: A study of 52 necropsy cases. Pediatr Pathol 1991;11:721.

Journois D, Israel-Biet D, Pouard P, et al. High-volume, zero-balanced hemofiltration to reduce delayed inflammatory response to cardiopulmonary bypass in children. Anesthesiology 1996;85:965.

Kagawa M, Takeshita M, Yato S, et al. Brain abscess in congenital heart disease. J Neurosurg 1983;58:913.

Kaplan P. Cerebral artery stenoses in Williams syndrome cause strokes in childhood. J Pediatr 1995;126:943.

Karademir S, Demirceken F, Atalay S, et al. Acute rheumatic fever in children in the Ankara area in 1990-1992 and comparison with a previous study in 1980-1989. Acta Paediatr 1994;83:862.

Kawai M, Nishikawa T, Tanaka M, et al. An autopsied case of Williams syndrome complicated by moyamoya disease. Acta Paediatr Jpn 1993;35:63.

Kent K, Moscucci M, Gallagher S, et al. Neuropathy after cardiac catheterization: Incidence, clinical patterns, and long-term outcome. J Vasc Surg 1994;19:1008.

Kim ES, Stolar CJ. ECMO in the newborn. Am J Perinatol 2000;17:345.

Kinney HC, Back SA. Human oligodendroglial development: Relationship to periventricular leukomalacia. Semin Pediatr Neurol 1998;5:180.

Kirklin JK, Westaby S, Blackstone EH, et al. Complement and the damaging effects of cardiopulmonary bypass. J Thorac Cardiovasc Surg 1983;86:845.

Komp D, Sparrow A. Polycythemia in cyanotic heart disease—a study of altered coagulation. J Pediatr 1970;76:231.

Krull F, Latta K, Hoyer P, et al. Cerebral ultrasonography before and after cardiac surgery in infants. Pediat Cardiol 1994;15:159.

Kupsky WJ, Drozd MA, Barlow CF. Selective injury of the globus pallidus in children with post-cardiac surgery choreic syndrome. Dev Med Child Neurol 1995;37:135.

Kurlan R, Griggs R. Cyanotic congenital heart disease with suspected stroke. Should all patients receive antibiotics? Arch Neurol 1983;40:209.

Lane JC, Tennison MB, Lawless ST, et al. Movement disorder after withdrawal of fentanyl infusion. J Pediatr 1991;119:649.

Lange R, Thielmann M, Schmidt K, et al. Spinal cord protection using hypothermic cardiocirculatory arrest in extended repair of recoarctation and persistent hypoplastic aortic arch. Eur J Cardiothorac Surg 1997;11:697.

Lanska M, Lanska D, Horwitz S, et al. Presentation, clinical course and outcome of childhood stroke. Pediatr Neurol 1991;7:333.

Laschinger J, Cunningham J, Isom O, et al. Definition of the safe lower limits of aortic resection during procedures on the thoracolumbar aorta: Use of somatosensory evoked potentials. J Amer Coll Cardiol 1983;2:959.

Laschinger J, Cunningham J, Cooper M, et al. Prevention of ischemic spinal cord injury following aortic cross-clamping: Use of corticosteroids. Ann Thorac Surg 1984;38:500.

Laschinger J, Izomoto H, Kouchoukos N. Evolving concepts in prevention of spinal cord injury during operations on the descending thoracic and thoracolumbar aorta. Ann Thorac Surg 1987;44:667.

Laschinger J, Owen J, Rosenbloom M, et al. Direct noninvasive monitoring of the spinal cord motor function during thoracic aortic occlusion: Use of motor evoked potentials. J Vasc Surg 1988;7:161.

LeBlanc F, Charrette E, Dobell A, et al. Neurological complications of aortic coarctation. Can Med Assoc J 1968;99:299.

Lederman RJ, Breuer AC, Hanson MR, et al. Peripheral nervous system complications of coronary artery bypass graft surgery. Ann Neurol 1982;12:297.

Lerberg D, Hardesty R, Siewers R, et al. Coarctation of the aorta in infants and children: 25 years of experience. Ann Thorac Surg 1982;33:159.

Leviton A, Gilles F. Astrocytosis without globules in infant cerebral white matter: An epidemiologic study. J Neurol Sci 1974;22:329.

Levy SR, Abroms IF, Marshall PC, et al. Seizures and cerebral infarction in the full-term newborn. Ann Neurol 1985;17:366.

Limperopoulos C, Majnemer A, Shevell MI, et al. Neurologic status of newborns with congenital heart defects before open heart surgery. Pediatrics 1999;103:402.

Limperopoulos C, Majnemer A, Shevell MI, et al. Neurodevelopmental status of newborns and infants with congenital heart defects before and after open heart surgery. J Pediatr 2000;137:638.

Linderkamp O, Klose H, Betke K, et al. Increased blood viscosity in patients with cyanotic congenital heart disease and iron deficiency. J Pediatr 1979;95:567.

Lindsay E, Goldberg R, Jurecic V, et al. Velo-cardio-facial syndrome: Frequency and extent of 22q11 deletions. Am J Med Genet 1995;57:514.

Ling F, Bao Y. Myelopathy and multiple aneurysms associated with aortic arch interruption: Case report. Neurosurgery 1994;35:310.

Lucchesi B. Complement activation, neutrophils, and oxygen radicals in reperfusion injury. Stroke 1993;24:I 41.

Lutas E, Roberts R, Devereux R, et al. Relation between the presence of echocardiographic vegetations and the complication rate in infective endocarditis. Am Heart J 1986;112:107.

Lutterman J, Scott M, Nass R, et al. Moyamoya syndrome associated with congenital heart disease. Pediatrics 1998;101:57.

Lynch B and Rust R. Natural history and outcome of neonatal hypocalcemic and hypomagnesemic seizures. Pediatr Neurol 1994;11:23.

Lyon G, Adams R, Kolodny E. Neurology of inherited metabolic diseases of children. New York: McGraw-Hill, 1996:327.

Mahle WT, Tavani F, Zimmerman RA, et al. An MRI study of neurological injury before and after congenital heart surgery. Circulation 2002;106:I109.

Mariotti C, Solari A, Torta D, et al. Idebenone treatment in Friedreich patients: One-year-long randomized placebo-controlled trial. Neurology 2003;60:1676.

Martelle R, Linde L. Cerebrovascular accidents with the tetralogy of Fallot. Am J Dis Child 1961;101:206.

Martin JJ, De Barsy T, van Hoof F, et al. Pompe's disease: An inborn lysosomal disorder with storage of glycogen. A study of brain and striated muscle. Act Neuropathol (Berl) 1973;23:229.

Massicotte P, Adams M, Marzinotto V, et al. Low-molecular weight heparin in pediatric patients with thrombotic disease: A dose finding study. J Pediatr 1996;128:313.

Mathews K, Bale J, Clark E, et al. Cerebral infarction complicating Fontan surgery for cyanotic congenital heart disease. Pediatr Cardiol 1986;7:161.

Medlock MD, Cruse RS, Winek SJ, et al. A 10-year experience with postpump chorea. Ann Neurol 1993;34:820.

Menache CC, du Plessis AJ, Wessel DL, et al. Current incidence of acute neurologic complications after open-heart operations in children. Ann Thorac Surg 2002;73:1752.

Millar AB, Armstrong L, van der Linden J, et al. Cytokine production and hemofiltration in children undergoing cardiopulmonary bypass. Ann Thorac Surg 1993;56:1499.

Miller G, Vogel H. Structural evidence of injury or malformation in the brains of children with congenital heart disease. Semin Pediatr Neurol 1999;6:20.

Miller G, Eggli K, Contant C, et al. Postoperative neurologic complications after open heart surgery on young infants. Arch Pediatr Adolesc Med 1995;149:764.

Miller SM, McQuillen PS, Vigneron DB, et al. Preoperative brain injury in newborns with transposition of the great arteries. Ann Thorac Surg 2004;77:1698.

Mizrahi E. Neonatal seizures: Problems in diagnosis and classification. Epilepsia 1987;28:S46.

Mok Q, Ross-Russell R, Mulvey D, et al. Phrenic nerve injury in infants and children undergoing cardiac surgery. Br Heart J 1991;65:287.

Moody D, Bell M, Challa V, et al. Brain microemboli during cardiac surgery or aortography. Ann Neurol 1990;28:477.

Mori E, Tabuchi M, Yoshida T, et al. Intracarotid urokinase with thromboembolic occlusion of the middle cerebral artery. Stroke 1988;19:802.

Morrow B, Goldberg R, Carlson C, et al. Molecular definition of the 22q11 deletions in velo-cardio-facial syndrome. Am J Hum Genet 1995;56:1391.

Moss E, Wang P, McDonald-McGinn D, et al. Characteristic cognitive profile in patients with a 22q11.2 deletion: Verbal IQ exceeds nonverbal IQ. Am J Hum Genet 1995;57:A20.

Nagai T, Tuchiya Y, Taguchi Y, et al. Fatal infantile mitochondrial encephalomyopathy with complex I and IV deficiencies. Pediatr Neurol 1993;9:151.

Newburger J, Silbert A, Buckley L, et al. Cognitive function and age at repair of transposition of the great arteries in children. N Engl J Med 1984;310:1495.

Newburger JW, Jonas RA, Wernovsky G, et al. A comparison of the perioperative neurologic effects of hypothermic circulatory arrest versus low-flow cardiopulmonary bypass in infant heart surgery. N Engl J Med 1993;329:1057.

Nussmeier N, McDermott J. Macroembolization: Prevention and outcome modification. In: Hilberman M, ed. Brain injury and protection during cardiac surgery. Boston: Martinus Nijhoff, 1988:85.

Nylander W, Plunkett R, Hammon J, et al. Thiopental modification of ischemic spinal cord injury in the dog. Ann Thorac Surg 1982;33:64.

O'Hare B, Bissonnette B, Bohn D, et al. Persistent low cerebral blood flow velocity following profound hypothermic circulatory arrest in infants. Can J Anaesth 1995;42:964.

Okada Y, Yamaguchi T, Minematsu K, et al. Hemorrhagic transformation in cerebral embolism. Stroke 1989;20:598.

Orsi P, Rosa G, Liberatori G, et al. Repair of two unruptured intracranial aneurysms in the presence of coarctation of the aorta-anesthetic implications and management. J Neurosurg Anesth 1993;5:48.

Padayachee T, Parsons S, Theobold R, et al. The detection of microemboli in the middle cerebral artery during cardiopulmonary bypass: A transcranial Doppler ultrasound investigation using membrane and bubble oxygenators. Ann Thorac Surg 1987;44:298.

Partridge BL, Abrams JH, Bazemore C, et al. Prolonged neuromuscular blockade after long-term infusion of vecuronium bromide in the intensive care unit. Crit Care Med 1990;18:1177.

Pelletier L, Petersdorf R. Infective endocarditis: A review of 125 cases from the University of Washington Hospitals, 1963-1972. Medicine 1977;6:287.

Pennington D, Liberthson R, Jacobs M, et al. Critical review of experience with surgical repair of coarctation of the aorta. J Thorac Cardiovasc Surg 1979;77:217.

Pessin M, Estol C, Lafranchise F, et al. Safety of anticoagulation after hemorrhagic infarction. Neurology 1993;43:1298.

Petzinger G, Mayer SA, Przedborski S. Fentanyl-induced dyskinesias. Mov Disord 1995;10:679.

Phornphutkul C, Rosenberg A, Nadas A, et al. Cerebrovascular accidents in infants and children with cyanotic congenital heart disease. Am J Cardiol 1973;32:329.

Plum F, Posner J. Multifocal, diffuse, and metabolic brain diseases causing stupor or coma. In: Plum F, Posner JB. The diagnosis of stupor and coma. Philadelphia: FA Davis, 1985:177.

Pruitt A, Rubin R, Karchmer A, et al. Neurologic complications of bacterial endocarditis. Medicine (Baltimore) 1978;57:329.

Pulver A, Nestadt G, Goldberg R, et al. Psychotic illness in patients diagnosed with velo-cardio-facial syndrome and their relatives. J Nerv Ment Dis 1994;182:476.

Puntis J, Green S. Ischemic spinal cord injury after cardiac surgery. Arch Dis Child 1985;60:517.

Rappaport LA, Wypij D, Bellinger DC, et al. Relation of seizures after cardiac surgery in early infancy to neurodevelopmental outcome. Boston Circulatory Arrest Study Group. Circulation 1998;97:773.

Redmond J, Gillinov A, Zehr K, et al. Glutamate excitotoxicity: A mechanism of neurologic injury associated with hypothermic circulatory arrest. J Thorac Cardiovasc Surg 1994;107:776.

Revenis ME, Glass P, Short BL. Mortality and morbidity rates among lower birth weight infants (2000 to 2500 grams) treated with extracorporeal membrane oxygenation. J Pediatr 1992;121:452.

Riela A, Roach E. Etiology of stroke in children. J Child Neurol 1993;8:201.

Robertson C, Foltz R, Grossman R, et al. Protection against experimental ischemic spinal cord injury. J Neurosurg 1986;64:633.

Robinson R, Samuels M, Pohl K. Choreic syndrome after cardiac surgery. Arch Dis Child 1988;63:1466.

Rodriguez R, Austin E, Audenaert S. Postbypass effects of delayed rewarming on cerebral blood flow velocities in infants after total circulatory arrest. J Thorac Cardiovasc Surg 1995;110:1686.

Rosenblum M, Hoff J, Norman D, et al. Nonoperative treatment of brain abscess in selected high-risk patients. J Neurosurg 1980;52:217.

Rosenthal DN, Bulbul ZR, Friedman AH, et al. Thrombosis of the pulmonary artery stump after distal ligation. J Thorac Cardiovasc Surg 1995a;110:1563.

Rosenthal DN, Friedman AH, Kleinman CS, et al. Thromboembolic complications after Fontan operations. Circulation 1995b;92 (Suppl II):287.

Rosenthal GR. Prevalence of congenital heart disease. In: Garson A, Bricker JT, Fisher DJ, Neish SR. Science and practice of pediatric cardiology. Baltimore: Williams & Wilkins, 1998:1083.

Rosman P, Shands K. Hydrocephalus caused by increased intracranial venous pressure: A clinicopathological study. Ann Neurol 1978;3:445.

Rousseau S, Metral S, Lacroix C, et al. Anterior spinal artery syndrome mimicking infantile spinal muscular atrophy. Am J Perinatol 1993;10:316.

Roy P, Tajik A, Giuliani E, et al. Spectrum of echocardiographic findings in bacterial endocarditis. Circulation 1976;53:474.

Rudack D, Baumgart S, Gross G. Subependymal (grade 1) intracranial hemorrhage in neonates on extracorporeal membrane oxygenation. Clin Pediatr 1994;33:583.

Rustin P, Lebidois J, Chretien D, et al. Endomyocardial biopsies for early detection of mitochondrial disorders in hypertrophic cardiomyopathies. J Pediatr 1994;124:224.

Saalouke M, Perry L, Breckbill D, et al. Cerebrovascular abnormalities in postoperative coarctation of the aorta. Four cases demonstrating left subclavian steal on aortography. Am J Cardiol 1978;42:97.

Saiman L, Prince A, Gersony W. Pediatric infective endocarditis in the modern era. J Pediatr 1993;122:847.

Sakamoto T, Jonas RA, Stock UA, et al. Utility and limitations of near-infrared spectroscopy during cardiopulmonary bypass in a piglet model. Pediatr Res 2001;49:770.

Sakamoto T, Zurakowski D, Duebener LF, et al. Interaction of temperature with hematocrit level and pH determines safe duration of hypothermic circulatory arrest. J Thorac Cardiovasc Surg 2004;128:220.

Satur C, Jennings A, Walker D. Hypomagnesemia and fits complicating pediatric cardiac surgery. Ann Clin Biochem 1993;30:315.

Scher MS, Painter MJ. Electroencephalographic diagnosis of neonatal seizures: Issues of diagnostic accuracy, clinical correlation, and survival. In: Wasterlain C, Vert P, eds. Neonatal seizures. New York: Raven Press, 1990:15.

Schoenberg B, Mellinger J, Schoenberg D. Cerebrovascular disease in infants and children: A study of incidence, clinical features, and survival. Neurology 1978;28:763.

Schumacher RE, Palmer TW, Roloff DW, et al. Follow-up of infants treated with extracorporeal membrane oxygenation for newborn respiratory failure. Pediatrics 1991;87:451.

Scotti G, Li M, Righi C, et al. Endovascular treatment of bacterial intracranial aneurysms. Neuroradiology 1996;38:186.

Sell LL, Cullen ML, Whittlesey GC, et al. Hemorrhagic complications during extracorporeal membrane oxygenation: Prevention and treatment. J Pediatr Surg 1986;21:1087.

Shearer W, Rutman J, Weinberg W, et al. Coarctation of the aorta and cerebrovascular accident: A proposal for early corrective surgery. J Pediatr 1970;77:1004.

Sherman D, Dyken M, Fisher M, et al. Antithrombotic therapy for cerebrovascular disorders. Chest 1992;102:529S.

Sheth RD, Bolton CF. Neuromuscular complications of sepsis in children. J Child Neurol 1995;10:346.

Shprintzen R, Goldberg R, Golding-Kushner K, et al. Late-onset psychosis in the velo-cardio-facial syndrome. Am J Med Genet 1992;42:141.

Shu-yuan Y. Brain abscess associated with congenital heart disease. Surg Neurol 1989;31:129.

Sladky JT, Rorke LB. Perinatal hypoxic/ischemic spinal cord injury. Pediatr Pathol 1986;6:87.

Solis R, Kennedy P, Beall A, et al. Cardiopulmonary bypass: Microembolization and platelet aggregation. Circulation 1975;52:103.

Soper R, Chaloupka JC, Fayad PB, et al. Ischemic stroke and intracranial multifocal cerebral arteriopathy in Williams syndrome. J Pediatr 1995;126:945.

Special Writing Group of the Committee on Rheumatic Fever, Endocarditis and Kawasaki Disease of the Council on Cardiovascular Disease in the Young of the American Heart Association. Guidelines for the diagnosis of rheumatic fever. Jones criteria, 1992 update. JAMA 1992;268:2069.

Steinberg JB, Kapelanski DP, Olson JD, et al. Cytokine and complement levels in patients undergoing cardiopulmonary bypass. J Thorac Cardiovasc Surg 1993;106:1008.

Stolar CJ, Snedecor SM, Bartlett RH. Extracorporeal membrane oxygenation and neonatal respiratory failure: Experience from the extracorporeal life support organization. J Pediatr Surg 1991;26:563.

Straussberg R, Shahar E, Gat R, et al. Delayed parkinsonism associated with hypotension in a child undergoing open-heart surgery. Dev Med Child Neurol 1993;35:1007.

Subramony SH, Carpenter DE, Raju S, et al. Myopathy and prolonged neuromuscular blockade after lung transplant. Crit Care Med 1991;19:1580.

Suzuki J, Kodama N. Moyamoya disease. A review. Stroke 1983;14:104.

Swedo SE. Sydenham's chorea: A model for childhood autoimmune neuropsychiatric disorders. JAMA 1994;272:1788.

Swedo SE, Kiessling LS. Speculations on antineuronal anti-body mediated neuropsychiatric disorders. Pediatrics 1994;93:323.

Swedo SE, Leonard HL, Mittleman BB, et al. Identification of children with pediatric autoimmune neuropsychiatric disorders associated with streptococcal infections by a marker associated with rheumatic fever. Am J Psychiatry 1997;154:110.

Swedo SE, Leonard HL, Schapiro MB, et al. Sydenham's chorea: Physical and psychological symptoms of St Vitus Dance. Pediatrics 1993;91:706.

Swenson M, Rubenstein R. Phrenic nerve conduction studies. Muscle Nerve 1992;15:597.

Tavani F, Zimmerman RA, Clancy RR, et al. Incidental intracranial hemorrhage after uncomplicated birth: MRI before and after neonatal heart surgery. Neuroradiology 2003;45:253.

Terplan K. Patterns of brain damage in infants and children with congenital heart disease: Association with catheterization and surgical procedures. Am J Dis Child 1973;125:175.

Terplan KL. Brain changes in newborns, infants and children with congenital heart disease in association with cardiac surgery. Additional observations. J Neurol 1976;212:225.

Tomlinson F, Piepgras D, Nichols D, et al. Remote congenital cerebral arteriovenous fistulae associated with aortic coarctation. J Neurosurg 1992;76:137.

Tyler R, Clark DB. Cerebrovascular accidents in patients with congenital heart disease. Arch Neurol Psychiatry 1957a;77:483.

Tyler R, Clark DB. Incidence of neurologic complications in congenital heart disease. Arch Neurol Psychiatry 1957b;77:17.

Utoh J, Miyauchi Y, Goto H, et al. Endovascular approach for an intracranial mycotic aneurysm associated with infective endocarditis. J Thorac Cardiovasc Surg 1995;110:557.

van Houten J, Rothman A, Bejar R. High incidence of cranial ultrasound abnormalities in full-term infants with congenital heart disease. Am J Perinatol 1996;13:47.

Vannucci R. Current and potentially new management strategies for perinatal hypoxic-ischemic encephalopathy. Pediatrics 1990;85:961.

Volpe JJ. Neurology of the newborn. Philadelphia: WB Saunders, 2001:482.

von Allmen D, Babcock D, Matsumoto J, et al. The predictive value of head ultrasound in the ECMO candidate. J Pediatr Surg 1992;27:36.

Waitling S, Dasta J. Prolonged paralysis in intensive care unit patients after use of neuromuscular blocking agents: A review of the literature. Crit Care Med 1994;22:884.

Wardle SP, Yoxall CW, Weindling AM. Cerebral oxygenation during cardiopulmonary bypass. Arch Dis Child 1998;78:26.

Watanabe T, Trusler GA, Williams WG, et al. Phrenic nerve paralysis after pediatric cardiac surgery. Retrospective study of 125 cases. J Thorac Cardiovasc Surg 1987;94:383.

Weese-Mayer DE, Hunt CE, Brouillette RT, et al. Diaphragm pacing in infants and children. J Pediatr 1992;120:1.

Wessel DL, du Plessis AJ. Choreoathetosis. In: Jonas RA, Newburger JW, Volpe JJ, eds. Brain injury and pediatric cardiac surgery. Boston: Butterworth-Heinemann, 1995:353.

Westaby S. Organ dysfunction after cardiopulmonary bypass: A systemic inflammatory reaction by the extracorporeal circuit. Intensive Care Med 1987;13:89.

Wical B, Tomasi L. A distinctive neurologic syndrome after profound hypothermia. Pediatr Neurol 1990;6:202.

Wilson W, Giuliani E, Danielson G, et al. Management of complications of infective endocarditis. Mayo Clin Proc 1982;57:162.

Wong PC, Barlow CF, Hickey PR, et al. Factors associated with choreoathetosis after cardiopulmonary bypass in children with congenital heart disease. Circulation 1992;86:118.

Yang J, Park Y, Hartlage P. Seizures associated with stroke in childhood. Pediatr Neurol 1995;12:136.

Yatsu F, Hart R, Mohr J, et al. Anticoagulation of embolic strokes of cardiac origin: An update. Neurology 1988;38:314.

Young R, Liberthson R, Zalneraitis E. Cerebral hemorrhage in neonates with coarctation of the aorta. Stroke 1982;13:491.

Zeviani M, Van Dyke D. Myopathy and fatal cardiopathy due to cytochrome c oxidase deficiency. Arch Neurol 1986;43:1198.

CHAPTER 89

Interrelationships between Renal and Neurologic Diseases and Therapies

Robert S. Rust and Raymond W. M. Chun

Diseases of the kidneys were among the first to be productively investigated with regard to pathophysiology, including deleterious effects secondarily produced on the nervous system by renal demise. Nearly 200 years ago, Richard Bright inaugurated this study as part of his great pioneering investigations of the correlation between disease manifestations and morbid anatomy [Bright, 1831].

The spectrum of neurologic disturbances that can result from renal failure has expanded considerably since the time of Bright. Fortunately, increased understanding of these consequences has engendered the development of strategies and treatments that prevent or ameliorate many of these neurologic abnormalities. The effects of kidney disease and treatments on the nervous system function constitute the initial and major portion of this chapter.

Heritable metabolic diseases are usefully classified on the basis of whether their predominant renal system effects are on the entire nephron or on only a portion (i.e., proximal tubule, distal tubule, or distal nephron). Most of the other systemic diseases that may acutely or chronically affect both the nervous and renal system function are vascular, inflammatory, or toxic processes. These various diseases that affect the nervous and renal systems are reviewed in the second section of this chapter. Greater detail is provided for diseases not considered in detail in other sections of this book.

A small number of primarily neurologic diseases produce renal dysfunction or injury. They are largely neuroendocrinologic (i.e., inappropriate antidiuretic hormone secretion, cerebral salt wasting, diabetes insipidus, dysautonomia). Renal injury may also be produced by neurologic drugs, by myoglobinuric muscle diseases, or as the consequences of a neurogenic bladder. Central hypertension may produce both dysfunctional renal responses and renal injury. Treatments for some neurologic diseases must be modified in the presence of renal dysfunction. These various associations are the subject of the final section of this chapter.

RENAL DISEASES SECONDARILY AFFECTING THE NERVOUS SYSTEM

Acute Renal Failure

Acute renal failure is a common problem. It occurs in as many as 4% of all hospital admittances in the United States or nearly 20% of those requiring critical care management [Schrier et al., 2004].

The two most important potential morbidities of acute renal failure are neurologic and renal. The most significant renal morbidity is the development of chronic renal failure. Risk for chronic renal failure is strongly influenced by the nature and severity of the underlying cause of acute renal failure. The morbidity of acute renal failure in newborns is greater if it occurs as a manifestation of hypoxic-ischemic injury with multiorgan failure (end-stage renal disease) and ensuing blood pressure instability [Andreoli, 2004]. The causes of neonatal acute renal failure are predominantly prerenal, particularly hypoxemic or asphyxial forms of hypoxic-ischemic stress. It usually results in a biphasic course of oliguria followed by diuresis. Sudden severe ischemia due to hemorrhage or cardiopulmonary arrest may produce multiorgan failure including not only kidney but also brain. The associated pattern of brain injury involves encephaloclastic injury to all cell types within the parasagittal watershed regions of the cerebral cortex or within the brainstem. Renal cortical necrosis may occur.

In such situations, protective cardiovascular reflexes preserve glomerular filtration in preference to some other organ systems [Schrier et al., 2004], but where possible these reflexes preserve cerebral perfusion at the cost of reducing renal perfusion. Reflexes designed to achieve hierarchal selection of flow to preserve cardiopulmonary and neurologic function work best in situations of hypoxemia or asphyxia, especially if partial and prolonged, but not in instances of sudden severe ischemic collapse.

The management of some of the important diseases that produce acute renal failure in children—those that have *independent* effects on the nervous system—are reviewed in the next section of this chapter. Many reviews of what is currently known about the benefits and risks of various medications and renal replacement strategies employed to treat acute renal failure are available [Hoste and Kellum, 2004; Schrier et al., 2004; Van Biesen et al., 2003; Williams, et al., 2002]. Few resources for optimal management of acute renal failure are available in developing nations, a situation that has necessitated circumscribed and adaptive application of often inadequate treatment strategies [Naicker, 2003].

Because the site of renal physiologic dysfunction determines selection of therapeutic interventions, it is important to be aware of diagnostic clues concerning the level at which initial renal dysfunction occurs [Andreoli, 2004; Moghal et al., 1998; Schrier and Wang, 2004; Stapleton et al., 1987]. Neurologic decompensation in association with acute intrinsic renal failure occurs with (1) fluid and electrolyte disturbances, (2) accumulation of toxins (e.g. uremia, medications), or (3) hypertension. Neurologic abnormalities secondary to acute renal failure may occur in patients who have normal blood urea nitrogen and creatinine levels. The likelihood, severity, and nature of the neurologic decompensation resulting from acute renal failure are functions of the rate and severity of uremia and oliguria, metabolic balance of the whole organism, and intake (alimentary or parenteral) of free water, salt, and protein [Mahoney and Arieff, 1982].

Acute onset of severe renal failure is more likely to cause neurologic dysfunction because slower development of renal failure permits compensatory mechanisms to blunt the effects of uremia, hypertension, or electrolyte disturbances. The likelihood that partial degrees of renal failure will engender neurologic dysfunction is determined by the concurrent metabolic state of the organism: the loads of solute, electrolytes, protein catabolites, and other potentially deleterious substances with which the nephron is expected to deal. These loads determine the likelihood that intrinsic renal adaptive capacity will be exceeded and that some ensuing neurotoxic combination of uremia, high anion gap acidosis, hyperkalemia, or hypertension will be achieved.

Water Intoxication

Neurologic abnormalities associated with water intoxication may arise in acute oliguric/anuric renal failure as well as in many other settings. The kidney's capacity to excrete from water in dilute urine is the chief mechanism for prevention of water intoxication. In acute renal failure this homeostatic mechanism is lost and neurologic dysfunction develops hours to days after the onset of renal failure, depending on initial water balance and the rate of additional free water intake. Individuals with sodium values as low as 120 to 125 mEq/L often remain asymptomatic. Symptoms become more prevalent once the serum sodium has fallen below 120 mEq/L.

Signs and symptoms of water intoxication may include headache, nystagmus, nausea, vomiting, diaphoresis, weakness, generalized tremulousness, ankle clonus, and the development of muscular irritability with coarse fibrillary twitching. Mental status changes range from apathy to progressive anxious restlessness, through agitation, confusion, or forgetfulness, to obtundation [Bhananker et al., 2004; Riggs, 2002]. It is possible that underlying predilections to migraine, anxiety, or other neurologic conditions may influence the symptomatic expression of water intoxication. The rate of deterioration in neurologic function ranges from gradual to rapid; the course ranges from linear to stepwise, and the severity ranges from mild to severe.

Children are at particularly high risk for the development of sudden decompensation due to brain edema at higher serum sodium concentration than adults because they usually have higher brain:skull ratios than adults. The immature brain often reaches adult size by 6 years of age, whereas adult skull size may not be achieved until 16 years of age [Moritz and Ayus, 2002]. Because of this vulnerability, the outcome of children whose water intoxication is overlooked may be worse than that for adults with similar duration and degree of excessive free water retention. Systemic aspects of water intoxication include cardiovascular compromise or pulmonary edema. These complications further jeopardize brain function owing to impaired oxygenation, provision of glucose, and removal of toxic metabolites of brain metabolism. Hyponatremia may result in seizures, increasing cerebral energy demand, and the rate at which toxic byproducts of metabolism accumulate. Brain edema may develop and increase intracranial pressure, further impairing cerebral circulation. The edema is due to osmotically mediated flow across the blood-brain barrier, diluting extracellular electrolytes and then intracellular electrolytes.

If hyponatremia associated with neurologic decompensation remains uncorrected, convulsions, coma, and death due to brain herniation or complications of generalized convulsions may follow in quick succession. The mortality rate for severe hyponatremia with associated cerebral edema may be greater than 50% [Baran and Hutchinson, 1984]. Under experimental conditions, the increase in brain water required to produce neurologic symptoms is about 3%, with an associated decrease in concentration of intracellular cations estimated to be 20% [Dodge et al., 1960].

Cerebral edema per se is unlikely to be the cause of many of the early neurologic signs and symptoms of water intoxication because these can be produced under experimental conditions without cerebral edema and because cerebral edema in isolation does not necessarily produce a similar constellation of signs and symptoms [Crawford and Dodge, 1964; Gutman et al., 1967; Kennedy et al., 1964; Wakim, 1969b]. It is far more likely that these abnormal findings are due to abnormal membrane excitability, enzymatic activity, or synaptic function. Similar findings develop in children with cystic fibrosis and heat prostration who are in a sodium-depleted state [Barbero and Sibinga, 1964]. Because correction of intracellular potassium concentration lags several hours behind that of sodium and because symptoms persist during this interval, it has been concluded by some authorities that dilution of intracellular potassium concentrations plays a more important direct role in neurologic dysfunction than sodium dilution. The water shifts that dilute intracellular potassium, however, are likely due to dilution of sodium—first in the intravascular and then in the interstitial brain compartments and finally the intracellular milieu [Dila and Pappius, 1972; Dodge et al., 1960]. Brain edema likely accounts for progressive headache and some of the focal signs of advanced water intoxication, including hemiparesis, ataxia, cranial nerve palsies, rigidity, and progressive obtundation [Riggs, 2002].

Treatment of hyponatremia in the patient with acute renal failure must be suited to the particular circumstances of the individual patient. Fluid restriction in early stages may be adequate for mild hyponatremia but can be dangerous if cerebral perfusion is compromised. Maintenance of circulation often requires judicious administration of isotonic or even hypertonic saline solutions. Dialysis may be necessary [Bhananker et al., 2004; Riggs, 2002]. The rate of sodium correction is a particularly important consideration. Excessively rapid correction poses the danger for development of central pontine myelinolysis.

In children, it is recommended that correction at the rate of approximately 1 mEq/L/hour be achieved until the patient becomes alert and seizure free, plasma sodium becomes 125 to 130 mEq/L, or serum sodium level is increased by 20 to 25 mEq/L, whichever occurs first. If seizures persist or there are signs of increased intracranial pressure (especially if these signs are worsening), the sodium concentration may be corrected at a rate of 4 to 8 mEq/L for 1 hour (if tolerated) or until seizures stop. Assuming that total body water comprises 50% of body mass, administration of 1 mL/kg of 3%

NaCl solution will increase plasma sodium by approximately 1 mEq/L [Moritz and Ayus, 2002].

Hyperkalemia

During the first 48 hours of anuric acute renal failure from prerenal causes there is loss of as much as 70% to 80% of renal outer medullary potassium secretory channel and 35% to 40% of the activity of potassium channel inducing factor.

Cardiac and pulmonary manifestations of hyperkalemia generally precede and are greater threats for survival than neurologic ones. Cardiac dysfunction is usually the earliest and most ominous clinical sign of hyperkalemia. Cardiac instability or arrest is virtually diagnostic of hyperkalemia in the setting of acute renal failure. Electrocardiography is an earlier and more sensitive indicator of the progressive effects of hyperkalemia that portend cardiac failure and should be performed promptly and monitored or repeated as indicated if hyperkalemia is suspected. In many cases of reversible acute renal failure, plasma potassium concentration peaks at about 48 hours and returns to normal in about 7 days. However, during the first 48 hours, it is critical to monitor and, if necessary, bind or redistribute existing potassium while at the same time preventing further intake. Rare instances of hyperkalemia of acute renal failure presenting as a neurologic sign (e.g., paralysis) rather than cardiac decompensation have been described [Cumberbatch and Hampton, 1999].

Elevation of serum potassium concentration reflects a complex set of equilibria. Factors include the degree of displacement of potassium from the intracellular compartment as the result of acidemia and the state of dilution or concentration of body fluids (the balance of free water intake and output). Hyperkalemia may provoke smooth or striated muscle weakness owing to lowered membrane resting potentials, delayed depolarization, rapid repolarization, or slowed cardiac and peripheral nerve conduction velocities [Chantler, 1988]. Correction of metabolic acidosis with infusion of calcium or glucose, insulin, and in some instances administration of an ∃-2 stimulant such as salbutamol may shift the circulating potassium excess to safer intracellular loci [Kemper et al., 1996]. Management may involve the use of ion exchange resins or dialysis.

Uremic Encephalopathy

Uremia is an extremely complicated, and as yet incompletely characterized, metabolic state that results from the failure of renal mechanisms for (1) regulation of fluid and electrolyte balance, (2) excretion of protein catabolites and other potentially toxic substances, and (3) endocrine regulation [Bergstrom, 1985]. It occurs when glomerular filtration rate has declined to less than 10% of normal. It is fatal if untreated. Most patients with acute uremia have experienced proportional injury to tubular and glomerular systems. Bicarbonate wasting occurs but is in part compensated for by the retention of nonchloride anions, such as sulfate and phosphate. The result is high anion gap acidosis with normal or increased serum potassium concentration. Sodium and chloride levels remain normal unless free water excretion is impaired. Brain edema is uncommon in uremic encephalopathy because most of the osmotically active molecules that accumulate in uremia are small molecules that equilibrate readily across the blood-brain barrier [Dettori et al., 1982; Mahoney and Arieff, 1983; Smogorzewski, 2001]. Occurrence and degree of uremic encephalopathy correlate poorly with renal function as measured by degree of blood urea nitrogen or creatinine abnormality.

Disturbances of endocrine function occur in uremia, with possible elevations, especially in chronic renal failure, of parathyroid hormone, insulin, growth hormone, glucagons, thyrotropin, prolactin, luteinizing hormone, or gastrin. Elevated concentrations of parathyroid hormone, associated particularly with cases of uremic decompensation of chronic renal failure, may activate second-messenger systems that alter cellular calcium hemostasis, the balance of which is viewed by many observers as a central element of the metabolic crisis that produces uremic encephalopathy [Arieff and Armstrong, 1980; D'Hooge et al., 2003; Fraser, 1992]. Parathyroid hormone concentration elevations have been clearly linked to the reduction of mental status and electroencephalographic (EEG) abnormalities associated with uremic encephalopathy [Cooper et al., 1978; Fraser, 1992; Guisado et al., 1975; Moe and Sprague, 1994; Smits et al., 1983]. In chronically uremic patients, EEG abnormalities and mental and psychiatric manifestations may improve with parathyroidectomy or chemical suppression of parathyroid function [Cogan et al., 1978]. Exogenous toxins, infectious and inflammatory disturbances, and particularities of glomerulotubular dysfunction may also play variable roles in exacerbating uremic encephalopathy but are not essential predisposing features for uremic encephalopathy.

Numerous lines of evidence suggest the considerable importance of disturbances of calcium homeostasis, membrane excitability, and neurotransmitter function as central functional abnormalities of uremic encephalopathy [Biasoli et al., 1984; Moe and Sprague, 1994]. It appears likely that some combination of effects produced by the presence of low-molecular-weight, fast-acting toxic solutes that are not excreted in renal failure are responsible for these disturbances. Among the dozens of unexcreted solutes that might produce such effects are urea, creatinine, hippuric acid, polyamines, polypeptides, guanidino compounds, acetoin, myoinositols, sulfates, aliphatic and aromatic amines, phenols, purines, indoles, glucuronates, spermine, DL-homocysteine, orotate, and glycine [Arieff et al., 1976; D'Hooge et al., 2003; Lubash et al., 1964; Ludwig et al., 1968; Morgan and Morgan, 1966]. These compounds have different capacities for the penetration of nervous tissues and may also have effects on blood vessels, membranes, enzymes, neurotransmitters, or receptors. Many of these potentially toxic chemicals, so quietly and efficiently removed by the normal kidney, are less efficiently removed from circulation by dialysis.

It has long been known that cerebral rates of utilization of glucose, oxygen, and high-energy phosphate compounds fall in uremic encephalopathy, apparently because of reduced demand rather than energy failure. To some extent this may be a protective adaptation [Mahoney et al., 1984; Scheinberg, 1954; Van den Noort et al., 1970], although it is possible that the reduction is due in part to failure of synaptic transmission. It is not as yet known whether this global reduction masks regional or focal excesses of utilization (in conjunction, for example, with focal seizure activity or "twitch-myoclonus") or whether some aspects of this reduction may injure rather than protect brain. Observed reduction in activity of the pentose phosphate shunt, an important source of reducing equivalents for maintenance of myelin and other synthetic tasks, may represent compensatory reduction of a temporarily dispensable energy expenditure. On the other hand, reduced flux in this pathway interferes with the maintenance of myelin. Interestingly, the uremic reduction in overall cerebral metabolic rate is not accompanied by reduction in cerebral blood flow, suggesting an unusual and as yet unexplained form of energy supply-demand uncoupling [Heyman et al., 1951; Scheinberg, 1954].

"Uremic" synaptosomal preparations have diminished activity of the metabolic pumps associated with Na^+/K^+ and Ca^{2+} adenosine triphosphatases and disturbances not only in calcium but also in cellular magnesium and potassium homeostasis. Evidence suggests that creatinine and acidic derivatives of guanidine metabolism (e.g., methyl guanidine and guanidinosuccinic acid) inhibit physiologic responses to γ-aminobutyric acid and glycine, disturb synaptic transmission in the CA1 region of the hippocampus, and elevate excitatory tone of certain neuronal populations. Guanidino compounds, phenol, and spermine, among the first uremic small molecules to have been proven to exert definable deleterious effects on brain, alter various membrane ionic conductances by means of voltage- or ligand-gated channels. These include the *N*-methyl-D-aspartate receptor complex, which variously enhances inward calcium or outward potassium currents [D'Hooge et al., 2003].

Sufficient concentrations of some of these various small-molecule compounds are capable of engendering clonic seizures under experimental conditions, and it is possible that they are responsible for such classic manifestations of uremic encephalopathy as uremic "twitch-myoclonus." Uremic myoclonus has also been associated with elevation of cerebrospinal fluid phosphate to concentrations in excess of 3.8 mg/mL, perhaps reflecting a particular sensitivity of the brainstem reticular formation to this chemical [Chadwick and French, 1979; Freeman et al., 1962]. Hypercalcemia (see later) is a known cause of myoclonic encephalopathy with seizures and dysarthria. Hypophosphatemia may also contribute to development of seizures in some patients [Rivera-Vazquez et al., 1980].

Toxicity of guanidinosuccinic acid is more marked in the post-hypoxic state [Torremans et al., 2004], owing to the generation of superoxides and hydroxyl free radicals that have been found to produce glial cell death under experimental conditions [Hiramatsu, 2003]. It is of interest that many of the small molecules associated with uremia may play important positive roles in normal brain, perhaps as free-radical scavengers. Factors that may account for toxicity of these same molecules during renal failure likely include loss of closely regulated and carefully compartmentalized concentrations and enhanced transformation of nontoxic and metabolically useful ones into toxic molecules. An important example of this is free radical-stimulated transformation of arginosuccinic acid into guanidinosuccinic acid [Cohen, 2003]. The generation of that toxic intermediate is enhanced in proportion to urea concentration [Aoyagi, 2003].

The complex state of uremia includes other pertinent and as yet incompletely understood or characterized metabolic and neurotransmitter disturbances, including the possible rise of glycine concentration in critical locations and fall in γ-aminobutyric acid concentrations in others. Uremic disturbance of tryptophan metabolism results in accumulation of kynurenine neurotransmitters that may provoke seizures, alter consciousness, or produce neuronal injury or cell death [Topczewska-Bruns et al., 2002]. Older data concerning uremic depression of metabolism of nucleotides, catecholamines, and amino acids involved in neurotransmitter synthesis [Fraser et al., 1985; Minkoff et al., 1972] may remain pertinent. Uremia may disturb the transport of amino and organic acids that activate excitatory or inhibitory synapses [Arieff et al., 1978; Biasioli et al., 1986; Deferrari et al., 1981; Fishman, 1970; Fishman and Raskin, 1967].

Pathologic studies of uremic encephalopathy suggest variable degrees of generalized neuronal degeneration. In some instances, perivascular necrosis and demyelinative changes are discerned. Abnormalities may be emphasized in cerebral cortex, subcortical and brainstem nuclei, or cerebellum. In persons dying of acute uremic encephalopathy, Alzheimer type II astrocytes may be found [Norenberg, 1994]. Subdural hemorrhages are found in less than 3% of cases of chronic renal failure with uremia [Fraser and Arieff, 1997].

Although uremic encephalopathy occurs in patients without a preceding history of serious renal disease, the majority of the 16,000 to 20,000 cases that occur in the United States annually occur in some of the more than 200,000 patients who are on chronic dialysis for end-stage renal disease. It is therefore important in caring for patients with chronic renal disease to be aware of the risk of this. Care should be taken before diagnoses such as for depression or frustration with chronic disease are used to explain behavioral changes. In patients with new-onset renal failure associated with uremia, an even wider differential diagnosis must be entertained as possible causes for neurologic deterioration. Difficulty may arise in instances in which new-onset renal disease with uremia pursues an indolent but subacutely progressive course. In each of these various groups, it must also be remembered that neurologic signs may precede definite clinical or biochemical evidence of renal failure.

Acute uremic encephalopathy produces deterioration of higher cortical function at a rate that varies from slowly progressive to fulminant. The earliest characteristic changes, often subtle or insidious, include inattention, indecisiveness, irritability, and diminished intellectual agility. These changes may be improperly ascribed to depression. They are often more apparent to caregivers than to the patient. They may be overlooked in children or may be falsely ascribed to uncooperativeness and irritability. Standardized assessment of vigilance with digit span or serial subtraction may be useful in following patients at risk. A peculiar dyspraxic hesitancy of speech is a common and distinctive clue, usually dyspraxia *without* dysnomia or other associated aphasia [Martinez et al., 1978; Raskin and Fishman, 1976a, 1976b].

Lethargy, somnolence, anorexia, nausea, vomiting, pruritus [Zucker et al., 2003] and disturbance of the sleep-wake cycle are other common early manifestations. Episodic confusion, disinterest in surroundings, or impairment of recent memory may develop, interspersed with more lucid intervals. Occasionally, especially in persons with fulminant renal failure, acute agitation, delirium, psychosis, coma, or catatonia suggests the presence of uremic encephalopathy [Souheaver et al., 1982]. In such instances, effects of an intoxicating drug (e.g., corticosteroids, propranolol, cimetidine, levetiracetam, phenobarbital, or tricyclic antidepressants) must be excluded [Stenback and Haapanen, 1967]. Uremic encephalopathy may produce signs suggestive of Wernicke-Korsakoff syndrome.

The development of tremor is a particularly reliable early sign of uremic encephalopathy and should prompt careful mental status evaluation. Both action (e.g., ataxic) and postural tremors of irregular amplitude may occur. Asterixis in persons with renal failure is another important sign of uremic encephalopathy but is seen in other metabolic encephalopathies that impair attentiveness [Adams and Foley, 1949, 1953]. The asterixic flap is not an active movement but appears to occur because patients fail to maintain voluntary motor extension of the wrists or feet. The rapidity of the flap does not, however, resemble the slower relaxation of effort seen with inattention. Central inhibition of sustained motor neuron activity has also been proposed in explanation, and the phenomenon has been called a variety of "negative myoclonus." Similar impersistence is observed with sustained eye closure or forced smiling [Adams, 1964; Tyler, 1964, 1965]. Truncal asterixis also occurs and may be so severe that it mimics epileptic drop attacks [Young and Shahani, 1986].

With progressive obtundation, encephalopathy becomes less intermittent and a wider variety of neurologic dysfunction is displayed. Along with more severe disturbances of orientation, memory, cognition, and judgment, primitive reflexes (e.g., snout, root, grasp) may emerge. Transient loss of hearing or vision (uremic amaurosis) may occur. Either may persist for several days. Visual loss may result from either optic nerve or cortical dysfunction, possibly owing to edema. The localization is readily ascertained by the absence or presence of the pupillary light reflex [Tyler, 1968]. Abducens palsy only occasionally complicates uremia. It is far more common in hypertensive encephalopathy. Seizures, usually generalized tonic-clonic, occur in 20% to 40% of children with uremic encephalopathy, typically at the time of onset of renal failure. They are especially common in cases in which renal failure is fulminant, as is seen in acute glomerulonephritis and other causes. Seizures are seldom the only sign of uremia. Their occurrence may, however, presage an ensuing rapid decline in renal function with multiple manifestations. In acute renal failure they are more commonly brief generalized motor than focal motor seizures. Epilepsia partialis continua may develop in some cases. Seizures occurring in the later stages of acute uremia generally signify the development of other complications such as infection or electrolytic disturbances during the diuretic phase of resolving acute renal failure or as consequences of overzealous dialysis.

Muscle twitching or fasciculation, especially in the distal extremities, is common in acute renal failure. Some patients report that such activity is preceded by distal extremity muscle ache or cramping. Multifocal uremic stimulus-sensitive myoclonus that Adams termed *twitch-convulsive* often emerges as uremic stupor develops [Tyler, 1968, 1976]. Restless leg phenomenon is not uncommon in uremic encephalopathy. Tetany (i.e., tonic muscle irritability, carpopedal spasm, Trousseau sign) may develop in uremia and may not respond to calcium supplementation [Tyler, 1968].

Choreoathetosis and even hemiballism may be observed. Moderate to severe motor weakness (including alternating hemiplegia) may follow. In patients with chronic renal failure/end-stage renal disease, acute weakness must be distinguished from preexisting changes related to neuropathy or hyperparathyroidism (see later). Hyperkalemia must be excluded. Rarely, signs of autonomic failure are noted [Levitan et al., 1982], some of which may be manifestations of uremic neuropathy [Yildiz et al., 1998]. Long-tract signs may be present and are often asymmetric and changeable. If coma deepens without treatment of uremia, progressive brainstem failure leading to death often follows [Chadwick and French, 1979; Dinapoli et al., 1966; Locke et al., 1961; Raskin and Fishman, 1976a; Schreiner, 1959; Stark, 1981]. No distinctive pathologic process has been identified in such cases [Olsen, 1961].

In the patient with new-onset renal disease, uremic encephalopathy must be distinguished from many other causes of acute encephalopathy, particularly if renal failure develops after inflammatory, infectious, cardiovascular, metabolic, or other diseases known to produce neurologic abnormalities whether or not renal failure develops. In the patient with known renal disease, the acuteness of uremic deterioration usually sets it apart from slower-onset neurologic deteriorations to which chronically dialyzed patients are also subject (see later). It may be more difficult in patients with chronic renal failure to clinically distinguish uremic encephalopathy from encephalopathy due to water intoxication or hypertension.

It is frequently difficult to ascertain exactly what metabolic stresses have provoked uremic encephalopathic decompensation in the patients with chronic renal disease. Among the influences or alternative diagnostic considerations that must be excluded are treatable conditions such as infection, endocrinopathy, vitamin deficiency states, or dialysis-related complications. Any question of increased intracranial pressure suggested by focal neurologic signs and symptoms of increased intracranial pressure must urgently be investigated and, if found, treated.

Given the complexity of the biochemical changes associated with uremic encephalopathy, great care must be taken to detect and fix readily correctable metabolic perturbations such as disturbances of sodium, potassium, phosphate, magnesium, and glucose. It should also be recognized that neurologic improvement may lag behind adequate correction of readily measurable metabolic parameters. Some abnormalities (e.g., emotional and intellectual) may respond quickly to dialysis, whereas others (e.g., motor and sensory) respond more slowly, persisting for an uncomfortable interval [Grushkin et al., 1972]. This latency may be related to the inefficiency of dialysis in the clearance of unmeasured toxic intermediates.

Drug screening, electroencephalography, evoked potentials, brain imaging, bacterial cultures, and lumbar puncture may be indicated in individuals with uremic encephalopathy to detect alternative or related diagnoses. In acute uremia, the electroencephalogram usually demonstrates generalized irregular but bisynchronous low-voltage slowing, particularly in patients whose blood urea nitrogen level is in excess of 60 mg/dL. The severity of these changes and prevalence of associated paroxysms roughly correlate with the further degrees of blood urea nitrogen elevation and degree of clinical encephalopathy. Slow alpha-dominant rhythm with occasional theta bursts and characteristic prolonged bursts of bisynchronous slow-sharp activity or spike and wave may be found. Bilateral spike discharges may accompany myoclonic jerks, and generalized electroconvulsive discharges in association with generalized convulsive seizures may also occur, possibly more commonly in patients with hypomagnesemia. Photomyoclonus and photic driving may be present.

Rarely, the electroencephalogram may be normal despite uremic encephalopathy [Raskin and Fishman, 1976a]. Bursts of high voltage 12- to 13-Hz vertex sharp activity may be seen in drowsiness, spindles may be absent in stage 2 sleep, and high-voltage slow bursts may occur with wakening. EEG abnormalities may persist for quite some time, especially in patients with chronic renal failure for whom many months of dialysis may be required before restoration of a normal EEG pattern is seen. Deteriorations in blood urea control or other indications of transient worsening of renal function may be associated with transient intrusion of diffuse delta and theta waves, generalized spike-wave discharges, or heightened sensitivity to photic stimulation [Kiley et al., 1976].

Infrequently, brain imaging in acute uremic encephalopathy may disclose subdural hemorrhage. Some patients manifest a gyriform increase in T2-weighted signal or similar abnormalities on magnetic resonance imaging (MRI) of parietal and occipital subcortical areas, changes that reverse with treatment and must be distinguished from changes suggesting hypertensive encephalopathy (see later). Generally, brain imaging is not of much practical value in straightforward uremic encephalopathy [Schmidt et al., 2001]. In uremic encephalopathy in individuals with preceding chronic renal failure, scans may indicate changes due to either atrophy or corticosteroid treatment–related pseudoatrophy. However, the scans of such persons are often normal.

Elevated lumbar cerebrospinal fluid pressure may be found in cases of uremic encephalopathy and usually resolves with dialysis. The decision to perform a lumbar puncture must be carefully weighed in individuals with severe encephalopathy given the risk for herniation. It is far from clear that lumbar puncture increases risk for herniation, but the performance of such a procedure represents a risk that is avoidable. Even without urgent performance of that test, appropriate broad-spectrum antibiotic therapy for possible infectious causes of deterioration can be undertaken. Cultures of blood and dialysate should be obtained when indicated, and lumbar puncture can be performed if still needed once it is clear that the risk of herniation has declined. Cerebrospinal fluid protein concentration may be elevated, and pleocytosis may be found. In such cases an underlying infectious cause, such as human immunodeficiency virus, can be sought. However, these changes may occur without identification of any treatable process and may be related to uremic alteration of blood-brain barrier function.

The primary treatment of uremic encephalopathy is dialysis, with scrupulous attention to water balance, electrolytes, blood pressure, and ventilation. Consideration must in some cases be given to parathyroidectomy or chemical parathyroid suppression. Response to dialysis may be rapid or may require many days [Locke et al., 1961]. Fixed deficits may develop, especially when uremic encephalopathy is complicated by hypertension or central nervous system (CNS) hemorrhage. Excessive or too rapid dialysis must be avoided because rapid shifts in water or solutes in various compartments may lead to alternative forms of neurologic decompensation.

Seizures should suggest reevaluation for hypertension, electrolyte or water imbalance, infection, or intoxication (commonly penicillin or a phenothiazine). Persistent seizures should be treated with antiepileptic drugs. Phenytoin, phenobarbital, and carbamazepine have been the most frequently employed antiseizure medicines in this setting, in part because of the considerable familiarity with the safe and effective use of such drugs in renal failure and dialysis. Phenytoin should be used cautiously. Uremia may increase phenytoin hepatic clearance while at the same time hypoalbuminemia may increase free phenytoin concentration owing to diminished protein binding. These effects often balance one another, but not invariably. It is wise to frequently assess free phenytoin concentrations in patients with uremic encephalopathy and seizures.

Hypertensive Encephalopathy

The designation *hypertensive encephalopathy* is generally reserved for hypertensive patients with alteration of consciousness and diffuse or multifocal CNS dysfunction in whom there is no better or more complex etiologic explanation [Chester et al., 1978]. Malignant hypertension as a cause of the neurologic abnormalities of hypertensive encephalopathy can arise in association with a number of underlying illnesses.

The causes of malignant hypertension in children vary according to age [Chantler, 1986]. Within the first month of life, two thirds of cases are related to renovascular thrombosis (spontaneous or associated with asphyxia, cyanotic heart disease, disseminated intravascular coagulopathy, or umbilical artery catheterization). Nearly 20% of cases are due to CNS disturbances, and approximately 8% are caused by tumors (e.g., Wilms' tumor, neuroblastoma) or coarctation. Malignant hypertension is rare in neonates, although it may arise as the consequence of renal failure or congenital adrenal hyperplasia [Spoudeas et al., 1993]. It is also not uncommon in infants 1 to 12 months of age. When it does occur in the first year of life, it carries high risk of morbidity and mortality, owing to the severity of the illnesses that typically underlie pressure elevation at this young age. These include aortic coarctation and polycystic kidneys (each accounting for about one third of such cases in young patients), nephritis (16%), and hemolytic-uremic syndrome (7%). The remaining cases are due to causes such as tumors that generate Cushing's syndrome (e.g., neuroblastoma, corticotropin-secreting ganglioneuroblastoma), high doses of adrenocorticotropic hormone used to treat infantile spasms, and various forms of renovascular disease. No cases of so-called central (primarily CNS-mediated) hypertension were described in the Boston Children's Hospital series of cases of malignant infantile hypertension [Ingelfinger, 1982].

In children older than 1 year of age, roughly two thirds of cases are caused by inflammatory or infectious parenchymal renal disease. These include hemolytic-uremic syndrome, acute glomerulonephritis, and collagen vascular diseases (particularly systemic lupus erythematosus). Renal or aortic vascular abnormalities such as renal artery stenosis, kidney malformations (multicystic or dysplastic kidneys), and tumors (Wilms' tumor, neuroblastoma, pheochromocytoma) account for the remaining one third in most centers. Renal graft rejection may be the most frequently encountered cause of hypertensive encephalopathy in centers that perform many kidney transplants, however. Immunosuppression employed in such cases may increase risk for acute hypertension even without graft rejection [Primavera et al., 2001; Proulx et al., 1993; Still and Cottom, 1967; Stocker et al., 2003; Zangeneh et al., 2003].

More than 40% of patients with malignant hypertension develop significant neurologic complications, including encephalopathy. In early reports, one or another of these neurologic complications were lethal in 20% of patients, particularly cerebral thrombosis or hemorrhage [Schottstaedt and Sokolow, 1953]. Although the fatality rate has undoubtedly declined, fatalities still occur, especially as the result of intracranial hemorrhage [Schwartz et al., 1995].

The risk for hypertensive encephalopathy is related to both the rapidity and severity of blood pressure increase from any given baseline [Dinsdale, 1983; Healton et al., 1982]. Thus, risk is higher in acute renal failure caused by acute glomerulonephritis or hemolytic-uremic syndrome than it is in essential hypertension or chronic renal failure/end-stage renal disease. Acute glomerulonephritis or hemolytic-uremic syndrome should be suspected in any child older than 1 month of age with unexplained hypertensive encephalopathy, even when initial laboratory findings are minimal [Hoyer et al., 1967]. Some inflammatory illnesses that cause acute hypertensive renal failure in children, such as hemolytic-uremic syndrome, may have direct effects on the CNS beyond those provoked by severe hypertension (see later).

Generalized severe headache is almost universal with severe hypertension. Seizures and visual loss are other common early manifestations of hypertensive encephalopathy [Wright and Mathews, 1996]. Headache develops hours to days after the initiating blood pressure crisis and may be accompanied by lethargy, projectile vomiting, meningismus, or edema of the eyelids and ankles. Papilledema is present in only one third of childhood cases of hypertensive encephalopathy. Retinal arteriolar spasm is a far more characteristic and important sign [Bar and Savir, 1982; McGregor et al., 1986]. Evidence of ischemic infarction of nerve fibers (white exudate or cotton-wool spots) is another important funduscopic indication [Pickering, 1968]. The earliest signs in newborns and infants include irritability, lethargy, and hypotonia.

Encephalopathy develops after 12 to 36 hours of headache and is heralded in most children by seizures, more commonly generalized than focal [Dedeoglu et al., 1996; Trompeter et al., 1982]. In virtually all cases of hypertensive encephalopathy with seizures, systolic and diastolic blood pressures are more than four standard deviations above the mean for age. Status epilepticus may further elevate systolic and diastolic blood pressures in more than 10% of cases. Elevation of blood pressure by four standard deviations above the mean for age should in no case, however, be ascribed to seizures alone [Proulx et al., 1993]. Seizures without persistently associated mental status changes occasionally occur as the sole initial clinical manifestation of hypertensive encephalopathy [Dinsdale, 1983].

Infants without hypertensive encephalopathy may exhibit opisthotonos, fever, and unresponsiveness. The level of consciousness in older children consists of fluctuating confusion, irritability, and restlessness that may progress to coma. Muscle twitching and myoclonus may occur. Focal neurologic signs occur in various combinations of aphasia, scotomas (retinal, optic nerve, or cortical), cranial neuropathy (especially abducens or facial nerves), and focal motor weakness (especially hemiparesis). In severe cases, rapidly progressive brainstem failure may precede death unless effective treatment is initiated [Jellinek et al., 1964; Lindfors-Lonnkvist and Jakobsson, 1994; Zangeneh et al., 2003].

Hypertension-associated occipital blindness with additional features such as headache, lethargy, transient motor deficits, confusion, visual hallucination, and convulsive seizures (generalized more commonly than focal) constitute a syndrome that has been termed *reversible posterior leukoencephalopathy* [Hinchey et al., 1996; Kwong et al., 1987; Saatci and Topaloglu, 1994; Sebire et al., 1995]. This clinically distinctive subcategory of hypertensive encephalopathy was first described in individuals receiving immunosuppression with cyclosporine. It occurs most commonly, however, in children or adults who develop acute hypertension in the setting of either acute or chronic nephrotic conditions.

Nephrotoxic (e.g., acyclovir) or cytotoxic (e.g., cyclosporine) drugs or treatment with high doses of methylprednisolone enhance risk, especially in patients receiving excessive fluid loads [Ikeda et al., 2001]. Cytotoxic drugs may enhance risk for reversible posterior leukoencephalopathy because they compromise the blood-brain barrier. The respiratory distress of fluid-overloaded patients may increase risk because of elevation of venous "back-pressure" of the cerebral venous circulation. Attention has been drawn to the development of MRI changes consistent with reversible posterior leukoencephalopathy in the hemisphere contralateral to predominantly hemiconvulsive seizures, suggesting that seizures themselves may have a role in the genesis and evolution of reversible posterior leukoencephalopathy [Obeid et al., 2004].

Brain imaging in reversible posterior leukoencephalopathy usually illustrates fairly symmetric and extensive abnormalities within 24 hours of clinical onset that are more apparent on MRI than on computed tomography (CT). With MRI, T2-weighted bright and T1-weighted dark abnormalities usually are due to edema rather than infarction and tend to be located in the posterior parietal/occipital cortical ribbon and especially the subadjacent white matter. Similar changes may be found in the frontal or temporal lobes, basal ganglia, brainstem, or cerebellum, representing more generalized changes of hypertensive encephalopathy. Gradient-echo techniques may demonstrate characteristic petechial hemorrhages [Kandt et al., 1995; Weingarten et al., 1994]. Because the parieto-occipital changes of reversible posterior leukoencephalopathy involve both gray and white matter in children, the designation occipital-parietal encephalopathy is favored by some investigators [Pavlakis et al., 1997]. In some instances, clinical and radiographic changes of reversible posterior leukoencephalopathy or of hypertensive encephalopathy do not resolve for days to as many as 8 weeks after control of hypertension. Reduction of dosage of medications such as cytotoxic or immunosuppressive agents may be required in persistent cases [Dedeoglu et al., 1996; Hinchey et al., 1996; Primavera et al., 2001].

The clinical findings and radiographic changes of reversible posterior leukoencephalopathy are virtually identical to those found in the syndrome of cyclosporine neurotoxicity (see later). In cases that promptly resolve after correction of blood pressure with medications or dialysis, the most likely pathogenesis is edema from hypertensive encephalopathy. Edema may be exacerbated by effects of cyclosporine on blood-brain barrier permeability [Lopez-Garcia et al., 2004; Primavera et al., 2001] rather than by any direct toxic effect of cyclosporine on brain. Intracranial hemorrhage is more typically associated with cyclosporine-induced than other forms of hypertensive encephalopathy, probably potentiated by cyclosporine-induced thrombocytopenia [Schwartz et al., 1995]. Changes resembling reversible posterior leukoencephalopathy develop in a minority of patients who have had long-term dialysis followed by administration of interferon alfa in preparation for renal transplantation. Some of these individuals have chronic hepatitis C infection.

Focal clinical features of hypertensive encephalopathy are not always transient. Aphasia, optic nerve scotomas, and hemiparesis may indicate the occurrence of brain, cranial nerve, or brainstem infarction. Unilateral infarction of some portion of the anterior optic pathways is especially characteristic. Infarction may be more common in patients who have had long-standing unrecognized hypertension. It also occurs in those who experience hypotensive episodes as the result of overly aggressive management of blood pressure elevation [Sebire et al., 1995]. It is as yet unclear if infarctions are due to vasculopathy or to impairment of blood flow related to edema and hypotension.

Information concerning the pathologic changes that occur in hypertensive encephalopathy is scant. Perivascular edema (with or without microhemorrhages) and swelling of astrocytes and myelin have been described [Lumsden, 1970]. The exact nature of the pathophysiology of hypertensive encephalopathy is not fully understood, but two major theories are advocated. An older view states that encephalopathy is the result of excessive cerebral vasoconstrictive autoregulation, stimulated to protect cerebral microvascularity from high pressure. This reduction of microcirculatory flow is believed to compromise capillary integrity and result in edema, vascular necrosis, microinfarction, and petechial hemorrhages. This sequence has been demonstrated in experimental models [Adams and Foley, 1953; Byrom, 1954; Finnerty, 1972; Myers et al., 1960].

A newer hypothesis suggests that hypertensive encephalopathy is actually the result of failure of cerebral autoregulation. In this model the vasoconstrictive threshold is exceeded and transudative perivascular edema develops, which may then compress the regional microvasculature. This process, perhaps in combination with back-pressure related to venous hypertension, may then result in proliferative endarteritis of retinal and cerebral arterioles with focal ischemic fibrinoid necrosis, petechial hemorrhages, and parenchymal microhemorrhages [Dinsdale, 1983; Goldby and Beilin, 1976; Gulliksen et al., 1983]. Loss of autoregulation, significantly impairing vascular compensation to intercurrent hypotensive episodes, may render the individual vulnerable to infarction in areas of vascular watershed across the parasagittal and deep gray regions of the cerebral hemispheres.

Neither theory has been proved, although experimental and clinical observations have been advanced supporting both. Although it is known that hypertension is necessary, it is not known whether it is sufficient to cause hypertensive encephalopathy or whether other inciting circumstances are required. Regardless of the initial event, microinfarction, edema, and loss of autoregulation do occur, necessitating caution in blood pressure reduction and manipulation of cardiac output because rapid changes may result in acute cerebral infarction [Healton et al., 1982]. Generally, intact cerebral autoregulatory mechanisms are capable of blunting systolic arterial pressure elevations as high as 200 mm Hg in adolescents and adults [Harper, 1966; Strandgaard et al., 1973].

These mechanisms can adapt to even greater pressures in patients with chronic hypertension [Lassen and Agnoli, 1972; Strandgaard et al., 1973]. On the other hand, children with chronic renal disease may experience particularly acute and severe episodes of hypertension. This vulnerability is ascribed to chronic volume expansion, renovascular constriction that results in increased plasma renin and angiotensin II, and increased vascular responsiveness to angiotensin II owing to increased plasma Na^+/K^+ adenosine triphosphatase inhibitor [de Wardener and MacGregor, 1988].

The upper limits of vascular autoregulation in the newborn are more uncertain than in older individuals, and little is known about cerebrovascular autoregulation in young children in a hypertensive state [Fraser and Arieff, 1988]. Autoregulatory responses become more complex when metabolic homeostasis is disturbed. Both acidosis and carbon dioxide accumulation prompt cerebral arteriolar dilatation and may permit higher pressure to be conveyed to the delicate microcirculation of the brain, perhaps lowering the pressure threshold for decompensation. This effect is best illustrated by the fact that only moderate blood pressure elevation is required to produce hypertensive encephalopathy in some children with acute pulmonary edema.

Abnormalities observed with magnetic resonance perfusion imaging support the concept that vasodilatation is an important aspect of vulnerability to hypertensive encephalopathy [Jones et al., 1997]. There is no clear explanation for the occipital preponderance of MRI-deprived changes in brain appearances, although it seems likely that there are physiologic or anatomic differences in the blood vessels or associated blood-brain barrier in posterior brain regions [Kandt et al., 1995].

Acute hypertension, severe headache, and encephalopathy progressing over several days is highly suggestive of hypertensive encephalopathy, particularly if there is funduscopic evidence of arteriolar spasm and/or ischemic infarction of nerve fibers. Inflammatory vasculitides (especially systemic lupus erythematosus) associated with a chronic hypertensive state often produce similar retinal changes even without hypertensive encephalopathy. Acute hypertensive encephalopathy associated with acute dependent edema and hematuria suggests the possibility of acute post-streptococcal glomerulonephritis. Diagnoses such as eclampsia, complications of immunosuppression, or acetaminophen-induced hepatorenal failure will be suggested by the clinical setting [Hinchey et al., 1996; Saatci and Topaloglu, 1994]. When appropriate, structural CNS lesions (tumor, hemorrhage, or stroke) should be excluded by unenhanced brain imaging because the presence of such lesions may influence blood pressure management.

In some cases it is difficult to exclude ischemic brain injury without serial imaging. Cerebral hemorrhage in hypertensive encephalopathy is usually petechial. In the preadolescent patient, any large brain hemorrhage is more likely the cause than the result of hypertension, except in patients with cyclosporine-induced thrombocytopenia [Schwartz et al., 1995]. Multiple infarctions are sometimes found in association with hypertensive encephalopathy. It may be important in some cases to exclude CNS infection by lumbar puncture. Both opening pressure and protein may be elevated in hypertensive encephalopathy, but cell count should be normal. The electroencephalogram is usually slow, resembling that of uremic encephalopathy. It may identify subclinical seizures. Focal EEG abnormalities may suggest infarction or subdural, intraparenchymal hemorrhages or tumor. However, focal clinical or EEG abnormalities may also be detected in hypertensive encephalopathy or uremic encephalopathy without identifiable structural lesions [Dinsdale, 1983].

Prompt remission with control of blood pressure is the most important confirmation of hypertensive encephalopathy [Healton et al., 1982; Hinchey et al., 1996; Kandt et al., 1995]. Medications employed in the management of blood pressure in children are shown in Table 89-1. Selection, utilization, side effects, and detailed dosage considerations for these medications fall outside the scope of this chapter. All patients should initially be managed as if cerebral edema is present. The fundamental steps include elevation of the head of the bed by 30 degrees and careful attention to free water balance. Further decisions about treatment depend on etiology. Unless hypertension is very severe, drug therapy should not be undertaken until space-occupying CNS lesions (stroke, tumor, hemorrhage) and the brittle dysautonomia of Guillain-Barré syndrome are excluded. Other important etiologic considerations for acute encephalopathy include intoxication, acute pulmonary edema, acute pancreatitis, and endocrine or metabolic diseases. Rarely, an acute anxiety reaction with hypertension and pseudoencephalopathy must be excluded. A careful history and examination should determine the selection of appropriate laboratory tests.

TABLE 89-1

Antihypertensive Medications Useful in Children

MEDICATION	ROUTE
Diazoxide	IV bolus
Hydralazine	IV/IM
Labetalol	IV
Sodium nitroprusside	IV
Captopril	PO
Chlorothiazide	PO
Furosemide	PO
Hydralazine	PO
Minoxidil	PO
Nifedipine	PO
Prazosin	PO
Propranolol	PO
Spironolactone	PO

If severe blood pressure elevation and the threat of permanent CNS injury (e.g., rapidly progressive visual loss) are present, blood pressure should be treated medically [Thien et al., 1979]. Care should be taken not to reduce the mean arterial pressure lower than the lower limit of cerebral blood flow autoregulation. Below this level, maximal autoregulatory vasodilatation fails to prevent cerebral ischemia and permanent nervous system injury may result [Brown et al., 1987; Graham, 1975; Hulse et al., 1979; Sebire et al., 1995]. Predicting this lower limit is difficult given age-related variation, as well as the fact that chronic hypertension may reduce the vasodilatory capacity of arterioles and thus raise the mean pressure at which decompensation occurs. Within these limits for blood pressure reduction, aggressive treatment is likely to be well tolerated except in the setting of increased intracranial pressure and dysautonomia, as in Guillain-Barré syndrome. The risk for neurologic sequelae (blindness, coma, pyramidal tract injury) from iatrogenic hypotension is related not only to the severity but also to the duration of hypotension [Franklin, 1984].

In most patients with childhood-accelerated hypertension, aggressive and safe blood pressure reduction can be achieved with intravenous sodium nitroprusside. This high-potency, brief-duration agent provides the considerable advantage of momentary titration to the responses of the individual patient. Sustained use in renal failure carries the risk of intoxication. Labetalol is another useful intravenous medication, but the longer duration of action is disadvantageous or even dangerous if hypotension develops. In patients with less severe elevations of blood pressure, hydralazine or nifedipine may be used [Kandt et al., 1995; Trompeter et al., 1982]. Captopril is a particularly useful agent in patients with renin-dependent hypertension (essential, renovascular, hemolytic-uremic syndrome or thrombotic thrombocytopenic purpura–related). Diazoxide is the medication most commonly associated with untoward hypotensive reduction of blood pressure with deleterious consequences. Large-bore venous access should be secured in every patient against the possibility of sudden hypotension, whatever therapeutic approach is undertaken. The appropriate medication choice and the dosage for use in the newborn are not well defined. Sodium nitroprusside may pose a greater risk for intoxication, and both methyldopa and reserpine may cause profound sedation.

Acute management of severe cerebral edema may involve mechanical hyperventilation, osmotic agents, or corticosteroids. In such instances, placement of an intracranial pressure monitor should be considered, especially with hyperventilation, because this action is associated with risk for reflexive cerebral capacitance vessel vasoconstriction that may worsen cerebral and brainstem perfusion defects. Osmotic agents may accumulate in acute renal failure and should be carefully dialyzed. Some patients respond slowly to treatment or develop permanent deficits, particularly visual and motor ones [Hulse et al., 1979]. Antiepileptic medications should be administered to children with acute, persistent seizures, but chronic anticonvulsant therapy is seldom required. Chronic hypertension carries a significant risk for seizures, cerebral thrombosis/hemorrhage, subarachnoid hemorrhage, and Bell's palsy even if acute hypertensive encephalopathy does not occur [Schottstaedt and Sokolow, 1953].

Some adults develop a subacute progressive hypertensive encephalopathy with pathologically identifiable changes in the deep cerebral microvasculature [Fisher, 1998]. It is unclear whether chronic hypertension or multiple episodes of acute blood pressure elevation produce similar changes in children. A number of antihypertensive medications may impair intellectual function of children and adults. Of particular importance are methyldopa, reserpine, propranolol, and clonidine. These changes may be due in part to sedation (usually transient), sleep disturbance, or depression [Light, 1980].

COMPLICATIONS OF CHRONIC RENAL FAILURE

The prevalence of chronic renal failure is 18 per 1 million children. End-stage renal disease is present in 1.5 per 1 million children [Leumann, 1976]. All of the neurologic complications observed in acute renal failure may occur as complications of chronic renal failure, particularly during acute uremic or hypertensive decompensations. However, other subacute forms of neurologic dysfunction not encountered in acute renal failure are characteristically observed in chronic renal failure and especially end-stage renal disease (defined as a glomerular filtration rate below 2.9 mL/minute/m^2, the level at which dialysis is required to maintain homeostasis) [Nissenson et al., 1977].

Chronic renal failure may be complicated by one of two different types of dementia. The first of these disorders is observed in young children with renal failure manifesting in infancy and is termed *congenital uremic encephalopathy.* The development of this dementia is independent of dialysis and is accompanied by microcephaly and severe growth failure. A second type of dementia, termed *progressive dialysis encephalopathy,* is found in dialyzed adolescent and adult patients with end-stage renal disease. Other complications of dialysis, chronic renal failure, and end-stage renal disease include headache, dialysis disequilibrium syndrome, dialysis-associated seizures, Wernicke's encephalopathy, cerebral hemorrhage, uremic neuropathy, and various neurologic complications of transplantation.

Congenital Uremic Encephalopathy

Severe chronic uremia (glomerular filtration rate ≤ 10% of normal) developing in the first year of life carries a very high risk for ensuing subacute progressive encephalopathy [Foley et al., 1981; Valanne et al., 2004]. Most of these infants have inherited forms of nephrosis, particularly congenital nephrosis of the Finnish type. It is possible that some of the neurologic abnormalities noted in these infants are independently inherited developmental abnormalities or due to the prenatal metabolic effects of nephrosis. The appearance of abnormalities may appear after a latent interval.

Early provision of dialysis has not prevented development of congenital uremic encephalopathy. Some children with genetically determined congenital nephroses have worse neurologic outcomes than others. There is emerging evidence concerning coexpression of defective enzymes in brain and kidney that may account for abnormal development and function of both organs. An important research priority remains that of discovering whether the neurologic abnormalities of congenital nephroses are (1) the inexorable result of unpreventable heritable neurodevelopmental defects or the effects of prenatal toxicity of the uremic state, or (2) whether and to what extent they may be due to postnatal course and treatment of the congenitally nephrotic child.

Older studies have tended to group all individuals with infantile onset of severe renal failure (those that survive the neonatal period) together for follow-up studies without consideration of varied genetic causes that are now appreciated. These studies have proved that more than two thirds of such children manifested seizures and developmental arrest in the first year of life, followed in the second year by developmental regression with acquired microcephaly [Polinsky et al., 1980, 1987; Sedman et al., 1984]. By several years of age, 60% to 80% have epilepsy (focal or generalized), as well as moderate-to-severe motor, cognitive, language, and psychosocial delay [McGraw et al., 1986; Rotundo et al., 1982]. By comparison, studies from the same era found that at least 90% of children who developed end-stage renal disease after early infancy enjoyed normal psychomotor development even if assessed after far greater durations of illness and dialysis [Rasbury et al., 1983].

Despite careful attention to nutrition and metabolic parameters, the linear growth of the majority of children with infantile-onset end-stage renal disease is retarded. More than two thirds of these children have acquired microcephaly. Craniosynostosis develops in a small number. Neurologic abnormalities include varied degrees of ataxia, choreoathetosis, facial myoclonus, hypotonicity, weakness, and hyperreflexia. If language develops, it is often compromised by dysarthria and lingual apraxia [Polinsky et al., 1987]. Most children with congenital uremic encephalopathy die within the first few years of life, often from progressive bulbar failure [Rotundo et al., 1982]. No evidence exists that renal transplantation reverses or even arrests progression of congenital uremic encephalopathy.

Improved neurologic function with dialysis remains a reliable way to distinguish acute infantile uremia with encephalopathy from congenital nephrosis with progressive uremic encephalopathy that does not manifest improvement [McGraw et al., 1986]. Inexorable decline in neurologic function and somatic growth despite careful attention to metabolic parameters is so characteristic that the diagnosis of congenital progressive uremic encephalopathy can usually be made on clinical grounds. The electroencephalogram initially indicates generalized slowing in either form of encephalopathy, but in the congenital progressive form the EEG organization deteriorates in a fashion parallel to observed neurologic deterioration despite treatment, with the development of paroxysmal sharp, rhythmic slow, or polyspike-wave discharges. The EEG findings improve in infantile uremia with encephalopathy in a fashion that roughly parallels improvement in the clinical capacities of the appropriately treated infant. These characteristic paroxysms resemble those observed in older children and adults with progressive dialysis encephalopathy [Guisado et al., 1975; Jacob et al., 1965].

Brain imaging of infants with progressive uremic encephalopathy due to congenital nephrosis usually reveals brain atrophy [Baluarte et al., 1977; McGraw and Haka-Ikse, 1985], although pseudoatrophy due to the concurrent use of corticosteroids in many of these children makes interpretation of scans difficult until encephalomalacia is fairly advanced. Pathologic examination of the brain of children with congenital nephrotic syndromes has confirmed that sulcal widening and enlarged ventricles are the result of neuronal loss greatest in the cerebral cortex, brainstem sensory nuclei, and reticular formation [Papageorgiou et al., 1982]. The volume loss is compounded by wallerian degeneration in the subcortical and brainstem fiber pathways.

Most children with congenital nephrosis have inherited the severe Finnish type. It is an autosomal recessive condition due to mutations in both nephrin gene (*NPHS1*) alleles. Many of these children are born a month or so before term and have low birth weight, microcephaly, ascites, edema, and massive proteinuria. Suspicion of this condition is raised by the detection of persistent elevation of amniotic fluid α-fetoprotein without evidence for neural tube defects. The severity of the Finnish type of congenital nephrosis has led to termination of some pregnancies [Overstreet et al., 2002]. Many infants with Finnish type congenital nephrosis die in the first few weeks or months of life. This genetic defect results in structural and functional abnormalities of the podocyte foot processes and slit-diaphragm structures of the developing kidney [Finn, 2003; Pollak, 2003; Valanne et al., 2004]. These infants lack expression in kidney of nephrin and have diminished kidney expression of synaptopodin and GLEPP1, proteins that are crucial to the assembly of the kidney podocyte and associated structures. It has recently been discovered that these proteins are also expressed in neurons. Their function in the nervous system is as yet uncertain, although they may play a role in synaptic plasticity [Deller et al., 2000, 2002, 2003; Mundell et al., 1997; Mundell and Kelly, 1998]. Some children with congenital nephrosis have corticosteroid-resistant focal segmental glomerulosclerosis. Often, these children also have neurologic abnormalities. This form of congenital nephrosis occurs as the result of mutations of both podocin gene (*NPHS2*) alleles. The relationship among nephrin, podocin, α-actinin-4 (*ACTN4*) and other genes whose proteins are coexpressed in kidney and brain to the poor neurologic development in many children with severe congenital renal disease remains unclear. Diminished expression of these various proteins is also found in renal conditions such as minimal change disease, which is not associated with neurologic abnormalities. In addition to genetic conditions that affect kidney structure, metabolic conditions such as type 1 carbohydrate-deficient glycoprotein disease may produce the phenotype of congenital renal failure with abnormal growth and neurologic dysfunction [Drouin-Garraud et al., 2001].

Galloway-Mowat, arthrogryposis, renal dysfunction, and cholestasis (ARC), and progressive encephalopathy with edema, hypsarrhythmia, and optic atrophy (PEHO) syndrome are among the heterogenous collection of phenotypes with early-onset nephropathy associated with various neurologic abnormalities. The Galloway-Mowat phenotype includes children with microcephaly, cerebellar atrophy or hypoplasia, and nephrosis due to focal segmental glomerulosclerosis that may not become clinically apparent until several years of age. End-stage renal disease may not develop until near the end of the first decade of life [Shiihara et al., 2003].

Certain potentially deleterious but preventable postnatal influences on neurologic development in children with congenital or early childhood chronic renal failure have been identified. These include aluminum toxicity, vascular accidents, chronic uremia, hypertension, malnutrition, circulatory disturbances, and psychosocial deprivation [Arieff and Armstrong, 1980; Chantler et al., 1981; Cogan et al., 1978; Elzouki et al., 1994].

ALUMINUM TOXICITY. Until recently, almost all infants with severe early-onset renal disease have received high doses of aluminum-containing phosphate binders indicated for the treatment of hyperphosphatemia that is the result of secondary hyperparathyroidism [Polinsky et al., 1980; Randall, 1983]. Aluminum is now known to be toxic, especially in the setting of hyperparathyroidism. Aluminum exposure has been identified in epidemiologic studies as a significant risk factor for encephalopathy in patients with end-stage renal disease at any age. Progressive dementia has been demonstrated in industrial aluminum exposure. Aluminum was proposed as a cause of Alzheimer's disease, although evidence has appeared increasingly unconvincing [Crapper et al., 1973, 1976].

It has been suggested, on the basis of limited information, that the known neurotoxicities of aluminum are due to alteration of cellular repair mechanisms, derangement of neurotransmitter or energy metabolism, or deleterious affects on vascular reactivity [Polinsky and Gruskin, 1984; Starkey, 1987; Wilson and Fearon, 1984]. It has also been suggested that aluminum may serve as an adjuvant for the toxic effects of other circulating toxins. It may alter membrane (e.g., blood-brain barrier) characteristics, permitting greater access of toxins to the CNS.

Sources of aluminum have included water (used in dialysate or commercially prepared infant formula), intravenous solutions, and parenteral medications, and especially the aluminum salts administered to control hyperphosphatemia [McGraw et al, 1986; Milliner et al., 1985; Sedman et al., 1985]. Bladder irrigation with alum as a treatment for hemorrhagic cystitis has resulted in acute encephalopathic deterioration of patients with chronic renal failure [Perazella and Brown, 1993]. Infants with congenital uremic encephalopathy have been found to have serum, bone, and brain concentrations of aluminum that exceed control values by up to 25-fold [Andreoli et al., 1984; Freundlich et al., 1985; Nathan and Pedersen, 1980]. Serum levels of aluminum do not correlate directly with degree of putative neurotoxicities observed in a given individual [Sedman et al., 1984].

Infants were at high risk for aluminum toxicity because of one or more of the following: (1) the total daily aluminum salt doses calculated for infants on a weight basis have been far higher than the total daily doses administered to older patients with end-stage renal disease (>100 mg/kg/day); (2) gut absorption and brain penetration by aluminum may be greater in infants, especially if they have hyperparathyroidism; and (3) cow's milk and infant formulas enriched in phosphate have prompted the use of higher doses of aluminum-containing phosphate binders [Polinsky et al., 1987].

Management of infantile chronic renal failure without the use of aluminum salts has greatly diminished the prevalence of progressive nephrotic encephalopathy. In one study, infants managed without these salts who receive vigorous nutritional and psychosocial support have demonstrated markedly improved neurologic outcome by 4 years of age. Neurologic examinations of such children may indicate only hypotonia. Microcephaly is found in approximately one third, brain atrophy in 20%, developmental delay in 20%, and neuropathy in less than 15% [Elzouki et al., 1994]. On the other hand, congenital uremic encephalopathy has developed in some infants who have never received aluminum-containing phosphate binders.

STROKES. Vascular accidents may cause acquired neurologic injuries in children with congenital nephroses. At 6 to 11 years of age, 50% of brains of children who have onset of nephrosis in the first year of life have vascular border zone abnormalities, mostly mild, suggesting prior ischemic brain injury. A smaller percentage has large artery territory or basal ganglia infarcts, and some have brain atrophy. The presence of lesions suggesting vascular territory infarctions appears to correlate with history of pretransplantation hemodynamic crises and with greater duration of management by dialysis before renal transplantation [Valanne et al., 2004]. Attention devoted to ensuring hemodynamic stability in infants undergoing dialysis for chronic renal failure and early consideration of transplantation may improve outcome.

MALNUTRITION. Head circumference is a reliable index of brain injury in malnourished infants with congenital uremic encephalopathy [Winick et al., 1971]. That severe encephalopathy does not develop in most patients with malabsorption syndromes despite poor somatic growth suggests that factors other than nutrition are of greater importance in producing this vulnerability to poor brain growth in children with congenital uremic encephalopathy [McGraw and Haka-Ikse, 1985]. Tube feedings and special formulas have improved growth but do not appear to prevent congenital uremic encephalopathy.

Nutritional disorders are difficult to dissociate from the metabolic and endocrine dysfunction of chronic renal failure. Recent information suggests that vitamin B_{12} deficiency with abnormality of methionine metabolism and hyperhomocystinuria may contribute to neurologic abnormalities [Herrmann and Knapp, 2002]. Renal osteodystrophy and hyperparathyroidism, routinely found in patients with congenital renal failure, have long been appreciated as factors of importance in developmental and growth delay. Osteodystrophy may secondarily impair gross motor function but does not explain the significant delay exhibited by these patients in other areas of development.

ENDOCRINOPATHY. Hyperparathyroidism and either hypercalcemia or hypocalcemia may directly injure the nervous system [Seyahi et al., 2004]. Uremia with hyperparathyroidism is associated with slowing of the EEG and may increase brain calcium to the extent that cerebral calcification results. This calcification is found in the subcortex and basal ganglia in children, rather than the cortical and hypothalamic calcification more typical of adults with end-stage renal disease. Parathyroid hormone excess may directly affect neurotransmission in brain [Smits et al., 1983]. Studies in animals and human adults have found that encephalopathy may be prevented or ameliorated with parathyroidectomy [Akmal et al., 1984; Mahoney and Arieff, 1983]. Poor somatic growth in congenital chronic renal failure has been ascribed in part to hypothalamic-pituitary dysfunction [Schmitz and Moller, 1983]. It has been found that normalization of parathyroid hormone leads to acceleration of growth velocity and "catch-up" growth in children with chronic renal failure [Waller et al., 2003].

Some patients with congenital onset of chronic renal failure have fulminant deterioration in neurologic function at some point in their course. Often, this deterioration occurs in association with infection, severe metabolic decompensation, or after surgery, including renal transplantation [Griswold et al., 1983]. In such patients, CNS infection, hemorrhage, electrolyte disturbances, intoxications, and hypertension must be excluded.

COMPLICATIONS OF DIALYSIS

Dialysis is efficacious in the remediation or prevention of acute uremic encephalopathy in patients with severe renal failure and is also beneficial in the treatment of uremic peripheral neuropathy and of some cases of acquired deafness [Mitschke et al., 1975].

Dialysis is associated with many potential complications of greater or lesser significance. Many are neurologic, including headache, dialysis disequilibrium syndrome, thiamine and carnitine deficiencies, intracranial hemorrhage, and progressive dialysis encephalopathy. Dialysis complications are three times as common during the first four dialysis sessions than later [Rosa et al., 1980]. Problems related to the preparation of dialysis fluids are now seldom encountered. When they do occur, they tend to manifest as seizures or decline in mental status. Once such improperly prepared fluids are identified, a satisfactory outcome may be achieved after gradual correction with properly prepared dialysate even after severe hypernatremia [Borrego Dominguez et al., 2003].

Prevalences of complications of dialysis vary from common to rare. Headache (2% to 25%) or cramps (15% to 50%) are common. Exceedingly rare complications in children include Wernicke's encephalopathy and dialysis-associated amyloidosis [Lopez and Collins, 1968; Rosa et al., 1980]. The incidence of many complications has decreased markedly in the past decade, particularly dialysis disequilibrium syndrome. Episodic hypertension is a common concern in dialysis and may be associated with hypertensive encephalopathy, brain hemorrhage, severe headache, and pulmonary edema. It is caused by extracellular fluid accumulation between dialysis sessions and the secretion of large amounts of renin, especially during and immediately after dialysis sessions. Hemodialyzed patients (especially blacks) may develop encephalopathy with hypertension related to acute pancreatitis [Avram, 1977].

Headache

The frequency of dialysis-associated headache is unclear, with various reports suggesting figures between 2% and 70% of patients with chronic renal failure/end-stage renal disease [Antoniazzi et al., 2002; Bana and Graham, 1976; Goksan et al., 2004; Rosa et al., 1980]. There is no reliable information concerning the frequency of headache in children who undergo dialysis. Mild-to-moderate headache is not uncommonly reported by older children. Criteria for diagnosis have been established by the International Headache Society and require headache related to dialysis to begin during hemodialysis and terminate within 24 hours of onset [Antoniazzi et al., 2003].

It is likely that dialysis headache is prompted by water and electrolyte shifts or by other aspects of dialysis disequilibrium (see later). Risk can be reduced by adjustment of dialysis parameters, including the use of sodium modeling programs during dialysis rather than administering a constant concentration of dialysate sodium [Sadowski et al., 1993]. Dialysis headache may share some of the mechanisms of water-deprivation headache [Blau et al., 2004]. Patients with higher predialysis systolic and diastolic blood pressure may be at greater risk for headache, as well as those who experience dialysis-related hypotension or weight loss [Antoniazzi et al., 2002; Goksan et al., 2004].

Our experience suggests that at least half the children who experience dialysis-associated headaches have historical evidence for a migrainous disorder, although their worst headaches may develop only with dialysis. Family history, occurrence of throbbing hemicrania, and relief with sleep support the diagnosis of migraine. Migrainous dialysis headache develops after several hours of dialysis, usually with bilaterally throbbing pain, but pain may have a viselike or dull quality. Headache is known to respond to administration of ergot or butalbital and rest [Bana and Graham, 1976]. Various other analgesics have been employed, including dipyrone [Antoniazzi et al., 2002]. There is as yet no information on the risks and benefits of triptans in this setting. Children or adolescents who do not have a history of migrainous headaches may also develop headaches of mild to moderate severity after 3 to 4 hours of dialysis. These headaches often respond to acetaminophen with or without butalbital.

Headache can result from readily detectable metabolic abnormalities (e.g., hypernatremic cellular dehydration or water intoxication), which must in some instances be excluded. Hypertension or subdural hemorrhage should be considered when headache is more severe or persistent, particularly if obtundation or new focal neurologic signs are present [Raskin and Fishman, 1976b]. Subdural hemorrhage associated with anticoagulation is a rare but important complication of dialysis. It causes progressive headache and obtundation, often with focal neurologic signs. Use of worn-out cellulose acetate dialysis membranes has been blamed for an outbreak of postdialysis headache and, in some instances, loss of hearing or vision (with corneal opacity) [Hutter et al., 2000].

Dialysis Disequilibrium Syndrome

Dialysis disequilibrium syndrome is a variable but distinctive mixture of neurologic symptoms and signs that are particularly likely to occur in the early phases of a dialysis program [Kiley, 1984]. In the early days of dialysis, disequilibrium syndrome occurred in nearly 10% of adults and more than 30% of children [Grushkin et al., 1972; Tyler and Tyler, 1984]. The most common manifestations are irritability or restlessness, fatigue, headache, nausea, blurred vision, muscle cramps, and, in some instances, twitching. Hypertension, tremulousness, vomiting, disorientation, agitated delirium, seizures, visual loss, elevated intraocular pressure, papilledema, and asterixis are sometimes seen [Kennedy et al., 1964; Peterson and Swanson, 1964]. Wernicke's encephalopathy has been reported rarely. Coma may develop, and death may occur from central herniation [Milutinovich et al., 1979]. EEG changes are usually limited to variable degrees of background slowing.

The syndrome is particularly likely to occur with recently initiated dialysis, utilization of rapid dialysis protocol, or dialysis with ultrafiltration [Kerr, 1980; Raskin and Fishman, 1976b; Tyler, 1968; Young et al., 1988]. The onset may be from 3 to 4 hours after initiation or as late as 20 hours after the completion of a dialysis session. Intellectual dysfunction, psychiatric symptoms, and visual abnormalities are usually self-limited, lasting for several hours. These problems may, in some instances, persist for several days. It is likely that subtle and unrecognized intellectual dysfunction occurs not infrequently in the early stages of dialysis as a manifestation of mild dialysis disequilibrium syndrome. Dialysis with rapid correction of hyponatremia has been blamed for one case of fatal pontine myelinolysis [Loo et al., 1995].

The term *osmotic demyelination* has been applied to some patients who experience deterioration of neurologic function after dialysis and are found to have hypointense abnormalities on T2-weighted MRI in the region of the pons. These changes may be found also in some patients with dialysis-associated seizures or mild disturbances of consciousness. Repeat scans usually demonstrate the rapid and complete disappearance of these changes, the imaging characteristics of which are consistent with edema. It is likely that many individuals with dialysis disequilibrium have merely developed transient dialysis-related brain edema rather than demyelination [Tarhan et al., 2004].

Dialysis removes osmotically active molecules from blood more rapidly than they can diffuse out of the brain. This movement results in an osmotic gradient that provokes net flow of water into the brain, resulting in cerebral edema, increased intracranial pressure, and encephalopathy [Arieff et al., 1973; Wakim, 1969a, 1969b]. These deleterious osmotic gradients were ascribed to effects of urea ("reverse urea syndrome") because dialysis disequilibrium syndrome did not appear to develop when nonuremic patients were dialyzed [Kennedy et al., 1963; Kleeman et al., 1962; Peterson and Swanson, 1964], but studies failed to provide convincing evidence of a significant urea gradient [Pappius et al., 1967; Wakim, 1969a]. Urea enters the brain at a very slow rate, but the use of a urea-containing dialysate has failed to prevent edema. Another theory suggested that osmotic activity is the result of retention within the brain or nonurea "middle molecules" or "idiogenic osmoles" [Arieff et al., 1973]. The fall in cerebrospinal fluid pH that may occur during dialysis was cited as indirect evidence for the accumulation of osmotically active organic acid and amine "middle molecules" in the CNS of patients with chronic renal failure [Arieff et al., 1978]. Another study found no evidence for any additional contribution by "idiogenic osmoles" to dialysis-induced cerebral edema [Silver et al., 1992]. Short echo-time magnetic resonance spectroscopy has documented changes in cerebral concentration of myo-inositol, choline-containing compounds, and water in brain during dialysis. These changes were greater in gray matter than in white matter [Michaelis et al., 1996].

Modifications in dialysis protocols have significantly reduced the frequency of dialysis disequilibrium. These modifications have included changes in dialysis priming, increased dialysate salt concentration, inclusion of colloids such as mannitol and albumin, limitation of dialysis to 10% of blood volume, and more gradual initial reduction of blood urea nitrogen to the range of 70 to 80 mg/dL. The most important element in preventing dialysis disequilibrium is early diagnosis and dialysis so that profound azotemia (blood urea nitrogen ≥ 200 mg/dL) is rarely encountered [Arieff et al., 1978; Port et al., 1973].

If dialysis disequilibrium is severe, mannitol administration may be beneficial. The use of mannitol must be carefully coordinated with dialysis to ensure that the mannitol and mobilized fluid are removed from the circulation with appropriate speed. Seizures due to dialysis disequilibrium are usually transient.

Dialysis-Associated Seizures

Dialysis-associated seizures occur in 7% to 10% of children (newborn to 21 years) with end-stage renal disease. Most are generalized tonic-clonic seizures that occur during or shortly after dialysis [Swartz et al., 1983]. They are more commonly associated with hemodialysis (8% to 9%) than peritoneal dialysis (0% to 4%) [Grushkin et al., 1972] and are likely due to chemical or osmotic disequilibria. The risk for dialysis-associated seizures is as high as 29% in children with a history of seizures [Glenn et al., 1992]. Other risk factors are young age, malignant hypertension, or encephalopathy due to uremia, dialysis disequilibrium, or congenital uremic encephalopathy [Swartz et al., 1983]. Seizures are more likely to occur during the early phases of a dialysis program when solute changes are the greatest. Increased risk with hemodialysis may be related to more rapid clearance of electrolytes and other osmotically active solutes by this method than by peritoneal dialysis [Glenn et al., 1992]. The frequency of dialysis-associated seizures in older children and in children who have undergone dialysis for more than 2 months may be accounted for by the greater likelihood of hemodialysis in those groups [Glenn et al., 1992; Polinsky et al., 1980]. Severe azotemia (blood urea nitrogen > 200 mg/dL), hypocalcemia (<6 mg/dL), hypomagnesemia (<1 mg/dL), anemia (hemoglobin < 5 mg/dL), hypertonicity, acidosis, and hypoxemia also increase the risk for dialysis-associated seizures [Swartz et al., 1983].

MRI abnormalities suggesting edema in the pons, as well as in extrapontine locations, may be present and resemble changes seen in dialysis disequilibrium syndrome [Tarhan et al., 2004]. The electroencephalogram may indicate frontal intermittent rhythmic delta and diffuse slowing with prominent photic activation [Watemberg et al., 2002]. These changes have been interpreted by some as representing the presence of old structural injury perhaps related to ischemic watershed infarction [Watemberg et al., 2002]. The efficacy of antiepileptic drugs in treating or preventing dialysis-associated seizures is poorly defined. The use of readily dialyzable medications may increase the risk for dialysis-associated seizures because these drugs are removed at the same time that the dialytic metabolic stress may induce seizures.

Vitamin and Cofactor Deficiencies

The B vitamins are water soluble, and most are readily dialyzable. A single dialysis session may reduce plasma thiamine concentration by as much as 40% [Lasker et al., 1963]. Patients with end-stage renal disease are therefore at risk for thiamine deficiency, which may present as confusion progressing rapidly to obtundation or coma. Associated findings may include chorea, visual loss, ophthalmoparesis, ataxia, myoclonus, or seizures. It has been estimated that this deficiency may account for as many as one third of all cases of unexplained acute encephalopathy in chronically dialyzed adults [Hung et al., 2001a, 2001b].

It is somewhat surprising that symptomatic thiamine deficiency has been reported only rarely in children, probably because stores of thiamine accumulated before the development of renal disease are only gradually depleted and considerable effort is expended by parents and caregivers to ensure good nutrition. Wernicke's encephalopathy has been described in a child undergoing dialysis who demonstrated the characteristic triad of ophthalmoplegia, encephalopathy, and ataxia [Faris, 1972]. Adult cases usually develop in the wake of prolonged malnutrition [Raskin and Fishman, 1976a]. Prompt recognition and treatment are important. Response to intravenous thiamine may confirm the diagnosis [Hung et al., 2001b].

Pyridoxine-deficiency seizures have been described in a child treated with peritoneal dialysis [Joshioka et al., 1984]. Deficiency of vitamin B_{12} may, in turn, provoke abnormal methionine metabolism. Hyperhomocystinuria is an important indicator of vitamin B_{12} deficiency. If found, it is associated with higher risk for preeclampsia, neural tube defects in offspring, atherosclerotic arterial disease (large and peripheral vessels), stroke, and venous thrombosis [Herrmann and Knapp, 2002]. Supplementation with B vitamins is routine to avoid these various complications [Kopple and Swendseid, 1975]. Dialysis may also result in depletion of serum carnitine; the possible clinical significance of this effect requires more investigation [Bartel et al., 1982].

Intracranial Hemorrhage

The incidence of subdural hematoma among children is unknown but is probably less than 10% [Grushkin et al., 1972]. Replacement of generalized with regional anticoagulation minimizes the risk of this serious complication. Subdural hematoma must be considered in renal patients with persistent drowsiness, headache, or vomiting, and particularly in those with persistent focal neurologic signs (typically hemiparesis) or meningismus. Signs and symptoms may fluctuate or progressively worsen [Bechar et al., 1972; Leonard and Shapiro, 1975].

Progressive Dialysis (Aluminum) Encephalopathy (Dementia)

A progressive and lethal dementia affecting patients with end-stage renal disease and manifesting dyspraxia and multifocal seizures at the onset was first described by Alfrey and associates in 1972. The entity quickly assumed epidemic proportions and caused considerable consternation in dialysis patients and their physicians [Mahurkar et al., 1973]. Aluminum exposure was the result of utilization of dialysate water purified with aluminum sulfate techniques and from the utilization of aluminum hydroxide as a phosphate binder [Dunea, 2001]. A largely unheeded warning of the potential toxicity of aluminum had been offered in 1970 [Berlyne et al., 1970], but the flurry of research that followed Alfrey's report of the clinical syndrome greatly enhanced recognition of the public health threat posed by this metal.

In the early stages, aluminum dementia must be distinguished from each of the many treatable forms of encephalopathy associated with chronic uremia (see earlier), including various metabolic disequilibria. It is especially important to consider thiamine deficiency, a condition for which all end-stage renal disease patients are at risk and which may present as confusion progressing rapidly to encephalopathy or coma (see earlier discussion). The chronically poor development and gradual decline of patients with congenital uremic encephalopathy is usually readily distinguishable from the abrupt deterioration of function that occurs early in aluminum dementia. Acquired speech dyspraxia is especially difficult to distinguish from the severe speech and language problems characteristically found in individuals with Finnish-type congenital renal failure.

Milder Forms of Encephalopathy

Neuropsychologic studies of adults have consistently documented subtle forms of cortical dysfunction in some patients with chronic renal failure, particularly low verbal IQ. Ability to concentrate may be reduced by even moderate azotemia [Teschan et al., 1983]. Little systematic information is available concerning subtle intellectual dysfunction and learning disability in children with end-stage renal disease. However, abnormalities of performance IQ, short-term visual and auditory memory, attention span, memory, and speed of decision making have been documented. The risk for such problems is greatest if end-stage renal disease developed in early childhood (particularly during the first year of life) or if the disease is of very long duration [Crittenden et al., 1985; Fennell et al., 1984; Osberg et al., 1982; Polinsky et al., 1980]. Subtle intellectual and behavioral abnormalities that are responsive to dialysis have been detected in older [Grushkin et al., 1972] but not all [Fennell et al., 1986] studies.

Evaluation of speech performance requires consideration of the high prevalence of depression, emotional stress, and hearing abnormalities in patients with chronic renal failure and exclusion of the confounding effects of prior developmental dysmaturity and chronic hospitalization. Sensorineural hearing abnormalities may be present in as many as half of patients with end-stage renal disease [Bergstrom and Thompson, 1983; Mirahmadi and Vaziri, 1980]. Drugs used for treatment of end-stage renal disease and its complications may provoke encephalopathy (see later). Seizures may interfere with school performance. The electroencephalogram must be interpreted cautiously because up to half of children with end-stage renal disease have bursts of spike-and-wave activity without evidence of clinical seizures [Foley et al., 1981].

Poor intellectual function should lead to identification and scrupulous correction of metabolic abnormalities. Moderate uremia may result in disturbances ranging from mild encephalopathy to mild chronic delirium or psychosis [Richet and Vachon, 1966]. In some patients, intellectual dysfunction, deafness, and neuropathy (see later discussion) unresponsive to optimal dialysis may improve after successful transplantation [Brown et al., 1987; Fennell et al., 1984; Mitschke et al., 1975]. Hypophosphatemia (especially serum phosphate < 1.0 mg/dL) is associated with delirium. A combination of aluminum binders, dialysis, and poor diet (often the consequence of anorexia in patients with chronic renal failure) may also provoke mental status changes. Neurologic dysfunction ranging from confusion to nonketotic hyperosmolar coma may occur as the result of using dialysate with a high glucose concentration.

Uremic Neuropathy (Neuropathy of Chronic Renal Failure)

Peripheral neuropathy, first reported more than 40 years ago [Hegstrom et al., 1962], occurs in some patients with advanced chronic renal failure. Asbury and colleagues [1963] provided the earliest detailed description. Somatic and autonomic nerves may be involved [Jedras et al., 2001]. Risk for neuropathy is not limited to any particular etiologic category of chronic renal failure. As with other neurologic complications, duration and severity of chronic renal failure (e.g., degree of loss of glomerular filtration) are the most important determinants of occurrence and severity of neuropathy [Jurcic et al., 1998]. In patients with congenital or early childhood onset of chronic renal failure, clinical manifestations of neuropathy have been detected as early as 8 years of age [Oh et al., 1978]. However, few well-documented childhood cases have been reported [Patten, 1984]. Although the term *uremic neuropathy* is commonly employed, the pathogenesis is complex and incompletely understood; and it may be preferable to refer to the condition as *neuropathy of chronic renal failure*.

Onset of this condition is usually insidious. It is not known how early in the course of the development of neuropathy that electrophysiologic abnormalities can be detected. Subclinical nerve conduction slowing is a not uncommon finding of patients with end-stage renal disease [Ackil et al., 1981; Arbus et al., 1975]. Electrophysiologic abnormalities consistent with neuropathy are ultimately detectable in as many as two thirds of adults with long-standing chronic renal failure, whether or not dialysis has been initiated [Hassan et al., 2003]. Occasionally, the onset of neuropathy is fulminant, suggesting the possibility of a nonuremic etiology [Asbury et al., 1963; Kondo et al., 1997].

Males are more likely to manifest sensorimotor uremic neuropathy than females and may develop somatic neuropathy in association with uremia of milder degree and briefer duration, but females are more likely to manifest autonomic neuropathy [Asbury et al., 1963; Jedras et al., 2001; Versaci et al., 1964]. A "restless legs" syndrome is among the most common presenting complaints of sensorimotor neuropathy, associated with an unpleasant sensation of "crawling skin" or a "dull ache" of legs that is worse in the evening. Dysesthesias tend to be relieved by leg movement. More convenient and sustained relief may be achieved with clonazepam [Callaghan, 1966]. Pruritus, which is complained of by as many as two thirds of patients who have had long-term dialysis for end-stage renal disease, may also be a sign of neuropathy in some cases. Likelihood is greatest in individuals who also complain of paresthesias, many of whom are found to have neurophysiologic symptoms and additional clinical evidence of neuropathy [Jedras et al., 1998].

Loss of deep tendon reflexes (especially the ankle jerk), diminished vibratory sensation, and weakness of great toe extension are among the earliest signs of uremic neuropathy [Tenckhoff et al., 1965]. Paradoxical heat sensation, the tendency to identify a low-temperature stimulus as "hot," is also a sensitive early sign of uremic polyneuropathy. This phenomenon appears to correlate not only with the degree of cold hypesthesia but also with the serum creatinine level [Yosipovitch et al., 1995]. As with other neuropathic forms of weakness, distal wasting of muscle is an important clinical sign that distinguishes neuropathic from myopathic causes of weakness. Early in the course of illness it may be difficult to discern either because wasting may be masked by obesity (due to inactivity, excessive caloric intake, or steroid use) or by excessive dependent fluid retention (due to inactivity, fluid shifts, or autonomic dysfunction).

Fully developed uremic neuropathy is a distal, symmetric polyneuropathy that involves both sensory and motor modalities in a length-dependent fashion. Greatest abnormality is detected in functions subserved by large, long peripheral nerve fibers. The legs are usually more severely affected than the arms [Bakke, 1970; Nielsen, 1971a, 1971b]. In most patients, uremic neuropathy so closely resembles nutritional, diabetic, or alcoholic neuropathies as to be clinically indistinguishable. Diminished sensitivity to all sensory modalities in a glove-stocking distribution gradually develops. Pressure palsies, to which chronic renal failure/neuropathic renal disease patients are particularly subject, may alter the expected distribution of abnormalities [Bolton et al., 1971].

Other forms of dysesthesia, nocturnal calf cramps, distal weakness, and atrophy may develop and vary considerably in severity [Callaghan, 1966; Tyler, 1976]. In adolescents and adults with dialysis for end-stage renal disease, sudomotor changes and postural hypotension are common consequences of autonomic neuropathy if it develops [Yildiz et al., 1998]. It is unknown how frequently autonomic neuropathy develops in children [Bach et al., 1979]. Successful renal transplantation may simultaneously and rapidly reverse both sympathetic and parasympathetic autonomic dysfunction that has developed in adult patients with end-stage renal disease [Yildiz et al., 1998]. Hearing loss, common in end-stage renal disease, may be the result of uremic axonal neuropathy, although other incompletely cleared endogenous or administered ototoxic substances may contribute to this and other neuropathic abnormalities. Uremic anemia might also contribute to the development of deafness [Shaheen et al., 1997].

Typical electrophysiologic abnormalities include slow motor nerve conduction velocities with reduced distal latencies and compound muscle action potentials of greater degree in the median, peroneal, and tibial nerves than in the ulnar nerves. Widespread reduction of sensory nerve conduction velocities and action potentials is found. Abnormalities of somatosensory-evoked potentials (including N9, N13, and N20 latencies and amplitudes) are commonly encountered, as are findings suggesting central and peripheral axonopathy. Abnormal leg F-waves, foot vibration detection thresholds, and sural nerve sensory action potential amplitude are among the most sensitive diagnostic tests for uremic neuropathy [Hassan et al., 2003; Jurcic et al., 1998; Makkar and Kochar, 1994].

If available, Von Frey hairs are excellent devices for assessment of peripheral nerve dysfunction. Quantitative assessment of vibratory sensation with a large tuning fork or especially a vibrometer (Somedic AB, Sweden) may be as sensitive as nerve conduction velocity testing in diagnosing uremic neuropathy. The persistence of apprehension of vibration of the tuning fork is assessed against the examiner's apprehension of this sensation (e.g., placing a finger beneath the joint of the great toe, the tuning fork above it). The vibrometer may be the most sensitive approach other than Von Frey hairs, although the findings of vibrometer testing do not entirely overlap with those identified by nerve conduction testing [Hilz et al., 1995].

Electrophysiologic evidence for phrenic nerve dysfunction is found in a majority of patients with uremic neuropathy and can be predicted by the prolonged peroneal nerve conduction velocities [Zifko et al., 1995]. Sex differences do not exist for electrophysiologic manifestations of parasympathetic (e.g., electrocardiographic RR interval variation) autonomic testing, although males more frequently manifest abnormal sympathetic skin responses [Jedras et al., 1998, 2001].

Changes found on biopsy are often more severe than anticipated on the basis of the conduction velocity results [Jennekens et al., 1971]. Pathologic features of uremic neuropathy are similar to those seen in other nutritional or toxic neuropathies and include primary axonopathy with secondary segmental demyelination and remyelination, all emphasized in distal portions of large, long nerve trunks. Muscle biopsy may indicate loss of type-2 fibers [Appenzeller et al., 1971; Dyck et al., 1971; Savazzi et al., 1980].

The mechanisms of nerve injury are unknown. They are not related to urea or creatinine concentrations and, except for "burning feet," do not involve deficiencies of vitamins or magnesium. Failure of certain energy-dependent axonal/perikaryonal functions, including ion pumps, axoplasmic transport, and neurofilament synthesis, have been alleged as causes of axonopathy [Bakke, 1970; Dyck et al., 1971; Nielsen, 1973]. Because "middle molecules" are removed more efficiently by peritoneal dialysis and because peripheral neuropathy is less common in peritoneal dialysis than in hemodialysis, deleterious effects of these compounds have been implicated. Sugar alcohols that accumulate in chronic renal failure (e.g., myoinositol) may also play a role [Oh et al., 1978]. Diminished occurrence of neuropathy in children managed without aluminum salt exposure suggests that aluminum may have played a role in uremic neuropathy [Elzouki et al., 1994].

After renal transplantation, some patients develop neuropathy as a manifestation of graft-versus-host disease [Kondo et al., 1997]. Burning dysesthesia of the feet was formerly more common than at present and was likely due to dialysis-induced depletion of thiamine [Bolton, 1980]. Some patients with end-stage renal disease develop combined system degeneration owing to vitamin B_{12} deficiency [Kondo et al., 1997]. With vitamin B supplementation, these latter two causes of neuropathy have become rare.

Many patients with uremic neuropathy become stable or slowly improve with long-term hemodialysis, although little if any improvement is seen after a single dialysis pass [Laaksonen et al., 2002]. Mild neuropathy may remit, but severe neuropathy seldom does. It is possible that increased hours of dialysis or initiation of peritoneal dialysis may provide benefit in some severe cases [el Aklouk et al., 2004]. Worsening of electrophysiologic but not clinical manifestations of neuropathy may be detected in patients who have had more than 10 years of hemodialysis [Jurcic et al., 1998].

Successful renal transplantation usually, but not invariably, leads to complete amelioration of neuropathy in 6 to 12 months, even in patients with severe neuropathy [Hodson, 1983; Nielsen, 1974a]. Improvement of motor conduction velocity can be documented within days [Oh et al., 1978] or months [Nielsen, 1974b] of transplantation. Sympathetic and parasympathetic autonomic dysfunctions remit fairly promptly after successful transplantation [Yildiz et al., 1998]. Femoral neuropathy is a rare complication of the transplant surgery itself [Probst et al., 1982; Yazbek et al., 1985]. The potential ameliorative effects of erythropoietin administration are under investigation [Hassan et al., 2003].

Uremic Myopathy (Myopathy of Chronic Renal Failure)

Weakness is a common and important source of morbidity in patients with chronic renal failure, especially those on long-term renal dialysis. The limitations that weakness may place on normal activities may produce one of the most significant negative impacts of chronic renal disease on quality of life. Untoward weight gain from a variety of causes may occur in renal patients and produce a vicious cycle of weakness-engendered inactivity, inactivity-engendered weight gain, and weight-related exacerbation of weakness. The effects of this cycle and its associated rate of functional decline may be worsened by mood disturbance or by such frequently encountered intermittent causes of exacerbation of muscular weakness such as hypokalemia.

In individuals with chronic advanced renal failure or end-stage renal disease, corticosteroids, uremic neuropathy (see later), or uremic osteodystrophy may also contribute to weakness. Corticosteroid myopathy tends to have a much more acute onset than uremic myopathy. The particularly abrupt and severe onset of so-called acute care myopathy may occur in patients with chronic renal failure. The wide variety of other conditions that may cause acute weakness must also be considered in patients with chronic renal disease with rapidly worsening weakness, including toxic, infectious, or inflammatory diseases of muscle [Berretta et al., 1986; Chazan et al., 1970].

Chronic and progressive muscular weakness may be the secondary consequence of uremic neuropathy, which has already been considered. Uremic vasculopathy is another cause of secondary myopathy of smooth or striated muscles. Vascular myopathy is a necrotic process that has been ascribed to severe hyperparathyroidism with calcification of blood vessels. This process may result in impaired muscle capillary oxygen transfer [Bardin, 2003; Goodhue et al., 1972]. As with many other myopathic conditions, proximal leg weakness is the predominant finding of the deleterious consequences of uremic vasculopathy on striated muscle function. Secondary hyperparathyroidism and the associated hyperphosphatemia contribute to this vascular calcification, which may involve the coronary arteries and produce coronary vascular disease, the "silent killer" of uremic patients. It has been suggested that excessive use of calcium-containing phosphate binders may increase the likelihood of uremic vasculopathy [Bardin, 2003]. Utilization of calcium-free and (for reasons noted earlier) aluminum-free phosphate binders is likely an important advance in the avoidance of not only renal osteodystrophy but also uremic vascular myopathy. Caution may need to be taken in the use of vitamin D derivatives as well because they may enhance hypercalcemia [Bardin, 2003].

Pelvic girdle myopathy may also develop despite the absence of significant vascular changes on biopsy or evidence of other processes noted earlier that may produce weakness. As with uremic neuropathy, the pathogenesis of the myopathy of chronic renal failure is complex and as yet incompletely understood. It may involve such disparate mediators as "uremic toxins," abnormalities of vitamin D metabolism, malnutrition, carnitine depletion, muscular energy failure, impaired protein synthesis or amino acid metabolism, hypophosphatemia, or impaired biochemical function of sarcolemma.

In uremic neuropathy the most striking finding in sampled muscle is moderate atrophy involving fast-twitch (type II) muscle fibers to a greater extent than slow-twitch (type I) fibers. Severe but nonspecific ultrastructural abnormalities may also be found with electron microscopy of human biopsy specimens, and milder degrees of type II atrophy may be found in muscle biopsy specimens of uremic patients who do not have clinical myopathy. Recent detailed reviews of uremic myopathy are available [Bardin, 2003; Campistol, 2002].

COMPLICATIONS OF TRANSPLANTATION

The quality of life, including certain aspects of neurologic function, of patients with end-stage renal disease is generally improved after transplantation. Dialysis-associated complications are avoided, and neuropathy usually improves. Higher cortical functions may also improve, including memory, concentration, vigilance, and even intelligence [Fennell, et al., 1986; Rasbury et al., 1983]. Transplantation improves head growth and psychomotor development of some children with end-stage renal disease [Kohaut et al., 1985; So et al., 1987]. Survival has improved with donor-related but not cadaver transplantation [Vollmer et al., 1983]. Transplantation is not helpful in some diseases that affect both the nervous system and the kidney, such as Fabry's disease or oxalosis.

Two major forms of encephalopathy (congenital uremic encephalopathy and progressive dialysis encephalopathy), once well established, do not improve after transplantation [Fennell and Rasbury, 1980]. For reasons noted earlier, the prevalence of progressive dialysis encephalopathy has been sharply reduced. It has not been clear why patients with congenital nephroses exhibit poor development, although emerging data suggest ischemic brain injury may play a role and that transplantation may reduce the risk for this complication.

A recent study considered 33 children aged 6 to 11, most of whom had Finnish-type congenital nephrosis, who underwent prior successful transplantation for end-stage renal disease before 5 years of age. It was found that more than half of these children had brain imaging evidence for cerebrovascular border zone ischemia, whereas a smaller number had evidence for major arterial territory infarctions. It appeared that the longer the latency to transplantation for individuals with severe congenital nephrosis, the more likely that they would manifest changes suggesting brain ischemia. Clinical histories of hemodynamic crises were documented in approximately 40% of these cases; and within the limits of the study, there was no clear evidence that prematurity, perinatal complications, or sepsis accounted for the imaging abnormalities [Valanne et al., 2004].

Transplantation entails risk for a particular set of neurologic complications. These complications can be divided into those related to graft failure and those related to immunosuppression. Immunosuppressive complications can further be divided into those related to the immunosuppressed state (in combination with chronic antigenic stimulation by the graft) and those related to immunosuppressive drugs [Ram Prasad et al., 1987].

Graft Failure or Rejection

A characteristic rejection encephalopathy with seizures occurs in children [Bates et al., 1986; Fine et al., 1971]. Rejection encephalopathy is clinically indistinguishable from hypertensive encephalopathy [Gross et al., 1982]. It is always important to check serum magnesium levels in patients with a recent or long-term kidney graft who manifest seizures because magnesium stores may be low in the pretransplantation epoch and after transplantation tubular reabsorption of magnesium may initially be inadequate despite maintenance of adequate glomerular filtration rate [Heering et al., 1996].

Infection

Infection is uncommon during the first month after transplantation. There is no evidence of difference in infection risk with immunosuppression due to either cyclosporine or tacrolimus [Woo et al., 1997]. When early infection does occur, it is usually fulminant bacterial infection by *Staphylococcus aureus* or by gram-negative organisms. After the first month, subacute and chronic meningoencephalitides or abscesses are more likely to develop. The pathogens are usually opportunistic organisms, such as *Listeria, Toxoplasma, Cryptococcus,* or *Aspergillus.* Infection with pneumococci, mycobacteria, *Pneumocystis, Nocardia, Histoplasma, Candida,* or *Mucor* occurs less commonly [Barmeir et al., 1981; Cohen and Raps, 1995; Hodson et al., 1978; Rifkind et al., 1967; Rubin et al., 1981; Tilney et al., 1982]. Of these, the agents that may present late (6 months or more after transplantation) tend to be *Nocardia* or *Toxoplasma.*

Listeria and *Toxoplasma gondii* are the most common causes of meningoencephalitis in transplant recipients. Fever is not necessarily prominent. *Listeria* should be suspected if profound cerebrospinal fluid monocytosis is found [Holden et al., 1980; Lechtenberg et al., 1979]. *Toxoplasma* infection may produce myocardial involvement, and clinical features closely resemble systemic cytomegalovirus infection (see later discussion) [Schmidt et al., 1995]. Brain abscess, which develops in slightly more than 1% of kidney transplant patients, is most often caused by *Nocardia* but may also be due to infection with *Aspergillus* or *Listeria* [Lechtenberg et al., 1979; Rubin et al., 1981]. Characteristic febrile pulmonary involvement may distinguish these and other opportunistic agents (e.g., *Gemella, Ochroconis gallopavum*) that may cause brain abscess from tumor [Murray et al., 1975; Rifkind, 1967; Selby et al., 1997; Wang et al., 2003].

Disseminated histoplasmosis may present in a myriad of ways, particularly as mass lesions of the brain or spinal cord. Cerebrospinal fluid may be normal; and, as with other fungal infections, biopsy may be necessary to confirm the diagnosis [Livas et al., 1995]. Cryptococcal or candidal septic-metastatic mycotic encephalitis may occur [Schwechheimer and Hashemian, 1995]. Cerebral or rhinocerebral aspergilloma has had a very poor outlook [Cuccia et al., 2000], but with early diagnosis the combination of surgical removal and aggressive antifungal therapy is occasionally curative [Mrowka et al., 1997]. Cerebral cysticercosis produces ring-enhancing lesions in transplant recipients and should be considered in the southwestern United States and in many developing countries as well as in migrants from such endemic areas [Gordillo-Paniagua et al., 1987].

These various opportunistic agents carry a mortality of 46% to 86%. They are often difficult to diagnose, with brain abscess presenting in many instances as personality change or withdrawal. Given the gravity of these infectious conditions, early biopsy of brain lesions should be considered. Treatment usually involves discontinuation of immunosuppression and reinstitution of dialysis [Selby et al., 1997; Wang et al., 2003].

Viral pathogens include Epstein-Barr, herpes simplex, and varicella-zoster viruses [Peterson and Ferguson, 1984]. The risk for cytomegalovirus infection is increased by both cyclosporine and tacrolimus [Woo et al., 1997]. Epstein-Barr virus may cause particularly malignant lymphoproliferative mononucleosis with encephalopathy and can lead to fatal multisystem failure. Acyclovir treatment with termination of immunosuppression may be lifesaving. Cytomegalovirus has been associated with systemic infection, encephalitis, retinitis, polyneuropathy, transverse myelitis, and graft loss [Bale et al., 1980; Chow, 1986; Fiala et al., 1975; Schneck, 1965; Spitzer et al., 1987].

Hepatitis C virus not uncommonly infects dialyzed patients with end-stage renal disease prior to transplantation. In such preinfected patients, few observable effects are noted either before or after transplantation with immunosuppression. However, infection with hepatitis C virus acquired during or after transplantation may provoke with unusual rapidity a fulminant hepatitis with or without cirrhosis. Hepatic encephalopathy develops in as many as half of these cases. Discontinuation of azathioprine, as well as in some cases cyclosporine and prednisolone, may be required to improve the ascites, jaundice, and encephalopathy. In some instances, discontinuation may be tolerated without change in graft function [Ok, 1998].

Progressive multifocal leukoencephalopathy and spongiform encephalopathy have been described in adult transplant recipients but not in children [ZuRhein and Varakis, 1974]. *Pneumocystis* is the most common protozoal cause of CNS infection after transplantation. Other rare pathogens include *Leishmania, Strongyloides, Sporothrix,* and *Schistosoma* [Gullberg et al., 1987; Tsanaclis and de Morais, 1986]. Tuberculosis is always a consideration, especially when no other pathogen is identified. Evaluation of cerebrospinal fluid should always be carefully considered in transplant recipients with otherwise unexplained lethargy.

Tumor

Renal transplant recipients have a 1.6% to 24% risk for malignancy, typically skin cancer (Kaposi sarcoma or malignant melanoma) or non-Hodgkin's malignant lymphoma [Penn, 1979; Tyler and Tyler, 1984]. Lymphoproliferative disorders are far more common in children than in adults who have received renal allografts and constitute the majority of neoplasms for which these children are at risk [Novello and Fine, 1982; Schneck and Penn, 1970]. The risk for reticulum cell sarcoma is increased 35-fold by transplantation [Hoover and Fraumeni, 1973]. Any of these forms of malignancy can involve the CNS. The risk for CNS glioma is also markedly increased after renal transplantation. The occurrence of these tumors may be related to reduced immune surveillance, chronic graft-related antigenic stimulation, oncogenic viruses (e.g., Epstein-Barr virus), or oncogenic effects of immunosuppressive drugs. Cyclosporine, azathioprine, and prednisone all appear to increase the risk of lymphoma [van Diemen-Steenvoorde et al., 1986; Wilkinson et al., 1989].

In a high percentage of the childhood transplant recipients who develop lymphoma, the neoplasm remains confined to the CNS. However, it is very rapidly progressive and poorly responsive to standard therapy for non-Hodgkin's lymphoma or acyclovir. Reduction or cessation of immunosuppression may be beneficial in some lymphoproliferative cases, but in most instances even this makes little difference to the grim outlook for this condition [Dean et al., 1997; Mirra et al., 1981]. Diagnosis may be difficult because changes observed on scans may resemble those produced by abscess or by such drugs as asparaginase or peg asparagase (Bushara and Rust, 1997). Persistent space-occupying lesions are more likely to be tumor than opportunistic abscess in patients without pulmonary infection or fever. The thrombotic changes induced by such compounds as asparaginase are transient and do not enhance with administration of a contrast agent.

In some cases, tumors and abscesses coexist [Schneck and Penn, 1970], and biopsy is frequently indicated. Precious stereotaxic biopsy material is best analyzed with a combination of immunocytochemistry and polymerase chain reaction. Benign polyclonal immune cell infiltrates may obscure tiny clones of malignant cells unless great care is taken in analyzing the specimen [Dean et al., 1997].

Stroke

Massive cerebral hemorrhages have been reported after renal transplantation [Schwechheimer and Hashemian, 1995]. The risk for vascular calcification in brain and in heart, the "silent killer" of adult uremic patients, is likely influenced by the complex interactions of hyperparathyroidism, hyperphosphatemia, osteodystrophy, and use of calcium-containing phosphate binders and of vitamin D derivatives [Bardin, 2003].

Drugs

Drug-related complications include hypertension, immunosuppression, oncogenesis, and direct neurotoxicity. Hypertension severe enough to result in hypertensive encephalopathy may result from corticosteroid or cyclosporine therapy. This complication usually occurs shortly after transplantation; acute graft rejection or renal artery thrombosis must be excluded [Fine et al., 1970; Hodson et al., 1978]. Immunosuppressive and oncogenic effects of drugs have already been considered. Cyclosporine, perhaps because it has been in use the longest, is the calcineurin inhibitor most commonly cited as producing neurologic side effects, including paresthesias, neuralgia, peripheral neuropathy, ataxia, tremor, stupor, coma, confusion, insomnia, psychosis, hallucinations, sympathetic overactivation, headaches, or seizures [Arns 1994; Peces et al., 1996; Shah et al., 1984].

One or more of these neurologic side effects are experienced by 10% to 38% of patients who receive cyclosporine [Beckstein, 2000]. In most instances the side effects disappear with dose reduction. The association of cyclosporine with reversible posterior leukoencephalopathy-associated seizures, stupor, and other findings has been considered in a previous section. The substrate for encephalopathy may include cyclosporine-induced vascular endothelial injury [Teshima et al., 1996].

There is recent evidence that tacrolimus, a more potent immunosuppressant than cyclosporine, may also have an even greater tendency to engender neurotoxicities of the same variety associated with cyclosporine use [Parvex et al., 2001; Primavera et al., 2001]. Either cyclosporine or tacrolimus may engender seizures or make it more difficult to control epilepsy in renal transplant recipients. Tacrolimus has been associated with a post-transplantation encephalopathy that includes MRI-discernible changes in both gray and white matter. This syndrome may subside without discontinuation of tacrolimus. A similar condition arose with sirolimus. It is not as yet known exactly what role the various drugs employed to prevent rejection of an implanted kidney play in these peculiar syndromes [Parvex et al., 2001].

Enzyme-inducing antiepileptic drugs may reduce expected serum levels of calcineurin-inhibiting immunosuppressive drugs. Corticosteroids such as methylprednisolone employed for graft-versus-host disease prophylaxis may produce headache, psychosis, bone demineralization, or spinal cord compression owing to extradural fat accumulation. Corticosteroids may interfere with myelination of the early developing brain [Lee et al., 1975; Polinsky et al., 1987]. Tacrolimus, an inhibitor of cytokine and T-cell function, may provoke tremor, headache, hyperkalemia, insomnia, confusion, lethargy, neuropathy, or hypertension.

Administration of the CD3 monoclonal antibody orthoclone OKT3 to prevent renal allograft rejection may variously provoke headache, fever, vomiting, a flulike syndrome, hypotension, seizure, or aseptic meningitis in as many as one third of patients. These changes may be severe and include obtundation or coma. Prompt investigation should exclude such alternative causes as CNS infection [Beaman et al., 1985; Capone and Cohen, 1991; Fernandez et al., 1993; Morris, 1999; Shihab et al., 1993]. OKT3-related encephalopathy has been associated with a cytokine release syndrome that involves elevation of concentrations of several CSF cytokines, including tumor necrosis factor and interleukin-6. Cerebral infarction may occur. Brain edema may develop and lead to brain herniation and death [Agarwal et al., 1993; Reiss et al., 1993; Shihab et al., 1993a, 1993b]. OKT3 may produce a state of akinetic mutism [Pittock et al., 2003], transient hemiparesis [Osterman et al., 1993], or blindness or optic disc swelling with abducens palsies due to increased intracranial pressure [Strominger et al., 1995].

DISEASES AFFECTING BOTH KIDNEY AND NERVOUS SYSTEM

These illnesses can be divided into four general categories: (1) inflammatory/vascular, (2) infectious, (3) toxic or metabolic, and (4) an increasing number of heritable disorders associated with static anomalies of brain and kidney. The inflammatory/vascular illnesses that are considered first in this section include thrombotic thrombocytopenic purpura, hemolytic-uremic syndrome, and other thrombocytopenic microangiopathies. In addition, the hepatorenal syndrome, Henoch-Schönlein syndrome, and familial amyloidosis are reviewed. Systemic lupus erythematosus, polyarteritis nodosa, and Wegener's granulomatosis are examples of other illnesses that produce inflammatory changes in both nervous and renal systems. The details of these illnesses are covered in Chapter 73.

Thrombotic Thrombocytopenic Purpura

Thrombotic thrombocytopenic purpura was first described by Moschcowitz in 1925 [Baehr et al., 1936], who noted that the combination of fever, hemolytic anemia, renal failure, and neurologic dysfunction could result from widespread hyaline thrombosis of small blood vessels. Subsequently, many hundreds of cases labeled *thrombotic thrombocytopenic purpura* have been reported. Formerly, clinical diagnosis required at least two major (thrombocytopenia, Coombs-negative microangiopathic anemia, or neurologic dysfunction) and two minor (fever, renal dysfunction, or circulating thrombi) manifestations [Bukowski, 1982]. In many cases (unlike hemolytic-uremic syndrome), there is associated fever at onset.

Hemolytic-uremic syndrome was first described by Gasser and colleagues in 1955. At that time it was usually fatal. Onset typically occurred in early childhood with Coombs-negative thrombocytopenic microangiopathic hemolytic anemia and irreversible acute renal failure that usually required dialysis. The outlook for survival has greatly improved, owing to therapeutic advances. However, hemolytic-uremic syndrome remains a leading cause of acute renal failure in North American children. It accounts for 7% of cases of hypertension in children younger than 12 months of age [de Chadarevian and Kaplan, 1978; Gianantonio et al., 1973; Lieberman et al., 1966]. The microangiopathic pathologic similarities to thrombotic thrombocytopenic purpura were recognized from the start. Kidney tropism *without* prominent neurologic abnormalities, onset before 10 years of age, and absence of associated fever were the common findings that permitted most cases of hemolytic-uremic syndrome to be readily distinguished from thrombotic thrombocytopenic purpura [Silverstein, 1968].

It became clear, however, that a minority of cases thought to be hemolytic-uremic syndrome (because kidney manifestations predominated) presented after 10 years of age whereas other cases with a predominant phenotype closely resembling thrombotic thrombocytopenic purpura occurred in small children.

A recent retrospective pathologic study has demonstrated that thrombotic thrombocytopenic purpura and hemolytic-uremic syndrome are pathologically distinct entities. In cases severe enough to prove fatal, thrombotic thrombocytopenic purpura–associated thrombi are platelet rich and are found in heart, pancreas, kidney, adrenal, and brain, in decreasing order of severity. Hemolytic-uremic syndrome–associated thrombi are fibrin/red cell rich and tend largely to be confined to the kidney [Hosler et al., 2003]. Other studies have found that thrombotic thrombocytopenic purpura thrombi are found in the brains and kidneys of 50% to 75% of individuals with fatal thrombotic thrombocytopenic purpura. These thrombi contained von Willebrand factor multimers. It has long been recognized that patients with thrombotic thrombocytopenic purpura have ultra-large von Willebrand factor multimers in circulation [Bell et al., 1991; Berkowitz et al., 1979; Chow et al., 1998). Brain thromboses of thrombotic thrombocytopenic purpura occur in small arterioles, capillaries, and venules and are associated with microinfarction. Small petechial hemorrhages may be widely scattered in gray matter [Adams, 1964].

Remarkable recent progress in the characterization of the pathogenesis of thrombotic thrombocytopenic purpura has explained the reasons that thrombotic thrombocytopenic purpura–associated thrombi differ from those of hemolytic-uremic syndrome. These advances have also provided diagnostic tests that reliably designate most heritable thrombotic thrombocytopenic purpura cases, as well as most individuals with acquired (autoimmune) thrombotic thrombocytopenic purpura [Raife, 2003]. On the basis of recent advances, thrombotic microangiopathies have been reclassified, as is shown in Table 89-2. Other as yet incompletely understood symptomatic thrombotic microangiopathies with a thrombotic thrombocytopenic purpura–like phenotype—conditions that tend to afflict adults and have predominantly neurologic manifestations—are now considered under their own headings in the new classification scheme for thrombotic microangiopathies.

Hemolytic-uremic syndrome constitutes a family of illnesses including at least one heritable (congenital) form,

TABLE 89-2

Thrombotic Microangiopathies

Congenital (idiopathic, ADMATS13-deficient) TTP
Acquired (inhibitory IgG-mediated) TTP
HUS not further specified
HUS with diarrhea prodrome
Atypical HUS
TMA not further specified
TMA associated with neoplasia or chemotherapy
TMA following hematopoietic stem cell transplantation
TMA with additional/alternative disorder
Other hematologic disorders

HUS, hemolytic-uremic syndrome; TMA, thrombotic microangiopathy; TTP, thrombotic thrombocytopenic purpura.
From MacWhinney JB, Packer JT, et al. Thrombotic thrombocytopenic purpura in childhood. Blood 1962;19:181.

as well as cases that are subclassified as atypical and symtomatic hemolytic-uremic syndrome. It is of interest to note that the prevalence of thrombotic microangiopathies appears to be increasing. In part, this increase is accounted for by the development of new symptomatic forms, such as that related to bone marrow transplantation. Population-based studies have found that the prevalence of hemolytic-uremic syndrome substantially increased in the decade of the 1980s [Martin et al., 1990; Tarr et al., 1989). More recently, an increase in prevalence of the acquired forms of thrombotic thrombocytopenic purpura has been discerned, an increase that is out of proportion to the development of novel provocations such as bone marrow transplant [Tsai and Shulman, 2003]. When considered against the background of increasing prevalence over the past 40 years of other autoimmune diseases in industrialized nations (e.g., juvenile rheumatoid arthritis, asthma, systemic lupus erythematosus, multiple sclerosis in women), it seems that some common set of influences is disturbing the development of immunoregulation and tolerance. Current research on the genetic and immunoexperiential factors that determine the competence of immunoregulatory T cells is likely to prove relevant to these worrisome observations.

Recent elegant studies have established the association of many cases of thrombotic thrombocytopenic purpura are due to congenital or acquired defects in the function of the zinc-dependent metalloproteinase ADAMTS13. This metalloproteinase is synthesized in liver. It is responsible for cleaving von Willebrand factor multimers. If properly cleaved, small multimers are capable, under highly regulated conditions, of binding to glycoprotein complexes Ib/IX/V and IIb/IIIa on the surface of platelets. Binding induces changes in platelet conformation from normal "clumping-resistant" globular form to an elongated form in which platelets tend readily to clump [Siedlecki et al., 1996]. The IIb/IIIa site, which in normal-sized multimers requires activation by circulating mediators or by sheer forces, may be particularly important in regulating platelet adhesiveness.

Ultra-large von Willebrand multimers persist in circulation if the plasma activity of ADAMTS13 is reduced to less than 5% of normal. Cleavage of the ultra-large multimers is a critical antithrombotic regulatory function that reduces and regulates Ib/IX/V and IIb/IIIa platelet receptor binding affinity. Without cleavage the large fragments are prothrombotic, tending to bind to platelets without appropriate activating signals. The ensuing platelet conformational change results in platelet clumping in arterioles and capillaries [Fujikawa et al., 2001; Furlan et al., 1997; Tsai et al., 1997; Zheng et al., 2001]. ADAMTS13 is not the only inducer of multimer cleavage. Calprins, leukocyte elastases, cathepsin G, plasmin, streptokinase, urokinase, and tissue-type plasminogen activator are others. These highly active substances are sequestered or inhibited under normal conditions and therefore play no role in physiologic von Willebrand factor cleavage.

Severe deficiency of ADAMTS13 is considered diagnostic of the acute idiopathic form of thrombotic thrombocytopenic purpura [Hovinga et al., 2004]. However, this deficiency is not found in all patients with a thrombotic thrombocytopenic purpura phenotype. In a series of 396 consecutive patients with various thrombotic microangiopathies, severe ADAMTS13 deficiency was found in 17% of the total. Moreover, it was found in at least 60% of congenital or acute idiopathic (sporadic) thrombotic thrombocytopenic purpura cases. It was not found in any of the 130 patients with hemolytic-uremic syndrome or in the 14 patients with hematopoietic stem cell transplantation–associated thrombotic microangiopathy. Severe ADAMTS13 deficiency was not invariably associated with microvascular platelet clumping and/or other cardinal features of thrombotic microangiopathies [Hovinga et al., 2004].

Certain generalizations about the clinical aspects of thrombotic thrombocytopenic purpura can be stated. Thrombotic thrombocytopenic purpura is slightly more common in females than in males (ratio 3:2). Although the peak incidence is in the third decade, it may occur in neonates and young children [Kennedy et al., 1980]. Cases occurring in adults are likely mostly acquired thrombotic thrombocytopenic purpura, whereas those in neonates or young children are most likely congenital thrombotic thrombocytopenic purpura. The old observation that tendency to recur cannot be predicted on either a clinical or laboratory basis remains true [Meacham et al., 1952].

Signs and symptoms of acute thrombotic thrombocytopenic purpura usually evolve quickly and quite noticeably over 7 to 10 days. Skin purpura is the initial manifestation in more than 90% of patients. Fever usually develops early in the course of the illness. Hemorrhage (retinal, choroidal, nasal, gingival, gastrointestinal, and genitourinary), pallor, abdominal pain, arthralgia, or pancreatitis may also develop. Neurologic findings are seen in most cases and include fatigue, confusion, headache, and varying degrees of dysfunction of vision or language. Significant laboratory findings include microangiopathic hemolytic anemia, thrombocytopenia, elevated lactate dehydrogenase, proteinuria, and microscopic hematuria. Cerebrospinal fluid chemistry, cell counts, and pressure are usually normal [Adams, 1964]. Other findings commonly associated with disseminated intravascular coagulopathy are not usually found. MRI of brain is often normal. Single-photon emission tomographic images may indicate diminished cerebral blood flow [Fiorani et al., 1995].

At the time of original description, thrombotic thrombocytopenic purpura was almost 100% fatal. The outlook for thrombotic thrombocytopenic purpura has considerably improved, but fatalities still occur in 10% to 40% of well-treated cases [Bukowski, 1982; Rock et al., 1991]. It is not clear whether the improved survival is the result of more efficacious specific therapies or the improvement in techniques for supporting patients during the acute stage of illness. To some extent the improved survival rates may reflect the inclusion of milder forms of illness that were formerly overlooked. Monotherapy with corticosteroids appears beneficial in milder cases, and these drugs may be valuable adjuvants when plasma exchange is undertaken in more severe cases. Response to plasmapheresis and plasma infusion is often so prompt and dramatic as to suggest that these treatments are the most important factors in the greatly improved outlook for the thrombotic thrombocytopenic purpura family of illnesses [Bukowski, 1982; Ridolfi and Bell, 1981; Rock et al., 1991]. Remarkably, only a minority of patients who recover from thrombotic thrombocytopenic purpura manifest any significant permanent organ damage [Tsai, 2003].

As has been suggested, plasma exchange may be more efficacious treatment than plasma infusion. In a controlled, prospective, double-blind crossover multicenter thrombotic thrombocytopenic purpura treatment trial [Rock et al., 1991], at least 80% survival was found for plasma exchange, compared with 60% survival for patients randomized to plasma infusion. A more recent report [Lawlor et al., 1997] suggests that the benefits of plasma exchange are related to infusion of larger volumes of plasma or better clearance of toxins, antibodies, multimers, or immune complexes compared with plasma infusion. Plasma infusions carry risk for transmission of infections, including hepatitis and possibly human immunodeficiency virus. Most thrombotic thrombocytopenic purpura patients have been treated with seven or eight exchanges (requiring blood from 200 or more donors), after which at least 60% of patients who had a more severe form of thrombotic thrombocytopenic purpura experienced relapse [Bell et al., 1991].

Most cases of thrombotic thrombocytopenic purpura are monophasic, but 11% to 28% of patients experience one or more recurrence. In some instances, chronic thrombotic thrombocytopenic purpura develops [Bell et al., 1991; Rock et al., 1991; Tsai and Shulman, 2003]. Relapses occur weeks to years after initial remission. For severe or recurrent cases, plasmapheresis and plasma infusion are useful, but the combination of both (plasma exchange) using fresh-frozen platelet-poor plasma appears to be the most beneficial form of therapy, sometimes in combination with corticosteroids [Moake et al., 1984; Moake, 1990]. Plasmapheresis may remove the large von Willebrand factor multimers and circulating antibodies, whereas infused fresh-frozen plasma may contribute ADAMTS13 and circulating antioxidants (e.g., prostacyclin) and may also dilute ADAMTS13-inhibiting IgG.

THROMBOTIC THROMBOCYTOPENIC PURPURA–LIKE THROMBOCYTOPENIC MICROANGIOPATHY SYMPTOMATIC OF OTHER ILLNESSES. The thrombotic thrombocytopenic purpura phenotype and other forms of thrombocytopenic microangiopathy may develop in association with the various categories shown in Table 89-2. Inflammatory vasculitic diseases (e.g., rheumatoid arthritis, polyarteritis nodosa, systemic lupus erythematosus, Sjögren's syndrome, HELLP syndrome) constitute one important category. Thrombocytopenic micoangiopathy with or without a thrombotic thrombocytopenic purpura phenotype may also develop in association with neoplasia (particularly lymphoma) or chemotherapy. Thrombocytopenic micoangiopathy associated with hematopoietic stem cell transplantation is yet another category. Remaining cases could be classified as (1) thrombocytopenic micoangiopathy with other conditions (endocarditis, during puerperium, factor H deficiency), (2) thrombocytopenic micoangiopathy due to drugs or poisons (i.e., sulfa, ticlopidine, cyclosporine, iodine, birth control pills, various other drugs and poisons), and the inevitable (3) thrombocytopenic micoangiopathy "not otherwise specified" [Hovinga et al., 2004; Remuzzi and Bertani, 1988; Teshima et al., 1996].

Hemolytic-Uremic Syndrome

Hemolytic-uremic syndrome is a Coombs-negative thrombocytopenic microangiopathy the onset of which is typically in early childhood. Two thirds of all cases occur in children younger than 3 years of age, and few cases occur after 5 years of age [Gianviti et al., 2003]. Hemolytic-uremic syndrome may occur in the neonate and occasionally occurs in adults, especially in the elderly. Manifestations tend to be much more focal than those of thrombotic thrombocytopenic purpura. In addition to microangiopathic hemolytic anemia, the characteristic and serious finding is that of acute renal failure, which is usually severe. If there are neurologic manifestations, they are usually mild. As has been noted, however, there is an area of clinical overlap between hemolytic-uremic syndrome and thrombotic thrombocytopenic purpura. Thrombotic thrombocytopenic purpura occasionally occurs in neonates, and hemolytic-uremic syndrome occasionally occurs in adults, especially the elderly. Hemolytic-uremic syndrome in the elderly may have a different pathogenesis from childhood cases because the disease of the elderly tends not to respond well to therapies that are effective in childhood cases [Blackall and Marques, 2004; Karlsber et al., 1997].

The venerable Drummond scheme [Drummond, 1985] of hemolytic-uremic syndrome classification has been greatly revised (Table 89-3) to more accurately subclassify the illness according to current understanding of the varied pathogenic bases on which hemolytic-uremic syndrome may arise. The new classification includes a "classic congenital" category and retains but redefines the "postinfectious," and "familial" categories. The postinfectious

TABLE 89-3

Classification of Hemolytic-Uremic Syndrome

FORMER	CURRENT
Classic infantile (D+)	Classic infantile (D+)
Postinfectious (D+ or D–)	Postinfectious (D+ *only*)
Familial	D+ familial
	D– familial
	H-factor positive subgroup
	H-factor negative subgroup
Immunologic	Sporadic
	D+ subgroup
	D– subgroup
Secondary	Subdivided into sporadic or familial categories
Endocrine	Subdivided into sporadic or familial categories

category is now restricted to individuals who manifest prodromal diarrhea (D+), despite the fact that some individuals without prodromal diarrhea harbor the same enteric Shiga-toxin–producing *Escherichia coli* bacteria that provoke the prodromal diarrhea in most postinfectious cases [Gianviti et al., 2003].

Familial cases are divided into those that do (D+) or do not (D–) have prodromal diarrhea. The former immunologic category is termed *sporadic* and is subdivided into D+ or D– subgroups. The former secondary and endocrine categories have been redistributed into the familial or sporadic groups depending on whether there is evidence for inheritance of the hemolytic-uremic syndrome predilection.

The primary event in the pathogenesis of hemolytic-uremic syndrome is damage to vascular endothelium, especially within the kidney. This mechanism may be shared by all categories of hemolytic-uremic syndrome, although it has been most thoroughly investigated and is now best understood for the postinfectious cases. Most of the children with postinfectious hemolytic-uremic syndrome harbor gastrointestinal Shiga-toxin–producing *Escherichia coli.* The Shiga toxin (verocytotoxin) elaborated by these bacteria enters the circulation and produces most of the ensuing injury in the vasculature of the kidney. The reason for this tropism is not entirely clear, nor is the age-related predilection, although both may be due to age-related expression of particular receptors in the kidney tubules (see later). Other causes of endothelial injury that results in hemolytic-uremic syndrome have been identified in children and especially in elderly adults with hemolytic-uremic syndrome and include cytotoxic drugs and systemic inflammatory illnesses.

The pathology of hemolytic-uremic syndrome is predominantly that of thrombotic microangiopathy that tends particularly to involve the capillary subendothelial space of the kidney. As has been noted, hemolytic-uremic syndrome–associated thrombi differ from those of thrombotic thrombocytopenic purpura in that they are fibrin/ erythrocyte-rich [Hosler et al., 2003] and do not contain von Willebrand factor multimers. Whereas thrombotic thrombocytopenic purpura thrombi are widespread, hemolytic-uremic syndrome thrombi are largely restricted to the renal microvasculature, particularly in children younger than 5 years of age [Blackall and Marques, 2004; Chow et al., 1998; Hosler et al., 2003]. In older children and adults, necrotizing arterial thrombosis may predominate. Direct injury to the glomerular endothelium has been observed in some patients [Remuzzi and Bertani, 1988].

Deficiency of ADAMTS13 activity is not a feature of hemolytic-uremic syndrome [Tsai, 2003; Tsai and Lian, 1998; Tsai et al., 2000]. Indeed, young children with Shiga-toxin–producing *Escherichia coli*–associated hemolytic-uremic syndrome may have elevated rates of ADAMTS13 cleavage of von Willebrand factor multimers, producing smaller than normal von Willebrand factor multimers. Enhanced cleavage may be due to greater availability of von Willebrand factor ADAMTS13 receptor sites. This availability may itself result from abnormal unfolding of the multimer receptor site areas owing to increased sheer stress to the von Willebrand factor multimers in the vicinity of hemolytic-uremic syndrome thrombi [Tsai, 2002]. Red blood cell fragmentation occurs in hemolytic-uremic syndrome [Tsai, 2002], in part explaining the erythrocyte enrichment of hemolytic-uremic syndrome thrombi. Fibrin deposition in clots has been explained, in Shiga-toxin-producing *E. coli*–related hemolytic-uremic syndrome cases, by activation of both prothrombin peptide F1+2 and D-dimer increase before the microangiopathic stage of Shiga-toxin–producing *E. coli*–associated hemolytic-uremic syndrome [Chandler et al., 2002].

Classic infantile hemolytic-uremic syndrome is the second largest category of hemolytic-uremic syndrome, accounting for approximately 10% of all hemolytic-uremic syndrome cases. These infants have a febrile prodrome with diarrhea but negative bacterial blood cultures. Viral cultures may also be negative, although echoviruses or coxsackieviruses, adenoviruses, and human immunodeficiency virus have been isolated in some instances. It is possible that viruses produce endothelial injury in the kidney vasculature, although currently there is little information concerning pathogenesis of classic infantile hemolytic-uremic syndrome. This type of hemolytic-uremic syndrome tends to be mild and to have a relatively good prognosis.

Postinfectious hemolytic-uremic syndrome is the largest hemolytic-uremic syndrome category. This group accounts for as many as 46% to 68% of all hemolytic-uremic syndrome cases [Gianviti et al., 2003; Martin et al., 1990]. The category that formerly bore this name included cases with or without a diarrheal prodrome. In the current scheme, only cases manifesting diarrhea are included and most cases are associated with Shiga-toxin–producing *E. coli.* In nearly 50% of Shiga-toxin–producing *E. coli* infections, the organism is *E. coli* O157:H7. However, other serotypes may be found, including *E. coli* O26 (25%), *E. coli* O111 (11%), *E. coli* O145 (11%), and *E. coli* O103 (6%). Other *E. coli* serotypes (O55, O86, O118, and O120) together account for less than 1% of postinfectious hemolytic-uremic syndrome cases [Gianviti et al., 2003]. Other pathogens associated with the development of postinfectious hemolytic-uremic syndrome include viruses (echoviruses, adenoviruses, human immunodeficiency virus, or coxsackieviruses) or bacteria *(Salmonella, Shigella, Streptococcus,* or *Yersinia).* Some of these bacteria, particularly *Shigella,* elaborate verotoxin.

The association of gastrointestinal *E. coli* O157-H7 with hemolytic-uremic syndrome, as well as with some cases of hemorrhagic colitis was first published in 1982 [Cimolai and Carter, 1991; Joh, 1997; Martin et al., 1990]. The implicated *E. coli* O157-H7 bacterial strains elaborate both an adhesion intimin and two verocytotoxins (VT-1 and VT-2, also known as *Shiga toxins*). The former mediates attachment of the ingested organism to colonocytes. The VT-2 verocytotoxins mediate attachment to circulating polymorphonuclear leukocytes, cells that, in turn, distribute the toxins throughout the body but particularly to the kidney [Te Loo et al., 2000]. The binding to leukocytes is of relatively low affinity, permitting reattachment to cell surfaces, particularly those of the kidney [Te Loo et al., 2001].

It is of interest that in several cases in adults with a thrombotic thrombocytopenic purpura rather than hemolytic-uremic syndrome phenotype there has been an associated *E. coli* O157:H7 infection [Kovacs et al., 1990]. The *E. coli* VT-2 verocytotoxin has been found to cause not only renal endothelial injury but also cerebral microcirculatory endothelial injury in piglets [Richardson et al., 1987; Tzipori et al., 1988]. This experimental model may include aspects that are pertinent to hemolytic-uremic syndrome and others that are pertinent to thrombotic thrombocytopenic purpura and suggests that there remains an area of pathophysiologic overlap between these two conditions.

It has been determined that as many as 82% of the household contacts of a child with postinfectious hemolytic-uremic syndrome also have verocytotoxin bound to their polymorphonuclear leukocytes, but despite this fact they are often asymptomatic. It is therefore hypothesized that an additional mediator is necessary for the development of postinfectious hemolytic-uremic syndrome, now presumed to be a lipopolysaccharide [Seigler et al., 2001]. The fact that the use of an antimotility agent increases the risk for hemolytic-uremic syndrome suggests the possibility that prolonged contact of organism with colonocytes or with inflammation-associated polymorphonuclear leukocytes may play an important role in pathogenesis [Joh, 1997].

It is also known that administration of antibiotics such as trimethoprim-sulfamethoxazole to children with *E. coli* O157–associated diarrhea may increase the risk for hemolytic-uremic syndrome [Joh, 1997; Wong et al., 2000]. The significance of this observation with regard to pathogenesis of hemolytic-uremic syndrome remains unclear. C3 complement levels are low in approximately half of all D+ hemolytic-uremic syndrome cases, suggesting that activation of the alternative complement pathway occurs in postinfectious hemolytic-uremic syndrome.

Postinfectious hemolytic-uremic syndrome tends to occur in the midsummer [Palomeque Rico et al., 1993]. It tends to be a much more severe illness than the classic infantile hemolytic-uremic syndrome and has a much more guarded prognosis. Undercooked hamburger appears to be a major vehicle for food-borne *E. coli* O157:H7 outbreaks in children, suggesting an epizootic reservoir [Riley et al., 1983].

Familial (atypical) hemolytic-uremic syndrome is defined clinically by the occurrence of hemolytic-uremic syndrome in two or more family members. The first description of familial hemolytic-uremic syndrome was provided in 1956, although the careful studies of Kaplan and associates made a considerable additional contribution in 1975 [Kaplan et al., 1975]. There are both autosomal-dominant and autosomal-recessive forms of familial hemolytic-uremic syndrome. The pathophysiology of familial hemolytic-uremic syndrome is less well understood than that of postinfectious hemolytic-uremic syndrome. Familial cases that lack a diarrheal prodrome are termed *D– familial hemolytic-uremic syndrome*. These cases are further classified according to whether there is an identifiable defect in factor H expression.

Ten to 20 percent of either familial or sporadic D– cases are associated with mutations in a region of chromosome 1 that encodes the expression of various complement regulatory proteins. Some familial cases are found to have heritable deficiencies of the third component of complement (C3), others of complement factor H [Noris et al., 1999; Warwicker et al., 1998]. Individuals with either of these deficiencies tend to have hemolytic-uremic syndrome of greater than average severity. A missense mutation in the gene that encodes factor H expression has been identified in some cases of familial hemolytic-uremic syndrome [Warwicker et al., 1998] with subsequent demonstration that there is genetic heterogeneity in affected individuals. It has further been demonstrated that mutations of this same gene may be associated with either familial or sporadic (defined by the absence of family history) varieties of D– hemolytic-uremic syndrome [Perez-Caballero et al., 2001].

Factor H is a fluid phase regulator of activation of the alternative complement pathway, a pathway that plays a critical role in regulation of the discernment of host from foreign tissues. Some of the various missense mutations associated with hemolytic-uremic syndrome result in abnormalities in the carboxyl terminal of factor H, a region that is important for binding to C3b complement and cell surface polyanionis. It is hypothesized that early procoagulant activation occurs, as in diarrheal cases, because of endothelial cell injury. Dysregulation of the alternative complement pathway, due to the abnormal binding function of factor H, then prolongs the abnormal procoagulant state.

Patients with hemolytic-uremic syndrome usually have normal levels of factor H with normal or low levels of complement or the C3 complement constituent [Noris et al., 1999; Richards et al., 2002]. A normal factor H level does not exclude the presence of mutation of the factor H gene. It is not yet clear how many D– hemolytic-uremic syndrome cases have demonstrable factor H gene abnormalities. One extensive recent literature review of severe hemolytic-uremic syndrome cases found reports of factor H gene abnormality in less than 15% of nondiarrheal cases requiring renal transplant. There is an inverse association between C3 levels and disease severity and outcome in both D+ and D– hemolytic-uremic syndrome [Fortin et al., 2004; Fremeaux-Bacchi et al., 2004; Rodriguez et al., 2004]. Although hemolytic-uremic syndrome occurs in individuals with specific abnormalities of the carboxyl terminus of factor H, complete absence of this factor in pigs, mice, and humans leads to mesangiocapillary glomerulonephritis rather than hemolytic-uremic syndrome [Alexander et al., 2005].

Sporadic hemolytic-uremic syndrome has replaced the former "immunologic" hemolytic-uremic syndrome category and includes cases of hemolytic-uremic syndrome associated with a fall in C3 component. These cases are subdivided into D+ or D– forms based on the presence or absence of diarrhea and other clinical features. As is noted earlier, very low C3 is a negative prognostic indicator for hemolytic-uremic syndrome. Some individuals with D+ sporadic hemolytic-uremic syndrome are found to harbor gastrointestinal Shiga-toxin–producing *Escherichia coli* infections [Gianviti et al., 2003], whereas other individuals classified as D– sporadic hemolytic-uremic syndrome are found to have factor H deficiency [Warwicker et al., 1998].

The most important associated underlying illnesses for sporadic D– hemolytic-uremic syndrome are vasculitic and inflammatory illnesses such as Henoch-Schönlein syndrome, systemic lupus erythematosus, scleroderma, polyarteritis nodosa, and Wegener's granulomatosis. Individuals with these underlying illnesses may, in some instances, develop thrombocytopenic microangiopathies with a thrombotic thrombocytopenic purpura phenotype. In many instances these diseases produce rapidly progressive vasculitic glomerulonephritis rather than the peculiar glomerulopathy of hemolytic-uremic syndrome. Other provocations include malignant hypertension, kidney radiation, bone marrow transplantation, medications employed for immunosuppression (cyclosporine, tacrolimus, methylprednisolone), snake venom or diethylene glycol intoxication, and cancer chemotherapy drugs such as mitomycin. Endocrine causes of hemolytic-uremic syndrome include pregnancy and oral contraceptives [Goldstein et al., 1979; Habib et al., 1958].

Tacrolimus-associated hemolytic-uremic syndrome, for which renal transplant patients are at risk, tends to arise in adults rather than children. It is representative of the generalization that hemolytic-uremic syndrome in adults tends to be more severe and difficult to treat than hemolytic-uremic syndrome in children that tends to afflict adults. It occurs slightly more often in men than women and has a mean onset at about 40 years of age or about 7 months after transplant. It is not dose related. Nearly 45% of cases improve with various mixtures of anticoagulation, antiplatelet agents, dialysis, and plasma exchange. Tacrolimus is usually replaced with cyclosporine, although in some instances an initial dose reduction of tacrolimus has been tried. Graft loss occurs in 25% of cases. Without successful retransplantation, all of these individuals die. Even with transplantation, approximately one third die. If there is associated liver failure, 60% die [Lin et al., 2003]; and these cases can be further subdivided between the sporadic or inherited forms of hemolytic-uremic syndrome, depending on whether there is a family history or demonstrated factor H or factor H gene defect.

CLINICAL ASPECTS OF HEMOLYTIC-UREMIC SYNDROME. Most diarrhea-associated (D+) hemolytic-uremic syndrome cases are preceded by days to weeks of varying degrees of abdominal pain, vomiting, diarrhea, and hematochezia. Abdominal pain may be severe and fever may be quite high. Children with a D– presentation who have a prodromal respiratory illness have a distinctly worse prognosis than those with a D+ presentation. Microangiopathic Coombs-negative hemolytic anemia and acute renal failure with microscopic hematuria and proteinuria (1 to 2 g/dL) abruptly mark the onset of hemolytic-uremic syndrome in nearly all patients. Leukocytosis may accompany this phase of illness, and elevated concentrations of α_1 and β_2 microglobulins may be found in the urine.

Neurologic manifestations of hemolytic-uremic syndrome—most commonly behavioral changes, motor seizures, stroke and varying degrees of encephalopathy—are seen in 30% to 40% of patients. Blindness, ataxia, hemiparesis, and decerebrate rigidity have also been reported [Kaplan et al., 1971; Martin et al., 1990; Sheth et al., 1986]. The occurrence of neurologic abnormalities predicts a worse outcome with enhanced risk for end-stage renal disease or death [Garg et al., 2003]. It is not always clear whether such neurologic changes are the result of cerebral microangiopathy or are secondary to metabolic disturbances and hypertension. MRI of brain may disclose focal areas of infarction with swelling and, in some cases, hemorrhage, especially in such areas as the internal capsule and deep gray nuclei [Jeong et al., 1994]. Children in whom neurologic signs develop are more likely to die or to have residual hypertension or chronic renal dysfunction [Palomeque Rico et al., 1993; Sheth et al., 1986]. Clinical features suggestive of hemolytic-uremic syndrome are noted in Table 89-4.

TABLE 89-4

Clinical Features Suggesting HUS Rather than TTP as Cause of Thrombocytopenic Microangiopathy

Age younger than 10 years
No other plausible explanation
Preceding diarrhea or colitis, pulmonary infiltrates, or respiratory disease
Absence of associated fever
Evidence for renal dysfunction
Oliguria or anuria
Hypertension (>140/90 mm Hg)
Serum creatinine > 3.5 mg/dL
Need for dialysis

HUS, hemolytic-uremic syndrome, TTP, thrombotic thrombocytopenic purpura.

Adapted from Tsai HM. Advances in the pathogenesis, diagnosis, and treatment of thrombotic thrombocytopenic purpura. J Am Soc Nephrol 2003;14:1072.

TREATMENT. Investigations have been undertaken concerning the efficacy of administering preparations containing inert adsorptive surfaces that are capable of binding circulating verocytotoxin, thereby preventing attachment to endothelial surfaces where they can engender injury. SYNSORB-pk ingestion was among the first approaches tried [Joh, 1997] but appears to have been abandoned. Other preparations are undergoing evaluation [Armstrong et al., 1995].

Improved supportive therapy, including transfusion, dialysis, and careful management of fluids, electrolytes, and hypertension, has reduced mortality from 50% half a century ago to what is variously estimated as 0% to 30% mortality, with recent pooled data suggesting roughly 10% [Garg et al., 2003; Gianantonio et al., 1973; Kaplan et al., 1976]. Adult mortality is much higher, probably because adult hemolytic-uremic syndrome more often occurs as a complication of much more severe systemic illnesses than are encountered in childhood hemolytic-uremic syndrome cases. Therapeutic options include anticoagulation, administration of antiplatelet or antioxidant agents, thrombolysis (streptokinase), plasmapheresis/plasma exchange, or infusions of plasma, prostacyclin, or gamma globulin [Arenson and August, 1975; Beattie et al., 1981].

None of these various approaches has well-established efficacy (beyond that achieved by excellent supportive care). Plasma manipulations appear to be less beneficial in hemolytic-uremic syndrome than in thrombotic thrombocytopenic purpura [Misiani et al., 1982; Moake, 1991; Powell, et al., 1984]. Trials of gamma globulin are in progress, and preliminary results are promising. Although it is undertaken in some adults with hemolytic-uremic syndrome, anticoagulation in childhood cases entails a certain risk in an illness that is frequently complicated by both bleeding and hypertension. Moreover, it does not appear to be beneficial even when combined with administration of oral antiplatelet agents. It is probably contraindicated [Proesmans et al., 1980].

Hemolytic-uremic syndrome–associated renal failure usually persists for several weeks. Dialysis is required in 30% to 50% of patients and is indicative of a poorer prognosis [Blaker et al., 1978; Ekberg et al., 1977; Garg et al., 2003; Martin et al., 1990]. Renal transplantation is necessary in severe hemolytic-uremic syndrome, amounting to approximately 25% of all childhood cases. Considerable interest is attached to the identification of reliable prognostic factors identifiable very early in the course of hemolytic-uremic syndrome. Such factors should be of importance in stratifying treatment groups for assessment of efficacy of various therapies and might permit aggressive novel strategies to be initiated early in the course of disease for cases with the poorest prognosis.

A review of 387 childhood cases of hemolytic-uremic syndrome has greatly contributed to this important objective. Among these cases, 68% of 276 tested were found to have Shiga-toxin–producing *Escherichia coli*–related hemolytic-uremic syndrome. Age at onset, leukocyte count, and evidence for CNS involvement did not predict time to recovery. However, the combined absence of prodromal diarrhea and Shiga-toxin–producing *Escherichia coli* infection was associated with poorer outcome. Only 34% of individuals who lacked *both* features recovered normal renal function as compared with 65% to 76% of those who did have one or both features [Gianviti et al., 2003].

For 118 cases in a study of postdiarrheal hemolytic-uremic syndrome with kidney transplantation, the recurrence rate was only 0.8%, causing graft loss in that single case. For 63 reported transplanted nondiarrheal hemolytic-uremic syndrome cases without factor H deficiency, 21% demonstrated recurrence with graft loss, whereas nearly 30% of seven transplanted nondiarrheal cases with factor H gene mutations demonstrated recurrence. In some transplanted cases without factor H deficiency or genetic defect, low C3 levels enhance risk for recurrence with graft loss. Disappointing as these statistics might be, they are better than the recurrence risk for heritable adult hemolytic-uremic syndrome, which is about 60% for both autosomal-recessive and autosomal-dominant forms [Loirat and Niaudet, 2003].

Adult hemolytic-uremic syndrome cases, constituting a tiny minority of all hemolytic-uremic syndrome cases, tend to result from a different pathogenesis than most childhood cases and may not be as responsive to therapies that are effective in children [Blackall and Marques, 2004; Karlsberg et al., 1977].

Vasculitic Diseases with Neurologic-Renal Presentations

Extended consideration of these various inflammatory disorders is to be found in Chapter 73.

Hepatorenal Syndrome

Hepatorenal syndrome is a widely accepted but controversial designation for the functional, potentially reversible renal failure that occurs in patients with various forms of liver failure [Bataller et al., 1998; Van Roey and Moore, 1996]. It is divided into two types, each with established diagnostic criteria [Arroyo et al., 1996]. Type 1 includes patients whose rapidly deteriorating renal function with hyponatremia and hyperkalemia develops in association with acute severe hepatic dysfunction (from various causes) or severe hepatic cirrhosis (chiefly alcoholic). It is usually fulminant and carries a high risk for death. Encephalopathy develops in most type 1 cases. Type 2 includes patients that manifest the combination of less severe liver and renal disease. Encephalopathy is less common in type 2 cases. Some form of hepatorenal syndrome develops in as many as 20% of patients who are in their first year of acute or subacute hepatic failure. It occurs in 40% of those who have experienced at least 5 years of chronic hepatic failure.

Cases of type 1 hepatorenal syndrome are rare in childhood. Half of all such cases occur in the wake of acute viral hepatitis with hepatic failure. It may also occur after other causes of liver failure (native or graft), particularly if portal hypertension is present and has produced gastrointestinal bleeding [Evans et al., 1995]. Liver necrosis (sometimes centrilobular) and fatty infiltration of liver may be found [Shida et al., 1996]. Some cases occur after liver transplantation for children who had chronic liver disease due to biliary atresia. One case has been reported in a 3-year-old child with α_1-antitrypsin deficiency. This child died with hepatorenal syndrome after developing hemorrhagic shock and encephalopathy, disseminated intravascular coagulopathy, metabolic acidosis, and nonketotic hypoglycemia [Shida et al., 1996]. Severe hepatorenal syndrome may also develop in children with hereditary fructose intolerance [Ali et al., 1993], with Wilson's disease, with liver malignancy, with autoimmune hepatitis, after shunting procedures for bleeding varices [Evans et al., 1995], or after administration of medications such as nonsteroidal anti-inflammatory drugs (NSAIDs) or minocycline [Arroyo et al., 1983; Boudreaux et al., 1993]. Spontaneous bacterial peritonitis may provoke the hepatorenal syndrome.

The understanding of the pathophysiology of hepatorenal syndrome is incomplete, and the available theories remain controversial. Renal failure probably occurs as the result of severe renal cortical arterial and arteriolar vasoconstrictive ischemia. Some believe that this is in response to the release hepatic substances that variously provoke vasoconstriction or vasodilation. Some believe that vasopressin, renin-angiotensin, or catecholamines may provoke intense selective vasoconstriction with ensuing renal failure [Neuschwander-Tetri, 1994]. Doppler ultrasonography has demonstrated increased renal vascular resistance in as many as 40% of patients with nonazotemic liver disease [Maroto et al., 1994; Sacerdoti et al., 1993]. Renal dysfunction subsequently develops in more than half of these at-risk individuals, half of whom in turn develop hepatorenal syndrome [Platt et al., 1994]. An inverse correlation has been observed between plasma-activated cytokine levels and improvement in renal function after treatment of hepatorenal syndrome with liver transplantation [Burke et al., 1993].

In patients who develop encephalopathy, it has been found that the cerebral circulation is also compromised by intense selective cerebral vasoconstriction [Better, 1983]. It is not known why the sustained vasoconstrictive sympathetic response may be so selective for vessels subserving kidney and brain circulation, whereas capacitance vessels in many other vascular beds dilate. Increased renal secretion of regional vascular modulators may enhance the vasoconstriction and produce additional deleterious effects on glomerular capillary ultrafiltration [Nijima, 1977; Van Roey and Moore, 1996]. Systemic hypotension frequently accompanies the onset of hepatorenal syndrome and may be due to the opening of portosystemic shunts with resulting splanchnic bed dilation, accompanied by blood pooling in that and possibly in other portions of the systemic circulation.

That hepatorenal syndrome may develop in children with septic or hemorrhagic shock suggests the importance of such vasoactive mediators as endotoxin, thromboxane A_2, or other prostaglandins that may alter circulatory balance [Henriksen, 1995; Shida et al., 1996]. Precipitation of hepatorenal syndrome by the administration of NSAIDs ingested by patients with cirrhosis has been regarded as evidence for the importance of prostaglandins in the maintenance of renal vascular tone when the liver is failing (Arroyo et al., 1983). Because of this presumed drug effect, many have thought it wiser to avoid these agents in patients with the hepatorenal syndrome. Some have proposed inadequate renal synthesis of vasodilating prostaglandin E_2 despite normal or increased renal thromboxane A_2 synthesis, and severe activation of endogenous vasoconstrictors is the cause of ischemic renal failure in hepatorenal syndrome [Laffi et al., 1997]. Whether the liver elaborates substances that provoke a dysfunctional "hepatorenal reflex" or fails to produce a much-needed counterregulatory substance, it is probable that failing liver cannot adequately clear circulating vasoactive substances (such as the false neurotransmitter octopamine or various cytokines) or other vascular regulatory substances from the circulation [Fischer and Baldessarini, 1971; Shida et al., 1996]. The performance of large-column paracentesis without compensatory replacement of plasma volume may contribute to the occurrence or severity of the hepatorenal syndrome. The initial renal response to the hepatorenal syndrome is hypermineralocorticoid (i.e., oliguric with retention of both water and salt). Salt wasting may supervene if acute tubular necrosis develops as a result of the intense vasoconstriction. The poor response of the oliguric phase of hepatorenal syndrome to volume expansion or exogenous vasodilators is among the reasons that some have questioned the primacy of renal cortical vasoconstrictive ischemia as the cause of renal failure.

Clinical features of hepatorenal syndrome include ascites, jaundice, and low arterial blood pressure despite increased plasma volume. Hepatomegaly is usually not present. A preexisting poor nutritional state is not uncommon. Laboratory findings often include hyponatremia, hyperkalemia, low urinary sodium clearance, low plasma but high urine osmolarity, high plasma renin activity, increased plasma norepinephrine, and moderately increased blood urea nitrogen and creatinine. Patients who develop acute encephalopathy with hepatorenal syndrome, probably due to severe cerebral vasoconstriction, may be found to have extensive symmetric ischemic brain injury suggestive of parasagittal infarction [Shida et al., 1996].

Most patients with type 1 hepatorenal syndrome are adults. Data on children with this condition are limited. Until recently, all age groups with hepatorenal syndrome had the same generally poor outlook, including a mortality rate of 80% to 95% depending on etiology [Van Roey and Moore, 1996]. Treatment has of necessity involved correction of hepatic failure and support. Some patients have responded to renal transplantation or performance of a shunt procedure to relieve the ascites that is found in 75% of patients with hepatorenal syndrome [Iwatsuki, 1973; Van Roey and Moore, 1996]. Resolution of renal dysfunction has required correction of hepatic dysfunction either by liver regeneration or by liver transplant. Coagulopathy must be corrected. It has been found that treatment with agonists of the vasopressin V(1) and α-adrenergic receptors, if combined with plasma expansion, may reverse both type 1 and 2 hepatorenal syndrome and improve survival. Current research is focusing on the best way to use the various novel drugs that work at these receptor sites [Barada, 2004].

Without effective treatment, patients with hepatorenal syndrome manifest progressive vascular pooling and edema, declining plasma oncotic pressure and blood pressure, and worsening circulatory failure. The outcome of this progressive failure is death. Before transplantation and other interventions, most patients with type 1 hepatorenal syndrome lived less than 2 weeks. Those with type 2 survived for 6 to 12 months. A wide variety of drug and circulating volume treatments aimed at reversing the systemic vasodilation and renal or cerebral vasoconstriction have failed or resulted in only modest improvement in survival. Misoprostol, a prostaglandin E_1 analog, has been touted as a treatment for hepatorenal syndrome, as well as for a wide variety of other toxic or inflammatory forms of hepatic or renal disease [Davies et al., 2001].

The use of systemic vasoconstrictors (terlipressin, ornipressin) with albumin has resulted in recovery of renal function in many patients or recovery of sufficient degree and duration of function to permit liver transplantation or a hepatic shunt procedure to be performed [Moreau, 2002; Ortega et al., 2002]. Liver transplantation has greatly improved survival rate [Restuccia et al., 2004]. However, the limited availability of grafts and the hesitancy to use them in the setting of a grave disease associated with so many predisposing medical conditions have limited the usefulness of this option. Transjugular intrahepatic portosystemic shunts have promise in management of hepatorenal syndrome [Angeli, 2004]. Among patients who experience hepatic recovery or have successful liver transplantation, approximately 7% develop end-stage renal disease [Gonwa et al., 1991].

Amyloidosis

Amyloidoses are divided into the heredofamilial (primary) and those that are the secondary (reactive) groups. Primary amyloidoses comprise a heterogeneous collection of conditions, many of which are rare and restricted to particular mutations shared by small isolated communities of individuals [Benson, 2003]. Identification of the specific gene defect underlying a particular family amyloidosis is of importance for selection of therapy, prognostication, and genetic counseling [Benson, 2003]. Reactive amyloidoses are associated with a wide variety of provocative circumstances, most of which are encountered only in adults. These include inflammatory arthritides or vasculitides, dialysis, and myeloma-associated immunoglobulin light chain deposition.

Table 89-5 lists selected amyloid-related disorders. Many forms of heredofamilial amyloidosis are chiefly cutaneous or do not involve the neurologic and renal systems. However, progressive nephrosis and neurologic disease (CNS tissues, nerve, or muscle) are among the most common manifestations

TABLE 89-5

Selected Heredofamilial (Primary) Amyloidoses

Type I (transthyretin methionine-30 amyloidosis)
Type II (Indiana-type amyloidosis)
Type III (Danish cardiac-type amyloidosis)
Type IV (Iowa-type amyloidosis)
Type V (amyloid cranial neuropathy with lattice corneal dystrophy, amyloidosis due to mutant gelsolin, Finnish-type amyloidosis, Meretoja-type amyloidosis)
Type VI (Icelandic-type amyloidosis)
Type VII (oculoleptomeningeal-type amyloidosis, Ohio-type amyloidosis)
Type VIII (familial renal/visceral amyloidosis; systemic non-neuropathic amyloidosis; Ostertag-type amyloidosis; German-type amyloidosis)
Type IX (familial cutaneous lichen amyloidosis; primary cutaneous amyloidosis; lichen amyloidosis, familial; primary localized cutaneous amyloidosis)
Amyloidosis of gingiva and conjunctiva, with mental retardation (Hornova-Dlurosova syndrome)

of either primary or secondary amyloidoses. Cardiac and gastrointestinal abnormalities are also common. Dysfunction in these various organ systems are the consequence of serositis and vasculitis associated with deposition of the insoluble beta-pleated sheet fibrils (low-molecular-weight peptides) that were long ago misnamed amyloid. Arterial and arteriolar wall deposition in affected organ systems is more common than capillary or venous.

Of the 24 amyloid proteins associated with disease in humans, 7 produce neurologic disease. Their genetic loci are shown in Table 89-6. As can be seen, most patients present in mid or late adulthood with dementia or stroke and many have little or no renal abnormality. Amyloid-β precursor protein may account for some aspects of the progressive dementia seen in Alzheimer's disease and Down syndrome, although this assertion remains controversial. CNS amyloid deposition in such individuals results in amyloid angiopathy that may produce visual disturbances (small or large, irregular, poorly reactive pupils; internal ophthalmoplegia; blindness), nerve deafness, bland or hemorrhagic cerebral infarction, dementia, seizures, polyneuropathy, weakness, or muscle wasting [Benson, 2002; Revesz, 2003; Rousset et al., 2000; Suhr et al., 2003]. The precursor protein is expressed in kidney and is a low concentration constituent of normal urine. The concentration of this soluble protein increases in certain forms of renal tubulopathy associated with a variety of metabolic diseases.

TABLE 89-6

Genetic Loci of Amyloid Proteins Associated with Human Central Nervous System Disease

PRECURSOR	CHROMOSOME	AMYLOID PROTEIN	DISEASE
Gelsolin	9	AGel	Familial amyloidosis, Finnish type
Transthyretin	18	ATTR	Meningovascular amyloidosis
Cystatin C	20	Acys	HCHWA-Icelandic type
Prion protein	20	AprP^{sc}	Creutzfeldt-Jakob disease, kuru, Gerstmann-Sträussler-Scheinker disease, fatal familial insomnia
Aβ precursor	21	Aβ	Alzheimer's, Down syndrome
ABri precursor	13	ABri	Familial British dementia
ADan precursor	13	ADan	Familial Danish dementia

Autosomal dominant familial amyloidotic polyneuropathy (type I amyloidosis) is most likely to occur in Portuguese, Spanish, Majorcan, Swedish, or Japanese kindreds. More than 80 identified missense mutations in the transthyretin gene produce variant transthyretins that account for various disease manifestations [Date et al., 1997; Falk et al., 1997; Uyama et al., 1997]. One of the mutations (Val121Ile) is found in about 3% of American blacks. This condition may present as lower extremity polyneuropathy at some point between the second and fourth decades of life. Individuals may develop fatal meningovascular angiopathy associated with early loss of short-term memory and in the advanced state with cerebral hemorrhage. Subsequently, hearing loss, autonomic or craniofacial polyneuropathy, ataxia, and pyramidal tract signs may be noted. Individuals with this condition may have abnormalities of kidney, liver, heart, gastrointestinal system, lungs, skin, and ovaries [Benson, 2002; Rousset, et al., 2000]. Treatment with early liver transplantation may improve neurologic manifestations, but cardiac and renal function may deteriorate somewhat after transplantation of liver [Suhr, 2003]. Chronic uremia may induce oxidative endothelial vascular damage that facilitates amyloid deposition and worsens the vasculopathy of various organ systems that this disease promotes [Sakashita et al., 2001].

A Hungarian variety of transthyretin gene mutation tends to be clinically restricted to the nervous system. Severe meningocerebrovascular changes are associated with memory disturbance, psychomotor deterioration, ataxia, hearing loss, migrainous headaches with vomiting and episodic disorientation, tremor, and nystagmus. Motor decline is associated with the development of pyramidal signs. Sleep disturbances and facial tics may be found. Peripheral nerve, heart, and kidney function are usually normal despite amyloid deposition, and vision remains normal [Garzuly et al., 1996].

Another autosomal dominant amyloidosis is termed *hereditary cerebral* (Icelandic type, type VI) *amyloidosis.* Mutations of codon 68 of cystatin C gene on chromosome 20 result in production of ACys. Affected normotensive Icelandic young adults have presented with hemorrhagic strokes that may recur or cause death. These are due to the particular tendency for the formation of heavy amyloid deposits on small arteries or arterioles of brain, although vessels of the kidney, spleen, lymph nodes, salivary glands, and seminal vesicles may be involved. Individuals who do not develop strokes may experience progressive middle-age onset of dementia [Olafsson et al., 1996].

Finnish-type (type V) amyloidosis is the result of mutations in the chromosome 9 gene that encodes gelsolin, a regulatory protein. This condition also occurs in Danish and Czech kindreds. There is disturbance of amyloid genesis but also of fusin proteolysis. The pathway that is involved with this disturbance is responsible for the production of *Pme117*-encoded fibrils, which are precursors for the biogenesis of melanosomes [Huff et al., 2003]. Individuals with this condition may have droopy-appearing eyes and protruding lips. Peculiar corneal "lattice" deposits may be seen. Neurologic abnormalities include peripheral or cranial neuropathy and progressive vasculopathy of blood vessels subserving brain, spine, and sensory ganglia. Homozygous Finnish-type amyloidosis due to the *ASN187* gelsolin mutation produces severe nephrotic syndrome. This syndrome may progress to end-stage renal disease owing to heavy glomerular deposits of gelsolin-derived amyloid, especially in tubular epithelium [Maury, 1993].

Among individuals of Middle Eastern ancestry, especially Sephardic Jews and Armenians, familial Mediterranean fever is the most important cause of secondary (AA) amyloidosis. This autosomal-recessive condition is common in the Middle East, with disease prevalence as high as 1:2600 and gene frequency as high as 1:50 in the Near Middle East. At least 30 different mutations of the *MEFV* gene on chromosome 16p13.3 have been linked to this disease [Aldea et al., 2004]. Typical recurrent manifestations develop between 4 months and 16 years of age and if untreated persist throughout life. They include short attacks of fever, abdominal or unilateral chest pain, erysipelas-like erythema, organomegaly, and serositis (pleuritic and arthritic).

Without adequate treatment secondary amyloidosis often develops, especially when there is a family history of amyloidosis. Affected persons are at risk of amyloidotic renal failure and neurologic complications. The risk for these eventualities is reduced by as much as 95% if chronic colchicine therapy is undertaken after early diagnosis [Aldea et al., 2004; Hojberg and Mertz, 1995]. If amyloidosis does develop, the 5-year risk for chronic renal failure ranges from 50% (type I amyloidosis) to greater than 80% (type II amyloidosis). Schönlein-Henoch purpura and polyarteritis nodosa may develop, as well as symptomatic thyroid and gastrointestinal amyloid deposition. Neurologic manifestations result either from CNS vasculitis or secondary to chronic renal failure [Kavukcu et al., 1995; Rawashdeh and Majeed, 1996; Saatci et al., 1993, 1997; Tinaztepe et al., 1993].

A severe form of autosomal-dominant familial secondary amyloidosis has been described in Spain, wherein intermittent bouts of joint pain occur. Progressive AA-associated renal failure may develop and is unresponsive to colchicine. All patients with this condition are heterozygotes for the newly described H4784 *MEFV* gene mutation. It is currently uncertain whether this condition ought to be classified with familial Mediterranean fever or with the newly described group of inherited autoinflammatory periodic syndromes seen in association with other gene mutations including *TNFRSF1A* and *CIAS1/PYPAF1/NALPO3* [Aldea et al., 2004].

There are a number of additional secondary or reactive forms of amyloidosis. One that has clinical similarities to Portuguese familial amyloidosis is Muckle-Wells syndrome. Like familial Mediterranean fever, it is an AA amyloidosis. Presentation may be in the second decade with corticosteroid-resistant nephrotic syndrome. Neurologic abnormalities include bilateral inner ear deafness and recurrent urticaria. Other findings are arthralgia, aphthosis, amyloid goiter, and skeletal abnormalities. Skin and joint abnormalities respond to immunosuppressive therapies including cyclophosphamide [Andrade et al., 1969; Berthelot et al., 1994; Black, 1969; Fuger et al., 1992; Muckle and Wells, 1962; Schwarz et al., 1989; Throssell et al., 1996].

Various chronic infectious or inflammatory conditions can provoke secondary amyloidosis. Examples include juvenile rheumatoid arthritis, systemic lupus erythematosus, granulomatous bowel disease, Takayasu's disease, tuberculosis, leprosy, osteomyelitis, and inadequately treated chronic suppurative infections such as subacute bacterial endocarditis. Hematuria, proteinuria, abnormal urinary sediment, diminished renal function, or hypertension may indicate the development of renal amyloidosis. However, such manifestations are not uncommonly the result of infectious glomerulonephritis or the administration of nephrotoxic drugs [Herbert et al., 1995; Kavukcu et al., 1995; Sieniawska et al., 1996; Tinaztepe, 1995].

A wide range of neurologic abnormalities may be seen in individuals with one or another of these secondary amyloidoses. Vasculopathy may result in neurologic consequences due to bland or infectious cardiogenic emboli, cerebral amyloid angiopathy, Takayasu's disease, or hypertensive encephalopathy [Sousa et al., 1993]. Close collaborative investigation and management of such complex patients by pediatric neurologists and nephrologists, rheumatologists, and infectious disease specialists is of great value in arriving at an accurate diagnosis. Decreased urinary excretion of glycosaminoglycans may be a marker for renal involvement in the amyloidoses. This finding is thought to be the result of (1) diminished number of functioning nephrons, (2) diminished glycosaminoglycans synthesis in functioning glomeruli, and (3) trapping of glycosaminoglycans by amyloid fibrils [Tencer et al., 1997]. The test may also prove valuable in the screening of patients with chronic inflammatory disorders, particularly those that affect the kidney and nervous system.

Metabolic Diseases Producing Generalized Nephron and Neurologic Dysfunction

Both acute and chronic generalized nephron dysfunction may result from metabolic diseases that have primary effects on both the kidney and nervous system. Diseases that are most likely to result in encephalopathy are those that produce the combination of a catabolic and acute renal failure. Under such conditions the metabolic perturbation worsens more rapidly and often achieves greater severity. Systemic diseases that can provoke encephalopathy even without renal failure (e.g., sepsis, burns, fever, ethylene glycol, lactic acidosis, or ketoacidosis) produce more fulminant, severe, and difficult-to-treat nervous system dysfunction when renal failure also occurs or was previously present. Therapeutic interventions undertaken in encephalopathic patients who have renal failure must be carried out with scrupulous attention to cerebrovascular dynamics because cardiac output is often low and cerebral autoregulation is often compromised. Administration of fluids or alkali may in some instances have deleterious effects on cerebral blood flow that must be considered.

Selective Tubular Dysfunction

Many inherited diseases and intoxications produce characteristic patterns of renal tubular acidosis in association with neurologic abnormalities; glomerular function is usually preserved in these diseases. Renal tubular acidosis is generally characterized by hyperchloremia and reduced plasma bicarbonate and is further divided into proximal (bicarbonate wasting) or distal (defective acid excreting) renal tubular varieties. Selective tubular dysfunction itself produces far fewer clinical manifestations than are observed in uremia. In many instances the neurologic dysfunction is more apparent than the associated renal dysfunction, which is often overlooked. The quite straightforward process of detecting and characterizing the renal tubular abnormality is often helpful in diagnosing the cause of observed neurologic dysfunction. Unfortunately the important diagnostic clues provided by selective tubular dysfunction may be overlooked because the renal defect itself may produce few signs or symptoms.

Important examples of diseases that produce neurologic dysfunction in association with proximal renal tubular acidosis are listed in Table 89-7. Those associated with distal renal tubular acidosis are listed in Table 89-8. Intense scrutiny is being paid to the molecular genetics and mechanisms of these various conditions, resulting in a rapidly evolving increase in understanding and a rich banquet of clinical and scientific data. Only a brief review can be provided here. Additional information can be obtained through the Online Mendelian Inheritance in Man (OMIM) available at http://www.ncbi.nlm.nih.gov/entrez/query.fcgi?db=OMIM.

TABLE 89-7

Heritable Nervous System Diseases with Proximal Renal Tubular Acidosis/Fanconi Syndrome

Amyloidosis (familial)
Carbonic anhydrase deficiency type II
Cystinuria
Galactosemia
Glycogen storage disease I
Hartnup disease
Hereditary fructose intolerance
Lowe (oculocerebrorenal) syndrome
Lysinuric protein intolerance
Methylmalonic aciduria
Nephropathic cystinosis
Nephrosialidosis
Primary mitochondrial cytopathies
Pyruvate carboxylase deficiency
Sjögren's syndrome
Tyrosinemia type I
Wilson's disease

TABLE 89-8

Diseases with Nervous System Dysfunction and Distal Renal Tubular Acidosis

Carnitine palmitoyltransferase deficiency
Chronic active hepatitis
Cryoglobulinemia
Fabry's disease
Glycogen storage disease type I
Hashimoto's thyroiditis
Hereditary fructose intolerance*
Leprosy
Lysinuric protein intolerance*
Neuraxonal dystrophy
Primary biliary cirrhosis
Primary hyperparathyroidism
Sickle cell anemia
Sjögren's syndrome*
Systemic lupus erythematosus
Type IV distal renal tubular acidemia
Wilson's disease*

*Also may cause proximal renal tubular acidosis/Fanconi syndrome.

Proximal Renal Tubular Acidosis

The function of the proximal tubule depends on maintenance of an electrical gradient across the tubular epithelium. The gradient requires low intracellular as compared with extracellular sodium concentration. As in the nervous system, the gradient is maintained by Na^+-K^+ adenosine triphosphatase pumps located in the basolateral membrane. It is clear that excessive generalized loss of solutes in urine produces a form of proximal renal tubular acidosis termed the de Toni-Debré-Fanconi ("renal" Fanconi, hereinafter Fanconi) syndrome. Associated serologic abnormalities suggest the presence of proximal renal tubular acidosis and the combination of these laboratory data with clinical findings may designate the presence of a particular underlying metabolic disorder.

A history of polyuria, polydipsia, and dehydration may be found if renal Fanconi syndrome is severe, although within the context of the early recognition of the diseases considered in this section such a history is uncommon. Febrile illnesses in infantile presentations may worsen dehydration. Detection of the characteristic urinary pattern of elevation of the concentrations of multiple amino acids, glucose, phosphate, bicarbonate, calcium, and protein is an especially convenient method of confirming proximal renal tubular acidosis. Characteristically, urine is often dilute despite the elevated concentrations of various solutes owing to a concentrating defect that is secondary to hypokalemia. Additional findings in most cases include stable but mildly reduced level of serum bicarbonate (15 to 20 mEq/L) and appropriate urine acidity on an early morning void (pH > 5.3) [McSherry, 1981]. Further diagnostic clues include normal anion gap acidosis, hypophosphatemia, and hypomagnesemia. Hypokalemia and bicarbonaturia worsen after administration of alkali.

Renal Fanconi syndrome may occur as a primary familial disorder. Of greater importance in this chapter is the secondary form of renal Fanconi syndrome that may occur in the setting of various heritable metabolic disorders (see Table 89-7), which also manifest neurologic abnormalities in addition to and not directly dependent on the presence of Fanconi syndrome. Indeed, in most of these metabolic conditions, Fanconi syndrome tends to be mild to moderate. In some of these diseases, most commonly nephropathic cystinosis, disease tends to progress to chronic renal failure. Almost all of these heritable metabolic conditions are autosomal recessive. The exceptions discussed in this section are X-linked recessive Lowe syndrome and maternally inherited mitochondropathies. Secondary renal Fanconi syndrome may also result from endocrinopathies, intoxications, and various other disorders.

Obviously, any disease that causes severe generalized proximal renal tubular acidosis, including familial Fanconi syndrome, may result in neurologic abnormalities when severe disturbances of potassium, glucose, or acid-base balance occur. This is particularly the case when poorly compensated chronic renal failure or end-stage renal disease develops. The occurrence of seizures in a patient with proximal renal tubular acidosis may be due to hypocalcemia or hypomagnesemia [Heering et al., 1996]. Some neurologic problems may be worsened by a proximal renal tubular leak. Carnitine loss in infantile renal Fanconi syndrome has been associated with poor muscle development and abnormal intramuscular lipid deposition. Hypokalemic muscle weakness is an important potential complication of alkali or thiazide treatment of proximal renal tubular acidosis from any cause. Individuals with inherited hyperkalemic periodic paralysis who have Fanconi syndrome may be vulnerable to an attack of their condition owing to those same interventions.

NEPHROPATHIC CYSTINOSIS. Nephropathic cystinosis, caused by a defective lysosomal membrane transport protein, is the most common identifiable cause of renal Fanconi syndrome in children. This autosomal recessive condition occurs almost exclusively in white individuals. The defective gene has been mapped to a 1-cM region of chromosome 17p13. Continued work, including the cloning of the responsible gene and studies of immortalized proximal tubule cells expressing the defect, should provide important information concerning the biology of lysosomal transport proteins [Jean et al., 1996; McDowell et al., 1996; Peters et al., 1997; Racusen et al., 1995; Stec et al., 1996].

Nephropathic cystinosis is one of the only lysosomal diseases for which there is effective therapy. Treatment is aimed at preventing the pathogenic accumulation of free intracellular cystine in various tissues, including kidney, cornea, thyroid, muscle, and brain [Gahl, 1997]. Cystine is a known nephrotoxin. Exposure of rat kidney slices or isolated tubule cells to cystine deimethylester is a commonly employed model of renal Fanconi syndrome. This compound accumulates in renal tubules and reduces the rate of mitochondrial respiration in association with decline in transporter activity, impaired glutamate-dependent mitochondrial oxygen consumption, and diminished concentrations of intracellular potassium and adenosine triphosphate [Foreman et al., 1995]. At present, diagnosis is usually established with the demonstration of elevated free cystine in polymorphonuclear white cells. This method also permits diagnosis of the heterozygous carrier state. Linkage studies should soon become the diagnostic method of choice. In the infantile form of cystinosis, biochemical evidence for proximal tubule cell dysfunction is usually detectable within the first few months of life. If untreated, frank renal failure usually develops within the first decade of life [Racusen et al., 1995]. The course of renal deterioration after the development of Fanconi syndrome is similar to that observed in other severely nephropathic diseases. Nephrocalcinosis and the formation of calcium oxalate stones are frequent occurrences in nephropathic cystinosis, related in part to supplementation of these patients with phosphate and alkalinizing agents [Theodoropoulos et al., 1995].

Evidence that cysteamine (or phosphocysteamine) administered in doses ranging from 33 to 51 mg/kg per day (or from 1.3 to 1.95 g/m^2 body surface area per day) significantly delays the onset of renal failure has prompted approval of this drug by the U.S. Food and Drug Administration for treatment of nephropathic cystinosis [van't Hoff and Gretz, 1995; Wu et al., 1995]. Although treatment is quite expensive, it delays the even greater expense and multiple complications of renal transplantation [Soohoo et al., 1997]. It may provide other benefits, including longer life expectancy. The potential efficacy of this drug is of further significance in that kidney transplantation does not prevent progressive injury because of the underlying disease to various organs, including the transplanted kidney [Almond et al., 1993].

Before renal transplantation was available, it was thought that neurologic abnormalities occurred only as consequences of renal dysfunction. With the prolonged survival that renal transplantation affords, it has become clear that the infantile and juvenile forms may be associated with visual, intellectual, and motor abnormalities that result from cystine accumulation in the eye (cornea, conjunctiva, retina) or brain (choroid plexus, cortex). Accumulation in the cornea causes progressive keratopathy. Recurrent corneal erosions may prove troublesome [Elder and Astin, 1994]. Cysteamine supplementation to deplete cystine does not influence the course of corneal keratopathy [Thoene, 1995].

Other neurologic consequences develop at various ages from childhood to adulthood. They may include headache; autonomic abnormalities (heat intolerance, hyperthermia, abnormal sweating); poor vision and deficient visual memory; short, raspy, repetitive speech; tremor; pyramidal or extrapyramidal motor defects; and weakness [Gahl et al., 1988; Jonas et al., 1987; Levine and Paparo, 1982]. Selective impairment of visual processing, such as inability to mentally rotate figures, is a frequent finding despite the typically normal intelligence and primary sensory function of these patients. Abnormality of tactile recognition with astereognosis has been discerned in some patients. These higher cortical deficits must be considered in the educational planning for children with this disorder. These subtle deficits are the likely basis of some of the school difficulties experienced by children with nephropathic cystinosis. In some instances the general level of intelligence may be slightly below that of parents or siblings. Intellectual deficits may be static or slowly progressive [Ballantyne et al., 1997; Colah and Trauner, 1997; Scarvie et al., 1996; Williams et al., 1994].

Some patients experience much more severe and strikingly progressive neurologic complications. Cystinosis-related encephalopathy is an entity characterized initially by manifesting cerebellar and pyramidal signs, with ensuing mental deterioration, and then development of pseudobulbar or bulbar palsy with a prominent swallowing disorder. Adults with nephropathic cystinosis may have strokelike episodes with coma and hemiplegia. In either of these clinical groupings, abnormalities may be discerned in MRI images [Broyer et al., 1996; Van Lierde et al., 1994]. These abnormalities correspond to demonstrable pathologic changes within the nervous system, which include nonobstructive hydrocephalus; calcification of the basal ganglia, periventricular zone, and internal capsule; and demyelination of the internal capsule and brachium pontis. Evidence suggests that cysteamine may reverse cystinosis-related encephalopathy, improve the radiologic appearance of brain, and prevent paroxysmal episodes [Broyer et al., 1996].

As has been noted in the section on uremic myopathy, approximately one fourth of patients with long-standing nephropathic cystinosis develop distal lipid inclusion myopathy and perhaps all such patients have subclinical electrophysiologic abnormalities. This result may be the direct effect of cystine toxicity, although carnitine deficiency and other potential causes may also contribute. It remains unclear whether replenishment of muscle carnitine with oral supplementation is beneficial [Gahl et al., 1993]. Patients with cystinosis-related myopathy develop weakness and wasting of small hand muscles, facial weakness, and muscular dysphagia. However, they retain sensation and tendon reflexes. Distal motor unit potentials may have reduced amplitude and duration, and biopsies may indicate a vacuolar myopathy of lysosomal origin [Charnas et al., 1994]. Cystine depletion with cysteamine has been advocated [Vester et al., 2000]. One case of anesthetic-induced malignant hyperthermia has been reported in a child with cystinosis, possibly related to myopathic changes [Purday et al., 1995]. Additional heritable diseases that may result in a combination of neurologic and renal manifestations are listed in Table 89-9.

Neurologic Drugs That May Affect Renal Function

Some drugs commonly used in the management of neurologic diseases may produce disturbances of renal function that range from mild transient effects on the regulation of free water clearance to severe parenchymal kidney injury. Important effects of selected neurologic drugs on renal function are summarized in Tables 89-10 and 89-11. It is well known that carbamazepine and oxcarbazepine produce hyponatremia in appreciable minorities of treated individuals. Prevalence with carbamazepine treatment is approximately 5% [Brewerton and Jackson, 1994]. Serum sodium concentrations in the 126- to 135-mM/L range are found in 18% to 25% of oxcarbazepine-treated children. They are less than 125 mM/L in no more than 3%. Symptomatic hyponatremia is found in 2% or less. No aspects of age, sex, or dose were predictive of risk for hyponatremia in either of two retrospective studies [Borusiak, 1998; Holtmann et al., 2002]. However, a study of institutionalized patients with intellectual disabilities found that more than 40% of those treated with carbamazepine had (largely asymptomatic) hyponatremia as compared with only about 5% of those who were not treated with this drug. Possible correlation of hyponatremic risk with higher carbamazepine levels was suggested [Kelly and Hillery, 2001].

TABLE 89-9

Syndromes with Kidney Malformation and Neurologic Disease

SYNDROME (INHERITANCE)	KIDNEY	NEUROLOGIC
Bardet-Biedl (AR)	CGN/HTN	MR/V
Beckwith/Wiedemann (Sp)	RD/RT	MR
Cat's eye	RA	MR/V
Cockayne's (AR)	RD/HTN	MR/D/A/PN
Fanconi pancytopenia (AR)	RH/RD	MR/CN/D
Fraser's (AR)	RA	MR
Johanson-Blizzard	RD/HN	MR/D
Joubert's	RC	CbD
Klippel-Feil (Sp)	RD	CN/NT/CD
Meckel-Gruber (AR)	RD	NT/M
Melnick-Fraser (AD)	RH/RD	D
MURCS	RA	CD/D
Orofaciodigital I	PCK	MR/M/HC/E
Pallister-Hall (Sp)	RD	T/M/NE
Partial trisomy 10S	RD	MR/M
Rubinstein-Taybi	RD	MR
Schinzel-Giedion	HN	MR/D/E
Short-rib polydactyly II	RD/PCK	CD/M
Townes'	RH/HN	D
Triploidy/mixoploidy	RD/PCK	MR/M/NT/HC
Trisomy 9 mosaic	D	MR/M/NT
Trisomy 18	HN/PCK	MR/M/NT/HC
Tuberous sclerosis (AD)	T	MR/T/MR/E
Turner's	RD/HTN	MR/D
Zellweger's (AR)	RC	MR/M

A, ataxia; AD, autosomal-dominant; AR, autosomal recessive; CbD, cerebellar dysplasia; CD, cervical dysplasia; CGN, congenital glomerulonephritis; CN, cranial neuropathy; D, deafness; E, encephalopathy; HC, hydrocephalus; HN, hydronephrosis; HTN, hypertension; M, central nervous system migrational abnormalities; MR, mental retardation; MURCS, müllerian duct renal and cervical vertebral defects; NT, neural tubule defects; PCK, polycystic kidneys; PN, peripheral neuropathy; RA, renal agenesis; RC, renal cysts; RD, renal dysplasia; RH, renal hypoplasia; Sp, sporadic; T, tumors; V, visual abnormalities.

TABLE 89-10

Neurologic Medications That May Produce Renal Dysfunction

Acetazolamide (PRTA/S/Postrenal failure)
Amphetamines (ARF/AIN)
Analgesics/NSAIDs (PRTA/F/DRTA/Prerenal failure)
Carbamazepine (ARF/AIN)
Cimetidine (ARF/AIN)
Indomethacin/NSAIDs (ARF/AIN/PN)
Phenobarbital (ARF/AIN)
Phenytoin (ARF/AIN)

AIN, acute interstitial nephritis; ARF, acute renal failure; DRTA, distal renal tubular acidosis; F, renal Fanconi; NSAIDs, nonsteroidal anti-inflammatory drugs; PN, papillary necrosis; PRTA, proximal renal tubular acidosis; S, seizures.

TABLE 89-11

Drugs/Toxins Affecting Nervous System and Kidney

DRUG	NEUROLOGIC	RENAL
Analgesics	E/H	PRTA/F/DRTA
Arsenic	E/H/PNM	PRTA/CRF
Burn toxin	E	PRTA
Cadmium	E/S/PNM	PRTA/F
Chromium	E	ARF/CRF
"Ecstasy"	E/S	ARF
Ethylene glycol	E	ARF/CRF
Gallium	B/PNM	ARF/CRF
Indium	E/S/PNM	ARF/CRF
Lead	E/PNM	PRTA/F
Lithium	E/D	DRTA
Mercury	E/M	PRTA/F
Mycotoxin	E	PRTA
Pentazocine	E/D/H	DRTA
Tellurium	E	ARF/CRF
Tetracycline	Ps	PRTA/F
Thallium	E/S/GBS	PRTA/F/DRTA
Toluene	E/L/S/D/Ps	PRTA < DRTA
Xylitol	E/S	ARF/CRF

ARF, acute renal failure; B, blindness; CRF, chronic renal failure; D, delirium; DRTA, distal renal tubular acidosis; E, encephalopathy; F, renal Fanconi; GBS, Guillain-Barré syndrome; H, headache; L, long-tract signs; M, myopathy; PNM, peripheral neuropathy and/or myopathy; PRTA, proximal renal tubular acidosis; Ps, pseudotumor; S, seizures.

The mechanism of hyponatremia with either of these drugs is in doubt. Although the syndrome of inappropriate secretion of antidiuretic hormone was formerly thought to explain the effect [Van Amelsvoort et al., 1994], it has recently been shown that this is not the case for carbamazepine. In patients with carbamazepine-associated hyponatremia, there is no compensatory rise in arginine vasopressin to a water load and there is a fall in free water clearance in response to declining serum sodium concentration. Alternative explanations include induction of enhanced renal response to normal circulating concentrations of antidiuretic hormone.

Clinical manifestations of hyponatremia are rare in children treated with either carbamazepine or oxcarbazepine [Flegel and Cole, 1977; Holtmann et al., 2002]. There is some evidence that co-treatment with demeclocycline or doxycycline may alleviate carbamazepine-associated hyponatremia when it is necessary to use the drug [Boutros et al., 1995; Brewerton and Jackson, 1994]. Combinations of oxcarbazepine with furosemide [Siniscalchi et al., 2004] or carbamazepine with thiazide diuretics [Ranta and Wooten, 2004] may result in acute hyponatremic encephalopathy.

Lamotrigine use in children with centrally mediated diabetes insipidus has been found to induce hyponatremia owing to change in desmopressin requirements [Mewasingh et al., 2000]. Acetazolamide may provoke a selective form of proximal renal tubular acidosis manifested by bicarbonate wasting without generalized proximal tubular dysfunction [Leaf et al., 1954]. Phenytoin, on the other hand, may inhibit the secretion of antidiuretic hormone, resulting in diabetes insipidus [Dousa and Hechter, 1970; Fichman and Bethune, 1968]. Phenytoin-induced lupus may, in turn, produce lupus-related nephropathy. Prolonged ethosuximide administration was associated with development of quite severe lupus in one individual. In addition to kidney dysfunction, this individual manifested cerebral abnormalities, an unusual development in drug-induced lupus. Weight loss, pancreatitis, and arthritis also occurred. Some authorities have discerned provocation of flares of preexisting lupus with initiation of ethosuximide treatment [Casteels et al., 1998]. Rarely, oral or parenteral barbiturates may cause nontraumatic rhabdomyolysis with ensuing acute tubular dysfunction.

Distal renal tubular acidosis with hyperkalemia (type IV distal renal tubular acidosis) may be caused by lithium or by indomethacin [Perez et al., 1975; Steele and Edwards, 1971]. Clinically significant nephrogenic diabetes insipidus develops in 20% to 30% of patients receiving long-term lithium carbonate therapy and may not be entirely irreversible. Subtler defects are found in more than 60% of chronically treated patients [Bucht and Wahlin, 1980]. NSAIDs may diminish renal perfusion because of selective inhibition of cyclooxygenase-2 with the occasional result of hyperkalemic renal failure [Brater, 1999].

There is considerable evidence that phenacetin and, to a lesser extent, aspirin, acetaminophen, and other NSAIDs are potentially nephrotoxic. Several forms of "analgesic nephropathy" have been described, particularly slowly progressive renal papillary necrosis, demonstrable on renal CT scans. There have been instances of acute or chronic interstitial nephritis associated with the use of NSAIDs. Likelihood of nephropathy is greater in individuals using analgesic combinations containing caffeine and/or codeine or individuals combining several different analgesics to achieve pain relief [Elseviers and De Broe, 1999]. Acetaminophen nephrotoxicity may be augmented by the co-administration of herbal remedies such as echinacea, kava, meadow sweet, or willow [Abebe, 2002]. Analgesic nephropathy is rare before 30 years of age. It has been suggested that nitric oxide-releasing NSAIDs may be devoid of nephrotoxicity. Indeed, it has been suggested that these NSAIDs may actually ameliorate kidney function [Fiorucci et al., 2001]. NSAIDs may blunt the response to antihypertensive agents [Brater, 1999].

In healthy individuals there is little evidence that aspirin used alone in therapeutic doses carries any significant risk for irreversible kidney injury. In individuals with glomerulonephritis, cirrhosis, chronic renal insufficiency, or children with congestive heart failure, short-term courses of aspirin have on occasion provoked reversible renal failure. Aspirin intoxication (>300 mg/kg) poses considerable risk for acute renal failure, and doses of more than 500 mg/kg may prove lethal [D'Agati, 1996]. Aspirin and other analgesic medications may produce hyperkalemia that is proportional to the degree and duration of renal failure [Lieberman et al., 1985]. Tricyclic drugs may interfere with the action of some antihypertensive medications and may provoke urine retention. Nifedipine may worsen the edema of renal failure.

Other drugs commonly employed for management of neurologic diseases can cause acute interstitial nephritis and include phenytoin, phenobarbital, carbamazepine, cimetidine, amphetamine, and interferon alfa [Sawaishi et al., 1992; Verrotti et al., 2000]. Phenobarbital appears even over several years of administration to pose a much smaller threat to kidney tubules than does valproate or carbamazepine [Verrotti et al., 2000]. Rarely, carbamazepine may cause membranous glomerulonephropathy or induce an acute hypersensitivity reaction with ensuing acute renal failure [Ray-Chaudhuri et al., 1989]. It is possible to assess whether renal injury is occurring by measurement of several urinary lysosomal hydrolases, *N*-acetyl glucosaminidase and β-galactosidase.

Valproic acid has direct effects on renal tubular ammonia metabolism, accelerating glutamine uptake, ammoniagenesis, and production of alanine, lactate, and pyruvate. These effects appear to be related to stimulation of renal tubular mitochondrial glutamine transport, increased flux of glutamate to malate, and/or reduction of the flux of pyruvate oxidation and carboxylation. In this manner, increased renal ammoniagenesis may combine with valproate-related inhibition of hepatic ureagenesis [Hjelm et al., 1986] to produce the hyperammonemia that is observed in some children with therapeutic serum valproate concentrations [Warter et al., 1983]. Liver enzyme levels remain normal [Gougoux and Vinay, 1988; Martin et al., 1987], and the only clear symptom may be sedation at the ammonia peak, especially after a high-protein meal [Gidal et al., 1997].

Chronic valproate administration may result in proximal renal tubular dysfunction [Gougoux and Vinay, 1989; Ponchaut et al., 1989; Verrotti et al., 2000]. Under experimental conditions, the observable reduction in glutathione (kidney > liver) associated with increased malondialdehyde concentration suggests that lipid peroxidation may play an important role in the development of tubular dysfunction [Raza et al., 1997]. Renal valproate toxicity appears to be a very gradual process that is both time and dose (i.e., "area under the dose/time curve") dependent. Long-term treatment with the combination of valproate and phenobarbital is particularly likely to produce this tubular dysfunction because larger doses of valproate are required to maintain therapeutic serum concentrations.

The development of tubulopathy may be suspected in patients who require unexpected increases in valproic dosage after long intervals of stable dosing to maintain a desirable serum level. An additional clue is the development of proteinuria of a modest degree. It is typically reversible after valproate discontinuation. Carbamazepine poses a smaller, although definite, risk to tubules than does valproate [Verrotti et al., 2000].

Acyclovir may result in acute renal failure; and although this drug has a high therapeutic index, high plasma concentrations increase the risk for this consequence. Coadministration of cephalosporins, which compete for tubular excretion, may increase the nephrotoxic risk of acyclovir administration. With acyclovir-associated renal failure, neurologic deterioration may follow, owing to accumulation of toxic substances as a consequence of renal failure, including high serum and CNS concentrations of acyclovir [Da Conceicao et al., 1999]. In renal transplant patients, the signs and symptoms of acyclovir-associated encephalopathy correlate poorly with acyclovir serum levels [de Knegt et al., 1995; Schwartz et al., 1995].

Drug Therapy in Renal Disease

Renal dysfunction may have significant effects on drug disposition, including many drugs commonly administered to treat neurologic complications of renal disease [Bennett et al., 1987]. Renal dysfunction may affect drug binding, hepatic biotransformation, or renal clearance either of the drug or its metabolites. Drug binding (especially of acidic drugs) may be affected by poor nutrition, by protein loss, or by the competition with the weak organic acids that accumulate in uremia. Biotransformation may be affected by changes in free fraction or, as is the case with phenytoin, by unknown mechanisms. Renal clearance is of little importance for some drugs but of great importance for others (e.g., barbiturates, levetiracetam, gabapentin, toxic metabolites of nitroprusside). Drug penetration into the CNS or systemic clearance may be altered in renal failure. These issues are the subject of several excellent reviews [Asconape and Penry, 1982; Reidenberg, 1977; Tyler, 1975]. Some of the most important problems are considered in the following sections.

DRUG-INDUCED ENCEPHALOPATHY IN RENAL FAILURE. Encephalopathy is the most common consequence of pharmacologic changes with renal failure, with manifestations ranging from subtle intellectual impairment to confusion, delirium, or coma. Hallucination and agitation should always suggest the possibility of intoxication in a patient with renal failure. Severe drug-related encephalopathy may closely resemble uremic encephalopathy, with seizures, myoclonus, and asterixis. Drugs most commonly implicated are antibiotics, antihistamines, antihypertensives, and neuropsychiatric medications [Richet et al., 1970]. Cyproheptadine may produce psychosis in patients with renal failure [Berger et al., 1977; McAllister et al., 1978]. Other commonly encountered drugs that produce encephalopathy in renal failure are listed in Table 89-12.

TABLE 89-12

Drugs That May Produce Unexpected* Encephalopathy in Individuals with Renal Failure

Antibiotics (penicillin G†, ticarcillin, aminoglycosides)
Antiepileptic drugs (barbiturates, benzodiazepines)
Antihistamines (cyproheptadine†, diphenhydramine)
Antihypertensives (prazosin)
Neuropsychiatric (chlorpromazine, haloperidol, phenothiazines)

*Within normal "therapeutic window" ranges of serum concentration.
†Described in children.
Data from Berger et al., 1977; Chin et al., 1986; McAllister et al., 1978; and Taclob and Needle, 1976.

Although a careful drug history is often of greater importance in ascertaining the deleterious drug than the symptom pattern or serum levels, some clinical findings are relevant. Agitation, emotional lability, and anticholinergic signs suggest antihistamines or neuroleptics. Anticholinergic effects may include life-threatening cardiorespiratory impairment. Myoclonus may result from penicillins, chelated aluminum, cyclosporine, nitroprusside, tricyclic antidepressants, phenothiazine, or meperidine. Prominent, recurrent seizures suggest penicillin toxicity. Established "toxic levels" of medications may not always represent reliable guides in renal failure where unmeasured toxic metabolites may accumulate. Therefore, trial withdrawal of expendable or especially toxic medications may be necessary. Recovery from medication effects may require weeks to months, as has been shown for phenothiazine and prazosin [Bloomer et al., 1967; Chin et al., 1986; Taclob and Needle, 1976].

ANTISEIZURE DRUGS. Seizures are common problems in children with renal disease. Most are brief and self-limited, resulting from transient, correctable metabolic disturbances (usually calcium, magnesium, sodium, or glucose) or acute hypertension. Management generally involves exclusion of a serious precipitating cause (e.g., CNS infection, hemorrhage, thrombosis, hypertensive crisis) and correction of metabolic disturbances. However, some individuals with renal disease experience prolonged seizures or develop epilepsy and require acute or chronic treatment with antiseizure medications. Treatment of prolonged seizures is based on seizure type [Rosenbloom and Upton, 1983]. Diazepam, phenobarbital, and phenytoin are the most commonly employed drugs. Acute short-term treatment may be accomplished by administration of loading doses without longer-term administration if clearance is low.

Longer-term or even chronic treatment with an antiseizure medication must be undertaken where risk for seizure recurrence is high. Such usage is guided by medication level, known pharmacokinetics and pharmacodynamics of the antiseizure medication, the extent to which these are likely to be altered at a given level of reduction of renal creatinine clearance or by dialysis, and the degree of hepatic dysfunction. Children with chronic renal failure who are at greater risk for seizure recurrence include those with potential seizure foci as suggested by clinical, imaging, or EEG abnormality. The EEG abnormalities of greatest concern are focal slowing and an active focus of spike discharge. These findings are of greatest concern if the focus corresponds to observed clinical semiology of seizures. Other groups with high risk for recurrence are children with epilepsy or underlying diseases known to provoke seizures.

Renal failure mandates adjustment of dosages and/or dosing intervals of many antiseizure medications. The effects of chronic renal failure on drug disposition are greatest for phenytoin [Letteri et al., 1971]. Protein binding of phenytoin may decrease by as much as threefold in uremia or nephrotic syndrome owing to hypoalbuminemia and the presence of competitive or noncompetitive inhibitors of binding (uremic or dialysis related). Conversely, the steady-state plasma concentration for a given dose of phenytoin also decreases by twofold to threefold as the result of an increase in the apparent volume of distribution and shortened half-time of elimination [Asconape and Penry, 1982]. It is particularly important to monitor carefully the phenytoin levels in patients with renal failure because the nonlinear kinetics of this drug, which are difficult to manage even without renal failure, are much more likely to produce subtherapeutic or supertherapeutic levels in patients with renal failure.

It is best to rely on published tables predicting free phenytoin concentrations as a function of serum creatinine in choosing a dosage [Reidenberg and Affrime, 1973] and to titrate dosage adjustments on the basis of free phenytoin levels. It should also be noted that enzyme-multiplied immunoassays for total phenytoin are unreliable in uremic serum [McDonald and Kabra, 1980; Sirgo et al., 1984]. Dosing intervals should be 8 hours or less because administration of larger, less-frequent doses may produce toxic symptoms as a result of the high free fraction. Hemodialysis has little effect on serum phenytoin concentration. In fact, heparinization for dialysis may displace bound phenytoin, resulting in transient toxicity [Steele et al., 1979]. Chronic phenytoin therapy may aggravate renal osteomalacia, but the same effect is produced by most, if not all, of the other antiepileptic drugs—especially when administered in combination.

Although few good studies are available, valproic acid is probably subject to pharmacokinetic changes similar to phenytoin when administered to patients with renal failure [Bruni et al., 1980]. The efficacy of dialysis in removing this drug is incompletely characterized [Orr et al., 1983]. However, the toxicity of valproate is generally quite low and the drug can be effective in controlling myoclonic and generalized uremic seizures [Asconape and Penry, 1982]. Theoretical considerations favor its use for seizures associated with cyclosporine therapy and renal graft rejection [Hillebrand et al., 1987].

Phenobarbital elimination depends in part on the glomerular filtration rate and urine pH, but there are surprisingly few data on the disposition of this drug in renal failure [Rust et al., 1989]. Over the short term, renal failure usually has little effect on serum phenobarbital levels [Fabre et al., 1966]. Long-term phenobarbital therapy in severe renal disease may require dosage reduction. Postdialysis doses are usually necessary because this drug is readily dialyzed, especially by hemodialysis. Doses should be adjusted according to postdialysis plasma levels. Pentobarbital, on the other hand, is poorly dialyzable. Primidone may prove toxic in renal failure and requires careful serum monitoring, particularly of the upstream intermediate, phenyl-ethylmalonic acid (PEMA).

Carbamazepine bioavailability and clearance are unlikely to be greatly affected by renal disease but have not been well studied. Reliable information regarding clearance by dialysis is lacking. The glucuronide metabolites of the new antiepileptic drug, oxcarbazepine, may accumulate in patients with severe renal dysfunction, but the concentration of the active monohydroxy derivative is less likely to do so. Additional studies are required [Lloyd et al., 1994; Rouan et al., 1994]. Ethosuximide has not been well studied, but it is seldom used in patients with renal disease. It is likely to be readily dialyzable.

As much as 90% of circulating levetiracetam is excreted in the urine—more than two thirds unchanged and the remainder as an inactive metabolite. It is not liver metabolized; hence, in patients with renal failure, dosage must be modified in a fairly linear fashion in accordance with the degree of decline in creatinine clearance. Approximately two thirds of zonisamide elimination is accomplished by the kidneys, either unchanged or as a glucuronide conjugate. Renal clearance of this drug also diminishes in an approximately linear relationship with diminished creatinine clearance. With severe renal failure (creatinine clearance < 20 mL/minute), zonisamide accumulation may result in serum concentrations approximately one third greater than otherwise anticipated. In assessing for this eventuality, it must be borne in mind that the very long elimination time of this drug means that steady-state elevation will not be achieved for a considerable interval after introduction or dose modification.

Lamotrigine inactivation is the result of hepatic conjugation with ensuing elimination of the predominantly 2-*N*-glucuronate adduct. At least 94% of elimination of this metabolite is renal; hence, accumulation occurs with renal failure. The mean plasma half-life of the drug is greater than 40 hours in renal failure as compared with 26 hours in patients who do not have renal or hepatic failure. Approximately 20% of the plasma concentration is removed by 4 hours of dialysis. The mean half-life is approximately 13 hours with hemodialysis but 57 hours without hemodialysis. These data suggest that, after normal initial dosing, increments should be half or less as great as would be employed without renal (or hepatic) failure with careful monitoring of predialysis and postdialysis trough concentrations. Given the prolonged upward dosage titration necessary to avoid allergy to this medication, its use in patients with renal failure may be a complicated undertaking. It has been suggested that lamotrigine (Lamictal) may elevate risk for renal stones by twofold to fourfold as compared with expected risk.

Gabapentin is not appreciably metabolized so that elimination is achieved almost entirely as unchanged drug in urine. Hence, there is a linear inverse relation of steady-state concentration to clearance. The usual elimination half-life of 5 to 7 hours is increased to a mean of 132 hours for creatinine clearance less than 30 mL/minute without dialysis or to approximately 50 hours in end-stage chronic renal failure with thrice-weekly dialysis. Published dosage tables for renal failure in adults receiving hemodialysis are available.

Individuals with creatinine clearance in the 30- to 60-mL/minute range usually require somewhat less than half of the expected daily maintenance doses (400 to 1400 mg/day as compared with 900 to 3600 mg/day), and the doses should again be cut in half (200 to 700 mg/day) if creatinine clearance is 15 to 29 mL/minute. Doses for individuals whose clearance is less than 15 mL/minute can be reduced linearly in proportion to fraction by which clearance is further reduced as compared to 15 mL/minute (i.e., dosage for clearance of 7.5 mL/minute is half that of 15 mL/minute). Approximate supplementary doses for adults after hemodialysis range, without regard to creatinine clearance, from 125 (total daily dose up to 700 mg/day) to 350 mg (total daily dosage > 700 mg/day). This treatment must be individualized, adjusted on the basis of peak and trough levels of gabapentin.

Benzodiazepines (especially clonazepam) are useful in controlling uremic myoclonus [Chadwick and French, 1979; Stark, 1981] and may not require dosage alteration for acute administration in renal failure, although protein binding may be reduced. Diazepam and lorazepam require reduction more often than clonazepam. Diazepam is not readily dialyzable. Little information is available concerning the dialysis of other benzodiazepines [Asconape and Penry, 1982]. These drugs may accumulate with repeated administration and produce encephalopathy or even myoclonus [Taclob and Needle, 1976]. Lidocaine may be useful in the treatment of uremic status epilepticus, but only limited information is available [Da Conceicao et al., 1999; Raskin and Fishman, 1976b].

OTHER NEUROLOGIC DRUGS. A number of other medications commonly used in the therapy of neurologic disease should be administered with caution in patients with renal failure. Acyclovir doses must be carefully adjusted in patients with renal insufficiency, including acyclovir-provoked renal insufficiency [Da Conceicao et al., 1999]. Both aspirin and acetaminophen require longer interdose intervals in renal failure. Aspirin should not be administered when the glomerular filtration rate is less than 10 mL/minute. Both of these analgesic drugs are readily cleared by dialysis.

Acetazolamide is entirely eliminated by renal mechanisms. The dosage should be reduced for renal failure and avoided in end-stage renal disease and in patients with acidosis, hypokalemia, or urolithiasis (all of which may be worsened by its administration).

Tricyclic drugs are not dialyzed well but usually do not require dosage changes in renal failure. They may have beneficial effects, increasing appetite and weight in end-stage renal disease. β Blockers and calcium-channel blockers are not readily cleared by dialysis. Dosage may require adjustment in severe renal failure. Haloperidol is not well dialyzed and may provoke hypotension in patients with renal failure. Lithium is a dialyzable drug that requires a longer interdose interval in renal failure. It should be avoided in patients with renal disease because of potential aggravation of renal tubular acidosis or provocation of nephrogenic diabetes insipidus or chronic interstitial fibrosis. Considerably greater detail concerning the management of drugs pertinent to neurologic and other forms of medical practice in children with renal failure is available in several recent reviews [Veltri et al., 2004].

REFERENCES

Abbassi V, Lowe CU, et al. Oculo-cerebro-renal syndrome: A review. Am J Dis Child 1968;115:145.

Abe T, Tamai M. Ocular changes of glycogen storage disease type I. Ophthalmologica 1995;209:92.

Abebe W. Herbal medication: Potential for adverse interactions with analgesic drugs. J Clin Pharm Ther 2002;27:391.

Accurso V, Shamsuzzaman AS, et al. Rhythms, rhymes, and reasons—spectral oscillations in neural cardiovascular control. Auton Neurosci 2001;90:41.

Ackil AA, Shahani BT, et al. Sural nerve conduction studies and late responses in children undergoing hemodialysis. Arch Phys Med Rehabil 1981;62:487.

Adams RD. Case records of the Massachusetts General Hospital. N Engl J Med 1964;271:200.

Adams RD, Foley JM. The neurologic changes in the more common type of severe liver disease. Trans Am Neurol Assoc 1949;74:217.

Adams RD, Foley JM. The neurologic disorders associated with liver disease. Res Path Assoc Res Dis 1953;32:198.

Agarwal RK, Ostaszewski ML, et al. Tumor necrosis factor and interleukin-6 in cerebrospinal fluid of a patient with recurrent adverse central nervous system events following OKT3. Transplant Proc 1993;25:2143.

Akasaki M, Fukui S, et al. Urinary excretion of a large amount of bound sialic acid and of under sulfated chondroitin sulfate A by patients with the Lowe syndrome. Clin Chim Acta 1978;89:119.

Akmal M, Goldstein DA, et al. Role of uremia, brain calcium, and parathyroid hormone on changes in electroencephalogram in chronic renal failure. Am J Physiol 1984;246:F575.

Al-Hazmi M, Ayoola EA, et al. Epidemic Rift Valley fever in Saudi Arabia: A clinical study of severe illness in humans. Clin Infect Dis 2003;36:245.

Aldea A, Campistol JM, et al. A severe autosomal-dominant periodic inflammatory disorder with renal AA amyloidosis and colchicine resistance associated to the MEFV H478Y variant in a Spanish kindred: An unusual familial Mediterranean fever phenotype or another MEFV-associated periodic inflammatory disorder? Am J Med Genet 2004;124A:67.

Alexander JJ, Pickering MC, et al. Complement Factor H limits immune complex deposition and prevents inflammation and scarring in glomeruli of mice with chronic serum sickness. J Am Soc Nephrol 2005;16:52.

Alfrey AC, LeGendre GR, et al. The dialysis encephalopathy syndrome: Possible aluminum intoxication. N Engl J Med 1976;294:184.

Ali M, Rellos P, et al. Hereditary fructose intolerance. J Med Genet 1998;35:353.

Ali M, Rosien U, et al. DNA diagnosis of fatal fructose intolerance from archival tissue. Q J Med 1993;86:25.

Almond PS, Matas AJ, et al. Renal transplantation for infantile cystinosis: Long-term follow-up. J Pediatr Surg 1993;28:232.

Amorosi EL, Karpatkin S. Antiplatelet treatment of thrombotic thrombocytopenic purpura [editorial]. Ann Intern Med 1977;86:102.

Amoroso E, Vitale C, et al. Spinal-cord compression due to extradural amyloidosis of the cervico-occipital hinge, in a hemodialysed patient: A case report. J Neurosurg Sci 2001;45:120.

Anderson RJ, Chung HM, et al. Hyponatremia: A prospective analysis of its epidemiology and the pathogenetic role of vasopressin. Ann Intern Med 1985;102:164.

Andrade C, Canijo M, et al. The genetic aspect of the familial amyloidotic polyneuropathy: Portuguese type of paramyloidosis. Humangenetik 1969;7:163.

Andreoli SP. Acute renal failure in the newborn. Semin Perinatol 2004;28:112.

Andreoli SP, Bergstein JM, et al. Aluminum intoxication from aluminum-containing phosphate binders in children with azotemia not undergoing dialysis. N Engl J Med 1984;310:1079.

Andreoli SP, Dunn D, et al. Intraperitoneal deferoxamine therapy for aluminum intoxication in a child undergoing continuous ambulatory peritoneal dialysis. J Pediatr 1985;107:760.

Angeli P. Prognosis of hepatorenal syndrome—has it changed with current practice? Aliment Pharmacol Ther 2004;20(Suppl 3):44.

Antoniazzi AL, Bigal ME, et al. [Headache and hemodialysis: evaluation of the possible triggering factors and of the treatment]. Arq Neuropsiquiatr (in Portuguese) 2002;60:614.

Antoniazzi AL, Bigal ME, et al. Headache associated with dialysis: The International Headache Society criteria revisited. Cephalalgia 2003;23:146.

Aoyagi K. Inhibition of arginine synthesis by urea: A mechanism for arginine deficiency in renal failure which leads to increased hydroxyl radical generation. Mol Cell Biochem 2003;244:11.

Appenzeller O, Kornfeld M, et al. Neuropathy in chronic renal disease: A microscopic, ultrastructural, and biochemical study of sural nerve biopsies. Arch Neurol 1971;24:449.

Arbus GS, Barnor NA, et al. Effect of chronic renal failure, dialysis and transplantation on motor nerve conduction velocity in children. Can Med Assoc J 1975;113:517.

Arenson EB Jr, August CS. Preliminary report: Treatment of the hemolytic-uremic syndrome with aspirin and dipyridamole. J Pediatr 1975;86:957.

Arieff AI, Armstrong DK. Parathyroid hormone and uremic neurotoxicity: An unproven association. Contrib Nephrol 1980;20:56.

Arieff AI, Guisado R, et al. Central nervous system pH in uremia and the effects of hemodialysis. J Clin Invest 1976;58:306.

Arieff AI, Lazarowitz VC, et al. Experimental dialysis disequilibrium syndrome: Prevention with glycerol. Kidney Int 1978;14:270.

Arieff AI, Massry SG, et al. Brain water and electrolyte metabolism in uremia: Effects of slow and rapid hemodialysis. Kidney Int 1973;4:177.

Arion WJ, Canfield WK. Glucose-6-phosphatase and type 1 glycogen storage disease: Some critical considerations. Eur J Pediatr 1993;152(Suppl 1):S7.

Arita J, Kajita T, et al. [Muscle fiber involvement in Lowe syndrome]. No To Hattatsu (in Japanese) 1994;26:423.

Armstrong GD, Rowe PC, et al. A phase I study of chemically synthesized verotoxin (Shiga-like toxin) Pk-trisaccharide receptors attached to chromosorb for preventing hemolytic-uremic syndrome. J Infect Dis 1995;171:1042.

Arns W. [Headaches in cyclosporine therapy]. Dtsch Med Wochenschr (in German) 1994;119:1135.

Arnutti P, Nathalang O, et al. Factor V Leiden and prothrombin G20210A mutations in Thai patients awaiting kidney transplant. Southeast Asian J Trop Med Public Health 2002;33:869.

Arroyo V, Gines P, et al. Definition and diagnostic criteria of refractory ascites and hepatorenal syndrome in cirrhosis. International Ascites Club. Hepatology 1996;23:164.

Arroyo V, Planas R, et al. Sympathetic nervous activity, renin-angiotensin system and renal excretion of prostaglandin E2 in cirrhosis: Relationship to functional renal failure and sodium and water excretion. Eur J Clin Invest 1983;13:271.

Asami T, Inano K, et al. Two families of Lowe oculocerebrorenal syndrome with elevated serum HDL cholesterol levels and *CETP* gene mutation. Acta Paediatr 1997;86:41.

Asbury AK, Victor M, et al. Uremic polyneuropathy. Arch Neurol 1963;8:413.

Asconape JJ, Penry JK. Use of antiepileptic drugs in the presence of liver and kidney diseases: A review. Epilepsia 1982;23(Suppl 1):S65.

Avram MM. High prevalence of pancreatic disease in chronic renal failure. Nephron 1977;18:68.

Awad M, Al-Ashwal AA, et al. Long-term follow up of carbonic anhydrase II deficiency syndrome. Saudi Med J 2002;23:25.

Bach C, Iaina A, et al. Autonomic nervous system disturbance in patients on chronic hemodialysis. Isr J Med Sci 1979;15:761.

Badawi N, Cahalane SF, et al. Galactosaemia—a controversial disorder: Screening & outcome. Ireland 1972-1992. Ir Med J 1996;89:16.

Baehr G, Klemperer P, et al. An acute febrile anemia and thrombocytopenic purpura with diffuse platelet thromboses of capillaries and arterioles. Trans Assoc Am Physicians 1936;51:43.

Baerlocher K, Gitzelmann R, et al. Hereditary fructose intolerance in early childhood: A major diagnostic challenge: Survey of 20 symptomatic cases. Helv Paediatr Acta 1978;33:465.

Bakke L. Uraemic polyneuropathy. Acta Neurol Scand 1970;46(Suppl):205.

Bale JF Jr, Siegler RL, et al. Encephalopathy in young children with moderate chronic renal failure. Am J Dis Child 1980;134:581.

Ballantyne AO, Scarvie KM, et al. Academic achievement in individuals with infantile nephropathic cystinosis. Am J Med Genet 1997;74:157.

Baluarte HJ, Gruskin AB, et al. Encephalopathy in children with chronic renal failure. Proc Clin Dial Transplant Forum 1977;7:95.

Bana DS, Graham JR. Renin response during hemodialysis headache. Headache 1976;16:168.

Bar S, Savir H. Renal retinopathy—the renewed entity. Metab Pediatr Syst Ophthalmol 1982;6:33.

Barada K. Hepatorenal syndrome: Pathogenesis and novel pharmacological targets. Curr Opin Pharmacol 2004;4:189.

Baran D, Hutchinson TA. The outcome of hyponatremia in a general hospital population. Clin Nephrol 1984;22:72.

Barbero GJ, Sibinga MS. The electrolyte abnormality in cystic fibrosis. Pediatr Clin North Am 1964;11:983.

Bardin T. Musculoskeletal manifestations of chronic renal failure. Curr Opin Rheumatol 2003;15:48.

Barmeir E, Mann JH, et al. Cerebral nocardiosis in renal transplant patients. Br J Radiol 1981;54:1107.

Baron DN, Dent CE, et al. Hereditary pellagra-like skin rash with temporary cerebellar ataxia: Constant renal amino-aciduria. And other bizarre biochemical features. Lancet 1956;2:421.

Barrueto F Jr, et al. A case of levetiracetam (Keppra) poisoning with clinical and toxicokinetic data. J Toxicol Clin Toxicol 2002;40:881.

Bartel LL, Hussey JL, et al. Effect of dialysis on serum carnitine, free fatty acids, and triglyceride levels in man and the rat. Metabolism 1982;31:944.

Bartter FC, Schwartz WB. The syndrome of inappropriate secretion of antidiuretic hormone. Am J Med 1967;42:790.

Basel-Vanagaite L, Marcus N, et al. New syndrome of simplified gyral pattern, micromelia, dysmorphic features and early death. Am J Med Genet 2003;119A:200.

Bataller R, Sort P, et al. Hepatorenal syndrome: Definition, pathophysiology, clinical features and management. Kidney Int Suppl 1998;66:S47.

Bates S, Nathan J, et al. Epilepsy in childhood renal transplantation: A 20 year experience in 135 patients. Ann Neurol 1986;20:426.

Beaman M, Parvin S, et al. Convulsions associated with cyclosporin A in renal transplant recipients. BMJ (Clin Res Ed) 1985;290:139.

Beattie TJ, Murphy AV, et al. Plasmapheresis in the haemolytic-uraemic syndrome in children. BMJ (Clin Res Ed) 1981;282:1667.

Becaria A, Campbell A, et al. Aluminum as a toxicant. Toxicol Ind Health 2002;18:309-320.

Bechar M, Lakke JP, et al: Subdural hematoma during long-term hemodialysis. Arch Neurol 1972;26:513.

Beigi B, O'Keefe M, et al. Ophthalmic findings in classical galactosaemia—prospective study. Br J Ophthalmol 1993;77:162.

Bell WR, Braine HG, et al. Improved survival in thrombotic thrombocytopenic purpura-hemolytic uremic syndrome: Clinical experience in 108 patients [see comments]. N Engl J Med 1991;325:398-403.

Bellomo R, Ronco C. Indications and criteria for initiating renal replacement therapy in the intensive care unit. Kidney Int Suppl 1998;66:S106.

Bennett WM, Aronoff GR, et al. Drug prescribing in renal failure: Dosing guidelines for adults. Am J Kidney Dis 1983;3:155.

Benson MD. Laboratory assessment of transthyretin amyloidosis. Clin Chem Lab Med 2002;40:1262.

Benson MD. The hereditary amyloidoses. Best Pract Res Clin Rheumatol 2003;17:909.

Berger M, White J, et al. Toxic psychosis due to cyproheptadine in a child on hemodialysis: A case report. Clin Nephrol 1977;7:43.

Bergeron A, Jorquera R, et al. [Hereditary tyrosinemia: An endoplasmic reticulum stress disorder?]. Med Sci (Paris) (in French) 2003;19:976.

Bergstrom J. Uremia is an intoxication. Kidney Int Suppl 1985;17:S2.

Bergstrom L, Thompson P. Hearing loss in pediatric renal patients. Int J Pediatr Otorhinolaryngol 1983;5:227.

Berkowitz LR, Dalldorf FG, et al. Thrombotic thrombocytopenic purpura: A pathology review. JAMA 1979;241:1709.

Berlyne GM, Ben-Ari J, et al. Hyperaluminaemia from aluminum resins in renal failure. Lancet 1970;2:494.

Berretta JS, Holbrook CT, et al. Chronic renal failure presenting as proximal muscle weakness in a child. J Child Neurol 1986;1:50.

Berry GT, Palmieri M, et al. The effect of dietary fruits and vegetables on urinary galactitol excretion in galactose-1-phosphate uridyltransferase deficiency. J Inherit Metab Dis 1993;16:91.

Berthelot JM, Maugars Y, et al. Autosomal dominant Muckle-Wells syndrome associated with cystinuria, ichthyosis, and aphthosis in a four-generation family. Am J Med Genet 1994;53:72.

Better OS. Bile duct ligation: An experimental model of renal dysfunction secondary to liver disease. In: Epstein M, ed. The kidney in liver disease. New York: Elsevier Biomedical, 1983;295.

Bhananker SM, Paek R, et al. Water intoxication and symptomatic hyponatremia after outpatient surgery. Anesth Analg 2004;98:1294, table of contents.

Biasioli S, D'Andrea G, et al. The role of neurotransmitters in the genesis of uremic encephalopathy. Int J Artif Organs 1984;7:101.

Biasioli S, D'Andrea G, et al. Uremic encephalopathy: An updating. Clin Nephrol 1986;25:57.

Binder DK, Oshio K, et al. Increased seizure threshold in mice lacking aquaporin-4 water channels. Neuroreport 2004;15:259.

Birgens H, Ernst P, et al. Thrombotic thrombocytopenic purpura: Treatment with a combination of antiplatelet drugs. Acta Med Scand 1979;205:437.

Bishop N, McGraw M, et al. Aluminium in infant formulas. Lancet 1989;1:565.

Black JT. Amyloidosis, deafness, urticaria, and limb pains: a hereditary syndrome. Ann Intern Med 1969;70:989.

Blackall DP, Marques MB. Hemolytic uremic syndrome revisited: Shiga toxin, factor H, and fibrin generation. Am J Clin Pathol 2004;121(Suppl):S81.

Blackburn CR, McLeod JG. CNS lesions in cystinuria. Arch Neurol 1977;34:638.

Blackman JA, Patrick PD, et al. Paroxysmal autonomic instability with dystonia after brain injury. Arch Neurol 2004;61:321.

Blaker F, Altrogge H, et al. [Treatment of severe haemolytic-uraemic syndrome by dialysis (author's transl)]. Dtsch Med Wochenschr (in German) 1978;103:1229.

Blau JN, Kell CA, et al. Water-deprivation headache: A new headache with two variants. Headache 2004;44:79.

Bloomer HA, Barton LJ, et al. Penicillin-induced encephalopathy in uremic patients. JAMA 1967;200:121.

Bohle A, Helmchen U, et al. Malignant nephrosclerosis in patients with hemolytic uremic syndrome (primary malignant nephrosclerosis). Curr Top Pathol 1977;65:81.

Bohu PA, Hannequin D, et al. [Late neurologic complications of galactosemia: Study of 3 cases]. Rev Neurol (Paris) (in French) 1995;151:136.

Boleda MD, Giros ML, et al. Severe neonatal galactose-dependent disease with low-normal epimerase activity. J Inherit Metab Dis 1995;18:88.

Bolton CF. Peripheral neuropathies associated with chronic renal failure. Can J Neurol Sci 1980;7:89.

Bolton CF, Baltzan MA, et al. Effects of renal transplantation on uremic neuropathy: A clinical and electrophysiologic study. N Engl J Med 1971;284:1170.

Boonpucknavig V, Soontornniyomkij V. Pathology of renal diseases in the tropics. Semin Nephrol 2003;23:88.

Borrego Dominguez RR, Imaz Roncero A, et al. [Severe hypernatremia: Survival without neurologic sequelae]. An Pediatr (Barc) (in Spanish) 2003;58:376.

Borusiak P, Korn-Merker E, et al. Hyponatremia induced by oxcarbazepine in children. Epilepsy Res 1998;30:241.

Bosch AM, Waterham HR, et al. [From gene to disease; galactosemia and galactose-1-phosphate uridyltransferase deficiency]. Ned Tijdschr Geneeskd 2004;148:80.

Boudreaux JP, Hayes DH, et al. Fulminant hepatic failure, hepatorenal syndrome, and necrotizing pancreatitis after minocycline hepatotoxicity. Transplant Proc 1993;25:1873.

Bourke E, Delaney VB, et al. Renal tubular acidosis and osteopetrosis in siblings. Nephron 1981;28:268.

Boutros NN, Guerra BM, et al. Carbamazepine-induced hyponatremia resolved with doxycycline. J Clin Psychiatry 1995;56:377.

Brady RO, Schiffmann R. Clinical features of and recent advances in therapy for Fabry disease. JAMA 2000;284:2771.

Branton M, Schiffmann R, et al. [alpha]-Galactosidase A activity influences renal disease course in Fabry disease. J Am Soc Nephrol 2000;11:403A.

Brater DC. Effects of nonsteroidal anti-inflammatory drugs on renal function: Focus on cyclooxygenase-2-selective inhibition. Am J Med 1999;107:65S; discussion 70S.

Bresolin N, Comi GP, et al. Clinical and biochemical evidence of skeletal muscle involvement in galactose-1-phosphate uridyl transferase deficiency. J Neurol 1993;240:272.

Brewer GJ, Turkay A, et al. Development of neurologic symptoms in a patient with asymptomatic Wilson's disease treated with penicillamine. Arch Neurol 1994;51:304.

Brewerton TD, Jackson CW. Prophylaxis of carbamazepine-induced hyponatremia by demeclocycline in six patients. J Clin Psychiatry 1994;55:249.

Bright R. Reports of medical cases with a view of illustrating the symptoms and cure of disease by reference to morbid anatomy. London: Longman, Rees, Brown and Green, 1831.

Brooks CC, Tolan DR. Association of the widespread A149P hereditary fructose intolerance mutation with newly identified sequence polymorphisms in the aldolase B gene. Am J Hum Genet 1993;52:835.

Brooks CC, Tolan DR. A partially active mutant aldolase B from a patient with hereditary fructose intolerance. Faseb J 1994;8:107.

Brown JJ, Sufit RL, et al. Visual evoked potential changes following renal transplantation. Electroencephalogr Clin Neurophysiol 1987;66:101.

Broyer M, Tete MJ, et al. Clinical polymorphism of cystinosis encephalopathy: Results of treatment with cysteamine. J Inherit Metab Dis 1996;19:65-75.

Bruni J, Wang LH, et al. Protein binding of valproic acid in uremic patients. Neurology 1980;30:557.

Brunner HR, Chang P, et al. Angiotensin II vascular receptors: Their avidity in relationship to sodium balance, the autonomic nervous system, and hypertension. J Clin Invest 1972;51:58.

Brunner JE, Redmond JM, et al. Central pontine myelinolysis and pontine lesions after rapid correction of hyponatremia: A prospective magnetic resonance imaging study. Ann Neurol 1990;27:61.

Buchanan WD. Toxicity of arsenic compounds. New York: Elsevier, 1962.

Bucht G, Wahlin A. Renal concentrating capacity in long-term lithium treatment and after withdrawal of lithium. Acta Med Scand 1980;207:309.

Buemi M, Allegra A, et al. Renal failure from mitochondrial cytopathies. Nephron 1997;76:249.

Bukowski RM. Thrombotic thrombocytopenic purpura: A review. Prog Hemost Thromb 1982;6:287.

Burchell A, Waddell ID. The molecular basis of the genetic deficiencies of five of the components of the glucose-6-phosphatase system: Improved diagnosis. Eur J Pediatr 1993;152(Suppl 1):S18.

Burke GW, Cirocco R, et al. Activated cytokine pattern in hepatorenal syndrome: Fall in levels after successful orthotopic liver transplantation. Transplant Proc 1993;25:1876.

Burks JS, Alfrey AC, et al. A fatal encephalopathy in chronic haemodialysis patients. Lancet 1976;1:764.

Burwen DR, Olsen SM, et al. Epidemic aluminum intoxication in hemodialysis patients traced to use of an aluminum pump. Kidney Int 1995;48:469.

Bushara KO, Rust RS. Reversible MRI lesions due to pegaspargase treatment of non-Hodgkin's lymphoma. Pediatr Neurol 1997;17:185.

Byrnes JJ, Khurana M. Treatment of thrombotic thrombocytopenic purpura with plasma. N Engl J Med 1977;297:1386.

Byrom FB. The pathogenesis of hypertensive encephalopathy and its relation to the malignant phase of hypertension: Experimental evidence from hypertensive rat. Lancet 1954;2:202.

Callaghan N. Restless legs syndrome in uremic neuropathy. Neurology 1966;16:359.

Calonge MJ, Gasparini P, et al. Cystinuria caused by mutations in *rBAT,* a gene involved in the transport of cystine [see comments]. Nat Genet 1994;6:420.

Calonge MJ, Volpini V, et al. Genetic heterogeneity in cystinuria: The *SLC3A1* gene is linked to type I but not to type III cystinuria. Proc Natl Acad Sci U S A 1995;92:9667.

Campistol JM. Uremic myopathy. Kidney Int 2002;62:1901.

Capone PM, Cohen ME. Seizures and cerebritis associated with administration of OKT3. Pediatr Neurol 1991;7:299.

Carroll WJ, Woodruff WW, et al. MR findings in oculocerebrorenal syndrome [see comments]. AJNR Am J Neuroradiol 1993;14:449.

Casteels K, Van Geet C, et al. Ethosuximide-associated lupus with cerebral and renal manifestations. Eur J Pediatr 1998;157:780.

Catto-Smith AG, Adams A. A possible case of transient hereditary fructose intolerance. J Inherit Metab Dis 1993;16:73.

Chacko BG, John T, et al. Dengue shock syndrome in a renal transplant recipient. Transplantation 2004;77:634.

Chadwick D, French AT. Uraemic myoclonus: An example of reticular reflex myoclonus? J Neurol Neurosurg Psychiatry 1979;42:52.

Chandler WL, Jelacic S, et al. Prothrombotic coagulation abnormalities preceding the hemolytic-uremic syndrome. N Engl J Med 2002;346:23.

Chang PF, Huang SF, et al. Metabolic disorders mimicking Reye's syndrome. J Formos Med Assoc 2002;99:295.

Chantler C. Systemic hypertension. In: Anderson RH, Tynan MJ, Shinebourne E, et al., eds. Paediatric cardiology. London: Churchill Livingstone, 1986.

Chantler C. Kidney disease in children. In: Schreier R, ed. Diseases of the kidney. 1988;2629.

Chantler C, Broyer M, et al. Growth and rehabilitation of long-term survivors of treatment for end-stage renal failure in childhood. Proc Eur Dial Transplant Assoc 1981;18:329.

Charnas LR, Luciano CA, et al. Distal vacuolar myopathy in nephropathic cystinosis. Ann Neurol 1994;35:181.

Chaves-Carballo E, Montes JE, et al. Hemorrhagic shock and encephalopathy: Clinical definition of a catastrophic syndrome in infants. Am J Dis Child 1990;144:1079.

Chazan JA, Ambler M, et al. Vascular deposits causing ischemic myopathy in uremia: Two brothers with hereditary nephritis. Ann Intern Med 1970;73:73.

Chen YT, Van Hove JL. Renal involvement in type I glycogen storage disease. Adv Nephrol Necker Hosp 1995;24:357.

Chester EM, Agamanolis DP, et al. Hypertensive encephalopathy: A clinicopathologic study of 20 cases. Neurology 1978;28:928.

Chik CL, Friedman A, et al. Pituitary-testicular function in nephropathic cystinosis. Ann Intern Med 1993;119:568.

Chin DK, Ho AK, et al. Neuropsychiatric complications related to use of prazosin in patients with renal failure. BMJ (Clin Res Ed) 1986;293:1347.

Chiu NC, Shen EY, et al. Hemorrhagic shock and encephalopathy syndrome: Report of two cases. Zhonghua Min Guo Xiao Er Ke Yi Xue Hui Za Zhi 1989;30:118.

Chow S. Acquisition of donor strains of cytomegalovirus by renal transplant recipients. N Engl J Med 1989;314:1418.

Chow TW, Turner NA, et al. Increased von Willebrand factor binding to platelets in single episode and recurrent types of thrombotic thrombocytopenic purpura. Am J Hematol 1998;57:293.

Cimolai N, Carter JE. Gender and the progression of *Escherichia coli* O157:H7 enteritis to haemolytic uraemic syndrome. Arch Dis Child 1991;66:171.

Clarkson EM, Talner LB, et al. The effect of plasma from blood volume expanded dogs on sodium, potassium and PAH transport of renal tubule fragments. Clin Sci 1970;38:617.

Cogan MG, Covey CM, et al. Central nervous system manifestations of hyperparathyroidism. Am J Med 1978;65:963.

Cohen BD. Methyl group deficiency and guanidino production in uremia. Mol Cell Biochem 2003;244:31.

Cohen JA, Raps EC. Critical neurologic illness in the immunocompromised patient. Neurol Clin 1995;13:659.

Colah S, Trauner DA. Tactile recognition in infantile nephropathic cystinosis. Dev Med Child Neurol 1997;39:409.

Cooper JD, Lazarowitz VC, et al. Neurodiagnostic abnormalities in patients with acute renal failure. J Clin Invest 1978;61:1448.

Cooper WC, Green IJ, et al. Cerebral salt-wasting associated with the Guillain-Barré syndrome. Arch Intern Med 1978;116:113.

Cori GT. Glycogen structure and enzyme deficiencies in glycogen storage disease. Harvey Lect 1954;48:145.

Corrigan JJ Jr. The "H" in hemorrhagic shock and encephalopathy syndrome should be "hyperpyrexia." Am J Dis Child 1990;144:1077.

Cox TM. Aldolase B and fructose intolerance. Faseb J 1994;8:62.

Crapper DR, Krishnan SS, et al. Brain aluminum distribution in Alzheimer's disease and experimental neurofibrillary degeneration. Science 1973;180:511.

Crapper DR, Krishnan SS, et al. Aluminium, neurofibrillary degeneration and Alzheimer's disease. Brain 1976;99:67-80.

Crawford JD, Dodge PR. Complications of fluid therapy in neurologic disease: Water intoxication and hypertonic dehydration. Pediatr Clin North Am 1964;11:1029.

Crittenden MR, Holliday MA, et al. Intellectual development of children with renal insufficiency and end stage disease. Int J Pediatr Nephrol 1985;6:275.

Cuccia V, Galarza M, et al. Cerebral aspergillosis in children: Report of three cases. Pediatr Neurosurg 2000;33:43.

Cumberbatch GL, Hampton TJ. Hyperkalaemic paralysis—a bizarre presentation of renal failure. J Accid Emerg Med 1999;16:230.

Cumming AD, Simpson G, et al. Acute aluminium intoxication in patients on continuous ambulatory peritoneal dialysis [letter]. Lancet 1982;1:103.

D'Agati V. Does aspirin cause acute or chronic renal failure in experimental animals and in humans? Am J Kidney Dis 1996;28(1 Suppl 1):S24.

D'Eufemia P, Giardini O, et al. Late onset of cystinuria in a case of gyrate atrophy. J Inherit Metab Dis 1993;16:904.

D'Hooge R, Van de Vijver G, et al. Involvement of voltage- and ligand-gated Ca^{2+} channels in the neuroexcitatory and synergistic effects of putative uremic neurotoxins. Kidney Int 2003;63:1764.

Da Conceicao M, Genco G, et al. [Cerebral and renal toxicity of acyclovir in a patient treated for meningoencephalitis]. Ann Fr Anesth Reanim (in French) 1999;18:996.

Damaraju SC, Rajshekhar V, et al. Validation study of a central venous pressure-based protocol for the management of neurosurgical patients with hyponatremia and natriuresis. Neurosurgery 1997;40:312; discussion 316.

Das AM, Schweitzer-Krantz S, et al. Absence of cytochrome c oxidase activity in a boy with dysfunction of renal tubules, brain and muscle. Eur J Pediatr 1994;153:267.

Date Y, Nakazato M, et al. Detection of three transthyretin gene mutations in familial amyloidotic polyneuropathy by analysis of DNA extracted from formalin-fixed and paraffin-embedded tissues. J Neurol Sci 1997;150:143.

David WS. Myoglobinuria. Neurol Clin 2000;18:215.

Davies NM, Longstreth J, et al. Misoprostol therapeutics revisited. Pharmacotherapy 2001;21:60-73.

Davies SC, Marcus RE, et al. Ocular toxicity of high-dose intravenous desferrioxamine. Lancet 1983;2:181.

de Chadarevian JP, Kaplan BS. The hemolytic uremic syndrome of childhood. Perspect Pediatr Pathol 1978;4:465-502.

de Klerk JB, Duran M, et al. Sudden infant death and lysinuric protein intolerance [letter; comment]. Eur J Pediatr 1996;155:256.

de Knegt RJ, van der Pijl H, et al. Acyclovir-associated encephalopathy, lack of relationship between acyclovir levels and symptoms. Nephrol 1995;10:1775.

de Wardener HE, MacGregor GA. Blood pressure and the kidney. In: Schreier R, Gottschalk CW, eds. Diseases of the kidney. Boston: Little, Brown, 1988;1543.

Dean AF, Diss TC, et al. Histologic, molecular, and radiologic characterization of resolving cerebral posttransplant lymphoproliferative disorder. Pediatr Res 1997;41:651.

Dedeoglu IO, Matanguihan ET, et al. Clinical quiz: Cerebral salt wasting syndrome. Pediatr Nephrol 1995;9:395.

Dedeoglu IO, Springate JE, et al. Hypertensive encephalopathy and reversible magnetic resonance imaging changes in a renal transplant patient. Pediatr Nephrol 1996;10:769.

Deferrari G, Garibotto G, et al. Brain metabolism of amino acids and ammonia in patients with chronic renal insufficiency. Kidney Int 1981;20:505.

Deller T, Haas CA, et al. Laminar distribution of synaptopodin in normal and reeler mouse brain depends on the position of spine-bearing neurons. J Comp Neurol 2002;453:33.

Deller T, Korte M, et al. Synaptopodin-deficient mice lack a spine apparatus and show deficits in synaptic plasticity. Proc Natl Acad Sci U S A 2003;100:10494.

Deller T, Merten T, et al. Actin-associated protein synaptopodin in the rat hippocampal formation: Localization in the spine neck and close association with the spine apparatus of principal neurons. J Comp Neurol 2000;418:164.

Demers SI, Phaneuf D, et al. Hereditary tyrosinemia type I: Strong association with haplotype 6 in French Canadians permits simple carrier detection and prenatal diagnosis. Am J Hum Genet 1994;55:327.

Demirkiran M, Jankovic J, et al. Neurologic presentation of Wilson disease without Kayser-Fleischer rings. Neurology 1996;46:1040.

Demiroglu H, Barista I, et al. The effect of desmopressin on platelet aggregation defect in systemic amyloidosis: A preliminary report. Eur J Haematol 1996;56:283.

Dettori P, La Greca G, et al. Changes of cerebral density in dialyzed patients. Neuroradiology 1982;23:95.

Di Rocco M. Interstitial lung disease in lysinuric protein intolerance [letter; comment]. J Pediatr 1994;124:655.

Diaz-Buxo JA. Peritoneal dialysis—60 years later [editorial]. Mayo Clin Proc 1983;58:687.

Dila CJ, Pappius HM. Cerebral water and electrolytes: An experimental model of inappropriate secretion of antidiuretic hormone. Arch Neurol 1972;26:85.

Dinapoli RP, Johnson WJ, et al. Experience with a combined hemodialysis-renal transplantation program: Neurologic aspects. Mayo Clin Proc 1966;41:809.

Dinsdale HB. Hypertensive encephalopathy. Neurol Clin 1983;1:3.

Diringer M, Ladenson PW, et al. Sodium and water regulation in a patient with cerebral salt wasting. Arch Neurol 1989;46:928.

DiRocco M, Garibotto G, et al. Role of haematological, pulmonary and renal complications in the long-term prognosis of patients with lysinuric protein intolerance. Eur J Pediatr 1993;152:437.

Dodge PR, Crawford JD, et al. Studies in experimental water intoxication. Arch Neurol 1960;3:513.
Donaldson MD, Warner AA, et al. Familial juvenile nephronophthisis, Jeune's syndrome, and associated disorders. Arch Dis Child 1985;60:426.
Donnell GN, Koch R, et al. Observations on results of management of galactosemic patients. In: Hsia DYY, ed. Galactosemia. Springfield, IL, Charles C Thomas, 1969;247.
Donzelli O, Nanni ML, et al. Lowe syndrome: General problems in a female patient. Chir Organi Mov 1993;78:183.
Dousa TP, Hechter G. The effect of NaCl and LiCl on vasopressin sensitive adenylate cyclase. Life Sci 1970;9:765.
Dreifuss FE, Stewart LF, et al. An epidemic of arsenic poisoning. Va Med Mon 1972;99:746.
Drouin-Garraud V, Belgrand M, et al. Neurological presentation of a congenital disorder of glycosylation CDG-Ia: Implications for diagnosis and genetic counseling. Am J Med Genet 2001;101:46.
Drummond KN. Hemolytic uremic syndrome—then and now [editorial]. N Engl J Med 1985;312:116.
Dubois J, Garel L, et al. Imaging features of type 1 hereditary tyrosinemia: A review of 30 patients. Pediatr Radiol 1996;26:845.
Dunea G. Dialysis dementia: An epidemic that came and went. Asaio J 2001;47:192.
Dyck PJ, Johnson WJ, et al. Segmental demyelination secondary to axonal degeneration in uremic neuropathy. Mayo Clin Proc 1971;46:400.
Dzido G, Sprague SM. Dialysis-related amyloidosis. Minerva Urol Nefrol 2003;55:121.
Ekberg M, Holmberg L, et al. Hemolytic uremic syndrome: Results of treatment with hemodialysis. Acta Paediatr Scand 1977;66:693.
el Aklouk I, Basic Kes V, et al. [Uremic polyneuropathy]. Acta Med Croatica (in Croatian) 2004;58:59.
Elder MJ, Astin CL. Recurrent corneal erosion in cystinosis. J Pediatr Ophthalmol Strabismus 1994;31:270.
Elliott HL, Dryburgh F, et al. Aluminium toxicity during regular haemodialysis. BMJ 1978;1:1101.
Elseviers MM, De Broe ME. Analgesic nephropathy: Is it caused by multi-analgesic abuse or single substance use? Drug Saf 1999;20:15–24.
Elzouki A, Carroll J, et al. Improved neurological outcome in children with chronic renal disease from infancy. Pediatr Nephrol 1994;8:205-210.
Erasmus RT, Kusnir J, et al. Hyperaluminemia associated with liver transplantation and acute renal failure. Clin Transplant 1995;9:307.
Esposito G, Vitagliano L, et al. Structural and functional analysis of aldolase B mutants related to hereditary fructose intolerance. FEBS Lett 2002;531:152.
Etheridge WB, O'Neill WM Jr. The "dialysis encephalopathy syndrome" without dialysis. Clin Nephrol 1978;10:250.
Evans D, Hansen JD, et al. Intellectual development and nutrition. J Pediatr 1980;97:358.
Evans S, Stovroff M, et al. Selective distal splenorenal shunts for intractable variceal bleeding in pediatric portal hypertension. J Pediatr Surg 1995;30:1115.
Fabre J, Rudhardt M, et al. [Influence of renal insufficiency on the excretion of diverse drugs (chloroquine, sedatives, methacycline)]. Helv Med Acta Suppl 1966;46:132.
Fairchild KD, Singh IS, et al. Hypothermia prolongs activation of NF-kappaB and augments generation of inflammatory cytokines. Am J Physiol Cell Physiol 2004;287:C422.
Falik-Borenstein ZC, Jordan SC, et al. Brief report: Renal tubular acidosis in carnitine palmitoyltransferase type 1 deficiency. N Engl J Med 1992;327:24.
Falk RH, Comenzo RL, et al. The systemic amyloidoses [see comments]. N Engl J Med 1997;337:898.
Fang JT, Chen YC. Systemic lupus erythematosus presenting initially as hydrogen ATPase pump defects of distal renal tubular acidosis. Renal Failure 2000;22:647.
Faris AA. Wernicke's encephalopathy in uremia. Neurology 1972;22:1293.
Farrington FH, Duncan LL, et al. Looking a gift horse in the mouth: Effects of cornstarch therapy and other implications of glycogen storage disease on oral hygiene and dentition. Pediatr Dent 1995;17:311.
Fathallah DM, Bejaoui M, et al. Carbonic anhydrase II (CA II) deficiency in Maghrebian patients: Evidence for founder effect and genomic recombination at the CA II locus. Hum Genet 1997;99:634.
Fennell EB, Fennell RS, et al. The effects of various modes of therapy for end stage renal disease on cognitive performance in a pediatric population—a preliminary report. Int J Pediatr Nephrol 1986;7:107–112.
Fennell RS III, Rasbury WC. Cognitive functioning of identical twins discordant for prune belly syndrome and end stage renal failure. Int J Pediatr Nephrol 1980;1:234.
Fennell RS III, Rasbury WC, et al. Effects of kidney transplantation on cognitive performance in a pediatric population. Pediatrics 1984;74:273.
Fernandes J, Berger R, et al. Lactate as a cerebral metabolic fuel for glucose-6-phosphatase deficient children. Pediatr Res 1984;18:335.
Fernandez O, Romero F, et al. [Neurologic complications induced by the treatment of the acute renal allograft rejection with the monoclonal antibody OKT3]. Neurologia 1993;8:277.
Fiala M, Payne JE, et al. Epidemiology of cytomegalovirus infection after transplantation and immunosuppression. J Infect Dis 1975;132:421.
Fichman MP, Bethune JE. The role of adrenocorticoids in the inappropriate antidiuretic hormone syndrome. Ann Intern Med 1968;68:806.
Fine RN, Korsch BM, et al. Renal homotransplantation in children. J Pediatr 1970;76:347.
Fine RN, Korsch BM, et al. Cadaveric renal transplantation in children. Lancet 1971;1:1087.
Finn LS. Genetic basis of congenital nephrotic syndrome. Pediatr Dev Pathol 2003;6:585.
Finnerty FA Jr. Hypertensive encephalopathy. Am J Med 1972;52:672.
Fiorani L, Vianelli N, et al. Brain MRI and SPET in thrombotic thrombocytopenic purpura. Ital J Neurol Sci 1995;16:149.
Fiorucci S, Antonelli E, et al. Nitric oxide-releasing NSAIDs: A review of their current status. Drug Saf 2001;24:801.
Fischer JE, Baldessarini RJ. False neurotransmitters and hepatic failure. Lancet 1971;2:75.
Fisher CM. Lacunes: Small, deep cerebral infarcts. 1965 [classical article]. Neurology 1998;50:841.
Fishman RA. Permeability changes in experimental uremic encephalopathy. Arch Intern Med 1970;12:835.
Fishman RA, Raskin NH. Experimental uremic encephalopathy: Permeability and electrolyte metabolism of brain and other tissues. Arch Neurol 1967;17:10.
Flegel KM, Cole CH. Inappropriate antidiuresis during carbamazepine treatment. Ann Intern Med 1977;87:722.
Foley CM, Polinsky MS, et al. Encephalopathy in infants and children with chronic renal disease. Arch Neurol 1981;38:656.
Folkow B, Rubinstein EG. Cardiovascular effects of acute and chronic stimulations of the hypothalamic defense area in the rat. Acta Physiol Scand 1965;68:48.
Fong JS, de Chadarevian JP, et al. Hemolytic-uremic syndrome: Current concepts and management. Pediatr Clin North Am 1982;29:835.
Fontana S, Gerritsen HE, et al. Microangiopathic haemolytic anaemia in metastasizing malignant tumours is not associated with a severe deficiency of the von Willebrand factor-cleaving protease. Br J Haematol 2001;113:100.
Foreman JW, Benson LL, et al. Metabolic studies of rat renal tubule cells loaded with cystine: The cystine dimethylester model of cystinosis. J Am Soc Nephrol 1995;6:269.
Fortin MC, Schurch W, et al. Complement factor H deficiency in acute allograft glomerulopathy and post-transplant hemolytic uremic syndrome. Am J Transplant 2004;4:270.
Fournier S, Liguory O, et al. Disseminated infection due to *Encephalitozoon cuniculi* in a patient with AIDS: Case report and review. HIV Med 2000;1:155.
Franklin SS. Hypertensive emergencies: The case for rapid reduction of blood pressure. In: Narins RG, ed. Controversies in nephrology and hypertension. New York: Churchill-Livingstone, 1984.
Fraser CL. Neurologic manifestations of the uremic state. In: Arieff A, Griggs R, eds. Metabolic brain dysfunction in systemic disorders. Boston: Little, Brown & Co, 1992;139.
Fraser CL, Arieff AI. Nervous system complications in uremia. Ann Intern Med 1988;109:143.
Fraser CL, Arieff AI. Epidemiology, pathophysiology, and management of hyponatremic encephalopathy. Am J Med 1997;102:67.
Fraser CL, Sarnacki P, et al. Abnormal sodium transport in synaptosomes from brain of uremic rats. J Clin Invest 1985;75:2014.
Freeman RB, Sheff MF, et al. The blood cerebrospinal fluid barrier in uremia. Ann Intern Med 1962;56:233.

Fremeaux-Bacchi V, Dragon-Durey MA, et al. Complement factor I: A susceptibility gene for atypical haemolytic uraemic syndrome. J Med Genet 2004;41:e84.

Freundlich M, Zilleruelo G, et al. Infant formula as a cause of aluminium toxicity in neonatal uraemia. Lancet 1985;2:527.

Freundlich M, Zilleruelo G, et al. Treatment of aluminum toxicity in infantile uremia with deferoxamine. J Pediatr 1986;109:140.

Friberg L, Piscator M, et al. Cadmium in the environment. Cleveland: Chemical Rubber Company Press, 1971.

Fried LF, Palevsky PM. Hyponatremia and hypernatremia. Med Clin North Am 1997;81:585.

Frohlich ED, Tarazi RC, et al. Hemodynamic and functional mechanisms in two renal hypertensions: Arterial and pyelonephritis. Am J Med Sci 1971;261:189.

Fuger K, Fleischmann E, et al. [Complications in the course of the Muckle-Wells syndrome]. Dtsch Med Wochenschr (in German) 1992;117:256.

Fujikawa K, Suzuki H, et al. Purification of human von Willebrand factor-cleaving protease and its identification as a new member of the metalloproteinase family. Blood 2001;98:1662.

Furlan M, Robles R, et al. Deficient activity of von Willebrand factor-cleaving protease in chronic relapsing thrombotic thrombocytopenic purpura. Blood 1997;89:3097.

Furlan M, Robles R, et al. von Willebrand factor-cleaving protease in thrombotic thrombocytopenic purpura and the hemolytic-uremic syndrome. N Engl J Med 1998;339:1578.

Furlan M, Robles R, et al. Acquired deficiency of von Willebrand factor-cleaving protease in a patient with thrombotic thrombocytopenic purpura. Blood 1998;91:2839.

Gahl WA. Nephropathic cystinosis. Pediatr Rev 1997;18:302.

Gahl WA, Bernardini IM, et al. Muscle carnitine repletion by long-term carnitine supplementation in nephropathic cystinosis. Pediatr Res 1993;34:115.

Gahl WA, Dalakas MC, et al. Myopathy and cystine storage in muscles in a patient with nephropathic cystinosis. N Engl J Med 1988;319:1461.

Gardner LB, Preston RA. University of Miami Division of Clinical Pharmacology Therapeutic Rounds: The water-intolerant patient and perioperative hyponatremia. Am J Ther 2000;7:23.

Garg AX, Suri RS, et al. Long-term renal prognosis of diarrhea-associated hemolytic uremic syndrome: A systematic review, meta-analysis, and meta-regression. JAMA 2003;290:1360.

Garty BZ, Levy I, et al. Sweet syndrome associated with G-CSF treatment in a child with glycogen storage disease type Ib. Pediatrics 1996;97:401-403.

Garzuly F, Vidal R, et al. Familial meningocerebrovascular amyloidosis, Hungarian type, with mutant transthyretin (TTR Asp18Gly). Neurology 1996;47:1562.

Gathof BS, Sommer M, et al. Characterization of two stop codon mutations in the galactose-1-phosphate uridyltransferase gene of three male galactosemic patients with severe clinical manifestation. Hum Genet 1995;96:721.

Geary DF, Fennell RS, et al. Encephalopathy in children with chronic renal failure. J Pediatr 1980;97:41.

George JN, Vesely SK, et al. The Oklahoma Thrombotic Thrombocytopenic Purpura-Hemolytic Uremic Syndrome (TTP-HUS) Registry: A community perspective of patients with clinically diagnosed TTP-HUS. Semin Hematol 2004;41:60.

Gianantonio CA, Vitacco M, et al. The hemolytic-uremic syndrome. Nephron 1973;11:174.

Gianviti A, Tozzi AE, et al. Risk factors for poor renal prognosis in children with hemolytic uremic syndrome. Pediatr Nephrol 2003;18:1229.

Gidal BE, et al. Diet- and valproate-induced transient hyperammonemia: Effect of L-carnitine. Pediatr Neurol 1997;16:301.

Gitzelmann R. Galactose-1-phosphate in the pathophysiology of galactosemia. Eur J Pediatr 1995;154(7 Suppl 2):S45.

Gleeson JG, Keeler LC, et al. Molar tooth sign of the midbrain-hindbrain junction: Occurrence in multiple distinct syndromes. Am J Med Genet 2004;125A:125; discussion 117.

Glenn CM, Astley SJ, et al. Dialysis-associated seizures in children and adolescents. Pediatr Nephrol 1992;6:182.

Goksan B, Karaali-Savrun F, et al. Haemodialysis-related headache. Cephalalgia 2004;24:284.

Gold RJ, Dobrinski MJ, et al. Cystinuria and mental deficiency. Clin Genet 1977;12:329.

Goldby FS, Beilin LJ. The microcirculation in malignant hypertension. In: Rorive G, ed. The arterial hypertensive diseases: A symposium. New York: Masson, 1976.

Goldstein MH, Churg J, et al. Hemolytic-uremic syndrome. Nephron 1979;23:263.

Gonwa TA, Morris CA, et al. Long-term survival and renal function following liver transplantation in patients with and without hepatorenal syndrome—experience in 300 patients. Transplantation 1991;51:428.

Goodhue WW, Davis JN, et al. Ischemic myopathy in uremic hyperparathyroidism. JAMA 1972;221:911.

Gordillo-Paniagua G, Munoz-Arizpe R, et al. Unusual complication in a patient with renal transplantation: Cerebral cysticercosis. Nephron 1987;45:65.

Gougoux A, Vinay P. Metabolic effects of valproate on dog renal cortical tubules. Can J Physiol Pharmacol 1989;67:88.

Goutieres F, Bourgeois M, et al. Moyamoya disease in a child with glycogen storage disease type Ia. Neuropediatrics 1997;28:133.

Goyer RA, May P, et al. Lead and protein content of isolated intranuclear inclusion bodies from kidneys of lead-poisoned rats. Lab Invest 1970;22:245.

Graf H, Stummvoll HK, et al. Dialysate aluminium concentration and aluminium transfer during haemodialysis [letter]. Lancet 1982;1:46.

Graham DI. Ischaemic brain damage of cerebral perfusion failure type after treatment of severe hypertension. BMJ 1975;4:739.

Griesdale DE, Honey CR. Aquaporins and brain edema. Surg Neurol 2004;61:418.

Griswold WR, Reznik V, et al. Accumulation of aluminum in a nondialyzed uremic child receiving aluminum hydroxide. Pediatrics 1983;71:56.

Grompe M, St-Louis M, et al. A single mutation of the fumarylacetoacetate hydrolase gene in French Canadians with hereditary tyrosinemia type I. N Engl J Med 1994;331:353.

Gross ML, Sweny P, et al. Rejection encephalopathy: An acute neurological syndrome complicating renal transplantation. J Neurol Sci 1982;56:23-34.

Gross P, Reimann D, et al. Treatment of severe hyponatremia: Conventional and novel aspects. J Am Soc Nephrol 2001;12(Suppl 17):S10.

Grushkin CM, Korsch B, et al. Hemodialysis in small children. JAMA 1982;221:869.

Guisado R, Arieff AI, et al. Changes in the electroencephalogram in acute uremia: Effects of parathyroid hormone and brain electrolytes. J Clin Invest 1975;55:738.

Gullberg RM, Quintanilla A, et al. Sporotrichosis: Recurrent cutaneous, articular, and central nervous system infection in a renal transplant recipient. Rev Infect Dis 1987;9:369.

Gulliksen G, Hojer-Pedersen E, et al. Autoregulation of cerebral blood flow in patients with malignant hypertension and hypertensive encephalopathy. Acta Med Scand Suppl 1983;678:43.

Gutman RA, Hickman RO, et al. Failure of high dialysis-fluid glucose to prevent the disequilibrium syndrome. Lancet 1967;1:295.

Guzzetta F, Mazzaglia E. [Hartnup disease. Observations on a further case]. Minerva Pediatr (in Italian) 1970;22:480.

Haber BA, Chuang E, et al. Variable gene expression within human tyrosinemia type 1 liver may reflect region-specific dysplasia. Hepatology 1996;24:65.

Habib R, Mathieu H, et al. Maladie thrombotique arteriolocapillaire du rein chez l'enfant. Rev Fr Etud Clin Biol 1958;3:891.

Hammond D, Lieberman E. The hemolytic uremic syndrome: Renal cortical thrombotic microangiopathy. Arch Intern Med 1970;126:816.

Hampers CL, Doak PB, et al. The electroencephalogram and spinal fluid during hemodialysis. Arch Intern Med 1966;118:340.

Hansen TW, Henrichsen B, et al. Neuropsychological and linguistic follow-up studies of children with galactosaemia from an unscreened population. Acta Paediatr 1996;85:1197.

Harper AM. Autoregulation of cerebral blood flow: influence of the arterial blood pressure on the blood flow through the cerebral cortex. J Neurol Neurosurg Psychiatry 1966;29:398.

Harrigan MR. Cerebral salt wasting syndrome: A review [see comments]. Neurosurgery 1996;38:152.

Harris RD, Campbell JK, et al. Neurovascular complications of dialysis and transplantation. Stroke 1974;5:725.

Hassan K, Simri W, et al. Effect of erythropoietin therapy on polyneuropathy in predialytic patients. J Nephrol 2003;16:121.

Hataya H, et al. Distal tubular dysfunction in lupus nephritis of childhood and adolescence. Pediatr Nephrol 1999;13:846.

Hayashi Y, Hanioka K, et al. Clinicopathologic and molecular-pathologic approaches to Lowe's syndrome. Pediatr Pathol Lab Med 1995;15:389.

Healton EB, Brust JC, et al. Hypertensive encephalopathy and the neurologic manifestations of malignant hypertension. Neurology 1982;32:127.

Heering P, Degenhardt S, et al. Tubular dysfunction following kidney transplantation. Nephron 1996;74:501.

Hegstrom RM, Murray JS, et al. Two years experience with periodic dialysis in treatment of chronic uremia. Trans Am Soc Artif Org 1962;8:266.

Henderson H. The clinical and molecular spectrum of glalactosemia in patients from the Cape Town region of South Africa. BMC Pediatrics 2002;2:7.

Henriksen JH. Cirrhosis: Ascites and hepatorenal syndrome: Recent advances in pathogenesis. J Hepatol 1995;23(Suppl 1):25-30.

Herbert MA, Milford DV, et al. Secondary amyloidosis from long-standing bacterial endocarditis. Pediatr Nephrol 1995;9:33.

Herrmann W, Knapp JP. Hyperhomocysteinemia: A new risk factor for degenerative diseases. Clin Lab 2002;48:471.

Hew TD, Chorley JN, et al. The incidence, risk factors, and clinical manifestations of hyponatremia in marathon runners. Clin J Sport Med 2003;13:41.

Heyman A, Patterson JL Jr, et al: Cerebral circulation and metabolism in uremia. Circulation 1951;3:558.

Heyman A, Pfeiffer JB Jr, et al. Peripheral neuropathy caused by arsenical intoxication: A study of 41 cases with observations on the effects of BAL (2, 3-dimercaptopropanol). N Engl J Med 1956;254:401.

Hillebrand G, Castro LA, et al. Valproate for epilepsy in renal transplant recipients receiving cyclosporine [see comments]. Transplantation 1987;43:915.

Hilz MJ, Zimmermann P, et al. Vibrameter testing facilitates the diagnosis of uremic and alcoholic polyneuropathy. Acta Neurol Scand 1995;92:486.

Hinchey J, Chaves C, et al. A reversible posterior leukoencephalopathy syndrome [see comments]. N Engl J Med 1996;334:494.

Hiramatsu M. A role for guanidino compounds in the brain. Mol Cell Biochem 2003;244:57.

Hjelm M, Oberholzer V, et al. Valproate-induced inhibition of urea synthesis and hyperammonaemia in healthy subjects. Lancet 1986;2:859.

Hodson AK. Peripheral neuropathy in childhood: An update in diagnosis and management. Pediatr Ann 1983;12:814.

Hodson EM, Najarian JS, et al. Renal transplantation in children ages 1 to 5 years. Pediatrics 1978;61:458.

Hojberg AS, Mertz H. [Nephrotic syndrome in familial Mediterranean fever—effect of colchicine therapy]. Ugeskr Laeger 1995;157:4035.

Holden FA, Kaczmer JE, et al. Listerial meningitis and renal allografts: A life-threatening affinity. Postgrad Med 1980;68:69.

Holliday MA. Calorie deficiency in children with uremia: Effect upon growth. Pediatrics 1972;50:590.

Holtmann M, Krause M, et al. Oxcarbazepine-induced hyponatremia and the regulation of serum sodium after replacing carbamazepine with oxcarbazepine in children. Neuropediatrics 2002;33:298.

Holton JB, de la Cruz F, et al. Galactosemia: The uridine diphosphate galactose deficiency-uridine treatment controversy [comment]. J Pediatr 1993;123:1009.

Honeyman MM, Green A, et al. Galactosaemia: Results of the British Paediatric Surveillance Unit Study, 1988-90. Arch Dis Child 1993;69:339.

Hoover R, Fraumeni JF Jr. Risk of cancer in renal-transplant recipients. Lancet 1973;2:55.

Horsford J, Saadi I, et al. Molecular genetics of cystinuria in French Canadians: Identification of four novel mutations in type I patients. Kidney Int 1996;49:1401.

Hory B, Billerey C, et al. Glomerular lesions in juvenile cystinosis: Report of 2 cases. Clin Nephrol 1994;42:327.

Hoshide R, Ikeda Y, et al. Molecular cloning, tissue distribution, and chromosomal localization of human cationic amino acid transporter 2 (HCAT2). Genomics 1996;38:174.

Hosler GA, Cusumano AM, et al. Thrombotic thrombocytopenic purpura and hemolytic uremic syndrome are distinct pathologic entities: A review of 56 autopsy cases. Arch Pathol Lab Med 2003;127:834.

Hoste EA, Kellum JA. Acute renal failure in the critically ill: Impact on morbidity and mortality. Contrib Nephrol 2004;144:1.

Hou JW, Wang TR. Transient tyrosinemia presenting as lactic acidosis in a term baby: Report of one case. Zhonghua Min Guo Xiao Er Ke Yi Xue Hui Za Zhi 1995;36:217.

Hovinga JA, Studt JD, et al. von Willebrand factor-cleaving protease (ADAMTS-13) activity determination in the diagnosis of thrombotic microangiopathies: The Swiss experience. Semin Hematol 2004;41:75.

Hoyer JR, Michael AF, et al. Acute poststreptococcal glomerulonephritis presenting as hypertensive encephalopathy with minimal urinary abnormalities. Pediatrics 1967;39:412.

Hu PY, Ernst AR, et al. Carbonic anhydrase II deficiency: Single-base deletion in exon 7 is the predominant mutation in Caribbean Hispanic patients. Am J Hum Genet 1994;54:602.

Huff ME, Balch WE, et al. Pathological and functional amyloid formation orchestrated by the secretory pathway. Curr Opin Struct Biol 2003;13:674.

Hulse JA, Taylor DS, et al. Blindness and paraplegia in severe childhood hypertension. Lancet 1979;2:553.

Humar A, Key N, et al. Kidney retransplants after initial graft loss to vascular thrombosis. Clin Transplant 2001;15:6.

Hung KL, Liao HT, et al. The spectrum of postinfectious encephalomyelitis. Brain Dev 2001a;23:42.

Hung SC, Hung SH, et al. Thiamine deficiency and unexplained encephalopathy in hemodialysis and peritoneal dialysis patients. Am J Kidney Dis 2001b;38:941.

Hurwitz LJ, Carson AJ, et al. Clinical, biochemical and histopathological findings in a family with muscular dystrophy. Brain 1967;90:799.

Hutter JC, Kuehnert MJ, et al. Acute onset of decreased vision and hearing traced to hemodialysis treatment with aged dialyzers. JAMA 2000;283:2128.

Igarashi T, Ishii T, et al. Persistent isolated proximal renal tubular acidosis—a systemic disease with a distinct clinical entity. Pediatr Nephrol 1994;8:70.

Ihara M, Tanaka H, et al. [Mitochondrial myopathy, encephalopathy, lactic acidosis, and stroke-like episodes (MELAS) with chronic renal failure: report of mother-child cases]. Rinsho Shinkeigaku (in Japanese) 1996;36:1069.

Ikeda M, Ito S, et al. Reversible posterior leukoencephalopathy in a patient with minimal-change nephrotic syndrome. Am J Kidney Dis 2001;37:E30.

Ingelfinger JR. Hypertension and the central nervous system. In: Infelfinger JR, ed. Pediatric hypertension. Philadelphia, WB Saunders, 1982;204.

Iwatsuki S, Popovtzer MM, et al. Recovery from "hepatorenal syndrome" after orthotopic liver transplantation. N Engl J Med 1973;289:1155.

Jackson M, Warrington EK, et al. Cognitive function in hemodialysis patients. Clin Nephrol 1987;27:26.

Jacob JC, Gloor P, et al. Electroencephalographic changes in chronic renal failure. Neurology 1965;15:419.

James WH. Review of the contribution of twin studies in the search for non-genetic causes of multiple sclerosis. Neuroepidemiology 1996;15:132.

Jayasinghe KS, Mendis BL, et al. Medullary sponge kidney presenting with hypokalaemic paralysis. Postgrad Med J 1984;60:303.

Jean G, Fuchshuber A, et al. High-resolution mapping of the gene for cystinosis, using combined biochemical and linkage analysis. Am J Hum Genet 1996;58:535.

Jedras M, Zakrzewska-Pniewska B, et al. [Uremic neuropathy—II. Is pruritus in dialyzed patients related to neuropathy?]. Pol Arch Med Wewn 1998;99:462.

Jedras M, Zakrzewska-Pniewska B, et al. [Uremic neuropathy is more frequent in male patients]. Pol Arch Med Wewn 2001;105:391.

Jellinek EH, Painter M, et al. Hypertensive encephalopathy with cortical disorders of vision. Q J Med 1964;33:239.

Jennekens FG, Mees EJ, et al. Clinical aspects of uraemic polyneuropathy. Nephron 1971;8:414.

Jeong YK, Kim IO, et al. Hemolytic uremic syndrome: MR findings of CNS complications. Pediatr Radiol 1994;24:585.

Joh K. [Predictive indicators for progression to severe complications (hemolytic-uremic syndrome and encephalopathy) and their prevention in enterohemorrhagic Escherichia coli infection]. Nippon Rinsho 1997;55:700.

Jonas AJ, Conley SB, et al. Nephropathic cystinosis with central nervous system involvement. Am J Med 1987;83:966.

Jones AC, Daniells CE, et al. Molecular genetic and phenotypic analysis reveals differences between TSC1 and TSC2 associated familial and sporadic tuberous sclerosis. Hum Mol Genet 1997;6:2155.

Joshioka T, Iitaka K, et al. Uncontrollable convulsions responsive to pyridoxal phosphate in a uremic child. Int J Pediatr Nephrol 1984;5:221.

Joy MD. The intramedullary connections of the area postrema involved in the central cardiovascular response to angiotensin II. Clin Sci 1971;41:89-100.

Jubinsky PT, Moraille R, et al. Thrombotic thrombocytopenic purpura in a newborn. J Perinatol 2003;23:85.

Jurcic D, Bago J, et al. Features of uremic neuropathy in long-term dialysis. Coll Antropol 1998;22:119.

Kadhom N, Baptista J, et al. Low efficiency of [^{14}C]galactose incorporation by galactosemic skin fibroblasts: Relationship with neurological sequelae. Biochem Med Metab Biol 1994;52:140.

Kadomitsu M, Murase M, et al. [Case of toluene poisoning associated with acute kidney failure]. Nippon Naika Gakkai Zasshi (in Japanese) 1994;83:120.

Kandt RS, Caoili AQ, et al. Hypertensive encephalopathy in children: Neuroimaging and treatment [see comments]. J Child Neurol 1995;10:236.

Kanematsu A, Segawa T, et al. [Multiple calcium oxalate stone formation in a patient with glycogen storage disease type I (von Gierke's disease) and renal tubular acidosis type I: A case report]. Hinyokika Kiyo (in Japanese) 1993;39:645.

Kaplan BS, Chesney RW, et al. Hemolytic uremic syndrome in families. N Engl J Med 1975;292:1090.

Kaplan BS, Katz J, et al. An analysis of the results of therapy in 67 cases of the hemolytic-uremic syndrome. J Pediatr 1971;78:420.

Kaplan BS, Thomson PD, et al. The hemolytic uremic syndrome. Pediatr Clin North Am 1976;23:761.

Kappy MS, Ganong CA. Cerebral salt wasting in children: The role of atrial natriuretic hormone. Adv Pediatr 1996;43:271.

Karlsberg RP, Lacher JW, et al. Adult hemolytic-uremic syndrome: Familial variant. Arch Intern Med 1997;137:1155.

Kaufman FR, McBride-Chang C, et al. Cognitive functioning, neurologic status and brain imaging in classical galactosemia. Eur J Pediatr 1995;154:S2.

Kaufman FR, Reichardt JK, et al. Correlation of cognitive, neurologic, and ovarian outcome with the Q188R mutation of the galactose-1-phosphate uridyltransferase gene. J Pediatr 1994;125:225.

Kavukcu S, Turkmen M, et al. Juvenile rheumatoid arthritis and renal amyloidosis (case report). Int Urol Nephrol 1995;27:251.

Kawajiri K, Matsuoka Y, et al. [Cerebral salt wasting syndrome secondary to head injury: A case report]. No Shinkei Geka (in Japanese) 1992;20:1003.

Keir G, Winchester BG, et al. Carbohydrate-deficient glycoprotein syndromes: Inborn errors of protein glycosylation. Ann Clin Biochem 1999;36(pt 1):20.

Kelly BD, Hillery J. Hyponatremia during carbamazepine therapy in patients with intellectual disability. J Intellect Disabil Res 2001;45(pt 2):152.

Kemper MJ, Harps E, et al. Hyperkalemia: Therapeutic options in acute and chronic renal failure. Clin Nephrol 1996;46:67.

Kennedy AC, Linton AL, et al. Electroencephalographic changes during haemodialysis. Lancet 1963;1:408.

Kennedy AC, Linton AL, et al. The pathogenesis and prevention of cerebral dysfunction during dialysis. Lancet 1964;1:790.

Kennedy SS, Zacharski LR, et al. Thrombotic thrombocytopenic purpura: Analysis of 48 unselected cases. Semin Thromb Hemost 1980;6:341.

Kenworthy L, Charnas L. Evidence for a discrete behavioral phenotype in the oculocerebrorenal syndrome of Lowe. Am J Med Genet 1995;59:283.

Kenworthy L, Park T, et al. Cognitive and behavioral profile of the oculocerebrorenal syndrome of Lowe. Am J Med Genet 1993;46:297.

Kerr DN. Clinical and pathophysiologic changes in patients on chronic dialysis: The central nervous system. Adv Nephrol Necker Hosp 1980;9:109.

Kiley JE. Neurological aspects of dialysis. In: Nissenson AR, Fine RN, Gentile DE, eds. Clinical dialysis. Norwalk, CT: Appleton-Century-Crofts, 1984;547.

Kiley JE, Pratt KL, et al. Techniques of EEG frequency analysis for evaluation of uremic encephalopathy. Clin Nephrol 1976;5:279.

Kirsztajn GM, Nishida SK, et al. Renal abnormalities in leprosy. Nephron 1993;65:381.

Klahr S, Miller SB. Acute oliguria. N Engl J Med 1998;338:671.

Kleeman CR, Davson H, et al. Urea transport in the central nervous system. Am J Physiol 1962;203:739.

Kloster R, Borresen HC, et al. Sudden death in two patients with epilepsy and the syndrome of inappropriate antidiuretic hormone secretion (SIADH). Seizure 1998;7:419.

Klujber V, Sallai A, et al. [Late onset type I tyrosinemia]. Orv Hetil (in Hungarian) 1997;138:1805.

Koch R, Acosta PB, et al. Nutritional therapy for pregnant women with a metabolic disorder. Clin Perinatol 1995;22:1.

Kodama H, Okabe I, et al. Renal tubular function of patients with classical Menkes disease. J Inherit Metab Dis 1992;51:157.

Kohaut EC, Whelchel JR, et al. Living-related donor renal transplantation in children presenting with end-stage renal disease in the first month of life. Transplantation 1985;40:725.

Kokame K, Matsumoto M, et al. Mutations and common polymorphisms in ADAMTS13 gene responsible for von Willebrand factor-cleaving protease activity. Proc Natl Acad Sci U S A 2002;99:11902.

Kondo H, Takeuchi M, et al. [Non-uremic neuropathy in hemodialysis patients]. No To Shinkei 1997;49:737.

Kopple JD, Swendseid ME. Vitamin nutrition in patients undergoing maintenance hemodialysis. Kidney Int Suppl 1975;(2):79.

Kovacs MJ, Roddy J, et al. Thrombotic thrombocytopenic purpura following hemorrhagic colitis due to *Escherichia coli* 0157:H7. Am J Med 1990;88:177.

Kretzschmar K, Nix W, et al. Morphologic cerebral changes in patients undergoing dialysis for renal failure. AJNR Am J Neuroradiol 1983;4:439.

Kroll M, Juhler M, et al. Hyponatraemia in acute brain disease. J Intern Med 1992;232:291.

Kumral E, Yuksel M, et al. Neurologic complications after deep hypothermic circulatory arrest: Types, predictors, and timing. Tex Heart Inst J 2001;28:83.

Kvittingen EA, Rootwelt H, et al. Hereditary tyrosinemia type I: Self-induced correction of the fumarylacetoacetase defect. J Clin Invest 1993;91:1816.

Kwong YL, Yu YL, et al. CT appearance in hypertensive encephalopathy. Neuroradiology 1987;29:215.

Laaksonen S, Metsarinne K, et al. Neurophysiologic parameters and symptoms in chronic renal failure. Muscle Nerve 2002;25:884.

Laffi G, La Villa G, et al. Arachidonic acid derivatives and renal function in liver cirrhosis. Semin Nephrol 1997;17:530.

Lai K, Langley SD, et al. A prevalent mutation for galactosemia among black Americans. J Pediatr 1996;128:89.

Laine J, Salo MK, et al. The nephropathy of type I tyrosinemia after liver transplantation. Pediatr Res 1995;37:640.

Langer RM, Kahan BD. Sirolimus does not increase the risk for postoperative thromboembolic events among renal transplant recipients. Transplantation 2003;76:318.

Lasker N, Harvey A, et al. Vitamin levels in hemodialysis and intermittent peritoneal dialysis. Trans Am Soc Artif Intern Organ 1963;9:51.

Laski ME, Kurtzman NA. Characterization of acidification in the cortical and medullary collecting tubule of the rabbit. J Clin Invest 1983;72:2050.

Lassen NA, Agnoli A. The upper limit of autoregulation of cerebral blood flow—on the pathogenesis of hypertensive encepholopathy. Scand J Clin Lab Invest 1972;30:113.

Lauteala T, Sistonen P, et al. Lysinuric protein intolerance (LPI) gene maps to the long arm of chromosome 14. Am J Hum Genet 1997;60:1479.

Lawlor ER, Webb DW, et al. Thrombotic thrombocytopenic purpura: A treatable cause of childhood encephalopathy. J Pediatr 1997;130:313.

Leaf A, Schwartz WB, et al. Oral administration of a potent carbonic anhydrase inhibitor ("Diamox"). N Engl J Med 1994;250:759.

Leahey AM, Charnas LR, et al. Nonsense mutations in the *OCRL-1* gene in patients with the oculocerebrorenal syndrome of Lowe. Hum Mol Genet 1993;2:461.

Lechtenberg R, Sierra MF, et al. *Listeria monocytogenes:* Brain abscess or meningoencephalitis? Neurology 1979;29:86-90.

Lederman RJ, Henry CE. Progressive dialysis encephalopathy. Ann Neurol 1978;4:199.

Lee DB, Drinkard JP, et al. The adult Fanconi syndrome: Observations on etiology, morphology, renal function and mineral metabolism in three patients. Medicine (Baltimore) 1972;51:107.

Lee KT, Little MD, et al. Intracellular (muscle-fiber) habitat of *Ancylostoma caninum* in some mammalian hosts. J Parasitol 1979;61:585.

Lee PJ, Chatterton C, et al. Urinary lactate excretion in type 1 glycogenosis—a marker of metabolic control or renal tubular dysfunction? J Inherit Metab Dis 1996;19:201.

Lee PJ, Dalton RN, et al. Glomerular and tubular function in glycogen storage disease. Pediatr Nephrol 1995;9:705.

Lee PJ, Patel JS, et al. Bone mineralisation in type 1 glycogen storage disease. Eur J Pediatr 1995;154:483.

Lee PT, Wu ML, et al. Rhabdomyolysis: an unusual feature with mushroom poisoning. Am J Kidney Dis 2001;38:E17.

Lee T, Bouhassira E, et al. ADAMTS13, the von Wilebrand factor cleaving metalloprotease, is expressed in the perisinusoidal cells of the liver. Blood 2002;100:497a.

Lei KJ, Chen YT, et al. Genetic basis of glycogen storage disease type 1a: Prevalent mutations at the glucose-6-phosphatase locus. Am J Hum Genet 1995;57:766.

Lei KJ, Shelly LL, et al. Mutations in the glucose-6-phosphatase gene are associated with glycogen storage disease types 1a and 1aSP but not 1b and 1c. J Clin Invest 1995;95:234.

Leonard A, Shapiro FL. Subdural hematoma in regularly hemodialyzed patients. Ann Intern Med 1975;82:650.

Letteri JM, Mellk H, et al. Diphenylhydantoin metabolism in uremia. N Engl J Med 1971;285:648.

Leumann EP. [Chronic juvenile kidney insufficiency: Results of a Swiss questionnaire]. Schweiz Med Wochenschr (in German) 1976;106:244.

Levin M. Syndromes with renal failure and shock. Pediatr Nephrol 1994;8:223.

Levin M, et al. Haemorrhagic shock and encephalopathy: A new syndrome with a high mortality in young children. Lancet 1983;2:64.

Levine S, Paparo G. Brain lesions in a case of cystinosis. Acta Neuropathol 1982;57:217.

Levitan D, Massry SG, et al. Autonomic nervous system dysfunction in patients with acute renal failure. Am J Nephrol 1982;2:213.

Levy GG, Nichols WC, et al. Mutations in a member of the *ADAMTS* gene family cause thrombotic thrombocytopenic purpura. Nature 2001;413:488.

Levy HL, Brown AE, et al. Vitreous hemorrhage as an ophthalmic complication of galactosemia. J Pediatr 1996;129:922.

Levy J, Abu-Ras MT, et al. Postnatal regression of glucose transport in a patient with glycogen storage disease type 1b. J Inherit Metab Dis 1994;17:16.

Lewis SE, Erickson RP, et al. *N*-ethyl-*N*-nitrosourea-induced null mutation at the mouse Car-2 locus: An animal model for human carbonic anhydrase II deficiency syndrome. Proc Natl Acad Sci U S A 1988;85:1962.

Lieberman E. Hemolytic-uremic syndrome. J Pediatr 1972;80:1.

Lieberman E, Heuser E, et al. Hemolytic-uremic syndrome: Clinical and pathological considerations. N Engl J Med 1966;275:227.

Lieberman JA, Cooper TB, et al. Tricyclic antidepressant and metabolite levels in chronic renal failure. Clin Pharmacol Ther 1985;37:301.

Light KC. Antihypertensive drugs and behavioral performance. In: Elias MF, Streeten DHP, eds. Hypertension and cognitive processes. Mt. Desert, ME, Beech Hill, 1980;119.

Lin CC, King KL, et al. Tacrolimus-associated hemolytic uremic syndrome: A case analysis. J Nephrol 2003;16:580.

Lin T, Orrison BM, et al. Spectrum of mutations in the OCRL1 gene in the Lowe oculocerebrorenal syndrome. Am J Hum Genet 1997;60:1384.

Lindfors-Lonnkvist K, Jakobsson B. [Facial paralysis in children. It may be hypertension—blood pressure determination should be conducted repeatedly!]. Lakartidningen (in Swedish) 1994;91:1420.

Lindgren A. Elevated serum methylmalonic acid: How much comes from cobalamin deficiency and how much comes from the kidneys? Scand J Clin Lab Invest 2002;62:15.

Livas IC, Nechay PS, et al. Clinical evidence of spinal and cerebral histoplasmosis twenty years after renal transplantation. Clin Infect Dis 1995;20:692.

Lloyd P, Flesch G, et al. Clinical pharmacology and pharmacokinetics of oxcarbazepine. Epilepsia 1994;35(Suppl 3):S10.

Locke S, Merrill JD, et al. Neurologic complications of acute uremia. Arch Intern Med 1961;108:75.

Loirat C, Niaudet P. The risk of recurrence of hemolytic uremic syndrome after renal transplantation in children. Pediatr Nephrol 2003;18:1095.

Longstreeth W, Rosenstock L, et al. Potroom palsy? Arch Intern Med 1985;145:1972.

Loo CS, Lim TO, et al. Pontine myelinolysis following correction of hyponatraemia. Med J Malaysia 1995;50:180.

Lopez RI, Collins GH. Wernicke's encephalopathy: A complication of chronic hemodialysis. Arch Neurol 1968;18:248.

Lopez-Garcia F, Amoros-Martinez F, et al. [A reversible posterior leukoencephalopathy syndrome]. Rev Neurol 2004;38:261.

Lorenz M, Hauser AC, et al. Anderson-Fabry disease in Austria. Wien Klin Wochenschr 2003;115:235.

Lowe CU, Terrey M, et al. Organic-aciduria, decreased renal ammonia production, hydrophthalmos, and mental retardation: A clinical entity. Am J Dis Child 1952;83:164.

Lubash GD, Stenzel KH, et al. Nitrogenous compounds in hemodialysate. Circulation 1964;30:848.

Ludwig GD, Senesky D, et al. Indoles in ureamia: identification by countercurrent distribution and paper chromatography. Am J Clin Nutr 1968;21:436.

Lumsden CE. Glia and myelin ischaemia, blood disorders and intoxications. In Vinken PK, Gruyn GW, eds. Handbook of Clinical Neurology. Amsterdam, North Holland, 1970;572.

Lyall H, Burchell A, et al. Early detection of metabolic abnormalities in preterm infants impaired by disorders of blood glucose concentrations. Clin Chem 1994;40:526.

MacWhinney JB, Packer JT, et al. Thrombotic thrombocytopenic purpura in childhood. Blood 1962;19:181.

Madani TA, Al-Mazrou YY, et al. Rift Valley fever epidemic in Saudi Arabia: Epidemiological, clinical, and laboratory characteristics. Clin Infect Dis 2003;37:1084.

Mahoney CA, Arieff AI. Uremic encephalopathies: Clinical, biochemical, and experimental features. Am J Kidney Dis 1983;2:324.

Mahoney CA, Arieff AI. Central and peripheral nervous system effects of chronic renal failure. Kidney Int 1983;24:170.

Mahoney CA, Sarnacki P, et al. Uremic encephalopathy: role of brain energy metabolism. Am J Physiol 1984;247(3 pt 2):F527.

Mahurkar SD, Salta S, et al. Dialysis dementia. Lancet 1973;1:1412.

Makkar RK, Kochar DK. Somatosensory evoked potentials (SSEPs); sensory nerve conduction velocity (SNCV) and motor nerve conduction velocity (MNCV) in chronic renal failure. Electromyogr Clin Neurophysiol 1994;34:295.

Malbrain ML, Lambrecht GL, et al. Acute renal failure in non-fulminant hepatitis A [letter; comment]. Clin Nephrol 1994;41:180.

Mangos JA, Lobeck CC. Studies of sustained hyponatremia due to central nervous system infection. Pediatrics 1964;34:503.

Manis FR, Cohn LB, et al. A longitudinal study of cognitive functioning in patients with classical galactosaemia, including a cohort treated with oral uridine. J Inherit Metab Dis 1997;20:549.

Maroto A, Gines A, et al. Diagnosis of functional kidney failure of cirrhosis with Doppler sonography: Prognostic value of resistive index. Hepatology 1994;20(4 pt 1):839.

Marotto MS, Marotto PC, et al. Outcome of acute renal failure in meningococcemia. Ren Fail 1997;19:807.

Marsh SE, Grattan-Smith P, et al. Neuroepithelial cysts in a patient with Joubert syndrome plus renal cysts. J Child Neurol 2004;19:227.

Martin DL, MacDonald KL, et al. The epidemiology and clinical aspects of the hemolytic uremic syndrome in Minnesota [see comments]. N Engl J Med 1990;323:1161.

Martin G, Durozard D, et al. Acceleration of ammonia-genesis in isolated rat kidney tubules by the antiepileptic drug: Valproic acid. In: Kovacevic Z, Guder W, eds. Molecular nephrology: Biochemical aspects of kidney function. Proceedings of the 8th International Symposium. Berlin: Walter de Gruyter, 1987;287.

Martin-Du Pan RC, Morris MA, et al. Mitochondrial anomalies in a Swiss family with autosomal dominant myoglobinuria. Am J Med Genet 1997;69:365.

Martinez WC, Rapin I, et al. Neurologic complications of renal failure. In: Edelman CM, ed. Pediatric kidney disease. Boston: Little, Brown, 1978;408.

Masramon J, Ricart MJ, et al. Dialysis encephalopathy [letter]. Lancet 1978;1:1370.

Matsumoto T, Okano R, et al. Hypergalactosaemia in a patient with portal-hepatic venous and hepatic arterio-venous shunts detected by neonatal screening. Eur J Pediatr 1993;152:990.

Mattern WD, Krigman MR, et al. Failure of successful renal transplantation to reverse the dialysis-associated encephalopathy syndrome. Clin Nephrol 1977;7:275.

Mayor GH, Keiser JA, et al. Aluminum absorption and distribution: Effect of parathyroid hormone. Science 1977;197:1187.

Mayor GH, Sprague SM, et al. Parathyroid hormone-mediated aluminum deposition and egress in the rat. Kidney Int 1980;17:40.

McAllister CJ, Scowden EB, et al. Toxic psychosis induced by phenothiazine administration in patients with chronic renal failure. Clin Nephrol 1978;10:191.

McDermott JR, Smith AI, et al. Brain-aluminium concentration in dialysis encephalopathy. Lancet 1978;1:901.

McDonald DM, Kabra PM. Renal disease may increase apparent phenytoin in serum as measured by enzyme-multiplied immunoassay [letter]. Clin Chem 1980;26:361.

McDowell G, Isogai T, et al. Fine mapping of the cystinosis gene using an integrated genetic and physical map of a region within human chromosome band 17p13. Biochem Mol Med 1996;58:135.

McGraw M, Bishop N, et al. Aluminium content of milk formulae and intravenous fluids used in infants [letter]. Lancet 1986;1:157.

McGraw ME, Haka-Ikse K. Neurologic-developmental sequelae of chronic renal failure in infancy. J Pediatr 1985;106:579.

McGregor E, Isles CG, et al. Retinal changes in malignant hypertension. BMJ (Clin Res Ed) 1986;292:233.

McManus DT, Moore R, et al. Necropsy findings in lysinuric protein intolerance. J Clin Pathol 1996;49:345.

McSherry E. Renal tubular acidosis in childhood. Kidney Int 1981;20:799.

McSherry E. Disorders of renal tubular transport. In: Rudolph AM, Hoffman JIE, eds. Pediatrics. New York: Appleton-Century-Crofts, 1982;1197.

McSherry E, Sebastian A, et al. Renal tubular acidosis in infants: The several kinds, including bicarbonate-wasting, classic renal tubular acidosis. J Clin Invest 1972;51:499.

Meacham GC, Orbiston JL, et al. Thrombotic thrombocytopenic purpura: A disseminated disease of arterioles. Blood 1952;6:706.

Mehta RP. Encephalopathy in chronic renal failure appearing before the start of dialysis. Can Med Assoc J 1979;120:1112.

Mendez A, Gonzalez G. [Dengue haemorrhagic fever in children: Ten years of clinical experience]. Biomedica (in Spanish) 2003;23:180.

Mewasingh L, Aylett S, et al. Hyponatraemia associated with lamotrigine in cranial diabetes insipidus. Lancet 2000;356:656.

Michaelis T, Videen JS, et al. Dialysis and transplantation affect cerebral abnormalities of end-stage renal disease. J Magn Reson Imaging 1996;6:341.

Miller RC, Wolf EC, et al. Fetal oculocerebrorenal syndrome of Lowe associated with elevated maternal serum and amniotic fluid alpha-fetoprotein levels. Obstet Gynecol 1994;84:77.

Milliner DS, Shinaberger JH, et al. Inadvertent aluminum administration during plasma exchange due to aluminum contamination of albumin-replacement solutions. N Engl J Med 1985;312:165.

Milutinovich J, Warren J, et al. Death caused by brain herniation during hemodialysis. South Med J 1979;72:418.

Minkoff L, Gaertner G, et al. Inhibition of brain sodium-potassium ATPase in uremic rats. J Lab Clin Med 1972;80:71.

Mirahmadi MK, Vaziri ND. Hearing loss in end-stage renal disease—effect of dialysis. J Dial 1980;4:159.

Mirra SS, Check IJ, et al. Rapid evolution of central nervous system lymphoma in renal transplant recipient [letter]. Lancet 1981;2:868.

Misiani R, Appiani AC, et al. Haemolytic uraemic syndrome: Therapeutic effect of plasma infusion. BMJ (Clin Res Ed) 1982;285:1304.

Mitschke H, Schmidt P, et al. Reversible uremic deafness after successful renal transplantation. N Engl J Med 1975;292:1062.

Miyabayashi H, Yamamori H, et al. [A case of rhabdomyolysis associated with *Salmonella* encephalopathy]. No To Hattatsu 2002;34:517.

Miyamoto K, Katai K, et al. Mutations of the basic amino acid transporter gene associated with cystinuria. Biochem J 1995;310(pt 3):951.

Moake JL. von Willebrand factor and the pathophysiology of thrombotic thrombocytopenia: From human studies to a new animal model. Lab Invest 1988;59:415.

Moake JL. The role of von Willebrand factor (vWF) in thrombotic thrombocytopenic purpura (TTP) and the hemolytic-uremic syndrome (HUS). Prog Clin Biol Res 1990;337:135.

Moake JL. TTP—desperation, empiricism, progress. N Engl J Med 1991;325:426.

Moake JL, Byrnes JJ, et al. Abnormal VIII: von Willebrand factor patterns in the plasma of patients with the hemolytic-uremic syndrome. Blood 1984;64:592.

Moammar H, Ratard R, et al. Incidence and features of galactosaemia in Saudi Arabs. J Inherit Metab Dis 1996;19:331-334.

Moe SM, Sprague SM. Uremic encephalopathy. Clin Nephrol 1994;42:251.

Moel DI, Kwun YA. Cortical blindness as a complication of hemodialysis. J Pediatr 1978;93:890.

Moghal NE, Ferreira MA, et al. The late histologic findings in diarrhea-associated hemolytic uremic syndrome. J Pediatr 1998;133:220.

Molitoris BA, Sandoval R, et al. Endothelial injury and dysfunction in ischemic acute renal failure. Crit Care Med 2002;30(5 Suppl):S235.

Moller HE, Ullrich K, et al. In vivo study of brain metabolism in galactosemia by 1H and 31P magnetic resonance spectroscopy. Eur J Pediatr 1995;154:S8.

Molteni KH, Oberley TD, et al. Progressive renal insufficiency in methylmalonic acidemia. Pediatr Nephrol 1991;5:323.

Moreau R. Hepatorenal syndrome in patients with cirrhosis. J Gastroenterol Hepatol 2002;17:739.

Morgan HG, Stewart WK, et al. Wilson's disease and the Fanconi syndrome. Q J Med 1962;31:361.

Morgan RE, Morgan JM. Plasma levels of aromatic amines in renal failure. Metabolism 1966;15:479.

Moritz ML, Ayus JC. Disorders of water metabolism in children: Hyponatremia and hypernatremia. Pediatr Rev 2002;23:371.

Morris A, Low DE. Nosocomial bacterial meningitis, including central nervous system shunt infections. Infect Dis Clin North Am 1999;13:735.

Morris AA, Taylor RW, et al. Neonatal Fanconi syndrome due to deficiency of complex III of the respiratory chain. Pediatr Nephrol 1995;9:407.

Mrowka C, Heintz B, et al. Isolated cerebral aspergilloma—long-term survival of a renal transplant recipient. Clin Nephrol 1997;47:394.

Muckle TJ, Wells M. Urticaria, deafness, and amyloidosis: A new heredo-familial syndrome. Q J Med 1962;31:235.

Muller D, Santer R, et al. Fanconi-Bickel syndrome presenting in neonatal screening for galactosaemia. J Inherit Metab Dis 1997; 20:607.

Mundell SJ, Benovic JL, et al. A dominant negative mutant of the G protein-coupled receptor kinase 2 selectively attenuates adenosine A2 receptor desensitization. Mol Pharmacol 1997;51:991.

Mundell SJ, Kelly E. Evidence for co-expression and desensitization of A2a and A2b adenosine receptors in NG108-15 cells. Biochem Pharmacol 1998;55:595.

Murcia FJ, Vazquez J, et al. Liver transplantation in type I tyrosinemia. Transplant Proc 1995;27:2301.

Murray HW, et al. Disseminated aspergillosis in a renal transplant patient: Diagnostic difficulties re-emphasized. Johns Hopkins Med J 1975;137:235.

Muruve DA, Steinman TI. Contrast-induced encephalopathy and seizures in a patient with chronic renal insufficiency. Clin Nephrol 1996;45:406.

Myers RN, Austin GM, et al. Solitary spinal cord tumors occurring in multiple members of a family. J Neurosurg 1960;17:783.

Naess PA, Bugge JF, et al. Lack of inhibitory effect of atrial natriuretic factor on renin release induced by renal hypotension. Scand J Clin Lab Invest 1996;56:665.

Naicker S. End-stage renal disease in sub-Saharan and South Africa. Kidney Int Suppl 2003;(83):S119.

Nakae H, Asanuma Y, et al. Cytokine removal by plasma exchange with continuous hemodiafiltration in critically ill patients. Ther Apher 2002;6:419.

Nakashita Y, Aoki M. [Mild brain hypothermia for influenza encephalitis/encephalopathy and its significance]. Nippon Rinsho (in Japanese) 2000;58:2333.

Nathan E, Pedersen SE. Dialysis encephalopathy in a non-dialysed uraemic boy treated with aluminium hydroxide orally. Acta Paediatr Scand 1980;69:793.

Nelson JS. The neuropathology of selected neurocutaneous diseases. Semin Pediatr Neurol 1995;2:192.

Nelson PB, Seif SM, et al. Hyponatremia in intracranial disease: Perhaps not the syndrome of inappropriate secretion of antidiuretic hormone (SIADH). J Neurosurg 1981;55:938.

Neuschwander-Tetri BA. Organ interactions in the hepatorenal syndrome. New Horiz 1994;2:527.

Niaudet P. Mitochondrial disorders and the kidney. Arch Dis Child 1998;78:387.

Niaudet P, Heidet L, et al. Deletion of the mitochondrial DNA in a case of de Toni-Debre-Fanconi syndrome and Pearson syndrome. Pediatr Nephrol 1994;8:164.

Niaudet P, Rotig A. The kidney in mitochondrial cytopathies. Kidney Int 1997;51:1000.

Nielsen VK. The peripheral nerve function in chronic renal failure: I. Clinical symptoms and signs. Acta Med Scand 1971a;190:105.

Nielsen VK. The peripheral nerve function in chronic renal failure:

II. Intercorrelation of clinical symptoms and signs and clinical grading of neuropathy. Acta Med Scand 1971b;190:113.
Nielsen VK. The peripheral nerve function in chronic renal failure: V. Sensory and motor conduction velocity. Acta Med Scand 1973;194:445.
Nielsen VK. The peripheral nerve function in chronic renal failure: IX. Recovery after renal transplantation: Electrophysiological aspects (sensory and motor nerve conduction). Acta Med Scand 1974a;195:171.
Nielsen VK. The peripheral nerve function in chronic renal failure: X. Decremental nerve conduction in uremia? Acta Med Scand 1974b;196:83.
Nijima A. Afferent discharges from venous pressoreceptors in liver. Am J Physiol 1977;232:C76.
Nissenson AR, Levin ML, et al. Neurological sequelae of end stage renal disease (ESRD). J Chronic Dis 1977;30:705.
Norenberg MD. Astrocyte responses to CNS injury. J Neuropathol Exp Neurol 1994;53:213.
Noris M, Ruggenenti P, et al. Hypocomplementemia discloses genetic predisposition to hemolytic uremic syndrome and thrombotic thrombocytopenic purpura: Role of factor H abnormalities. Italian Registry of Familial and Recurrent Hemolytic Uremic Syndrome/Thrombotic Thrombocytopenic Purpura. J Am Soc Nephrol 1999;10:281.
Novello AC, Fine RN. Renal transplantation in children—a review. Int J Pediatr Nephrol 1982;3:87-98.
Nussbaum RL, Orrison BM, et al. Physical mapping and genomic structure of the Lowe syndrome gene *OCRL1*. Hum Genet 1997;99:145.
Nyhan WL, Cooke RE. Symptomatic hyponatremia in acute infections of the central nervous system. Pediatrics 1956;18:604.
Nyhan WL, Gargus JJ, et al. Progressive neurologic disability in methylmalonic acidemia despite transplantation of the liver. Eur J Pediatr 2002;161:377.
Obara K, Saito T, et al. Renal histology in two adult patients with type I glycogen storage disease. Clin Nephrol 1993;39:59.
Obeid T, Shami A, et al. The role of seizures in reversible posterior leukoencephalopathy. Seizure 2004;13:277.
Oberholzer VG, Levin B, et al. Methylmalonic aciduria: An inborn error of metabolism leading to chronic metabolic acidosis. Arch Dis Child 1967;42:492.
Odievre M, Gentil C, et al. Hereditary fructose intolerance in childhood: Diagnosis, management, and course in 55 patients. Am J Dis Child 1978;132:605.
Ogier H, Lombes A, et al. de Toni-Fanconi-Debre syndrome with Leigh syndrome revealing severe muscle cytochrome c oxidase deficiency. J Pediatr 1988;112:734.
Ogier de Baulny H. Management and emergency treatments of neonates with a suspicion of inborn errors of metabolism. Semin Neonatol 2002;7:17-26.
Oh SJ, Clements RS Jr, et al. Rapid improvement in nerve conduction velocity following renal transplantation. Ann Neurol 1978;4:369.
Ohlsson A, Stark G, et al. Marble brain disease: Recessive osteopetrosis, renal tubular acidosis and cerebral calcification in three Saudi Arabian families. Dev Med Child Neurol 1980;22:72.
Ok E. Clinicopathological features of rapidly progressive hepatitis C virus infection in HCV antibody negative renal transplant recipients. Nephrol Dial Transplant 1998;13:103.
Olafsson I, Thorsteinsson L, et al. The molecular pathology of hereditary cystatin C amyloid angiopathy causing brain hemorrhage. Brain Pathol 1996;6:121.
Olivieri NF, Buncic JR, et al. Visual and auditory neurotoxicity in patients receiving subcutaneous deferoxamine infusions. N Engl J Med 1986;314:869.
Olivos-Glander IM, Janne PA, et al. The oculocerebrorenal syndrome gene product is a 105-kD protein localized to the Golgi complex. Am J Hum Genet 1995;57:817.
Olsen S. The brain in uremia. Acta Psychiatr Neurol Scand 1961;36:1.
Omori K, Kazama JJ, et al. Association of the MCP-1 gene polymorphism A-2518G with carpal-tunnel syndrome in hemodialysis patients. Amyloid 2002;9:175.
Ono J, Harada K, et al. MR findings and neurologic manifestations in Lowe oculocerebrorenal syndrome. Pediatr Neurol 1996;14:162.
Opastirakul S, Chartapisak W. Transient hyperkalemia and hypoaldosteronism in a patient with acute glomerulonephritis. J Med Assoc Thai 2002;85:509.
Oppenheimer BS, Fishberg AM. Hypertensive encephalopathy. Arch Intern Med 1925;41:264.
Orr JM, Farrell K, et al. The effects of peritoneal dialysis on the single dose and steady state pharmacokinetics of valproic acid in a uremic epileptic child. Eur J Clin Pharmacol 1983;24:387.
Ortega R, Gines P, et al. Terlipressin therapy with and without albumin for patients with hepatorenal syndrome: Results of a prospective, nonrandomized study. Hepatology 2002;36(4 pt 1):941.
Osberg JW, Meares GJ, et al. Intellectual functioning in renal failure and chronic dialysis. J Chronic Dis 1982;35:445.
Oshio T, Hino M, et al. Urologic abnormalities in Menker's kinky hair disease: Report of three cases. J Pediatr Surg 1992;32:782.
Osterman JD, Trauner DA, et al. Transient hemiparesis associated with monoclonal CD3 antibody (OKT3) therapy. Pediatr Neurol 1993;9:482.
Overstreet K, Benirschke K, et al. Congenital nephrosis of the Finnish type: Overview of placental pathology and literature review. Pediatr Dev Pathol 2002;5:179.
Palomeque Rico A, Pastor Duran X, et al. [Hemolytic uremic syndrome. Evaluation of clinical and prognostic factors]. An Esp Pediatr (in Spanish) 1993;39:391.
Papageorgiou C, Ziroyannis P, et al. A comparative study of brain atrophy by computerized tomography in chronic renal failure and chronic hemodialysis. Acta Neurol Scand 1982;66:378.
Pappius HM, Oh JH, et al. The effects of rapid hemodialysis on brain tissues and cerebrospinal fluid of dogs. Can J Physiol Pharmacol 1967;45:129.
Paradis K. Tyrosinemia: The Quebec experience. Clin Invest Med 1996;19:311.
Paradis K, D'Angata ID. Nephropathy of tyrosinemia and its long-term outlook. J Pediatr Gastroenterol Nutr 1997;24:113.
Parenti G, Sebastio G, et al. Lysinuric protein intolerance characterized by bone marrow abnormalities and severe clinical course. J Pediatr 1995;126:246.
Parvex P, Pinsk M, et al. Reversible encephalopathy associated with tacrolimus in pediatric renal transplants. Pediatr Nephrol 2001;16:537.
Pascoe MD. Clonazepam in dialysis encephalopathy [letter]. Ann Neurol 1981;9:200.
Patten BM. Neuromuscular complications. In: Eknoyan G, Knochel JP, eds. The systemic consequence of renal failure. Orlando, FL, Grune & Stratton, 1984;281.
Patzer L, Kentouche K, et al. Renal function following hematological stem cell transplantation in childhood. Pediatr Nephrol 2003;18:623.
Paut O, Remond C, et al. [Severe hyponatremic encephalopathy after pediatric surgery: Report of seven cases and recommendations for management and prevention]. Ann Fr Anesth Reanim (in French) 2000;19:467.
Pavlakis SG, Frank Y, et al. Occipital-parietal encephalopathy: A new name for an old syndrome [see comments]. Pediatr Neurol 1997;16:145.
Payton CD, Junor BJ, et al. Successful treatment of aluminium encephalopathy by intraperitoneal desferrioxamine [letter]. Lancet 1984;1:1132.
Peces R, de la Torre M, et al. Acyclovir-associated encephalopathy in haemodialysis [letter]. Nephrol Dial Transplant 1996;11:752.
Penn I. Tumor incidence in human allograft recipients. Transplant Proc 1979;11:1047.
Perazella M, Brown E. Acute aluminum toxicity and alum bladder irrigation in patients with renal failure. Am J Kidney Dis 1993;21:44.
Perez GO, Oster JR, et al. Incomplete syndrome of renal tubular acidosis induced by lithium carbonate. J Lab Clin Med 1975;86:386.
Perez-Caballero D, Gonzalez-Rubio C, et al. Clustering of missense mutations in the C-terminal region of factor H in atypical hemolytic uremic syndrome. Am J Hum Genet 2001;68:478.
Peters U, Senger G, et al. Nephropathic cystinosis (CTNS-LSB): Construction of a YAC contig comprising the refined critical region on chromosome 17p13. Eur J Hum Genet 1997;5:9.
Peterson H, Swanson AG. Acute encephalopathy occurring during hemodialysis. Arch Intern Med 1964;113:877.
Peterson LR, Ferguson RM. Fatal central nervous system infection with varicella-zoster virus in renal transplant recipients. Transplantation 1984;37:366.
Pfeiffer H, Weiss FU, et al. Fatal cerebro-renal oxalosis after appendectomy. Int J Legal Med 2004;118:98.
Pickering GW. High blood pressure. New York, Grune & Stratton, 1968.
Pitkanen S, Salo MK, et al. Serum levels of oncofetal markers CA 125, CA 19-9, and alpha-fetoprotein in children with hereditary tyrosinemia type I. Pediatr Res 1994;35:205.

Pittock SJ, Rabinstein AA, et al. OKT3 neurotoxicity presenting as akinetic mutism. Transplantation 2003;75:1058.
Platt JF, Ellis JH, et al. Renal duplex Doppler ultrasonography: A noninvasive predictor of kidney dysfunction and hepatorenal failure in liver disease. Hepatology 1994;20:362.
Platts MM. Dialysis encephalopathy [letter]. Lancet 1980;2:1035.
Platts MM, Anastassiades E. Dialysis encephalopathy: Precipitating factors and improvement in prognosis. Clin Nephrol 1981;15:223.
Ploos van Amstel JK, Bergman AJ, et al. Hereditary tyrosinemia type 1: novel missense, nonsense and splice consensus mutations in the human fumarylacetoacetate hydrolase gene; variability of the genotype-phenotype relationship. Hum Genet 1996;97:51.
Plum F, Posner JB. Multifocal, diffuse, and metabolic brain diseases causing stupor and coma. Philadelphia, FA Davis, 1980.
Polinsky MS, Gruskin AB. Aluminum toxicity in children with chronic renal failure. J Pediatr 1984;105:758.
Polinsky MS, Gruskin AB, et al. Aluminum in chronic renal failure. In: Strauss J, ed. Pediatric nephrology. New York: Plenum, 1984;315.
Polinsky MS, Kaiser BA, et al. Neurologic development of children with severe chronic renal failure from infancy. Pediatr Nephrol 1987;1:157.
Polinsky MS, Prebis JW, et al. A dialysis encephalopathy-like syndrome in childhood: An international survey. Pediatr Res 1980;14:1017.
Pollak MR. The genetic basis of FSGS and steroid-resistant nephrosis. Semin Nephrol 2003;23:141.
Ponchaut S, Draya J, et al. Influence of chronic administration of valproate on ultrastructure and enzyme content of peroxisomes in rat liver and kidney. Biochem Pharmacol 1989;38:3963.
Port FK, Johnson WJ, et al. Prevention of dialysis disequilibrium syndrome by use of high sodium concentration in the dialysate. Kidney Int 1973;3:327.
Potter D, Feduska N, et al. Twenty years of renal transplantation in children. Pediatrics 1986;77:465.
Powell HR, McCredie DA, et al. Vitamin E treatment of haemolytic uraemic syndrome. Arch Dis Child 1984;59:401.
Prickman LE, Millikan H. Hemorrhagic encephalopathy during arsenic therapy for asthma. JAMA 1953;153:1710.
Primavera A, Audenino D, et al. Reversible posterior leucoencephalopathy syndrome in systemic lupus and vasculitis. Ann Rheum Dis 2001;60:534.
Probst A, Harder F, et al. Femoral nerve lesion subsequent to renal transplantation. Eur Urol 1982;8:314.
Proesmans W, ki Muaka B, et al. The use of heparin in childhood hemolytic-uremic syndrome. In: Remuzzi G, Mecca G, de Gaetano G, eds. Hemostasis, prostaglandins, and renal disease. New York: Raven Press, 1980;407.
Proulx F, Lacroix J, et al. Convulsions and hypertension in children: Differentiating cause from effect. Crit Care Med 1993;21:1541.
Purday JP, Montgomery CJ, et al. Intraoperative hyperthermia in a paediatric patient with cystinosis. Paediatr Anaesth 1995;5:389.
Quek SC, Murugasu B, et al. Abnormal electrocardiographic patterns in renal failure. Ventricular tachycardia. Singapore Med J 1999;40:57.
Quimby BB, Alano A, et al. Characterization of two mutations associated with epimerase-deficiency galactosemia, by use of a yeast expression system for human UDP-galactose-4-epimerase. Am J Hum Genet 1997;61:590.
Qureshi F, Maalbared N. Unusual presentation of echinococcal cysts. Saudi Med J 2003;24:781.
Rabb H, Wang Z, et al. Possible molecular basis for changes in potassium handling in acute renal failure. Am J Kidney Dis 2000;35:871.
Racusen LC, Wilson PD, et al. Renal proximal tubular epithelium from patients with nephropathic cystinosis: Immortalized cell lines as in vitro model systems. Kidney Int 1995;48:536.
Raffel LJ, Cowan TM, et al. Transient neonatal galactosaemia identified by newborn screening. J Inherit Metab Dis 1993;16:894.
Raife TJ. Pathogenesis of thrombotic thrombocytopenic purpura. Curr Hematol Rep 2003;2:133.
Ram Prasad KS, Date A, et al. Central nervous system disease in renal transplant recipients. Nephron 1987;46:395.
Randall ME. Aluminium toxicity in an infant not on dialysis [letter]. Lancet 1983;1:1327.
Ranta A, Wooten GF. Hyponatremia due to an additive effect of carbamazepine and thiazide diuretics. Epilepsia 2004;45:879.
Rao YS, et al. Epilepsy after early-life seizures can be independent of hippocampal injury. Ann Neurol 2003;53:503.
Rasbury WC, Fennell RS, et al. Cognitive functioning of children with end-stage renal disease before and after successful transplantation. J Pediatr 1983;102:589.
Raskin NH, Fishman RA. Neurologic disorders in renal failure (first of two parts). N Engl J Med 1976a;294:143.
Raskin NH, Fishman RA. Neurologic disorders in renal failure (second of two parts). N Engl J Med 1976b;294:204.
Rathbun JK. Neuropsychological aspects of Wilson's disease. Int J Neurosci 1996;85:221.
Rawashdeh MO, Majeed HA. Familial Mediterranean fever in Arab children: The high prevalence and gene frequency. Eur J Pediatr 1996;155:540.
Ray-Chaudhuri K, Pye IF, et al. Hypersensitivity to carbamazepine presenting with a leukemoid reaction, eosinophilia, erythroderma, and renal failure. Neurology 1989;39:436.
Raza M, Al-Bekairi AM, et al. Biochemical basis of sodium valproate hepatotoxicity and renal tubular disorder: Time dependence of peroxidative injury. Pharmacol Res 1997;35:153.
Reidenberg MM. The binding of drugs to plasma proteins and the interpretation of measurements of plasma concentrations of drugs in patients with poor renal function. Am J Med 1977;62:466.
Reidenberg MM, Affrime M. Influence of disease on binding of drugs to plasma proteins. Ann NY Acad Sci 1973;226:115.
Reiss R, Makoff D, et al. Encephalopathy and cerebral infarction in OKT3-treated patients with concomitant elevation of cerebrospinal fluid tumour necrosis factor alpha. Nephrol Dial Transplant 1993;8:464.
Reitsma-Bierens WC. Renal complications in glycogen storage disease type I. Eur J Pediatr 1993;152(Suppl 1):S60.
Remuzzi G, Bertani T. Thrombotic thrombocytopenic purpura, hemolytic uremic syndrome, and acute cortical necrosis. In: Schrier RD, Gottschalk CW, eds. Diseases of the kidney. Boston: Little, Brown, 1988;2301.
Restaino I, Kaplan BS, et al. Nephrolithiasis, hypocitraturia, and a distal renal tubular acidification defect in type 1 glycogen storage disease. J Pediatr 1993;122:392.
Restuccia T, Ortega R, et al. Effects of treatment of hepatorenal syndrome before transplantation on posttransplantation outcome: A case-control study. J Hepatol 2004;40:140.
Revesz T. Cerebral amyloid angiopathies: A pathologic, biochemical, and genetic view. J Neuropathol Exp Neurol 2003;62:885.
Richards A, Goodship JA, et al. The genetics and pathogenesis of haemolytic uraemic syndrome and thrombotic thrombocytopenic purpura. Curr Opin Nephrol Hypertens 2002;11:431.
Richardson SE, Jagadha V, et al. Pathological effects of injected H.30 verotoxin (VT) in rabbits. Abstracts of the annual meeting of the American Society for Microbiology, Atlanta, March 1-6, 1987. Washington DC, American Society for Microbiology, 1987;42.
Richet G, Lopez de Novales E, et al. Drug intoxication and neurological episodes in chronic renal failure. BMJ 1970;2:394.
Richet G, Vachon F. [Neuropsychic disorders of chronic uremia]. Ann Biol Clin (Paris) (in French) 1966;24:565.
Rider LG, Buyon JP, et al. Treatment of neonatal lupus: case report and review of the literature [see comments]. J Rheumatol 1993;20:1208.
Ridolfi RL, Bell WR. Thrombotic thrombocytopenic purpura: Report of 25 cases and review of the literature. Medicine (Baltimore) 1981;60:413.
Rifkind D, Marchioro TL, et al. Systemic fungal infections complicating renal transplantation and immunosuppressive therapy: Clinical, microbiologic, neurologic and pathologic features. Am J Med 1967;43:28.
Riggs JE. Neurologic manifestations of electrolyte disturbances. Neurol Clin 2002;20:227, vii.
Rigoulot MA, et al. Neuroprotective properties of topiramate in the lithium-pilocarpine model of epilepsy. J Pharmacol Exp Ther 2004;308:787.
Riley LW, Remis RS, et al. Hemorrhagic colitis associated with a rare *Escherichia coli* serotype. N Engl J Med 1983;308:681.
Rivera-Vazquez AB, Noriega-Sanchez A, et al. Acute hypercalcemia in hemodialysis patients: Distinction from "dialysis dementia." Nephron 1980;25:243.
Robert JJ, Tete MJ, et al. Diabetes mellitus in patients with infantile cystinosis after renal transplantation. Pediatr Nephrol 1999;13:524.
Roberts MW, Blakey GH, et al. Enlarged dental follicles, a follicular cyst, and enamel hypoplasia in a patient with Lowe syndrome. Oral Surg Oral Med Oral Pathol 1994;77:264.
Robertson G. Vasopressin. In: Seldin D, Giebisch G, eds. The kidney: Physiology and pathophysiology. Philadelphia: Lippincott, Williams and Wilkins, 2000;1133.

Robertson JA, Salusky IB, et al. Sucralfate, intestinal aluminum absorption, and aluminum toxicity in a patient on dialysis. Ann Intern Med 1989;111:179.

Rock GA, Shumak KH, et al. Comparison of plasma exchange with plasma infusion in the treatment of thrombotic thrombocytopenic purpura. Canadian Apheresis Study Group. N Engl J Med 1991;325:393.

Rodriguez de Cordoba S, Esparza-Gordillo J, et al. The human complement factor H: Functional roles, genetic variations and disease associations. Mol Immunol 2004;41:355.

Rootwelt H, Berger R, et al. Novel splice, missense, and nonsense mutations in the fumarylacetoacetase gene causing tyrosinemia type 1. Am J Hum Genet 1994;55:653.

Ropper AH. Accelerated neuropathy of renal failure. Arch Neurol 1993;50:536.

Rosa AA, Fryd DS, et al. Dialysis symptoms and stabilization in long-term dialysis. Practical application of the CUSUM plot. Arch Intern Med 1980;140:804.

Rosenbloom D, Upton AR. Drug treatment of epilepsy: A review. Can Med Assoc J 1983;128:261.

Rossini PM, Pirchio M, et al. Checkerboard reversal pattern and flash VEPs in dialysed and non- dialysed subjects. Electroencephalogr Clin Neurophysiol 1981;52:435.

Rother KI, Schwenk WF. Glucose production in glycogen storage disease I is not associated with increased cycling through hepatic glycogen. Am J Physiol 1995;269:E774.

Rotig A, Bessis JL, et al. Maternally inherited duplication of the mitochondrial genome in a syndrome of proximal tubulopathy, diabetes mellitus, and cerebellar ataxia. Am J Hum Genet 1992;50:364.

Rotig A, Goutieres F, et al. Deletion of mitochondrial DNA in patient with chronic tubulointerstitial nephritis. J Pediatr 1995;126:597.

Rotundo A, Nevins TE, et al. Progressive encephalopathy in children with chronic renal insufficiency in infancy. Kidney Int 1982;21:486.

Rouan MC, Lecaillon JB, et al. The effect of renal impairment on the pharmacokinetics of oxcarbazepine and its metabolites. Eur J Clin Pharmacol 1994;47:161.

Rousset H, Sauron C, et al. [Clinical or biological symptoms leading to the search for amyloidosis]. Rev Med Interne 2000;21:161.

Rouviere O, Berger P, et al. Acute thrombosis of renal transplant artery: Graft salvage by means of intra-arterial fibrinolysis. Transplantation 2002;73:403.

Rubin RH, Wolfson JS, et al. Infection in the renal transplant recipient. Am J Med 1981;70:405.

Ruggenenti P, Remuzzi G, et al. Epidemiology of the hemolytic uremic syndrome [letter]. N Engl J Med 1991;15:1065.

Rust RS Jr. Infectious myositis. Philadelphia: Butterworth Heinemann, 2003.

Rust RS, Mathisen J, et al. Acute disseminated encephalomyelitis (ADE) and childhood multiple sclerosis (MS). Annals Neurol 1989;26:467.

Rust RS, Noetzel MJ, et al. An unusual movement disorder associated with tyrosinosis and elevated cerebrospinal fluid catecholamines. Ann Neurol 1985;19:399.

Saatci I, and Topaloglu R. Cranial computed tomographic findings in a patient with hypertensive encephalopathy in acute poststreptococcal glomerulonephritis. Turk J Pediatr 1994;36:325.

Saatci U, Bakkaloglu A, et al. Familial Mediterranean fever and amyloidosis in children. Acta Paediatr 1993;82:705.

Saatci U, Ozen S, et al. Familial Mediterranean fever in children: Report of a large series and discussion of the risk and prognostic factors of amyloidosis. Eur J Pediatr 1997;156:619.

Sacerdoti D, Bolognesi M, et al. Renal vasoconstriction in cirrhosis evaluated by duplex Doppler ultrasonography. Hepatology 1993;17:219.

Sadowski RH, Allred EN, et al. Sodium modeling ameliorates intradialytic and interdialytic symptoms in young hemodialysis patients. J Am Soc Nephrol 1993;4:1192-1198.

Salusky IB, Coburn JW, et al. Effects of oral calcium carbonate on control of serum phosphorus and changes in plasma aluminum levels after discontinuation of aluminum-containing gels in children receiving dialysis. J Pediatr 1986;108:767.

Sandvig K. Shiga toxins. Toxicon 2001;39:1629.

Santamaria R, Tamasi S, et al. Molecular basis of hereditary fructose intolerance in Italy: Identification of two novel mutations in the aldolase B gene. J Med Genet 1006;33:786.

Satsumi YN. [Recent abuse of 3,4-methylenedioxymethamphetamine ("yaoto-wang," "ecstasy")]. Seishin Shinkeigaku Zasshi (in Japanese) 2002;104:819.

Savazzi GM, Cambi V, et al. The influence of uraemic neuropathy on muscle: EMG, histoenzymatic and ultrastructural correlations. Proc Eur Dial Transplant Assoc 1980;17:312.

Savazzi GM, Cusmano F, et al. Cerebral imaging changes in patients with chronic renal failure treated conservatively or in hemodialysis. Nephron 2001;89:31.

Sawaishi Y, Komatsu K, et al. A case of tubulo-interstitial nephritis with exfoliative dermatitis and hepatitis due to phenobarbital hypersensitivity. Eur J Pediatr 1992;151:69.

Scarvie KM, Ballantyne AO, et al. Visuomotor performance in children with infantile nephropathic cystinosis. Percept Mot Skills 1996;82:67.

Scheinberg IH, Sternlieb I. Wilson's disease. Philadelphia, WB Saunders, 1984.

Scheinberg P. Effects of uremia on cerebral blood flow and metabolism. Neurology 1954;4:101.

Schmidt B, Wieneke H, et al. Encephalitic and myocardial toxoplasmosis masquerading as cytomegalovirus infection in a renal allograft recipient. Nephrol Dial Transplant 1995;10:284-286.

Schmidt M, Sitter T, et al. Reversible MRI changes in a patient with uremic encephalopathy. J Nephrol 2001;14:424.

Schmitz G, Hohage H, et al. Glucose-6-phosphate: A key compound in glycogenosis I and favism leading to hyper- or hypolipidaemia. Eur J Pediatr 1993;152(Suppl 1):S77.

Schmitz O, Moller J. Impaired prolactin response to arginine infusion and insulin hypoglycaemia in chronic renal failure. Acta Endocrinol (Copenh) 1983;102:486.

Schneck SA. Neuropathologic features of human organ transplantation: I. Probable cytomegalovirus infection. J Neuropathol Exp Neurol 1965;24:415.

Schneck SA, Penn I. Cerebral neoplasms associated with renal transplantation. Arch Neurol 1970;22:226.

Schottstaedt MF, Sokolow M. The natural history and course of hypertension with papilledema (malignant hypertension). Am Heart J 1953;45:331.

Schreier H, Dorfman C. Socially inept children. In: Aminoff MJ, Daroff RB, eds. Encyclopedia of the neurological sciences. San Diego, Calif: Academic Press, 2003;4:318.

Schreiner GE. Mental and personality changes in the uremic syndrome. Med Ann 1959;28:316.

Schrier RW. Acute renal failure. JAMA 1982;247:2518, 2524.

Schrier RW, Arnold PE, et al. Pathophysiology of cell ischemia. In Schrier RW, Gottschalk CW, eds. Diseases of the kidney, Boston: Little, Brown, 1988;1379.

Schrier RW, Wang W. Acute renal failure and sepsis. N Engl J Med 2004;351:159.

Schrier RW, Wang W, et al. Acute renal failure: Definitions, diagnosis, pathogenesis, and therapy. J Clin Invest 2004;114:5.

Schwartz CE, Cole BF, et al. Measuring patient-centered outcomes in neurologic disease: Extending the Q-TWIST method. Arch Neurol 1995;52:754.

Schwartz RB, Bravo SM, et al. Cyclosporine neurotoxicity and its relationship to hypertensive encephalopathy: CT and MR findings in 16 cases. AJR Am J Roentgenol 1995;165:627.

Schwarz RE, Dralle H, et al. Amyloid goiter and arthritides after kidney transplantation in a patient with systemic amyloidosis and Muckle-Wells syndrome. Am J Clin Pathol 1989;92:821.

Schwechheimer K, Hashemian A. Neuropathologic findings after organ transplantation: An autopsy study. Gen Diagn Pathol 1995;141:35.

Schweitzer S, Shin Y, et al. Long-term outcome in 134 patients with galactosaemia. Eur J Pediatr 1993;152:36.

Sebire G, Husson B, et al. [Encephalopathy induced by arterial hypertension: clinical, radiological and therapeutical aspects]. Arch Pediatr (in French) 1995;2:513.

Sedman AB, Klein GL, et al. Evidence of aluminum loading in infants receiving intravenous therapy. N Engl J Med 1985;312:1337.

Sedman AB, Miller NL, et al. Aluminum loading in children with chronic renal failure. Kidney Int 1984;26:201.

Sedman AB, Wilkening GN, et al. Encephalopathy in childhood secondary to aluminum toxicity. J Pediatr 1984;105:836.

Seigler RS, Avant MG, et al. A comparison of propofol and ketamine/midazolam for intravenous sedation of children. Pediatr Crit Care Med 2001;2:20-23.

Selby R, et al. Brain abscess in solid organ transplant recipients receiving cyclosporine-based immunosuppression. Arch Surg 1997;132:304.

Sengers RC, Stadhouders AM, et al. Mitochondrial myopathies: Clinical, morphological and biochemical aspects. Eur J Pediatr 1984;141:192.

Seyahi N, Apaydin S, et al. Intracranial calcification and tumoural calcinosis during vitamin D therapy. Nephrology (Carlton) 2004;9:89.

Shah D, Rylance PB, et al. Generalised epileptic fits in renal transplant recipients given cyclosporin A. BMJ (Clin Res Ed) 1984;289:1347.

Shaheen F, Mansuri N, et al. Reversible uremic deafness: Is it correlated with the degree of anemia? Ann Otol Rhinol Laryngol 1997;106:391.

Shenkman Z, Golub Y, et al. Anaesthetic management of a patient with glycogen storage disease type 1b. Can J Anaesth 1996;43:467.

Sheth KJ, Swick HM, et al. Neurologic involvement in hemolytic-uremic syndrome. Ann Neurol 1986;19:90.

Shida K, Matsuo M, et al. Extensive white matter involvement in hemorrhagic shock and encephalopathy syndrome. Acta Paediatr Jpn 1996;38:270.

Shihab F, Barry JM, et al. Cytokine-related encephalopathy induced by OKT3: Incidence and predisposing factors. Transplant Proc 1993a;25:564.

Shihab FS, Barry JM, et al. Encephalopathy following the use of OKT3 in renal allograft transplantation. Transplant Proc 1993b;25(2 Suppl 1):31.

Shiihara T, Kato M, et al. Microcephaly, cerebellar atrophy, and focal segmental glomerulosclerosis in two brothers: A possible mild form of Galloway-Mowat syndrome. J Child Neurol 2003;18:147.

Shimizu N, Suzuki M, et al. [A nation-wide survey for neurologic and hepato-neurologic type of Wilson disease: Clinical features and hepatic copper content]. No To Hattatsu (in Japanese) 1996;28:391.

Shin YS, Gathof BS, et al. Three missense mutations in the galactose-1-phosphate uridyltransferase gene of three families with mild galactosaemia. Eur J Pediatr 1996;155:393.

Shumov AM, Shutova LA, et al. [Hemodialysis in the treatment of acute kidney failure in hemorrhagic fever with renal syndrome]. Ter Arkh (in Russian) 1996;68:31.

Sidwell RW, Smee DF. Viruses of the Bunya- and Togaviridae families: Potential as bioterrorism agents and means of control. Antiviral Res 2003;57:101.

Siedlecki CA, Lestini BJ, et al. Shear-dependent changes in the three-dimensional structure of human von Willebrand factor. Blood 1996;88:2939.

Sieniawska M, Roszkowska-Blaim M, et al. Dialysis treatment in children with amyloidosis due to juvenile rheumatoid arthritis. Turk J Pediatr 1996;38:59.

Silver SM, DeSimone JA Jr, et al. Dialysis disequilibrium syndrome (DDS) in the rat: Role of the "reverse urea effect." Kidney Int 1992;42:161.

Silverstein A. Thrombotic thrombocytopenic purpura: The initial neurologic manifestations. Arch Neurol 1968;18:358.

Simell O, Perheentupa J, et al. Lysinuric protein intolerance. Am J Med 1975;59:229.

Singh S, Bohn D, et al. Cerebral salt wasting: Truths, fallacies, theories, and challenges. Crit Care Med 2002;30:2575.

Siniscalchi A, Mancuso F, et al. Acute encephalopathy induced by oxcarbazepine and furosemide. Ann Pharmacother 2004;38:509.

Sirgo MA, Green PJ, et al. Interpretation of serum phenytoin concentrations in uremia is assay- dependent. Neurology 1984;34:1250.

Sliman GA, Winters WD, et al. Hypercalciuria and nephrocalcinosis in the oculocerebrorenal syndrome. J Urol 1995;153:1244.

Sly WS. Recessive osteopetrosis: New clinical phenotype. Am J Hum Genet 1972;24:34A.

Sly WS, Hewett-Emmett D, et al. Carbonic anhydrase II deficiency identified as the primary defect in the autosomal recessive syndrome of osteopetrosis with renal tubular acidosis and cerebral calcification. Proc Natl Acad Sci U S A 1983;80:2752.

Smirk FH. The neurogenically maintained component in hypertension. Circ Res 1970;27(Suppl 2):55.

Smit GP. The long-term outcome of patients with glycogen storage disease type Ia. Eur J Pediatr 1993;152(Suppl 1):S52.

Smits MG, de Abreu RA, et al. Presence of cerebral parathyroid hormone—responsive adenylcyclase in humans [letter]. Ann Neurol 1983;14:348.

Smogorzewski MJ. Central nervous dysfunction in uremia. Am J Kidney Dis 2001;38(4 Suppl 1):S122.

So SKS, Chang R, et al. Growth and development in infants after renal transplantation. J Pediatr 1987;110:343.

Soda H. Carbonic anhydrase II deficiency syndrome—clinico-pathological, biochemical and molecular studies. Kurume Med J 1994;41:233.

Soda H, Yukizane S, et al. Carbonic anhydrase II deficiency in a Japanese patient produced by a nonsense mutation (TAT→TAG) at Tyr-40 in exon 2, Y40X). Hum Mutat 1995;5:348.

Solinas C, Briellmann RS, et al. Hypertensive encephalopathy: Antecedent to hippocampal sclerosis and temporal lobe epilepsy? Neurology 2003;60:1534.

Solomons NW. Diet and long-term health: An African Diaspora perspective. Asia Pac J Clin Nutr 2003;12:313.

Soni MG, White SM, et al. Safety evaluation of dietary aluminum. Regul Toxicol Pharmacol 2001;33:66.

Soohoo N, Schneider JA, et al. A cost-effectiveness analysis of the orphan drug cysteamine in the treatment of infantile cystinosis. Med Decis Making 1997;17:193.

Souheaver GT, Ryan JJ, et al. Neuropsychological patterns in uremia. J Clin Psychol 1982;38:490.

Sousa AE, Lucas M, et al. Takayasu's disease presenting as a nephrotic syndrome due to amyloidosis. Postgrad Med J 1993;69:488.

Sowunmi A. Clinical study of cerebral malaria in African children. Afr J Med Sci 1997;26:9.

Sperl W, Ruitenbeek W, et al. Mitochondrial myopathy with lactic acidaemia, Fanconi-De Toni-Debre syndrome and a disturbed succinate: Cytochrome c oxidoreductase activity. Eur J Pediatr 1988;147:418.

Spitzer PG, Tarsy D, et al. Acute transverse myelitis during disseminated cytomegalovirus infection in a renal transplant recipient. Transplantation 1987;44:151.

Spoudeas HA, Slater JD, et al. Deoxycorticosterone, 11 beta-hydroxylase and the adrenal cortex. Clin Endocrinol (Oxf) 1993;39:245.

Sprague SM, Corwin HL, et al. Encephalopathy in chronic renal failure responsive to deferoxamine therapy: Another manifestation of aluminum neurotoxicity. Arch Intern Med 1986;146:2063.

St-Louis M, Leclerc B, et al. Identification of a stop mutation in five Finnish patients suffering from hereditary tyrosinemia type I. Hum Mol Genet 1994;3:69.

Stapleton FB, Jones DP, et al. Acute renal failure in neonates: Incidence, etiology and outcome. Pediatr Nephrol 1987;1:314.

Stark RJ. Reversible myoclonus with uraemia. BMJ (Clin Res Ed) 1981;282:1119.

Starkey BJ. Aluminium in renal disease: Current knowledge and future developments. Ann Clin Biochem 1987;24:337.

Stec I, Peters U, et al. Yeast artificial chromosome mapping of the cystinosis locus on chromosome 17p by fluorescence in situ hybridization. Hum Genet 1996;98:321.

Steele TW, Edwards KD. Analgesic nephropathy: Changes in various parameters of renal function following cessation of analgesic abuse. Med J Aust 1971;1:181.

Steele WH, Lawrence JW, et al. Alterations of phenytoin protein binding with in vivo haemodialysis in dialysis encephalopathy. Eur J Clin Pharmacol 1979;15:69.

Steininger C, Popow-Kraupp T, et al. Acute encephalopathy associated with influenza A virus infection. Clin Infect Dis 2003;36:567.

Stenback A, Haapanen E. Azotemia and psychosis. Acta Psychiatr Scand 1967;43:1.

Still JL, Cottom D. Severe hypertension in childhood. Arch Dis Child 1967;42:34.

Stocker M, Gessler P, et al. Fatal hypertensive encephalopathy in a child with association of multicystic kidney and renal artery stenosis. Klin Padiatr 2003;215:205.

Strandgaard S. Autoregulation of cerebral blood flow in hypertensive patients: The modifying influence of prolonged antihypertensive treatment on the tolerance to acute, drug-induced hypotension. Circulation 1976;53:720.

Strandgaard S, Olesen J, et al. Autoregulation of brain circulation in severe arterial hypertension. BMJ 1973;1:507.

Strife CF, Zuroweste EL, et al. Tyrosinemia with acute intermittent porphyria: Aminolevulinic acid dehydratase deficiency related to elevated urinary aminolevulinic acid levels. J Pediatr 1977;90:400.

Strisciuglio P, Sartorio R, et al. Variable clinical presentation of carbonic anhydrase deficiency: Evidence for heterogeneity? Eur J Pediatr 1990;149:337.

Strominger MB, Liu GT, et al. Optic disk swelling and abducens palsies associated with OKT3. Am J Ophthalmol 1995;119:664.

Suchy SF, Olivos-Glander IM, et al. Lowe syndrome, a deficiency of phosphatidylinositol 4,5-bisphosphate 5-phosphatase in the Golgi apparatus. Hum Mol Genet 1995;4:2245.

Suhr OB, Svendsen IH, et al. Hereditary transthyretin amyloidosis from a Scandinavian perspective. J Intern Med 2003;254:225.

Suzuki H, Takahashi K, et al. Activation of the tyrosinase gene promoter by neurofibromin. Biochem Biophys Res Commun 1994;205:1984.

Swartz JD, Faerber EN, et al. CT demonstration of cerebral subcortical calcifications. J Comput Assist Tomogr 1983;7:476.

Swoboda K. HyperCKemia and rhabdomyolysis. Philadelphia: Butterworth Heinemann, 2003.

Taclob L, Needle M. Drug-induced encephalopathy in patients on maintenance haemodialysis. Lancet 1976;2:704.

Taes YE, Speeckaert M, et al. Effect of dietary creatine on skeletal muscle myosin heavy chain isoform expression in an animal model of uremia. Nephron Exp Nephrol 2004;96:e103.

Taher SM, Anderson RJ, et al. Renal tubular acidosis associated with toluene "sniffing." N Engl J Med 1974;290:765.

Tarhan NC, Agildere AM, et al. Osmotic demyelination syndrome in end-stage renal disease after recent hemodialysis: MRI of the brain. AJR Am J Roentgenol 2004;182:809.

Tarr PI, Neill MA, et al. The increasing incidence of the hemolytic-uremic syndrome in King County, Washington: Lack of evidence for ascertainment bias. Am J Epidemiol 1989;129:582.

Te Loo DM, Monnens LA, et al. Binding and transfer of verocytotoxin by polymorphonuclear leukocytes in hemolytic uremic syndrome. Blood 2000;95:3396.

Te Loo DM, van Hinsbergh VW, et al. Detection of verocytotoxin bound to circulating polymorphonuclear leukocytes of patients with hemolytic uremic syndrome. J Am Soc Nephrol 2001;12:800.

Tencer J, Torffvit O, et al. Decreased excretion of urine glycosaminoglycans as marker in renal amyloidosis. Nephrol Dial Transplant 1997;12:1161.

Tenckhoff HA, Boen FST, et al. Polyneuropathy in chronic renal insufficiency. JAMA 1965;192:1121.

Ter Meulen CG, et al. Flaccid paresis due to distal renal tubular acidosis preceding systemic lupus erythematosus. Neth J Med 2002;60:29.

Teschan PE, Bourne JR, et al. Electrophysiological and neurobehavioral responses to therapy: The National Cooperative Dialysis Study. Kidney Int Suppl 1983;13:S58.

Teshima T, Miyoshi T, et al. Cyclosporine-related encephalopathy following allogeneic bone marrow transplantation. Int J Hematol 1996;63:161.

Thabet F, Durand P, et al. [Severe Reye syndrome: report of 14 cases managed in a pediatric intensive care unit over 11 years]. Arch Pediatr (in French) 2002;9:581.

Theodoropoulos DS, Shawker TH, et al. Medullary nephrocalcinosis in nephropathic cystinosis. Pediatr Nephrol 1995;9:412.

Thien T, Huysmans FT, et al. Acute blood-pressure reduction in malignant hypertension [letter]. Lancet 1979;2:847.

Thoene JG. Cystinosis. J Inherit Metab Dis 1995;18:380.

Thomas GP, Grimm SE 3rd. Lowe's syndrome: Review of literature and report of case. ASDC J Dent Child 1994;61:68.

Throssell D, Feehally J, et al. Urticaria, arthralgia, and nephropathy without amyloidosis: Another variant of the Muckle-Wells syndrome? Clin Genet 1996;49:130.

Tierney WM, Martin DK, et al. The prognosis of hyponatremia at hospital admission. J Gen Intern Med 1986;1:380.

Tilney NL, Kohler TR, et al. Cerebromeningitis in immunosuppressed recipients of renal allografts. Ann Surg 1982;195:104.

Tinaztepe K. Renal amyloidosis in childhood: An overview of the topic with 25 years experience. Turk J Pediatr 1995;37:357.

Tinaztepe K, Gucer S, et al. The association between Henoch-Schonlein syndrome and renal amyloidosis: A proposal of a pathogenic mechanism. Turk J Pediatr 1993;35:249.

Tolan DR. Molecular basis of hereditary fructose intolerance: Mutations and polymorphisms in the human aldolase B gene. Hum Mutat 1995;6:210.

Topczewska-Bruns J, Pawlak D, et al. Increased levels of 3-hydroxykynurenine in different brain regions of rats with chronic renal insufficiency. Brain Res Bull 2002;58:423.

Torremans A, D'Hooge R, et al. Effect of NaCN on currents evoked by uremic retention solutes in dissociated mouse neurons. Brain Res 2004;1008:107.

Trapp G, Cannon J. Aluminum pots as a source of dietary aluminum. N Engl J Med 1981;304:172.

Trompeter RS, Smith RL, et al. Neurological complications of arterial hypertension. Arch Dis Child 1982;57:913.

Tsai HM. High titers of inhibitors of von Willebrand factor-cleaving metalloproteinase in a fatal case of acute thrombotic thrombocytopenic purpura. Am J Hematol 2000;65:251.

Tsai HM. Von Willebrand factor, ADAMTS13, and thrombotic thrombocytopenic purpura. J Mol Med 2002;80:639.

Tsai HM. Advances in the pathogenesis, diagnosis, and treatment of thrombotic thrombocytopenic purpura. J Am Soc Nephrol 2003;14:1072.

Tsai HM, Lian EC. Antibodies to von Willebrand factor-cleaving protease in acute thrombotic thrombocytopenic purpura. N Engl J Med 1998;339:1585.

Tsai HM, Rice L, et al. Antibody inhibitors to von Willebrand factor metalloproteinase and increased binding of von Willebrand factor to platelets in ticlopidine-associated thrombotic thrombocytopenic purpura. Ann Intern Med 2000;132:794.

Tsai HM, Shulman K. Rituximab induces remission of cerebral ischemia caused by thrombotic thrombocytopenic purpura. Eur J Haematol 2003;70:183.

Tsai HM, Sussman II, et al. Proteolytic cleavage of recombinant type 2A von Willebrand factor mutants R834W and R834Q: Inhibition by doxycycline and by monoclonal antibody VP-1. Blood 1997;89:1954.

Tsanaclis AM, de Morais CF. Cerebral toxoplasmosis after renal transplantation: Case report. Pathol Res Pract 1986;181:339.

Tsuchiya K. Epidemiological studies on cadmium in the environment in Japan: Etiology of itai-itai disease. Fed Proc 1976;35:2412.

Tyler HR. Studies in asterixis. Arch Neurol 1964;10:360.

Tyler HR. Asterixis. J Chron Dis 1965;18:409.

Tyler HR. Neurologic disorders in renal failure. Am J Med 1968;44:734.

Tyler HR. Neurological aspects of uremia: An overview. Kidney Int Suppl 1975;(2):188.

Tyler HR. Neurological disorders seen in renal failure. In: Vinkin PF, Bruyn GW, eds. Handbook of clinical neurology. Amsterdam: North Holland, 1976;321.

Tyler HR, Tyler KL. Neurologic complications. In: Eknoyan G, Knochel G, eds. The systemic consequences of renal failure. Orlando, FL: Grune & Stratton, 1984;311.

Tzipori S, Chow CW, et al. Cerebral infection with *Escherichia coli* 0.157:H7 in humans and gnotobiotic piglets. J Clin Pathol 1988;41:1099.

Uvnas B. Central cardiovascular control. In: Magoun HW, et al, eds. Handbook of physiology, vol. II, neurophysiology. Washington, DC: American Physiological Society, 1960;1131.

Uyama H, Shiiki H, et al. Primary amyloidosis complicated by systemic necrotizing arteritis [letter]. Histopathology 1997;31:203.

Vachharajani TJ, Zaman F, et al. Hyponatremia in critically ill patients. J Intensive Care Med 2003;18:3.

Valanne L, Qvist E, et al. Neuroradiologic findings in children with renal transplantation under 5 years of age. Pediatr Transplant 2004;8:44.

van't Hoff WG, Dixon M, et al. Combined liver-kidney transplantation in methylmalonic acidemia. J Pediatr 1998;132:1043.

van't Hoff WG, Gretz N. The treatment of cystinosis with cysteamine and phosphocysteamine in the United Kingdom and Eire. Pediatr Nephrol 1995;9:685.

Van Amelsvoort T, Bakshi R, et al. Hyponatremia associated with carbamazepine and oxcarbazepine therapy: A review. Epilepsia 1994;35:181.

Van Biesen W, Vanholder R, et al. Dialysis strategies in critically ill acute renal failure patients. Curr Opin Crit Care 2003;9:491.

Van Calcar SC, Harding CO, et al. Renal transplantation in a patient with methylmalonic acidaemia. J Inherit Metab Dis 1998;21:729.

Van den Noort S, Eckel RE, et al. Brain metabolism in experimental uremia. Arch Intern Med 1997;126:831.

van Diemen-Steenvoorde R, Donckerwolcke RA, et al. Epstein-Barr virus related central nervous system lymphoma in a child after renal transplantation. Int J Pediatr Nephrol 1986;7:55.

Van Lierde A, Colombo D, et al. Hemiparesis in a girl with cystinosis and renal transplant [letter]. Eur J Pediatr 1994;153:702.

Van Lierde S, van Leeuwen WJ, et al. Toxic shock syndrome without rash in a young child: Link with syndrome of hemorrhagic shock and encephalopathy? J Pediatr 1997;131:130.

Van Roey G, Moore K. The hepatorenal syndrome. Pediatr Nephrol 1996;10:100.

Vasconcelos PF, Luna EJ, et al. Serious adverse events associated with yellow fever 17DD vaccine in Brazil: A report of two cases. Lancet 2001;358:91.

Veltri MA, Neu AM, et al. Drug dosing during intermittent hemodialysis and continuous renal replacement therapy: Special considerations in pediatric patients. Paediatr Drugs 2004;6:45.

Verrotti A, Greco R, et al. Renal tubular function in patients receiving anticonvulsant therapy: A long-term study. Epilepsia 2000;41:1432.

Versaci AA, Olsen KJ, et al. Uremic polyneuropathy: and motor nerve conduction velocities. Trans Am Soc Artif Intern Organs 1964;10:328.

Vester U, Schubert M, et al. Distal myopathy in nephropathic cystinosis. Pediatr Nephrol 2000;14:36.

Visweswaran P, Guntupalli J. Rhabdomyolysis. Crit Care Clin 1999;15:415, ix.

Vollmer WM, Wahl PW, et al. Survival with dialysis and transplantation in patients with end-stage renal disease. N Engl J Med 1983;308:1553.

Von Gierke E. Hepato-nephro-megalia glykogenia (Glykogenspeicher-krankheit der Leber und Nieren). Beitr Pathol Anat 1929;82:497.

Wadelius C, Lagerkvist A, et al. Galactosemia caused by a point mutation that activates cryptic donor splice site in the galactose-1-phosphate uridyltransferase gene. Genomics 1993;17:525.

Wakayama I, Nerurkar VR, et al. Comparative study of chronic aluminum-induced neurofilamentous aggregates with intracytoplasmic inclusions of amyotrophic lateral sclerosis. Acta Neuropathol (Berl) 1996;92:545.

Wakim KG. The pathophysiology of the dialysis disequilibrium syndrome. Mayo Clin Proc 1969a;44:406.

Wakim KG. Predominance of hyponatremia over hypo-osmolality in simulation of the dialysis disequilibrium syndrome. Mayo Clin Proc 1969b;44:433.

Waller S, Ledermann S, et al. Catch-up growth with normal parathyroid hormone levels in chronic renal failure. Pediatr Nephrol 2003;18:1236.

Wang TK, et al. Disseminated ochroconis gallopavum infection in a renal transplant recipient: The first reported case and a review of trhe literature. Clin Nephrol 2003;60:415.

Warter JM, Brandt C, et al. The renal origin of sodium valproate-induced hyperammonemia in fasting humans. Neurology 1983;33:1136.

Warwicker P, Goodship TH, et al. Genetic studies into inherited and sporadic hemolytic uremic syndrome. Kidney Int 1998;53:836.

Watemberg N, Alehan F, et al. Clinical and radiologic correlates of frontal intermittent rhythmic delta activity. J Clin Neurophysiol 2002;19:535.

Weingarten K, Barbut D, et al. Acute hypertensive encephalopathy: Findings on spin-echo and gradient-echo MR imaging. AJR Am J Roentgenol 1994;162:665.

Weintraub R, Hams G, et al. High aluminium content of infant milk formulas. Arch Dis Child 1986;61:914.

Whittington LK, et al. Hemorrhagic shock and encephalopathy: Further description of a new syndrome. J Pediatr 1985;106:599.

Wilkinson AH, Smith JL, et al. Increased frequency of posttransplant lymphomas in patients treated with cyclosporine, azathioprine, and prednisone. Transplantation 1989;47:293.

Williams BL, Schneider JA, et al. Global intellectual deficits in cystinosis. Am J Med Genet 1994;49:83.

Williams DM, Sreedhar SS, et al. Acute kidney failure: A pediatric experience over 20 years. Arch Pediatr Adolesc Med 2002;156:893.

Wilson JG, Fearon DT. Altered expression of complement receptors as a pathogenetic factor in systemic lupus erythematosus. Arthritis Rheum 1984;27:1321.

Wilson SA. Neurology. Baltimore: Williams & Wilkins, 1940;2:806.

Winick M, Rosso P, Busel JA. Malnutrition and cellular growth in the brain: Existence of critical periods. In: Ciba Found Symp 1971;199.

Wolff JA, Strom C, et al. Proximal renal tubular acidosis in methylmalonic acidemia. J Neurogenet 1985;2:31.

Wolfsdorf JI, Crigler JF Jr. Cornstarch regimens for nocturnal treatment of young adults with type I glycogen storage disease. Am J Clin Nutr 1997;65:1507.

Wolfsdorf JI, Laffel LM, et al. Metabolic control and renal dysfunction in type I glycogen storage disease. J Inherit Metab Dis 1997;20:559.

Wong CS, Jelacic S, et al. The risk of the hemolytic-uremic syndrome after antibiotic treatment of *Escherichia coli* O157:H7 infections. N Engl J Med 2000;342:1930.

Woo M, Przepiorka D, et al. Toxicities of tacrolimus and cyclosporin A after allogeneic blood stem cell transplantation. Bone Marrow Transplant 1997;20:1095.

Woodrow G, Harnden P, et al. Acute renal failure due to accelerated hypertension following ingestion of 3,4-methylenedioxymeth-amphetamine ("ecstasy"). Nephrol Dial Transplant 1995;10:399.

Wright RR, Mathews KD. Hypertensive encephalopathy in childhood. J Child Neurol 1996;11:193.

Wu BL, Austin MA, et al. Deletion of the entire NF1 gene detected by the FISH: Four deletion patients associated with severe manifestations. Am J Med Genet 1995;59:528.

Yager C. Galactitol and galactonate in red blood cells of galactosemic patients. Mol Genet Metab 2003;80:283.

Yazbeck S, Larbrisseau A, et al. Femoral neuropathy after renal transplantation. J Urol 1985;134:720.

Yildiz A, Sever MS, et al. Improvement of uremic autonomic dysfunction after renal transplantation: A heart rate variability study. Nephron 1998;80:57.

Yokoyama K, Hayashi H, et al. Renal lesion of type Ia glycogen storage disease: The glomerular size and renal localization of apolipoprotein [see comments]. Nephron 1995;70:348.

Yoshida Y, Machigashira K, et al. Immunological abnormality in patients with lysinuric protein intolerance. J Neurol Sci 1995;134:178.

Yosipovitch G, Yarnitsky D, et al. Paradoxical heat sensation in uremic polyneuropathy. Muscle Nerve 1995;18:768.

Young JB, Ahmed-Jushuf IH, et al. The role of EEG monitoring and immobilization in dialysis encephalopathy. Dial Transpl 1988;17:15.

Young RR, Shahani BT. Asterixis: One type of negative myoclonus. Adv Neurol 1986;43:137.

Yuce A, Coskun T, et al. Type I glycogenosis with renal tubular dysfunction (presentation of two cases). Turk J Pediatr 1993;35:201.

Zangeneh F, Young WF Jr, et al. Cushing's syndrome due to ectopic production of corticotropin-releasing hormone in an infant with ganglioneuroblastoma. Endocr Pract 2003;9:394.

Zhang X, Jefferson AB, et al. The protein deficient in Lowe syndrome is a phosphatidylinositol-4,5-bisphosphate 5-phosphatase. Proc Natl Acad Sci U S A 1995;92:4853.

Zhao Q, et al. Detrimental effects of the ketogenic diet on cognitive function in rats. Pediatric Res 2004;55:368.

Zheng X, Chung D, et al. Structure of von Willebrand factor-cleaving protease (ADAMTS13), a metalloprotease involved in thrombotic thrombocytopenic purpura. J Biol Chem 2001;276:41059.

Zifko U, Auinger M, et al. Phrenic neuropathy in chronic renal failure. Thorax 1995;50:793.

Zimmerman BG, Gisslen J. Pattern of renal vasoconstriction and transmitter release during sympathetic stimulation in presence of angiotensin and cocaine. J Pharmacol Exp Ther 1968;163:320.

Zucker I, Yosipovitch G, et al. Prevalence and characterization of uremic pruritus in patients undergoing hemodialysis: Uremic pruritus is still a major problem for patients with end-stage renal disease. J Am Acad Dermatol 2003;49:842.

ZuRhein GM, Varakis J. Letter: Progressive multifocal leukoen-cephalopathy in a renal-allograft recipient. N Engl J Med 1974;291:798.

CHAPTER 90

Neurologic Disorders Associated with Gastrointestinal Diseases, Nutritional Deficiencies, and Fluid-Electrolyte Disorders

Yitzchak Frank and Stephen Ashwal

The association between the gastrointestinal (GI) tract and the nervous system is reciprocal. The central nervous system (CNS) depends on the GI system for a constant supply of glucose, the absorption and metabolism of a variety of other nutrients and vitamins required for normal brain function, and the removal of toxic metabolic wastes. The GI tract has an elaborate system of neurons and neural connections: the enteric nervous system, which controls motility, sphincter tone and activity, hormone secretion, and GI circulation. Although this system is partially independent, it has motor and sensory sympathetic and parasympathetic connections to the CNS [Goyal and Hirano, 1996]. Therefore, diseases of the GI tract and liver may cause neurologic abnormalities (e.g., hepatic encephalopathy), whereas neurologic abnormalities affecting the CNS or the enteric nervous system may give rise to GI abnormalities (e.g., achalasia, esophageal reflux, megacolon).

A significant number of GI disorders have neurologic manifestations or complications. Some of these are nutritional, related to malabsorption, and some are related to the toxic effects of waste products (e.g., ammonia). Other complications are not related to either of these (e.g., inflammatory bowel disease) and involve immunologic responses related to the underlying disease, genetic factors, vascular abnormalities, or infectious agents. In patients with celiac disease, complications that can develop include cerebellar ataxia, myelopathy, or cerebral, brainstem, and peripheral nerve abnormalities. In patients with Whipple's disease, possible complications include cognitive and psychiatric manifestations, supranuclear gaze palsy, upper motor neuron dysfunction signs, hypothalamic dysfunction, cranial nerve abnormalities, seizures, ataxia, and sensory deficits. Neurologic abnormalities in inflammatory bowel disease (e.g., Crohn's disease, ulcerative colitis) can be related to vascular changes, epilepsy, chronic inflammatory polyradiculoneuropathy, or myasthenia gravis. In patients with hepatitis C, neurologic abnormalities can develop because of vasculitis associated with hepatitis C virus–related cryoglobulinemia. Neurologic abnormalities in persons with GI disease also can be a consequence of vitamin B_1, nicotinamide, vitamin B_{12}, vitamin D, or other nutritional deficiencies. In some cases, onset of the neurologic manifestations may precede appearance of the GI abnormalities.

The first part of this chapter reviews neurologic complications of the most common GI and liver diseases. GI manifestations of enteric nervous system abnormalities are discussed for some of the common motility disorders. These manifestations are more comprehensively reviewed, as are the anatomy and physiology of the enteric nervous system, in Chapter 85. Several excellent reviews on this topic are available [Camilleri and Bharucha, 1996; Costa and Brookes, 1994; Ghezzi, 2001; Goyal and Hirano, 1996; Perkin, 1998; Quigley, 1997; Singaram, 1996; Skeen, 2002]. The second part of the chapter reviews disorders associated with malnutrition, vitamin deficiencies, and fluid and electrolyte disturbances.

Neurologic Complications of Common Gastrointestinal and Liver Diseases

DISORDERS ASSOCIATED WITH GASTROINTESTINAL DISEASES

Episodic Gastrointestinal Disease

Cyclic Vomiting Syndrome and Recurrent Abdominal Pain

Cyclic vomiting syndrome, described first by Gee [1882], is manifested by recurrent bouts of vomiting lasting for hours or days, which can cause dehydration, hypochloremic alkalosis, and ketosis [Abu-Arafeh and Russell, 1995]. The time of onset, during the day or night, and the duration of the episodes tend to be stereotypic for the affected person. Abdominal pain, weakness, and fever may be present, as well as pallor, skin blotching, and other autonomic features [Fleisher, 1997], and the patient may become drowsy and lethargic. Variable intervals of normal health between episodes are characteristic. Cyclic vomiting and recurrent abdominal pain (including abdominal migrane) are classified under childhood functional GI disorders [Rasquin-Weber, 1999]. The condition usually occurs in early childhood but can start later and usually resolves before adulthood [Fleisher and Matar, 1993]. Cyclic vomiting syndrome may affect up to 1.9% of school-aged children [Abu-Arafeh, 1995]. It causes a high degree of medical morbidity, with 50% of affected patients requiring intravenous rehydration and experiencing academic disruption. Complications of cyclic vomiting include esophagitis, which may be caused by the continued vomiting, hematemesis, electrolyte depletion, and hypertension [Fleisher, 1995].

The physiology of vomiting involves a number of systems at the level of the medulla including the area postrema and the nucleus tractus solitarius, all finally projecting to a central pattern generator for vomiting that controls the sequence of events during emesis. It receives efferent innervation from chemoreceptors in the area postrema in the floor of the fourth ventricle that are sensitive to different stimuli from vagal GI fibers, the vestibulo-ocular system, and the cortex. Vomiting, therefore, can be a result of GI, autonomic, or cerebral dysfunction secondary to tumors, hydrocephalus, toxins, hormonal changes, familial dysautonomia, or migraine [Johns, 1995]. Similarly, the treatment of vomiting differs according to the mechanism or underlying disorder. For instance, some of the antiemetics work through an effect on the vagal complex [Hornby, 2001]. Considerations in the differential diagnosis of cyclic vomiting syndrome include GI obstruction (i.e. malrotations, internal hernias, webs, atresias), inborn errors of metabolism such as urea cycle defects (e.g., ornithine transcarbamylase deficiency), organic acidemias (e.g., methylmalonicacademia), porphyria, fatty acid oxidation defects, and disorders of carbohydrate metabolism. The diagnosis is therefore not complete until established causes of cyclic vomiting syndrome have been investigated [Bu, 1998; Stein, 2001].

Other children have *recurrent abdominal pain* lasting for hours, with or without headaches, nausea, and vomiting. Some clinical and physiologic overlap exists among cyclic vomiting syndrome, abdominal migraine, and migraine headaches [Bu, 1999]. Exact pathophysiology is unknown, but mitochondrial DNA mutations, ion channelopathies, and excessive hypothalamic-pituitary-adrenal axis activation have been suggested [Bu, 2000]. Abnormal autonomic balance also has been suggested [Bu, 1999].

Recurrent abdominal pain has been referred to as *abdominal migraine* [Axon et al., 1991; Bentley et al., 1995; Fleisher and Matar, 1993; Symon and Russell, 1986]. A history of migraine headache in first-degree relatives is common [Symon and Russell, 1995]. An electroencephalographic pattern seen with migraine, consisting of posterior temporo-occipital delta slowing, was recorded in a patient with cyclic vomiting during an episode [Jernigan and Ware, 1991]. It also has been suggested that cyclic vomiting may be a manifestation of abdominal epilepsy [Lanzi et al., 1983], although good evidence to prove the existence of such a specific type of epilepsy is lacking.

Treatment of cyclic vomiting is with fluid and electrolyte replacement and treatment of esophagitis. Lorazepam has antiemetic and anxiolytic properties. Pharmacologic therapy includes antiemetic agents. Commonly used are chlorpromazine, butyrophenones, and metoclopramide. Serotonin (5-hydroxytryptamine-3) receptor antagonists such as ondansetron have been used recently as antiemetics for cyclic vomiting syndrome. Phenothiazines, butyrophenones, metoclopramide (Reglan), or trimethobenzamide (Tigan) may be effective as antiemetics but may cause extrapyramidal side effects. Prophylactic therapy with propranolol has been reported [Forbes and Withers, 1995]. At times, antiepileptic drugs, such as phenobarbital or valproic acid, may be of benefit. Prophylactic therapy with amitriptyline and with cyproheptadine was found to be effective in small, noncontrolled studies [Anderson, 1997], although treatment with tricyclic antidepressants was more effective in patients who had functional vomiting [Prakash, 1999]. Propranolol [Forbes, 1995], atenolol, and antiepileptic drugs including phenytoin and barbiturates [Gokhale, 1997] have been used. Trials of motilin agonist (erythromycin) have been performed [Vanderhoof, 1995]. Sumatriptan, a 5-hydroxytryptamine-1 agonist, may be effective when used early at the beginning of a cyclic vomiting syndrome episode [Huang, 1997].

Anatomic Disorders

Gastroesophageal Reflux

Gastroesophageal reflux occurs when an incompetent lower esophageal sphincter allows entry of gastric contents and acid into the esophagus, with the potential for aspiration and development of esophagitis [Hillemeier, 1996]. Some patients also may have a hiatal hernia [Mittal and Balaban, 1997]. Gastroesophageal reflux is common in infants and generally resolves spontaneously within the first year of life as the lower esophageal sphincter mechanism matures. Conservative management in these children involves thickened feedings and positional treatment. The reflux is considered a disease—gastroesophageal reflux disease—when it becomes symptomatic or causes pathologic consequences. Gastroesophageal reflux disease can be primary or secondary. Secondary gastroesophageal reflux disease is associated with a number of genetic syndromes, chromosomal anomalies, and esophageal atresia and also is seen in neurologically impaired children including those with myopathies [Berezin, 1988; Henry, 2004]. Therefore, in children in whom the etiology of gastroesophageal reflux is not established, evaluation for a neurologic cause should be considered.

Apnea in most preterm infants is unrelated to gastroesophageal reflux [Poets, 2004]. Factors contributing to the frequent occurrence of gastroesophageal reflux with neurologic conditions include esophageal muscle weakness, hypotonia, incoordination of the swallowing mechanism, scoliosis, and immobility.

Symptoms of gastroesophageal reflux include pain, discomfort, irritability, and vomiting. Anemia and recurrent aspiration pneumonia also may occur. Respiratory symptoms resulting from reflux, aspiration, and laryngospasm that cause apnea, cyanosis, and stiffening may be confused with seizures [Bray, 1977]. A relation among hiatal hernia, gastroesophageal reflux, and dystonic neck posture, described by Sandifer, was reported by Kinsbourne in 1964. The dystonic posture consists of extension and rotation of the neck. Other investigators have suggested that the dystonic posture allows for better peristalsis and clearance of acid from the distal esophagus [Puntis et al., 1989]. The same workers, however, could not reproduce these findings in two children with gastroesophageal reflux without dystonia or in normal adult controls.

The diagnosis of gastroesophageal reflux is made by upper GI contrast studies, endoscopy and esophageal manometry, and esophageal pH monitoring. Esophageal pH monitoring demonstrates intermittent periods of pH reduction, which indicates reflux of acid gastric contents into the distal esophagus [Hillemeier, 1996]. Esophageal manometry may demonstrate decreased sphincter pressure and reduced peristaltic activity. A barium swallow study of the upper intestinal tract also should be performed to determine the presence of other anatomic or functional abnormalities that may mimic reflux. In children whose symptoms are not ameliorated by being placed in an upright sitting position during and after feeding or by being given thickened feedings, medications that enhance GI motility (e.g., metoclopramide) may be beneficial [Cucchiara, 1996; Hillemeier, 1996; Jung, 2001]. In addition, antacids and the reduction of gastric acid production with histamine receptor type 2 antagonists such as cimetidine or ranitidine or proton pump inhibitors may be efficacious. The use of cisapride in childhood gastroesophageal reflux has been discontinued. These therapies are less effective in decreasing respiratory symptoms such as apnea in children with underlying neurologic disorders [Bagwell, 1995; Jolley et al., 1980; Smith et al., 1992].

In children with reflux refractory to aggressive medical treatment, fundoplication may be beneficial [Bagwell, 1995]. Indications for surgery include an established esophageal stricture, associated anatomic defect, and failure of medical therapy, or apneic spells secondary to documented reflux [Spitz, 2003]. A large proportion of children who undergo fundoplication for treatment of gastroesophageal reflux are helped by the operation [Bourne, 2003; Norrashidah, 2002]. Children with neurologic impairment tend to benefit from fundoplication, but they are at greater risk for postoperative complications (12% to 20%), are more likely to require gastrostomy tube placement, and are at greater risk for the development of recurrent reflux than are normal children [Bagwell, 1995; Pearl et al., 1990; Smith et al., 1992].

Hirschsprung's Disease

The enteric nervous system controls and modulates intestinal motility, sensation from the gut, mucosal secretion, and blood flow. It is a complex network of neurons within the wall of the intestine that originate in the neural crest.

Neurocristopathies are a group of diverse disorders that result from defective growth, differentiation, and migration of the neural crest cells [Bolande, 1997]. Hirschsprung's disease is a neurocristopathy with defective migration of neural crest cells to the colonic submucosa and failure to form enteric ganglia in the hindgut, resulting in aganglionic megacolon—the absence of the parasympathetic ganglion cells in the submucosal and myenteric plexuses of the gut, leading to narrowed distal segment and distention of the proximal portion of the bowel. A hypothesis for the pathogenesis of Hirschsprung's disease is that the migration of neuroenteric ganglion cells from the neural crest to the most distal part of the gut is incomplete, because the migrating neural crest cells confront a genetically determined segmental abnormal microenvironment in the colon [Sullivan, 1996]. The diagnosis is made by the absence of ganglion cells in a rectal biopsy. Increased acetylcholinesterase in the same segment also can be found.

Hirschsprung's disease has an incidence of 1 in 5000 live births. It has been described in conjunction with several syndromes, including Down syndrome, Smith-Lemli-Opitz syndrome, familial piebaldness, Goldberg-Shprintzen syndrome, Haddad's syndrome, and Waardenburg's syndrome, and with agenesis of the corpus callosum and other neurologic abnormalities [Kaplan, 1983; Shahar, 2003]. The Goldberg-Shprintzen syndrome includes the combination of unusual facial features (hypertelorism, cleft palate, and maxillary deficiency) and Hirschsprung's disease [Goldberg and Shprintzen, 1981; Yomo et al., 1991]. Mental retardation and epilepsy also are associated with this syndrome [Tanaka et al., 1993]. Computed tomography (CT) scanning demonstrates diffuse cerebral atrophy. This syndrome may be a manifestation of abnormal neuronal migration, because the parasympathetic ganglia involved in Hirschsprung's disease and the connective tissues of the face and affected oropharyngeal structures all are derived from the neural crest. Patients with Waardenburg's syndrome, which consists of dysmorphic facial features, partial or total heterochromia iridis, piebaldism of the skin or hair, and congenital deafness affecting one or both ears, also may have Hirschsprung's disease. Again, the embryonal defect may be a neural crest migration defect [Mallory et al., 1986].

Hirschsprung's disease also may occur in Haddad's syndrome, the combination of congenital alveolar hypoventilation requiring continuous mechanical ventilation in the neonate [Stern et al., 1981] and short-segment Hirschsprung's disease.

The existence of familial cases suggested that genetic factors are involved in the etiology of some cases of Hirschsprung's disease. The inheritance pattern was thought to be multifactorial or autosomal dominant. Recent genetic studies identified a number of genes that may be involved in the disease, including the tyrosine kinase receptor Ret, endothelin-B receptor, and endothelin-3 genes [Chakravarti, 1996; Edery et al., 1994]. In addition, mutations have been found in the gene encoding the glial cell line–derived neurotrophic factor [Wartiovaara, 1998], a factor that promotes the migration of neural crest stem cells in culture [Iwashita, 2003]. Recently, abnormalities of the *L1CAM* gene, a member of the immunoglobulin gene family of neural cell adhesion molecules localized at Xq28, have been described in cases of Hirschsprung's disease (and other idiopathic intestinal pseudo-obstruction syndromes) with X-linked hydrocephalus [Bott, 2004; Parisi, 2002; Okamoto, 2004].

Intestinal Pseudo-obstruction

Intestinal pseudo-obstruction is manifested by the clinical features of intestinal obstruction in the absence of mechanical blockage [Scott, 1996]. Infants with this condition do not have an anatomic-pathologic diagnosis (e.g., Hirschsprung's disease). Box 90-1 lists some of the common causes of intestinal pseudo-obstruction in children. Acute pseudo-obstruction (paralytic ileus) usually occurs postoperatively or secondary to the use of medications, including anticholinergic agents, phenothiazines, tricyclic antidepressants, narcotics, and certain antiepileptic drugs, particularly benzodiazepines and barbiturates. Chronic pseudo-obstruction may be due to a variety of abnormalities of the intestinal musculature (chronic myopathic intestinal pseudo-obstruction), such as muscular dystrophies [Barohn et al., 1988], myotonic dystrophies [Brunner et al., 1992], and disorders of intestinal innervation (chronic neuropathic intestinal pseudo-obstruction), including X-linked recessive neuronal forms [Auricchio et al., 1996]. Other syndromes associated with pseudo-obstruction include the POLIP (*p*olyneuropathy, *o*phthalmoplegia, *l*eukoencephalopathy, and *i*ntestinal *p*seudo-obstruction) syndrome, a familial, possibly autosomal-recessive, chronic neuropathic intestinal pseudo-obstruction that accompanies a progressive severe neuronal disease manifested by external ophthalmoplegia, ptosis, severe sensory and motor peripheral neuropathy, and neuronal hearing loss, without CNS or cognitive involvement [Faber et al., 1987; Steiner et al., 1987]. Postmortem examination in three cases revealed degenerative neuronal changes with eosinophilic intranuclear inclusion bodies and

Box 90-1 Causes of Intestinal Pseudo-obstruction in Children

I. Acute
   A. Postoperative
   B. Electrolyte disturbances
   C. Medication effects
   D. Acute infections or toxins
II. Chronic
   A. Disorders of the myenteric plexus
      1. Primary disorders of the myenteric plexus
         a. Developmental abnormalities
            1) Neuronal immaturity and developmental abnormalities
         b. Aganglionosis
            1) Hirschsprung's disease
            2) Segmental aganglionosis
      2. Familial visceral neuropathies—multiple subtypes
      3. Systemic disorders affecting the myenteric plexus
         a. Infectious—Chagas' disease, cytomegalovirus infection, infectious mononucleosis, zoster
         b. Neurologic disorders—familial dysautonomia
         c. Endocrine disorders—diabetes mellitus
         d. Gastrointestinal disorders—malabsorption syndromes
   B. Disorders of intestinal smooth muscle
      1. Primary disorders of smooth muscle
         a. Familial visceral myopathy—various inherited forms
         b. Sporadic childhood visceral myopathies
      2. Systemic disorders affecting visceral smooth muscle
         a. Muscular and myotonic dystrophies
         b. Hypothyroidism
         c. Connective tissue disorders—systemic lupus erythematosus, polymyositis/dermatomyositis
   C. Small intestinal diverticulosis
      1. With myopathic changes
      2. With neuropathic changes

Modified from Scott RB. Motility disorders. In: Walker WA, Durie PR, Hamilton JR, et al, eds. Pediatric gastrointestinal disease. St. Louis: Mosby, 1996.

demyelination in the myenteric plexus and the peripheral nervous system, possibly secondary to axonal atrophy. Cranial nerves and spinal roots were less severely involved, and neurons in the brainstem and spinal cord were intact [Simon et al., 1990].

Abnormal intestinal innervation can be the result of intestinal neuronal dysplasia. Evidence from animal models suggests that intestinal neuronal dysplasia is an entity caused by a genetic defect [Puri, 2004]. It also may exist in humans, in isolation or as a part of Hirschsprung's disease. Animal studies, however, have demonstrated histologic evidence that chronic intestinal obstruction can induce different degrees of enteric nervous system dysplasia [Galvez, 2004]. Therefore, it has not yet been clarified whether some of the pathologic features described for intestinal neural dysplasia are the result, rather than the cause, of impaired motility [Kapur, 2003].

The clinical manifestation of intestinal pseudo-obstruction is recurrent episodes of bowel obstruction without a mechanical obstructive cause. Symptoms and signs include poor feeding, vomiting, abdominal distention, megacolon, and constipation. Evaluation for pseudo-obstruction requires excluding structural, mechanical, and pharmacologic causes, followed by additional studies to evaluate motor activity and motility, including barium contrast studies of the GI tract, breath hydrogen determination, scintigraphy, and manometric studies [Scott, 1996; Vargas et al., 1988].

Intussusception

Intestinal intussusception with invagination of the gut into its distal segment is the most common cause of bowel obstruction in children between 2 months and 5 years of age. Presenting signs and symptoms are typically abdominal, but encephalopathy with irritability, lethargy, obtundation, or coma has been described. Impairment of mental status can precede the appearance of GI symptoms and signs [Pumberger, 2004]. Brainstem reflexes usually are normal, but extreme miosis may occur. Muscle tone and deep tendon reflexes may be decreased [Goetting et al., 1990; Hoisington et al., 1993]. Neurologic symptoms resolve after surgical reduction. The pathophysiology of this disorder is unknown; on the basis of an apparent response to naloxone, it has been suggested that pain may cause endorphin release, which accounts for miosis, hypotonia, hyporeflexia, and a generalized cortical depression that also could mask the abdominal pain [Tenenbein and Wiseman, 1987]. Alternatively, endotoxin release from intestinal mucosa may act as a CNS depressant [Conway, 1993].

Malabsorption Syndromes

A variety of well-known GI disorders are associated with malabsorption syndromes that can cause selected nutritional, biochemical, and vitamin deficiencies. Neurologic involvement in children is seen in some of these disorders. Various biochemical deficiencies, including vitamin E and vitamin B_{12} deficiency, that can occur as a result of GI disorders are reviewed later in this chapter.

Celiac Disease

Celiac disease is a malabsorption disorder characterized by permanent gluten intolerance. It is a common disorder with a prevalence of about 1%, caused by an inappropriate immune response to the gliadin component in dietary gluten [Dieterich, 1997]. Exposure to gluten perpetuates an enteropathy, leading to malabsorption with chronic diarrhea, weight loss, and abdominal distention. The small intestinal mucosa is abnormal, and jejunal biopsy demonstrates various degrees of villous atrophy, absence of surface mucosa, and crypt hyperplasia.

Abnormalities of humoral and cell-mediated immunity suggest that celiac disease is an immunologic disorder [Walker-Smith, 1996]. Anti–tissue transglutaminase antibody assay, an enzyme-linked immunoabsorbent assay, has been used clinically as a serologic screening test for celiac disease. Similarly, antiendomysial, antigliadin, and antireticulin immunoglobulin A antibodies are associated with celiac disease and can be used for serologic screening and monitoring, along with a duodenal biopsy. A large percentage of patients with celiac disease have the gene encoding HLA DQ2, and some have the HL A DR4 DQ8 gene [Hadjivassiliou et al, 1998; Skeen, 2002]. Treatment is by exclusion of gluten from the diet, resulting in healing of the enteropathy and normalization of small bowel function.

Gluten sensitivity also can be present in the absence of any symptoms or with neurologic abnormalities but without strictly defined celiac disease, which means that gluten sensitivity constitutes a large spectrum of disease [Fasano et al, 2001; Hadjivassiliou et al, 1998]. Studies report the development of neurologic or psychiatric problems in 10% to 50% of adults with celiac disease. These problems include most commonly ataxia [Luostarinen, 1999; Hadgivassiolou, 1996; Kieslich, 2001] but also depression, seizures, migraine, dementia, and, rarely, peripheral neuropathy or myopathy [Albers et al., 1989; Collin and Maki, 1994; Collin et al., 1991; Gobbi et al., 1992; Holmes, 1996]. Celiac disease occurs in 9% or more of patients with idiopathic cerebellar ataxia, in comparison with 2% of the healthy Finnish population. Patients can present with gait or limb ataxia, and/or dysarthria, oculomotor, sensory or bladder dysfunction [Hadjivassiliou, 2004; Luostarinen et al, 2001]. Because antigliadin antibodies are nonspecific, their presence in persons with ataxia may not necessarily prove the existence of gluten sensitivity [Hadjivassiliou, 2003; Willis, 2002]. Still, patients with idiopathic cerebellar ataxia should be evaluated for the possibility of gluten sensitivity.

Children with the disease are typically irritable. Seizures occur in 3.5% to 5.5% of patients with celiac disease [Holmes, 1996]. Neuropathy, manifested by paresthesias, numbness, reduced tendon reflexes, sensory ataxia, and weakness, usually occurs late in the disease, in adults with severe steatorrhea [Kaplan et al., 1988]. Nerve conduction velocity studies and nerve biopsies provide evidence of distal axonopathy. The neuropathy is believed to result from vitamin deficiency. Similarly, myopathy is a rare complication of celiac disease in childhood. CT may demonstrate cerebral calcifications, as well as cerebral and cerebellar atrophy.

Specific syndromes of occipital calcifications and epilepsy and cerebellar degeneration with or without epilepsy have been described in childen with celiac diseaese [Arroyo et al., 2002; Gobbi, 1992; Gordon, 2000; Labate et al., 2001]. Screening of patients with Down syndrome using immunoglobulin A (IgA) antiendomysium antibodies, IgA antigliadin antibodies, and total IgA level revealed that a high prevalence of these patients are positive for antiendomysium antibodies (1 in 14). In other studies, the prevalence of celiac disease in people with Down syndrome ranges from 1 in 6 to 1 in 14 [Zachor et al., 2000]. Neurologic disease may be the presenting sign of celiac disease [Finelli et al., 1980; Hardoff et al., 1980; Luostarinen, 1999]. In addition, celiac disease may be present in a significant number of patients with neurologic disease of unknown etiology [Hadjivassiliou, 1996]. Twenty percent of a group of children with biopsy-confirmed celiac disease were prospectively assessed for neurologic disease and were found on CT or MRI study to have white matter lesions, which may be the result of vascular or inflammatory demyelination [Kieslich, 2001].

Neuropathologic findings described in an adult patient with celiac disease who manifested a pancerebellar syndrome consisted of cerebellar and basal ganglia cell loss and fibrillary gliosis [Finelli et al., 1980]. Abnormalities also have been described in the cortex, spinal cord, and muscle [Steinberg and Frank, 1993]. The neuropathologic findings in patients with Down syndrome include degenerative changes and evidence of an autoimmune mechanism including inflammation and demyelination.

The pathogenesis of CNS or peripheral nervous system dysfunction in gluten enteropathy is not clear. Malabsorption with abnormalities of vitamins B_{12}, B_6, D, and E and folic acid, as well as hypocalcemia and hypokalemia, has been implicated [Ventura et al., 1991]. Although these abnormalities may cause neurologic changes and should be looked for in patients with celiac disease and neurologic abnormalities, evidence indicating that the neurologic complications are secondary to malabsorption is lacking in most patients. It has been suggested that the pathogenesis of neurologic abnormalities in celiac disease may be due to a vasculitis that involves the vascular endothelium. Biopsy-confirmed CNS vasculitis and a case of a stroke with CNS vasculitis were documented in association with celiac disease [Ozge, 2001; Rush, 1986]. The syndrome of occipital calcification reported with celiac disease may be the result of autoimmune endothelial inflammation [Gobbi, 1992]. In addition, occasional occurrence of cerebrospinal fluid oligoclonal bands and the presence of inflammatory necrosis, myelin loss, and prominent lymphocytic infiltration suggest an inflammatory immunomediated mechanism [Ghezzi, 2001]. Childhood stroke in association with celiac disease also has been reported [Goodwin, 2004]. CT study of the brain of a 3-year-old female with recurrent episodes of transient left arm weakness, ataxia, and prior history of recurrent diarrhea that subsided after reducing milk intake revealed a low-density enhancing lesion in the right caudate nucleus and two additional lesions, all of which were consistent with infarction. Results of antiendomesial IgA antibodies were positive, antitransglutaminase antibodies were elevated at over 200 U/mL, and duodenal biopsy confirmed the diagnosis of celiac disease. The authors of that report suggest that tissue transglutaminase may be important to the maintenance of vascular endothelial integrity [Kim, 2002]. The enzyme is present in the brain, most abundant in the caudate, putamen, and substantia nigra, and antiendomysial antibody has been reported to immunofluoresce with cerebral vasculature [Pratesi, 1998]. These findings may provide an explanation for the occurrence of vascular abnormalities, demyelination, and stroke in celiac disease.

A gluten-free diet or vitamin supplementation has not been found to reverse the CNS abnormalities, although improvement may follow gluten restriction in some patients with peripheral neuropathy or myopathy [Hardoff et al., 1980; Kaplan et al., 1988; Wills, 2000; Wills and Unsworth, 2002]. In a follow-up study of children with celiac disease, a greater frequency of symptoms was found in the group on an unrestricted diet [Bardella et al., 1994]. Neurologic complications, specifically epilepsy with cerebral calcifications, occurred only in patients who were not on a gluten-free diet.

Short Bowel Syndrome

Short bowel syndrome is a malabsorption syndrome that follows resection of a significant portion of the small bowel, usually for a congenital anomaly, necrotizing enterocolitis in the neonate, inflammatory bowel disease, or ischemic injury. The degree of malabsorption is related to the underlying cause for surgical resection, but the extent of bowel resection does not necessarily predict long-term outcome. If the malabsorption prevents normal growth on even specialized enteral feedings, then the child may require central intravenous hyperalimentation until bowel adaptation occurs. Eventual transition to full enteral feedings, however, is not possible in all children with short bowel syndrome who require intravenous nutrition.

An unusual complication of this syndrome is an encephalopathy that affects infants and is associated with hyperchloremic acidosis and increased blood and urine lactate. The encephalopathy has been attributed to elevated blood and presumably cerebral lactate concentrations [Gurevitch et al., 1993]. Early recognition, treatment with an intestinal antibiotic, and appropriate adjustment of enteral feedings facilitate correction of the hyperchloremic acidosis and recovery.

Inflammatory Bowel Disease

Inflammatory bowel disease, including Crohn's disease (regional enteritis) and ulcerative colitis, primarily affect young adults and occur infrequently in children. In 15% to 25% of affected persons, the disease starts in childhood [Kim, 2004]. The incidence of inflammatory bowel disease in Wisconsin children was found to be 7.05 per 100,000. The incidence of Crohn's disease was more than twice the rate of ulcerative colitis [Kugathasan et al, 2003].

Crohn's disease is a chronic, inflammatory process that can affect any region of the GI tract but mostly affects the small bowel in a discontinuous fashion [Hyams, 1996]. Inflammation involves all layers of the bowel in Crohn's disease. *Ulcerative colitis* is a chronic relapsing inflammatory disease involving the mucosa of the colon and rectum in a continuous manner [Kirschner, 1996]. The etiology of both diseases remains unknown, although they likely are of immune origin. Patients complain of diarrhea, rectal bleeding, abdominal pain, vomiting, and weight loss. The pathogenesis of inflammatory bowel disease is complex and involves a reaction to a putative persistent intestinal infection, defective mucosal barrier to luminal antigens, and a dysregulation of the immune response to ubiquitous antigens [Ghezzi, 2001]. Therapy is with anti-inflammatory agents, corticosteroids, and supportive nutritional management [Justinich and Hyams, 1994]. The increased understanding of the immunologic processes involved with inflammatory bowel disease has resulted in the increase of therapeutic agents used to treat the disease [Stein et al, 2001].

Extraintestinal manifestations occur in about 25% to 35% of patients with either disease. Neurologic manifestations are rare, occurring in about 3% of patients with inflammatory bowel disease, and are dominated by CNS vascular complications, including arterial occlusion, arteritis, and encephalopathy [Lloyd-Still and Tomasi, 1989; Lossos et al., 1995; Mezoff et al., 1990]. Seizures, focal neurologic deficits, and psychiatric disorders also are seen [Elsehery, 1997], as are myelopathy, myopathy, and myasthenia gravis. Peripheral neuropathy and disturbed autonomic functions occur infrequently in patients with long-standing Crohn's disease [Lindgren et al., 1991; Nemni et al., 1987]. Radiologic findings include arterial occlusion, sagittal sinus thrombosis, and cerebral arteritis. Increased T2 signal in the white matter on MRI scans appears in 40% to 50% of patients with inflammatory bowel disease [Geissler, 1995; Hart, 1998]. In a majority of patients, the onset of neurologic symptoms is within the first 5 to 6 years after the onset of inflammatory bowel disease symptoms [Lossos et al., 1995]. Because bowel fistulas to nearby organs are a complication of Crohn's disease, spinal infiltration can occur. Although rare, it is a serious complication of Crohn's disease and must be considered in every patient with significant back pain with or without obvious neurologic signs [Hershkowitz et al, 1990; Maggiore et al, 2004]. A comorbidity of Crohn's disease and multiple sclerosis also has been reported [Beaugerie, 1997; Kimura et al, 2000].

The pathophysiology of the neurologic manifestations in patients with Crohn's disease is unknown but may have a dysimmune basis, affecting cell-mediated and humoral immunity and inflammatory mechanisms. Elevated factor V and VIII levels and decreased antithrombin-3 have been found in inflammatory bowel disease. Children with inflammatory bowel disease and neurologic complications may have a family history of collagen-vascular disease (see Chapter 73).

Enteric Infections

Enteric bacterial and viral infections that cause primary CNS infection are reviewed in Chapters 68 and 69. A variety of systemic viral and bacterial infections, however, may cause an encephalopathy resulting from the presence of endotoxins or electrolyte and fluid disturbances (Chapter 89). Some of the more well-recognized entities are reviewed here.

Seizures and encephalopathy in infants with enteric infections and diarrhea can be caused by hyponatremia or hypernatremia. Hyponatremia may cause brain swelling because sodium and chloride ions cross the brain capillaries slower than water does. Treatment consists of rehydration with adequate sodium salts and avoidance of more dilute fluids [Finberg, 1986].

Hypokalemia can accompany diarrhea and may have neuromuscular manifestations, including hypotonia, diminished bowel sounds, weakness, lethargy, abdominal distention, and, in severe cases, rhabdomyolysis and myoglobinuria. Neuromuscular manifestations become more prominent with serum potassium levels lower than 3 mEq/liter. Severe hypokalemia occurs more frequently in children younger than 24 months and in infants receiving dextrose-containing intravenous fluids without electrolyte replacement and is related to the type of rehydration therapy [Chhabra et al., 1995]. The exact mechanism by which hypokalemia causes muscle weakness is still unclear, but hypokalemia has been demonstrated in experimental models to change the resting membrane potential, limit increases in blood flow in exercising muscles, and cause a reduction in muscle glycogen content.

Escherichia coli Infection

An outbreak of *Escherichia coli* hemorrhagic colitis in 1990 in Japan was associated with neurologic abnormalities, including generalized seizures, impaired consciousness, urinary incontinence, nystagmus, phrenic nerve palsy, action tremor, and vertigo. The neurologic manifestations were believed to be secondary to bacterial endotoxins [Hamano et al., 1993]. Additional similar cases have been described [Ephros et al., 1996].

Campylobacter jejuni Infection

Campylobacter jejuni, a frequently identified bacterial cause of gastroenteritis, has been associated with Guillain-Barré syndrome and encephalopathy [Duret et al., 1991; Nasaralla et al., 1993; Rees et al, 1995]. The incubation period for infections due to this organism usually is 24 to 72 hours but can be longer. Nonspecific prodromal symptoms of fever, myalgia, and headaches occur, and the diarrhea is typically watery but may become bloody. In approximately 30% to 40% of affected persons, Guillain-Barré syndrome develops following *C. jejuni* infection. Some evidence suggests that Guillain-Barré syndrome in these patients may be a more severe variant of the disease, with a more frequent need for ventilatory support and greater residual disability [Hughes et al, 1997; Rees et al, 1995]. *C. jejuni* infection with antibodies to GM_1 and GD_{1b} gangliosides are associated with a severe, pure motor form of Guillain-Barré syndrome. Cross-reactivity between neural antigens and *C. jejuni* may be one of the mechanisms by which Guillain-Barré syndrome is triggered [Rees et al., 1993]. An oral killed whole-cell vaccine is being tested [Scott, 1997].

Infant Botulism

Botulism can be acquired by ingesting contaminated food containing the toxin produced by the bacteria, and through wound infection. Infant botulism and other forms of the disease also have been described [Cherington, 2004]. Botulinum neurotoxin is the neuromuscular poison that is responsible for the disease botulism. The same toxin is being used as a treatment for an expanding list of disorders. Infant botulism, caused by the release of toxins (either type A, B, or E) from the bacterium *Clostridium botulinum*, occurs in young infants and is manifested by constipation, cranial nerve deficits, pupillary involvement, generalized hypotonia and weakness, and loss of deep tendon reflexes [Arnon, 1992; Clay et al., 1977; Cochran and Appleton, 1995; Hatheway, 1995]. The toxin blocks acetylcholine release by impairing calcium influx associated with membrane depolarization and causes an acute reversible motor unit disease. Affected infants have a history of lethargy, irritability, poor feeding, constipation, and generalized weakness of 12 hours to 7 days' duration. Examination may reveal ophthalmoplegia with sluggish pupillary responses and abnormal function of cranial nerves VII, IX, X, and XI. Other signs of autonomic dysfunction include delayed gastric emptying and a paralytic ileus. In moderate or severe cases of infant botulism, progressive respiratory failure occurs, with many patients requiring prolonged periods of mechanically assisted ventilation. Cardiovascular symptoms are absent.

Repetitive nerve stimulation studies document an unusual incremental response, and electromyography demonstrates a distinctive pattern consisting of brief small motor unit potentials. Treatment is supportive, focusing primarily on the need to maintain adequate ventilation and nutrition in a critical care setting.

Shigellosis

Shigellosis is an acute bacterial enteritis caused by *Shigella* bacteria and is characterized by intestinal and extraintestinal symptoms. Neurologic manifestations of dysentery caused by *Shigella* organisms are common and include convulsions, meningismus, lethargy, confusion, headache, and infrequently an encephalopathy, with hallucinations, delirium, or mutism [Selimoglu et al., 1995]. Neurologic abnormalities may appear before the onset of diarrhea and other GI symptoms [Ashkenazi et al., 1989]. Although seizures and encephalopathy usually are benign and rarely recur or have permanent sequelae [Ozturk et al., 1996], cases of severe fatal encephalopathy have been described [Sandyk and Brenna, 1983]. CT may demonstrate cerebral edema [Perles et al., 1995].

Convulsions occur in 12% to 45% of hospitalized patients with culture-proven shigellosis and are most common in children between 6 months and 4 years of age [Ashkenazi et al., 1983; Daoud et al., 1990]. In a large series, convulsions in a majority of the cases were generalized and lasted less than 10 minutes, and approximately 25% of the children had a history of previous febrile seizures [Ashkenazi et al., 1987]. In another study of 55 children with *Shigella* organism–associated convulsions who were followed for 6.9 to 14.1 years, none had subsequent nonfebrile seizures, and only 2 had subsequent febrile seizures [Lahat et al., 1990]. Therefore, chronic antiepileptic drug therapy usually is not indicated [Ozturk et al., 1996].

The mechanisms responsible for the neurologic complications of shigellosis have not been clearly elucidated. Some manifestations, especially seizures, may be related to fever, whereas others may not. Neurologic manifestations likely are not related to production of Shiga toxin [Ashkenazi et al., 1990]. A study from Bangladesh of 863 patients with diarrhea documented that clinical features of fever, severe dehydration, hypoglycemia, hyponatremia, or meningitis were present in 92% of the patients in whom a seizure was witnessed and in 92% of the patients who were unconscious [Kahn, 1999]. These findings suggested to the study authors that a majority of the cases of seizures or loss of consciousness were not related to Shiga toxin.

At postmortem examination in three patients with *Shigella* organism–related fatal encephalopathy, areas of necrosis were present throughout the brain; in one patient, pontine hemorrhages and demyelination were present [Sandyk and Brenna, 1983]. Studies in a mouse model of shigellosis demonstrated that local production of tumor necrosis factor-α and interleukin-1b in the brain may play a role in enhanced seizures in the animals infected with *Shigella dysenteriae* [Nofech-Mozes et al., 2000]. Other studies found that nitric oxide, induced by *S. dysenteriae*, and corticotropin-releasing hormone may be involved in enhancing the susceptibility to seizures caused by *Shigella* [Balter-Seri, 1999; Yuhas, 2004].

Rotavirus Infection

Enteric rotavirus infection causing gastroenteritis with concomitant afebrile seizures has also been described in infants [Lin et al., 1996; Tsai and Cho, 1996]. Seizures did not recur in these patients, and no long-term antiepileptic therapy was prescribed. Transient abnormalities on the electroencephalogram (EEG) also have been reported. The occurrence of exanthems in 4% of patients with rotavirus infection suggests the possibility of generalized viremia. It is possible, therefore, that the virus invades the CNS by a hematogenous route [Contino et al., 1994]. Direct inoculation of three strains of rotavirus, including human rotavirus strain 2, into monkey brain caused a neurologic syndrome including transient paresis, with pathologic evidence of viral invasion of the CNS.

Other Gastrointestinal Conditions

Whipple's Disease

Whipple's disease is a multisystem chronic granulomatous disease caused by the bacillus *Tropheryma whippelii* [Marth and Raoult, 2003]. The first case was reported by G. H. Whipple in 1907. It is described primarily in middle-aged adults (in males more often than in females) but can occur in childhood [Tan et al., 1995] and is manifested clinically by weight loss, steatorrhea, malabsorption, fever, arthritis, lymphadenopathy, and cardiac abnormalities. It involves mostly the small intestine. The diagnosis is based on the presence of periodic acid–Schiff–positive macrophages in duodenal or lymph node biopsy in patients with systemic involvement. Electron microscopy demonstrates gram-positive bacilli *(T. whippelii)* within the intestinal lamina propria. Periodic acid-Schiff-positive macrophages have been identified in body tissues including the CNS. Increased protein and lymphocytic pleocytosis are detected in the cerebrospinal fluid of patients with the disease.

Polymerase chain reaction studies have helped identify the *T. whippelii* organism [Relman et al, 1992] and have a high sensitivity and specificity. Attempts to culture the organism occasionally are successful. Gene sequencing of *T. whippelii* isolated from the cerebrospinal fluid of a patient diagnosed with Whipple's disease demonstrated a condensed genome with a lack of key biosynthetic pathways and a reduced capacity for energy metabolism [Bentley, 2003].

CNS abnormalities are found in 20% to 40% of the patients. In addition, cerebrospinal fluid polymerase chain reaction assay results are positive in 67% of patients with Whipple's disease without neurologic symptoms [von Herbay et al, 1997]. Signs of CNS infection include progressive dementia, supranuclear ophthalmoplegia, seizures, myoclonus and ataxia, and hypothalamic abnormalities including insomnia [Alba et al., 1995; Jovic and Jovic, 1996; Manzel, 2000]. Recurrent stroke-like episodes have been described, with multiple enhancing lesions on T2-weighted MRI. [Peters, 2002].

Oculomasticatory myorhythmia, possibly caused by brainstem tegmental abnormalities, is a movement disorder nearly unique to patients with Whipple's disease [Schwartz et al., 1983]. It consists of rhythmic convergence of the eyes and synchronous contractions of the eyelids, jaw, face, and neck with characteristics resembling spinal myoclonus.

Review of the 84 cases of CNS Whipple's disease revealed that 80% of the patients had systemic signs [Louis et al., 1996]. Cognitive changes were frequent (71%), and 47% of the patients with cognitive changes also had psychiatric signs. Oculomasticatory myorhythmia and oculofacial-skeletal myorhythmia, pathognomic for CNS Whipple's disease, were present in 20% of patients and were always accompanied by a supranuclear vertical gaze palsy. The possibility of CNS Whipple's disease should be entertained in the setting of unexplained systemic symptoms and neurologic signs (supranuclear vertical gaze palsy, rhythmic myoclonus, dementia with psychiatric symptoms, or hypothalamic manifestations), and in patients with such findings, small bowel biopsy should be considered.

CT and MRI demonstrate intracranial focal abnormalities, including low-density focal lesions in the pontine tegmentum and temporal lobe [Halperin et al., 1982; Schnider et al., 1995] and cortical and subcortical atrophy. In a pediatric patient with Whipple's disease, white matter lesions initially appeared as areas of very low signal intensity on T1-weighted images and hyperintensity on proton density-weighted and T2-weighted images and indicated slight peripheral enhancement on delayed contrast-enhanced T1-weighted images. MRI studies performed 3 and 5 months after antibiotic therapy demonstrated that the lesions had decreased in size and no longer enhanced [Duprez, 1996]. MRI features of single lesions may mimick a low-grade glioma [Lohr, 2004].

Neurologic abnormalities can be present without evidence of GI disease [Adams et al., 1987; Halperin et al., 1982; Jovic and Jovic, 1996; Schwartz et al., 1983]. Without treatment, the natural evolution of the disease is always fatal. It responds to antibiotics that cross the blood-brain barrier (such as parenteral penicillin with streptomycin, followed by oral trimethoprim-sulfamethoxazole) given for 1 year, with continuous monitoring of clinical signs and results of cerebrospinal fluid polymerase chain reaction assay [Alba et al., 1995]. Antibiotics, although effective for treating other systemic symptoms, may not affect the progression of neurologic complications [Adams et al., 1987; Halperin et al., 1982; Ratnaike, 2000]. CNS relapse usually is resistant to therapy. Antibiotics can be discontinued only when the results of cerebrospinal fluid polymerase chain reaction assay are negative. Appropriate therapy instituted earlier in the course of the disease is associated with a better neurologic outcome.

Porphyria

The porphyrias are a group of metabolic diseases characterized by abnormalities of porphyrin metabolism resulting from deficiencies in enzymes participating in their biosynthesis, the critical prosthetic group for numerous hemoproteins [Tefferi et al., 1994]. Accumulation of the heme precursor δ-aminolevulinic acid and other photoreactive byproducts, the porphyrins, is associated with neurologic manifestations, cutaneous photosensitivity, and dermatopathic manifestations [Bont et al., 1996; Ellefson and Ford, 1996; Lockwood, 1995]. Clinical manifestations may be neurovisceral or cutaneous, and patients may present with acute attacks or cutaneous lesions or both. Porphyrias are classified as erythropoietic or hepatic, depending on the primary enzyme defect.

Acute intermittent porphyria has an autosomal dominant pattern of inheritance [Schreiber, 1995]. This form of the disease is due to a mutation in the gene encoding porphobilinogen deaminase. Expression of symptoms ranges from mild to severe, and acute episodes of neuropathic porphyrias can progress to paralysis and life-threatening respiratory failure. During an acute attack, measurement of urinary porphobilinogen is the most reliable laboratory test and the method of choice for establishing a diagnosis. DNA mutation analysis is needed to confirm the diagnosis of acute intermittent porphyria [Kauppinen, 2002) and provides 95% sensitivity and approximately 100% specificity [Kauppinen, 2004].

Presentation in childhood is rare [Parsons et al., 1994]. Ten percent of children with DNA-verified acute intermittent porphyria followed prospectively had a clinical attack by the age of 15 years, but symptoms may be vague and of short duration, and urinary δ-aminolevulinic acid and porphobilinogen may be elevated only slightly [Hultdin, 2003]. Neurologic manifestations include abdominal pain, psychosis, and neuropathy [Suarez et al., 1997]. Abdominal pain, the most common complaint, likely results from an underlying autonomic neuropathy with dilatation of the bowel [Gupta and Dolwani, 1996]. Symptoms and signs of neuropathy and cerebrospinal fluid findings may develop acutely, resembling those of Guillain-Barré syndrome [Barohn et al., 1994]. Electrodiagnostic studies indicate axonal polyradiculopathy or neuropathy. Weakness may be asymmetric. CNS manifestations include neuropsychiatric symptoms [Crimlisk, 1997], seizures [Bylesjo et al., 1996], and focal abnormalities such as aphasia, hemiparesis, visual field abnormalities, [King and Bragdon, 1991], cortical blindness, and occipital brain lesions [Kupferschmidt, 1995].

MRI may demonstrate multiple high-signal-intensity abnormalities in the white matter on T2-weighted images [Bylesjo, 2004]. In a case study, a patient with an acute intermittent porphyria attack manifested by abdominal pain and seizures had bilateral lesions on T2-weighted images, especially on fluid-attenuated, inversion recovery (FLAIR) images, which completely resolved with clinical improvement [Utz, 2001]. The MRI abnormalities resemble those seen in patients with the posterior reversible encephalopathy syndrome [Celik, 2002].

The pathophysiology of the porphyric neuropathy is unknown but may relate to neurotoxicity of elevated δ-aminolevulinic acid [Albers, 2004]. Similarly, the pathophysiology of seizures may relate to intrinsic epileptic character of some of the porphyrins or to metabolic abnormalities such as hyponatremia [Solinas, 2004].

Treatment is primarily symptomatic and includes a high-carbohydrate diet, as well as prevention and treatment of water and electrolyte disorders that result from inappropriate antidiuretic hormone production. Long-term management consists of genetic counseling and avoidance of medications (e.g., barbiturates, phenytoin, sulfonamides, chloroquine) that precipitate acute attacks. Of the new antiepileptic drugs, lamotrigine has been reported to precipitate porphyric symptoms, whereas gabapentin has been used successfully to treat seizures in patients with acute intermittent porphyria [Gregersen et al., 1996; Krauss et al., 1995; Tatum and Zachariah, 1995].

NEUROLOGIC DISORDERS ASSOCIATED WITH HEPATOBILIARY DISEASES

Diseases of the liver may be associated with neurologic abnormalities, more commonly with CNS dysfunction, and less commonly with a disruption of the peripheral nervous system. Major neurologic syndromes discussed in this section are hepatitis, hepatic encephalopathy, Wilson's disease, acquired hepatocerebral degeneration (non-Wilsonian), Reye's syndrome, and bilirubin encephalopathy-kernicterus [Jones and Weissenborn, 1997; Lewis and Howdle, 2003; Lockwood, 2002; Raskin and Rowland, 1995; Rothstein and Herlong, 1989; Steinberg and Frank, 1993; Victor and Rothstein, 1992].

This section does not address some of the more specific conditions that affect the liver and the brain, including congenital hyperammonemia, galactosemia, and Zellweger's (cerebrohepatorenal) syndrome, because they are discussed elsewhere in the text. Other neurobehavioral manifestations of liver disease are pruritus in patients with cholestasis, and profound fatigue in patients with chronic cholestasis [Jones, 1995], which also may be associated with altered cerebral neurotransmitter function.

Hepatitis

Encephalitis, myelitis, Guillain-Barré syndrome, and polymyositis are infrequent complications of hepatitis A and B [Peters, 1989]. Similarly, hepatitis C virus infection may be associated with extrahepatic syndromes including those affecting the nervous system [Ghezzi, 2001]. Guillain-Barré syndrome infrequently complicates hepatitis [Tabor, 1987; Zimmerman and Lowry, 1947]. The co-occurrence of these disorders reported in the older literature may have represented cases of infectious mononucleosis or cytomegalovirus infection, both of which are capable of causing Guillain-Barré syndrome and hepatitis. Guillain-Barré syndrome has been reported to occur during the preicteric, icteric, or posticteric phase of the disease, although most patients have clinically apparent hepatitis at the time of onset of their polyneuritis. Circulating immune complexes containing hepatitis B antigens have been detected in serum and cerebrospinal fluid of adult patients at the height of neurologic symptoms, but it is unclear whether this finding is due to intrathecal synthesis or whether it reflects blood-brain barrier dysfunction [Penner et al., 1982; Peters, 1989; Tsukada et al., 1987]. The pattern of recovery appears similar to that in patients with Guillain-Barré syndrome associated with other etiologic disorders.

Other neurologic syndromes associated with viral hepatitis include mononeuritis, auditory neuritis, and seizures. Polymyositis can rarely occur [Mihas et al., 1978]. Clinical peripheral neuropathy is uncommon, but abnormal nerve conduction velocities have been reported [Chari et al., 1977].

The pathophysiology of peripheral nervous system abnormalities associated with hepatitis C may include vasculitis of the epineurial nerves [Heckermann, 1999 Khella, 1995]. The CNS also may be involved, with symptoms and signs including drowsiness, pyramidal signs, and myoclonus. Progressive encephalopathy, encephalomyelitis, and white matter abnormalities have been described [Heckermann, 1999]. Hepatitis C virus antibodies have been found in the cerebrospinal fluid [Propst, 1997]. The pathophysiology of CNS involvement is, similarly, vasculitis associated with hepatitis C virus-related cryoglobulinemia. Interferon-a, steroids, and plasmapheresis were reportedly effective in some cases [Propst, 1997].

Hepatic Encephalopathy

Hepatocellular failure may be complicated by the behavioral syndrome of hepatic encephalopathy characterized by an altered state of consciousness, abnormal mental status, and neurologic abnormalities [Butterworth, 1996]. Hepatic encephalopathy can complicate most liver diseases, whether acute, subacute, or chronic, and can occur with or without portosystemic shunting. Its symptoms and signs are related to the rapidity with which hepatic failure develops, and to its severity. It occurs frequently in patients with liver failure, although less often in affected children. Between 10% and 50% of patients with cirrhosis and/or portosystemic shunt will experience an episode of hepatic encephalopathy at some point during their illness.

Clinically, hepatic encephalopathy can be classified as one of three types—chronic portosystemic encephalopathy, cirrhosis with a precipitant, and acute liver failure [Sherlock, 1977]. Hepatic encephalopathy occurring in a patient with cirrhosis may be either acute or chronic. The acute form usually is associated with a clearly identifiable precipitating factor and usually resolves when the precipitating factor is removed or corrected.

Chronic portosystemic encephalopathy occurs in patients with chronic liver disease in association with the presence of a large portosystemic shunt, which may occur spontaneously when portal vein hypertension induces extensive portal collateral circulation or may be surgically created [Gonzales et al., 1990; Mutchnick et al., 1974]. Portal vein blood bypasses the impaired liver, which normally acts as a detoxification site, and drains directly into the systemic circulation to produce the cerebral intoxication. Hepatic encephalopathy also can occur when patients with underlying hepatic cirrhosis experience precipitating events that depress hepatocellular or cerebral function or increase intestinal nitrogenous material. Precipitating factors include oral protein load, GI bleeding, electrolyte imbalance, infection with consequent deteriorated liver function, and constipation [Basile, 1991].

Etiology

The most common cause of hepatic encephalopathy in the pediatric age group is fulminant viral hepatitis, accounting for 50% to 75% of cases. Other causes include ingestions of drugs and toxins such as paracetamol (acetaminophen), high-dose salicylate therapy, parenteral hyperalimentation, and ingestion of isoniazid, rifampicin, halothane, α-methyldopa, azathioprine, erythromycin, sodium valproate, or tetracycline [Alonso et al., 1995; Bhaduri and Mieli Vergani, 1996; Kalra and Murali, 1986]. In addition, chronic end-stage liver disease caused by biliary atresia, α_1-antitrypsin deficiency, autoimmune chronic active hepatitis, Wilson's disease, and Reye's syndrome also may cause a hepatic encephalopathy. Factors that precipitate hepatic encephalopathy in patients with liver disease include upper GI tract bleeding, usually from esophageal varices; excessive protein intake; use of diuretics, narcotics, sedatives, and hepatotoxic drugs; infections; constipation; hypovolemia and hypoxia. The etiology of hyperammonemia in children also includes disorders involving the urea cycle enzymes (Chapter 24).

Clinical Signs and Symptoms

The hallmark of hepatic encephalopathy is mental status change, including cognitive defects in orientation, memory, affect, perception, attention, and judgment, and deterioration of the level of consciousness [Kalra and Murali, 1986]. The earliest changes are subtle psychiatric and behavioral changes and mild impairments of intellectual function apparent to the patient's family and close friends, which reflect bilateral forebrain, parietal, and temporal dysfunction [Jones, 1997]. Sleep disturbances are a common early sign [Cordoba, 1998]. Initially, verbal ability is relatively well preserved. Later, performance both in work and at school deteriorates, motor functions become impaired, and consciousness decreases. Symptomatic hepatic encephalopathy is traditionally graded into four stages, with derangement of consciousness progressing from drowsiness to stupor and coma:

Grade I: Altered sleep cycle, altered affect (euphoria or belligerence, mild confusion, loss of spatial orientation)
Grade II: Drowsy, responding to simple commands
Grade III: Stuporous, responding only to painful stimuli
Grade IV: Unresponsive to pain, decorticate or decerebrate posturing

The neurologic examination may demonstrate pyramidal tract dysfunction including hypertonia, hyperreflexia, and extensor plantar responses, later changing to hypotonia when coma develops, and early parkinsonian syndrome, which may include hypomimia (i.e., masked facies), muscular rigidity, bradykinesia, monotony of speech, dyskinesia, and Parkinson's disease–like tremor [Spahr, 2000]. Other signs are ataxia, action tremor, dysarthria, and asterixis, a characteristic flapping tremor that consists of frequent involuntary flexion-extension movements of the hand associated electrophysiologically with periods of complete electrical silence in muscles. Asterixis can be elicited by having the patient extend the arms with dorsiflexion of the wrist, which elicits a "flap" [Rio et al., 1995]. Seizures are uncommon, occurring in 10% to 30% of patients [Decell et al., 1994]. Focal neurologic abnormalities may be findings [Cadranel, 2001], as can cerebral and retinal visual abnormalities [Miyata, 1988; Eckstein, 1997].

Cerebral edema is a frequent complication in late-stage hepatic encephalopathy in patients with acute liver failure and may be the cause of death. It is rarely seen in patients with encephalopathy resulting from chronic liver disease [Yanda, 1988]. Clinical signs are those of increased intracranial pressure and include dilated and sluggishly reactive pupils, respiratory changes, and increased muscle tone with decerebrate posturing.

Hepatic encephalopathy also can occur after the surgical placement of a portosystemic shunt. Symptoms and signs are similar to those of hepatic encephalopathy from other causes, but the occurrence of spastic paraparesis also has been described [Pantel et al, 1968b; Reskin et al., 1984]. On histopathologic examination, evidence of myelopathy with degeneration of the anterior and lateral corticospinal tracts is seen.

Some patients without liver disease who undergo portocaval shunting may have favorable neuropsychologic outcomes. In a study of portal vein obstruction without liver disease, 42 children were studied up to 24 years after surgery that had been performed between 2 and 14 years of age [Alagille et al., 1986]. Two control groups composed of children who had undergone other abdominal surgical procedures and children with portal vein obstruction that was not shunted also were studied. Serum ammonia levels were higher in the children with portosystemic shunts but little difference in scholastic achievement was found. Visual memory and spatial-temporal tests indicated slightly worse results in the portocaval shunt group. Findings on neurologic examination and EEG were similar in all groups.

Laboratory Tests

The diagnosis of hepatic encephalopathy is established clinically. No consistent correlation has been found between any specific laboratory test and the severity of symptoms caused by hepatic encephalopathy. Results of liver function tests usually are abnormal, but derangements may not be as drastic as expected from findings on the examination. Arterial blood ammonia may be elevated and correlates to some degree with the clinical state and the rate of ammonia uptake and metabolism by the brain, although the level does not correlate with the severity of encephalopathy [Kramer, 2000]. Cerebrospinal fluid glutamine concentration is more specific than blood ammonia and correlates better with the stage of hepatic encephalopathy. Neuropsychologic tests provide useful information, especially in patients with subclinical hepatic encephalopathy that would otherwise be overlooked.

Electrophysiologic Studies

The EEG is characteristic, although not specific, and correlates with clinical staging of hepatic encephalopathy. In the early stages, it demonstrates progressive slowing of the alpha rhythm, mixed with theta activity. With further clouding of consciousness, slower delta frequencies occur. As with other metabolic encephalopathies, triphasic waves may be present and are seen at a late stage of encepahopathy and usually carry a poor prognosis. These waves may, however, not be seen in young children [Sherlock, 1977]. Occasionally, triphasic waves occur before encephalopathy is clinically evident; this finding is useful in the differential diagnosis. Subsequently, wave amplitude decreases, and finally, cerebral activity ceases altogether. Brainstem and somatosensory evoked potential latencies are delayed [Chu, 1997; Jones, 2001; Kullmann et al., 1995; Sexana,, 2001], although the role of evoked potentials in patients with varying degrees of hepatic encephalopathy remains unclear.

Neuroimaging

CT scans may demonstrate cortical atrophy or cerebral edema, but findings may be normal early in the course of hepatic encephalopathy. Abnormalities detected by MRI in adults with non-Wilsonian chronic hepatic failure demonstrate increased signal in basal ganglia regions and in the anterior pituitary on T1-weighted images without corresponding abnormalities on T2-weighted images [Ballauff et al., 1994; Pujol et al., 1991; Weissenborn et al., 1995]. Significant abnormalities have not been demonstrated in the cerebral cortex or cerebellum. The MRI appearance does not correlate with laboratory indices of hepatic function, with histologic liver diagnosis, or with neurologic status at the time of MRI acquisition [Brunberg et al., 1991]. MR spectroscopy typically indicates depletion of myoinositol, preservation of *N*-acetylaspartate, and elevations in glutamine [Laubenberger et al, 1997].

Neuropathology

The neuropathologic characteristics of hepatic encephalopathy were initially described by Fredrichs in his "Treatise on Liver Disease" [1860] and later confirmed by Adams and Foley [1953]. The pathologic hallmark of hepatic encephalopathy in patients with cirrhosis and with portosystemic shunts is the presence of Alzheimer type II astrocytes, found in many brain regions, including the cortex and the lenticular, lateral thalamic, dentate, and red nuclei [Lockwood, 2001]. Although not specific to hepatic encephalopathy [Adams and Foley, 1952], these hypertrophic astrocytes are commonly found in the brains of patients who die with cirrhosis and portosystemic shunting, develop shortly after the onset of hepatic encephalopathy, and are related to the duration of coma; the neuropathologic changes are reversible [Sherlock, 1977; Norenberg, 1987]. Other significant parenchymal neuropathologic abnormalities are not present. In acute fulminant hepatic failure, the major finding is the presence of cerebral edema.

Pathophysiology

A major determinant causing hepatic encephalopathy is the metabolic effects of products toxic to the brain [Treem, 1996]. Such products, such as those related to bacterial action on proteins in the large intestine, normally are metabolized by the liver. In the presence of parenchymal liver disease or portosystemic shunting, these toxins accumulate in the extracellular fluid and reach the brain. In addition, the blood-brain barrier may be damaged in patients with liver failure, resulting in an increased permeability and increased access of such substances to the brain. Ammonia is regarded as the most likely toxin [Butterworth, 1987], although patients with hepatic encephalopathy may have normal blood ammonia levels. Multiple other agents have been implicated in the pathogenesis of hepatic encephalopathy, including short-chain fatty acids, mercaptans, false neurotransmitters, and γ-aminobutyric acid (GABA), a predominant CNS inhibitor. The relation between ammonia and hepatic encephalopathy is based on the following [Gabuzda, 1952]: (1) ammonia levels in serum and cerebrospinal fluid are elevated in hepatic failure; (2) a correlation exists between the degree of hyperammonemia and the depth of coma; (3) levels of glutamine and α-ketoglutarate (metabolites of ammonia) are elevated in the brain and cerebrospinal fluid of patients with hepatic encephalopathy; (4) hepatic encephalopathy results in neuropathologic damage (Alzheimer type II astrocytes) similar to that found in patients with congenital hyperammonemia caused by inherited defects of urea cycle enzymes or in animal models of hepatic portocaval encephalopathy [Cooper and Plum, 1987; Zieve, 1981]; and (5) the most effective treatments for hepatic encephalopathy involve lowering ammonia concentration.

Ammonia is produced in the intestinal tract by bacterial breakdown of ingested protein, transported to the liver by the hepatic portal vein, and converted to urea by the urea cycle enzymes; the urea is then excreted by the kidneys. Regardless of the etiology of elevated plasma ammonia levels, brain ammonia concentrations generally are increased in hepatic coma. This elevation may be due to increased permeability of the blood-brain barrier, allowing ammonia to more freely diffuse into the brain. This situation results in an ammonia-induced encephalopathy, although arterial ammonia levels are near normal or normal, and explains the emergence of toxin hypersensitivity as liver disease progresses [Lockwood, 1991].

In the brain, ammonia normally is detoxified by astrocytes, combining with α-ketoglutarate to form glutamic acid, which then forms glutamine, leading to elevated glutamine levels in the cerebrospinal fluid in cases of hepatic encephalopathy [Fraser and Arieff, 1985]. Elevated cerebrospinal fluid glutamine levels may be more specific than blood ammonia levels for hepatic encephalopathy. In addition, conversion of ammonia to glutamine requires ATP, and because of reduced ATP availability, slowing of the tricarboxylic cycle may occur.

Several mechanisms have been proposed to explain the neurotoxic action of ammonia, including modification of blood-brain barrier transport, effects on glucose metabolism and brain energy production, disruption of amino acid profiles in the brain (particularly glutamate), and alteration of the chloride pump and normal neuronal membrane physiology [Shields, 1992]. As previously discussed, however, hyperammonemia alone cannot explain the severity of hepatic encephalopathy[Kalra and Murali, 1986; Sherlock, 1977].

GABA, a principal neurotransmitter, is synthesized by intestinal bacteria. It is the major inhibitory neurotransmitter in the human brain. Increased GABA-mediated neurotransmission is known to cause impaired consciousness and psychomotor dysfunction. A few lines of evidence, some from studies in animal models, support the hypothesis that increased GABA-mediated neurotransmission contributes to the manifestations of hepatic encephalopathy [Basile, 1991; Jones, 1994]. Both increased GABA release and enhanced activation of the GABA receptor complex have been demonstrated [Albrecht, 1999]. GABA levels are markedly elevated in patients with fulminant hepatic failure and correlate well with the stage of encephalopathy [Ferenci et al., 1983]. Elevated plasma levels may be due to defective hepatic clearance by GABA transaminase. With impaired blood-brain barrier function, GABA accumulates postsynaptically, resulting in neuronal membrane inhibition. In a rabbit model, development of hepatic encephalopathy was associated with increased plasma levels of GABA, increased blood-brain barrier permeability, increased brain GABA and benzodiazepine binding sites, and a pattern of neuronal activity similar to that induced by drugs that activate the GABA neurotransmitter system [Schafer and Jones, 1982]. Similarly, patients who died with chronic liver disease and encephalopathy were found to have an increased density of brain GABA receptors, suggesting that symptoms were related to increased sensitivity of brain to GABAergic (mediated by GABA) neural inhibition [Jones and Schafer, 1986]. It was postulated that a combination of chronic low-grade glial edema and potentiation of the effect of GABA on the CNS by ammonia may be responsible for many of the symptoms of hepatic encephalopathy [Basile, 1997; Haussinger, 2002; Lewis, 2003].

In addition, benzodiazepine receptor ligands ameliorated both the behavioral depression and visual-evoked response abnormalities in the thioactamide-induced rat model of hepatic encephalopathy, suggesting involvement of the GABA/benzodiazepine receptor complex [Gammal et al., 1990]. Benzodiazepines can act at the type A GABA ($GABA_A$) receptor complex, and increased concentrations of endogenous benzodiazepines are found in the brain in liver failure [Basile, 1994]. Increased sensitivity of the brain of patients with cirrhosis to an exogenously administered benzodiazepine has been demonstrated [Jones, 1997]. Some patients with hepatic encephalopathy improve after administration of the $GABA_A$ receptor antagonist flumazenil.

Plasma levels of amino acids, short-chain free fatty acids, and substance P also are elevated in hepatic encephalopathy. False neurotransmitters, such as octopamine, are elevated in the brain and cerebrospinal fluid. Thus, it is possible that hepatic encephalopathy may be mediated by the synergistic actions of a number of agents, including ammonia, GABA, and mercaptans [Treem, 1996]. Neurotransmitters other than GABA may be involved in the pathogenesis of hepatic encephalopathy. These include glutamate, dopamine, serotonin, and opioid systems.

Therapy

Hepatic encephalopathy is reversible with medical treatment and is directed at removal or correction of any precipitating factors, reduction of absorption of nitrogenous substances from the intestinal tract, and reduction of increased portosystemic shunting [Jones, 1997]. Most effective therapies are based on reducing the ammonia concentration and treating various complications, including infections, renal and cardiovascular dysfunction, and bleeding secondary to ruptured varices, hypersplenism, or clotting factor deficiencies [Riordan and Williams, 1997]. Therapy also is effective for portosystemic encephalopathy but much less so for fulminant hepatic failure.

Ammonia production can be reduced by decreasing dietary protein, treating constipation, controlling GI tract bleeding, and reducing the bacterial content of the intestinal tract. Ammonia also can be removed from the gut by the osmotic action of nonabsorbable disaccharides such as lactulose. Lactulose is metabolized in the lower intestinal tract to lactic acid, reduces local pH (to 5.5), and inhibits growth of colonic organisms and the formation of ammonia. Ammonia is converted to the ammonium ion (NH_4) and is then excreted in the stool [Sherlock, 1987]. The resulting decrease in ammonia concentration is associated with improvements in mental status and correction of EEG abnormalities. Complications of lactulose therapy include dehydration and hypernatremia. Reduction of gut ammonia also can be achieved using antibiotics, such as neomycin, that are active against urease-producing bacteria. The efficacy of neomycin is similar to that of lactulose [Conn et al., 1977]. Treatments aimed at reversing the neurotransmitter defects, including the use of flumazenil, are still experimental. The imidazobenzodiazepine flumazenil, a benzodiazepine receptor antagonist, is a selective, high-affinity, competitive antagonist of central benzodiazepine receptors on the $GABA_A$-benzodiazepine receptor complex. It competes with high specificity with benzodiazepine receptor agonist ligands (for example, diazepam) for binding to those receptors. It is useful for the component of hepatic encephalopathy related to the effects of natural benzodiazepine receptor agonists. Flumazenil given as an intravenous bolus injection improved clinical and electrophysiologic signs of hepatic encephalopathy; some evidence suggests that it reduced the severity of hepatic encephalopathy [Ferenci, 1996; Gooday, 1995; Jones, 1990]

Management of acute severe cerebral edema involves restriction of intravenous fluids, use of hyperosmolar agents (e.g., mannitol, 3% normal saline), and in selected patients, intubation and hyperventilation [Murphy et al., 2004; Yanda, 1988;]. Cerebral edema is best controlled with mannitol (0.25 to 0.5 g/kg) infused rapidly over 20 minutes every 4 to 6 hours. Higher doses may cause a hyperosmolar state and result in decreased cerebral perfusion. Usually three to six doses are sufficient; prolonged use is not recommended. Intracranial pressure monitoring, although involving some risk, may in certain clinical situations be of value in assessing the effects of treatment and progression of the disease. Mannitol is contraindicated in patients with hepatorenal syndrome [Kalra and Murali, 1986]. A role for liver transplantation in fulminant hepatic failure has emerged over the past decade [Liu et al., 2003; Schafer and Shaw, 1989].

Prognosis

The prognosis for hepatic encephalopathy has not changed significantly over the past two decades, despite improvement in intensive medical support [Bustamante et al., 1999]. The 1-year survival rate is 40%, and the 3-year survival rate is 15%. Fulminant hepatic failure carries a mortality rate of 75%, and severe hepatic coma is associated with a substantial risk of permanent neurologic disability. On the other hand, the encephalopathy in patients who recover from acute liver failure can resolve without residual neurologic sequelae because, in most cases, brain structural lesions are reversible.

MINIMAL HEPATIC ENCEPHALOPATHY

Patients with cirrhosis of the liver are frequently cognitively impaired, even though they do not have evidence of overt encephalopathy. Minimal hepatic encephalopathy was known in the past as *subclinical hepatic encephalopathy* and refers to chronic liver disease in patients who are believed to be clinically non-encephalopathic but in fact have signs of cognitive impairment. Findings on the routine neurologic examination are normal, but application of psychometric and electrophysiologic tests discloses abnormal brain function [Groeneweg et al, 2000; Schmerus and Hamster, 1998]. Common findings on cognitive testing include impairments of visuospatial functioning, attention, and psychomotor speed [Weissenborn, 2001]. The neurophysiologic technique of critical flicker frequency was suggested to be an effective test of minimal hepatic encephalopathy [Kircheis, 2002]. This test establishes the frequency at which a flashing light appears to stop flashing and becomes continuous (fusion frequency). This finding suggests that hepatic encephalopathy represents a continuum, with variable degrees of impairment. Minimal hepatic encephalopathy has an impact on the patient's quality life; accordingly, appropriate treatment should be given [Groeneweg, 1998; Weissenborn, 2001]. Treatment of minimal hepatic encephalopathy is similar to treatment of overt hepatic encephalopathy, with dietary protein restriction and lactulose treatment. The prognostic significance of this condition is not clear [Amodio, 1999; Hartmann, 2000].

FULMINANT LIVER FAILURE

Fulminant liver failure is said to occur when hepatic encephalopathy occurs within 1 to several weeks of the first manifestation of liver disease [Bernuau, 1993]. Rapid loss of hepatocellular function favors the development of cerebral edema and raised intracranial pressure, which can lead to brain ischemia as a result of compression of cerebral vasculature, and to brainstem herniation. Raised intracranial pressure due to cerebral edema can contribute to neurologic deficits. Agitation and seizures are additional findings. Ammonia concentration higher than that usually associated with hepatic encephalopathy in cirrhotic patients can occur and may be responsible for symptoms of neurotoxicity such as psychomotor agitation, muscle twitching, mania, delirium, or seizures, especially in children. The higher ammonia concentrations also may contribute to the pathogenesis of cerebral edema and raised intracranial pressure by promoting increased conversion of glutamate to the organic osmolyte glutamine in astrocytes. From 70% to 80% of the patients with fulminant hepatic failure that progress to stage IV encephalopathy have cerebral edema. The mortality rate is high at 80% to 90% [Alper, 1998], although hepatic structure, histologic characteristics, and function can be completely restored in survivors [Yanda, 1988]. Survival rates have been improving, because many of the patients are receiving liver transplants [Bismuth, 1996; Hassanein, 1997]. Management includes monitoring for hypoglycemia and increased intracranial pressure and treatment as indicated [Donovan, 1992; Lidofsky, 1992] and maintenance of adequate cerebral perfusion pressure.

COGNITIVE ABNORMALITIES IN CHILDREN WITH LIVER DISEASE

Children with end-stage liver disease have cognitive delays relative to developmental gains made by children with cystic fibrosis or healthy children. Cognitive abnormalities are related to the age at onset and severity of disease [Stewart et al., 1991, 1992]. Nonverbal intelligence is affected more than verbal intelligence. Patients with intellectual impairment have an earlier onset and longer duration of illness, poorer nutritional status, and greater degree of vitamin E deficiency [Stewart et al., 1988]. When examined 1 year after transplantation, older children were more likely to have impairments of cognitive and social function [Stewart et al.,

1989]. With longer follow-up periods (up to 5 years), cognitive abilities remained unchanged, but gross motor function was better, and patients' behavior as judged by parental perceptions improved [Zitelli et al., 1988].

NEUROLOGIC COMPLICATIONS OF LIVER TRANSPLANTATION

Liver transplantation usually results in improved brain function in patients with hepatic encephalopathy, including a significant improvement in cognitive functioning, but patients do not return to normal, suggesting that hepatic encephalopathy is not completely reversible [Moore, 2000].

Neurologic complications also may arise after transplantation in a large percentage of patients [Blanco et al., 1995; Patchell, 1994]. Seventeen of 52 (33%) patients who underwent 56 orthotopic transplantation procedures had serious postoperative neurologic complications [Adams et al., 1987]. These complications included encephalopathy, seizures, involuntary movements, cortical blindness, brachial plexopathy, and peripheral neuropathy [Appleton et al., 1989; Estol et al., 1989a, 1989b; Garg et al., 1993]. Etiologic factors include air embolism, graft-versus-host reactions, coagulopathy-associated cerebral hemorrhage, seizures or central pontine myelinolysis resulting from severe electrolyte and metabolic changes, cerebral infarction resulting from perioperative hypotension, and meningoencephalitis or cerebral abscess resulting from opportunistic infection. Drug-induced neurologic disorders also may occur.

A common complication that occurs in 25% of patients, mostly within the first week after transplantation, is seizures [Adams et al., 1987]. Epileptiform activity seen on EEG is more frequent in patients who die than in survivors [Wszolek et al., 1991]. In one study, 21 patients who had seizures were found at postmortem examination to have combinations of the following: ischemic or hemorrhagic strokes in 18 patients, central pontine myelinosis in 5, and CNS infection in 5 [Estol et al., 1989a]. Multiple metabolic abnormalities were a contributing factor to the onset of seizures.

Immunosuppression may lead to opportunistic infections in the months after liver transplantation [Shields, 1992]. The most common organisms causing CNS infection include *Listeria monocytogenes*, *Cryptococcus neoformans*, disseminated *Nocardia* organisms, and disseminated *Aspergillus* organisms. Chronic dementia can be caused by progressive multifocal leukoencephalopathy.

Cyclosporine is an effective immunosuppressive agent, but it may have adverse effects on the CNS [Appleton et al., 1989]. It has been reported to cause a syndrome of encephalopathy without papilledema, cortical blindness, and seizures with white matter lesions that are sometimes hemorrhagic and are predominantly but not exclusively posterior [DeGroen et al., 1987; Rubin and Kang, 1987]. CT demonstrates nonenhancing areas of hypoattenuation, and MRI indicates T2 prolongation in these regions [Truwit et al., 1991]. A disorder of speech and language including mutism, dysarthria, and speech apraxia, with elements of aphasia, also has been described as a complication of orthotopic liver transplantation and may be related to cyclosporine therapy [Bird et al., 1990; Bronster et al., 1995; Stein et al., 1992]. Concurrent high-dose methylprednisolone treatment, hypertension, and possibly other metabolic abnormalities may be contributing factors to encephalopathy and seizures in such patients. Low total serum cholesterol also has been reported in some of these patients [Truwit et al., 1991]. Suggested mechanisms relating cholesterol to the cyclosporine-induced CNS toxicity include interference of cyclosporine with the transport of cholesterol and other lipids into the brain and an increase in cyclosporine concentration in lipoprotein particles resulting from low cholesterol levels, thereby increasing the brain uptake of cyclosporine. Symptoms and signs, as well as radiographic findings, are reversed after discontinuation or reduction in the dose of cyclosporine.

Other neurologic complications of liver transplantation include central pontine myelinolysis, especially with significant serum sodium changes. Careful monitoring of electrolytes in patients undergoing liver transplantation in the perioperative period is recommended [Estol et al., 1989a]. Increased intracranial pressure with reduced cerebral perfusion can occur during or within hours after liver transplantation, and therapy with mannitol may be necessary [Keays et al., 1991].

Chronic inflammatory demyelinating polyradiculoneuropathy or sensorimotor neuropathy has been reported after liver transplantation [Taylor et al., 1995] but is rare and has been tentatively linked to the use of immunosuppressive medications. A recent decrease in the incidence of neurologic complications after liver transplantation has been described and attributed to the immediate withdrawal of cyclosporine at the onset of a change in mental status or dysarthria and improvement in intraoperative and postoperative management [Stein et al., 1992].

Reye's Syndrome

Reye's syndrome is an uncommon syndrome characterized by an acute encephalopathy with fatty infiltration of various organs including the liver, kidney, and heart [Belay et al., 1999; Casteels-Van Daele et al., 2000; DeVivo, 1985; Glasgow and Middleton, 2001]. The syndrome typically is associated with viral illnesses such as influenza B and varicella, as well as salicylate therapy. Studies have established an increased risk for Reye's syndrome after aspirin use; in general, salicylates should be avoided in children [Hurwitz et al., 1985]. Some metabolic conditions (e.g., carnitine deficiency, organic acidurias, medium chain acyl-coenzyme A [CoA] dehydrogenase deficiency) can cause recurrent Reye-like syndrome. Therefore, patients with recurrent episodes should be evaluated for evidence of an underlying metabolic disorder (see Chapters 23 through 26 on metabolic disorders).

Patients with Reye's syndrome have abnormalities of mitochondrial function that cause a variety of metabolic derangements of carbohydrates, amino acids, fatty acids, clotting factors, ammonia, lactate, and acid-base balance. Insufficient energy availability to the brain results in massive cytotoxic edema [DeVivo, 1985].

Clinical presentation involves an antecedent viral infection followed by vomiting and marked changes in sensorium that may start with a hyperexcitable stage and progress to lethargy and coma with decorticate posturing. The latter symptoms are secondary to increased intracranial pressure and central herniation as a result of brain edema [Reye et al., 1963]. Clinical staging systems, consisting of four or five stages, have been reported and are based on the cephalocaudal progression of brainstem dysfunction secondary to increased intracranial pressure [Lovejoy et al., 1974] or on EEG criteria [Aoki and Lombroso, 1973].

Reported laboratory abnormalities include marked elevations of hepatic transaminases, prolongation of the prothrombin time, hyperammonemia, hypoglycemia, increases in plasma fatty acid levels, elevation of plasma lactate, and reduced phosphorus concentrations [DeVivo, 1985; Lockwood, 1995; Tonsgard et al., 1982]. Neuroimaging, MR spectroscopy, and single-photon emission computed tomography studies have been reported in several patients with Reye's syndrome, most of whom suffer severe sequelae [Kinoshita et al., 1996; Kreis et al., 1995; Ozawa et al., 1997].

The gross pathologic abnormalities described by Reye and colleagues [1963] consisted of "cerebral swelling, a slightly enlarged, firm, and uniformly bright-yellow liver, and pallor and slight widening of the renal cortex." Microscopic liver pathologic findings include microvesicular fatty infiltration, glycogen depletion, depleted Golgi membranes, proliferation of peroxisomes, and distorted mitochondria. Similar abnormalities of mitochondria together with lipid droplet accumulation and glycogen depletion have been seen in muscle biopsy specimens. Brain histopathologic examination demonstrates similar changes in mitochondria and abnormalities of myelin, as well as generalized cerebral edema. Biochemical studies demonstrate decreased activity of mitochondrial enzymes.

The most important therapeutic measure is reduction of intracranial pressure with intravenous mannitol or furosemide and hyperventilation (with carbon dioxide tension maintained at approximately 25 mm Hg). In selected patients, hypothermia or high-dose barbiturates can be used to control intracranial pressure elevations. Continuous measurements of intracranial pressure are helpful in monitoring the effects of therapy. Additional supportive treatments include the use of hypertonic glucose solution (15% to 20%) with intravenous insulin, fluid restriction, maintaining electrolyte balance and serum osmolality below 320 mOsm/L, correction of clotting factors, and fever reduction [Trauner, 1990]. Decompressive craniotomy may be beneficial in selected patients. Exchange transfusions, once popular in the 1970s and 1980s, are no longer used, provided that intracranial pressure is monitored and can be controlled by other conventional treatments.

Prognosis

Initial reports suggested that Reye's syndrome was associated with a high mortality rate, particularly in those patents with grade IV or V EEG abnormalities [Van Caillie et al., 1977]. Currently, the prognosis is much improved if the condition is recognized early and treated aggressively. Cognitive, neurologic, and psychological deficits that are frequently subtle but lasting can be found in some survivors [Meekin et al., 1999]. An international perspective reviewing etiologic and epidemiologic aspects of Reye's syndrome has been published [Stumpf, 1995].

Hepatolenticular Degeneration: Wilson's Disease

Wilson's disease is a rare defect of copper metabolism manifesting in late childhood or adolescence, with an autosomal-recessive pattern of inheritance [Pleskow and Grand, 1996]. Its manifestations are due to the toxic effects of copper deposition in various organs, including the brain, liver, kidneys, and corneas [Loudianos and Gitlin, 2000]. Copper is needed as a catalyst for numerous biologic processes, mainly those involving the utilization of oxygen. Mutations of genes that code for copper-transporting ATPase enzymes constitute the molecular basis for Wilson's and Menkes' diseases. Wilson's disease is characterized by excessive deposition of copper in the liver as a result of deficiency in biliary copper secretion, and subsequently throughout the body, mainly in the CNS and kidney, resulting in liver disease and in neuropsychiatric disease [El Youssef, 2003].

As with Menkes' disease, the Wilson's disease gene product has characteristics of a copper-transporting ATPase. It is located on 13q14 and encodes a copper-transporting ATPase [Schilsky, 1996]. It may serve a function in the export of copper from cells, whereas the Menkes' disease gene product has a role in the import of copper [Tanzi et al., 1993]. Another gene, the *MURR1* gene, also may be important for biliary copper excretion. [Wijmenga, 2004]. Ceruloplasmin functions in the enzymatic transfer of copper to copper-containing enzymes, such as cytochrome oxidase. Reduced activity of this enzyme has been reported in patients with Wilson's disease [Shokeir and Shreffler, 1969].

Liver disease can occur in the form of hepatitis and cirrhosis. Neurologic manifestations are gradual in onset and include cognitive abnormalities; dementia; movement disorders, including tremors of the hand or head, whole-body dystonia and rigidity, or other parkinsonian features; ataxia; and occasionally seizures [Lockwood, 1995; Steinberg and Frank, 1993]. Three subsets of patients with Wilson's disease have been recognized [Oder, 1993]: (1) pseudoparkinsonian patients, with dilatation of the third ventricle, who have signs of bradykinesia, rigidity, cognitive impairment, and an organic mood syndrome; (2) pseudosclerosis patients, with focal thalamic lesions, who exhibit ataxia, tremor, and reduced functional capacity; and (3) dyskinesia patients, with focal abnormalities of the putamen and globus pallidus, who exhibit dyskinesia, dysarthria, and an organic personality syndrome. Psychiatric symptoms often correlate with the severity of the neurologic disturbances [Akil, 1991; Dening, 1989, 1990]

In children, deterioration in school achievement and the development of abnormal behavioral or conduct disorders begin insidiously and progress slowly [Lingam et al., 1987]. Neurologic manifestations have been reported in children as young as 6 years of age, although traditionally, children younger than 10 years have the hepatic form of the disease and children older than 10 years have neurologic involvement, [Jones, 2000; Lingam et al., 1987; Scheinberg and Sternlieb, 1984; Walshe and Yealland, 1992]. Psychiatric disorders are common and include mania, psychosis, depression, and even schizophrenia. All patients with neurologic and psychiatric manifestations develop corneal Kayser-Fleischer rings, areas of granular brown pigmentation encircling the cornea caused by copper deposition in Descemet's membrane, which can be visualized by slit-lamp examination of the cornea.

Diagnosis is based on clinical and biochemical data [Sternleib, 1993]. In a patient with neurologic signs, a diagnosis of Wilson's disease can be made if Kayser-Fleischer rings are present and the ceruloplasmin concentration is less than 20 mg/dL. From 80% to 90% of patients with the disease have low serum ceruloplasmin concentration (less than 20 mg/dL). Other findings include increased urinary copper excretion and elevated liver copper concentration. Serum ceruloplasmin levels are low, and 24-hour urinary excretion is increased [Pleskow and Grand, 1996]. Liver biopsy and examination using radioactive ^{64}Cu or ^{67}Cu can be performed to study hepatic copper levels and metabolism.

Neuroimaging abnormalities are common in patients with Wilson's disease. CT scan abnormalities reported in 60 patients with Wilson's disease included ventriculomegaly (found in 73% of the patients), cortical atrophy (in 63%), brainstem atrophy (in 45%), hypodensities in the basal ganglia (in 45%), posterior fossa atrophy (in 10%), and no abnormalities (in 18%) [Williams and Walshe, 1981]. More recent studies have confirmed these CT observations [van Wassenaer–van Hall et al., 1996], and extended them to MRI [King et al., 1996]. MRI is more sensitive than CT in detecting abnormalities [Nazer, 1993]. CT findings are abnormal in 50% of asymptomatic patients. Cranial CT and MRI abnormalities other than brain atrophy can be reversed with chelation therapy [Roh, 1994]. Using positron emission tomography, changes in dopaminergic metabolic markers correlate with structural MRI changes but not with clinical symptoms [Westermark et al., 1995]. Proton MR spectroscopy in neurologically symptomatic patients with Wilson's disease indicates reduced *N*-acetylaspartate-to-creatine ratios and can determine the degree of neuronal loss in these patients [Van Den Heuvel et al., 1997].

Neuropathologic examination reveals diffuse copper deposition, atrophy of the caudate and putamen, neuronal loss, and Alzheimer type II astrocytes with cortical and basal ganglia demyelination [Yarze, 1992]. Abnormalities of the white matter and cerebral cortex occur in approximately 10% of cases [Brewer, 1992]. Copper concentrations in affected and unaffected regions of the brain are similar.

Treatment is directed at reducing systemic copper levels with a low-copper diet and with several anticopper medications. The four drugs currently used include (1) zinc, which blocks intestinal absorption of copper, (2) penicillamine and (3) trientine, both of which are chelators that increase urinary excretion of copper, and (4) tetrathiomolybdate, which forms a tripartite complex with copper and protein and can block copper absorption from the intestine or render blood copper nontoxic [Brewer, 1995; Ferenci, 2004]. Zinc is considered by some investigators to be the therapeutic agent of choice for maintenance therapy, for treatment of the presymptomatic patient from the beginning, and for treatment of the pregnant patient because of its efficacy and lack of toxicity [Brewer, 1995; Czlonkowska et al., 1996]. For patients with mild liver failure, combined treatment with trientine and zinc is effective [Brewer, 1995; Dahlman et al., 1995]. Trientine gives a strong, fast, negative copper balance, and zinc induces hepatic metallothionein, which sequesters hepatic copper. For patients with neurologic disease, tetrathiomolybdate is now preferred by some groups of investigators to penicillamine [Brewer et al., 1994; Schilsky, 1996]. Tetrathiomolybdate provides rapid, safe control of copper levels. Patients who receive penicillamine are at great risk of serious permanent neurologic worsening [Brewer, 1995] or side effects of this drug, which include rash, bone marrow suppression, immune complex disorders, nephrotic syndrome, optic neuropathy, and loss of taste. Pyridoxine should be given concurrently in those patients receiving penicillamine. Most of the psychiatric manifestations and cognitive abnormalities usually respond to copper chelation therapy [Dening, 1990; Lang, 1990; Lingam et al., 1987]. MRI abnormalities also may remit after treatment [Takahashi, 1996]. When patients with neurologic and psychiatric manifestations are diagnosed late in the course of the disease, some psychiatric dysfunction may remain.

In selected patients, primarily those with fulminant hepatitis or chronic hepatic insufficiency with or without neurologic symptoms, liver transplantation may be successful [Bellary et al., 1995; Chen et al., 1997; Schilsky et al., 1994]. Patients with neurologic Wilson's disease in the absence of hepatic insufficiency also may have clinical improvement [Bax et al., 1998]. Case reports of patients who underwent liver transplantation for Wilson's disease demonstrated an increase in ceruloplasmin level, disappearance of the Kayser-Fleischer ring, and normalization of urinary copper excretion. Neuropsychiatric abnormalities, as well as MRI abnormalities, tend to remit [Geissler, 2003; Stracciari, 2000], although not always [Kassam, 1998].

Acquired Hepatocellular Degeneration and Hepatic Myelopathy

Alpers' syndrome, described first by Alpers in 1931, is a heterogeneous group of disorders affecting young children manifested by progressive neurologic degeneration with seizures, brain atrophy with neuronal necrosis, and sometimes liver disease. It is discussed in detail in Chapter 59.

Bilirubin Encephalopathy: Kernicterus

Bilirubin is the end product of the catabolism of heme, the major source of which is circulating hemoglobin. Bilirubin is transported in plasma bound to albumin and converted in the liver to an excretable conjugated form. Conjugated bilirubin is then excreted into the bile, transported to the small intestine, further degraded by intestinal bacteria, and excreted in the stool.

Physiologic hyperbilirubinemia occurs in the first week of life as a result of increased bilirubin load to the liver and decreased bilirubin-conjugating capacity. A number of disorders in the newborn period, however, may lead to much higher concentrations of unconjugated bilirubin [Yao and Stevenson, 1995]. These include hemolytic diseases of the newborn caused by blood group incompatibility (but also some hemoglobinopathies), hemorrhage, polycythemia, inherited or acquired defects of conjugation, and hypothyroidism.

Some evidence suggests that bilirubin is injurious to neurons, particularly in its unconjugated form [Shapiro, 2003]. Acidosis and hypoalbuminemia facilitate the neurotoxicity of bilirubin and increase the risk of kernicterus. Bilirubin anions can bind to phospholipid. Bilirubin-phospholipid complexes are lipophilic, allowing bilirubin to move across the blood-brain barrier. Such mobility is increased when the blood-brain barrier is disrupted (e.g., with sepsis, asphyxia, or meningitis). In the full-term infant with marked hyperbilirubinemia secondary to hemolytic disease, a clear correlation can be established between the occurrence of kernicterus and the maximal recorded level of serum bilirubin [Maisels and Newman, 1995; Newman and Maisels, 1992; Penn et al., 1994]. In the preterm infant, kernicterus has occurred without marked hyperbilirubinemia [Watchko and Claassen, 1994]. These infants are more likely to have acidosis, asphyxia, hypothermia, or sepsis.

A distinctive regional topography and selective susceptibility of specific neurons to kernicterus have been described [Levine, 1988; Notter and Kendig, 1985]. In the brain, the bilirubin anion–phospholipid complex can attach to and destroy cellular membranes, thereby affecting multiple enzyme systems and organelles, particularly mitochondria, with resulting disturbances in mitochondrial respiration and oxidative phosphorylation, glycolysis, glycogen synthesis, citric acid cycle function, cyclic adenosine monophosphate synthesis, amino acid and protein metabolism, DNA synthesis, lipid metabolism, myelination, and synthesis and transport of neurotransmitters [Brann et al., 1987; Schiff et al., 1985; Wennberg et al., 1991].

The neuropathologic features of acute bilirubin encephalopathy consist of bilirubin staining followed by neuronal necrosis [Connolly and Volpe, 1990; Turkel, 1990]. Brain bilirubin staining and injury are selective. The regions most commonly stained by bilirubin are the basal ganglia, hippocampus, cranial nerve VIII nuclei and tracts, other brainstem and cerebellar nuclei, and the anterior horn cells of the spinal cord. The cerebral cortical neurons are mildly involved [Hayashi et al., 1991].

Early neuronal changes consist of swollen granular cytoplasm and disruption of neuronal and nuclear membranes, followed by neuronal loss with prominent astrocytosis. Distribution of neuronal injury is similar to that of the bilirubin staining. Little staining but severe neuronal loss occurs in Purkinje cells, especially in the preterm infant.

The sequence of acute bilirubin encephalopathy consists of three phases: (1) stupor, hypotonia, and poor sucking and feeding in the first days of life; (2) hypertonia, particularly in the extensor muscle groups, with backward arching of the neck or back (retrocollis-opisthotonos); (3) hypotonia, usually appearing after the first week of life [Van Praagh, 1961; Volpe, 1995]. A minority of infants with kernicterus may not demonstrate neurologic abnormalities in the neonatal period. Chronic bilirubin encephalopathy is manifested by auditory impairment, in most cases a high-frequency bilateral hearing loss [Hung, 1989]; extrapyramidal abnormalities (e.g., chorea, dystonia, or ballismus), which may fluctuate; and gaze abnormalities, which usually affect vertical gaze. Although affected children may manifest hypotonia and motor developmental delay, characteristic features may not become apparent until after 1 year of age. Severe intellectual deficits are encountered less commonly. In some patients, onset may be delayed for several years before development of a movement disorder [Scott and Jankovic, 1996; Volpe, 1995].

Determination of blood bilirubin, albumin, and pH levels may give an indication of the risk of kernicterus. Brainstem auditory-evoked response testing provides early detection of bilirubin neurotoxicity, demonstrating prolonged conduction times between waves I, III, and V [Nwaesei et al., 1984; Ozcelik et al., 1997; Perlman et al., 1983]. MRI may show high-intensity lesions in the globus pallidus on T2-weighted imaging [Martich Kriss et al., 1995; Yokochi, 1995].

The essential aspect of bilirubin encephalopathy management is the detection of the infant at risk for brain injury caused by bilirubin. Exchange transfusion is the treatment of choice for hyperbilirubinemia when urgent intervention is necessary [Yao and Stevenson, 1995]. Phototherapy refers to the exposure of the infant to light with high-energy output near the maximum absorption peak of bilirubin. This procedure exposes the bilirubin circulating in superficial capillaries to the light and stimulates photoisomerization of bilirubin to a form that is water soluble and can be excreted in bile without conjugation.

Hepatotoxicity of Antiepileptic Medications

Hepatotoxicity is one of the more alarming side effects of antiepileptic drugs and is reviewed in Chapter 49. Considered here is sodium valproate toxicity, because of all antiepileptic drugs, it has been most commonly associated with fatal toxicity. The pattern of occurrence in affected children suggests that the risk is highest in those younger than 2 years of age, on multiple antiepileptic drugs, with metabolic disorders, or with severe seizure disorders accompanied by mental retardation and organic brain diseases [Dreifuss et al., 1989; Willmore et al., 1991]. A Reye-like syndrome associated with valproic acid treatment also has been described [Gerber et al., 1979].

Sodium valproate therapy can be associated with decreased carnitine levels or with true carnitine deficiency. Carnitine is synthesized from dietary amino acids and has a role in long-chain fatty acid metabolism. Measurement of carnitine levels in patients who take carnitine, especially as one of multiple antiepileptic medications, is warranted, and carnitine supplements may be useful, although data are limited [Coulter, 1991].

Hepatic Tumors

Tuberous sclerosis is a disorder of autosomal-dominant inheritance characterized by seizures, mental retardation, and multiple hamartomas in many organ systems, including skin, brain, heart, kidneys, retina, and liver (see Chapter 31). Hamartomas of the liver (usually multiple) can occur in children with tuberous sclerosis and are more common in females (5:1) than in males and increase in incidence with age. They usually are benign and do not produce symptoms of hepatic dysfunction. On ultrasound studies, they appear as areas of increased echogenicity in comparison with the surrounding hepatic parenchyma [Jozwiak et al., 1992]. Brain metastasis from hepatocellular carcinoma is rare and occurs in less than 2% of patients [Tanabe et al., 1994].

Disorders of Nutrition, Including Fluid-Electrolyte Disturbances

OVERVIEW

Malnutrition remains a worldwide problem affecting a large number of children, and disorders of nutrition remain the most common environmental insult affecting the developing nervous system. Worldwide, the incidence of malnutrition in children decreased over the past decade, but it is estimated that still nearly 149 million children are undernourished [Bhan et al., 2005]. In the United States, less than 1% of all children have chronic malnutrition. Nevertheless, the incidence of malnutrition in some groups (e.g., children in homeless shelters or in rural areas) approaches 10% [Grigsby, 2003]. Studies of hospitalized children also suggest that as many as 25% of patients have some form of acute protein-energy malnutrition, and that 27% have chronic protein-energy malnutrition. Based on a national U.S. Census Bureau survey, 11.1% of all U.S. households (34.9 million people) in 2002 were categorized as "food insecure" because of lack of resources [http://www.frac.org/html/hunger_in_the_us/hunger_index.html]. Approximately 9.4 million of affected persons lived in households in the worst circumstances and experienced outright hunger. People living in 1 in 10 households (9.7%) with incomes below 185% of the federal poverty line also experienced hunger.

Disorders of nutrition include both states of undernutrition related to protein-energy malnutrition and deficiencies of vitamins, micronutrients, and minerals. The most common and clinically significant micronutrient deficiencies in children and women of childbearing age throughout the world include deficiencies of iron, iodine, folate, vitamin D, and vitamin A. In this second part of the chapter, some of the conditions that affect the developing nervous system are reviewed. Several excellent reviews discuss various aspects of the effects of undernutrition on brain development [Grantham-McGregor and Ani, 2001; Levitsky and Strupp, 1995; Olness, 2003; Uauya et al., 2001], cognition [Gorman, 1995; Grantham-McGregor, 1995], and behavior [Schurch, 1995]. Another aspect of malnutrion relates to the fact that a high prevalence of epilepsy is frequent among children in developing countries [Hackett and Iype, 2001]. It is likely that any of numerous vitamin, micronutrient, and electrolyte abnormalities of various causes might be a contributing factor in the pathogenesis of epilepsy in children with malnutrition. Conversely, the occurrence of epilepsy may have a detrimental effect on future development. In addition, still other, poverty-related factors in both developed and developing countries, as well as the AIDS pandemic, maternal depression, and the solely institutional care received by many malnourished infants and children, may affect long-term cognitive and behavioral outcomes [Richter, 2003].

PROTEIN-ENERGY MALNUTRITION

The World Health Organization (WHO) defines *malnutrition* as "the cellular imbalance between supply of nutrients and energy and the body's demand for them to ensure growth, maintenance, and specific functions" [Grigsby, 2003]. Kwashiorkor and marasmus are two forms of protein-energy malnutrition that have been described; the distinction between these entities is based on the presence (kwashiorkor) or absence (marasmus) of edema. *Kwashiorkor* is a chronic protein deficiency with adequate carbohydrate and often adequate caloric intake. Children are edematous, with swollen faces, ascites, hepatomegaly, and hair and skin depigmentation. If the condition is left untreated, death occurs as a result of infection or hepatic or cardiac failure. Kwashiorkor usually occurs in the latter part of the first to third years of life [Bhan et al., 2005].

Marasmus, a deficiency in both energy (i.e., calories) and protein, is characterized by extreme emaciation, growth failure, alternating apathy and irritability, and eventually obtundation and death. In most affected children, this disorder develops within the first year of life.

Because the developing brain reacts differently from the adult brain to severe chronic nutritional deficiencies, the risk for long-term irreversible anatomic, biochemical, and functional disorders is greater. These changes can be associated with intellectual and behavioral deficiencies that persist throughout life [Galler et al., 1986; Klein, 1980; Lloyd-Still, 1976].

Anatomic and Biochemical Effects of Undernutrition

Animal studies demonstrate that protein-calorie undernutrition in early life, during the accelerated period of brain development, can affect morphologic, physiologic, and biochemical maturation of the brain [de Souza, 2004; Marichich, 1979; Pinos, 2004; Rotta, 1999; Singh, 1999; Winick, 1976], as measured by growth parameters, synaptic development, myelination, and neurotransmitter levels. Early studies at the beginning of the last century demonstrated that undernutrition early in life had dramatic effects on brain growth. Undernourished animals had increased brain water content, decreased myelination and brain lipid content, and decreased cerebral cortical volume but no significant reductions in the total number of cells compared with age-matched control animals [Donaldson, 1911; Sugita, 1918]. These and later studies suggested that the primary effect of protein-energy deprivation is on the replication and growth of cells (rather than as a destructive process) and is strongest on those elements most actively proliferating during the insult [Dobbing, 1964, 1972; Dobbing and Sands, 1971; Dodge et al., 1975; Winick and Noble, 1966]. That is, the mammalian brain is most vulnerable to malnutrition during the period when the brain is growing most rapidly; consequently, those structures that develop postnatally, such as the cerebrum, hippocampus, and cerebellum, are the most susceptible to permanent morphologic changes [Levitsky and Strupp, 1995]. An alternative hypothesis is that the maximum period of critical vulnerability occurs when specific neurons are undergoing organizational development earlier in life, implying greater susceptibility prenatally than postnatally. The parameters of undernutrition may differ in various studies, and other factors definitely play a role and may modify the effect of undernutrition [Rajanna, 1987]. Although evidence exists for a causal relationship between severe early malnutrition and effects on brain development and functions, many variables are involved, including the duration of undernutrition, prenatal versus perinatal effects, time and extent of rehabilitation, the effects of lack of environmental stimulation, and early or late effects. The outcome also may depend on the quality of the subsequent environment [Grantham-McGregor, 1995]. Some animal studies suggest that the anatomic effects of early undernutrition may persist even if the animals are rehabilitated [Warren, 1988]

Box 90-2 lists some of the major neuropathologic abnormalities resulting from malnutrition described in animal experimental studies (see Levitsky and Strupp [1995] for a comprehensive review). Morphometric analysis of specific areas of cerebral cortex and of selected subcortical nuclei by

Box 90-2 Nutrition and Brain Development

Effects of Malnutrition on the Developing Brain

Reduction in brain volume
Sparing of cortical neurons
Increased cell packing
Disruption of cortical pyramidal cells
Reduction in cortical dendritic spines
Decrease in width of cortical neurons
Decreased dendritic branching in cortex
Reduced number of cortical glial cells
Reduced number of cortical synapses
Reduced number of synaptic reactive zones

Effects of Restoring Nutrition on Reversibility of Brain Lesions

Increase in brain weight and volume: "catch-up" head growth
Prolongation of period of mitotic activity
Prolongation of period of protein synthesis
Reversal of cell packing
Reduced cortical glial cell density
Persistence of reduced number of cortical dendrites and synaptic spines
Persistence of reduced myelination
Increase in number of mitochondria in neurons
Increase in synaptic density

Modified from Levitsky DA, Strupp BJ. Malnutrition and the brain: Changing concepts, changing concerns. J Nutr 1995;125:2212S.

Diaz-Cintra and colleagues [1981, 1984, 1990] suggests specific differences in the responses of selected neurons to undernutrition. For example, in the visual cortex of the protein-deprived rat, changes in the developmental pattern of the pyramidal cells of layer V differ from those in layers II and III [Diaz-Cintra et al., 1990].

Pregnant rats subjected to severe protein restriction from the fourth day of gestation give birth to litters that average a 15% decrease in the number of brain cells [Patel et al., 1973]. The reduction is most marked in the areas adjacent to the lateral ventricles and in the cerebellum [Guthrie and Brown, 1968; Shimada et al., 1977]. A similar decrease in cerebral protein has been reported [Zamenhof and Guthrie, 1977]. Activity of rat brain lactate dehydrogenase and of other brain enzymes is affected by food deprivation [Swaiman and Wolfe 1970; Swaiman et al., 1970].

Reductions in protein and calorie intake during the suckling period in rats produced a 10% to 30% reduction in brain weight, with a corresponding decrease in DNA [Fishman et al., 1971; Winick and Noble, 1966]. The major cellular change appears to involve oligodendroglial cells. These cells are reduced in number in both the cortex and the white matter, and their maturation is delayed [Bass et al., 1970]. No significant reduction in the number of neurons in the cerebral cortex is likely, although the number of neurons in the cerebellum, particularly granule cells, may be reduced [Clos et al., 1977]. In undernourished preweanling animals, the reduction of DNA content in the cerebellum is considerably greater than in the cerebrum [Chase et al., 1969]. This difference likely is secondary to the rapid proliferation of cerebellar neurons after birth in the rat. The effects of undernutrition on cell number are greatest when a nutritional insult is prolonged from early intrauterine life through the period of lactation, which results in a 60% reduction in cell number in human infants by the time of weaning [Winick, 1970]. Studies in Rhesus monkeys disclosed no effect on brain growth when the mother was adequately nourished during gestation and the infant was protein restricted at birth [Portman et al., 1987].

Myelination is another parameter of brain development that is easily measured in undernourished animals. Cholesterol, which is found in all membranes, is decreased in proportion to total lipids [Dobbing, 1964]; however, greater reductions occur in lipids, such as cerebrosides, that are found predominantly in myelin [Culley and Mertz, 1965]. Proteolipid protein, which also is a myelin constituent, is reduced disproportionately in comparison with other proteins and lipids [Benton et al., 1966].

The chemical composition of myelin from brains of undernourished animals does not differ markedly from that in control animals [Fishman et al., 1971]. Even with prolonged starvation in postnatal life, changes in the amount of myelin are not large. For example, in animals starved from birth to 21 days of age, total myelin quantity was reduced to only 86.5% of that in the control animals. In animals starved from birth to 53 days of age, myelin quantity was 71% of that in age-matched control animals [Fishman et al., 1971]. It is possible that the reduction in myelination is secondary to a reduction in the total number of oligodendroglial cells.

Reductions in both RNA and protein in the cerebral cortex of undernourished rats are greater than reductions in DNA. This finding suggests that the impairment in cell growth exceeds the reduction in cell number [Bass et al., 1970]. Levels of gangliosides also are a measure of cell size; these lipids are greatly reduced in undernourished piglets [Dickerson et al., 1971]. Cragg [1972] observed that the number of synapses in the cortex of undernourished rats was decreased. This reduction does not correspond with the general reduction in synaptic transmitters, however. For example, in the undernourished rat brain, serotonin is increased [Resnick and Morgane, 1984], acetylcholine is unchanged [Wiggins et al., 1984], and area-to-area variability in norepinephrine is apparent [Wiggins et al., 1984].

The major aspects of the anatomic and biochemical changes associated with severe protein-calorie malnutrition in animals have been observed in malnourished children. Brain weights are reduced, water content is increased, and a definite reduction in myelin is present that correlates with the length of starvation [Fishman et al., 1969]. DNA content also is reduced in the cerebrum and cerebellum and is related to a reduction in cell number, particularly of oligodendroglial cells [Winick and Rosso, 1969a, 1969b; Winick et al., 1970].

Animals may recover from periods of undernutrition as evidenced by normalization of brain weight and biochemical indices [Dobbing et al., 1971; Winick et al., 1968]. If the period of undernutrition persists during the entire period of cell replication, however, a deficit in cell numbers persists, regardless of the diet provided thereafter [Fish and Winick, 1969; Swaiman et al., 1970]. This deficit is indicated by reduced brain DNA in later life. Briefer insults ending before the age of 21 days in the rat (a period in which cell division is still programmed to occur in the rat brain) produce no permanent defects once the animal is re-fed [Culley and Lineberger, 1968; Winick and Noble, 1966].

Evidence in humans is less direct, but measurements of somatic growth and head size suggest that the length of the insult during development is an important factor in the production of permanent effects in humans as well [Chase and Martin, 1970; Hoorweg and Stanfield, 1976]. Physical growth also is decreased after long periods of kwashiorkor later in childhood [Bowie et al., 1980; Pereira et al., 1979]. At age 1 year, human preterm infants who were malnourished in utero, born small for gestational age, or undernourished in early extrauterine life had smaller head circumferences and poorer performances on the Bayley Infant Development scales than corresponding measurements in children of the same gestational age with normal birth weights who were undernourished in early extrauterine life [Georgieff et al., 1985]. This finding suggests that in animals and humans, a combination of intrauterine and extrauterine malnutrition produces the greatest effect on brain weight, chemical composition, and function.

The existence of a single common pathway by which lack of protein and calories affects growth of the nervous system is unlikely. It is certain, however, that for there to be significant effect on brain development, the insult occurs during a period of rapid nervous system growth or at a point when cell-cell interconnections are developing.

Effects of Protein-Calorie Undernutrition

As suggested earlier, the duration of the undernourished state and the time at which undernutrition occurs have complex effects on long-term cognitive function in children. These effects have been reviewed in detail, and the reader is referred to several sources [Gorman, 1995; Grantham-McGregor, 1995].

ACUTE EFFECTS ON BEHAVIOR AND COGNITION. Severely malnourished children demonstrate marked behavioral changes during the acute stages of malnutrition [Grantham-McGregor, 1995]. Apathy, reduced activity, decreased interest in and exploration of the environment, reduced stress responses, and impaired cognition all are well characterized. Brief postnatal insults lasting less than 4 to 5 months do not appear to have a permanent effect on mental function [Chase and Martin, 1970]. Starvation over a considerable period does have an effect on behavior and intelligence. Separating the effects of undernutrition from other variables, however, has made it difficult to categorize and quantify the nature and magnitude of deficits attributable to undernutrition. Numerous studies have demonstrated that the intellectual function, academic achievement, and behavior of persons malnourished for long periods differ from those in age-matched control subjects or in siblings in the same family [Cabak and Najdanvic, 1965; Cravioto et al., 1966; Galler et al., 1983; Grantham-McGregor, 1995; Ivanovic, 2000; Stoch and Smythe, 1976; Udani, 1992]. The environments in which malnourished children are reared, however, are almost always suboptimal. Overcrowding, poor education, lack of parental stimulation, and poverty are variables that cannot be confidently evaluated even in sibling studies.

TREATMENT. The only treatment of undernutrition is adequate food intake. An adequate protein and calorie intake certainly ends the acute insult, but it is not clear whether caloric supplements always improve growth and function. The use of dietary supplements, both in utero and during the suckling period, was attempted on several occasions with variable results [Herrera et al., 1980; Joos et al., 1983; Klein et al., 1976; Susser and Stein, 1980]. First, many of the supplements were not used or were used improperly [Beaton and Ghassemi, 1982]. Second, improved nutrition cannot compensate for the other problems of poverty, such as lack of parental interest and overcrowding. Third, it is not certain when improvement ceases or if differences between supplemented and control populations will be of less importance later in life. For example, the study of undernourished children in Bogata, which used both nutritional supplementation and environmental stimulation in different treatment groups, found that nutritionally supplemented children at 18 months of age had benefited in all tested aspects of development except language. At 36 months of age, however, the children's language skills also had benefited compared with those in nonsupplemented children of the same age. By contrast, the effects of early environmental stimulation lessened with age [Waber et al., 1981]. Nutritionally supplemented populations and their malnourished control subjects have now been followed for up to 9 years. The effects have been positive but small [Grantham-McGregor, 1987].

All facets of neurologic function do not need to recover in parallel. Celedon and DeAndraca [1979] reported that with feeding at the end of a period of protein-calorie undernutrition, psychomotor development improved, but the benefit was limited predominantly to social language and fine motor coordination. Gross motor coordination did not demonstrate any improvement during the 5 months in which the affected children received treatment. Other studies indicated the positive effects of psychosocial stimulation or relatively well-structured home environments during the recovery period [Beardslee et al., 1982; Cravioto and Arrieta, 1979; Grantham-McGregor et al., 1980]. In studies performed in underfed populations in New York City, no differences were disclosed in two groups—one supplemented and one eating the usual diet—using the Bayley Mental and Motor scales. These mothers, however, were supplemented only during pregnancy and not during lactation [Susser and Stein, 1980].

DISORDERS ASSOCIATED WITH VITAMIN DEFICIENCIES OR EXCESSES

Vitamins are organic compounds required by mammals in small amounts to sustain normal metabolism. They must be supplied from exogenous sources because they cannot be synthesized endogenously. The chemical structure, physiologic properties, and metabolic function of vitamins are quite diverse. In some instances, vitamins act as cofactors in defined enzymatic reactions; in others, they function by interacting with specific intracellular receptors in target organs or as reducing agents [Snodgrass, 1992]. The existence of vitamins became known through the study of disorders produced by vitamin deficiency in diets [Rosenfeld, 1997]. The almost complete eradication of nutritional vitamin deficiency disorders in developed countries marks one of the major advances in human health, but nutritional vitamin deficiency remains a public health problem in several developing countries and among the poor and aged worldwide. In addition, it is now estimated that about 40%

of the United States population consumes vitamin supplements, increasing the risk of hypervitaminosis [Meyers et al., 1996].

Clinical manifestations affecting the CNS and peripheral nervous system occur in most nutritional vitamin deficiency states. They also may occur in diseases affecting vitamin absorption, metabolism, and excretion. Iatrogenic vitamin deficiency has been associated with parenteral nutrition, chronic dialysis, and drug administration. An increasing number of inborn errors of metabolism, in which mutations lead to protein alterations that require pharmacologic rather than physiologic amounts of a vitamin, have been documented. These vitamin dependency states, although relatively rare, present a challenge to the clinician, because only through their recognition and the prompt initiation of specific therapy can severe neurologic consequences be prevented (Table 90-1). Ingestion or administration of excessive amounts of some vitamins also may cause neurologic abnormalities and other signs of intoxication.

Vitamin A (Retinol)

Vitamin A is the generic term for a group of fat-soluble compounds that possess the biologic activity of retinol (vitamin A_1) [Goodman, 1984]. This activity includes important physiologic roles in retinal function, growth and differentiation of epithelial tissue, bone growth, reproduction, embryonic development, and enhancement of the immune system [Snodgrass, 1992]. Physiologic functions of vitamin A are mediated through different forms of the compound. Retinol, the alcohol, serves as the transport molecule; retinal, the aldehyde, is active in the formation of visual pigments; and retinoic acid may be the active metabolite in the growth, maintenance, and differentiation of body tissues. Retinol esters function as storage material.

Vitamin A is necessary for the adaptation of the retinal rods and cones to dim light [O'Brien, 1982]. Rhodopsin, formed from the combination of the protein opsin and 11-*cis*-retinal, is the photosensitive pigment of the rods. After absorption of a photon of light, rhodopsin undergoes transformational changes through a series of intermediary steps that ultimately leads to the development of a retinal action potential [Stryer, 1986].

Retinol also has an important role in maintaining epithelial cell integrity by stimulating mucus production. Deprived of adequate amounts of retinol, goblet mucous cells disappear and epidermal basal cells proliferate, resulting in keratinization. The absence of normal mucous secretions promotes irritation and infection.

Animal work has suggested that vitamin A is required during early pregnancy and development [Zile, 2001]. In addition, major anatomic brain abnormalities occur in the absence of vitamin A [Maden, 1998]. Vitamin A and retinoids may play a role in CNS function. High levels of cellular retinol-binding protein type 1 immunoreactivity and an increased number of nuclear retinoid receptors were found in the CNS of the adult rodent. The vitamin and its derivatives, the retinoids, have been implicated in the synaptic plasticity of the hippocampus and in cognitive functions [Etchamendy, 2003].

Stored retinol esters are a dietary source of vitamin A. Carotenoids, pigmentary compounds present in all photosynthetic plant tissue, provide another major dietary source [Simpson and Chichester, 1981]. These retinol esters are hydrolyzed to retinol in the intestinal lumen and within the brush border of intestinal cells. Absorption mediated by cellular retinol-binding proteins depends on the presence of absorbable fat and bile and is considerably reduced in conditions associated with steatorrhea and other chronic diarrheas [Chytil and Ong, 1987]. Vitamin A is stored in the liver as retinol ester. In the plasma, retinol is bound to a specific retinol-binding protein that binds to specific cell surface sites [Ong, 1985]. The absorption, distribution, and metabolic fate of retinoic acid differ from those of retinol.

The recommended daily dietary requirement (i.e., the dietary reference intake) for vitamin A 500 µg/day is for infants younger than 1 year of age and 600 to 900 µg/day for children and adolescents. Under normal conditions, the liver concentration of retinol ester approximates 100 to 300 µg/g, and the normal plasma retinol concentration is 30 to 70 µg/dL.

TABLE 90-1

Vitamin Dependency Disorders

VITAMIN	DISORDER	DEFECTIVE ENZYME(S)
Thiamine	Lactic acidemia	Pyruvate carboxylase, pyruvate dehydrogenase
	Maple syrup urine disease	Branched-chain dehydrogenase complex
Riboflavin	Glutaricacidemia type I	Glutaryl-CoA dehydrogenase
	Glutaricacidemia type II	Multiple acyl-CoA dehydrogenase
Niacin	Hartnup's disease	—
Pyridoxine	Infantile convulsions	—
	Homocystinuria	Cystathionine synthase
	Cystathioninuria	Cystathionase
	Gyrate atrophy of retina (ornithinemia)	Ornithine-delta-aminotransferase
Cobalamin	Inherited transcobalamin II deficiency	—
	Methylmalonicacidemia	Methylmalonic-CoA mutase
	Homocystinuria with methylmalonicaciduria	Methyltetrahydrofolate reductase, methylmalonyl-CoA mutase
Folate	Congenital folate malabsorption	—
	Dihydrofolate reductase deficiency	Dihydrofolate reductase
	Formiminotransferase deficiency	Formiminotransferase
	Methylenetetrahydrofolate reductase deficiency	Methylenetetrahydrofolate reductase

CoA, coenzyme A

Vitamin A Deficiency

Dietary vitamin A deficiency continues to be a major cause of infantile blindness in some developing countries [Kello, 2003; Sommer, 1989; Sommer et al., 1981] and may be infrequently seen in developed countries [Rodrigues, 2004]. Reported estimates of the prevalence of inadequate vitamin A intake in several countries ranged from 32% to 68% [Calloway et al., 1993]. In one series, 11.6% of children had reduced blood concentrations [Wetherilt et al., 1992]. It is estimated that between 100 and 140 million children are vitamin A deficient and that an estimated 250,000 to 500,000 vitamin A–deficient children become blind every year, half of them dying within 12 months of losing their sight [WHO, 2004].

In developed countries, vitamin A is among the essential nutrients most likely to be ingested in marginal amounts by the poor. Signs and symptoms of vitamin A deficiency also occur in patients with steatorrhea and other forms of chronic diarrhea, hepatic and pancreatic disease, chronic infections, and hypermetabolic states (e.g., hyperthyroidism) [Abernathy, 1976; Main et al., 1983; Roos and Van Der Blij, 1985].

Clinical manifestations of vitamin A deficiency include night blindness (nyctalopia), corneal and conjunctival dryness (xerophthalmia), appearance of yellow patches on the bulbar conjunctivae (Bitot's spots), corneal ulcerations and scarring, and, if untreated, irreversible amblyopia [Sommer et al., 1980]. Keratinization of the skin and epithelial lining of the respiratory and urinary tracts leads to increased susceptibility to infection. Pseudotumor cerebri [Abernathy, 1976; Kasarkis and Bass, 1982; Lucidi et al., 1993; Roos and Van Der Blij, 1985] and facial nerve palsy [Sillman et al., 1985] also have been reported.

Because serum retinol levels are maintained for months at the expense of hepatic stores, low serum retinol concentrations imply that hepatic stores have been depleted. Clinical manifestations of deficiency may appear when the plasma concentration falls below 20 μg/dL. Clinical manifestations of deficiency should be treated with 6 to 15 mg of retinol (20,000 to 50,000 IU of vitamin A) per day for 4 to 5 days, followed by 0.6 to 1.5 mg per day for 1 to 2 months. In conditions interfering with intestinal vitamin absorption, aqueous preparations should be administered intramuscularly. Treatment initiated before the occurrence of corneal scarring leads to rapid and complete recovery.

Benign intracranial hypertension can occur with hypovitaminosis A and E [Lucidi, 1993].

A deficit in spatial learning and memory task was found in adult rats following 12 weeks of vitamin A–free diet, with this cognitive deficit fully reversed when vitamin A was restored in the diet. A reduction in the size of hippocampal nuclei of CA1 region in the vitamin-deficient rats, compared with rats fed with a vitamin A–sufficient diet, also has been reported. These findings suggest that vitamin A has a role in learning and memory processes [Cocco, 2002].

Vitamin A Intoxication

In the United States, about 10 to 15 cases of adult vitamin A toxicity are reported each year [Meyers et al., 1996]. This poisoning is due in part to increased vitamin A consumption because of its antioxidant properties [van Poppel and van den Berg, 1997]. Human sensitivity to excessive amounts of vitamin A is variable and more common in infants and children. Acute toxicity may occur after ingestion of 300,000 IU of vitamin A. Signs of chronic toxicity usually appear after the administration of 2500 IU/kg per day but may result after ingestion of smaller dosages [Bendich and Langseth, 1989]. Ingestion of such quantities of vitamin A is common in the treatment of acne or among megavitamin faddists [Lippe et al., 1981; Shaywitz et al., 1977]. Hepatitis may precipitate manifestations of toxicity [Hatoff et al., 1982]. The molecular basis of vitamin A toxicity is not known.

Acute toxicity is characterized by headache, vomiting, diplopia, papilledema (bulging fontanel in infants), stiff neck, and abducens nerve palsies caused by increased intracranial pressure (benign intracranial hypertension). In chronic exposure, manifestations of increased intracranial pressure may be preceded or accompanied by painful fissures at the corners of the mouth, a pruritic desquamating dermatitis, tender hyperostoses of the long bones and skull, limitations of joint motility, hepatomegaly, and failure to gain weight. Diagnosis is established from the dietary history and characteristic clinical findings. The plasma retinol concentration usually exceeds 100 to 600 μg/dL. Radiographs of the limbs may reveal periosteal new bone formation, metaphyseal cupping, and increased metaphyseal density. The uptake of technetium-99m polyphosphate is increased on bone scans. Removal of vitamin A from the diet invariably leads to resolution of symptoms and signs of toxicity within several days.

Vitamin A Teratogenesis

Retinoic acid is essential for both embryonic and adult growth, activating gene transcription by means of specific nuclear receptors. It is generated, through a retinaldehyde intermediate, from retinol. Evidence from several animal models indicates that retinoic acid participates in the regulation of the anterior-posterior axis of the hindbrain, the dorsal-ventral axis of the spinal cord, and certain gender-specific segments of the spinal cord [McCaffery et al., 2003]. Inappropriately high concentrations of retinoic acid result in abnormal development of cerebellum and hindbrain nuclei. Teratogenic effects with vitamin A toxicity during pregnancy include hydrocephalus, microcephaly, retinal and optic nerve defects, microtia or anotia, and conotruncal heart defects [Lammer et al., 1985]. Women should be warned preconceptionally about excessive intake of vitamins, especially products containing large amounts of vitamin A, including topical vitamin A derivatives (tretinoin) for acne and age-related skin damage, oral vitamin A derivatives for severe cystic acne (isotretinoin), and psoriasis (etretinate) [Steegers Theunissen, 1995; Swain and Kaplan, 1995].

Some evidence also suggests that low vitamin A levels during brain development interact with susceptibility genes to alter brain development, probably by epigenetic regulation that alters gene expression throughout adult life and may contribute to the development of schizophrenia [Mackay-Sim et al., 2004]. Induction between neural crest-derived, retinoic acid-producing mesenchyme, the anterior neural tube, and the anterior surface epithelium of the embryo guides regional differentiation and pathway formation during forebrain development. Furthermore, at least two mouse mutations—in the genes encoding Pax-6 and Gli-3—are known to cause peripheral malformations and specifically disrupt neural crest–mediated, retinoic acid–dependent induction and differentiation in the forebrain. These observations suggest that induction might provide a common target for genes that alter morphogenesis of peripheral structures. Disruption of retinoic acid signaling could potentially affect forebrain development, which might influence the numbers or cellular properties of neurons and circuits, possibly reflected in the aberrant forebrain function that characterizes schizophrenia [LaMantia, 1999].

Thiamine (Vitamin B_1)

Thiamine functions as a cofactor in oxidative decarboxylation and transketolation reactions [Davis and Leke, 1983]. Thiamine pyrophosphate, the physiologic active form, is an essential cofactor in the oxidative decarboxylation of pyruvate to acetyl-coenzyme A (CoA); α-ketoglutarate to succinyl-CoA; and the α-keto derivatives of isoleucine, leucine, and valine to their corresponding branched-chain CoA derivatives (see Chapters 23 and 28). Thiamine pyrophosphate also is the cofactor for the transketolase reaction in the hexose monophosphate shunt that provides pentose for nucleotide synthesis. In addition, thiamine has roles in cerebral metabolism, in which it is present as both a diphosphate and a triphosphate. Although the precise molecular basis of the nervous system function of thiamine is not known, experimental studies have implicated this factor in fatty acid synthesis [Volpe and Marasa, 1978], neuronal membrane transport [Voorhees et al., 1977], neuromuscular transmission [Waldehind, 1978], and axonal conduction [Schoffeniels, 1983].

Thiamine is readily available in meats, grains, and vegetables but is destroyed by heat. It is actively transported across the small intestine by a saturable process, limiting the amount that can be absorbed. In the blood, thiamine is bound to protein, predominantly albumin. Its transport into the CNS and cerebrospinal fluid is controlled by a rate-limiting process involving a specific membrane-bound phosphatase [Spector, 1976]. Excesses of the vitamin are excreted in the urine.

The requirement for thiamine depends on the metabolic rate and is increased when carbohydrates are the major energy source. The recommended daily dietary reference intake is 0.3 to 0.4 mg in infants younger than 1 year of age and 0.6 to 1.2 mg in older children and adolescents, amounts readily available in normal diets.

Thiamine Deficiency

Historically, clinical manifestations of dietary thiamine deficiency (beri-beri) occurred in populations in which polished rice formed the major dietary staple [Carpenter and Sutherland, 1995]. Signs of deficiency still occur in alcoholics and the aged, populations that use thiamine less effectively. Beri-beri also has been reported after ingestion of large amounts of raw freshwater fish, shellfish, and bracken foods that contain thiaminase-1, an enzyme promoting thiamine decomposition [Murata, 1965], and large quantities of tea, which contains another thiamine antagonist [Vimokesant et al., 1974]. An infantile form of beri-beri has been reported in breast-fed infants of thiamine-deficient mothers [Rao and Subrahmagam, 1964] and in infants fed a soybean formula in which the thiamine was presumably heat inactivated during preparation [Cochrane et al., 1961].

Early symptoms of thiamine deficiency are not specific and include apathy, fatigue, mental sluggishness, depression, anorexia, and abdominal discomfort. More prolonged and severe deficiency is associated with signs of peripheral neuropathy, nerve and muscle tenderness, and cardiomyopathy [Tojo et al., 1993]. Hoarseness caused by laryngeal nerve paralysis is a classic sign. Ptosis, optic atrophy, and encephalopathic features are other possible findings. As the deficiency persists, increased intracranial pressure, meningismus, seizures, and coma may progress rapidly to a fatal outcome from either neurologic or cardiac failure.

Vitamin B_1 deficiency also can cause Wernicke-Korsakoff syndrome. This syndrome usually is seen in adults with chronic alcoholism, pancreatitis, or carcinoma of the stomach or esophagus but also is found in children, in whom it is underdiagnosed. In a collected series of pediatric Wernicke's encephalopathy cases, 41.9% of patients were diagnosed at postmortem examination. The original patients with Wernicke's encephalopathy had a clinical triad comprising ocular abnormalities, mental status changes, and ataxia, but many of the patients do not present with this classic triad. In a review of a series of children and adolescents with this condition, only 6 of 30 presented with the Wernicke's encephalopathy clinical triad at the onset of their disease [Vasconcelos, 1999]. The most common symptom was mental state change, occurring in 82% of patients, followed by ocular signs (e.g., ophthalmoplegia, nystagmus, ptosis) in 68% and ataxia in 21%. CT abnormalities included hypodensities in the basal ganglia and medial thalami, whereas MRI demonstrated abnormalities in all tested patients manifested by increased signal in T2-weighted images and contrast enhancement of the basal ganglia, medial thalami, mammillary bodies, or periaqueductal gray matter. The most frequently underlying disorder in this series was malignancy. Symptoms of thiamine deficiency also can be seen in patients with GI disease who have malabsorption or vomiting and in patients on total parenteral nutrition [Hahn, 1998; Ming, 1990]. Single photon emission computed tomography in Wernicke's encephalopathy may reveal bilateral frontal and frontotemporal hypoperfusion and right basal ganglia hypoperfusion [Celik, 2004]. In children, MRI may be helpful in establishing the diagnosis of Wernicke's encephalopathy by demonstrating diencephalic and mesencephalic signal abnormalities on T2-weighted images and, in some patients, enhancement of the mammillary bodies and the floor of the hypothalamus [Coe et al., 2001; Ming et al., 1998; Sparacia et al., 1999]

Infantile beri-beri is characterized by vomiting, aphonia, abdominal distention, diarrhea, cyanosis, tachycardia, and convulsions. Death may occur suddenly. In less fulminant, more chronic depletions, infants fail to grow, and subsequently edema, oliguria, constipation, cardiomegaly, and hepatomegaly typically develop [Cochrane et al., 1961].

Neuropathologic features of beri-beri are fairly characteristic and consist of nerve cell degeneration, endothelial hyperplasia, and petechial hemorrhages localized to the periventricular gray matter around the third ventricle, sylvian aqueduct, fourth ventricle, and mammillary bodies [Cochrane et al., 1961]. Peripheral nerves manifest patchy areas of demyelination.

Diagnosis of thiamine deficiency depends primarily on suspicions raised by the dietary history and the presence of typical clinical manifestations. Determining serum thiamine concentrations is not of practical value. Urinary excretion of less than 120 μg of thiamine per gram of creatinine suggests thiamine deficiency. An increase of 25% or more in red cell ketolase activity after the addition of thiamine pyrophosphate also is characteristic of deficiency. Clinical response to the administration of thiamine is the best confirmatory test. Oral administration of 10 to 50 mg of thiamine daily will reverse clinical symptoms in a few weeks. Serious life-threatening neurologic manifestations or congestive heart failure should be treated with the parenteral administration of 5 to 20 mg of thiamine.

Thiamine Dependency

Pyruvate dysmetabolism disorders are among the varied causes of lactic acidosis [Evans, 1986]. Thiamine pyrophosphate is an essential cofactor in pyruvate decarboxylation. Several patients with documented thiamine-responsive lacticacidemia have been described [Duran and Wadman, 1985]. The age at onset of symptoms varies, ranging from the immediate postnatal period to 8 years. Mental retardation and episodic neurologic abnormalities, including intermittent ataxia, choreoathetosis, and hypotonia with areflexia, occur. Pyruvate carboxylase deficiency has been confirmed in one patient by liver biopsy, and a partial deficiency of the pyruvate dehydrogenase complex was confirmed in two others by enzymatic assay of cultured skin fibroblasts. Biochemical abnormalities normalized and episodic neurologic symptoms subsided after administration of pharmacologic amounts of thiamine (20 to 2400 mg per day). In view of the potential benefits, therapy with thiamine in pharmacologic amounts should be attempted in all patients with persistent lacticacidemia believed to be secondary to a primary metabolic defect. (See Chapters 23, 25, 28, and 81 for further discussion of the role of thiamine in metabolic diseases.)

Thiamine also is important in other inborn errors of metabolism, including a form of thiamine-dependent maple syrup urine disease and subacute necrotizing encephalomyelopathy (Leigh's disease) (see Chapter 23). A syndrome of thiamine-dependent megaloblastic anemia, sensorineural deafness, and diabetes mellitus also has been described [Haworth et al., 1982; Viana and Carvalho, 1978]. The finding that thiamine (20 to 25 mg per day) corrects the megaloblastic anemia was serendipitous. In one patient, it was possible to discontinue insulin use after the initiation of thiamine treatment. Hearing impairment was not reversible. The basis of the response to the thiamine in this syndrome is not known.

Riboflavin (Vitamin B_2)

Two coenzymes, flavin mononucleotide and flavin adenine dinucleotide, are the physiologically active forms of riboflavin. These nucleotides play a vital role in a variety of mitochondrial oxidation-reduction reactions involving flavoproteins, including amino acid oxidase, xanthine oxidase, glutathione reductase, and nitric oxide synthase [Neims and Helerman, 1970; Stuehr and Griffith, 1992]. Riboflavin is widely distributed in plant and animal tissues. Phosphorylation of riboflavin to flavin mononucleotide occurs in the intestinal mucosa through a reaction catalyzed by the cytosolic enzyme flavokinase, and both riboflavin and flavin mononucleotide are absorbed into the circulation [Jusko and Levy, 1975]. The upper limit of absorption is approximately 25 mg per dose. Only small amounts of riboflavin are stored, and unused riboflavin is excreted in the urine and feces. In the plasma, riboflavin and flavin mononucleotide are bound to protein, predominantly albumin. In tissues, riboflavin is converted to flavin mononucleotide in a reaction catalyzed by flavokinase. Flavin mononucleotide is subsequently converted to flavin adenine dinucleotide in a reaction catalyzed by flavin adenine dinucleotide pyrophosphorylase and then transported into the mitochondria. The recommended dietary reference intake for riboflavin is 0.3 to 0.4 mg in infants younger than 1 year of age and 0.5 to 1.8 mg in older children and adolescents.

Riboflavin Deficiency

Symptomatic riboflavin deficiency invariably occurs in association with deficiencies of other vitamins [Hoppel and Tandler, 1990]. Early symptoms include sore throat and angular stomatitis. Glossitis, cheilosis, seborrheic dermatitis of the face, and dermatitis over the trunk and limbs develop later. Other late effects include a normochromic, normocytic anemia with associated reticulocytopenia. A neuropathy characterizes the neurologic deficit.

Diagnosis rests primarily on suspicions raised by the dietary history and presence of characteristic symptoms. Serum riboflavin concentration determinations are of no practical value; urinary excretion rates below 30 μg per 24 hours suggest riboflavin depletion. The activity of the flavin-dependent erythrocyte glutathione reductase before and after flavin adenine dinucleotide activation is a good index of riboflavin status [Prentice and Bates, 1981]. Riboflavin in dosages of 5 to 10 mg per day readily reverses the manifestations of riboflavin deficiency.

Riboflavin Dependency

RIBOFLAVIN-DEPENDENT GLUTARICACIDEMIA TYPE I

Glutaryl-CoA dehydrogenase deficiency type I is an autosomal-recessive error of metabolism characterized by early acquired macrocephaly, severe mental retardation, seizures, progressive choreoathetosis, and dystonia associated with glutaricaciduria and 3-hydroxyglutaric-aciduria [Goodman et al., 1977; Stutchfield et al., 1985] (see Chapter 23). Neuropathologic features include severe symmetric destruction of the putamen and lateral margins of the caudate nuclei [Leibel et al., 1980]. The content of GABA in the basal ganglia and substantia nigra is markedly decreased, presumably because GABA synthetase is inhibited by glutaric acid [Bennett et al., 1986; Christensen and Brandt, 1978]. The activity of glutaryl-CoA dehydrogenase, an enzyme for which riboflavin is a cofactor, is deficient in leukocytes, cultured skin fibroblasts, and amniotic cells. The severity of the clinical manifestations, biochemical abnormalities, and amount of residual enzymatic activity vary considerably. Administration of riboflavin in pharmacologic dosages (200 to 300 mg per day) has led to clinical improvement and decreased the urinary excretion of glutaric acid in some patients [Brandt et al., 1979; Leibel et al., 1980; Stutchfield et al., 1985].

RIBOFLAVIN-DEPENDENT GLUTARICACIDEMIA TYPE II

Glutaricacidemia type II is characterized biochemically by nonketotic hypoglycemia, metabolic acidosis, and the accumulation and urinary excretion of a number of organic acids derived from saturated acyl-CoA esters, including C6 to C10 dicarboxylic acids and ethylmalonic, isobutyric, butyric, hexanoic, and glutaric acids. This organic aciduria is a direct consequence of a defect in the acyl-Co vitamin A dehydrogenase complex, which consists of several distinct acyl-CoA dehydrogenases, electron transfer flavoprotein, and electron transfer protein:ubiquinone oxidoreductase. The acyl-CoA dehydrogenase complex functions in the transfer of electrons from fatty acids and some branched-chain keto acids to coenzyme Q in the mitochondria [Gregerson, 1985]. In most cases the disorder is due to deficiency of electron transfer protein or electron transfer protein:ubiquinone oxidoreductase.

Considerable phenotypic variability in the clinical manifestations and quantitative pattern of urinary organic acids exists with this disorder. In the newborn, the illness is characterized by rapidly progressing respiratory difficulties, a "sweaty-feet" odor, convulsions, and severe metabolic acidosis without ketosis and leads to a fatal outcome in the first days or weeks of life [Przyrembel et al., 1976; Sweetman et al., 1980]. Some patients have dysmorphic clinical features and other congenital anomalies. Glutaricaciduria dominates in this form of the disease, although the other organic acids also are present in the urine. Administration of riboflavin is not beneficial in these patients.

A later-onset glutaricaciduria type II (ethylmalonic-adipicaciduria) manifests in older infants and children with repetitive episodes of acute encephalopathy, hepatomegaly, metabolic acidosis, and hypoglycemia, resembling Reye's syndrome [Gregerson et al., 1982; Mantagos et al., 1974]. Administration of riboflavin in pharmacologic dosages (300 mg per day in three equal doses) has resulted in dramatic metabolic improvement during the acute episode in such patients and appears to reduce the frequency of subsequent episodes.

In adolescents and young adults, ethylmalonic-adipicaciduria has been associated with a syndrome characterized by episodic symptoms of fatigue, lethargy, mild jaundice, hypoglycemia, and hepatomegaly precipitated by febrile illnesses or pregnancy [Dusheiko et al., 1979; Harpey et al., 1983]. In one such patient, prolonged periods of coma associated with protracted hypoglycemia occurred [Dusheiko et al., 1979]. In another, mild symptoms had occurred during the last trimester of several pregnancies and were associated with decreased fetal movements. One stillborn infant and six infants who died in the first month of life had been born to the affected patient before glutaricacidemia type II was diagnosed. After diagnosis, administration of riboflavin (20 mg per day) during the woman's ninth pregnancy led to symptomatic improvement and an increase in fetal movements [Harpey et al., 1983]. Riboflavin supplementation was continued for several months after birth, and the infant did well. Ethylmalonic-adipicaciduria also may be associated with a progressive lipid storage myopathy, which responded dramatically to administration of riboflavin 100 mg and carnitine 3 g per day [Brivet et al., 1991; DeVisser et al., 1986].

Niacin (Vitamin B_3)

The pyridine nucleotides nicotinamide adenine dinucleotide and nicotinamide adenine dinucleotide phosphate are the physiologically active forms of niacin (nicotinic acid), which is present in nucleotides in the form of an amide (nicotinamide) [Henderson, 1983]. These nucleotides function in a variety of oxidation-reduction reactions. The reduced nucleotides are subsequently reoxidized by flavoproteins [White, 1982].

Cellular nicotinamide-adenine dinucleotide and nicotinamide-adenine dinucleotide phosphate, found in a variety of foods, function as the dietary source of niacin. After ingestion, the nucleotides are hydrolyzed in the small intestine to niacin and nicotinamide by the mucosal enzyme nicotinamide-adenine dinucleotide glycohydrolase, a rate-limiting step in absorption. The released niacin and nicotinamide are then transported across the intestine by passive diffusion [Bernofsky, 1980]. The absorbed niacin is rapidly converted to nicotinamide adenine dinucleotide in erythrocytes, and in the liver, nicotinamide adenine dinucleotide glycohydrolases subsequently release nicotinamide for transport to other tissues, where it is reconverted into nicotinamide adenine dinucleotide and nicotinamide adenine dinucleotide phosphate.

Tryptophan is an important secondary dietary source of nicotinic acid [Horwitt et al., 1981]. Nicotinic acid is synthesized from tryptophan in a series of reactions through kynurenine, 3-hydroxy anthranilate, and quinolinate. Approximately 1 mg of nicotinic acid is derived from 60 mg of dietary tryptophan. That symptomatic niacin deficiency (pellagra) occurs predominantly in populations in which corn, which has a low content of tryptophan, serves as the major dietary staple attests to the importance of the substance as a dietary source of niacin.

The minimum amount of dietary niacin required to prevent symptomatic deficiency is 4.4 mg/1000 kcal. The recommended daily dietary reference intake for niacin is 2 to 4 mg/day niacin in children younger than 1 year of age and 6 to 16 mg/day in older children and adolescents.

Niacin Deficiency

The clinical manifestations of niacin deficiency (pellagra) are characterized by the triad of dermatitis, diarrhea, and dementia [Spivais and Jackson, 1977]. Cutaneous manifestations begin with an erythematous dermatitis on the hands; the forehead, neck, and feet are subsequently involved. Hyperpigmentation, desquamation, and scarring ultimately develop. Stomatitis, enteritis, recurrent diarrhea, and excessive salivation are the GI manifestations. CNS manifestations include headache, dizziness, insomnia, depression, and memory impairment. In severe cases, delusions, hallucinations, and dementia can occur. Motor and sensory peripheral nerve abnormalities also occur. Pellagra, caused by nicotinic acid deficiency, is seen mostly in relation to poverty and malnutrition and chronic alcoholism. Encephalopathy manifested by irritability, insomnia, and later hallucinations and delusions, followed by loss of consciousness and myoclonus, developed in an adult alcoholic patient with pellagra treated with B-complex vitamin tablets that did not contain niacin. The neurologic symptomatology resolved after treatment with nicotinic acid [Pitsavas, 2004].

The diagnosis rests predominantly on the dietary history, clinical findings, and a response to physiologic amounts of niacin. Measurement of urinary excretion of methylated metabolites of nicotinic acid is sometimes helpful in confirming the diagnosis.

Niacin Dependency

Hartnup's disease is a disorder of autosomal-recessive inheritance characterized by impairment of neutral amino acid transport by the kidneys and small intestine (see Chapter 23). A diagnostic feature is a striking neutral hyperaminoaciduria. Reduced intestinal absorption and increased renal excretion of tryptophan may lead to a reduced availability of this amino acid for niacin synthesis. Pellagra-like clinical features, including intermittent ataxia, psychotic behavior, and photosensitive skin rash, have been reported. Several reports document clinical but not biochemical improvement after daily administration of 50 to 300 mg of nicotinamide [Henderson, 1958; Herson and Rodnight, 1960].

Pyridoxine (Vitamin B_6)

Vitamin B_6 is the generic term for three naturally occurring pyridine derivatives—pyridoxine (an alcohol), pyridoxal (an aldehyde), and pyridoxamine (an amine) [Fowler, 1985]. Pyridoxal phosphate, the physiologically active form, functions as a cofactor for more than 50 enzymatic reactions, including the decarboxylation, transamination, and racemization of amino acids and reactions in the metabolism of tryptophan, sulfur-containing amino acids, and hydroxyamino acids. Several important interactions between pyridoxine and therapeutic drugs also have been identified [Bauernfeind and Miller, 1987]. Vitamin B_6 enhances the peripheral decarboxylation of levodopa, thereby reducing its therapeutic effectiveness. Isonicotinic acid hydrazide (isoniazid) acts as a potent inhibitor of pyridoxal kinase by combining with pyridoxal phosphate. Pyridoxine also interacts with cycloserine and hydralazine, and penicillamine promotes pyridoxine urinary excretion.

Pyridoxine, pyridoxal, and pyridoxamine are present in meats, liver, cereals, soybeans, and vegetables. Because all three compounds are degraded by heat, ultraviolet light, and oxidation, considerable losses may occur during food preparation. All three compounds are absorbed from the intestine by passive diffusion. In the blood, they are bound to proteins and hemoglobin. After passive uptake by the liver, they are converted to pyridoxal phosphate by the hepatic enzyme pyridoxal kinase. Plasma concentrations reflect concentrations in the liver [Lumeng et al., 1980]. The principal excretory product is pyridoxic acid, which is excreted in the urine after its formation in a reaction catalyzed by the hepatic enzyme aldehyde oxidase. Some unmetabolized pyridoxal also is excreted in the urine.

The requirement for pyridoxine increases with the amount of protein in the diet. The recommended daily dietary reference intake of pyridoxine is 0.1 to 0.3 mg in infants younger than 1 year of age and 0.5 to 1.7 mg in older children and adolescents.

Pyridoxine Deficiency

Clinical manifestations of vitamin B_6 deficiency affect the nervous system, skin, and blood. Neurologic abnormalities include seizures in infants and peripheral neuropathy in adolescents [Snodgrass, 1992]. In infants fed a formula deficient in pyridoxine, irritability, exaggerated startle responses, and generalized seizures developed [Coursin, 1954]. The convulsions may be a consequence of decreased brain concentrations of GABA, which is synthesized from glutamate in a reaction catalyzed by pyridoxal-dependent glutamic acid dehydrogenase [Kurleman et al., 1991; Lott et al., 1978]. Pyridoxine deficiency also leads to decreased brain concentrations of norepinephrine and serotonin [Lovenberg et al., 1962]. Cutaneous manifestations include a seborrheic dermatitis (predominantly about the eyes, nose, and mouth), glossitis, and stomatitis. Microcytic, hypochromic anemia is the characteristic hematologic abnormality.

The diagnosis of pyridoxine deficiency rests predominantly on the correlation of the dietary history, characteristic clinical findings, and prompt response of clinical symptoms with the administration of physiologic amounts of pyridoxine. An increase in the urinary excretion of the tryptophan metabolite xanthurenic acid after an oral load of tryptophan (100 mg/kg) serves as a possible confirmatory laboratory test.

Pyridoxine Dependency

Pyridoxine dependency is associated with an autosomal-recessive error of metabolism characterized by a severe neonatal (or prenatal) seizure disorder with the onset of generalized convulsions in the newborn period that is responsive to pharmacologic amounts of pyridoxine [Gospe, 2002; Haenggeli et al., 1991]. Seizures usually begin within the first hours of life, but their recognition may be delayed. An intrauterine onset also has been reported [Bejsovec et al., 1967]. Pyridoxine-dependent epilepsy is diagnosed clinically, but potentially more common presentations, with later onset and atypical features, widen the spectrum [Pearl and Gibson, 2004]. A majority of affected patients are mentally retarded [Burd, 2000] and may have other neuropsychiatric abnormalities [Baynes et al., 2003]. The EEG is severely abnormal, demonstrating a variety of abnormal paroxysmal patterns, including hypsarrhythmia [Mikati et al., 1991]. Cessation of seizures and normalization of the EEG occur promptly after the parenteral administration of pyridoxine (50 to 100 mg intravenously). Lifelong administration of pharmacologic amounts of pyridoxine (5 to 300 mg/kg per day) is necessary to prevent recurrence of convulsions [Haenggeli et al., 1991]. Neurologic damage usually can be prevented when appropriate therapy is initiated promptly.

The molecular basis of this disorder is not known. A mutation leading to defective binding of pyridoxal phosphate to glutamate decarboxylase, essential for GABA synthesis, has been suggested [Bonner et al., 1960]. No gene locus has been confirmed; the pathophysiology may involve alterations in pyridoxal phosphate transport, binding to glutamate decarboxylase, or other pyridoxal phosphate–dependent pathways [Pearl and Gibson, 2004]. An instability of plasma albumin pyridoxal binding also has been implicated [Heeley et al., 1978]. Pyridoxine dependency is also associated with one of the subtypes of homocystinuria (see Chapter 23). Recently, much interest has been focused on the role of B_6 and hyperhomocystinuria, particularly in relation to cerebrovascular disease and neuropsychiatric disorders in adults. No definite evidence exists for short-term benefit from vitamin B_6 in improving mood (depression, fatigue, and tension symptoms) or cognitive functions in adult patients [Malouf and Grimley, 2003], or for secondary prevention of stroke [Schwammenthal and Tanne, 2004].

Pyridoxine dependency also has been demonstrated in some patients with cystathioninuria. Deficient activity of cystathionase catalyzes the cleavage of cysteine to α-ketobutyrate and leads to cystathioninuria [Frimpter, 1965]. Cystathioninuria has been detected in patients suffering from retardation, seizures, nephrogenic diabetes insipidus, and diabetes mellitus; however, because cystathioninuria also is found in unaffected people, a causal association between the metabolic defect and clinical symptoms has not been substantiated [Nyhan, 1984]. Pyridoxal phosphate is a cofactor in the cystathionase reaction, and a dramatic reduction in the cystathioninuria occurs after administration of pyridoxine in pharmacologic dosages (up to 100 mg per day) in most instances [Pascal et al., 1975].

Another disorder associated with pyridoxine dependency involves ornithine metabolism. Ornithinemia (gyrate atrophy of the retina and choroid) and ornithinuria resulting from a deficiency in the activity of ornithine-delta-aminotransferase, for which pyridoxal phosphate is a cofactor, are associated with the autosomal-recessive syndrome of gyrate atrophy of the retina and choroid [Simell and Takki, 1973]. A variety of genetic mutations account for the disorder [Brody et al., 1992]. This disorder usually manifests with night blindness between the ages of 5 and 10 years and is gradually progressive, leading to blindness by the fourth decade of life. The name *gyrate atrophy* is derived from the early appearance of peripheral atrophic lesions of the retina that resemble cerebral gyri. The funduscopic abnormality, also progressive, eventually is characterized by retinitis pigmentosa and optic nerve atrophy. Although weakness is not a prominent symptom, type II muscle fibers are atrophic, and tubular aggregates are found in muscle biopsy specimens [Sipila et al., 1979]. Plasma ornithine concentrations are 10 to 20 times normal, and urinary ornithine excretion reaches 0.5 to 10 mmol per day. L-ornithin-2-oxoacid aminotransferase activity in cultured skin fibroblast from affected patients ranges from 0 to 5.7% of normal control subjects [O'Donnell et al., 1978]. Pharmacologic dosages of pyridoxine (500 to 1000 mg per day) substantially reduce the elevated plasma ornithine concentrations and appear to prevent further visual deterioration [Berson et al., 1981; Hayasaka et al., 1982; Weleber and Kennaway, 1981].

Penicillamine administration in persons with mild pyridoxine dependency can result in clinical symptoms [Swaiman and Milstein, 1970].

Pyridoxine Intoxication

Chronic pyridoxine intoxication produces a progressive axonal sensory neuropathy in experimental animals and human adults. Daily oral administration of 300 mg/kg of pyridoxine to adult beagles produced widespread neuronal degeneration in dorsal root ganglia [Krinke et al., 1980]. Smaller but still excessive amounts (50 to 200 mg per day) administered over longer periods produced a reversible axonal sensory neuropathy without demonstrable pathologic results in the dorsal root ganglia [Phillips et al., 1978; Windeback et al., 1985]. In the human adult, clinical manifestations of a sensory neuropathy occurred after the ingestion of 2 to 6 g per day for several months [Schaumburg et al., 1983]. Nerve conduction studies and histologic examination of sensory nerve biopsies limited the pathologic origin to sensory nerve axonal degeneration. Partial, gradual recovery followed cessation of pyridoxine ingestion. Subsequent reports indicated that sensory neuropathy could result from the ingestion of only 200 mg of pyridoxine per day [Berger and Schaumburg, 1984; Parry and Bredesen, 1985]. The molecular basis for the sensory neuropathy is unknown. A similar syndrome has not been reported in the pediatric age group.

Cobalamin (Vitamin B_{12})

Vitamin B_{12} is a generic term for organometallic compounds (cobalamins) in which a cobalt atom with a complex side chain is situated within a corrin ring [Davis, 1985]. The cobalamins are further differentiated by attachments to the cobalt atom. Hydroxycobalamin, methylcobalamin, and deoxyadenosylcobalamin have been isolated from mammalian tissue. Hydroxycobalamin is the major cobalamin in blood. Methylcobalamin and adenosylcobalamin function as cofactors in enzymatic reactions. Cyanocobalamin, a stable compound formed as an artifact of isolation, can be used in therapy because it is readily convertible to hydroxycobalamin. Methylcobalamin is a cofactor for cytoplasmic methionine synthase, the enzyme that catalyzes the transfer of a methyl group from 5-methyltetrahydrofolate in the remethylation of homocysteine to methionine. Deoxyadenosylcobalamin is a cofactor for mitochondrial methylmalonyl-CoA mutase, the enzyme that catalyzes the isomerization of methylmalonyl-CoA to succinyl-CoA.

Cobalamins can be synthesized only by certain microorganisms. Stored cobalamins in meats and dairy products provide the predominant dietary source for humans. Vitamin B_{12} absorption is a complex mechanism requiring several steps. Ingested cobalamin binds to intrinsic factor, a glycoprotein formed by gastric parietal cells, in the upper small intestine [Donaldson, 1981]. The cobalamin–intrinsic factor complex subsequently interacts with specific receptors on ileal brush border cells, where the complex is dissociated and free cobalamin is absorbed into the circulation. In blood, vitamin B_{12} is bound to several carrier proteins, the transcobalamins. Transcobalamin II is the predominant carrier protein for newly absorbed cobalamin, and the transcobalamin II–cobalamin complex is preferentially delivered to the liver, bone marrow, and other proliferating cells [Allen, 1976]. At the target tissue, the transcobalamin II-cobalamin complex attaches to specific surface receptors and subsequently is transported into the cells by pinocytosis.

Within the cell, proteolytic lysosomal enzymes degrade the carrier protein and release free cobalamin into the cytoplasm. Adenosylcobalamin is formed within mitochondria from hydroxycobalamin. The trivalent cobalt atom of hydroxycobalamin is successively reduced to monovalent cobalamin in enzymatic reactions catalyzed by reductase enzymes, and adenosylcobalamin is formed from monovalent cobalamin through a reaction catalyzed by adenosyltransferase. The recommended daily dietary reference intake for vitamin B_{12} is 0.4 to 0.5 μg in infants younger than 1 year of age and 0.9 to 2.4 μg for older children and adolescents.

Cobalamin Deficiency

Symptomatic cobalamin deficiency, although rare in childhood, can occur as a consequence of inadequate dietary intake, congenital or acquired intrinsic factor deficiency, removal of the vitamin from the intestine by bacteria or parasites, malabsorptive states resulting from surgical resection [Banerji and Hurwitz, 1971] or chronic disease [Pant et al., 1968a], or an inherited disease of the specific ileal receptor [Matthews and Linnell, 1982]. Vitamin B_{12} deficiency has been described primarily in adults, presumably because of the prolonged duration between surgery and the onset of neurologic symptoms [Williams et al., 1969]. Manifestations of cobalamin (vitamin B_{12}) deficiency are hematologic (pernicious anemia), GI, neurologic, and psychiatric [Carmel, 2003; Healton et al., 1991]. Characteristically, all of these systems are involved, but neurologic disease can occur in the absence of anemia or macrocytosis [Green and Kinsella, 1995; Lindenbaum et al., 1988]. The underlying biochemical abnormality associated with B_{12} deficiency is thought to be due to a defect in one of the two cobalamin-dependent enzymes, methionine synthase and methylmalonyl-CoA mutase [Beck, 1988].

Neurologic manifestations are caused by predominantly white matter degenerative lesions in the brain, spinal cord, and peripheral nerves and include optic neuropathy, progressive cerebellar ataxia, myelopathy, peripheral neuropathy, and gaze limitation. Most patients with pernicious anemia with neurologic dysfunction present with a mixed myelopathic-neuropathic picture. A description of "subacute combined degeneration" after partial gastrectomy was provided by Knox and Delamore [1960]. This entity involves degenerative changes in the posterior and lateral columns without proliferative glial changes. Degenerative changes in the cerebral white matter also may occur [Adams and Kubic, 1944; Pant, 1968a]. Clinical manifestations, seen primarily in adults, include paresthesias of the feet and fingers, disturbed vibratory and proprioceptive senses, and spasticity, caused by involvement of the peripheral nerves and spinal cord. Cognitive abnormalities include slow mentation, dementia, confusion, memory changes, and psychiatric symptoms including depression, acute psychosis, and manic and schizophrenic states [Lindenbaum et al., 1988]. Diffuse leukoencephalopathy is present on MRI, and a decrease in signs of subacute combined degeneration and neuropsychiatric abnormalities is observed after methylcobalamine therapy [Ahn, 2004; Healton, 1991; Lindenbaum et al., 1988; Morita, 2003; Williams et al., 1969]. MRI has been useful in detecting lesions in the spinal cord, brainstem, and cerebellum that appear as high-signal-intensity areas on T2-weighted images that can resolve with B_{12} treatment [Katsaros et al., 1998].

Inadequate cobalamin ingestion occurs predominantly in infants exclusively breast-fed by strictly vegetarian mothers [Cornejo et al., 2001; Grattan Smith et al., 1997; Higginbottom et al., 1978; Kuhne et al., 1991]. Two forms of intrinsic factor deficiency (pernicious anemia) occur in the pediatric age group [Arthur, 1972]. Congenital pernicious anemia is an inherited disorder in which intrinsic factor deficiency is not associated with other structural or functional gastric abnormalities, and antibodies to intrinsic factor are not detected. Symptoms usually begin before the age of 3 years. Juvenile pernicious anemia has characteristics similar to those of adult pernicious anemia—in both, the intrinsic factor deficiency is associated with gastric atrophy, achlorhydria, antibodies to intrinsic factor or gastric parietal cells, and other endocrinopathies. The juvenile form usually becomes symptomatic late in childhood or early in adolescence. A familial disorder in which cobalamin deficiency results from an impairment of transport across the specific ileal receptor also has been well documented [Grasbeck et al., 1960; Mackenzie et al., 1972]. An infant with mild symptoms of vitamin B_{12} deficiency secondary to the failure of the release of cobalamin into the cytoplasm from lysosomes also has been described [Rosenblatt et al., 1985].

Developmental regression is the presenting symptom in most infants with cobalamin (vitamin B_{12}) deficiency. A review of findings in six infants with nutritional B_{12} deficiency noted a consistent clinical pattern of irritability, anorexia, failure to thrive, marked developmental regression, and poor brain growth [Graham et al., 1992]. A recent report of 14 infants documented feeding difficulties, failure to thrive, hypotonia, seizures, microcephaly, and developmental delay with an unfavorable outcome, often with early death or significant neurologic impairment in survivors [Biancheri et al., 2001]. Cerebral white matter atrophy was detected by MRI in a majority of patients. Waking EEG exhibited epileptiform abnormalities, and a high incidence of seizures was reported in these cases. Increased latency of evoked responses and/or prolongation of central conduction time were the most significant neurophysiologic abnormalities. Irritability and lethargy may rapidly progress to coma. Mental retardation and signs of peripheral neuropathy [Renault et al., 1999] are common. Encephalopathy, seizures, and microcephaly were described in another infant with megaloblastic anemia, caused by a subclinical pernicious anemia of the mother [Korenke, 2004].

Involuntary movements are characteristic neurologic abnormalities in infants with B_{12} deficiency. In the case of an exclusively breast-fed infant of a vitamin B_{12}–deficient mother, symptoms and signs consisted of abnormal vigilance and a movement disorder. MRI of the brain demonstrated atrophy, or reduced brain volume, and a delay in myelination. Proton magnetic resonance spectroscopy revealed accumulation of lactate in the white and gray matter, suggesting an abnormality of oxidative energy metabolism [Horstmann, 2003]. In other infants with cobalamin deficiency caused by maternal cobalamin deficiency, abnormal movements developed a few days after the start of cobalamin therapy [Ozer, 2001]. The explanation for the timing of the onset of abnormal movements in these children is not clear. These abnormal movements were described as a combination of tremor and myoclonus and were treated with clonazepam. A case report of three infants with cobalamin deficiency and cognitive regression noted the onset of a movement disorder consisting of tremor and myoclonus, particularly involving the face, tongue, and pharynx, that appeared 48 hours after the initiation of treatment with intramuscular cobalamin [Grattan Smith et al., 1997]. Other neurologic symptoms subsided and the movements slowly abated 3 to 6 weeks after initiation of treatment. In general, vitamin B_{12} deficiency caused by maternal pernicious anemia needs to be considered in the differential diagnosis in infants with neurologic disease, especially if they have megaloblastic anemia. In older children, paresthesias, ataxia, hyperreflexia with a Babinski sign, ankle clonus, and distal loss of vibratory and position sense are common. These neurologic abnormalities likely result from deficient methionine synthase activity with deficiency of *S*-adenosylmethionine [Hall, 1990; Surtees, 1993]. Sensory ataxia, along with megaloblastic anemia and skin hyperpigmentation, was described in a young male patient with low serum B_{12} level and a family history of megaloblastic anemia. Spinal MRI demonstrated extensive demyelination of the posterior columns along the entire length of the cord. Treatment with cobalamin resulted in complete remission and normalization of the MRI appearance [Facchini, 2001].

Exposure to nitrous oxide, used during anesthesia, can be a precipitating factor for increased neurologic and other abnormalities in infants with megaloblastic anemia, because nitrous oxide depletes cobalamin [Felmet, 2000].

Macrocytic, megaloblastic anemia results from failure of erythrocytes to mature. Giant megakaryocytes and enlarged polymorphonuclear leukocytes are present in the peripheral smear. Characteristics of this anemia are similar to those of the macrocytic anemia secondary to folate deficiency: Cobalamin deficiency leads to a functional folate deficiency, because methyltetrahydrofolate cannot be demethylated to its active tetrahydrofolate form. Serum vitamin B_{12} concentration in this anemia is below 100 pg/mL (normal, 140 to 700 pg/mL). Methylmalonic acid is excreted in the urine. The amount of labeled vitamin B_{12} excreted in the urine after the ingestion of 1 to 2 μg of cobalt-57- or cobalt-60-labeled cyanocobalamin, followed by the intramuscular administration of 1 mg of unlabeled vitamin B_{12} (the Schilling test), is useful in assessing vitamin B_{12} absorption. Repeating the test with the addition of orally administered intrinsic factor will differentiate between pernicious anemia and other absorption defects.

Cobalamin neuropathy, in conjunction with low levels of cerebrospinal *S*-adenosylmethionine and abnormal myelination in inherited disorders affecting cobalamin and folate metabolism, also has been reported [Metz, 1993]. On rare occasions, neurologic complications of anorexia nervosa caused by vitamin B_{12} deficiency have been observed [Patchell et al., 1994].

Intramuscular injection of 1 to 5 μg of cobalamin results in prompt hematologic improvement and serves as a confirmatory test. Oral administration of 1000 μg of cobalamin at monthly intervals prevents recurrent deficiency; 1000 μg given at weekly intervals is suggested for the treatment of neurologic deficits.

Cobalamin Dependency

Transcobalamin II deficiency is an autosomal-recessive disorder characterized by failure to thrive, hypotonia, megaloblastic anemia, and recurrent infection [Hitzig et al., 1974]. Oral ulcerations and glossitis develop. The serum cobalamin concentration is normal despite the absence of transcobalamin II, the carrier protein for newly absorbed cobalamin. Oral or parenteral administration of cobalamin (1000 μg per week) results in remission of the clinical manifestations. When affected, other cobalamin-dependent enzyme pathways cause methylmalonicacidemia or homocystinuria with methylmalonicacidemia (see Chapter 23).

Vitamin B_{12} and Cognitive Functioning

Because animal products are the only source of vitamin B_{12}, infants breast-fed by mothers with low intakes of these products and children who do not consume them are at risk for vitamin B_{12} deficiency [Black, 2003]. Greater than two thirds of school-aged children from rural Kenya experience vitamin B_{12} deficiency [Siekmann et al., 2003], suggesting that the worldwide prevalence of B_{12} deficiency in developing countries may be substantial.

Most research examining the relation between B_{12} deficiency and cognitive functioning in children is limited to case studies of infants of mothers with pernicious anemia or vegan mothers [Black, 2003] or those who were on a macrobiotic diet (containing no meat or dairy products) during infancy and childhood. As recently reviewed, several studies have found delays in motor and language development, poorer cognitive performance, and delays in reaction time on neuropsychologic tests of perception, memory, and reasoning, along with academic problems including lower academic performance, lower teacher ratings, more attentional problems, and more delinquent behavior in children with B_{12} deficiency [Black, 2003; Bryan, 2004].

Vitamin C (Ascorbic Acid)

Vitamin C is a generic term for compounds that have the biologic activity of ascorbic acid [Englehard and Seifters, 1986; Levine, 1986]. Ascorbic acid, a six-carbon compound that is structurally related to glucose, can be synthesized by most vertebrates, but in humans and a few animals the last enzyme involved in ascorbate synthesis is missing. Ascorbic acid is reversibly oxidized in the body to dihydroascorbic acid, a compound that retains full vitamin C activity.

Vitamin C functions as a reducing agent in a variety of hydroxylation reactions, providing electrons to metal-containing enzymes to maintain the metal in the reduced form that is necessary for optimal activity. Known functions include the conversion of proline to hydroxyproline in collagen synthesis, the hydroxylation of lysine in carnitine synthesis, and the hydroxylation of dopamine to norepinephrine. Vitamin C also has a role in the synthesis of serotonin, several peptide hormones, and acetylcholine receptors [Block and Levine, 1991].

Ascorbic acid is available from fruits, vegetables, and potatoes. It is destroyed by heat, oxidation, and alkali but is stable in acid. Ascorbic acid is readily absorbed through the intestinal tract by simple diffusion, and its plasma concentration varies with the amount of intake. An active transport system in the choroid plexus maintains brain and cerebrospinal fluid ascorbic acid concentrations within a relatively narrow range [Spector and Lorenzo, 1973].

The recommended daily dietary reference intake for vitamin C is 40 to 50 mg for infants younger than 1 year of age and 15 to 75 mg for older children and adolescents. Consumption of ascorbic acid above the recommended daily allowance leads to increases in plasma concentrations and body stores, but because the renal threshold for ascorbic acid approximates 1.5 mg/dL, ingestion of amounts greater than 100 mg per day merely results in increased urinary excretion.

Vitamin C Deficiency

Symptomatic vitamin C deficiency (scurvy) is now quite rare but still occurs [Ratanachu-Ek et al., 2003]. In some developing countries, vitamin C deficiency has been reported in approximately 30% of children younger than 2 years of age and in 40% of women [Villalpando et al., 2003]. Even in developed countries, inadequate intake of vitamin C, defined as intake below two thirds of recommended values, has been reported in children [Serra-Majem et al., 2001]. In the United States, a study examining prevalence rates of vitamin C deficiency between 1984 and 1994 in adult and pediatric populations found that mean intakes and serum levels of vitamin C were normal but that vitamin C deficiency and depletion were common, occurring in 5% to 17% and 13% to 23%, respectively, of respondents [Hampl et al., 2004]. Infants fed exclusively cow's milk or unsupplemented evaporated milk formulas were the most prone to the development of scurvy [Grewar, 1959]. Occasional instances of scurvy in children with peculiar dietary habits continue to be reported [Douglas et al., 1973; Ellis et al., 1984]. Such habits have been observed in children with developmental delay [Weinstein et al., 2000], as well as those with autism [Monks et al., 2002]. Little correlation exists between clinical manifestations of vitamin C deficiency and known molecular functions on the vitamin.

The onset of symptoms is delayed for 4 to 9 months after the initiation of a deficient diet. Initial manifestations include irritability, tachypnea, anorexia, and pallor. The most striking subsequent manifestations are a consequence of musculoskeletal pain and a hemorrhagic diathesis [Akikusa et al., 2003; Ratanachu-Ek et al., 2003; Weinstein et al., 2000]. Bone pain leads to decreased voluntary movement, especially of the lower limbs (pseudoparalysis). Infants prefer to lie immobile in the supine position, with the hips partially flexed and externally rotated (pithed-frog position). Attempts at examination and passive movement cause considerable pain. Petechial hemorrhages secondary to capillary fragility appear in the skin, initially surrounding hair follicles, and at the gums and may lead to frank purpura. Subarachnoid and subdural hemorrhages may occur. Extraocular muscle palsy may result from intraocular hemorrhage. Radiographs of the long bones, especially around the knee, reveal characteristic abnormalities, including thinning of the cortex, rarefaction of the epiphyses, and trabecular atrophy. Epiphyseal separation may occur. During healing, the subperiosteal hemorrhages, not visualized in the acute stage, become calcified, and the healing bone assumes a characteristic dumbbell shape.

Plasma ascorbate levels reflect current intake rather than body stores. Leukocyte ascorbic acid concentrations below 30 mg/dL suggest depleted stores. Daily administration of 100 to 200 mg of ascorbic acid for 10 days leads to rapid reversal of clinical symptoms [Ratanachu-Ek et al., 2003]. Bone abnormalities resolve completely within a few months.

Transient Neonatal Tyrosinemia

Transient tyrosinemia is present in 0.2% to 10% of neonates and may persist for several months [Goldsmith, 1983]. It is more common in preterm infants and least common in breast-fed term neonates. Although the molecular basis of the disorder has not been fully elucidated, a combination of excessive protein intake and relative deficiency of the activity of the enzyme hydroxyphenylpyruvate oxidase likely is responsible. Ascorbic acid facilitates the activity of this hydroxylation enzyme.

Lethargy, feeding difficulties, hypotonia, and prolonged jaundice have been associated with tyrosinemia, although many infants are asymptomatic. Mild mental retardation may be a long-term sequela [Mamunes et al., 1976; Menkes et al., 1972]. In addition to hypertyrosinemia, the blood concentration of phenylalanine is increased in affected neonates, and urinary excretion of tyrosine and some of its metabolites is also increased. A reduction of daily protein intake to 2 to 3 g/kg usually corrects the hypertyrosinemia. In some infants, additional supplementation with ascorbic acid (100 to 400 mg per day) produces a dramatic response.

Vitamin D

Vitamin D is the generic term for a group of steroid compounds that function in the regulation of calcium and phosphate homeostasis by promoting the absorption of calcium and phosphorus from the intestine, enhancing calcium resorption by the kidney in conjunction with the parathyroid hormone, and mobilizing calcium from the bone [Bell, 1985; Henry and Norman, 1984]. Vitamin D_2 (calciferol) is derived from the plant sterol ergosterol, and vitamin D_3 (cholecalciferol) is derived from 7-dehydrocholesterol in skin. Calciferol and cholecalciferol are derived from respective provitamins by a nonenzymatic photochemical reaction activated by ultraviolet light, which results in the cleavage of the B-sterol ring to form a diene bridge. In humans, the metabolic fate and physiologic properties of vitamin D_2 and of vitamin D_3 are similar. 7-Dehydrocholesterol normally is present in the skin and is converted to cholecalciferol by solar ultraviolet radiation. Under optimal exposure to sunlight, dietary supplementation of vitamin D is not necessary because cholecalciferol is transported to the liver and stored.

The active form of vitamin D is calcitriol (1,25-dihydroxycholecalciferol), which is formed from cholecalciferol by two successive hydroxylations. The initial hydroxylation to calcidiol 25-hydroxycholecalciferol occurs in the liver, and the second hydroxylation to calcitriol occurs in the kidney. The activity of the kidney mitochondrial hydroxylase, which catalyzes the second hydroxylation, is stimulated by parathyroid hormone and increases with deficiencies of vitamin D, calcium, and phosphate. Dietary vitamin D and vitamin D_3 are absorbed from the small intestine. Bile is essential for absorption. After absorption, the vitamin, bound to a lipoprotein complex, is transported in lymph chylomicrons to the liver, where it is stored before its hydroxylation to calcidiol. Calcidiol is the major circulating form of vitamin D in the blood. Calcitriol is hydroxylated to 1,24,25-trihydroxycalciferol by a renal hydroxylase that also hydroxylates 25-hydroxycalciferol to 24,25-dihydroxycalciferol. These compounds have less vitamin D activity than calcitriol and probably represent excretory compounds excreted in the bile. The recommended daily dietary reference intake for vitamin D is 5.0 μg cholecalciferol for infants younger than 1 year of age and 5 to 15 μg for older children and adolescents.

Reports of nutritional rickets among U.S. children less than 18 years of age published between 1986 and 2003 found that the average age of children with rickets ranged from 4 to 54 months of age; that approximately 83% were black; and that 96% were breast-fed, and among those who were breast-fed, only 5% of records indicated vitamin D supplementation during breast-feeding [Weisberg et al., 2004]. In 1963, the American Academy of Pediatrics (AAP) recommended 400 IU of vitamin D per day for all infants and children [Greer, 2004]. In response to the 1997 Institute of Medicine recommendations, however, and after reports of increasing nutritional rickets in certain populations, the AAP in 2003 changed the dietary reference intake dose to 200 IU for all infants and children. In making these recommendations, several issues were considered, including the following: (1) Vitamin D deficiency is more than rickets, which is the final stage of the deficient state among growing children; (2) adequate sunlight exposure cannot be determined exactly; (3) ultraviolet B light exposure in childhood carries a risk for later development of skin cancer; and (4) intake of vitamin D-fortified food intake in older children and adolescents has been decreasing [Greer, 2004].

Vitamin D Deficiency

Symptomatic vitamin D deficiency can occur as a consequence of inadequate dietary intake [Edidin et al., 1980; Ladhani et al., 2004], inadequate exposure to sunlight, malabsorption states, chronic hepatic or renal disease, or administration of antiepileptic drugs, or from the chronic effects of severe burn injury [Klein et al., 2004]. Even in "dairy states" such as Wisconsin, vitamin D deficiency can occur, particularly in infants who were breast-fed and did not receive vitamin supplementation [Mylot et al., 2004]. Vitamin D deficiency remains the major cause of rickets among young infants in most developing countries because breast milk is low in vitamin D and its metabolites and because social and religious customs or climatic conditions often prevent adequate ultraviolet light exposure [Pettifor, 2004]. Also, mothers who are vitamin D–deficient in pregnancy are likely to be deficient postnatally, and their infants, especially if breast-fed, are at higher risk of vitamin D deficiency [Thompson et al., 2004].

Over the past several decades, antiepileptic drugs have been associated with rickets in children and osteomalacia in adults, but reports were primarily in institutionalized persons [Pack et al., 2004]. Studies in ambulatory adults and children taking antiepileptic drugs do not reveal rickets or osteomalacia but do report alterations of bone mineral metabolism and density and increased fracture rates. Antiepileptic drugs that induce the cytochrome P-450 enzyme system are most commonly associated with bone abnormalities, and data suggest that valproate, an enzyme inhibitor, also may affect bone metabolism [Pack et al., 2004]. Limited information is available on the newer antiepileptic drugs and the risk of developing rickets. Patients who are institutionalized are more vulnerable because of added factors including reduced physical activity and reduced exposure to light. Prophylactic supplementation with vitamin D is advised in such institutionalized patients chronically treated with antiepileptic drugs.

Clinical manifestations predominantly affect the bone, leading to rickets in children and osteomalacia in adults. The bone abnormalities in rickets are secondary to inadequate mineralization of osteoid tissue. Craniotabes, or thinning of the inner table of the skull, is an early manifestation in infants. Rickets is further characterized by epiphyseal enlargements at the wrists, ankles, and costochondral junctions; bending of the shafts of long bones; scoliosis; and kyphosis.

Neurologic manifestations are characterized by tetany, which occurs when the metabolic abnormality leads to hypocalcemia. Symptoms are not present in latent tetany, but elicitation of Chvostek's, Trousseau's, and Erb's signs constitutes evidence of increased neuromuscular irritability. Latent tetany is usually associated with serum calcium concentrations between 7 and 7.5 mg/dL. Manifest tetany, characterized by symptomatic carpopedal spasm, laryngospasm, or convulsions, usually is associated with serum calcium concentrations below 7 mg/dL. Vitamin D deficiency also causes muscle weakness and muscle aches and pains in both children and adults. Recent research has demonstrated that a large number of children and adults have deficient levels of vitamin D [Holick, 2003]. These patients may present with persistent musculoskeletal pain [Plotnikoff, 2003]. Limb-girdle muscle weakness secondary to vitamin D deficiency also has been recently reported [van der Heyden et al., 2004]. Hypocalcemia, elevated alkaline phosphatase, and low 25-hydroxycalciferol are found in patients receiving chronic antiepileptic therapy [Alderman, 1994]. Seizures can recur because of the hypocalcemia [Ali, 2004]. As reported in a recent study, the volume of the posterior fossa in children with rickets is significantly smaller than in normal children, and a significant number of them have a Chiari I malformation [Tubbs, 2004].

The diagnosis of rickets is confirmed by radiologic examination. Wrist radiographs are best for early diagnosis and demonstrate the characteristic widened, frayed, concave distal ends of the ulna and radius. The distance between the ends of these long bones and the carpal bones is increased, because the large rachitic metaphysis is not calcified. Plasma alkaline phosphatase level is elevated, and the serum phosphorus concentration usually is below 4 mg/dL. The serum calcium concentration may be normal or reduced. Daily administration of 0.2 to 0.5 μg of calcitriol leads to healing, demonstrable on radiographs within 2 to 4 weeks. In tetany, calcium supplementation also is necessary.

Vitamin D Dependency

VITAMIN D-DEPENDENT RICKETS TYPE I

Vitamin D-dependent rickets type I is transmitted as an autosomal-recessive trait and is characterized by hypotonia, weakness, failure to thrive, tetany, and convulsions in the first year of life [Rassmussen and Anast, 1983]. The disorder is caused by deficient activity of the renal 1-hydroxylase that catalyzes the synthesis of calcitriol from calcidiol. Bone radiographs are indistinguishable from those of vitamin D deficiency. The serum alkaline phosphatase level is elevated, and the phosphorus concentration is normal or low. Hypocalcemia is common. The serum calcidiol concentration is normal, but the calcitriol concentration is reduced. Treatment with pharmacologic dosages of vitamin D (vitamin D_3, 5000 to 40,000 units per day; calcitriol, 1 to 3 μg per day) reverses the manifestations of rickets and permits normal growth.

Vitamin D Intoxication

Symptoms of vitamin D intoxication develop 1 to 3 months after excessive intake of the vitamin. Clinical manifestations include irritability, hypotonia, polydipsia, polyuria, and constipation. Hypertension with retinopathy, aortic stenosis, corneal and conjunctival clouding, and nephropathy occur in chronic cases. Laboratory findings include hypercalcemia, hypercalciuria, and metastatic calcifications on radiographs of long bones. Treatment consists of discontinuing vitamin D ingestion and decreasing calcium intake.

Tocopherol (Vitamin E)

Vitamin E is the generic term for a group of fat-soluble compounds that function as scavengers of free radicals, protecting polyunsaturated fatty acids in subcellular organelles from oxidation by free radicals generated in normal metabolic reactions or by toxic compounds. α-Tocopherol is the most important of these compounds and is widely distributed in foods, especially vegetable oils. Absorption of vitamin E depends on the intestinal digestion and absorption of fat and the presence of bile. Once absorbed, the vitamin enters lymph channels and, in chylomicrons and very-low-density lipoproteins, is transported to the blood, where it equilibrates with plasma lipoproteins. It is stored predominantly in adipose tissue. Tissue stores will provide a source for the vitamin for long periods. Blood levels reflect recent dietary intake and absorption rather than body stores. The recommended daily dietary reference intake of vitamin E is 4 to 5 mg of α-tocopherol equivalents for infants younger than 1 year of age and 6 to 7 mg for older children and adolescents.

Vitamin E Deficiency

Vitamin E deficiency occurs predominantly in disorders associated with either chronic fat malabsorption (e.g., cystic fibrosis, celiac disease, chronic cholestatic hepatobiliary disorders including biliary atresia, short bowel syndrome, inflammatory bowel disease) or a deficiency of plasma lipoproteins (e.g., abetalipoproteinemia) [Gordon, 2000; Kayden, 1993; Koenig, 2003; Perkin, 1998; Sokol, 1990]. A neurologic degenerative syndrome associated with selective vitamin E deficiency not associated with fat malabsorption also has been documented [Harding et al., 1985; Krendel et al., 1987].

Infants are born in a state of relative vitamin E deficiency, with plasma α-tocopherol levels below 5 μg/mL (11.6 μmol/L) [Merck, 2005]. The smaller and more premature the infant, the greater the deficiency. Vitamin E deficiency in preterm infants persists during the first few weeks of life and can be attributed to limited placental transfer of vitamin E, low tissue levels at birth, relative dietary deficiency in infancy, intestinal malabsorption, and rapid growth. As the digestive system matures, vitamin E absorption improves, and blood vitamin E levels rise. In children and adults, malabsorption generally underlies vitamin E deficiency. Genetic abnormality in the transport of vitamin E also can play a role.

Clinical manifestations of vitamin E deficiency include progressive weakness, ataxia, ophthalmoplegia, loss of position and vibratory sense, neuropathy, dystonia, and in some instances, especially in abetalipoproteinemia, progressive visual impairment associated with retinitis pigmentosa [Aparicio et al., 2001; Koenig, 2003; Roubertie et al., 2003; Sokol, 1990]. Children with cystic fibrosis and low plasma α-tocopherol levels are at greater risk for long-term neurocognitive impairments unless the deficiency is treated with vitamin E supplementation [Koscik et al., 2004].

Neuropathologic features include cerebellar atrophy and loss of nerve cell bodies in the third and fourth cranial nerve nuclei and axonal dystrophy (e.g., swollen, dystrophic axons, spheroids) in the posterior columns, Clarke's column, and dorsal and ventral spinocerebellar tracts of the spinal cord [Rosenblum et al., 1981]. Premature lipofuscin accumulation in dorsal horn and peripheral nerve Schwann cell cytoplasm also has been reported [Werlin et al., 1983]. Nerve conduction studies [De Schepper et al., 1997] and brainstem evoked responses [Vaisman et al., 1996] also may be abnormal in some patients with vitamin E deficiency.

Early deficiency may not produce neurologic abnormalities. In children with chronic cholestasis and vitamin E deficiency, however, a slowly progressive neuromuscular disease with ataxia, dysmetria, dysarthria, areflexia, loss of vibratory sensation, and ophthalmoplegia, impaired vision, and a pigmentary retinopathy may develop [Guggenheim et al., 1982; Kayden, 1993; Satya-Murti et al., 1986]. The neuropathologic findings are similar to those in animals with experimental vitamin E deficiency and include posterior column degeneration; selective loss of peripheral nerve large-caliber, myelinated axons; and spheroids in the gracile and cuneate nuclei [Rosenblum et al., 1981]. Muscle histochemical studies demonstrate cytoplasmic inclusions and occasional necrotic fibers. Normal dosages of vitamin E for 6 to 14 months improved the neurologic disease in some but not all patients [Guggenheim et al., 1982]. Children with protein energy malnutrition and neurologic signs involving posterior column, spinocerebellar, retinal, and peripheral nerve deficits due to vitamin E deficiency can undergo significant improvement with supplementation [Kalra et al., 2001;

Patients with a familial disorder of vitamin E absorption, manifested by a normal absorption of vitamin E normally but an inability to conserve plasma α-tocopherol in very-low-density lipoproteins, had a neurologic syndrome resembling Friedreich's ataxia—ataxia, cerebellar signs, dysarthria, extensor plantar responses, pes cavus and scoliosis, absence of deep tendon reflexes in the lower extremities, and impaired proprioception [Gordon, 2001; Hamida, 1993]. The disease is genetically recessive and has been mapped to chromosome 8. It is suggested that patients presenting with a syndrome suggesting Friedreich's ataxia should have vitamin E levels measured.

Measurement of serum lipid concentrations documents most instances of vitamin E deficiency. The normal lower limit for adolescents is 5 mg/mL and is lower for younger children [Farrell et al., 1978]. Because vitamin E is bound to lipoproteins in the plasma, the ratio of vitamin E to total serum lipid concentration reflects vitamin E status more accurately in hyperlipidemic states. Limits of normal for this ratio of total tocopherol to total lipid are 0.8 mg/g in adolescents and 0.6 mg/g in infants and children. Serum vitamin E concentrations do not accurately reflect vitamin E states in patients with abetalipoproteinemia. In patients with abetalipoproteinemia, dietary supplementation with vitamin E (100 to 200 mg/kg per day) before the age of 1 year prevented the development of retinopathy and prevented, stabilized, or improved the neurologic disorder [Muller et al., 1977]. The neurologic function of children with vitamin E deficiency associated with chronic cholestasis also was significantly improved by large oral dosages (up to 10 mg/kg per day) or intramuscular injection of α-tocopherol (0.8 to 2.0 IU/kg per day) [Lemonnier et al., 1990; Perlmutter et al., 1987; Sokol et al., 1985].

Mutation of the gene for a-tocopherol transfer proteins, on chromosomal locus 8q13, an autosomal-recessive disorder, causes isolated vitamin E deficiency with ataxia (ataxia with vitamin E deficiency [AVED]) and responds to treatment with vitamin E [Federico, 2004; Mariotti, 2004]. Other neurologic abnormalities observed with these mutations include spasticity and retinitis pigmentosa. A male with vitamin E deficiency ataxia improved after treatment with vitamin E supplementation, but progressive dystonia developed subsequently [Roubertie, 2003].

Biotin (Vitamin H)

Biotin is a cofactor for four carboxylation enzymes: pyruvate carboxylase, acetyl-CoA carboxylase, propionyl-CoA carboxylase, and 3-methylcrotonyl carboxylase [Bartlett et al., 1985]. These enzymes all are involved in carbon chain elongation reactions: pyruvate carboxylase in gluconeogenesis, acetyl-CoA carboxylase in fatty acid synthesis, propionyl-CoA carboxylase in propionate metabolism, and 3-methylcrotonyl carboxylase in leucine catabolism. In these reactions, biotin is linked to a lysine residue of the apoenzyme, in a reaction catalyzed by the enzyme holocarboxylase synthetase, to form the functional carboxylase holoenzyme. Biotin is present in low concentrations in numerous foods [Roth, 1981]. The enzyme biotinidase cleaves biotin from biocytin (biotin-lysine) and from larger biotinyl peptide fragments formed in the degradation of the carboxylase, thereby allowing for biotin reuse.

Biotin-synthesizing bacteria in the small intestine also are a major nutritional source. Biotin is absorbed through the intestine by active transport mechanisms [Said et al., 1990]. In the blood, it is bound to proteins. It is excreted in the urine and feces. The recommended daily dietary reference intake is 5 to 6 μg for neonates and infants younger than 1 year of age and 8 to 25 μg for older children and adolescents.

Biotin Deficiency

Symptomatic biotin deficiency resulting from inadequate dietary intake is quite rare. Two children with symptomatic biotin deficiency associated with the ingestion of large quantities of raw albumin, which contains avidin (a glycoprotein that binds biotin so effectively that its intestinal absorption is prevented), have been described [Scott, 1958; Sweetman et al., 1981]. Biotin deficiency also has been reported as a consequence of parenteral hyperalimentation and chronic hemodialysis [Mock et al., 1981; Yatzidis et al., 1984].

Clinical manifestations of biotin deficiency include a generalized, scaly, erythematous rash resembling seborrheic dermatitis; alopecia totalis; anorexia; severe metabolic acidosis; and neurologic manifestations that include developmental delay or dementia, seizures, progressive ataxia, and hearing loss. In the neonate and young infant, the clinical manifestations may evolve rapidly, with vomiting, failure to thrive, hypotonia, and severe metabolic acidosis leading to coma and death, before other manifestations are evident.

Characteristic laboratory findings in addition to the metabolic acidosis include a specific organic aciduria; 3-methylcrotonylglycine, 3-hydroxyisovaleric acid, 3-hydroxypropionic acid, or 2-methylcitric acid may be detected in the urine. Symptoms and signs are rapidly reversed by the administration of 5 to 10 mg of biotin.

Changes in biotin levels in some children on antiepileptic drug therapy with carbamazepine, phenytoin, or phenobarbital have been described. The clinical significance of such changes remains unknown [Mock, 1998].

Biotin Dependency

The neurologic complications associated with biotin dependency, such as biotin-dependent propionicacidemia, biotin-dependent holocarboxylase synthetase deficiency (neonatal multiple carboxylase deficiency) and biotinidase deficiency (late-onset multiple carboxylase deficiency), are discussed in detail in Chapter 23.

Vitamin K

Vitamin K is a fat-soluble vitamin essential for the biosynthesis of several blood clotting factors, including prothrombin (factor II), proconvertin (factor VII), plasma-converting factor (Christmas factor, factor IX), and Stuart factor (factor X) [Corrigan, 1981; Olsen, 1984; Sutor, 2003]. Vitamin K_1 (phylloquinone), found in chloroplasts of plant leaves and in many vegetable oils, and vitamin K_2, comprising a series of compounds (menaquinones) in which the phytyl chain in vitamin K_1 has been replaced by a side chain containing 2 to 13 phytyl units, are synthesized predominantly by a gram-positive bacterium. Vitamin K_3 (menadione) is a synthetic compound with properties similar to those of phylloquinone.

Vitamin K acts as an essential cofactor for hepatic microsomal enzyme systems, which convert the biologically inactive precursors of prothrombin, proconvertin, and plasma thromboplastin components to the active compounds participating in the events necessary for normal blood clotting. In this process, vitamin K converts residues of phytic-bound glutamic acid in each of the precursors into γ-carboxyglutamyl residues. This conversion activates the blood clotting proteins by allowing them to bind calcium ions. The calcium-carboxyglutamyl proteins subsequently are bound to phospholipid surfaces.

In the process of γ-carboxylation of the glutamate residues, vitamin K quinone is converted to the 2,3-epoxide. An enzyme-dependent salvage mechanism for the regeneration of the active vitamin K catalyzed by the hepatic enzyme epoxide reductase is blocked by warfarin therapy. The recommended daily dietary reference intake for vitamin K is 2.0 to 2.5 μg for infants younger than 1 year of age and 30 to 75 μg for older children and adolescents. Such amounts are readily available when average diets are supplemented by the menaquinones produced by intestinal bacteria.

Vitamin K is absorbed through the small intestine. Bile salts and pancreatic secretions are necessary for optimal absorption. Once absorbed, vitamin K is incorporated into chylomicrons, transported to the liver, and bound to very-low-density lipoproteins, through which it is transported to other tissues.

Vitamin K Deficiency

Vitamin K deficiency results in a hemorrhagic diathesis known as *hemorrhagic disease of the newborn*. The newborn is particularly susceptible because vitamin K stores are deficient, and because factor II, IV, VII, IX, and X concentrations characteristically are only 50% of normal. These concentrations continue to decline for 48 to 72 hours after birth but subsequently increase slowly as a result of the absorption of dietary vitamin K and the initiation of synthesis by bacterial flora in the intestine. Breast-fed infants are particularly prone to development of the disorder, because the vitamin K content of breast milk is low. Hemorrhagic disease of the newborn can occur early (i.e., within the first 2 to 3 days of life) or late (between weeks 2 and 12) [Aydinli et al., 1998; Bor et al., 2000; Zipursky, 1999]. It is estimated that the median incidence of hemorrhagic disease of the newborn in developed countries is 7 per 100,000 births; it likely is much higher in developing countries [Victora and Van Haecke, 1998]. Presenting complaints in a recent study of the late form of the disease were seizures (in 91% of the patients), drowsiness (in 82%), poor sucking (in 64%), vomiting (in 46%), fever (in 46%), pallor (in 46%), acute diarrhea (in 27%), and irritability and high-pitched cry (in 18%); findings on examination included tense or bulging fontanel (in 73%), anisocoria (in 36%), weak neonatal reflexes (in 18%), and cyanosis (in 18%) [Aydinli et al., 1998]. Location of intracranial hemorrhage includes the following: intracerebral 91%, subarachnoid 46%, subdural 27%, and intraventricular 27%. At follow-up evaluation after periods ranging from 6 to 48 months, only three (27%) infants remained neurologically normal; seizures (in 73%), severe psychomotor retardation (in 46%), cerebral palsy (in 46%), microcephaly (in 46%), and hydrocephalus (in 27%) were observed in the remainder.

Vitamin K deficiency may occur in children with severe developmental disabilities [Yoshikawa et al., 2003]. Infection, use of antibiotics, and elemental nutrition are risk factors for vitamin K deficiency in severely disabled children, and vitamin K intake with enteral nutrition might be marginal.

Intracranial hemorrhage, the most serious neurologic consequence, rarely occurs without hemorrhage into other tissues. Hemorrhagic disease in the newborn is now rare because of the routine prophylactic administration of vitamin K on the first day of life but may occur in newborn infants and in older children in association with conditions impairing fat absorption and parenteral alimentation and after the chronic administration of broad-spectrum antibiotics, which sterilize the intestinal tract. Laboratory studies indicate prolonged prothrombin and partial thromboplastin times with normal platelet counts and fibrinogen concentrations.

Parenteral administration of 1 mg vitamin K usually is recommended, although 0.25 μg is sufficient in most instances. When vitamin K deficiency is associated with chronic disease, 1 to 5 mg of vitamin K_1 should be administered parenterally at weekly intervals.

Vitamin K may play a role in development of the CNS. Recently a congenital deficiency of vitamin K-dependent coagulation factors associated with CNS anomalies has been described [Puetz et al., 2004]. Vitamin K deficiency in the embryo secondary to maternal malabsorption has been suggested to cause severe malformations similar to those occurring with warfarin embryopathy and other related conditions [Menger et al., 1997]. It also has been demonstrated that vitamin K–dependent carboxylase expression is temporally regulated in a tissue-specific manner, with high expression in the CNS during early embryonic stages; a wide distribution of the novel vitamin K-dependent growth factor, Gas6, also was demonstrated [Tsaioun, 1999]. Studies with animals also support a role for vitamin K in the biosynthesis of sphingolipids, raising the possibility that vitamin K could be involved in major cellular events such as cell proliferation, differentiation, and survival [Carrie et al., 2004]. Taken together, these results suggest a possible role of vitamin K in nervous system development.

Folate (Vitamin M)

In the past 2 decades, recognition of the importance of folates in the developing nervous system has been increasing, based on its relation to formation of the neural tube (Chapter 19), its role in several of the pediatric neurotransmitter diseases (Chapter 30), and its role in cerebrovascular injury related to stroke risk and hyperhomocystinemia (Chapters 17 and 72).

The folates, a group of pteridine compounds composed of pteroic acid linked to a variable number of glutamate residues, have a fundamental role in cell growth and division [Stover, 2004]. Fully reduced methyltetrahydrofolate, formed from other folates in a reaction catalyzed by the enzyme dihydrofolate reductase, is the active cofactor. Known functions of folate include one-carbon transfer reactions in de novo purine synthesis and in the synthesis of methionine from homocysteine, serine from glycine, and deoxythymidylic acid from deoxyuridylic acid. Folate also is a cofactor in the conversion of formiminoglutamic acid to glutamic acid in the degradation of histidine.

Dietary folates consist predominantly of folate polyglutamates. During the process of absorption and transport across the jejunum, most polyglutamates are hydrolyzed to the monoglutamate, which is subsequently reduced and methylated to methyltetrahydrofolate [Halstead, 1980]. After absorption, methyltetrahydrofolate is rapidly transported to tissues and stored in the liver. Considerable liver methyltetrahydrofolate is excreted in the bile and resorbed in the small intestine. In the plasma, folates are transported either as the free form or loosely bound to protein. A specific folate-binding protein, which is found in low concentration in normal serum, is present in increased concentration in folate deficiency. A different folate-binding protein with a high affinity for methyltetrahydrofolate is present in umbilical cord blood, accounting for the preferential uptake of folate by the fetus, even in folate-depleted mothers. The choroid plexus also contains a folate-binding protein with a high affinity for methyltetrahydrofolate, reflecting the dependency of the CNS on methyltetrahydrofolate because of a low concentration of dihydrofolate reductase [Levitt et al., 1971; Spector and Lorenzo, 1975]. Methyltetrahydrofolate and other folate derivatives are excreted in the urine. Some folate is resorbed by the renal tubule.

The recommended dietary reference intake for folate is 2.0 to 2.5 µg for infants younger than 1 year of age and 30 to 75 µg for older children and adolescents. During pregnancy, lactation, and other conditions characterized by rapid cell division (e.g., hemolytic anemia), the folate requirement can increase to 400 µg per day.

Folate Deficiency

Inadequate dietary intake is rarely the sole cause of folate deficiency but can occur in populations fed exclusively well-boiled foods or in infants for whom goat's milk, which is deficient in folate, forms the major dietary staple. Folate deficiency more commonly results from conditions associated with increased folate requirements or diseases associated with abnormalities of folate absorption, use, or excretion. Pregnancy, prematurity, and diseases characterized by increased cell turnover (e.g., hemolytic anemia) are conditions associated with an increased folate requirement. The preterm infant is especially prone to develop this deficiency because the folate stores (normally formed during the third trimester) are inadequate, rapid growth is taking place, and renal tubular conservation mechanisms are not fully developed [Landon and Hey, 1974; Worthington-White et al., 1994]. Malabsorption defects and hepatic disease may interfere with folate absorption. Several drugs, including phenytoin, phenobarbital, oral contraceptives, and cycloserine, impede folate absorption and use [Waxman et al., 1970]. Methotrexate, trimethoprim, and triamterene specifically inhibit dihydrofolate reduction, preventing methyltetrahydrofolate synthesis [Winick et al., 1992].

A progressive megaloblastic anemia, irritability, diarrhea, and failure to gain weight are the clinical manifestations of folate deficiency in infants. A possible association between human immunodeficiency virus I (HIV) in children with folate deficiency presenting with neurologic symptoms of delayed development, developmental regression, seizures, hypotonia or spastic quadriplegia, and basal ganglia calcifications also has been reported [Habibi et al., 1989].

No single laboratory test is optimal for the documentation of folate deficiency. Megaloblastic anemia is associated with a low reticulocyte count. Nucleated erythrocytes may be present in peripheral blood. Neutropenia and thrombocytopenia also may be present. Vitamin B_{12} deficiency must be excluded because prolonged treatment with folic acid may reverse the megaloblastic anemia of vitamin B_{12} deficiency without affecting the neurologic abnormalities. The serum folate concentrations (normal, 5 to 12 ng/mL) and total red cell content (normal, 150 to 600 ng/mL) are low. The red cell content is a better measure of folate status than is the serum concentration. Formiminoglutamic acid is excreted in the urine, especially after an oral loading dose of histidine. Because the megaloblastic anemia improves within 72 hours, parenteral administration of 200 µg of folic acid can be used as a diagnostic test. Treatment with 2 to 5 mg of folic (pteroylglutamic) acid for 3 to 4 weeks usually is sufficient to reverse the clinical manifestations of deficiency. Disorders associated with cerebral folate deficiency recently have been reviewed [Ramaekers and Blau, 2004] and also are discussed in depth in Chapter 30.

Folate Deficiency and Neural Tube Defects

The mechanisms that underlie the relation between folate and neural tube defects have yet to be determined [Stover, 2004]. Folate-responsive neural tube defects are believed to result from impaired maternal and/or fetal folate metabolism, with the involved pathways being either deoxythymidine monophosphate (dTMP) or methionine synthesis. These metabolic disruptions can be overcome by elevating maternal folate levels. Proposed mechanisms for folate-responsive neural tube defects as reviewed by Stover [2004] include accumulation of homocysteine, decreased rates of DNA synthesis due to impaired dTMP synthesis, and elevations in the *S*-adenosylhomocysteine/methionine ratio. Some evidence indicates that homocysteine can react with and oxidize proteins and also bind to the *N*-methyl-D-aspartate (NMDA) receptor, but direct evidence that homocysteine inhibits closure of the neural tube is lacking. Impaired dTMP synthesis also has been proposed to affect cell proliferation or migration during the critical period of neural tube closure. Finally, increases in the *S*-adenosylhomocysteine/methionine ratio that result from impaired homocysteine remethylation can affect DNA methylation density and alter the expression of genes that are critical for the formation of the neural tube. The best evidence from human studies indicates that impairments in the homocysteine remethylation pathway, or in other affected methionine-dependent methylation reactions for which homocysteine serves as a marker, can impair normal embryonic development [Stover, 2004]. Moderate maternal hyperhomocysteinemia increases risks for neural tube defects.

Recommendations that all women capable of becoming pregnant should consume 400 µg of folic acid per day from supplements or fortified foods were made in the early 1990s, and subsequently the U.S. Food and Drug Administration (FDA) mandated the addition of folic acid to enriched cereal grain products. These changes have had a dramatic effect on improving folate status in this high-risk group and in reducing the incidence of neural tube defects [Hague et al., 2003]. Of additional concern is that increased maternal plasma homocysteine concentrations during pregnancy have been associated with the occurrence of diseases associated with placental vascular thrombosis—in particular, pre-eclampsia and placental abruption, conditions that are well know to potentially cause perinatal brain injury.

Since 1963, evidence from various studies has supported an association between antiepileptic drug and congenital malformations in the offspring of women with epilepsy [Oguni and Osawa, 2004]. Exposure to antiepileptic drug treatment in utero occurs in 1 of every 250 newborns. The absolute risk of major malformations in these infants is approximately 7% to 10%—approximately 3% to 5% higher than in the general population. In part, these teratogenic effects are related to folate deficiency [Lindhout et al., 1994]. Additional risk factors include high maternal daily dosage or serum concentrations of antiepileptic drug, polytherapy, and generalized seizures during pregnancy. Other factors that may contribute to the risk include concomitant diseases such as diabetes mellitus, occupational exposure to teratogens, excessive pre-pregnancy weight, and various nutrient deficiencies [Yerby, 2003]. Adverse pregnancy outcomes include neural tube defects and also congenital heart malformations, facial clefts, hypospadias, and growth and mental retardation [Lindhout et al., 1994]. Valproate and carbamazepine have been associated specifically with the development of neural tube defects. Data concerning the risk for congenital malformations associated with the newer antiepileptic drugs—gabapentin, felbamate, lamotrigine, leve-tiracetam, oxcarbazepine, tiagabine, topiramate, and zonisamide—are still limited. Several pregnancy registries for women taking antiepileptic drugs have been established. It is unclear whether the protective effect of folate supplementation is comparable for women with epilepsy and for pregnant women who do not have epilepsy and who are not on antiepileptic drugs. Despite uncertainty about the efficacy of periconceptional folate supplementation in women with epilepsy, it is recommended that folate supplementation be used (0.4 to 4 mg) [Lindhout et al., 1994; Morrell, 1998; Pennell, 2004; Yerby, 2003].

Hyperhomocysteinemia and Stroke

Hyperhomocysteinemia is an important risk factor for vascular disease, including stroke [Schwammenthal and Tanne, 2004]. Homocysteine is a metabolite of methionine, an essential amino acid derived from dietary protein. It is metabolized by one of two pathways: remethylation into methionine, catalyzed by the vitamin B_{12}–dependent enzyme methionine synthase, or trans-sulfuration to cysteine and glutathione by folate dependent methylene-tetrahydrofolate reductase. A role for homocysteine in the pathogenesis of atherosclerosis was first suggested in 1969; this possibility was based on observation of extensive atherosclerotic changes in two children with hyperhomocysteinemia and homocysteinuria [McCully, 1963]. Mechanisms that have been suggested for the atherothrombotic potential of homocysteine include endothelial dysfunction through oxidative damage (vascular toxicity), increased oxidation of low-density lipoprotein, stimulation of smooth muscle cell proliferation, prothrombotic effects, and impaired thrombolysis [Schwammenthal and Tanne, 2004].

Whether treatment of hyperhomocystinuria with B complex vitamins including folate reduces the risk of recurrent stroke remains somewhat controversial [Kaplan, 2003]. Results of the Vitamin Intervention for Stroke Prevention study (VISP) found that moderate reduction of total homocysteine after nondisabling cerebral infarction had no effect on recurrent stroke or coronary events [Toole, 2004]. Despite the absence of a treatment effect, however, a consistent association among baseline concentration, vascular risk, and the probability of stroke was found [Schwammenthal and Tanne, 2004].

The role of hyperhomocysteinemia in pediatric stroke is reviewed in Chapter 72 and in several recent studies [Cardo et al., 1999, 2000]. A higher prevalence of hyperhomocysteinemia and the nucleotide 677 cytosine-to-thymidine point mutation (677C>T) polymorphism was observed among 21 children with stroke than among 28 children without stroke (28.6% versus 14.3%) [Cardo et al., 2000]. Total plasma homocysteine levels were significantly increased in children aged 2 months to 15 years with stroke compared with reference values. Significant negative correlations also were found between total plasma homocysteine levels and folate and cobalamin levels. Overall, the studies demonstrated that the 677C>T genotype is a strong factor for predisposition to hyperhomocysteinemia and recurrent risk of stroke that also might be prevented with folate supplementation. The authors of these studies suggested that systematic screening for hyperhomocysteinemia should be included in protocols that investigate the etiology of stroke in children and that antiepileptic treatment in children with stroke may be responsible for the mild hyperhomocysteinemia observed in some patients [Cardo et al., 1999]. It also is suggested that dietary supplementation with folate may be of benefit in children with stroke and in those taking antiepileptic drugs.

Folate Dependency

CONGENITAL FOLATE MALABSORPTION SYNDROMES

Specific folate absorption defects have been described in several infants [Jebnoun et al., 2001; Malatack et al., 1999; Poncz and Cohen, 1999; Steinschneider et al., 1990]. In affected infants, selective deficiency occurs in the transport of folates in the intestinal tract and across the blood-brain barrier [Zittoun, 1995]. In addition to failure to thrive, diarrhea, and megaloblastic anemia, affected patients have CNS abnormalities of variable severity. Neurologic defects range from learning disability to profound mental retardation, seizures, progressive athetosis, and peripheral neuropathy. Basal ganglia calcifications may develop during adolescence. The megaloblastic anemia but not the progression of neurologic abnormalities responded to folate supplementation (10 to 40 mg/day of folic acid); parenteral administration was necessary in some patients [Jebnoun et al., 2001; Steinschneider et al., 1990]. Parenteral therapy with folinic acid, a reduced folate derivative more readily transported across the blood-brain barrier, decreased the CNS deficit and elevated the folate concentration in one patient [Steinschneider et al., 1990]. The variability in clinical presentation and responsiveness to folate therapy suggests that different genotypic mutations are involved.

METHYLENE-TETRAHYDROFOLATE REDUCTASE DEFICIENCY

Methylene-tetrahydrofolate reductase deficiency is the most common of the folate-dependent enzymatic disorders [Fattal-Valevski et al., 2000; Fowler, 1998; Haworth et al., 1993; Zittoun, 1995]. Symptoms are primarily neurologic and have included limb weakness, lack of coordination, paresthesias, and memory lapses, along with developmental delay, marked hypotonia, seizures, microcephaly, apnea, and coma and, rarely, schizophrenic syndromes. Vascular disease also may occur. Hematologic abnormalities are not observed. Low levels of folate in serum, red blood cells, and cerebrospinal fluid associated with homocystinuria are constant.

GLUTAMATE FORMIMINOTRANSFERASE DEFICIENCY

Formiminotransferase catalyzes the conversion of *N*-formiminoglutamic acid to glutamic acid, the final step in histidine catabolism. Several children in whom an excessive urinary excretion of formiminoglutamic acid suggested glutamate formiminotransferase deficiency have been reported [Fowler, 1998; Hilton et al., 2003]. This autosomal-recessive disorder is the second most common inborn error of folate metabolism and is presumed to be due to defects in the bifunctional enzyme glutamate formiminotransferase-cyclodeaminase. Two clinically and biochemically distinct syndromes emerge from these descriptions. In one, mild neurologic deficits (e.g., mild mental retardation, learning disabilities, attention-deficit disorder, hypotonia, clumsiness) are associated with massive urinary formiminoglutamic acid excretion, normal serum folate concentrations, and normal hematologic studies. In some of these patients, folate administered either orally as folic acid or intramuscularly as tetrahydrofolate decreased formiminoglutamic acid excretion [Fowler, 1998; Niederwieser et al., 1974; Perry et al., 1975]. In the other syndrome, severe mental retardation, diffuse cerebral atrophy, and increased serum folate concentrations and formiminoglutamic acid urinary excretion were associated with a partial deficit of formiminotransferase activity in liver biopsy specimens or erythrocytes. One of these children had a folate-responsive megaloblastic anemia [Zittoun, 1995].

FOLATE-DEPENDENT DIHYDROFOLATE REDUCTASE DEFICIENCY

Several patients with a suspected deficiency of dihydrofolate reductase, the enzyme catalyzing the reduction of folate derivatives to methyltetrahydrofolate, have been described [Fowler, 1998; Tauro et al., 1976; Walters, 1967]. The family history suggested that this enzyme defect may result in abortion or stillbirth. The patients first required treatment for failure to thrive and a severe megaloblastic anemia in early infancy. Mental retardation of variable degree was subsequently observed. The hematologic abnormality responded to the intramuscular administration of folinic acid (100 μg to 6 mg per day). Because therapy was delayed and intermittent, whether the neurologic deficit could have been prevented is not clear. Some investigators have suggested that the neurologic deficits seen in these patients may be due to reduced levels of *S*-adenosylmethionine [Bottiglieri and Hyland, 1994].

DISORDERS ASSOCIATED WITH MICRONUTRIENT DEFICIENCIES

Iron Deficiency

Overview

About 25% of the world's children younger than 3 years of age have iron deficiency anemia, with higher rates in developing countries; when iron deficiency without anemia is considered, rates are even higher [Black, 2003]. The WHO estimates that worldwide, 2 billion persons have anemia and up to 5 billion persons are iron deficient [WHO, 1992]. The estimated prevalence of iron deficiency in the United States, according to the 2002 Centers for Disease Control and Prevention report, is greatest in toddlers 1 to 2 years of age (7%) and in adolescent and adult females 12 to 49 years of age (9% to 16%) [From the Centers for Disease Control and Prevention, 2002]. The prevalence of iron deficiency is approximately twice as high among non-Hispanic black and Mexican-American females (19% to 22%) as it is among non-Hispanic white females (10%). Dietary deficiency is the most common cause of iron depletion in infants and children. Breast-feeding for less than 6 months' duration, the use of non–iron-fortified infant formula, the introduction of cow's milk before the age of 1 year, and a diet deficient in iron all are proven risk factors [Yager and Hartfield, 2002].

Iron is necessary for hemoglobin synthesis, and iron deficiency leads to reduced oxygen-carrying capacity and can have an impact on immunity, growth, and development. Clinical effects of iron deficiency include anemia, weakness, failure to thrive, and breath-holding spells [Leung and Chan, 2001]. Iron deficiency results in decreased heme proteins, iron-containing enzymes, and reactions in which iron is involved as a cofactor. Consequently, changes in nucleic acid biosynthesis, oxidative respiration and mitochondrial function, detoxification of metabolic byproducts, and catecholamine metabolism occur [Yager and Hartfield, 2002].

The brain is sensitive to dietary iron depletion and repletion and reacts to changes by means of homeostatic regulatory mechanisms regulated by the blood-brain barrier in response to iron status [Beard et al., 2001; Bryan et al., 2004]. Brain tissue is overall very rich in iron, with concentrations differing according to brain region and stage of development [Youdim and Yehuda, 2000]. Some areas of the brain that are important for cognition—such as the cortex, hippocampus, and striatum—are more sensitive to iron deficiency than others. Iron affects myelination during development and is an important cofactor for dopaminergic, serotoninergic, and noradrenergic neurotransmitter synthesis [Bryan et al., 2004]. Studies in rats have found that iron deficiency results in a reduction of dopamine D_2 receptor densities and inadequate dopamine reuptake [Ashkenazi et al., 1982], suggesting that alterations in frontal cortical dopamine levels may be associated with deficits in executive function, attention, perception, memory, motivation, and motor control [Beard, 2003].

Evidence of CNS structural abnormalities in children with iron deficiency anemia is limited [Grantham-McGregor and Ani, 2001; Yager and Hatfield, 2002]. Auditory-evoked brainstem responses have suggested impaired myelin synthesis, based on prolongation of the central conduction time [Roncagliolo et al., 1998]. Other studies have found that children who received treatment for iron deficiency anemia also have longer P100 latencies on visual-evoked potential testing compared with control subjects, again suggesting that iron deficiency anemia alters myelination [Algarin et al., 2003].

The relation of iron deficiency and cognitive development in children has received much attention in the past 3 decades and has been recently reviewed [Bryan et al., 2004; Gordon, 2003; Grantham-McGregor and Ani, 2001]. Studies have found a correlation between hemoglobin concentrations and cognitive performance or school achievement scores, especially in iron-deficient persons [Sungthong et al., 2002]. Children with iron deficiency anemia early in life demonstrate lower academic performance during their school years, even after the anemia had been treated. Comparisons of iron-deficient, anemic, and nonanemic children have demonstrated that anemic children perform more poorly on tests assessing development, cognitive performance, and school achievement in areas such as mathematics [Halterman et al., 2001]. Longitudinal studies examining associations between iron status in children younger than 2 years of age and later measures of cognitive performance suggest that early anemia, even if treated, is associated with impaired long-term development [Bryan et al., 2004; Lozoff et al., 2000].

A Cochrane Review examined the impact of iron therapy in children younger than 3 years of age with iron deficiency anemia and found positive and negative correlations [Logan et al., 2001]. Several clinical trials also have examined whether iron supplementation in children younger than 3 is beneficial. About half of the studies found improved cognitive performance [Black, 2003]. In the trials in which improvement was observed, mental and motor development and language skills were better and lessening of symptoms such as wariness and irritability was reported. Evidence is scarce regarding the efficacy of short-term iron supplementation on the cognitive development of anemic children younger than 2 years of age, or of longer-term treatment to help anemic children catch up with nonanemic children in development level [Bryan, 2004]. Studies in developing countries, however, have found a beneficial effect of longer-term treatment of anemic older children [Idjradinata and Pollitt, 1993; Stoltzfus et al., 2001]. The results of nine randomized, controlled trials in children older than 2 years and in adolescents recently have been summarized and demonstrated inconsistent findings [Bryan, 2004; Grantham-McGregor and Ani, 2001]. Overall, although little evidence exists for the efficacy of short-term iron supplementation in children younger than 2 years of age, reasonable evidence suggests a beneficial effect of longer-term iron supplementation on the cognitive performance of older children. A detailed discussion of these studies is beyond the scope of this chapter but is presented in the review by Grantham-McGregor and Ani [2001]. Currently, no practice guidelines have been published on screening for iron deficiency or use of iron supplementation to prevent cognitive or behavioral defects.

The foregoing findings must be tempered by an appreciation of the ongoing controversy regarding the relative effects that micronutrient deficiencies such as iron are responsible for a majority of observed impairments that occur. As reviewed by Pollit [2000], (1) studies of protein-energy malnutrition suggest that environmental factors can moderate the relation between early nutritional insult and later developmental disadvantage; (2) profound developmental changes can occur after the age of fastest brain growth when the environment changes and the child's basic needs are met without interruption; (3) no data are available to suggest that the observed delays of cognition reported for children in middle or late childhood, who were iron deficient as infants, were not a result of familial variables; and (4) documentation is lacking that the cerebral alterations produced by experimentally induced iron-deficiency anemia in rat models are the reasons for cognitive delays of children.

Specific Neurologic Effects of Iron Deficiency

Three neurologic problems have been associated with iron deficiency: stroke, breath-holding spells, and benign intracranial hypertension [Yager and Hartfield, 2002].

STROKE

Stroke occurring in association with iron deficiency has been reported in both children and adults [Belman et al., 1990; Bruggers et al., 1990]. In some children, an antecedent viral infection was reported [Hartfield et al., 1990], whereas in others, congenital heart disease in conjunction with venous thrombosis also was present [Cottrill et al., 1973]. Several mechanisms have been proposed to explain the association between iron deficiency anemia and stroke and include (1) development of thrombocytosis due to loss of iron regulation of platelet production; (2) development of a hypercoagulable state consequent to increased blood viscosity from the microcytic, poorly deformable red blood cells resulting from the iron deficiency, with increased risk of venous thrombosis; and (3) development of anemic hypoxia, which has been associated with transient hemiplegia and cerebellar infarcts [Yager and Hartfield, 2002].

BREATH-HOLDING SPELLS

Breath-holding episodes also have been associated with iron deficiency and can occur in up to 27% of affected children [Colina et al., 1995; Daoud et al., 1997]. Autonomic dysregulation resulting in vagally mediated cardiac arrest or bradycardia has been proposed [Holowach and Thurston, 1965], as have the effects of anemia on reducing oxygen-carrying capacity. Iron-deficient children also are known to be more irritable; presumably, this may increase the likelihood of an event. Treatment with iron supplementation has been shown to significantly reduce or eliminate the risk of recurrence [Daoud et al., 1997].

BENIGN INTRACRANIAL HYPERTENSION

Iron deficiency as a cause of benign intracranial hypertension has been recognized for more than a century [Yager and Hartfield, 2002]. It is most common in young females. Although the underlying mechanism is unknown, it has been proposed that tissue hypoxia leads to increased capillary permeability and development of brain edema or abnormalities in cerebrovascular hemodynamics that increase cerebral blood flow, leading to increased intracranial pressure. Depletion of iron-containing enzymes also may contribute to the development of cerebral edema. Several studies report that benign intracranial hypertension due to iron deficiency is reversible with iron supplementation [Tugal et al., 1994].

IODINE DEFICIENCY

Iodine deficiency is the most preventable cause of mental retardation in the world [Black, 2003]. It is a major problem that affects children in geographic areas in which iodine is depleted from the soil, primarily mountainous regions, such as the Himalayas and Andes, and in flood plains. A 1996 WHO report estimates that 2.2 billion persons are at risk for iodine deficiency [WHO, 1996]. People consuming iodine-deficient foods grown in these areas become iodine deficient unless iodine can be consumed from external sources [Bryan, 2004]. Public health measures such as use of iodized salt, injections of iodinated oil, and oral iodine supplementation have been effective in preventing congenital hypothyroidism and the associated mental retardation [Stanbury, 1994].

Iodine is required for synthesis of the thyroid hormones triiodothyronine (T_3) and thyroxine (T_4), which are necessary for skeletal growth and for growth and development of the brain [Reavley, 1998]. Iodine deficiency in utero results in fetal hypothyroidism and irreversible neurologic and cognitive deficits manifested as cretinism, characterized by mental retardation, primitive reflexes, visual problems, facial deformities, stunted growth, and impaired motor function [Halpern, 1994]. In addition to cognitive delays, primitive reflexes, and pyramidal signs, features of myxedematous cretinism include severe growth retardation, dry skin, and electrocardiographic abnormalities [Black, 2003]. Chronic hypothyroidism also can have ongoing effects across all ages, and affected persons can have epilepsy, motor dysfunction, dementia, depression, and disorders of vigilance, visuomotor planning, and abstract thinking [Bryan, 2004]. Patients who are most severely affected are those who have congenital cretinism and postnatal hypothyroidism that extends into childhood and adulthood.

Summaries of studies on the effects of iodine deficiency on cognitive development and the effects of iodine supplementation have recently been published [Black, 2003; Bryan, 2004]. A meta-analysis of 18 studies completed by Bleichrodt and Born [1994] indicated a general loss of 13.5 IQ points in chronically iodine-deficient populations compared with non–iodine-deficient groups. Another study found that children with mild hypothyroidism had deficits in spelling and reading compared with control subjects [Huda et al., 1999]. Some studies indicate that children with goiter perform significantly less well on tests of nonverbal reasoning ability, whereas other studies have found no difference between groups on measures of general intelligence [Bryan, 2004]. One difficulty with comparing children on the basis of the presence of goiter is that no clear relation between goiter and the degree of hypothyroidism has been described. A number of studies have used other biomarkers of iodine deficiency, such as urinary iodine status, which has been found to correlate with cognitive performance studies [van den Briel et al., 2000].

Randomized iodine supplementation trials from iodine-deficient areas found that children whose mothers were supplemented before conception or early in pregnancy have better developmental outcomes than those in children born to unsupplemented mothers. Clinical trials also have examined the impact of iodine supplementation on cognitive performance of infants and children in iodine-deficient areas [Black, 2003]. The results have been inconsistent. Most studies were performed in iodine-deficient populations, and about half of the studies found positive effects on mental performance [Bryan, 2004]. In some studies, improvements in mental performance were seen only in those children who also had an improved iodine status [Bryan, 2004]. In studies in which cognitive improvement was not detected, problems with study design or other factors may have been present [Bryan, 2004]. In a recent longitudinal follow-up study of school-age children, all of whom received iodine, those whose mothers received iodine before the third trimester had better scores on a measure of psychomotor performance than corresponding scores in children whose mothers received iodine later in pregnancy or who received iodine at age 2 years [O'Donnell et al., 2002]. The effects of postnatal iodine deficiency on children's cognitive performance are less clear than the effects of prenatal iodine deficiency.

As noted by Black [2003], universal salt iodization is a public health priority for women of childbearing age to protect their unborn children from the severe consequences of hypothyroidism. In geographic regions in which iodine deficiency is common, but iodized salt is either not consumed or unavailable, iodized oil can be used. Although iodine supplementation reduces the incidence of goiter in children, the impact on their cognitive development requires further investigation.

ZINC DEFICIENCY

Zinc deficiency remains a serious health problem worldwide, affecting developed as well as developing countries. Zinc deprivation during periods of rapid growth negatively affects cognitive function, growth, and development [Gibson, 1998; Oken and Duggan, 2002; Rivera et al., 2003; Salgueiro et al., 2004]. Zinc deficiency has been demonstrated in animal models to affect cognitive development by decreasing activity, increasing emotional behavior, and impairing memory and the capacity to learn [Bhatnagar and Taneja, 2001].

Zinc has a critical role in the function of several structural, regulatory, and catalytic proteins [Hambidge, 2000; McCall et al., 2000]. Zinc is known to play an important molecular role in processes of gene replication, activation, and repression, as well as in DNA transcription and translation and protein synthesis [Bryan et al., 2004; Walsh et al., 1994]. Prompted by early reports of birth defects in the offspring of zinc-deficient rats in the 1980s, more recent investigations have examined the effects of zinc deficiency. Zinc may be an important modulator of neuronal excitability, because it is present in high concentrations in the synaptic vesicles of "zinc-containing" neurons in the forebrain, and it also plays important roles in myelination and GABA and glutamate release. Zinc also is important for neurogenesis, neuronal migration, and synaptogenesis, and its deficiency could interfere with neurotransmission and neurophysiologic development [Bhatnagar and Taneja, 2001]. Zinc also is involved in the metabolism of thyroid hormones and receptor function and transport of other hormones that could influence the CNS.

Indirectly, zinc deficiency may affect cognitive performance through its interactions with other nutrients [Bryan et al., 2004. Because iron and zinc are most bioavailable from many of the same foods and their absorption is inhibited by many of the same dietary substances, iron and zinc deficiencies often occur simultaneously [Bryan et al., 2004]. Zinc also is known to affect vitamin A metabolism, and zinc deficiency might thereby contribute to the consequences of vitamin A deficiency.

Biologic measures of zinc status, such as plasma and hair zinc concentrations, are imperfect indicators of functional impairment due to zinc deficiency, and response to randomized trials of zinc supplementation conducted in zinc-deficient populations has been an important means to examine the consequences of zinc deficiency [Black, 2003]. Supplementation trials among nutritionally deficient infants have demonstrated beneficial effects of zinc on growth, diarrhea and pneumonia morbidity, and on mortality. A majority but not all of the zinc supplementation studies in pregnant women, infants, and toddlers have shown improved activity and motor development [Bentley et al., 1997; Castillo-Duran et al., 2003; Sazawa et al., 1996; Tamura et al., 2003]. Zinc supplementation trials have resulted in alteration in fetal neurobehavior, better motor development in infants of very low birth weight, more vigorous and functional activity in malnourished infants and toddlers, and improved neuropsychologic functions in school-aged children.

Although evidence from supplementation trials in infants and toddlers suggests that zinc deficiency may compromise early motor development, the evidence linking zinc deficiency to cognitive development is inconclusive [Black, 2003, 1998]. Several randomized trials of zinc supplementation measuring cognitive development in school-aged children have found mixed results [Black, 2003]. In two studies, however, one from China [Penland et al., 1997] and one involving Mexican-American children from Texas [Penland et al., 1999], found improved neuropsychologic performance, particularly in reasoning, in zinc-supplemented children. Additional studies will be needed to determine the indications for zinc supplementation, the correct populations that require treatment, the optimal intensity and duration of treatment, and how this should be combined with treatment for other micronutrient deficiencies.

Fluid and Electrolyte Abnormalities

Fluid and electrolyte abnormalities may cause severe acute injury that results in long-term neurologic and developmental sequelae, particularly in children. This section reviews the more common clinically encountered conditions [Gullans and Verbalis, 1993] and their effect on the developing nervous system. Aspects of the neurologic complications of renal disease are extensively reviewed in Chapter 89. Management of fluid and electrolyte disorders is reviewed in standard textbooks of pediatrics [Behrman et al., 1996; Hoekelman et al., 1997; Oski et al., 1994; Rudolph et al., 1996] and elsewhere [Jospe and Forbes, 1996; Mahalanabis and Snyder, 1996; Meyers, 1994]. Other reviews have considered fluid and electrolyte disorders in neurologic [Riggs, 2002], neurosurgical [Andrews, 1994], or pediatric surgical patients [Filston, 1992]; in patients with bacterial meningitis [Brown and Feigin, 1994]; in children with other critical care illnesses [Khilnani, 1992]; after anesthesia in the perioperative and postoperative periods [Gold, 1992]; and in the neurologically impaired patient [Parobek and Alaimo, 1996]. In addition, new technologies, such as proton MR spectroscopy, which allows measurement of myoinositol, a key brain osmol [Haussinger et al., 1994], or diffusion-weighted imaging, which determines early water movement after injury [Nomura et al., 1994], may allow better understanding of many of the common fluid and electrolyte disorders (also see Chapter 89).

SODIUM, WATER, AND CHLORIDE ABNORMALITIES

Sodium and Water

The regulation of sodium and water metabolism is closely integrated. Sodium is the principal cation in the extracellular fluid and, through its osmotic properties, determines extracellular volume. Sodium content depends on dietary intake, intestinal absorption, and renal and extrarenal (e.g., in sweat or feces) excretion. The kidneys play a pivotal role in sodium homeostasis. Sodium excreted in the glomerular filtrate is subsequently reabsorbed in the renal tubular system. An increased sodium load promotes an increase in glomerular filtration and a decrease in renal tubular sodium reabsorption, whereas a decreased sodium load leads to a decrease in glomerular filtration and an increase in tubular reabsorption of sodium. These processes are mediated through complex interactions of multiple hormones, including the cardiac hormone atrial natriuretic factor, the adrenal hormone aldosterone, and the hypophyseal antidiuretic hormone. Atrial natriuretic factor, stored in the atrial cardiocyte, is activated in response to volume expansion (e.g., sodium content excess), leading to an increase in glomerular filtration and renal tubular sodium excretion. Aldosterone promotes renal tubular sodium reabsorption. It is released from the adrenal medulla in response to the activation of angiotensin II by the stimulation of juxtaglomerular cells in afferent renal arterioles by small decreases in plasma volume (e.g., sodium content depletion). Extracellular sodium concentration is regulated primarily by antidiuretic hormone. Synthesized in the supraoptic nuclei of the hypothalamus and subsequently stored in synaptic vesicles in the posterior pituitary, antidiuretic hormone is released into the plasma in response to stimulation by hypothalamic osmoreceptors and promotes the reabsorption of water by the distal renal tubules.

Hyponatremia

Hyponatremia may result from excessive sodium loss, excessive water intake or retention, a shift of water from cells to extracellular fluid, or a shift of sodium from extracellular fluid into cells (Table 90-2) [Berry and Belsha, 1990]. Combinations of mechanisms occur frequently. In the pediatric age group, hyponatremia most commonly results from either sodium loss or water retention.

As hyponatremia develops, an associated reduction of plasma osmolality with a rapid shift of water into the brain occurs. Subsequent homeostatic mechanisms, including the shift of water into the cerebrospinal fluid and the shift of intracellular potassium and organic cations into the interstitial cerebral space, provide protection against fulminant cerebral edema [Fishman, 1974; Rymer and Fishman, 1973]. The neurologic effects of chronic hyponatremia reflect the

TABLE 90-2

Causes of Hyponatremia

MECHANISM	SOURCE	CAUSATIVE FACTOR/ DISORDER
Excessive NaCl loss	Gastrointestinal tract	Diarrhea
	Skin	Cystic fibrosis
		Heat stress
	Urinary tract	Salt-losing renal disease
		Adrenal insufficiency
		Diabetes mellitus
Excessive water intake	Oral	Psychogenic
		Acute renal failure
	Parenteral	Therapeutic error
		Coma
	Rectal	Tap water enema
Defective water excretion	Inappropriate antidiuretic hormone secretion	Anesthetic drugs
		Craniocerebral trauma
		Infection

electrolyte depletion of brain cells and may be secondary to the inhibition of transmitter release [Hajtha and Shersin, 1975] or abnormalities in energy metabolism [Fishman, 1974].

Symptomatic hyponatremia invariably develops only after the plasma sodium concentration has decreased below 120 mEq/L and involves the CNS. An alteration in mental status is the most common neurologic manifestation of hyponatremia and ranges in degree from mild confusion to coma. The severity of clinical manifestations depends on the degree of hyponatremia and the rapidity by which the sodium concentration has decreased. Mild symptoms are relatively nonspecific and include malaise, fatigue, listlessness, and muscle cramping. The rapid onset of severe hyponatremia may lead to confusion, disorientation, delirium, weakness, ataxia, and seizures, frequently followed by prolonged coma. Rare descriptions of rhabdomyolysis associated with hyponatremia exist [Rizzieri, 1995].

The treatment of symptomatic hyponatremia consists of the correction of serum osmolality by the intravenous administration of a hypertonic saline solution. The optimum rate for correction remains controversial [Oh and Carroll, 1992]. Excessively rapid correction may shrink the volume of adapted brain cells [Sterns et al., 1989] and has been implicated in the pathogenesis of *central pontine myelinolysis*, a fulminating demyelinative disorder of the body of the pons, clinically characterized by quadriparesis, pseudobulbar palsy, and the "locked-in" state [Arieff, 1981; Brunner et al., 1990; Pirazda and Ali, 2001; Sterns et al., 1986]. A 17-month-old infant with kwashiorkor and hyponatremia had a central pontine lesion on MRI with a clinical presentation of acute massive myoclonus [Tan, 2004]. Central pontine myelinolysis, as well as osmotic demyelination syndrome, may complicate the correction of hyponatremia. *Osmotic demyelination syndrome* is the term used to describe the combination of pontine and extrapontine myelinolysis [Martin, 2004]. Most cases of central pontine myelinolysis occur in alcoholics, about 20% occur after the correction of hyponatremia, and 17% occur in patients who underwent liver transplantation, in whom the disorder is attributed to treatment with the immunosuppressive medication cyclosporine [Lampl, 2002]. Osmotic demyelination syndrome, manifested clinically mostly as an altered level of consciousness and convulsions, can develop in patients with hyponatremia after hemodialysis. With this syndrome, MRI abnormalities are seen in the pons in most cases, and in the pons along with extrapontine sites in a minority. Prospective MRI studies demonstrated the development of characteristic pontine lesions in patients who recieived treatment for hyponatremia in relation to rapid correction of the hyponatremia (more than 12 mEq/liter per day) [Brunner et al, 1990]. Diffusion-weighted MRI identified pontine abnormalities within 24 hours of onset of symptoms [Ruzek, 2004]. The lesions usually resolved rapidly, suggesting that they represent edema rather than demyelination [Tarhan, 2004].

The correction of hyponatremia can cause central pontine myelinolysis or osmotic demyelination syndrome. Therefore, treatment should take into consideration a number of factors, including whether the hyponatremia is symptomatic, the patient's volume status, and the severity and duration of the hyponatremia and hypo-osmolarity [Han, 2002].

Hypernatremia

Hypernatremia, defined as an increase in serum sodium concentration above 150 mEq/L, may result from excessive sodium intake or retention, excessive water loss, a shift of water into cells, or a shift of sodium out of cells (Table 90-3). Hypernatremia can occur in association with increased, decreased, or normal body sodium content. In the pediatric age group, the loss of hypotonic fluid with gastroenteritis is among the more common causes of hypernatremia [Finberg, 1967, 1973; Finberg et al., 1963].

Neurologic manifestations of hypernatremia include restlessness and irritability, followed by lethargy, seizures, spasticity, and coma. Hypernatremia in a child was associated with transient thalamic signal changes [Hartfield et al, 1999]. Permanent neurologic sequelae are frequent because acute hypernatremia leads to cellular dehydration and brain shrinkage, which may be associated with venous thrombosis and subdural or parenchymal intracerebral hemorrhage [Arieff and Guisado, 1976; Korkmaz et al, 2000]. Permanent brain damage was reported in one third of children with severe

TABLE 90-3

Causes of Hypernatremia

MECHANISM	CAUSATIVE FACTOR/DISORDER
Excess sodium intake	Improperly mixed formula or rehydration solution
	Excessive sodium bicarbonate administration during resuscitation
	Saltwater drowning
Water deficit	Diabetes insipidus
	Diabetes mellitus
	Excessive sweating
	Increased water loss
	Adipsia
	Inadequate water intake
Water deficit in excess of sodium deficit	Diarrhea
	Osmotic diuretics
	Obstructive uropathy
	Renal dysplasia

hypernatremia [Morris-Jones et al, 1967]. The production of "idiogenic osmols"—the amino acids taurine, glutamine, alanine, and aspartic acid, derived from the catabolism of intracellular protein—subsequently restores the quantity of intracellular water to near normal [Trachtman et al., 1988].

Treatment should be directed toward correcting the basic disease process whenever possible, preserving perfusion, and restoring normal sodium concentration. Excessively rapid restoration of the sodium concentration to normal in chronic hypernatremia may lead to cerebral edema and should be avoided. A rate of reduction of the serum sodium concentration by 10 to 15 mEq/L per day is recommended [Conley, 1990].

Chloride

Chloride is the major anion in intracellular fluid and plays an important role in maintaining electrochemical neutrality in the extracellular fluid and blood plasma. Chloride input and output parallel those of sodium; chloride transport is predominantly passive along an electrochemical gradient created by sodium, although a site for the active transport of chloride in the thick ascending loop of Henle specifically blocked by furosemide has been established [Rochas and Kokko, 1973]. In most circumstances, alterations in plasma chloride concentrations parallel those of sodium and are most frequently observed in dehydration from diarrhea.

Hypochloremia

Hypochloremia is associated with metabolic alkalosis and occurs as a consequence of excessive chloride loss or deficient intake [Roy, 1984]. Excessive loss may occur from the upper GI tract (e.g., vomiting, pyloric stenosis), the skin (e.g., cystic fibrosis), or the urine (e.g., administration of diuretics, Bartter's syndrome). A rare congenital disorder characterized by a chloride-losing diarrhea also has been reported [Holmberg, 1986]. Chloride depletion also has resulted from the feeding of a chloride-deficient formula [Grossman et al., 1980; Roy and Arant, 1979]. Affected infants developed muscular weakness, delayed motor development, anorexia, and constipation associated with hypochloremic metabolic acidosis, hyponatremia, hypokalemia, hypoaldosteronuria, and microscopic hematuria. In a majority of affected infants, these symptoms and signs were associated with failure to thrive and microcephaly. Clinical and laboratory abnormalities disappeared promptly after the restoration of normal chloride intake, and on subsequent studies the children were normal at 4 to 5 years of age, except for persistent behavioral problems in a few [Hellerstein et al., 1985].

Hyperchloremia

Hyperchloremia occurs in several forms of metabolic acidosis and may be a consequence of bicarbonate loss from the GI or urinary tract, the administration of drugs (e.g., acetazolamide, ammonium chloride), or renal tubular acidosis.

POTASSIUM CONCENTRATION ABNORMALITIES

Potassium is the principal intracellular cation; the intracellular potassium concentration approximates 150 mEq/L, whereas the potassium concentration in the extracellular fluid varies, ranging from 3.5 to 5.5 mEq/L. Because extracellular fluid contains only 2% of the total body potassium and the potassium content of adipose tissue is negligible, total body potassium correlates closely with lean body mass.

Dietary potassium is absorbed in the upper GI tract. Although some potassium is excreted in the feces and sweat, the kidney is the principal organ responsible for potassium balance. Because potassium filtered through the renal glomeruli is almost completely resorbed in the proximal tubules, urinary potassium excretion is principally a consequence of the amount of potassium secreted by the distal renal tubular system. This process is controlled by multiple interrelated factors, including electrochemical and concentration gradients between the distal tubular cells and the lumen, sodium-potassium adenosine triphosphatase pumps, and plasma aldosterone concentration [Giebish, 1980]. Acute changes in the ratio of intracellular to extracellular concentration of potassium are influenced by epinephrine and insulin, which promote potassium uptake by liver and muscle cells [Brem, 1990].

The neurologic manifestations of potassium disturbances involve mostly the peripheral nervous system and only rarely the CNS.

Hypokalemia

Hypokalemia, defined as serum potassium concentrations less than 3.5 mEq/L, may result from decreased potassium intake, renal or extrarenal potassium loss, or a shift of plasma potassium into cells (Table 90-4). Clinical manifestations associated with hypokalemia include skeletal muscle weakness, areflexia, decreased intestinal peristalsis and paralytic ileus, and loss of the ability of the kidney to concentrate urine. Paralysis and death from respiratory failure can occur. Prolonged hypokalemia may lead to perman-

TABLE 90-4

Causes of Hypokalemia

MECHANISM	CAUSATIVE FACTOR/DISORDER
Deficient intake	Protein-calorie malnutrition
	Parenteral nutrition
Renal loss	Distal tubular acidosis
Renal disease	Proximal tubular acidosis (Fanconi's syndrome)
	Bartter's syndrome
	Interstitial nephritis
	Pyelonephritis
Extrarenal disease	Diabetes mellitus
	Cushing's syndrome
	Aldosteronism
	Drug administration (diuretic, aspirin, steroids)
	Hypomagnesemia
	Hypercalcemia
Shift (extracellular to intracellular)	Alkalosis
	Drugs (insulin, catecholamines)
	Parenteral nutrition
Extrarenal loss	Vomiting, diarrhea
	Fistula drainage
	Laxative abuse
	Ion-exchange resins
	Congenital alkalosis

TABLE 90-5

Causes of Hyperkalemia

MECHANISM	CAUSATIVE FACTOR/DISORDER
Excessive intake	Potassium-containing salt substitutes
	Parenteral administration (excessive infusion, outdated blood)
	Gastrointestinal bleeding
Decreased renal excretion	
Renal disease	Oliguric renal failure
	Chronic hydronephrosis
	Potassium-sparing diuretics
Extrarenal causes	Addison's disease
	Congenital adrenal hyperplasia
	Diabetes mellitus
	Drugs (beta blockers, heparin)
Shift (intracellular to extracellular)	Rapid cell breakdown (trauma, infection, cytotoxic agents)
	Acidosis
	Freshwater drowning

ent impairment of renal function associated with vacuolar changes in the tubular epithelium that can persist even after potassium repletion. Treatment consists of the administration of potassium with serial monitoring of electrolytes.

Hyperkalemia

Hyperkalemia, defined as a serum potassium concentration greater than 5.5 mEq/L, may result from excessive potassium intake or administration, decreased renal excretion, or a shift of potassium from the intracellular to the extracellular space (Table 90-5). Clinical manifestations primarily affect neuromuscular transmission and result from a reduction of action potentials toward threshold levels, leading to delayed depolarization, rapid repolarization, and slowing of conduction velocity. These responses lead to paresthesias, weakness, and ultimately flaccid paralysis. The heart is particularly vulnerable to hyperkalemia; serum concentration greater than 6.5 mEq/L must be considered a medical emergency because ventricular fibrillation and death may ensue rapidly.

Emergency therapeutic measures include the rapid administration of sodium bicarbonate (up to 2 mEq/kg over 5 to 10 minutes) or of glucose and insulin (glucose in a dose of 0.5 g/kg and regular insulin in a dose of 0.3 unit/g, given over 2 hours). Intravenous calcium gluconate (a 10% solution in a dose of up to 0.5 mL/kg, given over 2 to 4 minutes) will counter the cardiac toxicity but must be accompanied by electrocardiographic monitoring. These emergency methods do not remove excess potassium and should be accompanied by cessation of all potassium intake and, if necessary, the use of an ion exchange resin (e.g., Kayexalate), hemodialysis, or peritoneal dialysis.

CALCIUM CONCENTRATION ABNORMALITIES

Calcium is the fifth most abundant element in the body; approximately 99% of the body calcium content is in bone. Despite the large calcium reserve in bone, extracellular calcium concentration is maintained remarkably constant at approximately 5 mEq/L (10 mg/dL) under normal conditions. Approximately 40% of extracellular calcium is bound to protein, predominantly albumin; 10% is diffusible but complexed to anions such as citrate and phosphate; and the remaining 50% (2.5 mEq/L) is freely diffusible as calcium ions. The freely diffusible fraction is responsible for the physiologic effects of calcium in neuromuscular transmission, in which calcium functions as a coupling agent for excitation-transmission in the nervous system and excitation-contraction in muscle [Lynch, 1990; Rassmussen, 1986]. The absorption of calcium in the intestinal tract is mediated by an active carrier process [DeLuca and Schnoes, 1983], which is enhanced by vitamin D and parathyroid hormone. In addition to intestinal calcium absorption, plasma calcium concentration also is controlled through renal calcium reabsorption and bone resorption [Bushinsky and Monk, 1998]. Calcium absorption is increased in sarcoidosis, carcinomatosis, and multiple myeloma and is decreased by increased GI motility, with decreased bowel length, and in the presence of phytate, oxalate, and phosphate, which promote the formation of unabsorbable complexes. Diffusible calcium is excreted by the kidney. Almost 99% of the calcium filtered by renal glomeruli is resorbed. Renal calcium resorption is enhanced by 1,25-dihydroxyvitamin D and parathyroid hormone and is inhibited by thyrocalcitonin. Renal calcium excretion also is increased by osmotic diuretics, growth hormone, thyroid hormone, glucagon, metabolic acidosis, prolonged fasting, and prolonged physical activity.

The cerebrospinal fluid concentration of calcium varies, ranging from 2 to 3 mEq/L, roughly approximating the diffusible fraction in the extracellular fluid. Transport of calcium into the cerebrospinal fluid is determined by a carrier-mediated transport process [Goldstein et al., 1979; Graziani et al., 1965].

Hypocalcemia

Although hypocalcemia may occur at any age, it most commonly is observed in the neonatal period (Box 90-3) [Juan, 1977]. Relatively uncommon in breast-fed infants, it may occur in otherwise healthy, non–breast-fed newborns as a consequence of transient physiologic hypoparathyroidism and after ingestion of the relatively high phosphate load of cow's milk for several days. Neonatal hypocalcemia also may occur in the first 36 hours of life, particularly in preterm infants born to mothers who have diabetes and in association with conditions leading to perinatal encephalopathy.

Excessive secretion of thyrocalcitonin may cause persistent hypocalcemia in preterm infants [Tsang et al., 1973]. More persistent neonatal hypocalcemia also may be a consequence of maternal hypoparathyroidism or a manifesta-

Box 90-3 Causes of Hypocalcemia

- Vitamin D deficiency
- Hypoparathyroidism
- Pseudohypoparathyroidism
- Hyperphosphatemia
- Magnesium deficiency
- Acute pancreatitis
- Alkalosis
- Rapid correction of acidosis

tion of agenesis of the parathyroid glands (DiGeorge's syndrome). In later life, hypocalcemia can occur in nutritional rickets, in chronic malabsorption states, during the treatment of dehydration as a manifestation of hypoparathyroidism or pseudohypoparathyroidism, and rarely as a consequence of chronic antiepileptic drug therapy.

In the newborn, convulsions are the most characteristic manifestation of tetany. Laryngospasm with cyanosis and apneic episodes also may occur. Poor feeding, vomiting, and lethargy are frequent, nonspecific associated manifestations. Bradycardia with heart block is rarely observed. Treatment of neonatal symptomatic tetany consists of the slow intravenous administration of 10% calcium gluconate in a dose of 2 mL/kg. Concurrent monitoring of the cardiac rate to prevent excessive bradycardia is advised. The intravenous dose can be repeated at 6- to 8-hour intervals.

In older children, clinical manifestations associated with symptomatic hypocalcemic tetany include paresthesias, stiffness, and cramping of limb muscles; stridor; and convulsions. Convulsions may be the sole clinical abnormality associated with hypocalcemia. Carpopedal spasms may occur spontaneously or be precipitated by hyperventilation or application of a constricting blood pressure cuff (Trousseau's sign). Myotatic stretch reflexes are characteristically hyperactive, and the hyperirritability of peripheral nerves can be elucidated by observing muscle contraction after tapping of the peroneal nerve at the lateral margin of the knee (peroneal sign) or tapping of the facial nerve in front of the ear (Chvostek's sign). Mental status abnormalities include irritability, anxiety, confusion, and psychosis. Calcifications of the basal ganglia are seen in patients with chronic hypoparathyroidism.

Hypercalcemia

Hypercalcemia may result from hyperparathyroidism, vitamin D intoxication, hyperthyroidism, prolonged immobilization, malignancies (especially in bone), sarcoidosis, Williams' syndrome, and the use of diuretics. Clinical manifestations include anorexia, nausea, vomiting, polydipsia and polyuria, and muscle weakness. Hypercalcemia has been associated with apnea in infants [Kooh and Binet, 1990]. Chronic hypercalcemia leads to nephrocalcinosis and renal failure.

MAGNESIUM CONCENTRATION ABNORMALITIES

Magnesium, the fourth most abundant cation in the body, plays an important role in neuronal and muscle excitability and is essential for the normal activity of the various enzyme systems, including all those requiring adenosine triphosphate [Rude and Singer, 1981]. Almost all magnesium is located intracellularly, predominantly in bone, muscle, and liver; only 1% of the total body magnesium content is distributed in extracellular spaces. Under normal conditions, plasma magnesium concentrations range from 1.5 to 2.2 mEq/L.

Magnesium is absorbed in the small intestine through an active transport process linked to calcium absorption and is excreted predominantly by the kidney. Most of the magnesium filtered by the renal glomeruli is resorbed in the proximal tubules; only approximately 3% to 5% of filtered magnesium is excreted in the urine.

Box 90-4 Causes of Hypomagnesemia

- Malabsorption
- Hypoparathyroidism
- Renal tubular acidosis
- Diuretic therapy
- Primary aldosteronism
- Neonatal tetany

Hypomagnesemia

Although cellular depletion of magnesium can occur without demonstrable hypomagnesemia [Montgomery, 1960], clinical manifestations of magnesium depletion usually are associated with hypomagnesemia (serum concentration of 1.3 mEq/L or less). Hypomagnesemia can occur in chronic diarrhea or vomiting, sprue, or celiac disease; with prolonged parenteral nutrition therapy; and in hypoaldosteronism (Box 90-4). Tetany that is clinically indistinguishable from hypocalcemic tetany is the most distinctive symptom of magnesium depletion, but muscle tremors, fasciculations, weakness, choreoathetosis or tremor, dysphagia, ataxia, vertigo, nystagmus, and mental changes including irritability and confusion also may occur [Fishman, 1965; Hamed and Lindeman, 1978; Langley and Mann, 1991]. Cardiac dysrhythmias may occur. Hypocalcemia resistant to vitamin D therapy caused by impaired parathyroid function [Rude et al., 1976] and hypokalemia caused by impaired renal potassium resorption [Shils, 1969] also have been reported. Because of the similarity between the neurologic manifestations of hypomagnesemia and those of hypocalcemia, it is important to assess both calcium and magnesium status in treating patients with these manifestations.

Hypermagnesemia

Hypermagnesemia usually signifies impaired renal function. Clinical manifestations of hypermagnesemia rarely occur unless the serum magnesium concentration is greater than 4 mEq/L. Neuromuscular and cardiac symptoms and signs predominate. The neuromuscular manifestations are a consequence of decreased impulse transmission across the neuromuscular junction, decreased responsiveness of the postsynaptic membrane, and an increased threshold for axonal excretion [Mordes and Walker, 1978; Rude and Singer, 1981]. Hyporeflexia or areflexia may be observed with serum magnesium concentrations greater than 4 mEq/L, somnolescence at concentrations of 4 to 7 mEq/L, and paralysis at concentrations greater than 10 mEq/L. Cardiac conduction deficits characterized by prolonged P-R and R-T intervals and increased T wave amplitude are observed at serum concentrations of 5 to 10 mEq/L. Complete heart block and cardiac arrest in diastole may occur with serum concentrations greater than 15 mEq/L. Although rare, symptomatic hypermagnesemia can occur in patients with renal failure, Addison's disease after excessive parenteral administration, or iatrogenic poisoning (Box 90-5). Hypermagnesemia has been reported in newborns after magnesium

Box 90-5 Causes of Hypermagnesemia

- Decreased renal function
- Magnesium-containing laxatives or enema preparations
- Maternal magnesium sulfate treatment

sulfate treatment of preeclampsia in their mothers [Donovan et al., 1980; Lipsitz, 1971]. Intravenous administration of calcium gluconate rapidly reverses the clinical manifestations of hypermagnesemia.

REFERENCES

Abernathy RS. Bulging fontanelle as a presenting sign in cystic fibrosis. Am J Dis Child 1976;130:1360.

Abrahams P, Burkitt BFE. Hiatus hernia and gastrooesophageal reflux in children and adolescents with cerebral palsy. Aust Paediatr J 1970;6:41.

Abu-Arafeh I, Russell G. Cyclic vomiting syndrome in children: A population-based study. J Pediatr Gastroenterol Nutr 1995;21:454.

Adams DH, Ponsford S, Gunson B, et al. Neurological complications following liver transplantation. Lancet 1987;1:949.

Adams M, Rhyner PA, Day J, et al. Whipple's disease confined to the central nervous system. Ann Neurol 1987;21:104.

Adams RD, Foley JM. The neurological disorder associated with liver disease. Proc Assoc Res Nerv Ment Dis 1952;32:198.

Adams RD, Kubik CS. Subacute degeneration of the brain in pernicious anemia. N Engl J Med 1944;231:2.

Ahn TB, Cho JW, Jeon BS. Unusual neurological presentations of vitamin B_{12} deficiency. Eur J Neurol 2004;11:339.

Akikusa JD, Garrick D, Nash MC. Scurvy: Forgotten but not gone. J Paediatr Child Health 2003;39:75.

Akil M, Schwartz JA, Dutchak D, et al. The psychiatric presentation of Wilson's disease. J Neuropsychiatr Clin Neurosci 1991;3:377.

Alagille D, Curlier S, Chiva M, et al. Long-term neuropsychological outcome in children undergoing portal-systemic shunts for portal vein obstruction without liver disease. J Pediatr Gastroenterol Nutr 1986;5:861.

Alba D, Molina F, Vazquez JJ. Neurologic manifestations of Whipple disease. Ann Med Intern 1995;12:508.

Albers JW, Nostrant TT, Riggs JE. Neurologic manifestations of gastrointestinal disease. Neurol Clin 1989;7:525.

Albrecht J, Jones EA. Hepatic encephalopathy: Molecular mechanisms underlying the clinical syndrome. J Neurol Sci 1999;170:138.

Alderman CP, Hill CL. Abnormal bone mineral metabolism after long-term anticonvulsant treatment. Ann Pharmacother 1994;28:47.

Algarin C, Peirano P, Garrido M, et al. Iron deficiency anemia in infancy: Long-lasting effects on auditory and visual system functioning. Pediatr Res 2003;53:217.

Ali FE, Al-Bustan MA, Al-Busairi WA, et al. Loss of seizure control due to anticonvulsant-induced hypocalcemia. Ann Pharmacother 2004;38:1002.

Allen RH. The plasma transport of vitamin B_{12}. Br J Haematol 1976;33:161.

Alonso EM, Sokol RJ, Hart J, et al. Fulminant hepatitis associated with centrilobular hepatic necrosis in young children. J Pediatr 1995;127:888.

Alper G, Jarjour IT, Reyes JD, et al. Outcome of children with cerebral edema caused by fulminant hepatic failure. Pediatr Neurol 1998;18:299.

Alpers BJ. Diffuse progressive degeneration of gray matter of the cerebrum. Arch Neurol Psychiatry 1931;25:469.

Amodio P, Del Piccolo F, Marchetti P, et al. Clinical features and survival of cirrhotic patients with subclinical cognitive alterations detected by the number connection test and computerized psychometric tests. Hepatology 1999;29:1662.

Anderson J, Sugerman K, Lockhart JR, et al. Effective prophylactic therapy for cyclic vomiting syndrome in children using amitriptyline or cyproheptadine. Pediatrics 1997;100:977.

Andrews BT. Fluid and electrolyte disorders in neurosurgical intensive care. Neurosurg Clin North Am 1994;5:707.

Aoki Y, Lombroso CT. Prognostic value of electroencephalography in Reye's syndrome. Neurology 1973;23:333.

Aparicio JM, Belanger-Quintana A, Suarez L, et al. Ataxia with isolated vitamin E deficiency: Case report and review of the literature. J Pediatr Gastroenterol Nutr 2001;33:206.

Appleton RE, Farrell K, Teal P, et al. Complex partial status epilepticus associated with cyclosporin A therapy. J Neurol Neurosurg Psychiatry 1989;52:1068.

Arieff AI, Guisado R. Effects on central nervous system hypernatremia and hyponatremia states. Kidney Int 1976;10:104.

Arieff AI. Rapid correction of hyponatremia: Cause for pontine myelinolysis. Am J Med 1981;71:846.

Arnon SS. Infant botulism. In: Feigin RD, Cherry JD, eds. Textbook of pediatric infectious diseases. Philadelphia: WB Saunders, 1992.

Arroyo HA, De Rosa S, Ruggieri V, et al. Epilepsy, occipital calcifications, and oligosymptomatic celiac disease in childhood. J Child Neurol 2002;17:800.

Arthur LJH. Juvenile pernicious anemia. Proc R Soc Med 1972;65:728.

Ashkenazi R, Ben-Shachar D, Youdim MB. Nutritional iron and dopamine binding sites in the rat brain. Pharmacol Biochem Behav 1982;17:43.

Ashkenazi S, Bellah G, Cleary TG. Hallucinations as an initial manifestation of childhood shigellosis. J Pediatr 1989;14:95.

Ashkenazi S, Cleary KR, Pickering LK, et al. The association of Shiga toxin and other cytotoxins with the neurologic manifestations of shigellosis. J Infect Dis 1990;161:961.

Ashkenazi S, Dinari G, Weitz B, et al. Convulsions in shigellosis: Evaluation of possible risk factors. Am J Dis Child 1983;137:1985.

Ashkenazi S, Dinari G, Zevulunov A, et al. Convulsions in childhood shigellosis: Clinical and laboratory features in 153 children. Am J Dis Child 1987;141:208.

Auricchio A, Brancolini V, Casari G, et al. The locus for a novel syndromic form of neuronal intestinal pseudo-obstruction maps to Xq28. Am J Hum Genet 1996;58:743.

Axon ATR, Long DE, Jones SC. Abdominal migraine: Does it exist? J Clin Gastroenterol 1991;13:615.

Aydinli N, Citak A, Caliskan M, et al. Vitamin K deficiency—late onset intracranial haemorrhage. Eur J Paediatr Neurol 1998;2:199.

Bagwell CE. Gastroesophageal reflux in children. Surg Ann 1995;27:133.

Ballauff A, Engelbrecht V, Voit T. Hyperintense lesions of the globus pallidus on MRI in children with chronic liver disease. Eur J Pediatr 1994;153:802.

Balter-Seri J, Yuhas Y, Weizman A, et al. Role of nitric oxide in the enhancement of pentylentetrazole-induced seizures caused by *Shigella dysenteriae*. Infect Immun 1999;67:6364.

Banerji NK, Hurwitz LJ. Nervous system manifestations after gastric surgery. Acta Neurol Scand 1971;47:485.

Bardella MT, Molteni N, Prampolini L, et al. Need for follow up in coeliac disease. Arch Dis Child 1994;70:211.

Barohn RJ, Levine EJ, Olson JO, et al. Gastric hypomotility in Duchenne's muscular dystrophy. N Engl J Med 1988;319:15.

Barohn RJ, Sanchez JA, Anderson KE. Acute peripheral neuropathy due to hereditary coproporphyria. Muscle Nerve 1994;17:793.

Bartlett K, Ghneim HK, Stirk HK, et al. Enzyme studies in biotin-responsive disorders. J Inherit Metab Dis 1985;8 (Suppl 1):46.

Basile AS, Jones EA. Ammonia and GABA-ergic neurotransmission: Interrelated factors in the pathogenesis of hepatic encephalopathy. Hepatology 1997;25:1303.

Basile AS, Harrison PM, Hughes RD, et al. Relationship between plasma benzodiazepine receptor ligand concentrations and severity of hepatic encephalopathy. Hepatology 1994;19:112.

Basile AS, Hughes RD, Harrison PM, et al. Elevated brain concentrations of 1,4-benzodiazepines in fulminant hepatic failure. N Engl J Med 1991;325:473.

Basile AS, Jones EA, Skolnick P. The pathogenesis and treatment of hepatic encephalopathy: Evidence for the involvement of benzodiazepine receptor ligands. Pharmacol Rev 1991;43:27.

Bass NH, Netsky MG, Young E. Effect of neonatal malnutrition on the developing cerebrum. Arch Neurol 1970;23:289.

Bauernfeind JC, Miller ON. Vitamin B_6: Nutritional and pharmacologic usage, stability, bioavailability, antagonists and safety. In: Human vitamin B_3 requirements. Washington, DC: National Academy of Sciences, 1987.

Bax RT, Hassler A, Luck W, et al. Cerebral manifestation of Wilson's disease successfully treated with liver transplantation. Neurology 1998;51:863.

Baynes K, Farias ST, Gospe SM Jr. Pyridoxine-dependent seizures and cognition in adulthood. Dev Med Child Neurol 2003;45:782.

Beard JL. Iron biology in immune function, muscle metabolism and neuronal functioning. J Nutr 2001;131:568S.

Beard JL. Iron deficiency alters brain development and functioning. J Nutr 2003;133:1468S.

Beardslee WR, Wolff PH, Hurwitz I, et al. The effects of infantile malnutrition on behavioral development: A follow-up study. Am J Clin Nutr 1982;35:1437.

Beaton GH, Ghassemi H. Supplementary feeding programs for young children in developing countries. Am J Clin Nutr 1982;35:864.

Beck WS. Cobalamin and the nervous system. N Engl J Med 1988;318:1752.

Behrman RE, Kliegman RM, Arvin AM, eds. Nelson textbook of pediatrics, 15th ed. Philadelphia: WB Saunders, 1996.

Bejsovec M, Kulenda Z, Ponca E. Familial intrauterine convulsions in pyridoxine dependency. Arch Dis Child 1967;42:201.

Belay ED, Bresee JS, Holman RC, et al. Reye's syndrome in the United States from 1981 through 1997. N Engl J Med 1999;340:1377.

Bell NH. Vitamin D—endocrine system. J Clin Invest 1985;76:1.

Bellary S, Hassanein T, Van Thiel DH. Liver transplantation for Wilson's disease. J Hepatol 1995;23:373.

Belman AL, Roque CT, Ancona R, et al. Cerebral venous thrombosis in a child with iron deficiency anemia and thrombocytosis. Stroke 1990;21:488.

Bendich A, Langseth L. Safety of vitamin A. Am J Clin Nutr 1989;49:385.

Bennett MJ, Marlow N, Pollin RJ, et al. Glutaric aciduria type I: Biochemical and postmortem findings. Eur J Pediatr 1986;145:403.

Bentley D, Kehely A, Al-Bayaty M, et al. Abdominal migraine as a cause of vomiting in children: A clinician's view. J Pediatr Gastroenterol Nutr 1995;21:549.

Bentley ME, Caulfield LE, Ram M, et al. Zinc supplementation affects the activity patterns of rural Guatemalan infants. J Nutr 1997;127:1333.

Bentley SD, Maiwald M, Murphy LD, et al. Sequencing and analysis of the genome of the Whipple's disease bacterium *Tropheryma whippelii*. Lancet 2003;361:637.

Benton JW, Moser HW, Dodge PR, et al. Modification of the schedule of myelination in the rat by early nutritional deprivation. Pediatrics 1966;38:801.

Berezin S, Newman LS, Schwarz SM, et al. Gastroesophageal reflux associated with nemaline myopathy of infancy. Pediatrics 1988;81:111.

Berger A, Schaumburg HH. Move on neuropathy from pyridoxine abuse. N Engl J Med 1984;311:986.

Bernofsky C. Physiologic aspects of pyridine nucleotide regulation in mammals. Mol Cell Biochem 1980;33:135.

Bernuau J, Benhamou JP. Classifying acute liver failure. Lancet 1993;342:252.

Berry PL, Belsha CW. Hyponatremia. Pediatr Clin North Am 1990;37:351.

Berson EL, Shih VE, Sullivan PL. Ocular findings in patients with gyrate atrophy on pyridoxine and low protein, low arginine diets. Ophthalmology 1981;88:311.

Bhaduri BR, Mieli Vergani G. Fulminant hepatic failure: Pediatric aspects. Semin Liver Dis 1996;16:349.

Bhan MK, Bhandari N, Bahl R. Management of the severely malnourished child: Perspective from developing countries. BMJ 2003;326;146.

Bhatnagar S, Taneja S. Zinc and cognitive development. Br J Nutr 2001;85 (Suppl 2):S139.

Biancheri R, Cerone R, Schiaffino MC, et al. Cobalamin (Cbl) C/D deficiency: Clinical, neurophysiological and neuroradiologic findings in 14 cases. Neuropediatrics 2001;32:14.

Bicknese AR, May W, Hickey WF, et al. Early childhood hepatocerebral degeneration misdiagnosed as valproate hepatotoxicity. Ann Neurol 1992;32:767.

Bird GLA, Meadows J, Goka J, et al. Cyclosporin-associated akinetic mutism and extrapyramidal syndrome after liver transplantation. J Neurol Neurosurg Psychiatry 1990;53:1068.

Bismuth H, Azoulay D, Samuel D, et al. Auxiliary partial orthotopic liver transplantation for fulminant hepatitis. The Paul Brousse experience. Ann Surg 1996;224:712.

Black MM. Zinc deficiency and child development. Am J Clin Nutr 1998;68:464S.

Black MM. Micronutrient deficiencies and cognitive functioning: 1, 2. J Nutrition 2003;133:3927S.

Blanco R, De Girolami U, Jenkins RL, et al. Neuropathology of liver transplantation. Clin Neuropathol 1995;14:109.

Blei AT. Diagnosis and treatment of hepatic encephalopathy. Baillieres Best Pract Res Clin Gastroenterol 2000;14:959.

Bleichrodt N, Born MP. A meta-analysis of research on iodine and its relationship to cognitive development. In: Stanbury J, ed. The damaged brain of iodine deficiency: Cognitive, behavioral, neuromotor and educative aspects. Elmsford, NY: Cognizant Communication Corporation, 1994.

Block G, Levine M. Vitamin C: A new look. Ann Intern Med 1991;114:909.

Bolande RP. Neurocristopathy: its growth and development in 20 years. Pediatr Pathol Lab Med 1997;17:1.

Boles RG, Adams K, Ito M, et al. Maternal inheritance in cyclic vomiting syndrome with neuromuscular disease. Am J Med Genetics A 2003;120:474.

Bonner DM, Suyama Y, Domoss A. Genetic fine structure and enzyme formation. Fed Proc 1960;19:926.

Bont A, Steck AJ, Meyer UA. Acute hepatic porphyria and its neurological syndrome. Schweiz Med Wochenschr 1996;126:6.

Bor O, Akgun N, Yakut A, et al. Late hemorrhagic disease of the newborn. Pediatr Int 2000;42:64.

Bott L, Boute O, Mention K, et al. Congenital idiopathic intestinal pseudo-obstruction and hydrocephalus with stenosis of the aqueduct of Sylvius. Am J Med Genet A 2004;130:84.

Bottiglieri T, Hyland K. *S*-adenosylmethionine levels in psychiatric and neurological disorders: A review. Acta Neurol Scand Suppl 1994;154:19.

Bourne MC, Wheeldon C, MacKinlay GA, et al. Laparoscopic Nissen fundoplication in children: 2-5-year follow-up. Pediatr Surg Int 200;19:537.

Bowie MD, Moodie AD, Mann MD, et al. A prospective 15-year follow up study of kwashiorkor patients. Part I. Physical growth and development. South Afr Med J 1980;58:671.

Brandt NJ, Gregerson N, Christensen E, et al. Treatment of glutaryl-CoA dehydrogenase deficiency (glutaric aciduria). J Pediatr 1979;94:669.

Brann BS, Stonestreet BS, Oh W, et al. The in vivo effect of bilirubin and sulfisoxazole on cerebral oxygen, glucose, and lactate metabolism in newborn piglets. Pediatr Res 1987;22:135.

Bray PF, Herbst JJ, Johnson DG, et al. Childhood gastroesophageal reflux: Neurologic and psychiatric syndromes mimicked. JAMA 1977;237:1342.

Brem AS. Disorders of potassium homeostasis. Pediatr Clin North Am 1990;37:419.

Brewer GJ. Practical recommendations and new therapies for Wilson's disease. Drugs 1995;50:240.

Brewer GJ, Yuzbasiyan-Gurkan V. Wilson's disease. Medicine 1992;71:139.

Brewer GJ, Dick RD, Johnson V, et al. Treatment of Wilson's disease with ammonium tetrathiomolybdate. I. Initial therapy in 17 neurologically affected patients. Arch Neurol 1994;51:545.

Brivet M, Tardicu M, Khellaf A, et al. Riboflavin responsive ethylmalonic-adipic aciduria in a 9 month old boy with liver cirrhosis, myopathy, and encephalopathy. J Inherit Metab Dis 1991;14:333.

Brody LC, Mitchell GA, Obie C, et al. Ornithine delta aminotransferase mutations in gyrate atrophy. J Biol Chem 1992;267:3302.

Bronster DJ, Boccagni P, D'Rourke M, et al. Loss of speech after orthotopic liver transplantation. Transpl Int 1995;8:234.

Brown LW, Feigin RD. Bacterial meningitis: Fluid balance and therapy. Pediatr Ann 1994;23:93.

Brown WD. Osmotic demyelination disorders: Central pontine and extrapontine myelinolysis. Curr Opin Neurol 2000;13:691.

Bruggers CS, Ware R, Altman AJ, et al. Reversible focal neurologic deficits in severe iron deficiency anemia. J Pediatr 1990;117:430.

Brunberg JA, Kanal E, Hirsch W, et al. Chronic acquired hepatic failure: MR imaging of the brain at 1.5 T. AJNR Am J Neuroradiol 1991;12:909.

Brunner HG, Hamel BCJ, Rieu P, et al. Intestinal pseudo-obstruction in myotonic dystrophy. J Med Genet 1992;29:791.

Brunner JE, Redmund LM, Hagger AM, et al. Central pontine myelinolysis and pontine lesions after rapid correction of hyponatremia: A prospective magnetic resonance imaging. Ann Neurol 1990;27:61.

Bryan J, Osendarp S, Hughes D, et al. Nutrients for cognitive development in school-aged children. Nutr Rev 2004;62:295.

Burd L, Stenehjem A, Franceschini LA, et al. A 15-year follow-up of a boy with pyridoxine (vitamin B_6)-dependent seizures with autism, breath holding, and severe mental retardation. J Child Neurol 2000;15:763.

Bushinsky DA, Monk RD. Calcium. Lancet 1998;352:306.

Bustamante J, Rimola A, Ventura PJ, et al. Prognostic significance of hepatic encephalopathy in patients with cirrhosis. J Hepatol 1999;30:890.

Butterworth RF, Giguere J, Michaud J, et al. Ammonia: Key factor in the pathogenesis of hepatic encephalopathy. Neurochem Pathol 1987;6:1.

Butterworth RF. The neurobiology of hepatic encephalopathy. Semin Liver Dis 1996;16:235.

Bylesjo I, Brekke OL, Prytz J, et al. Brain magnetic resonance imaging white-matter lesions and cerebrospinal fluid findings in patients with acute intermittent porphyria. Eur Neurol 2004;51:1.

Bylesjo I, Forsgren L, Lithner F, et al. Epidemiology and clinical characteristics of seizures in patients with acute intermittent porphyria. Epilepsia 1996;37:230.

Cabak V, Najdanvic R. Effect of undernutrition in early life on physical and mental development. Arch Dis Child 1965;40:532.

Cadranel JF, Lebiez E, Di Martino V, et al. Focal neurological signs in hepatic encephalopathy in cirrhotic patients: An underestimated entity? Am J Gastroenterol 2001;96:515.

Calloway DH, Murphy SP, Beaton GH, et al. Estimated vitamin intakes of toddlers: Predicted prevalence of inadequacy in village populations in Egypt, Kenya, and Mexico. Am J Clin Nutr 1993;58:376.

Camilleri M, Bharucha AE. Gastrointestinal dysfunction in neurologic disease. Semin Neurol 1996;16:203.

Cardo E, Monros E, Colome C, et al. Children with stroke: Polymorphism of the *MTHFR* gene, mild hyperhomocysteinemia, and vitamin status. J Child Neurol 2000;15:295.

Cardo E, Vilaseca MA, Campistol J, et al. Evaluation of hyperhomocysteinaemia in children with stroke. Eur J Paediatr Neurol 1999;3:113.

Carmel R, Green R, Rosenblatt DS, et al. Update on cobalamin, folate, and homocysteine. Hematology (Am Soc Hematol Educ Program) 2003:62.

Carpenter KJ, Sutherland B. Eijkman's contribution to the discovery of vitamins. J Nutr 1995;125:155.

Carrie I, Portoukalian J, Vicaretti R, et al. Menaquinone-4 concentration is correlated with sphingolipid concentrations in rat brain. J Nutr 2004;134:167.

Casteels-Van Daele M, Van Geet C, Wouters C, et al. Reye syndrome revisited: A descriptive term covering a group of heterogeneous disorders. Eur J Pediatr 2000;159:641.

Castillo-Duran C, Perales CG, Hertrampf ED, et al. Effect of zinc supplementation on development and growth of Chilean infants. J Pediatr 2001;138:229.

Catello MA, Operamolla P, Clerico A. Nonfamilial intestinal polyposis and brain tumor in a 5 year old girl. Pediatr Hematol Oncol 1987;4:247.

Celedon JM, DeAndraca I. Psychomotor development during treatment of severely marasmic infants. Early Hum Dev 1979;3:267.

Celic Y, Kaya M. Brain SPECT findings in Wernicke's encephalopathy. Neurol Sci 2004;25:23.

Celik M, Forta H, Dalkilic T, et al. MRI reveals reversible lesions resembling posterior reversible encephalopathy in porphyria. Neuroradiology 2002;44:839.

Chakravarti A. Endothelin receptor-mediated signaling in Hirschsprung disease. Hum Mol Genet 1996;5:303.

Chari VR, Katiyar BL, Rastogi BL, et al. Neuropathy in hepatic disorders: A clinical, electrophysiological and histopathological appraisal, J Neurol Sci 1977;31:93.

Chase HP, Martin HP. Undernutrition and child development. N Engl J Med 1970;282:933.

Chase HP, Lindsley WFB Jr, O'Brien D. Undernutrition and cerebellar development. Nature 1969;221:554.

Chen CL, Chen YS, Lui CC, et al. Neurological improvement of Wilson's disease after liver transplantation. Transplant Proc 1997;29:497.

Cherington M. Botulism: Update and review. Semin Neurol 2004;24:155.

Chhabra A, Patwari AK, Aneja S, et al. Neuromuscular manifestations of diarrhea related hypokalemia. Indian Pediatr 1995;32:409.

Christensen E, Brandt NJ. Studies on glutaryl-CoA dehydrogenase in leukocytes, fibroblasts and amniotic fluid cells: The normal enzymes and the mutant form in patients with glutaric aciduria. Clin Chim Acta 1978;88:267.

Chu NS, Yang SS, Liaw YF. Evoked potentials in liver diseases. J Gastroenterol Hepatol 1997;12:S288.

Chytil F, Ong D. Intracellular vitamin A–binding proteins. Annu Rev Nutr 1987;7:321.

Clay SA, Ramseyer C, Fishman LS, et al. Acute infantile motor unit disorder. Infantile botulism? Arch Neurol 1977;34:246.

Clos J, Favre C, Selme-Matrat M, et al. Effects of undernutrition on cell formation in the rat brain and especially cellular composition of the cerebellum. Brain Res 1977;123:13.

Cocco S, Diaz G, Stancampiano R, et al. Vitamin A deficiency produces spatial learning and memory impairment in rats. Neuroscience 2002;115:475.

Cochran DP, Appleton RE. Infant botulism: Is it that rare? Dev Med Child Neurol 1995;37:274.

Cochrane WA, Collins-Williams C, Donahue WL. Superior hemorrhagic polioencephalitis (Wernicke's disease) occurring in an infant: Probably due to thiamine deficiency from use of a soybean product. Pediatrics 1961;28:771.

Coe M, Carfagnini F, Tani G, et al. Wernicke's encephalopathy in a child: Case report and MR findings. Pediatr Radiol 2001;31:167.

Colina KF, Abelson HT. Resolution of breath-holding spells with treatment of concomitant anemia. J Pediatr 1995;126:395.

Collin P, Maki M. Associated disorders in coeliac disease: Clinical aspects. Scand J Gastroenterol 1994;29:769.

Collin P, Pirittila T, Hurmikko T, et al. Celiac disease, brain atrophy, and dementia. Neurology 1991;41:372.

Conley SB. Hypernatremia. Pediatr Clin North Am 1990;37:365.

Conn HO, Leevy CM, Vlahcevic AR, et al. Comparison of lactulose and neomycin in the treatment of chronic portal-systemic encephalopathy: A double-blind controlled trial. Gastroenterology 1977;72:573.

Connolly AM, Volpe JJ. Clinical features of bilirubin encephalopathy. Clin Perinatol 1990;17:371.

Contino MF, Lebby T, Arcinue EL. Rotaviral gastrointestinal infection causing afebrile seizures in infancy and childhood. Am J Emerg Med 1994;12:94.

Conway EE Jr. Central nervous system findings and intussusception: How are they related? Pediatr Emerg Care 1993;9:15.

Cooper AJL, Plum F. Biochemistry and physiology of brain ammonia. Physiol Rev 1987;67:440.

Cordoba J, Blei AT. Brain edema and hepatic encephalopathy. Semin Liver Dis 1996;16:271.

Cordoba J, Cabrera J, Lataif L, et al. High prevalence of sleep disturbance in cirrhosis. Hepatology 1998;27:339.

Cornejo W, Gonzalez F, Toro ME, et al. Subacute combined degeneration. A description of the case of a strictly vegetarian child. Rev Neurol 2001;33:1154.

Corrigan JJ. The vitamin K dependent proteins. Adv Pediatr 1981;28:57.

Costa M, Brookes SJ. The enteric nervous system. Am J Gastroenterol 1994;89:S129.

Cottrill CM, Kaplan S. Cerebral vascular accidents in cyanotic congenital heart disease. Am J Dis Child 1973;125:484.

Coulter D. Carnitine, valproate, and toxicity. J Child Neurol 1991;6:7.

Coursin DB. Convulsive seizures in infants with pyridoxine deficient diets. JAMA 1954;213:1867.

Cowan MJ, Wara DW, Packman S, et al. Multiple biotin dependent carboxylase deficiency associated with defects in T-cell and B-cell immunity. Lancet 1979;2:115.

Cragg BG. The development of cortical synapses during starvation in the rat. Brain 1972;95:143.

Cravioto J, Arrieta R. Stimulation and mental development of malnourished infants. Lancet 1979;2:899.

Cravioto J, DeLicardie ER, Birch HC. Nutrition, growth and neurointegrative development: an experimental and ecologic study. Pediatrics 1966;38:319.

Crimlisk HL. The little imitator—porphyria: A neuropsychiatric disorder. J Neurol Neurosurg Psychiatry 1997;62:319.

Cucchiara S. Cisapride therapy for gastrointestinal disease. J Pediatr Gastroenterol Nutr 1966;22:259.

Culley WJ, Lineberger RO. Effect of undernutrition on the size and composition of the rat brain. J Nutr 1968;96:375.

Culley WJ, Mertz ET. Effect of restricted food intake on growth and composition of preweanling rat brain. Proc Soc Exp Biol Med 1965;118:233.

Czlonkowska A, Gajda J, Rodo M. Effects of long-term treatment in Wilson's disease with D-penicillamine and zinc sulphate. J Neurol 1996;243:269.

Dabbagh O, Brismar J, Gascon GG, et al. The clinical spectrum of biotin-treatable encephalopathies in Saudi Arabia. Brain Dev 1994;16 (Suppl):72.

Dahlman T, Hartvig P, Lofholm M, et al. Long-term treatment of Wilson's disease with triethylene tetramine dihydrochloride (trientine). Q J Med 1995;88:609.

Daoud AS, Batieha A, Al-sheyyab M, et al. Effectiveness of iron therapy on breath-holding spells. J Pediatr 1997;130:547.

Daoud AS, Zaki M, al-Mutairi G, et al. Childhood shigellosis: Clinical and bacteriological study. J Trop Med Hyg 1990;93:275.

Davis RE. Clinical chemistry of vitamin B_{12}. Adv Clin Chem 1985;24:163.

Davis RE, Leke GC. Clinical chemistry of thiamine. Adv Clin Chem 1983;23:93.

De Schepper J, Hachimi-Idrissi S, Dab I, et al. Nerve conduction in vitamin E deficient cystic fibrosis patients. Eur J Pediatr 1997;156:251.

Decell MK, Gordon JB, Silver K, et al. Fulminant hepatic failure associated with status epilepticus in children: Three cases and a review of potential mechanisms. Intensive Care Med 1994;20:375.

DeGroen PC, Askamit AJ, Rakela J, et al. Central nervous system toxicity after liver transplantation: The role of cyclosporine and cholesterol. N Engl J Med 1987;317:861.

DeLuca HF, Schnoes HK. Vitamin D: Recent advances. J Biochem 1983;52:411.

Denning TR, Berrios GE. Wilson's disease: Psychiatric symptoms in 195 cases. Arch Gen Psychiatry 1989;46:1126.

Denning TR, Berrios GE. Wilson's disease: A longitudinal study of psychiatric symptoms. Biol Psychiatry 1990;28:255.

DeVisser M, Scholte HR, Schutgens RBH. Riboflavin responsive lipid storage myopathy and glutaric aciduria of early adult onset. Neurology 1986;36:367.

DeVivo DC. Reye syndrome. Neurol Clin 1985;3:95.

Diamantopoulos N, Painter MJ, Wolf B, et al. Biotinidase deficiency: Accumulation of lactate in brain and response to physiologic doses of biotin. Neurology 1986;36:1107.

Diaz-Cintra S, Cintra L, Kemper T, et al. The effects of protein deprivation on the nucleus raphe dorsalis: A morphometric Golgi study in rats of three age groups. Brain Res 1981;221:243.

Diaz-Cintra S, Cintra L, Kemper T, et al. The effects of protein deprivation on the nucleus locus coeruleus: A morphometric Golgi study in rats of three age groups. Brain Res 1984;304:243.

Diaz-Cintra S, Cintra L, Ortega A, et al. Effects of protein deprivation on pyramidal cells of the visual cortex in rats of three age groups. J Comp Neurol 1990;292:117.

Dickerson JWT, Merat A, Widdowson EM. Intrauterine growth retardation in the pig. Biol Neonate 1971;19:354.

Dietrich W, Ehnis T, Bauer M, et al. Identification of tissue transglutaminase as the autoantigen of celiac disease. Nature Med 1997;3:707.

Dobbing J. The influence of early nutrition on the development and myelination of the brain. Proc R Soc Lond (Biol) 1964;159:503.

Dobbing J. Vulnerable periods of brain development. In: Ciba Foundation. Lipids, malnutrition and the developing brain. Amsterdam: Elsevier, 1972.

Dobbing J, Sands J. Vulnerability of developing brain. IX. The effect of nutritional growth retardation on the timing of the brain growth spurt. Biol Neonate 1971;19:363.

Dobbing J, Hopewell JW, Lynch A. Vulnerability of developing brain. VII. Permanent deficit of neurons in cerebral and cerebellar cortex following early mild undernutrition. Exp Neurol 1971;32:439.

Dodge PR, Prensky AL, Feigin RD. Nutrition and the developing nervous system. St. Louis: Mosby, 1975.

Donaldson HH. The effect of underfeeding on the percentage of water, on the ether-alcohol extract, and on medullation in the central nervous system of the albino rat. J Comp Neurol 1911;21:139.

Donaldson RM Jr. Intrinsic factor and the transport of cobalamin. In: Jowson LR, ed. Physiology of the gastrointestinal tract. New York: Raven Press, 1981.

Donovan EF, Tsang RC, Steichen JJ, et al. Neonatal hypermagnesium: Effect on parathyroid hormone and calcium homeostasis. J Pediatr 1980;96:305.

Donovan JP, Shaw BW Jr, Langnas AN, et al. Brain water and acute liver failure: The emerging role of intracranial pressure monitoring Hepatology 1992;16:267.

Douglas NL, Liakos D, Vlachos P. Scurvy in a 4 year old child. Am J Dis Child 1973;126:712.

Dreifuss FE, Langer DH, Moline KA, et al. Valproic acid hepatic fatalities. II. U.S. experience since 1984. Neurology 1989;39:201.

Duprez TP, Grandin CB, Bonnier C, et al. Whipple disease confined to the central nervous system in childhood. AJNR Am J Neuroradiol 1996;17:1589.

Duran M, Wadman SK. Thiamine responsive inborn errors of metabolism. J Inherit Metab Dis 1985;8 (Suppl 1):70.

Durand DV, Lecomte C, Cathebras P. Whipple's disease: Clinical review of 52 cases. Medicine 1997;76:170.

Duret M, Herbaut AG, Flamme F, et al. Another case of atypical acute axonal polyneuropathy following *Campylobacter* enteritis. Neurology 1991;41:2008.

Dusheiko G, Kew MC, Joffe BI, et al. Recurrent hypoglycemia associated with glutaric aciduria type II in an adult. N Engl J Med 1979;301:1405.

Eckstein AK, Reichenbach A, Jacobi P, et al. Hepatic retinopathia. Changes in retinal function. Vision Res 1997;37:1699.

Edery P, Pelet A, Mulligan LM, et al. Long segment and short segment familial Hirschsprung's disease: Variable clinical expression at the *RET* locus. J Med Genet 1994;31:602.

Edidin DV, Levitsky LL, Schey W, et al. Resurgence of nutritional rickets associated with breast feeding and special dietary practices. Pediatrics 1980;65:232.

Ellefson RD, Ford RE. The polyphyrias: Characteristics and laboratory tests. Regul Toxicol Pharmacol 1996;24:S119.

Ellis CN, Vanduveen EE, Rassmussen JE. Scurvy: A case caused by peculiar dietary habits. Arch Dermatol 1984;120:1212.

Elsehety A, Bertorini TE. Neurologic and neuropsychiatric complications of Crohn's disease. South Med J 1997;90:606.

El-Youssef M. Wilson disease. Mayo Clin Proc 2003;78:1126.

Englehard S, Seifters S. The biochemical functions of ascorbic acid. Annu Rev Nutr 1986;6:365.

Ephros M, Cohen D, Yavzori M, et al. Encephalopathy associated with enteroinvasive *Escherichia coli* O144:NM infection. J Clin Microbiol 1996;34:2432.

Estol CJ, Faris AA, Martinez AJ, et al. Central pontine myelinolysis after liver transplantation. Neurology 1989a;39:493.

Estol CJ, Lopez O, Brenner ZP, et al. Seizures after liver transplantation: A clinicopathologic study. Neurology 1989b;39:1297.

Etchamendy N, Enderlin V, Marighetto A, et al. Vitamin A deficiency and relational memory deficit in adult mice: Relationships with changes in brain retinoid signalling. Behav Brain Res 2003;145:37.

Evans OB. Lactic acidosis in childhood. Pediatr Neurol 1986;2:5.

Faber J, Fich A, Steinberg A, et al. Familial intestinal pseudo-obstruction dominated by a progressive neurologic disease at a young age. Gastroenterology 1987;92:786.

Facchini SA, Jami MM, Neuberg RW, et al. A treatable cause of ataxia in children. Pediatr Neurol 2001;24:135.

Farrell PM, Levine SL, Murphy D, et al. Plasma tocopherol levels and tocopherol-lipid relationship in a normal population of children as compared to healthy adults. Am J Clin Nutr 1978;31:1720.

Fasano A, Catassi C. Current approaches to diagnosis and treatment of celiac disease: An evolving spectrum. Gastroenterology 2001;120:636.

Fattal-Valevski A, Bassan H, Korman SH, et al. Methylenetetrahydrofolate reductase deficiency: Importance of early diagnosis. J Child Neurol 2000;15:539.

Federico A. Ataxia with isolated vitamin E deficiency: A treatable neurological disorder resembling Friedreich's ataxia. Neurol Sci 2004;25:119.

Felmet K, Robins B, Tilford DAA, et al. Acute neurologic decompensation in an infant with cobalamin deficiency exposed to nitric oxide. J Pediatr 2000;137:427.

Ferenci P. Review article: Diagnosis and current therapy of Wilson's disease. Aliment Pharmacol Ther 2004;19:157.

Ferenci P, Covell D, Schafer DF, et al Metabolism of the inhibitory neurotransmitter gamma-aminobutyric acid in a rabbit model of fulminant hepatic failure. Hepatology 1983;3:507.

Ferenci P, Herneth A, Steindl P. Newer approaches to therapy of hepatic encephalopathy. Semin Liver Dis 1996;16:329.

Filston HC. Fluid and electrolyte management in the pediatric surgical patient. Surg Clin North Am 1992;72:1189.

Finberg L. Hypernatremic dehydration. Adv Pediatr 1967;16:325.

Finberg L. Hypernatremia (hypertonic) dehydration in infants: Current concepts. N Engl J Med 1973;289:196.

Finberg L. Too little water has become too much: The changing epidemiology of water balance and convulsions in infant diarrhea. Am J Dis Child 1986;140:524.

Finberg L, Kiley J, Hutrell C. Mass accidental salt poisoning in infancy. JAMA 1963;184:121.

Finelli PF, McEntee WS, Ambler M, et al. Adult celiac disease presenting as cerebellar syndrome. Neurology 1980;30:245.

Fish I, Winick M. Cellular growth in various regions of the developing rat brain. Pediatr Res 1969;3:407.

Fishman MA, Madyastha P, Prensky AL. The effect of undernutrition on the development of myelin in the rat central nervous system. Lipids 1971;6:458.

Fishman MA, Prensky AL, Dodge PR. Low content of cerebral lipids in infants suffering from malnutrition. Nature 1969;221:552.

Fishman RA. Neurologic aspects of magnesium metabolism. Arch Neurol 1965;12:562.

Fishman RA. Cell volume pumps and neurologic function: brain's adaptation to somatic stress. In: Plum F, ed. Brain dysfunction in metabolic disorders. Vol. 53. New York: Raven Press, 1974.

Fleisher DR. Management of cyclic vomiting syndrome. J. Pediatr Gastroenterol Nutr 1995;21 (Suppl 1):S52.

Fleisher DR. Cyclic vomiting syndrome: A paroxysmal disorder of brain-gut interaction. J Pediatr Gastroenterol Nutr 1997;25:S13.

Fleisher DR, Matar M. The cyclic vomiting syndrome: A report of 71 cases and literature review. J Pediatr Gastroenterol Nutr 1993;17:361.

Forbes D, Withers G. Prophylactic therapy in cyclic vomiting syndrome. J Pediatr Gastroenterol Nutr 1995;21:S57.

Fowler B. Recent advances in the mechanism of pyridoxine responsive disorders. J Inherit Metab Dis 1985;8 (Suppl 1):76.

Fowler B. Genetic defects of folate and cobalamin metabolism. Eur J Pediatr 1998;157 (Suppl 2):S60.

Fraser CL, Arieff AI. Hepatic encephalopathy. N Engl J Med 1985;313:865.

Fredrich SFT. Clinical treatise on disease of the liver. Vol. 1. Murchison C, trans. London: New Sydenham Soc, 1961.

Frimpter GW. Cystathioninuria: Nature of the defect. Science 1965;149:1095.

From the Centers for Disease Control and Prevention. Iron deficiency—United States, 1999-2000. MMWR Morb Mortal Wkly Rep 2002;51:897.

Gabuzda GJ, Phillips GB, Davidson CS. Reversible toxic manifestations in patients with cirrhosis of the liver given cation-exchange resins. N Engl J Med 1952;246:124.

Galler J, Ramsey F, Solimano G, et al. The influence of early malnutrition on subsequent behavioral development. I. Degree of impairment in intellectual performance. J Am Acad Child Psychiatry 1983;22:8.

Galler JR, Ramsey F, Forde V. A follow-up study of the influence of early malnutrition on subsequent development. 4. Intellectual performance during adolescence. Nutr Behav 1986;3:211.

Galvez Y, Skaba R, Vajtrova R, et al. Evidence of secondary neuronal intestinal dysplasia in a rat model of chronic intestinal obstruction. J Invest Surg 2004;17:31.

Gammal SH, Basile AS, Geller A, et al. Reversal of the behavioral and electrophysiological abnormalities of an animal model of hepatic encephalopathy by benzodiazepine receptor ligands. Hepatology 1990;11:371.

Garg BP, Walsh LE, Pescovitz MD, et al. Neurologic complications of pediatric liver transplantation. Pediatr Neurol 1993;9:444.

Gee S. On fitful or recurrent vomiting. St Bart Hosp Rep 1882;18:1.

Geissler I, Heinemann K, Rohm S, et al. Liver transplantation for hepatic and neurological Wilson's disease. Transplant Proc 2003;35:1445.

Georgieff MK, Hoffman JS, Pereira GR, et al. Effect of neonatal caloric deprivation on head growth and 1-year developmental status in preterm infants. J Pediatr 1985;107:581.

Gerard A, Sarrot-Reynauld F, Liozon E, et al. Neurological presentation of Whipple disease: Report of 12 cases and review of the literature. Medicine (Baltimore) 2002;81:443.

Gerber N, Dickinson RG, Harland RC, et al. Reye-like syndrome associated with valproic acid therapy. J Pediatr 1979;95:142.

Ghezzi A, Zaffaroni M. Neurological manifestations of gastrointestinal disorders, with particular reference to the differential diagnosis of multiple sclerosis. Neurol Sci 2001;22 (Suppl 2):S117.

Gibson RS. Zinc: A critical nutrient in growth and development. NZ Med J 1998;111:63.

Giebish G. Newer aspects of renal tubular potassium transport. Contrib Nephrol 1980;21:106.

Ginat Israeli T, Hurvitz H, Klar A, et al. Deteriorating neurological and neuroradiological course in treated biotinidase deficiency. Neuropediatrics 1993;24:103.

Glasgow JF, Middleton B. Reye syndrome—insights on causation and prognosis. Arch Dis Child. 2001;85:351.

Gobbi G, Bouquet F, Greco L, et al. Coeliac disease, epilepsy and cerebral calcifications. The Italian working group on celiac disease and epilepsy. Lancet 1992;340:439.

Goetting MG, Tiznado-Garcia E, Bakdash TF. Intussusception encephalopathy: An underrecognized cause of coma in children. Pediatr Neurol 1990;6:419.

Gokhale R, Huttenlocher PR, Brady L, et al. Use of barbiturates in the treatment of cyclic vomiting during childhood. J Ped Gastroenterol Nutr 1997;25:64.

Gold MS. Perioperative fluid management. Crit Care Clin 1992;8:409.

Goldberg RB, Shprintzen RJ. Hirschsprung megacolon and cleft palate in two sibs. J Craniofac Genet Dev Biol 1981;1:185.

Goldblum JR, Whyte RI, Orringer MB, et al. Achalasia: A morphologic study of 42 resected specimens. Am J Surg Pathol 1994;18:327.

Goldsmith LA. Tyrosinemia and related disorders. In: Stanbury JB, Wyngaarden JB, Frederickson DS, et al, eds. Metabolic basis of inherited disease, 5th ed. New York: McGraw-Hill, 1983.

Goldstein GW, Romoff M, Bogin F, et al. Relationship between the concentration of calcium and phosphorus in blood and cerebrospinal fluid. J Clin Endocrinol Metab 1979;49:58.

Gonzales ER, Hastings C, Morton D Jr, et al. Hepatic encephalopathy induced by small bowel obstruction in a noncirrhotic child with portal vein thrombosis. J Pediatr Surg 1990;25:1276.

Gonzalez-Heydrich J, Kerner JA Jr, Steiner H. Testing the psychogenic vomiting diagnosis. Am J Dis Child 1991;145:913.

Gooday R, Hayes PC, Bzeisi K, et al. Benzodiazepine receptor antagonism improves reaction time in latent hepatic encephalopathy. Psychopharmacology 1995;119:295.

Goodman DS. Vitamin A and retinoids in health and disease. N Engl J Med 1984;310:1023.

Goodman SI, Morenberg MD, Shikes RH, et al. Glutaric aciduria: Biochemical and morphologic considerations. J Pediatr 1977;90:746.

Goodwin FC, Beattie RM, Millar J, et al. Celiac disease and childhood stroke. Pediatr Neurol 2004;31:139.

Gordon N. Cerebellar ataxia and gluten sensitivity: A rare but possible cuase of ataxia, even in childhood. Dev Med Child Neurol 2000;42:283.

Gordon N. Hereditary vitamin-E deficiency. Dev Med Child Neurol 2001;43:133.

Gordon N. Iron deficiency and the intellect. Brain Dev 2003;25:3.

Gorman KS. Malnutrition and cognitive development: evidence from experimental/quasi-experimental studies among the mild-to-moderately malnourished. J Nutr 1995;125:2233S.

Gospe SM. Pyridoxine-dependent seizures: Findings from recent studies pose new questions. Pediatr Neurol 2002;26:181.

Goyal RK, Hirano I. The enteric nervous system. N Engl J Med 1996;334: 1106.

Graham SM, Arvela OM, Wise GA. Long-term neurologic consequences of nutritional vitamin B_{12} deficiency in infants. J Pediatr 1992;121:710.

Grantham-McGregor S. Field studies in early nutrition and later achievement. In: Dobbing J, ed. Early nutrition and later achievement. New York: Academic Press, 1987.

Grantham-McGregor S. A review of studies of the effect of severe malnutrition on mental development. J Nutr 1995;125:2233S.

Grantham-McGregor S, Ani C. A review of studies on the effect of iron deficiency on cognitive development in children. J Nutr 2001;131:649S.

Grantham-McGregor SM, Ani CC. Undernutrition and mental development. Nestle Nutrition Workshop Series Clinical and Performance Program. Vol. 54. Nestec Ltd. Vevey/S. Basel: Karger AG, 2001, pp 1-72.

Grantham-McGregor S, Stewart ME, Schofield WN. Effect of long-term psychosocial stimulation on mental development of severely malnourished children. Lancet 1980;2:785.

Grasbeck R, Gordin R, Kantero I, et al. Selective vitamin B_{12} malabsorption and proteinuria in young people: A syndrome. Acta Med Scand 1960;167:289.

Grattan-Smith PJ, Wilcken B, Procopis PG, et al. The neurological syndrome of infantile cobalamin deficiency: Developmental regression and involuntary movements. Mov Disord 1997;12:39.

Graziani LK, Escriva A, Katzman R. Exchange of calcium between blood, brain and cerebrospinal fluid. Am J Physiol 1965;208:1058.

Green R, Kinsella LJ. Current concepts in the diagnosis of cobalamine deficiency. Neurology 1995;45:1435.

Greer FR. Issues in establishing vitamin D recommendations for infants and children. Am J Clin Nutr 2004;80:1759S.

Gregersen H, Nielsen JS, Peterslund NA. Acute porphyria and multiple organ failure during treatment with lamotrigine. Ugeskr Laeger 1996;158:4091.

Gregerson N. Riboflavin responsive deficits of beta oxidation. J Inherit Metab Dis 1985;8 (Suppl 1):65.

Gregerson N, Wintzensen H, Kolvraa S, et al. C6-C10 dicarboxylic aciduria: Investigation of a patient with riboflavin responsive multiple acyl-CoA dehydrogenation defects. Pediatr Res 1982;16:861.

Grewar D. Scurvy and its prevention by vitamin C fortified evaporated milk. Can Med Assoc J 1959;80:977.

Grigsby DG. Malnutrition. 2003. Available at http://www.emedicine.com/ped/topic1360.htm.

Groeneweg M, Moerland W, Quero JC, et al. Screening of subclinical hepatic encephalopathy. J Hepatol 2000;32:748.

Groeneweg M, Quero JC, De Bruijn I, et al. Subclinical hepatic encephalopathy impairs daily functioning. Hepatology 1998;28:45.

Grossman H, Duggan E. McCamman S, et al. The dietary chloride deficiency syndrome. Pediatrics 1980;66:366.

Grunewald S, Champion MP, Leonard JV, Schaper J, Morris AA. Biotinidase deficiency: A treatable leukoencephalopathy. Neuropediatrics 2004;35:211.

Guggenheim MA, Ringel SP, Silverman A, et al. Progressive neuromuscular disease in children with chronic cholestasis and vitamin E deficiency: Diagnosis and treatment with alpha tocopherol. J Pediatr 1982;100:51.

Gullans SR, Verbalis JG. Control of brain volume during hyperosmolar and hypo-osmolar conditions. Annu Rev Med 1993;44:289.

Gupta S, Dolwani S. Neurological complications of porphyria. Postgrad Med J 1996;72:631.

Gurevitch J, Sela B, Jonas A, et al. D-Lactic acidosis: A treatable encephalopathy in pediatric patients. Acta Paediatr 1993;82:119.

Guthrie HA, Brown ML. Effect of severe undernutrition in early life on growth, brain size and composition in adult rats. J Nutr 1968;94:419.

Habibi P, Strobel S, Smith I, et al. Neurodevelopmental delay and focal seizures as presenting symptoms of human immunodeficiency virus I infection. Eur J Pediat 1989;148;315.

Hackett R, Iype T. Malnutrition and childhood epilepsy in developing countries. Seizure 2001;10:554.

Hadjivassilioun M, Grunewald R. Reply to: Gluten ataxia "in perspective." Brain 2003;126:685.

Hadjivassiliou M, Gruenwald RA, Chattopadhyay AK, et al. Clinical, radiological, neurophysiological, and neuropathological characteristics of gluten ataxia. Lancet 1998;352:1582.

Hadjivassiliou M, Grunewald R, Chattopadhyay AK, et al. Gluten ataxia and gluten neuropathy: The effect of a gluten-free diet. J Neurol Neurosurg Pscychiatry 2002;72:129.

Hadjivassiolou M, Gibson A, Davies-Jones GA, et al. Does cryptic gluten sensitivity play a part in neurological illness? Lancet 1999;347:369.

Hadjivassiliou M, Grunewald R, Sharrack B, et al. Gluten ataxia in perspective: Epidemiology, genetic susceptibility and clinical characteristics. Brain 2003;126:685.

Haenggeli CA, Girardin E, Paunier L. Pyridoxine-dependent seizures, clinical and therapeutic aspects. Eur J Pediatr 1991;150:452.

Hague WM. Homocysteine and pregnancy. Best Pract Res Clin Obstet Gynaecol. 2003;17:459

Hahn JS, Berquest W, Alcorn DM, et al. Wernicke encephalopathy and beriberi during total parenteral nutrition attributable to multivitamin infusion shortage. Pediatrics 1998;101:E10.

Hajtha A, Shersin H. Inhibition of amino acid uptake by the absence of sodium in slices of brain. J Neurochem 1975;24:667.

Hall CA. Function of vitamin B_{12} in the central nervous system revealed by congenital defects. Am J Hematol 1990;34:121.

Halperin JJ, Landis DMD, Kleinman GM, et al. Whipple disease of the nervous system. Neurology 1982;32:612.

Halpern, J. The neuromotor deficit in endemic cretinism and its implications for the pathogenesis of the disorder. In: Stanbury JB, ed. The damaged brain of iodine deficiency. Elmsford, NY: Cognizant Communication, 1994.

Halstead CH. Intestinal absorption and malabsorption of folates. Annu Rev Med 1980;31:79.

Halterman JS, Kaczorowski JM, Aligne CA, et al. Iron deficiency and cognitive achievement among school-aged children and adolescents in the United States. Pediatrics 2001;107:1381.

Hamano S, Nakanishi Y, Nara T, et al. Neurological manifestations of hemorrhagic colitis in the outbreak of *Escherichia coli* O157:H7 infection in Japan. Acta Paediatr 1993;82:454.

Hambidge M. Human zinc deficiency. J Nutr 2000;130 (5S Suppl):1344S.

Hamed IA, Lindeman RD. Dysphagia and vertical nystagmus in magnesium deficiency. Ann Intern Med 1978;89:222.

Hampl JS, Taylor CA, Johnston CS. Vitamin C deficiency and depletion in the United States: The Third National Health and Nutrition Examination Survey, 1988 to 1994. Am J Public Health 2004;94:870.

Harding AE, Matthews S, Jones S, et al. Spinocerebellar degeneration associated with selective defect of vitamin E absorption. N Engl J Med 1985;313:32.

Harding B, Alsanjari H, Smith SJM, et al. Progressive neuronal degeneration of childhood with liver disease (Alpers disease) presenting in young adults. J Neurol Neurosurg Psychiatry 1995;58:320.

Harding BN. Progressive neuronal degeneration of childhood with liver disease (Alpers-Huttenlocher syndrome): A personal review. J Child Neurol 1990;5:273.

Hardoff D, Sharf B, Berger A. Myopathy as a presentation of coeliac disease. Dev Med Child Neurol 1980;22:781.

Harper CG, Giles M, Finley-Jones R. Clinical signs in the Wernicke-Korsakoff complex. A retrospective analysis of 131 cases diagnosed at necropsy. J Neurol Neurosurg Psychiatry 1986;49:341.

Harpey IP, Charpentier C, Goodman SI, et al. Multiple acyl-CoA dehydrogenase deficiency in pregnancy and caused by a defect in riboflavin metabolism in the mother. J Pediatr 1983;103:394.

Hart PE, Gould SR, MacSweeney JE, et al. Brain white matter lesions in inflammatory bowel disease. Lancet 1998;351:1558.

Hartfield DS, Loewy JA, Yager JY. Transient thalamic changes on MRI in a child with hypernatremia. Pediatr Neurol 1999;20:60.

Hartfield DS, Lowry NJ, Keene DL, et al. Iron deficiency: A cause of stroke in infants and children. Pediatr Neurol 1997;16:50.

Hartmann IJ, Groenweg M, Quero JC, et al. The prognostic significance of subclinical hepatic encephalopathy. Am J Gastroenterol 2000;95:2029.

Hassanein TI, Wahlstrom HE, Samora JU, et al. Conventional care of fulminant hepatic failure. Am Surg 1991;57:546.

Hatheway CL. Botulism: The present status of the disease. Curr Top Microbiol Immunol 1995;195:55.

Hatoff DE, Gertler SL, Miya K, et al. Hypervitaminosis A unmasked by acute viral hepatitis. Gastroenterology 1982;82:124.

Haussinger D, Laubenberger J, von Dahl S, et al. Proton magnetic resonance spectroscopy studies on human brain myo-inositol in hypo-osmolarity and hepatic encephalopathy. Gastroenterology 1994;107:1475.

Haussinger D, Schliess F, Kircheis G. Pathogenesis of hepatic encephalopathy. J Gastroenterol Hepatol 2002;17 (Suppl 3):S256.

Haworth C, Evans DIK, Mitra I, et al. Thiamine responsive anemia: Study of two further cases. Br J Haematol 1982;50:549.

Haworth JC, Dilling LA, Surtees RA, et al. Symptomatic and asymptomatic methylenetetrahydrofolate reductase deficiency in two adult brothers. Am J Med Genet. 1993;45:572.

Hayasaka S, Saito T, Nakajima H. Gyrate atrophy with hyperornithemia: Different types of responsiveness to vitamin B_6. Br J Ophthalmol 1982;65:478.

Hayashi M, Satoh J, Sakamoto K, et al. Clinical and neuropathological findings in severe athetoid cerebral palsy: A comparative study of globo-Luysian and thalamo-putaminal groups. Brain Dev 1991;13:47.

Healton EB, Savage DB, Brust JC, et al. Neurologic aspects of cobalamin deficiency. Medicine 1991;70:229.

Heeley A, Pugh RJP, Clayton BE, et al. Pyridoxal metabolism in vitamin B–responsive convulsions of early infancy. Arch Dis Child 1978;53:794.

Hellerstein S, Duggan E, Merveille O, et al. Follow-up studies on children with dietary chloride deficiency during infancy. Pediatrics 1985;75:1.

Henderson LM. Niacin. Annu Rev Nutr 1983;3:289.

Henderson W. Case of Hartnup disease. Arch Dis Child 1958;33:114.

Henry HL, Norman AW. Vitamin D: Metabolism and biologic actions. Annu Rev Nutr 1984;4:493.

Henry SM. Discerning differences: Gastroesophageal reflux and gastroesophageal reflux disease in infants. Adv Neonatal Care 2004;4:235.

Herrera MG, Mora JO, Christiansen N, et al. Effects of nutritional supplementation and early education on physical and cognitive development. In: Turner RR, Reese HW, eds. Lifespan psychology: Intervention. New York: Academic Press, 1980.

Hershkowitz S, Link R, Radven M, et al. Spinal empyema in Crohn's disease. J Clin Gastroenterol 1990;12:69.

Herson LA, Rodnight R. Hartnup disease in psychiatric practice: Clinical and biochemical features of three cases. J Neurol Neurosurg Psychiatry 1960;23:40.

Higginbottom MC, Sweetman L, Nyhan WL. A syndrome of methylmalonic aciduria, homocystinuria, megaloblastic anemia and neurologic abnormalities in a vitamin B_{12}–deficient breastfed infant of a strict vegetarian. N Engl J Med 1978;299:317.

Higgins JJ, Glasgow AM, Lusk M, et al. MRI, clinical, and biochemical features of partial pyruvate carboxylase deficiency. J Child Neurol 1994;9:436.

Hillemeier AC. Gastroesophageal reflux. Diagnostic and therapeutic approaches. Pediatr Clin North Am 1996;43:197.

Hilton JF, Christensen KE, Watkins D, et al. The molecular basis of glutamate formiminotransferase deficiency. Hum Mutat 2003;22:67.

Hitzig WH, Dohmann U, Pluss HI. Hereditary transcobalamin II deficiency: Clinical findings in a new family. J Pediatr 1974;85:622.

Hoekelman RA, Friedman SB, Nelson NM, et al. Primary pediatric care, 3rd ed. Philadelphia: Mosby, 1997.

Hoisington G, Bartlett W, Kelly T. Intussusception presenting as encephalopathy. Iowa Med 1993;83:107.

Holmberg C. Congenital chloride diarrhea. Clin Gastroenterol 1986;15:583.

Holmes GK. Non-malignant complications of coeliac disease. Acta Paediatr Suppl 1996;412:68.

Holowach J, Thurston DL. Breath-holding spells and anemia. N Engl J Med 1963;268:21.

Hoorweg J, Stanfield JP. The effects of protein energy malnutrition in early childhood on intellectual and motor abilities in later childhood and adolescence. Dev Med Child Neurol 1976;18:330.

Hoppel CL, Tandler B. Riboflavin deficiency. Prog Clin Biol Res 1990;321:233.

Horstmann M, Neumaier-Probst E, Lukacs Z, et al. Infantile cobalamin deficiency with cerebral lactate accumulation and sustained choline depletion. Neuropediatrics 2003;34:261.

Horwitt MK, Harper AE, Henderson LM. Tryptophan relationships for measuring niacin equivalents. Am J Clin Nutr 1981;84:423.

Hsu YS, Chang YC, Lee WT, et al. A diagnostic value of sensory evoked potentials in pediatric Wilson disease. Pediatr Neurol 2003;29:42.

Huang S, Lavine J. Efficacy of sumatriptan in aborting attacks of cyclic vomiting. Gastroenterology 1997;112:A751.

Huda SN, Grantham-McGregor SM, Rahman KM, et al. Biochemical hypothyroidism secondary to iodine deficiency is associated with poor school achievement and cognition in Bangladeshi children. J Nutr 1999;129:980.

Hughes RAC, Rees JH. Clinical and epidemiologic features of Guillain-Barré syndrome. J Infect Dis 1997;176 (Suppl 2):S92.

Hultdin J, Schmauch A, Wikberg A, et al. Acute intermittent porphyria in childhood: A population-based study. Acta Paediatr 2003;92:562.

Hung KL. Auditory brainstem responses in patients with neonatal hyperbilirubinemia and bilirubin encephalopathy. Brain Dev 1989;11:297.

Hurwitz ES, Barrett MJ, Bregman D, et al. Public health service study on Reye's syndrome and medications. N Engl J Med 1985;313:849.

Huttenlocher PR, Solitaire GB, Adams G. Infantile diffuse cerebral degeneration with hepatic cirrhosis. Arch Neurol 1976;33:186.

Hyams JS. Crohn's disease in children. Pediatr Clin North Am 1996;43:255.

Idjradinata P, Pollitt E. Reversal of developmental delays in iron-deficient anaemic infants treated with iron. Lancet 1993;341:1.

Itoh H, Hirata K, Ohsato K. Turcot's syndrome and familial adenomatous polyposis associated with brain tumor: Review of related literature. Int J Colorect Dis 1993;8:87.

Iwashita T, Kruger GM, Pardal R, et al. Hirschsprung disease is linked to defects in neural crest stem cell function. Science 2003;301:972.

Jacobs BC, Rothbarth PH, van der Meche FGA, et al. The spectrum of antecedent infections in Guillain-Barré syndrome. A case-control study. Neurology 1998;51:1110.

Jebnoun S, Kacem S, Mokrani CH, et al. A family study of congenital malabsorption of folate. J Inherit Metab Dis 2001;24:749.

Jernigan SA, Ware LM. Reversible quantitative EEG changes in a case of cyclic vomiting: Evidence for migraine equivalent. Dev Med Child Neurol 1991;33:80.

Johns D. Disorders of the central and autonomic nervous systems as a cause of emesis in infants. Semin Pediatr Surg 1995;4:152.

Jolley SG, Herbst JJ, Johnson DG, et al. Surgery in children with gastroesophageal reflux and respiratory symptoms. J Pediatr 1980;96:194.

Jones EA, Basile AS, Mullen KD, et al. Flumazenil: Potential implications for hepatic encephalopathy. Pharmacol Ther 1990;45:331.

Jones EA, Giger-Mateeva VI, Reits D, et al. Visual event-related potentials in cirrhotic patients without overt encephalopathy: The effects of flumaxenil. Metab Brain Dis 2001;16:43.

Jones EA, Schafer DF. Hepatic encephalopathy: A neurochemical disorder. Prog Liver Dis 1986;8:525.

Jones EA, Weisenborn K. Neurology and the liver. J Neurol Neurosurg Psychiatry 1997;63:279.

Jones EA, Yurdaydin C, Basile AS. The GABA hypothesis—state of the art. Adv Exp Med Biol 1994;368:89.

Jones EA. Fatigue associated with chronic liver disease: A riddle wrapped in a mystery inside an enigma. Hepatology 1995;25:492.

Joos SK, Pollitt E, Mueller WH, et al. The Bacon Chow Study: Maternal nutritional supplementation and infant behavioral development. Child Dev 1983;54:669.

Jospe N, Forbes G. Fluids and electrolytes: Clinical aspects. Pediatr Rev 1996;17:395.

Jovic NS, Jovic JZ. Neurologic disorders in Whipple's disease. Srp Arh Celok Lek 1996;124:98

Jozwiak S, Pedich M, Rajszys P, et al. Incidence of hepatic hamartomas in tuberous sclerosis. Arch Dis Child 1992;67:1363.

Juan D. Hypocalcemia: Differential diagnosis and mechanisms. Arch Intern Med 1977;139:1166.

Jung AD. Gastroesophageal reflux in infants and children. Am Fam Physician 2001;64:1853.

Jusko WJ, Levy G. Absorption, protein bindings and elimination of riboflavin. In: Rivlin RS, ed. Riboflavin. New York: Plenum, 1975.

Justinich CJ, Hyams JS. Inflammatory bowel disease in children and adolescents. Pediatr Endoscopy 1994;4:39.

Kalra V, Grover JK, Ahuja GK, et al. Vitamin E administration and reversal of neurological deficits in protein-energy malnutrition. J Trop Pediatr 2001;47:39.

Kalra V, Murali MV. Fulminant hepatic failure and hepatic encephalopathy. Indian Pediatr 1986;23:139.

Kaplan ED. Association between homocyst(e)ine levels and risk of vascular events. Drugs Today (Barc) 2003;39:175.

Kaplan JG, Pack D, Horoupian D, et al. Distal axonopathy associated with chronic gluten enteropathy: A treatable disorder. Neurology 1988;38:642.

Kaplan P. X-linked recessive inheritance of agenesis of the corpus callosum. J Med Genet 1983;20:122.

Kapur RP. Neuronal dysplasia: A controversial pathological correlate of intestinal pseudo-obstruction. Am J Med Genet A 2003;122:287.

Kasarkis EJ, Bass NH. Benign intracranial hypertension induced by deficiency of vitamin A during infancy. Neurology 1982;32:1292.

Kassam N, Witt N, Kneteman N, et al. Liver transplantation for neuropsychiatric Wilson disease. Can J Gastroenterol 1998;12:65.

Katsaros VK, Glocker FX, Hemmer B, et al. MRI of spinal cord and brain lesions in subacute combined degeneration. Neuroradiology 1998;40:716.

Kauppinen R, von, Fraunberg M. Molecular and biochemical studies of acute intermittent porphyria in 196 patients and their families. Clin Chem 2002;48:1891.

Kauppinen R. Molecular diagnostics of acute intermittent porphyria. Expert Rev Mol Diagn 2004;4:243.

Kayden HJ. The neurologic syndrome of vitamin E deficiency: A significant cause of ataxia. Neurology 1993;43:2167.

Keays R, Potter D, O'Grady J, et al. Intracranial and cerebral perfusion pressure changes before, during and immediately after orthotopic liver transplantation for fulminant hepatic failure. Q J Med 1991;79:425.

Kello AB, Gilbert C. Causes of severe visual impairment and blindness in children in schools for the blind in Ethiopia. Br J Ophthalmol 2003;87:526.

Khasawinah TA, Ramirez A, Berkenbosch JW, et al. Preliminary experience with dexmedetomidine in the treatment of cyclic vomiting syndrome. Am J Ther 2003;10:303.

Khilnani P. Electrolyte abnormalities in critically ill children. Crit Care Med 1992;20:241.

Kieslich M, Errazuriz G, Posselt HG, et al. Brain white matter lesions in celiac disease: A prospective study of 75 diet treated patients. Pediatrics 2001;108:E21.

Kim SC, Feery GD. Inflammatory bowel diseases in pediatric and adolescent patients: Clinical, therapeutic and psychosocial considerations. Gastroenterology 2004;126:1550.

Kim SY, Jeitner TM, Steinert PM. Transglutaminase in disease. Neurochem Int 2002;40:85.

Kimura K, Hunter SF, Thollander MS, et al. Concurrence of inflammatory bowel disease and multiple sclerosis. Mayo Clin Proc 2000;75:802.

King AD, Walshe JM, Kendall BE, et al. Cranial MR imaging in Wilson's disease. AJR Am J Roentgenol 1996;167:1579.

King, PH, Bragdon AC. MRI reveals multiple reversible cerebral lesions in an attack of acute intermittent porphyria. Neurology 1991;41:1300.

Kinoshita T, Takahashi S, Ishii K, et al. Reye's syndrome with cortical laminar necrosis: MRI. Neuroradiology 1996;38:269.

Kinsbourne M. Hiatus hernia with contortions of the neck. Lancet 1964;1:1058.

Kirchreis G, Wettstein M, Timmermann L, et al. Critical flicker frequency for quantification of low-grade hepatic encephalopathy. Hepatology 2002;35:357.

Kirschner BS. Ulcerative colitis in children. Pediatr Clin North Am 1996;43:235.

Klein GL, Chen TC, Holick MF, et al. Vitamin D deficiency in burned children: Causes and consequences. Asia Pac J Clin Nutr 2004;13:S152.

Klein PS. Nutritional deprivation and retardation of cognitive functions. In: Mittler P, ed. Frontiers of knowledge of mental retardation. Vol. 2. Biomedical Aspects. Baltimore: University Park Press, 1980.

Klein RE, Arenales P, Delgado H, et al. Effects of maternal nutrition on fetal growth and infant development. Bull Pan Am Health Org 1976;10:301.

Knox JDE, Delamore WI. Subacute combined degeneration of the cord after partial gastrectomy. BMJ 1960;2:1494.

Koenig M. Rare forms of autosomal recessive neurodegenerative ataxia. Semin Pediatr Neurol 2003;10:183.

Kooh SW, Binet A. Hypercalcemia in infants presenting with apnea. Can Med Assoc J 1990;143:509.

Korenke GC, Hunneman DH, Eber S, et al. Severe encephalopathy with epilepsy in an infant caused by subclinical maternal pernicious anaemia: Case report and review of the literature. Eur J Pediatr 2004;163:196.

Korkmaz A, Yigit S, Firat M, et al. Cranial MRI in neonatal hypernatraemic dehydration. Pediatr Radiol 2000;30:323.

Korson M. Metabolic etiologies of cyclic or recurrent vomiting. J Pediatr Gastroenterol Nutr 1995;21 (Suppl 1):S15.

Koscik RL, Farrell PM, Kosorok MR, et al. Cognitive function of children with cystic fibrosis: Deleterious effect of early malnutrition. Pediatrics 2004;113:1549.

Kramer L, Tribl G, Gendo A, et al. Partial pressure of ammonia versus ammonia in hepatic encephalopathy. Hepatology 2000;31:30.

Krauss GL, Simmons O'Brien E, Campbell M. Successful treatment of seizures and porphyria with gabapentin. Neurology 1995;45:594.

Kreis R, Pfenninger J, Herschkowitz N, et al. In vivo proton magnetic resonance spectroscopy in a case of Reye's syndrome. Intensive Care Med 1995;21:266.

Krendel DA, Gilchrist JM, Johnson AO, et al. Isolated deficiency of vitamin E with progressive neurology deterioration. Neurology 1987;37:538.

Krinke G, Schaumburg HH, Spencer PS, et al. Pyridoxine megavitaminosis produces degeneration of peripheral sensory neurons (sensory neuropathy) in the dog. Neurotoxicology 1980;2:13.

Kugathasan S, Judd RH, Hoffmann RG, et al. Epidemiologic and clinical characteristics of children with newly diagnosed inflammatory bowel disease in Wisconsin: A statewide population-based study. J Pediatr 2003;143:525.

Kuhne T, Bubl R, Baumagartner R. Maternal vegan diet causing a serious infantile neurological disorder due to vitamin B_{12} deficiency. Eur J Pediatr 1991;150:205.

Kullmann F, Hollerbach S, Holstege A, et al. Subclinical hepatic encephalopathy: The diagnostic value of evoked potentials. J Hepatol 1995;22:101.

Kupferschmidt H, Bont A, Schnorf H, et al. Transient cortical blindness and bioccipital brain lesions in two patients with acute intermittent porphyria. Ann Intern Med 1995;123:598.

Kurleman G, Menges EM, Palm DG. Low level of GABA in CSF in vitamin B_6–dependent seizures. Dev Med Child Neurol 1991;33:749.

Labate A, Gambardella A, Messina D, et al. Silent celiac disease in patients with childhood localization-related epilepsies. Epilepsia 2001;42:1153.

Ladhani S, Srinivasan L, Buchanan C, et al. Presentation of vitamin D deficiency. Arch Dis Child 2004;89:781.

Lahat E, Katz Y, Bistritzer T, et al. Recurrent seizures in children with *Shigella*-associated convulsions. Ann Neurol 1990;28:393.

LaMantia AS. Forebrain induction, retinoic acid, and vulnerability to schizophrenia: Insights from molecular and genetic analysis in developing mice. Biol Psychiatry 1999;46:19.

Lammer EJ, Chen DT, Hoar RM, et al. Retinoic acid embryopathy. N Engl J Med 1985;313:837.

Landon MI, Hey FN. Renal loss of folate in the preterm infant. Arch Dis Child 1974;49:292.

Lang C, Muller D, Clalus D, et al. Neuropsychological findings in treated Wilson's disease. Acta Neurol Scand 1990;81:75.

Langley WF, Mann D. Central nervous system magnesium deficiency. Arch Intern Med 1991;151:593.

Lanzi G, Balottin V, Ottolini F, et al. Cyclic vomiting and recurrent abdominal pains as migraine or epileptic equivalent. Cephalalgia 1983;3:115.

Lardy HA, Adler J. Synthesis of succinate from proprionate and bicarbonate by soluble enzymes from liver mitochondria. J Biol Chem 1956;219:935.

Laubenberger J, Haussinger D, Bayer S, et al. Proton magnetic resonance spectroscopy of the brain in symptomatic and asymptomatic patients with liver cirrhosis. Gastroenterology 1997;112:1610.

Leibel RL, Shih VE, Goodman SI, et al. Glutaric aciduria: A metabolic disorder causing progressive choreoathetosis. Neurology 1980;30:1163.

Lemonnier F, Alvarez F, Babin F, et al. Effects of vitamin E treatment in cholestatic children. Adv Exp Med Biol 1990;264:143.

Leung AKC, Chan KAW. Iron deficiency anemia. Adv Pediatr 2001;48:385.

Levine M. New concepts in the biology and biochemistry of ascorbic acid. N Engl J Med 1986;314:892.

Levine RL. Neonatal jaundice. Acta Paediatr Scand 1988;77:177.

Levitsky DA, Strupp BJ. Malnutrition and the brain: Changing concepts, changing concerns. J Nutr 1995;125:2212S.

Levitt M, Nixon PF, Pincus IH, et al. Transport of folates in cerebrospinal fluid. J Clin Invest 1971;50:1301.

Lewis M, Howdle PD. The neurology of liver failure. Q J Med 2003;96:623.

Lewis MB, MacQuillan G, Bamford JM, et al. Delayed myelopathic presentation of the acquired hepatocerebral degeneration syndrome. Neurology 2000;54:1011.

Li BU, Balint JP. Cyclic vomiting syndrome: Evolution in our understanding of a brain-gut disorder. Adv Pediatr 2000;47:117.

Li BU, Murray RD, Heitlinger LA, et al. Heterogeneity of diagnoses presenting as cyclic vomiting. Pediatrics 1998;102:583.

Li BU, Murray RD, Heitlinger LA, et al. Is cyclic vomiting syndrome related to migraine? J Pediatr 1999;134:567.

Li BUK. Consensus statement. Proceedings of the International Scientific Symposium on Cyclical Vomiting Syndrome. Diagnosis criteria for cyclic vomiting syndrome. J Pediatr Gastroenterol Nutr 1995;21 (Suppl 1):vi.

Li BUK. Cyclic vomiting: New understanding of an old disorder. Contemp Pediatr 1996;13:48.

Li BUK. Heterogeneity of diagnoses presenting as cyclic vomiting. Pediatrics 1998;102:583.

Lidofsky SD, Bass NM, Prager MC, et al. Intracranial pressure monitoring and liver transplantation for fulminant heptic failure. Hepatology 1992;16:1.

Lin S, Hsu H, Wang P, et al. Rotavirus gastroenteritis associated with afebrile seizure in childhood. Acta Paediatr Scand 1996;37:204.

Lindenbaum J, Healton EB, Savage DG, et al. Neuropsychiatric disorders caused by cobalamin deficiency in the absence of anemia or macrocytosis. N Engl J Med 1988;318:1720.

Lindgren S, Lilja B, Rosen I, et al. Disturbed autonomic nerve function in patients with Crohn's disease. Scand J Gastroenterol 1991;26:361.

Lindhout D, Omtzigt JG.Teratogenic effects of antiepileptic drugs: Implications for the management of epilepsy in women of childbearing age. Epilepsia 1994;35 (Suppl 4):S19.

Lingam S, Wilson J, Nazer H, et al. Neurological abnormalities in Wilson's disease are reversible. Neuropediatrics 1987;18:11.

Lippe B, Hensen L, Menoza G, et al. Chronic vitamin A intoxication. Am J Dis Child 1981;135:634.

Lipsitz PJ. The clinical and biochemical effects of excess magnesium in the newborn. Pediatrics 1971;47:501.

Liu CL, Fan ST, Lo CM, et al. Live donor liver transplantation for fulminant hepatic failure in children. Liver Transpl 2003;9:1185.

Lloyd-Still JD. Malnutrition and intellectual development. Littleton, Mass: Publishing Sciences Group, 1976.

Lloyd-Still JD, Tomasi L. Neurovascular and thromboembolic complications of inflammatory bowel disease in childhood. J Pediatr Gastroenterol Nutr 1989;9:461.

Lockwood AH. Hepatic encephalopathy and other neurological disorders associated with gastrointestinal disease. In: Aminoff MJ, ed. Neurology and general medicine. The neurological aspects of medical disorders, 2nd ed. New York: Churchill Livingstone, 1995.

Lockwood AH. Hepatic encephalopathy. Neurol Clin 2002;20:241.

Lockwood AH, Yap EWH, Wong W. Cerebral ammonia metabolism in patients with severe liver disease and hepatic encephalopathy. J Cereb Blood Flow Metab 1991;11:337.

Logan S, Martins S, Gilbert R. Iron therapy for improving psychomotor development and cognitive function in children under the age of three with iron deficiency anaemia. Cochrane Database Syst Rev 2001;CD001444.

Lohr M, Stenzel W, Plum G, et al. Whipple disease confined to the central nervous system presenting as a solitary frontal tumor. Case report. J Neurosurg 2004;101:336.

Lossos A, River Y, Eliakim A, et al. Neurologic aspects of inflammatory bowel disease. Neurology 1995;45:416.

Lott IT, Coulombe T, DiPaolo RY, et al. Vitamin B_6–dependent seizures: pathology and chemical findings in brain. Neurology 1978;28:47.

Loudianos G, Gitlin JD. Wilson's disease. Semin Liver Dis 2000;20:353.

Louis ED. Whipple disease. Curr Neurol Neurosci Rep 2003;3:470.

Louis ED, Lynch T, Kaufmann P, et al. Diagnostic guidelines in central nervous system Whipple's disease. Ann Neurol 1996;40:561.

Lovejoy FJ Jr, Smith AL, Bresnan MJ, et al. Clinical staging in Reye syndrome. Am J Dis Child 1974;128:36.

Lovenberg W, Weissbach H, Udenfriend S. Aromatic L-amino acid decarboxylase. J Biol Chem 1962;237:89.

Lozoff B, Jimenez E, Hagen J, et al. Poorer behavioral and developmental outcome more than 10 years after for iron deficiency in infancy. Pediatrics 2000;105:E51.

Lucidi V, Di Capua M, Rosati P, et al. Benign intracranial hypertension in an older child with cystic fibrosis. Pediatr Neurol 1993;9:494.

Lumeng L, Lui A, Li T. Plasma content of B_6 vitamins and its relationship to hepatic vitamin B_6 metabolism. J Clin Invest 1980;66:688.

Luostarinen L, Pirttila T, Collin P. Coeliac disease presenting with neurological disorders. Eur Neurol 1999;42:132.

Luostarinen LK, Collin PO, Peraaho MJ, et al. Coeliac disease in patients with cerebellar ataxia of unknown origin. Ann Med 2001;33:445.

Lynch RE. Ionized calcium: Pediatric perspective. Pediatr Clin North Am 1990;37:373.

Mackay-Sim A, Feron F, Eyles D, et al. Schizophrenia, vitamin D, and brain development. Int Rev Neurobiol 2004;59:351.

Mackenzie IL, Donaldson RM, Trier JS. Ileal mucosa in familial selective vitamin B_{12} malabsorption. N Engl J Med 1972;286:1021.

Maden M, Gale E, Zile M. The role of vitamin A in the development of the central nervous system. J Nutr 1998;128 (Suppl):471S.

Maggiore R, Miller F, Stryker S, et al. Meningitis and epidural abscess associated with fistulizing Crohn's disease. Dig Dis Sci 2004;49:1461.

Mahalanabis D, Snyder JD. Fluid and dietary therapy of diarrhea. In: Walker WA, Durie PR, Hamilton JR, et al, eds. Pediatric gastrointestinal disease. St. Louis: Mosby, 1996.

Main ANH, Mills PR, Russel RI, et al. Vitamin A deficiency in Crohn's disease. Gut 1983;24:1169.

Maisels MJ, Newman TB. Kernicterus in otherwise healthy, breast-fed term newborns. Pediatrics 1995;96:730.

Malatack JJ, Moran MM, Moughan B. Isolated congenital malabsorption of folic acid in a male infant: Insights into treatment and mechanism of defect. Pediatrics 1999;104:1133.

Mallory SB, Wiener E, Hordlund JJ. Waardenburg's syndrome with Hirschsprung's disease: A neural crest defect. Pediatr Dermatol 1986;3:119.

Malouf R, Grimley Evans J. The effect of vitamin B_6 on cognition. Cochrane Database Syst Rev 2003;CD004393.

Mamunes P, Prince PE, Thornton NH, et al. Intellectual deficits after transient tyrosinemia in the term neonate. Pediatrics 1976;57:675.

Mantagos S, Genel M, Tanaka K. Ethylmalonic adipic aciduria. J Clin Invest 1974;64:1580.

Manzel K, Tranel D, Cooper G. Cognitive and behavioral abnormalities in a case of central nervous system Whipple disease. Arch Neurol 2000;57:399.

Mardach R, Zempleni J, Wolf B, et al. Biotin dependency due to a defect in biotin transport. J Clin Invest 2002;109:1617.

Mariotti C, Gellera C, Rimoldi M, et al. Ataxia with isolated vitamin E deficiency: Neurological phenotype, clinical follow-up and novel mutations in *TTPA* gene in Italian families. Neurol Sci 2004;25:130.

Marsac C, Gaudry M, Augereaw C, et al. Biotin dependent carboxylase activity in normal human and multicarboxylase deficient patient fibroblasts: Relationship of biotin content of the culture medium. Clin Chim Acta 1983;129:119.

Marth T, Raoult D. Whipple's disease. Lancet 2003;361:239.

Martich Kriss V, Kollias SS, Ball WS Jr. MR findings in kernicterus. AJNR Am J Neuroradiol 1995;16:819.

Martin RJ. Central pontine and extrapontine myelinolysis: The osmotic demyelination syndromes. J Neurol Neurosurg Psychiatry 2004;75 (Suppl 3):iii.

Matthews DM, Linnell JC. Cobalamin deficiency and related disorders in infancy and childhood. Eur J Pediatr 1982;138:6.

McCaffery PJ, Adams J, Maden M, et al. Too much of a good thing: Retinoic acid as an endogenous regulator of neural differentiation and exogenous teratogen. Eur J Neurosci 2003;18:457.

McCall KA, Huang C, Fierke CA. Function and mechanism of zinc metalloenzymes. J Nutr 2000;130 (5S Suppl):1437S.

McCully KS. Vascular pathology of homocysteinemia: implications for the pathogenesis of arteriosclerosis. Am J Pathol 1969;56:111.

Meekin SL, Glasgow JF, McCusker CG, et al. A long-term follow-up of cognitive, emotional, and behavioural sequelae to Reye syndrome. Dev Med Child Neurol 1999;41:549.

Menger H, Jorg J. Outcome of central pontine and extra-pontine myelinolysis (n = 44). J Neurol 1999;246:700.

Menger H, Lin AE, Toriello HV, et al. Vitamin K deficiency embryopathy: A phenocopy of the warfarin embryopathy due to a disorder of embryonic vitamin K metabolism. Am J Med Genet 1997;72:129.

Menkes JH, Welcher DW, Levi HS, et al. Relationship of elevated blood tyrosine to the ultimate intellectual performance of premature infants. Pediatrics 1972;49:218.

Merck, 2005. Available at http://www.merck.com/mrkshared/mmanual/section1/chapter3/3f.jsp.

Metz J. Pathogenesis of cobalamin neuropathy: Deficiency of nervous system *S*-adenosylmethionine? Nutr Rev 1993;51:12.

Meyers A. Fluid and electrolyte therapy for children. Curr Opin Pediatr 1994;6:303.

Meyers DG, Maloley PA, Weeks D. Safety of antioxidant vitamins. Arch Intern Med 1996;156:925.

Mezoff AG, Cohen MB, Maisel SS, et al. Crohn disease in an infant with central nervous system thrombosis and protein-losing enteropathy. J Pediatr 1990;117:436.

Mihas, A, Kirby JD, Kent SP. Hepatitis B antigen and polymyositis. JAMA 1978;239:221.

Mikati MA, Trevatrian E, Krishnamoorthy KS, et al. Pyridoxine-dependent epilepsy: EEG investigations and long-term follow-up. Electroencephalogr Clin Neurophysiol 1991;78:215.

Ming X, Wang MM, Zee D, et al. Wernicke's encephalopathy in a child with prolonged vomiting. J Child Neurol 1998;13:187.

Mittal RK, Balaban DH. The esophagogastric junction. N Engl J Med 1997;336:924.

Miyata Y, Motomura S, Tsuji Y, et al. Hepatic encephalopathy and reversible cortical blindness. Am J Gastroenterol 1988;83:780.

Mock DM, DeLorimer AA, Liebman WM, et al. Biotin deficiency: An unusual complication of parental alimentation. N Engl J Med 1981;304:820.

Mock DM, Mock NI, Nelson RP, Lombard KA. Disturbances in biotin metabolism in children undergoing long-term anticonvulsant therapy. J Pediatr Gastroenterol Nutr 1998;26:245.

Monks G, Juracek L, Weigand D, et al. A case of scurvy in an autistic boy. J Drugs Dermatol 2002;1:67.

Montgomery RD. Magnesium metabolism in infantile protein malnutrition. Lancet 1960;2:74.

Moore KA, McL Jones R, Burrows GD. Quality of life and cognitive function of liver transplant patients: A prospective study. Liver Transpl 2000;6:633.

Mordes JP, Walker WE. Excess magnesium. Pharmacol Rev 1978;29:273.

Morita S, Miwa H, Kihira T, et al. Cerebellar ataxia and leukoencephalopathy associated with cobalamin deficiency. J Neurol Sci 2003;216:183.

Morrell MJ. Guidelines for the care of women with epilepsy. Neurology 1998;51 (5 Suppl 4):S21.
Morris-Jones PH, Houston IB, Evans RC. Prognosis of the neurological complications of acute hypernatremia. Lancet 1967;2:1385.
Mortimer MJ, Kay J, Jaron A. Clinical epidemiology of childhood abdominal migraine in an urban general practice. Dev Med Child Neurol 1993;35:243.
Moslinger D, Muhl A, Suormala T, et al. Molecular characterisation and neuropsychological outcome of 21 patients with profound biotinidase deficiency detected by newborn screening and family studies. Eur J Pediatr 2003;162 (Suppl 1):S46.
Mueller C, Patel S, Irons M, et al. Normal cognition and behavior in a Smith-Lemli-Opitz syndrome patient who presented with Hirschsprung disease. Am J Med Genet A 2003; 123A:100.
Muller DPR, Lloyd JK, Bird AC. Long-term management of abetalipoproteinemia: Possible role for vitamin E. Arch Dis Child 1977;52:209.
Murata K. Thiaminase. In: Shimazono N, Katsura E, eds. Review of Japanese literature on beri-beri and thiamine. Tokyo: Igaku-Shoin, 1965.
Murphy N, Auzinger G, Bernel W, et al. The effect of hypertonic sodium chloride on intracranial pressure in patients with acute liver failure. Hepatology 2004;39:464.
Mutchnick MG, Lerner E, Conn HO. Portal-systemic encephalopathy and portocaval anastomosis: A prospective, controlled investigation. Gastroenterology 1974;66:1005.
Mylott BM, Kump T, Bolton ML, Greenbaum LA. Rickets in the Dairy State. World Med J 2004;103:84.
Nasralla CA, Pay N, Goodpasture HC, et al. Postinfectious encephalopathy in a child following *Campylobacter jejuni* enteritis. AJNR Am J Neuroradiol 1993;14:444.
Nazer H, Brismar J, Al-Kawi MZ, et al. Magnetic resonance imaging of the brain in Wilson's disease Neuroradiology 1993;35:130.
Neims AH, Helerman L. Flavoenzyme catalysis. Annu Rev Biochem 1970;39:867.
Nemni R, Fazio R, Corbo M, et al. Peripheral neuropathy associated with Crohn's disease. Neurology 1987;37:1414.
Newman TB, Maisels MJ. Evaluation and treatment of jaundice in the term newborn: A kinder, gentler approach. Pediatrics 1992;89:809.
Niederwieser A, Giliberti P, Matasovic A, et al. Folic acid non-dependent formimino glutamic aciduria in two siblings. Clin Chim Acta 1974;54:293.
Nofech-Mozes Y, Yuhas Y, Kaminsky E, et al. Induction of mRNA for tumor necrosis factor-alpha and interleukin-1 beta in mice brain, spleen and liver in an animal model of Shigella-related seizures. Isr Med Assoc J 2000 2:86–90.
Nomura Y, Sakuma H, Takeda K, et al. Diffusional anisotropy of the human brain assessed with diffusion-weighted MR: Relation with normal brain development and aging. AJNR Am J Roentgenol 1994;15:231.
Norenberg MD. The role of astrocytes in hepatic encephalopathy. Neurochem Pathol 1987;6:13.
Norrashidah AW, Henry RL. Fundoplication in children with gastro-oesophageal reflux disease. J Paediatr Child Health 2002;38:156.
Notter MF, Kendig JW. Differential sensitivity of neural cells to bilirubin toxicity. Pediatr Res 1985;19:393.
Nwaesei C, VanAerde J, Boyden M, et al. Changes in auditory brainstem responses in hyperbilirubinemic infants before and after exchange transfusion. Pediatrics 1984;74:800.
Nyhan WL. Cystathioninuria. In: Nyhan WL. Abnormalities in amino acid metabolism in clinical medicine. New York: Appleton Century Crofts, 1984.
O'Donnell KJ, Rakeman MA, Zhi-Hong D, et al. Effects of iodine supplementation during pregnancy on child growth and development at school age. Dev Med Child Neurol 2002;44:76.
O'Brien DF. The chemistry of vision. Science 1982;218:961.
Oder W, Prayer L, Grimm G, et al. Wilson's disease: Evidence of subgroups derived from clinical findings and brain lesions. Neurology 1993;43:120.
O'Donnell JJ, Sandman RP, Martin SR. Gyrate atrophy of the retina: Inborn error of L-ornithine 2-oxoacid aminotransferase. Science 1978;200:200.
Oguni M, Osawa M. Epilepsy and pregnancy. Epilepsia 2004;45 (Suppl 8):37.
Oh MS, Carroll HJ. Disorders of sodium metabolism: Hypernatremia and hyponatremia. Crit Care Med 1992;20:94.
Okamoto N, Del Maestro R, Valero R, et al. Hydrocephalus and Hirschsprung's disease with a mutation of *L1CAM*. J Hum Genet 2004;49:334.
Oken E, Duggan C. Update on micronutrients: Iron and zinc. Curr Opin Pediatr 2002;14:350.
Olness K. Effects on brain development leading to cognitive impairment: A worldwide epidemic. J Dev Behav Pediatr 2003;24:120.
Olsen RE. The function and metabolism of vitamin K. Annu Rev Nutr 1984;4:281.
Ong DE. Vitamin A–binding proteins. Nutr Rev 1985;43:225.
Oski FA, DeAngelis CD, McMillan JA, et al. Principles and practice of pediatrics, 2nd ed. Philadelphia: JB Lippincott, 1994.
Ozand PT, Gascon GG, Al Essa M, et al. Biotin-responsive basal ganglia disease: A novel entity. Brain 1998;121:1267.
Ozawa H, Sasaki M, Sugai K, et al. Single-photon emission CT and MR findings in Kluver-Bucy syndrome after Reye syndrome. AJNR Am J Roentgenol 1997;18:540.
Ozcelik T, Onerci M, Ozcelik U, et al. Audiological findings in kernicteric patients. Acta Otorhinolaryngol Belg 1997;51:31.
Ozer EA, Turker M, Bakiler AR, et al. Involuntary movements in infantile cobalamin deficiency appearing after treatment. Pediatr Neurol 2001;25:81.
Ozge A, Karakelle A, Kaleagasi H. Celiac disease associated with recurrent stroke: A coincidence or cerebral vasculitis? Eur J Neurol 2001;8:373.
Ozturk MK, Caksen H, Sumerkan B. Convulsions in childhood shigellosis and antimicrobial resistance patterns of *Shigella* isolates. Turk J Pediatr 1996;38:183.
Pack AM, Gidal B, Vazquez B. Bone disease associated with antiepileptic drugs. Cleve Clin J Med 2004;71 (Suppl 2):S42.
Pant SS, Asbury AK, Richardson EP Jr. The myelopathy of pernicious anemia: A neuropathological reappraisal. Acta Neurol Scand 1968a;44:7.
Pant SS, Rebeiz JJ, Richardson EP Jr. Spastic paraparesis following portocaval shunts. Neurology 1968b;8:134.
Parisi MA, Kapur RP, Neilson I, et al. Hydrocephalus and intestinal aganglionosis: Is *L1CAM* a modifier gene in Hirschsprung disease? Am J Med Genet 2002;108:51.
Parobek V, Alaimo I. Fluid and electrolyte management in the neurologically-impaired patient. J Neurosci Nurs 1996;28:322.
Parry GJ, Bredesen DE. Sensory neuropathy with low dose pyridoxine. Neurology 1985;35:1466.
Parsons JL, Sahn EE, Holden KR, et al. Neurologic disease in a child with hepatoerythropoietic porphyria. Pediatr Dermatol 1994;11:216.
Pascal TA, Gaull GE, Beratis NG, et al. Vitamin B_6-responsive and unresponsive cystathioninuria: Two variant molecular forms. Science 1975;190:1209.
Patchell RA, Fellows HA, Humphries LL. Neurologic complications of anorexia nervosa. Acta Neurol Scand 1994;89:111.
Patchell RA. Neurological complications of organ transplantation. Ann Neurol 1994;36:688.
Patel AJ, Balazs R, Johnson AL. Effect of undernutrition on cell formation in the rat brain. J Neurochem 1973;20:1151.
Pearl PL, Gibson KM. Clinical aspects of the disorders of GABA metabolism in children. Curr Opin Neurol 2004;17:107.
Pearl RH, Robie DK, Ein SH, et al. Complications of gastroesophageal antireflux surgery in neurologically impaired versus neurologically normal children. J Pediatr Surg 1990;25:1169.
Penland JG, Sandstead HH, Alcock NW, et al. A preliminary report: Effects of zinc and micronutrient repletion on growth and neuropsychological function of urban Chinese children. J Am Coll Nutr 1997;16:268.
Penland J, Sanstead H, Egger N, et al. Zinc, iron and micronutrient supplementation effects on cognitive and psychomotor function of Mexican-American school children. FASEB J 1999;13:A921.
Penn AA, Enzmann DR, Hahn JS, et al. Kernicterus in a full term infant. Pediatrics 1994;93:1003.
Pennell PB. Pregnancy in women who have epilepsy. Neurol Clin 2004;22:799.
Penner E, Malda E, Mamdi B, et al. Serum and cerebrospinal fluid immune complexes containing hepatitis B surface antigen in Guillain-Barré syndrome. Gastroenterology 1982;82:576.
Pereira SM, Sundarar JR, Begum A. Physical growth and neurointegrative performance of survivors of protein-energy malnutrition. Br J Nutr 1979;42:165.
Perkins GD, Murray-Lyon I. Neurology and the gastrointestinal system. J Neurol Neurosurg Psychiatry 1998;65:291.
Perles Z, Bar-Ziv J, Granot E. Brain edema: An underdiagnosed complication of *Shigella* infection. Pediatr Infect Dis J 1995;14:1114.

Perlman M, Fainmesser P, Sohmer H, et al. Auditory nerve brainstem evoked responses in hyperbilirubinemic neonates. Pediatrics 1983;72:658.

Perlmutter DH, Gross P, Jones HR, et al. Intramuscular vitamin E repletion in children with chronic cholestasis. Am J Dis Child 1987;141:170.

Perry TL, Applegarth DE, Evans ME, et al. Metabolic studies of a family with massive formimino glutamic aciduria. Pediatr Res 1975;9:117.

Peters ACB. Hepatitis B: Nervous system complications. Handbook Clin Neurol 1989;12:295.

Peters G, du Plessis DG, Humphry PR. Cerebral Whipple's disease with a stroke-like presentation and cerebrovascular pathology. J Neurol Neurosurg Psychiatry 2002;73:336.

Pettifor JM. Nutritional rickets: Deficiency of vitamin D, calcium, or both? Am J Clin Nutr 2004;80:1725S.

Pfau BT, Li BUK. Differentiating cyclic from chronic vomiting patterns in children—quantitative criteria and diagnostic implications. Pediatrics1996;97:367.

Phillips WEJ, Mills JHL, Charbonneau SM, et al. Subacute toxicity of pyridoxine-hydrochloride in the beagle dog. Toxicol Appl Pharmacol 1978;44:323.

Pirzada NA, Ali II. Central pontine myelinolysis. Mayo Clinic Proc 2001;76:559.

Pitsavas S, Andreou C, Mascialla F, et al. Pellagra encephalopathy following B-complex vitamin treatment without niacin. Int J Psychiatry Med 2004;34:91.

Pleskow RG, Grand RJ. Wilson's disease. In: Walker WA, Durie PR, Hamilton JR, et al, eds. Pediatric gastrointestinal disease. St. Louis: Mosby, 1996.

Poets CF. Gastroesophageal reflux: A critical review of its role in preterm infants. Pediatrics 2004;113:e128.

Pollitt E. Developmental sequel from early nutritional deficiencies: Conclusive and probability judgments. J Nutr 2000;130 (2S Suppl):350S.

Poncz M, Cohen A. Long-term treatment of congenital folate malabsorption. J Pediatr. 1996;129:948.

Portman OW, Neuringer M, Alexander M. Effects of maternal and long-term postnatal protein malnutrition on brain size and composition in Rhesus monkeys. J Nutr 1987;117:1844.

Prakash C, Clouse RE. Cyclic vomiting syndrome in adults: Clinical features and response to tricyclic antidepressants. Am J Gastroenterol 1999;94:2855.

Prakash C, Staiano A, Rothbaum RJ, et al. Similarities in cyclic vomiting syndrome across age groups. Am J Gastroenterol 2001;96: 684.

Pratesi R, Gandolfi L, Friedman H, et al. Serum IgA antibodies from patients with coeliac disease react strongly with human brain blood-vessel structures. Scand J Gastrol 1998;33:817.

Prentice AM, Bates CJ. A biochemical evaluation of the erythrocytic glutathione reductase test for riboflavin status. Br J Nutr 1981;45:37.

Przyrembel H, Wendel IJ, Becker K, et al. Glutaric aciduria type II: Report of a previously undescribed metabolic disorder. Clin Chim Acta 1976;66:277.

Puetz J, Knutsen A, Bouhasin J. Congenital deficiency of vitamin K–dependent coagulation factors associated with central nervous system anomalies. Thromb Haemost 2004;91:819.

Pujol A, Graus F, Peri J, et al. Hyperintensity in the globus pallidus on T1-weighted and inversion-recovery MRI: A possible marker of advanced liver disease. Neurology 1991;41:1526.

Pujol A, Pujol J, Graus F, et al. Hyperintense globus pallidus on TI-weighted MRI in cirrhotic patients associated with severity of liver failure. Neurology 1993;43:65.

Pumberger W, Dinhobl I, Dremsek P. Altered consciousness and lethargy from intestinal blood flow in children. Am J Emerg Med 2004;22:307.

Puntis JWL, Smith HL, Buick RG, et al. Effect of dystonic movements on esophageal peristalsis in Sandifer's syndrome. Arch Dis Child 1989;64:113.

Puri P, Shinkai T. Pathogenesis of Hirschsprung's disease and its variants: Recent progress. Semin Pediatr Surg 2004;13:18.

Quigley EM. Enteric neuropathology: Recent advances and implications for clinical practice. Gastroenterologist 1997;5:233.

Rahman S, Standing S, Dalton RN, et al. Late presentation of biotinidase deficiency with acute visual loss and gait disturbance. Dev Med Child Neurol 1997;39:830.

Ramaekers VT, Blau N. Cerebral folate deficiency. Dev Med Child Neurol 2004;46:843.

Rao RR, Subrahmagam I. Investigation of thiamine content of mother's milk in relation to infantile convulsions. Indian J Med Res 1964;52:1198.

Raskin NH, Bredesen D, Ehrenfeld WK, et al. Periodic confusion caused by congenital extrahepatic portocaval shunt. Neurology 1984;34:666.

Raskin NH, Rowland LP. Hepatic disease. In: Rowland LP, ed. Merrit's textbook of neurology, 9th ed. Baltimore: Williams & Wilkins, 1995.

Rasquin-Weber A, Hyman PE, Cucchiara S, et al. Childhood functional gastrointestional disorders. Gut 1999;45 (Suppl 2):II60.

Rassmussen H, Anast C. Familial hypophosphatemic rickets and vitamin D–dependent rickets. In: Stanbury JB, Wyngaarden JB, Fredrickson DS, et al, eds. Metabolic basis of inherited disease, 5th ed. New York: McGraw-Hill, 1983.

Rassmussen H. The calcium messenger system. N Engl J Med 1986;314:1094.

Ratanachu-Ek S, Sukswai P, Jeerathanyasakun Y, Wongtapradit L. Scurvy in pediatric patients: A review of 28 cases. J Med Assoc Thai 2003;86 (Suppl 3):S734.

Ratnaike RN. Whipple's disease. Postgrad Med J 2000;76:760.

Reavley N. Vitamins, etc. Melbourne: Bookman Media Pty Ltd, 1998.

Rees JH, Gregson HA, Griffiths PL, et al. *Campylobacter jejuni* and Guillain-Barré syndrome. Q J Med 1993;86:623.

Relman DA, Schmidt TM, Mac Dermott RP, et al. Identification of the uncultured bacillus of Whipple's disease. N Eng J Med 1992;327:293.

Renault F, Verstichel P, Ploussard JP, et al. Neuropathy in two cobalamin-deficient breast-fed infants of vegetarian mothers. Muscle Nerve 1999;22:252.

Resnick O, Morgane PJ. Ontogeny of the levels of serotonin in various parts of the brain in severely protein malnourished rats. Brain Res 1984;303:163.

Reye RDK, Morgan G, Baral J. Encephalopathy and fatty degeneration of the viscera: A disease entity in childhood. Lancet 1963;2:749.

Reynolds FH, Rothfeld P, Pincus JH. Neurological disease associated with folate deficiency. BMJ 1973;3:398.

Richter LM. Poverty, underdevelopment and infant mental health. J Paediatr Child Health 2003;39:243.

Riggs JE, Schochet SS. Neurological dysfunction in Whipple's disease. In: Goetz CG, Aminoff MJ, eds. Handbook of clinical neurology. Amsterdam: Elsevier Science, 1998.

Riggs JE. Neurologic manifestations of electrolyte disturbances. Neurol Clin 2002;20:227.

Rio J, Montalban J, Pujadas F, et al. Asterixis associated with anatomic cerebral lesions: A study of 45 cases. Acta Neurol Scand 1995;91:377.

Riordan SM, Williams R. Treatment of hepatic encephalopathy. N Engl J Med 1997;337:473.

Rivera JA, Hotz C, Gonzalez-Cossio T, et al. The effect of micronutrient deficiencies on child growth: A review of results from community-based supplementation trials. J Nutr 2003;133:4010S.

Rizzieri DA. Rhabdomyolysis after correction of hyponatremia due to psychogenic polydypsia. Mayo Clin Proc 1995;70:473.

Rochas AS, Kokko JP. Sodium chloride and water transport in the medullary thick ascending limb of Henle: Evidence for active chloride transport. J Clin Invest 1973;52:612.

Rodrigues MI, Dohlman CH. Blindness in an American boy caused by unrecognized vitamin A deficiency. Arch Ophthalmol 2004;122:1228.

Rohe JK, Lee TG, Wie BA, et al. Initial and follow-up brain MRI findings and correlation with the clinical course in Wilson's disease. Neurology 1994;44:1064.

Roncagliolo M, Garrido M, Walter T, et al. Evidence of altered central nervous system development in infants with iron deficiency anemia at 6 mo: Delayed maturation of auditory brainstem responses. Am J Clin Nutr 1998;68:683.

Roos RAC, Van Der Blij JF. Pseudotumor cerebri associated with hypovitaminosis A and hyperthyroidism. Dev Med Child Neurol 1985;27:246.

Rosenblatt DS, Hosack A, Matiaszuk NV. Defect in vitamin B_{12} release from lysosomes: Newly described inborn error of vitamin B_{12} metabolism. Science 1985;228:1319.

Rosenblum JL, Keating JP, Prensky AL, et al. A progressive neurologic syndrome in children with chronic liver disease. N Engl J Med 1981;304:503.

Rosenfeld L. Vitamine—vitamin. The early years of discovery. Clin Chem 1997;43:680.

Roth KS. Biotin in clinical medicine: A review. Am J Clin Nutr 1981;34:1967.

Rothstein JD, Herlong HF. Neurologic manifestations of hepatic disease. Neurol Clin 1989;7:463.
Roubertie A, Biolsi B, Rivier F, et al. Ataxia with vitamin E deficiency and severe dystonia: Report of a case. Brain Dev 2003;25:442.
Roy S III, Arant BS Jr. Alkalosis from chloride deficient Neo-Mull-Soy. N Engl J Med 1979;301:615.
Roy S III. The chloride depletion syndrome. Adv Pediatr 1984;31:235.
Rubin AM, Kang H. Cerebral blindness and encephalopathy with cyclosporin A toxicity. Neurology 1987;37:1072.
Rude RK, Oldham SB, Singer FR. Functional hypoparathyroidism and parathyroid end-organ resistance in human magnesium deficiency. Clin Endocrinol 1976;5:209.
Rude RK, Singer FR. Magnesium deficiency and excess. Annu Rev Med 1981;32:245.
Rudolph AM, Hoffman JLE, Rudolph CD. Rudolph's pediatrics, 20th ed. Stamford, Conn: Appleton & Lange, 1996.
Rush PJ, Inman R, Bernstein M, et al. Isolated vasculitis of the central nervous system in a patient with celiac disease. Am J Med 1986;81:1092.
Ruzek KA, Campeau NG, Miller GM. Early diagnosis of central pontine myelinolysis with diffusion-weighted imaging. Am J Neuroradiol 2004;25:210.
Rymer MM, Fishman RA. Protective adaption of brain to water intoxication. Arch Neurol 1973;28:49.
Said HM, Sharifian A, Bagherzade H. Transport of biotin in the ileum of suckling rats: Characteristics and ontogeny. Pediatr Res 1990;28:266.
Sakai T, Wakizaka A, Nirasawa Y. Congenital central hypoventilation syndrome associated with Hirschsprung's disease: Mutation analysis of the RET and endothelin-signaling pathways. Eur J Pediatr Surg 2001;1:335.
Sakamoto O, Suzuki Y, Li X, et al. Relationship between kinetic properties of mutant enzyme and biochemical and clinical responsiveness to biotin in holocarboxylase synthetase deficiency. Pediatr Res 1999;46:671.
Salgueiro MJ, Weill R, Zubillaga M, et al. Zinc deficiency and growth: Current concepts in relationship to two important points: Intellectual and sexual development. Biol Trace Elem Res 2004;99:49.
Sandyk R, Brenna MJW. Fulminating encephalopathy associated with *Shigella flexneri* infection. Arch Dis Child 1983;58:70.
Santer R, Muhle H, Suormala T, et al. Partial response to biotin therapy in a patient with holocarboxylase synthetase deficiency: Clinical, biochemical, and molecular genetic aspects. Mol Genet Metab 2003;79:160.
Satya-Murti S, Howard L, Krohel G, et al. The spectrum of neurologic disorder from vitamin E deficiency. Neurology 1986;36:917.
Saxena N, Bhatia M, Joshi YK, et al. Auditory P399 event-related potentials and number connection test for evaluation of subclinical hepatic encephalopathy in patients with cirrhosis of the liver: A follow-up study. J Gastroenterol Hepatol 2001;16:322.
Sazawal S, Bentley M, Black RE, et al. Effect of zinc supplementation on observed activity in preschool children in an urban slum population. Pediatrics 1996;98:1132.
Schafer DF, Jones EA. Hepatic encephalopathy and the gamma-aminobutyric-acid neurotransmitter system. Lancet 1982;1:18.
Schafer DF, Shaw BW. Fulminant hepatic failure and orthotopic liver transplantation. Semin Liver Dis 1989;9:189.
Schaumburg H, Kaplan J, Windebank A, et al. Sensory neuropathy from pyridoxine abuse. N Engl J Med 1983;309:445.
Scheinberg IH, Sternlieb J. Wilson's disease. Philadelphia: WB Saunders, 1984.
Schiff D, Chan G, Poznansky M. Bilirubin toxicity of neural cells in culture. Pediatr Res 1985;19:362.
Schiff D, Chan G, Poznansky MJ. Bilirubin toxicity in neural cell lines N115 and NBR10A. Pediatr Res 1985;19:908.
Schilsky ML. Identification of the Wilson's disease gene: Clues for disease pathogenesis and potential for molecular diagnosis. Hepatology 1994;20:529.
Schilsky ML. Wilson disease: Genetic basis of copper toxicity and natural history. Semin Liver Dis 1996;16:83.
Schilsky ML, Scheinberg IH, Sternlieb I. Liver transplantation for Wilson's disease: Indications and outcome. Hepatology 1994;19:583.
Schnider P, Trattnig S, Kollegger H, et al. MR of cerebral Whipple disease. AJNR Am J Neuroradiol 1995;16:1328.
Schoffeniels E. Thiamine phosphorylated derivates and bioelectrogenesis. Arch Int Physiol Biochem 1983;91:223.
Schomerus H, Hamster W. Neuropsychological aspects of portal-systemic encephalopathy. Metab Brain Dis 1998;13:361.
Schreiber WE. Acute intermittent porphyria: laboratory diagnosis by molecular methods. Clin Lab Med 1995;15:943.
Schurch B. Malnutrition and behavioral development: The nutrition variable. J Nutr 1995;125:2255S.
Schwammenthal Y, Tanne D. Homocysteine, B-vitamin supplementation, and stroke prevention: From observational to interventional trials. Lancet Neurol 2004;3:493.
Schwartz MA, Selhorst JB, Ochs AL, et al. Oculomasticatory myorhythmia: A unique movement disorder occurring in Whipple's disease. Ann Neurol 1983;20:677.
Scott BL, Jankovic J. Delayed-onset progressive movement disorders after static brain lesions. Neurology 1996;46:68.
Scott D. Clinical biotin deficiency ("egg white injury"): Report of a case with some remarks on serum cholesterol. Acta Med Scand 1958;162:69.
Scott DA. Vaccines against *Campylobacter jejuni.* J Infect Dis 1997;176 (Suppl 2):S183.
Scott RB. Motility disorders. In: Walker WA, Durie PR, Hamilton JR, et al, eds. Pediatric gastrointestinal disease. St. Louis: Mosby, 1996.
Selimoglu M, Akday R, Kirpinar I. A case of childhood shigellosis with mutism. Turkish J Pediatr 1995;37:431.
Serra-Majem L, Ribas L, Ngo J, et al. Risk of inadequate intakes of vitamins A, B_1, B_6, C, E, folate, iron and calcium in the Spanish population aged 4 to 18. Int J Vitam Nutr Res 2001;71:325.
Shahar E, Shinawi M. Neurocristopathies presenting with neurologic abnormalities associated with Hirschsprung's disease. Pediatr Neurol 2003;28:385.
Shapiro SM. Bilirubin toxicity in the developing nervous system. Pediatr Neurol 2003;29:410.
Shaywitz BA, Siegel NJ, Pearson HA. Megavitamins for minimal cerebral dysfunction: A potentially dangerous therapy. JAMA 1977;238:1749.
Sherlock S. Chronic portal systemic encephalopathy: Update 1987. Gut 1987;28:1043.
Sherlock S. Hepatic encephalopathy. Br J Hosp Med 1977;17:144.
Shields WD. Disorders of gastrointestinal tract and liver. In: Berg BO, ed. Neurologic aspects of pediatrics. Boston: Butterworth-Heinemann, 1992.
Shils ME. Experimental human magnesium depletion. Medicine 1969;48:61.
Shimada M, Wamano T, Nakamura T, et al. Effect of maternal malnutrition on matrix cell proliferation in cerebrum of mouse embryo: An autoradiographic study. Pediatr Res 1977;11:728.
Shokeir MHK, Shreffler DC. Cytochrome oxidase deficiency in Wilson's disease: A suggested ceruloplasmin function. Proc Natl Acad Sci USA 1969;62:867.
Siekmann JH, Allen LH, Bwibo NO, et al. Micronutrient status of Kenyan school children: Response to meat, milk, or energy supplementation. J Nutr 2003;133:3972S.
Sillman JS, Evay RD, Reardon EJ, et al. Metabolic facial palsy in an infant. Arch Otolaryngol 1985;111:822.
Simell O, Takki K. Raised plasma ornithine and gyrate atrophy of the choroid and retina. Lancet 1973;2:1031.
Simon L, Horoupian DS, Dorfman LJ, et al. Polyneuropathy, ophthalmoplegia, leukoencephalopathy, and intestinal pseudo-obstruction: POLIP syndrome. Ann Neurol 1990;28:349.
Simpson KL, Chichester CO. Metabolism and nutritional significance of carotenoids. Annu Rev Nutr 1981;1:351.
Singaram C. Neuropathology of the gut. Semin Neurol 1996;16:227.
Sipila I, Simell O, Rapola J, et al. Gyrate atrophy of the choroid and retina with hyperornithemia: Tubular aggregates and type 2 fiber atrophy in muscle. Neurology 1979;29:996.
Skeen MB. Neurologic manifestations of gastrointestinal disease. In: Riggs JE, ed. Neurologic manifestations of systemic disease. Neurol Clin 2002;20:195.
Skeham S, Norris S, Hegarty J, et al. Brain MRI chanes in chronic liver disease. Eur Radiol 1997;7:905.
Smith CD, Othersen HB, Gogan NJ, et al. Nissen fundoplication in children with profound neurologic disability. High risks and unmet goals. Ann Surg 1992;215:654.
Smith FE, Goodman DS. Vitamin A transport in human vitamin A toxicity. N Engl J Med 1976;294:805.
Snodgrass SR. Vitamin neurotoxicity. Mol Neurobiol 1992;6:41.
Sokol RJ. Vitamin E and neurologic deficits. Adv Pediatr 1990;37:119.

Sokol RJ, Guggenheim MA, Iannoccone ST, et al. Improved neurologic function after long-term correction of vitamin E deficiency in children with chronic cholestasis. N Engl J Med 1985;313:1580.

Solinas C, Vajda FJ. Epilepsy and porphyria: New perspectives. J Clin Neurosci 2004;11:356.

Sommer A. New imperatives for an old vitamin (A). Symposium: Biological actions of carotenoids. J Nutr 1989;119:96.

Sommer A, Hussaini G, Muhilal, et al. History of night blindness: A simple tool for xerophthalmia screening. Am J Clin Nutr 1980;33:887.

Sommer A, Tarwotjo I, Hussaini G, et al. Incidence scale of blinding malnutrition. Lancet 1981;1:1407.

Sondheimer JM, Morris BA. Gastroesophageal reflux among severely retarded children. J Pediatr 1979;94:710.

Soto-Moyano R, Ruiz S, Perez H, et al. Early undernutrition and long-lasting functional derangement of the noradrenergic system projecting to the cerebral cortex. Nutr Rep Int 1987;36:309.

Spahr L, Vingerhoets F, Lazeyras F et al. Magnetic resonance imaging and proton spectroscopic alterations correlate with parkinsonian signs in patients with cirrhosis. Gasterenterology 2000;119:774.

Sparacia G, Banco A, Lagalla R. Reversible MRI abnormalities in an unusual paediatric presentation of Wernicke's encephalopathy. Pediatr Radiol 1999;29:581.

Spector R. Thiamine transport in the central nervous system. Am J Physiol 1976;230:1101.

Spector R, Lorenzo AV. Ascorbic acid homeostasis in the central nervous system. Am J Physiol 1973;225:775.

Spector R, Lorenzo AV. Folate transport by the choroid plexus in vivo. Science 1975;187:540.

Spitz L, McLeod E. Gastroesophageal reflux. Semin Pediatr Surg 2003;12:237.

Spivais JL, Jackson DL. Pellagra: An analysis of 18 patients and a review of the literature. Johns Hopkins Med J 1977;140:295.

Stanbury JB. The damaged brain of iodine deficiency. Elmsford, NY: Cognizant Communication, 1994.

Steegers Theunissen BP. Maternal nutrition and obstetric outcome. Baillieres Clin Obstet Gynaecol 1995;9:431.

Stein DP, Lederman RJ, Vogt DP, et al. Neurologic complications following liver transplantation. Ann Neurol 1992;31:644.

Stein MT, ed. Cyclical vomiting. J Develop Behav Pediatr 2001;22 (2 Suppl):S139.

Stein RB, Lichtenstein GR. Medical therapy for Crohn's disease: The state of the art. Surg Clin North Am 2001;81:71.

Steinberg A, Frank Y. Neurological manifestations of systemic diseases in children. New York: Raven Press, 1993.

Steiner I, Steinberg A, Argov Z, et al. Familial progressive neuronal disease and chronic idiopathic intestinal pseudo-obstruction. Neurology 1987;37:1046.

Steinschneider M, Sherbany A, Pavlakis S, et al. Congenital folate malabsorption: Reversible clinical and neurophysiologic abnormalities. Neurology 1990;40:1315.

Stern M, Hellwege HH, Gravinghoff L, et al. Total aganglionosis of the colon (Hirschsprung's disease) and congenital failure of automatic control of ventilation (Ondine's curse). Acta Paediatr Scand 1981;70:121.

Sternlieb I. The outlook for the diagnosis of Wilson's disease. J Hepatol 1993;17:263.

Sterns RH, Riggs JE, Schochetl SS Jr. Osmotic demyelination syndrome following correction of hyponatremia. N Engl J Med 1986;314:1535.

Sterns RH, Thomas DJ, Herndon RM. Brain dehydration and neurologic deterioration after rapid correction of hyponatremia. Kidney Int 1989;35:69.

Stewart SM, Campbell RA, McCallon D, et al. Cognitive patterns in school-age children with end-stage liver disease. Dev Behav Pediatr 1992;13:331.

Stewart SM, Hiltebeitel C, Nici J, et al. Neuropsychological outcome of pediatric liver transplantation. Pediatrics 1991;87:367.

Stewart SM, Uauy R, Kennard BD, et al. Mental development and growth in children with chronic liver disease of early and late onset. Pediatrics 1988;82:167.

Stewart SM, Vavy R, Waller DA, et al. Mental and motor development, social competence, and growth one year after successful pediatric liver transplantation. J Pediatr 1989;114:574.

Stoch MB, Smythe PM. 15-year developmental study on effects of severe undernutrition during infancy on subsequent physical growth and intellectual functioning. Arch Dis Child 1976;54:327.

Stojeba N, Meyer C, Jeanpierre C, et al. Recovery from a variegate porphyria by a liver transplantation. Liver Transpl 2004;10:935.

Stoltzfus RJ, Kvalsvig JD, Chwaya HM, et al. Effects of iron supplementation and anthelmintic treatment on motor and language development of preschool children in Zanzibar: Double blind, placebo controlled study. BMJ 2001;323:1389.

Stracciari A, Tempestini A, Borghi A, et al. Effect of liver transplantation on neurological manifestations in Wilson disease. Arch Neurol 2000;57:384.

Straussberg R, Shorer Z, Weitz R, et al. Familial infantile bilateral striatal necrosis: Clinical features and response to biotin treatment. Neurology 2002;59:983.

Stryer L. Cyclic GMP cascade of vision. Annu Rev Neurosci 1986;9:87.

Stuehr DJ, Griffith OW. Mammalian nitric oxide synthases. Adv Enzymol Relat Areas Mol Biol 1992;65:287.

Stumpf DA. Reye syndrome: An international perspective. Brain Dev 1995;17:77.

Stutchfield P, Edwards ME, Gray RGF, et al. Glutaric aciduria type I misdiagnosed as Leigh's encephalopathy and cerebral palsy. Dev Med Child Neurol 1985;27:514.

Suarez JI, Cohen ML, Larkin J, et al. Acute intermittent porphyria: Clinicopathologic correlation. Report of a case and review of the literature. Neurology 1997;48:1678.

Sugita N. Comparative studies on the growth of the cerebral cortex. VII. On the influence of starvation at an early age upon the development of the cerebral cortex: Albino rat. J Comp Neurol 1918;29:177.

Sullivan PB, Hirschprung's disease. Arch Dis Child 1996;74:5.

Sungthong R, Mo-suwan L, Chongsuvivatwong V. Effects of haemoglobin and serum ferritin on cognitive function in school children. Asia Pac J Clin Nutr 2002;11:117.

Surtees R. Biochemical pathogenesis of subacute combined degeneration of the spinal cord and brain. J Inherit Metab Dis 1993;16:762.

Susser N, Stein ZA. Human development and prenatal nutrition: An overview of epidemiological experiments, quasi-experiments, and natural experiments in the past decade. In: Mittler P, ed. Frontiers of knowledge in mental retardation. Vol. 2. Biomedical aspects. Baltimore: University Park Press, 1980.

Sutor AH. New aspects of vitamin K prophylaxis. Semin Thromb Hemost 2003;29:373.

Swaiman KF, Milstein JM: Pyridoxine-dependency and penicillamine. Neurology 1970;20:78.

Swaiman KF, Wolfe RN: The effect of food-deprivation on lactic dehydrogenase activity in immature rat brain. Proc Soc Exp Biol Med 1970;134:185.

Swaiman KF, Daleiden JM, Wolfe RN: The effect of food deprivation on enzyme activity in immature rat brain. Brain Res 1972;43:296.

Swain R, Kaplan B. Vitamins as therapy in the 1990s. J Am Board Fam Pract 1995;8:206.

Sweetman L, Nyhan WL, Trauner DA, et al. Glutaric aciduria type II. J Pediatr 1980;96:1020.

Sweetman L, Surh IL, Baker H, et al. Clinical and metabolic abnormalities in a boy with dietary deficiency of biotin. Pediatrics 1981;68:553.

Symon DNK, Russell G. Abdominal migraine: A childhood syndrome defined. Cephalalgia 1986;6:223.

Symon DNK, Russell G. The relationship between cyclic vomiting syndrome and abdominal migraine. J Pediatr Gastroenterol Nutr 1995;21:542.

Szerb JC, Butterworth RF. Effect of ammonium ions on synaptic transmission in the mammalian central nervous system. Prog Neurobiol 1992;39:135.

Tabor E. Guillain-Barré syndrome and other neurologic syndromes in hepatitis A, B, and non-A, non-B. J Med Virol 1987;21:207.

Takahashi W, Yoshii F, Shinohara Y. Reversible magnetic resonance imaging lesions in Wilson's disease: Clinical-anatomical correlation. J Neuroimaging 1996;6:246.

Tamura T, Goldenberg RL, Ramey SL, et al. Effect of zinc supplementation of pregnant women on the mental and psychomotor development of their children at 5 y of age. Am J Clin Nutr 2003;77:1512.

Tan H, Onbas O. Central pontine myelinolysis manifested with massive myoclonus. Pediatr Neurol 2004;31:64.

Tan TQ, Vogel H, Tharp BR, et al. Presumed central nervous system Whipple's disease in a child: Case report. Clin Infect Dis 1995;20:883.

Tanabe H, Kondo A, Kinuta Y, et al. Unusual presentation of brain metastasis from hepatocellular carcinoma: Two case reports. Neurol Med Chir (Tokyo) 1994;34:748.

Tanaka H, Ito J, Cho K, et al. Hirschsprung disease, unusual face, mental retardation, epilepsy, and congenital heart disease: Goldberg-Shprintzen syndrome. Pediatr Neurol 1993;9:479.

Tanzi RE, Petrukhin K, Chernov I, et al. The Wilson disease gene is a copper transporting ATPase with homology to the Menkes disease gene. Nature Genet 1993;5:344.

Tatum WO 4th, Zachariah SB. Gabapentin treatment of seizures in acute intermittent porphyria. Neurology 1995;45:1216.

Tauro GP, Danks DM, Rowe PB, et al. Dihydrofolate reductase deficiency causing megaloblastic anemia in two families. N Engl J Med 1976;294:466.

Taylor BV, Wijdicks EFM, Polerncha JJ, et al. Chronic inflammatory demyelinating polyneuropathy complicating liver transplantation. Ann Neurol 1995;38:828.

Tefferi A, Colgan JP, Solberg LA Jr. Acute porphyrias: Diagnosis and management. Mayo Clin Proc 1994;69:991.

Tenenbein M, Wiseman NE. Early coma in intussusception: Endogenous opioid induced? Pediatr Emerg Care 1987;3:22.

Thompson K, Morley R, Grover SR, et al. Postnatal evaluation of vitamin D and bone health in women who were vitamin D–deficient in pregnancy, and in their infants. Med J Aust 2004;181:486.

To J, Issenman RM, Kamath MV. Evaluation of neurocardiac signals in pediatric patients with cyclic vomiting syndrome through power spectral analysis of heart rate variability. J Pediatr. 1999;135:363.

Tojo M, Nitta H, Matsui T, et al. A case with severe neurological involvement due to vitamin B_1 deficiency associated with megaduodenum. No To Hattatsu 1993;25:169.

Toki F, Suzuki N, Inoue K, et al. Intestinal aganglionosis associated with the Waardenburg syndrome: Report of two cases and review of the literature. Pediatr Surg Int 2003;19:725.

Tonsgard JH, Huttenlocher PR, Thisted RA. Lactic acidemia in Reye's syndrome. Pediatrics 1982;69:64.

Toole JF, Malinow MR, Chambless LE, et al. Lowering homocysteine in patients with ischemic stroke to prevent recurrent stroke, myocardial infarction, and death: The Vitamin Intervention for Stroke Prevention (VISP) randomized controlled trial. JAMA 2004;291:565.

Trachtman H, Barbour R, Sturman JA. Taurine and osmoregulation: Taurine is a cerebral osmoprotective molecule in chronic hypernatremic dehydration. Pediatr Res 1988;23:35.

Trauner DA. Treatment of Reye syndrome. Ann Neurol 1990;7:2.

Treem WR. Hepatic failure. In: Walker WA, Durie PR, Hamilton JR, et al, eds. Pediatric gastrointestinal disease. St. Louis: Mosby, 1996.

Truwit CL, Denaro CP, Luke JZ, et al. MR imaging of reversible cyclosporin A–induced neurotoxicity. AJNR Am J Neuroradiol 1991;12:651.

Tsai CH, Cho CT. Rotavirus and non-febrile convulsions. Chung Hua Min Kuo Hsiao Erh Ko I Hsueh Hui Tsa Chih 1996;37:165.

Tsang RC, Light IJ, Sutherland JM, et al. Possible pathogenic factors in neonatal hypercalcemia of prematurity. J Pediatr 1973;82:423.

Tsukada N, Koh CS, Inoue A, et al. Demyelinating neuropathy associated with hepatitis B virus infection: detection of immune complexes composed of hepatitis B virus surface antigen. J Neurol Sci 1987;77:203.

Tubbs RS, Webb D, Abdullatif H, et al. Posterior cranial fossa volume in patients with rickets: Insights into the increased occurrence of Chiari I malformation in metabolic bone disease. Neurosurgery 2004;55:380.

Tugal O, Jacobson R, Berezin S, et al. Recurrent benign intracranial hypertension due to iron deficiency anemia: Case report and review of the literature. Am J Pediatr Hematol Oncol 1994;16:266.

Turkel SB. Autopsy findings associated with neonatal hyperbilirubinemia. Clin Perinatol 1990;17:381.

Uauy R, Mena P, Peirano P. Nutrition and brain: Mechanisms for nutrient effects on brain development and cognition. In: Fernstrom JD, Uauy R, Arroyo PC, eds. Nestle nutrition workshop series clinical and performance program. Vol. 5. Nestec Ltd, Vevey/S. Basel: Karger, 2001.

UNICEF. The state of the world's children. Available at http://www.unicef.org/sowc02/fullreport.htm.

Utz N, Kinkel B, Hedde JP, et al. MR imaging of acute intermittent porphyria mimicking reversible posterior leukoencephalopathy syndrome. Neuroradiology 2001;43:1059.

Vaisman N, Tabachnik E, Shahar E, et al. Impaired brainstem auditory evoked potentials in patients with cystic fibrosis. Dev Med Child Neurol 1996;38:59.

van Caillie M, Morin CL, Roy CC, et al. Reye's syndrome: Relapse and neurological sequelae. Pediatrics 1977;59:244.

van den Briel T, West CE, Bleichrodt N, et al. Improved iodine status is associated with improved mental performance of schoolchildren in Benin. Am J Clin Nutr 2000;72:1179.

Van Den Heuvel AG, Van der Grond J, Van Rooij LG, et al. Differentiation between portal-systemic encephalopathy and neurodegenerative disorders in patients with Wilson disease: ^{1}H-MR spectroscopy. Radiology 1997;203:539.

van der Heyden JJ, Verrips A, ter Laak HJ, et al. Hypovitaminosis D–related myopathy in immigrant teenagers. Neuropediatrics 2004;35:290.

van Poppel G, van den Berg H. Vitamins and cancer. Cancer Lett 1997;114:195

Van Praagh R. Diagnosis of kernicterus in the neonatal period. Pediatrics 1961;28:870.

van Wassenaer-van Hall HN. Neuroimaging in Wilson disease. Metab Brain Dis 1996;12:1.

Vanderhoof JA, Young R, Kaufman SS, et al. Treatment of cyclic vomiting in childhood with erythromycin. J Pediatr Gastroenterol Nutr 1995;21 (Suppl 1):S60.

Vargas JH, Sachs P, Ament ME. Chronic intestinal pseudo-obstruction syndrome in pediatrics. Results of a national survey by members of the North American Society of Pediatric Gastroenterology and Nutrition. J Pediatr Gastroenterol Nutr 1988;7:323.

Vasconcelos MM, Silva KP, Vidal G, et al. Early diagnosis of pediatric Wernicke's encephalopathy. Pediatr Neurol 1999;20:289.

Ventura A, Bouquet F, Surtorelli C, et al. Coeliac disease, folic acid deficiency and epilepsy with cerebral calcifications. Acta Paediatr Scand 1991;80:559.

Viana MB, Carvalho RT. Thiamine responsive megaloblastic anemia, sensorineural deafness and diabetes mellitus: A new syndrome? J Pediatr 1978;93:235.

Victor M, Rothstein JD. Neurologic manifestations of hepatic and gastrointestinal diseases: In: Asbury AK, Mckhann GM, McDonald WI, eds. Diseases of the nervous system: Clinical neurobiology. Philadelphia: WB Saunders, 1992.

Victora CG, Van Haecke P. Vitamin K prophylaxis in less developed countries: Policy issues and relevance to breastfeeding promotion. Am J Public Health 1998;88:203.

Villapando S, Montalvo-Velarde I, Zambrano N, et al. Vitamins A, and C and folate status in Mexican children under 12 years and women 12-49 years: A probabilistic national survey. Salud Publica Mex 2003;45 (Suppl 4):S508.

Vimokesant SL, Nakornchi S, Dhanalllitta S, et al. Effect of tea consumption. Nutr Rep Int 1974;9:371.

Volpe JJ, Marasa JC. A role for thiamine in the regulation of fatty acid and cholesterol biosynthesis in cultured cells of neural origin. J Neurochem 1978;3:975.

Volpe JJ. Neurology of the Newborn: Bilirubin and brain injury, 3rd ed. Philadelphia: WB Saunders, 1995.

Von Herbay A, Ditton HJ, Schumacher F, et al. Whipple's disease: Staging and monitoring by cytology and polymerase chain reaction analysis of cerebrospinal fluid. Gastroenterology 1997;113:434.

Voorhees CV, Schmidt DE, Barrett RJ, et al. Effects of thiamine deficiency on acetylcholine levels and utilization in rat brain. J Nutr 1977;107:1902.

Waber DP, Vuori-Christiansen L, Ortiz N, et al. Nutritional supplementation, maternal education and cognitive development of infants at risk of malnutrition. Am J Clin Nutr 1981;34:801.

Waldehind L. Studies on thiamine and neuromuscular transmission. Acta Physiol Scand 1978;459 (Suppl):1.

Walker-Smith JA. Celiac disease. In: Walker WA, Durie PR, Hamilton JR, et al, eds. Pediatric gastrointestinal disease. St. Louis: Mosby, 1996.

Walsh CT, Sandstead HH, Prasad AS, et al. Zinc: Health effects and research priorities for the 1990s. Environ Health Perspect 1994;102:5.

Walshe, JM, Yealland M. Wilson's disease: The problem of delayed diagnosis. J Neurol Neurosurg Psychiatry 1992;55:692.

Walters TR. Congenital megaloblastic anemia responsive to *N*-5-formyl-tetrahydrofolic acid administration. J Pediatr 1967;7:686.

Wang Q, Ito M, Adams K, et al. Mitochondrial DNA control region sequence variation in migraine headache and cyclic vomiting syndrome. Am J Med Genet A 2004;131:50.

Wartiovaara K, Salo M, Sariola H. Hirschsprung's disease genes and the development of the enteric nervous system. Ann Med 1998;30:66.

Watchko JF, Claassen D. Kernicterus in premature infants: Current prevalence and relationship to NICHD Phototherapy Study exchange criteria. Pediatrics 1994;93:996.

Waxman S, Corcino JJ, Herbert V. Drugs, toxins and dietary amino acids affecting vitamin B_{12} and folic acid absorption and utilization. Am J Med 1970;48:599.

Weber P, Scholl S, Baumgartner ER. Outcome in patients with profound biotinidase deficiency: Relevance of newborn screening. Dev Med Child Neurol 2004;46:481.

Weinstein M, Babyn P, Zlotkin S. An orange a day keeps the doctor away: Scurvy in the year 2000. Pediatrics 2001;108:E55

Weisberg P, Scanlon KS, Li R, et al. Nutritional rickets among children in the United States: Review of cases reported between 1986 and 2003. Am J Clin Nutr 2004;80:1697S.

Weissenborn K, Ehrenheim C, Hori A, et al. Basal ganglia lesions in patients with liver cirrhosis: Clinical and MRI evaluation. Metab Brain Dis 1995;10:219.

Weissenborn K, Ennen JC, Schomerus H, et al. Neuropsychological characterization of hepatic encephalopathy. J Hepatol 2001;34:768.

Weleber RG, Kennaway NG. Clinical trial of vitamin B_6 for gyrate atrophy of the choroid and retina. Ophthalmology 1981;88:316.

Wennberg RP, Johansson BB, Folbergrova J, et al. Bilirubin-induced changes in brain energy metabolism after osmotic opening of the blood-brain barrier. Pediatr Res 1991;30:473.

Werlin SL, Harb JM, Swick H, et al. Neuromuscular dysfunction and ultrastructural pathology in children with chronic cholestasis and vitamin E deficiency. Ann Neurol 1983;13:291.

Westermark K, Tedroff J, Thuomas KA, et al. Neurological Wilson's disease studied with magnetic resonance imaging and with positron emission tomography using dopaminergic markers. Mov Disord 1995;10:596.

Wetherilt H, Ackurt F, Brubacher G, et al. Blood vitamin and mineral levels in 7-17 year old Turkish children. Int J Vitam Nutr Res 1992;62:21.

White HB. Biosynthetic and salvage pathways of pyridine nucleotide coenzymes. In: Everse J, Anderson B, You KS, eds. Pyridine nucleotide coenzymes. New York: Academic Press, 1982.

Wiggins RC, Fuller G, Enna SJ. Undernutrition and the development of brain neurotransmitter systems. Life Sci 1984;35:2085.

Wijmenga C, Klomp LW. Molecular regulation of copper excretion in the liver. Proc Nutr Soc 2004;63:31.

Williams FJB, Walshe JM. Wilson's diseases. An analysis of the cranial computerized tomographic appearances found in 60 patients and the changes in response to treatment with chelating agents. Brain 1981;104:735.

Williams JA, Hall GS, Thompson AG, et al. Neurologic disease after partial gastrectomy. BMJ 1969;3:210.

Willmore LJ, Triggs WJ, Pellock JM. Valproate toxicity: Risk-screening strategies. J Child Neurol 1991;6:3.

Wills AJ. The neurology and neuropathology of coeliac disease. Neuropathol Appl Neurobiol 2000;26:493.

Wills AJ, Unsworth DJ. The neurology of gluten sensitivity: Separating the wheat from the chaff. Curr Opin Neurol 2002;15:519.

Wills AJ, Unsworth DJ. Gluten ataxia "in perspective." Brain 2003;126:E4.

Windeback AJ, Low PA, Blexrud MC, et al. Pyridoxine neuropathy in rats: Specific degeneration of sensory axons. Neurology 1985;35:1617.

Winick M. Nutrition and nerve cell growth. Fed Proc 1970;29:1510.

Winick M. Malnutrition and brain development. New York: Oxford University Press, 1976.

Winick M, Noble A. Cellular responses in rats during malnutrition at various ages. J Nutr 1966;89:300.

Winick M, Rosso P. The effect of severe early malnutrition on cellular growth of the human brain. Pediatr Res 1969a;3:181.

Winick M, Rosso P. Head circumference and cellular growth of the brain in normal and marasmic children. J Pediatr 1969b;74:774.

Winick NJ, Bowman WP, Kamen BA, et al. Unexpected acute neurological toxicity in the treatment of children with acute lymphoblastic leukemia. J Natl Cancer Inst 1992;84:252.

Winick M, Fish I, Rosso P. Cellular recovery in rat tissues after a brief period of neonatal malnutrition. J Nutr 1968;95:623.

Winick M, Rosso P, Waterlow J. Cellular growth of cerebrum, cerebellum and brainstem in normal and marasmic children. Exp Neurol 1970;26:363.

Withers GD, Siburn SR, Forbes DA. Precipitants and aetiology of cyclic vomiting syndrome. Acta Paediatr 1998;87:272.

Wiznitzer M, Bangert BA. Biotinidase deficiency: Clinical and MRI findings consistent with myelopathy. Pediatr Neurol 2003;29:56.

Wolf B, Feldman GL. The biotin dependent carboxylase deficiencies. Am J Hum Genet 1982;34:699.

Wolf B, Grier RE, Allen RJ, et al. Phenotypic variations in biotinidase deficiency. J Pediatr 1983;103:233.

Wolf B, Heard GS, Jefferson LG, et al. Clinical findings in four children: Biotinidase deficiency detected through a statewide neonatal screening program. N Engl J Med 1985;313:16.

Wolf B, Hsia YE, Sweetman L, et al. Multiple carboxylase deficiency: Clinical and biochemical improvement following neonatal biotin treatment. Pediatrics 1981;68:113.

World Health Organization. The prevalence of anemia in women: A tabulation of available information, 2nd ed. Maternal Health and Safe Motherhood Programme. WHO/MCH/MSM/92.2. Geneva: World Health Organization, 1992.

World Health Organization. Global prevalence of iodine deficiency disorders. MDIS Working Paper No. 1. Geneva: World Health Organization, 1993.

World Health Organization. Essential trace elements: Iodine. In: World Health Organization. Trace elements in human nutrition and health. Geneva: World Health Organization, 1996.

World Health Organization. Vitamin A. 2004. Available at http://www.who.int/nut/vad.htm.

Worthington-White DA, Behnke M, Gross S. Premature infants require additional folate and vitamin B-12 to reduce the severity of the anemia of prematurity. Am J Clin Nutr 1994;60:930.

Wszolek ZK, Aksamit AJ, Ellingson RJ, et al. Epileptiform electroencephalographic abnormalities in liver transplant recipients. Ann Neurol 1991;30:37.

Yager JY, Hartfield DS. Neurologic manifestations of iron deficiency in childhood. Pediatr Neurol 2002;27:85.

Yanda RJ. Fulminant hepatic failure. West J Med 1988;149:586.

Yao TC, Stevenson DK. Advances in the diagnosis and treatment of neonatal hyperbilirubinemia. Clin Perinatol 1995;22:741.

Yarze JC, Martin P, Munoz SJ, et al. Wilson's disease: Current status. Am J Med 1992;92:643.

Yatzidis H, Koutsicos D, Agroyannis B, et al. Biotin in the management of uremic neurologic disorders. Nephron 1984;36:183.

Yerby MS. Management issues for women with epilepsy: Neural tube defects and folic acid supplementation. Neurology 2003;61 (6 Suppl 2):S23.

Yokochi K. Magnetic resonance imaging in children with kernicterus. Acta Paediatr 1995;84:937.

Yomo A, Taira T, Kondo I. Goldberg-Shprintzen syndrome: Hirschsprung disease, hypotonia, and ptosis in sibs. Am J Med Genet 1991;41:188.

Yoshikawa H, Yamazaki S, Watanabe T, et al. Vitamin K deficiency in severely disabled children. J Child Neurol 2003;18:93.

Youdim MB, Yehuda S. The neurochemical basis of cognitive deficits induced by brain iron deficiency: involvement of dopamine-opiate system. Cell Mol Biol 2000;46:491.

Yuhas Y, Weizman A, Chrousos GP, et al. Involvement of the neuropeptide corticotropin-releasing hormone in an animal model of *Shigella*-related seizures. J Neuroimmunol 2004;153:36.

Zachor D, Mroczek-Musulman E, Brown P. Prevalence of celiac disease in Down syndrome in the United States. J Pediatr Gastroenterol Nutr 2000;31:275.

Zaffanello M, Zamboni G, Fontana E, et al. A case of partial biotinidase deficiency associated with autism. Neuropsychol Dev Cogn C Child Neuropsychol 2003;9:184.

Zamenhof S, Guthrie D. Differential responses to prenatal malnutrition among neonatal rats. Biol Neonate 1977;32:205.

Zieve L. The mechanism of hepatic coma. Hepatology 1981;1:360.

Zile MH. Function of vitamin A in vertebrate embryonic development. J Nutr 2001;131:705.

Zimmerman HJ, Lowry CF. Encephalomyeloradiculitis (Guillain-Barré syndrome) as a complication of infectious hepatitis. Ann Intern Med 1947;26:934.

Ziporin ZZ, Nunes WT, Powell RC, et al. Thiamine requirement in the adult human as measured by urinary excretion of thiamine metabolites. J Nutr 1965;85:297.

Zipursky A. Prevention of vitamin K deficiency bleeding in newborns. Br J Haematol 1999;104:430.

Zitelli BJ, Miller JW, Gartner JC, et al. Changes in life style after liver transplantation. Pediatrics 1988;82:173.

CHAPTER 91

Neurologic Complications of Immunization

Claudia A. Chiriboga

Immunization programs are undoubtedly cost-effective public health measures that protect against infectious disease. Recommendations on immunization schedules are made by the Advisory Committee on Immunization Practices (ACIP) of the Centers for Disease Control and Prevention to the Surgeon General. New recommendations of the ACIP are published in *Morbidity and Mortality Weekly Report*, and they are the standard of care for immunization practices (Table 91-1).

Vaccination programs have proved successful in eradicating diseases worldwide. For instance, smallpox was eradicated in 1980, and a World Health Organization (WHO) vaccination program to eradicate poliomyelitis by the year 2000 has made steady progress, with cases decreasing from 4000 in 1994 to 600 in 2003. Efforts have been thwarted by mistrust of vaccines in Nigeria, where the government stopped vaccinating against polio because of unfounded fears that it caused sterilization. As of July 2004, Nigeria accounted for 78% of 440 polio cases worldwide. Vaccine mistrust is not just a problem in Third World countries. Increasingly, antivaccine movements are afoot in the United States and other industrialized countries. These types of movements have potential for harming children by not affording them needed protection against infections at a biologically vulnerable age. For instance, countries such as the United States that have strong antivaccine movements have rates of pertussis that are 10 to 100 times higher than rates in countries such as Hungary without such antivaccine movements, where levels of vaccination are very high [Gangarosa et al., 1998]. Antivaccine movements are fueled by ignorance, lack of scientific scrutiny of the Internet, anecdotal reports, and frustration among parents by the lack of well-defined causes to explain neurologic or developmental disorders (e.g., autism) that may temporally coincide with vaccination. The high rates of complications of earlier vaccines (e.g., rabies) may also contribute to this mistrust.

TABLE 91-1

Schedule of Routine Immunization of Healthy Infants and Children

RECOMMENDED AGE	IMMUNIZATIONS
Birth	HBV
2 months	DTaP, HBV, HIB, OPV or eIPV
4 months	DTaP, Hib, eIPV
6 months	DTaP, HBV, Hib
12–15 months	DTaP, Hib, MMR, eIPV, Var, PCV
4–6 years	DTaP, MMR, eIPV
11–12 years	DT, MMR, and Var if not given at or after 12 months

DT, diphtheria-tetanus; DTaP, pertussis vaccine combined with diphtheria and tetanus toxoids; eIPV, enhanced-potency trivalent inactivated polio vaccine; HBV, hepatitis B virus; Hib, *Haemophilus influenzae* type b; MMR, measles, mumps, and rubella vaccine; OPV, oral polio vaccine; Var, live-attenuated varicella vaccine.

ASSESSING CAUSALITY

Events that are temporally associated are not necessarily causally linked. Determining causal relationships between vaccinations and specific disorders with certainty is difficult. Among existing methods, the one least helpful in assessing causality is the case report, which relies on simple temporal associations that may easily have occurred by coincidence. For example, any exposure (e.g., vaccinations) that affects an entire population (e.g., children) is bound to be associated with an outcome, even a rare outcome, by simple chance. When the outcomes are common (e.g., developmental disorders), associations by chance are expected to occur and do not denote causality.

Clinical trials and epidemiologic population-based studies are more robust in assessing links between vaccines and adverse outcomes. Clinical trials, not usually employed to assess vaccine safety and efficacy in the United States, compare adverse outcomes in an exposed (i.e., vaccinated) and unexposed (i.e., not vaccinated or vaccinated with a different preparation) group of randomly selected individuals. Findings resulting from such studies are valid, but they are limited by their relatively small sample size that precludes identifying associations with rare outcomes. Population-based studies are useful, especially if large, because they can assess even rare outcomes. The risks of adverse outcomes in one population can then be compared with risk among the nonvaccinated populations or rates of the naturally occurring disease. However, causality cannot be determined with certainty, only suspected, unless there is a biologic marker. Further complicating assigning causality is the administration of several vaccines at one time [Fenichel, 1999; Howe et al., 1997].

The U.S. Institute of Medicine was charged with undertaking the first reviews of vaccine-related complications, and it continues to review vaccine safety. Given the lack of a “smoking gun” to attribute causality and because absence of proof is not proof of absence, the Institute of Medicine takes into account level of proof and does not make determination based on lack of evidence. Instead, the literature is reviewed, biologic mechanisms are taken into account, and causality is classified into the following five levels of proof: (1) no evidence bearing on a causal relationship, (2) evidence is inadequate to accept or reject a causal relationship, (3) evidence favors rejection of a causal relationship, (4) evidence favors acceptance of a causal relationship, and

Box 91-1 Types of Vaccines

Whole-Killed Organisms
- Influenza
- Pertussis
- Poliomyelitis (i.e., inactivated polio vaccine)
- Rabies

Live-Attenuated Viruses
- Measles
- Mumps
- Poliomyelitis (i.e., oral poliovirus vaccine)
- Rubella
- Varicella
- Influenza (i.e., nasal vaccine)

Components of Organisms
- Acellular pertussis
- *Haemophilus influenzae* type b
- Pneumococcal conjugate
- Diphtheria
- Tetanus

Recombinant
- Hepatitis B

(5) evidence establishes a causal relationship [Institute of Medicine, 1991, 1993].

In determining causality, biologic mechanisms (formerly defined as biologic plausibility), should first be taken into account (i.e., whether there is a plausible mechanism by which the vaccine could cause the complication or disease in question). For example, a measles vaccine cannot elicit vaccine-associated polio. Next, the method of vaccine preparation should be considered. Four types of vaccines are available: vaccines composed of whole-killed organisms, vaccines composed of live-attenuated viruses, vaccines composed of components of organisms, and recombinant vaccines (Box 91-1). Adverse events should be congruent with the vaccine preparation. For example, vaccines made of components of organisms cannot cause the disease being vaccinated against, but live-attenuated viruses can do so in the right host (e.g., vaccine-associated polio).

VACCINE INJURY COMPENSATION PROGRAM

The U.S. Vaccine Injury Compensation Program (VICP), effective since 1988, is a federal no-fault system designed to compensate individuals or families of individuals who have been injured by childhood vaccines. Vaccines covered under the VICP are diphtheria, tetanus, and pertussis (DTP, DTaP, DT, TT, or Td); measles, mumps, and rubella (MMR or any components); polio (OPV or IPV); hepatitis B; *Haemophilus influenzae* type b; varicella (chickenpox); rotavirus; and pneumococcal conjugate, whether administered individually or in combination. A table of injuries was established outlining known injuries to covered vaccines (Table 91-2). The injuries listed are presumed to be caused by the vaccine unless an alternate cause is established.

TYPES OF VACCINES

Vaccines Composed of Whole-Killed Organisms

Vaccines composed of whole-killed organisms were the first laboratory-produced vaccines. They provoke an antibody response that provides temporary immunity. Some vaccines made from whole-killed organisms may cause immune-mediated disorders.

Inactivated Polio Vaccine

The Salk inactivated polio vaccine (IPV) was licensed in 1955 and immediately led to a drop in the incidence of paralytic poliomyelitis. The Salk vaccine has been highly effective, with a 70% to 90% protection rate. It was replaced in 1963 by Sabin's oral poliovirus vaccine (OPV), which resulted in polio eradication in the United States by 1979, the time of the last documented wild type poliovirus infection.

Because OPV is prepared with a live-attenuated virus, it is associated with a low risk of eliciting polio in healthy individuals and a larger risk in immune-suppressed people (see "Vaccines Composed of Live-Attenuated Viruses"). An enhanced-potency trivalent polio vaccine (eIPV) was licensed in the United States in 1987, which was initially indicated for immunodeficient individuals. After a successful transition from OPV, eIPV has become the vaccine used to immunize children in the United States [CDC, 1997]. It is easier to administer, and it is not associated with vaccine-associated poliomyelitis.

Influenza Virus Vaccine

Epidemic human influenza illness is caused by influenza A and B. Influenza A viruses are categorized into subtypes based on two surface antigens: hemagglutinin (H) and neuraminidase (N). New influenza virus variants result from changes in antigens (i.e., antigenic drift) due to point mutations arising during viral replication. Every year, a new influenza vaccine is developed to protect against the prevalent virus strains that are expected to appear in the United States the following winter. Each vaccine contains three influenza viruses: one A (H3N2) virus, one A (H1N1) virus, and one B virus.

Two types of flu vaccines are available: the inactivated flu vaccine (discussed later) and the nasal-spray flu vaccine (i.e., live-attenuated influenza vaccine [LAIV]). The "flu shot" vaccine is prepared from inactivated flu virus and is approved for use in all high-risk groups. The LAIV is prepared from live, attenuated flu viruses that do not cause disease in humans. This nasal preparation is cold adapted to replicate best at 25° C, and it is temperature sensitive so that it cannot replicate in lower airways. LAIV was licensed for use in the United States in 2003 and is approved for use in healthy people 5 to 49 years of age who are not pregnant. Trials in children have found comparable efficacy and safety profile between inactivated flu vaccine and LAIV in children [Zangwill et al., 2003, 2004]. Annual vaccination against influenza with inactivated virus is recommended for both extremes of life: children age 6 to 23 months (as of 2002) and the elderly (>65 years). It is also recommended for people of all ages with chronic diseases.

TABLE 91-2

National Childhood Vaccine Injury Act: Vaccine Injury Table

VACCINE	ADVERSE EVENT*	TIME INTERVAL
Tetanus toxoid-containing vaccines (e.g., DTaP, DTP-Hib, DT; Td, or TT)	A. Anaphylaxis or anaphylactic shock	0–4 hours
	B. Brachial neuritis	2–28 days
	C. Any acute complication or sequela (including death) of above events	Not applicable
Pertussis antigen-containing vaccines (e.g., DTaP, DTP, P, DTP-Hib)	A. Anaphylaxis or anaphylactic shock	0–4 hours
	B. Encephalopathy (or encephalitis)	0-72 hours
	C. Any acute complication or sequela (including death) of above events	Not applicable
Measles, mumps and rubella virus-containing vaccines in any combination (e.g., MMR, MR, M, R)	A. Anaphylaxis or anaphylactic shock	0–4 hours
	B. Encephalopathy (or encephalitis)	5–15 days
	C. Any acute complication or sequela (including death) of above events	Not applicable
Rubella virus-containing vaccines (e.g., MMR, MR, R)	A. Chronic arthritis	7–42 days
	B. Any acute complication or sequela (including death) of above event	Not applicable
Measles virus-containing vaccines (e.g., MMR, MR, M)	A. Thrombocytopenic purpura	7–30 days
	B. Vaccine-strain measles viral infection in an immunodeficient recipient	0-6 months
	C. Any acute complication or sequela (including death) of above events	Not applicable
Polio live virus-containing vaccines (OPV)	A. Paralytic polio	
	In a non-immunodeficient recipient	0–30 days
	In an immunodeficient recipient	0–6 months
	In a vaccine-associated community case	Not applicable
	B. Vaccine-strain polio viral infection	
	In a non-immunodeficient recipient	0–30 days
	In an immunodeficient recipient	0–6 months
	In a vaccine-associated community case	Not applicable
	C. Any acute complication or sequela (including death) of above events	Not applicable
Polio inactivated-virus containing vaccines (e.g., IPV)	A. Anaphylaxis or anaphylactic shock	0–4 hours
	B. Any acute complication or sequela (including death) of above event	Not applicable
Hepatitis B antigen–containing vaccines	A. Anaphylaxis or anaphylactic shock	0–4 hours
	B. Any acute complication or sequela (including death) of above event	Not applicable
Vaccines containing live, oral, rhesus-based rotavirus	A. Intussusception	0–30 days
	B. Any acute complication or sequela (including death) of above event	Not applicable

*Information effective as of August 26, 2002; see http://www.hrsa.gov/osp/vicp/table.htm for full definition of each adverse event. No condition specified for compensation for *Haemophilus influenzae* type b, pneumococcal conjugated vaccine, rotavirus vaccine, or varicella vaccine.
DT, diphtheria-tetanus vaccine; DTaP, acellular pertussis vaccine combined with diphtheria and tetanus toxoids; Hib, *Haemophilus influenzae* type b; IPV, inactivated polio vaccine; MMR, measles, mumps, and rubella vaccine; MR, mumps and rubella vaccine; OPV, oral polio vaccine; Td, tetanus and diphtheria toxoid; TT, tetanus toxoid.

GUILLAIN-BARRÉ SYNDROME

Increased rates of Guillain-Barré syndrome (GBS) were reported to be associated with the swine vaccine of 1976, with rates of GBS among vaccinees found to exceed the background rate of less than 10 cases per 1 million persons vaccinated. However, subsequent influenza seasons studied have not found a significant increase risk of GBS after influenza vaccination [Hurwitz et al., 1981]. The Institute of Medicine has determined a causal relationship between GBS and influenza vaccination for 1976 but not for other years. Nevertheless, because individuals with a history of GBS have a substantially greater likelihood of subsequently experiencing GBS than individuals without such a history, it has been recommended that influenza vaccination be avoided among individuals with a history of GBS and who are known to have experienced GBS within 6 weeks of a previous influenza vaccination (http://www.cdc.gov/flu/protect/vaccine.htm). Whether influenza vaccination truly increases the risk for recurrence of GBS or is coincidental is unknown. Even if GBS were a true complication of influenza vaccination, the risk of GBS attributable to the vaccine would be only about 1 additional case per 1 million persons vaccinated, a figure that is substantially less than the risk for severe influenza, especially among high-risk individuals. No cases of GBS are reported in vaccinated children [Institute of Medicine, 2003].

MULTIPLE SCLEROSIS

There is no evidence that influenza vaccination increases the risk of multiple sclerosis relapse. Several studies, including a double-blind clinical trial [Miller et al., 1997] and a cohort study [Confavreux et al., 2001], have failed to find an association between multiple sclerosis relapse and vaccination. Influenza vaccination does not induce relapse and should be used in affected individuals.

BELL'S PALSY

Higher rates of Bell's palsy were reported after intranasal vaccination with inactivated influenza virus in a case-control study in Switzerland [Mutsch et al., 2004]. Such reports have not been replicated elsewhere.

Rabies Vaccine

Rabies was the first manufactured vaccine to be used in humans. Early vaccines were grown in the central nervous system of animals and contained myelin basic protein [Hemachudha et al., 1987]. These vaccines, still in use in underdeveloped countries, have been associated with encephalomyelitis, polyradiculitis, and polyneuritis [Tullu et al., 2003]. The rabies vaccine licensed for use in the United States is prepared from rabies virus grown on human diploid cells, and it has an excellent safety record. Rare cases of an atypical GBS are the only reported reactions [Boe and Nyland, 1980].

Whole-Cell Pertussis Vaccine

Before 1992, pertussis vaccination was composed of a suspension of formalin-inactivated *Bordetella pertussis* bacteria (i.e., whole-cell pertussis vaccine). A more purified acellular vaccine was subsequently introduced, and it is the primary vaccine in use (see "Acellular Pertussis Vaccine").

Whole-cell pertussis vaccine has been routinely combined with diphtheria and tetanus toxoids (DTwP). The endotoxin contained in the whole-cell vaccine causes fever and pain at the injection site. Whole-cell pertussis immunization also has been associated with seizures, especially febrile and hypotonic hyporesponsiveness in about 1 case per 1750 doses and with a rare (0 to 10.5 cases per 1 million doses administered) acute encephalopathy, characterized by persistent crying [Cody et al., 1981]. The Institute of Medicine review of combined pertussis vaccine (DwPT) concluded that the evidence, although not probative, was consistent with a causal relationship between DwPT and an acute encephalopathy in the children who experience a serious acute neurologic illness within 7 days after receiving DwPT vaccine [Institute of Medicine, 1994]. Several detailed reviews of available studies by a number of countries, including those by the U.S. Institute of Medicine, have concluded that the data did not support a causal relationship between DTwP and chronic nervous dysfunction [American Academy of Pediatrics, 1996; Cowan et al., 1993].

Vaccines Composed of Live-Attenuated Viruses

Live-attenuated virus vaccines are intended to cause an asymptomatic infection. However, properly constituted vaccines can cause symptomatic infection and the expected complications of the natural disease. The immunity provided by live-attenuated virus vaccines is similar to that from natural diseases, and it may persist for life.

Measles: Rubeola

Measles vaccinations have been in use since 1963. Before routine vaccinations, approximately 3 to 4 million cases of measles and 450 deaths occurred annually in the United States, where no endemic measles currently exists. Most reported measles cases in the United States are imported. Occasionally, outbreaks have occurred in populations that refuse vaccination (e.g., communities in Utah and Nevada, Christian Scientist schools in Missouri and Illinois). To avoid outbreaks in adolescents, a second measles booster is recommended at 10 to 12 years of age [Wittler et al., 1991].

The licensed measles vaccine uses the Edmonton B measles virus attenuated by prolonged passage in chick embryo cell culture that is combined with mumps and rubella vaccines (MMR). Children who receive live-attenuated measles vaccines are expected to develop an asymptomatic case of measles. Some children develop fever, rash, and conjunctivitis in the second week after immunization (i.e., the incubation period is at least 5 days).

Children with vaccine-induced measles can develop any of the known complications of natural infection. The main neurologic complication of measles immunization is a febrile seizure during the second week after immunization [Griffin et al., 1991]. In a large Danish study, MMR vaccination was associated with a transient increased rate of febrile seizures, but the risk difference was small, even among high-risk children. The rate of epilepsy, however, was not increased in such children compared with children who had febrile seizures of a different cause [Vestergaard et al., 2004]. Rare cases of measles encephalitis with neurologic sequelae have been reported to the VICP [Fenichel, 1982]. Isolated cases of subacute sclerosing panencephalitis, a chronic form of measles encephalitis, have been reported among measles vaccinees in countries where measles is endemic, suggesting prior subclinical measles infection [Bonthius, 2000]. Studies that have genetically characterized the viral material from brains of patients with subacute sclerosing panencephalitis have all reported wild type of measles sequences [Barrero et al., 2003; Jin et al., 2000]. Moreover, cases of subacute sclerosing panencephalitis in individuals who did not recall having measles all have identified the wild type of measles. In developed countries with scant or no endemic measles, subacute sclerosing panencephalitis has disappeared in tandem with the disappearance of measles [Bloch et al., 1985; CDC, 1982].

Mumps

The mumps vaccine is administered with MMR vaccination. It is prepared by passage of the Jeryl Lynn strain of mumps virus in chick embryo cell culture. Mumps vaccine has eliminated natural mumps infection, including mumps encephalitis. No adverse neurologic events are associated with the mumps vaccine used in the United States. Aseptic meningitis has been associated with the mumps vaccine used in other countries that use a different viral strain [Arruda and Kondageski, 2001; Suigura and Yamada, 1991]. A total of 10 isolated cases of sensorineural deafness has been reported after immunization with MMR [Kaga et al., 1998; Stewart and Prabhu, 1993]. Three of these cases could be explained from other causes; the remaining cases were unexplained.

Rubella

Earlier rubella vaccines that were grown in various animal kidneys were associated with high rates of neuropathy and arthritis. Since 1979, the rubella vaccine used in the United States is prepared from human diploid cells. The immunologic response it produces parallels that of the natural infection. Up to 25% of people receiving the current rubella vaccine may develop transient arthralgias and paresthesias. Other chronic illnesses that have been reported after rubella vaccination include painful limb syndrome, blurred vision, fibromyalgia, and fatigue [Morton-Kute, 1985; Tingle et al., 1985]. In 1991, the Institute of Medicine reviewed the available scientific evidence and determined it to be consistent with, but not probative of, a causal relationship between rubella vaccination and chronic arthritis in women [Institute of Medicine, 1991]. Studies designed to address this question have not identified an association between chronic arthritis and rubella vaccination [Ray et al., 1997; Slater et al., 1995]. Rubella virus vaccine has been highly successful and has nearly eradicated rubella embryopathy.

Oral Polio Vaccine

Sabin's OPV, introduced in 1963, was successful in eradicating polio in the United States. Because the greatest risk of contracting polio in the United States was vaccine associated (i.e., the risk of wild polio is nil), OPV has been replaced by an enhanced-potency trivalent IPV (eIPV). The overall risk for vaccine-associated paralytic poliomyelitis (VAPP) after OPV administration is approximately 1 case per 2.4 million doses distributed. Among immunocompetent persons, 82% of cases among vaccine recipients and 65% of cases among contacts occur after administration of the first dose. After administration of the first dose among immunocompetent children, 82% of cases occur among vaccine recipients, and 65% of cases occur among contact persons. The risk for VAPP is 1 case per 750,000 first doses of OPV distributed [Nathanson et al., 1979]. Immunodeficient patients, particularly those who have B-lymphocyte disorders that inhibit synthesis of immune globulins (i.e., agammaglobulinemia and hypogammaglobulinemia), are at greatest risk for VAPP (3200-fold to 6800-fold greater than the risk for immunocompetent OPV recipients) [Sutter and Prevots, 1994].

There is no scant evidence that administration of OPV or IPV increases the risk for GBS [Kinnunen et al., 1989]. A population-based study found that GBS in children was not associated with OPV vaccination, because no cases had developed within a month of the vaccination. Moreover, 70% of cases of GBS were preceded by an intercurrent infection [Rantala et al., 1984].

Varicella

A live-attenuated varicella virus (Oka strain) vaccine was licensed in 1995 in the United States, and it is currently recommended for routine childhood immunization for susceptible children between 12 and 24 months of age [American Academy of Pediatrics, 2000]. It is safe and effective in normal and immunocompromised children, and it is being used to protect children with acute lymphocytic leukemia [White et al., 1991] and HIV-infected children (before immune suppression) [Levin et al., 2001]. The vaccine produces a mild case of chickenpox. Varicella vaccination can cause herpes zoster among vaccine recipients, but incidence rates of vaccine-associated herpes zoster are much lower (approximately 2.6 per 100,000 vaccine doses distributed [CDC, unpublished data, 1998]) than rates reported among immunocompetent children (<20 years) with natural varicella infection (68 per 100,000 person-years) [Guess et al., 1986]. Serious adverse events, such as encephalitis, ataxia, seizures, neuropathy, and death, have been reported in temporal association with varicella vaccine. In some cases, the wild type of varicella-zoster virus or another causal agent has been identified. In most cases, data are insufficient to determine a causal association.

Smallpox

Eradicated in 1980, smallpox has again emerged as a potential risk in the wake of recent terrorist events because of its potential use as a biologic weapon. The United States has commissioned the manufacture of vaccinia vaccines in preparation for possible intentional release of smallpox among the populace. In case of an outbreak, individuals of all ages would be vaccinated. The smallpox vaccine currently is recommended only for high-risk personnel (i.e., laboratory workers and at-risk military personnel) and is contraindicated for children and individuals with cutaneous disorders and immune suppression [Wharton et al., 2004].

The smallpox vaccine is prepared from vaccinia, a live poxvirus that causes mild disease, including rash, fever, and aches. The main neurologic complication of smallpox vaccination is post-vaccinal encephalomyelitis [CDC, 2003]. Neuropathologic reports describe cerebral edema and perivenular and leptomeningeal inflammation, findings that are consistent with an immune-mediated response [Perdrau, 1928]. However, vaccinia has been cultured [Angulo et al., 1964], as well as antigen recovered from affected brains [Kurata, 1977].

A comprehensive review based on data collected before 1970 estimates the risk of postvaccinal encephalomyelitis to be at least 3 cases per 1 million primary vaccinations and vaccinia necrosum to be 1 case per 1 million primary vaccinations [Aragon et al., 2003]. The highest risk for developing postvaccinial encephalomyelitis was among infants younger than 1 year (risk ratio = 2.80, compared with vaccinees 1 year or older). The mortality rate among patients with postvaccinial encephalomyelitis was 29%, and among patients with vaccinia necrosum, it was 15%. Among revaccinees, the risk of postvaccinial encephalomyelitis was reduced 26-fold, the risk of generalized vaccinia was reduced 29-fold, and the risk of eczema vaccinatum was reduced 12-fold. Clinical trials of recombinant smallpox vaccine are being carried out. The recombinant smallpox vaccine was designed to be safer for patients with cutaneous disorders, and it is expected to be associated with a lower risk of postvaccinial encephalomyelitis. Compensation for smallpox vaccination complications are covered under a separate congressional act [Health Resources and Services Administration, 2003).

Component Vaccines

Acellular pertussis vaccine and *Haemophilus influenzae* type b vaccine are made from components of the bacteria. Toxoids are composed of denatured bacterial toxins. Toxoids prevent disease but not infection.

Acellular Pertussis Vaccine

Since 1997, acellular pertussis vaccines have been recommended for initial vaccination of children beginning at 5 weeks of age [CDC, 1997]. Acellular pertussis vaccines contain substantially fewer proteins (five) and less endotoxin than whole-cell pertussis vaccines. Acellular pertussis vaccination is associated with fewer local adverse events and systemic adverse events compared with DwPT [Rosenthal et al., 1996]. Fewer rates of serious neurologic disorders are also reported [Geier and Geier, 2004]. In a large Canadian study, no encephalopathy could be identified attributable to acellular pertussis after the administration of more than 6.5 million doses of vaccines [Moore et al., 2004].

Haemophilus influenzae Type b

Haemophilus influenzae type b (Hib) vaccines in use in the United States are based on Hib polysaccharide conjugated to a protein carrier, such as a tetanus toxoid (PRP-T), a meningococcal outer membrane protein (PRP-OMP), a diphtheria toxoid (PRP-D), or a diphtheria toxoid–like protein (PRP-HbOC). The conjugation of PRP to the protein induces a T-cell-dependent immune response to the Hib polysaccharide. The vaccine is administered in the United States during infancy concomitantly with DTaP as repeated doses. Hypersensitivity to the vaccine components is the only contraindication to its administration. No neurologic adverse events have been attributed to the vaccine in the United States.

Pneumococcal Conjugated Vaccine

The first conjugate pneumococcal vaccine was licensed in the United States in 2000. It is composed of purified capsular polysaccharide of seven serotypes of streptococcal pneumonia conjugated to a nontoxic strain of diphtheria toxoid. Pneumococcal conjugated vaccine is indicated for routine vaccination of children younger than 2 years. Before routine vaccination, *Streptococcus* pneumonia was responsible for invasive disease in 188 per 100,000 children younger than 2 years, accounting for 20% of all invasive pneumococcal disease. Rates of invasive disease have fallen 95% after vaccination. The vaccine produces local side effects, fever, and myalgias. No serious neurologic side effects have been attributed to pneumococcal conjugated vaccine.

Tetanus and Diphtheria

Tetanus and diphtheria are toxoids that are produced by formalin inactivation of the toxins elaborated by the two organisms. Both have low rates of complications [Lloyd et al., 2003]. Tetanus toxoid is given alone to children and adults after injury or burn exposure. The only contraindication for either toxoid is a history of a neurologic or severe hypersensitivity reaction after a previous dose.

GBS associated with tetanus toxoid has been reported in one child and one adult. The adult patient developed recurrent episodes of GBS after three doses of tetanus toxoid separated by many years and later developed chronic inflammatory demyelinating polyneuropathy without prior vaccination [Pollard and Selby, 1978].

Infants have been reported who developed brachial neuritis after DTP immunization, and in such cases, the tetanus toxoid has been implicated [Hamati-Haddad and Fenichel, 1997]. The Institute of Medicine had concluded that a causal relationship exists in adults between tetanus toxoid and brachial neuritis based on repeated reports (class III).

Recombinant Vaccines

Recombinant vaccines are genetically engineered vaccines. Hepatitis B is the only recombinant vaccine in use.

Hepatitis B Vaccine

Hepatitis B vaccine is prepared by introducing DNA coding for the hepatitis B surface antigen into yeasts for cloning. The original plasma-derived vaccine is also safe and effective, and it is still used elsewhere in the world. Multiple sclerosis has been temporally associated with hepatitis B vaccine. Initial reports occurred when hepatitis B immunization became mandatory for health care workers in France [Gout et al., 1997]. A few cases of GBS, Bell's palsy, acute cerebellar ataxia, and brachial plexitis have been reported after use of the plasma-derived vaccine [Deisenhammer et al., 1994; Shaw et al., 1988]. Controlled studies found no association between hepatitis B vaccine with new-onset multiple sclerosis in adults [Ascherio et al., 2001; Verstraeten et al., 2001] or adolescents [Sadovnik and Scheifele, 2000] or with multiple sclerosis relapse [Confavreux et al., 2001]. The Institute of Medicine has determined that the evidence is insufficient to support a cause-and-effect association [Institute of Medicine, 1993].

COMBINATION VACCINES AND ADDITIVES

Most vaccination preparations involve combination vaccines. Concerns have been raised that combination vaccines (e.g., MMR) or vaccine additives (e.g., thimerosal) could elicit specific developmental disorders of childhood.

Mumps, Measles, and Rubella Vaccine and Autism

A major debate arose after publication of a small gastroenterology study in Britain of a link between the MMR vaccine and autism. The study of 12 patients found gastrointestinal complaints among patients with autistic regression, 8 of whom had been vaccinated with MMR as determined retrospectively [Wakefield et al., 1998]. The authors have since retracted their conclusion of a causal link with autism [Murch et al., 2004], but not before causing broad repercussions throughout Britain and the United States. Subsequently, several studies [Chen et al., 2004; Madsen et al., 2002; Verstraeten et al., 2001] have found that MMR is not associated with pervasive developmental delay or autistic regression. The Institute of Medicine has concluded after a careful review of existing studies that data do not support a causal relationship between MMR and autism [Institute of Medicine, 2004].

Thimerosal-Containing Vaccines and Developmental Disorders of Childhood

Thimerosal is an organic mercury compound preservative that has been in use since the 1930s. It was contained in more than 30 vaccines licensed and marketed in the United States, including some of the vaccines administered to infants for protection against diphtheria, tetanus, pertussis, *Haemophilus influenzae* type b, and hepatitis B. Thimerosal is metabolized to ethylmercury and thiosalicylate. Theoretical concerns were raised that cumulative exposure to ethylmercury, a known neurotoxin, could have developmental side effects [Thimerosal in vaccines, 1999]. In 1999, thimerosal was removed from vaccines to trace amounts (<3 μg). Several studies [Hviid et al., 2003; Verstraeten et al., 2001] have found no association between thimerosal-containing vaccines and autism. Subsequent ecologic studies reported that after discontinuation of thimerosal-containing vaccines, rates of autism remained unchanged or increased [Madsen et al., 2003]. The Institute of Medicine has concluded that thimerosal-containing vaccines are not associated with neurodevelopmental disorders, including autism, attention-deficit–hyperactivity disorder, and developmental delay [Institute of Medicine, 2004].

REFERENCES

American Academy of Pediatrics. Varicella vaccine update. American Academy of Pediatrics Committee on Infectious Diseases. Pediatrics 2000;105;136-141.

American Academy of Pediatrics. The relationship between pertussis vaccine and central nervous system sequelae: Continuing assessment. American Academy of Pediatrics Committee on Infectious Diseases. Pediatrics 1996;97:279-281.

Angulo JJ, Pimenta-de-Campos E, de-Salles-Gomes LF. Postvaccinial meningo-encephalitis. Isolation of the virus from the brain. JAMA 1964;187:151–153.

Aragon TJ, Ulrich S, Fernyak S, et al. Risks of serious complications and death from smallpox vaccination: A systematic review of the United States experience, 1963–1968. BMC Public Health 2003;3:3–26.

Arruda WO, Kondageski C. Aseptic meningitis in a large MMR vaccine campaign (590,609 people) in Curitiba, Parana, Brazil, 1998. Rev Inst Med Trop Sao Paulo 2001;3:301–302.

Ascherio A, Zhang SM, Hernan MA, et al. Hepatitis B vaccination and the risk of multiple sclerosis. N Engl J Med 2001;344:327–332.

Barrero PR, Grippo J, Viegas M, et al. Wild-type measles virus in brain tissue of children with subacute sclerosing panencephalitis, Argentina. Emerg Infect Dis 2003;9:1333–1336.

Bloch AB, Orenstein WA, Stetler HC, et al. Health impact of measles vaccination in the United States. Pediatrics 1985;6:524.

Boe E, Nyland H. Guillain-Barré syndrome after vaccination with human diploid cell rabies vaccine. Scand J Infect Dis 1980;12:231–232.

Bonthius DJ, Stanek N, Grose C. Subacute sclerosing panencephalitis, a measles complication, in an internationally adopted child. Emerg Infect Dis 2000;6:377–381.

Centers for Disease Control and Prevention (CDC). Subacute sclerosing panencephalitis surveillance—United States. MMWR Morb Mortal Wkly Rep 1982;31:585–588.

Centers for Disease Control and Prevention (CDC). Vaccination: Use of acellular pertussis vaccines among infants and young children: Recommendations of the Advisory Committee on Immunization Practices (ACIP). MMWR Morb Mortal Wkly Rep 1997;46:1–25.

Centers for Disease Control and Prevention (CDC). Smallpox vaccination and adverse reactions. Guidance for clinicians [Dispatch]. MMWR Morb Mortal Wkly Rep 2003;52(RR04):1–28.

Chen W, Landau S, Sham P, et al. No evidence for links between autism, MMR and measles virus. Psychol Med 2004;34:543–553.

Cody CL, Baraff LJ, Cherry JD, et al. Nature and rates of adverse reactions associated with DTP and DT immunizations in infants and children. Pediatrics 1981;68:650–659.

Confavreux C, Suissa S, Saddier P, et al, for the Vaccines in Multiple Sclerosis Study Group. Vaccinations and the risk of relapse in multiple sclerosis. Vaccines in Multiple Sclerosis Study Group. N Engl J Med 2001;344:319–326.

Cowan LD, Griffin MR, Howson CP, et al. Acute encephalopathy and chronic neurological damage after pertussis vaccine. Vaccine 1993;11:1371–1379.

Deisenhammer F, Pohl P, Bösch S, et al. Acute cerebellar ataxia after immunisation with recombinant hepatitis B vaccine. Acta Neurol Scand 1994;89:462–463.

Fenichel GM. Assessment: Neurologic risk of immunization. Report of the Therapeutics and Technology Assessment Subcommittee of the American Academy of Neurology. Neurology 1999;52:1546–1552.

Fenichel GM. Neurological complications of immunization. Ann Neurol 1982;12:119–128.

Gangarosa EJ, Galazka AM, Wolfe CR, et al. Impact of anti-vaccine movements on pertussis control: The untold story. Lancet 1998;351:356–361.

Geier DA, Geier MR. An evaluation of serious neurological disorders following immunization: A comparison of whole-cell pertussis and acellular pertussis vaccines. Brain Dev 2004;26:296–300.

Guess HA, Broughton DD, Melton LJ, et al. Population-based studies of varicella complications. Pediatrics 1986;78:723–727.

Gout O, Théodorou I, Liblau R, et al. Central nervous system demyelination after recombinant hepatitis B vaccination: Report of 25 cases. Neurology 1997;48 (Suppl 3):A424.

Griffin MR, Ray WA, Mortimer EA, et al. Risk of seizures after measles-mumps-rubella immunization. Pediatrics 1991;88:881.

Hamati-Haddad A, Fenichel GM. Brachial neuritis following routine childhood immunization for diphtheria, tetanus, and pertussis (DTP): Report of two cases and review of the literature. Pediatrics 1997;99:602–603.

Hemachudha T, Griffin DE, Giffels JJ, et al. Myelin basic protein as an encephalitogen in encephalomyelitis and polyneuritis following rabies vaccination. N Engl J Med 1987;316:369–374.

Health Resources and Services Administration (HHS). Smallpox Vaccine Injury Compensation Program: Administrative implementation. Interim final rule. Fed Regist 2003;68:70079–70106.

Hurwitz ES, Schonberger LB, Nelson DB, et al. Guillain-Barré syndrome and the 1978–1979 influenza vaccine. N Engl J Med 1981;304:1557–1561.

Howe CJ, Johnston RB, Fenichel GM. Detecting and responding to adverse events following vaccination: Workshop summary. In: Institute of Medicine Vaccine Safety Forum: Summary of two workshops. Washington, DC: National Academy Press, 1997.

Hviid A, Stellfeld M, Wohlfahrt J, et al. Association between thimerosal-containing vaccine and autism. JAMA 2003;290:1763–1766.

Institute of Medicine. Adverse effects of pertussis and rubella vaccines. Washington, DC: National Academy Press, 1991.

Institute of Medicine. Adverse events associated with childhood vaccines: Evidence bearing on causality. Washington, DC: National Academy Press, 1993.

Institute of Medicine. DPT vaccine and chronic nervous system dysfunction: A new analysis. Washington, DC: National Academy Press, 1994.

Institute of Medicine. Immunization safety review: Influenza vaccine and neurological complications. Washington, DC: National Academy Press, 2003.

Institute of Medicine. Immunization safety review: Vaccine and autism. Washington, DC: National Academy Press, 2004.

Jin L, Beard S, Brown DWG, et al. Characterization of measles virus strains causing SSPE: A study of 11 cases. J Neurovirol 2002;8:335–344.

Kaga K, Ichimura K, Ihara M. Unilateral total loss of auditory and vestibular function as a complication of mumps vaccination. Int J Pediatr Otorhinolaryngol 1998;43:73–75.

Kinnunen E, Färkkilä M, Hovi T, et al: Incidence of Guillain-Barré syndrome during a nationwide oral poliovirus vaccine campaign. Neurology 1989;39:1036.

Kurata T, Aoyama Y, Kitamura T. Demonstration of vaccinia virus antigen in brains of postvaccinial encephalitis cases. Jpn J Med Sci Biol 1977;30:137–147.

Levin MJ, Gershon AA, Weinberg A, et al, for the AIDS Clinical Trials Group 265 Team. Immunization of HIV-infected children with varicella vaccine. J Pediatr 2001;139:305–310.

Lloyd JC, Haber P, Mootrey GT, et al., for the VAERS Working Group. Adverse event reporting rates following tetanus-diphtheria and tetanus toxoid vaccinations: Data from the Vaccine Adverse Event Reporting System (VAERS), 1991–1997. Vaccine 2003;21:3746–3750.

Madsen KM, Hviid A, Vestergaard M, et al. A population-based study of measles, mumps, and rubella vaccination and autism. N Engl J Med 2002;347:1477–1482.

Madsen KM, Lauritsen MB, Pedersen CB, et al. Thimerosal and the occurrence of autism: Negative ecological evidence from Danish population-based data. Pediatrics 2003;112:604-606.

Miller AE, Morgante E, Buchwald LY, et al. A multicenter, randomized, double-blind, placebo-controlled trial of influenza immunization in multiple sclerosis. Neurology 1997;48:312–314.

Morton-Kute L. Rubella vaccine and facial paresthesias [Letter]. Ann Intern Med 1985;102:563.

Moore DL, Le Saux N, Scheifele D, et al., Members of the Canadian Paediatric Society/Health Canada Immunization Monitoring Program Active (IMPACT). Lack of evidence of encephalopathy related to pertussis vaccine: Active surveillance by IMPACT, Canada, 1993–2002. Pediatr Infect Dis J 2004;23:568–571.

Murch SH, Anthony A, Casson DH, et al. Retraction of an interpretation. Lancet 2004;363:7506.

Mutsch M, Zhou W, Rhodes P, et al. Use of the inactivated intranasal influenza vaccine and the risk of Bell's palsy in Switzerland. N Engl J Med 2004;350:896–903.

Nathanson N, Martin JR. The epidemiology of poliomyelitis: Enigmas surrounding its appearance, epidemicity, and disappearance. Am J Epidemiol 1979;110:672–692.

Perdrau JR. The histology of post-vaccinal encephalitis. J Pathol Bacteriol 1928;31:17–32.

Pollard JD, Selby G. Relapsing neuropathy due to tetanus toxoid. J Neurol Sci 1978;37:113.

Rantala H, Cherry JD, Shields WD, et al. Epidemiology of Guillain-Barré syndrome in children: Relationship of oral polio vaccine administration to occurrence. J Pediatr 1994;124:220–223.

Ray P, Black S, Shinefield H, et al. Risk of chronic arthropathy among women after rubella vaccination. JAMA 1997;278:551–556.

Rosenthal S, Chen R, Hadler S. The safety of acellular pertussis vaccine vs whole-cell pertussis vaccine: A postmarketing assessment. Arch Pediatr Adolesc Med 1996;150:457–460.

Sadovnik AD, Scheifele DW. School-based hepatitis B vaccination programme and adolescent multiple sclerosis. Lancet 2000;355:549–550.

Slater PE, Tirtsa B, Fogel A, et al. Absence of an association between rubella vaccination and arthritis in underimmune postpartum women. Vaccine 1995;13:1529–1532.

Shaw FE, Graham DJ, Guess HA, et al. Postmarketing surveillance for neurological adverse events reported after hepatitis B vaccination. Am J Epidemiol 1988;127:337–352.

Stewart BJ, Prabhu PU. Reports of sensorineural deafness after measles, mumps, and rubella immunization. Arch Dis Child 1993;69:153–154.

Sugiura A, Yamada A. Aseptic meningitis as a complication of mumps vaccination. Pediatr Infect Dis J 1991;10:209–213.

Sutter RW, Prevots DR. Vaccine-associated paralytic poliomyelitis among immunodeficient persons. Infect Med 1994;11:426,429–430, 435–438.

Thimerosal in vaccines: A joint statement of the American Academy of Pediatrics and the Public Health Service. MMWR Morb Mortal Wkly Rep 1999;48:563–565.

Tingle AJ, Chantler JK, Pot KH, et al. Postpartum rubella immunization: Association with development of prolonged arthritis, neurological sequelae, and chronic rubella viremia. J Infect Dis 1985;152:606–612.

Tullu MS, Rodrigues S, Muranjan MN, et al. Neurological complications of rabies vaccines. Indian Pediatr 2003;40:150–154.

Vestergaard M, Hviid A, Madsen KM, et al. MMR vaccination and febrile seizures: Evaluation of susceptible subgroups and long-term prognosis. JAMA 2004;21:351–357.

Verstraeten T, DeStefano F, Jackson L, et al. Risk of demyelinating disease after hepatitis B vaccination—West Coast, United States, 1995–1999. Paper presented at the 50th Annual Epidemic Intelligence Service Conference, Atlanta, GA, 2001.

Wakefield AJ, Murch SH, Anthony A, et al. Ileal-lymphoid-nodular hyperplasia, non-specific colitis, and pervasive developmental disorder in children. Lancet 1998;351:637–641.

Wharton M, Strikas RA, Harpaz R, et al. Recommendations for using smallpox vaccine in a pre-event vaccination program. Supplemental recommendations of the Advisory Committee on Immunization Practices (ACIP) and the Healthcare Infection Control Practices Advisory Committee (HICPAC). MMWR Morb Mortal Wkly Rep 2004:52(RR-7):1–16.

White CJ, Kuter BJ, Hildebrand CS, et al. Varicella vaccine (Varivax) in healthy children and adolescents: Results from clinical trials, 1987 to 1989. Pediatrics 1991;87:604–610.

Wittler RR, Veit BC, McIntyre S, et al. Measles revaccination response in a school-age population. Pediatrics 1991;88:1024–1030.

Zangwill KM, Greenberg DP, Chiu CY, et al. Safety and immunogenicity of a heptavalent pneumococcal conjugate vaccine in infants. Vaccine 2003;21:1894–1900.

Zangwill KM. Belshe RB. Safety and efficacy of trivalent inactivated influenza vaccine in young children: A summary for the new era of routine vaccination. Pediatr Infect Dis J 2004;23:189–197.

PART XVI

Care of the Child with Neurologic Disorders

CHAPTER 92

Pediatric Neurorehabilitation Medicine

Ann H. Tilton and Maria B. Weimer

Within the scope of pediatric neurorehabilitation, distinct diseases can produce specific complications; these complications, however, can also occur in association with many other disorders. For example, spasticity from injury to the upper motor neuron unit can develop in many neurologic disorders in children. Several of these complications can be quite severe and potentially life-threatening—for example, autonomic dysreflexia, deep vein thrombosis, and heterotopic ossification. In this chapter the major conditions encountered in pediatric neurorehabilitation are reviewed, as well as complications seen in these and other common disorders. Additional information is available in several recently published reference texts [DeLisa and Gans, 2005; Dobkins, 2003; Lazar, 1998; Umphred, 2001].

COMMON CONDITONS CAUSING BRAIN INJURY IN CHILDREN

Traumatic Brain Injury

Traumatic brain injury is a common cause of morbidity and mortality in adults and children. The incidence of traumatic brain injury is 180 per 100,000 in the general population, with 70 per 100,000 considered moderate to severe brain injury (see Chapter 62). Childhood traumatic brain injury results in an estimated 3000 deaths, 29,000 hospitalizations, and 400,000 emergency department visits annually in the United States (children 0–14 years old) [Thurman, 2000, 2001]. Males and adolescents ages 15 to 24 represent the largest group of patients. Although a majority of persons with traumatic brain injury are considered mildly affected, symptoms nonetheless interrupt daily activities [Dombovy, 1997; Thompson and Irby, 2003]. The definition of mild, moderate, and severe head injury is classically based on the Glasgow Coma Scale score or the duration of post-traumatic amnesia (the lack of memory for ongoing events) [Thompson and Irby, 2003]. The Glasgow Coma Scale score examines three variables: eye opening, motor response, and verbal response. A score of 8 or less indicates severe injury, 9 to 12 moderate injury, and 13 to 15 mild head injury. Post-traumatic amnesia is considered to be mild if the duration is less than 24 hours, moderate if 1 to 7 days in duration, and severe if lasting 8 days or longer [Levin et al., 1982]. A complicating factor in determining the consequences of traumatic brain injury is that persons with preexisting behavioral or cognitive difficulty or with prior head injury, are more likely to have a traumatic brain injury [Dombovy, 1997; Luis and Mittenberg, 2002].

In children, the cause of traumatic brain injury is age-dependent. Nonaccidental trauma is more common in children younger than 2 years of age. In children younger than 5 years of age, falls predominate, whereas motor vehicle and bicycle accidents are more common in children ranging in age from 5 to 14 years [Goldstein and Levin, 1987].

The pathophysiology of traumatic brain injury involves a complex combination of forces that has been a subject of substantial debate [Drew and Drew, 2004]. Immediate injury to the brain is followed by metabolic derangements and secondary injury. In addition, there are direct impact injuries and injuries related to transitional forces from acceleration and deceleration. These forces may be linear or rotational. In the classic theory of coup-contrecoup injury, the hard surfaces of the skull cause contusional injury, and cavitation or vaporization of the brain also occurs as negative–pressure gradients form in the opposite poles. Shearing forces are responsible for diffuse axonal injury. In this setting, the patient may not demonstrate major abnormalities on neuroimaging yet clinically will have a very significant head injury with immediate loss of consciousness. The metabolic cascade that follows diffuse axonal injury progresses for hours and is responsible for the often-associated prolonged coma. Following head injuries, regardless of the mechanism, there is release of excitatory neurotransmitters that contribute to the injury [Dombovy, 1997]. The pathophysiology of traumatic brain injury is reviewed in detail in Chapter 62.

Medical Issues

Although the acute issues are largely resolved before the patient is transferred for rehabilitation, there is still a need to ensure that all aspects of general medical care are provided. Patients with traumatic brain injury often have non-neurologic injuries that may be obscured by the patient's inability to indicate discomfort. Bone scans have been helpful in detecting fractures that require orthopedic evaluation [Heinrich et al., 1994].

During the rehabilitation process, patients with traumatic brain injury are at risk for other complications of their injuries. Tone abnormalities and spasticity due to upper motor neuron lesions, as well as the development of deep vein thrombosis and heterotopic ossification, can develop and are a major focus of rehabilitation.

Before discharge, repeat neuroimaging studies should be considered. This repetition provides follow-up of known abnormalities such as previous hemorrhage or diffuse axonal injury. Additionally, chronic subdural hematomas may develop and necessitate intervention if symptoms of increased intracranial pressure are present. A plateau in improvement may suggest the development of hydrocephalus that also requires surgical intervention and may affect long-term outcome.

Behavioral Aspects

Children who have had a traumatic brain injury often have behavioral disturbances, even when their intelligence has not been affected, although in most individuals the behavioral abnormalities correlate with the severity of injury. Post-traumatic amnesia is helpful in gauging the probability of future behavioral problems. With post-traumatic amnesia of less than 1 week duration, permanent and more serious behavioral problems are less frequent than in patients in whom the duration of amnesia is longer. Frontal lobe injury commonly results in emotional dysregulation and cognitive abnormalities [Dombovy, 1997]. Frequently, motor recovery far exceeds behavioral recovery.

Other psychiatric disorders have been described following head injury in children, including depression, mania, and anxiety. Agitation is an expected component of recovery and may be difficult to control. Providing structure and familiar surroundings is helpful as is frequently reorienting the patient to the environment, family members, and others. Close medical and rehabilitation supervision is critical in assessing and managing these problems. Medications most often prescribed by head injury specialists include beta-blockers, carbamazepine, and tricyclic antidepressants. Sedating medications such as the benzodiazepines and haloperidol are used much less frequently [Fugate et al., 1997]. Although stimulants are recommended in the setting of attention-deficit disorder, antipsychotic medications are not routinely recommended for children unless there is an established diagnosis of psychosis (although they are now more commonly being used) [Dombovy, 1997].

A major difficulty for many patients is memory loss. Families should be counseled that long-term memory is better preserved. Short-term memory is a significant issue in the rehabilitation setting and in the community as the patient tries to incorporate new information and strategies. Another well-recognized cognitive problem is the onset or accentuation of an attention-deficit disorder following injury, a complication that can be improved with the use of stimulant medications such as methylphenidate. Use of these medications is reviewed in Chapter 36. Clonidine also has been employed and may have the additional benefit of evening sedation that will help with sleeping. There are few well-controlled studies to help guide clinicians in the optimal choices of medications to use for the different types of neuropsychiatric problems that occur in children with traumatic brain injury [Dombovy, 1997].

Post-traumatic Seizures

A question that frequently arises is whether it is appropriate to continue antiepileptic drugs in children with head injuries. Recommendations in the literature address this issue in adults. If an individual does not have a seizure during the first week after injury, the risk of developing seizures approaches 1% (see Chapter 62). If a seizure is witnessed within the first week, the risk for lifetime occurrence increases to 25%. Structural lesions such as depressed skull fractures, open injuries, hematomas, and brain contusions also increase the risk [Dombovy, 1997]. Children overall do have a higher risk of early post-traumatic seizures than adults but nevertheless have a good prognosis for resolution of the seizures. Five percent of all children have a focal or major motor seizure in the first week after head trauma. The long-term risk of seizure recurrence is 17% within 4 years after injury [Rosman et al., 1979]. Data about adults support the recommendation that seizure prophylaxis does not need to be continued past the first few weeks in individuals who remain seizure-free. One practice parameter addressed post-traumatic seizures in adults with severe traumatic brain injury and found that phenytoin prophylaxis was effective in decreasing the risk of early post-traumatic seizures but that prophylaxis with antiepileptic drugs was probably not effective in decreasing the risk of late post-traumatic seizures [Chang and Lowenstein, 2003]. It was recommended that additional investigations were needed to evaluate patients with milder forms of traumatic brain injury for the risk of epilepsy and the need for antiepileptic drugs. In addition, use of the newer antiepileptic drugs for the treatment of post-traumatic seizures, the role of the EEG, and the relevance of these findings to children were also reviewed. EEGs are helpful in identifying focal epileptiform abnormalities and, if they are present, use of carbamazepine and valproic acid should be considered if the decision to treat is recommended [Hauser, 1990].

Rehabilitation Approach

Rehabilitation of children with traumatic brain injury is similar to that of adults. Therapy is focused on addressing functional skills and the use of strategies or retraining to perform daily living skills, as well as to advance mobility. Whereas the focus in adult patients is on reentering the workplace, the focus in children is on returning to school. An extensive team evaluation of children regarding motor needs along with behavioral, cognitive, and communication requirements is important as they make the transition from the rehabilitation facility to the home and school setting. School personnel need to be included in this transitional reentry process. Support and education of all persons involved in the patient's life are vital, because the patient's relationship with family and peers is frequently dramatically altered by the injury.

Prognosis

Prognosis directly correlates with the severity of injury. Several factors have been cited as prognostic risk factors after major head injury in childhood. These include a post-traumatic vigilance disturbance for longer than 24 hours, a Glasgow Coma Scale score less than 7, increased intracranial pressure with cerebral perfusion pressure less than 50 mm Hg, age younger than 2 years at the time of the injury, physical abuse, and the development of post-traumatic epilepsy [Kirshblum et al., 2003].

Spinal Cord Injury

The annual incidence of spinal cord injuries in the United States is estimated to be 30 to 40 new cases per million individuals. About 3% to 5% of cases each year occur in children younger than 15 years of age [Price et al., 1994]. The male-to-female ratio of patients is 4:1 in the general population, but in younger age groups the ratio is approximately 1.5:1 [Zidek and Srinuvasan, 2003]. Chapter 66 contains a detailed discussion of spinal cord injuries in children.

Etiology and Pathophysiology

Motor vehicle accidents are the most frequent cause of spinal cord injury, although injuries associated with sports activities or related to violent behavior are becoming more common. There has been an increase in violent behaviors as a cause of spinal cord injury in children during the past 20 years from approximately 10% to more than 35% [Zidek and Srinuvasan, 2003]. Spinal cord injury without radiologic abnormality is uniquely seen in children usually younger than age 10 because of the flexibility of the ligaments and lack of stability of the spine. The most sensitive test in this setting is magnetic resonance imaging [Hamilton and Myles, 1992].

Clinical Evaluation

Clinical evaluation of a patient with a suspected spinal cord injury is based on sensory and motor evaluation. Scores are generated by the responses elicited from 28 dermatomes for pinprick and dull and light touch based on a 3-point scale, with a motor strength grading of 10 key muscles bilaterally—5 in the upper extremities and 5 in the lower extremities on each side. The neurologic level is the most caudal level at which sensory and motor responses are evident bilaterally. The American Spinal Injury Association (ASIA) criteria provide international standards for neurologic classifications for spinal cord injuries based on levels A to E (Table 92-1). Key muscle groups, when injured and weak, are helpful in determining the level of spinal cord injury (Table 92-2). Additional information about using the neurologic examination to localize spinal cord injury is provided in Chapters 2 to 4.

Outcome after spinal cord injury is based on the functional motor level. Other variables such as concomitant injuries, the patient's medical history, and degree of home and social support also affect outcome. Regardless of whether damage to the spinal cord is complete or incomplete, the majority of recoveries occur during the first 6 months following injury [Yarkony, 1997]. Individuals with high cervical injuries (C1-C4) almost always require ventilatory support and adaptive equipment, such as sip-and-puff switches, mouth sticks, and head controls. A power wheelchair is needed in addition to a manual backup wheelchair. The patient with a C5 lesion has the capability of having functional arm flexion because of use of the biceps muscles.

TABLE 92-1

American Spinal Injury Association Classification of Spinal Cord Injury

A	Complete: No motor or sensory function preserved, including sacral segments S4-S5.
B	Incomplete: Sensory but no motor function below the neurologic level, including the sacral segments S4-S5.
C	Incomplete: Motor function is preserved below the neurologic level, and more than half of the key muscles have a muscle grade <3.
D	Incomplete: Motor function is preserved below the neurologic level, and at least half of the key muscles below the neurologic level have a muscle grade >3.
E	Motor and sensory functions are normal

TABLE 92-2

Key Muscle Groups for Determining the Spinal Level of Injury

SPINAL LEVEL	KEY MUSCLES
C5	Elbow flexors
C6	Wrist extensors
C8	Finger flexors
L2	Hip flexors
L3	Knee extensors
L5	Long toe extensors
S1	Ankle plantar flexors

Therapists are active in strategies to increase independence and function that are often facilitated with orthotics. Children can be trained so that they can feed themselves and use communication devices. Control of a power wheelchair is possible with use of a joystick or other hand-held controls. A reclining wheelchair is helpful because of the need for pressure relief to prevent skin breakdown. In patients with a C6 spinal lesion, radial wrist extension expands functional use. Orthotics are important to improve tenodesis for independence. Children with a C6 lesion are often able to feed themselves and perform some dressing activities. Power wheelchairs are valuable, and manual wheelchairs can be independently propelled. Patients with injuries at the C7-C8 level have adequate arm extension and improved hand function, which is helpful for improving self-reliance. This functionality is critical for mobility and being able to transfer, as well as for bowel and bladder training programs. The ability to ambulate improves in patients with injury at lower levels [Yarkony, 1997].

The ASIA motor score has been used to predict ambulation as early as 1 month after injury [Waters et al., 1994]. If there is hip or knee extension of at least a trace or of poor quality, the potential for ambulation at 1 year is good. If patients demonstrate incomplete paraplegia below T12, they have a 20% chance of becoming a community ambulator using orthotic devices [Yarkony, 1997]. In some individuals, devices such as reciprocating gait orthoses may be helpful on a limited basis. Because of the high energy and time consumption needed for ambulation, weaker patients often prefer to use wheelchairs for community activities and reserve ambulation for shorter distances. It is difficult emotionally for the child and family to accept the loss of being able to walk independently. A wheelchair may be more acceptable to children, who often place a high priority on keeping up with friends, and they may tire of the limitations imposed by orthotic devices.

Major concerns in the medical care of patients with spinal cord injury are spasticity, deep vein thrombosis, autonomic dysreflexia, and heterotopic ossification. Because of the significance they hold in the care of children with spinal cord injuries, they are discussed in detail later in this chapter.

Other medical care issues that must be addressed include pulmonary function, hypercalcemia, bowel and bladder management, avoidance of pressure ulcers, and prevention of joint contractures and scoliosis. Pulmonary complications are seen acutely and also chronically. In patients with injury above the C3 level, apnea may occur and ventilatory support is required. With high cervical lesions, diaphragm function is partially or completely impaired and the intercostal muscles are needed to assist during inspiration. If the patient has an injury at the C6-C7 level, weaning from a ventilator is usually possible [Yarkony, 1997].

Hypercalcemia is seen in almost 25% of patients 1 to 12 weeks after injury and is due to bone resorption [Maynard, 1986]. Clinically, nausea, vomiting, and lack of appetite occur, and calcium levels frequently are higher than 12 mg/dL. Diuretics are commonly used to treat this problem [Meythaler et al., 1996; Tori and Hill, 1978].

Bladder dysfunction is another common complication, and anticipatory care of the problems associated with a neurogenic bladder is extremely important [Decter and Bauer, 1993; Zidek and Srinuvasan, 2003]. During the acute period of spinal shock, the bladder is atonic or hypotonic, a phenomenon that persists for the first 6 to 12 weeks after injury. As this resolves, bladder tone increases to a more spastic state. Uninhibited contractions are seen and detrusor sphincter dyssynergy is common. This lack of coordination results in decreased bladder emptying capacity, high intravesicular pressures, and damage to the upper urinary tract. Urodynamic evaluation is important, as is recognition that there will be a transition from spinal shock to spasticity. Initially, indwelling catheters are helpful but transition to a program of intermittent catheterization every 4 to 6 hours is much preferred once the patient is stable and is weaned from intravenous fluids. There are numerous advantages to intermittent catheterization, including the reduced risk of urinary tract infection. Colonization of the bladder is common but usually should not be treated unless the patient has symptoms of a urinary tract or systemic infection.

Symptoms associated with a neurogenic bladder may benefit from treatment with anticholinergic medications such as oxybutynin (in children 1 to 5 years, 0.2 mg/kg orally two to four times daily; in children older than 5 years, 5 mg two to three times daily to a maximum of 15 mg/day) or imipramine (in children 6 to 12 years, 10 to 50 mg daily; in children older than 12 years, 10 to 75 mg/day). Botulinum toxin is used to alleviate increased bladder pressure related to sphincter dyssynergy [Dykstra and Sidi, 1990]. In patients who are unable to tolerate these medications or who have persistent bladder overdistention, high voiding pressures, or progressive upper urinary tract deterioration due to persistent vesicoureteral reflux or poor bladder emptying, urologic surgical procedures may be required.

A bowel program should be instituted. Typically, this requires the use of glycerin suppositories every other day, digital stimulation, and administration of a stool softener and, at times, laxative agents. To prevent formation of sacral decubiti, which occur in approximately a third of patients, pressure relief is necessary, and the individual and family must be educated about the importance of avoiding this complication.

As a consequence of muscle imbalance and orthopedic injuries that may accompany spinal cord injury, children are at high risk for scoliosis. If a child sustains a spinal injury before skeletal maturation occurs, the probability of developing scoliosis approaches almost 100%, with 70% of children requiring surgery [Dearoff et al., 1990]. Scoliosis needs to be radiographically monitored every 6 months and orthopedic consultation is recommended. Orthotics are often used when the spinal curve is less than 40 degrees, but spinal fusion is usually required once the child is skeletally mature (older than10 years of age) and the spinal curve is greater than 35 to 40 degrees [Massagli, 2000].

Another common concern that needs to be evaluated and treated is the pain that often accompanies spinal cord injury. This includes radicular pain, musculoskeletal pain, dysesthesias, and physical discomfort such as that related to wheelchair positioning. Multiple medications have been recommended, of which the most recent addition is gabapentin [Zidek and Srinuvasan, 2003].

Orthotics and Wheelchair Requirements

Children with injuries below C6 often have recovery of hand function, and splints may not be necessary [Zidek and Srinuvasan, 2003]. However, wrist extension splints are recommended when there is extensor muscle weakness and if the patient is unable to do a pincer grasp. Adaptations include use of mobile arm supports and universal cuffs for activities of daily living skills. Walkers are helpful for lower-extremity weakness. A swivel walker provides a substantial amount of support in the trunk area and allows the patient to have a swivel gait but does limit the patient to a standing position. A parapodium walker provides truncal support and a swivel gait and also allows the patient to sit. The Louisiana State University (LSU) reciprocating gait orthosis can be used to provide a swing-through gait pattern in patients who have injury at a lower level (Fig. 92-1). It can be used on uneven surfaces but does require independent leg movements. Ankle-foot orthoses are appropriate for patients with paraplegia due to lesions below T6. It was reported that at least 10 degrees of hip extension and 5 to 10 degrees of ankle dorsiflexion are needed to utilize them appropriately. Ankle-foot orthoses are frequently used to assist ambulation in a child with an L5 or lower injury and also for support and positioning of the foot in patients with injuries at higher levels. There are substantial psychologic benefits for a child to be at eye level with peers. However, because of increased

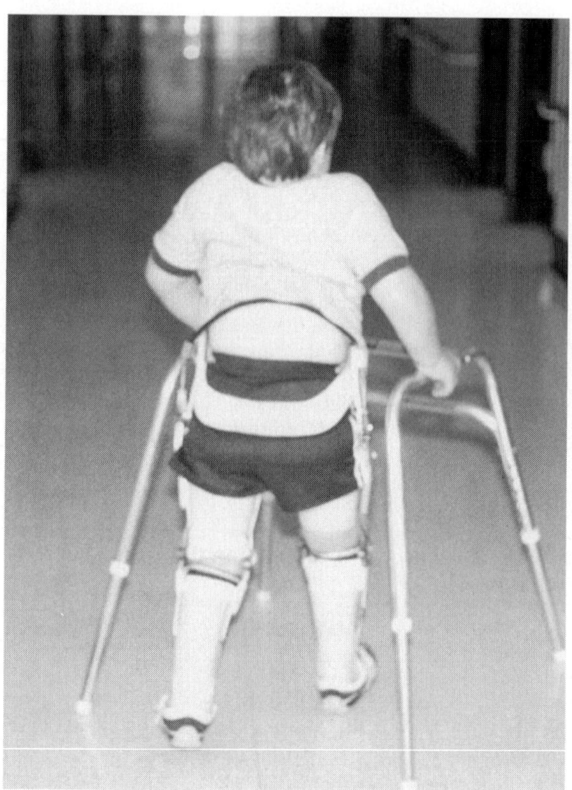

FIGURE 92–1. The Louisiana State University (LSU) reciprocating gait orthosis.

energy requirements needed for the use of complicated orthotics, children often choose to use the most efficient means of transportation, the manual or power wheelchair. A good wheelchair is expensive and often needs multiple modifications to meet current and anticipated needs of the patient. Typically, a manual wheelchair can be used by children when they reach 18 to 24 months of age, and a power wheelchair can be operated quite well by cognitively appropriate children as young as 24 months. A child with C6 level or lower injuries should be able to use a light manual wheelchair, whereas children or adults with injuries above C6 will require power wheelchairs for mobility.

Cerebral Palsy

Comprehensive rehabilitation of children with cerebral palsy integrates the contributions of multiple care providers, the educational and recreational setting, the family, and, most important, the child. The common goal is to maximize the functional and emotional independence of the child and facilitate the steps necessary to accomplish these goals.

In clinical practice, *cerebral palsy* is often a term of convenience, defining a clinical condition [Nelson and Ellenberg, 1978]. Inherent in the diagnosis is that the disorder is static and not progressive. This statement is not to imply that the child's clinical course is not changing, because for most children this evolves to meet new needs, demands, and associated complications. Chapter 20 reviews aspects of the epidemiology, etiology, diagnosis, and management of children with cerebral palsy.

Recent studies have suggested that neurorehabilitation has the potential to affect subsequent brain development. Studies in animal models and humans have found that experience such as specific motor training before the age of 12 years results in increased cortical representation and differentiation [Farmer et al., 1991; Gingold and Iannaccone, 1998]. The developing nervous system may have greater capability for repair, or may possess alternative mechanisms related to innervation and plasticity. This has been suggested by studies that have found spontaneous resolution of motor deficits in patients with cerebral palsy [Nelson and Ellenberg, 1982].

Traditionally, subtypes of cerebral palsy are defined by the pattern of motor impairments that are the main focus as the clinician addresses patient independence. There are now more treatment options to address spasticity, dystonia, and other motor disorders. Certain deficits that affect motor development and influence rehabilitation occur more commonly in children with cerebral palsy [Russman et al., 1997]. The contribution to impairment by the underlying weakness in addition to the symptoms of tone abnormalities cannot be underestimated (Table 92-3).

Physical Therapy

Physical therapy is required to improve muscle function and activities of daily living in children with cerebral palsy as well as other central nervous system disorders such as traumatic brain injury. Regular stretching of involved muscles to maintain full range of motion and prevention of contractures is necessary and, in addition to improving function, can reduce pain. Stretching of the relaxed muscle at least 1 minute every 12 hours is necessary for muscles to grow and preserve elasticity [Reimers, 1991]. Children with mild and moderate disabilities normally are active and want to move, and with parental education many range-of-motion exercises can be met by daily recreational activities [Russman, 1986]. However, impairments may lead to use of compensatory strategies that minimize movement of the affected joint. As a result, the muscles become overcontracted and relatively shorter. This problem is functionally magnified as the bones grow and may increase the potential for a fixed contracture. To minimize this potential, regular stretching of all affected limbs is recommended. Stretching can reduce the severity of tone for several hours, providing a short-term, but not long-term, antispasticity action.

Physical therapy may encompass a regular exercise program, hydrotherapy, horseback riding, use of a hand-propelled tricycle (Fig. 92-2), and other modalities, including cold, heat, biofeedback, and electrical stimulation. The intensity of physical therapy needed to maximize gains has

TABLE 92-3

Specific Motor and Functional Deficits in Children with Cerebral Palsy

MOTOR DEFICIT	FUNCTIONAL DEFICIT
Loss of selective motor control	Impairment in the development of sequential motor skills with difficulty in individualizing and coordinating motor movements
Abnormal muscle tone influenced by abnormal body posture	Persistent abnormal developmental reflexes interfere with appropriate movements
Imbalance between muscle agonists and antagonists	Multiple treatments focus on decreasing tone to allow more functional growth and balance
Symptoms due to impaired balance	Orthotics and mobility devices may be required

Adapted from Russman BS, Tilton A, Gormley ME Jr. Cerebral palsy: A rational approach to a treatment protocol, and the role of botulinum toxin in treatment. Muscle Nerve Suppl 1997;6:S181.

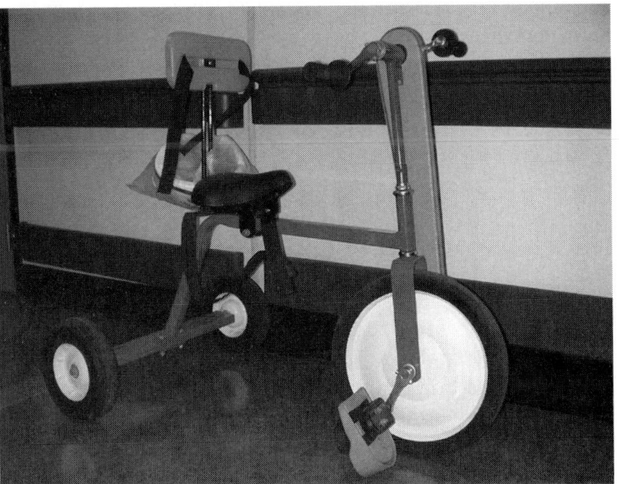

FIGURE 92–2. A hand-propelled tricycle used for exercise activities and mobility.

been the subject of several studies. Bower and colleagues [2001] compared the effects of the usual amount of physical therapy to intensive therapy (1 hour per day, 5 days per week) in children between ages 3 and 12 years over a 6-month period. Differences in function or performance between groups were not found.

Ankle-foot orthoses are commonly used to treat dynamic equinovarus foot deformities in children with cerebral palsy. Gait analysis studies have shown that ankle-foot orthoses can reduce ankle excursion and increase the dorsiflexion angle at foot strike but may not improve stride length or walking speed [Carlson et al., 1997]. Ankle-foot orthoses can also improve sit-to-stand transition in preambulatory children whose standing is impaired by equinovarus foot deformities [Wilson et al., 1997].

In patients with spastic diplegia, posterior balance is a major problem. If balance can be maintained while the patient leans forward, independent walking is possible. If anterior balance is also abnormal, crutches are required. If lateral balance is abnormal, a walker is usually necessary [Russman et al., 1997]. Children with spasticity frequently can walk better with a reverse walker, which offers increased speed while helping with posture [Gingold and Iannaccone, 1998].

Other equipment is also appropriate. Standing frames place the non–weight-bearing child in an appropriate position to help prevent contractures. Inhibitive or serial casting is used for immobilization or prolonged passive stretch. In a child with increased tone and contractures, frequent revision of the casts allows stretching of the contracture to the desired angle. Then the cast can be bivalved and used as a splint to prevent or slow the rate of recurrence. An ankle-foot orthosis may be fabricated to maintain the new range of motion. Serial casting is now frequently used in conjunction with botulinum toxin to treat spasticity and associated contractures.

Treatment Planning

Caregivers play a central role in the day-to-day management of children with motor impairment and should participate in each stage of goal setting, treatment planning, and plan modification. Additionally, the age of the child, the presence of coexistent conditions such as seizures or cognitive impairment, and the ability of the family to implement treatments at home, continue ongoing outpatient care, and manage the financial costs of care and other issues need to be balanced in determining the best treatment.

MEMBERS OF THE NEUROREHABILITATION TEAM

Physical Medicine and Rehabilitation Physicians

Physical medicine and rehabilitation physicians play an important role in the evaluation and management of children with acquired brain injury as well as those with disorders that are genetic or due to other conditions. These specialists provide integrated care in the treatment of neurologic and musculoskeletal disabilities and focus on the restoration of function in patients with problems ranging from simple physical mobility issues to those with complex cognitive involvement [DeLisa and Gans, 2005]. When treating patients with severe physical problems, physiatrists often serve as leaders of an interdisciplinary team that may include medical professionals from multiple disciplines as well as allied health professionals such as physical and occupational therapists, speech pathologists, vocational counselors, psychologists, and social workers. The American Academy of Physical Medicine and Rehabilitation is the national medical society representing more than 7000 physical medicine and rehabilitation physicians; its website is http://www.aapmr.org/.

Child Neurologists

Child neurologists frequently are actively involved in the care of children with rehabilitation needs, and in some centers the child neurologist functions as the primary neurorehabilitationist. Child neurologists frequently assist in the assessment of patients to help determine long-term prognosis, to determine whether patients may have epilepsy, and often to provide input into use of medications to manage some of the complications that infants and children with rehabilitation needs have. The Child Neurology Society is the national medical society representing more than 1500 child neurologists; its website is http://www.childneurologysociety.org/.

Physical Therapists

Physical therapists are very active in the care of children with developmental issues and gross motor delays and have special skills in the selection and modification of orthotics and mobility devices [Campbell et al., 2000]. In addition to contributing emotional support and education of caregivers and patients, therapists emphasize the importance of regular stretching to maintain full range of motion and prevention of contractures. The American Physical Therapy Association (APTA) is the national professional organization representing more than 63,000 members; its website is www.apta.org.

Occupational Therapists

Occupational therapists can help children with deficits in fine motor control, feeding, oral motor function, and activities of daily living. They can help to improve functional deficits related to dressing, eating, and upper extremity function and can also assist with modification of equipment to improve patients' access to their environment [Neistadt and Crepeau, 1998; Pedretti and Early, 2001]. Occupational therapists have roles similar and complementary to those of physical therapists in care of the child younger than 3 years, in which the focus is mainly on family support and the child's development of appropriate postural control and patterns of movement. The American Occupational Therapy Association is the national professional organization in the United States, with approximately 35,000 occupational therapists; its website is http://www.aota.org.

Speech Therapists and Audiologists

Speech therapists and audiologists are important in ensuring the maximum independence of the child by developing communication skills, including both verbal skills and the use of alternative modalities [Owens et al., 2003]. Often children's cognitive abilities are underestimated because of their inability to use traditional testing techniques. Communication boards, sign language, and computer modifications may offer new ways to communicate. Audiologic screening is important to ensure that hearing impairment is not an additional contributing factor to language delay. The American Speech-Language-Hearing Association is the national professional and scientific association of more than 115,000 speech-language pathologists, audiologists, and scientists in the United States and internationally; its website is http://www.asha.org/.

Other Team Members

Psychologists can provide insight into the appropriate educational setting that a child needs and can help the child and family with counseling. Psychologists may address the impact that the diagnosis has on the family and the multiple transitions that the children experience as they become teenagers and young adults. The American Psychological Association, with more than 150,000 members, is the professional organization that represents psychology in the United States and internationally (http://www.apa.org/). The National Association of School Psychologists is another active organization of psychologists involved in the care of children (http://www.nasponline.org/).

Social workers are important in identifying resources in the community to help with therapy, equipment, and funding. Music and recreational therapists utilize leisure activities and music to fulfill the therapeutic goals identified for the patient by the rehabilitation team. The National Association of Social Workers, the national organization of professional social workers, has more than 153,000 members; its website is http://www.naswdc.org/.

SELECTED ASPECTS OF NEUROREHABILITATION

Autonomic Dysreflexia

Autonomic dysreflexia is the acute and potentially life-threatening syndrome of excessive and uncontrolled sympathetic output that occurs in patients with spinal cord injury at or above level T6. Correct and early recognition of this syndrome is critical to avoid the serious consequences inherent in the untreated disorder. Although the best treatment is prevention, if autonomic dysreflexia is addressed appropriately, it can be effectively managed.

Clinical Findings

The estimated lifetime frequency of autonomic dysreflexia varies widely (from 19% to 70%) in patients with spinal cord injuries [Blackmer, 2003]. Symptoms include diffuse, pounding headache with associated nasal congestion, nausea, and sweating in areas above the spinal cord lesion. Hypertension is common and is associated with increased morbidity. When hypertension is present, patients may experience seizures, intracranial hemorrhage, cardiac and pulmonary complications, coma, and death [Blackmer, 2003]. In the practical management of patients with spinal cord lesions, blood pressure during the recovery phase after injury often is low (in the range of 90/60 mm Hg in adults). A pressure that is 20 to 30 mm Hg above baseline should be considered elevated [Blackmer, 2003]. Reports of "silent autonomic dysreflexia" have raised awareness that during routine bowel programs, substantial elevation in blood pressure may occur without other clinical symptoms [Kirshblum et al., 2003]. In some patients, autonomic dysreflexia may occur even if the level of spinal injury is below T6 [Krassioukov et al., 2003].

Virtually any noxious stimulus that occurs below the level of spinal injury may precipitate symptoms. Urinary tract infections and bladder dysfunction due to insufficient catheterization or catheter blockage are the most common stimuli, accounting for 75% to 85% of cases. Bowel distention is responsible for an additional 10% to 20% of cases [Lindan et al., 1980]. Pressure sores and ingrown toenails may also trigger autonomic dysreflexia; fractures, joint dislocations, and heterotopic ossification can also precipitate symptoms in patients with multiple traumas. Lower, extremely deep vein thrombosis, which may be asymptomatic, can be recognized by the swelling and redness that often accompany the disorder. A review of the patient's medications is important to determine if sympathomimetics may be an additional contributing factor.

Pregnant patients are also at risk for autonomic dysreflexia. During labor and delivery, approximately 85% to 90% of mothers with a lesion at T6 or above may suffer from these symptoms [Blackmer, 2003]. On occasion, autonomic dysreflexia may occur after an intramuscular injection, although this is relatively rare [Selcuk et al., 2004].

Autonomic dysreflexia occurs between 1 and 6 months after injury in patients with complete or incomplete tetraplegia [Helkowski et al., 2003], but it may occur as early as 7 to 31 days after acute cord transection, a point when even the deep tendon reflexes are still absent [Silver, 2000]. Autonomic dysreflexia often occurs after patients have been discharged to outpatient care. Anticipatory patient education is very important.

Pathophysiology

Autonomic dysreflexia is associated with the preservation of normal spinal reflex mechanisms below the injury site. Any noxious afferent stimulus, such as a urinary tract infection, distended bladder, or even an ingrown toenail, generates a substantial and generalized sympathetic response. Vasoconstriction below the neurologic lesion follows, with a resultant elevation of blood pressure that stimulates the vascular baroreceptors. Normally, brainstem-mediated afferent inhibitory signals regulate this sympathetic response. However, in patients with spinal cord injury, inhibition of this sympathetic chain response is blocked. Unopposed parasympathetic output above the level of the lesion and the ensuing peripheral vasodilation trigger symptoms of headaches, flushing, sweating, and nasal congestion [Blackmer, 2003].

Treatment

Understanding the etiology and providing education and anticipatory care underlie effective management of autonomic dysreflexia. If symptoms occur, early identification is important. The following approach to treatment [Blackmer, 2003] is recommended:

1. Sit the patient in the upright position.
2. Loosen any clothing or restrictive devices.
3. Monitor blood pressure every 2 to 5 minutes during the episode.
4. If no indwelling catheter is present, perform intermittent catheterization.
5. If an indwelling catheter is present, check for obstruction and irrigate the bladder.
6. If symptoms are present and systolic blood pressure is elevated, treat with antihypertensive pharmacologic agents.
7. If symptoms persist and the systolic blood pressure is elevated but less than 150 mm Hg in the "adult," manually disimpact the bowel. If catheterization or disimpaction is attempted, the application of lidocaine jelly is important.
8. If symptoms persist, search for other precipitants.
9. If the patient is an outpatient, admit to evaluate for other etiologies.

The choice of pharmacologic agent to control hypertension is unclear because randomized trials have not been performed. Nifedipine has been used in a bite-and-swallow technique; more recently, captopril also has been found to be of benefit [Esmail et al., 2002].

Education of the patient and family is helpful and effective. Information regarding recognition of the clinical symptoms and treatment of autonomic dysreflexia is crucial. Because children spend a substantial portion of their day at school, education of school personnel is beneficial.

Sialorrhea

Sialorrhea, or drooling, in children older than 4 years of age, is considered pathologic; when it occurs in conjunction with developmental impairment and disability, it leads to further social isolation and barriers to the successful integration of the child in the home and school environment [Crysdale, 1989]. Between 10% and 37% of children with cerebral palsy have persistent drooling [Bachrach et al., 1998; Bothwell et al., 2002]. Studies of swallowing in cerebral palsy patients revealed incomplete lip closure, low suction pressure, and prolonged delay between the sucking stage and the stage in which foods are propelled into the gastrointestinal tract [Blasco and Allaire, 1992; Lespargot et al., 1993]. Affected children and caregivers often report this as a major source of anxiety. Associated difficulties can range from skin breakdown to life-threatening consequences secondary to aspiration. When families request assistance, the treating physician is faced with the need to find an effective treatment not associated with significant side effects.

Although numerous approaches have been used individually and in combination to treat drooling, none have been universally successful. Behavioral programs and oral appliances have been employed but are not very effective [Harris and Purdy, 1987]. Anticholinergic drugs, such as glycopyrrolate, scopolamine, and benztropine, have been administered orally or transdermally to reduce formation of secretions [Brodtkorb et al., 1988]. The anticholinergic drugs have little selectivity for the parasympathetic receptor sites; as a result, the majority of patients experience systemic side effects, including constipation, irritability, and urinary retention [Bachrach et al., 1998; Blasco and Stansbury, 1996; Mier et al., 2000].

More invasive treatment methods, such as irradiation of the parotid gland, are rarely used because of the secondary risk of malignancy. Surgical approaches have had variable results, with benefits in only two thirds of patients [Burton, 1991; Webb et al., 1995].

Botulinum toxin A has been used for the treatment of many neurologic disorders [Blitzer and Sulica, 2001; Yablon, 2001]. Its ability to chemodenervate at the neuroglandular junction has been recognized, and it has been used therapeutically for the treatment of hyperhidrosis and vasomotor rhinorrhea [Kim et al., 1998; Shaari et al., 1998; Wilkie and Broady, 1977]. Botulinum toxin A has been used recently for the treatment of sialorrhea based on a presumed similar mechanism of action. The duration of the clinical effect of botulinum toxin A at the neuromuscular junction is approximately 3 to 4 months. A longer duration of effect was reported at the glandular level [Jongerius et al., 2004; Suskind and Tilton, 2002].

Several studies have reported the successful use of botulinum toxin A for the treatment of drooling in children with cerebral palsy using injection into the submandibular or parotid glands alone or in combination with other agents [Bothwell et al., 2002; Jongerius et al., 2001, 2004; Suskind and Tilton, 2002]. In some studies the beneficial effects have lasted for up to 4 months [Jongerius et al., 2004] without serious side effects or disturbances of oral function [Jongerius et al., 2001, 2004; Suskind and Tilton, 2002].

Prevention of Deep Vein Thrombosis and Pulmonary Embolism

Deep vein thrombosis and pulmonary embolism in children are rare but may have considerable morbidity and occasional mortality. The incidence in Canada of deep vein thrombosis in children is 5.3 per 10,000 hospital admissions [Andrew et al., 1994].

Clinical Findings

Symptoms of deep vein thrombosis include pain, swelling, and discoloration in the affected extremity. Although it may occur spontaneously, one study demonstrated that 98% of children with deep vein thrombosis had an underlying disorder or predisposing factor [David and Andrew, 1993]. Of 308 children evaluated for venous thrombosis, the most common etiologies were indwelling catheter (21%), surgery (13%), trauma (8.8%), systemic lupus erythematosus (7.5%), infection (6.2%), tumor (5.8%), total parenteral nutrition (5.5%), and unknown (5.5%). Deep vein thrombosis in the upper venous system was usually due to central venous catheters, whereas deep vein thrombosis in the lower extremities was often related to non-catheter thrombotic complications. Children with spinal cord injury are at risk for developing deep vein thrombosis; in adolescents older than 15 years, the incidence was 10%, a percentage much lower than that reported in adults [Radecki and Gaebler-Spira, 1994].

A retrospective analysis of pulmonary embolism revealed an incidence of 78 per 100,000 in hospitalized adolescents

[Bernstein et al., 1986]. The most common risk factors were oral contraceptive use (26%), recent trauma to the lower extremities without fracture (21%), and elective abortion (21%). Symptoms of pulmonary embolism include pleuritic pain, dyspnea, and cough. In children, pulmonary embolism results more often from cardiac emboli rather than from a peripheral vein; therefore, prophylactic placement of a caval filter is not necessary [McBride et al., 1994]. A ventilation-perfusion scan should be obtained to evaluate children for the possibility of pulmonary embolism when clinical symptoms are present [David and Andrew, 1993].

Detection of deep vein thrombosis may be done with invasive techniques such as venous angiography or non-invasively with ultrasonography. Some authors consider that an angiographic study should be done for most pediatric patients with thrombotic complications [David and Andrew, 1993]. In a retrospective review of children clinically suspected of having deep vein thrombosis, only 18% of venograms demonstrated abnormalities indicative of deep vein thrombosis [Perlmutt and Fellows, 1983]. In a prospective study in children, it was concluded that only periodic venous duplex studies accurately diagnosed the disorder in patients with increased risk for deep vein thrombosis [Rohrer et al., 1996]. There are no studies comparing the sensitivity and specificity of duplex ultrasonography and venography in children [Andrew et al., 1994].

Treatment

Treatment of thromboses in children may include heparin therapy followed by oral anticoagulant therapy or thrombolytic therapy followed by anticoagulants [David and Andrew, 1993]. This topic is reviewed in greater detail in Chapter 72. Heparin therapy should be started with a dose of 75 units/kg (maximum 5000 units) for 10 minutes followed by an infusion at 20 units/kg/hour [David and Andrew, 1993]. Approximately 4 to 6 hours after the initial dose, the activated partial thromboplastin time should be obtained to measure the effects of heparin. Except for patients with extensive thrombosis or pulmonary embolism, heparin therapy for 5 to 7 days is sufficient [David et al., 1995]. In children younger than 1 year of age, maintenance heparin requirements are 25% higher compared with older children [Andrew et al., 1994]. Anticoagulant (warfarin) therapy is initiated within the first 2 days of heparin therapy. The protocol for warfarin is a loading dose of 0.2 mg/kg/day (maximum 10 mg) for 2 consecutive days if the baseline international normalized ratio is 1.0 to 1.3; however, if liver dysfunction is present, the initial loading dose should be decreased to 0.1 mg/kg [Andrew et al., 1994]. Subsequent loading doses depend on the international normalized ratio. Heparin therapy is continued with warfarin until a stable therapeutic international normalized ratio is obtained. A protocol and guidelines advocating additional loading doses and long-term warfarin therapy to maintain an international normalized ratio of 2 to 3 have been proposed [Andrew et al., 1994]. The average daily dosing of warfarin and the intensity of laboratory observation are age-dependent. Additional factors affecting the required dosage depend on the nature of the underlying disorder. Warfarin may be discontinued after 3 months unless the thrombosis is recurrent or the underlying cause of the thrombosis is still present [David et al., 1995]. In such circumstances, the duration of warfarin therapy needs to be individualized.

More recently, low-molecular-weight heparin therapy has been used for prophylaxis and treatment of deep vein thrombosis in children. For prophylaxis, the dosing of enoxaparin is 0.75 mg/kg subcutaneously every 12 hours for infants younger than 2 months of age and 0.5 mg/kg subcutaneously every 12 hours for children older than 2 months [Massicotte, 2001]. The dose for prophylactic reviparin is 30 units/kg every 12 hours in children younger than 3 months of age and 50 units/kg every 12 hours for children 3 months and older [Massicotte, 2001]. Target antifactor Xa levels are not needed for prophylaxis unless renal failure is present.

Enoxaparin dosing for treatment of deep vein thrombosis is higher than that used to prevent its occurrence and is age-dependent: 1.5 mg/kg every 12 hours for children younger than 2 months and 1 mg/kg every 12 hours for older children [Massicotte, 2001]. Reviparin dosing for children weighing more than 5 kg is 100 units/kg every 12 hours [Massicotte et al., 1997; Michelson et al., 1998]. There are no published data for the dosing of reviparin for children who weigh 5 kg or less [Massicotte, 2001]. Placement of a subcutaneous catheter may reduce local tissue trauma resulting from frequent subcutaneous dosing [Dix et al., 2000].

When children are receiving low-molecular-weight heparin therapy, antifactor Xa monitoring and dose recalculations are required as they grow and gain weight [Massicotte, 2001]. Target antifactor Xa levels are 0.5 to 1.2 units/ml. Monitoring is also necessary when an underlying disease may intermittently put a child at increased risk for bleeding, renal failure, or thrombocytopenia [Massicotte, 2001].

Heterotopic Ossification

Heterotopic ossification indicates true bone formation in an atypical location such as soft tissue. It frequently occurs in patients with central nervous system insults, such as traumatic brain injury, cerebral anoxia, and spinal cord injury, but can occur after soft tissue trauma or surgical insults [Garland, 1991; Kluger et al., 2000]. Approximately 20% to 30% of adults with spinal cord injury will develop heterotopic ossification [Stover et al., 1991]. In one study of 643 pediatric patients, the incidence of heterotopic ossification was 5%, which included all central nervous system etiologies [Kluger et al., 2000]. In a separate 11-year prospective study of 145 comatose and head-injured children and adolescents, the incidence of heterotopic ossification was 15% [Mital et al., 1987]. Overall, the incidence is lower in children than in adults [Garland et al., 1989].

Clinical Findings

The initial onset of symptoms of heterotopic ossification is variable. In one pediatric study, the average time of onset of symptoms after the initial insult was 4 months (range, 4 weeks to 20 months) [Kluger et al., 2000]. In another study, the peak onset was 2 months (range, 1 to 4 months) after the initial insult, irrespective of etiology [Garland, 1991].

Symptoms include pain, fever, swelling, erythema, and decreased joint mobility [Shehab et al., 2002]. These symptoms may mimic those of a septic joint or thrombophlebitis.

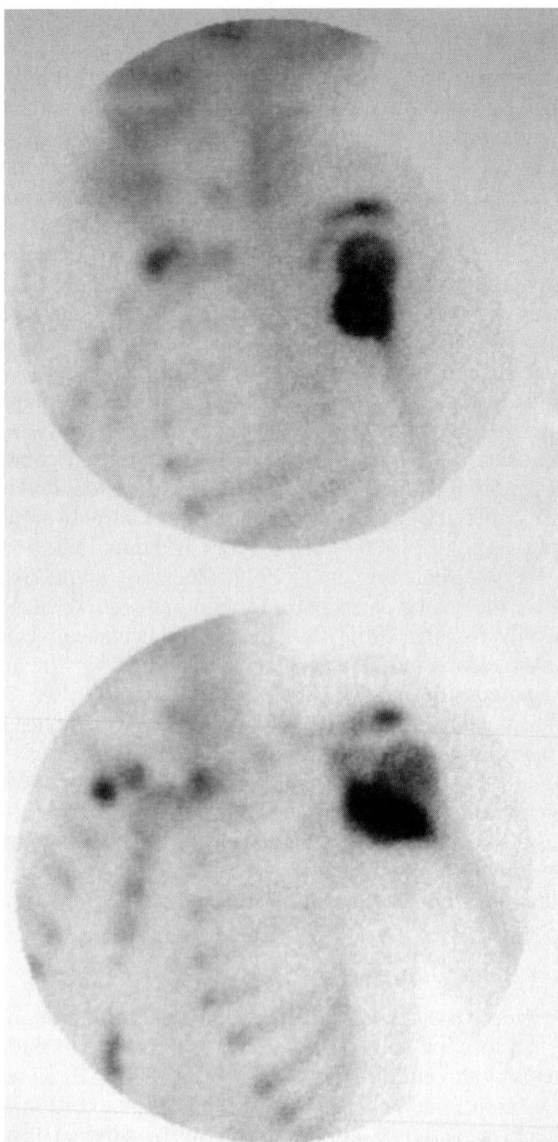

FIGURE 92–3. Bone scan of heterotopic ossification demonstrating radionuclide uptake in the shoulder area where the ossification is located.

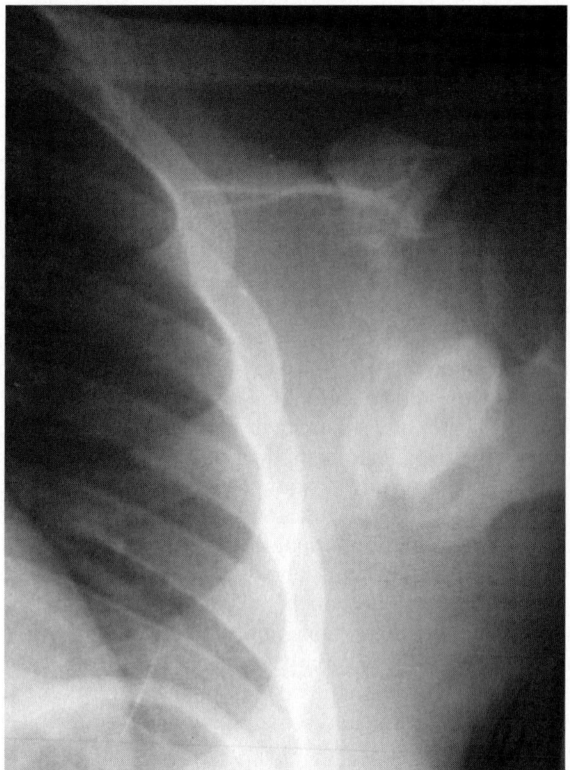

FIGURE 92–4. Heterotopic ossification in formation.

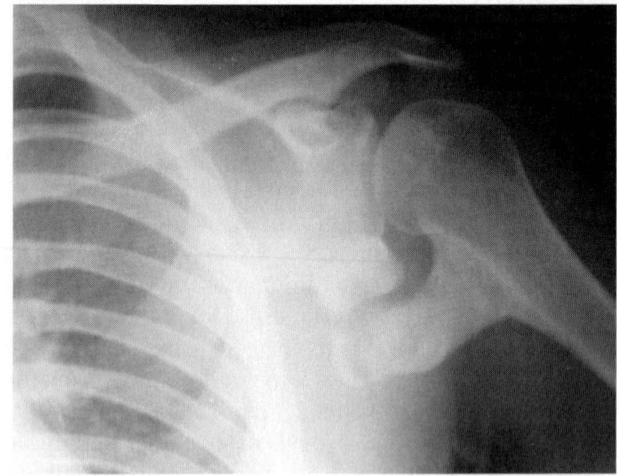

FIGURE 92–5. Heterotopic ossification in the mature phase.

The most common locations for heterotopic ossification are the axial musculature and proximal limbs, but multiple areas may be affected [Garland, 1991]. In spinal cord injury, heterotopic ossification develops only in sites distal to the level of injury [Shehab et al., 2002].

Elevation of the alkaline phosphatase level is a sensitive indicator of heterotopic ossification and precedes radiologic findings of ectopic bone [Mital et al., 1987]. However, alkaline phosphatase levels, which are mildly elevated in children because of incomplete bone growth, may not be a reliable marker [Kluger et al., 2000]. Triple-phase bone scans appear to be the most sensitive method for detecting heterotopic ossification (Fig. 92-3). Radiographic abnormalities lag behind clinical symptoms and may not reveal heterotopic ossification for 4 to 6 weeks, in contrast with triple-phase bone scans on which such changes are evident much earlier [Freed et al., 1982]. This is shown in Figure 92-4, in which early formation of heterotopic ossification is depicted, and in Figure 92-5, which shows a mature heterotopic ossification.

Pathophysiology

Although the pathophysiology of heterotopic ossification is unknown, there does appear to be conversion of soft tissue mesenchymal cells to cells with the capability to form bone. This capability is thought to occur in response to multiple factors including local trauma, spasticity, variations in blood flow with stasis, and anoxia independent of the degree of mobility (i.e., complete immobilization to mobilization with physical therapy) [Kluger et al., 2000]. There appears to be a cumulative effect when local trauma is associated with a head injury, especially if surgery is required [Garland, 1991].

Treatment

Treatment modalities for heterotopic ossification include medication, radiation, and surgery. Salicylates at a daily dose of 60 mg/kg/day for a 6-week period, maintaining a drug level of 15 to 20 mg/100 mL, appear to be a safe and successful measure to avert recurrence of heterotopic ossification [Mital et al., 1987]. Salicylates prevent the continued development of heterotopic ossification when initiated early. Contraindications to salicylate therapy include kidney disease, coagulopathies, blood dyscrasias, and salicylate intolerance. Corticosteroids and indomethacin have been used in adults, but these medications have not been tried in children because of potential adverse effects in already fragile patients [Mital et al., 1987]. Because of the lack of adequate placebo-controlled studies, the use of biphosphates in treating heterotopic ossification has not been justified [Kluger et al., 2000]. Radiation therapy in children with recurrence of heterotopic ossification is not considered safe [Kluger et al., 2000]. Additional evidence points toward the benefit of an aggressive approach to spasticity, including the use of botulinum toxin and intrathecal baclofen [Kluger et al., 2000].

A debate exists as to the benefits and risks associated with manipulation of the affected area. One argument is that mobilization increases the inflammatory response and contributes to heterotopic ossification formation, whereas the opposing view is that manipulation does not affect heterotopic ossification formation but does maintain mobility. Manipulation under anesthesia is sometimes required and provides the necessary range of motion after the procedure [Garland, 1991].

Surgical excision is most favorable when the patient begins to demonstrate neurologic recovery and when the heterotopic ossification is a hindrance to rehabilitation [Mital et al., 1987]. It is important to recognize that to reduce the risk of recurrent surgical procedures, resections should not be performed until complete maturation of the heterotopic ossification occurs, which is usually 1 to 2 years after the initial manifestation (see Figs. 92-4 and 92-5) [Garland and Orwin, 1989; Kluger et al., 2000]. However, when heterotopic ossification severely impedes rehabilitation, earlier resection may be indicated, and in that setting salicylates are important for preventive therapy [Kluger et al., 2000].

Spasticity and Other Forms of Muscle Overactivity

Brain or spinal cord injury may lead to the upper motor neuron syndrome, whose characteristic signs include paresis, loss of fine motor control, and muscle overactivity. The predominant forms of muscle overactivity include spasticity, clonus, flexor and extensor spasms, and co-contraction. In addition, rheologic changes in muscle occur, with prolonged distortion of the normal range of motion that may restrict motion further and complicate assessment and treatment. The combination of these findings varies with each individual and even within the same individual depending on activity, treatment, and other factors. Reduction of muscle overactivity may be beneficial to the patient, but the determination of whether to treat, what to treat, and how to treat muscle overactivity requires a comprehensive evaluation. Setting of realistic functional goals and involvement of the family and caregivers is very important for a successful outcome.

Spasticity

Spasticity is defined as a velocity-dependent increase in resistance to passive stretch. In the clinic, spasticity is elicited when the examiner moves the limb passively through its range of motion; as the speed of the passive movement increases, there is increasing resistance or stiffness. For the patient engaged in normal activities at home, passive stretch may occur during transfers, dressing, and similar activities. Spasticity may interfere with such activities and therefore may become an appropriate object of treatment. On the other hand, some spasticity, especially in the lower limbs, may be useful to the patient—for example, providing limb stiffness for transfers when muscle control is lacking.

Flexor and Extensor Spasms

Spasms of the flexor and/or extensor muscles can occur spontaneously or in response to stimuli. The exaggerated motor responses emanate from abnormal spinal cord circuitry as it is influenced by proprioceptive, nociceptive, and extraceptive input, as well as the descending inputs from the suprasegmental areas [Mayer, 1997]. Stimuli may be external, such as from tight clothing or excessive pressure against the arm of a wheelchair, and may be internal, such as from a full bladder, pressure sores, ingrown toenail, or heterotopic ossification. Spasms may affect an individual muscle, a small group of muscles, or an entire limb. Spasms are often painful and may last from seconds to minutes. They may interfere with the full range of daily functions, including sleep.

Co-contraction

Co-contraction occurs when an antagonist is activated together with an agonist. Co-contraction is a normal feature of fine motor control but becomes pathologic when activated at inappropriate times or excessively. Patients with co-contraction move slowly and with effort and may have difficulty with full range of motion of limbs.

Rheologic Changes

Changes in muscle plasticity or viscoelasticity, collectively called *rheologic changes*, may have a significant impact on muscle function. Immobilization or reduced range of motion can lead to muscle shortening and fibrosis, which together lead to a static contracture, or permanent shortening and stiffening of the muscle [Herman, 1970; Hufschmidt, 1985]. Contractures are among the most difficult consequences of muscle overactivity to treat, often requiring orthopedic intervention, physical therapy, and bracing. Avoidance of contracture is a major goal of treatment.

Treatment Planning for Muscle Overactivity

Multiple factors must be considered in devising a treatment plan for muscle overactivity in children. The first consideration is whether to treat at all, since mild overactivity may not be disabling, and even moderately increased tone may be acceptable if it does not interfere with function, comfort, or care or is not predicted to lead to future orthopedic problems. In most cases, some form of treatment is appropriate.

Factors that must be considered in devising a treatment plan include the distribution of overactivity (focal, regional, or global), degree of overactivity, coexistent conditions such as mental retardation or feeding difficulties, family involvement and abilities, physical and financial access to medical care, and social factors such as educational needs. For example, a child who lives many miles from a treatment center may not be a candidate for intrathecal baclofen, and a child who is going to school may not benefit from oral medications with cognitive side effects.

A hierarchy of treatment goals may provide a framework in which to develop a treatment plan. One such hierarchy [Pierson, 1997] is as follows:

- Reduce pain.
- Decrease decubiti and contracture formation.
- Promote safe and comfortable seating.
- Promote the plantigrade foot under the pelvis for gait, and the plantigrade hand under the shoulder for weight-bearing.
- Promote motor control development.
- Minimize cost, invasiveness, and required maintenance of treatment.

With this hierarchy in mind, choices can be made among the available treatment options (Fig. 92-6). Such options [Tilton and Maria, 2001] include the following:

- Physical and occupational therapy
- Orthotics and casting
- Oral medications
- Nerve and motor point blocks
- Botulinum toxin
- Selective dorsal rhizotomy
- Intrathecal baclofen
- Orthopedic interventions

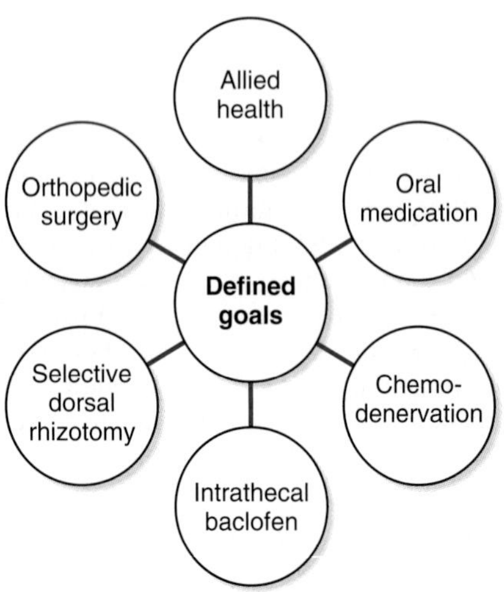

FIGURE 92–6. Treatment options for a child with muscle overactivity. (Modified from Tilton AH, Maria BL. Consensus statement on pharmacotherapy for spasticity, J Child Neurol 2001;16:66-67.)

PHYSICAL AND OCCUPATIONAL THERAPY

Physical therapy begins with stretching, which is an essential part of any spasticity treatment program. Stretching maintains range of motion and reduces the occurrence of contractures. Therapy programs may include motor retraining, sensory reintegration, and strengthening. Occupational therapy includes use of seating and standing devices, communication aids, and other adaptive equipment, as well as upper extremity training. Modalities employed by physical therapists and occupational therapists may include transcutaneous electrical stimulation, biofeedback, and use of heat and cold, as well as the more familiar types of equipment, including orthotics, braces, and casting. Efficacy of any of these techniques is variable, and few clinical trials have been conducted to assess their indications and efficacy. The duration of gains from such treatments is usually several months after treatment is stopped; benefits are not permanent for any intervention [Bower et al., 2001].

ORAL MEDICATIONS

A wide variety of medications are used for reduction of muscle overactivity. The most common are diazepam and other benzodiazepines, dantrolene sodium, tizanidine, and baclofen. Sedation is a common side effect and is dose-limiting. Because they have a global effect on tone, oral medications are most appropriate for a child with widespread muscle overactivity.

The benzodiazepines act as postsynaptic γ-aminobutyric acid A (GABA-A) agonists. Diazepam is the most commonly used agent. A major component of its action is generalized relaxation [Marsh, 1965]. Double-blind, placebo-controlled studies of cerebral palsy have found significant improvement in spasticity, especially in younger children and in those children with athetosis [Denhoff, 1964; Engle, 1966; Holt, 1964; Pranzatelli, 1996]. Diazepam in combination with dantrolene has also been found to be superior to either medication used alone [Nogen, 1979]. Side effects include excessive somnolence, dizziness, mild weakness, and a withdrawal syndrome that may limit its use [Gracies et al., 1997]. Clorazepate and clonazepam also have demonstrated anti-spasticity action in adult studies, with sedation being a limiting factor with clonazepam [Gracies et al., 1997]. Clorazepate is less sedating, but studies of this medication in children with spasticity have not been conducted [Gracies et al., 1997]

Baclofen is a pre-synaptic inhibitor of GABA-B. It is most effective for spinal cord lesions and less effective for spasticity of cerebral origin. A placebo-controlled, double-blind crossover study of oral baclofen in children with cerebral palsy reported significant reduction in spasticity and improved use of extremities [Milla and Jackson, 1977; Pranzatelli, 1996]. Side effects of baclofen include central nervous system depression, confusion, and weakness.

Dantrolene is a unique medication that acts directly on muscle, inhibiting calcium release from the sarcolemmal membrane causing uncoupling of excitation and contraction. Because of its peripheral action, it is less sedating than other centrally acting agents. Dantrolene's side-effect profile has limited its use in children despite proven benefits in placebo-controlled studies of children with cerebral palsy [Haslam et al., 1974; Joynt and Leonard, 1980]. Side effects

TABLE 92-4

Oral Anti-Spasticity Medications

DRUG	MECHANISM	DOSAGE	SIDE EFFECT	STUDIES
Baclofen Oral	GABA-B agonist inhibits at spinal cord level	2–7 yr, max 40 mg; 8–11 yr, max 60 mg; >12 yr, max 80 mg; divided tid to qid; increase q3days	2+ sedation, confusion, 2+ weakness, ± seizure control	DBPC (adult)
Clorazepate	Facilitates GABA	>9–12 yr, max 60 mg/day; >12 yr, max 90 mg/day; divided bid to tid; increase weekly	1–2+ sedation, 1–2+ weakness	DBPC (adult)
Clonazepam	Facilitates GABA	<10 yr or 30 mg, max 0.1–0.2 mg/kg/day; >10 yr or 30 kg, max 20 mg/g/day; divided bid to tid; increase q3days	3++ sedation, 2+ weakness	Open trial only
Diazepam	Facilitates GABA	<12 yr, 0.1–0.8 mg//kg/day; >12 yr, 6–30 mg/day divided tid to qid; increase weekly	3+ sedation, 2+ weakness, dizziness	DBPC (child/adult)
Dantrolene	Interferes with skeletal muscle contraction by interruption of calcium release from sarcoplasmic reticulum	>5 yr, 12 mg/kg/day; divided bid to qid; adult max 400 mg/day; increase q4–7days	1+ sedation, 3+ weakness, hepatotoxicity, GI complaints	DBPC (child/adult)
Tizanidine	Alpha-2 adrenergic agonist with presynaptic inhibition	0.2–0.3 mg/kg/day divided tid to qid; night dosing helpful for sleep; adult max 36 mg; increase weekly	2++ sedation, 1+ weakness, hypotension	DBPC (adult)

DBPC, double-blind, placebo-controlled; GABA, γ-aminobutyric acid; GI, gastrointestinal.

include excessive weakness and gastrointestinal complaints. Hepatotoxicity was reported in 1% of patients. Monitoring of hepatic function should be considered in children taking dantrolene [Katz, 1988; Young and Delwaide, 1981].

Tizanidine is an alpha-2 agonist that inhibits the release of excitatory amino acids and facilitates the action of glycine at spinal and supraspinal levels. There have been numerous controlled studies in adults with spasticity of multiple etiologies, but controlled studies of tizanidine have not been performed in children [Lataste et al., 1994]. Side effects include dry mouth and sedation. Sedation can be beneficial when the medication is administered at bedtime in a child who has difficulty initiating sleep or who has spasms at night. Although tizanidine does not cause hypotension as often as clonidine, it may occasionally have this side effect. Caution should be exercised when using it with antihypertensive agents. Hallucinations have been reported with its use (Table 92-4) [Gracies et al., 1997].

NERVE AND MOTOR POINT BLOCKS

A nerve block is a perineural injection targeting a motor nerve, whereas a motor point block is an intramuscular injection that targets individual branches near nerve terminals. A nerve block offers complete blockade and reduction in tone, whereas a motor point block gives a graded but highly variable response. Phenol and ethyl alcohol are commonly used for nerve and motor point blocks. Electrical stimulation is used to target the nerve or motor point. Because the injection requires precision and may be painful and stressful in children, an anxiolytic or sedation may be appropriate. The duration of effect for motor blockade with phenol averages 4 to 8 months but is highly variable in individual patients [Yadav et al., 1994]. Painful dysesthesia is a known adverse effect, occurring most commonly when mixed nerves are targeted. A randomized, double-blind comparative trial of phenol and botulinum toxin type A for treatment of the sequelae of stroke produced similar efficacy but more ambulation-limiting dysesthesias in those receiving phenol [Kirazli et al., 1998].

BOTULINUM TOXIN

Botulinum toxin is injected into overactive muscle, where it provides a dose-dependent reduction in tone for up to 3 months. The beneficial effect usually begins within 1 week after injection and the peak benefit occurs at 2 weeks. Electromyography may aid in site selection, better targeting, and dose reduction [Ajax et al., 1998]. Botulinum toxin is commercially available in the United States as Botox (serotype A) or Myobloc (serotype B). The two serotypes have different unit potencies, side-effect profiles, and dilution schedules. Both have been used in children with cerebral palsy, although serotype A has been used more extensively. Dosing guidelines have been suggested for botulinum toxin A (as Botox) for adult and pediatric patients. Adult recommendations are available for botulinum toxin B, but studies are ongoing for pediatric patients (Table 92-5) [Tilton, 2003].

Botulinum toxin can be used for reduction of focal spasticity. Its effects are localized but may extend beyond the injected muscle, probably through interruption of synergy

TABLE 92-5

Dosing Guidelines for BTX-A (specifically Botox)

DOSE	DOSING FACTORS	TOTAL DOSE	DILUTION	SITES	REINJECTION
Small muscles: 1–3 units/kg (pronators) Large muscles: 3–6 units/kg (hamstrings)	Muscle mass Degree of spasticity Number of muscles to be injected Prior response to injections Injector's experience	Typical maximum dose: 12–15 units/kg 300 units (child); 400 units (adult) LD_{50} = 39 units/kg	100 units/mL or 100 units/2 mL; 0.9% Preservative-free saline	4–5 cm apart if possible; 1–2 sites/muscle; 0.5 mL max per site	≥3 months

Modified with permission from Tilton, A.H., Butterbaugh, G. Mental retardation and cerebral palsy. In: Noseworthy, JH, ed. Neurological Therapeutics: Principles and Practice, Vol 2. New York: Martin Dunitz, 2003;1617–1629.

TABLE 92-6

Optimal Candidate for Botulinum Toxin

AGE	STRENGTH	LIMITATION OF MOVEMENT	MUSCLE INVOLVEMENT
1 to 6 yrs for lower extremity; ≥4 yrs for upper extremity; 5 to 15 yrs for hemiplegia (younger age recommendations are being studied)	Sufficient underlying strength to allow weakening of the injected muscles	Due to spasticity and not a fixed contracture; demonstrates some degree of selective motor control; has applications for care and comfort	Focal involvement of ≤4 muscle groups or specific muscle involvement with a generalized treatment approach

patterns that replace selected muscle control in the upper motor neuron syndrome. Tone reduction has been demonstrated repeatedly in children with cerebral palsy, but functional benefits have been more difficult to demonstrate [Edgar, 2000; Kirschner et al., 2001; Yablon, 2001]. This difficulty may be due to the inadequacy of current rating scales to measure the highly localized improvements associated with focal injections (Table 92-6). Side effects include development of localized muscle weakness, injection site discomfort, and mild flulike symptoms. Dry mouth has been reported more often for serotype B than for serotype A. Dysphagia is a common problem in the cervical dystonia population, but not in individuals receiving treatment for spasticity.

SELECTIVE DORSAL RHIZOTOMY

Selective dorsal rhizotomy is a surgical procedure in which selected afferent fibers in the dorsal roots are dissected and cut in an attempt to reduce aberrant muscle spindle input believed to trigger muscle overactivity. Nerve rootlets from L1 to S2 are exposed and stimulated. Those rootlets exhibiting abnormal responses (40% to 60 % of the rootlets in the L4 to S1 distribution) are cut [Lazareff et al., 1999]. The operation may be appropriate in children with spastic diplegia, usually between the ages of 4 and 6, and in patients with pure spasticity, isolated leg movements, and good strength and trunk control [Engsberg et al., 1999]. Ability to walk after selective dorsal rhizotomy is best in children who are diplegic and who had good gait scores before the operation [Chicoine et al., 1996]. Intensive therapy is recommended after rhizotomy, including physical therapy 4 to 5 times a week and occupational therapy once or twice a week for 6 months to return motor function to preoperative levels. Randomized studies of selective dorsal rhizotomy have demonstrated improvement in tone and motor function, with evidence that the procedure may be most efficacious in marginal ambulators [Lin, 1998; McLaughlin et al., 1998; Wright et al., 1998].

The side-effect profile of rhizotomy includes complications associated with the surgical procedure. Long-term concerns regarding the development of lordosis and scoliosis have been raised [Crawford et al., 1996]. The risk of developing a structural spinal deformity ranges from 24% to 36% for scoliosis and is 50% for lordosis for an average of 4 to 11 years after selective dorsal rhizotomy [Johnson et al., 2004; Turi and Kalen, 2000]. Although laminectomy and laminoplasty had no impact, older age, more severe neurologic impairment, and preexisting spinal deformity were reported to increase this risk [Johnson et al., 2004; Turi and Kalen, 2000].

INTRATHECAL BACLOFEN

Intrathecal delivery of baclofen allows a much lower dose of drug than oral delivery, greatly reducing cognitive and systemic side effects [Gracies et al., 1997]. At the same time, the dose reaching the target in the spinal cord is much higher, resulting in better tone control. Intrathecal baclofen is delivered via a catheter, whose tip is placed in the intrathecal space, usually at the T11-T12 level. The pump containing the medication reservoir is implanted in the abdomen and is battery-powered and programmable via telemetry from a hand-held computer. The pump has a reservoir that stores enough medication for approximately 3 to 6 months and emits an audible alarm when the reservoir is low. It can be refilled percutaneously. Batteries must be replaced approximately every 7 years.

Patients who benefit most from intrathecal baclofen therapy are those with generalized spasticity and lower-extremity weakness whose spasticity is interfering with function, comfort, or care and those with movement disorders and dystonia [Albright et al., 1991;Gilmartin et al., 2000; Van Schaeybroeck et al., 2000]. A catheter trial or bolus-screening dose may be used to gauge response, but this trial is not necessarily predictive of the functional benefit that may be achieved with continuous infusion. Likewise, the response to oral baclofen is not a predictor of the potential benefit from intrathecal baclofen.

Adverse effects include weakness, nausea, vomiting, and hypotonia, as well as changes in urinary and bowel function. Human error in programming and equipment malfunction are potentially life threatening. Symptoms of an overdose are consistent with those seen in oral baclofen overdose: sedation leading to coma and respiratory compromise. Families must be trained to recognize symptoms of the withdrawal syndrome. Initially, mild symptoms include pruritus, nausea, and return of the pretreatment spasticity. Unrecognized, the syndrome may rarely advance to hyperthermia, severe spasticity, and seizures. Case reports have included rhabdomyolysis, multisystem organ failure, and death [Gilmartin et al., 2000; Green and Nelson, 1999]. As a precaution, families are prescribed Valium or Diastat as well as oral baclofen to have at home. If there is evidence of withdrawal, one of these medications is administered, and the patient is instructed to go immediately to the emergency department. Although aggressive use of benzodiazepines and oral baclofen may be helpful, recognition and return of the appropriate intrathecal baclofen dosage is essential for rapid recovery [Alden et al., 2002].

The withdrawal syndrome is sometimes confused with an intercurrent illness such as a urinary tract infection. An illness or noxious stimuli can increase spasticity and result in fever, but a catheter or pump malfunction must always be considered. Because of inherent risks, families must be fully committed to scheduled refilling of the pump.

ORTHOPEDIC SURGERY

Surgery can be beneficial for selected patients to correct deformities induced by force imbalances across a joint [Morrissy and Weinstein, 2001]. Uncorrected deformities cause pain, interfere with mobility or care, and lead to subluxation. The most common deformity is an equinovarus deformity of the foot. Subluxation, or partial dislocation of the hip joints, is also frequent. Correction of equinovarus deformity is usually accomplished by tendon lengthening or by splitting the tendon and transferring the distal end of the lateral half to the cuneiform and cuboid bones, where it exerts a corrective pull across the joint. Hip joint dislocation correction involves multiple tenotomies and transfers of the thigh adductors, and in severe cases, femoral osteotomy. Surgery may also be helpful in correcting deformities of the knee and the upper extremities, depending on the degree of deformity in these joints.

The best time to perform orthopedic procedures is after a child's gait has matured, usually between the ages of 6 and 10 years [Renshaw et al., 1995]. It is preferable to perform all procedures at the same time to minimize postsurgical recovery and immobility. Postoperative physical therapy is essential to improve strength and range of motion.

REFERENCES

Ajax T, Ross MA, Rodnitzky RL. The role of electromyography in guiding botulinum toxin injections for focal dystonia and spasticity. J Neuro Rehab 1998;12:1.

Albright AL, Cervi A, Singletary J. Intrathecal baclofen for spasticity in cerebral palsy. JAMA 1991;265:1418.

Alden TD, Lytle RA, Park T, et al. Intrathecal baclofen withdrawal: A case report and review of the literature. Childs Nerv Sys 2002;18:522.

Andrew M, David M, Adams M, et al. Venous thromboembolic complications (VTE) in children: First analysis of the Canadian Registry of VTE. Blood 1994;83:1251.

Andrew M, Marzinotto V, Brooker LA, et al. Oral anticoagulation therapy in pediatric patients: A prospective study. Thromb Haemost 1994;71:265.

Andrew M, Marzinotto V, Massicotte MP, et al. Heparin therapy in pediatric patients: A prospective cohort study. Pediatr Res 1994;35:78.

Bachrach SJ, Walters RS, Trzcinski K. Use of glycopyrrolate and other anticholinergic medications for sialorrhea in children with cerebral palsy. Clin Pediatr 1998;37:485.

Bernstein D, Coupey S, Schonberg SK. Pulmonary embolism in adolescents. Am J Dis Child 1986;140:667.

Blackmer J. Rehabilitation medicine: 1. Autonomic dysreflexia. CMAJ 2003;169:931.

Blasco PA, Allaire JH. Drooling in the developmentally disabled: Management practices and recommendations. Dev Med Child Neurol 1992;34:849.

Blasco PA, Stansbury JC. Glycopyrrolate treatment of chronic drooling. Arch Pediatr Adolesc Med 1996;150:932.

Blitzer A, Sulica L. Botulinum toxin: Basic science and clinical uses in otolaryngology. Laryngoscope 2001;111:218.

Bothwell JE, Clarke K, Dooley JM, et al. Botulinum toxin A as a treatment for excessive drooling in children. Pediatr Neurol 2002;27:18.

Bower E, Michell D, Campbell MJ, et al. Randomized controlled trial of physiotherapy in 56 children with cerebral palsy followed for 18 months. Dev Med Child Neurol 2001;43:4.

Brodtkorb E, Wyzocka-Bakawska MM, Lillevold PE, et al. Transdermal scopolamine in drooling. J Ment Defic Res 1988;32:233.

Burton MJ. The surgical management of drooling. Dev Med Child Neurol 1991;33:1110.

Campbell SK, Vander Linden DW, Palsiano RJ. Physical Therapy for Children. Philadelphia: WB Saunders, 2000.

Carlson WE, Vaughan CL, Damiano DL, et al. Orthotic management of gait in spastic diplegia. Am J Phys Med Rehab 1997;76:219.

Chang BS, Lowenstein DH. Practice parameter: Antiepileptic drug prophylaxis in severe traumatic brain injury: Report of the Quality Standards Subcommittee of the American Academy of Neurology. Neurology 2003;60:10.

Chicoine MR, Park TS, Voger GP, et al. Predictors of ability to walk after selective dorsal rhizotomy in children with cerebral palsy. Neurosurgery 1996;38:711.

Crawford K, Karol LA, Herring JA. Severe lumbar lordosis after dorsal rhizotomy. J Pediatr Orthop 1996;16:336.

Crysdale WS. Management options for the drooling patient. Ear Nose Throat J 1989;68:820.

David M, Andrew M. Venous thromboembolic complications in children. J Pediatr 1993; 123:337.

David M, Manco-Johnson M, Andrew M. Diagnosis and treatment of venous thromboembolism in children and adolescents. On behalf of the Subcommittee on Perinatal Haemostasis of the Scientific and Standardization Committee of the ISTH. Thromb Haemost 1995;74:791.

Dearoff WW 3rd, Betz RR, Vogel LC, et al. Scoliosis in pediatric spinal cord injured patients. J Pediatr Orthop 1990;10:214.

Decter RM, Bauer SB. Urologic management of spinal cord injury in children. Urol Clin N Am 1993;20:475.

DeLisa JA, Gans BM. Physical Medicine and Rehabilitation: Principles and Practice. Philadelphia: Lippincott Williams & Wilkins, 2005.

Denhoff E. Cerebral palsy—a pharmacologic approach. Clin Pharmacol Ther 1964; 5:947.

Dikmen SS, McLean A Jr, Temkin NR, et al. Neuropsychologic outcome at one-month post injury. J Neurol Neurosurg Psychiatry 1986;49:1227.

Dix D, Andrew M, Marzinotto V, et al. The use of low molecular weight heparin in pediatric patients: A prospective cohort study. J Pediatr 2000;136:439.

Dobkins BH. The Clinical Science of Neurologic Rehabilitation. London: Oxford University Press, 2003.

Dombovy ML. Traumatic brain injury. In: Lazar RB, ed. Principles of Neurologic Rehabilitation. New York: McGraw-Hill, 1997.

Drew LB, Drew WE. The contrecoup-coup phenomenon: A new understanding of the mechanism of closed head injury. Neurocrit Care 2004;1:385.

Dykstra DD, Sidi AA. Treatment of detrusor-sphincter dyssynergia with botulinum A toxin: A double blind study. Arch Phys Med Rehab 1990;71:24.

Edgar T. Clinical utility of botulinum toxin in the treatment of cerebral palsy: Comprehensive review. J Child Neurol 2000;16:37.

Engle HA. The effects of diazepam (Valium) in children with cerebral palsy: A double blind study. Dev Med Child Neurol 1966;8:661.

Engsberg JR, Ross SA, Park TS. Changes in ankle spasticity and strength following selective dorsal rhizotomy and physical therapy for spastic cerebral palsy. J Neurosurg 1999;91:727.

Esmail Z, Shalansky KF, Sunderji R, et al. Evaluation of captopril for the management of hypertension in autonomic dysreflexia: A pilot study. Arch Phys Med Rehab 2002;83:604.

Farmer SF, Harrison LM, Ingram D, et al. Plasticity of central motor pathways in children with hemiplegic cerebral palsy. Neurology 1991;41:1505.

Freed J, Hahn H, Menter R, et al. The use of the three-phase bone scan in the early diagnosis of heterotopic ossification (HO) and in the evaluation of Didronel therapy. Paraplegia 1982;20:208.

Fugate LP, Spacek LA, Kresty LA, et al. Measurement and treatment of agitation following traumatic brain injury: II. A survey of the Brain Injury Special Interest Group of the American Academy of Physical Medicine and Rehabilitation. Arch Phys Med Rehabil 1997; 78:924.

Garland D. A clinical perspective on common forms of acquired heterotopic ossification. Clin Orthop 1991;263:13.

Garland D, Orwin J. Resection of heterotopic ossification in patients with spinal cord injuries. Clin Orthop 1989;242:169.

Garland D, Shimoyama S, Lugo C, et al. Spinal cord insults and heterotopic ossification in the pediatric population. Clin Orthop 1989;245:303.

Gilmartin R, Bruce D, Abbott R, et al. Intrathecal baclofen for the management of spastic cerebral palsy: Multicenter trial. J Child Neurol 2000;15:71.

Gingold M, Iannaccone ST. Cerebral palsy and developmental disabilities. In: Lazar RB, ed. Principles of Neurologic Rehabilitation. New York: McGraw-Hill, 1998.

Goldstein F, Levin HS. Epidemiology of pediatric closed head injury: Incidence, clinical characteristics and risk factors. J Learn Dis 1987;20:518.

Gracies JM, Elovic E, McGuire J, et al. Traditional pharmacological treatments for spasticity part I: Local treatments. Muscle Nerve 1997;20:S61.

Gracies JM, Nance P, Elovic E, et al. Traditional pharmacological treatments for spasticity part II: general and regional treatments. Muscle Nerve 1997;20:S92.

Green LB, Nelson VS. Death after withdrawal of intrathecal baclofen: Case report and literature review. Arch Phys Med Rehabil 1999;80:1600.

Hamilton MG, Myles ST. Pediatric spinal injury: Review of 174 hospital admissions. J Neurosurg 1992;77:700.

Harris SR, Purdy AH. Drooling and its management in cerebral palsy. Dev Med Child Neurol 1987;29:805.

Haslam RH, Walcher JR, Leitman PS. Dantrolene sodium in children with spasticity. Arch Phys Med Rehabil 1974;55:384.

Hauser WA. Prevention of post-traumatic epilepsy. N Eng J Med 1990;323:540.

Heinrich SD, Gallagher D, Harris M, et al. Undiagnosed fractures in severely injured children and young adults. Identification with technetium imaging. J Bone Joint Surg 1994;76:561.

Helkowski WM, Ditunno JF Jr, Boninger M. Autonomic dysreflexia: Incidence in persons with neurologically complete and incomplete tetraplegia. J Spinal Cord Med 2003;26:244.

Herman R. The myotactic reflex: Clinicophysiological aspects of spasticity and contracture. Brain 1970;93:273.

Holt KS. The use of diazepam in childhood cerebral palsy. Report of a small study including electromyographic observations. Ann Phys Med 1964;Suppl:16.

Hufschmidt A. Chronic transformation of muscle in spasticity: A peripheral contribution to increased tone. J Neurol Neurosurg Psychiatry 1985;48:676.

Johnson M, Goldstein L, Thomas S, et al. Spinal deformity after selective dorsal rhizotomy in ambulatory patients with cerebral palsy. J Pediatr Orthop 2004;24:529.

Jongerius PH, Rotteveel JJ, van den Hoogen F, et al. Botulinum toxin A: A new option for treatment of drooling in children with cerebral palsy. Presentation of a case. Eur J Pediatr 2001;160:509.

Jongerius PH, van den Hoogen F, van Limbeek J, et al. Effect of botulinum toxin in the treatment of drooling: A controlled clinical trial. Pediatrics 2004;114:620.

Joynt RL, Leonard JA. Dantrolene sodium suspension in treatment of spastic cerebral palsy. Dev Med Child Neurol 1980;22:755.

Katz RT. Management of spasticity. Am J Phys Med Rehabil 1988;67:108.

Kim KS, Kim SS, Yoon JH, et al. The effects of botulinum toxin type A injections for intrinsic rhinitis. J Laryngol Otol 1998;112.

Kirazli Y, Yagiz A, Kismali B, et al. Comparison of phenol block and botulinum toxin type A in the treatment of spastic foot after stroke. Am J Phys Med Rehabil 1998;77:510.

Kirschner J, Berweck S, Mall V, et al. Botulinum toxin treatment in cerebral palsy: Evidence for a new option. J Neurol 2001;248:28.

Kirshblum SC, House JG, O'Connor KC. Silent autonomic dysreflexia during a routine bowel program in persons with traumatic spinal cord injury: A preliminary study. Arch Phys Med Rehabil 2003;83:1774.

Kluger G, Kochs A, Holthausen H. Heterotopic ossification in childhood and adolescence. J Child Neurol 2000;15:406.

Krassioukov AV, Furlan JC, Fehlings MG. Autonomic dysreflexia in acute spinal cord injury: An under-recognized clinical entity. J Neurotrama 2003;20:707.

Lataste X, Emre M, Davis C, et al. Comparative profile of tizanidine in the management of spasticity. Neurosurgery 1994;44:S53.

Lazar RB. Principles of Neurologic Rehabilitation. New York: McGraw-Hill, 1998.

Lazareff JA, Garcia-Mendez MA, De Rosa R, et al. Limited (L4-S1, L5-S1) selective dorsal rhizotomy for reducing spasticity in cerebral palsy. Acta Neurochirurgica 1999;141:743.

Lespargot A, Langevin MF, Muller S, et al. Swallowing disturbances associated with drooling in cerebral palsied children. Dev Med Child Neurol 1993;35:298.

Levin HS, Benton AL, Grossman RG. Neurobehavioral Consequences of Closed Head Injury. New York: Oxford University Press, 1982.

Lin JP. Dorsal rhizotomy and physical therapy. Dev Med Child Neurol 1998;40:219.

Lindan R, Joiner E, Freehafer A, et al. Incidence and clinical features of autonomic dysreflexia in patients with spinal cord injury. Paraplegia 1980;18:285.

Luis CA, Mittenberg W. Mood and anxiety disorders following pediatric traumatic brain injury: a prospective study. J Clin Exp Neuropsychol 2002;24:270.

Marsh HO. Diazepam in incapacitating cerebral palsied children. JAMA 1965;191:797.

Massagli TL. Medical and rehabilitation issues in the care of children with spinal cord injury. Phys Med Rehabil Clin N Am 2000;11:169.

Massicotte MP. Low-molecular-weight heparin therapy in children. J Pediatr Hematol Oncol 2001;23:189.

Massicotte MP, Adams M, Leaker M, et al. A nomogram to establish therapeutic levels of the low molecular weight heparin (LMWH), Clivarine in children requiring treatment for venous thromboembolism (VTE). Thromb Haemost 1997;Suppl:282.

Mayer NH. Clinicophysiologic concepts of spasticity and motor dysfunction in adults with an upper motor neuron lesion. Muscle Nerve Suppl 1997; 6:S1.

Maynard FM. Immobilization hypercalcemia following spinal cord injury. Arch Phys Med Rehabil 1986;67:41.

McBride WJ, Gadowski GR, Keller MS, et al. Pulmonary embolism in pediatric trauma patients. J Trauma 1994;37:913.

McLaughlin JF, Bjornson KF, Astley SJ, et al. Selective dorsal rhizotomy: Efficacy and safety in an investigator-masked randomized clinical trial. Dev Med Child Neurol 1998;40:220.

Meythaler JM, DeVivo MJ, Hadley MN. Prospective study on the use of bolus intrathecal baclofen for spastic hypertonia due to acquired brain injury. Arch Phys Med Rehabil 1996;77:461.

Michelson AD, Bovill E, Monagle P, et al. Antithrombotic therapy in children. Chest 1998;114:748S.

Mier RJ, Bachrach SJ, Lakin RC, et al. Treatment of sialorrhea with glycopyrrolate. A double-blind, dose-ranging study. Arch Pediatr Adolesc Med 2000;154:1214.

Milla PJ, Jackson ADM. A controlled trial of baclofen in children with cerebral palsy. J Int Med Res 1977;5:398.

Mital M, Garber J, Stinson J. Ectopic bone formation in children and adolescents with head injuries: Its management. J Pediatr Orthop 1987;7:83.

Morrissy R, Weinstein SL. Lovell and Winter's Pediatric Orthopaedics. Philadelphia: Lippincott Williams & Wilkins, 2001.

Neistadt ME, Crepeau E. Occupational Therapy. Philadelphia: Lippincott Williams & Wilkins, 1998.

Nelson K, Ellenberg J. Children who "outgrew" cerebral palsy. Pediatrics 1982:69:529.

Nelson KB, Ellenberg JH. Epidemiology of cerebral palsy. Adv Neurol 1978;19:421.

Nogen AG. Effect of dantrolene sodium on the incidence of seizures in children with spasticity. Childs Brain 1979;5:420.

Owens RE, Metz DE, Haas A. Introduction to Communication Disorders: A Life Span Perspective. In: Dragin SD, ed. Boston: Pearson Education, 2003.

Pedretti L, Early MB. Occupational Therapy—Practice for Physical Dysfunction. St Louis: Mosby, 2001.

Perlmutt L, Fellows K. Lower extremity deep vein thrombosis in children. Pediatr Radiol 1983;13:266.

Pierson SH. Outcome measures in spasticity management. Muscle Nerve 1997;20:S36.

Pranzatelli MR. Oral pharmacotherapy for the movement disorders of cerebral palsy. J Child Neurol 1996;11:S13.

Price C, Makintubee S, Herndon W, et al. Epidemiology of traumatic spinal cord injury and acute hospitalization and rehabilitation charges for spinal cord injuries in Oklahoma, 1988-1990. Am J Epidemiol 1994;139:37.

Radecki RT, Gaebler-Spira DJ. Deep vein thrombosis in the disabled pediatric population. Arch Phys Med Rehabil 1994;75:248.

Reimers J. Clinically based decision making for surgery. In: Sussman MD, ed. The Diplegic Child: Evaluation and Management. Rosemont: American Academy of Orthopedic Surgeons, 1991.

Renshaw TS, Green NE, Griffin PP, et al. Cerebral palsy: Orthopaedic management. J Bone Joint Surg 1995;77-A:1590.

Rohrer MJ, Cutler BS, MacDougall E, et al. A prospective study of the incidence of deep venous thrombosis in hospitalized children. J Vasc Surg 1996;24:46.

Rosman NP, Herskowitz J, Carter AP, et al. Acute head trauma in infancy and childhood. Pediatr Clin N Am 1979;26:707.

Russman BS. Are infant stimulation programs useful ? Arch Neurol 1986;43:282.

Russman BS, Tilton A, Gormley ME Jr. Cerebral palsy: A rational approach to a treatment protocol, and the role of botulinum toxin in treatment. Muscle Nerve Suppl 1997;6:S181.

Selcuk B, Inanir M, Kurtaran A, et al. Autonomic dysreflexia after intramuscular injection in traumatic tetraplegia: A case report. Am J Phys Med Rehabil 2004;83:61.

Shaari CM, Wu B, Biller HF, et al. Botulinum toxin decreases salivation from canine submandibular glands. Otolaryngol Head Neck Surg 1998;118:452.

Shehab D, Elgazzar A, Collier B. Heterotopic ossification. J Nucl Med 2002;43:346.

Silver JR. Early autonomic dysreflexia. Spinal Cord 2000;38:229.

Stover SL, Niemann KM, Tulloss JR. Experience with surgical resection of heterotopic bone in spinal cord injury patients. Clin Orthop 1991;263:71.

Suskind DL, Tilton AH. Clinical study of botulinum-A toxin in the treatment of sialorrhea in children with cerebral palsy. Laryngoscope 2002;112:73.

Thompson MD, Irby JW. Recovery from mild head injury in pediatric populations. Semin Pediatr Neurol 2003;10:130.

Thurman DJ. Traumatic brain injury (TBI) in the United States: Assessing outcomes in children. Appendix B. Centers for Disease Control and Prevention, 2000.

Thurman DJ. Epidemiology and economics of head trauma. In: Miller LP, Hayes R, eds. Head trauma: Basic preclinical and clinical directions, New York: Wiley-Liss, 2001.

Tilton AH. Injectable neuromuscular blockade in the treatment of spasticity and movement disorders. J Child Neurol 2003;18:S50.

Tilton AH, Maria BL. Consensus statement on pharmacotherapy for spasticity. J Child Neurol 2001;16:66.

Tori JA, Hill LL. Hypercalcemia in children with spinal cord injury. Arch Phys Med Rehabil 1978;59:444.

Turi M, Kalen V. The risk of spinal deformity after selective dorsal rhizotomy. J Pediatr Orthop 2000;20:104.

Umphred DA. Neurologic rehabilitation. Philadelphia: WB Saunders, 2001, p 1038.

Van Schaeybroeck P, Nuttin B, Lagae L, et al. Intrathecal baclofen for intractable cerebral spasticity: A prospective placebo-controlled, double-blind study. Neurosurgery 2000;46:603.

Waters RL, Adkins RH, Yarkur JS. Motor and sensory recovery following incomplete paraplegia. Arch Phys Med Rehabil 1994;75:67.

Webb K, Reddihough DS, Johnson H, et al. Long-term outcome of saliva-control surgery. Dev Med Child Neurol 1995;37:755.

Wilkie TF, Broady GS. The surgical treatment of drooling: A ten-year review. Plast Reconstr Surg 1977;59:791.

Wilson H, Haideri N, Song K, et al. Ankle foot orthoses for preambulatory children with spastic diplegia. J Pediatr Orthop 1997;17:370.

Wright F, Sheil EM, Drake JM, et al. Evaluation of selective dorsal rhizotomy for the reduction of spasticity in cerebral palsy: A randomized control study. Dev Med Child Neurol 1998;40:239.

Yablon S. Botulinum neurotoxin intramuscular chemodenervation. Role in the management of spastic hypertonia and related motor disorders. Phys Med Rehabil Clin N Am 2001;12:833.

Yadav SL, Singh U, Dureja GP. Phenol block in the management of spastic cerebral palsy. Indian J Pediatr 1994;61:249.

Yarkony GM. Spinal cord injury rehabilitation. In: Lazar RB, ed. Principles of Neurologic Rehabilitation. New York: McGraw-Hill, 1997, p 121.

Young RR, Delwaide PJ. Drug therapy: Spasticity (first of two parts). N Engl J Med 1981;304:28.

Zidek K, Srinuvasan R. Rehabilitation of a child with spinal cord injury. Semin Pediatr Neurol 2003;10:140.

CHAPTER 93

Pain Management and Palliative Care

John Colin Partridge

PAIN MANAGEMENT

Pain has been defined as "an unpleasant sensory and emotional experience associated with actual or potential tissue damage, or described in terms of such damage" [International Association for the Study of Pain, 1979]. The stimulus can be thermal (heat or cold), chemical (acid or alkali), or mechanical (torsion, stretch, pinch, or prick). Nociception, or pain perception, is the series of electrochemical events following tissue damage or injury, excluding any emotional correlates of the noxious sensation. Acute pain occurs in a wide variety of pediatric medical encounters, and chronic pain in one form or another affects an estimated 15% to 20% of children [Goodman and McGrath, 1991]. Pain can be effectively relieved in 90% of patients; nevertheless, only 20% of patients achieve effective pain relief [Ferrel and Rhiner, 1991]. Many studies demonstrate that neonates, infants, and children can safely receive analgesia and anesthesia [Anand et al., 1999; Polaner, 2001; Shah and Ohlsson, 2002; Stevens et al., 2000; Taddio, 2002].

Historical Background

Studies from the 1970s into the 1990s documented undertreatment of pediatric patients undergoing uncomfortable diagnostic (e.g., lumbar puncture) or major surgical procedures (e.g., amputations, nephrectomies, and atrial septal defect repairs) [Bauchner, 1991; Schechter, 1989; Schechter et al., 1986]. Despite an increased number of studies documenting adverse effects of pain over the past two decades, misinformation about pain and nociception in very young children and neonates prevailed until recently. Contrary to prevalent myths, newborn infants have the neurophysiologic basis necessary to experience and remember pain [Anand and Hickey, 1992; Grunau et al., 1994a, 1994b; Taddio et al., 1997]. Fortunately, pain assessment and attention to treatment of painful symptoms are now standards of care for patients of all ages [Joint Commission on Accreditation of Healthcare Organizations, 2001].

Physiology

The physiology of pain perception has been reviewed [Anand and Carr, 1989]. Nociceptors present in mucosal membranes, cornea, subcutaneous tissue, bone and teeth, joints, and muscle detect noxious or potentially noxious thermal, chemical, and mechanical stimuli. A noxious stimulus is translated into electrical sensory nerve activity, and the sensory information is transmitted to the central nervous system via several fiber types: (1) A-beta (moderately myelinated, fast-conducting) fibers carry impulses from pressure/position sensors; (2) A-delta (moderately myelinated, fast-conducting) fibers carry impulses from high-threshold mechanoreceptors and polymodal peripheral sensory neurons that respond to pressure and temperature; and (3) C-fibers (unmyelinated, slow-conducting) carry impulses from cutaneous and deep, low-threshold mechanoreceptors, chemoreceptors, and thermoreceptors. A-delta fibers carry sharp, spatially distinct pain signals, whereas C-fibers carry diffuse pain signals. A-beta fibers signal nonpainful touch and pressure that can compete with nociception. Peripherally, the sensory process can be influenced by local release of inflammatory mediators that sensitize neurons and recruit silent receptors, resulting in hyperalgesia. The majority of peripheral sensory neurons have cell bodies in the dorsal root ganglion, with some afferent input transmitted through the ventral root. Entering through the dorsal root, these fibers separate into A and C fiber bundles in the medial and lateral divisions of the dorsolateral fasciculus and form synapses within the laminae of spinal cord gray matter. Neurons within the laminae synapse with the peripheral sensory neurons and relay information via ascending tracts to various portions of the brain. The long ascending tracts make monosynaptic or polysynaptic reflex connections with lower motor neurons in the ventral horns and have projections to higher brain centers. In the brain, secondary neurons terminate in the medulla, midbrain, periaqueductal gray matter, hypothalamus, thalamus, and cortex. Sensory signals can be amplified by neuronal activation in the periphery or the spinal cord by inflammatory mediators (bradykinin, cytokines, catecholamines, and substance P) or they can be attenuated by competitive stimulation of A-beta fibers. Afferent impulses can be amplified in the spinal cord by substance P or neurokinin A or they can be attenuated by endogenous opioids (endorphins, dynorphins and enkephalins) and serotonergic, noradrenergic, cholinergic and GABA-ergic compounds. Opioid receptors, present in the spinal cord, limbic system, midbrain respiratory centers, and periphery, respond to stereospecific endogenous opioids to produce analgesia, as well as side effects (euphoria/dysphoria, respiratory depression, decreased gastrointestinal motility, bradycardia/tachycardia, and dependency). Several anatomic pathways also inhibit peripheral sensory input, including the cortex, thalamus, periaqueductal gray matter, medulla and dorsolateral funiculus via inhibitory effects of norepinephrine, endogenous opioids, GABA, and acetylcholine.

Developmental Differences

Fetal stress responses to painful stimuli have been documented as early as 18 weeks of gestation, with peripheral, spinal, and suprapinal capacity for afferent pain transmission by 26 weeks [Klimach and Cooke, 1988]. At this age, newborns can mount behavioral, autonomic, and metabolic stress responses to tissue injury [Anand et al., 1987]. Neonates demonstrate characteristic facial expressions, aversive body movements, alterations in cardiac activity, and changes in their cry in response to painful stimuli [Fitzgerald and Anand, 1993]. Nociceptive nerve endings are fewer in number in children than in adults; therefore, tissue damage may be more significant before a pain response is elicited. Young infants may perceive pain more intensely than older children or adults because descending inhibitory pathways develop later than afferent excitatory pathways [Fitzgerald and Koltenburg, 1986; Franck et al., 2000]. Inadequately treated pain in premature infants is associated with adverse short-term effects (e.g., more postoperative complications) [Anand and Hickey, 1992]; the accompanying physiologic changes (increased heart rate and blood pressure, cardiac variability, hypoxemia, changes in autonomic tone, increased venous pressure, increased cerebral blood flow and intracranial pressure) may augment risks of intraventricular hemorrhage or white matter injury in the immature brain [Low et al., 1992]. Inadequately treated repetitive pain in the developing brain may accentuate neuronal apoptosis [Bhutta and Anand, 2002], foster wind-up (in which unmodified afferent transmission enhances *N*-methyl-D-aspartate [NMDA] receptors and facilitates hyperalgesia) [Dickenson, 1995], foster hyperreactive pain responses to subsequent stimuli [Weisman et al., 1998], and cause long-term behavioral changes [Grunau et al., 1994a, 1994b; Taddio et al., 1997]. Use of opioids in the first week of life after perinatal asphyxia has been found to increase the brain's resistance to hypoxic-ischemic insults [Angeles et al., 2005].

TABLE 93–1

Responses to Painful Stimuli

Behavioral Responses to Pain

1. Crying, whimpering
2. Facial expressions: brow bulge, eye squeeze, and deepening of the nasolabial folds
3. Active movement and attempts to withdraw from the painful stimulus
   a. Thrashing
   b. Tremulousness
   c. Limb withdrawal, flexion
   d. Bicycling
   e. Arching
4. Disorganized behavior; limp and flaccid
5. Flexor responses; leg withdrawal
6. Exaggerated reactivity
7. Changes in state
   a. Decrease in sleep periods
   b. Rapid changes in state cycles
   c. Decreased rapid eye movement (REM) sleep

Physiologic/Autonomic Responses

1. Changes in heart rate and variability
2. Changes in respiratory rate and quality
3. Fluctuations in blood pressure
4. Decreased transcutaneous oxygen and carbon dioxide levels
5. Oxygen desaturation
6. Increased intracranial pressure
7. Palmar sweating
8. Pallor
9. Flushing
10. Pupillary dilation
11. Increased catabolic state

Clinical Assessment

Pain is a subjective and variable experience with no direct relation between "pain experience" and pain intensity or between physical pathology and pain intensity. Responses to pain vary widely, depending on gestational age, chronologic age, developmental state, initial behavioral state, prior experience of pain, and the ability to respond to and become habituated to sensory stimuli. There is no single uniform, standard technique for assessing pain in neonates or children. Biochemical responses to pain (elevations in cortisol, catecholamines, beta-endorphins, insulin, glucagon, renin-aldosterone, growth hormone, and prolactin) are rarely useful to clinicians. Infants and children demonstrate a variety of nonspecific but consistent behavioral, physiologic, and autonomic responses to pain (Table 93-1) [Anand and Carr,1989]. These signs have been used by clinicians to recognize pain in nonverbal infants and to quantitate severity of the pain experience.

Self-report, usually by use of a linear analog scale, is regarded as most reliable but only for children who have the cognitive capacity to respond appropriately. Infants and preverbal children cannot self-report pain, quantify its severity, or inform providers as to the efficacy of analgesic treatments. For preverbal patients, pain assessment is best achieved using multidimensional scales including behavioral, physiologic, and autonomic responses (Table 93-2). Behavioral observational scales are used for pain assessment in neonates, children younger than 4 years of age, and cognitively impaired children. Neonatal scales used include the NIPS (Neonatal Infant Pain Scale), PIPP (Premature Infant Pain Profile), and pain assessment score sheet [Franck et al., 2000]. Toddlers and pre-school children who cannot effectively communicate pain quality or intensity can often use structured questioning or standardized semiquantitative pain assessment tools (poker chips in increasing numbers, cartoon drawings of faces, a pain thermometer, and colors or words) to consistently and reliably rate pain intensity. Children 8 years or older are able to effectively communicate pain intensity and quality using questionnaires or visual analog scales designed for adults. Behavioral assessment tools, such as FLACC (see Table 93-2), have been used to evaluate children with developmental delay who are at particular risk for acute or chronic undiagnosed or untreated pain [McGrath et al., 1999; Oberlander et al., 1999; Voepel-Lewis et al., 2002].

Management

Pain should be regularly assessed and aggressively treated with nonpharmacologic methods and appropriate analgesic therapies. Effective pain management schemes use the simplest effective regimen, dose around the clock for on-going painful conditions, and tailor the regimen to fit individual patient needs. Oral medications are preferred whenever possible, and regular repeated doses should be ordered with appropriate dosing intervals. Additional medication should be made available on an as needed basis for breakthrough pain. Doses should be titrated according to the patient's

TABLE 93–2

Examples of Pain Assessment Scales for Differing Developmental Ages

1. Modified Neonatal Infant Pain Scale (NIPS)*

PARAMETER		FINDING	POINTS
Facial expression	Relaxed	Restful face, neutral expression	0
	Grimace	Tight facial muscles, furrowed brow, chin, jaw	1
Cry	No cry	Quiet, not crying	0
	Whimper	Mild moaning, intermittent	1
	Vigorous crying	Loud scream, shrill, continuous (silent cry may be scored if intubated)	2
Breathing pattern	Relaxed	Usual pattern for infant	0
	Change in breathing	Irregular, faster than usual, gagging, breath holding	1
Arms	Relaxed	No muscular rigidity, occasional random movements	0
	Flexed/extended	Tense, straight arms, rigid and/or rapid extension, flexion	1
Legs	Relaxed	No muscular rigidity, occasional random movements	0
	Flexed/extended	Tense, straight legs, rigid and/or rapid extension, flexion	1
State of arousal	Sleeping/awake	Quiet, peaceful, sleeping or alert and settled	0
	Fussy	Alert, restless and thrashing	1
Heart rate	Within 10% of baseline		0
	Within 11–20% of baseline		1
	>20% of baseline		2
Oxygen saturation	No additional oxygen needed to maintain saturation		0
	Additional oxygen needed to maintain saturation		1

2. FLACC Scale†

CATEGORIES	SCORING 0	1	2
Face	No particular expression or smile	Occasional grimace or frown, withdrawn, disinterested	Frequent to constant quivering chin, clenched jaw
Legs	Normal position or relaxed	Uneasy, restless, tense	Kicking, or legs drawn up
Activity	Lying quietly, normal position, moves easily	Squirming, shifting back and forth, tense	Arched, rigid or jerking
Cry	No cry (awake or asleep)	Moans or whimpers; occasional complaining	Crying steadily, screams or sobs, frequent complaints
Consolability	Content, relaxed	Reassured by occasional touching, hugging or being talked to, distractible	Difficult to console or comfort

3. FACES Scale‡

0	1	2	3	4	5
No hurt	Hurts little bit	Hurts little more	Hurts even more	Hurts whole lot	Hurts worst

4. Visual Analog Scale§

0	1	2	3	4	5	6	7	8	9	10
No pain				Moderate pain					Worst possible pain	

5. Numerical Analog Scale||

If "0" is no pain and "10" is the worst possible pain, how would you rate your pain?

6. Verbal Descriptive Scale||

0 = no pain; 1–3 = mild pain; 4–6 = moderate pain; 7–10 = worst possible pain

*For preterm and term infants; scored on a 0-10 point system.

†For infants 4 months of age to children 3 years of age. Each of the five categories—(**F**) Face; (**L**) Legs; (**A**) Activity; (**C**) Cry; (**C**) Consolability—is scored from 0 to 2, resulting in a total score between zero and 10.

‡For children 3 to 11 years of age.

§For children ≥7 years of age.

||For children older than 11 years of age.

Example 1, Neonatal Infant Pain Scale (NIPS), modified from Lawrence J, Alcock D, McGrath P, et al. The development of a tool to assess neonatal pain. Neonatal Netw 1993;6:59-66.

Example 2, FLACC Scale, from Merkel SI, Voepel-Lewis T, Shayevitz JR, Malviya S. The FLACC: A behavioral scale for scoring postoperative pain in young children. Pediatr Nurs 1997;23:293-297.

Example 3, FACES Scale, from Wong DL, Hockenberry-Eaton M, Wilson D, et al. Wong's Essentials of Pediatric Nursing, 6th ed. St Louis: Mosby, 2001;1301.

response, with close attention to the developmental changes in physiology and pharmacokinetics occurring between birth and childhood.

A four-step approach to painful conditions, initially intended as a model for cancer pain management but applicable to other diseases, has been advocated by the World Health Organization [Schug et al.,1990]. Mild pain can be treated with cognitive techniques and weak analgesics (e.g., nonsteroidal anti-inflammatory drugs [NSAIDs] and acetaminophen). For moderate pain, oral "weaker" opioids or combinations of opioids and NSAIDs or acetaminophen can be used. Severe pain requires more aggressive, parenteral opioids such as morphine or fentanyl. Intractable pain or unacceptable toxicities of pain management may require invasive interventions such as nerve blocks and intraspinal anesthetic infusions. A multimodal approach to pain relief allows drug synergy or potentiation and can reduce single drug doses, minimizing side effects [Galloway and Yaster, 2000]. Common side effects of opiates such as drowsiness, constipation, nausea, and pruritus should be treated prophylactically or when they occur without reducing analgesic doses. Sucrose (given orally as a 24% or 30% solution) is effective in reducing mild procedural pain (such as circumcision and immunizations) in neonates and infants; however, an association between poor neurodevelopmental outcomes and repeated sucrose analgesia has been reported [Johnston et al., 2002].

Anticipatory pain control (administering analgesics before to a painful procedure) can reduce hyperexcitability, diminish the total amount of drug required to treat pain, and prevent later behavioral changes. Nonpharmacologic techniques that may be effective include comfort measures (swaddling, pacifiers, contralateral tactile stimulation for newborns), soothing sounds, gentle handling and proper positioning, rest periods between procedures, reduced environmental stimuli, heat and cold, massage, transcutaneous electrical nerve stimulation, cognitive approaches, guided imagery, and distraction. Consultation with or referral to a multidisciplinary pain service may be indicated for unexpected pain duration, neuropathic pain, concerns about addiction, previous use of drugs or alcohol, or complicated family psychosocial issues.

Types of Pain Medication

Aspirin, Acetaminophen, and Nonsteroidal Anti-inflammatory Drugs

Except for specific indications in rheumatologic diseases and for inhibition of platelet adhesion, aspirin is not commonly used as an analgesic in pediatrics because of its association with Reye's syndrome. NSAIDs are most effective as preemptive agents or for treatment of mild-to-moderate pain of somatic origin. Acetaminophen is widely

TABLE 93–3

Dosage Guidelines for Analgesics

DRUG	DOSE	INTERVAL (hr)	ROUTE	COMMENTS
Sucrose	0.2 ml of 30% solution		PO	Optimal dose not established
Acetaminophen	10–15 mg/kg	4	PO, PR	
	Maximum daily dose:			
	Infants, <75 mg/kg			
	Neonates, >32 wks, 60 mg/kg			
	Neonates, 28–32 wks, 40 mg/kg			
Ibuprofen	6–10 mg/kg	6	PO	
Naproxen	5–6 mg/kg	8–12	PO	
Aspirin	10–15 mg/kg	4–6	PO	Restricted use for anti-platelet or anti-inflammatory effect
Ketorolac	0.5 mg/kg	8	IV	
Opioid Analgesics*				
Morphine	Bolus: 0.1 mg/kg	2–4	IV	No ceiling effect for severe pain
	Infusion:			
	Children, 0.03 mg/kg/hr	IV		
	Infants, 0.01–0.03 mg/kg/hr	IV		
	Term neonates, 0.005–0.02 mg/kg/hr	IV		
	Preterm neonates, 0.002–0.01 mg/kg/hr	IV		
	Oral immediate release: 0.3 mg/kg	3–4	PO	
	Oral sustained release:			
	Infants 20-35 kg, 10–15 mg/kg	8–12	PO	
	Infants 35–50 kg, 15–30 mg/kg	8–12	PO	
Oxycodone	0.1–0.2 mg/kg	3–4	PO	
Methadone	0.1mg/kg	4–8	IV, PO	
Fentanyl	Bolus: 0.5–1.0 μg/kg	1–2	IV	
	Infusion:			
	Children, 0.05–2.0 μg/kg/hr		IV	
	Infants, 1–2 μg/kg/hr		IV	
	Term neonates, 0.05–2 μg/kg/hr		IV	
	Preterm neonates, 0.05–1 μg/kg/hr		IV	
Hydromorphone	Bolus: 0.02 mg/kg	2–4	IV	
	Infusion: 0.006 mg/kg/hr		IV	
	Oral: 0.04–0.08 mg/kg	3–4	PO	

*Initial doses and intervals.

Adapted from Berde CB, Sethna NF. N Engl J Med 2004;347:1094-1103; Stevens B, Gibbons S, Franck LS. Pediatr Clin North Am, 2000;47:633-650; Holder KA, Patt RB. Pediatr Ann 1995;24:164-168; Tobias JD. Pediatr Clin North Am 2000;47:527-543.

used for minor pain and discomfort. Dosage guidelines for aspirin and other analgesics are summarized in Table 93-3. Because excess dosing can cause hepatic failure in infants and children, maximum daily doses are also listed. Other NSAIDs, most commonly ibuprofen and naproxen, have gained wide acceptance for pediatric use and are equally effective. For children who cannot tolerate oral dosing, ketorolac is available.

NSAIDs provide a weak analgesia effect that tends to be more effective for pain that has an inflammatory component, as in postoperative pain. The concurrent use of NSAIDs can reduce opioid doses needed for effective pain management. The use of more than one NSAID concurrently offers little therapeutic advantage and increases the risk of side effects. NSAIDs used in conjunction with corticosteroids augment the risk of serious gastrointestinal complications.

Opioids

Opioids are the mainstay of treatment of severe pain, operative procedures, postoperative pain relief, and management of chronic painful medical conditions in neonates and children [Berde and Sethna, 2002; Golianu et al., 2000; Stevens et al., 2000]. Opioids bind to brain and spinal cord opiate receptors to block neurotransmitter production. Mu-receptor agonists such as morphine, codeine, fentanyl, hydrocodone, and hydromorphone are effective for all pain intensities and are first-line choices for pain management. Agonist-antagonist drugs are not recommended because they have an analgesic ceiling, may precipitate withdrawal, and have limited routes of administration. Suggested guidelines for opiate-naïve patients are listed in Table 93-3.

Because opiate-agonists have no therapeutic ceiling, doses should be adjusted to meet the patient's individual needs. The overall safety and efficacy of opioids are well established. In children, as in adults, the risks of addiction after receiving opioids for pain are low [McCaffery and Pasero, 1999]; thus, clinicians should not hesitate to treat pain aggressively. However, increased risks for respiratory depression in infants younger than 6 months of age require close cardiorespiratory and saturation monitoring in settings in which emergent airway management is feasible. Fentanyl is the drug used most often for short procedures because of its rapid onset (1 to 2 minutes), peak effect (3 to 5 minutes), and short duration of action (2 to 4 hours). Morphine has a somewhat slower onset (5 minutes), with a peak response at 10 to 30 minutes, and longer duration of action (3 to 8 hours).

Intravenous bolus or continuous infusions allow more rapid and reliable onset of analgesia that can be easily titrated and quickly reversed by narcotic antagonists. Patient-controlled analgesia can be used in children (generally older than 7 years of age), but younger children should be under parent or nurse control. Opioids may also be administered subcutaneously, orally, rectally, transdermally, or intranasally. For some procedures, oral transmucosal fentanyl citrate provides an alternative for conscious sedation, although emesis is a frequent side effect. Rectal administration can be used when oral dosing is contraindicated; intramuscular injection should be used only as a last resort.

Adverse effects of opioids include respiratory depression, sedation, vasodilation, hypotension, bradycardia (Fentanyl), muscle rigidity, urinary retention, ileus, seizures, and rigid chest (Fentanyl given rapidly). Tolerance may develop more rapidly with continuous infusions and with use of synthetic opioids [Arnold et al., 1990; Katz et al., 1994]. Characteristic withdrawal symptoms including irritability, hypertonicity, diaphoresis, fever, and emesis can occur when opioids are abruptly discontinued after several days' exposure.

Procedural Sedation and Analgesia

Most minor procedures that are minimally invasive can be performed using a mild analgesic and sedation. More uncomfortable procedures require deeper sedation appropriately performed by anesthesiologists, intensivists, or emergency physicians trained in advanced life-support and experienced in deep sedation techniques and monitoring. The American Academy of Pediatrics (AAP) has defined two levels of sedation less deep than general anesthesia [AAP, 2002]. Conscious sedation is a medically controlled state of depressed consciousness that: (1) allows protective reflexes to be maintained, (2) retains ability to maintain airway independently and continuously, and (3) permits appropriate response by the patient to physical stimulation or verbal commands. Deep sedation is a medically controlled state of depressed consciousness or unconsciousness from which the patient is not easily aroused, loses protective airway reflexes, and cannot maintain an airway or respond purposefully to physical stimulation or verbal command. Guidelines for sedating children undergoing therapeutic or diagnostic procedures have been reviewed by Krauss and Green [2000].

Analgesia

Topical analgesia can reduce the discomfort of minor procedures or the local infiltration of anesthetic agents used for lumbar punctures, difficult intravenous cannulation, and suturing. Useful topical compounds when skin is intact include TAC (tetracaine, epinephrine, and cocaine), LET (lidocaine, epinephrine, and tetracaine), and EMLA (eutectic mixture of topical anesthetics, prilocaine and lidocaine). For brief procedures, ethyl chloride or fluoromethane can be used to cool the skin and provide a limited analgesic effect. For procedures involving deeper structures or prolonged painful interventions, local anesthetics or peripheral nerve blocks are required. For such procedures, fentanyl is preferred because of its faster onset, shorter duration, and lack of a histamine-inducing effect; transmucosal fentanyl (lozenges or lollipops) offers procedural analgesia but often causes emesis. For procedures of longer duration, morphine and meperidine remain the preferable agents. For painful procedures, ketamine (given by the IM, IV, or enteral route) induces profound analgesia, sedation, and immobilization whereas spontaneous respiratory activity, airway tone, and protective reflexes are maintained. It may be the drug of choice for emergency procedures when the patient has not fasted. Side effects such as hallucinations, dreams, and dysphoria are seen less commonly in younger children than in adults.

Sedation

Benzodiazepines are the most commonly used drugs for sedating children, particularly in pediatric intensive care units. Midazolam is the preferred drug for procedural sedation [McCaffery and Pasero, 1999]. It has a rapid onset of action (1 to 5 minutes), and a short half-life (1 to 12 hours). Given by the IV, IM, intratracheal, or enteral route, it provides potent sedation, some muscle relaxation, memory loss, and anxiolysis. Oral or intravenous routes are preferable for children; nasal administration causes an intense irritant response. As it has shorter duration than diazepam or lorazepam, it is a more appropriate choice for brief procedural sedation. Oral diazepam avoids the pain of intravenous injection and the variable absorption of intramuscular doses. For painful procedures, benzodiazepine sedation should be accompanied by opioid analgesia, and the patient should be monitored for hypoxia or respiratory depression. Midazolam can be reversed by flumazenil.

Barbiturates are considered the sedatives of choice for diagnostic imaging in children older than 3 years of age, but they do not provide analgesia. Barbiturates lower the pain threshold, especially when pain is already present. Intravenous pentobarbital, rectal methohexital, and thiopental are the most extensively used drugs for procedural sedation. Chloral hydrate, an acceptably safe alternative sedative without analgesic efficacy, can be used for nonpainful procedures; the oral or rectal dose is 25 to 100 mg/kg (maximum dose, 2 g). Its use is largely restricted to sedation for electroencephalograms and diagnostic imaging in children younger than 3 years of age. Its extremely long half-life in neonates mitigates against repeated administration (Mayer et al., 1991), and other concerns have been raised because of potential carcinogenicity and genotoxicity in mice, even when given as a single low dose (Salmon et al., 1995). Given at subanesthetic doses, intravenous ultra-short-acting agents (etomidate, methohexital, propofol, remifentanil, and thiopental) can be used for procedural pain management, but they should be used only by practitioners experienced in dealing with the potential for oversedation or rapid swings in consciousness.

Types of Pain

Neuropathic Pain

A variety of neuromuscular and neurodegenerative diseases can cause both nociceptive pain (e.g., contractures or osteoarthritis) and neuropathic pain (e.g., nerve injury or entrapment) [Galloway and Yaster, 2000]. Neuropathic pain is difficult to treat with opioids and often requires multiple modalities for effective pain relief. Infiltration or compression of nerves by tumors responds to varying degrees to palliative radiation, steroids, surgical decompression, adjuvant drugs (tricyclic antidepressants, antiepileptics), neurolytic nerve blocks, epidural and intrathecal blocks, and opioids (which are often ineffective) [Galloway and Yaster, 2000]. Phantom pain after amputation may respond to preemptive regional anesthesia, antiepileptics, tricyclic antidepressants, calcitonin, topical agents, and intrathecal medication. Nerve trauma may be treated with injected local anesthetics, steroids, neurolysis, antiepileptics, tricyclics, or mexiletine. Neuropathies after chemotherapy can be treated with antiepileptics, tricyclics, or mexiletine.

Tricyclic antidepressants (most commonly amitryptilene, doxepin, and sertraline) are used as adjuvants to inhibit norepinephrine and serotonin uptake, thereby increasing neurotransmitter tone at the spinal cord level. Pain relief is achieved more quickly than the slower antidepressant effect of these drugs, with a response in 1 to 2 weeks. Given the quinidine-like effects of tricyclic antidepressants on cardiac conduction, baseline and periodic ECGs are recommended. Antiepileptic agents (carbamazepine and gabapentin) have been used to a limited extent in children to treat lancinating pain from peripheral nerve compression or injury and for peripheral neuropathies [Galloway and Yaster, 2000]. Mexiletine, an oral antiarrhythmic drug with potent analgesic effects, may be useful for neuropathic pain resistant to tricyclic antidepressants and antiepileptic medications. Because it also enhances the efficacy of other agents, it is generally used in combination with other drugs.

Pain in Children with Significant Neurologic Impairment

Children with cerebral palsy or developmental delays experience pain, despite some reports of blunted pain responses or insensitivity to pain [Oberlander et al., 1999]. Patients with neurodevelopmental impairments have a variety of conditions or procedures that may cause pain, including splinting and casting, dislocations and joint contractures, spasticity, pressure sores, feeding tubes, constipation, diagnostic tests and specific treatments. Pain from spasticity and muscle spasms can be treated with diazepam, dantrolene, or oral baclofen. Oral analgesia is the least invasive method of administration and therefore the preferred route; intramuscular injections may be more painful in children with decreased muscle mass. Subcutaneous and transdermal administration can be used for chronic administration.

Patients with neurologic impairment are more likely to have pain discounted or denied by caregivers and thus may have pain ineffectively treated. In patients too impaired to communicate their experience of pain, behavioral responses should be regarded as surrogate measures of pain and the pain treated appropriately. To avoid over- or undertreatment when self-report is uncertain, it is important to choose a measure appropriate to the individual patient that can be ascertained over time. For children with significant neurologic impairments, the need for analgesia for acute procedural pain must be balanced by the recognition that systemic opioids may have undesirable side effects, such as respiratory depression and constipation.

Migraine and Headache

Symptomatic pain relief from headache can be obtained by oral, rectal, or intravenous routes and has been reviewed elsewhere [Annequin et al., 2000] (see Chapter 53). NSAIDs or weak analgesics can be given in adequate doses for mild-to-moderate pain from tension headaches and migraine attacks. For intractable migraine, dihydroergotamine and sumatriptan have been used in preference to opioids, because of the potential for abuse or dependence in patients with recurrent attacks. The hallmark of effective control of migraine is treatment early in an attack. Intranasal administration of sumatriptan [Lewis et al., 2004] or possibly dihydroergotamine may be preferable because of the nausea and vomiting associated with some migraine headaches. The condition of children with tension headaches improves with simple analgesia and relief of any precipitating stressors. Once a chronic pattern is established, cognitive-behavioral techniques such as biofeedback and relaxation therapy may help alleviate headaches.

Summary

Relief of pain is one of the most important aspects of ethical medical care, especially in young children and children with neurologic handicaps who cannot communicate their experience of pain [Oberlander et al., 1999]. The success of nonpharmacologic means in reducing anxiety or fear should not dissuade physicians from giving pediatric patients appropriate analgesics.

PALLIATIVE CARE

Over 50,000 children die each year in the United States from trauma, lethal congenital conditions, extreme prematurity, heritable disorders, and acquired illness [Catlin and Carter, 2002; Himelstein et al., 2004]. At least 500,000 children suffer life-threatening medical conditions that put them at high risk for not surviving into adulthood [Himelstein et al., 2004]. Nearly half of pediatric deaths occur in the hospital, and over 70% of deaths from chronic complex conditions are in hospital; of these, nearly half occur in intensive care settings [Feudtner et al., 2002]. Although children younger than 1 year of age have a higher death rate than any other pediatric age group [Behrman et al., 1996; Guyer et al., 1999], it is estimated that only 5000 to 7000 children (1% of dying children) receive hospice care or formal palliative care services. It is thought that another 10,000 to 15,000 children could benefit from hospice services [World Health Organization, 1998]. Currently, approximately 60% of deaths in pediatric intensive care units and nearly 75% of deaths in neonatal intensive care units follow limitation of care or withdrawal of life-sustaining treatments when therapy appears to offer no benefits or when quality of life appears unacceptable [Garros et al., 2003; Wall and Partridge, 1997]. Recent population-based studies have documented that 15% of pediatric hospital deaths are from neurologic or neuromuscular diseases [Feudtner et al., 2002]. Neuromuscular disorders cause 3% to 4% of childhood deaths in all age groups but account for 15% to 20% of deaths of children with complex chronic conditions. A variety of severe neurologic diagnoses fit into four broad categories of life-limiting conditions for which palliative care may be indicated (Box 93-1) [Dangel, 2002].

Deficiencies in provision of end-of-life care have been well documented [Wolfe et al., 2000] in other subspecialty fields. Some neurologists believe that they lack the training and experience required to manage the complex needs of dying children, to treat pain and other end-of-life symptoms, or to communicate bad news to young patients and their families.

Box 93-1 Examples of Neurologic Conditions That May Be Appropriate for Pediatric Palliative Care

Life-Threatening Conditions

Curative treatment may be feasible but can fail.

- Cancer
- Meningitis
- Encephalitis (herpes simplex virus)
- Extreme prematurity

Chronic Conditions

Long periods of intensive treatment aimed at prolonging life and allowing participation in normal childhood activities are required, but premature death is still possible.

- Neurofibromatosis
- Tuberous sclerosis
- Hydrocephalus
- Muscular dystrophy and progressive neuropathies
- Neurodegenerative diseases
- Metabolic disorders with neurologic manifestations, including inborn errors of metabolism
- Stroke, including moyamoya disease

Progressive Conditions

Treatment is exclusively palliative and commonly extends over many years.

- Severe congenital myopathies
- Spinal muscular atrophy
- Anencephaly
- Rachischisis
- Intraventricular hemorrhage
- Periventricular leukomalacia
- Progressive metabolic disorders

Nonprogressive Conditions

Severe neurologic disability may cause weakness and susceptibility to health complications, but the patient may deteriorate unpredictably.

- Unresponsive seizure disorders
- Severe/high meningomyelocele
- Central nervous system trauma
- Hypoxic-ischemic encephalopathy
- Chromosomal abnormalities with neurodevelopmental consequences (e.g., trisomy 13 or 18)
- Holoprosencephaly or other severe brain malformations
- Severe static encephalopathies with recurrent infections or symptoms difficult to control
- Profound mental retardation

Historical Background

Palliative care as an adjunct to modern medical care began with the founding of St. Christopher's Hospice by Cecily Saunders in 1967 [Saunders, 1988]. Whitfield later adapted models for care of adults to care of dying infants and their families, recommending changes in the intensive care environment [Whitfield et al., 1982]. Although the first pediatric hospices were started in 1982, it is only recently that widespread institution of pediatric palliative care has been recommended [American Academy of Pediatrics, 1996, 2000; World Health Organization, 1998].

Pediatric palliative care offers a cost-effective means to care for dying children [Pierucci et al., 2001]. It decreases the number of procedures that patients receive, increases the use of support services, shifts deaths to less-intensive settings, and increases the incidence of withholding or withdrawing aggressive measures [Pierucci et al., 2001]. Increasing emphasis on understanding patients' and their families' experience of death and dying can improve the care of critically ill children [Kirschbaum, 1990; Wolfe et al., 2000]. End-of-life care has more recently become a national focus for national quality improvement initiatives.

Definitions of Palliative Care

Encompassing more than end-of-life care, palliative care embraces a philosophy of care that extends beyond and complements the aims of curing and healing children with life-limiting conditions. Dying pediatric patients (or their proxy decision-makers) have the same basic concerns as adults with terminal disease: (1) relief of pain and suffering, (2) avoiding inappropriate prolongation of dying, (3) achieving a sense of control, (4) relieving burdens, and (5) strengthening relationships with loved ones [Singer et al., 1999]. Typically provided by a multidisciplinary team, palliative care seeks to ensure the quality of living and of dying for the child for whom curative efforts are not (or are no longer) considered appropriate (Box 93-2) [Catlin and Carter, 2002]. The primary focus is to provide comprehensive, compassionate, and developmentally appropriate care that meets the physical, psychologic, emotional, social, and spiritual needs of the child as the disease progresses [American Academy of Pediatrics, 2000; Institute of Medicine, 1997; World Health Organization, 1998]. Additionally, palliative care optimally provides support and respite for parents during the illness, death, and bereavement in ways appropriate to their values, upbringing, religion, culture, and community. The intent is a decent or "good" death—free from avoidable distress and suffering for patients, families, and caregivers.

Box 93-2 Interdisciplinary Team for Palliative Care

- Primary care provider, community pediatricians, subspecialists
- Pediatric registered nurses/case managers
- Pediatric social worker
- Child life therapist
- Spiritual care counselor
- Home health aides
- Pediatric medical consultants
- Physical/occupational therapists
- Clinical pharmacist
- Clinical dietitian
- Volunteers
- Insurers/payers
- Other providers
- Regional centers
- Durable medical equipment companies
- Community pharmacies

Components of Palliative Care

Identifying the Need

Whether providing primary care or subspecialty consultation, neurologists must learn when to address the palliative care needs of their patients and the family members. Children with neuromuscular diseases, and their family members, have a diverse range of medical, psychologic and emotional needs that differ from those of dying adults. Providers should learn to recognize when the need for palliative care is becoming more salient with neurodegenerative diseases and progressive neuropathies and when medical complications from a static encephalopathy impinge on the quality of life (e.g., aspiration in patients with spastic quadriplegia). Medical information about expected outcome and services should be appropriate for the child's developmental age, current cognitive capacity, and emotional stage, as well as sensitive to the parents' ability to accept their child's clinical deterioration.

Providers should allow time for the parents to nurture their child, while recognizing the difficult emotional stresses that parents face when seeing the acute change in their child's condition or coming to grips with a certainty of neurologic compromise or death in the future. Providers should attempt to give parents—and when appropriate, children—some sense of control when they feel helpless and overwhelmed. Even when critically ill or dying, children benefit from being with and comforted by their parents. Although to an extent remaining strangers at the bedside [Rothman, 1991], physicians and nurses often become powerful and meaningful sources of support to parents [Meyer et al., 2002].

Transition in Goals of Care

Palliative care for children does not need to be restricted to those expected to die soon when therapeutic interventions fail or are withdrawn. Some neurologic conditions are associated with a predictably shortened life span (e.g., trisomy 13 and 18, neurodegenerative diseases, anencephaly, severe hydrocephalus, and many inborn errors of metabolism), and the primary focus of care is limited to optimizing quality of life when a cure is not possible. Other diseases make prediction of life expectancy and quality of life more difficult (e.g., traumatic or hypoxic brain injury, some central nervous sytem or spinal tumors, congenital myopathies and neuropathies, muscular dystrophy, and storage diseases). Because it can be difficult to tell who will die early as a result of certain central nervous system and neuromuscular disease processes, it seems appropriate to offer palliative care to children with progressive conditions early, transitioning from curative efforts to palliative care as their condition worsens [Simpson Sligh, 1993]. Accordingly, palliative care efforts can and should coincide with therapies aimed to cure the disease or limit its progression. With children old enough to express their preferences, it is important to address future choices for care before neurologic status deteriorates to the extent that the child is no longer able to participate in health-care decisions. Parents must be given information necessary for decision making but must also understand the limits of the provider's ability

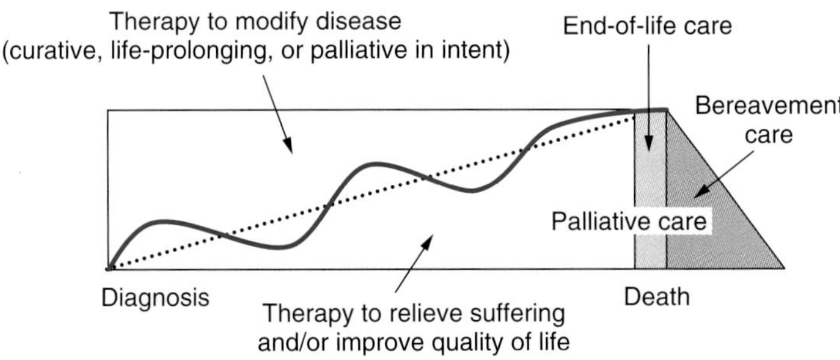

FIGURE 93-1. Model for transition to palliative care. (Adapted from Ferris et al., 2002).

to prognosticate treatment efficacy and outcome. Mention of palliative therapies, supportive care, or levels of non-intervention early in the course of a chronic or progressive life-threatening disease can soften the impact of non-intervention discussions later in the disease trajectory. An essential step is to clarify, and periodically reassess, the goals of continuing, rather than limiting, on-going interventions as the chances for cure lessen (Figure 93-1).

Providers should facilitate the transition from curative or life-extending care to supportive efforts intended to improve quality of life. They may need to initiate discussions about changing treatment goals when parents have difficulty admitting that end-of-life care is needed [Callahan, 2000], particularly when parents have adapted to the demands of caring for children with life-threatening chronic conditions and to the diminished quality of life associated with many of these conditions (e.g., spinal muscular atrophy, unresponsive central nervous system tumors, and states of minimal consciousness). Acute brain injury (e.g., perinatal asphyxia and other sudden catastrophic deteriorations in neurologic status) can make the transition to palliative care difficult, because physicians often cannot offer clear prognostic certainty on survival or later neurodevelopmental functioning. With emergent conditions, there is often little time for difficult decisions or coping with complex emotions, and the transition from curative interventions to palliative care can seem abrupt [Frager, 1996; Sahler et al., 2000].

Levels of Care

The shift in treatment goals, however, does not imply that ongoing medical interventions aimed at treating or curing the child's disease (such as administration of blood products, oxygen, and antibiotics) must be abandoned, as they typically are in adult hospice care [Children's Hospice International, 1989]. Some potentially beneficial treatments entail significant burdens, and it becomes important to clarify which specific measures will continue to be used as well as which level of nonintervention is most appropriate. An order proscribing all or selected resuscitative measures in the event of a cardiac or respiratory arrest ("Do not resuscitate" [DNR] or "Do not attempt resuscitation" [DNAR] order) is often the first step. This order represents a selective nonintervention order in the event of respiratory or cardiac arrest, not a half-hearted resuscitation ("slow code") of a child deemed likely to die. When providers and parents perceive that further medical therapy offers no benefit, that on-going interventions are inappropriate, or that the present quality of life is untenable, more extensive discussions about withholding or withdrawing specific life-sustaining therapies may be indicated [Wall and Partridge, 1997].

Withholding of life-sustaining measures involves an agreement not to institute specific medical measures that would otherwise be indicated. This level of nonintervention is usually reserved for children with a grim prognosis or whose quality of life would not be improved by more aggressive interventions. Such a level of nonintervention might be deemed appropriate for infants with trisomy 13 or 18, cerebral or spinal tumors, severe central nervous system malformations, or severe hydrocephalus. Interventions deemed futile are not required and should be discontinued [Paris et al., 1999]—for example in patients with brain death, anencephaly, lethal neuropathies and myopathies, and untreatable inborn errors of metabolism.

Withdrawal of life-sustaining measures involves the discontinuation of medical interventions currently in use but deemed either futile or no longer appropriate to the child's best interests, accepting the possibility that death may be hastened. Although ethically equivalent, withholding and withdrawing treatment often feels different at the bedside and can raise emotional responses in parents and providers. Whenever support is withheld or withdrawn, it is appropriate for the primary physician to discuss DNAR status with parents and the healthcare team before writing the order.

Communication

Patterns of communication sensitive to the child's developmental age and neurologic status and to the parents' emotional state are critical to good palliative care for children. The degree to which the child can participate in decision making increases with older children (older than 7 years of age). The use of pictures, stories, toys, and music can help younger children communicate their preferences. On the other hand, infections of the nervous system, hypoxia-ischemia, neurodegenerative diseases, or traumatic brain injury can diminish an older child's decision-making capacity. Whenever the child has the cognitive capacity to participate, it is important for providers to allow the child the time to express hopes, dreams, and fears [Back, 2003].

Discussions about treatment options should review the child's current status, estimate the presumed disease

Box 93-3 Protocol for Palliative Care Communications—SPIKES: A Protocol for Delivering Bad News and Negotiating Goals of Care

- **S**etting: Create environment conducive to communication.
- **P**erception: Determine what the family knows.
- **I**nvitation: Determine how the family would like information delivered.
- **K**nowledge: Provide information.
- **E**motions: Empathetically support patient.
- **S**ummarize: Set realistic goals, make a treatment plan, and follow through.

From Buckman R. Breaking bad news: A guide for health care professionals. Baltimore: Johns Hopkins University Press, 1992.

trajectory, characterize the quality of life that each treatment choice entails, and finally assist the child and parents in selecting which measures should and should not be carried out. The primary focus is to determine what is important to the child and the family—for example, longer life, freedom from pain, time with family members, specific desires, choice of environment and setting, and time to say goodbye.

The next step is to devise a collaborative care plan that respects the patient's emotional and spiritual needs, incorporates family values, and supports family involvement in health-care decisions. When time allows, such planning is best done by parents and primary care providers working together over a period of time, giving cognitively capable patients and parents time for questions, second-opinion consultations, talks among family members, reflection, deliberation, and informed decision making. Repeated discussions empower informed decision making and help minimize the guilt some parents feel about their decisions after their child dies.

A structured approach can help physicians deliver difficult news and negotiate goals of care (Box 93-3). Critical aspects of the communication process include simple, direct, clear, and honest explanations that relate the expected outcomes of each treatment option without prejudicing or constraining the parents' choices. It is important that the information neither overwhelms the parents nor leaves them in despair. Providers should avoid promising outcomes that they do not believe are feasible.

Neurologists play a key role in communicating the expected neurologic outcome after a life-threatening illness; neurology consultation can help parents understand expected functional status when there is little chance for an acceptable outcome. To minimize the sense of giving up or abandoning their child, it is critical that parents understand that the goal of care is to do everything that *should* be done rather than everything that *can* be done.

Health-Care Decision Making

Because children usually have no previously documented preferences for health-care decisions, parents and physicians must assess when the burdens of care are no longer in the best interests of the child. The first issue is to identify and involve those who will be making health-care decisions. To the level of their developmental capacity, older children themselves have the right to determine what quality of life means to them, with support from their parents and physicians. Younger children necessarily depend on their parents as the predominant decision makers.

Parents (or the competent adolescent) determine the quantity of information necessary for them to make an informed decision. If decisions seem not to reflect a full understanding of the disease, the goals of care, or expected outcomes, further discussions facilitate review of the information and reflection on treatment options. Decisions that do not concur with the provider's choices should be respected when made in the child's best interests. Advanced directives specifying care preferences of once-competent adults, or identifying proxy decision makers should an adult become incapacitated have no legal relevance in pediatric patients [Pierucci et al., 2001]. In general, parents are assumed to be the primary proxy decision-makers for young children; however, their discretion is not unlimited. When consensus is difficult to reach, ethics committee consultation can help clarify impediments to decision making. In rare situations in which parents' judgment may be questionable or the child's best interests remain uncertain, providers may need to advocate for the child or even refer to child welfare services. A process of guided autonomy can support the involvement of the child and the parents in treatment decisions while preserving some autonomy and minimizing the undue emotional strain of making decisions to limit care.

VEGETATIVE STATE

A small proportion of children who survive critical illnesses continue for varying periods of time in a vegetative or a minimally conscious state. Although the exact incidence is unknown, an estimated 4000 to 10,000 infants and children in the United States live in this condition and present a special challenge to clinicians and ethicists alike [Ashwal et al., 1992]. Although there is no consensus about whether children in a vegetative state experience pain and suffering, it seems prudent to treat signs or symptoms in children in a vegetative state that may mimic or appear like pain and suffering. Decisions to withdraw or withhold life-sustaining measures should be made in collaboration with parents only when neurodiagnostic testing and a sufficient period of observation suggest there is no chance for a meaningful recovery [AAN Quality Standards Subcommittee, 1995]. Decisions to forego supportive care, especially those involving withholding fluids or hydration, remain controversial even when deemed appropriate responses to the child's medical situation. Such decisions present complex emotional and ethical challenges to clinicians and family members [Carter and Leuthner, 2003].

Environment for Death and Dying

Some parents may prefer continued care in the hospital, where skilled nursing and medical care offsets limitations to privacy and the inhospitable ambience of most in-patient settings. A private space for families to gather before and after the child's death is recommended (e.g., a screen for privacy or, better, a separate comfort-care room) and should not impede nursing care or medical attention to pain and symptoms. Other in-patient options include transfer to a lower level of care or to a hospice, although some parents may feel abandoned by changes in care providers late in the course of their child's disease. Death at home is preferred by a significant number of children and parents [Pierucci et al., 2001]. Parents who opt for home care must be adequately supported in managing terminal care for the child outside the hospital. Plans for a death at home require a care provider skilled in managing pain and suffering and able to provide 24-hour coverage from discharge through the child's death and the parents' bereavement.

Support during Dying

When death is near, providers can prepare parents for the child's imminent death by envisioning expected changes in the child's appearance, advising them as to likely timing, and assuring them that pain will continue to be aggressively treated. Parents usually choose to hold their dying child, and this choice should be facilitated and the parents' well-being ensured as best as possible. Mention can be made of discussions that will be required after the child dies, such as autopsy or organ donation. Some families perceive organ donation as a positive aspect within the tragedy of their child's death (e.g., after traumatic brain death or sudden infant death syndrome). In other cases, such as anencephalic infants, organ donation continues to pose difficult medicolegal issues for clinicians [Walters, 2001]. Overall support of a family when a child dies involves a balance between respect for privacy and close but noninvasive attention to the child's and the family members' needs. Neurologists caring for terminal patients can turn to primary care pediatricians, social workers, clergy, psychologists, psychiatrists, and other sources of support, as the parents' adjustment dictates.

Assessment and Treatment of Symptoms

A primary focus of palliative care is the relief of distressing symptoms that detract from the child's quality of life. Providers should discuss in advance symptom management to reassure patients and parents and to educate them about what may occur as the disease progresses. Providers should reevaluate the efficacy of pain and symptom management as the disease progresses. Some neurologists feel comfortable managing pain and other end-of-life symptoms and will follow the child throughout the course of the disease. Others may prefer to consult the primary care pediatrician or a pediatric palliative care specialist with expertise in symptom management.

Pain should be aggressively treated with analgesics. When there is severe or unremitting pain at the end of life, terminal sedation with opioids is used to alleviate suffering, recognizing that opioids may suppress respiratory drive in debilitated patients and may thereby hasten death. The risk of death is justified because there is no alternative that alleviates suffering while lessening the risk of death [Fleischman, 1998]. Fears of addiction to opioids, the mainstay of pain management at the end-of-life care, on the part of providers or family members are unwarranted. Paralytics are not appropriate when life support is being withdrawn [Pierucci et al., 2001]. Anxiolytics may help terminal agitation and perhaps air hunger experienced in the terminal phases.

Many neurologists are comfortable treating seizures, insomnia, and depression in dying patients but may prefer to have primary care pediatricians or palliative care specialists manage other frequently encountered end-of-life symptoms such as dyspnea, anxiety, fatigue, fever, bleeding, nausea, skin breakdown, anorexia, dehydration, and constipation. Despite shared concerns for patient well-being, treatment of symptoms experienced by dying patients has been inconsistent [Partridge and Wall, 1997; Pierucci et al., 2001; Wolfe et al., 2000]. Attempts should be made to organize a care plan allowing death without suffering (either at home or in hospital) for any child in need, regardless of socioeconomic circumstances.

Developmental, Emotional, and Spiritual Concerns

Care for a dying child requires candor, openness, and emotional availability to the child's experience of illness and imminent death. Children need to understand death and dying in terms of their developmental age. Research indicates that they begin to understand it as a change of being by age 3 and as a universal fact of living by age 5 or 6 and have gained a concept of their personal mortality by age 8 or 9 [Himelstein et al., 2004]. Spirituality is one way that patients and families cope with death and dying whether or not they adhere to any specific religion. Approaches that respect the child's spiritual nature at varying developmental stages allow providers to explore issues of love, hope, security, and loneliness and concepts of the legacy that the child will leave to surviving parents, siblings, friends, and schoolmates. Family routines and rituals add familiar structure and a sense of normality as the child's medical condition worsens and should be encouraged whenever possible.

Bereavement

Children are aware of dying and disease; they understand much more about death and dying than adults realize. Parents who sense that the child is aware of imminent death more often regret not having talked with the child than do parents who do not sense this awareness in the child, and typically parents who talk with a child about death do not regret doing so [Kreicbergs et al., 2004]. Children grieve as much as adults, although in different ways. Dying children may grieve their impending death, the loss of functional status, or the inability to participate in current or future events. They may worry about how family members will cope after their death. Dying children and their siblings do not need to be protected from death and dying as much as they need help making it understandable. When heritable neuromuscular disorders pose a future risk for affected siblings, particular care is necessary to deal with parents' sense of guilt, parents' and siblings' grief, concerns about subsequent pregnancies, and family fears of illness in the future.

In general, the grieving process should not be rushed. Providers should allow family members the opportunity to spend time grieving with their deceased child alone. In the immediate moment, there is a time to talk and a time to be silent; it may be helpful to celebrate their child's life, recap the family's experience, value their loss and their emotional responses, and help them contact other family members and friends. Parents should be offered access to religious observances, social services support, family support groups, or other measures to help them cope.

Excluding children from the grieving process may foster a loss of trust or a sense of resentment. Attending the funeral can be a way in which children can participate in remembering and valuing the dead child. In some cases, psychologic counseling may be offered as a way to help parents and siblings work through the emotional trauma.

Follow-up Conference

Many physicians arrange a conference after the child's death to see how the parents are coping and help them resume more normal functioning in the aftermath of the child's death. A meeting can review postmortem examination results and

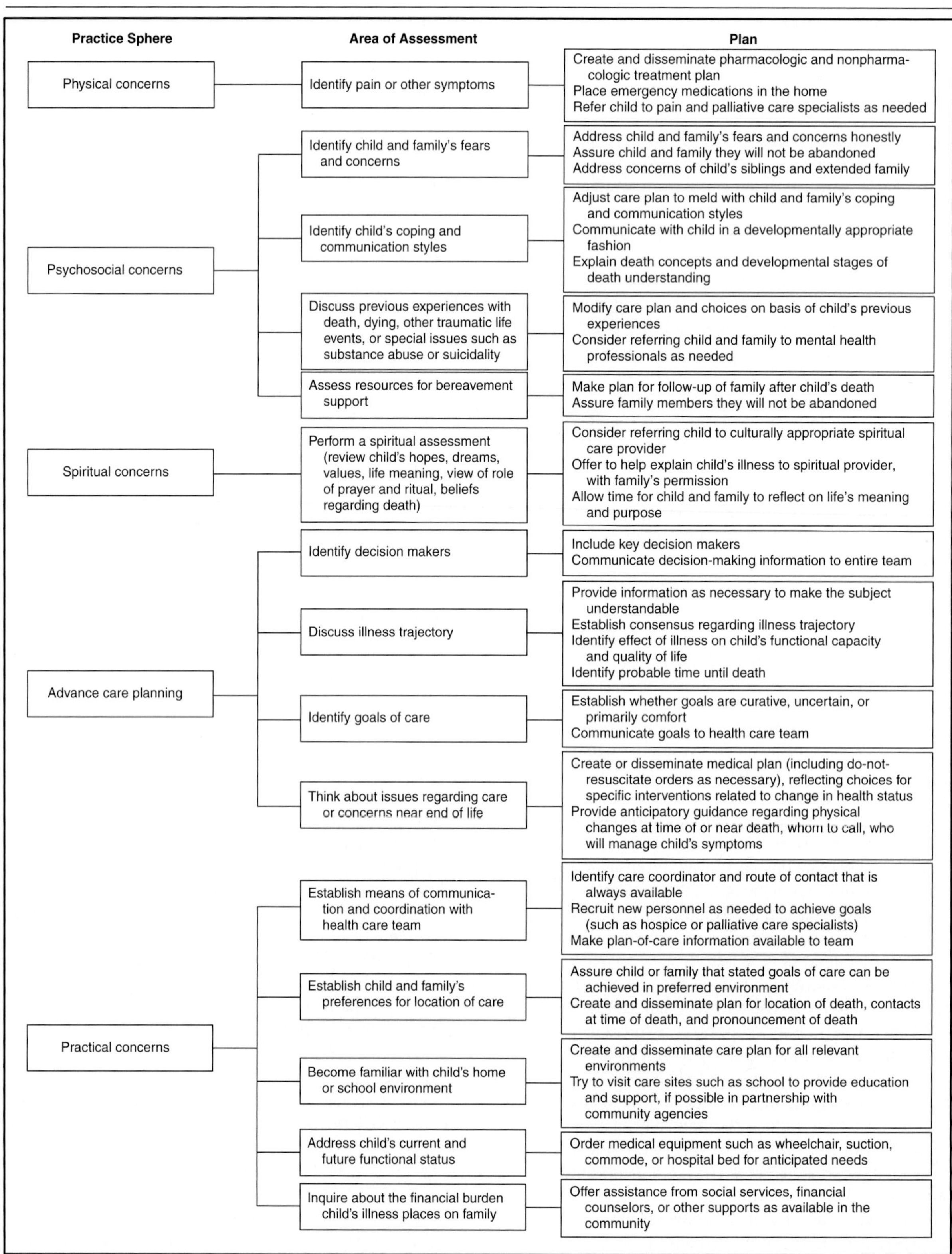

FIGURE 93–2. Essential elements in the approach to pediatric palliative care. (From Himelstein BP, Hilden JM, Boldt AM, Weissman D. Pediatric palliative care. N Engl J Med 2000 350;1752–1762.

clarify aspects of the diagnosis, etiology, and end-of-life events; it can provide a measure of solace by demonstrating that providers remember their child and continue to care about the family. Often it is an opportunity to put to rest parents' questions about "what might have been," to minimize tendencies to blame themselves or their child's providers, to detail the implications of heritable neurologic disorders for siblings or subsequent pregnancies, and to offer referrals to counseling or support groups.

Barriers to Palliative Care

The remarkable success of medicine in treating many medical conditions can make it difficult to abandon attempts to cure the primary disease. Providers may overtly or tacitly encourage treatments with little or no hope of a favorable outcome, abandoning them only when death seems inevitable. In pediatrics, a late transition from curative to palliative care is a frequent problem. Some providers may conceive of palliative care as a second-string treatment regimen, to be offered and used only for patients who cannot be cured and only very near the end of life [Pierucci et al., 2001]. In many pediatric neurologic diagnoses, it is difficult to predict the course of the disease, which children will die from the disease, or the quality of life as the disease progresses. Parents' recognition that death is inevitable often lags behind their understanding of the diagnosis. Both parents and providers may feel that the death of a child is inexplicable, unnatural, something that should not happen. Palliative care requires increased time and staff to provide for the many needs of the dying patient and of family members.

Summary

When cure of a life-threatening disease is not expected, neurologists can offer children and their families other benefits: the best medical information on diagnosis, current status, and expected outcome; adequate analgesia and treatment of other symptoms; medical and emotional support; perspective and referrals; assistance in decision-making partnership; open discussion about ways to "optimize" the dying process; follow-up meetings; and opportunities/referrals for grief counseling.

Palliative care offers many ways to improve children's and families' experience of end-of-life care (Figure 93-2). Neurologists should develop expertise in palliative care of children with life-threatening neurologic and neuromuscular conditions. When serving as a consultant, neurologists should work with primary pediatric providers and palliative care specialists to meet their patients' needs for end-of-life care. With an interdisciplinary team approach and the use of medical technology only when benefits outweigh burdens, providers and parents ensure the best possible life while the child lives and a death that is comfortable, peaceful, and dignified.

REFERENCES

AAN Quality Standards Subcommittee. Practice parameters: Assessment and management of patients in the persistent vegetative state. Neurology 1995;45:1015.

American Academy of Pediatrics Committee on Bioethics. Ethics and the care of critically ill infants and children. Pediatrics 1996;98:149.

American Academy of Pediatrics Committee on Bioethics and Committee on Hospital Care. Palliative care for children. Pediatrics 2000;106:351.

Anand KJS, Barton BA, McIntosh N, et al. Analgesia and sedation in preterm neonates who require ventilatory support: Results from the NOPAIN trial. Neonatal Outcome and Prolonged Analgesia in Neonates. Arch Pediatr Adolesc Med 1999;153:331. [Erratum in Arch Pediatr Adolesc Med 1999;153:895.]

Anand KJS, Carr DB. The neuroanatomy, neurophysiology, and neurochemistry of pain, stress, and analgesia in newborns and children. Pediatr Clin North Am 1989;36:795.

Anand KJS, Hickey P. Halothane-morphine compared with high-dose sufentanil for anesthesia and postoperative analgesia in neonatal cardiac surgery. N Engl J Med 1992; 326:1.

Anand KJS, Sippell WG, Aynsley-Green A. A randomised trial of fentanyl anaesthesia in preterm babies undergoing surgery: Effects on the stress response. Lancet 1987;1:62. [Erratum in Lancet 1987; 1:234]

Anand KJS, Thrivikraman KV, Engelmann M, et al. Long-term behavioral effects of repetitive pain in neonatal rat pups. Physiol Behav 1999;66:627.

Angeles DM, Wycliffe N, Michelson D, et al. Use of opioids in asphyxiated term neonates: Effects on neuroimaging and clinical outcome. Pediatr Res 2005;57:873.

Annequin D, Tourniare B, Massiou H. Migraine and headache in childhood and adolescence. Pediatr Clin North Am 2000;47:617.

Arnold JH, Truog RD, Orav EJ, et al. Tolerance and dependence in neonates sedated with fentanyl during extracorporeal membrane oxygenation. Anesthesiology 1990;73:1136.

Ashwal S, Bale JF, Coulter DL, et al. The persistent vegetative state in children: Report of the Child Neurology Society Ethics Committee. Ann Neurol 1992;32:570.

Back AL, Arnold RM, Quill TE. Hope for the best, and prepare for the worst. Ann Int Med 2003;138:439.

Bauchner H. Procedures, pain, and parents. Pediatrics 1991;87:563.

Behrman RE. Overview of pediatrics. In: Behrman RE, Kleigman RM, Arvin AM, eds. Nelson's textbook of pediatrics, 16th ed. Philadelphia: WB Saunders, 2000.

Berde CB, Sethna NF. Analgesics for the treatment of pain in children. N Engl J Med 2002;347:1094.

Beyer JE, McGrath PJ, Berde CB. Discordance between self-report and behavioral pain measures in children aged 3-7 years after surgery. J Pain Symptom Manage 1990;5:350.

Bhutta AT, Anand KJ. Vulnerability of the developing brain. Neuronal mechanisms. Clin Perinatol 2002;29:357.

Callahan D. Death and the research imperative. New Engl J Med 2000;342:654.

Cancer Pain Relief and Palliative Care: Technical Report Series 804. Geneva: World Health Organization, 1990.

Carter BS, Leuthner SR. The ethics of withhold/withdrawing nutrition in the newborn. Semin Perinatol 2003;27:480.

Catlin A, Carter B. Creation of a neonatal end-of-life palliative care protocol. J Perinatol 2002;22:184.

Children's Hospice Care: Differences between hospice care for children and adults. Alexandria, VA: Children's Hospice International, 1989.

Committee on Drugs, American Academy of Pediatrics. Guidelines for monitoring and management of pediatric patients during and after sedation for diagnostic and therapeutic procedures. Pediatrics 2002;110:836.

Dangel T. The status of pediatric palliative care in Europe. J Pain Symptom Manage 2002;24:160.

Davies B, Brenner P, Orloff S, et al. Addressing spirituality in pediatric hospice and palliative care. J Palliat Care 2002;18:59.

Dickenson A. Spinal cord pharmacology of pain. Br J Anaesth 1995;75:193.

Ferrell BR, Rhiner M. High-tech comfort: Ethical issues in cancer pain management for the 1990s. J Clin Ethics 1991; 2:108.

Ferris FD, Balfour HM, Bowen K, et al. A model to guide patient and family care. J Pain Sympt Manage 2002;24:106.

Feudtner C, Christakis DA, Zimmerman FJ, et al. Characteristics of deaths occurring in children's hospitals: Implications for supportive services. Pediatrics 2002;109:887.

Fitzgerald M, Anand KJS. Development neuroanatomy and neurophysiology of pain, In: Schechter NL, Berde CB, Yaster M, eds. Pain in infants, children, and adolescents. Baltimore: Williams & Wilkins, 1993.

Fitzgerald M, Koltzenburg M. The functional development of descending inhibitory pathways in the dorsolateral funiculus of the newborn rat spinal cord. Brain Res 1986;389:261.

Fleischman AR. Commentary: Ethical issues in pediatric pain management and terminal sedation. J Pain Symptom Manage 1998;15:260.

Frager G. Pediatric palliative care: Building the model, bridging the gaps. J Palliat Care 1996;12:9.

Franck LS, Greenberg CS, Stevens B. Pain assessment in infants and children. Pediatr Clin North Am 2000;47:487.

Galloway KS, Yaster M. Pain and symptom control in terminally ill children. Pediatr Clin North Am, 2000;47:711.

Garros D, Rosychuk RJ, Cox PN. Circumstances surrounding end of life in a pediatric intensive care unit. Pediatrics 2003;112:e371.

Golianu B, Krane EJ, Galloway KS, et al. Pediatric acute pain management. Pediatr Clin North Am, 2000;47:559.

Goodman JE, McGrath PJ. The epidemiology of pain in children and adolescents: A review. Pain 1991;46:247.

Grunau RVE, Whitfield M, Petrie P, et al. Early pain experience, child and family factors, as precursors of somatization: A prospective study of extremely premature and full-term children. Pain 1994a;56:353.

Grunau RVE, Whitfield M, Petrie J. Pain sensitivity and temperament in extremely low-birth-weight premature toddlers and preterm and full-term controls. Pain 1994b:58:341.

Guyer B, Hoyert DL, Martin JA, et al. Annual summary of vital statistics—1998. Pediatrics 1999;104:1229.

Himelstein BF, Hilden JM, Boldt AM, Weissman D. Pediatric palliative care. N Engl J Med 2004;350:1752.

Holder KA, Patt RB. Taming the pain monster: Pediatric postoperative pain management. Pediatr Ann 1995;24:164.

Howard RF. Current status of pain management in children. N Engl J Med 2003;290:2464.

Institute of Medicine, Committee on Care at the End of Life. Approaching death: Improving care at the end of life. Washington, DC: National Academy Press,1997.

Institute of Medicine. Field MJ, Behrman R, eds. When children die: Improving palliative and end-of-life care for children and their families. Washington, DC: National Academy Press, 2003.

International Association for the Study of Pain, Subcommittee on Taxonomy. Pain terms: A list with definitions and notes on usage. Pain 1979;6:249.

Joint Commission on Accreditation of Healthcare Organizations. Pain assessment and management standards—hospitals. Oakbrook Terrace, IL: Joint Commission Resources, 2001.

Johnston CC, Filion F, Snider L, et al. Routine sucrose analgesia during the first week of life in neonates younger than 31 weeks' postconceptional age. Pediatrics 2002;110:523.

Katz R, Kelly HW, His A. Prospective study on the occurrence of withdrawal in critically ill children who receive fentanyl by continuous infusion. Crit Care Med 1994;22:763.

Kirschbaum MS. Needs of parents of critically ill children. Dimens Crit Care Nurs 1990;9:344.

Klimach VJ, Cooke RW. Maturation of the neonatal somatosensory evoked response in preterm infants. Dev Med Child Neurol 1988;30:208.

Krauss B, Green SM. Sedation and analgesia for procedures in children. N Engl J Med 2000;342:938.

Kreicbergs U, Valdimarsdottir U, Onelov E, et al. Talking about death with children who have severe malignant disease. N Engl J Med 2004;351:1175.

Lawrence J, Alcock D, McGrath P, et al. The development of a tool to assess neonatal pain. Neonatal Netw 1993;122:59.

Lewis D, Ashwal S, Hershey A, et al. Practice parameter: Pharmacological treatment of migraine headache in children and adolescents. Neurology 2005, in press.

Mayer D, Hindmarsh KW, Sankaran K, et al. Chloral hydrate disposition following single dose administration to critically ill neonates and children. Dev Pharmacol Ther 1991;16:71.

McCaffery M, Pasero C. Teaching patients to use a numerical pain-rating scale. Am J Nurs 1999;99:22.

McGrath PJ, Rosmus C, Camfield C, et al. Behaviors caregivers use to determine pain in non-verbal cognitively impaired children. Dev Med Child Neurol 1999;40:340.

Merkel SI, Voepel-Lewis T, Shayevitz JR, Malviya S. The FLACC: A behavioral scale for scoring postoperative pain in young children. Pediatr Nurs 1997;23:293.

Meyer EC, Burns JP, Griffith JL, et al. Parental perspective on end-of-life care in the pediatric intensive care unit. Crit Care Med 2002;30:226.

Paris JJ, Singh J, Schreiber MD, et al. Unilateral do-not-resuscitate order in the neonatal intensive care unit. J Perinatol 1999;19:383.

Partridge JC, Wall SN. Analgesia for dying infants whose life support is withdrawn or withheld. Pediatrics 1997;99:76.

Pierucci RL, Kirby RS, Leuthner SR. End-of-life care for neonates and infants: The experience and effects of a palliative care consultation service. Pediatrics 2001;108:653.

Polaner DM. Sedation-analgesia in the pediatric intensive care unit. Pediatr Clin North Am 2001;48:695.

Rothman DJ. Strangers at the bedside: A history of how law and bioethics transformed medical decision making. New York: BasicBooks, Harper Collins, 1991.

Sahler OJ, Frager G, Levetown M, et al. Medical education about end-of-life care in the pediatric setting: Principles, challenges, and opportunities. Pediatrics 2000;105:575.

Salmon AG, Kizer KW, Zeise L, et al. Potential carcinogenicity of chloral hydrate—a review. J Toxicol Clin Toxicol 1995;33:115.

Saunders CM, ed. St. Christopher's in celebration: Twenty-one years at Britain's first modern hospice. London: Hodder and Stoughton, 1988.

Schechter NL, Allen DA, Hanson K. Status of pediatric pain control: A comparison of hospital analgesic usage in children and adults. Pediatrics 1986;77:11.

Schechter NL. The undertreatment of pain in children: An overview. Pediatr Clin North Am 1989;36:781.

Schug SA, Zech D, Dorr U. Cancer pain management according to WHO analgesic guidelines. J Pain Symptom Manage 1990;5:27.

Shah V, Ohlsson A. The effectiveness of premedication for endotracheal intubation in mechanically ventilated neonates. A systematic review. Clin Perinatol 200;29:535.

Simpson Sligh J. An early model of care. In: Armstrong-Dailey A, Zarbock Goltzer S, eds. Hospice care for children. New York, Oxford: Oxford University Press, 1993.

Singer PA, Martin DK, Kelner M. Quality end-of-life care: Patients' perspectives. JAMA 1999;281:163.

Stevens B, Gibbins S, Franck LS. Treatment of pain in the neonatal intensive care unit. Pediatr Clin North Am 2000;47:633.

Taddio A. Opioid analgesia for infants in the neonatal intensive care unit. Clin Perinatol 2002;29:493.

Taddio A, Katz J, Ilersich AL, et al. Effect of neonatal circumcision on pain responses during subsequent routine vaccination. Lancet 1997;349:599.

Tobias JD. Weak analgesics and nonsteroidal anti-inflammatory agents in the management of children with acute pain. Pediatr Clin North Am 2000;47:527.

Voepel-Lewis T, Merkel S, Tait AR, et al. The reliability and validity of the Face, Legs, Activity, Cry, Consolability observational tools as a measure of pain in children with cognitive impairment. Anesth Analg 2002;95:1224.

Wall SN, Partridge JC. Death in the intensive care nursery: Physician practice of withdrawing and withholding life support. Pediatrics 1997;99:64.

Walters JW. Anencephalic infants as organ sources. Bioethics 1991;5:326.

Weisman SJ, Bernstein B, Schechter NL. Consequences of inadequate analgesia during painful procedures in children. Arch Pediatr Adolesc Med 1998;152:147.

Whitfield JM, Siegel RE, Glicken AD, et al. The application of hospice concepts to neonatal care. Am J Dis Child 1982;136:421.

Wolfe J, Grier HE, Klar N, et al. Symptoms and suffering at the end of life in children with cancer. N Engl J Med 2000;342:326.

Wong DL, Hockenberry-Eaton M, Wilson D, et al. Wong's Essentials of pediatric nursing, 6th ed. St. Louis: Mosby, 2001.

World Health Organization. Cancer pain relief and palliative care in children. Geneva: World Health Organization, 1998.

CHAPTER 94

Ethical Issues in Child Neurology

David L. Coulter

The "task" of ethics in general is to understand how human beings should behave in regard to other persons and to society [Slote, 1995] or to understand what is right and what is wrong. The philosophical study of ethics is as old as civilization itself and parallels the growth and development of human society. Morality is understood as the set of generally accepted rules and guidelines for acceptable conduct in society. These social conventions about what is right and wrong constitute the "common morality" [Beauchamp and Childress, 1994]. Philosophical ethics can be thought of as the attempt to develop a rational basis for morality. Although ethics (as a form of philosophy) strives for universal truth, it is inextricably linked to the realities of the human societies whose morality it seeks to understand [Slote, 1995]. Distinguishing between "moral" and "ethical" behavior is often difficult [Bernat, 1994]. Perhaps moral behavior may be thought of as a personal attempt to conduct one's life in conformity with the common morality, whereas ethical behavior may be thought of as a more theoretical or rational attempt to apply philosophical thinking to what is right and wrong. In other words, ethics is a systematic attempt to understand how to live and act morally in a social context.

Ethics addresses all aspects of human behavior. Bioethics considers the interaction between biology and ethics. It is defined as "the systematic study of the moral dimensions of the life sciences and health care" and includes consideration of "the health-related and science-related moral issues in the areas of public health, environmental health, population ethics and animal care" [Reich, 1995]. Clinical ethics is a subcategory of bioethics that refers to the day-to-day moral decision making of those caring for patients [Callahan, 1995]. More specifically, clinical ethics refers to the identification, analysis, and resolution of moral problems that arise in the care of a particular patient [Jonsen et al., 1998]. Medical ethics is a subcategory of clinical ethics that refers to the moral behavior of physicians (and is thus distinguishable from nursing ethics, social work, and pastoral/spiritual ethics).

Neuroethics is a new concept that cuts across most of these distinctions. As an area of bioethics, it considers the interaction between the neurosciences and ethics in all of the same areas of study as bioethics noted previously [Pfaff, 1983]. As a clinical discipline, it addresses the care of patients with neurologic disorders. As an area of medical ethics, it refers most directly to the moral behavior of neurologists and neurosurgeons. Thus, child neurologists interested in ethics need to be knowledgeable about the general approaches to ethics, the emerging scope of bioethics, and the more specific approaches to ethics in medicine, nursing, and other health-related disciplines.

This edition of this textbook on pediatric neurology is the first to include a chapter on ethics. Although many articles and books have been published on ethical topics of interest to child neurologists, few provide a systematic approach to ethics in child neurology. A recent collection of articles covered a number of important topics [Shevell, 2002], and a recent casebook presented a number of illustrative cases whose analyses illuminate many of the important ethical issues in child neurology [Freeman and McDonnell, 2001]. The best general, systematic resource on ethics in neurology is the classic text by Bernat [1994], but it mainly covers topics of interest in adult neurology. This chapter follows the general structure of Bernat's book and seeks to apply its concepts specifically to the area of pediatric neurology. The goal of the chapter is to provide child neurologists interested in ethics with the tools they need to identify, analyze, and resolve moral problems they may encounter in the care of children and adolescents with neurologic disorders.

The first part of this chapter covers the most significant theoretical approaches to ethics as they apply to child neurology. The second part considers the varied duties of the child neurologist caring for patients with morally problematic issues. The third part discusses several specific ethical problems in child neurology. The discussion of these specific problems is broadly conceptual to identify issues and raise questions whose answers will need to be elaborated in the context of caring for a particular patient and family.

THEORETICAL APPROACHES TO ETHICS

Philosophy may be a search for truth, but the fact is that there is no one, true, universal approach to ethics. Physicians who want to act ethically should be aware of the several major ethical theories that compete for attention in contemporary medical practice. Two ethical theories in particular dominate thinking in Western philosophy. *Utilitarianism* is derived from the writings of Jeremy Bentham [Bentham, 1982] and John Stuart Mill [Mill, 1971]. *Deontology* is derived mainly from the writings of Immanuel Kant [Kant, 1959]. Elements of both theories persist in modern ethical approaches to clinical problems, usually in somewhat modified form. Most physicians will find themselves using utilitarian thinking on some occasions and deontologic thinking on other occasions, or using some combination of both when it is necessary to resolve an ethical dilemma in clinical practice. A number of other ethical approaches have been developed more recently and also deserve consideration. As a general statement, probably no one theory or approach is optimal in every case in medical practice. A skillful physician will recognize which approach is best suited to the challenges of a specific ethical situation.

Utilitarianism

The essence of utilitarian theory is the idea that the morality of an action is determined mainly by its consequences: the morally right action is the one that produces the best result [Beauchamp and Childress, 1994]. Of course, the result of an action may be quite complex. An action that helps one person may harm another person. Withdrawing support from a child in a vegetative state undoubtedly harms the child, since it results in the child's death, but the action may help the family grieve and may allow society to use limited medical resources to help other patients. The utility principle states that one should act to produce the best overall balance of positive and negative consequences of the act. This idea is embedded in the concept of balancing risks and benefits to achieve the best overall result.

Utilitarian theory is often cited to justify actions that are most likely to increase happiness, but other desirable results are also possible. Individuals may wish to act in such a way so as to increase personal quality of life, enjoyment of and satisfaction with life, success in a preferred career, and general knowledge and understanding or to strengthen personal relationships. Lawyers and policymakers use the utility principle to produce the best overall balance of justice and fairness for society.

Utilitarian thinking is almost intuitive in many aspects of ordinary life. Understanding this form of thinking is important because it may help avoid the potential pitfalls that can result from uncritical application of the theory. Perhaps the most familiar situation is the use of utilitarian theory to justify the killing of defective newborns [Kuhse and Singer, 1985]. Although theoretically logical, such arguments are morally repugnant to persons who apply a different moral standard based on some other approach to ethics. Another problem with utilitarian theory is its failure to protect minorities, which results from its emphasis on producing the most good for the majority. The needs of children with rare neurologic disorders can be overlooked if utilitarian thinking allocates scarce medical resources primarily to children with more common disorders.

Deontology

Deontologic theory is based on the importance of "deon," or duty. Duty is based more on the intentions that lead a person to act than on the outcomes or consequences of the action. Utilitarian thinking is mostly situational and depends on the specific aspects of a given situation; deontologic thinking strives to be more universal and to emphasize decisions that would apply in all relevant situations. Thus, Kant's categorical imperative states that *we* should act only in a way that is consistent with a universal law or obligation [Kant, 1959]. Using people as means to an end implies that different actions (or reactions) are needed, depending on the end or outcome that is desired; therefore, the actions are not universally applicable. For this reason, deontologic thinking stipulates that we should treat all people as "ends" and not as means to an end. This could cause problems in thinking about the morality of organ transplantation if the organ donor is thought of only as a means to the end of survival for the recipient. Clearly, deontologic thinking imposes a duty to respect the rights and value of the donor as much as those of the recipient because anyone could be either a donor or a recipient.

Deontologic thinking emphasizes duties and obligations, but these may conflict. For example, physicians may have different and competing obligations toward patients, families, hospitals, insurance companies, and society. The attempt to describe duties leads to formulation of general or universal rules for moral action, but these rules may also conflict. Rules may be too abstract and impractical to apply to real-life situations. Deontologically based rules do not take into account the messiness of human relationships, a point that is essential to keep in mind when considering the ethics of care discussed later in this chapter.

Common Morality and Natural Law

What are the universal rules that spring from deontologic thinking? Most Western philosophers would argue that these rules can be derived from the application of reason—from rational, logical thinking about the nature of human existence. The general argument is that "all rational persons would agree that these rules are essential to govern and guide the moral actions of individuals in a cohesive society" [Beauchamp and Childress, 1994]. Beauchamp and Childress [1994] describe the "common morality" as socially approved norms of human conduct that form the basis of ethical theory This common-sense understanding of what is needed for individuals to behave in society is not derived from theory but rather forms the basis for potentially competing theories.

Natural law theory is an ancient approach to deriving universal rules through the application of reason [Simon, 1992]. For Thomas Aquinas, natural law sprang from man's participation in God's eternal law and was brought into being by the application to action of human intelligence and reasoning [May, 1991]. This application leads first to the principle that all things desire that which is good; therefore, good is to be pursued and evil is to be avoided. Good things are those to which man has a natural inclination, such as life (existence), social interaction, family life, and civil government. To pursue these good things, one should act fairly, love God, and love other persons. Secondary precepts or rules (such as the Ten Commandments) follow from these basic principles.

Secular interpretations of natural law are as old as Aristotle and are still used in some forms of legal theory. Bernard Gert [2000] defined two sets of rules that he believed all rational persons would accept as natural and essential, without relying explicitly on natural law theory. Many of his rules are in fact similar to the Ten Commandments. Gert also emphasized that the rules are not absolute and that violations may be considered in specific circumstances. Beauchamp and Childress [1994] do not define any specific rules as part of their common morality, but they do define four principles that are not absolute and that need to be specified based on actual circumstances. Nonetheless, their four principles may be seen to correlate with the precepts of natural law:

1. Do good (beneficence)
2. Avoid evil (nonmaleficence)
3. Act fairly (justice)
4. Love one another (autonomy)

Whatever the source of the common morality, it is the basis for *principlism*, the ethical theory based on the application of principles to specific situations.

Principlism

Principlism is an approach to ethical problems that is based on the application of the four principles of beneficence, nonmaleficence, justice, and autonomy. It is more of a practical guide than an abstract theory, and it has found widespread acceptance in a variety of settings [Beauchamp and Childress, 1994]. It was adopted explicitly in the Belmont Report, which forms the foundation for research ethics in the United States [Belmont Report, 1979]. Although principlism is perhaps the best known approach to clinical ethical problems, it is by no means the only approach. Understanding principlism is necessary to consider these alternative systems.

The principle of *autonomy* has become pre-eminent in Western society, although it may be less prominent in Eastern societies that place a greater value on social harmony. Physicians need to keep this in mind when caring for patients from other cultures. An autonomous choice is one that is based on sufficient knowledge of the facts involved, the ability to understand the situation, and the independence to choose without undue influence from other people. An autonomous person can determine for himself what he thinks is best, and this principle states that other people should respect these choices even when they do not agree with or approve of them. Autonomy is the basis for the concept of informed consent, which requires that a patient has the capacity or competence to understand the issues, full disclosure of all of the information needed to make a decision, and freedom from any coercion that might influence the decision.

In general, persons younger than 18 years of age are not considered to have the capacity to make fully autonomous choices, although their preferences should be considered and respected if possible. American law recognizes that persons 18 years of age and older are fully competent unless a judge has determined otherwise. This recognition is critically important for young adults with neurologic disorders that may affect their capacity to make fully autonomous decisions. If capacity is in doubt, the family will need to initiate legal proceedings to obtain guardianship when the person becomes 18 years old. A young adult (over 18 years) with a neurologic disorder that results in limited competence is unable to give informed consent, but his parents cannot give consent for him or her unless they have obtained guardianship. Failure to obtain guardianship when it is necessary can interfere seriously with medical treatment.

The principle of *beneficence* encourages physicians to do good or to act in the best interest of the patient whenever possible. This principle can also be interpreted to suggest that physicians should seek to promote an optimal quality of life or satisfaction with life. Considerable debate exists about how to measure quality of life [Nordenfelt, 1994; Nussbaum and Sen, 1993; Schalock, 1996]. Objective measures are based on the judgments of others, whereas subjective measures are based on the opinions of the patient about what constitutes a satisfying life. In general, preference is given to subjective judgments when they can be known.

The principle of *nonmaleficence* encourages physicians to avoid doing harm to patients and dates back to Hippocrates. It is related logically to the principle of beneficence. Both principles are considered when physicians attempt to strike a balance between providing a benefit for the patient (doing good) and not imposing a burden (avoiding harm). This balance may become especially problematic when the same action could produce both a good, or desired, effect, as well as a bad, or undesired effect. The classic example is prescription of sufficient medicine to reduce pain while knowing that it may also cause the patient to stop breathing. This problem is known as the "situation of double effect" [Beauchamp and Childress, 1994]. In Catholic moral theory (which contains the most explicit analysis of such situations), an action that causes double effects is morally justifiable only if it meets all of the following criteria:

1. The action itself is not morally wrong (such as killing).
2. The intent is to produce the good effect, even though the bad effect may be expected.
3. The good effect is not based on achieving the bad effect.
4. The benefit to be obtained is greater than the harm that might occur.

This concept is admittedly difficult to apply in practice. Evaluation of each criterion may be arguable in a specific situation. Perhaps the best that can be expected is that physicians will make a good-faith effort to adhere to the principles involved and seek to obtain the optimal balance between benefit and harm for the patient and family.

The principle of *justice* requires that equals be treated equally, but the basis for an equal distribution of resources may be arguable. Should resources be distributed according to need, effort, merit, contribution to society, or some other factor? Utilitarian, libertarian, communitarian, and egalitarian approaches have been proposed to answer this question [Beauchamp and Childress, 1994]. Rawls [1971] suggests that resources should be distributed to ameliorate the effects of life's natural and social lotteries. It may be simply bad luck ("losing the lottery") that a child is born with a disabling condition or is born into poverty. If the child is not responsible for this condition, then society should act to remedy the situation. According to this rule, unfair situations would presumably have priority over merely unfortunate situations. How many resources should be provided to those who have been unfairly deprived? The limits of this redistribution policy may be the extent to which it disables or impoverishes the rest of society [Veatch, 1986].

Jonsen and colleagues [1998] suggest that ethical issues can be analyzed by asking the following four questions (which are in fact practical applications of the four principles discussed previously):

1. What are the medical indications for treatment? (principle of beneficence)
2. What are the patient's preferences? (principle of autonomy)

3. What impact on the patient's quality of life can be reasonably anticipated? (principle of beneficence)
4. What are the burdens and benefits that may affect the family and society? (principles of justice and nonmaleficence)

The questions may be somewhat hierarchic, in the sense that medical indications and patient preferences are usually more important than potential social burdens, but physicians should not be too rigid about this. In fact, asking (and answering) these four questions in a particular case is an excellent way to make sure that the relevant issues are identified and evaluated. These issues can then be considered by the caregiving team, patient, and family. Resolution of the issues may vary from case to case, but at least everyone involved will be able to see how the decision was made.

Virtue or Character Ethics

Virtue can be described as a trait that has moral or social value. According to Aristotle, virtuous behavior requires both the right motive and the right action. In other words, wanting (or intending) to do the right thing is not enough by itself. This idea is somewhat at variance with pure deontologic thinking, as described previously. In virtue theory, following a presumably universal rule is not necessarily a moral or virtuous act if it produces a bad result. Similarly, doing right for the wrong reason is not necessarily a moral or virtuous act if the motive itself was not virtuous.

The catalog of virtues is not exhaustive and varies from one writer to another. Pellegrino and Thomasma [1993] suggest eight virtues that are necessary for sound medical practice:

1. Fidelity to trust (trustworthiness)
2. Compassion (understanding the patient's feelings)
3. Prudence (clinical judgment)
4. Justice (in the sense of love and altruism)
5. Fortitude (sustained courage in the face of difficulty or despair)
6. Temperance (balance in one's life, perhaps also Osler's sense of equanimity)
7. Integrity (personal honesty and wholeness)
8. Effacement of self-interest (putting the patient's interests first)

They argue that these eight virtues are necessary but not sufficient for physicians to practice ethically. Possessing these virtues provides evidence of good intent but they must be linked to ethical action. They suggest that principlism, although not specifically part of virtue theory, can provide a guide for virtue-based ethical action.

Ethics of Care

Care-based ethical thinking is prominent in nursing practice but may be somewhat unfamiliar to physicians. It arose as somewhat of an alternative to deontologic, rule-based thinking that depends on adherence to more or less rigid principles. It also arose from feminist research studies comparing male and female approaches to ethical dilemmas. Gilligan [1982] found that males were more likely to look for rules to follow and to insist on adherence to these rules. Females were more likely to look for some situation-based way to resolve a dilemma, taking into consideration the person's feelings and significant relationships [Gilligan, 1982]. This "feminine" way is not exclusively reserved for women (or for nurses), of course. Rather, it provides an alternative and perhaps more subjective way to evaluate an ethical problem that is especially relevant when a rule-based approach seems to be inappropriate or unhelpful [Taylor and Watson, 1989].

Somewhat obviously, care-based ethics does not have any fixed rules. In fact, it challenges the idea that impartial or universal rules should guide ethical action. Instead, it looks at the particularity of the patient and the clinical situation and seeks to find answers that fit this unique case. Care-based ethics accepts the fact that emotions have important moral value and must be considered carefully. It also emphasizes the patient's human relationships and the mutual interdependence of the patient, family, and all members of the caregiving team. A care-based approach to an ethical dilemma would say something like, "That can't be the only possible ethical solution. There must be another way to resolve this problem that is acceptable to everyone here. We all want to do what's best for the patient, so let's think about what that means. Maybe we could start by understanding what the patient is feeling and by talking to the family. We should also talk about how *we* feel about all of this. Let's brainstorm some ideas and think about what they would involve. Maybe we need to talk to some more people and get more information. If we keep working at it, we'll find a way."

This approach will sound familiar to anyone who has been involved in difficult cases in the intensive care unit (ICU), which emphasizes the ubiquity and usefulness of this way of thinking in clinical practice. Perhaps an awareness of the sound ethical foundation of care-based ethics will also help clinicians give this way of thinking the respect it deserves.

Casuistry

Casuistry, or case-based ethics, is another alternative to utilitarian or rule-based ethical approaches [Jonsen and Toulmin, 1988]. It rejects the very idea of a "moral calculus" that can be analyzed impartially, based on abstract concepts. Instead of a "top-down" approach based on pure theory, it takes a "bottom-up" approach based on the particularity of specific cases. Casuistry looks at specific cases and emphasizes points of agreement about those cases. It recognizes that moral intuition may be more important than adherence to principles. It is common knowledge that members of hospital ethics committees often agree on what needs to be done but cannot always say with clarity why they feel that way (or what ethical theory they relied on to make a particular judgment). This moral intuition may also reflect the influence of the "common morality" described previously. By looking at the particularities of a specific case, casuistry is also sensitive to contextual influences and individual differences.

The method of casuistry is somewhat analogous to the method of case law used in the United States. One first identifies several key cases about which there is a consensus regarding the proper ethical approach. These are cases that have had careful scrutiny in the past and are still believed to be instructive. New cases are then compared with these key cases, selecting those past cases that have the greatest similarity to the current case. One then seeks to develop a consensus about how to resolve the current case, based on how these past cases were resolved. Each new case that is resolved in this way goes into the body of case experience, so that the consensus is revised and modified incrementally in the light of clinical experience.

One can see that casuistry is very similar to what an experienced clinician does naturally, drawing on his or her experience in past cases to sort out the issues in a new case. One has to be careful about which past cases to consider and to what extent the decisions made in those cases apply to the current case. Experience in past cases may also be conflicting, and it may be difficult to sort out the similarities and differences compared with the current case. One also has to be careful about how much weight should be given to one past case compared with another past case. In a very real sense, every new case is different (as every clinician knows), but there is still much to be learned from past experience. Casuistry provides a sound ethical foundation for using this clinical experience in resolving ethical dilemmas.

Spirituality

Spirituality is variously defined, but it can be understood as a belief system that focuses on intangible elements that impart vitality and meaning to one's life [Koenig, 2002]. Because it is based on beliefs, or faith statements, it is not provable through logical argument. Spirituality in medicine is often based on religious beliefs [Sulmasy, 1997], but it need not be. As an expression of ultimate concern, it reflects the elements of our lives that are the most important and make life worth living. Most people have some spiritual beliefs that become prominent when their health is threatened; yet these beliefs are often not considered by physicians and other health-care providers. Physicians may anticipate that patients would have certain beliefs based on knowledge of their religious background [Numbers and Amundsen, 1998], but individual differences exist even within a religious tradition. A more direct understanding of the patient's spirituality would be preferable.

One approach to understanding the patient's spirituality is the "three ways of looking" [Coulter, 2001]. The *first look* is to see the person subjectively as an individual human being. Compassion requires distance and objectivity [Pellegrino and Thomasma, 1993], but this first look requires closeness and subjectivity. It is an attempt to understand the patient's spiritual beliefs. The *second look* is to recognize in the other person that which we know to be central to our own existence. With the second look, we can value in the patient that which we most value in ourselves. These values include living, freedom, tolerance, respect, happiness, and satisfaction with life. Physicians would then seek to protect for their patients the values that they would protect for themselves. The *third look* is more elusive and is an attempt to grasp through our relationship with another person the transcendence or divinity that is the basis of our spiritual existence. This third look comes when it is least expected, often in the vulnerability of a frustrating or challenging ethical situation. When we are open to it, it can provide insight, enrichment, and ethical guidance.

The three ways of looking can be the basis for a spiritual approach to medical ethics. Three precepts can be identified:

1. Respect in others what I value in myself. This precept is similar to the principle of autonomy but is based on the mutuality of spiritual sharing between physician and patient.
2. Do the most loving thing possible. When we love in the patient what we love in ourselves, we will strive to do that which is best for all. Love—not just duty, convention, rules, or cost containment—is the basis for action.
3. Seek guidance from the source of my own and the other person's being, through deep reflection, prayer, advice, or sharing. Thoughtful physicians often do this in difficult ethical situations but may not recognize the spiritual nature of these reflections.

These precepts do not appear to depend on any specific religious tradition and should be applicable in all cultures and religions. One need not be religious to apply them to one's practice. They avoid the relativity of accepting cultural practices at face value by providing a general structure for applying differing cultural beliefs to specific clinical situations. Spirituality cannot and must not be coerced or imposed on others, but physicians who are open to the role of spirituality in the lives of their patients may find these precepts useful in considering difficult ethical challenges.

ETHICAL RESPONSIBILITIES

Child neurologists have duties as physicians, as pediatricians, and as neurologists. These categories overlap to some extent. Physicians in general have duties that are reflected in the Hippocratic Oath and the Code of Ethics of the American Medical Association (AMA). Pediatricians have duties as primary care physicians and as caregivers for minor children in a family context. Neurologists have duties as specialists to provide consultation and to maintain expertise in the field.

Duties as a Physician

The AMA Code of Ethics is a document that has been revised over the years and includes opinions and statements on a variety of current issues. It incorporates the current version of the Principles of Medical Ethics [American Medical Association, 2001]:

1. A physician shall be dedicated to providing competent medical care, with compassion and respect for human dignity and rights.
2. A physician shall uphold the standards of professionalism, be honest in all professional interactions, and strive to report physicians deficient in character or competence, or engaging in fraud or deception, to appropriate entities.
3. A physician shall respect the law and recognize a responsibility to seek changes in those requirements which are contrary to the best interests of the patient.
4. A physician shall respect the rights of patients, colleagues, and other health professionals, and shall

safeguard patient confidences and privacy within the constraints of the law.

5. A physician shall continue to study, apply, and advance scientific knowledge, maintain a commitment to medical education, make relevant information available to patients, colleagues, and the public, obtain consultation, and use the talents of other health professionals when indicated.
6. A physician shall, in the provision of appropriate patient care, except in emergencies, be free to choose whom to serve, with whom to associate, and the environment in which to provide medical care.
7. A physician shall recognize a responsibility to participate in activities contributing to the improvement of the community and the betterment of public health.
8. A physician shall, while caring for a patient, regard responsibility to the patient as paramount.
9. A physician shall support access to medical care for all people.

Additional guidance may be found in descriptions of the virtues needed for medical practice [Pellegrino and Thomasma, 1993]. These include the need for trustworthiness, compassion, empathy, prudent clinical judgment, altruism, fortitude, temperance, integrity, and primacy of the patient's interest. Indeed, many of these virtues are implicit in the principles delineated by the AMA.

Many professional societies have developed ethical codes or guidelines that are specific for their field. The websites of the American Academy of Pediatrics (www.aap.org), the American Academy of Neurology (www.aan.com), and the Child Neurology Society (www.childneurologysociety.org) may be consulted for the most up-to-date statements about the ethical responsibilities of members of these societies.

Conflicts may arise in applying these principles during ordinary practice. For example, physicians should generally tell the truth, but what if truth-telling would appear to be harmful to the patient? There are no easy answers. The application of a care-based ethical approach may be useful in such situations. A carefully considered amount of information may be provided in such a way and in a particular context, taking into account the physician-patient relationship, so that all involved will understand the information being conveyed and be able to use it to benefit the patient.

Consider this example: A 6-month-old infant is up for adoption and the agency wants an opinion about the child's developmental potential. The child's mother was an alcoholic, but the child does not meet criteria for a diagnosis of fetal alcohol syndrome. Should the agency be told that the child is at risk for alcohol-related neurodevelopmental delay (fetal alcohol effects), which could jeopardize the potential adoption and relegate the child to prolonged and potentially damaging foster care? Or should the physician accentuate the positive and simply say there is no evidence of fetal alcohol syndrome? How much truth needs to be told, and how certain can the physician be that others will be able to use the information for the benefit of the patient?

Physicians are often called upon to write letters for patients. These letters may be used to secure benefits for the patient in school, work, or other settings. Letters may also be requested to assist the patient or family in obtaining insurance coverage for tests or treatments, or in obtaining help with housing and utilities (heat, electricity, or telephone services). In general, physicians would seem to be required to do what is best for the patient, but what if this seems to conflict with a duty to respect the law and to do what is best for the community?

Consider this example: A 17-year-old boy with Klein-Levin syndrome has been difficult to treat but did best when he was involved in competitive sports in school. Unfortunately, his grades are now not good enough for him to participate in varsity football. Should the physician write a letter to the school principal stating that it is medically necessary for him to play football, even though this would violate the school's rules about eligibility for sports? Or should the physician and the principal negotiate a way for the patient to obtain the benefit of vigorous exercise and competition in some other format?

Physicians are often requested by insurance companies to prescribe older, cheaper drugs or to use generic products instead of new brand-name products. Indeed, in some insurance arrangements (such as full capitation), physicians may receive a financial benefit by limiting the cost of the patient's care. Should a physician order expensive tests or prescribe expensive treatments anyway, if they are believed to be in the patient's best interest? How much is a physician responsible for the overall cost of health care in society, and how should this responsibility be balanced against the responsibility to do what is best for the patient?

Consider this example: A physician believes that atomoxetine would be a better choice to treat a child with attention-deficit-hyperactivity disorder instead of a stimulant drug such as methylphenidate or dextroamphetamine. However, Medicaid refuses to pay for atomoxetine unless the child has already failed a trial of stimulant drugs. Should the physician prescribe a generic stimulant and wait for the child to have adverse effects from it, or should the physician "shade the truth" in requesting Medicaid coverage for atomoxetine?

Clearly, application of general principles of medical ethics to complicated clinical situations is anything but straightforward. Nonetheless, physicians should make a genuine effort to do the best they can. The requirement to make the patient's interests paramount would appear to be the defining standard in most cases. In doubtful or difficult situations, consultation or discussion with one's colleagues (either formally or informally) is probably a good idea.

Duties as a Pediatrician

Many (but not all) child neurologists have trained as pediatricians and have some experience with the roles and responsibilities of a pediatrician. Most also have frequent contact with referring pediatricians who provide primary care for the patients seen in neurologic practice. The role of a pediatrician often involves primary care in the United States, but in other countries and other settings the pediatrician is a specialist who manages diseases involving other parts of the body. Child neurologists interact regularly with pediatric specialists involved in the care of children with complex disorders. Thus, there is an overlap between the duties of the child neurologist and the pediatrician that warrants some exploration.

Primary care involves the longitudinal management of all of the health issues of the child and family and requires a commitment to being accessible, available, and capable. Effective primary care is compassionate, culturally competent, and comprehensive and includes coordination and oversight of all of the child's health problems [Tonniges and Palfrey, 2004]. Most child neurologists do not provide this type of primary care. Many do, however, provide many of the same elements of care for children whose neurologic problems constitute the main health issues. These include older children and adolescents who are otherwise healthy but have ongoing neurologic problems, as well as patients with complex neurologic problems whose general health problems are fairly straightforward. Child neurologists have no obligation to take on this role and may confine their role to that of a consultant. Those who do take on this role would seem to have the same duties as those of a primary care physician listed above, except that their duties are limited to management of the child's neurologic problems.

All physicians who care for children (including pediatricians and child neurologists) have a duty to understand and respect the child's status as a minor. This duty has two elements: one involves promoting the child's emerging development into an adult, and the other involves protecting the child from harm. Promoting the child's development involves an understanding of normal child development and helping the child succeed as much as possible. Child neurologists ordinarily monitor the child's progress in school and provide whatever assistance is possible to secure special education and therapeutic resources needed to promote the child's development. Although the primary responsibility rests with the parents and the school, the child neurologist should be available and capable of providing help when needed.

Because children are not capable of making sound judgments about their own best interests, others must judge for them what is in their best interests. Social convention and the law generally recognize that parents are the best judge of what is in the child's best interest, but this recognition is not absolute. A substantial body of law and regulation governs when and in what circumstances a parent's rights may be superseded. Consideration of these laws and regulations is beyond the scope of this chapter [see Beauchamp and Childress, 1994; Bernat, 1994]. Child neurologists may be called upon to give an opinion about what medical care is in the child's best interest. They may also be asked about whether they believe the child is capable of independent judgment. Persons who are 18 years old are usually assumed to be fully autonomous adults who are capable of giving informed consent for medical treatment. Many neurologic patients with significant intellectual disabilities are not capable, however; therefore, others must be designated as guardians for them. The child neurologist should be aware of what is involved in determining the need for guardianship and assist the patient and family in whatever way is appropriate.

The United Nations [1990] has formulated a declaration on the rights of children, the Convention on the Rights of the Child, which contains 54 Articles that stipulate the rights of the child to life, safety, health, education, and a decent standard of living. Article 23 states that a mentally or physically disabled child should enjoy a full and decent life in conditions which ensure dignity, promote self-reliance, and facilitate the child's active participation in the community. It further recognizes the rights of the disabled child to special care. Article 24 states that the child should have access to quality health services, including primary care, preventive health care, and treatment of health conditions. Although the Convention's declaration is not legally binding, it provides a strong moral statement about the internationally accepted obligations of states to protect the best interests of all children. Awareness of this international consensus may be helpful to physicians who are advocating for children under their care.

Duties as a Neurologist

Child neurologists are specialists or subspecialists and have duties that correspond to this role. They provide longitudinal care for children and adolescents with chronic neurologic disorders that includes corresponding duties that resemble those of primary care, as described previously. They also provide consultative opinions about diagnosis and treatment, both in outpatient and inpatient settings. As a consultant, the child neurologist has a duty to provide a fair, impartial, accurate, and (as much as possible) evidence-based statement about the facts of the case. The child neurologist's principal role in evaluating ethical dilemmas is to clarify the facts. This is a critical role, because accurate data are essential for making sound ethical decisions [Coulter et al., 1988]. Indeed, poor or questionable ethical decisions are often due to inadequate specialized medical information regarding the diagnosis, treatment, and/or prognosis of a case. This problem is illustrated well in cases when the patient is in a vegetative state. Some may consider such a state permanent and hopeless after only a few weeks and seek to withdraw life-sustaining treatment. The child neurologist, acting as a consultant in such a case, would inform the family and caregivers about the published data suggesting that the vegetative state is not considered permanent until 3 months after an anoxic injury and 12 months after a traumatic brain injury [Multi-Society Task Force on PVS, 1994]. The family may be given some hope for possible recovery of consciousness before these time periods, which may call for continued treatment and rehabilitation.

The role of an expert consultant has certain limitations. For the most part, child neurologists are experts in child neurology and not in ethics. The child neurologist should distinguish between opinions regarding the neurologic data and opinions regarding the ethical issues involved in cases that present ethical dilemmas. The child neurologist's opinion about the ethical issues is one voice among many and is not necessarily the most important or determining opinion. Normally, the family's opinion about the ethical issues is the most important. The views of the extended family and the family's religious or faith community are often important. In many cases, the views of individuals who have had long-term, close and personal relationships with the patient (e.g., friends, personal attendants, or group home staff) also deserve consideration. Child neurologists, as well as other physicians and nurses involved in such cases, should be careful not to impose their own ethical opinions or attempt to override the expressed opinions of the patient's family and friends.

The child neurologist also has a duty to maintain expertise in the field. This is a duty that is shared with all medical specialists. Expertise is maintained through continuing education, which may involve reading journals, attending conferences, and discussing issues or cases with colleagues who may have more knowledge or experience regarding the issues in question.

Research

Many child neurologists are involved in research, which carries additional ethical duties. One of the challenges for child neurologists involved in clinical research is to separate their ethical obligations as investigators from their ethical obligations as physicians responsible for treating patients who may be enrolled as subjects in the neurologist's research study. This challenge is harder than it may seem. In the United States, research ethics is based on the Belmont Report [1979], which adopted the principles of autonomy, beneficence, and justice (see earlier discussion) as the basis of research ethics. In general, the researcher's principal ethical obligation is to protect the rights and welfare of the research subject [Dunn and Chadwick, 1999]. Poorly designed research studies are inherently unethical because they are not likely to produce sound scientific results, and thus they place the patient-subject at risk for harm without the prospect of benefit. The researcher's ethical obligation as an investigator to pursue well-designed scientific studies is secondary to his or her obligation to protect the subject involved in the research. When the research subject is also a patient, this means that the child neurologist-investigator's clinical duties to the patient are ordinarily stronger than his or her duties to enroll subjects in the research study.

In the United States, federally sponsored research is governed by the Code of Federal Regulations, which stipulates the roles and responsibilities of researchers and institutions involved in clinical research [see Dunn and Chadwick, 1999]. Researchers are required to obtain review and approval of the research study by a properly constituted Institutional Review Board for the Protection of Human Subjects in Research (IRB). Child neurologists involved in clinical research have legal and ethical obligations to follow these rules and regulations. In general, ethical issues in research should be considered when the study is being designed, not just at the end of the study when IRB review and approval are requested. The researcher should be knowledgeable about ethical issues in research. If the researcher has questions about ethical aspects of study design or protocol development, most IRBs will provide assistance. Building ethics into the study from the beginning will usually prevent problems later during the process of IRB approval, as well as during continuing review and oversight of the study.

ETHICAL PROBLEMS

Personhood

Critical ethical problems in child neurology often center on the question of *personhood*. Some authorities [Field and Behrman, 2004], consider this the most important problem in bioethics. Indeed, the history of the concept of personhood can be traced to Plato and Aristotle [Mahowald, 1995]. This history includes many rich and varied discussions based on several key questions. Should all human beings be considered persons, in a moral sense, to whom ethical duties are owed? Or are some human beings (such as fetuses or infants with anencephaly) "nonpersons" who can be treated differently than "real persons"? Is personhood absolute or are there degrees of personhood, and thus degrees of ethical obligations? Can personhood be lost while human existence persists—for example, in a vegetative state? Are there reliable and valid criteria that one can use to determine whether a human being is a person?

The capacity for rational thought is often considered to be what separates human persons from nonpersons, yet rationality may not be sufficient by itself. Plato, Aristotle, Augustine, Aquinas, and other classical philosophers emphasized the unity of reason and spirit, or soul [Mahowald, 1995]. Current religious and theologic arguments maintain this position by arguing that all human beings have a God-given soul, which confers moral personhood and that requires ethical respect. Berrigan wrote that the presence of God is most apparent when we are with those who are unable to respond to us [Berrigan, 2000]. Enlightenment philosophers such as Locke and Kant redefined the issue to emphasize self-consciousness, or the rational ability to have a concept of oneself as a unique being and thus to exercise autonomy or free will. This definition would suggest that human beings who do not have this ability may not be fully human persons in a moral sense. Modern thinkers have sought to identify criteria by which one may determine whether personhood is present. Fletcher [1979] identified a number of such criteria, including self-awareness, self-control, a sense of one's history and future, the capacity to relate to others, and the ability to communicate. For Fletcher, IQ could be used as a surrogate measure of these abilities, so that an IQ below 20 meant that one was not a person. Utilitarian theory has been used to arrive at essentially the same position [Kuhse and Singer, 1985]. This position has been criticized on philosophical grounds [Byrne, 2000]. Hauerwas considered the question of developing criteria for personhood "fundamentally wrong-headed" because it ignores the real question, which is how others should relate to those who may not meet these criteria: "I suspect that we are human exactly to the extent we can reach out and provide care to those who have no right to it" [Swinton, 2004].

The question of what it means to be human can be considered from an anthropologic and historical perspective. Fernandez-Armesto [2004] identified six challenges to our understanding of human personhood:

1. The similarity between humans and nonhuman primates
2. The presence of "human" qualities (such as language or tool-making) in other animals
3. The indistinct boundary between modern humans (*Homo sapiens*) and prehistoric ancestors (such as Neanderthals)
4. The evolutionary mutability of all species
5. The problem of artificial intelligence and "humanoid" robots
6. The ability to modify the human genome by addlng or subtracting characteristics and abilities.

Considering these challenges leads to the conclusion that the boundaries of what physicians consider "humankind" or human personhood, from an anthropologic perspective, are by definition necessarily indistinct [Fernandez-Armesto, 2004].

What does this mean for child neurologists? Many patients (such as infants with severe neurologic disabilities, children with profound intellectual disabilities, and adolescents in a persistent vegetative state) would not meet the criteria of personhood advocated by Fletcher. Are physicians' ethical obligations to them any less than to other patients who are more obviously human persons, or do theories of justice require physicians to provide more compensatory resources to help them function more effectively in society [Veatch, 1986]? Theories of beneficence argue that physicians should attempt to promote and protect the patient's quality of life as perceived by the patient, regardless of what physicians may think of it [Beauchamp and Childress, 1994]. From a clinical perspective, parents rarely regard their children with severe disabilities as nonpersons. Child neurologists, working together with parents and other caregivers, will want to focus on doing what is best for the child and family. Distinguishing between moral status and moral agency [Mahowald, 1995], physicians may conclude that patients whose moral status is questionable because of presumed limited personhood are still moral agents with human rights to whom those with greater moral status have ethical obligations as members of human society.

Euthanasia

The challenge of euthanasia is one of the most important ethical issues in neurology and medicine today. Conventional thinking distinguishes between passive euthanasia (not doing something to preserve life) and active euthanasia (doing something to end life). Passive euthanasia is generally considered acceptable medical practice in some situations, whereas active euthanasia is not (and is illegal in most situations). However, this distinction may be vague and confusing in some cases. Legitimate and illegitimate applications of both passive and active euthanasia can be identified. In their discussion of the ethical principle of nonmaleficence, Beauchamp and Childress [1994] argue for recasting the distinction in terms of respect for autonomy and serving the patient's best interests. They argue that in some carefully specified situations, physicians may legitimately assist patients in dying (active euthanasia) if the action responds to the patients' wishes and serves their interests.

Passive euthanasia (withdrawal of life-sustaining treatment) is often considered for persons who are in a persistent vegetative state (PVS). Consensus exists regarding the medical aspects of a vegetative state in children and adults [Multi-Society Task Force on PVS, 1994], but the ethical and legal issues are more contentious [Jennett, 2002]. With respect to children and adolescents, two questions arise: (1) What are the boundaries of the diagnosis of the vegetative state? (2) How confident can we be about the prognosis for patients in a vegetative state?

The Multi-Society Task Force on PVS included representation from the Child Neurology Society and reviewed the literature to address these questions. The Task Force concluded that the concept of the vegetative state cannot be applied to preterm infants, and the diagnosis of a vegetative state is difficult to make before three months of life. An exception to this statement may be made for infants with true anencephaly who by definition are in a vegetative state. Caregivers are often confused when patients demonstrate subtle or minimal signs of responsiveness, which would suggest that the diagnosis of PVS is no longer accurate. Patients who demonstrate minimal but definite behavioral evidence of self or environmental awareness may be diagnosed instead as being in a minimally conscious state, which is distinct from the vegetative state. Diagnostic criteria exist for distinguishing between a minimally conscious state and a vegetative state in children [Ashwal and Cranford, 2002]. Data also exist regarding the prognosis for children and adolescents in a minimally conscious state or a vegetative state. It is possible to distinguish between a mobile (ability to lift the head, roll over, or sit) and an immobile minimally conscious state, but studies have found little difference in survival between children in either state [Strauss et al., 2000]. For children 3 years of age in a vegetative state or an immobile minimally conscious state, 12% to 18% had evolved to a state better than a minimally conscious state after 3 additional years. For children in a vegetative state from birth to 1 year of age, median survival was 4.2 years and life expectancy was 7.2 additional years. For adolescents still in a vegetative state 1 year after onset, median survival was 5.2 years and life expectancy was 10.5 additional years [Strauss et al., 1999].

Withdrawal of life-sustaining treatment (including nutrition and hydration) is generally considered legally and ethically appropriate for children and adults who are in a permanent vegetative state [Jennett, 2002]. This view has been challenged recently for Roman Catholics because of the statement by Pope John Paul II [2004], that the withdrawal of assisted (artificial) nutrition and hydration "has to be considered a genuine act of euthanasia by omission, which is morally unacceptable." The Pope's statement was not delivered under the doctrine of infallibility and thus is not binding in the strict sense. Catholic theologians consider it to represent an important opinion to be discussed carefully in the ongoing debate about the care of patients in a vegetative state [Shannon and Walter, 2004]. The legal and ethical standards for withdrawing life-sustaining treatment from patients in a minimally conscious state are much less clear, since such patients theoretically could feel pain and suffering [Ashwal and Cranford, 2002].

The concept of futility implies that a proposed treatment or course of action offers negligible potential for overall patient benefit, whether that potential is considered quantitatively in terms of the probability of success or qualitatively in terms of the expected impact on the patient's quality of life. The question often arises when patients or families request treatment that caregivers do not believe is appropriate. Rather than focus on strict guidelines or policies to follow in such cases, physicians are encouraged to develop fair and transparent procedures for decision-making that encompass the views of all parties involved in these difficult situations [Shevell, 2002].

Voluntary active euthanasia is much more controversial than passive euthanasia [Smith, 1997]. Often called *mercy killing* or *physician-assisted suicide*, it is opposed by the American Medical Association and is illegal in all of the United States except in Oregon. On the other hand, it is legal in some countries, most visibly in The Netherlands, where it has recently been extended to include children younger than 12 years of age. Following Beauchamp and Childress [1994], many people wish to be able to exercise their autonomy rights and to choose death (with or without medical assistance) when this is a conscious, carefully considered, noncoerced, personal decision they make for themselves. Whether it is ever ethical for others to make this decision on behalf of nonautonomous persons (such as children and adolescents) is not at all clear (even in The Netherlands), and no convincing ethical argument has been advanced so far to support a consensus on this point.

Perfection and Neuroethics

The attempt to create more perfect children is universal and perhaps understandable. Parents do not wish to create a child whom they believe to be imperfect [Murray, 1996]. Some deaf parents may wish to create a child whom others might consider imperfect because of deafness but whom they consider more perfect because of the child's ability to participate in deaf society [Middleton et al., 2001]. Even parents who love and accept their child's imperfections would likely still prefer to have those imperfections disappear if possible. In asking whether "the retarded suffer from being retarded," Hauerwas [1986] argues that individuals project on them their own fears of what it would be like to have an intellectual disability and thus fail to imagine what living with such a disability is really like. Obversely, people desire perfection for their children because they value perfection in ourselves.

The desire for perfection may be a relevant consideration when parents must make decisions about life-sustaining treatment for infants and young children faced with the prospect of lifelong severe disability. Often the child is still dependent on life-sustaining technology, which, if withdrawn, will result in the child's death. The prognosis may be somewhat uncertain and likely to become clearer with time [Coulter, 1987]. Yet if the parents wait, the child's medical situation may stabilize and no longer require life-sustaining technology. Parents who are relatively intolerant of imperfection (lifelong severe disability) may thus choose to withdraw life-sustaining treatment before the exact prognosis is clarified, rather than wait and lose the opportunity to choose. This situation is very difficult for the child neurologist caring for the patient, whose principal duties are to provide accurate data about diagnosis and prognosis and to support the family's decision [Glass, 2002]. Although some observers think that parents may be making these choices earlier and withdrawing support more often than they did in the past, little or no published data are available to verify this observation or to explore why this might be true. Literature on the social and spiritual significance of disability [Eiesland, 1994; Vehmas, 2004] points out that individuals with disabilities often perceive their quality of life to be better than those without disabilities might expect. On the other hand, some contemporary philosophers argue that personhood is limited in the presence of severe disability, and withdrawal of life support is appropriate [Kuhse and Singer, 1985]. Perhaps child neurologists can do no more than be aware of these issues and discuss them with families who are faced with these difficult choices.

The issue of perfection is framed more starkly when considering what has been termed *cosmetic neurology* [Dees, 2004]. Chatterjee [2004] distinguished between the goal of medicine to treat disease and the goal to enhance quality of life by improving normal functions. Should drugs be prescribed to enhance strength, coordination, attention, learning, memory, mood, and affect in those who are neurologically normal? He identified four ethical dilemmas related to cosmetic neurology:

1. What degree of risk should be acceptable when enhancing normal brain function (when the alternative is normality)?
2. How does enhancement of normal brain function alter our views of what it means to be a person [as suggested by Fernandez-Armesto]?
3. Should enhancement of normal brain function be available to all or only to those who can afford it?
4. Are persons subject to coercion from employers and others who would value enhanced brain function and reward those who have it?

Furthermore, if the advent of cosmetic neurology is inevitable, how will neurologists respond when their patients request it? Child neurologists will be faced with an additional ethical question: Should parents be able to request cosmetic neurology for their children? Clearly much ethical thought will be needed to address these questions.

Cosmetic neurology is one aspect of what has been termed *neuroethics*. This is a new concept that incorporates the application of modern neuroscientific research to clinical problems and to general society. Related to this, the term *neurotheology* has been coined to encompass the application of neuroscientific research to understanding religious and spiritual experience [Joseph, 2002]. Functional neuroimaging now allows us to evaluate personal information such as personality traits, social and moral attitudes, individual preferences, deception, guilt, and thoughts [Farah and Wolpe, 2004]. The principal ethical challenges of these applications of neuroimaging relate to privacy, autonomy, and respect for the person.

Another aspect of neuroethics is the use of new genetic knowledge to diagnose and treat neurogenetic disorders. Ethical issues in genetic diagnosis include stigma and privacy, whereas gene therapy raises ethical issues similar to those of cosmetic neurology [Avard and Knoppers, 2002]. Scientific progress is inevitable and desirable and the challenges of neuroethics will become even more important in the near future. All neurologists must be aware of these ethical challenges and become informed about appropriate responses as they are developed.

SYNTHESIS

The child neurologist striving to do the right thing and to avoid doing the wrong thing will listen to many voices conveying a variety of messages. Some of these voices are internal and reflect the several theoretical approaches that provide a "best fit" for the patient's problem. The neurologist's mind will hear different ways of conceptualizing the problem, perhaps from an ethics of care or a utilitarian perspective or some other approach. Experience teaches that clinical ethics is not procrustean, that no theory or approach will fit every clinical situation. Every case is unique and provides lessons that can be stored away in memory and called upon another day. Drawing upon his or her knowledge about ethics derived from careful study, as well as the knowledge that can only come from having been at the bedside of many sick children over the years, the neurologist will struggle to derive a sense of harmony that will be helpful when a decision must be made.

The child neurologist also listens to the external voices of others who are involved in the clinical situation. Foremost among them is the voice of the family. When love is present, families usually find a way to deal with whatever life hands them. It may not be the "right" way (the way others want them to take), but it is a way that works for them and deserves respect. At any given point in time most people are doing the best they can, given their skills and abilities and the pressures and limitations they face. When physicians seek to understand the situation from the family's point of view, they may be able to help them do the best they can for themselves and for their child [Coulter, 2002]. The neurologist will also hear the voices of other patients and families he or she has treated and followed over the years, who were in a similar situation in the past and whose subsequent history speaks to the wisdom of decisions that were made [Freeman, 2004].

The child neurologist also will hear the voices of other caregivers involved in a particular case, especially those of the nurses who have a more intimate relationship with the patient and family. In some cases, the voices of long-time friends, pastoral ministers, and staff who have cared for the patient before the present situation arose will need to be heard and considered carefully. The soft but insistent voices of insurance administrators and utilization reviewers may also be audible.

Synthesizing all of these arguments and perspectives is never easy and perhaps benefits most from a deep sense of humility. Reflecting on the lessons he had learned in a long and distinguished career as one of the foremost child neurologists in the United States, John Freeman concluded:

"One lesson I believe I have learned is that decision-making should be a process, and the process for arriving at a decision is far more important than the decision arrived at. This process cannot be left solely to the family, or to relatives and friends, with their biases and prejudices, any more than it can be left solely to the physician. Physicians and families together must learn to work out a plan for the handicapped or potentially handicapped newborn—and likewise for the premature infant, for the person with late-stage Alzheimer's disease, for the critically ill patient, and for individuals at both ends of life." [Freeman, 2004]

REFERENCES

American Medical Association. Principles of medical ethics. Chicago: American Medical Association, 2001.

Ashwal S, Cranford R. The minimally conscious state in children. Semin Pediatr Neurol 2002;9:19.

Avard DM, Knoppers BM. Ethical dimensions of genetics in pediatric neurology: A look into the future. Semin Pediatr Neurol 2002;9:53.

Beauchamp TL, Childress JF. Principles of biomedical ethics, 4th ed. New York: Oxford University Press, 1994.

Bentham J. An Introduction to the principles of morals and legislation. New York: Methuen, 1982.

Bernat JL. Ethical issues in neurology. Boston: Butterworth-Heinemann, 1994.

Berrigan D. God is love. Noah Homes Newsletter 2000;Spring issue:2.

Byrne P. Philosophical and ethical problems in mental handicap. New York: Palgrave, 2000.

Callahan D. Bioethics. In: Reich W, ed. Encyclopedia of bioethics. New York: Simon and Schuster Macmillan, 1995.

Chatterjee A. Cosmetic neurology: The controversy over enhancing movement, mentation and mood. Neurology 2004;63:968.

Coulter DL, Murray TH, Cerreto M. Practical ethics in pediatrics. Curr Probl Pediatr 1988;18:139.

Coulter DL. Neurological uncertainty in neonatal intensive care. N Engl J Med 1987;316:840.

Coulter DL. Recognition of spirituality in health care: Personal and universal implications. J Religion Disability Health 2001;5:1.

Coulter DL. The strength of families and individuals. J Religion Disability Health 2002;6:1.

Dees RH. Slippery slopes, wonder drugs, and cosmetic neurology: The neuroethics of enhancement. Neurology 2004;63:951.

Dunn CM, Chadwick G. Protecting study subjects in research. Boston: CenterWatch, 1999.

Eiesland NL. The disabled god: Toward a liberatory theology of disability. Nashville, TN: Abingdon Press, 1994.

Farah MJ, Wolpe PR. Monitoring and manipulating brain function: New neuroscience technologies and their ethical implications. Hastings Cent Rep 2004;34:35.

Fernandez-Armesto F. Humankind: A brief history. New York: Oxford University Press, 2004.

Field MJ, Behrman RE, eds, Ethical conduct of clinical research involving children. Washington, DC: National Academy Press, 2004.

Fletcher J. Humanhood: Essays in biomedical ethics. Buffalo, NY: Prometheus Books, 1979.

Freeman JF, McDonnell K. Tough decisions: Cases in medical ethics, 2nd ed. New York: Oxford University Press, 2001.

Freeman JM. On learning humility: A thirty-year journey. Hastings Cent Rep 2004;34:13.

Gert B. The relevance of moral theory to pediatric neurology. Semin Pediatr Neurol 2002;9:2.

Gilligan C. In a different voice. Cambridge, MA: Harvard University Press, 1982.

Glass KC. Ethical issues in neonatal intensive care: Perspectives for the neurologist. Semin Pediatr Neurol 2002;9:35.

Hauerwas S. Suffering presence: theological reflections on medicine, the mentally handicapped, and the church. Notre Dame, IN: University of Notre Dame Press, 1986.

Jennett B. The vegetative state: Medical facts, ethical and legal dilemmas. New York: Cambridge University Press, 2002.

Jonsen AR, Siegler M, Winslade WJ. Clinical ethics: A practical approach to ethical decisions in clinical medicine, 4th ed. New York: McGraw-Hill, 1998.

Jonsen AR, Toulmin S. The abuse of casuistry: A history of moral decision-making. Berkeley, CA: University of California Press, 1988.

Joseph R, ed. Neurotheology: Brain, science, spirituality, religious experience. San Jose, CA: University Press, 2002.

Kant I. Foundations of the metaphysics of morals. Indianapolis, IN: Bobbs-Merrill, 1959.

Koenig HG. Spirituality in patient care: Why, how, when and what. Philadelphia: Templeton Foundation Press, 2002.

Kuhse H, Singer P. Should the Baby Live? The problem of handicapped infants. New York: Oxford University Press, 1985.

Mahowald M. The person. In: Reich W, ed. Encyclopedia of bioethics. New York: Simon and Schuster Macmillan, 1995.

May WE. An introduction to moral theology. Huntington, IN: Our Sunday Visitor Publications, 1994.

Middleton A, Hewison J, Mueller R. Prenatal diagnosis for inherited deafness—what is the potential demand? J. Genet Couns 2001;10:121.

Mill JS. Utilitarianism. Indianapolis, IN: Bobbs-Merrill, 1971.

Murray TH. The worth of a child. Berkeley, CA: University of California Press, 1996.

Nordenfelt L, ed. Concepts and measurement of quality of Life in health care. Boston: Kluwer Academic, 1994.

Numbers RL, Amundsen DW, eds. Caring and curing: Health and medicine in the western religious traditions. Baltimore: Johns Hopkins University Press, 1998.

Nussbaum MC, Sen A, eds. The quality of life. Oxford: Clarendon Press, 1993.

Pellegrino E, Thomasma D. The virtues in medical practice. New York: Oxford University Press, 1993.
Pfaff DW, ed. Ethical questions in brain and behavior. New York: Springer-Verlag, 1983.
Pope John Paul II. Joint statement on the vegetative state, 2004. www.vatican.va.
Rawls J. A Theory of justice. Cambridge, MA: Harvard University Press, 1971.
Reich W: Introduction. In: Reich W, ed. Encyclopedia of bioethics. New York: Simon and Schuster Macmillan, 1995.
Schalock RL, ed. Quality of Life, Vol 1: Conceptualization and measurement. Washington, DC: American Association on Mental Retardation, 1996.
Shannon TA, Walter JJ. Implications of the papal allocution on feeding tubes. Hastings Cent Rep 2004;34:18.
Shevell MI, ed. Ethical issues in pediatric neurology. Semin Pediatr Neurol 2002;9:1.
Shevell MI. Reflections on futility. Semin Pediatr Neurol 2002;9:41.
Simon YR. The tradition of natural law. New York: Fordham University Press, 1992.
Slote M. The task of ethics. In: Reich W, ed. Encyclopedia of bioethics. New York: Simon and Schuster Macmillan, 1995.
Smith WJ. Forced exit. New York: Random House, 1997.
Strauss DJ, Ashwal S, Day SM, et al. Life expectancy of children in vegetative and minimally conscious states. Pediatr Neurol 2000;23:312.
Strauss DJ, Shavelle RM, Ashwal S. Life expectancy and median survival time in the permanent vegetative state. Pediatr Neurol 1999;21:626.
Sulmasy DP. The healer's calling: A spirituality for physicians and other health care professionals. New York: Paulist Press, 1997.
Swinton J, ed. Disabling society, enabling theology: Critical reflections of Stanley Hauerwas' theology of disability. Binghamton, NY: Haworth Press, 2004.
Taylor RL, Watson J, eds. They shall not hurt: Human suffering and human caring. Boulder, CO: University of Colorado Press, 1989.
The Belmont Report. Ethical principles and guidelines for the protection of human subjects in research. Washington, DC: Federal Register Document 79-12065, 1979.
The Multi-Society Task Force on PVS. Medical aspects of the persistent vegetative state. N Engl J Med 1994; 330:499(Part 1), 1572 (Part 2).
Tonniges TF, Palfrey JS. The medical home. Pediatrics 2004;113:1471.
United Nations. Convention on the Rights of the Child. New York: Office of the United Nations High Commissioner for Human Rights, 1990.
Veatch RV. The foundations of justice: why the retarded and the rest of us have claims to equality. New York: Oxford University Press, 1986.
Velmas S. Ethical analysis of the concept of disability. Ment Retard 2004;42:209.

CHAPTER 95

The Internet and Its Resources for the Child Neurologist

Kenneth J. Mack and Steven M. Leber

The rapid explosion of the Internet has created a plethora of opportunities and challenges in the field of child neurology, both for practitioners and for patients and their families. Not only is clinical and scientific information more rapidly and universally available, but new forms of information now exist only because of the power of electronic communication. Libraries of all sorts are now literally at our fingertips, and clinical consultation and research collaboration with distant colleagues have never been easier. In this chapter, many of the potential applications of the Internet for pediatric neurology are reviewed. Obtaining and learning to use the new software and hardware require time and money, and some of the potential costs of the new methodologies are also noted.

Just as the well-informed physician needs continuing medical education to keep pace with the rapid growth of clinical knowledge, he or she must invest time and energy in "continuing informatics education" to keep up with the explosion of computer methods available to assist in the care of patients. For those who are proficient in the use of computers and the Internet, the challenge will be to apply the methodology creatively to clinical practice. For others who find learning to use computers like trying to learn a new language well past the critical period, the challenge is simply to keep up with the changes. For still others around the world, access to the hardware required for any of these applica-tions is severely limited. The greatest challenge to all, however, may be in developing the wisdom and experience necessary to determine the quality of information being communicated.

THE INTERNET

The Internet was initially established in the 1960s as a U.S. military communication system with the goal of providing a reliable communication system in the event of a nuclear war. Over time, multiple regional and academic connections were made to the initial network, and the Internet became a network of multiple computers. Currently, the Internet consists of hundreds of millions of connected computers all around the world. Similar to telephone services, no central organization is currently responsible for the entire Internet. The strength of this design is that it is nearly impossible for the Internet to break down. The disadvantage is that the Internet can seem poorly organized.

In the previous edition of this book, this chapter focused on how to access the Internet. In the ensuing years, access has become almost trivial, and the Internet is now a tool used by most clinicians.

THE INTERNET'S POTENTIAL USEFULNESS

Electronic Mail

Electronic mail (e-mail) provides a connection between two computers on the Internet. Data, typically as text files such as letters, are sent from one computer to another. Other computer files, such as graphic files, audio files, video files, or even computer programs, can be attached to an e-mail message. For instance, if one wanted to confer with a colleague about an intriguing magnetic resonance scan or an unusual histologic specimen, he or she could scan the image into a file and then e-mail that file across the country or around the world within seconds. E-mail addresses are typically in the following form: username@domain.top-domain (e.g., president@whitehouse.gov). Among the top-domain codes in the United States are *edu* (educational), *com* (commercial), *gov* (government), and *org* (organization). Outside of the United States, two-letter suffixes usually identify the country (e.g., uk for United Kingdom).

An e-mail message can be sent to a central computer, which distributes the messages to everyone on a "mailing list." Typically, mailing lists are organized by topics, so that there are separate mailing lists for child neurology, adult neurology, child psychiatry, epilepsy, and so forth (see Neurosciences on the Internet [http://www.neuroguide.com/neurolist.html] for some). Most medical mailing lists are either "closed" or "monitored." In closed lists, access is restricted (e.g., to physicians only). In monitored lists, the messages are screened by the system operator to decrease the probability that inappropriate messages are sent out in the mailings. Many lists now have a "digest" option, so that all the e-mail of a single day can be incorporated into a daily digest. This digest option significantly cuts down on the clutter in many e-mail inboxes.

When using a mailing list, note that there are generally two mailing addresses. For instance, in the "Child-Neuro" mailing list, mail sent to child-neuro@waisman.wisc.edu will go out to all the subscribers to the list [Hernandez-Borges et al., 1997; Mack and Leber, 1996]. In contrast, the e-mail address listserv@waisman.wisc.edu is used to address the computer managing the Child-Neuro list and acts as a command—for example, to add a name (subscribe) to the list.

Two issues of recurrent concern for physicians discussing individual patients in e-mail discussion groups are patient confidentiality and professional liability. As with case reports in published journals, anonymity is imperative when patients are discussed, and names and other identifying protected health information must be deleted when imaging studies are shared. Although breaches are possible in unmonitored lists, generally this has not been a problem for most groups. If potentially identifying information is shared (e.g., facial photographs), informed consent must be obtained. In situations in which patient databases are created for intra- or inter-institutional studies, adequate security controls must be installed and anonymity maintained. The issue of liability for online consultation is quite complex and beyond the scope of this discussion, but many attorneys believe that advice provided online is similar to that given in phone consultation: When a physician advises another health care provider without establishing a direct doctor-patient contact or expecting payment for services, that physician is not held liable for the advice given [De Ville, 1996; Elliot and Elliot, 1996].

Even if the legal aspects of this issue become clarified as Internet law evolves, the question of quality of advice will remain. Many postings are unsigned, and the numerous "I treat disease X this way" postings, which may not be based on scientifically controlled trials, are certainly subject to legitimate caution, if not criticism. However, rigorously proved answers are not available for many of the questions pediatric neurologists pose, and this type of practical advice often is exactly what is being sought. Furthermore, although postings to e-mail lists are not subject to any direct peer-review prescreening, the ability of any reader to reply to the original message creates the possibility of a post facto review from clinicians with a broader diversity of expertise than might be found in the traditional two- or three-person review process used in journal publications.

Mailing lists can also be useful in providing notification of publication of articles related to specified medical topics and subspecialties. For example, MDLinx (http://www.mdlinx.com/) has a variety of neurology and pediatric subspecialty mailing lists (including pediatric neurology), supplying brief summaries and links to entire articles. Amedeo (http://www.amedeo.com/) allows subscribers to choose particular areas of neurology and specific journals and then sends out regular lists of new publications, along with links to the articles in PubMed (see later). Both are free services.

USENET Groups

USENET, the user's network, is dedicated to topic-specific discussion groups. These are "bulletin boards" where anyone can post or place a message, and where others can read that message at their convenience, similar to postings on a "real" bulletin board. An initial comment and the responses it prompts are known as a thread. More than 10,000 news groups exist, arranged in a hierarchical fashion. At least 20 of these discuss neurology or neuroscience-related topics, and many are dedicated to particular diseases. USENET is an excellent forum for obtaining the opinion of people with an interest in a particular topic even when one has no way of knowing in advance who these "experts" may be. Because access is open to everyone, the nature and quality of the discussions vary considerably from group to group and thread to thread, but discussions that professionals might not find medically useful (e.g., many in the general medicine news group *sci.med*) can be quite educational in giving clinicians a glimpse of the concerns of patients and families expressed outside the office setting. Similar discussion forums exist on private online services, such as America Online. Neurosciences on the Internet (http://www.neuroguide.com/neuronews.html) lists many of these groups.

Access to USENET can be through dedicated software called *newsreaders* (see http://users.rcn.com/kateshort/nnq/nnewsreader.html for an overview) or through World Wide Web browsers (see later discussion). New users are urged to begin with the group *news.announce.newusers*.

World Wide Web

Access to the Internet became available for people without a strong computer science background when browsers such as Mosaic, Netscape, and Internet Explorer became available. The World Wide Web (WWW) originated as a project to connect researchers in the high-energy physics community. Originally, the basic algorithm for the WWW was developed by researchers at CERN (the European Laboratory for Particle Physics in Switzerland) in 1989. This initial Web was a consortium of computer users who implemented a standardized, nonproprietary syntax termed *hypertext markup language* (HTML). HTML is a standardized method for including images, videos, and audio in documents that can be displayed on a variety of computers, including Apple Macintosh, IBM PCs, and UNIX-based computers [McEnery, 1995]. Later, an NSF-funded effort at the University of Illinois (National Center for Supercomputer Applications) developed Mosaic, a browser program that allows easy access to the large number of text, video, and audio files on the web.

The web has its own specific jargon. A *homepage* is a virtual or computer home. Often a homepage contains links to other useful pages containing text or graphic files. These pages are connected by *hypertext*, a highlighted word or icon that allows one to switch to a new page, regardless of whether that page is on the same computer, in the same city, or across the world. In this way, the web can link a variety of information on a single topic from different information sources around the world. The name or location of a page is called its *URL*, or *uniform resource locator*. Most begin with the code *http://*, which stands for *h*yper*t*ext *t*ransfer *p*rotocol and tells the reading program the mode of access it will use to read the information on the page. This information is followed by a series of characters that specify the location of the host computer and of the file within that computer. Although URLs generally consist of almost unmanageably long lists of letters, web browsers have bookmark features that allow users to save URLs of interest for future reference. In addition to the multimedia and hypertext features, another use of the web involves its capacity for interaction: The reader can fill out forms, respond to questions, and run searches for specific information.

Numerous web browsers are available. Among the more popular are Netscape and Microsoft Internet Explorer. Most are extremely easy to use, and all are in rapid evolution. In addition, numerous helper applications or plug-ins are being developed that expand the capacities of these browsers for audio, video, and interactivity, including three-dimensional virtual reality features.

Many universities, private companies, and other groups are developing their own Intranets. These consist of Web-like pages and documents that are accessible via web browsers but only internally, and that are intended for intra-institutional communication. These may be used for accessing medical records, laboratory data and radiographic images, patient schedules, and medical references; for listing telephone, paging, and e-mail directories; and for posting a wide variety of documents previously printed on paper, such as meeting minutes, call schedules, and practice parameters. Current physiologic data, such as blood pressure and intracranial pressure, can also be placed online in a format accessible from home or office by a physician with a web browser. Because information can flow both to and from the documents and because the documents can be linked to databases, online equipment and supply catalogs can be combined with ordering forms. Interactive intranets can be set up to schedule meetings by coordinating individual schedules. Furthermore, since intra-institutional USENET-like discussion groups can be set up, the need for face-to-face meetings may actually decrease.

Academy and Societal Web Sites

The Child Neurology Society formed an Electronic Communication Committee to facilitate access to useful information on the Internet. In addition, a new Child Neurology Society website (http://www.childneurologysociety.org/) contains information about meetings, fellowship and job opportunities, practice parameters, society publications, a membership directory, and a variety of society business affairs. The Child Neurology Society can be contacted by e-mail at nationaloffice@childneurologysociety.org. Before the completion of the Society's website, a Child-Neuro website was organized (http://www-personal.umich.edu/~leber/c-n/) by the authors of this chapter in an attempt to consolidate useful Internet information of interest to child neurologists and parents of children with neurologic diseases. This site contains supplemental information of value to child neurologists, including listing of research studies seeking patients, research opportunities in child neurology, and patient education resources. The International Child Neurology Association has also developed a site (http://www.child-neuro.net/) for the field of child neurology.

The American Academy of Child and Adolescent Psychiatry site (http://www.aacap.org/) is also worth visiting. The most innovative part of this site is its "Facts For Families," a series of fact sheets for patients and their families on common clinical problems in the field, such as autism, tics, and depression.

The American Academy of Pediatrics has a well-designed site (http://www.aap.org/) that features patient and professional information. This site includes information on "Professional Education" and includes other useful Internet resources for pediatrics.

The American Academy of Neurology is aggressively expanding its website (http://www.aan.com/). Plans include having searchable text documents on the site, useful cross-listing of other sites, and academy information. One of the publications of the American Psychiatric Association site (http://www.psych.org/) is available online (*Psychiatric News*), as well as a continuing medical education program that includes text, audio, and graphic materials.

Journal Sites

Most journals are now available online. A few examples are listed in Table 95-1. An expanding number of journals allow online access to full articles and text, although a paid subscription (either personal or through a library) is usually required. Articles are generally available either in plain text format with links to figures or as print-format PDF files, which can be viewed with special readers, such as Adobe Acrobat Reader, available at no cost from http://www.adobe.com/products/acrobat/readstep2.html. The Highwire Press (http://www.highwire.org/) of Stanford University is a leader in moving journals toward electronic publishing. Both abstracts and full-text articles are available.

Online journals can make current medical and scientific information readily accessible to the third world, and the Health InterNetwork (http://www.healthinternetwork.net/) is leading efforts to provide this free of charge.

The advantages of online journals include the ability to publish quickly and ease of access. Other potential advantages include search capabilities, forums for discussions of articles, links to related articles, and the ability to include supplemental resources and data too extensive to include in a print format. Furthermore, audio and video components can be included in publications without difficulty, which should be of tremendous utility to neurologists discussing language or movement disorders, for example.

Electronic Textbooks

Electronic books are available both online and as purchasable CD-ROM volumes (see Table 93-1). Online Mendelian Inheritance in Man (OMIM) (http://www.ncbi.nlm.nih.gov/entrez/query.fcgi?db=OMIM) is a federally funded project run through the National Center for Biotechnology Information that provides searchable information on human genes and genetic syndromes. It is based in part on McKusick's excellent book on genetic syndromes [McKusick, 1998] but has the advantage of being continually updated. Clinical, historical, and genetic information, with hypertext links available to the abstracts of the cited references, is provided for a vast number of disorders. Currently, this is perhaps the single most useful site for a child neurologist. For example, if a neurologist sees a patient with ataxia and albinism, a search of OMIM reveal eight disorders in which this combination has been seen and describes the clinical and genetic features of each. Other useful book sites include online versions of the *Physicians Desk Reference* and the *Merck Manual.*

More than 40 peer-reviewed topics in child neurology and many more topics in general neurology and other areas of medicine are contained in the electronic text "eMedicine" (http://www.emedicine.com/). The Neuromuscular Disease Center at Washington University (http://www.neuro.wustl.edu/neuromuscular/) is a comprehensive and up-to-date outline covering many aspects of neuromuscular disease in a searchable format. Neuropathology and Neuroanatomy on the Internet (http://www.neuropat.dote.hu/) features an online neuropathology atlas, as well as a tutorial on normal brain structures.

A search of an online bookstore in early 1998 found eight neurology books available or soon-to-be available as CD-

TABLE 95-1

Selected Websites of Interest to Pediatric Neurologists

Name	URL (Address)	Description
Academy Sites		
American Academy of Neurology	http://www.aan.com/	Academic and administrative publications (e.g., AAN News), practice parameters, directory information, neurology rating scales, and clinical trials.
American Academy of Child and Adolescent Psychiatry	http://www.aacap.org/	"Facts for Families" gives parents information on a variety of topics. Useful for office handouts.
American Academy of Pediatrics	http://www.aap.org/	A variety of patient and professional information.
American Association of Neurological Surgeons	http://www.aans.org/	A well-designed web site that features society information.
American Psychiatric Association	http://www.psych.org/	CME program via the Internet, as well as publications, news.
Child Neurology Education and Research Foundation	http://childneurologyfoundation.org/	Research arm of the Child Neurology Society; information about funding opportunities.
Child Neurology Society	http://childneurologysociety.org/	Academy meeting and employment information.
International Child Neurology Association	http://www.child-neuro.net/icna.htm	Academy meeting information. This site address will soon be changed to icna.be.
Society for Neuroscience	http://web.sfn.org/	Largest neuroscience research association.
Clinical Decision-Making Software		
Isabel	http://www.isabel.org.uk/	Commercial, pediatric decision-making software
Simulconsult	http://simulconsult.com/	Free; source for neurologic syndromes; Peer-reviewed, frequently updated.
Clinical Testing Information		
Gene tests	http://www.genetests.org/	A very in-depth database of available molecular testing.
CME Sites		
American Medical Association (AMA)	http://www.ama-assn.org/ama/pub/category/2797.html	Includes database of CME sites.
NIH Consensus Program	http://odp.od.nih.gov/consensus/cme/cme.htm	Program based on NIH consensus statements.
Virtual Lecture Hall	http://www.vlh.com/	Large listing of online CME courses.
Electronic Texts		
eMedicine	http://www.emedicine.com/	Peer-reviewed texts on a variety of neurologic topics.
Medcyclopaedia	http://www.amershamhealth.com/medcyclopaedia/about.asp	Based on the *Encyclopaedia of Medical Imaging*.
Merck Manual	http://www.merck.com/mrkshared/mmanual/home.jsp	Searchable editions of the Merck Manuals.
Neurologic Exam	http://medstat.med.utah.edu/neurologicexam/	Text, illustrations, and videos are provided to illustrate various elements of the neurologic exam.
PediNeuroLogicExam	http://medstat.med.utah.edu/pedineurologicexam/	Pediatric neurologic examination, with movies.
Neuromuscular Disease Center	http://www.neuro.wustl.edu/neuromuscular/	Comprehensive site on neuromuscular disease.
Neuropathology and Neuroanatomy	http://www.neuropat.dote.hu/	Excellent directory of neurology web sites, as well as pathology and anatomy contents.
OMIM: Online Mendelian Inheritance in Man	http://www3.ncbi.nlm.nih.gov/entrez/query.fcgi?db=OMIM	Superb, continuously updated online version of Victor A. McKusick's book*; disorders searchable by symptoms and signs, with references.
Physicians Desk Reference	http://www.medecinteractive.com/	
Whole Brain Atlas	http://www.med.harvard.edu/AANLIB/home.html	Excellent MRI images.
Journal Sites		
Annals of Neurology	http://www3.interscience.wiley.com/cgi-bin/jhome/76507645	
Archives of Neurology	http://archneur.ama-assn.org/	
BMC Neurology	http://www.biomedcentral.com/1471-2377	Free access; totally electronic journal.
British Medical Journal	http://www.bmj.com/bmj	
Brain and Development	http://www.sciencedirect.com/science/journal/03877604	
Developmental Medicine and Child Neurology	http://titles.cambridge.org/journals/journal_catalogue.asp?mnemonic=DMC	
European Journal of Child Neurology	http://www.sciencedirect.com/science/journal/10903798	
Highwire Press	http://www.highwire.org/	Collection of biomedical journals available on the Internet.
Journal of the American Medical Association	http://jama.ama-assn.org/	
Journal of Child Neurology	http://www.bcdecker.com/productDetails.aspx?BJID=69	

TABLE 95-1, *cont'd*

Selected Websites of Interest to Pediatric Neurologists

Name	URL (Address)	Description
Lancet	http://www.thelancet.com/	
Nature	http://www.nature.com/	
Neuroguide	http://www.neuroguide.com/neurojour_5.html	Electronic guide to neurology and neuroscience journals available on the web.
Neurology	http://www.neurology.org/	
New England Journal of Medicine	http://www.nejm.org/	
Pediatrics	http://www.pediatrics.org/	Includes access to electronic articles.
Pediatric Neurology	http://www.sciencedirect.com/science/journal/08878994	
Science	http://science-mag.aaas.org/science/	
Medical Education Resources		
Brain Pathology	http://www.brainpathology.com/	Interesting cases that include actual MRI images, as well as histologic sections.
Medical Student WebSite	http://www.medicalstudent.com/	Links to many online medical texts.
Stanford University Medworld	http://www-med.stanford.edu/medworld/home	Frequently updated; edited by medical students at Stanford University.
Visible Human Project	http://www.nlm.nih.gov/research/visible/visible_human.html	
Medline Browsers		
PubMed	http://www.ncbi.nlm.nih.gov/PubMed/	Extremely useful and updated search engine of the Medline database.
Miscellaneous		
Child-Neuro	http://www-personal.umich.edu/~leber/c-n/	Linkage to other relevant sites and mailing lists, clinical trials, specialized laboratories, etc.
Neurology and Pediatrics Patient and Physician Resources		
American Academy of Neurology	http://www.aan.com/public/index.cfm	Includes information for patients.
BrainTalk Communities	http://brain.hastypastry.net/forums/	Interactive, online discussion about various neurology-related topics, through the Massachusetts General Hospital.
GeneralPediatrics.com	http://www.generalpediatrics.com/	Very thorough directory and search engine for pediatric resources.
Harriet Lane Links	http://www.med.jhu.edu/peds/neonatology/poi.html	Catalog of pediatric information available on the Internet.
Library of The Family Village	http://www.familyvillage.wisc.edu/library.htm	The ultimate catalog of Internet resources concerning neurologic diseases and developmental disabilities.
NIH	http://www.nih.gov/	National Institutes of Health home page.
NINDS	http://www.ninds.nih.gov/	National Institute of Neurological Diseases and Stroke home page.
U.S. Department of Health and Human Services	http://www.healthfinder.org/	A good gateway site for patient-related information.
Research Studies		
Basic Science in Child Neurology Departments	http://www-personal.umich.edu/~leber/c-n/cnlist.htm	Listing of basic science studies.
Center Watch "Clinical Trials In Neurology"	http://www.centerwatch.com/patient/studies/area10.html	A searchable listing for patients and physicians.
NCI Clinical Trials	http://cancernet.nci.nih.gov/	From the U.S. National Cancer Institute.
NIH Clinical Trial Database	http://clinicaltrials.gov/	
Search Engines In Neurology		
Neuroguide	http://www.neuroguide.com/	
Disease-Related Sites		
Ataxia Telangiectasia	http://www.atcp.org/	
Autism Society of America	http://www.autism-society.org/	
Brain Tumor: OncoLink: Pediatric	http://oncolink.upenn.edu/disease/ped_brain/index.html	
Centers for Disease Control	http://www.cdc.gov/	
Cerebral Palsy	http://www.ucp.org/	
Dystonia	http://www.dystonia-foundation.org/	
Epilepsy Foundation of America	http://www.efa.org/	
Headache	http://ahsnet.org/	American Headache Society.
Ketogenic Diet Site	http://www.stanford.edu/group/ketodiet/	From Stanford University.
Leukodystrophy	http://www.ulf.org/	United Leukodystrophy Foundation.
Mental Retardation	http://www.aamr.org/	American Association on Mental Retardation.
Movement Disorders	http://www.wemove.org/	We Move.

continued

TABLE 95-1, *cont'd*

Selected Websites of Interest to Pediatric Neurologists

Name	URL (Address)	Description
Muscular Dystrophy Association	http://www.mdausa.org/	
Neurofibromatosis	http://www.nf.org/	National Neurofibromatosis Foundation.
Neuropathy	http://www.neuropathy.org/	Neuropathy Association.
Rett Syndrome	http://www.rettsyndrome.org/	International Rett Syndrome Association.
Tourette Syndrome	http://www.tsa-usa.org/	Tourette Syndrome Association.
Tuberous Sclerosis Association	http://www.tsalliance.org/	National Tuberous Sclerosis Association.

CME, continuing medical education; NIH, National Institutes of Health.
From McKusick VA, 1998.

ROMs. In contrast, a search in 2004 revealed nearly 2000. The computerized versions generally have an advantage over traditional texts in that they allow searches by keywords, phrases, chapter titles, authors, and so forth; have hyperlinks between topics and to images and references; and are frequently updated at minimal expense. In addition, they have the capacity for color images and multimedia files. For example, video is extremely useful in discussing movement disorders and eye movements. Many anatomy and radiology books also are available as CD-ROM editions.

The Bookshelf (http://www.ncbi.nlm.nih.gov/entrez/query.fcgi?db=Books), produced by the National Center for Biotechnology Information, is a collection of biomedical books, searchable by concept or keyword and linked to terms in PubMed abstracts. The site organizes the books into units of content rather than mirroring a textbook in print, and is designed so that the reader can begin browsing with a search on the PubMed link rather than reading a book sequentially from beginning to end. Once browsing the book page, it is possible to navigate around a whole unit of content.

Other Interesting Reference Sites

It is estimated that the web consists of hundreds of millions of documents and resources. Trying to navigate to an area of interest is a formidable task. A wide variety of search engines, such as Google and Yahoo, are available to help with this task. These can either allow direct searches or searches via a hierarchical categorization of topics (known as *web directories*). One can prompt any of these search engines to provide website information on topics as diverse as medicine, gardening, space, and art. These search engines have simple interfaces and are easy to use, but also have advanced features (including the use of Boolean logic) that are worth spending a few minutes learning, allowing both more focused and more comprehensive searches.

One of the most useful web functions is access to the MEDLINE database. The MEDLINE file contains bibliographic citations and author abstracts from more than 4800 current biomedical journals published in the United States and 70 other countries. The file contains more than 12 million records dating back to 1966. This database can be accessed through a variety of browsers. One such browser, PubMed (http://www.ncbi.nlm.nih.gov/PubMed/), was developed at the National Library of Medicine. It has been developed in conjunction with publishers of biomedical literature as a search tool for accessing literature citations and linking to full-text journals at websites of participating publishers. It has the advantage of ease of use, a frequently updated database, and no charge to users. PubMed also allows access to OLDMEDLINE, which has 2 million citations of articles published between 1951 and 1965, as well as to new publications not yet indexed in MEDLINE.

The Visible Human Project (http://www.nlm.nih.gov/research/visible/visible_human.html) features a collection of images (cryopreserved, computed tomography, and magnetic resonance imaging) of an entire male and female [Lindberg and Humphreys, 1995]. Harvard University provides a whole brain atlas (http://www.med.harvard.edu/AANLIB/home.html) that provides imaging examples of normal structures, as well as pathologic findings.

Several excellent websites aim at teaching the neurologic examination using both text and video. NeuroLogicExam (http://medstat.med.utah.edu/neurologicexam/) and Neuroexam.com (http://www.neuroexam.com/) each use videos to illustrate various elements of a neurologic examination. The former also features helpful anatomic diagrams. A new site, PediNeuroLogicExam (http://medstat.med.utah.edu/pedineurologicexam/) provides videos and text, demonstrating the changing examination as the child matures and the approach to examining the young patient. GeneralPediatrics.Com (http://www.generalpediatrics.com) is a compilation of Internet resources useful both to pediatricians and to parents.

The explosion of research in pediatric neurology has made it difficult to keep up with genetic testing and research studies. Two sites, both sponsored by the National Institutes of Health, are exceptionally helpful. Gene Tests (http://www.genetests.org/), from the University of Washington, contains information about clinical and research tests available for genetic diseases, including where to send the specimens, as well as clinical summaries about some of the conditions. Clinical Trials (http://clinicaltrials.gov/), from the National Library of Medicine, provides information about federally and privately supported clinical research on human volunteers, including the purpose of the trial, inclusion and exclusion criteria, location, and contact information. For example, in September, 2004, input of "leukodystrophy" revealed 5 ongoing trials, and "epilepsy" (further restricted to trials in children), 27. Privately sponsored sites, such as Center Watch's "Clinical Trials In Neurology" (http://www.centerwatch.com/patient/studies/area10.html), also list trials seeking patients.

Several directories of neurology and neuroscience sites provide excellent starting points in searching for information. Two such directories are "Neurosciences on The Internet" (http://www.neuroguide.com/) and the Internet Handbook on Neurology (http://www.neuropat.dote.hu/neurology.htm).

Clinical Decision-Making Software

SimulConsult (http://simulconsult.com/) is a free, medical-decision-support application developed by Dr. Michael Segal. It allows users to input information about a patient's age, symptoms, age at which symptoms began, and laboratory findings and generates a differential diagnosis. It then suggests additional findings and laboratory tests that will be useful in reaching a diagnosis. The database used to generate this information is provided by a large peer-reviewed community of experts and is being continually updated. Recently, Segal and his colleagues have also developed web-based tools to generate and share educational cases over the web (http://simulconsult.com/neurologicalsyndromes/edu/).

ISABEL (http://www.isabel.org.uk/) is a commercial, online clinical decision information system covering a broader spectrum of pediatrics, including pediatric neurology.

THE PROBLEMS

In a recent editorial, concern was expressed that any "preprint" posted on the Internet (like those in the physics community) is "incomplete until it undergoes peer review" [Kassirer and Angell, 1995]. Certainly, anyone can post almost any item of information on the Internet, and currently there are no safeguards to ensure that the information is accurate. Some websites, like those for the journal *Science* or for the American Academy of Neurology, have high credibility because the postings have gone through some form of review. However, the quality of a web site on headaches cannot be controlled. Web sites cannot be deemed reputable simply because they are associated with a university department or patient organization. Physicians cannot trust an e-mail or a bulletin board posting, especially if such communications are unsigned or are signed by unknown individuals. Certainly, as when reading any journal article, the physician must be critical and take into account the source of that article or information. In the future, a few sites may distinguish themselves by their usability and accuracy in our field [Hernandez-Borges et al., 1997]. Codes of conduct for medical publishing on the Internet do exist, such as Health on The Net Foundations's Code of Conduct (http://www.hon.ch/HONcode/Conduct.html) and new methods are being assessed for measuring quality [Eysenbach and Diepgen, 1999].

Issues of payment and copyright arise when journals or academics place information on the Internet. The technology is available to restrict access to certain websites so that only (paying) members can enter. One can transfer credit card information, although this is generally not considered to be risk free. In terms of copyright, there is concern about how information is downloaded and reproduced by other individuals [Stern and Westenberg, 1995; Taubes, 1995]. The biggest problems for medical resources on the Internet seem not to be of a technical nature but rather of quality of information, accessibility, and appropriate reimbursement (e.g., for access to journal subscriptions).

A PATIENT EDUCATION RESOURCE

The Internet and forums on private services (such as America Online) are rapidly becoming major sources of information for patients and their families. Websites, e-mail lists, and USENET groups dedicated to particular diseases provide a wealth of factual information, as well as contact with patients, families, and (less commonly) health care providers sharing similar interests. The Family Village (http://www.familyvillage.wisc.edu/) is an example of a website that attempts to catalog useful Internet information for families of patients with developmental disabilities. Some medical centers and departments are using the Web to advertise their particular areas of expertise to other clinicians and patients. Be aware, however, that these Internet resources provide excellent supplements to the information provided by the patient's doctor but cannot substitute for it. The quality of information shared is variable, and rumors and word of purported treatments occasionally run wild. Sometimes, of course, some of these rumors contain truth, and the dissemination of this information is highly desired. Who is to determine truth or quality, however? An interesting development in the United States is that the Federal Trade Commission is starting to regulate promotions on the web and USENET for products and services claiming to help cure, treat, or prevent a variety of diseases. The problem lies not only in the lack of a peer-review type of process but also in limited physician involvement in many patient-centered discussion groups. These problems are hardly surprising, given time constraints, the absence of compensation for this type of work, and appropriate fears of misguiding patients and of contradicting their own physicians. Physicians interested in Internet resources for patients are often caught in a bind between trying to provide families with reliable information over the Internet, quelling rumors in the making, and returning patients to their best resources, their own doctors. These issues are likely to become even more significant in the future as Internet access becomes more universal and routine.

COMMUNICATING WITH PATIENTS VIA E-MAIL

Although the actual office or hospital visit is the gold standard of medical care, many patients choose to interact with physicians via phone or fax. Typically, these interactions are for simple requests, such as prescription refills, but also can involve diagnostic, management, and triaging decisions. E-mail has the advantage to the physician and patient of avoiding the time-consuming and sometimes expensive "phone tag," of allowing questions and responses to be formulated carefully in advance, and of providing documentation of the interaction for future reference and for the medical record. However, the use of e-mail raises concerns about breaches of confidentiality, the authenticity of the senders and recipients of e-mail, and the risk of missed e-mail messages. Guidelines have been developed to minimize the risks and maximize the benefit of e-mail [Bovi, 2003; Gerstle, 2004; Kane et al., 1998]. Unsolicited e-mail from patients unknown to the physician also poses potential moral and legal problems [Eysenbach, 2000].

Some of these problems may be addressed by the development of secure servers, web-based portals that "triage" patient messages [Gerstle, 2004; Katz et al., 2003]. Patients are given passwords, log into a web site as they might for online banking, and are notified by e-mail when a new message from their health-care provider waits for them on the web site. Messages coming into the doctor's office via the web site are triaged in ways similar to incoming phone calls. The use of such a secure server has been found to increase the amount and, in the eyes of the physicians, the quality of communication between patients and providers but did not reduce the number of telephone calls, office visits, or missed appointments [Katz et al., 2003].

PERSONAL DIGITAL ASSISTANTS

Miniaturization has made it practical for the physician to carry a small, handheld computer into the examination room. The personal digital assistant (PDA) may soon be as necessary a piece of equipment as the reflex hammer, particularly as hospital and office medical records evolve from being paper-based to electronic and as connectivity between these handheld devices and hospital computers improves. Many medical programs for these PDAs already exist, and the variety of uses is likely to expand as use becomes routine and wireless connectivity becomes standard. As of 2002, more than one third of pediatricians used PDAs in their clinical practice [Carroll and Chistakis, 2004].

Patient encounters can be tracked, with automated access to demographic information and laboratory data on the main office or hospital computer. Prior records and laboratory values available at the bedside in a searchable fashion would be extremely helpful. Conversely, information obtained at the bedside can be entered into the main computer. This information can include charge entries, such as diagnoses and procedures, each with automated coding. Information entered at the bedside, such as vital signs, patient orders, and admission and progress notes, can become part of an electronic medical record or, as an intermediate step, can be printed out to become part of the paper chart. Entry of orders and progress notes may be faster and more complete if a word processing program with diagnosis-specific templates and menu selections is used (e.g., "headache" could lead to entries for location, frequency, quality, and positional dependence).

In addition to information flow between PDAs and main computers, medical resources available at the bedside, such as practice parameters, medical references, and drug information, can also be a boon for both the doctor and patient. Other organizational tools can aid in patient management. These include applications to perform clinical calculations, to digitalize "scut lists," to write prescriptions and communicate them online to the patient's pharmacy, and to manage patient schedules and interface them with physicians' personal schedules. Many of these tasks could also be performed with computer terminals located in examination rooms or on small laptops or tablet computers. The advantages of bigger screens are their usefulness in the display of anatomic images, as well as in multimedia displays that could be used in patient education.

The Handheld Computing Center (http://aan.com/pda.cfm) of the American Academy of Neurology aims to help the neurologist expand his or her understanding and use of handheld devices. A recent review of handheld computers [Al-Ubaydii, 2004] lists more likely uses, and calls attention to versions of PubMed (http://pubmedhh.nlm.nih.gov/nlm/pubmed/index.html and http://archive.nlm.nih.gov/proj/pmot/pmot.php) and evidenced-based medicine resources (www.infopoems.com), as well as many other resources, customized for PDAs. The review also discusses the security concerns brought about by the use of these devices.

TELEMEDICINE

Telemedicine is a rapidly expanding set of applications in which electronic communication is applied directly to patient care. Still images, live video, audio, text, and quantitative data can be transmitted between physician and physician, physician and patient, imaging center and physician, and so forth. The methods are promising, but cost-effectiveness is not yet proved, and many legal and administrative issues need to be worked out before they gain widespread use.

In addition to videoconferencing, which is gaining widespread use as an educational tool, pediatric neurologists are likely to see telemedicine applications evolve in several patient care areas in the coming decade:

1. Electronic storage of patients' medical records and laboratory data, with improved dissemination between specialists and primary caretakers
2. Transmission of radiology and pathology images from the sites where these images were created both to specialized interpreters (e.g., neuroradiologists and neuropathologists), and to the physicians (e.g., pediatric neurologists) caring for the patients
3. Transmission of these images in the opposite direction—attachment of relevant radiographic and even video images to electronic consultation letters and discharge summaries "may be worth a thousand words."
4. Remotely accessible databases for research, teaching, and patient care (e.g., outcomes research, practice parameters)
5. Transmission of data from patients' homes (e.g., remote electroencephalogram monitoring)
6. Consultations—perhaps the most important, and certainly the most challenging application. Both physician-to-physician and physician-to-patient consultations would expand on the telephone conversations now common and accepted. Allowing geographically separated physicians to discuss patients with specialists while looking at radiographic images or even live video of the patients themselves could allow more efficient triaging and improved

recommendations for patient care. For patients in rural or other settings remote from specialty centers, at least limited pediatric neurology "office" evaluations could be performed without requiring traveling long distances. Similarly, one specialist could easily consult another, even in another country.

Many obvious difficulties are associated with these types of consultations:

1. Neurologic examinations would, by necessity, be limited (e.g., inadequate evaluation of strength and tone), and the criteria by which these video visits could replace face-to-face evaluations need to be determined.
2. In a similar vein, although sound and image quality are rapidly improving, they are not consistently equivalent to personal examination, and the brief delays often associated with transmission can be annoying.
3. Although one goal of this type of consultation would be to lower health-care costs by improving centralization of specialty care, the initial costs of setting up such systems can be quite high.
4. The means by which a physician can bill for electronic consultations remain to be determined.
5. It remains to be proved that electronic consultations truly improve efficacy in a cost-effective manner. For example, two studies comparing television and telephone consultations found that the former took more time and was more expensive without any improvement in diagnostic accuracy, the number of tests requested, or referral rates [Dunn et al., 1977; Moore et al., 1975].
6. Finally, numerous legal, liability, and privacy issues arise, particularly when care is being shared across state or even national boundaries. The issue of out-of-state licensing needs to be addressed when the physician and patient are in different locales. Malpractice liability becomes confusing when care is shared by physicians, particularly if different rules apply in different states. The confidentiality of medical records, whether video images transmitted electronically or patient databases, needs to be maintained and may be complicated by different privacy laws in different states.

WHAT DOES THE FUTURE HOLD?

The question for our field is whether the Internet is something that can make our careers easier, more efficient, and more effective. From our personal standpoint, the answer is yes because specific programs or web sites are identifiable, can be used, and have been helpful. In a certain sense, the Internet is a fluid, expanding library of information. Since the last version of this chapter was published in 1999, geographically dispersed centers have begun pooling patient data for descriptions of rare disorders and for designing and managing trials; electronic medical records and radiographic data have become the norm; physicians have begun to use medical decision-making software after seeing a patient and before writing their consultation notes; and textbooks themselves are becoming continually updated, with online versions that include audio and video data and linkage to outside references and websites.

It is likely that all of this information will become more portable as wireless, handheld computers become standard tools. As more information and programs are made available, the usefulness to the profession will increase. Certain organizations, such as the American Academy of Neurology and the Child Neurology Society, are trying to take the lead and help organize and review the information that is available. The best is yet to come. As child neurologists, the usefulness of the Internet should not be judged on what it contains now but what it will contain in the near future.

REFERENCES

Al-Ubaydii M. Handheld computers. BMJ 2004;15:1181.

Bovi AM; Council on Ethical and Judicial Affairs of the American Medical Association. Ethical guidelines for use of electronic mail between patients and physicians. Amer J Bioethics 2003;3:W43.

Carroll AE, Chistakis, DA. Pediatricians' use of and attitudes about personal digital assistants. Pediatrics 2004;113:238.

De Ville KA. Internet listservers and pediatrics: Newly emerging legal and clinical practice issues. II. Pediatrics 1996;98:453.

Dunn EV, Conrath DW, Bloor WG, et al. An evaluation of four telemedicine systems for primary care. Health Serv Res 1977;12:19.

Elliot SJ, Elliot RG. Internet listservers and pediatrics: Newly emerging legal and clinical practice issues. Pediatrics 1996;97:399.

Eysenbach G. Towards ethical guidelines for dealing with unsolicited patient emails and giving teleadvice in the absence of a pre-existing patient-physician relationship: Systematic review and expert survey. J Med Internet Res 2000;2:e1. (http://www.jmir.org/2000/1/e1/).

Eysenbach G, Diepgen TL. Labeling and filtering of medical information on the Internet. Methods Inf Med 1999;38:80.

Gerstle RS. E-mail communication between pediatricians and their patients. Pediatrics 2004;114:317.

Hernandez-Borges AA, Pareras LG, Jimenez A. Comparative analysis of pediatric mailing lists on the internet. Pediatrics 1997;100:E8.

Kane B, Sands DZ, for the AMIA Internet Working Group, Task Force on Guidelines for the Use of Clinic-Patient Electronic Mail. Guidelines for the clinical use of electronic mail with patients. J Am Med Inform Assoc 1998;5:104 (http://www.amia.org/pubs/other/email_guidelines.html).

Kassirer JP, Angell M. The Internet and the journal. N Engl J Med 1995;332:1709.

Katz SJ, Moyer CA, Cox DT, et al. Effect of a triage-based e-mail system on clinical resource use and patient and physician satisfaction in primary care. J Gen Intern Med 2003;18:734.

Lindberg DA, Humphreys BL. Computers in medicine. JAMA 1995;273:1667.

Mack KJ, Leber SM. Child neurology and the Internet. Pediatr Neurol 1996;15:283.

McEnery KW. The Internet, World-Wide Web, and Mosaic: An overview. AJR Am J Roentgenol 1995;164:469.

McKusick VA. Mendelian inheritance in man, 12th ed. Baltimore: John Hopkins University Press, 1998.

Moore GT, Willemain RT, Bonanno R, et al. Comparison of television and telephone for remote medical consultation. N Engl J Med 1975;292:729.

Stern EJ, Westenberg L. Copyright law and academic radiology: Rights of authors and copyright owners and reproduction of information. AJR Am J Roentgenol 1995;164:1083.

Taubes G. Indexing the Internet. Science 1995;269:1354.

INDEX

Page numbers followed by *b, f,* or *t* denote boxes, figures, and tables, respectively.

C

F

G

M

T

U